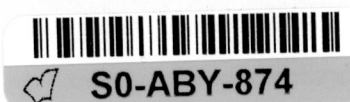
S0-ABY-874

ARTHRITIS AND ALLIED CONDITIONS

A Textbook of Rheumatology

FOURTEENTH EDITION

ARTHRITIS AND ALLIED CONDITIONS

A Textbook of Rheumatology

FOURTEENTH EDITION

Edited by

William J. Koopman

Professor and Chairman
Department of Medicine
University of Alabama at Birmingham
Birmingham, Alabama

VOLUME TWO

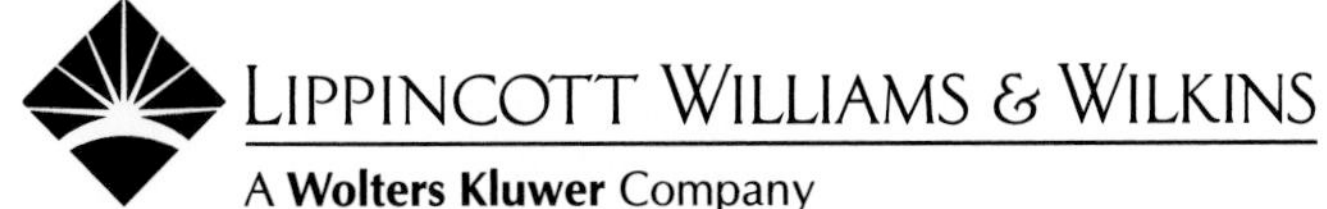

Philadelphia • Baltimore • New York • London
Buenos Aires • Hong Kong • Sydney • Tokyo

Acquisitions Editor: Richard Winters
Developmental Editor: Michael Standen
Production Editor: Robin E. Cook
Manufacturing Manager: Benjamin Rivera
Cover Designer: Q.T. Design
Compositor: Lippincott Williams & Wilkins Desktop Division
Printer: Courier Kendalville

530 Walnut Street
Philadelphia, PA 19106-3780 USA
www.LWW.com

Printed in the USA

Library of Congress Cataloging-in-Publication Data

Arthritis and allied conditions.–14th ed. / editor, William J. Koopman.
p. ; cm.
Includes bibliographical references and index.
ISBN 0-7817-2240-3
1. Arthritis. 2. Rheumatism. I. Koopman, William J.
[DNLM: 1. Arthritis. 2. Rheumatic Diseases. WE 344 A7866 2000]
RC933 .A64 2000
616.7'22–dc21

00-028724

Care has been taken to confirm the accuracy of the information presented and to describe generally accepted practices. However, the authors, editors, and publisher are not responsible for errors or omissions or for any consequences from application of the information in this book and make no warranty, expressed or implied, with respect to the currency, completeness, or accuracy of the contents of the publication. Application of this information in a particular situation remains the professional responsibility of the practitioner.

The authors, editors, and publisher have exerted every effort to ensure that drug selection and dosage set forth in this text are in accordance with current recommendations and practice at the time of publication. However, in view of ongoing research, changes in government regulations, and the constant flow of information relating to drug therapy and drug reactions, the reader is urged to check the package insert for each drug for any change in indications and dosage and for added warnings and precautions. This is particularly important when the recommended agent is a new or infrequently employed drug.

Some drugs and medical devices presented in this publication have Food and Drug Administration (FDA) clearance for limited use in restricted research settings. It is the responsibility of the health care provider to ascertain the FDA status of each drug or device planned for use in their clinical practice.

10 9 8 7 6 5 4 3 2 1

CONTENTS

VOLUME ONE

VI. OTHER INFLAMMATORY ARTHRITIS SYNDROMES

VOLUME TWO

VII. SYSTEMIC RHEUMATIC DISEASES

CONTRIBUTING AUTHORS

Graciela S. Alarcón, M.D., M.P.H. Jane Knight Lowe Professor, Division of Rheumatology, Department of Medicine, University of Alabama, Associate Director, Multipurpose Arthritis and Musculoskeletal Disease Center, Birmingham, Alabama

Roy D. Altman, M.D. Professor of Medicine and Chief, Director Clinical Research, GRECC, Miami Veterans Affairs Medical Center, Department of Rheumatology and Immunology, University of Miami Medical Center, Miami, Florida

Frank C. Arnett, M.D. Professor, Department of Internal Medicine, University of Texas-Houston Medical School, Chief, Rheumatology Service, Department of Internal Medicine, Memorial Hermann Hospital, Houston, Texas

Gene V. Ball, M.D. Professor of Medicine, Division of Clinical Immunology and Rheumatology, University of Alabama, Birmingham, Alabama,

J. D. Bartleson, M.D. Associate Professor, Department of Neurology, Mayo Clinic, Rochester, Minnesota

Michael J. Battistone, M.D. Assistant Professor, Department of Internal Medicine, University of Utah College of Medicine, Staff Physician, Medical Care Center, Salt Lake City Veterans Affairs Medical Center, Salt Lake City, Utah

Michael A. Becker, M.D. Professor, Department of Medicine, University of Chicago, Chicago, Illinois

Nicholas Bellamy, M.D., F.R.C.P. Director, Centre of National Research on Disability and Rehabilitation Medicine, Department of Medicine, Block 6-F Floor, Royal Brisbane Hospital, Brisbane, Queensland, Australia

Robert M. Bennett, M.D. Professor, Department of Medicine, Chairman, Division of Arthritis and Rheumatic Disease, Oregon Health Sciences University, Portland, Oregon

Merrill D. Benson, M.D. Professor, Departments of Medicine and Pathology and Laboratory Medicine, Indiana University School of Medicine, and, Departments of Medicine and Pathology, Indiana University Medical Center, Indianapolis, Indiana

Joseph J. Biundo, M.D. Chief, Section of Physical Medicine and Rehabilitation, Department of Physical Medicine and Rehabilitation, Louisiana State University Medical Center, New Orleans, Louisiana

Warren D. Blackburn, Jr., M.D. Clinical Professor, Rheumatology Section VA 111-F, Birmingham Veterans Affairs Medical Center, Birmingham, Alabama

Harry Blair, M.D. Associate Professor, Department of Pathology, The University of Alabama, Birmingham, Alabama

Marcy B. Bolster, M.D. Assistant Professor, Department of Medicine, Division of Rheumatology and Immunology, Medical University of South Carolina, Charleston, South Carolina

Dennis W. Boulware, M.D. Professor, Department of Medicine, University of Alabama, Birmingham, Alabama

Dimitrios Boumpas, M.D. Arthritis and Rheumatism Branch, NIAMS, National Institutes of Health, Bethesda, Maryland

Laurence A. Bradley, M.D. Professor of Medicine, Division of Clinical Immunology and Rheumatology, University of Alabama, Birmingham, Alabama

Victoria A. Brander, M.D. Assistant Professor of Physical Medicine and Rehabilitation, Northwestern University Medical School, Director, Arthritis Center, Rehabilitation Institute of Chicago, Chicago, Illinois

S. Louis Bridges, Jr., M.D., Ph.D. Assistant Professor, Departments of Medicine and Microbiology, University of Alabama, Staff Physician, Departments of Medicine and Rheumatology, Birmingham Veterans Affairs Medical Center, Birmingham, Alabama

Paul H. Brion, M.D. Clinical Instructor, Division of Rheumatology, UCLA School of Medicine, Los Angeles, California

W. Watson Buchanan, M.D. Emeritus Professor and Consultant Physician, Department of Medicine, McMaster University, Hamilton, Ontario, Canada

Daniel C. Bullard, Ph.D. Assistant Professor, Department of Comparative Medicine, University of Alabama, Birmingham, Alabama

Grant W. Cannon, M.D. Professor, Division of Rheumatology, Department of Medicine, University of Utah, Associate Chief of Staff for Academic Affiliations, Veterans Affairs Medical Center, Salt Lake City, Utah

Juan J. Canoso, M.D. Adjunct Professor, Department of Medicine, Tufts University School of Medicine, Boston, Massachusetts, and, Rheumatologist, American-British Cowdray Hospital, Mexico City, Mexico

Robert H. Carter, M.D. Associate Professor of Medicine, Division of Clinical Immunology and Rheumatology, Department of Medicine, University of Alabama, Birmingham, Alabama

Rowland W. Chang, M.D., M.P.H. Professor of Preventive Medicine, Medicine and Physical Medicine and Rehabilitation, Northwestern University Medical School, Chicago, Illinois

W. Winn Chatham, M.D. Associate Professor, Departments of Medicine and Rheumatology, University of Alabama, Staff Physician, Veterans Affairs Medical Center, Birmingham, Alabama

Albert C. Chen, Ph.D. Post-Doctoral Researcher, Department of Bioengineering, University of California at San Diego, La Jolla, California

Silvia S. Chen, Ph.D. Post-Doctoral Researcher, Department of Bioengineering, University of California at San Diego, La Jolla, California

Daniel O. Clegg, M.D. Professor and Chief, Division of Rheumatology, Department of Medicine, University of Utah School of Medicine, Chief, Rheumatology Section, Medical Service, Salt Lake City Veterans Affairs Medical Center, Salt Lake City, Utah

John R. Couchman, Ph.D. Professor, Department of Cell Biology, University of Alabama, Birmingham, Alabama

Leslie J. Crofford, M.D. Associate Professor, Department of Internal Medicine, University of Michigan Health System, Ann Arbor, Michigan

Mary E. Cronin, M.D. Associate Professor of Medicine Division of Rheumatology, Medical College of Wisconsin, Milwaukee, Wisconsin

Bruce N. Cronstein, M.D. Professor of Medicine and Pathology, Department of Medicine, New York University School of Medicine, New York, New York

Mary K. Crow, M.D. Professor of Medicine, Department of Medicine, Weill Medical College of Cornell University, New York, New York, Attending Physician, Department of Rheumatology, Hospital for Special Surgery, New York, New York

John M. Cuckler, M.D. Professor and Director, Division of Orthopedics, University of Alabama, Birmingham, Alabama

Marta L. Cuéllar, M.D. Assistant Professor, Section of Rheumatology, Department of Medicine, Tulane University School of Medicine, Tulane Hospital and Clinic, New Orleans, Louisiana

Martha R. Curry, M.S., R.N.C., P.N.P. Instructor, Division of Rheumatology, Texas Children's Hospital, Houston, Texas

John J. Cush, M.D. Associate Professor, Division of Rheumatic Diseases, University of Texas Southwestern Medical Center, Arthritis Center, Presbyterian Hospital/Dallas, Dallas, Texas

Filip de Keyser, M.D. Department of Rheumatology, University Hospital, Gent, Belgium

Ara H. Dikranian, M.D. Fellow, Division of Rheumatology, University of California, San Diego, La Jolla, California

Michael A. DiMicco, M.S. Graduate Student, Department of Bioengineering, University of California at San Diego, La Jolla, California

M. Franklin Dolwick, D.M.D., Ph.D. Professor, Department of Oral and Maxillofacial Surgery, University of Florida, Gainesville, Florida

Joseph Duffy, M.D. Associate Professor of Medicine, Division of Rheumatology, Department of Internal Medicine, Mayo Medical School, Mayo Clinic, Rochester, Minnesota

N. Lawrence Edwards, M.D. Professor of Medicine, Department of Medicine, Division of Rheumatology, University of Florida, Gainesville Florida

Michael H. Ellman, M.D. Professor of Clinical Medicine, Department of Medicine, University of Chicago, Chicago, Illinois

Luis R. Espinoza, M.D. Professor and Chief, Section of Rheumatology, Department of Medicine, Louisiana State University Health Sciences Center, New Orleans, Louisiana

David T. Felson, M.D., M.Ph. Professor, Departments of Medicine and Public Health, Boston University School of Medicine, Boston, Massachusetts

Robert H. Fitzgerald, Jr., M.D. Paul B. Magnuson Professor, Department of Orthopedic Surgery, University of Pennsylvania, Hospital of the University of Pennsylvania, Philadelphia, Pennsylvania

David A. Fox, M.D. Professor, Department of Internal Medicine, Chief, Division of Rheumatology, University of Michigan, Ann Arbor, Michigan

Robert I. Fox, M.D., Ph.D. Associate Member, Department of Immunology, The Scripps Research Institute, Rheumatologist, Department of Rheumatology, Scripps Memorial Hospital, La Jolla, California

Daniel E. Furst, M.D. Clinical Professor, Department of Medicine, Division of Rheumatology, University of Washington, Director, Arthritis Clinical Research Unit, Virginia Mason Research Center, Seattle, Washington

Renate E. Gay, M.D. Chief of Staff, Dean's Office, Medical Faculty, University of Zurich, Zurich, Switzerland

Robert M. Gay, Jr., M.D. Cornerstone Medical Specialties, High Point, North Carolina

Steffen Gay, M.D. Professor, Department of Rheumatology, University Hospital, Zurich, Switzerland

Harry K. Genant, M.D. Professor of Radiology, Medicine, Epidemiology and Orthopaedic Surgery, Department of Radiology, Executive Director, Osteoporosis and Arthritis Research Group, University of California San Francisco, San Francisco, California

Edward H. Giannini, M.Sc., Dr.PH. Professor, Department of Pediatrics, University of Cincinnati College of Medicine, Clinical Epidemiology, Department of Rheumatology, Children's Hospital Medical Center, Cincinnati, Ohio

Allan Gibofsky, M.D. Professor, Departments of Medicine and Public Health, Weill Medical College of Cornell University, Attending Rheumatologist, Department of Rheumatology, Hospital for Special Surgery, New York, New York

Gary S. Gilkeson, M.D. Associate Professor of Medicine/Microbiology and Immunology, Medical University of South Carolina, Charleston, South Carolina

Jean G. Gispen, M.D. Private Practice, Internal Medicine Associates, Oxford, Mississippi

Don L. Goldenberg, M.D. Private Practice, Division of Rheumatology, Newton-Wellesley Hospital, Boston, Massachusetts

Tom P. Gordon, M.D., Ph.D. Professor and Director, Department of Immunology, Allergy, and Arthritis, Flinders University of South Australia, Flinders Medical Centre, Bedford Park, South Australia, Australia

Jörg J. Goronzy, M.D. Professor of Medicine and Immunology, Division of Rheumatology, Department of Medicine, Mayo Clinic, Rochester, Minnesota

Jan Tore Gran, M.D. Professor and Head of Department, Department of Rheumatology, University of Tromso, Tromso, Norway

Courtney Gray-McGuire, M.D. Predoctoral Fellow, Arthritis and Immunology Program, Oklahoma Medical Research Foundation, Oklahoma City, Oklahoma

Barry L. Gruber, M.D. Associate Professor of Medicine and Dermatology, Chief, Division of Rheumatology, State University of New York at Stony Brook, Northport Veterans Affairs Medical Center, Stony Brook, New York

Nortin M. Hadler, M.D. Professor of Medicine and Microbiology/Immunology, Department of Medicine, University of North Carolina School of Medicine, Chapel Hill, North Carolina

Hans-Jacob Haga, M.D. Professor, Division of Rheumatology, University of Bergen, Consultant, Department of Rheumatology, Haubeland Hospital, Bergen, Norway

Laura P. Hale, M.D. Assistant Professor, Department of Pathology, Duke University Medical Center, Durham, North Carolina

James T. Halla, M.D. Private Practice, Abilene, Texas

Paul B. Halverson, M.D. Professor of Medicine, Department of Rheumatology, Medical College of Wisconsin, Milwaukee, Wisconsin

Joe G. Hardin, Jr., M.D. Professor, Department of Medicine, University of South Alabama, Attending Physician, Department of Medicine, University of South Alabama Medical Center, Mobile, Alabama

John B. Harley, M.D., Ph.D. Professor, Department of Medicine, Member, Arthritis and Immunology Program, University of Oklahoma, Oklahoma Medical Research Foundation, Staff Physician, Medical Service, U.S. Department of Veterans Affairs Medical Center, Oklahoma City, Oklahoma

Barton F. Haynes, M.D. Chair, Department of Medicine, Duke University Medical Center, Durham, North Carolina

Louis W. Heck, Jr., M.D. Professor, Department of Medicine, University of Alabama School of Medicine, University of Alabama Hospitals, Birmingham, Alabama

Jan Hillson, M.D. Arthritis Clinical Research Unit, Virginia Mason Research Center, Seattle, Washington

Daniel Holderbaum, M.D. Senior Research Unit, Associate, Division of Rheumatology, Department of Medicine, Adjunct Assistant Professor, Case Western Reserve University School of Medicine, University Hospitals, Cleveland, Ohio

James P. Hollowell, M.D. Associate Professor, Department of Neurosurgery, Medical College of Wisconsin, Milwaukee, Wisconsin

Greg A. Horton, M.D. Assistant Professor, Orthopaedic Surgery, Kansas University Medical Center, Kansas City, Kansas

Aubrey J. Hough, Jr., M.D. Professor and Chairman, Department of Pathology, University of Arkansas for Medical Sciences, Chief of Services, Department of Pathology, University Hospital, Little Rock, Arkansas

David S. Howell, M.D. Emeritus Professor of Medicine, Division of Immunology and Rheumatology, Department of Medicine, University of Miami School of Medicine, Staff Physician, Division of Immunology and Rheumatology, Department of Medicine, University of Miami Health Center/Jackson Memorial Hospital, Miami, Florida

Gunnar Husby, M.D. Professor, Rikshospitalet, University of Oslo, Head, Center for Rheumatic Diseases, The National Hospital, Oslo, Norway

Robert W. Ike, M.D. Associate Professor, Division of Rheumatology, Department of Medicine, University of Michigan Medical Center, Ann Arbor, Michigan,

Robert D. Inman, M.D. Professor of Medicine and Immunology, University of Toronto, Director, Arthritis Center of Excellence, Department of Medicine, Toronto Western Hospital, Toronto, Ontario, Canada

Christopher G. Jackson, M.D. Associate Professor, Director of Clinical Trials, Division of Rheumatology, University of Utah School of Medicine, University of Utah Health Sciences Center, Salt Lake City Department of Veterans Affairs Medical Center, Salt Lake City, Utah

Hugo E. Jasin, M.D. Professor of Internal Medicine, Department of Medicine, Division of Rheumatology, University of Arkansas, Medical Sciences Center, Little Rock, Arkansas

John Paul Jones Jr., M.D. President, Diagnostic Osteonecrosis Center and Research Foundation, Kelseyville, California

Roland Jonsson, D.M.D., Ph.D. Professor, Broegelman Research Laboratory, University of Bergen, Consultant, Department of Otolaryngology, Haukeland University Hospital, Bergen, Norway

Bruce A. Julian, M.D. Professor of Medicine and Transplant Surgery, The University of Alabama, Birmingham, Alabama

Kenneth C. Kalunian, M.D. Associate Professor of Clinical Medicine, Department of Medicine, Division of Rheumatology, UCLA School of Medicine, Los Angeles, California

Allen P. Kaplan, M.D. Professor and Co-Director, Asthma and Allergy Center, Department of Medicine, Medical University of South Carolina, Charleston, South Carolina

Daniel L. Kastner, M.D., Ph.D. Chief, Genetics Section, Arthritis and Rheumatism Branch, National Institute of Arthritis and Musculoskeletal and Skin Diseases, National Institutes of Health, Bethesda, Maryland

Christopher G. Kevil, Ph.D. Research Fellow, Department of Comparative Medicine, University of Alabama, Birmingham, Alabama

Robert P. Kimberly, M.D. Howard L. Holley Professor of Medicine, Department of Medicine, University of Alabama, Director, Division of Clinical Immunology and Rheumatology, Director, Multipurpose Arthritis and, Musculoskeletal Diseases Center, University of Alabama Hospital, Birmingham, Alabama

Lynell W. Klassen, M.D. Stokes-Shackleford Professor, Department of Internal Medicine, University of Nebraska Medical Center, Omaha, Nebraska

William J. Koopman, M.D. Professor and Chairman, Department of Medicine, Spencer Chair in Medical Science Leadership, University of Alabama, Birmingham, Alabama

Joseph H. Korn, M.D. Professor, Department of Medicine, Boston University School of Medicine, Chief, Rheumatology Division, Department of Medicine, Boston Medical Center, Boston, Massachusetts

Joel M. Kremer, M.D. Professor of Medicine, Head, Division of Rheumatology, Department of Medicine, Albany Medical College, Attending Physician, Albany Medical Center Hospital, Albany, New York

Melissa S. Kurtis, M.S. Graduate Student, Department of Bioengineering, University of California at San Diego, La Jolla, California

Sanford J. Larson, M.D., Ph.D. Professor of Neurosurgery, Department of Neurosurgery, Medical College of Wisconsin, Milwaukee, Wisconsin

Kelvin W. Li, M.S Graduate Student, Department of Bioengineering, University of California at San Diego, La Jolla, California

Peter E. Lipsky, M.D. Scientific Director, National Institute of Arthritis and Musculoskeletal and Skin Diseases, National Institutes of Health, Bethesda, Maryland

Albert F. LoBuglio, M.D. Director, Comprehensive Cancer Center, Evalina B Spencer Professor of Oncology, Associate Dean, University of Alabama, Wallace Tumor Center, Birmingham, Alabama

Michael D. Lockshin, M.D. Professor, Department of Medicine, Weill Medical College of Cornell University, Director, Barbara Volcker Center, Hospital for Special Surgery, New York, New York

Lisa M. Lottman, B.S. Staff Research Associate II and Lab Manager, Department of Bioengineering, University of California at San Diego, La Jolla, California

Martin K. Lotz, M.D. Professor and Head, Division of Arthritis Research, Department of Molecular and Experimental Medicine, Scripps Research Institute, La Jolla, California

Carlos J. Lozada, M.D. Assistant Professor of Medicine, Director, Rheumatology Fellowship Program, Division of Rheumatology and Immunology, University of Miami School of Medicine, Attending Physician, Department of Medicine, Jackson Memorial Hospital, Miami, Florida

Harvinder S. Luthra, M.D Professor of Medicine, Mayo Medical School, Chair, Division of Rheumatology, Department of Internal Medicine, Mayo Clinic, Rochester, Minnesota

Maren L. Mahowald, M.D. Professor of Medicine, Department of Internal Medicine, University of Minnesota, Chief, Rheumatology Section, Department of Medicine, Minneapolis Veterans Affairs Medical Center, Minneapolis, Minnesota

Stephen E. Malawista, M.D. Professor of Medicine, Yale University School of Medicine, Department of Internal Medicine, Section of Rheumatology, New Haven, Connecticut

Johanne Martel-Pelletier, Ph.D. Professor of Medicine, Department of Medicine, University of Montreal, Director, Osteoarthritis Research Unit, Notre Dame Hospital, Montreal, Quebec, Canadac

Richard Mayne, Ph.D. Professor, Department of Cell Biology, University of Alabama, Birmingham, Alabama

Daniel J. McCarty, M.D. Will and Cava Ross Professor of Medicine, Department of Medicine, Medical College of Wisconsin, Senior Attending Physician, Department of Medicine, Froedtent Memorial Lutheran Hospital, Milwaukee, Wisconsin

Thomas A. Medsger, Jr., M.D. Gerald P. Rodnan Professor of Medicine, Department of Medicine, University of Pittsburgh School of Medicine, Pittsburgh, Pennsylvania

Clement J. Michet, M.D., M.P.H. Consultant, Mayo Clinic, Rochester, Minnesota

Herman Mielants, M.D. Professor, Department of Rheumatology, Ghent University, Ghent University Hospital, Ghent, Belgium

Frederick W. Miller, M.D. Senior Investigator, Laboratory of Molecular and Developmental Immunology, Center for Biologics Evaluation and Research, Food and Drug Administration, Bethesda, Maryland

Gerald F. Moore, M.D. Professor of Medicine, Department of Internal Medicine, University of Nebraska Medical Center, Omaha, Nebraska

Larry W. Moreland, M.D. Professor of Medicine, Department of Medicine, University of Alabama, Birmingham, Alabama

Sarah L. Morgan, M.D., R.D., F.A.D.A., F.A.C.P. Associate Professor, Departments of Nutrition Sciences and Medicine, University of Alabama at Birmingham, Medical Director, Osteoporosis Prevention and Treatment Clinic, The Kirklin Clinic, Birmingham, Alabama

Roland W. Moskowitz, M.D. Professor of Medicine, Division of Rheumatology, Department of Medicine, Case Western Reserve University School of Medicine, Director, Division of Rheumatic Diseases, University Hospitals, Cleveland, Ohio

John D. Mountz, M.D., Ph.D. Professor, Department of Medicine, University of Alabama, Birmingham, Alabama

Ulf Müller-Ladner, M.D. Attendant, Department of Internal Medicine I, University of Regendsburg, Regensburg, Bavaria, Germany

Barry L. Myones, M.D. Associate Professor, Departments of Pediatrics and Microbiology/Immunology, Baylor College of Medicine, Director of Research, Pediatric Rheumatology Center, Texas Children's Hospital, Houston, Texas

Stanley J. Naides, M.D. Thomas B. Hallowell Professor of Medicine, Professor of Microbiology and Immunology, Chief, Division of Rheumatology, Milton S. Hershey Medical Center, Pennsylvania State University College of Medicine, Hershey, Pennsylvania

Charles L. Nelson, M.D. Assistant Professor, Attending Surgeon, Department of Orthopaedic Surgery, University of Pennsylvania, Hospital of the University of Pennsylvania, Philadelphia, Pennsylvania

Barbara S. Nepom, M.D. Research Associate Member, Immunology Program, Virginia Mason Research Center, Research Associate Professor, Department of Pediatrics, University of Washington School of Medicine, Seattle, Washington

James R. O'Dell, M.D. Professor of Medicine, Department of Internal Medicine, University of Nebraska Medical Center, Omaha, Nebraska

Shawn W. O'Driscoll, M.D., Ph.D. Professor of Orthopedics, Department of Orthopedics, Mayo Clinic, Rochester, Minnesota

J. Desmond O'Duffy, M.B. Sarasota, Florida

Richard S. Panush, M.D. Clinical Professor of Medicine Mount Sinai School of Medicine, New York, New York, and, Chairman, Department of Medicine, Saint Barnabas Medical Center, Livingston, New Jersey

Jean-Pierre Pelletier, M.D. Professor, Department of Medicine, University of Montreal, Head, Arthritis Division, Notre Dame Hospital, Montreal, Quebec, Canada

Maria D. Perez, M.D. Assistant Professor, Division of Rheumatology, Texas Children's Hospital, Houston, Texas

Andras Perl, M.D., Ph.D. Professor of Medicine and of Microbiology and Immunology, Department of Medicine, State University of New York Upstate Medical University, Syracuse, New York

Charles G. Peterfy, M.D., Ph.D. Assistant Clinical Professor of Radiology, Osteoporosis and Arthritis Research Group, University of California at San Francisco, Chief Scientific Officer, Synarc, Inc., San Francisco, California

Karin S. Peterson, M.D. Assistant Professor, Department of Pediatrics, Columbia University, New York New York

Michelle A. Petri, M.D., M.P.H. Associate Professor of Medicine, Division of Rheumatology, Department of Medicine, Johns Hopkins University School of Medicine, Director, Lupus Center, Johns Hopkins Hospital, Baltimore, Maryland

Ross E. Petty, M.D., Ph.D. Professor, Department of Pediatrics, British Columbia's Childrens Hosptial, Vancouver, British Columbia, Canada

Mark R. Philips, M.D. Assistant Professor of Medicine and Cell Biology, Division of Rheumatology, Department of Medicine, New York University Medical Center, New York, New York

Paul E. Phillips, M.D. Professor, Departments of Medicine and Pediatrics, Chief, Rheumatology Division, State University of New York Upstate Medical University, Syracuse, New York

Robert S. Pinals, M.D. Professor and Vice Chairman, Department of Medicine, University of Medicine and Dentistry of New Jersey, Robert Wood Johnson Medical School, New Brunswick, New Jersey, and, Attending Physician, Department of Medicine, Medical Center at Princeton, Princeton, New Jersey

A. Robin Poole, Ph.D., D.S.C. Director, Joint Diseases Laboratory, Shriners Hospital for Crippled Children, Montreal Unit, McGill University, Montreal, Quebec, Canada

Reed Edwin Pyeritz, M.D., Ph.D. Professor of Human Genetics, Medicine, and Pediatrics, Chair, Department of Human Genetics, MCP Hahnemann School of Medicine, Philadelphia, Pennsylvania, and, Director, Center for Medical Genetics, Allegheny General Hospital, Pittsburgh, Pennsylvania

Eric L. Radin, M.D. Director, Bone and Joint Center, Henry Ford Hospital, Clinical Professor of Surgery (Orthopedics), University of Michigan, Ann Arbor, Michigan, Detroit, Michigan

Westley H. Reeves, M.D. Marcia Whitney Schott Professor of Medicine, Chief, Division of Rheumatology and Clinical Immunology, Department of Medicine, University of Florida, Shands Hospital, Gainesville, Florida

Antonio J. Reginato, M.D. Professor and Chief, Division of Rheumatology, University of Medicine and Dentistry of New Jersey, Robert Wood Johnson Medical School, Cooper Hospital, Camden, New Jersey

Morris Reichlin, M.D. George Lynn Cross Research Professor of Medicine and Chief of the Rheumatology, Immunology and Allergy Section, Oklahoma University Health Sciences Center, Head, Arthritis and Immunology Program, Department of Arthritis and Immunology, Oklahoma Medical Research Foundation, Oklahoma City, Oklahoma

John D. Reveille, M.D. George S. Bruce Jr. Professor in Arthritis and Other Rheumatic Diseases, Division of Rheumatology and Clinical Immunogenetics, The University of Texas at Houston Health Science Center, Houston, Texas

Ann K. Rosenthal, M.D. Associate Professor and Chief, Division of Rheumatology, Department of Medicine, Medical College of Wisconsin, Zablocki Veterans Affairs Medical Center, Milwaukee, Wisconsin

Robert A. S. Roubey, M.D. Research Assistant Professor, Division of Rheumatology, Department of Medicine, University of North Carolina School of Medicine, Chapel Hill, North Carolina

Perry J. Rush, M.D., F.R.C.P.C. Assistant Professor of Medicine, Department of Medicine, Division of Rheumatology and Physical Medicine and Rehabalitation, University of Toronto, North York, Ontario, Canada

Lawrence M. Ryan, M.D. Will and Cava Ross Professor and Chief, Department of Rheumatology, Medical College of Wisconsin, Milwaukee, Wisconsin

Kenneth Saag, M.D., M.Sc. Associate Professor, Department of Medicine, The University of Alabama at Birmingham, University Hospital, Birmingham, Alabama

Kenneth E. Sack, M.D. Professor of Clinical Medicine, Attending Physician, Division of Rheumatology, Department of Medicine, University of California at San Francisco, San Francisco, California

Robert. L. Sah, M.D. Associate Professor, Department of Bioengineering, University of California at San Diego, La Jolla, California

Mansoor N. Saleh, M.D. Professor of Medicine and Pathology, Associate Director for Clinical Network, Division of Hematology/Oncology, University of Alabama, Birmingham, Alabama

Charles L. Saltzman, M.D. Associate Professor, Department of Orthopaedic Surgery, University of Iowa, University of Iowa Hospitals and Clinics, Iowa City, Iowa

John D. Sandy, Ph.D. Associate Professor, Department of Pharmacology and Therapeutics, University of South Florida, Senior Investigator, Center for Research in Skeletal Development and Pediatric Orthopedics, Shriners Hospital for Children, Tampa, Florida

Minoru Satoh, M.D. Research Associate Professor, Department of Medicine, University of Florida, Gainesville, Florida

Allen D. Sawitzke, M.D. Assistant Professor of Medicine, Department of Medicine, University of Utah School of Medicine, Salt Lake City, Utah

Harry W. Schroeder, Jr., M.D., Ph.D. Professor of Microbiology, Professor of Medicine, Division of Clinical and Developmental Immunology, Department of Medicine, University of Alabama, Birmingham, Alabama

H. Ralph Schumacher, Jr., M.D. Professor of Medicine, Department of Medicine, Division of Rheumatology, University of Pennsylvania School of Medicine, Director, Arthritis/Immunology Center, Department of Medicine, Veterans Affairs Medical Center, Philadelphia, Pennsylvania

Charles N. Serhan, Ph.D. Professor of Anesthesia (Biochemistry and Molecular Pharmacology), Harvard Medical School, Director, Center for Experimental Therapeutic and Reperfusion Injury, Department of Anesthesia, Perioperative, and Pain Medicine, Brigham and Women's Hospital, Boston, Massachusetts

Randy R. Sibbitt, M.D. Private Practice, Helena, Montana

Wilmer L. Sibbitt, Jr., M.D. Professor, Departments of Internal Medicine and Neurology, University of New Mexico Health Sciences Center, Albuquerque, New Mexico

Leonard H. Sigal, M.D., F.A.C.P., F.A.C.R. Professor and Chief, Division of Rheumatology, Department of Medicine, University of Medicine and Dentistry of New Jersey, Robert Wood Johnson Medical School, Robert Wood Johnson University Hospital, New Brunswick, New Jersey

Richard M. Silver, M.D. Director, Division of Rheumatology and Immunology, Professor of Medicine and Pediatrics, Department of Medicine, Medical University of South Carolina, Professor of Medicine and Pediatrics, Department of Medicine, Medical University Hospital, Charleston, South Carolina

Peter A. Simkin, M.D. Professor of Medicine, Department of Medicine, Division of Rheumatology, University of Washington, Seattle, Washington

Robert A. Terkeltaub, M.D. Professor, Department of Medicine, University of California at San Diego, Chief, Department of Rheumatology, Veterans Affairs Medical Center, San Diego, California

Eric M. Veys, M.D. Department of Rheumatology, University of Ghent, Ghent University Hospital, Ghent, Belgium

John E. Volanakis, M.D. Professor, Department of Medicine, University of Alabama School of Medicine, Birmingham, Alabama, and Director, Biomedical Sciences Research Center "A. Fleming", Vari, Greece

Angela A. Wang, M.D. Instructor, Department of Orthopedics, University of Utah, Salt Lake City, Utah

Robert W. Warren, M.D., Ph.D., M.P.H. Associate Professor, Department of Pediatrics-Rheumatology, Baylor College of Medicine, Chief, Rhematology Section, Department of Pediatric Rheumatology, Texas Children's Hospital, Houston, Texas

Casey T. Weaver, M.D. Associate Professor of Pathology, Department of Pathology, University of Alabama at Birmingham, Birmingham, Alabama

Andrew J. Weiland, M.D. Professor of Orthopaedic and Plastic Surgery, Hospital for Special Surgery, New York, New York

Michael E. Weinblatt, M.D. Professor of Medicine, Department of Medicine, Harvard Medical School, Co-Director of Clinical Rheumatology, Brigham and Women's Hospital, Boston, Massachusetts

Michael H. Weisman, M.D. Professor of Medicine, Division of Rheumatology, Department of Medicine, University of California at San Diego, La Jolla, California, and, Director, Division of Rheumatology, Cedars-Sinai Medical Center, Los Angeles, California

Peter F. Weller, M.D. Professor of Medicine, Department of Medicine, Harvard Medical School, Chief, Allergy and Inflammation Division, Co-Chief, Infectious Disease Division, Beth Israel Deaconess Medical Center, Boston, Massachusetts

Cornelia M. Weyand, M.D., Ph.D. Professor of Medicine, Division of Rheumatology, Department of Medicine, Mayo Clinic and Foundation, Rochester, Minnesota

Ronald L. Wilder, M.D., Ph.D. Chief, Inflammatory Joint Diseases Section, National Institute of Arthritis and Musculoskeletal and Skin Diseases, National Institutes of Health, Bethesda, Maryland

Andrew P. Wilking, M.D. Associate Professor, Department of Pediatrics, Baylor College of Medicine, Texas Children's Hospital, Houston, Texas

H. James Williams, M.D. Professor and Associate Chairman, Department of Internal Medicine, Division of Rheumatology, University of Utah College of Medicine, University of Utah Medical Center, Salt Lake City, Utah

Robert J. Winchester, M.D. Professor, Departments of Pediatrics, Medicine, and Pathology, Columbia University, and, Attending Physician, Departments of Pediatrics and Medicine, New York Hospital, New York, New York

Robert L. Wortmann, M.D. Chairman, Department of Medicine, University of Oklahoma Health Sciences Center, Tulsa Campus, Tulsa, Oklahoma

David E. Yocum, M.D. Professor of Medicine, Arizona Arthritis Center, University of Arizona, Chief, Department of Rheumatology and Immunology, University of Arizona Medical Center, Tucson, Arizona

John B. Zabriskie, M.D. Associate Professor, Head, Laboratory of Clinical Microbiology and Immunology, Rockefeller University, New York, New York

Huang-Ge Zhang, D.V.M., Ph.D. Research Assistant Professor, Department of Medicine/Rheumatology, University of Alabama, Birmingham, Alabama

Tong Zhou, M.D. Assistant Professor of Medicine, Division of Clinical Immunology and Rheumatology, Department of Medicine, University of Alabama, Birmingham, Alabama

FOREWORD

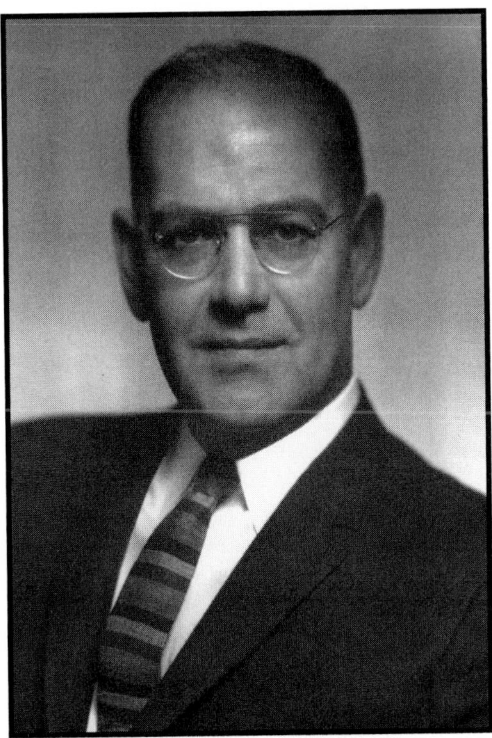

JOE HOLLANDER

I am grateful to Bill Koopman for the opportunity to write this Foreword for the fourteenth edition of this remarkable textbook. I recently learned of Joe Hollander's death, and so I write with heavy heart. Joe was my medical father and a mighty link in the evolutionary chain of progress in rheumatology as recorded in the successive editions of this textbook. Taken together, these books arguably represent the best available history of our field.

Bernard Isaac Comroe, one of two gifted physician brothers (the other was Julius Comroe, father of modern pulmonology), wrote the first three editions as sole author. Although he used the term "rheumatologist" in the preface to the first edition in 1940, the subtitle "A Textbook of Rheumatology" did not appear until the sixth edition in 1960. According to Hollander's preface to this edition, Comroe had used the "Rheumatism Reviews" edited by Philip S. Hency of the Mayo Clinic, which had been published at yearly intervals in the *Annals of Internal Medicine* since 1935, as the basis for his texts. Most contributors to the "Rheumatism Reviews" were in service together in World War II, and they became the nucleus of the multiauthored textbooks under Hollander's editorship, beginning with the fourth edition in 1949. After Bernard Comroe's untimely death in 1945, Joe was appointed chief of the Arthritis Clinic of the Hospital of the University of Pennsylvania by O. H. Perry Pepper, the department chairman.

Dr. Pepper, now emeritus chairman, wrote the first ever foreword in the fifth edition (1953) as a eulogy to Bernard Comroe. The foreword to the sixth edition (1960) was written by Dr. Russell L. Cecil. Dr. Cecil was an Alabama native who had been chairman of medicine at Cornell and who, together with Dr. Robert Loeb, founded a textbook of medicine. Robert M. Stecher from Western Reserve University, a pioneer of genetics in the rheumatic diseases, wrote the forewords to both the seventh and eighth editions. Joe Hollander himself wrote the Foreword to editions nine through twelve as editor emeritus. Bob Stecher and Joe Hollander were the driving forces behind the founding of the *Arthritis and Rheumatism* journal in 1958. Apparently what goes around comes around—both Bill Koopman and I have served as editors of this journal!

The practice of rheumatology has become both more complex and more rational in the years since Dr. Comroe's 1940 preface, in which he posed such questions as: "Should tonsils be removed routinely in all cases of infectious arthritis?" "Should all devitalized teeth be removed in the patient with rheumatoid arthritis?" "How often do accessory nasal sinus infection, chronic prostatitis, chronic cholecystitis, chronic non-specific cervicitis etc. actually play a role in the etiology of arthritis?" "May the intestinal tract act as a focus in this condition?"

Although the answers to some of these important queries remain unclear, I believe Dr. Comroe would have enjoyed reading the fourteenth edition of his textbook, with 131 chapters by over 100 authors dealing with our current understandings and contemporary controversies. How he would have marveled at the clinical and laboratory science that produced specific COX-2 inhibitors, anti-cytokine molecules, and immunoregulatory drugs! Progress has been made in small steps in rheumatology. In the aggregate, however, this text is as different from the first edition as Sanskrit is from Swahili.

Daniel J. McCarty, M.D.
Milwaukee, Wisconsin

PREFACE

The fourteenth edition of *Arthritis and Allied Conditions* records the impressive advances made during the last four years of the twentieth century in fundamental insights and clinical knowledge relevant to the field. Several of the changes in this edition are consistent with the dynamic nature of our discipline. There are seven chapters addressing new topics (nitric oxide, genetic basis of the rheumatic diseases, minocycline, lefluonomide, bone marrow transplantation, therapy of systemic lupus erythematous, pregnancy and the rheumatic diseases, and Paget's disease) and 37 chapters authored by new contributors. Definitive chapters on the epidemiology of the rheumatic diseases and analytic methods for their clinical evaluation have been updated. Such changes reflect the sustained commitment to scholarly excellence and authoritativeness established by my predecessors, Dan McCarty and the late Joe Hollander.

Since the last edition, there have been extraordinary advances in understanding of the structure of the joint and its constituent molecules, mechanisms underlying the inflammatory response, and the effector pathways that contribute to the pathogenesis of tissue injury in the rheumatic diseases. Each chapter covering the scientific basis of the rheumatic diseases has been authored by a leader in the field who is well-positioned to interpret the significance of these advances.

A new chapter on proteoglycans, together with extensively updated chapters on collagen, cartilage, and synovial cells, provide cutting-edge treatments of these important topics. Chapters on apoptosis, cytokines and their receptors, immune complexes, nitric oxide, and eicosanoids capture the substantial progress in these important fields that contribute substantially to the pathogenesis of this group of diseases. The molecular basis of immunoglobulin and T-cell receptor diversity is concisely presented. Several updated and new chapters convey new insights regarding the cellular basis of the inflammatory response, including the role of neutrophils, macrophages, lymphocytes, mast cells, eosinophils, and platelets. A new chapter covers the active role of adhesive molecules in directing cellular participants to sites of inflammation. Other new chapters on the HLA complex and the role of non-HLA genes in the pathogenesis of rheumatic disease highlight substantial progress in understanding of the genetic bases of these diseases.

The substantial interim advances in understanding of the pathogenesis of several rheumatic diseases have fostered explosive progress in the development of new therapeutic approaches. Chapters on biologic agents, immunomodulatory agents, gene therapy, and bone marrow transplantation record the considerable excitement and promise these approaches engender. The recent availability of cyclooxygenase-2 inhibitors and lefluonomide for therapeutic use is reflected in an extensively updated chapter on nonsteroidal, antiinflammatory drugs and a new chapter on lefluonomide, respectively.

Rheumatoid arthritis, as the prototypic chronic inflammatory arthritide, is the focus of the first clinical section in this edition. Progress in understanding of the pathology, pathogenesis, clinical expression, and therapy of this disease is lucidly presented in new and updated chapters by authorities in the field. Impressive developments in surgical approaches for rheumatoid arthritis are extensively covered in a separate section.

Rapid advances in the delineation of the role of bacteria in the pathogenesis of reactive arthritis, enteropathic arthritis, and Lyme disease are emphasized in revised chapters. Systemic lupus erythematosus continues to capture the interest of clinicians and investigators alike. Chapters on the pathogenesis, clinical manifestations, and therapy of this disease comprehensively discuss new insights. Updated chapters on vasculitis and its mimics reflect a wealth of clinical insights and provide an experienced perspective for the consulting rheumatologist. A separate chapter on scleroderma variants complements a new chapter on the clinical picture and treatment of the disease. Remarkable advances in understanding of the pathogenesis and treatment of osteoporosis, both in women and men, are captured in a new chapter on this topic. Progress in defining mechanisms underlying the pathogenesis of osteroarthritis holds great promise for new therapeutic approaches, including induction of cartilage repair, which is concisely discussed in a new chapter.

I deeply appreciate the efforts of the many authors who have faithfully captured the vitality of this field in their contributions and my predecessors for establishing this textbook as the forum for recording advances in our discipline.

William J. Koopman, M.D.
Birmingham, Alabama

ACKNOWLEDGMENTS

My sincere appreciation to Ms. Cynthia Shepard, Managing Editor, for her superb efforts in coordinating the preparation of this textbook. Her attention to detail and commitment to the highest quality are evident throughout the book. Many thanks for the outstanding efforts of Ms. Gloria Purnell in keeping this effort on track. I am deeply indebted to my many colleagues, staff, and faculty in the Division of Clinical Immunology and Rheumatology at the University of Alabama at Birmingham for their enormous support over the years and their many contributions to the field (and to this textbook). I also wish to acknowledge the outstanding efforts of the staff of Lippincott Williams & Wilkins in the preparation of this edition. Above all, I want to thank my cherished wife and companion of 33 years, Lilliane, and my beloved children (Benjamin, Anna, Rebecca, and Steven) and grandchildren (Margaret and William) for their love, patience, understanding, and support over so many years. This book is dedicated to them.

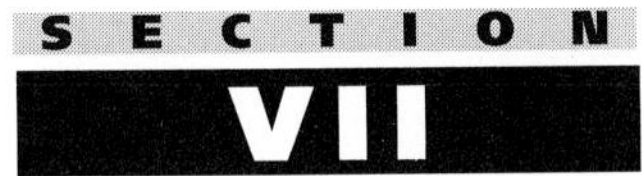

SYSTEMIC RHEUMATIC DISEASES

72

UNDIFFERENTIATED CONNECTIVE TISSUE DISEASES, OVERLAP SYNDROMES, AND MIXED CONNECTIVE TISSUE DISEASES

MORRIS REICHLIN

Systemic rheumatic diseases share several properties that often make a specific diagnosis difficult. The diseases in question are rheumatoid arthritis (RA), systemic lupus erythematosus (SLE), progressive systemic sclerosis (PSS) or systemic scleroderma, polymyositis (PM), dermatomyositis (DM), and Sjögren's syndrome (SS; keratoconjunctivitis sicca and xerostomia due to lymphocytic infiltration of the lacrimal and salivary glands), which exists in a primary form or in association with one of the four diseases mentioned, in which case it is called secondary. Of most importance is the occurrence of several clinical features that are shared to a variable extent by all of these diseases. These include Raynaud's phenomenon, polyarthritis, anemia, interstitial lung disease, pleuropericarditis, and vasculitis. Patients with one or more of these features often do not satisfy criteria for any of the recognized systemic rheumatic diseases. Additionally, evolution to a recognizable connective tissue disease may require years, may never occur, or the signs and symptoms may disappear, eliminating the necessity for any disease designation. Serologic features also are shared to a variable extent by all of these diseases, particularly antinuclear antibodies and rheumatoid factors (RFs). These and several other serologic markers to be discussed are listed in Table 72.1. Frequent sharing of clinical features and serologic findings renders diagnosis difficult in the early stages of this group of diseases, for which no etiology has been established. Moreover, no definitive diagnostic tests exist for the clinician in the absence of a cluster of clinical features that comprise the diagnostic features of the differentiated form of each of these diseases. Moreover, there is the additional problem that each of the systemic rheumatic diseases is extremely heterogeneous. It is very clear that, especially for SLE, PSS, PM, and DM, numerous subsets can be classified on the basis of a combination of clinical characteristics and the recognition of specific autoantibodies directed to well-defined molecular target antigens. These disease-specific autoantibodies are listed in Table 72.2.

TABLE 72.1. SEROLOGIC TESTS FREQUENTLY POSITIVE IN UNDIFFERENTIATED CONNECTIVE TISSUE DISEASE OR OVERLAP SYNDROMES

Antinuclear antibodies detected by indirect immunofluorescence (especially with speckled or homogeneous patterns)
Rheumatoid factors
Anti-ssDNA
Anti-U_1RNP, Anti-U_2RNP
Anti-chromatin

TABLE 72.2. DISEASE-SPECIFIC AUTOANTIBODIES

Disease	Antigens
Systemic lupus erythematosus (SLE)	dsDNA
	Ribosomal "P" proteins
	Ro/SSA, La/SSB (also in Sjögren's syndrome)
	Sm
Progressive systemic sclerosis (PSS)	Topoisomerase I (Scl 70)
	Centromere antigens
	RNA polymerase II, III
	Nucleolar antigens Pm/Scl, RNA polymerase I
	Fibrillarin (U_1RNA), NOR 90
Polymyositis (PM)	Myositis-specific targets tRNA synthetases (histidyl, threonyl, alanyl, glycyl, isoleucyl)
	Other cytoplasmic targets
	SRP (signal recognition particle)
	Mas
	Fer (elongation factor E1α)
	KJ (translation factor, molecular nature unknown)
Dermatomyositis (DM)	Mi_2 nuclear antigen

TABLE 72.3. OVERLAP SYNDROMES

Systemic rheumatic diseases with Sjögren's syndrome
Rheumatoid arthritis with systemic lupus erythematosus, Rhupus
Progressive systemic sclerosis, systemic lupus erythematosus, polymyositis or mixed connective tissue diseases
Scleroderma, polymyositis without anti-U_1RNP or systemic lupus erythematosus
Primary biliary cirrhosis, Sjögren's syndrome, limited forms of scleroderma (CREST)

This great heterogeneity of the systemic rheumatic diseases, their frequent incomplete expression, especially in the early phases, and the tendency for overlap among them has created the necessity for a concept that is one of the major themes of this chapter: undifferentiated connective tissue disease. Two early articles set this problem in perspective (1,2), and this "problem" has spawned a multicenter collaborative study to define the clinical boundaries of early undifferentiated connective tissue disease (UCTD) syndrome and to study its natural history (3–5). Articles continue to be written about the clinical problems posed by these patients (6,7), but the multicenter trial addressed several fundamental questions about the nature of UCTD and the fate of individual patients over time with respect to course, prognosis, and the frequency of evolution to differentiated forms of the systemic rheumatic diseases.

Finally, in numerous instances, there is the concurrent presence of two or more diseases that are more or less fully expressed. Examples are listed in Table 72.3. The most controversial of these is mixed connective tissue disease (MCTD), in which there are features of SLE, PM or DM, and PSS in various combinations in association with high titers of autoantibodies to the nRNP or U1RNP antigen (8,9). There are, however, many known instances of overlap among and between these diseases unaccompanied by antibodies to U1RNP; conversely, these specific antibodies occur to a variable extent with each of these diseases when they occur alone. Reports that antibodies to the 70-kd polypeptide of the U1RNP antigen are characteristic of MCTD have been confirmed, but these autoantibodies also occur in at least half the SLE patients with anti-U1RNP precipitins who do not have overlap features (10). The present view of MCTD is discussed in a later section of this chapter.

RECOGNITION OF DIFFERENTIATED CONNECTIVE TISSUE DISEASES

Clinical investigation in the systemic rheumatic diseases requires that criteria be established to classify patients for the purposes of clinical research. Clinical findings are characteristic of each of the systemic rheumatic diseases, and these comprise the most important criteria used to classify the diseases, with the help of statistical analysis. Some of these disease-specific findings are listed in Table 72.4, and, wherever appropriate, nonspecific clinical findings frequently present in UCTD are listed in parallel fashion. These and other disease criteria eventually form the basis for the classification criteria for RA, SLE, and PSS, as determined by committees of the American College of Rheumatology. Similar approaches have been used for PM, DM, and SS. The primary function of these criteria is to identify patients who are to be entered into clinical trials.

TABLE 72.4. CLINICAL AND LABORATORY MANIFESTATIONS OF SYSTEMIC RHEUMATIC DISEASE WITH HIGH DISEASE SPECIFICITY CONTRASTED WITH NONSPECIFIC MANIFESTATIONS OF UNDIFFERENTIATED CONNECTIVE TISSUE DISEASE

Disease	Specific	Undifferentiated Connective Tissue Disease
SLE	Photosensitive rashes, malar distribution Subacute cutaneous LE	Pleuropericardial disease
SLE	Glomerulonephritis with hypocomplementemia	Proteinuria
SLE	Coombs-positive hemolytic anemia	Normochromic normocytic anemia
SLE/APL Syndrome	Thrombocytopenia	Normal platelet count
DM	Heliotrope, Gottron's papules	Muscle atrophy
PM & DM	Proximal muscle weakness associated with elevated myogenic enzymes in serum with characteristic muscle biopsy and electromyographic findings	Weight loss, fatigue, generalized weakness
RA	Symmetric erosive destructive polyarthritis associated with positive rheumatoid factors	Nondestructive polyarthritis
RA	Caplan's syndrome	Interstitial lung disease
PSS	Skin thickening proximal to the wrist, telangiectasia, sclerodactyly, calcinosis	Raynaud's phenomenon

APL, antiphospholipid syndrome.

In the evaluation of individual patients for clinical diagnosis, characteristic specific features are sought whose pattern comprises the disease picture for each of the systemic rheumatic diseases. Whereas these are discussed in detail in other chapters of this book, a brief review is presented so that the specific clinical and serologic features of these diseases can be contrasted with the nonspecific clinical and serologic findings that lead to the designation of UCTD: a way station for the numerous incomplete connective tissue syndromes that cannot be classified.

Systemic Lupus Erythematosus

In SLE, "differentiated" features rarely seen in the other connective tissue diseases include glomerulonephritis, photosensitivity, characteristic skin rashes, central nervous system (CNS) disease, and various cytopenias such as Coombs' positive hemolytic anemia, leukopenia, and thrombocytopenia. These are all very unusual in PSS, RA, and PM or DM. Pleuropericarditis and peritonitis are common in SLE, but are seen to a variable extent in the other systemic rheumatic diseases. Serologically, antibodies to native DNA, Sm, and ribosomal "P" proteins are seen almost exclusively in SLE, whereas precipitating antibodies to U1RNP, Ro/SSA, and La/SSB, although present in aggregate in 85% of SLE patients, are present in other rheumatic diseases. Precipitating antibodies to Ro/SSA and La/SSB are seen more commonly in primary SS than in SLE. There are numerous combinations of these clinical findings in association with several defined autoantibodies that would definitively make the diagnosis of SLE. Patients with SLE in early phases of the disease may exhibit only nonspecific clinical features and a positive antinuclear antibody without any of the disease-specific autoantibodies. One of the very common, positive serologic tests frequently present in early (and late) phases of the disease is antibody to chromatin, manifest as a positive antinuclear antibody with a diffuse homogeneous pattern. These antibodies, although present in the majority of patients with SLE, also are found in variable numbers of patients with RA and PSS (11). In a recent study in murine SLE, it has been shown that antibodies to chromatin (or nucleosomes) are an early feature of the evolving autoimmunity to nuclear antigens, and antibodies to dsDNA (the most specific of the serologic tests for SLE) appear later in the disease (12,13).

Progressive Systemic Sclerosis

There is less heterogeneity in PSS than in SLE, but the diagnosis depends strongly on the presence of thickened skin due to dermal collagen accumulation in a diffuse pattern, in which the thickening extends proximal to the wrists and also involves the trunk and face. Patients with diffuse skin involvement, as defined earlier, have an increased risk of sclerosis of the internal organs such as the heart, lungs, and bowel, as well as renal nephrosclerosis with malignant hypertension. Virtually all patients with PSS have Raynaud's phenomenon, and a subset has limited skin involvement restricted to the hands (sclerodactyly) and face, calcinosis, esophageal motility disturbances, and telangiectasia (CREST syndrome). Patients with limited skin disease may have various combinations of these findings (e.g., REST, RST, constituting limited forms of the CREST syndrome).

There also is a family of antinuclear antibodies, which are highly specific for PSS, which include antibodies to various nucleolar antigens, Scl70, or topoisomerase I, and the centromere antigens. These are listed in Table 72.2. Antibodies to the centromere antigens correlate highly with the presence of the CREST variant of PSS. Until recently there has been no serologic marker that occurs in the majority of patients with diffuse skin disease, although antibodies to topoisomerase I occur more frequently in diffuse disease than in patients with limited skin disease or CREST (14–16). In recent publications, autoantibodies to RNA polymerase III appear to be the most prevalent of the class of enzymes that are disease specific and may be a marker for diffuse disease (17). Additionally, antibodies to RNA polymerase II (18,19) and its phosphorylated form (20) are highly specific for PSS, with a preference for diffuse disease. Antibodies to RNA polymerase I have long been noted to occur in a small percentage of patients with PSS (18,19), to be responsible for a speckled nucleolar staining pattern, and to be associated with diffuse disease (21).

Polymyositis and Dermatomyositis

The differentiated forms of these diseases exhibit the features of inflammatory myopathy with its attendant proximal weakness, elevated myogenic enzymes, and characteristic electromyograph (EMG) and muscle biopsy findings. Additionally, a family of disease-specific autoantibodies are associated with clinical subsets. These are listed in Table 72.2. Patients with PM and interstitial lung disease produce antibodies to a set of translation-related proteins, including Jo_1, Pl_7, and Pl_{12}, which are histidyl, threonyl, and alanyl tRNA synthetases, respectively, as well as the translation component KJ. Also included in this group are antibodies to the glycyl and isoleucyl tRNA synthetases, as well as the antigens Mas and Fer, which are molecular components of the translation apparatus. Antibodies to signal-recognition particles occur in patients with PM without interstitial lung disease, and antibodies to Mi_2 a nuclear protein complex occur in patients with DM. These antibodies have not been reported in the other connective tissue diseases to any significant extent, even when sensitive tests are used for their detection (22). A detailed discussion of the clinical significance of these myositis-specific antibodies has appeared (23).

Rheumatoid Arthritis

The two most common differentiated systemic rheumatic diseases are RA and SS. The diagnostic features of RA rest in the recognition of its clinical features and the exclusion of other defined diseases that can mimic it. Thus RA is diagnosed when chronicity and symmetry of polyarthritis are featured in a destructive process that causes cartilage destruction and bone erosions in characteristic locations. RFs, antibodies [particularly immunoglobulin M (IgM)] directed to the Fc fragment of IgG are present in elevated titers in 70% to 80% of clinically typical cases. The fraction of otherwise typical RA patients who lack RFs in their entire course probably have other diseases whose etiologies are not apparent. The heterogeneity of "true" RA is great, with a spectrum of severity ranging from Felty's syndrome at one extreme, with vasculitis and numerous extraarticular features, to chronic polyarthritis with a fairly benign course and little systemic involvement. In the early phases of RA, it is easy to appreciate the confusion that may confront clinicians as they ponder the diagnosis.

Sjögren's Syndrome

Sjögren's syndrome exists in two forms. In the so-called "primary" disease, lymphocytic infiltration and destruction of the lacrimal and salivary glands, leads to the combined signs and symptoms of the disease, which are keratoconjunctivitis sicca (dry eyes) and xerostomia (dry mouth). RFs are present in at least 80% of the patients, and precipitating antibodies to the small ribonucleoproteins Ro/SSA and La/SSB occur in 50% to 80% and 20% to 30% of the patients, respectively. Sensitive enzyme-linked immunosorbent assay (ELISA) procedures put the prevalence of these autoantibodies even higher, although some unknown percentage of patients with primary SS are always negative (24). Perhaps like the seronegative RA patients, these otherwise typical primary SS patients have another disease underlying their sicca syndrome such as acquired immunodeficiency syndrome (AIDS) (25) or other as yet unidentified viruses or retroviruses. As in RA, with its extraarticular disease, primary SS patients are known to exhibit numerous extraglandular features such as polyarthritis, nonthrombocytopenic purpura, and a broad range of CNS and peripheral nervous system complications, often in association with vasculitis. A subset of these patients develops the lesions of subacute cutaneous LE and are said to have Sjögren's–SLE overlap, in which shared immunogenetic features (DR2 and DR3, HLA-DQ1/DQ2 heterozygosity) and antibodies to Ro/SSA and La/SSB are almost uniformly present (26–28). These observations reemphasize the strong overlap among and between the various systemic rheumatic diseases.

UNDIFFERENTIATED CONNECTIVE TISSUE DISEASE

The designation UCTD arose because many patients do not clearly express the clinical features of any single disease. Such patients probably compose as much as 50% of tertiary referrals in patients with suspected systemic rheumatic diseases. An example of this conundrum is illustrated by the patients with Raynaud's phenomenon with no other clinical findings. The first issue here is whether the Raynaud's phenomenon is an isolated phenomenon or is the harbinger of a systemic rheumatic disease. Should a thorough laboratory and physical examination fail to reveal evidence of a systemic rheumatic disease, the presence or absence of a positive antinuclear antibody test is useful, because its presence indicates high risk for the development of a systemic rheumatic disease (29). In addition, the characteristic changes of dropout and dilatation in the nailfold capillary bed are associated primarily with scleroderma but also occur in a fraction of SLE and PM/DM patients (30). If the positive antinuclear antibody is anticentromere antibody or anti–topoisomerase I, it is likely that PSS will develop in those patients (31,32). A large prospective study of this type is in progress; and in the coming years, data will become available to enable clinicians to tell patients with isolated Raynaud's phenomenon and anticentromere or anti–topoisomerase I (or other disease-specific autoantibodies) what their risk and time frame are for the development of PSS (3–5). We can deduce from the studies thus far reported that certain associated factors predict the development of a systemic rheumatic disease in patients with Raynaud's phenomenon. These factors, listed in Table 72.5, include older age at onset, high severity from the onset, positive antinuclear antibody, and abnormal capillary microscopy. Because the frequency of Raynaud's phenomenon in normal women and men is 8% and 2% to 3%, respectively, the availability of predictive clinical and serologic features is valuable.

Recent follow-up of a cohort of patients with UCTD found the following initial findings conferred substantial predictive value for SLE after analysis in a COX regression model: discoid lupus (relative risk = 15.8), serositis (4.1), homogeneous ANA (4.8) and anti-Sm positivity (28.2) (51). Another follow-up study of 91 patients with UCTD revealed a long-term stability of 79 of the patients (mean period, 3 years), whereas 12 evolved to the definite diagnosis of SLE (52). These 79 stable patients exhibited a limited

TABLE 72.5. FACTORS IN PATIENTS WITH RAYNAUD'S PHENOMENON THAT PREDICT DEVELOPMENT OF A DIFFERENTIATED SYSTEMIC RHEUMATIC DISEASE

1. Older age at onset
2. Severe Raynaud's phenomenon
3. Presence of antinuclear antibodies
4. Abnormal patterns of dilatation and dropout on nailfold capillary microscopy

Prevalence data shown from and calculated from incidence data listed in Masi AT, Medsger TA Jr. Epidemiology of the rheumatic diseases. In: McCarty DJ Jr, ed. *Arthritis and other conditions.* 11th ed. Philadelphia: Lea & Febiger, 1989:16–55, with permission.

autoimmune repertoire with distinct but limited clinical findings, as 30% had anti-Ro/SSA alone; 28%, anti-U1RNP alone; and, in all, 82% were characterized by a single autoantibody specificity. Anti-U1RNP antibodies alone were associated with Raynaud's phenomenon and arthritis, whereas anti-Ro/SSA antibodies alone were correlated with xerostomia and xeropthalmia (52).

Another common conundrum is the patient with an inflammatory polyarthritis without bone erosions with or without a positive antinuclear antibody, no RF, and no disease-specific autoantibodies or other clinical findings that define a clinical syndrome. This is one of the largest groups in the recently recruited cohort of patients with early UCTD (3). Some of the patients will evolve into RA, SLE, or PSS. Of the 67 patients with unexplained polyarthritis, 57% have a positive antinuclear antibody, five have anti-U1RNP, and one has anti-Ro/SSA. It is likely that the five patients with anti-U1RNP will develop either PSS or SLE, and the patient with anti-Ro/SSA will develop SS or SLE if these patients follow the pattern seen in the study of Kallenberg et al. (31).

Among the 115 patients in the cohort (3) designated UCTD, 68 (59%) had a positive antinuclear antibody, and 40 (35%) had disease-specific autoantibodies (4). Thus one might predict that the six patients with anti-DNA and the three patients with anti-Sm would develop SLE. The 16 patients with anti-U1RNP are likely to develop either PSS or SLE or an overlap of these diseases with PM, and the 14 patients with anti-Ro/SSA would develop either SS, SLE, or an overlap between those two diagnoses. One patient had anti-Jo, a myositis-specific autoantibody, yet must not have satisfied criteria for either PM or DM. This is a very rare event but has been previously reported (51). This reemphasizes that, for most of these disease-specific autoantibodies, their appearance almost always antedates the development of clinical disease, a point emphasized in two articles previously mentioned with respect to both PSS and SLE (31,32). Predictive power is inherent in this knowledge. Based on records of the Finnish Social Security Institution population register, it has also been shown that positive antinuclear antibody tests precede the development of SLE (33), as do positive RF tests and the onset of RA (34). It is well known that a significant minority of RA patients convert to seropositivity well into their disease course, but the previously described situation (RF positivity preceding clinical disease expression) is likely more common.

The presence of these autoantibodies, almost invariably preceding disease, means that they are not secondary to tissue damage or disease expression but are either etiopathogenic or are tightly associated with the pathogenic process.

Patients with any of the incompletely expressed rheumatic diseases accompanied by autoantibodies that are not diagnostic are best designated UCTD. Such patients are not well served by making a definitive diagnosis before the clinical data indicate the nature of the disease. In many instances, the "disease" remits permanently, or the undifferentiated nature of the malady may be long lasting, requiring only that symptomatic therapy be given because the prognosis and course are unknown. Figure 72.1 summarizes the course of patients designated UCTD. We hope, as our knowledge expands, that etiologies and additional autoantibodies with certain disease specificity, which antedate clinical disease, will be discovered.

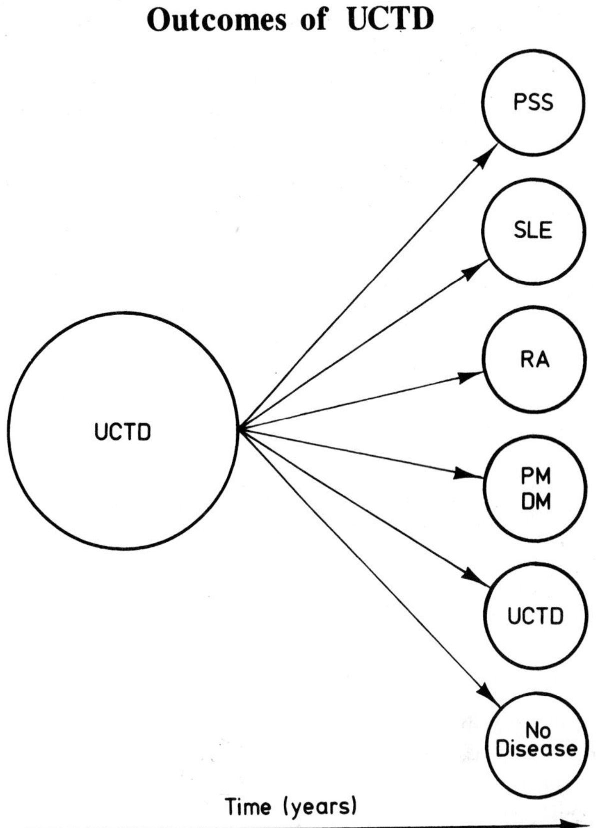

FIGURE 72.1. The evolution of undifferentiated connective tissue disease into various differentiated rheumatic diseases or remission of symptoms.

OVERLAP SYNDROMES

A major reason to be interested in the occurrence of overlap syndromes is to uncover clues about etiology and pathogenesis. Of equal importance is to gather information about course and prognosis by studying the natural history of defined syndromes. These issues can be illustrated by discussing any of the overlap syndromes listed in Table 72.3. The overlap of PSS and PM provides a fertile starting point. Excluding for the moment the diagnosis of this disease association in the context of MCTD or in tandem with high titers of antibody to U1RNP, there are now substantial numbers of patients with the overlap PSS–PM. If one examines these patients from a serologic standpoint, there is an interesting relation of PM with various other autoantibodies. Thus this overlap can occur with autoantibodies to topoisomerase I (Scl_{70}), centromere, various nucleolar antigens, and most remarkably with the nucleolar antigen PM-Scl (22,23). HLA-DR or -DQ associations in the systemic rheumatic diseases are almost always much stronger with specific autoantibody responses than with the disease in question. This is exemplified by the relation of HLA-DR1 with anticentromere, HLA-DR5 with anti–topoisomerase I, and HLA-DR3 with anti–PM-Scl (35–37). However, from the reciprocal standpoint, PM occurs in a minority (5–10%) of the cases of PSS associated with anti–topoisomerase I and anticentromere. However, 44% to 90% of cases of PM exhibiting anti–PM-Scl are associated with PSS (36,37). This suggests a very tight and special relation of the anti–PM-Scl response to the overlap syndrome of PM–PSS controlled in part by the HLA-DR3 allele associated with the anti–PM-Scl response (35–37). One is then tempted to speculate that when PM occurs in PSS in association with anti–PM-Scl, it has either a different etiology or a different pathogenesis, marked by the presence of anti–PM-Scl.

Thus there appear to be at least two types (i.e., differing in etiopathogenesis) of PM associated with PSS: one associated with the anti–PM-Scl response, and the other in the remaining PSS population. Scholars of PM believe that the mechanism of this disease resides in an autoimmune attack (either T or B cell–mediated) on antigenic targets yet to be characterized, in or on muscle cells. Clearly, definition of these targets is a central goal for future research and likely will hold the keys to understanding the various mechanisms involved in the pathogenesis of PM and DM.

It is of great interest that the so-called myositis-specific antibodies (MSAs) have never been reported to occur in PM associated with PSS outside of the PM–PSS cases associated with PM-Scl. Additionally, MSAs have not been reported in cases of PM associated with SLE or RA. This high disease specificity, at the minimum, suggests the presence of an etiopathogenesis for the PM patients who have MSAs that is distinct from that of patients with PM-PSS.

Although they have not been excluded as the targets responsible for the immunopathogenesis of PM, the MSA targets are not thought to be responsible for the myositis *per se* for the following reasons. First, the MSAs do not fluctuate with disease activity; and second, the antigens are intracellular, and as none has been reported to occur on cell surfaces, they make unlikely targets for an immune-based organ-specific pathogenic pathway. These antibodies are, therefore, viewed as important markers of disease expression but not directly involved in the muscle injury.

Another phenomenon suggested by the frequent overlap of systemic rheumatic diseases is the existence of as yet unidentified factors that are shared by the various defined diseases. As an example, one can consider the overlap of SLE and PSS. The prevalence of SLE in the United States is estimated at about 1 in 1,000, whereas that of PSS is 10 times less or 1 in 10,000. The prevalence of the two independent diseases occurring together would be 1 in 107, so that one would expect only 25 such cases in the U.S. Although no one knows how many such cases exist, many times this number of such cases are reported in the literature. PM and DM have a prevalence similar to that of PSS (1/10,000), so that the combined prevalence of PM–PSS should be 1 in 108, predicting the existence of only two to three such patients in the U.S. if that overlap represented the concurrence of two independent diseases. I have seen more than 20 such patients, which must represent an infinitesimal fraction of the number of overlap patients with PM and scleroderma. In any case, the message is clear that these diseases must share many underlying unidentified genetic or nongenetic factors that underlie their pathogenesis.

Examples of shared genetic factors might include genes controlling immune tolerance, antigen processing, reticuloendothelial function, thymic development, cytokine regulation, and the probable large number of regulatory genes that operate on the processes of B-and T-cell development and maturation. Environmental factors include the many drugs that can induce these diseases such as pronestyl and hydralazine for SLE, penicillamine for PM and pemphigus vulgaris, the contaminant in rape seed oil and past lots of contaminated L-tryptophan that induced PSS and eosinophilia myalgia syndrome, respectively, to mention only some of the more dramatic examples. Might there not be pervasive ubiquitous materials in our environment that play a crucial role in the development of systemic rheumatic diseases? These might be chemicals, food additives, and other environmental agents as well as a range of infectious agents that could initiate immune responses that trigger autoimmunity through molecular mimicry or direct interactions (such as superantigens) with elements of the immune system. Although genetic factors are very important, identical twin studies, as in SLE, show concordance rates of from 24% to 60%, indicating a role for nongenetic or environmental factors (38).

MIXED CONNECTIVE TISSUE DISEASE

Mixed connective tissue disease was first described by Sharp in 1972 as a mixture of features of several diseases including SLE, PSS, PM, DM, and RA. A defining characteristic was the presence of antibody to the ribonuclease-sensitive component of extractable nuclear antigen (ENA) (8). This was shown to be associated with precipitating antibodies to nRNP (39), later demonstrated to be the U1RNP particle (40). Finally, 68-kd, one of three U1RNP-specific polypeptides, was identified as the disease-defining target of autoimmunity for patients with MCTD (41,42). There has been endless controversy concerning whether MCTD is a "disease" or a "syndrome," about the early contention that the course was largely benign and the disease generally steroid responsive, and what ultimate course patients with MCTD would follow.

Observations that raised doubts about the existence of MCTD as a distinct entity arose from many quarters. On the clinical nosology side, for example, a careful study of 27 patients with overlap syndromes from a single large clinic in Argentina contrasted the clinical features of 17 anti-U1RNP$^+$ and 10 anti-U1RNP$^-$ patients (43). The patients were very similar in all regards, with more than half of the patients in both groups exhibiting skin rashes and lung abnormalities, and 80% to 95% of both groups having puffy hands, Raynaud's phenomenon, and myositis. This study clearly showed that the pleomorphic clinical picture of MCTD lacked specificity. Second, the overlap features that defined the disease in the early phases of the first cohort described by Sharp et al. (44) gave way to a picture of PSS in 10 of the patients (i.e., the overlap syndrome differentiated into a well-defined rheumatic disease). Additionally, large doses of corticosteroids were occasionally required for the control of the disease, and finally, several features of the syndrome were serious and ultimately fatal. Long-term outcomes of 47 patients with MCTD from the clinic of Dr. Sharp were recently published (53). Whereas 62% had a favorable outcome, 38% either had active disease (7% or 15%) or died (11% or 23%). The most common cause of death was pulmonary hypertension (nine of 11), a finding not seen or appreciated in the original cohort. Other findings included both renal failure associated with malignant hypertension and immune complex glomerulonephritis, a rapidly fatal pulmonary hypertension associated with a proliferative vasculopathy that could occur without pulmonary fibrosis, and numerous serious CNS complications, as well as vasculitis. The recognition of these issues has spawned an acerbic view of MCTD as embodied in the title "Mixed Connective Tissue Disease—Goodbye to All That" (45). In that same article, review of the literature indicated that these serious complications result in a mortality (13% dead in 12 years) that belies the original concept of a benign prognosis (45). Finally, although the specificity of the immune response to the 68-kd peptide is indeed characteristic of MCTD, this response occurs in a large proportion of SLE patients who produce antibodies to the U1RNP particle (10,46).

In the face of these new developments, the concept of MCTD has not withered and died but has undergone modification and evolution. The various contrasting viewpoints concerning MCTD may be undergoing an interesting convergence. This convergence is particularly germane to one of the major themes of this chapter: the concept of UCTD. A consensus has emerged that resembles the concept of UCTD proposed by LeRoy in 1980. This conceptualization of MCTD was described recently by Mairesse et al. (47) as "a core of minor symptoms (Raynaud's phenomenon, puffy fingers, mild myositis, and arthritis) associated significantly with anti–U1-68-kD antibody, defining an undifferentiated connective tissue disease that may ultimately overlap with features of major connective tissue diseases" (47). If that description were extended slightly to say, "may ultimately differentiate and mainly be expressed as a major connective tissue disease," it would address most of the criticisms of MCTD as an entity raised by Black and Isenberg (45). A slight amendment to this concept would incorporate the patients described by Mosca et al. (52) with anti-Ro/SSA alone and features of SS, who stably have a limited clinical and serologic expression. Indeed, these authors proposed renaming MCTD "undifferentiated autoimmune rheumatic/connective tissue disorder." The idea that the presence of anti-U1RNP (and anti–68-kd) is closely related to the occurrence of Raynaud's phenomenon, which is seen in all the published series of MCTD, has been further strengthened by the report of an informative family. In that instance, one sister had PSS–PM overlap with anti-U1RNP (and Raynaud's phenomenon), and a second sister several years later had a clinical picture of SLE (seizures, polyarthritis, and Raynaud's phenomenon) in association with the development of autoantibodies to U1RNP, including a strong response to the 68-kd peptide in Western blot (48). This longitudinal temporal relation of anti–68-kd and Raynaud's phenomenon suggests either a causal relation between anti–68-kd and Raynaud's phenomenon or a common factor controlling the expression of Raynaud's phenomenon and the production of anti–68-kd antibodies.

A recent paper added new evidence supporting the concept of MCTD as a distinct entity: the description of autoantibodies to the constitutive 73-kd heat-shock protein in MCTD (47). In that study, very high levels of antibodies to HSP 73 were seen in MCTD but not in RA, SLE, PSS, or PM/DM. There was no overlap between the levels of anti–HSP 73 in MCTD and these other diseases. There was no increase of anti–HSP 73 levels above those of healthy controls in SLE and PM/DM, but there was in RA and PSS, although levels in these latter two diseases did not overlap with those seen in the MCTD patients. Furthermore, although the anti–HSP 73 antibodies were associated with high levels of anti–68-kd antibodies, no cross-reactions were seen between these systems, although the data were not presented. The authors themselves are cautious in interpreting these results because a previous study from a group long experienced in studying autoimmunity to heat-shock proteins failed to find any reactivity in eight MCTD sera for HSP 73 (49).

In summary, it seems reasonable to view MCTD as one component of UCTD, which is anticipated either to differentiate into one of its component diseases or to remain in an "ambiguous" state for long periods. The relation of the various systemic rheumatic diseases including MCTD is depicted in Fig. 72.2.

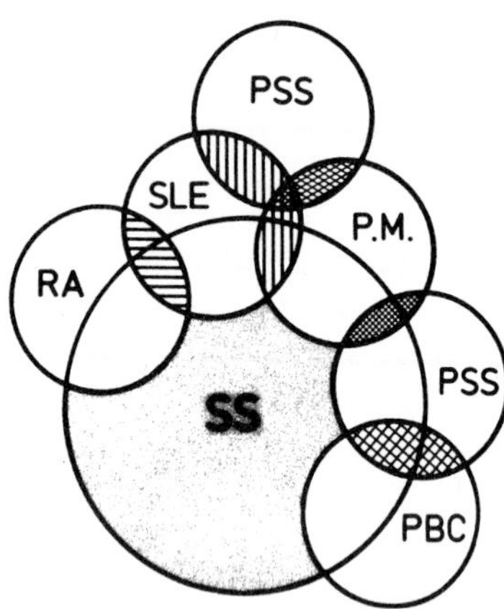

FIGURE 72.2. Overlap of diseases represented by different line patterns: horizontal lines designate Rhupus, vertical lines designate mixed connective tissue disease (*MTCD*); three types of polymyositis–progressive systemic sclerosis (*PM-PSS*) overlap designated with vertical lines (*MCTD*); two other line patterns recognized by (a) presence of anti–PM-Scl and (b) presence of other progressive systemic sclerosis–specific antibodies, overlap of progressive systemic sclerosis–primary biliary cirrhosis (*PSS-PBC*) and Sjögren's syndrome (*SS*) as well as the overlap of Sjögren's syndrome with all the systemic rheumatic diseases.

MANAGEMENT OF AND THERAPY FOR UNDIFFERENTIATED CONNECTIVE TISSUE DISEASE AND OVERLAP SYNDROMES

Management of the patient with UCTD is a prototype for dealing with uncertainty. Prospective natural history trials and investigations into clinical factors, autoantibodies, and genetic factors that may predict disease differentiation and expression are all aimed at reducing uncertainty and providing data that permit clinicians to give sound advice to patients.

An approach that makes good sense is to suggest the safest therapies that may be empirically given to patients with the component disease manifestations of UCTD. In patients with polyarthritis, who are undifferentiated, it is reasonable to prescribe nonsteroidal antiinflammatory drugs (NSAIDs), combined with a program of physical therapy and exercise. If the arthritis is not responsive to these basic measures, one could consider drugs such as plaquenil or sulfasalazine. In the absence of a diagnosis, the disease may be characterized by early erosions despite the measures used; and if the diagnosis is still not clear, more aggressive therapy with drugs such as methotrexate or azathioprine (Imuran) is indicated. This resembles the pyramid approach to the therapy of RA (and it is). Although many clinicians now propose inverting the pyramid for the therapy for RA and starting with methotrexate early, usually accompanied by some use of corticosteroids, I doubt that anyone would propose such a therapeutic strategy for the polyarthritis of UCTD, because the course and prognosis are unknown in individual patients, and it is likely that many patients will have a benign course. This is, of course, the kind of information that will emerge from the natural history trials of early UCTD now under way (3–5,52).

One would deal similarly with each component of the disease as it evolved. One's response to Raynaud's phenomenon would be little different from the management of primary Raynaud's phenomenon, in which keeping warm and prescribing vasodilators such as calcium channel blockers or α-blockers are standard therapies. If, however, one knew that either the antinuclear antibody were positive or the capillary microscopy were abnormal, it would be prudent to advise the patient to at least take a monthly blood pressure reading and to have a yearly measurement of carbon dioxide diffusion in the lung (DLCO), which decreases sharply in patients who develop pulmonary hypertension, as happens in patients with PSS, especially the limited form. For the patients with Raynaud's phenomenon destined to develop scleroderma renal disease, early treatment of blood pressure elevations with angiotensin-converting enzyme (ACE) inhibitors is undoubtedly useful. It is not yet clear that there are effective therapies for the pulmonary hypertension of MCTD or PSS, although a recent case report describes the successful treatment of such a case by the sequential use of cyclophosphamide and cyclosporine over a 10-year period (50). The frequency of such developments will be revealed by the natural history trials. These complications are so serious, it seems that the type of surveillance described is conservative and well advised.

The development of myositis, interstitial lung disease, hematologic disease, serositis, or nephritis would be approached in the same manner as if these complications appeared or developed in the context of the differentiated diseases in which they occur.

Managing patients with systemic rheumatic disease requires an understanding of their great heterogeneity, the frequent overlaps that occur between them, and an appreciation of the uncertainty felt by patients who are told their diagnosis is not clear and that the best diagnosis is UCTD. I am uncertain whether patients previously given the diagnosis MCTD would feel better or worse if they were told instead that they had UCTD.

What is clear, however, is that in our present state of knowledge, patients will ultimately benefit from our continued efforts to unravel the mysteries of these fascinating yet still obscure diseases. In the meantime, we cannot and must not tell them more than we really know.

ACKNOWLEDGMENT

This work was supported by the National Institutes of Health grant R01 AR43975 and a Biomedical Research Grant from the Arthritis Foundation.

REFERENCES

1. LeRoy EC, Maricq HR, Kahaleh MB. Undifferentiated connective tissue syndromes. *Arthritis Rheum* 1980;23:341–343.

2. Christian CL. Connective tissue disease: overlap syndromes. In: Cohen A, Bennett JC, eds. *Rheumatology and immunology.* 2nd ed. New York: Grune & Stratton, 1986:175–179.
3. Alarcón GS, Williams GV, Singer JZ, et al. Early undifferentiated connective tissue disease. I. Early clinical manifestations in a large cohort of patients with undifferentiated connective tissue diseases compared to cohorts of well established connective tissue diseases. *J Rheumatol* 1991;18:1332–1339.
4. Clegg DO, Williams HJ, Singer JZ, et al. Early undifferentiated connective tissue disease. II. The frequency of circulating antinuclear antibodies in patients with early rheumatic diseases. *J Rheumatol* 1991;18:1340–1343.
5. Bulpitt KJ, Clements PJ, Lackenbruch PA, et al. Early undifferentiated connective tissue disease. III. Outcome and prognostic indicators in early scleroderma (systemic sclerosis). *Ann Intern Med* 1993;118:602–609.
6. Mukerji B, Hardin JG. Undifferentiated overlapping and mixed connective tissue diseases. *Am J Med Sci* 1993;305:114–119.
7. Kallenberg CGM. Overlapping syndromes, undifferentiated connective tissue disease, and other fibrosing conditions. *Curr Opin Rheumatol* 1993;5:809–815.
8. Sharp GC, Irvin WS, Tan EM, et al. Mixed connective tissue disease: an apparently distinct rheumatic disease syndrome associated with a specific antibody to extractable nuclear antigen (ENA). *Am J Med* 1972;52:148–159.
9. Sharp GC, Irwin WS, May CH, et al. Association of antibodies to ribonucleoprotein and Sm antigens with connective tissue disease, systemic lupus erythematosus, and other rheumatic diseases. *N Engl J Med* 1976;295:1149–1154.
10. Reichlin M, van Venrooij WJ. Autoantibodies to the URNP particles: relationship to clinical diagnosis and nephritis. *Clin Exp Immunol* 1991;83:286–290.
11. Wallace DJ, Lin HC, Shen GQ, et al. Antibodies to histone (H2A-H2B) DNA complexes in the absence of antibodies to double stranded DNA or to H2A-H2B complexes are more sensitive and specific for scleroderma related disorders than for lupus. *Arthritis Rheum* 1994;37:1795–1797.
12. Burlingame RW, Rubin RL, Balderas RS, et al. Genesis and evolution of anti-chromatin autoantibodies in murine lupus indicates T-dependent immunization with self-antigen. *J Clin Invest* 1993;91:1687–1696.
13. Amoura Z, Chalere H, Koutouzov S, et al. Nucleosome-restricted antibodies are detected before anti-ds DNA and/or antihistone antibodies in serum of MRL-MP lpr/lpr and +/+ mice, and are present in kidney eluates of lupus mice with proteinuria. *Arthritis Rheum* 1994;37:1684–1688.
14. van Venrooij WJ, Stapel SO, Houben H, et al. Scl-86, a marker antigen for diffuse scleroderma. *J Clin Invest* 1985;75:1053–1060.
15. Weiner ES, Earnshaw WC, Senecal JH, et al. Clinical association of anticentromere antibodies and antibodies to topoisomerase I. *Arthritis Rheum* 1988;31:378–385.
16. Steen VD, Powell DL, Medsger TA Jr. Clinical correlations and prognosis based on serum autoantibodies in patients with systemic sclerosis. *Arthritis Rheum* 1988;31:196–203.
17. Okano Y, Steen VD, Medsger TA Jr. Autoantibody reactive with RNA polymerase III in systemic sclerosis. *Ann Intern Med* 1993;119:1005–1013.
18. Kuwana M, Kaburaki J, Mimori T, et al. Autoantibody reactive with three classes of RNA polymerases in sera from patients with systemic sclerosis. *J Clin Invest* 1993;91:1399–1404.
19. Hirakata M, Okano Y, Pati U, et al. Identification of autoantibodies to RNA polymerase II. *J Clin Invest* 1993;91:2665–2672.
20. Satoh M, Kuwana M, Ogasawara T, et al. Association of autoantibodies to topoisomerase I and the phosphorylated form of RNA polymerase II in Japanese scleroderma patients. *J Immunol* 1994;153:5838–5848.
21. Reimer G, Steen VD, Penning CA, et al. Correlates between autoantibodies to nucleolar antigen and clinical features in patients with systemic sclerosis (scleroderma). *Arthritis Rheum* 1985;31:525–532.
22. Targoff IN. Polymyositis. In: Bigazzi PL, Reichlin M, eds. *Systemic autoimmunity.* New York: Marcel Dekker, 1991:201–246.
23. Targoff IN. Autoantibodies associated with polymyositis and dermatomyositis. *Clin Aspects Autoimmun* 1993;5:5–18.
24. Harley JB, Alexander E, Bias WB, et al. Anti-Ro/SSA and La/SSB in patients with Sjögren's syndrome. *Arthritis Rheum* 1988; 29:196–206.
25. Itescu S, Winchester R. Diffuse infiltrative lymphocytosis syndrome: a disorder occurring in human immunodeficiency virus-I infection that may present as a sicca syndrome. *Rheum Dis Clin North Am* 1993;18:683–697.
26. Provost TT, Alexander EL, Reichlin M. The relationship between anti-Ro positive lupus erythematosus and Sjögren's syndrome. In: Talal N, Moutsopoulous H, eds. *Sjögren's syndrome.* Heidelberg: Springer-Verlag, 1987:244–257.
27. Provost TT, Talal N, Harley JB, et al. The relationship between anti-Ro(SSA) antibody positive Sjögren's syndrome and anti-Ro(SS-A) antibody positive lupus erythematosus. *Arch Dermatol* 1988;124:63–71.
28. Provost TT, Talal N, Bias W, et al. Ro(SSA) positive Sjögren's/lupus erythematosus (SCLE) overlap patients are associated with the HLA-DR3 and/or DRw6 phenotypes. *J Invest Dermatol* 1988;91:369–371.
29. Kallenberg CGM, Wouda AA, The TH, et al. Systemic involvement and immunologic findings in patients presenting with Raynaud's phenomenon. *Am J Med* 1980;69:675–680.
30. Harper FE, Maricq HR, Turner RE, et al. A prospective study of Raynaud's phenomenon and early connective tissue disease. *Am J Med* 1982;72:883–888.
31. Kallenberg CGM, Wouda AA, Hoet MH, et al. Development of connective tissue disease in patients presenting with Raynaud's phenomenon: a six year follow-up with emphasis on the predictive value of antinuclear antibodies as detected by immunoblotting. *Ann Rheum Dis* 1988;147:634–641.
32. Weiner ES, Hildebrandt S, Senecal JL, et al. Prognostic significance of anticentromere antibodies and anti-topoisomerase I antibodies in Raynaud's disease. *Arthritis Rheum* 1988;34:68–77.
33. Aho K, Koskela P, Mäkitalo R, et al. Antinuclear antibodies heralding the onset of systemic lupus erythematosus. *J Rheumatol* 1992;19:1377–1379.
34. Aho K, Heliövaara M, Maatela J, et al. Rheumatoid factors antedating clinical rheumatoid arthritis. *J Rheumatol* 1991;18: 1282–1284.
35. Genth E, Mierau R, Genetzky P, et al. Immunogenetic association of scleroderma related antinuclear antibodies. *Arthritis Rheum* 1990;33:657–665.
36. Marguerie C, Bunn CC, Copier J, et al. The clinical and immunogenetic features of patients with autoantibodies to the nucleolar antigen PM-Scl. *Medicine* 1992;71:327–336.
37. Oddis CV, Okano Y, Rudert WA, et al. Serum autoantibody to the nucleolar antigen PM-Scl. *Arthritis Rheum* 1992;35: 1211–1217.
38. Deapen D, Escalante A, Weinrib L, et al. A revised estimate of twin concordance in systemic lupus erythematosus. *Arthritis Rheum* 1992;35:311–318.
39. Mattioli M, Reichlin M. Characterization of a soluble nuclear ribonucleoprotein antigen reactive with SLE sera. *J Immunol* 1971;107:1281–1290.
40. Lerner MR, Steitz JA. Antibodies to small nuclear RNAs complexed with proteins are produced by patients with systemic lupus erythematosus. *Proc Natl Acad Sci U S A* 1979;76:5495–5499.
41. Habets WJ, DeRooij J, Salden MH, et al. Antibodies against distinct nuclear matrix proteins are characteristic for MCTD. *Clin Exp Immunol* 1983;54:268–276.

42. Petterson I, Wang G, Smith EL, et al. The use of immunoblotting and immunoprecipitation of small nuclear ribonucleoproteins in the analysis of sera of patients with mixed connective tissue disease and systemic lupus erythematosus. *Arthritis Rheum* 1986;29:986–996.
43. Lazaro MA, Maldonado Cocco JA, Catoggio LJ, et al. Clinical and serologic characteristics of patients with overlap syndrome: is mixed connective tissue disease a distinct clinical entity? *Medicine* 1989;68:58–65.
44. Nimmelstein SH, Brody S, McShane D, et al. Mixed connective tissue disease: a subsequent evaluation of the original 25 patients. *Medicine* 1980;59:239–248.
45. Black C, Isenberg DA. Mixed connective tissue disease—goodbye to all that. *Br J Rheumatol* 1992;31:695–700.
46. McHugh N, James I, Maddison P. Clinical significance of antibodies to a 68 kDa U1RNP polypeptide in connective tissue disease. *J Rheumatol* 1990;17:1320–1328.
47. Mairesse N, Kahn MF, Appelboom T. Antibodies to the constitutive 73 kD heat shock protein: a new marker of mixed connective tissue disease? *Am J Med* 1993;95:595–600.
48. Reichlin M, Abumohor P, Itoh Y. Two sisters producing anti-U1RNP exhibit serological concordance and clinical discordance. *Lupus* 1992;1:249–254.
49. Jarjour WN, Jeffries BD, Davis JS, et al. Autoantibodies to human stress proteins. *Arthritis Rheum* 1991;34:1133–1138.
50. Dahl M, Chalmers A, Wade J, et al. Ten-year survival of a patient with advanced pulmonary hypertension and mixed connective tissue disease treated with immunosuppressive therapy. *J Rheumatol* 1992;19:1807–1809.
51. Calvo-Alén J, Alarcón GS, Burgard SL, et al. Systemic lupus erythematosus: predictors of its occurrence among a cohort of patients with early undifferentiated connective tissue disease: multivariate analyses and identification of risk factors. *J Rheumatol* 1996;23:469–475.
52. Mosca M, Tavoni A, Neri R, et al. Undifferentiated connective tissue diseases: the clinical and serological profiles of 91 patients followed for at least 1 year. *Lupus* 1998;7:95–100.
53. Burdt MA, Hoffman RW, Deutscher SL, et al. Long-term outcome in mixed connective tissue disease. *Arthritis Rheum* 1999;42:899–909.

73

SYSTEMIC LUPUS ERYTHEMATOSUS: CLINICAL ASPECTS

MICHELLE A. PETRI

Systemic lupus erythematosus (SLE) remains the classic example of a systemic autoimmune disease, given its capacity to encompass every organ system. The term "lupus," Latin for wolf, was initially used because facial lesions were thought to resemble animal bites. Kaposi recognized that cutaneous lupus could be associated with systemic disease including fever, neurologic symptoms, pleuropneumonia, and anemia (1). The breadth of systemic manifestations, including arthritis, pneumonia, central nervous system disease, gastrointestinal crises, endocarditis, pericarditis, nephritis, and hemorrhage was described by Osler. Osler also described the natural history of recurrent exacerbations, or flares (2). Important clinical descriptions of lupus were compiled by Ropes (3) and the Hopkins group (4).

The varied clinical manifestations of SLE remain a challenge to the most astute clinician today, as they did 150 years ago. Although four major organ systems, cutaneous, musculoskeletal, hematologic, and renal, continue to dominate the clinical presentation of lupus, the importance of other organ system involvement (such as neurologic disease, including cognitive function deficits) and the secondary antiphospholipid antibody syndrome (APS), is more appreciated today.

In this chapter, the clinical features of SLE are reviewed. In addition to highlighting classic and instructive past studies, the experience of the Hopkins Lupus Cohort longitudinal study will be cited.

CLASSIFICATION OF LUPUS

SLE is one of several forms of lupus (Table 73.1). Other forms include chronic cutaneous (discoid) lupus (without other systemic features), drug-induced lupus (a self-limited form of lupus, predominantly arthritis and serositis, which resolves when the offending drug is discontinued), subacute cutaneous lupus, and neonatal lupus (a transient rash or permanent congenital heart block in a newborn exposed by placental transfer of maternal anti-Ro). Patients with features of lupus, but not sufficient to warrant a diagnosis of lupus, are usually diagnosed with undifferentiated connective tissue disease (UCTD). Only 13% of those initially diagnosed with UCTD evolve to a true diagnosis of SLE over the next 5 years. Those who later develop SLE are more likely to have discoid lupus, serositis, homogeneous pattern antinuclear antibody (ANA), and a positive anti-Sm (5).

Classification criteria for lupus were revised by a committee in 1982 (6) and again, by a letter to the editor, in 1997 (7). Four of these criteria (Table 73.2) are required for classification of SLE. Although not designed as diagnostic criteria, these criteria are frequently used for that purpose. They do emphasize that SLE is a multisystem disease and that a positive ANA alone is not sufficient to diagnose SLE. However, it is possible to have SLE and not meet four criteria (such as a patient with lupus nephritis, positive ANA, and anti-dsDNA), and vice versa, to have four criteria and not have SLE (such as a primary APS patient with anticardiolipin, ANA, seizures from a stroke, and thrombocytopenia).

Chronic cutaneous (discoid) lupus occurs in 27% of our SLE patients, more frequently in African-American SLE patients (38%) than whites (18%). Chronic cutaneous (discoid) lupus also can occur without other manifestations of SLE. Only 5% of chronic cutaneous lupus patients progress to true SLE.

Subacute cutaneous lupus erythematosus (SCLE) can occur in patients with SLE, although it is quite rare (5%). Patients labeled with SCLE alone, without SLE, may have serologic or laboratory features suggestive of SLE, but do not meet classification criteria for SLE (8).

TABLE 73.1. TYPES OF LUPUS ERYTHEMATOSUS

Systemic lupus erythematosus (SLE)
Chronic cutaneous (discoid) lupus (CLE)
Subacute cutaneous lupus erythematosus (SCLE)
Drug-induced lupus erythematosus (DILE)
Neonatal lupus erythematosus (NLE)

TABLE 73.2. THE 1997 REVISED AMERICAN COLLEGE OF RHEUMATOLOGY CRITERIA FOR SYSTEMIC LUPUS ERYTHEMATOSUS

Criterion	Definition
1. Malar rash	Fixed malar erythema, flat or raised
2. Discoid rash	Erythematous raised patches with keratotic scaling and follicular plugging; atrophic scarring may occur in older lesions
3. Photosensitivity	Skin rash as an unusual reaction to sunlight, by patient history or physician observation
4. Oral ulcers	Oral or nasopharyngeal ulcers, usually painless, observed by physician
5. Arthritis	Nonerosive arthritis involving two or more peripheral joints, characterized by tenderness, swelling, or effusion
6. Serositis	a. Pleuritis (convincing history of pleuritic pain or rub heard by physician or evidence of pleural effusion) OR b. Pericarditis (documented by ECG or rub or evidence of pericardial effusion)
7. Renal disorder	a. Persistent proteinuria >0.5 g/day or >3+ OR b. Cellular casts of any type
8. Neurologic disorder	a. Seizures (in the absence of other causes) b. Psychosis (in the absence of other causes)
9. Hematologic disorder	a. Hemolytic anemia b. Leukopenia (<4,000/mm^3 on two or more occasions) c. Lymphopenia (<1,500/mm^3 on two or more occasions) d. Thrombocytopenia (<100,000/mm^3 in the absence of offending drugs)
10. Immunologic disorder	a. Anti-dsDNA OR b. Anti-Sm OR c. Positive finding of anti-phospholipid antibodies based on 1) An abnormal serum level of IgG or IgM anti-cardiolipin antibodies, OR 2) A positive test result for lupus anticoagulant using a standard method, OR 3) A false-positive serologic test for syphilis known to be positive for ≥6 months and confirmed by *Treponema pallidum* immobilization or fluorescent treponemal antibody absorption test
11. Antinuclear antibody	An abnormal titer of ANA by immunofluorescence or an equivalent assay at any time and in the absence of drugs known to be associated with "drug-induced lupus syndrome"

Drug-induced lupus erythematosus (DILE) occurs in 15,000 to 20,000 people yearly in the United States. The most common precipitants are hydralazine and procainamide, followed by chlorpromazine, isoniazid, methyldopa, penicillamine, quinidine, and sulfasalazine, but many other drugs have been associated with drug-induced ANAs or true drug-induced lupus. Some drugs that cause drug-induced lupus, including procainamide and hydralazine, are aromatic amines or hydrazines. However, these medications can be used safely in SLE. Environmental agents with aromatic amines or hydrazine compounds (such as hair dyes or hair straighteners), which contain potential oxidants of sulfide bonds and glycerol monothioglycolate, have not been associated with SLE (9,10). The slow acetylator phenotypes that are associated with DILE are not increased in SLE.

The most common presentations of DILE are arthralgias, arthritis, myalgias, serositis, and fever. Nephritis and central nervous system (CNS)-SLE are rarely seen. Antihistone antibodies are commonly found. For biologic agents associated with SLE, such as interferons and antibodies to tumor necrosis factor-α (TNF-α), it is speculated that a disruption of the cytokine network leads to lupus (11). Clinical manifestations of DILE resolve on drug cessation, although short-term corticosteroid treatment is sometimes required.

Neonatal lupus erythematosus (NLE) presents as a transient lupus rash or as permanent congenital heart block. Other manifestations, such as cytopenias and hepatitis, are very rare. It is caused by the transplacental transfer of maternal anti-Ro (12).

EPIDEMIOLOGY

Female Predominance

One of the most striking features of SLE is its female predominance. The importance of female hormones in the pathogenesis of SLE has been elegantly studied in murine models (13). In humans, the ratio of women to men is 9:1, although in a recent study from Rochester, Minnesota, the ratio was less (14). Women with SLE may metabolize estrogen by using pathways that lead to elevated levels of the more active metabolite 16α-hydroxyestrone (15), which would accentuate the effect of estrogen on the immune system (16). First-degree relatives are more likely to express increased levels of 16α-hydroxylation as well (17). Under-production of androgens, excessive transformation of androgens to estrogens, and low levels of dehydroepiandrosterone (DHEA), the major adrenal steroid, also occur. Male SLE patients can have decreased androgen levels (18). Thus in both sexes, an imbalance of estrogen-to-androgen ratio predisposes to lupus. The mechanism by which this imbalance leads to autoimmunity is less clear, because sex hormones could act at multiple levels. Sex hormones bind to receptors in the thymus and spleen (19) and to receptors on lymphocytes (20,21), and increase mitogen-induced immunoglobulin production (22).

Age at Onset

SLE is usually a postpubertal disease, with onset of clinical symptoms usually in the 20s to 30s. Childhood and older-onset lupus differ from the classic presentation, with less female predominance and different clinical presentations. In the Hopkins Lupus Cohort, younger-onset lupus (before age 20) has an increase in cutaneous and renal lupus and is more likely have low serum C4 than older-onset lupus. In a retrospective study of 31 children with SLE, arthritis, anemia, and seizures were associated with a poor prognosis (23). Older-onset (older than 40 years), lupus is less likely to have malar rash, proteinuria, and low serum C4, but more likely to have secondary Sjögren's syndrome.

Race

In both the U.S. (24,25) and the United Kingdom (26), SLE is more common in African-Americans and African-Caribbeans, yet SLE is not a common autoimmune disease in Africa. SLE does appear to be common in Asia (27,28) and Latin America (29), but comparisons of Asian-American and Hispanic-American incidence rates have not been done. The LUMINA study in the United States has begun a comparison of SLE in whites, Hispanics, and African-Americans (30,31).

Race affects both the presentation and the course of SLE. African-Americans with SLE are more likely than whites to have discoid lupus (32), lupus nephritis (32–34), lymphadenopathy, myositis, and pericarditis, but less likely to have malar rash and mouth ulcers. African-Americans are more likely to have antiribonucleoprotein (anti-RNP) and anti-Sm, but less likely to have anticardiolipin and lupus anticoagulant than are white patients.

Socioeconomic Factors

Differences in SLE presentation and course that are ascribed to socioeconomic status may actually be due to other factors. In a prospective study of predictors of poor renal outcome (renal insufficiency, renal failure, and chronic nephrotic syndrome), socioeconomic status and race were not found to be significant predictors. Instead, compliance with visits and medication and hypertension were the major explanatory variables for poor renal outcomes (33).

Education, however, was associated with major co-morbidities of SLE, such as cataracts, hypertension, peptic ulcer, and thrombosis, even after adjustment for race, in the Hopkins Lupus Cohort. Education also was associated with several clinical manifestations, including discoid rash, psychosis, and seizures. The apparent association of education with these factors may be due to confounding variables such as diet and social habits.

Incidence and Prevalence

Recent work from Rochester, Minnesota, indicates that the incidence of lupus has tripled since the 1970s, from 1.51 in 100,000 (1950–1979) to 5.56 in 100,000 (1980–1992). Because the proportion with lupus nephritis is steady, this increase in incidence appears to be a valid finding and not due to earlier diagnosis or to the inclusion of milder cases. Studies comparing the incidence and prevalence of SLE are shown in Table 73.3.

Environmental and Hormonal Triggers of SLE

Previous case–control studies have found statistically significant risk factors for SLE, starting with hair dyes in the study of Freni-Titulaer et al. (50) in Georgia in 1986. Other factors found to be significant in previous case–control studies include herpes zoster and allergy (50,51); smoking,

TABLE 73.3. INCIDENCE AND PREVALENCE OF SLE

Author, Year	Incidence[a]	Prevalence[b]
Siegel and Lee, 1973 (35)	2.0	14.6
Fessel, 1974 (24)	7.6	50.8
Meddings and Grennan, 1980 (39)		15.0
Helve, 1985 (36)		28.0
Michet et al., 1985 (38)	2.2	40.0
Nived et al., 1985 (40)	4.6	
Hochberg, 1987 (41)		12.0
Nakae et al., 1987 (42)		21.0
Gudmundsson and Steinsson, 1990 (46)	5.8	
Samanta et al., 1992 (44)		26.1
Nossent, 1992 (45)	4.6	47.0
Hopkinson et al., 1994 (26)	4.4	24.0
Maskarinec and Katz, 1995 (43)		41.8
Hochberg et al., 1995 (37)	4.6	
McCarty et al., 1995 (47)	2.8	
Johnson et al., 1995 (48)	3.8	27.7
Gourley et al., 1997 (49)		25.4
Uramoto et al., 1999 (14)	5.8	12.2

[a]Expressed as number of cases per 100,000 per year.
[b]Expressed as number of cases per 100,000.

age at menarche, asthma, and dusty work (28,52); and meat and menstrual irregularity (53). The largest published case–control study, that of Nagata et al. (28,52), contained 282 patients (and 292 controls) in Japan.

Ultraviolet Light

Ultraviolet light remains the classic trigger, not only of the induction of lupus, but of flares in patients with established disease as well. Although it was originally thought that UV-B was the responsible wavelength, both UV-B and UV-A can induce cutaneous lupus lesions. In one study, 33% of patients responded to UV-B, 14% to UV-A, and 53% to both (54). Although clinicians rely on the patient's history to determine photosensitivity, recent work has shown that history alone may not be sufficient. Of patients who reported photosensitivity, only 16% had a cutaneous lupus flare on provocation, whereas 48% had a reaction consistent with polymorphous light eruption. The patients who had a true cutaneous lupus reaction were more likely to have anti-Ro and anti-La (55). Ultraviolet light is capable of inducing noncutaneous flares, as well, even neurologic ones (56).

Even a single exposure to UV-B can induce cutaneous lupus lesions (57). Multiple groups have demonstrated that UV-B exposure increases binding of Ro to cultured epidermal keratinocytes. Perturbation of calreticulin may be responsible (58). UV-B induces binding of U_1RNP, Sm, and Ro, especially when autologous sera are present (59,60). UV-B also induces lymphocyte apoptosis (61). There is a 65% increase in DNA synthesis after exposure to UV-B (62).

In one study, 78% of SLE patients also reacted to UV-A (63). UV-A increases the accumulation of oxygen radicals in SLE splenocytes (64). It also increases both interleukin-6 (IL-6) and TNF in keratinocytes and fibroblasts (65). There is some increase in binding of immunoglobulin G (IgG) autoantibodies after exposure to UV-A, but less than that seen with UV-B (66). Some SLE patients also are sensitive to unshaded fluorescent lights, which can emit UV-B wavelengths (67). McGrath (68) has demonstrated that fluorescent lights can induce the immunomodulator *cis*-urocanic acid.

Not all UV-A wavelengths are harmful in SLE. McGrath (69) has studied the role of UV-A1 (340–400 nm) as a potential treatment of SLE. Benefit was shown in six patients with mean follow-up of 3.4 years. Improvement in autoantibodies has been demonstrated (70). In the most rigorous study, a two-phase study with the first 6 weeks blinded, improvement was again noted (71). Fluorescent light may be beneficial in animal models of lupus (72).

Hormones

The hormonal influence of SLE has been shown most clearly in the murine model, with improvement with androgens and worsening with estrogens (22). SLE patients have low levels of androgens, including DHEA (73). Lahita et al. (74) have shown an increase in 16α-hydroxylation of estrogen in some SLE patients, leading to more active metabolites. These metabolic pathways, including P-450 oxidation, can be influenced by diet and smoking (75,76).

Exogenous Estrogen

Multiple case reports have suggested a temporal association between use of oral contraceptives or estrogen replacement therapy and onset of SLE (77). Several prospective studies have suggested that exogenous estrogen plays a role in the induction of human SLE. In the Nurses' Health Study, oral contraceptives had a borderline risk (78), and estrogen replacement therapy, a statistically significant risk (79) in SLE development. Oral contraceptives were not a statistically significant risk for SLE in the case–control studies of Grimes et al. (80) in Atlanta or Strom et al. (51,81) in Philadelphia.

Endogenous Estrogen

Endogenous estrogen exposure also may be important. Younger age at menarche (with increased length of estrogen exposure), shorter menstrual periods (with more unopposed estrogen exposure), and later menopause might all be possible promoting factors for SLE. A cohort effect would be expected for age at menarche, which has decreased significantly in the U.S., perhaps because of better nutrition. However, age at menarche was actually later in the SLE cases in the case–control study of Nagata et al. (28, 52) in Japan and was not found to be a risk factor in the case–control study of Grimes et al. (80) in Atlanta. Menstrual irregularity was increased, however, in a case–control study from Japan (28,52).

Pregnancy

Pregnancy leads to increased exposure to both estrogens and prolactin. Prolactin may be an important immunomodulator in SLE (82). Earlier pregnancies could be a potential trigger of SLE. However, the previous case–control studies, including those of Grimes et al. (80) in Atlanta, and Nagata et al. (28,52) and Minami et al. (53) in Japan, did not find an association of pregnancy, age at first pregnancy, or miscarriages with onset of SLE. This seems contrary to the conventional wisdom of rheumatologists, who recognize the entity of "gestational lupus," with onset of typical SLE nephritis during pregnancy.

Smoking

The role of smoking in autoimmune disease is complex. Smoking has been found to be a risk factor for both rheumatoid arthritis (RA) (83) and SLE. In RA, smoking is associated with rheumatoid factor seropositivity, radiographic erosions, rheumatoid nodules, and interstitial lung disease (84). Smoking has a complex effect on immune function, leading to a decrease in T-suppressor function (85), natural killer cells (85,86), immunoglobulins (86,87), antibody response to sheep red cells (88), and cell-mediated responses to transplanted tumors (89). It raises rheumatoid factor titers (90,91) in addition to inducing antibodies to substances in cigarette smoke (92). However, several of the effects of smoking might be hypothesized to be helpful in SLE, such as its antiestrogenic effect (93,94) and an increase in DHEA levels (95).

Five case–control studies have addressed the association of smoking and SLE. Three case–control studies; the Black Women's Health Study (96), a case–control study in Japan (28), and a case–control study in the United Kingdom (97) found a statistically significant association of smoking and SLE, with odds ratios of about 2.0. A fourth study, in Sweden, with only 56 SLE cases, found an odds ratio of 1.8, but failed to achieve statistical significance (98). However, one study in Philadelphia of 195 SLE cases found no association at all (51). Smoking is increased in African-American women and could be a potential explanation for the increased prevalence of SLE in African-Americans versus whites.

In the Hopkins Lupus Cohort study, smoking before cohort entry is an independent risk factor for discoid lupus, leg ulcers, and pulmonary hypertension. A study by Gallego et al. (99) found a similar association of discoid lupus and smoking in patients with chronic cutaneous lupus. In Toronto, SLE patients who smoke are more resistant to antimalarial therapy, suggesting that smoking leads to more severe disease (100).

Hair Products

Hair products were initially suggested as a risk factor for SLE in a case–control study of autoimmune disease patients (50). The scientific rationale included the chemical similarities to aromatic amines known to cause drug-induced lupus, based on the "slow acetylator" hypothesis. Slow acetylation is no longer thought to explain idiopathic SLE, however (81). Our case–control study (9) and another (81) did not find any association of hair products (hair dyes or hair straighteners) with SLE. The prospective cohort Nurses' Health Study also did not find an association of hair products with SLE (10).

Drugs and Diet

Our case–control study found an increase in penicillin and sulfonamide allergy in SLE, with trimethoprim/sulfamethoxazole also leading to an increase in SLE flares in patients with established disease (101). Several subsequent studies have demonstrated an increase in allergies (including insect allergies) in SLE (102). A similar increase in antibiotic allergies also has been shown in Sjögren's syndrome.

Minocycline, the antibiotic commonly prescribed for acne vulgaris, is associated with SLE (103). Eleven cases were reported by Gough et al. (104), followed by 60 cases reported by Angulo et al. (105). Minocycline lupus has some characteristics of drug-induced lupus, in that it resolves on drug cessation. However, it is not associated with antihistone antibodies, but with antineutrophile cytoplasm antibody (p-ANCA) (106) and sometimes with anti-dsDNA (107).

Over-the-counter nutriceuticals are widely used by the general population (108). Echinacea has been touted as an immune stimulant for the common cold. Within our cohort, we have two examples of echinacea use before onset of SLE, and one of echinacea use before a major nephritis flare in a patient with previously quiescent lupus.

In murine models, alteration of the amount of protein, fat, trace minerals, vitamins, or calories can affect the development of SLE (109). Antioxidants and omega-3 fatty acids may be protective in murine lupus, whereas high total fat accelerates the disease (110,111). In the case–control study of Nagata et al. (28) in Japan, alcohol and milk intake were inversely associated with SLE risk. Similarly, McAlindon et al. found that alcohol use was protective against lupus nephritis (112). Monkeys fed alfalfa sprouts develop an SLE-like illness (113). This may be due to L-canavanine, which is destroyed by heat (114).

Infections

Multiple infections have been invoked as potential triggers of SLE, including Epstein–Barr (EB) virus (115–117), hepatitis C, cytomegalovirus (CMV), and parvovirus. EB virus has the most scientific rationale. SLE patients are more likely to make an IgG anti-p542 after EB viral infection (118) and antiviral antibodies that cross-react with autoantigens such as SmD (119,120). An association of EB virus with SLE in children has been reported (121,122). An initial EB viral infection, followed by epitope spreading, is thought to be the pathogenetic connection (123).

Several cases of hepatitis C before SLE onset have been reported (124,125). Hepatitis B also has been reported before SLE in other countries (126). In a case–control study, past herpes zoster was found to be a risk factor for SLE (51).

A major concern has been a possible association of hepatitis B vaccine with SLE (127–131). In two patients in the Hopkins Lupus Cohort, SLE developed after hepatitis B vaccine. Given the safety of other vaccines, including pneumococcal vaccine and influenza vaccine (132), it is not obvious why the hepatitis B vaccine should precipitate SLE.

Environmental Toxins

Well water contaminated with trichloroethylene was shown to lead to more SLE symptoms and higher ANAs in exposed versus unexposed subjects in a case–control study (133). Silica dust also has been reported to be associated with SLE, as well as other autoimmune diseases (134–137).

Prognosis

Survival studies in SLE have several sources of bias, often dictated by study entry criteria, such as attendance at an academic center, or inclusion of prevalent cases with long disease duration. However, even given these limitations, it is obvious that survival in SLE has improved dramatically. Five-year survival in Baltimore in 1954 was 51% (138), but by 1981 had improved to 97% (139). Some centers now report 10-year survival of 90% or better (140). However, a recent study from the Mayo Clinic was sobering in its lower 10-year survival (14).

Prognosis studies in the U.S. are confounded by two major variables, African-American race and socioeconomic status. African-American race is associated with shorter survival in most studies (141–143). In a 1982 multicenter study, shorter survival in African-Americans was explained by lack of private insurance and more severe disease (142). However, two studies found that African-American race was associated with greater mortality, even after adjustment for medical insurance (141,143). In contrast, in a large study of 609 private patients with SLE, African-Americans did not differ in survival from other races (white, Hispanic, Asian) (144). No effect of socioeconomic status on SLE health status was found in Canada (145).

National statistics on survival in SLE have been instructive. In the National Center for Health Statistics mortality data for 1968 through 1972, mortality in African-American SLE patients, especially female patients, increased and then declined during the early and middle adult ages (whereas whites had increasing mortality with age) (146). Data from 1972 to 1976 showed greater mortality rates for African-American women during early and middle adulthood (147).

Lupus nephritis has had the major negative impact on survival in most studies. In the 1960s, the 5-year survival of SLE patients with nephritis was 50%, versus 77% in those without nephritis (148). Both nephritis and seizures were associated with SLE-related mortality in a cohort of 408 patients (149). The large prospective multicenter study of SLE in Europe found a 5-year survival of 95%, with renal disease leading to decreased survival. Renal damage, thrombocytopenia, high SLE Disease Activity Index (SLEDAI) score, pulmonary lupus, and older-age onset of lupus predicted mortality in a 20-year study of 665 patients (150). The 10-year survival of SLE patients with renal insufficiency is only 12% versus 80% in those with normal creatinine levels (142). Nephrotic syndrome also has a negative impact on survival (151).

In a multivariate analysis of survival of 566 patients between 1959 and 1992, independent risk factors for mortality included male gender, abnormal electrocardiogram (ECG), hypocomplementemia, and high corticosteroid dose. The early occurrence of a low C3 level reduced the probability of survival (152). A poorer prognosis for male patients was similarly found in a second study (153). Major causes of death in SLE include active SLE (29%), infections (29%), and thromboses (27%) (154).

Domains of SLE

To describe adequately the natural history and impact of SLE, it is necessary to define and measure three domains of SLE: disease activity, disease damage, and health status. The Systemic Lupus International Cooperating Clinics (SLICC) group has been instrumental in validation and reliability studies of instruments to measure these domains. Recently the importance of measuring all three domains in clinical studies of SLE was ratified by the OMERACT group, as well (155,156).

Disease Activity

Three major patterns of SLE exist. The classic pattern, one of exacerbations, or "flares" of disease activity, is now called the "relapsing remitting pattern" (157) (Fig. 73.1). This pattern was found in 53% of our cohort patients (158). To define this pattern numerically , we designated that a 1.0 change occurring on a 0 to 3 visual analogue scale of disease activity, over the last 3 months, would be a flare. The distribution of flares in different organ systems was then calculated (Table 73.4).

Predictors of the relapsing remitting pattern in the Hopkins Lupus Cohort have included female sex (vs. male) and premenopausal (vs. postmenopausal status). Serologic tests, such as C3, C4, and anti-dsDNA (usually done on a quarterly basis in the Hopkins Lupus Cohort) were not predic-

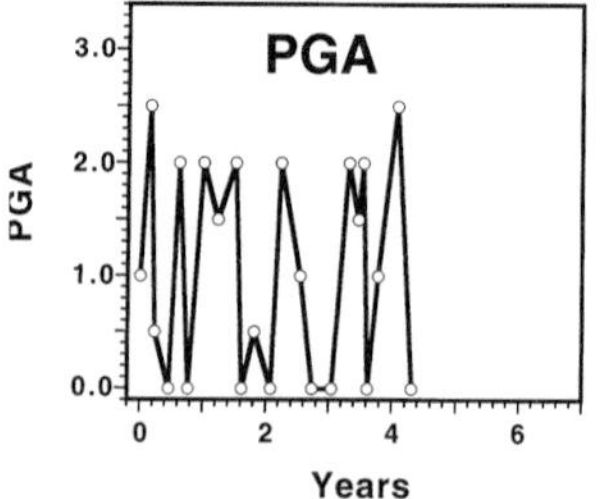

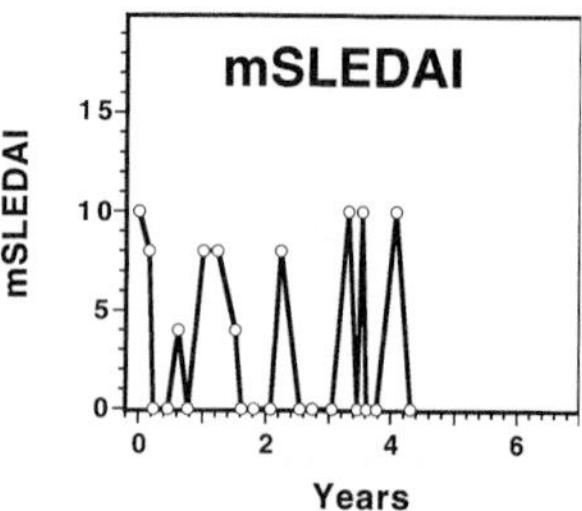

FIGURE 73.1. The "flare" or "relapsing remitting" pattern can be graphically demonstrated by using disease activity measures, such as the Physician's Global Assessment (PGA) (0–3 scale) and Systemic Lupus Erythematosus Disease Activity Index (SLEDAI).

TABLE 73.4. ORGAN SYSTEM INVOLVEMENT IN FLARES IN THE HOPKINS LUPUS COHORT

	Percentage of Patients
Constitutional	66
Dermatologic	47
Musculoskeletal	58
Serositis	12
Neurologic	21
Renal	22
Pulmonary	7
Hematologic	17

tive of a flare. The natural history of the relapsing remitting or flare pattern is not clear. We have seen the flare pattern in patients with established disease. In contrast, in studies of Dutch and Swedish SLE patients, the flare pattern was characteristic of the early disease course (159,160).

The second pattern, one of chronic (or continuous) activity, is equally common. The third pattern is more accurately called "long quiescence," rather than remission, because many patients have a later reappearance of lupus activity. Long quiescence is a rare pattern in our cohort. In another study of remission, 156 (23%) of 667 patients had a 1 year or longer period of treatment-free clinical remission. The mean duration of remission was 4.6 years. Remissions occurred even in patients with renal or CNS involvement (161).

To measure disease activity in either longitudinal or clinical trial settings, several validated and reliable disease activity measures are available, including SLEDAI (162), Systemic Lupus Activity Measure (SLAM) (163), Lupus Activity Index (LAI) (164), and British Isles Lupus Activity Group (BILAG) (165). These indices differ in the number of organ system descriptors, in whether severity within an organ descriptor is captured, and in inclusion/exclusion of serologic measures such as complement and anti-dsDNA. They correlate highly with each other.

Clinical trials in SLE require instruments that adequately capture change in disease activity, both improvement and worsening, between study visits. Although the existing disease activity instruments have been used in clinical trials, construction of, and validation of, a true "responder index" in SLE clinical trials has become a priority. In a multicenter trial of DHEA in SLE, the responder index accepted as the primary outcome was a compilation of improvement/stability in the SLEDAI or SLAM (with no worsening in the second index) and no worsening in the Krupp Fatigue Severity Scale (166) or patient's visual analogue scale. Recently a responder index that captures all important organ descriptors and defines worsening, partial response, and complete response, the RIFLE (Responder Index for Lupus Erythematosus) has been used in several clinical trials.

Disease Spread, "Evolution"

Longitudinal follow-up of SLE patients demonstrates that new organ system involvement can occur over time. We have coined the term evolution to describe this spread of SLE. The pathogenesis of this evolution of SLE is not understood, although it is attractive to invoke the concept of "epitope spreading" to explain it (123). An example of the evolution of SLE in the renal system is shown in Table 73.5. In the Hopkins Lupus Cohort, 43% of patients developed new symptoms or signs of SLE more than 5 years after diagnosis. However, in Dutch SLE patients, evolution of SLE was unlikely after the first 5 years (160). The evolution of SLE is one of several factors mandating that SLE patients receive routine follow-up (usually on a quarterly basis), even if they appear to feel well, to identify new organ involvement at an early and treatable stage.

Laboratory Testing in SLE

Laboratory testing is essential to make the diagnosis of SLE. Several of the classification criteria, including positive ANA, antiphospholipid antibodies, anti-Sm, leukopenia, lymphopenia, hemolytic anemia, and nephritis, are entirely dependent on laboratory tests. Other tests that are not part of the classification criteria, especially low levels of the complement components C3 and C4, are very helpful in suggesting or in helping to confirm the diagnosis of SLE and related connective tissue diseases.

Laboratory monitoring is crucial in the follow-up of lupus patients, to determine adequacy of treatment, to detect new organ system involvement (such as hematologic or nephritis), to monitor for corticosteroid or other immunosuppressive drug toxicity, and to evaluate the febrile SLE patient for infection.

Biomarkers in SLE

Although both low complement and anti-dsDNA are very useful in making the diagnosis of SLE, it is controversial whether they are good biomarkers of disease activity. Several groups (158,167,168) have not found low complement or high anti-dsDNA to be predictive of disease flare. In contrast,

TABLE 73.5. DEVELOPMENT OF NEW SLE NEPHRITIS OVER TIME

	Duration of SLE		
	<1 yr (*n* = 322)	1–5 yr (*n* = 211)	>5 yr (*n* = 138)
Proteinuria	36%	24.2%	20.3%
Hematuria	14%	19.4%	18.8%

SLE, systemic lupus erythematosus.

an increase in anti-dsDNA (with the Farr assay being most useful) was predictive of a flare in another study (169). In a prospective study with monthly follow-up, we demonstrated that a decrease in anti-dsDNA [with either enzyme-linked immunosorbent assay (ELISA) or Crithidia assays] occurred at the time of disease flare, suggesting deposition in tissues.

Complement components are inherently limited as biomarkers because their levels reflect production, genetic null alleles, catabolism, dilution, and elimination. Complement split products may be more useful, but are not commonly available (170). Ultimately, cytokines and adhesion cell molecules may have some role as biomarkers of disease (171). Markers of T- and B-cell activation and/or antigen-dependent T-cell responses are other future possibilities.

Disease Damage

More than 50% of our SLE patients have been permanently damaged by the disease and its treatments. The SLICC group developed and validated the Damage Index for SLE, which was later adopted by the American College of Rheumatology. The SLICC/ACR Damage Index captures permanent organ damage, occurring since disease onset, and lasting for at least 6 months (Table 73.6). The Damage Index has been used worldwide (172). In our cohort, the most common damage is musculoskeletal, defined by using the SLICC/ACR Damage Index as osteoporosis with fracture, avascular necrosis of bone, Jaccoud's arthropathy, and/or tendon ruptures (the latter being very rare).

By using Cox proportional hazards analysis of time to the occurrence of organ damage, we investigated the role of corticosteroid therapy, either the cumulative dose, the highest dose, or pulse methylprednisolone. Pulse methylprednisolone therapy was associated only with cognitive impairment. This association may be a spurious one, because intravenous pulse methylprednisolone therapy is routinely used for CNS-lupus. Cumulative prednisone use was associated with development of cataract, osteoporosis, and coronary artery disease. High-dose prednisone use was associated with development of cataract, osteoporosis, hypertension, and diabetes mellitus (173).

The association of corticosteroid use with coronary artery disease is controversial. We believe the role of prednisone is explained by its effect in worsening known traditional risk factors for coronary artery disease, such as hyperlipidemia, hypertension, and weight. In a longitudinal regression analysis, we demonstrated that a small increase in prednisone (10 mg), led to significant increases in cholesterol, mean arterial pressure, and weight at the next visit (174).

Health Status

In general, SLE patients report poor health status, similar in degree to patients with RA (175) and human immunodeficiency virus (HIV). The SLICC group adopted the Medical Outcomes Study SF-36 (176) as their instrument to assess health status in SLE. This instrument assesses multiple facets of health status, including fatigue.

Fatigue is such an important component of health status that some studies have used additional instruments, such as the Krupp Fatigue Severity Scale (177) to capture it. However, it is not clear that chronic fatigue represents activity of SLE (178). Multiple centers have shown that fibromyalgia is more common in SLE than in the general population (179–181), and it explains a significant proportion of the chronic fatigue that leads to poor health status.

CLINICAL MANIFESTATIONS OF SLE

Initial versus Cumulative Symptoms/Signs of SLE

The most common initial symptoms/signs of SLE are cutaneous, musculoskeletal, renal, and hematologic. Because of lupus "spread" to other organ systems over time, cumulative frequencies are higher than initial ones (Table 73.7).

TABLE 73.6. PERMANENT ORGAN DAMAGE IN SLE IN THE HOPKINS LUPUS COHORT

Organ System	Percentage with Damage
Musculoskeletal	25.2
Neuropsychiatric	15.0
Ocular	12.6
Renal	11.7
Pulmonary	10.4
Cardiovascular	10.1
Gastrointestinal	7.4
Skin	7.4
Peripheral vascular	5.5
Diabetes	6.1
Malignancy	2.5
Premature gonadal failure	1.2

TABLE 73.7. PRESENTING AND CUMULATIVE SYMPTOMS/SIGNS OF SLE

Manifestation	Percentage with Symptom/Sign	Cumulative Percentage
Malar (butterfly) rash	30	56
Discoid lupus	14	27
Photosensitivity	29	54
Arthritis	40	70
Proteinuria	21	53
Seizures	4	10
Psychosis	2	5
Pericarditis	6	18
Pleurisy	16	38
Leukopenia	18	46
Thrombocytopenia	9	20

Cutaneous

Cutaneous manifestations of SLE are extremely frequent in the Hopkins Lupus Cohort (Table 73.8). Four of the manifestations, malar rash, discoid lupus, photosensitivity, and aphthous ulceration, are included in the classification criteria for SLE. Several of the manifestations are affected by race, with discoid lupus and alopecia more common in African-Americans and malar rash and aphthous ulcer more common in whites with SLE.

Malar, or butterfly rash, remains the classic cutaneous sign of SLE. It is defined as a "fixed erythema, flat or raised, over the malar eminences, tending to spare the nasolabial folds." Facial rashes not due to SLE are frequently misdiagnosed as a malar rash. Patients correctly diagnosed with SLE can develop other facial rashes as well. Common rashes to be considered in the differential diagnosis of malar rash include acne rosacea, seborrheic dermatitis, acne vulgaris, actinic damage with telangiectasias, and chloasma of pregnancy. Malar rash commonly coexists with a similar maculopapular erythematosus rash on other sun-exposed areas, especially the V-region of the neck and the forearms.

Discoid lupus lesions can occur alone as part of chronic cutaneous lupus or as part of SLE. Discoid lesions are most commonly found on the face, scalp, ears, and arms. Scarring alopecia can be a result of discoid lupus. Active discoid lupus is an erythematosus, plaque-like, slightly elevated lesion. With resolution, the inner central area will scar with either hypo- or hyperpigmentation that can be extremely disfiguring, especially in darkly pigmented patients. The differential diagnosis of discoid lupus includes psoriasis and fungal infections.

Photosensitivity is defined as "skin rash as a result of unusual reaction to sunlight, by patient history or physician observation." Photosensitivity also can occur in Sjögren's syndrome and dermatomyositis, often as the first presenting sign. Some SLE patients are sensitive to fluorescent lighting, as well, especially if unshielded (67). However, the differential diagnosis of photosensitivity is broad, and many patients may be misclassified. Five conditions, polymorphous light eruption (PMLE), solar urticaria, lupus, drug and/or chemical photosensitivity, and porphyria, are the most common causes of photosensitivity. PMLE is most commonly mistaken for lupus photosensitivity. PMLE occurs in 10% of whites, as a rash that appears in hours to a day after sun exposure and that can persist for several days. Solar urticaria, in which hives begin within minutes of sun exposure, but resolve within hours, is less likely to be confused with SLE (182). Some drugs frequently used in SLE patients, such as nonsteroidal antiinflammatory drugs (NSAIDs), also may cause photosensitivity.

TABLE 73.8. CUTANEOUS MANIFESTATIONS IN THE HOPKINS LUPUS COHORT

Manifestation	Percentage with Manifestation
Malar (butterfly) rash	56
Discoid lupus	27
Photosensitivity	54
Aphthous ulceration	41
Subacute cutaneous lupus (SCLE)	5
Alopecia	51
Livedo reticularis	22
Cutaneous vasculitis	17
Leg ulcers	4
Bullous lupus	<1
Lupus panniculitis/profundus	2
Verrucous lupus	<1
Nailfold capillary changes	Not studied
Raynaud's phenomenon	52
Angioedema	<1

Aphthous ulceration is defined as "oral or nasopharyngeal ulceration, usually painless, observed by the physician." In SLE, aphthous ulcers are found on the buccal mucosa, but also on the palate, gingiva, and tongue. Mucosal lupus also can include erythematous and discoid lesions (183). The differential diagnosis of aphthous ulcers includes trauma, iron and vitamin deficiencies, infections (such as herpes simplex), drugs, and other diseases, such as Behcet's disease and inflammatory bowel disease.

SCLE can occur as an isolated entity, but it also occurs, although uncommonly, in patients with SLE. SCLE occurs as a papulosquamous and as an annular/polycyclic form. It is a photosensitive rash, associated with anti-Ro. Discoid lupus causes a dense, deep infiltrate, whereas SCLE has a sparse superficial infiltrate. Unlike discoid lupus, SCLE lesions rarely scar. Some drugs, such as thiazide diuretics, may precipitate SCLE. On biopsy, a particulate epidermal IgG deposition is found in SCLE (184).

Alopecia has multiple causes in SLE. Lupus can cause a diffuse nonscarring alopecia and chronic scarring alopecia from discoid lesions. Scalp discoid lupus is usually present at SLE onset and responds poorly to treatment (185). Alopecia areata can occur in patients who also have SLE. Biopsies in SLE show a continuous granular deposition of IgG at the dermoepidermal junction (which is unusual in idiopathic alopecia areata) (186). Alopecia also can be secondary to drugs, including corticosteroids, azathioprine, methotrexate, and cyclophosphamide. Telogen effluviums can occur in SLE patients after infections. Hirsutism can occur in SLE patients treated with DHEA or cyclosporine.

Cutaneous vasculitis is the most common type of vasculitis in SLE. In one series, 194 of 540 SLE patients had vasculitis. The vasculitis was cutaneous in 160 patients, visceral in 24 patients, or both in ten patients. In the first episode of cutaneous vasculitis in these patients, punctate lesions occurred in 111, 32 had palpable purpura, six had urticaria, six had ulcers, eight had papules, five had erythematous plaques, two had erythema with necrosis, and one had panniculitis (187).

TABLE 73.9. CUTANEOUS MANIFESTATIONS OF ANTIPHOSPHOLIPID ANTIBODIES

Livedo reticularis
Superficial thrombophlebitis
Leg ulcers
Digital gangrene
Cutaneous necrosis
Blue-toe syndrome
Splinter hemorrhages
Porcelain white scars
Acrocyanosis

Antiphospholipid antibodies are associated with multiple cutaneous manifestations (Table 73.9). The classic antiphospholipid rash, livedo reticularis, is a purple lace-like reticular rash. It also can occur in SLE patients with vasculitis, or cryoglobulinemia, or even in SLE patients without antiphospholipid antibodies. It is not specific for SLE; a benign reversible form occurs in children and young women on cold exposure, and a fixed form can occur in older people with arteriosclerosis. In a case–control study, acrocyanosis, capillaritis, Raynaud's phenomenon, and superficial thrombophlebitis were also more common in APS (188).

Urticarial lesions, persisting for longer than a day, can occur as a result of lupus. Biopsy may reveal vasculitis. Hypocomplementemic urticarial vasculitis is a separate syndrome seen as urticaria, cutaneous vasculitis, and arthritis, often with anti-C1q antibodies. Some patients with hypocomplementemic urticarial vasculitis progress to true SLE. Angioedema can occur in SLE. C1 esterase inhibitor deficiency is usually not found. Leg ulcers in SLE can be due to vasculitis, thrombosis from antiphospholipid antibodies, pyoderma gangrenosum, or infection.

Bullous lupus, one of the rarest cutaneous manifestations, has blistering lesions. Biopsies often also show leukocytoclastic vasculitis (189). Some but not all bullous lupus responds to dapsone.

Lupus panniculitis (formerly called lupus profundus) is rare (190). Patients have multiple painful deep subcutaneous nodules, often with overlying discoid lupus (191). Lupus panniculitis causes necrosis of fat with lymphocytic aggregates. On rare occasions, fasciitis occurs, especially when the cutaneous involvement is extensive and firm (192).

Verrucous lupus (also called hypertrophic lupus) is very rare in SLE and is sometimes confused with wart infection (which also is increased in SLE) (193).

Common nail and hand changes in SLE include peringual erythema, nailfold capillary changes, nail changes, and palmar erythema. Raynaud's phenomenon is frequent in SLE, but rarely is severe enough to cause digital gangrene.

Musculoskeletal

Polyarthralgias and polyarthritis are two of the most frequent initial signs of SLE. SLE arthritis usually starts in the small joints of the hand [proximal interphalangeals (PIPs), metacarpophalangeals (MCPs), and wrist], in a symmetric fashion. Early lupus arthritis and RA are indistinguishable clinically. However, over time, SLE arthritis is less likely to be erosive. The subset of SLE arthritis that is destructive and erosive is nicknamed "Rhupus" and is often associated with rheumatoid factor (194,195). Rheumatoid nodules can be found in SLE (196).

Lupus arthritis can lead to deformity, but unlike RA, the deformities, including subluxations and ulnar deviation, are usually reducible. This "Jaccoud's arthropathy" is caused by periarticular fibrosis and ligamentous laxity (197). A similar deforming arthritis also can occur in the feet of SLE patients (198). In addition to true arthritis, tenosynovitis occurs in SLE. A rare complication of SLE (and corticosteroid therapy) is spontaneous tendon rupture. Radiographs of SLE joints affected by arthritis often show soft tissue swelling, diffuse osteopenia, and occasionally joint-space narrowing and erosions.

SLE can cause myositis. This is more common in patients with anti-RNP. Muscle biopsy may show perivascular, interstitial, and perifascicular inflammation, atrophy, and nonspecific changes, or polymyositis. SLE myositis can be either relapsing remitting or persisting, and can be as severe as primary myositis (199). Corticosteroid-induced myopathy also can be seen, usually with doses of prednisone greater than 20 mg daily. SLE patients with muscle weakness and elevated creatine phosphokinase (CPK) also should be evaluated for hypothyroidism.

The most common cause of muscle pain in SLE is fibromyalgia, occurring in 10% to 30% of SLE patients (180). Some SLE patients with fibromyalgia and chronic pain have neurally mediated hypotension on tilt-table testing.

Renal

In the Hopkins Lupus Cohort, 75% of African-American SLE patients and 50% of white SLE patients have renal involvement over time. The American College of Rheumatology (ACR) classification criterion for renal disorder is (a) persistent proteinuria greater than 0.5 g per day, or greater than 3+ if quantification is not performed; or (b) cellular casts: red cell, hemoglobin, granular, tubular, or mixed. Renal involvement can be found in renal biopsies of SLE patients who have no proteinuria or normal urine sediment (200).

Lupus nephritis can be classified according to light microscopy, electron microscopy, and immunofluorescent findings. The World Health Association (WHO) classification is most commonly used. In one study, 11% of patients had mesangial glomerulonephritis IIA, and 28% had IIB; 27% had focal proliferative; 16%, diffuse proliferative; and 18%, membranous glomerulonephritis (201). In a study of 158 renal biopsies from one center, mesangial was found in 22%, focal proliferative in 22%, diffuse proliferative in

27%, membranous in 20%, chronic sclerosing in 1%, other nephritis in 6.5%, and normal kidney in 1.5%. Transformation from one histologic pattern to another was found in 50% of serial biopsies (202).

Mesangial glomerulonephritis is usually a mild nephritis, with mesangial deposits and mild cellular proliferation on biopsy. Focal and diffuse proliferative glomerulonephritis are two ends of a spectrum. In severe diffuse proliferative glomerulonephritis, renal function is impaired, and nephrotic syndrome, hematuria, and red blood cell casts are found. The renal biopsy shows highly active proliferative and necrotizing changes, with subendothelial and mesangial deposits in addition to subepithelial and intramembranous deposits (203). Membranous glomerulonephritis has a slower course, with normal renal function for years, even with nephrotic syndrome. The renal biopsy shows mild cellular proliferation, with subepithelial and a few mesangial deposits.

The renal biopsy can also be used to grade activity and chronicity. Serial renal biopsies are sometimes necessary to evaluate chronic proteinuria and to determine the need for further therapy. Detection of reduced glomerular filtration rate (GFR) in SLE is important clinically, because such patients may benefit from angiotensin-converting enzyme (ACE)-inhibitor therapy and low-protein diets. Tubular secretion of creatinine makes creatinine and creatinine clearance imperfect markers of GFR. For that reason, nuclear medicine GFR measurements, with technetium-DTPA, isothalamate, or other markers, are recommended (204). Because cimetidine blocks tubular secretion of creatinine, it can be given to a patient to improve the creatinine clearance as a measure of GFR (205).

Multiple studies have shown that lupus activity can persist after both hemodialysis and peritoneal dialysis (206,207). However, recurrence of lupus nephritis after transplant is very rare (208).

Pulmonary

Pleurisy, with or without pleural effusion, occurs in 41% of the Hopkins Lupus Cohort. Pleurisy frequently co-occurs with pericardial pain. Pleuritic pain can be unilateral or bilateral, lasting days or weeks. Pleural effusions are usually exudative, with low to moderate volumes.

Acute lupus pneumonitis is rare, occurring in fewer than 5% of SLE patients. Pneumonitis presents as fever, dyspnea, cough, hemoptysis, and pleuritic pain. Chest radiographs may show a diffuse infiltrate, with biopsies demonstrating an interstitial lymphocytic infiltrate. Anti-Ro is associated with interstitial pneumonitis (209,210). Bronchoscopy may be necessary to rule out infection. Prompt treatment is essential, but many SLE patients still progress to chronic interstitial lung disease (211). Some pregnancy and postpartum SLE flares have begun as pleuritis and progressed to adult respiratory distress syndrome (212). Pulmonary hemorrhage, which appears similar to pneumonitis, may be life threatening (213).

A rare condition, shrinking lung, associated with diaphragmatic dysfunction, occurs (214,215). Two patients in the Hopkins Lupus Cohort have developed bronchiolitis obliterans with organizing pneumonia (BOOP), a very rarely reported pulmonary manifestation of SLE (216).

Cardiac

Pericarditis is the most common cardiac manifestation of active lupus, although often it is not evident clinically. Although pericarditis can occur at any time during the course of SLE, it tends to be one of the earlier cardiac manifestations and can even be the first manifestation of lupus (217) (Table 73.10). Coexistent pleurisy and/or effusions are common, occurring in 14 of 28 cases in one series (218). Pericarditis usually appears as an isolated attack or as recurrent episodes, with or without symptoms (219). In a French series, of 28 cases of pericarditis, 23 had pain, 12 had a rub, and four required pericardiocentesis because of tamponade (218).

Patients with pericardial effusion (as opposed to thickening) are more likely to have pericardial pain and active lupus elsewhere (220,221). In one study, only the patients with moderate or severe pericardial effusion had clinical or ECG evidence of pericarditis (221). When present, pericardial effusions are usually small and do not cause hemodynamic problems. Pericardial tamponade has been reported, however, even in treated patients (217). In the modern era, most pericardial effusions do not cause hemodynamic problems (220). Constrictive pericarditis is very rare (222–225). Pericardial fluid in SLE is usually exudative, the amount of fluid varying from 100 to more than 1,000 ml (5). Although not helpful in patient management, the fluid may contain anti-dsDNA and exhibit low complement levels (46).

Myocarditis, as recognized clinically, is rare in SLE. The clinical detection of myocarditis ranges from 3% to 15%, although it appears to be much more common in autopsy studies, suggesting the largely subclinical nature of the myocardial pathology. Myocardial abnormalities were found

TABLE 73.10. CARDIAC MANIFESTATIONS IN THE HOPKINS LUPUS COHORT

Manifestation	Percentage with Manifestation
Pericarditis	18
Pericardial tamponade	<1
Cardiac murmur	49
Left ventricular diastolic dysfunction	Not studied
Coronary artery vasculitis with myocardial infarction	0
Hypertension	42

in 20% of patients by using echocardiograms, but only one patient with an echocardiographic pattern of myocarditis developed myocardial dysfunction clinically (221).

More recent series that relied on clinical detection suggest that the frequency does not exceed 14% (218,226). Echocardiographic studies cannot definitively diagnose myocarditis, but global hypokinesis, in the absence of other known causes, is strongly suggestive. Large echo series have found frequencies of global hypokinesis between 5% and 20%. However, segmental areas of hypokinesis on echocardiogram can also be indicative of myocarditis (227).

The diagnosis of subtle degrees of left ventricular diastolic or systolic dysfunction is made echocardiographically. Echocardiographic studies (220,228–231) consistently show that 5% to 31% of SLE patients have some degree of left ventricular dysfunction. Initially, it was thought that left ventricular systolic function was not affected or affected only mildly by SLE (228,230,232,233), or, if it did occur, that it was due to hypertension, coronary artery disease, or other co-morbid processes (234). SLE patients may have systolic dysfunction that becomes apparent only with exercise (235).

Diastolic dysfunction, although subclinical, is found more consistently (230,233). Giunta et al. (230) found that disease duration was longer in patients with diastolic dysfunction. Similarly, Enomoto et al. (233) found that diastolic function deteriorated progressively with age. In contrast, several groups have found that disease activity is a major determinant of diastolic dysfunction (220,232,236,237).

Verrucous endocarditis can affect valve leaflets, papillary muscles, and the mural endocardium, as initially described by Libman and Sacks (238). However, Libman and Sacks (238) and Gross (239) found the tricuspid valve involved most often, whereas recent studies have found the mitral valve (followed by aortic) to be most affected. In the corticosteroid era, valvular vegetations are found less frequently.

It is rare for valvular disease in SLE to be clinically significant. In a series of 421 patients, only 1% to 2% had significant morbidity or mortality. Of the 14 cases with available pathology, only six had evidence of SLE valvulopathy, either verrucous vegetations or valvulitis with necrosis and vasculitis (240). Transesophageal echocardiogram is the modality of choice in terms of sensitivity in detecting valvular disease due to either lupus or APS (231,241).

Studies are conflicting on the role that antiphospholipid antibodies play in the development of the vegetations of Libman–Sacks endocarditis (242). Valvulopathy is common in the primary APS, usually found in about a third of patients in large series (231,243–250). Thrombus formation, usually on the mitral valve, can be massive and require valve replacement (251).

The strongest association of SLE with conduction disturbance is congenital heart block, usually in the setting of maternal anti-Ro and anti-La (252,253). The most common cardiac arrhythmia in adult SLE is sinus tachycardia (148,254).

Coronary arteritis is extremely rare in SLE. The most common clinical presentation is angina and/or myocardial infarction, in a child or young adult who does not have a long history of corticosteroid therapy. There is no clear correlation with extracardiac disease activity, although it has been present in some cases (255–258). Three of eight SLE patients who had a coronary artery aneurysm had no physical or laboratory evidence of active SLE (257). Arteritis is suggested when coronary aneurysms are found, if there are smooth focal lesions, or if there are rapidly developing stenoses (255,259).

Pulmonary hypertension is unusual in SLE patients, in contrast to mixed connective tissue disease and scleroderma, particularly limited scleroderma ("CREST"). It is usually asymptomatic, discovered on a screening echo Doppler. In one series of SLE patients, those with pulmonary hypertension by Doppler (14% of the group) had a shorter duration of SLE and corticosteroid therapy and a higher prevalence of Raynaud's phenomenon (260). A 5-year follow-up study of these patients documented a gradual worsening (261).

Hypertension was not a major feature of early series of SLE patients. Today, however, it is a major clinical challenge. Several studies found that hypertension was more common in those with underlying lupus nephropathy (217). All patients with hypertension in the series of Armas-Cruz et al. (262), and 86% of those in the series of Estes and Christian (148) had lupus nephritis. Pollack et al. (263) found a correlation of mean diastolic blood pressure and increasing renal damage. Others have found an association with corticosteroids (264), and, specifically, a worsening of hypertension by corticosteroids (217,219). Hypertension is especially likely to develop or worsen when patients with nephropathy are given corticosteroids (265).

We examined the relation of prednisone and blood pressure by using the Hopkins Lupus Cohort database, in which patients are seen on a quarterly basis. Using regression methods appropriate for longitudinal data, we found that an increase in prednisone dose of 10 mg led to an increase in mean arterial pressure, adjusting for all other factors that affect blood pressure (174).

Myocardial infarction was not common in the early autopsy series (266), but was a major feature of the Bulkley and Roberts (267) and subsequent autopsy series (268), especially those from Toronto (269,270). Angina and/or myocardial infarction, occurs in 7% to 9% of most SLE series (159,218,220,223,226,228,266–278). Cross-sectional or retrospective studies using more sensitive screening studies for atherosclerosis (such as nuclear medicine myocardial scans), have found reversible (exercise-induced) ischemia in 11% to 23% (228,273), suggesting that this is a more realistic estimate.

Our work has found that routine coronary artery disease (CAD) risk factors are very frequent in SLE patients (Table 73.11). In fact, the average SLE patient in our cohort study

TABLE 73.11. PREVALENCE OF CAD RISK FACTORS IN THE HOPKINS LUPUS COHORT

Characteristic	All Females	White	Black
Number of patients	199	88	109
Hypertension history, by questionnaire	46%	43%	49%
Hypertension, requiring treatment during cohort	39%	40%	39%
Hypercholesterolemia (>200 mg/dL)	55%	58%	52%
Hypercholesterolemia (>240 mg/dL)	28%	24%	30%
Obesity (NHANES definition)	39%	30%	48%
Smoking ever	58%	67%	61%
Smoking current	37%	29%	44%
Sedentary life style	70%	53%	83%
Diabetes	6%	5%	7%
Mean number of risk factors (±SD)	3.7 ± 1.4	3.6 ± 1.4	3.8 ± 1.3

has three or more of these routine CAD risk factors (279). Some of these risk factors could be due to SLE. Hypertension, for example, is more prevalent in SLE patients with renal disease (148,262). Hyperlipidemia in SLE has two major patterns. One pattern occurs in active disease, especially in pediatric patients. These patients have low high-density lipoprotein (HDL) cholesterol and apoprotein A_1 with elevated very low density lipoprotein (VLDL) cholesterol and triglyceride levels (280). Lahita et al. (281) have found a similar dyslipoproteinemia in SLE patients with anticardiolipin antibody. The second pattern occurs in SLE patients taking corticosteroids, with higher levels of triglyceride, cholesterol, and LDL cholesterol (282).

Neurologic

The 1982 neurologic classification criterion for SLE is seizures or psychosis (in the absence of offending drugs or known metabolic derangements), but this barely touches the surface of neurologic lupus (Table 73.12). CNS involvement occurred in 37% to 55% of patients in the 1960s and 1970s (283). Today, cognitive function deficits are recognized as the most common CNS problem in SLE.

Although the term *CNS vasculitis* is often used synonymously with CNS lupus, this is not supported by pathologic studies. Vasculitis is uncommonly found in neurologic lupus, even the subgroup with stroke, by arteriogram (284) or by pathology. Small vessel vasculopathy, thought to be mediated by immune complexes, leading to microinfarcts and small hemorrhages, is the predominant finding (285). Embolic brain infarcts, secondary to Libman–Sacks endocarditis, chronic valvulitis, and mural thrombus, are another pathophysiologic mechanism of stroke. Cerebral infarcts in SLE also can result from hypertension, atherosclerosis, antiphospholipid antibody–mediated thrombosis, or vasculitis.

Seizures have been reported in as many as 24% to 45% of SLE patients with neurologic involvement, but in the Hopkins Lupus Cohort, only 10% are affected. Most commonly, seizures occur in the setting of active systemic disease, although they can be an isolated finding. Other potential causes of seizures, including infection, uremia, hypertension, or past cerebral infarct, always must be excluded.

Psychosis occurs predominantly within the first year of diagnosis of SLE, although it also may occur after long duration of illness. In the Hopkins Lupus Cohort, 5% have had psychosis due to SLE. An association of anti-P antibodies with lupus psychosis has been found in some but not all studies (286–288). Psychosis in SLE patients can also be due to corticosteroid therapy, co-morbid conditions such as schizophrenia, drug reactions, and infection.

Transverse myelitis, usually with numbness, weakness, or both, is rare in SLE, but is sometimes the initial sign of lupus. Patients with transverse myelitis and SLE ("lupoid sclerosis") may sometimes show overlapping features with demyelinating disease. Some of these patients may have

TABLE 73.12. NEUROLOGIC MANIFESTATIONS IN THE HOPKINS LUPUS COHORT

Manifestation	Percentage with Manifestation
Seizures	10
Psychosis	5
Organic brain syndrome	8
Visual scotomata	<1
Retinopathy	<1
Cranial neuropathy	<1
Lupus headache	17
Stroke	7
Transverse myelitis	<1
Mononeuritis multiplex	2
Peripheral neuropathy	Not studied
Chorea	<1
Pseudotumor cerebri	<1
Meningitis	3
Syndrome of inappropriate ADH secretion	<1
Cognitive impairment	Not studied

ADH, antidiuretic hormone.

antiphospholipid antibodies. Magnetic resonance imaging (MRI) scans of the spinal cord may show inflammation, shrinkage, or actual infarcts. Pathologic examination of the spinal cord can reveal ischemic necrosis or vascular lesions.

Optic neuritis can occur in SLE, even as the presenting sign, but is rare. Retinopathy, a more common ophthalmologic sign, occurs in several patterns, including disc vasculitis, cotton-wool spots, and normal fundus with leakage of fluorescein on angiogram. Retinopathy is associated with active SLE (289).

Peripheral neuropathy occurs in as many as 10% of SLE patients. One type, mononeuritis multiplex, is attributed to ischemic damage secondary to vasculitis (290). In fact, mononeuritis multiplex is the most common presentation of visceral vasculitis in SLE (187). Other peripheral neuropathies include an acute symmetric demyelinating polyneuropathy of the Guillain–Barré type, a subacute symmetric sensorimotor polyneuropathy, and a chronic demyelinating polyneuropathy. The differential diagnosis would include diabetes mellitus, renal failure, and drug causes (such as thalidomide).

Cognitive impairment occurs frequently in SLE, but lack of standardization of testing has led to differences in prevalence estimates (291). In several studies, cognitive impairment has been independent of other manifestations of active CNS lupus or systemic disease activity (292), but has been associated with a history of neurologic lupus (293). An association with prednisone dose also has been found (294). Several recent studies have found that SLE patients with antiphospholipid antibodies have more cognitive function deficits or more deterioration (295,296).

Headache can occur because of lupus meningitis, CNS-SLE, intracranial hypertension, and dural sinus thrombosis. Most headaches in SLE patients are not due to active SLE (297).

The evaluation of a lupus patient with new neurologic symptoms and signs is often complex. It is necessary to exclude nonlupus pathology, including infection, tumor, drug reaction (including the rare association of antiinflammatory agents, especially ibuprofen, with meningitis and hydroxychloroquine with seizure), hypertension, atherosclerosis, uremia, and other metabolic processes. There is no gold standard test to diagnose neurologic lupus. Potentially useful tests include the lumbar puncture (which may show an elevated cell count, low glucose, elevated protein, elevated IgG index, or oligoclonal bands), EEG (especially the quantitated EEG), brain scan [with MRI, especially with gadolinium, generally more sensitive than computed tomography (CT)], evoked potentials, and angiography.

Hematologic

Classification criteria for SLE include hemolytic anemia with reticulocytosis, leukopenia less than 4,000/mm^3 on two or more occasions, lymphopenia with less than 1,500/mm^3 on two or more occasions, and thrombocytopenia with less than 100,000/mm^3, in the absence of offending drugs.

Although anemia is the most common hematologic abnormality in SLE, occurring in more than 50%, it is not usually of the autoimmune type. The most common anemia is the anemia of chronic disease. Other nonimmune causes of anemia include hypersplenism, iron deficiency, peptic ulcer disease, or renal disease. Autoimmune hemolytic anemia is of the "warm variety," usually due to IgG. Patients with SLE can have a positive Coomb's test to antibody, to complement on the erythrocyte, or to both (298).

The incidence of thrombocytopenia in SLE ranges from 15% to 50%. Shortened platelet survival is responsible for the thrombocytopenia. Bone marrow aspirates show normal or increased numbers of megakaryocytes. Idiopathic thrombocytopenic purpura (ITP) may be the initial manifestation of SLE. In one series, one of eight patients who underwent splenectomy for ITP later developed SLE (299). SLE patients with antiphospholipid antibodies also may have thrombocytopenia, although it is usually mild. Evaluation of a thrombocytopenic SLE patient would include antiplatelet antibodies and antiphospholipid antibodies. Severe thrombocytopenia may require a bone marrow aspirate/biopsy. The differential diagnosis of thrombocytopenia would include drug causes (especially immunosuppressive drugs), infections, malignancies, thrombotic thrombocytopenic purpura, and disseminated intravascular coagulation.

Rare manifestations of SLE include thrombotic thrombocytopenic purpura (300), myelofibrosis (301), and aplastic anemia (302,303).

Constitutional

Lymphadenopathy occurs in 12% to 59% of SLE patients (304). The most common nodal groups involved are cervical, mesenteric, axillary, and inguinal. On biopsy, a paracortical focus of necrosis and inflammatory infiltration is found, with "hematoxylin bodies," which are classic for lupus lymphadenitis. The pathology of necrotizing lymphadenitis in SLE is similar to that in Kikuchi–Fujomoto disease, a self-limited form (305).

Fever is a common sign of SLE flare. However, infection must always be considered, as well.

Gastrointestinal

In the past, gastrointestinal symptoms were frequently found in SLE patients. Today, most nonspecific gastrointestinal symptoms are secondary to the side effects of treatment. NSAIDs are well-recognized causes of gastropathy (306). Salicylate hepatitis is rarely seen today. Azathioprine can cause nausea and vomiting, hepatitis, and pancreatitis.

Methotrexate causes nausea and elevated liver-function tests, but the incidence is low when daily folic acid is given. Hydroxychloroquine, especially the generic form, may cause nausea, abdominal cramps, and diarrhea.

Lupus serositis limited to the peritoneum ("primary lupus peritonitis") (3,307) can occur both acutely and chronically. Acute ascites can occur because of lupus peritonitis, lupus pancreatitis, bowel infarction, or infection. Chronic ascites is most often due to congestive heart failure, nephrotic syndrome, or cirrhosis, but chronic lupus peritonitis (308), constrictive pericarditis, Budd–Chiari syndrome, and protein-losing enteropathy (309) are in the differential diagnosis.

In early series, acute surgical abdomen in SLE patients was frequently due to intestinal vasculitis (310–312). Clinical associates included peripheral vasculitis, CNS-SLE, osteonecrosis, thrombocytopenia, and rheumatoid factor (311). Vasculitis also can lead to bowel hemorrhage, intraperitoneal hemorrhage, intestinal perforation (313), and colonic pneumatosis cystoides intestinalis.

Secondary APS can lead to hepatic (including Budd–Chiari syndrome), splenic, or intestinal infarcts (314). Adrenal infarction or hemorrhage also is seen in APS.

The term "lupus enteritis" encompasses SLE bowel disease, including small vessel and occasionally large vessel vasculitis with mucosal ulcers (4,315,316). Some SLE patients appear to have inflammatory bowel disease without vasculitis (317). Sulfasalazine, used to treat idiopathic inflammatory bowel disease, can cause a drug-induced lupus.

Protein-losing enteropathy is seen with edema and hypoalbuminemia. Other causes include pericarditis, lymphangiectasia, and celiac disease. Immunopathology may demonstrate deposition of C3 in the villous capillary wall (318).

Pancreatitis due to SLE can occur as a result of arteritis, other vascular lesions, necrotizing pancreatitis, inspissated concretions attributable to corticosteroids, and thrombus (319,320). In animal models, corticosteroids can cause pancreatic lesions and peripancreatic fat necrosis. However, corticosteroids are rarely the cause of SLE pancreatitis.

The most common hepatic problem in SLE is elevation of liver function test results, occurring in 25% to 50% (321). A pathologic series of 52 patients found hepatic congestion in 38, arteritis in 11, cholestasis in nine, peliosis hepatitis in six, chronic persistent hepatitis in six, reactive hepatitis in five, cholangiolitis in three, nodular regenerative hyperplasia in three, and hemangioma in three (322). Fatty liver is usually associated with glucocorticoid therapy. Both hepatomegaly and splenomegaly can occur because of SLE.

Esophageal manometric studies are frequently abnormal in SLE (323), but severe esophageal dysmotility is rare. Gastroesophageal reflux disease is common, as it is in the general population, and may be aggravated by use of NSAIDs.

COMPLICATIONS OF SLE

Corticosteroid-induced Osteoporosis

In the Hopkins Lupus Cohort, 22% of patients have osteoporosis, and 13% have had an osteoporotic fracture. In a Cox proportional-hazards model of time to an osteoporotic fracture, both cumulative prednisone and the highest prednisone dose used were predictive. Because most SLE patients are premenopausal, management of corticosteroid-induced osteoporosis presents special challenges. Of course, reduction of corticosteroid doses is helpful. Bisphosphonates cannot be used during pregnancy. In postmenopausal women with SLE, a safety study of estrogen replacement therapy ("SELENA") is currently under way.

Avascular Necrosis of Bone/Osteonecrosis

Avascular necrosis of bone (AVN) occurs in 12% of the Hopkins Lupus Cohort. Risk factors include use of prednisone in a dose greater than 20 mg daily, Raynaud's phenomenon, and vasculitis. AVN is more common in African-Americans than in whites (324). Although we have not found an association with antiphospholipid antibodies in the entire cohort, an association with markers of hypercoagulability was found in a case–control study (325). Other centers have failed to find an association with corticosteroid dose or Raynaud's phenomenon (326).

AVN of bone occurs most commonly in hips, followed by knees and shoulders. It is usually bilateral. Early detection is best achieved by MRI scan. Management of early stages of AVN is by core decompression of bone, which can relieve pain and either save the joint or at least delay the need for total joint replacement (327).

Stroke

Stroke in SLE is often not due to active CNS-SLE. Strokes in SLE can be thrombotic, due to APS; embolic, due to heart valve lesions (Libman–Sacks endocarditis); hypertensive; and atherosclerotic. SLE patients frequently have elevated levels of homocysteine, a risk factor for atherothrombosis (328). B-vitamin supplementation, especially with folic acid, can reduce levels of homocysteine.

Accelerated Atherosclerosis

The major cause of death in many series of SLE patients is cardiovascular disease. Women with SLE aged 35 to 44 years were 50 times more likely to have a myocardial infarction than are control women in the Framingham offspring study (329). The bimodal pattern of mortality (early deaths due to active disease, later deaths due to atherosclerosis) (274) has now, because of better treatment of atherosclerosis, become a saga of cardiovascular morbidity as well.

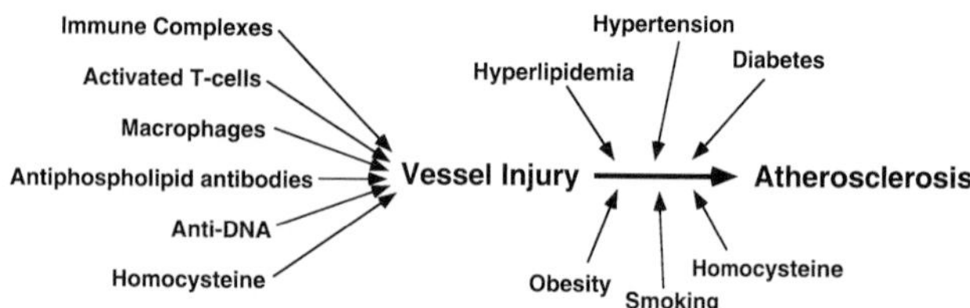

FIGURE 73.2. Two-stage model of accelerated atherosclerosis in systemic lupus erythematosus (SLE).

Accelerated atherosclerosis in SLE is multifactorial. We have adopted a two-stage model. The first stage is vessel injury, due to immune-complex deposition, activated lymphocytes, cytokines, anti–endothelial cell antibodies, and antiphospholipid antibodies, and the second stage is accelerated atherosclerosis mediated by elevated levels of traditional cardiovascular risk factors, such as hypertension, hyperlipidemia, obesity, diabetes mellitus, smoking, and nontraditional risk factors such as antiphospholipid antibodies and homocysteine (Fig. 73.2). Because most SLE patients have a pattern of frequent exacerbations or of chronic (continuous) activity, there may be many opportunities for vessel injury, leading to a vicious cycle.

Antiphospholipid antibodies have been found to be a prospective risk factor for atherosclerosis in the Hopkins Lupus Cohort and a risk factor in many (but not all) studies in the general population as well (330,331). Recent work has shown that β_2-glycoprotein-1 inhibits uptake of oxidized LDL, but, in the presence of anticardiolipin, it undergoes a conformational change that then increases oxidized LDL uptake (332).

Secondary Antiphospholipid Antibody Syndrome

Criteria for the APS have recently been revised (333) (Table 73.13). These new criteria expand thrombosis to include the vasculopathic events that especially characterize catastrophic APS and enlarge the definition of pregnancy morbidity to include severe preeclampsia and placental insufficiency.

Lupus anticoagulant, anticardiolipin, and anti–β_2-glycoprotein-1 occur frequently in SLE patients. Levels may fluctuate with disease activity or treatment with corticosteroids and other immunosuppressive drugs. In prospective work, both the lupus anticoagulant and anticardiolipin antibody predict later venous and arterial thrombosis in SLE (334). Of the two antibodies, several studies (335,336) have found that the lupus anticoagulant is a more specific predictor. In addition to antiphospholipid antibodies, serologic markers of active lupus and traditional cardiovascular risk factors are predictive of later thrombosis. In our cohort, 10% have had sequelae of APS; although other series report a higher frequency. SLE patients, with or without antiphospholipid antibodies, frequently exhibit biochemical markers of ongoing coagulation, such as *d* dimers, thrombin–antithrombin III complexes, and prothrombin fragment 1.2.

TABLE 73.13. REVISED CRITERIA FOR THE ANTIPHOSPHOLIPID ANTIBODY SYNDROME

Clinical criteria
Vascular thrombosis
Arterial
Venous
Small vessel
Pregnancy morbidity
One or more fetal losses after week 10
One or more premature births (<34 weeks)
Preeclampsia
Placental insufficiency
Three or more consecutive spontaneous abortions
Laboratory criteria
Confirmed presence of lupus anticoagulant or moderate-to-high anticardiolipin.

From Wilson WA, Gharavi AE, Koike T, et al. International consensus statement on preliminary classification criteria for definite antiphospholipid syndrome: report of an international workshop. *Arthritis Rheum* 1999;42:1309–1311, with permission.

Infections

Infection remains one of the leading causes of death in SLE in both older (337) and newer (338) series. It is likely that current series underestimate mortality due to infection in SLE. The few studies that include autopsies (270,339) have highlighted that fatal opportunistic infections are often missed before death. The infection rate in SLE patients is 10 times that in RA patients and 5 times that in nephrotic patients (340). In a Swedish series, SLE patients differed most from normal controls in their increased risk for bacterial infections (341). Infection is a major cause of hospitalization in SLE (342–344).

Risk factors for infection in SLE include active lupus, renal lupus activity, renal insufficiency/failure, proteinuria, low albumin, corticosteroid use, and immunosuppressive drug use. Both azathioprine (345) and cyclophosphamide predispose to herpes zoster. Cyclophosphamide predisposes to opportunistic infections, which are more likely to be fatal (339,346). In our prospective analysis of hospitalization for infection, we found that disease activity, corticosteroid use, and immunosuppressive drug use were all independent predictors (343). SLE itself is a well-recognized cause of immune dysfunction that can predispose to infection.

Infections in SLE patients usually are caused by common bacterial pathogens. Skin or other infections caused by *Staphylococcus aureus* are frequently reported (341). Gram-negative infections are prevalent in SLE patients with renal failure (347). SLE patients appear to be at special risk for pneumococcal infection because of splenic dysfunction (348–350). Neisserial infection may be increased in SLE because of complement deficiencies, reticuloendothelial system dysfunction, and functional asplenia (351,352). Salmonella infection, with bacteremia and septic arthritis, is overrepresented in SLE (340,353). Outside of the U.S., tuberculosis remains a major issue in SLE (27,354).

Virtually all known opportunistic infections have been reported in SLE, with special emphasis on fungal infections (340,354–356), *Pneumocystis carinii* (27,339,357,358), herpes zoster (339,359), and cytomegalovirus (27,353, 359). In a series of 44 SLE patient deaths, opportunistic infections were as common as bacterial infections, with Candida in six and Pneumocystis in three (339). Complications of infections in SLE patients include multiple infections (340), deep tissue infections, bacteremia (340,353, 356), disseminated intravascular coagulation (360), and adult respiratory distress syndrome (361).

No perfect formula exists for differentiating fever due to infection from that due to SLE flare. However, in one series, leukocytosis, elevated polymorphonuclear leukocytes, shaking chills, and normal anti-dsDNA levels were indicative of infection (344).

ACKNOWLEDGMENTS

The Hopkins Lupus Cohort is supported by NIH RO-1 AR 43727 and by the Hopkins Outpatient Clinical Research Center. The research was supported by the American Heart Association Grant-in-Aid.

REFERENCES

1. Hebra F, Kaposi M. On diseases of the skin, including the exanthemata. In: Hitlon FC, ed. *The new Sydenham Society*. London: 1874:1866–1880.
2. Osler W. On the visceral manifestations of the erythema group of skin diseases. *Trans Assoc Am Physicians* 1903;18:599–624.
3. Ropes MW. *Systemic lupus erythematosus.* Cambridge, MA: Harvard University Press, 1976.
4. Harvey AM, Shulman LE, Tumulty PA, et al. Systemic lupus erythematosus: review of the literature and clinical analysis of 138 cases. *Medicine* 1954;33:291–437.
5. Calvo-Alen J, Bastian HM, Straaton KV, et al. Identification of patient subsets among those presumptively diagnosed with, referred, and/or followed up for systemic lupus erythematosus at a large tertiary care center. *Arthritis Rheum* 1995;38:1475–1484.
6. Tan EM, Cohen AS, Fries JF, et al. The 1982 revised criteria for the classification of systemic lupus erythematosus. *Arthritis Rheum* 1982;25:1271–1277.
7. Hochberg MC. Updating the American College of Rheumatology revised criteria for the classification of systemic lupus erythematosus. *Arthritis Rheum* 1997;40:1725.
8. Sontheimer RD, Thomas JR, Gilliam JN. Subacute cutaneous lupus erythematosus: a cutaneous marker for a distinct subset. *Arch Dermatol* 1979;115:1409–1415.
9. Petri M, Allbritton J. Hair product use in systemic lupus erythematosus: a case-control study. *Arthritis Rheum* 1992;35:625–629.
10. Sanchez-Guerrero J, Karlson EW, Colditz GA, et al. Hair dye use and the risk of developing systemic lupus erythematosus: a cohort study. *Arthritis Rheum* 1996;39:657–662.
11. Price EJ, Venables PJ. Drug-induced lupus. *Drug Saf* 1995;12: 283–290.
12. Buyon JP. Neonatal lupus syndromes. *Am J Reprod Immunol* 1992;28:259–263.
13. Steinberg AD, Melez KA, Raveche ES, et al. Approach to the study of the role of sex hormones in autoimmunity. *Arthritis Rheum* 1979;22:1170–1176.
14. Uramoto KM, Michet CJJ, Thumboo J, et al. Trends in the incidence and mortality of systemic lupus erythematosus, 1950-1992. *Arthritis Rheum* 1999;42:46–50.
15. Lahita RG, Bradlow HL, Kunkel HG, et al. Alterations of estrogen metabolism in systemic lupus erythematosus. *Arthritis Rheum* 1979;22:1195–1198.
16. Bucala R, Lahita RG, Fishman J, et al. Anti-oestrogen antibodies in users of oral contraceptives and in patients with systemic lupus erythematosus. *Clin Exp Immunol* 1987;67:167–175.
17. Lahita RG. Sex and age in systemic lupus erythematosus. In: Lahita RG, ed. *Systemic lupus erythematosus.* New York: Wiley, 1984:523–539.
18. Lavalle C, Loyo E, Paniagua R, et al. Correlation study between prolactin and androgens in male patients with systemic lupus erythematosus. *J Rheumatol* 1987;14:268–272.
19. Stimson WH. Sex steroids, steroid receptors and immunity. In: Berczi I, Kovacs K, eds. *Hormones and immunity.* Lancaster: MTP Press, 1987:45–53.
20. Cohen JHM, Davel L, Cordier G, et al. Sex steroid receptors in peripheral T cells: absence of androgen receptors and restriction of estrogen receptors to OKT8 positive cells. *J Immunol* 1983;131:2767–2771.
21. Holdstock GI, Chastenay BF, Krawitt EL. Effects of testosterone, estradiol and progesterone on immune regulation. *Clin Exp Immunol* 1982;47:449–456.
22. Ahmed SA, Penhale WJ, Talal N. Sex hormones, immune responses and autoimmune diseases: mechanisms of sex hormone action. *Am J Pathol* 1985;121:531–551.
23. Rood MJ, ten Cate R, van Suijlekom-Smit LWA, et al. Childhood-onset systemic lupus erythematosus: clinical presentation and prognosis in 31 patients. *Scand J Rheumatol* 1999;28: 222–226.
24. Fessel WJ. Systemic lupus erythematosus in the community: incidence, prevalence, outcome, and first symptoms; the high prevalence in black women. *Arch Intern Med* 1974;134:1027–1035.
25. Hochberg MC. Racial differences in the descriptive and clinical epidemiology of systemic lupus erythematosus in the United States. In: *Proceedings of the Second International Conference on Systemic Lupus Erythematosus.* Singapore: Professional Postgraduate Services, KK, 1989:32–34.
26. Hopkinson ND, Doherty M, Powell RJ. Clinical features and race-specific incidence/prevalence rates of systemic lupus erythematosus in a geographically complete cohort of patients. *Ann Rheum Dis* 1994;53:675–680.
27. Wong KL. Pattern of SLE in Hong Kong Chinese: a cohort study. *Scand J Rheumatol* 1992;21:289–296.
28. Nagata C, Fujita S, Iwata H, et al. Systemic lupus erythematosus: a case-control epidemiologic study in Japan. *Int J Dermatol* 1995;34:333–337.
29. Alarcón-Segovia D, Osmundson PJ. Peripheral vascular syndromes associated with systemic lupus erythematosus. *Ann Intern Med* 1965;62:907–919.
30. Alarcon GS, Friedman AW, Straaton KV, et al. Systemic lupus erythematosus in three ethnic groups: III. A comparison of characteristics early in the natural history of the LUMINA cohort: lupus in minority populations: nature vs nurture. *Lupus* 1999;8:197–209.

31. Alarcón GS, Roseman JM, Bartolucci AA, et al. Systemic lupus erythematosus in three ethnic groups: II. Features predictive of disease activity early in its course: LUMINA Study Group: lupus in minority populations: nature vs nurture. *Arthritis Rheum* 1998;41:1173–1180.
32. Hochberg MC, Boyd RE, Ahearn JM, et al. Systemic lupus erythematosus: a review of clinico-laboratory features and immunogenetic markers in 150 patients with emphasis on demographic subsets. *Medicine* 1985;64:285–295.
33. Petri M, Perez-Gutthann S, Longenecker JC, et al. Morbidity of systemic lupus erythematosus: role of race and socioeconomic status. *Am J Med* 1991;91:345–353.
34. Reveille JD, Schrohenloher RE, Acton RT, et al. DNA analysis of HLA-Dr and Dq genes in American blacks with systemic lupus erythematosus. *Arthritis Rheum* 1989;32:1243–1251.
35. Siegel M, Lee SL. The epidemiology of systemic lupus erythematosus. *Semin Arthritis Rheum* 1973;3:1–54.
36. Helve T. Prevalence and mortality rates of systemic lupus erythematosus and causes of death in SLE patients in Finland. *Scand J Rheumatol* 1985;14:43–46.
37. Hochberg MC, Perlmutter SL, Medsger TA, et al. Prevalence of self-reported physician-diagnosed systemic lupus erythematosus in the USA. *Lupus* 1995;4:454–456.
38. Michet CJ Jr, McKenna CH, Elveback LR, et al. Epidemiology of systemic lupus erythematosus and other connective tissue diseases in Rochester, Minnesota, 1950 through 1979. *Mayo Clin Proc* 1985;60:105–113.
39. Meddings J, Grennan DM. The prevalence of systemic lupus erythematosus (SLE) in Dunedin. *N Z Med J* 1980;91:205.
40. Nived O, Sturfelt G, Wollheim F. Systemic lupus erythematosus in an adult population in Southern Sweden: incidence, prevalence and validity of ARA revised classification criteria. *Br J Rheumatol* 1985;24:147–154.
41. Hochberg MC. Prevalence of systemic lupus erythematosus in England and Wales, 1982-2. *Ann Rheum Dis* 1987;46:664–666.
42. Nakae K, Furusawa F, Kasukawa R, et al. A nationwide epidemiological survey on diffuse collagen diseases: estimation of prevalence rate in Japan. In: Kasukawa R, Sharp GC, eds. *Mixed connective tissue disease and anti-nuclear antibodies.* Amsterdam: Elsevier Science Publishers BV, 1987:9.
43. Maskarinec G, Katz AR. Prevalence of systemic lupus erythematosus in Hawaii: is there a difference between ethnic groups? *Hawaii Med J* 1995;54:406–409.
44. Samanta A, Roy S, Peehally J, et al. The prevalence of diagnosed systemic lupus erythematosus in whites and Indian Asian immigrants in Leicester City, UK. *Br J Rheumatol* 1992;31:679–682.
45. Nossent JC. Systemic lupus erythematosus on the Caribbean island of Curacao: an epidemiological investigation. *Ann Rheum Dis* 1992;51:1197–1201.
46. Gudmundsson S, Steinsson K. Systemic lupus erythematosus in Iceland 1975 through 1984: a nationwide epidemiological study in an unselected population. *J Rheumatol* 1990;17:1162–1167.
47. McCarty DJ, Manzi S, Medsger TA Jr, et al. Incidence of systemic lupus erythematosus: race and gender differences. *Arthritis Rheum* 1995;38:1260–1270.
48. Johnson AE, Gordon C, Palmer RG, et al. The prevalence and incidence of systemic lupus erythematosus in Birmingham, England. *Arthritis Rheum* 1995;38:551–558.
49. Gourley IS, Patterson CC, Bell AL. The prevalence of systemic lupus erythematosus in Northern Ireland. *Lupus* 1997;6: 399–403.
50. Freni-Titulaer LWJ, Kelley DB, Grow AG, et al. Connective tissue disease in southeastern Georgia: a case-control study of etiologic factors. *Am J Epidemiol* 1989;130:404–409.
51. Strom BL, Reidenberg MM, West S, et al. Shingles, allergies, family medical history, oral contraceptives, and other potential risk factors for systemic lupus erythematosus. *Am J Epidemiol* 1994;140:632–642.
52. Nagata C, Yoshida H, Fujita S, et al. A case-control SLE study based on patients receiving financial aid for treatment. In: Yanagawa H, Sasaki R, Nagai M, eds. *Recent progress of epidemiologic study of intractable diseases in Japan.* Tokyo: Ministry of Health and Welfare of Japan, 1992:113–116.
53. Minami Y, Sasaki T, Komatsu S, et al. Female systemic lupus erythematosus in Miyagi prefecture, Japan: a case-control study of dietary and reproductive factors. *Tohoku J Exp Med* 1993; 169:245–252.
54. Lehmann P, Holzle E, Kind P, et al. Experimental reproduction of skin lesions in lupus erythematosus by UVA and UVB radiation. *J Am Acad Dermatol* 1990;22:181–187.
55. Hasan T, Nyberg F, Stephansson E, et al. Photosensitivity in lupus erythematosus, UV photoprovocation results compared with history of photosensitivity and clinical findings. *Br J Dermatol* 1997;136:699–705.
56. Nived O, Sturfelt G, Ryberg B. Two UV-induced episodes of myelitis in a patient with systemic lupus erythematosus. *J Intern Med* 1992;232:461–463.
57. Higuchi D, Ogura Y, Watanabe H, et al. Experimental production of DLE lesion with a single exposure to UVB (2.7 MEDs) radiation. *J Dermatol* 1991;18:545–548.
58. Kawashima T, Zappi EG, Lieu TS, et al. Impact of ultraviolet irradiation on expression of SSA/Ro autoantigenic polypeptides in transformed human epidermal keratinocytes. *Lupus* 1994; 3:493–500.
59. Furukawa F, Kanauchi H, Imamura S. Susceptibility to UVB light in cultured keratinocytes of cutaneous lupus erythematosus. *Dermatology* 1994;189(suppl 1):18–23.
60. Jones SK. Ultraviolet radiation (UVR) induces cell-surface Ro/SSA antigen expression by human keratinocytes in vitro: a possible mechanism for the UVR induction of cutaneous lupus lesions. *Br J Dermatol* 1992;126:546–553.
61. Abe M, Ishikawa O, Miyachi Y, et al. In vitro spontaneous and UVB-induced lymphocyte apoptosis are not specific to SLE. *Photodermatol Photoimmunol Photomed* 1997;13:204–207.
62. Golan TD, Foltyn V, Roueff A. Increased susceptibility to in vitro ultraviolet B radiation in fibroblasts and lymphocytes cultured from systemic lupus erythematosus patients. *Clin Immunol Immunopathol* 1991;58:289–304.
63. Nived O, Johansen PB, Sturfelt G. Standardized ultraviolet-A exposure provokes skin reaction in systemic lupus erythematosus. *Lupus* 1993;2:247–250.
64. Golan TD, Dan S, Haim H, et al. Solar ultraviolet radiation induces enhanced accumulation of oxygen radicals in murine SLE-derived splenocytes in vitro. *Lupus* 1994;3:103–106.
65. Avalos-Diaz E, Alvarado-Flores E, Herrera-Esparza R. UV-A irradiation induces transcription of IL-6 and TNF alpha genes in human keratinocytes and dermal fibroblasts. *Rev Rhum Engl Ed* 1999;66:13–19.
66. Golan TD, Elkon KB, Gharavi AE, et al. Enhanced membrane binding of autoantibodies to cultured keratinocytes of systemic lupus erythematosus patients after ultraviolet B/ultraviolet A irradiation. *J Clin Invest* 1992;90:1067–1076.
67. Rihner M, McGrath H Jr. Fluorescent light photosensitivity in patients with systemic lupus erythematosus. *Arthritis Rheum* 1992;35:949–952.
68. McGrath H Jr, Bell JM, Haycock JW. Fluorescent light activates the immunomodulator cis-urocanic acid in vitro: implications for patients with systemic lupus erythematosus. *Ann Rheum Dis* 1994;53:396–399.
69. Molina JF, McGrath H Jr. Longterm ultraviolet-A1 irradiation therapy in systemic lupus erythematosus. *J Rheumatol* 1997;24: 1072–1074.

70. McGrath H Jr. Ultraviolet-A1 irradiation decreases clinical disease activity and autoantibodies in patients with systemic lupus erythematosus. *Clin Exp Rheumatol* 1994;12:129–135.
71. McGrath H Jr, Martinez-Osuna P, Lee FA. Ultraviolet-A1 (340-400 nm) irradiation therapy in systemic lupus erythematosus. *Lupus* 1996;5:269–274.
72. McGrath H Jr, Bak E, Zimny ML, et al. Fluorescent light decreases autoimmunity and improves immunity in B/W mice. *J Clin Lab Immunol* 1990;32:113–116.
73. Folomeev M, Dougados M, Beaune J, et al. Plasma sex hormones and aromatase activity in tissues of patients with systemic lupus erythematosus. *Lupus* 1992;1:191–195.
74. Lahita RG, Bradlow L, Fishman J, et al. Estrogen metabolism in systemic lupus erythematosus: patients and family members. *Arthritis Rheum* 1982;25:843–846.
75. Martucci CP, Fishman J. P450 enzymes of estrogen metabolism. *Pharmacol Ther* 1993;57:237–257.
76. Parke AL, Parke DV, Jones FA. Diet and nutrition in rheumatoid arthritis and other chronic inflammatory diseases. *J Clin Biochem Nutr* 1996;20:1–26.
77. Petri M, Robinson C. Oral contraceptives and systemic lupus erythematosus. *Arthritis Rheum* 1997;40:797–803.
78. Sanchez-Guerrero J, Karlson EW, Liang MH, et al. Past use of oral contraceptives and the risk of developing systemic lupus erythematosus. *Arthritis Rheum* 1997;40:804–808.
79. Sanchez-Guerrero J, Liang MH, Karlson EW, et al. Postmenopausal estrogen therapy and the risk for developing systemic lupus erythematosus. *Ann Intern Med* 1995;122:430–433.
80. Grimes DA, LeBolt SA, Grimes KR, et al. Systemic lupus erythematosus and reproductive function: a case-control study. *Am J Obstet Gynecol* 1985;153:179–186.
81. Reidenberg MM, Drayer DE, Lorenzo B, et al. Acetylation phenotypes and environmental chemical exposure of people with idiopathic systemic lupus erythematosus. *Arthritis Rheum* 1993;36:971–973.
82. Walker SE, Allen SH, Hoffman RW, et al. Prolactin: a stimulator of disease activity in systemic lupus erythematosus. *Lupus* 1995;4:3–9.
83. Deighton C. Smoke gets in your joints? *Ann Rheum Dis* 1997; 56:453–454.
84. Saag KG, Cerhan JR, Kolluri S, et al. Cigarette smoking and rheumatoid arthritis severity. *Ann Rheum Dis* 1997;56: 463–469.
85. Hughes DA, Haslam PL, Townsend PJ, et al. Numerical and functional alterations in circulatory lymphocytes in cigarette smokers. *Clin Exp Immunol* 1985;61:459–466.
86. Ferson M, Edwards A, Lind A, et al. Low natural killer-cell activity and immunoglobulin levels associated with smoking in human subjects. *Int J Cancer* 1979;23:603–609.
87. Miller LG, Goldstein G, Murphy M, et al. Reversible alterations in immunoregulatory T cells in smoking: analysis by monoclonal antibodies and flow cytometry. *Chest* 1982;82:526–529.
88. Thomas WR, Holt PG, Keast D. Recovery of immune system after cigarette smoking. *Nature* 1974;248:358–359.
89. Chalmer J, Holt PG, Keast D. Cell-mediated immune responses to transplanted tumors in mice chronically exposed to cigarette smoke. *J Natl Cancer Inst* 1975;55:1129–1134.
90. Mathews JD, Whittingham S, Hooper BM, et al. Association of autoantibodies with smoking, cardiovascular morbidity, and death in the Busselton population. *Lancet* 1973;2:754–758.
91. Tuomi T, Heliovaara M, Palosuo T, et al. Smoking, lung function, and rheumatoid factors. *Ann Rheum Dis* 1990;49:753–756.
92. Hersey P, Lawrence S, Prendergast D, et al. Association of Sjögren's syndrome with C4 deficiency, defective reticuloendothelial function and circulating immune complexes. *Clin Exp Immunol* 1983;52:551–560.
93. Baron JA. Smoking and estrogen-related disease. *Am J Epidemiol* 1984;119:9–22.
94. Michnovicz JJ, Hershcopf RJ, Naganuma H, et al. Increased 2-hydroxylation of estradiol as a possible mechanism for the antiestrogenic effect of cigarette smoking. *N Engl J Med* 1986;315: 1305–1309.
95. Khaw KT, Tazuke S, Barrett-Connor E. Cigarette smoking and levels of adrenal androgens in postmenopausal women. *N Engl J Med* 1988;318:1705–1709.
96. McAlindon T, Felson D, Palmer J, et al. Associations of cigarette smoking and alcohol with systemic lupus erythematosus among participants in the Black Women's Health Study [abstract]. *Arthritis Rheum* 1997;40:S162.
97. Hardy CJ, Palmer BP, Muir KR, et al. Smoking history, alcohol consumption, and systemic lupus erythematosus: a case-control study. *Ann Rheum Dis* 1998;57:451–455.
98. Benoni C, Nilsson A, Nived O. Smoking and inflammatory bowel disease: comparison with systemic lupus erythematosus: a case-control study. *Scand J Gastroenterol* 1990;25:751–755.
99. Gallego H, Crutchfield CE 3rd, Lewis EJ, et al. Report of an association between discoid lupus erythematosus and smoking. *Cutis* 1999;63:231–234.
100. Rahman P, Gladman DD, Urowitz MB. Efficacy of antimalarial therapy in cutaneous lupus in smokers versus nonsmokers. *Arthritis Rheum* 1997;40(suppl 9):S58(abst).
101. Petri M, Allbritton J. Antibiotic allergy in SLE: a case-control study. *J Rheumatol* 1992;19:265–269.
102. Petri M, Allbritton J. Antibiotic allergy in systemic lupus erythematosus: reply [Letter]. *J Rheumatol* 1992;19:1994.
103. Pointud P. Minocycline related lupus [Letter]. *J Rheumatol* 1997;24:1851–1852.
104. Gough A, Chapman S, Wagstaff K, et al. Minocycline induced autoimmune hepatitis and systemic lupus erythematosus-like syndrome. *Br Med J* 1996;312:169–172.
105. Angulo JM, Sigal LH, Espinoza LR. Coexistent minocycline-induced systemic lupus erythematosus and autoimmune hepatitis. *Semin Arthritis Rheum* 1998;28:187–192.
106. Elkayam O, Yaron M, Caspi D. Minocycline-induced autoimmune syndromes: an overview. *Semin Arthritis Rheum* 1999;28: 392–397.
107. Tubach F, Kaplan G, Berenbaum F. Highly positive dsDNA antibodies in minocycline-induced lupus [Letter]. *Clin Exp Rheumatol* 1999;17:124–125.
108. Moore AD, Petri MA, Manzi S, et al. The use of alternative medical therapies in patients with systemic lupus erythematosus (SLE). *Arthritis Rheum* 2000; submitted.
109. Carr R, Forsyth S, Sadi D. Abnormal responses to ingested substances in murine systemic lupus erythematosus: apparent effect of a casein-free diet on the development of systemic lupus erythematosus in N2B/Wn mice. *J Rheumatol* 1987;14:158–165.
110. Weimann BJ, Weiser H. Effects of antioxidant vitamins C, E, and β-carotene on immune functions in MRL/lpr mice and rats. *Ann N Y Acad Sci* 1992;669:390–392.
111. Fernandes G. Dietary lipids and risk of autoimmune disease. *Clin Immunol Immunopathol* 1994;72:193–197.
112. McAlindon T, Giannotta L, Taub N, et al. Environmental factors predicting nephritis in systemic lupus erythematosus. *Ann Rheum Dis* 1993;52:720–724.
113. Malinow MR, Bardana EJ, Pirofsky B, et al. Systemic lupus erythematosus-like syndrome in monkeys fed alfalfa sprouts: role of a nonprotein amino acid. *Science* 1982;216:415–417.
114. Montanaro A, Bardana EJ Jr. Dietary amino acid-induced systemic lupus erythematosus. *Rheum Dis Clin North Am* 1991;17:323–332.
115. Keen GA, Yeats J. Epstein-Barr virus-induced systemic lupus erythematosus? [Letter]. *S Afr Med J* 1996;86:850.

116. Matsukawa Y. Epstein-Barr virus-induced systemic lupus erythematosus [Letter]. *S Afr Med J* 1996;86:850–851.
117. Bhimma R, Adhikari M, Coovadia HM. Epstein-Barr virus-induced systemic lupus erythematosus. *S Afr Med J* 1995;85:899–900.
118. Vaughan JH, Nguyen MD, Valbracht JR, et al. Epstein-Barr virus-induced autoimmune responses. II. Immunoglobulin G autoantibodies to mimicking and nonmimicking epitopes: presence in autoimmune disease. *J Clin Invest* 1995;95:1316–1327.
119. Incaprera M, Rindi L, Bazzichi A, et al. Potential role of the Epstein-Barr virus in systemic lupus erythematosus autoimmunity. *Clin Exp Rheumatol* 1998;16:289–294.
120. Marchini B, Dolcher MP, Sabbatini A, et al. Immune response to different sequences of the EBNA I molecule in Epstein-Barr virus-related disorders and in autoimmune diseases. *J Autoimmun* 1994;7:179–191.
121. Harley JB, James JA. Epstein-Barr virus infection may be an environmental risk factor for systemic lupus erythematosus in children and teenagers [Letter]. *Arthritis Rheum* 1999;42:1782–1783.
122. James JA, Kaufman KM, Farris AD, et al. An increased prevalence of Epstein-Barr virus infection in young patients suggests a possible etiology for systemic lupus erythematosus. *J Clin Invest* 1997;100:3019–3026.
123. James JA, Harley JB. B-cell epitope spreading in autoimmunity. *Immunol Rev* 1998;164:185–200.
124. Nepveu K, Libman B. Hepatitis C as another possible cause of porphyria cutanea tarda and systemic lupus erythematosus: comment on the article by Kutz and Bridges [Letter]. *Arthritis Rheum* 1996;39:352–354.
125. McMurray RW, Elbourne K. Hepatitis C virus infection and autoimmunity. *Semin Arthritis Rheum* 1997;26:689–701.
126. Chng HH, Fock KM, Chew CN, et al. Hepatitis B virus infection in patients with systemic lupus erythematosus. *Singapore Med J* 1993;34:325–326.
127. Senecal JL, Bertrand C, Coutlee F. Severe exacerbation of systemic lupus erythematosus after hepatitis B vaccination and importance of pneumococcal vaccination in patients with autosplenectomy: comment on the article by Battafarano et al. [Letter]. *Arthritis Rheum* 1999;42:1307–1308.
128. Grezard P, Chefai M, Philippot V, et al. [Cutaneous lupus erythematosus and buccal aphthosis after hepatitis B vaccination in a 6-year-old child]. *Ann Dermatol Venereol* 1996;123:657–659.
129. Guiserix J. Systemic lupus erythematosus following hepatitis B vaccine [Letter]. *Nephron* 1996;74:441.
130. Mamoux V, Dumont C. [Lupus erythematosus disseminatus and vaccination against hepatitis B virus (Letter)]. *Arch Pediatr* 1994;1:307–308.
131. Tudela P, Marti S, Bonal J. Systemic lupus erythematosus and vaccination against hepatitis B [Letter]. *Nephron* 1992;62:236.
132. Petri M. Infection in systemic lupus erythematosus. *Rheum Dis Clin North Am* 1998;24:423–456.
133. Kilburn KH, Warshaw RH. Prevalence of symptoms of systemic lupus erythematosus (SLE) and of fluorescent antinuclear antibodies associated with chronic exposure to trichloroethylene and other chemicals in well water. *Environ Res* 1992;57:1–9.
134. Steenland K, Goldsmith DF. Silica exposure and autoimmune diseases. *Am J Ind Med* 1995;28:603–608.
135. Steenland K, Brown D. Mortality study of gold miners exposed to silica and nonasbestiform amphibole minerals: an update with 14 more years of follow-up. *Am J Ind Med* 1995;27:217–229.
136. Brown LM, Gridley G, Olsen JH, et al. Cancer risk and mortality patterns among silicotic men in Sweden and Denmark. *J Occup Environ Med* 1997;39:633–638.
137. Wilke RA, Salisbury S, Abdel-Rahman E, et al. Lupus-like autoimmune disease associated with silicosis. *Nephrol Dial Transplant* 1996;11:1835–1838.
138. Merrill M, Shulman LE. Determination of prognosis in chronic disease, illustrated by systemic lupus erythematosus. *J Chronic Dis* 1955;1:12–32.
139. Hochberg MC, Dorsch CA, Feinglass EJ, et al. Survivorship in systemic lupus erythematosus: effect of antibody to extractable nuclear antigen. *Arthritis Rheum* 1981;24:54–59.
140. Hochberg MC, Perez-Gutthann S, Roubenoff R. *Prognosis in systemic lupus erythematosus:* postgraduate advances in rheumatology. Forum Medicum, 1990:1–9.
141. Reveille JS, Bartolucci A, Alarcón GS. Prognosis in systemic lupus erythematosus: negative impact of increasing age at onset, black race, and thrombocytopenia, as well as causes of death. *Arthritis Rheum* 1990;33:37–48.
142. Ginzler EM, Diamond HS, Weiner M, et al. A multicenter study of outcome in systemic lupus erythematosus. I. Entry variables as predictors of prognosis. *Arthritis Rheum* 1982;25:601–611.
143. Studenski S, Allen NB, Caldwell DS, et al. Survival in systemic lupus erythematosus: a multivariate analysis of demographic factors. *Arthritis Rheum* 1987;30:1326–1332.
144. Pistiner M, Wallace DJ, Nessim S, et al. Lupus erythematosus in the 1980s: a survey of 570 patients. *Semin Arthritis Rheum* 1991;21:55–64.
145. Esdaile JM, Sampalis JS, Lacaille D, et al. The relationship of socioeconomic status to subsequent health status in systemic lupus erythematosus. *Arthritis Rheum* 1988;31:423–427.
146. Kaslow RA, Masi AT. Age, sex, and race effects on mortality from systemic lupus erythematosus in the United States. *Arthritis Rheum* 1978;21:473–478.
147. Gordon MF, Stolley PD, Schinnar R. Trends in recent systemic lupus erythematosus mortality rates. *Arthritis Rheum* 1981;24:762–765.
148. Estes D, Christian CL. The natural history of systemic lupus erythematosus by prospective analysis. *Medicine* 1971;50:85–95.
149. Ward MM, Pyun E, Studenski S. Mortality risks associated with specific clinical manifestations of systemic lupus erythematosus. *Arch Intern Med* 1996;156:1337–1344.
150. Abu-Shakra M, Urowitz MB, Gladman DD, et al. Mortality studies in systemic lupus erythematosus: results from a single center. II. Predictor variables for mortality. *J Rheumatol* 1995;22:1265–1270.
151. Wallace DJ, Podell TE, Weiner JM, et al. Lupus nephritis: experience with 230 patients in a private practice from 1950 to 1980. *Am J Med* 1982;72:209–217.
152. Xie SK, Feng SF, Fu H. Long term follow-up of patients with systemic lupus erythematosus. *J Dermatol* 1998;25:367–373.
153. Chang CC, Shih TY, Chu SJ, et al. Lupus in Chinese male: a retrospective study of 61 patients. *Chung Hua I Hsueh Tsa Chih Taipei* 1995;55:143–150.
154. Cervera R, Khamashta MA, Font J, et al. Morbidity and mortality in systemic lupus erythematosus during a 5-year period: a multicenter prospective study of 1,000 patients: European Working Party on Systemic Lupus Erythematosus. *Medicine* 1999;78:167–175.
155. Strand V, Gladman D, Isenberg D, et al. Outcome measures to be used in clinical trials in systemic lupus erythematosus. *J Rheumatol* 1999;26:490–497.
156. Smolen JS, Strand V, Cardiel M, et al. Randomized clinical trials and longitudinal observational studies in systemic lupus erythematosus: consensus on a preliminary core set of outcome domains. *J Rheumatol* 1999;26:504–507.
157. Petri M, Barr SG, Zonana-Nach A, et al. Measures of disease activity, damage, and health status: the Hopkins Lupus Cohort Experience. *J Rheumatol* 1999;26:502–503.
158. Petri M, Genovese M, Engle E, et al. Definition, incidence and clinical description of flare in systemic lupus erythematosus: a prospective cohort study. *Arthritis Rheum* 1991;34:937–944.

159. Jonsson H, Nived O, Sturfelt G. Outcome in systemic lupus erythematosus: a prospective study of patients from a defined population. *Medicine* 1989;68:141–150.
160. Swaak AJG, Nossent JC, Bronsveld W, et al. Systemic lupus erythematosus. II. Observations on the occurrence of exacerbations in the disease course: Dutch experience with 110 patients studied prospectively. *Ann Rheum Dis* 1989;48:455–460.
161. Drenkard C, Villa AR, Garcia-Padilla C, et al. Remission of systematic lupus erythematosus. *Medicine* 1996;75:88–98.
162. Bombardier C, Gladman DD, Urowitz M, et al. Derivation of the SLEDAI: a disease activity index for lupus patients. *Arthritis Rheum* 1992;35:630–640.
163. Liang MH, Stern S, Esdaile JM. Towards an operational definition of SLE activity for clinical research. *Clin Rheum Dis* 1988; 14:57–66.
164. Petri M, Hellmann D, Hochberg M. Validity and reliability of lupus activity measures in the routine clinic setting. *J Rheumatol* 1992;19:53–59.
165. Hay EM, Bacon PA, Gordon C, et al. The BILAG index: a reliable and valid instrument for measuring clinical disease activity in systemic lupus erythematosus. *Q J Med* 1993;86:447–458.
166. Krupp LB, LaRocca NC, Muir-Nash J, et al. The Fatigue Severity Scale applied to patients with multiple sclerosis and systemic lupus erythematosus. *Arch Neurol* 1989;46:1121–1123.
167. Walz LeBlanc BAE, Gladman DD, Urowitz MB. Serologically active clinically quiescent systemic lupus erythematosus: predictors of clinical flares. *J Rheumatol* 1994;21:2239–2241.
168. Esdaile JM, Abrahamowicz M, Joseph L, et al. Laboratory tests as predictors of disease exacerbations in systemic lupus erythematosus. Why some tests fail. *Arthritis Rheum* 1996;39:370–378.
169. ter Borg EJ, Horst G, Hummel EJ, et al. Measurement of increases in anti-double-stranded DNA antibody levels as a predictor of disease exacerbation in systemic lupus erythematosus: a long-term, prospective study. *Arthritis Rheum* 1990;33:634–643.
170. Manzi S, Riarie JE, Carpenter B, et al. Sensitivity and specificity of plasma and urine complement split products as indicators of lupus disease activity. *Arthritis Rheum* 1996;39:1178–1188.
171. Janssen BA, Luqmani RA, Gordon C, et al. Correlation of blood levels of soluble vascular cell adhesion molecule-1 with disease activity in systemic lupus erythematosus and vasculitis. *Br J Rheumatol* 1994;33:1112–1116.
172. Gladman D, Ginzler E, Goldsmith C, et al. The development and initial validation of the Systemic Lupus International Collaborating Clinics/American College Rheumatology damage index for systemic lupus erythematosus. *Arthritis Rheum* 1996; 39:363–369.
173. Zonana-Nacach A, Barr SG, Magder LS, et al. *Damage in systemic lupus erythematosus and its association with corticosteroids.* submitted 2000.
174. Petri M, Lakatta C, Magder L, et al. Effect of prednisone and hydroxychloroquine on coronary artery disease risk factors in systemic lupus erythematosus: a longitudinal data analysis. *Am J Med* 1994;96:254–259.
175. Gilboe IM, Kvien TK, Husby G. Health status in systemic lupus erythematosus compared to rheumatoid arthritis and healthy controls. *J Rheumatol* 1999;26:1694–1700.
176. Ware JE Jr, Sherbourne CD. The MOS 36-item Short-Form Health Survey (SF-36). I. Conceptual framework and item selection. *Med Care* 1992;30:473–483.
177. Krupp LB, LaRocca NG, Muir-Nash J, et al. The Fatigue Severity Scale: application to patients with multiple sclerosis and systemic lupus erythematosus. *Arch Neurol* 1989;46:1121–1123.
178. Bruce IN, Mak VC, Hallett DC, et al. Factors associated with fatigue in patients with systemic lupus erythematosus. *Ann Rheum Dis* 1999;58:379–381.
179. Gladman DD, Urowitz MB, Gough J, et al. Fibromyalgia is a major contributor to quality of life in lupus. *J Rheumatol* 1997; 24:2145–2148.
180. Middleton GD, McFarlin JE, Lipsky PE. The prevalence and clinical impact of fibromyalgia in systemic lupus erythematosus. *Arthritis Rheum* 1994;37:1181–1188.
181. Akkasilpa S, Minor M, Goldman D, et al. Association of coping responses with fibromyalgia tender points in systemic lupus erythematosus patients. *Arthritis Rheum* 1997;40:S209(abst).
182. Bickers DR. Treatment of selected photosensitivity diseases. *Med Clin North Am* 1982;66:927–939.
183. Jorizzo JL, Salisbury PL, Rogers RS III, et al. Oral lesions in systemic lupus erythematosus: do ulcerative lesions represent a necrotizing vasculitis? *J Am Acad Dermatol* 1992;27:389–394.
184. David-Bajar KM, Bennion SD, DeSpain JD, et al. Clinical, histologic, and immunofluorescent distinctions between subacute cutaneous lupus erythematosus and discoid lupus erythematosus. *J Invest Dermatol* 1992;99:251–257.
185. Wilson CL, Burge SM, Dean D, et al. Scarring alopecia in discoid lupus erythematosus. *Br J Dermatol* 1992;126:307–314.
186. Werth VP, White WL, Snachez MR, et al. Incidence of alopecia areata in lupus erythematosus. *Arch Dermatol* 1992;128:368–371.
187. Drenkard C, Villa AR, Reyes E, et al. Vasculitis in systemic lupus erythematosus. *Lupus* 1997;6:235–242.
188. Naldi L, Locati F, Marchesi L, et al. Cutaneous manifestations associated with antiphospholipid antibodies in patients with suspected primary antiphospholipid syndrome: a case-control study. *Ann Rheum Dis* 1993;52:219–222.
189. Lance NJ, Blaszak W, Swartz TJ. Bullous skin lesions in systemic lupus erythematosus. *Semin Arthritis Rheum* 1991;20:396–404.
190. Kundig TM, Trueb RM, Krasovec M. Lupus profundus/panniculitis. *Dermatology* 1997;195:99–101.
191. Caproni M, Palleschi GM, Papi C, et al. Discoid lupus erythematosus lesions developed on lupus erythematosus profundus nodules [see comments]. *Int J Dermatol* 1995;34:357–359.
192. Carsuzaa F, Pierre C, De Jaureguiberry JP, et al. [Panniculitis-fasciitis syndrome disclosing systemic erythematous lupus]. *Ann Dermatol Venereol* 1996;123:259–261.
193. Perniciaro C, Randle HW, Perry HO. Hypertrophic discoid lupus erythematosus resembling squamous cell carcinoma. *Dermatol Surg* 1995;21:255–257.
194. Panush RS, Edwards L, Longley S, et al. "Rhupus" syndrome. *Arch Intern Med* 1988;148:1633–1636.
195. Richter Cohen M, Steiner G, Smolen JS, et al. Erosive arthritis in systemic lupus erythematosus: analysis of a distinct clinical and serological subset. *Br J Rheumatol* 1998;37:421–424.
196. Hahn BH, Yardley JH, Stevens MB. "Rheumatoid" nodules in systemic lupus erythematosus. *Ann Intern Med* 1970;72:49–58.
197. Bywaters EGL. Jaccoud's syndrome: a sequel to the joint involvement of systemic lupus erythematosus. *Clin Rheum Dis* 1975;1:125–148.
198. Mizutani W, Quismorio FP. Lupus foot: deforming arthropathy of the feet in systemic lupus erythematosus. *J Rheumatol* 1984;11:80–82.
199. Garton MJ, Isenberg DA. Clinical features of lupus myositis versus idiopathic myositis: a review of 30 cases. *Br J Rheumatol* 1997;36:1067–1074.
200. Gladman DD, Urowitz MB, Cole E, et al. Kidney biopsy in SLE. I. A clinical-morphologic evaluation. *Q J Med* 1989;272: 1125–1133.
201. Appel GB, Cohen DJ, Pirani CL, et al. Long-term follow-up of patients with lupus nephritis: a study based on the classification of the World Health Organization. *Am J Med* 1987;83:877–885.
202. Huong DL, Papo T, Beaufils H, et al. Renal involvement in systemic lupus erythematosus: a study of 180 patients from a single center. *Medicine* 1999;78:148–166.
203. Tateno S, Kobayashi Y, Shigematsu H, et al. Study of lupus

nephritis: its classification and the significance of subendothelial deposits. *Q J Med* 1983;207:311–331.

204. Petri M, Bockenstedt L, Colman J, et al. Serial assessment of glomerular filtration rate in lupus nephropathy. *Kidney Int* 1988;34:832–839.
205. Roubenoff R, Drew H, Moyer M, et al. Oral cimetidine improves the accuracy and precision of creatinine clearance in lupus nephritis. *Ann Intern Med* 1990;113:501–506.
206. Krane NK, Burjak K, Archie M, et al. Persistent lupus activity in end-stage renal disease. *Am J Kidney Dis* 1999;33:872–879.
207. Rodby RA, Korbet SM, Lewis EJ. Persistent of clinical and serological activity in patients with systemic lupus erythematosus undergoing peritoneal dialysis. *Am J Med* 1987;83:613–618.
208. Stone JH, Millward CL, Olson JL, et al. Frequency of recurrent lupus nephritis among ninety-seven renal transplant patients during the cyclosporine era. *Arthritis Rheum* 1998;41:678–686.
209. Mochizuki T, Aotsuka S, Satoh T. Clinical and laboratory features of lupus patients with complicating pulmonary disease [In Process Citation]. *Respir Med* 1999;93:95–101.
210. Magro CM, Crowson AN. The cutaneous pathology associated with seropositivity for antibodies to SSA (Ro): a clinicopathologic study of 23 adult patients without subacute cutaneous lupus erythematosus. *Am J Dermatopathol* 1999;21:129–137.
211. Matthay RA, Schwartz MI, Petty TL, et al. Pulmonary manifestations of systemic lupus erythematosus: review of twelve cases of acute lupus pneumonitis. *Medicine* 1975;54:397–409.
212. Katz VL, Kuller JA, McCoy MC, et al. Fatal lupus pleuritis presenting in pregnancy: a case report. *J Reprod Med* 1996;41: 537–540.
213. Koh WH, Thumboo J, Boey ML. Pulmonary haemorrhage in Oriental patients with systemic lupus erythematosus. *Lupus* 1997;6:713–716.
214. Hoffbrand BI, Beck ER. "Unexplained" dyspnoea and shrinking lungs in systemic lupus erythematosus. *Br Med J* 1965;1: 1273–1277.
215. Walz Leblanc BA, Urowitz MB, Gladman DD, et al. The "shrinking lungs syndrome" in systemic lupus erythematosus: improvement with corticosteroid therapy. *J Rheumatol* 1992; 19:1970–1972.
216. Min JK, Hong YS, Park SH, et al. Bronchiolitis obliterans organizing pneumonia as an initial manifestation in patients with systemic lupus erythematosus. *J Rheumatol* 1997;24: 2254–2257.
217. Shearn M. The heart in systemic lupus erythematosus. *Am Heart J* 1959;58:452–466.
218. Godeau P, Guilleven L, Fechner J, et al. Manifestations cardiques du lupus erythemateaux aigu dissemine. *Nouv Presse Med* 1981;10:2175–2178.
219. Brigden W, Bywaters EGL, Lessof MH, et al. The heart in systemic lupus erythematosus. *Br Heart J* 1960;22:1–16.
220. Leung W-H, Wong K-L, Lau C-P, et al. Cardiac abnormalities in systemic lupus erythematosus: a prospective M-mode, cross-sectional and Doppler echocardiographic study. *Int J Cardiol* 1990;27:367–375.
221. Cervera R, Font J, Paré C, et al. Cardiac disease in systemic lupus erythematosus: prospective study of 70 patients. *Ann Rheum Dis* 1992;51:156–159.
222. Jacobson EJ, Reza MJ. Constrictive pericarditis in systemic lupus erythematosus. *Arthritis Rheum* 1978;21:972–974.
223. Hejtmancik MR, Wright JC, Quint R. The cardiovascular manifestations of systemic lupus erythematosus. *Am Heart J* 1964; 68:119–130.
224. Yurchak PM, Levine SA, Gorlin R. constrictive pericarditis complicating disseminated lupus erythematosus. *Circulation* 1965;31:113–118.
225. Starkey RH, Hahn BH. Rapid development of constrictive pericarditis in a patient with systemic lupus erythematosus. *Chest* 1973;63:448–450.
226. Badui E, Garcia-Rubi D, Robles E, et al. Cardiovascular manifestations in systemic lupus erythematosus: prospective study of 100 patients. *Angiology* 1985;36:431–441.
227. Berg G, Bodet J, Webb K, et al. Systemic lupus erythematosus presenting as isolated congestive heart failure. *J Rheumatol* 1985;12:1182–1185.
228. Sturfelt G, Eskilsson J, Nived O, et al. Cardiovascular disease in systemic lupus erythematosus: a study of 75 patients from a defined population. *Medicine* 1992;71:216–223.
229. Nihoyannopoulos P, Gomez PM, Joshi J, et al. Cardiac abnormalities in systemic lupus erythematosus: association with raised anticardiolipin antibodies. *Circulation* 1990;82:369–375.
230. Giunta A, Picillo U, Maione S, et al. Spectrum of cardiac involvement in systemic lupus erythematosus: echocardiographic, echo-Doppler observations and immunological investigation. *Acta Cardiol* 1993;48:183–197.
231. Roldan CA, Shively BK, Lau CC, et al. Systemic lupus erythematosus valve disease by transesophageal echocardiography and the role of antiphospholipid antibodies. *J Am Coll Cardiol* 1992; 20:1127–1134.
232. Murai K, Oku H, Takeuchi K, et al. Alterations in myocardial systolic and diastolic function in patients with active systemic lupus erythematosus. *Am Heart J* 1987;113:966–971.
233. Enomoto K, Kaji Y, Mayumi T, et al. Left ventricular function in patients with stable systemic lupus erythematosus. *Jpn Heart J* 1991;32:445–453.
234. Winslow TM, Ossipov MA, Fazio GP, et al. The left ventricle in systemic lupus erythematosus: initial observations and a five-year follow-up in a university medical center population. *Am Heart J* 1993;125:1117–1122.
235. Bahl VK, Aradhye S, Vasan RS, et al. Myocardial systolic function in systemic lupus erythematosus: a study based on radionuclide ventriculography. *Clin Cardiol* 1992;15:433–435.
236. Strauer BE, Brune I, Schenk H, et al. Lupus cardiomyopathy: cardiac mechanics, hemodynamics, and coronary blood flow in uncomplicated systemic lupus erythematosus. *Am Heart J* 1976;92:715–722.
237. Ito M, Kagiyama Y, Omura I, et al. Cardiovascular manifestations in systemic lupus erythematosus. *Jpn Circ J* 1979;43:985–994.
238. Libman E, Sacks B. A hitherto undescribed form of valvular and mural endocarditis. *Arch Intern Med* 1924;33:701–737.
239. Gross L. The cardial lesions in Libman-Sacks disease with a consideration of its relationship to acute diffuse lupus erythematosus. *Am J Pathol* 1940;16:375–407.
240. Straaton KV, Chatham WW, Reveille JD, et al. Clinically significant valvular heart disease in systemic lupus erythematosus. *Am J Med* 1988;85:645–650.
241. Klinkhoff AV, Thompson CR, Reid GD, et al. M-mode and two dimensional echocardiographic abnormalities in systemic lupus erythematosus. *JAMA* 1985;253:3273–3277.
242. Nesher G, Ilany J, Rosenmann D, et al. Valvular dysfunction in antiphospholipid syndrome: prevalence, clinical features, and treatment. *Semin Arthritis Rheum* 1997;27:27–35.
243. Gabrielli F, Alcini E, Di Prima MA, et al. Cardiac valve involvement in systemic lupus erythematosus and primary antiphospholipid syndrome: lack of correlation with antiphospholipid antibodies. *Int J Cardiol* 1995;51:117–126.
244. Vianna JL, Khamashta MA, Ordi-Ros J, et al. Comparison of the primary and secondary antiphospholipid syndrome: a European multicenter study of 114 patients. *Am J Med* 1994;96:3–9.
245. Galve E, Ordi J, Barquinero J, et al. Valvular heart disease in the primary antiphospholipid syndrome. *Ann Intern Med* 1992;116:293–298.
246. Gleason CB, Stoddard MF, Wagner SG, et al. A comparison of

cardiac valvular involvement in the primary antiphospholipid syndrome versus anticardiolipin-negative systemic lupus erythematosus. *Am Heart J* 1993;125:1123–1129.
247. Brenner B, Blumenfeld Z, Markiewicz W, et al. Cardiac involvement in patients with primary anti-phospholipid syndrome. *J Am Coll Cardiol* 1991;18:931–936.
248. Garcia-Torres R, Amigo MC, de la Rossa A, et al. Valvular heart disease in primary antiphospholipid syndrome: clinical and morphological findings. *Lupus* 1996;5:56–61.
249. Badui E, Solorio S, Martinez E, et al. The heart in the primary antiphospholipid syndrome. *Arch Med Res* 1995;26:115–120.
250. Cervera R, Khamashta MA, Font J, et al. High prevalence of significant heart valve lesions in patients with the primary antiphospholipid syndrome. *Lupus* 1991;1:43–47.
251. Ford PH, Ford SE, Lillicrap DP. Association of lupus anticoagulant with severe valvular heart disease in SLE. *J Rheumatol* 1988;15:597–600.
252. Buyon JP, Winchester RJ, Slade SG, et al. Identification of mothers at risk for congenital heart block and other neonatal lupus syndromes in their children: comparison of enzyme-linked immunosorbent assay and immunoblot for measurement of anti-SS-A/Ro and anti-SS-B/La. *Arthritis Rheum* 1993;36:1263–1273.
253. Petri M, Watson R, Hochberg MC. Anti-Ro antibodies and neonatal lupus. *Rheum Dis Clin North Am* 1989;15:335–360.
254. Guzman J, Cardiel MH, Arce-Salinas A, et al. The contribution of resting heart rate and routine blood tests to the clinical assessment of disease activity in systemic lupus erythematosus. *J Rheumatol* 1994;21:1845–1848.
255. Homcy CJ, Liberthson RR, Fallon JT, et al. Ischemic heart disease in systemic lupus erythematosus in the young patient: report of 6 cases. *Am J Cardiol* 1982;49:478–484.
256. Bonfiglio TA, Botti RE, Hagstrom JWC. Coronary arteritis, occlusion and myocardial infarction due to lupus erythematosus. *Am Heart J* 1972;83:153–158.
257. Wilson VE, Eck SL, Bates ER. Evaluation and treatment of acute myocardial infarction complicating systemic lupus erythematosus. *Chest* 1992;101:420–424.
258. Bor I. Cardiac infarction in the Libman-Sacks endocarditis [Letter]. *N Engl J Med* 1968;279:164.
259. Heibel RH, O'Toole JD, Curtiss EI, et al. Coronary arteritis in systemic lupus erythematosus. *Chest* 1976;69:200–203.
260. Simonson JS, Schiller NB, Petri M, et al. Pulmonary hypertension in systemic lupus erythematosus. *J Rheumatol* 1989;16:918–925.
261. Winslow TM, Ossipov MA, Fazio GP, et al. Five-year follow-up study of the prevalence and progression of pulmonary hypertension in systemic lupus erythematosus. *Am Heart J* 1995;129:510–515.
262. Armas-Cruz R, Harnecker J, Ducach G, et al. Clinical diagnosis of systemic lupus erythematosus. *Am J Med* 1958;25:409–419.
263. Pollack VE, Kant KS. Diffuse and focal proliferative lupus nephritis: treatment approaches and results. *Nephron* 1991;59:177–183.
264. Sofer LJ, Bader R. Corticotropin and cortisone in acute disseminated lupus erythematosus. *JAMA* 1952;149:1002–1008.
265. Dubois EL, Commons RR, Starr P, et al. Corticotropin and cortisone treatment for systemic lupus erythematosus. *JAMA* 1952;149:995.
266. Kong TQ, Kellum RE, Haserick JR. Clinical diagnosis of cardiac involvement in systemic lupus erythematosus: a correlation of clinical and autopsy findings in thirty patients. *Circulation* 1962;26:7–11.
267. Bulkley BH, Roberts WC. The heart in systemic lupus erythematosus and the changes induced in it by corticosteroid therapy: a study of 36 necropsy patients. *Am J Med* 1975;58:243–264.
268. Haider YS, Roberts WC. Coronary arterial disease in systemic lupus erythematosus: quantification of degree of narrowing in 22 necropsy patients (21 women) aged 16 to 37 years. *Am J Med* 1981;70:775–781.
269. Abu-Shakra M, Urowitz MB, Gladman DD, et al. Mortality studies in systemic lupus erythematosus: results from a single center. I. Causes of death. *J Rheumatol* 1995;22:1259–1264.
270. Rubin LA, Urowitz MB, Gladman DD. Mortality in systemic lupus erythematosus: the bimodal pattern revisited. *Q J Med* 1985;55:87–98.
271. Shome GP, Sakauchi M, Yamane K, et al. Ischemic heart disease in systemic lupus erythematosus: a retrospective study of 65 patients treated with prednisone. *Jpn J Med* 1989;28:599–603.
272. Hearth-Holmes M, Baethge BA, Broadwell L, et al. Dietary treatment of hyperlipidemia in patients with systemic lupus erythematosus. *J Rheumatol* 1995;22:450–454.
273. Hospenpud JD, Montanaro A, Hart MV, et al. Myocardial perfusion abnormalities in asymptomatic patients with systemic lupus erythematosus. *Am J Med* 1984;77:286–292.
274. Urowitz MB, Bookman AAM, Koehler BE, et al. The bimodal mortality pattern of systemic lupus erythematosus. *Am J Med* 1976;60:221–225.
275. Gladman DD, Urowitz MB. Morbidity in systemic lupus erythematosus. *J Rheumatol* 1987;14:223–226.
276. Petri M, Perez-Gutthann S, Spence D, et al. Risk factors for coronary artery disease in patients with systemic lupus erythematosus. *Am J Med* 1992;93:513–519.
277. Griffith GC, Vural IL. Acute and subacute disseminated lupus erythematosus: a correlation of clinical and postmortem findings in eighteen cases. *Circulation* 1951;3:492.
278. Bidani AK, Roberts JL, Schwartz MM, et al. Immunopathology of cardiac lesions in fatal systemic lupus erythematosus. *Am J Med* 1980;69:849–858.
279. Petri M, Spence D, Bone LR, et al. Coronary artery disease risk factors in the Hopkins Lupus Cohort: prevalence, patient recognition, and preventive practices. *Medicine* 1992;71:291–302.
280. Ilowite NT, Samuel P, Ginzler E, et al. Dyslipoproteinemia in pediatric systemic lupus erythematosus. *Arthritis Rheum* 1988;31:859–863.
281. Lahita RG, Rivkin E, Cavanagh I, et al. Low levels of total cholesterol, high-density lipoprotein, and apolipoprotein A1 in association in patients with systemic lupus erythematosus. *Arthritis Rheum* 1993;36:1566–1574.
282. Ettinger WH, Goldberg AP, Applebaum-Bowden D, et al. Dyslipoproteinemia in systemic lupus erythematosus: effect of corticosteroids. *Am J Med* 1987;83:503–508.
283. Feinglass EJ, Arnett FC, Dorsch CA, et al. Neuropsychiatric manifestations of systemic lupus erythematosus: diagnosis, clinical spectrum, and relationships to other features of the disease. *Medicine* 1976;55:323–329.
284. Scharre D, Petri M, Engman E, et al. Large cell arteritis with giant cells in systemic lupus erythematosus. *Ann Intern Med* 1986;104:661.
285. Johnston RT, Richardson EP. The neurologic manifestations of systemic lupus erythematosus: a clinical pathological study of 24 cases and review of the literature. *Medicine* 1968;47:337–369.
286. Bonfa E, Golombek SJ, Kaufman LD, et al. Association between lupus psychosis and anti-ribosomal P protein antibodies. *N Engl J Med* 1987;317:265–271.
287. Georgescu L, Mevorach D, Arnett FC, et al. Anti-P antibodies and neuropsychiatric lupus erythematosus. *Ann N Y Acad Sci* 1997;823:263–269.
288. Yoshio T, Masuyama JI, Minota S, et al. A close temporal rela-

tionship of liver disease to antiribosomal P0 protein antibodies and central nervous system disease in patients with systemic lupus erythematosus. *J Rheumatol* 1998;25:681–688.

289. Lanham JG, Barrie T, Kohner EM, et al. SLE retinopathy: evaluation by fluorescein angiography. *Ann Rheum Dis* 1982;41:473–478.
290. Hellmann DB, Laing TJ, Petri M, et al. Mononeuritis multiplex: the yield of evaluations for occult rheumatic diseases. *Medicine* 1988;67:145–153.
291. Denburg SD, Carbotte RM, Denburg JA. Psychological aspects of systemic lupus erythematosus: cognitive function, mood, and self-report. *J Rheumatol* 1997;24:998–1003.
292. Carbotte RM, Denburg SD, Denburg JA. Cognitive dysfunction in systemic lupus erythematosus is independent of active disease. *J Rheumatol* 1995;22:863–867.
293. Hay EM, Black D, Huddy A, et al. Psychiatric disorder and cognitive impairment in systemic lupus erythematosus. *Arthritis Rheum* 1992;35:411–416.
294. Hanly JG, Fisk JD, Sherwood G, et al. Cognitive impairment in patients with systemic lupus erythematosus. *J Rheumatol* 1992;19:562–567.
295. Hanly JG, Hong C, Smith S, et al. A prospective analysis of cognitive function and anticardiolipin antibodies in systemic lupus erythematosus. *Arthritis Rheum* 1999;42:728–734.
296. Menon S, Jameson-Shortall E, Newman SP, et al. A longitudinal study of anticardiolipin antibody levels and cognitive functioning in systemic lupus erythematosus. *Arthritis Rheum* 1999;42:735–741.
297. Sfikakis PP, Mitsikostas DD, Manoussakis MN, et al. Headache in systemic lupus erythematosus: a controlled study. *Br J Rheumatol* 1998;37:300–303.
298. Budman DR, Steinberg AD. Hematologic aspects of systemic lupus erythematosus: current concepts. *Ann Intern Med* 1977;86:220–229.
299. Mestanza-Peralta M, Ariza-Ariza R, Cardiel MH, et al. Thrombocytopenic purpura as initial manifestation of systemic lupus erythematosus. *J Rheumatol* 1997;24:867–870.
300. Musio F, Bohen EM, Yuan CM, et al. Review of thrombotic thrombocytopenic purpura in the setting of systemic lupus erythematosus. *Semin Arthritis Rheum* 1998;28:1–19.
301. Konstantopoulos K, Terpos E, Prinolakis H, et al. Systemic lupus erythematosus presenting as myelofibrosis. *Haematologia (Budap)* 1998;29:153–156.
302. Pereira RM, Velloso ER, Menezes Y, et al. Bone marrow findings in systemic lupus erythematosus patients with peripheral cytopenias. *Clin Rheumatol* 1998;17:219–222.
303. Liu H, Ozaki K, Matsuzaki Y, et al. Suppression of haematopoiesis by IgG autoantibodies from patients with systemic lupus erythematosus (SLE). *Clin Exp Immunol* 1995;100:480–485.
304. Shapira Y, Weinberger A, Wysenbeek AJ. Lymphadenopathy in systemic lupus erythematosus: prevalence and relation to disease manifestations. *Clin Rheumatol* 1996;15:335–338.
305. Eisner MD, Amory J, Mullaney B, et al. Necrotizing lymphadenitis associated with systemic lupus erythematosus. *Semin Arthritis Rheum* 1996;26:477–482.
306. Lichtenstein DR, Syngal S, Wolfe MM. Nonsteroidal antiinflammatory drugs and the gastrointestinal tract. *Arthritis Rheum* 1995;38:5–18.
307. Miller MH, Urowitz MB, Gladman DD, et al. Chronic adhesive lupus serositis as a complication of systemic lupus erythematosus. *Arch Intern Med* 1984;144:1863–1864.
308. Mier A, Weir W. Ascites in systemic lupus erythematosus. *Ann Rheum Dis* 1985;44:778–779.
309. Schousboe JT, Koch AE, Chang RW. Chronic lupus peritonitis with ascites? Review of the literature with a case report. *Semin Arthritis Rheum* 1988;18:121–126.
310. Pollak VE, Grove WJ, Kark RM, et al. Systemic lupus erythematosus simulating acute surgical condition of the abdomen. *N Engl J Med* 1958;259:258–266.
311. Zizic TM, Classen JN, Stevens MB. Acute abdominal complications of systemic lupus erythematosus and polyarteritis nodosa. *Am J Med* 1982;73:525–531.
312. Prouse PJ, Thompson EM, Gumpel JM. Systemic lupus erythematosus and abdominal pain. *Br J Rheumatol* 1983;22:172–175.
313. Ozeki I, Abe T, Sakai H, et al. [A case of systemic lupus erythematosus developed with intestinal perforation]. *Ryumachi* 1998;38:523–528.
314. Sβnchez-Guerrero J, Reyes E, Alarcón-Segovia D. Primary antiphospholipid syndrome as a cause of intestinal infarction. *J Rheumatol* 1992;19:623–625.
315. Gladman DD, Ross T, Richardson B, et al. Bowel involvement in systemic lupus erythematosus: Crohn's disease or lupus vasculitis. *Arthritis Rheum* 1985;28:466–470.
316. Kistin MG, Kaplan MM, Harrington JT. Diffuse ischemic colitis associated with systemic lupus erythematosus response to subtotal colectomy. *Gastroenterology* 1978;75:1147–1151.
317. Font J, Bosch X, Ferre RJ, et al. Systemic lupus erythematosus and ulcerative colitis. *Lancet* 1988;1:770.
318. Tsutsumi A, Sugiyama T, Matsumura R, et al. Protein losing enteropathy associated with collagen diseases. *Ann Rheum Dis* 1991;50:178–181.
319. Petri M. Pancreatitis: a rare manifestation of systemic lupus erythematosus. *Rheumatol Rev* 1992;1:75–79.
320. Petri M. Pancreatitis, in search of a mechanism [Editorial]. *J Rheumatol* 1992;19:1014–1016.
321. van Hoek B. The spectrum of liver disease in systemic lupus erythematosus. *Neth J Med* 1996;48:244–253.
322. Matsumoto T, Yoshimine T, Shimouchi K, et al. The liver in systemic lupus erythematosus: pathologic analysis of 52 cases and review of Japanese autopsy registry data. *Hum Pathol* 1992;23:1151–1158.
323. Ramirez-Mata M, Reyes PA, Alarcon-Segovia D, et al. Esophageal motility in systemic lupus erythematosus. *Am J Dig Dis* 1974;19:132–136.
324. Petri M. Musculoskeletal complications of systemic lupus erythematosus in the Hopkins Lupus Cohort: an update. *Arthritis Care Res* 1995;8:137–145.
325. Petri M, Fairbank A, Jinnah R, et al. Progression of avascular necrosis (AVN) of the femoral head in SLE: long-term follow-up report. *Arthritis Rheum* 1993;36:S184.
326. Rascu A, Manger K, Kraetsch HG, et al. Osteonecrosis in systemic lupus erythematosus, steroid-induced or a lupus-dependent manifestation? *Lupus* 1996;5:323–327.
327. Mont MA, Fairbank AC, Petri M, et al. Core decompression for osteonecrosis of the femoral head in systemic lupus erythematosus. *Clin Orthop* 1997;Jan(334):91-97.
328. Petri M, Roubenoff R, Dallal GE, et al. Plasma homocysteine as a risk factor for atherothrombotic events in systemic lupus erythematosus. *Lancet* 1996;348:1120–1124.
329. Manzi S, Meilahn EN, Rairie JE, et al. Age-specific incidence rates of myocardial infarction and angina in women with systemic lupus erythematosus: comparison with the Framingham Study. *Am J Epidemiol* 1997;145:408–415.
330. Hamsten A, Norberg R, Bj÷rkholm M, et al. Antibodies to cardiolipin in young survivors of myocardial infarction: an association with recurrent cardiovascular events. *Lancet* 1986;1:113–116.
331. Petri M. Epidemiology of the antiphospholipid syndrome. In:

Asherson RA, Cervera R, Piette J-C, eds. *The antiphospholipid syndrome.* Boca Raton: CRC Press, 1996:13–28.

332. Matsuura E, Hasunuma Y, Makita Z, et al. Oxidatively modified LDL as a target for β_2-glycoprotein I antibodies. *Lupus* 1996;5:517(abst).
333. Wilson WA, Gharavi AE, Koike T, et al. International consensus statement on preliminary classification criteria for definite antiphospholipid syndrome: report of an international workshop. *Arthritis Rheum* 1999;42:1309–1311.
334. Petri M. Thrombosis and systemic lupus erythematosus: the Hopkins Lupus Cohort perspective. *Scand J Rheumatol* 1996;25:191–193.
335. Derksen RHWM, Hasselaar P, Blokzijl L, et al. Coagulation screen is more specific than the anticardiolipin antibody ELISA in defining a thrombotic subset of lupus patients. *Ann Rheum Dis* 1988;47:364–371.
336. Ghirardello A, Doria A, Ruffatti A, et al. Antiphospholipid antibodies (aPL) in systemic lupus erythematosus: are they specific tools for the diagnosis of aPL syndrome? *Ann Rheum Dis* 1994;53:140–142.
337. Klemperer P, Pollack AD, Baehr G. Pathology of disseminated lupus erythematosus. *Arch Pathol* 1941;32:569–631.
338. Ichikawa Y, Tsunematsu T, Yokohari R, et al. [Multicenter study of causes of death in systemic lupus erythematosus: a report from the Subcommittee for Development of Therapy, the Research Committee for Autoimmune Diseases Supported by the Ministry of Health and Welfare]. *Ryumachi* 1985;25:258–264.
339. Hellmann DB, Petri M, Whiting-O'Keefe Q. Fatal infections in systemic lupus erythematosus: role of opportunistic organisms. *Medicine* 1987;66:341–348.
340. Staples PJ, Gerding DN, Decker JL, et al. Incidence of infection in systemic lupus erythematosus. *Arthritis Rheum* 1974;17:1–10.
341. Nived O, Sturfelt G, Wollheim F. Systemic lupus erythematosus and infection: a controlled and prospective study including an epidemiological group. *Q J Med* 1985;55:271–287.
342. Nies KM, Louie JS. Impaired immunoglobulin synthesis by peripheral blood lymphocytes in systemic lupus erythematosus. *Arthritis Rheum* 1978;21:51–57.
343. Petri MP, Genovese M. Incidence of and risk factors for hospitalizations in systemic lupus erythematosus: a prospective study of the Hopkins Lupus Cohort. *J Rheumatol* 1992;19:1559–1565.
344. Stahl NI, Klippel JH, Decker JL. Fever in systemic lupus erythematosus. *Am J Med* 1979;67:935–940.
345. Ginzler EM, Diamond HS, Kaplan D, et al. Computer analysis of factors influencing frequency of infection in systemic lupus erythematosus. *Arthritis Rheum* 1978;21:37–44.
346. Janwityanuchit S, Krachangwongchai K, Totemchokchyakarn K, et al. Infection in systemic lupus erythematosus. *J Med Assoc Thai* 1993;76:542–548.
347. Duffy KN, Duffy CM, Gladman DD. Infection and disease activity in systemic lupus erythematosus: a review of hospitalized patients. *J Rheumatol* 1991;18:1180–1184.
348. Piliero P, Furie F. Functional asplenia in systemic lupus erythematosus. *Semin Arthritis Rheum* 1990;20:185–189.
349. Van der Straeten C, Wei N, Rothschild J, et al. Rapidly fatal pneumococcal septicemia in systemic lupus erythematosus. *J Rheumatol* 1987;14:1177–1180.
350. Webster J, Williams BD, Smith AP, et al. Systemic lupus erythematosus presenting as pneumococcal septicaemia and septic arthritis. *Ann Rheum Dis* 1990;49:181–183.
351. Schenfeld L, Gray RG, Poppo MJ, et al. Bacterial monoarthritis due to neisseric meningitis in systemic lupus erythematosus. *J Rheumatol* 1981;8:145–148.
352. Edelen JS, Lockshin MD, Leroy EC. Gonococcal arthritis in two patients with active systemic lupus erythematosus: a diagnostic problem. *Arthritis Rheum* 1971;14:557–559.
353. de Luis A, Pigrau C, Pahissa A, et al. [Infections in 96 cases of systemic lupus erythematosus]. *Med Clin (Barc)* 1990;94: 607–610.
354. Feng PH, Tan TH. Tuberculosis in patients with systemic lupus erythematosus. *Ann Rheum Dis* 1982;41:11–14.
355. Harisdangkul V, Nilganuwonge S, Rockhold L. Cause of death in systemic lupus erythematosus: a pattern based on age at onset. *South Med J* 1987;80:1249–1253.
356. Yuhara T, Takemura H, Akama T, et al. Predicting infection in hospitalized patients with systemic lupus erythematosus [see comments]. *Intern Med* 1996;35:629–636.
357. Porges AJ, Beattie SL, Ritchlin C, et al. Patients with systemic lupus erythematosus at risk for *Pneumocystis carinii* pneumonia. *J Rheumatol* 1992;19:1191–1194.
358. Godeau B, Coutant V, Huong DLT, et al. *Pneumocystis carinii* pneumonia in the course of connective tissue disease: report of 34 cases. *J Rheumatol* 1994;21:246–251.
359. ter Borg EJ, Horst G, Limburg PC, et al. C-reactive protein levels during disease exacerbations and infections in systemic lupus erythematosus: a prospective longitudinal study. *J Rheumatol* 1990;17:1642–1648.
360. Shimamoto Y, Suga K, Ohta A, et al. Risk factors for the development of acute disseminated intravascular coagulation in patients with systemic lupus erythematosus. *Clin Rheumatol* 1995;14:176–179.
361. Andonopoulos AP. Adult respiratory distress syndrome: an unrecognized premortem event in systemic lupus erythematosus. *Br J Rheumatol* 1991;30:346–348.

74

AUTOANTIBODIES IN SYSTEMIC LUPUS ERYTHEMATOSUS

WESTLEY H. REEVES
MINORU SATOH

The LE cell phenomenon (phagocytosis of relatively intact nuclear material by polymorphonuclear leukocytes) reported by Hargraves et al. (1) in 1948 provided the first evidence that systemic lupus erythematosus (SLE) is an autoimmune disease. This was followed by the discovery of antinuclear antibodies (ANAs) specific for DNA and/or histones [reviewed in (2)]. The discovery by Tan and Kunkel (3) in 1966 that anti-Sm antibodies are specific for SLE, and the characterization of autoantibody markers for polymyositis, scleroderma, biliary cirrhosis, and other autoimmune syndromes (2,4) revolutionized the serologic diagnosis of systemic autoimmune disease. This chapter reviews these markers and their clinical use. The goal is to provide a conceptual framework for understanding the humoral autoimmune response in SLE as well as a practical approach to the diagnostic use of autoantibody markers.

LABORATORY EVALUATION OF AUTOANTIBODIES

A variety of assays are used for detecting and quantifying autoantibodies in human sera, including immunofluorescence, enzyme-linked immunosorbent assays (ELISAs), double immunodiffusion, counterimmunoelectrophoresis (CIE), immunoblotting, and immunoprecipitation. The LE cell test (1) is used infrequently at present. The advantages and disadvantages of these assays are summarized later.

Immunofluorescence

Immunofluorescence is used for detecting ANAs and anti-DNA antibodies (Crithidia test). The fluorescent antinuclear antibody test (FANA) detects autoantibodies in a test serum against cell antigens. Although originally performed by using mouse liver or kidney sections as substrate, more reliable results are obtained by using adherent human cell lines such as HEp-2 (human laryngeal carcinoma). As illustrated in Fig. 74.1, the cells are allowed to adhere to a microscope slide, fixed and permeabilized with methanol, and then incubated with the patient's serum. The slide is washed to remove unbound antibodies, followed by incubation with fluorescent antiimmunoglobulin antibodies. The slide is then viewed by using a fluorescence microscope, and nuclear staining intensity and pattern are scored at various serum dilutions (Figs. 74.2 and 74.3).

Enzyme-Linked Immunosorbent Assay

ELISA is a simple, rapid, and sensitive approach used widely for screening (5). Plastic wells of a microtiter plate are coated

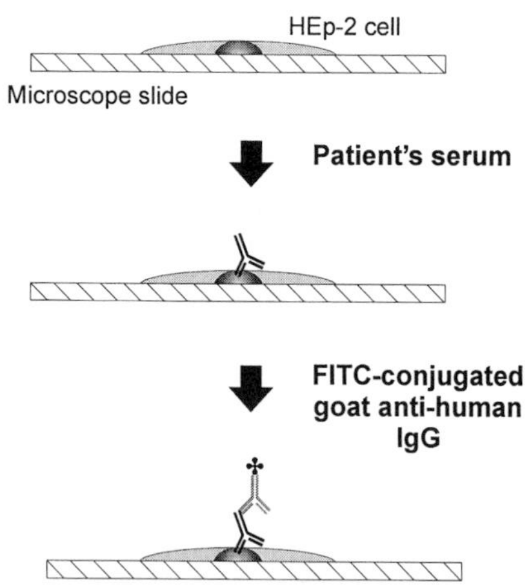

FIGURE 74.1. Fluorescent antinuclear antibody technique. Adherent human cells (HEp-2 or HeLa) are grown on a microscope slide or coverslip until about two thirds confluent. They are then fixed with methanol and incubated with medium containing bovine calf serum to block nonspecific sticky sites. The cells then are incubated sequentially with diluted serum from a patient, followed by fluorescein isothiocyanate (FITC)-conjugated goat anti-human immunoglobulin G (IgG) antibodies. The slides are washed and viewed by using an epifluorescence microscope equipped with an FITC filter.

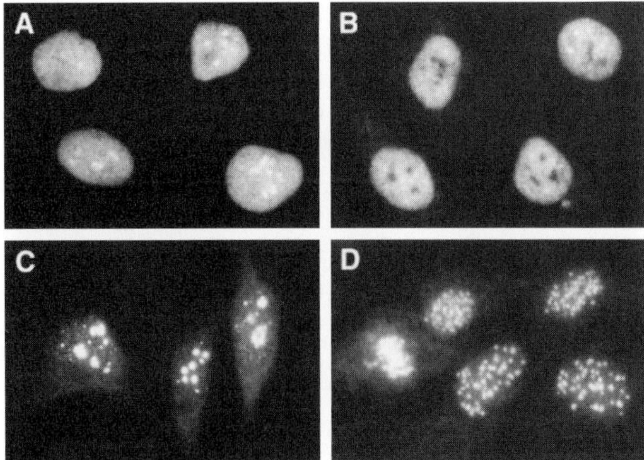

FIGURE 74.2. Nuclear immunofluorescence patterns. HeLa cells were stained with patient sera at a 1:40 dilution followed by FITC-conjugated goat anti-human IgG antibodies. **A:** Diffuse (homogeneous) pattern produced by anti-DNA antibodies. **B:** Speckled pattern, produced by anti-Sm antibodies. **C:** Nucleolar pattern produced by anti-fibrillarin (U3 RNP) antibodies. **D:** Centromere pattern produced by anti-CENP-B antibodies. [From Reeves WH, Richards HB, Satoh M. Autoantibodies. In: Lahita RG, Chiorazzi N, Reeves WH, eds. *Textbook of the autoimmune diseases.* Philadelphia: Lippincott-Raven (in press)].

with a purified antigen, and diluted test serum is added, followed by enzyme-labeled antiimmunoglobulin antibodies. Binding of the second antibody is detected by adding a substrate for the enzyme, forming a colored product. The product is quantified by determining absorbance in a spectrophotometer. In view of their high sensitivity, ELISAs must be standardized carefully to avoid measuring nonspecific binding. The major drawback is that standard ELISAs depend on

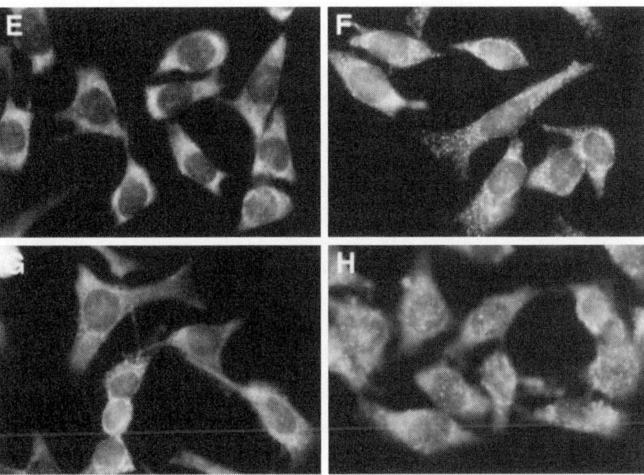

FIGURE 74.3. Cytoplasmic immunofluorescence patterns. HeLa cells were stained with patient sera at a 1:40 dilution followed by FITC-conjugated goat anti-human IgG antibodies. **E:** Anti-ribosomal P antibodies. **F:** Anti-signal recognition particle (SRP) antibodies. **G:** Anti-Jo-1 (histidyl tRNA synthetase) antibodies. **H:** Anti-mitochondrial antibodies.

the availability of pure autoantigens for coating the wells. This problem can be circumvented by using a double-sandwich or antigen-capture assay (5), in which antigen is affinity purified onto the wells by using a monoclonal antibody. This allows the antigen to be highly purified, but has the disadvantage that sera containing antiimmunoglobulin antibodies (rheumatoid factor) may bind to the immobilized monoclonal antibody, leading to false positives.

Double Immunodiffusion and Counterimmunoelectrophoresis

Double immunodiffusion (Ouchterlony) is performed by placing antigen and antibody into wells in an agarose gel (6). Each reactant diffuses radially through the gel, with concentration decreasing as a geometric function of distance from the well. An insoluble precipitin line, consisting of immune complexes, forms where the antigen and antibody meet in approximately equal concentrations. The precipitin line can be viewed directly in the gel. If two serum samples contain the same specificity, their precipitin lines will fuse, forming a curved "line of identity." Double immunodiffusion is used extensively to test for anti-Sm, nRNP, Ro (SS-A), La (SS-B), topoisomerase I, ribosomal P, and other autoantibodies (2). However, it is labor intensive, it is difficult to interpret multiple lines, and the sensitivity is lower than alternatives, such as ELISA.

CIE is more sensitive than double immunodiffusion in gels. Acidic antigens and serum immunoglobulins are electrophoresed toward one another, forming precipitin lines. The advantage is that multiple lines that may not resolve in double-immunodiffusion testing can be distinguished. However, nonimmunologic precipitin lines can form, complicating interpretation.

Immunoblot (Western Blot)

The immunoblot or Western blot technique is analogous to ELISA. Proteins in a crude or purified antigen preparation are separated according to molecular weight by sodium dodecylsulfate (SDS)-polyacrylamide gel electrophoresis and transferred electrophoretically to a membrane such as nitrocellulose (7). The membrane is incubated with diluted test serum, followed by an enzyme-labeled second antibody. The enzyme substrate forms a colored, insoluble reaction product that is deposited on the membrane. Radioactive or chemiluminescent detection also may be used. This allows reactivity of the test serum with individual proteins in a complex mixture to be assessed. The technique is very sensitive, but more demanding technically than other assays. A major drawback is that Western blot assays are performed after dissociating the antigen into its individual constituents. Many antigenic determinants are conformational and may be destroyed by the harsh conditions used in SDS–polyacrylamide gel electrophoresis.

Immunoprecipitation

Immunoprecipitation of radiolabeled cell extracts has become an important research tool for examining autoantibody specificities. Radiolabeled antigens are allowed to form immune complexes with autoantibodies, which are purified onto protein A–Sepharose beads. The proteins are eluted from the beads, separated by SDS–polyacrylamide gel electrophoresis, and detected by autoradiography. This test can be used to detect a wide variety of autoantibodies associated with SLE (Fig. 74.4A), scleroderma (Fig. 74.4B), or polymyositis (Fig. 74.4C). The identity of the [^{35}S]-methionine–labeled antigen(s) immunoprecipitated by a serum is established by comparing the molecular weight(s) with those of the proteins immunoprecipitated by reference sera. A similar approach can be used to analyze the [^{32}P]-labeled nucleic acid components of small ribonucleoprotein particles recognized by these autoantibodies (8).

Antinuclear Antibodies

Antinuclear antibody testing is usually the first step in the immunodiagnosis of systemic autoimmune diseases such as SLE. Immunofluorescence is the standard approach, but alternatives such as ELISA have become available and are more amenable to automation.

Fluorescent Antinuclear Antibody (FANA) Test

Several prototype nuclear FANA patterns, including diffuse (homogeneous), speckled, nucleolar, and centromere, may be seen depending on the location of the target antigen (Fig. 74.2A–D, respectively). These patterns correspond with the presence of autoantibodies against different nuclear antigens. A nucleolar pattern (Fig. 74.2C) is suggestive of the diagnosis of scleroderma (2,9). A centromere pattern (Fig. 74.2D) is associated with limited scleroderma, in particular the CREST syndrome (calcinosis, Raynaud's phenomenon, esophageal dysmotility, sclerodactyly, telangiectasias), a scleroderma variant. Other patterns (Fig. 74.2A and B) are less disease specific.

The FANA technique also is useful for detecting autoantibodies against cytoplasmic antigens. Figure 74.3 (A–D) illustrates the patterns characteristic of antiribosomal P (Fig. 74.3A), anti–signal recognition particle (SRP, Fig. 74.3B), antihistidyl tRNA synthetase (Jo-1; Fig. 74.3C), and antimitochondrial (Fig. 74.3D) antibodies.

Sensitivity And Specificity

The FANA assay is an ideal screening assay for SLE because of its sensitivity and simplicity. The sensitivity ranges from 90% to 95% or more by using human cultured cells as substrate (10,11). Even the entity of "ANA-negative lupus" is associated with autoantibodies against cytoplasmic autoantigens, such as Ro (SS-A) or ribosomal P.

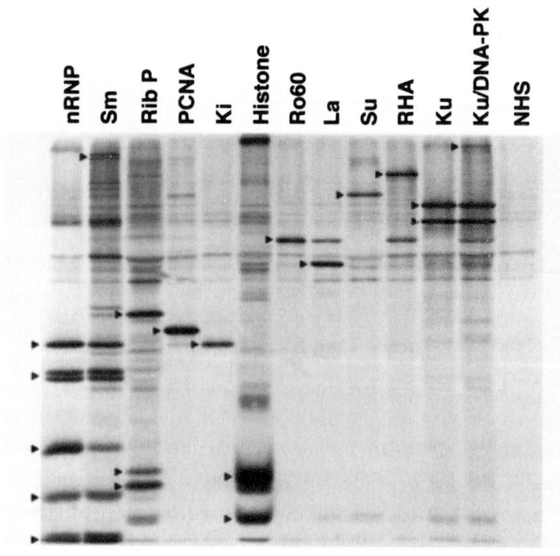

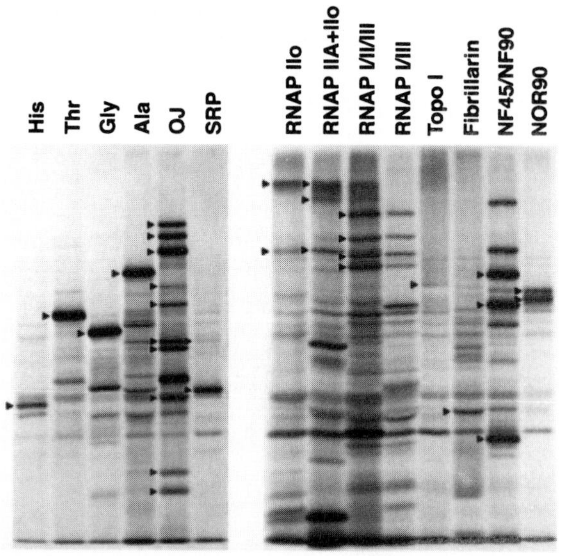

FIGURE 74.4. Immunoprecipitation analysis of autoantibody specificities. Human K562 cells were labeled with [^{35}S]-methionine and cysteine, and an extract was immunoprecipitated by using prototype human autoimmune sera. Immune complexes were absorbed onto protein A-Sepharose beads, washed, and analyzed by sodium dodecylsulfate (SDS)-polyacrylamide gel electrophoresis. Positions of specific bands immunoprecipitated by the sera are indicated with *arrowheads*. **A:** SLE sera. Specificities illustrated include anti-nRNP, Sm, ribosomal P (*Rib P*), proliferating cell nuclear antigen (*PCNA*), Ki, histone, Ro60, La (SS-B), Su, RNA helicase A (*RHA*), Ku, and Ku plus DNA-PK catalytic subunit. Pattern using normal human serum (*NHS*) is shown for comparison. **B:** Polymyositis sera. Specificities illustrated include anti-Jo-1 (histidyl tRNA synthetase), PL-7 (threonyl tRNA synthetase), EJ (glycyl tRNA synthetase), PL-12 (alanyl tRNA synthetase), OJ (multiprotein complex containing isoleucyl and other tRNA synthetases), and signal recognition particle (SRP). **C:** Scleroderma sera. Specificities illustrated include anti-RNA polymerase sera specific for the phosphorylated form of RNA polymerase II (*IIO*), the phosphorylated as well as the unphosphorylated forms of RNA polymerase II, RNA polymerases I, II, and III, and RNA polymerases I and III. Also shown are anti-topoisomerase I (*Topo I*), fibrillarin, nuclear factors 45 and 90 (*NF45/NF90*), and NOR90.

In contrast, the specificity of the FANA for SLE is relatively low (12,13). Of 276 FANA-positive individuals studied by Shiel and Jason (12), 18.8% had SLE; 10.9%, drug-induced lupus; and 21.7%, other collagen vascular diseases, such as scleroderma or polymyositis; 10.1%, autoimmune thyroiditis; 5.8%, other organ-specific autoimmune diseases; 8.3%, infections; 2.9%, neoplasms; and 24.3%, other conditions or "idiopathic" autoantibodies. Similarly, others have reported a positive predictive value of 11% to 13% of the FANA test for SLE (11,14). In addition, some healthy individuals produce low-titer ANAs (15,16). The prevalence of a positive FANA is 3% to 5% in randomly selected healthy whites (16). The production of ANAs is strongly age-dependent, increasing to 10% to 37% in healthy individuals older than 65 years (Fig. 74.5) (15). However, although ANAs are not unusual in healthy individuals, the titers are generally lower (≤1:40) than those in systemic autoimmune diseases. It has been reported that 3.3% of normal individuals are FANA positive at a 1:320 serum dilution versus 31.7% at a 1:40 dilution (17) (Fig. 74.6).

In contrast to the low positive predictive value of ANA testing, a patient with a negative FANA has less than a 3% chance of having SLE. Thus although of limited utility in confirming the diagnosis of SLE, the lack of ANAs by FANA testing is a useful criterion for excluding the diagnosis.

Correct interpretation of FANA staining depends on the experience of the microscopist. Distinguishing between negative and positive staining is subjective, resulting in a degree of variability between laboratories. In one study, interlaboratory coefficients of variation ranged from 36% at a 1:320 dilution to 51% at a 1:40 dilution (17). Nevertheless, the test can discriminate normal individuals from those with SLE, scleroderma, or Sjögren's syndrome most of the time. The optimal balance between sensitivity and specificity is at a serum dilution of approximately 1:160. At this dilution, SLE is correctly classified in 95% of patients, scleroderma in 87%, and Sjögren's syndrome in 74%, and normal individuals are correctly classified in 95% of controls (17). Thus it has been recommended that FANA test results be reported at both 1:40 and 1:160 dilutions. A more recent approach has been the use of computer-aided image analysis to determine an ANA "titer" with a single serum dilution (Y. Kobe, Medical & Biological Laboratories Co., Ltd., personal communication). This approach may help to limit the subjectivity of interpreting immunofluorescence data.

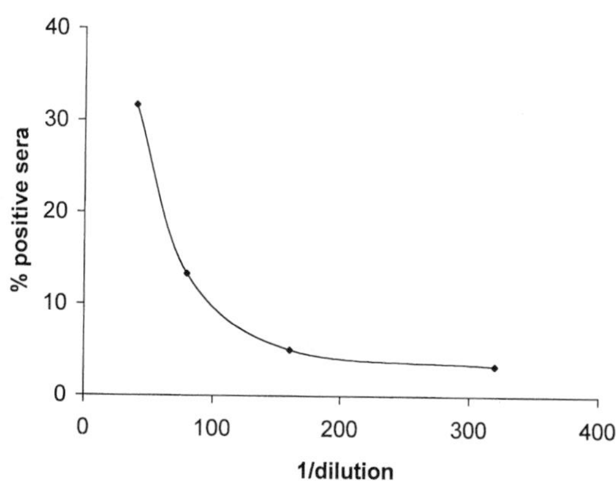

FIGURE 74.6. Positive FANA test in normal individuals as a function of serum dilution. Sera from 125 normal individuals were tested by FANA assay at dilutions of 1:40, 1:80, 1:160, and 1:320. The frequency of a positive reading is plotted as a function of serum dilution. (Adapted from Tan EM, Feltkamp TE, Smolen JS, et al. Range of antinuclear antibodies in "healthy" individuals. *Arthritis Rheum* 1997;40:1601, with permission.

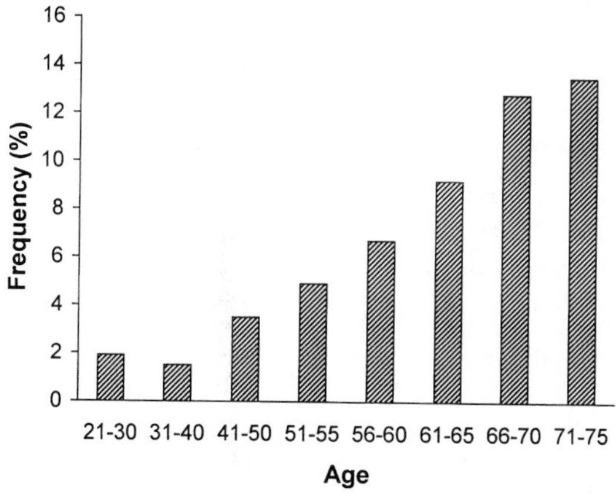

FIGURE 74.5. Prevalence of antinuclear antibodies as a function of age. Sera from 3,492 healthy individuals from rural Australia were tested for antinuclear antibodies. The frequency of a positive FANA test is plotted as a function of age. (Adapted from Hooper B, Whittingham S, Mathews JD, Mackay IR, Curnow DH. Autoimmunity in a rural community. *Clin Exp Immunol* 1972; 12:79, with permission.).

Antinuclear Antibody ELISA

Commercially available ELISAs for automated ANA testing use one of two approaches for coating the microtiter wells: crude nuclear extracts or mixtures of purified antigens recognized by autoantibodies associated with lupus or other diseases. The use of crude nuclear extracts for ANA ELISA testing has the drawback that the binding of individual antigens to the polystyrene wells cannot be monitored readily. Moreover, insoluble nuclear autoantigens, such as the nuclear lamins A, B, and C (18), are lost during the extraction process and do not bind to the plastic. The binding of DNA to the wells also is variable (11). Another disadvantage of using crude nuclear extract is that the information provided by ANA patterns is unavailable. In one comparison of six ELISAs with the FANA test, the results differed substantially (11). However, others have reported good agreement (19).

ANA ELISAs with purified nuclear antigens are limited by the inability to detect autoantibodies against antigens not included in the assay. Further studies are needed to compare the value of ANA ELISA versus the FANA for screening. At present, it is difficult to recommend discarding the standard, but more labor-intensive, immunofluorescent test.

CLINICAL APPLICATIONS OF AUTOANTIBODY TESTING

The discovery that certain types of ANAs are specific for the diagnosis of SLE or for other systemic autoimmune diseases was a major advance in the diagnosis of systemic autoimmunity. Autoantibodies specific for SLE, scleroderma, polymyositis, and primary biliary cirrhosis (PBC) are of considerable use clinically (Tables 74.1, 74.2, and 74.3; Fig. 74.4) [reviewed in (2,4)]. More recently, autoantibodies specific for rheumatoid arthritis (RA) have been reported, as well (20–23). The ensuing discussion focuses on autoantibodies that are useful in the clinical evaluation of SLE (Table 74.1; Fig. 74.4A). Most of the antigens are multicomponent complexes consisting of proteins plus nucleic acids (see later). Antiphospholipid antibodies, another serologic marker of considerable importance in SLE, are discussed in Chapter 77, and are not dealt with further here.

Anti-DNA, -Histone, -Nucleosome, and -Chromatin Antibodies

The nucleosome, a complex of DNA and histones, was the first lupus autoantigen to be identified (1,24). A subset of autoantibodies specific for this structure is responsible for the LE phenomenon (24). Autoantibodies against nucleosomes and their constituents, as well as chromatin, are an important component of the autoimmune response in lupus (25). Immune responses against chromatin also are characteristic of the lupus-like syndrome induced by certain drugs, such as procainamide, hydralazine, quinidine, and isoniazid (26).

TABLE 74.1. AUTOANTIBODY MARKERS SPECIFIC FOR SLE

Autoantibody	Prevalence[a]	Clinical Associations
α-dsDNA	40–70%	Nephritis, active disease
α-Sm	7–30%	Highly specific for SLE
α-Ribosomal P	15%	Neuropsychiatric involvement
α-PCNA	2–5%	Nephritis
α-RNA helicase A[b]	10–15%	Not known

[a]Approximate prevalence of autoantibody in SLE.
[b]Tentative association with SLE, data incomplete.

TABLE 74.2. AUTOANTIBODY MARKERS FOR SCLERODERMA

Autoantibody	Prevalence[a]	Clinical Associations
α-Topoisomerase I	15%	Proximal (severe) scleroderma
α-RNA polymerase (RNAP) I, II, III	20%	Severe disease; anti-RNAP I/III more specific than II
α-Fibrillarin	5%	Highly specific for scleroderma
α-NOR90	Rare	Also seen in other disorders (247)
α-Th	5%	Highly specific for scleroderma
α-NF45/NF90	Rare	Scleroderma–rheumatoid arthritis overlap

[a]Approximate prevalence of autoantibody in associated disease subset.

The Antigen

Chromatin is a complex of double-stranded DNA with histones and nonhistone proteins. DNA is packaged in a complex of histones consisting of 145 base pairs of double-stranded DNA wound around the core histone octamer consisting of two molecules each of H2A/H2B, H3, and H4 (27,28). A single unit is called a nucleosome. Nucleosomes are connected by linker DNA, which is associated with histone H1. At this level of organization, the DNA strand resembles beads on a string. Higher level folding results in the formation of chromatin fibers of increasing complexity.

TABLE 74.3. AUTOANTIBODY MARKERS FOR POLYMYOSITIS OR DERMATOMYOSITIS

Autoantibody	Prevalence[a]	Clinical Associations
α-Jo-1 ($tRNA^{his}$ synthetase)	20%	Antisynthetase syndrome (see Chapter 78)
α-PL-7 ($tRNA^{thr}$ synthetase)	3%	Antisynthetase syndrome
α-EJ ($tRNA^{gly}$ synthetase)	2%	Antisynthetase syndrome
α-PL-12 ($tRNA^{ala}$ synthetase)	3%	Antisynthetase syndrome
α-OJ (complex of isoleucyl and other tRNA synthetases)	2%	Antisynthetase syndrome
α-KS ($tRNA^{asn}$ synthetase)	<1%	Interstitial lung disease
α-SRP[b]	4%	Severe myositis without antisynthetase features
α-PM-Scl	8%	Polymyositis–scleroderma overlap syndrome

[a]Approximate prevalence of autoantibody in associated disease subset.
[b]SRP, signal recognition particle.

Antichromatin and Antinucleosomal Antibodies

Chromatin is a major target of the autoimmune response in SLE (25). However, autoantibodies to chromatin are found in a variety of disorders, including drug-induced lupus and other forms of systemic autoimmune disease, and thus are not specific for SLE. They produce a homogeneous FANA pattern (Fig. 74.2A). Chromatin is a complex mixture of DNA plus both histones and nonhistone proteins. Although autoantibodies to high-mobility group (HMG) proteins, a major nonhistone constituent of chromatin, and histone H1 have been reported in lupus (29,30), the major target antigen appears to be the H2A–H2B–DNA complex (26,31).

Autoantibodies against chromatin or H2A–H2B–DNA complexes are assayed by ELISA (32). Detection of immunoglobulin G (IgG) autoantibodies to the H2A–H2B–DNA complex in an individual taking one of the medications associated with drug-induced lupus is consistent with that diagnosis. However, they are not a specific marker because of the high prevalence in SLE and their occurrence in a subset of patients with scleroderma or related diseases. The sensitivity of IgG anti–H2A-H2B-DNA for procainamide-induced lupus is 84% at the time of diagnosis, with significantly elevated levels detectable as early as 1 year before the onset of symptoms (33). Interestingly, the levels of anti–H2A-H2B-DNA diminish with decreasing disease activity and disappear altogether in most individuals with drug-induced lupus on cessation of the medication. The most important clinical application of antichromatin antibodies may be in monitoring patients taking drugs known to precipitate a lupus-like syndrome.

Antihistone and Anti–Single-Stranded (SS) DNA Antibodies

Autoantibodies to ssDNA and individual histones are common in drug-induced as well as in idiopathic lupus. Their significance is similar to that of anti–H2A-H2B-DNA, but sensitivity is less. Like antichromatin and antinucleosomal antibodies, they are not specific. Antihistone antibodies can be detected by ELISA or Western blot, and anti-ssDNA antibodies, by ELISA.

Anti–Double-Stranded (ds) DNA Antibodies

Anti-dsDNA antibodies are found in up to 70% of SLE patients' sera at some point during the disease and are 95% specific for SLE, making them a valuable disease marker (13,34). In animal models, the progression from antichromatin to anti-dsDNA antibodies is associated with the development of renal disease (35). Conversely, both renal disease and anti-dsDNA antibodies are extremely unusual in drug-induced lupus. Anti-dsDNA antibodies can be eluted specifically from glomerular immune deposits of lupus patients, suggesting that immune complexes containing anti-DNA antibodies are pathogenic (36). The precise mechanism by which they promote renal injury remains controversial. Three main hypotheses have been proposed: (a) preformed DNA–anti-DNA immune complexes may deposit in the glomerular basement membrane (GBM), resulting in inflammation; (b) DNA or nucleosomes may become trapped in the GBM and bind anti-DNA antibodies *in situ* (37); and (c) a subset of anti-DNA antibodies may cross-react with endogenous glomerular antigens (38,39).

Consistent with the immune complex–mediated pathogenesis of lupus, anti-dsDNA antibody and complement levels frequently exhibit a reciprocal pattern, with high levels of anti-dsDNA antibodies and hypocomplementemia during exacerbations and the reverse pattern during remissions (40). However, some asymptomatic patients have persistently high levels of anti-dsDNA antibodies (41).

Nephritogenicity of Anti-dsDNA Antibodies

Injection of some, but not all, mouse monoclonal anti-ds or -ssDNA antibodies induces renal disease in recipient mice, consistent with the possibility that they are nephritogenic (42,43). The features that make some anti-DNA antibodies nephritogenic are not known with certainty. The ability to cross-react with endogenous renal antigens is one possibility (38,44,45). Efficient complement fixation also may be important (46,47). However, this could be merely a consequence of the close correlation between anti-dsDNA titer and complement fixing anti-dsDNA titer (48). Pathogenicity also may be a function of the avidity for DNA (49,50), although in (NZB × NZW)F_1 mice, the severity of lupus correlates with low-avidity anti-DNA antibodies (51).

Testing for Anti-DNA Antibodies

These considerations make it difficult to recommend a definitive approach for identifying potentially pathogenic anti-DNA autoantibodies. Several assays are in common use, including radioimmunoassay (Farr), Millipore filter assay, polyethylene glycol (PEG) assay, *Crithidia luciliae* kinetoplast staining assay, and ELISA (Table 74.4). It is

TABLE 74.4. TESTS FOR ANTI-DNA ANTIBODIES

Assay	Avidity of Antibodies Detected	References
Radioimmunoassay (Farr)	High	(54, 248)
Millipore assay	High	(249)
PEG assay	Intermediate to high	(250)
Crithidia luciliae kinetoplast staining	Intermediate to high	(53, 248)
ELISA	Low to high	(248, 251)

important to discriminate between anti-ssDNA and anti-dsDNA antibodies because only the latter are associated strongly with disease activity. This could reflect the fact that anti-ssDNA antibodies are of lower affinity than anti-dsDNA (50). There are two main approaches to ensure specificity for dsDNA. One is to remove single-stranded DNA from DNA preparations by S1 nuclease treatment or absorbing on hydroxyapatite (52). An alternative approach is to use closed circular DNA, which has no ends that could unravel. This forms the basis of the *Crithidia luciliae* kinetoplast staining assay. The kinetoplast contains a single closed circular DNA molecule that can be stained with patient serum followed by fluorescein isothiocyanate (FITC)-labeled goat anti–human Ig antibodies (53).

Monitoring Disease Activity with the Farr Assay

In the Farr assay, immune complexes of radiolabeled DNA and anti-DNA antibodies are precipitated by using ammonium sulfate and quantified (54). This assay is relatively specific for high-avidity anti-DNA antibodies (50,55) and may be a better predictor of disease activity than are assays that detect lower avidity antibodies, such as ELISA (50). It has been shown to be predictive of relapses as early as 10 weeks before a flare (56). Serial (prospective) measurement of anti-dsDNA may be preferable to measuring C3 or C4 levels. Moreover, treatment with prednisone, as soon as a significant increase in the anti-dsDNA antibody level is documented by Farr assay, can prevent relapse (57). This approach to the management of relapse based on early serologic changes alone warrants further study, but remains controversial.

Anti-nRNP and Sm Antibodies

The anti-Sm antibody system was discovered by Tan and Kunkel in 1966 (3), and its close relation with anti-nRNP (ribonuclease sensitivity and line of partial identity in double immunodiffusion) was established by Mattioli and Reichlin (58). Anti-Sm antibodies are produced by 7% to 30% of lupus patients depending on ethnicity and, like anti-dsDNA, also are virtually pathognomonic of SLE (3,59). Anti-nRNP antibodies are strongly associated with anti-Sm, but are not disease specific and are of limited utility in diagnosing SLE or in predicting its course. The frequency of anti-nRNP antibodies in SLE is 20% to 40% (60–62). There is little evidence that either anti-nRNP or anti-Sm antibodies cause disease.

The Sm and nRNP Antigens

Anti-Sm and anti-nRNP antibodies recognize different subsets of the protein components of the U1 small nuclear ribonucleoprotein (snRNP) particle (Fig. 74.7A). The U1 snRNP is an RNA–protein complex consisting of proteins designated U1-70K (70 kd), A (33 kd), B′/B (29 and 28 kd, respectively), C (23 kd), D1/2/3 (16 kd), E (12 kd), F (11 kd), and G (10 kd) associated with a single U1 small nuclear RNA molecule (8,59). The proteins B′/B, D, E, F, and G assemble into a stable 6S particle (the Sm core particle) reactive with anti-Sm, but not anti-nRNP, antibodies (63). The U1-A and 70K proteins interact directly with U1 RNA through RNA recognition motifs (64), whereas the RNA-dependent association of U1-C with the U1 snRNP is mediated through interactions with the B′/B components of the Sm core particle (65). In addition to the U1 snRNP, other snRNPs, each with a unique uridine-rich (U) RNA species as well as unique proteins, carry the Sm core particle (Table 74.5). These include the U2, U4/U6, and U5 snRNPs, as well as other less abundant U snRNPs (59).

Autoantibodies from patients' sera (8) made it possible to define the critical role of U1, U2, U4-6, and U5 snRNPs

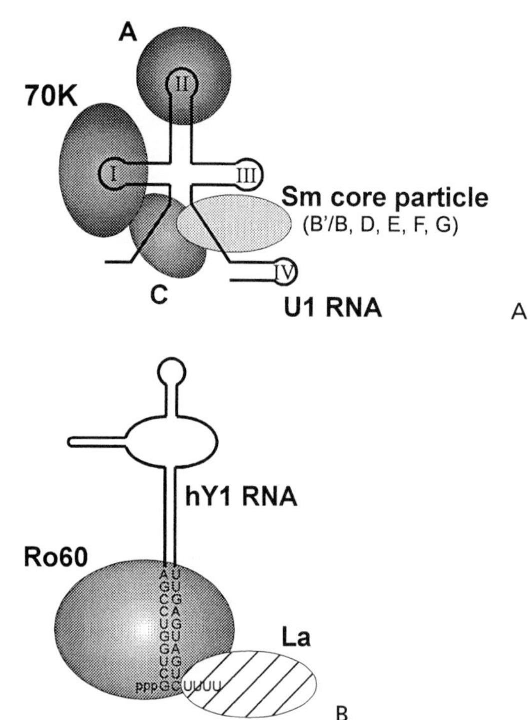

FIGURE 74.7. Structure of the U1 and Ro ribonucleoprotein particles. **A:** The U1 small nuclear ribonucleoprotein consists of three unique polypeptides (70K, A, and C) that are recognized by anti-nRNP sera, the Sm core particle (proteins B′/B, D, E, F, and G, reactive with anti-Sm antibodies), and a single molecule of U1 RNA. Locations of stem-loops I–IV of U1 RNA are indicated. Autoantibodies against stem-loops II and IV have been reported. **B:** The Ro ribonucleoprotein consists of the Ro60 protein (reactive with anti-Ro/SS-A antibodies) and a single molecule of hY1, hY3, hY4, or hY5 RNA (hY1 RNA is illustrated). Newly synthesized particles carry the La polypeptide bound to a U-rich sequence located at the 3′ end of the RNA. The 47-kd La protein is reactive with anti-La (SS-B) antibodies. Autoantibodies specific for the hY5 RNA have been reported, but not antibodies against the hY1 molecule.

TABLE 74.5. PROTEIN AND RNA COMPONENTS OF THE MAJOR U SNRNPS

snRNP Particle	RNA	Shared Proteins	Unique Proteins	Autoantibodies
U1 snRNP	U1	Sm core particle[a]	70 K, A, C	Sm, nRNP
U2 snRNP	U2	Sm core particle[a]	A′, B"	Sm, A′, B"
U5 snRNP	U5	Sm core particle[a]	8 proteins	Sm, 100 K, 102 K, 200 K (doublet)
U4/U6 snRNP	U4 and U6	Sm core particle[a]	150 K	Sm, 150 K

[a]Proteins B′/B, D (D1, D2, D3), E, F, and G form the 6S Sm core particle, which is shared by all of the U snRNPs listed.

in the splicing of precursor heterogeneous nuclear RNA into messenger RNA (66,67). During splicing, the U snRNPs and other proteins assemble into an even larger structure termed a spliceosome (68), which mediates recognition of sequences at intron–exon junctions, cleavage of the intervening sequences, and rejoining of the mature mRNA (67). The U1 small RNA base pairs with the 5′ splice site of a precursor RNA, leading to its cleavage and leaving an invariant guanosine residue at the 5′ end of the intron, which subsequently forms a lariat-like structure. Formation of the lariat structure requires binding of the U2 snRNP to the branch point (67). After cleavage at the 3′ end of the intron, the U5 and U4/U6 snRNPs bind near the 3′ splice site, and the exons are re-ligated to produce mature mRNA. The individual spliceosomes, comprising arrays of snRNPs involved in the splicing reaction, are responsible for the fine speckled immunofluorescence pattern associated with anti-nRNP or anti-Sm autoantibody activity (Fig. 74.2B).

Anti-Sm Versus Anti-nRNP Antibodies

Distinguishing the clinically important anti-Sm antibodies from anti-nRNP is simplified by understanding the structure of the U1 snRNP particle (Fig. 74.7A). Anti-Sm and anti-nRNP antibodies immunoprecipitate a similar set of polypeptides (Fig. 74.4A) because the Sm core particle is associated with the anti-nRNP reactive proteins U1-A and U1-C in the abundant U1 snRNP (the methionine-deficient U1-70K protein is poorly visualized by immunoprecipitation). However, the two patterns can be distinguished by the immunoprecipitation of a characteristic doublet of proteins at 200 kd by anti-Sm (Fig. 74.4A, Sm lane, *arrowhead*) but not anti-nRNP sera. These proteins are unique components of the U5 snRNP, which carries the Sm core particle but not the nRNP proteins A, C, or 70K (Table 74.5). The different fine specificities of anti-nRNP and anti-Sm antibodies become clear if immunoprecipitation is carried out after dissociating the U1 snRNP into its individual components by $MgCl_2$ or ribonuclease treatment (69,70). They also can be demonstrated by Western blotting (71).

Anti-Sm and anti-nRNP sera also immunoprecipitate distinctive subsets of small RNAs, as shown by analysis of the [^{32}P]-labeled RNAs (8). Thus both anti-nRNP and anti-Sm sera immunoprecipitate U1 RNA, whereas the U2, U4, U5, and U6 small RNAs are immunoprecipitated by sera containing anti-Sm, but not by sera having only anti-nRNP activity. This is because the Sm core particle is a component of each of the U snRNPs, whereas the U1-70K, U1-A, and U1-C proteins recognized by anti-nRNP antibodies are unique to the U1 snRNP.

Anti-nRNP and Anti-Sm Antibodies Constitute a Linked Autoantibody Set

Nearly all sera containing anti-Sm antibodies contain anti-nRNP antibodies, as well (72,73). Usually the levels of anti-nRNP antibodies in human autoimmune sera greatly exceed the levels of anti-Sm (73). Most sera with autoantibodies to the U1 snRNP recognize multiple polypeptides. In one study, only one of 29 sera containing anti-nRNP or Sm antibodies recognized a single protein by Western blot, and the majority recognized three or more of the proteins U1-70K, U1-A, U1-C, and Sm-B′/B, Sm-D, and Sm-E (71).

Another class of autoantibodies is specific for antigenic sites present only on the native antigen, such as anti–native U1-C (69) or epitopes formed by the association of the E, F, and G Sm polypeptides (74). Autoantibodies that stabilize the interactions between the U1-C protein and the Sm core particle or between U1-A and the Sm core particle also have been reported (70). All human sera with anti-nRNP activity stabilize the interaction between U1-C and the Sm core particle, whereas "stabilizing antibodies" are not seen in the small subset of human sera with anti-Sm but not anti-nRNP antibodies or in the anti-Sm sera from MRL/lpr mice (70).

The U1 small RNA molecule also is recognized by autoantibodies in many sera (75,76). Although initially thought to be unusual, autoantibodies to U1 RNA are found in about 40% of anti-nRNP/Sm–positive sera (77). The antibodies recognize the stem of stem-loop II and the loop of stem-loop IV of U1 RNA (Fig. 74.7A) (75,76).

Interestingly, these antibodies are uniquely reactive with U1 RNA, even though stem-loop II of U1 RNA differs in only a few nucleotides from the fourth loop of U2 RNA. Autoantibodies to the U1 RNA molecule are linked strongly to the production of anti-nRNP antibodies, and are absent in sera containing anti-Sm, but not nRNP, antibodies (77).

In summary, autoimmune responses to the U1 snRNP and to chromatin are similar in several respects: (a) both target nucleic acid–protein complexes, (b) autoantibodies recognize both the proteins and the nucleic acid components, and (c) autoantibodies against multiple components are produced tandemly as part of a so-called "linked set" (78).

Cross-Reactions of Anti-nRNP and Anti-Sm Antibodies

Although autoantibodies against constituents of the U1 snRNP often are exquisitely specific for that antigen, clinically significant examples of immunologic cross-reactivity have been reported. Epitope sharing between the individual protein components of the U1 snRNP has been noted (79,80). In addition, some anti-Sm antibodies cross-react with the ribosomal protein S10 (81,82) or with ribosomal P (83). Cross-reactivity of anti-Sm-D or U1-A with DNA has been reported (84,85). The frequency of clinically significant cross-reactivity is not certain at present.

CLINICAL SIGNIFICANCE OF THE ANTIBODIES

Autoantibodies to the Sm core particle are found exclusively in SLE (3,60). In contrast, anti-nRNP antibodies recognize proteins A, C, and 70K and may be found in sera from patients with scleroderma, polymyositis, and other subsets of systemic autoimmune disease, as well as SLE (60,72,86). Extremely high levels of anti-nRNP antibodies without anti-Sm are seen in mixed connective tissue disease (MCTD) (87). Although highly specific, anti-Sm antibodies are found only in about 7% to 30% of lupus patients (60,61). In view of their specificity, anti-Sm and anti-dsDNA antibodies are included among the American Rheumatism Association's 1982 revised diagnostic criteria for SLE (10).

The frequency of anti-Sm varies markedly depending on ethnicity: they are found in fewer than 10% of Europeans but 25% to 30% of African-Americans or Chinese (61,62). Although there are reports of anti-Sm antibodies in other diseases, including organic brain syndrome secondary to lupus (88), schizophrenia (89), and uveitis (90), the presence of these autoantibodies was determined by ELISA and not verified by double immunodiffusion or immunoprecipitation. Thus the association of anti-Sm with other disease entities is controversial. There also are reports that anti-Sm antibodies are associated with an increased frequency of Raynaud's phenomenon and mild renal or central nervous system disease (91,92), but this is controversial (93). Although not as dramatic as the changes in levels of anti-DNA antibodies, it has been suggested that anti-Sm or nRNP antibody levels may reflect disease activity (94). Antibodies specific for stem-loop IV of U1 RNA also increase and decrease in parallel with disease activity, suggesting that this subset may provide an independent marker of disease activity in SLE (95). However, it is widely accepted that once anti-nRNP or anti-Sm antibodies develop, they remain at relatively constant levels and do not disappear during periods of disease quiescence, unlike anti-DNA antibodies (96).

Tests for anti-Sm and nRNP Antibodies

Immunoprecipitation assays should probably be considered the "gold standard" for detecting anti-nRNP/Sm antibodies, but are technically demanding, require the use of radioactive isotopes, and are not widely available. Clinical testing for anti-nRNP or Sm antibodies relies largely on the following assays: (a) double immunodiffusion, (b) CIE, (c) ELISA, and (d) immunoblotting. All of these assays have drawbacks, however. Immunodiffusion is specific and easily performed without special instrumentation or purified antigens, but is relatively insensitive. At present, this and the more sensitive CIE test (60) probably represent the most reliable approach for the routine detection of anti-Sm and anti-nRNP. ELISAs can provide valuable information if properly standardized. Highly purified antigen is essential, and in view of the high frequency of autoantibodies against conformational determinants of the U1 snRNP, it is best to use intact snRNPs for coating the polystyrene wells instead of individual recombinant U snRNP proteins. As is true of anti-DNA ELISAs, the significance of low-affinity antibodies reactive in ELISA is uncertain. Some sera contain immunoglobulins that bind to Sm antigen–coated wells in commercial assays at levels above background, yet do not immunoprecipitate the U1 snRNP particle (H. Yoshida, M. Satoh, and W.H. Reeves, unpublished observations, 1999). Whether such antibodies are designated "anti-Sm" is a semantic issue similar to the question of whether low-affinity "natural" autoantibodies reactive with DNA by ELISA should be considered true anti-DNA antibodies (97). Finally, Western blotting can provide useful information about antibodies reactive with linear determinants found on individual proteins, but it does not readily distinguish anti-Sm from anti-nRNP antibodies and cannot detect certain autoantibodies against conformational determinants. In general, it is less suitable than the other approaches.

Anti-Ro (SS-A) and La (SS-B) Antibodies

The Ro (SS-A)/La (SS-B) autoantibody system was discovered independently by Anderson et al. (98), Clark et al.

(99), and Alspaugh and Tan (100). It was later recognized that the antigen systems were the same (101). Anti-Ro (SS-A) and anti-La (SS-B) antibodies are produced by 10% to 50% and 10% to 20% of SLE patients, respectively, but are not specific markers for the disease (102–104). The variability in frequency of detection reflects differences in the assays as well as the ethnicity of the subjects. There are three antigens in the Ro (SS-A)-La (SS-B) system.

The Antigens

One of the SS-A/Ro antigens is a 60-kd protein (Ro60) that binds to the stem of four small RNAs designated hY1, hY3, hY4, and hY5 (Fig. 74.7B) (105). An additional protein of 52 kd (Ro52) (106) is reactive with many sera containing anti-Ro (SS-A) antibodies. It is controversial whether Ro52 interacts with Ro60 or the Y RNAs (107,108). The functions of the 60K Ro and 52K Ro antigens remain uncertain.

The La (SS-B) antigen is a 47-kd phosphoprotein that associates transiently with the precursors of several small RNAs synthesized by RNA polymerase III (109,110). It binds to a short stretch of uridylate residues at the 3′ end of these RNAs (Fig. 74.7B) through an RNA recognition motif shared with other autoantigens including the U1-70K protein (111,112). The La (SS-B) protein is a transcription-termination factor for RNA polymerase III and has an adenosine triphosphatase (ATPase) activity that melts DNA/RNA hybrids (113,114).

The subcellular localization of the Ro antigens is not known with certainty. Both a cytoplasmic and a nuclear distribution have been reported (99,100,115). La (SS-B), conversely, is generally believed to have primarily a nuclear location.

Anti-Ro (SS-A) and Anti-La (SS-B) Antibodies Constitute a Linked Autoantibody Set

Mattioli, Wasicek, and Reichlin (104,116) established that anti-La (SS-B) antibodies virtually always are associated with anti-Ro (SS-A), whereas anti-Ro (SS-A) occurs relatively frequently in the absence of anti-La (SS-B). Of 55 anti-Ro/La sera studied, 23 had both specificities and 30 had anti-Ro (SS-A) alone, whereas only two had anti-La (SS-B) antibodies alone (104). Thus like the anti-nRNP/Sm system, anti-Ro (SS-A) and La (SS-B) constitute a linked autoantibody set (78). Autoantibodies specific for the hY5 RNA moiety of Ro ribonucleoproteins also occur in tandem with anti-Ro (SS-A) (117).

CLINICAL SIGNIFICANCE

Anti-Ro (SS-A) and La (SS-B) antibodies both are present at very high frequency in Sjögren's syndrome sera (103). They are important because they are associated with sicca syndrome as well as subacute cutaneous lupus and neonatal lupus syndromes, including congenital complete heart block. The transplacental transfer of these antibodies in neonatal lupus argues that they are pathogenic.

Primary and Secondary Sjögren's Syndrome

Anti-Ro (SS-A) antibodies are present in 60% to 80% of sera from patients with primary Sjögren's syndrome and 10% to 50% of SLE sera by double immunodiffusion (102,118,119). They are found at a lower frequency in sera from patients with RA and in some sera from otherwise healthy individuals (103). Anti-Ro52 and Ro60 antibodies can be associated with either disorder, but there are different patterns. Anti-Ro52 without anti-Ro60 antibodies is most commonly associated with primary Sjögren's syndrome, whereas anti-Ro60 without anti-Ro52 usually is associated with SLE (102). Patients with SLE and anti-Ro (SS-A) antibodies frequently have secondary Sjögren's syndrome (103) or subacute cutaneous lupus (120). The prevalence of anti-Ro (SS-A) in SLE patients with secondary Sjögren's syndrome is 70% (121), whereas the prevalence in the annular subgroup of subacute cutaneous lupus is 60% to 80% (122). A direct role for anti-Ro (SS-A) antibodies in the pathogenesis of these skin lesions has been suggested (123). Anti-La (SS-B) antibodies also are found at high frequency in both primary Sjögren's syndrome (prevalence, 47%) (102) and SLE with secondary Sjögren's syndrome (prevalence, 50% compared with 10% to 20% in unselected SLE patients) (102,121).

Neonatal Lupus Syndrome and Congenital Complete Heart Block

Neonatal lupus syndrome consists of skin rashes resembling subacute cutaneous lupus and other abnormalities, including congenital complete heart block (124,125). The skin rash is transient, disappearing concomitant with the disappearance of maternal IgG from the circulation of the neonate. There is a very strong association with maternal anti-Ro (SS-A) antibodies (126).

Congenital complete heart block, appearing usually late in the second trimester (>22 weeks' gestation), is a more ominous complication associated with autoantibodies to Ro (SS-A) as well as La (SS-B) (127,128). Interestingly, the cardiac lesion affects the fetus selectively, with few adverse effects on the mother (128). The presence of either anti-Ro52 or anti-La is associated with a higher risk of developing this complication than that of anti-Ro60. The combination of antibodies to Ro52 and to La is increased in neonatal lupus mothers, with an odds ratio of 35 (127). Anti-Ro52 antibodies were concentrated in the heart tissue eluate of an infant with complete heart block (129). Cross-reactivity of the autoantibodies with cardiac antigens may be responsible for the development of cardiomyopathy and complete heart block secondary to fibrosis of the conduction system (130–132). However, the risk of the neonate born to a mother with anti-Ro52 or La (SS-B) developing complete heart block is low. How the autoantibodies cause complete heart block is an area of active investigation. The strong association of congenital complete heart block with anti-Ro52 or anti-La (SS-B) antibodies has led to proposals for fetal cardiac monitoring in seropositive mothers. Plasmapheresis can reduce antibody titers, with amelioration of the cardiac disease (128). Corticosteroid therapy also may play a role in suppressing the manifestations of fetal carditis. Dexamethasone is the preferred agent because it is not metabolized by the placenta and therefore is available to the fetus in active form (see Chapter 89).

Tests for Anti-Ro (SS-A) and Anti-La (SS-B) Antibodies

A variety of tests can be used to detect anti-Ro52, anti-Ro60, and anti-La antibodies. CIE and double immunodiffusion have been used to detect anti-Ro (SS-A) and La (SS-B) autoantibodies for many years. It is important to use a human substrate, such as spleen or Wil-2 cell extract, for detecting anti-Ro (SS-A). CIE and double immunodiffusion cannot detect anti-Ro52 antibodies, which generally are nonprecipitating (133). Some anti-La antibodies also are nonprecipitating (134).

Anti-Ro52 and Ro60 specificities can be distinguished by Western blotting. For anti-Ro52, Western blot is an excellent detection method (106). However, the detection of anti-Ro60 by this technique is unreliable because many sera contain primarily autoantibodies against the native form of the antigen (135,136). Western blot is a highly efficient and sensitive approach for detecting anti-La (SS-B) antibodies (134). Anti-recombinant La ELISAs are reliable and widely used (137). Recombinant antigen-based ELISAs for anti-Ro52 and anti-Ro60 are used in a research setting (138,139) and increasingly in the clinical arena. However, the sensitivity of the anti-Ro60 ELISA may be higher with biochemically purified cellular antigens (133,139).

Immunoprecipitation of [^{35}S]-labeled proteins or [^{32}P]-labeled small RNAs is the gold standard for detecting anti-Ro60 and anti-La antibodies. Anti-Ro60 antibodies immunoprecipitate a protein of 60 kd (Fig. 74.4A) and a characteristic group of small RNAs (hY1, hY3, hY4, and hY5) (2,4,140). Anti-La (SS-B) antibodies immunoprecipitate a protein of 47 kd (Fig. 74.4A) as well as a series of small RNAs, including 7SL, 5S, transfer RNAs, and other species synthesized by RNA polymerase III (109). Although anti-Ro52 antibodies recently have been shown to be capable of immunoprecipitating the native protein (133,141), Western blotting should be considered the gold standard for detecting anti-Ro52.

Antiribosomal Antibodies

Antiribosomal antibodies in sera from SLE patients were reported by several groups in the 1960s and 1970s (142–144). It was not until 1985, however, that the nature of the antigens was determined (145,146).

The Antigens

Ribosomes are critical components of the cell's protein-synthesis machinery and consist of a 40S and a 60S subunit. Together the two ribosomal subunits contain 80 proteins and four RNA molecules. The most common antiribosomal antibodies recognize three phosphoproteins of 38, 19, and 17 kd (P0, P1, and P2) that are components of the 60S ribosomal subunit (Fig. 74.4A, RibP). Anti-P autoantibodies recognize primarily a conserved epitope contained on the C-terminal portion of P0, P1, and P2 (147). Other ribosomal proteins, including the S10 (148), L5 (149), and L12 (149) proteins, also are autoantigens, as is the 28S ribosomal RNA molecule (150).

Clinical Significance

Antibodies to the ribosomal P0, P1, and P2 antigens are highly specific for the diagnosis of SLE (144,151), but less sensitive than anti-Sm or anti-dsDNA, with a prevalence of about 15% (Table 74.1). The major epitope recognized by lupus sera resides on the C-terminal 22 amino acids (151). Anti-P antibodies have been linked retrospectively with neuropsychiatric manifestations, especially lupus psychosis, and their levels may be useful in predicting a relapse of lupus psychosis (151–153). However, their association with neuropsychiatric manifestations remains controversial (154,155). The basis for these discrepancies is unclear, but may reflect differences in race or ethnicity, the assays used, or the diagnostic criteria for neuropsychiatric disease. At present, antiribosomal P antibodies can be regarded as a useful marker for SLE, but the utility of measuring these antibodies as a diagnostic or prognostic marker for neuropsychiatric disease will require further study.

Tests for Antiribosomal Antibodies

Antiribosomal P antibodies can be detected by immunoprecipitation (Fig. 74.4A) and immunodiffusion. An ELISA using a C-terminal peptide of the human P2 antigen and immunoblotting also is used (155,156).

Other Specificities (Anti-PCNA, RNA Polymerase II, Su, Ku, and RNA Helicase A)

Other autoantibodies associated with SLE are less valuable from a diagnostic or prognostic standpoint. Some of the more important are antibodies against proliferating cell nuclear antigen (PCNA), RNA polymerase II, Su, Ku, and RNA helicase A. Immunoprecipitation analysis of these antibodies is illustrated in Fig. 74.4A.

Anti-PCNA

The PCNA antigen is a 36-kd protein (Fig. 74.4A) that exhibits variable immunofluorescence staining using methanol-fixed cells (157,158). It is an auxiliary factor for DNA polymerase δ (159,160). Rapidly proliferating or mitogen-stimulated cells exhibit nuclear staining, whereas resting (G0) cells remain unstained. The lack of staining in G_0 cells is not due to the absence of the antigen, but rather to the ease of extraction during methanol fixation (161). With formalin fixation, anti-PCNA antibodies stain cells at all phases of the cell cycle.

Antibodies to PCNA appear to be highly specific for SLE but are uncommon (4,157,158). Their frequency in SLE is about 2% to 5% (157,162). There is insufficient information on the frequency of anti-PCNA antibodies in other diseases to make a definitive statement about their specificity for lupus, but nearly all reports of this antibody are in SLE patients, often in association with diffuse proliferative glomerulonephritis (157,162). Retrospective longitudinal analyses suggest that titers may correlate with disease activity, but further study is needed to answer this question (162). Autoantibodies to PCNA can be detected by using double immunodiffusion, CIE, or immunoprecipitation.

Anti-RNA Polymerase II

RNA polymerase II is a multiprotein complex consisting of eight to 12 proteins that synthesizes messenger RNA. The two largest subunits (220 and 140 kd) carry the catalytic site of the enzyme. The C-terminal domain of the largest subunit is phosphorylated in the transcriptionally active form of the enzyme (163). RNA polymerases I and III are involved in the synthesis of ribosomal RNA and a subclass of small RNA molecules, respectively. These enzymes have different large subunits from RNA polymerase II, but some of the smaller subunits are shared by polymerases I, II, and III (163). Thus some sera with anti-RNA polymerase antibodies immunoprecipitate all three enzymes (Fig. 74.4C; RNAP I/II/III).

Although autoantibodies to RNA polymerases are usually thought to be associated primarily with scleroderma (164,165), autoantibodies against RNA polymerase II are found in about 10% of SLE patients' sera (166). A subset of these sera exhibits remarkable specificity for a transcriptionally active form of the enzyme in which the large subunit is hyperphosphorylated (Fig. 74.4C; RNAP IIO) (166). In scleroderma patients, anti-RNA polymerase IIO antibodies may be associated with anti–topoisomerase I antibodies and with more severe disease (167). In contrast to anti-RNA polymerase II, autoantibodies to RNA polymerases I and III are highly specific for scleroderma (168). At present, the only reliable assay for anti-RNA polymerase I, II, or III is immunoprecipitation.

Anti-Ku and DNA-Dependent Protein Kinase (DNA-PK)

Autoantibodies to Ku and the catalytic subunit of DNA-dependent protein kinase ($DNA\text{-}PK_{cs}$) recognize a multiprotein complex involved in DNA repair, V(D)J recombination, and transcriptional activation (169). DNA-PK binds to DNA through the Ku (p70/p80 heterodimer) antigen (170,171). The association of Ku, $DNA\text{-}PK_{cs}$, and DNA is relatively tenuous. In the presence of 0.5 *M* NaCl, Ku, $DNA\text{-}PK_{cs}$, and DNA dissociate from one another, and can be immunoprecipitated separately (Fig. 74.4A; cf. "Ku" and "Ku/DNA-PK" lanes), whereas at lower salt concentrations, these antigens are co-immunoprecipitated as a complex (169).

Autoantibodies to Ku70, Ku80, and $DNA\text{-}PK_{cs}$ frequently coexist, suggesting that these autoantibodies compose a linked set (172–174). Autoantibodies that stabilize the interaction of $DNA\text{-}PK_{cs}$ with Ku and the interaction of p70 with p80 are common (172,174).

Anti-Ku autoantibodies are found in a variety of autoimmune conditions. They originally were reported in sera of 55% of Japanese patients with polymyositis–scleroderma overlap syndrome (175). In American and European patients, anti-Ku antibodies are associated mainly with SLE or overlap syndromes, but also have been reported in scleroderma, polymyositis, Sjögren's syndrome, RA, and primary pulmonary hypertension (170,176,177). Estimates of the prevalence of anti-Ku antibodies vary widely (169,170,176), possibly reflecting differences in the prevalence of these antibodies in different racial groups (178). Anti-Ku antibodies can be detected by double immunodiffusion, ELISA, Western blot, or immunoprecipitation techniques (169).

Anti-Su

The Su antigen consists of proteins of 100, 102, and 200 kd (Fig. 74.4A) (179). The function and subcellular distribution of the Su antigen remain unknown. Although originally thought to be specific for SLE (180), anti-Su autoantibodies are found in other disease subsets, as well (179). The frequency of these autoantibodies is about 20% in SLE, scleroderma, and overlap syndromes, including MCTD, and lower in polymyositis, Sjögren's syndrome, or RA. Thus anti-Su antibodies are not a marker for any particular disease, nor is there evidence that they are associated with a particular clinical manifestation or that their levels fluctuate with disease activity.

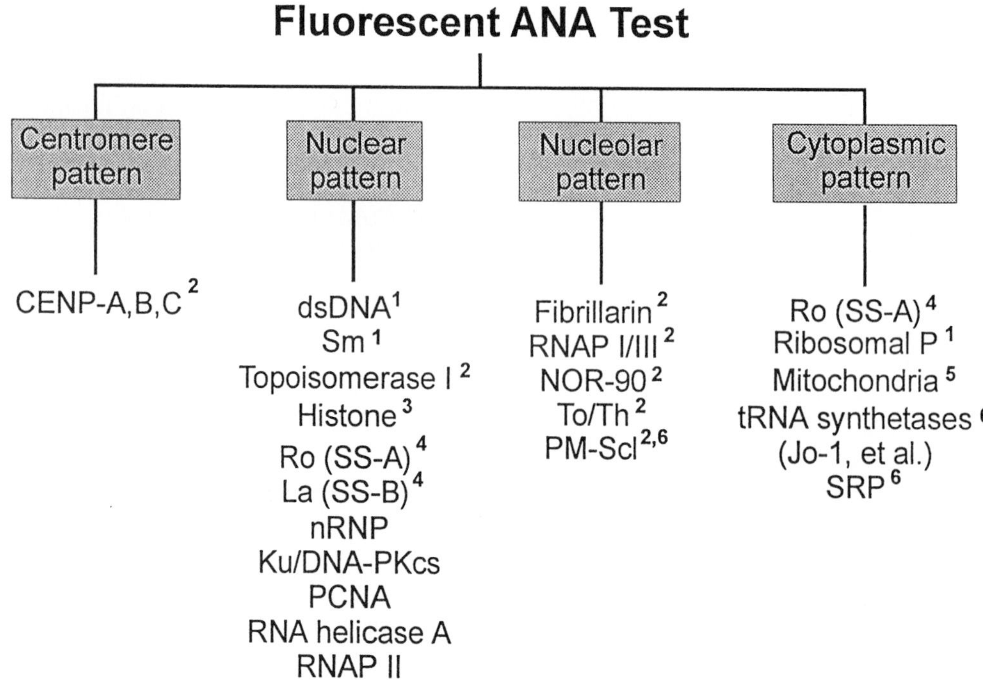

FIGURE 74.8. Algorithm for the evaluation of a positive fluorescent ANA test. Differential diagnoses for various patterns including centromere, nuclear (nucleoplasmic), nucleolar, and cytoplasmic are listed. Only autoantibody specificities with particular clinical relevance are shown. Disease associations are as follows: *1*, systemic lupus erythematosus; *2*, scleroderma or variants; *3*, drug-induced lupus; *4*, primary or secondary Sjögren's syndrome; *5*, primary biliary cirrhosis; *6*, polymyositis or dermatomyositis.

Anti-RNA Helicase A

RNA helicase A is a 140-kd double-stranded RNA binding factor that interacts selectively with the adenovirus virus–associated (VA) RNAII and certain other highly structured viral RNAs (181). It has been found to be the target of autoantibodies in lupus (Fig. 74.4A; RHA; H. Yoshida, M. Satoh, R. Lenfestey, and W.H. Reeves, unpublished data, 1999). Anti-RNA helicase A autoantibodies represent a new and potentially disease-specific serologic marker for lupus-like disease. However, larger numbers of patients must be evaluated to verify the prevalence and disease specificity of anti-RNA helicase antibodies in SLE.

Why Are Some Autoantibodies Disease Specific?

It is not certain why anti-dsDNA, Sm, and ribosomal P antibodies are found only in lupus, whereas anti–topoisomerase I, fibrillarin, and RNA polymerases I/III are specific for systemic sclerosis, and anti-tRNA synthetase antibodies are specific for myositis. Similar disease associations are found in mice: anti-dsDNA antibodies are produced by (NZB×W)F_1 mice (182), anti-dsDNA, Sm, and ribosomal P by MRL mice (182,183), and anti-Sm, DNA, and ribosomal P by BALB/c and SJL mice, respectively, which develop a lupus-like syndrome after pristane treatment (184,185). Autoantibodies could contribute directly to the disease process, as in the case of glomerulonephritis induced by certain anti-DNA antibodies (43). Alternatively, marker autoantibodies could reflect disease-specific immune mechanisms. The unanswered question of whether disease marker autoantibodies cause disease or reflect a unique aspect of the disease process is key to understanding the pathogenesis of SLE.

CLINICAL APPROACH TO A POSITIVE ANA

Testing for specific autoantibodies often is more useful clinically than is standard ANA testing. Nevertheless, the FANA is a useful screening test that can be used as a basis for further evaluation in much the same way as the hemoglobin and mean red cell volume are used to direct an anemia evaluation. Further evaluation of a high-titer positive ANA is warranted for both diagnostic and prognostic purposes. A flow chart based on the ANA pattern is illustrated in Fig. 74.8.

Centromere Pattern

Centromere staining (large punctate staining in the nucleus of interphase cells and of the condensed chromosomes of mitotic cells, (Fig. 74.4D) is a distinctive pattern that generally does not require further evaluation. However, it should be kept in mind that rare sera may produce a similar pattern without recognizing the major centromere autoantigens (CENP-B, 80 kd; CENP-A, 17 kd; or CENP-C, 140 kd) (186). Patients with limited clinical manifestations in the presence of anticentromere antibodies have a relatively high likelihood of developing additional manifestations of scleroderma over time, making their detection useful for assessing prognosis (187–189).

Nuclear (Nucleoplasmic) Pattern

A wide variety of ANAs produce nucleoplasmic staining of different patterns, including the diffuse (homogeneous) and speckled patterns illustrated in Fig. 74.4A and B. Because of the common occurrence of mixed patterns (e.g., diffuse plus speckled) and occasional difficulty classifying the staining pattern, we have combined all nucleoplasmic staining into a single differential diagnosis, which includes anti-dsDNA, Sm, topoisomerase I (Scl-70), histone, Ro (SS-A), and La (SS-B) (Fig. 74.8). Although the list is far from complete, the specificities indicated are the most useful ones clinically. As discussed earlier, anti-dsDNA and anti-Sm are of diagnostic value in SLE, and anti-dsDNA has been used for monitoring disease activity. Anti–topoisomerase I is a diagnostic marker for scleroderma, and its production may precede the onset of disease (188). Anti-Ro (SS-A) and La (SS-B) are included because of their utility in diagnosing primary or secondary Sjögren's syndrome and in monitoring lupus pregnancies. Anti-nRNP antibodies, although not disease specific, can be added to this list because of their association with overlap features (87). Antihistone and antichromatin antibodies may be useful in the evaluation of drug-induced lupus, as indicated earlier. Tests for anti-Ku/DNA-PK_{cs}, anti-PCNA, anti-RNA polymerase II, and anti-RNA helicase A may potentially be of value, but are best considered research procedures at present.

Nucleolar Pattern

Isolated nucleolar staining usually is associated with the diagnosis of scleroderma (9), although autoantibodies to a 100-kd nucleolar RNA helicase have been reported in patients with "watermelon stomach" (190). Clinically useful autoantibodies producing isolated nucleolar staining include antifibrillarin or U3 RNP (a 34-kd protein; Fig. 74.4C), anti-NOR-90 (94- and 96-kd doublet, Fig. 74.4C), and anti-Th or 7-2 and 8-2 RNP (RNase P and RNase MRP, respectively) (191,192). Anti-RNA polymerase I antibodies also produce an isolated nucleolar pattern. Finally, autoantibodies to the PM-Scl antigen, a complex of 10 or more nucleolar proteins including prominent 75- and 100-kd subunits, give nucleolar staining. These autoantibodies are associated with a subset of patients having an autoimmune syndrome with features of both polymyositis and scleroderma (193).

Cytoplasmic Pattern

The differential diagnosis of cytoplasmic staining includes anti-Ro (SS-A), ribosomal P, signal-recognition particle SRP, and a variety of tRNA synthetase antibodies (Table 74.3), as well as antimitochondrial antibodies. Most of the autoantibodies associated with polymyositis give a cytoplasmic pattern. These antibodies are predictive of disease in polymyositis (194). Their occurrence in a lupus patient may herald the onset of an overlap syndrome or a change in the disease course (195). In some cases, the appearance of myositis-specific autoantibodies in SLE may predate the onset of muscle disease by several years (196). Similarly, antimitochondrial antibodies specific for the dihydrolipoamide acetyltransferase component (E2) of pyruvate dehydrogenase can precede the onset of biliary cirrhosis by many years and may develop in patients with other autoimmune diseases, including lupus (197,198). A high percentage of asymptomatic individuals with these autoantibodies will go on to develop primary biliary cirrhosis (PBC) (197,198). We recently observed a lupus patient in whom the FANA pattern changed from nuclear to cytoplasmic (unpublished data). Further evaluation revealed the onset of antimitochondrial antibodies and a mildly elevated alkaline phosphatase. Liver biopsy was consistent with PBC.

Early detection of specific ANAs opens the door to timely clinical intervention. For example, treatment of early primary biliary cirrhosis with ursodeoxycholic acid may delay disease progression (199), and myositis is more responsive to steroid therapy if initiated early in the disease course (200). Early detection and treatment as well as information regarding prognosis are strong arguments for considering further evaluation of a positive ANA, especially in a young individual with a high titer on screening.

ORIGINS OF AUTOANTIBODIES

An understanding of the origins of ANAs remains elusive, despite intensive study. The B-cell subsets responsible for autoantibody production are heterogeneous, as is the requirement for T cells, antigen drive, and somatic hypermutation.

B-Cell Subsets

Two B-cell subsets have been defined. Conventional B cells are responsible for most high-affinity IgG antibodies. They are derived from the bone marrow, but undergo antigen-induced differentiation in the germinal centers of peripheral lymphoid organs. The B1 subset is thought to be a distinct lineage enriched in the peritoneal cavity that is self-renewing, and characterized by a unique phenotype ($CD23^-$, IgM^{hi}, IgD^{lo}, often but not always $CD5^+$). B1 cells produce mainly low-affinity, polyreactive, IgM antibodies (201).

Autoantibodies are produced by both B-cell subsets, but their characteristics differ. Anti-DNA antibodies and rheumatoid factors produced by the conventional B-cell subset tend to be high-affinity, monospecific IgG autoantibodies, whereas autoantibodies produced by the CD5$^+$ B-cell subset tend to be low-affinity, polyreactive IgMs (97,202). The CD5$^+$ B-cell subset is expanded in human rheumatoid arthritis and Sjögren's syndrome in association with rheumatoid factor production (203–205).

GENERATION OF AUTOANTIBODIES

Autoantibodies can be created during V(D)J recombination, or can arise as a consequence of antigen-stimulated and T cell–dependent somatic mutation and affinity maturation of the immunoglobulin variable regions (206). The relative importance of each mechanism in generating pathogenic autoantibodies is controversial. Once autoreactive B cells are generated, they are censored in the bone marrow or the periphery by a variety of mechanisms including anergy and deletion (207).

Unlike low-affinity, polyreactive anti-ssDNA autoantibodies produced by the B1 subset, which frequently bear germline Ig variable region sequences and may be only weakly dependent on T-cell help, conventional autoantibodies bear numerous somatic mutations and do not develop in the absence of T cells. Conventional autoantibodies, which are dependent on antigen-driven B-cell activation and T-cell help appear to be of major importance in lupus (208,209).

Role of T Cells

There is considerable evidence for the importance of T cells in autoantibody formation in murine lupus models (210–212). Autoantibodies and nephritis do not develop in T cell–deficient lupus mice (213,214). Moreover, treatment of MRL/lpr or (NZB/W)F_1 mice with anti-CD4 antibodies abrogates the production of anti-DNA antibodies (210,215), and these antibodies fail to develop in CD4-deficient lupus-prone mice (216). Autoreactive T cells specific for various autoantigens also have been identified in human SLE (217–220).

B7-CD28

Ligation of the T cell–antigen receptor signals cell death or anergy unless a co-stimulatory signal delivered by antigen-presenting cells also is delivered (221). The best-characterized co-stimulatory molecules are B7-1 and B7-2 (222). The CD28 molecule is the only receptor for B7-1 and B7-2 on naive T cells, but after activation, the higher affinity CTLA-4 receptor also is expressed (222,223). The primary role of CTLA-4 may be to downregulate antigen-specific T-cell responses, although it also can have stimulatory effects (223). CTLA-4–deficient or CD28-deficient mice have impaired IgG responses to T cell–dependent antigens (222), and humoral immune responses to exogenous antigens are profoundly inhibited by a fusion protein consisting of the extracellular domain of CTLA-4 bound to the immunoglobulin Cγ1 chain (CTLA4Ig) (224). Treatment of (NZB/W)F_1 mice with CTLA4Ig before the onset of autoimmunity dramatically reduces anti-dsDNA autoantibodies and prolongs survival (211).

CD40-CD40 Ligand (CD40L)

The CD40-CD40L system also plays an important role in autoantibody responses. CD40 is a surface receptor belonging to the tumor necrosis receptor family that is expressed constitutively on B cells. It binds to CD40 ligand (CD154), a T-cell surface protein related to tumor necrosis factor that is expressed on activated CD4$^+$ T cells (225). CD40L is essential for the formation of germinal centers in response to thymus-dependent antigens (225). CD40L deficiency abrogates the production of anti-dsDNA autoantibodies and ameliorates glomerulonephritis in MRL/lpr mice (226). Of potential therapeutic significance, when anti-CD40L treatment is combined with CTLA4Ig treatment, long-lasting inhibition of autoantibody production as well as glomerulonephritis can be achieved in (NZB/W)F_1 mice (227). The efficacy of therapy directed against B7-CD28 or CD40-CD40L now is being tested in SLE patients.

Role of Cytokines

Cytokines produced by two classes of helper T cells, designated T helper 1 (Th1) and T helper 2 (Th2) also influence autoantibody production. Cytokines produced by the Th1 subset include IL-2 and interferon-γ (IFN-γ), whereas those produced by the Th2 subset include IL-4 and IL-5, and IL-10 (228,229). The two subsets are regulated reciprocally by cytokines: IL-4 and IL-10 favor Th2 cytokine production, whereas IFN-γ and IL-12 favor Th1 cytokine production. In (NZB/W)F_1 mice, treatment with anti–IL-10 antibodies reduces the production of IgG anti-dsDNA antibodies and delays the onset of renal disease, suggesting that Th2 cytokines may contribute to autoantibody production (230). Overproduction of IL-4 also is linked with autoantibody production (231). However, the Th1 cytokine IFN-γ is likely to enhance autoantibody production and renal disease in other circumstances (232,233).

IL-6 also has been implicated in the pathogenesis of anti-DNA antibodies and nephritis in lupus mice (234,235). Moreover, patients with IL-6–secreting tumors, such as atrial myxomas, produce autoantibodies (236,237). Interestingly, elderly individuals produce increased amounts of IL-6 (238) and have a higher frequency of ANAs.

TRIGGERS OF AUTOANTIBODY PRODUCTION

How autoantibody production is initiated remains poorly understood. Several potential explanations have been offered, and multiple mechanisms could be at work. Three of the more popular hypotheses are molecular mimicry, altered self, and abnormal apoptosis.

Molecular Mimicry

Immunologic cross-reactivity of a self antigen with a non-self antigen can generate autoantibodies. This has been termed "molecular mimicry" (239). For example, immunologic cross-reactivity has been shown between a retroviral $p30^{gag}$ protein and the U1-70K component of the U1 snRNP (240). Autoantibodies that recognize phosphoamino acids or other common posttranslational modifications also have been reported. This may be relevant to the strong association of autoantibodies against the phosphorylated form of RNA polymerase II with antibodies to the phosphoprotein topoisomerase I in scleroderma patients (167).

Altered Self Hypothesis

Tolerance to self antigens is incomplete. Immunization with cryptic self peptides not usually presented by antigen-processing cells can elicit anti self T-cell responses (241). The binding of a foreign antigen to a self protein also can induce autoimmunity. For example, autoantibodies against the p53 tumor suppressor protein can be induced by immunizing mice with complexes of p53 with the simian virus 40 (SV40) large T antigen (242). The binding of SVT to self p53 may alter its processing by antigen-presenting cells, leading to the presentation of cryptic self peptides.

The "cryptic epitope" hypothesis could have far-reaching implications for autoimmunity because there are so many ways of generating altered self. These include the binding of a metal ion or drug to a self protein (243), abnormal degradation of self proteins (244), and alteration of a protein's structure by somatic mutation, as in the case of certain neoplastic diseases associated with autoantibody production (245).

Apoptotic Bleb Hypothesis

Several antigens recognized by lupus or scleroderma autoantibodies are sequestered in apoptotic blebs and degraded by interleukin (IL)-1β–converting enzyme-like proteases. Cleavage by these enzymes may define a class of autoantigens (246). Because apoptosis is a normal part of embryonic development, it might be predicted that only abnormal apoptosis events lead to autoimmunity, possibly by generating cryptic self peptides. The scleroderma autoantigens topoisomerase I, RNA polymerase II, and NOR-90 are uniquely fragmented by reactive oxygen species in an iron- or copper-dependent manner, raising the possibility that metal-catalyzed oxidation reactions might target a subset of antigens for autoimmunity (244).

CONCLUSION

Autoantibodies are important early markers of specific disease processes. Some may be involved directly in disease pathogenesis. They can induce disease by binding to their target antigens and initiating immune injury or indirectly through immune complex formation. Many of the specific autoantibodies associated with autoimmune diseases appear to be antigen selected and require T-cell help, characteristics most commonly associated with conventional B-cell responses. How these autoantibody responses are initiated and regulated is an area of active investigation. Therapy designed to interfere with autoantibody formation shows promise in mouse models and is undergoing human testing.

ACKNOWLEDGMENT

This work was supported by grants from the Arthritis Foundation and the United States Public Health Service (R01 AR40391). We thank Ms. Melody Shaw for expert technical assistance and Dr. Daniel McCauliffe (University of North Carolina, Department of Dermatology) for useful comments on the manuscript.

REFERENCES

1. Hargraves MM, Richmond H, Morton R. Presentation of two bone-marrow elements: the Tart cell and LE cell. *Proc Staff Meetings Mayo Clin* 1948;23:25.
2. Tan EM. Autoantibodies to nuclear antigens (ANA): their biology and medicine. *Adv Immunol* 1982;33:167.
3. Tan EM, Kunkel HG. Characteristics of a soluble nuclear antigen precipitating with sera of patients with systemic lupus erythematosus. *J Immunol* 1966;96:464.
4. Tan EM. Antinuclear antibodies: diagnostic markers for autoimmune diseases and probes for cell biology. *Adv Immunol* 1989;44:93.
5. Carpenter AB. Enzyme-linked immunoassays. In: Rose NR, Conway de Macario E, Folds JD, Lane HC, Nakamura RM, eds. *Manual of clinical laboratory immunology.* Washington, DC: ASM Press, 1997:20–29.
6. Johnson AM. Immunoprecipitation in gels. In: Rose NR, Friedman H, Fahey JL, eds. *Manual of clinical laboratory immunology.* Washington, DC: American Society for Microbiology, 1986: 14–24.
7. Towbin H, Staehelin T, Gordon J. Electrophoretic transfer of proteins from polyacrylamide gels to nitrocellulose sheets: pro-

cedure and some applications. *Proc Natl Acad Sci U S A* 1979;76:4350.
8. Lerner MR, Steitz JA. Antibodies to small nuclear RNAs complexed with proteins are produced by patients with systemic lupus erythematosus. *Proc Natl Acad Sci U S A* 1979;76:5495.
9. Reimer G, Steen VD, Penning CA, Medsger TA, Tan EM. Correlates between autoantibodies to nucleolar antigens and clinical features in patients with systemic sclerosis (scleroderma). *Arthritis Rheum* 1988;31:525.
10. Tan EM, Cohen AS, Fries JF, et al. The 1982 revised criteria for the classification of systemic lupus erythematosus. *Arthritis Rheum* 1982;25:1271.
11. Emlen W, O'Neill L. Clinical significance of antinuclear antibodies: comparison of detection with immunofluorescence and enzyme-linked immunosorbent assays. *Arthritis Rheum* 1997; 40:1612.
12. Shiel WC, Jason M. The diagnostic associations of patients with antinuclear antibodies referred to a community rheumatologist. *J Rheumatol* 1989;16:782.
13. Edworthy SM, Zatarain E, McShane DJ, Bloch DA. Analysis of the 1982 ARA lupus criteria data set by recursive partitioning methodology: new insights into the relative merit of individual criteria. *J Rheumatol* 1988;15:1493.
14. Slater CA, Davis RB, Schmerling RH. Antinuclear antibody testing. *Arch Intern Med* 1996;156:1421.
15. Hooper B, Whittingham S, Mathews JD, Mackay IR, Curnow DH. Autoimmunity in a rural community. *Clin Exp Immunol* 1972;12:79.
16. Hawkins BR, O'Connor KJ, Dawkins RL, Dawkins B, Rodger B. Autoantibodies in an Australian population. I. Prevalence and persistence. *J Clin Lab Immunol* 1979;2:211.
17. Tan EM, Feltkamp TE, Smolen JS, et al. Range of antinuclear antibodies in "healthy" individuals. *Arthritis Rheum* 1997; 40:1601.
18. Reeves WH, Chaudhary N, Salerno A, Blobel G. Lamin B autoantibodies in sera of certain patients with systemic lupus erythematosus. *J Exp Med* 1987;165:750.
19. Jaskowski TD, Schroder C, Martins TB, Mouritsen CL, Litwin CM, Hill HR. Screening for antinuclear antibodies by enzyme immunoassay. *Am J Clin Pathol* 1996;105:468.
20. Despres N, Boire G, Lopez-Longo FJ, Menard HA. The Sa system: a novel antigen-antibody system specific for rheumatoid arthritis. *J Rheumatol* 1994;21:1027.
21. Skriner K, Sommergruber WH, Tremmel V, et al. Anti-A2/RA33 autoantibodies are directed to the RNA binding region of the A2 protein of the heterogeneous nuclear ribonucleoprotein complex. *J Clin Invest* 1997;100:127.
22. Girbal-Neuhauser E, Durieux JJ, Arnaud M, et al. The epitopes targeted by the rheumatoid arthritis-associated antifilaggrin autoantibodies are posttranslationally generated on various sites of (pro)filaggrin by deimination of arginine residues. *J Immunol* 1999;162:585.
23. Schellekens GA, De Jong BA, van den Hoogen FH, Van de Putte LB, van Venrooij WJ. Citrulline is an essential constituent of antigenic determinants recognized by rheumatoid arthritis-specific autoantibodies. *J Clin Invest* 1998;101:273.
24. Friou GJ. Identification of the nuclear component of the interaction of lupus erythematosus globulin with nuclei. *J Immunol* 1958;80:476.
25. Burlingame RW, Boey ML, Starkebaum G, Rubin RL. The central role of chromatin in autoimmune responses to histones and DNA in systemic lupus erythematosus. *J Clin Invest* 1994; 4:184.
26. Burlingame RW, Rubin RL. Drug-induced anti-histone autoantibodies display two patterns of reactivity with substructures of chromatin. *J Clin Invest* 1991;88:680.
27. Monestier M, Kotzin BL. Antibodies to histones in systemic lupus erythematosus and drug-induced lupus syndromes. *Rheum Dis Clin North Am* 1992;18:415.
28. Rubin RL. Histone (H2A-H2B)-DNA autoantibodies. In: Peter JB, Shoenfeld Y, eds. *Autoantibodies.* Amsterdam: Elsevier Science, 1996:364–372.
29. Bustin M, Reisch J, Einck L, Klippel JH. Autoantibodies to nucleosomal proteins: antibodies to HMG-17 in autoimmune diseases. *Science* 1982;215:1245.
30. Monestier M, Fasy TM, Bohm L. Monoclonal anti-histone H1 autoantibodies from MRL lpr/lpr mice. *Mol Immunol* 1989; 26:749.
31. Totoritis MC, Tan EM, McNally EM, Rubin RL. Association of antibody to histone complex H2A-H2B with symptomatic procainamide-induced lupus. *N Engl J Med* 1988;318:1431.
32. Burlingame RW, Rubin RL. Histones. In: van Venrooij WJ, Maini RN, eds. *Manual of biological markers of disease.* Dordrecht: Kluwer Academic Publishers, 1994:1–28.
33. Rubin RL, Burlingame RW, Arnott JE, Totoritis MC, McNally EM, Johnson AD. IgG but not other classes of anti-[(H2A-H2B)-DNA] is an early sign of procainamide-induced lupus. *J Immunol* 1995;154:2483.
34. Weinstein A, Bordwell B, Stone B, Tibbetts C, Rothfield NF. Antibodies to native DNA and serum complement (C3) levels: application to diagnosis and classification of systemic lupus erythematosus. *Am J Med* 1983;74:206.
35. Yoshida H, Kohno A, Ohta K, Hirose S, Maruyama N, Shirai T. Genetic studies of autoimmunity in New Zealand mice. III. Associations among anti-DNA antibodies, NTA, and renal disease in (NZB×NZW)F_1 × NZW backcross mice. *J Immunol* 1981;127:433.
36. Koffler D, Agnello V, Carr RI, Kunkel HG. Anti-DNA antibodies and the renal lesions of patients with systemic lupus erythematosus. *Transplant Proc* 1969;1:933.
37. Rumore PM, Steinman CR. Endogenous circulating DNA in systemic lupus erythematosus: occurrence as multimeric complexes bound to histone. *J Clin Invest* 1990;86:69.
38. Raz E, Brezis M, Rosenmann E, Eilat D. Anti-DNA antibodies bind directly to renal antigens and induce kidney dysfunction in the isolated perfused rat kidney. *J Immunol* 1989;142:3076.
39. Lefkowith JB, Gilkeson GS. Nephritogenic autoantibodies in lupus: current concepts and continuing controversies. *Arthritis Rheum* 1996;39:894.
40. Schur PH, Sandson J. Immunologic factors and clinical activity in systemic lupus erythematosus. *N Engl J Med* 1968;278:533.
41. Gladman DD, Urowitz MB, Keystone EC. Serologically active clinically quiescent systemic lupus erythematosus: a discordance between clinical and serological features. *Am J Med* 1979; 66:210.
42. Vlahakos DV, Foster MH, Adams S, et al. Anti-DNA antibodies form immune deposits at distinct glomerular and vascular sites. *Kidney Int* 1992;41:1690.
43. Ohnishi K, Ebling FM, Mitchell B, Singh RR, Hahn BH, Tsao BP. Comparison of pathogenic and non-pathogenic murine antibodies to DNA: antigen binding and structural characteristics. *Int Immunol* 1994;6:817.
44. Sabbaga J, Line SRP, Potocnjak P, Madaio MP. A murine nephritogenic monoclonal anti-DNA autoantibody binds directly to mouse laminin, the major non-collagenous protein component of the glomerular basement membrane. *Eur J Immunol* 1989;19:137.
45. D'Andrea DM, Coupaye-Gerard B, Kleyman TR. Lupus autoantibodies interact directly with distinct glomerular and vascular cell surface antigens. *Kidney Int* 1996;49:1214.
46. Rothfield NF, Stollar BD. The relation of immunoglobulin class, pattern of anti-nuclear antibody, and complement-fixing

antibodies to DNA in sera from patients with systemic lupus erythematosus. *J Clin Invest* 1967;46:1785.
47. Beaulieu A, Quismorio FP, Kitridou RC, Friou GJ. Complement fixing antibodies to ds-DNA in systemic lupus erythematosus: a study using the immunofluorescent *Crithidia luciliae* method. *J Rheumatol* 1979;6:389.
48. Esparza RH, Swaak T, Aarden L, Smeenk R. Complement-fixing antibodies to dsDNA detected by the immunofluorescence technique on *Crithidia luciliae: a critical appraisal.* J Rheumatol 1985;12:1109.
49. Leon SA, Green A, Ehrlich GE, Poland M, Shapiro B. Avidity of antibodies in SLE: relation to severity of renal involvement. *Arthritis Rheum* 1977;20:23.
50. Smeenk RJT, Berden JHM, Swaak AJG. dsDNA autoantibodies. In: Peter JB, Shoenfeld Y, eds. *Autoantibodies.* Amsterdam: Elsevier Science, 1996:227–236.
51. Steward MW, Katz FE, West NJ. The role of low affinity antibody in immune complex disease: the quantity of anti-DNA antibodies in NZB/W F_1 hybrid mice. *Clin Exp Immunol* 1975; 21:121.
52. Locker JD, Medof ME, Bennett RM, Sukhupunyaraksa S. Characterization of DNA used to assay sera for anti-DNA antibodies; determination of the specificities of anti-DNA antibodies in SLE and non-SLE rheumatic disease states. *J Immunol* 1977;118:694.
53. Sontheimer RD, Gilliam JN. An immunofluorescence assay for double-stranded DNA antibodies using *Crithidia luciliae* kinetoplast as a double-stranded DNA substrate. *J Lab Clin Med* 1978;91:550.
54. Wold RT, Young FE, Tan EM, Farr RS. Deoxyribonucleic acid antibody: a method to detect its primary interaction with deoxyribonucleic acid. *Science* 1968;161:806.
55. Emlen W, Pisetsky DS, Taylor RP. Antibodies to DNA: a perspective. *Arthritis Rheum* 1986;29:1417.
56. ter Borg EJ, Horst G, Hummel EJ, Limburg PC, Kallenberg CGM. Measurement of increases in anti-double-stranded DNA antibody levels as a predictor of disease exacerbation in systemic lupus erythematosus. *Arthritis Rheum* 1990;33:634.
57. Bootsma H, Spronk P, Derksen R, et al. Prevention of relapses in systemic lupus erythematosus. *Lancet* 1995;345:1595.
58. Mattioli M, Reichlin M. Characterization of a soluble nuclear ribonucleoprotein antigen reactive with SLE sera. *J Immunol* 1971;107:1281.
59. Craft J. Antibodies to snRNPs in systemic lupus erythematosus. *Rheum Dis Clin North Am* 1992;18:311.
60. Kurata N, Tan EM. Identification of antibodies to nuclear acidic antigens by counterimmunoelectrophoresis. *Arthritis Rheum* 1976;19:574.
61. Bernstein RM, Bunn CC, Hughes GRV, Francoeur AM, Mathews MB. Cellular protein and RNA antigens in autoimmune disease. *Mol Biol Med* 1984;2:105.
62. Arnett FC, Hamilton RG, Roebber MG, Harley JB, Reichlin M. Increased frequencies of Sm and nRNP autoantibodies in American blacks compared to whites with systemic lupus erythematosus. *J Rheumatol* 1988;15:1773.
63. Fisher DE, Conner GE, Reeves WH, Wisniewolski R, Blobel G. Small nuclear ribonucleoprotein particle assembly in vivo: demonstration of a 6S RNA-free core precursor and posttranslational modification. *Cell* 1985;42:751.
64. Query CC, Bentley RC, Keene JD. A common RNA recognition motif identified within a defined U1 RNA binding domain of the 70K U1 snRNP protein. *Cell* 1989;57:89.
65. Nelissen RLH, Will CL, van Venrooij WJ, Luhrmann R. The association of the U1-specific 70K and C proteins with U1 snRNPs is mediated in part by common U snRNP proteins. *EMBO J* 1994;13:4113.
66. Padgett RA, Mount SM, Steitz JA, Sharp PA. Splicing of messenger RNA precursors is inhibited by antisera to small nuclear ribonucleoproteins. *Cell* 1983;35:101.
67. Padgett RA, Grabowski PJ, Konarska MM, Seiler S, Sharp PA. Splicing of messenger RNA precursors. *Annu Rev Biochem* 1986;55:1119.
68. Grabowski PJ, Seiler SR, Sharp PA. A multicomponent complex is involved in the splicing of messenger RNA precursors. *Cell* 1985;42:345.
69. Satoh M, Langdon JJ, Hamilton KJ, et al. Distinctive immune response patterns of human and murine autoimmune sera to U1 small nuclear ribonucleoprotein C protein. *J Clin Invest* 1996;97:2619.
70. Satoh M, Richards HB, Hamilton KJ, Reeves WH. Human anti-nRNP autoimmune sera contain a novel subset of autoantibodies that stabilizes the molecular interaction of U1RNP-C protein with the Sm core proteins. *J Immunol* 1997;158:5017.
71. Pettersson IM, Hinterberger M, Mimori T, Gottlieb E, Steitz JA. The structure of mammalian small nuclear ribonucleoproteins: identification of multiple protein components reactive with anti-(U1)RNP and anti-Sm antibodies. *J Biol Chem* 1984; 259:5907.
72. Mattioli M, Reichlin M. Physical association of two nuclear antigens and mutual occurrence of their antibodies: the relationship of the Sm and RNA protein (Mo) systems in SLE sera. *J Immunol* 1973;110:1318.
73. Reeves WH, Fisher DE, Lahita RG, Kunkel HG. Autoimmune sera reactive with Sm antigen contain high levels of RNP-like antibodies. *J Clin Invest* 1985;75:580.
74. Brahms H, Raker VA, van Venrooij WJ, Luhrmann R. A major, novel systemic lupus erythematosus autoantibody class recognizes the E, F, and G Sm snRNP proteins as an E-F-G complex but not in their denatured states. *Arthritis Rheum* 1997;40:672.
75. Deutscher SL, Keene JD. A sequence-specific conformational epitope on U1 RNA is recognized by a unique autoantibody. *Proc Natl Acad Sci U S A* 1988;85:3299.
76. Hoet RM, de Weerd P, Gunnewiek JK, Koornneef I, van Venrooij WJ. Epitope regions of U1 small nuclear RNA recognized by anti-U1RNA-specific autoantibodies. *J Clin Invest* 1992; 90:1753.
77. van Venrooij WJ, Hoet R, Hageman B, Mattaj IW, Van de Putte LB. Anti-(U1) small nuclear RNA antibodies in anti-small nuclear ribonucleoprotein sera from patients with connective tissue diseases. *J Clin Invest* 1990;86:2154.
78. Hardin JA. The lupus autoantigens and the pathogenesis of SLE. *Arthritis Rheum* 1986;29:457.
79. Habets WJ, Sillekens PTG, Hoet MH, McAllister G, Lerner MR, van Venrooij WJ. Small nuclear RNA-associated proteins are immunologically related as revealed by mapping of autoimmune reactive B-cell epitopes. *Proc Natl Acad Sci U S A* 1989; 86:4674.
80. James JA, Harley JB. Linear epitope mapping of an Sm B/B′ polypeptide. *J Immunol* 1992;148:2074.
81. Nojima Y, Minota S, Yamada A, Takaku F. Identification of an acidic ribosomal protein reactive with anti-Sm autoantibody. *J Immunol* 1989;143:1915.
82. Hasegawa H, Uchiumi T, Sato T, Arakawa M, Kominami R. Anti-Sm autoantibodies cross-react with ribosomal protein S10: a common structural unit shared by the small nuclear RNP proteins and the ribosomal protein. *Arthritis Rheum* 1998;41:1040.
83. Caponi L, Bombardieri S, Migliorini P. Anti-ribosomal antibodies bind the Sm proteins D and B/B′. *Clin Exp Immunol* 1998;112:139.
84. Bloom DD, Davignon JL, Cohen PL, Eisenberg RA, Clarke SH. Overlap of the anti-Sm and anti-DNA responses of MRL/Mp-lpr/lpr mice. *J Immunol* 1993;150:1579.

85. Reichlin M, Martin A, Taylor Albert E, et al. Lupus autoantibodies to native DNA cross-react with the A and D SnRNP polypeptides. *J Clin Invest* 1994;93:443.
86. Northway JD, Tan EM. Differentiation of antinuclear antibodies giving speckled staining patterns in immunofluorescence. *Clin Immunol Immunopathol* 1972;1:140.
87. Sharp GC, Irvin WS, Tan EM, Gould RG, Holman HR. Mixed connective tissue disease: an apparently distinct rheumatic disease syndrome associated with a specific antibody to an extractable nuclear antigen (ENA). *Am J Med* 1972;52:148.
88. Hirohata S, Kosaka M. Association of anti-Sm antibodies with organic brain syndrome secondary to systemic lupus erythematosus. *Lancet* 1994;343:796.
89. Sirota P, Firer M, Schild K, et al. Increased anti-Sm antibodies in schizophrenic patients and their families. *Prog Neuropsychopharmacol Biol Psychiatry* 1993;17:793.
90. Amital H, Klemperer I, Blank M, et al. Analysis of autoantibodies among patients with primary and secondary uveitis: high incidence in patients with sarcoidosis. *Int Arch Allergy Appl Immunol* 1992;99:34.
91. Winn DM, Wolfe JF, Lindberg DA, Fristoe FH, Kingsland L, Sharp GC. Identification of a clinical subset of systemic lupus erythematosus by antibodies to the Sm antigen. *Arthritis Rheum* 1979;22:1334.
92. Homma M, Mimori T, Takeda Y, et al. Autoantibodies to the Sm antigen: immunological approach to clinical aspects of systemic lupus erythematosus. *J Rheumatol* 1987;14(suppl):188.
93. Gulko PS, Reveille JD, Koopman JP, Burgard SL, Bartolucci AA, Alarcon GS. Survival impact of autoantibodies in systemic lupus erythematosus. *J Rheumatol* 1994;21:224.
94. Barada FAJ, Andrews BS, Davis JSI, Taylor RP. Antibodies to Sm in patients with systemic lupus erythematosus: correlation of Sm antibody titers with disease activity and other laboratory parameters. *Arthritis Rheum* 1981;24:1236.
95. Hoet RM, Koornneef I, de Rooij DJ, Van de Putte LB, van Venrooij WJ. Changes in anti-U1 RNA antibody levels correlate with disease activity in patients with systemic lupus erythematosus overlap syndromes. *Arthritis Rheum* 1992;35:1202.
96. Nishikai M, Okano Y, Mukohda Y, Sato A, Ito M. Serial estimation of anti-RNP antibody titers in systemic lupus erythematosus, mixed connective tissue disease and rheumatoid arthritis. *J Clin Lab Immunol* 1984;13:15.
97. Casali P, Burastero SE, Balow JE, Notkins AL. High-affinity antibodies to ssDNA are produced by CD-5 cells in systemic lupus erythematosus patients. *J Immunol* 1989;143:3476.
98. Anderson JR, Gray KG, Beck JS, Kinnear WF. Precipitating autoantibodies in Sjögren's disease. *Lancet* 1961;2:456.
99. Clark G, Reichlin M, Tomasi TB. Characterization of a soluble cytoplasmic antigen reactive with sera from patients with systemic lupus erythematosus. *J Immunol* 1969;102:117.
100. Alspaugh MA, Tan EM. Antibodies to cellular antigens in Sjögren's syndrome. *J Clin Invest* 1975;55:1067.
101. Alspaugh M, Maddison P. Resolution of the identity of certain antigen-antibody systems in systemic lupus erythematosus and Sjögren's syndrome: an interlaboratory collaboration. *Arthritis Rheum* 1979;22:796.
102. Ben-Chetrit E, Fox RI, Tan EM. Dissociation of immune responses to the SS-A (Ro) 52-kd and 60-kd polypeptides in systemic lupus erythematosus and Sjögren's syndrome. *Arthritis Rheum* 1990;33:349.
103. Tzioufas AG, Moutsopoulos HM. Clinical significance of autoantibodies to Ro/SSA and La/SSB. In: van Venrooij WJ, Maini RN, eds. *Autoantibody manual.* Dordrecht: Kluwer Academic Publishers, 1999:1–14.
104. Wasicek CA, Reichlin M. Clinical and serological differences between systemic lupus erythematosus patients with autoantibodies to Ro versus patients with antibodies to Ro and La. *J Clin Invest* 1982;69:835.
105. Chan EKL, Buyon JP. The SS-A/Ro antigen. In: van Venrooij WJ, Maini RN, eds. *Manual of biological markers of disease.* Dordrecht: Kluwer Academic Publishers, 1994:1–18.
106. Ben-Chetrit E, Chan EKL, Sullivan KF, Tan EM. A 52 kd protein is a novel component of the SS-A/Ro antigenic particle. *J Exp Med* 1988;167:1560.
107. Kelekar A, Saitta MR, Keene JD. Molecular composition of Ro small ribonucleoprotein complexes in human cells: intracellular localization of the 60- and 52-kD proteins. *J Clin Invest* 1994; 93:1637.
108. Slobbe RL, Pluk W, van Venrooij WJ, Pruijn GJM. Ro ribonucleoprotein assembly in vitro identification of RNA-protein and protein-protein interactions. *J Mol Biol* 1992;227:361.
109. Rinke J, Steitz JA. Precursor molecules of both human 5S ribosomal RNA and transfer RNAs are bound by a cellular protein reactive with anti-La lupus antibodies. *Cell* 1982;29:149.
110. Stefano JE. Purified lupus antigen La recognizes an oligouridylate stretch common to 3′ termini of RNA polymerase III transcripts. *Cell* 1984;36:145.
111. Kenan DJ, Query CC, Keene JD. RNA recognition: towards identifying determinants of specificity. *Trends Biochem Sci* 1991;16:214.
112. Pruijm GJM, Slobbe RL, van Venrooij WJ. Structure and function of La and Ro RNPs. *Mol Biol Rep* 1990;14:43.
113. Gottlieb E, Steitz JA. The RNA binding protein La influences both the accuracy and the efficiency of RNA polymerase III transcription in vitro. *EMBO J* 1989;8:841.
114. Bachmann M, Pfeifer K, Schroder HC, Muller EG. Characterization of the autoantigen La as a nucleic acid-dependent ATPase/dATPase with melting properties. *Cell* 1990;60:85.
115. Yell JA, Wang L, Yin H, McCauliffe DP. Disparate locations of the 52- and 60-kDa Ro/SS-A antigens in cultured human keratinocytes. *J Invest Dermatol* 1996;107:622.
116. Mattioli M, Reichlin M. Heterogeneity of RNA protein antigens reactive with sera of patients with systemic lupus erythematosus: description of a cytoplasmic nonribosomal antigen. *Arthritis Rheum* 1974;17:421.
117. Boulanger C, Chabot B, Menard H, Boire G. Autoantibodies in human anti-Ro sera specifically recognize deproteinized hY5 Ro RNA. *Clin Exp Immunol* 1995;99:29.
118. Alspaugh MA, Talal N, Tan EM. Differentiation and characterization of autoantibodies and their antigens in Sjögren's syndrome. *Arthritis Rheum* 1976;19:216.
119. Harley JB, Alexander EL, Bias WB, et al. Anti-Ro (SS-A) and anti-La (SS-B) in patients with Sjögren's syndrome. *Arthritis Rheum* 1986;29:196.
120. McCauliffe DP. Cutaneous diseases in adults associated with anti-Ro/SS-A autoantibody production. *Lupus* 1997;6:158.
121. Andonopoulos AP, Skopouli FN, Dimou GS, Drosos AA, Moutsopoulos HM. Sjögren's syndrome in systemic lupus erythematosus. *J Rheumatol* 1990;17:201.
122. Sontheimer RD, Maddison PJ, Reichlin M, Jordon RE, Stastny P, Gilliam JN. Serologic and HLA associations in subacute cutaneous lupus: a clinical subset of lupus erythematosus. *Ann Intern Med* 1982;97:664.
123. Lee LA, Gaither KK, Coulter SN, Norris DA, Harley JB. Pattern of cutaneous immunoglobulin G deposition in subacute cutaneous lupus erythematosus is reproduced by infusing purified anti-Ro (SSA) autoantibodies into human skin-grafted mice. *J Clin Invest* 1989;83:1556.
124. Buyon JP. Congenital complete heart block. *Lupus* 1993;2:291.
125. Petri M. Systemic lupus erythematosus and pregnancy. *Rheum Dis Clin North Am* 1994;20:87.
126. McCauliffe DP. Neonatal lupus erythematosus: a transplacen-

tally acquired autoimmune disorder. *Semin Dermatol* 1995; 14:47.
127. Buyon JP, Ben-Chetrit E, Karp S, et al. Acquired congenital heart block: pattern of maternal antibody response to biochemically defined antigens of the SSA/Ro-SSB/La system in neonatal lupus. *J Clin Invest* 1989;84:627.
128. Buyon JP, Swersky SH, Fox HE, Bierman FZ, Winchester RJ. Intrauterine therapy for presumptive fetal myocarditis with acquired heart block due to systemic lupus erythematosus. *Arthritis Rheum* 1987;30:44.
129. Reichlin M, Brucato A, Frank MB, et al. Concentration of autoantibodies to native 60-kd Ro/SS-A and denatured 52-kd Ro/SS-A in eluates from the heart of a child who died with congenital complete heart block. *Arthritis Rheum* 1994;37:1698.
130. Li JM, Horsfall AC, Maini RN. Anti-La(SS-B) but not anti-Ro52 (SS-A) antibodies cross-react with laminin: a role in the pathogenesis of congenital heart block? *Clin Exp Immunol* 1995;99:316.
131. Litsey SE, Noonan JA, O'Connor WN, Cottrill CM, Mitchell B. Maternal connective tissue disease and congenital heart block. *N Engl J Med* 1985;312:98.
132. Scott JS, Maddison PJ, Taylor PV, Esscher E, Scott O, Skinner RP. Connective-tissue disease, antibodies to ribonucleoprotein, and congenital heart block. *N Engl J Med* 1983;309:209.
133. McCauliffe DP, Wang L, Satoh M, Reeves WH, Small D. Recombinant 52 kDa Ro(SSA) ELISA detects autoantibodies in Sjögren's syndrome sera that go undetected by conventional serologic assays. *J Rheumatol* 1997;24:860.
134. Pruijn GJM. The La (SS-B) antigen. In: van Venrooij WJ, Maini RN, eds. *Manual of biological markers of disease.* Dordrecht: Kluwer Academic Publishers, 1994:1–14.
135. Itoh Y, Reichlin M. Autoantibodies to the Ro/SSA antigen are conformation dependent. I: anti-60 kD antibodies are mainly directed to the native protein: anti-52 kD antibodies are mainly directed to the denatured protein. *Autoimmunity* 1992;14:57.
136. Tzuzaka K, Fujii T, Akizuki M, et al. Clinical significance of antibodies to native or denatured 60-kd or 52-kd Ro/SS-A proteins in Sjögren's syndrome. *Arthritis Rheum* 1994;37:88.
137. St. Clair EW, Pisetsky DS, Reich CF, Chambers JC, Keene JD. Quantitative immunoassay of anti-La antibodies using purified recombinant La antigen. *Arthritis Rheum* 1988;31:506.
138. Chan EK, Hamel JC, Buyon JP, Tan EM. Molecular definition and sequence motifs of the 52-kD component of human SS-A/Ro autoantigen. *J Clin Invest* 1991;87:68.
139. McCauliffe DP, Yin H, Wang LX, Lucas L. Autoimmune sera react with multiple epitopes on recombinant 52 and 60 kDa Ro(SSA) proteins. *J Rheumatol* 1994;21:1073.
140. Wolin SL, Steitz JA. The Ro small cytoplasmic ribonucleoproteins: identification of the antigenic protein and its binding site on the Ro RNAs. *Proc Natl Acad Sci U S A* 1984;81:1996.
141. Buyon JP, Slade SG, Reveille JD, Hamel JC, Chan EKL. Autoantibody responses to "native" 52 kD SS-A/Ro protein in neonatal lupus syndromes, systemic lupus erythematosus, and Sjögren's syndrome. *J Immunol* 1994;152:3675.
142. Sturgill BC, Carpenter RR. Antibody to ribosomes in systemic lupus erythematosus. *Arthritis Rheum* 1965;8:213.
143. Schur PH, Moroz LA, Kunkel HG. Precipitating antibodies to ribosomes in the serum of patients with systemic lupus erythematosus. *Immunochemistry* 1967;4:447.
144. Miyachi K, Tan EM. Antibodies reacting with ribosomal ribonucleoprotein in connective tissue diseases. *Arthritis Rheum* 1979;22:87.
145. Elkon KB, Parnassa AP, Foster CL. Lupus autoantibodies target ribosomal P proteins. *J Exp Med* 1985;162:459.
146. Francoeur A-M, Peebles CL, Heckman KJ, Lee JC, Tan EM. Identification of ribosomal protein autoantigens. *J Immunol* 1985;135:2378.
147. Elkon K, Skelly S, Parnassa A, et al. Identification and chemical synthesis of a ribosomal protein antigenic determinant in systemic lupus erythematosus. *Proc Natl Acad Sci U S A* 1986; 83:7419.
148. Bonfa E, Parnassa AP, Rhoads DD, Roufa DJ, Wool IG, Elkon KB. Antiribosomal S10 antibodies in humans and MRL/lpr mice with systemic lupus erythematosus. *Arthritis Rheum* 1989; 32:1252.
149. Steitz JA, Berg C, Hendrick JP, et al. A 5S rRNA/L5 complex is a precursor to ribosome assembly in mammalian cells. *J Cell Biol* 1988;106:545.
150. Chu J-L, Brot M, Weissbach H, Elkon K. Lupus antiribosomal P antisera contain antibodies to a small fragment of 28S rRNA located in the proposed ribosomal GTPase center. *J Exp Med* 1991;174:507.
151. Elkon KB, Bonfa E, Brot N. Antiribosomal antibodies in systemic lupus erythematosus. *Rheum Dis Clin North Am* 1992; 18:377.
152. Bonfa E, Golombek SJ, Kaufman LD, et al. Association between lupus psychosis and anti-ribosomal P protein antibodies. *N Engl J Med* 1987;317:265.
153. Schneebaum AB, Singleton JD, West SG, Blodgett JK, Allen LG, Cheronis JC. Association of psychiatric manifestations with antibodies to ribosomal P proteins in systemic lupus erythematosus. *Am J Med* 1991;90:54.
154. Teh LS, Isenberg DA. Antiribosomal P protein antibodies in systemic lupus erythematosus. *Arthritis Rheum* 1994;37:307.
155. van Dam A, Nossent H, de Jong J, et al. Diagnostic value of antibodies against ribosomal phosphoproteins: a cross sectional and longitudinal study. *J Rheumatol* 1991;18:1026.
156. Arnett FC, Reveille JD, Moutsopoulos HM, Georgescu L, Elkon KB. Ribosomal P autoantibodies in systemic lupus erythematosus. *Arthritis Rheum* 1996;39:1833.
157. Miyachi K, Fritzler MJ, Tan EM. Autoantibody to a nuclear antigen in proliferating cells. *J Immunol* 1978;121:2228.
158. Takasaki Y, Fishwild D, Tan EM. Characterization of proliferating cell nuclear antigen recognized by autoantibodies in lupus sera. *J Exp Med* 1984;159:981.
159. Bravo R, Frank R, Blundell PA, Macdonald-Bravo H. Cyclin/PCNA is the auxiliary protein of DNA polymerase-delta. *Nature* 1987;326:515.
160. Prelich G, Tan KK, Kostura M, et al. Functional identity of proliferating cell nuclear antigen and a DNA polymerase-delta auxiliary protein. *Nature* 1987;326:517.
161. Bravo R, Macdonald-Bravo H. Existence of two populations of cyclin/proliferating cell nuclear antigen during the cell cycle: association with DNA replication sites. *J Cell Biol* 1987; 105:1549.
162. Fritzler MJ, McCarty GA, Ryan JP, Kinsella TD. Clinical features of patients with antibodies directed against proliferating cell nuclear antigen. *Arthritis Rheum* 1983;26:140.
163. Young RA. RNA polymerase II. *Annu Rev Biochem* 1991; 60:689.
164. Kuwana M, Okano Y, Kaburaki J, Medsger TA, Wright TM. Autoantibodies to RNA polymerases recognize multiple subunits and demonstrate cross-reactivity with RNA polymerase complexes. *Arthritis Rheum* 1999;42:275.
165. Hirakata M, Okano Y, Pati U, et al. Identification of autoantibodies to RNA polymerase II: occurrence in systemic sclerosis and association with autoantibodies to RNA polymerase I and III. *J Clin Invest* 1993;91:2665.
166. Satoh M, Ajmani AK, Ogasawara T, et al. Autoantibodies to RNA polymerase II are common in systemic lupus erythematosus and overlap syndrome: specific recognition of the phospho-

rylated (IIO) form by a subset of human sera. *J Clin Invest* 1994;94:1981.
167. Satoh M, Kuwana M, Ogasawara T, et al. Association of autoantibodies to topoisomerase I and the phosphorylated (IIO) form of RNA polymerase II in Japanese scleroderma patients. *J Immunol* 1994;153:5838.
168. Reimer G, Rose KM, Scheer U, Tan EM. Autoantibody to RNA polymerase I in scleroderma sera. *J Clin Invest* 1987; 79:65.
169. Reeves WH, Wang J, Ajmani AK, Stojanov L, Satoh M. The Ku autoantigen. In: Zanetti M, Capra JD, eds. *The antibodies.* Amsterdam: Harwood Academic Publishers, 1997:33–84.
170. Reeves WH. Use of monoclonal antibodies for the characterization of novel DNA-binding proteins recognized by human autoimmune sera. *J Exp Med* 1985;161:18.
171. Mimori T, Hardin JA, Steitz JA. Characterization of the DNA-binding protein antigen Ku recognized by autoantibodies from patients with rheumatic disorders. *J Biol Chem* 1986;261:2274.
172. Wang J, Dong X, Stojanov L, Kimpel D, Satoh M, Reeves WH. Human autoantibodies stabilize the quaternary structure of Ku antigen. *Arthritis Rheum* 1997;40:1344.
173. Suwa A, Hirakata M, Takeda Y, et al. Autoantibodies to DNA-dependent protein kinase: probes for the catalytic subunit. *J Clin Invest* 1996;97:1417.
174. Satoh M, Ajmani AK, Stojanov LP, et al. Autoantibodies that stabilize the molecular interaction of Ku antigen with DNA dependent protein kinase catalytic subunit. *Clin Exp Immunol* 1996;105:460.
175. Mimori T, Akizuki M, Yamagata H, Inada S, Yoshida S, Homma M. Characterization of a high molecular weight acidic nuclear protein recognized by autoantibodies from patients with polymyositis-scleroderma overlap. *J Clin Invest* 1981;68: 611.
176. Yaneva M, Arnett FC. Antibodies against Ku protein in sera from patients with autoimmune diseases. *Clin Exp Immunol* 1989;76:366.
177. Isern RA, Yaneva M, Weiner E, et al. Autoantibodies in patients with primary pulmonary hypertension: association with anti-Ku. *Am J Med* 1992;93:307.
178. Kuwana M, Okano Y, Kaburaki J, Tojo T, Medsger TA. Racial differences in the distribution of systemic sclerosis-related serum antinuclear antibodies. *Arthritis Rheum* 1994;37:902.
179. Satoh M, Langdon JJ, Chou CH, et al. Characterization of the Su antigen: a macromolecular complex of 100/102 and 200 kDa proteins recognized by autoantibodies in systemic rheumatic diseases. *Clin Immunol Immunopathol* 1994;73:132.
180. Treadwell EL, Alspaugh MA, Sharp GC. Characterization of a new antigen-antibody system (Su) in patients with systemic lupus erythematosus. *Arthritis Rheum* 1984;27:1263.
181. Liao HJ, Kobayashi R, Mathews MB. Activities of adenovirus virus-associated RNAs: purification and characterization of RNA binding proteins. *Proc Natl Acad Sci U S A* 1998;95:8514.
182. Theofilopoulos AN, Dixon FJ. Murine models of systemic lupus erythematosus. *Adv Immunol* 1985;37:269.
183. Elkon KB, Bonfa E, Llovet R, Eisenberg RA. Association between anti-Sm and anti-ribosomal P protein autoantibodies in human systemic lupus erythematosus and MRL/lpr mice. *J Immunol* 1989;143:1549.
184. Satoh M, Reeves WH. Induction of lupus-associated autoantibodies in BALB/c mice by intraperitoneal injection of pristane. *J Exp Med* 1994;180:2341.
185. Satoh M, Hamilton KJ, Ajmani AK, et al. Autoantibodies to ribosomal P antigens with immune complex glomerulonephritis in SJL mice treated with pristane. *J Immunol* 1996; 157:3200.
186. Casiano CA, Landberg G, Ochs RL, Tan EM. Autoantibodies to a novel cell cycle-regulated protein that accumulates in the nuclear matrix during S phase and is localized in the kinetochores and spindle midzone during mitosis. *J Cell Sci* 1993; 106:1045.
187. Tramposch HD, Smith CD, Senecal JL, Rothfield N. A long-term longitudinal study of anticentromere antibodies. *Arthritis Rheum* 1984;27:121.
188. Weiner ES, Hildebrandt S, Senecal JL, et al. Prognostic significance of anticentromere antibodies and anti-topoisomerase I antibodies in Raynaud's disease. *Arthritis Rheum* 1991;34:68.
189. Fritzler MJ, Kinsella TD, Garbutt E. The CREST syndrome: a distinct serologic entity with anticentromere antibodies. *Am J Med* 1980;69:520.
190. Arnett FC, Reveille JD, Valdez BC. Autoantibodies to a nucleolar RNA helicase protein in patients with connective tissue diseases. *Arthritis Rheum* 1997;40:1487.
191. Gold HA, Topper JN, Clayton DA, Craft J. RNA processing enzyme RNase MRP is identical to the Th RNP and related to RNase P. *Science* 1989;245:1377.
192. Okano Y, Medsger TA. Autoantibody to Th ribonucleoprotein (nucleolar 7-2 RNA protein particle) in patients with systemic sclerosis. *Arthritis Rheum* 1990;33:1822.
193. Alderuccio F, Chan EKL, Tan EM. Molecular characterization of an autoantigen of PM-Scl in the polymyositis/scleroderma overlap syndrome: a unique and complete human cDNA encoding an apparent 75-kD acidic protein of the nucleolar complex. *J Exp Med* 1991;173:941.
194. Miller FW, Twitty SA, Biswas T, Plotz PH. Origin and regulation of a disease-specific autoantibody response: antigenic epitopes, spectrotype stability, and isotype restriction of anti-Jo-1 autoantibodies. *J Clin Invest* 1990;85:468.
195. Satoh M, Miyazaki K, Mimori T, et al. Changing autoantibody profiles with variable clinical manifestations in a patient with relapsing systemic lupus erythematosus and polymyositis. *Br J Rheumatol* 1995;34:915.
196. Stojanov L, Satoh M, Hirakata M, Reeves WH. Correlation of anti-synthetase antibody levels with disease course in a patient with interstitial lung disease and elevated muscle enzymes: quantitation of anti-glycyl tRNA synthetase antibodies by immunoprecipitation. *J Clin Rheumatol* 1996;2:89.
197. Metcalf JV, Mitchison HC, Palmer JM, Jones DE, Bassendine MF, James OFW. Natural history of early primary biliary cirrhosis. *Lancet* 1996;348:1399.
198. Mitchison HC, Lucey MR, Kelly PJ, Neuberger JM, Williams R, James OFW. Symptom development and prognosis in primary biliary cirrhosis: a study in two centers. *Gastroenterology* 1990;99:778.
199. Poupon RE, Balkau B, Eschwege E, Poupon R, UDCA-PBC Study Group. A multicenter, controlled trial of ursodiol for the treatment of primary biliary cirrhosis. *N Engl J Med* 1991; 324:1548.
200. Joffe MM, Love LA, Fraser DD, Hicks JE, Plotz PH, Miller FW. Drug therapy of the idiopathic inflammatory myopathies: predictors of response to prednisone, azathioprine, and methotrexate and a comparison of their efficacy. *Am J Med* 1993;94:379.
201. Hardy RR, Hayakawa K. CD5 B cells, a fetal B cell lineage. *Adv Immunol* 1994;55:297.
202. Casali P, Notkins AL. $CD5^+$ B lymphocytes, polyreactive antibodies and the human B-cell repertoire. *Immunol Today* 1989;10:364.
203. Hardy RR, Hayakawa K, Shimizu M, Yamasaki K, Kishimoto T. Rheumatoid factor secretion from human $Leu\text{-}1^+$ B cells. *Science* 1987;236:81.
204. Plater-Zyberk C, Maini RN, Lam K, Kennedy TD, Janossy G. A rheumatoid arthritis B cell subset expresses a phenotype sim-

ilar to that in chronic lymphocytic leukemia. *Arthritis Rheum* 1985;28:971.

205. Dauphinee M, Tovar Z, Talal N. B cells expressing CD5 are increased in Sjögren's syndrome. *Arthritis Rheum* 1988;31:642.
206. Davidson A, Shefner R, Livneh A, Diamond B. The role of somatic mutation of immunoglobulin genes in autoimmunity. *Annu Rev Immunol* 1987;5:85.
207. Goodnow CC, Cyster JG, Hartley SB, et al. Self-tolerance checkpoints in B lymphocyte development. *Adv Immunol* 1995; 59:279.
208. Shlomchik M, Mascelli M, Shan H, et al. Anti-DNA antibodies from autoimmune mice arise by clonal expansion and somatic mutation. *J Exp Med* 1990;171:265.
209. Reap EA, Sobel ES, Cohen PL, Eisenberg RA. Conventional B cells, not B-1 cells, are responsible for producing autoantibodies in lpr mice. *J Exp Med* 1993;177:69.
210. Wofsy D, Seaman WE. Successful treatment of autoimmunity in NZB/NZW F_1 mice with monoclonal antibody to L3T4. *J Exp Med* 1985;161:378.
211. Finck BK, Linsley PS, Wofsy D. Treatment of murine lupus with CTLA4Ig. *Science* 1994;265:1225.
212. Sobel ES, Kakkanaiah VN, Kakkanaiah M, Cheek RL, Cohen PL, Eisenberg RA. T-B collaboration for autoantibody production in lpr mice is cognate and MHC-restricted. *J Immunol* 1994;152:6011.
213. Mihara M, Ohsugi Y, Saito K, et al. Immunologic abnormality in NZB/NZW F_1 mice: thymus-independent occurrence of B cell abnormality and requirement for T cells in the development of autoimmune disease, as evidenced by an analysis of the athymic nude individuals. *J Immunol* 1988;141:85.
214. Richards HB, Satoh M, Jennette JC, Okano T, Kanwar YS, Reeves WH. Disparate T cell requirements of two subsets of lupus-specific autoantibodies in pristane-treated mice. *Clin Exp Immunol* 1999;115:547.
215. Santoro TJ, Portanova JP, Kotzin BL. The contribution of L3T4$^+$ T cells to lymphoproliferation and autoantibody production in MRL-lpr/lpr mice. *J Exp Med* 1988;167:1713.
216. Koh DR, Ho A, Rahemtulla A, Fung-Leung WP, Griesser H, Mak TW. Murine lupus in MRL/lpr mice lacking CD4 or CD8 T cells. *Eur J Immunol* 1995;25:2558.
217. Hoffman RW, Takeda Y, Sharp GC, et al. Human T cell clones reactive against U-small nuclear ribonucleoprotein autoantigens from connective tissue disease patients and healthy individuals. *J Immunol* 1993;151:6460.
218. Okubo M, Yamamoto K, Kato T, et al. Detection and epitope analysis of autoantigen-reactive T cells to the U1-small nuclear ribonucleoprotein A protein in autoimmune disease patients. *J Immunol* 1993;151:1108.
219. Crow MK, DelGuidice-Asch G, Zehetbauer JB, et al. Autoantigen-specific T cell proliferation induced by the ribosomal P2 protein in patients with systemic lupus erythematosus. *J Clin Invest* 1994;94:345.
220. Rajagopalan S, Zordan T, Tsokos GC, Datta SK. Pathogenic anti-DNA autoantibody-inducing T helper cell lines from patients with active lupus nephritis: isolation of CD4-8$^-$ T helper cell lines that express the gamma delta T-cell antigen receptor. *Proc Natl Acad Sci U S A* 1990;87:7020.
221. Harding FA, McArthur JG, Gross JA, Raulet DH, Allison JP. CD28-mediated signalling co-stimulates murine T cells and prevents induction of anergy in T-cell clones. *Nature* 1992; 356:607.
222. Lenschow DJ, Walunas TL, Bluestone JA. CD28/B7 system of T cell costimulation. *Annu Rev Immunol* 1996;14:233.
223. Bluestone JA. Is CTLA-4 a master switch for peripheral T cell tolerance? *J Immunol* 1997;158:1989.
224. Linsley PS, Wallace PM, Johnson J, et al. Immunosuppression in vivo by a soluble form of the CTLA-4 T cell activation molecule. *Science* 1992;257:792.
225. Laman JD, Claassen E, Noelle RJ. Functions of CD40 and its ligand, gp39 (CD40L). *Crit Rev Immunol* 1996;16:59.
226. Ma J, Xu J, Madaio MP, et al. Autoimmune lpr/lpr mice deficient in CD40 ligand: spontaneous Ig class switching with dichotomy of autoantibody responses. *J Immunol* 1996;157:417.
227. Daikh DI, Finck BK, Linsley PS, Hollenbaugh D, Wofsy D. Long-term inhibition of murine lupus by brief simultaneous blockade of the B7/CD28 and CD40/gp39 costimulation pathways. *J Immunol* 1997;159:3104.
228. Romagnani S. Lymphokine production by human T cells in disease states. *Annu Rev Immunol* 1994;12:227.
229. Hagiwara E, Klinman DM. Abnormalities in cytokine production and responsiveness in autoimmune disease. In: Snapper CM, ed. *Cytokine regulation of humoral immunity:* basic and clinical aspects. Chichester, UK: John Wiley & Sons, 1996: 409–430.
230. Ishida H, Muchamuel T, Sakaguchi S, Andrade S, Menon S, Howard M. Continuous administration of anti-interleukin 10 antibodies delays onset of autoimmunity in NZB/W F_1 mice. *J Exp Med* 1994;179:305.
231. Erb KJ, Ruger B, von Brevern M, Ryffel B, Schimpl A, Rivett K. Constitutive expression of interleukin (IL)-4 in vivo causes autoimmune-type disorders in mice. *J Exp Med* 1997;185:329.
232. Jacob CO, van der Meide PH, McDevitt HO. In vivo treatment of (NZB × NZW)F_1 lupus-like nephritis with monoclonal antibody to gamma interferon. *J Exp Med* 1987;166:798.
233. Ozmen L, Roman D, Fountoulakis M, Schmid G, Ryffel B, Garotta G. Experimental therapy of systemic lupus erythematosus: the treatment of NZB/W mice with mouse soluble interferon-gamma receptor inhibits the onset of glomerulonephritis. *Eur J Immunol* 1995;25:6.
234. Alarcón Riquelme ME, Moller G, Fernandez C. Macrophage depletion decreases IgG anti-DNA in cultures from (NZB × NZW)F_1 spleen cells by eliminating the main source of IL-6. *Clin Exp Immunol* 1993;91:220.
235. Richards HB, Satoh M, Shaw M, Libert C, Poli V, Reeves WH. IL-6 dependence of anti-DNA antibody production: evidence for two pathways of autoantibody formation in pristane-induced lupus. *J Exp Med* 1998;188:985.
236. Hirano T, Taga T, Yasukawa K, et al. Human B-cell differentiation factor defined by an anti-peptide antibody and its possible role in autoantibody production. *Proc Natl Acad Sci U S A* 1987;84:228.
237. Jourdan M, Bataille R, Seguin J, Zhang XG, Chaptal PA, Klein B. Constitutive production of interleukin-6 and immunologic features in cardiac myxomas. *Arthritis Rheum* 1990;33:398.
238. Fagiolo U, Cossarizza A, Scala E, et al. Increased cytokine production in mononuclear cells of healthy elderly people. *Eur J Immunol* 1993;23:2375.
239. Oldstone MBA. Molecular mimicry and autoimmune disease. *Cell* 1987;50:819.
240. Query CC, Keene JD. A human autoimmune protein associated with U1 RNA contains a region of homology that is cross-reactive with retroviral p30^{gag} antigen. *Cell* 1987;51:211.
241. Cibotti R, Kanellopoulos JM, Cabaniols JP, et al. Tolerance to a self protein involves its immunodominant but does not involve its subdominant determinants. *Proc Natl Acad Sci U S A* 1992;89:416.
242. Dong X, Hamilton KJ, Satoh M, Wang J, Reeves WH. Initiation of autoimmunity to the p53 tumor suppressor protein by complexes of p53 and SV40 large T antigen. *J Exp Med* 1994; 179:1243.
243. Griem P, Gleichmann E. Metal ion induced autoimmunity. *Curr Opin Immunol* 1995;7:831.

244. Casciola-Rosen L, Wigley F, Rosen A. Scleroderma autoantigens are uniquely fragmented by metal-catalyzed oxidation reactions: implications for pathogenesis. *J Exp Med* 1997;185:71.
245. Soussi T. The humoral response to the tumor-suppressor gene-product p53 in human cancer: implications for diagnosis and therapy. *Immunol Today* 1996;17:354.
246. Casciola-Rosen LA, Anhalt GJ, Rosen A. DNA-dependent protein kinase is one of a subset of autoantigens specifically cleaved early during apoptosis. *J Exp Med* 1995;182:1625.
247. Fujii T, Mimori T, Akizuki M. Detection of autoantibodies to nucleolar transcription factor nor 90/hUBF in sera of patients with rheumatic diseases, by recombinant autoantigen-based assays. *Arthritis Rheum* 1996;39:1313.
248. Werle E, Blazek M, Fiehn W. The clinical significance of measuring different anti-dsDNA antibodies by using the Farr assay, an enzyme immunoassay and a *Crithidia luciliae* immunofluorescence test. *Lupus* 1992;1:369.
249. Ginsberg B, Keiser H. A Millipore filter assay for antibodies to native DNA in sera of patients with systemic lupus erythematosus. *Arthritis Rheum* 1973;16:199.
250. Smeenk RJT. DNA as antigen in SLE. In: van Venrooij WJ, Maini RN, eds. *Manual of biological markers of disease.* Dordrecht: Kluwer Academic Publishers, 1994:1–15.
251. Brinkman K, Termaat R, Van den Brink H, Berden J, Smeenk R. The specificity of the anti-dsDNA ELISA: a closer look. *J Immunol Methods* 1991;91.

75

SYSTEMIC LUPUS ERYTHEMATOSUS: PATHOGENESIS

KARIN S. PETERSON
ROBERT J. WINCHESTER

Systemic lupus erythematosus (SLE) is a distinctive chronic, immune-mediated multisystem disease, occurring in a genetically predisposed individual, that results from an autoimmune recognition event in which T cells play a critical initiating role. The characteristic immune response is driven by certain self antigens and involves cells of both the T- and B-cell compartments (Table 75.1). This immune activation results in the conspicuous production of certain autoantibodies, and accordingly SLE has been considered a classic immune complex–mediated autoimmune disorder. However, evidence is increasing for a separate role of the T cell as a direct effector of some tissue injury.

This chapter synthesizes the pathogenic events underlying SLE that are initiated by the inheritance of susceptibility genes and culminate in the production of a sustained and injurious autoimmune response. The discussion begins with an approach to conceptualizing the etiology and pathogenesis of SLE, followed by a description of the immunologic phenomena in the autoimmune response contributing to tissue injury. The current understanding of susceptibility genes and how they may operate to cause this inappropriate but otherwise physiologic immune response is then discussed, followed by sections on the development and nature of the pathogenic immune response and how it mediates tissue injury.

TABLE 75.1. IMMUNOLOGIC CHARACTERISTICS THAT DEFINE SYSTEMIC LUPUS ERYTHEMATOSUS (SLE)

Evidence of a coordinated cognitive autoimmune response in both T- and B-cell compartments centered on an immune recognition event involving self peptide presented by MHC molecules to T cells
Driven by a limited number of self antigens composing elements of one or a few cellular organelle particles, notably, nucleochromatin, Sm and related snRNPs composing the spliceosome, and the SS-A/Ro, SS-B/La hYRNA species
Results in the production of high concentrations of pathogenic IgG autoantibodies, immune complexes or antibody-mediated cellular attack; activated autoreactive T cells are present and found infiltrating tissues in areas of inflammation
Genetic susceptibility involves several genes including ones identified as MHC class II alleles, and others that are still incompletely defined

IgG, immunoglobulin G; hYRNA, human RNAs Y-5; MHC, major histocompatibility complex; snRNP, small nuclear ribonucleoprotein.

CURRENT PARADIGM

Conceptualizing the complex events in the pathogenesis of SLE is aided by distinguishing several theoretic stages through which an individual progresses until a point is arrived where SLE can be diagnosed. This begins with a genetic predisposition and culminates in the production of pathogenic autoantibodies and autoreactive effector T cells. Based on clinical and laboratory information, four main theoretic stages can be postulated (Fig. 75.1).

Predisposition

An individual in this stage has inherited the susceptibility genes for SLE but is without any evidence of disease or immunologic abnormalities. The genetic basis includes certain allelic major histocompatibility complex (MHC) molecules and several other genes that are still incompletely or entirely unidentified. The MHC genes appear to act to influence the shaping of the T-cell repertoire toward one capable of self recognition through presentation of self peptides that result in the autoimmune state recognized clinically as SLE. The predisposition state likely also includes genes that either promote a sustained autoimmune response following the initial activation or, in some way, lower the threshold for self reactivity. Apart from the presence of certain MHC alleles, this stage is currently difficult to identify. An example would be a healthy identical twin whose sib has

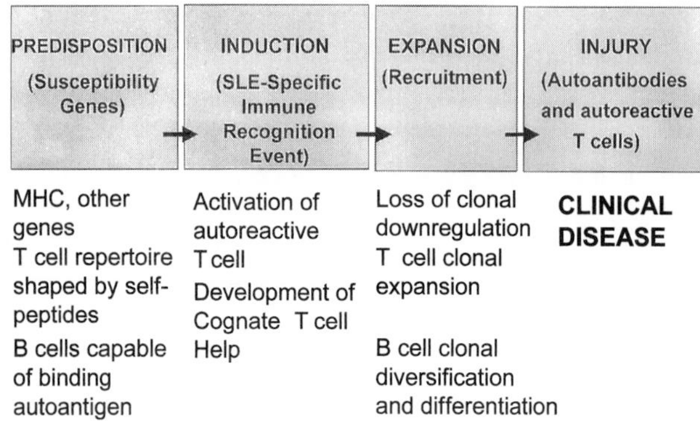

FIGURE 75.1. Four theoretic stages of systemic lupus erythematosus (SLE) through which an individual progresses, beginning with a genetic predisposition and culminating in the production of pathogeneic antibodies and autoreactive T cells. Based on clinical and laboratory information, these four main theoretic stages can be postulated.

developed SLE. The conversion of the predisposition phase into the next phase involves abrogation of the still incompletely understood phenomenon of "self tolerance."

Induction Phase

This precursor state to SLE is characterized by the development of autoreactive T cells that no longer remain "tolerized" to self. These initially expand slowly. Limited T-cell help for B cells having surface immunoglobulin (Ig) specific for autoantigens may be demonstrable. The individual in this phase of the development of the disease may produce small amounts of IgM autoantibodies to one or perhaps two members of a linked set of autoantigens. The titer and affinity of these antinuclear autoantibodies is likely to be very low, and sequence studies would show that the genes encoding the autoantibodies are in, or near to, the germ line configuration. Effector or memory autoreactive T cells may be present but in numbers too low to cause damage or be readily detected. This individual is without any overt disease and exhibits, at most, minimal evidence of autoimmunity.

Expansion Phase

The expansion phase is another preclinical SLE state and is characterized by considerable clonal expansion of B and T cells capable of autorecognition. The clonal expansion and activation are produced as a result of autoantigen drive. This phase includes development of considerable T-cell help to shift autoantibody isotype to IgG, likely occurring through presentation of self peptides to T cells by B cells reactive to autoantigen. Antibodies are of higher affinity and titer and include evidence of B-cell somatic diversification. This reflects cognitive interactions of T and B cells that occur in germinal centers. Autoreactive T cells are present in higher numbers, and there may be evidence of epitope spreading among the reactive B and T cells. By definition, although these patients have an autoimmune state, they are symptom-free and do not have an autoimmune disease. Regulatory interactions likely operate in this and the previous inductive phase to allow the autoreactive immune response to decay.

Injury Phase

In this phase, the disease of clinical SLE develops with the provision of autoantibodies of the appropriate specificity, IgG class, and maturing affinity as well as an accessible autoantigen molecule for initiation of immune complex–mediated injury. The number of autoreactive T cells is increased and may display a predominance of either a T-helper 1 (Th1)- or a Th2-type cytokine profile. The nature of the infiltrating T cell is likely to show correlation with the clinical pattern of disease (e.g., autoreactive Th1 cells having the potential to mediate direct tissue injury alone or in concert with cells of the monocytic lineage). The role of cellular immune effector responses in the injury phase of SLE is likely to be very important, but represents an evolving area of active research and is less well documented than immune complex–mediated injury. Secondary immunologic alterations appear, and the process of injury begets more autoimmune injury. Certain of the phenomena involved in the injury phase may spontaneously revert to an earlier level of disease evolution, resulting in a clinical remission through the action of mechanisms that regulate immune responsiveness. Antiinflammatory and potent immunosuppressive therapies are employed to control the processes of autoimmune injury. Of central importance, newer therapies are being developed to modulate, specifically, the immune response by affecting cognitive interactions, regulatory circuits, and the repertoire of responsible cells. These therapies hold singular promise to fundamentally improve the outlook of a patient with SLE.

THE DIAGNOSIS, RELATIONSHIP TO OTHER AUTOIMMUNE DISEASES, AND CLINICAL HETEROGENEITY OF SLE

While there is little doubt about the major characteristics of SLE, which have been highlighted by the syndromic classification criteria (1) and discussed in Chapter 73, some patients clearly challenge our understanding of what is and is not SLE. The criteria have been developed for accurate classification of series of patients (1). Accordingly, they have sacrificed sensitivity for specificity and are not designed to be a sensitive tool useful to either the physician or the investigator in determining whether a given person has or does not have SLE. For example, application of the classification criteria likely underestimates the prevalence of SLE in the population, the number of affected relatives, and the concordance rates in twins, and also effectively excludes other pathogenically irrelevant disorders with different autoimmune features.

There are two contrasting objectives in development of classification criteria. The clinical investigator requires a highly sensitive set of criteria to identify SLE and the presence of incomplete forms of the disorder. On the other hand, from the viewpoint of the patient and the treating physician, it is highly inappropriate to brand a patient as having SLE, with its associated set of defined serious outcomes, if the patient does not meet the same criteria as those with SLE who were used to identify these outcomes. The diagnosis "undifferentiated autoimmune state" is sometimes useful in this circumstance (see Chapter 72). The classification criteria for SLE aim at distinguishing SLE from entities included in the loosely applied terms *lupus* or *lupus-like. Lupus* is perhaps too often used to denote a disease with some general laboratory features of autoimmunity and clinical findings that do not meet the classification criteria. For example, the relationship of discoid lupus to SLE is still incompletely resolved. Although few patients with discoid lupus meet the criteria for classification as SLE, with the passage of time about 10% develop an illness that meets the criteria for SLE. In contrast, although drug-induced lupus is placed under the broad grouping of lupus, the various drug-induced lupus disorders are sharply distinguished from SLE by differences in epidemiology, autoantibody profile, clinical features, and genetic susceptibility.

A more challenging problem is found in the relationship of SLE to the clinical overlap syndromes that exhibit some features of SLE. This suggests that SLE is heterogeneous and may contain several clinical subsets such as subacute cutaneous SLE. Patients with subacute cutaneous SLE usually meet all of the SLE criteria and share common features of genetic susceptibility. Mixed connective tissue disease (MCTD) is less closely related to SLE. The syndrome of MCTD appears to result from the production of one of a group of specific autoantibodies including those directed to U1 ribonucleoprotein (RNP) species (2). Some members of this group of antibodies occur in SLE where they may be associated with features of the syndrome of MCTD, although this is not always the case. These antibodies also occur in other conditions that clearly have a different etiology (3), likely accounting for the nosologic uncertainty associated with MCTD. With time, a person who presents with findings of MCTD may evolve either into SLE or another illness (4). This problem of diagnostic sensitivity and heterogeneity in classification is of central importance in our thinking about SLE, because it ultimately defines the patients who are included in studies to determine the mechanism of disease.

Although the criteria for the classification of SLE have been established to facilitate the identification of patients with SLE in studies, it is also clear that SLE encompasses many different phenotypes. These vary from a mild disease, characterized by skin rash and joint pain that requires little medication, to life-threatening involvement of the brain, kidney, and blood vessels. In a particular patient with SLE, the pattern of organ involvement and autoantibody production tends to remain in the same clinical category, especially after the initial years of disease (5).

The question of what phenotype should be taken as the starting point for clinical investigation remains unanswered. This is important in the characterization of the proband, and especially so in the ascertainment of affected family members, where different phenotypes may exist. In view of the increasing evidence of immunologic subphenotypes, which has received clear support from murine studies, it is likely that future genetic epidemiologic studies will use various immunologic markers or features that define subphenotypes rather than rely exclusively on the occurrence of disease that meets classification criteria.

EPIDEMIOLOGIC FEATURES AND THE INSIGHTS THEY PROVIDE INTO SLE PATHOGENESIS

Epidemiologic information highlights the potential phenotypic and genetic complexity of the disease described above, while directing attention to the factors acting to determine susceptibility and induction of the autoimmune state. In the future, this information should be useful for providing additional insight into pathogenesis and for identifying candidate genes.

Incidence and Prevalence

The influence of sex, age at onset, and ethnicity on the relative risk of developing SLE provide major clues to still incompletely identified genes affecting susceptibility to the disease. This subject has been informatively reviewed by Hochberg (6). The female preponderance is reflected by incidence rates of SLE in a study performed in Baltimore from 1970 to 1977 revealing 0.4 cases per 100,000 Caucasian males and 3.9 cases per 100,000 Caucasian females. In contrast, among African Americans the rates are 2.5 and 11.4 per 100,000 males and females, respectively.

Age of onset is influenced by both ethnicity and sex. In instances of SLE occurring in individuals over 65 years of age, the female to male predominance drops to a less than three to one ratio. Black females primarily develop SLE in early adulthood. The maximal age-specific incidence rate is 20 per 100,000 in those 25 to 34 years of age. But in Caucasians, SLE is not a disease of young women, since Caucasian females primarily develop SLE in late middle life, with a maximal age-specific incidence rate of 15.9 per 100,000 in the 45- to 64-year-old age group (6).

These ethnic differences in incidence and prevalence of SLE might at first be thought to involve environmental events such as socioeconomic factors; however, the most probable explanation is that the African American and Caucasian races differ in their frequencies of particular susceptibility genes mapping outside the MHC that regulate the immune response. For example, ethnicity influences the development of tertiary neurosyphilis in the opposite sense. General paresis is 28 times more likely to occur in a syphilis-infected Caucasian male than in an infected African American female (7).

Female Preponderance of SLE Remains a Puzzle

The nature of the trait that predisposes women to develop SLE is still the subject of intense inquiry. There are two general explanations for the distorted sex ratio in SLE. The first is based on the role of sex determination and female hormones on the immune response. The second focuses on an undefined gene on the X chromosome that exerts its effect either by being present in a double dose or through a recessive-dominant effect (8). If the latter were found, the random inactivation of portions of the X chromosome could contribute to the divergence in concordance rates in female identical twins.

Although the pattern of age-specific incidence in women certainly does not precisely parallel age-related alterations in the levels of female hormones and differs between African American and Caucasian females, it is still difficult to avoid an obvious explanation of the female preponderance based on hormones. Lahita and co-workers (9,10) have argued that female sex hormones selectively predispose to SLE, and that males develop SLE only when they exhibit hormonal patterns similar to those found in females. Males with SLE are reported to have levels of 16α-hydroxyestrone and prolactin resembling those in females (11). Both of these hormones have been reported to upmodulate certain immunologic functions that may be relevant to SLE (12). Other hormones like glucocorticoids and prolactin are also known to have immunomodulatory effects. Glucocorticoids that are also produced in the thymus may have a role on negative and positive selection, and tolerance to self antigens (13).

INSIGHTS INTO SLE FROM ANIMAL MODELS OF AUTOIMMUNITY

Although none of the murine autoimmune diseases appears to represent a precise equivalent of SLE, these spontaneous diseases of autoimmunity provide major insights into the genetic regulation of autoimmunity and into disease processes that may operate in SLE (14–17). The F1 hybrid of New Zealand black and New Zealand white mice, (NZB × NZW)F1, has a markedly accelerated development of glomerulonephritis compared to either of the parental strains. The F1 exhibits a pattern of autoantibody production similar to that found in some patients with SLE. The Medical Research Laboratory lymphoproliferative (MRL-*lpr/lpr*) mouse and the BXSB mouse which carries the disease-associated gene, Yaa, on the Y chromosome, are two other models of spontaneous murine autoimmunity that also have certain similarities to SLE.

Studies of the (NZB × NZW)F1 mouse have been particularly informative in delineating the genetic complexity of the predisposition to autoimmunity and the relationship of genetic control to the immunologic elements composing the autoimmune phenotype in these mice (16). These genetic approaches are only possible in experimental animal studies. Experimental crosses among these mice have been performed, generating hundreds of meioses from a single set of parents, with low genetic heterogeneity (parental inbred strains), and have allowed the study of more complex interactions. Through back-crosses and other breeding approaches, the number of genes determining susceptibility are beginning to emerge. Several quantitative trait loci (QTL) controlling aspects of the autoimmune processes in each strain have been identified (18,19), some overlapping the same genomic regions in different crosses, and some overlapping with genomic regions involved in the regulation of other experimental models of autoimmunity (17). The results of this approach have provided interesting candidate genes and have identified some 31 susceptibility regions or suppressor regions in the murine genome that control autoimmunity (16). The relative importance of these regions and the precise genes responsible for susceptibility have largely not yet been identified.

Several conclusions are evident from the studies on the (NZB × NZW)F1 mouse. First, the autoimmune phenotype is under the control of multiple genes acting to foster or suppress its expression. Second, epistatic interactions among genes are important in the development of autoimmune disease. Third, many genetic regions identified are syntenic to regions in the human chromosome that contain candidate genes potentially relevant to SLE (Table 75.2) (17). Fourth, the primary autoimmune phenotype can be deconstructed into a number of clinical and immunologic subphenotypes or autoimmune states that are under separate genetic control, and which together account for the primary phenotype. By extrapolation to SLE, these data also indicate the potential for genetically controlled mechanisms to be identified, which help to explain how different clinical patterns of disease develop in individuals from the same family and how a subclinical state of disordered autoimmunity is sometimes found in still other members of the family.

The MLR-*lpr/lpr* strain carries a mutation in the death receptor, Fas. Engagement of the Fas receptor by Fas ligand (FasL) is the first step in one of the best-studied pathways of apoptosis. Homozygosity for this mutation in the mouse leads to the accumulation of double negative ($CD4^-$, $CD8^-$) T cells through the failure of thymocytes to undergo apop-

TABLE 75.2. SUSCEPTIBILITY LOCI IN MURINE LUPUS AND THEIR HOMOLOGOUS HUMAN CYTOGENETIC LOCATION[a]

Mouse Chromosome	Murine Locus[b]	Mouse Chromosome Location (centimorgan, cM)	Homologous Human Cytogenetic Band
1	*Sle1*	66–106	1q31-q32, 1q25-q25, 1q21-q23, 1q41-q43[c]
1	*Lbw7*	66–92.3	1q32,[e] 1q23
1	*Nba2*	94–95.8	1q21-q23
1	Drake et al.[d]	80–92.5	1q31-q32, 1q23
4	*Sle2*	27.8–45	9q31-q32, 1p31-p32
4	*Lbw2*	44.9–59.1	1p32-p31, 1p33-p32
4	*Nba1;* Rozzo et al.[f]	55.6–69.8	1p35, 1p35-p34, 1p36
4	Drake et al.[d]	62.3	1p36-p35
7	*Sle3*	23–37	19q13-q13, 15q11-q13, 15q26[e]
7	Drake et al.[d]	51	11p15
11	*Lbw8*	28–40	5q31, 17p11-p12[e]
11	Rozzo et al.[f]	2–17	16p13 or 5q31,[e] 7p13-p12
17	*Lbw1*	24.5	6p21[c]
17	*Sle4*	24.5	6p21[c]
17	Rozzo et al.[f]	24.5	6p21[c]
18	*Lbw6*	24–47	5q22 or 5q23,[e] 18q21-q21

[a]Mouse-human homologies based on the Mouse Genome Database (http://www.informatics.jax.org/mgd.html), and the National Institutes of Health Human-Mouse Homology Relationships (http://www.ncbi.nlm.nih.gob/homology).
[b]Murine lupus loci reviewed in ref. 16.
[c]Location of loci linked to human SLE; only regions with a logarithm of odds (lod) above 3 are indicated in table. Linkage between 1q41 and SLE shows variation between different ethnic groups (128). The human MHC region (6p11-6p21) showed the strongest evidence of linkage (lod = 3.9) to SLE in a recent study (100). The murine MHC is located on chromosome 17.
[d]*See* ref. 18.
[e]Precise location could not be estimated based on homology data.
[f]Described in Rozzo SJ, Vyse TJ, Drake CG, et al. Effect of genetic background on the contribution of New Zealand Black loci to autoimmune lupus nephritis. *Proc Natl Acad Sci U S A* 1996;93:15164–15168.
Modified from Gulko P, Winchester R. The genetics of systemic lupus erythematosus. In: Kammer GM, Tsokos GC, eds., *Lupus: molecular and cellular pathogenesis*. Totowa, NJ: Humana Press, 1999:101–123.

tosis after they have not been positively selected. A state of autoimmunity ensues with production of autoantibodies to erythrocytes and platelets and, finally, development of immune complex–mediated glomerulonephritis. Mutations in the Fas-FasL–induced pathway have been identified in humans with an autoimmune proliferative syndrome (ALPS) or the Canale-Smith syndrome (20). However, this disorder is clinically distinct from SLE. So far only two patients with SLE have been reported that carry mutations in the Fas pathway and, these as well as other studies suggest that defects of apoptosis, at least those in the Fas-FasL pathway, rarely lead to the clinical picture of SLE (21,22). When the MRL-*lpr* mouse is crossed to other strains, congenic for the Fas-*lpr* mutation, several additional loci have been identified that contribute to the development of autoimmunity in the MRL-*lpr* model.

Genome-wide linkage studies, currently being conducted in models of other major autoimmune disorders such as experimental autoimmune encephalitis and the spontaneous autoimmune diabetes of the nonobese diabetic (NOD) strain of mice, have demonstrated that multiple susceptibility loci are present in every model and, interestingly, that some susceptibility loci or regions appear to be shared between different disease models.

MAJOR IMMUNOLOGIC ALTERATIONS IN SLE

This section highlights the major immunologic alterations that characterize individuals with SLE.

T-Cell–Specific Autoimmune Recognition Is at the Center of the Pathogenesis of SLE

There is compelling indirect evidence for the participation of the T cell in the autoimmune response of SLE (Table 75.3). This includes the particular features of the autoantibody response in SLE that imply the existence of cognate, autoantigen-specific T-cell help. The association of susceptibility with class II MHC alleles indicates that a specific antigen presentation event to CD4-positive T cells occurs in the context of a specific class II MHC molecule and/or that these molecules acted earlier in ontogeny to select the T-cell repertoire, including those that are capable of autoantigenic recognition. Furthermore, the nature of the autoantibody response bears unmistakable evidence of the presence of help by CD4 T cells in lymph node germinal centers, including their IgG isotype, extent of somatic mutation away from germline Ig genes, and

TABLE 75.3. EVIDENCE THAT AN AUTOIMMUNE CD4 T-CELL COGNATE IMMUNE RESPONSE IN SLE REGULATES THE PRODUCTION OF AUTOANTIBODIES

Autoantibody B-cell response reflects existence of antigen specific T-cell help
Direct demonstration of T-cells reactive to same peptide autoantigens that are targets of autoantibodies
Structure of the T-cell receptor α and β chains implies antigenic selection and drive
Association of susceptibility with MHC class II alleles suggesting that MHC class II molecules present autoantigenic peptides to CD4 lineage T-cells
Amelioration of disease with T-cell specific therapy and selective immunodeficiency of AIDS

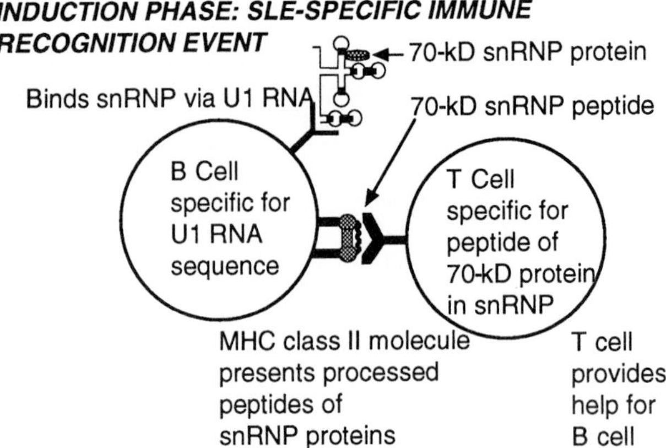

FIGURE 75.2. Participation of T cells with specificity for autologous peptides in the autoimmune response of systemic lupus erythematosus (SLE), indicating that it is an autoantigen-driven process centered on the presentation of autoantigens by antigen-presenting cells (e.g., a B cell) to a CD4+ T cell. These, in turn, provide T cell help to the B cells, resulting in their differentiation into cells that produce pathogenic autoantibodies. A hypothetic example illustrating an immune recognition event involving a T-cell and a B-cell response to U1 small nuclear ribonucleoprotein (snRNP) with the B cell specific for a ribonucleic acid moiety is depicted.

the broadening of the autoantibody immune response to epitopes on the same autoantigen and to members of "linked sets" of physically interrelated molecules. These features suggest that presentation of autoantigens to these T cells occurs through B cells that are specific for autoantigens in a manner resembling that of the physiologic secondary immune response. In addition, the significant therapeutic response to T-cell–specific therapy in SLE, and remissions in association with the immunodeficiency of advanced human immunodeficiency virus type 1 (HIV-1) infection argue for the importance of the T cell in the pathogenesis of SLE. Taken together, these phenomena indicate that the autoimmune response of SLE is an autoantigen-driven process centered on the presentation of autoantigens by B cells to CD4-positive T cells. These autoantigens, in turn, provide T-cell help to the B cells, resulting in their differentiation into cells that produce pathogenic autoantibodies (Fig. 75.2).

One of the most interesting aspects to emerge in the study of the pathogenesis of SLE has been the direct identification of T cells with specificity for autologous peptides (Table 75.4). These cells are candidates for the cells postulated to exist in the previous paragraph. Several groups of investigators have now successfully demonstrated antigen-specific T-cell responses to both cytoplasmic and nuclear autoantigens, including U1 small nuclear RNP (snRNP) (23–26), ribosomal P2 protein (27), histones (28,29), and to both the SS-A/Ro (30) and SS-B/La ribonucleoprotein (26) (Table 75.4). Similar responses have been identified in the SNF_1 (NZB × SWR) murine model of SLE studied by Mohan and colleagues (31), in which autoantigen-specific T cells reactive against nucleosomes (histone-DNA) have been identified that are capable of augmenting the production of anti-DNA autoantibodies by syngeneic B cells. In general, these autoantigen-specific T-cell clones or lines have been predominantly $CD4^+$ and MHC class II restricted (primarily DR), and are capable of providing the requisite "help" to B cells that produce pathogenic anti–double-stranded DNA (dsDNA) autoantibodies. Perhaps most important in implicating these autoreactive T cells as specifically central to the autoimmune response is the finding that autoantigen-specific T cells have been demonstrated only in those individuals who also demonstrate a corresponding antigen-specific autoantibody.

In all patients with SLE who make autoantibodies to elements of the U1 snRNP particle, there is a T-cell response to two proteins composing the U1 snRNP complex, protein A (25) and the 70-kd protein (23), and this is directed to the same C-terminal region of the molecules (Table 75.4). T-cell immune responses to these protein antigens were not found in patients with SLE who did not have autoantibodies directed to the U1 snRNP. This suggests a model of T-cell cooperation with B cells in the formation of the autoantibodies of SLE (Fig. 75.2). A similar pattern has been shown by Crow and co-workers (27) to exist in the T-cell response to the ribosomal P2 protein in that only those patients who demonstrated antiribosomal P2 autoantibodies made an antigen-specific response in the T-cell compartment (Table 75.4) (27).

TABLE 75.4. AUTOANTIGEN SPECIFICITY OF MHC CLASS II RESTRICTED AUTOIMMUNE T-CELL RESPONSES IN SLE

Autoantigen Specificity	Reference Number
U1 snRNP protein A	25
U1 snRNP 70-kd protein	23
Histone	28,29
SS-A/Ro	30
SS-B/La	26
Ribosomal P2 protein	27

Further, structural analysis of the T-cell receptor (TCR) α (32) and β chains (33) in antigen-specific T-cell clones directed to histone epitopes revealed a biased Vβ usage and a preference for somatically encoded negatively charged residues in the third complementarity-determining region (CDR3), the region of the TCR that interacts with antigenic peptides presented by MHC molecules. The cationic histone moieties may contribute the complementary positively charged peptides to which these T-cell clones are reactive. In similar studies of nucleosomal-reactive T-cell clones in human SLE, Datta's group (28) found a distinctive structural motif of charged residues in the CDR3 region of the TCR as well as a significantly biased utilization of the Vβ8 variable region. Talken and co-workers (34) calculated and inferred the three-dimensional structure of an αβ CD4 TCR from the sequence of αβ chains of clones that recognized U1 RNP. These authors concluded that the dominant interaction between the TCR and the peptide–MHC class II complex depended on the α chain CDR3 region.

The T-Cell Compartment in SLE Is Characterized by Extensive and Unexplained Activation

Prior to the identification of autoantigen-specific T cells, studies of the T-cell compartment in SLE revealed abnormalities reflecting a combination of the ongoing autoantigen-driven and specific immune response, as well as the consequences of the state of SLE, including an autoantibody-mediated attack on the cells of the immune system. The number of circulating T cells is decreased in parallel with increases in disease activity (35,36) and with increased levels of antilymphocyte antibodies, some of which possess specificities for T cells (37–39).

The entire T-cell repertoire in SLE revealed statistically significant differences of β chain CDR3 length distribution between SLE patients and normal subjects, for both active and inactive SLE using spectratyping (40). These results suggest that clonal activation of peripheral T cells correlates with disease activity and exhibits features of a secondary antigen-driven immune response. This study did not define whether the abnormalities were primarily in the CD4 or CD8 T-cell populations. The T-cell repertoire has also been the subject of detailed study in murine models of lupus (41). These findings provide additional evidence of specific T-cell responses in SLE.

Early investigations into T-cell function and phenotype in SLE revealed a strikingly enhanced activation phenotype of circulating lymphocytes, characterized by expression of human leukocyte antigen HLA-DR and CD69, along with increased levels of integrin expression and other molecules associated with a mature antigen-reactive T cell (42). Paradoxically, this inappropriate activation was found together with a diminished delayed hypersensitivity skin test and diminished responses in most *in vitro* responses of T-cell function, including proliferation to test antigens, compared to healthy controls. The events responsible for the high level of endogenously activated T cells in SLE have not been characterized, nor has it been ascertained whether these T cells are polyclonal or represent oligoclonal expansions. In any event, the presence of activated cells, regardless of the route of activation, suggests the possibility that they have a decreased requirement for co-stimulatory signals and could directly react with the autoantigens with which they were originally selected. More recent studies have shown that, in patients with active SLE, there is an increased and prolonged cell surface expression of CD40L.

After the cognate recognition of antigen by the T cell, co-stimulatory recognition is necessary for T-cell activation to proceed. CD40L is transiently expressed on the T cell with a maximum expression at about 6 hours after initial antigen recognition, and it mediates the cognate co-stimulation. In a spontaneous murine autoimmune nephritis animal, (NZB × SWR)F1, the percentage of splenic CD40L-positive T cells is elevated even at an age when clinically there were no signs of autoimmunity (43).

The evidence of frank immune impairment in SLE is as pervasive as the evidence of inappropriate T-cell activation. The mixed lymphocyte culture (MLC) reaction is impaired in the ability of SLE cells both to stimulate and to respond (44,45), as is the autologous mixed lymphocyte response (AMLR) (44,45). CD8-positive T-cell–mediated cytotoxic mechanisms are also decreased (46). There is a decrease in interleukin-2 (IL-2) release in most assays of *in vitro* T-cell stimulation (47). In each of these studies, there is a direct correlation between the severity of disease activity and the level of hyporesponsiveness demonstrated *in vitro* (48).

Biochemical TCR-mediated signaling abnormalities have also been identified in T cells isolated from patients with active SLE or when in clinical remission. After engagement of the TCR, these T cells exhibit an increased intracellular Ca^{2+} response and an increased production of tyrosine phosphorylated proteins, the initial step in TCR/CD3 signaling (49). The CD3 γ, δ, and ε chains are present as monomers, noncovalently associated with the TCR αβ heterodimer and with each other. CD3 ζ and η chains are present as ζ dimers or ζη heterodimers, and these chains may associate noncovalently with the TCR or other CD3 chains. Analysis of antigen-induced signaling by tyrosine phosphorylation revealed that in 77% of patients with SLE, the 16-kd CD3 ζ chain fails to phosphorylate due to reduced amounts of the corresponding protein and messenger RNA (mRNA) (50). The CD3 ζ chain is also a signal-transducing subunit of the FcG3R (CD16) molecule. The CD3 ζ chain can be reversibly downregulated in activated T cells from healthy individuals; however, in T cells from patients with SLE, the absence of the ζ chain does not correlate with disease activity or any treatment regimens.

The Ca^{2+}-mediated signaling pathway, initiated by engagement of the TCR, activates nuclear factor-activated

T cells (NF-AT)–mediated transcription of several genes, among them HLA-DR and CD40L. Thus, an increase in the Ca^{2+}-activated pathway will enhance the expression of CD40L, and this was shown to be the case in studies of lupus B and T cells when compared to healthy individuals. This observation seems to be at odds with the finding of decreased levels of CDR3-ζ chain expression and signaling described above.

The basis of the entire set of phenomena described in this section remains unexplained. However, they could be of central importance in the pathogenesis of SLE, because they appear to provide a means for the T cells in this disease to bypass or reduce the requirement for a second activating signal. This point is discussed subsequently. The basis of the diminished response to conventional antigens remains incompletely understood, but might be a consequence of the events associated with the inappropriate and presumably autoimmune activation described above.

Cytokines

An elevated level of certain cytokines has been well recognized, especially during periods of clinical activity (47,51). This may account for some of the characteristic fatigue and fever of the illness, as well as the enhancement of the sustained B-cell response in SLE through noncognate mechanisms, a role that could be partially played by the IL-6 elevations (51). Elevated levels of cytokines could account for certain of the nonlocalized neuropsychiatric alterations in SLE. Cytokines may also play a role in predisposing to immune complex injury in vessels and in the sclerotic response in glomeruli. The "lupus storm" of hyperpyrexia and vascular collapse seen more in the presteroid era of SLE might also have had a component of a cytokine release syndrome.

Following activation by antigen, the $CD4^+$ T cell becomes polarized into either of two main subsets, Th1 or Th2, each defined by its unique cytokine profile. The Th1 cell, which characteristically secretes IL-2, interferon-γ (IFN-γ), IL-12, and tumor necrosis factor-α (TNF-α), mainly promotes cellular immune responses via IFN-γ action on macrophages, but is also characterized by IFN-γ–mediated antibody class switching to particular isotypes. The Th2 cell secretes IL-4, IL-5, IL-6, IL-10, and IL-13, and mainly protects against extracellular antigens by promoting a humoral immune response. The dichotomy of Th1 and Th2 is somewhat less clear when cells of human rather than murine sources are studied.

Polarization of CD4 T Cells into Th1 and Th2 Responses

A Th2-type response has been postulated in the pathogenesis of SLE because of the central role that autoantibody production and immune complex formation have had in understanding the pathogenesis of the disease. However, recent studies, both in the area of immune complex–mediated tissue damage and in the evaluation of cytokine profiles found in patients with SLE or the corresponding mouse models, have suggested that the picture may have been oversimplified. Five lines of study shed additional light on this aspect of autoimmunity.

First, in mouse models it has been shown that a Th1 response, as indicated by IFN-γ production, is necessary for the spontaneous autoimmune disease to develop (52). The isotype of the important anti-DNA antibodies in nephritis are predominantly of the IFN-γ–induced type both in murine and human glomerulonephritis; moreover, in the BXSB mouse model the development of disease is independent of IL-4 production (53). IFN-γ is an important cytokine in amplifying the local immune response that could function through its effects on activating infiltrating mononuclear cells, or by an effect on resident cells in the kidney.

Second, *in vitro* antigen activation of T cells, isolated from patients with SLE, using peptides derived from histone proteins to which the individual is producing autoantibodies, leads to the production of a pattern of cytokines that reflects an origin in either a predominantly Th1 or Th2 response, depending on the particular patient (29). The Th1 response, characterized by the production of IFN-γ was preponderant. The significance of these cytokine profiles to the clinical manifestations of disease in the individual patients is unknown.

Third, in SLE glomerulonephritis, one of the best histopathologic predictors of renal outcome is the presence of mononuclear cells in the interstitium of the kidney (54,55). A mononuclear influx of cells into the glomeruli and the interstitium is a feature predominantly of active class III and IV nephritis. Both monocytes and lymphocytes are present in these infiltrates, but the proportion in relation to each other and to the class of nephritis has not been well documented. These cells would not necessarily be expected to predominate in an Arthus-type Th2-immune complex–mediated lesion.

Fourth, a large proportion of the infiltrating lymphocytes in SLE glomerulonephritis express CD40L, a cell surface activation marker normally expressed on the antigen-activated T cell, but which has been demonstrated in increased amounts on T cells, as well as B cells of patients with SLE (56). The CD40L expression pattern in SLE correlates with activity of disease and further suggests the importance of Th1 activation mechanisms.

Fifth, a study by Massengill and co-workers (57) has recently provided evidence of an oligoclonal TCR expansion in renal tissue obtained from five patients with SLE. This further supports an antigen-specific T-cell immune recognition event in the lupus kidney. Taken together, these five points emphasize the importance of CD4 T cells in SLE nephritis and suggest that they largely function as if they were Th1. Thus, in addition to the classic role of immune complex–mediated injury, evidence is increasing for the potential of autoantigen-reactive CD4 T cells to injure the kidney directly by release of cytokines such as IFN-γ, or by modulation of gene expression in the kidney parenchyma, or, indirectly, via macrophage activation.

Antilymphocyte Autoantibodies and Functional Derangement

An intriguing feature of SLE is the production of IgM and IgG antilymphocyte autoantibodies directed against separate and shared determinants on the membrane of autologous T and B lymphocytes (38,58). The antilymphocyte autoantibodies may appear early in the development of SLE. A consequence of the IgM isotype is increased avidity due to multivalency. This is reflected by their greatly enhanced binding at temperatures below that of 37°C, resulting in lymphocytotoxicity.

These autoantibodies have been demonstrated to affect a variety of *in vitro* functional tests of immune responsiveness (59), although it is unclear whether they affect *in vivo* immune function. The titers of antilymphocyte antibodies correlate with the development of lymphopenia during disease flares, suggesting that antilymphocyte autoantibodies may either cause abnormalities in lymphocyte trafficking or directly lead to lymphocyte destruction (60). The presence of antilymphocyte antibodies on the surface of B cells during periods of clinical activity may be a secondary pathway leading to additional B-cell activation or dysfunction (58). Autoantibodies are concentrated in cryoprecipitates during clinical flares in disease activity (61). These interesting antibodies have not recently received much attention, but may play a role in initiating some of the immunologic abnormalities discussed previously.

T-Cell Dependent B-Cell Autorecognition in SLE

An analysis of the detailed pattern of autoantibodies in SLE reveals this response to be indistinguishable from any physiologic antigen-driven immune response of B cells (Table 75.5) as shown by the high titers of autoantibodies, the presence of an isotype switch to antibodies of the IgG class, and the involvement of a number of structurally related B-cell clones, indicating affinity maturation (3,62,63). Thus, the autoantibody production in SLE is driven by self antigens and involves both T-cell and B-cell recognition, identical to the immune responses to exogenous antigens (Table 75.3).

TABLE 75.5. FEATURES CHARACTERISTIC OF AUTOANTIBODY PRODUCTION IN SLE REFLECTS AN ONGOING IMMUNE RESPONSE DIRECTED TO AND DRIVEN BY SELF ANTIGENS

Oligoclonality but not monoclonality or polyclonality of autoantibodies
Somatic diversification and affinity maturation of autoantibodies
Extremely high titers of autoantibodies
Isotype switching of autoantibody immunoglobulin from IgM to IgG with predominance of IgG1
Autoantigenic targets are associated with components of functional particles
B cells lack CD5 and are not of B1 phenotype

Linked Sets of Autoantibodies in SLE Imply a Limited Autoantigen Drive

The diverse collection of autoantibodies that are found in SLE, described in Chapter 74, raised conceptual problems about their origin and the nature of the autoimmunity state in SLE. In the past, the diversity of the autoantibodies was thought to reflect a global disorder in immunologic self recognition leading to polyclonal B-cell activation. This led to the interesting idea, fitting with the then prevalent concept of "horror autotoxicus," that SLE was due to a single major non-MHC genetic locus that determined either global dominant autoimmunity or normal immunity.

However, quite a different explanation for the diversity of autoantibodies in SLE has resulted from the progress in understanding the immunologic features of autoantibody production and the cellular and molecular biologic organization of the molecules that are the autoantigenic targets. As shown by the work of Tan (3) and Hardin (62), it is now clear that most of the autoantibodies in SLE serum can be grouped into three major related, or linked, sets based on their reactivity with components of three different intracellular aggregates of physically interrelated molecules. These three macromolecular particles appear to be the target of the SLE immune response (Table 75.6) (3,62). These findings demonstrate that the autoantibody response in SLE is oligoclonal, not polyclonal, and in this respect further resembles a physiologic antibody response to exogenous antigen. This simplifies the problem of understanding autoantibodies in SLE in that rather than having to account for the many dozens of seemingly different autoantigenic specificities that may be found in one or another patient with SLE, it is necessary only to account for how three, or fewer, major sets of autoantibodies develop from a distinct immune response to these macromolecular particles. Lim-

TABLE 75.6. AUTOANTIBODY PRODUCTION TO LINKED SETS OF AUTOANTIGENS SUGGESTS A SINGLE INITIATING EVENT IN EACH GROUP: GENERAL CORRELATION WITH DIFFERENT CLINICAL MANIFESTATIONS

Particle Initiating Autoantibodies	Clinical Manifestations
Nucleochromatin	Nephritis
snRNP	Mixed connective tissue disease features
SS-A/Ro, SS-B/La, hYRNA	CCHB, skin disease

CCHB, congenital complete heart block.

ited evidence suggests that the control of these autoantibodies may be related to particular genetic subphenotypes.

One set of molecules responsible for a linked set of autoantibodies found in about one-third of patients with SLE includes the targets of the Sm and U1 snRNP autoantibodies. The target particulate antigen consists of both the RNA and protein components of a variety of molecules, including U2, U4-6, and U5 snRNPs, that function together as a complex structure. The production of these autoantibodies has not been associated with a readily apparent genetic background involving MHC alleles (64). However, the occurrence of antibodies to elements of this particle correlates with the presence of certain clinical features (Table 75.6). The detailed associations of these antibodies and their clinical correlates are discussed in Chapter 74.

One of the earliest observations of this correlation was the description of the clinical entity of MCTD based on the uniform presence of antibodies to U1 snRNP (2) in patients exhibiting Raynaud's phenomenon, microangiopathy, and myositis (Table 75.6). These patients appeared to have a disorder with overlapping clinical features of systemic sclerosis, SLE, and polymyositis. A follow-up of the initial group of patients identified as having MCTD revealed that the illness ultimately evolved into one of several well-recognized autoimmune diseases, such as SLE or scleroderma. This suggests that the clinical features of MCTD result from the presence of particular autoantibodies that act through a still undefined mechanism to cause a uniform pattern of disease, rather than reflecting factors that result in a separate disease (4), in that the presence of the clinical findings predicts the presence of autoantibodies of this linked set rather than the presence of a distinctive disease.

A second major set of linked autoantibodies that are found in over half of the patients with SLE consists of DNA and certain of the related DNA-binding proteins that compose chromatin, such as the histones. This set of antibodies can be grouped into several subsets of related multimolecular complexes including nucleosomes, transcription complexes, and DNA replication complexes that also include polymerases (31,60). The production of dsDNA antibodies is strongly, although again not absolutely, associated with the development of glomerulonephritis.

The SS-A/Ro and SS-B/La molecules compose a third set of molecular complexes that is targeted in about one-third of patients with SLE. Nearly all of these molecules are associated with a single hYRNA species, a small uridine-rich oligonucleotide (65–67). As reflected by the SS in the designation of these autoantibodies, they are characteristic of both Sjögren's syndrome and SLE. In SLE, these autoantibodies are associated with the presence of the typical photosensitive skin rash and the subacute cutaneous lupus clinical subset of SLE, although they may be found in equally high titer in asymptomatic individuals. Regardless of the clinical disease state or symptoms associated with these autoantibodies, their presence in pregnant women indicates a significantly greater risk that the fetus will develop congenital complete heart block (CCHB) by passively acquired autoimmunity (68). Intriguingly, these antibodies are often the major, or only, autoantibodies found in those with certain homozygous complement deficiencies.

A few additional linked sets of autoantibodies will probably be identified, such as that postulated by Roubey (69) to consist of physically and functionally related macromolecules, containing phospholipids and various phospholipid-binding proteins that are targeted in the anticardiolipin syndrome (Chapter 77).

B-Cell Abnormalities

Despite their role in the production of autoantibodies, the numbers of circulating B cells in SLE are not increased (58). However, the state of B-cell differentiation is altered, with increased numbers of plasmacytoid B cells characterized by cytoplasmic Ig and the secretion of IgG immunoglobulin, particularly in periods of heightened clinical activity (70,71).

Biochemical abnormalities in B-cell receptor–mediated signaling, similar to those described above for TCR signaling, have been documented in SLE. After engagement of the cell surface IgG or IgM receptor, the SLE B cell responds with increased intracellular Ca^{2+} release and enhanced production of tyrosine phosphorylated cellular proteins compared to the response in normal B cells (49). These signaling defects are reported to be independent of disease state, treatment, or clinical type of SLE, although their significance remains unclear.

After binding antigen and receiving the first signal for immune activation, several sets of co-stimulatory molecules, such as the CD40:CD40L and the CD28/CTLA4: B7-1/B7-2 pairs, need to be brought into action for an immune response to occur. Lack of a second signal will abrogate the immune response, whereas aberrant second signal engagement can lead to an inappropriate immune response (Fig. 75.3).

Quantitative differences in co-stimulatory receptor expression can influence the magnitude of the immune response. Studies of B cells isolated from patients with SLE have identified dysregulated expression patterns for some of these cell surface molecules, even at times of quiescent disease. Increased expression of B7-1 and B7-2 have been documented on subsets of B cells obtained from patients in remission (72). NZB and NZB/W mice also have an increased proportion of splenic B cells expressing elevated levels of B7-1 and B7-2 (73). This raises the possibility that activated B cells provide co-stimulatory signals to self-reactive T cells, leading to loss of tolerance. This could serve as a mechanism for fostering the induction of an autoimmune response in the progression of SLE.

The CD40L molecule, normally transiently expressed on activated T cells, has been found to be expressed also on

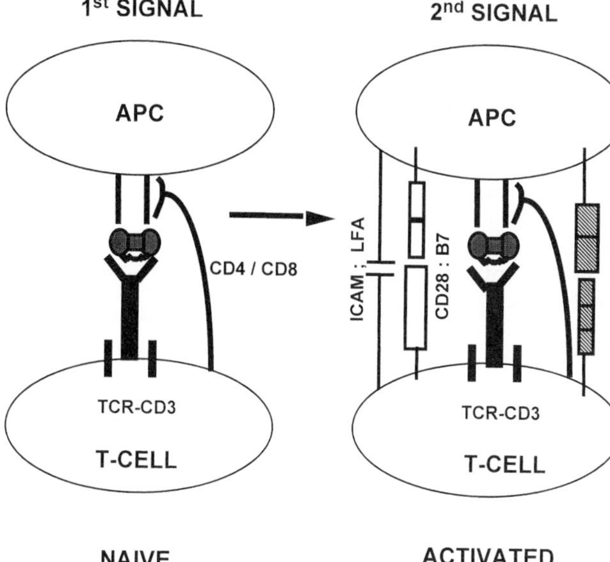

FIGURE 75.3. T-cell activation normally requires co-stimulatory signaling. An antigen-presenting cell (APC)—macrophage, dendritic cell, or B cell—delivers the first signal to the T cell by presenting an antigenic peptide bound to a major histocompatibility complex (MHC) class I or II molecule. B cells capture antigen via their surface-immunoglobulin (Ig) receptors, as shown in Figs. 75.2, 75.4, and 75.5, whereas other APCs take up antigen via non–antigen-specific receptors or through endocytosis. Low-affinity interactions among MHC, CD4/CD8, intercellular adhesion molecules (ICAMs), lymphocyte function–associated antigens (LFA), help to stabilize the antigen-specific interaction. The second signal is mediated by pairs of cell surface molecules—CD40:CD40L, CD28/CTLA4:B7–1/B7–2—that cluster around the MHC–T-cell receptor (TCR) complex in the plane of the cell membrane. If a second signal is not received, the T cell may develop immunologic tolerance to the peptide. CD3 is the signaling molecule noncovalently associated with the TCR.

SLE B cells obtained from patients with active disease in levels as high as on the activated T cell. B cells isolated from patients in remission express normal levels of CD40L (74,75).

These abnormalities imply that B-cell activation and autoantibody production may be enhanced. It is unlikely that any of these quantitative differences in cell surface expression can act to cause development of SLE by themselves, but they may act in an additive manner to lower the threshold at which the B cells are activated. The increased understanding of the importance of these co-stimulatory molecules for a successful activation of the immune system has also led to the development of therapeutic interventions aimed at abrogating the pathologic immune response in SLE. It is also evident that individuals with SLE differ in their expression pattern of these molecules. Whether the dysregulated expression patterns observed above occur on a genetic basis or whether they are secondary to other immune abnormalities in SLE is also an unresolved issue. Currently, it appears that intrinsic abnormalities of the SLE B cell have not been conclusively identified and that the B cell appears to act appropriately in response to abnormal signals from other cells of the immune system.

Apoptosis

Several features in SLE direct attention to the potential importance of the phenomenon of apoptosis to the disease (76) (see Chapter 27). These include the role of apoptotic cells in initiating an immune response (77); the production of autoantibodies to linked sets of macromolecules; down-regulating an immune response, which involves T-cell apoptosis; and, lastly, defects in Fas-FasL signaling, which are associated with autoimmunity.

During the orderly process of apoptosis, the cell undergoes nuclear condensation, enzymatic digestion, and shrinkage, followed by the formation of at least two distinct types of surface blebs, structures that are bound by plasma membrane and visible by light microscopy. A striking finding in apoptotic cells is that a variety of autoantigens selectively aggregate together in blebs on the surface of the stressed and dying cell. The large blebs contain nucleosomal DNA, Ro/La, and snRNP. The small blebs contain Ro, components of the endoplasmic reticulum, and ribosomes (76). Other molecules have also been identified in apoptotic blebs depending on the particular cell type they originate from. Phospholipids, an integral part of the plasma membrane, are associated with the outer leaflet of apoptotic blebs (78). When DNA is purified from the serum of patients with active SLE, it is found to be present largely as double-stranded, small fragments with discrete molecular weights typically of 150 to 200, 400, 600, and 800 base pair (bp) (79). This resembles the characteristic "DNA ladder" that can be demonstrated by agarose-gel electrophoresis, after apoptotic degradation of DNA into histone-containing nucleosomes (80,81).

Taken together, these data provide strong evidence that apoptotic blebs are a potential source of nearly all of the autoantigens that are targets in SLE. Attention has been drawn toward apoptosis as a mechanism for presentation of autoantigens in novel contexts that may influence peptide processing and presentation (76). The apoptotic process may contribute to development of autoimmunity by affecting the physical compartmentalization of these protein-DNA/RNA autoantigen complexes, by altering the endosomal processing pathway of phagocytes resulting from the unusual physical interaction of certain autoantigenic peptides, or by the release of the apoptotic bodies and their specific binding to preexisting B cells directed to one component in the apoptotic body, resulting in an enriched presentation of certain self peptides on a single antigen-presenting cell. These processes might reveal previously cryptic regions of the peptide that had not been presented to the T-cell repertoire and to which it is not tolerant, as discussed subsequently.

During physiologic conditions, cellular components degraded by apoptosis are rapidly cleared by phagocytic cells, without initiating an inflammatory or immune response. However, recent studies of antigen presentation by dendritic cells have clearly demonstrated the capacity of the differentiated dendritic cell to present apoptotic cell components to the T cell with resulting immune activation, although the physiologic significance of this is not yet fully understood (77). The differentiated dendritic cell can then process endogenous proteins through the lysosome for presentation on class II molecules, the classic pathway, but interestingly, also on class I molecules, termed "cross-presentation." Autoantigen presentation by dendritic cells in the setting of SLE has not been delineated, but these new findings make for interesting hypotheses regarding the source of autoantigens in SLE and the mechanisms by which immune activation can be initiated and propagated.

However, as discussed above in the section on murine disease (see Insights into SLE from Animal Models of Autoimmunity), there is yet no evidence that SLE results from a defect in the apoptotic pathway. On the contrary, it has been reported that patients with SLE have increased numbers of circulating apoptotic cells and exhibit accelerated lymphocyte apoptosis *in vitro*. This raises the possibility that dysregulation of the cellular machinery, including macrophage phagocytosis, which mediates removal of apoptotic fragments could be a mechanism whereby increased quantities of autoantigens could be made available for presentation to the immune system in the individual predisposed to developing SLE, perhaps by shunting to dendritic cells where it might serve to initiate or accelerate autoimmunity.

Lymphadenopathy is a common finding in active SLE, often seen at presentation of disease, as emphasized by Klemperer (82) many years ago. The histopathology of SLE lymph node biopsies obtained from patients with lymphadenopathy reveals follicular and paracortical hyperplasia with foci of necrosis, nuclear debris, and a large number of apoptotic cells. Immunophenotyping revealed a predominance of histiocytes and CD8 T cells in the region (83–84). The peptide specificity of these CD8 T cells is unknown. It is possible that this either reflects CD8 T cells mediating apoptosis through the perforin-granzyme pathway after recognition of antigenic peptides presented on a class I molecule, or dendritic cell cross-presentation of antigens to the CD8 T cells.

GENETIC BASIS OF THE SLE SUSCEPTIBILITY STATE

When SLE develops in an adult patient, the disorder appears in what seems a sporadic manner that does not immediately suggest a genetic etiology. However, both formal genetic studies of the occurrence of the disease in families and the concordance between identical twins, along with studies on the association of susceptibility with certain genes, have shown SLE to be a heritable disorder. The pattern of inheritance depends on the interaction of several relatively common alleles. This multigenic, or complex, inheritance of susceptibility along with a predisposition that only reveals itself with the passage of time, accounts for the seeming sporadic character of the illness (85). This section addresses the genetic determinants that result in susceptibility to SLE and how epidemiology provides clues for potential susceptibility genes. These findings are based on the study of twins, familial aggregations, and population studies of associations with candidate genes (Table 75.7).

TABLE 75.7. FORMAL GENETICS OF SLE: INSIGHTS FROM TWIN STUDIES AND FAMILIAL AGGREGATION

Heritability >0.95 implying, a very strong genetic influence and minimal contribution from environment
Oligogenic inheritance, a minimum of three to four major genes define susceptibility
Nonmendelian inheritance, likely additive
Penetrance rate increases with time, exceeding 60%
Ascertainment and criteria for diagnosis influence quantitative estimates

Insights from Studies of Twin Concordance and Familial Aggregation

Concordance, the frequency of both members of a twinship being affected by the same disease, will be relatively similar in identical and fraternal twins, if the disease is predominantly environmentally induced. In contrast, it is markedly higher in the identical twinship if the disease is genetic. This difference in concordance rates reflects the fact that both members of an identical (monozygotic) twin pair are identical at the level of their germline endowment of genes. In contrast, the members of a fraternal twin pair differ from each other by an average of 50% of their genetic information, and correspondingly at each locus there is a 50% chance that each twin will have inherited a different allele. If susceptibility to the disorder is specified by several genes, the concordance rates will differ in proportion to $1/2$ raised to the power of the number of genes. The difference in concordance rates is used to measure the relative roles of genetic versus environmental phenomena in the index termed "heritability." Heritability has a value of 0 if only environment is important, and 1.0 if the disease is purely genetic.

The application of this approach offered a way to evaluate the relative influence of heredity and environment on the development of SLE (86–88) (Table 75.7). In an early study by Block and colleagues (89), the concordance rate in monozygotic twins was found to be 57%, compared to approximately 5% in dizygotic twins. This tenfold difference in concordance rates is used to calculate that the heritability of SLE is >0.95 (86–88), implying SLE is a genetic disease with little, if any, role played by specific environmental events. The absolute observed rates of concordance in any twin group varies according to how the presence of disease is ascertained and, most importantly, the duration of the period of observation of the second twin after the first member of the twinship developed SLE. Interestingly, affected identical twins have a much greater concordance of specific autoantibody profiles and disease manifestations than dizygotic twins, even though a number of years may separate the onset of disease in each member of the twinship (5).

The data on familial SLE is in agreement with that found in the twin studies and leads to the same conclusions about the genetics of SLE. The frequency of SLE among first- or second-degree relatives of an adult propositus with SLE ranges from 1.7% to 12%, while the frequency of SLE among a normal control population was 0.18%. Thus, the relative risk of developing SLE if a first- or second-degree relative has the disease ranges from 9.0 to more than 50. The percentage of affected first-degree relatives is 1.7% to 3%, making the clustering of disease in families common (estimated from the ratio of the risk for relatives of patients with disease and the population prevalence of that disease, λ_R = 20–75) (17). The frequency of involved relatives in instances of childhood-onset SLE is reported to approach 25%, emphasizing the role of heightened genetic "dose" in early-onset SLE and the effect of this heightened load of susceptibility alleles on increasing the frequency of SLE in relatives of the propositus (5).

The Number of Genes Determining SLE Susceptibility

The same differences in the concordance rates of monozygotic and dizygotic twins also provide an estimate of the number and nature of the genes determining SLE susceptibility. If the trait of SLE were due to a single dominant gene, one would expect to find concordance for the trait at one-half the rate observed in the identical twin pairs. If it were due to the independent segregation of two genes, then the SLE would be found four times more frequently among identical than fraternal twinships. The approximately tenfold observed difference in prevalence between these two types of twins suggests that a minimum of three to four genes encode the trait of susceptibility to SLE. This would be in the range of what is designated as oligogenic control (86–88), making the inheritance of SLE an example of a genetically complex disease.

Mode of Inheritance

While pedigrees with parent–child involvement are plentiful, it is clear that the mode of inheritance is not a simple mendelian dominant pattern. Multigenic inheritance fully explains both instances of parent–child inheritance as well as what appears to be sporadic development of the disease. The possible models of multigenic heritability include either a multifactorial inheritance, in which each gene contributes an equal liability to develop SLE, with a threshold set at three to four genes; an alternative model with one or possibly two major genes and associated modifying genes; and a third model in which each susceptibility gene specifies an autoimmune subphenotype that, taken together, results in SLE. It has not yet been possible to distinguish between these possibilities.

IDENTIFICATION OF GENES DEFINING THE SUSCEPTIBILITY STATE OF SLE

The identification of the genes that determine susceptibility to SLE is far from complete. Multiple approaches have been tried in a very extensive and ongoing research effort.

Candidate Genes Mapping in the MHC

Because SLE involves a misdirected immune response that targets certain autoantigens, genes regulating the immune response were the first obvious candidate genes to be studied. MHC genes are immensely polymorphic, and the different alleles regulate the immune response at the level of selection of the TCR repertoire through their different peptide binding properties. As discussed in Chapters 15 and 28, during the process of T-cell development various self peptides bound to self MHC molecules expressed on the thymic epithelium select the T-cell repertoire in a positive manner. Thus, MHC molecules first act to select the repertoire of T cells with which they will subsequently interact, and subsequently, during an immune response, the MHC molecules present peptides to the T cell to initiate the T-cell response. Perhaps equally important, the MHC molecules containing self peptides act to maintain the naive T cells in the repertoire (90). Immune events illustrated in Figs. 75.2, 75.4, and 75.5 place

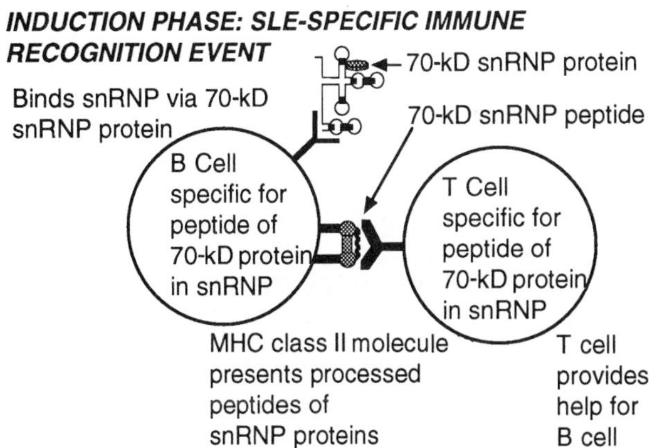

FIGURE 75.4. A second equivalent scenario for participation of T cells with specificity for autologous peptides in the autoimmune response of systemic lupus erythematosus (SLE) involving B cells specific for the protein moiety of snRNP particles. The B cell binds the particle through a protein epitope and presents the peptides of the particle to T cells with the same properties as shown in Fig. 75.2.

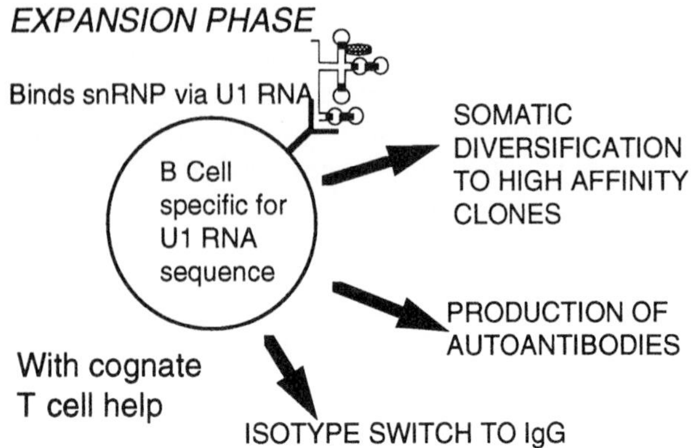

FIGURE 75.5. Expansion of the autoimmune response. T-cell and B-cell clonal expansion is driven by the available supply of autoantigen presented by the semicognate or cognate B cell. Recruitment of additional B cells producing antibodies to physically interrelated molecules and recruitment and diversification of the T cells in an exact parallel of a physiologic secondary immune response is shown.

demands and constraints on the ability of MHC class II molecules to bind peptides for presentation and to define the T-cell repertoire and perhaps require the specific effects of certain DR2 and DR3 allelic products to result in SLE.

Following this paradigm, genes mapping in the MHC were studied to determine whether they were involved in specifying SLE susceptibility. Fifteen years ago, the first strong association between SLE and certain serologically determined MHC class II DR specificities was reported, with a significant increase in Caucasian SLE patients typing for either HLA-DR2 or HLA-DR3 (91–93) (Table 75.8).

The use of DNA typing methods confirmed and extended the early serologic observations by finding an increase of HLA-DR2 (DRB1*1501) and -DR3 (DRB1*0301) haplotypes in SLE (94–96). These data also explained the weaker earlier associations with class I alleles, since many of the alleles encoding the HLA-DR2 or HLA-DR3 specificities were found on two haplotypes exhibiting strong linkage disequilibrium, HLA-A3-B7-DR2 (DRB1*1501) and HLA-A1-B8-DR3 (DRB1*0301). The molecular genetics of SLE have been analyzed in various populations. HLA-DR2 is significantly increased among both Japanese and Chinese patients with SLE (97). In Japanese patients, some limited evidence also was found for an effect contributed by DR4-containing haplotypes (98), which may act in concert with DR2 haplotypes to increase susceptibility. The first extensive study of DQ and DP alleles identified an increase of DQw2.1(DQB1*0201), part of the HLA-B8-DRB1*0301-DQB1*0201 haplotype (95). Particularly detailed studies of the DR2 and DR3 haplotypes associated with SLE susceptibility have been performed by a European collaborating group (99,100). The complex history of the molecular genetics of SLE is summarized in several reviews (88,101), of which Arnett and Reveille's (101) is particularly comprehensive.

Importantly, genome-wide scans of microsatellites in linkage studies have also implicated the MHC (6p11-p21) as the site of the single greatest genetic predisposition, using multipoint nonparametric methods. This was found at the D6S257 microsatellite allele, located at 6p11-6p12, centromeric to the MHC class II region, logarithm of odds (lod) = 3.90, p = .000011 (102). This effect was much stronger than other non-MHC loci identified in this study.

Implication of HLA Associations for Disease Pathogenesis

The central implication of the fact that susceptibility to SLE is associated with HLA-DR alleles is that the T-cell repertoire contains CD4 T cells that have been selected on, and are capable of recognizing, particular self peptides that are efficiently bound and presented by these MHC molecules. This suggests that an immune recognition event critical to SLE pathogenesis occurs that involves presentation of one or several specific self peptides to T cells capable of their recognition. Presumably, the T-cell repertoire of the susceptible individual differs from that of the person who lacks the MHC susceptibility allele, in that the latter does not contain T cells that can recognize self peptides capable of initiating immune recognition events that underlie SLE. This would also suggest that there are other MHC alleles

TABLE 75.8. COMPOSITE DATA ILLUSTRATING THAT ALLELES ENCODING THE SEROLOGIC SPECIFICITIES OF HLA-DR2 AND HLA-DR3 ARE ASSOCIATED WITH SUSCEPTIBILITY TO SLE

HLA-DR Specificity	Patients (% positive) (n = 82)	Controls (% Positive) (n = 788)	Chi Square (Yates)	Rel. Risk
DR1	26.8	14.1	9.3	2.2
DR2	53.7	26.1	27.5	3.3
DR3	45.1	20.4	25.8	3.2
DR4	19.5	35.3	6.8	–2.2
DR5	10.9	22.3	5.1	–2.3
DR7	18.9	10.3	4.5	2.1

HLA, human leukocyte antigen.

that would exert a dominant inhibitory effect on development of the autoreactive clone or clones.

The presence in the T-cell repertoire of clones with this recognition ability is a necessary, but not sufficient, step in the development of SLE. The second key element, the regulation of clonal responsiveness, is determined by entirely different systems. The regulation of this latter aspect of the immune response is determined by a number of alternative signaling pathways activated during the "immunologic synapses" between antigen-presenting cells, such as dendritic cells or B cells, and the T-cell clone. This is so because, although the specificity of T-cell recognition is determined by the antigen-specific TCR, whether or not the clone is activated by the presented peptide is largely a function of additional signaling pathways mediated by the interaction of additional receptor-ligand pairs (Fig. 75.3).

However, there are a large number of unanswered questions. The particular clone or clones involved in the immune recognition event underlying SLE have not been identified and their peptide specificity is also unknown. The molecular basis of susceptibility provided by the MHC genes is still not well understood. It is possible that one or more of the T-cell clones that recognize autoantigens that are targets of the autoantibody response such as Ro/SSA or ribonucleoproteins could be the clone that participates in the immune recognition that underlies SLE as described above in the induction and expansion phase. Alternatively, the critical immune recognition event could involve an entirely different peptide that currently is not surmised to play a role in SLE, because there is no significant autoantibody produced to the protein containing the peptide. That there is no ready explanation for this critical aspect of SLE is not surprising in view of the relatively limited knowledge of the intricate events occurring in this aspect of the immune system (90).

Interaction of Ethnicity, Sex, and Onset Age with MHC Alleles

Certain HLA alleles are often distinctive features of an ethnic group, and over the course of history there have been multiple events that affect the composition of the gene pool in a given area. In the instance of individuals of European background, HLA-A1-B8-DRB1*0301 and HLA-A3-B7-DRB1*1501(DR2) are both relatively recent introductions into much of the Northern European Caucasian gene pool as illustrated in Fig. 75.6. It has been speculated that these

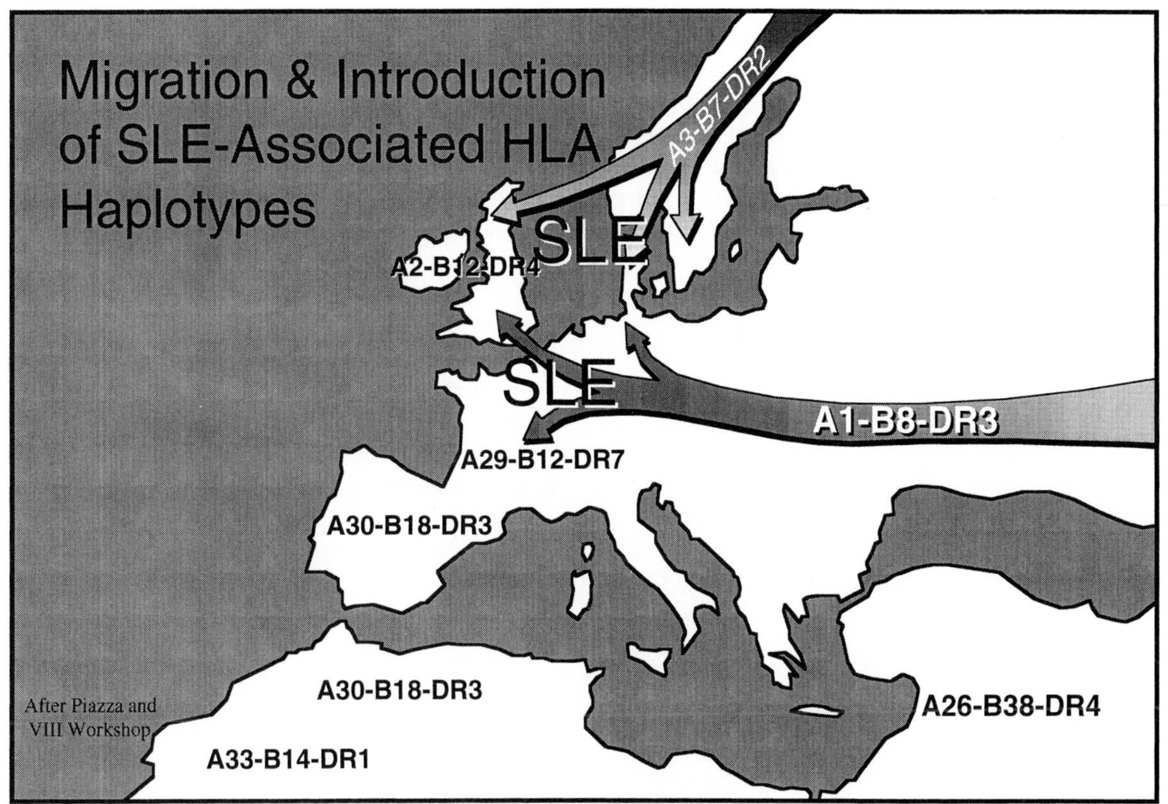

FIGURE 75.6. A genetic map of Europe showing that Northern European Caucasian populations have two HLA haplotypes, HLA-A1-B8-DRB1*0301 and HLA-A3-B7-DRB1*1501(DR2), which are both relatively recent introductions into their gene pool. The HLA-A1-B8-DRB1*0301 may have been introduced earlier by invasions by cultures such as the Visigoths and Huns, whereas the HLA-A3-B7-DRB1*1501 haplotype was spread more recently by the Vikings.

haplotypes were disseminated in their present distribution by the invading Visigoths and Huns for the HLA-A1-B8-DRB1*0301 haplotype and by the Norsemen for the HLA-A3-B7-DRB1*1501(DR2) haplotype. The particularly strong association of SLE with HLA-DR3 is principally found in individuals of Northern European origin and largely reflects an association that is primarily with the HLA-A1-B8-DRB1*0301 haplotype.

In view of the increased frequency of SLE among African Americans, the molecular genetics of this group hold a place of special importance. Two groups identified a higher frequency of the HLA-DR3 specificity in African Americans from Washington, D.C., and Chicago (103,104), which was in the range of 57% to 62% compared to a frequency of 18% to 27% in a control group. Support for the concept that genetic admixture of Caucasian and African gene pools acts as a predisposing factor is provided by the observations of Arnett and colleagues (105), who examined a subset of individuals with antibodies to SS-A/Ro. They asked the interesting question as to whether the increase in the HLA-DR3 serologic specificity was accounted for by haplotypes containing the Caucasoid DRB1*0301 allele or the African haplotypes containing the DRB1*0302 allele. The answer was that only the Caucasian haplotype with the DRB1*0301 allele was increased in frequency among these African Americans with SLE. This suggests that the epistasis between a Caucasian haplotype containing DRB1*0301 and other background African genes results in the high frequency of SLE among American blacks. It is possible that this same epistatic effect is present in Northern European Caucasians because the two HLA haplotypes, HLA-A1-B8-DRB1*0301 and HLA-A3-B7-DRB1*1501(DR2), are both relatively recent introductions into the Northern European Caucasian gene pool (Fig. 75.6).

Age of Onset, HLA-DR Alleles, and Genetic Heterogeneity

Since a general tenet of genetics holds that in multigenic diseases, individuals with the larger dose of stronger susceptibility genes will manifest the disease earlier than those with a lesser dose, the question of the influence of HLA alleles on the age at which SLE develops is of interest. Hochberg (6) found that the frequency of HLA-DR2 is 48% in the youngest disease-onset quartile, which developed disease before age 22, falling to 23% in the oldest quartile, which developed disease after age 44, and to 16% in those in whom SLE appeared after age 50, a value lower than that of 24% found in the healthy control population.

A more unexpected observation was made by Bell and colleagues (106), who found that HLA-DR3, and by implication the haplotype containing the DRB1*0301 allele, was increased in frequency among Caucasoid females with late-onset SLE (mean age 48 years), compared to early-onset SLE (mean age 22 years), suggesting this haplotype acts more slowly to cause disease. In one series, HLA-DRw8 was found in 39% of African American SLE patients with onset before 20 years of age versus 0% in patients over 40 years of age at onset (107).

DR Alleles and Specific Manifestations In SLE

In view of the heterogeneity in clinical and laboratory manifestations of SLE, combined with the insight from murine autoimmune disease of the genetic control of subphenotypes, it has been of continuing interest to determine whether this heterogeneity could be associated with any genetic polymorphisms found in patients. Using autoantibodies as indirect markers of T-cell recognition of autoantigens, only a limited association has been found between MHC genotype and the production of antibodies to dsDNA and the small cytoplasmic ribonucleoprotein system (e.g., Ro/SS-A). dsDNA antibodies are strongly related to HLA-DR3 or HLA-DR2 (Table 75.9) (108). Griffing and colleagues (109) reported that 67% of patients with SLE with anti-dsDNA antibodies were HLA-DR3, whereas only 13% of patients lacking HLA-DR3 had these antibodies. In contrast, in a different population, 68% of SLE patients with anti-dsDNA antibodies were HLA-DR2 (110). The presence of autoantibodies to Ro/SS-A, especially in clinical subsets such as subacute cutaneous SLE, is associated with DR3 in 65% of patients (111). Anti-Ro/SS-A antibodies are found in 70% of patients with subacute cutaneous lupus erythematosus (111). It is likely that T-cell responses will provide a clearer insight into the identity of the peptide recognized in the context of the MHC susceptibility alleles.

TABLE 75.9. GENERAL CHARACTERISTICS OF AUTOIMMUNE RESPONSE ASSOCIATED WITH EITHER DR2 OR DR3 HAPLOTYPES

Haplotype	DR2	DR3
DR allele	DRB1*1501	DRB1*0301
Autoantibodies	Anti-dsDNA	Anti-dsDNA
	Anti-SSA/Ro	Anti-SSA/Ro
	Anti-Sm	
Clinical syndrome	Glomerulonephritis?	Subacute SLE
		Neonatal SLE

Similarly, the neonatal lupus syndrome of thrombocytopenia, hemolytic anemia, annular erythematous rash, vasculitis, and sometimes cardiac conduction and other developmental abnormalities, is also strongly associated with the presence in the mother of both DR3 and anti-Ro/SSA antibodies (112). The anti-RNP antibody system and the highly disease specific anti-Sm antibodies are associated with HLA-DR2 (DRB1*1501) and with the DQAI*0102 and DQB1*0602 alleles that are present on certain HLA-DR2 and DRw6 haplotypes (113).

One of the paradoxical observations concerning the association of MHC alleles, notably HLA-DR3, with susceptibility to autoimmune disease is that different diseases, such as gluten-sensitive enteropathy, myasthenia gravis, insulin-dependent diabetes mellitus (IDDM), and SLE are associated with similar, if not the same, DR3 haplotypes, yet these diseases are not found strongly clustered together in epidemiologic studies. This emphasizes the point that the predisposition for one autoimmune disease is not simply a predisposing immunologic environment for the development of other autoimmune diseases and that the specific interaction of other MHC genes, nonclassic MHC genes, or genes outside the MHC region are important in the development of susceptibility for a particular autoimmune disease.

Other Genes of the MHC Not Involved in Antigen Presentation

The MHC class II genes are likely to be only one group of susceptibility alleles for SLE in the class II or III region of the MHC, and it is possible that MHC genes not directly involved in presenting peptides to T cells will also be involved in specifying susceptibility for SLE (114). For example, the TNFB*1 allele of TNF is overrepresented in the SLE population, perhaps because of the presence of this allele in the HLA-A1-B8-DR3 haplotype. A polymorphism in the promoter-enhancer region of the *Tnf-α* gene was identified in this haplotype that correlates with elevated secretion of TNF-α.

Complement Polymorphisms

The C4Q0 null alleles for C4 are associated with an increased risk of SLE, but because this allele is a component of the HLA-A1-B8-DRB1*0301-C4AQ0-C4B haplotype, it does not appear that the C4Q0 null alleles are responsible for driving the association with this haplotype and that DR3 is more central, based on a large study of over 300 central Europeans (115).

The Relationship of Homozygous C2 Deficiency to Classic SLE

Several of the homozygous complete complement deficiencies that involve different components of the classic and alternative pathways, notably C2 or C4, are associated with a greatly increased risk for the development of a lupus-like autoimmune syndrome. The null gene responsible for C2 deficiency is very often associated with the haplotype HLA-A25-B18-C2(null)-DR2 (DRB1*1501)-DQw1 (116). A proportion of individuals with this deficiency have a lupus-like illness characterized by the onset during adult life of constitutional symptoms, nondestructive polyarthritis, pericarditis, photosensitivity, and other rashes (116). Antinuclear antibodies and antibodies to the Ro/SS-A are sometimes present, although at a lower frequency and in lower titer than is found in classic SLE.

Non-MHC Genes

Cytokine Genes

As reviewed by Gulko and Winchester (17), several cytokine, cytokine receptor, and signal transduction genes that regulate B- and T-cell activity and maturation may have a regulatory role in SLE and are thus attractive candidate genes, although a definitive relationship to susceptibility has not yet been found. For example, IL-10 is produced at high levels by B lymphocytes and monocytes of SLE patients, and regulates anti-dsDNA antibody production (117). IL-10 levels are under genetic control, and relatives of SLE patients have higher IL-10 levels than controls (118). While IL-10 promoter polymorphisms are not associated with SLE, an allelic imbalance in SLE of microsatellite alleles in the IL-10 region has been reported (119). Increased spontaneous production or serum levels of other proinflammatory cytokines such as IL-1 and IL-6 are found in SLE. An IL-6 restriction fragment length polymorphism (RFLP) allele is reported to be increased in one series of SLE patients (120), as has an IL-1 receptor antagonist gene polymorphism (IL1RN*2), particularly in association with photosensitivity and discoid skin lesions (121).

Genes Involved in Clearance of Immune Complexes

Genes involved in clearance of immune complexes by the mononuclear phagocyte system, including Fc-receptors, complement receptor-1 (CR1), and mannose-binding proteins (MBPs), have been studied (17). The FcGR2A-H131 allele of the FcGR2A locus residing on chromosome 1 is the only human FcR that recognizes IgG2 efficiently, and the presence of this allele was reported as protective for renal disease among African American SLE patients, with the R131 genotype increasing the risk for renal disease (122). This area has been informatively reviewed (123). CR1 expression is decreased on erythrocytes of SLE patients. Some of the early interest in the erythrocyte CR1 levels has been tempered by the demonstration that the reduction in levels of this receptor is secondary to the load of immune complexes, though interest persists in the role of polymorphisms of this molecule (124). However, erythrocyte CR1 levels are not correlated with any CR1 gene polymorphisms (125). MBP binds hypoglycosylated IgG Fc region and activates complement. MBP has two polymorphic codons (Glu57 and Asp54) that correlate with decreased serum levels of the protein, and both codons are present in increased frequency in African American SLE patients, when compared to normal controls (126). Ig allotypes have long been considered as possible candidate genes in SLE susceptibility. However, their relevance has now been excluded by the findings obtained in a large case series (127).

Genome-Wide Scans

The availability of microsatellite polymorphisms, which are simple polymorphic nucleotide repeat patterns scattered at frequent intervals throughout the genome, has greatly facilitated the search for loci relevant to autoimmunity and has been reviewed (128). Linkage analysis has been used in SLE by several groups (reviewed in ref. 17). The use of linkage techniques allows an unbiased assessment of novel genes not previously thought to be relevant to disease. In complex trait disease, though, the mode of inheritance is usually not mendelian, and techniques that do not require assumption of the mode of transmission are better applied. Linkage studies done so far by Tsao and colleagues (129) using this approach have identified a potential locus at human chromosome 1q41-q42. This locus is far from the FcG2RA gene [>60 centimorgan (cM)], spans 15 cM, and may contain 500 genes. It is not clear which is the gene responsible for this locus, and it may well be one that has not been identified yet. Kearns' group (102) identified regions on 1p36, 1p13, and 1q41-q42. Candidate genes for the 1p36 locus include TNFR2 and IL-14. Additional support for a susceptibility locus in this region was provided by the study of a large cohort (130).

POTENTIAL MECHANISMS FOR INITIATING THE INDUCTION PHASE OF SLE

Figure 75.1 depicts a model for SLE pathogenesis in which the susceptibility state is followed by the induction phase characterized by the development of autoreactive T cells that reflect loss of self tolerance. The delayed appearance of SLE implies that the susceptibility genes require a set of subsequent events to proceed through the stages of clonal induction and expansion that lead to loss of tolerance and, ultimately, to mechanisms of tissue injury and the disease of SLE. The occurrence of these events likely also accounts for lack of perfect twin concordance rates and apparent partial penetrance of the trait for SLE.

There are several ways of classifying events that may explain the development of SLE in a genetically susceptible person many years after birth. One way, which focuses on the origin of the event, distinguishes external nongenetic precipitating events such as sun exposure or endogenous effects that act slowly. In another classification, the mechanisms leading to the loss of T-cell tolerance are placed in two groups. The first group are those that involve induction of a novel peptide structure that potentially stimulates quiescent, but not previously tolerized, T cells that are in the torpid state (sometimes termed clonal ignorance). The second group includes those in which previously established T-cell tolerance is broken.

Normalcy of Susceptibility Genes

One potential explanation that has been ruled out, at least in the case of the MHC susceptibility genes, is that there is nothing inherently pathologic or abnormal about the DRB1*0301 or DR2 MHC alleles associated with SLE. Indeed, the identification of additional SLE susceptibility genes will most likely result in the identification of otherwise "normal" alleles that influence aspects of immune responsiveness and that are not intrinsically deleterious. As knowledge grows about the immune system, the line is becoming increasingly blurred between autorecognition, upon which the physiologic action of the immune system is based, and autoimmunity upon which the development of autoimmune disease is based. Importantly also, because the same T cells selected on self peptides are involved in both physiologic and autoimmune responses, the events are not likely to wholly depend on the structure of the TCR.

Alterations in Peptide Presentation or Processing

Anomalous Processing of Peptide in Apoptosis

The potential of apoptosis to present peptides in an anomalous manner has been emphasized above (76). Anomalous peptide presentation is a general mechanism for stimulating quiescent, but not previously tolerized, T cells. The premise is that the self-tolerant state is abrogated by the anomalous presentation of peptides (Table 75.10). An incisive approach to the analysis of self determinants recognized by the T-cell repertoire has been taken by Sercarz and Datta (131). They and workers in several other laboratories have distinguished regions of self peptides to which the T-cell immune system has become tolerant, the immunodominant regions, and other regions to which the immune system does not become tolerant, the so-called cryptic regions for which there are T cells in the repertoire that can recognize, but do not respond to, these regions. The peptides composing the dominant self are processed and presented in the thymus, leading to central and, probably, peripheral tolerance. However, the major portion of any given peptide avoids this process and seemingly escapes the attention of

TABLE 75.10. HYPOTHETICAL MECHANISMS OF HOW GENETIC PREDISPOSITION TO AN IMMUNE RECOGNITION EVENT LEADS TO THE INDUCTION PHASE OF SLE

Peptide presentation abrogates tolerance
Self antigen presented in the context of different MHC molecules
Induction of ectopic MHC class II expression
Altered processing/apoptosis of self peptide
Hormone-induced alteration in cellular expression
Non–self antigen presentation
Mimicry
T-cell repertoire bias
Allele-specific selection differences
Drift due to non–antigen-specific or superantigen clonal stimulation
Effect of cytokine balance
Shift to Th2 or Th1 environment

Th, T-helper.

the T cells. Novel antigen-processing events, such as those mediated by caspases in apoptosis, that draw the attention of the T cell to cryptic determinants likely could arise from expression of aggregates of autoantigens in apoptotic blebs as discussed above.

Ectopic Expression of MHC Class II Molecules

The second major mechanisms for altering peptide antigen presentation is de novo expression of MHC class II molecules on cells that normally do not express them (Table 75.10). This concept is based on the novel presentation of a cell-specific peptide in the context of MHC class II molecules to CD4 T cells that may only have been tolerized to self peptides normally encountered in the context of class I molecules. Co-stimulation is not usually provided by cells that are not professional antigen presenters; however, because of the enhanced state of activation of the T-cell repertoire in SLE, this co-stimulation requirement may be reduced.

Stimulation of "Tolerant" or "Ignorant" T-Cell Clones

Tolerance Disruption Through Mimicry of Self Peptide and a Microorganism Peptide

One of the nongenetic explanations for the delayed appearance of SLE is infection with a particular inciting agent. This is perhaps the most simple and intrinsically appealing of all etiologic hypotheses to attempt to account for the delayed development of SLE. Crow and Christian (7) critically evaluated the data favoring an infectious etiology, pointing out some of the similarities of the host autoimmune response of SLE to that found in immune response to infection. The theory that Epstein-Barr virus (EBV) infection is somehow implicated has had a resurgence of interest with the observation that virtually all, 99%, of young SLE patients had seroconverted against EBV, as compared with only 70% of their controls (132). However, there is no unambiguous direct or indirect evidence in support of the role of any specific infectious agent. Moreover, the general epidemiologic and genetic findings of SLE are not consistent with specific infection as a possible mechanism, specific organisms have not been identified on culture, and there has been no consistent serologic evidence of an immune response to a known infectious agent in extensive laboratory studies. Furthermore, even the murine models of autoimmunity are spontaneous endogenous processes that do not have an evident specific infectious trigger. Thus, the hypothesis of a specific infection initiating SLE remains a conjecture unsupported by any data.

In contrast, cross-reactive mechanisms for tolerance disruption through mimicry by a commensal microorganism have been identified in animal experiments. Studies in organ-specific autoimmune diseases such as multiple sclerosis and the animal model of autoimmune encephalomyelitis reveal that the candidate autoimmunity-inducing peptide need have only five residues of the native peptide to induce reactivity or autoimmunity (133,134). In SLE, there are diverse theoretic examples of this as a potential mechanism, based on sequence homologies, but none has as yet been established as being directly implicated. These examples include sharing of conformational epitopes between a structure on the U1 snRNP-C protein and a protein encoded by the herpes simplex virus (135), and the Sm-D protein and Epstein-Barr encoded EBNA-1 protein (136).

Superantigen or Other Mechanisms of Polyclonal Activation

Superantigens capable of non–antigen-specific activation of cells bearing particular TCRs formed from particular Vβ elements act in a manner analogous to that of the mimicry mechanism described above. The importance of the state of the T-cell repertoire is illustrated by the fact that superantigen exposure stimulates autoimmunity if it occurs after autoreactivity is induced, possibly through its Th1-like effect, but decreases the likelihood of autoimmunity if superantigen exposure occurs before induction of autoreactivity (137). The infection of B cells by EBV is a special example, perhaps because it is a pandemic virus that initiates a prolonged illness with marked host responsiveness. Although neither EBV nor other viruses have been implicated as specific causative agents, prior EBV infections have been described more often in young-age–onset SLE than in controls (132). B-cell activation could alter presentation of self antigens by affecting the basal level of antigen processing and presentation. The polyclonal B-cell activation phase could fortuitously affect a B cell with a B-cell receptor specific for a self structure that in turn leads to T-cell clonal activation sufficient to disrupt tolerance.

Cytokine Environment

A second major effect is the cytokine environment in which the particular immune response is occurring. A Th1 environment favors the production of autoimmunity that is characterized by T-cell mechanisms, while autoimmunity involving antibody formation is fostered by a Th2 environment. A shift in the cytokine balance to one favoring a Th2 response is a well-recognized effect of the immune response to parasitic infections (138). The genetic effect that contributes to the regulation of the Th1-Th2 balance most likely acts through promotion of the qualitative tendency of the T-cell repertoire to recognize autoantigens and, possibly, through the particular pattern of cytokines elaborated during the autoimmune recognition events (139). Even in the absence of a specific infectious etiology, non–autoantigen-specific infections could act to modifying either the T-cell repertoire or the cytokine environment in a way that encourages the evolution of autoimmunity (140).

Bias and Qualitative Features of the T Cell Repertoire

Stoichastic events enter into several aspects of the generation of the immune system and an immune response. The genes composing the Ig and TCR recognition structures are generated by a process of combinatorial and junctional diversity that involves random nucleotide deletion and addition. This is followed by positive and negative clonal selection that involves chance encounters with other cells presenting self peptides in the context of MHC molecules. Furthermore, the maintenance of the naive repertoire requires continued interaction with the same peptide-MHC structures (90).

The effect of the general microorganism environment on susceptibility to autoimmune disease has been studied in several murine models. On the one hand, the presence of environmental microorganisms diminished the penetrance of the genetically determined autoimmune insulinitis in NOD mice, suggesting a protective role of environmental antigen challenge, while it increases susceptibility to neurologic disease in a myelin basic protein transgenic mouse model (141,142). This effect could be produced at the level of altering the relative preponderance of certain T-cell clones in the repertoire or by affecting the cytokine balance (143). Infection by a microbial agent bearing a superantigen could also, in theory, significantly shift the repertoire in a direction leading to enhanced autoreactivity of SLE (Table 75.10).

Activation of Dendritic Cells

Dendritic cells play a powerful role in the regulation of immunity, with their "natural adjuvant"-like action (142). An understanding of the events associated with the induction of clonal anergy rather than clonal deletion, both centrally and peripherally, and its reversal during the induction of an autoimmune response is rapidly evolving (88). There is increasing appreciation that anergization, itself, proceeds through multiple mechanisms. Signals provided by dendritic cells play a large role in determining whether a particular peptide will become the object of an immune response. The absence of co-stimulatory molecules on a cell expressing a self peptide may result in a passive anergic clonal response that is characterized by the inability of the T cell to respond to the self peptide with the release of IL-2 (145). Alternatively, the provision of co-stimulatory signals by a dendritic cell to a quiescent clone may activate it to sustained self reactivity. Little is currently known about the role of dendritic cells in initiating recognition of self peptides, although it is clear that these cells are powerfully stimulated by apoptotic cells (77).

Noninfectious Agents in the Environment as an Explanation for Development of SLE

Sun exposure is an exogenous environmental effect that clearly plays a role in the biology of SLE in view of the high frequency of the light-sensitive butterfly rash and other cutaneous manifestations of SLE. Indeed, in some individuals the skin component appears first, or is clearly exacerbated following sun exposure. Occasionally, the first clinical evidence of SLE affecting other organs develops in the weeks following severe sun exposure. Sun exposure could simply reveal an already existing state of autoimmunity by provoking autoantigen release from a damaged keratinocyte. Alternatively, sun exposure could affect localization of preexisting autoantibody-containing immune complexes through the direct injury of endothelium or the nonspecific release by the injured keratinocyte of cytokines and other mediators of inflammation that affect endothelial permeability to circulating complexes (146). Sun exposure might also act much earlier in the pathogenic sequence in the induction phase to initiate a *de novo* autoimmune response. There are three main possibilities. In experimental animals, ultraviolet (UV) irradiation has been shown to alter cellular DNA through the formation of novel nucleotide adducts and dimers leading to evidence of autoimmunity. Second, sun-induced injury of the keratinocyte induces an apoptotic response that includes redistribution of autoantigenic molecules, such as DNA- and RNA-binding proteins, to the cell surface (147). This may promote a large local concentration of complexed and unusually processed molecules serving to initiate autoimmune reactivity, perhaps through presentation by dendritic cells. Third, by inducing expression of class II MHC molecules, the response to sun injury may result in the appearance of peptides presented in the context of MHC class II molecules to which the individual may not have been tolerized in the thymus.

Chemicals and Drugs: Drug-Induced Lupus

Drug-induced lupus is caused by a variety of specific chemical agents that initiate a number of different autoimmune states. The development of autoimmunity in a predisposed person serves as a possible model for events in SLE. There has been considerable interest in the possibility of a relationship between drug-induced lupus and classic idiopathic SLE, as well as in the mechanisms involved in initiating the changes in immune recognition induced by the drug. Despite some limited clinical similarities, the drug-induced lupus syndromes are now understood to be entirely distinct from idiopathic SLE in terms of the differences in susceptibility genes, including genes that regulate drug biotransformation and pharmacokinetics, as well as quite different MHC allele associations. The profile of autoantibodies also differs considerably, indicating that the autoantigenic targets of the immune response initiated by the drug are different. Little is known about the T-cell response involved in the response. Furthermore, epidemiologic studies do not indicate an increased frequency of untoward reactions to these drugs in SLE or in their family members. Exposure to silicone in breast implants or other prostheses also has been investigated as a putative agent for initiating SLE-like responses with entirely negative results (148). However, if considered as potential subphenotypes of autoimmune responsiveness, the drug-induced responses may provide significant insight into the mechanisms operating in SLE.

INVOLVEMENT OF T CELLS AND B CELLS IN THE INDUCTION PHASE OF SLE

This section discusses some of the potential immune recognition events that convert the susceptibility state to the induction phase of SLE, as illustrated in Fig. 75.2. The critical immune recognition event that is central to the development of SLE occurs when a CD4 T cell binds to, and is activated by, an autoantigen presented in the context of MHC class II molecules. The development of an autoimmune response to snRNP particles is used as an illustration of an immune recognition event (Fig. 75.2). The T cell of the CD4 lineage is specific for a self peptide found in one of the subcellular particles responsible for initiating linked sets of autoantibodies. The B cell that is the clonal antecedent of an autoantibody producing cell, but which acts to bind the subcellular particle through recognition of a specific epitope on a molecule of the particle such as the RNA moiety, internalizes and processes the peptides of the particle and presents them in the context of a class II molecule to the T cell. In this example, a B cell has been used to illustrate the antigen-presenting cell, but it is increasingly possible that it would be more correct to depict a dendritic cell serving to induce the initial autorecognition event that activates the CD4 T cell. The B cell directed to a cognate autoantigen specificity would then be capable of maintaining the activation status of the autoreactive T cell.

B Cells Specific for the RNA Moiety of snRNP Particles

Several scenarios for the immune recognition of snRNP particles may be envisioned, according to the fine specificities of the B cell. One such scenario is that the entire snRNP response is initiated by the presence of a B-cell clone specific for the RNA moiety, as shown in Fig. 75.2 (62,149). The autoantibody response to the U1-specific snRNPs, which include the 70-kd protein and protein A and protein C of this complex, as well as to conformationally distinctive regions on the RNA molecule itself has been studied (150). Because a large proportion of autoantibodies are reactive with various conformational entities on the U1 molecule, it has been suggested that RNA molecules may be a special target driving the initiation phase of the autoimmune reaction to the U1 snRNP complex, rather than a late consequence of primary recognition at another site (150,151).

It is likely that the B-cell clone that initiates or amplifies this early step in the induction of autoimmunity has a low affinity for U1 RNA species and might be part of the normal B-cell repertoire. The putative U1-specific B-cell clone would bind not only free U1 RNA species, but also the entire snRNP particle on its IgM surface Ig receptor. The complex would be endocytosed and the associated peptides expressed on the surface of the B cell, where they await the chance arrival of a member of an autoimmune CD4-positive T-cell clone endowed with the capacity to recognize these self-peptides presented in the context of class II MHC molecules for initiation of the induction phase of the autoimmune response of SLE. Once this T-cell recognition occurs, semicognate help is provided for the B-cell clone and some members of the B-cell clone differentiate into antibody producing cells, while others proliferate to expand the clone and differentiate into memory cells. The B-cell repertoire may not, itself, be unbiased, since there is evidence from transgenic mice that some selection against autoreactive B cells occurs during the formation of the repertoire by a process designated receptor editing that occurs during light chain selection (152).

B Cells Specific for the Protein Moiety of SNRNP Particles

A second equivalent scenario begins with B cells specific for the protein moiety of snRNP particles rather than a B cell specific for a nucleic acid. This B cell binds the particle through a protein epitope and presents the peptides of the particle to T cells with the same properties that have just been described (Fig. 75.4).

INVOLVEMENT OF T AND B CELLS IN THE EXPANSION PHASE OF SLE

Following the induction of autoreactive T cells in the induction phase of SLE, the immune system responds by progressively enlarging and strengthening the autoimmune response (Fig. 75.1). It is likely that only one or a few B-cell clones or other antigen-presenting cells play a central role in initiating the presentation of self antigen to T cells during the expansion of the autoimmune response. This accounts for recruitment of the production of additional antibodies to physically interrelated molecules and by recruitment and diversification of the T cells in the physiologic secondary immune response. Evidence for the participation of this system has been presented by Mamula and colleagues (151,153). The T-cell clone expands, being driven by the available supply of autoantigen presented by the semicognate or cognate B cell, and the B-cell clones similarly expand (Fig. 75.5).

In the case of the DNA binding B cell, site-directed mutagenesis has established the importance of somatic hypermutation of the autoantigen-specific B-cell immunoglobulin receptor in increasing the weak intrinsic affinity of an antibody for DNA. This occurs especially by the addition of positively charged arginine residues (154). The physiologic maturation of affinity of B cells is driven by T-cell help and is a part of the normal immune response. However, the selective change in the B-cell compartment appears critical for the subsequent development of T-cell autoimmunity by driving the process toward B cells that are capable of eliciting enhanced cognate T-cell help, thus reinforcing the cycle leading to a full-fledged autoimmune response.

This first component of the expansion process sets the next stage in this process of recruitment, in which the autoimmune response can expand to include other B cells that have IgM receptors separately specific for different molecular epitopes in the snRNP particle. The inciting particle behaves as an immunogen with the focus of the autoimmune response spreading to other elements of the particle. In the instance of the mechanism in Fig. 75.2, B cells specific for other nucleic acid moieties are recruited, whereas in the case of the mechanism shown in Fig. 75.4, B cells specific for additional proteins are recruited. The expanding number of T cells in the autoimmune clone provide help to these new B cells, which, in common with the originating (e.g., U1-specific) B cell, present the self peptide recognized by the autoimmune T cells, although they bind different elements of the snRNP particle. It can be imagined that this binding is of a lower order than that of the originating (e.g., U1-specific) B cell. The spreading of the immune response is a strikingly evident finding in several other autoimmune responses in SLE, including the formation of autoantibodies to SS-A/Ro and SS-B/La (155) and the Sm antigen B/B′ peptide of the spliceosome (156).

T-Cell Repertoire Determinant Spread

It remains uncertain whether the disruption of immunity initiated by T-cell autoimmune clones described above undergoes an expansion to recruit additional clones. In some murine disease models, and in human diseases such as multiple sclerosis, in which the autoantigen is sequestered, the response of the immune system to a break in tolerance is progressive broadening of the immune response to additional determinants on the peptide that breached the tolerant state and to molecules associated with it. In the case of murine immunization with myelin basic protein, the response of the T-cell repertoire is initially directed to a single stretch of 11 amino acids, but progressively the T-cell response broadens to different determinants and includes several additional regions on the molecule (157). In this sense, the state of autoimmunity is seen as dynamic and evolving rather than fixed, an observation that is particularly consistent with the changing pattern of autoantibodies seen in SLE.

There are several features of SLE that can be explained by events postulated to occur in this hypothetical phase. Clearly, as in the induction phase, the process in the expansion phase is stochastic in that the chance meeting of the appropriate B cell, T cell, and antigen is required, a meeting that becomes more likely with the passage of time. This phase accounts for the shift in autoantibody isotype to IgG, which also greatly enhances the pathogenic properties of the autoantibodies by allowing them to readily leave the circulation. The likelihood that the B-cell and T-cell events of the expansion and selection process take considerable time may explain several clinical features of SLE. These include, for example, the delay into late childhood or adulthood of the onset of SLE, the incomplete penetrance of the trait as seen from the less than 100% concordance of identical twins for SLE, and the progressive increase in severity of SLE.

Because the selection process in the B-cell and T-cell compartments in SLE is driven by the combination of B-cell antigen presentation and T-cell recognition, which ultimately reduces to the provision of cognate help, this process does not select for pathogenicity of the resulting autoantibodies. Thus, the development of autoantibodies that are particularly pathogenic, for example those that are highly active in forming immune complexes that are injurious to the kidney, is a stochastic outcome of the autoimmune response and not an objective for which there appears to be intrinsic selection.

Regulatory T Cells

There is renewed interest in the active regulatory role of T-cell subsets in the dynamic anergization of autoreactive T cells (158). This is visualized to occur through a variety of cytokine networks involving CD4 and CD8 T cells (139). Some of these mechanisms may involve interactions mediated by class I MHC molecules, or even the nonclassic variety of class I molecules (159,160). In the aggregate, mechanisms such as these may account for anergization and the conversion of this state to active self recognition.

Cognate Interactions of T Cells and B Cells as Therapeutic Targets

In view of the importance of the CD40-CD40L pathway in regulating the cognate interaction of T and B cells, as well as the clear abnormalities in expression of members of this ligand receptor pair, interruption of this pathway is a potential target for immunomodulation of SLE. Treatment with antibodies that blocked the CD40-CD40L interaction could considerably delay the development of fatal lupus nephritis, if given early (43,161). Trials in SLE are currently under way to determine the safety and efficacy of monoclonal antibodies to CD40L.

ROLE OF AUTOANTIBODIES AND FORMATION OF IMMUNE COMPLEXES IN PATHOGENESIS OF THE DESTRUCTIVE PHASE

The destructive phase of SLE is characterized by the expression of this coordinated autoimmune response that results in significant and clinically evident immunologic injury. This injury is largely, although not exclusively, attributed to the action of autoantibodies resulting from the autoimmune response. The antibodies cause injury through their ability to bind to molecules that are or become accessible on the cell membrane, that are normally found in plasma, or that are released into blood or connective tissue from intracellular sites of injured cells.

Direct Binding of Autoantibodies to Target Molecules

Autoantibodies may cause immune injury or impairment of function by directly binding to target autoantigenic structures that are either normally found on the cell surface, induced to traffic to that location, or that usually circulate as plasma proteins. There are four main consequences of this binding:

1. The function of the target molecule may be impaired by blockade of its active region by the antibody, as is the case for some of the anticardiolipin group of antibodies (Chapter 77), or antilymphocyte autoantibodies that impair, for example, mixed lymphocyte reactivity (58,59).
2. The binding of an autoantibody may act as a stimulating surrogate ligand. Direct activation of circulating polymorphonuclear leukocytes (PMNs) in fluid phase may be induced by antileukocyte antibodies or by soluble immune complexes, cytokines, and other mediators of acute inflammation. This results in cell–cell adhesion and clumping of PMNs, an event termed leukergy. This is a somewhat uncommon, but serious, event in SLE that is distinguished from vasculitis by the absence of localized deposition of circulating immune complexes and the absence of primary inflammation of the vessel wall. In its extreme form, it is responsible for a form of adult respiratory distress syndrome. Similarly, some instances of the thrombotic thrombocytopenic purpura syndrome that occasionally develops in SLE may be due to a similar platelet activation mechanism mediated by certain antiplatelet antibodies.
3. Another consequence is cellular destruction. Thrombocytopenia and Coombs-positive anemia result from antibody binding to differentially expressed surface structures on these two cell types through the uptake of the antibody-coated cell or molecule by phagocyte Fc receptors.
4. Lastly, the bound antibodies may initiate activation of effector systems such as complement that may result in cellular injury and inflammation and also contribute to the cytopenias of the disease through opsonization followed by phagocytosis (3). A particularly interesting feature of SLE is the formation of IgG antibodies to C1q that appear to activate this component and thus initiate activation of the classic pathway of the complement system (162).

Neonatal SLE Syndrome Suggests How Autoantibodies May Cause Injury

Is there a pathogenic role for autoantibodies directed to intracellular autoantigens such as nucleic acids or their binding proteins when these autoantigens are still in an intact cell? Apart from direct binding to molecules normally accessible to the plasma, such as in immune complex formation, a direct pathogenic role for these autoantibodies is very difficult to demonstrate. However, the striking clinical observations on the events in autoantibody-mediated congenital complete heart block (CCHB) in neonatal SLE suggests that our understanding of how autoantibodies cause injury is still very incomplete (163). In CCHB, antibodies from the mother that are directed to snRNPs of the SS-A/Ro, SS-B/La group are passively transferred across the placenta to the gestating infant. These maternally derived autoantibodies, which are specific for autoantigens that we consider intracellular, have been implicated as proximate causes of the neonatal SLE syndrome. This syndrome consists of the typical rash of SLE, hepatitis, and carditis with gross impairment of the conduction system that results in CCHB. Its occurrence serves as strong evidence for an injurious role of the autoantibodies of SLE.

However, the mechanism by which these passively acquired autoantibodies result in a fetal disease that does not have the appearance of immune complex injury is still unclear. Nonetheless, the biology of CCHB reminds us to keep an open mind regarding how autoantibodies cause injury in SLE, apart from the well-documented immune complex mechanism. One interesting observation has shown that the neonatal heart expresses a different isotype of the 52-kd Ro/SSA molecule involving alternative splicing of an exon (164). In view of the striking alteration in the location of autoantigenic particles in cells undergoing apoptosis (76), and if the fetus is considered as metabolically stressed due to its relative hypoxemia, then apoptosis or stress is another potential mechanism for the initiation of autoantigen accessibility.

Immune Complex Injury

Autoantibodies also may mediate injury either by forming circulating complexes or by binding to released autoantigens that have first bound to components of connective tissue. There is clear evidence for a role of both of these types of immune complexes in mediating at least part of the systemic nature of the manifestations of SLE, including inflammation of the small blood vessels and organs such as the kidney. The identification of the role of immune complexes in SLE has primarily been the achievement of Kunkel and his colleagues (165,166). Beginning with studies that identified the serum factors responsible for the lupus erythematosus (LE) cell phenomenon as autoantibodies directed to nuclear components, workers in that laboratory characterized the specificity of the autoantibodies by identifying a number of the autoantigen molecules and demonstrated the clinical utility of following their levels (167). The current understanding of the mechanisms of renal injury and their pathologic concomitants have been comprehensively reviewed (168).

Pathogenesis of Immune Complex Injury

Insight into the pathophysiologic role of immune complex clearance and the appearance of immune injury, including vasculitis and glomerulonephritis, came from studies of experimental serum sickness conducted by Dixon (165). Greater glomerular proliferative and infiltrative alterations were observed in animals with higher titers of antibodies, while mesangial alterations predominated in those with lower titers, suggesting that the clinical classification of glomerulonephritis largely reflected the chronicity and intensity of immune complex injury. Mannik and colleagues (170,171) studied the stoichiometry of antigen and antibody in the formation of a circulating immune complex and its pathophysiologic consequences. Large complexes containing greater than three antibody molecules were preferentially removed by the liver and other elements of the phagocytic system, including the spleen and lymph nodes, leaving the smaller complexes in circulation, where they were ultimately deposited in tissue sites.

The World Health Organization (WHO) classification of SLE nephritis reflects the immune complex–mediated changes that occur in the glomerulus and is entirely based on assessment of glomerular alterations (168).

Fc receptors and complement receptors both participate in the clearance of immune complexes. In the case of complexes that have activated and fixed components of complement, the opsonized complexes bind to C3b receptors (CD21 molecules) present on erythrocytes, which then circulate to the liver where the complexes and the CD21 molecules are removed by Kupffer cells (172). Activation of the complement system consumes some of the early complement components, notably C2 and C4, thereby lowering the total hemolytic complement activity. Immune complexes of DNA and antibodies to dsDNA are particularly effective in binding to C1q and initiating complement activation. Some circulating complexes gain access to tissue, a process influenced by the stoichiometry of autoantigen to autoantibody, the net charge of the antigen or antibody, the level of vasoactive amines and cytokines, and the activation state of the endothelium. Organs with a fenestrated capillary network, such as the skin, synovium, choroid plexus, and glomeruli, are particularly likely to exhibit immune complex deposition. Negatively charged sulfate side chains on glycosaminoglycan components of the glomerular basement membrane, skin, and vessel wall cause positively charged cationic antigens or antibodies to adhere to these oppositely charged sites, whereas neutral complexes of equivalent size do not bind (173).

The action of histamine on the endothelium results in the expression of P-selectin, which interacts with a counterreceptor on the PMN, causing the cell to roll along the endothelium (174). Activation steps in the PMN result in upregulation of certain integrin molecules such as CD11b/CD18 from cytoplasmic stores, as well as activation of these molecules to a state of enhanced adherence through pathways involving phosphorylation on cytoplasmic domains. These leukocyte integrins interact with endothelial molecules, such as intercellular adhesion molecules (ICAMs), to attach the cell firmly to the endothelium and, ultimately, mediate its leaving the vascular compartment to mediate injury in an inappropriate attempt to ingest the immune complexes. Vasoactive amines, such as histamine, released from mast cells influence the process by enhancing vascular permeability, a phenomenon seen in the "wheal and flare" component of immune injury, and by altering the microarchitecture of the vessel. Platelet-derived factors, as well as cytokines from reacting T cells, alter the endothelial cell interactions with themselves and the underlying basement membrane, resulting in the formation of newly exposed surfaces in a subendothelial location where complexes may localize (175). Cytokines may also play an important role in regulating the influx of PMNs through leukocyte-endothelial interactions.

When PMNs are attracted to a region containing immune complexes, tissue injury, leukocytoclasis, and endothelial changes may result as the PMNs attempt to phagocytose the immune complexes. The chemoattractants include C5a; other mediators of inflammation including leukotrienes, such as LTB_4; and chemokines, such as IL-8, released by activated monocytes or other cells. Some of the injury may be attributable to release of enzymes normally restricted to phagocytic vacuoles, whereas other elements of the injury reflect various bioactive products elaborated by the activated PMN, such as superoxide radicals.

Rheumatoid Factor Response in SLE

As studied in detail by Agnello and colleagues (172), the IgM, but not the IgG, class of cold-reactive rheumatoid factors are a curious feature of SLE. Rheumatoid factors in SLE are more often seen in association with HLA-DR3 and the presence of Ro/SS-A antibodies, possibly suggesting a relationship to events occurring in the pathogenesis of Sjögren's syndrome. The rheumatoid factor response in SLE, unlike that in rheumatoid arthritis, varies from oligoclonal to monoclonal, with the antibodies remaining close to germline configuration, suggesting that they are not produced as a consequence of T-cell help. The presence of these antiglobulins is associated with a mixed cryoprecipitate that may contain enriched levels of IgG autoantibodies to a variety of non-IgG autoantigens. The appearance of a cold-reactive rheumatoid factor in SLE often heralds the development of glomerulonephritis and, when present, could be an indication for plasmapheresis. Evidence of the presence of IgM rheumatoid factors in the glomerulus has been obtained in several patients using antiidiotypic staining (176).

Immune Complex Clearance

Individuals with SLE have substantial alterations in the mechanisms of immune complex clearance. Both Fc receptor function and erythrocyte clearance via complement receptors are reduced (177,178). The use of labeled IgG-coated erythrocytes as a technique for measuring Fc receptor function reveals a significant diminution in clearance in a large proportion of patients (179). These abnormalities are largely independent of the genetic variation in FcR function that has been associated with increased susceptibility to developing SLE (122). The function of the C3b receptors (CR1) on erythrocytes is decreased in active SLE (180). Both the Fc and complement receptor deficits improve considerably with therapy, emphasizing that they are secondary consequences of the immune alterations of SLE. These defects, regardless of their etiology, not only potentially exacerbate the problem of clearance of autoantibody-containing immune complexes in SLE, but also likely affect the entire process of immune clearance during an immune response to an exogenous antigen.

The central role of the Fc-receptor pathway for elimination of immune complexes in the kidney has been elegantly demonstrated by Ravetch and colleagues (181,182) in a series of experiments in which the lupus mouse model (NZB × NZW)F1 was studied after genetic elimination of either the C3 complement factor or the FcγR. Elimination of C3 in these mice did not prevent the development of severe immune complex–mediated glomerulonephritis, suggesting that the glomerular injury is caused not merely by complement activation, but also by influx of PMNs that attempt to phagocytose the complexes, but in the process injure the tissue. When the common γ chain of the FcγR, on the other hand, was eliminated, these mice exhibited a complete resistance to the development of nephritis, even in the presence of high levels of circulating immune complexes. This clearly demonstrates the requirement for immune complex ingestion by phagocytic or dendritic cells in order for the manifestations of immune complex injury to occur in the kidney. The intracellular fate of the ingested immune complex has not been studied in any detail, but it is interesting to speculate that it actually may be processed and presented to activated T cells. A subpopulation of the resident mesangial phagocytes in rat has been shown to express MHC class II molecules (54), thus making them capable of antigen presentation. During the development of glomerulonephritis in a rat model, there is an influx of monocytes and lymphocytes into the glomerulus, and the monocytes differentiate and become indistinguishable from the resident mesangial phagocyte (54,183).

CONCLUSION

Systemic lupus erythematosus, perhaps because of its unpredictable course and the lack of effective therapy, has raised increasingly penetrating questions as to the nature of autoimmunity. What is the critical immune recognition event that initiates the chain of autoimmune responsiveness? How does the genetic predisposition influence the immune system to make this recognition event possible? What are the self molecules that are the initial targets of autoimmune recognition, and is there a particular event that triggers this recognition or is it a progressive evolution of the predisposition state? What is the meaning of tolerance to a self-molecule? Which genes influence the likelihood of this recognition and how do they act? What are the relative contributions of the T- and B-cell compartments to the initiating and amplification stages of autoimmune recognition? What transforms the presence of a pattern of autoimmunity characteristic of SLE into the autoimmune disease of SLE? These questions are still not fully answered, but the accumulated research of the past four decades has taken us quite far in our understanding of the processes underlying SLE.

REFERENCES

1. Tan EM, Cohen AS, Fires J, et al. The 1982 revised criteria for the classification of systemic lupus erythematosus (SLE). *Arthritis Rheum* 1982;25:1272–1277.
2. Sharp GC, Irvin WS, Tan EM, et al. Mixed connective tissue

disease—an apparently distinct rheumatic disease syndrome associated with a specific antibody to an extractable nuclear antigen (ENA). *Am J Med* 1972;52:148–159.

3. Tan EM. Antinuclear antibodies: diagnostic markers for autoimmune diseases and probes for cell biology. *Adv Immunol* 1989;44:93–151.
4. Nimelstein SH, Brody S, McShane D, et al. Mixed connective tissue disease: a subsequent evaluation of the original 25 patients. *Medicine* 1980;59:239–248.
5. Arnett FC, Shulman LE. Studies in familial systemic lupus erythematosus. *Medicine* 1976;55:313.
6. Hochberg MC. Systemic lupus erythematosus [review]. *Rheum Dis Clin North Am* 1990;16:617–639.
7. Crow MK, Christian CL. Etiologic hypotheses for systemic lupus erythematosus. In: Lahita RG, ed. *Systemic lupus erythematosus.* New York: Churchill Livingstone, 1992:51–64.
8. Gregersen PK. Discordance for autoimmunity in monozygotic twins. Are "identical" twins really identical? *Arthritis Rheum* 1993;36:1185–1192.
9. Lahita RG. Sex steroids and the rheumatic diseases. *Arthritis Rheum* 1985;28:121.
10. Lahita RG, Bradlow HL, Ginzler E, et al. Low plasma androgens in women and systemic lupus erythematosus. *Arthritis Rheum* 1987;30:241.
11. Lahita RG, Bucala R, Bradlow HL, et al. Determination of 16 alpha-hydroxyestrone by radioimmunoassay in systemic lupus erythematosus. *Arthritis Rheum* 1985;28:1122–1127.
12. Lavalle C, Loyo E, Paniagua R, et al. Correlation study between prolactin and androgens in male patients with systemic lupus erythematosus [see comments]. *J Rheumatol* 1987;14:268–272.
13. Vacchio MS, Ashwell JD. Thymus-derived glucocorticoids regulate antigen-specific positive selection. *J Exp Med* 1997;185: 2033–2038.
14. Theofilopoulos AN. The basis of autoimmunity: Part I. Mechanisms of aberrant self-recognition [review]. *Immunol Today* 1995;16:90–98.
15. Theofilopoulos AN. The basis of autoimmunity: Part II. Genetic predisposition [review]. *Immunol Today* 1995;16:150–159.
16. Wakeland EK, Wandstrat AE, Liu K, et al. Genetic dissection of systemic lupus erythematosus. *Curr Opin Immunol* 1999;11: 701–707.
17. Gulko P, Winchester R. The genetics of systemic lupus erythematosus. In: Kammer GM, Tsokos GC, eds. *Lupus: molecular and cellular pathogenesis*, Totowa, NJ: Humana Press, 1999: 101–123.
18. Drake CG, Rozzo SJ, Hirschfeld HF, et al. Analysis of the New Zealand black contribution to lupus-like renal disease. Multiple genes that operate in a threshold manner. *J Immunol* 1995;154: 2441–2447.
19. Vyse TJ, Todd JA. Genetic analysis of autoimmune disease. *Cell* 1996;85:311–318.
20. Drappa J, Vaishnaw AK, Sullivan KE, et al. Fas gene mutations in the Canale-Smith syndrome, an inherited lymphoproliferative disorder associated with autoimmunity [see comments]. *N Engl J Med* 1996;335:1643–1649.
21. Kojima T, Horiuchi T, Nishizaka H, et al. Analysis of fas ligand gene mutation in patients with systemic lupus erythematosus. *Arthritis Rheum* 2000;43:135–139.
22. Wu J, Wilson J, He J, et al. Fas ligand mutation in a patient with systemic lupus erythematosus and lymphoproliferative disease. *J Clin Invest* 1996;98:1107–1113.
23. O'Brien RM, Cram DS, Coppel RL, et al. T-cell epitopes on the 70-kDa protein of the (U1)RNP complex in autoimmune rheumatologic disorders. *J Autoimmun* 1990;3:747–757.
24. Hoffman RW, Takeda Y, Sharp GC, et al. Human T cell clones reactive against U-small nuclear ribonucleoprotein autoantigens from connective tissue disease patients and healthy individuals. *J Immunol* 1993;151:6460–6469.
25. Okubo M, Yamamoto K, Kato T, et al. Detection and epitope analysis of autoantigen-reactive T cells to the U1–small nuclear ribonucleoprotein A protein in autoimmune disease patients. *J Immunol* 1993;151:1108–1115.
26. Pham BN, Prin L, Gosset D, et al. T lymphocyte activation in systemic lupus erythematosus analysed by proliferative response to nucleoplasmic proteins on nitrocellulose immunoblots. *Clin Exp Immunol* 1989;77:168–174.
27. Crow MK, DelGiudice-Asch G, Zehetbauer JB, et al. Autoantigen-specific T cell proliferation induced by the ribosomal P2 protein in patients with systemic lupus erythematosus. *J Clin Invest* 1994;94:345–352.
28. Desai-Mehta A, Mao C, Rajagopalan S, et al. Structure and specificity of receptors expressed by pathogenic anti-DNA autoantibody-inducing T cells in human lupus. *Arthritis Rheum* 1994;37(9):S282.
29. Lu L, Kaliyaperumal A, Boumpas DT, et al. Major peptide autoepitopes for nucleosome-specific T cells of human lupus. *J Clin Invest* 1999;104:345–355.
30. Karsh J, Scofield RH, Harley JB. Ro reactive T cells in systemic lupus erythematosus. *Arthritis Rheum* 1993;36(5):R34.
31. Mohan C, Adams S, Stanik V, et al. Nucleosome: a major immunogen for pathogenic autoantibody-inducing T cells of lupus. *J Exp Med* 1993;177:1367–1381.
32. Mao C, Osman GE, Adams S, et al. T cell receptor alpha-chain repertoire of pathogenic autoantibody-inducing T cells in lupus mice. *J Immunol* 1994;152:1462–1470.
33. Adams S, Leblanc P, Datta SK. Junctional region sequences of T-cell receptor beta-chain genes expressed by pathogenic anti-DNA autoantibody-inducing helper T cells from lupus mice: possible selection by cationic autoantigens. *Proc Natl Acad Sci U S A* 1991;88:11271–11275.
34. Talken BL, Lee DR, Caldwell CW, et al. Analysis of T cell receptors specific for U1-70kD small nuclear ribonucleoprotein autoantigen: the alpha chain complementarity determining region three is highly conserved among connective tissue disease patients. *Hum Immunol* 1999;60:200–208.
35. Messner RP, Lindstrom FD, Williams RC Jr. Peripheral blood lymphocyte cell surface markers during the course of systemic lupus erythematosus. *J Clin Invest* 1973;52:3046–3056.
36. Glinski W, Gershwin ME, Steinberg AD. Fractionation of cells on a discontinuous Ficoll gradient. Study of subpopulations of human T cells using anti-T-cell antibodies from patients with systemic lupus erythematosus. *J Clin Invest* 1976;57:604–614.
37. Searles RP, Williams RC Jr. Anti-lymphocyte antibodies in the pathogenesis of SLE [review]. *Clin Exp Rheumatol* 1986;4: 175–182.
38. Winfield JB. Anti-lymphocyte antibodies in systemic lupus erythematosus [review]. *Clin Rheum Dis* 1985;11:523–549.
39. Winchester RJ, Fu SM, Winfield JB, et al. An immunofluorescent demonstration of autoantibodies directed to a buried membrane structure present in lymphocytes and erythrocytes. *J Immunol* 1975;114:410–414.
40. Kolowos W, Herrmann M, Ponner BB, et al. Detection of restricted junctional diversity of peripheral T cells in SLE patients by spectratyping. *Lupus* 1997;6:701–707.
41. Singer PA, Theofilopoulos AN. T-cell receptor V beta repertoire expression in murine models of SLE [review]. *Immunol Rev* 1990;118:103–127.
42. Yu DT, McCune JM, Fu SM, et al. Two types of Ia-positive T cells. *J Exp Med* 1980;152:89–98.
43. Mohan C, Shi Y, Laman JD, et al. Interaction between CD40 and its ligand gp39 in the development of murine lupus nephritis. *J Immunol* 1995;154:1470–1480.

44. Kuntz MM, Innes JB, Weksler ME. The cellular basis of the impaired autologous mixed lymphocyte reaction in patients with systemic lupus erythematosus. *J Clin Invest* 1979;63:151–153.
45. Sakane T, Steinberg AD, Green I. Failure of autologous mixed lymphocyte reactions between T and non-T cells in patients with systemic lupus erythematosus. *Proc Natl Acad Sci U S A* 1978;75:3464–3468.
46. Fauci AS, Steinberg AD, Haynes BF, et al. Immunoregulatory aberrations in systemic lupus erythematosus. *J Immunol* 1978; 121:1473–1479.
47. Friedman RM, Preble O, Black R, et al. Interferon production in patients with systemic lupus erythematosus. *Arthritis Rheum* 1982;25:802–803.
48. Bermas BL, Petri M, Goldman D, et al. T helper cell dysfunction in systemic lupus erythematosus (SLE): relation to disease activity. *J Chem Immunol* 1994;14:169–177.
49. Tsokos GC, Liossis SN. Immune cell signaling defects in lupus: activation, anergy and death. *Immunol Today* 1999;20:119–124.
50. Liossis SN, Ding XZ, Dennis GJ, et al. Altered pattern of TCR/CD3-mediated protein-tyrosyl phosphorylation in T cells from patients with systemic lupus erythematosus. Deficient expression of the T cell receptor zeta chain. *J Clin Invest* 1998; 101:1448–1457.
51. Linker-Israeli M, Deans RJ, Wallace DJ, et al. Elevated levels of endogenous IL-6 in systemic lupus erythematosus. A putative role in pathogenesis. *J Immunol* 1991;147:117–123.
52. Kuroiwa T, Lee EG. Cellular interactions in the pathogenesis of lupus nephritis: the role of T cells and macrophages in the amplification of the inflammatory process in the kidney. *Lupus* 1998;7:597–603.
53. Kono DH, Balomenos D, Park MS, et al. Development of lupus in BXSB mice is independent of IL-4. *J Immunol* 2000; 164:38–42.
54. Rovin BH, Schreiner GF. Cell-mediated immunity in glomerular disease. *Annu Rev Med* 1991;42:25–33.
55. Kashgarian M. Lupus nephritis: lessons from the path lab. *Kidney Int* 1994;45:928–938.
56. Yellin MJ, D'Agati V, Parkinson G, et al. Immunohistologic analysis of renal CD40 and CD40L expression in lupus nephritis and other glomerulonephritides. *Arthritis Rheum* 1997;40: 124–134.
57. Massengill SF, Goodenow MM, Sleasman JW. SLE nephritis is associated with an oligoclonal expansion of intrarenal T cells. *Am J Kidney Dis* 1998;31:418–426.
58. Winchester RJ, Wernet P, Winfield J, et al. Lymphocyte populations in patients with rheumatoid arthritis and systemic lupus erythematosus. Occurrence of cold reactive anti-lymphocyte antibodies that interfere with the determination of surface markers. *J Clin Invest* 1974;54:1082.
59. Wernet P, Kunkel HG. Demonstration of specific T-lymphocyte membrane antigens associated with antibodies inhibiting the mixed leukocyte culture in man. *Transplant Proc* 1973;5: 1875–1881.
60. Reeves WH, Satoh M, Wang J, et al. Antibodies to DNA, DNA-binding proteins, and histones. *Rheum Dis Clin North Am* 1994;20:1–17.
61. Winfield JB, Koffler D, Kunkel HG. Specific concentration of polynucleotide immune complexes in the cryoprecipitates of patients with systemic lupus erythematosus. *J Clin Invest* 1975;56:563–570.
62. Hardin JA. The lupus autoantigens and the pathogenesis of systemic lupus erythematosus. *Arthritis Rheum* 1986;29:457–460.
63. Chen PP, Olsen NJ, Yang PM, et al. From human autoantibodies to fetal antibody repertoire to B-cell malignancy: it's a small world after all [review]. *Int Rev Immunol* 1990;5(34):239–251.
64. Yao Z, Seelig HP, Ehrfeld H, et al. HLA class II genes and antibodies against recombinant U1-nRNP proteins in patients with systemic lupus erythematosus. SLE Study Group. *Rheumatol Int* 1994;14:63–69.
65. Ben Chetrit E, Chan EK, Sullivan KF, et al. A 52-kD protein is a novel component of the SS-A/Ro antigenic particle. *J Exp Med* 1988;167:1560–1571.
66. Buyon JP, Slade SG, Chan EKL, et al. Effective separation of the 52 kDa SSA/Ro polypeptide from the 48 kDa SSB/La polypeptide by altering conditions of polyacrylamide gel electrophoresis. *J Immunol Methods* 1990;129(2):207–210.
67. Maddison PJ, Isenberg DA, Goulding NJ, et al. Anti La(SSB) identifies a distinctive subgroup of systemic lupus erythematosus. *Br J Rheumatol* 1988;27:27–31.
68. Buyon JP, Swersky S, Parke A, et al. Complete congenital heart block: risk of occurrence and therapeutic approach to prevention. *J Rheumatol* 1988;15:1104–1108.
69. Roubey RA. Antigenic specificities of "antiphospholipid autoantibodies." *Springer Sem Immunopathol* 1994;16:211–222.
70. Ginsburg WW, Finkelman FD, Lipsky PE. Circulating and pokeweed mitogen-induced immunoglobulin-secreting cells in systemic lupus erythematosus. *Clin Exp Immunol* 1979;35:76–88.
71. Budman DR, Merchant EB, Steinberg AD, et al. Increased spontaneous activity of antibody-forming cells in the peripheral blood of patients with active SLE. *Arthritis Rheum* 1977;20:829–833.
72. Folzenlogen D, Hofer MF, Leung DY, et al. Analysis of CD80 and CD86 expression on peripheral blood B lymphocytes reveals increased expression of CD86 in lupus patients [see comments]. *Clin Immunol Immunopathol* 1997;83:199–204.
73. Wither JE, Roy V, Brennan LA. Activated B cells express increased levels of costimulatory molecules in young autoimmune NZB and (NZB × NZW)F(1) mice. *Clin Immunol* 2000; 94:51–63.
74. Koshy M, Berger D, Crow MK. Increased expression of CD40 ligand on systemic lupus erythematosus lymphocytes. *J Clin Invest* 1996;98:826–837.
75. Desai-Mehta A, Lu L, Ramsey-Goldman R, et al. Hyperexpression of CD40 ligand by B and T cells in human lupus and its role in pathogenic autoantibody production. *J Clin Invest* 1996; 97:2063–2073.
76. Casciola-Rosen LA, Anhalt G, Rosen A. Autoantigens targeted in systemic lupus erythematosus are clustered in two populations of surface structures on apoptotic keratinocytes [see comments]. *J Exp Med* 1994;179:1317–1330.
77. Albert ML, Sauter B, Bhardwaj N. Dendritic cells acquire antigen from apoptotic cells and induce class I-restricted CTLs. *Nature* 1998;392:86–89.
78. Casciola-Rosen L, Rosen A, Petri M, et al. Surface blebs on apoptotic cells are sites of enhanced procoagulant activity: implications for coagulation events and antigenic spread in systemic lupus erythematosus. *Proc Natl Acad Sci U S A* 1996;93:1624–1629.
79. Rumore PM, Steinman CR. Endogenous circulating DNA in systemic lupus erythematosus. Occurrence as multimeric complexes bound to histone. *J Clin Invest* 1990;86:69–74.
80. Herrmann M, Lorenz HM, Voll R, et al. A rapid and simple method for the isolation of apoptotic DNA fragments. *Nucleic Acids Res* 1994;22:5506–5507.
81. Herrmann M, Zoller OM, Hagenhofer M, et al. What triggers anti-dsDNA antibodies? *Mol Biol Rep* 1996;23:265–267.
82. Klemperer P, Pollack AD, Baehr G. Diffuse collagen disease. Acute disseminated lupus erythematosus and diffuse scleroderma. *JAMA* 1942;119:331–339.
83. Medeiros LJ, Kaynor B, Harris NL. Lupus lymphadenitis: report of a case with immunohistologic studies on frozen sections. *Hum Pathol* 1989;20:295–299.
84. Case records of the Massachusetts General Hospital. Weekly clinicopathological exercises. Case 33—a 29-year-old woman

with necrotizing lymphadenitis, the nephrotic syndrome, and acute renal failure [clinical conference]. *N Engl J Med* 1998;339: 1308–1317.

85. Winchester R. Genetics of autoimmune diseases. *Curr Opin Immunol* 1989;1:199–204.
86. Shen HH, Winchester RJ. Susceptibility genetics of systemic lupus erythematosus. *Springer Semin Immunopathol* 1986;9: 143–159.
87. Winchester RJ, Nunez-Roldan A. Some genetic aspects of systemic lupus erythematosus. *Arthritis Rheum* 1982;25:833–837.
88. Winchester R. Genetic susceptibility to systemic lupus erythematosus. In: Lahita RG, ed. *Systemic lupus erythematosus,* 2nd ed. New York: Churchill Livingstone, 1992:65–85.
89. Block SR, Winfield JB, Lockshin MD, et al. Studies of twins with systemic lupus erythematosus. A review of the literature and presentation of 12 additional sets [review]. *Am J Med* 1975; 59:533–552.
90. Goldrath AW, Bevan MJ. Selecting and maintaining a diverse T-cell repertoire. *Nature* 1999;402:255–262.
91. Reinertsen JL, Klippel JH, Johnson AH, et al. B-lymphocyte alloantigens associated with systemic lupus erythematosus. *N Engl J Med* 1978;299:515.
92. Gladman DD, Terasaki PI, Park MS, et al. Increased frequency of HLA-DRW2 in SLE. *Lancet* 1979;2:902.
93. Gibofsky A, Winchester R, Hansen J, et al. Contrasting patterns of newer histocompatibility determinants in patients with rheumatoid arthritis and systemic lupus erythematosus. *Arthritis Rheum* 1978;21:S134–S138.
94. Dunckley H, Gatenby PA, Serjeantson SW. DNA typing of HLA-DR antigens in systemic lupus erythematosus. *Immunogenetics* 1986;24:158–162.
95. Reveille JD, Anderson KL, Schrohenloher RE, et al. Restriction fragment length polymorphism analysis of HLA-DR, DQ, DP and C4 alleles in Caucasians with systemic lupus erythematosus. *J Rheumatol* 1991;18:14–18.
96. So AK, Fielder AH, Warner CA, et al. DNA polymorphism of major histocompatibility complex class II and class III genes in systemic lupus erythematosus. *Tissue Antigens* 1990;35:144–147.
97. Kawai T, Katoh K, Tani K, et al. HLA antigens in Japanese patients with central nervous system lupus. *Tissue Antigens* 1990;35:45–46.
98. Nishikai M, Sekiguchi S. Relationship of autoantibody expression and HLA phenotype in Japanese patients with connective tissue diseases. *Arthritis Rheum* 1985;28:579–581.
99. Bettinotti MP, Hartung K, Deicher HR, et al. DR2 haplotypes (DRB1, DQA1, DQB1) associated with systemic lupus erythematosus. *Immunogenetics* 1993;38:74–77.
100. Hartung K, Ehrfeld H, Lakomek HJ, et al. The genetic basis of Ro and La antibody formation in systemic lupus erythematosus. Results of a multicenter study. The SLE Study Group. *Rheumatol Int* 1992;11:243–249.
101. Arnett FC, Reveille JD. Genetics of systemic lupus erythematosus [review]. *Rheum Dis Clin North Am* 1992;18:865–892.
102. Gaffney PM, Kearns GM, Shark KB, et al. A genome-wide search for susceptibility genes in human systemic lupus erythematosus sib-pair families. *Proc Natl Acad Sci U S A* 1998;95: 14875–14879.
103. Alarif LI, Ruppert GB, Wilson R Jr, et al. HLA-DR antigens in blacks with rheumatoid arthritis and systemic lupus erythematosus. *J Rheumatol* 1983;10:297–300.
104. Kachru RB, Sequeira W, Mittal KK, et al. A significant increase of HLA-DR3 and DR2 in systemic lupus erythematosus among blacks. *J Rheumatol* 1984;11:471–474.
105. Arnett FC, Bias WB, Reveille JD. Genetic studies in Sjogren's syndrome and systemic lupus erythematosus [review]. *J Autoimmun* 1989;2:403–413.
106. Bell DA, Rigby R, Stiller CR, et al. HLA antigens in systemic lupus erythematosus: relationship to disease severity, age at onset, and sex. *J Rheumatol* 1984;11:475–479.
107. Reveille JD, Schrohenloher RE, Acton RT, et al. DNA analysis of HLA-DR and DQ genes in American blacks with systemic lupus erythematosus. *Arthritis Rheum* 1989;32(10): 1243–1251.
108. Bell DA, Maddison PJ. Serologic subsets in systemic lupus erythematosus: an examination of autoantibodies in relationship to clinical features of disease and HLA antigens. *Arthritis Rheum* 1980;23:1268–1273.
109. Griffing WL, Moore SB, Luthra HS, et al. Associations of antibodies to native DNA with HLA-DRw3. A possible major histocompatibility complex-linked human immune response gene. *J Exp Med* 1980;152:319s-325s.
110. Ahearn JM, Provost TT, Dorsch CA, et al. Interrelationships of HLA-DR, MB and MT phenotypes, autoantibody expression, and clinical features in systemic lupus erythematosis. *Arth Rheum* 1982;25:1031–1040.
111. Sontheimer RD, Stastny P, Gilliam JN. Human histocompatibility antigen associations in subacute cutaneous lupus erythematosus. *J Clin Invest* 1981;67:312–316.
112. Buyon JP. Congenital complete heart block [review]. *Lupus* 1993;2:291–295.
113. Olsen ML, Arnett FC, Reveille JD. Anti-Sm and anti-RNP antibodies are associated with distinct and different HLA-DQ alpha and Beta chain genes. *Arthritis Rheum* 1990;33(suppl):S100.
114. Campbell RD, Milner CM. MHC genes in autoimmunity [review]. *Curr Opin Immunol* 1993;5:887–893.
115. Hartung K, Baur MP, Coldewey R, et al. Major histocompatibility complex haplotypes and complement C4 alleles in systemic lupus erythematosus. Results of a multicenter study. *J Clin Invest* 1992;90:1346–1351.
116. Agnello V. Complement deficiency states [review]. *Medicine* 1978;57:1–23.
117. Llorente L, Zou W, Levy Y, et al. Role of interleukin 10 in the B lymphocyte hyperactivity and autoantibody production of human systemic lupus erythematosus. *J Exp Med* 1995;181: 839–844.
118. Llorente L, Richaud-Patin Y, Couderc J, et al. Dysregulation of interleukin-10 production in relatives of patients with systemic lupus erythematosus. *Arthritis Rheum* 1997;40:1429–1435.
119. Eskdale J, Wordsworth P, Bowman S, et al. Association between polymorphisms at the human IL-10 locus and systemic lupus erythematosus [published erratum appears in *Tissue Antigens* 1997;50(6):699]. *Tissue Antigens* 1997;49:635–639.
120. Linker-Israeli M, Wallace DJ, Prehn JL, et al. A greater variability in the 3′ flanking region of the IL-6 gene in patients with systemic lupus erythematosus (SLE). *Autoimmunity* 1996;23: 199–209.
121. Blakemore AI, Tarlow JK, Cork MJ, et al. Interleukin-1 receptor antagonist gene polymorphism as a disease severity factor in systemic lupus erythematosus. *Arthritis Rheum* 1994;37: 1380–1385.
122. Salmon JE, Millard S, Schachter LA, et al. Fc gamma RIIA alleles are heritable risk factors for lupus nephritis in African Americans. *J Clin Invest* 1996;97:1348–1354.
123. Vyse TJ, Kotzin BL. Genetic basis of systemic lupus erythematosus. *Curr Opin Immunol* 1996;8:843–851.
124. Cornillet P, Gredy P, Pennaforte JL, et al. Increased frequency of the long (S) allotype of CR1 (the C3b/C4b receptor, CD35) in patients with systemic lupus erythematosus. *Clin Exp Immunol* 1992;89:22–25.
125. Cohen JH, Caudwell V, Levi-Strauss M, et al. Genetic analysis of CR1 expression on erythrocytes of patients with systemic lupus erythematosus. *Arthritis Rheum* 1989;32:393–397.

126. Sullivan KE, Wooten C, Goldman D, et al. Mannose-binding protein genetic polymorphisms in black patients with systemic lupus erythematosus. *Arthritis Rheum* 1996;39:2046–2051.
127. Hartung K, Coldewey R, Rother E, et al. Immunoglobulin allotypes in systemic lupus erythematosus—results of a central European multicenter study. SLE Study Group. *Exp Clin Immunogenet* 1991;8:11–15.
128. Garchon HJ. Non-MHC-linked genes in autoimmune diseases. [Review]. *Curr Opin Immunol* 1993;5:894–899.
129. Tsao BP, Cantor RM, Kalunian KC, et al. Evidence for linkage of a candidate chromosome 1 region to human systemic lupus erythematosus. *J Clin Invest* 1997;99:725–731.
130. Moser KL, Gray-McGuire C, Kelly J, et al. Confirmation of genetic linkage between human systemic lupus erythematosus and chromosome 1q41. *Arthritis Rheum* 1999;42:1902–1907.
131. Sercarz EE, Datta SK. Mechanisms of autoimmunization: perspective from the mid-90s [review]. *Curr Opin Immunol* 1994; 6:875–881.
132. James JA, Kaufman KM, Farris AD, et al. An increased prevalence of Epstein-Barr virus infection in young patients suggests a possible etiology for systemic lupus erythematosus. *J Clin Invest* 1997;100:3019–3026.
133. Gautam AM, Pearson CI, Smilek DE, et al. A polyalanine peptide with only five native myelin basic protein residues induces autoimmune encephalomyelitis. *J Exp Med* 1992;176:605–609.
134. Valli A, Sette A, Kappos L, et al. Binding of myelin basic protein peptides to human histocompatibility leukocyte antigen class II molecules and their recognition by T cells from multiple sclerosis patients. *J Clin Invest* 1993;91:616–628.
135. Misaki Y, Yamamoto K, Yanagi K, et al. B cell epitope on the U1 snRNP-C autoantigen contains a sequence similar to that of the herpes simplex virus protein. *Eur J Immunol* 1993;23: 1064–1071.
136. Sabbatini A, Bombardieri S, Migliorini P. Autoantibodies from patients with systemic lupus erythematosus bind a shared sequence of SmD and Epstein-Barr virus-encoded nuclear antigen EBNA I. *Eur J Immunol* 1993;23:1146–1152.
137. Brocke S, Gaur A, Piercy C, et al. Induction of relapsing paralysis in experimental autoimmune encephalomyelitis by bacterial superantigen. *Nature* 1993;365:642–644.
138. Greenwood BM. Autoimmune disease and parasitic infections in Nigerians. *Lancet* 1968;2:380–382.
139. O'Garra A, Murphy K. Role of cytokines in determining T-lymphocyte function [review]. *Curr Opin Immunol* 1994;6: 458–466.
140. Mosmann TR, Coffman RL. TH1 and TH2 cells: different patterns of lymphokine secretion lead to different functional properties [review]. *Annu Rev Immunol* 1989;7:145–173.
141. Todd JA. A protective role of the environment in the development of type 1 diabetes? [review]. *Diabet Med* 1991;8:906–910.
142. Goverman J, Woods A, Larson L, et al. Transgenic mice that express a myelin basic protein-specific T cell receptor develop spontaneous autoimmunity. *Cell* 1993;72:551–560.
143. O'Garra A, Murphy K. T-cell subsets in autoimmunity [review]. *Curr Opin Immunol* 1993;5:880–886.
144. Steinman RM, Inaba K, Turley S, et al. Antigen capture, processing, and presentation by dendritic cells: recent cell biological studies. *Hum Immunol* 1999;60:562–567.
145. Oldstone MB, Nerenberg M, Southern P, et al. Virus infection triggers insulin-dependent diabetes mellitus in a transgenic model: role of anti-self (virus) immune response. *Cell* 1991;65: 319–331.
146. Tan EM, Stoughton RB. 1969. Ultraviolet light alteration of cellular deoxyribonucleic acid in vivo. *Proc Natl Acad Sci U S A* 1969;62:708–714.
147. Casciola-Rosen L, Rosen A. Ultraviolet light-induced keratinocyte apoptosis: a potential mechanism for the induction of skin lesions and autoantibody production in LE. *Lupus* 1997;6: 175–180.
148. Sanchez-Guerrero J, Schur PH, Sergent JS, et al. Silicone breast implants and rheumatic disease. Clinical, immunologic, and epidemiologic studies [review]. *Arthritis Rheum* 1994;37: 158–168.
149. van Venrooij WJ, Hoet R, Castrop J, et al. Anti-(U1) small nuclear RNA antibodies in anti-small nuclear ribonucleoprotein sera from patients with connective tissue diseases. *J Clin Invest* 1990;86:2154–2160.
150. Tsai DE, Keene JD. In vitro selection of RNA epitopes using autoimmune patient serum. *J Immunol* 1993;150:1137–1145.
151. Mamula MJ, Fatenejad S, Craft J. B cells process and present lupus autoantigens that initiate autoimmune T cell responses. *J Immunol* 1994;152:1453–1461.
152. Radic MZ, Erikson J, Litwin S, et al. B lymphocytes may escape tolerance by revising their antigen receptors. *J Exp Med* 1993; 177:1165–1173.
153. Mamula MJ, Craft J. The expression of self antigenic determinants: implications for tolerance and autoimmunity. [Review]. *Curr Opin Immunol* 1994;6:882–886.
154. Radic MZ, Mackle J, Erikson J, et al. Residues that mediate DNA binding of autoimmune antibodies. *J Immunol* 1993;150: 4966–4977.
155. Topfer F, Gordon T, McCluskey J. Intra- and intermolecular spreading of autoimmunity involving the nuclear self-antigens La (SS-B) and Ro (SS-A). *Proc Natl Acad Sci U S A* 1995;92: 875–879.
156. James JA, Gross T, Scofield RH, et al. Immunoglobulin epitope spreading and autoimmune disease after peptide immunization: Sm B/B′-derived PPPGMRPP and PPPGIRGP induce spliceosome autoimmunity. *J Exp Med* 1995;181:453–461.
157. Lehmann PV, Sercarz EE, Forsthuber T, et al. Determinant spreading and the dynamics of the autoimmune T-cell repertoire [see comments]. *Immunol Today* 1993;14:203–208.
158. Mason D, Fowell D. T-cell subsets in autoimmunity [review]. *Curr Opin Immunol* 1992;4:728–732.
159. Jiang H, Ware R, Stall A, et al. Murine CD8+ T cells that specifically delete autologous CD4+ T cells expressing V beta 8 TCR: a role of the Qa-1 molecule. *Immunity* 1995;2:185–194.
160. Ware R, Jiang H, Braunstein N, et al. Human CD8+ T lymphocyte clones specific for T cell receptor V beta families expressed on autologous CD4+ T cells. *Immunity* 1995;2:177–184.
161. Kalled SL, Cutler AH, Datta SK, et al. Anti-CD40 ligand antibody treatment of SNF1 mice with established nephritis: preservation of kidney function. *J Immunol* 1998;160:2158–2165.
162. Agnello V, Winchester RJ, Kunkel HG. Precipitin reactions of the C1q component of complement with aggregated gammaglobulin and immune complexes in gel diffusion. *Immunology* 1970;19:909–919.
163. Buyon JP, Winchester RJ, Slade SG, et al. Identification of mothers at risk for congenital heart block and other neonatal lupus syndromes in their children. Comparison of enzyme-linked immunosorbent assay and immunoblot for measurement of anti-SS-A/Ro and anti-SS-B/La antibodies. *Arthritis Rheum* 1993;36:1263–1273.
164. Buyon JP, Tseng CE, Di Donato F, et al. Cardiac expression of 52beta, an alternative transcript of the congenital heart block-associated 52-kd SS-A/Ro autoantigen, is maximal during fetal development. *Arthritis Rheum* 1997;40:655–660.
165. Kunkel HG. Mechanisms of renal injury in systemic lupus erythematosus. *Arthritis Rheum* 1966;9:725–727.
166. Koffler D, Agnello V, Thoburn R, et al. Systemic lupus erythematosus: prototype of immune complex nephritis in man. *J Exp Med* 1971;134(suppl):169S.

167. Tan EM. Autoantibodies to nuclear antigens (ANA): their immunobiology and medicine [review]. *Adv Immunol* 1982;33: 167–240.
168. D'Agati VD. Renal disease in systemic lupus erythematosus, mixed connective tissue disease, Sjogren's syndrome and rheumatoid arthritis. In: Jennette JC, Olson JL, Schwartz MM, eds. *Heptinstall's pathology of the kidney.* Philadelphia: Lippincott-Raven, 1998:541–624.
169. Dixon FJ. The role of antigen-antibody complexes in disease. *Harvey Lect* 1963;58:21.
170. Mannik M, Arend MP, Hall AP, et al. Studies on antigen-antibody complexes. I. Elimination of soluble complexes from rabbit circulation. *J Exp Med* 1971;133:713–739.
171. Arend WP, Mannik M. Studies on antigen-antibody complexes. II. Quantification of tissue uptake of soluble complexes in normal and complement-depleted rabbits. *J Immunol* 1971;107: 63–75.
172. Cornacoff JB, Hebert LA, Smead WL, et al. Primate erythrocyte-immune complex-clearing mechanism. *J Clin Invest* 1983; 71:236–247.
173. Joselow SA, Mannik M. Localization of preformed, circulating immune complexes in murine skin. *J Invest Dermatol* 1984;82: 335–340.
174. Lawrence MB, Springer TA. Leukocytes roll on a selectin at physiologic flow rates: distinction from and prerequisite for adhesion through integrins. *Cell* 1991;65:859–873.
175. Cochrane CG. Mechanisms involved in the deposition of immune complexes in tissues. *J Exp Med* 1971;134(suppl): 75s–89s.
176. Agnello V, Koffler D, Kunkel HG. Immune complex systems in the nephritis of systemic lupus erythematosus [review]. *Kidney Int* 1973;3:90–99.
177. Kimberly RP, Parris TM, Inman RD, et al. Dynamics of mononuclear phagocyte system Fc receptor function in systemic lupus erythematosus. Relation to disease activity and circulating immune complexes. *Clin Exp Immunol* 1983;51:261–268.
178. Salmon JE, Kimberly RP, Gibofsky A, et al. Defective mononuclear phagocyte function in systemic lupus erythematosus: dissociation of Fc receptor-ligand binding and internalization. *J Immunol* 1984;133:2525–2531.
179. Frank MM, Lawley TJ, Hamburger MI, et al. NIH Conference: immunoglobulin G Fc receptor-mediated clearance in autoimmune diseases. *Ann Intern Med* 1983;98:206–218.
180. Miyakawa Y, Yamada A, Kosaka K, et al. Defective immune-adherence (C3b) receptor on erythrocytes from patients with systemic lupus erythematosus. *Lancet* 1981;2:493–497.
181. Ravetch JV, Clynes RA. Divergent roles for Fc receptors and complement in vivo. *Annu Rev Immunol* 1998;16:421–432.
182. Clynes R, Maizes JS, Guinamard R, et al. Modulation of immune complex-induced inflammation in vivo by the coordinate expression of activation and inhibitory Fc receptors. *J Exp Med* 1999;189:179–185.
183. Van Goor H, Ding G, Kees-Folts D, et al. Macrophages and renal disease. *Lab Invest* 1994;71:456–464.

76

THE TREATMENT OF SYSTEMIC LUPUS ERYTHEMATOSUS

JOHN D. REVEILLE

There is no disagreement that the prognosis of systemic lupus erythematosus (SLE) has improved remarkably since the early 1950s, when less that 50% of patients survived more than 5 years from diagnosis. There are many reasons for this, including increasing awareness of the disease and many serologic tests for SLE that have been developed. The result is that more patients are being diagnosed, many earlier and with less severe disease. But the treatment of SLE has also changed, from the introduction of antimalarials (1) and corticosteroids in the early 1950s, to the popularization of cytotoxic agents (themselves introduced in the 1950s) in the early 1980s, and to the introduction of biologic agents in the 1990s. One of the most important results of the advances in our molecular understanding of SLE has been the introduction of new treatments based on the molecular mechanisms of disease pathogenesis. A new era in SLE treatment has been ushered in, and it is explored in this chapter.

Our new knowledge has resulted not only in novel medical treatments, but also in the realization that outcome in SLE is influenced by a number of host factors, such as depression, disease education, and cardiovascular fitness, all of which must be addressed at the same time.

GENERAL PRINCIPLES

Education

While it is unrealistic to assume that all SLE patients can be comprehensively taught about their disease (and it may be disconcerting for the physician to hear a patient inquiring about new treatment information obtained from a support group or the Internet, information about which the physician may be unaware), at the very least the treating physician should inquire about the patient's expectations and fears. The risks and benefits of planned treatments should be addressed, as well as alternate regimens. Similarly, the implications of pregnancy should be discussed, a crucial concern to a patient population that includes young women of childbearing age (see Chapter 89). The improved outcome now seen in many SLE patients should be emphasized, as well as the need for patients to participate in the management of their disease. It is important to give the patient a measure of control in choosing a treatment plan; actively involving the patient not only improves compliance, but also potentially improves outcome.

Rest and Exercise

Although not studied in any controlled manner, it has been long held that adequate rest is important during periods of disease activity. Given the significant fatigue that frequently accompanies disease flares, this is a sensible consideration. However, with weight gain, muscular and cardiac deconditioning, and osteoporosis, all of which can accompany disease flares or the treatment thereof, the need for a regular exercise program to combat these accompaniments of the disease (and its therapy) cannot be overemphasized.

Avoidance of Sun

Given the high proportion of patients with SLE who develop photosensitive rashes on exposure to ultraviolet (UV) light, avoidance of exposure to sunlight is important in SLE treatment. Patients should use sunscreens with an SPF of greater than 15 and wear long sleeves and broad-brimmed hats when venturing out into sunlight.

Social Support

Most studies of outcome in SLE have shown that poor social support contributes negatively to outcomes (2). Admittedly, much of the concept of social support resides in the patient's perception; however, education of family members and follow-up phone calls by the medical staff can help to reinforce this support.

Diet

In general there is no specific diet that has been found to be particularly efficacious in controlling active SLE. Food restriction has been shown to lower disease activity in murine SLE (3), but this may not be practical for patients with SLE. Nevertheless, patients should be encouraged to maintain a healthy diet, especially during periods of disease activity, taking care to avoid extra calories while on high doses of glucocorticoids. Fish oil (eicosapentaenoic acid) has been reported to lower disease activity in both murine and human SLE (4–6), although the amount required and the nature of such a diet may be unrealistic for many patients.

APPROACHES TO MEDICAL TREATMENT

Nonsteroidal Antiinflammatory Drugs

Nonsteroidal antiinflammatory drugs (NSAIDs) are useful for their analgesic, antipyretic, and antiinflammatory properties. They are particularly useful in the treatment of SLE-associated fevers and arthralgia/arthritis. Their limitation and major toxicity is gastrointestinal (GI), specifically bleeding and ulceration. It is hoped that the significantly lower GI complications seen with newer cyclooxygenase-2 (COX-2) inhibitors (celecoxib, rofecoxib) will at least minimize this problem. However, with their higher cost, COX-2 inhibitors should be reserved for those patients with prior GI complications from NSAIDs or when other treatments have failed. Other side effects seen with NSAIDs are central nervous system (CNS) symptoms (especially with indomethacin), including dizziness, headache, and feelings of confusion and disorientation that can mimic CNS lupus. Although these complications are less common, a role of NSAIDs should be kept in mind in SLE patients presenting with these complaints and the drug withheld until its contribution to the CNS complaint is ruled out. Another concern is the fall in the glomerular filtration rate (GFR), albeit transient, that can result from NSAID use, especially in those with compromised renal function due to lupus nephritis.

Antimalarial Drugs (Hydroxychloroquine, Chloroquine, Quinacrine)

The efficacy of antimalarials has long been established for the skin and joint manifestations of SLE (Table 76.1), and these drugs are regarded as the first line of treatment for cutaneous lupus erythematosus (LE), particularly discoid and subacute cutaneous LE. As a whole, antimalarials constitute a safe and well-tolerated treatment alternative (7) (see Chapter 34). They are thought to exert their therapeutic effect by interfering with antigen processing in macrophages and other antigen-presenting cells by increasing the pH within the lysosomal vacuoles (8). Antimalarial drugs also inhibit phagocytosis, neutrophil migration, and membrane phospholipid metabolism. Long-term outcome studies have suggested hydroxychloroquine (200–400 mg/day) to protect against major disease flares (9,10). In addition to protecting against disease flares, hydroxychloroquine has been shown to lower blood lipid levels, including cholesterol (11–13).

The most common toxicities of antimalarials are gastrointestinal, including nausea, bloating, and diarrhea. Other toxicities also seen are dizziness, skin rashes, and hyperpigmentation of the skin. These usually improve on discontinuation of the drug.

Retinal toxicity is the most feared complication of antimalarial treatment, although it is uncommon. Blurred vision, photophobia, and visual halos, owing to deposition of the drug in the cornea, can occur in the first few weeks after starting hydroxychloroquine or chloroquine and tend to resolve even with continuation of therapy. True retinal toxicity is associated with loss of night vision and scotomata. It seems to be dose related, occurring with doses of hydroxychloroquine of greater than 6 mg/kg per day, or with cumulative doses of greater than 800 g, or in older patients (14–16). Numerous studies, however, have shown this to be extremely rare (16). Most rheumatologists and ophthalmologists recommend semiannual examinations to screen for the retinal hyperpigmentation characteristic of antimalarial retinopathy (17).

TABLE 76.1. ANTIMALARIAL MEDICATIONS CURRENTLY AVAILABLE

Medication	Dosage	Side Effects
Hydroxychloroquine (Plaquenil)	200–400 mg/day	Malaise, nausea, vomiting, abdominal cramps, diarrhea, hepatic dysfunction, blood dyscrasias (including aplastic anemia), pruritus, rashes, alopecia, bleaching of hair, irritability, dizziness, headache, tinnitus, neuromyopathy, blurred vision, photophobia, visual halos around objects (the latter three transient symptoms), visual field defects, blurred distance vision, difficulty reading, visual light flashes or streaks
Chloroquine (Aralen)	250 mg/day	Same as hydroxychloroquine except with greater tendency for retinal damage
Quinacrine (Atabrine)	100 mg/day	Yellow (common) to bluish-black skin pigmentation, otherwise same as hydroxychloroquine, except that retinopathy is extremely rare

Advanced retinal lesions demonstrate an area of depigmentation of the macula surrounded by a concentric ring of hyperpigmentation (the classic "bull's-eye" lesion).

Previously there were concerns regarding the use of antimalarials during pregnancy because of fears of teratogenicity. However, a number of groups have shown an absence of adverse effects in women with SLE who continued chloroquine or hydroxychloroquine during pregnancy (18–20). On the other hand, active SLE during pregnancy can be associated with significant fetal and maternal morbidity. Hence, it is possible, perhaps even advisable, to continue these drugs in pregnant patients rather than to risk a disease flare.

Quinacrine (Atabrine), in doses of 65 mg t.i.d., is another antimalarial agent that is also effective against cutaneous manifestation of SLE and lacks the ocular toxicity of other antimalarials. Its use is limited, however, by the common side effect of yellowish (or, more rarely, bluish-black) discoloration of the skin. One study demonstrated that the combination of quinacrine and hydroxychloroquine was superior to the latter used alone in treatment-resistant chronic and subacute subcutaneous LE (21).

Corticosteroids

Since the landmark discovery of the effectiveness of corticosteroids in the treatment of SLE in the early 1950s, they have been the mainstay of SLE treatment (see Chapter 40). The actions of corticosteroids in treating SLE are both antiinflammatory and immunosuppressive. Corticosteroids cause altered leukocyte migration, modulation of cytokine synthesis and release, reduction in cytokine receptors and major histocompatibility complex (MHC) class II surface expression, and induction of lymphocyte apoptosis. Ingestion of glucocorticoids results in a lymphopenia that reaches its lowest point 4 to 6 hours after administration and resolves within 24 to 48 hours.

Of the variety of corticosteroids available (Table 76.2), the most commonly used are prednisone or methylprednisolone. The effectiveness of corticosteroids in treating SLE is not disputed, despite the lack of controlled trials in this disease. The challenge comes in minimizing their usage to avoid, as much as possible, their devastating complications. This has led to the concept of "steroid-sparing" medications (methotrexate, azathioprine, etc.), which is discussed in more detail below. Deflazacort was developed over 20 years ago and has slightly less negative effects on glucose and calcium metabolism than equipotential doses of prednisone. Despite this, it has not found widespread usage.

TABLE 76.2. RELATIVE POTENCIES OF ORAL/PARENTERAL CORTICOSTEROID PREPARATIONS CURRENTLY AVAILABLE

Type	Potency (Compared to Prednisone)*	Plasma Half-Life
Hydrocortisone	4:1	60 minutes
Prednisone	NA	60 minutes
Methylprednisolone	4:5	80–180 minutes
Triamcinolone	4:5	2–5 hours
Dexamethasone	1:7	2–5 hours
Betamethasone	1:7	1–6 hours
Deflazacort	5:6	28 hours

*Ratios indicate milligrams of drug to have equipotency with prednisone, for example, 4 mg of methylprednisone is equivalent in dose to 5 mg of prednisone.

The use of alternate-day steroids avoids suppression of the hypothalamic-pituitary-adrenal axis and has significantly fewer side effects. Unfortunately, this regimen is frequently inadequate to control active SLE, and mainly should be used as part of a steroid-tapering regimen once disease control is achieved.

Complications of corticosteroid usage in patients with SLE are well described and can cause great distress. Facial swelling, weight gain, and development of the "buffalo hump" can cause alterations in body image that can contribute to a patient's depression. Other sequelae of long-term corticosteroid use, such as the development of diabetes due to the "antiinsulin" properties of glucocorticoids and alterations in lipid metabolism, can result in major cardiovascular complications over time. Many complications of corticosteroids, however, are dose-related. For example, osteonecrosis is not commonly seen in SLE patients who have not undergone protracted courses of high-dose corticosteroids (i.e., 60 mg of prednisone/day for 1 month or more), although it nonetheless can occur. On the other hand, even low doses of steroids (10–15 mg/day) can cause weight gain, facial swelling, osteoporosis, or increased risk of cataract formation.

The efficacy of corticosteroids in treating active lupus nephritis has been well documented for nearly 40 years. Generally, a dose of 1 to 2 mg/kg per day is used, with tapering occurring as either clinical or laboratory improvement occurs (lowering of the serum creatinine, decreasing proteinuria).

Intravenous pulse methylprednisolone (30 mg/kg/day) in daily pulses, given in a variety of schedules, from alternate day to daily over 3 days, has been shown to be effective in acute exacerbations of lupus nephritis and other SLE complications (22,23). However, this beneficial effect has been found to be transient, limiting the usefulness of this modality in the long-term management of SLE patients (24).

Topical steroids are principally used for cutaneous LE. The use of occlusive dressings (such as plastic wrap or steroid-impregnated tape) can further enhance the localized antiinflammatory effect. Chronic administration can result in localized atrophy of the skin, with telangiectasia. Localized purpura and striae can also occur. It is generally advised that topical steroids with greater potency, such as fluorinated compounds, not be used on the face and intertriginous regions, where the skin is thinner and atrophy has greater cosmetic implications.

Intralesional steroids are indicated for the same purposes as in other rheumatic diseases, such as injection into an inflamed joint or bursa not responsive to NSAIDs or moderate doses of corticosteroids, or the injection of an aqueous steroid suspension into discoid LE (DLE) lesions. There is little indication for intramuscular steroids, except where intravenous access cannot be easily achieved.

Methotrexate

Low-dose weekly methotrexate (MTX), in doses up to 15 mg, has been shown to be effective as a steroid-sparing agent and is well tolerated in patients with SLE, particularly in the cutaneous and musculoskeletal manifestations of the disease (25–27) (Chapter 35). At these doses, it is not clear whether MTX is acting more as an antiinflammatory agent, increasing adenosine release at sites of inflammation, which diminishes local leukocyte accumulation, or as an immunosuppressive agent (28). One study reported minor asymptomatic alterations in pulmonary function tests in SLE patients taking MTX, but found no overall higher risk of MTX-associated pneumonitis in these patients (29). The other complications of MTX are well described and are well known to the practicing clinician (oral ulcers, gastrointestinal toxicity, hepatotoxicity). As in patients with rheumatoid arthritis (RA), the advisability of obtaining a liver biopsy after prolonged use of MTX is controversial, although hepatic transaminases should be regularly monitored and care should be taken in using this drug in patients with prior liver disease.

Intravenous Immunoglobulin

Initially introduced as a treatment for immune thrombocytopenia associated with SLE (30), intravenous immunoglobulin (IVIg) has also been reported as efficacious in suppressing disease activity (31,32). The dosing varies, with some using 2 g/kg in a single dose (probably the most widely used) and others using 0.4 g/kg per day for five consecutive days on a monthly basis The mechanism of this effect is not entirely clear, although reticuloendothelial system Fc receptor blockade, with prevention of platelet phagocytosis, is most widely held. Side effects are mild, although transient neutropenia has been reported. The major limiting factors in using IVIg are availability (it is currently in short supply at most medical centers) and its cost ($1,800–$3,500 per dose for a 70-kg patient) (33). Thus, IVIg should be reserved for those patients with active SLE resistant to standard therapy or to situations of fulminant SLE.

Immunosuppressive Agents

Azathioprine

Azathioprine is an imidazolyl derivative of 6-mercaptopurine that is metabolized into the latter drug by sulfhydral compounds (Table 76.3). Subsequent metabolism of the drug yields methylthiopurines, which alter cellular purine biosynthesis and cellular DNA function. Azathioprine is also oxidized by xanthine oxidase to form 6-thiouric acid, which is subsequently metabolized to uric acid. Thus, the concomitant administration of allopurinol, which inhibits breakdown of the drug and can enhance the effect of the drug, should be viewed with concern. Patients taking both allopurinol and azathioprine should have the dosage of the latter reduced by one-third (see Chapter 38).

The use of azathioprine has been extensively studied in patients with SLE. Although described as effective in many SLE manifestations, the most extensive literature is in lupus nephritis, where it has been shown to stabilize renal function, decrease proteinuria, and even improve findings on

TABLE 76.3. IMMUNOSUPPRESSIVE/CYTOTOXIC MEDICATIONS

Medications	Dosage	Most Common Side Effects
Azathioprine	Oral: 1–3 mg/kg/day	Nausea, vomiting, hepatotoxicity, cervical atypia, lymphoma
Cyclophosphamide	Oral: 1–3 mg/kg/day	Nausea, vomiting, malaise, irritability, alopecia, bone marrow suppression, aplastic anemia, sterility, hemorrhagic cystitis, bladder carcinoma, higher frequency of other malignancies, opportunistic infection
	IV: 0.5–1.0 mg/kg/m × 6 months	Same as for oral route, except hemorrhagic cyctic and bladder carcinoma less common
Chlorambucil	Oral: 0.1–0.2 mg/kg/day	Same as for cyclophosphamide except for absence of bladder toxicity and probability of myelosuppression and leukemia higher
Fludarabine	IV: 20 mg/m^2/day over 2–3 days	Myelosuppression, opportunistic infection, nausea and vomiting, malaise, fatigue, fever, chills
Cladribine	Oral: 0.05 mg/kg/day	Lymphopenia, myelosuppression
Mycophenylate mofetil	Oral: 1 to 2 g p.o. b.i.d.	Nausea, vomiting, diarrhea
Cyclosporine	Oral: 3–5 mg/kg/day	Hypertrichosis, paresthesias, gingival hyperplasia, hypertension, nephrotoxicity, gout

serial renal biopsies. However, its benefit even in this setting has not been consistently seen, although one meta-analysis showed it to be effective (34). With reports of superior efficacy of intravenous pulse cyclophosphamide, the use of azathioprine is more limited now, although it is still recommended as a steroid-sparing agent, particularly after a course of intravenous pulse cyclophosphamide (35).

The major toxicities are constitutional, gastrointestinal (which is dose-related), dermatologic, hematologic, and neurologic. A hypersensitivity reaction has been described (36), consisting of fever and severe malaise, and, rarely, hypotension and oliguria. Under these circumstances, the drug should be discontinued immediately. Azathioprine is much less likely to produce abnormalities in liver function tests than methotrexate, although the possibility still exists and should be monitored. Pancreatitis resulting from azathioprine usage has been described and can be difficult to distinguish from pancreatitis due to SLE; hence, when abdominal pain and elevations in serum amylases occur in an SLE patient, azathioprine should be discontinued. The drug can also cause chromosomal abnormalities; hence, its use is contraindicated during pregnancy (even though successful pregnancies have occurred even when the drug has been continued). Patients taking azathioprine are at increased risk for non-Hodgkin's lymphoma (37). A fourfold risk of cervical atypia has been reported in women taking azathioprine (38), necessitating regular gynecologic examinations.

Cyclophosphamide

The use of alkylating agents in SLE dates back over 50 years (39). Nitrogen mustard was the first used, although its early introduction was largely supplanted by the introduction of corticosteroids in the early 1950s. Cyclophosphamide has been the most extensively used of the immunosuppressive agents with numerous studies spanning nearly four decades (40).

Cyclophosphamide results from the insertion of a cyclic phosphamide moiety in the *N*-methyl group of methchlorethamine. It is ultimately metabolized in the liver to the alkylating agent phosphoramide mustard. It can be administered either orally (as commonly used for Wegener's granulomatosis) or by intravenous pulses. The demonstration of lower toxicity by the latter route has made this the preferred method of administration of this drug. The pulses are given monthly, at doses of 0.5 to 1.0 g per square meter surface area for 6 months.

A number of published studies have shown that the combination of pulse cyclophosphamide and high-dose glucocorticoids is effective in the treatment of proliferative lupus nephritis, especially in reducing proteinuria, maintaining renal function, and improving the histologic picture in both adults and children (41). Parenteral pulse cyclophosphamide has also been reported as efficacious in uncontrolled series of patients with severe neuropsychiatric SLE (42), interstitial lung disease, (43) and refractory autoimmune thrombocytopenia (44). However, this benefit comes at significant cost. Nausea and vomiting are common during the 12 to 24 hours after administration of the IV pulse, making pretreatment with antiemetics [such as ondanserton (Zofran)] advisable. During the pulse therapy (as well as during oral administration) alopecia is especially common, to the degree that the patient may need to wear a wig or hairpiece. It is reassuring that the hair loss is reversible with completion of the pulse or of the oral therapy.

Cytopenias commonly occur after cyclophosphamide administration, with the peripheral white blood count (WBC) reaching its lowest point 8 to 12 days after administration of the drug and returning to baseline after day 14. If the total WBC falls below 2,000/mm^3, the dose should be adjusted downward. With chronic cyclophosphamide therapy, particularly orally, bone marrow hypoplasia may ensue, necessitating discontinuation of the drug.

The increased frequency of malignancies after cyclophosphamide administration is well established, particularly lymphoreticular neoplasms, leukemias, and transitional cell carcinoma of the bladder. The patient should be warned about this before cytotoxic therapy is begun. The risk is thought to be lower if intermittent pulse cyclophosphamide is used (as compared to daily oral therapy).

One result of the cytopenias is an increased frequency of infections that can complicate cyclophosphamide treatment, including viral (herpes zoster), fungal *(Aspergillus)*, and parasitic *(Pneumocystis carinii)*, to which concomitant high-dose glucocorticoid therapy can further contribute (45).

Pregnancy should be avoided while taking cyclophosphamide, due to its high teratogenic potential. Ovarian failure is also a well-described complication of cyclophosphamide therapy (46,47). Hemorrhagic cystitis is a feared complication that is rare with IV pulse and more likely to occur with daily oral administration of the drug. This is thought to result from chronic exposure of the bladder epithelium to the toxic metabolite acrolein (48), which occurs only intermittently with monthly pulses but chronically with oral therapy. Hemorrhagic cystitis can be prevented, at least in part, by treatment with mesna (Mesnex), which binds acrolein (49). The dose of mesna is 20% of the total cyclophosphamide dose given either intravenously or orally, starting immediately before administration of cyclophosphamide and every 3 hours thereafter for a total of four doses. Acrolein is also thought to be involved in the pathogenesis of bladder carcinoma.

Chlorambucil

Chlorambucil is another alkylating agent that has also been used in patients with SLE. It is given orally at doses of 0.1 to 0.2 mg/kg daily. Although not studied to the same extent as cyclophosphamide, it has been reported as being effective in patients with aggressive multisystem disease. One advantage that chlorambucil has is the lack of bladder toxicity compared to cyclophosphamide. Otherwise, the toxicity profiles of the two drugs are similar. However, bone marrow suppression is particularly a problem with chlorambucil and limits the use of this medication. Thus, its use is probably limited to situations where an immunosuppressive treatment is necessary and cyclophosphamide use is otherwise not tolerated or contraindicated.

Cyclosporine

Cyclosporine, at doses of 3 to 5 mg/kg, has been shown to be effective in reducing disease activity and the degree of proteinuria in patients with SLE (51–53). Its effect is usually seen within 4 to 8 weeks after starting the drug (see Chapter 42).

Perhaps the most limiting side effect of cyclosporine is nephrotoxicity. The toxic effect of this drug on the distal collecting system of the kidney can result in gouty arthritis, and should be kept in mind in the SLE patient taking this medication who presents with an acute monoarthritis.

Tacrolimus (FK506)

Tacrolimus is a fungal-derived cyclic molecule similar to cyclosporine both in its action [by inhibiting production of cytokines such as interferon-γ (IFN-γ) and interleukin-2 (IL-2)] and in its toxicity (renal). It has also been shown in small studies to be effective in controlling active SLE refractory to conventional therapy (54). The usual dosage range is 0.06 to 0.18 mg/kg per day.

Mycophenolate Mofetil

Initially developed for prophylaxis against organ rejection in transplant patients, mycophenolate mofetil (CellCept) has been shown to be well tolerated and effective in relapsing and resistant proliferative glomerulonephritis (55) (see Chapter 42). It inhibits the enzyme inosine monophosphate dehydrogenase, which acts in the synthesis of the nucleoside guanine. Its biologic actions include suppression of lymphocyte proliferation, and antibody synthesis, cytokine antagonism, and depressed leukocyte recruitment to inflammatory sites. The dosage varies between 1 and 2 g b.i.d.. Adverse effects include herpes stomatitis, nausea, and vomiting. Although controlled trials are in progress, this may represent a new approach to the treatment of SLE, especially in patients resistant to or intolerant of cyclophosphamide.

Fludarabine

Fludarabine (Fludara) is a purine nucleoside with selective activity against both dividing and resting lymphocytes. Used at doses of 20 mg/m^2 per day over 2 to 3 days for up to 6 monthly cycles, it has been shown to be effective in treating membranous nephropathy (50) by targeting both naive and memory T cells. Myelosuppression is the limiting toxicity, with consequent infections. Its use is largely investigational at this point, although it shows promise as a possible alternative to more potent immunosuppressive agents.

Cladribine(Chloro-2′-Deoxyadenosine)

Cladribine (chloro-2′-deoxyadosine) (Leustatin) is a purine nucleoside analogue that was initially introduced as an antineoplastic agent. In one study, 2-chloro-2′-deoxyadenosine (0.05 mg/kg/day) was safely administered to 12 patients with lupus nephritis, and was efficacious when given as a continuous 7-day infusion, despite inducing prolonged reductions in lymphocyte counts (56). In higher doses, it can cause profound myelosuppression and concomitant opportunistic infection.

Hormonal Treatments

Dehydroxyepiandrosterone Sulfate

Both men and women with SLE are known to oxidize and eliminate testosterone at a faster rate than normal individuals (57). Dehydroxyepiandrosterone sulfate (DHEAS) is a weakly androgenic adrenal steroid, that, given at doses of 50 to 200 mg/day, has been found in controlled studies to be useful in improving generalized symptoms, reducing disease activity, and allowing reduction in the dose of prednisone in mild-to-moderate SLE (58). In addition, DHEAS may diminish the severity of certain glucocorticoid side effects, such as myopathy, osteoporosis, and avascular necrosis (59). Mild acneiform dermatitis is the most common side effect, and hirsutism is less commonly seen.

Danazol

Danazol is a synthetic steroid derived from ethisterone with attenuated androgenic activity that has been found to be particularly effective in the treatment of autoimmune thrombocytopenia and hemolytic anemia associated with SLE (60,61). The mechanism of action in ameliorating SLE is unknown. Case reports suggest that it also may be effective in some of the milder generalized symptoms of SLE, especially in males. Virilizing symptoms, such as hirsutism, hair loss, and voice changes, do not commonly occur, but can limit the use of the drug in women with SLE. Other side effects are maculopapular rash, amenorrhea, emotional lability, elevations in liver function tests, and hyperlipidemia.

Bromocriptine

Prolactin has been shown to stimulate inflammation and immunity. High prolactin concentrations were associated with early death from autoimmune renal disease in New Zealand black/New Zealand white (NZB/NZW)F1 mice, and women with SLE have been reported as having high serum prolactin levels. Because of the prolongation of life that was found in (NZB/NZW)F1 mice treated with bromocriptine, which is a prolactin suppressor, this drug has been tried in patients with SLE (62). In one controlled study, a daily dose of 2.5 mg of prolactin over a 6-month trial period was found to be safe and effective in decreasing SLE flares (63). The most common side effect is depression. It is probably premature to recommend this treatment for general use in SLE, although it is clearly indicated for SLE patients with prolactin-secreting pituitary adenomas.

Other Treatments

Dapsone

Available for more than 50 years for use in leprosy, dapsone has been employed successfully for cutaneous LE, particularly bullous LE, DLE, and urticarial vasculitis in doses of 50 to 150 mg/day (64–66). It is also effective against leukopenia and thrombocytopenia in patients with SLE (67,68). Nearly all patients receiving dapsone will undergo a low-grade hemolytic anemia, usually dose-related in severity. Those with glucose-6-phosphate dehydrogenase (G6PD) deficiency may massively hemolyze and develop methemoglobulinemia; thus patients should be screened for this before therapy is initiated.

Clofazimine (Lamprene)

Clofazimine is another drug used for the treatment of leprosy that has been shown to be effective in refractory cutaneous LE. Used at doses of 100 to 200 mg/day, the major side effects are pink or brownish-black discoloration of the skin, dryness of the skin, and pruritus. Nausea, diarrhea, and abdominal pain also occur. Rarer complications include mesenteric vascular thrombosis. Given these possibilities, clofazimine should probably be reserved for those intolerant to dapsone, thalidomide (see below), or other treatments.

Thalidomide

Thalidomide, at starting doses of 50 to 100 mg/day and maintenance doses of 25 to 50 mg/day, is effective in the treatment of refractory cutaneous LE (69,70). It is thought to act as an inhibitor of tumor necrosis factor-α (TNF-α). The principal side effect is peripheral neuropathy, which improves on drug cessation. With the well-publicized reports of fetal malformations (such as phocomelia) associated with the use of thalidomide, this drug is contraindicated in pregnancy. Relapses are common on drug withdrawal. Nevertheless, with its relatively low side-effect profile and apparent effectiveness, this once-feared drug is gaining new respect and application in the treatment of cutaneous LE.

External Devices

Plasmapheresis

Plasmapheresis is commonly utilized for thrombotic thrombocytopenic purpura (TTP) or cryoglobulinemia. The rationale is to remove "offending" autoantibodies that may be contributing to disease activity and to replace them with saline or other "neutral" components. Despite a great deal of enthusiasm in the late 1970s and early 1980s, however, few data support a role for pheresis in the treatment of SLE; in fact, a controlled trial of plasmapheresis therapy in lupus nephritis found no beneficial effect of this modality on outcome (71). Thus, plasmapheresis has been largely abandoned for more effective treatments. It still has an accepted place in the treatment of TTP, cryoglobulinemia, or hyperviscosity syndrome in patients with SLE.

Photopheresis

Although there is no evidence of benefit in SLE of leukapheresis or lymphapheresis per se, in this variant of plasmapheresis, lymphocytes are separated from peripheral blood, sensitized with methoxypsoralen, treated with UVA light, and reinfused back into the patient. In one small pilot study, modest improvement was seen in seven of ten patients with mild SLE (72). However, the rather cumbersome nature and significant expense of this procedure, its questionable scientific rationale, and its marginal efficacy make it impractical for most SLE patients.

Immunoadsorption

This is another refinement of plasmapheresis in which anti-DNA, anticardiolipin, and other SLE-related autoantibodies are removed from a patient's circulation by passing blood or serum through a variety of columns or membranes. Several uncontrolled trials and small series of patients with SLE have been reported thus far, with some promising results. Recent data have shown a variation of this technique to be effective in patients with RA (73). Its usefulness to patients with SLE remains to be determined.

UVA1 Light

Despite the fact that many SLE patients are photosensitive, UVA radiation in the 340- to 400-nm wavelength range has been found to have immunomodulatory effects. After anecdotal reports suggested that this may be of benefit in patients with SLE, one double-blind crossover study of 26 SLE patients showed UVA1 irradiation (340–400 nm) to actually reduce disease activity and anti–double-stranded DNA (dsDNA) levels (74).

Total Lymphoid Irradiation

Total lymphoid irradiation was introduced in the early 1980s at two centers for treatment of severe and refractory SLE. While effective, it results in long-standing immunosuppression, severe infections (including with herpes zoster and fungi), as well as malignancies, which occurred in many patients afterward (75,76). Thus, this treatment has not gained widespread acceptance even though it could be speculated that other aggressive immunosuppressive treatment may have resulted in similar outcomes (i.e., infections and malignancies).

Experimental Biologic Treatments

In view of the effectiveness of TNF-α antagonists in RA, it is safe to assume that the era of biologic treatments for the rheumatic diseases has arrived. In SLE, the effectiveness of TNF-α antagonists has yet to be demonstrated. In fact, the demonstration that TNF gene polymorphisms associated with low TNF production are associated with lupus nephritis (77) raises concern about this treatment modality in SLE. Studies of monoclonal antibodies have not shown convincing results to date, although CD154 receptor agents in murine lupus have shown promising results (78). The possibility that this anti-CD40 ligand might be an effective approach is further heightened by the recent finding that levels of soluble CD154 (sCD154) correlate with anti-dsDNA antibody levels and disease activity (79). Results from clinical trials in humans are pending.

LJP 394 is a novel immunomodulant designed to lower anti-dsDNA antibodies by inducing highly selective B lymphocyte tolerance. One pilot study showed it to be effective and well tolerated in four SLE patients (80), although anti-dsDNA antibodies returned to baseline levels in two of the patients within 4 weeks of the infusion. Larger trials are pending.

Bone Marrow Transplantation/Reconstitution

Based on descriptions of patients with severe SLE going into remission following bone marrow transplantation (BMT) (81,82) (usually done as treatment for concomitant leukemias or lymphomas), both autologous and allogeneic BMT are being tried in SLE patients with life-threatening disease refractory to other treatments. Given the significant morbidity (graft-versus-host disease, infection), mortality, and considerable expense of this treatment, as well as the report of a new SLE manifestation occurring 3 years after autologous BMT (immune thrombocytopenia) (81), BMT should still be regarded as an experimental approach and should be reserved only for the most aggressive and refractory cases of SLE.

TREATMENT OF MILD SYSTEMIC LUPUS ERYTHEMATOSUS FLARES

Not uncommonly, the physician will be faced with patients with active SLE without evidence of major organ involvement. There is no indication for prophylactic treatment of SLE that is only "chemically" active, such as the presence of elevated anti-dsDNA titers, hypocomplementemia, leukopenia, or even mild thrombocytopenia (platelet count of 100,000 to 150,000/mm^3) in the absence of other clinical evidence of disease activity. Fatigue can occur with and without active SLE, and without more specific symptoms of active SLE, it responds poorly to treatment. Exacerbation of certain "milder" SLE symptoms (arthritis, rash, etc.) can be treated with NSAIDs or antimalarials without necessarily having to initiate or increase corticosteroid or cytotoxic therapy.

TREATMENT OF LIFE-THREATENING SYSTEMIC LUPUS ERYTHEMATOSUS

One of the greatest challenges facing the clinician is the patient presenting with rapidly progressive multiorgan failure due to active SLE. Because of the absence of a uniform definition of what constitutes life-threatening SLE and the uncommon occurrence of this condition, there are few data, controlled trials, or systematic approaches. It is clear that prevention by careful vigilance and monitoring is the most effective approach. However, this circumstance can often characterize the initial presentation of SLE, and cannot be foreseen. Moreover, most clinicians realize that it is not possible always to monitor patients as closely as would be preferred.

What is clear, however, is the need for rapid and aggressive intervention. Most of the drugs used in the treatment of SLE have the onset of their action in days to weeks, and may not be effective in an emergent or rapidly progressing situation. Intravenous high-dose pulse corticosteroids are frequently used in fulminantly active or rapidly progressing SLE. Given its effectiveness in many of the more severe manifestations of the disease, intravenous pulse cyclophosphamide is also advocated (although the presence of infection, which can mimic an SLE flare, should be ruled out first). IVIg is also recommended, particularly where immune thrombocytopenia is part of the clinical picture. Finally, plasmapheresis may be tried, although its lack of proven clinical efficacy in most SLE manifestations should limit its use unless a component of TTP is suspected. It is disappointing that, despite these interventions, a high mortality still frequently accompanies the setting of "fulminant"

SLE. The impact of biologic agents currently under investigation remains to be seen.

TREATMENT OF SPECIFIC SYSTEMIC LUPUS ERYTHEMATOSUS MANIFESTATIONS

Difficult Cutaneous Lupus Erythematosus

In most patients, the cutaneous manifestations of the disease (malar rashes, alopecia) occur mainly during disease flares and improve with "standard" treatment (Table 76.4). The rashes of subacute cutaneous LE or DLE can exacerbate or worsen with little evidence of systemic disease. In addition, many therapies effective for systemic involvement (high-dose glucocorticoids, methotrexate, cyclophosphamide), which have significant toxicity, have not been shown to be definitively effective in this setting.

The treatment of difficult cutaneous LE should involve a partnership between the rheumatologist and the dermatologist. The first line of treatment should consist of antimalarials, such as hydroxychloroquine, as well as topical corticosteroids (taking precautions not to use potent steroid preparations on the face and intertriginous areas in order to minimize risk of skin atrophy and telangiectasia) as noted above. The use of occlusive agents such as plastic wrap or tape can further potentiate the steroid effect. Intralesional steroids can also be used in recalcitrant areas.

In cases in which topical corticosteroids and antimalarials are not effective, second-line drugs should be added. The addition of quinacrine (although many patients may not tolerate the yellowish skin pigmentation that accompanies therapy) or dapsone should be attempted. Retinoids, given orally, such as isotretinoin (Accutane) and etretinate (Tegison) are also effective, at least temporarily. Thalidomide, as noted above, is also effective in anti–malarial-resistant cutaneous LE, particularly in those intolerant or unresponsive to dapsone. Cofazimine (Lamprene), can also be efficacious in this setting. Gold, administered either orally or parenterally, has also been reported as effective, although blood counts and urinalyses should be monitored to safeguard against bone marrow toxicity or renal involvement. Laser treatment, administered locally for cutaneous LE, is effective for telangiectasia and DLE lesions.

It is only when these measures fail that systemic immunosuppression (high-dose corticosteroids, cytotoxic agents, i.e., third-line agents) should be added to the treatment regimen of the patient with primarily cutaneous LE.

Neuropsychiatric Systemic Lupus Erythematosus

Neuropsychiatric disease represents a real challenge in treatment due to the lack of objective monitoring measures and the multifactorial etiology of neuropsychiatric involvement in SLE (see Chapter 73) (Table 76.5). A functional deficit, such as hemiparesis, could result from active SLE (i.e., vasculitis or vasculopathy), from vessel occlusion from antiphospholipid antibody syndrome, or from accelerated atherosclerosis and stroke due to dyslipidemias resulting from SLE or the treatment thereof. Depression and other affective disorders may be the direct result of active SLE or a manifestation of the patient's reaction to alterations of body image, function, or other lifestyle changes from SLE, or may even be the direct result of factors unrelated to SLE. Seizures may be a manifestation of active SLE or stem from a scar in the brain from a previous episode of active SLE or atherosclerotic stroke. Neurocognitive dysfunction can also be a manifestation of endocrine or other metabolic disorders, such as thyroid disease or diabetes mellitus. Thus, it is necessary

TABLE 76.4. THE TREATMENT OF DIFFICULT CUTANEOUS LUPUS ERYTHEMATOSUS (LE)

General care
Sunscreen (SPF >15)
Broad-brimmed hats, long sleeves, other protective clothing
First-line treatment
Antimalarials (hydroxychloroquine, chloroquine)
Topical and intralesional steroids
Second-line treatment
Addition of a second antimalarial (quinacrine)
Dapsone
Thalidomide
Retinoids
Clofazimine
Third-line treatment
High-dose systemic steroids
Immunosuppressive agents
Other treatments
Laser (for telangiectasia)
UVA1 radiation

TABLE 76.5. TREATMENT OF NEUROPSYCHIATRIC LE

General Principles
Rule out infection, metabolic causes (e.g., uremia, hyper- or hypoglycemia)
Rule out exacerbation related to prior increase in steroid dosage (steroid psychosis)
High doses of glucocorticoids (60–120 mg of prednisone or its equivalent per day)
Intravenous high-dose pulse corticosteroids
Immunosuppressive agents (pulse cyclophosphamide)
Intravenous immunoglobulin (IVIg) (limited experience, anecdotal evidence for benefit)
Plasmapheresis (anecdotal)
Antipsychotic drugs (for affective disorders)
Anticonvulsants (if no evidence of a cortical scar, or EEG is negative and seizures do not recur, discontinue after 1 year; otherwise, long-term anticonvulsant therapy)
Anticoagulants (where thrombotic episode attributed to antiphospholipid antibody syndrome)

first to discern whether the neuropsychiatric event in question is attributable to active SLE.

If the neuropsychiatric disease is thought to be due to active SLE, then immunosuppressive therapy is indicated. High doses of glucocorticoids should be initiated immediately, starting at doses of 1 to 2 mg/kg per day. For rapidly progressive or severe CNS involvement, high-dose intravenous glucocorticoids may be used, although there are no controlled trials to suggest they are superior to high-dose oral glucocorticoids in this setting. Intravenous pulse cyclophosphamide is recommended for severe neuropsychiatric involvement, although controlled trials are also lacking.

Affective disorders should also be treated with antidepressants, such as tricyclics or selective serotonin uptake inhibitors; psychosis should be treated with antipsychotic drugs such as haloperidol. Psychiatric consultation can be invaluable in planning specific drugs and dosages.

Seizures attributed to active CNS lupus should be treated with anticonvulsants, as well as immunosuppressive therapy. If there is no evidence of a cortical scar such as from a cerebrovascular accident, or if the EEG is negative and seizures do not recur, then they can be discontinued after 1 year. Otherwise, long-term anticonvulsant therapy may be required.

If the CNS event is thought to be due to thrombosis of intracranial vessels in the setting of anticardiolipin antibodies or the lupus anticoagulant, then systemic anticoagulation should be begun (see Chapter 77).

Lupus Nephritis

The relatively poor prognosis of long-term hemodialysis and reports of high failure rates in patients undergoing renal transplantation underscore the need for control of lupus nephritis before significant renal damage occurs (Table 76.6). For nearly two decades, the recommendation has been to biopsy the patient with SLE presenting with proteinuria early in the disease course in order to determine the histopathology. Those patients with proliferative lesions—especially diffuse proliferative glomerulonephritis, or World Health Organization (WHO) class IV—or mixed membranous/proliferative lesions are recommended to receive a course of intravenous pulse cyclophosphamide along with high-dose corticosteroids, possibly followed by oral azathioprine. Pulse intravenous methylprednisolone has limited usefulness in lupus nephritis, but should be considered for rapidly progressive renal failure/crescentic glomerulonephritis. For patients intolerant or unresponsive to standard immunosuppressive therapy, newer agents such as mycophenolate mofetil or tacrolimus should be considered, although the experience with them is limited.

Membranous glomerulonephritis (WHO class V) classically is treated less aggressively, since it has been thought to be a less severe type of lupus nephritis. It should be stressed, however, that membranous disease frequently will have a proliferative component, and these patients should be treated as though they have a class IV lesion. Where the proteinuria is massive (>3 g/24 hours), long-term atherosclerotic or thrombotic complications may occur as a result of hypercholesterolemia and perturbation of the clotting cascade from urinary loss of such factors as anti–thrombin III. Pulse cyclophosphamide, clorambucil, fludarabine, and cyclosporine have all been used in this setting with some success (50,83,84).

TABLE 76.6. TREATMENT OF LUPUS NEPHRITIS

Where proteinuria and/or "active urinary sediment," especially WBC or RBC casts, occur, begin prednisone treatment at 1 mg/kg/day
Consider renal biopsy early where cellular casts or 24 hour protein excretion is >1 g
Consider pulse cyclophosphamide therapy for a proliferative [World Health Organization (WHO) III–IV] glomerulonephritis (GN) or mixed membranous/proliferative (V/III–IV) lesion, especially with a high activity index
IV pulse methylprednisolone for rapidly progressive renal failure/crescentic glomerulonephritis
Consider azathioprine as alternative (albeit less desirable) to cyclophosphamide or as adjunct therapy (steroid-sparing) after IV cyclophosphamide induction
Cyclosporine for refractory membranous GN
Newer therapies
- Mycophenolate mofetil—especially for patients intolerant or nonresponsive to other immunosuppressive agents
- Tacrolimus—still largely experimental, experience limited
- Fludarabine—still largely experimental, experience limited
- Cladribine (2-chloro-2′-deoxyadenosine) still largely experimental, experience limited
- Bone marrow transplantation—still largely experimental, experience limited

Treat comorbid conditions that mimic or worsen renal disease (diabetes, hyperlipidemia, hypertension)

Uncontrolled hypertension in patients with lupus nephritis can lead to irreversible renal damage independent of disease activity, and rigorous control is mandatory. Hypercholesterolemia should be managed with appropriate lipid-lowering therapy.

While not a treatment of SLE per se, the unfortunate progression of lupus nephritis to end-stage renal disease is being increasingly managed with allograft transplantation. As noted above, many of the drugs routinely used in organ transplantation to prevent organ rejection, such as cyclosporine and tacrolimus, can themselves suppress lupus activity. Nonetheless, recent evidence that renal transplantation patients with SLE exhibit inferior transplantation outcomes, with more than twice the risk of allograft loss, should be treated with concern (85).

Other Complications of Systemic Lupus Erythematosus or Its Treatment

Treatment of the antiphospholipid antibody syndrome, which occasionally occurs in patients with SLE, as well as management of complications of treatment of SLE, such as avascular necrosis or steroid-related osteoporosis, are more comprehensively covered in other chapters of this textbook (see Chapters 77, 108, and 122).

CONCLUSION

The best approach to treatment of the patient with SLE is both multidisciplinary and individualistic, keeping in mind the patient's own preferences and needs, the benefit of involving the patient in planning the treatment program, and the requirements of the clinical situation. Moreover, especially when the involvement of one organ system is more severe than the systemic disease, treatment approaches may be quite different. The side effects of the treatment should always be weighed against the side effects of the disease process untreated. For instance, the complications of using a high dose of prednisone for a long period of time may not justify using it to suppress persistent constitutional symptoms, arthralgias, or myalgias. A plethora of new medications has been introduced in the past few years that can provide less toxic alternatives. The physician should become knowledgeable and comfortable in their use. We have more to offer patients than ever before, and the menu is growing ever more rapidly.

ACKNOWLEDGMENT

We are grateful for the secretarial assistance of Margaret Dougherty in the completion of this chapter.

REFERENCES

1. Dubois EL. Quinacrine (atabrine) in treatment of systemic and discoid lupus erythematosus. *Arch Intern Med* 1954;94:131.
2. Alarcón GS, Roseman J, Bartolucci AA, et al. Systemic lupus erythematosus in three ethnic groups. II. Features predictive of disease activity early in its course. *Arthritis Rheum* 1998;41:1173–1180.
3. Urao M, Ueda G, Abe M, et al. Food restriction inhibits an autoimmune disease resembling systemic lupus erythematosus in (NZB × NZW) F1 mice. *J Nutr* 1995;125:2316–2324.
4. Walton AJ, Snaith ML, Locniskar M, et al. Dietary fish oil and the severity of symptoms in patients with systemic lupus erythematosus. *Ann Rheum Dis* 1991;50:463–466.
5. Chandrasekar B, Troyer DA, Venkatraman JT, et al. Dietary omega-3 lipids delay the onset and progression of autoimmune lupus nephritis by inhibiting transforming growth factor beta mRNA and protein expression. *J Autoimmun* 1995;8:381–393.
6. Clark WF, Parbtani A, Huff MW, et al. Omega-3 fatty acid dietary supplementation in systemic lupus erythematosus. *Kidney Int* 1989;36:653–660.
7. Morand EF, McCloud PI, Littlejohn GO. Continuation of long treatment with hydroxychloroquine in systemic lupus erythematosus and rheumatoid arthritis. *Ann Rheum Dis* 1992;51:1318–1321.
8. Fox RI. Mechanism of action of hydroxychloroquine as an antirheumatic drug. *Semin Arthritis Rheum* 1993;23:82–91.
9. Tsakonas E, Joseph L, Esdaile JM, et al. A randomized study of the effect of withdrawing hydroxychloroquine sulfate in systemic lupus erythematosus. The Canadian Hydroxychloroquine Study Group. *N Engl J Med* 1991;324:150–154.
10. Tsakonas E, Joseph L, Esdaile JM, et al. A long term study of hydroxychloroquine withdrawal on exacerbations in systemic lupus erythematosus. *Lupus* 1998;7:80–85.
11. Petri M, Lakatta C, Magder L, et al. Effect of prednisone and hydroxychloroquine on coronary artery disease risk factors in systemic lupus erythematosus: a longitudinal data analysis. *Am J Med* 1994;96:254–259.
12. Hodis HN, Quismorio FP Jr, Wickham E, et al. The lipid, lipoprotein, and apolipoprotein effects of hydroxychloroquine in patients with systemic lupus erythematosus. *J Rheumatol* 1993; 20:661–665.
13. Wallace DJ, Metzger AL, Stecher VJ, et al. Cholesterol-lowering effect of hydroxychloroquine in patients with rheumatic disease: reversal of deleterious effects of steroids on lipids. *Am J Med* 1990; 89:322–326.
14. Johnson MW, Vine AK. Hydroxychloroquine therapy in massive total doses without retinal toxicity. *Am J Ophthalmol* 1982;104: 104–139.
15. Rynes RI. Ophthalmologic safety of long-term hydroxychloroquine sulfate treatment. *Am J Med* 1983;75:35.
16. Levy GD, Munz SJ, Paschal J, et al. Incidence of hydroxychloroquine retinopathy in 1207 patients in a large multicenter outpatient practice. *Arthritis Rheum* 1997;40:1482–1486.
17. Mazzuca S, Yung R, Brandt KD, et al. Current practices for monitoring ocular toxicity related to hydroxychloroquine (plaquenil) therapy. *J Rheumatol* 1994;21:59–63.
18. Levy M, Buskila D, Gladmann DD, et al. Pregnancy outcome following first trimester exposure to chloroquine. *Am J Perinatol* 1991;8:174–178.
19. Khamashta MA, Buchanan NM, Hughes GR. The use of hydroxychloroquine in lupus pregnancy: the British experience. *Lupus* 1996;5:65–66.
20. Parke AL, Rothfield NF. Antimalarial drugs in pregnancy—the North American experience. *Lupus* 1996;5:67–69.
21. Feldmann R, Salomon D, Saurat JH. The association of the two antimalarials chloroquine and quinacrine for treatment-resistant chronic and subacute cutaneous lupus erythematosus. *Dermatology* 1995;190:257–258.
22. Hoch S, Schur PH. Methylprednisolone pulse therapy for lupus nephritis: a followup study. *Clin Exp Rheumatol* 1984;2:313–320.
23. Kimberly RP. Pulse methylprednisolone in SLE. *Clin Rheum Dis* 1982;8:261–278.
24. Ballou SP, Khan MA, Kushner I. Intravenous pulse methylprednisolone followed by alternate day corticosteroid therapy in lupus erythematosus: a prospective evaluation. *J Rheumatol* 1985;12: 944–948.
25. Rothenberg RJ, Graziano FM, Grandone JT, et al. The use of methotrexate in steroid resistant systemic lupus erythematosus. *Arthritis Rheum* 1988;31:612–615.
26. Kipen Y, Littlejohn GO, Morand EF. Methotrexate use in systemic lupus erythematosus. *Lupus* 1997;6:385–389.
27. Wise CM, Vuyyuru S, Roberts WN. Methotrexate in nonrenal lupus and undifferentiated connective tissue disease—a review of 36 patients. *J Rheumatol* 1996;23:1005–1010.
28. Cronstein BN, Naime D, Ostad E. The antiinflammatory mechanism of methotrexate: increased adenosine release at inflamed sites diminishes leukocyte accumulation in an in vivo model of inflammation. *J Clin Invest* 1993;92:2675–2682.
29. Cottin V, Tebib J, Massonnet B, et al. Pulmonary function in patients receiving long-term low-dose methotrexate. *Chest* 1996; 9:933–938.
30. Maier WP, Gordon DS, Howard RF, et al. Intravenous

immunoglobulin therapy in systemic lupus erythematosus-associated thrombocytopenia. *Arthritis Rheum* 1990;33:1233–1239.
31. Francioni C, Galeazzi M, Fioravanti A, et al. Long-term i.v. Ig treatment in systemic lupus erythematosus. *Clin Exp Rheumatol* 1994;12:163–168.
32. Schroeder JO, Zeuner RA, Euler HH, et al. High dose intravenous immunoglobulins in systemic lupus erythematosus: clinical and serological results of a pilot study. *J Rheumatol* 1996;23:71–75.
33. Heyneman CA, Gudger CA, Beckwith JV. Intravenous immune globulin for inducing remissions in systemic lupus erythematosus. *Ann Pharmacother* 1997;31:242–244.
34. Felson DT, Anderson J. Evidence for the superiority of immunosuppressive drugs and prednisone over prednisone alone in lupus nephritis. Results of a pooled analysis. *N Engl J Med* 1984;311:1528–1533.
35. Chan TM, Li FK, Wong RW, et al. Sequential therapy for diffuse proliferative and membranous lupus nephritis: cyclophosphamide and prednisolone followed by azathioprine and prednisolone. *Nephron* 1995;71:321–327.
36. Knowles SR, Gupta AK, Shear NH, et al. Azathioprine hypersensitivity-like reactions—a case report and a review of the literature. *Clin Exp Dermatol* 1995;20:353–356.
37. Kinlen LJ, Sheil AG, Peto J, et al. Collaborative United Kingdom–Australasian study of cancer in patients treated with immunosuppressive drugs. *Br Med J* 1979;2:1461–1466.
38. Nyberg G, Eriksson O, Westberg NG. Increased incidence of cervical atypia in women with systemic lupus erythematosus treated with chemotherapy. *Arthritis Rheum* 1981;24:648–650.
39. Rohn RJ, Bond WH. Some effects of nitrogen mustard and triethylene melamine in acute disseminated lupus erythematosus. *Am J Med Sci* 1950;226:179.
40. Seah CS, Wong KL, Chew AGK, et al. Cyclophosphamide in the treatment of systemic lupus erythematosus. *Br Med J* 1966;1:333.
41. Austin HA, Klippel JH, Balow JE, et al. Therapy of lupus nephritis: controlled trial of prednisone and cytotoxic drugs. *N Engl J Med* 1986;314:614–619.
42. Neuwelt CM, Lacks S, Kaye BR, et al. Role of intravenous cyclophosphamide in the treatment of severe neuropsychiatric systemic lupus erythematosus. *Am J Med* 1995;98:32–41.
43. Eiser AR, Shanies HM. Treatment of lupus interstitial lung disease with intravenous cyclophosphamide. *Arthritis Rheum* 1994;37:428–431.
44. Boumpas DT, Barez S, Klippel JH, et al. Intermittent cyclophosphamide for the treatment of autoimmune thrombocytopenia in systemic lupus erythematosus. *Ann Intern Med* 1990;112:674–677.
45. Pryor BD, Bologna SG, Kahl LE. Risk factors for serious infection during treatment with cyclophosphamide and high-dose corticosteroids for systemic lupus erythematosus. *Arthritis Rheum* 1996;39:1475–1482.
46. Warne GL, Fairley KF, Hobbs JB, et al. Cyclophosphamide-induced ovarian failure. *N Engl J Med* 1973;289:1159–1162.
47. Boumpas DT, Austin HA, Vaughan EM, et al. Risk for sustained amenorrhea in patients with systemic lupus erythematosus receiving intermittent pulse cyclophosphamide therapy. *Ann Intern Med* 1993;119:366–369.
48. Cox PJ. Cyclophosphamide cystitis-identification of acrolein as the causative agent. *Biochem Pharmacol* 1979;28:2045–2049.
49. Hows J, Mehta A, Ard L, et al. Comparison of mesna with forced diuresis to prevent cyclophosphamide induced haemorrhagic cystitis in marrow transplantation: a prospective randomized study. *Br J Cancer* 1984;50:753–756.
50. Caccavo D, Lagana B, Mitterhofer AP, et al. Long-term treatment of systemic lupus erythematosus with cyclosporin A. *Arthritis Rheum* 1997;40:27–35.
51. Radhakrishnan J, Junis CL, D'Agati V, et al. Cyclosporine treatment of lupus membranous nephropathy. *Clin Nephrol* 1994;42:147–154.
52. Dostal C, Tesar V, Rychilik I, et al. Effect of 1 year cyclosporine A treatment on the activity and renal involvement of systemic lupus erythematosus: a pilot study. *Lupus* 1998;7:29–36.
53. Duddridge M, Powell RJ. Treatment of severe and difficult cases of systemic lupus erythematosus with tacrolimus. A report of three cases. *Ann Rheum Dis* 1997;56:690–692.
54. Dooley MA, Cosio FG, Nachman PH, et al. Mycophenolate mofetil therapy in lupus nephritis: clinical observations. *J Am Soc Nephrol* 1999;10:833–839.
55. Boumpas DT, Tassiulas IO, Fleisher TA, et al. A pilot study of low dose fludarabine in membranous nephropathy refractory to therapy. *Clin Nephrol* 1999;52:67–75.
56. Davis JCJ, Austin H, Boumpas D, et al. A pilot study of 2-chloro-2′-deoxyadenosine in the treatment of systemic lupus erythematosus associated glomerulonephritis. *Arthritis Rheum* 1998;41:335–343.
57. Lahita RG, Bradlow L, Ginzler E, et al. Low androgen levels in females with active systemic lupus erythematosus. *Arthritis Rheum* 1984;30:241–248.
58. van Vollenhoven RF, Park JL, Genovese MC, et al. A double-blind placebo-controlled, clinical trial of dehydroepiandrosterone in severe systemic lupus erythematosus. *Lupus* 1999;8:181–187.
59. Robinzon B, Cutolo M. Should dehydroepiandrosterone replacement therapy be provided with glucocorticoids? *Rheumatology (Oxf)* 1999;38:488–495.
60. West SG, Johnson SC. Danazol for the treatment of refractory autoimmune thrombocytopenia in systemic lupus erythematosus. *Ann Intern Med* 1988;108:703–706.
61. Agnello V, Pariser K, Gell J, et al. Preliminary observations on danazol therapy of systemic lupus erythematosus: effects on DNA antibodies thrombocytopenia and complement. *J Rheumatol* 1983;10:682–687.
62. Walker SE, McMurray RW, Houri JM, et al. Effects of prolactin in stimulating disease activity in systemic lupus erythematosus. *Ann NY Acad Sci* 1998;840:762–772.
63. Alvarez NJ, Cobarrubias-Cobos A, Escalante-Triay F, et al. Bromocriptine in systemic lupus erythematosus: a double-blind, randomized, placebo-controlled study. *Lupus* 1998;7:414–419.
64. Nishijima C, Hatta N, Inaoki M, et al. Urticarial vasculitis in systemic lupus erythematosus: fair response to prednisolone/dapsone and persistent hypocomplementemia. *Eur J Dermatol* 1999;9:54–56.
65. Holtman JH, Neustadt DH, Klein J, et al. Dapsone is an effective therapy for the skin lesions of subacute cutaneous lupus erythematosus and urticarial vasculitis in a patient with C2 deficiency. *J Rheumatol* 1990;17:1222–1225.
66. Hall RP, Lawley TJ, Smith HR, et al. Bullous eruption of systemic lupus erythematosus. Dramatic response to dapsone therapy. *Ann Intern Med* 1982;97:165–170.
67. Nishina M, Saito E, Kinoshita M. Correction of severe leukocytopenia and thrombocytopenia in systemic lupus erythematosus by treatment with dapsone. *J Rheumatol* 1997;24:811–812.
68. Moss C, Hamilton PJ. Thrombocytopenia in systemic lupus erythematosus responsive to dapsone. *Br Med J* 1988;297:266–266.
69. Knop J, Bonsmann G, Happle R, et al. Thalidomide in the treatment of sixty cases of chronic discoid lupus erythematosus. *Br J Dermatol* 1983;108:461–466.
70. Stevens RJ, Andujar C, Edwards CJ, et al. Thalidomide in the treatment of the cutaneous manifestations of lupus erythematosus: experience in sixteen consecutive patients. *Br J Rheumatol* 1997;36:353–359.

71. Lewis EJ, Hunsicker LG, Lan SP, et al. A controlled trial of plasmapheresis therapy in severe lupus nephritis. *N Engl J Med* 1992;326:1373–1379.
72. Knobler RM, Graninger W, Lindmaier A, et al. Extracorporeal photochemotherapy for the treatment of systemic lupus erythematosus. A pilot study. *Arthritis Rheum* 1992;35:319–324.
73. Felson DT, LaValley MP, Baldassare AR, et al. The prosorba column for treatment of refractory rheumatoid arthritis. *Arthritis Rheum* 1999;42:2153–2159.
74. McGrath H, Martinez-Osuna P, Lee FA. Ultraviolet-A1 (340–400 nm) irradiation therapy in systemic lupus erythematosus. *Lupus* 1996;5:269–274.
75. Strober S, Field E, Hoppe RT, et al. Treatment of intractable lupus nephritis with total lymphoid irradiation. *Ann Intern Med* 1985;102:450–458.
76. Ben-Chetrit E, Gross DJ, Braverman A, et al. Total lymphoid irradiation in refractory systemic lupus erythematosus. *Ann Intern Med* 1986;105:58–60.
77. Jacob CO, Fronek Z, Lewis GD, et al. Heritable major histocompatibility complex class II-associated differences in production of tumor necrosis factor alpha: relevance to genetic predisposition to systemic lupus erythematosus. *Proc Natl Acad Sci U S A* 1990;87:1233–1237.
78. Early GS, Zhao W, Burns CM. Anti-CD40 ligand antibody treatment prevents the development of lupus-like nephritis in a subset of New Zealand black × New Zealand white mice. Response correlates with the absence of an anti-antibody response. *J Immunol* 1996;157:3159–3164.
79. Kato K, Santana-Sahagun E, Rassenti LZ, et al. The soluble CD40 ligand sCD154 in systemic lupus erythematosus. *J Clin Invest* 1999;104:947–955.
80. Weisman MH, Bluestein HG, Berner CM, et al. Reduction in circulating dsDNA antibody titer after administration of LJP 394. *J Rheumatol* 1997;24:314–318.
81. Snowden JA, Patton WN, O'Donnell JL, et al. Prolonged remission of longstanding systemic lupus erythematosus after autologous bone marrow transplant for non-Hodgkin's lymphoma. *Bone Marrow Transplant* 1997;19:1247–1250.
82. Marmont AM. Stem cell transplantation for severe autoimmune disorders, with special reference to rheumatic diseases. *J Rheumatol Suppl* 1997;48:13–18.
83. Moroni G, Maccario M, Banfi G, et al. Treatment of membranous lupus nephritis. *Am J Kidney Dis* 1998;31:681–686.
84. Radhakrishnan J, Junis CL, D'Agati V, et al. Cyclosporine treatment of lupus membranous nephropathy. *Clin Nephrol* 1994;42:147–154.
85. Stone JH, Amend WJ, Criswell LA. Outcome of renal transplantation in ninety-seven cyclosporine-era patients with systemic lupus erythematosus and matched controls. *Arthritis Rheum* 1998;41:1438–1445.

77

ANTIPHOSPHOLIPID ANTIBODY SYNDROME

ROBERT A. S. ROUBEY

The association of autoantibodies having an apparent specificity for anionic phospholipids with venous and arterial thrombosis, recurrent fetal loss, and thrombocytopenia is recognized as the antiphospholipid antibody (aPL) syndrome (1,2) (Table 77.1). Patients with the aPL syndrome often have systemic lupus erythematosus (SLE) or related autoimmune diseases. The syndrome may also occur in the absence of such diseases as the primary aPL syndrome. A multicenter study suggests that there is little fundamental difference between the primary and secondary syndromes (3).

TABLE 77.1. PRELIMINARY CLASSIFICATION CRITERIA FOR DEFINITE (aPL) SYNDROME (2)[a]

Clinical criteria (at least one must be present)

1. Vascular thrombosis
   One or more clinical episodes of arterial, venous, or small-vessel thrombosis in any tissue or organ, confirmed by imaging or Doppler studies, or histopathology (except for superficial venous thrombosis); for histopathologic confirmation, thrombosis should be present without significant evidence of inflammation in the vessel wall
2. Pregnancy morbidity
   a. One or more unexplained deaths of a morphologically normal fetus at or beyond the 10th week of gestation, with normal fetal morphology documented by ultrasound or direct examination; or
   b One or more premature births of a morphologically normal neonate at or before the 34th week of gestation because of severe preeclampsia or eclampsia, or severe placental insufficiency; or
   c. Three or more unexplained consecutive spontaneous abortions before the 10th week of gestation, with maternal anatomic or hormonal abnormalities and parental chromosome causes excluded

Laboratory criteria (at least one must be present)

1. Anticardiolipin antibody
   IgG and/or IgM isotype in blood, present in medium or high titer, on two or more occasions, at least 6 weeks apart, measured by a standardized ELISA for β_2-GPI-dependent anticardiolipin antibodies
2. Lupus anticoagulant
   Present in plasma, on two or more occasions at least 6 weeks apart, detected according to the guidelines of the Internation Society on Thrombosis and Haemostasis Scientific Standardization Subcommittee on Lupus Anticoagulants/Phospholipid-Dependent Antibodies (220)

[a]These classification criteria focus on the essential features of the syndrome, supported by prospective studies, in order to facilitate clinical studies. They are not designed for routine diagnostic use outside of such studies.
ELISA, enzyme-linked immunosorbent assay; GPI, glycoprotein I; Ig, immunoglobulin.

TERMINOLOGY

Traditionally, aPL has been classified based on the three types of clinical laboratory assays used to detect it. First, aPL may give false-positive reactions in nontreponemal screening tests for syphilis. Tests such as the Venereal Disease Research Laboratory (VDRL) and Rapid Plasma Reagin (RPR) are flocculation assays in which the anionic phospholipid cardiolipin is a constituent of the antigenic mixture. Second, antibodies that are detected by their ability to prolong certain *in vitro* phospholipid-dependent coagulation reactions, for example, the conversion of prothrombin to thrombin, are termed lupus anticoagulants. Third, anticardiolipin antibodies are detected in enzyme-linked immunosorbent assays (ELISAs) in which cardiolipin is immobilized on microtiter plates.

This classification and nomenclature is cumbersome and problematic in that most autoantibodies associated with the aPL syndrome may not actually recognize anionic phospholipids, as had previously been thought. In patients with the aPL syndrome, the large majority of autoantibodies detected in lupus anticoagulant and anticardiolipin assays are directed against one or more phospholipid-binding plasma proteins and/or complexes of these proteins with phospholipids (4). At this time, the best characterized autoantibodies with "anticardiolipin" and/or lupus anticoagulant activity are those directed against the plasma protein β_2-glycoprotein I (β2GPI) (5–10) and prothrombin (11–16). Additionally, autoantibodies to other phospholipid-bound proteins (e.g., protein C and protein S) (14,17), and endothelial cell surface molecules (e.g., thrombomodulin) (18), not detectable in standard aPL assays, may also be associated with the antiphospholipid syndrome. For ease of discussion, the terms *aPL* and *anticardiolipin* are used in this chapter, with the understanding that they do not accurately describe the antigenic specificities of the autoantibodies associated with the aPL syndrome.

HISTORICAL OVERVIEW

Our understanding of the aPL syndrome dates to the development of serologic tests for syphilis, beginning with the Wassermann test in 1907. In 1941, Pangborn (19) identified the essential antigenic component of tissue extracts used in these tests as a novel phospholipid, which she named cardiolipin, because it had been isolated from beef heart. Beginning in the late 1930s, widespread screening for syphilis led to the identification of individuals with false-positive serologic tests (20,21). Transient false-positive tests were found to occur in association with a variety of infectious diseases, whereas persistently false-positive tests were associated with a high risk for the subsequent development of SLE and related disorders. In the early 1950s, acquired coagulation inhibitors were observed in a number of patients with lupus, some of whom had false-positive serologic tests for syphilis (22–24). These circulating inhibitors blocked certain phospholipid-dependent coagulation reactions and were subsequently termed lupus anticoagulants (25).

Although lupus anticoagulants prolonged clotting *in vitro,* no association with abnormal bleeding was observed, even in patients undergoing surgery (26). In 1963, Bowie et al. (27) was the first to report an increased incidence of thrombosis in patients with lupus anticoagulants. In his 1974 review, Lechner (28) described the clinical association of chronic false-positive syphilis serology, arterial or venous thrombosis, and thrombocytopenia in patients with systemic lupus and the lupus anticoagulant. Despite an early report by Alagille et al. (29), the association of lupus anticoagulants with recurrent fetal losses was not generally recognized until somewhat later (30–33). Much of the current interest in, and awareness of, the aPL syndrome derives from the work of Hughes and colleagues (34,35) in the 1980s, including the development of a solid-phase immunoassays for anticardiolipin antibodies (36,37).

In retrospect, a number of early reports suggested that certain plasma proteins played an important role in the expression of lupus anticoagulant activity. Loeliger (38) was among the first to describe the lupus anticoagulant "cofactor" phenomenon, i.e., normal plasma contains a cofactor that potentiates lupus anticoagulant activity, and concluded that the cofactor was most likely prothrombin itself. Several case reports of the coexistence of hypoprothrombinemia and lupus anticoagulants suggested that these anticoagulants might be directed against prothrombin (39–41). In 1965, Yin and Gaston (42) purified a lupus anticoagulant and, in an assay system using purified components, demonstrated that its anticoagulant activity required a protein cofactor. Although not fully characterized, this cofactor was present in normal and patient plasma and was not prothrombin.

IMMUNOLOGIC FEATURES

Specificities of Autoantibodies Associated with the aPL Syndrome

Phospholipid-Binding Plasma Proteins

β2GPI

In 1990 three groups of investigators reported that immunoglobulin G (IgG) anticardiolipin antibodies affinity-purified from patient sera did not bind to solid-phase cardiolipin or cardiolipin liposomes in serum-free assay systems (5,8,43). Addition of normal serum restored antibody binding. The serum component required for the binding of anticardiolipin autoantibodies to cardiolipin was found to be β2GPI, a phospholipid-binding plasma protein.

β2GPI, a 50-kd glycoprotein, is a noncomplement member of the complement control protein family (44). It has five of the consensus repeats, or so-called sushi domains, characteristic of such proteins. The fifth domain contains a major phospholipid-binding region (45–47). β2GPI has also been termed apolipoprotein H (48), as up to 40% may circulate bound to lipoproteins. However, β2GPI bears no structural similarity to other apolipoproteins. The plasma level of β2GPI is under genetic control (49). Approximately 94% of the population is homozygous for the normal allele, with a mean plasma concentration of ~200 >gm>g/mL, whereas approximately 6% are heterozygous with a mean concentration of ~100 μg/mL. Homozygous deficiency of β2GPI is rare (<1 in 1,000).

Although its physiologic role is not known, *in vitro* data suggest that β2GPI may play a role in coagulation. β2GPI binds to anionic phospholipids (50) and inhibits the contact phase of intrinsic blood coagulation (51,52), adenosine diphosphate (ADP)-dependent platelet aggregation (53), and the prothrombinase activity of platelets (54). Although these data imply an anticoagulant role for β2GPI, the binding of β2GPI to phospholipid membranes under physiologic conditions is actually quite weak, relative to that of coagulation factors (55), and it is unlikely that β2GPI functions as a physiologic anticoagulant based on its phospholipid binding properties. Additionally, deficiency of this protein is not a clear risk factor for thrombosis. A study of familial thrombophilia demonstrated that heterozygous partial β2GPI deficiency (plasma levels of ~60 to 140 μg/mL) is not associated with thrombosis (56). Two brothers with homozygous β2GPI deficiency were identified; one had a history of venous thrombosis, while the other was asymptomatic at age 35. Two additional individuals with homozygous deficiency and essentially normal coagulation profiles have recently been reported (57). Patients with the aPL syndrome have normal or somewhat elevated levels of β2GPI (58,59).

Interestingly, the requirement for β2GPI clearly distinguishes the anticardiolipin antibodies that occur in the setting of autoimmune disease and the aPL syndrome from those that occur in the setting of syphilis and other infectious diseases (43,60–62). Syphilis-associated anticardiolipin antibodies bind to cardiolipin in the absence of β2GPI, and this binding to cardiolipin is inhibited by human β2GPI, presumably because the antibodies and β2GPI bind to similar phospholipid structures. This difference in antigenic specificity may explain why the autoimmune type of anticardiolipin antibody is associated with the lupus anticoagulant and thrombosis, fetal loss, etc., while anticardiolipin antibodies associated with infection are not (63).

Most autoimmune anticardiolipin antibodies recognize epitopes expressed on β2GPI, and antibody binding to β2GPI in the absence of phospholipid has been observed by several groups (5–7,9,10,64–66). Similarly, certain human monoclonal anticardiolipin antibodies derived from patients with the aPL syndrome recognize β2GPI (67). The majority of anti-β2GPI autoantibodies in patient sera recognize epitopes on native β2GPI (9,10). One or more major epitopes are located on the first domain of β2GPI (6). The antibodies have low intrinsic affinity, and the observed high avidity binding to β2GPI is dependent on multivalent attachment to immobilized antigen (9,10). Other data suggest that certain anti-β2GPI autoantibodies may be specific for conformational epitopes of β2GPI, formed when the protein binds to anionic phospholipids or certain synthetic surfaces (7,68).

Certain autoantibodies to β2GPI have lupus anticoagulant activity (61,69–71). β2GPI itself inhibits prothrombinase activity *in vitro* (54), and β2GPI-dependent lupus anticoagulants appear to enhance this anticoagulant effect of β2GPI. A number of monoclonal and polyclonal antibodies to β2GPI have similar anticoagulant activity (61,72). Autoantibody enhancement of β2GPI's anticoagulant activity is likely due to cross-linking of surface bound β2GPI (73,74). Cross-linking increases the strength of the β2GPI-phospholipid interaction, thereby effectively decreasing the amount of phospholipid available to participate in the prothrombinase complex. The reason why some anti-β2GPI antibodies have lupus anticoagulant activity while others do not is unclear, but may be related to avidity and/or epitope specificity.

Prothrombin

Autoantibodies directed against prothrombin are the other major specificity of lupus anticoagulants in patients with the aPL syndrome (11,13,16,75). Antiprothrombin autoantibodies were first demonstrated by Bajaj et al. (76) in two patients with the lupus anticoagulant and acquired hypoprothrombinemia. Hypoprothrombinemia in these patients was thought to be due to the clearance of prothrombin immune complexes. Circulating prothrombin-antibody complexes have been observed in patients with lupus anticoagulants and normal prothrombin levels as well (12,77). Although autoantibodies to prothrombin were thought initially to be distinct from lupus anticoagulants, it is now clear that certain affinity-purified antiprothrombin autoantibodies have lupus anticoagulant activity (12,15). As with autoantibodies to β2GPI, antiprothrombin antibodies may be of intrinsically low affinity and/or recognize conformational epitopes formed when prothrombin binds to anionic phospholipid. The occurrence of hypoprothrombinemia in a small subset of patients with lupus anticoagulant suggests that the antiprothrombin antibodies in this group of patients are of high affinity and recognize native prothrombin.

Other Phospholipid-Binding Proteins

Limited data suggest that certain patients with the aPL syndrome may have autoantibodies to other phospholipid-binding plasma proteins. These include components of the protein C pathway, protein C, and protein S (14,17). Although inhibition of this pathway is associated with venous thrombosis and fetal loss (78), the functional and clinical significance of such antibodies is unclear (79,80). There are case reports of patients with the aPL syndrome and autoantibodies to factor V (81) and factors XI and XII (82). Rarely, anticardiolipin assays may detect autoantibodies recognizing complement factor H, complement C4b-binding protein, thrombin-modified antithrombin, or lipopolysaccharide binding protein, although it is not clear whether such antibodies are associated with the aPL syndrome (83). Annexins are a family of calcium-dependent phospholipid-binding proteins thought to play important roles in membrane processes such as exocytosis and membrane fusion. Autoantibodies directed against annexin V have been reported in patients with the aPL syndrome (84–86). This protein may play a role in the pathophysiology of the syndrome, as discussed below.

Autoantibodies with an apparent specificity for phosphatidylethanolamine have been reported in certain patients with the aPL syndrome (87–90). These antibodies are directed against a complex of phosphatidylethanolamine and high and/or low molecular weight kininogens (91,92).

Endothelial Cell Surface Proteins

Certain molecules expressed on the luminal surface of vascular endothelial cells may be antigenic targets in patients with the aPL syndrome. Thrombomodulin, an endothelial cell receptor for thrombin, plays a critical role in protein C activation. Autoantibodies to thrombomodulin have been identified in some patients (18,93,94). Vascular heparan sulfate proteoglycan is expressed on endothelial cells and plays an important role in vascular structure and function, including hemostasis. Importantly, vessel wall heparan sulfate is required for the activation of antithrombin III. Fillit and coworkers have demonstrated autoantibodies to both heparan sulfate (95) and the protein core of vascular heparan sulfate proteoglycan (96) in the sera of certain patients with SLE.

Anionic Phospholipids

Previous studies indicating the phospholipid specificity of lupus anticoagulants and anticardiolipin autoantibodies are difficult to interpret due to the fact that most experiments were performed in the presence of serum or plasma. Therefore, the possible role of plasma proteins and/or protein-phospholipid complexes may not have been appreciated. Additionally, contamination of purified antibodies and other reagents with plasma proteins now known to be important (e.g., β2GPI), was not directly evaluated. For example, it has recently been demonstrated that prothrombin plays a key role in the previously reported specificity of lupus anticoagulants for hexagonal (II) phase phosphatidylethanolamine (97,98). Anionic phospholipids do appear to be the target of anticardiolipin antibodies associated with syphilis (43,60,61).

Anionic phospholipids may play an important role *in vivo* in the binding of autoantibodies to phospholipid-bound plasma proteins. As discussed, antibody binding may depend on the phospholipid surface to provide a high local concentration of antigen, thereby promoting high-avidity bivalent binding of intrinsically low-affinity antibodies. Further, certain antibodies may be specific for protein conformations induced when the proteins bind to phospholipids.

Anticardiolipin assays may detect antibodies directed against oxidized lipids. The fatty acid chains of cardiolipin derived from natural sources are readily oxidizable, and some degree of oxidation is likely under the conditions used in most anticardiolipin ELISAs (99). It is also possible that β2GPI or certain other serum proteins may bind covalently to oxidized cardiolipin. The presence of oxidized lipids in anticardiolipin assays is intriguing in view of some reports suggesting cross-reactivity between anticardiolipin antibodies and antibodies to oxidized lipoproteins (100). It is unclear whether there is true cross-reactivity or if this observation is due to detection of antibodies to β2GPI or other proteins in both assays.

Relationship to Antiplatelet and Antiendothelial Cell Antibodies

Antiplatelet and antiendothelial cell antibodies have been reported to occur in patients with the aPL syndrome (101–103). The exact relationship of these autoantibodies to those detected in standard lupus anticoagulant and anticardiolipin assays is not clear. In patients with the aPL syndrome, the binding of certain antibodies to platelets (104) and to endothelial cells (105,106) is dependent on β2GPI. Antibodies to thrombomodulin and heparan sulfate proteoglycan have been discussed above.

Relationship to the Traditional Classification of aPL

The relationship of some of the antigenic specificities outlined above to the traditional classification of aPL is shown in Table 77.2. Currently used clinical laboratory tests for aPL detect some, but not all, of these autoantibodies. Standard anticardiolipin ELISAs detect both autoantibodies to β2GPI and authentic anticardiolipin antibodies that are associated with syphilis and other infections. In this assay, β2GPI present in the bovine serum used in the blocking buffer and in the patient's serum sample binds to the cardiolipin-coated microtiter plate and can subsequently be engaged by anti-β2GPI autoantibodies. Certain autoantibodies to β2GPI, as well as autoantibodies to prothrombin, demonstrate lupus anticoagulant activity in assays such as the activated partial thromboplastin time (aPTT) and the dilute Russell viper venom time (dRVVT). The dRVVT is relatively more sensitive to the lupus anticoagulant effect of anti-β2GPI autoantibodies, whereas the kaolin clotting time is relatively more sensitive to the effects of antiprothrombin antibodies (107). Neither type of aPL assay detects autoantibodies to protein C and protein S. Thus, the reactivity of autoantibodies with different antigenic specificities in the currently used aPL assays appears to explain much of the heterogeneity and inconsistent overlap of anticardiolipin antibodies and lupus anticoagulants. For example, it clarifies why, in some patients, anticardiolipin antibodies and lupus anticoagulants are the same antibodies (anti-β2GPI antibodies with anticoagulant activity), while in others they are clearly distinct (anti-β2GPI antibodies without anticoagulant activity and antiprothrombin antibodies).

TABLE 77.2. RELATIONSHIP OF AUTOANTIBODY SPECIFICITIES TO REACTIVITY IN STANDARD aPL ASSAYS

	Reactivity in	
Autoantibody Specificity	Anticardiolipin ELISA	Lupus Anticoagulant
Anti-β2GPI	Positive	Positive and negative
Antiprothrombin	Negative	Positive and negative
Anti–protein C	Negative	Negative
Anti–protein S	Negative	Negative

Significance of Autoantibody Heterogeneity

Immunologically, it is of interest that autoantibodies to different phospholipid-binding proteins occur together, in various combinations (17). Speculatively, this is similar to certain linked sets of antinuclear antibodies that occur in patients with SLE (e.g., antibodies to constituents of small nuclear ribonucleoprotein particles). Antibodies may be directed against several different protein components of such particles, such as Sm and U1-RNP proteins, suggesting that the immune response is antigen-driven (108). By analogy, the co-occurrence of antibodies to different phospholipid-binding proteins suggests that the relevant antigenic particle in this instance may consist of proteins bound in close proximity to one another on an anionic phospholipid surface, perhaps a vascular endothelial cell, activated platelet, or apoptotic cell.

CLINICAL FEATURES

Prevalence of aPL and the aPL Syndrome

The prevalence of anticardiolipin antibodies in patients with SLE is approximately 40% (1). Lupus anticoagulants are present in approximately 30%. Clinical manifestations of the aPL syndrome probably affect 30% to 40% of patients with these antibodies or about 10% to 15% of lupus patients.

The prevalence of the primary aPL syndrome is unknown. Retrospective studies have identified aPL in 7% to 30% of patients with a history of thrombosis but without SLE (109–111). Ginsburg and co-workers (112) studied banked sera from a prospectively followed cohort of male physicians 40 years of age or older, without a prior history of thrombosis. Of 90 subjects who subsequently experienced an episode of deep venous thrombosis or pulmonary embolism over a 5-year period, 19 (21%) had IgG anticardiolipin levels above the 95th percentile (≥33 GPL units). No association with ischemic stroke was found, perhaps due to the study design and the age of the subjects. In contrast, data analyzed by Kittner and Gorelick (113) indicate that aPL may account for approximately one-third of new strokes in patients under the age of 50. Recurrent idiopathic fetal losses in apparently healthy women are probably attributable to the aPL syndrome in approximately 5% to 15% of cases (114,115). The frequency of aPL in normal controls is approximately 2% (116), and may increase with age.

Thrombosis

Thrombotic events in nearly all sites of the vascular tree have been reported to occur in association with aPL. The deep and superficial veins of the lower extremity are the most common sites of the venous thrombosis (34,117,118). Deep venous thrombosis may be complicated by pulmonary embolism in a third of cases. Stroke is the most common form of arterial thrombosis seen in patients with aPL (34,117–120). Thrombosis may be the underlying disease process in a number of clinical events in patients with aPL, for example, pregnancy loss (placental thrombosis and infarction) (121), renal dysfunction (thrombosis of intrarenal blood vessels) (122), cutaneous ulcers (thrombosis of dermal blood vessels) (123), certain forms of central nervous system disease (multiinfarct dementia) (124,125), and pulmonary hypertension (recurrent pulmonary emboli) (126).

Recurrent Fetal Loss

The presence of aPL in pregnant women is strongly associated with fetal deaths occurring from the late first trimester onward (127–129). The association of aPL with spontaneous abortion occurring at less than 10 weeks' gestation is less well established due to the high incidence of such losses in the general population (130). In addition to fetal loss, aPL is also associated with an increased incidence of obstetric and postnatal complications, including preeclampsia, fetal distress, fetal growth impairment, and premature delivery, and maternal thrombotic events in the postpartum period (127,131). Most cases of fetal death related to aPL are preceded by fetal growth impairment and oligohydramnios (130).

Thrombocytopenia

Thrombocytopenia in patients with SLE is associated with aPL. It occurs in nearly 40% of lupus patients with aPL and only 10% of patients without these antibodies (132). aPL is present in 70% to 80% of lupus patients with thrombocytopenia, and about 30% of patients with chronic autoimmune thrombocytopenia. In patients with the aPL syndrome, thrombocytopenia is usually moderate (platelet counts ≥50 × 10^9/L) and not associated with hemorrhage. Patients with aPL and low platelet counts are still at risk for thrombosis (133).

Other Clinical Features

Valvular Heart Disease

Valvular heart disease is associated with the presence of aPL both in patients with systemic lupus (134–136) and in patients with the primary aPL syndrome (137,138). In particular, a number of patients have been reported with noninfective verrucous vegetations (Libman-Sacks endocarditis). Embolization arising from endocardial lesions may account for some of the cerebral ischemic events in these patients (139,140).

Neurologic Syndromes

Cerebrovascular thrombosis and embolic stroke are the major neurologic manifestations of the aPL syndrome. Transient ischemic attack may also occur (141). Nonstroke neurologic events that have been reported in patients with aPL include transverse myelitis (142), Guillain-Barré syndrome, chorea (143), migraine headache (144), and syndromes resembling multiple sclerosis (145,146).

Dermatologic Manifestations

Cutaneous ulcers, usually involving the lower extremities, have been reported in several series (147,148). Livedo reticularis, a latticework of blue to red subcutaneous mottling, is often present in patients with aPL (149). Certain patients with Sneddon's syndrome, the association of livedo reticularis and cerebrovascular disease, are recognized as having the aPL syndrome (150,151). Skin necrosis has also been reported in association with aPL (152).

Drug-Induced aPL

A number of medications, including chlorpromazine, hydralazine, phenytoin, and procainamide, may induce aPL (153–157). Drug-induced aPL is often of the IgM isotype, and exhibits the same dependence on β2GPI as autoimmune aPL (157,158). Thrombosis and thrombocytopenia have occurred in some patients with drug-induced aPL (154,156).

Catastrophic aPL Syndrome

An acute syndrome of widespread, multiple vascular occlusions associated with aPL has been reported in over 50 patients (159). Common features include occlusive vascular disease involving kidney, lungs, brain, heart, and/or liver; hypertension; thrombocytopenia; and hemolytic anemia. Most patients with the catastrophic syndrome have a prior history of SLE, lupus-like disease, or the primary aPL syndrome. Both high-titer IgG anticardiolipin antibodies and a lupus anticoagulant are usually present. Apparent precipitating events including infections, medications, withdrawal of anticoagulant therapy, minor surgical procedures, and the postpartum period have been identified in some cases. This syndrome was fatal in half the cases reviewed by Asherson (159).

PATHOPHYSIOLOGY

Several general observations are compatible with the hypothesis that autoantibodies play a direct role in the pathogenesis of the aPL syndrome: (a) unlike antinuclear autoantibodies, autoantibodies in the aPL syndrome target plasma proteins or components of cells surface membranes that are accessible to circulating antibodies; (b) a number of the antigens are involved in hemostasis; (c) animal models of the aPL syndrome have been developed via passive transfer of immunoglobulins from patients with the aPL syndrome (160–162); (d) the presence of aPL has been shown to precede the first episode of thrombosis, rather than develop as a sequela of a thrombotic event (112); and (e) the risk of developing clinical manifestations of the aPL syndrome correlates directly with the level of aPL (112,163).

There are a limited number of mechanisms by which autoantibodies to phospholipid-binding plasma proteins, such as β2GPI and prothrombin, could interact with their respective antigens. First, high-affinity, neutralizing autoantibodies may directly inhibit an antigen's function and/or decrease plasma antigen levels via clearance of antigen-antibody complexes. This type of interaction is characteristic of acquired inhibitors to coagulation factors. With the exception of the small subset of patients with lupus anticoagulants and hypoprothrombinemia, antibodies associated with the aPL syndrome tend to be of relatively low affinity and do not decrease plasma antigen levels. A second possibility is that autoantibodies and antigens may form immune complexes that deposit in vessel walls, leading to inflammation and tissue injury. This occurs in serum sickness and many vasculitides, but does not appear to occur with either acquired factor inhibitors or the aPL syndrome.

Two other possibilities may be particularly relevant to the aPL syndrome. As previously mentioned, intrinsically low-affinity autoantibodies to phospholipid-binding plasma proteins may bind with high avidity, via bivalent or multivalent attachment, to antigens on membranes. This autoantibody cross-linking of membrane-bound antigens will markedly decrease the rate at which the antigens dissociate from the membrane, causing dysregulation of phospholipid-dependent reactions. This is the likely mechanism by which certain anti-β2GPI autoantibodies exhibit lupus anticoagulant activity (73,74,164). Alternatively, if the target antigens are bound to receptor proteins on the cell surface, cross-linking by antibodies may trigger signal transduction and certain cellular responses. This may well be the mechanism by which anti-β2GPI autoantibodies stimulate the upregulation of adhesion molecules on endothelial cells (105,106).

If autoantibodies play a role in the pathogenesis of the aPL syndrome, the spectrum of antigenic specificities may offer an explanation for the heterogeneity of clinical manifestations of the syndrome, as well as the confusing variety of proposed pathophysiologic mechanisms. It is reasonable to speculate that antibodies to different phospholipid-bound proteins or cell surface molecules would have different effects. For example, it has been suggested that antibodies that alter the prostacyclin/thromboxane balance may be associated with arterial thrombosis, whereas antibodies that inhibit the protein C pathway may be associated with venous thrombosis (165). Some specificities may not be related to any disease manifestation, thus explaining why many patients are asymptomatic. The possible relationship of certain autoantibodies to proposed mechanisms of thrombosis is shown in Table 77.3.

Autoantibody-Mediated Thrombosis: Potential Mechanisms

Dysregulation of Hemostatic Reactions

Inhibition of the Protein C Pathway

The clinical importance of the protein C pathway in normal hemostasis is evidenced by the association of inherited deficiencies of protein C and protein S with thrombosis, and by the identification of resistance to activated protein C as one

TABLE 77.3. RELATIONSHIP OF AUTOANTIBODY SPECIFICITIES TO SOME PROPOSED MECHANISMS OF ANTIBODY-MEDIATED THROMBOSIS

Proposed Mechanism	Autoantibodies that May Be Involved
Inhibition of the protein C pathway	
Protein C activation	Anti–protein C, antithrombomodulin
Inactivation of factors Va and VIIIa	Anti–protein C, anti–protein S, anti-β2GPI
Inhibition of antithrombin III activation	Anti–heparan sulfate, anti–β_2-GPI
Displacement of annexin V	Anti–annexin V, anti–β_2-GPI
Inhibition of β_2-GPI	Anti–β_2-GPI
Impaired fibrinolysis	Anti–β_2-GPI, anti–factor XII, anti–PE/HMWK*
Increased monocyte TF expression	Anti–β_2-GPI
Increased expression of adhesion molecules on endothelial cells	Anti–β_2-GPI
Enhanced platelet activation	Anti–β_2-GPI
Increased platelet thromboxane A_2	Anti–β_2-GPI

PE/HMWK, phosphatidylethanolamine/high molecular weight kininogen; TF, tissue factor.

of the most common inherited cause of thrombosis cause of thrombosis (166). Autoantibodies may inhibit phospholipid-dependent reactions of the protein C anticoagulant pathway: (a) the activation of protein C by thrombin bound to thrombomodulin, and/or (b) the inactivation of factors Va and VIIIa by activated protein C and its cofactors protein S and factor V with APC (activated protein C) (14,167–171) (Fig. 77.1). Anti-β2GPI autoantibodies may be involved, although data are equivocal (172–174). There is also evidence that autoantibodies directed against protein C pathway components (i.e., thrombomodulin, protein C, and protein S) may play a role (14,18). Decreased levels of protein S have been reported in a small number of patients with the antiphospholipid antibody syndrome (80,175,176).

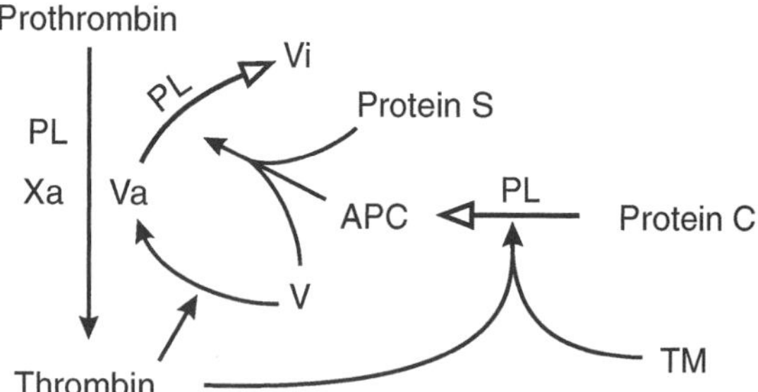

FIGURE 77.1. Relation between the procoaglant prothrombinase reaction and the anticoagulant protein C pathway. Prothrombin is cleaved to form thrombin by the enzyme factor Xa and its cofactor, factor Va, on an anionic phospholipid (PL) surface in the presence of Ca^{2+} ions. In a positive feedback reaction, thrombin activates factor V to form more factor Va. Thrombin also binds to thrombomodulin (TM) on the surface of vascular endothelial cells leading to the activation of protein C. Activated protein C (APC) then exerts an anticoagulant effect by inactivating membrane bound factors Va (to Vi) and Villa (not shown). Protein S and factor V (but not Va) act as cofactors for activated protein C. *Open arrowheads* denote reactions of the protein C pathway.

Inhibition of Antithrombin III

Antithrombin III is the major plasma inhibitor of factor IXa, factor Xa, and thrombin. To optimally inhibit these factors, antithrombin III must bind to heparan sulfate expressed on vascular endothelium. Autoantibodies to vascular heparan sulfate proteoglycan and/or heparin may contribute to a thrombotic tendency by blocking the activation of antithrombin III (177–179). In view of the fact that β2GPI binds to heparin, anti-β2GPI antibodies could have a similar effect.

Displacement of Annexin V

It is proposed that annexin V bound to the luminal surface of vascular endothelial cells functions as a physiologic anticoagulant, although data supporting such a role is limited. Displacement of annexin V from cell surfaces by certain aPL (perhaps in the presence of β2GPI) might contribute to hypercoagulability in the aPL syndrome (180).

Inhibition of β2GPI

Certain *in vitro* data suggest that β2GPI may be a natural anticoagulant, although, as discussed above, the phospholipid binding properties of β2GPI (55) and studies of β2GPI-deficient individuals (56,57) do not support such a function. One study suggests that β2GPI acts as inhibitor of factor Xa generation on the surface of platelets and that autoantibodies to β2GPI block this activity (181).

Impaired Fibrinolysis

Studies of tissue plasminogen activator levels, before and after venous occlusion, have generally been inconclusive. The most consistent finding is an elevated level of plasminogen activator inhibitor-1 (PAI-1) in patients with systemic lupus (182–185). However, PAI-1 is an acute-phase reactant and there is no strong correlation among increased PAI-1, the presence or level of aPL, and a history of thrombosis.

The contact system may play an important role in fibrinolysis (186), and inhibition of the factor XII–dependent fibrinolytic pathway has been observed in patients with the aPL syndrome (187,188). In view of the fact that β2GPI inhibits factor XII and prekallikrein activation on anionic phospholipid surfaces (51,189,190), anti-β2GPI autoantibodies may amplify this inhibitory activity. Autoantibodies to high molecular weight kininogen (91) or factor XII (82) could also influence this pathway.

Effects on Cells

Monocytes

Tissue factor (TF) is the major initiator of normal and pathologic coagulation and is not normally expressed by cells in contact with blood. There is increasing evidence that increased expression of TF on circulating blood monocytes is an important mechanism of hypercoagulability in the aPL syndrome (191–194). Anticardiolipin (anti-β2GPI) antibodies from patient sera and patient-derived monoclonal anti-β2GPI autoantibodies induce TF expression on normal blood monocytes *in vivo,* and TF expression is increased on monocytes from patients with IgG anticardiolipin antibodies and a history of thrombosis.

Endothelial Cells

There are several mechanisms by which autoantibodies may enhance the procoagulant activity of vascular endothelial cells. Sera and IgG fractions from certain patients increase the expression of TF (195,196), the production of endothelin 1 (197), and the expression of the adhesion molecules E-selectin, vascular cell adhesion molecule-1 (VCAM-1), and intercellular adhesion molecule-1 (ICAM-1) (105,106). The latter activities have been shown to be dependent on β2GPI and anti-β2GPI autoantibodies.

Another mechanism involves dysregulation of eicosanoid metabolism. There is some evidence that autoantibodies associated with the aPL syndrome inhibit production of endothelial cell prostacyclin (PGI_2), a potent vasodilator and platelet inhibitor (198,199). Autoantibody effects on platelet eicosanoids may be more important, however, as discussed below.

Platelets

Autoimmune thrombocytopenia is part of the aPL syndrome and thought to be due to the antiplatelet activity of a subset of these antibodies. Potential antigenic targets include β2GPI bound to platelet membranes (104) and CD36, an 88-kd membrane glycoprotein (200).

Some studies suggest that aPL induces platelet aggregation (201), whereas others have observed inhibition (202), perhaps due to differences in antibody subsets. Monoclonal anti-β2GPI antibodies bind to platelets in a β2GPI-dependent fashion and lead to platelet activation in the presence of subthreshold concentrations of weak agonists (203). There is consistent evidence that aPL enhances platelet thromboxane A_2 production (204–207). Increased levels of platelet-derived thromboxane urinary metabolites were associated with anti-β2GPI autoantibodies (207).

Fetal Loss: Potential Mechanisms

Fetal losses related to the aPL syndrome are most likely due to hypoxia caused by insufficient uteroplacental blood flow (130). Pathophysiologic findings include maternal spiral artery vasculopathy leading to placental infarction, chronic villitis, atherosis, a decreased number or syncytiovascular membranes, an increased number of syncytial knots, and fetal thrombi (121,208,209). Placental infarction may result from decreased amounts of annexin V on the surface of placental villi of women with the aPL syndrome and recurrent fetal losses (210–213).

EVALUATION AND TREATMENT

Laboratory Evaluation

Patients with recurrent arterial or venous thrombotic events, a family history of thrombosis, thrombosis at a young age (≤45 years), venous thrombosis in locations other than the deep veins of the legs, arterial thrombosis in the absence of atherosclerosis, one or more fetal deaths, or unexplained thrombocytopenia, should be evaluated for the aPL syndrome. It is not clear that women with a history of one or two early spontaneous abortions require testing. In some centers all patients with SLE are screened for the presence of aPL as part of their serologic evaluation. Tests for both anticardiolipin antibodies and the lupus anticoagulant may need to be performed as the assays are discordant in up to 35% of patients with the aPL syndrome (116). Although the strongest clinical associations have been established with IgG anticardiolipin antibodies, isolated IgM or IgA antibodies may be associated with the syndrome. The presence of aPL should be confirmed by repeating a positive test in 6 to 8 weeks.

Important strides have been made in the standardization of the anticardiolipin ELISA, including the establishment of positive standards for IgG, IgM, and IgA isotypes and corresponding GPL, MPL, and APL units (214,215). Significant interlaboratory variation remains a problem, however (216). In light of the importance of β2GPI in the antigenic specificity of anticardiolipin autoantibodies, anti-β2GPI ELISAs have been introduced (7,9,64,65,68,217). Compared to anticardiolipin assays, anti-β2GPI assays may be more specific for clinical manifestations of the aPL syndrome and may detect species specific autoantibodies that recognize human, but not bovine, β2GPI (218). Standardization, interlaboratory comparisons, and prospective clinical studies are needed to define the role of anti-β2GPI assays in clinical practice. Immunoassays for antiprothrombin antibodies are being developed (13,16,75).

Screening tests for the lupus anticoagulant include an appropriately sensitive aPTT, the Russell viper venom time, and the kaolin clotting time (219–221). If prolongation of one of these tests is observed, confirmation of a lupus anticoagulant requires demonstration of an inhibitor (failure of the abnormal screening test to correct when patient plasma is mixed with normal plasma) and demonstration of phospholipid dependence (the inverse relationship of phospholipid concentration to prolongation of the coagulation test). In the tissue thromboplastin inhibition test and the dilute phospholipid aPTT, reduced phospholipid in the assay accentuates the anticoagulant activity. Conversely, in the platelet neutralization procedure, excess phospholipid, in the form of platelet membranes, tends to neutralize the anticoagulant activity.

Differential Diagnosis

Patients with thrombosis should also be evaluated for hereditary and acquired hypercoagulable conditions other than the aPL syndrome, including deficiencies of protein C, protein S, antithrombin III, and plasminogen, resistance to activated protein C (222), the prothrombin G20210A mutation (223), dysfibrinogenemias, excess PAI-1, homocysteinemia (224), malignancies, myeloproliferative disorders, nephrotic syndrome, and Behçet's syndrome. A basic laboratory evaluation would include a complete blood count and smear, genetic tests for activated protein C resistance and the prothrombin G20210A mutation, protein C, protein S, and antithrombin III activities, and a thrombin or reptilase time. If the diagnosis is still obscure, measurement of plasminogen, PAI-1, and homocysteine may be indicated. Similarly, patients with a history of fetal deaths should be evaluated by an obstetrician skilled in high risks to determine if there is an obstetrical cause for the failed pregnancies. Other medical conditions, including thyroid disease and diabetes mellitus, should also be excluded.

The differential diagnosis of the catastrophic aPL syndrome typically includes lupus vasculitis, disseminated intravascular coagulopathy, and thrombotic thrombocytopenic purpura.

Treatment

The risks associated with moderate to high levels of aPL may be substantial. The relative risk of deep venous thrombosis, pulmonary embolism, or stroke (age ≤50) is in the range of 7 to 8 (112,113). Unfortunately, there are few controlled therapeutic trials in the aPL syndrome, and treatment remains largely empirical. A number of principles have emerged from retrospective studies and case reports that offer the clinician some guidance.

Thrombosis

Patients with a history or arterial or venous thrombosis and significant levels of aPL have a high risk of recurrent thrombosis (225–227). Following immediate therapy with heparin, warfarin anticoagulation at relatively high levels (international normalized ratio ≥2.6 to 3.0) is probably required to prevent recurrent thrombotic events (225–227). Lifelong anticoagulation may be necessary. Given the risks of such treatment, the decision regarding long-term anticoagulation should be individualized, and numerous factors should be considered including the level of aPL, the type of thrombotic event, the temporal distance from the event, and the age and reliability of the patient. In certain patients, autoantibodies may interfere with accurate determination of the international normalized ratio (INR), requiring other tests to assess the level of anticoagulation (228,229).

Fetal Loss

Women with a history of two or more fetal deaths (>10 weeks' gestation) and moderate to high levels of aPL are candidates for treatment. Treatment with heparin and low-dose aspirin (~80 mg/day) or prednisone and aspirin is equally efficacious, resulting in delivery of a viable infant in approximately 75% of patients (131,230–234). Because prednisone is associated with a higher frequency of adverse side effects, including infection, preeclampsia, gestational diabetes, and osteonecrosis (231), most experts favor heparin therapy. A typical regimen is subcutaneous heparin, 5,000 to 10,000 units every 12 hours, and low-dose aspirin. The lower dose of heparin appears to be equally efficacious (232,234). Treatment is begun as soon as a viable pregnancy is diagnosed, usually at 5 to 6 weeks' gestation. Heparin is held at the time of delivery, and then reinstituted for 4 to 6 weeks after delivery, due to the risk of thrombosis in the postpartum period. Intravenous immunoglobulin therapy is an option if heparin and prednisone fail (235–237).

Thrombocytopenia

Modest thrombocytopenia (platelet counts ≥50 × 10^9/L) usually does not require treatment. Lower counts may require treatment with corticosteroids.

Catastrophic aPL Syndrome

Based on case reports, the combination of plasmapheresis and anticoagulation appears to be the treatment of choice for the catastrophic aPL syndrome (159,238). Immunosuppressive therapy, including high-dose and pulse corticosteroids, may be ineffective. Two cases suggest that fibrinolytic agents may be useful.

Asymptomatic Patients

Many experienced clinicians recommend that asymptomatic patients with aPL receive low-dose aspirin prophylactically, with the understanding that supporting data are lacking.

CONCLUSION

A clear picture of the aPL syndrome has emerged over the past decade. Autoantibodies associated with the syndrome are directed mainly against a number of phospholipid-binding proteins, and possibly certain cell surface molecules expressed on vascular endothelium and platelets. These data have led to a reevaluation of the pathophysiology of aPL syndrome, particularly with regard to mechanisms of autoantibody-mediated thrombosis. The spectrum of antigenic specificities appears to explain the heterogeneity of lupus anticoagulants and anticardiolipin antibodies in clinical laboratory testing, and may ultimately explain the heterogeneity of the clinical manifestations of the syndrome. There is a continued need for well-controlled therapeutic trials. At the present time anticoagulation, rather than immunosuppression, is the mainstay of treatment.

REFERENCES

1. Kandiah DA, Sali A, Sheng Y, et al. Current insights into the "antiphospholipid" syndrome: clinical, immunological, and molecular aspects. *Adv Immunol* 1998;70:507–563.
2. Wilson WA, Gharavi AE, Koike T, et al. International consensus statement on preliminary classification criteria for definite antiphospholipid syndrome. *Arthritis Rheum* 1999;42: 1309–1311.
3. Vianna JL, Khamashta MA, Ordi-Ros J, et al. Comparison of the primary and secondary antiphospholipid syndrome: a European multicenter study of 114 patients. *Am J Med* 1994;96:3–9.
4. Roubey RAS. Immunology of the antiphospholipid antibody syndrome. *Arthritis Rheum* 1996;39:1444–1454.
5. Galli M, Comfurius P, Maassen C, et al. Anticardiolipin antibodies directed not to cardiolipin but to a plasma protein cofactor. *Lancet* 1990;335:1544–1547.
6. Iverson GM, Victoria EJ, Marquis DM. Anti-β_2-glycoprotein I (β2GPI) autoantibodies recognize an epitope on the first domain of β2GPI. *Proc Natl Acad Sci U S A* 1998;95:15542–15546.
7. Matsuura E, Igarashi Y, Yasuda T, et al. Anticardiolipin antibodies recognize β_2-glycoprotein I structure altered by interacting with an oxygen modified solid phase surface. *J Exp Med* 1994;179:457–462.
8. McNeil HP, Simpson RJ, Chesterman CN, et al. Anti-phospholipid antibodies are directed against a complex antigen that includes a lipid-binding inhibitor of coagulation: β_2-glycoprotein I (apolipoprotein H). *Proc Natl Acad Sci U S A* 1990;87: 4120–4124.
9. Roubey RAS, Eisenberg RA, Harper MF, et al. "Anticardiolipin" autoantibodies recognize β_2-glycoprotein I in the absence of phospholipid. Importance of antigen density and bivalent binding. *J Immunol* 1995;154:954–960.
10. Tincani A, Spatola L, Prati E, et al. The anti-2-glycoprotein I activity in human anti-phospholipid syndrome sera is due to monoreactive low-affinity autoantibodies directed to epitopes located on native 2-glycoprotein I and preserved during species evolution. *J Immunol* 1996;157:5732–5738.
11. Bevers EM, Galli M, Barbui T, et al. Lupus anticoagulant IgG's (LA) are not directed to phospholipids only, but to a complex of lipid-bound human prothrombin. *Thromb Haemost* 1991;66: 629–632.
12. Fleck RA, Rapaport SI, Rao LV. Anti-prothrombin antibodies and the lupus anticoagulant. *Blood* 1988;72:512–519.
13. Galli M, Beretta G, Daldossi M, et al. Different anticoagulant and immunological properties of anti-prothrombin antibodies in patients with antiphospholipid antibodies. *Thromb Haemost* 1997;77:486–491.
14. Oosting JD, Derksen RHWM, Bobbink IWG, et al. Antiphospholipid antibodies directed against a combination of phospholipids with prothrombin, protein C, or protein S: an explanation for their pathogenic mechanism? *Blood* 1993;81:2618–2625.
15. Permpikul P, Rao LVM, Rapaport SI. Functional and binding studies of the roles of prothrombin and β_2-glycoprotein I in the expression of lupus anticoagulant activity. *Blood* 1994;83: 2878–2892.
16. Arvieux J, Darnige L, Caron C, et al. Development of an ELISA for autoantibodies to prothrombin showing their prevalence in patients with lupus anticoagulants. *Thromb Haemost* 1995;74: 1120–1125.
17. Pengo V, Biasiolo A, Brocco T, et al. Autoantibodies to phospholipid-binding plasma proteins in patients with thrombosis and phospholipid-reactive antibodies. *Thromb Haemost* 1996; 75:721–724.
18. Carson CW, Comp PC, Esmon NL, et al. Thrombomodulin antibodies inhibit protein C activation and are found in patients with lupus anticoagulant and unexplained thrombosis. *Arthritis Rheum* 1994;37:S296(abst).
19. Pangborn MC. A new serologically active phospholipid from beef heart. *Proc Soc Exp Biol Med* 1941;48:484–486.
20. Moore JE, Mohr CF. Biologically false positive serologic tests for syphilis. *JAMA* 1952;150:467–473.
21. Moore JE, Lutz WB. The natural history of systemic lupus erythematosus: an approach to its study through chronic biologic false positive reactors. *J Chron Dis* 1955;1:297–316.
22. Conley CL, Hartmann RC. A hemorrhagic disorder caused by circulating anticoagulant in patients with disseminated lupus erythematosus. *J Clin Invest* 1952;31:621–622.
23. Frick PG. Acquired circulating anticoagulants in systemic "collagen disease." *Blood* 1955;10:691–706.
24. Laurell A-B, Nilsson IM. Hypergammaglobulinemia, circulating anticoagulant, and biologic false positive Wassermann reaction. *J Lab Clin Med* 1957;49:694–707.
25. Feinstein DI, Rapaport SI. Acquired inhibitors of blood coagulation. *Prog Hemost Thromb* 1972;1:75–95.
26. Margolius A Jr, Jackson DP, Ratnoff OD. Circulating anticoagulants: a study of 40 cases and a review of the literature. *Medicine* 1961;40:145–202.
27. Bowie EJW, Thompson JH Jr, Pascuzzi CA, et al. Thrombosis in systemic lupus erythematosus despite circulating anticoagulants. *J Lab Clin Med* 1963;62:416–430.
28. Lechner K. Acquired inhibitors in nonhemophilic patients. *Haemostasis* 1974;3:65–93.

29. Alagille D, Crosnier J, Soulier JP. Anticoagulant circulant à activité antithromboplastique. *Rev Fr Clin Biol* 1956;1: 335–345.
30. Carreras LO, DeFreyn G, Machin SJ, et al. Arterial thrombosis, intrauterine death and "lupus" anticoagulant: detection of immunoglobulin interfering with prostacyclin formation. *Lancet* 1981;1:244–246.
31. Firkin BG, Howard MA, Radford N. Possible relationship between lupus inhibitor and recurrent abortion in young women. *Lancet* 1980;2:366.
32. Nilsson IM, Åstedt B, Hedner U, et al. Intrauterine death and circulating anticoagulant ("antithromboplastin"). *Acta Med Scand* 1975;197:153–159.
33. Soulier JP, Boffa MC. Avortements à répétition, thrombose et anticoagulant circulant anti-thromboplastine. *Nouv Presse Med* 1980;9:859–864.
34. Boey ML, Colaco CB, Gharavi AE, et al. Thrombosis in systemic lupus erythematosus: striking association with the presence of circulating lupus anticoagulant. *Br Med J* 1983;287: 1021–1023.
35. Hughes GRV. Thrombosis, abortion, cerebral disease and the lupus anticoagulant. *Br Med J* 1983;287:1088–1089.
36. Harris EN, Gharavi AE, Boey ML, et al. Anticardiolipin antibodies: detection by radioimmunoassay and association with thrombosis in systemic lupus erythematosus. *Lancet* 1983;ii: 1211–1214.
37. Loizou S, McCrea JD, Rudge AC, et al. Measurement of anticardiolipin antibodies by an enzyme-linked immunosorbent assay (ELISA): standardization and quantitation of results. *Clin Exp Immunol* 1985;62:738–745.
38. Loeliger A. Prothrombin as co-factor of the circulating anticoagulant in systemic lupus erythematosus? *Thromb Diath Haemorrh* 1959;3:237–256.
39. Bonnin JA, Cohen AK, Hicks ND. Coagulation defects in a case of systemic lupus erythematosus with thrombocytopenia. *Br J Haematol* 1956;2:168–179.
40. Hougie C. Naturally occurring species specific inhibitor of human prothrombin in lupus erythematosus. *Proc Soc Exp Biol Med* 1964;116:359–361.
41. Medal LS, Lisker R. Circulating anticoagulant in disseminated lupus erythematosus. *Br J Haematol* 1959;5:284–293.
42. Yin ET, Gaston LW. Purification and kinetic studies on a circulating anticoagulant in a suspected case of lupus erythematosus. *Thromb Diath Haemorrh* 1965;14:89–115.
43. Matsuura E, Igarashi Y, Fujimoto M, et al. Anticardiolipin cofactor(s) and differential diagnosis of autoimmune disease. *Lancet* 1990;336:177–178.
44. Reid KBM, Bentley DR, Campbell RD, et al. Complement system proteins which interact with C3b or C4b: a superfamily of structurally related proteins. *Immunol Today* 1986;7:230–234.
45. Steinkasserer A, Barlow PN, Willis AC, et al. Activity, disulphide mapping and structural modelling of the fifth domain of human β_2-glycoprotein I. *FEBS Lett* 1992;313:193–197.
46. Hunt JE, Simpson RJ, Krilis SA. Identification of a region of β_2-glycoprotein I critical for lipid binding and anti-cardiolipin cofactor activity. *Proc Natl Acad Sci U S A* 1993;90:2141–2145.
47. Hagihara Y, Goto Y, Kato H, et al. Role of the N- and C-terminal domains of bovine β_2-glycoprotein I in its interaction with cardiolipin. *J Biochem* 1995;118:129–136.
48. Lee NS, Brewer HB Jr, Osborne JC Jr. Beta-2-glycoprotein I: molecular properties of an unusual apolipoprotein, apolipoprotein H. *J Biol Chem* 1983;258:4765–4770.
49. Cleve H. Genetic studies on the deficiency of β_2-glycoprotein I of human serum. *Humangenetik* 1968;5:294–304.
50. Wurm H. β_2-glycoprotein I (apolipoprotein H) interactions with phospholipid vesicles. *Int J Biochem* 1984;16:511–515.
51. Schousboe I. β_2-glycoprotein I: a plasma inhibitor of the contact activation of the intrinsic blood coagulation pathway. *Blood* 1985;66:1086–1091.
52. Henry ML, Everson B, Ratnoff OD. Inhibition of the activation of Hageman factor (factor XII) by β_2-glycoprotein I. *J Lab Clin Med* 1988;111:519–523.
53. Nimpf J, Wurm H, Kostner GM. β_2-glycoprotein-I (apo H) inhibits the release reaction of human platelets during ADP-induced aggregation. *Atherosclerosis* 1987;63:109–114.
54. Nimpf J, Bevers EM, Bomans PHH, et al. Prothrombinase activity of human platelets is inhibited by β_2-glycoprotein I. *Biochim Biophys Acta* 1986;884:142–149.
55. Harper MF, Hayes PM, Lentz BR, et al. Characterization of β_2-glycoprotein I binding to phospholipid membranes. *Thromb Haemost* 1998;80:610–614.
56. Bancsi LFJMM, van der Linden IK, Bertina RM. β_2-glycoprotein I deficiency and the risk of thrombosis. *Thromb Haemost* 1992;67:649–653.
57. Takeuchi R, Yasuda S, Atsumi T, et al. Coagulation and fibrinolytic characteristics in a β_2-glycoprotein I deficiency. *Lupus* 1998;7:S191(abst).
58. De Benedetti E, Reber G, Miescher PA, et al. No increase of β_2-glycoprotein I levels in patients with antiphospholipid antibodies. *Thromb Haemost* 1992;68:624.
59. Galli M, Cortelazzo S, Daldossi M, et al. Increased levels of beta-2-glycoprotein I (aca-cofactor) in patients with lupus anticoagulant. *Thromb Haemost* 1992;67:386.
60. Matsuura E, Igarashi Y, Fujimoto M, et al. Heterogeneity of anticardiolipin antibodies defined by the anticardiolipin cofactor. *J Immunol* 1992;148:3885–3891.
61. Roubey RAS, Pratt CW, Buyon JP, et al. Lupus anticoagulant activity of autoimmune antiphospholipid antibodies is dependent upon β_2-glycoprotein I. *J Clin Invest* 1992;90:1100–1104.
62. McNally T, Purdy G, Mackie IJ, et al. The use of an anti-β_2-glycoprotein-I assay for discrimination between anticardiolipin antibodies associated with infection and increased risk of thrombosis. *Br J Haematol* 1995;91:471–473.
63. Johansson AE, Lassus A. The occurrences of circulating anticoagulants in patients with syphilitic and biologically false positive antilipoidal antibodies. *Ann Clin Res* 1974;6:105–108.
64. Arvieux J, Roussel B, Jacob MC, et al. Measurement of antiphospholipid antibodies by ELISA using β_2-glycoprotein I as an antigen. *J Immunol Methods* 1991;143:223–229.
65. Viard J-P, Amoura Z, Bach J-F. Association of anti-β_2 glycoprotein I antibodies with lupus-type circulating anticoagulant and thrombosis in systemic lupus erythematosus. *Am J Med* 1992; 93:181–186.
66. Hunt J, Krilis S. The fifth domain of β_2-glycoprotein I contains a phospholipid binding site (cys281-cys288), and a region recognised by anticardiolipin antibodies. *J Immunol* 1994;152: 653–659.
67. Ichikawa K, Khamashta MA, Koike T, et al. β_2-glycoprotein I reactivity of monoclonal anticardiolipin antibodies from patients with the antiphospholipid syndrome. *Arthritis Rheum* 1994;37:1453–1461.
68. Pengo V, Biasiolo A, Fior MG. Autoimmune antiphospholipid antibodies are directed against a cryptic epitope expressed when β_2-glycoprotein I is bound to a suitable surface. *Thromb Haemost* 1995;73:29–34.
69. Oosting JD, Derksen RHWM, Entjes HTI, et al. Lupus anticoagulant activity is frequently dependent on the presence of β_2-glycoprotein I. *Thromb Haemost* 1992;67:499–502.
70. Galli M, Comfurius P, Barbui T, et al. Anticoagulant activity of β_2-glycoprotein I is potentiated by a distinct subgroup of anticardiolipin antibodies. *Thromb Haemost* 1992;68:297–300.
71. Keeling DM, Wilson AJG, Mackie IJ, et al. Lupus anticoagulant

activity of some antiphospholipid antibodies against phospholipid-bound β_2 glycoprotein I. *J Clin Pathol* 1993;46:665–667.
72. Arvieux J, Pouzol P, Roussel B, et al. Lupus-like anticoagulant properties of murine monoclonal antibodies to β_2-glycoprotein I. *Br J Haematol* 1992;81:568–573.
73. Willems GM, Janssen MP, Pelsers MMAL, et al. Role of divalency in the high-affinity binding of anticardiolipin antibody-β_2-glycoprotein I complexes to lipid membranes. *Biochemistry* 1996;35:13833–13842.
74. Arnout J, Wittevrongel C, Vanrusselt M, et al. Beta-2-glycoprotein I dependent lupus anticoagulants form stable bivalent antibody beta-2-glycoprotein I complexes on phospholipid surfaces. *Thromb Haemost* 1998;79:79–86.
75. Horbach DA, van Oort E, Derksen RH, et al. The contribution of anti-prothrombin-antibodies to lupus anticoagulant activity—discrimination between functional and non-functional anti-prothrombin-antibodies. *Thromb Haemost* 1998;79:790–795.
76. Bajaj SP, Rapaport SI, Fierer DS, et al. A mechanism for the hypoprothrombinemia of the acquired hypoprothrombinemia-lupus anticoagulant syndrome. *Blood* 1983;61:684–692.
77. Edson JR, Vogt JM, Hasegawa DK. Abnormal prothrombin crossed-immunoelectrophoresis in patients with lupus inhibitors. *Blood* 1984;64:807–816.
78. Sanson B-J, Friederich PW, Simioni P, et al. The risk of abortion and stillbirth in antithrombin-, protein C-, and protein S-deficient women. *Thromb Haemost* 1996;75:387–388.
79. Ruiz-Argüelles A, Vazquez-Prado J, Deleze M, et al. Presence of serum antibodies to coagulation protein C in patients with systemic lupus erythematosus is not associated with antigenic or functional protein C deficiencies. *Am J Hematol* 1993;44:58–59.
80. Parke AL, Weinstein RE, Bona RD, et al. The thrombotic diathesis associated with the presence of phospholipid antibodies may be due to low levels of free protein S. *Am J Med* 1992; 93:49–56.
81. Kapur A, Kelsey PR, Isaacs PE. Factor V inhibitor in thrombosis. *Am J Hematol* 1993;42:384–388.
82. Åberg H, Nilsson IM. Recurrent thrombosis in a young woman with a circulating anticoagulant directed against factors XI and XII. *Acta Med Scand* 1972;192:419–425.
83. Arvieux J, Pernod G, Regnault V, et al. Some anticardiolipin antibodies recognize a combination of phospholipids with thrombin-modified antithrombin, complement C4b-binding protein, and lipopolysaccharide binding protein. *Blood* 1999; 93:4248–4255.
84. Kaburaki J, Kuwana M, Yamamoto M, et al. Clinical significance of anti-annexin V antibodies in patients with systemic lupus erythematosus. *Am J Hematol* 1997;54:209–213.
85. Matsuda J, Saitoh N, Gohchi K, et al. Anti-annexin V antibody in systemic lupus erythematosus patients with lupus anticoagulant and/or anticardiolipin antibody. *Am J Hematol* 1994;47: 56–58.
86. Matsuda J, Gotoh M, Saitoh N, et al. Anti-annexin antibody in the sera of patients with habitual fetal loss or preeclampsia. *Thromb Res* 1994;75:105–106.
87. Falcón CR, Hoffer AM, Carreras LO. Evaluation of the clinical and laboratory associations of antiphosphatidylethanolamine antibodies. *Thromb Res* 1990;59:383–388.
88. Staub HL, Harris EN, Khamashta MA, et al. Antibody to phosphatidylethanolamine in a patient with lupus anticoagulant and thrombosis. *Ann Rheum Dis* 1989;48:166–169.
89. Karmochkine M, Cacoub P, Piette JC, et al. Antiphosphatidylethanolamine antibody as the sole antiphospholipid antibody in systemic lupus erythematosus with thrombosis. *Clin Exp Rheumatol* 1992;10:603–605.
90. Berard M, Chantome R, Marcelli A, et al. Antiphosphatidylethanolamine antibodies as the only antiphospholipid antibodies. I. Association with thrombosis and vascular cutaneous diseases. *J Rheumatol* 1996;23:1369–1374.
91. Sugi T, McIntyre JA. Autoantibodies to phosphatidylethanolamine (PE) recognize a kininogen-PE complex. *Blood* 1995;86:3083–3089.
92. Boffa MC, Berard M, Sugi T, et al. Antiphosphatidylethanolamine antibodies as the only antiphospholipid antibodies detected by ELISA. II. Kininogen reactivity. *J Rheumatol* 1996; 23:1375–1379.
93. Ruiz-Argüelles GJ, Ruiz-Argüelles A, Deleze M, et al. Acquired protein C deficiency in a patient with primary antiphospholipid syndrome. Relationship to reactivity of anticardiolipin antibody with thrombomodulin. *J Rheumatol* 1989;16:381–383.
94. Oosting JD, Preissner KT, Derksen RHWM, et al. Autoantibodies directed against the epidermal growth factor-like domains of thrombomodulin inhibit protein C activation in vitro. *Br J Haematol* 1993;85:761–768.
95. Fillit H, Lahita R. Antibodies to vascular heparan sulfate proteoglycan in patients with systemic lupus erythematosus. *Autoimmunity* 1991;9:159–164.
96. Fillit H, Shibata S, Sasaki T, et al. Autoantibodies to the protein core of vascular basement membrane heparan sulfate proteoglycan in systemic lupus erythematosus. *Autoimmunity* 1993;14: 243–249.
97. Rauch J, Tannenbaum M, Janoff AS. Distinguishing plasma lupus anticoagulants from anti-factor antibodies using hexagonal (II) phase phospholipids. *Thromb Haemost* 1989;62:892–896.
98. Rauch J, Tannenbaum M, Neville C, et al. Inhibition of lupus anticoagulant activity by hexagonal phase phosphatidylethanolamine in the presence of prothrombin. *Thromb Haemost* 1998;80:936–941.
99. Hörkkö S, Miller E, Branch DW, et al. The epitopes for some antiphospholipid antibodies are adducts of oxidized phospholipid and β_2-glycoprotein I (and other proteins). *Proc Natl Acad Sci U S A* 1997;94:10356–10361.
100. Hörkkö S, Miller E, Dudl E, et al. Antiphospholipid antibodies are directed against epitopes of oxidized phospholipids. *J Clin Invest* 1996;98:815–825.
101. Harris EN, Asherson RA, Gharavi AE, et al. Thrombocytopenia in SLE and related autoimmune disorders: association with anticardiolipin autoantibody. *Br J Haematol* 1985;59:227–230.
102. Jouhikainen T, Kekomaki R, Leirisalo Repo M, et al. Platelet autoantibodies detected by immunoblotting in systemic lupus erythematosus: association with the lupus anticoagulant, and with history of thrombosis and thrombocytopenia. *Eur J Haematol* 1990;44:234–239.
103. Walker TS, Triplett DA, Javed N, et al. Evaluation of lupus anticoagulants: antiphospholipid antibodies, endothelium associated immunoglobulin, endothelial prostacyclin secretion, and antigenic protein S levels. *Thromb Res* 1988;51:267–281.
104. Shi W, Chong BH, Chesterman CN. β_2-glycoprotein I is a requirement for anticardiolipin antibodies binding to activated platelets: differences with lupus anticoagulants. *Blood* 1993;81: 1255–1262.
105. Simantov R, LaSala JM, Lo SK, et al. Activation of cultured vascular endothelial cells by antiphospholipid antibodies. *J Clin Invest* 1995;96:2211–2219.
106. Del Papa N, Guidali L, Spatola L, et al. Relationship between anti-phospholipid and anti-endothelial cell antibodies III: β_2-glycoprotein I mediates the antibody binding to endothelial membranes and induces the expression of adhesion molecules. *Clin Exp Rheumatol* 1995;13:179–185.
107. Galli M, Finazzi G, Bevers EM, et al. Kaolin clotting time and dilute Russell's viper venom time distinguish between prothrombin-dependent and β_2-glycoprotein I-dependent antiphospholipid antibodies. *Blood* 1995;86:617–623.

108. Hardin JA. The lupus autoantigens and the pathogenesis of systemic lupus erythematosus. *Arthritis Rheum* 1986;29:457–460.
109. Kapiotis S, Speiser W, Pabinger Fasching I, et al. Anticardiolipin antibodies in patients with venous thrombosis. *Haemostasis* 1991;21:19–24.
110. Exner T, Koutts J. Autoimmune cardiolipin-binding antibodies in oral anticoagulant patients. *Aust NZ J Med* 1988;18:669–673.
111. Chu P, Pendry K, Blecher TE. Detection of lupus anticoagulant in patients attending an anticoagulation clinic. *Br Med J* 1988; 297:1449.
112. Ginsburg KS, Liang MH, Newcomer L, et al. Anticardiolipin antibodies and the risk for ischemic stroke and venous thrombosis. *Ann Intern Med* 1992;117:997–1002.
113. Kittner SJ, Gorelick PB. Antiphospholipid antibodies and stroke: an epidemiological perspective. *Stroke* 1992;23(suppl I): I-19–I-22.
114. Love PE, Santoro SA. Antiphospholipid antibodies: anticardiolipin and the lupus anticoagulant in systemic lupus erythematosus (SLE) and in non-SLE disorders. Prevalence and clinical significance. *Ann Intern Med* 1990;112:682–698.
115. Reece EA, Gabrielli S, Cullen MT, et al. Recurrent adverse pregnancy outcome and antiphospholipid antibodies [see comments]. *Am J Obstet Gynecol* 1990;163:162–169.
116. Petri M. Diagnosis of antiphospholipid antibodies. *Rheum Dis Clin North Am* 1994;20:443–469.
117. Lechner K, Pabinger Fasching I. Lupus anticoagulants and thrombosis. A study of 25 cases and review of the literature. *Haemostasis* 1985;15:254–262.
118. Gastineau DA, Kazmier FJ, Nichols WL, et al. Lupus anticoagulant: an analysis of the clinical and laboratory features of 219 cases. *Am J Hematol* 1985;19:265–275.
119. Levine SR, Deegan MJ, Futrell N, et al. Cerebrovascular and neurologic disease associated with antiphospholipid antibodies: 48 cases. *Neurology* 1990;40:1181–1189.
120. Asherson RA, Khamashta MA, Gil A, et al. Cerebrovascular disease and antiphospholipid antibodies in systemic lupus erythematosus, lupus-like disease, and the primary antiphospholipid syndrome. *Am J Med* 1989;86:391–399.
121. De Wolf F, Carreras LO, Moerman P, et al. Decidual vasculopathy and extensive placental infarction in a patient with repeated thromboembolic accidents, recurrent fetal loss and a lupus anticoagulant. *Am J Obstet Gynecol* 1982;142:829–834.
122. Asherson RA, Kant KS. Antiphospholipid antibodies and the kidney. *J Rheumatol* 1993;20:1268–1272.
123. Grattan CE, Burton JL. Antiphospholipid syndrome and cutaneous vasoocclusive disorders. *Semin Dermatol* 1991;10:152–159.
124. Coull BM, Bourdette DN, Goodnight SHJ, et al. Multiple cerebral infarctions and dementia associated with anticardiolipin antibodies. *Stroke* 1987;18:1107–1112.
125. Asherson RA, Mercey D, Phillips G, et al. Recurrent stroke and multi-infarct dementia in systemic lupus erythematosus: association with antiphospholipid antibodies. *Ann Rheum Dis* 1987; 46:605–611.
126. Asherson RA, Higenbottam TW, Dinh Xuan AT, et al. Pulmonary hypertension in a lupus clinic: experience with twenty-four patients. *J Rheumatol* 1990;17:1292–1298.
127. Lockshin MD. Pregnancy loss and antiphospholipid antibodies. *Lupus* 1998;7(suppl 2):S86–S89.
128. Lockshin MD, Druzin ML, Goei S, et al. Antibody to cardiolipin as a predictor of fetal distress or death in pregnant patients with systemic lupus erythematosus. *N Engl J Med* 1985;313:152–156.
129. Branch DW, Scott FR, Kochenour NK, et al. Obstetric complications associated with the lupus anticoagulant. *N Engl J Med* 1985;313:1322–1326.
130. Branch DW. Thoughts on the mechanism of pregnancy loss associated with the antiphospholipid syndrome. *Lupus* 1994;3: 275–280.
131. Branch DW, Silver RM, Blackwell JL, et al. Outcome of treated pregnancies in women with antiphospholipid syndrome: an update of the Utah experience. *Obstet Gynecol* 1992;80:614–620.
132. McNeil HP, Chesterman CN, Krilis SA. Immunology and clinical importance of antiphospholipid antibodies. *Adv Immunol* 1991;49:193–280.
133. Alarcón-Segovia D, Sanchez-Guerrero J. Correction of thrombocytopenia with small dose aspirin in the primary antiphospholipid syndrome. *J Rheumatol* 1989;16:1359–1361.
134. Khamashta MA, Cervera R, Asherson RA, et al. Association of antibodies against phospholipids with heart valve disease in systemic lupus erythematosus. *Lancet* 1990;335:1541–1544.
135. Chartash EK, Lans DM, Paget SA, et al. Aortic insufficiency and mitral regurgitation in patients with systemic lupus erythematosus and the antiphospholipid syndrome. *Am J Med* 1989; 86:407–412.
136. Leung W-H, Wong K-L, Lau C-P, et al. Association between antiphospholipid antibodies and cardiac abnormalities in patients with systemic lupus erythematosus. *Am J Med* 1990;89:411–419.
137. Galve E, Ordi J, Barquinero J, et al. Valvular heart disease in the primary antiphospholipid syndrome. *Ann Intern Med* 1992; 116:293–298.
138. Espinola-Zavaleta N, Vargas-Barron J, Colmenares-Galves T, et al. Echocardiographic evaluation of patients with primary antiphospholipid syndrome. *Am Heart J* 1999;137:973–978.
139. Pope JM, Canny CL, Bell DA. Cerebral ischemic events associated with endocarditis, retinal vascular disease, and lupus anticoagulant. *Am J Med* 1991;90:299–309.
140. Barbut D, Borer JS, Gharavi A, et al. Prevalence of anticardiolipin antibody in isolated mitral or aortic regurgitation, or both, and possible relation to cerebral ischemic events. *Am J Cardiol* 1992;70:901–905.
141. Tietjen GE, Levine SR, Brown E, et al. Factors that predict antiphospholipid immunoreactivity in young people with transient focal neurological events. *Arch Neurol* 1993;50:833–836.
142. Lavalle C, Pizarro S, Drenkard C, et al. Transverse myelitis: a manifestation of systemic lupus erythematosus strongly associated with antiphospholipid antibodies. *J Rheumatol* 1990;17:34–37.
143. Cervera R, Asherson RA, Font J, et al. Chorea in the antiphospholipid syndrome—clinical, radiologic, and immunologic characteristics of 50 patients from our clinics and the recent literature. *Medicine* 1997;76:203–212.
144. Brey RL, Gharavi AE, Lockshin MD. Neurologic complications of antiphospholipid antibodies. *Rheum Dis Clin North Am* 1993;19:833–850.
145. Ijdo JW, Conti-Kelly AM, Greco P, et al. Anti-phospholipid antibodies in patients with multiple sclerosis and MS-like illnesses: MS or APS? *Lupus* 1999;8:109–115.
146. Tourbah A, Clapin A, Gout O, et al. Systemic autoimmune features and multiple sclerosis: a 5-year follow-up study. *Arch Neurol* 1998;55:517–521.
147. Johansson EA, Niemi KM, Mustakallio KK. A peripheral vascular syndrome overlapping with systemic lupus erythematosus. *Dermatologica* 1977;155:257–267.
148. Naldi L, Locati F, Marchesi L, et al. Cutaneous manifestations associated with antiphospholipid antibodies in patients with suspected primary antiphospholipid syndrome: a case-control study. *Ann Rheum Dis* 1993;52:219–222.
149. Englert HJ, Loizou S, Derue GG, et al. Clinical and immunologic features of livedo reticularis in lupus: a case-control study. *Am J Med* 1989;87:408–410.
150. Levine SR, Langer SL, Albers JW, et al. Sneddon's syndrome: an antiphospholipid antibody syndrome? *Neurology* 1988;38: 798–800.

151. Frances C, Papo T, Wechsler B, et al. Sneddon syndrome with or without antiphospholipid antibodies. A comparative study in 46 patients. *Medicine* 1999;78:209–219.
152. Paira S, Roverano S, Zunino A, et al. Extensive cutaneous necrosis associated with anticardiolipin antibodies. *J Rheumatol* 1999;26:1197–2000.
153. Harrison RL, Alperin JB, Kumar D. Concurrent lupus anticoagulants and prothrombin deficiency due to phenytoin use. *Arch Pathol Lab Med* 1987;111:719–722.
154. Asherson RA, Zulman J, Hughes GR. Pulmonary thromboembolism associated with procainamide induced lupus syndrome and anticardiolipin antibodies. *Ann Rheum Dis* 1989;48:232–235.
155. Canoso RT, De Oliveira RM. Chlorpromazine-induced anticardiolipin antibodies and lupus anticoagulant: absence of thrombosis. *Am J Hematol* 1988;27:272–275.
156. Morgan M, Chesterman CN, Downs K, et al. Clinical analysis of 125 patients with the lupus anticoagulant. *Aust NZ J Med* 1993;23:151–156.
157. Merrill JT, Shen C, Gugnani M, et al. High prevalence of antiphospholipid antibodies in patients taking procainamide. *J Rheumatol* 1997;24:1083–1088.
158. Gharavi AE, Sammaritano LR, Wen J, et al. Characteristics of human immunodeficiency virus and chlorpromazine induced antiphospholipid antibodies: effect of β_2 glycoprotein I on binding to phospholipid. *J Rheumatol* 1994;21:94–99.
159. Asherson RA, Cervera R, Piette JC, et al. Catastrophic antiphospholipid syndrome. Clinical and laboratory features of 50 patients. *Medicine* 1998;77:195–207.
160. Branch DW, Dudley DJ, Mitchell MD. IgG fractions from patients with antiphospholipid antibodies cause fetal death in BALB/c mice: a model for autoimmune fetal loss. *Am J Obstet Gynecol* 1990;163:210–216.
161. Blank M, Cohen J, Toder V, et al. Induction of anti-phospholipid syndrome in naive mice with mouse lupus monoclonal and human polyclonal anti-cardiolipin antibodies. *Proc Natl Acad Sci U S A* 1991;88:3069–3073.
162. Pierangeli SS, Barker JH, Stikovac D, et al. Effect of human IgG antiphospholipid antibodies on an in vivo thrombosis model in mice. *Thromb Haemost* 1994;71:670–674.
163. Harris EN, Chan JKH, Asherson RA, et al. Thrombosis, recurrent fetal loss, thrombocytopenia: predictive value of IgG anticardiolipin antibodies. *Arch Intern Med* 1986;146:2153–2156.
164. Takeya H, Mori T, Gabazza EC, et al. Anti-β_2-glycoprotein I (β2GPI) monoclonal antibodies with lupus anticoagulant-like activity enhance the β2GPI binding to phospholipids. *J Clin Invest* 1997;99:2260–2268.
165. Triplett DA. Antiphospholipid antibodies: proposed mechanisms of action. *Am J Reprod Immunol* 1992;28:211–215.
166. Dahlbäck B. Physiological anticoagulation: resistance to activated protein C and venous thromboembolism. *J Clin Invest* 1994;94:923–927.
167. Borrell M, Sala N, de Castellarnau C, et al. Immunoglobulin fractions isolated from patients with antiphospholipid antibodies prevent the inactivation of factor Va by activated protein C on human endothelial cells. *Thromb Haemost* 1992;68: 268–272.
168. Cariou R, Tobelem G, Bellucci S, et al. Effect of lupus anticoagulant on antithrombogenic properties of endothelial cells - inhibition of thrombomodulin-dependent protein C activation. *Thromb Haemost* 1988;60:54–58.
169. Comp PC, DeBault LE, Esmon NL, et al. Human thrombomodulin is inhibited by IgG from two patients with non-specific anticoagulants. *Blood* 1983;62(suppl 1):299a(abst).
170. Malia RG, Kitchen S, Greaves M, et al. Inhibition of activated protein C and its cofactor protein S by antiphospholipid antibodies. *Br J Haematol* 1990;76:101–107.
171. Marciniak E, Romond EH. Impaired catalytic function of activated protein C: a new in vitro manifestation of lupus anticoagulant. *Blood* 1989;74:2426–2432.
172. Keeling DM, Wilson AJG, Mackie IM, et al. β_2-glycoprotein I inhibits the thrombin/thrombomodulin dependent activation of protein C. *Blood* 1991;78:184a(abst).
173. Oosting JD, Derksen RHWM, Hackeng TM, et al. In vitro studies of antiphospholipid antibodies and its cofactor, beta-2-glycoprotein I, show negligible effects on endothelial cell mediated protein C activation. *Thromb Haemost* 1991;66:666–671.
174. Matsuda J, Gohchi K, Kawasugi K, et al. Inhibitory activity of anti-β_2-glycoprotein I antibody on factor Va degradation by activated-protein C and its cofactor protein S. *Am J Hematol* 1995;49:89–91.
175. Ruiz-Argäelles GJ, Ruiz-Argäelles A, Alarcón-Segovia D, et al. Natural anticoagulants in systemic lupus erythematosus. Deficiency of protein S bound to C4bp associates with recent history of venous thromboses, antiphospholipid antibodies, and the antiphospholipid syndrome. *J Rheumatol* 1991;18:552–558.
176. Moreb J, Kitchens CS. Acquired functional protein S deficiency, cerebral venous thrombosis, and coumarin skin necrosis in association with antiphospholipid syndrome: report of two cases. *Am J Med* 1989;87:207–210.
177. Shibata S, Sasaki T, Harpel P, et al. Autoantibodies to vascular heparan sulfate proteoglycan in systemic lupus erythematosus react with endothelial cells and inhibit the formation of thrombin-antithrombin III complexes. *Clin Immunol Immunopathol* 1994;70:114–123.
178. Chamley LW, McKay EJ, Pattison NS. Inhibition of heparin/antithrombin III cofactor activity by anticardiolipin antibodies: a mechanism for thrombosis. *Thromb Res* 1993;71: 103–111.
179. Shibata S, Harpel PC, Gharavi A, et al. Autoantibodies to heparin from patients with antiphospholipid antibody syndrome inhibit formation of antithrombin III-thrombin complexes. *Blood* 1994;83:2532–2540.
180. Rand JH, Wu XX, Andree HA, et al. Antiphospholipid antibodies accelerate plasma coagulation by inhibiting annexin-V binding to phospholipids: a "lupus procoagulant" phenomenon. *Blood* 1998;92:1652–1660.
181. Shi W, Chong BH, Hogg PJ, et al. Anticardiolipin antibodies block the inhibition by β_2-glycoprotein I of the factor Xa generating activity of platelets. *Thromb Haemost* 1993;70:342–345.
182. Tsakiris DA, Marbet GA, Makris PE, et al. Impaired fibrinolysis as an essential contribution to thrombosis in patients with lupus anticoagulant. *Thromb Haemost* 1989;61:175–177.
183. Violi F, Ferro D, Valesini G, et al. Tissue plasminogen activator inhibitor in patients with systemic lupus erythematosus and thrombosis. *Br Med J* 1990;300:1099–1102.
184. Jurado M, Páramo JA, Gutierrez-Pimentel M, et al. Fibrinolytic potential and antiphospholipid antibodies in systemic lupus erythematosus and other connective tissue disorders. *Thromb Haemost* 1992;68:516–520.
185. Ames PR, Tommasino C, Iannaccone L, et al. Coagulation activation and fibrinolytic imbalance in subjects with idiopathic antiphospholipid antibodies—a crucial role for acquired free protein S deficiency. *Thromb Haemost* 1996;76:190–194.
186. Wachtfogel YT, DeLa Cadena RA, Colman RW. Structural biology, cellular interactions and pathophysiology of the contact system. *Thromb Res* 1993;72:1–21.
187. Sanfelippo MJ, Drayna CJ. Prekallikrein inhibition associated with the lupus anticoagulant: a mechanism of thrombosis. *Am J Clin Pathol* 1982;77:275–279.
188. Killeen AA, Meyer KC, Vogt JM, et al. Kallikrein inhibition and C1-esterase inhibitor levels in patients with lupus inhibitor. *Am J Clin Pathol* 1987;88:223–228.

189. Schousboe I. Inositol phospholipid-accelerated activation of prekallikrein by activated factor XII and its inhibition by β_2-glycoprotein I. *Eur J Biochem* 1988;176:629–636.
190. Schousboe I. In vitro activation of the contact activation system (Hageman factor system) in plasma by acidic phospholipids and the inhibitory effect of β_2-glycoprotein I on this activation. *Int J Biochem* 1988;20:309–315.
191. Amengual O, Atsumi T, Khamashta MA, et al. The role of the tissue factor pathway in the hypercoagulable state in patients with the antiphospholipid syndrome. *Thromb Haemost* 1998; 79:276–281.
192. Cuadrado MJ, López-Pedrera C, Khamashta MA, et al. Thrombosis in primary antiphospholipid syndrome: a pivotal role for monocyte tissue factor expression. *Arthritis Rheum* 1997;40: 834–841.
193. Kornberg A, Blank M, Kaufman S, et al. Induction of tissue factor-like activity in monocytes by anti-cardiolipin antibodies. *J Immunol* 1994;153:1328–1332.
194. Reverter JC, Tassies D, Font J, et al. Effects of human monoclonal anticardiolipin antibodies on platelet function and on tissue factor expression on monocytes. *Arthritis Rheum* 1998;41: 1420–1427.
195. Oosting JD, Derksen RHWM, Blokzijl L, et al. Antiphospholipid antibody positive sera enhance endothelial cell procoagulant activity—studies in a thrombosis model. *Thromb Haemost* 1992;68:278–284.
196. Tannenbaum SH, Finko R, Cines DB. Antibody and immune complexes induce tissue factor production by human endothelial cells. *J Immunol* 1986;137:1532–1537.
197. Atsumi T, Khamashta MA, Haworth RS, et al. Arterial disease and thrombosis in the antiphospholipid syndrome: a pathogenic role for endothelin 1. *Arthritis Rheum* 1998;41:800–807.
198. Carreras LO, Maclouf J. The lupus anticoagulant and eicosanoids. *Prostaglandins Leukot Essent Fatty Acids* 1993;49: 483–488.
199. Carreras LO, Martinuzzo ME, Maclouf J. Antiphospholipid antibodies, eicosanoids and expression of endothelial cyclooxygenase-2. *Lupus* 1996;5:494–497.
200. Rock G, Chauhan K, Jamieson GA, et al. Anti-CD36 antibodies in patients with lupus anticoagulant and thrombotic complications. *Br J Haematol* 1994;88:878–880.
201. Escolar G, Font J, Referter JC, et al. Plasma from systemic lupus erythematosus patients with antiphospholipid antibodies promotes platelet aggregation. *Arterioscler Thromb* 1992;12:196–200.
202. Ostfeld I, Dadosh-Goffer N, Borokowski S, et al. Lupus anticoagulant antibodies inhibit collagen-induced adhesion and aggregation of human platelets in vitro. *J Clin Immunol* 1992;12:415–423.
203. Arvieux J, Roussel B, Pouzol P, et al. Platelet activating properties of murine monoclonal antibodies to β_2-glycoprotein I. *Thromb Haemost* 1993;70:336–341.
204. Hasselaar P, Derksen RHWM, Blokzijl L, et al. Thrombosis associated with antiphospholipid antibodies cannot be explained by effects on endothelial and platelet prostanoid synthesis. *Thromb Haemost* 1988;59:80–85.
205. Maclouf J, Lellouche F, Martinuzzo M, et al. Increased production of platelet-derived thromboxane in patients with lupus anticoagulants. *Agents Actions Suppl* 1992;37:27–33.
206. Martinuzzo ME, Maclouf J, Carreras LO, et al. Antiphospholipid antibodies enhance thrombin-induced platelet activation and thromboxane formation. *Thromb Haemost* 1993;70:667–671.
207. Forastiero R, Martinuzzo M, Carreras LO, et al. Anti-β_2-glycoprotein I antibodies and platelet activation in patients with antiphospholipid antibodies: association with increased excretion of platelet-derived thromboxane urinary metabolites. *Thromb Haemost* 1998;79:42–45.
208. Magid MS, Kaplan C, Sammaritano LR, et al. Placental pathology in systemic lupus erythematosus: a prospective study. *Am J Obstet Gynecol* 1998;179:226–234.
209. Levy RA, Avvad E, Oliveira J, et al. Placental pathology in antiphospholipid syndrome. *Lupus* 1998;7(suppl 2):S81–S85.
210. Rand JH, Wu XX, Guller S, et al. Reduction of annexin-V (placental anticoagulant protein-I) on placental villi of women with antiphospholipid antibodies and recurrent spontaneous abortion. *Am J Obstet Gynecol* 1994;171:1566–1572.
211. Rand JH, Wu XX, Guller S, et al. Antiphospholipid immunoglobulin G antibodies reduce annexin-V levels on syncytiotrophoblast apical membranes and in culture media of placental villi. *Am J Obstet Gynecol* 1997;177:918–923.
212. Rand JH, Wu XX, Andree HAM, et al. Pregnancy loss in the antiphospholipid-antibody syndrome—a possible thrombogenic mechanism. *N Engl J Med* 1997;337:154–160.
213. Lakasing L, Campa JS, Poston R, et al. Normal expression of tissue factor, thrombomodulin, and annexin V in placentas from women with antiphospholipid syndrome. *Am J Obstet Gynecol* 1999;181:180–189.
214. Harris EN, Gharavi AE, Patel SP, et al. Evaluation of the anti-cardiolipin test: report of an international workshop held 4 April 1986. *Clin Exp Immunol* 1987;68:215–222.
215. Harris EN. Special report. The Second International Anti-cardiolipin Standardization Workshop/the Kingston Anti-Phospholipid Antibody Study (KAPS) group. *Am J Clin Pathol* 1990;94:476–484.
216. Peaceman AM, Silver RK, MacGregor SN, et al. Interlaboratory variation in antiphospholipid antibody testing. *Am J Obstet Gynecol* 1992;166:1780–1787.
217. Lewis S, Keil LB, Binder WL, et al. Standardized measurement of major immunoglobulin class (IgG, IgA, and IgM) antibodies to β_2-glycoprotein I in patients with antiphospholipid syndrome. *J Clin Lab Anal* 1998;12:293–297.
218. Arvieux J, Darnige L, Hachulla E, et al. Species specificity of anti-β_2-glycoprotein I autoantibodies and its relevance to anticardiolipin antibody quantitation. *Thromb Haemost* 1996;75: 725–730.
219. Triplett DA. Coagulation assays for the lupus anticoagulant: review and critique of current methodology. *Stroke* 1992;23 (suppl I):11–14.
220. Brandt JT, Triplett DA, Alving B, et al. Criteria for the diagnosis of lupus anticoagulants: an update. *Thromb Haemost* 1995; 74:1185–1190.
221. Brandt JT, Barna LK, Triplett DA. Laboratory identification of lupus anticoagulants: results of the Second International Workshop for Identification of Lupus Anticoagulants. On behalf of the Subcommittee on Lupus Anticoagulants/Antiphospholipid Antibodies of the ISTH. *Thromb Haemost* 1995;74:1597–1603.
222. Dahlbäck B. Resistance to activated protein C caused by the factor V R506Q mutation is a common risk factor for venous thrombosis. *Thromb Haemost* 1997;78:483–488.
223. Bertina RM. The prothrombin 20210 G to A variation and thrombosis. *Curr Opin Hematol* 1998;5:339–342.
224. Welch GN, Loscalzo J. Mechanisms of disease: homocysteine and atherothrombosis. *N Engl J Med* 1998;338:1042–1050.
225. Rosove MH, Brewer PMC. Antiphospholipid thrombosis: clinical course after the first thrombotic event in 70 patients. *Ann Intern Med* 1992;117:303–308.
226. Derksen RHWM, De Groot PG, Kater L, et al. Patients with antiphospholipid antibodies and venous thrombosis should receive long term anticoagulant treatment. *Ann Rheum Dis* 1993;52:689–692.
227. Khamashta MA, Cuadrado MJ, Mujic F, et al. The management of thrombosis in the antiphospholipid-antibody syndrome. *N Engl J Med* 1995;332:993–997.

228. Della Valle P, Crippa L, Safa O, et al. Potential failure of the international normalized ratio (INR) system in the monitoring of oral anticoagulation in patients with lupus anticoagulants. *Ann Med Interne (Paris)* 1996;147 Suppl 1:10–14.
229. Moll S, Ortel TL. Monitoring warfarin therapy in patients with lupus anticoagulants. *Ann Intern Med* 1997;127:177–185.
230. Rosove MH, Tabsh K, Wasserstrum N, et al. Heparin therapy for pregnant women with lupus anticoagulant or anticardiolipin antibodies. *Obstet Gynecol* 1990;75:630–634.
231. Cowchock FS, Reece EA, Balaban D, et al. Repeated fetal losses associated with antiphospholipid antibodies: a collaborative randomized trial comparing prednisone to low-dose heparin treatment. *Am J Obstet Gynecol* 1992;166:1318–1323.
232. Rai R, Cohen H, Dave M, et al. Randomised controlled trial of aspirin and aspirin plus heparin in pregnant women with recurrent miscarriage associated with phospholipid antibodies. *Br Med J* 1997;314:253–257.
233. Kutteh WH. Antiphospholipid antibody-associated recurrent pregnancy loss: treatment with heparin and low-dose aspirin is superior to low-dose aspirin alone. *Am J Obstet Gynecol* 1996;174:1584–1589.
234. Kutteh WH, Ermel LD. A clinical trial for the treatment of antiphospholipid antibody-associated recurrent pregnancy loss with lower dose heparin and aspirin. *Am J Reprod Immunol* 1996;35:402–407.
235. Scott JR, Branch DW, Kochenour NK, et al. Intravenous immunoglobulin treatment of pregnant patients with recurrent pregnancy loss caused by antiphospholipid antibodies and Rh immunization. *Am J Obstet Gynecol* 1988;159:1055–1056.
236. Spinnato JA, Clark AL, Pierangeli SS, et al. Intravenous immunoglobulin therapy for the antiphospholipid syndrome in pregnancy. *Am J Obstet Gynecol* 1995;172:690–694.
237. Clark AL, Branch DW, Silver RM, et al. Pregnancy complicated by the antiphospholipid syndrome: outcomes with intravenous immunoglobulin therapy. *Obstet Gynecol* 1999;93:437–441.
238. Neuwelt CM, Daikh DI, Linfoot JA, et al. Catastrophic antiphospholipid syndrome: response to repeated plasmapheresis over three years [see comments]. *Arthritis Rheum* 1997;40:1534–1539.

78

INFLAMMATORY MYOPATHIES: POLYMYOSITIS, DERMATOMYOSITIS, AND RELATED CONDITIONS

FREDERICK W. MILLER

Diseases characterized by acquired muscle inflammation are designated *inflammatory myopathies.* This term encompasses a large number of disorders that include viral, fungal, and parasitic infections of muscle; toxic myopathies; and other causes of muscle damage (Table 78.1). Patients with these conditions often present with nonspecific signs and symptoms such as fatigue, fever, and myalgias that can result in misdiagnosis and delays in therapy. When the appropriate clinical, laboratory, and pathologic studies eliminate known causes of muscle inflammation, however, a diagnosis of idiopathic inflammatory myopathy (IIM) can be made (1).

The most common forms of IIM are polymyositis, in which patients have inflammation of multiple muscles, and dermatomyositis, in which inflammatory changes occur in the skin as well as muscles. Yet, the IIM themselves are a heterogeneous group of rare syndromes that differ considerably in their clinical presentations, pathologic findings, disease courses, responses to therapy, and prognoses (2). This heterogeneity has delayed progress in the field and almost certainly reflects multiple etiologies and pathogenic mechanisms that result in a final common path of muscle inflammation (2,3).

The presence of mononuclear cell infiltration in muscle and frequent immune abnormalities, including autoantibodies, in patients with IIM has resulted in most of these disorders being thought of as autoimmune or immune-mediated diseases. This has also been the basis for the major therapeutic approaches for IIM that have been directed toward decreasing inflammation in the many organs that may be affected in these diseases (4).

HISTORICAL OVERVIEW

It is not known how long IIMs have existed, but published reports in the German medical literature first appeared more than 100 years ago. The first descriptions of polymyositis appear to be those of Wagner in 1863 (5) and 1887 (6), with Potain (7) and Hepp (8) describing similar cases at about the same time, and Unverricht (9,10) naming dermatomyositis as an entity shortly thereafter. Nonetheless, the early literature is confused by indiscriminate use of the terms *polymyositis* and *dermatomyositis* without regard to skin involvement. The first reported American cases were in 1887 and 1888 (11,12).

Important milestones in the history of myositis include a critical review and elegant description of the then known cases by Steiner (13) in 1903; development of corticosteroid therapy (14,15); publication of the classic text on polymyositis by Walton and Adams (16); recognition of the pathology of childhood dermatomyositis (17); use of methotrexate in resistant disease (18); proposed criteria and classifications of Bohan, Peter, and Pearson (19,20); recognition of the distinct clinical entity of inclusion body myositis (21–23); definition of different mononuclear cell subsets in the muscle infiltrates occurring in polymyositis and dermatomyositis (24); usefulness of serology in defining distinct groups of patients (25); and publication of comprehensive and authoritative texts on myology (26,27).

DIFFERENTIAL DIAGNOSIS AND CRITERIA

Patients presenting with complaints of weakness or muscle pain are very common in clinical practice. Because the differential diagnosis of muscle complaints is quite large, many disorders must be carefully considered in evaluating such patients (Table 78.2). The evaluation should involve a directed history, physical examination, and laboratory tests that in most cases result in a diagnosis and plan for therapy.

TABLE 78.1. INFLAMMATORY MYOPATHIES

Infectious myopathies
- Bacterial
  - Staphylococcus
  - Streptococcus
  - Clostridia
  - Borrelia
  - *Mycoplasma pneumoniae*
  - *Serratia marcescens*
  - *Citrobacter freundii*
  - Salmonella
- Viral
  - Influenza
  - Adenovirus
  - Epstein-Barr virus
  - Coxsackievirus
  - Echovirus
  - Hepatitis B
  - Hepatitis C
  - HIV
  - Human T-cell leukemia (HTLV-1)
- Fungal
  - Candida
  - Coccidioidomycosis
- Protozoal
  - Toxoplasmosis
  - Sarcocystis
  - Trypanosomiasis
  - Microsporidia, increasingly described in AIDS
  - Malaria
- Cestode infections
  - Cysticercosis
  - Echinococcosis
- Nematode infections
  - Trichinosis
  - Toxocariasis

Toxic myopathies
- Adulterated rapeseed oil (toxic oil syndrome)
- Cimetidine
- Cocaine-heroin
- D-penicillamine
- Ethanol
- L-tryptophan (eosinophilia myalgia syndrome)

Myositis associated with graft-versus-host disease
Myositis ossificans
Myositis associated with the vasculitides
Idiopathic inflammatory myopathies (see Table 78.6 and 78.8)

TABLE 78.2. A DIFFERENTIAL DIAGNOSIS OF MUSCLE WEAKNESS/PAIN

Inflammatory myopathies (see Table 78.1)
Noninflammatory myopathies
- Congenital—nemaline rod, centronuclear, central core
- Mitochondrial—with genetic defects
- Metabolic—acid maltase deficiency, McArdle's phosphofructokinase deficiency, carnitine and carnitine palmityltransferase deficiency, uremia
- Endocrine—hypo- and hyperthyroidism, acromegaly, diabetes, Cushing's, Addison's, hypo- and hyperparathyroidism, hypocalcemia, hypokalemia
- Toxic—from many drugs, including ethanol, corticosteroids, cocaine, colchicine, clofibrate, chloroquine, lovastatin, emetine, ipecac, zidovudine (AZT)
- Nutritional—vitamin E deficiency, malabsorption syndromes

Malignant hyperthermia
Muscular dystrophies
- Duchenne's
- Becker's
- Fascioscapulohumeral
- Limb-girdle
- Emery-Dreifuss
- Distal
- Oculopharyngeal

Myotonia
Neuropathies
- Denervating conditions
  - Spinal muscular atrophy
  - Amyotrophic lateral sclerosis
- Proximal neuropathies
  - Guillain-Barré syndrome
  - Autoimmune polyneuropathy
  - Diabetic plexopathy
  - Acute intermittent porphyria

Neuromuscular junction disorders
- Eaton-Lambert syndrome
- Myasthenia gravis

Overuse syndromes
Periodic paralyses
Paraneoplastic syndromes
- Carcinomatous neuropathy
- Cachexia
- Myonecrosis

Rhabdomyolysis
Rheumatic syndromes
- Giant cell arteritis/polymyalgia rheumatica
- Wegener's granulomatosus
- Polyarteritis nodosa
- Fibromyalgia syndromes

Tendonitis-fasciitis syndromes
Trauma

The first priority is to define clearly the patient's primary problems and any associated features. A careful history may reveal the diagnosis. Questions should focus on (a) the exact nature and location of weakness, myalgias, or other muscle symptoms; (b) any exacerbating or ameliorating factors; (c) the time frame and tempo of the progression of symptoms; and (d) the development of any associated nonmuscular symptoms such as fatigue, rashes, breathing or swallowing difficulties, arthralgias, or arthritis. After the patient's problems are clearly defined, one needs to consider the possible causes for these problems. Has the individual been exposed to any myotoxins, licit or illicit drugs, botanical or other over-the-counter preparations that could result in myopathy, or had any unusual environmental exposure or infections, or returned from foreign travel? Are there any symptoms or findings that suggest hypothyroidism or hyperthyroidism? Is there a family history of a similar muscle disorder that would suggest a dystrophy or other inherited myopathy?

When most of the known causes of myopathy are excluded by the clinical context and nature of the symptoms, the physical examination and laboratory testing should be directed at narrowing further the diagnostic possibilities and determining if more invasive procedures are needed. Muscle weakness needs to be distinguished from fatigability or pain that might limit function. The distribution of skeletal muscle tenderness or atrophy should be noted. Involvement of other muscles, including the heart, oropharynx, gastrointestinal tract, or ocular and respiratory muscles, as well as any other nonmuscle abnormalities, should be documented. Rashes need to be carefully evaluated and in some cases biopsied. Unfortunately, the distinctions among many of the disorders associated with myopathy are not well defined, and in many cases the diseases remain constellations of signs, symptoms, and laboratory abnormalities. Although molecular genetic studies are identifying the genes responsible for more of the dystrophies, metabolic, and mitochondrial myopathies each year (28–32), some patients, even after the most thorough evaluations, continue to defy diagnostic evaluations and remain enigmas. They should be fully educated about the limitations of our understanding of muscle disease and the risk-benefits of possible empiric therapy.

Criteria that define the IIM syndromes and distinguish them from the many other myopathies were proposed over 20 years ago (20). Although in need of reassessment, given findings regarding the role of autoantibodies and magnetic resonance imaging (MRI) in the diagnosis of myositis (33), they remain useful today (Table 78.3). After excluding other causes of myopathy, the presence of the following abnormalities usually establishes a diagnosis of IIM: proximal muscle weakness; elevated serum levels of sarcoplasmic enzymes; myopathic changes on electromyography; muscle biopsy showing myofiber degeneration and regeneration with chronic inflammatory infiltrates; and, in the case of dermatomyositis, the presence of a heliotrope rash, Gottron's sign, or papules. In a significant minority of cases, however, all the muscle-associated enzyme levels will be normal, and the biopsy or electromyography findings will be neither diagnostic nor characteristic of IIM. These findings may occur because of technical limitations, misinterpretations of the studies, or the focal nature of the pathology in these conditions. In such cases, additional clues that can assist in making the diagnosis of an IIM, and that need to be studied as possible criteria in the future, include the presence of antinuclear or myositis-specific autoantibodies (34,35), a strong family history of autoimmune disease (36), inflammatory changes in proximal muscles on MRI (37–41), and a clinical response to immunosuppressive therapy (42) (Table 78.4).

Criteria are not well established to distinguish among the different forms of IIM. Regarding the recently defined entity of inclusion body myositis, the finding of IIM criteria in the context of slowly progressive proximal and distal weakness, serum creatine kinase (CK) levels less than 12 times the upper limits of normal, with characteristic rimmed vacuoles by light microscopic evaluation of stained sections of frozen muscle specimens, with or without filaments present by ultrastructural analysis (43–45),

TABLE 78.3. CRITERIA FOR THE DIAGNOSIS OF IDIOPATHIC INFLAMMATORY MYOPATHY (IIM)[a]

1 Symmetric weakness, usually progressive, of the limb-girdle muscles
2. Muscle biopsy evidence of myositis
   - Necrosis of type I and type II muscle fibers
   - Phagocytosis
   - Degeneration and regeneration of myofibers with variation in myofiber size
   - Endomysial, perimysial, perivascular, or interstitial mononuclear cells
3. Elevation of serum levels of muscle-associated enzymes
   - Creatine kinase
   - Aldolase
   - Lactate dehydrogenase
   - Transaminases (ALT/SGPT and AST/SGOT)
4. Electromyographic triad of myopathy
   - Short, small, low-amplitude polyphasic motor unit potentials
   - Fibrillation potentials, even at rest
   - Bizarre high-frequency repetitive discharges
5. Characteristic rashes of dermatomyositis
   - Heliotrope rash—a lilac discoloration of the eyelids and periorbital area
   - Gottron's papules—scaly erythematous eruptions over the metacarpophalangeal and interphalangeal joints, or over other extensor surfaces (knees, elbows, and medial malleoli)
   - Gottron's sign—erythema in the distribution of Gottron's papules but without papules

[a]In patients in whom all known causes of myopathy have been excluded.
Definite IIM = 4 of the above criteria 1–4; or 4 of the above (including the rash) for dermatomyositis.
Probable IIM = 3 of the above criteria 1–4; or 3 of the above (including the rash) for dermatomyositis.
Possible IIM = 2 of the above criteria 1–4; or 2 of the above (including the rash) for dermatomyositis
ALT/SGPT, alanine aminotransferase/serum glutamic-pyruvic transaminase; AST/SGOT, aspartate aminotransferase/serum glutamic-oxaloacetic transaminase.
Modified from Bohan A, Peter JB. Polymyositis and dermatomyositis (parts 1 and 2). N Engl J Med 1975;292:344–347, 403–407, with permission.

TABLE 78.4. USEFUL DISCRIMINATORS FOR MYOSITIS IN CONFUSING CASES OF MYOPATHY

Features Leading Toward Myositis	Features Leading Away from Myositis
Family history of autoimmune disease	Family history of a similar syndrome as the patient's signs/symptoms
Symmetric, chronic, proximal > distal weakness*	Weakness related to exercise, eating or fasting, or of the face
Muscle atrophy after chronic symptoms	Muscle atrophy early or hypertrophy ever
Absence of neuropathy by exam or EMG/NCV*	Presence of neuropathy
Lack of fasciculations and little muscle cramping	Fasciculations or prominent muscle cramping
Gottrons*, Heliotrope*, V sign, shawl-sign rashes, linear extensor erythema, cuticular overgrowth, or vasculitis	No rash or vasculitis
Features of CTD—fevers, arthritis, ILD, Raynaud's, etc.	No CTD symptoms
CK, AST, ALT, LD, aldolase levels 2–100× normal*	Enzymes <2× normal range, or >100× normal
Positive ANA, MSA, or ENA	Negative autoantibodies
Muscle biopsy evidence of myofiber degeneration-regeneration with inflammation*, strong alkaline phosphatase staining of the interstitium	Myofiber vacuoles, ragged red fibers, parasites—neither inflammation nor alkaline phosphatase staining in the interstitium
MRI—spotty bright symmetric areas in muscle by STIR	MRI normal or only shows atrophy
Clinical response to immunosuppressives	No clinical response to immunosuppressives

*Accepted criteria for the diagnosis of idiopathic inflammatory myopathy (IIM) per Table 78.3. *CTD,* connective tissue disease; *ILD,* interstitial lung disease; *ANA,* antinuclear antibody; *MSA,* myositis-specific autoantibody; *ENA,* antibody to extractable nuclear antigens (Ro, La, RNP, etc.); *STIR,* short tau inversion repeat.

is usually adequate for a diagnosis of inclusion body myositis. Patients who meet criteria for both IIM and another connective tissue disease are considered to have an overlap syndrome associated with myositis. As discussed later, the association of cancer with myositis remains controversial (46). Yet, in view of data from population-based studies (47) and many other clinical series and anecdotes, most investigators consider a patient to have cancer-associated myositis if both diagnoses are made within 2 years of one another.

CLINICAL CHARACTERISTICS AND THEIR EVALUATION

Consideration of the primary pathologic processes operative in a disease may be useful in predicting the major clinical manifestations to be expected in a given disorder. In the myositis syndromes, inflammation and the subsequent death of muscle cells are hallmarks of the disorders and will delimit the expected clinical manifestations. Because IIMs are systemic connective tissue diseases, however, other organ systems can be involved with inflammation or other pathologic processes (Table 78.5). Additionally, secondary events that result from the inflammation or its therapy, including regeneration and atrophy of myocytes, the replacement of muscle and other affected tissues by fibrous tissue and fat, and immunosuppression and secondary infections, can each alter the course of the disease.

Skeletal Muscle Involvement

Most patients present with acute or subacute onset of proximal weakness. This is usually manifested by complaints of hip muscle weakness, which may include increasing difficulty getting up from a chair or out of a car, or climbing stairs. The shoulder muscles often become symptomatic later, resulting in difficulty combing or styling the hair, putting on heavy clothing, or retrieving objects from high shelves. Because misdiagnosis is common in IIM, patients with poor responses to therapy should be carefully reevaluated for alternate diagnoses, such as dystrophies or metabolic myopathies, which would not respond well to immunosuppressive treatment. The physical examination should complement the history in defining the extent of involvement of disease and ruling out cancer, infection, or other effects of myositis or of immunosuppression, that may complicate the course and treatment. Special attention should be focused on the evaluation of muscle strength using standard manual muscle strength testing, noting how a patient rises from a squatting or sitting position, how rapidly the patient is able to dress or undress, walk times, and noting what the patient can and cannot do compared to a previous time point (48). A simple questionnaire about activities of daily living that can be easily scored is often useful in this regard (49).

TABLE 78.5. SYSTEMIC MANIFESTATIONS OF THE IDIOPATHIC INFLAMMATORY MYOPATHIES

General
- Fatigue
- Fevers
- Weight loss
- Voice changes—nasal speech, hoarseness
- Raynaud's phenomenon and other vasomotor instability

Musculoskeletal system
- Muscle weakness-proximal > distal, upper and lower limbs, neck muscles, rare facial weakness
- Unexpected falling
- Myalgia
- Muscle tenderness
- Muscle atrophy
- Contractures
- Arthralgias
- Arthritis
- Deforming arthropathy*

Respiratory system
- Dyspnea at rest and on exertion
- Dry cough
- Wheezing/rales/rhonchi
- Atelectasis
- Interstitial lung disease
- Pneumonia secondary to immunosuppression and poor clearing of secretions
- Pneumothorax*
- Pneumomediastinum*
- Cricopharyngeal obstruction*

Cardiac system
- Myocarditis
- Arrhythmias
- Congestive failure
- Pericarditis*

Gastrointestinal system
- Dysarthria—poor tongue propulsions
- Dysphagia—upper and lower esophagus
- Odynophagia
- Nasal regurgitation
- Reflux esophagitis
- Poorly coordinated peristalsis
- Constipation/diarrhea
- Ulcerations (particularly in juvenile dermatomyositis)
- Pneumatosis intestinalis*

Skin
- Dermatomyositis-specific rashes—Gottron's papules, Gottron's sign, heliotrope
  - Less specific rashes—diffuse rashes, erythroderma, V sign, shawl sign, mechanic's hands, linear extensor erythema, acrosclerosis
  - Poikiloderma vasculare atrophicans
  - Photosensitivity
- Mucin deposition
- Panniculitis
- Scleredema
- Calcifications
- Vasculitis and ulceration
- Periungual capillary changes
- Cuticular overgrowth
- Alopecia*
- Purpura*

Renal
- Membranous nephropathy*
- Insufficiency from myoglobinuria*

*Rare manifestations.

Extraskeletal Muscle Involvement

When performing the physical examination, it is important to evaluate the forms and extent of extraskeletal muscle involvement (Table 78.5). The location and nature of arthritis, skin rashes, subcutaneous tenderness, vasomotor instability, and pulmonary, cardiac, and gastrointestinal abnormalities should all be documented (Figs. 78.1 and 78.2), and consideration given to further evaluation of any positive findings by radiologic studies, electrocardiography, biopsy, or other laboratory testing (Table 78.6).

The rashes of dermatomyositis may precede, follow, or develop concurrently with muscle weakness. None of the many skin lesions that have been described in dermatomyositis patients (50,51) is pathognomonic except Gottron's papules. These are palpable lesions overlying the extensor surfaces of the hand joints, elbows, knees, or malleoli with an erythematous base (Fig. 78.1). Several other rashes are so characteristic for dermatomyositis, however, that they may be considered adequate for meeting the skin criterion for the IIM. These include the purplish discoloration around the eyes, known as the heliotrope rash (Fig. 78.1), and Gottron's sign, scaling erythema without papules in the same distribution as Gottron's papules. Other common rashes include linear extensor erythema that overlies the extensor surface of the hands beyond the usual location of Gottron's papules or sign, periungual vasculitic changes and cuticular overgrowth, photosensitive diffuse erythroderma with accentuated erythema in the V of the neck (V sign), and a drying and cracking of the skin over the lateral and palmar surfaces of the fingers, known as "mechanic's hands" (Fig. 78.1).

Pulmonary, cardiac, and gastrointestinal involvement can present in a variety of ways and have a more significant impact on morbidity and mortality than the skeletal muscle involvement itself. Dyspnea on exertion and dry cough are common symptoms usually caused by weakness of the intercostal muscles and diaphragm. Respiratory muscle weakness can result in atelectasis and pulmonary infections in myositis patients, especially after the initiation of immunosuppressive therapy. Pulmonary fibrosis, also known as interstitial lung disease, is often associated with pulmonary hypertension and is the most worrisome of the pulmonary findings because of its poor response to therapy and dismal prognosis. Pulmonary fibrosis can lead to cor pulmonale. Myocarditis is usually subclinical, but occasionally can result in cardiac failure or life-threatening intractable arrhythmias. Dysphagia is the most common gastrointestinal symptom and is caused by weakness of the tongue, oropharynx, or esophagus, disordered peristalsis, or cricopharyngeal dysfunction. Patients also complain of symptoms of reflux esophagitis, abdominal bloating, and constipation that may result from mucosal inflammation or vascular changes in the intestines.

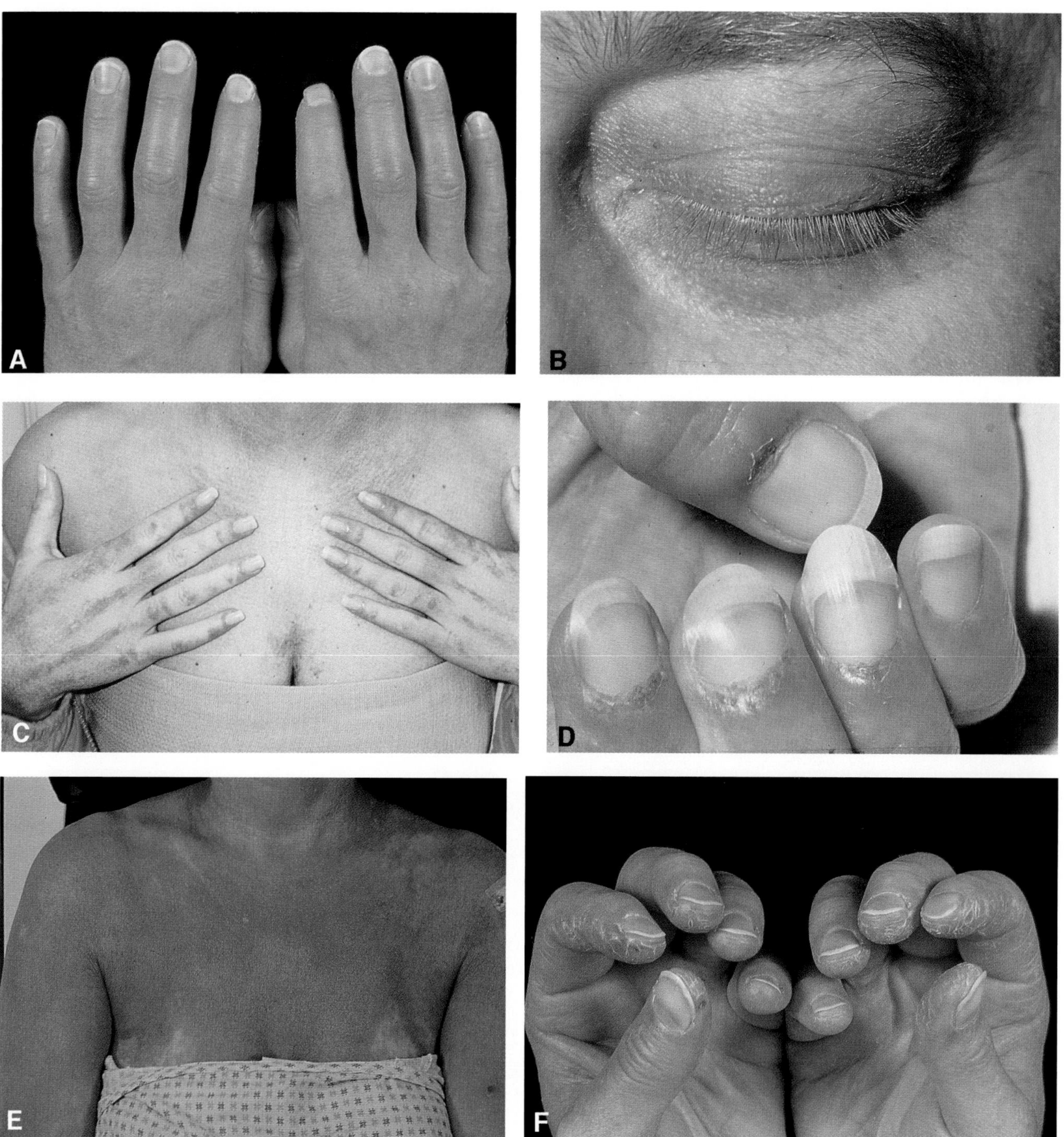

FIGURE 78.1. Skin changes seen in dermatomyositis. **A:** Gottron's papules are scaly papules overlying the extensor surfaces of the hands (over the metacarpophalangeal and proximal interphalangeal joints in this case), elbows, knees, or malleoli. This patient also has sclerodactyly and arthritis of the metacarpophalangeal and proximal interphalangeal joints. **B:** The heliotrope rash is a purplish discoloration around the eyes, especially on the upper lids. **C:** Linear extensor erythema overlies the extensor surface of the hands beyond the usual location of Gottron's papules or sign. **D:** Periungual vasculitic changes and cuticular overgrowth. **E:** Photosensitive diffuse erythroderma with accentuated erythema in the V of the neck (V sign) in a patient with cancer-associated dermatomyositis. **F:** Drying and cracking of the skin over the lateral and palmar surfaces of the fingers, known as "mechanic's hands," is seen frequently in patients with autoantibodies to aminoacyl-tRNA synthetases (the antisynthetase syndrome).

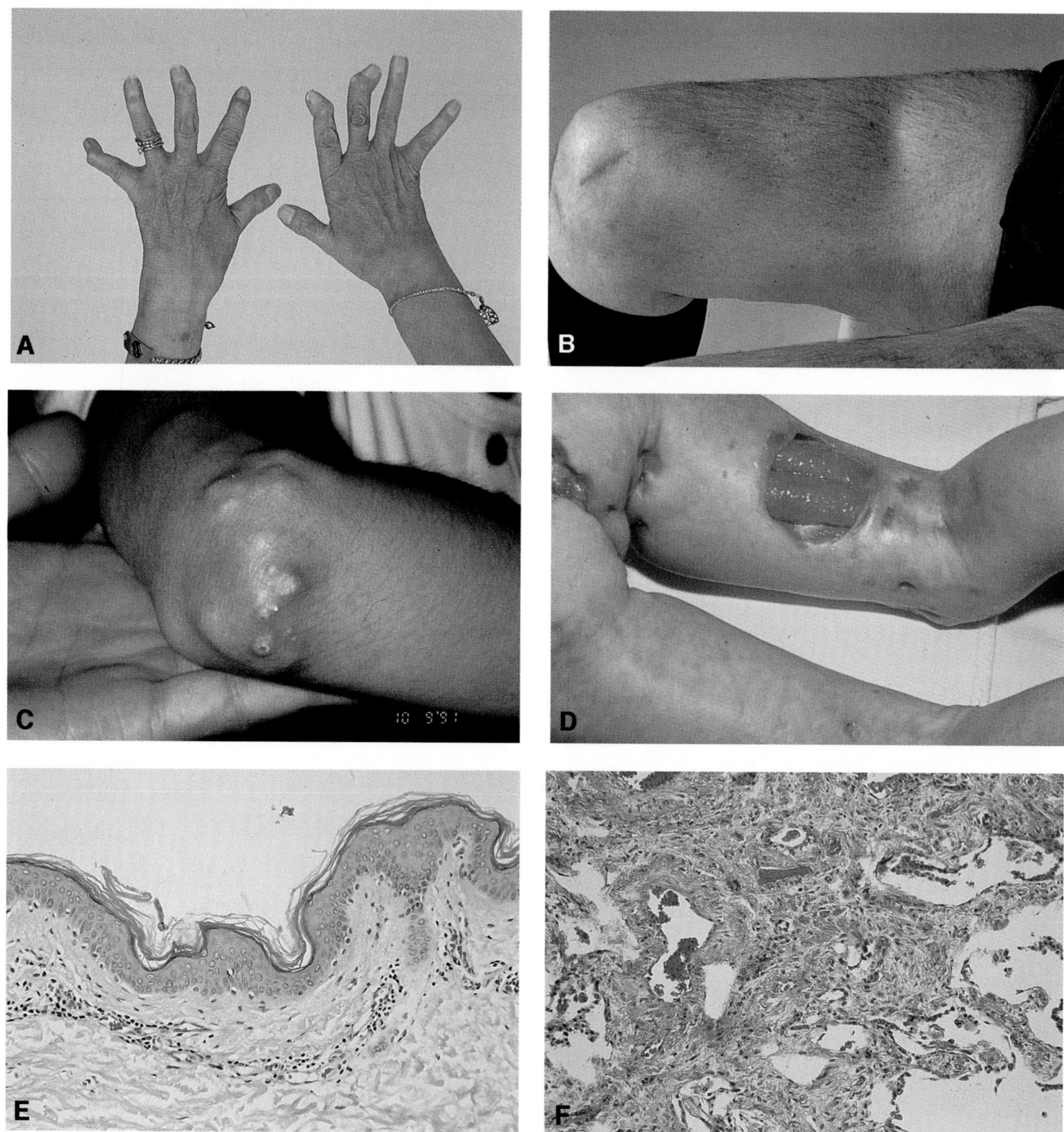

FIGURE 78.2. Manifestations of idiopathic inflammatory myopathy (IIM). **A:** A deforming arthropathy is occasionally seen in polymyositis patients as a manifestation of the antisynthetase syndrome as seen in this patient with anti–Jo-1 autoantibodies. **B:** Irregular and asymmetric muscle atrophy, often in the anterior thigh muscles, is often seen in patients with inclusion body myositis. **C:** Extensive calcifications over the elbow in a child with juvenile dermatomyositis (courtesy of Dr. Robert Rennebohm). **D:** Severe vasculitis with erosions into muscle in a patient with dermatomyositis (courtesy of Dr. Robert Rennebohm). **E:** Biopsy from affected skin demonstrating surface scaling, vacuolization, and subcutaneous perivascular mononuclear cells characteristic, but not diagnostic, of dermatomyositis [hematoxylin and eosin (H&E)stain] (courtesy of Dr. Lori A. Love). **F:** Lung biopsy from a patient with antisynthetase syndrome and interstitial lung disease demonstrating destruction of the normal architecture and extensive replacement by inflammatory cells and fibrotic tissue (H&E) (courtesy of Dr. Lori A. Love).

TABLE 78.6. LABORATORY ABNORMALITIES IN MYOSITIS PATIENTS

Laboratory Test	Comments
Muscle-associated enzymes	CK, AST, ALT, LD, aldolase—generally useful to assess the presence and degree of myositis, but may not always correlate with disease activity. May be normal in 5–10% of IIM patients at myositis onset and may become normal later despite active disease because of loss of muscle mass or circulating inhibitors of enzyme activity. Elevations may predate clinical flares of disease by weeks to months and, conversely, decreases may precede clinical responses to therapy by a similar time period. Levels also relate to muscle mass, so are higher in men compared to women and blacks compared to whites. Elevation of transaminases often result in the misdiagnosis of non-A non-B hepatitis in myositis patients.
CK MB fraction	A correlate of disease activity and a common source of misdiagnosis of myocardial infarction. Probably arises from myoblasts rather than from cardiac muscle in most myositis patients.
Creatinuria	Increased urinary exretion of creatine indicates muscle damage.
Creatinine	Decreased serum levels often reflect long-standing myositis and muscle atrophy.
Myoglobin serum/urine	May correlate with muscle strength better than muscle enzymes and may predict clinical relapse. Due to diurnal variation, myoglobin levels should be measured at the same time of day.
Heme + urine without red blood cells	Usually indicates myoglobinuria.
White blood cell and platelet counts	Elevated values sometimes seen with active myositis.
Hypergammaglobulinemia	Seen in about 10% of IIM patients in whom the level correlates with myositis activity. Elevated IgE can be seen in juvenile myositis.
Hypo- or agammaglobulinemia	A rare finding except in echovirus-associated cases of juvenile dermatomyositis.
Monoclonal gammopathy	Rare but sometimes seen in cancer-associated myositis.
IgA deficiency	Increased frequency in some series of myositis patients.
ESR	Elevated in less than half of IIM patients. Does not correlate with disease activity.
C-reactive protein	Normal in most IIM patients. Elevation often indicative of bacterial infection.
↑ Factor VIII related antigen	Elevated in active juvenile dermatomyositis and correlates with disease activity, but elevation occurs in only a subset of patients.
↑ Neopterin	Correlates with disease activity in many juvenile dermatomyositis patients.
+ ANA	Seen in 60–90% of IIM patients and a good discriminator of IIM from other forms of myopathy, in which ANAs are much less frequent. Cytoplasmic staining in a diffuse pattern suggests the presence of another autoantibody, often a myositis-specific autoantibody.
Other autoantibodies	See Table 78.7.

ANA, antinuclear autoantibody; CK, creatine kinase; ESR, erythrocyte sedimentation rate; Ig, immunoglobulin; LD, lactate dehydrogenase.
Modified from Rider LG, Miller FW. Laboratory evaluation of the inflammatory myopathies. *Clin Diag Lab Immunol* 1995;2:1–9, with permission.

LABORATORY FINDINGS

Clinical Chemistry

The laboratory plays an important role in evaluating IIM (52,53), and many abnormalities may be detected in routine screening blood tests (Table 78.6). One of the primary laboratory clues to a myopathy is the presence in the serum of elevated levels of enzymes originating from the cytoplasm of the muscle cell (sarcoplasm). The most frequently measured enzyme in this regard is CK due to its high sensitivity, muscle specificity, and relatively good correlation with disease activity and muscle strength. Nonetheless, in IIM patients lactate dehydrogenase, serum glutamic-oxaloacetic transaminase (SGOT)/aspartate aminotransferase, serum glutamic-pyruvic transaminase (SGPT)/alanine aminotransferase, and aldolase serum levels all tend to correlate with CK levels, but their elevations occur less frequently and to a lesser extent than CK (52). Unfortunately, elevated serum transaminase levels without a CK determination in myositis patients may be mistakenly attributed to hepatic disease and lead to an inappropriate liver biopsy.

At the onset of illness, serum CK levels may be elevated as much as 10 to 100 times the upper limit of normal. CK levels are elevated in over 95% of adult patients with myositis at presentation or during the course of disease, making it the most frequently elevated sarcoplasmic enzyme in the serum of myositis patients. The serum levels of CK and other muscle-derived enzymes are generally useful in following myositis activity and responses to therapy, although the magnitude of elevation does not always correlate with global disease activity, especially in children. Therefore, CK levels alone can never substitute for a thorough evaluation of the patient, which includes functional assessment. The lack of correlation of CK levels with disease activity is partly due to the 3- to 8-week delay between normalization of CK and improvement in muscle strength, and the 5- to 6-week lag between elevation of CKs and clinical relapse (54). Enzyme levels also do not reflect the degree of pulmonary, gastrointestinal, articular, and other nonmuscular involvement in IIM.

The presence of a normal CK level in the face of active disease, demonstrated by muscle weakness and accompanied by inflammation on muscle biopsy or MRI, may be related to suppression of CK by corticosteroids, the presence of serum inhibitors of CK enzyme activity (55), or the presence of extensive muscle atrophy due to chronic disease. Because muscle mass is the major determinant of CK values in normal resting subjects, men tend to have higher baseline levels than women, and African Americans higher CK levels than Hispanics, who in turn have higher levels than Caucasians (56). Also, patients with systemic lupus erythematosus (SLE), rheumatoid arthritis (RA), and other connective tissue diseases tend to have abnormally low CK levels (52); thus, a normal CK level in these patients may indicate active myositis. For all these reasons, the serum CK level needs to be interpreted in the context of prior levels in an individual patient, and serial levels should ideally be performed in a single laboratory using the same assay. In the majority of patients, most of the elevation of serum CK levels is due to increases in the MM isoenzyme fraction, which is released from skeletal muscle. Elevation of the MB isoenzyme, found primarily in myocardium, may also occur not only as a result of myocarditis but also as an indicator of skeletal muscle regeneration (52).

A problem that physicians often encounter after initiating corticosteroid therapy in myositis patients is deciding the relative contribution of steroid myopathy versus active myositis to the patient's weakness. One clue to steroid myopathy is the presence of an elevated urinary creatine excretion with simultaneously normal serum muscle enzymes (52).

Abnormalities of nonspecific markers of inflammation, such as leukocytosis, elevated platelet counts, C-reactive protein (CRP), and erythrocyte sedimentation rate (ESR), may be found in myositis patients. These are generally not useful in assessing myositis activity, but usually reflect coexisting processes in IIM patients. The 24-hour urinary creatine excretion, which reflects muscle mass and damage, is elevated in most patients with muscle diseases. In fact, creatinuria may be a more sensitive indicator of active myositis than serum CK (52). Abnormally low serum creatinine levels may be the result of loss of muscle mass and should alert one to the presence of chronic myositis.

Immunology

Immunologic abnormalities are sometimes the first clue that a patient has IIM and can be helpful in making the diagnosis in difficult or atypical cases. The most frequent abnormalities are hypergammaglobulinemia or the presence of an autoantibody. Antinuclear autoantibodies (ANAs) are the most common autoantibodies seen in IIM. The ANA usually displays a speckled pattern, although any other pattern can also be present. Other immune abnormalities, however, may also be present including hypogammaglobulinemia, hypergammaglobulinemia, monoclonal gammopathy, cryoglobulinemia, and a variety of autoantibodies, some of which are specific for myositis (Tables 78.6 and 78.7).

Electromyography and Other Tests

Electromyography (EMG) and nerve conduction velocity (NCV) measurements are often performed to distinguish neuropathies from myopathies. They also can add to the probability that the patient has an inflammatory myopathy when characteristic abnormalities are present (Table 78.3). As mentioned earlier, radiographs, electrocardiograms, and other laboratory studies should be performed based on the nature and severity of the symptoms and findings, and concern for the presence of cancer, which may be associated with IIM, particularly in older persons with dermatomyositis.

Current research techniques for assessment of myositis activity that seem promising for the future include measurement of serum levels of myosin light chains (57), cellular markers of inflammation such as soluble (s) interleukin-2 receptors (sIL-2R), sCD4, and sCD8 (58,59), IL-1a, IL-2 (59–61), and IL-1 receptor antagonist (60).

Muscle Biopsy

Although physicians may be reluctant to perform a muscle biopsy in what would appear to be straightforward cases of myositis, a biopsy should be included early in the evaluation of most patients. Muscle biopsy may reveal an unexpected disease, sometimes with important therapeutic, prognostic, or reproductive implications (Fig. 78.3E,F). In the author's experience, dystrophies, metabolic abnormalities, amyloidosis, neuropathic features, toxic changes, unusual cellular infiltrates, and inclusion body myositis have each been diagnosed by muscle biopsy in otherwise "typical" polymyositis patients. Nonetheless, a muscle biopsy may not always be diagnostic. Inflammation in typical myositis may be missed because of its spotty nature or as a result of therapy. Conversely, muscle inflammation can be present in some dystrophies, especially fascioscapulohumeral dystrophy, and toxic myopathies. Inclusions are not always present in the first biopsy in what appears clinically as inclusion body myositis.

To optimize the yield from the muscle biopsy, it is important to choose a weak, but not atrophied, muscle that has not undergone recent injections, electromyogram (EMG) evaluation, or other trauma that may cause artifacts. The discovery that MRI can detect muscle inflammation and damage may improve the yield of biopsy diag-

TABLE 78.7. A SEROLOGIC CLASSIFICATION OF THE INFLAMMATORY MYOPATHIES

Serologic Category	Associations and Comments
Myositis-specific autoantibodies[a]	
Antisynthetase[b]	High frequency of symmetric nonerosive arthritis, interstitial lung disease, fever, mechanic's hands, Raynaud's phenomenon; often occurs as an acute, severe myositis with onset in the spring, moderate response to therapy, myositis flare with tapering of therapy; seen in 20–25% of all myositis cases
Antisignal recognition particle	Cardiac involvement with frequent palpitations and myalgias; very acute onset of severe polymyositis in the fall; most often in black women; poor response to therapy; seen in <5% of myositis patients
Anti-Mi-2	Classic dermatomyositis with V sign, shawl sign, and cuticular overgrowth; good response to therapy; seen in 5–10% of myositis patients
Anti-Mas[c]	Polymyositis following alcoholic rhabdomyolysis
Anti-Fer[c]	Seen in <1% of myositis patients
Anti-KJ[c]	Polymyositis interstitial lung disease, Raynaud's phenomenon
None of the above (MSA negative)	A heterogeneous group of patients
Myositis-associated autoantibodies[b]	
Anti-PM-Scl	Scleroderma/myositis overlap syndromes
Anti-Ku[c]	Scleroderma/myositis overlap syndromes
Anti-U1RNP[c]	Myositis overlap syndromes
Ani-U2RNP[c]	Scleroderma/myositis overlap syndromes
Anti-U5RNP[c]	Myositis overlap syndromes

[a]Myositis-specific autoantibodies are only seen in myositis patients; myositis-associated autoantibodies are seen in myositis patients and those with other autoimmune disorders.
[b]Includes patients with anti-Jo-1 autoantibodies (directed against histidyl-tRNA synthetase) and those with autoantibodies to threoryl-(PL-7), alanyl-(PL-12), isoleucyl-(OJ), and glycyl-(EJ) tRNA synthetases.
[c]Possibly distinct entities for which less substantiating data exist than do for the other categories.
Modified from Miller FW. Classification and prognosis of inflammatory muscle disease. *Rheum Dis Clin North Am* 1994;20:811–826, with permission.

nosis by directing the site of biopsy. The muscle biopsy should be collected and processed for histochemistry by experienced persons using special stains to rule out many of the forms of myopathy previously listed. The pathologic findings of myositis are seen best in hematoxylin and eosin– and Masson trichrome–stained cross sections of muscle snap frozen by immersion into isopentane cooled by liquid nitrogen. Figure 78.3A–D illustrates some of the typical findings on muscle biopsy of IIM. When a muscle cell dies for any reason, a secondary inflammatory process may occur. What distinguishes IIM, however, is that the inflammation is primary and chronic. Chronic inflammatory cells, mononuclear cells that are predominantly lymphocytes, may be found not only in direct relation to a dying cell (endomysial), but between unaffected cells and fascicles (perimysial), or in the adjacent interstitial tissue. Most importantly for the diagnosis of a primary inflammatory myopathy, lymphocytes may be found around or within normal-appearing cells. Patients with polymyositis tend to have more inflammatory cells in endomysial locations, whereas those with dermatomyositis have more perivascular and perimysial inflammation. Predominance of neutrophils or perineural inflammation usually points to a process other than IIM, whereas predominant plasma cells, eosinophils, or granulomata in an otherwise typical myositis suggest the type of IIM present (Fig. 78.3F).

In addition to the types of cells found in the biopsy, vacuoles, inclusions, and other tinctorial properties of individual myocytes with certain stains help distinguish myositis from other entities (62). Irregular red-rimmed inclusions on the Masson's trichrome stain can identify the most common form of IIM in persons over 50 years of age—inclusion body myositis (Fig. 78.3C). Strong activity of the alkaline phosphatase stain in the interstitium suggests an IIM even if inflammation is not prominent (Fig. 78.3D). The finding of prominent glycogen [by periodic acid-Schiff (PAS) stain], fat (by oil red O stain), abnormal mitochondria (the ragged red fiber on hematoxylin and eosin stain), or other inclusions should suggest not IIM but rather other syndromes that can mimic myositis. Small angulated cells are more commonly seen in neurogenic disorders. In myopathy secondary to nerve damage, the abnormal fibers are often grouped together. When the damage or atrophy of myofibers is most severe around the edge of the fascicle (perifascicular), it may be a reflection of a primary vascular process located in connective tissue. Vascular pathology and perifascicular atrophy are most prominent in dermatomyositis, suggesting that the primary pathology is a vasculopathy (Fig. 78.3B).

Electron microscopy is rarely necessary for assessing patients with clinical myositis. One possible exception is the evaluation of suspected inclusion body myositis when the characteristic rimmed vacuoles are not present by

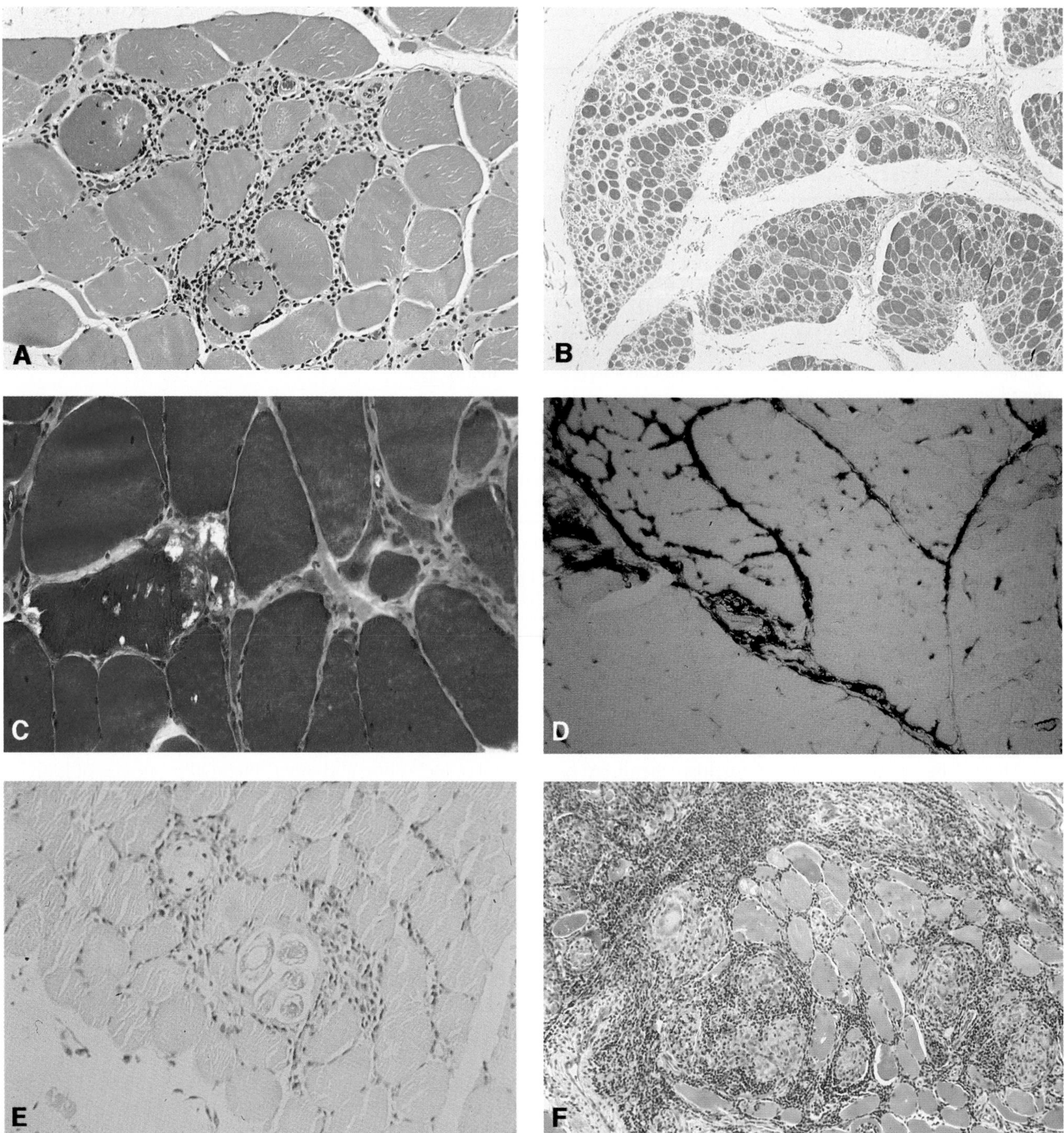

FIGURE 78.3. Histopathology of inflammatory myopathies. **A,B:** Muscle biopsies from polymyositis patients tend to show focal endomysial infiltration by mononuclear cells (A: H&E), while those from dermatomyositis patients show more perivascular and interstitial inflammation with perifascicular myofiber atrophy (**B:** modified trichrome stain). **C:** Transverse fresh-frozen section of muscle from a patient with inclusion body myositis displaying purplish granular material lining the multiple vacuoles in several myofibers and the presence of angulated myofibers (modified trichrome stain). **D:** Strong alkaline phosphatase staining of the interstitium is common in the IIM and can help distinguish this condition from other myopathies even in the absence of inflammation. **E:** Trichinosis parasites in a myofiber surrounded by mononuclear inflammatory cells in a patient originally misdiagnosed with polymyositis (courtesy Dr. Lori A. Love). **F:** Intensely inflammatory granulomatous myositis is characterized by the presence of granulomata and endomysial inflammation in this patient with sarcoidosis (H&E).

light microscopic evaluation. In such cases, the presence of typical nuclear or cytoplasmic microtubular filaments can be useful in making a diagnosis (44). Special stains, enzyme assays, and molecular genetic testing for metabolic and dystrophic conditions are available in referral centers and are sometimes essential to avoid the mistake of treating a noninflammatory disease with immunosuppressive drugs.

Imaging Studies

Routine radiographic studies are useful in screening for and assessing gastrointestinal, cardiac, and pulmonary disease; erosive arthropathy; or calcifications (Fig. 78.4). There is increasing interest in using computed tomography (CT), ultrasound, MRI, and a related technique called magnetic resonance spectroscopy (MRS) to assess muscle disease because these techniques are noninvasive and can sample larger volumes of muscle than EMG and muscle biopsy. Most investigators agree that MRI is superior to CT or ultrasound scanning because it provides additional information about inflammation (Fig. 78.5). Studies suggest that a combination of the T1-weighted image and the STIR (short tau inversion repeat) or other fat-suppressed image provides the best overall assessment of muscle disease in IIM patients (37,63,64). Multiple cross sections of the thighs are the most useful views in the majority of patients, but the location to be evaluated should depend on the signs and symptoms of the individual. T1-weighted MRI best evaluates the anatomy and degree of atrophy and fatty replacement of muscle, and thus gives the best assessment of disease damage due to chronicity of the disease. STIR-MRI is a fat-suppressed image suitable for assessing the degree of inflammation, and thus the current activity of the disease. Despite the expense of MRI, it may be a cost-effective adjunct for diagnosing and assessing selected patients (65). The newer and less available modality of MRS evaluates the levels of different high-energy phosphates in muscle. These are abnormal in the IIM and other myopathies and this technique should provide more sensitive means of assessing myopathies in the future (66,67). A potential confounder in these analyses is that active exercise can cause muscle changes that result in transient elevations in serum CK levels (68) and inflammatory changes on MRI (69,70). Therefore, patients should avoid vigorous exercise and rest for at least an hour prior to these studies (71).

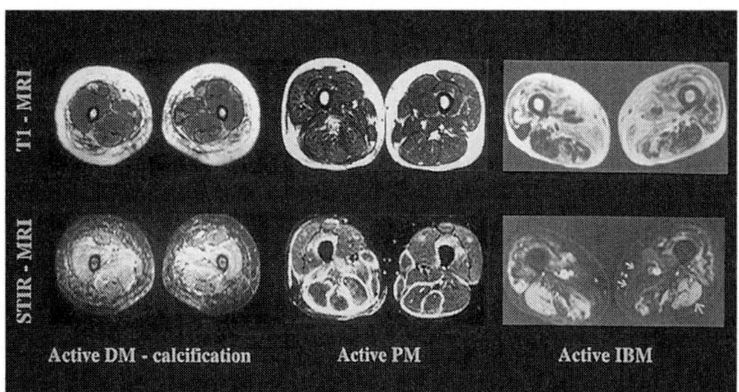

FIGURE 78.5. Magnetic resonance imaging (MRI) of the thighs is a useful modality to quantitate and distinguish IIM disease activity (muscle inflammation) from disease damage (muscle atrophy and fibrosis). The MRIs from three patients with both disease activity and damage are shown: dermatomyositis with subcutaneous calcifications (which appear black) on the left, polymyositis in the middle, and inclusion body myositis on the right. The T1-weighted MRIs (**top**) define anatomic details and show disease damage represented by severe muscle atrophy and replacement of muscle by fat. The STIR (short tau inversion recovery) MRIs (**bottom**) help quantitate inflammation demonstrated by bright areas in muscle (active myositis), subcutaneous tissue (panniculitis), and skin (active dermatitis). (Courtesy of Dr. Elizabeth Adams.)

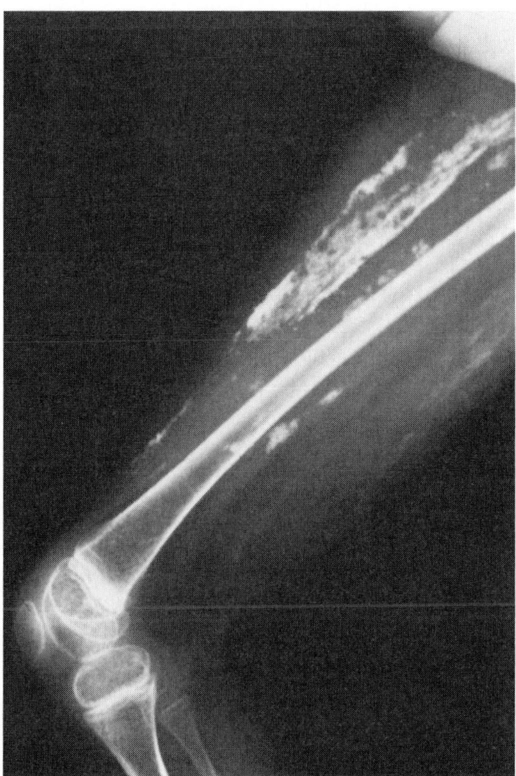

FIGURE 78.4. Subcutaneous and perimuscular calcifications in a patient with juvenile dermatomyositis.

CLASSIFICATION

A number of classification schemes have been proposed for IIM as our understanding of these conditions has evolved (72,73). Although the simplest differentiation of these syndromes is into polymyositis, dermatomyositis, and inclusion body myositis (74), this classification approach

TABLE 78.8. A CLINICOPATHOLOGIC CLASSIFICATION OF THE INFLAMMATORY MYOPATHIES[a]

Clinicopathologic Category	Associations and Comments
Primary idiopathic polymyositis	A diagnosis of exclusion—defined by the absence of all below[b]
Primary Idiopathic dermatomyositis	Heliotrope rash, Gottron's papules or sign is present, but other rashes may coexist; myositis may be clinically silent (dermatomyositis sine myositis)
Myositis associated with another connective tissue disease	Mild myositis, good response to therapy; rheumatoid arthritis, systemic sclerosis, and systemic lupus erythematosus most common as overlaps
Juvenile myositis	More frequent calcifications and gastrointestinal vasculitis than seen in adults; may be more heterogeneous than previously thought
Myositis associated with malignancy	Myositis onset often within 2 years of cancer; ovarian cancer may be overrepresented
Inclusion body myositis	Occurs mainly in older white men with insidious onset and progression; poor response to therapy; rimmed inclusions in myocytes
Granulomatous myositis	Granulomas prominent and frequent in muscle biopsy; can be seen in sarcoidosis
Eosinophilic myositis	Eosinophils prominent in muscle; can be a part of hypereosinophilic syndrome or eosinophilic fasciitis
Vasculitic myositis	Vasculitis prominent in muscle; can be part of other vasculitides, including polyarteritis nodosa
Orbital or ocular myositis	Involvement of extraocular muscles only; often diagnosed by computerized tomography or magnetic resonance imaging
Focal or nodular myositis[c]	Focal involvement of one or more limbs; can progress to polymyositis, remain isolated or resolve
Myositis ossificans[c]	Occurs as a local limited phenomenon or more generalized excessive proliferation of connective tissue and replacement by bone

[a]Categories are not mutually exclusive.
[b]In a patient meeting criteria for definite or probable myositis (18).
[c]Possibly distinct entities for which less substantiating data exist than do for the other categories.
Modified from Miller FW. Classification and prognosis of inflammatory muscle disease. *Rheum Dis Clin North Am* 1994;20:811–826, with permission.

does not capture all the useful information that divisions into the more specific clinicopathologic and serologic groups can generate (75). Nonetheless, classification is one of the more controversial areas in the study of myositis today and all schemes suffer from deficiencies. More rational ways of distinguishing these increasingly recognized syndromes are needed to facilitate understanding of pathogenic processes and causes. Additionally, newer approaches, integrating genetics and environmental exposure histories, may be necessary to create even more homogeneous and understandable groups of patients. Two major classification systems have proved the most useful to date in terms of research and patient care: serologic (Fig. 78.6, Table 78.7) and clinicopathologic (Fig. 78.6, Table 78.8) divisions.

Clinicopathologic Groups

Primary idiopathic polymyositis differs from primary idiopathic dermatomyositis in adults in clinical presentation (25), histopathology (1,26), the number and distribution of both circulating and muscle-infiltrating CD4+ and CD8+ T cells and B cells (76–78), and responses to therapy (79). Some physicians believe that a distinct entity known as dermatomyositis without myositis (dermatomyositis sine myositis) exists (80–82); however, it remains unclear whether this is a separate entity or simply at one end of a continuum in myositis severity. Factors contributing to this dilemma include lag time (as much as a decade) between the development of the rash and muscle involvement in dermatomyositis, the relatively mild muscle weakness and lower serum CK levels in dermatomyositis, and the understandable reluctance of physicians to perform muscle biopsy or electromyography to confirm muscle disease in a patient without clinical evidence of weakness. MRI and spectroscopy (64), as well as histopathologic studies (83), suggest that there are abnormalities in the muscles of some patients who exhibit typical dermatomyositis rash but do not have clinical evidence of muscle weakness.

Overlap myositis syndromes refer to the occurrence of myositis in association with criteria for other connective tissue diseases such as systemic sclerosis, RA, SLE, or Sjögren's syndrome. These overlap diseases tend to be characterized by a higher frequency of Raynaud's; myalgias; arthritis (25); higher frequencies and titers of ANAs; anti-Ro, anti-La, and anti-U1 ribonucleoprotein (RNP) autoantibodies (25); possible histopathologic differences (62); and less severe myositis with a better response to therapy (79,84), compared to other forms of myositis.

Juvenile myositis, or myositis in children, is being recognized as an increasingly heterogeneous group of disorders, and it may be that there are fewer differences from the adult forms of myositis than previously believed (85–88). Polymyositis, dermatomyositis, cancer-associated myositis, overlap myositis, focal myositis, and even inclusion body myositis have all been diagnosed in children. The same serologic groups are also seen in children as adults, and both groups appear to have similar genetic risk factors (88). For these reasons, the author prefers not to consider the myositis that develops in children as a separate category. Nonetheless, juvenile dermatomyositis patients seem to have more frequent vasculitic complications and soft tissue calcifications (Figs. 78.2 and 78.4), and a better response to therapy than that seen in most adult myositis patients (89).

Cases of myositis developing in association with malignancy, responding to simple resection of the cancer, and returning to herald the recurrence of the cancer have anecdotally supported a cancer-associated form of myositis. While this has been a controversial area, there appears to be an increased risk of a variety of cancers with certain forms of IIM. A population survey has demonstrated a significantly increased risk of cancer in patients with either polymyositis or dermatomyositis, with most, but not all cancers, developing within 2 years of the onset of myositis (90). Cancer-associated myositis patients have fewer serologic abnormalities and a poorer prognosis compared to other myositis patients (25). While many forms of cancer have been associated with myositis in case series, and the distribution is similar to that observed in the general population, it may be that gastric and ovarian cancers are over-represented (90–94).

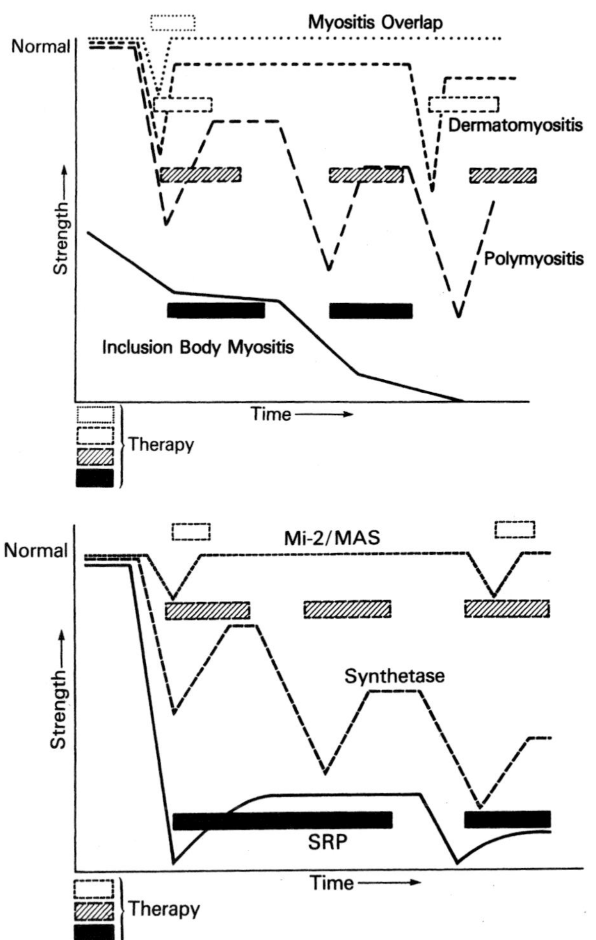

FIGURE 78.6. Generalized myositis courses differ in different IIM clinical (**top**) and serologic (**bottom**) subgroups.

The association of myositis with cancer in population studies raises the difficult question of how to address cancer screening in the individual IIM patient. A careful history, physical examination, and routine laboratory screening, with rigorous follow-up of any abnormalities suspicious of cancer, is preferable to a nondirected series of radiologic or invasive studies (1). Increased vigilance for cancer is warranted in myositis patients over 50 years old, in those with other risk factors for cancer, in IIM patients without autoantibodies, and those with severe or unresponsive skin rashes, erythroderma, or vasculitis (95). Because of the heightened concern about ovarian cancer, the author believes that most women with dermatomyositis, including those with normal pelvic examinations and pap smears, should undergo testing with CA-125 or ovarian CT/MRI evaluations.

Yunis and Samaha (23) were the first to apply the term *inclusion body myositis* to a myopathy that resembled polymyositis but could be distinguished on muscle biopsy by the appearance of cytoplasmic inclusions. Following publication of several hundred such cases, it is becoming clear that inclusion body myositis is perhaps the most underdiagnosed form of IIM. The inclusion body myopathy syndromes consist of two major groups of disorders: (a) inflammatory conditions in which activated lymphocytes infiltrating normal muscle are seen in muscle biopsies, making these entities a form of IIM (these are referred to as the inclusion body myositis syndromes); and (b) noninflammatory disorders (the noninflammatory inclusion body myopathy syndromes). Both the inflammatory and noninflammatory forms can be either sporadic or familial. A continuing confusion in the field relates to the unfortunate use by many workers in this area of a similar abbreviation—IBM—to represent both types of these disorders.

Recent progress has been made in identifying a number of proteins in vacuolated muscle fibers of inclusion body myopathy patients including ubiquitin, β-amyloid precursor protein, prion protein, presinilin 1, and phosphorylated tau (96). These are particularly of interest because these proteins that accumulate in the muscle of both the hereditary and sporadic forms of inclusion body myopathy are identical to those that accumulate in the brain of both the hereditary and sporadic forms of Alzheimer's disease. Because inclusion body myopathy and Alzheimer's disease also share slowly progressive target organ damage that mainly affects older individuals, it is tempting to speculate that a similar process is at work in both of these increasingly recognized and costly diseases. Unfortunately, it is still unclear if these findings represent primary or secondary events in disease pathogenesis. Nevertheless, the use of a variety of immunohistochemical and ultrastructural methods facilitates making more definitive diagnoses regarding IBM and assists in separating these entities from other clinically similar myopathies. Inclusion body myositis differs clinically, pathologically, serologically, and prognostically from all the other forms of IIM (44,97). When an elderly white man presents with a slowly progressive, often asymmetric proximal and distal weakness, unexpected falling, quadriceps atrophy, few serologic abnormalities or extraskeletal manifestations, serum CK levels less than 12-fold the upper limits of normal, and a poor response to corticosteroids, the diagnosis of inclusion body myositis should be strongly considered (25).

Eosinophilic, granulomatous, and vasculitic myositis have distinctive muscle pathology features (26,98); however, because they are extremely rare, little is known about them. Another unusual inflammatory myopathy is termed ocular or orbital myositis and involves chronic inflammation of structures within the orbit. Individuals with this form of IIM usually present with unilateral periorbital pain that is often made worse with eye movement, as well as proptosis, diplopia, and swelling of the eyelid (99–101). The diagnosis is often made by orbital ultrasonography, high-resolution CT, or MRI (102); evidence of inflammation of the extraocular muscles or surrounding tissues is readily apparent in most symptomatic patients. To make the diagnosis, Graves' disease should be excluded by appropriate laboratory and radiologic studies (103).

Syndromes defined by local areas of pain, swelling, or weakness, but which on biopsy show the typical features of IIM, have been variously called focal, nodular, or focal nodular myositis (104,105). Although trauma has been implicated in some of these cases, in other cases there has been no evidence of trauma. It is likely that these disorders represent a number of diseases with heterogeneous etiologies and pathogeneses inasmuch as they can either progress to systemic polymyositis, remain chronically focal, or spontaneously resolve. MRI is a particularly useful modality for the diagnosis and follow-up evaluation of these conditions (106).

Serologic Groups

The past decade has seen an explosion of immunologic studies that has redefined our thinking about IIM. This is largely the result of identifying particular autoantibodies only in myositis patients, the myositis-specific autoantibodies (MSAs), which define relatively homogeneous groups of patients with similar signs and symptoms, immunogenetics, disease course, and prognoses. Other autoantibodies that are frequently, but not exclusively, found in myositis patients, the myositis-associated autoantibodies, have also been identified recently. Thus, a new serologic classification of the inflammatory myopathies using the myositis-specific and myositis-associated autoantibodies has been proposed (Table 78.7).

The more common MSAs—the antisynthetase, anti–signal recognition particle (SRP), and anti–Mi-2 autoantibodies—each appear to define a syndrome sufficiently different from the others in epidemiology, clinical features, severity of myositis, immunogenetics, responses to therapy, and prognosis as to be considered a distinct disorder (2,25,35,107). Dividing IIMs into serologic groups may also prove useful in investigative approaches to the etiologies and pathogeneses of these syndromes. Many of the assays for the MSAs are still research procedures only available in a few centers. Currently, only anti–Jo-1 autoantibody testing by Ouchterlony double-immunodiffusion or enzyme-linked immunosorbent assay (ELISA) is widely available, although an increasing number of other MSA assays are becoming available through commercial laboratories. These assays, however, may not be as sensitive or specific as the immunoprecipitation and enzyme inhibition techniques that originally defined these specificities (108,109). The cloning and expression of the genes for the autoantigens targeted by these autoantibodies (110,111), and further identification of their epitopes (112–114), should allow testing for these autoantibodies to become standardized and routine in the future.

A number of autoantibodies, found both in myositis patients and those without myositis appear to have clinical and immunogenetic associations. These so-called myositis-associated autoantibodies are usually seen in myositis-overlap patients. The most common of this group of autoantibodies are the anti–PM-Scl autoantibodies. They have been associated with scleroderma-myositis overlap syndromes, human leukocyte antigens HLA-DR3 and HLA-DQw2, and a good response to therapy (115–118). Anti-Ku autoantibodies also have been associated with myositis-scleroderma overlap syndromes and are found in patients with primary pulmonary hypertension (119).

EPIDEMIOLOGY AND POSSIBLE ETIOLOGIES

Epidemiology

The syndromes collectively designated as IIM have probably existed for well over 100 years, are now found worldwide, and affect every race. They are, however, among the least common systemic connective tissue disorders, with annual incidences estimated in the United States at 5 to 10 cases per million adults and 0.6 to 3.2 cases per million children per year (2). Yet this is an increasingly recognized group of diseases with a nearly twofold increased incidence recorded during the last several decades (120). Factors that are known to slightly increase risk for the development of IIM include race, gender, and immunogenetics. For example, the incidence ratio of blacks to whites is about 2–4:1. The female to male incidence is about 2:1 in children, but rises to 5:1 during the childbearing years in the United States (120). Alterations in sex hormone levels, including pregnancy itself, may be risk factors for the development of myositis (121–129). Although the disease can be acquired at any age, there is a bimodal distribution of onset with a first peak in childhood at 5 to 14 years of age and a second peak in adults between 45 to 64 years of age (130). Polymyositis appears to be more common than dermatomyositis in adults. In children, however, dermatomyositis is far more common than polymyositis by about 20:1 (2). Although the myositis syndromes occur worldwide, there is increasing evidence that the distribution of phenotypes and genotypes for IIM may differ in different regions of the world (131).

Genetic Risk Factors for Idiopathic Inflammatory Myopathy

The strongest genetic risk factor for IIM is the HLA haplotype A1-B8-DR3 (DRB1*0301)-DQA1*0501 (132–135), which also increases risk for a number of other systemic connective tissue diseases (136). Other risk factors for all the clinical forms of myositis include HLA DQA1*0501, HLA DRB1*0301 (which is linked to DQA1*0501), and other DRB1 alleles that share a common amino acid sequence motif with DRB1*0301 in the second hypervariable region (134). Each serologic group, and some environmentally triggered forms of myositis, however, appear to have different HLA risk and protective alleles that may differ among different races (25,134). Given that family members share many genes and environmental exposures, one might expect a higher incidence of myositis among family members of IIM patients. Indeed, over 30 pedigrees of familial myositis have been reported, but their rarity suggests that the development of myositis requires multiple genes and multiple environmental exposures (137,138). The strongest genetic risk factor for familial IIM is homozygosity at the DQA1 locus, a risk factor not seen in sporadic IIM. Of interest, the same clinical form of myositis was usually found within a given multiplex family (137,138).

Possible Environmental Triggers for Idiopathic Inflammatory Myopathy

Anecdotal reports of the clustering in onset of myositis cases have suggested strong environmental influences in the development of IIM. Additionally, a meta-analysis of all published pedigrees of familial myositis demonstrated that the differences in the time of onset of myositis (median 1.1 years) were significantly less than the differences in age at myositis onset (median 7.5 years) in the affected family members (137,138). These data are consistent with the hypothesis that genetically susceptible family members shared common environmental exposures within a short time frame that may have triggered IIM in that family. Animal model and patient studies have also implicated a number of infectious agents as initiators of myositis (139–147). Yet, because of the lack of evidence for persistence of viral genomes in target tissues of myositis patients (148), a growing number of noninfectious agents are being investigated as possible triggers of disease as well (Table 78.9). The latter include selected foods and dietary supplements, drugs, occupational exposures, and medical devices (149). The boundary between an idiopathic and environmentally associated myopathy is thus blurred and sometimes difficult to define. Environmentally associated disorders may be similar to idiopathic rheumatic disorders in clinical presentation, pathology, serology, and response to immunosuppressive therapy, but more often they differ from them in genetic risk factors or expression (149–151). Although there may be a temporal association between the putative environmental exposure and the myositis, the pathophysiologic mechanisms involved in the evolution of the inflammation and a cause-effect relationship with the exposure are often not clear.

A careful attribution analysis of each case of a suspected environmentally associated rheumatic disease should be conducted to assure an appropriate temporal association with the

TABLE 78.9. POSSIBLE ENVIRONMENTAL TRIGGERS FOR IIM

- Infections
  - Viruses
    - Hepatitis B
    - Hepatitis C
    - HIV
    - HTLV-1
    - Echovirus
    - Coxsackievirus
  - Parasites
    - Lyme
    - Toxoplasmosis
  - Bacteria
    - Staph/streptococcus
- Noninfectious agents
  - Drugs
    - D-penicillamine
    - Cimetidine
    - Gemfibrozil
    - Tiopronin
  - Foods
    - L-tryptophan
    - Adulterated rapeseed oil
    - Ciguatera toxin
  - Biologics
    - Human growth hormone therapy
    - Interleukin-2 therapy
    - Vaccines
  - Medical devices
    - Silicone implants
    - Collagen implants
  - Occupational exposures
    - Silica
    - Polyvinyl chloride
    - Dyes and organic solvents
  - Ultraviolet light

exposure, lack of alternative explanations, biologic plausibility, improvement in the syndrome if the agent is removed (dechallenge), and deterioration if it is clinically appropriate to reexpose the patient to the environmental agent (rechallenge). Cases of drug-associated myositis are the clearest examples of environmentally associated myositis syndromes. The prototypic example of penicillamine-induced myositis is well documented as a potentially fatal entity that can exhibit similar clinical, serologic, laboratory, and pathologic findings as idiopathic myositis (150–153). Interestingly, the immunogenetic risk factors for the development of myositis after penicillamine exposure appear to differ from those of idiopathic myositis (154,155). This example suggests that perhaps other, as yet unidentified, environmental agents may be responsible for some cases of IIM.

Etiology

While the causes of IIM are by definition unknown, evidence suggests that they likely result from one or more environmental stimuli acting on genetically susceptible individuals to induce chronic immune activation and subsequent myositis. Recent clinical (156) and molecular (157) data suggest that the same group of common genes may predispose to many different autoimmune diseases. These and other findings imply that gene-environment interactions may lead to different pathophysiologic processes that result in unique syndromes—each of which may be distinguished by a distinct matrix of signs, symptoms, or laboratory abnormalities—that all share myositis. Each of these syndromes has been referred to as an elemental disorder (138,151), and has been defined by the minimal necessary and sufficient environmental exposures and genes that result in the pathology that leads to a given sign-symptom complex (Fig. 78.7). The heterogeneity of the myositis syndromes suggests that they, like most autoimmune diseases, are composed of many elemental disorders, the definition of which could have an important impact on the treatment and possible prevention of some cases of myositis.

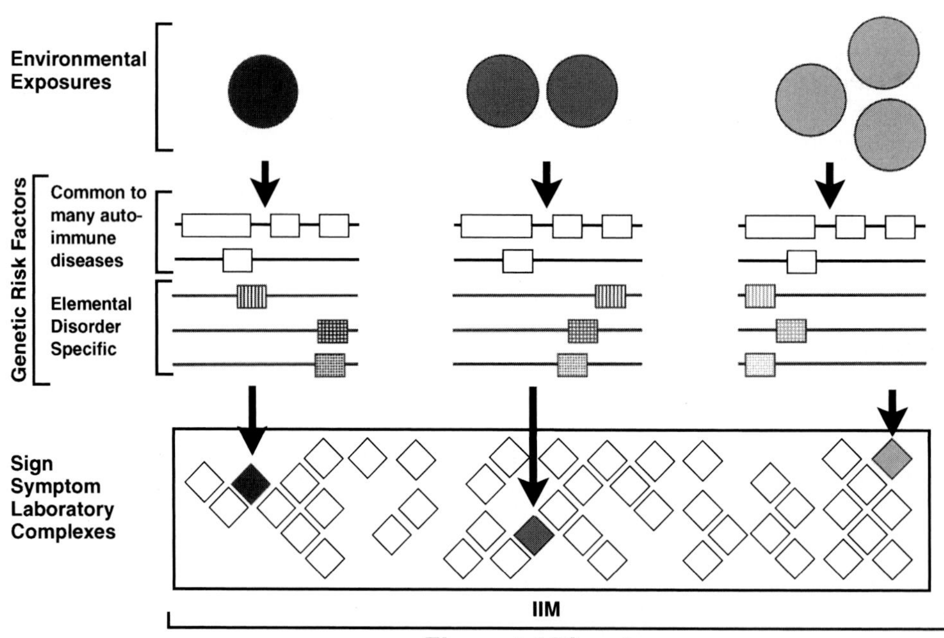

FIGURE 78.7. Possible mechanisms by which IIM subgroups (elemental disorders) may arise. The elemental disorder hypothesis posits that each autoimmune disease, as currently classified, is a heterogeneous collection of clinical signs, symptoms, and laboratory findings composed of many elemental disorders. Elemental disorders are recognized clinically by selected cardinal signs, symptoms, and laboratory findings, and are defined by the minimal necessary and sufficient environmental exposures and genes that need to be present in individuals to induce a common pathology that results in the given sign-symptom-lab complex. The environmental risk factors in this hypothetical construct could be single exposures or multiple sequential or concomitant exposures. The genetic risk factors for autoimmunity would consist of two forms: those that are common to many autoimmune diseases and those that are specific for a given elemental disorder.

PATHOGENESIS

Whatever genetic and environmental factors are responsible for the etiology of IIM syndromes and subsets, their pathogeneses center on activation of both the cellular and humoral arms of the immune system (62,158).

Cellular Immunity

Many lines of indirect evidence suggest that cellular immune activation is responsible for the pathologic effects seen in myositis (Table 78.10). Evaluation of biopsy specimens by immunologic techniques suggests a role for both cellular and humoral immune systems in muscle damage as well as differences among some of the clinical groups that may point to different pathogenic mechanisms (78,159–162). For example, in dermatomyositis, B cells are relatively abundant, especially in perivascular regions, and the late components of complement, C5–9 [the membrane attack complex (MAC)] is also found in perivascular regions and within damaged intrafascicular capillaries. Endomysial T cells are mostly activated and are cytotoxic (DR^+ and $CD8^+$) by phenotype. In the perimysial and perivascular regions, there is a higher proportion of helper ($CD4^+$) T cells (78). Furthermore, there is a decrease of intrafascicular capillaries even before myocyte or other capillary damage is evident (163).

In contrast, in both polymyositis and inclusion body myositis, individual myocytes that appear otherwise normal may be invaded by T cells of which a proportion are activated (DR^+). The dominant T cells in the inflammatory infiltrates are also $CD8^+$. In the perimysium and perivascular region, the relative proportion of helper T cells rises, but in contrast to dermatomyositis, B cells are not prominent. Natural killer (NK) cells are not abundant in either disease. Analyses of the T-cell receptors utilized by myocyte-infiltrating cells suggest that dermatomyositis patients have more polyclonal T-cell receptor patterns, while polymyositis and inclusion body myositis patients exhibit more oligoclonal T-cell receptor patterns (164,165). Additionally, there is increasing molecular evidence that the T-cell receptors expressed in muscle are restricted as a result of being antigen-driven (164,166–168). Consistent with these findings are data suggesting that the types of circulating lymphocytes also differ in different groups of IIM patients. Dermatomyositis patients have more activated B lymphocytes, whereas patients with polymyositis and inclusion body myositis have more activated T lymphocytes (77). If circulating lymphocytes are removed, radiolabeled, and returned to patients with IIM, they tend to home to mus-

TABLE 78.10. IMMUNOLOGIC ABNORMALITIES IN THE IDIOPATHIC INFLAMMATORY MYOPATHIES

Cellular abnormalities	
Activated mononuclear cells in muscle	
Restricted T-cell receptor expression in muscle	
Common motifs found in putative T-cell receptor antigen-binding regions in muscle of some clinical and serologic groups	
Altered expression of activation markers on myocytes	
Elevated levels of soluble CD8, IL-2 receptors, and cytokines in serum	
Altered peripheral mononuclear cell immunophenotypes	
Altered peripheral mononuclear cell trafficking to muscle	
Decreased autologous mixed lymphocyte and mitogenic responses	
Proliferative responses of peripheral lymphocytes to autologous muscle	
Humoral abnormalities	
Autoantibodies	
Myositis-specific	Antisynthetases [directed against histidyl-(Jo-1), alanyl-, glycyl-, threonyl-, and isoleucyl-tRNA synthetases]
	Anti-MI-2
	Antisignal recognition particle (SRP) and others
Not specific to myositis	Antinuclear antibodies
	Rheumatoid factor
	Antimuscle
	Antithyroid
	Anti-nRNP
	Anti-Ro/La
	Anti-PM-ScL
	Anti-Ku and others
Immunoglobulin and complement deposition in muscle	
Hypergammaglobulinemia, hypogammaglobulinemia, and agammaglobulinemia	
Monoclonal gammopathies	
Circulating immune complexes	

cle (169). Studies of myositis associated with graft-versus-host disease also implicate T cells as playing a role in pathogenesis of this form of myositis (170–172).

Despite these data suggesting that lymphocytes are involved in the pathogenesis of myositis, their precise role is unclear. This is partly attributable to difficulties in determining primary versus secondary immune events, and partly because the antigen or antigens driving T-cell responses remain unknown.

Humoral Immunity

Considerable evidence indicates abnormalities of the humoral arm of the immune system exist in patients with myositis (Table 78.10). Early damage and loss of capillaries in dermatomyositis prior to the development of muscle weakness suggest that a vasculopathy may be the primary event responsible for the later muscle damage. Additionally, localization of the membrane attack complex to the damaged vessels implicates a humoral immune response(s) in the process. Although IIM patients in all clinical groups may have a variety of autoantibodies, they are most common in those with an associated connective tissue disease, and least common in those with inclusion body myositis or a cancer-associated myositis. The discovery of the MSAs, however, has led to a more critical analysis of humoral autoimmunity in this clinically heterogeneous family of diseases (34,35).

The myositis-specific antibodies share a number of important and probably telling characteristics (34,132,173–175). First, they are directed at cellular components—usually proteins of a ribonucleoprotein complex—that are common to all types of cells. Second, they are directed at intracellular, usually intracytoplasmic, molecules, not cell surface molecules. Third, the target molecules (autoantigens) are usually parts of the protein synthetic machinery, and the regions of these autoantigens that autoantibodies target are conserved among species, often among quite distant species. Fourth, they are directed against the functional site of the molecule and, in all cases that have been tested, inhibit the recognized function of the molecule or particle. Finally, and of perhaps greatest importance, in the few cases studied so far, the myositis-specific antibodies appear to antedate the clinical illness, and their levels correlate with clinical or other laboratory evidence of disease activity (173,174,176,177). This implies that whatever process is responsible for the continuing production of these disease-specific autoantibodies, it is closely linked to the pathogenic mechanisms in myositis itself.

Of further importance, each of the myositis-specific antibodies is associated with a particular clinical syndrome defined by common clinical features, a predominant HLA type, a characteristic onset, response to therapy, and prognosis. Patients expressing any of these myositis-specific antibodies may therefore be referred to as having a distinct syndrome, for example the antisynthetase syndrome (176), that for practical purposes may be considered a separate disease. These strong disease correlations with each autoantibody suggest that each myositis-specific antibody syndrome results from the interaction of one or more environmental agents with a particular, individual, genetic background (Fig. 78.7). Although the genetic risk factors are becoming more clearly defined, except for seasonal and geographic associations with some of the myositis-specific antibodies (178,179) and anecdotal cases of myositis following certain environmental exposures (149), there are no hints as to what the triggering environmental agents might be.

In summary, despite intense investigation, the pathogenesis of the IIM syndromes is poorly understood. Numerous clues imply that immune-mediated events are central to the evolution of these diseases, but because immunologic characteristics vary from one group to another, different pathogenic mechanisms are likely to be operative in each syndrome. In dermatomyositis, the primary immune target appears to be the muscle blood vessel endothelium that may be damaged by humoral effector mechanisms. In polymyositis, and inclusion body myositis, however, antigen-driven cytotoxic T cells directed against antigens expressed on the myocyte surface may be the primary immune event. All the genetic, clinical, and immunologic investigations discussed above, taken together with information from the study of other autoimmune diseases, suggest that environmental agents may induce different immune responses in individuals with different genetic backgrounds and result in distinct syndromes called elemental disorders. The critical questions to be answered are: Which environmental events are triggers in which individuals? And what antigenic structures are specifically targeted in which patients?

PROGNOSIS

The idiopathic inflammatory myopathies are serious and sometimes life-threatening diseases. Survival of myositis patients has been increasing during the past few decades from 50% prior to the introduction of corticosteroid therapy (180), to 5-year survival rates of 65% in 1947–1968 (181), to approximately 80% in the 1980s (182). This improvement is probably the result of many factors, including better general medical care, earlier diagnosis, and improved treatment of the myositis syndromes. The rarity and heterogeneity of myositis has limited the collection of such data, yet a number of studies have attempted to define prognostic factors in Table 78.11.

Certain centers have reported different experiences that are difficult to reconcile. Nonetheless, studies have implied that poor prognostic factors include polymyositis as opposed to dermatomyositis (183), older age (184,185), associated malignancy or cardiac disease (186), severe weakness (185), and longer duration of weakness prior to diagnosis (185,186). It is often not clear from these studies how each

TABLE 78.11. POOR PROGNOSTIC FACTORS IN THE INFLAMMATORY MYOPATHIES

Based on demographics
African-American (versus Caucasian) race
Old (versus young)
Female (versus male) gender
Based on sign-symptom complex
Severe myositis
Dysphagia
Pulmonary involvement
Cardiac involvement
Delay to diagnosis and therapy
Normal CK
Based on clinicopathologic group
Polymyositis versus dermatomyositis
Cancer-associated myositis
Adult versus juvenile myositis
Inclusion body myositis
Based on serologic group
Antisynthetase autoantibodies
Antisignal recognition particle autoantibodies

Modified from Miller FW. Classification and prognosis of inflammatory disease. *Rheum Dis Clin North Am* 1994;20:811–826, with permission.

of these factors may have impacted the outcome of the others. More sophisticated studies, some using mortality as the outcome and multivariate analytical methods, have identified fever (187), dysphagia or aspiration (187,188), black race and female gender (189), pulmonary infiltration (181), cardiac involvement (182), delay in instituting therapy (79,190,191), failure to induce remission, leukocytosis over 10,000/mm^3, older age (187,189), the diagnosis of inclusion body myositis, or the presence of antisynthetase or antisignal recognition particle autoantibodies (79) as adversely affecting prognosis. Some of the signs and symptoms associated with a poor response to therapy, for example pulmonary or cardiac disease, may relate to the presence of the MSA syndromes, which have been shown to be indicators of a poor prognosis (79). Some serologic findings predict a more benign myositis course. These include anti–Mi-2, anti–PM-Scl, and anti-U1RNP autoantibodies (4,35).

Morbidity is more difficult to quantify than mortality and less data have been reported on this aspect of myositis. Early literature on morbidity suggested that perhaps one-third of children and nearly one-half of adults with IIM suffered significant impairment (192). Other studies have found less severe functional impairment (190); however, because there are no validated measures of disease damage and its long-term impact on patient functioning, it is difficult to assess the validity of such reports.

Limitations exist for all the studies attempting to estimate the mortality and morbidity of the inflammatory myopathies. To obtain a large enough cohort of patients for evaluation, referral populations at tertiary care centers are needed, and these are more likely to include patients with more severe disease who might be more refractory to therapy than typical myositis patients seen in the community (193). Prognostic studies are often retrospective, thereby limiting the quality of the data compared to prospective, blinded measurements of response to treatment. Specific criteria for measuring responses to treatment are often not defined, and it may be that they were not consistently applied. Despite these limitations, available studies do suggest some prognostic factors that should be confirmed and extended in more definitive future studies.

MANAGEMENT

General Considerations

Before discussing specific therapies, some general management considerations need to be reviewed. First, therapy needs to be individualized, taking into account prognostic factors, severity of disease, and risk factors for the adverse events associated with each therapeutic agent. Second, it is more difficult to assess disease severity, especially in chronic cases, than is often appreciated. This is because of the absence of generally accepted validated tools to assess and distinguish myositis disease activity (defined as inflammatory changes that may respond to immunosuppressive therapy) from disease damage (defined as irreversible changes that result from prior disease activity). Also, there are few validated tools to assess any of the extramuscular manifestations of myositis and there is a lack of a "gold standard" for disease activity. Other factors that complicate disease assessment include the lack of correlation of enzyme levels with disease activity in many subjects, the variable effects of past inflammation resulting in scarring or atrophy, and possible adverse effects of the therapies themselves (194).

Optimal therapy is based on the correct diagnosis, a physician's thorough understanding of the patient, and a patient's thorough understanding of the disease. Reassessment of the diagnosis should be a priority in evaluating atypical cases, unresponsive patients, and those developing new or unusual signs or symptoms. Patients should be counseled and educated about myositis generally and the specific manifestations they are likely to experience based on their prognostic features. The past decade has seen a shift from the traditional approach of stepped therapy—in which a structured series of first-line, second-line, and third-line agents are prescribed in rigid chronologic order as disease severity increases—to more individualized, and often more aggressive, forms of therapy that take into account the risk profile for poor prognostic outcomes. This latter integrating approach now seems more appropriate in the treatment of myositis patients.

Role of Rehabilitation

The goal of all therapy is to optimize the functional levels of patients and, if possible, to return them to normal. In this regard, physical and occupational therapy remain underutilized modalities. Graded rehabilitation that takes into account the stage and severity of the patient's myositis is the best approach (195). Although bed rest is often necessary during periods of severe disease, passive range of motion exercises and stretching should be initiated early in the course of the disease, especially in very debilitated, hospitalized patients to prevent the formation of contractures. Massage and heat treatment for painful muscles, collars, splints, or braces for support of extremely weak muscles, and assistive devices for self-care may be helpful. As the degree of myositis decreases, patients should increase their activity through stages: active-assisted range-of-motion, followed by isometric, then isotonic, and finally aerobic exercise. In our (196) and others' (197) experience, this approach has resulted not in disease flares but rather in strength and functional improvements without CK rising.

Therapeutic Approaches for Myositis

Despite nearly half a century of drug development, corticosteroids remain the primary therapy for IIM and should be initiated as early as possible in nearly all patients. Factors important in determining corticosteroid responses are an adequate initial dose (at least 1 mg/kg/day), continuation of prednisone until or after the serum CK becomes normal, and a slow rate of prednisone tapering (198). When deciding on the rate of reduction of prednisone therapy, one should take into account a number of individual prognostic features, as well as risk factors for its use. Nonetheless, in my experience, the rate of decrease most likely to minimize a flare of myositis averages about 10 mg/month or 25% of the existing dose per month, whichever is less, from the first reduction until such time that a maintenance dose is achieved. In patients with poor prognostic factors, the author usually maintains the dose of prednisone at 0.25 mg/kg every other day for periods of 6 to 12 months before further reductions in the dose. The role of pulse corticosteroids and alternate-day therapy as initial treatment remains unclear. Some investigators believe that high-dose intravenous pulse corticosteroid therapy results in more rapid responses with fewer side effects. This may be true for juvenile dermatomyositis patients, as several small uncontrolled trials have suggested (199,200). The author's experience strongly suggests that those individuals with poor prognostic factors (Table 78.11) should be considered for more aggressive therapy using corticosteroids with an added cytotoxic agent from the very beginning of their disease.

Because the clinical and serologic groups differ in the rapidity of myositis onset, severity of disease, responses to therapy, and clinical course (25,79), this information can be useful in deciding how quickly and aggressively to initiate treatment and how to alter subsequent therapy (Fig. 78.6). Regarding the clinical groups, myositis overlap patients tend to have the mildest muscle disease with the best responses to therapy and the fewest flares of disease over time. Myositis overlap syndromes are followed by dermatomyositis and then polymyositis in terms of ascending disease severity. The treatment of inclusion body myositis remains controversial and most patients with inclusion body myositis do not respond to therapy as well as patients in the other clinical groups (44). Some patients with inclusion body myositis, however, may benefit from corticosteroid and cytotoxic therapy in terms of slowing the rate of progression of disease (201,202). The serologic groups also differ in their disease courses in a similar way. Patients with anti–Mi-2 autoantibodies tend to have mild myositis with good responses to therapy and few flares of disease, whereas patients with the antisynthetase syndrome tend to have more severe and persistent disease. Finally, patients with antisignal recognition particle autoantibodies have the most acute onset and the most severe myositis, with the least response to therapy and the most persistent disease (25,203).

Although most patients have at least a partial response to corticosteroids, some do not respond adequately, many more experience disease activity increases during steroid tapering, and most eventually suffer from the toxicities of corticosteroids. Little is known about optimal therapy in corticosteroid-resistant patients. Oral methotrexate, at doses of 7.5 to 25 mg/week, and azathioprine, at 50 to 150 mg/day (204), are the major therapeutic options for corticosteroid-resistant patients (79), with the choice regarding the particular agent primarily determined by the relevant adverse event risk factors for each patient. One study suggested that males, in general, and patients with the antisynthetase syndrome, in particular, may respond better to methotrexate than azathioprine (79). A combination of methotrexate and azathioprine leads to improvement in some patients who have had inadequate responses to either agent given alone (205). Intravenous immunoglobulin (IVIg), cyclophosphamide, cyclosporine, FK506, chlorambucil, high-dose intravenous methotrexate with leucovorin rescue, or other combinations of cytotoxics may be beneficial in some patients and warrant further evaluation.

A number of uncontrolled series using different outcomes, end points, and IIM patient groups implied that IVIg therapy was beneficial (172,206–216). A double-blind, placebo-controlled trial has shown that IVIg at least transiently increases strength and decreases CK, rash, and muscle inflammation (217). In addition, IVIg alters the level of circulating complement components (218) in some patients with dermatomyositis. Nonetheless, the long-term efficacy, safety, usefulness in other groups of IIM patients, and cost-effectiveness of IVIg have been questioned (219–227). Given the expense, current scarcity, and adverse events associated with IVIg, my approach is to reserve this therapy for children with moderate to severe dermatomyositis; adult patients who have not responded to corticosteroids, methotrexate, and azathioprine; those who have poor prognostic factors; and patients who are severely ill, infected, or immunocompromised.

The role of cyclophosphamide in myositis therapy is unclear, but several small uncontrolled studies imply that it may be particularly useful in intravenous pulse form in adult patients with the antisynthetase syndrome (228–230), and orally in children with severe vasculitic complications. Chlorambucil (4–6 mg/d) may be effective in treating some IIM patients, but concern about the long-term carcinogenic potential of this alkylating agent is high. Interest in using combination therapies of methotrexate with either azathioprine, chlorambucil, or cyclosporine has increased, particularly in very refractory cases (202,231,232). Cyclosporine and FK506 have been reportedly effective in treating small series of adults and children with myositis; however, the narrow therapeutic window and concern about nephrotoxicity have limited their use.

A randomized double-blinded sham-controlled trial of apheresis has failed to show any significant benefit for plasma exchange or leukapheresis in steroid-resistant myositis patients not taking cytotoxics (233). Past therapies reported to be of benefit in small numbers of patients but that are not being pursued at present include total body irradiation, thymectomy, and photophoresis (4,234). Novel therapies using biologic antiinflammatory agents and autologous stem cell transplants are now under study and may represent important advances in the treatment of myositis in the future (235).

The treatment of inclusion body myositis is controversial. Although many texts in the past have stated that inclusion body myositis was untreatable and patients suffered a slowly inexorable deterioration despite therapy, several recent studies provide some hope that a subset of patients may respond to treatment. Retrospective reviews of corticosteroid and cytotoxic therapy (202,236), a prospective open trial of IVIg (212), and a randomized trial of combination oral methotrexate-azathioprine versus high-dose methotrexate with leucovorin rescue (202) suggest that the rate of deterioration may be decreased or stabilized and strength improved in a subset of inclusion body myositis patients. Characteristics that identify inclusion body myositis patients more likely to respond are CKs greater than five times the upper limits of the normal range, active inflammation on MRI or muscle biopsy, and associated autoimmune phenomena.

Treatment of Extramuscular Manifestations

Many organ systems may be affected in IIM with resultant significant morbidity and mortality. General symptoms of fatigue, fever, and weight loss often respond to corticosteroid or cytotoxic therapy for the underlying myositis. Raynaud's phenomenon may respond to avoidance of the cold or calcium channel blockers.

The rash of dermatomyositis may be a very troublesome problem for the patient and may persist long after the myositis has resolved. Avoidance of sun and photosensitizers, as well as topical sunscreens and steroids may be helpful, but often the use of hydroxychloroquine (237) or methotrexate is required. Some authors have used quinacrine successfully, and isotretinoin, despite teratogenic concerns, may be useful in the treatment of IIM rashes (4). Subcutaneous calcifications, more common in children than adults, can be very troubling. No treatment, other than therapy for the underlying myositis, has been shown to improve the calcifications, although a number of approaches have been tried. In severe cases in which the calcifications impinge on critical structures or cause chronic pain, surgery may be necessary to remove them.

Dyspnea can result from respiratory muscle weakness, atelectasis, aspiration, secondary infections, and interstitial pulmonary fibrosis. Pulmonary fibrosis is a worrisome complication in IIM patients and some patients do not improve with any therapy. Yet, methotrexate, pulse corticosteroids, and cyclophosphamide are often tried in an attempt to treat this cause of great morbidity and mortality. The role of pulmonary transplantation in pulmonary dysfunction associated with systemic autoimmune disease remains unclear, but anecdotal reports suggest successful outcomes in some patients (238,239). Symptomatic cardiac disease should be treated with diuretics or digitalis to resolve heart failure, antiarrhythmics as needed, and corticosteroids and cytotoxics if evidence of myocarditis is present (192). Despite aggressive therapy, cardiac disease is a major cause of mortality in the IIM, especially in the antisignal recognition particle autoantibody group.

Gastrointestinal involvement may be severe and difficult to manage in some patients. Some patients have such severe dysphagia and are at such risk of aspiration that tube feedings are necessary. Reflux esophagitis is common and should be treated by the usual approaches of elevating the head of the bed and prescribing antacids or H2-receptor antagonists. Cricopharyngeal dysfunction can be the cause of significant dysphagia and odynophagia and may improve with myotomy (240). An unusual but life-threatening complication, seen more commonly in children with dermatomyositis, is mucosal ulceration or perforation of the lower gastrointestinal tract because of active vasculitis that can lead to severe hemorrhage. This manifestation often requires emergent surgery and aggressive therapy with high-dose intravenous corticosteroids and cytotoxic therapy.

CURRENT QUESTIONS AND FUTURE DIRECTIONS

The diagnosis, classification, and treatment of inflammatory muscle disease have improved as our technologies and understanding of the etiopathogenesis of the idiopathic inflammatory myopathies have evolved over the last century. Yet, critical unanswered questions remain. For example, what changes in the current criteria, such as adding genetic or serologic markers or MRI findings, would maximize our capacity to diagnose IIM and separate the idiopathic myositis syndromes from the many other myopathies? What are the primary events or antigens driving the cellular and humoral immune responses? If interactions of environmental agents and genetics are responsible for distinct myositis syndromes, what are the agents, the genes, and the number of distinct elemental disorders to be identified? Can some forms of myositis be prevented via the avoidance of certain environmental exposures in genetically susceptible individuals or by gene therapy? How can we assess prognostic factors, disease activity, and morbidity more accurately? In addition, what are the optimal therapies for each of the clinical and serologic groups of patients? Answers to these questions will require significant resources and the dedication and cooperation of patients, physicians, and investigators working in many fields of research over the coming decades.

ACKNOWLEDGMENTS

The author is indebted to Lisa Rider, M.D., and Lori A. Love, M.D., Ph.D., for their useful comments after critically reviewing the manuscript.

REFERENCES

1. Plotz PH, Dalakas M, Leff RL, et al. Current concepts in the idiopathic inflammatory myopathies: polymyositis, dermatomyositis, and related disorders. *Ann Intern Med* 1989;111: 143–157.
2. Targoff IN. Dermatomyositis and polymyositis. *Curr Probl Dermatol* 1991;3:131–180.
3. Plotz PH, Rider LG, Targoff IN, et al. Myositis: immunologic contributions to understanding cause, pathogenesis, and therapy. *Ann Intern Med* 1995;122:715–724.
4. Oddis CV. Therapy of inflammatory myopathy. *Rheum Dis Clin North Am* 1994;20:899–918.
5. Wagner E. Fall einer seltenen Muskelkranheit. *Arch Heilkd* 1863;4:282.
6. Wagner E. Ein Fall von acuter Polymyositis. *Dtsch Arch Klin Med* 1887;40:241–266.
7. Potain R. Morve chronique de forme anormale. *Bull Soc Med Hop* 1895;12:314–320.
8. Hepp P. Ueber einen Fall von acuter parenchymatoser Myositis, welche Geschwulste bildete und Fluctuation, Vortauschte. *Klin Wochenschr* 1887;24:389–398.
9. Unverricht H. Polymyositis acuta progressiva. *Z Klin Med* 1887;12:533.
10. Unverricht H. Dermatomyositis acuta. *Dtsch Med Wochenschr* 1891;17:41–49.
11. Jackson H. Myositis universalis acuta infectiosa, with a case. *Boston Med Surg J* 1887;116–121.
12. Jacoby GW. Subacute progressive polymyositis. *J Nerv Ment Dis* 1888;15:697–711.
13. Steiner WR. Dermatomyositis, with report of a case which presented a rare muscle anomaly but once described in man. *J Exp Med* 1903;6:407–442.
14. Opel TW, Cohen C, Milhorat AT. Effect of pituitary adrenocorticotropin (ACTH) in dermatomyositis. *Ann Intern Med* 1950;32:318–322.
15. Wedgwood RJP, Cook CD, Cohen J. Dermatomyositis. Report of 26 cases in children with a discussion of endocrine therapy in 13. *Pediatrics* 1953;12:447–465.
16. Walton JN, Adams RD. *Polymyositis.* London: E.S. Livingstone, 1958.
17. Banker BO, Victor M. Dermatomyositis (systemic angiopathy) of childhood. *Medicine* 1966;45:261.
18. Sokoloff MC, Goldberg LS, Pearson CM. Treatment of corticosteroid-resistant polymyositis with methotrexate. *Lancet* 1971;1: 14–16.
19. Bohan A, Peter JB, Bowman RL, et al. Computer-assisted analysis of 153 patients with polymyositis and dermatomyositis. *Medicine (Baltimore)* 1977;56:255–286.
20. Bohan A, Peter JB. Polymyositis and dermatomyositis (parts 1 and 2). *N Engl J Med* 1975;292:344–347,403–407.
21. Chou SM. Myxovirus-like structures and accompanying nuclear changes in chronic polymyositis. *Arch Pathol* 1968;86: 649–658.
22. Sato T, Walker DL, Peters HA, et al. Myxovirus-like inclusion bodies in chronic polymyositis: electron microscopic and viral studies. *Trans Am Neurol Assoc* 1969;94:339–341.
23. Yunis EJ, Samaha FJ. Inclusion body myositis. *Lab Invest* 1971; 25:240–248.
24. Engel AG, Arahata K. Mononuclear cells in myopathies: quantitation of functionally distinct subsets, recognition of antigen-specific cell-mediated cytotoxicity in some diseases, and implications for the pathogenesis of the different inflammatory myopathies. *Hum Pathol* 1986;17:704–721.
25. Love LA, Leff RL, Fraser DD, et al. A new approach to the classification of idiopathic inflammatory myopathy: myositis-specific autoantibodies define useful homogeneous patient groups. *Medicine* 1991;70:360–374.
26. Engel AG, Banker BQ. *Myology,* 1st ed. New York: McGraw-Hill 1986:1385–1524.
27. Engel AG, Franzini-Armstrong C. *Myology,* 2nd ed. New York: McGraw-Hill, 1994:1–1937.
28. Zeviani M, Antozzi C. Defects of mitochondrial DNA. *Brain Pathol* 1992;2:121–132.
29. Sarnat HB. New insights into the pathogenesis of congenital myopathies. *J Child Neurol* 1994;9:193–201.
30. Cooper JM, Mann VM, Krige D, et al. Human mitochondrial complex I dysfunction. *Biochim Biophys Acta* 1992;1101: 198–203.
31. Raben N, Sherman J, Miller F, et al. A 5′ splice junction mutation leading to exon deletion in an Ashkenazic Jewish family with phosphofructokinase deficiency (Tarui disease). *J Biol Chem* 1993;268:4963–4967.
32. Sherman JB, Raben N, Nicastri C, et al. Common mutations in the phosphofructokinase-M gene in Ashkenazi Jewish patients with glycogenesis VII—and their population frequency. *Am J Hum Genet* 1994;55:305–313.
33. Targoff IN, Miller FW, Medsger TAJ, et al. Classification criteria for the idiopathic inflammatory myopathies. *Curr Opin Rheumatol* 1997;9:527–535.
34. Miller FW. Myositis-specific autoantibodies. Touchstones for understanding the inflammatory myopathies (clinical conference). *JAMA* 1993;270:1846–1849.
35. Targoff IN. Immune manifestations of inflammatory muscle disease. *Rheum Dis Clin North Am* 1994;20:857–880.
36. Mbauya AL, Plotz PH, Wilder RL, et al. Increased prevalence of autoimmune disease in first degree relatives of patients with

idiopathic inflammatory myopathy. *Arthritis Rheum* 1993;36 (suppl):D139(abst).

37. Fraser DD, Frank JA, Dalakas M, et al. Magnetic resonance imaging in the idiopathic inflammatory myopathies. *J Rheumatol* 1991;18:1693–1700.
38. Huppertz HI, Kaiser WA. Serial magnetic resonance imaging in juvenile dermatomyositis—delayed normalization. *Rheumatol Int* 1994;14:127–129.
39. Stonecipher MR, Jorizzo JL, Monu J, et al. Dermatomyositis with normal muscle enzyme concentrations. A single-blind study of the diagnostic value of magnetic resonance imaging and ultrasound. *Arch Dermatol* 1994;130:1294–1299.
40. Reimers CD, Schedel H, Fleckenstein JL, et al. Magnetic resonance imaging of skeletal muscles in idiopathic inflammatory myopathies of adults. *J Neurol* 1994;241:306–314.
41. Park JH, Olsen NJ, King L Jr, et al. Use of magnetic resonance imaging and P-31 magnetic resonance spectroscopy to detect and quantify muscle dysfunction in the amyopathic and myopathic variants of dermatomyositis. *Arthritis Rheum* 1995;38:68–77.
42. Love LA, Miller FW. Understanding the idiopathic inflammatory myopathies. *Contemp Int Med* 1995;7:29–43.
43. Lotz BP, Engel AG, Nishino H, et al. Inclusion body myositis. Observations in 40 patients. *Brain* 1989;112:727–747.
44. Calabrese LH, Chou SM. Inclusion body myositis. *Rheum Dis Clin North Am* 1994;20:955–972.
45. Griggs RC, Askanas V, DiMauro S, et al. Inclusion body myositis and myopathies. *Ann Neurol* 1995;38:705–713.
46. Callen JP. Relationship of cancer to inflammatory muscle diseases. Dermatomyositis, polymyositis, and inclusion body myositis. *Rheum Dis Clin North Am* 1994;20:943–953.
47. Sigurgeirsson B, Lindel÷f B, Edhag O, et al. Risk of cancer in patients with dermatomyositis or polymyositis. A population-based study. *N Engl J Med* 1992;326:363–367.
48. Moxley RT. Evaluation of neuromuscular function in inflammatory myopathy. *Rheum Dis Clin North Am* 1994;20:827–843.
49. Kagen LJ. Inflammatory muscle disease. Management. In: Klippel JH, Dieppe PA, eds. *Rheumatology.* Boston: Mosby, 1994; 14.1–14.4.
50. Franks AG. Important cutaneous markers of dermatomyositis. *J Musculoskeletal Med* 1988;5:39–63.
51. Kasteler JS, Callen JP. Scalp involvement in dermatomyositis. Often overlooked or misdiagnosed. *JAMA* 1994;272:1939–1941.
52. Rider LG, Miller FW. Laboratory evaluation of the inflammatory myopathies. *Clin Diag Lab Immunol* 1995;2:1–9.
53. Bohlmeyer TJ, Wu AH, Perryman MB. Evaluation of laboratory tests as a guide to diagnosis and therapy of myositis. *Rheum Dis Clin North Am* 1994;20:845–856.
54. Kroll M, Otis J, Kagen L. Serum enzyme, myoglobin and muscle strength relationships in polymyositis and dermatomyositis. *J Rheumatol* 1986;13:349–355.
55. Kagen LJ, Aram S. Creatine kinase activity inhibitor in sera from patients with muscle disease. *Arthritis Rheum* 1987;30: 213–217.
56. Black HR, Quallich H, Gareleck CB. Racial differences in serum creatine kinase levels. *Am J Med* 1986;81:479–487.
57. Mader R, Nicol PD, Turley JJ, et al. Inflammatory myopathy—early diagnosis and management by serum myosin light chains measurements. *Isr J Med Sci* 1994;30:902–904.
58. Miller FW, Love LA, Twitty SA, et al. Soluble CD8 and interleukin-2 receptor levels are measures of disease activity in the idiopathic inflammatory myopathies (IIM). *Arthritis Rheum* 1989;32:S33(abst).
59. Wolf RE, Baethge BA. Interleukin-1 alpha, interleukin-2, and soluble interleukin-2 receptors in polymyositis. *Arthritis Rheum* 1990;33:1007–1014.
60. Gabay C, Gay-Croisier F, Roux-Lombard P, et al. Elevated serum levels of interleukin-1 receptor antagonist in polymyositis/dermatomyositis. A biologic marker of disease activity with a possible role in the lack of acute-phase protein response. *Arthritis Rheum* 1994;37:1744–1751.
61. Kalovidouris AE, Horn CA, Plotkin Z. The role of cytokines in polymyositis. III. Recombinant human interferon-gamma enhances T cell adhesion to cultured human muscle cells. *Arthritis Rheum* 1994;37:907–914.
62. Engel AG, Hohlfeld R, Banker BQ. The polymyositis and dermatomyositis syndromes. In: Engel AG, Franzini-Armstrong C, eds. *Myology.* New York: McGraw-Hill, 1994:1335–1383.
63. Park JH, Vital TL, Ryder NM, et al. Magnetic resonance imaging and P-31 magnetic resonance spectroscopy provide unique quantitative data useful in the longitudinal management of patients with dermatomyositis. *Arthritis Rheum* 1994;37: 736–746.
64. Park JH, Olsen NJ, King L Jr, et al. Use of magnetic resonance imaging and P-31 magnetic resonance spectroscopy to detect and quantify muscle dysfunction in the amyopathic and myopathic variants of dermatomyositis. *Arthritis Rheum* 1995;38: 68–77.
65. Schweitzer ME, Fort J. Cost-effectiveness of MR imaging in evaluating polymyositis. *AJR* 1995;165:1469–1471.
66. Kent-Braun JA, Miller RG, Weiner MW. Magnetic resonance spectroscopy studies of human muscle. *Radiol Clin North Am* 1994;32:313–335.
67. Slopis JM, Jackson EF, Narayana PA, et al. Proton magnetic resonance imaging and spectroscopic studies of the pathogenesis and treatment of juvenile dermatomyositis. *J Child Neurol* 1993;8:242–249.
68. Nuviala RJ, Roda L, Lapieza MG, et al. Serum enzymes activities at rest and after a marathon race. *J Sports Med Phys Fitness* 1992;32:180–186.
69. Le Rumeur E, Carre F, Bernard AM, et al. Multiparametric classification of muscle T1 and T2 relaxation times determined by magnetic resonance imaging. The effects of dynamic exercise in trained and untrained subjects. *Br J Radiol* 1994;67:150–156.
70. Jenner G, Foley JM, Cooper TG, et al. Changes in magnetic resonance images of muscle depend on exercise intensity and duration, not work. *J Appl Physiol* 1994;76:2119–2124.
71. Summers RM, Brune AM, Choyke PL, et al. Juvenile idiopathic inflammatory myopathy: exercise-induced changes in muscle at short inversion time inversion-recovery MR imaging. *Radiology* 1998;209:191–196.
72. Research Group on Neuromuscular Diseases of the World Federation of Neurology. Classification of the neuromuscular disorders. *J Neurol* 1968;19:545–566.
73. Bohan A, Peter JB, Bowman RL, et al. Computer-assisted analysis of 153 patients with polymyositis and dermatomyositis. *Medicine (Baltimore)* 1977;56:255–286.
74. Dalakas MC. Polymyositis, dermatomyositis and inclusion-body myositis. *N Engl J Med* 1991;325:1487–1498.
75. Miller FW. Classification and prognosis of inflammatory muscle disease. *Rheum Dis Clin North Am* 1994;20:811–826.
76. Arahata K, Engel AG. Monoclonal antibody analysis of mononuclear cells in myopathies V: identification and quantitation of $T8^+$ cytotoxic and $T8^+$ suppressor cells. *Ann Neurol* 1988;23:493–499.
77. Miller FW, Love LA, Barbieri SA, et al. Lymphocyte activation markers in idiopathic myositis: changes with disease activity and differences among clinical and autoantibody subgroups. *Clin Exp Immunol* 1990;81:373–379.
78. Engel AG, Arahata K, Emslie-Smith A. Immune effector mechanisms in inflammatory myopathies. *Res Publ Assoc Res Nerv Ment Dis* 1990;68:141–157.
79. Joffe MM, Love LA, Leff RL, et al. Drug therapy of the idio-

pathic inflammatory myopathies: predictors of response to prednisone, azathioprine, and methotrexate and a comparison of their efficacy. *Am J Med* 1993;94:379–387.
80. Stonecipher MR, Jorizzo JL, White WL, et al. Cutaneous changes of dermatomyositis in patients with normal muscle enzymes: dermatomyositis sine myositis? *J Am Acad Dermatol* 1993;28:951–956.
81. Euwer RL, Sontheimer RD. Amyopathic dermatomyositis: a review. *J Invest Dermatol* 1993;100:124S-127S.
82. Euwer RL, Sontheimer RD. Amyopathic dermatomyositis (dermatomyositis sine myositis). Presentation of six new cases and review of the literature. *J Am Acad Dermatol* 1991;24:959–966.
83. Emslie-Smith AM, Engel AG. Microvascular changes in early and advanced dermatomyositis: a quantitative study. *Ann Neurol* 1990;27:343–356.
84. Tsokos GC, Moutsopoulos HM, Steinberg AD. Muscle involvement in systemic lupus erythematosus. *JAMA* 1981;246: 766–768.
85. Serratrice G, Schiano A, Pellissier JF, et al. Anatomoclinical expressions of polymyositis in the child. 23 cases. *Ann Pediatr (Paris)* 1989;36:237–243.
86. Rider LG, Miller FW, Targoff IN, et al. A broadened spectrum of juvenile myositis. Myositis-specific autoantibodies in children. *Arthritis Rheum* 1994;37:1534–1538.
87. Rider LG, Miller FW. New perspectives on the idiopathic inflammatory myopathies of childhood. *Curr Opin Rheumatol* 1994;6:575–582.
88. Rider LG, Miller FW. Classification and treatment of the juvenile idiopathic inflammatory myopathies. *Rheum Dis Clin North Am* 1997;23:619–655.
89. Pachman LM, Miller FW. Idiopathic inflammatory myopathies: dermatomyositis, polymyositis and related disorders. In: Frank MM, Austin KF, Claman HN, eds. *Samter's immunologic diseases.* Boston: Little, Brown, 1995:791–803.
90. Barnes BE, Mawr B. Dermatomyositis and malignancy. A review of the literature. *Ann Intern Med* 1976;84:68–76.
91. Sakon M, Monden M, Fujimoto Y, et al. Gastric carcinoma associated with dermatomyositis. *Acta Chir Scand* 1989;155: 365–366.
92. Whitmore SE, Rosenshein NB, Provost TT. Ovarian cancer in patients with dermatomyositis. *Medicine (Baltimore)* 1994;73: 153–160.
93. Cherin P, Piette JC, Herson S, et al. Dermatomyositis and ovarian cancer: a report of 7 cases and literature review. *J Rheumatol* 1993;20:1897–1899.
94. Zantos D, Zhang Y, Felson D. The overall and temporal association of cancer with polymyositis and dermatomyositis. *J Rheumatol* 1994;21:1855–1859.
95. Basset-Seguin N, Roujeau JC, Gherardi R, et al. Prognostic factors and predictive signs of malignancy in adult dermatomyositis. A study of 32 cases. *Arch Dermatol* 1990;126:633–637.
96. Askanas V, Engel WK. Sporadic inclusion-body myositis and hereditary inclusion-body myopathies: current concepts of diagnosis and pathogenesis. *Curr Opin Rheumatol* 1998;10:530–542.
97. Figarella-Branger D, Pellissier JF, Pouget J, et al. Inclusion body myositis and neuromuscular diseases with rimmed vacuoles. *Rev Neurol (Paris)* 1992;148:281–290.
98. Pickering MC, Walport MJ. Eosinophilic myopathic syndromes. *Curr Opin Rheumatol* 1998;10:504–510.
99. Serratrice G, Pellissier JF, Desnuelle C, et al. Mitochondrial and ocular myopathies (62 cases). *Rev Neurol (Paris)* 1991;147: 474–475.
100. Yoritaka A, Kogahara K, Yoshino H, et al. Clinical and neuroradiological studies on orbital myositis and Tolosa-Hunt syndrome. *Rinsho Shinkeigaku* 1992;32:593–599.
101. Scott IU, Siatkowski RM. Idiopathic orbital myositis. *Curr Opin Rheumatol* 1997;9:504–512.
102. Casteels I, De Bleecker C, Demaerel P, et al. Orbital myositis following an upper respiratory tract infection: contribution of high resolution CT and MRI. *J Belge Radiol* 1991;74:45–47.
103. George JL, Raspiller A, Lesure P, et al. Oculomotor disorders and enlargement of the extraocular muscles. *Ophtalmologie* 1989;3:167–168.
104. Noel E, Tebib J, Walch G, et al. Focal myositis: a pseudotumoral form of polymyositis. *Clin Rheumatol* 1991;10: 333–338.
105. Kransdorf MJ, Temple HT, Sweet DE. Focal myositis. *Skeletal Radiol* 1998;27:283–287.
106. Moreno-Lugris C, Gonzalez-Gay MA, Sanchez-Andrade A, et al. Magnetic resonance imaging: a useful technique in the diagnosis and follow up of focal myositis. *Ann Rheum Dis* 1996; 55:856
107. Targoff IN, Arnett FC. Clinical manifestations in patients with antibody to PL-12 antigen (alanyl-tRNA synthetase). *Am J Med* 1990;88:241–251.
108. Mathews MB, Bernstein RM. Myositis autoantibody inhibits histidyl-tRNA synthetase: a model for autoimmunity. *Nature* 1983;304:177–179.
109. Targoff IN, Reichlin M. Measurement of antibody to Jo-1 by ELISA and comparison to enzyme inhibitory activity. *J Immunol* 1987;138:2874–2882.
110. Hong TJ, Escribano J, Coca-Prados M. Isolation of cDNA clones encoding the 80-kd subunit protein of the human autoantigen Ku (p70/p80) by antisera raised against ciliary processes of human eye donors. *Invest Ophthalmol Vis Sci* 1994; 35:4023–4030.
111. Ge Q, Trieu EP, Targoff IN. Primary structure and functional expression of human Glycyl-tRNA synthetase, an autoantigen in myositis. *J Biol Chem* 1994;269:28790–28797.
112. Raben N, Nichols R, Dohlman J, et al. A motif in human histidyl-tRNA synthetase which is shared among several aminoacyl-tRNA synthetases is a coiled-coil that is essential for enzymatic activity and contains the major autoantigenic epitope. *J Biol Chem* 1994;269:24277–24283.
113. Ge Q, Wu Y, Trieu EP, et al. Analysis of the specificity of anti-PM-Scl autoantibodies. *Arthritis Rheum* 1994;37:1445–1452.
114. Nilasena DS, Trieu EP, Targoff IN. Analysis of the Mi-2 autoantigen of dermatomyositis. *Arthritis Rheum* 1995;38: 123–128.
115. Marguerie C, Bunn CC, Copier J, et al. The clinical and immunogenetic features of patients with autoantibodies to the nucleolar antigen PM-Scl. *Medicine (Baltimore)* 1992;71:327–336.
116. Oddis CV, Okano Y, Rudert WA, et al. Serum autoantibody to the nucleolar antigen PM-Scl. Clinical and immunogenetic associations. *Arthritis Rheum* 1992;35:1211–1217.
117. Blaszczyk M, Jablönska S, Szymanska-Jagiello W, et al. Childhood scleromyositis: an overlap syndrome associated with PM-Scl antibody. *Pediatr Dermatol* 1991;8:1–8.
118. Hausmanowa-Petrusewicz I, Kowalska-Oltedaka E, Miller FW, et al. Clinical, serologic, and immunogenetic features in Polish patients with idiopathic inflammatory myopathies. *Arthritis Rheum* 1997;40:1257–1266.
119. Isern RA, Yaneva M, Weiner E, et al. Autoantibodies in patients with primary pulmonary hypertension: association with anti-Ku. *Am J Med* 1992;93:307–312.
120. Oddis CV, Conte CG, Steen VD, et al. Incidence of polymyositis-dermatomyositis: a 20-year study of hospital diagnosed cases in Allegheny County, PA 1963–1982. *J Rheumatol* 1990;17: 1329–1334.
121. Houck W, Melnyk C, Gast MJ. Polymyositis in pregnancy. A case report and literature review. *J Reprod Med* 1987;32:208–210.

122. England MJ, Perlmann T, Veriava Y. Dermatomyositis in pregnancy. A case report. *J Reprod Med* 1986;31:633–636.
123. King CR, Chow S. Dermatomyositis and pregnancy. *Obstet Gynecol* 1985;66:589–592.
124. Gutierrez G, Dagnino R, Mintz G. Polymyositis/dermatomyositis and pregnancy. *Arthritis Rheum* 1984;27:291–294.
125. Spiera H. The clinical picture of connective tissue diseases in pregnancy. *Prog Clin Biol Res* 1981;70:303–307.
126. Katz AL. Another case of polymyositis in pregnancy [letter]. *Arch Intern Med* 1980;140:1123.
127. Rosenzweig BA, Rotmensch S, Binette SP, et al. Primary idiopathic polymyositis and dermatomyositis complicating pregnancy: diagnosis and management. *Obstet Gynecol Surv* 1989; 44:162–170.
128. Ishii N, Ono H, Kawaguchi T, et al. Dermatomyositis and pregnancy. Case report and review of the literature. *Dermatologica* 1991;183:146–149.
129. Satoh M, Ajmani AK, Hirakata M, et al. Onset of polymyositis with autoantibodies to threonyl-tRNA synthetase during pregnancy. *J Rheumatol* 1994;21:1564–1566.
130. Medsger TA, Dawson WN, Masi AT. The epidemiology of polymyositis. *Am J Med* 1970;48:715–723.
131. Rider LG, Shamim E, Okada S, et al. Genetic risk and protective factors for idiopathic inflammatory myopathy in Caucasians and Koreans: A tale of two loci. *Arthritis Rheum* 1999; 42:1285–1290.
132. Miller FW. Humoral immunity and immunogenetics in the idiopathic inflammatory myopathies. *Curr Opin Rheumatol* 1991;3:902–910.
133. Garlepp MJ. Immunogenetics of inflammatory myopathies. *Baillieres Clin Neurol* 1993;2:579–597.
134. Arnett FC, Targoff IN, Mimori T, et al. Interrelationship of major histocompatibility complex class II alleles and autoantibodies in four ethnic groups with various forms of myositis. *Arthritis Rheum* 1996;39:1507–1518.
135. Garlepp MJ, Laing B, Zilko PJ, et al. HLA associations with inclusion body myositis. *Clin Exp Immunol* 1994;98:40–45.
136. Arnett FC. Histocompatibility typing in the rheumatic diseases. Diagnostic and prognostic implications. *Rheum Dis Clin North Am* 1994;20:371–390.
137. Rider LG, Gurley RC, Pandey JP, et al. Clinical, serologic, and immunogenetic features of familial idiopathic inflammatory myopathy. *Arthritis Rheum* 1998;41:710–719.
138. Shamim E, Miller FW. Familial Autoimmunity and the Idiopathic Inflammatory Myopathies. *Curr Rheum Rep* 2000 *(in press).*
139. Strongwater SL, Dorovini-Zis K, Ball RD, et al. A murine model of polymyositis induced by coxsackievirus B1 (Tucson strain). *Arthritis Rheum* 1984;27:433–442.
140. Miller FW, Love LA, Biswas T, et al. Viral and host genetic factors influence encephalomyocarditis virus-induced polymyositis in adult mice. *Arthritis Rheum* 1987;30:549–556.
141. Cronin ME, Love LA, Miller FW, et al. The natural history of encephalomyocarditis virus-induced myositis and myocarditis in mice. Viral persistence demonstrated by in situ hybridization. *J Exp Med* 1988;168:1639–1648.
142. Ytterberg SR, Mahowald ML, Messner RP. Coxsackievirus B1-induced polymyositis. Lack of disease expression in nu/nu mice. *J Clin Invest* 1987;80:499–506.
143. Neu N, Beisel KW, Traystman MD, et al. Autoantibodies specific for the cardiac myosin isoform are found in mice susceptible to Coxsackievirus B3-induced myocarditis. *J Immunol* 1987;138:2488–2492.
144. Magid SK, Kagen LJ. Serologic evidence for acute toxoplasmosis in polymyositis-dermatomyositis. Increased frequency of specific anti-toxoplasmosis IgM antibodies. *Am J Med* 1983;75: 313–320.
145. Plotz PH, Miller FW. Animal models of myositis. *Mt Sinai J Med (NY)* 1988;55:501–505.
146. Dalakas MC. Retroviruses and inflammatory myopathies in humans and primates. *Baillieres Clin Neurol* 1993;2:659–691.
147. Ytterberg SR. The relationship of infectious agents to inflammatory myositis. *Rheum Dis Clin North Am* 1994;20:995–1015.
148. Leff RL, Love LA, Miller FW, et al. Viruses in idiopathic inflammatory myopathies: absence of candidate viral genomes in muscle. *Lancet* 1992;339:1192–1195.
149. Love LA, Miller FW. Noninfectious environmental agents associated with myopathies. *Curr Opin Rheumatol* 1993;5:712–718.
150. Takahashi K, Ogita T, Okudaira H, et al. D-penicillamine-induced polymyositis in patients with rheumatoid arthritis. *Arthritis Rheum* 1986;29:560–564.
151. Miller FW. Genetics of environmentally-associated rheumatic disease. In: Kaufman LD, Varga J, eds. *Rheumatic diseases and the environment.* London: Arnold, 1999:33–45.
152. Halla JT, Fallahi S, Koopman WJ. Penicillamine-induced myositis. Observations and unique features in two patients and review of the literature. *Am J Med* 1984;77:719–722.
153. Christensen PD, Sörensen KE. Penicillamine-induced polymyositis with complete heart block. *Eur Heart J* 1989;10:1041–1044.
154. Taneja V, Mehra N, Singh YN, et al. HLA-D region genes and susceptibility to D-penicillamine-induced myositis [letter]. *Arthritis Rheum* 1990;33:1445–1447.
155. Carroll GJ, Will RK, Peter JB, et al. Penicillamine induced polymyositis and dermatomyositis. *J Rheumatol* 1987;14: 995–1001.
156. Ginn LR, Lin JP, Plotz PH, et al. Familial autoimmunity in pedigrees of idiopathic inflammatory myopathy patients suggests common genetic risk factors for many autoimmune diseases. *Arthritis Rheum* 1998;41:400–405.
157. Becker KG, Simon RM, Bailey-Wilson JE, et al. Clustering of non-major histocompatibility complex susceptibility candidate loci in human autoimmune diseases. *Proc Natl Acad Sci U S A* 1998;95:9979–9984.
158. Kalovidouris AE. Mechanisms of inflammation and histopathology in inflammatory myopathy. *Rheum Dis Clin North Am* 1994;20:881–897.
159. Engel AG, Arahata K. Monoclonal antibody analysis of mononuclear cells in myopathies II: phenotypes of autoinvasive cells in polymyositis and inclusion body myositis. *Ann Neurol* 1984;16:209–215.
160. Engel AG, Arahata K. Mononuclear cells in myopathies: quantitation of functionally distinct subsets, recognition of antigen-specific cell-mediated cytotoxicity in some diseases, and implications for the pathogenesis of the different inflammatory myopathies. *Hum Pathol* 1986;17:704–721.
161. Pluschke G, Ruegg D, Hohlfeld R, et al. Autoaggressive myocytotoxic T lymphocytes expressing an unusual gamma/delta T cell receptor. *J Exp Med* 1992;176:1785–1789.
162. Hohlfeld R, Goebels N, Engel AG. Cellular mechanisms in inflammatory myopathies. *Baillieres Clin Neurol* 1993;2:617–635.
163. De Visser M, Emslie-Smith AM, Engel AG. Early ultrastructural alterations in adult dermatomyositis. Capillary abnormalities precede other structural changes in muscle. *J Neurol Sci* 1989;94:181–192.
164. O'Hanlon TP, Dalakas MC, Plotz PH, et al. Predominant TCR-alpha beta variable and joining gene expression by muscle-infiltrating lymphocytes in the idiopathic inflammatory myopathies. *J Immunol* 1994;152:2569–2576.
165. O'Hanlon TP, Dalakas MC, Plotz PH, et al. The alpha beta T-cell receptor repertoire in inclusion body myositis: diverse pat-

terns of gene expression by muscle-infiltrating lymphocytes. *J Autoimmun* 1994;7:321–333.

166. Mantegazza R, Andreetta F, Bernasconi P, et al. Analysis of T cell receptor repertoire of muscle-infiltrating T lymphocytes in polymyositis. Restricted V alpha/beta rearrangements may indicate antigen-driven selection. *J Clin Invest* 1993;91: 2880–2886.
167. Pluschke G, Ruegg D, Hohlfeld R, et al. Autoaggressive myocytotoxic T lymphocytes expressing an unusual gamma/delta T cell receptor. *J Exp Med* 1992;176:1785–1789.
168. Lindberg C, Oldfors A, Tarkowski A. Restricted use of T cell receptor V genes in endomysial infiltrates of patients with inflammatory myopathies. *Eur J Immunol* 1994;24:2659–2663.
169. Miller FW, Read EJ, Carrasquillo JA, et al. Abnormal lymphocyte trafficking to muscle in patients with idiopathic inflammatory myopathy. *Arthritis Rheum* 1988;31:S60(abst).
170. Prussick R, Brain MC, Walker IR, et al. Polymyositis: a manifestation of chronic graft-versus-host disease. *J Am Acad Dermatol* 1991;25:560–562.
171. Gartner JG, Halliday WC, Merry AC, et al. Inflammatory myopathy in F1 hybrid mice with acute graft-versus-host reactions. *Transplantation* 1989;48:328–331.
172. Hanslik T, Jaccard A, Guillon JM, et al. Polymyositis and chronic graft-versus-host disease: efficacy of intravenous gammaglobulin. *J Am Acad Dermatol* 1993;28:492–493.
173. Miller FW, Twitty SA, Biswas T, et al. Origin and regulation of a disease-specific autoantibody response: antigenic epitopes, spectrotype stability, and isotype restriction of anti-Jo-1 autoantibodies. *J Clin Invest* 1990;85:468–475.
174. Miller FW, Waite KA, Biswas T, et al. The role of an autoantigen, histidyl-tRNA synthetase, in the induction and maintenance of autoimmunity. *Proc Natl Acad Sci U S A* 1990;87:9933–9937.
175. Targoff IN. Humoral immunity in polymyositis/dermatomyositis. *J Invest Dermatol* 1993;100:116S–123S.
176. Targoff IN, Trieu EP, Plotz PH, et al. Antibodies to glycyl-transfer RNA synthetase in patients with myositis and interstitial lung disease. *Arthritis Rheum* 1992;35:821–830.
177. Targoff IN, Trieu EP, Miller FW. Reaction of anti-OJ autoantibodies with components of the multi-enzyme complex of aminoacyl-tRNA synthetases in addition to isoleucyl-tRNA synthetase. *J Clin Invest* 1993;91:2556–2564.
178. Leff RL, Burgess SH, Miller FW, et al. Distinct seasonal patterns in the onset of adult idiopathic inflammatory myopathy in patients with anti-Jo-1 and anti-signal recognition particle autoantibodies. *Arthritis Rheum* 1991;34:1391–1396.
179. Love LA, Burgess SH, Hill PC, et al. Geographical and seasonal clustering in the onset of idiopathic inflammatory myopathy in groups defined by myositis-specific autoantibodies. *Arthritis Rheum* 1992;35(suppl):S22(abst).
180. O'Leary PA, Waisman M. Dermatomyositis. *Arch Dermatol* 1940;41:1001–1018.
181. Medsger TA, Robinson H, Masi AT. Factors affecting survivorship in polymyositis. *Arthritis Rheum* 1971;14:249–258.
182. Hochberg MC, Feldman D, Stevens MB. Adult onset polymyositis/dermatomyositis: an analysis of clinical and laboratory features and survival in 76 patients with a review of the literature. *Semin Arthritis Rheum* 1986;15:168–178.
183. Moyer RA, Phillips CA, Torretti D, et al. Clinical features and outcome in inflammatory myopathy. *Arthritis Rheum* 1989;32(suppl):S32(abst).
184. McKendry RJ. Influence of age at onset on the duration of treatment in idiopathic adult polymyositis and dermatomyositis. *Arch Intern Med* 1987;147:1989–1991.
185. Tymms KE, Webb J. Dermatopolymyositis and other connective tissue diseases: a review of 105 cases. *J Rheumatol* 1985;12: 1140–1148.
186. Henriksson KG, Sandstedt P. Polymyositis—treatment and prognosis. A study of 107 patients. *Acta Neurol Scand* 1982;65: 280–300.
187. Benbassat J, Gefel D, Larholt K, et al. Prognostic factors in polymyositis/dermatomyositis. A computer-assisted analysis of ninety-two cases. *Arthritis Rheum* 1985;28:249–255.
188. Carpenter JR, Bunch TW, Engel AG, et al. Survival in polymyositis: corticosteroids and risk factors. *J Rheumatol* 1977; 4:207–214.
189. Hochberg MC, Lopez-Acuna D, Gittelsohn AM. Mortality from polymyositis and dermatomyositis in the United States, 1968–1978. *Arthritis Rheum* 1983;26:1465–1471.
190. DeVere R, Bradley WG. Polymyositis: its presentation, morbidity and mortality. *Brain* 1975;98:637–666.
191. Fafalak RG, Peterson MG, Kagen LJ. Strength in polymyositis and dermatomyositis: best outcome in patients treated early. *J Rheumatol* 1994;21:643–648.
192. Gottdiener JS, Sherber HS, Hawley RJ, et al. Cardiac manifestations in polymyositis. *Am J Cardiol* 1978;41:1141–1149.
193. Hoffman GS, Franck WA, Raddatz DA, et al. Presentation,treatment, and prognosis of idiopathic inflammatory muscle disease in a rural hospital. *Am J Med* 1983;75:433–438.
194. Rider LG. Assessment of disease activity and its sequelae in children and adults with myositis. *Curr Opin Rheumatol* 1996;8: 495–506.
195. Hicks JE. Rehabilitation of patients with myositis. In: Klippel JH, Dieppe PA, eds. *Rheumatology.* Boston: Mosby, 1994; 15.4–15.6.
196. Hicks JE, Miller F, Plotz P, et al. Isometric exercise increases strength and does not produce sustained creatinine phosphokinase increases in a patient with polymyositis. *J Rheumatol* 1993; 20:1399–1401.
197. Wiesinger GF, Quittan M, Graninger M, et al. Benefit of 6 months long-term physical training in polymyositis/dermatomyositis patients. *Br J Rheumatol* 1998;37:1338–1342.
198. Oddis CV. Therapy for myositis. *Curr Opin Rheumatol* 1993;5: 742–748.
199. Laxer RM, Stein LD, Petty RE. Intravenous pulse methylprednisolone treatment of juvenile dermatomyositis. *Arthritis Rheum* 1987;30:328–334.
200. Malleson PN. Controversies in juvenile dermatomyositis [editorial]. *J Rheumatol* 1990;17:731–732.
201. Cohen MR, Sulaiman AR, Garancis JC, et al. Clinical heterogeneity and treatment response in inclusion body myositis. *Arthritis Rheum* 1989;32:734–740.
202. Leff RL, Miller FW, Hicks J, et al. The treatment of inclusion body myositis: a retrospective review and a randomized, prospective trial of immunosuppressive therapy. *Medicine (Baltimore)* 1993;72:225–235.
203. Targoff IN, Johnson AE, Miller FW. Antibody to signal recognition particle in polymyositis. *Arthritis Rheum* 1990;33: 1361–1370.
204. Bunch TW, Worthington JW, Combs JJ, et al. Azathioprine with prednisone for polymyositis. A controlled, clinical trial. *Ann Intern Med* 1980;92:365–369.
205. Villalba L, Hicks JE, Adams EM, et al. Treatment of refractory myositis: a randomized crossover study of two new cytotoxic regimens. *Arthritis Rheum* 1998;41:392–399.
206. Cherin P, Herson S, Wechsler B, et al. Intravenous immunoglobulin for polymyositis and dermatomyositis [letter] (published erratum appears in *Lancet* 1990;336:518). *Lancet* 1990; 336:116.
207. Dalakas MC. High-dose intravenous immunoglobulin and serum viscosity: risk of precipitating thromboembolic events. *Neurology* 1994;44:223–226.
208. Bussel A, Boulechfar H, Naim R. Immunoglobulins or plasma exchange? Synchronization of plasma exchange and intravenous

polyvalent immunoglobulins. A consecutive study of 11 patients. *Ann Med Interne (Paris)* 1993;144:532–538.

209. Cherin P, Herson S. Indications for intravenous gammaglobulin therapy in inflammatory myopathies. *J Neurol Neurosurg Psychiatry* 1994;57(suppl):50–54.
210. Collet E, Dalac S, Maerens B, et al. Juvenile dermatomyositis: treatment with intravenous gammaglobulin. *Br J Dermatol* 1994;130:231–234.
211. Lang BA, Laxer RM, Murphy G, et al. Treatment of dermatomyositis with intravenous gammaglobulin. *Am J Med* 1991;91: 169–172.
212. Soueidan SA, Dalakas MC. Treatment of inclusion-body myositis with high-dose intravenous immunoglobulin. *Neurology* 1993;43:876–879.
213. Morita R, Nakano K, Hirano Y, et al. Dramatic effects of high-dose intravenous gammaglobulin in each patient with intractable dermatomyositis and polymyositis. *No To Hattatsu* 1989;21: 523–528.
214. Saito Y, Hamamura K, Sugimoto T. A case of dermatomyositis complicated by thrombotic thrombocytopenic purpura (TTP) which responded to combination of gamma globulin and vincristine—clinical analysis on TTP cases in the Japanese literatures. *Rinsho Ketsueki* 1993;34:68–73.
215. Misbah SA, Spickett GP, Ryba PC, et al. Chronic enteroviral meningoencephalitis in agammaglobulinemia: case report and literature review. *J Clin Immunol* 1992;12:266–270.
216. Crennan JM, Van Scoy RE, McKenna CH, et al. Echovirus polymyositis in patients with hypogammaglobulinemia. Failure of high-dose intravenous gammaglobulin therapy and review of the literature. *Am J Med* 1986;81:35–42.
217. Dalakas MC, Illa I, Dambrosia JM, et al. A controlled trial of high-dose intravenous immune globulin infusions as treatment for dermatomyositis. *N Engl J Med* 1993;329:1993–2000.
218. Basta M, Dalakas MC. High-dose intravenous immunoglobulin exerts its beneficial effect in patients with dermatomyositis by blocking endomysial deposition of activated complement fragments. *J Clin Invest* 1994;94:1729–1735.
219. Cherin P, Piette JC, Wechsler B, et al. Intravenous gamma globulin as first line therapy in polymyositis and dermatomyositis: an open study in 11 adult patients. *J Rheumatol* 1994;21:1092–1097.
220. Reimold AM, Weinblatt ME. Tachyphylaxis of intravenous immunoglobulin in refractory inflammatory myopathy. *J Rheumatol* 1994;21:1144–1146.
221. Misbah SA, Chapel HM. Adverse effects of intravenous immunoglobulin. *Drug Safety* 1993;9:254–262.
222. Litzman J, Wiedermannova D, Lokaj J, et al. Side effects of administration of gamma globulin preparations in patients with primary agammaglobulinemia. *Vnitr Lek* 1992;38:490–494.
223. Minchinton RM, Cunningham I, Cole-Sinclair M, et al. Autoreactive platelet antibody in post transfusion purpura. *Aust NZ J Med* 1990;20:111–115.
224. Bussel JB, Fitzgerald-Pedersen J, Feldman C. Alternation of two doses of intravenous gammaglobulin in the maintenance treatment of patients with immune thrombocytopenic purpura: more is not always better. *Am J Hematol* 1990;33:184–188.
225. Nixon RR, Smith SA, Johnson RL, et al. Misleading hepatitis C serology following administration of intravenous immunoglobulin. *Am J Clin Pathol* 1994;101:327–328.
226. Duhem C, Dicato MA, Ries F. Side-effects of intravenous immune globulins. *Clin Exp Immunol* 1994;97(suppl):1:79–83.
227. Sekul EA, Cupler EJ, Dalakas MC. Aseptic meningitis associated with high-dose intravenous immunoglobulin therapy: frequency and risk factors. *Ann Intern Med* 1994;121:259–262.
228. Cronin ME, Miller FW, Hicks JE, et al. The failure of intravenous cyclophosphamide therapy in refractory idiopathic inflammatory myopathy. *J Rheumatol* 1989;16:1225–1228.
229. Bombardieri S, Hughes GR, Neri R, et al. Cyclophosphamide in severe polymyositis [letter]. *Lancet* 1989;1:1138–1139.
230. Leroy JP, Drosos AA, Yiannopoulos DI, et al. Intravenous pulse cyclophosphamide therapy in myositis and Sjögren's syndrome. *Arthritis Rheum* 1990;33:1579–1581.
231. Wallace DJ, Metzger AL, White KK. Combination immunosuppressive treatment of steroid-resistant dermatomyositis/polymyositis. *Arthritis Rheum* 1985;28:590–592.
232. Cagnoli M, Marchesoni A, Tosi S. Combined steroid, methotrexate and chlorambucil therapy for steroid-resistant dermatomyositis [letter]. *Clin Exp Rheumatol* 1991;9:658–659.
233. Miller FW, Leitman SF, Cronin ME, et al. Controlled trial of plasma exchange and leukapheresis in polymyositis and dermatomyositis. *N Engl J Med* 1992;326:1380–1384.
234. Engel WK, Lichter AS, Galdi AP. Polymyositis: remarkable response to total body irradiation [letter]. *Lancet* 1981;1:658.
235. Brodsky RA, Smith BD. Bone marrow transplantation for autoimmune diseases. *Curr Opin Oncol* 1999;11:83–86.
236. Sayers ME, Chou SM, Calabrese LH. Inclusion body myositis: analysis of 32 cases. *J Rheumatol* 1992;19:1385–1389.
237. Woo TY, Callen JP, Voorhees JJ, et al. Cutaneous lesions of dermatomyositis are improved by hydroxychloroquine. *J Am Acad Dermatol* 1984;10:592–600.
238. Pigula FA, Griffith BP, Zenati MA, et al. Lung transplantation for respiratory failure resulting from systemic disease. *Ann Thorac Surg* 1997;64:1630–1634.
239. Levine SM, Anzueto A, Peters JI, et al. Single lung transplantation in patients with systemic disease. *Chest* 1994;105:837–841.
240. Kagen LJ, Hochman RB, Strong EW. Cricopharyngeal obstruction in inflammatory myopathy (polymyositis/dermatomyositis). Report of three cases and review of the literature. *Arthritis Rheum* 1985;28:630–636.

79

SYSTEMIC SCLEROSIS (SCLERODERMA): CLINICAL ASPECTS

THOMAS A. MEDSGER, JR.

Systemic sclerosis is a chronic disorder of connective tissue characterized by inflammation and fibrosis and by degenerative changes in the blood vessels, skin, synovium, skeletal muscle, and certain internal organs, notably the gastrointestinal tract, lung, heart, and kidney (1). Although there is an early, often clinically unappreciated, inflammatory component, the hallmark of the disease is thickening of the skin (scleroderma) and other organs caused by excessive accumulation of connective tissue. Subintimal proliferative vascular changes are prominent and lead to Raynaud's phenomenon and obliterative arteriolar and capillary lesions.

The term scleroderma traditionally has been applied to the cutaneous changes of both systemic sclerosis and a heterogeneous group of conditions designated collectively as localized scleroderma. In the latter disorders, dermal fibrosis is more circumscribed, both vascular and internal organ involvement are absent, and the characteristic serologic abnormalities of systemic sclerosis are not found (see Chapter 80). Coexistence of these entities is rare. Although "evolution" of localized scleroderma to systemic sclerosis has been suggested by some case reports, it is more likely that these are instances in which a single patient has two coexistent autoimmune diseases. Many other conditions with systemic features exhibit scleroderma-like, but often distinctive, skin changes and lack the typical visceral manifestations and characteristic serologic abnormalities of systemic sclerosis (see Chapter 80).

CLASSIFICATION OF SYSTEMIC SCLEROSIS

Clinical Subsets

Systemic sclerosis is divided into two major clinical variants, diffuse cutaneous and limited cutaneous disease, distinguished from one another primarily by the degree and extent of skin involvement (2). The term *overlap syndrome* is used when features commonly encountered in other connective tissue diseases also are present (Table 79.1) (3). A similar spectrum of disease is recognized in the classification systems proposed by other authors.

The diffuse cutaneous variant is characterized by distal and proximal extremity and truncal skin thickening, whereas in the limited cutaneous subtype, skin thickening is most often restricted to the fingers, hands, and face. Most often the elbows and knees are considered the dividing line; a patient has diffuse cutaneous involvement if skin thickening affects the upper arms, thighs, or trunk (anterior chest, abdomen, back). Acrosclerosis (skin thickening limited to the most distal portions of the extremities) and CREST syndrome (an acronym referring to the findings of calcinosis, Raynaud's phenomenon, esophageal hypomotility, sclerodactyly, and telangiectasia) (4) are closely analogous to

TABLE 79.1. CLASSIFICATION OF SCLERODERMA

I. Systemic (systemic sclerosis)
   - With diffuse cutaneous scleroderma: symmetric widespread skin fibrosis, affecting the distal and proximal extremities and often the trunk and face; tendency to rapid progression of skin changes; and early appearance of visceral involvement
   - With limited cutaneous scleroderma: symmetric restricted skin fibrosis affecting the distal extremities (often confined to the fingers) and face; prolonged delay in appearance of distinctive internal manifestations (e.g., pulmonary arterial hypertension); and prominence of calcinosis and telangiectasis
   - With "overlap": having either diffuse or limited skin fibrosis and typical features of one or more of the other connective tissue diseases

II. Localized
   - Morphea: single or multiple plaques of skin fibrosis
   - Linear scleroderma: single or multiple bands of skin fibrosis; includes scleroderma *en coup de sabre* (with or without facial hemiatrophy)
   - Eosinophilic fasciitis: fascial and deep subcutaneous fibrosis
   - Eosinophilia-myalgia syndrome
   - Toxic oil syndrome

limited cutaneous scleroderma. Some patients with systemic sclerosis have no detectable skin thickening (systemic sclerosis sine scleroderma) (5); in my experience, these individuals are otherwise indistinguishable from those with limited cutaneous disease in their clinical, laboratory, and serologic findings and natural history of disease. Additionally, many demographic, clinical, and laboratory features help to distinguish diffuse cutaneous from limited cutaneous diseases (Table 79.2).

Disease subtype classification is particularly important to the patient and managing physician because it serves to predict the subsequent natural history of disease, identifying potential complications and the time frame during which they are most likely to occur. Diffuse cutaneous disease is associated with palpable tendon friction rubs, arthritis with joint contractures, serum anti–topoisomerase I (anti-Scl 70) or anti-RNA polymerase antibodies, and earlier, more frequent occurrence of visceral disease affecting the gastrointestinal tract, lung, heart, and kidney. In contrast, limited cutaneous disease is correlated with calcinosis, telangiectasia, serum anticentromere antibodies, and the occasional late development of pulmonary arterial hypertension or small bowel malabsorption. Systemic sclerosis in overlap includes patients with either diffuse or limited cutaneous involvement who also have convincing evidence of another connective tissue disease, such as polymyositis (myositis, dermatomyositis rash) or systemic lupus erythematosus (SLE; leukopenia, glomerulonephritis, pleuropericarditis, typical rash). Overlap with rheumatoid arthritis (RA) is surprisingly rare (6). Other subsets of systemic sclerosis undoubtedly exist, but their distinctive features have not been clearly delineated.

Serologic Subsets

Since the identification of anti–topoisomerase I and anticentromere antibodies and their strong associations with diffuse cutaneous and limited cutaneous disease, respectively, the concept of serologic subsets within the spectrum of systemic sclerosis has been popular. Other serum autoantibodies relatively specific for scleroderma also have been described. The proportion of patients having one of the seven scleroderma-associated autoantibodies is nearly 85% (Fig. 79.1). Persons with the limited cutaneous variant most frequently have anticentromere or anti-Th (7) antibody. Individuals with diffuse cutaneous involvement have anti–topoisomerase I or anti–RNA polymerase I and III antibody (8,9). Patients with systemic sclerosis in overlap most often have anti-U1RNP (10), anti-PM-Scl (11,12), or anti-U3RNP antibodies (13). Clinical features and genetic factors associated with these autoantibodies are described later in the section on serum autoantibodies.

TABLE 79.2. COMPARISON OF CLINICAL AND LABORATORY FEATURES FOUND AT ANY TIME DURING THE COURSE OF SYSTEMIC SCLEROSIS (UNIVERSITY OF PITTSBURGH, 1989–1998)

	Diffuse Scleroderma (n = 534)	Limited Scleroderma (n = 543)	Overlap Syndrome (n = 128)
Demographic features			
Age at onset (<40)	38%	48%	63%
Race (nonwhite)	12%	6%	15%
Sex (female)	75%	86%	84%
Duration of symptoms at first visit (years)	3.8	11.3	6.9
Organ system involvement			
Skin thickening (maximal total skin score)	28.0	5.4	8.0
Telangiectases	53%	70%	44%
Calcinosis	12%	32%	29%
Raynaud's phenomenon	93%	96%	94%
Arthralgias or arthritis	93%	47%	81%
Tendon friction rubs	52%	4%	14%
Joint contractures	86%	29%	45%
Skeletal myopathy	10%	1%	57%
Esophageal hypomotility	60%	59%	52%
Pulmonary fibrosis	28%	31%	29%
Cardiac involvement	10%	5%	18%
Scleroderma renal crisis	16%	2%	5%
Laboratory data			
Antinuclear antibody positive (1:16^{+})	98%	98%	95%
Anticentromere antibody positive	3%	41%	7%
Anti-Scl 70 antibody positive	29%	16%	4%
Cumulative survival after first physician diagnosis			
5 yr	80%	90%	93%
10 yr	68%	78%	81%

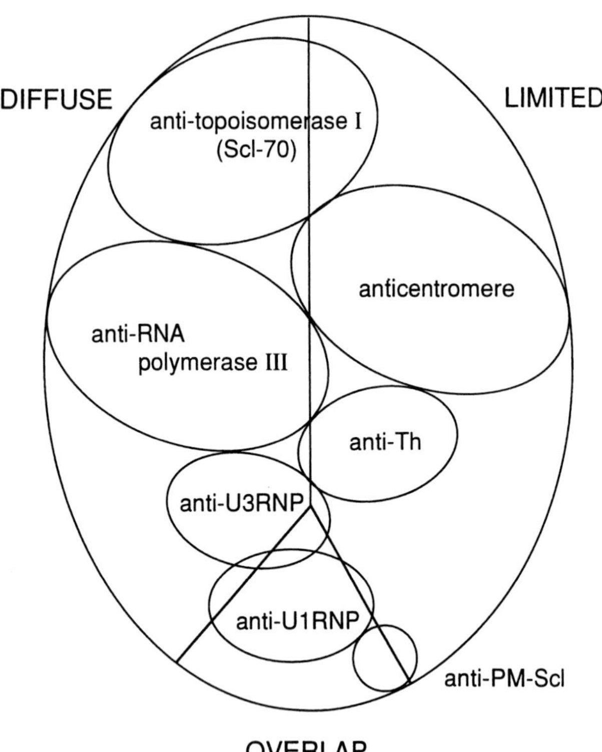

FIGURE 79.1. Classification of systemic sclerosis by clinical subsets and autoantibody types.

Criteria for Classification

These criteria are intended for description of large series of patients in research studies and not for diagnosis of an individual patient. A prospective multicenter study by the American College of Rheumatology (ACR) compared 264 systemic sclerosis patients with 413 persons having polymyositis–dermatomyositis, SLE, or Raynaud's disease for the purpose of developing classification criteria (14). Sclerodermatous skin change in any location proximal to the digits was found to be the major discriminating criterion for definite systemic sclerosis. Such thickening was present in 91% of systemic sclerosis cases and in fewer than 1% of comparison patients. With the addition of any two of three minor criteria (sclerodactyly, digital pitting scars, or bibasilar pulmonary interstitial fibrosis on chest radiograph), sensitivity increased to 97% and specificity was maintained at 98%.

In our experience, however, nearly 10% of individuals with definite systemic sclerosis do not satisfy these criteria (15). All are patients with limited cutaneous disease who have other convincing evidence of systemic sclerosis such as esophageal or small bowel hypomotility or pulmonary arterial hypertension. Whether to modify the ACR criteria to include patients with limited cutaneous involvement more adequately, or to develop separate subset criteria, presents a challenge for the future.

EPIDEMIOLOGY

The epidemiology of systemic sclerosis is discussed in Chapter 1. The disease has been described in all races and is global in distribution. A United States community study detected nearly 20 new hospital-diagnosed cases per million population at risk annually (16). Overall, women are affected approximately three times as often as men, and this ratio is increased during the childbearing years. No significant overall racial differences have been found. Systemic sclerosis usually begins in persons between ages 30 and 50 years. Onset during childhood and after age 80 has been reported, but is uncommon. In African-American women, disease onset occurs at a younger age, diffuse disease is more common, and survival poor (17). Prevalence estimates for systemic sclerosis have been in the range of 200 per million population (18).

Several environmental factors have been implicated as predisposing to or precipitating systemic sclerosis (19,20), including occupational organic solvent exposure (18,21). The resulting disorders and other scleroderma-like illnesses attributed to environmental agents are described in Chapter 80. After a flurry of interest in the possible association of silicone breast implants and systemic sclerosis, numerous retrospective case–control studies have failed to demonstrate any sizeable increased risk (22–25).

An increased prevalence of familial systemic sclerosis has been detected in three U.S. cohorts (26). Relatives of patients with systemic sclerosis are often affected by other connective tissue diseases, suggesting a heritable predisposition to this family of disorders. In multicase families, affected siblings shared human leukocyte antigen (HLA) haplotypes, but the development of disease could not be entirely accounted for by HLA genes, suggesting that major histocompatibility complex (MHC) genes are important, but not sufficient, for disease expression (27).

CLINICAL FEATURES

Initial Symptoms

In most cases of limited cutaneous disease, the initial complaint is Raynaud's phenomenon. In contrast, patients with diffuse cutaneous disease most often have diffuse swelling of the hands, skin thickening, or arthritis as the first manifestation. Occasionally, the earliest clue is that of visceral involvement, such as esophageal symptoms (dysphagia, heartburn) or dyspnea from pulmonary fibrosis.

Features of Organ Systemic Involvement

Skin

Easily recognized phases are present in the evolution of skin involvement. Initially, patients complain about tight, puffy fingers, especially on rising in the morning (edematous phase). Pitting or nonpitting edema of the fingers ("sausaging") and hands may occur, also frequently involving the forearms, legs, feet, and face. These changes extend beyond joints rather than being restricted to periarticular areas, assisting in the distinction from arthritis. Edema may last indefinitely (e.g., fingers in limited cutaneous disease) or may be replaced gradually by thickening and tightening of the skin (indurative phase) after several weeks or months. In the limited cutaneous subset, these changes are generally restricted to the fingers, hands, and face, whereas diffuse cutaneous disease first affects the fingers and hands but then spreads with variable rapidity to the forearms, upper arms, thighs, chest, and abdomen. Involved skin becomes increasingly shiny, taut, thickened, and tightly adherent to the underlying subcutis. During this phase, the dermis is markedly thickened, but the epidermis is thinned, leading to loss of skin creases, hair, sweat, and oils. Facial changes may result in the development of a characteristic pinched, immobile, expressionless appearance, with thin, tightly pursed lips, vertical folds around the mouth, and reduced oral aperture (Fig. 79.2). The limited oral opening interferes with eating and with proper dental care. After several years, the dermis tends to soften somewhat, and in many cases, reverts to normal thickness or actually becomes thinner than normal (atrophic phase). At that time, the most striking finding is digital and facial telangiectases, which consist of widely dilated capillary loops and distended venules (Fig. 79.3).

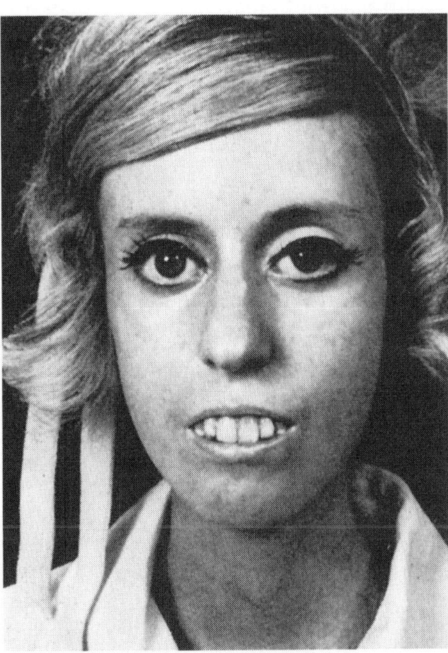

FIGURE 79.2. Face of a 19-year-old woman with diffuse cutaneous systemic sclerosis. Note loss of normal skin folds and retraction of lips.

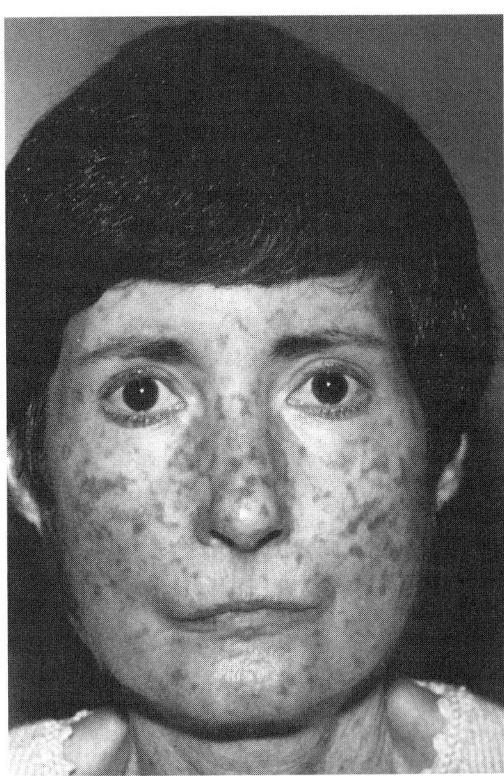

FIGURE 79.3. Face of a 45-year-old woman with limited cutaneous systemic sclerosis who had no skin thickening but had multiple telangiectases.

The natural history of skin involvement in the two major variants of systemic sclerosis is notably different when one of several reported semiquantitative methods is used to measure the degree and extent of cutaneous thickening in multiple sites (Fig. 79.4) (28,29). In limited cutaneous disease, skin thickening is either absent or remains minimal over many years and bears no relation to visceral sequelae. In contrast, in diffuse cutaneous scleroderma, early, rapid increase in skin thickness is the rule, reaching a peak after 1 to 2 years. A common mistake is to classify a patient with new sclerodactyly alone prematurely as having limited cutaneous involvement. Close observation over the next 3 to 6 months is necessary because many such patients will have proximal evolution and obvious diffuse skin thickening during that interval. Rapid progression of skin thickness is associated with the development of joint contractures and internal organ problems, including involvement of the gastrointestinal tract, lung, heart, and kidney. Thus although extensive skin thickening *per se* does not influence prognosis, the associated visceral disease is clearly life threatening. After maximal skin thickening has developed in diffuse scleroderma, slow but definite regression of this abnormality ensues and, in some cases, is remarkable (30). The classic pattern of improvement is that the most recently affected areas (usually the anterior chest and abdomen) are the first to improve.

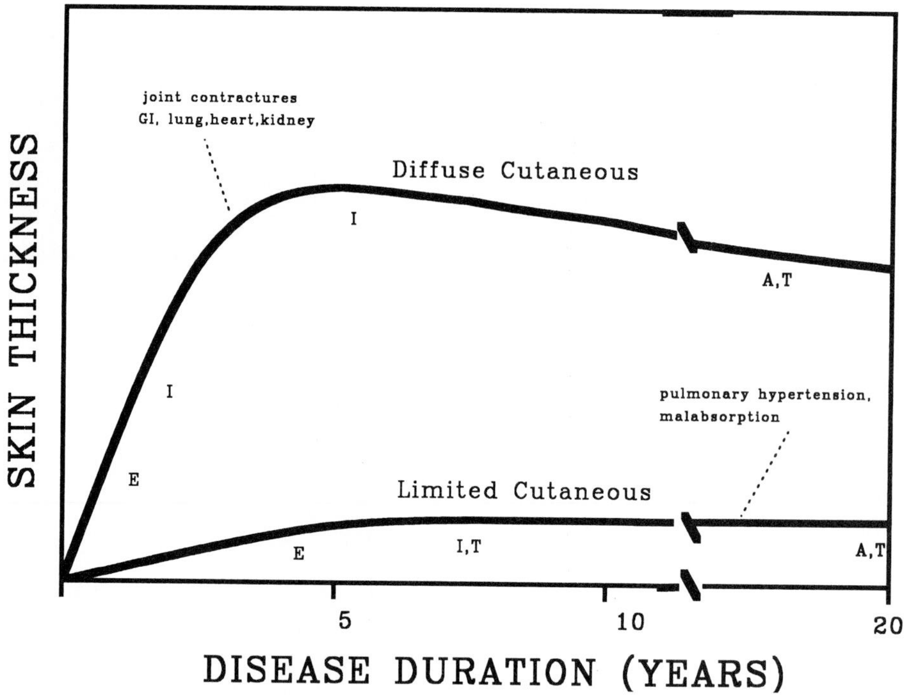

FIGURE 79.4. Natural history of skin thickness and timing of some serious complications during the course of systemic sclerosis with the two major disease variants. *E*, edema; *I*, induration; *A*, atrophy; *T*, telangiectasia.

Skin thickening is frequently accompanied by, and in some instances preceded by, impressive hyperpigmentation that spares the mucous membranes. This change is most prominent in the area of hair follicles, with surrounding hypopigmentation leading to a "salt-and-pepper" appearance. Hyperpigmentation is most striking over the course of superficial blood vessels (31) and tendons (32).

In early disease, skin biopsy is a less reliable method of establishing a diagnosis than is physical examination. Skin thickness "scores" are simple, inexpensive, correlate closely with skin biopsy thickness (33), and are reliable and reproducible (34,35). High-frequency ultrasound (20 MHz) and a plicometer test also have been reported to be feasible methods with very low interobserver variability (36,37). Skin biopsy specimens, obtained during the active indurative phase, disclose a striking increase of compact collagen fibers in the reticular dermis and hyalinization and fibrosis of arterioles. Simultaneously, thinning of the epidermis occurs with loss of rete pegs and atrophy of dermal appendages. Variably large accumulations of mononuclear cells, chiefly T lymphocytes, are encountered in the lower dermis and upper subcutis (Fig. 79.5) (38). Direct immunofluorescence is negative for immunoglobulins and complement components at the dermal–epidermal junction and in blood vessels (39). Degranulated mast cells, which have been linked to many fibrosing conditions, are found in increased numbers and density in clinically involved skin from patients with early diffuse cutaneous disease (40).

The skin overlying bony prominences, and especially over extensor surfaces of the proximal interphalangeal joints and elbows, becomes tightly stretched as a result of contractures and is extremely vulnerable to trauma. In such areas, cutaneous thinning (atrophy) occurs rather than thickening.

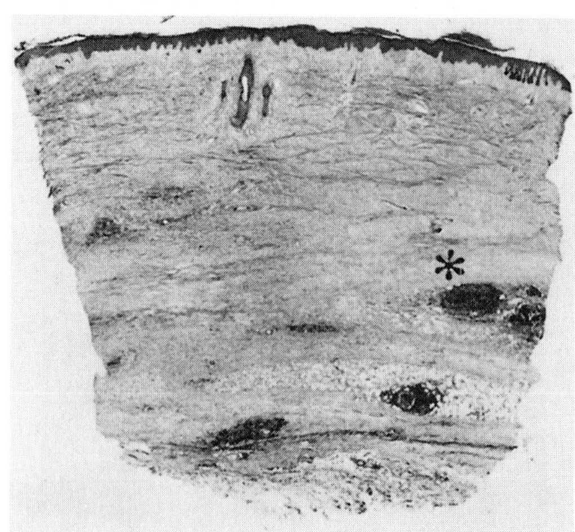

FIGURE 79.5. Photomicrograph of a skin-punch biopsy from the dorsum of the forearm of a 53-year-old woman with diffuse cutaneous systemic sclerosis. Skin appendages are atrophic, the dermis is thickened as a result of deposition of dense collagenous connective tissue, and there are prominent collections of small round cells (*asterisk*) that were identified as T lymphocytes.

Patients are often plagued by painful ulcerations at these sites and, less commonly, over the bony prominences about the shoulders and ankles. These ulcers heal extremely slowly and frequently become secondarily infected. Except for the tips of the digits, healing of skin in other locations, including sites of surgical incisions, is normal.

Calcinosis

Patients with limited scleroderma or late-stage diffuse disease commonly develop intracutaneous and/or subcutaneous calcifications composed of hydroxyapatite. These deposits occur chiefly in the digital pads and periarticular tissues, along the extensor surfaces of the forearms, and in the olecranon bursae, prepatellar areas, and buttocks. They vary in size from tiny punctate lesions of the fingers (Fig. 79.6) to large conglomerate masses in the forearms. Symptomatic cervical and lumbar spine calcinosis has been reported (41). Calcinosis may be complicated by ulceration of overlying skin, intermittent extrusion of calcareous material, and secondary bacterial infection (typically staphylococcal). Trauma and microvascular insufficiency are believed to be important predisposing factors.

Peripheral Vascular System

Raynaud's phenomenon is defined as paroxysmal vasospasm in response to cold exposure or emotional stress, leading to pallor and cyanosis of the digits, which also become cold, numb, and painful. During rewarming, reactive hyperemia is common. The toes are often affected, and less frequently involved sites include the tip of the nose, earlobes, and tongue. Raynaud's phenomenon occurs at some time during the disease in more than 95% of persons with systemic sclerosis.

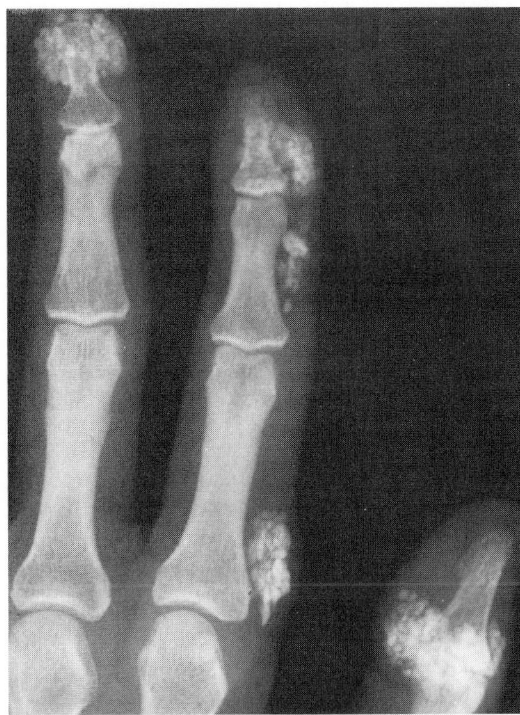

FIGURE 79.6. Close-up hand radiograph of a 46-year-old woman with limited cutaneous systemic sclerosis. Note extensive subcutaneous calcinosis.

Many patients with bilateral Raynaud's phenomenon without obvious symptoms or signs of underlying connective tissue disease are referred to internists or rheumatologists for evaluation. In some of these individuals, a connective tissue disorder will develop within the first 2 years after the onset of Raynaud's phenomenon (42). After 2 years, few patients (<5%) do so, and they almost all ultimately have scleroderma with limited skin thickening (43). Clinical clues predicting the subsequent appearance of systemic sclerosis in patients with only Raynaud's phenomenon include sclerodactyly, puffy fingers, digital pitting scars, capillary microscopic abnormalities (44), and systemic sclerosis–related serum autoantibodies (7,45).

In most cases of systemic sclerosis, Raynaud's phenomenon begins at the same time as skin changes and/or rheumatic complaints or precedes the latter by a few months to a year. In patients with the limited cutaneous variant, Raynaud's phenomenon may antedate other evidence of disease by many years. In contrast, in up to 20% of patients with the diffuse cutaneous subtype, skin thickening is noted before Raynaud's phenomenon occurs. This "reverse" order of events, with skin thickening preceding Raynaud's phenomenon, has been found to predict subsequent diffuse skin thickening and renal involvement (46). Because it is almost universal in systemic sclerosis, the presence or absence of Raynaud's phenomenon has little prognostic importance.

Small areas of fingertip ischemic necrosis or ulceration are frequent, often leaving pitted scars. Gangrene of the terminal portions of the phalanges occurs in a few patients. Angiographic and autopsy studies have disclosed narrowing and obstruction of the digital arteries (47). At necropsy, these vessels typically show prominent intimal and adventitial fibrosis without evidence of inflammation (Fig. 79.7). When severe, such pathologic changes lead to considerable luminal narrowing or occlusion. Recent or old thrombosis is frequently found, and 25% of vessels have a distinctive lesion: telangiectases of the vasa vasorum (47). Similar alterations have been noted in larger arteries (e.g., radial, ulnar, or popliteal) and are not due to atherosclerosis (47,48). A Doppler study identified the ulnar artery as particularly narrow compared with those in matched control subjects (49), and a case–control analysis implicated peripheral vascular but not coronary artery or cerebrovascular disease (50). Arterial occlusions occur in limited cutaneous scleroderma (48) and have been associated with anticardiolipin antibody (51). A subset of patients has been described with limited skin thickening, ischemia, and amputations of mul-

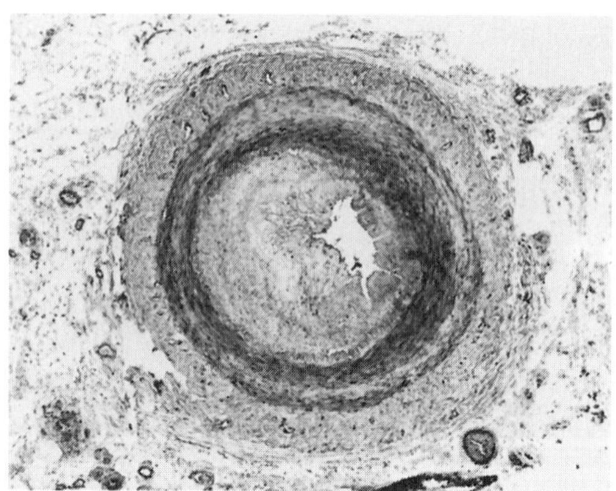

FIGURE 79.7. Photomicrograph of a digital artery obtained at autopsy from a 45-year-old woman with diffuse cutaneous systemic sclerosis who had Raynaud's phenomenon for more than 20 years before her death. Near occlusion of the lumen is due to subintimal proliferation and striking periadventitial fibrosis.

tiple digits, anticentromere antibody, immunoglobulin M (IgM) anticardiolipin antibodies, and "vasculitis" on histologic examination of their digital vessels (52).

On microscopic examination, the capillary circulation is altered by the appearance of dilated or "giant" loops, and in diffuse scleroderma, by a paucity of nailfold vessels or "dropout" (Fig. 79.8) (53). Complete arrest of blood flow in these vessels has been observed after cold exposure (54). Capillary microscopic patterns are interpreted from photographs (55), and semiquantitative grading scales have been devised for both capillary size and extent of "avascularity" (56). These observations are a useful permanent record of the state of the microvasculature in a given patient. Nailfold biopsy has confirmed the accuracy of *in vivo* microscopy (57). In addition to the vascular changes, including multilayering of the basal lamina, a high proportion of patients have perivascular mononuclear cell collections and immunoglobulin deposits (58), as well as increased perivascular fibroblasts and mast cells (59). Such capillary abnormalities are an early predictor of evolution to scleroderma in persons who clinically appear to have Raynaud's phenomenon alone (60). Differences in nailfold capillary patterns help to identify patients with other diseases, such as SLE and RA (61). Although a relation between reduced number and increased size of nailfold capillaries and visceral organ involvement in systemic sclerosis has been claimed (62), not all authors agree (63).

Patients with Raynaud's phenomenon, with or without scleroderma, have a persistently reduced digital pad temperature in the basal state and subnormal capillary blood flow in the fingers in both warm and cool environments (64). Reduction in finger systolic blood pressure (65), unaltered by blockade of the sympathetic nervous system (66), has been observed. Together with delay in rewarming of the fingers after cold exposure, these findings suggest structural as well as functional narrowing of blood vessels. A progressive depletion of peripheral sensory nervous system fibers

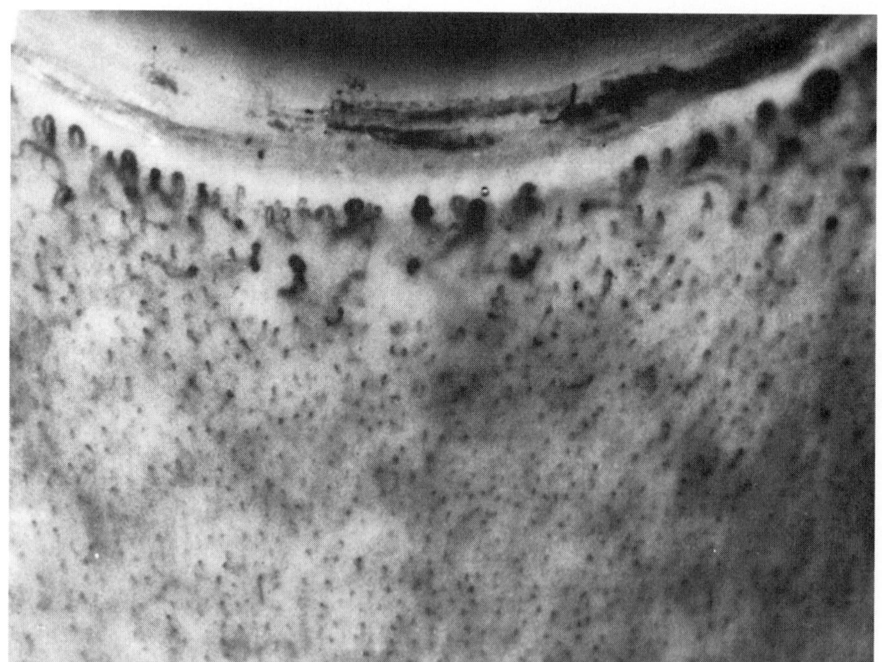

FIGURE 79.8. Nailfold capillary pattern of a patient with diffuse cutaneous systemic sclerosis (×18). Note extensive avascular area along the edge of the nailfold and grossly enlarged capillary loops. (Reproduced with permission from Maricq HR, LeRoy EC. Capillary blood flow in scleroderma. *Bibl Anat* 1973;11:352–358).

has been postulated, leading to impaired neuronal input into vascular tone control, resulting in unopposed vasoconstricting effects of endothelial cell injury and platelet factors (67). Endothelin-1, a potent vasoconstrictor peptide released by endothelial cells, is increased in plasma of patients with scleroderma-related but not primary Raynaud's phenomenon or other connective tissue disease–associated secondary Raynaud's phenomenon (68,69). However, blood levels of endothelin-1 could not be increased by inducing Raynaud's phenomenon in patients with scleroderma (69).

The plasma activity of a product of endothelial cells, factor VIII/von Willebrand factor antigen (VWF), was increased under basal conditions (70) and even more after cold exposure (71) in patients with scleroderma. Elevated plasma VWF levels have been associated with reduced ethylenediaminetetraacetic acid (EDTA) creatinine clearance and pulmonary arterial hypertension in the absence of pulmonary fibrosis (72). Also observed were decreased platelet serotonin content, presumably secondary to its release (73), increased serotonin-induced platelet aggregation (74), and increased levels of circulating platelet aggregates and plasma β-thromboglobulin, presumed to reflect vascular injury and repair (75,76). Measurement of β-thromboglobulin may differentiate patients with systemic sclerosis from those with primary Raynaud's phenomenon (76).

Joints, Tendons, and Bones

Symmetric polyarthralgias and joint stiffness of the fingers, wrists, knees, and ankles are frequent initial or early complaints. Generalized swelling of the fingers also occurs. It is difficult to ascertain the degree to which limitation of interphalangeal joint motion is caused by joint, periarticular, or tenosynovial disease, or by changes in the skin. Synovitis mimicking that of RA is uncommon, but may be the first manifestation of diffuse cutaneous disease. Larger peripheral joints are occasionally slightly warm or swollen, and contain scanty synovial fluid with predominantly mononuclear leukocytes numbering less than 3,000/mm^3. Pathologic examination of involved synovium reveals variable numbers of chronic inflammatory cells, either in focal aggregates or scattered diffusely (77). Fibrin deposition on the synovial surface is frequent. Patients with typical subcutaneous calcinosis also may develop extensive calcification of the synovium and tendon sheaths (78). The synovial fluid in such cases is milky or chalky and contains large numbers of hydroxyapatite crystals (79).

Some patients are aware of a "squeaking" sensation on movement of their extremities. A distinctive coarse, leathery crepitus (tendon friction rub) may be palpated over such areas during joint motion, particularly over the olecranon bursae, wrist and finger flexor and extensor tendons, distal quadriceps tendons superior to the knees, anterior tibial tendons above the ankles, and Achilles tendons. Such rubs are due to fibrinous deposits on the surfaces of tendon sheaths and overlying fascia and are relatively specific for scleroderma with diffuse cutaneous involvement. Friction rubs often antedate an explosive increase in skin thickening and are associated with reduced survival (80). Carpal tunnel syndrome is caused by flexor tenosynovitis at the wrist.

Flexion contractures ("bowed fingers") are attributed, at least in part, to tendinous and periarticular fibrosis and shortening (81) and true arthritis. These contractures, which occur commonly in the fingers, wrists, elbows, and ankles, usually become apparent within several months of the onset of diffuse disease and may rapidly result in significant disability (82).

The most frequent bony radiographic abnormality is partial resorption of the tufts of the terminal phalanges of the fingers; complete dissolution of the terminal phalanx is rare. The cause of tuft resorption is unknown but is presumed to be ischemic. In a few patients, severe erosive changes of the finger joints develop, which radiographically most closely resemble osteoarthritis (OA) (83). Overlap with the radiographic features of classic RA also is recognized (84). Other examples of bone resorption include "notching" of the superior margins of the posterior ribs (85) and dissolution of the condyle and ramus of the mandible (86), both of which have been reported exclusively in patients with diffuse scleroderma.

Skeletal Muscle

In most instances, weakness and atrophy of skeletal muscle result from disuse because of joint contractures or chronic disease. Approximately 20% of patients have a primary myopathy (87). Typically, this is a subtle process, with weakness noted by the examining physician but not the patient, mild or no serum muscle enzyme elevation, and muscle biopsy showing focal replacement of myofibrils with collagenous connective tissue and perimysial and epimysial fibrosis without inflammatory changes. This bland myopathy is distinctive in that it seldom occurs in patients with other connective tissue diseases. It is nonprogressive and does not warrant intervention. In contrast, a minority of patients exhibit more pronounced proximal muscle weakness and electrophysiologic, biochemical, and pathologic evidence of polymyositis (87,88). These persons have been classified as having either systemic sclerosis with myositis or systemic sclerosis in overlap with polymyositis.

Gastrointestinal Tract

Oral Cavity

Thinning of the lips (microcheilia) and reduced oral aperture (microstomia) are frequent. Temporomandibular joint involvement may also limit mouth opening in some patients (86). In the CREST variant, numerous lip and buccal mucosa telangiectases are common. Atrophy of the mucous membrane and tongue papillae with impaired taste perception has been reported (89). Thickening of the periodontal membrane occurs in up to 30% of patients and is due to fibrosis (90). Loss of the lamina dura with gingivitis and subsequent loosening of the teeth also has been noted. These problems are compounded by the mechanical difficulty of maintaining good oral hygiene (finger contractures, limited oral opening) and by associated Sjögren's syndrome.

Esophagus and Stomach

Esophageal dysfunction eventually develops in nearly 80% of patients, thus constituting the most common visceral manifestation. No predilection for either the diffuse or limited disease subtype has been noted. In some instances, this abnormality, usually accompanied by Raynaud's phenomenon, occurs long before evidence of cutaneous involvement.

As a result of incoordination of the normal propulsive peristalsis of distal esophageal smooth muscle, solids (meat, bread) become transiently "stuck" in the mid or lower esophagus. Patients appreciate this problem in a retrosternal location during food ingestion and often need to drink liquids for relief. A second abnormality is incomplete closure of the lower esophageal sphincter, which leads to gastroesophageal reflux with peptic esophagitis. Although some patients have no symptoms, most complain about retrosternal burning pain, postprandial fullness, or acid regurgitation, especially after eating too close to bedtime or on reclining at night, when the protective effect of gravity is absent. Despite the frequency of peptic esophagitis, and the presence of mucosal telangiectases in that area, esophageal hemorrhage is surprisingly unusual. After years of inadequately treated reflux esophagitis, distal esophageal stricture is likely to develop, leading to reduced oral intake and, on occasion, loss of appreciable amounts of weight. Pharyngoesophageal dysphagia, caused by dysfunction of upper esophageal striated muscle, may occur with or without associated polymyositis (91). The result is incoordination of the initiation of swallowing, leading to regurgitation of liquids through the nose and occasionally aspiration into the tracheobronchial tree (92). This complication is most likely to develop in patients with severe esophageal reflux.

Radiographic abnormalities are found in three fourths of patients studied, including some who have no esophageal symptoms, irrespective of their classification as having diffuse or limited cutaneous disease. Cinefluoroscopic examination, the standard method of evaluation, reveals diminished or absent peristaltic activity in the distal esophagus and gastroesophageal reflux. Esophageal pH monitoring may be useful in documenting the presence of reflux (93). Esophagitis has been found to be more frequent in patients with diffuse cutaneous involvement (94). Chronic reflux predisposes to Barrett's metaplasia (95) and thus, theoretically, to adenocarcinoma of the esophagus, although there is no published support for this sequence of events in systemic sclerosis (96). Incoordination and loss of contractile power and a reduction in the tone of the gastroesophageal sphincter can be confirmed by manometric measurements, which are more sensitive but less well tolerated than standard barium radiography (97). Radionuclide scintigraphy has the advantages of being quantitative and easy for patients to complete; it gives results that correlate highly with manometric measurements (98). Specificity for systemic sclerosis is lacking, however, because abnormal radionuclide studies also have been reported in other connective tissue diseases and in normal subjects (99).

Gastric atony and dilatation may occur, but involvement of the stomach is uncommon compared with other portions of the alimentary tract. Gastric acid secretion is unimpaired, but both hyperchlorhydria and increased basal and/or stimulated gastric acid output have been reported (100). In rare instances, telangiectases have been considered the source of serious bleeding from the distal esophagus, stomach, or other gastrointestinal tract sites, especially in persons with limited cutaneous disease (101). Heavy bleeding may result from an unusual condition termed "watermelon stomach," in which ectatic capillaries and dilated submucosal vessels are so prominent that they are grossly visible as broad "stripes" at endoscopy (102). Watermelon stomach has been reported as the initial manifestation of systemic sclerosis in two patients (103).

Histologic changes are most significant in the lower two thirds of the esophagus, where thinning of the mucosa and cellular infiltrates in the submucosa have been noted. There is increased collagen in the lamina propria and the muscularis, which may be almost totally replaced by fibrous tissue. The walls of small arteries and arterioles are thickened and often surrounded by periadventitial deposits of collagen, but physiologic and pharmacologic studies of esophageal blood flow have not been performed. The myenteric plexuses of Auerbach, which may be conspicuously lacking in ganglion cells, usually appear to be normal.

Small Intestine

In a small proportion of patients, the illness is dominated by intestinal complaints consisting of severe postprandial bloating and abdominal cramps. These symptoms occur because of hypomotility of the small intestine and may result in a functional ileus (pseudo-obstruction) with symptoms simulating mechanical obstruction.

Hypomotility favors the overgrowth of intestinal microorganisms that consume large amounts of vitamin B_{12} and interfere with normal fat absorption as a result of their deconjugation of bile salts. Profuse watery diarrhea, weight loss, and extreme wasting can ensue despite adequate caloric intake, resulting in malabsorption (104). Other deficiencies encountered in this circumstance include iron (duodenal malabsorption) and calcium. Radiographic findings consist of prolonged retention of barium in the atonic and widely dilated second and third portions of the duodenum (loop sign) and irregular flocculation or hypersegmentation of barium or localized areas of dilatation of the jejunum and/or ileum. The mucosa of the distended jejunum is arranged in prominent transverse folds (Fig. 79.9). The first case of extensive small intestinal telangiectasia has recently been reported (105). The valvulae conniventes remain close to one another despite pronounced dilatation of the lumen ("closed accordion" sign), presumably owing to excessive fibrosis of the submucosa. Similar changes occasionally are found in the ileum. Celiac disease may mimic malabsorption in scleroderma (106). Volvulus of a greatly dilated small intestine has been observed (107).

Pneumatosis intestinalis is an occasional complication of systemic sclerosis. Gas enters from the bowel lumen through small defects in the mucosa and muscularis mucosae and appears as numerous radiolucent cysts or linear streaks within the bowel wall. Rupture of these collections of air into the peritoneal space is occasionally accompanied by symptoms of partial bowel obstruction or by those mimicking a perforated viscus. Most often, however, such an event results only in asymptomatic pneumoperitoneum.

With the addition of serosal fibrosis, the pathologic changes in the small intestine are similar to those described for the esophagus (i.e., normal mucosa or mild villous atrophy, infiltration of the lamina propria by lymphocytes and plasma cells, fibrous thickening of the submucosa, atrophy of smooth muscle with collagenous replacement, and thickening of the walls of small arteries and arterioles). Peroral biopsy specimens of the duodenum have revealed increased amounts of collagen surrounding and infiltrating Brunner's glands. Similar periglandular fibrosis is seen involving the esophageal, minor salivary, nasal mucosal, and thyroid glands (108–110).

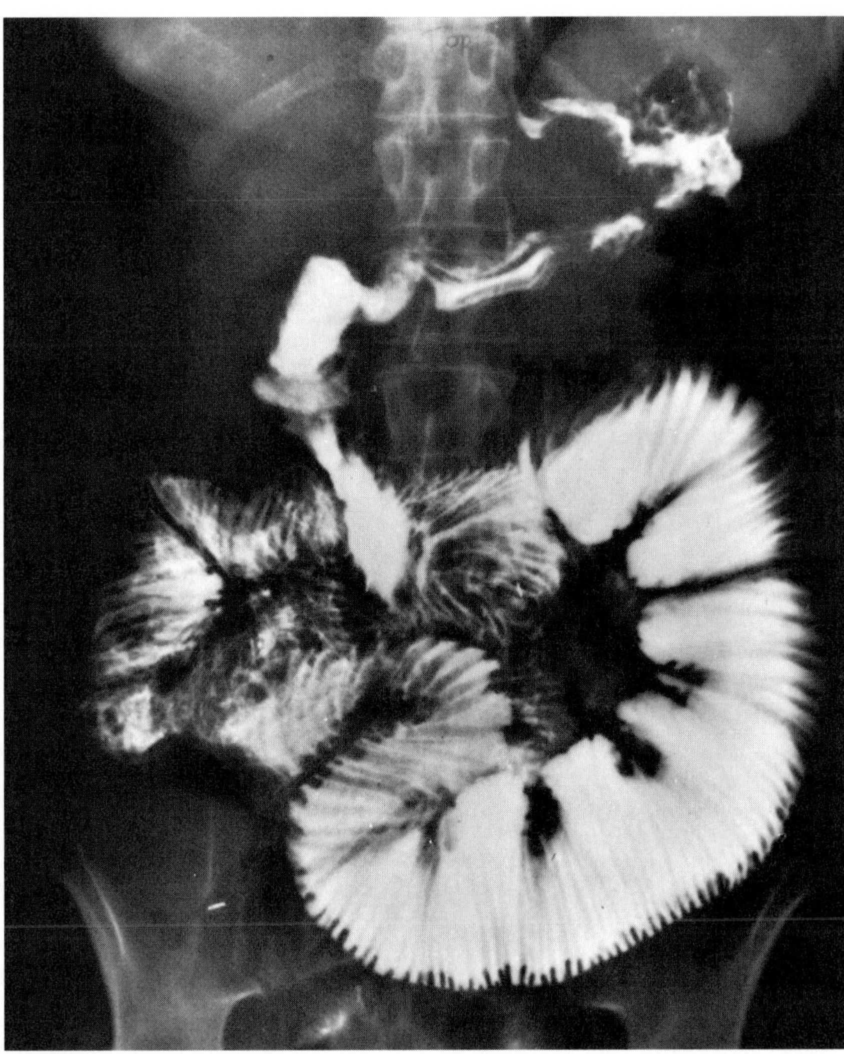

FIGURE 79.9. Upper gastrointestinal tract roentgenogram in a 46-year-old woman with diffuse cutaneous systemic sclerosis. Although dilatation of the jejunum is striking, its valvulae conniventes remain closely approximated (*closed accordion sign*).

Colon

Constipation, either alone or alternating with diarrhea, may signal colonic involvement. Reduced anorectal capacity, motility, compliance, and sphincter pressure have been reported (111,112), and in one study, the frequencies of anorectal and esophageal dysmotility were similar (113). Rectal incontinence and prolapse are uncommon but disabling problems (114). Patchy atrophy of the muscularis leads to the development of wide-mouthed diverticula, which usually occur along the antimesenteric border of the transverse and descending colon (Fig. 79.10). They are almost entirely unique to systemic sclerosis, having been described only in a single patient with amyloidosis (115). Ordinarily, these outpouchings cause no difficulty, but rarely they may perforate or become impacted with fecal matter, producing obstruction (116).

Lung

Lung involvement occurs in more than 70% of patients (117) and during the past 15 years has emerged as the most common disease-related cause of death. The most prominent symptom is exertional dyspnea, which is present in nearly half of patients. Less often, there is a chronic cough, which is nonproductive unless associated with superimposed infection. Many patients remain entirely asymptomatic, despite radiographic and functional evidence of pulmonary interstitial fibrosis, possibly because their physical activity is restricted by musculoskeletal disease. Limited exercise tolerance may be independent of both lung and heart involvement, occurring instead because of diffuse microvascular damage with impaired oxygen diffusion (118). Occasionally, pleuritic chest pain is appreciated, but pleural friction rubs are uncommon, and exudative pleural effusions are rare.

Pulmonary function abnormalities occur in more than two thirds of all patients, irrespective of disease variant (85,119). A restrictive ventilatory defect, indicated by a reduction in forced vital capacity and decreased lung compliance, is most common and generally accompanies interstitial lung disease. Impairment in gas exchange, evidenced by a reduced diffusing capacity for carbon monoxide, also is usually present in patients with restrictive lung disease, but may occur as an isolated defect without significant alteration in ventilation or roentgenographic evidence of fibrosis. A few patients have obstructive disease, but this finding is most often attributable to cigarette smoking (120). In longitudinal studies of pulmonary function, no excessive deterioration occurred in patients with scleroderma compared with a normal population (121,122).

Interstitial Fibrosis

In more than one third of patients with both diffuse and limited cutaneous scleroderma, the chest radiograph discloses interstitial thickening in a reticular pattern of linear, nodular, and lineonodular densities most pronounced in the lower lung fields. The radiographic appearance is that of diffuse mottling or "honeycombing," indicative of fibrosis with cystic lesions. Dry bibasilar end-inspiratory "fibrotic" rales are frequently heard in these persons. In some patients with interstitial involvement, progressive, fatal respiratory failure

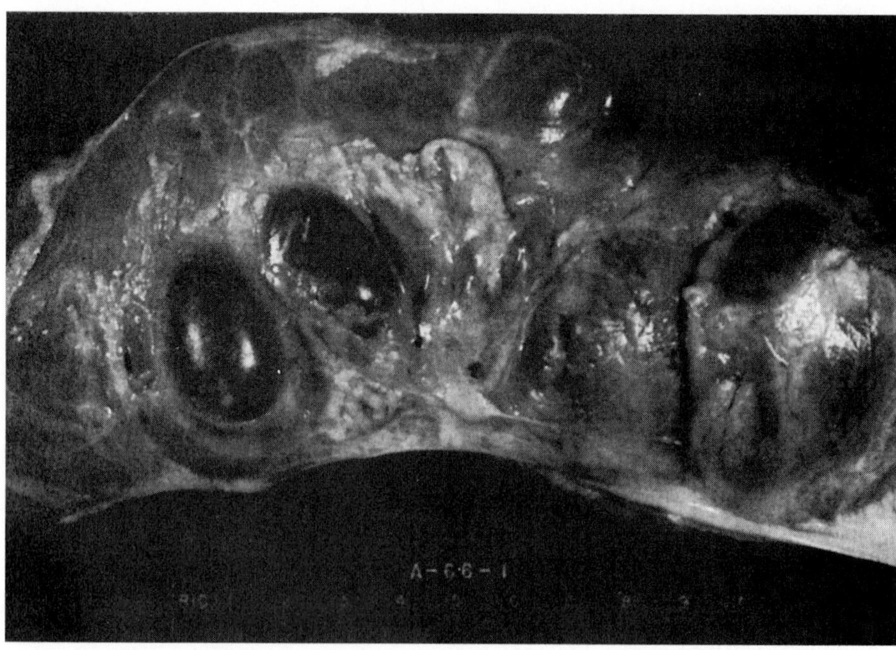

FIGURE 79.10. Gross appearance of the transverse colon from a patient with limited cutaneous systemic sclerosis showing numerous wide-mouthed colonic diverticula, which had been demonstrated previously on barium enema.

develops. At greatest risk are younger individuals, blacks, and male patients, as well as those with diffuse cutaneous disease and serum anti–topoisomerase I antibody (123).

High-resolution computerized tomography (HRCT) is a more sensitive method for detecting interstitial lung disease and is abnormal in 75% of patients with systemic sclerosis with normal chest radiographs (124,125). This technique may identify a "ground-glass" appearance, which is believed to represent inflammation (alveolitis), as indicated in two studies in which the HRCT grade was compared with that of open lung biopsy specimens (126,127). At this stage, HRCT (126) and/or gallium scanning (128,129) are abnormal in many patients. Alveolitis has been documented by bronchoalveolar lavage, with large numbers of macrophages and lymphocytes and increased proportions of neutrophils and/or eosinophils in the lavage fluid (130–133). It is believed that mononuclear cell products, particularly platelet-derived growth factor (PDGF) and transforming growth factor-β (TGF-β) are important stimulants of the proliferation of lung fibroblasts (134) and that certain cytokines produced by $CD8^+$ T cells in bronchoalveolar lavage fluid [interferon-γ (IFN-γ), interleukin-4 (IL-4), IL-5] are associated with reduced pulmonary function over time (135).

The predominant histologic changes in interstitial fibrosis, present in nearly all cases at postmortem examination, consist of diffuse alveolar, interstitial, peribronchial, and pleural fibrosis (Fig. 79.11). A moderate degree of "secondary" pulmonary hypertension, with a relatively slow progression, follows widespread pulmonary interstitial fibrosis, because the fibrotic process very gradually obliterates more and more of the pulmonary vascular bed.

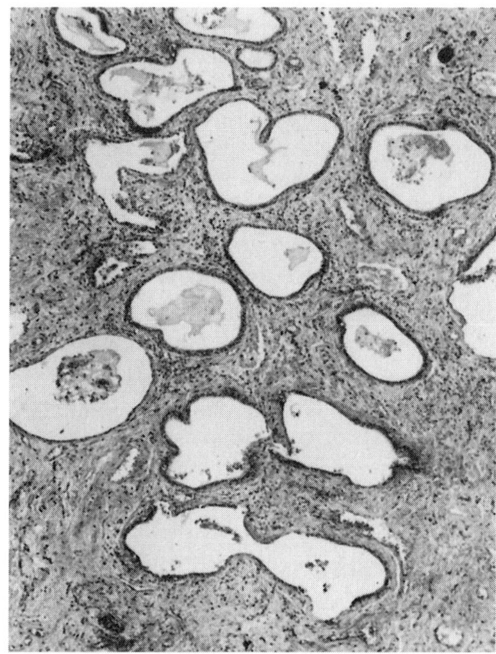

FIGURE 79.11. Photomicrograph of the lung of a 52-year-old woman with diffuse cutaneous systemic sclerosis who died as the result of respiratory insufficiency. Note the dramatic interstitial fibrosis and dilatation of air sacs (honeycomb lung).

Pulmonary Arterial Hypertension

A very different clinical entity is severe "primary" pulmonary arterial hypertension with minimal or no pulmonary interstitial fibrosis. This complication is encountered predominantly in a subset of patients with limited cutaneous involvement followed up for 10 to 30 years (136), but occasionally is found in individuals with diffuse skin thickening who also have anti-U3RNP antibody (137). The rate of progression of dyspnea is alarmingly rapid in this circumstance. A patient may go from normal exercise tolerance to oxygen dependence in 6 to 12 months. In contrast, individuals with interstitial lung disease have a similar degree of disability develop over 2 to 10 years. There is frequently accentuation of the pulmonic component of the second heart sound, and ultimately, signs of right-sided cardiac failure. The diffusing capacity is extremely low, consistent with impaired gas exchange across thickened small pulmonary blood vessels (138). Diagnosis is confirmed by echocardiogram or by right heart catheterization with direct measurement of the pulmonary artery pressure. The mean duration of survival from detection of primary pulmonary hypertension is 2 years, emphasizing its serious nature (136). Pathologic findings include medial smooth muscle hypertrophy and uniform narrowing and/or occlusion of small pulmonary arteries caused by subintimal proliferative changes without evidence of vasculitis (Fig. 79.12) (136,139). The existence of "pulmonary Raynaud's phenomenon" is controversial (140).

As expected, reduced diffusing capacity (40% or less of predicted normal) and an obstructive ventilatory defect have been found to be associated with increased mortality (141). Lung cancer occurs with increased frequency in late-stage systemic sclerosis, generally in the setting of long-standing pulmonary fibrosis with intense bronchiolar epithelial proliferation and cellular atypia and is independent of cigarette smoking (142,143).

Heart

Cardiac involvement may be classified as primary or secondary (144–146). Primary disease consists of pericarditis with or without effusion, left ventricular or biventricular congestive failure, or a serious supraventricular or ventricular arrhythmia. Patients with scleroderma develop atherosclerosis and hypertensive heart disease with frequencies similar to their occurrence in the general population. For this reason, one should assume that scleroderma is the cause of heart disease only after an appropriate search has excluded common etiologies.

Small pericardial effusions and pericardial thickening are detected frequently by echocardiography. Acute sympto-

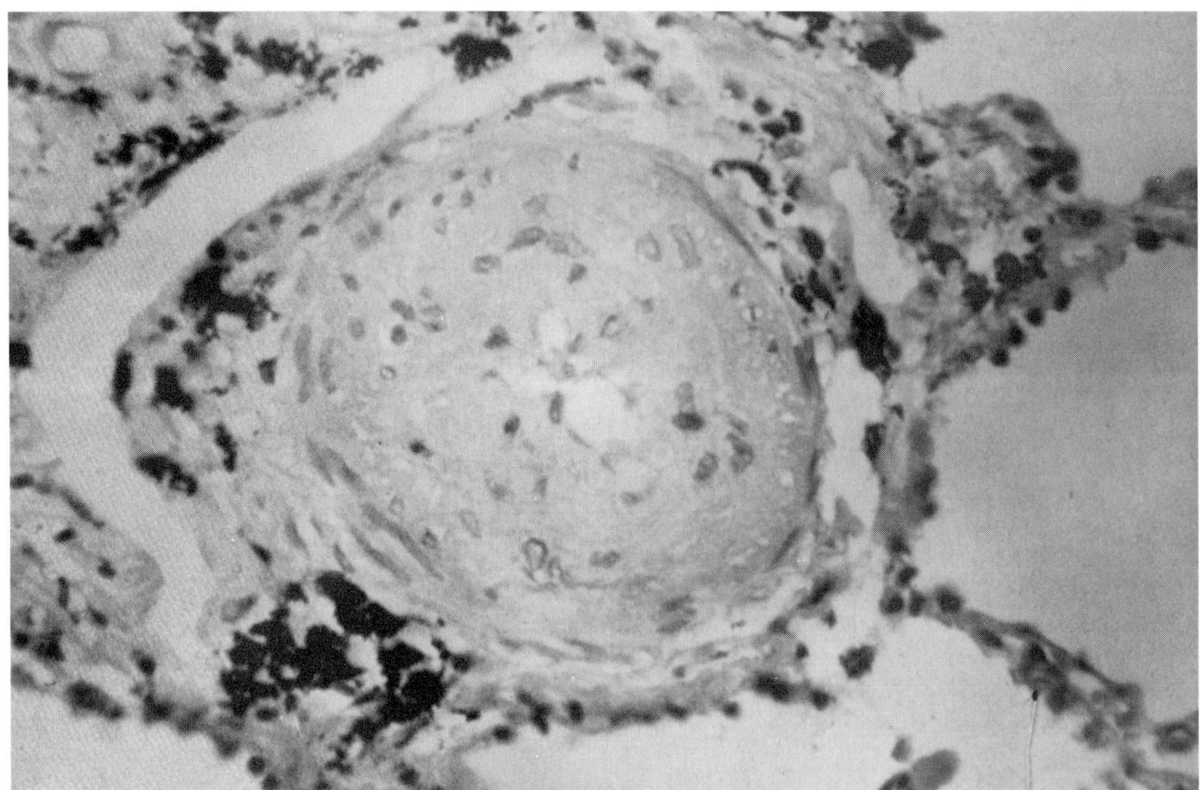

FIGURE 79.12. Photomicrograph of the lung of a 61-year-old woman with systemic sclerosis and limited scleroderma who died as the result of pulmonary arterial hypertension with cor pulmonale. There is significant intimal proliferation and medial hypertrophy of this small pulmonary artery and no interstitial fibrosis.

matic pericarditis is unusual, and cardiac tamponade is rare. Pericardial effusion may antedate renal involvement (147, 148), and massive effusions have been noted to occur in persons with diffuse scleroderma and anti–topoisomerase I antibody (148). The few reported pericardial fluids were exudates with low white blood cell counts and no evidence of immune complexes or complement activation.

Clinical evidence of left-sided congestive failure secondary to myocardial fibrosis occurs in fewer than 5% of patients, nearly all of whom have diffuse cutaneous involvement. New noninvasive radionuclide studies, however, show that subtle abnormalities of ventricular function, including diastolic dysfunction, are frequent and may be associated with diminished cardiac functional reserve (149–151). These changes have been associated with a long duration of Raynaud's phenomenon (151) and have been attributed to microvascular obliteration and diffuse atrophy and fibrous replacement of functioning myocardium. Myocarditis has been reported in four patients with scleroderma who also had typical polymyositis (152,153). Based on abnormal myocardial gallium scans, a larger proportion of older patients with systemic sclerosis may have subtle myocardial interstitial inflammation (154). The relation between skeletal and cardiac muscle involvement is emphasized by a report of the strong association of these findings in 25 patients, many of whom died suddenly, presumably due to cardiac arrhythmias (155).

Although a few patients have exertional chest pain that mimics angina pectoris, coronary angiograms are most often normal. Electrocardiographic evidence of myocardial ischemia and/or necrosis in the absence of the clinical syndrome of myocardial infarction has been noted (156). Both resting and reversible exercise and cold-induced myocardial perfusion defects and left ventricular dysfunction have been detected (157,158), especially in patients with diffuse disease (150) and long-standing Raynaud's phenomenon (158), raising the possibility that multiple vasospastic ischemic episodes can lead to myocardial fibrosis. These resting defects are reversible after administration of oral nifedipine (159) or intravenous dipyridamole (160). The latter potent vasodilator also was used to determine coronary blood flow and resistance reserve, which were reduced in patients with scleroderma cardiomyopathy compared with controls (161). These studies should be interpreted with caution, however, because the changes reported may not represent improvements in myocardial perfusion but, instead, may represent selective redistribution of blood flow to more healthy subepicardial regions (162).

Autopsies of patients with diffuse scleroderma may show extensive degeneration of myocardial fibers with replacement by irregular patches of fibrosis that are prominent in, but not limited to, perivascular areas (Fig. 79.13). Mast cells, recognized for their presence in increased numbers in areas of fibrosis, were prominent in three fatal cases of scleroderma heart disease (163). The pathologic finding of "contraction band necrosis" is consistent with the concept that heart damage may be due to intermittent vascular spasm or "intramyocardial Raynaud's phenomenon" (164). The large extramural coronary arteries are typically normal, but focal infiltrates of round cells and considerable thickening of smaller coronary vessels may occur (165). Myocardial infarction is unusual.

Cardiac arrhythmias, including complete heart block and other electrocardiographic abnormalities, are encountered, as expected, in cardiomyopathy regardless of cause. During 24-hour continuous electrocardiography (Holter monitor), one fifth of patients with scleroderma had conduction defects in a point-prevalence study (166). Arrhythmias may limit exercise performance in up to one third of patients (167). Careful dissection of the conduction system of several patients with rhythm disturbances, including complete heart block, has revealed fibrous replacement of the sinus node; atrioventricular node, particularly in its proximal segment (168); and bundle branches (169). In most cases, however, no specific morphologic changes have been identified in this specialized tissue, and arrhythmias have been attributed to disturbances of the myocardium.

Valvular heart disease is uncommonly encountered, but, when present, may be associated with the antiphospholipid antibody syndrome (170), akin to Libman–Sacks endocarditis in SLE.

Secondary causes of heart disease in scleroderma are pulmonary and systemic arterial hypertension. The former occurs chiefly in the limited cutaneous variant, as noted previously. Severe systemic arterial hypertension associated with renal involvement frequently leads to acute myocardial dysfunction, which is typically reversible with control of blood pressure.

Kidney

Renal disease is an important aspect of systemic sclerosis and in previous decades has been the major cause of death (171). Clinically evident renal involvement is restricted almost exclusively to persons with diffuse cutaneous disease, especially those with rapidly progressive skin thickening of less than 3 years' duration (172). Rarely is a person with the limited cutaneous variant or systemic sclerosis sine scleroderma (173) affected; most such cases are misclassified during an early stage in the evolution of diffuse disease.

In 20% of patients with diffuse cutaneous scleroderma, a dramatic complication termed *scleroderma renal crisis*

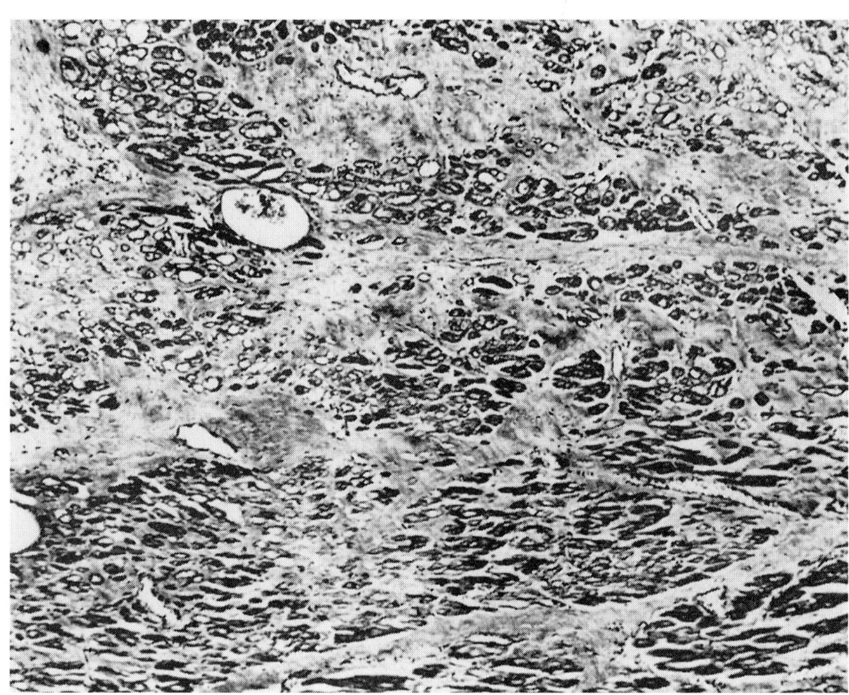

FIGURE 79.13. Photomicrograph of myocardium of a 52-year-old woman with diffuse cutaneous systemic sclerosis who died of congestive heart failure. Loss of normal myocardial fibers is extensive, and interstitial fibrosis is severe.

develops, with the abrupt onset of accelerated hypertension, followed promptly by rapidly progressive oliguric renal failure. In some populations, renal crisis is considerably less frequent for unknown reasons (174). The presenting symptoms are varied and include headache, visual blurring from hypertensive retinopathy, seizures, and acute dyspnea due to sudden left ventricular failure. Within several days or weeks, microscopic hematuria and low-grade proteinuria are noted, along with rapidly increasing azotemia, and finally, oliguria or anuria. Severe hypertension is typically associated with extremely high plasma renin levels, but baseline plasma renin levels do not predict outcome (175).

On occasion, the blood pressure may remain within normal limits, and azotemia and severe microangiopathic hemolytic anemia become the dominant features (176). Prior administration of corticosteroids has been associated with the normotensive type (176). A recent retrospective case–control study identified an increased risk of renal crisis associated with antecedent corticosteroid therapy with prednisone [15 mg/day or the equivalent (177)]. Sudden, severe volume depletion also may trigger renal crisis in the susceptible patient, who often has had clinically undetected reduced renal blood flow.

Renal angiography, during life and postmortem injection studies, has demonstrated a striking constriction of interlobular arteries and afferent arterioles and a sharp decrease in glomerular perfusion (Fig. 79.14) (178). When microangiopathic hemolysis is the dominant clinical feature, the possibility of concomitant thrombotic thrombocytopenic purpura is inevitably raised (179). All clinical manifestations in such cases can be comfortably accounted for by "scleroderma renal crisis," however, suggesting that only one disease is present.

Before the 1980s, survival for more than 3 to 6 months after the onset of renal crisis was almost unknown. Control of malignant hypertension was difficult or impossible, and nearly all patients died of renal or cardiac failure or cerebral hemorrhage. Today the aggressive use of potent new drugs that block the renin–angiotensin system is uniformly successful in controlling hypertension, although renal insufficiency may nevertheless progress, requiring dialysis. In many instances, it has been possible to discontinue dialysis after several months (180). Simultaneous impressive reduction in skin thickness has been noted in some, but not all, patients who have survived renal crisis (181).

Numerous small cortical infarcts are seen grossly in the affected kidneys. Focal microscopic alterations consist of subintimal proliferative changes in the intralobular arteries, intimal hyperplasia with acid mucopolysaccharide deposition, and necrosis of the walls of these vessels, afferent arterioles, and glomerular tufts (Fig. 79.15). Only prominent fibrosis of the adventitia of the small vessels may distinguish this lesion from that of nonsclerodermatous malignant nephrosclerosis (178). Identical histopathologic changes have been observed in the absence of hypertension (182). These alterations are reminiscent of those encountered in the digital vessels, as discussed earlier.

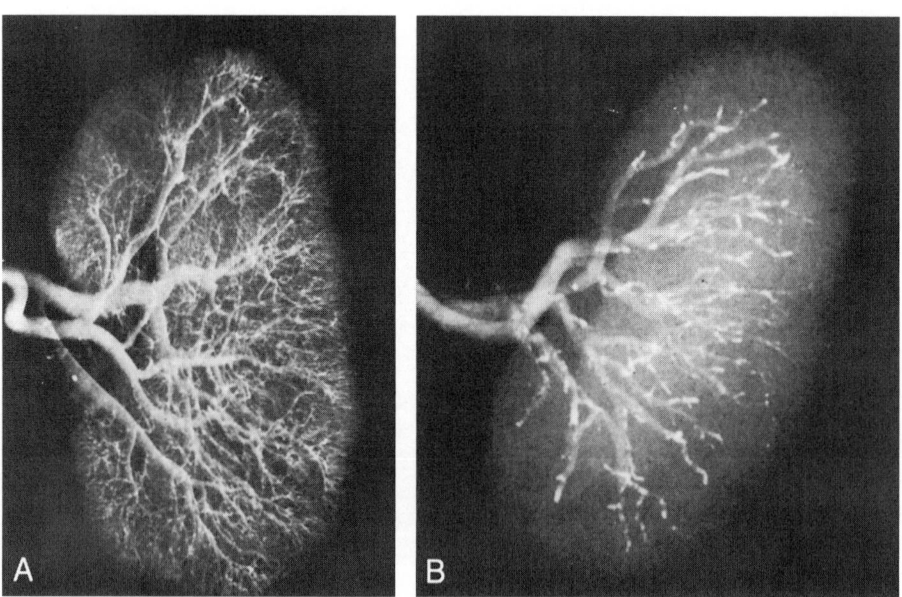

FIGURE 79.14. Radiographs of kidneys, injected postmortem, of two patients with diffuse cutaneous systemic sclerosis. **A:** Kidney of a man who died of cardiac disease without clinical evidence of renal involvement. Filling of the interlobular and small cortical vessels is normal. **B:** Kidney of a man in whom "scleroderma renal crisis" with malignant hypertension and renal failure developed. There is irregular narrowing of the interlobular vessels and little filling of smaller vessels supplying the renal cortex.

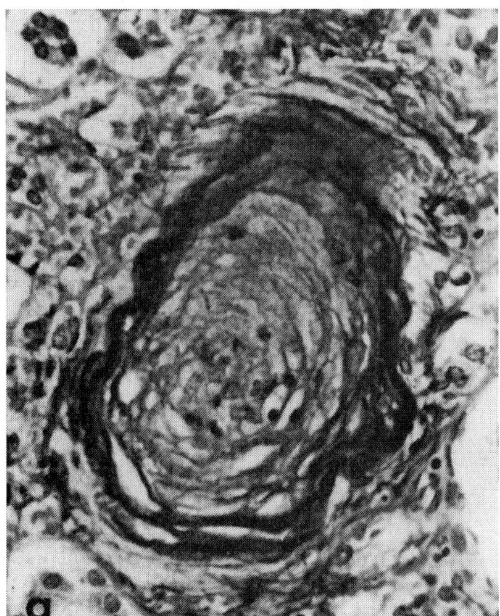

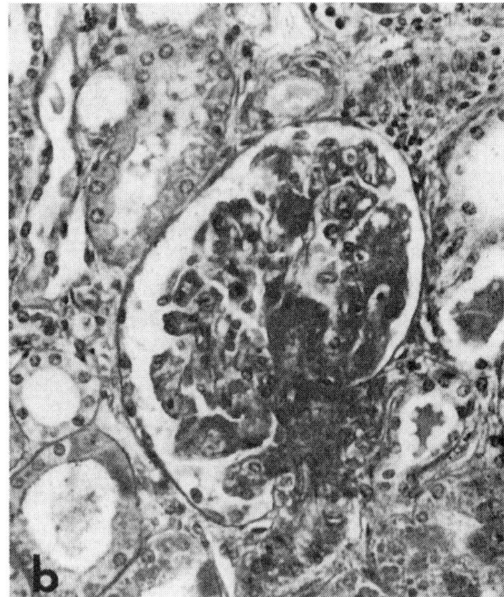

FIGURE 79.15. Photomicrographs of kidneys of two women who died of malignant arterial hypertension and renal insufficiency complicating diffuse cutaneous systemic sclerosis. **A:** Intimal hyperplasia with complete luminal occlusion of an interlobular artery. Note reduplication and fraying of the internal elastic lamina (orcein stain). **B:** Fibrinoid necrosis of blood vessels in the glomerulus.

Immunohistologic examination has revealed the regular presence of immunoglobulins (chiefly IgM), complement components (also reported in malignant hypertension not associated with systemic sclerosis), and fibrinogen in the walls of affected vessels (183,184), but these changes also are seen in accelerated essential hypertension. Electron-microscopic examination, however, has failed to reveal discrete electron-dense deposits or other features indicative of the presence of immune complexes (183).

Genitourinary Tract

Symptomatic sclerodermatous involvement of the lower urinary tract is rare, although histologic evidence of increased bladder wall connective tissue deposition and proliferative vascular lesions has been reported (185). Vaginal symptoms are common, including dryness, dyspareunia, and difficulty achieving orgasm (186). Vaginal tightness and constricted introitus contribute to these problems. Impotence without other obvious cause has been described and is most likely due to reduced penile blood flow (187). Detailed studies on a single patient have suggested another mechanism, venoocclusive disease and reduced penile length due to excessive synthesis of extracellular matrix proteins by trabecular smooth muscle cells (188).

Liver and Pancreas

Primary biliary cirrhosis occurs in some women with the limited cutaneous variant (189), most frequently in association with Sjögren's syndrome (190). In these patients, pruritus, jaundice, and hepatomegaly develop, with a pronounced elevation of serum alkaline phosphatase. Almost all have serum antimitochondrial antibodies, which are most often directed against the 72-kd M2 autoantigen (191). Nodular regenerative hyperplasia of the liver also has been reported (192). There is no convincing clinical evidence of pancreatic exocrine or endocrine dysfunction or increased pancreatic fibrosis at autopsy in systemic sclerosis cases compared with controls (193).

Blood

In typical systemic sclerosis, hematologic studies are normal. Abnormalities suggest either a specific complication or an associated illness (194). Only a few patients have anemia, the most common causes of which are chronic disease, gastrointestinal tract blood loss (peptic esophagitis or telangiectatic bleeding), excessive destruction (microangiopathic hemolysis), or metabolic (intestinal malabsorption). The peripheral blood and bone marrow reflect these circumstances, and the marrow is not fibrotic. Autoimmune hemolytic anemia (195) and neutropenia (196) have been noted. Leukopenia is occasionally present when systemic sclerosis exists in overlap with SLE or with mixed connective tissue disease (194). Impressive eosinophilia (>500 cells/mm^3) is unusual (197); its presence should alert the physician to the possibility that the correct diagnosis is one of the localized forms of scleroderma, such as eosinophilic fasciitis (see Chapter 80).

Nervous System

Primary symptomatic disorders of the nervous system are seldom encountered. Most neurologic abnormalities in patients with systemic sclerosis are either coincidental or represent secondary compressive phenomena (e.g., carpal tunnel syndrome). One study documented electrophysiologic abnormalities of sensory nerve conduction in the majority of patients tested (198). Trigeminal sensory neuropathy, an infrequent finding, is associated most closely with myositis and serum anti-U1RNP antibodies (199). Isolated central nervous system vasculitis has been reported but never proven histologically (200) and may represent the coexistence of systemic sclerosis and isolated angiitis of the central nervous system. Peripheral vasculitis believed due to coexisting Sjögren's syndrome has been described (201). Sjögren's syndrome has been implicated in patients with systemic sclerosis with sensorimotor polyneuropathy and myelopathy (202). Autonomic dysfunction has been observed, particularly affecting the gastrointestinal tract (203), in decreased parasympathetic control of heart rate (204), and in a syndrome characterized by sympathetic overactivity (205,206).

Eyes and Ears

With the exception of keratoconjunctivitis sicca, most symptomatic ocular disease in patients with systemic sclerosis is due to nonautoimmune conditions (207). Hypertensive retinopathy found in persons with renal crisis has already been described. Patchy areas of nonperfusion have been noted in the choroidal capillary bed (208). Sensorineural hearing loss was found in the majority of patients in one study and was not attributable to factors such as age, drugs, or noise (209).

Sjögren's Syndrome

Dry eyes and dry mouth are frequent complaints voiced by patients with systemic sclerosis. Dry mouth may be attributed to either lymphocytic infiltration of minor salivary glands on labial biopsy (15–20% of patients) (110) or to periglandular and intraglandular fibrosis (a similar proportion). A few affected persons have serum anti-SSA/Ro and/or anti-SSB/La antibodies, consisting almost exclusively of those with glandular lymphocytic infiltration rather than fibrosis (110). As in primary Sjögren's syndrome, vasculitis involving the skin (palpable purpura and leg ulcers) and peripheral nervous system (sensory neuropathy and mononeuritis multiplex) may occur (201). Those at risk for this complication have limited cutaneous changes, anti-SSA and/or anti-SSB antibodies, and hypocomplementemia (201).

Thyroid Gland

Hypothyroidism, often clinically unrecognized, occurs in one fourth of patients with systemic sclerosis and is frequently accompanied by serum antithyroid antibodies (210). As in the salivary glands, the histologic picture is varied. Fibrosis is a prominent histologic finding (109), whereas lymphocytic infiltration typical of Hashimoto's thyroiditis is unusual. Hyperthyroidism also has been noted (211).

Childhood Disease

Systemic sclerosis is rare in childhood (212). Most reported children have diffuse cutaneous disease (213) or overlap syndrome (214). Clinical findings are similar to those in adults except for an increased frequency of "renal crisis" among children (213,215–218). Serum antinucleolar antibodies may be more commonly detected in children than in adults (219).

Pregnancy

There is controversy concerning both fertility and the frequency of spontaneous abortion (220–222). Pregnancy appears to exert no consistent effect on the course of systemic sclerosis (221–224). Moreover, the disease ordinarily does not interfere with pregnancy or parturition. Nevertheless, participation in a high-risk obstetric monitoring program is recommended (225). Similar to those with other connective tissue diseases, women with established systemic sclerosis have a higher frequency of delayed conception, infertility, perinatal loss, and low birth weight in pregnancies that occurred before scleroderma onset, compared with healthy controls (226), for unknown reasons. Instances of hypertension alone (221), serious and fatal third trimester or postpartum renal involvement with severe hypertension (227,228), and nephrotic syndrome (229) have been reported but are likely unrepresentative. Women with early diffuse disease should be advised not to become pregnant until after skin thickening has peaked and has begun to improve.

Malignancy

The published frequency of cancer in large clinical series has varied from 3% to 7% (230–232). In the only studies in which population denominators and comparison groups have been used, several important associations have been detected. In two case series (230,233) and an epidemiologic study (142), breast cancer developed in a subset of women at or near the time of onset of scleroderma. Lung cancer is significantly more frequent than in the age- and sex-matched general population, occurs in the setting of longstanding scleroderma with pulmonary interstitial fibrosis, and is independent of cigarette smoking (142,143). Alveolar cell carcinoma, for many years believed to be a specific sequel of scleroderma, is only one of the pulmonary malignancies found and does not itself occur more often than expected (142). Surprisingly few lymphoproliferative malignancies have been reported in systemic sclerosis patients. As might be expected, however, the use of immunosuppressive agents may be followed by an excessive number of late lymphoproliferative neoplasms (234).

Radiation Therapy

Patients with systemic sclerosis may be extremely sensitive to the adverse effects of radiation therapy. Extensive local fibrosis has been observed in six patients 2 to 4 months after standard doses of radiation were delivered (235,236). Because radiation therapy is recognized to cause vascular damage, it seems likely that both disease and radiation combine to cause vascular obliteration and to intensify the sclerodermatous process.

Serum Autoantibodies

Moderate hypergammaglobulinemia (1.4–2.0 g/dL) occurs in more than one fourth of patients, most often in those with overlap syndromes. Typically, IgG is increased, but IgM elevation also has been observed (237). Monoclonal gammopathy and immunoglobulin deficiency are rare (238,239). Serum complement levels are normal except when Sjögren's syndrome with vasculitis coexists (201). One third of patients have positive tests for rheumatoid factor, usually in low titer.

With the use of multiple substrates, antinuclear antibodies have been found in the sera of more than 90% of patients with systemic sclerosis (240). The titers are typically low as compared with those found in SLE, but titers of 1:1,000 or greater are seen occasionally. In most instances, the pattern of nuclear fluorescence is that of fine or large speckles or threads, but nucleolar and occasionally diffuse (homogeneous) nuclear staining also occur. It is widely accepted that certain autoantibodies are highly specific for systemic sclerosis and also define clinically homogeneous patient subsets. In aggregate, one of seven autoantibodies are present in nearly 85% of all patients with scleroderma. Their immunofluorescence patterns on routine antinuclear antibody testing and their clinical and immunogenetic associations are shown in Table 79.3.

Anti–topoisomerase I antibodies are detected in 20% to more than 50% of systemic sclerosis sera, but rarely in control specimens (241,242), and are associated with diffuse cutaneous involvement and pulmonary interstitial fibrosis (123). Originally designated anti-Scl 70 (241), this antibody is now known to recognize the nuclear enzyme DNA toposiomerase I (243). It is clear that this antibody is directed against multiple epitopes on the topoisomerase I molecule (244). Furthermore, reactivity to one of the epitope regions (ER4) identifies a subgroup of patients with diffuse skin thickening, a higher frequency of pulmonary interstitial fibrosis, and reduced long-term survival (245).

Anticentromere antibodies appear morphologically as fine, discrete speckles (246) and are directed against three distinct antigens in the centromeric portion of chromosomes present in dividing cells (247). They identify patients with limited skin thickening, occurring in more than 50% of such individuals, but are uncommon in persons with diffuse cutaneous disease, where they are present in fewer than 5% of patients (248,249). These antibodies are found in some patients with Raynaud's phenomenon alone, who are at increased risk for limited scleroderma development during follow-up (250). A few patients with other diagnoses, including SLE, RA, other rheumatic diseases, and nonrheumatic disorders have been reported to have anticentromere antibodies (251–254), although Raynaud's phenomenon is almost universally present in these cases. These predominantly IgG antibodies tend to persist in the serum for prolonged periods (255). Immunoelectron microscopy has pinpointed the antigen as residing in the

TABLE 79.3. CLINICAL AND LABORATORY CHARACTERISTICS OF PATIENTS WITH SYSTEMIC SCLEROSIS ACCORDING TO SERUM AUTOANTIBODY

	Autoantibody Subtype						
Characteristics	ACA	Th	U1RNP	PM-Scl	U3RNP	RNA POL I, III	Scl-70
ANA staining pattern	Centromere	Nucleolar	Speckled	Nucleolar	Nucleolar	Speckled/ nucleolar	Speckled/ nucleolar
Proportion of all patients	25%	5%	10%	5%	5%	20%	15%
Clinical classification	Limited	Limited	Limited, overlap	Mixed, overlap	Mixed, overlap	Diffuse	Diffuse
Organ involvement	PHT	PHT, small bowel	Muscle	Muscle	Muscle, PHT	Skin, renal	Lung fibrosis
HLA association	None			DR3, w52			DR5

ANA, antinuclear antibody; HLA, human leukocyte antigen; PHT, "primary" pulmonary hypertension; ACA, anticentromere; RNA POL, RNA polymerase; RNP, ribonucleoprotein.

kinetochore region of the chromosome, but its precise identity is not yet known (256). The clinical relevance of antibodies directed at one or more of the three centromere antigens also is unknown (257). Antibodies to other components of dividing cells such as metaphase chromatin (258) and centrioles (259) also have been noted in sera of patients with systemic sclerosis. The latter were reported in two patients with systemic sclerosis (260,261) and in one with Raynaud's phenomenon (260). The coexistence of anti–topoisomerase I and anticentromere antibodies was reported in two of 121 patients (262), but must be rare indeed, as we have found only four such occurrences in more than 1,000 positive tests.

Some patients have high titers of antibody to nuclear ribonucleoprotein (anti-U1RNP); these persons tend to have myositis more frequently than those without high-titer anti-U1RNP (263). Antibody directed against the nuclear antigen Ku, distinct from nRNP, was found in a small proportion of Japanese patients, nearly all of whom had a scleroderma–polymyositis overlap syndrome (264). Anti-Ku also has been observed in patients with SLE, RA, and undifferentiated connective tissue disease (265,266). Both of these autoantibodies produce speckled staining in routine antinuclear antibody testing.

Nucleolar immunofluorescence is relatively specific for systemic sclerosis, particularly in patients with associated Sjögren's syndrome. Several of the responsible nucleolar antigens have now been identified and include families of small ribonucleoproteins considered important in messenger RNA processing. Patients with anti–topoisomerase I antibody display nucleolar staining (9), and anti–RNA polymerase I antibody is typically nucleolar (267). The latter identifies a group of women with otherwise typical diffuse cutaneous disease (9). Anti–PM-Scl (previously termed anti–PM-1), which also is directed against a nucleolar antigen (11), is associated with limited skin thickening and polymyositis (12), but also occurs in persons with other diseases or no diseases (268). Several newly described autoantibodies have helped to complete the profile of antinucleolar antibodies in systemic sclerosis. Anti-Th antibody may account for 10% to 20% of patients with limited cutaneous disease and is much less frequently encountered in the diffuse disease variant (7,269). Anti-U3RNP, directed against the nucleolar protein fibrillarin, identifies patients with both diffuse and limited skin disease, but two interesting subsets include black women with skeletal myopathy and a small group of individuals with diffuse disease and pulmonary arterial hypertension without pulmonary fibrosis (13). New data have shown that a large group of persons with diffuse disease have anti–RNA polymerase III antibodies, some of whom also have anti–RNA polymerase I or I and II antibodies (8,270,271). In contrast to the anti–RNA polymerase I sera, those with only anti–RNA polymerase III activity display nuclear rather than nucleolar staining. Among patients with diffuse disease, those with anti–RNA polymerase III antibody have more severe and extensive skin thickening, increased likelihood of renal crisis, and less interstitial lung disease (8) compared with patients who are anti–topoisomerase I positive.

Anticardiolipin antibody in low concentration has been detected in as many as one third of patients without vascular disease or other clinical associations (272) and as low as 7% in another study, barely more than the 4% reported in controls (273). One study suggested that anticardiolipin antibodies identified a subset of patients with more severe diffuse cutaneous involvement and myocardial ischemia or necrosis (274). A "lupus anticoagulant" has been reported infrequently, but several cases suggest its association with vascular thrombosis (51,52). Anti–proteinase 3 (cANCA) and antimyeloperoxidase (pANCA) in systemic sclerosis patients are rarely detected (275); if encountered, the latter may be associated with renal vasculitis rather than typical scleroderma renal involvement (276). Antibodies to high-mobility group (HMG) proteins, believed to play a role in transcription, have been found in scleroderma patients (277), as have antiubiquitin antibodies, which are closely correlated with antihistone antibodies (278,279). Anti–endothelial cell antibodies are increased in systemic sclerosis and are associated with diffuse cutaneous disease, digital infarcts with gangrene, and pulmonary arterial hypertension (280).

Immunogenetics of the Autoantibody Response

In the first reports of HLA antigens in patients with systemic sclerosis, published nearly 30 years ago, no immunogenetic associations were found. More recent work using oligotyping suggests, however, that if this heterogenous disease is divided according to serologic subsets, definite HLA relations are evident. The anticentromere response is most strongly associated with HLA-DQB1*0501, *0301, and *0402 (281). These alleles share a polar amino acid at position 26. Anti–topoisomerase I is associated with HLA-DQB1*0301 in several populations (282–284). The considerable difference in genetic background is illustrated by the finding of a striking increase in the HLA-DRB1*1502-DRB5*0102 haplotype in anti–topoisomerase I–positive Japanese patients with systemic sclerosis, who also have an uncharged polar amino acid residue at position 30 of the HLA-DQB1 allele because of DQB1*0601 linkage (285), but do not have the previously noted position 26 association (286). The autoantibody profile of patients with systemic sclerosis also varies considerably from population to population (287), most likely related to the underlying frequency of certain HLA genes in the population. For example, Japanese patients with systemic sclerosis were found not to have anti–PM-Scl antibody (287), which is strongly linked to HLA-DR3 (288), probably because HLA-DR3 is extremely rare in Japanese persons.

DISEASE COURSE

The course of systemic sclerosis is extremely variable. Early in the illness, it is difficult to judge prognosis with respect to either survival or disability. Many patients with diffuse cutaneous involvement experience steadily increasing sclerosis of the fingers and hands, leading to deforming flexion contractures. In others, mobility is maintained despite advancing skin changes. The most reliable early signs predicting subsequent severe diffuse skin involvement are the appearance of cutaneous thickening before the onset of Raynaud's phenomenon, rapid progression of scleroderma toward the more proximal parts of the extremities, palpable tendon friction rubs, and serum anti–topoisomerase I or anti–RNA polymerase I or III antibodies. Often, later in the disease, spontaneous improvement in skin thickening occurs, and thus, the prefix "progressive" is not uniformly applicable and should be abandoned (30).

Limited cutaneous scleroderma was initially considered to represent a benign variant associated with a relatively favorable prognosis. Raynaud's phenomenon, alone or in combination with swollen, puffy fingers, may be present for up to a decade or more before the diagnosis of systemic sclerosis is evident. The life span of patients with limited cutaneous involvement is significantly longer than that of patients with diffuse scleroderma, in part because the former patients rarely, if ever, develop myocardial or renal disease. Anticentromere antibody itself is often a clue to a good prognosis (289). As noted previously, however, a small number of patients with limited cutaneous involvement develop severe pulmonary arterial hypertension, which is independent of the presence of anticentromere antibody and is almost uniformly fatal (136).

At present there are no consensus guidelines for determining disease activity. Clinical evidence of active disease consists of increase in the extent and severity of skin thickness, as well as worsening of clinical or laboratory features of musculoskeletal or visceral involvement. Considering the pathophysiology of disease, several newly described laboratory studies may provide useful guides to disease activity. Microvascular damage is paralleled by the release into the plasma of factor VIII/von Willebrand factor antigen from injured endothelium (71,290). Thrombomodulin, an endothelium-specific glycoprotein, is increased in the plasma of systemic sclerosis patients and may be a molecular marker of endothelial cell injury (291). Serum levels of the soluble adhesion molecules intercellular adhesion molecule-1 (ICAM-1), vascular cell adhesion molecule-1 (VCAM-1), E-selectin, and P-selectin have been shown to be elevated (292,293) and correlate with clinical evidence of disease activity and progression, as well as with the *in situ* expression of these adhesion molecules in affected skin (293). Lymphocyte activation is reflected by increased serum levels of IL-2 (294) and soluble IL-2 receptors (sIL-2Rs) (295), and one longitudinal study has demonstrated correlation of sIL-2R levels with disease activity (296). A fibroblast activity surrogate, serum procollagen III peptide concentration, has been reported (297). Urinary excretion of amino acid markers of elastin and collagen are increased in patients with systemic sclerosis compared with controls, but their correlations with clinical evidence of disease activity are not strong (298). These laboratory studies also have the potential to be useful adjuncts in the performance of clinical trials. Because of the difficulty in defining disease activity by current clinical or laboratory means, a validated disease severity index based on tissue damage and malfunction has been developed (299).

Several large survival studies have been reported and summarized (300). During the 1960s to 1980s, the 5-year cumulative survival rate after either first physician diagnosis or entry to study ranged from 34% to 73%, and most authors agreed that male sex, older age, and involvement of the kidney, heart, and lung adversely affected outcome (Fig. 79.16). However, by using an inception cohort, one group found that female subjects had a higher age-adjusted mortality (301). It is probable that survival has improved during recent decades for a variety of reasons, especially the successful management of renal crisis (180). In one study, the 6-year cumulative survival rate was 76% (302). Our overall figures for patients first evaluated during 1989 through 1998 are 86% at 5 years and 74% at 10 years after first physician diagnosis (see subset details in Table 79.2).

Anemia and the early occurrence of pericarditis and abnormal skin pigmentation are reported to be poor prog-

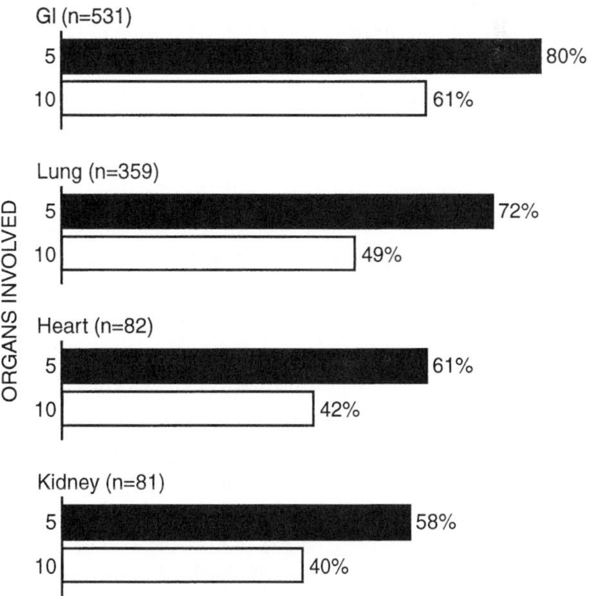

FIGURE 79.16. Cumulative survival rates in patients with systemic sclerosis 5 and 10 years after the first detection of certain types of visceral involvement (University of Pittsburgh, 1981–1990).

nostic signs (303,304). Long-term follow-up studies indicate continued excess mortality overall (305), especially among patients with diffuse cutaneous disease compared with the general population (304,306). In a Danish mortality study, there was a twofold increased risk due to causes apparently unrelated to scleroderma, including cancer, suggesting that the excess mortality is more appropriately termed "indirectly related" to scleroderma (307). Serum autoantibodies also are useful in predicting prognosis, because they have the earlier mentioned associations with serious visceral disease (308).

Disability in systemic sclerosis has been the subject of several recent publications (309). The Health Assessment Questionnaire (HAQ), a patient self-report measure of functional status used extensively in evaluation of RA, has been validated in scleroderma patients (310). A modified HAQ also has been validated, and the HAQ disability index was found to correlate directly with skin and many visceral involvements, to parallel skin thickness score over time, and to predict survival (311). Another disability-assessment instrument suitable for administration by either the patient or a trained observer was proposed and performed well in preliminary studies (312). Despite its low prevalence, systemic sclerosis has annual direct and indirect costs estimated to be 1.5 billion dollars in the U.S. (313).

TREATMENT

The first responsibility of the physician is to discuss the nature of the disease with the patient and family, who are often unreasonably pessimistic. Classification as diffuse cutaneous or limited cutaneous systemic sclerosis is helpful in understanding the future risk of developing visceral complications and which ones they may be. Such discussion aids in establishing a good relationship between physician and patient, which is particularly important in this chronic, demanding disease. Diagrams of the blood vessels, skin, esophagus, and other appropriate illustrations are useful in instruction. Several excellent publications geared to lay persons are available, and these should be recommended (314, 315). Finally, many scleroderma patients and their family members benefit greatly from participation in support groups, which are now widely available.

Numerous vitamins, hormones, pharmaceuticals, and surgical procedures have been used to treat systemic sclerosis; nearly all of these therapies have been abandoned after initial enthusiasm and later critical evaluation. Improvement can hardly be expected in those manifestations that are the result of far-advanced tissue fibrosis. Too often, success has been claimed solely on the basis of a diminution in subjective complaints (e.g., a reduction in frequency of Raynaud's phenomenon, which occurs with virtually any new treatment, and poorly documented "softening" of the skin).

Evaluation of the effectiveness of treatment has proved difficult for several reasons (316). Conceptually, fibrosis can be reversed only very slowly; a therapeutic agent should be given a minimum of 18 to 24 months if fibrosis (skin, other sites) is one of the end points to be studied. There has been disagreement about the accuracy of skin-thickness examination, but a review of three independent studies has shown that within-patient variability is low, and reproducibility is good (317). Because spontaneous improvement often occurs after several years, controlled trials are necessary. Systemic sclerosis is variable in its severity and in its rate of progression; therefore the classification of patients into subsets and disease stages is important in interpreting the results of therapy. The disease occurs infrequently enough that multicenter trials must have adequate power to answer the important morbidity questions. Significant mortality differences between treated and untreated patient cohorts may require 3 to 4 years of follow-up to establish. There are limitations in the availability of valid outcome measures and the application of objective criteria for ascertaining improvement (or deterioration) in the condition, thus making decisions about therapeutic efficacy in clinical trials most difficult (318,319). Finally, the influence of psychological factors on many of the symptoms is important. Because of these numerous problems, a set of guidelines has been developed for clinical trials of potential disease-modifying agents in systemic sclerosis (320).

Drugs

The pathogenesis of systemic sclerosis is discussed in detail in Chapter 81. Figure 79.17 indicates those points at which therapeutic intervention might be considered (321,322). In the past, no drug or combination of drugs has been proven to be of value in adequately controlled prospective trials (323). Antiinflammatory agents and corticosteroids have been disappointing. Because of their potential toxicity, corticosteroids are typically restricted to patients with inflam-

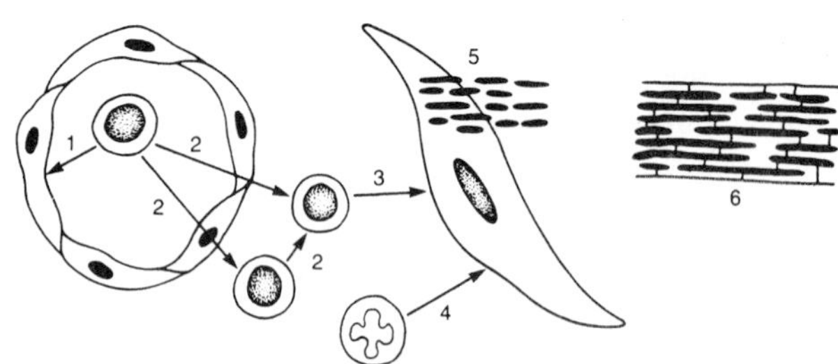

FIGURE 79.17. Pathophysiology of systemic sclerosis with possible sites for therapeutic intervention. Rational therapy would be designed to (1) prevent endothelial cell damage, (2) alter communication between mononuclear cells, (3) prevent mononuclear cell stimulation of fibroblasts, (4) prevent mast cell degranulation, (5) block fibroblast production of extrusion of procollagen, or (6) increase solubilization of preformed collagen.

matory myopathy or symptomatic serositis inadequately controlled with NSAIDs. On occasion, refractory arthritis and the "edematous" phase of skin involvement respond favorably to relatively small doses of corticosteroids, such as prednisone, 5 to 10 mg/day. Myositis, however, may require higher doses. There is concern that high-dose corticosteroid therapy may precipitate acute renal failure (324), and thus daily oral doses of prednisone greater than 15 mg/day should be avoided. It is possible that high-dose intermittent (pulse) corticosteroid therapy could be beneficial and safe (325).

In the past, attention has been focused on D-penicillamine, a compound that interferes with the intermolecular cross-linking of collagen and also possesses immunosuppressive activity. Reports from England (326), Denmark (327), and the former U.S.S.R. (328) have been optimistic. In two retrospective U.S. studies of early diffuse disease (28,329), one with an untreated "comparison" group (28), there was striking improvement in skin thickening, reduced frequency of subsequent renal involvement, and increased survival using drug doses up to 1,000 to 1,500 mg/day. Another uncontrolled study showed significant improvement in baseline skin thickness and other objective measures and absence of serious visceral sequelae during follow-up (330). In a recent double-blind randomized multicenter study of early diffuse disease patients, high-dose (mean, 833 mg/day) and low-dose (mean, 72 mg/day) D-penicillamine were compared (331). Both groups had a mean improvement in skin score of 30% after 2 years, similar frequency of renal crisis, and similar survival, but adverse effects (none fatal) occurred more frequently in the high-dose group. D-Penicillamine also may improve mild interstitial lung disease when given for a prolonged period (332,333). Its use may be accompanied by a variety of side effects, including some that are autoimmune, such as nephrotic syndrome, glomerulonephritis (334), pemphigus, and myasthenia gravis (335). As in RA, proteinuria is more frequent in HLA-DR3–positive individuals (336). Up to one fourth of patients may be forced to discontinue the drug because of toxicity (336). Adverse reactions occur with lower frequency when the D-penicillamine dose is increased slowly over a 6- to 8-month period. Careful monitoring of the white blood cell and platelet counts and urine protein are recommended. Chemically related compounds such as *N*-acetylcysteine (337) and *S*-adenosylmethionine (338) also have been used with limited success.

Relaxin, believed important in "remodeling" the connective tissue of the female pelvis during pregnancy, has been studied in a 6-month multicenter double-blind placebo-controlled fashion in stable diffuse disease (339). Recombinant human relaxin was administered subcutaneously twice weekly and was well tolerated; the results were encouraging.

Colchicine inhibits the accumulation of collagen by blocking the conversion of procollagen to collagen, probably through interference with microtubule-mediated transport or perhaps by stimulation of collagenase production. In one long-term open trial (mean follow-up, 39 months), improvement in skin thickening occurred in 17 of 19 patients who received colchicine, 10 mg/week (340). Several other negative studies have been published, however (341,342). In none of these trials was colchicine toxicity a serious limiting factor. Aminobenzoate potassium, an antifibrotic agent, was recently studied and found not to affect skin thickening in patients with long-standing stable disease (343).

A variety of potential beneficial effects can be hypothesized from the use of immunosuppressive drugs, including alterations in interactions between immunocompetent cells and inhibition of the effects of soluble mediators on fibroblast function. Azathioprine was considered beneficial in an uncontrolled study (344), and 5-fluorouracil was reported to result in some cutaneous improvement but had unacceptable gastrointestinal toxicity (345). Chlorambucil results have been mixed, but a 3-year double-blind controlled trial was negative (346). As in RA (347), late-developing malignancy is a limiting feature of the use of alkylating agents (348). Plasmapheresis has been advocated (348–350), but its effects are not uniformly beneficial (351) and are difficult to evaluate because of confounding immunosuppressive and corticosteroid therapy. Cyclosporine (Cyclosporin A) has been used in a limited number of patients and may improve skin thickening (352–354). No cyclosporine trials are currently ongoing because, even at doses less than 5 mg/kg/day, there has been some suggestion of an unacceptably high frequency of hypertension and renal insufficiency, which could be attributable either to the drug or to scleroderma (355). The effects of recombinant IFN-γ, an "immunomodulating" drug, are promising on the basis of five uncontrolled open trials (356–360). In contrast, interferon-α did not improve skin thickness in diffuse disease after a 1-year trial (361). Anti–thymocyte globulin has been recommended on the basis of a few case reports in which most patients exhibited prompt improvement after its administration (362,363), along with nearly complete elimination of peripheral blood $CD4^+$ and $CD8^+$ T lymphocytes (363). Several reports have been published on the beneficial effects of methotrexate (364,365). A controversial new treatment, extracorporeal photochemotherapy, was studied in comparison with D-penicillamine and found to be effective (366), but these results have been challenged on methodologic grounds (367,368). There is no general agreement regarding the effectiveness of immunosuppressive or immunomodulating forms of therapy. Additional adequately controlled therapeutic trials are needed (315). The use of immunosuppressive measures seems justified in patients with early, rapidly progressive, life-threatening, and/or disabling diffuse disease, provided there is informed consent and close surveillance for adverse effects.

Agents designed to protect injured endothelial cells and to prevent platelet aggregation and subsequent release of platelet-derived growth factors are a logical extension of the vascular hypothesis of scleroderma. Although increased circulating platelet aggregates and plasma β-thromboglobulin levels were reduced by treatment with dipyridamole and aspirin (369), a randomized, double-blind 2-year trial of these agents versus placebo showed no significant clinical improvement in the treatment group (370). Lower doses of dipyridamole in the latter study could conceivably account for the ineffectiveness. This approach to systemic sclerosis should be investigated further.

Supportive Measures

Proper management of individual organ system complications of systemic sclerosis may prolong survival and enhance the quality of life in this serious chronic disease (371).

Raynaud's Phenomenon

Common-sense self-management includes avoiding undue cold exposure, dressing warmly, and abstaining from tobacco use. Induced vasodilation (372) and biofeedback (373,374) also may be helpful. Various vasodilating drugs have been used, including topical glyceryl nitrate (375), intraarterial reserpine (376), methyldopa (377), and α-receptor–blocking and β-receptor–stimulating adrenergic drugs (378). In general, these compounds have proved disappointing, probably because structural damage and narrow arterioles rather than excessive vasospasm are most responsible for secondary Raynaud's phenomenon.

Several pharmacologic agents have been effective in double-blind studies, including the calcium channel blocker nifedipine (379,380); a direct vasodilator, prazosin (381); an oral serotonin antagonist, ketanserin (382,383); pentoxifylline (384); prostaglandin E_1 (PGE_1) (385); and prostacyclin (386). Iloprost, a prostacyclin analogue administered by intravenous infusion, led to prolonged improvement in Raynaud's phenomenon and healing of digital ulcers (387), but oral Iloprost failed (388). In a preliminary report, infusion of calcitonin gene–related peptide had a dramatic effect on digital blood flow and ulcer healing (389). Whether renin–angiotensin blockade benefits vascular disease in organs other than the kidney is unknown, although captopril did not ameliorate Raynaud's phenomenon or alter digital plethysmographic findings during cold challenge in one study (390). Plasmapheresis, an unusual form of treatment for Raynaud's phenomenon in systemic sclerosis, was reported to be effective (391).

Thoracic sympathectomy may be followed by partial (usually transient) improvement in Raynaud's phenomenon, but not by significant or sustained influence on the course of cutaneous changes or visceral sclerosis (378). Digital sympathectomy has been used successfully in some difficult cases (392–394), but these observations are uncontrolled and lack long-term follow-up. When large vessels are involved, such as the radial or ulnar arteries, microvascular surgical reconstruction should be considered (395,396). Digital tip amputation occasionally may be required, although the demarcation of tissue achieved by autoamputation is preferred (396,397). Thus if pain can be controlled with narcotic analgesics for the time necessary for such demarcation, tissue loss may be minimized. If "wet" gangrene with osteomyelitis develops, surgical amputation is required.

Calcinosis

Unfortunately, reliable treatment to eradicate calcinosis is not available. Surgical excision of large calcareous masses may be helpful in selected instances (396). Soft tissue calcinotic deposits contain increased amounts of the amino acid 4-carboxyl-L-glutamic acid (Gla) (398). Thus long-term inhibition of Gla with low-dose anticoagulant therapy has been considered theoretically attractive, but this form of therapy remains unproven (399). The successful use of diltiazem for treatment of calcinosis has been reported (400,401). Suppression of local sterile inflammation surrounding these hydroxyapatite deposits has been achieved with colchicine, which is given in 7- to 10-day courses rather than as long-term therapy (402).

Skin

Special lotions, soaps, and bath oils should be used to relieve excessive skin dryness; those containing a high glycerine content are the most effective penetrants. Taking unduly frequent baths and using household detergents may aggravate dryness. Pruritus is a frequent and occasionally dominant problem in early diffuse cutaneous disease. There is no adequate therapy for pruritus, but fortunately it disappears later in the course of the illness.

Digital tip ulcerations can be protected by plastic finger "cages." Noninfected ulcers respond rapidly to the use of occlusive dressings, such as Duoderm, which also are protective. If these lesions become infected (almost always with staphylococci), half-strength hydrogen peroxide soaks and gentle local debridement are used, and oral antibiotics are sometimes needed. Deeper soft tissue infections, septic arthritis, and osteomyelitis must be treated vigorously with intravenous antibiotics, excision of infected and devitalized tissue, joint fusion, and rarely, amputation (403).

Joints and Muscles

Articular complaints may be treated with salicylates or other NSAIDs, with careful attention to their potential to aggravate gastroesophageal reflux and to reduce renal blood flow. Corticosteroids are seldom necessary, but patients with true synovitis may benefit from prednisone (5 to 7.5

mg/day), during the first 6 to 12 months of disease. Persons with diffuse cutaneous involvement often develop digital contractures with deformity. Dynamic splinting does not prevent the progression of this process (404), but a vigorous twice-daily range-of-motion exercise program should be recommended. Liberal use of analgesics before each exercise session will maximize the results.

Proximal interphalangeal joint replacement arthroplasties have been performed later in disease, with improvement in hand function and appearance (405). When severe finger contractures have occurred, excessive flexion of the proximal interphalangeal joints leaves them vulnerable to trauma with repeated skin breakdown and infection, including septic arthritis. In this circumstance, joint replacement will not be effective, and proximal interphalangeal joint fusion is preferred (396). After such fusions, hand function depends on the amount of motion present at the metacarpophalangeal joints. Surgical wound healing has been excellent.

Active polymyositis with proximal muscle weakness that is due to systemic sclerosis or attributable to an overlap syndrome should be treated with moderate doses of corticosteroids (prednisone, 15–20 mg/day). Methotrexate, azathioprine, or another immunosuppressive agent can be added if the response is incomplete. In contrast, bland myopathy with minimal or no elevation of serum creatine kinase and little or no progression of weakness should not be treated pharmacologically.

Gastrointestinal Tract

Maintenance of the oral opening requires mouth-stretching exercises (406); the patient also must maintain good oral hygiene and make regular visits to a dentist for prophylaxis. For edentulous individuals with microstomia, a flexible prosthesis has been designed to augment the exercise program (407).

Patients who have difficulty in swallowing should learn to masticate carefully and/or avoid foods likely to cause substernal dysphagia, such as meat and bread. Metoclopramide improves esophageal motility and is useful in some patients (408), and cisapride stimulates both gastric and esophageal emptying (409). Erythromycin functions as a prokinetic drug and was reported to stimulate gastric and gallbladder motility and emptying (410); it may improve gastroparesis in scleroderma (411). Octreotide, a somatostatin analogue, also has prokinetic properties, which have been shown to increase gastrointestinal muscular activity in short-term trials (412). Because nifedipine is capable of decreasing lower esophageal sphincter pressure and contraction amplitude in the body of the esophagus (413), it may aggravate esophageal symptoms. In this situation, diltiazem may be a preferable agent (414).

Reflux esophagitis can be minimized by appropriate common-sense measures, such as complete mastication, more frequent, smaller-sized meals, sitting upright during and after eating, avoiding food before bedtime, and raising the head of the bed on blocks to prevent nocturnal reflux. Antacids, 45 to 60 minutes after meals and at bedtime, and histamine (H_2) receptors are useful. The most dramatic results are achieved with the hydrogen ion exchange inhibitor, omeprazole, which virtually eliminates gastric acidity in doses of 20 to 60 mg/day (415). Esophageal stricture may require periodic endoscopic dilatation. Successful excision of strictures and correction of gastroesophageal reflux by gastroplasty combined with fundoplication have been reported (416). Bleeding telangiectases and the ectatic vessels of watermelon stomach can be treated with sclerotherapy (417) and laser coagulation (102), respectively.

Transient improvement in steatorrhea and other signs of intestinal malabsorption may follow the administration of tetracycline or other broad-spectrum antibiotics, but the underlying hypomotility is unaffected. Two-week rotations of tetracycline, ampicillin, metronidazole, trimethoprim–sulfamethoxazole, and ciprofloxacin, for example, interspersed with 2-week rest periods with no antibiotics, have proven useful in many patients. An alternate cause of small bowel bacterial overgrowth in a few patients is omeprazole (418). Metoclopramide significantly increases small bowel motility (419) but is not effective in patients with gross malabsorption. Cisapride, also a direct stimulant of intestinal motor activity, has been used with variable results (409). In advanced circumstances, one must replace calcium and fat-soluble vitamins, use more easily absorbed medium-chain triglycerides, and often resort to parenteral hyperalimentation (420). In the latter circumstance, adequate nutrition (increased weight, hematocrit, and serum albumin), as well as improved quality of life, can generally be achieved (421). In severe malabsorption, the likelihood of septicemia of catheter origin, serious bacterial infection, and premature death from other causes is high.

Lung

Patients with pulmonary interstitial fibrosis who have bacterial bronchitis or pneumonitis require prompt and vigorous antibiotic treatment. Prophylactic influenza and *Streptococcus pneumoniae* vaccinations should be given. In persons with documented inflammatory alveolitis, which has been shown to predict subsequent decline in pulmonary function (422), high-dose corticosteroids, with or without immunosuppressive drugs (particularly cyclophosphamide), may be efficacious short-term therapy (423–425). D-Penicillamine may be useful for interstitial lung disease (426–428), but recent evidence suggests that the most beneficial response in active alveolitis is achieved with cyclophosphamide (429). When there is resting or exercise-precipitated hypoxia, supplemental oxygen should be administered.

"Primary" pulmonary arterial hypertension unassociated with interstitial fibrosis typically comes to attention at an advanced stage. Numerous pharmacologic measures have been suggested, but only the serotonin antagonist ketanserin (430), calcium channel antagonists (431), and captopril (432) are capable of lowering pulmonary artery pressure after direct pulmonary artery instillation. Both intermittent and continuous intravenous use of the prostacyclin analogues iloprost and epoprostenol have resulted in improvement of pulmonary hypertension in systemic sclerosis while being administered, but recurrence of pulmonary hypertension promptly follows their discontinuation (433–435). The high cost of such therapies is a serious limitation. Unfortunately, the subsequent oral administration of these agents does not appear to alter the inexorably fatal course. It would thus appear that structural narrowing is a more important determinant of pulmonary vascular flow than is intermittent vasospasm (436). Corticosteroids have been recommended (437), but no reports of their successful use have been published. Because those in whom right-sided cardiac failure develops often respond poorly to digitalis and easily become digitalis intoxicated, greater reliance is placed on the use of diuretics. Anticoagulation is often prescribed in patients with right-sided failure and venous stasis, which may predispose to venous thrombosis. Anticoagulation also should be used in individuals with one or more of the laboratory features of the antiphospholipid antibody syndrome because of the association of this disorder with venous and/or arterial thrombosis and pulmonary hypertension (438). Heart–lung or single-lung transplantation is an option that has not been adequately explored. One center has performed eight such procedures, and five of the patients are living after 18 to 84 months (J. Dauber, personal communication, 1999).

Heart

Symptomatic pericarditis is treated with NSAIDs or corticosteroids. Hemodynamically significant pericardial effusion should be managed with pericardiocentesis or, if recurrent, with an open pericardial window procedure. If myocarditis can be identified clinically or by endomyocardial biopsy, high-dose glucocorticoids should be tried. The typical progressive left ventricular failure caused by myocardial fibrosis is unaffected by any therapy and is uniformly fatal, unless some correctable nonsclerodermatous problem also is present. Serious arrhythmias complicate myocardial fibrosis and respond inconsistently to antiarrhythmic drugs.

Kidney

The most important aspect of therapy for renal involvement is early detection. A vulnerable patient is one with rapidly progressive diffuse skin thickening (172). If the 24-hour creatinine clearance decreases to less than 60 mL/min, or decreases by more than 20 mL/min from one determination to the next, the patient is clearly at increased risk. If any one of a number of markers of renal disease, such as hypertension, microscopic hematuria or proteinuria, azotemia, or microangiopathic hemolytic anemia develops in such a person, it is recommended that stimulated plasma renin levels be obtained, and if they are elevated, treatment begun immediately (439). The availability of new and more potent antihypertensive agents and of improved dialysis procedures and care has dramatically increased survival in patients having "renal crisis." The angiotensin-converting enzyme (ACE) inhibitors are the drugs of choice (180), but early aggressive therapy with other potent antihypertensive agents can be successful. Regardless, some individuals require dialysis (440). Theoretically, scleroderma patients may have inadequate vascular access and thus ineffective hemodialysis, but we have not encountered this problem. Likewise, poor peritoneal clearance has been described (441), but continuous ambulatory peritoneal dialysis has been successfully used (442).

Many patients with renal failure maintained on ACE inhibitors have a slow reversal of renal vascular damage and can discontinue dialysis after 3 to 24 months (180). A remarkable reduction in the degree of dermal thickening and induration has been observed in some, but not all, of these patients during dialysis (181,443). Numerous successful renal transplants have now been reported (444), but typical scleroderma kidney histologic changes have been reported in transplanted organs (445,446).

REFERENCES

1. Medsger TA Jr. Systemic sclerosis (scleroderma): clinical aspects. In: Koopman WJ, ed. *Arthritis and allied conditions.* 13th ed. Philadelphia: Lea & Febiger, 1997:1433–1464.
2. LeRoy EC, Black C, Fleischmajer R, et al. Scleroderma (systemic sclerosis): classification, subsets, and pathogenesis. *J Rheumatol* 1980;152:202–205.
3. Sharp GC. Association of progressive systemic sclerosis with other connective tissue diseases ("overlap syndromes"). In: Black CM, Myers AR, eds. *Systemic sclerosis (scleroderma).* New York: Gower Medical Publishing, 1985:33.
4. Winterbauer RH. Multiple telangiectasia, Raynaud's phenomenon, sclerodactyly, and subcutaneous calcinosis: a syndrome mimicking hereditary hemorrhagic telangiectasia. *Bull Johns Hopkins Hosp* 1964;114:361–383.
5. Poormoghim H, Lucas M, Fertig N, et al. Systemic sclerosis sine scleroderma: demographic, clinical, and serologic features and survival in forty-eight patients. *Arthritis Rheum* 2000;43: 444–451.
6. Terumi H, Junko M, Masatoshi T, et al. The coexistence of systemic sclerosis and rheumatoid arthritis in five patients: clinical and immunogenetic features suggest a distinct entity. *Arthritis Rheum* 1996;39:152–156.
7. Okano Y, Medsger TA Jr. Antibody to Th ribonucleoprotein (nucleolar 7-2 RNA protein particle) in patients with systemic sclerosis (scleroderma). *Arthritis Rheum* 1990;33:1822–1828.
8. Okano Y, Steen VD, Medsger TA Jr. Antibody reactive with RNA polymerase III in systemic sclerosis. *Ann Intern Med* 1993; 119:1005–1013.
9. Reimer G, Steen VD, Penning CA, et al. Correlates between autoantibodies to nucleolar antigens and clinical features in

patients with systemic sclerosis (scleroderma). *Arthritis Rheum* 1988;31:525–532.
10. Sharp GC, Irvin WS, Tan EM, et al. Mixed connective tissue disease: an apparently distinct rheumatic disease syndrome associated with a specific antibody to an extractable nuclear antigen (ENA). *Am J Med* 1972;52:148–159.
11. Targoff IN, Reichlin M. Nucleolar localization of the PM-Scl antigens. *Arthritis Rheum* 1985;28:226–230.
12. Treadwell EL, Alspaugh MA, Wolfe JF, et al. Clinical relevance of PM-1 antibody and physiochemical characterization of PM-1 antigen. *J Rheumatol* 1984;11:658–662.
13. Okano Y, Steen VD, Medsger TA Jr. Autoantibody to U3 nucleolar ribonucleoprotein (fibrillarin) in patients with systemic sclerosis. *Arthritis Rheum* 1992;35:95–100.
14. Masi AT, Rodnan GP, Medsger TA Jr, et al. Preliminary criteria for the classification of systemic sclerosis (scleroderma). *Arthritis Rheum* 1980;23:581–590.
15. Medsger TA Jr. Comment on scleroderma criteria cooperative study. In: Black CM, Myers AR, eds. *Current topics in rheumatology:* systemic sclerosis. New York: Gower Medical Publishing, 1985:16–17.
16. Steen V, Oddis CV, Conte CG, et al. Incidence of systemic sclerosis: a twenty year study of hospital diagnosed cases in Allegheny County, PA, 1963-1982. *Arthritis Rheum* 1997;40: 441–445.
17. Laing TJ, Gillespie BW, Toth MB, et al. Racial differences in scleroderma among women in Michigan. *Arthritis Rheum* 1997; 40:734–742.
18. Lawrence RV, Helmick CG, Arnett FC, et al. Estimates of the prevalence of arthritis and selected musculoskeletal disorders in the United States. *Arthritis Rheum* 1998;41:778–799.
19. Silman H, Hochberg MC. Occupational and environmental influences on scleroderma. *Rheum Dis Clin North Am* 1996;22: 737–749.
20. Haustein U-F, Herrmann K. Environmental scleroderma. *Clin Dermatol* 1994;12:467–473.
21. Nietert PJ, Sutherland SE, Silver RM, et al. Is occupational organic solvent exposure a risk factor for scleroderma. *Arthritis Rheum* 1998;41:1111–1118.
22. Hochberg MC, Perlmutter DL, Medsger TA Jr. Lack of association between augmentation mammopathy and systemic sclerosis (scleroderma). *Arthritis Rheum* 1996;39:1125–1131.
23. Sanchez-Guerrero J, Colditz GA, Karlson EW, et al. Silicone breast implants and the risk of connective tissue diseases and symptoms. *N Engl J Med* 1995;332:1666–1670.
24. Gabriel SE, O'Fallon WM, Korland LJ, et al. Risk of connective tissue diseases and other disorders after breast implantation. *N Engl J Med* 1994;330:1697–1702.
25. Hennekens CH, Lee I-M, Cook NR, et al. Self-reported breast implants and connective tissue diseases in female health professionals: a retrospective cohort study. *JAMA* 1996;275:616–621.
26. Aguilar MB, Cho M, Reveille JD, et al. Prevalences of familial systemic sclerosis and other autoimmune diseases in three U.S. cohorts. *Arthritis Rheum* 1999;42:S186.
27. Mandios N, Dunckley H, Chivers T, et al. Immunogenetic analysis of 5 families with multicase occurrence of scleroderma and/or related variants. *J Rheumatol* 1995;22:85–92.
28. Steen VD, Medsger TA Jr, Rodnan GP. D-Penicillamine therapy in progressive systemic sclerosis (scleroderma). *Ann Intern Med* 1982;97:652–658.
29. Kahaleh MB, Sultany GL, Smith EA, et al. A modified scleroderma skin scoring method. *Clin Exp Rheumatol* 1986;4: 367–369.
30. Black C, Dieppe PK, Huskisson T, et al. Regressive systemic sclerosis. *Ann Rheum Dis* 1986;45:384–388.
31. Jawitz JC, Albert MK, Nigra TP, et al. A new skin manifestation of progressive systemic sclerosis. *J Am Acad Dermatol* 1984;2: 265–268.
32. Sukenik S, Kleiner-Baumgarten A, Horowitz J. Hyperpigmentation along tendons in progressive systemic sclerosis [Letter]. *J Rheumatol* 1986;13:474–475.
33. Rodnan GP, Lipinski E, Luksick J. Skin thickness and collagen content in progressive systemic sclerosis (scleroderma) and localized scleroderma. *Arthritis Rheum* 1979;22:130–140.
34. Clements P, Lachenbruch P, Seibold J, et al. Inter- and intraobserver variability of total skin thickness score (modified Rodnan TSS) in systemic sclerosis. *J Rheumatol* 1995;22:1281–1285.
35. Silman AJ, Harrison M, Brennan P, et al. Is it possible to reduce the observer variability in skin score assessment of scleroderma? *J Rheumatol* 1995;22:1277–1280.
36. Scheja A, Akesson A. Comparison of high frequency (20 MHz) ultrasound and palpation for the assessment of skin involvement in systemic sclerosis (scleroderma). *Clin Exp Rheumatol* 1997;15:283–288.
37. Nives Parodi M, Castagneto C, Filaci G, et al. Plicometer skin test: a new technique for the evaluation of cutaneous involvement in systemic sclerosis. *Br J Rheumatol* 1997;36:244–250.
38. Roumm AD, Whiteside TL, Medsger TA Jr, et al. Lymphocytes in the skin of patients with progressive systemic sclerosis: quantification, subtyping and clinical correlations. *Arthritis Rheum* 1984;27:645–653.
39. Connolly SM, Winkelmann RK. Direct immunofluorescent findings in scleroderma syndromes. *Acta Derm Venereol (Stockh)* 1981;61:29–36.
40. Hawkins RA, Claman HN, Clark RAF, et al. Increased dermal mast cell populations in progressive systemic sclerosis: a link in chronic fibrosis? *Ann Intern Med* 1985;102:182–186.
41. Ward M, Cure J, Schabel S, et al. Symptomatic spinal calcinosis in systemic sclerosis (scleroderma). *Arthritis Rheum* 1997;40: 1892–1895.
42. Sheiner NM, Small P. Isolated Raynaud's phenomenon: a benign disorder. *Ann Allergy* 1987;58:114–117.
43. Gerbracht DD, Steen VD, Ziegler GL, et al. Evolution of primary Raynaud's phenomenon (Raynaud's disease) to connective tissue disease. *Arthritis Rheum* 1985;28:87–92.
44. Fitzgerald O, Hess EV, O'Connor GT, et al. Prospective study of the evolution of Raynaud's phenomenon. *Am J Med* 1988;84: 718–726.
45. Kallenberg CGM, Wouda AA, Hoet MH, et al. Development of connective tissue disease in patients presenting with Raynaud's phenomenon: a six year follow-up with emphasis on the predictive value of antinuclear antibodies as detected by immunoblotting. *Ann Rheum Dis* 1988;47:634–641.
46. Young EA, Steen V, Medsger TA Jr. Systemic sclerosis without Raynaud's phenomenon. *Arthritis Rheum* 1986;29(suppl):S51 (abst).
47. Rodnan GP, Myerowitz RL, Justh GO. Morphologic changes in the digital arteries of patients with progressive systemic sclerosis (scleroderma) and Raynaud's phenomenon. *Medicine* 1980;59: 393–408.
48. Merino J, Casanueva B, Piney E, et al. Hemiplegia and peripheral gangrene secondary to large and medium size vessels involvement in C.R.E.S.T. syndrome. *Clin Rheumatol* 1982;1: 295–299.
49. Stafford L, Englert H, Gover J, et al. Distribution of macrovascular disease in scleroderma. *Ann Rheum Dis* 1998;57:476–479.
50. Youssef P, Brama T, Englert H, et al. Limited scleroderma is associated with increased prevalence of macrovascular disease. *J Rheumatol* 1995;22:469–472.
51. Shapiro LS. Large vessels, arterial thrombosis in systemic sclerosis associated with antiphospholipid antibodies. *J Rheumatol* 1990;17:685–688.

52. Herrick AL, Oogarah PK, Freemont AJ, et al. Vasculitis in patients with systemic sclerosis and severe digital ischaemia requiring amputation. *Ann Rheum Dis* 1994;53:323–326.
53. Maricq HR, Spencer-Green G, LeRoy EC. Skin capillary abnormalities as indicators of organ involvement in scleroderma (systemic sclerosis). *Am J Med* 1976;61:862–870.
54. Maricq HR, LeRoy EC. Capillary blood flow in scleroderma. *Bibl Anat* 1973;11:352–358.
55. Kenik JG, Maricq HR, Bole GG. Blind evaluation of the diagnostic specificity of nailfold capillary microscopy in the connective tissue diseases. *Arthritis Rheum* 1981;24:885–891.
56. Maricq HR. Comparison of quantitative and semiquantitative estimates of nailfold capillary abnormalities in scleroderma spectrum disorders. *Microvasc Res* 1986;32:271–276.
57. Thompson RP, Harper FE, Maize JC, et al. Nailfold biopsy in scleroderma and related disorders: correlation of histologic, capillaroscopic, and clinical data. *Arthritis Rheum* 1984;27:97–103.
58. Von Vierbrauer AFG, Mennel HD, Schmidt JA, et al. Intravital microscopy and capillaroscopically guided nailfold biopsy in scleroderma. *Ann Rheum Dis* 1996;55:305–310.
59. von Bierbrauer A, Barth P, Willert J, et al. Electron microscopy and capillaroscopically guided nailfold biopsy in connective tissue diseases: detection of ultrastructural changes of the microcirculatory vessels. *Br J Rheumatol* 1998;37:1272–1278.
60. Zufferey P, Depairon M, Chamot A-M, et al. Prognostic significance of nailfold capillary microscopy in patients with Raynaud's phenomenon and scleroderma-pattern abnormalities: a six-year follow-up study. *Clin Rheumatol* 1992;11:536–541.
61. McGill NW, Gow PJ. Nailfold capillaroscopy: a blinded study of its discriminatory value in scleroderma, systemic lupus erythematosus, and rheumatoid arthritis. *Aust N Z J Med* 1986; 16:457–460.
62. Houtman PM, Kallenberg CGM, Wouda AA, et al. Decreased nailfold capillary density in Raynaud's phenomenon: a reflection of immunologically mediated local and systemic vascular disease? *Ann Rheum Dis* 1985;44:603–609.
63. Lovy M, MacCarter D, Steigerwald JC. Relationship between nailfold capillary abnormalities and organ involvement in systemic sclerosis. *Arthritis Rheum* 1985;28:496–501.
64. Coffman JD, Cohen AS. Total and capillary fingertip blood flow in Raynaud's phenomenon. *N Engl J Med* 1971;285: 259–263.
65. Maricq HR, Diat F, Weinrich MC, et al. Digital pressure responses to cooling in patients with suspected early vs. definite scleroderma (systemic sclerosis) vs. primary Raynaud's phenomenon. *J Rheumatol* 1994;21:1472–1476.
66. Hendriksen O, Kristensen JK. Reduced systolic blood pressure in fingers of patients with generalized scleroderma (acrosclerosis). *Acta Derm Venereol (Stockh)* 1981;61:531–534.
67. Kahaleh B, Matucci-Cerinic M: Raynaud's phenomenon and scleroderma: dysregulated neuroendothelial control of vascular tone. *Arthritis Rheum* 1995;38:1–4.
68. Yamane D, Miyauchi T, Suzuki N, et al. Elevated plasma levels of endothelin-1 in systemic sclerosis [Letter]. *Arthritis Rheum* 1991;34:243–244.
69. Yamane D, Miyauchi T, Suzuki N, et al. Significance of plasma endothelin-1 levels in patients with systemic sclerosis. *J Rheumatol* 1992;19:1566–1571.
70. Belch JJF, Zoma AA, Richards IM, et al. Vascular damage and factor-VIII-related antigen in the rheumatic diseases. *Rheumatol Int* 1987;7:107–111.
71. Kahaleh MB, Osborn I, LeRoy EC. Increased factor VIII/von Willebrand factor antigen and von Willebrand factor activity in scleroderma and in Raynaud's phenomenon. *Ann Intern Med* 1981;94:482–484.
72. Scheja A, Eskilsson J, Akesson A, et al. Inverse relation between plasma concentration of von Willebrand factor and CrEDTA clearance in systemic sclerosis. *J Rheumatol* 1994;21:639–642.
73. Zeiler J, Weissbarth E, Baruth B, et al. Serotonin content of platelets in inflammatory rheumatic diseases: correlation with clinical activity. *Arthritis Rheum* 1983;26:532–540.
74. Friedhoff LT, Seibold JR, Kim HC, et al. Serotonin induced platelet aggregation in systemic sclerosis. *Clin Exp Rheumatol* 1984;2:119–123.
75. Kahaleh MB, Osborn I, LeRoy EC. Elevated levels of circulating platelet aggregates and beta-thromboglobulin in scleroderma. *Ann Intern Med* 1982;96:610–613.
76. Seibold JR, Harris JN. Plasma β-thromboglobulin in the differential diagnosis of Raynaud's phenomenon. *J Rheumatol* 1985; 12:99–103.
77. Rodnan GP. The nature of joint involvement in progressive systemic sclerosis (diffuse scleroderma): clinical study and pathological examination of synovium in twenty-nine patients. *Ann Intern Med* 1962;56:422–439.
78. Devogelaer JP, Huaux JP, Maldague B, et al. Intra-articular calcification in progressive systemic sclerosis. *Clin Rheumatol* 1986;5:262–267.
79. Brandt KD, Krey PR. Chalky joint effusion: the result of massive synovial deposition of calcium apatite in progressive systemic sclerosis. *Arthritis Rheum* 1977;20:792–796.
80. Steen VD, Medsger TA Jr. The palpable tendon friction rub: an important physical examination finding in patients with systemic sclerosis. *Arthritis Rheum* 1997;40:1146–1151.
81. Palmer DG, Hale EM, Grennan DM, et al. Bowed fingers: a helpful sign in the early diagnosis of systemic sclerosis. *J Rheumatol* 1981;8:266–272.
82. Poole JL, Steen VD. The use of the health assessment questionnaire to determine physical disability in systemic sclerosis. *Arthritis Care Res* 1991;4:27–31.
83. Blocka KLN, Bassett LW, Furst DE, et al. The arthropathy of advanced progressive systemic sclerosis: a radiographic survey. *Arthritis Rheum* 1981;24:874–884.
84. Armstrong RD, Gibson T. Scleroderma and erosive polyarthritis: a disease entity? *Ann Rheum Dis* 1982;41:141–146.
85. Owens GR, Fino GJ, Herbert DL, et al. Pulmonary function in progressive systemic sclerosis: comparison of CREST syndrome variant with diffuse scleroderma. *Chest* 1983;84:546–550.
86. Osial TA Jr, Avakian A, Sassouni V, et al. Resorption of the mandibular condyles and coronoid processes in progressive systemic sclerosis (scleroderma). *Arthritis Rheum* 1981;24:729–733.
87. Medsger TA Jr. Progressive systemic sclerosis: skeletal muscle involvement. *Clin Rheum Dis* 1979;5:103–113.
88. Clements PJ, Furst DE, Campion DS, et al. Muscle disease in progressive systemic sclerosis: diagnostic and therapeutic considerations. *Arthritis Rheum* 1978;21:62–71.
89. Foster TD, Fairburn EA. Dental involvement in scleroderma. *Br Dent J* 1968;124:353–356.
90. Rowell NR, Hopper FE. The periodontal membrane in systemic sclerosis. *Br J Dermatol* 1977;96:15–20.
91. Rajapakse CNA, Bancewicz J, Jones CJP, et al. Pharyngoesophageal dysphagia in systemic sclerosis. *Ann Rheum Dis* 1981;40:612–614.
92. Takebayashi S, Matsui K, Ozawa Y, et al. Cervical esophageal motility: evaluation with US in progressive systemic sclerosis. *Radiology* 1991;179:389–393.
93. Stentoft P, Hendel L, Aggestrup S. Esophageal manometry and pH-probe monitoring in the evaluation of gastroesophageal reflux in patients with progressive systemic sclerosis. *Scand J Gastroenterol* 1987;22:499–504.
94. Bassotti G, Bataglia E, Debernardi V, et al. Esophageal dysfunction in scleroderma: relationship with disease subsets. *Arthritis Rheum* 1997;40:2252–2259.

95. Katzka DA, Reynolds JC, Saul SH, et al. Barrett's metaplasia and adenocarcinoma of the esophagus in scleroderma. *Am J Med* 1987;82:46–52.
96. Segel MC, Campbell WL, Medsger TA Jr, et al. Systemic sclerosis (scleroderma) and esophageal adenocarcinoma: is increased patient screening necessary? *Gastroenterology* 1985;89:485–488.
97. Garrett JM, Winkelmann RK, Schlegel JF, et al. Esophageal deterioration in scleroderma. *Mayo Clin Proc* 1971;46:92–96.
98. Davidson A, Russell C, Littlejohn GO. Assessment of esophageal abnormalities in progressive systemic sclerosis using radionuclide transit. *J Rheumatol* 1985;12:472–477.
99. Tsianos EB, Drosos AA, Chiras CD, et al. Esophageal manometric findings in autoimmune rheumatic disease: is scleroderma esophagus a specific entity? *Rheumatol Int* 1987;7:23–27.
100. Akesson A, Akesson B, Gustafson T, et al. Gastrointestinal function in patients with progressive systemic sclerosis. *Clin Rheumatol* 1985;4:441–448.
101. Rosenkrans PC, de Rooy DJ, Bosman FT, et al. Gastrointestinal telangiectasia as a cause of severe blood loss in systemic sclerosis. *Endoscopy* 1980;12:200–204.
102. Scolapio J, Matteson EL. The watermelon stomach in scleroderma. *Arthritis Rheum* 1993;36:724–725.
103. Carbone L, McKown KM, St. Hilaire RJ, et al. Scleroderma and the watermelon stomach. *Ann Rheum Dis* 1996;55:560–561.
104. Lundberg A-C, Akesson A, Akesson B. Dietary intake and nutritional status in patients with systemic sclerosis. *Ann Rheum Dis* 1992;51:1143–1148.
105. Vautier G, McDermott E, Carty JE, et al. Small bowel telangiectasia in scleroderma. *Ann Rheum Dis* 1995;54:78.
106. Marguerie C, Kaye S, Vyse T, et al. Malabsorption caused by coeliac disease in patients who have scleroderma. *Br J Rheumatol* 1995;34:858–861.
107. Hendy MS, Torrance HB, Warnes TW. Small-bowel volvulus in association with progressive systemic sclerosis. *Br Med J* 1979;1:1051–1052.
108. Elwany S, Talaat M, Kamel N, et al. Further observations on nasal mucosal changes in scleroderma. *J Laryngol Otol* 1984;98:979–986.
109. Gordon MB, Klein I, Dekker A, et al. Thyroid disease in progressive systemic sclerosis (PSS): increased frequency of glandular fibrosis and hypothyroidism. *Ann Intern Med* 1981;95:431–435.
110. Osial TA Jr, Whiteside TL, Buckingham RB, et al. Clinical and serologic study of Sjögren's syndrome in patients with progressive systemic sclerosis. *Arthritis Rheum* 1983;26:500–508.
111. Battle WM, Snape WJ Jr, Wright S, et al. Abnormal colonic motility in progressive systemic sclerosis. *Ann Intern Med* 1981;94:749–752.
112. Leighton JA, Valdovinos MA, Pemberton JH, et al. Anorectal dysfunction and rectal prolapse in progressive systemic sclerosis. *Dis Colon Rectum* 1993;36:182–185.
113. Hamel-Roy J, Devroede G, Ashan P, et al. Comparative esophageal and anorectal motility in scleroderma. *Gastroenterology* 1985;88:1–7.
114. D'Angelo G, Stern HS, Myers E. Rectal prolapse in scleroderma: case report and review of the colonic complications of scleroderma. *Can J Surg* 1985;28:62–63.
115. Kemp-Harper RA, Jackson DC. Progressive systemic sclerosis. *Br J Radiol* 1965;38:825–834.
116. Robinson JC, Teitelbaum SL. Stercoral ulceration and perforation of the sclerodermatous colon: report of two cases and review of the literature. *Dis Colon Rectum* 1974;17:622–632.
117. Owens GR, Follansbee WP. Cardiopulmonary manifestations of systemic sclerosis. *Chest* 1987;91:118–127.
118. Sudduth CD, Strange C, Cook WR, et al. Failure of the circulatory system limits exercise performance in patients with systemic sclerosis. *Am J Med* 1993;95:413–418.
119. Guttadauria M, Ellman H, Emmanuel G, et al. Pulmonary function in scleroderma. *Arthritis Rheum* 1977;20:1071–1079.
120. Bjerke RD, Tashkin DP, Clements PJ, et al. Small airways in progressive systemic sclerosis (PSS). *Am J Med* 1979;66:201–209.
121. Peters-Golden M, Wise RA, Schneider P, et al. Clinical and demographic predictors of loss of pulmonary function in systemic sclerosis. *Medicine* 1984;63:221–231.
122. Greenwald GI, Tashkin DP, Gong H, et al. Longitudinal changes in lung function and respiratory symptoms in progressive systemic sclerosis. *Am J Med* 1987;83:83–92.
123. Steen VD, Conte C, Owens G, et al. Severe restrictive lung disease in systemic sclerosis. *Arthritis Rheum* 1994;37:1283–1289.
124. Schurawitzki H, Stigbauer R, Graninger W. Interstitial lung disease in progressive systemic sclerosis: high-resolution CT versus radiography. *Radiology* 1990;176:755–759.
125. Warrick JH, Bhalla M, Schabel SI, et al. High resolution computed tomography in early scleroderma lung disease. *J Rheumatol* 1991;18:1520–1528.
126. Wells AU, Hansell DM, Corrin B, et al. High resolution computed tomography as a predictor of lung histology in systemic sclerosis. *Thorax* 1992;47:738–742.
127. Wells AU, Hansell DM, Rubens MB, et al. The predictive value of appearances on thin-section computed tomography in fibrosing alveolitis. *Am Rev Respir Dis* 1993;148:1076–1082.
128. Baron M, Feiglin D, Hyland R, et al. ^{67}Gallium lung scans in progressive systemic sclerosis. *Arthritis Rheum* 1983;26:969–974.
129. Furst DE, Davis JA, Clements PJ, et al. Abnormalities of pulmonary vascular dynamics and inflammation in early progressive systemic sclerosis. *Arthritis Rheum* 1981;24:1403–1408.
130. Silver RM, Metcalf JF, Stanley JH, et al. Interstitial lung disease in scleroderma: analysis by bronchoalveolar lavage. *Arthritis Rheum* 1984;27:1254–1261.
131. Konig G, Lunderschmidt C, Hammer C, et al. Lung involvement in scleroderma. *Chest* 1984;85:318–324.
132. Rossi GA, Bitteman PB, Rennard SI, et al. Evidence for chronic inflammation as a component of the interstitial lung disease associated with progressive systemic sclerosis. *Am Rev Respir Dis* 1985;131:612–617.
133. Edelson JS, Hyland RH, Ramsden M, et al. Lung inflammation in scleroderma: clinical, radiographic, physiologic and cytopathological features. *J Rheumatol* 1985;12:957–963.
134. Silver RM. Scleroderma: clinical problems: the lungs. *Rheum Dis Clin North Am* 1996;22:825–840.
135. Atamas SP, Yurovsky VV, Wise R, et al. Production of type 2 cytokines by $CD8^+$ lung cells is associated with greater decline in pulmonary function in patients with systemic sclerosis. *Arthritis Rheum* 1999;42:1168–1178.
136. Stupi A, Steen VD, Medsger TA Jr, et al. Pulmonary hypertension (PHT) in the CREST syndrome variant of progressive systemic sclerosis (PSS). *Arthritis Rheum* 1986;29:515–524.
137. Sacks DG, Okano Y, Steen VD, et al. Isolated pulmonary hypertension in systemic sclerosis with diffuse cutaneous involvement: association with anti-U3RNP antibody. *J Rheumatol* 1996;23:639–642.
138. Steen VD, Graham G, Conte C, et al. Isolated diffusing capacity reduction in systemic sclerosis. *Arthritis Rheum* 1992;35:765–770.
139. Yousem SA. The pulmonary pathologic manifestations of the CREST syndrome. *Hum Pathol* 1990;21:467–474.
140. Shuck JW, Oetgen WJ, Tesar JT. Pulmonary vascular response during Raynaud's phenomenon in progressive systemic sclerosis. *Am J Med* 1985;78:221–227.

141. Peters-Golden M, Wise RA, Hochberg MC, et al. Carbon monoxide diffusing capacity as predictor of outcome in systemic sclerosis. *Am J Med* 1984;77:1027–1034.
142. Roumm AD, Medsger TA Jr. Cancer and systemic sclerosis. *Arthritis Rheum* 1985;28:1336–1340.
143. Abu-Shakra M, Guillemin F, Lee P. Cancer in systemic sclerosis. *Arthritis Rheum* 1993;36:460–464.
144. Deswal A, Follansbee WF. Cardiac involvement in scleroderma. *Rheum Dis North Am* 1996;22:841–860.
145. Follansbee W. The cardiovascular manifestations of systemic sclerosis (scleroderma). *Curr Probl Cardiol* 1986;11:242–298.
146. Bulkley BH. Progressive systemic sclerosis: cardiac involvement. *Clin Rheum Dis* 1979;5:131–149.
147. McWhorter JE, LeRoy EC. Pericardial disease in scleroderma (systemic sclerosis). *Am J Med* 1974;57:566–574.
148. Satoh M, Tokuhira M, Hama N, et al. Massive pericardial effusion in scleroderma: a review of five cases. *Br J Rheumatol* 1995; 34:564–567.
149. Valentini G, Vitale DF, Giunta A, et al. Diastolic abnormalities in systemic sclerosis: evidence for associated defective cardiac functional reserve. *Ann Rheum Dis* 1996;55:455–460.
150. Follansbee WP, Curtiss EI, Medsger TA Jr, et al. Physiologic abnormalities of cardiac function in progressive systemic sclerosis with diffuse scleroderma. *N Engl J Med* 1984;310:142–148.
151. Armstrong GP, Whalley GA, Doughty RN, et al. Left ventricular function in scleroderma. *Br J Rheumatol* 1996;35:983–988.
152. West SG, Killian PJ, Lawless DJ. Association of myositis and myocarditis in progressive systemic sclerosis. *Arthritis Rheum* 1981;24:662–667.
153. Carette S, Turcotte J, Mathon G. Severe myositis and myocarditis in progressive systemic sclerosis. *J Rheumatol* 1985;12: 997–999.
154. Gaal J, Hegedus I, Devenyi K, et al. Myocardial gallium-67 citrate scintigraphy in patients with systemic sclerosis. *Ann Rheum Dis* 1995;54:856–858.
155. Follansbee WP, Zerbe TR, Medsger TA Jr. Cardiac and skeletal muscle disease in systemic sclerosis (scleroderma): a high risk association. *Am Heart J* 1993;125:194–203.
156. Todesco S, Gatta A, Glorioso S, et al. Cardiac involvement in progressive systemic sclerosis. *Acta Cardiol* 1979;5:311–322.
157. Ellis WW, Baer AN, Robertson RM, et al. Left ventricular dysfunction induced by cold exposure in patients with systemic sclerosis. *Am J Med* 1986;80:385–392.
158. Lekakis J, Mavrikakis M, Emmanuel M, et al. Cold-induced coronary Raynaud's phenomenon in patients with systemic sclerosis. *Clin Exp Rheumatol* 1998;16:135–140.
159. Kahan A, Devaux J, Amor B, et al. Nifedipine and thallium-201 myocardial perfusion in progressive systemic sclerosis. *N Engl J Med* 1986;314:1397–1402.
160. Kahan A, Devaux J, Amor B, et al. Pharmacodynamic effect of dipyridamole on thallium-201 myocardial perfusion in progressive systemic sclerosis with diffuse scleroderma. *Ann Rheum Dis* 1986;45:718–725.
161. Nitenberg A, Foult J-M, Kahan A, et al. Reduced coronary flow and resistance reserve in primary scleroderma myocardial disease. *Am Heart J* 1986;112:309–315.
162. McCarthy G, Kenny D. Nicardipine in systemic sclerosis [Letter]. *J Rheumatol* 1989;16:415.
163. Lichtbroun AS, Sandhaus LM, Giorno RC, et al. Myocardial mast cell in systemic sclerosis: a report of three fatal cases. *Am J Med* 1990;89:372–376.
164. Smith JW, Clements PJ, Levisman J, et al. Echocardiographic features of progressive systemic sclerosis (PSS): correlation with hemodynamic and postmortem studies. *Am J Med* 1979;66: 28–33.
165. James TN. De subitaneis mortibus: VIII. Coronary arteries and conduction system in scleroderma heart disease. *Circulation* 1974;50:844–956.
166. Clements PJ, Furst DE, Cabeen W, et al. The relationship of arrhythmias and conduction disturbances to other manifestations of cardiopulmonary disease in progressive systemic sclerosis (PSS). *Am J Med* 1981;71:38–46.
167. Blom-Bulow B, Jonson B, Bauer K. Factors limiting exercise performance in progressive systemic sclerosis. *Semin Arthritis Rheum* 1983;13:174–181.
168. Roberts NK, Cabeen WR. Atrioventricular nodal function in progressive systemic sclerosis: electrophysiological and morphological findings. *Br Heart J* 1980;44:529–533.
169. Ridolfi RL, Bulkley BH, Hutchins GM. The cardiac conduction system in progressive systemic sclerosis: clinical and pathologic features of 35 patients. *Am J Med* 1976;61:361–366.
170. Penmetcha M, Rosenbush SW, Harris CA. Cardiac valvular disease in scleroderma and systemic lupus erythematosus/scleroderma overlap associated with antiphospholipid antibodies. *J Rheumatol* 1996;23:2171–2174.
171. Steen VD. Scleroderma renal crisis. *Rheum Dis Clin North Am* 1996;22:861–878.
172. Steen VD. Factors predicting the development of renal involvement in progressive systemic sclerosis. *Am J Med* 1984;76: 779–786.
173. Molina JF, Anaya JM, Cabrera GE, et al. Systemic sclerosis sine scleroderma: an unusual presentation in scleroderma renal crisis. *J Rheumatol* 1995;22:557–560.
174. Sundar AS, Malhotra KK, Bhuyan UN, et al. Kidney in progressive systemic sclerosis. *Indian J Med Res* 1985;82:534–539.
175. Clements PJ, Lachenbruch PA, Furst DE, et al. Abnormalities of renal physiology in systemic sclerosis: a prospective study with 10-year follow-up. *Arthritis Rheum* 1994;37:67–74.
176. Salyer WR, Salyer DC, Heptinstall RH. Scleroderma and microangiopathic hemolytic anemia. *Ann Intern Med* 1973;78: 895–897.
177. Steen VD, Medsger TA Jr. Case-control study of corticosteroids and other drugs that either precipitate or protect from the development of scleroderma renal crisis. *Arthritis Rheum* 1998; 41:1613–1619.
178. Cannon PJ, Hassar M, Case DB, et al. The relationship of hypertension and renal failure on scleroderma (progressive systemic sclerosis) to structural and functional abnormalities of the renal cortical circulation. *Medicine* 1974;53:1–46.
179. Cookson S, Krueger ML, Bennett RM. Fulminant thrombotic thrombocytopenic purpura in a patient with the limited form of scleroderma: successful outcome using plasma exchange. *J Rheumatol* 1991;18:900–901.
180. Steen VD, Costantino JP, Shapiro AP, et al. Outcome of renal crisis in systemic sclerosis: relation to availability to angiotensin converting enzyme (ACE) inhibitors. *Am Intern Med* 1990; 113:352–357.
181. Beckett VL, Donadio JV, Brennan LA, et al. Use of captopril as early therapy for renal scleroderma: a prospective study. *Mayo Clin Proc* 1985;60:763–771.
182. Moore HC, Sheehan HL. The kidney of scleroderma. *Lancet* 1952;1:68–70.
183. Lapenas D, Rodnan GP, Cavallo T. Immunopathology of the renal vascular lesion of progressive systemic sclerosis (scleroderma). *Am J Pathol* 1978;91:243–258.
184. McGiven AR, deBoer WGRM, Barnett AJ. Renal immune deposits in scleroderma. *Pathology* 1971;3:145–150.
185. Lally EV, Kaplan SR, Susset JG, et al. Pathologic involvement of the urinary bladder in progressive systemic sclerosis. *J Rheumatol* 1985;12:778–781.

186. Bhadauria S, Moser DK, Clements PJ, et al. Genital tract abnormalities and female sexual function impairment in systemic sclerosis. *Am J Obstet Gynecol* 1995;172:580–587.
187. Nowlin NS, Brick JE, Weaver DJ, et al. Impotence in scleroderma. *Ann Intern Med* 1986;104:794–798.
188. Nehra A, Hall SJ, Basile G, et al. Systemic sclerosis and impotence: a clinicopathological correlation. *J Urol* 1995;153:1140–1146.
189. Culp KS, Fleming CR, Duffy J, et al. Autoimmune association of primary biliary cirrhosis. *Mayo Clin Proc* 1982;57:365–370.
190. Clarke AK, Galbraith RM, Hamilton EDB, et al. Rheumatic disorders in primary biliary cirrhosis. *Ann Rheum Dis* 1978;37:42–47.
191. Alderuccio F, Toh B-H, Barnett AJ, et al. Identification and characterization of mitochondria autoantigens in progressive systemic sclerosis: identity with the 74,000 dalton autoantigen in primary biliary cirrhosis. *J Immunol* 1986;137:1855–1859.
192. Russell ML, Kahn JJ. Nodular regenerative hyperplasia of the liver associated with progressive systemic sclerosis: a case report with ultrastructural observation. *J Rheumatol* 1983;10:748–752.
193. D'Angelo WA, Fries JF, Masi AT, et al. Pathologic observations in systemic sclerosis (scleroderma): study of 58 autopsy cases and 58 matched controls. *Am J Med* 1969;46:428–440.
194. Frayha RA, Shulman LE, Stevens MB. Hematological abnormalities in scleroderma: a study of 180 cases. *Acta Haematol* 1980;64:25–30.
195. Sumithran E. Progressive systemic sclerosis and autoimmune haemolytic anemia. *Postgrad Med J* 1976;52:173–176.
196. Waugh D, Ibels L. Malignant scleroderma associated with autoimmune neutropenia. *Br Med J* 1980;280:1577–1578.
197. Falanga V, Medsger TA Jr. Frequency, levels and significance of blood eosinophilia in systemic sclerosis, localized scleroderma and eosinophilic fasciitis. *J Am Acad Dermatol* 1987;17:648–656.
198. Schady W, Sheard A, Hassell A, et al. Peripheral nerve dysfunction in scleroderma. *Q J Med* 1991;80:661–675.
199. Farrell DA, Medsger TA Jr. Trigeminal neuropathy in progressive systemic sclerosis. *Am J Med* 1982;73:57–62.
200. Blanche P, Lamy C, Zuber M, et al. Cerebral arteriopathy in scleroderma. *Clin Exp Rheumatol* 1996;14:700–701.
201. Oddis CV, Eisenbeis CH Jr, Reidbord HE, et al. Vasculitis in systemic sclerosis: association with Sjögren's syndrome and the CREST syndrome variant. *J Rheumatol* 1987;14:942–948.
202. Averbuch-Heller L, Steiner I, Abramsky O. Neurologic manifestations of progressive systemic sclerosis. *Arch Neurol* 1992;49:1292–1295.
203. Cerinic MM, Generini S, Pignone A, et al. The nervous system in systemic sclerosis (scleroderma): clinical features and pathogenetic mechanisms. *Rheum Dis Clin North Am* 1996;22:879–892.
204. Hermosillo AG, Ortiz R, Dabague J, et al. Autonomic dysfunction in diffuse scleroderma vs. CREST: an assessment by computerized heart rate variability. *J Rheumatol* 1994;21:1849–1854.
205. Sonnex C, Paice E, White AG. Autonomic neuropathy in systemic sclerosis: a case report and elevation of six patients. *Ann Rheum Dis* 1986;45:957–960.
206. Dessein PH, Joffe BI, Metz RM, et al. Autonomic dysfunction in systemic sclerosis: sympathetic overactivity and instability. *Am J Med* 1992;93:143–150.
207. West RH, Barnett AJ. Ocular involvement in scleroderma. *Br J Ophthalmol* 1979;63:845–847.
208. Grennan DM, Forrester JA. Involvement of the eye in SLE and scleroderma. *Ann Rheum Dis* 1977;36:152–156.
209. Tosti A, Patrizi A, Veronesi S. Audiologic involvement in systemic sclerosis. *Dermatologica* 1984;168:206.
210. Kahl LE, Medsger TA Jr, Klein I, et al. Prospective evaluation of thyroid function in patients with systemic sclerosis (scleroderma). *J Rheumatol* 1986;12:103–107.
211. Nicholson D, White S, Lipson A, et al. Progressive systemic sclerosis and Graves' disease: report of 3 cases. *Arch Intern Med* 1986;146:2350–2352.
212. Medsger TA Jr, Masi AT. Epidemiology of systemic sclerosis (scleroderma). *Ann Intern Med* 1971;74:714–721.
213. Suarez-Almazor ME, Catoggio LJ, Maldonado-Cocco JA, et al. Juvenile progressive systemic sclerosis: clinical and serologic findings. *Arthritis Rheum* 1985;28:699–702.
214. Blaszczyk M, Jablonska S, Szymanska-Jagiello W, et al. Childhood scleromyositis: an overlap syndrome associated with PM-Scl antibody. *Pediatr Dermatol* 1991;8:1–8.
215. Singsen BH. Scleroderma in childhood. *Pediatr Clin North Am* 1986;33:1119–1139.
216. Hanson V. Dermatomyositis, scleroderma and polyarteritis nodosa. *Clin Rheum Dis* 1976;2:455–464.
217. Cassidy JT, Sullivan DB, Dabich L, et al. Scleroderma in children. *Arthritis Rheum* 1977;20(suppl):351–354.
218. Ansell BM, Falcini F, Woo P. Scleroderma in childhood. *Clin Dermatol* 1994;12:299–307.
219. Bernstein RM, Pereira RS, Holden AJ, et al. Autoantibodies in childhood scleroderma. *Ann Rheum Dis* 1985;44:503–506.
220. Giordano M, Valentini G, Lupoli S, et al. Pregnancy and systemic sclerosis. *Ann Rheum Dis* 1985;28:237–238.
221. Ballou SP, Morley JJ, Kushner I. Pregnancy and systemic sclerosis. *Arthritis Rheum* 1984;27:295–298.
222. Steen VD, Medsger TA Jr. Fertility and pregnancy outcome in women with systemic sclerosis. *Arthritis Rheum* 1999;42:763–768.
223. Mor-Yosef S, Navot D, Rabinowitz R, et al. Collagen diseases in pregnancy. *Obstet Gynecol Surg* 1984;39:67–84.
224. Steen VD, Conte C, Day N, et al. Pregnancy in women with systemic sclerosis. *Arthritis Rheum* 1989;32:151–157.
225. Steen VD. Scleroderma and pregnancy. *Rheum Dis Clin North Am* 1997;23:133–147.
226. Englert H, Brennan P, McNeil P, et al. Reproductive function prior to disease onset in women with scleroderma. *J Rheumatol* 1992;19:1575–1579.
227. Scarpinato L, MacKenzie AH. Pregnancy and progressive systemic sclerosis: case report and review of the literature. *Cleve Clin Q* 1985;52:207.
228. Sood SV, Kohler HG. Maternal death from systemic sclerosis: report of a case of renal scleroderma masquerading as pre-eclamptic toxaemia. *J Obstet Gynecol Br Commw* 1970:77:1109–1112.
229. Palma A, Sanchez-Palencia A, Armas JR, et al. Progressive systemic sclerosis and nephrotic syndrome. *Arch Intern Med* 1981;141:520–521.
230. Duncan SC, Winkelmann RK. Cancer and scleroderma. *Arch Dermatol* 1979;115:950–955.
231. Medsger TA Jr, Masi AT. The epidemiology of systemic sclerosis (scleroderma) among male U.S. veterans. *J Chronic Dis* 1978;31:73–85.
232. Black KA, Zilko PJ, Dawkins RL, et al. Cancer in connective tissue disease. *Arthritis Rheum* 1982;25:1130–1133.
233. Lee P, Alderdice C, Wilkinson S, et al. Malignancy in progressive systemic sclerosis: association with breast carcinoma. *J Rheumatol* 1983;10:665–666.
234. Medsger TA Jr. Systemic sclerosis and malignancy: are they related? *J Rheumatol* 1985;12:1041–1043.
235. Varga J, Haustein UF, Creech R, et al. Exaggerated radiation-

induced fibrosis in patients with systemic sclerosis. *JAMA* 1991;265:3292–3295.

236. Robertson JM, Clarke DH, Pevzner MM, et al. Breast conservation therapy: severe breast fibrosis after radiation therapy in patients with collagen vascular disease. *Cancer* 1991;68: 502–508.
237. Barnett AJ. Some observations on the immunological status in scleroderma (progressive systemic sclerosis). *Aust N Z J Med* 1978;8:622–627.
238. Kogo Y, Yamaguchi I, Tamura M, et al. A case of the progressive systemic sclerosis (PSS) with high serum concentration of M protein. *Jpn Soc Intern Med* 1975;64:1167–1173.
239. Ja S, Helm S, Wary BB. Progressive systemic scleroderma with IgA deficiency in a child. *Am J Dis Child* 1981;135:965–966.
240. Bernstein RM, Steigerwald JC, Tan EM. Association of antinuclear and antinucleolar antibodies in progressive systemic sclerosis. *Clin Exp Immunol* 1982;48:43–51.
241. Douvas AS, Achten M, Tan EM. Identification of a nuclear protein (Scl-70) as a unique target of human antinuclear antibodies in scleroderma. *J Biol Chem* 1979;254:10514–10522.
242. Catoggio LJ, Bernstein RM, Black CM, et al. Serological markers in progressive systemic sclerosis: clinical correlations. *Ann Rheum Dis* 1983;42:23–27.
243. Shero JH, Bordwell B, Rothfield NF, et al. High titers of autoantibodies to topoisomerase I (Scl-70) in sera from scleroderma patients. *Science* 1986;231:737–740.
244. D'Arpa P, White-Cooper H, Cleveland D, et al. Use of molecular cloning methods to map the distribution of epitopes on topoisomerase I (Scl-70) recognized by sera of scleroderma patients. *Arthritis Rheum* 1990;33:1501–1511.
245. Kuwana M, Kaburaki J, Mimori T, et al. Autoantigenic epitopes on DNA topoisomerase I: clinical and immunogenetic associations in systemic sclerosis. *Arthritis Rheum* 1993;36: 1406–1413.
246. Burnham TK, Kleinsmith D'AM. The "true speckled" antinuclear antibody (ANA) pattern: its tumultuous history. *Semin Arthritis Rheum* 1983;13:155–159.
247. Weiner ES, Earnshaw WC, Senecal J-L, et al. Clinical associations of anticentromeric antibodies and antibodies to topoisomerase I: a study of 355 patients. *Arthritis Rheum* 1988;31: 378–385.
248. Catoggio LJ, Rodrigué S, Laborde H, et al. Autoantibodies in Argentine patients with systemic sclerosis (scleroderma). *Arthritis Rheum* 1985;28:715–717.
249. Steen VD, Ziegler GL, Rodnan GP, et al. Clinical and laboratory associations of anticentromere antibody (ACA) in patients with progressive systemic sclerosis (scleroderma). *Arthritis Rheum* 1984;27:125–131.
250. Kallenberg CGM, Pastoor GW, Wouda AA, et al. Antinuclear antibodies in patients with Raynaud's phenomenon: clinical significance of anticentromere antibodies. *Ann Rheum Dis* 1982; 41:382–387.
251. Migliaresi S. Infrequency of anticentromere antibody in patients without systemic sclerosis and without Raynaud's phenomenon. *Arthritis Rheum* 1987;30:358–359.
252. Goldman JA. Anticentromere antibody in patients without CREST and scleroderma: association with active digital vasculitis, rheumatic and connective tissue disease. *Ann Rheum Dis* 1989;48:771–775.
253. Genth E, Mierau R, Genetzky P, et al. Immunogenetic associations of scleroderma-related antinuclear antibodies. *Arthritis Rheum* 1990;33:657–665.
254. Zuber M, Gotzen R, Filler J. Clinical correlation of anticentromere antibodies. *Clin Rheumatol* 1994;13:427–432.
255. McCarty GA, Rice JR, Bembe ML, et al. Anticentromere antibody: clinical correlations and association with favorable prognosis in patients with scleroderma variants. *Arthritis Rheum* 1983;26:1–7.
256. Brenner S, Pepper D, Berns MW, et al. Kinetochore structure, duplication, and distribution in mammalian cells: analysis by human autoantibodies from scleroderma patients. *J Cell Biol* 1981;91:95–102.
257. Earnshaw W, Bordwell B, Marino C, et al. Three human chromosomal autoantigens are recognized by sera from patients with anti-centromere antibodies. *J Clin Invest* 1986;77:426–430.
258. Fritzler MJ, Ayer LM, Gohill J, et al. An antigen in metaphase chromatin and the midbody of mammalian cells binds to scleroderma sera. *J Rheumatol* 1987;14:291–294.
259. Osborn TG, Ryerse JS, Bauer NE, et al. Anticentriole antibody in a patient with progressive systemic sclerosis. *Arthritis Rheum* 1986;29:142–146.
260. Moroi Y, Murata I, Takevchi A, et al. Human anticentriole autoantibody in patients with scleroderma and Raynaud's phenomenon. *Clin Immunol Immunopathol* 1983;29:381–390.
261. Osborn TG, Patel NJ, Ross SC, et al. Antinuclear antibody staining only centrioles in a patient with scleroderma. *N Engl J Med* 1982;307:253–254.
262. Ruffatti A, Calligaro A, Ferri C, et al. Association of anti-centromere and anti-Scl 70 antibodies in scleroderma: report of two cases. *J Clin Lab Immunol* 1985;16:227–229.
263. Furst DE, Obrodovic M, Barnett EV, et al. Case control study of antibodies to ENA in progressive systemic sclerosis patients. *J Rheumatol* 1984;11:298–305.
264. Mimori T, Akizuki M, Yamagata H, et al. Characterization of a high molecular weight acidic nuclear protein recognized by autoantibodies in sera from patients with polymyositis-scleroderma overlap. *J Clin Invest* 1981;68:611–620.
265. Yaneva M, Arnett FC. Antibodies against Ku protein in sera from patients with autoimmune diseases. *Clin Exp Immunol* 1989;76:366–372.
266. Cooley HM, Melny BJ, Gleeson R, et al. Clinical and serological associations of anti-Ku antibody. *J Rheumatol* 1999;26: 563–567.
267. Reimer G, Rose KM, Scheer U, et al. Autoantibody to RNA polymerase I in scleroderma sera. *J Clin Invest* 1987;79:65–72.
268. Schnitz W, Taylor-Albert E, Targott IN, et al. Anti-PM/Scl autoantibodies in patients with clinical polymyositis or scleroderma. *J Rheumatol* 1996;23:1729–1733.
269. Kipnis R, Craft J, Hardin J. The analysis of antinuclear and antinucleolar antibodies of scleroderma by radioimmunoprecipitation assays. *Arthritis Rheum* 1990;33:1431–1437.
270. Hirakata M, Okano Y, Pati U, et al. Identification of autoantibodies to RNA polymerase II: occurrence in systemic sclerosis and association with autoantibodies to RNA polymerases I and III. *J Clin Invest* 1993;91:2665–2672.
271. Kuwana M, Kaburaki J, Mimori T, et al. Autoantibody reactive with three classes of RNA polymerases in sera from patients with systemic sclerosis. *J Clin Invest* 1993;91:1399–1404.
272. Seibold JR, Knight PJ, Peter JB. Anticardiolipin antibodies in systemic sclerosis [Letter]. *Arthritis Rheum* 1986;29: 1052–1053.
273. Merkel PA, Chang YC, Pierangeli SS, et al. The prevalence and clinical associations of anticardiolipin antibodies in a large inception cohort of patients with connective tissue diseases. *Am J Med* 1996;101:576–583.
274. Picillo U, Migliaresi S, Marcialis MR, et al. Clinical setting of patients with systemic sclerosis by serum autoantibodies. *Clin Rheumatol* 1997;16:378–383.
275. Merkel PA, Polisson RP, Chang YC, et al. Prevalence of antineutrophil cytoplasmic antibodies in a large inception cohort of patients with connective tissue disease. *Ann Intern Med* 1997; 126:866–873.

276. Locke JC, Worrall JG, Leaker B, et al. Autoantibodies to myeloperoxidase in systemic sclerosis. *J Rheumatol* 1997;24: 86–89.
277. Ayer LM, Senecal JL, Martin L, et al. Antibodies to high mobility group proteins in systemic sclerosis. *J Rheumatol* 1994;21: 2071–2075.
278. Fujimoto M, Sato S, Ihn H, et al. Antiubiquitin antibody in localized and systemic scleroderma. *Ann Rheum Dis* 1996;55: 399–402.
279. Wallace DJ, Lin HC, Shen GQ, et al. Antibodies to histone (H2A-H2B)-DNA complexes in the absence of antibodies to double-stranded DNA or to (H2A-H2B) complexes are more sensitive and specific for scleroderma-related disorders than for lupus. *Arthritis Rheum* 1994;37:1795–1797.
280. Negi VS, Tripathy NK, Misra R, et al. Antiendothelial cell antibodies in scleroderma correlate with severe digital ischemia and pulmonary arterial hypertension. *J Rheumatol* 1998;25:462–466.
281. Reveille JD, Owerbach D, Goldstein R, et al. Association of polar amino acids at position 26 of the HLA-DQB1 first domain with the anticentromere autoantibody response in systemic sclerosis (scleroderma). *J Clin Invest* 1992;89:1208–1213.
282. Reveille JD, Durban E, MacLeod MJ, et al. Association of amino acid sequences in the HLA-DQB1 first domain with the anti-topoisomerase I autoantibody response in scleroderma (progressive systemic sclerosis). *J Clin Invest* 1992;90:973–980.
283. Kuwana M, Kaburaki J, Okano Y, et al. Molecular immunogenetic association with an autoantigenic epitope on topoisomerase I. *Arthritis Rheum* 1992;35(suppl):S83(abst).
284. Tan FK, Howard RF, Reveille JD, et al. Case control study of systemic sclerosis among Choctaw Native Americans in southeastern Oklahoma. *Arthritis Rheum* 1994;73(suppl):S282(abst).
285. Takeuchi F, Nakano K, Yamada H, et al. Association of HLA-DR with progressive systemic sclerosis in Japanese. *J Rheumatol* 1994;21:857–863.
286. Kuwana M, Okano Y, Kaburaki J, et al. HLA class II genes associated with anticentromere antibody in Japanese patients with systemic sclerosis (scleroderma). *Ann Rheum Dis* 1995;54: 983–987.
287. Kuwana M, Okano Y, Kuburaki J, et al. Racial differences in distribution of systemic sclerosis-related serum antinuclear antibodies. *Arthritis Rheum* 1994;37:902–906.
288. Oddis CV, Okano Y, Rudert WA, et al. Serum autoantibody to the nucleolar antigen PM-Scl: clinical and immunogenetic associations. *Arthritis Rheum* 1992;35:1211–1217.
289. Miller MH, Littlejohn GO, Davidson A, et al. The clinical significance of the anticentromere antibody. *Br J Rheumatol* 1987; 26:17–21.
290. Greaves M, Malia RG, Ward AM, et al. Elevated von Willebrand factor antigen in systemic sclerosis: relationship to visceral disease. *Br J Rheumatol* 1988;27:281–285.
291. Soma Y, Takahara K, Sato S, et al. Increase in plasma thrombomodulin in patients with systemic sclerosis. *J Rheumatol* 1993; 20:1444–1445.
292. Kiener H, Graninger W, Machold K, et al. Increased levels of circulating intercellular adhesion molecule 1 in patients with systemic sclerosis. *Clin Exp Rheumatol* 1994;12:483–487.
293. Gruschwitz MS, Hornstein OP, von den Driesch P. Correlation of soluble adhesion molecules in the peripheral blood of scleroderma patients with their in situ expression and with disease activity. *Arthritis Rheum* 1995;38:184–189.
294. Kahaleh MB, LeRoy EC. Interleukin-2 in scleroderma: correlation of serum level with extent of skin involvement and disease duration. *Ann Intern Med* 1989;110:446–450.
295. Degiannis D, Seibold JR, Czarnecki M, et al. Soluble interleukin-2 receptors in patients with systemic sclerosis. *Arthritis Rheum* 1990;33:375–380.
296. Steen VD, Charley MS, Medsger TA Jr, et al. Soluble serum interleukin-2 receptors in patients with systemic sclerosis. *J Rheumatol* 1996;23:446–449.
297. Black CM, McWhirter A, Harrison NK, et al. Serum type III procollagen peptide concentrations in systemic sclerosis and Raynaud's phenomenon: relationship to disease activity and duration. *Br J Rheumatol* 1989;28:98–103.
298. Stone PJ, Korn JH, North H, et al. Cross-linked elastin and collagen degradation products in the urine of patients with scleroderma. *Arthritis Rheum* 1995;38:517–524.
299. Medsger TA Jr, Silman AJ, Steen VD, et al. Development of a severity index for systemic sclerosis. *Arthritis Rheum* 1994;37 (suppl):S260.
300. Medsger TA Jr, Masi AT. Epidemiology of progressive systemic sclerosis. *Clin Rheum Dis* 1979;5:15–25.
301. Bryan C, Howard Y, Brennan P, et al. Survival following the onset of scleroderma: results from a retrospective inception cohort study of the UK patient population. *Br J Rheumatol* 1996;35:1122–1126.
302. Lee P, Langevitz P, Alderdice CA, et al. Mortality in systemic sclerosis (scleroderma). *Q J Med* 1992;82:139–148.
303. Nagy Z, Czirjak L. Predictors of survival in 171 patients with systemic sclerosis (scleroderma). *Clin Rheumatol* 1997;16: 454–460.
304. Altman RD, Medsger TA Jr, Bloch D, et al. Predictors of survival in systemic sclerosis (scleroderma). *Arthritis Rheum* 1991; 34:403–413.
305. Silman AJ. Scleroderma and survival. *Ann Rheum Dis* 1991;50: 267–269.
306. Spooner MS, LeRoy EC. The changing face of severe scleroderma in five patients. *Clin Exp Rheumatol* 1990;8:101–105.
307. Jacobsen S, Halberg P, Ullman S. Mortality and causes of death of 344 Danish patients with systemic sclerosis (scleroderma). *Br J Rheumatol* 1998;37:750–755.
308. Giordano M, Valentini G, Migliaresi S, et al. Different antibody patterns and different prognoses in patients with scleroderma with various extent of skin sclerosis. *J Rheumatol* 1986;13: 911–916.
309. Merkel PA. Measurement of functional status, self-assessment and psychological well-being in scleroderma. *Curr Opin Rheumatol* 1998;10:589–594.
310. Poole JL, Williams CA, Bloch DA. Concurrent validity of the Health Assessment Questionnaire Disability Index in scleroderma. *Arthritis Care Res* 1995;8:189–193.
311. Steen VD, Medsger TA Jr. The value of the Health Assessment Questionnaire and special patient-generated scales to demonstrate change in systemic sclerosis patients over time. *Arthritis Rheum* 1997;40:1984–1991.
312. Silman A, Akesson A, Newman J, et al. Assessment of functional ability in patients with scleroderma: a proposed new disability assessment instrument. *J Rheumatol* 1998;25:79–83.
313. Wilson L. Cost-of-illness of scleroderma: the case for rare diseases. *Semin Arthritis Rheum* 1997;27:73–84.
314. Mayes MD. *The scleroderma book: a guide for patients and families.* New York: Oxford University Press, 1999.
315. Flapan M. *Perspectives of living with scleroderma. Voicing the hidden emotions of the chronically ill.* Danvers, MA: Scleroderma Federation, 1997.
316. Medsger TA Jr. Progressive systemic sclerosis. *Clin Rheum Dis* 1983;9:655–670.
317. Clements PJ, Lachenbruch PA, Seibold JR, et al. Skin thickness score in systemic sclerosis: an assessment of interobserver variability in 3 independent studies. *J Rheumatol* 1993;20: 1892–1896.
318. Pope JE, Bellamy N. Outcome measurement in scleroderma clinical trials. *Semin Arthritis Rheum* 1993;23:22–33.

319. Seibold JR, McCloskey DA. Skin involvement as a relevant outcome measure in clinical trials of systemic sclerosis. *Curr Opin Rheumatol* 1997;9:571–575.
320. Medsger TA Jr, Silman AF, Steen VD, et al. A disease severity scale for systemic sclerosis. Development and testing. *J Rheumatol* 1999;26:2159–2167.
321. Medsger TA Jr. Treatment of systemic sclerosis. *Rheum Dis Clin North Am* 1989;15:513–531.
322. Ghersetich I, Matucci-Cerinic M, Lotti T. A pathogenetic approach to the management of systemic sclerosis (scleroderma). *Int J Dermatol* 1990;29:616–622.
323. Pope JE. Treatment of systemic sclerosis. *Rheum Dis Clin North Am* 1996;22:893–907.
324. Helfrich DJ, Banner B, Steen VD, et al. Normotensive renal failure in systemic sclerosis. *Arthritis Rheum* 1989;32: 1128–1134.
325. Sharada B, Kumar A, Kakker R, et al. Intravenous dexamethasone pulse therapy in diffuse systemic sclerosis: a randomized placebo-controlled study. *Rheumatol Int* 1994;14:91–94.
326. Jayson MIV, Lovell C, Black CM. Penicillamine therapy in systemic sclerosis. *Proc R Soc Med* 1977;70:82–88.
327. Asboe-Hansen G. Treatment of generalized scleroderma: updated results. *Acta Derm Venereol* 1979;59:465–467.
328. Ivanova MM, Guseva NG, Balabanova RM, et al. Treatment of systemic sclerosis with D-penicillamine. *Ther Arch* 1977;7: 91–99.
329. Jimenez SA, Andrews RP, Myers AR. Treatment of rapidly progressive scleroderma (PSS) with D-penicillamine: a prospective study. In: Black CM, Myers AR, eds. *Systemic sclerosis (scleroderma):* current topics in rheumatology. New York: Gower Medical Publishing, 1985:387–393.
330. Sattar MA, Guindi TR, Sugathan TN. Penicillamine in systemic sclerosis: a reappraisal. *Clin Rheumatol* 1990;9:517–522.
331. Clements PJ, Furst DE, Wong W-K, et al. High-dose versus low-dose D-penicillamine in early diffuse systemic sclerosis: analysis of a two-year, double-blind, randomized, controlled clinical trial. *Arthritis Rheum* 1999;42:1194–1203.
332. Steen VD, Owens G, Redmond C, et al. The effect of D-penicillamine on pulmonary findings in systemic sclerosis. *Arthritis Rheum* 1985;28:882–888.
333. deClerck LS, Dequeker J, Francx L, et al. D-Penicillamine therapy and interstitial lung disease in scleroderma: a long-term followup study. *Arthritis Rheum* 1987;30:643–650.
334. Ntoso KA, Tomaszweski JE, Jiminez SA, et al. Penicillamine-induced rapidly progressive glomerulonephritis in patients with progressive systemic sclerosis: successful treatment of two patients and a review of the literature. *Am J Kidney Dis* 1986;8: 159–163.
335. Torres CF, Griggs RC, Baum J, et al. Penicillamine-induced myasthenia gravis in progressive systemic sclerosis. *Arthritis Rheum* 1980;23:505–508.
336. Steen VD, Blair S, Medsger TA Jr. The toxicity of D-penicillamine in systemic sclerosis. *Ann Intern Med* 1986;104: 699–705.
337. Furst DE, Clements PJ, Harris R, et al. Measurement of clinical change in progressive systemic sclerosis: a 1 year double-blind placebo-controlled trial of *N*-acetylcysteine. *Ann Rheum Dis* 1979;38:356–361.
338. Oriente P, Scarpa R, Biondi C, et al. Progressive systemic sclerosis and *S*-adenosylmethionine. *Clin Rheum* 1985;4:360–361.
339. Seibold JR, Clements PJ, Furst DE, et al. Safety and pharmacokinetics of recombinant human relaxin in systemic sclerosis. *J Rheumatol* 1998;25:302–307.
340. Alarcon-Segovia D. Progressive systemic sclerosis: management. Part IV: Colchicine. *Clin Rheum Dis* 1979;5:294–302.
341. Steigerwald JC, Lynch D. Colchicine therapy versus placebo: a double-blind study in progressive systemic sclerosis: abstract from the XIV International Congress of Rheumatology, San Francisco, 1977:163.
342. Guttadauria M, Diamond H, Kaplan D. Colchicine in the treatment of scleroderma. *J Rheumatol* 1977;4:272–275.
343. Clegg DO, Reading JC, Mayes MD, et al. Comparison of aminobenzoate potassium and placebo in the treatment of scleroderma. *J Rheumatol* 1994;21:105–110.
344. Jansen GT, Baraza DF, Ballard JL, et al. Generalized scleroderma: treatment with an immunosuppressive agent. *Arch Dermatol* 1968;97:690–698.
345. Casas J, Saway PA, Villarreal I, et al. 5-Fluorouracil in the treatment of scleroderma: a randomised, double-blind, placebo controlled international collaborative study. *Ann Rheum Dis* 1990; 49:926–928.
346. Furst DE, Clements PJ, Hillis S, et al. Immunosuppression with chlorambucil vs. placebo for scleroderma: results of a three-year, parallel, randomized, double-blind study. *Arthritis Rheum* 1989; 32:584–593.
347. Baker GL, Kahl LE, Zee BC, et al. Malignancy following treatment of rheumatoid arthritis with cyclophosphamide. *Am J Med* 1987;83:1–9.
348. Dau PC, Kahalen MD, Sagebiel RW. Plasmapheresis and immunosuppressive drug therapy in scleroderma. *Arthritis Rheum* 1981;24:1128–1136.
349. Schmidt C, Schooneman F, Siebert P, et al. Traitement de la sclerodermie generalisee par echanges plasmatiques. *Ann Med Interne (Paris)* 1988;139(suppl 1):20–22.
350. Capodicasa G, DeSanto NG, Galione A, et al. Clinical effectiveness of apheresis in the treatment of progressive systemic sclerosis. *Int J Artif Organs* 1983;6:81–86.
351. Guillevin L, Amoura Z, Merviel PH, et al. Treatment of progressive systemic sclerosis by plasma exchange: long-term results in 40 patients. *Int J Artif Organs* 1990;13:125–128.
352. Zachariae H, Halkier-Sorensen L, Heickendorff L, et al. Cyclosporin A treatment of systemic sclerosis. *Br J Dermatol* 1990;122:677–681.
353. Vayssairat M, Baudot N, Boitard C, et al. Cyclosporin therapy for severe systemic sclerosis associated with anti-Scl-70 autoantibody. *J Am Acad Dermatol* 1990;22:695–696.
354. Clements PJ, Lachenbruch PA, Sterz M, et al. Cyclosporine in systemic sclerosis: results of a forty-eight-week open safety study in ten patients. *Arthritis Rheum* 1993;36:75—83.
355. Denton CP, Sweny P, Abdulla A, et al. Acute renal failure occurring in scleroderma treated with cyclosporin A: a report of three cases. *Br J Rheumatol* 1994;33:90–92.
356. Kahan A, Amor B, Menkes CJ, et al. Recombinant interferon-gamma in the treatment of systemic sclerosis. *Am J Med* 1989; 87:237–277.
357. Freundlich B, Jiminez SA, Steen VD, et al. Treatment of systemic sclerosis with recombinant interferon-γ. *Arthritis Rheum* 1992;35:1134–1142.
358. Hein R, Behr J, Hundgen M, et al. Treatment of systemic sclerosis with γ-interferon. *Br J Dermatol* 1992;126:496–501.
359. Vlachoyiannopoulos PG, Tsifetaki N, Dimitriou I, et al. Safety and efficacy of recombinant gamma interferon in the treatment of systemic sclerosis. *Ann Rheum Dis* 1996;55:761–768.
360. Polisson RP, Gilkeson GS, Pyun EH, et al. A multicenter trial of recombinant human interferon gamma in patients with systemic sclerosis: effects on cutaneous fibrosis and interleukin-2 receptor levels. *J Rheumatol* 1996;23:654–658.
361. Black CM, Silman AJ, Herrick AI, et al. Interferon-α does not improve outcome at one year in patients with diffuse cutaneous scleroderma: results of a randomized, double-blind, placebo-controlled trial. *Arthritis Rheum* 1999;42:299–305.
362. Tarkowski A, Lindgren I. Beneficial effects of antithymocyte

globulin in severe cases of progressive systemic sclerosis. *Transplant Proc* 1994;26:3197–3199.
363. Goronzy JJ, Weyand CM. Long-term immunomodulation effects of T-lymphocyte depletion in patients with systemic sclerosis. *Arthritis Rheum* 1990;33:511–519.
364. van den Hoogen FH, Boerbooms AM, Swaak AJ, et al. Comparison of methotrexate with placebo in the treatment of systemic sclerosis: a 24-week randomized double-blind trial, followed by a 24-week observational trial. *B J Rheumatol* 1996; 35:364–372.
365. Bode BY, Yocum DE, Gall EP, et al. Methotrexate (MTX) in scleroderma: experience in 10 patients. *Arthritis Rheum* 1990; 33:566(abst).
366. Rook AH, Freundlich B, Jegasothy BV, et al. Treatment of systemic sclerosis with extracorporeal photochemotherapy: results of a multicenter trial. *Arch Dermatol* 1992;128:337–346.
367. Trentham D. Photochemotherapy in systemic sclerosis: the stage is set [Editorial]. *Arch Dermatol* 1992;128:389–390.
368. Fries JF, Seibold JR, Medsger TA Jr. Photopheresis for scleroderma? No! [Editorial]. *J Rheumatol* 1992;19:1011–1013.
369. Kahaleh MD, Sherer DL, LeRoy EC. Endothelial injury in scleroderma. *J Exp Med* 1979;149:1326–1335.
370. Beckett VL, Conn DL, Fuster V, et al. Trial of platelet-inhibiting drug in scleroderma: double-blind study with dipyridamole and aspirin. *Arthritis Rheum* 1984;27:1137–1143.
371. Legerton CW 3rd, Smith EA, Silver RM. Systemic sclerosis (scleroderma): clinical management of its major complications. *Rheum Dis Clin North Am* 1995;21:203–216.
372. Jobe JB, Sampson JB, Roberts DE, et al. Induced vasodilation as treatment for Raynaud's disease. *Ann Intern Med* 1982;97: 706–709.
373. Yocum DE, Hodes R, Sundstrom WR, et al. Use of biofeedback training in treatment of Raynaud's disease and phenomenon. *J Rheumatol* 1985;12:90–93.
374. Freedman RR. Quantitative measurements of finger blood flow during behavioral treatments for Raynaud's disease. *Psychophysiology* 1989;26:437–444.
375. Herrick AL, Gush RJ, Tully M, et al. A controlled trial of the effect of topical glyceryl trinitrate on skin blood flow and skin elasticity in scleroderma. *Ann Rheum Dis* 1994;53:212.
376. McFayden IJ, Housley E, MacPherson AIS. Intra-arterial reserpine administration in Raynaud's syndrome. *Arch Intern Med* 1973;132:526–528.
377. Varadi DP, Lawrence AM. Suppression of Raynaud's phenomenon by methyldopa. *Arch Intern Med* 1969;124:13–18.
378. Blunt RJ, Porter JM. Raynaud's syndrome. *Semin Arthritis Rheum* 1981;10:282–308.
379. Rodeheffer RJ, Rommer JA, Wigley F, et al. Controlled double-blind trial of nifedipine in the treatment of Raynaud's phenomenon. *N Engl J Med* 1983;308:880–883.
380. Finch MB, Dawson J, Johnston GD. The peripheral vascular effects of nifedipine in Raynaud's syndrome associated with scleroderma: a double-blind crossover study. *Clin Rheumatol* 1986;5:493–498.
381. Surwit RS, Gilgor RS, Allen LM, et al. A double-blind study of prazosin in the treatment of Raynaud's phenomenon in scleroderma. *Arch Dermatol* 1984;120:329–331.
382. Seibold JR, Jageneau AHM. Treatment of Raynaud's phenomenon with ketanserin: a selective antagonist of the serotonin 2 (5-HT2) receptor. *Arthritis Rheum* 1984;27:139–146.
383. Coffman JD, Clement DL, Creager MA, et al. International study of ketanserin in Raynaud's phenomenon. *Am J Med* 1989; 87:264–268.
384. Goodfield MJD, Rowell NR. Treatment of peripheral gangrene due to systemic sclerosis with intravenous pentoxifylline. *Clin Exp Dermatol* 1989;14:161–162.
385. Mizushima Y, Shiokawa Y, Homma M, et al. A multicenter double-blind controlled study of lipo-PGE_1, PGE_1 incorporated in lipid microspheres, in peripheral vascular disease secondary to connective tissue disorders. *J Rheumatol* 1987;14: 97–101.
386. Keller J, Kaltenecker A, Schricker KT, et al. Inhibition of platelet aggregation by a new stable prostacyclin introduced in therapy of patients with progressive scleroderma. *Arch Dermatol Res* 1985;277:323–325.
387. Wigley FM, Wise RA, Seibold JR, et al. A multi-center placebo-controlled double-blind study of intravenous iloprost infusion in patients with Raynaud's phenomenon secondary to systemic sclerosis (scleroderma). *Ann Intern Med* 1994;120:199–206.
388. Wigley FM, Korn JH, Csuka ME, et al. Oral iloprost treatment in patients with Raynaud's phenomenon secondary to systemic sclerosis: a multicenter, placebo-controlled, double-blind study. *Arthritis Rheum* 1998;41:670–677.
389. Bunker CB, Reavley C, O'Shaughnessy DJ, et al. Calcitonin gene-related peptide in treatment of severe peripheral vascular insufficiency in Raynaud's phenomenon. *Lancet* 1993;342: 80–82.
390. Tosi S, Marchesoni A, Messina K, et al. Treatment of Raynaud's phenomenon with captopril. *Drugs Exp Clin Res* 1987;13: 37–42.
391. Jacobs MJ, Jorning PJ, Van Rede van der Kloot EJ. Plasmapheresis in Raynaud's phenomenon in systemic sclerosis: a microcirculatory study. *Int J Microcirc Clin Exp* 1991;10:1–11.
392. Flatt AE. Digital artery sympathectomy. *J Hand Surg* 1980;5: 550–556.
393. Drake DB, Kesler RW, Morgan RF. Digital sympathectomy for retracting Raynaud's phenomenon in an adolescent. *J Rheumatol* 1992;18:1286–1288.
394. Stratton R, Howell K, Goddard N, et al. Digital sympathectomy for ischaemia in scleroderma. *Br J Rheumatol* 1997;36: 1338–1339.
395. O'Brien BMC, Kluman PAU, Mellow CG, et al. Radial microarteriolysis in the treatment of vasospastic disorders of the hand, especially scleroderma. *J Hand Surg [Br]* 1992;17: 447–452.
396. Jones NF, Raynor SC, Medsger TA Jr. Microsurgical revascularisation of the hand in scleroderma. *Br J Plast Surg* 1987;40: 264–269.
397. Gahhos F, Ariyan S, Frazier WH, et al. Management of sclerodermal finger ulcers. *J Hand Surg [Am]* 1984;9:320–327.
398. Lian JB, Skinner M, Glimcher MJ, et al. The presence of g-carboxyglutamic acid in the proteins associated with ectopic calcification. *Biochem Biophys Res Commun* 1976;73:349–355.
399. Berger RG, Featherstone GL, Raasch RH, et al. Treatment of calcinosis universalis with low-dose warfarin. *Am J Med* 1987; 83:72–76.
400. Dolan AL, Kassimos D, Gibson T, et al. Diltiazem induces remission of calcinosis in scleroderma. *Br J Rheumatol* 1995;34: 576–578.
401. Palmieri GMA, Sebes JI, Aelion JA, et al. Treatment of calcinosis with diltiazem. *Arthritis Rheum* 1995;38:1646–1654.
402. Fuchs D, Fruchter L, Fishel B, et al. Colchicine suppression of local inflammation due to calcinosis in dermatomyositis and progressive systemic sclerosis. *Clin Rheumatol* 1986;5:527–530.
403. Jones NF, Raynor SC, Medsger TA Jr. Surgery for scleroderma of the hand. *J Hand Surg Am* 1987;12:391–400.
404. Seeger MW, Furst DE. Effects of splinting in the treatment of hand contractures in progressive systemic sclerosis. *Am J Occup Ther* 1987;41:118–121.
405. Norris RW, Brown HG. The proximal interphalangeal joint in systemic sclerosis and its surgical management. *Br J Plast Surg* 1985;38:526–531.

406. Naylor WP. Oral management of the scleroderma patient. *J Am Dent Assoc* 1982;105:814.
407. Naylor WP, Manor RC. Fabrication of a flexible prosthesis for the edentulous scleroderma patient with microstomia. *J Prosthet Dent* 1983;50:536–538.
408. Ramirez-Mata M, Ibanez G, Alarcon-Segovia D. Stimulatory effect of metaclopramide on the esophagus and lower esophageal sphincter of patients with PSS. *Arthritis Rheum* 1977;20:30–34.
409. Horowitz M, Maddem GJ, Maddox A, et al. Effects of cisapride on gastric and esophageal emptying in progressive systemic sclerosis. *Gastroenterology* 1987;93:311–315.
410. Fiorucci S, Distrutti E, Bassotti G, et al. Effect of erythromycin administration on upper gastrointestinal motility in scleroderma patients. *Scand J Gastroenterol* 1994;29:807–813.
411. Dull JS, Raufman J-P, Zakai MD, et al. Successful treatment of gastroparesis with erythromycin in a patient with progressive systemic sclerosis. *Am J Med* 1990;89:528–530.
412. Soudah H, Hasler W, Owyang C. Effect of octreotide on intestinal motility and bacterial overgrowth in scleroderma. *N Engl J Med* 1991;325:1461–1509.
413. Kahan A, Bour B, Couturier D, et al. Nifedipine and esophageal dysfunction in progressive systemic sclerosis: a controlled manometric study. *Arthritis Rheum* 1985;28:490–495.
414. Jean F, Aubert A, Bloch F, et al. Effects of diltiazem versus nifedipine on lower esophageal sphincter pressure in patients with progressive systemic sclerosis. *Arthritis Rheum* 1986;29:1054–1055.
415. Olive A, Maddison PJ, Davis M. Treatment of oesophagitis in scleroderma with omeprazole. *Br J Rheumatol* 1989;28:553.
416. Orringer MB, Orringer JS, Dabich L, et al. Combined Collis gastroplasty-fundoplication operations for scleroderma reflux esophagitis. *Surgery* 1981;90:624–630.
417. Gates C, Morand EF, Davis M, et al. Sclerotherapy as treatment of recurrent bleeding from upper gastrointestinal telangiectasia in chest syndrome. *Br J Rheumatol* 1993;32:760–761.
418. Gough A, Andrews D, Bacon PA, et al. Evidence of omeprazole-induced small bowel bacterial overgrowth in patients with scleroderma. *Br J Rheumatol* 1995;34:976–977.
419. Rees WD, Leigh RJ, Christofides ND, et al. Interdigestive motor activity in patients with systemic sclerosis. *Gastroenterology* 1982;83:575–580.
420. Levien DH, Fiallos F, Barone R, et al. The use of cyclic home hyperalimentation for malabsorption in patients with scleroderma involving the small intestines. *J Parenter Enter Nutr* 1985;9:623–625.
421. Cheng S, Clements PJ, Berquist WE, et al. Home central venous hyperalimentation in fifteen patients with severe scleroderma bowel disease. *Arthritis Rheum* 1989;32:212–216.
422. Silver RM, Miller KS, Kinsella MB, et al. Evaluation and management of scleroderma lung disease using bronchoalveolar lavage. *Am J Med* 1990;88:470–476.
423. Kallenberg CGM, Jansen HM, Elema JD, et al. Steroid-responsive interstitial pulmonary disease in systemic sclerosis: monitoring by bronchoalveolar lavage. *Chest* 1984;86:489–492.
424. Silver RM, Warrick JH, Kinsella MB, et al. Cyclophosphamide and low-dose prednisone therapy in patients with systemic sclerosis (scleroderma) with interstitial lung disease. *J Rheumatol* 1993;20:838–844.
425. Akesson A, Scheja A, Lundin A, et al. Improved pulmonary function in systemic sclerosis after treatment with cyclophosphamide. *Arthritis Rheum* 1994;37:729–735.
426. Medsger TA Jr. D-Penicillamine treatment of lung involvement in patients with systemic sclerosis (scleroderma). *Arthritis Rheum* 1987;30:832–834.
427. Steen VD, Owens G, Redmond C, et al. The effect of D-penicillamine on pulmonary findings in systemic sclerosis. *Arthritis Rheum* 1985;28:882–888.
428. deClerck LS, Dequeker J, Franc L, et al. D-Penicillamine therapy and interstitial lung disease in scleroderma: a long-term followup study. *Arthritis Rheum* 1987;30:643–650.
429. Steen VD, Lanz JK, Conte C, et al. Therapy for severe interstitial lung disease in systemic sclerosis: a retrospective study. *Arthritis Rheum* 1994;37:1290–1296.
430. Seibold JR, Molony RR, Turkevich D, et al. Acute hemodynamic effects of ketanserin in pulmonary hypertension secondary to systemic sclerosis. *J Rheumatol* 1987;14:519–524.
431. O'Brien JT, Hill JA, Pepine CJ. Sustained benefit of verapamil in pulmonary hypertension with progressive systemic sclerosis. *Am Heart J* 1985;109:380–382.
432. Rouse PJ, Lahiri A, Gumpel JM. The CREST syndrome—successful reduction of pulmonary hypertension by captopril. *Postgrad Med J* 1984;60:672–674.
433. de la Mata J, Gomez-Sanchez MA, Aranzana M, et al. Long-term iloprost infusion therapy for severe pulmonary hypertension in patients with connective tissue diseases. *Arthritis Rheum* 1994;37:1528–1533.
434. Bartosik I, Eskilsson J, Scheja A, et al. Intermittent iloprost infusion therapy of pulmonary hypertension in scleroderma: a pilot study. *Br J Rheumatol* 1996;35:1187–1190.
435. Badesch DB, Tapson VF, McGoon MD, et al. Continuous intravenous epoprostenol for pulmonary hypertension due to scleroderma spectrum of disease. *Ann Intern Med* 2000;132:424–434.
436. Al-Sabbagh R, Steen V, Zee B, et al. Pulmonary arterial histology and morphometry in systemic sclerosis: a case-control autopsy study. *J Rheumatol* 1989;16:1038–1042.
437. LeRoy EC. Sentinel signs and symptoms of systemic sclerosis. *Curr Opin Rheumatol* 1989;1:499–504.
438. Asherson RA, Khamashta MA, Orti-Ros J, et al. The primary antiphospholipid syndrome: major clinical and serological features. *Medicine (Baltimore)* 1989;68:366–374.
439. LeRoy EC. Systemic sclerosis (scleroderma). In: Kelley WN, Harris ED Jr, Ruddy S, Sledge CB, eds. *Textbook of rheumatology.* Philadelphia: WB Saunders, 1985:1183–1205.
440. Brown EA, MacGregor GA, Maini RN. Failure of captopril to reverse the renal crisis of scleroderma. *Ann Rheum Dis* 1983;42:52–53.
441. Nolph KD, Stolz ML, Maher JL. Altered peritoneal permeability in patients with systemic vasculitis. *Ann Intern Med* 1971;75:753–755.
442. Copley JB, Smith BJ. Continuous ambulatory peritoneal dialysis and scleroderma. *Nephron* 1985;40:353–356.
443. Barker DJ, Farr MJ. Resolution of cutaneous manifestations of systemic sclerosis after hemodialysis. *Br Med J* 1976;1:501.
444. LeRoy EC, Fleischmann RM. The management of renal scleroderma: experience with dialysis, nephrectomy and transplantation. *Am J Med* 1978;64:974–978.
445. Merino GE, Sutherland DE, Kjellstrand CM, et al. Renal transplantation for progressive systemic sclerosis with renal failure. *Am J Surg* 1977;133:745–749.
446. Woodhall PB, McCoy RC, Gunnells JC, et al. Apparent recurrence of progressive systemic sclerosis in a renal allograft. *JAMA* 1976;236:1032–1034.

80

VARIANT FORMS OF SCLERODERMA

RICHARD M. SILVER
MARCY B. BOLSTER

Several idiopathic, toxin-associated, or metabolic disorders may be accompanied by dermal sclerosis and, thus, may be considered variant forms of scleroderma. In some instances, these conditions differ from systemic sclerosis (idiopathic scleroderma) by the distribution of skin sclerosis, type of internal organ involvement, and presence of unique clinical or histopathologic lesions not generally associated with systemic sclerosis. Such conditions have been termed *pseudoscleroderma,* or variant forms of scleroderma. Some of these pseudoscleroderma conditions bear a striking resemblance to one another, suggesting a common etiology or pathogenesis. For example, eosinophilic fasciitis, toxic oil syndrome, and eosinophilia-myalgia syndrome (EMS) are similar in many respects, yet differ from idiopathic scleroderma.

Environmental and occupational exposure to a variety of chemicals and toxins may induce either a variant form of scleroderma or, in some instances, an illness that appears to be identical to systemic sclerosis. An understanding of the pathogenesis and the basis for susceptibility to such conditions might provide insight into the pathogenesis of idiopathic scleroderma and other forms of abnormal fibrosis. This chapter reviews the clinical, histologic, and epidemiologic aspects of the variant forms of scleroderma, and discusses localized forms of scleroderma. Table 80.1 lists the diseases with cutaneous features resembling scleroderma. Systemic sclerosis is discussed in Chapters 79 and 81.

TABLE 80.1. DISEASES WITH CUTANEOUS FEATURES RESEMBLING SCLERODERMA

- Fasciitis with eosinophilia
  - Idiopathic diffuse fasciitis with eosinophilia (DFE)
  - Toxic oil syndrome (TOS) associated with adulterated rapeseed oil
  - Eosinophilia-myalgia syndrome (EMS) associated with contaminated L-tryptophan
- Silica and silicone associated scleroderma
- Other chemicals associated with fibrosis
  - Bleomycin
  - Vinyl chloride
  - Pentazocine
  - Biogenic amines other than L-tryptophan
    - 5-hydroxy-L-tryptophan
    - Appetite suppressants
    - Bromocriptine
  - Epoxy resin vapor
  - Organic solvents
    - Trichloroethylene (TCE)
    - Trichloroethane
    - Perchloroethylene
    - Toluene
    - Benzene
    - Xylene
    - Methylene chloride
    - Metaphenylenediamine
- Graft-versus-host disease
- Digital sclerosis of diabetes mellitus
- Scleredema adultorum of Buschke
- Scleromyxedema
- Rare metabolic conditions
  - Carcinoid syndrome
  - Phenylketonuria
  - Porphyria cutanea tarda
  - Acromegaly
- Other rare conditions
  - Werner's syndrome
  - Progeria
  - Rothmund's syndrome
  - Lichen sclerosis et atrophicus
  - Acrodermatitis chronica atrophicans
  - Amyloidosis
- Neurologic disorders with dystrophic skin
  - Reflex sympathetic dystrophy syndrome
  - Hemiplegia or paraplegia

SCLERODERMA VARIANTS CHARACTERIZED BY FASCIITIS WITH EOSINOPHILIA

Diffuse fasciitis with eosinophilia, toxic oil syndrome, and EMS are characterized by fascial inflammation, fibrosis, and eosinophilia. Fibrosis within the dermis and subcutaneous tissue results in hardening of the skin that may mimic systemic sclerosis, yet various clinical, serologic, and histopathologic features serve to distinguish these conditions from systemic sclerosis. In these variant forms, for example, sclerosis of the fingers and face generally does not

TABLE 80.2. CLINICAL MANIFESTATIONS OF ACUTE DFE, TOS, AND EMS[a]

Clinical Features	DFE	TOS	EMS
Gender	F = M	F > M	F ≥ M
Age of onset, mean (years)	45	47	49
Precipitant (% cases)	Exercise (30%)	Adulterated rapeseed oil (~100%)	Contaminated L-tryptophan (98%)
Occurrence	Sporadic	Epidemic	Epidemic
Peak onset	N/A	1981	1989
Fever	+/–	++++	++
Myalgia	+	++++	++++
Alopecia	+/–	++++	++
Rash	+/–	+++	+++
Scleroderma-like lesions	++++	++	++
Arthralgia/arthritis	++	++++	+++
Dyspnea/infiltrate	+/–	++++	+++
Peripheral neuropathy	+/–	++	++
Cardiac disease	+/–	+	+
Pulmonary hypertension	+/–	+	+/–
Hepatic disease	+/–	+	+/–
Thromboemboli	+/–	+	+/–

[a]Compiled from refs. 24, 27, 80.
DFE, diffuse fasciitis with eosinophilia; TOS, toxic oil syndrome; EMS, eosinophilia-myalgia syndrome; N/A, not applicable.
++++, >75% cases; +++, >50–75% cases; ++, >25–50% cases; +, <25% cases; +/– <5% or absent.

occur, nor are these conditions associated with other findings common to systemic sclerosis, e.g., Raynaud's phenomenon, abnormalities of nailfold capillaries, antinuclear antibodies (ANAs), and visceral organ disease. Although these conditions have occurred sporadically (diffuse fasciitis with eosinophilia) or as epidemics separated temporally and geographically (toxic oil syndrome and EMS), as a group they closely resemble one another (Table 80.2) in terms of myalgia, fasciitis, and eosinophilia, suggesting a common cause or pathogenesis. They differ from one another in certain aspects, however, particularly extracutaneous features (Table 80.2).

Diffuse Fasciitis with Eosinophilia

Described initially in 1974, diffuse fasciitis with eosinophilia is also termed eosinophilic fasciitis or Shulman's syndrome and is characterized by abrupt onset of edema and stiffness of extremities accompanied by eosinophilia (1). Its cause is unknown. A role for *Borrelia burgdorferi* infection has been suggested in some cases (2). In approximately one-third of patients, the onset of diffuse fasciitis with eosinophilia follows physical activity that is unusual or excessive. Two cases were reported to have occurred in association with prolonged exposure to the organic solvent trichlorethylene (3), a chemical that has also been associated with systemic sclerosis (see Table 80.1). In diffuse fasciitis with eosinophilia, the skin of the legs and arms (usually sparing the fingers and toes) becomes taut and woody, often with a *peau d'orange* appearance (Fig. 80.1). The skin is restricted by the subcutaneous tissue and patients often have a "groove sign" that also has been observed in patients with toxic oil syndrome or EMS. Unlike the latter conditions, diffuse fasciitis with eosinophilia predominantly affects the dermis and subcutaneous tissues, generally sparing visceral organs (Table 80.2) and rarely requires hospitalization. Some patients with diffuse fasciitis with eosinophilia develop thrombocytopenia or aplastic anemia, and, in rare cases, diffuse fasciitis with eosinophilia may occur as a paraneoplastic syndrome associated with myeloid or lymphoid malignant neoplasms (4). Hypergammaglobulinemia accompanies the peripheral blood eosinophilia in many patients. ANAs may be detected, but they exhibit different specificities than those occurring in patients with systemic sclerosis.

The diagnosis is established by a full-thickness skin biopsy revealing fascia that is markedly thickened by collagen deposition and an associated inflammatory cell infiltrate consisting of lymphocytes, plasma cells, and, often, eosinophils (Fig. 80.2) (1,5). Inflammation and fibrosis of the fascia may be demonstrated by magnetic resonance imaging (MRI), which has been suggested as a noninvasive tool for diagnosis (6). Lesional fibroblasts secrete abnormally large amounts of collagen *in vitro*. Additionally, *in situ* hybridization analysis reveals elevated signals for messenger RNA (mRNA) of type I collagen and transforming growth factor-β_1 (TGF-β_1) mRNA (7,8), as observed in EMS (9,10). An alteration in L-tryptophan metabolism, similar to that demonstrated in patients with EMS and toxic oil syndrome, has been reported in patients with diffuse fasciitis with eosinophilia and in patients lacking a history of L-tryptophan ingestion, suggesting a common

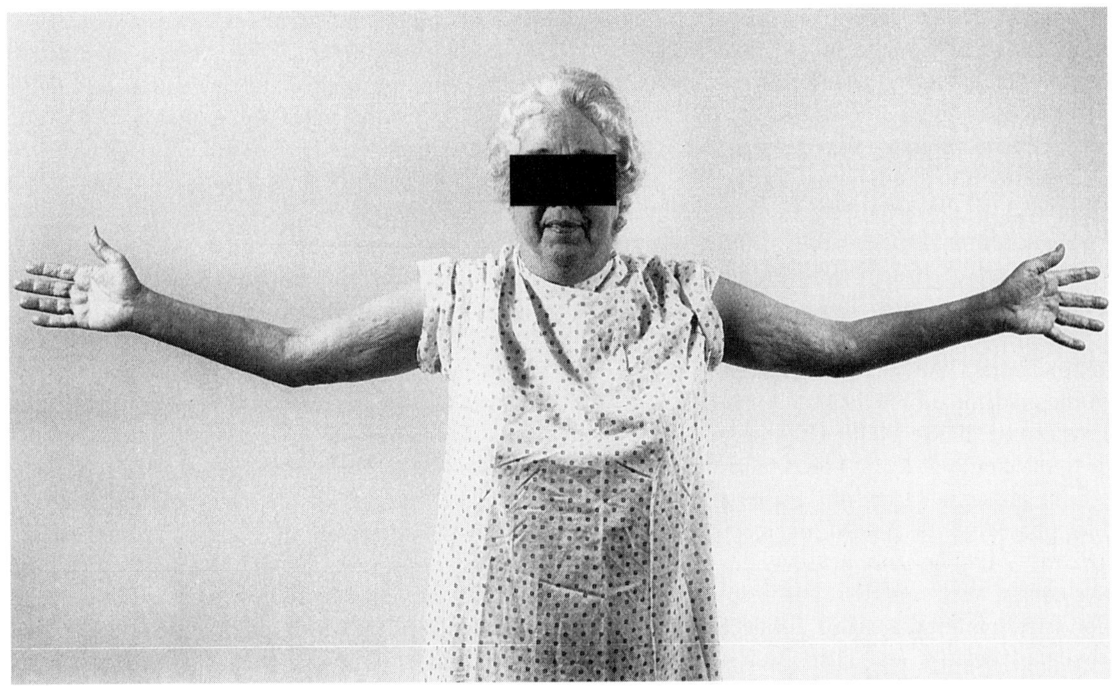

FIGURE 80.1. Taut skin with *peau d'orange* appearance and flexion contractures affecting the arms of a patient with diffuse fasciitis with eosinophilia.

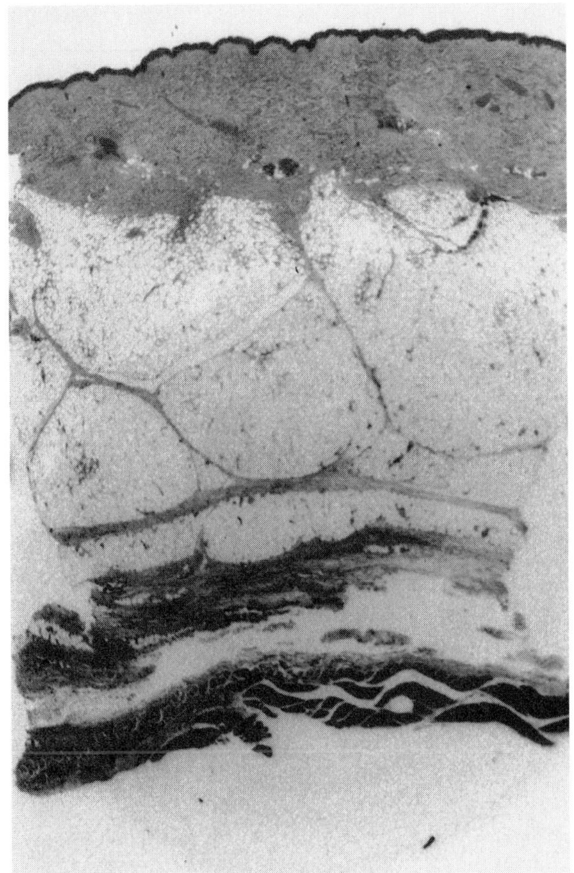

FIGURE 80.2. Full-thickness skin biopsy specimen from the distal lower extremity of a patient with diffuse fasciitis with eosinophilia. There is dermal thickening accompanied by septal panniculitis and marked sclerosis of the fascia.

pathogenesis, which may be cytokine-driven and involve interferon-γ (IFN-γ) (11).

The majority of patients with diffuse fasciitis with eosinophilia respond favorably to oral corticosteroid therapy with or without the addition of hydroxychloroquine (5). Other agents that have been reported to be of therapeutic benefit include cimetidine (12), ketotifen (13), and cyclosporin A (14). Spontaneous remissions also have been reported (5,12,15). Consequently, all uncontrolled reports of therapeutic success are difficult to interpret.

Toxic Oil Syndrome

In 1981, a new food-borne disease that came to be known as the toxic oil syndrome occurred in epidemic proportions in Spain (16). Approximately 20,000 persons were affected, with more than 800 deaths reported. The majority of those surviving continue to display symptoms and signs to varying degrees. Epidemiologic studies of toxic oil syndrome showed a strong association with the ingestion of adulterated rapeseed oil (17). Rapeseed oil denatured with aniline was sold door to door or in weekly open-air markets as olive oil in 5-L plastic containers (18). Although the precise agent was never identified, virtually all studies support the conclusion that adulterated rapeseed oil was the vehicle of the toxic oil syndrome agent. Case-associated oils were contaminated with fatty acid anilides and aniline and a dose-response relationship existed between the level of aniline and anilide contamination and the risk of developing toxic oil syndrome (19).

Virtually all toxicity studies of case-associated oils in experimental animals have been negative (20).

One possible etiologic agent, 3-(*N*-phenylamino)-1,2-propanediol (PAP), was present in some case-associated oils. Fatty acid esters of this compound were present after simulated refining procedures with oils containing aniline, indicating that esters of PAP were products of the refining process and were not formed spontaneously during storage (21). PAP produced tissue toxicity when administered to mice in only one toxicology study, however (22). Of interest is the identification of a similarly structured compound, 3-(phenylamino)alanine (PAA), in batches of L-tryptophan implicated in the epidemic of EMS (23).

Toxic oil syndrome affected both children and adults, with a female to male ratio of 1.5:1. The clinical course was divided into three phases: an acute phase (months 1 to 2), an intermediate phase (months 3 to 4), and a chronic phase (month 5 onward) (24). The acute phase was marked by a nonproductive cough, chest tightness, and dyspnea. Other symptoms consisted of fever, malaise, headache, edema, myalgia, arthralgia, pruritus, and rash. Eosinophilia was observed in more than 85% of patients during this phase. Serum levels of immunoglobulin E (IgE), triglycerides, and hepatic transaminases were often elevated. Chest radiography revealed generalized alveolar-interstitial infiltrates and pleural effusions. The clinical picture was consistent with noncardiogenic pulmonary edema. Respiratory failure was a frequent cause of death during the acute phase.

In those patients who survived the acute phase, the disease evolved to an intermediate phase 3 to 4 months after onset. Edema of the skin and subcutaneous tissue, a prominent feature of this phase, often progressed to fibrosis with contracture formation. Other cutaneous manifestations included alopecia and hyperpigmented papules. Severe myalgias and muscle cramps occurred. In some patients a sensory neuropathy developed. Thromboembolic complications occurred also and in some patients were fatal. The chronic phase was marked by peripheral neuropathy (37%), hepatomegaly (32%), scleroderma-like skin changes (22%), and pulmonary hypertension (10%) (25). Skin changes more closely resembled those of diffuse fasciitis with eosinophilia and EMS than systemic sclerosis. The eosinophilia resolved and the fibrosis of the skin and subcutis evolved to an atrophic stage. Death attributable to pulmonary hypertension was reported during the chronic phase. Although severe neuromuscular sequelae, scleroderma-like skin changes, and pulmonary hypertension were not observed in one cohort studied 12 years after the onset of toxic oil syndrome, a significant percentage of patients continued to have symptoms of muscle cramping (60%), fatigue (55%), arthralgias (43%), subjective cognitive impairment (44%), psychiatric disease (27%), and soft tissue tenderness (22.5%) (26).

The distinctive lesion of toxic oil syndrome was a non-necrotizing vasculitis affecting mainly the intima (an "endovasculitis") and involving vessels of every type and size in nearly every organ (27). Damage extended from the intima into the media and adventitia without fibrinoid necrosis, but with a mixed inflammatory cell infiltrate (lymphocytes, histiocytes, and eosinophils). Subintimal fibrosis ensued, and thromboembolic complications were related to the endovasculitis.

Skin lesions in the acute phase were marked by edema of the papillary dermis with superficial and deep perivascular inflammatory infiltrates. In the intermediate phase, scleroderma-like lesions were characterized by fibrosis and vascular changes in the deep dermis and panniculus. Mucin deposits were present in papular lesions. Eventually, dermal sclerosis occurred with loss of hair follicles and sebaceous glands.

Empiric treatment consisted of antibiotics, corticosteroids, D-penicillamine, immunosuppressive agents, plasmapheresis, vasodilators, and antioxidants. No convincing effect was noted with any of these therapies. Corticosteroid therapy may have ameliorated the acute pulmonary edema and eosinophilia, but did not appear to prevent chronic disease. Chronic pulmonary hypertension and neuromuscular disease remain difficult problems with no effective treatment.

Eosinophilia-Myalgia Syndrome

A seemingly new illness was first described in the United States in 1989, when physicians in New Mexico reported the occurrence of generalized myalgias and eosinophilia in three women with a history of ingesting the amino acid L-tryptophan (28). The illness reached epidemic proportions in 1989 and subsided when L-tryptophan–containing products were recalled (Fig. 80.3) (29). This illness, now known as the EMS, frequently was complicated by scleroderma-like hardening of the skin and subcutaneous tissues and shared many features with diffuse fasciitis with eosinophilia and toxic oil syndrome (1,16,26,30). The Centers for Disease Control (CDC) established the following case definition for surveillance purposes: (a) eosinophil count $>1 \times 10^9$/L; (b) generalized myalgias of sufficient severity to limit activity; and (c) exclusion of neoplasm or infection to account for the syndrome (31). More than 1,500 cases of EMS and 38 deaths from neurologic, cardiac, and pulmonary complications have been reported (32).

A number of case-control studies showed a strong association of EMS with the ingestion of L-tryptophan (33–35). In fact, the CDC national surveillance revealed that only 2% of persons with EMS reported never having used L-tryptophan (36). A study from Minnesota found that 29 of 30 (97%) EMS patients and 21 of 35 controls (60%) had consumed L-tryptophan manufactured by a single manufacturer (odds ratio 19.3, $p < .001$) (33). A study of 418 L-tryptophan users from a single psychiatry practice showed that the risk of developing EMS was dose-related and age-

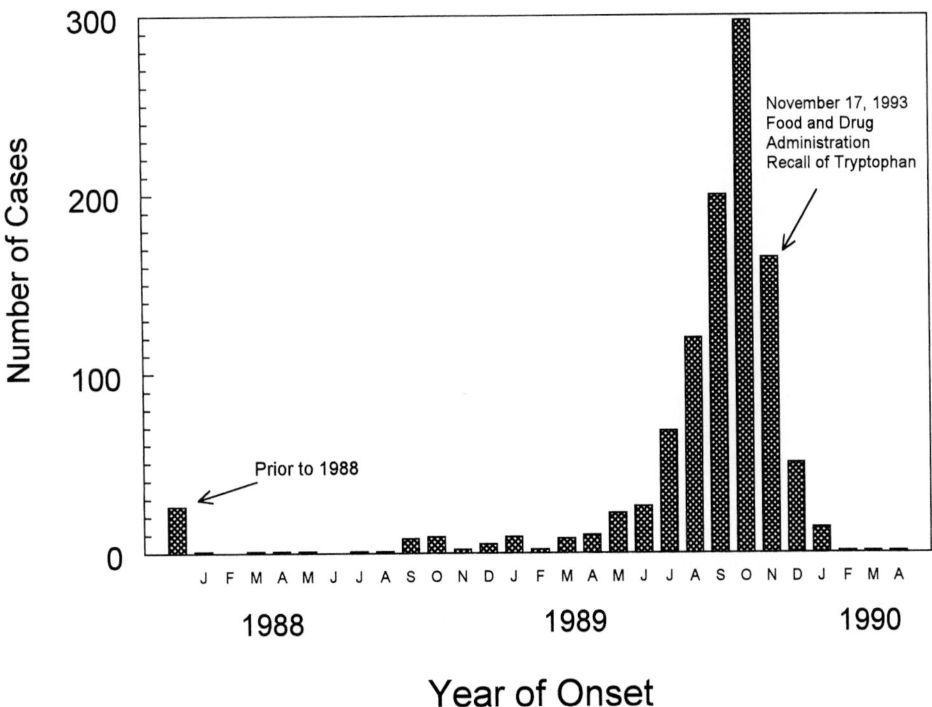

FIGURE 80.3. Reported dates of onset of eosinophilia-myalgia syndrome (EMS) by month and year, as reported to the Centers for Disease Control, Atlanta, GA. (From Swygert LA, Maes EF, Sewell LE, et al. Eosinophilia-myalgia syndrome. Results of national surveillance. *JAMA* 1990;264:1698–1703, with permission.)

related (37). These and other studies suggested that contamination during the manufacture of L-tryptophan was responsible for the epidemic and that the attack rate might have been influenced by cofactors such as age.

The manufacturing process employed by the implicated company involved a bacterial fermentation process with subsequent filtration and purification. In 1988, a genetically modified strain of *Bacillus amyloliquefaciens* that yielded increased amounts of L-tryptophan was introduced, and the filtration process was modified to reduce the amount of activated carbon and bypass a reverse osmosis membrane filter. A significant association between lots used by case patients and changes in the manufacturing process was confirmed (33). High-performance liquid chromatography of the L-tryptophan demonstrated several peaks, including one (peak E) that was strongly associated with the syndrome (33).

The structure of peak E was confirmed as 1,1′-ethylidenebis(L-tryptophan) (EBT) (Fig. 80.4) (38). One case-control study revealed an attack rate of 2.2% and a significant association between EMS and ingestion of L-tryptophan containing a high concentration of EBT (70

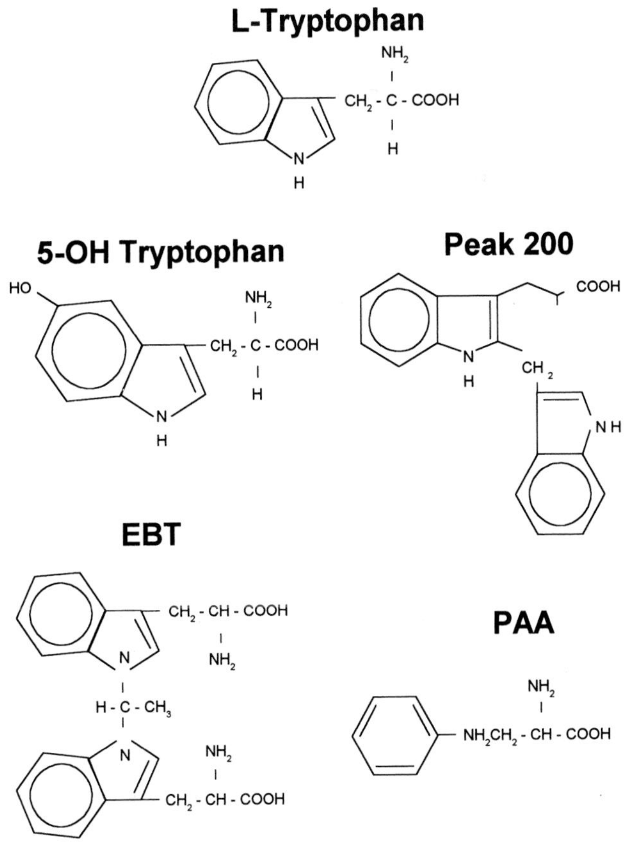

L-Tryptophan

5-OH Tryptophan

Peak 200

EBT

PAA

FIGURE 80.4. Chemical structure of L-tryptophan and related compounds associated with EMS.

mg/g) (adjusted odds ratio = 35.9; 95% confidence interval, 1.9–675.3; $p = .02$) (39). UV-5, a second trace contaminant in implicated batches of L-tryptophan, was identified as PAA, and it also has been linked to the EMS epidemic (23). Its structure is similar to a putative etiologic agent of toxic oil syndrome, PAP (21,23). Other trace contaminants in implicated batches of L-tryptophan, including 2[3-indolymethyl]-L-tryptophan (also designated peak 200), were also associated with the EMS epidemic (40).

Implicated L-tryptophan lots and synthesized EBT have been shown to induce inflammation and fibrosis of the fascia and perimysium of female Lewis rats (41,42). Another rodent model has been proposed in which daily intraperitoneal administration of EBT to C57BL/6 mice yields significant inflammation and fibrosis of the dermis, fascia, and perimysium, consistent with changes observed in patients with EMS (43). Mast cells, also seen in EMS lesions, have been observed in both of these proposed models. In neither model, however, has tissue or blood eosinophilia been observed. *In vitro* studies indicate that EBT stimulates human fibroblasts to proliferate and increase collagen synthesis (44).

Eosinophilia-myalgia syndrome is a multisystem disease often with a flu-like onset and an acute phase with fever, rash, arthralgias, and dyspnea, as well as the characteristic myalgias and eosinophilia. Nearly one-third of patients required hospitalization. The majority of patients were Caucasian women, probably a reflection of the ingestion patterns of L-tryptophan rather than race- or sex-related susceptibility. The median daily dose of L-tryptophan ingested was 1.5 g. Myalgias were nearly universal and often diffuse and debilitating (45,46). Serum levels of creatine kinase were usually normal, but aldolase levels were mildly elevated as in some cases of toxic oil syndrome. Severe muscle cramps occurred, and for many patients this has been a persistent and debilitating feature of the chronic phase of EMS, as in toxic oil syndrome. Ischemia and neuropathic changes may underlie their pathogenesis, but myonecrosis has not been observed. An acquired metabolic abnormality is also possible, given the observation of abnormal P-31 magnetic resonance spectroscopy of skeletal muscle (47).

Eosinophilia is one of the criteria for the case definition of EMS and was present in most but probably not all patients. The median eosinophil count was more than 5×10^9/L (48). Serum and urine levels of eosinophil major basic protein and eosinophil-derived neurotoxin and tissue levels of eosinophil granule proteins were elevated in some patients, consistent with eosinophil activation and degranulation (49). Interleukin-5 (IL-5), a cytokine that stimulates eosinophil production and enhances eosinophil survival (see Chapter 17), was detectable in the serum of some EMS patients (50). The eosinophilia resolved promptly after the administration of glucocorticoids.

Skin rash or induration was present in the majority of patients with EMS (45,46,51). During the acute phase, erythematous macules, sometimes pruritic, were often present on the trunk and extremities. Papular eruptions (papular mucinosis) occurred in some patients (52). Subcutaneous edema, sometimes massive, occurred in many patients, affecting the upper and lower extremities. Edema often evolved to a tense, woody induration with a *peau d'orange* quality similar to that seen in patients with diffuse fasciitis with eosinophilia or toxic oil syndrome. Unlike scleroderma, the face and the acral portions of the body were usually spared by the indurative process. Alopecia affecting the scalp and the body was sometimes present in the early phase of EMS.

Many patients with EMS had dyspnea and cough during the early phase of the illness (53–56), but respiratory complaints were both less frequent and less severe than in toxic oil syndrome in which noncardiogenic pulmonary edema was severe and sometimes fatal. Linear opacities with or without pleural effusions were frequently seen on chest radiographs and usually resolved with corticosteroid therapy. Interstitial pneumonitis with eosinophilia and perivascular inflammation was evident in lung biopsy specimens. In some patients, pulmonary vascular disease was present and sometimes fatal. Unlike toxic oil syndrome, few cases of late-onset pulmonary hypertension have been reported during the follow-up of patients with EMS.

Peripheral neuropathy with diffuse and localized paresthesias or hyperesthesia occurred in many patients with EMS (46,57–60). An ascending polyneuropathy occurred rarely. Two-thirds of the known deaths from EMS were related to complications of progressive polyneuropathy and myopathy such as respiratory failure, pneumonia, and sepsis (32). Central nervous system (CNS) involvement was described in a few patients (61–64). MRI revealed multiple white-matter lesions in some cases, and the results of one autopsy showed a perivascular lymphocytic infiltrate and meningitis (64). In several patients, CNS signs and symptoms appeared long after the eosinophilia had resolved.

Neurocognitive dysfunction such as memory impairment, difficulty concentrating, or difficulty remembering words or names of persons has been reported in as many as 60% of EMS patients (65,66). Neither the actual prevalence nor the pathogenesis of this aspect of EMS is known at this time. Potential neurotoxic mediators in EMS include eosinophil-derived neurotoxin and the kynurenine metabolite, quinolinic acid. Significant elevations of quinolinic acid were detected not only in the plasma (51), but also in the cerebrospinal fluid of patients with EMS (58,67).

Cardiac involvement was implicated in the death of some patients with EMS, although cardiac disease was not a major clinical feature of the illness. Lesions in the coronary arteries, neural structures, and conducting system in three patients suggested a basis for significant cardiac electrical instability and sudden death (68). Similar lesions were observed in cardiac tissue of patients with toxic oil syndrome (69). One case of severe restrictive cardiomyopathy in association with eosinophil major basic protein deposits along the fibrotic endocardial-myocardial interface was reported (70).

Full-thickness biopsy specimens of skin lesions showed an inflammatory and fibrosing process affecting the dermis and subcutaneous tissue. The process involved the fascia and extended to the perimysium, accompanied by a perivascular mononuclear cell infiltrate (with or without eosinophils) (Fig. 80.5). Endothelial cells appeared swollen, but true vasculitis was rare. Similar lesions were seen in patients with toxic oil syndrome, although the results of examination of full-thickness biopsy specimens were seldom reported. Inflammation and fibrosis affecting the subcutaneous fat, septa, and fascia also occurred in diffuse fasciitis with eosinophilia, but dermal changes appear to have been more prominent in EMS (71,72).

Reactive mesenchymal cells sharing features of histiocytes and fibroblasts were observed in the deep fascia (73). Expression of mRNA for types I and VI collagen, as well as TGF-β_1, was increased in affected fascia (9,10), supporting a role for cytokine-driven fibrosis. In addition to the increased expression of TGF-β, there was evidence of increased production of other cytokines, including IFN-γ (74), IL-4 (75), and IL-5 (50). The nature of the dermal lymphocytic infiltrate has not been well characterized. Fascial and muscle cellular infiltrates were composed predominantly of T lymphocytes (most are $CD8^+$) and macrophages; B lymphocytes and eosinophils were present, but accounted for only a small fraction of the cellular infiltrate (76).

Alteration in L-tryptophan metabolism has been described in a number of inflammatory and rheumatic conditions, including scleroderma and diffuse fasciitis with eosinophilia (77). Sternberg et al. (78) first described altered metabolism of L-tryptophan in a patient with a scleroderma-like illness associated with the ingestion of 5-hydroxy-L-tryptophan. Several similar cases have been described (79,80), all closely resembling EMS. Although elevated levels of kynurenine were initially attributed to a possible inborn error of metabolism, subsequent studies suggest that, in these conditions, it is caused by the induction of indoleamine-2,3-dioxygenase (IDO), with shunting of L-tryptophan via the kynurenine pathway. During the active, eosinophilic phase of the illness, untreated patients with EMS had a low plasma level of L-tryptophan and a high plasma level of kynurenine and its breakdown product, quinolinic acid (51). Plasma neopterin was elevated and correlated with quinolinic acid (74). When given a loading dose of L-tryptophan, these patients demonstrated enhanced kynurenine and quinolinic acid synthesis (67). Corticosteroid-treated patients with EMS metabolized L-tryptophan similar to age- and sex-matched healthy controls. Thus, the handling of L-tryptophan in EMS and related conditions is likely the result of cytokine induction of IDO and not related to an inborn error of metabolism. Identical findings have been reported in patients with toxic oil syndrome and diffuse fasciitis with eosinophilia (11,74).

Optimal treatment of EMS, as well as its natural history, remains to be determined. As with toxic oil syndrome, for many patients EMS has become a chronic disease; more than 50% of patients reported myalgias, muscle cramps, fatigue, paresthesias, and scleroderma-like skin changes 18 to 24 months after disease onset (81–83). Myalgias and

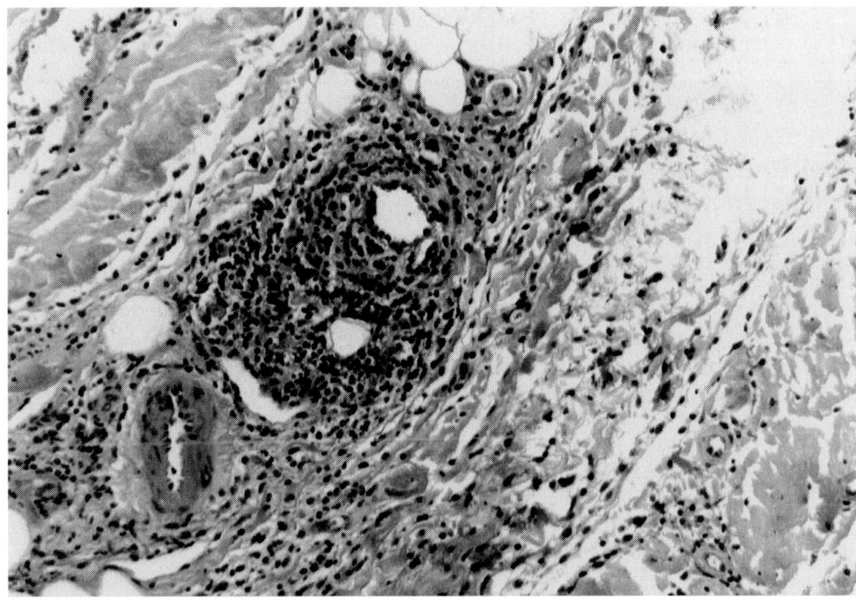

FIGURE 80.5. Perivascular inflammatory cell infiltrate within the thickened fascia of a patient with EMS.

fatigue also persisted in the majority of patients, and only 26% reported that they were able to perform all normal daily activities (84). Cognitive difficulties appear to have developed later in the course of the disease, and significant improvement in these symptoms has not been observed (81). In one cohort, age- and sex-adjusted mortality (19%) was three times higher than that of the general population or that of asymptomatic L-tryptophan users (85).

Treatment has generally been empiric and uncontrolled. Eosinophilia, edema, and pneumonitis usually resolved promptly after the initiation of glucocorticoid therapy, but disease duration does not appear to have been affected, and symptoms often returned after withdrawal of glucocorticoids. A variety of other agents including nonsteroidal anti-inflammatory drugs, cyclophosphamide, azathioprine, cyclosporin A, methotrexate, plasmapheresis, D-penicillamine, antimalarials, and octreotide have been employed, but none has shown consistent beneficial effects (86).

SCLERODERMA VARIANTS ASSOCIATED WITH EXPOSURE TO SILICA AND SILICONE

Exposure to elemental silicon has been associated with a variety of connective tissue diseases, most notably scleroderma. This association was first made in 1914, in Scottish workers exposed to silica dust (silicon dioxide, SiO_2), when Bramwell (87) reported the occurrence of scleroderma in nine of 27,000 patients in his general medical practice, six of whom were exposed to silica by virtue of their occupation, five as stonemasons, and one as a coal miner (87). Typical features of scleroderma were described, including Raynaud's phenomenon, digital ulcers, swollen and hidebound skin over the hands, telangiectasia, and arthralgias. The association of scleroderma and silica exposure received little attention until 1957, when Erasmus (88) reported the occurrence of scleroderma among 17 South African gold miners exposed to high concentrations of silica. Later, the association of scleroderma with silica exposure and silicosis was confirmed in American and German coal miners (89,90). German investigators estimated the likelihood of developing scleroderma to be 25-fold higher in persons exposed to silica and 110-fold higher in persons with actual silicosis (91). Although a later study of 79 South African gold miners with scleroderma failed to confirm the association between scleroderma and silicosis (radiographically defined), it did find a significantly higher cumulative lifetime silica exposure in scleroderma patients than in controls (90). Despite differences in methods and controls, reports spanning many years and from many geographic locales support an association between silica exposure, particularly in the mining industry, and scleroderma. No excess mortality from systemic sclerosis has been observed in subjects with nonmining occupational silica exposure (91). The illness is typical of systemic sclerosis and in some patients there may be a fulminant pulmonary component of the disease (92). Antibodies to topoisomerase I (anti–Scl-70) are detectable in as many as 50% of silica-associated scleroderma patients (93–95). Anticentromere antibodies also have been reported (94). Silica dust is capable of activating microvascular endothelial cells, mononuclear cells and dermal fibroblasts *in vitro,* simulating the changes observed in these cells from patients with systemic sclerosis (92).

The relationship between silicone (dimethylpolysiloxane) and connective tissue disease, especially scleroderma, has generated much controversy and is one of the most litigious issues of our time. Silicone has been used extensively in medicine and surgery, e.g., Silastic or silicone gel, and was exempted from the regulations of the Medical Device Amendment to the Federal Food, Drug, and Cosmetics Act (96). The long-term safety of silicone gel-filled breast implants was subsequently questioned and, in 1992, the U.S. Food and Drug Administration required the manufacturers of breast implants to provide proof of safety of these prostheses (97).

The earliest report suggesting an association between augmentation mammoplasty and connective tissue disease was in 1964, when Miyoshi et al. (98) reported two cases of arthritis after paraffin and silicone injections for cosmetic breast augmentation. The term *human adjuvant disease* was coined by these Japanese investigators. Before the 1970s, direct injection of paraffin, silicone, or processed petroleum jelly was performed to augment breast size. Later, implantable Silastic envelopes containing silicone gel or saline were developed. A review of the Japanese experience with silicone injections identified 46 patients with various disorders, including 24 with connective tissue disease such as scleroderma, rheumatoid arthritis (RA), systemic lupus erythematosus, and polymyositis (99). The relative risk for scleroderma was estimated to be increased threefold (99). Subsequently, there have been numerous case reports or small series reporting connective tissue disease in women after silicone gel breast implantation, with an average latency period of 10 years. Of 85 patients reported in the literature before 1993, 50 had a definite connective tissue disease (25 scleroderma, 13 RA, 8 systemic lupus erythematosus, 4 mixed connective tissue disease), and the remainder had a poorly defined disorder often referred to as human adjuvant disease (100). The validity of the association of augmentation mammoplasty with scleroderma remains uncertain, but the claimed preponderance of scleroderma among silicone-exposed subjects with connective tissue disease is intriguing and has raised the question of a possible role for silicone exposure in triggering scleroderma in a susceptible individual, although this has not been proven. A retrospective cohort study involving nearly 400,000 female health professionals concluded there was no evidence of large risks of connective tissue diseases following breast implants, but there was perhaps a small increased risk of scleroderma in this self-report study (relative risk, 1.84; 95% confidence interval, 0.98–3.46, $p = .06$) (101).

A multicenter case control study noted a frequency of 1.31% for augmentation mammoplasty before diagnosis of scleroderma, which is not different from the frequency of 1.24% observed in controls (102). A case-control study from Michigan also found no increased risk of scleroderma among women with silicone breast implants (103).

Cases of scleroderma occurring in individuals with a history of silicone exposure resemble those of idiopathic scleroderma, with skin fibrosis in a limited (acrosclerosis) or diffuse (truncal) cutaneous distribution (104–111) or, occasionally, as morphea without systemic involvement (112,113). Raynaud's phenomenon, digital ulceration, arthralgia or arthritis, and visceral involvement have been reported. In at least two patients with scleroderma, renal crises have been reported (114,115), with apparent reversal after silicone implant removal in one (114).

Overall, the clinical response to removal of silicone implants has been variable; some patients have shown dramatic improvement in skin and visceral organ involvement, whereas others have had progressive, sometimes fatal, disease (111). Esophageal dysmotility similar to that observed in scleroderma but without skin changes, relapsing polychondritis, or ANA has been reported in a few selected children breast-fed by mothers with silicone breast implants (116). There is no evidence that silicone is present in breast milk (117). Present data do not support a ban against breast-feeding by mothers with silicone implants (118).

Positive ANAs occur in a variable percentage of women with silicone breast implants, depending in part on the substrate or method employed and irrespective of clinical presentation (reviewed in ref. 119). Western blot analysis is more sensitive than indirect immunofluorescence tests, but even with the former the frequency of recognized ANAs may be lower than in systemic sclerosis (120). Generally, the more well defined the connective tissue disease, the higher the likelihood of finding a positive ANA. Scleroderma-specific autoantibodies, e.g., antitopoisomerase I, anticentromere, and anti-RNA polymerase I, have been detected in some scleroderma patients with silicone exposure (120,121).

Fibrous encapsulation and contracture may occur around the intact breast prosthesis. Surrounding tissue may be the site of a chronic inflammatory response with numerous macrophages, multinucleated giant cells, lymphocytes, and fibroblasts (96). Silicone implants leak silicone gel, even without frank rupture. Elemental silicon is present in the fibrous breast capsule, as well as in regional lymph nodes and tissues involved by connective tissue disease (Fig. 80.6) (109,122,123). Using electron probe x-ray microanalysis, a spectroscopic technique that measures the emission of x-rays unique to each element during electron microscopy, elemental silicon was detected in skin involved by scleroderma, but not in clinically uninvolved skin (122). In a second patient with interstitial lung disease and features of scleroderma and systemic lupus erythematosus, silicon was present in alveolar macrophages (122). Silicon also was identified within macrophages present in synovial tissue of four women with chronic synovitis following silicone gel breast augmentation (123). Foamy macrophages in the capsule surrounding breast implants contained vacuoles with small residual fragments of refractile, nonpolarizable material containing silicon (109,122,123) (Fig. 80.7). Similar histologic and electron microscopic features have been described in axillary lymph nodes (109). Taken together, these studies demonstrate that silicone or elemental silicon may escape from breast implants (even without frank rupture) and migrate (perhaps within macrophages) beyond the capsule to regional lymph nodes and distant sites of inflammation and fibrosis (123). The role of silicone in this process is unknown, but experimental evidence indicates that elemental silicon can trigger persistent inflammatory and fibrotic reactions. Subcutaneous injection of silicone in animals is followed by a local inflammatory response with

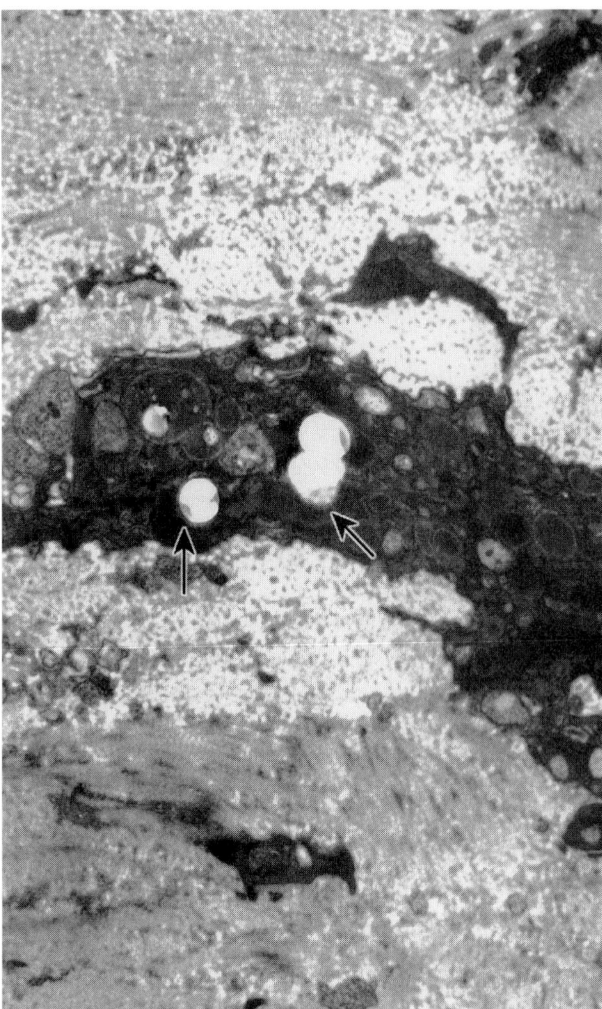

FIGURE 80.6. Electron micrograph (×10,000) showing an amorphous deposit of silicon in a macrophage *(arrows)*. (Courtesy of Dr. William Greene.)

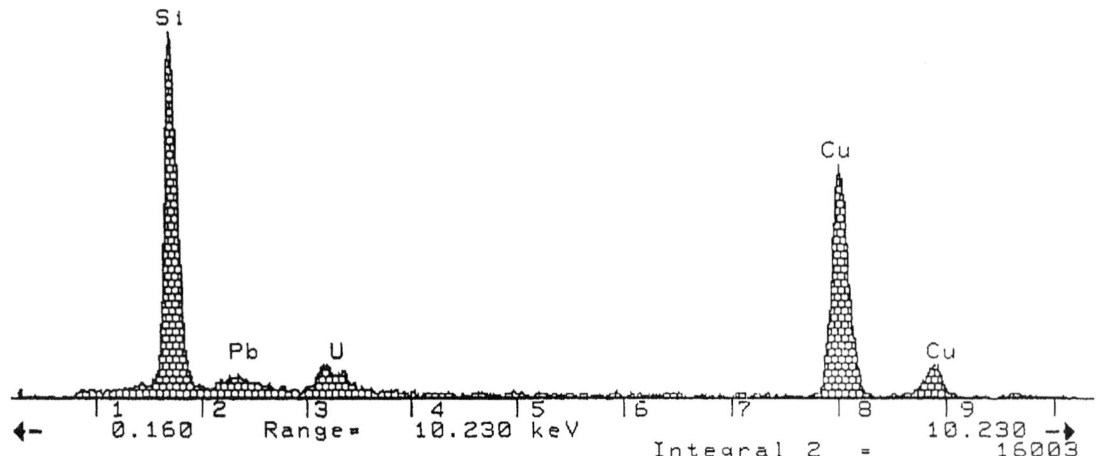

FIGURE 80.7. Representative electron probe microanalysis spectra of silicon identified in the macrophage shown in Figure 80.6. Si is the peak for the silicon inclusions shown at the *arrows* in Figure 80.6. Pb and U are the peaks of lead citrate and urynal acetate stain, respectively, used to gain electron contrast. The two Cu peaks arise from the copper grid on which the sections were mounted. Background was subtracted. (Courtesy of Dr. William Greene.)

accumulation of vacuolated macrophages that ingest silica, followed by chronic inflammation and fibrosis (124).

Macrophages that have ingested silicone may convert it to a more toxic form, i.e., silica, by the action of powerful oxidizing free radicals (125). Silica can affect both cellular and humoral immune processes; inhalation exposure is associated with subsequent development of pulmonary fibrosis and in some cases scleroderma. Macrophages exposed to silica may release fibrogenic cytokines and stimulate collagen synthesis (126,127). It remains to be determined whether the inflammatory or immunologic response to silicone and silica are related to the immunogenetic background of the host.

Although the above results are intriguing, the currently available epidemiologic data do not establish a significant association between breast implants and a defined autoimmune disease.

SCLERODERMA VARIANTS ASSOCIATED WITH CHEMICAL OR DRUG EXPOSURE

Vinyl Chloride Disease

Exposure to vinyl chloride ($CH_2 = CHCl$) has been associated with a scleroderma-like illness referred to as occupational acro-osteolysis (128). Large-scale production of polyvinyl chloride (PVC) began in the 1930s in the United States and Germany (129), and reports of the health hazards of chronic occupational exposure to vinyl chloride monomer (VCM) were first reported in the mid-1950s. Workers at plants producing VCM presented with symptoms of Raynaud's phenomenon ("toxic angioneurosis") (130). Findings included vasospasm of the digital arteries; swollen fingers; induration of the skin on the volar surface of the forearms; paresthesias; CNS symptoms such as headache, decreased memory, and insomnia; mild hemolysis; and a destructive lesion of the distal phalanges in the hands (acro-osteolysis). On wide-field capillary microscopy, microvascular abnormalities resembling those seen in idiopathic scleroderma were noted in many patients with vinyl chloride disease (131).

Less than 3% of exposed workers developed acro-osteolysis (132). Long-term reactor cleaning was most frequently associated with Raynaud's phenomenon and acro-osteolysis. Susceptibility to vinyl chloride disease was reported to be associated with the presence of human leukocyte antigen HLA-DR5, and progressive disease was linked to the presence of the A1,B8,DR3 haplotype in workers in the United Kingdom (133,134). The ANA was generally negative, and neither anticentromere nor antitopoisomerase I antibodies were detected (133).

Skin changes suggestive of scleroderma included thickening of the skin of the fingers, hands, and forearms, sometimes accompanied by puffiness or coarsening of the face. Raised nodules or ivory-colored plaques of indurated skin were seen in the hands and forearms (135). Biopsy specimens showed dermal sclerosis without epidermal atrophy (136). Unlike idiopathic scleroderma, digital pitting scars, esophageal dysmotility, renal disease, and cardiac disease were generally absent. Pulmonary disease was noted in some patients (133), but its relationship to vinyl chloride exposure is uncertain (129). Noncirrhotic portal hypertension and hepatic angiosarcoma occurred as late sequelae in some cases.

Skin lesions regressed after cessation of exposure to vinyl chloride. Serious cases of vinyl chloride disease can be avoided by controlling exposure to VCM and screening exposed employees for Raynaud's phenomenon and radiographic signs of early acro-osteolysis.

Organic Solvents

Since the initial report in 1957 of scleroderma in a woman with a 2-year history of exposure to trichloroethylene (137), more than 50 such patients have been described (138). A case-control study confirmed occupational exposure to solvents to be a risk factor for scleroderma, especially for male patients and for patients with anti–Scl-70 autoantibodies (139). Solvent exposure from hobbies may also increase the risk of scleroderma (140). Two cases of eosinophilic fasciitis have been reported in association with trichloroethylene exposure (3).

Organic solvents reported to be associated with scleroderma include trichloroethylene, trichloroethane, benzene, xylene, methylene chloride, toluene, perchlorethylene, and metaphenylenediamine. The organic solvent implicated most often is trichloroethylene ($CHCl = CCl_2$). It and perchlorethylene ($CCl_2 = CCl_2$) are similar in structure to vinyl chloride.

Scleroderma in patients with solvent exposure is generally indistinguishable from cases of idiopathic systemic sclerosis. Duration and intensity of exposure before onset of disease vary. Most cases are characterized by diffuse cutaneous involvement and are accompanied by Raynaud's phenomenon and visceral organ disease. The nailfold capillaries are abnormal and the ANA is positive. The disease usually does not subside following avoidance of solvent exposure, and fatalities have been reported.

AMINES

Workers engaged in the polymerization of epoxy resins have been reported to develop a scleroderma-like condition. In 1980, Japanese investigators first described this illness in six of 233 workers with a history of brief exposure to the vapor of epoxy resins (141). The patients had erythema and edema that evolved to generalized dermal sclerosis and alopecia. Skin changes were accompanied by weakness and muscle atrophy. Raynaud's phenomenon was not present, and tests for ANA were negative. Skin biopsy specimens revealed deposits of melanin in the epidermis and increased collagen deposition in the dermis, as well as panniculitis that evolved to fibrosis of the subcutaneous adipose tissue. Thickening of the fascia and a low-grade inflammation of the perimysium were seen. Skin and muscle abnormalities improved gradually with avoidance of exposure to the resin together with protease and corticosteroid therapy.

Nine chemicals were present in the epoxy resin vapor. Intraperitoneal injection of one compound, bis(4-amino-3-methyl-cyclohexyl)methane, produced dermal sclerosis in a murine model (141). Although three additional compounds also produced skin changes in some animals, bis(4-amino-3-methyl-cyclohexyl)methane was suspected to be the etiologic agent as it had been added to the polymerization process as a plasticizer at the time of the occurrence of the illness.

Further outbreaks of scleroderma or morphea related to epoxy resin exposure have not been reported, but other amines have been linked to the development of scleroderma-like conditions. EMS is the most recent example. The similar illness associated with 5-hydroxytryptophan also has been discussed. Other amines associated with morphea or scleroderma-like conditions include bromocriptine (142,143), various appetite suppressants (144,145), and 5-hydroxytryptamine (serotonin) in patients with carcinoid syndrome (146,147). Fibrosis is a complication of ingestion of other amines (e.g., methysergide), and pulmonary hypertension has been reported to occur in association with certain appetite suppressants, e.g., aminorex and fenfluramine (148–150).

BLEOMYCIN

Raynaud's phenomenon and scleroderma occur in some cancer patients treated with bleomycin (151–153). Bleomycins are a group of related glycopeptide antibiotics isolated from *Streptomyces verticillus* that differ from one another in the terminal amine. Cutaneous lesions in cases associated with bleomycin are identical to idiopathic scleroderma, and lesional fibroblasts synthesize increased quantities of glycosaminoglycan and collagen (152). Rats injected with bleomycin develop weight loss, alopecia, hyperpigmentation, and skin tightness (154). Histologic findings are consistent with those of systemic sclerosis. Features of systemic sclerosis may not be present, and the ANA is variably positive (153). Partial resolution occurs after cessation of bleomycin therapy and may be hastened by the addition of corticosteroids (153).

The mechanism whereby bleomycin induces scleroderma is unknown. The possibility that vascular injury may be the primary process is suggested by the observation that endothelial injury is the earliest pathologic lesion in experimental animal models of bleomycin-induced pulmonary fibrosis (155). Vascular abnormalities (e.g., Raynaud's phenomenon) occur frequently in men treated for testicular carcinoma with bleomycin and vinblastine (156). Even low-dose bleomycin injected locally may be followed by the development of Raynaud's phenomenon (157).

PENTAZOCINE

Cutaneous sclerosis complicating intramuscular injections of the analgesic pentazocine is readily distinguishable from systemic sclerosis. Brawny induration and deep penetrating ulcers around the sites of injection are characteristic. These changes may be accompanied by a fibrous myopathy, joint contractures, neuropathy, and soft tissue calcification (158–160). The skin of the face and fingers is spared, and patients do not have visceral organ involvement. Histologic findings include dermal fibrosis extending to the panniculus with varying degrees of inflammation, small vessel thrombosis, intimal proliferation, and lymphohistiocytic perivascular inflammation.

LOCALIZED SCLERODERMA

Localized scleroderma is characterized by induration of the skin, pigmentary changes, and reduced elasticity, which may progress to scarring. There are three main variants of localized scleroderma: morphea, generalized morphea, and linear scleroderma. Morphea and linear scleroderma have a three- to fourfold increased incidence in females. The incidence of morphea is estimated at 2.7 per 100,000 population (161). Linear scleroderma occurs in a younger age group of patients, with most patients being younger than 18 years of age.

Morphea

Morphea may occur in one of several forms including plaque, guttate, morphea profundus, and generalized. Most commonly, morphea occurs as one or more plaques, typically on the trunk. The lesions are characterized by central skin hardening associated with edema, and pigmentary changes (hyper- or hypo-). Active or progressive lesions typically have a violaceous border (Fig. 80.8). Late changes include scarring with white or yellow indurated plaques. Guttate morphea lesions are similar in appearance to plaque morphea, but are smaller and multiple and have been described as "confetti." Generalized morphea begins as multiple patches of morphea but becomes pansclerotic and may involve large areas of the body, though typically without sclerodactyly or facial involvement. It most commonly affects the trunk and extremities. Patients with generalized morphea lack Raynaud's phenomenon and internal organ involvement, and only rare cases progress to systemic sclerosis. It may be difficult to differentiate generalized morphea from diffuse fasciitis with eosinophilia, as both may involve nearly the entire body surface area, yet on a deep incisional biopsy the patient with generalized morphea will not demonstrate inflammation and fibrosis of the fascia.

The histopathology of localized scleroderma is identical to that of patients with systemic sclerosis, exhibiting an inflammatory cell infiltrate of the dermis composed of lymphocytes, plasma cells, eosinophils, and mast cells. Excessive collagen deposition and fibroblast proliferation occur. Small arteries may be occluded as a result of collagen deposition and damage to endothelial cells. Morphea profundus is similar to lupus profundus in that the pathologic changes involve many levels in the skin and subcutaneous tissues, in particular from the dermis to the level of muscle, and thus the lesion appears to involve a deeper level of induration.

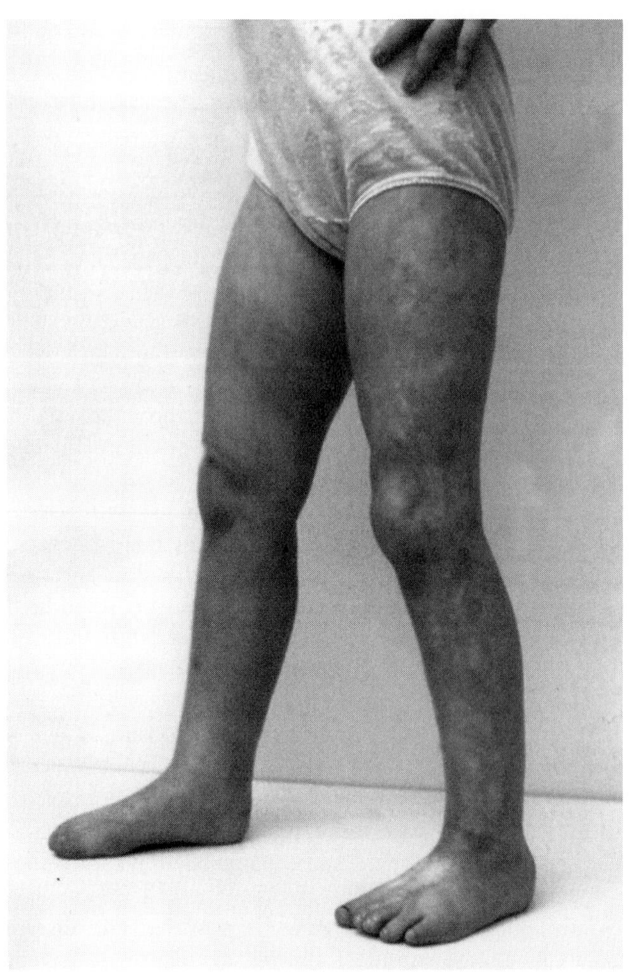

FIGURE 80.8. A child with linear scleroderma involving the left lower extremity with evidence of a left knee flexion contracture. There is a plaque of morphea on the right thigh.

Linear Scleroderma

Linear scleroderma presents as a band of sclerosis with pigmentary alterations, typically unilateral and affecting a longitudinal portion of an extremity (Fig. 80.8). This variant of localized scleroderma usually develops in the first or second decade of life and may lead to significant morbidity by affecting limb growth. In addition to the cutaneous sclerosis, there may be involvement of muscle and bone, resulting in muscle atrophy, joint contractures, and growth retardation of the involved bone. Involvement of the face by linear scleroderma is termed *en coup de sabre,* resulting in hemifacial atrophy and disfigurement. Similar to morphea, the development of systemic sclerosis from linear scleroderma has only rarely been reported.

Laboratory Features

The laboratory abnormalities seen in localized scleroderma include a positive ANA and/or rheumatoid factor (RF), peripheral eosinophilia, and elevated levels of serum immunoglobulin G (IgG). Other specific connective tissue disease serologies, for example antitopoisomerase I or anti-DNA antibodies, are notably negative. The peripheral eosinophilia reflects disease activity in localized scleroderma (162) and, in contrast, is not typically seen in systemic sclerosis. In patients with active linear scleroderma, a peripheral eosinophilia may be present in 50% of patients (162). A polyclonal gammopathy occurs in nearly 50% of patients and also reflects disease severity. Nailfold capillaroscopy findings are normal in patients with localized scleroderma, unlike the changes that occur characteristically in systemic sclerosis (163).

Etiology

The etiology of localized scleroderma is not known. Several groups have studied a possible association between *B. burgdorferi* and morphea. A study of ten Swiss patients with localized scleroderma described the presence of *Borrelia* antibodies in all patients (164). However, studies using polymerase chain reaction and enzyme-linked immunosorbent assay techniques have found no evidence to support a link between *Borrelia* infections and localized scleroderma (165,166).

Therapy

Plaque morphea may be asymptomatic and may disappear within 3 to 5 years from onset. However, if symptomatic or cosmetically displeasing, topical steroids are useful. Both morphea profundus and generalized morphea are likely to be more symptomatic than plaque morphea, often due to pruritus or flexion contractures. In these instances, systemic therapy may be warranted. In addition to topical corticosteroids, systemic corticosteroids in moderate (0.25 to 0.50 mg/kg) to high doses can be used (167). Although not studied systematically, hydroxychloroquine is used as a second-line agent for plaque morphea or generalized morphea. Open trials with oral calcitriol (1,25-dihydroxyvitamin D_3) have shown efficacy in patients with generalized morphea (168). Although the mechanism of action is unknown, it is believed to relate to fibroblast inhibition and cytokine modulation.

D-penicillamine (2 to 5 mg/kg/day) may be of benefit in linear scleroderma or generalized morphea, but no controlled trials have been reported (169). Other anecdotal reports have shown efficacy with cyclosporin A (170) or plasmapheresis in conjunction with high-dose glucocorticoids (171). Psoralen-ultraviolet A irradiation (PUVA) therapy has also been reported to be effective in some patients with localized scleroderma (172–174).

PSEUDOSCLERODERMA

Scleredema

Scleredema adultorum (Buschke's disease) is a rare connective tissue disease characterized by the sudden onset of rapidly progressive induration of the skin. In many cases, it is preceded by a febrile illness (streptococcal most often) and it is sometimes associated with diabetes mellitus. It is not to be confused with the digital sclerosis of juvenile-onset diabetes mellitus (diabetic cheirarthropathy) (175), in which there is an increase in dermal collagen due to nonenzymatic glycosylation interfering with normal collagen turnover. Scleredema usually begins as a brawny, painless induration at the nape of the neck and may spread to involve the scalp, face, and trunk. Unlike idiopathic scleroderma, the hands and feet are spared. A skin biopsy specimen reveals intradermal mucopolysaccharide deposits. Like scleromyxedema, some cases have been associated with myeloma and monoclonal gammopathies (176). However, in most patients regression of the skin induration occurs within 6 to 18 months.

Scleromyxedema

Scleromyxedema (papular mucinosis) is a rare condition characterized by papular skin lesions associated with sclerosis and monoclonal gammopathy (177). It is a chronic disease that occurs in the third to fifth decade of life (178). Papular lesions occur most commonly on the face and arms; the lesions consist of large amounts of dermal acid mucopolysaccharide (mostly hyaluronic acid) and proliferating fibroblasts with irregularly arranged bundles of collagen (177). The serum of nearly all patients with scleromyxedema contains an IgG λ paraprotein. Although clinical involvement is generally restricted to the skin and bone marrow, some patients may have involvement of muscle, nerve, esophagus, and lung that may mimic scleroderma (177). The absence of Raynaud's phenomenon and the clinical and histopathologic cutaneous differences distinguish this condition from systemic sclerosis. Immunosuppressive therapy is successful in some patients but the response is variable.

Other Conditions

A number of other rare conditions (Table 80.1) may be accompanied by taut skin, thus mimicking scleroderma (178). In some, the skin is indurated (e.g., amyloidosis), whereas in others the skin is atrophic (e.g., lichen sclerosis et atrophicus or neurologic disorders). These conditions are usually readily distinguishable from scleroderma by the absence of characteristic microvascular morphologic changes, the absence of typical ANAs, and the absence of typical visceral organ involvement seen in scleroderma (systemic sclerosis).

GRAFT-VERSUS-HOST DISEASE

Chronic graft-versus-host disease after allogeneic bone marrow transplantation is associated with several clinical and histopathologic features resembling autoimmune diseases, including sicca syndrome and scleroderma. Three or more months after transplantation, up to 50% of patients develop a lichenoid eruption characterized by a lymphocytic infiltrate in the epidermis and upper dermis. Some patients progress from lichenoid to sclerodermatous lesions (179) in which there is diffuse dermal fibrosis, basal cell vacuolization, basement membrane thickening, and a band-like dermal lymphohistiocytic infiltrate (180). Rarely, patients may develop fasciitis resembling diffuse fasciitis with eosinophilia (181). Chronic graft-versus-host disease with scleroderma-like manifestations can be associated with the occurrence of scleroderma-specific autoantibodies, including anti–Scl-70 antibodies (182).

A similar cutaneous disease can be induced in animal models of graft-versus-host disease following allogeneic bone marrow transplantation (183) or syngeneic bone marrow transplantation after withdrawal of cyclosporin A. A role for T-helper cells has been postulated in these models (184,185). Microvascular disease resembling that in systemic sclerosis has been observed in experimental models of graft-versus-host disease (186). Similarly, intercellular cell adhesion molecule type 1 (ICAM-1) expression is enhanced in chronic graft-versus-host disease (187). HLA class II compatibility of mother and child, together with evidence of microchimerism in female scleroderma patients, suggests a role for graft-versus-host mechanisms in the pathogenesis of idiopathic scleroderma (188).

Early treatment of chronic graft-versus-host disease with an alternating regimen of cyclosporin A and prednisone has led to improved survival, and the incidence of disabling scleroderma-like disease has decreased dramatically (189). Some patients have reportedly benefited from treatment with thalidomide, extracorporeal photopheresis, PUVA, or etretinate.

REFERENCES

1. Shulman LE. Diffuse fasciitis with eosinophilia: a new syndrome? *Trans Assoc Am Phys* 1975;88:70–86.
2. Granter SR, Barnhill RL, Duray PH. *Borrelia* fasciitis: diffuse fasciitis and peripheral eosinophilia associated with *Borrelia* infection. *Am J Dermatopathol* 1996;18:465–473.
3. Waller PA, Clauw D, Cupps T, et al. Fasciitis (not scleroderma) following prolonged exposure to an organic solvent (trichloroethylene): a report of two cases. *J Rheumatol* 1994;21:1567–1570.
4. Chan LS, Hanson CA, Cooper KD. Concurrent eosinophilic fasciitis and cutaneous T-cell lymphoma. *Arch Dermatol* 1991; 127:862–865.
5. Lakhanpal S, Ginsburg WW, Michet CJ, et al. Eosinophilic fasciitis: clinical spectrum and therapeutic response in 52 cases. *Semin Arthritis Rheum* 1988;17:221–231.
6. Al-Shaikh A, Freeman C, Avruch L, et al. Use of magnetic resonance imaging in diagnosing eosinophilic fasciitis. Report of two cases. *Arthritis Rheum* 1994;11:1602–1608.
7. Peltonen J, Kahari L, Jaakkola S, et al. Evaluation of transforming growth factor beta and type I procollagen gene expression in fibrotic skin diseases by in situ hybridization. *J Invest Dermatol* 1990;94:365–371.
8. Kahari VM, Heino J, Niskanen L, et al. Eosinophilic fasciitis. Increased collagen production and type I procollagen messenger RNA levels in fibroblasts cultured from involved skin. *Arch Dermatol* 1990;126:613–617.
9. Varga J, Peltonen J, Uitto JM, et al. Development of diffuse fasciitis with eosinophilia during L-tryptophan treatment: demonstration of elevated type I collagen gene expression in affected tissues. A clinicopathologic study of four patients. *Ann Intern Med* 1990;112:344–351.
10. Peltonen J, Varga J, Sollberg S, et al. Elevated expression of the genes for transforming growth factor-1 and type VI collagen in diffuse fasciitis associated with the eosinophilia-myalgia syndrome. *J Invest Dermatol* 1991;96:20–25.
11. Bolster MB, Allen N, Heyes M, et al. Kynurenine pathway of L-tryptophan metabolism in eosinophilic fasciitis. *Arthritis Rheum* 1993;36(suppl):R17.
12. Naschitz JE, Yeshurun D, Zuckerman E, et al. The fasciitis-panniculitis syndrome: clinical spectrum and response to cimetidine. *Semin Arthritis Rheum* 1992;21:211–220.
13. Ching DWT, Leibowitz MR. Ketotifen—a therapeutic agent of eosinophilic fasciitis? *J Intern Med* 1992;231:555–559.
14. Laneuville P. Cyclosporin A induced remission of CD4⁺ T-CLL associated with eosinophilia and fasciitis. *Br J Haematol* 1992;80:252–254.
15. Gaffney K, Kearns G, Moraes D, et al. Eosinophilic fasciitis: a good response with conservative treatment. *Irish J Med Sci* 1993;162:256–257.
16. Toxic Epidemic Syndrome Study Group. Toxic epidemic syndrome, Spain, 1981. *Lancet* 1982;2:697–702.
17. Tabuenca JM. Toxic-allergic syndrome caused by ingestion of rapeseed oil denatured with aniline. *Lancet* 1981;2:567–568.
18. Kilbourne EM, Posada de la Paz M, Abaitua Borda I. Current knowledge and future perspectives. In: *Toxic oil syndrome.* WHO regional publications, European series, no. 42. Copenhagen: World Health Organization, 1992:5–26.
19. Kilbourne EM, Bernert JT Jr, Posada de la Paz M, et al. Chemical correlates of pathogenicity of oils related to the toxic oil syndrome in Spain. *Am J Epidemiol* 1988;127:1210–1227.
20. Aldridge WN. Current knowledge and future perspectives. In: *Toxic oil syndrome.* WHO regional publications, European series, no. 42. Copenhagen: World Health Organization, 1992:67–98.
21. Hill RH Jr, Schurz H, Posada de la Paz M, et al. Possible etiologic agents for toxic oil syndrome: fatty acid esters of 3-(N-phenylamino)-1,2-propanediol. *Arch Environ Contam Toxicol* 1995;28:259–264.
22. Pagani R, Portoles MT, Gavilanes FG, et al. The microviscosity of liver plasma membranes of rats fed with oleoylanilide. *Biochem J* 1984;218:125–129.
23. Mayeno AN, Belongia EA, Lin F, et al. 3-(Phenylamino)alanine, a novel aniline-derived amino acid associated with the eosinophilia-myalgia syndrome: a link to the toxic oil syndrome? *Mayo Clin Proc* 1992;67:1134–1139.
24. Philen RM, Posada M. Toxic oil syndrome and eosinophilia-myalgia syndrome: May 8–10, 1991, World Health Organization meeting report. *Semin Arthritis Rheum* 1993;23:104–124.
25. Abaitua Borda I, Posada de la Paz M. Current knowledge and future perspectives. In: *Toxic oil syndrome.* WHO regional publications, European series, no. 42. Copenhagen: World Health Organization, 1992:27–38.

26. Kaufman LD, Martinez MI, Serrano JM, et al. Twelve year followup study of epidemic Spanish toxic oil syndrome. *J Rheumatol* 1995;22:282–288.
27. Martinez-Tello FJ, Tellez I. Current knowledge and future perspectives. In: *Toxic oil syndrome.* WHO regional publications, European series, no. 42. Copenhagen: World Health Organization, 1992:39–66.
28. Hertzman PA, Blevins WL, Mayer J, et al. Association of the eosinophilia-myalgia syndrome with the ingestion of L-tryptophan. *N Engl J Med* 1990;322:869–873.
29. Swygert LA, Maes EF, Sewell LE, et al. Eosinophilia-myalgia syndrome. Results of national surveillance. *JAMA* 1990;264:1698–1703.
30. Varga J, Griffin R, Newman JH, et al. Eosinophilic fasciitis is clinically distinguishable from the eosinophilia-myalgia syndrome and is not associated with L-tryptophan use. *J Rheumatol* 1991;18:259–263.
31. Centers for Disease Control. Eosinophilia-myalgia syndrome—New Mexico. *JAMA* 1989;262:3116.
32. Swygert LA, Back EE, Auerbach SB, et al. Eosinophilia-myalgia syndrome: mortality data from the US national surveillance system. *J Rheumatol* 1993;20:1711–1717.
33. Belongia EA, Hedberg CW, Gleich GJ, et al. An investigation of the cause of the eosinophilia-myalgia syndrome associated with tryptophan use. *N Engl J Med* 1990;323:357–365.
34. Slutsker L, Hoesly FC, Miller L, et al. Eosinophilia-myalgia syndrome associated with exposure to tryptophan from a single manufacturer. *JAMA* 1990;264:213–217.
35. Eidson M, Philen RM, Sewell CM, et al. L-tryptophan and eosinophilia-myalgia syndrome in New Mexico. *Lancet* 1990;335:645–648.
36. Sullivan EA, Staehling N, Philen RM. Eosinophilia-myalgia syndrome among the non-L-tryptophan users and pre-epidemic cases. *J Rheumatol* 1996;23:1784–1787.
37. Kamb ML, Murphy JJ, Jones JL, et al. Eosinophilia-myalgia syndrome in L-tryptophan-exposed patients. *JAMA* 1992;267:77–82.
38. Mayeno AN, Lin F, Foote CS, et al. Characterization of "peak E," a novel amino acid associated with eosinophilia-myalgia syndrome. *Science* 1990;250:1707–1708.
39. Henning KJ, Jean-Baptiste E, Singh T, et al. Eosinophilia-myalgia syndrome in patients ingesting a single source of L-tryptophan. *J Rheumatol* 1993;20:273–278.
40. Hill RH Jr, Caudill SP, Philen RM, et al. Contaminants in L-tryptophan associated with eosinophilia myalgia syndrome. *Arch Environ Contam Toxicol* 1993;25:134–142.
41. Crofford LJ, Rader JI, Dalakas MC, et al. L-tryptophan implicated in human eosinophilia-myalgia syndrome causes fasciitis and perimyositis in the Lewis rat. *J Clin Invest* 1990;86:1757–1763.
42. Love LA, Rader JI, Crofford LJ, et al. Pathological and immunological effects of ingesting L-tryptophan and 1,1′-ethylidenebis(L-tryptophan) in Lewis rats. *J Clin Invest* 1993;91:804–811.
43. Silver RM, Ludwicka A, Hampton M, et al. A murine model of the eosinophilia-myalgia syndrome induced by 1,1′-ethylidenebis(L-tryptophan). *J Clin Invest* 1994;93:1473–1480.
44. Takagi H, Ochoa MS, Zhou L, et al. Enhanced collagen synthesis and transcription by peak E, a contaminant of L-tryptophan preparations associated with the eosinophilia-myalgia syndrome epidemic. *J Clin Invest* 1995;96:2120–2125.
45. Clauw DJ, Nashel DJ, Katz P. Tryptophan-associated eosinophilic connective-tissue disease. A new clinical entity? *JAMA* 1990;263:1502–1506.
46. Kaufman LD, Seidman RJ, Gruber BL. L-tryptophan-associated eosinophilic perimyositis, neuritis, and fasciitis. A clinicopathologic and laboratory study of 25 patients. *Medicine* 1990;69:187–199.
47. Clauw DJ, Hewes B, Nelson M, et al. P-31 magnetic resonance spectroscopy of skeletal muscle in the eosinophilia myalgia syndrome. *J Rheumatol* 1994;21:654–657.
48. Hertzman P, Falk H, Kilbourne EM, et al. The eosinophilia-myalgia syndrome: the Los Alamos conference. *J Rheumatol* 1991;18:867–873.
49. Martin RW, Duffy J, Engel AG, et al. The clinical spectrum of the eosinophilia-myalgia syndrome associated with L-tryptophan ingestion. Clinical features in 20 patients and aspects of pathophysiology. *Ann Intern Med* 1990;113:124–134.
50. Owen WF Jr, Petersen J, Sheff DM, et al. Hypodense eosinophils and interleukin-5 activity in the blood of patients with the eosinophilia-myalgia syndrome. *Proc Natl Acad Sci U S A* 1990;87:8647–8651.
51. Silver RM, Heyes MP, Maize JC, et al. Scleroderma, fasciitis, and eosinophilia associated with the ingestion of tryptophan. *N Engl J Med* 1990;322:874–881.
52. Kaufman L, Seidman R, Phillips M, et al. Cutaneous manifestations of the L-tryptophan-associated eosinophilia-myalgia syndrome: a spectrum of sclerodermatous skin disease. *J Am Acad Dermatol* 1990;23:1063–1069.
53. Tazelaar HD, Myers JL, Drage CW, et al. Pulmonary disease associated with L-tryptophan-induced eosinophilic myalgia syndrome. Clinical and pathologic features. *Chest* 1990;97:1032–1036.
54. Strumpf IJ, Drucker RD, Anders KH, et al. Acute eosinophilic pulmonary disease associated with the ingestion of L-tryptophan-containing products. *Chest* 1991;99:8–13.
55. Banner A, Borochovitz D. Acute respiratory failure caused by pulmonary vasculitis after L-tryptophan ingestion. *Am Rev Respir Dis* 1991;143:661–664.
56. Read CA, Clauw D, Weir C, et al. Dyspnea and pulmonary function in the L-tryptophan-associated eosinophilia-myalgia syndrome. *Chest* 1992;101:1282–1286.
57. Smith BE, Dyck PJ. Peripheral neuropathy in the eosinophilia-myalgia syndrome associated with L-tryptophan ingestion. *Neurology* 1990;40:1035–1040.
58. Heiman-Patterson TD, Bird, SJ, Parry GJ, et al. Peripheral neuropathy associated with eosinophilia-myalgia syndrome. *Ann Neurol* 1990;28:522–528.
59. Donofrio PD, Stanton C, Miller VS, et al. Demyelinating polyneuropathy in eosinophilia-myalgia syndrome. *Muscle Nerve* 1992;15:796–805.
60. Tolander LM, Bamford CR, Yoshino MT, et al. Neurologic complications of the tryptophan-associated eosinophilia myalgia syndrome. *Arch Neurol* 1991;48:436–438.
61. Adair JC, Rose JW, Digre KB, et al. Acute encephalopathy associated with the eosinophilia-myalgia syndrome. *Neurology* 1992;42:461–462.
62. Greenfield BM, Mayer JW, Sibbitt RR. The eosinophilia myalgia syndrome and the brain. *Ann Intern Med* 1991;115:159–160.
63. Lynn J, Rammohan KW, Bornstein RA, et al. Central nervous system involvement in the eosinophilia-myalgia syndrome. *Arch Neurol* 1992;49:1082–1085.
64. Pixley JS, Eaton JM, Zweig RM. Central nervous system inflammation in the eosinophilia-myalgia syndrome. *Br J Rheumatol* 1992;32:174.
65. Anonymous. Eosinophilia-myalgia syndrome: follow-up survey of patients—New York, 1990–1991. *MMWR* 1991;40:401–403.
66. Krupp LB, Masur DM, Kaufman LD. Neurocognitive dysfunction in the eosinophilia-myalgia syndrome. *Neurology* 1993;43:931–936.

67. Silver RM, McKinley K, Smith EA, et al. Tryptophan metabolism via the kynurenine pathway in patients with the eosinophilia myalgia syndrome. *Arthritis Rheum* 1992;35: 1097–1105.
68. James TN, Kamb ML, Sandberg GA, et al. Postmortem studies of the heart in three fatal cases of the eosinophilia-myalgia syndrome. *Ann Intern Med* 1991;115:102–110.
69. James TN, Gomez-Sanchez MA, Martinez-Tello FJ, et al. Cardiac abnormalities in the toxic oil syndrome, with comparative observations on the eosinophilia-myalgia syndrome. *J Am Coll Cardiol* 1991;18:1367–1379.
70. Berger PB, Duffy J, Reeder GS, et al. Restrictive cardiomyopathy associated with the eosinophilia-myalgia syndrome. *Mayo Clin Proc* 1994;69:162–165.
71. Feldman SR, Silver RM, Maize JC. A histopathologic comparison of Shulman's syndrome (diffuse fasciitis with eosinophilia) and the fasciitis associated with the eosinophilia-myalgia syndrome. *J Am Acad Dermatol* 1992;26:95–100.
72. Umbert I, Winkelmann RK, Wegener L. Comparison of the pathology of fascia in eosinophilic myalgia syndrome patients and idiopathic eosinophilic fasciitis. *Dermatology* 1993;186:18–22.
73. Lin JD, Phelps RG, Gordon ML, et al. Pathologic manifestations of the eosinophilia myalgia syndrome: analysis of 11 cases. *Hum Pathol* 1992;23:429–437.
74. Silver RM, Sutherland SE, Carreira P, et al. Alterations in tryptophan metabolism in the toxic oil syndrome and in the eosinophilia-myalgia syndrome. *J Rheumatol* 1992;19:69–73.
75. Kaufman LD, Gruber BL, Needleman BW. Interleukin-4 levels in the eosinophilia-myalgia syndrome. *Am J Med* 1991;91 :664–665.
76. Emslie-Smith AM, Engel AG, Duffy J, et al. Eosinophilia myalgia syndrome: I. Immunocytochemical evidence for a T-cell-mediated immune effector response. *Ann Neurol* 1991;29: 524–528.
77. Houpt JB, Ogryzlo MA, Hunt M. Tryptophan metabolism in man (with special reference to rheumatoid arthritis and scleroderma). *Semin Arthritis Rheum* 1973;2:333–353.
78. Sternberg EM, van Woert MH, Young SN, et al. Development of a scleroderma-like illness during therapy with L-5-hydroxytryptophan and carbidopa. *N Engl J Med* 1980;303:782–787.
79. Auffranc JC, Berbis P, Fabre JF, et al. Syndrome sclerodermiforme et poikilodermique observe au cours d'un traitement par carbidopa et 5–hydroxy-tryptophanne. *Ann Dermatol Venereol* 1985;112:691–692.
80. Joly P, Lampert A, Thomine E, et al. Development of pseudobullous morphea and scleroderma-like illness during therapy with L-5-hydroxytryptophan and carbidopa. *J Am Acad Dermatol* 1991;25:332–333.
81. Hertzman P, Clauw D, Kaufman L, et al. Status of 205 patients and results of treatment with eosinophilia-myalgia syndrome (EMS) two years after onset. *Ann Intern Med* 1995;22:161–163.
82. Campbell DS, Morris PD, Silver RM. Eosinophilia-myalgia syndrome: a long-term follow-up study. *South Med J* 1995; 88:953–958.
83. Culpepper RC, Williams RG, Mease PJ, et al. Natural history of the eosinophilia-myalgia syndrome. *Ann Intern Med* 1991; 115:437–442.
84. Hedberg K, Urbach D, Slutsker L, et al. Eosinophilia-myalgia syndrome. Natural history in a population-based cohort. *Arch Intern Med* 1992;152:1889–1892.
85. Sullivan EA, Kamb ML, Jones JL, et al. The natural history of eosinophilia-myalgia syndrome in a tryptophan-exposed cohort in South Carolina. *Arch Intern Med* 1996;156:973–979.
86. Kaufman LD, Seidman RJ. L-tryptophan-associated eosinophilia-myalgia syndrome: perspective of a new illness. *Rheum Dis Clin North Am* 1991;17:427–441.
87. Bramwell B. Diffuse sclerdermia: its frequency; its occurrence in stone-masons; its treatment by fibrolysin—elevations of temperature due to fibrolysin injections. *Edinburgh Med J* 1914; 12:387–401.
88. Erasmus LD. Scleroderma in gold-miners on the Witwatersrand with particular reference to pulmonary manifestations. *S Afr J Lab Clin Med* 1957;3:209–231.
89. Rodnan GP, Benedek TG, Medsger Jr TA, et al. The association of progressive systemic sclerosis (scleroderma) with coal miners' pneumoconiosis and other forms of silicosis. *Ann Intern Med* 1967;66:323–334.
90. Sluis-Cremer GK, Hessel P, Nizdo EH, et al. Silica, silicosis, and progressive systemic sclerosis. *Br J Ind Med* 1985;42:838–843.
91. Walsh SJ. Effects of non-mining occupational silica exposure on proportional mortality from silicosis and systemic sclerosis. *J Rheumatol* 1999;26:2179–2185.
92. Haustein UF, Anderegg V. Silica induced scleroderma—clinical and experimental aspects. *J Rheumatol* 1998;25:1917–1926.
93. Gabay C, Kahn M-Fr. Les sclerodermies masculines: role de l'exposition professionnelle. *Schweiz Med Wochenschr* 1992;122: 1746–1752.
94. Haustein U-F, Ziegler V, Herrmann K, et al. Silica-induced scleroderma. *J Am Acad Dermatol* 1990;22:444–448.
95. McHugh NJ, Whyte J, Harvey G, et al. Anti-topoisomerase-1 antibodies are found in the majority of males with silica-associated systemic sclerosis and all inhibit topoisomerase-1 function. *Arthritis Rheum* 1992;35:S67(abst).
96. Spiera RF, Gibofsky A, Spiera H. Silicone gel filled breast implants and connective tissue disease: an overview. *J Rheumatol* 1994;21:239–245.
97. Galb LN. Panel recommendations on silicone gel-filled breast implants follow moratorium. *FDA Med Bull* 1992;22:3.
98. Miyoshi K, Miyaoka T, Kobayashi Y, et al. Hypergamma-globulinemia by prolonged adjuvanticity in man: disorders developed after augmentation mammoplasty. *Ijishimpo* 1964; 2122:9–14.
99. Kumagai Y, Shiokawa Y, Medsger TA Jr, et al. Clinical spectrum of connective tissue disease after cosmetic surgery. Observations on eighteen patients and a review of the Japanese literature. *Arthritis Rheum* 1984;27:1–12.
100. Hochberg MC. Cosmetic surgical procedures and connective tissue disease: the Cleopatra syndrome revisited. *Ann Intern Med* 1993;118:981–983.
101. Hennekens CH, I-Min L, Cook NR, et al. Self-reported breast implants and connective-tissue diseases in female health professionals. A retrospective cohort study. *JAMA* 1996;275: 616–621.
102. Hochberg MC, Perlmutter DL, Medsger TA Jr, et al. Lack of association between augmentation mammoplasty and systemic sclerosis (scleroderma). *Arthritis Rheum* 1996;9:1125–1131.
103. Burns LJ, Laing TJ, Gillespie BW, et al. The epidemiology of scleroderma among women: assessment of risk from exposure to silicone and silica. *J Rheumatol* 1996;23:1904–1911.
104. Kumagai Y, Abe C, Shiokawa Y. Scleroderma after cosmetic surgery. Four cases of human adjuvant disease. *Arthritis Rheum* 1979;22:532–537.
105. Kondo H, Kumagai Y, Shiokawa Y. Scleroderma following cosmetic surgery ("adjuvant disease"): a review of nine cases reported in Japan. In: Black C, Myers AR, eds. *Current topics in rheumatology—systemic sclerosis (scleroderma).* New York: Gower, 1985:135–137.
106. Endo LP, Edwards NL, Longley S, et al. Silicone and rheumatic diseases. *Semin Arthritis Rheum* 1987;17:112–118.
107. Brozena SJ, Fenske NA, Cruse CW, et al. Human adjuvant disease following augmentation mammoplasty. *Arch Dermatol* 1988;124:1383–1386.

108. Spiera H. Scleroderma after silicone augmentation mammoplasty. *JAMA* 1988;260:236–238.
109. Varga J, Schumacher R, Jimenez SA. Systemic sclerosis after augmentation mammoplasty with silicone implants. *Ann Intern Med* 1989;111:377–383.
110. Marik PE, Kark AL, Zambakides A. Scleroderma after silicone augmentation mammoplasty. A report of 2 cases. *S Afr Med J* 1990;77:212–213.
111. Spiera H, Kerr LD. Scleroderma following silicone implantation: a cumulative experience of 11 cases. *J Rheumatol* 1993;20: 958–961.
112. Sahn EE, Garen PD, Silver RM, et al. Scleroderma following augmentation mammoplasty. Report of a case and review of the literature. *Arch Dermatol* 1990;126:1198–1202.
113. Lazar AP, Lazar P. Localized morphea after silicone gel breast implantation: more evidence for a cause and effect relationship. *Arch Dermatol* 1991;127:263.
114. Gutierrez V, Espinoza LR. Progressive systemic sclerosis complicated by severe hypertension: reversal after silicone implant removal. *Am J Med* 1990;89:390–392.
115. Hitoshi S, Ito Y, Takehara K, et al. A case of malignant hypertension and scleroderma after cosmetic surgery. *Jpn J Med* 1991; 30:97–100.
116. Levine JJ, Ilowite NT. Scleroderma-like esophageal disease in children breast-fed by mothers with silicone breast implants. *JAMA* 1994;271:213–216.
117. Liau M, Ito S, Koren G. Letter to the editor. *JAMA* 1994;272: 769.
118. Flick AJ. Silicone implants and esophageal dysmotility: are breast-fed infants at risk? *JAMA* 1994;271:240–241.
119. Cuellar ML, Scopelitis E, Tenenbaum SA, et al. Serum ANA in women with silicone breast implants. *J Rheumatol* 1995;22: 236–240.
120. Bridges AJ, Conley C, Wang G, et al. A clinical and immunologic evaluation of women with silicone breast implants and symptoms of rheumatic disease. *Ann Intern Med* 1993;118: 929–936.
121. Press RI, Peebles CL, Kumagai Y, et al. Antinuclear autoantibodies in women with silicone breast implants. *Lancet* 1992; 340:1304–1307.
122. Silver RM, Sahn EE, Allen JA, et al. Demonstration of silicon in sites of connective tissue disease in patients with silicone-gel breast implants. *Arch Dermatol* 1993;129:63–68.
123. Greene WB, Raso DS, Walsh LG, et al. Electron probe microanalysis of silicone and the role of the macrophages in proximal "capsule" and distant site migration in post-mammoplasty patients. *Plast Reconst Surg* 1995;95:513–519.
124. Ballantyne DL, Rees TD, Seidman I. Silicone fluid: response to massive subcutaneous injections of dimethylpolysulfoxone fluid in animals. *Plast Reconst Surg* 1965;36:629–631.
125. Heggers JP, Kossofsky N, Parsons RW, et al. Biocompatibility of silicone implants. *Ann Plast Surg* 1983;11:38–41.
126. Lugano EM, Dauber JH, Elias JA, et al. The regulation of lung fibroblast proliferation by alveolar macrophages in experimental silicosis. *Am Rev Respir Dis* 1984;129:767–771.
127. Dauber JH, Rossman MD, Pietra GG, et al. Experimental silicosis: morphologic and biochemical abnormalities produced by instillation of quartz into guinea pig lungs. *Am J Pathol* 1980; 101:595–612.
128. Straniero NR, Furst DE. Environmentally-induced systemic sclerosis-like illness. *Baillieres Clin Rheum* 1989;3:63–79.
129. Lelbach WK, Marsteller HJ. Vinyl chloride-associated disease. *Ergeb Inn Med Kinderheilkd* 1981;47:1–110.
130. Kubota J. Occupational diseases in synthetic resin and fibre industries (Japanese text). *J Sci Labour* 1957;33:1–22.
131. Maricq HR, Johnson MN, Whetstone CL, et al. Capillary abnormalities in polyvinyl chloride production workers. Examination by in vivo microscopy. *JAMA* 1976;236:1368–1371.
132. Wilson RH, McCormick WE, Tatum CF, et al. Occupational acroosteolysis. Report of 31 cases. *JAMA* 1967;201:577–581.
133. Black CM, Walker AE, Catoggio LJ, et al. Genetic susceptibility to scleroderma-like syndrome induced by vinyl chloride. *Lancet* 1983;1:53–55.
134. Black C, Pereira S, McWhirter A, et al. Genetic susceptibility to scleroderma-like syndrome in symptomatic and asymptomatic workers exposed to vinyl chloride. *J Rheumatol* 1986;13: 1059–1062.
135. Veltman G, Lange CE, Juhe S, et al. Clinical manifestations and course of vinyl chloride disease. *Ann NY Acad Sci* 1975;246:6–17.
136. Jayson MIV, Bailey AJ, Black C, et al. Collagen studies in acroosteolysis. *Proc R Soc Med* 1976;69:295–297.
137. Reinl W. Scleroderma caused by trichloroethylene? *Bull Hyg* 1957;32:678–679.
138. Owens GR, Medsger TA Jr. Systemic sclerosis secondary to occupational exposure. *Am J Med* 1988;85:114–116.
139. Nietert PJ, Sutherland SE, Silver RM, et al. Is occupational organic solvent exposure a risk factor for scleroderma? *Arthritis Rheum* 1998;41:1111–1118.
140. Nietert PJ, Sutherland SE, Silver RM, et al. Solvent oriented hobbies and the risk of systemic sclerosis. *J Rheumatol* 1999;26: 2369–2372.
141. Yamakage A, Ishikawa H, Saito Y, et al. Occupational scleroderma-like disorder occurring in men engaged in the polymerization of epoxy resins. *Dermatologica* 1980;161:33–44.
142. Dupont E, Olivarius B, Strong MJ. Bromocriptine-induced collagenosis-like symptomatology in Parkinson's disease. *Lancet* 1982;1:850–851.
143. Leshin B, Piette WW, Caplan RM. Morphea after bromocriptine therapy. *Int J Dermatol* 1989;28:177–179.
144. Tomlinson IW, Jayson MIV. Systemic sclerosis after therapy with appetite suppressants. *J Rheumatol* 1984;11:254.
145. Aeschlimann A, de Truchis P, Kahn MF. Scleroderma after therapy with appetite suppressants. Report of four cases. *Scand J Rheumatol* 1990;19:87–90.
146. Zarafonetis CJD, Lorber SH, Hanson SM. Association of functioning carcinoid syndrome and scleroderma. I. Case report. *Am J Med Sci* 1958;236:1–14.
147. Fries JF, Lindgren, JA, Bull JM. Scleroderma-like lesions and the carcinoid syndrome. *Arch Intern Med* 1973;131:550–553.
148. Graham JR, Suby HI, LeCompte PR, et al. Fibrotic disorders associated with methysergide therapy for headaches. *N Engl J Med* 1966;274:359–368.
149. Follath F, Burkart F, Schweizer W. Drug-induced pulmonary hypertension? *Br Med J* 1971;1:265–266.
150. Douglas JG, Munro JF, Kitchin AH, et al. Pulmonary hypertension and fenfluramine. *Br Med J* 1981;283:881–883.
151. Cohen IS, Mosher MB, O'Keefe EJ, et al. Cutaneous toxicity of bleomycin therapy. *Arch Dermatol* 1973;107:553–555.
152. Finch WR, Rodnan GP, Buckingham RB, et al. Bleomycin-induced scleroderma. *J Rheumatol* 1980;7:651–659.
153. Kerr LD, Spiera H. Scleroderma in association with the use of bleomycin. A report of 3 cases. *J Rheumatol* 1992;19:294–296.
154. Mountz JD, Downs Minor MB, Turner R, et al. Bleomycin-induced cutaneous toxicity in the rat: analysis of histopathology and ultrastructure compared with progressive systemic sclerosis. *Br J Dermatol* 1983;108:679–686.
155. Fasske E, Morgenroth K. Experimental bleomycin lung in mice. A contribution to the pathogenesis of pulmonary fibrosis. *Lung* 1983;161:133–146.
156. Vogelzang NJ, Bosl GJ, Johnson K, et al. Raynaud's phenomenon: a common toxicity after combination chemotherapy for testicular cancer. *Ann Intern Med* 1981;95:288–292.

157. Smith EA, Harper FE, LeRoy EC. Raynaud's phenomenon of a single digit following local intradermal bleomycin sulfate injection. *Arthritis Rheum* 1985;28:459–461.
158. Hertzman A, Toone E, Resnik CS. Pentazocine induced myocutaneous sclerosis. *J Rheumatol* 1986;13:210–214.
159. Furner BB. Parenteral pentazocine: cutaneous complications revisited. *J Am Acad Dermatol* 1990;22:694–695.
160. Palestine RF, Millns JL, Spigel GT, et al. Skin manifestations of pentazocine abuse. *J Am Acad Dermatol* 1980;2:47–55.
161. Peterson LS, Nelson AM, Su WP, et al. The epidemiology of morphea (localized scleroderma) in Olmstedt County 1960–1993. *J Rheumatol* 1997;24:73–80.
162. Falanga V, Medsger TA Jr. Frequency, levels, and significance of blood eosinophilia in systemic sclerosis, localized scleroderma, and eosinophilic fasciitis. *J Am Acad Dermatol* 1987;17:648–656.
163. Maricq HR. Nailfold capillary abnormalities in patients with connective tissue diseases. In: Manabe H, Zweifach BW, Messmer K, eds. *Microcirculation in circulatory disorders.* New York: Springer-Verlag, 1988:389–394.
164. Buechner SA, Winkelmann RK, Lautenschlager S, et al. Localized scleroderma associated with Borrelia burgdorferi infection: Clinical, histologic, and immunohistochemical observations. *J Am Acad Dermatol* 1993;29:190–196.
165. Wienecke R, Schlüpen E-M, Zöchling N, et al. No evidence for *burgdorferi*-specific DNA in lesions of localized scleroderma. *J Invest Dermatol* 1995;104:23–26.
166. Tuffanelli DL. Do some patients with morphea and lichen sclerosis et atrophicans have a *Borrelia* infection? *Am J Dermatopathol* 1987;9:371–373.
167. Joly P, Bamberger N, Crickx B, et al. Treatment of severe forms of localized scleroderma with oral corticosteroids: Follow up study on 17 patients. *Arch Dermatol* 1994;130:663–664.
168. Hulshof MM, Pavel S, Breedveld FC, et al. Oral calcitriol as a new therapeutic modality for generalized morphea. *Arch Dermatol* 1994;130:1290–1293.
169. Falanga V, Medsger TA. D-penicillamine in the treatment of localized scleroderma. *Arch Dermatol* 1990;126:609–612.
170. Peter RU, Ruzicka T, Eckert F. Low-dose cyclosporine in the treatment of disabling morphea. *Arch Dermatol* 1991;127: 1420–1421.
171. Wach F, Ullrich H, Schmitz G, et al. Treatment of severe localized scleroderma by plasmapheresis: report of three cases. *Br J Dermatol* 1995;133:605–609.
172. Stege H, Berneburg M, Humke S, et al. High-dose UVA radiation therapy for localized scleroderma. *J Am Acad Dermatol* 1997;36:938–944.
173. Kerscher M, Meurer M, Sander C, et al. PUVA bath photochemotherapy for localized scleroderma. *Arch Dermatol* 1996; 132:1280–1282.
174. Kanekura T, Fukumaru S, Matsushita S, et al. Successful treatment of scleroderma with PUVA therapy. *J Dermatol* 1996; 23:455–459.
175. Brik R, Berant M, Vardi P. The scleroderma-like syndrome of insulin-dependent diabetes mellitus. *Diabetes Metab Rev* 1991; 7:121–128.
176. Angeli-Besson C, Koeppel MC, Jacquet P, et al. Electron-beam therapy in scleredema adultorum with associated monoclonal hypergammaglobulinaemia. *Br J Dermatol* 1994;130:394–397.
177. Gabriel SE, Perry HO, Oleson GB, et al. Scleromyxedema: a scleroderma-like disorder with systemic manifestations. *Medicine* 1988;67:58–65.
178. Rocco VK, Hurd ER. Scleroderma and scleroderma-like disorders. *Semin Arthritis Rheum* 1986;16:22–69.
179. Furst DE, Clements PJ, Graze P, et al. A syndrome resembling progressive systemic sclerosis after bone marrow transplantation. A model for scleroderma? *Arthritis Rheum* 1979;22: 904–910.
180. Wick MR, Moore SB, Gastineau DA, et al. Immunologic, clinical, and pathologic aspects of human graft-versus-host disease. *Mayo Clin Proc* 1983;58:603–612.
181. Janin A, Socie G, Devergie A, et al. Fasciitis in chronic graft-versus-host disease. A clinicopathologic study in 14 cases. *Ann Intern Med* 1994;120:993–998.
182. Bell SA, Faust H, Mittermuller J, et al. Specificity of antinuclear antibodies in scleroderma-like chronic graft-versus-host disease. *Br J Dermatol* 1996;134:848–854.
183. Jaffee BD, Claman HN. Chronic graft-versus-host disease (GVHD) as a model for scleroderma. I. Description of model systems. *Cell Immunol* 1983;77:1–12.
184. Bos GMJ, Majoor GD, Willighagen RGJ, et al. Chronic cyclosporine-induced autoimmune disease in the rat: a new experimental model for scleroderma. *J Invest Dermatol* 1989;93: 610–615.
185. Bos GMJ, Majoor GD, van de Gaar MJ, et al. T-Helper lymphocytes and syngeneic graft-versus-host disease. *Transplant Proc* 1989;21:3016–3017.
186. Bos G, Majoor G, Slaaf D, et al. In vivo demonstration of microvascular pathology by intravital microscopy in experimental chronic graft-versus-host disease: analogy with scleroderma. *J Rheumatol* 1988;15:1339–1345.
187. Schiltz PM, Giorno RC, Claman HN. Increased ICAM-1 expression in the early stages of murine chronic graft-versus-host disease. *Clin Immunol Immunopathol* 1994;71:136–141.
188. Nelson JL, Furst DE, Maloney S, et al. Microchimerism and HLA-compatible relationships of pregnancy in scleroderma. *Lancet* 1998;351:559–562.
189. Siadak M, Sullivan KM. The management of chronic graft-versus-host disease. *Blood Rev* 1994;8:154–160.

81

PATHOGENESIS OF SYSTEMIC SCLEROSIS

JOSEPH H. KORN

The clinical expression of systemic sclerosis (SSc) is the result of an interplay among at least three pathogenetic processes: immune activation, vascular injury and obliteration, and fibroblast activation with synthesis of increased extracellular matrix components. The precise way in which these processes interact is unclear, but considerable knowledge has been gained regarding the cellular and molecular basis for each. Also unclear is the etiology of the disease, i.e., the events that initiate immune cell activation, vascular pathology, and fibrosis. It would appear, from the evidence discussed below, that in an individual with the right (or wrong) genetic background, infectious or other environmental agents might trigger the expression of the scleroderma phenotype.

GENETIC AND ENVIRONMENTAL FACTORS

Genetic Factors

Although families with multiple cases of SSc have been described (1,2), familial occurrence is unusual. Approximately 1% of individuals with SSc will have a first-degree relative with the disease (3,4). However, the clustering of multiple autoimmune diseases, including SSc, systemic lupus erythematosus, and rheumatoid arthritis (RA), in the same family is more frequently seen. Approximately 5% of patients will have a first-degree relative with an autoimmune disease, such as RA, systemic lupus erythematosus, or autoimmune myositis (3–5). This would suggest that there is a genetic predisposition to autoimmune disease but that genetic factors may not be sufficient to determine the outcome. Other influences, genetic and/or environmental, affect whether a disease will be expressed and what the pattern of expression will be, i.e. what particular disease entity, if any, will be observed. This interpretation is supported by the results of family and twin studies. Family members of patients with SSc are much more likely to have antinuclear antibodies than healthy controls (6,7). In genetic studies of families with multiple cases of SSc, there is disease linkage to human leukocyte antigen (HLA), but possession of the disease-linked HLA type is not sufficient for disease expression (8). In monozygotic twins where one has SSc, there is 100% concordance for autoantibodies. Nonetheless, concordance for the disease is only 6%, a rate comparable to that in dizygotic twins (5,9).

Studies by Arnett and co-workers (10) provide even stronger evidence for a role of genetics in the pathogenesis of SSc. They found a very high incidence of SSc in the Chocktaw Indian tribe in Oklahoma; the rate of SSc in the Choctaws was at least 20-fold greater than in the general population. The tribe originated in Mississippi and migrated to Oklahoma in the early 1800s; the prevalence of scleroderma is not increased in Mississippi Choctaws, suggesting a "founder" gene effect. The clinical picture is remarkably homogeneous in affected individuals: almost all have diffuse skin disease, interstitial lung involvement, and antibodies to topoisomerase I. The HLA haplotype DQ7, DR2 (DRB1 1602) is strongly associated with antitopoisomerase antibodies and disease (11). However, the prevalence of autoantibodies is far higher than the prevalence of the disease. Further genetic studies have shown a highly significant linkage of SSc in Chocktaws to chromosome markers very close to the fibrillin 15 gene (12). Not all individuals carrying the "marker" had SSc nor did all affected individuals carry the chromosomal marker, suggesting that other genes or factors were involved. An actual role for fibrillin is suggested by studies in the tight skin (Tsk) mouse, a model for scleroderma. In the Tsk mouse, thickened and tight skin is inherited as an autosomal-dominant trait. A mutation in the fibrillin gene results in duplication of a portion of the gene and is presumed responsible for the tight skin phenotype (13). It is hypothesized that the abnormal fibrillin may "bind" increased amounts of growth factors, particularly transforming growth factor-β (TGF-β) or that the abnormal protein may lead to formation of an abnormal extracellular matrix scaffold that signals inappropriately to the fibroblast.

Environmental Factors

Infectious Agents

As already noted, the low twin concordance for SSc and low familial association indicate that genetic factors alone cannot entirely explain disease expression. Although autoimmunity, in the form of autoantibodies, is more strongly linked to genetic factors, environmental factors also appear to be important. Spouses of patients with SSc have an increased incidence of autoantibodies compared to controls (2,7). Both infectious and chemical triggers have been hypothesized to play a role. Viral or other infections could alter self antigens or, by causing tissue damage or immune cell activation, engender an inflammatory and immune response. It has been suggested that latent viral infection might accelerate or promote disease expression in the susceptible host. Cytomegalovirus (CMV) can, by its effects on endothelial cells, fibroblasts, and immune cells, affect the vascular, fibrotic, and immunologic features of the disease (14). Thus, CMV infection of endothelial cells can lead to subsequent immune-mediated injury, and CMV can inhibit normal immune responses and promote fibrosis by stimulating TGF-β production (14).

A role for a possible viral trigger for SSc is also suggested by the studies of Maul and co-workers (15), who showed that there was a shared epitope (i.e., a similarity in protein sequence), between topoisomerase 1 and certain retroviruses that serve as tumor viruses in animals. The anti-topoisomerase response seen in SSc might really represent reactivity to viral antigens, suggesting prior infection with retroviruses, and might not play a direct pathogenetic role. Alternatively, shared antigens between virally encoded and host proteins, what has been called molecular mimicry, might result in an immune response to the infectious agent that cross-reacts with host proteins and thus becomes an autoimmune response. Such an event might occur only in a genetically susceptible host, a host unable to eliminate a particular virus, or one tilted to a particular kind of immune response. These explanations are supported by studies that show an association between certain HLA genes and antitopoisomerase antibodies as well as an association of HLA with other autoantibodies in SSc, including antifibrillarin and anti-RNA polymerase (16,17).

Noninfectious Environmental Factors

A number of environmental agents have been implicated in the etiology of SSc either based on case clustering or on formal epidemiologic studies. One of the earliest observations was the presence of a high number of cases of SSc in stonemasons (18). Similar "clustering" was noted among gold miners in South Africa and coal miners in the United States, suggesting that exposure to silica dust might be playing a role in disease pathogenesis in these individuals (19,20). However, later case-control epidemiologic studies, one in the United Kingdom and one in Michigan, have not supported an association of SSc with silica exposure (21,22). The occupations noted above also have in common the use of vibrating instruments that have been shown to be associated with Raynaud's phenomenon and even sclerodactyly (23). As silica exposure may cause interstitial lung disease (silicosis), the possibility exists that some of the patients identified as having scleroderma may have had a fortuitous confluence of two entities. Silicone, a polymer of dimethyl siloxane, is used as a lubricant in medical devices and prosthetics and, most famously, in breast implants. Although there have been claims that breast implants have led to the development of SSc, several good epidemiologic studies, including case-control studies, have uniformly failed to support a causal relationship (22,24–27). A relationship of scleroderma-like syndromes to toxic exposures to environmental agents appears fairly convincing. In most cases, the epidemic nature of the illness, or the proximity of exposure to symptom onset, is clearly indicative of a cause-and-effect relationship.

The development of scleroderma-like disease among workers exposed to vinyl chloride monomer was appreciated as unusual in frequency because of the predominantly male population and the coincident discovery of hepatic angiosarcomas, a rare tumor, in this population (28). The exposure occurs in the manufacturing process of vinyl chloride polymer and not in connection with any finished product. Affected individuals had vascular features of scleroderma such as Raynaud's, telangiectasia, and nailfold capillary changes, but not characteristic skin changes. A scleroderma-like syndrome also was seen in an acute epidemic associated with ingestion of contaminated rapeseed oil. The clinical picture, called toxic oil syndrome, was characterized by acute myalgia, fever, neuropathy, scleroderma-like skin disease, and pulmonary hypertension (29). A third convincing toxic exposure was the development of eosinophilia myalgia syndrome with fasciitis and dermal induration in individuals consuming the nutritional supplement L-tryptophan (30,31). The syndrome was clinically similar to the toxic oil syndrome described above. Development of the syndrome appears related to the ingestion of 1,1′-ethylidenebis(L-tryptophan), a contaminant in some batches of L-tryptophan produced by bacterial fermentation (32). However, an association of eosinophilic fasciitis with L-tryptophan produced by other means, and presumably without the suspect contaminant, had been reported much earlier and may be related to abnormalities of tryptophan metabolism in affected individuals. All three syndromes described are "scleroderma-like" in that Raynaud's is generally absent as is the characteristic gastrointestinal pathology, including esophageal hypomotility. In addition, the pattern of skin involvement differs, being more truncal in distribution and sparing the hands.

Convincing evidence linking typical SSc to other chemical exposures is lacking. Scattered reports have linked SSc to certain industrial solvents. Trichloroethane (TCA), trichloroethylene (TCE), toluene, and xylene are among those most often cited. Interestingly, trichloroethylene has a similar structure to vinyl chloride. A recent epidemiologic study found an association between exposure to petroleum distillates and development of undifferentiated connective tissue disease (33). Implicated compounds included hydrocarbons such as paint thinners and benzene and chlorinated solvents such as TCA and TCE. Odds ratios for exposed versus unexposed individuals were small but statistically significant, generally indicating a twofold increase in risk.

Several drugs have been implicated in the genesis of scleroderma-like syndromes. The antitumor agent bleomycin induces pulmonary fibrosis in animal models, and several cases of scleroderma with Raynaud's syndrome have been reported to occur in patients undergoing cancer chemotherapy (34). The mechanism of bleomycin toxicity is unclear, but bleomycin is known to cause acute tissue damage as well as chromosome breaks in exposed cells (35). In separate studies, scleroderma patients have been shown to have an abnormally high frequency of chromosome breaks, an abnormality shared by unaffected family members (36,37). Chromosome breaks may occur in response to oxidative stress, and such oxidative stress may also preferentially lead to formation and release of unique autoantigens in scleroderma (38,39). Thus, genetic and environmental factors may interact through overlapping pathways to initiate or perpetuate pathogenetic processes in SSc.

It thus appears that genetic factors, infectious agents, and environmental toxins or other exposures might interplay to initiate and perpetuate the pathogenesis of scleroderma. The broad and varied clinical spectrum may reflect the wide range of initiating events and multiple genes that may be important in modulating disease expression.

IMMUNE CELL FUNCTION IN SYSTEMIC SCLEROSIS

Multiple findings suggest that the immune system and its activation play a central role in pathogenesis of SSc (Table 81.1). The clinical association of SSc with other autoimmune diseases in both families and individuals suggests that genetic factors are present that predispose to autoimmune disease. Early studies have demonstrated the presence of autoantibodies in patients with SSc, often with unique patterns on immunofluorescence and characteristic antigenic specificities (reviewed in refs. 40 and 41). This includes antibodies to topoisomerase I seen predominantly in diffuse cutaneous SSc and antibodies to centromeric proteins seen predominantly in limited cutaneous SSc. Autoantibody formation, in particular, is strongly linked to the major human histocompatibility locus (HLA), particularly HLA-DQ, suggesting a relationship to immune response genes. However, although autoantibodies provide some useful diagnostic and prognostic information in SSc, there is a paucity of evidence that autoantibodies per se play a pathogenetic role. In contrast, considerable evidence has accumulated showing that T cells are activated in SSc and that T cells, macrophages, and their secreted products play an important role in pathogenesis.

TABLE 81.1. EVIDENCE FOR IMMUNE SYSTEM INVOLVEMENT IN PATHOGENESIS OF SYSTEMIC SCLEROSIS (SSC)

T-cell infiltrates in skin
Inflammatory interstitial lung disease
T-cell infiltrates
T cells in bronchoalveolar lavage fluid
Circulating cytokines, CD4, IL-2R
Autoantibodies
Linkage to HLA
Family members with other autoimmune diseases
Overlapping syndromes with systemic lupus erythematosus, dermatomyositis
Similarity to GVHD

HLA, human leukocyte antigen; IL-2R: interleukin-2 receptor; GVDH:graft-versus-host disease.

Evidence of Mononuclear Cell Activation

The study of organ pathology in SSc places immune cells at sites of connective tissue activation and clinical fibrosis, particularly in the skin and lungs. Dermal infiltrates of mononuclear cells are sometimes quite prominent and often found in a perivascular distribution (Fig. 81.1). Infiltrates are most common in early disease and are also seen in localized scleroderma or morphea. Direct study of infiltrating lymphocytes shows evidence of T-cell activation with expression of DR antigens. In the blood, increased levels of interleukin-2 (IL-2), interferon-γ, and IL-4, and the T cell surface molecules IL-2 receptor (IL-2R) and CD4 and CD8 are seen (42,43). In addition, there are increased levels of IL-1, tumor necrosis factor-α (TNF-α), and IL-6, indicating monocyte recruitment and activation.

The initiating events for T-cell activation have not been established. The resemblance of graft-versus-host disease to SSc (44), in both its cutaneous and vascular features, raises the possibility that SSc reflects an immune response to self antigens. Recent studies of "microchimerism" in SSc lend support to this hypothesis. A chimera possesses two separate cell lineages. For example, the recipient of a bone marrow graft has cells of both host and donor origin. Studies have shown that women who have been pregnant and given birth to sons have, in their circulation, immune cells containing Y chromosomes (45) suggesting a fetal origin. Using HLA typing, it has been established that these cells are of fetal origin, i.e., the HLA type matches the son's. Using similar typing, it is clear that cells from daughters also circulate in the mother. Furthermore, fetal cells circulate for periods as

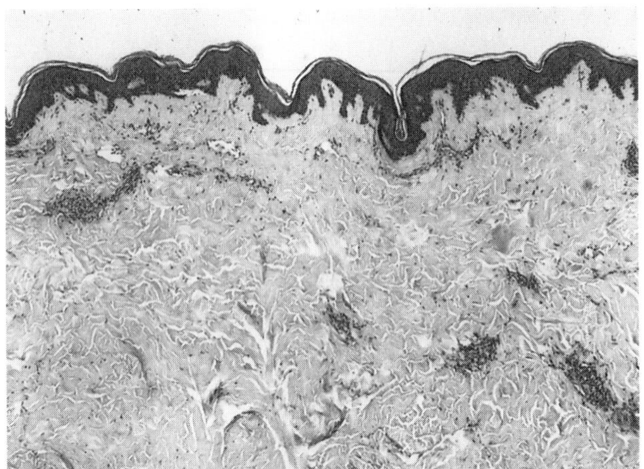

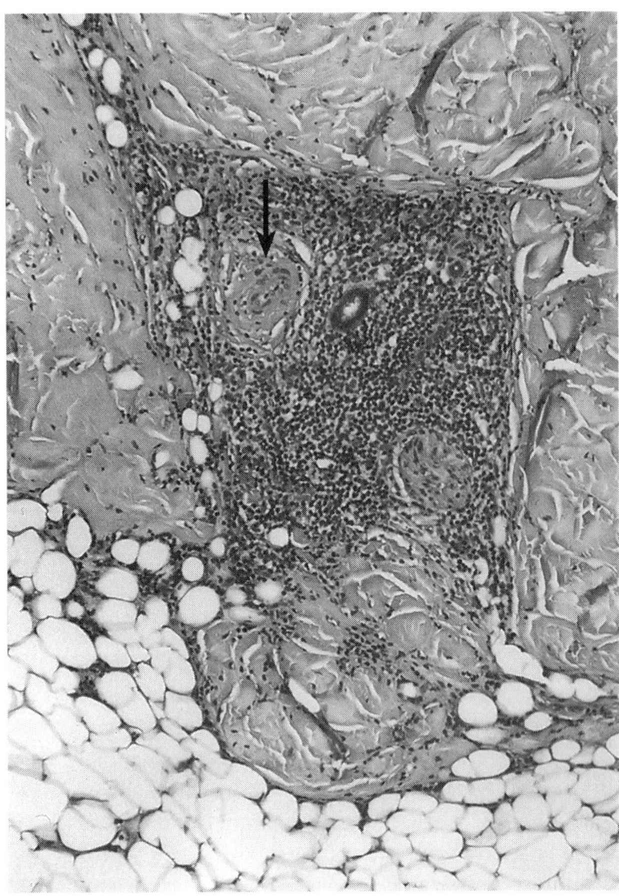

FIGURE 81.1. **A:** Mononuclear cell infiltrates in the skin of a patient with localized scleroderma. The infiltrates are predominantly, but not exclusively, perivascular. There is marked thickening of the dermis. (H&E; 40× original magnification.) **B:** High-power view of lymphoid and monocytic infiltrate in the same patient. The infiltrate is in the deep dermis and extends into the loose fatty tissue. An occluded vessel is present in the midst of the lesion *(arrow)*. (H&E; 40× original magnification.)

long as 20 years after a pregnancy. Conversely, maternal cells are found in the circulation of children well after birth (46). Much higher numbers of fetal cells are found in the circulation of women with SSc than in normal individuals; moreover, cells of fetal origin may be found in tissue sites such as the skin (47,48). In SSc female patients, compared to controls, a higher incidence of materno-child histocompatibility was found; that is, HLA of scleroderma female patients was more likely to match the paternal HLA carried by their children than observed in controls (47,49). This match might lead to longer persistence of fetal cells as the mother is less able to "reject" them.

How might microchimerism lead to autoimmune disease? First, fetal cells might generate a graft-versus-host response directed against unique maternal antigens; however, the small number of cells present and the "naive" nature of the transferred cells make this unlikely. Alternatively, the mother might mount an immune response to the graft, a response that is weak and may ultimately become self-directed (i.e., autoimmune). Indeed, chronic graft-versus-host disease resembling SSc is elicited by transfer of immune cells that are a good match at major histocompatibility loci but a mismatch at minor loci (44).

The particular antigenic targets for ongoing T-cell reactivity are not established. T-cell reactivity to epitopes on topoisomerase I has been demonstrated (50), but its role in disease pathogenesis is unclear. It has been suggested that particular nuclear autoantigens are generated in response to oxidative injury and apoptosis (39). Reactivity to such antigens might be responsible for ongoing immune stimulation. The genetic background may determine the nature and breadth of immune responses generated. During the course of the disease, other neoantigens are likely generated that engender new and specific immune responses. For example, pulmonary bronchoalveolar lavage yields γ/δ T cells that show clonality based on T-cell receptor analysis (51). The clonality suggests expansion of a T-cell subset in response to a particular antigenic stimulus; the antigens to which these T cells are reactive are as yet unknown.

ENDOTHELIAL CELL ALTERATIONS IN SYSTEMIC SCLEROSIS

Vascular abnormalities are the most common initial manifestations of SSc, which suggests an early role in pathogenesis. The earliest vascular abnormalities are functional, with increased and abnormal reactivity to cold (i.e., Raynaud's phenomenon). The abnormal vascular reactivity is not only cutaneous but also visceral, since renal vessels have also been shown to constrict in response to cold exposure (52). What begins as a functional abnormality becomes structural; vessels in multiple tissues show vascular obliteration with proliferation of intimal endothelial cells and smooth muscle cells and matrix deposition, as well as perivascular fibrosis or "cuffing" (Figs. 81.2 and 81.3). The vascular obliteration leads to tissue ischemia and damage. Cutaneous ulcers and infarcts, renal disease, cardiomyopathy, and intestinal hypomotility (with ischemic damage to myenteric plexuses) are all manifestations of vascular scleroderma.

Biochemical and pathologic investigations suggest that endothelial cell injury is the initial event leading to impaired vascular function. Circulating plasma levels of factor VIII/von Willebrand factor are elevated in the large majority of SSc patients (53); factor VIII/von Willebrand factor is released by endothelial cells in experimental models of injury. Angiotensin-converting enzyme, also released by endothelial cells, is similarly increased. Ultrastructural studies show early evidence of endothelial injury; in SSc lung disease, such injury precedes fibrotic events (54–56). The intimal changes seen on light microscopy, with cellular proliferation and fibrosis, resemble those seen in experimental mechanical injury or immunologic injury in graft-versus-host disease. They differ in this regard from the necrotizing vasculitis seen in immune complex diseases and other vasculitides.

The precise causes of endothelial cell injury are unclear. Possibilities include immune complex injury, antibody-mediated injury, cell-mediated cytotoxicity, and infectious or nonimmune toxic factors. Circulating immune complexes have been reported in a minority of SSc patients but immune complex deposition in the vessel walls is not a feature of the disease. Similarly, evidence of local binding of antibody to endothelial cells that might mediate cytotoxicity is lacking. Although perivascular immune cell infiltration is seen, this may be part of the process of immune localization rather than immune responses to endothelial or other vascular antigens. Cellular immunity to laminin, a basement membrane component, has been reported, as have antibodies to endothelial cells and basement membrane proteins (57); however, their pathogenetic role is unclear and they may well arise consequent to vascular injury. As noted earlier, viral infection has been suggested as a potential early event that renders endothelial cells in SSc susceptible to later injury (14). A possible mediator of such injury includes an endothelial cytotoxic factor described in the serum of a large number of scleroderma patients (58). Although not definitively explained, the toxicity could be secondary to granzyme A, a T-cell serine protease, other T-cell products, and/or lipid oxidation products (59–61). Granzyme A levels are increased in the serum of SSc patients (60). Activated T cells may bind to adhesion molecules on endothelial cells, release granzyme A, and cause or propagate endothelial injury. T-cell–mediated cytotoxicity could also result from induction of endothelial cell apoptosis by interaction of T-cell surface Fas ligand (FasL) with Fas on the endothelial cell surface. Once injury begins and there is tissue ischemia, hypoxia and reperfusion can lead to release of free radicals that promote further injury and tissue damage. Once injured, endothelial cells express higher levels of adhesion molecules, promoting increased immune cell adhesion and localization.

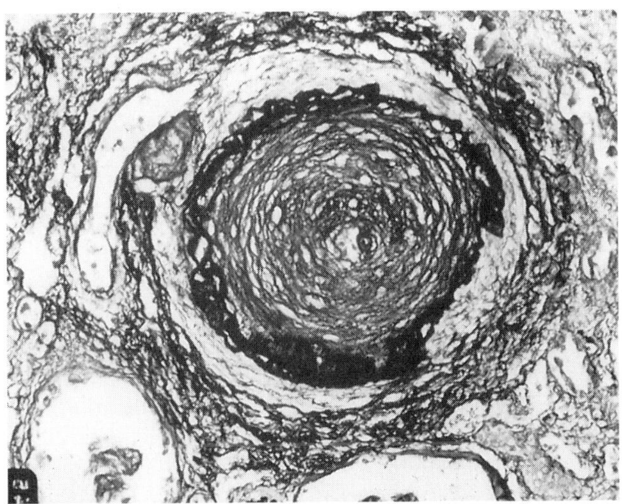

FIGURE 81.2. Vascular obliteration in the kidney in systemic sclerosis (SSc). There is intimal occlusion of the vessel with deposition of matrix components. The media of the vessel are thinned and there is a perivascular cuff of connective tissue that is characteristic of SSc and differs from the lesion of malignant hypertension. (Trichrome stain; 400× original magnification.)

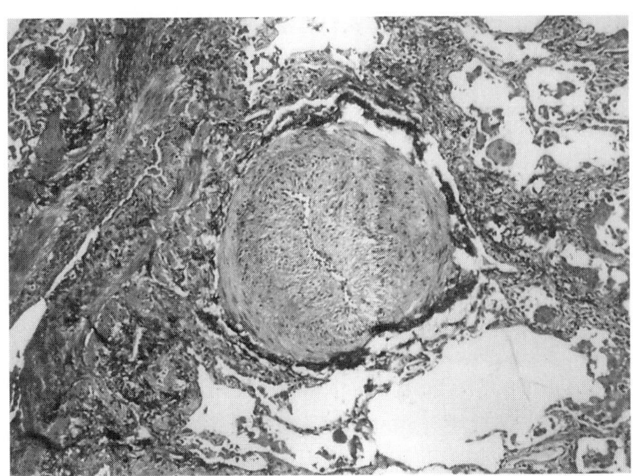

FIGURE 81.3. Vascular obliteration in a pulmonary vessel of a patient with interstitial lung disease. There is intimal thickening with both cellular proliferation and matrix deposition. The vessel lumen is nearly completely occluded. A perivascular cuff of connective tissue is present. (Trichrome stain; 400× original magnification.) (Courtesy of Dr. James D. Faix, Beth Israel Deaconess Medical Center, Boston.)

FIBROBLAST ACTIVATION AND MATRIX DEPOSITION

Fibrosis is the culmination of multiple immune, vascular, and biochemical processes in the skin and visceral organs in SSc. Fibrosis, once fully developed, leads to organ dysfunction not only by its constrictive effect (e.g., cutaneous or pulmonary fibrosis) but also by replacement of cellular components of tissue and of normal tissue architecture. Thus, lung fibrosis can lead to remodeling of alveolar architecture to an extent that even reversal of fibrosis cannot restore normal function (Fig. 81.4). In the gastrointestinal tract, replacement of smooth muscle in the submucosa leads to irreversible loss of motility. Although the exact relationship of immune and vascular events to pathologic fibrosis is unclear, it is evident that they play a critical role. Understanding the early and continuing processes promoting tissue fibrosis is critical to prevention and management strategies in the disease.

Examination of skin and other fibrotic tissues in SSc demonstrates markedly increased accumulation of extracellular matrix without much increase in fibroblast number. Type I collagen, composed of two α_1(I) chains and one α_2(I) chain, is the most abundant extracellular matrix protein in skin and in fibrotic tissues in general, and regulation of its metabolism has been the most extensively studied. Discussions of increased matrix metabolism in SSc have focused on increased deposition of type I collagen, although other matrix proteins, including other collagens, fibronectin, and glycosaminoglycans, are similarly increased (62). Except in situations of regeneration and repair, in normal individuals, collagen synthesis and degradation proceed at a low rate and are in balance. Excess deposition of connective tissue could result from disturbance of either process—biosynthesis or degradation. Although there is some evidence in SSc for decreased activity of collagenase, i.e., the enzyme that initiates collagen degradation, the preponderance of evidence suggests that the principal defect is increased de novo synthesis of collagen and other matrix components. The phenotype of increased matrix biosynthesis could be an abnormality intrinsic to the fibroblast (i.e., an inherent metabolic defect), or due to fibroblast activation resulting from modulatory factors in the fibroblast microenvironment. Included among these would be factors released by immune and vascular cells, alterations in oxygen tension, and changes in the interstitial matrix per se that regulate fibroblast behavior by interactions with fibroblast cell surface integrins (Table 81.2).

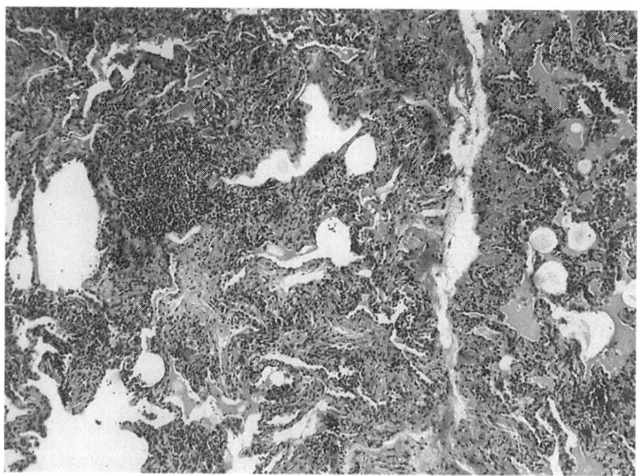

FIGURE 81.4. Interstitial lung disease in a patient with SSc. There is an extensive inflammatory cell infiltrate, interstitial cell proliferation, and matrix deposition. The entire pulmonary architecture is destroyed. (H&E; 100× original magnification.)

TABLE 81.2. FIBROBLAST ACTIVATION IN SSC

Exogenous Factors	Intrinsic Factors
Immune cell activation	Increased sensitivity to cytokines
T-cell factors	TGF receptor function
Macrophage products	Membrane/cytoskeletal signaling
Cytokines/growth factors	Integrins, focal adhesion kinases, cytoskeletal proteins
TGF-β, PDGF	Clonal selection
Matrix signaling	Immune factors, apoptosis, hypoxia
Fibronectin, fibrillin, collagen	Autocrine factors
Hypoxia	TGF-β
Mast cells	
Tryptase	
Endothelial cell products	
Endothelin	

TGF, transforming growth factor; PDGF, platelet-derived growth factor.

IMMUNE BASIS OF FIBROSIS

As already noted, immune cells are commonly found in close proximity to sites of active matrix deposition in SSc, including the skin and lungs (Figs. 81.1 and 81.4). This association is also characteristic of other fibrotic disorders including chronic active hepatitis leading to cirrhosis, granulomas associated with parasitic diseases, and foreign body reactions. It has been appreciated for many years that immune cells are critical to the scar formation that characterizes normal wound repair (63). *In vitro* studies attempting to clarify the role of immune cells in fibrosis have shown that immune cells can stimulate fibroblast reparative processes, which include regulation of proliferation and biosynthesis of matrix components such as interstitial collagens, glycosaminoglycans, and fibronectin (64). Regulation occurs chiefly through the release of specific proteins, called cytokines, that act in a paracrine fashion to modulate behavior of nearby cells. The delineation of the precise molecular nature and mechanism of action of these cytokines has clarified how the immune system is involved in reparative and fibrotic processes.

The regulation of collagen synthesis is chiefly at the transcriptional level [i.e., actions on the promoter region of the collagen gene (and the first intron)] to increase transcription of collagen messenger RNA (mRNA). Multiple intracellular proteins have been identified that bind to various regions on the collagen promoter to regulate its activity. Included among these are proteins such as Sp1, AP-1, AP-2, and NF-1 that are known to act on the promoter of a wide variety of genes (65,66). There are also factors that transcriptionally control a much more limited set of genes such as cKROX, which acts principally to regulate matrix proteins (67). In some cases, complex intracellular pathways have been identified that link the action of a particular cytokine with a particular stretch of DNA in the gene promoter. This generally involves multiple steps: (a) binding of the cytokine to its receptor; (b) receptor activation (usually via phosphorylation), receptor translocation, or receptor association with another signaling molecule; (c) activation of a series of intracellular signaling proteins along a specific pathway; and (d) translocation of a DNA binding molecule to the nucleus and its interaction with stretches of DNA in the gene promoter. The various proteins in a signaling pathway are generally kinases (phosphorylating proteins) that sequentially activate the next protein in the pathway. In some cases, cytokine receptor engagement may lead to new synthesis of a protein that, in turn, binds to DNA directly or activates a new pathway.

In the setting of inflammation, multiple mediators are present, often with opposing effects on collagen biosynthesis and generally activating multiple signaling pathways. A simple sum of net profibrotic and antifibrotic cytokines is clearly not possible. What is clear, however, is that *in vivo,* the net effect is in favor of increased collagen production. This is evidenced not only by increased accumulation of collagen but also by increased signal for procollagen mRNA in skin fibroblasts, detected by *in situ* hybridization.

The immune system appears to play an important direct role in the genesis of cutaneous and visceral fibrosis in SSc by regulating collagen gene transcription and the synthesis of other matrix components. T-cell localization at inflammatory sites is a result of migration through the endothelium and binding, via receptor engagement, to tissues. T cells attach to the matrix via β_1 integrins that bind to collagen and fibronectin, and to fibroblasts via lymphocyte functional antigen-1 (LFA-1), a β_2 integrin, that binds intercellular cell adhesion molecule-1, -2, and -3 (ICAM-1, -2, and -3) on fibroblasts. Endothelial cell injury and activation (see below) probably result in increased lymphocyte migration at inflammatory sites. There is increased ICAM-1 expression by SSc fibroblasts (68,69), likely a result of activation by IL-1 and interferon-γ, leading to increased T-cell adhesion. T cells isolated from the blood of patients with SSc display increased adhesion to fibroblasts, and scleroderma fibroblasts, cultured from skin biopsies, support increased adhesion of normal T cells (69).

Once localized to tissue sites, immune cells release a variety of cytokines that influence fibroblast behavior. Included among these are cytokines that regulate synthesis of matrix components as well as synthesis and release of matrix metalloproteinases, enzymes that degrade collagen and other interstitial proteins. IL-4, IL-1, and TGF-βs (including TGF-β_1, -β_2, and -β_3) are among the principal profibrotic cytokines released by immune cells. IL-4 is released by CD4$^+$ T cells of the T-helper 2 (Th2) type and stimulates fibroblast proliferation, chemotaxis, and collagen synthesis (70) as well as ICAM-1 synthesis and expression on fibroblasts (71). IL-1 is principally a monocyte product and has similar activities, stimulating proliferation, collagen synthesis, and ICAM-1 expression (72). IL-1 and TNF-α stimulate fibroblast proliferation probably by stimulating production of platelet-derived growth factor-AA (PDGF-AA) homodimer (73) and also stimulate PDGF-$\beta\beta$ receptor (74). TNF-α and IL-1 also stimulate collagenase production, and TNF-α is a major stimulus for production of other metalloproteinases. TGF-β is likely the most important profibrotic cytokine; it is a potent stimulator of fibroblast collagen synthesis and synthesis of other matrix components (75,76). TGF-β stimulates collagen gene transcription, at least in part, by activating the Smad signaling pathway (77), and also stimulates collagen synthesis at the posttranscriptional level (78). TGF-β also stimulates expression of PDGF receptors, further promoting the fibrotic response. TGF-β is released by platelets as well as by fibroblasts and immune cells, and is generally present in a latent or inactive form. It binds to the interstitial matrix that forms a reservoir for the cytokine.

Immune cells also release cytokines that inhibit collagen synthesis and promote its degradation. Interferon-γ is likely the most important suppressor of collagen synthesis; it is a product of Th1 T cells. Interferon-γ also activates monocyte function, stimulates adhesion molecule expression on fibroblasts and other cells, and in general, activates the immune system. TNF-α is a potent stimulus for production of collagenase and other matrix metalloproteinases and it has a variable effect on collagen synthesis.

Nonimmune Factors

Mast cells may also play a role in the pathogenesis of scleroderma, in particular in stimulating fibrosis. Degranulated mast cells are found in the skin of patients with SSc, including skin that is clinically normal, possibly in a prefibrotic state (79). When mast cells are cocultured with fibroblasts, stimuli that lead to mast cell degranulation lead to increased fibroblast collagen synthesis (80). Tryptase, an abundant protein in mast cells that is released following degranulation, directly increases collagen synthesis. The stimuli for mast cell degranulation in SSc are unknown.

Endothelial cells can also elaborate factors that modulate the accumulation of extracellular matrix. Endothelin, released by endothelial cells in response to injury or activation, stimulates fibroblast collagen synthesis and also vasoconstriction. Endothelin levels are increased in SSc (81). Endothelial cells also elaborate other as yet unidentified factors that stimulate collagen synthesis in fibroblasts (82). Hypoxia, resulting from decreased tissue perfusion due to endothelial cell injury or vasoconstriction, stimulates fibroblast collagen synthesis as well, in part by stimulating endogenous TGF-β production by fibroblasts (83).

It is possible that vascular and immune events, whether linked or independent in their genesis, interact in their effects on fibroblast function. Immune perturbations of endothelial cell function, via injury or cytokine release, may ultimately lead to increased matrix synthesis.

Intrinsic Fibroblast Abnormalities

The actions of immune cell cytokines, mast cells, and endothelial cells do not, however, completely explain increased matrix biosynthesis in scleroderma. Studies by LeRoy (84) showed that fibroblasts from scleroderma patients synthesize increased amounts of matrix *in vitro,* a defect that persisted for multiple cell generations *in vitro* and is not dependent on the continuing presence of other cell types. Studies with cultured fibroblasts, long after removal from the *in vivo* environment, also have shown increased mRNA for collagen with both increased rates of transcription and increased message stability (85,86). This suggests that there is either a genetic metabolic abnormality or that, at some point in the disease, abnormal fibroblast behavior has become autonomous of extracellular signals and plays a role in continuing disease pathogenesis.

Fibroblast genetic defects might not become manifest until (or unless) fibrotic events are initiated by exogenous triggers, including immune, vascular, and other factors. Such genetic abnormalities would include abnormal responses to signals from the extracellular matrix that would normally attenuate and terminate fibrotic processes. Cell surface integrins bind to specific sequences on collagen and fibronectin and regulate the cytoskeleton, focal adhesion kinases, intracellular signals, and matrix production. $\alpha_1\beta_1$ and $\alpha_2\beta_1$ integrins bind to collagen, and their engagement leads to downregulation of collagen synthesis and upregulation of collagenase production, respectively (87). Abnormally low expression of both integrin receptors has been reported in SSc, and SSc fibroblasts do not downregulate collagen synthesis normally when grown in collagen gels (88–90). Structural abnormalities of fibrillin or quantitative changes in expression of the fibrillin gene might lead to abnormal organization of the extracellular matrix and to abnormal signals to the fibroblast.

Even in the absence of genetic defects, long-term changes in gene expression could result if the same stimuli that induce initial abnormalities in lymphocyte and/or endothelial cell behavior also alter fibroblast metabolism. Thus, viral infection, immune cytokines, endothelial cell products, or hypoxia could turn on certain genes that continually upregulate matrix biosynthesis. These genes may either persist in an activated state or lead to activation of autocrine loops, in other words, production of self-stimulatory factors that lead to increased matrix biosynthesis. For example, SSc fibroblasts have been shown to have an increased expression of type 2 high-affinity receptors for TGF-β, potentially leading to increased collagen synthesis (91). Since TGF-β can induce its own receptor, increased receptor function could be self-amplifying and perpetuating. Other potential candidates for mediating persistently increased collagen synthesis are protease nexin 1 and IL-1, both expressed in increased amounts by SSc fibroblasts and both capable of upregulating collagen production (92,93).

An alternative hypothesis for the induction of long-term phenotypic changes in SSc fibroblasts is based on the con-

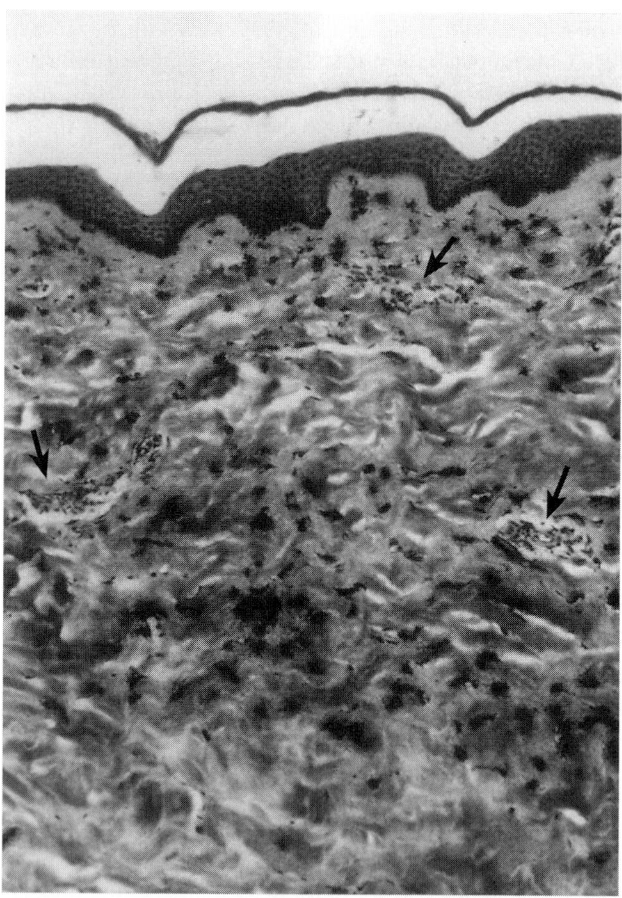

FIGURE 81.5. *In situ* hybridization for collagen messenger RNA (mRNA) in the skin of a patient with scleroderma. The dermis is quite thickened and small mononuclear infiltrates are seen *(arrows). Black areas* represent collagen mRNA detected by autoradiographic emulsion after hybridization to radiolabeled Col1A1 probe (α_1 chain of type I collagen). There is considerable heterogeneity in the signal detected in different fibroblasts. (H&E counterstain; 400× original magnification.) (Courtesy of Dr. A. Jelaska, Boston University School of Medicine).

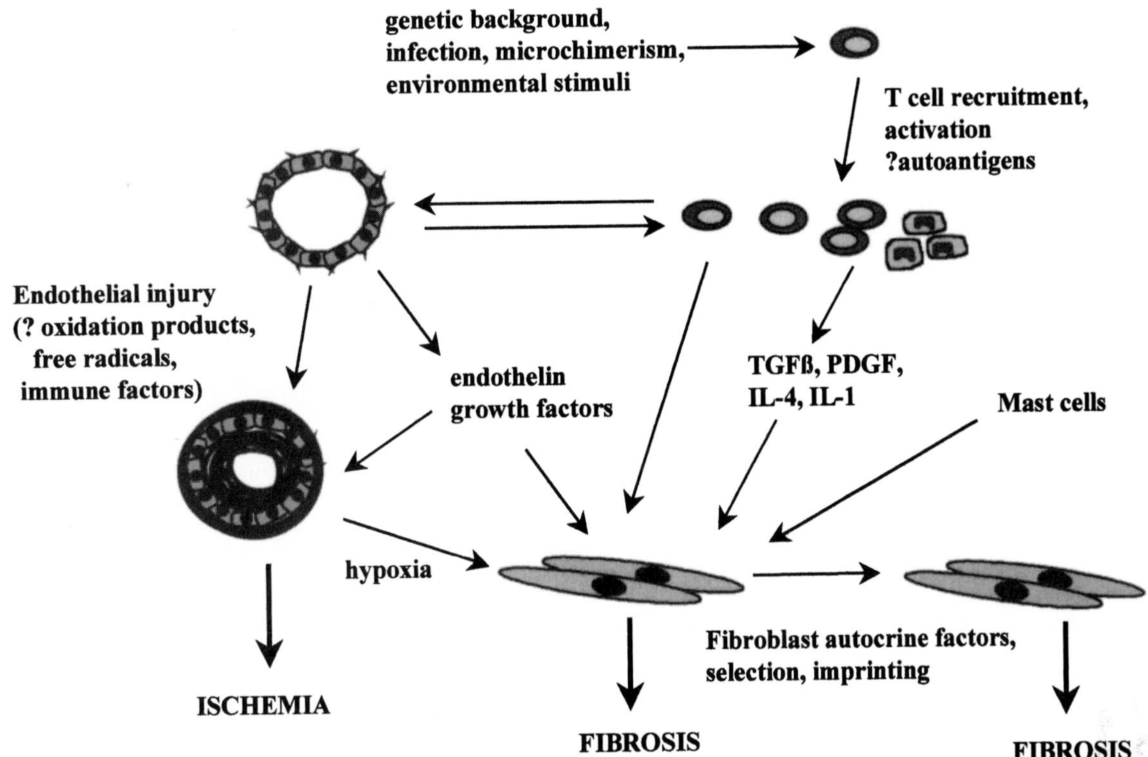

FIGURE 81.6. Pathways leading to vascular injury and fibrosis in SSc. TGF-β, transforming growth factor-β; PDGF, platelet-derived growth factor; IL-4, interleukin-4; IL-1, interleukin-1.

cept of clonal selection. Normal fibroblasts are heterogeneous with regard to collagen synthesis, proliferative capacity, and other metabolic parameters (94,95). In response to immune cytokines, endothelial cell factors, hypoxia, or other stimuli, preferential growth of some high collagen-producing fibroblast subsets might lead to a change in the makeup of the overall population to a high collagen phenotype. Indeed, when one examines scleroderma fibroblasts either by *in situ* hybridization of the skin or in culture, only a modest proportion show high expression of collagen mRNA (85) (Fig. 81.5). What distinguishes SSc from normal is an increase in the normally small proportion of cells with high expression of the procollagen gene. Alternative mechanisms for clonal selection include selective apoptosis of low collagen producing cells with persistence of the high collagen phenotype. This apoptosis can be mediated by Fas ligand on activated T cells interacting with Fas on the fibroblast cell membrane (96). Selected populations may persist long after initiating events have ceased. Thus, fibrosis initiated by immunologic processes may persist even in the absence of continuing immune cell activation.

CONCLUSION

The clinical expression of SSc includes vascular, fibrotic, and immunologic features. This reflects pathogenetic events that include endothelial cell injury and vascular obliteration, increased matrix deposition by dermal and visceral fibroblasts, and activation of cellular and humoral immune responses. Although these three arms of pathogenesis are mutually interdependent, the precise nature of the interactions and the initiating events are incompletely understood. In addition, it is clear that genetic and/or environmental factors play a role in disease susceptibility and in triggering disease expression (Fig. 81.6).

REFERENCES

1. McGregor AR, Watson A, Yunis E, et al. Familial clustering of scleroderma spectrum disease. *Am J Med* 1988;84:1023–1032.
2. Stephens CO, Briggs DC, Whyte J, et al. Familial scleroderma—evidence for environmental versus genetic trigger. *Br J Rheumatol* 1994;33:1131–1135.
3. Mayes MD. Epidemiology of systemic sclerosis and related diseases. *Curr Opin Rheumatol* 1997;9:557–561.
4. Aguilar MB, Cho M, Reveille JD, et al. Prevalences of familial systemic sclerosis and other autoimmune diseases three U.S. cohorts. *Arthritis Rheum* 1999;42:S186(abst).
5. Englert H, Small-McMahon J, Chambers P, et al. Familial risk estimation in systemic sclerosis. *Aust NZ J Med* 1999;29:36–41.
6. Maddison PJ, Skinner RP, Pereira RS, et al. Antinuclear antibodies in the relatives and spouses of patients with systemic sclerosis. *Ann Rheum Dis* 1986;45:793–799.
7. Maddison PJ, Stephens C, Briggs D, et al. Connective tissue disease and autoantibodies in the kindreds of 63 patients with sys-

temic sclerosis. The United Kingdom Systemic Sclerosis Study Group. *Medicine* 1993;72:103–112.

8. Manolios N, Dunckley H, Chivers T, et al. Immunogenetic analysis of 5 families with multicase occurrence of scleroderma and/or related variants. *J Rheumatol* 1995;22:85–92.
9. Feghali CA, Wright TM. Epidemiologic and clinical study of twins with scleroderma. *Arthritis Rheum* 1995;38:S308(abst).
10. Arnett FC, Howard RF, Tan F, et al. Increased prevalence of systemic sclerosis in a Native American tribe in Oklahoma. Association with an Amerindian HLA haplotype. *Arthritis Rheum* 1996;39:1362–1370.
11. Tan FK, Stivers DN, Arnett FC, et al. HLA haplotypes and microsatellite polymorphisms in and around the major histocompatibility complex region in a Native American population with a high prevalence of scleroderma (systemic sclerosis). *Tissue Antigens* 1999;53:74–80.
12. Tan FK, Stivers DN, Foster MW, et al. Association of microsatellite markers near the fibrillin 1 gene on human chromosome 15q with scleroderma in a Native American population. *Arthritis Rheum* 1998;41:1729–1737.
13. Siracusa LD, McGrath R, Ma Q, et al. A tandem duplication within the fibrillin 1 gene is associated with the mouse tight skin mutation. *Genome Res* 1996;6:300–313.
14. Pandey JP, LeRoy EC. Human cytomegalovirus and the vasculopathies of autoimmune diseases (especially scleroderma), allograft rejection, and coronary restenosis. *Arthritis Rheum* 1998;41:10–15.
15. Maul GG, Jimenez SA, Riggs E, et al. Determination of an epitope of the diffuse systemic sclerosis marker antigen DNA topoisomerase I: sequence similarity with retroviral gag protein suggests a possible role in autoimmunity in systemic sclerosis. *Proc Natl Acad Sci U S A* 1989;86:8492–8496.
16. Arnett FC, Reveille JD, Goldstein R, et al. Autoantibodies to fibrillarin in systemic sclerosis (scleroderma). An immunogenetic, serologic, and clinical analysis. *Arthritis Rheum* 1996;39:1151–1160.
17. Fanning GC, Welsh KI, Bunn C, et al. HLA associations in three mutually exclusive autoantibody subgroups in UK systemic sclerosis patients. *Br J Rheumatol* 1998;37:201–207.
18. Bramwell B. Diffuse scleroderma: its frequency; its occurrence in stonemasons; its treatment by fibrolysin-elevations of temperature due to fibrolysin injections. *Edinburgh Med J* 1914;12:387–401.
19. Erasmus LD. Scleroderma in gold-miners on the Witwatersrand with particular reference to pulmonary manifestations. *S Afr J Lab Clin Med* 1957;3:209–231.
20. Rodnan GP, Benedek TG, Medsger TA, et al. The association of progressive systemic sclerosis (scleroderma) with coal miners' pneumoconiosis and other forms of silicosis. *Ann Intern Med* 1966;66:323–334.
21. Silman AJ, Jones S. What is the contribution of occupational environmental factors to the occurrence of scleroderma in men? *Ann Rheum Dis* 1992;51:1322–1324.
22. Burns CJ, Laing TJ, Gillespie BW, et al. The epidemiology of scleroderma among women: assessment of risk from exposure to silicone and silica. *J Rheumatol* 1996;23:1904–1911.
23. Blair HM, Headington IT, Lynch PJ. Occupational trauma, Raynaud's phenomenon and sclerodactylia. *Arch Environ Health* 1974;28:80–81.
24. Edworthy SM, Martin L, Barr SG, et al. A clinical study of the relationship between silicone breast implants and connective tissue disease. *J Rheumatol* 1998;25:254–260.
25. Gabriel SE, Woods JE, O'Fallon WM, et al. Complications leading to surgery after breast implantation. *N Engl J Med* 1997;336:677–682.
26. Hochberg MC, Perlmutter DL, Medsger TA, et al. Lack of association between augmentation mammoplasty and systemic sclerosis (scleroderma). *Arthritis Rheum* 1996;39:1125–1131.
27. Hennekens CH, Lee IM, Cook NR, et al. Self-reported breast implants and connective-tissue diseases in female health professionals. A retrospective cohort study [published erratum appears in *JAMA* 1998;279(3):198]. *JAMA* 1996;275:616–621.
28. Veltman G, Lange CE, Juhe S, et al. Clinical manifestations and course of vinyl chloride disease. *Ann NY Acad Sci* 1975;246:6–17.
29. Tabuenca JM. Toxic-allergic syndrome caused by ingestion of rapeseed oil denatured with aniline. *Lancet* 1981;2:567–568.
30. Belongia EA, Hedberg CW, Gleich GJ, et al. An investigation of the cause of the eosinophilia-myalgia syndrome associated with tryptophan use. *N Engl J Med* 1990;323:357–365.
31. Silver RM, Heyes MP, Maize JC, et al. Scleroderma, fasciitis, and eosinophilia associated with the ingestion of tryptophan. *N Engl J Med* 1990;322:874–881.
32. Silver RM, Ludwicka A, Hampton M, et al. A murine model of the eosinophilia-myalgia syndrome induced by 1,1′-ethylidenebis (L-tryptophan). *J Clin Invest* 1994;93:1473–1480.
33. Lacey JV, Garabrant DH, Laing TJ, et al. Petroleum distillate solvents as risk factors for undifferentiated connective tissue disease (UCTD). *Am J Epidemiol* 1999;149:761–770.
34. Kerr LD, Spiera H. Scleroderma in association with the use of bleomycin: a report of 3 cases. *J Rheumatol* 1992;19:294–296.
35. Finch WR, Rodnan GP, Buckingham RB, et al. Bleomycin-induced scleroderma. *J Rheumatol* 1980;7:651–659.
36. Emerit I, Housset E, Feingold J. Chromosomal breakage and scleroderma: studies in family members. *J Lab Clin Med* 1976;88:81–86.
37. Wolff DJ, Needleman BW, Wasserman SS, et al. Spontaneous and clastogen induced chromosomal breakage in scleroderma. *J Rheumatol* 1991;18:837–840.
38. Emerit I, Filipe P, Meunier P, et al. Clastogenic activity in the plasma of scleroderma patients: a biomarker of oxidative stress. *Dermatology* 1997;194:140–146.
39. Casciola-Rosen L, Wigley F, Rosen A. Scleroderma autoantigens are uniquely fragmented by metal-catalyzed oxidation reactions: implications for pathogenesis. *J Exp Med* 1997;185:71–79.
40. Vasquez-Abad D, Rothfield NF. Autoantibodies in systemic sclerosis. *Int Rev Immunol* 1995;12:145–157.
41. Lee B, Craft JE. Molecular structure and function of autoantigens in systemic sclerosis. *Int Rev Immunol* 1995;12:129–144.
42. Needleman BW, Wigley FM, Stair RW. Interleukin-1, interleukin-2, interleukin-4, interleukin-6, tumor necrosis factor alpha, and interferon-gamma levels in sera from patients with scleroderma. *Arthritis Rheum* 1992;35:67–72.
43. Kahaleh MB. Soluble immunologic products in scleroderma sera. *Clin Immunol Immunopathol* 1991;58:139–144.
44. Claman HN. Graft-versus-host disease and animal models for scleroderma [review]. *Curr Opin Rheumatol* 1990;2:929–931.
45. Bianchi DW, Zickwolf GK, Weil GJ, et al. Male fetal progenitor cells persist in maternal blood for as long as 27 years post-partum. *Proc Natl Acad Sci U S A* 1996;93:705–708.
46. Maloney S, Smith A, Furst DE, et al. Microchimerism of maternal origin persists into adult life. *J Clin Invest* 1999;104:41–47.
47. Nelson JL, Furst DE, Maloney S, et al. Microchimerism and HLA-compatible relationships of pregnancy in scleroderma. *Lancet* 1998;351:559–562.
48. Artlett CM, Smith JB, Jimenez SA. Identification of fetal DNA and cells in skin lesions from women with systemic sclerosis. *N Engl J Med* 1998;338:1186–1191.
49. Artlett CM, Welsh KI, Black CM, et al. Fetal-maternal HLA compatibility confers susceptibility to systemic sclerosis. *Immunogenetics* 1997;47:17–22.
50. Kuwana M, Medsger TA, Wright TM. Highly restricted TCR-

alpha beta usage by autoreactive human T cell clones specific for DNA topoisomerase I: recognition of an immunodominant epitope. *J Immunol* 1997;158:485–491.
51. Yurovsky VV, Sutton PA, Schulze DH, et al. Expansion of selected V delta 1+ gamma delta T cells in systemic sclerosis patients. *J Immunol* 1994;153:881–891.
52. Cannon PJ, Hassar M, Case DB, et al. The relationship of hypertension and renal failure in scleroderma (progressive systemic sclerosis) to structural and functional abnormalities of the renal cortical circulation. *Medicine* 1974;53:1–46.
53. Kahaleh MB, Osborn I, LeRoy EC. Increased factor VIII/von Willebrand factor antigen and von Willebrand factor activity in scleroderma and in Raynaud's phenomenon. *Ann Intern Med* 1981;94:482–484.
54. Winchurch RA. Activation of thymocyte responses to interleukin-1 by zinc. *Clin Immunol Immunopathol* 1988;47: 174–180.
55. Madtes DK, Raines EW, Sakariassen KS, et al. Induction of transforming growth factor-α in activated human alveolar macrophages. *Cell* 1988;53:285–293.
56. Briggs DC, Vaughan RW, Welsh KI, et al. Immunogenetic prediction of pulmonary fibrosis in systemic sclerosis. *Lancet* 1991; 338:661–662.
57. Huffstutter JE, DeLustro FA, LeRoy EC. Cellular immunity to collagen and laminin in scleroderma. *Arthritis Rheum* 1985;28: 775–780.
58. Kahaleh MB, Sherer GK, LeRoy EC. Endothelial injury in scleroderma. *J Exp Med* 1979;149:1326–1335.
59. Kahaleh MB, LeRoy EC. Endothelial injury in scleroderma. A protease mechanism. *J Lab Clin Med* 1983;10:553–560.
60. Kahaleh MB, Fan PS. Mechanism of serum-mediated endothelial injury in scleroderma: identification of a granular enzyme in scleroderma skin and sera. *Clin Immunol Immunopathol* 1997;83: 32–40.
61. Bruckdorfer KR, Hillary JB, Bunce T, et al. Increased susceptibility to oxidation of low-density lipoproteins isolated from patients with systemic sclerosis. *Arthritis Rheum* 1995;38: 1060–1067.
62. Bashey RI, Millan A, Jimenez SA. Increased biosynthesis of glycosaminoglycans by scleroderma fibroblasts in culture. *Arthritis Rheum* 1984;27:1040–1045.
63. Leibovich SJ, Ross R. A macrophage dependent factor that stimulates the proliferation of fibroblasts in vitro. *Am J Pathol* 1976; 84:501–514.
64. Strehlow D, Korn JH. Biology of the scleroderma fibroblast. *Curr Opin Rheumatol* 1998;10:572–578.
65. Li L, Artlett CM, Jimenez SA, et al. Positive regulation of human a1(I) collagen promoter activity by transcription factor Sp1. *Gene* 1995;164:229–234.
66. Jimenez SA, Hitraya E, Varga J. Pathogenesis of scleroderma: collagen. *Rheum Dis Clin North Am* 1999;22:647–674.
67. Widom RL, Culic I, Lee JY, et al. Cloning and characterization of hcKrox, a transcriptional regulator of extracellular matrix gene expression. *Gene* 1997;198:407–420.
68. Needleman BW. Increased expression of intercellular adhesion molecule 1 on the fibroblasts of scleroderma patients. *Arthritis Rheum* 1990;33:1847–1851.
69. Abraham D, Lupoli S, McWhirter A, et al. Expression and function of surface antigens on scleroderma fibroblasts. *Arthritis Rheum* 1991;34:1164–1172.
70. Postlethwaite AE, Katai H, Raghow R. Human fibroblasts synthesize elevated levels of extracellular matrix in response to interleukin 4. *J Clin Invest* 1992;90:1479–1485.
71. Piela-Smith TH, Broketa G, Hand A, et al. Regulation of ICAM-1 expression and function in human dermal fibroblasts by IL-4. *J Immunol* 1992;148:1375–1381.
72. Postlethwaite AE, Raghow R, Stricklin GP, et al. Modulation of fibroblast functions by interleukin 1: increased steady-state accumulation of type I procollagen messenger RNAs and stimulation of other functions but not chemotaxis by human recombinant interleukin 1α and β. *J Cell Biol* 1988;106:311–318.
73. Raines EW, Dower SK, Ross R. Interleukin 1 mitogenic activity for fibroblasts and smooth muscle cells is due to PDGF-AA. *Science* 1989;243:393–396.
74. Tingstrom A, Reuterdahl C, Lindahl P, et al. Expression of platelet-derived growth factor-β receptors on human fibroblasts. Regulation by recombinant platelet-derived growth factor-BB, IL-1, and tumor necrosis factor-α. *J Immunol* 1992;148: 546–554.
75. Roberts AB, Sporn MB, Assoian RK, et al. Transforming growth factor-beta: rapid induction of fibrosis and angiogenesis in vivo and stimulation of collagen formation in vitro. *Proc Natl Acad Sci U S A* 1986;83:4167–4171.
76. Varga J, Jimenez SA. Stimulation of normal human fibroblast collagen production and processing by transforming growth factor-beta. *Biochem Biophys Res Commun* 1986;138:974–980.
77. Chen SJ, Yuan W, Mori Y, et al. Stimulation of type I collagen transcription in human skin fibroblasts by TGF-beta: involvement of Smad 3. *J Invest Dermatol* 1999;112:49–57.
78. Raghow R, Postlethwaite AE, Keski-Oja J, et al. Transforming growth factor-beta increases steady state levels of type I procollagen and fibronectin messenger RNAs posttranscriptionally in cultured human dermal fibroblasts. *J Clin Invest* 1987;79: 1285–1288.
79. Claman HN, Giorno RC, Seibold JR. Endothelial and fibroblastic activation in scleroderma. The myth of the "uninvolved skin." *Arthritis Rheum* 1991;34:1495–1501.
80. Gruber BL, Kew RR, Jelaska A, et al. Human mast cells activate fibroblasts: tryptase is a fibrogenic factor stimulating collagen messenger ribonucleic acid synthesis and fibroblast chemotaxis. *J Immunol* 1997;158:2310–2317.
81. Levin ER. Endothelins. *N Engl J Med* 1995;333:356–363.
82. Denton CP, Shiwen X, Welsh KI, et al. Scleroderma fibroblast phenotype is modulated by co-culture with human endothelial cells. *J Rheumatol* 1996;23:633–638.
83. Falanga V, Qian SW, Danielpour D, et al. Hypoxia upregulates the synthesis of TGF-beta 1 by human dermal fibroblasts. *J Invest Dermatol* 1991;97:634–637.
84. LeRoy EC. Increased collagen synthesis by scleroderma skin fibroblasts in vitro. *J Clin Invest* 1974;54:880–889.
85. Jelaska A, Arakawa M, Broketa G, et al. Heterogeneity of collagen synthesis in normal and systemic sclerosis skin fibroblasts. *Arthritis Rheum* 1996;39:1338–1346.
86. Jimenez SA, Feldman G, Bashey RI, et al. Co-ordinate increase in the expression of type I and type III collagen genes in progressive systemic sclerosis fibroblasts. *Biochem J* 1986;237: 837–844.
87. Langholz O, Rockel D, Mauch C, et al. Collagen and collagenase gene expression in three-dimensional collagen lattices are differentially regulated by alpha 1 beta 1 and alpha 2 beta 1 integrins. *J Cell Biol* 1995;131:1903–1915.
88. Kozlowska E, Sollberg S, Mauch C, et al. Decreased expression of alpha 2 beta 1 integrin in scleroderma fibroblasts. *Exp Dermatol* 1996;5:57–63.
89. Ivarsson M, McWhirter A, Black CM, et al. Impaired regulation of collagen pro-alpha 1(I) mRNA and change in pattern of collagen-binding integrins on scleroderma fibroblasts. *J Invest Dermatol* 1993;101:216–221.
90. Mauch C, Kozlowska E, Eckes B, et al. Altered regulation of collagen metabolism in scleroderma fibroblasts grown within three-dimensional collagen gels. *Exp Dermatol* 1992;1:185–190.
91. Kawakami T, Ihn H, Xu W, et al. Increased expression of TGF-

beta receptors by scleroderma fibroblasts: evidence for contribution of autocrine TGF-beta signaling to scleroderma phenotype. *J Invest Dermatol* 1998;110:47–51.

92. Strehlow D, Jelaska A, Strehlow K, et al. A potential role for protease nexin 1 overexpression in the pathogenesis of scleroderma. *J Clin Invest* 1999;103:1179–1190.
93. Kawaguchi Y, Hara M, Wright TM. Endogenous IL-1alpha from systemic sclerosis fibroblasts induces IL-6 and PDGF-A. *J Clin Invest* 1999;103:1253–1260.
94. Botstein GR, Sherer GK, LeRoy EC. Fibroblast selection in scleroderma: an alternative model of fibrosis. *Arthritis Rheum* 1982; 25:189–195.
95. Goldring SR, Stephenson ML, Downie E, et al. Heterogeneity in hormone responses and patterns of collagen synthesis in cloned dermal fibroblasts. *J Clin Invest* 1990;85:798–803.
96. Jelaska A, Korn JH. Anti-Fas induces apoptosis and proliferation in human dermal fibroblasts: differences between foreskin and adult fibroblasts. *J Cell Physiol* 1998;175:19–29.

82

VASCULITIS

GENE V. BALL
ROBERT M. GAY, JR.

Vasculitis is defined pathologically as inflammation of blood vessels, leading to variable degrees of occlusion and tissue ischemia. The simplicity of this pathologic definition belies its value in clinical practice, given the heterogeneous nature of vasculitis. It may be a solitary manifestation of disease, such as cutaneous polyarteritis, or one of several manifestations of a specific disease such as virus-related cryoglobulinemia and vasculitis. Moreover, vasculitis may be systemic or isolated to one organ. The overlapping features of vasculitic syndromes further confound its classification.

CLASSIFICATION OF VASCULITIS

In the absence of accurate knowledge of the causes and pathogenesis of the various kinds of vasculitis, schemes for their classification should be viewed as provisional. Fitting a patient into any of the categories may be difficult because of the ambiguities of clinical presentations, the limited number of diagnostic laboratory tests, and the difficulty in obtaining appropriate tissue for histologic examination (which may not provide categoric information). Features of more than one type of vasculitis may be present in a given patient, and a given type is not immutable. For example, leukocytoclastic vasculitis may "evolve" into polyarteritis or other ominous systemic disease. Nevertheless, a classification scheme is necessary to facilitate treatment and research.

In 1866, Küssmaul and Maier (1) described the pathology of classic periarteritis nodosa (polyarteritis nodosa; PAN). Thereafter, the term periarteritis nodosa was used generically to encompass a variety of vascular conditions, despite the authors' detailed description of the gross and microscopic histology of PAN. Other distinct vasculitic disorders were recognized later: Wegener's granulomatosis (WG) and allergic granulomatosis were described in 1936 and 1951, respectively (2,3). The first classification of vasculitis was proposed in 1952 when Zeek (4) critically reviewed "periarteritis nodosa." Zeek introduced the inclusive term "necrotizing angiitis" and differentiated five types of systemic vasculitis: hypersensitivity angiitis, allergic granulomatous angiitis, rheumatic arteritis, periarteritis nodosa, and temporal arteritis. WG and Takayasu arteritis were omitted, probably because neither was mentioned in the English language medical literature until after 1953 (5). Despite its obvious limitations, this classification scheme has served as the model for its successors.

Vasculitis has been classified according to features such as size, type, and distribution of blood vessel involvement; the histology of vessel walls and extravascular lesions (e.g., granulomatous reactions); clinical and laboratory features; and whether primary or secondary (6–10). The Chapel Hill Consensus Conference on the Nomenclature of Systemic Vasculitides has proposed nomenclature that defines PAN as necrotizing inflammation of medium or small arteries without glomerulonephritis or vasculitis in arterioles, capillaries, or venules. In their system, microscopic polyangiitis is defined as necrotizing vasculitis of small vessels, with minimal immune deposits, and variable involvement of small or medium-sized arteries. Applying these definitions, PAN is rare compared with microscopic polyangiitis. This nomenclature does not seem to accommodate PAN with hepatitis B virus (HBV) antigenemia, in which both glomerulonephritis and immune deposits are common (11). None of these classifications has gained universal acceptance. Because few, if any, of the vasculitides have consistent clinical or laboratory features, a definitive diagnosis of vasculitis still depends on histologic confirmation. Therefore until the etiology and pathogenesis of the different syndromes are better elucidated, it is probably best to rely heavily on histologic features for classification. Lie (5) has proposed an expanded and modified version of Zeek's histopathologic classification based on the predominant type and size of blood vessel involvement in the primary disorders. In addition, the segregation of primary vasculitis from secondary vasculitis as proposed by Tervaert and Kallenburg (12) is useful from a clinical standpoint. Problems still arise, however, because of the significant overlap within and between the major vasculitic syndromes with respect to the predominant size of the affected vessel. Furthermore, the acquisition of adequate tissue from visceral organs is often difficult and sometimes impossible in clinical practice. The recognition of distinct clinical subsets of vasculitis also limits the utility of a pathologic classification of vasculitis.

In 1990, the American College of Rheumatology (ACR) Subcommittee on Classification of Vasculitis chose to analyze seven distinct clinical vasculitic syndromes prospectively rather than attempt to formulate a new classification (13). The Committee established clinical criteria to differentiate PAN, Churg–Strauss syndrome (CSS), WG, hypersensitivity vasculitis, Henoch–Schönlein purpura (HSP), temporal arteritis, and Takayasu arteritis. Rao et al. (14) evaluated the ACR criteria for diagnosis of WG, giant cell arteritis (GCA), PAN, and hypersensitivity vasculitis among 198 patients who were referred to university and Veterans Affairs medical centers with diagnoses of possible vasculitis or related disorders. Vasculitis was ultimately diagnosed in 51 patients, of whom only 38 met the ACR criteria for one or more types of vasculitis; the criteria also were fulfilled in 31 of the 147 patients without vasculitis. Of the 51 patients with vasculitis, 15 met two or more sets of ACR criteria, and 13 met none. Furthermore, when the criteria were applied to all 198 patients, the positive predictive values of the criteria for WG, GCA, PAN, and hypersensitivity vasculitis ranged from only 17% to 29%. These findings reinforce the admonition that the criteria were not meant to be used for diagnostic purposes, and underscore the importance of histopathologic diagnoses. Types of vasculitis are listed in Table 82.1.

TABLE 82.1. TYPES OF VASCULITIS

- Primary vasculitis
  - Affecting large, medium, and small arteries
    - Takayasu's arteritis
    - Giant cell arteritis/temporal arteritis
    - Isolated CNS angiitis
    - Cogan's syndrome
  - Affecting predominantly medium and small blood vessels
    - Polyarteritis nodosa and cutaneous polyarteritis nodosa
    - Wegener's granulomatosis
    - Churg–Strauss syndrome
    - Kawasaki disease
    - Buerger's disease
  - Affecting predominantly small blood vessels
    - Microscopic polyarteritis (angiitis)
    - Cutaneous leukocytoclastic angiitis (including erythema elevatum diutinum)
    - Henoch–Schönlein purpura
    - Serum sickness
    - Hypocomplementemic urticarial vasculitis
    - Essential mixed cryoblobulinemia
    - Degos' syndrome
    - Behçet's disease
- Secondary vasculitis
  - Infection-related vasculitis
  - Vasculitis associated with connective tissue diseases
  - Drug-induced vasculitis
  - Vasculitis associated with malignancy
  - Organ-transplant vasculitis
  - Vasculitis associated with systemic diseases

Please note that Behçet's disease and isolated angiitis of the central nervous system have been omitted from this chapter because they are covered in Chapter 83.
CNS, central nervous system.

PATHOGENESIS

The pathogenesis of vasculitis is complex, involving more than one mechanism. Immune complexes appear to initiate the inflammation of leukocytoclastic vasculitis related to infections and medications, of HSP, and of some cryoglobulinemias. Antineutrophil cytoplasmic antibodies are probably major actors in the pathogenesis of "pauciimmune" vasculitis, and pathologic responses of T cells may be involved in others. Most types of vasculitis undoubtedly reflect the interaction of more than one of these. The concept that immunologic mechanisms play an active role in the pathogenesis of vasculitis is supported by the response of patients with vasculitis to antiinflammatory and immunosuppressive therapy. Proposed mechanisms incorporate pathogenic immune complex formation and deposition in vessel walls, antineutrophil cytoplasmic antibodies, antiendothelial antibodies, cellular immune responses and granuloma formation, and damaged or altered endothelial cell function due to infectious organisms, tumors, or toxins. Rapid expansion of our knowledge of the molecules that regulate interactions between immune cells and interactions between leukocytes and endothelial cells promises greater insight into the pathogenesis of vessel damage and potential sites for drug intervention. Cytokines (see Chapter 20) and adhesion molecules (see Chapter 21) involved in normal immune responses are the major mediators of pathogenic immune responses in vasculitis syndromes.

Immune Complexes in Vasculitis

Deposition of immune complexes in blood vessels has long been implicated as the instigating mechanism of vascular inflammation: animal models of serum sickness and the Arthus reaction provide most of the support for this role of immune complexes. In the acute serum sickness model, the single injection of a large amount of a heterologous serum protein is followed 10 to 14 days later by the development of arteritis, glomerulonephritis, and endocarditis. The vasculitic lesions, which appear when circulating antigen–antibody complexes are formed in slight antigen excess, contain antigen, immunoglobulin, and complement (15). After immune complexes deposit, the vasculitis of acute serum sickness resembles PAN histologically with segmental infiltration of arterial walls by neutrophils and mononuclear cells, intimal proliferation, and fibrinoid necrosis. Antigen has not been detected in glomeruli, arteries, or the endocardium by fluorescent antibody techniques before immune complex deposition, suggesting that *in situ* formation is not the mechanism involved, as it is in the Arthus reaction (15).

Vasculitis is absent in animal models of chronic serum sickness. There is a variable host response to intravenous injections of foreign protein given daily for several weeks. The majority of animals rapidly clear antigen; others acquire immunologic tolerance; and 10% to 20% form immune complexes that are slowly removed from the circulation, resulting in chronic glomerulonephritis (16). An explanation of the difference between acute and chronic serum sickness with respect to the development of arteritis has not been forthcoming.

It is likely that other factors contribute to the quantity and quality of the host immune response, accounting for the inconsistent expression of vasculitis in animal and human immune complex disease. Cytokines and adhesion molecules released by neutrophils and endothelial cells are undoubtedly necessary for generation of the inflammatory response in pathogenesis of immune vasculitis. The role of antibodies in specific pathologic processes is uncertain. The mere presence of circulating immune complexes is not sufficient to produce vasculitis, as indicated by the paucity of vasculitis in animals injected with preformed immune complexes (10). Cochrane et al. (17) demonstrated that the release of vasoactive amines from platelets is necessary for the tissue deposition of immune complexes in experimental acute serum sickness. Pretreatment with antihistamines or depletion of platelets clearly suppressed the deposition of immune complexes and prevented vasculitis. Physical properties of the immune complexes also are important as only those with a sedimentation coefficient greater than 19S are deposited in vessel walls (17). Other specific factors that influence their proinflammatory nature include the ability of the immune complex to activate complement, the antigen–antibody combining ratio, and structural and hemodynamic differences between various blood vessels (18). The tendency for immune complexes to deposit at vessel branching sites, heart valves, and dependent areas is partly explained by hydrostatic forces.

Detection of immunoglobulin and complement in human vasculitic lesions by immunofluorescent or immunochemical techniques provides circumstantial evidence of immune complex–mediated disease. These proteins are most readily detected in cutaneous vasculitis, but inconsistently in systemic vasculitis. Definitive support for a pathogenetic role for immune complexes requires the detection of a relevant antigen and specific antibody simultaneously in the circulation and in sites of vascular injury. This has been a fruitless pursuit in most cases of vasculitis because the inciting antigen is seldom known, and it is not usually possible to elute sufficient material from vasculitic lesions to isolate and quantify specific antibodies (10). Failure to detect immunoglobulins in vasculitic lesions argues against their pathogenic role only when early lesions are examined, because neutrophils have been shown to degrade immune complexes within 24 to 48 hours after their deposition (19).

Prospective evaluation of human serum sickness has confirmed the immunologic observations made in experimental animals. After treatment of patients with bone marrow failure with horse antithymocyte globulin, serum sickness appeared, coincident with increased circulating immune complexes, decreased serum complement, and localization of immunoglobulin and complement in affected small cutaneous blood vessels (20). Current evidence also implicates immune complex deposition as the primary pathogenic mechanism in some forms of vasculitis such as HSP and vasculitis associated with hepatitis B, hepatitis C, and cryoglobulinemia, which primarily affect small or medium-sized vessels (21).

In the 1970s, persistent hepatitis B infection was linked to some cases of PAN, and essential mixed cryoglobulinemia with vasculitis (22,23). Several vasculitic syndromes, cutaneous and systemic, have been associated with hepatitis B infection. Hepatitis B surface antigen (HBsAg)–antibody complexes have been found in the circulation (22,24), and deposits of HBsAg, immunoglobulin, and complement have been found in lesions of muscular arteries (22,25), dermal vessels (26), glomeruli (27), and vasa nervorum (28). Hypocomplementemia may accompany vasculitis associated with hepatitis B infection, and cryoglobulins have been shown to contain HBsAg and particles resembling the virus (23). Several investigators were able to elute all of the HBsAg and part of the immunoglobulin from vascular deposits by treatment with buffers known to dissociate antigen–antibody bonds but not with phosphate-buffered saline, arguing against nonspecific binding to preexisting lesions (25). Substantial evidence therefore correlates the immunopathologic events of hepatitis B–associated vasculitis with experimental serum sickness.

For several years, the presumed pathogenesis of leukocytoclastic vasculitis has been that circulating immune complexes are deposited in the small blood vessels of the skin, with inflammation after complement activation. Activated neutrophils release collagenase and elastase, which, in conjunction with free oxygen radicals, result in necrosis of vessels. Cytokines from T cells and endothelial cells are involved, and various antibodies such as those reacting with endothelial cells may contribute to the complex phenomena of inflammation (29). Immunoglobulins and complement are seen on direct immunofluorescence of vasculitic skin lesions. Circulating immune complexes may be detected, but serum complement levels are not usually decreased (30). Intradermal injection of histamine and epinephrine into uninvolved skin of patients with cutaneous vasculitis reproduces the histopathologic findings of spontaneous lesions. Although deposition of immunoreactants can be demonstrated in normal-appearing skin of patients with leukocytoclastic vasculitis, increased deposition of immunoglobulin and complement follows the injection of histamine in a few hours, but neither is detected after 24 hours (31,32). By using direct immunofluorescence, Grunwald et al. (33) were able to demonstrate immunoreactants in skin biopsies of vasculitis of various causes and of early, mature, and healing ages. Biopsies from 92% of patients were positive, in increasing concentration, for fibrinogen, albumin, immunoglobulin G (IgG), IgM, IgA, and C4. Gower et al. (32) also demonstrated that the deposition of immune complexes and complement precedes the inflammatory infiltrate. IgA and complement play a primary role in HSP. IgA deposits have been found in vasculitic lesions obtained simultaneously from skin, kidney, and small intestine (34). IgA, C3, and fibrin have been found together in affected skin and glomeruli (35). There are increased numbers of IgA-producing lymphocytes in HSP (36,37), and high levels of circulating IgA-containing immune complexes (38). The data are consistent with the concept of impaired clearance of IgA immune complexes by the reticuloendothelial system. IgA immune complexes do not activate the classic complement pathway and are ineffective in fixing C3 (39). There has been little evidence of classic pathway activation in HSP, as C1q, C3, and C4 are usually not depressed (40). Waxman et al. (41) also have shown that IgA complexes bind poorly to erythrocytes, are inefficiently cleared by the liver, and become deposited in the kidney and lungs. The membrane-attack complex, C5b-9, is a component of IgA and C3 deposits in vessel walls of the skin and in capillary walls and mesangium of glomeruli of patients with HSP nephritis (42). C5b-9 appears to damage dermal vascular endothelial cells in the absence of polymorphonuclear cells.

Role of Complement in the Elimination of Immune Complexes

The frequent conjunction of genetic deficiencies of complement and immune complex diseases implies an important pathogenetic interaction between the two. Activation of the classic and alternative complement pathways results in the adherence of C3b to immune complexes, facilitating their clearance by the reticuloendothelial system and modifying their structure and biologic activity. An intact classic complement pathway is required for this binding of C3b, which inhibits precipitation of the complexes. Activation of the alternative pathway may solubilize precipitated immune complexes (39,43). This conceivably allows diffusion of antigen–antibody complexes from the site of their formation and minimizes the local inflammatory response (39).

The C3b component of immune complexes binds to a specific receptor, complement receptor type 1 (CR1). This binding prevents immune complex interaction with other structures such as vascular endothelium. Ninety percent to 95% of the CR1 in humans is located on the surface of erythrocytes (39), but it also is found on polymorphonuclear leukocytes, macrophages, B lymphocytes, some T lymphocytes, dendritic reticular cells in germinal centers, and glomerular podocytes. Immune complexes bound to CR1 on red blood cells are then removed from the circulation by spleen and liver macrophages (44). CR1 also is a potent inhibitor of the complement cascade, serving as a cofactor for the enzyme (factor 1) that inactivates C3b by cleavage (45,46).

Thus experimental evidence corroborates the critical role of complement in processing immune complexes so that they remain soluble and can be transported to tissue macrophages for elimination. There are several plausible reasons for failure of the normal processes for eliminating immune complexes that could lead to the development of vasculitis and other manifestations of immune complex disease: (a) depletion or deficiency of complement components, (b) failure of various antibody classes within immune complexes to bind complement, (c) depletion or blockade of CR1, and (d) impairment of tissue macrophage function (18).

Antineutrophil Cytoplasmic Antibodies

Antineutrophil cytoplasmic antibodies (ANCAs) are specific for cytoplasmic antigens located in primary granules of neutrophils and lysosomes of monocytes. By indirect immunofluorescence (IIF), they are identified as cytoplasmic (cANCA) or perinuclear (pANCA). The antigens responsible for cytoplasmic IIF are usually proteinase 3 (PR3) and those detected as perinuclear are often myeloperoxidase (MPO). Antibodies to other neutrophil constituents such as elastase and lactoferrin produce a pANCA pattern, but the ANCAs of diagnostic significance are those directed against PR3 and MPO. A comprehensive review of the clinical aspects of ANCAs has been published recently (47). The current recommendation for the testing and reporting of ANCAs is that screening should be done with IIF for newly investigated patients. Sera positive for ANCAs, or for any cytoplasmic fluorescence, or homogeneous or peripheral nuclear fluorescence, should then be tested in enzyme-linked immunosorbent assays (ELISAs) for PR3 and MPO ANCAs (48).

Two major hypotheses have been advanced to elucidate the role of ANCAs in the development of vasculitis. These assume that the antibodies are of pathogenic importance, although this has not been proven. The first proposes that the release of PR3 or MPO antigenic targets of ANCAs from neutrophil primary granules or monocyte lysosomes results in binding of these antigens to blood vessel walls, with subsequent *in situ* immune complex formation and its consequences. Evidence to support this hypothesis is tenuous because of the paucity of immunoglobulin or complement deposits in ANCA-positive vasculitis. The other hypothesis is based on *ex vivo* evidence that ANCAs are directly involved in the pathogenesis of vasculitis through interaction with primed neutrophils, which are then capable of injuring endothelial cells. Neutrophils exposed to tumor necrosis factor (TNF) express both MPO and PR3 on their cell surface where they may interact with ANCAs. This interaction stimulates a respiratory burst and degranulation in the primed neutrophils (49,50). Cytokine priming of neutrophils, as might occur with infection, may not be necessary for translocation of primary granules to their surface. This translocation also occurs during neutrophil apoptosis, and experiments have shown that ANCA$^+$ sera will react with the apoptotic neutrophils, but not with viable neutrophils (51). For ANCA-activated neutrophils to cause vasculitis, they must adhere to and injure endothelial cells, as has been shown to occur *in vitro* by using cultured human umbilical vein endothelial cells (52,53). Incubation of endothelial cells with anti-PR3 antibodies also leads to an increase in vascular cell adhesion molecule-1 (VCAM-1) expression, and increased adhesion of T lymphocytes to the cells. Thus ANCAs can contribute to regulation of T-lymphocyte migration (54).

Jennette and Falk (55), who first described pANCA in patients with necrotizing glomerulonephritis and microscopic polyangiitis, and who identified the antigen as MPO, have summarized their views of the role of ANCA in pathogenesis, as well as the evidence supporting their pathogenicity. A partial listing of the clinical evidence they adduce includes (a) the frequent occurrence of ANCA in the sera of patients with vasculitis and necrotizing crescentic glomerulonephritis, (b) the response of these diseases to immunosuppressive drugs, (c) their pauciimmune nature, and (d) the induction of ANCAs and vasculitis by medications such as propylthiouracil and hydralazine. The disease and ANCAs may disappear with cessation of the offending medication. Thus considerable evidence supports a role for ANCAs in pathogenesis of disease. A plausible yet hypothetical diagram of the induction of vasculitis by ANCAs is depicted in Fig. 82.1. Muller Kobold et al. (56) have found increased expression of PR3 on neutrophils from patients with active WG but not from those with quiescent disease or from healthy controls. The expression correlated with disease activity. They concluded that the availability of PR3 and the interaction of ANCAs and PR3 are central to WG. The same investigators reported that markers of monocyte activation, including neopterin, interleukin-6 (IL-6), and CD11b, were increased with active disease (57).

ANCAs are detected in diseases other than vasculitis. For example, pANCAs are found in sera from persons with ulcerative colitis and in a higher than expected number of unaffected relatives. Twenty-seven of 50 sera from patients with ulcerative colitis contained ANCAs, none of which were reactive with MPO, elastase, or PR3 (58). Seibold et al. (59) have concluded that pANCAs in ulcerative colitis patients and in colitic mice are cross-reactive with enteric bacterial antigens. ANCAs reacting with PR3 have been found in sera from a few patients with bacterial endocarditis (60). Sera from almost half of patients with rheumatoid arthritis (RA) and systemic lupus erythematosus (SLE) contain ANCAs reactive with elastase or MPO, or lactoferrin (61).

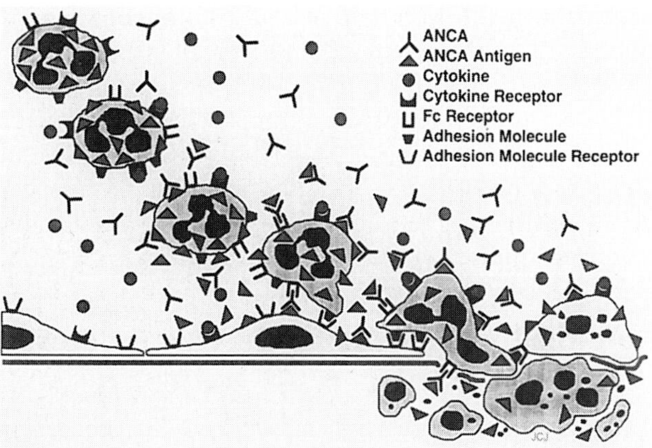

FIGURE 82.1. A hypothetical cartoon of the induction of vasculitis by antineutrophil cytoplasmic antibodies (ANCAs). (Reproduced with permission from Jeannett JC. Pathogenesis of the vascular and glomerular damage in ANCA-positive vasculitis. *Nephrol Dial Transplant* 1998;13(suppl 1):16–20.)

Vasculitides in which ANCAs have diagnostic significance include WG, microscopic polyangiitis, and CSS, all typically diseases of small vessels. These usually have variable, and potentially lethal courses, with frequent involvement of the lungs, upper respiratory tracts, and kidneys. They have in common their occurrence with little or no demonstrable immune complex deposition, and without complement consumption, hence the term "pauciimmune," which does not imply the absence of an immunologic pathogenesis. ANCAs are not present in all persons with any of these diseases, and both cANCAs and pANCAs may be present in sera from patients with any of these entities. This concept is relevant to diagnosis. For example, the clinical and pathologic similarities between microscopic polyangiitis and WG are such that extrarenal granulomatous inflammation may at times represent the only significant difference between them. Granulomas may be missed on biopsy, and biopsies may be restricted to the kidney, resulting in an inappropriate diagnosis, by default, of microscopic polyangiitis. These clinical similarities are reflected in overlapping results of testing for ANCAs. Thus of 66 patients with biopsy-proven vasculitis, 12 with microscopic polyangiitis were anti-MPO positive, but 22 given this diagnosis were anti-PR3 positive (62). The specificities of ANCAs were examined in another group consisting of 98 patients with vasculitis diagnosed on clinical and histologic grounds. Thirty-eight patients had anti-PR3 antibodies. Of these, WG was diagnosed in 19; microscopic polyangiitis, in 15; necrotizing and crescentic glomerulonephritis, in two; and relapsing polychondritis, in two. Of the 45 patients with anti-MPO, 26 had microscopic polyangiitis; three had PAN; five, WG; eight, glomerulonephritis; two, SLE; and one had CSS (63). In regard to the significance of IIF ANCAs, they seem to be comparable to antinuclear antibodies in their lack of specificity; PR3 cANCAs are more specific for vasculitic diseases, analogous to the specificity of certain subsets of antinuclear antibodies in other rheumatic diseases.

Role of Antiendothelial Cell Antibodies in Vasculitis

A role for antiendothelial cell antibodies in the pathogenesis of vasculitis has been inferred from their presence in WG, microscopic polyangiitis, and Kawasaki disease, as well as in vasculitis associated with SLE and RA. High titers of these antibodies have been found in 18 of 19 patients with Takayasu's arteritis. It was unclear whether they were markers for vasculitis or contributors to its pathogenesis (64). Salojin et al. (65) also have found increased levels of anti–endothelial cell antibodies in patients with vasculitis of large and medium-sized arteries. Brasile (66) detected anti–endothelial cell antibodies in 86% of 21 patients with systemic necrotizing vasculitis, correlating these with disease activity. He also reported preferential binding of the anti–endothelial cell antibodies to splenic and inferior mesenteric endothelium in comparison to aortic endothelium, findings that are compatible with visceral arterial involvement in vasculitis. Other investigators have reported anti–endothelial cell antibodies in 19% of 27 patients with WG and in 2% of 43 patients with microscopic polyangiitis (67).

Anti–endothelial cell antibodies can induce endothelial cell injury and lysis through complement-mediated cytotoxicity or antibody-dependent cellular cytotoxicity (ADCC). By using sera from patients with Kawasaki disease and systemic vasculitis, anti–endothelial cell antibodies have been shown to participate in complement-mediated cytotoxicity of cultured human umbilical vein endothelial cells (66,68,69), an observation not confirmed by all investigators (70). ADCC is a process by which specific antibody binds to a target cell and engages a natural killer cell through its Fc receptor, resulting in lysis of the cell. Its role in systemic vasculitis is unclear, but ADCC has been demonstrated *in vitro* against endothelial cells (71). These activities of anti–endothelial cell antibodies may account for observed elevations of von Willebrand factor–related and factor VIII–related antigen in the sera of patients with vasculitis.

Direct Vessel Damage by Infectious Agents

It is conceivable that any infectious agent or foreign antigen that induces an immune response might result in vasculitis, but some infectious agents probably cause vasculitis through nonimmunologic mechanisms. In equine viral arteritis, evidence supports viral infection of the vascular endothelium (72). A more convincing example of an arteritis without immunologic mediation has come from experimental central nervous system (CNS) arteritis in turkeys infected with *Mycoplasma gallisepticum* (73). Inoculation of a large dose of organisms resulted in arteritic lesions within 24 hours, implicating a direct toxic effect of mycoplasma organisms, or their products, on vascular endothelium. Numerous exotic parasites and microbes also cause animal, and less often human, vasculitis.

In humans, invasion by infectious organisms resulting in direct vascular injury is seen with bacteria, including mycobacteria, spirochetes, and rickettsia. Varicella-zoster virus, herpes simplex virus (HSV), and cytomegalovirus appear to cause human vasculitis. Viral inclusion bodies have been detected within and closely adjacent to vessel walls in several patients (74–76). HSV-1 infection of human endothelial cells results in expression of C3b and Fc receptors on the cell surface (77). The human retrovirus human T-cell leukemia virus-1 (HTLV-1) has been shown to infect human endothelial cells *in vitro,* which may explain the cutaneous vasculitis associated with HTLV-1–induced T-cell leukemia (18). Human immunodeficiency virus (HIV) appears to cause vasculitis directly; however, other causes of vasculitis, such as medications and opportunistic infections, may be identified in persons with acquired immunodeficiency syndrome (AIDS) (78).

Tumor Cell–Mediated Vascular Damage

Vasculitis has been associated primarily with lymphomatoid and myeloproliferative malignancies. Because of its rarity, there is a paucity of data on the pathogenesis of vasculitis in the setting of malignancy. It is assumed a tumor antigen activates cellular immunity or participates in immune complex formation. The vasculitis of hairy cell leukemia is the best studied of these. Of 42 persons with this disease, 17 had polyarteritis, 21 had leukocytoclastic vasculitis, and four had vessel wall infiltration by hairy cells. Immune complexes were found in three of four patients tested. Three patients, of 12 tested, were HBsAg positive. Vasculitis most often occurred after splenectomy (79–81). Unidentified viral infections also may play a role through either immune complex disease or direct infection of endothelial cells. Direct invasion of vascular walls also has been documented in mycosis fungoides, in HTLV-1–associated T-cell leukemia, and in the premalignant syndrome of lymphomatoid granulomatosis (18).

Cell-Mediated Immune Responses and Granuloma Formation in Vasculitis

The occurrence of granulomas in WG and CSS is indicative of activation of lymphocytes and macrophages. It has been hypothesized that CD4+ T cells are triggered by antigens in the circulation or within vascular walls, and release cytokines chemotactic for monocytes. Monocytes transformed into macrophages are then capable of releasing lysosomal enzymes that damage endothelial cells (9). Experimental evidence for this comes from mice that were injected with syngeneic T cells sensitized *in vitro* to cultured vascular smooth muscle cells (82). Twenty percent of the mice developed granulomatous vasculitis of the pulmonary arterioles.

In human vasculitis, cell-mediated immunity has been studied primarily in WG. Activated T cells, both CD4+ and CD8+ subtypes, have been found in biopsies from the upper and lower respiratory tracts and kidneys (83–85). The expanded populations show high expression of activation markers HLA-DR and CD25, independent of activity of disease, and there are high levels of intracellular and secreted interferon-γ (IFN-γ) and IL-2 (86). Patients with active WG had higher percentages of activated CD38+ B cells than did those in remission or control subjects; however, activated T cells persisted during remission of the vasculitis (87). Earlier studies found significant elevations of soluble IL-2 receptor (sIL-2R) in active generalized WG (88). Peripheral blood mononuclear cells from patients with WG proliferate *in vitro* on exposure to proteinase 3 (PR3), suggesting the presence of antigen-primed memory T cells (89). A sustained response to monoclonal antibodies directed against CD4+ T cells (Campath 1-H and anti-CD4) also has been observed in four patients with life-threatening systemic vasculitis that had been unresponsive to conventional immunosuppressive agents (90).

RECOGNITION OF AND CLINICAL APPROACH TO SYSTEMIC VASCULITIS

The irreversible loss of kidney function within a few days from the symptomatic onset of WG is uncommon, but it exemplifies the importance of prompt recognition and treatment of vasculitis. The nonspecific symptoms of vasculitis may imitate more benign connective tissue disease or even malignant and infectious diseases. Key features suggestive of vasculitis include fever, malaise, skin lesions, peripheral neuropathy, nondestructive oligoarthritis, and the symptom complex of polymyalgia rheumatica. Jaw claudication is almost pathognomonic of vasculitis, and although it is most common in temporal arteritis, it has been described in PAN, CSS, and WG, as well as in amyloidosis (91). Common laboratory findings include anemia, leukocytosis, thrombocytosis, elevation of the erythrocyte sedimentation rate (ESR), an abnormal urinary sediment, and proteinuria. The overlapping features of the vasculitic syndromes that may hinder classification can thus facilitate recognition of systemic vasculitis as the cause of an illness.

The majority of persons with systemic vasculitis will have constitutional symptoms such as fatigue, weight loss, fever, arthralgias, myalgias, and anorexia. Polymyalgia rheumatica may be noted in any systemic vasculitis. The cutaneous manifestations are variable and nonspecific but of great diagnostic value and include palpable purpura, urticaria, ulcerations, infarctions, nodules, livedo reticularis, and maculopapular rashes.

TABLE 82.2. CONDITIONS THAT MAY PRODUCE THE SYNDROME OF MULTIPLE MONONEUROPATHIES

Vasculitis
Diabetes mellitus
Sarcoidosis
Inherited susceptibility to pressure palsies
Leprosy
Lymphomatoid granulomatosis
Human immunodeficiency virus (HIV) infection
Malignant infiltration of nerve trunks
Lyme disease
Multifocal motor neuropathy with conduction block
Neurofibromatosis
Subacute bacterial endocarditis

Reproduced with permission from Chalk CH, Dyck PJ, Conn DL. *Peripheral neuropathy.* 3rd ed. Philadelphia: WB Saunders, 1993:1426.

Moore and Fauci (92) reported peripheral neuropathies in 60% and CNS abnormalities in 40% of patients with systemic vasculitis. Mononeuritis multiplex is classically associated with PAN but may complicate any systemic vasculitis. This peripheral neuropathy is characterized by asymmetric and asynchronous sensorimotor deficits in named nerve roots. Mononeuritis multiplex, in the absence of diabetes and trauma, has often been considered diagnostic of vasculitis, but there are other causes (Table 82.2), and evaluations of unselected patients identified a cause in only 50% of 57 patients (93). These studies provide evidence that the association of systemic vasculitis and mononeuritis multiplex is not so strong as has been previously thought. Nevertheless, if it occurs in combination with another systemic symptom, mononeuritis multiplex is one of the more specific and early clinical signs of systemic vasculitis. In general, mononeuritis multiplex develops as a late complication of SLE and RA, whereas it occurs early in the course of PAN (94). Extensive mononeuritis, cutaneous neuropathy, and polyneuropathy are other patterns of peripheral neuropathy occurring in systemic vasculitis. Vasculitis confined to the peripheral nervous system also has been described (95,96).

Diagnosis of Systemic Vasculitis

Definitive diagnosis of systemic vasculitis requires histologic confirmation when involved tissue is accessible, although angiography may be an acceptable alternative approach. Angiography is an appropriate substitute for histologic diagnosis in suspected cases of Takayasu's arteritis, Buerger's disease, PAN, and some cases of GCA. The distribution of arterial lesions is most useful from a diagnostic standpoint because stenosis, occlusion, aneurysms, or irregularities may occur in nonvasculitic diseases.

A biopsy should be performed on any otherwise unexplained skin lesion when vasculitis is suspected. The yield from skin biopsy is increased by sampling early lesions and avoiding necrotic areas. The presence of cutaneous vasculitis often correlates poorly with systemic involvement, but a positive biopsy in the company of multisystem disease is confirmatory for systemic vasculitis.

Sural nerve biopsy, although of unproven sensitivity and specificity, is probably the least invasive and safest alternative to skin biopsy for tissue diagnosis, as abnormal sural nerve conduction correlates well with vasculitis on biopsy (Fig. 82.2). Furthermore, a significant number of asymptomatic peripheral neuropathies may be detected in systemic vasculitis by electromyography and nerve-conduction studies (97).

The yield from muscle biopsies is greater from painful areas, but blind biopsies also may reveal vasculitis (Fig. 82.3) (98). In general, kidney biopsies usually demonstrate a nonspecific segmental necrotizing glomerulonephritis, and these should probably be reserved for patients who have renal involvement only. Necrotizing vasculitis also has been found on rectal biopsy, and this might be considered before proceeding to more invasive procedures (99). Open testicular biopsies to diagnose PAN have been used primarily in symptomatic persons, but are not widely performed because of the requirement for general anesthesia.

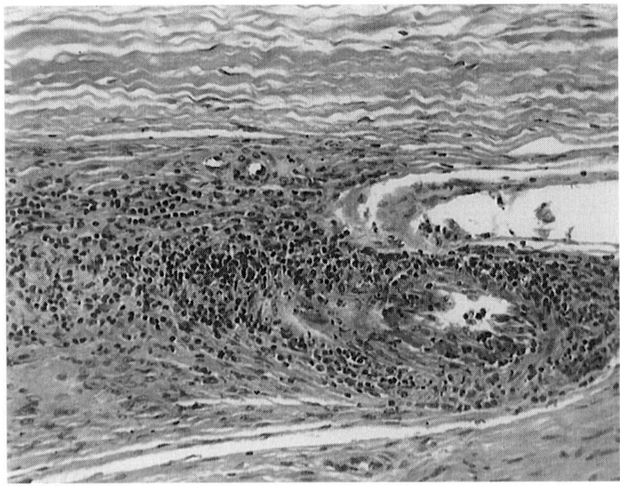

FIGURE 82.2. Sural nerve biopsy with an inflammatory infiltrate and nuclear debris within a small vessel wall, areas of segmental fibrinoid necrosis, and a prominent perivascular infiltrate. (Courtesy of Dr. Shin J. Oh.)

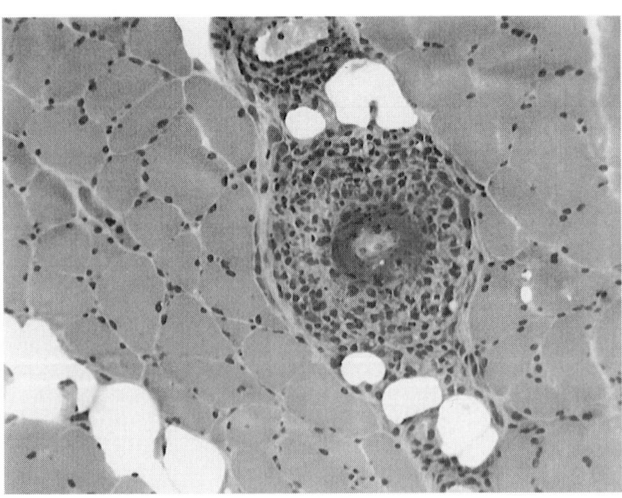

FIGURE 82.3. Muscle biopsy from a patient with polyarteritis showing inflammatory cells within a vessel wall, eccentric fibrinoid necrosis, and near-total occlusion of the lumen. There also is a marked perivascular infiltrate. (Courtesy of Dr. Shin J. Oh.)

Polyarteritis Nodosa

The description by Küssmaul and Maier in 1866 of focal, inflammatory, arterial nodules accounts for the original name, periarteritis nodosa (1). This term has been superseded by the more anatomically accurate polyarteritis, which refers to inflammation of the entire arterial wall. After Küssmaul and Maier's eloquent description of the disease, all forms of vasculitis were labeled periarteritis until Zeek's classification of vasculitis in 1952 (4). PAN remains the prototype of vasculitis and continues to confound physicians, as evidenced by the relatively poor sensitivity and specificity of the ACR diagnostic classification criteria (100).

PAN is a disease of small and medium-sized muscular arteries, involving any organ, but in particular, joints, muscles, peripheral nerves, gastrointestinal tract, and skin. Affecting persons of any age, but most often those between 40 and 60 years, PAN is more common in the United States in men, with a male-to-female ratio of 2:1. Accurate determinations of its incidence are thwarted by its rarity and varying approaches to classification; for instance, microscopic polyangiitis may, or may not, be separated from PAN by a given investigator. PAN may be a feature of hepatitis B infection, RA, Sjögren's syndrome, mixed cryoglobulinemia, and hairy cell leukemia. There are numerous anecdotal reports of various medications causing PAN, and, as an illustration of its association with a variety of disorders, it has been ascribed to familial Mediterranean fever in four of 302 children with this syndrome (101,102).

The highly variable signs and symptoms of PAN are primarily attributable to diffuse vascular inflammation and resulting ischemia of affected organs. Most often, the presenting complaints are nonspecific: fever, malaise, weight loss, anorexia, and abdominal pain. PAN also has been reported to occur as a benign self-limited condition involving a single organ, including skin, skeletal muscle (103), peripheral nerves (96), and visceral organs. Asymptomatic arteritis limited to the appendix, found in 88 cases by Plaut (104), fosters speculation that episodes of focal vasculitis are a normal occurrence.

The reported prevalence of specific organ involvement in PAN comes mainly from studies that do not distinguish between PAN and microscopic polyangiitis, which only recently has been recognized as a separate entity. Looked at in this inclusive way, the most frequently affected internal organs in PAN are kidneys, heart, and liver (105). (Severe kidney disease manifested as rapidly progressive glomerulonephritis is more typical of microscopic polyangiitis than of PAN). PAN seldom leads to renal failure, as does microscopic polyangiitis. Hypertension is common and is associated with abnormal urinary sediment (106). Rupture of aneurysms can cause intrarenal, perirenal, and retroperitoneal hemorrhage. In one study, only two of 165 patients progressed to end-stage renal disease and chronic hemodialysis or renal transplant (107). Among 47 patients with polyarteritis–microscopic polyangiitis, necrotizing glomerulonephritis was found in 11, crescentic glomerulonephritis in 13, and small and medium-sized arteritis in six. Six patients had rapidly progressive renal failure, and 18 had protein excretion greater than 2 g/24 h, which is uncommon in classic PAN (108).

Although as many as 90% of persons with PAN have abnormal hearts at autopsy, clinical manifestations of heart involvement are uncommon. Congestive heart failure is most frequent, and is indicative of coronary arteritis and hypertension (109). Myocardial infarction is usually clinically silent, even though 62% of 66 autopsied persons with PAN harbored vasculitis of the coronary arteries and myocardial infarcts (110). Acute pericarditis and arrhythmias are encountered occasionally (111).

Gastrointestinal involvement in PAN is evident most often as abdominal pain, and when there is gastrointestinal bleeding, PAN may be mistaken for inflammatory bowel disease. However, gastrointestinal lesions have been reported to occur only when there is other clinical evidence of systemic vasculitis (112). Hemorrhage, bowel infarction, and perforation are usually fatal. As mentioned, the liver is frequently involved on postmortem examination; however, clinical evidence is usually absent except for occasional elevations of alkaline phosphatase. Abnormalities in transaminases may be associated with chronic active hepatitis B. There also are reports of isolated PAN affecting the intestine (113), gallbladder, pancreas (114), and liver (115), as well as the appendix (104).

Peripheral neuropathies are present in 50% to 70% of patients (116), and despite increased recognition of CNS involvement, appear to be more common than CNS disease (92,107). Manifestations of peripheral neuropathies include mononeuritis multiplex, extensive mononeuritis, distal sensorimotor polyneuropathy, and sensory neuropathy. The onset of peripheral neuropathies is usually early in the course of the disease, with equal distribution between the upper and lower extremities. In general, the lesions occur distally rather than proximally, and are a direct result of occlusion of vasa nervorum or nutrient arteries (117). With appropriate therapy, the prognosis for improvement and recovery of peripheral neuropathies is good (92).

Unlike peripheral neuropathies, CNS lesions tend to become evident 2 to 3 years after the onset of PAN (92,118). The major signs of these include diffuse encephalopathy, focal neurologic deficits, and seizures (92,119). Usually insidious in onset, diffuse encephalopathy is more common than the other two and is characterized by cognitive dysfunction and decreased level of alertness. Formal psychologic testing has detected abnormalities in patients without clinically evident neurologic disease (120). The pathogenesis of the encephalopathy is unclear, but it appears to occur during episodes of acute vasculitis. On the other hand, cerebrovascular accidents, a leading cause of death, occur more frequently when there is scant evidence of systemic disease. Focal and generalized seizures may occur, but electroencephalograms are either normal or reveal nonspecific slowing. Chronic seizure disorders ascribable to PAN have not been reported. It is therefore necessary to treat with anticonvulsants only during periods of active vasculitis.

Skin abnormalities occur in about 40% of patients, usually as nonspecific maculopapular eruptions, purpura, livedo reticularis, urticaria, and ulcerations, and less often as nailfold and digital vasculitis, ecchymoses secondary to ruptured aneurysms, gangrene, and Raynaud's phenomenon. Subcutaneous nodules are observed much less frequently in systemic PAN (about 15% of cases) than in cutaneous polyarteritis (105,121). About half of patients complain of arthralgia and myalgia. Myalgias usually involve the lower extremities and may or may not be related to vasculitis of muscles. An asymmetric, nondeforming polyarthritis characteristically appears early in the course of the disease.

The usual nonspecific laboratory abnormalities of systemic inflammatory diseases are encountered in cases of PAN, and immunologic abnormalities include low titers of rheumatoid factor, circulating immune complexes, and diminished serum complement. Low complement levels are usually associated with rheumatoid factors and cryoglobulins and may indicate active vasculitis (122). HBsAg has been detected in the past in 10% to 54% of patients with PAN (116).

Inflammation of the entire vessel wall consists of a mixture of mononuclear cells and variable numbers of neutrophils and eosinophils, and fibrinoid necrosis is an invariable feature (123). Inflammation typically occurs in a focal and segmental fashion, with a predilection for bifurcations.

The principles discussed previously in the section on clinical approach and diagnosis apply to PAN. A single

TABLE 82.3. CLASSIFICATION CRITERIA FOR POLYARTERITIS NODOSA

1. Weight loss of >4 kg since beginning of illness
2. Livedo reticularis
3. Testicular pain or tenderness
4. Myalgias, weakness, or leg tenderness
5. Mononeuropathy or polyneuropathy
6. Development of hypertension
7. Elevated BUN or creatinine unrelated to dehydration or obstruction
8. Presence of hepatitis B surface antigen or antibody in serum
9. Arteriogram demonstrating aneurysms or occlusions of the visceral arteries
10. Biopsy of small or medium artery containing granulocytes

For classification purposes, a patient shall be said to have PAN if at least three of these 10 criteria are present.
BUN, blood urea nitrogen; PAN, polyarteritis nodosa.
Reproduced and adapted with permission from Lightfoot RW, Michel BA, Bloch DA, et al. The American College of Rheumatology 1990 criteria for the classification of polyarteritis nodosa. *Arthritis Rheum* 1990;33:1091.

biopsy procedure, followed by angiographic evaluation if necessary, was calculated to have a sensitivity of 85% and a specificity of 96% in a literature-based decision analysis approach (124) (Table 82.3).

Awareness of conditions allied with PAN and those that imitate vasculitis (Table 82.4) is important from a clinical standpoint to ensure institution of appropriate therapy. Diseases that may mimic PAN include sepsis, endocarditis, malignancy, left atrial myxoma, and cholesterol embolization. A detailed discussion of these is found in Chapter 84. In a prospective angiographic study of PAN, there was no association between the presence of clinical findings and the presence of aneurysms. Sixty percent of patients with clinical PAN had aneurysms. In most persons, more than ten aneurysms were present, and there was no case of a solitary aneurysm. This study also suggested that patients with aneurysms have more severe visceral involvement and an increased mortality. Cases with only occlusive small vessel disease are more difficult to interpret; however, diagnosis of PAN is strongly suggested if stenoses and occlusions are present in arteries of the small intestine, liver, and kidneys (125). It is therefore appropriate to proceed with angiographic evaluation even in the absence of clinical evidence of hepatic, gastrointestinal, or renal involvement in patients whose illness suggests systemic vasculitis. The presence of multiple intraparenchymal microaneurysms on angiography (Fig. 82.4) has been considered pathognomonic of PAN (126), but the angiographic appearance of embolization secondary to atrial myxoma may be identical (127), as may necrotizing angiitis resulting from parenteral amphetamine abuse (128). Microaneurysms have been reported infrequently in other types of vasculitis, including microscopic polyangiitis, WG, SLE, RA, CSS, and Behçet's syndrome.

Systemic PAN in the pretreatment era had a miserable prognosis, with a 5-year survival rate of approximately 10% (106,129). The prognosis may be worse than was observed in early reports because of the possible inclusion of cutaneous polyarteritis. Glucocorticoids and cytotoxic agents, especially cyclophosphamide, have had a major impact on the treatment and prognosis of this condition. An increase of 5-year survival rates to around 50% has been seen with the use of glucocorticoids alone (129,130). The systematic inclusion of cyclophosphamide in the initial treatment regimen is controversial; cyclophosphamide is not needed to induce remission in all cases. Unfortunately, there is no way to predict which cases will completely respond to treatment solely with glucocorticoids. Management decisions must be individualized, taking into account the extent of visceral involvement and the rate of progression of disease.

Persons with systemic disease should be treated initially with high doses of glucocorticoids, such as 60 mg of prednisone per day in divided doses. Gradual tapering of the prednisone dose may begin after a clinical response is

TABLE 82.4. DISEASES ASSOCIATED WITH OR CAUSALLY IMPLICATED IN POLYARTERITIS NODOSA

Infection	Rheumatic	Other
Hepatitis B	Systemic lupus erythematosus	Hairy cell leukemia
Acute otitis media	Rheumatoid arthritis	Amphetamine drug abuse
Streptococcal infection	Sjögren's syndrome	Inflammatory bowel disease
Hepatitis C	Dermatomyositis	Allergic hyposensitization therapy
	Scleroderma	Mesenteric arteritis after surgical repair of aortic coarctation
	Essential mixed cryoglobulinemia	
	Relapsing polychronditis	
	Giant cell arteritis	

Reproduced and adapted with permission from Cupps TR, Fauci AS. *The vasculitides.* 1st ed. Philadelphia: WB Saunders, 1981:37.

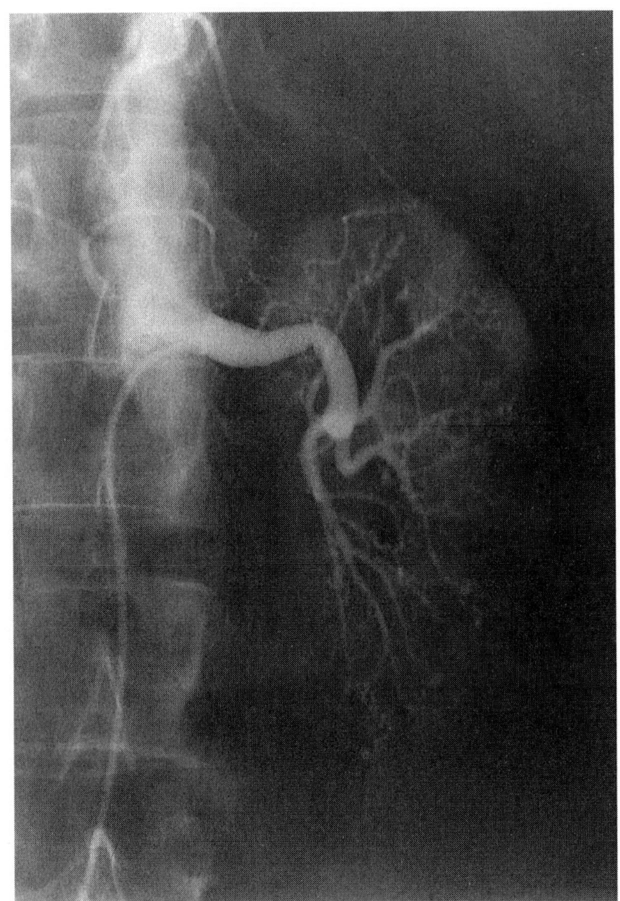

FIGURE 82.4. Renal arteriogram with multiple aneurysms. (Courtesy of Dr. Marc Schwartzberg.)

observed and the ESR returns to normal. Despite histologic evidence of effective control of vascular inflammation, occlusion may result from fibrosis (131). In particular, elderly persons with preexisting atherosclerosis may have an increased tendency to develop occlusive arteriopathy. Thus, careful clinical evaluation often is necessary to differentiate between ischemia secondary to active vasculitis and that due to other vascular disease. In the latter, vasodilators and antiplatelet drugs may be beneficial.

Although glucocorticoid therapy results in complete remissions of disease activity in many cases of PAN, insidious progression to end-organ damage may ensue when active disease is only partially suppressed. Addition of a cytotoxic agent is then indicated for control of disease activity. Cyclophosphamide has become the preferred immunosuppressive agent because of its rapid onset of action and its documented efficacy in WG. Fauci et al. (132) have demonstrated improvement in control of PAN when cyclophosphamide is added to steroid-resistant cases. Conflicting results have been observed in uncontrolled, retrospective analyses regarding the long-term prognosis of patients treated with glucocorticoids alone versus combination therapy. Leib et al. (130) reported improvement in the 5-year survival rate to 80% when patients were treated with an immunosuppressive agent in addition to glucocorticoids. In contrast, Cohen et al. (122) observed no beneficial effects on survival in patients who received a combination of glucocorticoids and cytotoxic agents compared with the former alone. Interpretation of these survival data is difficult because of the uncontrolled nature of these retrospective reports and the variety of immunosuppressive drugs used.

In another retrospective analysis, Guillevin et al. (133) reported that combination therapy at the onset of disease was of no more benefit than steroids alone. Subsequently, these investigators conducted the first randomized evaluation of cyclophosphamide for the treatment of PAN. The administration of cyclophosphamide and glucocorticoids at the onset of disease provided better disease control and lower relapse rates; however, there was no improvement in the 10-year survival rate (134). Cyclophosphamide was administered orally at an initial dose of 2 mg/kg and continued for 1 year. The French Cooperative Study Group in Polyarteritis (135) evaluated the effect of adding plasma exchange to corticosteroid therapy, without immunosuppressive drugs, in the initial treatment of PAN. The study was discontinued because of higher rates of relapse, in comparison to those observed earlier. Plasma exchange appeared to have little effect on disease control or survival in this study, but it may benefit a subgroup of patients with severe renal disease (136). See the section on WG for further discussion of glucocorticoid and cyclophosphamide use.

The most frequent immediate causes of death due to PAN are gastrointestinal hemorrhage and perforation, congestive heart failure, and infections. The four factors that appear to have the greatest impact on prognosis include age older than 50 years, cardiomyopathy, and renal and gastrointestinal involvement (107,122,130). Deaths occurring more than 1 year after diagnosis are usually attributed to myocardial infarction or cerebrovascular accidents (122). The clinical course and response to treatment of patients with PAN associated with HBsAg has been thought to be no different from that of uninfected patients (137,138); however, a retrospective study demonstrated that 1-year survival rates were significantly lower for persons with HBsAg (70%) than for persons without infection (85%) (139). The increase in mortality was related to gastrointestinal complications, including hemorrhage and perforation. The long-term effects of immunosuppressive therapy on chronic hepatitis in PAN patients are unknown. Steroids and immunosuppressive agents increase viral replication and enhance progression to cirrhosis in chronic hepatitis B, despite their beneficial effects on vasculitis (140,141). Guillevin et al. (142) have retrospectively observed an improved outcome in PAN related to HBV from treatment with short-term prednisone followed by vidarabine and plasma exchanges, compared with standard immunosuppressive treatment. The combination of the nucleoside analogue famciclovir and interferon-α2b has been used to reduce viral replication and symptoms (143). Guillevin et al. (144) have asserted that HBV-related PAN can be cured with the combination of antiviral agents and plasma exchanges. The frequency with which HBV was found in PAN patients in France decreased from 20% in the years 1980 to 1990 to 7.3% in 1992, a decline attributed to vaccination for HBV in the population at risk (145).

Microscopic Polyangiitis (Microscopic Polyarteritis)

In its tendency to involve medium arteries, and also arterioles, venules, and capillaries, microscopic polyangiitis (MPA) has been considered a variant of PAN. Separation of the two on anatomic grounds has been based on the presence of segmental, necrotizing glomerulonephritis, and involvement of the lung in MPA, both of which are uncommon in PAN. Segmental necrosis of glomerular tufts, and capillary rupture and bleeding ultimately result in formation of crescents and glomerular dropout. Without treatment, renal function declines rapidly. Immunoglobulin deposits are uncommon. In the lungs, vasculitis leads to widespread alveolar hemorrhage in as many as one fourth of patients (others may have interstitial disease mimicking idiopathic pulmonary fibrosis). Early symptoms of MPA are fever, myopathies, night sweats, and neuropathy (146). Diverse systemic symptoms are similar to those of PAN and the other pauciimmune vasculitides, emphasizing the problems of categorizing patients with these diseases. Ear, nose, and throat involvement is more common in MPA than in PAN, and arterial aneurysms are seldom found in patients with MPA. A more distinguishing feature vis-à-vis PAN is the occurrence of ANCAs in sera of as many as 75% of patients with MPA. Lhote et al. (147) based diagnosis of MPA on lung involvement, glomerulonephritis, ANCA positivity, negative tests for HBV and HCV, and small vessel disease. The same group later reported on 85 patients who fulfilled their criteria for MPA. Seventy-nine percent of them had signs of renal disease; fever was recorded in 55%; mononeuritis multiplex in 58%; and arthralgias in 50%. Heart failure, in 18% of patients, was almost as common as lung disease and was more common than alveolar hemorrhage, seen in 12% of patients. The 5-year survival rate was 74%; prognosis was better in those treated with glucocorticoids and immunosuppressive drugs than in those treated without the latter (148).

Although rare, MPA was estimated to be more common than PAN in a single district hospital in the United Kingdom. The estimate of annual incidence for the former was 3.6/million, and for PAN was 2.4/million (149). In contrast, el-Reshaid et al. (150) estimated a combined annual incidence of MPA and PAN of 45/million adult Kuwaitis. Most reports of MPA have come from outside North America.

Churg–Strauss Syndrome (Allergic Granulomatosis)

Allergic granulomatosis and angiitis was described in 1951 by Churg and Strauss as a syndrome consisting of asthma, eosinophilia, fever, and accompanying vasculitis of various organ systems (3). Characteristic histologic findings within blood vessels were a necrotic eosinophilic exudate and severe fibrinoid changes of collagen, and granulomatous proliferation of epithelioid and giant cells in connective tissue. The syndrome was noted to share a number of clinical and pathologic features with PAN; however, the presence of granulomas was thought to separate these disorders. Churg and Strauss reviewed 15 cases of PAN without asthma and found no granulomas.

It has since been recognized that the "Churg–Strauss granuloma" is not pathognomonic of the syndrome. For example, a review from the Mayo Clinic of 27 skin biopsies with extravascular, necrotizing granulomas reported an association with autoimmune disease, lymphoproliferative disease, and systemic vasculitis not limited to CSS (151). Reports have since mentioned the infrequency with which all three major histologic lesions are found together in antemortem tissue biopsies.

Lanham et al. (152) emphasized the distinct clinical presentation rather than the pathologic findings. A phasic pattern of disease progression was described, which began with allergic disease (nasal polyposis and allergic rhinitis along with asthma) and was followed by eosinophilia with tissue infiltration (resembling Löffler's syndrome, chronic eosinophilic pneumonia, or eosinophilic gastroenteritis) and finally vasculitis. All three "phases" have occurred simultaneously (153). Keeping in mind caveats pertaining to the limitations of classification criteria, the clinical, radiologic, and pathologic variables listed in Table 82.5 provide

TABLE 82.5. TRADITIONAL FORMAT CLASSIFICATION OF CHURG–STRAUSS SYNDROME

1. Asthma
2. Eosinophilia >10% on differential WBC count
3. Mononeuropathy (including multiplex) or polyneuropathy
4. Nonfixed pulmonary infiltrates on radiography
5. Paranasal sinus abnormalities
6. Biopsy containing a blood vessel with extravascular eosinophils

For classification purposes, a patient shall be said to have Churg–Strauss syndrome (CSS) if at least four or more of the six criteria are positive.
WBC, white blood cell.
Reproduced and adapted from Masi AT, Hunder GG, Lie JT, et al. The American College of Rheumatology 1990 criteria for the classification of Churg-Strauss syndrome (allergic granulomatosis and angiitis). *Arthritis Rheum* 1990;33:1098, with permission.

a framework for diagnosis (154). Guillevin et al. (155) diagnosed CSS on the basis of asthma, hypereosinophilia, and clinical manifestations consistent with systemic vasculitis. In their retrospective study of 96 patients, they observed asthma as the most common manifestation followed by mononeuritis multiplex. Other common manifestations were fever, rashes, myalgia and arthralgia, weight loss, and pulmonary infiltrates. Some patients had paranasal sinusitis, evoking again the difficulties in differentiating CSS and WG in an atopic patient. Hattori et al. (156) confirmed a pattern of mononeuritis multiplex initially, evolving into asymmetric polyneuropathy confined to the limbs. Like Guillevin, they reported a good long-term prognosis.

The cause or causes of CSS are not known. A provocative report identified the leukotriene modifier, zafirlukast, used for the treatment of asthma, as a possible cause in nine asthma patients whose vasculitis appeared while they were taking this drug, and being weaned from oral corticosteroids (157).

Although asthma is the single best discriminator for this disease among the vasculitides, it often subsides with the onset of vasculitis (3,152,153). Pulmonary infiltrates are a central feature of CSS and commonly include transient patchy infiltrates, nodular infiltrates without cavitation, and diffuse interstitial disease. Less common radiographic abnormalities include hilar adenopathy and pleural effusions, which frequently contain large numbers of eosinophils. Prominent, but nonspecific, skin manifestations are erythematous maculopapular rashes, palpable purpura, and cutaneous or subcutaneous nodules (158). The infrequency of significant renal disease tends to distinguish CSS from other forms of vasculitis. In the combined experience of the Mayo Clinic and the Hammersmith Hospital, in only one of 46 patients had renal failure. The predominant glomerular lesion of CSS appears to be focal segmental glomerulonephritis. There are no distinctive laboratory features; however, elevated levels of IgE have been detected in a substantial number of patients. Hypocomplementemia and circulating immune complexes are rarely noted. A definitive pathologic diagnosis depends on demonstration of vasculitis (granulomatous or nongranulomatous) and extravascular necrotizing granulomas, usually with eosinophilic infiltrates (123). The inflammation targets small arteries and veins, with extrapulmonary lesions most commonly found in the gastrointestinal tract, spleen, and heart.

Differentiation from WG, and MPA, may be difficult. This is confounded by the detection of ANCAs in as many as half of patients given the diagnosis of CSS. Furthermore, ANCA may be cytoplasmic by IIF, and PR3 positive by ELISA. For example, Schmitt et al. (159) found cANCAs in four, and pANCAs in three of 16 patients with CSS. The same investigators found increased concentrations of soluble IL-2 receptors indicating T-cell activation, and of eosinophil cationic protein in sera of patients with active CSS. If confirmed, this could greatly facilitate differential diagnosis of diseases with similar symptoms.

Before the use of glucocorticoids, CSS was thought to be uniformly fatal, the majority of deaths occurring as a result of congestive heart failure or myocardial infarction. A short interval from the onset of asthma to the development of vasculitis has been identified as a poor prognostic sign (3,152,153). Symptoms of CSS usually abate during treatment with an initial dose of 40 to 60 mg/day of prednisone. Azathioprine and cyclophosphamide have been used successfully in persons with an inadequate response to glucocorticoids. Dramatic responses have been reported with the use of intravenous cyclophosphamide (160) and pulse methylprednisolone (161) in persons unresponsive to oral corticosteroids. Clinical improvement also has been reported after intravenous immune globulin (162).

Resolution of constitutional signs, improvement of cardiac and renal function, and stabilization of neuropathy are the primary clinical signs of response to therapy. The most reliable laboratory indicators of response include decrease of eosinophil and white blood cell counts and a decrease in the ESR. The duration of required treatment of vasculitis appears to be less than 1 year (152); however, the length of therapy needs to be individualized. Major disease sequelae include hypertension, residual peripheral neuropathy, and, infrequently, renal insufficiency. In the study cited earlier of 96 patients followed from 1963 to 1995, it was found that despite clinical remission in 91%, 11 patients died of causes attributed to the vasculitis. Severe gastrointestinal and heart involvement augured a poor prognosis. Persistent asthma may require continuing glucocorticoids after recovery from vasculitis (155). In comparison to PAN, long-term follow-up of CSS patients has shown an improved prognosis with respect to end-organ damage, disability, and mortality (163). Survival has been reported as 90% at 1 year, 76% at 3 years, and 62% at 5 years (153).

Wegener's Granulomatosis

Klinger (164) described the first patient with what is now called WG in 1931, and a few years later, Wegener recognized it as a distinct form of vasculitis, describing the triad of (a) necrotizing granulomatous vasculitis of the upper and lower respiratory system, (b) systemic vasculitis, and (c) focal necrotizing glomerulonephritis. Over the past few years, the association with ANCAs has intensified interest in this fascinating disease, the course of which can be rapidly progressive and life threatening. Although WG usually responds to treatment with low-dose cyclophosphamide and glucocorticoids, extended follow-up studies of patients have emphasized its chronic relapsing nature, and the permanent morbidity related to both the disease and its treatment.

WG is a rare disease with an annual incidence of 8.5/million population estimated for a cohort of 414,000 adults in the U.K. (165), and an estimated prevalence of 33/million persons in the United States (166). A similar prevalence of 53/million persons was found in a small Norwegian county (167). It occurs at any age, but most commonly in the fourth and fifth decades. Distribution among the sexes is roughly equal with a slight male predominance, and it is significantly more common in whites than in other races. A genetic predisposition has not been identified consistently. Commentary on WG and its putative relation to infection has appeared recently (168).

Since the first description of this disease, there has been a realization that every organ system may be affected by granulomas or vasculitis, and that the majority of patients will have respiratory tract involvement. Although spread to both upper (92%) and lower respiratory tracts (85%) occurs in most cases during the course of disease (169), initial patient complaints usually refer to the nose, sinuses, ears, or trachea (170,171). The most common initial problems are persistent sinusitis and rhinitis that have not responded to conventional therapies, and which may be accompanied by serosanguinous drainage, epistaxis, nasal pain, and mucosal ulcerations. Serous otitis media is the most frequent ear manifestation, but sensorineural hearing loss also is common and is usually associated with a conductive component due to otitis or perforation of the tympanic membrane (170). Characteristic upper airway manifestations of the disease are saddle-nose deformity and tracheobronchial stenosis (usually subglottic).

In most persons with nasal and sinus involvement, secondary bacterial infections are common, and *Staphylococcus aureus* is the most frequently identified pathogen. Antibiotics often do not eradicate sinus infections, and surgical drainage procedures may be necessary. The distinction between sinus infections and granulomatous inflammation of WG in the sinuses may pose a difficult management issue. Colonization of the nares with *S. aureus* possibly predisposes WG patients to relapses of disease activity (172).

After the upper respiratory tract, the lungs are most commonly affected in WG. Clinical and physical signs are nonspecific; symptoms reported in descending order of frequency include cough, dyspnea, hemoptysis, and pleuritic chest pain (173). Approximately 34% of persons reported from the National Institutes of Health had (NIH) asymptomatic pulmonary involvement (169). The most common radiographic abnormalities are nodules and infiltrates in the mid and lower lung zones, both of which may cavitate (Figs. 82.5 and 82.6). Pleural effusions have also been observed in as many as 20% of patients (169), and may be indicative of subclinical disease activity predicting relapse, thus warranting consideration of immunosuppressive therapy (174). There is infrequent hilar and mediastinal lymphadenopathy or calcification. By pulmonary function testing, obstructive airway disease is most common; however, decreased lung volumes and diffusion capacity are also found (169).

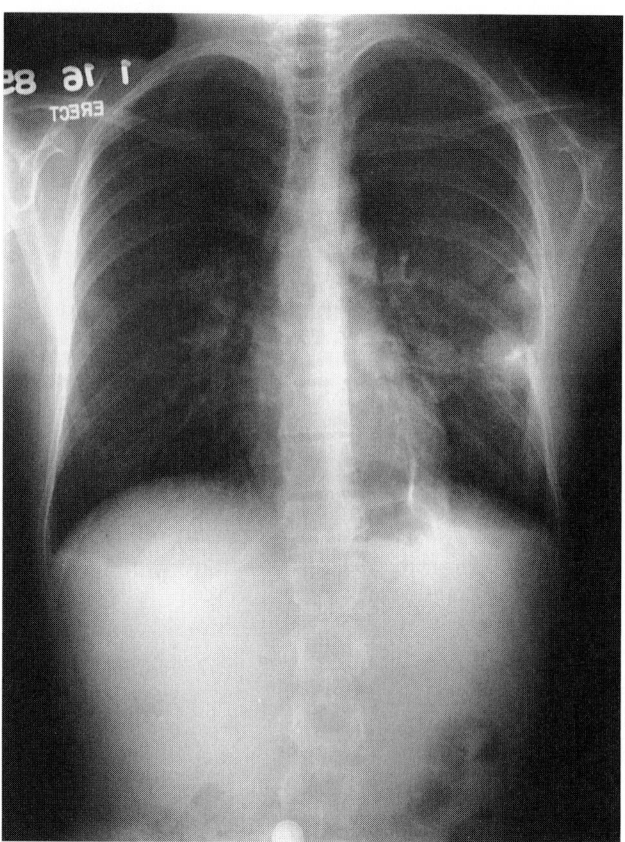

FIGURE 82.5. Chest radiograph from a Wegener's granulomatosis patient with multiple nodules. (Courtesy of Dr. Myung S. Shin.)

A rapidly progressive course of WG, culminating in death, has been well documented. In the pretreatment era, average survival was only 5 months after the onset of disease, and there was an 83% mortality rate at 1 year, with the majority of deaths attributed to renal failure (175). A subset of patients with a slower course of disease has since been recognized. Thirty percent of the patients described from the NIH had a delay in diagnosis of greater than 1 year (169). Nine patients have been described whose prediagnostic symptoms recurred over a period of more than 3 years, and in one person, as long as 20 years (176). The concept of a "limited form of WG" embodies an absence of clinical renal disease, an improved prognosis, and better responsiveness to glucocorticoids (177,178). Granulomas and focal angiitis were noted in a few kidney biopsy specimens in patients with limited WG, but glomerulonephritis was absent. Others have observed focal glomerulonephritis on renal biopsy in greater than 50% of cases with limited WG (179). Whether or not limited WG is a separate entity or merely reflects less widespread disease remains speculative. The absence of clinically detectable renal disease, however, seems to portend a disease course with a much better prognosis.

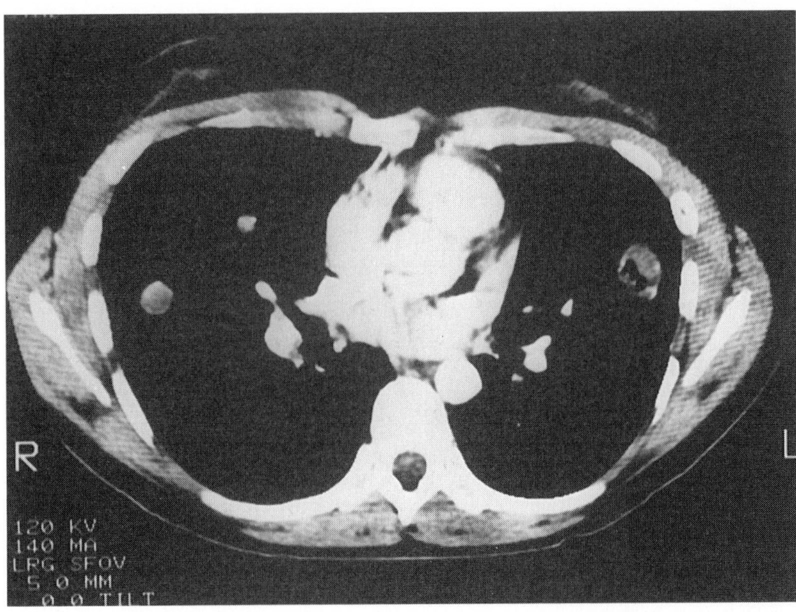

FIGURE 82.6. Computed tomography of the chest in a patient with Wegener's granulomatosis demonstrating multiple nodules, one of which is cavitating. (Courtesy of Dr. Myung S. Shin.)

In general, other manifestations of WG precede the renal manifestations. Urinary abnormalities are usually those of glomerulonephritis with hematuria, proteinuria, pyuria, and erythrocyte casts. Eighteen percent of NIH patients initially had renal involvement, and 70% of these developed glomerulonephritis during the course of the disease, the majority occurring within the first 2 years of disease onset. The common renal lesion is a focal and segmental necrotizing glomerulonephritis. Vasculitis and granuloma formation are infrequent findings on renal biopsy specimens (169). There also has been minimal immunoglobulin and complement deposition in these (171,180). The progression from mild to severe glomerulonephritis may occur within several days in some patients with WG, resulting in abrupt loss of renal function (170,181). In contrast to other systemic necrotizing vasculitides with renal involvement, hypertension is uncommon, even in the presence of severe renal failure (182,183).

Eye signs are common and are ascribed to contiguous granulomatous sinus disease and focal vasculitis (169). The spread of disease from the sinuses causes proptosis, nasolacrimal duct obstruction, and ocular muscle or nerve lesions. Focal vasculitis may cause conjunctivitis, episcleritis, scleritis, corneoscleral ulceration, uveitis, and lesions of the optic nerve or retina. Proptosis, which occurs in 15% to 22% of patients, is the most diagnostically useful sign and is due to pseudotumor or orbital cellulitis. Retroorbital pseudotumors are the primary cause of loss of vision in about 8% of persons with WG (184).

The other prominent disease features are fever and arthralgias/myalgias. Patients may have persistent or recurrent monarticular or polyarticular arthritis, which often leads to diagnostic confusion when other classic features of WG are absent. Skin lesions found in WG include palpable purpura, ulcers, vesicles, papules, and subcutaneous nodules. The most common cardiac complication is pericarditis, encountered in 6% of 158 NIH patients. Neurologic signs and symptoms are rarely seen at the onset of disease, but about 15% of patients have mononeuritis multiplex during the course of disease (169). Frequencies of disease manifestations are shown at presentation and during the course of disease in Fig. 82.7.

Hallmark pathologic features are necrotizing granulomatous inflammation and vasculitis within the upper and lower respiratory tract, and glomerulonephritis (175,185). Earlier clinical recognition and the use of tissue biopsy procedures, particularly of the lung, have broadened the recognized spectrum of pathologic manifestations in WG. The three major pathologic features reported in a review of lung biopsy specimens from 67 patients were (a) parenchymal necrosis, including microabscesses; (b) vasculitis in arteries, veins, and capillaries; and (c) granulomatous inflammation with a mixed inflammatory infiltrate (186) (Fig. 82.8). Several nonspecific changes in lung biopsy tissue were sometimes the predominant finding. These so-called minor pathologic features of WG included tissue eosinophilia, alveolar hemorrhage, interstitial fibrosis, lipoid pneumonia, and a variety of bronchial or bronchiolar lesions. Of note, some degree of tissue eosinophilia was present on nearly all the biopsy specimens, although it was usually graded as mild. Acute and chronic hemorrhage also was seen in nearly half of the lung biopsies (186). Over the past few years, diffuse pulmonary hemorrhage has been increasingly recognized as a complication of this disease; WG has been reported to be the most common cause of diffuse pulmonary hemorrhage (187).

The diagnosis of WG is clinicopathologic, requiring careful interpretation of the clinical, laboratory, and patho-

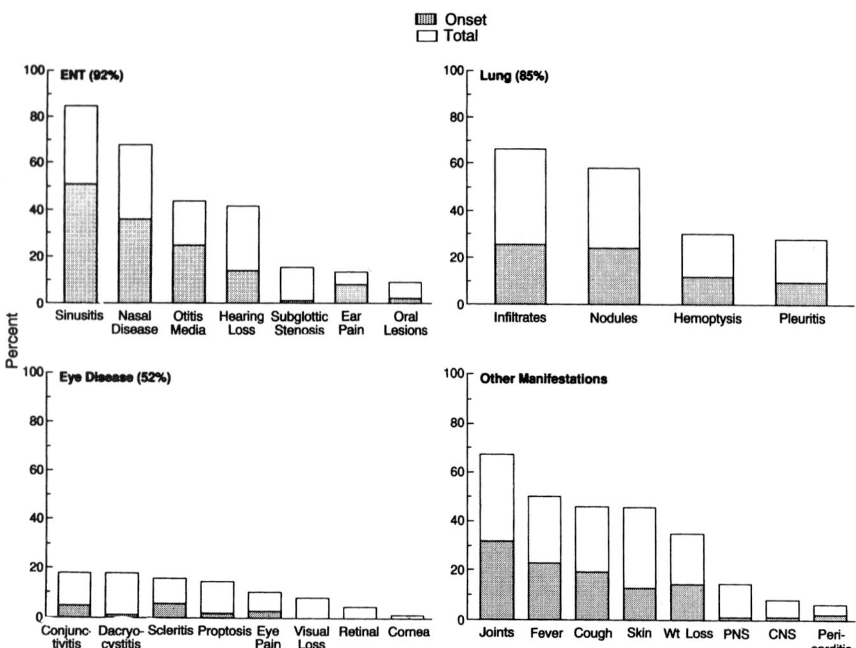

FIGURE 82.7. Type and frequency of disease manifestations are represented at the time of presentation and as they may have occurred during the course of illness. *ENT*, ear, nose, and throat involvement. (Reproduced with permission from Hoffman GS, Kerr GS, Leavitt RY, et al. Wegener granulomatosis: an analysis of 158 patients. *Ann Intern Med* 1992;116: 490.)

logic data. In the absence of the full-blown clinical syndrome, the diagnosis may be difficult because of similarities to other entities. A significant achievement in the study of vasculitis has been the identification of ANCAs. The high sensitivity and specificity of cANCAs for WG was first recognized by Van der Woude et al. in 1985 (188) and confirmed by others (189,190). As mentioned elsewhere, it is now obvious that cANCAs are seen occasionally in other disorders. Several studies of WG have observed significant variation in the sensitivity of cANCAs with the activity and extent of disease. In patients with active generalized WG, the sensitivity of cANCAs has surpassed 90% (189,190).

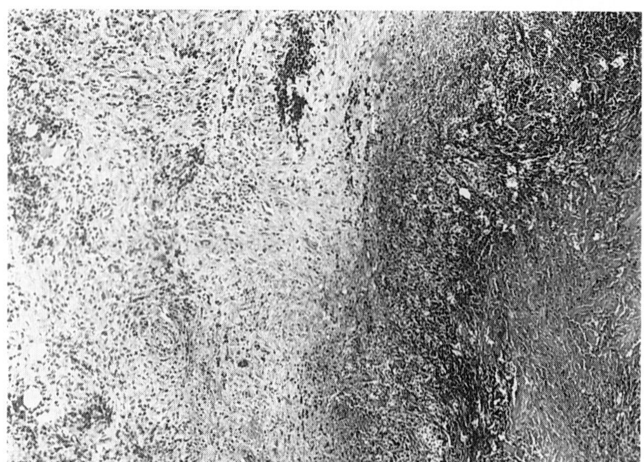

FIGURE 82.8. Open lung biopsy specimen revealing layers of geographic necrosis and scattered giant cells in a patient with Wegener's granulomatosis. (Courtesy of Dr. Robert M. Gay.)

The positivity of cANCAs drops off, however, in cases with active but localized involvement. A tendency of cANCA titers to parallel disease activity also has been reported by a number of investigators, resulting in studies to determine its reliability as a gauge of disease activity. Although exceptions have been noted, the majority of these studies have reported changes of cANCA titers in tandem with disease activity (174,188,190,191). At least one study indicated that an increase in titer in the absence of clinical deterioration may be indicative of subclinical disease activity predicting relapse, and warrants consideration of immunosuppressive therapy (174). Others have determined that the relation between disease activity and cANCA titers is unpredictable. For example, among 106 patients, an increase in titers preceded relapses in only 24%, whereas there was no direct correlation between titer and disease activity in 27% of patients (192). Lang et al. (193) have described a patient with WG whose illness remitted after some period of treatment, but whose anti-PR3 antibody titers remained "excessively" high for 3 years. These data bolster the argument against initiation or increase of potentially dangerous immunosuppressive therapy based solely on an increased ANCA titer.

Pathologic confirmation of the diagnosis is mandated by the life-threatening nature of WG and the toxicity of immunosuppressive therapy. Open lung biopsy often is required, and is the procedure of highest diagnostic usefulness. For example, diagnostic tissue specimens were obtained in 91% of open lung biopsies (169). Because of the high specificity of cANCAs, it could be argued that a positive result in the proper clinical setting would obviate the need for biopsy. In a given patient, excluding mycobacterial and fungal infections in both the lung and upper airways is necessary because these may mimic WG by causing necrotizing granulomas and vasculitis (170,186). Skin biopsies usually reveal changes of leukocytoclastic vasculitis, and renal biopsies rarely show granulomatous inflammation or vasculitis (169).

Diagnosis of early WG is complicated by the absence of the "classic triad" of clinical manifestations, or pathognomonic tissue abnormalities. Granulomatous involvement of the head and neck without vasculitis has been described as the first phase of disease (194). The interpretation of nasal and sinus biopsies has been scrutinized recently in an attempt to refine their diagnostic usefulness (195–197). The small size of specimens has made it difficult to obtain histologic evidence of vasculitis from these and other head and neck biopsies; thus emphasis has been placed on other features including mucosal ulceration, acute and chronic inflammation, necrosis, and granulomatous changes. In general, the number of pathologic manifestations required to confirm the diagnosis should be inversely related to the extent of clinical symptoms. Biopsies from the paranasal sinuses usually have a higher diagnostic yield than those of the nasal mucosa (195,197).

The use of glucocorticoids alone to treat WG prolongs the survival rate from 5 months without therapy to 12.5 months (198). Since the advent of treatment with cytotoxic agents, its prognosis has improved significantly. Cyclophosphamide is now considered the treatment of choice because its efficacy has been prospectively documented in a group of 158 patients treated at the NIH (126) and confirmed by others (169–171,199,200). Full remission was achieved in 75% and significant improvement in 91% of patients treated with low-dose cyclophosphamide and prednisone. Relapses are common.

A treatment protocol has been recommended by investigators at the NIH for combined cyclophosphamide and prednisone use in WG and other forms of systemic vasculitis (Table 82.6) (169,181). It is designed to treat the vasculitis effectively without severely compromising the immune system. Specifically, maintenance of the total white blood cell and neutrophil counts above arbitrarily defined levels, and the use of alternate-day prednisone dosing, are likely to reduce the number of infectious complications. Nevertheless, 73 (46%) of 158 persons treated with this regimen experienced one or more serious infections (169). Infectious complications also have been reported in 10 of 15 patients treated with a similar regimen for WG, PAN, or isolated angiitis of the CNS (201). The need to taper the prednisone to alternate-day dosing as soon as possible, and to follow the leukocyte counts closely, should be emphasized. Fifty percent of serious infections occur during periods of daily glucocorticoid therapy. Patients with less fulminant or slowly progressive disease also may be treated effectively with cyclophosphamide alone (9,132). Despite a stable dose of cyclophosphamide, leukocyte counts should be checked as often as every 2 to 4 weeks to avoid leukopenia. Glucocorticoids counter the bone marrow suppression induced by cyclophosphamide, and therefore, neutropenia may develop when prednisone is reduced. Although there are no definite guidelines regarding the duration of treatment with cyclophosphamide, it seems reasonable to taper and discontinue its use after 1 year of clinical remission. In lieu of daily oral cyclophosphamide, monthly pulse doses have been used in an attempt to reduce toxicity, which includes induction of various tumors as well as infection and bone marrow failure. Although this issue is controversial, the opinion favoring the use of maintenance oral drug seems more persuasive (202). Relapses are common in WG, and chronic, continuous, treatment with cyclophosphamide should be avoided if possible because of cumulative drug toxicity. Judged by a therapeutic trial at the NIH, methotrexate may represent an alternative drug for some patients. Forty-two patients were given 17.5- to 20-mg weekly doses of methotrexate in addition to the usual dose of prednisone. Patients with rapidly progressive renal or pulmonary failure were given the cyclophosphamide/prednisone regimen. Sixty per cent of those treated with methotrexate had signs of disease activity in three or more organ systems, and 50% had active glomerulonephritis. Complete remission

TABLE 82.6. COMBINED CYCLOPHOSPHAMIDE–PREDNISONE THERAPY FOR SEVERE SYSTEMIC VASCULITIS

Cyclophosphamide: Initial dose of 2 mg/kg/day orally; adjust so that white blood cell count remains >3,000–3,500/mm^3 (neutrophil count, 1,000–1,500/mm^3); continue therapy with frequent downward adjustments of dosage, to prevent severe neutropenia; continue therapy for a year after induction of complete remission, and then taper dose by 25-mg decrements every 2 mo until discontinued.

Prednisone: Initial dose of 1 mg/kg/day in three to four divided doses for 7–10 days; consolidate to single morning dose by 2–3 weeks; continue single morning daily dose until patient has had 1 mo total corticosteroid treatment; convert to alternate-day regimen for the second month; maintain alternate-day regimen for the third month, followed by gradual tapering of alternate-day dose for the next 3–6 mo

Reproduced with permission from Fauci AS, Leavitt RY. Systemic vasculitis. In: Lichtenstein LM, Fauci AS, eds. *Current therapy in allergy, immunology, and rheumatology.* 3rd ed. Philadelphia: BC Decker, 1988:1308.

was achieved in 33 of the 42 patients; however, three patients had progressive disease requiring institution of cyclophosphamide. Signs of relapse appeared in 19 of the 33 who achieved remission; in all but two, these appeared when methotrexate was either discontinued or decreased (203). Less satisfactory results with a similar regimen of methotrexate and prednisone have been reported by Stone et al. (204). Although 14 of 19 patients achieved remission, seven of them relapsed, and there were no sustained, complete remissions. This was a retrospective study, and the data for dosages were incomplete. The methotrexate dose at relapse was available for only seven patients; it varied from 0 in one, to 20 mg in one. The mean dose at relapse for the six patients taking the drug was 10.8 mg/week.

The exact role of trimethoprim/sulfamethoxazole in the treatment of WG has not been established. There have been enough anecdotal reports of patients achieving remissions while taking trimethoprim/sulfamethoxazole, as well as relapse after discontinuation, to consider its use as prophylaxis in selected patients (205). Conversely, a prospective study of trimethoprim/sulfamethoxazole therapy for maintenance of remission in patients with systemic WG determined that this combination was inferior to low-dose methotrexate, and in fact, appeared to increase the chance of remission (206). There may be a role for this drug in treatment of selected patients with limited disease that spares the kidneys. The National Institute of Allergy and Infectious Diseases is currently conducting a study of etanercept in treatment of WG.

Kawasaki Disease

Kawasaki disease, first described by Tomasaka Kawasaki in 1967, and also known as mucocutaneous lymph node syndrome, is an acute form of systemic vasculitis that affects primarily infants and children. In this illness, there is a proclivity for coronary artery vasculitis as well as a characteristic clinical pattern consisting of persistent fever, cutaneous lesions, mucosal inflammation, and cervical lymphadenopathy. It occurs worldwide, but is most prevalent in Japan. Community-wide epidemics occur most often in the winter and spring, and their pattern suggests an infectious cause in genetically susceptible children. Leung et al. (207) have reviewed studies pertaining to the immunopathogenesis of this disease and the grounds for indicting staphylococcal and streptococcal toxins as its primary cause. Symptoms of Kawasaki disease are usually self-limited, but the development of coronary artery aneurysms may lead to myocardial infarction, sudden death, and chronic coronary insufficiency. Autopsy studies of children dying with the disease invariably reveal inflammation of small and medium-sized blood vessels.

In the absence of a diagnostic laboratory test, diagnostic guidelines have been promulgated (Table 82.7). Diagnosis is considered definite if five of six of the principal signs are met, or four of six when coronary artery aneurysms are documented by echocardiography or angiography. High spiking fevers of 103°F to 105°F usually mark the onset of the illness, and on average, persist for 10 to 12 days in the absence of therapy. The typical clinical progression to conjunctivitis and oropharyngeal lesions follows within the first 3 days of illness. Swelling of the hands and feet, erythema of the palms and soles, and rash subsequently develop within 5 days of the onset of the fever (208,209). The erythematous rash is not associated with vesicles or crusts. At approximately 2 weeks after the onset of fever, there is desquamation of the fingertips. Cervical lymphadenopathy is the least reliable clinical marker, occurring in just over 50% of patients. Some nonspecific features of Kawasaki disease and their frequencies are CNS abnormalities, 90%; urethral inflammation with sterile pyuria, 70%; arthritis, 40%; aseptic meningitis, 20%; severe abdominal pain and diarrhea, 20%; and obstructive jaundice with hepatic dysfunction usually due to hydrops of the gallbladder, 10% (209). Common laboratory abnormalities include leukocytosis, anemia, thrombocytosis, elevated liver transaminase levels, and sterile pyuria.

TABLE 82.7. PRINCIPAL SIGNS OF KAWASAKI DISEASE

1. Fever persisting for ≥5 days
2. Bilateral conjunctival injection
3. Changes of lips and oropharynx
   - Erythema, fissuring, or crusting of lips
   - Strawberry tongue
   - Diffuse erythema of oropharynx
4. Cervical lymphadenopathy
5. Changes of peripheral extremities
   - Erythema of palms or soles
   - Edema of hands or feet
   - Desquamation of fingertips and toetips

Practitioners are faced with the clinical dilemma of establishing an early diagnosis before the onset of coronary complications. Many of the features of Kawasaki disease are present in other pediatric illnesses, and some patients with fewer than four of the principal signs develop coronary aneurysms. Burns et al. (210) have compared the physical findings and laboratory studies of 280 Kawasaki disease patients with 42 children referred for evaluation of possible Kawasaki disease in whom alternative diagnoses were established. Infectious disease, particularly measles and group A β-hemolytic streptococcal infections, followed by presumed self-limited viral infections, drug reactions, and juvenile RA, most often mimicked Kawasaki disease. Forty-six percent of the comparison group fulfilled diagnostic criteria for Kawasaki disease; however, discrete intraoral lesions, exudative conjunctivitis and pharyngitis, and generalized adenopathy were much less common in patients with Kawasaki disease. Laboratory abnormalities more common in Kawasaki disease were anemia, an elevated ESR, and increased serum alanine aminotransferase activity.

Kawasaki disease has emerged as the leading cause of acquired heart disease in the pediatric population in Japan and the U.S. During the initial stages of Kawasaki disease, myocarditis can be inferred from electrocardiographic, echocardiographic, radiographic, and clinical abnormalities in 50% of patients. A direct relation between myocarditis and coronary aneurysm formation has not been observed (211). As determined by coronary arteriography, the percentage of Kawasaki disease patients who develop coronary artery lesions has varied from 15% to 25% in large numbers of Japanese patients. Aneurysms are significantly more common than stenosis or occlusion within 1 year of disease onset, whereas after 1 year, stenoses and occlusions become more apparent (212). Disappearance of coronary aneurysms was demonstrated in 21 of 42 patients in one angiographic study (213). Coronary angiography is now done less often because of the high sensitivity and specificity (100% and 97%, respectively) of two-dimensional echocardiography for detection of aneurysms within the first 4 weeks of disease onset (214). Despite the significant number of patients with coronary artery lesions, myocardial infarction occurs in only 0.9% to 1.3%, mainly within the first year (215). It is unknown if Kawasaki disease patients are predisposed to premature development of coronary atherosclerosis, but pathologic examination has revealed fibrous intimal thickening in vessels of normal caliber obtained from Kawasaki disease patients who died of other causes (216). Other cardiac complications include pericardial effusions in as many as 35% of patients during the acute stage (213), and residual mitral valvular disease in 1% (217).

The two primary goals in the management of Kawasaki disease are reduction of inflammation in the myocardium and coronary vessels and prevention of thrombosis. Despite a lack of understanding of the etiology and pathogenesis, aspirin and high-dose intravenous gammaglobulin have emerged as effective therapy. There is no clear evidence that the antiinflammatory properties of aspirin retard the development of coronary lesions; however, it is now well established that intravenous gammaglobulin treatment administered within the first 10 days of disease onset significantly reduces the prevalence of coronary artery abnormalities. Treatment with intravenous gammaglobulin at 400 mg/kg/day for 4 days plus aspirin at 80 to 100 mg/kg/day was demonstrated to be more effective than aspirin alone in reducing coronary artery abnormalities detected by echocardiogram in the first 2 months after illness (218) and 1 to 2 years later (219). A single infusion of 2 g/kg of intravenous gammaglobulin is now thought to be more effective in reducing coronary abnormalities at 2 months than the 4-day regimen. Patients treated with the single-infusion regimen defervesced more rapidly, and there was a more rapid return to normal of laboratory indicators of acute inflammation (220).

Thromboangiitis Obliterans (Buerger's Disease)

Thromboangiitis obliterans, better known as Buerger's disease, has received little attention in the literature of vasculitis and was not included in the 1990 ACR criteria for the classification of vasculitis. Buerger first described the disease in 1908 and later defined it as, "A disease in which an acute inflammatory lesion and occlusive thrombosis of the arteries and veins are the characteristic lesions" (221).

The exact prevalence of thromboangiitis obliterans is unknown, but it varies in different geographic regions. It is more common in Southeast Asia, India, and the Middle East, and appears to be highest in populations with the largest percentage of cigarette smokers. In these regions, thromboangiitis obliterans is not uncommon [e.g., 39 patients were admitted to a general hospital in Bangladesh during a 2-month period in 1989 (222)]. It appears to be uncommon in blacks, and fewer than 2% of patients reported earlier were older than 50 years, or women; however, among patients at the Cleveland Clinic from 1970 to 1987, 32 (29%) of 112 were older than 50 years, and 23% were women (223). Thromboangiitis obliterans also has been reported to occur in users of smokeless tobacco (224).

The clinical picture of thromboangiitis obliterans is distinct from that of premature atherosclerosis. Initial symptoms are usually intermittent claudication of the arch of the foot and sometimes the hands. Unlike atherosclerosis, the disease begins in the distal circulation of the extremities and then progresses proximally in either a contiguous or skip-zone fashion. The interval from the onset of symptoms to development of ischemic complications is short, ranging from a few months to a couple of years. At initial medical evaluation, rest pain was present in 81%, and ischemic ulcers in 76% of patients reported from the Cleveland Clinic (223). Other frequent manifestations include thrombophlebitis, Raynaud's phenomenon, and paresthesiae. Ischemic neuropathy is the most obvious explanation for the sensory findings, but secondary fibrotic encasement of nerve fibers is another proposed explanation. Involvement of two or more limbs is the rule, and Shionoya (225) has found that approximately 75% of patients have three or four limbs affected. Although legs are more frequently involved than forearms, evaluation of upper extremity circulation should be routine for a person with lower extremity ulcers and a clinical picture compatible with thromboangiitis obliterans. More than 20 persons with intestinal artery lesions have been reported (226).

A variety of disorders affecting the peripheral circulation should be considered in the differential diagnosis. The two most common of these are atherosclerosis and embolization; thus patients suspected of having thromboangiitis obliterans should be evaluated with an arteriogram and an echocardiogram. Connective tissue diseases, other types of vasculitis, antiphospholipid antibody syndrome, blood dyscrasias such as polycythemia vera, ergotamine abuse, frequent use of vibratory tools, hypothenar hammer syndrome, Ehlers–Danlos syndrome, pseudoxanthoma elasticum, calciphylaxis, and thrombosed aneurysms are other diagnostic considerations (227). Multiple, bilateral, focal segments of stenosis or occlusions with more severe changes distally are the characteristic arteriographic abnormalities. Collateral vessels are abundant and often have a corkscrew configuration. Although none of the angiographic features is pathognomonic for thromboangiitis obliterans, the pattern of involvement can often be distinguished from that of other peripheral vascular diseases, with the exception of atherosclerosis in some diabetic patients. The digital, pedal, and calf arteries on both sides are affected in nearly all patients (228,229). In 105 patients studied by Shionoya (228), bilateral infrapopliteal occlusions were seen with this distribution: 90% anterior tibial artery; 80% posterior tibial artery; and 50% peroneal artery. Progression to the suprapopliteal region occurred in about 40% of patients; iliac disease is encountered in only 10% of cases (230).

The histopathology of acute lesions, especially of veins, is distinct and specific for thromboangiitis obliterans. It comprises thrombosis and vasculitis, with microabscesses containing a variable number of multinucleated giant cells within the thrombus (123). The inflammatory infiltrate of the vessel wall is primarily lymphocytic, and there is an absence of fibrinoid necrosis. It has been uncommon to obtain such specimens, however, because of the fear that biopsy of an already ischemic extremity will lead to new skin ulcerations.

Abstinence from tobacco in all forms is the only way to prevent progression of disease. Olin et al. (223) reported that 42% of amputations in their patients occurred in those who continued to smoke, but there were only two amputations among persons who discontinued cigarette smoking, and both of these already had critical ischemia with gangrene at the time they discontinued smoking. Other medical treatments such as glucocorticoids, vasodilators, antiplatelet agents, and anticoagulants have proven ineffective. Intraarterial infusion of prostaglandin E_1 and thrombolytic therapy may help avoid amputation in selected patients who have discontinued tobacco use (227). Oral iloprost may be more effective than placebo in relieving rest pain. Surgical revascularization is usually not a feasible alternative because of distal occlusive arterial disease, and long-term results have been poor for the few patients who have undergone arterial bypass procedures.

Because of the strong association with tobacco use, thromboangiitis obliterans has been considered an autoimmune reaction triggered by tobacco use. One group of investigators has shown that patients with thromboangiitis obliterans exhibit increased cellular sensitivity to types I and III collagen (constituents of human arteries) and produce significant levels of anticollagen antibodies (231). The same group was unable to demonstrate any differences in the humoral and cellular responses to tobacco glycoprotein between thromboangiitis obliterans patients and smokers without the disease (232), suggesting that other factors may be involved in its pathogenesis. ANCAs were found in sera of 15 of 27 patients with this disorder; six of the 15 ANCAs were MPO positive, and four were positive for lactoferrin (233). Anti–endothelial cell antibodies may play a role in the pathogenesis of thromboangiitis obliterans; high titers of these were found in seven patients with active disease (234).

Cutaneous Vasculitis (Hypersensitivity Vasculitis)

Leukocytoclastic vasculitis is the most common type of cutaneous vasculitis and is often the first indication that a person has systemic vasculitis, although approximately 50% of cases are limited to the skin (Fig. 82.9). It is histopathologically defined as fibrinoid necrosis of the vessel wall accompanied by a neutrophilic infiltrate within and around

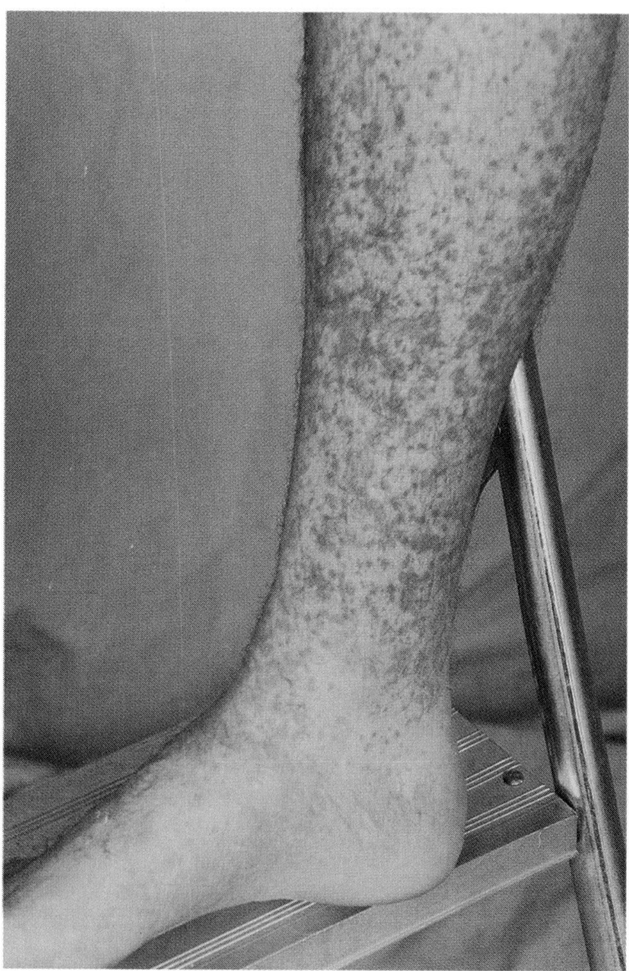

FIGURE 82.9. Leukocytoclastic vasculitis in a 40-year-old man with type II cryoglobulinemia and circulating hepatitis C virus RNA.

the vessel, leukocytoclasis, extravasation of erythrocytes, and endothelial swelling. Palpable purpura of the lower extremities and buttocks is present in more than half of leukocytoclastic vasculitis cases, but other clinical manifestations include, in descending order of frequency, urticaria-like lesions, ulceration, nodules, vesiculobullous lesions, erythematous plaques, livedo reticularis, erythematous papules, and necrosis (235).

Autoimmune diseases, lymphoproliferative disorders or malignancies, systemic vasculitis, infections, and hypersensitivity drug reactions all appear to cause leukocytoclastic vasculitis at times. Table 82.8 summarizes the prevalence of associated conditions from a report of 101 cases of cutaneous necrotizing vasculitis. Many drugs have been implicated as etiologic agents, and in most cases, the vasculitic eruption begins a few days after their initiation. Penicillin and its derivatives and sulfa drugs are the most common offenders. Palpable purpura usually develops acutely, appearing in crops, with individual lesions measuring from 3 to 6 mm in diameter. Small lesions may lack palpability but may progress to as large as 1 cm in diameter or become confluent with adjacent lesions to form plaques. Individual lesions usually persist from 1 to 4 weeks and often heal with residual hyperpigmentation. The ESR is frequently increased, but this does not separate systemic vasculitis from disease limited to the skin. Other laboratory data may suggest a type of vasculitis or reflect involved organ systems.

TABLE 82.8. DISORDERS ASSOCIATED WITH CUTANEOUS VASCULITIS

Disorder
Necrotizing vasculitis associated with coexistent disease
Autoimmune (33%)
Rheumatoid arthritis (12%)
Polyarteritis nodosa (7%)
Systemic lupus erythematosus (6%)
Sjögren's syndrome (3%)
Cryoglobulinemia (3%)
Hypergammaglobulinemic purpura (2%)
Malignancy (8%)
Systemic granulomatous vasculitis (5%)
Wegener's granulomatosis (3%)
Allergic granulomatosis (Churg–Strauss, 2%)
Miscellaneous (3%)
Granuloma faciale
Necrotizing vasculitis associated with precipitating events (22%)
Drug reaction (13%)
Bacterial infection (8%)
Viral infection (1%)
Necrotizing vasculitis of uncertain cause (30%)
Idiopathic palpable purpura (13%)
Chronic urticaria or angioedema (10%)
Henoch–Schönlein purpura (4%)
Idiopathic vasculitis with nodules (3%)

Reproduced with permission from Sanchez NP, Van Hale HM, Su WPD, et al. Clinical and histopathologic spectrum of necrotizing vasculitis: report of findings in 101 cases. *Arch Dermatol* 1985;121:220–221.

Approximately 50% of patients with leukocytoclastic vasculitis will have lesions in other organ systems, usually the musculoskeletal, renal, gastrointestinal, pulmonary, and peripheral nervous systems (235).

Biopsy is necessary to confirm the presence of leukocytoclastic vasculitis in all cases because nonvasculitic skin lesions may closely resemble palpable purpura (Fig. 82.10). For example, purpura simplex is a group of clinical syndromes in which leakage of erythrocytes from postcapillary venules is present without any evidence of blood vessel destruction (236). Thrombosis of small dermal blood vessels is a feature of septic vasculitis (237), but when this is the primary histologic feature, coagulation disorders such as thrombotic thrombocytopenic purpura, cryoglobulinemia and cryofibrinogenemia, coumarin-induced necrosis, and antiphospholipid syndrome must be excluded. Special stains to detect infectious organisms such as Neisseria species, cytomegalovirus, and spirochetes that can cause direct blood vessel damage should be done in all cases of leukocytoclastic vasculitis.

Direct immunofluorescence of leukocytoclastic vasculitis most commonly reveals deposition of IgM, C3, and fibrin, and is more sensitive if lesions of less than 24-hour duration

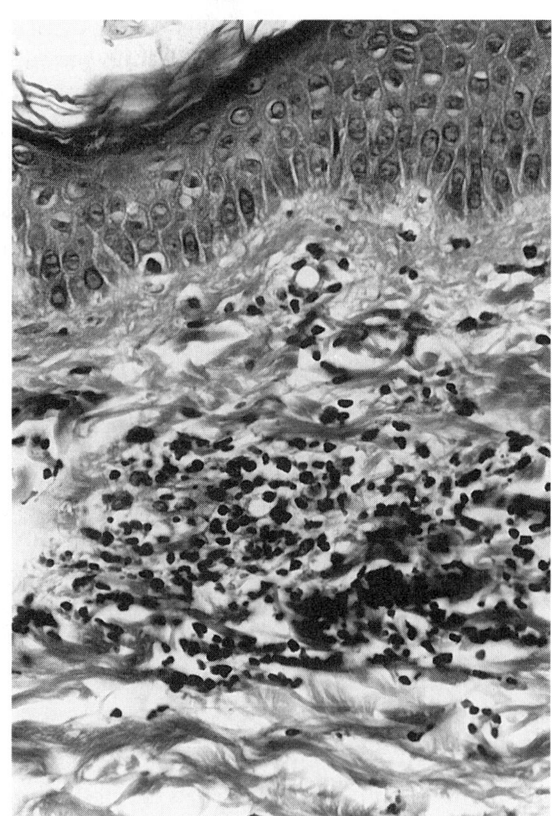

FIGURE 82.10. Skin biopsy of a patient with leukocytoclastic vasculitis, as demonstrated by involvement of postcapillary venules and leukocytoclasis (nuclear debris). (Courtesy of Dr. Robert M. Gay.)

are sampled. In addition to confirming the presence of leukocytoclastic vasculitis, a biopsy also may provide information suggesting a specific etiology [e.g., IgA deposits are characteristic for but not diagnostic of HSP; they are found in streptococcal infections (238)]. Patients with SLE frequently have dermal mucin deposition and an inflammatory infiltrate at the dermoepidermal junction. Vascular plugging with eosinophilic material also has been demonstrated frequently in cryoglobulinemia (237). Although it has not been emphasized, the infiltrate in leukocytoclastic vasculitis is usually mixed with equal numbers of neutrophils and mononuclear cells. Sanchez et al. (238) have reported that a biopsy with an overwhelming predominance of neutrophils is characteristic of hypocomplementemic vasculitis. They also correlated greater extent and depth of the vasculitic process in the skin with the presence of systemic vasculitis.

If there is no evidence of systemic vasculitis on first evaluation, the likelihood of its occurrence is low (235,239). The prognosis of leukocytoclastic vasculitis in a community setting is remarkably better than has been reported from tertiary medical centers, with only two fatalities among 82 consecutive cases. Approximately 50% of leukocytoclastic vasculitis patients will have no discernible associated disease or causative factor. Urticaria-like lesions and livedo reticularis are more likely to be complicated by a chronic course (235). Management decisions for leukocytoclastic vasculitis patients should be individualized because no therapeutic approach is consistently effective. Simple measures include avoidance of cold and prolonged standing. In patients taking an identifiable precipitating drug, its removal may be all that is necessary. Treatment of associated conditions also may have a beneficial effect on leukocytoclastic vasculitis. Patients with recurrent cutaneous vasculitis limited to the skin seldom have progression of their disease, and aggressive management is not warranted. Furthermore, Cupps et al. (240) observed poor responses to aggressive therapy with glucocorticoids and cyclophosphamide in such patients. Their observations are contrary to those of physicians who believe that glucocorticoids are clearly indicated. It is probably wise to reserve the prolonged use of immunosuppressive agents for patients in whom skin necrosis develops (239). In patients with cutaneous vasculitis limited to the lower legs without ulceration, appropriate initial therapy is colchicine at a dose of 0.6 mg, two to three times daily (241). Dapsone, 75 to 150 mg daily, is an alternative treatment in unresponsive or progressive cases (242).

Henoch–Schönlein Purpura

HSP, a systemic disease of small vessels, is the most common pediatric vasculitis syndrome, with an estimated incidence in a pediatric population of 13.5/100,000/year (243). There are descriptions of adults with HSP, but the majority of patients are boys between the ages of 2 to 11 years. Blanco et al. (244) studied 303 patients with cutaneous vasculitis. The absence of suitable criteria for differentiating hypersensitivity vasculitis and HSP was emphasized. They diagnosed HSP when patients had three or more of the following: palpable purpura, abdominal angina, gastrointestinal bleeding, hematuria, age at onset younger than 20 years, and no medications as a precipitating factor. Within these boundaries, 14 children and 70 adults were thought to have hypersensitivity vasculitis, and 116 children and 39 adults had HSP. These classic signs and symptoms develop in a variable time sequence and in different combinations. The long-term prognosis is determined largely by the degree of renal involvement, but the majority of HSP patients have a benign and self-limited condition.

Although it is the presenting sign in only 50% of patients, palpable nonthrombocytopenic purpura is a prerequisite for the diagnosis of HSP. The appearance of petechiae and purpura within areas of urticarial or erythematous maculopapular lesions is classic, but the rash may present as erythema multiforme. Gravity-dependent areas such as the buttocks and the lower extremities are characteristic sites for the purpuric rash, but it also may be seen on the face, arms, and trunk. The rash may be transient or persist for several weeks, and has been reported to recur in almost half of patients (245). Skin biopsy reveals leukocytoclastic vasculitis, with characteristic findings on direct immunofluorescence of IgA, C3, and fibrin/fibrinogen within the involved vessels (35). Localized angioedema of the face, hands, arms, feet, and scrotum is the other prominent cutaneous manifestation of HSP, occurring in 45% of patients (246).

Joint symptoms are the second most common feature of HSP, and swelling of joints is the initial manifestation in 25% of children (245). Swelling is usually due to periarticular inflammation rather than effusion or hemarthrosis. The knees and ankles are most commonly affected, whereas finger and wrist involvement is unusual. In most patients, the arthritis is nonmigratory, of short duration, and nondamaging.

Cramping abdominal pain is the third most common sign of HSP and is usually attributed to submucosal and intramural extravasation of fluid or blood caused by mesenteric vasculitis. Occult gastrointestinal bleeding occurs in more than half the patients (247), but only 5% develop serious gastrointestinal hemorrhage. Vomiting frequently accompanies the abdominal pain, but hematemesis is noted in fewer than 10% of patients. Although gastrointestinal manifestations usually followed onset of rash, abdominal pain preceded the rash in 19 (14%) of 131 patients (245). The pain may be severe enough to suggest a surgical abdomen; however, lesions requiring operation seldom precede the typical rash. Otherwise, an increase in severity of abdominal pain or its acute onset in HSP may be caused by intussusception, bowel infarction, bowel perforation, pancreatitis, or hydrops of the gallbladder. Surgical abdominal lesions appear in 2% to 6% of HSP patients, with intussusception most common, whereas intestinal infarction and perforation are infrequent (248). Almost all intussusceptions are ileocolic in the general population, but 66% of HSP intussusceptions are confined to the small intestine (247). Ultrasound is a useful tool for evaluating abdominal pain, as it rapidly and reliably detects surgical complications such as intussusception and perforation, as well as edematous hemorrhagic infiltration of the intestinal wall (249). Endoscopic lesions are largely nonspecific, although hemorrhagic erosive duodenitis involving the second portion of the duodenum may suggest the diagnosis in patients in whom gastrointestinal symptoms develop before the pathognomonic rash (250,251).

Renal disease is the major source of morbidity and mortality in HSP. The exact prevalence of glomerulonephritis in HSP has not been established, although, based on the detection of renal abnormalities in 55 of 270 unselected patients, 20% is probably a close estimate (243). Clinical expression ranges from transient, isolated microscopic hematuria to rapidly progressive glomerulonephritis. Asymptomatic microscopic or gross hematuria is the most common finding, and is frequently accompanied by proteinuria. Nephritis precedes the purpura in only about 3% of patients (247) and is usually evident within 3 months of the onset of rash (252). There has been no consistent relation between the severity of glomerulonephritis and other disease manifestations; however, gastrointestinal disease usually coincides with renal disease, and exacerbations of nephritis may coincide with episodes of recurrent purpura.

In general, the severity of the initial nephritis correlates with the long-term renal outcome. Nearly all HSP patients with isolated hematuria or with proteinuria of less than 1 g/day have complete recovery (253), whereas the majority of children with progressive glomerulonephritis have had acute nephritis or nephrotic syndrome (254). Several studies also have determined that the prognosis depends on the severity of the pathologic process in the kidneys, the proportion of glomeruli with crescents being the best prognostic guide. For example, Niaudet (253) has reported that among 68 patients who had had biopsies showing greater than 50% crescentic glomeruli, 13 had a persistent nephropathy, and 25 progressed to end-stage renal disease. Persistent nephrotic syndrome and the presence of crescents in more than 50% of glomeruli are the two most reliable prognostic indicators of a poor renal outcome. The overall prognosis in HSP has been reported as excellent, as only 1% to 2% of patients have residual nephropathy, and fewer than 1% have end-stage renal disease (243). Prolonged follow-up of 78 HSP nephritis patients (mean duration, 23.4 years after onset) has shown that the renal outcome may not be as benign as was thought (255). Of these patients, 17 deteriorated clinically, among whom seven were judged to have had a complete recovery 10 years after disease onset. Furthermore, 36% of successful pregnancies in this group were complicated by hypertension, persistent proteinuria, or both.

HSP may also be complicated by hemorrhage in other organs. Scrotal swelling and hemorrhage, sometimes involving the testis and epididymis, is encountered in fewer than 10% of male patients (256). Diagnostic confusion with testicular torsion is usually not a problem because testicular involvement is rarely the initial presenting sign of HSP. CNS lesions are uncommon. Headache is the most common CNS symptom, but seizures, subarachnoid and intracerebral hemorrhage, infarction, and hypertensive encephalopathy have all been reported infrequently (257). Pulmonary manifestations of HSP also are unusual, but include severe pulmonary hemorrhage (258).

No laboratory abnormalities have been judged to be sufficiently sensitive or specific for inclusion among diagnostic criteria (259). Anemia secondary to gastrointestinal blood loss, and hematuria and proteinuria from glomerulonephritis, are the most common findings. An elevated ESR and thrombocytosis reflect acute inflammation. Hemorrhagic complications may be related to vitamin K deficiency or diminished factor XIII activity (258). More specific tests for HSP include an elevated serum IgA and skin biopsy revealing leukocytoclastic vasculitis. An increased serum IgA level was detected in all 12 patients tested within 2 weeks of disease onset and suggested the diagnosis (37). IgA is detected on skin biopsies of more than 70% of patients and aids in differentiating HSP from other types of cutaneous vasculitis (260). Renal histopathologic changes range from minimal to those of severe crescentic glomerulonephritis. Mesangial deposits predominate on electron microscopy, but subepithelial and subendothelial deposits may be more prominent in biopsies with marked cellular proliferation. Immunofluorescence detects IgA in 90% of renal biopsies, followed in descending frequency by C3, fibrin, IgG, properdin, and IgM (252). IgA deposits have been found simultaneously in involved skin, kidney, and intestine (34).

Because HSP is most often a self-limited illness, treatment is largely supportive. Glucocorticoids have been useful in managing joint, testicular, and gastrointestinal pain and are recommended for treatment of localized vasculitis of the lungs, testes, and CNS (247). Management of HSP nephritis is highly controversial because there is no clear evidence that any form of therapy alters the course of kidney disease (252,253). Various combinations of steroids, alkylating agents, anticoagulants, and plasmapheresis have been used to treat nephrotic syndrome or nephritis (261), which has been reported to subside with intravenous high-dose immunoglobulin (262). Evaluation of efficacy is clouded by the lack of controlled studies. In one controlled study, factor XIII administration was reported to improve gastrointestinal symptoms (263).

Cutaneous Polyarteritis Nodosa

Although its existence as a distinct disease entity separate from systemic PAN has been debated, cutaneous polyarteritis appears to be distinguished by a benign course and lack of discernible visceral damage. It is thus considered a localized disease process with sparing of visceral arteries; however, the disease is not strictly confined to the skin, as there may be "systemic" features including fever, regional neuropathy, myositis, arthralgias, and arthritis. In 1932, Lindberg recognized polyarteritis confined to the skin. The concept of cutaneous polyarteritis was strengthened by descriptions of 52 patients observed as long as 27 years, who had no clinical evidence of systemic involvement (265,266,268).

Cutaneous polyarteritis has a variable age of onset and no gender predilection. The prevalence of the disease has not been established, but it is not particularly rare, as more than 100 cases have been reported (264). No reports of death have been attributed to cutaneous polyarteritis, and autopsies of patients dying of other causes have not revealed systemic vasculitis (265,266). There is one report of a patient initially with skin disease and a normal urinalysis, CBC, and ESR, in whom systemic PAN was found later (267). Lesions of cutaneous polyarteritis include nodules, livedo reticularis, ulcerations, and gangrene. Nodules are usually painful and tend to occur in crops, ranging from 0.5 to 3.0 cm in diameter. Usually the first sign of the disease, the nodules are predominantly localized to the lower legs below the knee but may involve any part of the body except mucosal surfaces. In comparison, nodules are rarely observed in systemic PAN (122). Livedo reticularis usually occurs later than nodules and is confined to areas of nodulation. This pattern of patchy livedo reticularis with inflammatory nodules within the branches has been considered a unique dermatologic feature of cutaneous polyarteritis and is described as a starburst lesion (Fig. 82.11) (266).

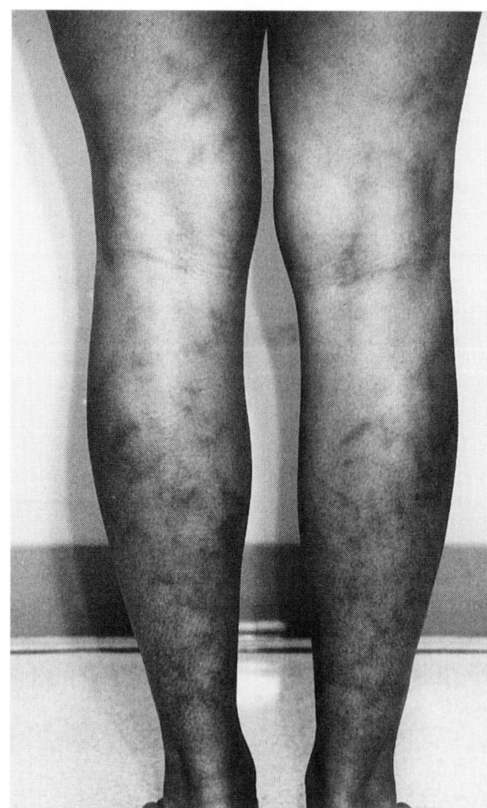

FIGURE 82.11. Numerous postinflammatory hyperpigmented macules in a patient with cutaneous polyarteritis nodosa.

Extracutaneous features have been documented in a significant percentage of cases despite the predominance of cutaneous manifestations (265,266,268). Neuromuscular symptoms are usually localized to areas of skin involvement. Aching pain and stiffness in the calves due to myositis are common, as are peripheral neurologic symptoms, which include numbness, paresthesias, painful neuritis, and mononeuritis multiplex. In contrast to the neuromuscular manifestations, arthralgias may occur in joints remote from areas of skin lesions (266). There also have been a few examples of well-documented nondestructive arthritis (269,270).

The diagnosis is confirmed by excisional biopsy, which must sample the deep dermis and subcutaneous tissue. Inflammation of small and medium-sized arteries is histologically identical to that seen in visceral lesions of systemic PAN and occurs at the dermal–subcutaneous border (271). An elevated ESR is the only consistent laboratory abnormality, although anemia, leukocytosis, and thrombocytosis have been reported.

The etiology of cutaneous polyarteritis is unknown, but IgM, C3, and fibrin deposition within affected vessels on direct immunofluorescent staining suggests that immune complexes are involved in the pathogenesis of the disease (266,270,272,273); however, circulating immune complexes have been detected infrequently. Concurrent streptococcal upper respiratory infections and tuberculosis also suggest immune complex mediation. Cutaneous polyarteritis with hepatitis B antigenemia has been reported (274), and cutaneous polyarteritis has accompanied inflammatory bowel disease (273,275).

Cutaneous polyarteritis has a variable course with frequent relapses and spontaneous remissions, complicating assessment of treatment. The benign prognosis of cutaneous polyarteritis justifies conservative management with analgesics, nonsteroidal antiinflammatory drugs (NSAIDs), and low to moderate doses of glucocorticoids. Salicylates will relieve pain in the majority of patients. More bothersome lesions have been treated with immunosuppressive drugs, colchicine, dapsone, and intravenous immunoglobulins. Myositis and neuritis have been reported to respond to treatment within a period of months (265). Patients with repeated streptococcal infections and recurrences of cutaneous polyarteritis have reportedly benefited from prolonged penicillin therapy (266). Low doses of sulfapyridine also have been reported to induce remissions and may be most effective in cases associated with inflammatory bowel disease (275).

Mixed Cryoglobulinemia and Vasculitis

Cryoglobulins have been classified as type I, consisting of a single monoclonal immunoglobulin; type II, comprising an IgM monoclonal rheumatoid factor plus polyclonal immunoglobulin; and type III, polyclonal immunoglobulins of various isotypes. In 1966, Meltzer et al. (276) described in patients with mixed cryoglobulinemia, a syndrome of purpura, arthralgia, and weakness, which was sometimes accompanied by diffuse glomerulonephritis. This entity, sometimes known as the Meltzer–Franklin syndrome, was designated essential mixed cryoglobulinemia in the absence of other known causes of mixed cryoglobulins such as infectious, autoimmune, or lymphoproliferative disease (two of nine patients had sicca symptoms possibly related to primary Sjögren's syndrome). Although leukocytoclastic vasculitis is the predominant clinical manifestation of all types, postmortem examination has revealed visceral arteritis in some patients. Decreased serum complement and deposition of IgM, IgG, and complement within affected blood vessel walls of skin and glomeruli have provided evidence that the cryoprecipitable immune complexes are directly related to the pathogenesis (276–279).

The largest number of patients with this syndrome has been reported by The Italian Group for the Study of Cryoglobulinaemias. They looked retrospectively at clinical and laboratory features of 913 patients in whom cryoglobulinemia was diagnosed. Six hundred fifty-four were classified as essential cryoglobulinemia, and 259 were associated with other diseases, chief among them being chronic liver disease in 107 persons. Purpura, as the most common manifestation of all types, was found in 75.6% overall, and in 80% of patients with essential cryoglobulinemia. The triad of purpura, weakness, and arthralgia appeared in 30% of those with essential, in 14% of those with chronic liver disease, and in 27% of those whose cryoglobulins were secondary to lymphoproliferative disease. The next two most common symptoms were Raynaud's phenomenon in 19.5%, and those related to the kidney (mainly membranoproliferative glomerulonephritis) in 20% of all patients. Renal involvement and Raynaud's were observed in only 14% and 4.6%, respectively, of patients with chronic liver disease. Biochemical or histologic evidence of hepatitis or cirrhosis was present at some time in their illness in 288 of the 654 patients classified as having essential cryoglobulinemia, in 26 of those with lymphoproliferative diseases, and in eight of 49 patients with connective tissue diseases.

Anti–hepatitis C antibodies, sought in sera from 224 patients, were detected in 79.5% of patients with essential cryoglobulinemia; in 70.3% of those with chronic liver disease; in 87.5% of those with lymphoproliferative disease; and in 40% of patients with connective tissue diseases. The clinical and laboratory features of patients with type II and type III essential cryoglobulinemias were found to be similar in most regards. Both types are associated with various lymphoproliferative disorders, e.g., Waldenström's disease, myeloma, and lymphoma. The differences were a slightly higher prevalence of purpura in type II and significantly greater renal involvement, with more frequent cryocrits greater than 3% and decreased C4 concentrations in type II. They were similar in numbers with regard to liver involvement, rheumatoid factors, neurologic symptoms, and anti-HCV antibodies (280).

A study of 79 patients in Germany detected anti-HCV antibodies in only 17, and HCV-RNA in 11, leading the investigators to conclude there is a south–north gradient in the prevalence of HCV-related cryoglobulinemia in Europe (281). Extending observations of the frequent association of HCV and cryoglobulinemia, Agnello and Gyorgy (282) have detected HCV in the cutaneous vasculitis of persons with type II cryoglobulinemia, the severity of the rash correlating with the level of viremia. Rheumatologic symptoms in patients with chronic hepatitis C infection were similar in those with and without cryoglobulinemia (283).

Essential mixed cryoglobulinemia is most prevalent in middle-aged women, whose illness begins with recurrent episodes of lower extremity purpura of 3 to 10 days' duration. Other prominent cutaneous manifestations include Raynaud's phenomenon in 25% of patients and ulcers over the malleoli in 30%. Symmetric polyarthralgias have been reported in more than half of some patients, and in the rare instances when arthritis does occur, it is nondeforming. The prevalence of renal involvement is from 20% to 50%, and the most common renal histopathology is diffuse proliferative glomerulonephritis. Twelve of 40 patients reported by Gorevic et al. (277) required management of congestive heart failure during the course of their disease. Rheumatic heart disease probably accounted for heart failure in five patients; however, coronary vasculitis was demonstrated in two of nine autopsies from this large patient group. Generalized lymphadenopathy, peripheral neuropathy, and thyroiditis were observed less frequently (284).

Mixed cryoglobulins are seen during the acute phases of viral illnesses and a variety of chronic hepatic diseases. Levo (23) was the first to emphasize the high prevalence of liver abnormalities found in essential mixed cryoglobulinemia patients, which suggested a role for hepatotropic viruses in the production of the mixed cryoglobulins. The same group then reported the presence of HBsAg or its antibody in 15 of 25 serum samples and 14 of 19 cryoprecipitates from patients with essential mixed cryoglobulinemia. Particles resembling hepatitis B also were seen in all four cryoprecipitates examined by electron microscopy. Subsequent studies found less evidence of either hepatitis B infection in essential mixed cryoglobulinemia or increased concentration of HBsAg and antibody in the cryoprecipitate versus serum; there was no HBsAg or antibody in the sera of 12 patients with essential mixed cryoglobulinemia, and only one of these had anti-HBs in the cryoprecipitate (285,286). Galli and Invernizzi (287) found HBV antigens or antibodies in

60% of 40 essential mixed cryoglobulinemia patients, but only 32% had these in their cryoprecipitates. Moreover, there was no statistically significant difference between the essential mixed cryoglobulinemia patients and controls or the general population in the prevalence of exposure to hepatitis B. It is now clear that in some populations, HBV infection is associated less often with cryoglobulinemia than is HCV infection, and that co-infection occurs (288). Significant numbers of cases labeled essential mixed cryoglobulinemia are caused by HBV and HCV and should be reclassified as secondary mixed cryoglobulinemia. Long-term follow-up of patients initially thought to have essential mixed cryoglobulinemia has also led to a diagnosis of autoimmune disease or hematologic malignancy in 10 of 22 patients (284).

Laboratory abnormalities in essential mixed cryoglobulinemia include moderate anemia, an elevated ESR, polyclonal hypergammaglobulinemia, and hypocomplementemia in more than 60% of patients. Selective depression of C4 accompanying a low CH50, with relatively normal levels of C3, is a characteristic finding. Hypocomplementemia, cryocrit, and serum levels of cryoglobulins do not correlate well with disease activity. Renal involvement usually follows the onset of purpura and is the primary determinant of the prognosis. Fourteen of 20 patients with renal involvement followed up by Gorevic et al. (277) died compared with four of 13 without this. Other deaths have been attributed to systemic vasculitis and infection.

A benign course has been observed in up to 50% of essential mixed cryoglobulinemia patients, making treatment decisions difficult. The primary indications for therapy include deterioration in renal and neurologic function. Controlled drug trials are lacking in this uncommon disease, but corticosteroids, cytotoxic agents, and plasmapheresis have been used with variable success. Interferon-α has become standard treatment for hepatitis C–associated cryoglobulinemia; however, there are a few reports of increased ischemia after such treatment (289–291). Ribavirin may decrease manifestations of HCV-related cryoglobulinemia but benefits may disappear when the drug is discontinued. For patients with serious symptoms related to the cryoglobulin, cryofiltration apheresis is a specific therapy, and deserves further study (292).

Urticarial Vasculitis

Urticarial vasculitis is defined as recurrent episodes of persistent urticarial lesions due to vasculitis of postcapillary venules. In 1973, McDuffie et al. (293) described an immune complex syndrome in four patients of urticaria, arthralgia or synovitis, and hypocomplementemia. Three of the four patients had leukocytoclastic vasculitis identified on biopsy of urticarial lesions. It has since been recognized that urticarial vasculitis occurs in patients with varied clinical (localized cutaneous disease to multisystem disease) and immunopathologic features. Among all patients with chronic urticaria, the prevalence of vasculitis has not been well established, but a large prospective study identified leukocytoclastic vasculitis in 12 of 100 cases of chronic idiopathic urticaria (293). Urticarial vasculitis has been recognized in connective tissue diseases, particularly SLE, and also Sjögren's syndrome, mixed connective tissue disease, PAN, and WG (294). Furthermore, urticarial vasculitis has been described with viral infections such as hepatitis B, with drug reactions and sun exposure, as well as exercise, although most patients do not have an identifiable risk factor.

No physical signs differentiate urticarial vasculitis from chronic idiopathic urticaria. The skin lesions begin as typical wheals or erythematous papules that may be accompanied by angioedema. Clinical features suggestive of urticarial vasculitis include a burning or painful sensation, persistence of lesions for more than 24 hours, and healing with evidence of red cell extravasation such as purpura or hyperpigmentation. Approximately 64% of patients have individual lesions lasting longer than 1 day, and about one third have residual purpura or hyperpigmentation or associated pain (295).

Musculoskeletal symptoms, fever, abdominal or chest pain, obstructive pulmonary disease, renal disease, and inflammatory eye disease have been reported in connection with urticarial vasculitis. The systemic features are more frequent and severe in patients with hypocomplementemia than in those without (292). Approximately half of all patients with urticarial vasculitis complain of arthralgias, but only 28% have definite arthritis. Obstructive pulmonary disease is present in roughly 20% of patients and may be due to pulmonary vasculitis; two patients with urticarial vasculitis and obstructive pulmonary disease have been shown to have vasculitis on open lung biopsy. Low-grade microscopic hematuria occurs in about one third of patients and is often accompanied by proteinuria. The presence of glomerulonephritis on renal biopsies is as low as 5% (235), and significant elevations of serum creatinine are rare; however, patients with lupus nephritis sometimes have hypocomplementemic urticarial vasculitis. Systemic disease features of urticarial vasculitis from the two largest reported groups of patients include fever (10–15%), abdominal or chest pain (17–25%), and episcleritis and uveitis (4–17%) (295,296). There also may be a relation to pseudotumor cerebri, as three of 40 patients reported by Sanchez et al. (297) had this unusual disorder.

The histologic demonstration of vessel damage in the form of leukocytoclastic or necrotizing vasculitis distinguishes urticarial vasculitis from common urticaria, which is characterized by dermal edema, vascular dilatation, and a sparse perivascular lymphocytic infiltrate. Nevertheless, a few investigators have emphasized the continuum of histologic changes between common urticaria and urticarial vasculitis, identifying a subgroup of patients with a prominent perivascular infiltrate but no vasculitis (297,298). The pathogenesis of urticarial vasculitis is unknown but is thought to be directly related to immune complex deposition. Direct immunofluorescence of involved skin has revealed immunoglobulin and complement (primarily C3 and IgM) in blood vessel walls and the dermal–epidermal border in more than 50% of some patients (295,296,299). Glomerulonephritis has been detected on kidney biopsies, but the results of immunofluorescent staining have not been reported. Circulating immune complexes in 44% of patients (297) and hypocomplementemia in 32% to 40% (295,296) provide further indirect proof of immune complex disease. In hypocomplementemic urticarial vasculitis, Fab-dependent binding of IgG antibodies to C1q may play a role in the pathogenesis of the disease (300).

Records of 132 patients seen between 1975 and 1995 at the Mayo Clinic with urticarial vasculitis were reviewed by Davis et al. (302). Twenty-four (female) patients were hypocomplementemic. They all had generalized urticarial plaques and a course of illness characterized by exacerbations and remission. Fifty-four percent of them met the ACR criteria for the classification of SLE. One hundred eight patients were normocomplementemic; 43 of them were men. Except for equal numbers with fever, patients with hypocomplementemia had significantly more signs of disease. For example, arthritis was seen in 75% of these patients in contrast to 24% of normocomplementemic patients. Autoantibodies were more common in hypocomplementemic patients. The most consistent laboratory difference was in the prevalence of the "lupus band," defined by two conjugates, on skin biopsy. This was found in all but one of the hypocomplementemic group, and in none whose serum complement levels were normal. The authors of this report concluded that hypocomplementemic urticarial vasculitis should be considered a subset of SLE.

Despite evidence of systemic disease in many patients, idiopathic urticarial vasculitis typically has a benign, yet chronic, course. Inconsistent results have been obtained with a variety of treatments. A response to NSAIDs and/or antihistamines has been observed in about half of patients, and the majority of persons with urticarial vasculitis will obtain symptomatic relief with glucocorticoids or antimalarials, although high doses of prednisone may be required (>40 mg/day) (295,296). The course of patients with hypocomplementemic vasculitis is apt to be more severe, as in SLE, and to require glucocorticoids in moderate amounts for control. Dapsone has been cited as a possible drug of choice for hypocomplementemic urticarial vasculitis (302).

Takayasu's Disease

Takayasu's disease is a chronic inflammatory vasculitis that affects primarily the aorta and its major branches and the pulmonary arteries. Synonyms such as aortic arch syndrome, pulseless disease, and aortitis syndrome mirror this anatomic localization. The disease affects mainly women younger than 40 years. Reported worldwide, Takayasu's disease appears to be most common in East Asia and rare in the U.S. and Europe. A population study of Olmsted County, Minnesota, yielded a yearly incidence of 2.6 cases/million persons (303). Its cause is unknown, and there is scant evidence of immunopathology. Antibodies to human aorta extract and components have not been found when looked for in 35 sera from patients with this disease (304). Hoffman and Ahmed (305) have compared results of tests in 29 patients and controls. The tests were ESR, C-reactive protein (CRP), tissue factor, von Willebrand factor, thrombomodulin, tissue plasminogen activator, intercellular adhesion molecule-1 (ICAM-1), VCAM-1, E-selectin, and platelet–endothelial cell adhesion molecule-1 (PECAM-1). There were no diagnostically significant differences between patients and controls. A genetic predilection for Takayasu's arteritis is suggested by significantly increased frequency of HLA-B52 and B39 in Japanese patients compared with controls (306).

The variable symptoms of many patients with this disease account for the difficulties in establishing a diagnosis—the shortest median delay from the onset of symptoms to the time of diagnosis for a large number of patients has been 10 months (307). Nonspecific complaints include dizziness, headaches, arthralgias, myalgias, malaise, fever, and weight loss. Early reports emphasized a two-stage disease process: a "prepulseless" phase characterized by nonspecific symptoms, followed by a late "pulseless" or occlusive phase (308,309). Prospective evaluation of 60 Takayasu's patients revealed significant disease course diversity rather than distinct stages of disease. Constitutional symptoms at the onset of disease were present in only one third of patients and in an additional 10% throughout the disease course (307).

Symptoms and signs of extremity or organ ischemia are the hallmark clinical features; bruits, absent or reduced pulses, systolic blood pressure discrepancy of more than 30 mm Hg between the arms, and carotodynia are all suggestive physical findings. Vascular bruits are detected in more than 80% of patients, and pulses are diminished or absent in more than half (307). Gradual progression of arterial obstruction allows the development of collateral vessels and probably accounts for the variability in frequency of claudication (29–70%), which is much more common in the upper than the lower extremities. Severe occlusive disease of the carotid and vertebrobasilar systems is strongly associated with postural dizziness and visual disturbances (303,307,309). Early funduscopic changes of Takayasu's disease, sometimes pointing to the diagnosis, are microaneurysms in the peripheral retina, venous dilatation, and beading. Peripapillary arteriovenous anastomoses, as described by Takayasu (310), develop later, as do retinal hemorrhages, cotton-wool exudates, optic atrophy, retinal detachment, retinitis proliferans, and vitreous hemorrhage. Hypertensive retinopathy is more common than Takayasu's retinopathy (311).

Although aortic regurgitation from dilatation of the aortic root and separation of the valve leaflets is the most common cardiac complication of Takayasu's disease in the U.S., occurring in 20% of patients (307), there has been increasing recognition elsewhere of other cardiac features. Constitutional symptoms and congestive heart failure seem to be more common in children than in adults (309). Congestive heart failure has been attributed to hypertension, aortic regurgitation, and mitral regurgitation; however, myocarditis may contribute to cardiac dysfunction and has been prospectively identified by endomyocardial biopsy in about half of 54 patients in India (312). Coronary artery disease is present in about 10% of persons; the distribution of coronary lesions by angiography was 72% ostial and 18.5% proximal (313).

Pulmonary vascular arteritis was evident in about half of 66 patients studied with angiography (314,315). The symptoms of mild-to-moderate pulmonary hypertension, present in the majority of these patients, were usually subtle. During the course of disease, systemic hypertension also is detected in more than 50% of persons. Detection of hypertension is difficult in persons with ischemia of all four extremities because of falsely low peripheral blood pressure readings, and can be reliably assessed only by central systemic recording. Hypertension is usually directly related to stenosis of one or both renal arteries, but may also be due to reduced elasticity of arterial walls, narrowing of the thoracic or abdominal aorta, brain ischemia, and disruption of carotid baroreceptors (316). Severe hypertension contributes significantly to morbidity and death, as was apparent in autopsy studies of 10 persons with a mean age of 22.6 years. Multiple lesions were identified. Eight persons had stenosis of the aorta, six had dilatation, two had aneurysms, and one had dissection of the aorta. The abdominal aorta was involved in nine persons, and renal arteries in six. Left ventricular hypertrophy was present in nine persons, and four had congestive heart failure. Two persons had chronic renal failure, and four had tuberculosis. Active inflammation was found even though the disease had been chronic and "silent," confounding treatment issues (317).

Myalgia and arthralgia are experienced by approximately 50% of Takayasu's disease patients, whereas synovitis has been recognized in only 19% of patients (303). Skin lesions also are prominent in Takayasu's disease. There is an association with erythema nodosum and more commonly, with leukocytoclastic vasculitis, and in Japan, Takayasu's disease is the most common systemic disease associated with pyoderma gangrenosum (318).

Delay in diagnosis has been attributed primarily to the nonspecific nature of the initial symptoms. Takayasu's disease should be suspected in a young girl or woman with evidence of a systemic illness and vascular ischemia. Its onset at an early age was illustrated in a review from South Africa, where 31 patients were seen in a pediatric nephrology unit over a 15-year period. The mean age at time of diagnosis was 8.42 years. The most common sign at presentation was hypertension, followed by heart failure. An interesting finding, which has been alluded to by others, was the 90% positive rate for tuberculin skin testing versus 5% for a control group (319). During periods of inflammation, an elevated ESR is found more frequently than anemia, leukocytosis, hypoalbuminemia, and hypergammaglobulinemia. Chest radiographic abnormalities suggestive of Takayasu's disease include widening of the ascending aorta, contour irregularities of the descending aorta, aortic calcification, pulmonary artery hypertensive changes, and rib notching (320). Confirmation of diagnosis in all suspected cases requires comprehensive invasive or magnetic resonance angiography of the entire aorta and its major branches, looking for stenoses or aneurysms (the latter in 27% of patients) (307). The greatest geographic variation in disease expression has been a higher frequency of aortic arch disease in Japanese patients vis-à-vis disease of the thoracic and abdominal aorta in most other countries (307,309). In the U.S., the most frequently affected arteries are the left subclavian, superior mesenteric, and abdominal aorta (each in approximately 80% of patients) followed by the right renal and left carotid (Fig. 82.12) (303). Although temporal arteritis may have

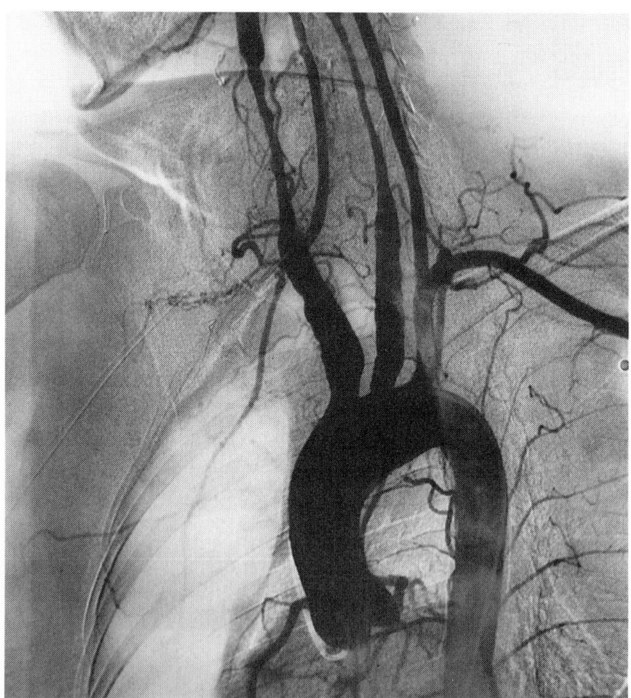

FIGURE 82.12. Arteriogram of Takayasu's disease showing irregularity of the brachiocephalic, and absence of the right subclavian, with extensive stenosis of the right common carotid, and poststenotic dilatation. The left common carotid also shows a long segment of stenosis with poststenotic dilatation. (Courtesy of Dr. Marc Schwartzberg.)

identical angiographic abnormalities, correlation of these with clinical data is usually sufficient to establish the diagnosis of Takayasu's disease. In an unblinded study, magnetic resonance imaging adequately detected lesions of the aorta (particularly long axis images) and proximal branches of the aortic arch (321). It also was thought to provide better visualization of aortic wall thickening and mural thrombi than did conventional angiography.

The clinical features that best distinguish Takayasu's disease from other forms of vasculitis include age of onset younger than 40, claudication of extremities, decreased brachial artery pulse, systolic blood pressure difference more than 10 mm Hg between arms, bruit over subclavian arteries, and arteriographic abnormalities (322). The histopathologic features of Takayasu's disease are diagnostic only when areas of active inflammation are sampled. Granulomatous arteritis with a predominantly lymphoplasmacytic infiltrate confined to the media, variable numbers of giant cells, and patchy areas of medial musculoelastic lamellae destruction are characteristic findings (123).

Glucocorticoids are customary initial medication for active arteritis. Prednisone, at a dose of 30 to 60 mg/day, is usually effective in suppressing systemic symptoms such as fever and arthralgias and reducing the ESR. Efficacy of glucocorticoid treatment also has been demonstrated in selected cases by return of absent pulses (303) and regression of arterial lesions (323). Prolonged therapy is often required because of the chronic, relapsing nature of Takayasu's disease, and tapering of prednisone to a maintenance dose has been based primarily on the ESR level and the clinical response. Fever, arthralgias, symptoms or signs of progressive vascular ischemia or inflammation, and new angiographic lesions, as well as the elevation of the ESR, all may influence treatment plans. Investigators at the NIH have reported an inadequate response to glucocorticoid treatment in 50% of patients (307). They also noted a poor correlation between clinical assessment and disease activity, as 44% of arterial biopsy specimens from patients thought to have inactive disease revealed active vasculitis. Whether glucocorticoid treatment reduces the mortality of Takayasu's disease has not been firmly established; however, improvement in survival from 25% at 2 years in early reports (324) to greater than 94% at 5 years in two recent patient groups suggests that it does (303,307). Although the role of cytotoxic drugs in the treatment of Takayasu's disease is not well defined, beneficial effects have been seen with cyclophosphamide (325) and methotrexate (326) in glucocorticoid-resistant cases and in patients in whom prednisone could not be tapered to a maintenance dose. Cyclosporine has less ovarian toxicity than other cytotoxic agents and has proved to be effective in patients who wish to retain fertility (327). Mycophenolate mofetil also has been used with apparent success in a few patients (328).

The main causes of death among Takayasu's disease patients are congestive heart failure and cerebrovascular accidents, emphasizing the need for blood pressure control. Prognosis has been directly related to the presence, degree, and number of complications of Takayasu's disease (Takayasu's retinopathy, secondary hypertension, aortic valvular insufficiency, and aortic/arterial aneurysms) (329,330). Surgical procedures have therefore been aimed primarily at relieving brain ischemia, renovascular hypertension unresponsive to medical therapy, and coronary artery ischemia, and at correction of arteriovenous insufficiency and aneurysms. It is advisable to control systemic inflammation before surgery when feasible, because active vasculitis has resulted in a higher incidence of suture failure, aneurysmal formation, and graft occlusion (331). Selected patients have been treated with percutaneous artery stenting (332).

Giant Cell Arteritis (Temporal Arteritis)

Giant cell arteritis (GCA) was recognized as a disease entity in 1932 by Horton et al. (334), who reported temporal artery biopsy results for the first time. Since their landmark case report, the disease's clinical spectrum has broadened considerably with its inclusion as a systemic arteritis involving any large or medium-sized elastic artery, although branches of the carotid artery primarily are affected. Blindness was recognized as a complication of the disease in 1938 by Jennings (335). It has since been learned that this and other complications can most often be prevented by prompt diagnosis and treatment with corticosteroids. Preventable complications and its recognition as one of the most common forms of vasculitis underscore its importance.

There is considerable variation in the incidence of GCA in different geographic regions. Highest rates are seen in northern areas, with the majority of reports from the northern United States and Europe. In patients older than 50 years with biopsy-proven disease, comparable incidence rates for 1980 through 1985 have been determined in the county of Ribe, Denmark (335), and Olmsted County, Minnesota (336) (23.3/100,000 and 24.1/100,000, respectively). The cause of GCA is unknown; however, there are reports suggesting a possible link with parainfluenza viruses and parvoviruses (337,338). Significantly lower incidence rates have been found in nonendemic areas (339). Once considered to occur exclusively in whites, GCA has been reported in blacks, Asians, and Hispanics (340,341). This vasculitis is rare in individuals younger than 50 years (342,343), and the prevalence increases with advancing age. Most reports also have noted a slight female predilection. Several reports of familial cases of temporal arteritis, as well as polymyalgia rheumatica, have been documented, providing evidence that genetic factors are associated with the disease (344). An increased prevalence of HLA-DRB104 alleles has been noted in various population groups [e.g., these alleles were found in 48.78% of 41 persons with biopsy-confirmed GCA and 19.79% of controls (345)].

An elderly patient with headache, painful indurated temporal arteries, polymyalgia rheumatica, and an increased ESR presents little diagnostic uncertainty. The majority of patients will have fewer overt signs of GCA, and it is these in whom a tissue or angiographic diagnosis should be required. One of the most vexing problems pertaining to GCA that the authors have had to contend with is that of patients who are aged 50 years or older, with ESRs of 50 or 60 mm/h, and who may have headaches, and who are then begun and maintained on prednisone until complications from the drug require reevaluation. Or the patients continue to have the same manifestations that led to empiric glucocorticoid treatment, and the physician must decide whether this represents inadequate treatment of GCA, or improper diagnosis. Color duplex ultrasonography has been proposed as a noninvasive way of diagnosing temporal arteritis, but this has not been validated adequately (346). Patients often have subtle symptoms such as fever, anorexia, weight loss, malaise, or depression, which mimic infectious disease, psychiatric illness, or an underlying malignancy (Table 82.9). Constitutional symptoms were the initial disease manifestations in 38% of a group of 34 patients, leading to significant delays in diagnosis (347). The majority of symptoms are related to involvement of the medium-sized branches of the carotid arteries; however, GCA also may affect the aorta and its major branches in 10% to 15% of patients (348). The carotid, subclavian, axillary, and brachial arteries are most commonly affected. The most frequent symptoms are upper extremity claudication, paresthesias, Raynaud's phenomenon, and muscular weakness with corresponding physical findings, including absent or reduced pulses, bruits, and decreased humoral blood pressure. Inflammation of the coronary arteries also may occur, leading to angina and myocardial infarction, although the prevalence is unknown. An interesting prospective study of the relative values of certain clinical signs and laboratory data has been reported for 106 patients with temporal artery biopsies positive for GCA. The values were compared with those of 257 patients referred for GCA, but who had negative temporal artery biopsies. The odds of having a positive biopsy were 9.1 times greater with jaw claudication, 3.4 times with neck pain, 3.2 times greater with a C-reactive protein (CRP) greater than 2.45 mg/dL, and 2.0 times greater with an ESR exceeding 47 mm/h. This study of large numbers of patients confirmed the specificity of jaw claudication for vasculitis (usually GCA), and the superiority of CRP for diagnosis (349).

TABLE 82.9. EARLY MANIFESTATIONS OF TEMPORAL ARTERITIS

Frequent (>50% cases)	Occasional (10–50%)	Unusual (<10% cases)
Headache	Jaw claudication	Blindness
Abnormal temporal artery	Polymyalgia rheumatica	Claudication of extremities
	Scalp tenderness	Claudication of tongue
	Weight loss	Vertigo
	Fever	Stroke
	Depression	Angina
	Facial neuralgia	

Reproduced and adapted with permission from Allen NB, Studenski SA. Polymyalgia rheumatica and temporal arteritis. *Med Clin North Am* 1986;70:373.

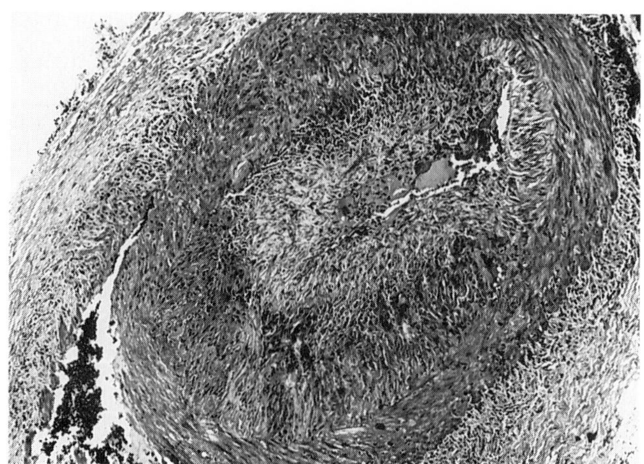

FIGURE 82.13. Biopsy specimen from a patient with temporal arteritis. (Courtesy of Dr. Robert M. Gay.)

Prevention of blindness is the most important treatment issue because there are no effective means to reverse visual loss. Prednisone, 40 to 60 mg in divided doses, is generally regarded as effective initial treatment of patients with clinical signs of temporal arteritis without visual symptoms or evidence of large artery involvement (350). Histologic confirmation should be obtained by temporal artery biopsy in all patients within 1 week of beginning prednisone so that the inflammation within the vessel is not significantly altered (Fig. 82.13). The initial dose of prednisone should be 60 to 80 mg/day in divided doses for patients with visual symptoms or those with large-artery involvement. Several reports attribute the reversal of acute visual loss to high-dose corticosteroids (350,351). There are also reports of progression of ischemic optic neuropathy in one eye and appearance of ischemia in the other despite large doses of glucocorticoids (352). After 1 month of treatment, the initial dose of prednisone can be gradually tapered to a maintenance dose of 5 to 7.5 mg/day. The majority of patients with temporal arteritis will require treatment for only 2 to 3 years. See elsewhere in this volume for a more complete discussion.

VASCULITIS ASSOCIATED WITH CONNECTIVE TISSUE DISEASE

Vasculitis may complicate all of the connective tissue diseases, most commonly RA, SLE, and Sjögren's syndrome. In most cases, small vessels are affected; however, there may be systemic necrotizing vasculitis that is indistinguishable from PAN. Vasculitis associated with RA classically occurs in seropositive male patients with erosions, nodules, quiescent synovitis, and disease duration greater than 10 years, and usually affects the skin and nerves. Periungual infarctions are relatively common in RA with or without other evidence of vasculitis, but often coexist with other skin lesions in patients with systemic vasculitis. Lower extremity ulcers are the most common cutaneous feature of rheumatoid vasculitis, followed by gangrene and purpura or petechiae. Unusual cutaneous manifestations of rheumatoid vasculitis have included pyoderma gangrenosum and erythema elevatum diutinum. Mononeuritis multiplex usually involves more than one extremity and is present in nearly half of rheumatoid vasculitis patients. Except for weight loss, other organ system involvement and constitutional symptoms are uncommon. Gastrointestinal involvement has been observed in only one tenth of cases but may be the initial manifestation of rheumatoid vasculitis (353–355). Two large series, totalling 102 patients, found abnormal urinary sediments in approximately 10% of rheumatoid vasculitis patients (353,354). Despite its clinical rarity, renal arteritis or glomerulonephritis was found on autopsy in nearly half of 18 patients with systemic rheumatoid vasculitis (356).

Vasculitis is more common in patients with other extraarticular features of RA and Felty's syndrome, as well as higher titers of rheumatoid factors, cryoglobulins, diminished serum complement, and an increased prevalence of HLA-DR4 alleles. Diagnostic confirmation of rheumatoid vasculitis is usually acquired by either skin or sural nerve biopsy, but a presumptive diagnosis can be made in patients with typical cutaneous or neurologic features.

The choice of therapy should be based on the extent and degree of organ involvement. Isolated digital vasculitis is benign and requires no specific treatment. Progressive ischemic and ulcerative cutaneous disease, neuropathy, and visceral vasculitis warrant aggressive therapy. There is only one randomized, double-blind controlled trial assessing therapy of rheumatoid vasculitis; therefore, medical management is derived from treatment of other types of vasculitis and experience with uncomplicated RA. Glucocorticoids are the mainstay of treatment, in doses equivalent to 0.5 to 1.0 mg/kg/day (357). A substantial number of RA patients evaluated at the Mayo Clinic with vasculitis had not received disease-modifying drugs, implying that standard therapy directed against arthritis may protect against vasculitis (354), and institution of methotrexate at a dose of 10 to 20 mg once weekly has resulted in resolution of cutaneous ulcers and neuropathy (358). The single reported randomized trial of therapy for rheumatoid vasculitis included only 15 patients and did not show any benefit for azathioprine over placebo (359). Use of cyclophosphamide has been advocated in uncontrolled case series, and results from an open clinical trial suggested that intermittent intravenous cyclophosphamide plus methylprednisolone is more effective than a variety of other treatments in healing cutaneous infarcts, vasculitic ulcers, and neuropathy (360).

VASCULITIS ASSOCIATED WITH MALIGNANCY

Vasculitis has been reported to precede or follow the appearance of malignancies. There are numerous anecdotal, single-case reports of congruent vasculitis and malignancy; some may be coincidental. Greer et al. (361) reported their experience with 13 patients and reviewed the literature, finding a significant association between vasculitis and lymphomyeloproliferative malignancies compared with other malignancies. Review of the Florida tumor registry from 1970 through 1987 uncovered eight cases of vasculitis among 1,730 lympho- and myeloproliferative disorders. In contrast, no cases of vasculitis were found among 13,160 other malignancies. Review of the American medical literature revealed that vasculitis had been reported in 41 persons with blood or lymphatic malignancies but in only 11 with other cancers. A more recent review of the literature found 44 persons with vasculitis and myelodysplastic syndrome, and a patient was described who had myelodysplasia and vasculitis causing toe necrosis (362).

The majority of patients have had cutaneous vasculitis, often antedating the diagnosis of malignancy (361,363) and, occasionally, polyarthritis. Laboratory tests for HBsAg, Coomb's antibodies, rheumatoid factors, ANA, cryoglobulins, complement, and circulating immune complexes are generally normal or negative. Greer et al. (361,363) did not observe any leukemic cells in skin biopsy specimens, and immunofluorescent staining was negative for immunoglobulin and complement in all of their 13 cases. There also was no consistent response of the vasculitic lesions to NSAIDs, antihistamines, or chemotherapy, although improvement did accompany chemotherapy in several instances. The most favorable response of vasculitic skin lesions has been to glucocorticoid therapy.

Vasculitis resembling PAN or cutaneous vasculitis has been found most frequently in association with hairy cell leukemia, often after splenectomy (361,364). Arthritis occurs frequently in this syndrome, but circulating immune complexes, cryoglobulinemia, and hypocomplementemia are usually not detected. Perivascular and mural wall hairy cell infiltration have been documented in a few patients (80,81), suggesting that these cells are directly involved in vascular damage.

MISCELLANEOUS SYNDROMES WITH VASCULITIS

Cogan's syndrome is an unusual disorder typically consisting of interstitial keratitis, sensorineural hearing loss, tinnitus, and vertigo. Initial symptoms may be referable to either the eyes or ears, but both organs are affected within 5 months in the majority of patients (365). Eye symptoms are redness, photophobia, pain, and a change in visual acuity. Deafness occurs in approximately 50% of affected ears despite appropriate treatment, but blindness occurs in only about 5% of involved eyes. Fever, weight loss, and fatigue are reported in 50% of patients. A mixed, transmural infiltrate affecting either large, medium, or small arteries and veins has been found in 15% of patients in the aorta, coronary arteries, kidney, muscle, and skin. Aortic insufficiency is the most frequent cardiac complication of Cogan's syndrome and is frequently associated with vasculitis. Topical glucocorticoids are used to treat the interstitial keratitis, and systemic glucocorticoids are recommended for otologic and systemic manifestations as well as keratitis not responding to topical therapy (365,366). Early glucocorticoid treatment may be necessary to prevent or reverse hearing loss in patients with vestibuloauditory signs. Cochlear implants can improve auditory function (367). Cytotoxic–immunosuppressive agents are of no confirmed value as treatment of Cogan's syndrome.

Erythematous papules with atrophic white centers ("porcelain-white") scattered on the trunk and extremities are distinct skin lesions found in Degos' syndrome. In the past, wedge-shaped infarctions and thrombotic occlusion of small vessels in the dermis were described as the characteristic histologic findings, leading to classification as a thrombotic vasculopathy. Further investigation has uncovered lymphocytic vasculitis in the majority of patients and infrequent thrombosis, which is now thought to be a late event (368,369). This syndrome may be associated with catastrophic abdominal and CNS manifestations as a result of vasculitis of these organs. Necrotizing inflammation of the central retinal artery and smaller arteries in the optic nerve has been described in one patient (369) and lymphocytic vasculitis in the CNS and gastrointestinal tract in another (368). The most common cause of death is intestinal perforation, with mortality reported to be as high as 50% (370,371). Nevertheless, patients have also been followed for up to 14 years without evidence of systemic involvement (368). No effective treatment for this rare form of vasculitis has been identified.

Primary vasculitis of the CNS (PACNS; see Chapter 83) is probably more common than of CNS vasculitis due to Degos' syndrome. As described by Calabrese et al. (372,373), it involves meningeal and cortical small or medium-sized arteries and veins, and is unusual for the varied patterns that might be seen in one biopsy specimen. These include those of granulomatous arteritis, polyarteritis, or lymphocytic vasculitis. The dominant symptoms are headache, neurologic dysfunction, decreased cognition, seizure, and stroke. It has been suggested that patients who have acute focal neurologic signs and minimal cerebrospinal fluid abnormalities are apt to have angiographic abnormalities and a benign course, hence the designation benign angiopathy of the central nervous system or BACNS. The sensitivity and specificity of cerebral angiography are low, and angiograms are not without risk of infarction. Diagnosis in those patients with a chronic meningitis-like picture requires CNS biopsy, if only to exclude those diseases such as tuberculous meningitis, which can mimic PACNS. Premortem biopsies were negative in 25% of autopsy-proven cases. The diagnosis is difficult, the course unpredictable, and the treatment unsettled. Calabrese et al. (373) recommended aggressive treatment with high-dose glucocorticoids and an immunosuppressive drug for patients with progressive neurologic illness, and those with confirmed primary granulomatous angiitis (372,373).

REFERENCES

1. Küssmaul A, Maier R. Ueber eine bisher nicht beschriebene eigenthümliche arterienerkrankung (periarteritis nodosa), die mit morbus brightii und rapid fortschreitender allgemeiner muskellähmung einhergeht. *Dtsch Arch Klin Med* 1866;1:484–518.
2. Wegener F. Über generalisierte, septische gefasserkrankungen. *Verh Dtsch Ges Pathol* 1936;29:202–210.
3. Churg J, Strauss L. Allergic granulomatosis, allergic angiitis, and periarteritis nodosa. *Am J Pathol* 1951;27:277–301.
4. Zeek PM. Periarteritis nodosa: a critical review. *Am J Clin Pathol* 1952;22:777–790.
5. Lie JT. Nomenclature and classification of vasculitis: plus ça change plus c'est la meme chose. *Arthritis Rheum* 1994;37:181–186.
6. Alarcón-Segovia D, Brown AL Jr. Classification and etiologic aspects of necrotizing angiitides: an analytic approach to a confused subject with a critical review of the evidence for hypersensitivity in polyarteritis nodosa. *Mayo Clin Proc* 1964;39:205–222.
7. Deshazo RD. The spectrum of systemic vasculitis: a classification to aid diagnosis. *Postgrad Med J* 1975;58:78–82.
8. Gilliam JN, Smiley JD. Cutaneous necrotizing vasculitis and related disorders. *Ann Allergy* 1976;37:328–339.
9. Fauci AS, Haynes BF, Katz P. The spectrum of vasculitis: clinical, pathologic, immunologic, and therapeutic considerations. *Ann Intern Med* 1978;89:660–676.
10. McCluskey RT, Fienberg R. Vasculitis in primary vasculitides, granulomatoses, and connective tissue diseases. *Hum Pathol* 1983;14:305–315.
11. Jennette JC, Falk RJ, Andrassy K, et al. Nomenclature of systemic vasculitides: proposal of an international consensus conference. *Arthritis Rheum* 1994;37:187–192.
12. Cohen P, Tervaert JW, Kallenburg C. Neurologic manifestations of systemic vasculitides. *Rheum Dis Clin North Am* 1993;19:913–940.
13. Hunder GG, Arend WP, Bloch DA, et al. The American College of Rheumatology 1990 criteria for the classification of vasculitis: introduction. *Arthritis Rheum* 1990;33:1065–1067.
14. Rao JK, Allen NB, Pincus, T. Limitations of the 1990 American College of Rheumatology Classification Criteria in the Diagnosis of Vasculitis. *Ann Intern Med* 1998;129:345–352.
15. Dixon FJ, Vazquez JJ, Weigle WO, Cochrane CG. Pathogenesis of serum sickness. *Arch Pathol* 1958;65:18–28.
16. Christian CL, Sergent JS. Vasculitis syndromes: clinical and experimental models. *Am J Med* 1976;61:385–392.

17. Cochrane CG. Mechanisms involved in the deposition of immune complexes in tissues. *J Exp Med* 1971;134:75S–89S.
18. Haynes BF. Vasculitis: pathogenic mechanisms of vessel damage. In: Gallin JI, Goldstein IM, Snyderman R, eds. *Inflammation:* basic principles and clinical correlates. 2nd ed. New York: Raven Press, 1992:921–941.
19. Cochrane CG, Weigle WO, Dixon FJ. The role of polymorphonuclear leukocytes in the initiation and cessation of the Arthus vasculitis. *J Exp Med* 1959;110:481–494.
20. Lawley TJ, Bielory L, Gascon P, Yancey KB, Young NS, Frank MM. A prospective clinical and immunologic analysis of patients with serum sickness. *N Engl J Med* 1984;311: 1407–1413.
21. Hoffman GS. Vasculitic syndromes: editorial overview. *Curr Opin Rheumatol* 1994;6:1–2.
22. Gocke DJ, Hsu K, Morgan C, Bombardieri S, Lockshin M, Christian CL. Association between polyarteritis and Australia antigen. *Lancet* 1970;2:1149–1153.
23. Levo Y, Gorevic PD, Kassab HJ, Zucker-Franklin D, Franklin EC. Association between hepatitis B virus and essential mixed cryoglobulinemia. *N Engl J Med* 1977;296:1501–1504.
24. Trepo CG, Zuckerman AJ, Bird RC, Prince AM. The role of circulating hepatitis B antigen/antibody immune complexes in the pathogenesis of vascular and hepatic manifestations in polyarteritis nodosa. *J Clin Pathol* 1974;27:863–868.
25. Michalak T. Immune complexes of hepatitis B surface antigen in the pathogenesis of periarteritis nodosa: a study of seven necroscopy cases. *Am J Pathol* 1978;90:619–632.
26. Gower RG, Sausker WF, Kohler PF, Thorne GE, McIntosh RM. Small vessel vasculitis caused by hepatitis B virus immune complexes. *J Allergy Clin Immunol* 1978;62:222–228.
27. Combes B, Stastny P, Shorey J, et al. Glomerulonephritis with deposition of Australia antigen-antibody complexes in glomerular basement membrane. *Lancet* 1971;1:234–237.
28. Tsukada N, Koh CS, Owa M, Yanagisawa N. Chronic neuropathy associated with immune complexes of hepatitis B virus. *J Neurol Sci* 1983;61:193–211.
29. Claudy A. Pathogenesis of leukocytoclastic vasculitis. *Eur J Dermatol* 1998;8:75–79.
30. Kammer GM, Soter NA, Schur PH. Circulating immune complexes in patients with necrotizing vasculitis. *Clin Immunol Immunopathol* 1980;15:658–672.
31. Braverman IM, Yen A. Demonstration of immune complexes in spontaneous and histamine-induced lesions and in normal skin of patients with leukocytoclastic angiitis. *J Invest Dermatol* 1975;64:105–112.
32. Gower RG, Sams WM Jr, Thorne EG, Kohler PF, Claman HN. Leukocytoclastic vasculitis: sequential appearance of immunoreactants and cellular changes in serial biopsies. *J Invest Dermatol* 1977;69:477–484.
33. Grunwald MH, Avinoach I, Amichai B, Halevy S. Leukocytoclastic vasculitis-correlation between different histologic stages and direct immunofluorescence results. *Int J Dermatol* 1997;36: 349–352.
34. Stevenson JA, Leong LA, Cohen AH, Border WA. Henoch-Schönlein purpura: simultaneous demonstration of IgA deposits in involved skin, intestine, and kidney. *Arch Pathol Lab Med* 1982;106:192–195.
35. Giangiacomo J, Tsai CC. Dermal and glomerular deposition of IgA in anaphylactoid purpura. *Am J Dis Child* 1977;131: 981–983.
36. Kuno-Sakai H, Sakai H, Nomoto Y, Takakura I, Kimura M. Increase of IgA-bearing peripheral blood lymphocytes in children with Henoch-Schönlein purpura. *Pediatrics* 1979;64: 918–922.
37. Kondo N, Kasahara K, Shinoda S, Orii T. Accelerated expression of secreted alpha-chain gene in anaphylactoid purpura. *J Clin Immunol* 1992;12:193–196.
38. Kauffmann RH, Herrmann WA, Meyer CJLM, Daha MR, Van Es LA. Circulating IgA-immune complexes in Henoch-Schönlein purpura. *Am J Med* 1980;69:859–866.
39. Schifferli JA, Yin CN, Peters DK. The role of complement and its receptor in the elimination of immune complexes. *N Engl J Med* 1986;315:488–495.
40. Garcia-Fuentes M, Martin A, Chantler C, Williams DG. Serum complement components in Henoch-Schönlein purpura. *Arch Dis Child* 1978;53:417–419.
41. Waxman FJ, Hebert LA, Cosio FG, et al. Differential binding of immunoglobulin A and immunoglobulin G1 immune complexes to primate erythrocytes in vivo: immunoglobulin A immune complexes bind less well to erythrocytes and are preferentially deposited in glomeruli. *J Clin Invest* 1986;77:82–89.
42. Kawana S, Nishiyama S. Serum SC5b-9 (terminal complement complex) level, a sensitive indicator of disease activity in patients with Henoch-Schönlein purpura. *Dermatology* 1992; 184:171–176.
43. Miller GW, Nussenzweig V. A new complement function: solubilization of antigen-antibody aggregates. *Proc Natl Acad Sci U S A* 1975;72:418–422.
44. Cornacoff JB, Hebert LA, Smead WL, VanAman ME, Birmingham DJ, Waxman FJ. Primate erythrocyte-immune complex-clearing mechanism. *J Clin Invest* 1983;71:236–247.
45. Medof ME, Iida K, Mold C, Nussenzweig V. Unique role of the complement receptor CR1 in the degradation of C3b associated with immune complexes. *J Exp Med* 1982;156:1739–1754.
46. Fearon DT. Cellular receptors for fragments of the third component of complement. *Immunol Today* 1984;5:105–110.
47. Hoffman GS, Specks U. Antineutrophil cytoplasmic antibodies. *Arthritis Rheum* 1998;41:1521–1537.
48. Savage J, Gillis D, Benson E, et al. International Consensus Statement on Testing and Reporting of Antineutrophil Cytoplasmic Antibodies (ANCA). *Am J Clin Pathol* 1999;111: 507–513.
49. Charles LA, Caldas MLR, Falk RJ, Terrell RS, Jennette JC. Antibodies against granule proteins activate neutrophils in vitro. *J Leukoc Biol* 1991;50:539–546.
50. Falk RJ, Terrell RS, Charles LA, Jennette JC. Anti-neutrophil cytoplasmic autoantibodies induce neutrophils to degranulate and produce oxygen radicals in vitro. *Proc Natl Acad Sci U S A* 1990;87:4115–4119.
51. Gilligan HM, Bredy B, Brady HR, et al. Antineutrophil cytoplasmic autoantibodies interact with primary granule constituents on the surface of apoptotic neutrophils in the absence of neutrophil priming. *J Exp Med* 1996;184:2231—2241.
52. Savage COS, Pottinger BE, Gaskin G, Pusey CD, Pearson JD. Autoantibodies developing to myeloperoxidase and proteinase 3 in systemic vasculitis stimulate neutrophil cytotoxicity toward cultured endothelial cells. *Am J Pathol* 1992;141:335–342.
53. Ewert BH, Jennette JC, Falk RJ. Antibodies against myeloperoxidase stimulate primed neutrophils to damage human endothelial cells in vitro. *Kidney Int* 1992;41:375–383.
54. Mayet WJ, Schwarting A, Orth T, et al. Antibodies to proteinase 3 mediate expression of vascular cell adhesion molecule-1 (VCAM-1). *Clin Exp Immunol* 1996;103:259–267.
55. Jennette CJ, Falk RJ. Pathogenesis of the vascular and glomerular damage in ANCA-positive vasculitis. *Nephrol Dial Transplant* 1998;13(suppl 1):16–20.
56. Muller Kobold AC, Kallenberg CG, Tervaert JW. Leucocyte membrane expression of proteinase 3 correlates with disease activity in patients with WG. *Br J Rheumatol* 1998;37: 901–907.
57. Muller Kobol AC, Kallenberg CG, Tervaert JW. Monocyte acti-

vation in patients with Wegener's granulomatosis. *Ann Rheum Dis* 1999;58:237–245.
58. Cambridge G, Rampton DS, Stevens TR, et al. Anti-neutrophil antibodies in inflammatory bowel disease: prevalence and diagnostic role. *Gut* 1992;33:668–674.
59. Seibold F, Brandwein S, Simpson S, et al. pANCA represents a cross-reactivity to enteric bacterial antigens. *J Clin Immunol* 1998;18:153–160.
60. Subra JF, Michelet C, Laporte J, et al. The presence of cytoplasmic antineutrophil cytoplasmic antibodies (cANCA) in the course of subacute bacterial endocarditis with glomerular involvement: coincidence of association? *Clin Nephrol* 1998;49: 15–8.
61. de Bandt M, Meyer O, Haim T, Kahn MF. Antineutrophil cytoplasmic antibodies in rheumatoid arthritis patients. *Br J Rheumatol* 1996;35:38–43.
62. Franssen C, Gans R, Kallenberg C, et al. Disease spectrum of patients with antineutrophil cytoplasmic autoantibodies of defined specificity: distinct differences between patients with anti-proteinase 3 and anti-myeloperoxidase autoantibodies. *J Intern Med* 1998;244:209–216.
63. Geffriaud-Ricouard C, Noel LH, Chauveau D, et al. Clinical spectrum associated with ANCA of defined antigen specificities in 98 selected patients. *Clin Nephrol* 1993;39:125–136.
64. Eichhorn J, Dagmar S, Thiele B, et al. Anti-endothelial cell antibodies in Takayasu arteritis. *Circulation* 1996;94:2396–2400.
65. Salojin KV, LeTonqueze M, Nassovov EL et al. Anti-endothelial cell antibodies in patients with various forms of vasculitis. *Clin Exp Rheumatol* 1996;14:163–169.
66. Brasile L, Kremer JM, Clarke JL, Cerilli J. Identification of an autoantibody to vascular endothelial cell-specific antigens in patients with systemic vasculitis. *Am J Med* 1989;87:74–80.
67. Varagunam M, Nwosu Z, Adu D, et al. Little evidence for anti-endothelial cell antibodies in microscopic polyarteritis and Wegener's granulomatosis. *Nephrol Dial Transplant* 1992;8: 113–117.
68. Leung DYM, Geha RS, Newburger JW, et al. Two monokines, interleukin-1 and tumor necrosis factor, render cultured vascular endothelial cells susceptible to lysis by antibodies circulating during Kawasaki syndrome. *J Exp Med* 1986;164:1958–1972.
69. Leung DYM, Collins T, Lapierre LA, Geha RS, Pober JS. Immunoglobulin M antibodies present in the acute phase of Kawasaki syndrome lyse cultured vascular endothelial cells stimulated by gamma interferon. *J Clin Invest* 1986;77: 1428–1435.
70. Savage COS, Pottinger BE, Gaskin G, Lockwood CM, Pusey CD, Pearson JD. Vascular damage in Wegener's granulomatosis and microscopic polyarteritis: presence of anti-endothelial cell antibodies and their relation to anti-neutrophil cytoplasm antibodies. *Clin Exp Immunol* 1991;85:14–19.
71. Del Papa N, Meroni PL, Barcellini W, et al. Antibodies to endothelial cells in primary vasculitides mediate in vitro endothelial cytotoxicity in the presence of normal peripheral blood mononuclear cells. *Clin Immunol Immunopathol* 1992; 63:267–274.
71. Del Papa N, Meroni PL, Barcellini W, et al. Antibodies to endothelial cells in primary vasculitides mediate in vitro endothelial cytotoxicity in the presence of normal peripheral blood mononuclear cells. *Clin Immunol Immunopathol* 1992; 63:267–274.
72. Estes PC, Cheville NF. The ultrastructure of vascular lesions in equine viral arteritis. *Am J Pathol* 1970;58:235–253.
73. Thomas L, Davidson M, McCluskey RT. Studies of PPLO infection I. The production of cerebral polyarteritis by *Mycoplasma gallisepticum* in turkeys; the neurotoxic property of the mycoplasma. *J Exp Med* 1966;123:897–912.
74. Reyes MG, Fresco R, Chokroverty S, Salud EQ. Viruslike particles in granulomatous angiitis of the central nervous system. *Neurology* 1976;26:797–799.
75. Linnemann CC, Alvira MM. Pathogenesis of varicella-zoster angiitis in the CNS. *Arch Neurol* 1980;37:239–240.
76. Doyle PW, Gibson G, Dolman CL. Herpes zoster ophthalmicus with contralateral hemiplegia: identification of cause. *Ann Neurol* 1983;14:84–85.
77. Cines DB, Lyss A, Mahin B, Corkey R, Kefalides NA, Friedman HM. Fc and C3 receptors induced by herpes simplex virus on cultured human endothelial cells. *J Clin Invest* 1982;69: 123–128.
78. Gisselbrecht M. Les vascularites au cours de l'infection par le virus de l'immunodeficience acquise. *Pathol Biol* 1999;47: 245–247.
79. Hasler P, Kistler H, Gerber H. Vasculitides in hairy cell leukemia. *Semin Arthritis Rheum* 1995;25:134–142.
80. Krol T, Robinson J, Bekeris L, Messmore H. Hairy cell leukemia and a fatal periarteritis nodosa-like syndrome. *Arch Pathol Lab Med* 1983;107:583–585.
81. Klima M, Waddell CC. Hairy cell leukemia associated with focal vascular damage. *Hum Pathol* 1984;15:657–659.
82. Hart MN, Tassell SK, Sadewasser KL, Schelper RL, Moore SA. Autoimmune vasculitis resulting from in vitro immunity of lymphocytes to smooth muscle. *Am J Pathol* 1985;119: 448–455.
83. Rasmussen N, Petersen J, Ralfkiaer E, Avnstrom S, Wiik A. Spontaneous and induced immunoglobulin synthesis and anti-neutrophil cytoplasm antibodies in Wegener's granulomatosis: relation to leukocyte subpopulations in blood and active lesions. *Rheumatol Int* 1988;8:153–158.
84. Gephardt GN, Ahmad M, Tubbs RR. Pulmonary vasculitis (Wegener's granulomatosis): immunohistochemical study of T and B cell markers. *Am J Med* 1983;74:700–704.
85. Ten Berge IJM, Wilmink JM, Meyer CJLM, et al. Clinical and immunological follow-up of patients with severe renal disease in Wegener's granulomatosis. *Am J Nephrol* 1985;5:21–29.
86. Giscombe R, Nityanand S, Lewin N, Grunewald J, Lefvert AK. Expanded T cell populations in patients with Wegener's granulomatosis: characteristics and correlates with disease activity. *J Clin Immunol* 1998;18:404–413.
87. Popa ER, Stegeman CA, Bos NA, Kallenberg CG, Tervaert JW. Differential B- and T-cell activation in Wegener's granulomatosis. *J Allergy Clin Immunol* 1999;103:885–894.
88. Schmitt WH, Heesen C, Csernok E, Rautmann A, Gross WL. Elevated serum levels of soluble interleukin-2 receptor in patients with Wegener's granulomatosis: association with disease activity. *Arthritis Rheum* 1992;35:1088–1096.
89. Kallenberg CGM, Cohen P, Tervaert JW, et al. Autoimmunity to lysosomal enzymes: new clues to vasculitis and glomerulonephritis? *Immunol Today* 1991;12:61–64.
90. Lockwood CM, Thiru S, Isaacs JD, Hale G, Waldmann H. Long-term remission of intractable systemic vasculitis with monoclonal antibody therapy. *Lancet* 1993;341:1620–1622.
91. Conn DL. Update on systemic necrotizing vasculitis. *Mayo Clin Proc* 1989;64:535–543.
92. Moore PM, Fauci AS. Neurologic manifestations of systemic vasculitis: a retrospective and prospective study of the clinicopathologic features and responses to therapy in 25 patients. *Am J Med* 1981;71:517–524.
93. Hellman DB, Laing TJ, Petri M, Whiting-O'Keefe Q, Parry GJ. Mononeuritis multiplex: the yield of evaluation for occult rheumatic diseases. *Medicine* 1988;67:145–153.
94. Brune MB, Walton SP, Varga D. Extensive mononeuritis multiplex as a solitary presentation of polyarteritis nodosa. *J Ky Med Assoc* 1995;93:15–18.

95. Kissel JT, Slivka AP, Warmolts JR, Mendell JR. The clinical spectrum of necrotizing angiopathy of the peripheral nervous system. *Ann Neurol* 1985;18:251–257.
96. Dyck PJ, Benstead TJ, Conn DL, Stevens JC, Windebank AJ, Low PA. Nonsystemic vasculitic neuropathy. *Brain* 1987;110: 843–854.
97. Wees SJ, Sunwoo IN, Oh SJ. Sural nerve biopsy in systemic necrotizing vasculitis. *Am J Med* 1981;71:525–532.
98. Dahlberg PJ, Lockhart JM, Overholt EL. Diagnostic studies for systemic necrotizing vasculitis: sensitivity, specificity, and predictive value in patients with multisystem disease. *Arch Intern Med* 1989;149:161–165.
99. Tribe CR, Scott DGI, Bacon PA. Rectal biopsy in the diagnosis of systemic vasculitis. *J Clin Pathol* 1981;34:843–850.
100. Lightfoot RW Jr, Michel BA, Bloch DA, et al. The American College of Rheumatology 1990 criteria for the classification of polyarteritis nodosa. *Arthritis Rheum* 1990;33:1088–1093.
101. Schrodt BJ, Callen JP. Polyarteritis nodosa attributable to minocycline treatment for acne vulgaris. *Pediatrics* 1999;103: 503–504.
102. Tekin M, Yalcinkaya F, Tumer N, et al. Familial Mediterranean fever: renal involvement by diseases other than amyloid. *Nephrol Dial Transplant* 1999;14:475–479.
103. Garcia F, Pedrol E, Casademont J, et al. Polyarteritis nodosa confined to calf muscles. *J Rheumatol* 1992;19:303–305.
104. Plaut A. Asymptomatic focal arteritis of the appendix: eighty-eight cases. *Am J Pathol* 1951;27:247–263.
105. Nuzum JW Jr, Nuzum JW Sr. Polyarteritis nodosa: statistical review of one hundred seventy-five cases from the literature and report of a typical case. *Arch Intern Med* 1954;94: 942–955.
106. Rose GA, Spencer H. Polyarteritis nodosa. *Q J Med* 1957;101: 43–81.
107. Guillevin L, Huong LTD, Godeau P, Jais P, Wechsler B. Clinical findings and prognosis of polyarteritis nodosa and Churg-Strauss angiitis: a study in 165 patients. *Br J Rheumatol* 1988; 27:258–264.
108. el-Reshaid K, Kapoor MM, el-Reshaid W, et al. The spectrum of renal disease associated with microscopic polyangiitis and classic polyarteritis nodosa in Kuwait. *Nephrol Dial Transplant* 1997;12:1874–1882.
109. Schrader ML, Hochman JS, Bulkley BH. The heart in polyarteritis nodosa: a clinicopathologic study. *Am Heart J* 1985; 109:1353–1359.
110. Holsinger DR, Osmundson PJ, Edwards JE. The heart in periarteritis nodosa. *Circulation* 1962;25:610–618.
111. Hu PJ, Shih IM, Hutchins GM, Hellman DB. Polyarteritis nodosa of the pericardium: antemortem diagnosis in a pericardiectomy specimen. *J Rheumatol* 1997;24:2042–2044.
112. Camilleri M, Pusey CD, Chadwick VS, Rees AJ. Gastrointestinal manifestations of systemic vasculitis. *Q J Med* 1983;206: 141–149.
113. Freilich BL, Bernstein CN. Vasculitis possibly confined to the small and large intestine. *West J Med* 1995;162:63–65.
114. Ito M, Sano K, Inaba H, Hotchi M. Localized necrotizing arteritis: a report of two cases involving the gallbladder and pancreas. *Arch Pathol Lab Med* 1991;115:780–783.
115. Cowan RE, Mallinson CN, Thomas GE, Thomson AD. Polyarteritis nodosa of the liver: a report of two cases. *Postgrad Med J* 1977;53:89–93.
116. Conn DL. Polyarteritis. *Rheum Dis Clin North Am* 1990;16: 341–362.
117. Dyck PJ, Conn DL, Okazaki H. Necrotizing angiopathic neuropathy: three-dimensional morphology of fiber degeneration related to sites of occluded vessels. *Mayo Clin Proc* 1972;47: 461–475.
118. Moore PM, Cupps TR. Neurological complications of vasculitis. *Ann Neurol* 1983;14:155–167.
119. Rosenberg MR, Parshley M, Gibson S, Wernick R. Central nervous system polyarteritis nodosa. *West J Med* 1990;153: 553–556.
120. Ford RG, Siekert RG. Central nervous system manifestations of periarteritis nodosa. *Neurology* 1965;15:114–122.
121. Cupps TR, Fauci AS. Systemic necrotizing vasculitis of the polyarteritis nodosa group. In: Smith LHJ, ed. *The vasculitides.* Philadelphia: WB Saunders, 1981:26–49.
122. Cohen RD, Conn DL, Ilstrup DM. Clinical features, prognosis, and response to treatment in polyarteritis. *Mayo Clin Proc* 1980;55:146–155.
123. Lie JT. Illustrated histopathologic classification criteria for selected vasculitis syndromes. *Arthritis Rheum* 1990;33: 1074–1087.
124. Albert DA, Rimon D, Silverstein MD. The diagnosis of -polyarteritis nodosa. I. A literature-based decision analysis approach. *Arthritis Rheum* 1988;31:1117–1127.
125. Travers RL, Allison DJ, Brettie RP, Hughes GRV. Polyarteritis nodosa: a clinical and angiographic analysis of 17 cases. *Semin Arthritis Rheum* 1979;8:184–199.
126. Bron KM, Strott CA, Shapiro AP. The diagnostic value of angiographic observations in polyarteritis nodosa. *Arch Intern Med* 1965;116:450–454.
127. Leonhardt ETG, Kullenberg KPG. Bilateral atrial myxomas with multiple arterial aneurysms: a syndrome mimicking polyarteritis nodosa. *Am J Med* 1977;62:792–794.
128. Citron BP, Peters RL. Angiitis in drug abusers. *N Engl J Med* 1971;284:112.
129. Frohnert PP, Sheps SG. Long-term follow-up study of periarteritis nodosa. *Am J Med* 1967;43:8–14.
130. Leib ES, Restivo C, Paulus HE. Immunosuppressive and corticosteroid therapy of polyarteritis nodosa. *Am J Med* 1979;67: 941–947.
131. Baggenstoss AH, Shick RM, Polley HF. The effect of cortisone on the lesions of periarteritis nodosa. *Am J Pathol* 1951;27: 537–559.
132. Fauci AS, Katz P, Haynes BF, Wolff SM. Cyclophosphamide therapy of severe systemic necrotizing vasculitis. *N Engl J Med* 1979;301:235–238.
133. Guillevin L, Fechner J, Godeau P, et al. Périartérite noueuse: étude clinique et thérapeutique de 126 malades étudiés en 23 ans. *Ann Med Interne* 1985;136:6–12.
134. Guillevin L, Jarrousse B, Lok C, et al. Longterm followup after treatment of polyarteritis nodosa and Churg-Strauss angiitis with comparison of steroids, plasma exchange and cyclophosphamide to steroids and plasma exchange: a prospective randomized trial of 71 patients. *J Rheumatol* 1991;18:567–574.
135. Guillevin L, Fain O, Lhote F, et al. Lack of superiority of steroids plus plasma exchange to steroids alone in the treatment of polyarteritis nodosa and Churg-Strauss syndrome. *Arthritis Rheum* 1992;35:208–215.
136. Pusey CD, Rees AJ, Evans DJ, Peters DK, Lockwood CM. Plasma exchange in focal necrotizing glomerulonephritis without anti-GBM antibodies. *Kidney Int* 1991;40:757–763.
137. Sergent JS, Lockshin MD, Christian CL, Gocke DJ. Vasculitis with hepatitis B antigenemia: long-term observations in nine patients. *Medicine* 1976;55:1–18.
138. Duffy J, Lidsky MD, Sharp JT, et al. Polyarthritis, polyarteritis and hepatitis B. *Medicine* 1976;55:19–37.
139. Guillevin L, Le THD, Gayraud M. Systemic vasculitis of the polyarteritis nodosa group and infection with hepatitis B virus: a study in 98 patients. *Eur J Intern Med* 1989;1:97–105.
140. Wood JR, Czaja AJ, Taswell HF, Ludwig J, Rakela J, Chase R. Hepatitis B virus deoxyribonucleic acid in serum during hepati-

tis Be antigen clearance in corticosteroid-treated severe chronic active hepatitis B. *Gastroenterology* 1987;93:1225–1230.
141. Lam KC, Lai CL, Ng RP, Trepo C, Wu PC. Deleterious effect of prednisolone in HBsAg-positive chronic active hepatitis. *N Engl J Med* 1981;304:380–386.
142. Guillevin L, Lhote F, Jarrousse B, et al. Polyarteritis nodosa related to hepatitis B virus: a retrospective study of 66 patients. *Ann Med Interne* 1992;143(suppl):63–74.
143. Kruger M, Boker KH, Zeidler H, Manns MP. Treatment of hepatitis B-related polyarteritis nodosa with famciclovir and interferon alfa-2b. *J Hepatol* 1997;26:935–939.
144. Guillevin L, Lhote F, Gherardi R. The spectrum and treatment of virus-associated vasculitides. *Curr Opin Rheumatol* 1997;9:31–36.
145. Mouthon L. Periarterite noueuse liee au virus de l'hepatite B. *Pathol Biol* 1999;47:237–244.
146. Kirkland GS, Saige J, Wilson D et al. Classical polyarteritis nodosa and microscopic polyarteritis with medium vessel involvement: a comparison of the clinical and laboratory features. *Clin Nephrol* 1997;47:176–180.
147. Lhote F, Cohen P, Genereau T, et al. Microscopic polyangiitis: clinical aspects and treatment. *Ann Med Interne* 1996;147: 165–177.
148. Guillevin L, Durand-Gasselin B, Cevallos R, et al. Microscopic polyangiitis: clinical and laboratory findings in eighty-five patients. *Arthritis Rheum* 1999;42:421–430.
149. Watts RA, Jolliffe VA, Carruthers DM, Lockwood M, Scott DG. Effect of classification on the incidence of polyarteritis nodosa and microscopic polyangiitis. *Arthritis Rheum* 1996;39: 1208–1212.
150. el-Reshaid K, Kapoor MM, el-Reshaid W, et al. The spectrum of renal disease associated with microscopic polyangiitis and classic polyarteritis nodosa in Kuwait. *Nephrol Dial Transplant* 1997;12:1874–1882.
151. Finan MC, Winkelmann RK. The cutaneous extravascular necrotizing granuloma (Churg-Strauss granuloma) and systemic disease: a review of 27 cases. *Medicine* 1984;62:142–158.
152. Lanham JG, Elkon KB, Pusey CD, Hughes GR. Systemic vasculitis with asthma and eosinophilia: a clinical approach to the Churg-Strauss syndrome. *Medicine* 1984;63:65–81.
153. Chumbley LC, Harrison EG Jr, DeRemee RA. Allergic granulomatosis and angiitis (Churg-Strauss syndrome): report and analysis of 30 cases. *Mayo Clin Proc* 1977;52:477–484.
154. Masi AT, Hunder GG, Lie JT, et al. The American College of Rheumatology 1990 criteria for the classification of Churg-Strauss syndrome (allergic granulomatosis and angiitis). *Arthritis Rheum* 1990;33:1094–1100.
155. Guillevin L, Cohen P, Gayraud M, et al. Churg-Strauss syndrome: clinical study and long-term followup of 96 patients. *Medicine* 1999;78:26–37.
156. Hattori N, Ichimura M, Nagamatsu M, et al. Clinicopathological features of Churg-Strauss syndrome associated neuropathy. *Brain* 1999;122:427–439.
157. Holloway J, Ferriss J, Groff J, Craig TJ, Klinik M. Churg-Strauss syndrome associated with zafirlukast: review. *J Am Osteopath Assoc* 1998:98:275–278.
158. Churg J. Allergic granulomatosis and granulomatous-vascular syndromes. *Ann Allergy* 1963;21:619–628.
159. Schmitt WH, Csernok E, Kobayashi S, et al. Churg-Strauss syndrome: serum markers of lymphocyte activation and endothelial damage. *Arthritis Rheum* 1998;41:445–452.
160. Chow CC, Li EKM, Lai FM. Allergic granulomatosis and angiitis (Churg-Strauss syndrome): response to pulse intravenous cyclophosphamide. *Ann Rheum Dis* 1989;48:605–608.
161. MacFadyen R, Tron V, Keshmiri M, Road JD. Allergic angiitis of Churg and Strauss syndrome: response to pulse methylprednisolone. *Chest* 1987;91:629–631.
162. Levy Y, George J, Fabbrizzi F, et al. Marked improvement of Churg-Strauss vasculitis with intravenous gammaglobulins. *South Med J* 1999;92:412–414.
163. Abu-Shakra M, Smythe H, Lewtas J, Badley E, Weber D, Keystone E. Outcome of polyarteritis nodosa and Churg-Strauss syndrome: an analysis of twenty-five patients. *Arthritis Rheum* 1994;37:1798–1803.
164. Klinger H. Grenzformen der periarteritis nodosa. *Frankf Z Pathol* 1931;42:455–480.
165. Watts RA, Carruthers DM, Scott DG. Epidemiology of systemic vasculitis: changing incidence or definition? *Semin Arthritis Rheum* 1995;25:28–34.
166. Cotch MF, Hoffman GS, Yerg DE, et al. The epidemiology of Wegener's granulomatosis: estimates of the five-year period prevalence, annual mortality, and geographic disease distribution from population-based data sources. *Arthritis Rheum* 1996;39:87–92.
167. Haugeberg G, Bie R, Bendvold A, Larsen AS, Johnsen V. Primary vasculitis in a Norwegian community hospital: a retrospective study. *Clin Rheumatol* 1998;17:364–368.
168. George J, Levy Y, Kallenberg CGM, Schoenfeld Y. Infections and Wegener's granulomatosis: a cause and effect relationship? *Q J Med* 1997;90:367–373.
169. Hoffman GS, Kerr GS, Leavitt RY, et al. Wegener granulomatosis: an analysis of 158 patients. *Ann Intern Med* 1992;116: 488–498.
170. McDonald TJ, DeRemee RA. Wegener's granulomatosis. *Laryngoscope* 1983;93:220–231.
171. Romas E, Murphy BF, d'Apice AJF, Kennedy JT, Niall JF. Wegener's granulomatosis: clinical features and prognosis in 37 patients. *Aust N Z J Med* 1993;23:168–175.
172. Stegeman CA, Tervaert JWC, Sluiter WJ, Manson WL, De Jong PE, Kallenberg CGM. Association of chronic nasal carriage of *Staphylococcus aureus* and higher relapse rates in Wegener granulomatosis. *Ann Intern Med* 1994;120:12–17.
173. Cordier JF, Valeyre D, Guillevin L, Loire R, Brechot JM. Pulmonary Wegener's granulomatosis: a clinical and imaging study of 77 cases. *Chest* 1990;97:906–912.
174. Cohen P, Tervaert JW, Huitema MG, et al. Prevention of relapses in Wegener's granulomatosis by treatment based on antineutrophil cytoplasmic antibody titre. *Lancet* 1990;336: 709–711.
175. Walton EW. Giant-cell granuloma of the respiratory tract (Wegener's granulomatosis). *Br Med J* 1958;2:265–270.
176. Schleiffer T, Burkhard B, Klooker P, Brass H. Clinical course and symptomatic prediagnostic period of patients with Wegener's granulomatosis and microscopic polyangiitis. *Renal Fail* 1998;20:519–532.
177. Carrington CB, Liebow AA. Limited forms of angiitis and granulomatosis of Wegener's type. *Am J Med* 1966;41:497–527.
178. Cassan SM, Coles DT, Harrison EG Jr. The concept of limited forms of Wegener's granulomatosis. *Am J Med* 1970;49: 366–379.
179. Fauci AS, Wolff SM. Wegener's granulomatosis: studies in eighteen patients and a review of the literature. *Medicine* 1973;52: 535–560.
180. Wolff SM, Fauci AS, Horn RG, Dale DC. Wegener's granulomatosis. *Ann Intern Med* 1974;81:513–525.
181. Fauci AS, Haynes BF, Katz P, Wolff SM. Wegener's granulomatosis: prospective clinical and therapeutic experience with 85 patients for 21 years. *Ann Intern Med* 1983;98:76–85.
182. Pinching AJ, Lockwood CM, Pussell BA, et al. Wegener's granulomatosis: observations on 18 patients with severe renal disease. *Q J Med* 1983;208:435–460.
183. Andrassy K, Erb A, Koderisch J, Waldherr R, Ritz E. Wegener's granulomatosis with renal involvement: patient survival and

correlations between initial renal function, renal histology, therapy and renal outcome. *Clin Nephrol* 1991;35:139–147.

184. Haynes BF, Fishman ML, Fauci AS, Wolff SM. The ocular manifestations of Wegener's granulomatosis: fifteen years experience and review of the literature. *Am J Med* 1977;63:131–141.
185. Fahey JL, Leonard E, Churg J, Godman G. Wegener's granulomatosis. *Am J Med* 1954;17:168–179.
186. Travis WD, Hoffman GS, Leavitt RY, Pass HI, Fauci AS. Surgical pathology of the lung in Wegener's granulomatosis: review of 87 open lung biopsies from 67 patients. *Am J Surg Pathol* 1991;15:315–333.
187. Travis WD, Colby TV, Lombard C, Carpenter HA. A clinicopathologic study of 34 cases of diffuse pulmonary hemorrhage with lung biopsy confirmation. *Am J Surg Pathol* 1990;14: 1112–1125.
188. Van der Woude FJ, Rasmussen N, Lobatto S, et al. Autoantibodies against neutrophils and monocytes: tool for diagnosis and marker of disease activity in Wegener's granulomatosis. *Lancet* 1985;1:425–429.
189. N÷lle B, Specks U, Lüdemann J, Rohrbach MS, DeRemee RA, Gross WL. Anticytoplasmic autoantibodies: their immunodiagnostic value in Wegener granulomatosis. *Ann Intern Med* 1989; 111:28–40.
190. Specks U, Wheatley CL, McDonald TJ, Rohrbach MS, DeRemee RA. Anticytoplasmic autoantibodies in the diagnosis and follow-up of Wegener's granulomatosis. *Mayo Clin Proc* 1989; 64:28–36.
191. Cohen P, Tervaert JW, Van der Woude FJ, et al. Association between active Wegener's granulomatosis and anticytoplasmic antibodies. *Arch Intern Med* 1989;149:2461–2465.
192. Kerr GS, Fleisher TA, Hallahan CW, Leavitt RY, Fauci AS, Hoffman GS. Limited prognostic value of changes in antineutrophil cytoplasmic antibody titer in patients with Wegener's granulomatosis. *Arthritis Rheum* 1993;36:365–371.
193. Lang SM, Astner S, Fischer R, Schiffl H, Huber RM. Dissociation between high anti-PR3 titers (c-ANCA) and the clinical course of disease in a case of Wegener granulomatosis. *Wien Klin Wochenschr* 1998;110:691–694.
194. Gross WL, Csernok E, Flesch BK. Classic anti-neutrophil cytoplasmic autoantibodies (cANCA), Wegener's autoantigen and their immunopathogenic role in Wegener's granulomatosis. *J Autoimmun* 1993;6:171–184.
195. Devaney KO, Travis WD, Hoffman G, Leavitt R, Lebovics R, Fauci AS. Interpretation of head and neck biopsies in Wegener's granulomatosis: a pathologic study of 126 biopsies in 70 patients. *Am J Surg Pathol* 1990;14:555–564.
196. Del Buono EA, Flint A. Diagnostic usefulness of nasal biopsy in Wegener's granulomatosis. *Hum Pathol* 1991;22:107–110.
197. Colby TV, Tazelaar HD, Specks U, DeRemee RA. Nasal biopsy in Wegener's granulomatosis. *Hum Pathol* 1991;22:101–104.
198. Hollander D, Manning RT. The use of alkylating agents in the treatment of Wegener's granulomatosis. *Ann Intern Med* 1967; 67:393–398.
199. Reza MJ, Dornfeld L, Goldberg LS, Bluestone R, Pearson CM. Wegener's granulomatosis: long-term followup of patients treated with cyclophosphamide. *Arthritis Rheum* 1975;18: 501–506.
200. Illum P, Thorling K. Wegener's granulomatosis: long-term results of treatment. *Ann Otol Rhinol Laryngol* 1981;90: 231–235.
201. Bradley JD, Brandt KD, Katz BP. Infectious complications of cyclophosphamide treatment for vasculitis. *Arthritis Rheum* 1989;32:45–53.
202. Langford CA, Sneller MC. Pulse versus oral cyclophosphamide in the treatment of Wegener's granulomatosis: comment on the article by Guillevin et al. *Arthritis Rheum* 1998;41:1706–1707.
203. Langford CA, Klippel JH, Balow JE, James SP, Sneller MC. Use of cytotoxic agents and cyclosporine in the treatment of autoimmune disease. Part 2: Inflammatory bowel disease, systemic vasculitis, and therapeutic toxicity. *Ann Intern Med* 1998;129: 49–58.
204. Stone JH, Tun W, Hellman DB. Treatment of non-life threatening Wegener's granulomatosis with methotrexate and daily prednisone as the initial therapy of choice. *J Rheumatol* 1999; 26:1134–9.
205. DeRemee RA, McDonald TJ, Weiland LH. Wegener's granulomatosis: observations on treatment with antimicrobial agents. *Mayo Clin Proc* 1985;60:27–32.
206. deGroot K, Reinhold-Keller E, Tatsis E, et al. Therapy for the maintenance of remission in sixty-five patients with generalized Wegener's granulomatosis. *Arthritis Rheum* 1996;39:2052–2061.
207. Leung DYM, Schlievert PM, Meissner CH. The immunopathogenesis and management of Kawasaki syndrome. *Arthritis Rheum* 1998;41:1538–1547.
208. Kawasaki T, Kosaki F, Okawa S, Shigematsu I, Yanagawa H. A new infantile acute febrile mucocutaneous lymph node syndrome (MLNS) prevailing in Japan. *Pediatrics* 1974;54: 271–276.
209. Melish ME. Clinical and epidemiologic aspects of Kawasaki disease. *Clin Cardiol* 1991;14(suppl II):3–10.
210. Burns JC, Mason WH, Glade MP, et al. Clinical and epidemiologic characteristics of patients referred for evaluation of possible Kawasaki disease. *J Pediatr* 1991;118:680–686.
211. Hiraishi S, Yashiro K, Oguchi K, Kusano S, Ishii K, Nakazawa K. Clinical course of cardiovascular involvement in the mucocutaneous lymph node syndrome: relation between clinical signs of carditis and development of coronary arterial aneurysm. *Am J Cardiol* 1981;47:323–330.
212. Suzuki A, Kamiya T, Kuwahara N, et al. Coronary arterial lesions of Kawasaki disease: cardiac catheterization findings of 1100 cases. *Pediatr Cardiol* 1986;7:3–9.
213. Kato H, Ichinose E, Yoshioka F, et al. Fate of coronary aneurysms in Kawasaki disease: serial coronary angiography and long-term follow-up study. *Am J Cardiol* 1982;49:1758–1766.
214. Capannari TE, Daniels SR, Meyer RA, Schwartz DC, Kaplan S. Sensitivity, specificity and predictive value of two-dimensional echocardiography in detecting coronary artery aneurysms in patients with Kawasaki disease. *J Am Coll Cardiol* 1986;7: 355–360.
215. Wortmann DW, Nelson AM. Kawasaki syndrome. *Rheum Dis Clin North Am* 1990;16:363–375.
216. Tanaka N, Naoe S, Masuda H, Ueno T. Pathological study of sequelae of Kawasaki disease (MCLS): with special reference to the heart and coronary arterial lesions. *Acta Pathol Jpn* 1986;36: 1513–1527.
217. Akagi T, Kato H, Inoue O, Sato N, Imamura K. Valvular heart disease in Kawasaki syndrome: incidence and natural history. *Am Heart J* 1990;120:366–372.
218. Newburger JW, Takahashi M, Burns JC, et al. The treatment of Kawasaki syndrome with intravenous gamma globulin. *N Engl J Med* 1986;315:341–347.
219. Takahashi M, Newburger JW. Long-term follow-up of coronary abnormalities in Kawasaki syndrome treated with and without IV gamma globulin. *Circulation* 1990;82(suppl):717.
220. Newburger JW, Takahashi M, Beiser AS, et al. A single intravenous infusion of gamma globulin as compared with four infusions in the treatment of acute Kawasaki syndrome. *N Engl J Med* 1991;324:1633–1639.
221. Buerger L. Recent studies in the pathology of thromboangiitis obliterans. *J Med Res* 1914;31:181–194.
222. Grove WJ, Stansby GP. Buerger's disease and cigarette smoking in Bangladesh. *Ann R Coll Surg Engl* 1992;74:115–118.

223. Olin JW, Young JR, Graor RA, Ruschhaupt WF, Bartholomew JR. The changing clinical spectrum of thromboangiitis obliterans (Buerger's disease). *Circulation* 1990;82(suppl IV):3–8.
224. Lie JT. The rise and fall and resurgence of thromboangiitis obliterans (Buerger's disease). *Acta Pathol Jpn* 1989;39: 153–158.
225. Shionoya S. What is Buerger's disease. *World J Surg* 1983;7: 544–551.
226. Lie JT. Visceral Intestinal Buerger's disease. *Int J Cardiol* 1998; 66(suppl 1):S249–256.
227. Olin JW. Thromboangiitis obliterans. *Curr Opin Rheumatol* 1994;6:44–49.
228. Shionoya S, Hirai M, Kawai S, Seko T, Ban I. Pattern of arterial occlusion in Buerger's disease. *Angiology* 1982;33:375–384.
229. Suzuki S, Mine H, Umehara I, Yoshida T, Okada Y. Buerger's disease (thromboangiitis obliterans): an analysis of the arteriograms of 119 cases. *Clin Radiol* 1982;33:235–240.
230. Joyce JW. Buerger's disease (thromboangiitis obliterans). *Rheum Dis Clin North Am* 1990;16:463–470.
231. Adar R, Papa MZ, Halpern Z, et al. Cellular sensitivity to collagen in thromboangiitis obliterans. *N Engl J Med* 1983;308: 1113–1116.
232. Papa M, Bass A, Adar R, et al. Autoimmune mechanisms in thromboangiitis obliterans (Buerger's disease): the role of tobacco antigen and the major histocompatibility complex. *Surgery* 1992;111:527–531.
233. Halacheva KS, Manolova IM, Petkov DP, Andreev AP. Study of anti-neutrophil cytoplasmic antibodies in patients with thromboangiitis obliterans (Buerger's disease). *Scand J Immunol* 1998; 48:544–550.
234. Eichhorn J, Sima D, Lindschau C, et al. Antiendothelial cell antibodies in thromboangiitis obliterans. *Am J Med Sci* 1998; 315:17–23.
235. Ekenstam E, Callen JP. Cutaneous leukocytoclastic vasculitis: clinical and laboratory features of 82 patients seen in private practice. *Arch Dermatol* 1984;120:484–489.
236. Gibson LE, Su WPD. Cutaneous vasculitis. *Rheum Dis Clin North Am* 1990;16:309–324.
237. Smoller BR, McNutt NS, Contreras F. The natural history of vasculitis: what the histology tells us about pathogenesis. *Arch Dermatol* 1990;126:84–89.
238. Sanchez NP, Van Hale HM, Su WPD. Clinical and histopathologic spectrum of necrotizing vasculitis: report of findings in 101 cases. *Arch Dermatol* 1985;121:220–224.
239. Sams WM Jr. Hypersensitivity angiitis. *J Invest Dermatol* 1989; 93:78S–81S.
240. Cupps TR, Springer RM, Fauci AS. Chronic, recurrent small-vessel cutaneous vasculitis: clinical experience in 13 patients. *JAMA* 1982;247:1994–1998.
241. Hazen PG, Michel B. Management of necrotizing vasculitis with colchicine: improvement in patients with cutaneous lesions and Behçet's syndrome. *Arch Dermatol* 1979;115: 1303–1306.
242. Fredenberg MF, Malkinson FD. Sulfone therapy in the treatment of leukocytoclastic vasculitis: report of three cases. *J Am Acad Dermatol* 1987;16:772–778.
243. Stewart M, Savage JM, Bell B, McCord B. Long term renal prognosis of Henoch-Schönlein purpura in an unselected childhood population. *Eur J Pediatr* 1988;147:113–115.
244. Blanco R, Martinez-Taboada VM, Rodriguez-Valverde V, Garcia-Fuentes M. Cutaneous vasculitis in children and adults: associated diseases and etiologic factors in 303 patients. *Medicine* 1998;77:403–418.
245. Allen DM, Diamond LK, Howell DA. Anaphylactoid purpura in children (Schönlein-Henoch syndrome). *Am J Dis Child* 1960;99:833–854.
246. Ansell BM. Henoch-Schönlein purpura with particular reference to the prognosis of the renal lesion. *Br J Dermatol* 1970;82: 211–215.
247. Lanzkowsky S, Lanzkowsky L, Lanzkowsky P. Henoch-Schönlein purpura. *Pediatr Rev* 1992;13:130–137.
248. Martinez-Frontanilla LA, Haase GM, Ernster JA, Bailey WC. Surgical complications in Henoch-Schönlein purpura. *J Pediatr Surg* 1984;19:434–436.
249. Couture A, Veyrac C, Baud C, Galifer RB, Armelin I. Evaluation of abdominal pain in Henoch-Schönlein syndrome by high frequency ultrasound. *Pediatr Radiol* 1992;22:12–17.
250. Kato S, Shibuya H, Naganuma H, Nakagawa H. Gastrointestinal endoscopy in Henoch-Schönlein purpura. *Eur J Pediatr* 1992;151:482–484.
251. Tomomasa T, Hsu JY, Itoh K, Kuroume T. Endoscopic findings in pediatric patients with Henoch-Schönlein purpura and gastrointestinal symptoms. *J Pediatr Gastroenterol Nutr* 1987;6:725–729.
252. Austin HA III, Balow JE. Henoch-Schönlein nephritis: prognostic features and the challenge of therapy. *Am J Kidney Dis* 1983;2:512–520.
253. Niaudet P, Murcia I, Beaufils H, Broyer M, Habib R. Primary IgA nephropathies in children: prognosis and treatment. *Adv Nephrol Necker Hosp* 1993;22:121–140.
254. Meadow SR, Glasgow EF, White RHR, Moncrieff MW, Cameron JS, Ogg CS. Schönlein-Henoch nephritis. *Q J Med* 1972;41:241–258.
255. Goldstein AR, White RHR, Akuse R, Chantler C. Long-term follow-up of childhood Henoch-Schönlein nephritis. *Lancet* 1992;339:280–282.
256. Clark WR, Kramer SA. Henoch-Schönlein purpura and the acute scrotum. *J Pediatr Surg* 1986;21:991–992.
257. Belman AL, Leicher CR, Moshe SL, Mezey AP. Neurologic manifestations of Schönlein-Henoch purpura: report of three cases and review of the literature. *Pediatrics* 1985;75:687–692.
258. Clark JH, Fitzgerald JF. Hemorrhagic complications of Henoch-Schönlein syndrome. *J Pediatr Gastroenterol Nutr* 1985;4:311–315.
259. Mills JA, Michel BA, Bloch DA, et al. The American College of Rheumatology 1990 criteria for the classification of Henoch-Schönlein purpura. *Arthritis Rheum* 1990;33:1114–1121.
260. Gibson LE. Cutaneous vasculitis: approach to diagnosis and systemic associations. *Mayo Clin Proc* 1990;65:221–229.
261. Hattori M, Ito K, Konomoto T, et al. Plasmapheresis as the sole therapy for rapidly progressive Henoch-Schönlein purpura nephritis in children. *Am J Kidney Dis* 1999;33:427–433.
262. Kusuda A, Migita K, Tsuboi M, et al. Successful treatment of adult-onset Henoch-Schönlein purpura nephritis with high-dose immunoglobulins. *Intern Med* 1999;38:376–9.
263. Fukui H, Kamitsuji H, Nagao T, et al. Clinical evaluation of a pasteurized factor XIII concentrate administration in Henoch-Schönlein purpura. *Thromb Res* 1989;56:667–675.
264. Moreland LW, Ball GV. Cutaneous polyarteritis nodosa. *Am J Med* 1990;88:426–430.
265. Borrie P. Cutaneous polyarteritis nodosa. *Br J Dermatol* 1972; 87:87–95.
266. Diaz-Perez JL, Winkelmann RK. Cutaneous periarteritis nodosa. *Arch Dermatol* 1974;110:407–414.
267. Dyk T. Cutaneous polyarteritis. *Br Med J* 1973;1:551.
268. Lindgren I, Lundmark C. Periarteritis nodosa as a skin disease. *Acta Derm Venereol* 1956;36:343–354.
269. Smukler NM, Schumacher HR Jr. Chronic nondestructive arthritis associated with cutaneous polyarteritis. *Arthritis Rheum* 1977;20:1114–1120.
270. Mekori YA, Awai LE, Wiedel JD, Kohler PF. Cutaneous polyarteritis nodosa associated with rapidly progressive arthritis. *Arthritis Rheum* 1984;27:574–578.

271. Lever W, Shaumberg-Lever G. Vascular diseases. In: Lever W, Shaumberg-Lever G, eds. *Histopathology of the skin.* 7th ed. Philadelphia: JB Lippincott, 1990:196–197.
272. Diaz-Perez JL, Schroeter AL, Winkelmann RK. Cutaneous periarteritis nodosa: immunofluorescence studies. *Arch Dermatol* 1980;116:56–58.
273. Goslen JB, Graham W, Lazarus GS. Cutaneous polyarteritis nodosa: report of a case associated with Crohn's disease. *Arch Dermatol* 1983;119:326–329.
274. Whittaker SJ, Dover JS, Greaves MW. Cutaneous polyarteritis nodosa associated with hepatitis B surface antigen. *J Am Acad Dermatol* 1986;15:1142–1145.
275. Solley GO, Winkelmann RK, Rovelstad RA. Correlation between regional enterocolitis and cutaneous polyarteritis nodosa. *Gastroenterology* 1975;69:235–239.
276. Meltzer M, Franklin EC, Elias K, McCluskey RT, Cooper N. Cryoglobulinemia: a clinical and laboratory study. II. Cryoglobulins with rheumatoid factor activity. *Am J Med* 1966;40: 837–856.
277. Gorevic PD, Kassab HJ, Levo Y, et al. Mixed cryoglobulinemia: clinical aspects and long-term follow-up of 40 patients. *Am J Med* 1980;69:287–308.
278. Giannetti A, Serri F, Bernasconi C. Immunofluorescent studies of the skin in mixed cryoglobulinaemia and Schönlein-Henoch purpura. *Acta Derm Venereol* 1976;56:211–216.
279. Sinico RA, Winearls CG, Sabadini E, Fornasieri A, Castiglione A, D'Amico G. Identification of glomerular immune deposits in cryoglobulinemia glomerulonephritis. *Kidney Int* 1988;34: 109–116.
280. Monti G, Galli M, Invernizzi F, et al. Cryoglobulinaemias: a multi-centre study of the early clinical and laboratory manifestations of primary and secondary disease. *Q J Med* 1995;88: 115–126.
281. Weiner SM, Berg T, Berthold H, et al. A clinical and virological study of hepatitis C virus-related cryoglobulinemia in Germany. *J Hepatol* 1998;29:375–384.
282. Agnello V, Gyorgy A. (Localization of hepatitis C virus in cutaneous vasculitic lesions in patients with type II cryoglobulinemia. *Arthritis Rheum* 1997;40:2007–2015.
283. Lee YH, Ji JD, Yeon JE, et al. Cryoglobulinaemia and rheumatic manifestations in patients with hepatitis C virus infection. *Ann Rheum Dis* 1998;57:728–731.
284. Brouet JC, Clauvel JP, Danon F, Klein M, Seligmann M. Biologic and clinical significance of cryoglobulins: a report of 86 cases. *Am J Med* 1974;57:775–788.
285. Shusterman N, London WT. Hepatitis B and immune-complex disease. *N Engl J Med* 1984;310:43–46.
286. Popp JW, Dienstag JL, Wands JR, Bloch KJ. Essential mixed cryoglobulinemia without evidence for hepatitis B virus infection. *Ann Intern Med* 1980;92:379–383.
287. Galli M, Invernizzi F. Hepatitis B virus and cryoglobulinemia. *Ann Intern Med* 1981;95:522.
288. Levey JM, Bjornsson B, Banner B, et al. Mixed cryoglobulinemia in chronic hepatitis C infection: a clinicopathologic analysis of 10 cases and review of recent literature. *Medicine* 1994;73:53–67.
289. Cohen P. Cryoglobulinemia related to the hepatitis B and C viruses. *Pathol Biol* 1999;47:232–236.
290. Gordon ACH, Edgar JDM, Finch RG. Acute exacerbation of vasculitis during interferon-α therapy for hepatitis C-associated cryoglobulinaemia. *J Infect* 1998;36:229–230.
291. Cid MC, Hernandez-Rodriguez J, Robert J, et al. Interferon-alpha may exacerbate cryoglobulinemia-related ischemic manifestations: an adverse effect potentially related to its anti-angiogenic activity. *Arthritis Rheum* 1999;42:1051–1055.
292. Siami FS, Siami GA. Cryofiltration apheresis in the treatment of cryoprecipitate induced diseases. *Ther Apher* 1997;1:58–62.
293. McDuffie FC, Sams WM Jr, Maldonado JE, Andreini PH, Conn DL, Samayoa EA. Hypocomplementemia with cutaneous vasculitis and arthritis. *Mayo Clin Proc* 1973;48:340–348.
294. Peteiro C, Toribio J. Incidence of leukocytoclastic vasculitis in chronic idiopathic urticaria: study of 100 cases. *Am J Dermatopathol* 1989;11:528–533.
295. Asherson RA, D'Cruz D, Stephens CJM, McKee PH, Hughes GRV. Urticarial vasculitis in a connective tissue disease clinic: patterns, presentations, and treatment. *Semin Arthritis Rheum* 1991;20:285–296.
296. Mehregan DR, Hall MJ, Gibson LE. Urticarial vasculitis: a histopathologic and clinical review of 72 cases. *J Am Acad Dermatol* 1992;26:441–448.
297. Sanchez NP, Winkelmann RK, Schroeter AL, Dicken CH. The clinical and histopathologic spectrums of urticarial vasculitis: study of forty cases. *J Am Acad Dermatol* 1982;7:599–605.
298. Monroe EW, Schulz CI, Maize JC, Jordan RE. Vasculitis in chronic urticaria: an immunopathologic study. *J Invest Dermatol* 1981;76:103–107.
299. Jones RR, Bhogal B, Dash A, Schifferli J. Urticaria and vasculitis: a continuum of histological and immunopathological changes. *Br J Dermatol* 1983;108:695–703.
300. Aboobaker J, Greaves MW. Urticarial vasculitis. *Clin Exp Dermatol* 1986;2:436–444.
301. Wisnieski JJ, Naff GB. Serum IgG antibodies to C1q in hypocomplementemic urticarial vasculitis syndrome. *Arthritis Rheum* 1989;32:1119–1127.
302. Davis MD, Daoud MS, Gibsone LE, Rogers RS III. Clinicopathologic correlation of hypocomplementemic and normocomplementemic urticarial vasculitis. *J Am Acad Dermatol* 1998;38:899–905.
303. Eiser AR, Singh P, Shanies HM. Sustained dapsone-induced remission of hypocomplementemic urticarial vasculitis: a case report. *Angiology* 1997;48:1019–1022.
304. Hall S, Barr W, Lie JT, Stanson AW, Kazmier FJ, Hunder GG. Takayasu arteritis: a study of 32 North American patients. *Medicine* 1985;64:89–99.
305. Baltazares M, Mendoza F, Dabague J, Reyes PA. Antiaorta antibodies and Takayasu arteritis. *Int J Cardiol* 1998;66(suppl 1): S183–S188.
306. Hoffman GS, Ahmed AE. Surrogate markers of disease activity in patients with Takayasu arteritis: a preliminary report from The International Network for the Study of the Systemic Vasculitides (INSSYS). *Int J Cardiol* 1998;66(suppl 1): S191–S194.
307. Kitamura H, Kobayashi Y, Kimura A, Numano F. Association of clinical manifestations with HLA-B alleles in Takayasu arteritis. *Int J Cardiol* 1998;66(suppl 1):121–126.
308. Kerr GS, Hallahan CW, Giordano J, et al. Takayasu arteritis. *Ann Intern Med* 1994;120:919–929.
309. Strachan RW. The natural history of Takayasu's arteriopathy. *Q J Med* 1964;33:57–69.
310. Lupi-Herrera E, Sanchez-Torres G, Marcushamer J, Mispireta J, Horwitz S, Vela JE. Takayasu's arteritis: clinical study of 107 cases. *Am Heart J* 1977;93:94–103.
311. Spencer R, Tolentino FI, Doyle GJ. Takayasu's arteritis: case report and review emphasizing ocular manifestations. *Ann Ophthalmol* 1980;12:935–938.
312. Hall S, Buchbinder R. Takayasu's arteritis. *Rheum Dis Clin North Am* 1990;16:411–422.
313. Talwar KK, Kumar K, Chopra P, et al. Cardiac involvement in nonspecific aortoarteritis (Takayasu's arteritis). *Am Heart J* 1991;122:1666–1670.
314. Amano J, Suzuki A. Coronary artery involvement in Takayasu's arteritis: collective review and guideline for surgical treatment. *J Thorac Cardiovasc Surg* 1991;102:554–560.

315. Lupi E, Sanchez G, Horwitz S, Gutierrez E. Pulmonary artery involvement in Takayasu's arteritis. *Chest* 1975;67:69–74.
316. Sharma S, Kamalakar T, Rajani M, Talwar KK, Shrivastava S. The incidence and patterns of pulmonary artery involvement in Takayasu's arteritis. *Clin Radiol* 1990;42:177–182.
317. Ask-Upmark E. On the pathogenesis of the hypertension in Takayasu's syndrome. *Acta Med Scand* 1961;169:467–477.
318. Sharma BK, Jain S, Radotra BD. An autopsy study of Takayasu's arteritis in India. *Int J Cardiol* 1998;66(suppl 1):85–90.
319. Perniciaro CV, Winkelmann RK, Hunder GG. Cutaneous manifestations of Takayasu's arteritis: a clinicopathologic correlation. *J Am Acad Dermatol* 1987;17:998–1005.
320. Hahn D, Thomson PD, Kala U, et al. A Review of Takayasu's arteritis in children in Gauteng, South Africa. *Pediatr Nephrol* 1998;12:68–75.
321. Berkmen YM, Lande A. Chest roentgenography as a window to the diagnosis of Takayasu's arteritis. *Am J Roentgenol Radium Ther Nucl Med* 1975;125:842–846.
322. Yamada I, Numano F, Suzuki S. Takayasu arteritis: evaluation with MR imaging. *Radiology* 1993;188:89–94.
323. Arend WP, Michel BA, Bloch DA, et al. The American College of Rheumatology 1990 criteria for the classification of Takayasu arteritis. *Arthritis Rheum* 1990;33:1129–1134.
324. Ishikawa K. Effects of prednisolone therapy on arterial angiographic features in Takayasu's disease. *Am J Cardiol* 1991;68: 410–413.
325. Fraga A, Mintz G, Valle L, Flores-Izquierdo G. Takayasu's arteritis: frequency of systemic manifestations (study of 22 patients) and favorable response to maintenance steroid therapy with adrenocorticosteroids (12 patients). *Arthritis Rheum* 1972; 15:617–624.
326. Shelhamer JH, Volkman DJ, Parrillo JE, Lawley TJ, Johnston MR, Fauci AS. Takayasu's arteritis and its therapy. *Ann Intern Med* 1985;103:121–126.
327. Hoffman GS, Leavitt RY, Kerr GS, Rottem M, Sneller MC, Fauci AS. Treatment of glucocorticoid-resistant or relapsing Takayasu arteritis with methotrexate. *Arthritis Rheum* 1994;37:578–582.
328. Anonymous. Case records of the Massachusetts General Hospital (case 4-1995). *N Engl J Med* 1995;332:380–386.
329. Daina E, Schieppati A, Remuzzi G. Mycophenolate mofetil for the treatment of Takayasu arteritis: report of three cases. *Ann Intern Med* 1999;130:422–426.
330. Ishikawa K. Survival and morbidity after diagnosis of occlusive thromboaortopathy (Takayasu's disease). *Am J Cardiol* 1981;47: 1026–1032.
331. Subramanyan R, Joy J, Balakrishnan KG. Natural history of aortoarteritis (Takayasu's disease). *Circulation* 1989;80: 429–437.
332. Kimoto S. The history and present status of aortic surgery in Japan particularly for aortitis syndrome. *J Cardiovasc Surg* 1979; 20:107–126.
333. Sharma S, Bahl Vk, Saxena A, et al. Stenosis in the aorta caused by non-specific aortitis: results of treatment by percutaneous stent placement. *Clin Radiol* 1999;54:46–50.
334. Horton BT, Magath TB, Brown GE. An undescribed form of arteritis of the temporal vessels. *Mayo Clin Proc* 1932;7:700–701.
335. Jennings GH. Arteritis of the temporal vessels. *Lancet* 1938;1: 424–428.
336. Boeson P, Sorensen SF. Giant cell arteritis, temporal arteritis, and polymyalgia rheumatica in a Danish county: a prospective investigation, 1982-1985. *Arthritis Rheum* 1987;30:294–299.
337. Machado EBV, Michet CJ, Ballard DJ, et al. Trends in incidence and clinical presentation of temporal arteritis in Olmsted County, Minnesota, 1950-1985. *Arthritis Rheum* 1988;31: 745–749.
338. Duhaut P, Bosshard S, Calvet A, et al. Giant cell arteritis, polymyalgia rheumatica, and viral hypotheses: a multicenter, prospective case-control study: Groupe de Recherche sur l'Arterite a Cellules Geantes. *J Rheumatol* 1999;26:361–369.
339. Gabriel SE, Espy M, Erdman DD, et al. The role of parvovirus B19 in the pathogenesis of giant cell arteritis: a preliminary evaluation. *Arthritis Rheum* 1999;42:1255–1258.
340. Smith CA, Fidler WJ, Pinals RS. The epidemiology of giant cell arteritis: report of a ten-year study in Shelby County, Tennessee. *Arthritis Rheum* 1983;26:1214–1219.
341. Bielory L, Ogunkoya A, Frohman LP. Temporal arteritis in blacks. *Am J Med* 1989;86:707–708.
342. Gonzalez EB, Varner WT, Lisse JR, Daniels JC, Hokanson JA. Giant-cell arteritis in the southern United States: an 11-year retrospective study from the Texas Gulf Coast. *Arch Intern Med* 1989;149:1561–1565.
343. Lie JT, Gordon LP, Titus JL. Juvenile temporal arteritis: biopsy study of four cases. *JAMA* 1975;234:496–499.
344. Bethlenfalvay NC, Nusynowitz ML. Temporal arteritis: a rarity in the young adult. *Arch Intern Med* 1964;114:487–489.
345. Mathewson JA, Hunder GG. Giant cell arteritis in two brothers. *J Rheumatol* 1986;13:190–192.
346. Rauzy O, Fort M, Nourhashemi F, et al. Relation between HLA DRB1 alleles and corticosteroid resistance in giant cell arteritis. *Ann Rheum Dis* 1998;57:380–382.
347. Schmidt WA, Kraft HE, Vorpahl K, et al. Color duplex ultrasonography in the diagnosis of temporal arteritis. *N Engl J Med* 1998;11:760.
348. Desmet GD, Knockaert DC, Bobbaers HJ. Temporal arteritis: the silent presentation and delay in diagnosis. *J Intern Med* 1990;227:237–240.
349. Klein RG, Hunder GG, Stanson AW, Sheps SG. Large artery involvement in giant cell (temporal) arteritis. *Ann Intern Med* 1975;83:806–812.
350. Hayreh SS. Masticatory muscle pain: an important indicator of giant cell arteritis. *Spec Care Dentist* 1998;18:60–65.
351. Gardner GC. Polymyalgia rheumatica, temporal arteritis, and Takayasu's arteritis. In: Weisman MH, Weinblatt ME, eds. *Treatment of the rheumatic diseases:* companion to textbook of rheumatology. Philadelphia: WB Saunders, 1995:158–171.
352. Kupersmith MJ, Langer R, Mitnick H, et al. Visual performance in giant cell arteritis (temporal arteritis) after 1 year of therapy. *Br J Ophthalmol* 1999;83:796–801.
353. Hwang JM, Girkin CA, Perry JD, et al. Bilateral ocular ischemic syndrome secondary to giant cell arteritis progressing despite corticosteroid treatment. *Am J Ophthalmol* 1999;127:102–104.
354. Scott DGI, Bacon PA, Tribe CR. Systemic rheumatoid vasculitis: a clinical and laboratory study of 50 cases. *Medicine* 1981; 60:288–297.
355. Vollertsen RS, Conn DL, Ballard DJ, Ilstrup DM, Kazmar RE, Silverfield JC. Rheumatoid vasculitis: survival and associated risk factors. *Medicine* 1986;65:365–375.
356. Geirsson AJ, Sturfelt G, Truedsson L. Clinical and serological features of severe vasculitis in rheumatoid arthritis: prognostic implications. *Ann Rheum Dis* 1987;46:727–733.
357. Boers M, Croonen AM, Dijkmans BAC. Renal findings in rheumatoid arthritis: clinical aspects of 132 necropsies. *Ann Rheum Dis* 1987;46:658–663.
358. Vollertsen RS, Conn DL. Vasculitis associated with rheumatoid arthritis. *Rheum Dis Clin North Am* 1990;16:445–461.
359. Espinoza LR, Espinoza CG, Vasey FB, Germain BF. Oral methotrexate therapy for chronic rheumatoid arthritis ulcerations. *J Am Acad Dermatol* 1986;15:508–512.
360. Nicholls A, Snaith ML, Maini RN, Scott JT. Controlled trial of azathioprine in rheumatoid vasculitis. *Ann Rheum Dis* 1973;32: 589–591.
361. Scott DGI, Bacon PA. Intravenous cyclophosphamide plus

methylprednisolone in treatment of systemic rheumatoid vasculitis. *Am J Med* 1984;76:377–383.
362. Greer JM, Longley S, Edwards NL, Elfenbein GJ, Panush RS. Vasculitis associated with malignancy: experience with 13 patients and literature review. *Medicine* 1988;67:220–230.
363. Pirayesh A, Verbunt RJ, Kluin PM, et al. Myelodysplastic syndrome with vasculitic manifestations: review. *J Intern Med* 1997;242:425–431.
364. Sánchez-Guerrero J, Gutiérrez-Ureóna S, Vidaller A, Reyes E, Iglesias A, Alarcón-Segovia D. Vasculitis as a paraneoplastic syndrome: report of 11 cases and review of the literature. *J Rheumatol* 1990;17:1458–1462.
365. Farcet JP, Weschsler J, Wirquin V, Divine M, Reyes F. Vasculitis in hairy-cell leukemia. *Arch Intern Med* 1987;147:660–664.
366. Vollertsen RS, McDonald TJ, Younge BR, Banks PM, Stanson AW, Ilstrup DM. Cogan's syndrome: 18 cases and a review of the literature. *Mayo Clin Proc* 1986;61:344–361.
367. Cote DN, Molony TB, Waxman J, Parsa D. Cogan's syndrome manifesting as sudden bilateral deafness: diagnosis and management. *South Med J* 1993;86:1056–1060.
368. St. Clair EW, McCallum RM. Cogan's syndrome. *Curr Opin Rheumatol* 1999;11:47–52.
369. Su WPD, Schroeter AL, Lee DA, Hsu T, Muller SA. Clinical and histologic findings in Degos' syndrome (malignant atrophic papulosis). *Cutis* 1985;35:131–138.
370. Soter NA, Murphy GF, Mihm MC. Lymphocytes and necrosis of the cutaneous microvasculature in malignant atrophic papulosis: a refined light microscope study. *J Am Acad Dermatol* 1982;7:620–630.
371. Burrow JN, Blumbergs PC, Iyer PV, Hallpike JF. Kohlmeier-Degos disease: a multisystem vasculopathy with progressive cerebral infarction. *Aust N Z J Med* 1991;21:49–51.
372. Fruhwirth J, Mischinger JH, Werkgartner G, et al. Kohlmeier-Degos's disease with primary intestinal manifestation. *Scand J Gastroenterol* 1997;32:1066–1070.
373. Calabrese LH, Duna GF, Lie JT. Vasculitis in the central nervous system. *Arthritis Rheum* 1997;40:1189–1201.
374. Schachna L, Ryan PF. Angiography in cerebral vasculitis: caveat emptor: comment on the article by Calabrese et al. [Letter]. *Arthritis Rheum* 1998;41:2086–2087.

83

CEREBRAL VASCULITIS

LEONARD H. SIGAL

Central nervous system (CNS) abnormalities are common in vasculitic and rheumatic syndromes. The underlying diagnosis can usually be made on the basis of the associated clinical and laboratory findings. Occasionally, however, there is no apparent underlying disease in a patient with only neurologic complaints. In this circumstance, the clinician must differentiate between the isolated neurologic presentation of a (then clinically silent) systemic inflammatory disease and an isolated CNS process. The systemic necrotizing vasculitides (1) and their CNS manifestations (2–4) have been reviewed.

The purpose of this chapter is to discuss the clinical, laboratory, and pathologic findings of *isolated CNS vasculitis* (ICNSV), also known as *isolated angiitis of the CNS* (IACNS), *granulomatous angiitis of the nervous system* (GANS) or *primary angiitis of the central nervous system* (PACNS), and to offer suggestions on efficient and proper evaluation and management of patients with possible CNS vasculitis. The term GANS is based on the histopathologic description of affected tissue and should be reserved for only those cases of apparent CNS vasculitis confirmed pathologically. The preferred nomenclature AICNSV or APACNS are more general terms for a vasculitis restricted to the CNS, but not necessarily granulomatous. The "isolated" in ICNSV refers to the fact that there is no clinically apparent vasculitis in any other organ system; the "primary" in PACNS suggests that the vasculitis is initially or fundamentally of the CNS.

This chapter also compares ICNSV with *herpes zoster ophthalmicus* (HZO) *with delayed contralateral hemiplegia,* more properly known as *herpes zoster–associated cerebral angiitis* (HZO-CA). Other primary CNS vasculitides, the systemic vasculitides, other rheumatic diseases that can produce CNS symptoms, and mimics of ICNSV also are discussed briefly. These subjects have been reviewed previously (3,5,6).

ICNSV is an angiitis, often granulomatous (thus GANS, the older name for this syndrome) that often affects the cerebral and spinal cord leptomeningeal and parenchymal small arteries. It occurs in the absence of clinically significant or symptomatic systemic necrotizing vasculitis. In the past decade, more experience with ICNSV has added to the view that this is not a disease *sui generis,* but rather a pathologic process due to a number of inciting influences, including a variety of infections (7,8), and often associated with an underlying lymphoid malignancy, suggesting that an immune deficiency state may play a role.

There is an emerging consensus that ICNSV may be a more benign process than previously thought. Part of the problem in better defining ICNSV is the heterogeneity of documentation: some cases are based on purely clinical grounds, others on only angiographic appearance, and still others are biopsy proven. At the extreme end of the clinical spectrum is a self-limited entity termed *benign angiopathy of the CNS* (BACNS) that requires no treatment. As well, certain drugs have been implicated as causing a usually monophasic angiopathy that angiographically resembles ICNSV. In the past, HZO-CA has often been considered a form of ICNSV/GANS. Postherpetic angiitis superficially resembles the latter, but HZO-CA is less severe, more limited in extent, related to a known pathogenic agent, and more likely to resolve. A history of herpes infection, and the differences in severity and extent of involvement, help differentiate these two conditions. The experience with ICNSV in the 1950s through 1970s suggested that aggressive therapy was usually warranted. Based on the experience of the last two decades (the favorable natural history in many cases and the unreliability of angiography and other diagnostic tools), it has become apparent that aggressive evaluation and individualization of treatment is warranted.

CENTRAL NERVOUS SYSTEM VASCULITIS ASSOCIATED WITH SYSTEMIC VASCULITIS

CNS vasculitis associated with other rheumatic diseases can occur with or without systemic vasculitis. A description of the primary CNS presentations of these syndromes can be found elsewhere (9). There is usually evidence of systemic rheumatic disease or of systemic vasculitis to suggest the proper diagnosis. In few circumstances will there be no systemic extracranial manifestations, but cases of systemic lupus erythematosus, progressive systemic sclerosis, Sjögren's syndrome, Behçet's syndrome, cryoglobulinemia, and lymphomatoid granulomatosis have been reported without extracerebral manifestations. The diagnosis has sometimes been delayed up to 5 years before the extracranial disease became manifest. In most circumstances, however, a thorough clinical evaluation will reveal the underlying disease.

Until recently, the diagnosis of CNS vasculitis in patients with known systemic vasculitis was often made clinically, without proof that vasculitis was actually the cause of CNS dysfunction. Because CNS dysfunction is often due to damage to other organs such as the lung or kidney in systemic lupus erythematosus, progressive systemic sclerosis, rheumatoid arthritis (RA), or systemic vasculitides, rather than vasculitis, it is imperative that a more precise evaluation of CNS dysfunction be completed in these settings. Angiography and biopsy are now considered essential for diagnosis and proper management (2). The angiographic findings of cerebral arteritis include narrowing and dilatation of vessels, changes in blood flow, and associated masses (2). "Vasculitic" angiographic changes can be seen in a variety of inflammatory, infectious, and noninflammatory diseases (2). A basilar artery distribution of vasculitis may be a clue that the cause is actually infectious (e.g., tuberculosis or fungal) or sarcoidosis. Occlusion of a single arterial sub-branch should suggest possible embolic disease. Angiographically diagnosed CNS vasculitis may occasionally spontaneously resolve within days, suggesting that the changes were probably due to vasospasm rather than true vasculitis (2) (e.g., BACNS). Leptomeningeal biopsy is necessary to differentiate true vasculitis from vasospasm, benign vasculopathies, or other causes of these angiographic changes. Thus angiographic results are no longer considered proof of vasculitis. Given the gravity of the therapeutic decision and prognostic considerations, biopsy is indicated.

Many vasculitic, rheumatologic, and noninflammatory diseases can damage the nervous system, usually in systemic disease. Table 83.1 lists these as four separate classes. The primary CNS vasculitides (e.g., Cogan's syndrome) usually are not associated with systemic disease (Table 83.2).

TABLE 83.1. CAUSES OF CENTRAL NERVOUS SYSTEM VASCULITIS

Primary CNS vasculitides
1. Granulomatous angiitis of the nervous system
2. Herpes zoster ophthalmicus–associated cerebral angiitis
3. Cogan's syndrome
4. Eales' disease
5. Isolated spinal cord arteritis

Systemic necrotizing vasculitides that often affect the CNS
1. Polyarteritis nodosa group
   a. Classic polyarteritis nodosa
   b. Churg–Strauss vasculitis
   c. Drug-associated vasculitis
   d. Hepatitis B virus–associated vasculitis
2. Giant cell arteritis
3. Takayasu aortitis
4. Wegener's granulomatosis
5. Lymphomatoid granulomatosis
6. Henoch–Schönlein purpura
7. Cryoglobulinemia

Rheumatologic diseases associated with CNS involvement, due to vasculitis or other mechanisms
1. Systemic lupus erythematosus
2. Progressive systemic sclerosis
3. Mixed connective tissue disease
4. Sjögren's syndrome
5. Rheumatoid disease
6. Juvenile rheumatoid arthritis
7. Polymyositis/dermatomyositis
8. Behçet's syndrome
9. Lyme disease
10. Ankylosing spondylitis
11. Reiter's syndrome

Nonrheumatologic/vasculitic disease
1. Sarcoidosis
2. Inflammatory bowel disease
3. Drugs
   a. Allopurinol
   b. Amphetamines
   c. Cocaine
   d. Heroin
   e. Ephedrine
4. Local infections: bacteria, viruses, protozoa, rickettsia, mycoplasma
5. Mimics of vasculitis: moyamoya, acute hypertension, radiation vasculopathy, anticardiolipin antibody syndrome, sickle cell disease, thrombotic thrombocytopenic purpura

CNS, central nervous system.

Primary Central Nervous System Vasculitides

Cogan's syndrome is defined by episodes of acute interstitial keratitis or scleritis/episcleritis with vestibuloauditory dysfunction, usually in young adults (2). Interstitial keratitis and vestibuloauditory abnormalities are found in other diseases including polyarteritis nodosa, Wegener's granulomatosis, and RA. Interstitial keratitis can be caused by congenital syphilis, tuberculosis, and viral infections, each of which must be excluded. A syndrome of subacute encephalopathy, sensorineural hearing loss, and retinal arteriolar occlusions in young adults due to occlusive nonvasculitic vasculopathy also has been described (2). The presence of retinal and neuropsychiatric findings and the absence of interstitial keratitis or other inflammation of the anterior segment of the eye differentiates this syndrome from Cogan's syndrome.

Eales' disease is an isolated peripheral retinal vasculitis in young adults, often leading to visual loss (2). It must be distinguished from the retinal vasculitis of other syndromes such as Wegener's granulomatosis, systemic lupus erythematosus, Behçet's syndrome, sickle cell disease, sarcoidosis, and tuberculosis. Retinal vasculitis rarely accompanies anterior uveitis (2).

Spinal cord arteritis, occurring with myelopathy, can be the first manifestation of a systemic disease, or can represent an isolated vasculitis (2,10).

TABLE 83.2. PRIMARY CENTRAL NERVOUS SYSTEM VASCULITIDES

Disease	Age at Onset (yr)	Sex (M:F)	% with CNS Disease	Isolated or Predominant CNS Presentation	Other Reported CNS Manifestations	Other Features of the Syndrome	Tests of Diagnostic Value
ICNSV	30–50	4:3	100%	Headache Cerebrovascular syndromes Confusion/Psychiatric disorders Aphasia/Dysphasia Seizures Ataxia Cranial Neuropathy Transverse myelopathy			Angiography Leptomeningeal and cortical biopsy
Cogan's syndrome	15–30	1:1.2	2–5%	Meningoencephalitis Seizures Ataxia Cerebrovascular syndromes Cranial neuropathy Organic mental syndrome	Inferior cerebellar artery occlusion Headache	Nonsyphilitic interstitial keratitis (90–100%) or scleritis/episcleritis Vestibulo-auditory abnormalities (100%) Systemic necrotizing vasculitis—in "atypical" cases (30%) Aortic insufficiency	Ophthalmologic examination Auditory evaluation
Eales' disease	25–45	1.5:1	Rare	Optic disc vasculitis			Ophthalmologic examination Fluorescein angiography
Isolated spinal cord arteritis	25–60			Myelopathy		Heroin addiction	Myelography Angiography Biopsy

Isolated Central Nervous System Vasculitis

ICNSV was first described as a separate entity by Cravioto and Feigin in 1959 (11). Two cases described by Harbitz in 1922 in his review of cerebral arteritis are compatible with this diagnosis (3). A review of the English literature in 1987 summarized 61 cases of GANS (3), and 55 cases have been collected since then (9,10,12,13). In 1987, 39 cases of HZO-CA were reviewed (3), and 11 cases have been collected since then (2,10).

The presenting signs and symptoms of these cerebral angiitides are usually nonspecific, often suggesting global CNS dysfunction, often with focal changes superimposed with a more gradual onset. The acute or subacute onset of confusion, headache, change in personality, paresis, cranial neuropathy, or loss of consciousness suggests a variety of diagnoses at first evaluation. Patients with ICNSV have been mistakenly diagnosed as having severe migraine headaches, idiopathic seizure disorder, stroke due to atherosclerosis, viral encephalitis, primary or metastatic tumor, syphilis, tuberculosis, sarcoidosis, and multiple sclerosis.

Calabrese et al. (14) suggested four major subsets of ICNSV (they preferred the term PACNS): (a) GANS; (b) mass lesions (15% of PACNS in their series, usually seen as headache); (c) spinal cord arteritis [14% of PACNS, seen as myelopathy progressing to paraparesis, most with elevated protein or cell count in the cerebrospinal fluid (CSF)]; and (d) CNS hemorrhage (11% of PACNS, seen as intracerebral, subarachnoid or spinal subdural hemorrhage, often from an underlying aneurysm, in their series associated with an underlying lymphoproliferative disorder in ~30% of cases).

The critical features of reported cases of ICNSV are summarized in Table 83.3. Men outnumbered women by 4 to 3. The mean age was 42 years, with a range from 3 to 78 years. Presenting symptoms included headache (64%), weakness (38%), and confusion or "possible psychiatric disorder" (40%). Aphasia or dysphasia, nausea or vomiting, disorders of memory, lethargy, seizure disorder, or frank loss of consciousness were seen in approximately 15% to 30% of cases. Presentation as a stroke is relatively uncommon (15). Associated or antecedent disorders included hypertension, renal failure, diabetes mellitus, ileitis, upper respira-

TABLE 83.3. CLINICAL FEATURES OF ISOLATED CENTRAL NERVOUS SYSTEM VASCULITIS (ICNSV) AND HERPES ZOSTER OPHTHALMICUS-ASSOCIATED CEREBRAL ANGIITIS (HZO-CA)

	ICNSV (*n* = 116)	HZO-CA (*n* = 50)
Age (yr)	42.1	61.0
Sex (male/female)	67/49	31/19
Clinical symptoms (% of total cases)		
Headache	64	14
Confusion/psychiatric disorder	40	40
Weakness	38	70
Aphasia/dysphasia/dysarthria	28	8
Nausea/vomiting	23	5
Seizure	20	6
Incoordination	18	6
Lethargy	17	14
Memory disturbance	17	4
Loss of consciousness	13	2
Numbness	13	6
Stiff neck/back	10	0
Physical findings (% of total cases)		
Hemiplegia/single-limb paresis/paraplegia	48	70
Pathologic lower extremity reflexes	30	18
Fever	17	6
Hypertension	16	4
Funduscopic abnormalities	16	0
Myelopathy	8	0
Ataxia	6	10
Maculopapular rash	3	0
Tremor	2	2
Cranial nerve disorder	29	45
II	2	8
III	4	18
IV	1	0
V	1	11
VI	8	11
VII	13	39
VIII	3	2
IX	1	0
X	1	2
XI	0	4
XII	0	8
Horner's syndrome	0	4
Preceding or associated diseases (number of cases reported)		
Hodgkin's disease	9	3
Hypertension	8	1
Chronic renal failure	8	1
Recent upper respiratory infection	4	0
Trauma	4	0
Non-Hodgkin's lymphoma	2	1
Diabetes mellitus	2	0
Ileitis	1	0
Postpartum	1	0
Chronic lymphocytic leukemia	0	2
Renal transplant	0	2
Colonic cancer	0	1
Breast cancer	0	1
Tonsillar cancer	0	1
Sarcoidosis	0	1

tory infection, Hodgkin's disease or non-Hodgkin's lymphoma, and other malignancies in a small proportion of cases; no causal relation with the vasculitis can be inferred. A recent report documents CNS vasculitis in association with selective IgA deficiency (16). ICNSV has occurred during pregnancy and in the postpartum period (17).

Fever and elevated blood pressure were noted in about one sixth of patients; dermatologic abnormalities were described in only two cases. Neurologic evaluation was remarkable for muscle weakness in about half of patients; pathologic lower extremity reflexes were elicited in most patients with lower extremity motor findings. Funduscopy revealed papilledema or vascular changes in 13% of patients. Cranial neuropathy, usually facial or abducens, occurred in 25%.

The erythrocyte sedimentation rate (ESR) was usually elevated, but in many cases, the ESR was normal (Table 83.4). Serologies for syphilis were uniformly negative, an important finding because meningovascular syphilis can be clinically indistinguishable from ICNSV (2). CSF analysis was abnormal in 93% of patients tested, usually revealing increased pressure and total protein, lymphocytic pleocytosis, but normal glucose levels (Table 83.4). Electroencephalograms were abnormal in 65% of patients tested, usually diffusely slow, often with superimposed lateral or focal findings. Antinuclear antibody (ANA) and antineutrophil cytoplasmic antibody (ANCA) are usually of no value in the evaluation of this syndrome unless there is evidence of an underlying systemic disorder. Cerebral angiography, computed axial tomography (CAT), and radionu-

TABLE 83.4. LABORATORY FEATURES OF ISOLATED CENTRAL NERVOUS SYSTEM VASCULITIS (ICNSV) AND HERPES ZOSTER OPHTHALMICUS–ASSOCIATED CEREBRAL ANGIITIS (HZO-CA)

Laboratory Test (% of total cases)	ICNSV (*n* = 93)	HZO-CA (*n* = 47)
Increased sedimentation rate	58	27
Cerebrospinal fluid		
Normal	7	2
Increased pressure	60	33
Lymphocytic pleocytosis	71	95
Increased protein	62	63
Decreased glucose	27	7
Electroencephalogram		
Normal	33	14
Diffuse slowing	43	32
Diffuse slowing, unilateral predominance	14	2
Unilateral slowing	6	37
Diffuse slowing, plus focal abnormality	12	10
Focal abnormality	10	17
Other		
Radionuclide brain scan abnormal	54	50
Brain computed tomography abnormal	65	68
Cerebral angiography abnormal	82	96

clide brain scan were valuable, in that order, in identifying disease. The potential use of magnetic resonance imaging (MRI) in the evaluation of CNS vasculitis is described in the section on diagnostic testing.

Postmortem and biopsy examinations in ICNSV reveal an inflammatory process involving small arteries and arterioles (typically 200 to 500 μm in diameter) affecting parenchymal and leptomeningeal more than subcortical vessels (Fig. 83.1; Table 83.5). Multinucleate giant cells of the Langhans and foreign-body type, granulomata, macrophages, and lymphocytes are present, often adjacent to a disrupted elastic lamella. Intimal proliferation and fibrosis are frequent. Relative sparing of the media compared with the other vessel wall layers is often cited in descriptions of GANS, in contradistinction to giant cell arteritis, which GANS resembles histologically (3). Veins are affected about half the time, but usually far less severely than the arteries.

Significant vasculitis is rarely seen outside of the cranium, although spinal cord, temporal arteries, and cranial nerves are affected rarely. Eleven of the postmortem examinations showed pathologic changes outside the nervous system, most notably in lung and kidney. In none of these cases were the lesions of any clinical significance or noted before death (Table 83.5).

ETIOPATHOGENESIS OF ISOLATED CENTRAL NERVOUS SYSTEM VASCULITIS

The cause of ICNSV is unknown. Infectious agents as the cause of CNS vasculitis is the subject of two recent reviews (7,8). The relative sparing of media and intima suggests that in ICNSV, a causative agent might reach the vessel from an extravascular site, rather than hematogenously. Intracranial spread of an agent is compatible with the distribution and nonsystemic nature of ICNSV. The disrupted elastica might be the focus of inflammation, as has been suggested in giant cell arteritis (3). An angiitis similar to GANS can be produced in turkeys inoculated intravenously with *Mycoplasma gallisepticum,* with organisms found attached to or in the cerebral arterial wall at the lesional sites (2). Two patients with GANS had mycoplasma-like inclusion bodies within giant cells in the vasculitis lesion, located near the internal elastica, but cultures for mycoplasma were negative (2).

Alternatively, a preceding viral infection could be the culprit. In one case of GANS, electron-microscopic studies of glial cells revealed intranuclear virus-like particles in an aggregate of about 100 nm in diameter. A few appeared to be budding from the nuclear membrane, and some had electron-dense cores. No cytoplasmic particles were found (9). Complement consumption in the intrathecal space suggested a role for local immune reactivity in ICNSV (2). Human immunodeficiency virus can produce CNS vasculitis histologically similar to ICNSV (see Chapter 131) (2). Viral or other infection within the brain can elicit the local production of cytokines, which might then play a role in the pathogenesis of CNS vasculitis. Injection of γ-interferon into rat brain is associated with the induction of a CNS vasculitis (18). Tumor necrosis factor may play a role in the development of neurovascular lesions (19). Elevated levels of interleukin-6 have been found in the CSF of three patients with CNS vasculitis (one each with polyarteritis nodosa, giant cell arteritis, and Behçet's syndrome); levels decreased in parallel with successful therapy (20).

DIAGNOSTIC EVALUATION OF THE PATIENT WITH SUSPECTED ISOLATED CENTRAL NERVOUS SYSTEM VASCULITIS

There is certainly clinical (and likely etiologic) heterogeneity of the syndrome known as ICNSV. As noted earlier, the mainstays of diagnosing ICNSV are angiography and leptomeningeal and cortical biopsy. The angiographic images of the internal carotid artery and its branches are numbered, the lowest number being assigned to the regions nearest the bifurcation of the internal carotid artery, the origin of the anterior and middle cerebral arteries (Fig. 83.2). Cerebral angiography in ICNSV reveals diffuse or localized abnormalities of large, intermediate, and small arteries in the distribution of several of the cerebral arteries (Fig. 83.3). These changes include beading, aneurysms, circumferential or eccentric vessel irregularities, and avascular mass effect. However, none of these findings, either separately or in combination, is diagnostic of vasculitis; any can be due to malignancy, infection, drugs, or can be a benign self-limited process. Conversely, angiography can be normal in biopsy-proven cerebral vasculitis, because angiography is unable to detect changes in vessels smaller than 100 to 200 μm in diameter. Thus biopsy is imperative to prove that the process is truly inflammatory (i.e., a vasculitis).

In a serial angiography study of patients with ICNSV, progressive worsening of the angiogram before therapy was noted, with improvement described after therapy. The earlier the therapy is started, the higher the likelihood that the angiogram will revert to normal (21). Comparison of standard angiography with magnetic resonance angiography (MRA) suggested that the latter was not sufficiently sensitive for use in evaluation of ICNSV (21). Standard MRI was usually abnormal in ICNSV patients, but changes were less extensive than those seen in angiography (13). In another study of seven patients with ICNSV, the MRI abnormalities usually correlated with the changes seen on angiogram, but normal MRI studies were found in some cases of vasculitis (22). There are no pathognomonic findings of vasculitis on MRI. Changes include single or multiple territorial infarcts and hemorrhages and nonspecific T2 hyperintense lesions in the cortex, basal ganglia, and white matter (23,24). Cloft et al. (25) concurred that MRI is a poor indicator of cerebral vasculitis and cannot be used as a substitute for angiography.

The relative sensitivity of CSF analysis, CT, and MRI were compared in a study of CNS vasculitis; seven patients

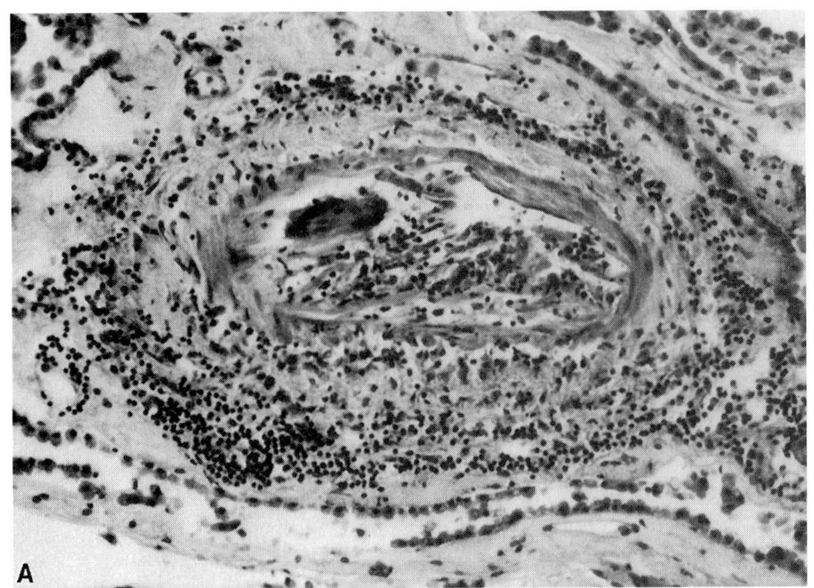

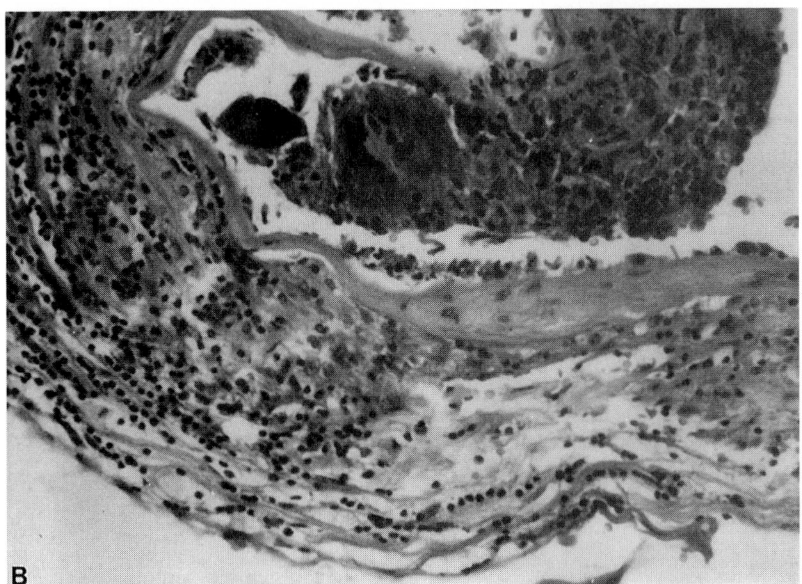

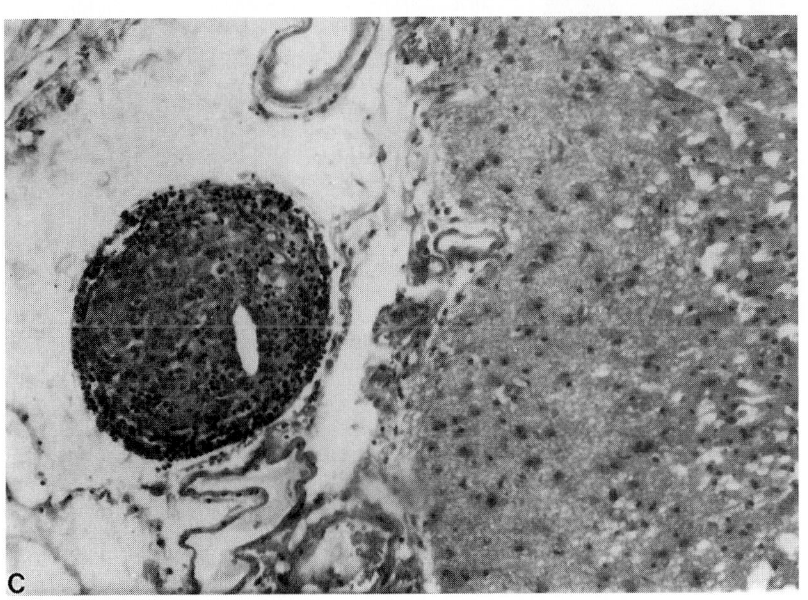

FIGURE 83.1. A: Photomicrograph of a postmortem specimen from the choroid plexus of a patient with isolated central nervous system vasculitis (ICNSV). Near occlusion of the vessel is secondary to subintimal reaction. Inflammatory infiltrate in the media and adventitia with lymphocytes and a giant cell is seen (magnification ×205). **B:** Photomicrograph of a postmortem specimen from the subarachnoid space of a patient with ICNSV. A more fully developed mononuclear cell reaction is seen with a giant cell and more vessel wall damage than in **A**. Damage to the internal elastic lamella is seen (magnification ×256). **C:** Photomicrograph of a postmortem specimen from the cerebral cortex of a patient with ICNSV. A vessel with severe wall damage and near total loss of the lumen is seen. Damage of the external granular layer is seen, with necrosis and reactive gliosis in the molecular layer of the cortex (magnification ×160). (Reproduced with permission from Sigal LH. The neurologic presentation of vasculitic and rheumatologic syndromes: a review. *Medicine* 1987;66:157–180.)

TABLE 83.5. MICROSCOPIC TISSUE EXAMINATION OF PATIENTS WITH ISOLATED CENTRAL NERVOUS SYSTEM VASCULITIS (ICNSV) AND HERPES ZOSTER–ASSOCIATED CEREBRAL ANGIITIS (HZ-CA)

	ICNSV		HZ-CA	
	Biopsy (*n* = 16)	Autopsy (*n* = 43)	Biopsy (*n* = 39)	Autopsy (*n* = 9)
Type of cellular infiltrate in vessels (number of cases reported)				
Granulomata	5	30		4
Epithelial cells	6	11	11	0
Multinucleate giant cells	14	40	38	4
Lymphocytes	14	39	37	7
Histiocytes	6	14		6
Type of vessels affected (number of cases reported)				
Arterioles	9	14	1	1
Small arteries	9	17	1	3
Medium arteries	1	9		2
Large arteries	0	6		2
Disrupted elastic lamelle	5	15	1	5
Veins	4	20	1	0
Arteries more affected than veins		13/19		
Veins more affected than arteries		1/19		
Peripheral nerves affected		0		0
Spinal cord affected		7		
Cranial nerves affected		3		1
Nonnervous system foci of vasculitis noted at autopsy		11		0
Lung		7		
Kidney		7		
Coronary vessels		5		
Liver		3		
Lymph nodes		2		
Spleen, stomach, prostate, testis, uterus		1		

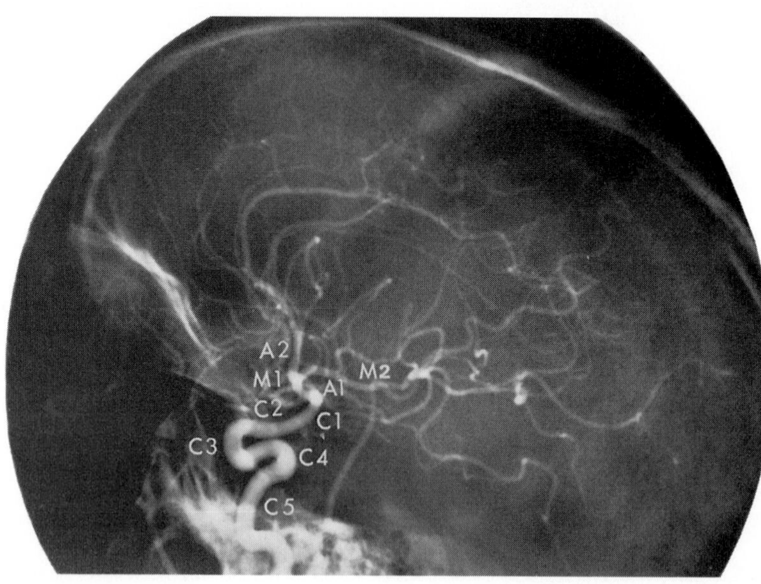

FIGURE 83.2. Angiogram of the internal carotid artery and its branches. The omega-shaped loop consisting of *C2*, *C3*, and *C4* is called the carotid siphon. The internal carotid enters the skull at the carotid foramen, passes anteromedially, and then rises vertically (*C5*) to pass forward opposite the sella turcica (*C4*). The artery then passes upward within the dura (*C3*) and emerges below and medial to the anterior clinoid (*C2*) and gives rise to the ophthalmic artery. The gasserian nucleus lies immediately adjacent to the siphon and to the initial branches of the anterior and middle cerebral arteries. The carotid then bifurcates (*C1*) to form the anterior and middle cerebral arteries. The anterior cerebral artery is directed anteromedially (*A1*) until it reaches the midline, where it turns upward (*A2*) to be joined by the anterior communicating artery. Thereafter, the frontopolar and pericallosal arteries arise. The medial portions of the frontal and parietal lobes and the corpus callosum are supplied by these vessels. The middle cerebral artery extends laterally (*M1*) and gives off three branches (*M2*), which supply the basal ganglia, internal capsule, and lateral aspects of the frontal, parietal, and temporal lobes.

had ICNSV, eight had underlying rheumatologic conditions (four with lupus, two with polyarteritis nodosa, one with giant cell arteritis, and one with Sjögren's syndrome), and four had other disorders (two with malignancy, one with infection, and one with prior radiation therapy to the head). CT was positive in 16 (94%) of 17 patients, and MRI was positive in 12 (92%) of 13 patients. CSF abnormalities were found in eight of 15 angiographically proven cases for a sensitivity of 53% (95% confidence interval, 27–79%). The sensitivity of CT scan was 65% (11 of 17; confidence interval, 38–86%), and that of MRI, 75% (12 of 16; confidence interval, 48–93%). Combining spinal fluid analysis and CT or MRI was more sensitive than fluid analysis alone: for fluid analysis and CT, the sensitivity was 92% (11 of 12; confi-

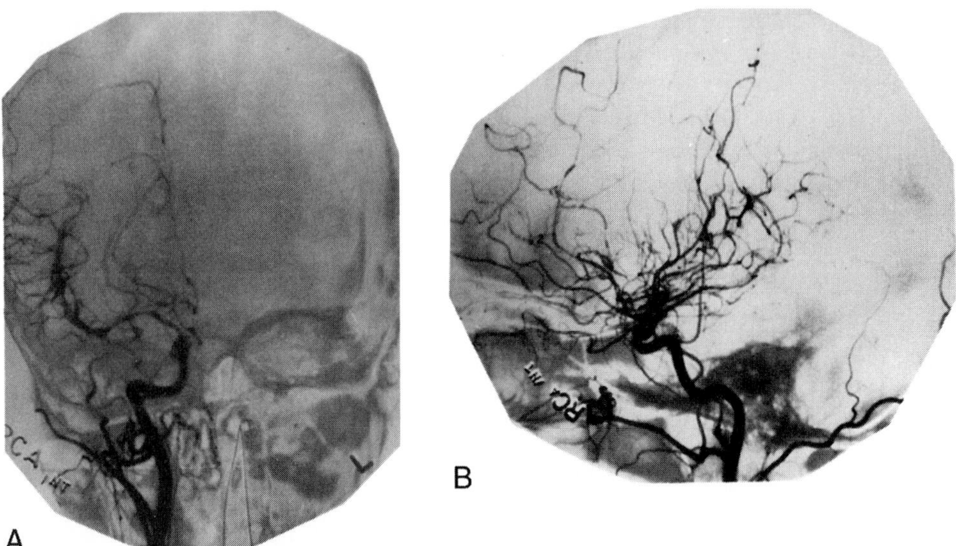

FIGURE 83.3. A: Right carotid angiogram (anteroposterior view) in a patient with isolated central nervous system vasculitis (ICNSV). Focal narrowing of multiple vessels is seen in both the anterior and posterior cerebral arterial systems. **B:** Right carotid angiogram (lateral view) in a patient with ICNSV. Beading and multiple irregularities are seen both proximally and distally. (Reproduced with permission from Sigal LH. The neurologic presentation of vasculitic and rheumatologic syndromes: a review. *Medicine* 1987;66:157–180.)

dence interval, 62–100%), and for fluid analysis and MRI, it was 100% (12 of 12; confidence interval, 74–100%). On the basis of this study, one can state that angiography in a patient with possible CNS vasculitis is unlikely to be abnormal if the CSF and either CT or MRI are normal (26). Harris et al. (27) found that a normal MRI virtually excludes angiographic abnormalities. Chu et al. (23) found that leptomeningeal enhancement and/or periventricular white matter lesions increased the positive predictive value (from 43% to 50–70%) and specificity (from 19% to 75–81%) of MRI remarkably; the periventricular changes in ICNSV were less numerous and milder than usually seen in multiple sclerosis. Another study found that the angiographic changes correlated with the clinical findings in nine of 16 CNS vasculitis patients, whereas seven of 16 had a normal CT or radionuclide brain scan despite an abnormal angiogram (28). Neither MRI nor CT scan is sufficiently sensitive or specific to be diagnostic. Enhancement in contrast studies is nonspecific. MRA has not proven to be a substitute for angiography in the evaluation of cerebral vasculitis, perhaps because MRA lacks resolution. There is insufficient experience with single-photon emission computed tomography (SPECT) and positron emission tomography (PET) scanning to rely on either in the evaluation of possible ICNSV; although either can be useful to document cerebral blood flow alterations, it is unlikely that either will be of great utility. Defects seen in these functional imaging techniques do not necessarily relate to specific clinical changes or even to vascular changes, inflammatory or otherwise. The study by Meusser et al. (29) suggested that SPECT might be useful for the documentation of early changes that might then lead to a more definitive evaluation.

Concern is often raised about the safety of angiography in a patient with possible cerebral vessel inflammation. In a review of 125 cerebral angiograms, of which 16 were positive for CNS vasculitis (eight ICNSV, four with systemic lupus erythematosus, and one each with Sjögren's syndrome, Takayasu's arteritis, giant cell arteritis, and cutaneous vasculitis), there was no greater risk of complications in the patients with proven CNS vasculitis than in the patients with negative studies. With a logistic model, the predictors of complications due to angiography were the presence of a previous stroke (relative risk, 3.47) and an abnormal CSF (relative risk, 3.24). With similar analysis, predictors of an abnormality on angiogram were an abnormal fluid analysis and a history of a previous rheumatic disease. Five deaths were recorded in the group, none due to the angiogram. One stroke and one carotid dissection occurred (30).

As noted earlier, angiography by itself is not sufficient to make the specific diagnosis of vasculitis. Angiograms have been described as normal in biopsy-proven cases of ICNSV (2). Conversely, biopsies of angiographically abnormal vessels have been reported as normal (2), perhaps a testament to the patchy distribution of ICNSV, an example of "benign cerebral vasculitis" or, perhaps, reversible vasospasm (2). Biopsies thought to be compatible with vasculitis also can be seen in the region of cerebral lymphoma (31). As well, Chu et al. (23) reported the case of a 47-year-old man with a mass lesion due to a focal monophasic vasculitis that was apparently cured by excision of that region of the brain, there being no recurrences elsewhere. Thus even the presence of vasculitis on biopsy does not predict outcome or indicate how aggressive therapy should be.

The report of transient cerebral angiographic abnormalities in a patient with acute postpartum hypertension accentuates the difficulty of interpreting abnormal CNS angiograms (32). Transient narrowing and dilatation of cerebral vessels also has been reported in eclampsia (33). Even after the arbitrary 2 days postpartum time limit set for eclampsia, there have been cases of cerebral angiitis in women without concomitant proteinuria or edema, suggesting to some authors that the definition of eclampsia should be expanded (17). Thus biopsy is a crucial part of the evaluation of an individual with isolated CNS disease due to presumed vasculitis. Many reports suggest that the leptomeningeal vessels often are affected, so that a combined cortical and leptomeningeal biopsy offers the best chance of diagnosis. The diagnostic yield can be increased by using an angiogram to guide the biopsy to the affected area (3). If no focal angiographic abnormalities are accessible, biopsy of the temporal tip of the nondominant hemisphere is often preferred (i.e., an area of "ineloquent cortex") (34); biopsy of the basilar meninges can be useful in the evaluation of possible sarcoidosis or chronic meningitis (e.g., tuberculous or fungal). Temporal artery biopsy is not indicated in the diagnostic evaluation of likely ICNSV, as the temporal vessels are usually not affected and are certainly not involved in the pathogenesis of the patient's findings. An abnormal angiogram followed by a normal biopsy raises the possibility of vasospasm or of having missed the focus of vasculitis (i.e., "sampling error"). In this circumstance, therapeutic decisions should be dictated by the overall clinical status of the patient, exclusion of other conditions that might mimic ICNSV, and the progression of the neurologic abnormalities (31). It is clear that control of hypertension, if present, will accelerate the resolution of vasospasm. Given that certain viruses, fungi, and bacteria can cause a syndrome quite similar to ICNSV, brain tissue and spinal fluid should be subjected to appropriate microbiologic analysis.

There are only two reports of positive ANCA determinations in patients with CNS vasculitis. In the first, pANCA was present in a patient with CNS vasculitis and Crohn's disease (35). A second patient had a systemic necrotizing vasculitis and a brain MRI with findings "compatible with vascular lesions," which resolved after corticosteroid and cyclophosphamide therapy was reported (36). Thus ANCA has not been reported in true ICNSV (or in HZO-CA) and should not be part of the routine evaluation.

THERAPEUTIC APPROACHES IN ISOLATED CENTRAL NERVOUS SYSTEM VASCULITIS

The early reports of cerebral vasculitis suggested a uniformly dismal prognosis, with death inexorably following the diagnosis by 1 day to 9.5 months (mean, 45 days; median, 16.5 days). In more recent experience, there have been therapeutic successes in patients with ICNSV by using high-dose corticosteroids (dexamethasone or prednisone) and cytotoxic agents (cyclophosphamide or azathioprine; Table 83.6). In one case, radiotherapy and corticosteroid treatment of underlying Hodgkin's disease was associated with resolution of cerebral vasculitis (2). Response of ICNSV (in the absence of an underlying malignancy) to radiotherapy has been reported in a single case; once the patient had received a maximal dose of radiation, therapy with corticosteroids and cyclophosphamide proved ineffective (12). The successful use of cyclosporine in the treatment of a patient with CNS vasculitis complicating progressive systemic sclerosis was reported; of note, the authors stated that both neurologic and skin manifestations responded (37). A recent review of GANS concluded that there was no evidence that the addition of cyclophosphamide was of benefit, a message tempered by the fact that this historical review included a small number of patients, unmatched for age or severity, with nonuniform follow-up (38).

TABLE 83.6. CLINICAL OUTCOME OF PATIENTS WITH ISOLATED CENTRAL NERVOUS SYSTEM VASCULITIS (ICNSV) AND HERPES ZOSTER–ASSOCIATED CEREBRAL ANGIITIS (HZ-CA)

	ICNSV (n = 103)	HZ-CA (n = 50)
No followup available	1	4
Treatment: none		
Fatal or progressive	38	17
No progression	1	8
Improved	2	18
Treatment: steroids		
Fatal or progressive	5	0
Temporary response	4	1
No progression	4	0
Improved	23	2
Treatment: steroids + cytotoxic agent		
Fatal or progressive	3	0
No progression	3	0
Improved	20	0
Treatment: radiation therapy		
Transient response[a]	1	

[a]Prior corticosteroid and cyclophosphamide had been unsuccessful; on relapse, patient could not receive further radiation therapy.

The more recent reports of a more benign outcome in many patients, often with a monophasic illness, suggests that immediate recourse to cytotoxic therapy is not always warranted. Therapy should, of course, be individualized based on the severity of clinical findings and progression. Use of calcium channel blockers and avoidance of oral contraceptives, sympathomimetics, and caffeine has been suggested for such patients and, although not of proven value, seem prudent steps to take (14).

HERPES ZOSTER OPHTHALMICUS–ASSOCIATED CEREBRAL ANGIITIS

In HZO-CA, a 5:3 male predominance is seen, but the patients are somewhat older (average age, 61 years; range,

7–96 years), probably because zoster infections are more common in an older population. Vasculopathy-associated neurologic sequelae follow the HZO by 1 week to 2 years. There were five patients in whom the delays were 117 days, 4, 5, and 6 months, and 2 years; if these are excluded, the mean and median delay were both about 31 days. A report documented a CNS vasculitis shortly after varicella infection in a child (39). Herpes zoster–associated neurologic system dysfunction also includes these entities: zoster radiculopathy, zoster myelitis, cranial neuropathy (including Ramsay Hunt syndrome), zoster meningoencephalitis, and remote leukoencephalitis.

The clinical presentation of HZO-CA differs from that of ICNSV, however. With the exception of more frequent and severe weakness, HZO-CA is usually a milder illness (Table 83.3). Only four (36%) of 11 ESRs reported were elevated. The CSF findings were also usually abnormal. Focal or unilateral electroencephalographic abnormalities were more common in HZO-CA than in ICNSV. The angiographic findings in HZO-CA are characteristic (2), with segmental, unilateral involvement of vessels in the distribution of the middle cerebral artery, and occasionally of the internal carotid artery (Fig. 83.4). The results of tissue examination in 16 patients (five biopsy specimens and 11 autopsies) revealed similarities with results of examinations of patients with ICNSV (Fig. 83.5).

The pathogenesis of HZO-CA is still unclear, and theories relating to this syndrome have been summarized elsewhere (2). Virus can spread from the eye by intraaxonal or

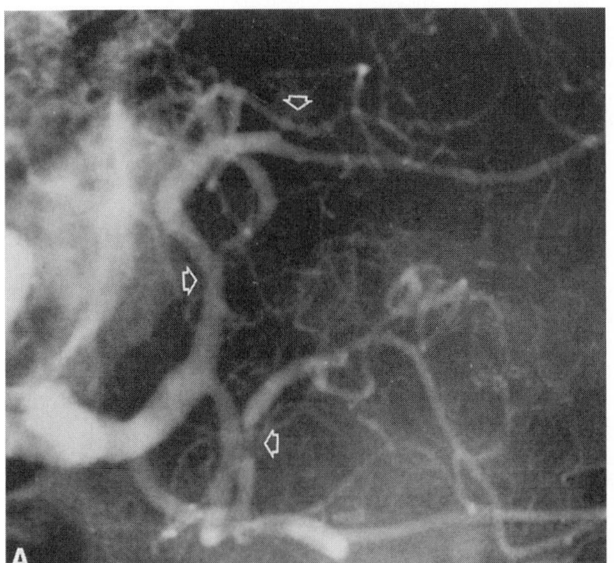

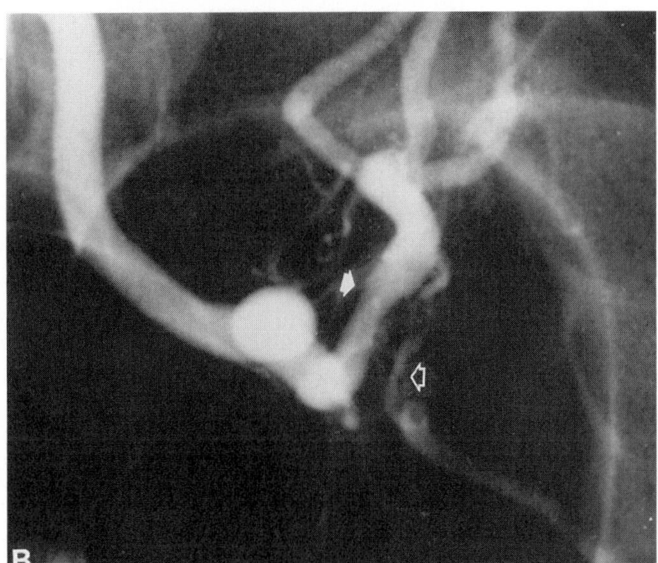

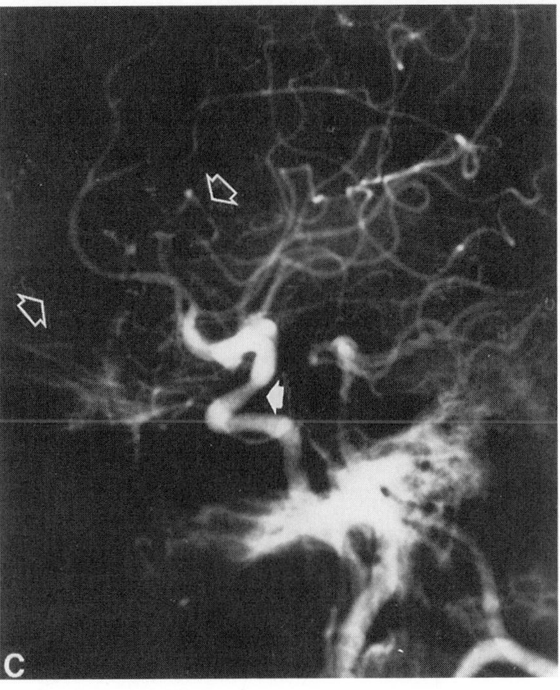

FIGURE 83.4. A: Left internal carotid angiogram (anteroposterior view) in a patient with contralateral hemiplegia after herpes zoster ophthalmicus. Note narrowing of the M1 portion of the left middle cerebral artery and the A1 portion of the left anterior cerebral artery (*open arrow*). Segmental beading is seen more distally. **B:** Right internal carotid angiogram (oblique view) in a patient with contralateral hemiplegia after herpes zoster ophthalmicus. Note narrowing of the right intracranial carotid artery (*solid arrow*) and irregularity of the A1 portion of the right anterior cerebral artery (*open arrow*). **C:** Right retrograde brachial cerebral angiogram (lateral view) in a patient with contralateral hemiplegia after herpes zoster ophthalmicus. Of note is narrowing of the right intracranial carotid artery in the region of the carotid siphon (*solid arrow*) and irregularities of the distal anterior and middle cerebral arteries (*open arrow*). (Reproduced with permission from Sigal LH. The neurologic presentation of vasculitic and rheumatologic syndromes: a review. *Medicine* 1987;66:157–180.)

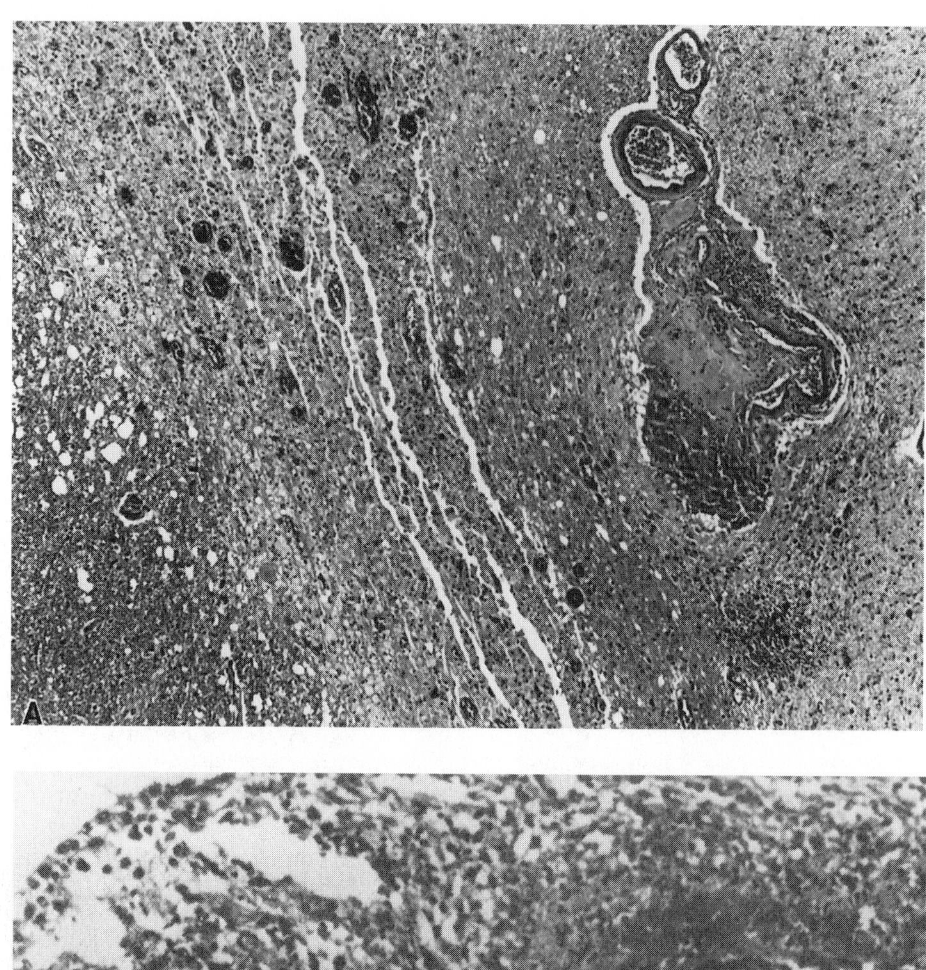

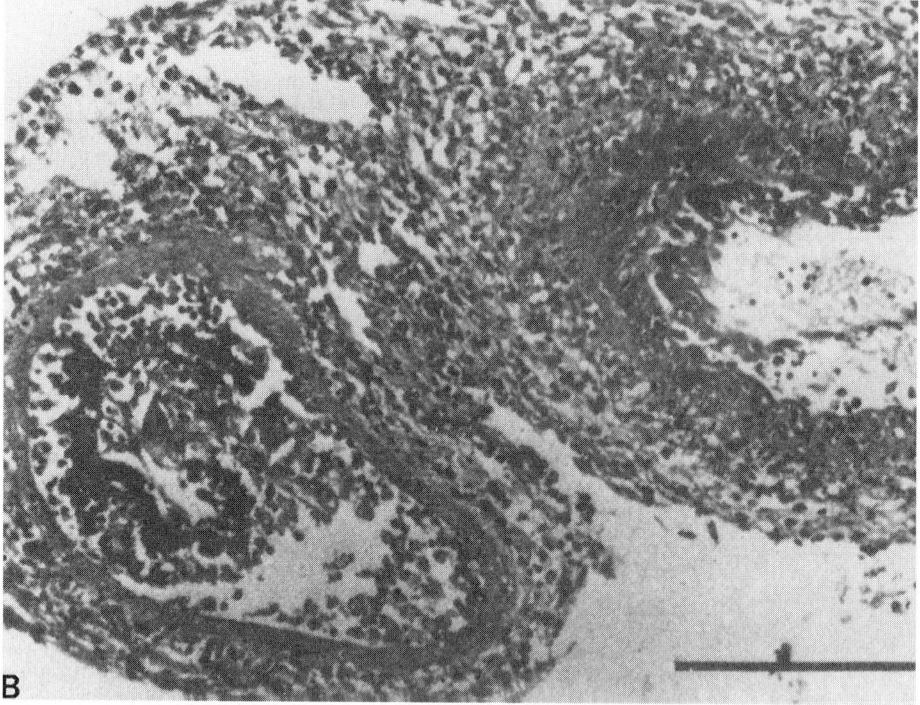

FIGURE 83.5. A: Photomicrograph of a postmortem specimen from a patient with contralateral hemiplegia after herpes zoster ophthalmicus. Necrotizing histiocytic angiitis is seen in the vessel on the right; histiocytes and giant cells infiltrate the vessel wall. **B:** Photomicrograph of a postmortem specimen from a patient with contralateral hemiplegia after herpes zoster ophthalmicus. Two small basilar arteries are shown with heavy mononuclear and histiocytic infiltrate. Granulomatous inflammatory process is segmental; fibrinoid necrosis also is seen involving the wall of one artery. (Reproduced with permission from Sigal LH. The neurologic presentation of vasculitic and rheumatologic syndromes: a review. *Medicine* 1987;66:157–180.)

neuroglial pathways to the Gasserian nucleus, where it elicits inflammation. Contiguous inflammation can then spread to the overlying vessels, causing tissue damage downstream (2). Virus-like particles have been described in smooth muscle cells in the walls of affected vessels (Fig. 83.6).

The prognosis in HZO-CA is encouraging (Table 83.6). Only two reported cases were treated with corticosteroids. Corticosteroid and acyclovir therapy was associated with improvement in one case. Corticosteroid therapy was thought to be beneficial in a second case, but death due to intracranial hemorrhage from a vasculitic aneurysm supervened. An additional patient was treated with aspirin, 500 mg daily, and dipyridamole, 75 mg t.i.d., with no disease progression (2).

OTHER NOTABLE MIMICS OF ISOLATED CENTRAL NERVOUS SYSTEM VASCULITIS

The use of intravenous (2) and oral (40) methamphetamine or cocaine [intravenous (2, 41), "snorted" (2, 41), or inhaled "crack" (41, 42)] also can cause CNS vasculitis in the absence of any systemic vascular abnormality. CNS vasculitis also has accompanied ephedrine abuse (2) and the use of phenylpropanolamine, a major ingredient in many over-the-counter diet pills, decongestants, and stimulants. Most of these patients took the drug at the recommended dose and had no systemic manifestation of vascular damage (2). Certain herbal preparations, e.g., ma huang, contain ephedrine-like compounds; use of herbal remedies should be a matter of inquiry in such cases. The resulting CNS syndrome could represent severe CNS vascular spasm rather than true vasculitis (2).

With the addition of transesophageal echocardiography to the diagnostic armamentarium, atheromata protruding into the thoracic aorta are now appreciated as a potential cause of atheromatous embolism to the brain, which can mimic CNS vasculitis, if no systemic embolization occurs (43–47). The discharge of embolic material is probably much more common than currently appreciated (e.g., after angiography or carotid surgery). Emboli originate more often from vessels other than the carotids than previously thought (especially the aorta), with a predilection to occlude the middle cerebral artery (47). Transesophageal echocardiography has already proven to be more sensitive for the diagnosis of atrial myxoma (another mimic of vasculitis) than is transthoracic echocardiography (48).

BENIGN ANGIOPATHY OF THE CENTRAL NERVOUS SYSTEM

Occasional cases of what seems to be ICNSV occur and resolve spontaneously. These cases, often in young women, are usually acute monophasic focal events. The CSF is usually normal or only slightly abnormal. Angiography reveals changes compatible with vasculitis. Such patients apparently have a form of benign angiopathy, perhaps vascular spasm rather than a vasculitis, and do well without therapy (49,50). In all such cases, a thorough history should include reference to use of medications that can induce vascular spasm, as

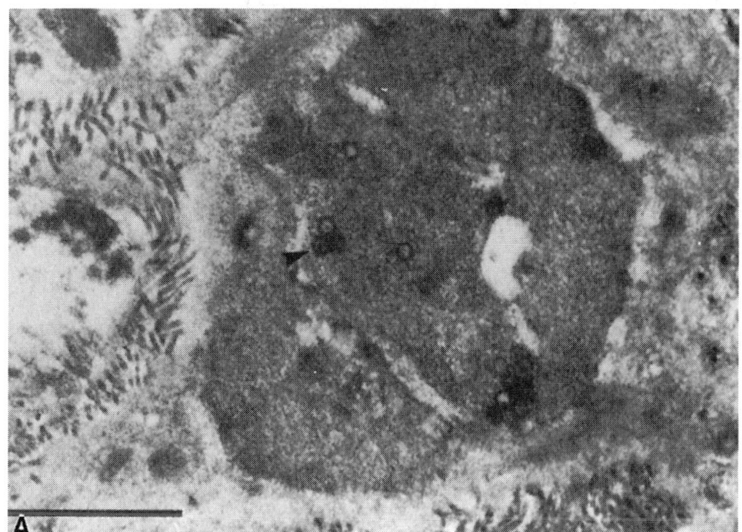

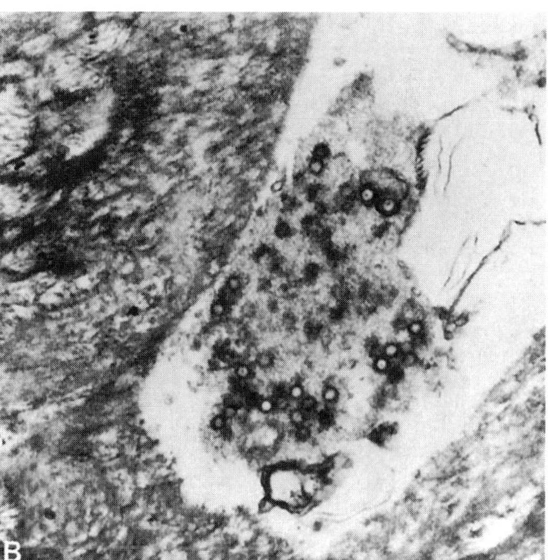

FIGURE 83.6. A: Electron micrograph of a postmortem specimen from a patient with contralateral hemiplegia after herpes zoster ophthalmicus. This area of granulomatous angiitis reveals intranuclear particles characteristic of herpes virus nucleocapsids, which are found in smooth muscle cells but not in endothelial cells. **B:** Electron micrograph of a postmortem specimen from a patient with contralateral hemiplegia after herpes zoster ophthalmicus. The nucleus of a smooth muscle is seen as a clear space, with darker cytoplasm around it. Hexagonal virions measuring 115 nm in diameter, consistent with herpesvirus, are seen within an inclusion body composed of debris. (Reproduced with permission from Sigal LH. The neurologic presentation of vasculitic and rheumatologic syndromes: a review. *Medicine* 1987;66:157–180.)

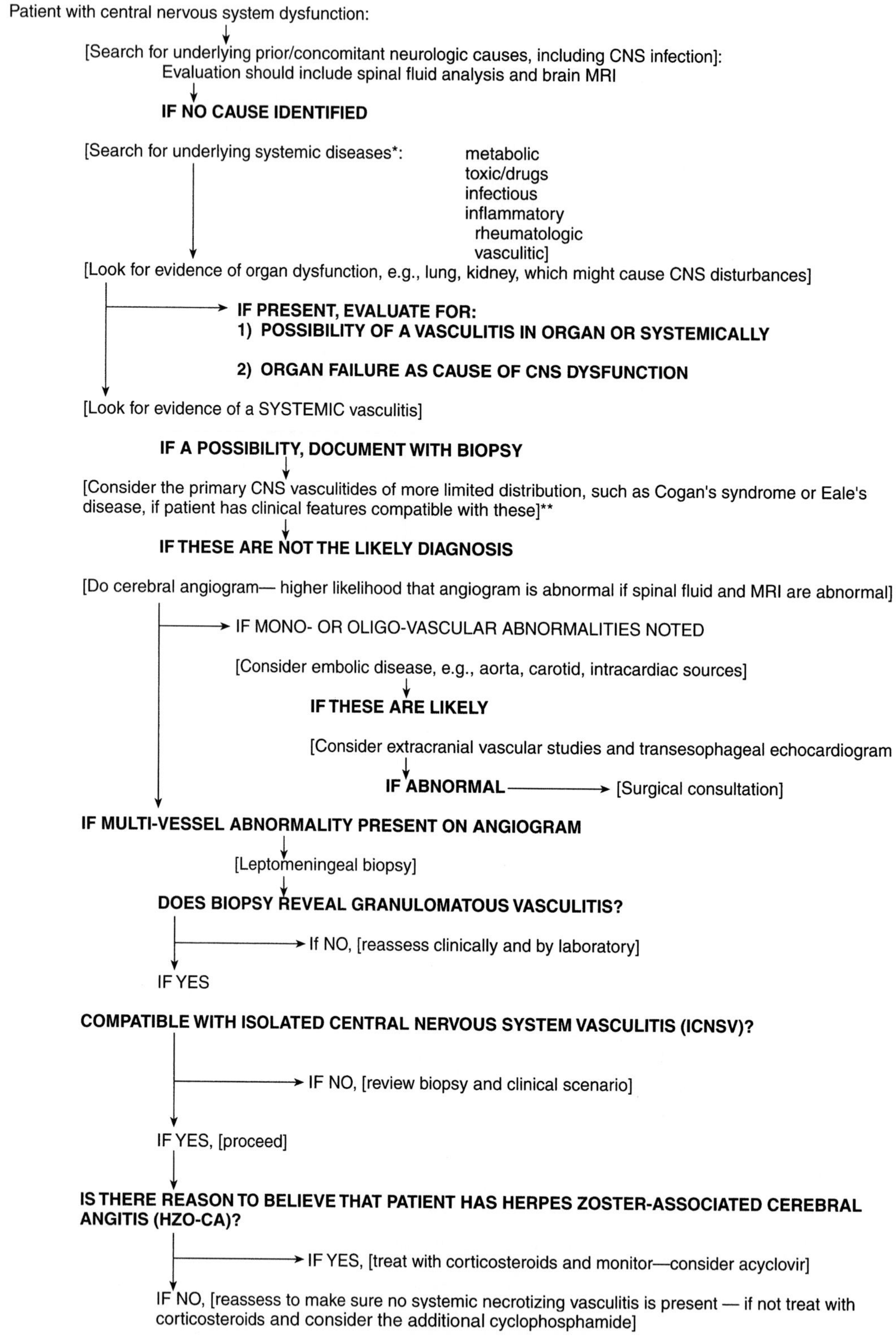

Patient with central nervous system dysfunction:

↓

[Search for underlying prior/concomitant neurologic causes, including CNS infection]:
Evaluation should include spinal fluid analysis and brain MRI

↓

IF NO CAUSE IDENTIFIED

[Search for underlying systemic diseases*: metabolic
toxic/drugs
infectious
inflammatory
rheumatologic
vasculitic]

↓

[Look for evidence of organ dysfunction, e.g., lung, kidney, which might cause CNS disturbances]

→ **IF PRESENT, EVALUATE FOR:**
1) POSSIBILITY OF A VASCULITIS IN ORGAN OR SYSTEMICALLY
2) ORGAN FAILURE AS CAUSE OF CNS DYSFUNCTION

↓

[Look for evidence of a SYSTEMIC vasculitis]

IF A POSSIBILITY, DOCUMENT WITH BIOPSY

↓

[Consider the primary CNS vasculitides of more limited distribution, such as Cogan's syndrome or Eale's disease, if patient has clinical features compatible with these]**

↓

IF THESE ARE NOT THE LIKELY DIAGNOSIS

[Do cerebral angiogram— higher likelihood that angiogram is abnormal if spinal fluid and MRI are abnormal]

→ IF MONO- OR OLIGO-VASCULAR ABNORMALITIES NOTED

[Consider embolic disease, e.g., aorta, carotid, intracardiac sources]

↓

IF THESE ARE LIKELY

[Consider extracranial vascular studies and transesophageal echocardiogram

↓

IF ABNORMAL → [Surgical consultation]

↓

IF MULTI-VESSEL ABNORMALITY PRESENT ON ANGIOGRAM

↓

[Leptomeningeal biopsy]

↓

DOES BIOPSY REVEAL GRANULOMATOUS VASCULITIS?

→ If NO, [reassess clinically and by laboratory]

↓

IF YES

COMPATIBLE WITH ISOLATED CENTRAL NERVOUS SYSTEM VASCULITIS (ICNSV)?

→ IF NO, [review biopsy and clinical scenario]

↓

IF YES, [proceed]

↓

IS THERE REASON TO BELIEVE THAT PATIENT HAS HERPES ZOSTER-ASSOCIATED CEREBRAL ANGITIS (HZO-CA)?

→ IF YES, [treat with corticosteroids and monitor—consider acyclovir]

↓

IF NO, [reassess to make sure no systemic necrotizing vasculitis is present — if not treat with corticosteroids and consider the additional cyclophosphamide]

*See Table 83.1 for a partial list of possible syndromes; search should not be limited to these syndromes.
**See Table 83.2 for clinical features of these syndromes.

FIGURE 83.7. Algorithm for use in the approach to the patient with possible central nervous system vasculitis.

noted previously. The mild and nonprogressive quality of their defects can differentiate such patients from true ICNSV.

CONCLUSIONS

Although histologically similar, ICNSV and HZO-CA are clearly distinct clinical entities. ICNSV is diffuse, as demonstrated both by angiography and by its clinical manifestations, with a poor prognosis. Angiitis associated with HZO is localized, less severe, and has a somewhat better prognosis even in the absence of therapy. The known antecedent infection with herpes zoster suggests the pathogenesis of HZO-CA, whereas the etiology of ICNSV remains unknown (2).

A patient with suspected ICNSV should be evaluated quickly. Potentially reversible phenomena should always be sought before institution of systemic therapy. A syndrome similar to ICNSV can be seen in patients with uncontrolled hypertension (e.g., pheochromocytoma) or history of complex headaches, in the postpartum period, and due to certain drugs. Questioning should be directed toward determination of prior use of sympathomimetic agents, including ephedrine and phenylpropanolamine and illicit chemicals like amphetamines and cocaine. If the neurologic defects are mild and nonprogressive and a BACNS is suspected, one can withhold therapy during the evaluation.

If the diagnosis of ICNSV is confirmed by biopsy, treatment with high doses of corticosteroids is indicated. The addition of a cytotoxic agent might be warranted, but further experience is needed before a definitive opinion can be rendered. Cyclophosphamide also has been used in 26 patients, only three of whom deteriorated. Recent experience with a series of 15 patients would suggest that cytotoxic agents might not be necessary, however (10). A management approach for patients with nervous system vasculitis has been proposed (51). The usually less severe, self-limited, neurologic sequelae in HZO-CA and its better outcome suggest that in most mild cases, therapy is not necessary. Of the 43 cases receiving no therapy, 17 died, however. In severe cases, corticosteroid therapy is probably indicated. Whether acyclovir should also be given remains to be investigated. Figure 83.7 presents an algorithm summarizing the approach suggested in this chapter.

REFERENCES

1. Gay RM Jr, Ball GV. Vasculitis. In: Koopman WJ, ed. *Arthritis and allied conditions.* 13th ed. Philadelphia: Lea & Febiger, 1997: 1491–1524.
2. Sigal LH. Isolated central nervous system vasculitis. In: Koopman WJ, ed. *Arthritis and allied conditions.* 13th ed. Philadelphia: Lea & Febiger, 1997:1547–1560.
3. Sigal LH. The neurologic presentation of vasculitic and rheumatologic syndromes: a review. *Medicine* 1987;66:157–180.
4. Calabrese LH, Mallek JA. Primary angiitis of the central nervous system: report of 8 new cases, review of the literature, and proposal for diagnostic criteria. *Medicine* 1987;67:20–39.
5. Ferro JM. Vasculitis of the central nervous system. *J Neurol* 1998;245:766–776.
6. Fieschi C, Rasura M, Anzini A, et al. Central nervous system vasculitis. *J Neurol Sci* 1998;153:159–171.
7. Somer T, Finegold SM. Vasculitides associated with infectious immunization and antimicrobial drugs. *Clin Infect Dis* 1995;20: 1010–1036.
8. Coyle PK, Gerber O, Roque C. Vasculitis owing to infection. *Neurol Clin* 1997;15:903–926.
9. Crane R, Kerr LD, Spiera H. Clinical analysis of isolated angiitis of the central nervous system. *Arch Intern Med* 1991;151: 229–294.
10. Lie JT. Primary (granulomatous) angiitis of the central nervous system: a clinicopathologic analysis of 15 new cases and a review of the literature. *Hum Pathol* 1992;23:164–171.
11. Cravioto H, Feigin I. Noninfectious granulomatous angiitis with a predilection for the nervous system. *Neurology* 1959;9:599–609.
12. Sanchez de Toledo Codina J, Rodriguez Galindo C, Moraga Llop F, et al. Response of central nervous system vasculitis to irradiation. *Lancet* 1991;337:1105–1106.
13. Kattah JC, Cupps TR, Di Chiro G, Manz HJ. An unusual case of central nervous system vasculitis. *J Neurol* 1987;234:344–347.
14. Calabrese LH, Duna GF, Lie JT. Vasculitis in the central nervous system. *Arthritis Rheum* 1997;40:1189–1201.
15. Vollmer TL, Guarnaccia J, Harrington W, et al. Idiopathic granulomatous angiitis of the central nervous system. *Arch Neurol* 1993;50:925–930.
16. Liu M-F, Li J-S, Tsao C-J, et al. Selective IgA deficiency with recurrent vasculitis of the central nervous system. *Clin Exp Rheumatol* 1998;16:77–79.
17. Raps EC, Galetta SL, Broderick M, et al. Delayed perpartum vasculopathy: cerebral eclampsia re-visited. *Ann Neurol* 1993;33: 222–225.
18. Sethna MP, Lampson LA. Immune modulation within the brain: recruitment of inflammatory cells and increased major histocompatibility antigen expression following intracerebral injection of interferon-gamma. *J Neuroimmunol* 1991;34:121–132.
19. Grau GF, Piguet P-F, Vassalli P, Lambert P-H. Involvement of tumour necrosis factor and other cytokines in immune-mediated vascular pathology. *Int Arch Allergy Appl Immunol* 1989;88: 34–39.
20. Hirohata S, Tanimoto K, Ito K. Elevation of cerebrospinal fluid interleukin 6 activity in patients with vasculitides and central nervous system involvement. *Clin Immunol Immunopathol* 1993; 66:225–229.
21. Alhalabi M, Moore PM. Serial angiography in isolated angiitis of the central nervous system. *Neurology* 1994;44:1221–1226.
22. Greenan TJ, Grossman RI, Goldberg HI. Cerebral vasculitis: MR imaging and angiographic correlation. *Radiology* 1992;182:65–72.
23. Chu CT, Gray L, Goldstein LB, Hulette CM. Diagnosis of intracranial vasculitis: a multi-disciplinary approach. *J Neuropathol Exp Neurol* 1998;57:30–38.
24. Wynne PJ, Younger DS, Khandji A, Silver AJ. Radiographic features of central nervous system vasculitis. *Neurol Clin* 1997;15: 779–804.
25. Cloft HJ, Phillips CD, Dix JE, McNulty BC, Zagardo MT, Kallmes DF. Correlation of angiography and MR imaging in cerebral vasculitis. *Acta Radiol* 1999;40:83–87.
26. Stone JH, Pomper MG, Roubenoff R, Miller TJ, Hellmann DB. Sensitivities of noninvasive tests for central nervous system vasculitis: a comparison of lumbar puncture, computed tomography, and magnetic resonance imaging. *J Rheumatol* 1994;21:1277–1282.
27. Harris KG, Tran DD, Sickels WJ, Cornell SH, Yuh WTC. Diag-

nosing intracranial vasculitis: the roles of MR and angiography. *AJNR Am J Neuroradiol* 1994;15:317–330.
28. Bryant GL, Weinblatt ME, Rumbaugh C, Coblyn JS. Cerebral vasculopathy: an analysis of sixteen cases. *Semin Arthritis Rheum* 1986;15:297–302.
29. Meusser S, Rubbert A, Manger B, et al. 99m-Tc-HMPAO-SPECT in diagnosis of early cerebral vasculitis. *Rheumatol Int* 1996;16:37–42.
30. Hellmann DB, Roubenoff R, Healy RA, Wang H. Central nervous system angiography: safety and predictors of a positive result in 125 consecutive patients evaluated for possible vasculitis. *J Rheumatol* 1992;19:568–572.
31. Duna GF, Calabrese LH. Limitations of invasive modalities in the diagnosis of primary angiitis of the central nervous system. *J Rheumatol* 1995;22:662–667.
32. Garner BF, Burns P, Bunning RD, Laureno R. Acute blood pressure elevation can mimic arteriographic appearance of cerebral vasculitis (a postpartum case with relative hypertension). *J Rheumatol* 1990;17:93–97.
33. Trommer BL, Homer D, Mikhael MA. Cerebral vasospasm and eclampsia. *Stroke* 1988;3:326–329.
34. Nadeau SE. Diagnostic approach to central and peripheral nervous system vasculitis. *Neurol Clin* 1997;15:759–778.
35. Adamek RJ, Wegener M, Wedmann B, Buttner T, Ricken D. Cerebral vasculitis in Crohn's disease. *Leber Magen Darm* 1993; 23:91–93.
36. Stumvoll M, Schnauder G, Overkamp D, Buettner UW, Grodd W, Eggstein M. Systemic vasculitis positive for circulating antineutrophil cytoplasmic antibodies and with predominantly neurological presentation. *Clin Invest* 1993;71:613–615.
37. Ishida K, Kamata T, Tsukagoshi H, Tanizak Y. Progressive systemic sclerosis with CNS vasculitis and cyclosporin A therapy. *J Neurol Neurosurg Psychiatry* 1992;56:720.
38. Younger DS, Calabrese LH, Hays AP. Granulomatous angiitis of the central nervous system. *Neurol Clin* 1997;15:821–834.
39. Shuper A, Vining EPG, Freeman JM. Central nervous system vasculitis after chickenpox: cause or coincidence? *Arch Dis Child* 1990;65:1245–1248.
40. Matick H, Anderson D, Brumlik J. Cerebral vasculitis associated with oral amphetamine overdose. *Arch Neurol* 1983;40:253–254.
41. Daras M, Tuchman AJ, Marks S. Central nervous system infarction related to cocaine abuse. *Stroke* 1991;22:1320–1325.
42. Krendel DA, Ditter SM, Frankel MR, Ross WK. Biopsy proven cerebral vasculitis associated with cocaine abuse. *Neurology* 1990; 40:1092–1094.
43. Karalis DG, Chandrasekharan K, Victor MF, Ross JJ Jr, Mintz GS. Recognition and embolic potential of intraortic atherosclerotic debris. *J Am Coll Cardiol* 1991;17:73–78.
44. Tunick PA, Perez JL, Kronzon I. Protruding atheromas in the thoracic aorta and systemic embolization. *Ann Intern Med* 1991; 115:423–427.
45. Masuda J, Yutani C, Ogata J, Kuriyama Y, Yamaguchi T. Atheromatous embolization in the brain: a clinicopathologic analysis of 15 autopsy cases. *Neurology* 1994;44:1231–1237.
46. Horowitz DR, Tuhrim S, Bud J, Goldman ME. Aortic plaque in patients with brain ischemia: diagnosis by transesophageal echocardiography. *Neurology* 1992;42:1602–1604.
47. Caplan LR. Brain embolism revisited. *Neurology* 1993;43: 1281–1287.
48. Sigal LH. Pseudovasculitis syndromes. In: McCarty DJ, ed. *Arthritis and allied conditions.* 12th ed. Philadelphia: Lea & Febiger, 1993:1323.
49. Calabrese LH, Gragg LA, Furlan AJ. Benign angiopathy: a distinct subset of angiographically defined primary angiitis of the central nervous system. *J Rheumatol* 1993;20:2046–2050.
50. Berger JR, Romano J, Menkin M, Norenberg M. Benign focal cerebral vasculitis: case report. *Neurology* 1995;45:1731–1734.
51. Kissel JT, Rammohan KW. Review: pathogenesis and therapy of nervous system vasculitis. *Clin Neuropharmacol* 1991;14: 28–48.

84

MIMICKERS OF VASCULITIS

KENNETH E. SACK

The term vasculitis encompasses an extraordinarily heterogeneous group of disorders (1,2) that have diverse etiologies and overlapping clinical manifestations (3–30). As a consequence, understanding vasculitis at the bedside, in the laboratory, and in the medical literature can be daunting. If, however, one categorizes the mechanisms by which vascular damage can occur, the concept of vasculitis and its mimickers becomes easier to comprehend.

MECHANISMS OF VASCULAR INJURY

The etiology of vascular injury is elusive because different stimuli can produce identical responses in the vessel wall. Furthermore, vessels damaged from whatever cause accumulate immune complexes readily and clear fibrin poorly. These factors further obscure the initial insult, and rather than representing a primary event, the vascular injury may simply reflect inflammation in neighboring tissues (31).

Pathways to vascular injury are numerous. In addition to immune-mediated mechanisms, they include direct infection (10,32–38); trauma from external injury (39–43), internal injury [e.g., hypertension (31)], occlusive processes (1,44,45), deposition of damaging substances (1,44, 46–50), or exposure to cold (51,52); ischemia from obstruction of vasa vasorum; neoplasia, either primary (53–62) or secondary (54,55,63–67); and congenital defects in the vessel wall (68–70).

RELATION OF VESSEL SIZE TO CLINICAL MANIFESTATIONS

Involvement of arterioles or venules underlies palpable purpura or urticaria; it also may cause macules, papules, vesicles, or pustules (71,72). Diseases of small arteries tend to produce nodules or livedo reticularis (a red–blue mottling of the skin in a net-like configuration; Fig. 84.1) (71,73). If medium-

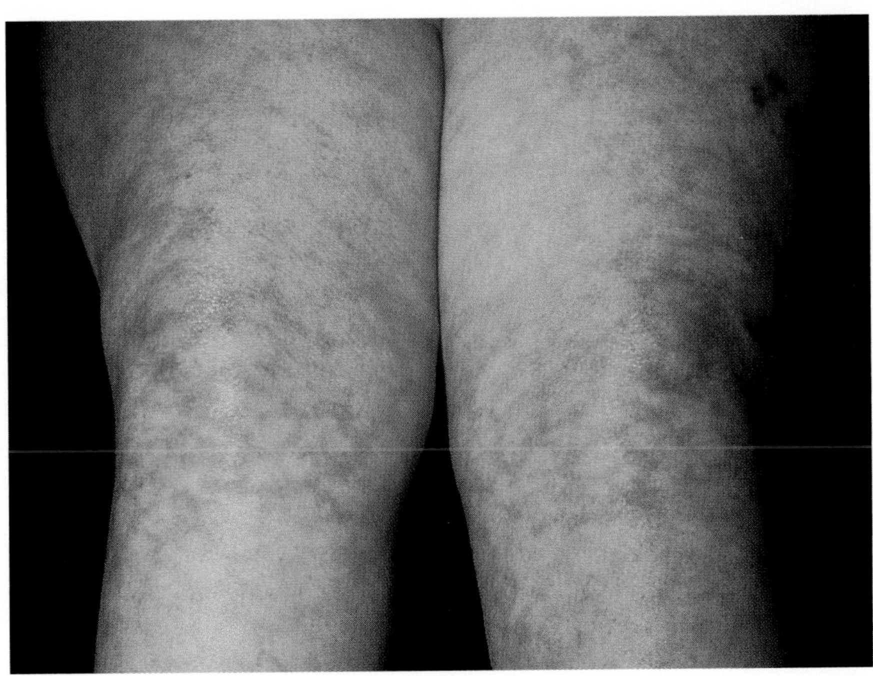

FIGURE 84.1. Livedo reticularis. (Courtesy of Dr. Kenneth Fye.)

sized arteries are affected, the lesions range from nodules to ulcerations, and peripheral gangrene or organ infarction may ensue (74). Large-vessel involvement typically induces claudication or injury to major organs (71).

Clinical signs do not allow one to predict the cause of the vascular abnormality. For instance, livedo reticularis can occur in autoimmune disorders, atheromatous disease, hyperviscosity and thrombotic states, after drug use, or after exposure to heat or cold (75–89).

PITFALLS IN DIAGNOSIS

On gross inspection, a variety of cutaneous lesions can look as though they reflect vasculitis. Examples of such lesions are erythema nodosum (a septal panniculitis) (90), pyoderma gangrenosum (a nonspecific inflammatory process) (91,92), the bite of the brown recluse spider (93), neoplasia (94), infection (95–98), and Sweet's syndrome (neutrophilic dermatosis) (99,100).

Histopathologic examination of vascular tissues also can be confusing. Acute arterial hypertension may cause fibrinoid changes in vessel walls, usually without cellular infiltration. In areas such as the lower leg, where stasis occurs, a mild degree of perivascular cellular infiltration and vascular hypertrophy is the rule (31). Vascular inflammation can result not only from immunologic events, but also from infection (10,27,34,36–38,101–107), neoplasia (63,108), embolic phenomena (45,109–112), or cold-induced injury (52).

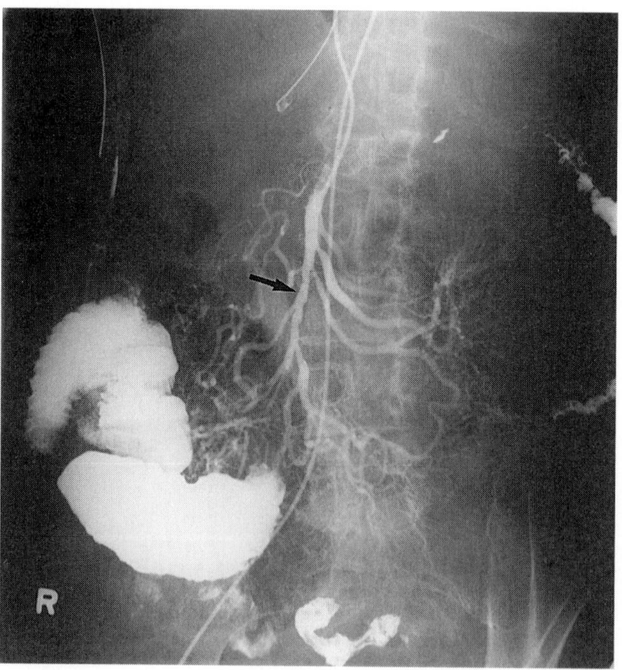

FIGURE 84.2. Beading of the superior mesenteric artery resulting from encasement by a carcinoid tumor. (Courtesy of Dr. Ernest Ring.)

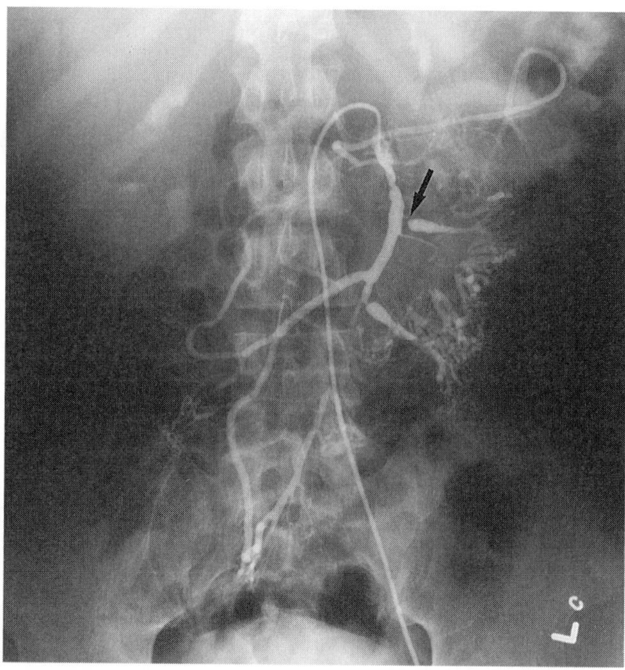

FIGURE 84.3. Stenosis of a jejunal branch (*arrow*) of the superior mesenteric artery in a patient who abused amphetamines. (Courtesy of Dr. Ernest Ring.)

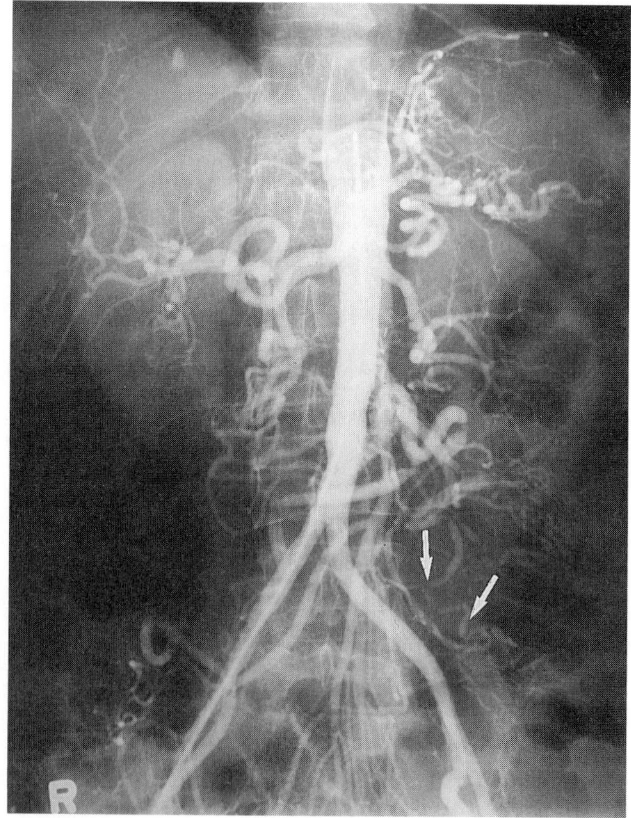

FIGURE 84.4. Beading in left colic artery (*arrows*) after repair of an occluded superior mesenteric artery. (Courtesy of Dr. Ernest Ring.)

The findings in any histopathologic specimen are a function of the time between the original insult and the biopsy. Anoxia, for example, can severely damage vascular smooth muscle within 2 hours (31). By contrast, the atherosclerotic changes and periarterial fibrosis caused by radiation injury may have a latency of 20 years (113).

Typical angiographic manifestations of vasculitis include irregularities in vessel walls, segmental occlusions, and vascular dilatations, yet similar abnormalities may be seen with neoplasia (55,114) (Fig. 84.2), infection (115,116), neurofibromatosis (117,118), fibromuscular dysplasia (119), pseudoxanthoma elasticum (120), hypertension (121), migraine (122,123), trauma (124–126), amyloidosis (127), atrial myxoma (128,129), pheochromocytoma (130), drug abuse (Fig. 84.3) (131), thrombotic thrombocytopenic purpura (132), Ehlers–Danlos syndrome (70), and moyamoya disease (133,134). To complicate the matter further, these same angiographic features also can appear after injection of dye, exposure to radiation (135) or cold (136), or reperfusion of normal vessels (Fig. 84.4).

DISEASES THAT MIMIC VASCULITIS

The following disorders may be confused with commonly recognized "vasculitis" syndromes.

Atheroembolic Disease

The atherosclerotic plaque consists of lipid-laden smooth muscle cells surrounded by lipid, collagen, elastic fibers, and proteoglycans (137). Together these components provide a veritable storehouse of "ammunition" to fire on major organs.

More than 100 years ago, pathologists recognized that atheromatous material could embolize (138), but they did not appreciate the importance of this phenomenon until 1945, when Flory (139) described characteristic findings in affected vessels at autopsy (*vide infra*). He correctly surmised that the findings resulted from emboli and that their occurrence correlated with the degree of atherosclerosis in the aorta. He reproduced these findings by injecting rabbits with suspensions of atheromatous material from a human aorta (139). Over the ensuing years, reports accumulated of atheroemboli affecting the extremities (140), eye (141), skin (142,143), pancreas (144), kidney (145–147), and central nervous system (148,149). Atheroembolic disease thus became a recognized mimicker of systemic vasculitis (150). In a review of 842 cases filed in the Dutch National Pathology Information System over a 20-year period, Moolenaar and Lamers (151) estimated an average frequency of 6.2 cases/million/year. Autopsy studies (152,153), however, indicated a prevalence of 2% to 4%. Furthermore, recent reports suggested that cholesterol emboli may account for 4% of unexplained cases of renal failure (83,154).

Pathophysiology

Atheromatous plaques may dislodge and embolize in fragments or may ulcerate and release cholesterol crystals or other components (155,156). In some instances, thrombi overlying the plaque constitute the main embolic material (157). The emboli typically lodge in arteries with diameters of 150 to 200 μm (156).

Vessels affected by atheroemboli undergo successive pathologic changes (114,141,152,157). Soon after cholesterol crystals and amorphous atheromatous material lodge in the arterial lumen, an acute inflammatory response occurs. Intimal hyperplasia and a panarteritis follow rapidly, often accompanied by foreign-body giant cells. Intimal fibrosis ensues along with complete encasement of the cholesterol crystals by collagenous tissue. The vessel lumen, which initially contained slit-like passages (Fig. 84.5), may eventually become completely occluded. Superimposed thrombosis is uncommon (145,157).

Usual methods for preparing histologic specimens dissolve cholesterol crystals, leaving characteristic clefts (Fig. 84.5) (156). In some cases, necrotizing angiitis is the dom-

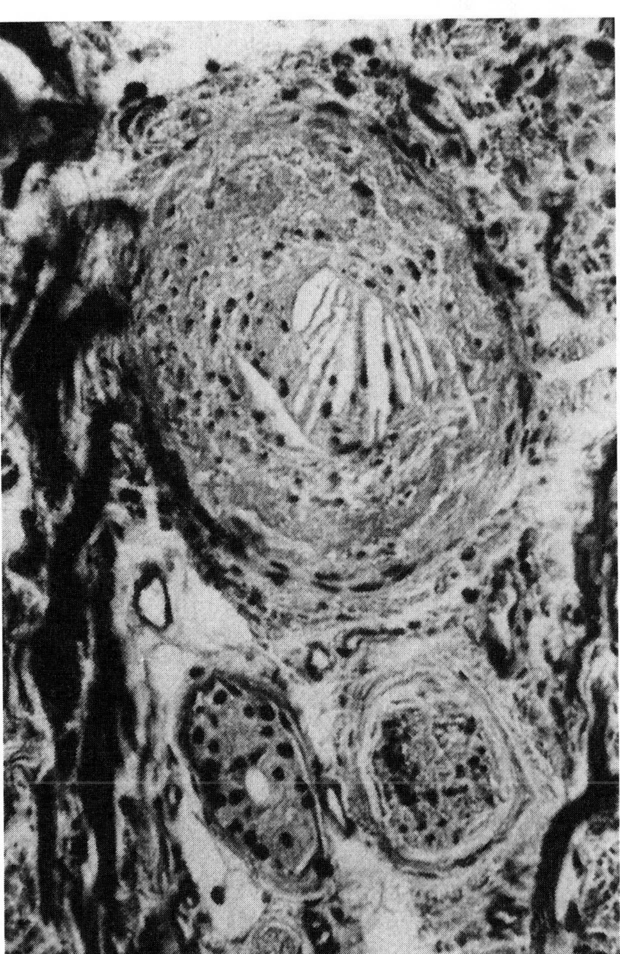

FIGURE 84.5. Cholesterol clefts in a small renal artery.

inant pathologic finding, and only careful scrutiny of serial sections or examination of other vessels will uncover the tell-tale signs (109,158–160). Many cholesterol emboli go unnoticed when the involved vessels are small and collateral circulation prevents infarction (156). In the appropriate setting, biopsy of a skin lesion (143) or the kidney (87,161) usually yields the diagnosis. Occasionally, random biopsy of muscle (158) or bone marrow (162) is diagnostic.

Crystalline cholesterol, as well as lipids from atheromata, can fix complement (163,164). This process not only produces hypocomplementemia but also results in the production of C5a (163), a potent chemotactic factor for eosinophils and neutrophils (164). Consequently, atheroembolic disease frequently causes eosinophilia (82,164–169). Eosinophiluria also occurs and is easily identified by using Hansel's instead of Wright's stain to analyze urine sediment (170).

A variety of laboratory abnormalities may accompany atheroembolic disease (Table 84.1). It is easy, therefore, to mistake this disease for an immune-mediated condition when tests for antinuclear antibody (ANA) (45,165,171, 172) or rheumatoid factor (RF) (165) are positive, the serum creatine phosphokinase (CPK) level (165,169) is elevated, or the urine contains protein or cells or both (165, 168–170,173).

Clinical Syndromes

Atheroembolic disease is manifested in numerous ways and often simulates systemic vasculitis (45,150,165,172,174). Typically, symptoms follow catheterization or surgical manipulation of an artery during which plaques become disrupted and embolize distally (76,78,82,83,85,146,147, 155,169,175–177). Curiously, angioplasty does not add to the risk of catheterization (178). Anticoagulation may prevent formation of a "protective" thrombus over an atheromatous plaque, thereby predisposing to subsequent embolization (138,179–182). Thrombolytic therapy might also initiate embolization (183,184), but in many such reported cases, the patient also had received an anticoagulant (161,185–187). When the syndrome occurs without an obvious triggering event, other signs and symptoms of atherosclerotic disease or an aortic aneurysm are present (45,80,83,87,169,173,188–190).

Atheroembolic disease can affect almost any organ (144,151,156,157,165,173,191). Autopsy studies suggest that such emboli are common but often asymptomatic (144,157,169). The kidney is the most frequently affected organ, followed closely by the pancreas and spleen (142,169). Involvement of the skin, gastrointestinal tract, and central nervous system also is common (83,109,151,192).

Perhaps the most frequent visible manifestation of atheroembolic disease is purple discoloration of the toes, progressing at times to ulceration and gangrene. In this situation, the patient typically has normal peripheral pulses and livedo reticularis that symmetrically affects the lower part of the body (80,142,143,159). Many cases of "blue toe" syndrome after the administration of an anticoagulant may be caused by atheroemboli (111,142,179,180,182). Rarely, such emboli cause gangrene in unusual areas [e.g., scrotum and penis (160, 193) or splinter hemorrhages in the fingers or toenails (194)].

Unexplained acute or progressive renal failure (82,83,87, 146,147,161,175,189,192,195,196) or hypertension (45, 145,192,193) also suggests atheroembolic disease. The urinary sediment may be normal or show varying amounts of red cells, white cells [including eosinophils (159)], casts, and proteinuria (169,170) (rarely, in the nephrotic range (173,197,198). Renal angiography occasionally shows stenosis and dilatation of medium-sized and small arteries (165), but renal biopsy characteristically shows atheroembolic material occluding arcuate and interlobular arteries (87,161). Most reports describe an unrelenting downhill course (82,161,193), but spontaneous resolution of renal insufficiency may occur (87).

Other clinical conditions caused by atheroembolic disease include acute pancreatitis (144,177), amaurosis (172, 192,199), transient ischemic attacks (165,172,173), stroke syndromes (109,148,149,165,172), abdominal pain (78, 150,199,200) (with or without gastrointestinal bleeding), occult gastrointestinal bleeding (200,201), angina pectoris (165), and myocardial infarction (199). Occasionally nonspecific symptoms such as fever, weight loss, or myalgias occur. Arthritis and mononeuritis multiplex are distinctly unusual (157,169). Rarely atheroemboli produce the picture of disseminated intravascular coagulation (DIC) (202).

Treatment of atheroembolic disease is largely supportive. Use of low-molecular-weight dextran, antiplatelet drugs, or

TABLE 84.1. LABORATORY ABNORMALITIES ASSOCIATED WITH ATHEROEMBOLIC DISEASE

Common
Anemia
Leukocytosis
Eosinophilia
Thrombocytopenia
Elevated erythrocyte sedimentation rate (ESR)
Azotemia
Hyperamylasemia
Hypocomplementemia
Positive antinuclear antibody or rheumatoid factor
Proteinuria
Granular or hyaline urinary casts
Eosinophiluria
Uncommon
Elevated creatine phosphokinase or aldolase
Cryoglobulinemia
Glycosuria
Hematuria
Pyuria
Cellular urinary casts

vasodilators does not alter the course substantially (78,80, 165). Anticoagulants can precipitate the syndrome, and patients may improve after discontinuing these agents (203). Corticosteroids can temporarily alleviate some manifestations of atheroembolic disease, but their use does not affect the outcome (78). Treatment with lipid-lowering drugs can sometimes halt or reverse the atheromatous process (204–206), and some reports suggested that such therapy may have clinical benefit (188,191,196). Pentoxifylline has reportedly led to clinical improvement (207). Presumably, agents with the potential to stabilize atherosclerotic plaques (208) could effect similar benefit.

Prognosis is poor. Some series show a mortality of 70% to 90% (78,143,169,200), and the need for long-term dialysis is not uncommon (82). Outcome probably relates to the cause and extent of the disease (87). Thus a patient with limited emboli from a discrete source (e.g., aneurysm or localized atheromatous plaque) may do well, particularly on removal of the offending lesion (199,209). The incidence of this lethal disease should decrease if we can prevent or reduce atherosclerosis, detect plaques by noninvasive means (210), and manipulate intravascular catheters cautiously.

Cardiac Myxoma

More than 100 years have passed since the initial description of atrial myxoma (211), but confirmation of its neoplastic nature (129,212–215) and the ability to diagnose it before death (216–219) are relatively recent. Myxomas compose more than 50% of cardiac neoplasms. Most of them occur in the atria, especially the left (219,220), and only about 5% involve the ventricles (219). These tumors are typically pedunculated and attached to the atrial septum near the fossa ovalis (217,219,221), but they can appear anywhere (e.g., on a valve or the chordae tendineae) (219). They usually affect patients between the ages of 30 and 60 years, are uncommon in blacks (219), and rarely are familial (222,223).

Pathophysiology

Cardiac myxomas are typically single (occasionally multiple), pedunculated, soft, friable masses ranging from a few millimeters to greater than 10 cm in diameter (218,219). Rarely they calcify (217). Microscopic examination shows a paucicellular collection of polygonal and stellate cells in an amorphous mucopolysaccharide matrix with variable vascularity (219,220). Although the cells contain few mitotic figures, the fact that atrial myxomas sometimes recur locally or in peripheral sites confirms their neoplastic nature (129,212–215). On immunohistochemical and ultrastructural study, myxoma cells may show endothelial, epithelial, smooth muscle, fibroblastic, and histiocytic features, suggesting that they originate from a multipotential mesenchymal cell (221,224,225).

The location of these pedunculated tumors explains their ability to obstruct flow across the atrioventricular valve. The rarer sessile (and relatively immobile) tumors produce valve obstruction only when quite large (219). In addition to their ability to block or damage cardiac valves, atrial myxomas may fragment and embolize to peripheral vascular beds or produce cytokines such as interleukin-6 (IL-6), a potent B lymphocyte–stimulating and hepatocyte-stimulating factor (221,226–228). Thrombus overlying the myxoma (219) or infection of the tumor (229–232) can alter the clinical presentation.

Clinical Manifestations

Although sometimes asymptomatic (219,233), myxomas usually cause systemic, obstructive, and embolic symptoms (217,219,221,234–236). Patients may complain of fever, weight loss, arthralgia, myalgia, or Raynaud's phenomenon (128,217–219,221,234–241). Occasionally a skin rash occurs that ranges from erythematous (or livedoid) macules or papules to frank ulcerations or even telangiectasia (110, 221,226,242–244). Clubbing also may develop (217,221). Obstruction of the mitral valve can cause shortness of breath (which may improve during recumbency), fatigue, weakness, or syncope (219,221,234–237,239,245–248).

In a review of 24 consecutive cases of atrial myxomas, new-onset congestive heart failure, chest pain, and episodic pulmonary edema were the most common cardiac-related symptoms (233). When shortness of breath improves in the supine position or when syncope occurs during reclining, atrial myxoma merits strong consideration (219). One fourth to half of the patients will have one or more embolic events (217,218,221,233,234,236), 50% of which affect the central nervous system (219,249) causing focal neurologic abnormalities (129,250–252). Emboli may travel to almost any arterial bed, resulting in a variety of clinical syndromes including mononeuritis multiplex (243). Right-sided myxomatous emboli typically produce symptoms and signs of acute pulmonary thromboemboli; occasionally their manifestations simulate those of constrictive pericarditis (221). Recurrent emboli can produce pulmonary hypertension (212,218,219,234). Rarely atrial myxomas are associated with spotty skin pigmentation and tumors of other organs (e.g., adrenal gland, breast, testicle) (253).

Physical examination of the heart may show no abnormality (233,243). Some patients, however, have an accentuated first heart sound, an increased pulmonic component of the second heart sound, and a diastolic rumble suggesting mitral stenosis (217,219,234,236,245,247). In such cases, however, enlargement of the left atrium and atrial fibrillation are unusual (219). A unique but infrequent finding is a low-frequency sound ("tumor plop") heard 0.08 to 0.15 seconds after the second heart sound and occasionally mistaken for an S_3 or opening snap (217,219,236,245). Rarely a cardiac rub that has a to-and-fro "crunching" quality may appear (217).

Right-sided myxomas can produce the murmurs of tricuspid stenosis or regurgitation, jugular venous distention, hepatomegaly, edema, or ascites (219). Ventricular myxomas can cause signs of ventricular outflow obstruction (218,219).

Laboratory Findings

Before 1952, autopsy was the only means of diagnosing atrial myxoma (254). Now echocardiography confirms the diagnosis virtually 100% of the time (219,232). A two-dimensional echocardiogram shows not only the size, shape, and location of the tumor, but also estimates the tumor's mobility (219,255,256). Computed tomography (CT) and magnetic resonance imaging (MRI) also detect myxomas if the lesions are at least 0.5 to 1 cm in diameter (221).

Embolic fragments of a myxoma are sometimes visible in tissue specimens (217,219,241), but at other times, one sees only "vasculitis" (257). Angiographic findings of vascular irregularities, dilatations, or aneurysms (128,129,219,241, 250,251,257) enhance the diagnostic confusion.

The immune-stimulating properties of myxomas (e.g., the production of IL-6) no doubt account for the common findings of anemia, leukocytosis, thrombocytopenia, hypocomplementemia, elevated erythrocyte sedimentation rate (ESR), acute-phase reactants, and formation of autoantibodies (217,218,221,226,236,237,243,247,258,259). For unclear reasons, polycythemia may accompany right atrial myxomas (217–219,236). An infected myxoma that yields positive blood cultures can lead to an erroneous diagnosis of infective endocarditis (229,232).

Treatment

The first successful resection of an atrial myxoma took place in the 1950s (260). Since then, the prognosis for surviving a myxoma has vastly improved (217,219,221,233,235,236, 248,261). Because the tumor is occasionally multicentric, direct visualization of all four cardiac chambers is important (219). Full-thickness excision of the tumor at the base of its pedicle is usually curative. The operative mortality is 0 to 2.7%. The recurrence rate is 0 to 14% (219,221,236,248, 261), but may reach 22% for complex myxomas (221). Most recurrences are local and occur within 1 to 2 years of diagnosis. In some cases, however, the interval is longer (215,219, 236,262). The tumor also may recur at extracardiac sites (215, 262), presumably from slow growth of myxomatous emboli.

Occlusive Processes

Thrombotic Disorders

Thrombosis in multiple vessels can create widespread damage mimicking "vasculitis." In turn, inflammation in a vessel wall can injure the endothelium and predispose to thrombosis (263). Determining which came first—inflammation or thrombosis—can be difficult.

Of the more than 25 "hypercoagulable states" (264, 265), the antiphospholipid antibody syndrome most often simulates vasculitis. The antibodies in this syndrome occasionally induce widespread thrombosis, causing ischemia in single (266–269) or multiple (270) organs. A variety of skin manifestations also may occur (79,272,270,271,273), the most characteristic being livedo reticularis (79,84,86,89, 272–279), often accompanied by acrocyanosis (84). Other cutaneous manifestations include small, nonblanching erythematous or cyanotic areas on the hands and feet, as well as localized or scattered hemorrhages, ulcers, and gangrene (272,273,276,277,279,280). Although histopathologic examination of the skin may show inflammation of small vessels (84,281,282), thrombosis is probably the primary event (79,266,275,277–279,283–285). Angiograms occasionally demonstrate vascular narrowing or multiple occlusions of the involved vessels (286).

Thrombotic thrombocytopenic purpura (TTP) characteristically causes a pentad of microangiopathic hemolytic anemia, thrombocytopenic purpura, neurologic abnormalities, renal dysfunction, and fever (287,288). Histologic examination of tissues such as gingiva or kidney shows hyaline thrombi, microaneurysm formation, and endothelial cell proliferation in small arteries and arterioles (132,287,288).

Changes similar to those of TTP occur when injury to vascular endothelium results in disseminated intravascular coagulation (289). Additionally, thrombocythemia can cause digital gangrene and livedo reticularis without demonstrable arterial disease (290). Sickle cell anemia can give rise to vascular narrowing (291,292).

Malignant atrophic papulosis (Kohlmeier–Degos' syndrome) is a thrombotic vasculopathy (293–295) that typically is seen as small pink or grey–yellow papules that rapidly umbilicate, and then acquire a white, porcelain-like center and a narrow rose or violaceous border, crisscrossed by fine telangiectases. These papules tend to appear in crops, spread over the trunk and upper limbs, and never resolve completely (296). Whereas they are virtually pathognomonic of Kohlmeier–Degos' syndrome, similar cutaneous findings may accompany systemic lupus erythematosus (297) and scleroderma (298). Histologic examination characteristically shows thrombosed dermal vessels (with little inflammatory reaction) underlying an atrophic and hyperkeratotic epidermis (294,296,299). Some authors have noted a lymphocytic infiltrate in and around arterioles and venules (300). Within months or years, similar vascular changes occur in other organs (294,296,299,301,302) (e.g., gastrointestinal tract, central nervous system). Involvement of internal organs rarely precedes the cutaneous lesions (299,302–304).

The cause of Kohlmeier–Degos' syndrome is unknown. No consistent pattern of complement or immunoglobulin deposition occurs in the walls of affected vessels (302), and theories regarding a viral etiology (305) remain unproven. The association of this illness with anticardiolipin antibodies (295) raised hopes that use of anticoagulants or platelet inhibitors would be beneficial (293), but unfortunately, such antibodies are not a consistent finding (306). Treatment with various immunosuppressive agents (296,304) does not alter the usual fatal outcome, which typically results from sepsis consequent to peritonitis (303).

Thromboembolism

Thromboembolism can simulate vasculitis by occluding multiple arterial beds (307). The embolic material ordinarily comes from the heart (e.g., *in situ* thrombi, marantic valvular lesions) or a large artery (77), but venous thrombi can embolize "paradoxically" through a patent foramen ovale (308). The emboli occasionally consist of air, fat, or neoplastic tissue (309).

Embolic disease is one of the many causes of "blue toe syndrome" (i.e., the sudden onset of one or more discrete painful, blue or purple discolorations on the foot or toes). Other reported causes of this phenomenon include thrombi, true vasculitis, infection, cyanotic heart disease, hyperviscosity, calciphylaxis, and pheochromocytoma (111, 179,310,311).

Other Occlusive Diseases

Substances other than thrombotic and atheromatous debris can occlude vessels and mimic systemic vasculitis. In some of these cases, temperature plays an important role. For example, cryoglobulins and cryofibrinogens precipitate in cold temperature and can occlude vessels (312,313), causing cutaneous ulcerations and acral purpura (247,248,250, 251). Cryofibrinogens occur most commonly in patients with neoplasia or diabetes mellitus (81,314). The characteristic histopathologic feature is eosinophilic thrombi in dermal vessels associated with minimal signs of inflammation (315,316). Because the process of clotting consumes fibrinogen, testing for cryofibrinogen requires anticoagulation of the patient's blood with oxalate, citrate, or ethylenediaminetetraacetic acid (EDTA) (314,315). Whole immunoglobulins or light chains rarely can form occlusive crystals at cool temperatures (317–320). The clinical manifestations include polyarthralgia, palpable purpura, necrotic cutaneous ulcers, digital infarcts, and nerve palsies (317–320).

Noncryoprecipitable paraproteins also may cause an occlusive vasculopathy. This vasculopathy occasionally accompanies multiple myeloma (321), but it also appears in a condition termed POEMS (polyneuropathy, organomegaly endocrinopathy, M protein, and skin changes) (322–329). The cardinal feature is severe, progressive sensorimotor polyneuropathy. Other common findings are plasma cell dyscrasia in association with osteosclerotic bone lesions, production of an M protein, hepatosplenomegaly, lymphadenopathy, thickening and hyperpigmentation of the skin, and endocrine dysfunction (e.g., diabetes mellitus, hypothyroidism, adrenal insufficiency, amenorrhea, gynecomastia, and impotence).

Infection

Direct infection of vessel walls or infection-initiated immune processes can compromise vascular integrity and simulate vasculitis (34,36,103,330). Several organisms have been implicated (Table 84.2). Clinical manifestations range from nonspecific systemic complaints and a variety of skin lesions to infarction of major organs. Additionally, bacterial endocarditis (331), viral infection (36,332), basilar meningitis(116,291, 333–343) (e.g., secondary to bacteria, mycobacteria, fungi, or spirochetes), and brain abscess sometimes evoke changes suggestive of "vasculitis" on cerebral angiograms.

Erythema induratum manifests as chronic tender, ulcerating nodules on the lower extremities, predominantly in

TABLE 84.2. INFECTIOUS CAUSES OF VASCULITIS

Bacteria (101, 230, 244, 263, 265, 272, 273, 276–278, 513)
Neisseria
Hemophilus
Salmonella
Yersinia
Actinomycetes
Pseudomonas pseudomallei
Pyogenic organisms
Mycobacteria (35, 279, 280, 344)
M. tuberculosis
Spirochetes (281–284, 514–518)
Toponemia pallidum
Borellia burgdorferi
B. garinii
Rickettsiae (11, 285)
Fungi (45, 102, 230, 276, 287, 509, 512, 519–521)
Mucormycosis
Aspergillosis
Sporotrichosis
Histoplasmosis
Cryptococcosis
Fusarium
Viruses (7, 10, 27, 32, 33, 37, 55, 105, 106, 115, 288–294, 522–532)
Herpes virus
Human immunodeficiency virus (HIV)
Human T-lymphotrophic virus III (HTLV-III)
Cytomegalovirus
Parvovirus
Rabies
Rubella
Parasites (244, 533–536)
Schistosomiasis mansoni
Visceral larva migrans
Ameba
Trypanosomiasis
Cysticercosis
Protozoa (104)
Toxoplasmosis

young or middle-aged women. *Mycobacterium tuberculosis* is the cause (344–347).

Infections with organisms such as *Strongyloides stercoralis* (348) trichinella (9), acanthamoeba (96,98,349), human immunodeficiency virus (HIV) (36,115,330,350–352), and rabies virus occasionally produce symptoms and signs identical to those of vasculitis. Additionally, I have observed a patient with myalgias, scalp tenderness, jaw pain, and a markedly elevated ESR, whose subsequent orbital swelling, proptosis, and gaze paralysis yielded the correct diagnosis of orbital cellulitis.

Trauma

External

The "hypothenar hammer syndrome" exemplifies how external trauma can affect a blood vessel (40,123,124, 353–355). Patients with this syndrome invariably give a history of striking or pushing hard surfaces with the hypothenar aspect of the hand. In this circumstance, the hand is the "hammer," the hook of the hamate bone is the "anvil," and the unprotected superficial palmar branch of the ulnar artery is the "horseshoe." What typically ensues is intermittent lancinating pain, followed by a dull ache over the hypothenar eminence. The subsequent ischemic symptoms often lead to a diagnosis of Raynaud's phenomenon, but careful questioning reveals that neither a triphasic color change nor involvement of the thumb occurs (40). An angiogram will show either an irregularity, an aneurysm, or an occlusion of the ulnar artery, sometimes associated with occlusion of the more distal arteries (40,123,124,354). Histopathologic examination of the affected vessels often demonstrates thrombosis on the intimal surface and fibrosis in the media (354). Similar histopathologic changes in the vessel wall could be responsible for some of the vascular narrowing seen on cerebral angiograms after severe head trauma; however, cerebral vasospasm consequent to intracranial hemorrhage may be a factor in those cases (125).

Trauma to the carotid artery can mimic cerebral vasculitis by causing dissection of the vessel wall (42) or formation of a thrombus that embolizes distally (356). Likewise, if atlantoaxial subluxation causes injury to the vertebral arteries, multiple cerebellar infarctions may ensue (43).

Internal

Brief elevations of blood pressure can produce angiographic findings of vasoconstriction and dilatation in cerebral vessels (121). Segmental narrowing of these vessels also may occur before, during, or after episodes of migraine (122, 123,357–360) and in the postpartum period (359,360). Dissections of extracranial and intracranial arteries, and occasionally of visceral arteries, can cause long foci of arterial narrowing on angiograms, resulting in the erroneous diagnosis of arteritis (361).

Exposure to Damaging Substances

Amyloid

Amyloid angiopathy can appear as an isolated phenomenon in the central nervous system (49,362–365) or as a manifestation of systemic amyloidosis with an associated paraprotein (366,367). Clinical manifestations range from those typical of temporal arteritis (127,368,369) to those of progressive dementia or multiple cerebral infarctions (49, 362–365). Intracerebral hemorrhage is common (363–365), and when such hemorrhage occurs in a patient with dementia, amyloid cerebrovascular disease is an important consideration (364). Amyloid also can affect peripheral vessels and produce ischemic organ damage or purpura (366,367). Renal failure or hematuria, with or without proteinuria, may reflect amyloidosis (370). Vascular narrowing or occlusion is an occasional angiographic finding (368); histopathologic examination of vessels demonstrates infiltration with amyloid, accompanied at times by obliterative intimal changes, aneurysm formation, perivascular or transmural inflammatory infiltrates, and fibrinoid necrosis (362, 365–367).

α_1-Antitrypsin Deficiency

α_1-Antitrypsin, the most abundant proteinase inhibitor in human plasma, plays a major role in protecting tissues (including blood vessels) from endogenous toxins (371). Thus when this protease inhibitor is deficient, there is an increased incidence of fibromuscular dysplasia (372), intracranial aneurysm (373), spontaneous dissection of cervical or peripheral arteries (374), panniculitis (373), and antineutrophil cytoplasmic antibody–associated vasculitis (375). Some of these associations, however, remain unproven (376).

Calciphylaxis

In 1962, Selye (377) showed that tissues could be rendered sensitive to calcification and termed this phenomenon calciphylaxis. He found that exposure to a "sensitizer," followed by a critical latent period and then contact with a "challenger," could lead to local or widespread calcification. Most patients who demonstrate this process have end-stage renal disease and hyperparathyroidism, resulting in a high serum calcium × phosphorous product (the sensitizer) (378–385). Some infections (i.e., granulomatous, HIV) also may serve as sensitizers (386). Postulated challengers include iron, albumen, corticosteroids, vitamin D, intramuscular tobramycin, calcium heparinate, erythropoietin, insulin, and immunosuppressive agents (379,384–389).

In patients with calciphylaxis, a livedo reticularis–like rash typically develops that becomes plaque-like, nodular, or bullous, progressing at times to necrosis with ulceration (Fig. 84.6A) (378,382–385,390,391). Calcification may

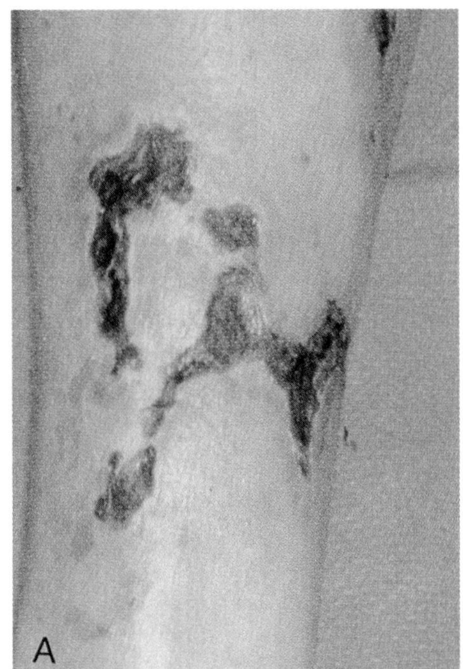

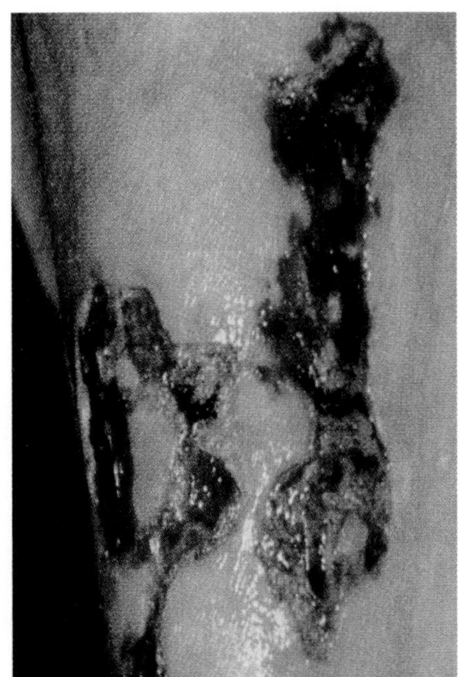

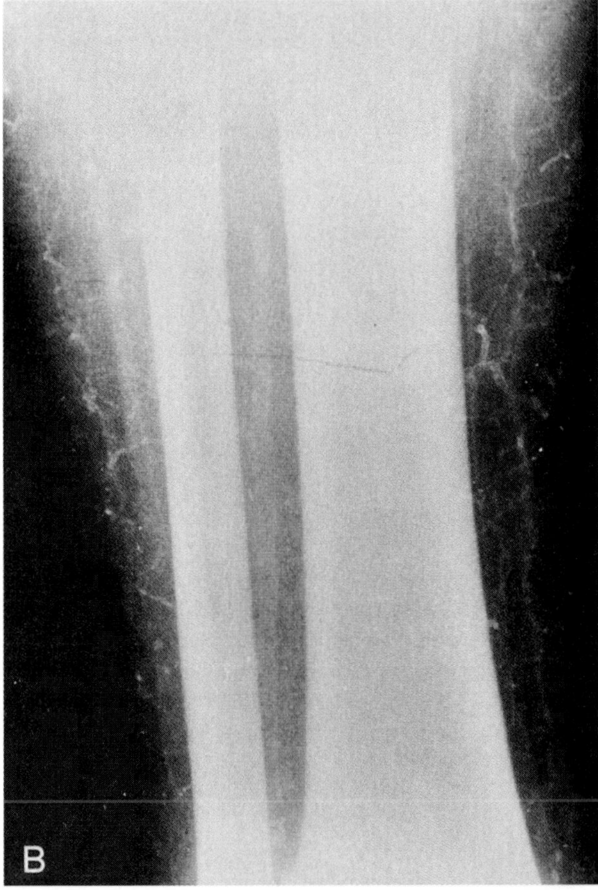

FIGURE 84.6. Calciphylaxis. **A:** Necrotic skin lesions on the calves. **B:** Roentgenogram of the lower leg showing calcified subcutaneous vessels. (Reproduced with permission from Ivker RA, Woosley J, Briggaman RA. Calciphylaxis in three patients with end-stage renal disease. *Arch Dermatol* 1995;131:63–68.)

appear in the lungs and be mistaken for interstitial fibrosis (384). Infarction of major organs is rare (392). Radiographs of an affected extremity show calcium deposits outlining small and large vessels (Fig. 84.6B) (379,380,385). Punch biopsy of the skin may demonstrate no abnormality, but histologic examination of tissue from a deep incisional biopsy usually shows calcification in the media of subcutaneous vessels (384,385). Although parathyroidectomy is sometimes successful in halting this process, the course is often relentlessly downhill (378,380–382,384,385,393). A report suggested hyperbaric oxygen as a potential therapy for this condition (394).

Anderson–Fabry Disease (Angiokeratoma Corporis Diffusum)

Anderson–Fabry disease is unique among the sphingolipid storage diseases because it is X-linked recessive and may cause symptoms in female carriers (122). A deficiency in the lysosomal enzyme, α-galactosidase, results in wide-

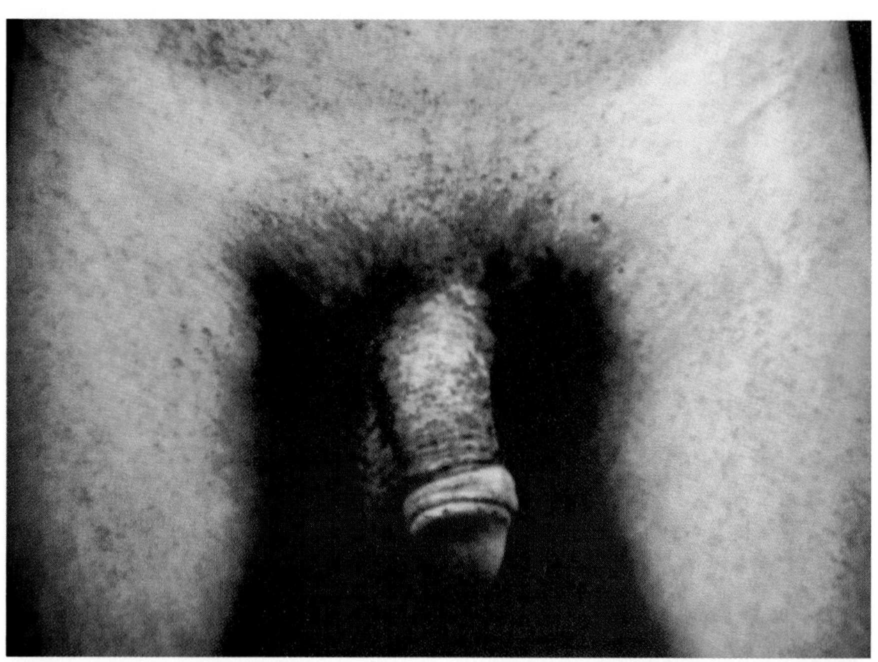

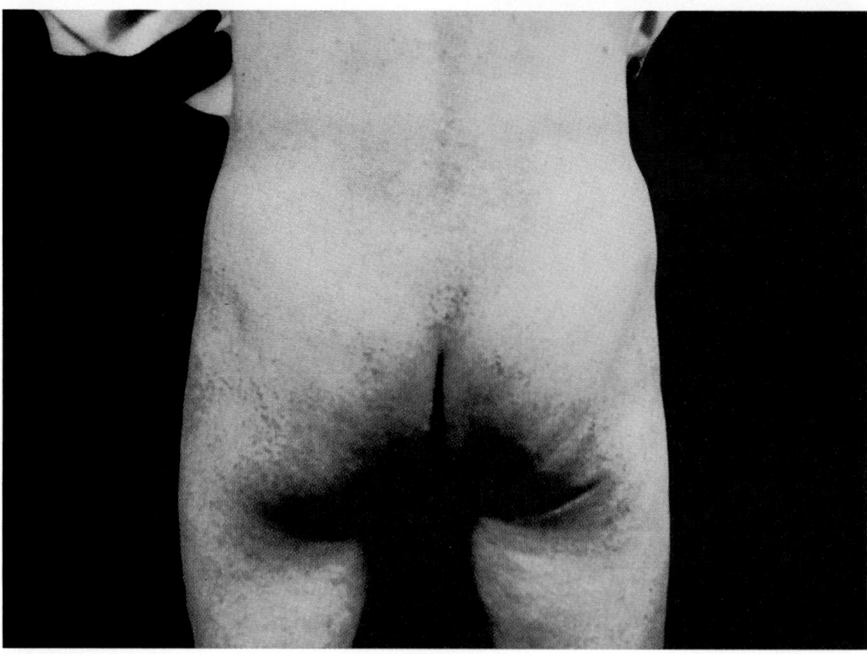

FIGURE 84.7. Angiokeratomas in a "bathing suit" distribution in a young man with Anderson–Fabry disease. (Courtesy of Dr. Herbert Fred.)

spread deposition of uncleaved glycosphingolipids, primarily trihexosylceramide (395). Clinical manifestations are protean and nonspecific. The characteristic skin lesion is an angiokeratoma (Fig. 84.7), a red–purple papule that blanches on pressure if not thrombosed. These lesions typically appear in a "bathing suit" distribution (e.g., genitalia, buttocks, and lower abdomen) during childhood or adolescence. They also may affect the elbows, thighs, fingers, lips, and mucous membranes (122,174,395).

In adult men, virtually any organ system may be involved. A painful autonomic neuropathy is a frequent early symptom. It manifests as burning paresthesias, which may intensify with exertion or fever, and be accompanied by hypohidrosis (122,396). Abnormalities of thermal sensation, especially cold sensitivity, are common, even in otherwise asymptomatic carriers (397). A characteristic finding on slit-lamp examination of the cornea is a whorl-like lesion similar to that occasionally seen after use of phenothiazines, chloroquine, or indomethacin. Other ocular findings are cataracts, corneal opacities, and aneurysmal dilatations of conjunctival and retinal vessels (398). Additional manifestations include cerebrovascular occlusions (122), myocardial or cardiac valvular dysfunction (399–401), obstructive airway disease (402), nondestructive arthropathy (403), avascular necrosis of bone (404), bowel dysfunction (405), vertigo, sensorineural hearing loss, and, rarely, lymphadenopathy (395). Without dialysis or kidney transplant, most patients die of renal failure by age 50 years (395).

Elevated serum levels of ceramide trihexoside help confirm the diagnosis (122). Detecting deficient α-galactosidase A activity in plasma, tears, or cultured fibroblasts can help detect carriers (396). Biopsy of an angiokeratoma typically shows ectatic cutaneous capillaries protruding into a hyperkeratotic epidermis. Similar lesions appear in other inherited lysosomal disorders (50,406) and, rarely, as an isolated finding (407,408).

Treatment is largely symptomatic. Renal transplantation, although occasionally of temporary benefit (409), does not appear to supply enough of the missing enzyme to stop progression of the disease. However, the isolation and characterization of the α-galactosidase gene offer promise of enzyme replacement or gene therapy (395).

Homocystinuria

Homocysteine can injure vascular endothelium, potentiate the oxidation of low-density lipoprotein cholesterol, and promote thrombosis (410–414). Patients who are homozygous for deficiency of cystathionine γ-synthase have hyperhomocysteinemia (and homocystinuria) and are thereby susceptible to premature atherosclerosis and thromboembolism (414). Heterozygote patients (approximately 1–2% of the population) have milder elevations of homocysteine levels but also are predisposed to occlusive vascular disease (411,413,415–418). Low serum levels of folate and B_{12} may accompany hyperhomocysteinemia (419). Folate supplementation can decrease serum homocysteine levels and conceivably could ameliorate the associated vasculopathy (410,418,419).

Hyperoxaluria

Hyperoxaluria is an autosomal recessive condition that causes build-up of oxalic acid, an end product of glycine metabolism (75). Patients with this disorder typically have a history of nephrocalcinosis, often beginning before age 5 years (75,420,421). Renal failure may eventually ensue, after which calcium oxalate accumulates in extrarenal tissues such as heart, skin, bone, joints, blood vessels, and eyes. Vascular complications are common (75,420,421) and consist of acrocyanosis, Raynaud's phenomenon, livedo reticularis, decreased pulses, and peripheral gangrene. Oxalate crystals may deposit in the media of the vessel wall or physically occlude smaller vessels (75,420,421). Calcium oxalate activates complement and thus may trigger neutrophil-mediated endothelial cell injury (422). An elevated total oxalate measurement in a 24-hour urine collection establishes the diagnosis of hyperoxaluria; biopsy of affected tissues reveals the vascular oxalosis (75,420). With the onset of renal failure, serum oxalate levels are difficult to interpret (75). Consequently, distinguishing primary from secondary forms of oxalosis may require specific enzyme assays. Oxalate is readily dialyzable; however, hemodialysis and peritoneal dialysis cannot keep up with its synthesis. Thus most effective approaches for preserving renal function enhance oxalate solubility in the urine (e.g., with phosphate, magnesium oxide, or citrate supplementation) or decrease its production (e.g., with high doses of pyridoxine) (420,423).

Polyvinyl Chloride

Exposure to polyvinyl chloride tubing during hemodialysis can cause a necrotizing dermatitis. Histopathologic examination reveals thrombosis of vessels in the corium, fibrin deposits in the walls of arterioles, and inflammatory infiltrates without leukocytoclasis. Precipitates of immunoglobulin G (IgG) and complement occur in small vessels, but serum immunoglobulin and complement levels are normal. The rash does not occur when polyurethane tubing is used (424).

Radiation

External radiation can injure vascular endothelial cells within hours (425,426). Subsequently there may be thickening and irregularity of the intima as well as focal fibrosis and necrosis of the media. Exposure to 3,600 to 6,800 rads (135) can cause rupture or occlusion of an artery within several weeks or after many years (113,135).

Exposure To Cold

Prolonged exposure to nonfreezing cold, particularly when the humidity is high, can cause the condition known as pernio (or chilblains) (52,136,426). In the acute, self-limited form of this condition, pruritic or painful purplish swellings appear on the extremities (or, rarely, the face) about 24 hours after the exposure. Tender blue nodules, and occasionally ulcerations, follow and persist for 10 to 14 days (52). Some patients acquire a chronic form of pernio. In this circumstance, the characteristic lesions recur during winter months. The ulcerations are slow to heal and may leave scarring or postinflammatory pigmentation (52). Middle-aged women seem especially predisposed (52,136), perhaps because of hyperreactivity of their arterial circulation to cold, or because of diminished temperature in skin overlying a relatively thick layer of subcutaneous fat (136,426). Other factors that may play a causative role include systemic illness, nutritional deficiences, neuromuscular dysfunction, and genetic traits (51,52,427,428).

Histopathologic examination demonstrates nonspecific inflammation and edema in the papillary dermis along with perivascular mononuclear cell infiltrates around dermal arterioles (52,426,429). Proliferation of the vessel intima (426), deposition of fibrin, and a true lymphocytic vasculitis (52) also may appear. Angiograms may show occlusions and aneurysms of affected vessels (136).

Treatment of pernio can be difficult. Protection from the cold is essential (136,426). Additionally, a weight-loss program could theoretically reduce the insulating layer of subcutaneous fat and raise skin temperature (426). Use of calcium channel blockers is occasionally successful (430), and corticosteroid creams can reduce itching (431).

Ischemia

Obstruction of vasa vasorum by any mechanism can produce ischemic necrosis of an arterial wall. This may be a mechanism by which mycotic aneurysms form (69).

Neoplasia

Neoplasms can injure vessels in several ways. Some forms of leukemia, lymphoma, myeloma, and solid tumors induce vascular inflammation (14,15,17,18,22,23,25,292,432–439), presumably by immune-mediated processes (18,25,54,65, 439,440). In other instances, the neoplasm causes vascular occlusion, either by direct embolization [e.g., atrial myxoma (12,217,219,241), choriocarcinoma (60), and malignant melanoma (441)], induction of a hypercoagulable state (12,111,265,442,443), or elaboration of an abnormal protein (12,320,321,438). Solid tumors and lymphomas may invade vessel walls directly (24,67,94,114,291,333,444–447) or the microscopic nerves supplying the vessels (448). By contrast, some lymphomas invade major nerves, creating the picture of mononeuritis multiplex (449) and thereby simulating vasculitis. Pheochromocytoma, perhaps by releasing catecholamines, sometimes produces ischemic lesions and angiographic findings typical of vasculitis (130,450).

Angiotropic lymphomas and the related condition, lymphomatoid granulomatosis, can easily mimic vasculitis (63, 64,66,94,108,451,452). Malignant angioendotheliomatosis, once considered a vascular neoplasm of endothelial cell origin (453,454), is probably an angiotropic lymphoma (53,55,56,58–62,455) with a predilection for vessels of the central nervous system (57,456). Primary vascular sarcomas tend to obstruct vessels or embolize distally (457); occasionally they induce aneurysms (458).

Congenital Abnormalities

Congenital weakness in an arterial wall may eventually result in an aneurysmal dilatation (69) or dissection (68) of the vessel.

Pseudoxanthoma elasticum, an inherited disorder of elastic tissue, causes premature vascular disease (459,460): accelerated atherosclerosis, friable blood vessels, and formation of aneurysms (120). Arterial aneurysms also occur in Ehlers–Danlos syndrome (70), a heritable disorder of connective tissue.

Neurofibromatosis, a hamartomatous disorder of neural crest tissue, can affect the intima and adventitia of arteries, producing stenoses (117,461) or aneurysms (118). These abnormalities typically involve the renal arteries (118,461), but other major arteries may be affected as well (117,461).

Miscellaneous

Drug Effects

Drugs commonly associated with vascular abnormalities include ergot derivatives (462,463) and sympathomimetic agents (464–472). Of the latter, amphetamines and ephedrine are the usual offenders (434), but other related compounds, as well as cocaine and the opiates, may be the culprits (471,473). The cause of vasculopathy in these cases is probably multifactorial. Vasospasm plays a role, as evidenced by the angiographic findings of transient segmental arterial constrictions soon after exposure to the offending drug (131,462,463). In some instances, histopathologic studies show true vasculitic lesions (465,471), and angiograms occasionally show more permanent changes [e.g., formation of aneurysms (465,467)]. Vasoconstriction may be the initial event, followed by ischemia of the vessel wall (131,468,473–475). Some drugs, however, may stimulate the release of toxic mediators or cause a coagulopathy (131). Concomitant infection or emboli of drug contaminants also may play a role (131,465).

Intimal proliferation reportedly occurs in the vessel walls of women during or after pregnancy, or while taking oral contraceptives (476). This observation suggests a toxic effect of female reproductive hormones on the vasculature and might explain the transient “cerebrovascular disease of pregnancy” (477).

Moyamoya Disease

Moyamoya disease is an occlusive vasculopathy primarily affecting the arteries of the circle of Willis (134,478).

Although first recognized in Japan (479), it occurs in virtually all races (134). The onset of disease has two peaks, one in the first and the other in the fourth decade of life, with a striking male predominance (134). Children typically have ischemic attacks, whereas cerebral hemorrhage is the common adult manifestation. In the early stages, angiograms show bilateral stenoses of the carotid arteries at their suprasellar positions. As these arteries progressively narrow, a characteristic network of moyamoya ("hazy puff of smoke") vessels appears. These increase in prominence as major trunks of the anterior circle of Willis become occluded. With involvement of all the components (including the posterior cerebral arteries), the moyamoya vessels diminish in size and may completely disappear as collaterals develop from the extracranial circulation (478). Histopathologic examination of stenotic vessels shows fibrous intimal thickening; dilated vessels have attenuation of the media and fragmentation of the elastic lamina (480).

The pathogenesis is unclear, and multiple factors have been implicated (481–483). Case reports describe familial occurrences, an increased incidence in Down syndrome (134), and antibodies to Ro (SS-A) and La (SS-B) (133).

The disease usually progresses and has a high mortality rate, especially in adults. Anastomotic surgical procedures may be beneficial (134,484).

Fibromuscular Dysplasia

Fibromuscular dysplasia can affect the intima, media, or adventitia, causing stenosis, dilatation, or the formation of aneurysms (119,485–488). The renal arteries are the usual targets, but any artery can be involved (485,486,489–492). A recently described condition, segmental arterial mediolysis, may be a form of fibromuscular dysplasia (493).

Sarcoidosis

Vascular involvement in sarcoidosis is uncommon (434,494), but when it does occur, there is usually only perivascular inflammation (495). Occasionally, a true granulomatous vasculitis develops (496–500), and angiograms may show segmental arterial narrowing and dilatations (495,499).

Nonvascular Diseases

Here, the list is endless. Already mentioned were such cutaneous mimickers as the neutrophilic dermatoses (99,100, 501,502), pyoderma gangrenosum (91,92), insect bites (93), and panniculitis (including erythema nodosum) (90, 344). Others include familial leg ulcers (503–505), neoplasms (506) or infections (95–98,507–509) of the skin, and the perifollicular hemorrhages of scurvy (510). Finally, a report of occult subacute thyroiditis masquerading as giant cell arteritis (511) and an article describing cavitary pulmonary sporotrichosis in association with an antineutrophil cytoplasmic antibody (cANCA) (512) demonstrate that nonvascular diseases of almost any organ can fool us.

CONCLUSIONS

The list in Table 84.3 is a sobering reminder that a broad range of disparate processes can injure vessels or make them appear injured.

TABLE 84.3. MIMICKERS OF VASCULITIS

- Infectious causes
  - Bacteria
  - Mycobacteria
  - Spirochetes
  - Rickettsiae
  - Fungi
  - Viruses
  - Parasites
- Vascular trauma
  - External
    - Hypothenar hammar syndrome
  - Internal
    - Hypertension
    - Migraine
    - Dissections
- Occlusive processes
  - Atheroembolic disease
  - Thromboembolism
  - Other emboli (air, fat, tumor)
  - Thrombotic disorders
  - Paraproteins
- Damaging substances
  - α_1-Antitrypsin deficiency
  - Amyloidosis
  - Anderson–Fabry disease
  - Calciphylaxis
  - Homocystinuria
  - Hyperoxaluria
  - Pernio (chilblains)
  - Polyvinylchloride
  - Radiation
- Neoplasia
  - Cardiac myxoma
  - Leukemia
  - Lymphoma (including malignant angioendotheliomatosis)
  - Myeloma
  - Solid tumors
  - Primary vascular neoplasm
  - Pheochromocytoma
- Congenital defects
  - Ehlers–Danlos syndrome
  - Neurofibromatosis
  - Pseudoxanthoma elasticum
- Miscellaneous conditions
  - Drug effects
  - Moyamoya disease
  - Fibromuscular dysplasia
  - Pregnancy
  - Sarcoidosis
  - Nonvascular disease
    - Neutrophilic dermatoses
    - Pyoderma gangrenosum
    - Insect bites
    - Erythema nodosum
    - Familial leg ulcers
    - Scurvy

REFERENCES

1. Lie JT. Nomenclature and classification of vasculitis: plus ca change, plus c'est la meme chose [Editorial]. *Arthritis Rheum* 1994;37:181–186.
2. Lie JT. The Canadian Rheumatism Association, 1991 Dunlop-Dottridge Lecture: Vasculitis, 1815 to 1991: classification and diagnostic specificity. *J Rheumatol* 1992;19:83–89.
3. Mader R, Keystone EC. Infections that cause vasculitis. *Curr Opin Rheumatol* 1992;4:35–38.
4. Marcellin P, Calmus Y, Takahashi H, et al. Latent hepatitis B virus HBV infection in systemic necrotizing vasculitis. *Clin Exp Rheumatol* 1991;9:23–28.
5. Carson CW, Conn DL, Czaja AJ, et al. Frequency and significance of antibodies to hepatitis C virus in polyarteritis nodosa. *J Rheumatol* 1993;20:304–309.
6. Quint L, Deny P, Guillevin L, et al. Hepatitis C virus in patients with polyarteritis nodosa: prevalence in 38 patients. *Clin Exp Rheumatol* 1991;9:253–257.
7. Finkel TH, Teoreok TJ, Ferguson PJ, et al. Chronic parvovirus B19 infection and systemic necrotising vasculitis: opportunistic infection or aetiological agent? [see comments]. *Lancet* 1994; 343:1255–1258.
8. Pile K, Kwong T, Fryer J, et al. Polyarteritis associated with *Yersinia enterocolitica* infection. *Ann Rheum Dis* 1992;51: 678–680.
9. Frayha RA. Trichinosis-related polyarteritis nodosa. *Am J Med* 1981;71:307–312.
10. Golden MP, Hammer SM, Wanke CA, et al. Cytomegalovirus vasculitis: case reports and review of the literature. *Medicine* 1994;73:246–255.
11. Wenzel RP, Hayden FG, Greoschel DH, et al. Acute febrile cerebrovasculitis: a syndrome of unknown, perhaps rickettsial cause. *Ann Intern Med* 1986;104:606–615.
12. Mertz LE, Conn DL. Vasculitis associated with malignancy. *Curr Opin Rheum* 1992;4:39–46.
13. Sanchez-Guerrero J, Gutierrez-Urena S, Vidaller A, et al. Vasculitis as a paraneoplastic syndrome: report of 11 cases and review of the literature. *J Rheumatol* 1990;17:1458–1462.
14. Greer JM, Longley S, Edwards NL, et al. Vasculitis associated with malignancy: experience with 13 patients and literature review. *Medicine* 1988;67:220–230.
15. Longley S, Caldwell JR, Panush RS. Paraneoplastic vasculitis: unique syndrome of cutaneous angiitis and arthritis associated with myeloproliferative disorders. *Am J Med* 1986;0: 1027–1030.
16. Callen JP. Cutaneous leukocytoclastic vasculitis in a patient with an adenocarcinoma of the colon. *J Rheumatol* 1987;14: 386–389.
17. Petri M, Fye KH. Digital necrosis: a paraneoplastic syndrome. *J Rheumatol* 1985;12:800–802.
18. O'Donnell JR, Keaveny TV, O'Connell LG. Digital arteritis as a presenting feature of malignant disease. *Ir J Med Sci* 1980; 149:386–390.
19. O'Shea JJ, Jaffe ES, Lane HC, et al. Peripheral T cell lymphoma presenting as hypereosinophilia with vasculitis: clinical, pathologic, and immunologic features. *Am J Med* 1987;82:539–545.
20. Kurzrock R, Cohen PR, Markowitz A. Clinical manifestations of vasculitis in patients with solid tumors: a case report and review of the literature. *Arch Intern Med* 1994;154:334–340.
21. Lacour JP, Castanet J, Perrin C, et al. Cutaneous leukocytoclastic vasculitis and renal cancer: two cases. *Am J Med* 1993;94: 104–108.
22. Fernandez AM, Abeles M, Wong RL. Recurrent leukocytoclastic vasculitis as the initial manifestation of acute myelomonocytic leukemia. *J Rheumatol* 1994;21:1972–1974.
23. Stahl RL, Silber R. Vasculitic leg ulcers in chronic myelogenous leukemia. *Am J Med* 1985;78:869–872.
24. Gabriel SE, Conn DL, Phyliky RL, et al. Vasculitis in hairy cell leukemia: review of literature and consideration of possible pathogenic mechanisms. *J Rheumatol* 1986;13:1167–1172.
25. Farcet JP, Weschsler J, Wirquin V, et al. Vasculitis in hairy-cell leukemia. *Arch Intern Med* 1987;147:660–664.
26. Lie JT. Primary granulomatous angiitis of the central nervous system: a clinicopathologic analysis of 15 new cases and a review of the literature. *Hum Pathol* 1992;23:164–171.
27. Calabrese LH. Vasculitis and infection with the human immunodeficiency virus. *Rheum Dis Clin North Am* 1991;17:131–147.
28. Conn DL. Polyarteritis. *Rheum Dis Clin North Am* 1990;16: 341–362.
29. Gibson LE, Su WP. Cutaneous vasculitis. *Rheum Dis Clin North Am* 1990;16:309–324.
30. Calabrese LH, Clough JD. Hypersensitivity vasculitis group HVG: a case-oriented review of a continuing clinical spectrum. *Cleve Clin Q* 1982;49:17–42.
31. Ryan TJ, Wilkinson DS. Cutaneous vasculitis: "angiitis." In: Rook A, Wilkinson DS, Ebling FJG, Champion RH, Burton JL, eds. *Textbook of dermatology.* 4th ed. Oxford: Blackwell Scientific, 1986:1121–1185.
32. Harmon DC, Mark EJ. Case records of the Massachusetts General Hospital. *N Engl J Med* 1999;340:1099–1106.
33. Hogarth MB, Qureshi T, Lloyd J, et al. A blistering rash and swollen knees. *Lancet* 1999;353:978.
34. Somer T, Finegold SM. Vasculitides associated with infections, immunization, and antimicrobial drugs. *Clin Infect Dis* 1995; 20:1010–1036.
35. Blanco FJ, Blas MS, Gonzalez MF. Histopathologic features of cerebral vasculitis associated with *Mycobacterium tuberculosis. Arthritis Rheum* 1999;42:383.
36. Lie JT. Vasculitis associated with infectious agents. *Curr Opin Rheumatol* 1996;8:26–29.
37. Pandey JP, LeRoy EC. Human cytomegalovirus and the vasculopathies of autoimmune diseases (especially scleroderma), allograft rejection, and coronary restenosis. *Arthritis Rheum* 1998; 41:10–15.
38. Walker DH, Mattern WD. Rickettsial vasculitis. *Am Heart J* 1980;100:896–906.
39. Olivero JJ. Case in point. *Hosp Pract* 1997;32:30.
40. Pineda CJ, Weisman MH, Bookstein JJ, et al. Hypothenar hammer syndrome: form of reversible Raynaud's phenomenon. *Am J Med* 1985;79:561–570.
41. Martens PB, Levine JA, Hunder GG. Splinter hemorrhages following arterial puncture. *Arthritis Rheum* 1996;39:169–170.
42. Nance J, Abbott K, Morris L, et al. An unfortunate consequence of being tickled. *Lancet* 1997;349:1142.
43. Shim SC, Yoo DH, Lee JK, et al. Multiple cerebellar infarction due to vertebral artery obstruction and bulbar symptoms associated with vertical subluxation and atlanto-occipital subluxation in ankylosing spondylitis. *J Rheumatol* 1998;25:2464–2468.
44. Albert L, Inman R, Gordon DA, et al. Cryocrystalglobulinemia mimicking rheumatoid arthritis and vasculitis. *J Rheumatol* 1996;23:1272–1277.
45. Sack KE. The difficulties of differentiating vasculitis from its mimics. *Cleve Clin J Med* 1998;65:550–552.
46. Estrada A, Stenzel TT, Burchette JL, et al. Multiple myeloma-associated amyloidosis and giant cell arteritis. *Arthritis Rheum* 1998;41:1312–1317.
47. Greenberg SM, Edgar MA. Case records of the Massachusetts General Hospital. *N Engl J Med* 1996;335:189–196.
48. Rodon P, Friocort P, Blanchet S, et al. Temporal artery involvement revealing AL amyloidosis and IgD monoclonal gammopathy. *J Rheumatol* 1996;23:189–190.

49. Silbert PL, Bartleson JD, Miller GM, et al. Cortical petechial hemorrhage, leukoencephalopathy, and subacute dementia associated with seizures due to cerebral amyloid angiopathy. *Mayo Clin Proc* 1995;70:477–480.
50. Kanzaki T, Yokota M, Irie F, et al. Angiokeratoma corporis diffusum with glycopeptiduria due to deficient lysosomal alpha-*N*-acetylgalactosaminidase activity: clinical, morphologic, and biochemical studies. *Arch Dermatol* 1993;129:460–465.
51. Millard LG, Rowell NR. Chilblain lupus erythematosus Hutchinson: a clinical and laboratory study of 17 patients. *Br J Dermatol* 1978;98:497–506.
52. Herman EW, Kezis JS, Silvers DN. A distinctive variant of pernio: clinical and histopathologic study of nine cases. *Arch Dermatol* 1981;117:26–28.
53. Bhawan J, Wolff SM, Ucci AA, et al. Malignant lymphoma and malignant angioendotheliomatosis: one disease. *Cancer* 1985; 55:570–576.
54. Fortin PR. Vasculitides associated with malignancy. *Curr Opin Rheumatol* 1996;8:30–33.
55. Fredericks RK, Walker FO, Elster A, et al. Angiotropic intravascular large-cell lymphoma (malignant angioendotheliomatosis): report of a case and review of the literature. *Surg Neurol* 1991; 35:218–223.
56. Kao NL, Broy S, Tillawi I. Malignant angioendotheliomatosis mimicking systemic necrotizing vasculitis. *J Rheumatol* 1992; 19:1133–1135.
57. Lie JT. Malignant angioendotheliomatosis: intravascular lymphomatosis clinically simulating primary angiitis of the central nervous system [see comments]. *Arthritis Rheum* 1992;35: 831–834.
58. Otrakji CL, Voigt W, Amador A, et al. Malignant angioendotheliomatosis, a true lymphoma: a case of intravascular malignant lymphomatosis studied by Southern blot hybridization analysis. *Hum Pathol* 1988;19:475–478.
59. Petroff N, Koger OW, Fleming MG, et al. Malignant angioendotheliomatosis: an angiotropic lymphoma. *J Am Acad Dermatol* 1989;21:727–733.
60. Sheibani K, Battifora H, Winberg CD, et al. Further evidence that "malignant angioendotheliomatosis" is an angiotropic large-cell lymphoma. *N Engl J Med* 1986;314:943–948.
61. Sienknecht CW, Whetsell WO, Pollock P. Intravascular malignant lymphoma ("malignant angioendotheliomatosis") mimicking primary angiitis of the central nervous system. *J Rheumatol* 1995;22:1769–1770.
62. Wick MR, Mills SE, Scheithauer BW, et al. Reassessment of malignant "angioendotheliomatosis": evidence in favor of its reclassification as "intravascular lymphomatosis." *Am J Surg Pathol* 1986;10:112–123.
63. Roux S, Grossin M, De Brandt M, et al. Angiotropic large cell lymphoma with mononeuritis multiplex mimicking systemic vasculitis. *J Neurol Neurosurg Psychiatry* 1995;58:363–366.
64. Kleinschmidt-DeMasters BK, Filley CM, Bitter MA. Central nervous system angiocentric, angiodestructive T-cell lymphoma (lymphomatoid granulomatosis). *Surg Neurol* 1992;37: 130–137.
65. Hasler P, Kistler H, Gerber H. Vasculitides in hairy cell leukemia. *Semin Arthritis Rheum* 1995;25:134–142.
66. Glass J, Hochberg FH, Miller DC. Intravascular lymphomatosis. *Cancer* 1993;71:3156–3164.
67. Webster E, Corman LC, Braylan RC. Syndrome of temporal arteritis with perivascular infiltration by malignant cells in a patient with follicular small cleaved cell lymphoma. *J Rheumatol* 1986;13:1163–1166.
68. Schievink WI. A surgeon with a nasty taste in his mouth. *Lancet* 1997;350:260.
69. Olmsted WW, McGee TP. The pathogenesis of peripheral aneurysms of the central nervous system: a subject review from the AFIP. *Radiology* 1977;123:661–666.
70. Imahori S, Bannerman RM, Graf CJ, et al. Ehlers-Danlos syndrome with multiple arterial lesions. *Am J Med* 1969;47:967–977.
71. Fan PT, Davis JA, Somer T, et al. A clinical approach to systemic vasculitis. *Semin Arthritis Rheum* 1980;9:248–304.
72. Soter NA, Mihm MC Jr, Gigli I, et al. Two distinct cellular patterns in cutaneous necrotizing angiitis. *J Invest Dermatol* 1976; 66:344–350.
73. Jennette CJ, Milling DM, Falk RJ. Vasculitis affecting the skin: a review [Editorial]. *Arch Dermatol* 1994;130:899–906.
74. Jorizzo JL. Classification of vasculitis. *J Invest Dermatol* 1993; 100:106S–110S.
75. Baethge BA, Sanusi ID, Landreneau MD, et al. Livedo reticularis and peripheral gangrene associated with primary hyperoxaluria. *Arthritis Rheum* 1988;31:1199–1203.
76. Gaines PA, Cumberland DC, Kennedy A, et al. Cholesterol embolisation: a lethal complication of vascular catheterisation. *Lancet* 1988;1:168–170.
77. Halasz CLG, Strauss EB. Unilateral livedo reticularis. *N Engl J Med* 1998;338:1127.
78. Hendel RC, Cuenoud HF, Giansiracusa DF, et al. Multiple cholesterol emboli syndrome: bowel infarction after retrograde angiography. *Arch Intern Med* 1989;149:2371–2374.
79. Ingram SB, Goodnight SH Jr, Bennett RM. An unusual syndrome of a devastating noninflammatory vasculopathy associated with anticardiolipin antibodies: report of two cases. *Arthritis Rheum* 1987;30:1167–1172.
80. Kalter DC, Rudolph A, McGavran M. Livedo reticularis due to multiple cholesterol emboli. *J Am Acad Dermatol* 1985;13: 235–242.
81. Kirsner RS, Eaglstein WH, Katz MH, et al. Stanozolol causes rapid pain relief and healing of cutaneous ulcers caused by cryofibrinogenemia. *J Am Acad Dermatol* 1993;28:71–74.
82. Lye WC, Cheah JS, Sinniah R. Renal cholesterol embolic disease. *Am J Nephrol* 1993;13:489–493.
83. Mayo RR, Swartz RD. Redefining the incidence of clinically detectable atheroembolism. *Am J Med* 1996;100:524–529.
84. Naldi L, Locati F, Marchesi L, et al. Cutaneous manifestations associated with antiphospholipid antibodies in patients with suspected primary antiphospholipid syndrome: a case-control study. *Ann Rheum Dis* 1993;52:219–222.
85. Pai RG, Heywood JT. Atheroembolism. *N Engl J Med* 1995; 333:852.
86. Sammaritano LR, Gharavi AE, Lockshin MD. Antiphospholipid antibody syndrome: immunologic and clinical aspects. *Semin Arthritis Rheum* 1990;20:81–96.
87. Smith MC, Ghose MK, Henry AR. The clinical spectrum of renal cholesterol embolization. *Am J Med* 1981;71:174–180.
88. Klahr S. Clinicopathologic conference: cyanotic feet and renal failure in a 67-year-old man. *Am J Med* 1983;5:509–517.
89. Weinstein C, Miller MH, Axtens R, et al. Livedo reticularis associated with increased titers of anticardiolipin antibodies in systemic lupus erythematosus. *Arch Dermatol* 1987;123: 596–600.
90. De Almeida Prestes C, Winkelmann RK, Su WP. Septal granulomatous panniculitis: comparison of the pathology of erythema nodosum migrans migratory panniculitis and chronic erythema nodosum. *J Am Acad Dermatol* 1990;22:477—483.
91. Callen JP. Pyoderma gangrenosum and related disorders. *Med Clin North Am* 1989;73:1247–1261.
92. Shore RN. New look at pyoderma gangrenosum. *Cutis* 1977;20:209–213, 217–219.
93. Rees RS, Fields JP, King LE Jr. Do brown recluse spider bites induce pyoderma gangrenosum? *South Med J* 1985;78: 283–287.

94. Thomas R, Vuitch F, Lakhanpal S. Angiocentric T cell lymphoma masquerading as cutaneous vasculitis. *J Rheumatol* 1994;21:760–762.
95. Supparatpinyo K, Chiewchanvit S, Hirunsri P, et al. *Penicillium marneffei* infection in patients infected with human immunodeficiency virus. *Clin Infect Dis* 1992;14:871–874.
96. Murakawa GJ, McCalmont T, Altman J, et al. Disseminated acanthamebiasis in patients with AIDS. *Arch Dermatol* 1995; 131:1291–1296.
97. Greene SL, Su WPD, Muller SA. Ecthyma gangrenosum: report of clinical, histopathologic, and bacteriologic aspects of eight cases. *J Am Acad Dermatol* 1984;11:781–787.
98. Chandrasekar PH, Nandi PS, Fairfax MR, et al. Cutaneous infections due to Acanthamoeba in patients with acquired immunodeficiency syndrome. *Arch Intern Med* 1997;157: 569–572.
99. Von Den Driesch P. Sweet's syndrome (acute febrile neutrophilic dermatosis). *J Am Acad Dermatol* 1994;31:535–556.
100. Moreland LW, Brick JE, Kovach RE, et al. Acute febrile neutrophilic dermatosis Sweet syndrome: a review of the literature with emphasis on musculoskeletal manifestations. *Semin Arthritis Rheum* 1988;17:143–153.
101. Torrens JK, McWhinney PHM, Tompkins DS. A deadly thorn: a case of imported melioidosis. *Lancet* 1999;353:1016.
102. Nelson PE, Dignani MC, Anaissie EJ. Taxonomy, biology, and clinical aspects of Fusarium species. *Clin Microbiol Rev* 1994; 7:479–504.
103. Sundy JS, Haynes BF. Pathogenic mechanisms of vessel damage in vasculitis syndromes. *Rheum Dis Clin North Am* 1995;21: 861–881.
104. Huang TE, Chou SM. Occlusive hypertrophic arteritis as the cause of discrete necrosis in CNS toxoplasmosis in the acquired immunodeficiency syndrome. *Hum Pathol* 1988;19: 1210–1214.
105. Morgello S, Block GA, Price RW, et al. Varicella-zoster virus leukoencephalitis and cerebral vasculopathy. *Arch Pathol Lab Med* 1988;112:173–177.
106. Murakami K, Oshawa M, Hu SX, et al. Large-vessel vasculitis associated with chronic active Epstein-Barr virus infection. *Arthritis Rheum* 1998;41:369–373.
107. Weigand DA, Burgdorf WH, Tarpay MM. Vasculitis in cytomegalovirus infection. *Arch Dermatol* 1980;116: 1174–1176.
108. Walker UA, Herbst EW, Ansorge O, et al. Intravascular lymphoma simulating vasculitis. *Rheumatol Int* 1994;14:131–133.
109. Sijpkens Y, Westendorp R, Van Kemenade F, et al. Vasculitis due to cholesterol embolism. *Am J Med* 1997;102:302–303.
110. Navarro PH, Bravo FP, Beltran GG. Atrial myxoma with livedoid macules as its sole cutaneous manifestation. *J Am Acad Dermatol* 1995;32:881–883.
111. O'Keeffe ST, Woods BO, Breslin DJ, et al. Blue toe syndrome: causes and management [see comments]. *Arch Intern Med* 1992; 152:2197–2202.
112. Snyder HE, Shapiro JL. A correlative study of atheromatous embolism in human beings and experimental animals. *Surgery* 1961;49:195–204.
113. Lie JT. Vasculitis simulators and vasculitis look-alikes. *Curr Opin Rheumatol* 1992;4:47–55.
114. Leeds NE, Rosenblatt R. Arterial wall irregularities in intracranial neoplasms: the shaggy vessel brought into focus. *Radiology* 1972;103:121–124.
115. Marks C, Kuskov S. Pattern of arterial aneurysms in acquired immunodeficiency disease. *World J Surg* 1995;19:127–132.
116. Ferris EJ, Rudikoff JC, Shapiro JH. Cerebral angiography of bacterial infection. *Radiology* 1968;90:727–734.
117. Tomsick TA, Lukin RR, Chambers AA, et al. Neurofibromatosis and intracranial arterial occlusive disease. *Neuroradiology* 1976;11:229–234.
118. Finley JL, Dabbs DJ. Renal vascular smooth muscle proliferation in neurofibromatosis. *Hum Pathol* 1988;19:107–110.
119. Meyers DS, Grim CE, Keitzer WF. Fibromuscular dysplasia of the renal artery with medial dissection: a case simulating polyarteritis nodosa. *Am J Med* 1974;56:412–416.
120. Travers RL, Allison DJ, Brettle RP, et al. Polyarteritis nodosa: a clinical and angiographic analysis of 17 cases. *Semin Arthritis Rheum* 1979;8:184–199.
121. Garner BF, Burns P, Bunning RD, et al. Acute blood pressure elevation can mimic arteriographic appearance of cerebral vasculitis: a postpartum case with relative hypertension. *J Rheumatol* 1990;17:93–97.
122. Serdaru M, Chiras J, Cujas M, et al. Isolated benign cerebral vasculitis or migrainous vasospasm? *J Neurol Neurosurg Psychiatry* 1984;47:73–76.
123. Masuzawa T, Shinoda S, Furuse M, et al. Cerebral angiographic changes on serial examination of a patient with migraine. *Neuroradiology* 1983;24:277–281.
124. Savader SJ, Savader BL, Drewry GR. Hypothenar hammer syndrome with embolic occlusion of digital arteries. *Clin Radiol* 1988;39:324–325.
125. Suwanwela C, Suwanwela N. Intracranial arterial narrowing and spasm in acute head injury. *J Neurosurg* 1972;36:314–323.
126. Pepe J. A construction worker with a digital eschar. *Hosp Pract Office Ed* 1992;27:120.
127. Salvarani C, Gabriel SE, Gertz MA, et al. Primary systemic amyloidosis presenting as giant cell arteritis and polymyalgia rheumatica [see comments]. *Arthritis Rheum* 1994;37: 1621–1626.
128. Thomas MH. Myxoma masquerading as polyarteritis nodosa. *J Rheumatol* 1981;8:133–137.
129. New PF, Price DL, Carter B. Cerebral angiography in cardiac myxoma: correlation of angiographic and histopathological findings. *Radiology* 1970;96:3350–345.
130. Armstrong FS, Hayes GJ. Segmental cerebral arterial constriction associated with pheochromocytoma: report of a case with arteriograms. *J Neurosurg* 1961:843–846.
131. Rumbaugh CL, Bergeron RT, Fang HC, et al. Cerebral angiographic changes in the drug abuse patient. *Radiology* 1971;101: 335–344.
132. Orbison JL. Morphology of thrombocytopenic purpura with demonstration of aneurysms. *Am J Pathol* 1952;28:129–143.
133. Provost TT, Moses H, Morris EL, et al. Cerebral vasculopathy associated with collateralization resembling moya moya phenomenon and with anti-Ro/SS-A and anti-La/SS-B antibodies. *Arthritis Rheum* 1991;34:1052–1055.
134. Ueki K, Meyer FB, Mellinger JF. Moyamoya disease: the disorder and surgical treatment. *Mayo Clin Proc* 1994;69:749–757.
135. McCready RA, Hyde GL, Bivins BA, et al. Radiation-induced arterial injuries. *Surgery* 1983;93:306–312.
136. Jacob JR, Weisman MH, Rosenblatt SI, et al. Chronic pernio: a historical perspective of cold-induced vascular disease. *Arch Intern Med* 1986;146:1589–1592.
137. Ross R, Glomset JA. The pathogenesis of atherosclerosis first of two parts. *N Engl J Med* 1976;295:369–377.
138. Panum PL. Experimentelle beitrage zur lehre von der embolie. *Virchows Arch Pathol Anat* 1862;25:308–331.
139. Flory CM. Arterial occlusions produced by emboli from eroded aortic atheromatous plaques. *Am J Pathol* 1945;21:549–565.
140. Hoye SJ, Teitelbaum S, Gore I, et al. Atheromatous embolization: a factor in peripheral gangrene. *N Engl J Med* 1959; 261:128–131.
141. Hollenhorst RW. Significance of bright plaques in the retinal arterioles. *JAMA* 1961;178:123–129.

142. Fisher ER, Hellstom HR, Myers JD. Disseminated atheromatous emboli. *Am J Med* 1960;29:176–180.
143. Falanga V, Fine MJ, Kapoor WN. The cutaneous manifestations of cholesterol crystal embolization. *Arch Dermatol* 1986; 122:1194–1198.
144. Probstein JG, Joshi RH, Blumenthal HT. Atheromatous embolization: an etiology of acute pancreatitis. *AMA Arch Surg* 1957;75:566–572.
145. Handler FP. Clinical and pathological significance of atheromatous embolization with emphasis on an etiology of renal hypertension. *Am J Med* 1956;20:366–373.
146. Thurlbeck WM, Castleman B. Atheromatous emboli to the kidneys after aortic surgery. *N Engl J Med* 1957;257:442–447.
147. Harrington JT, Sommers SC, Kassirer JP. Atheromatous emboli with progressive renal failure: renal arteriography as the probable inciting factor. *Ann Intern Med* 1968;68:152–160.
148. Meyer WW. Cholesterinkrystallemboli kleiner organarterien und ihre Folgen. *Virchows Arch Path Anat* 1947;314:616–638.
149. Winter WJ. Atheromatous emboli: a cause of cerebral infarction. *AMA Arch Pathol* 1957;64:137–142.
150. Richards AM, Eliot RS, Kanjuh VI, et al. Cholesterol embolism: a multiple-system disease masquerading as polyarteritis nodosa. *Am J Cardiol* 1965;15:696–707.
151. Moolenaar W, Lamers BHW. Cholesterol crystal embolization in the Netherlands: a review of 842 cases filed in the Dutch National Pathology Information System from 1973 through 1994. *Arch Intern Med* 1996;156:653–657.
152. Cross SS. How common is cholesterol embolism? *J Clin Pathol* 1991;44:859–861.
153. Maurizi CP, Barker AE, Trueheart RE. Atheromatous emboli: a postmortem study with special reference to the lower extremities. *Arch Pathol* 1968;86:528–534.
154. Preston RA, Stemmer CL, Materson BJ, et al. Renal biopsy in patients 65 years of age or older: an analysis of the results of 334 biopsies. *J Am Geriatr Soc* 1990;38:669–674.
155. Kennedy A, Cumberland D, Gaines P. The pathology of cholesterol embolism arising as a complication of intra-aortic catheterization. *Histopathology* 1989;15:515–521.
156. Eliot RS, Kanjuh VI, Edwards JE. Atheromatous embolism. *Circulation* 1964;30:611–618.
157. Retan JW, Miller RE. Microembolic complications of atherosclerosis: literature review and report of a patient. *Arch Intern Med* 1966;118:534–545.
158. Anderson WR. Necrotizing angiitis associated with embolization of cholesterol: case report, with emphasis on the use of the muscle biopsy as a diagnostic aid. *Am J Clin Pathol* 1965; 43:65–71.
159. Anderson WR, Richards AM. Evaluation of lower extremity muscle biopsies in the diagnosis of atheroembolism. *Arch Pathol* 1968;86:535–541.
160. Rosansky SJ. Multiple cholesterol emboli syndrome. *South Med J* 1982;75:677–680.
161. Gupta BK, Spinowitz BS, Charytan C, et al. Cholesterol crystal embolization-associated renal failure after therapy with recombinant tissue-type plasminogen activator. *Am J Kidney Dis* 1993;21:659–662.
162. Pierce JR Jr, Wren MV, Cousar JB Jr. Cholesterol embolism: diagnosis antemortem by bone marrow biopsy. *Ann Intern Med* 1978;89:937–938.
163. Hammerschmidt DE, Greenberg CS, Yamada O, et al. Cholesterol and atheroma lipids activate complement and stimulate granulocytes: a possible mechanism for amplification of ischemic injury in atherosclerotic states. *J Lab Clin Med* 1981; 98:68–77.
164. Cosio FG, Zager RA, Sharma HM. Atheroembolic renal disease causes hypocomplementaemia. *Lancet* 1985;2:118–121.
165. Cappiello RA, Espinoza LR, Adelman H, et al. Cholesterol embolism: a pseudovasculitic syndrome. *Semin Arthritis Rheum* 1989;18:240–246.
166. Kay AB, Shin HS, Austen KF. Selective attraction of eosinophils and synergism between eosinophil chemotactic factor of anaphylaxis ECF-A and a fragment cleaved from the fifth component of complement C5a. *Immunology* 1973;24:969–976.
167. Kasinath BS, Lewis EJ. Eosinophilia as a clue to the diagnosis of atheroembolic renal disease [Editorial]. *Arch Intern Med* 1987; 147:1384–1385.
168. Ebert TH, McCluskey RT. Clinicopathological conference. *N Engl J Med* 1986;315:308–315.
169. Fine MJ, Kapoor W, Falanga V. Cholesterol crystal embolization: a review of 221 cases in the English literature. *Angiology* 1987;38:769–784.
170. Wilson DM, Salazer TL, Farkouh ME. Eosinophiluria in atheroembolic renal disease. *Am J Med* 1991;91:186–189.
171. Goldman M, Goldman A, Dereume JP, et al. Aortic atheromatosis presenting as a cutaneous vasculitis with antinuclear antibody [Letter]. *Arthritis Rheum* 1980;23:1407–1408.
172. Young DK, Burton MF, Herman JH. Multiple cholesterol emboli syndrome simulating systemic necrotizing vasculitis. *J Rheumatol* 1986;13:423–426.
173. Stanton RC, Nickeleit V. Case records of the Massachusetts General Hospital. *N Engl J Med* 1996;334:973–979.
174. Sack KE. When vasculitis is not vasculitis. *Hosp Pract Office Ed* 1993;28:94–97, 100–103.
175. Thadhani RI, Camargo CA, Xavier RJ, et al. Atheroembolic renal failure after invasive procedures: natural history based on 52 histologically proven cases. *Medicine* 1995;74:350–358.
176. Colt HG, Begg RJ, Saporito JJ, et al. Cholesterol emboli after cardiac catheterization: eight cases and a review of the literature. *Medicine* 1988;67:389–400.
177. Orvar K, Johlin FC. Atheromatous embolization resulting in acute pancreatitis after cardiac catheterization and angiographic studies. *Arch Intern Med* 1994;154:1755–1761.
178. Sanborn TA, Faxon DP, Waugh D, et al. Transluminal angioplasty in experimental atherosclerosis: analysis for embolization using an in vivo perfusion system. *Circulation* 1982;66: 917–922.
179. Nevelsteen A, Kutten M, Lacroix H, et al. Oral anticoagulant therapy: a precipitating factor in the pathogenesis of cholesterol embolization? *Acta Chir Belg* 1992;92:33–36.
180. Moldveen-Geronimus M, Merriam JC Jr. Cholesterol embolization: from pathological curiosity to clinical entity. *Circulation* 1967;35:946–953.
181. Teepe RG, Broekmans AW, Vermeer BJ, et al. Recurrent coumarin-induced skin necrosis in a patient with an acquired functional protein C deficiency. *Arch Dermatol* 1986;122: 1408–1412.
182. Hyman BT, Landas SK, Ashman RF, et al. Warfarin-related purple toes syndrome and cholesterol microembolization. *Am J Med* 1987;82:1233–1237.
183. Queen M, Biem HJ, Moe GW, et al. Development of cholesterol embolization syndrome after intravenous streptokinase for acute myocardial infarction. *Am J Cardiol* 1990;65:1042–1943.
184. Rivera-Manrique E, Castro-Solomo A, Azon-Masoliver A, et al. Cholesterol embolism: a fatal complication after thrombolytic therapy for acute myocardial infarction. *Arch Intern Med* 1998; 158:1575.
185. Bhardwaj M, Goldweit R, Erlebacher J, et al. Tissue plasminogen activator and cholesterol crystal embolization [Letter]. *Ann Intern Med* 1989;111:687–688.
186. Mendia R, D'Aloya G, Cavaliere G, et al. Does thrombolysis produce cholesterol embolisation? [Letter]. *Lancet* 1992;339: 562.

187. Case records of the Massachusetts General Hospital. Weekly clinicopathological exercises: case 38-1993: renal failure and a painful toe in a 70-year-old man after an acute myocardial infarct. *N Engl J Med* 1993;329:948–955.
188. Cabili S, Hochman I, Goor Y. Reversal of gangrenous lesions in the blue toe syndrome with lovastatin: a case report. *Angiology* 1993;44:821–825.
189. Jones DB, Iannaccone PM. Atheromatous emboli in renal biopsies: an ultrastructural study. *Am J Pathol* 1975;78:261–276.
190. Karmody AM, Powers SR, Monaco VJ, et al. "Blue toe" syndrome: an indication for limb salvage surgery. *Arch Surg* 1976; 111:1263–1268.
191. Kawakami Y, Hirose K, Watanabe Y, et al. Management of multiple cholesterol embolization syndrome: a case report. *Angiology* 1990;41:248–252.
192. Bradley M. Spontaneous atheroembolism. *N Engl J Med* 1995; 332:998.
193. Dahlberg PJ, Frecentese DF, Cogbill TH. Cholesterol embolism: experience with 22 histologically proven cases. *Surgery* 1989;105:737–746.
194. Turakhia AK, Khan MA. Splinter hemorrhages as a possible clinical manifestation of cholesterol crystal embolization. *J Rheumatol* 1990;17:1083–1086.
195. Spring MW, Hartley B, Scoble JE, et al. A man with diabetes and unexplained renal failure. *Lancet* 1998;352:956.
196. Woolfson RG, Lachmann H. Improvement in renal cholesterol emboli syndrome after simvastatin. *Lancet* 1998;351: 1331–1332.
197. Williams HH, Wall BM, Cooke CR. Reversible nephrotic range proteinuria and renal failure in atheroembolic renal disease. *Am J Med Sci* 1990;299:58–61.
198. Gress DR, Eichhorn JH. Clinicopathological conference. *N Engl J Med* 1991;324:113–120.
199. Darsee JR. Cholesterol embolism: the great masquerader. *Southern Med J* 1979;72:174–180.
200. Moolenaar W, Lamers CBHW. Cholesterol crystal embolization to the alimentary tract. *Gut* 1996;38:196–200.
201. Bourdages R, Prentice RS, Beck IT, et al. Atheromatous embolization to the stomach: an unusual cause of gastrointestinal bleeding. *Am J Dig Dis* 1976;21:889–894.
202. Thibault GE. Clinical problem-solving: one more hypothesis [see comments]. *N Engl J Med* 1993;329:38–42.
203. Bruns FJ, Segel DP, Adler S. Control of cholesterol embolization by discontinuation of anticoagulant therapy. *Am J Med Sci* 1978;275:105–108.
204. Mercuri M, Bond G, Sirtori CR, et al. Pravastatin reduces carotid intima-media thickness progression in an asymptomatic hypercholesterolemic Mediterranean population: the carotid atherosclerosis Italian ultrasound study. *Am J Med* 1996; 101:627–634.
205. Kane JP, Malloy MJ, Ports TA, et al. Regression of coronary atherosclerosis during treatment of familial hypercholesterolemia with combined drug regimens. *JAMA* 1990;264:3007–3012.
206. Lee BI. Regression of CAD: a review of the angiographic evidence. *Drug Ther* 1993;23:35–42.
207. Carr ME, Sanders K, Todd WM. Pain relief and clinical improvement temporally related to the use of pentoxifylline in a patient with documented cholesterol emboli: a case report. *Angiology* 1994;45:65–69.
208. Kullo IJ, Edwards WD, Schwartz RS. Vulnerable plaque: pathobiology and clinical implications. *Ann Intern Med* 1998;129: 1050–1060.
209. Kazimer FJ, Sheps SG, Bernatz PE, et al. Livedo reticularis and digital infarcts: a syndrome due to cholesterol emboli arising from atheromatous abdominal aortic aneurysms. *Vasc Dis* 1966; 3:12–24.
210. Celermajer DS. Noninvasive detection of atherosclerosis. *N Engl J Med* 1998;339:2014–2015.
211. King TW. On simple vascular growths in the left auricle of the heart. *Lancet* 1845;5:488–529.
212. Heath D, Mackinnon J. Pulmonary hypertension due to myxoma of the right atrium: with special reference to the behavior of emboli of myxoma in the lung. *Am Heart J* 1964;68: 227–235.
213. Price DL, Harris JL, New PF, et al. Cardiac myxoma: a clinicopathologic and angiographic study. *Arch Neurol* 1970;236: 558–567.
214. Read RC, White HJ, Murphy ML, et al. The malignant potentiality of left atrial myxoma. *J Thorac Cardiovasc Surg* 1974;68: 857–868.
215. Desousa AL, Muller J, Campbell R, et al. Atrial myxoma: a review of the neurological complications, metastases, and recurrences. *J Neurol Neurosurg Psychiatry* 1978;41:1119–1124.
216. Goldberg HP, Glenn F, Dotter CT, et al. Myxoma of the left atrium: diagnosis made during life with operative and postmortem findings. *Circulation* 1952;6:762–767.
217. Greenwood WF. Profile of atrial myxoma. *Am J Cardiol* 1968; 21:367–375.
218. Wold LE, Lie JT. Cardiac myxomas: a clinicopathologic profile. *Am J Pathol* 1980;101:219–240.
219. Markel ML, Waller BF, Armstrong WF. Cardiac myxoma: a review. *Medicine* 1987;66:114–125.
220. Tazelaar HD, Locke TJ, McGregor CG. Pathology of surgically excised primary cardiac tumors. *Mayo Clin Proc* 1992;67: 957–965.
221. Reynen K. Cardiac myxomas. *N Engl J Med* 1995;333: 1610–1617.
222. Siltanen P, Tuuteri L, Norio R, et al. Atrial myxoma in a family. *Am J Cardiol* 1976;38:252–256.
223. Liebler GA, Magovern GJ, Park SB, et al. Familial myxomas in four siblings. *J Thorac Cardiovasc Surg* 1976;71:605–608.
224. Landon G, Ordaoanez NG, Guarda LA. Cardiac myxomas: an immunohistochemical study using endothelial, histiocytic, and smooth-muscle cell markers. *Arch Pathol Lab Med* 1986;110:116–120.
225. Goldman BI, Frydman C, Harpaz N, et al. Glandular cardiac myxomas: histologic, immunohistochemical, and ultrastructural evidence of epithelial differentiation. *Cancer* 1987;59: 1767–1775.
226. Gravallese EM, Waksmonski C, Winters GL, et al. Fever, arthralgias, skin lesions, and ischemic digits in a 59-year-old man: clinicopathologic conference. *Arthritis Rheum* 1995;38: 1161–1168.
227. Hirano T, Taga T, Yasukawa K, et al. Human B-cell differentiation factor defined by an anti-peptide antibody and its possible role in autoantibody production. *Proc Natl Acad Sci U S A* 1987;84:228–231.
228. Jourdan M, Bataille R, Seguin J, et al. Constitutive production of interleukin-6 and immunologic features in cardiac myxomas. *Arthritis Rheum* 1990;33:398–402.
229. Revankar SG, Clark RA. Infected cardiac myxoma: case report and literature review. *Medicine* 1998;77:337–344.
230. Rogers EW, Weyman AE, Noble RJ, et al. Left atrial myxoma infected with *Histoplasma capsulatum*. *Am J Med* 1978;64: 683–690.
231. Graham HV, Von Hartitzsch B, Medina JR. Infected atrial myxoma. *Am J Cardiol* 1976;38:658–661.
232. Rajpal RS, Leibsohn JA, Liekweg WG, et al. Infected left atrial myxoma with bacteremia simulating infective endocarditis. *Arch Intern Med* 1979;139:1176–1178.
233. Bulkley BH, Hutchins GM. Atrial myxomas: a fifty year review. *Am Heart J* 1979;97:639–643.

234. Goodwin JF. Diagnosis of left atrial myxoma. *Lancet* 1963; 1:464–468.
235. Nasser WK, Davis RH, Dillon JC, et al. Atrial myxoma. I. Clinical and pathologic features in nine cases. *Am Heart J* 1972; 83:694–704.
236. St. John Sutton MG, Mercier LA, Giuliani ER, et al. Atrial myxomas: a review of clinical experience in 40 patients. *Mayo Clin Proc* 1980;55:371–376.
237. MacGregor GA, Cullen RA. The syndrome of fever, anemia, and high sedimentation rate with an atrial myxoma. *Br Med J* 1959;2:991–997.
238. Fitzpatrick AP, Lanham JG, Doyle DV. Cardiac tumours simulating collagen vascular disease. *Br Heart J* 1986;55:592–595.
239. Cohen AI, McIntosh HD, Orgain ES. The mimetic nature of left atrial myxomas: report of a case presenting as a severe systemic illness and simulating massive mitral insufficiency at cardiac catheterization. *Am J Cardiol* 1963;11:802–807.
240. Kaminsky ME, Ehlers KH, Engle MA, et al. Atrial myxoma mimicking a collagen disorder. *Chest* 1979;75:93–95.
241. Boussen K, Moalla M, Blondeau P, et al. Embolization of cardiac myxomas masquerading as polyarteritis nodosa. *J Rheumatol* 1991;18:283–285.
242. Huston KA, Combs JJ Jr, Lie JT, et al. Left atrial myxoma simulating peripheral vasculitis. *Mayo Clin Proc* 1978;53:752–756.
243. Byrd WE, Matthews OP, Hunt RE. Left atrial myxoma presenting as a systemic vasculitis. *Arthritis Rheum* 1980;23: 240–243.
244. Bridges BF, Hector DA. Possible association of cutaneous telangiectasia with cardiac myxoma. *Am J Med* 1989;87: 483–485.
245. Harvey WP. Clinical aspects of cardiac tumors. *Am J Cardiol* 1968;21:328–343.
246. Symbas PN, Abbott OA, Logan WD, et al. Atrial myxomas: special emphasis on unusual manifestations. *Chest* 1971;59: 504–510.
247. Selzer A, Sakai FJ, Popper RW. Protean clinical manifestations of primary tumors of the heart. *Am J Med* 1972;52:9–18.
248. Peters MN, Hall RJ, Cooley DA, et al. The clinical syndrome of atrial myxoma. *JAMA* 1974;230:695–701.
249. Schmidley JW. Neurological presentations of atrial myxoma. *Heart Dis Stroke* 1993;2:483–486.
250. Stoane L, Allen JH Jr, Collins HA. Radiologic observations in cerebral embolization from left heart myxomas. *Radiology* 1966; 87:262–266.
251. Schwarz GA, Schwartzman RJ, Joyner CR. Atrial myxoma: cause of embolic stroke. *Neurology* 1972;22:1112–1121.
252. Yufe R, Karpati G, Carpenter S. Cardiac myxoma: a diagnostic challenge for the neurologist. *Neurology* 1976;26:1060–1065.
253. Carney JA, Gordon H, Carpenter PC, et al. The complex of myxomas, spotty pigmentation, and endocrine overactivity. *Medicine* 1985;64:270–283.
254. Prichard RW. Tumors of the heart: review of the subject and report of one hundred and fifty cases. *AMA Arch Pathol* 1951; 51:98–128.
255. DePace NL, Soulen RL, Kotler MN, et al. Two dimensional echocardiographic detection of intraatrial masses. *Am J Cardiol* 1981;48:954–960.
256. Alam M, Sun I. Transesophageal echocardiographic evaluation of left atrial mass lesions. *J Am Soc Echocardiogr* 1991;4: 323–330.
257. Leonhardt ET, Kullenberg KP. Bilateral atrial myxomas with multiple arterial aneurysms: a syndrome mimicking polyarteritis nodosa. *Am J Med* 1977;62:792–794.
258. Goodwin JF. The spectrum of cardiac tumors. *Am J Cardiol* 1968;21:307–314.
259. Savige JA, Yeung SP, Davies DJ, et al. Anti-neutrophil cytoplasmic antibodies associated with atrial myxoma [Letter]. *Am J Med* 1988;85:755–756.
260. Crawford C. *Discussion on late results of mitral commissurotomy. International Symposium on Cardiovascular Surgery.* Philadelphia: WB Saunders, 1955:202–211.
261. Richardson JV, Brandt BD, Doty DB, et al. Surgical treatment of atrial myxomas: early and late results of 11 operations and review of the literature. *Ann Thorac Surg* 1979;28:354–358.
262. Markel ML, Armstrong WF, Waller BF, et al. Left atrial myxoma with multicentric recurrence and evidence of metastases. *Am Heart J* 1986;111:409–413.
263. Jordan JM, Allen NB, Pizzo SV. Defective release of tissue plasminogen activator in systemic and cutaneous vasculitis. *Am J Med* 1987;82:397–400.
264. Cervera R, Font J, Asherson RA. Antiphospholipid antibodies: guidelines for determination. *J Clin Rheumatol* 1997;3:368–373.
265. Nachman RL, Silverstein R. Hypercoagulable states [see comments]. *Ann Intern Med* 1993;119:819–827.
266. Dessailloud R, Papo T, Vaneecloo S, et al. Acalculous ischemic gallbladder necrosis in the catastrophic antiphospholipid antibody syndrome. *Arthritis Rheum* 1998;41:1318–1320.
267. Gertner E. Diffuse alveolar hemorrhage in the antiphospholipid syndrome: spectrum of disease and treatment. *J Rheumatol* 1999;26:805–807.
268. Marie I, Levesque H, Heron F, et al. Acute adrenal failure secondary to bilateral infarction of the adrenal glands as the first manifestation of primary antiphospholipid antibody syndrome. *Ann Rheum Dis* 1997;56:567–568.
269. Sneddon IB. Cerebro-vascular lesions and livedo reticularis. *Br J Dermatol* 1965;77:180–185.
270. Asherson RA, Cervera R, Piette JC, et al. Catastrophic antiphospholipid antibody syndrome: clinical and laboratory features of 50 patients. *Medicine* 1998;77:195–207.
271. Asherson RA, Jacobelli S, Rosenberg H, et al. Skin nodules and macules resembling vasculitis in the antiphospholipid syndrome: a report of two cases. *Clin Exp Dermatol* 1992;17:266–269.
272. Asherson RA. The catastrophic antiphospholipid syndrome [Editorial]. *J Rheumatol* 1992;19:508–512.
273. Hughes GR. The antiphospholipid syndrome: ten years on [see comments]. *Lancet* 1993;342:341–344.
274. Alarcon-Segovia D, Mestanza M, Cabiedes J, et al. The antiphospholipid/cofactor syndromes. II. A variant in patients with systemic lupus erythematosus with antibodies to beta$_2$-glycoprotein I but no antibodies detectable in standard antiphospholipid assays. *J Rheumatol* 1997;24:1545–1551.
275. Fessler BJ. Thrombotic syndromes and autoimmune diseases. *Rheum Dis Clin North Am* 1997;23:461–479.
276. Alegre VA, Gastineau DA, Winkelmann RK. Skin lesions associated with circulating lupus anticoagulant. *Br J Dermatol* 1989; 120:419–429.
277. Bowles CA. Vasculopathy associated with the antiphospholipid antibody syndrome. *Rheum Dis Clin North Am* 1990;16:471–490.
278. Smith KJ, Skelton HGd, James WD, et al. Cutaneous histopathologic findings in "antiphospholipid syndrome": correlation with disease, including human immunodeficiency virus disease. *Arch Dermatol* 1990;126:1176–1183.
279. Stephens CJ. The antiphospholipid syndrome: clinical correlations, cutaneous features, mechanism of thrombosis and treatment of patients with the lupus anticoagulant and anticardiolipin antibodies. *Br J Dermatol* 1991;125:199–210.
280. Grob JJ, San Marco M, Aillaud MF, et al. Unfading acral microlivedo: a discrete marker of thrombotic skin disease associated with antiphospholipid antibody syndrome [see comments]. *J Am Acad Dermatol* 1991;24:53–58.
281. Grob JJ, Bonerandi JJ. Cutaneous manifestations associated with the presence of the lupus anticoagulant: a report of two

cases and a review of the literature. *J Am Acad Dermatol* 1986; 15:211–219.

282. Goldberger E, Elder RC, Schwartz RA, et al. Vasculitis in the antiphospholipid syndrome: a cause of ischemia responding to corticosteroids [see comments]. *Arthritis Rheum* 1992;35: 569–572.
283. Lie JT. Vasculitis in the antiphospholipid syndrome: culprit or consort? [Editorial; see comments]. *J Rheumatol* 1994;21: 397–399.
284. Gertner E, Lie JT. Systemic therapy with fibrinolytic agents and heparin for recalcitrant nonhealing cutaneous ulcer in the antiphospholipid syndrome. *J Rheumatol* 1994;21:2159–2161.
285. Klein KL, Pittelkow MR. Tissue plasminogen activator for treatment of livedoid vasculitis [see comments]. *Mayo Clin Proc* 1992;67:923–933.
286. Roberts WN, De Meo JH, Breitbach SA. Well-imaged large vessel vasculitis attributed to anticardiolipin antibody. *Arthritis Rheum* 1994;37:1254–1257.
287. Fox DA, Faix JD, Coblyn J, et al. Thrombotic thrombocytopenic purpura and systemic lupus erythematosus. *Ann Rheum Dis* 1986;45:319–322.
288. Jain R, Chartash E, Susin M, et al. Systemic lupus erythematosus complicated by thrombotic microangiopathy. *Semin Arthritis Rheum* 1994;24:173–182.
289. Gilbert JA Jr, Scalzi RP. Disseminated intravascular coagulation. *Emerg Med Clin North Am* 1993;11:465–480.
290. Singh AK, Wetherley-Mein G. Microvascular occlusive lesions in primary thrombocythaemia. *Br J Haematol* 1977;36: 553–564.
291. Liebeskind A, Cohen S, Anderson R, et al. Unusual segmental cerebrovascular changes. *Radiology* 1973;106:119–122.
292. Calabrese LH, Furlan AJ, Gragg LA, et al. Primary angiitis of the central nervous system: diagnostic criteria and clinical approach. *Cleve Clin J Med* 1992;59:293–306.
293. Stahl D, Thomsen K, Hou-Jensen K. Malignant atrophic papulosis: treatment with aspirin and dipyridamole. *Arch Dermatol* 1978;114:1687–1689.
294. Dastur DK, Singhal BS, Shroff HJ. CNS involvement in malignant atrophic papulosis, Kohlmeier-Degos disease: vasculopathy and coagulopathy. *J Neurol Neurosurg Psychiatry* 1981;44: 156–160.
295. Englert HJ, Hawkes CH, Boey ML, et al. Degos' disease: association with anticardiolipin antibodies and the lupus anticoagulant. *Br Med J Clin Res Ed* 1984;289:576.
296. Degos R. Malignant atrophic papulosis. *Br J Dermatol* 1979; 100:21–35.
297. Dubin HV, Stawiski MA. Systemic lupus erythematosus resembling malignant atrophic papulosis. *Arch Intern Med* 1974;134: 321–323.
298. Durie BG, Stroud JD, Kahn JA. Progressive systemic sclerosis with malignant atrophic papulosis. *Arch Dermatol* 1969;100:575–581.
299. McFarland HR, Wood WG, Drowns BV, et al. Papulosis atrophicans maligua (Kohlmeier-Degos disease): a disseminated occlusive vasculopathy. *Ann Neurol* 1978;3:388–392.
300. Su WPD, Schroeter AL, Lee DA, et al. Clinical and histologic findings in Degos' syndrome (malignant atrophic papulosis). *Cutis* 1985;35:131–138.
301. Pierce RN, Smith GJ. Intrathoracic manifestations of Degos' disease malignant atrophic papulosis. *Chest* 1978;73:79–84.
302. Case records of the Massachusetts General Hospital. Weekly clinicopathological exercises: case 44-1980. *N Engl J Med* 1980; 303:1103–1111.
303. Lankisch MR, Johst P, Scolapio JS, et al. Acute abdominal pain as a leading symptom for Degos' disease (malignant atrophic papulosis). *Am J Gastroenterol* 1999;94:1098–1099.
304. Fruhwirth J, Mischinger HJ, Werkgartner G, et al. Kohlmeier-Degos' disease with primary intestinal manifestation. *Scand J Gastroenterol* 1997;32:1066–1070.
305. Gajdusek D, Gibbs C, Earle K, et al. Transmission of subacute spongiform encephalopathy to the chimpanzee and squirrel monkey from a patient with papulosis atrophicans maligna of Kohlmeier-Degos. In: Subirana A, Espadaler J, Burrows E, eds. *Proceedings of the Tenth International Congress of Neurology.* Amsterdam: Excerpta Medica, 1974:390–392.
306. Assier H, Chosidow O, Piette JC, et al. Absence of antiphospholipid and antiendothelial antibodies in malignant atrophic papulosis. *J Am Acad Dermatol* 1996;33:831–833.
307. Sprabery AT, Newman K, Lohr KM. Aortic mural thrombus presenting as pseudovasculitis. *Chest* 1994;106:282–283.
308. Karl M. Clinicopathologic conference. *Am J Med* 1975;59: 837–843.
309. Lee KF, Hodes PJ. Intracranial ischemic lesions. *Radiol Clin North Am* 1967;5:363–393.
310. Abdelmalek MF, Spittel PC. 79-year-old woman with blue toes. *Mayo Clin Proc* 1995;70:292–295.
311. Federman DG, Valdivia M, Kirsner RS. Syphilis presenting as the "blue toe syndrome." *Arch Intern Med* 1994;154: 1029–1031.
312. Korst DR, Kratochvil CH. "Cryofibrinogen" formation in a cse of lung neoplasm associated with thrombophlebitis migrans. *Blood* 1955;10:945–953.
313. Waxman S, Dove JT. Cryofibrinogenemia aggravated during hypothermia. *N Engl J Med* 1969;281:1291–1292.
314. Smith SB, Arkin C. Cryofibrinogenemia: incidence, clinical correlations, and a review of the literature. *Am J Clin Pathol* 1972;58:524–530.
315. Beightler E, Diven DG, Sanchez RL, et al. Thrombotic vasculopathy associated with cryofibrinogenemia. *J Am Acad Dermatol* 1991;24:342–345.
316. Burruss JB, Fabrae VC, Callen JP. Painful acral purpuric nodules. *Arthritis Rheum* 1994;37:1812–1815.
317. Von Bonsdorff B, Groth H, Packalen T. On the presence of a high-molecular crystallizable protein in blood serum in myeloma. *Folia Haematol Leipz* 1938;59:184–208.
318. Grossman J, Abraham GN, Leddy JP, et al. Crystalglobulinemia. *Ann Intern Med* 1972;77:395–400.
319. Dotten DA, Pruzanski W, Olin J, et al. Cryocrystalglobulinemia. *Can Med Assoc J* 1976;114:909–912.
320. Stone GC, Wall BA, Oppliger IR, et al. A vasculopathy with deposition of lambda light chain crystals. *Ann Intern Med* 1989; 110:275–278.
321. Dornan TL, Blundell JW, Morgan AG, et al. Widespread crystallisation of paraprotein in myelomatosis. *Q J Med* 1985;57: 659–667.
322. Lesprit P, Authier FJ, Gherardi R, et al. Acute arterial obliteration: a new feature of the POEMS syndrome? *Medicine* 1996;75:226–232.
323. Soubrier M, Guillon R, Dubost JJ, et al. Arterial obliteration in POEMS syndrome: possible role of vascular endothelial growth factor. *J Rheumatol* 1998;25:813–815.
324. Takatsuki K, Uchiyama T, Sagawa K, et al. Plasma cell dyscrasia with polyneuropathy and endocrine disorder: review of 32 patients: In: *Internation Congress Series No. 415, Topic of Haemotoogy:* Proceeding of the 16th International Congress of Haemotology. Kyoto, Japan: 1976:454.
325. Trentham DE, Masi AT, Marker HW. Polyneuropathy and anasarca: evidence for a new connective-tissue syndrome and vasculopathic contribution. *Ann Intern Med* 1976;84:271–274.
326. Bardwick PA, Zvaifler NJ, Gill GN, et al. Plasma cell dyscrasia with polyneuropathy, organomegaly, endocrinopathy, M protein, and skin changes: the POEMS syndrome: report on two cases and a review of the literature. *Medicine* 1980;59:311–322.

327. Viard JP, Lesavre P, Boitard C, et al. POEMS syndrome presenting as systemic sclerosis: clinical and pathologic study of a case with microangiopathic glomerular lesions. *Am J Med* 1988; 84:524–528.
328. Manning WJ, Goldberger AL, Drews RE, et al. POEMS syndrome with myocardial infarction: observations concerning pathogenesis and review of the literature. *Semin Arthritis Rheum* 1992;22:151–161.
329. Soubrier MJ, Dubost JJ, Sauvezie BJ. POEMS syndrome: a study of 25 cases and a review of the literature: French Study Group on POEMS Syndrome. *Am J Med* 1994;97:543–553.
330. Mandel BF, Calabrese LH. Infections and systemic vasculitis. *Curr Opin Rheumatol* 1998;10:51–57.
331. Leeds NE, Goldberg HI. Angiographic manifestations in cerebral inflammatory disease. *Radiology* 1971;98:595–604.
332. Victor DI, Green WR. Temporal artery biopsy in herpes zoster ophthalmicus with delayed arteritis. *Am J Ophthalmol* 1976;82: 628–630.
333. Leeds NE, Rosenblatt R, Zimmerman HM. Focal angiographic changes of cerebral lymphoma with pathologic correlation: a report of two cases. *Radiology* 1971;99:595–599.
334. Greitz T. Angiographyin tuberculous meningitis. *Acta Radiol* 1964;2:369–378.
335. Lehrer H. The angiographic triad in tuberculous meningitis: a radiographic and clinicopathologic correlation. *Radiology* 1966; 87:829–835.
336. Wickbom GI, Davidson AJ. Angiographic findings in intracranial actinomycosis: a case report and consideration of pathogenesis. *Radiology* 1967;88:536–537.
337. El Gammal T. Extra-ventricular communicating hydrocephalus: some observations on the midline ventricles. *A J Roentgenol Radium Ther Nucl Med* 1969;106:308–328.
338. Thomas VH, Hopkins IJ. Arteriographic demonstration of vascular lesions in the study of neurologic deficit in advanced *Haemophilus influenzae* meningitis. *Dev Med Child Neurol* 1972;14:783–787.
339. Vatz KA, Scheibel RL, Keiffer SA, et al. Neurosyphilis and diffuse cerebral angiopathy: a case report. *Neurology* 1974;24: 472–476.
340. Tjia TL, Yeow YK, Tan CB. Cryptococcal meningitis. *J Neurol Neurosurg Psychiatry* 1985;48:853–858.
341. Veenendaal-Hilbers JA, Perquin WV, Hoogland PH, et al. Basal meningovasculitis and occlusion of the basilar artery in two cases of *Borrelia burgdorferi* infection. *Neurology* 1988;38: 1317–1319.
342. Wheat LJ, Batteiger BE, Sathapatayavongs B. *Histoplasma capsulatum* infections of the central nervous system: a clinical review. *Medicine* 1990;69:244–260.
343. Williams PL, Johnson R, Pappagianis D, et al. Vasculitic and encephalitic complications associated with *Coccidioides immitis* infection of the central nervous system in humans: report of 10 cases and review. *Clin Infect Dis* 1992;14:673–682.
344. Baselga E, Margall N, Barnadas MA, et al. Detection of *Mycobacterium tuberculosis* in lobular granulomatous panniculitis erythema induratum-nodular vasculitis. *Arch Dermatol* 1997;133:457–462.
345. Lebel M, Lassonde M. Erythema induratum of Bazin. *J Am Acad Dermatol* 1986;14:738–742.
346. Rademaker M, Lowe DG, Munro DD. Erythema induratum Bazin's disease. *J Am Acad Dermatol* 1989;21:740–745.
347. Ollert MW, Thomas P, Korting HC, et al. Erythema induratum of Bazin: evidence of T-lymphocyte hyperresponsiveness to purified protein derivative of tuberculin: report of two cases and treatment. *Arch Dermatol* 1993;129:469–473.
348. Wachter RM, Burke AM, MacGregor RR. *Strongyloides stercoralis* hyperinfection masquerading as cerebral vasculitis. *Arch Neurol* 1984;41:1213–1216.
349. Slater CA, Sickel JZ, Visvesvara GS, et al. Brief report: successful treatment of disseminated acanthamoeba infection in an immunocompromised patient [see comments]. *N Engl J Med* 1994;331:85–87.
350. Roh SS, Gertner E. Digital necrosis in acquired immune deficiency syndrome vasculopathy treated with recombinant tissue plasminogen activator. *J Rheumatol* 1997;24:2258–2261.
351. Lipton SA, Ma MJ. Case records of the Massachusetts General Hospital. *N Engl J Med* 1996;335:1587–1595.
352. Simpson DM, Tagliati M. Neurologic manifestations of HIV infection [published erratum appears in *Ann Intern Med* 1995;122:317] [see comments]. *Ann Intern Med* 1994;121: 769–785.
353. Laroche GP. Traumatic vasospastic disease in chain-saw operators. *Can Med Assoc J* 1976;115:1217–1221.
354. Vayssairat M, Debure C, Cormier JM, et al. Hypothenar hammer syndrome: seventeen cases with long-term follow-up. *J Vasc Surg* 1987;5:838–843.
355. Wernick R, Smith DL. Bilateral hypothenar hammer syndrome: an unusual and preventable cause of digital ischemia. *Am J Emerg Med* 1989;7:302–306.
356. Thomas P, Lowitt NR. A traumatic experience. *N Engl J Med* 1995;333:307–310.
357. Dukes HT, Vieth RG. Cerebral arteriography during migraine prodrome and headache. *Neurology* 1964;14:636–639.
358. Ekbom K, Greitz T. Carotid angiography in cluster headache. *Acta Radiol Diagn* 1970;10:177–186.
359. Call GK, Fleming MC, Sealfon S, et al. Reversible cerebral segmental vasoconstriction. *Stroke* 1988;19:1159–1170.
360. Bogousslavsky J, Despland PA, Regli F, et al. Postpartum cerebral angiopathy: reversible vasoconstriction assessed by transcranial Doppler ultrasounds. *Eur Neurol* 1989;29:102–105.
361. Caplan DN, Louis DN. Case records of the Massachusetts General Hospital. *N Engl J Med* 1996;335:952–959.
362. Okazaki H, Reagan TJ, Campbell RJ. Clinicopathologic studies of primary cerebral amyloid angiopathy. *Mayo Clin Proc* 1989; 54:22–31.
363. Vanley CT, Aguilar MJ, Kleinhenz RJ, et al. Cerebral amyloid angiopathy. *Hum Pathol* 1981;12:609–616.
364. Gilbert JJ, Vinters HV. Cerebral amyloid angiopathy: incidence and complications in the aging brain. I. Cerebral hemorrhage. *Stroke* 1983;14:915–923.
365. Mandybur TI. Cerebral amyloid angiopathy: the vascular pathology and complications. *J Neuropathol Exp Neurol* 1986; 45:79–90.
366. Breathnach SM, Wells GC. Amyloid vascular disease: cord-like thickening of mucocutaneous arteries, intermittent claudication and angina in a case with underlying myelomatosis. *Br J Dermatol* 1980;102:591–595.
367. Jennette JC, Sheps DS, McNeill DD. Exclusively vascular systemic amyloidosis with visceral ischemia. *Arch Pathol Lab Med* 1982;106:323–327.
368. Gertz MA, Kyle RA, Griffing WL, et al. Jaw claudication in primary systemic amyloidosis. *Medicine* 1986;65:173–179.
369. Rao JK, Allen NB. Primary systemic amyloidosis masquerading as giant cell arteritis: case report and review of the literature. *Arthritis Rheum* 1993;36:422–425.
370. Friman C, Pettersson T. Amyloidosis. *Curr Opin Rheumatol* 1996;8:62–71.
371. Cox DW. Alpha 1-antitrypsin: a guardian of vascular tissue [Editorial; comment]. *Mayo Clin Proc* 1994;69:1123–1124.
372. Schievink WI, Bjeornsson J, Parisi JE, et al. Arterial fibromuscular dysplasia associated with severe alpha 1-antitrypsin deficiency [see comments]. *Mayo Clinic Proc* 1994;69:1040–1043.

373. Schievink WI, Prakash UB, Piepgras DG, et al. Alpha 1-antitrypsin deficiency in intracranial aneurysms and cervical artery dissection [see comments]. *Lancet* 1994;343:452–453.
374. Cattan S, Mariette X, Labrousse F, et al. Iliac artery dissection in alpha 1-antitrypsin deficiency [Letter; comment]. *Lancet* 1994;343:1371–1372.
375. Esnault VL, Testa A, Audrain M, et al. Alpha 1-antitrypsin genetic polymorphism in ANCA-positive systemic vasculitis. *Kidney Int* 1993;43:1329–1332.
376. Elzouki AN, Eriksson S. Severe alpha 1-antitrypsin deficiency and intracranial aneurysms [Letter; comment]. *Lancet* 1994; 343:1037.
377. Seyle H. *Calciphylaxis.* Chicago: University of Chicago Press, 1962:1–16.
378. Roe SM, Graham LD, Brock WB, et al. Calciphylaxis: early recognition and management. *Am Surg* 1994;60:81–86.
379. Anderson DC, Stewart WK, Piercy DM. Calcifying panniculitis with fat and skin necrosis in a case of uraemia with autonomous hyperparathyroidism. *Lancet* 1986;2:323–325.
380. Winkelmann RK, Keating FR Jr. Cutaneous vascular calcification, gangrene and hyperparathyroidism. *Br J Dermatol* 1970; 83:263–268.
381. Conn J Jr, Krumlovsky FA, Del Greco F, et al. Calciphylaxis: etiology of progressive vascular calcification and gangrene? *Ann Surg* 1973;177:206–210.
382. Gipstein RM, Coburn JW, Adams DA, et al. Calciphylaxis in man: a syndrome of tissue necrosis and vascular calcification in 11 patients with chronic renal failure. *Arch Intern Med* 1976; 136:1273–1280.
383. Mehregan DA, Winkelmann RK. Cutaneous gangrene, vascular calcification, and hyperparathyroidism. *Mayo Clin Proc* 1989; 64:211–215.
384. Khafif RA, DeLima C, Silverberg A, et al. Calciphylaxis and systemic calcinosis: collective review [published erratum appears in *Arch Intern Med* 1990;150:2592]. *Arch Intern Med* 1990;150: 956–959.
385. Ivker RA, Woosley J, Briggaman RA. Calciphylaxis in three patients with end-stage renal disease. *Arch Dermatol* 1995;131: 63–68.
386. Young PC, Cuozzo DW, Seidman AJ, et al. Widespread livedo reticularis with painful ulcerations. *Arch Dermatol* 1995;131: 786–788.
387. Ruggian JC, Maesaka JK, Fishbane S. Proximal calciphylaxis in four insulin-requiring diabetic hemodialysis patients. *Am J Kidney Dis* 1996;28:409–414.
388. Pan D, Hsu K, Ray SC. Ecchymoses and eschars at sites of injection. *Lancet* 1997;349:1364.
389. Khafif RA, Delima C, Silverberg A, et al. Acute hyperparathyroidism with systemic calcinosis: report of a case. *Arch Intern Med* 1989;149:681–684.
390. Golitz LE, Field JP. Metastatic calcification with skin necrosis. *Arch Dermatol* 1972;106:398–402.
391. Bargman JM. Calciphylaxis, calcinosis and calcergy—separate but not equal [Editorial; comment]. *J Rheumatol* 1995;22:5–7.
392. Adroguae HJ, Frazier MR, Zeluff B, et al. Systemic calciphylaxis revisited. *Am J Nephrol* 1981;1:177–183.
393. Blumberg A, Weidmann P. Successful treatment of ischaemic ulceration of the skin in azotaemic hyperparathyroidism with parathyroidectomy. *Br Med J* 1977;1:552–553.
394. Vassa N, Twardowski ZJ, Campbell JJ. Hyperbaric oxygen therapy in calciphylaxis-induced skin necrosis in a peritoneal dialysis patient. *Am J Kidney Dis* 1994;23:878–881.
395. Anderson-Fabry disease [editorial]. *Lancet* 1990;336:24–25.
396. Desnick RJ, Astrin KH, Bishop DF. Fabry disease: molecular genetics of the inherited nephropathy. *Adv Nephrol* 1989;18: 113–128.
397. Morgan SH, Rudge P, Smith SJM, et al. The neurological complications of Anderson-Fabry disease (alpha-galactosidase A deficiency): investigation of symptomatic and presymptomatic patients. *Q J Med* 1990;75:491–504.
398. Klein P. Ocular manifestations of Fabry's disease. *J Am Optometr.. Assoc* 1986;57:672–674.
399. Nakao S, Takenaka T, Maeda M, et al. An atypical variant of Fabry's disease in men with left ventricular hypertrophy. *N Engl J Med* 1995;333:288–293.
400. Becker AE, Schoorl R, Balk AG, et al. Cardiac manifestations of Fabry's disease: report of a case with mitral insufficiency and electrocardiographic evidence of myocardial infarction. *Am J Cardiol* 1975;36:829–835.
401. Fisher EA, Desnick RJ, Gordon RE, et al. Fabry disease: an unusual cause of severe coronary disease in a young man. *Ann Intern Med* 1992;117:221–223.
402. Rosenberg DM, Ferrans VJ, Fulmer JD, et al. Chronic airflow obstruction in Fabry's disease. *Am J Med* 1980;68:898–905.
403. Sheth KJ, Bernhard GC. The arthropathy of Fabry disease. *Arthritis Rheum* 1979;22:781–783.
404. Ross G, Kuwamura F, Goral A. Association of Fabry's disease with femoral head avascular necrosis. *Orthopedics* 1993;16: 471–473.
405. Rowe JW, Gilliam JI, Warthin TA. Intestinal manifestations of Fabry's disease. *Ann Intern Med* 1974;81:628–631.
406. Rodriguez-Serna M, Botella-Estrada R, Chabas A, et al. Angiokeratoma corporis diffusum associated with beta-mannosidase deficiency. *Arch Dermatol* 1996;132:1219–1222.
407. Holmes RC, Fensom AH, McKee P, et al. Angiokeratoma corporis diffusum in a patient with normal enzyme activities. *J Am Acad Dermatol* 1984;10:384–387.
408. Calzavara-Pinton PG, Colombi M, Carlino A, et al. Angiokeratoma corporis diffusum and arteriovenous fistulas with dominant transmission in the absence of metabolic disorders. *Arch Dermatol* 1995;131:57–62.
409. Mosnier JF, Degott C, Bedrossian J, et al. Recurrence of Fabry's disease in a renal allograft eleven years after successful renal transplantation. *Transplantation* 1991;51:759–762.
410. Stein JH, McBride PE. Hyperhomocysteinemia and atherosclerotic vascular disease: pathophysiology, screening, and treatment. *Arch Intern Med* 1998;158:1301–1306.
411. Welch GN, Loscalzo J. Homocysteine and atherothrombosis. *N Engl J Med* 1998;338:1042–1050.
412. Chambers JC, McGregor A, Jean-Marie J, et al. Acute hyperhomocysteinemia and endothelial cell dysfunction. *Lancet* 1998; 351:36–37.
413. Clarke R, Daly L, Robinson K, et al. Hyperhomocysteinemia: an independent risk factor for vascular disease [see comments]. *N Engl J Med* 1991;324:1149–1155.
414. Robinson K, Mayer E, Jacobsen DW. Homocysteine and coronary artery disease. *Cleve Clin J Med* 1994;61:438–450.
415. Faszbender K, Mielke O, Bertsch T, et al. Homocysteine in cerebral macroangiography and microangiopathy. *Lancet* 1999; 353:1586–1587.
416. Graham IM, Daly LE, Refsum HM, et al. Plasma homocysteine as a risk factor for vascular disease: the European concerted action project. *JAMA* 1997;277:1775–1781.
417. Boers GH, Smals AG, Trijbels FJ, et al. Heterozygosity for homocystinuria in premature peripheral and cerebral occlusive arterial disease [see comments]. *N Engl J Med* 1985;313: 709–715.
418. Selhub J, Jacques PF, Bostom AG, et al. Association between plasma homocysteine concentrations and extracranial carotid-artery stenosis [see comments]. *N Engl J Med* 1995;332: 286–291.

419. Stampfer MJ, Malinow MR. Can lowering homocysteine levels reduce cardiovascular risk? [Editorial; comment]. *N Engl J Med* 1995;332:328–329.
420. Kuiper J. Initial manifestation of primary hyperoxaluria type I in adults. *West J Med* 1996;164:42–53.
421. Blackburn WE, McRoberts JW, Bhathena D, et al. Severe vascular complications in oxalosis after bilateral nephrectomy. *Ann Intern Med* 1975;82:44–46.
422. Boogaerts MA, Hammerschmidt DE, Roelant C, et al. Mechanisms of vascular damage in gout and oxalosis: crystal induced, granulocyte mediated, endothelial injury. *Thromb Haemost* 1983;50:576–580.
423. Milliner DS, Eickholt JT, Bergstralh EJ, et al. Results of long-term treatment with orthophosphate and pyridoxine in patients with primary hyperoxaluria. *N Engl J Med* 1994;331: 1553–1558.
424. Bommer J, Ritz E, Andrassy K. Necrotizing dermatitis resulting from hemodialysis with polyvinylchloride tubing. *Ann Intern Med* 1979;91:869–870.
425. Fonkalsrud EW, Sanchez M, Zerubavel R, et al. Serial changes in arterial structure following radiation therapy. *Surg Gynecol Obstet* 1977;145:395–400.
426. Page EH, Shear NH. Temperature-dependent skin disorders [see comments]. *J Am Acad Dermatol* 1988;18:1003–1019.
427. Thomas EWP. Chapping and chilblains. *Practitioner* 1964;193: 755–760.
428. Kelly JW, Dowling JP. Pernio: a possible association with chronic myelomonocytic leukemia. *Arch Dermatol* 1985;121: 1048–1052.
429. Wall LM, Smith NP. Perniosis: a histopathological review. *Clin Exp Dermatol* 1981;6:263–271.
430. Dowd PM, Rustin MH, Lanigan S. Nifedipine in the treatment of chilblains. *Br Med J Clin Res Ed* 1986;293:923–924.
431. Ganor S. Corticosteroid therapy for pernio [Letter]. *J Am Acad Dermatol* 1983;8:136.
432. Wright GD, McCullagh CD, Walsh IK, et al. Digital necrosis with Ogilvie's syndrome. *Ann Rheum Dis* 1997;56:224–225.
433. Madiedo JMA, Murthy A, Cortese DA, et al. An unusual case of carcinoma polyarthritis with associated vasculitis. *Arthritis Rheum* 1997;40:779–782.
434. Calabrese LH, Mallek JA. Primary angiitis of the central nervous system: report of 8 new cases, review of the literature, and proposal for diagnostic criteria. *Medicine* 1988;67:20–39.
435. Krol T, Robinson J, Bekeris L, et al. Hairy cell leukemia and a fatal periarteritis nodosa-like syndrome. *Arch Pathol Lab Med* 1983;107:583–585.
436. Friedman SA, Bienenstock H, Richter IH. Malignancy and arteriopathy: a report of two cases. *Angiology* 1969;20:136–143.
437. Greco FA, Kolins J, Rajjoub RK, et al. Hodgkin's disease and granulomatous angiitis of the central nervous system. *Cancer* 1976;38:2027–2032.
438. Kois JM, Sexton FM, Lookingbill DP. Cutaneous manifestations of multiple myeloma. *Arch Dermatol* 1991;127:69–74.
439. Tolosa-Vilella C, Ordi-Ros J, Vilardell-Tarres M, et al. Raynaud's phenomenon and positive antinuclear antibodies in a malignancy [see comments]. *Ann Rheum Dis* 1990;49: 935–936.
440. Burnham TK. Antinuclear antibodies in patients with malignancies. *Lancet* 1972;2:436.
441. Primka EJD, King C, O'Keefe EJ. Malignant melanoma of unknown origin presenting as a systemic vasculitis [Letter]. *Arch Dermatol* 1993;129:1205–1207.
442. Taylor LM, Hauty MG, Edwards JM, et al. Digital ischemia as a manifestation of malignancy. *Ann Surg* 1987;206:62–68.
443. Fengler SA, Berenberg JL, Lee YT. Disseminated coagulopathies and advanced malignancies. *Am Surg* 1990;56:335–338.
444. Kanno J, Takemura T, Kasaga T. Malignant endothelioma of the aorta. *Virchows Arch A* 1987;412:183–188.
445. Lin JP, Siew FP. Glioblastoma multiforme presenting angiographically as intracranial atherosclerotic vascular disease. *Radiology* 1971;101:353–354.
446. Garces M, Gosink B. Aneurysm of the right iliac artery associated with fibrosarcoma. *Radiology* 1972;102:583–584.
447. Krieger C, Robitaille Y, Jothy S, et al. Intravascular malignant histiocytosis mimicking central nervous system vasculitis: an immunopathological diagnostic approach. *Ann Neurol* 1982; 12:489–492.
448. O'Connor B. Symmetrical gangrene. *Br Med J* 1884;1:460.
449. Jones HR, Edgar MA. Case records of the Massachusetts General Hospital. *N Engl J Med* 1995;332:730–737.
450. McColl GJ, Fraser K. Pheochromocytoma and pseudovasculitis [Letter]. *J Rheumatol* 1995;22:1442–1443.
451. Anders KH, Latta H, Chang BS, et al. Lymphomatoid granulomatosis and malignant lymphoma of the central nervous system in the acquired immunodeficiency syndrome. *Hum Pathol* 1989;20:326–334.
452. Lipford EH Jr, Margolick JB, Longo DL, et al. Angiocentric immunoproliferative lesions: a clinicopathologic spectrum of post-thymic T-cell proliferations. *Blood* 1988;72:1674–1681.
453. Petito CK, Gottlieb GJ, Dougherty JH, et al. Neoplastic angioendotheliosis: ultrastructural study and review of the literature. *Ann Neurol* 1978;3:393–399.
454. Braverman IM, Lerner AB. Diffuse malignant proliferation of vascular endothelium: a possible new clinical and pathological entity. *Arch Dermatol* 1961;84:22–30.
455. DiGiuseppe JA, Nelson WG, Seifter EJ, et al. Intravascular lymphomatosis: a clinicopathologic study of 10 cases and assessment of response to chemotherapy. *J Clin Oncol* 1994;12: 2573–2579.
456. Kamesaki H, Matsui Y, Ohno Y, et al. Angiotropic lymphoma with histologic features of neoplastic angioendotheliomatosis presenting with predominant respiratory and hematologic manifestations: report of a case and review of the literature [corrected] [published erratum appears in *Am J Clin Pathol* 1992; 98:650] [see comments]. *Am J Clin Pathol* 1990;94:768–772.
457. Mason MS, Wheeler JR, Gregory RT, et al. Primary tumors of the aorta: report of a case and review of the literature. *Oncology* 1982;39:167–172.
458. Case records of the Massachusetts General Hospital. Weekly clinicopathological exercises: case 26-1993: a 73-year-old man with an enlarging inguinal mass 10 years after treatment for prostate and colon cancers. *N Engl J Med* 1993;329:43–48.
459. Nishida H, Endo M, Koyanagi H, et al. Coronary artery bypass in a 15-year-old girl with pseudoxanthoma elasticum. *Ann Thorac Surg* 1990;49:483–485.
460. Lebwohl M, Halperin J, Phelps RG. Brief report: occult pseudoxanthoma elasticum in patients with premature cardiovascular disease [see comments]. *N Engl J Med* 1993;329: 1237–1239.
461. DiPrete DA, Abuelo JG, Abuelo DN, et al. Acute renal insufficiency due to renal infarctions in a patient with neurofibromatosis. *Am J Kidney Dis* 1990;15:357–360.
462. Kapoor OP. Iatrogenic ergot vasospastic angiitis: a case report. *Vasc Surg* 1976;10:58–60.
463. Henry PY, Larre P, Aupy M, et al. Reversible cerebral arteriopathy associated with the administration of ergot derivatives. *Cephalalgia* 1984;4:171–178.
464. Fallis RJ, Fisher M. Cerebral vasculitis and hemorrhage associated with phenylpropanolamine. *Neurology* 1985;35:405–407.

465. Citron BP, Halpern M, McCarron M, et al. Necrotizing angiitis associated with drug abuse. *N Engl J Med* 1970;283: 1003–1011.
466. Kalant H, Kalant OJ. Death in amphetamine users: causes and rates. *Can Med Assoc J* 1975;112:299–304.
467. Matick H, Anderson D, Brumlik J. Cerebral vasculitis associated with oral amphetamine overdose. *Arch Neurol* 1983;40: 253–254.
468. Lake CR, Gallant S, Masson E, et al. Adverse drug effects attributed to phenylpropanolamine: a review of 142 case reports. *Am J Med* 1990;89:195–208.
469. Sloan MA, Kittner SJ, Rigamonti D, et al. Occurrence of stroke associated with use/abuse of drugs. *Neurology* 1991;41: 1358–1364.
470. Pearlson GD, Jeffery PJ, Harris GJ, et al. Correlation of acute cocaine-induced changes in local cerebral blood flow with subjective effects. *Am J Psychiatry* 1993;150:495–497.
471. Tapia JF, Schumacher JM. Case records of the Massachusetts General Hospital. *N Engl J Med* 1993;329:117–124.
472. Kaye BR, Fainstat M. Cerebral vasculitis associated with cocaine abuse. *JAMA* 1987;258:2104–2106.
473. Fredericks RK, Lefkowitz DS, Challa VR, et al. Cerebral vasculitis associated with cocaine abuse. *Stroke* 1991;22: 1437–1439.
474. Rumbaugh CL, Bergeron RT, Scanlan RL, et al. Cerebral vascular changes secondary to amphetamine abuse in the experimental animal. *Radiology* 1971;101:345–351.
475. Karch SB, Billingham ME. The pathology and etiology of cocaine-induced heart disease. *Arch Pathol Lab Med* 1988;112: 225–230.
476. Irey NS, Norris HJ. Intimal vascular lesions associated with female reproductive steroids. *Arch Pathol* 1973;96:227–234.
477. Brick JF. Vanishing cerebrovascular disease of pregnancy. *Neurology* 1988;38:804–806.
478. Suzuki J, Takaku A. Cerebrovascular "moyamoya" disease: disease showing abnormal net-like vessels in base of brain. *Arch Neurol* 1969;20:288–299.
479. Takeuchi K, Shimizu K. Hypogenesis of bilateral internal carotid arteries. *No To Shinkei* 1957;9:37–43.
480. Yamashita M, Oka K, Tanaka K. Histopathology of the brain vascular network in moyamoya disease. *Stroke* 1983;14:50–58.
481. Hoshimaru M, Takahashi JA, Kikuchi H, et al. Possible roles of basic fibroblast growth factor in the pathogenesis of moyamoya disease: an immunohistochemical study. *J Neurosurg* 1991;75: 267–270.
482. Yamamoto M, Aoyagi M, Fukai N, et al. Differences in cellular responses to mitogens in arterial smooth muscle cells derived from patients with moyamoya disease. *Stroke* 1998;29: 1188–1193.
483. Masuda J, Ogata J, Yutani C. Smooth muscle cell proliferation and localization of macrophages and T cells in the occlusive intracranial major arteries in moyamoya disease. *Stroke* 1993; 24:1960–1967.
484. Kinugasa K, Mandai S, Kamata I, et al. Surgical treatment of moyamoya disease: operative technique for encephalo-duro-arterio-myo-synangiosis, its follow-up, clinical results, and angiograms. *Neurosurgery* 1993;32:527–531.
485. Jones HJ, Staud R, Williams RC. Rupture of a hepatic artery aneurysm and renal infarction: 2 complications of fibromuscular dysplasia that mimic vasculitis. *J Rheumatol* 1998;25: 2015–2018.
486. Chan RJ, Goodman TA, Aretz TH, et al. Segmental mediolytic arteriopathy of the splenic and hepatic arteries mimicking systemic necrotizing vasculitis. *Arthritis Rheum* 1998;41:935–938.
487. Najafi H. Fibromuscular hyperplasia of the external iliac arteries: an unusual cause of intermittent claudication. *Arch Surg* 1966;92:394–396.
488. Den Butter G, Van Bockel JH, Aarts JC. Arterial fibrodysplasia: rapid progression complicated by rupture of a visceral aneurysm into the gastrointestinal tract. *J Vasc Surg* 1988;7:449–453.
489. Iwai T, Konno S, Hiejima K, et al. Fibromuscular dysplasia in the extremities. *J Cardiovasc Surg* 1985;26:496–501.
490. Rybka SJ, Novick AC. Concomitant carotid, mesenteric and renal artery stenosis due to primary intimal fibroplasia. *J Urol* 1983;129:798–800.
491. Stokes JB, Bonsib SM, McBride JW. Diffuse intimal fibromuscular dysplasia with multiorgan failure. *Arch Intern Med* 1996;156:2611–2614.
492. Malek AM, Higashida RT, Phatouros CC, et al. A strangled wife. *Lancet* 1999;353:1324.
493. Slavin RE, Saeki K, Bhagavan B, et al. Segmental arterial mediolysis: a precursor to fibromuscular dysplasia? *Mod Pathol* 1995; 8:287–294.
494. Johns CJ, Michele TM. The clinical management of sarcoidosis: a 50-year experience at the Johns Hopkins Hospital. *Medicine* 1999;78:65–111.
495. Lawrence WP, El-Gammal T, Pool WH Jr, et al. Radiological manifestations of neurosarcoidosis: report of three cases and review of literature. *Clin Radiol* 1974;25:343–348.
496. Reske-Mielson E, Harmsen A. Periangiitis and panangiitis as manifestation of sarcoidosis of the brain: report of a case. *J Nerv Ment Dis* 1962;135:399–412.
497. Herring AB, Urich H. Sarcoidosis of the central nervous system. *J Neurol Sci* 1969;9:405–422.
498. Caplan L, Corbett J, Goodwin J, et al. Neuro-ophthalmologic signs in the angiitic form of neurosarcoidosis. *Neurology* 1983; 33:1130–1135.
499. Maeda S, Murao S, Sugiyama T, et al. Generalized sarcoidosis with "sarcoid aortitis." *Acta Pathol Jpn* 1983;33:183–188.
500. Stern BJ, Krumholz A, Johns C, et al. Sarcoidosis and its neurological manifestations. *Arch Neurol* 1985;42:909–917.
501. Scherbenske JM, Benson PM, Lupton GP, et al. Rheumatoid neutrophilic dermatitis. *Arch Dermatol* 1989;125:1105–1108.
502. Lowe L, Kornfeld B, Clayman J, et al. Rheumatoid neutrophilic dermatitis. *J Cutan Pathol* 1991;19:48–53.
503. Angle B, Burton BK. Familial leg ulcers. *Lancet* 1998;351: 1031–1032.
504. Ganor S, Cohen T. Leg ulcers in a family with both beta thalassaemia and glucose-6-phosphate dehydrogenase deficiency. *Br J Dermatol* 1976;95:203–206.
505. Winkler E, Levertowsky D, Shvoron A, et al. Familial leg ulcers of juvenile onset [see comments]. *Lancet* 1991;337:15–16.
506. Husak R, Blume-Peytaki U, Orfanos CE. Aleukemic leukemia cutis in an adolescent boy. *N Engl J Med* 1999;340:893–894.
507. Orth B, Frei R, Itin PH, et al. Outbreak of invasive mycoses caused by *Paecilomyces lilacinus* from a contaminated skin lotion. *Ann Intern Med* 1996;125:799–806.
508. Cuende E, Almeida V, Portu J, et al. Poncet's disease and papulonecrotic tuberculid in a patient infected with the human immunodeficiency virus. *Arthritis Rheum* 1998;41:1884–1888.
509. Benedict LM, Kusne S, Torre-Cisneros J, et al. Primary cutaneous fungal infection after solid-organ transplantation: report of five cases and review. *Clin Infect Dis* 1992;15:17–21.
510. Case records of the Massachusetts General Hospital. Weekly clinicopathological exercises: case 33-1986: a 62-year-old alcoholic man with confusion, ataxia, and a rash. *N Engl J Med* 1986;315:503–508.
511. Rosenstein ED, Kramer N. Occult subacute thyroiditis mimicking classic giant cell arteritis. *Arthritis Rheum* 1994;37: 1618–1620.

512. Byrd RP, Hourany J, Cooper C, et al. False-positive antineutrophil cytoplasmic antibodies in a patient with cavitary pulmonary sporotrichosis. *Am J Med* 1998;104:101–103.
513. Mastrolonardo M, Loconsole F, Conte A, et al. Cutaneous vasculitis as the sole manifestation of disseminated gonococcal infection: case report. *Genitourin Med* 1994;70:130–131.
514. Peters M, Gottschalk D, Boit R, et al. Meningovascular neurosyphilis in human immunodeficiency virus infection as a differential diagnosis of focal CNS lesions: a clinicopathological study. *J Infect* 1993;27:57–62.
515. May EF, Jabbari B. Stroke in neuroborreliosis. *Stroke* 1990; 21:1232–1235.
516. Johnston YE, Duray PH, Steere AC, et al. Lyme arthritis. spirochetes found in synovial microangiopathic lesions. *Am J Pathol* 1985;118:26–34.
517. Fontana PE, Gabutti L, Piffaretti JC, et al. Antibiotic treatment for giant cell arteritis? *Lancet* 1996;348:1630.
518. Camponovo F, Meier C. Neuropathy of vasculitic origin in a case of Garin-Boujadoux-Bannwarth syndrome with positive Borrelia antibody response. *J Neurol* 1986;233:69–72.
519. Woods GL, Goldsmith JC. Aspergillus infection of the central nervous system in patients with acquired immunodeficiency syndrome. *Arch Neurol* 1990;47:181–184.
520. Stone JH, Pomper MG, Hellmann DB. Histoplasmosis mimicking vasculitis of the central nervous system. *J Rheumatol* 1998;25:1644–1648.
521. Aberfeld DC, Gladstone JL. Cryptococcal meningoencephalitis presenting with hemiplegia of sudden onset. *JAMA* 1967; 202:90–91.
522. Yankner BA, Skolnik PR, Shoukimas GM, et al. Cerebral granulomatous angiitis associated with isolation of human T-lymphotrophic virus type III from the central nervous system. *Ann Neurol* 1986;20:362–364.
523. Weck KE, Dal Canto AJ, Gould JD, et al. Murine gamma-herpes virus 68 causes severe large-vessel arteritis in mice lacking interferon-gamma responsiveness: a new model for virus-induced vasculitis. *Nat Med* 1997;3:1346–1353.
524. Pumarola-Sune T, Navia BA, Cordon-Carlo C, et al. HIV antigen in the brains of patients with the AIDS dementia complex. *Ann Neurol* 1987;21:490–496.
525. Mizusawa H, Hirano A, Llena JF, et al. Cerebrovascular lesions in acquired immune deficiency syndrome (AIDS). *Acta Neuropathol* 1988;76:451–457.
526. Linnemann CC, Alvira MM. Pathogenesis of varicella-zoster angiitis in the CNS. *Arch Neurol* 1980;37:239–240.
527. Joshi VV, Pawel B, Connor E, et al. Arteriopathy in children with acquired immune deficiency syndrome. *Pediatr Pathol* 1987;7:261–275.
528. Gruber BL, Schranz JA, Fuhrer J, et al. Isolated pulmonary microangiitis mimicking pneumonia in a patient infected with human immunodeficiency virus. *J Rheumatol* 1997;24: 759–762.
529. Gray F, Belec L, Lescs MC, et al. Varicella-zoster virus infection of the central nervous system in the acquired immune deficiency syndrome. *Brain* 1994;117:987–999.
530. Esterly JR, Oppenheimer EH. Vascular lesions in infants with congenital rubella. *Circulation* 1967;36:544–550.
531. Erhard H, Runger TM, Kreienkamp M, et al. Atypical varicella-zoster virus infection in an immunocompromised patient: result of a virus-induced vasculitis. *J Am Acad Dermatol* 1995;32: 908–911.
532. Berger JR, Harris JO, Gregorios J, et al. Cerebrovascular disease in AIDS: a case-control study. *AIDS* 1990;4:239–244.
533. Salgado P, Rojas R, Sotelo J. Cysticercosis: clinical classification based on imaging studies. *Arch Intern Med* 1997;157: 1991–1997.
534. Oddo D, Casanova M, Acuna G, et al. Acute Chagas' disease (*Trypanosomiasis americana*) in acquired immune deficiency syndrome: report of two cases. *Hum Pathol* 1992;23:41–44.
535. Martinez AJ, Guerra AE, Garcia-Tamayo J, et al. Granulomatous amebic encephalitis: a review and report of a spontaneous case from Venezuela. *Acta Neuropathol* 1994;87:430–434.
536. Kraus A, Valencia X, Cabral AR, et al. Visceral larva migrans mimicking rheumatic diseases. *J Rheumatol* 1995;22:497–500.

85

SJÖGREN'S SYNDROME

ROLAND JONSSON
HANS-JACOB HAGA
TOM P. GORDON

Sjögren's syndrome is a chronic inflammatory and lymphoproliferative disease with autoimmune features characterized by a progressive mononuclear cell infiltration of exocrine glands, notably the lacrimal and salivary glands (autoimmune exocrinopathy). These lymphoid infiltrations lead to dryness of the eyes (keratoconjunctivitis sicca), dryness of the mouth (xerostomia), and frequently, dryness of the nose, throat, vagina, and skin. Sjögren's syndrome is associated with the production of autoantibodies because B-cell activation is a consistent immunoregulatory abnormality. The spectrum of the disease extends from an organ-specific autoimmune disorder to a systemic process (musculoskeletal, pulmonary, gastric, hematologic, dermatologic, renal, and nervous system involvement). Sjögren's syndrome may occur alone (primary) or in association with almost any of the autoimmune rheumatic diseases (secondary), the most frequent being rheumatoid arthritis (RA) and systemic lupus erythematosus (SLE). Sjögren's syndrome also is associated with an increased risk of B-cell lymphoma development.

KEY ADVANCES: MILESTONES AND HISTORIC OVERVIEW

Between 1882 and 1924, a number of case reports described Sjögren's syndrome with various combinations of dry mouth, dry eyes, and chronic arthritis (1–5). In 1892, Mikulicz (6) reported a man with bilateral parotid and lacrimal gland enlargement associated with massive round cell infiltration. Gourgerot (7), in 1925, described three patients with salivary and mucous gland atrophy and insufficiency. In 1927 Mulock Houwer (8) reported the association of filamentary keratitis, the major ocular manifestation of the syndrome, with chronic arthritis. In 1933 Henrik Sjögren (9), a Swedish ophthalmologist, reported, in his classic doctoral dissertation, detailed clinical and histologic findings in 19 women with xerostomia and keratoconjunctivitis sicca, of whom 13 had chronic arthritis. Later, in 1953, Morgan and Castleman (10) established that Sjögren's syndrome and Mikulicz's disease were the same entity. The link between Sjögren's syndrome and malignant lymphoma was described in a classic article in 1964 (11). The distinction between primary and secondary Sjögren's syndrome was suggested in 1965 (12) and the Sjögren's syndrome–associated autoantibodies (Ro/SSA) in the sera were described in 1969 (13). From the diagnostic point of view, the first histologic grading assessing the infiltration of labial glands was described in 1968 (14). A set of preliminary classification criteria was identified by a European Concerted Action in 1993, which has been widely accepted (15).

EPIDEMIOLOGY

Sjögren's syndrome is a worldwide disease and may occur in individuals of all ages. However, the peak incidence is in the fourth and fifth decades of life, with a female/male ratio of 9:1.

The studies performed on the prevalence of primary Sjögren's syndrome differ slightly from one another because of the controversies involving different classification criteria. Fox et al. (16) reviewed the patient records in their clinic in San Diego, and found that the prevalence of Sjögren's syndrome was as low as 1 (0.08%) in 1,250 by using the California criteria. Conversely, a Canadian study of 2,500 sera obtained from female blood donors between the ages of 20 and 50 years revealed a frequency of 0.44% for the Sjögren-associated anti-Ro/SSA autoantibodies, with the highest frequency (0.72%) in the 45- to 50-year age group (17). Because anti-Ro/SSA autoantibodies are not specific for Sjögren's syndrome, only a proportion of the primary Sjögren's syndrome patients have this autoantibody, depending on the criteria used.

In a Swedish population-based study, 35% of the participating persons between ages 52 and 72 years complained about dry mouth and/or dry eyes (18). The symptomatic individuals had a higher frequency of abnormal measurements of exocrine gland function, and they had a 1.54- to 2.88-fold increase of Ro/SSA and La/SSB autoantibodies compared with asymptomatic persons, suggesting that exocrine gland dysfunction and serologic findings in primary Sjögren's syndrome affect a substantial proportion of the general population (19). The same group found a minimal prevalence of primary Sjögren's syndrome as high as 2.7% in the same study population, by using the Copenhagen criteria (18). In a recent study from Denmark including 504 persons aged 30 to 60 years, the frequency of keratoconjunctivitis sicca was estimated to be 11% and 8% when using the Copenhagen and the preliminary European criteria, respectively (20). The frequency of primary Sjögren's syndrome was estimated to be 0.2% to 0.8% when using the Copenhagen criteria, and 0.6% to 2.1% when using the preliminary European criteria, confirming the high prevalence found in the Swedish study (18).

Whereas the Scandinavian studies estimated the prevalence of primary Sjögren's syndrome mainly in middle-aged subjects, a population-based study in Beijing, involving 2,060 individuals, estimated the prevalence of primary Sjögren's syndrome in a younger population older than 16 years. By using the Copenhagen criteria, the prevalence of primary Sjögren's syndrome was estimated to be 0.77%, whereas the prevalence was 0.29% by using the California criteria (21). The results of this study were limited because none of the participants agreed to have a biopsy of the minor salivary glands. With the European criteria, the prevalence of primary Sjögren's syndrome in 837 women aged 18 years or older in a closed Greek rural community was studied (22). The classification criteria for definite Sjögren's syndrome were satisfied by five women, corresponding to an estimated prevalence of 0.60%, whereas probable primary Sjögren's syndrome was diagnosed in 2.99% of the women (22). The women with definite Sjögren's syndrome were older than 60 years, and none had signs or symptoms of extraglandular manifestations. These women had mild complaints of dry eyes and mouth for several years but were not aware of the disease.

Several studies have estimated the prevalence of primary Sjögren's syndrome in elderly subjects. In the elderly, there are several reasons for dryness of the eye and mouth, such as diabetes and use of drugs affecting the glandular secretions. The prevalence of dry-mouth symptoms has been shown to increase with age, especially in women, and correlates with decreased salivary production (23). In a population of 103 white women with an average age of 81 years, 39% had sicca symptoms, and 24% had an abnormal Schirmer's tear test, whereas 2% satisfied criteria for primary Sjögren's syndrome, and 12% were thought to have possible Sjögren's syndrome (24). In a Greek study of nursing home residents older than 65 years, four (6.5%) of 62 persons could be classified as having primary Sjögren's syndrome, and the authors concluded that Sjögren's syndrome in elderly people is subclinical, benign, and relatively common (25).

The peak incidence of primary Sjögren's syndrome is in the forties (26), and the preliminary results from a study performed on subjects in their forties in Bergen, Norway, suggested a prevalence of 0.60% for definite primary Sjögren's syndrome, and 2.77% for probable primary Sjögren's syndrome (unpublished observations). These estimates were based on the presence of at least three items in the European criteria including questionnaires about dry eyes and mouth, Shirmer I test, and the collection of unstimulated whole saliva.

The prevalence studies demonstrate that sicca symptoms and primary Sjögren's syndrome affect a considerable portion of the population, influenced by the age group studied and by the criteria used. However, one must keep in mind the distinction between criteria used for classification and the criteria used in daily practice for diagnostic purposes. Subjects identified as having primary Sjögren's syndrome in population studies often have mild to moderate complaints, and many of them have been found to be unaware of the disease.

CLINICAL FEATURES

Sjögren's syndrome expresses a varied clinical spectrum, extending from an organ-specific autoimmune exocrinopathy to a systemic disease affecting several organs. The disease is characterized by insidious onset, with dry eyes and mouth as the most common clinical presentation in adults. The patients may often have difficulty in specifying the time of the onset of the disease (27,28). Sjögren's syndrome is rare in children, and bilateral parotid swelling may be the most common sign at onset (29) and during the course (30). The disease manifestations are not influenced by age (27) or sex (31), but several studies have demonstrated that young adults with primary Sjögren's syndrome have a higher frequency of autoantibodies than do middle-aged and elderly patients, indicating a more active immunologic disease (27,32–34). It has been demonstrated that younger-aged patients with primary Sjögren's syndrome, diagnosed according to the European criteria, had a higher prevalence of lymphadenopathy and monoclonal immunoglobulins, and higher incidence of lymphomas than did patients with later onset (33).

There are currently no measures of disease activity in primary Sjögren's syndrome, but a model for grading disease manifestations according to their clinical significance has recently been proposed (35). By using this model, quantitative and qualitative assessment of organ involvement in primary Sjögren's syndrome at specific, group, and global levels can be performed, giving a detailed analysis of the clinical presentation of Sjögren's syndrome. A damage index for primary Sjögren's syndrome also has been proposed (36).

Sicca Manifestations

Oral dryness is caused mainly by a decrease in the flow of saliva, but qualitative changes also should be considered. As saliva plays an important role in mastication and in the maintenance of the oral soft and hard tissues, reduction of saliva may result in changes in the oral cavity and its functions. These changes may result in an increased incidence of dental caries, predominantly located on the cervical and incisal surfaces (37); dysphagia (38); angular cheilitis, abnormalities of taste and smell; fissures of the tongue and lips; and difficulty with chewing and phonation (Fig. 85.1). In about one third of the patients, chronic erythematous oral candidiasis may be present (39), and this complication is even more common in patients taking steroids. These oral manifestations cause considerable disability and are the second most common subjective sign leading to consultation after keratoconjunctivitis sicca (28).

Dryness also may affect the upper respiratory tract, causing hoarseness, dryness of the nose, bronchitis, and pneumonitis. Dryness of the skin may be a result of decreased secretory capacity of the sebaceous and sweat glands.

Oral and ocular complaints tend to be more severe in patients whose onset occurs late in life (28). The ocular symptoms are caused by both reduced tear flow and a qualitative change of the mucinous tear secretions. These changes may induce decreased tear film stability, resulting in a rapid tear break-up time. The symptoms associated with dry eyes often are nonspecific, such as foreign-body sensation in the eyes ("gritty" or "sandy" feeling), burning eyes, decreased tearing, photosensitivity, itching, blepharitis, and fluctuating vision. These symptoms typically are reported by patients with primary Sjögren's syndrome, but they also may be reported in other conditions and in healthy individuals. Long-standing, severely reduced tear flow may eventually be complicated by corneal ulceration, vascularization, and corneal opacification.

Decrease in ocular tear flow and saliva production can occur as a consequence of aging, and also occur in patients who are taking medications with anticholinergic side effects, such as antidepressants.

Enlargement of the parotid (Fig. 85.2) and/or submandibular glands is apparent in about one third to half of patients with primary Sjögren's syndrome. Usually the glands are firm and nontender, and the swelling commonly fluctuates. A rapid increase of salivary gland size or pain should suggest the possibility of a retrograde infection caused by the normal bacterial flora of the oral cavity or a sialolith. Long-standing swelling or a hard or nodular gland should suggest a neoplasm. In a recent European study of malignant lymphoma in primary Sjögren's syndrome patients, the majority (84%) of non-Hodgkin's lymphoma patients with primary Sjögren's syndrome had bilateral parotid gland enlargement (40). Salivary gland involvement can occur in diseases other than Sjögren's syndrome, such as sarcoidosis, amyloidosis, and infections with accompanying inflammation.

Up to half of the female patients complain about vaginal dryness, and 45% have dyspareunia (26). This problem, which can be eradicated by treatment of infections and with topical lubricants, seems to be underdiagnosed by physicians (41).

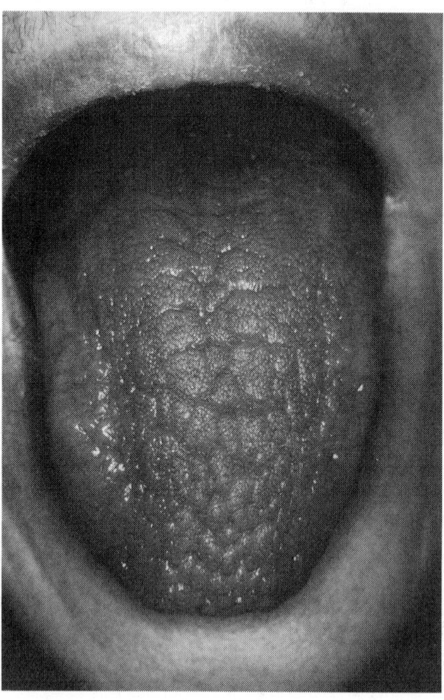

FIGURE 85.1. Oral dryness illustrated by severe dry tongue and lips in Sjögren's syndrome.

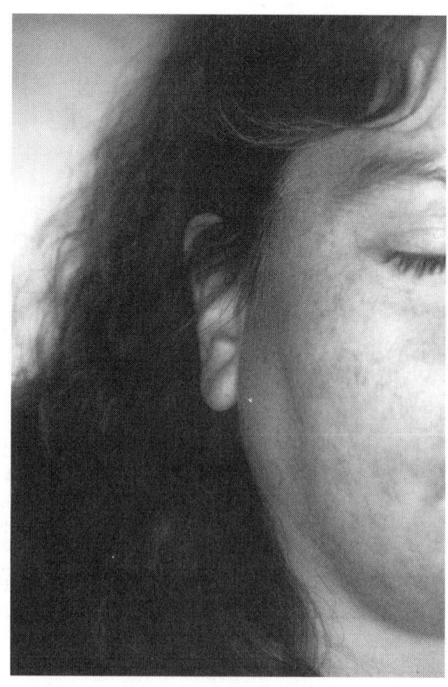

FIGURE 85.2. Parotid gland enlargement in Sjögren's syndrome.

Systemic Manifestations

Patients with primary Sjögren's syndrome experience significant fatigue, regardless of age (26,28). Sleep disturbances may contribute to the fatigue associated with Sjögren's syndrome, as patients have difficulties both in initiating and maintaining sleep (42). Sleep disturbance also may be due to nocturia caused by excessive water intake during the daytime to reduce oral symptoms of dryness. Arthralgias and myalgias are other major symptoms, and are most severe in patients in whom disease started at an early age (28). Arthralgias are present primarily in the finger joints, and are usually present only periodically (43). However, arthritis may be observed in up to 18% of the patients (26), affecting knees, ankles, metacarpophalangeal joints, shoulders, and wrists. It is usually mild and fluctuating, and rarely results in joint deformity or erosions.

When the main symptoms are fatigue and arthralgia/myalgia, primary Sjögren's syndrome easily may be misdiagnosed as fibromyalgia. In addition, these two conditions may be overlapping, as the prevalence of fibromyalgia has been reported to be as high as as 6.9% for probable and 11.0% for possible Sjögren's syndrome (44). However, in a study of 80 patients with Sjögren's syndrome, fibromyalgia was diagnosed in only about 5% of patients (A. Giles and D. Isenberg, personal communication, 1999).

Raynaud's phenomenon is a common extraglandular disease manifestation present in 54% of patients with Sjögren's syndrome diagnosed according to the European criteria (27), and up to 84% of patients diagnosed according to a modified version of the California criteria (45).

Lung Involvement

The most common forms of lung involvement in Sjögren's syndrome are tracheobronchitis sicca, bronchitis/bronchiolitis, and interstitial pulmonary fibrosis. In a longitudinal study of patients with primary Sjögren's syndrome in England, chest symptoms were common, with the highest frequency being 68% in Ro/SSA- and La/SSB- positive patients with Sjögren's syndrome (45). Involvement of the bronchial glands by the inflammatory process may result in drying of secretions causing tracheobronchitis sicca and dry cough. Periodic dry cough is reported by 54% of patients with primary Sjögren's syndrome (26), and has been reported to be the only pulmonary symptom in 17% of patients (46). Dry cough also may be the presenting complaint of patients with pulmonary fibrosis and pulmonary lymphoma. The frequency of dyspnea in large cross-sectional studies of patients with Sjögren's syndrome varies from 25% to 40% (46–48), and this symptom is usually closely related to abnormal pulmonary function. Abnormal lung function has been reported in 24% of patients with Sjögren's syndrome (48), and most authors have reported a predominantly restrictive pattern (46,47,49).

Pleural disease is uncommon (50) and may coexist with other lung disease. Lung fibrosis has been reported in 7% to 8% of patients with Sjögren's syndrome (51,52), and the main symptom is dyspnea. In the early stages, high-resolution computed tomography is suitable for detection of pulmonary fibrosis, whereas standard chest radiographs will usually detect advanced fibrosis.

A variety of lymphoproliferative disorders can be found in the lungs of patients with Sjögren's syndrome. "Pseudolymphoma" has been used to describe nodular lymphocytic infiltrates, whereas diffuse infiltrates consisting mainly of plasma cells are given the term lymphocytic interstitial pneumonitis. Lymphocytic interstitial pneumonitis has been described in five of 18 patients with Sjögren's syndrome (53), whereas lymphoma in the lung was found in two of 33 patients with Sjögren's syndrome and lymphoma (40). Patients with lymphoma and pseudolymphoma may be asymptomatic, but dyspnea and dry cough are the most frequent symptoms (54).

Pulmonary hypertension is an uncommon complication in patients with Sjögren's syndrome (55). The clinical, pathologic, radiographic, and physiologic characteristics of lung disease in the setting of Sjögren's syndrome and sarcoidosis can be very similar, and the pulmonary involvement in these two conditions may coexist and be difficult to distinguish (56).

Renal Involvement

When the kidney is involved in primary Sjögren's syndrome, renal histopathology mainly shows tubulointerstitial nephritis with interstitial infiltration by lymphocytes, tubular atrophy, and fibrosis (57,58). An important sign of tubular dysfunction is distal renal tubular acidosis, which is common in patients with Sjögren's syndrome (59–62). In distal renal tubular acidosis, the distal tubule exhibits diminished hydrogen ion transport, resulting in potassium depletion and acidosis. Distal renal tubular acidosis is associated with an inability to reduce the urine pH below 5.5 and hypocitraturia, both of which represent risk factors for the development of urolithiasis. Proximal renal tubular acidosis is characterized by an abnormality in resorption of bicarbonate by the proximal nephron, whereas the hydrogen ion transport at the distal nephron is normal (63). In summary, renal tubular acidosis is characterized by hyperchloremic acidosis and an inability to excrete a highly acidic urine. In addition to renal tubular acidosis, interstitial nephritis may present clinically as hyposthenuria (58,60) and the rare Fanconi syndrome (64). The prevalence of renal tubular acidosis in patients with Sjögren's syndrome has been reported to be between 22% and 30% (60,61), and many of these cases were latent and detected only after acid-loading test. By studying Sjögren's syndrome patients diagnosed according to the European criteria, our group has recently found a much lower prevalence of distal renal tubular acidosis of 11.3% (K. Aasarød et al., unpublished observations, 1999).

Glomerulonephritis is uncommon in patients with Sjögren's syndrome and has been described mainly in case reports (58,65). The pathogenesis may be associated with immune complex deposition, cryoglobulinemia, and macroglobulinemia.

Bladder symptoms are a common and poorly understood feature of Sjögren's syndrome and include frequency of micturition, nocturia, urgency, and incomplete bladder emptying. Bladder biopsy may reveal interstitial cystitis (66).

The Nervous System

Peripheral neuropathy occurs in Sjögren's syndrome, and the most common manifestation is sensory polyneuropathy involving mainly the lower extremities, whereas sensorimotor polyneuropathy and polyradiculoneuropathy are less common (67). Understanding of the pathogenesis is incomplete, but nonspecific epineural inflammation has been demonstrated in 70% of nerve biopsies, whereas vasculitic neuropathy is uncommon (67). Peripheral neuropathy has been reported in 10% to 20% of patients with Sjögren's syndrome (68,69).

Cranial nerve involvement may be peripheral or central. Episodic unilateral or bilateral numbness or paraesthesia in the distribution of the maxillary and/or mandibular division of the trigeminal nerve is the most well recognized cranial nerve syndrome (68). This cranial nerve syndrome can exacerbate sicca symptoms and increase the risk of corneal ulceration, and has been reported to alter taste perception (70). Entrapment syndromes in the carpal, ulnar, and tarsal distribution are common, even in the absence of synovitis.

Major central nervous system involvement is rare. The clinical manifestations of central nervous system disease are focal deficits such as hemiparesis, hemisensory deficits, seizure disorders, and movement disorders (71). Diffuse manifestations include encephalopathy and aseptic meningoencephalitis (72,73). Progressive dementia in primary Sjögren's syndrome has been reported, and was treated successfully with high-dose prednisone (120 mg/day orally) (74). The spinal cord may be involved in Sjögren's syndrome central nervous system disease, and transverse myelitis, neurogenic bladder, chronic progressive myelopathy, and Brown–Sequard syndrome, mimicking multiple sclerosis, have been reported (75). Cerebral white matter lesions detected by magnetic resonance imaging (MRI) were significantly more frequent in patients with primary Sjögren's syndrome than in age- and sex-matched control subjects, yet did not appear to be associated with significant clinical manifestations (76).

Patients with primary Sjögren's syndrome may have signs of vagal (parasympathetic) nerve disturbances (77), as indicated by low E/I ratio (heart-rate reaction due to deep breathing), which is a sensitive test of vagal neuropathy.

Gastrointestinal Involvement

Gastrointestinal complaints are common in patients with primary Sjögren's syndrome, but few have severe problems, and it is rarely the first symptom of the disease (28). Difficulty in swallowing is a frequent problem, however, and may be due to decreased saliva production (78) or abnormal esophageal motility (79). One study has shown that esophageal dysfunction is altered in approximately one third of patients with primary Sjögren's syndrome (80).

Dyspepsia is common, and gastric biopsies have shown chronic atrophic gastritis and lymphocytic infiltrates mainly of T lymphocytes (81–84). These changes may be associated with decreased volume and acid content of gastric secretions (82), reduced level of pepsinogen, and elevated serum gastrin (85,86).

Acute pancreatitis is rare in patients with Sjögren's syndrome, but moderately increased levels of serum amylase have been described in 24% of patients and may indicate a subclinical pancreatitis (87). A state of hyposecretion with decreased volume of exocrine secretion in response to secretin has been reported (88), and a deficient secretion of pancreatic juice and bicarbonate also has been noted in patients with Sjögren's syndrome (89). Pancreatic insufficiency seen as diabetes mellitus or malabsorption is uncommon, however.

Various forms of chronic liver diseases have been associated with primary Sjögren's syndrome. In a total of 63 patients with chronic liver disease, the "sicca complex" was detected in 42% of patients with chronic active hepatitis, 72% of patients with primary biliary cirrhosis, and 38% of those with nonspecific cirrhosis, whereas none were detected in the group with alcoholic cirrhosis (90). Clinical or biochemical evidence of liver disease is found in 5% to 10% of patients with Sjögren's syndrome (91,92). Usually the liver enzymes are only moderately increased and without clinical significance, but when the biochemical liver dysfunction is associated with the presence of antimitochondrial antibodies, primary biliary cirrhosis should be suspected. Primary biliary cirrhosis is the liver disease most closely associated with Sjögren's syndrome.

Cutaneous Manifestations

Allergic drug eruptions are common in primary Sjögren's syndrome, and it has been reported that 18% of patients diagnosed according to the European criteria are allergic to penicillin, whereas 15% are allergic to sulfur compounds (26). It has been shown that at least one manifestation of allergic manifestation was seen in 65% of patients with primary Sjögren's syndrome, and drug allergy and skin-contact allergy were found to be more prevalent than in the control groups (93). Vasculitis is often seen clinically as hypergammaglobulinemic purpura that occurs symmetrically in the lower extremities, often being indistinguishable from the lesions of Waldenström's benign hypergammaglobulinemia (94). This purpura may be precipitated by physical activity and alcohol, and repeated rashes may give a brownish discoloration of the skin on the legs.

Leukocytoclastic vasculitis is often associated with the presence of cryoglobulins in the sera of patients with primary Sjögren's syndrome, together with hypocomplementemia and hepatitis C virus (HCV) infection (95).

Endocrine Disturbances

Thyroid disorders have been reported in association with Sjögren's syndrome. A recent study confirmed that thyroid disorders are more common in primary Sjögren's syndrome than in patients with RA and healthy controls (96). Thyroid gland dysfunction and/or presence of antithyroid antibodies were noted in 28.9% of the patients with primary Sjögren's syndrome. It was found that 17.6% of the patients had antimicrosomal antibodies, and patients with both primary Sjögren's syndrome and RA were more likely to have antithyroglobulin antibodies (13.4% and 10.9%, respectively). The prevalence of hypothyroidism was more common among primary Sjögren's syndrome patients than in patients with RA (13.4% vs. 3.1%). Another study concluded that, compared with the population at large, the prevalence of primary Sjögren's syndrome was increased ten-fold in patients with autoimmune thyroiditis, and the prevalence of autoimmune thyroiditis was increased ninefold in patients with Sjögren's syndrome (97).

In a recent study, it was found that patients with Sjögren's syndrome have moderately increased levels of serum prolactin compared to controls, and this difference was especially evident in patients diagnosed at a young age with active immunologic disease (98). Prolactin is an immunomodulatory pituitary hormone that may be of pathogenic importance in autoimmune diseases. A high level of prolactin may precede the development of Sjögren's syndrome by several years (98).

AUTOANTIBODIES IN DIAGNOSIS AND PATHOGENESIS

Several autoantibodies have been reported in both primary and secondary Sjögren's syndrome, reflecting both B-cell activation and a loss of immune tolerance in the B-cell compartment in these conditions. Over the past few years, there have been significant advances in defining the fine specificity of these antibodies and characterizing their target autoantigens. In some cases, the antibodies are correlated with the extent and severity of disease in Sjögren's syndrome and are potentially involved in the pathogenic process of the autoimmune exocrinopathy.

Anti-Ro and Anti-La

The linked non–organ-specific autoantibodies anti-Ro/SSA and anti-La/SSB (see Chapter 74) are the most clinically important and best characterized autoantibodies in primary Sjögren's syndrome. The Ro autoantigen was first found as a precipitin in Ouchterlony assay and later shown to be a 60-kd protein existing as a ribonucleoprotein complex with four small hY (human cytoplasmic) RNA molecules (13,99,100). Sera with anti-Ro precipitins preferentially react with the native 60-kd Ro molecule (101), with some sera reacting additionally with continuous epitopes mapped with recombinant Ro60 fragments (102). The majority of anti–Ro-positive sera also react with the denatured form of a 52-kd protein termed Ro52, which is structurally distinct protein from Ro60 and probably does not directly associate with the Ro ribonucleoprotein particle (103,104). However, the two Ro proteins co-localize to surface membrane blebs on apoptotic cells, where they may become targets of an autoimmune response (105). Human monoclonal antibodies reactive with continuous and conformation-dependent epitopes on Ro52 have recently been cloned from a patient with primary Sjögren's syndrome (106).

Anti-La/SSB antibodies were first defined by immunodiffusion in association with anti-Ro60 precipitins (13). Recent studies have shown that up to 40% of anti–La-positive sera are negative on immunodiffusion and detectable only by immunoblot or enzyme-linked immunosorbent assay (ELISA). These are termed nonprecipitating anti-La antibodies (99,107). The 47-kd La molecule associates with a variety of small RNAs derived from RNA polymerase III, including the Ro hY RNAs as well as viral RNAs, and appears to be a transcription termination factor for RNA polymerase (108,109). Anti-La are invariably accompanied by anti-Ro, reflecting the physical association of these molecules in Ro/La ribonucleoprotein particles, but anti-Ro frequently occurs in the absence of anti-La. B-cell epitope mapping experiments have shown that precipitating anti-La antibodies are polyclonal and recognize three immunodominant epitopes located at the amino-terminus, the RNA recognition motif in the middle of the molecule, and the carboxy-terminus (110,111,112). Conversely, nonprecipitating anti-La antibodies show a more restricted epitope recognition with sparing of the carboxy-terminal epitope (107).

The reported frequencies of anti-Ro and anti-La depend on the methods of detection and the referral bias of the center performing the study. Overall, anti-Ro precipitins occur in approximately 60% to 75% of patients with primary Sjögren's syndrome and also are observed in cases of secondary

Sjögren's syndrome whether the associated disease is SLE, progressive systemic sclerosis, RA, or primary biliary cirrhosis (113). Anti-La autoantibodies were initially reported to occur in up to 40% of patients with primary Sjögren's syndrome, and at higher frequencies when measured by ELISA or immunoblotting (114). The association of antibodies to La or Ro with symptoms of dry eyes, xerostomia, and a positive rose bengal staining or Schirmer's test has a sensitivity and specificity of 94% for primary Sjögren's syndrome (15). Further studies have shown that anti-La (with anti-Ro) antibodies have a higher diagnostic specificity for primary Sjögren's syndrome than does anti-Ro alone (115). Various correlations between Ro52 and Ro60 epitope recognition in Sjögren's syndrome and SLE have been reported, but the results are conflicting and not sufficiently discriminating to be of diagnostic value (116). Occasional patients with primary Sjögren's syndrome can have serum anti-Ro52 antibodies in the absence of antibodies to Ro60 and La. These monospecific anti-Ro52 sera are negative when tested by routine immunodiffusion, and are detected by using recombinant Ro52 on ELISA or immunoblot (117,118).

Considerations regarding the pathogenetic role of anti-Ro and anti-La in Sjögren's syndrome include (a) their association with a high frequency of palpable purpura, leukopenia, lymphopenia, and hypergammaglobulinemia, and with more severe salivary gland disease (119–121); (b) surface expression of La on conjunctival cells and an aberrant expression pattern of La in labial salivary glands of patients with Sjögren's syndrome (122,123); (c) salivary enrichment of anti-Ro and anti-La in patients with Sjögren's syndrome, suggesting local production in salivary glands (124,125); and (d) presence of Ro52, Ro60, and La autoantibody-producing cells in salivary gland biopsy samples from patients with Sjögren's syndrome (126,127).

B-cell epitopes on the Ro and La antigens can be mapped by using recombinant protein fragments or short synthetic peptides, with the latter mimicking linear determinants on the surface of native proteins. Both types of antigenic probes are required to determine the major and minor epitopes on these autoantigens (102). This knowledge may lead to the design of refined diagnostic tools, and such peptides may be useful in immunomodulation of the autoimmune response.

Recent studies in a model of murine experimental autoimmunity have shown that reciprocal spreading to the Ro52, Ro60, and La polypeptides occurs after immunization with a single component. This intermolecular epitope spreading suggests that there is little or no tolerance to Ro and La in the B-cell compartment and limited tolerance in the T-cell compartment (128–131). Other studies have reported that the response also spreads to molecular chaperones and the Sm and U1RNP antigens, suggesting the presence of cross-reactive determinants on these molecules and Ro60 (132,133).

Anti–La-positive sera give a speckled antinuclear antibody (ANA) pattern on cultured cells, whereas sera with anti-Ro60 alone may be ANA negative because of the low abundance and variable expression of the Ro60 antigen. This problem may be overcome by using HEp-2 cells, which overexpress the human Ro60 protein, as a substrate (134).

Other Autoantibodies

Antithyroid microsomal and antigastric parietal cell antibodies occur in about one third of patients with both primary and secondary Sjögren's syndrome, but other organ-specific antibodies are infrequent (135). Anti–salivary duct antibodies were described more than 30 years ago as an organ-specific antibody in Sjögren's syndrome but have remained poorly characterized, and their clinical significance is uncertain. It appears that these antibodies are relatively uncommon in primary Sjögren's syndrome and are seen more often in RA with secondary Sjögren's syndrome; however, there is considerable variability in reported frequency of anti–salivary duct antibodies in Sjögren's syndrome, possibly reflecting technical problems with the indirect immunofluorescence assay on salivary gland substrate (136,137).

Several other autoantibodies have been reported to be present frequently in the sera of patients with primary Sjögren's syndrome including antibodies directed against carbonic anhydrase (138,139), proteasomal subunits (140), and α-fodrin (141). These results are intriguing but await independent confirmation in larger groups of Sjögren's syndrome patients. Antiphospholipid antibodies of the immunoglobulin A (IgA) isotype were reported in 20% of patients with primary Sjögren's syndrome, but were not associated with clinical manifestations of antiphospholipid syndrome (142). The finding of serum autoantibodies directed against the muscarinic M3 receptor (expressed in salivary and lacrimal glands) in the majority of patients is an important advance in understanding the pathogenesis of impaired glandular function in Sjögren's syndrome (143,144). Recent studies in the nonobese diabetic (NOD) mouse have indicated that muscarinic receptor autoantibodies are directed against the agonist binding site of the molecule on the cell surface and interfere with secretory function of exocrine tissues in Sjögren's syndrome (145). The clinical significance of these antibodies in Sjögren's syndrome remains to be elucidated.

Rheumatoid factor (RF) (see Chapter 61) is found in the serum and saliva of 60% to 80% of primary Sjögren's syndrome patients (146,147). There appears to be little role for somatic hypermutation in their generation, in contrast to RF in patients with RA (148). A significant number of patients with primary Sjögren's syndrome have mixed monoclonal cryoglobulins containing an IgM monoclonal RF (149). The latter frequently possess cross-reactive idiotypes, notably the 17.109 (VκIIIb) and G-6 (VH1 related) idiotypes, which may serve as markers for lymphoma development in primary Sjögren's syndrome (150,151).

GENETICS

A role for genetic factors in the pathogenesis of Sjögren's syndrome is suggested by a strong tendency toward familial aggregation and the presence of autoantibodies and other autoimmune diseases in family members (152). However, apart from the influence of the major histocompatibility complex (MHC) on autoantibody production, little is known about the genetics of Sjögren's syndrome. Genetic studies in primary Sjögren's syndrome twins have not been performed, and only a few case reports describing twins have been published (153,154). Considerable effort has been put into the collection of data on affected families by the European Concerted Action on Sjögren's syndrome group, and linkage analysis with microsatellite genetic markers and candidate gene analysis is expected within the next few years (155).

The development of primary Sjögren's syndrome is strongly associated with MHC class II genes, most specifically human leukocyte antigen (HLA)-DR and -DQ alleles. Because of the strong linkage disequilibrium between these alleles, it has not been possible to determine whether the disease association is primarily with DR or DQ alleles. The HLA-mediated risk appears to be more strongly linked with the anti-Ro/La antibody response rather than with the disease itself. In white populations, the HLA class II associations with primary Sjögren's syndrome can be adequately described in terms of HLA-DR2, -DR3, or -DR5, or alternatively, DQA1*0102 or DQA1*0501. Both HLA-DR3 and HLA-DR5 have been reported to be associated with primary Sjögren's syndrome in different populations, and as both these alleles are in linkage disequilibrium with DQA1*0501, this DQA1 allele has been implicated as the common HLA risk factor for primary Sjögren's syndrome (156–160). Recently, the DR3-DQ2 haplotype has been correlated with the degree of anti-Ro/La antibody diversification and implicated as a marker for a more active immune response in primary Sjögren's syndrome patients (161,162).

Studies of HLA haplotypes in multiplex families and differences between ethnic groups indicate that HLA-DR and -DQ alleles are probably not the primary disease-associated alleles. Several non-MHC genes that collectively may contribute to disease susceptibility and are presently under investigation in Sjögren's syndrome include cytokine genes and their promoters such as interleukin-10 (IL-10) and tumor necrosis factor-α (TNF-α); genes involved in innate immunity and clearance of immune complexes such as mannose-binding lectin, complement components, and Fcγ receptors; and genes and promoters involved in apoptosis such as Fas and its ligand, FasL. Mutations in TAP2 genes encoding transporters associated with antigen processing may be involved in anti-Ro antibody production in both primary Sjögren's syndrome and SLE and could be a genetic factor that determines susceptibility to Sjögren's syndrome (163,164). A few studies of small populations of patients with secondary Sjögren's syndrome suggest that the HLA associations may be with the associated disease. This issue requires clarification with DNA-typing techniques on larger populations (135).

DIAGNOSIS AND DIAGNOSTIC TESTS

The delay from start of symptoms to final diagnosis has been reported to be as long as 11 years for primary Sjögren's syndrome (26), probably illustrating the slow progression of the disease, but also low awareness of the disease among health personnel. Patients with undiagnosed Sjögren's syndrome usually see their physician because of nonspecific symptoms such as arthralgias, fatigue, and extraglandular complications associated with the disease, and the large variety of symptoms can be misinterpreted. Patients rarely report dry eyes and mouth spontaneously, and it is therefore important for their doctor to interview about mucosal dryness to be aware of the diagnosis.

There is no straightforward and simple diagnostic test for Sjögren's syndrome, and currently there are no universally accepted diagnostic criteria for the disease. However, there are several classification criteria designed for research purposes. The application of these classification criteria in the daily routine in the clinic is not always suitable, as they are based partly on theoretic considerations and the general opinions of experts in the field. Given the lack of diagnostic criteria, they are still widely used. During the last 15 years, several classification criteria have been suggested, notably the California (16), Japanese (165), Copenhagen (166), Greek, (167), and most recently, the European criteria (15). The latest European criteria from 1993 differ from the other criteria by the inclusion of a questionnaire to identify symptomatic dry eyes and dry mouth, thereby placing more emphasis on the patient's subjective complaints (Table 85.1). The criteria include six items, and the diagnosis is based on the presence of at least four of the items listed in Table 85.1. The criteria set has been tested on primary Sjögren's syndrome patients and non–Sjögren's syndrome controls, and the accuracy of the criteria for correctly classifying primary Sjögren's syndrome patients has been confirmed by sensitivity and specificity calculations (168). The European criteria may include up to 10 times more patients than the California criteria, however, and the European criteria have therefore been criticized for including patients without immunologically active disease (169). Initiatives have therefore been taken to propose a new set of classification criteria in a joint effort by the European and American research groups in this field. Nevertheless, an algorithm based on the European criteria (15) has been suggested for the diagnosis of Sjögren's syndrome (Fig. 85.3) (170).

TABLE 85.1. THE EUROPEAN PRELIMINARY CLASSIFICATION CRITERIA FOR PRIMARY SJÖGREN'S SYNDROME

I. Ocular symptoms: a positive response to at least one of three selected questions:
   1. Have you had daily, persistent, troublesome dry eyes for >3 months?
   2. Do you have recurrent sensation of sand or gravel in the eyes?
   3. Do you use tear substitutes >3 times a day?

II. Oral symptoms: a positive response to at least one of the three selected questions:
   1. Have you had a daily feeling of dry mouth for >3 months?
   2. Have you had recurrently or persistently swollen salivary glands as an adult?
   3. Do you frequently drink liquids to aid swallowing dry food?

III. Ocular signs: objective evidence of ocular involvement defined as a positive result in at least one of the following two tests:
   1. Schirmer's I test (≤5 mm/5 min)
   2. Rose bengal score (≥4 according to van Bijsterveld's scoring system)

IV. Histopathology: a focus score ≥1 per 4 mm^2 in minor salivary gland biopsy

V. Salivary gland involvement: objective evidence of salivary gland involvement defined by a positive result in at least one of the following three diagnostic tests:
   1. Salivary scintigraphy
   2. Parotid sialography
   3. Unstimulated salivary flow (≤1.5 mL/15 min)

VI. Autoantibodies: presence of at least one of the following serum autoantibodies:
   1. Antibodies to Ro/SSA or La/SSB antigens
   2. Antinuclear antibodies
   3. Rheumatoid factor

Diagnosis of Sjögren's syndrome requires that at least four of six categories be present.

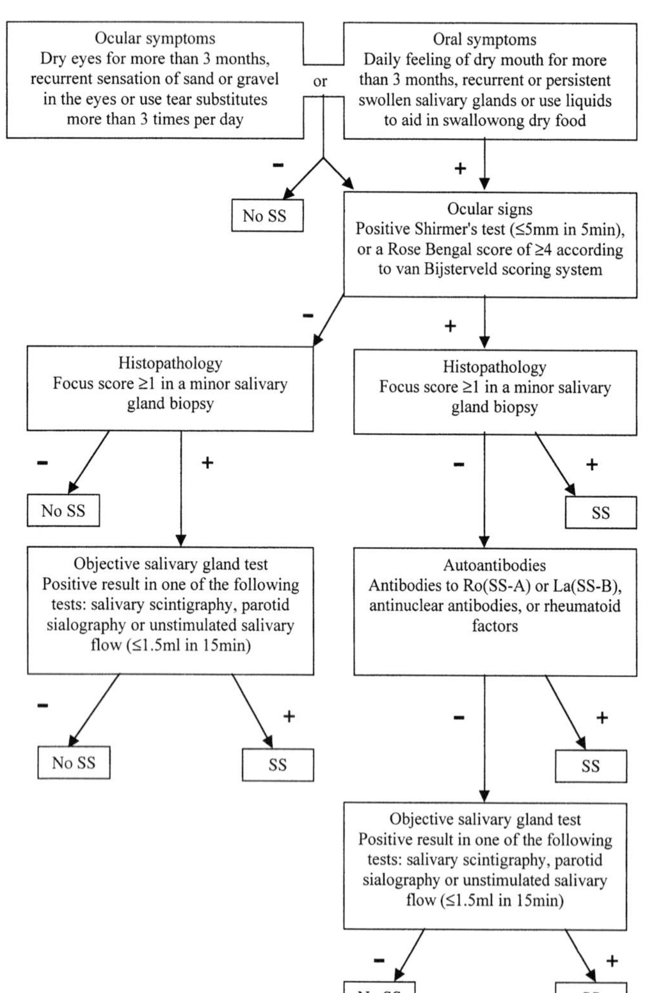

FIGURE 85.3. An algorithm for the diagnosis of Sjögren's syndrome based on the European criteria (From Vitali C, Bombardieri S, Moutsopoulos H, et al. Preliminary criteria for the classification of Sjögren's syndrome: results of a prospective concerted action supported by the European Community. *Arthritis Rheum* 1993;36:340–347; and Tzioufas AG, Moutsopoulos HM. Sjögren's syndrome. In: Klippel J, Dieppe P, eds. *Rheumatology.* London: Mosby, 1998:32:1–12, with permission).

Objective Evaluation of Sicca Symptoms

The most commonly used tests for the detection of dry eyes are the Schirmer I and the rose bengal score. Schirmer I is performed by using standardized tear test strips, placed for 5 minutes between the eyeball and the most lateral part of the inferior lid, without using anesthetic eyedrops. The patient sits in a resting position with the eyes closed, but not squeezed tight. After 5 minutes, the length of the damped area of the strip is measured, starting from the notch corresponding to the inferior lid margin. In the European classification criteria, the Schirmer I test is positive when the wetting is less than 5 mm/5 minutes. A positive Schirmer I test in patients with primary Sjögren's syndrome is highly reproducible in both eyes when retested after 1 year (84.2%), and the sensitivity of the test may increase by repeated testing (171).

Another test for keratoconjunctivitis sicca is the rose bengal score, detecting destroyed conjunctival epithelium induced by desiccation. The test is performed by placing 25 μL of Rose Bengal solution in the inferior fornix of each eye, and a slit-lamp is used for evaluating red spots resulting from destroyed epithelium. The red spots are counted and scored: 1 (sparsely scattered), 2 (densely scattered), or 3 (confluent). The red spots are counted in three different regions, the lateral and nasal conjunctiva and the cornea. If the sum of the scores is more than 4 in the three regions in at least one eye, the test is considered abnormal (172).

Saliva-production tests are simple screening tests for salivary gland involvement in Sjögren's syndrome. Saliva, which is produced by three major and numerous minor salivary glands, exhibits great flow variations among healthy individuals, and in the same individual under diverse conditions (173,174). The test should therefore be standardized to be performed in the morning or midmorning after the patient has been fasting overnight, and brushing of teeth, mouth rinsing, or tobacco smoking must be avoided the last 1 hour before the test is performed. The unstimulated whole saliva collection test is performed by collecting saliva for 15 minutes, and the test is considered positive when less than 1.5 mL whole saliva is collected, which is well below the normal mean range. A positive test in primary Sjögren's syndrome patients is found to be highly reproducible (84.2%) when repeated over a 1-year interval under standardized conditions (171). Moreover, this functional test has been shown to have a high specificity (80.7%) for patients with primary Sjögren's syndrome (172).

Other tests used to evaluate salivary gland involvement include parotid sialography and salivary gland scintigraphy. Sialography typically shows sialectasis in contrast to the fine arborization seen in normal parotid ductules. In the scintigraphic test, ^{99m}Tc-pertechnetate is given intravenously, and in patients with primary Sjögren's syndrome, the typical finding is decreased uptake and release in response to stimulation in the parotid and submandibular salivary glands. This test is a sensitive and valid method to measure abnormalities in salivary gland function in the hands of skilled personnel (175). The specificity of these two tests in patients with Sjögren's syndrome is 78.9% for salivary gland scintigraphy and 100% for parotid sialography, whereas the sensitivity is 87.2% and 78.6%, respectively (172).

The labial salivary gland biopsy has an important role in establishing the diagnosis of Sjögren's syndrome. It is performed preferentially according to the procedure described by Daniels (Fig. 85.4) (176,177). After local anesthesia, a 1.5- to 2-cm incision is made parallel to the vermilion border in the middle of the lower lip, between the midline and the corner of the mouth. At least five lobes of labial glands are then obtained by blunt dissection. After routine histologic fixation and preparation, the biopsy is evaluated according to a method in which a focus is defined as an accumulation of at least 50 inflammatory cells per 4 mm^2 (Fig. 85.5A) (177). According to the European criteria, a biopsy is positive if the focus score is more than or equal to one per 4 mm^2, whereas the California criteria define a positive biopsy as more than one focus per 4 mm^2. Occasionally epimyoepithelial islands are seen in labial gland biopsies (Fig. 85.5B), but these are more common in the major glands. One differential diagnostic feature is the presence of granulomatous inflammation, which is seen with sarcoidosis but not Sjögren's syndrome (Fig. 85.5C).

The specificity of a positive labial salivary gland biopsy is 86.2%, and the sensitivity is 82.4% in patients with primary Sjögren's syndrome diagnosed according to the European criteria (172). The focal infiltration of lymphoid cells in the salivary glands is a progressive process in Sjögren's syndrome, as demonstrated by an increase in the focus score over time (178). The focus score is associated with the presence of keratoconjunctivitis sicca and autoantibodies (179,180), whereas the correlation with xerostomia is less evident (178). Another pattern of inflammation in labial salivary gland biopsy is chronic sialadenitis, characterized

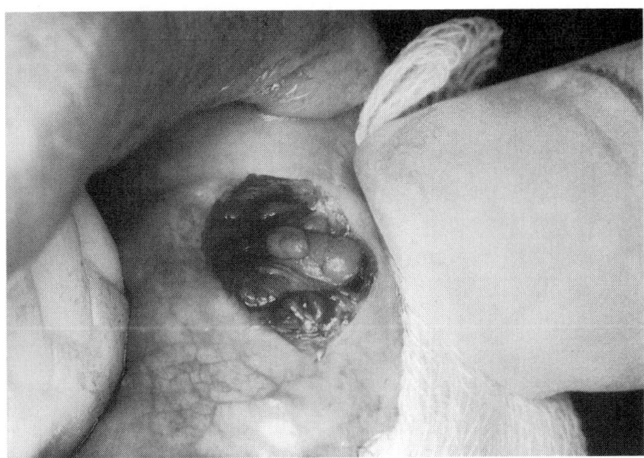

FIGURE 85.4. Labial salivary gland biopsy after initial incision through oral mucosa and blunt dissection, revealing individual minor salivary glands.

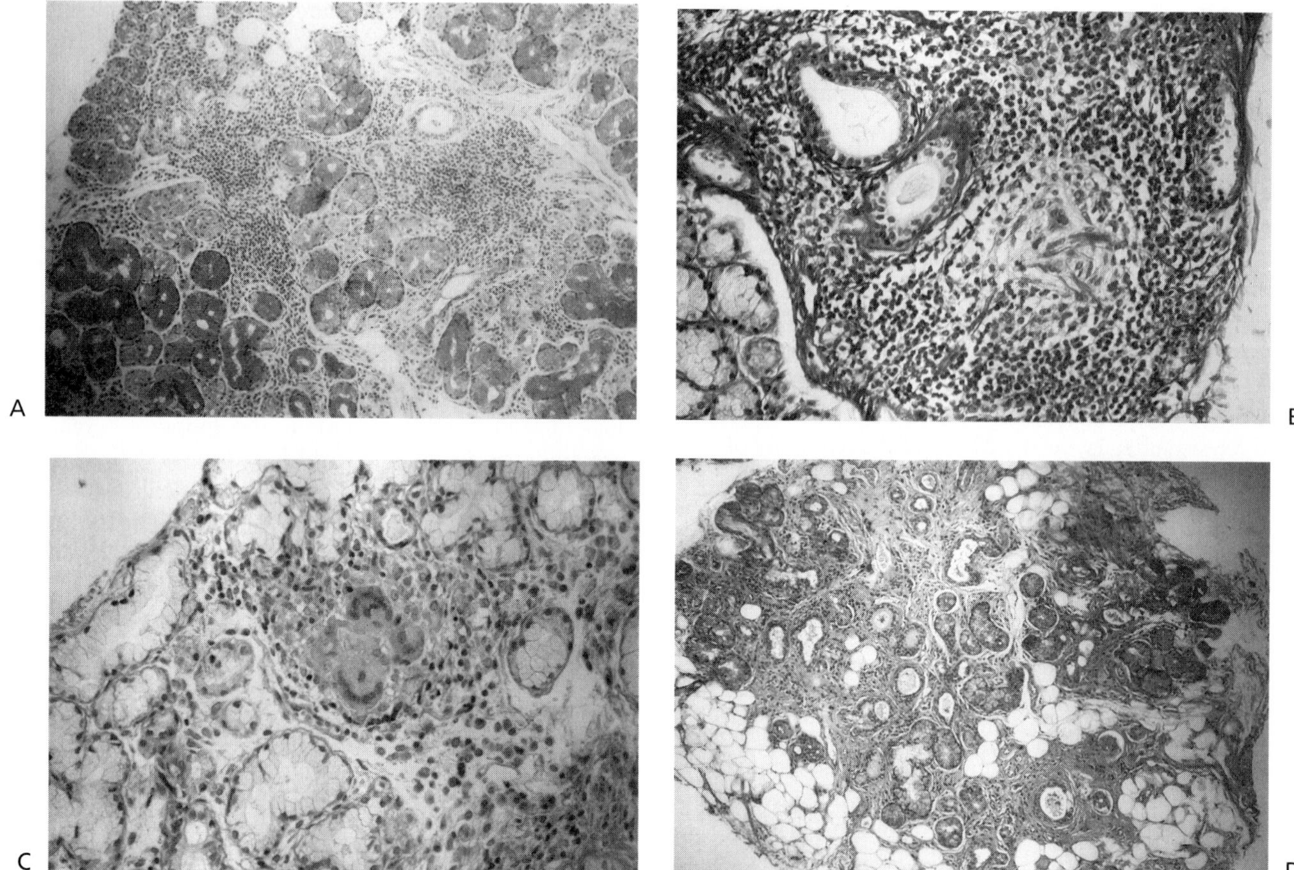

FIGURE 85.5. Histopathologic features in labial salivary gland biopsy specimens. **A:** Focal sialadenitis in a gland with normal-appearing parenchyma in a patient with Sjögren's syndrome. **B:** Epimyoepithelial island in Sjögren's syndrome. **C:** Granulomatous inflammation in sarcoidosis. **D:** Degenerative changes illustrated by parenchymal atrophy, fibrosis, some ductal hyperplasia, and fatty replacement.

by scattered mononuclear cell infiltration without focal aggregates and accompanied by degenerative changes (acinar atrophy, ductal hyperplasia, fibrosis and/or fatty infiltration; Fig. 85.5D). This pattern is not considered to be associated with primary Sjögren's syndrome, and often leads to glandular atrophy and xerostomia.

The presence of autoantibodies usually also is important for the diagnosis of Sjögren's syndrome. The titers of anti-Ro60, anti-Ro52, and anti-La have been shown to stay relatively stable over long periods in many patients with Sjögren's syndrome (181). In addition, the presence of ANA, anti-Ro, anti-La, and RF have been shown to be highly reproducible in Sjögren's syndrome when tested over a 1-year interval (171).

Routine laboratory tests usually yield little diagnostic information in primary Sjögren's syndrome. In 72 patients diagnosed according to the preliminary European criteria, it was found that 45.7% of the patients had a normal hemoglobin, erythrocyte sedimentating rate (ESR), C-reactive protein (CRP), and leukocyte count (Table 85.2) (26), which are the standard screening tests in general practice.

TABLE 85.2. PERCENTAGE DISTRIBUTION OF OBSERVED LABORATORY FINDINGS AND SEROLOGIC TESTS IN 72 PRIMARY SJÖGREN'S SYNDROME PATIENTS DIAGNOSED ACCORDING TO THE EUROPEAN CRITERIA

Finding	Percentage
Anemia (<13.2 g/100 mL men, <11.6 g/100 mL women)	12
Leukopenia (<4 × 10^9/L)	20
High ESR (>20 mm/h)	33
High CRP (>10 mg/L)	5
ANA	51
RF	44
Elevated serum IgG	44

ESR, erythrocyte sedimentation rate; CRP, C-reactive protein; ANA, antinuclear antibody; RF, rheumatoid factor; Ig, immunoglobulin. From Vitali C, Bombardieri S, Moutsopoulos H, et al. Preliminary criteria for the classification of Sjögren's syndrome: results of a prospective concerned action supported by the European community. *Arthritis Rheum* 1993;36:340–347, with permission.

Identification of new genetic markers and better characterization of novel autoantibodies (e.g., those directed against muscarinic receptors in exocrine glands) may lead to the development of better diagnostic and prognostic tests in Sjögren's syndrome. With regard to differential diagnosis, a number of conditions have to be considered (Table 85.3).

ETIOLOGY AND PATHOGENESIS

Etiologic Considerations

Interest in the relation between viruses and autoimmunity began some decades ago. However, the epidemiology of relevant viruses must be taken into consideration when interpreting the association between a virus and disease. Possible mechanisms related to Sjögren's syndrome whereby viruses might induce tolerance bypass include, among others, polyclonal activation of B cells and molecular mimicry between viral epitopes and autoantigens.

The potential etiologic role of different viruses in Sjögren's syndrome also might be explained by the fact that salivary glands are a site of latent infection by certain viruses. Sjögren's syndrome may result from an abnormal immune response to a ubiquitous virus, such as Epstein–Barr virus (EBV) (182). A higher prevalence of human herpesvirus-6 (HHV-6) antibodies also has been detected in patients with Sjögren's syndrome than in normal individuals (36% vs. 10%) (183). By contrast, some investigators found normal antibody prevalence to HHV-6 (184). Difficulties in analyzing the significance of these viruses is related to the high prevalence of both herpesviruses (EBV and HHV-6) in the normal population.

Retroviruses are known to infect cells of the immune system and cause abnormalities in immune regulation (185). High serum titers of antibodies directed against human T lymphotropic virus type I (HTLV-I) and a high prevalence of salivary IgA-class anti–HTLV-I antibodies in patients with Sjögren's syndrome have been reported (186).

HCV infection also has, in some populations, been frequently detected (14%) in patients with primary Sjögren's syndrome, and liver involvement was found to be present in all of these patients (187). Analysis of the association between chronic lymphocytic sialadenitis and chronic HCV liver disease showed that histologic features of Sjögren's syndrome were significantly more common in HCV-infected patients (57%) compared with controls (5%) (188).

The Ro/SSA and La/SSB autoantigens have been found to share sequence similarities with some viral proteins. It has been shown that there is a homology between six regions of the 60-kd Ro/SSA and the nucleocapsid protein of vesicular stomatitis virus (189). Some of the immunoreactive regions within the La/SSB protein have been found to have homology with proteins of EBV, HHV-6, and human immunodeficiency virus-1 (HIV-1) (190). It seems possible that these viruses might promote autoantibody production (particularly anti-La/SS-B) through molecular mimicry. However, it is important to remember that these homologies may simply have occurred by chance and be of no etiologic relevance.

TABLE 85.3. DIFFERENTIAL DIAGNOSIS IN SJÖGREN'S SYNDROME

Infections	Senile xerostomia
Influenza	Oral breathing
Mumps	Neurologic diseases
EBV	Cranial nerve V and VII involvement
HIV	Cystic fibrosis
Coxsackie virus	Drugs
HTLV-1	β-blockers
Cytomegalovirus	Psychotherapeutic
Streptococcus	Parasympatholytic
Staphylococcus	Phenylbutazone
Sarcoidosis	Irradiation
Tumors	Congenital
Amyloidosis	Ocular diseases
Metabolic/Endocrine	Chronic conjunctivitis
Chronic pancreatitis	Bullous dermatitis
Hepatic cirrhosis	Chronic blepharitis
Acromegaly	Graft-versus-host disease
Diabetes mellitus	
Hypovitaminosis A	
Chronic sialoadenitis	
Psychogenic	
Dehydration	

EBV, Epstein–Barr virus; HIV, human immunodeficiency virus; HTLV-1, human T-cell lymphotropic virus-1.

Not only viruses have been considered as etiologic candidates. More recently the presence of antibodies against *Helicobacter pylori* and its heat-shock protein 60 has been reported (191), and the possibility that such an infection might trigger a widespread clonal B-cell disorder in these patients has been postulated (192).

Another potential etiologic factor is the role of hormones, but the precise reason that it is principally women who have Sjögren's syndrome remains unclear.

Immunopathologic Features

Immunohistologic analysis of salivary gland lymphoid cell infiltrates in exocrine glands in Sjögren's syndrome shows a predominance of T cells (Fig. 85.6A) with fewer B cells, macrophages, and mast cells (135,170). Adhesion molecules including activated lymphocyte function–associated antigen type-1 (LFA-1) promote homing and occasional characteristic cell clustering similar to follicular structures of lymph nodes with evidence of antigen-driven clonal proliferation of B cells (193). Expression of the mucosal lymphocyte integrin $\alpha_E\beta_7$ and its ligand E-cadherin suggest a mucosal origin of a portion of the infiltrating cells (194). There is an aberrant and differentiated expression of HLA-DR/DP/DQ molecules on acinar and ductal epithelial cells

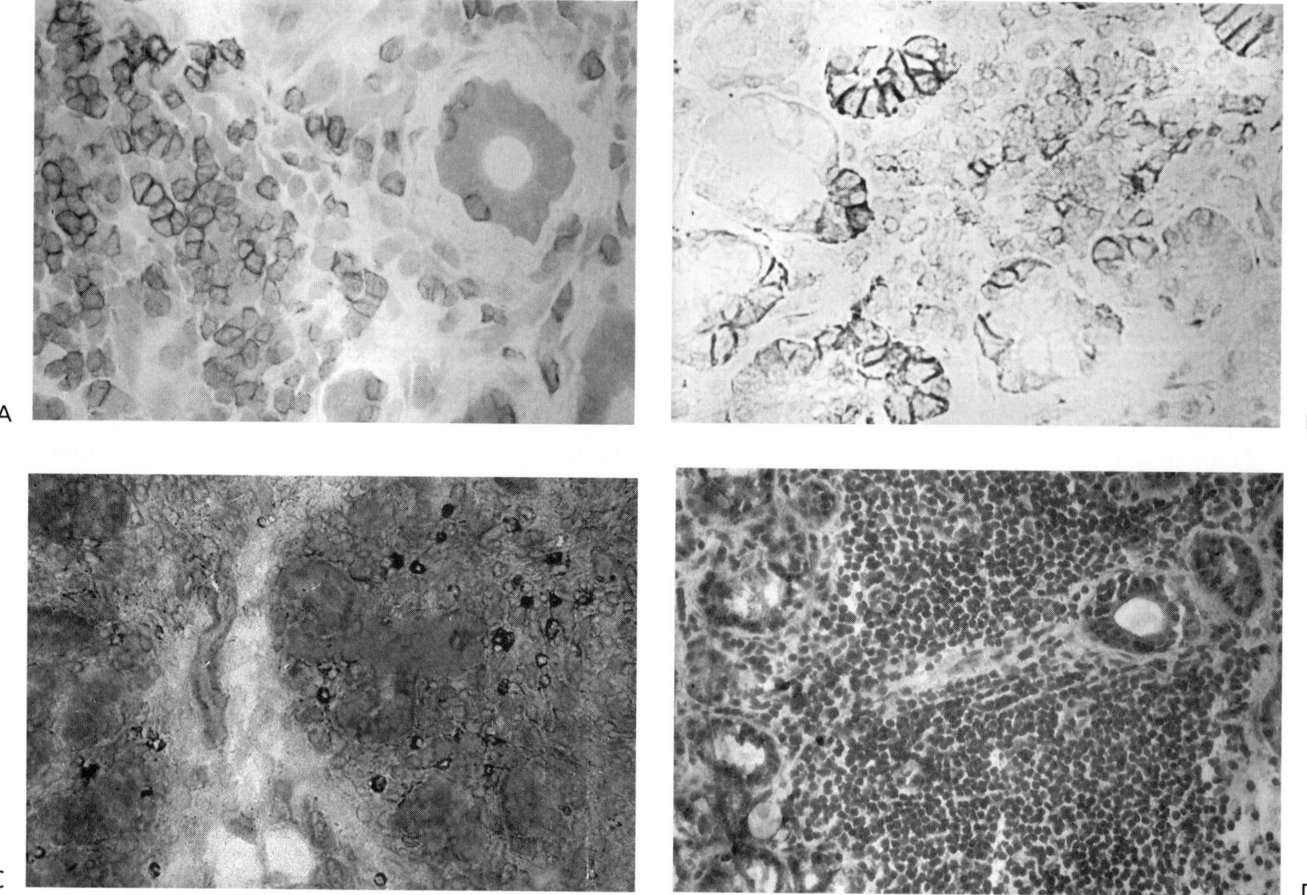

FIGURE 85.6. Immunohistologic features seen in labial salivary gland biopsy specimens from patients with Sjögren's syndrome. **A:** A large proportion of CD3-positive T cells in focal sialadenitis. **B:** Aberrant HLA-DR expression on glandular epithelium. **C:** Local anti-Ro production by individual B cells. **D:** Apoptosis detection by TUNEL; only a few cells are positively stained (<1%).

(195), presumably due to local production of interferon-γ (IFN-γ) by activated T cells. The majority of T cells in the lymphocytic infiltrates are $CD4^+$ T-helper cells with a CD4/CD8 ratio well over 2. Most of these T cells bear the memory phenotype $CD45RO^+$ and express the α/β T-cell receptor (TCR) and LFA-1, and may contribute significantly to B-cell hyperactivity. Some studies have indicated oligoclonal expansion of certain TCR Vβ family expressing lymphocytes (196). Natural killer cells are rarely observed in salivary gland infiltrates.

Aberrant expression of HLA molecules (Fig. 85.6B), and the more recently demonstrated B7 co-stimulatory molecules (197), by salivary gland epithelium in Sjögren's syndrome, suggests that these cells may function as nonprofessional antigen-presenting cells interacting with $CD4^+$ T cells. Such interaction may lead to further production of cytokines and stimulation of B-cell proliferation and differentiation. High levels of IL-1β, IL-6, and TNF-α are produced by epithelial cells, whereas IL-10 and IFN-γ are produced mainly by infiltrating T cells (135,170). IL-6 and IL-10 also are produced in increased amounts in peripheral blood (198). The low level of IL-2 observed in Sjögren's syndrome might be due to absence of T-cell co-stimulatory signals, resulting in the induction of anergy in the responding T-cell population, but other explanations are quite plausible.

B-cell activation is a consistent immunoregulatory abnormality in Sjögren's syndrome, in which the B cells make up roughly 20% of the infiltrating cell population in exocrine glands. The B cells produce increased amounts of immunoglobulins with autoantibody activity for IgG (RF), Ro, and La (Fig. 85.6C) (126). A substantial number of the B cells are $CD5^+$ (B-1 cells) (199). IgG is the predominant isotype expressed by the infiltrating B cells (127) in contrast to IgA, which dominates in normal salivary glands.

Among the infiltrating T cells, some express activation markers such as CD25, proto-oncogene products, and HLA-DR, but few T cells proliferate, as determined by cell-cycle studies and autoradiography. It has been difficult to stimulate the T lymphocytes in Sjögren's syndrome with the autoantigens Ro and La (200). This might suggest that memory T cells in the infiltrates may be semiactivated and engaged in low-grade responses to persisting antigen(s).

Immunologic studies of the peripheral blood of patients with primary Sjögren's syndrome have yielded findings similar to those in salivary glands, although a difference in magnitude is occasionally evident.

Role of Cell Destruction and Apoptosis

Even though the actual mechanism(s) behind the characteristic glandular destruction of Sjögren's syndrome salivary glands remains obscure, immunopathologic findings demonstrate that infiltrating cytotoxic T cells could play a major role in this event. On recognition of an appropriate MHC–antigen complex presented by a target cell, cytotoxic T cells induce cell death through one of two independent pathways, the perforin-mediated or the Fas-mediated pathway. In the Fas-mediated pathway, apoptotic death signals are transmitted to the target cell on cross-linkage of two cell-surface molecules, Fas ligand (FasL) on the cytotoxic T cell and Fas on the target cell. Fas (APO1 antigen, CD95) is a member of the TNF-α receptor family and is expressed constitutively or induced after activation on a variety of cell types, including epithelial cells (201). FasL, a type II transmembrane protein, is expressed in nonlymphoid sites such as the cornea and testis, and on activated T lymphocytes (202). Interestingly, signalling for apoptosis seems to be nonfunctional in salivary glands of autoimmune MRL/lpr mice since these mice are devoid of apoptotic cells among the infiltrating mononuclear cells (203).

Expression of Fas, FasL, Bcl-2, and other apoptosis-associated genes/proteins has been detected by reverse transcriptase–polymerase chain reaction (RT-PCR) and immunohistochemical staining of minor salivary glands from patients with Sjögren's syndrome (204,205). In particular, ductal and acinar epithelial cells, and to some extent infiltrating mononuclear cells, express abnormal levels of Fas and FasL in Sjögren's syndrome, especially in cases with severe mononuclear cell infiltration. Upregulation of different apoptosis-inducing/promoting molecules such as Fas and Bax (206) in ductal and acinar cells suggests that these cells are capable of undergoing apoptosis. Most *in situ* DNA nick-end-labeling (TUNEL) studies have clearly shown a low rate or even absence of apoptosis among infiltrating mononuclear cells (Fig. 85.6D) (204,205). Upregulated Bcl-2 expression has been detected which may contribute to the inhibition of apoptosis in these cells (206).

The presence of granzyme A in Sjögren's syndrome salivary glands (207) suggests that the perforin pathway of cytotoxic T-cell killing also may be involved in glandular destruction. However, there have been some contradictions concerning expression studies of apoptosis-associated genes, especially in acinar cells. In two preliminary studies of salivary gland apoptosis using several methods of tissue processing and apoptosis detection, no increase in acinar or ductal epithelial apoptosis was observed in patients with Sjögren's syndrome compared with healthy controls (208,209).

Glandular hypofunction, however, is not solely a result of glandular destruction because normal acinar cells may be observed in Sjögren's syndrome salivary glands, and lymphocytic glandular infiltration is not always accompanied by hyposalivation. Consequently, other mechanisms in addition to immunologic pathways are likely involved in the pathogenesis of the disease (210).

Animal Models

As noted previously, there are genetic associations that may predispose to Sjögren's syndrome, in particular, the genes encoding products of the MHC and immune receptors, but other candidate genes also are relevant. It is thus natural to seek more knowledge in genetically well-characterized, inbred, and controlled animal models that are available for study (211). In particular, the current challenge will be to find links between a particular genetic background and phenotypic expression(s).

Any proposed animal model should fulfill criteria and features found in the human disease. Moreover, the clinical symptoms of Sjögren's syndrome in humans usually appear relatively late in life, thus making examination of early events difficult. An animal model of the disease would make it possible to study earlier events and to identify potentially important immune reactions in the pathogenesis of this disease. Finally, both immune manipulation and the effects of drug therapy can be studied in animals (211).

The earlier reports on attempts to induce Sjögren's syndrome in animals by injection with salivary gland extracts, with or without adjuvants, largely produced a transient inflammation that was self-limiting and did not mirror the human disease in either the temporal course of events or in the serologic profile. The better models are mice with spontaneous autoimmune disease with long-lasting and progressive exocrinopathy, but even in these examples, the disorder has, at best, represented only secondary Sjögren's syndrome (211). Both anti-Ro (212) and anti-La (213) autoantibodies have been detected in spontaneous murine models. Because these autoantibodies are the dominant serologic markers in patients with primary Sjögren's syndrome, this finding is an important starting point for future work.

Interesting observations were made in the MRL/lpr mouse, in which the lpr genotype has been identified as a mutation in the gene encoding Fas. Apoptotic cells are absent or appear at very low frequency among the infiltrating mononuclear cells in salivary glands. Based on analysis of apoptotic activity, the T cells were rescued from apoptosis because of a failure in signaling (203).

To analyze Fas and TNF receptor I apoptosis pathways in inflammatory salivary gland disease induced by murine cytomegalovirus (MCMV) infection, different strains of mice were infected (214). Although acute salivary gland inflammation developed in all MCMV-infected mice, only one strain, the B6-lpr/lpr, showed chronic inflammation.

Apoptotic cells were detected during the acute but not the chronic phase of inflammation. Both Fas-mediated and TNF receptor I–mediated apoptosis was found to contribute to the clearance of MCMV-infected cells in salivary glands. However, because Fas-mediated apoptosis is necessary for the downmodulation of the immune response, a defect in this process can lead to a postinfectious, chronic inflammatory response that resembles Sjögren's syndrome.

In order to better understand the role of IL-10 in Sjögren's syndrome, transgenic mice were constructed (215). The transgenic expression of IL-10 induced apoptosis of glandular tissue and infiltration of lymphocytes consisting of primarily FasL$^+$, CD4$^+$ T cells as well as *in vitro* upregulation of FasL expression on T cells. Altogether, this suggested that glandular overexpression of IL-10 and the subsequent Fas/FasL-mediated bystander tissue destruction may be a causal factor in the development of Sjögren's syndrome.

The appearance of autoimmune diabetes before autoimmune exocrinopathy in the NOD mouse suggests that it is a model of secondary, but not primary, autoimmune sicca complications. Because the unique MHC I-A(g7) expression in NOD mice is essential for the development of insulitis and diabetes in these animals, the exocrine gland function in NOD.B10.H2b mice, which have an MHC congenic to NOD, were investigated as a potential model for primary Sjögren's syndrome (216). NOD.B10.H2b mice exhibited exocrine gland lymphocytic infiltration typical of Sjögren's syndrome–like disease observed in NOD mice, but without the insulitis and diabetes. This suggests that the unique MHC I-A(g7) is not essential for exocrine tissue autoimmunity. Furthermore, these findings indicate that murine sicca syndrome occurs independent of autoimmune diabetes and that the congenic NOD.B10.H2b mouse represents a novel murine model of primary Sjögren's syndrome.

In conclusion, the etiology of Sjögren's syndrome is still a matter of conjecture, although several hypotheses prevail. Nevertheless, there is considerable evidence that an (as yet unknown) initiating factor set against the appropriate genetic background may invoke immunologically mediated inflammatory mechanisms that result in the chronic exocrine lesions. T cell–mediated autoimmune responses in the glandular tissue as well as apoptotic events are currently considered to be of central importance in the pathogenesis of Sjögren's syndrome.

MONOCLONALITY AND LYMPHOMA

Oligoclonal or monoclonal B-cell expansion has been reported to occur in 14% to 100% of Sjögren's syndrome patients, arising mainly from salivary glands but also from visceral organs and lymph nodes (217). Sjögren's syndrome appears to be a crossroad between autoimmunity and malignancy, and it is suggested that patients with evidence of clonal expansions of B cells in their salivary glands are at high risk of developing lymphoma (218–220). As already mentioned, patients with monoclonal RFs expressing certain cross-reactive idiotypes are associated with non-Hodgkin's lymphoma. Various studies have reported that between 25% and 80% of salivary lymphoepithelial lesions in Sjögren's syndrome have morphologic and/or immunophenotypic evidence of low-grade lymphoma (221). However, there is no absolute correlation between monoclonality and the development of lymphoma. Although a high proportion of lymphoepithelial lesions may show evidence of clonal immunoglobulin gene rearrangements, clonality does not necessarily predict progression to clinically overt lymphoma. The practical role of immunogenotypic analysis in the clinical diagnosis of salivary gland lymphoma in Sjögren's syndrome remains to be defined (222,223). A recent study reported that a history of swollen salivary glands, lymphadenopathy, and leg ulcers predicted lymphoma development in patients with primary Sjögren's syndrome (224).

Malignant lymphoma was first reported in patients with Sjögren's syndrome in 1963, and the risk later estimated to be 44 times that of the normal population (225,226). A recent European multicenter study has reported the largest series of patients to date, describing the histologic diagnosis and clinical characteristics of lymphoma in 33 patients with primary Sjögren's syndrome (40). The estimated prevalence of malignant lymphoma in Sjögren's syndrome was 4.3%, with the majority being low-grade marginal zone B-cell lymphomas, particularly of mucosa-associated lymphoid tissue (MALT) origin (227). The latter are indolent neoplasms characterized by a prolonged clinical course and persistent disease at the site of origin (228). Extranodal localization of lymphoma was observed in 26 of the 33 cases, most often in the salivary gland. Lymphadenopathy, cutaneous vasculitis, peripheral neuropathy, low-grade fever, anemia, and lymphopenia were significantly more frequent than in the general Sjögren's syndrome population. The median survival for patients with intermediate-grade lymphoma was 1.83 years compared with 6.33 years for low-grade lymphoma, with survival of low-grade lymphoma being similar in treated versus untreated cases (40).

SECONDARY SJÖGREN'S SYNDROME

Sjögren's syndrome is associated with other inflammatory rheumatic disorders, such RA, SLE, systemic sclerosis, polymyositis, mixed cryoglobulinemia, and polyarteritis nodosa (135). The sicca symptoms are usually mild compared with the symptoms associated with the inflammatory rheumatic disease, and secondary Sjögren's syndrome is therefore often underdiagnosed.

Secondary Sjögren's syndrome often appears late in the course of the primary rheumatic disease, but may precede the disease by several years in children (29). Sicca symptoms have been reported by a high proportion of patients with RA (229). RA patients with sicca symptoms have a more active and severe disease with higher scores for disability, fatigue, and tender joints than patients without such symptoms (229). Another study demonstrated reduced tear production in 29% of patients with RA, and reduced saliva production in 17% (230). The minimal frequency of secondary Sjögren's syndrome in the same study was 7%, but biopsy of the minor salivary glands was not part of the diagnostic procedure. Other studies estimated a clearly higher prevalence of secondary Sjögren's syndrome among patients with RA from 31% (231,232) and 55% to 62% (233,234).

The prevalence of the sicca syndrome in patients with SLE has been reported in a large cohort of patients to be 5% at onset of the disease, and 12% during evolution (average, 8 years) (235). The sicca syndrome was more frequently found in older patients with SLE with onset after age 50 years, the frequency being 6% at onset and 33% during evolution (235). Elderly SLE patients have a lower frequency of malar rash, arthritis, and nephropathy as the first symptom. Due to considerable overlap of symptoms and findings, the distinction between primary Sjögren's syndrome and SLE may be difficult in some patients.

TREATMENT

It is important that patients with primary Sjögren's syndrome are informed about the nature of their disease to cope with a chronic disorder that rarely is disabling, but still gives the patient considerable distress. The patient should be seen regularly by a rheumatologist as well as an ophthalmologist and dentist to access functional and physical deteriorations, extraglandular complications, and other associated conditions that may be treatable and preventable.

Artificial tears often alleviate ocular complaints and are of importance in preventing corneal damage and conjunctivitis (236). Artificial tears should be used as often as possible, at least every 2 to 3 hours, as topical treatment given regularly may improve the status of keratoconjunctivitis with time (237). Artificial tears often contain preservatives, stabilizers, and salt that may cause irritation and sensitivity in patients with Sjögren's syndrome, requiring different preparations (238,239). If relief does not last long enough, then an artificial tear preparation with greater viscosity can be tried. The patients should be informed that dusty environments, tobacco smoke, and low humidity may worsen their symptoms and require more frequent use of artificial tears and lubricants. Ointments are particular useful at night, as they reduce the rate of tear evaporation but tend to cause blurring of the vision. Slow-release artificial tear inserts (Lacrisert) require some residual tear production and is not suitable for use in a completely dry eye. The use of topical steroids is not recommended because these patients have a high risk of secondary bacterial and viral infections in the eye, and because of the serious complications associated with long-term use.

Another treatment option for keratoconjunctivitis sicca is "punctal occlusion" by using a variety of "plugs" to occlude the punctal openings at the inner aspects of the eyelids (239). After this procedure, instilled artificial tears remain in the eye for a longer time.

Management of dry mouth (xerostomia) aims to prevent and treat infections, gum disease, and caries (240). The patients should be encouraged to keep good dental hygiene and use sugarless sweets and chewing gums to stimulate residual salivary flow, thereby reducing the risk of caries. Various forms of artificial saliva products and special toothpaste also are of benefit for some patients (236,238,239), and fluoride supplementation is advocated. Adequate treatment for oral candidiasis usually provides significant improvement of oral symptoms, in spite of continuing oral dryness. Patients should be informed that consuming large quantities of water does not reduce oral dryness and does cause nocturia. Drinking small sips of water during the day may help reduce oral symptoms.

Acupuncture may be a useful adjunct for the stimulation of salivary flow in some patients with xerostomia (241). Systemic treatment with high doses of the expectorant bromhexine have suggested a modest beneficial response in both tear (237) and saliva flow, but controlled trials have failed to improve salivary output (242,243). Oral pilocarpine has recently been shown to be safe and to produce subjective and objective benefits for patients with primary Sjögren's syndrome with symptoms associated with dry eyes and dry mouth (244,245). This drug may be associated with systemic side effects (246). Interferon-α may be of benefit for the symptoms associated with xerostomia (247). Cevimeline, a novel quinuclidine derivate of acetylcholine exhibiting high affinity for the muscarinic M3 receptor, has long-lasting sialogogic action and few side effects (248).

Vaginal dryness may be treated by lubricant jellies, and dry lips and skin, with moisturizing lotions.

At present, treatment for most patients is essentially symptomatic. The effect of antimalarials has been studied by several research groups. Hydroxychloroquine may be effective as an immunomodulating agent in reducing immune activation and lymphoproliferation, which may be beneficial for patients with Sjögren's syndrome (249). In a prospective, placebo-controlled, 2-year double-blind crossover trial, the use of hydroxychloroquine at a dose of 400 mg daily, taken over a 12-month period, did not have a worthwhile clinical benefit despite an improvement in hyperglobulinemia and slight changes in the ESR and serum IgM levels (250). In a retrospective study with patients fulfilling the California criteria for primary Sjögren's syndrome, treatment with hydroxychloroquine, 6 to 7 mg/kg/day over a 3-year period, resulted in sustained improvement of local symptoms such as painful eyes and mouth, and improvement of systemic manifestations such as arthralgias and myalgias (251). In the same study, a significant improvement in the ESR and IgG levels in serum was observed. No effect on sicca symptoms have been documented after the use of antimalarials in patients with Sjögren's syndrome. The efficacy of hydroxychloroquine in reducing the risk of extraglandular complications in primary Sjögren's syndrome remains to be studied.

Systemic steroids have been shown to improve the signs and symptoms of primary Sjögren's syndrome (252), but are used mainly for the treatment of severe extraglandular complications such as pulmonary and renal involvement. A 6-month randomized, double-blinded, placebo-controlled study examined the effect of 30 mg prednisone on alternate days, and found no improvement in histologic or functional parameters of salivary and lacrimal glands in patients with primary Sjögren's syndrome (253). In the same study, no effect was obtained by treatment with piroxicam, 20 mg daily.

Cyclosporine (Cyclosporin A) and nandrolone decanoate also have been evaluated as therapeutic agents, without great success (254,255). Cyclosporine improved only the symptom of dryness of the mouth. Weekly administration of methotrexate, 0.2 mg/kg body weight, resulted in improvement of subjective symptoms such as dry eyes and mouth, as well as the frequency of parotid gland enlargement, dry cough, and purpura (256). Methotrexate had no effect on the objective parameters of dry eyes and dry mouth, however, and double-blind trials are needed for further evaluation of this agent. Medication is associated with increased risk of gastrointestinal side effects and esophageal discomfort. These problems can be reduced by using enteric-coated tablets that are less likely to adhere to dry mucosa, and by taking the medication with a large volume of fluid while sitting upright.

PROGNOSIS

There are few studies regarding the natural course of primary Sjögren's syndrome, but it has been described as a stepwise, gradual progression from a disorder mainly of exocrine glands, to systemic extraglandular features and finally to lymphoid neoplasia development (170,257). Primary Sjögren's syndrome is generally characterized by a stable and rather mild course of glandular and extraglandular manifestations, in contrast to the increased risk for development of malignant lymphoma in some patients (Table 85.4).

End-organ damage is uncommon in primary Sjögren's syndrome when compared with SLE, with the exception of damage in the oral region, which is seen in up to 62% of the patients with Sjögren's syndrome (36). The degree of functional disability as evaluated by measures for quality of life and well-being is as great as in those with SLE, however.

TABLE 85.4. SYSTEMIC MANIFESTATIONS IN PRIMARY SJÖGREN'S SYNDROME

Systemic manifestation(s)	Range (%)
Arthralgias	24–94
Arthritis	0–17
Myalgias	0–54
Cutaneous vasculitis	3–26
Systemic vasculitis	0–13
Raynaud's phenomenon	20–81
Pulmonary disease	8–44
Renal disease	0–38
Anemia	0–10
Leukopenia	6–42
Lymphadenopathy	6–50
Splenomegaly	4–23
Malignant lymphoma	2–14
Neurologic CNS manifestations	0–13
Neurologic peripheral manifestations	0–15
Gastrointestinal	2–24

Results are based on cumulative frequencies during the course of the disease in 601 patients diagnosed according to different classification criteria (35, 50, 258–263).
CNS, central nervous system.

Serology can be useful in predicting the subsequent outcome and complications in patients with primary Sjögren's syndrome. The presence of anti-Ro/SSA antibodies identifies patients with more systemic disease, with increased incidence of parotid swelling, lymphadenopathy, and lymphoma (50). Although seronegative patients (ANA, RF, Ro/SSA, and La/SSB negative) usually remain polysymptomatic, they do not develop systemic complications (45). About one third of ANA- or RF-positive Sjögren's syndrome patients who were negative for Ro/SSA and La/SSB were given revised diagnosis during a follow-up period, including RA, SLE, mixed connective tissue disease, and scleroderma (45). In Ro/La-positive patients, the relative risk of developing non-Hodgkin's lymphoma has been reported as 49.7 after 10 years of follow-up (45).

Patients with isolated keratoconjunctivitis sicca without autoantibodies do not seem to have an increased risk of developing malignant lymphoma, and this subgroup has reduced risk of developing extraglandular disease, in contrast to patients with primary and secondary Sjögren's syndrome, respectively (264). Some researchers have not identified factors predictive for developing extraglandular manifestations in patients with primary Sjögren's syndrome (45), whereas others have found that plasma IgG levels predict the long-term course of primary Sjögren's syndrome (265). The development of extraglandular manifestations seems to be influenced by a number of factors including the MHC. Both HLA-B8 and -DR3 are associated with an increased frequency of extraglandular complications (36,266).

Spontaneous symptomatic improvement has been described in 12% of patients with primary Sjögren's syndrome, sometimes after a long history of severe sicca features (50). This tended to occur in older female patients, all of whom were postmenopausal, with some clinical overlap among these patients with SLE. In a recent study on survivorship in a population-based cohort of patients with Sjögren's syndrome from 1976 to 1992, the authors did not demonstrate increased mortality (267). However, mortality may have been increased in patients with secondary Sjögren's syndrome, the majority of whom had RA.

ACKNOWLEDGMENT

This work was supported by grants from the European BIOMED program (BMH4-CT96-0595), the Research Council of Norway (115563/320), and the Broegelmann Foundation.

SUGGESTED READINGS

1. Shearn M. *Sjögren's syndrome.* Philadelphia: WB Saunders, 1971.
2. Talal N, Moutsopoulos HM, Kassan SS, eds. *Sjögren's syndrome:* clinical and immunological aspects. Berlin: Springer-Verlag, 1987.
3. Isenberg DA, Horsfall AC, eds. *Autoimmune diseases:* focus on Sjögren's syndrome. Oxford: Bios Scientific Publishers, 1994.
4. Proceedings of First International Seminar on Sjögren's syndrome. *Scand J Rheumatol Suppl* 1986;61:1–291.
5. Proceedings of the Second International Symposium on Sjögren's syndrome. *J Autoimmun* 1989;2:309–611.
6. Workshop on Diagnostic Criteria for Sjögren's syndrome (proceedings). *Clin Exp Rheumatol* 1989;7:111–219.
7. Third International Symposium on Sjögren's syndrome (abstracts). *Clin Exp Rheumatol* 1991;9:311–340.
8. Homma M, Sugai S, Tojo T, et al. eds. *Sjögren's syndrome:* state of the art (Proceedings of the Fourth International Symposium). Amsterdam: Kugler Publications, 1994.
9. Vth International Symposium on Sjögren's syndrome (proceedings + abstracts). *Clin Rheumatol* 1995;14 suppl 1:3–62.
10. VIth International Symposium on Sjögren's syndrome (proceedings + abstracts). *J Rheumatol* 1997;24(suppl 50):1–54.
11. International Conference on Immunopathology of Mucous Membranes and Exocrine Glands (abstracts). *Scand J Immunol* 1997;45:557–580.
12. Eriksson P, Jonsson R, eds. The 100-year anniversary of Henrik Sjögren (proceedings + abstracts). *Hygiea* 1999;108(suppl 1): 1–114.

REFERENCES

1. Leber T. Präparate zu dem vortrag über entstehung der netzhautablösung und über verschiedene hornhautaffektionen. *Ophthalm Ges Heidelb Klin Mbl Augenheilk* 1882;xx:165.
2. Hadden WB. On "dry mouth" or suppression of the salivary and buccal secretions. *Trans Clin Soc Lond* 1888;21:176.
3. Hutchinson J. A case of "dry mouth" (aptyalism). *Trans Clin Soc Lond* 1888;21:180.
4. Fischer E. Über Fädchenkeratitis. *Graefes Arch* 1889;35:201.
5. Stock W. *Die pathologie der tränenorgane:* Graefe-Saemisch Handbdges Augenheilk, *1924.* Vol IX, Berlin.
6. Mikulicz J. Über eine eigenartige symmetrische erkrankung der tränen- und mundspeicheldrüsen. *Beitr z Chir Festscr f Theodor Billrodt.* Stuttgart, 1892:610–630.
7. Gourgerot H. Insufficance progresive et atrophie des glands salivaires er muqueuses de la bouche, des conjonctives (et parfois des muqueuses nasale, laryngée, vulvaire) sécheresse de la bouche, des conjonctives. *Bull Med (Paris)* 1926;40:360–368.
8. Mulock Houwer AW. Keratitis filamentosa and chronic arthritis. *Trans Ophthal Soc U K* 1927;47:88–95.
9. Sjögren H. Zur kenntnis der keratoconjunctivitis sicca. *Acta Ophthalmol* 1933;11(suppl II):1–151.
10. Morgan WS, Castleman B. A clinicopathologic study of Mikulicz's disease. *Am J Pathol* 1953;29:471–503.
11. Talal N, Bunim JJ. Development of malignant lymphoma in the course of Sjögren's syndrome. *Am J Med* 1964;36:529–540.
12. Bloch KJ, Buchanan WW, Wohl MJ, et al. Sjögren's syndrome: a clinical, pathological and serological study of sixty-two cases. *Medicine* 1965;44:187–231.
13. Clark G, Reichlin M, Tomasi TB. Characterization of a soluble cytoplasmic antigen reactive with sera from patients with systemic lupus erythematosus. *J Immunol* 1969;102:117–122.
14. Chrisholm DM, Mason DK. Labial salivary gland biopsy in Sjögren's disease. *J Clin Pathol* 1968;21:656–660.
15. Vitali C, Bombardieri S, Moutsopoulos H, et al. Preliminary criteria for the classification of Sjögren's syndrome: results of a prospective concerted action supported by the European Community. *Arthritis Rheum* 1993;36:340–347.
16. Fox RI, Robinson C, Curd J, et al. Suggested criteria for classification of Sjögren's syndrome. *Scand J Rheumatol* 1986;61: 28–30.
17. Fritzler MJ, Pauls JD, Kinsella TD, et al. Antinuclear, anticytoplasmic, and anti-Sjögren's syndrome antigen A (SS-A/Ro) antibodies in female blood donors. *Clin Immunol Immunopathol* 1985;36:120–128.
18. Jacobsson LTH, Axell TE, Hansen BU, et al. Dry eyes or mouth: an epidemiological study in Swedish adults, with special reference to primary Sjögren's syndrome. *J Autoimmun* 1989; 2:521–527.
19. Jacobsson LTH, Hansen BU, Manthorpe R, et al. Association of dry eyes and dry mouth with anti-Ro/Sjögren's syndrome-A and anti-Sjögren's syndrome-La/Sjögren's syndrome-B autoantibodies in normal adults. *Arthritis Rheum* 1992;35:1492–1501.
20. Bjerrum K. Keratoconjunctivitis sicca and primary Sjögren's syndrome in a Danish population aged 30-60 years. *Acta Ophthalmol Scand* 1997;75:281–286.
21. Zhang NZ. Primary Sjögren's syndrome, a highly misrecognized disease in China. In: Nasution AR, Darmawan J, Isbagio H, eds. *APLAR rheumatology.* Edinburgh: Churchill Livingstone, 1992:199–202.
22. Dafni UG, Tzioufas G, Staikos P, et al. Prevalence of Sjögren's syndrome in a closed rural community. *Ann Rheum Dis* 1997; 56:521–525.
23. Hochberg MC, Tielsch J, Munoz B, et al. Prevalence of symptoms of dry mouth and their relationship to saliva production in community dwelling elderly: the SEE project. *J Rheumatol* 1998;25:486–491.
24. Strickland RW, Tesar JT, Berne BH, et al. The frequency of sicca syndrome in an elderly female population. *J Rheumatol* 1987; 14:766–771.
25. Drosos AA, Andonopoulos AP, Costopoulos JS, et al. Prevalence of primary Sjögren's syndrome in an elderly population. *Br J Rheumatol* 1988;27:123–127.
26. Haga H-J, Rygh T, Jacobsen H, et al. Sjögren's syndrome: new diagnostic aspects. *Tidsskr Nor Laegeforen* 1997;117: 2197–2200.
27. Haga H-J, Jonsson R. The influence of age on disease manifes-

tations and serological characteristics in primary Sjögren's syndrome. *Scand J Rheumatol* 1999;28:227–232.

28. Bjerrum K, Prause JU. Primary Sjögren's syndrome: a subjective description of the disease. *Clin Exp Rheumatol* 1990;8: 283–288.
29. Anaya JM, Ogawa N, Talal N. Sjögren's syndrome in childhood. *J Rheumatol* 1995;22:1152–1158.
30. Ostuni PA, Ianniello A, Sfrisco P, et al. Juvenile onset of primary Sjögren's syndrome: report of 10 cases. *Clin Exp Rheumatol* 1996;14:689–693.
31. Anaya JM, Talal N. Primary Sjögren's syndrome in men. *Ann Rheum Dis* 1995;54:748–751.
32. Whaley K, Williamson J, Wilson T, et al. Sjögren's syndrome and autoimmunity in a geriatric population. *Age Ageing* 1972;1:197.
33. Ramos-Casals M, Cervera R, Font J, et al. Young onset of primary Sjögren's syndrome: clinical and immunological characteristics. *Lupus* 1998;7:202–206.
34. Manoussakis MN, Tzioufas AG, Pange PJE, et al. Serological profiles in subgroups of patients with Sjögren's syndrome. *Scand J Rheumatol* 1986;15(suppl 61):89–92.
35. Assmussen K, Andersen V, Bendixen G, et al. Quantitative assessment of clinical disease status in primary Sjögren's syndrome. *Scand J Rheumatol* 1997;26:197–205.
36. Sutcliffe N, Stoll T, Pyke S, et al. Functional disability and end organ damage in patients with systemic lupus erythematosus (SLE), SLE and Sjögren's syndrome (Sjögren's syndrome) and primary Sjögren's syndrome. *J Rheumatol* 1998;25:63–68.
37. Daniels TE, Silverman S, Michalski JP, et al. The oral component of Sjögren's syndrome. *Oral Surg Oral Med Oral Pathol* 1975;39:875–885.
38. Caruso AJ, Sonies BC, Atkinson JC, et al. Objective measures of swallowing in patients with primary Sjögren's syndrome. *Dysphagia* 1989;4:101–105.
39. Hernandez YL, Daniels TE. Oral candidiasis in Sjögren's syndrome: prevalence, clinical correlations and treatment. *Oral Surg Oral Med Oral Pathol* 1989;8:324–329.
40. Voulgarelis M, Dafni UG, Isenberg DA, et al. Malignant lymphoma in primary Sjögren's syndrome: a multicenter, retrospective, clinical study by the European concerted action on Sjögren's syndrome. *Arthritis Rheum* 1999;42:1765–1772.
41. Mulherin DM, Sheeran TP, Kumararatne DS, et al. Sjögren's syndrome in women presenting with chronic dyspareuni. *Br J Obstet Gynaecol* 1997;104:1019–1023.
42. Gudbjörnsson B, Broman JE, Hetta J, et al. Sleep disturbances in patients with primary Sjögren's syndrome. *Br J Rheumatol* 1993;32:1072–1076.
43. Peace CT, Shattles W, Barrett NK, et al. The arthropathy of Sjögren's syndrome. *Br J Rheumatol* 1993;32:609–613.
44. Bonafede RP, Downey DC, Bennett RM. An association of fibromyalgia with primary Sjögren's syndrome: a prospective study of 72 patients. *J Rheumatol* 1995;22:133–136.
45. Davidson KS, Kelly CA, Griffiths ID. Primary Sjögren's syndrom in the north east of England: a long-term follow-up study. *Rheumatology* 1999;38:245–253.
46. Constantopoulos SH, Papadimitriou CS, Moutsopoulos HM. Respiratory manifestations in primary Sjögren's syndrome. *Chest* 1985;88:226–229.
47. Oxholm P, Bundgaard A, Birk Madsen E, et al. Pulmonary function in patients with primary Sjögren's syndrome. *Rheumatol Int* 1982;2:179–181.
48. Kelly C, Gardiner P, Pal B, et al. Lung function in primary Sjögren's syndrome: a cross-sectional and longitudinal study. *Thorax* 1991;46:180–183.
49. Vitali C, Tavoni A, Viegi G, et al. Lung involvement in Sjögren's syndrome: a comparison between patients with primary and with secondary syndrome. *Ann Rheum Dis* 1985;44:455–461.
50. Kelly CA, Foster H, Pal B. et al. Primary Sjögren's syndrome in northeast England: a longitudinal study. *Br J Rheumatol* 1991; 30:437–442.
51. Alarcón-Segovia D, Divertie MB, Brown AL. Pleuropulmonary manifestations associated with Sjögren's syndrome. *Arthritis Rheum* 1965;8:427–428.
52. Gardiner P, Ward C, Allison A, et al. Pleuropulmonary abnormalities in primary Sjögren's syndrome. *J Rheumatol* 1993;20: 831–837.
53. Liebow AA, Carrington CB. Diffuse pulmonary lymphoreticular infiltrations associated with dysproteinaemia. *Med Clin North Am* 1973;57:809–843.
54. Hansen LA, Prakash UBS, Colby TV. Pulmonary lymphoma in Sjögren's syndrome. *Mayo Clinic Proc* 1989;64:920–931.
55. Sato T, Matsubara O, Tanaka Y, et al. Association of Sjögren's syndrome with pulmonary hypertension: report of two cases and review of the literature. *Hum Pathol* 1993;24:199–205.
56. Lois M, Roman J, Holland W, et al. Coexisting Sjögren's syndrome and sarcoidosis in the lung. *Semin Arthritis Rheum* 1998; 28:31–40.
57. Shioji R, Furuyama T, Onodera S, et al. Sjögren's syndrome and renal tubular acidosis. *Am J Med* 1970;48:456–463.
58. Tu WH, Shearn MA, Lee JC, et al. Interstitial nephritis in Sjögren's syndrome. *Ann Intern Med* 1968;69:1163–1170.
59. Pokorny G, Sonkodi S, Ivanyi B, et al. Renal involvement in patients with primary Sjögren's syndrome. *Scand J Rheumatol* 1989;18:231–234.
60. Shearn MA, Tu WH. Latent renal tubular acidosis in Sjögren's syndrome. *Ann Rheum Dis* 1968;27:27–32.
61. Talal N, Zisman E, Shur PH. Renal tubular acidosis, glomerulonephritis and immunologic factors in Sjögren's syndrome. *Arthritis Rheum* 1968;11:774–786.
62. Vitali C, Tavoni A, Sciutyo M, et al. Renal involvement in primary Sjögren's syndrome: a retrospective-prospective study. *Scand J Rheumatol* 1991;20:132–136.
63. Glassock RJ, Feinstein EE, Tannen R, et al. Metabolic acidosis in a young woman. *Am J Nephrol* 1984;4:58–65.
64. Shearn M, Tu W. Nephrogenic diabetes insipidus and other defects of renal tubular function in Sjögren's syndrome. *Am J Med* 1965;39:312–318.
65. Moutsopoulos HM, Balow JE, Cawley TJ, et al. Immune complex glomerulonephritis in sicca syndrome. *Am J Med* 1978;64: 955–960.
66. Van de Merwe J, Kamerling R, Arendsen E, et al. Sjögren's syndrome in patients with interstitial cystitis. *J Rheumatol* 1993;20: 962–966.
67. Grant IA, Hunder GG, Homburger HA, et al. Peripheral neuropathy associated with sicca complex. *Neurology* 1997;48: 855–862.
68. Kaltreider HB, Talal N. The neuropathy in Sjögren's syndrome: trigeminal nerve involvement. *Ann Intern Med* 1969;70: 751–762.
69. Alexander EL, Provost TT, Stevens MB, et al. Neurologic complications in primary Sjögren's syndrome. *Medicine* 1982;61: 247–257.
70. Von Bekesy G. Duplicity theory of taste. *Science* 1964;145: 834–835.
71. Alexander EL. Neurologic disease in Sjögren's syndrome: mononuclear inflammatory vasculopathy affecting central/peripheral nervous system and muscle: a clinical review and update of immunopathogenesis. *Rheum Dis Clin North Am* 1993;19: 869–908.
72. Caselli RJ, Scheithauer BW, O'Duffy JD, et al. Chronic inflammatory meningoencephalitis should not be mistaken for Alzheimer's disease. *Mayo Clin Proc* 1993;68:846–853.
73. Gerraty RP, McKelvie PA, Byrne E. Aseptic meningoencephali-

tis in primary Sjögren's syndrome: response to plasmapheresis and absence of CNS vasculitis at autopsy. *Acta Neurol Scand* 1993;88:309–311.

74. Caselli RJ, Scheithauer BW, Bowles CA, et al. The treatable dementia of Sjögren's syndrome. *Ann Neurol* 1991;30:98–101.
75. Alexander EL, Malinow K, Lijewski JE, et al. Primary Sjögren's syndrome with central nervous system dysfunction mimicking multiple sclerosis. *Ann Intern Med* 1986;104:323–330.
76. Coates T, Slavotinek JP, Reischmueller M, et al. Cerebral white matter lesions in primary Sjögren's syndrome: a controlled study. *J Rheumatol* 1999;26:1301–1305.
77. Mandl T, Jacobsson L, Lilja B, et al. Disturbances of autonomic nervous function in primary Sjögren's syndrome. *Scand J Rheumatol* 1997;26:401–406.
78. Kjellen G, Fransson SG, Lindström F, et al. Esophageal function, radiography, and dysphagia in Sjögren's syndrome. *Dig Dis Sci* 1986;31:225.
79. Ramirez-Mata M, Pena-Acir F, Alarcon-Segovia D. Abnormal esophageal motility in Sjögren's syndrome. *J Rheumatol* 1976;3: 63.
80. Tsianos EB, Chiras CD, Drosos AA, et al. Oesophageal dysfunction in patients with primary Sjögren's syndrome. *Ann Rheum Dis* 1985;44:610–613.
81. Maury CPJ, Tornroth T, Teppo A-M. Atrophic gastritis in Sjögren's syndrome: morphologic, biochemical and immunologic findings. *Arthritis Rheum* 1985;28:388–389.
82. Buchanan WW, Cox AG, Harden RMcG, et al. Gastric studies in Sjögren's syndrome. *Gut* 1966;7:351–354.
83. Van Jebavy M, Hradsky M, Herout V. Gastric biopsy in patients with Sjögren's syndrome. *Z Med Lab Diagn* 1961;16:930–940.
84. Kilpi A, Bergroth V, Konttinen Y, et al. Lymphocyte infiltrations of the gastric mucosa in Sjögren's syndrome. *Arthritis Rheum* 1983;26:1196–1200.
85. Maury CPJ, Rasanen V, Teppo A-M, et al. Serum pepsinogen I in rheumatic diseases: reduced level in Sjögren's syndrome. *Arthritis Rheum* 1982;25:1059–1063.
86. Mulders AV, Van Den Bergh H, Dequeker J. Hypergastrinemia in rheumatoid arthritis related to Sjögren's syndrome [Letter]. *J Rheumatol* 1984;11:246–247.
87. Tsianosis EB, Tzioufas AG, Kita MD, et al. Serum isoamylases in patients with autoimmune rheumatic diseases. *Clin Exp Rheumatol* 1984;2:235–238.
88. Fenster FL, Buchanan WW, Laster L, et al. Studies of pancreatic function in Sjögren's syndrome. *Ann Intern Med* 1964;61: 498–508.
89. Hradsky M, Bartos V, Keller O. Pancreatic function in Sjögren's syndrome. *Gastroenterology* 1967;108:252–260.
90. Golding PL, Brown R, Mason AMS, et al. "Sicca complex" in liver disease. *Br Med J* 1970;4:340–342.
91. Whaley K, Williamson J, Dick W, et al. Liver disease in Sjögren's syndrome. *Lancet* 1970;1:861.
92. Webb J, Whaley K, MacSween R, et al. Liver disease in rheumatoid arthritis and Sjögren's syndrome. *Ann Rheum Dis* 1975;34: 70.
93. Tishler M, Paran D, Yaron M. Allergic disorders in primary Sjögren's syndrome. *Scand J Rheumatol* 1998;27:166–169.
94. Kyle R, Gleich G, Baynd E, et al. Benign hyperglobulinemic purpura of Waldenström. *Medicine (Baltimore)* 1971;50:113.
95. Ramos-Casals M, Cervera R, Yagüe J, et al. Cryoglobulinemia in primary Sjögren's syndrome: prevalence and clinical characteristics in a series of 115 patients. *Semin Arthritis Rheum* 1998;28:200–205.
96. Punzi L, Ostuni PA, Betterle C, et al. Thyroid gland disorders in primary Sjögren's syndrome. *Rev Rhum* 1996;63:809–814.
97. Hansen BU, Ericsson UB, Henricsson V, et al. Autoimmune thyroiditis and primary Sjögren's syndrome: clinical and laboratory evidence of the coexistence of the two diseases. *Clin Exp Rheumatol* 1991;9:137–141.
98. Haga H-J, Rygh T. The prevalence of hyperprolactinemia in patients with primary Sjögren's syndrome. *J Rheumatol* 1999; 26:1291–1295.
99. Alspaugh MA, Tan EM. Antibodies to cellular antigens in Sjögren's syndrome. *J Clin Invest* 1975;55:1067–1073.
100. Wolin SL, Steitz J. The Ro small cytoplasmic ribonucleoproteins: identification of the antigenic protein binding site on the Ro RNAs. *Proc Natl Acad Sci U S A* 1985;81:1990–2000.
101. Boire G, Lopez-Longo FJ, Lapointe S, et al. Sera from patients with autoimmune disease recognise conformational determinants on the 60-kD Ro/SSA protein. *Arthritis Rheum* 1991;34: 722–730.
102. Wahren-Herlenius M, Muller S, Isenberg D. Analysis of B-cell epitopes of the Ro/SS-A autoantigen. *Immunol Today* 1999;20: 234–240.
103. Ben-Chetrit E, Chan EK, Sullivan KF, et al. A 52-kD protein is a novel component of the SS-A/Ro antigenic particle. *J Exp Med* 1988;167:1560–1571.
104. Boire G, Gendron M, Monast N, et al. Purification of antigenically intact Ro ribonucleoproteins: biochemical and immunological evidence that the 52-kD protein is not a Ro protein. *Clin Exp Immunol* 1995;100:489–498.
105. Casciola-Rosen LA, Anhalt G, Rosen A. Autoantigens targeted in systemic lupus erythematosus are clustered in two populations of surface structures on apoptotic keratinocytes. *J Exp Med* 1994;179:1317–1330.
106. Elagib KEE, Tengnér P, Levi M, et al. Immunoglobulin variable genes and epitope recognition of human monoclonal anti-Ro 52-kd from primary Sjögren's syndrome. *Arthritis Rheum* 1999; 42:2471–2481.
107. Gordon T, Mavrangelos C, McCluskey J. Restricted epitope recognition by precipitin-negative anti-La/SS-B-positive sera. *Arthritis Rheum* 1992;35:663–666.
108. Rinke J, Steitz JA. Precursor molecules of both human SS ribosomal RNA and transfer RNAs are bound by a cellular protein reactive with anti-La lupus antibodies. *Cell* 1982;29:149–159.
109. Gottlieb E, Steitz JA. Function of mammalian La protein: evidence for its action in transcription termination by RNA polymerase III. *EMBO J* 1989;8:851–861.
110. St. Clair EW. Anti-La antibodies. *Rheum Dis Clin North Am* 1992;18:359–377.
111. McNeilage LJ, Umapathysivam K, Macmillan E, et al. Definition of a discontinuous immunodominant epitope at the NH2 terminus of the La(SS-B) ribonucleoprotein autoantigen. *J Clin Invest* 1992;89:1652–1656.
112. Rischmueller M, McNeilage LJ, McCluskey J, et al. Human autoantibodies directed against the RNA recognition motif of La(SS-B) bind to a conformational epitope present on the intact La(SS-B) ribonucleoprotein particle. *Clin Exp Immunol* 1995; 101:39–44.
113. Reichlin M, Scofield RH. SS-A(Ro) autoantibodies. In: Peter JB, Schoenfeld Y, eds. *Autoantibodies*. Amsterdam: Elsevier, 1996:783–788.
114. Keech CL, McCluskey J, Gordon TP. SS-B(La) autoantibodies. In: Peter JB, Schoenfeld Y, eds. *Autoantibodies*. Amsterdam: Elsevier, 1996:789–797.
115. Venables PJ, Shattles W, Pease CT, et al. Anti-La(SS-B): a diagnostic criterion for Sjögren's syndrome. *Clin Exp Rheumatol* 1989;7:181–184.
116. Scofield RH, Farris AD, Horsfall AC, et al. Fine specificity of the autoimmune response to the Ro/SSA and La/SSB ribonucleoproteins. *Arthritis Rheum* 1999;42:199–209.
117. McCauliffe DP, Wang L, Satoh M, et al. Recombinant 52kDa Ro(SS-A) ELISA detects autoantibodies in Sjögren's syndrome

sera that go undetected by conventional serologic assays. *J Rheumatol* 1997;24:860–866.
118. Beer RG, Rischmueller M, Coates T, et al. Non-precipitating anti-La(SS-B) autoantibodies in primary Sjögren's syndrome. *Clin Immun Immunopathol* 1996;79:314–318.
119. Harley JB. Autoantibodies in Sjögren's syndrome. *J Autoimmun* 1989;2:283–294.
120. Atkinson JC, Travis WD, Slocum L, et al. Serum anti-SS-B/La and IgA rheumatoid factor are markers of salivary gland disease activity in primary Sjögren's syndrome. *Arthritis Rheum* 1992; 35:1368–1372.
121. Gerli R, Muscat C, Giansanti M, et al. Quantitative assessment of salivary gland inflammatory infiltration in primary Sjögren's syndrome. *Br J Rheumatol* 1997;36:969–975.
122. Yannopoulos DI, Roncin S, Lamour A, et al. Conjunctival epithelial cells from patients with Sjögren's syndrome inappropriately express major histocompatibility complex molecules, La(SS-B) antigen and heat-shock proteins. *J Clin Immunol* 1992;12:259–265.
123. De Wilde PCM, Kater L, Bodeutsch C, et al. Aberrant expression pattern of the SS-B/La antigen in the labial salivary glands of patients with Sjögren's syndrome. *Arthritis Rheum* 1996;39: 783–791.
124. Horsfall AC, Rose LM, Maini RN. Autoantibody synthesis in salivary glands of Sjögren's syndrome patients. *J Autoimmun* 1989;2:559–568.
125. Halse A-K, Marthinussen MC, Wahren-Herlenius, et al. Isotype distribution of anti-Ro/SS-A and anti-La/SS-B antibodies in plasma and saliva of patients with Sjögren's syndrome. *Scand J Rheumatol* 2000;29:13–19.
126. Tengnér P, Halse A-K, Haga H-J, et al. Detection of anti-Ro/SSA and anti-La/SSB autoantibody-producing cells in salivary glands from patients with Sjögren's syndrome. *Arthritis Rheum* 1998;41:2238–2248.
127. Halse A-K, Harley JB, Kroneld U, et al. Ro/SS-A-reactive B lymphocytes in salivary glands and peripheral blood of patients with Sjögren's syndrome. *Clin Exp Immunol* 1999;115:203–207.
128. Topfer F, Gordon T, McCluskey J. Intra- and intermolecular spreading of autoimmunity involving the nuclear self-antigens La(SS-B) and Ro(SS-A). *Proc Natl Acad Sci U S A* 1995;92: 875–879.
129. Keech CL, Gordon TP, McCluskey J. The immune response to 52-kDa Ro and 60-kDa Ro is linked in experimental autoimmunity. *J Immunol* 1996;157:3694–3699.
130. Tseng C-E, Chan EKL, Miranda E, et al. The 52-kd protein as a target of intermolecular spreading of the immune response to components of the SS-A/Ro-SS-B/La complex. *Arthritis Rheum* 1997;49:936–944.
131. Reynolds P, Gordon TP, Purcell AW, et al. Hierarchical self-tolerance to T cell determinants within the ubiquitous nuclear self-antigen La(SS-B) permits induction of systemic autoimmunity in normal mice. *J Exp Med* 1996;184:1857–1870.
132. Kinoshita G, Purcell AW, Keech CL, et al. Molecular chaperones are targets of autoimmunity in Ro(SS-A) immune mice. *Clin Exp Immunol* 1999;115:268–274.
133. Deshmukh BUS, Lewis JE, Gaskin F, et al. Immune responses to Ro60 and its peptides in mice. I. The nature of the immunogen and endogenous autoantigen determine the specificities of the induced autoantibodies. *J Exp Med* 1999;189:531–540.
134. Keech CL, McCluskey J, Gordon TP. Transfection and overexpression of the human 60-kDa Ro/SS-A autoantigen in HEp-2 cells. *Clin Immun Immunopathol* 1994;73:146–151.
135. Sjögren's syndrome. In: Morrow J, Nelson L, Watts R, et al. eds. *Autoimmune rheumatic disease.* Oxford: University Press, 1999:147–169.
136. MacSween RNM, Govidie RB, Anderson JR, et al. Occurrence of antibody to salivary duct epithelium in Sjögren's disease, rheumatoid arthritis and other arthritides: a clinical and laboratory study. *Ann Rheum Dis* 1967;26:402–411.
137. Feltkamp TEW, Van Rossum AL. Antibodies to salivary duct cells and other autoantibodies in patients with Sjögren's syndrome and other idiopathic autoimmune diseases. *Clin Exp Immunol* 1968;3:1–16.
138. Inagak Y, Jinno-Yoshida Y, Hamasaki Y, et al. A novel autoantibody reactive with carbonic anhydrase in sera from patients with systemic lupus erythematosus and Sjögren's syndrome. *J Dermatol Sci* 1991;2:147–154.
139. Kino-Ohsaki J, Nishimori I, Morita M, et al. Serum antibodies to carbonic anhydrase I and II in patients with idiopathic chronic pancreatitis and Sjögren's syndrome. *Gastroenterology* 1996;10:1579–1586.
140. Freist E, Kuckelkorn U, Dorner T, et al. Autoantibodies in primary Sjögren's syndrome are directed against proteasomal subunits of the α and β type. *Arthritis Rheum* 1999;42:697–702.
141. Haneji N, Nakamura T, Takio K, et al. Identification of α-fodrin as a candidate autoantigen in primary Sjögren's syndrome. *Science* 1997;276:604–607.
142. Asherson RA, Fei H-M, Stab HL, et al. Anti-phospholipid antibodies and HLA associations in primary Sjögren's syndrome. *Ann Rheum Dis* 1992;51:495–498.
143. Bacman S, Sterin-Borda L, Camusso JJ, et al. Circulating antibodies against rat parotid gland M3 muscarinic receptors in primary Sjögren's syndrome. *Clin Exp Immunol* 1996;104: 454–459.
144. Bacman S, Perez Leiros C, Sterin-Borda L, et al. Autoantibodies against lacrimal gland M3 muscarinic acetylcholine receptors in patients with primary Sjögren's syndrome. *Invest Ophthalmol Vis Sci* 1998;39:151–156.
145. Robinson CP, Brayer J, Yamachika S, et al. Transfer of human serum IgG to NOD.Igμ^{null} mice reveals a role for autoantibodies in the loss of secretory function of exocrine tissues in Sjögren's syndrome. *Proc Natl Acad Sci U S A* 1998;95:7538–7543.
146. Markusse HM, Otten HG, Vroom TM, et al. Rheumatoid factor isotypes in serum and salivary fluid of patients with primary Sjögren's syndrome. *Clin Immunol Immunopathol* 1993;66: 26–32.
147. Atkinson JC, Fox PC, Travis WD, et al. IgA rheumatoid factor and IgA containing immune complexes in primary Sjögren's syndrome. *J Rheumatol* 1989;16:1205–1210.
148. Elagib KEE, Borretzen M, Jonsson R, et al. Rheumatoid factors in primary Sjögren's syndrome (pSS) use diverse VH region genes, the majority of which show no evidence of somatic hypermutation. *Clin Exp Immunol* 1999;117:388–394.
149. Tzioufas AG, Manoussakis MN, Costello R, et al. Cryoglobulinaemia in autoimmune rheumatic diseases. *Arthritis Rheum* 1986;29:1098–1104.
150. Tzioufas AG, Bouma DS, Skopouli FN, et al. Mixed monoclonal cryoglobulinemia and monoclonal rheumatoid factor cross-reactive epitopes as predictive factors for the development of lymphoma in primary Sjögren's syndrome. *Arthritis Rheum* 1996;39:767–772.
151. Fox RI, Chen P, Carson DA, et al. Expression of a cross-reactive idiotype on rheumatoid factor in patients with Sjögren's syndrome. *J Immunol* 1986;136:477–483.
152. Reveille JD, Arnett FC. The immunogenetics of Sjögren's syndrome. *Rheum Dis Clin North Am* 1992;101:748–756.
153. Besana C, Salmaggi C, Pellegrino C, et al. Chronic bilateral dacryo-adenitis in identical twins: a possible incomplete form of Sjögren's syndrome. *Eur J Pediatr* 1991;150:652–655.
154. Scofield RH, Kurien BT, Reichlin M. Immunologically restricted and inhibitory anti-Ro/SSA in monozygotic twins. *Lupus* 1997;6:395–398.

155. Bolstad AI, Nakken B. Genetics of Sjögren's syndrome. In: Eriksson R, Jonsson R, eds. The 100-year anniversary of Henrik Sjögren. *Hygiea* 1999;108:74–77.
156. Reveille JD. The molecular genetics of systemic lupus erythematosus and Sjögren's syndrome. *Curr Opin Rheumatol* 1992; 4:644–656.
157. Roitberg-Tambur A, Friedmann A, Safirman C, et al. Molecular analysis of HLA class II genes in primary Sjögren's syndrome: a study of Israeli Jewish and Greek non-Jewish patients. *Hum Immunol* 1993;36:235–242.
158. Hinzova E, Ivanyi D, Sula K. HLA-Dw3 in Sjögren's syndrome. *Tissue Antigens* 1997;37:10–15.
159. Chused TM, Kassan SS, Opelz G, et al. Sjögren's syndrome associated with Dw3. *N Engl J Med* 1977;296:895–897.
160. Papasteriades C, Skopouli FN, Drosos AA, et al. HLA alloantigen associations in Greek patients with Sjögren's syndrome. *J Autoimmun* 1988;1:85–91.
161. Rischmueller M, Lester S, Chen Z, et al. HLA class II phenotype controls diversification of the autoantibody response in primary Sjögren's syndrome. *Clin Exp Immunol* 1998;111: 365–371.
162. Kerttula TO, Collin P, Polvi A, et al. Distinct immunologic features of Finnish Sjögren's syndrome patients with HLA alleles DRB1*0301, DQA1*0501 and DQB1*0201. *Arthritis Rheum* 1996;39:1733–1739.
163. Kumagai S, Kanagawa S, Morinobu A, et al. Association of a new allele of the TAP2 gene, TAP2*Bky2 (Val577), with susceptibility to Sjögren's syndrome. *Arthritis Rheum* 1997;40: 1685–1692.
164. Martin-Villa JM, Martinez-Laso J, Moreno-Pelayo MA, et al. Differential contribution of HLA-DR, DQ and TAP2 alleles to systemic lupus erythematosus susceptibility in Spanish patients: role of TAP2*01 alleles in Ro autoantibody production. *Ann Rheum Dis* 1998;57:214–219.
165. Homma M, Tojo T, Akizuki M, et al. Criteria for Sjögren's syndrome in Japan. *Scand J Rheumatol* 1986;61:26–27.
166. Manthorpe R, Oxholm P, Prause JU, et al. The Copenhagen criteria for Sjögren's syndrome. *Scand J Rheumatol* 1986;61: 19–21.
167. Skopouli FN, Drosos AA, Papaioannou T, et al. Preliminary diagnostic criteria for Sjögren's syndrome. *Scand J Rheumatol* 1986;61:22–25.
168. Vitali C, Bombardieri S, Moutsopoulos HM, et al. Assessment of the European classification criteria for Sjögren's syndrome in a series of clinically defined cases: results of a prospective multicentre study. *Ann Rheum Dis* 1996;55:116–121.
169. Daniels TE. Sjögren's syndrome: clinical spectrum and current diagnostic controversies. *Adv Dent Res* 1996;10:3–8.
170. Tzioufas AG, Moutsopoulos HM. Sjögren's syndrome. In: Klippel J, Dieppe P, eds. *Rheumatology.* London: Mosby, 1998: 32:1–12.
171. Haga H-J, Hulten B, Bolstad AI, et al. Reliability and sensitivity of diagnostic tests for primary Sjögren's syndrome. *J Rheumatol* 1999;26:604–608.
172. Vitali C, Moutsopoulos HM, Bombardieri S, et al. The European community study group on diagnostic criteria for Sjögren's syndrome: sensitivity and specificity of tests for ocular and oral involvement in Sjögren's syndrome. *Ann Rheum Dis* 1994;53: 637–647.
173. Dawes C. Physiological factors affecting salivary flow rate, oral sugar clearance and the sensation of dry mouth in men. *J Dent Res* 1987;66:648–653.
174. Tishler M, Yaron I, Shirazi I, et al. Saliva: an additional diagnostic tool in Sjögren's syndrome. *Semin Arthritis Rheum* 1997; 27:173–179.
175. Håkansson U, Jacobsson L, Lilja B, et al. Salivary gland scintigraphy in subjects with and without symptoms of dry mouth/or eyes, and in patients with primary Sjögren's syndrome. *Scand J Rheumatol* 1994;23:326–333.
176. Daniels TE. Labial salivary gland biopsy in Sjögren's syndrome: assessment as a diagnostic criterion in 362 suspected cases. *Arthritis Rheum* 1984;27:147–156.
177. Daniels TE. Salivary histopathology in diagnosis of Sjögren's syndrome. *Scand J Rheumatol* 1986;(suppl 61):36–43.
178. Jonsson R, Kroneld U, Bäckman K, et al. Progression of sialoadenitis in Sjögren's syndrome. *Br J Rheumatol* 1993;32: 578–581.
179. Atkinson JC, Travis WD, Slocum L, et al. Serum anti-Sjögren's syndrome-B/La and IgA rheumatoid factor are markers of salivary gland disease activity in primary Sjögren's syndrome. *Arthritis Rheum* 1992;35:1368–1372.
180. Daniels TE, Whitcher JP. Association of patterns of labial salivary gland inflammation with keratoconjunctivitis sicca: analysis of 618 patients with suspected Sjögren's syndrome. *Arthritis Rheum* 1994;37:869–877.
181. Wahren M, Tengner P, Gunnarsson I, et al. Ro/Sjögren's syndrome-A and La/Sjögren's syndrome-B antibody level variation in patients with Sjögren's syndrome systemic lupus erythematous. *J Autoimmun* 1998;11:29–38.
182. Wen S, Shimizu N, Toshiyama H, et al. Association of Epstein-Barr virus (EBV) with Sjögren's syndrome. *Am J Pathol* 1996; 149:1511–1517.
183. Biberfeld P, Petren AL, Eklund A, et al. Human herpesvirus-6 (HHV-6, HBLV) in sarcoidosis and lymphoproliferative disorders. *J Virol Methods* 1988;21:49–59.
184. Baboonian C, Venables PJW, Maini R, et al. Antibodies to human herpesvirus-6 in Sjögren's syndrome [Letter]. *Arthritis Rheum* 1990;33:1749–1750.
185. Yamano S, Renard JN, Mizuno F, et al. Retrovirus in salivary glands from patients with Sjögren's syndrome. *J Clin Pathol* 1997;50:223–230.
186. Terada K, Katamine S, Egushi K, et al. Prevalence of serum and salivary antibodies to HTLV-1 in Sjögren's syndrome. *Lancet* 1994;344:1116–1119.
187. Garsia-Carrasco M, Ramos M, Cervera R, et al. Hepatitis C virus infection in primary Sjögren's syndrome: prevalence and clinical significance in a series of 90 patients. *Ann Rheum Dis* 1997;56:173–175.
188. Haddad J, Deny P, Munz-Gotheil C, et al. Lymphocytic sialadenitis of Sjögren's syndrome associated with chronic hepatitis C virus liver disease. *Lancet* 1992;339:321–323.
189. Scofield RH, Harley JB. Autoantigenicity of Ro/SSA antigen is related to nucleocapsid protein of vesicular stomatitis virus. *Proc Natl Acad Sci U S A* 1991;88:3343–3347.
190. Haaheim LR, Halse A-K, Kvakestad R, et al. Serum antibodies from patients with primary Sjögren's syndrome and systemic lupus erythematosus recognize multiple epitopes on the La (Sjögren's syndrome-B) autoantigen resembling viral protein sequences. *Scand J Immunol* 1996;43:115–121.
191. Aragona P, Magazzu G, Macchia G, et al. Presence of antibodies against *Helicobacter pylori* and its heat-shock protein 60 in the serum of patients with Sjögren's syndrome. *J Rheumatol* 199;26:1306–1311.
192. De Vita S, Ferraccioli G, Avellini C, et al. Widespread clonal B-cell disorder in Sjögren's syndrome predisposing to *Helicobacter pylori*-related gastric lymphoma. *Gastroenterology* 1996;110: 1969–1974.
193. Stott DI, Hiepe F, Hummel M, et al. Antigen-driven clonal proliferation of B cells within the target tissue of an autoimmune disease: the salivary glands of patients with Sjögren's syndrome. *J Clin Invest* 1998;102:938–946.
194. Kroneld U, Jonsson R, Carlsten H, et al. Expression of the

mucosal lymphocyte integrin $\alpha^E\beta_7$ and its ligand E-cadherin in salivary glands of patients with Sjögren's syndrome. *Scand J Rheumatol* 1998;27:215–218.

195. Jonsson R, Klareskog L, Bäckman K, et al. Expression of HLA-D locus (DP, DQ, DR) coded antigens, β_2-microglobulin, and the interleukin 2 receptor in Sjögren's syndrome. *Clin Immunol Immunopathol* 1987;45:235–243.
196. Sumida T, Yonaha F, Maeda T, et al. T-cell receptor repertoire of infiltrating T-cells in lips of Sjögren's syndrome patients. *J Clin Invest* 1992;89:681–685.
197. Manoussakis MN, Dimitriou ID, Kapsogeorgou EK, et al. Expression of B7 costimulatory molecules by salivary gland epithelial cells in patients with Sjögren's syndrome. *Arthritis Rheum* 1999;42:229–239.
198. Halse A-K, TengnΘr P, Wahren-Herlenius M, et al. Increased frequency of IL-6 and IL-10 secreting cells in peripheral blood from patients with primary Sjögren's syndrome. *Scand J Immunol* 1999;49:533–538.
199. Dauphinee M, Tovar Z, Talal N. B cells expressing CD5 are increased in Sjögren's syndrome. *Arthritis Rheum* 1988;31: 642–647.
200. Halse A-K, Wahren M, Jonsson R. Peripheral blood in Sjögren's syndrome does not contain increased levels of T lymphocytes reactive with the recombinant Ro/SSA 52 kD and La/SSB 48 kD autoantigens. *Autoimmunity* 1996;23:25–34.
201. Oehm A, Behrmann I, Falk W, et al. Purification and molecular cloning of the APO-1 cell surface antigen, a member of the tumor necrosis factor/nerve growth factor receptor superfamily. *J Biol Chem* 1992;267:10709–10715.
202. Suda T, Takahashi T, Golstein P, et al. Molecular cloning and expression of the fas ligand: a novel member of the tumor necrosis factor family. *Cell* 1993;75:1169–1175.
203. Skarstein K, Nerland AH, Eidsheim M, et al. Lymphoid cell accumulation in salivary glands of autoimmune MRL mice can be due to impaired apoptosis. *Scand J Immunol* 1997;46: 373–378.
204. Kong L, Ogawa N, Nakabayashi T, et al. Fas and Fas ligand expression in the salivary glands of patients with primary Sjögren's syndrome. *Arthritis Rheum* 1997;40:87–97.
205. Nakamura H, Koji T, Tominaga M, et al. Apoptosis in labial salivary glands from Sjögren's syndrome (SS) patients: comparison with human T lymphotropic virus-I (HTLV-I)-seronegative and -seropositive SS patients. *Clin Exp Immunol* 1998:114:106–112.
206. Kong L, Ogawa N, McGuff HS, et al. Bcl-2 family expression in salivary glands from patients with primary Sjögren's syndrome: involvement of Bax in salivary gland destruction. *Clin Immunol Immunopathol* 1998;88:133–141.
207. Alpert S, Kang H-I, Weissan I, et al. Expression of granzyme A in salivary gland biopsies from patients with Sjögren's syndrome. *Arthritis Rheum* 1994;37:1046–1054.
208. Rischmueller M, Scott J, Beroukas D, et al. Salivary gland apoptosis in primary Sjögren's syndrome: a controlled study. *Arthritis Rheum* 1998;41:S325.
209. Ohlsson M, Bolstad AI, Johannessen AC, et al. Low incidence of Fas-induced apoptosis in Sjögren's syndrome. *Scand J Immunol* 1999;50:336/I7.
210. Humphreys-Beher MG, Brayer J, Yamachika S, et al. An alternative perspective to the immune response in autoimmune exocrinopathy: induction of functional quiescence rather than destructive autoaggression. *Scand J Immunol* 1999;49:7–10.
211. Jonsson R, Skarstein K. Experimental models of Sjögren's syndrome. In: Theofilopoulos B, Bona G, eds. *The molecular pathology of autoimmune diseases,* 2nd ed. Chur: Harwood Academic Publishers (in press).
212. Wahren M, Skarstein K, Blange I, et al. MRL/lpr mice produce anti-Ro 52kD antibodies: detection, analysis of specificity and site of production. *Immunology* 1994;83:9–15.
213. St. Clair EW, Kenan D, Burch JA, et al. Anti-La antibody production by MRL-lpr/lpr mice: analysis of fine specificity. *J Immunol* 1991;146:1885–1892.
214. Fleck M, Kern ER, Zhou T, et al. Murine cytomegalovirus induces a Sjögren's syndrome-like disease in C57Bl/6-lpr/lpr mice. *Arthritis Rheum* 1998;41:2175–2184.
215. Saito I, Haruta K, Shimuta M, et al. Fas ligand-mediated exocrinopathy resembling Sjögren's syndrome in mice transgenic for IL-10. *J Immunol* 1999;162:2488–2494.
216. Robinson CP, Yamachika S, Bounous DI, et al. A novel NOD-derived murine model for primary Sjögren's syndrome. *Arthritis Rheum* 1998;41:150–156.
217. Anaya JM, McGuff S, Banks PM, et al. Clinicopathological factors relating malignant lymphoma with Sjögren's syndrome. *Semin Arthritis Rheum* 1996;25:337–346.
218. Hyjek E, Smith WJ, Isaacson PG. Primary B-cell lymphoma of salivary glands and its relationship to myoepithelial sialadenitis. *Hum Pathol* 1988;19:766–776.
219. Jordan R, Diss TC, Lench NJ, et al. Immunoglobulin gene rearrangements in lymphoplasmacyctic infiltrates of labial salivary glands in Sjögren's syndrome: a possible predictor of lymphoma development. *Oral Surg Oral Med Oral Pathol* 1995;79: 723–729.
220. Diss TC, Wotherspoon AD, Speight PM, et al. B-cell monoclonality, Epstein Barr virus and t(14;18) translocations in myoepithelial sialadenitis and low grade MALT lymphoma of the parotid gland. *Am J Surg Pathol* 1995;19:531–536.
221. Harris NL. Lymphoid proliferations of the salivary glands. *Am J Clin Pathol* 1999;111(suppl 1):S94–S103.
222. Quintana PG, Kapadia SB, Bahler SW, et al. Salivary gland lymphoid infiltrates associated with lymphoepithelial lesions: a clinicopathologic, immunophenotypic, and genotypic study. *Hum Pathol* 1997;28:850–861.
223. His ED, Siddique J, Schnitzer B, et al. Analysis of immunoglobulin heavy chain gene arrangement in myoepithelial sialadenitis by polymerase chain reaction. *Am J Clin Pathol* 1996;106: 498–503.
224. Sutcliffe N, Inanc M, Speight PM, et al. Predictors of lymphoma development in primary Sjögren's syndrome. *Semin Arthritis Rheum* 1998;28:80–87.
225. Bunim JJ, Talal N. Development of malignant lymphoma in the course of Sjögren's syndrome. *Trans Assoc Am Physicians* 1963;76:45–56.
226. Kassan SS, Thomas TL, Moutsopoulos HM, et al. Increased risk of lymphoma in sicca syndrome. *Ann Intern Med* 1978; 89:888–892.
227. Isaacson PG, Spencer J. Malignant lymphoma of mucosa-associated lymphoid tissue. *Histopathology* 1987;11:445–462.
228. Isaacson PG. Lymphomas of mucosa in associated lymphoid tissue (MALT). *Histopathology* 1990;16:617–619.
229. Jensen JL, Uhlig T, Kvien TK, et al. Characteristics of rheumatoid arthritis patients with self-reported sicca symptoms: evaluation of medical, salivary and oral parameters. *Oral Dis* 1997; 3:254–261.
230. Uhlig T, Kvien TK, Jensen JL, et al. Sicca symptoms, saliva and tear production, and disease variables in 636 patients with rheumatoid arthritis. *Ann Rheum Dis* 1999;58:1–8.
231. Andonopoulos AP, Drosos AA, Skopouli FN, et al. Sjögren's syndrome in rheumatoid arthritis and progressive systemic sclerosis: a comparative study. *Clin Exp Rheumatol* 1989;7: 203–205.
232. Ericson S, Sundmark E. Studies on the sicca syndrome in patients with rheumatoid arthritis. *Acta Rheumatol Scand* 1970;16:60–80.

233. Castro EM, Marques AO, Llorach MB, et al. Rheumatoid arthritis and Sjögren's syndrome, with special reference to the duration of rheumatoid arthritis. *Med Clin (Barc)* 1990;94: 655–659.
234. Coll J, Rives A, Grino MC, et al. Prevalence of Sjögren's syndrome in autoimmune diseases. *Ann Rheum Dis* 1987;46: 286–289.
235. Cervera R, Munther MA, Font J, et al. Systemic lupus erythematosus: clinical and immunologic patterns of disease expression in a cohort of 1000 patients. *Medicine* 1993;72:113–123.
236. Oxholm P, Prause JU, Schiødt M. Rational drug therapy recommendations for the treatment of patients with Sjögren's syndrome. *Drugs* 1998;56:345–353.
237. Kriegbaum NJ, von Linstow M, Oxholm P, et al. Keratoconjunctivitis sicca in patients with primary Sjögren's syndrome: a longitudinal study of ocular parameters. *Acta Ophthalmol* 1988; 66:481–484.
238. Foster HE, Gilroy JJ, Kelly CA, et al. Treatment of sicca features in Sjögren's syndrome: a clinical review. *Br J Rheumatol* 1994; 33:278–282.
239. Fox RI. Treatment of the patient with Sjögren's syndrome. *Rheum Dis Clin North Am* 1992;18:699–709.
240. Wright WE. Management of oral sequel. *J Dent Res* 1987;66: 699–702.
241. Blom M, Dawidson I, Angmar-Mansson B. The effect of acupuncture on salivary flow rates in patients with xerostomia. *Oral Surg Oral Med Oral Pathol* 1992;73;293–298.
242. Frost-Larsen K, Isager H, Manthorpe R. Sjögren's syndrome treated with bromhexine: a randomised clinical study. *Br Med J* 1978;i:1579–1581.
243. Prause JU, Frost-Larsen K, Høj L, et al. Lacrimal and salivary secretion in Sjögren's syndrome: the effect of systemic treatment with bromhexine. *Acta Ophthalmol* 1984;62:489–497.
244. Papas A, Chamey M, Golden H, et al. The effectiveness of oral pilocarpine HCL tablets for the treatment of dry mouth symptoms associated with Sjögren's syndrome. *Arthritis Rheum* 1997; 40(suppl S202):1026.
245. Nusair S, Rubinow A. The use of oral pilocarpine in xerostomia and Sjögren's syndrome. *Semin Arthritis Rheum* 1999;6:360–367.
246. Fox PC, Van der Ven PF, Baum BJ, et al. Pilocarpine for the treatment of xerostomia associated with salivary gland dysfunction. *Oral Surg* 1986:61:243–248.
247. Shiozawa S, Morimoto I, Tanaka Y, et al. A preliminary study on interferon-alpha treatment for xerostomia of Sjögren's syndrome. *Br J Rheumatol* 1993;32:52–54.
248. Ninomiya T, Iga Y, Fukui K, et al. The pharmacological profile of cevimeline: a novel muscarinic agonist for treatment in various models. *Arthritis Rheum* 1998;41(suppl):S329.
249. Panayi GS, Neill WA, Duthie JJ, et al. Action of chloroquin phosphate in rheumatoid arthritis. I. Immunosuppressive effect. *Ann Rheum Dis* 1973;32:316–318.
250. Kruize AA, Hené RJ, Kallenberg CGM, et al. Hydroxychloroquine treatment for primary Sjögren's syndrome: a two year double blind crossover trial. *Ann Rheum Dis* 1993;52:360–364.
251. Fox RI, Guarrasi V, Krubel S. Treatment of primary Sjögren's syndrome with hydroxychloroquine: a retrospective, open-label study. *Lupus* 1996;5(suppl 1):S31–S36.
252. Tabbara KF, Frayha RA. Alternate-day steroid therapy for patients with primary Sjögren's syndrome. *Ann Ophthalmol* 1983;15:358–361.
253. Fox PC, Datiles M, Atkinson JC, et al. Prednisone and piroxicam for treatment of primary Sjögren's syndrome. *Clin Exp Rheumatol* 1993;11:149–156.
254. Drosos AA, Skopouli FN, Costopoulos JS, et al. Cyclosporin A in primary Sjögren's syndrome: a double blind study. *Ann Rheum Dis* 1986;45:732–735.
255. Drosos AA, Van Vliet-dascalopoulou E, Andonopoulos AP, et al. Nandrolone decanoate in primary Sjögren's syndrome: a double blind pilot study. *Clin Exp Rheumatol* 1988;6:53–57.
256. Skopouli FN, Jagiello P, Tsifetaki N, et al. Methotrexate in primary Sjögren's syndrome. *Clin Exp Rheumatol* 1996;14:555–558.
257. Moutsopoulos HM, Manoussakis MN. Immunopathogenesis of Sjögren's syndrome: "facts and fancy." *Autoimmunity* 1989;5:17–24.
258. Moutsopoulos HM, Webber BI, Vlagopoulos TP, et al. Differences in the clinical manifestations of sicca syndrome and absence of rheumatoid arthritis. *Am J Med* 1979;66:733–736.
259. Pavlidis NA, Karsh J, Moutsopoulos HM. The clinical picture of primary Sjögren's syndrome: a retrospective study. *J Rheumatol* 1982;9:685–690.
260. Fox RI, Howell FV, Bone RC, et al. Primary Sjögren's syndrome: clinical and immunopathological features. *Semin Arthritis Rheum* 1984;14:77–105.
261. Markusse HM, Oudkerk M, Vroom ThM, et al. Primary Sjögren's syndrome: clinical spectrum and mode of presentation based on analysis of 50 patients selected from a department of rheumatology. *Neth J Med* 1992;40:125–134.
262. Patiente D, Anaya JM, Combe B, et al. Non-Hodgkin's lymphoma associated with primary Sjögren's syndrome. *Eur J Med* 1992;1:337–342.
263. Tishler M, Aharon A, Ehrenfeld M, et al. Sjögren's syndrome in Israel: primary versus secondary disease. *Clin Rheumatol* 1994; 13:438–441.
264. Kruize AA, Henà RJ, van der Heide A, et al. Long-term followup of patients with Sjögren's syndrome. *Arthritis Rheum* 1996;39:297–303.
265. Asmussen K, Andersen V, Bendixen G, et al. Plasma immunoglobulin G predicts the long term course of primary Sjögren's syndrome. In: Homma M, Sugai S, Tojo T, Miyasaka N, Akizuki M, eds. *Sjögren's syndrome:* state of the art. Amsterdam: Kugler Publications, 1994:361–363.
266. Pease CT, Charles PJ, Shattles W, et al. Serological and immunogenetic markers of extraglandular primary Sjögren's syndrome. *Br J Rheumatol* 1993;32:574–577.
267. Martens PB, Pillemer SR, Jacobsson LTH, et al. Survivorship in a population based cohort of patients with Sjögren's syndrome,1976-1992. *J Rheumatol* 1999;26:1296–1300.

86

RHEUMATIC FEVER: ETIOLOGY, DIAGNOSIS, AND TREATMENT

ALLAN GIBOFSKY
JOHN B. ZABRISKIE

Acute rheumatic fever (ARF) is a delayed, nonsuppurative sequela of a pharyngeal infection with the group A streptococcus. Following the initial streptococcal pharyngitis, there is a latent period of 2 to 3 weeks. The onset of disease is usually characterized by an acute febrile illness that may manifest itself in one of three classic ways: (a) migratory arthritis predominantly involving large joints; (b) clinical and laboratory signs of carditis and valvulitis; and (c) involvement of the central nervous system, manifesting itself as Sydenham's chorea. The clinical episodes are self-limiting, but damage to the valves may be chronic and progressive, resulting in cardiac decompensation and death.

Although there has been a dramatic decline in both the severity and mortality of the disease since the turn of the century, there have been reports of resurgence in this country (1) and in many military installations around the world, indicating that the disease remains a public health problem even in developed countries. Additionally, the disease continues essentially unabated in many of the developing countries—estimates suggest there will be 10 to 20 million new cases per year in those countries where two-thirds of the world population lives.

EPIDEMIOLOGY

The incidence of ARF actually began to decline long before the introduction of antibiotics, decreasing from 250 to 100 patients/100,000 population between 1862 and 1962 in Denmark (2). The introduction of antibiotics in 1950 rapidly accelerated this decline, until by 1980 the incidence ranged from 0.23 to 1.88 patients per 100,000, primarily in children and teenagers. A notable exception to this has been in the native Hawaiian and Maori populations (both of Polynesian ancestry) where the incidence continues to be 13.4/100,000 hospitalized children/year (3).

Only a few M serotypes (types 5, 14, 18, and 24) have been identified with outbreaks of ARF, suggesting that certain strains of group A streptococci may be more "rheumatogenic" than others (4). In Trinidad, however, types 41 and 11 have been the most common strains isolated from the oropharynx of patients with ARF. In our own series, gathered over a 20-year period (Table 86.1) a large number of different M serotypes were isolated, including six strains that could not be typed. Kaplan et al. (5) isolated several M types from patients seen during an outbreak of ARF in Utah, and these strains were both mucoid and nonmucoid in character. Thus, whether or not certain strains are more rheumatogenic than others remains unresolved. What is true, however, is that a streptococcal strain capable of causing a well-documented pharyngitis is generally capable of causing ARF, although notable exceptions have been reported (reviewed in ref. 6).

TABLE 86.1. POSITIVE THROAT CULTURES—GROUP A β-HEMOLYTIC STREPTOCOCCI AMONG ROCKEFELLER UNIVERSITY HOSPITAL RHEUMATIC FEVER PATIENTS (N = 87)

M Type	RHD	No RHD	Total
Nontypable	1	5	6
1	1	1	2
2	0	1	1
5	1	1	2
6	1	1	2
12	0	2	2
18	2	2	4
19	2	1	3
28	1	0	1
Total	9	11	23

RHD, patients with rheumatic heart disease.
No RHD, patients without rheumatic heart disease.

PATHOGENESIS

While there is little evidence of the direct involvement of group A streptococci in the affected tissues of patients with ARF, there is a large body of epidemiologic and immunologic evidence indirectly implicating the group A streptococcus in the initiation of the disease process: (a) It is well known that outbreaks of ARF closely follow epidemics of either streptococcal sore throats or scarlet fever (6). (b) Adequate treatment of a documented streptococcal pharyngitis markedly reduces the incidence of subsequent ARF (7). (c) Appropriate antimicrobial prophylaxis prevents the recurrences of disease in known patients with acute ARF (8). (d) If one tests the sera of the majority of patients with ARF for three antistreptococcal antibodies (streptolysin "O," hyaluronidase, and streptokinase), the vast majority of ARF patients (whether or not they recall an antecedent streptococcal sore throat) will have elevated antibody titers to these antigens (9).

A note of caution is necessary concerning documentation (either clinical or microbiologic) of an antecedent streptococcal infection. The frequency of isolation of group A streptococci from the oropharynx is extremely low even in populations with limited access to microbial antibiotics. Further, there appears to be an age-related discrepancy in the clinical documentation of an antecedent sore throat. In older children and young adults, the recollection of a streptococcal sore throat approaches 70%; in younger children, this rate approaches only 20% (1). Thus, it is important to have a high index of suspicion of ARF in children or young adults presenting with signs of arthritis or carditis even in the absence of a clinically documented sore throat.

Another intriguing, and as yet unexplained, observation has been the invariable association of ARF only with streptococcal pharyngitis. While there have been many outbreaks of impetigo, ARF almost never occurs following infection with these strains. Furthermore, in Trinidad, where both impetigo and ARF are concomitant infections, the strains colonizing the skin are different from those associated with ARF, and they did not influence the incidence of ARF (10).

The explanations for these observations remain obscure. It is clear that group A streptococci fall into two main classes based on differences in the C repeat regions of the M protein (11). One class is clearly associated with streptococcal pharyngeal infection, the other (with some exceptions) is commonly associated with impetigo. Thus, the particular strain of streptococcus may be crucial in initiating the disease process. The pharyngeal site of infection with its large repository of lymphoid tissue may also be important in the initiation of the abnormal humoral response by the host to those antigens cross-reactive with target organs. Finally, while impetigo strains do colonize the pharynx, they do not appear to elicit as strong an immunologic response to the M protein moiety as do the pharyngeal strains (12,13). This may prove to be an important factor, especially in light of the known cross-reactions between various streptococcal structures and mammalian proteins.

GROUP A STREPTOCOCCUS

Figure 86.1 is a schematic cross-section of the group A streptococcus. The capsule is composed of equimolar concentrations of *N*-acetylglucosamine and glucuronic acid and is structurally identical to hyaluronic acid of mammalian tissues (14).

Although numerous attempts to produce antibodies to this capsule have been unsuccessful (15,16), Fillit et al. (17) were able to demonstrate high antibody titers to hyaluronic acid using techniques designed to detect nonprecipitating antibodies in the sera of immunized animals. Similar antibodies have been noted in humans (18). The data establishing the importance of this capsule in human infections have been almost nonexistent, although Stollerman (19) has commented on the presence of a large mucoid capsule as being one of the more important characteristics of certain rheumatogenic strains.

With respect to the M protein moiety, investigations by Lancefield and others spanning almost 70 years (reviewed in ref. 20) have established that the M protein molecule (at least 80 distinct serologic types) is perhaps the most important virulence factor in group A streptococcal infections of humans. The protein is a helical coiled-coil structure and bears a striking structural homology to the cardiac cytoskeletal proteins, tropomyosin and myosin, as well as to

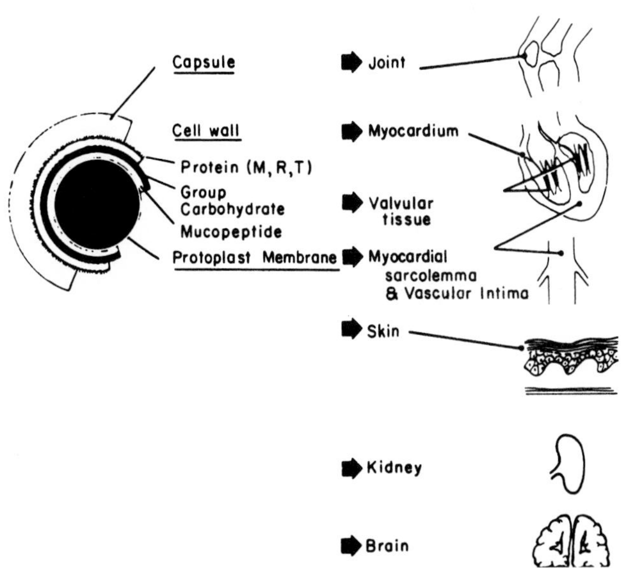

FIGURE 86.1. Various structures of the group A streptococcus. Note the wide variety of cross-reactions between its antigens and mammalian tissues.

many other coiled-coil structures including keratin, DNA, lamin, and vimentin.

Once the amino acid sequence of a number of M proteins was delineated, it was possible to specifically localize cross-reactive areas of the molecules. The studies of Dale and Beachey (21) showed that the segment of the M protein involved in the opsonic reaction also cross-reacted with human sarcolemma antigens. Sargent and co-workers (22) more precisely localized this cross-reaction to the M protein amino acid residues 164 to 197.

The evidence implicating cross-reactions in the pathogenesis of ARF remains scant. Antibodies to myosin have been detected in the sera of ARF patients, but they are also present in a high percentage of sera obtained from individuals who had a streptococcal infection but did not subsequently develop ARF (23). The significance of this observation is unclear, since myosin is an internal protein of cardiac muscle cells and therefore not easily exposed to M protein cross-reacting antibodies.

The group-specific carbohydrate of the streptococcus is a polysaccharide chain consisting of repeating units of rhamnose capped by *N*-acetylglucosamine molecules. The *N*-acetylglucosamine is immunodominant and gives rise to the serologic group specificity of group A streptococci (24). The cross-reaction between group A carbohydrate and valvular glycoproteins was first described by Goldstein et al. (25), and the reactivity was related to the *N*-acetylglucosamine moiety present in both structures. Goldstein and Caravano (26) noted that ARF sera reacted to the heart valve glycoprotein. Fillit (unpublished data) has observed strong reactivity of ARF sera with purified proteoglycan material. Thus, these cross-reactions could involve the sugar moiety present in both the proteoglycan portion of the glycoprotein and the carbohydrate.

It has generally been assumed that group A anticarbohydrate antibodies do not play a role in phagocytosis of group A streptococci. However, Salvadori and co-workers (27) demonstrated that human sera containing high titers of antigroup A carbohydrate antibody promoted opsonization and phagocytosis of a number of different M protein specific strains, and the opsonophagocytic antibodies were directed to the *N*-acetylglucosamine moiety of the group A carbohydrate.

The mucopeptide portion of the cell wall is the "backbone" of the organism and thus quite rigid in structure. It consists of repeating units of muramic acid and *N*-acetylglucosamine, cross-linked by peptide bridges (28). It is particularly difficult to degrade and induces a wide variety of lesions when injected into various animal species, including arthritis in rats (29) and myocardial granulomas in mice resembling (but not identical to) ARF Aschoff lesions (30).

The relationship of cell wall mucopeptides to the pathogenesis of ARF remains obscure. Elevated levels of antimucopeptide antibody have been detected not only in the sera of patients with ARF, but also in the sera of patients with rheumatoid arthritis (RA) and juvenile rheumatoid arthritis (31); however, its pathogenetic relationship to clinical disease has been difficult to establish. There is no evidence that cell wall antigens are present either in the Aschoff lesion or in the myocardial tissue obtained from patients with ARF.

Perhaps the most significant cross-reactions lie in the streptococcal membrane structure. We have shown that immunization with membrane material (32) elicited antibodies that bound to heart sections in a pattern similar to that observed with acute RF sera (Fig. 86.2).

Kingston and Glynn (33) were the first to show that animals immunized with streptococcal antigens developed

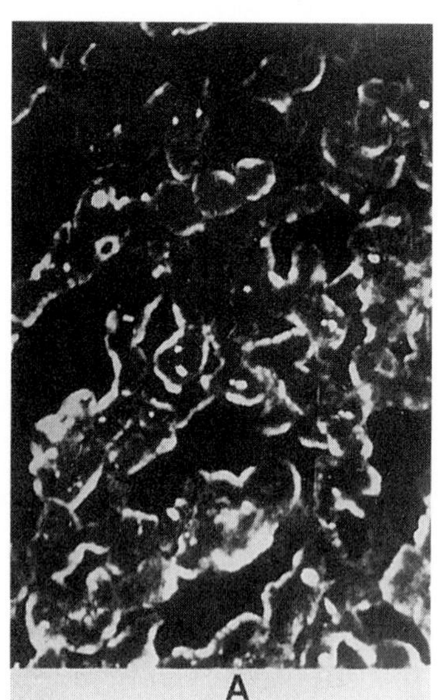

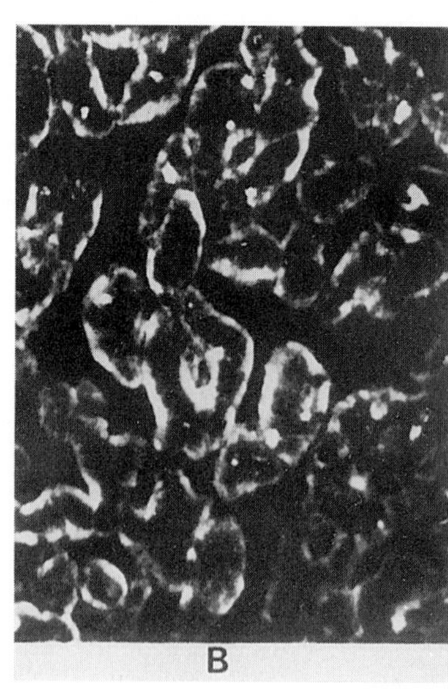

FIGURE 86.2. Photomicrographs of immunofluorescent staining of heart sections with **(A)** rabbit serum immunized with group A streptococcal membranes and **(B)** human serum obtained from a patient with acute rheumatic fever (RF). Note the identical sarcolemmal staining patterns of both sera.

antibodies in their sera that stained astrocytes. Husby and co-workers (34) demonstrated that sera from ARF patients with chorea contained antibodies that were reactive with caudate cells. Absorption of the sera with streptococcal membrane antigens eliminated the reactivity with caudate cells.

Numerous other cross-reactions between streptococcal membranes and other organs have also been reported (e.g., renal basement membranes, basement membrane proteoglycans, and skin, particularly keratin). In the context of this chapter, space does not permit an exhaustive discussion of these cross-reactions, and the reader is referred to our previous review (35) for a more detailed discussion. Whether or not these cross-reactions (especially those seen with basement membranes and skin) play a role in the disease awaits further study.

GENETICS

The concept that ARF might be the result of a host genetic predisposition has intrigued investigators for over a century (36). It has been variously suggested that the disease gene is transmitted in an autosomal-dominant fashion (37), or autosomal-recessive fashion with limited penetrance (38), or that it is possibly related to the genes conferring blood group secretor status (39).

Renewed interest in the genetics of ARF occurred with the recognition that gene products of the human major histocompatibility complex (MHC) were associated with certain clinical disease states. Using an alloserum from a multiparous donor, an increased frequency of a B-cell alloantigen was reported in several genetically distinct and ethnically diverse populations of ARF individuals and was not MHC-related (40).

More recently, a monoclonal antibody (D8/17) was prepared by immunizing mice with B cells from an ARF patient (41). A B-cell antigen identified by this antibody was found to be expressed on increased numbers of B cells in 100% of rheumatics of diverse ethnic origins, and in only 10% of normal individuals. This antigen showed no association with or linkage to any of the known MHC alleles, nor did it appear to be related to B-cell activation antigens.

Studies with D8/17 have been expanded to a larger number of patients with RF (Table 86.2) of diverse ethnic origins with essentially the same results. As will be discussed below, the presence or absence of elevated levels of D8/17$^+$ B cells in cases of questionable RF has been helpful in establishing or ruling out the diagnosis.

These studies contrast with other reports in which an increased frequency of human leukocyte antigens HLA-DR4 and HLA-DR2 was seen in Caucasian and black patients with rheumatic heart disease (42). Other studies have implicated DR1 and DR6 as susceptibility factors in South African black patients with rheumatic heart disease (43). More recently, Guilherme and associates (44) reported an increased frequency of HLA-DR7 and DR53 in ARF patients in Brazil. These seemingly conflicting results concerning HLAs and ARF susceptibility raise the possibility that these reported associations might be of class II genes close to (or in linkage disequilibrium with), but not identical to, the putative ARF susceptibility gene. Alternatively, and more likely, susceptibility to ARF is polygenic, and the D8/17 antigen might be associated with only one of the genes. While the explanation remains to be determined, the presence of the D8/17 antigen does appear to identify a population at increased risk for contracting ARF.

TABLE 86.2. FREQUENCY OF THE D8/17 MARKER IN PATIENTS WITH RHEUMATIC FEVER, OTHER DISEASES, AND CONTROLS IN VARIOUS GEOGRAPHICAL POPULATIONS

	Number	Percent Positive
Rheumatic Fever Patients		
New York (USA)	43/45	93
New Mexico (USA)	30/31	97
Utah (USA)[a]	18/18	100
Russia (Georgian)	27/30	90
Russia (Moscow)	50/52	96
Mexico	35/39	89
Chile	45/50	90
Normals		
Russia	4/78	5
New York	8/68	8
Chile	8/50	16
Mexico	6/72	8
Other diseases		
Rheumatoid arthritis	2/42	4
Ischemic heart disease	0/10	0
Multiple sclerosis	1/25	4
Lupus erythematosus	1/12	9

[a]Acute patients.

ETIOLOGIC CONSIDERATIONS

While a large body of immunologic and epidemiologic evidence has implicated the group A streptococcus in the induction of the disease process, the precise pathologic mechanisms involved still remain obscure. At least three main theories have been proposed.

The first theory is concerned with the question of whether persistence of the organism is important. Despite several controversial reports, no investigators have been able to consistently and reproducibly demonstrate live organisms in rheumatic cardiac tissues or valves (45).

The second theory revolves around the question of whether deposition of toxic products is required. Although an attractive hypothesis, little or no experimental evidence has been obtained to support this concept. For example, Halbert et al. (46) suggested that streptolysin O (an extracellular product of group A streptococci) is cardiotoxic and might be carried to the site by circulating complexes containing streptolysin O and antibody. However, in spite of an intensive search for these products, no such complexes *in situ* have been identified (47) (Zabriskie JB, unpublished data, 1959).

Renewed interest in extracellular toxins has emerged with the observation by Schlievert et al. (48) that certain streptococcal pyrogenic toxins (A and C) may act as superantigens. These antigens may stimulate large numbers of T cells through their unique bridging interaction with T-cell receptors of specific V_β types and class II MHC molecules. This interaction is clearly distinct from conventional antigen presentation in the context of the MHC complex. Once activated, these T cells elaborate tumor necrosis factor, interferon-γ, and a number of interleukin moieties, thereby contributing to the initiation of pathologic damage. Furthermore, it has been suggested (49) that in certain disease states such as RA, autoreactive cells of specific V_β lineage may "home" to the target organ. Although an attractive hypothesis, no data concerning the role of superantigens in ARF have as yet been forthcoming.

Perhaps the best evidence to date favors the theory of an abnormal host immune response (both humoral and cellular) in the genetically susceptible individual to those streptococcal antigens cross-reactive with mammalian tissues. The evidence supporting this theory is drawn from three broad categories:

1. Employing a wide variety of methods, numerous investigators have documented the presence of heart reactive antibodies in ARF sera. The prevalence of these antibodies has varied from a low of 33% to a high of 85% in various series. While these antibodies occur in other individuals (notably those with uncomplicated streptococcal infections that do not go on to ARF and patients with poststreptococcal glomerulonephritis), the titers are always lower than that seen in ARF and decrease with time during the convalescent period (Table 86.3).

   An important point both in terms of diagnosis and prognosis has been the observation (50) that these heart-reactive antibody titers decline over time. By the end of 3 years, titers are essentially undetectable in those patients who had only a single attack (Fig. 86.3). This pattern is consistent with the well-known clinical observations that recurrences of ARF most often occur within the first 2 to 3 years after the initial attack and become rarer 5 years after an initial episode.

   As illustrated in Fig. 86.4 this pattern of titers also has prognostic value. During the 2- to 5-year period after the initial attack, patient M.P.'s titers dropped to undetectable levels. However, with a known break in prophylaxis starting in year 6, at least two streptococcal infections occurred, as evidenced by rise in anti-streptolysm O (ASO) titers during that period. Of note was the concomitant rise in heart-reactive antibody titers. The final infection was followed by a clinical recurrence of classic rheumatic carditis complete with isolation of the organism, elevated heart-reactive antibodies, and acute-phase reactants 11 years after the initial attack.
2. Sera from patients with ARF also contain increased levels of antibodies to both myosin and tropomyosin, as compared to sera from patients with pharyngeal streptococcal infections that do not go on to develop ARF. These myosin-affinity purified antibodies also cross-react with M protein epitopes, suggesting this molecule could be the antigenic stimulus for the production of myosin antibodies in these sera (23).
3. Finally, as indicated earlier, autoimmune antibodies are a prominent finding in another major clinical manifestation of ARF, chorea, and these antibodies are directed against cells in the caudate nucleus. The titer of these antibodies corresponds with clinical disease activity (34).

While not necessarily autoimmune in nature, the presence of immune complexes in ARF has been well documented both in the sera and in the joints of ARF patients (51). Elevated levels of immune complexes, which may be

TABLE 86.3. HEART-REACTIVE ANTIBODY TITERS IN THE SERA OF PATIENTS WITH ACUTE RHEUMATIC FEVER AS COMPARED TO UNCOMPLICATED STREPTOCOCCAL INFECTIONS AND OTHER ARTHRITIC DISEASES

Clinical Disorder	Number of Patients	Serum Dilutions			Average ASO Titer
		1:5	1:10	1:20	
Acute rheumatic fever[a]	34	4+	2+	+	700
Uncomplicated streptococcal infection[a]	40	1+	0	0	560
Acute poststreptococcal glomerulonephritis	20	+/–	0	0	520
Rheumatoid arthritis[b]	10	0	0	0	ND
Systemic lupus erythematosus	10	0	0	0	ND

[a]Serum samples obtained at onset of rheumatic fever and at a comparable time in the group with uncomplicated scarlet fever.
[b]Sera obtained during active disease.
ND, not determined.

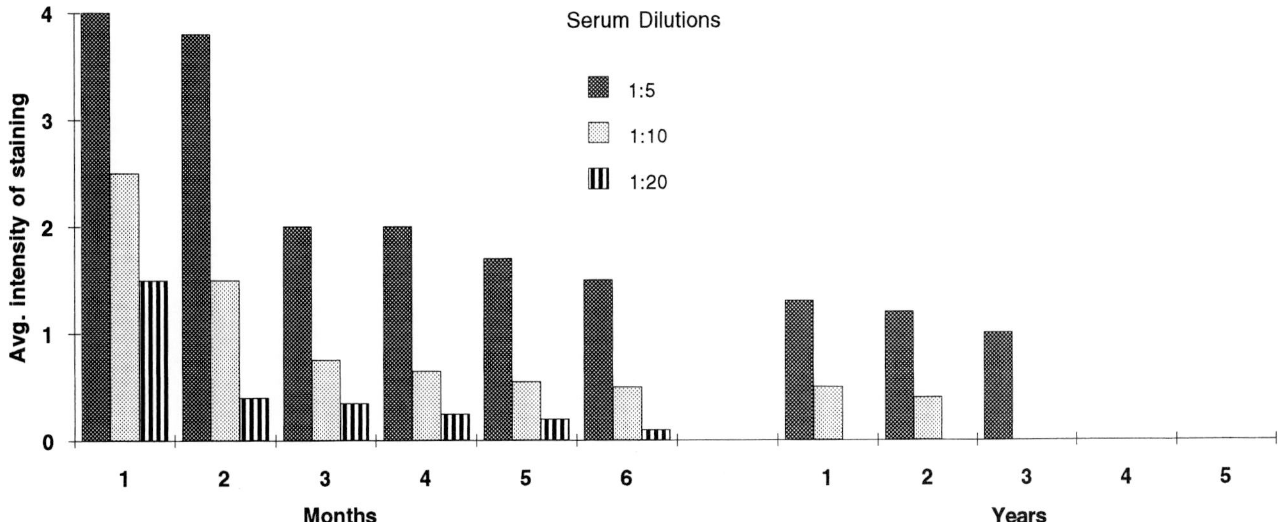

FIGURE 86.3. Serial heart reactive antibody titers in 40 patients with documented ARF. Note the slow decline of these titers over the first 2 years after the initial episode and the absence of these antibodies 5 years after the initial attack.

as high as those seen in classic, acute, poststreptococcal glomerulonephritis, may be responsible for the immune complex vasculitis seen in ARF tissues and may provide the initial impetus for vascular damage followed by the secondary penetration of autoreactive antibodies. Support for the concept is the close clinical similarity of arthritis in ARF to experimentally induced serum sickness in animals or secondary to drug hypersensitivity. Deposition of host immunoglobulin and complement is also seen in the cardiac tissues of ARF patients, suggesting deposition of autoreactive immunoglobulins in or near the Aschoff lesions.

At a cellular level, there is convincing evidence of the presence of both lymphocytes and macrophages at the site of pathologic damage in the heart of patients with ARF (52). The cells are predominantly $CD4^+$ helper lymphocytes (ratio of $CD4^+/CD8^+$ lymphocytes = 4:1) during acute stages of the disease. In chronic valvular specimens, the ratio of $CD4^+/CD8^+$ lymphocytes (2:1) more closely approximates the normal ratio (Table 86.4). A majority of

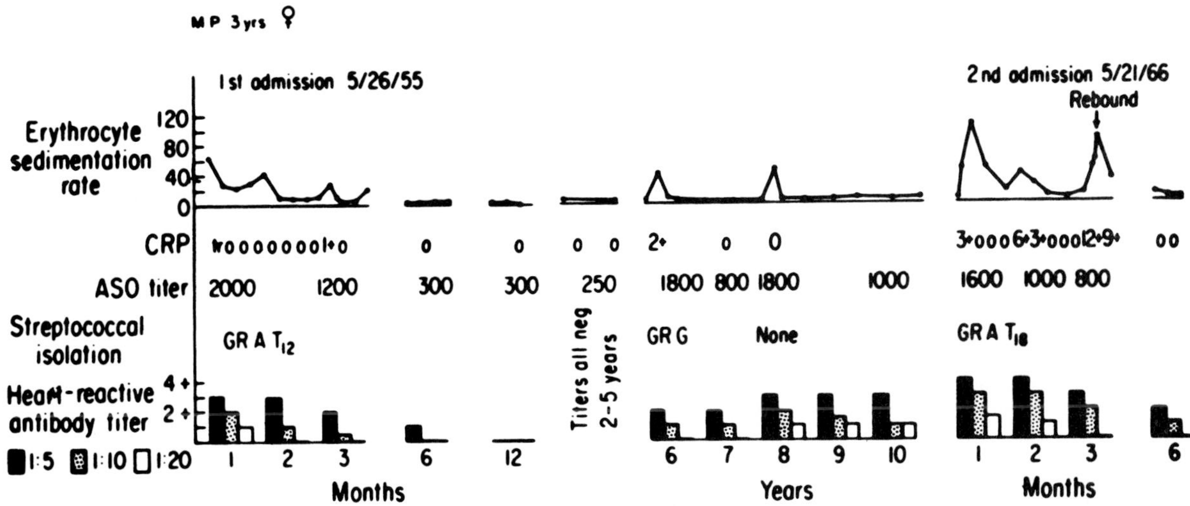

FIGURE 86.4. Heart reactive antibody titers and laboratory data obtained from a patient with ARF who had two well-documented acute attacks 11 years apart. Note absence of the heart reactive antibody during years 2 to 5 and its reappearance during years 6 to 10 after evidence of two intercurrent streptococcal infections secondary to breaks in penicillin prophylaxis (see anti-streptolysm O [ASO] titers). High titers of heart reactive antibody appeared with the second attack. CRP, C-reactive protein.

TABLE 86.4. COMPOSITION OF MONONUCLEAR CELLULAR INFILTRATES IN ACUTE AND CHRONIC ACTIVE RHEUMATIC VALVULITIS

Patients	Type of Valve	Type of Valvulitis[a]	Composition of Infiltrate (%)						CD4/CD8 ratio
			HLA-DR$^+$	CD14^{+b}	CD20^{+c}	CD3^{+d}	CD4^{+e}	CD8^{+f}	
Acute valvulitis									
1	Mitral	Acute	58.9	42.6	5.1	49.5	75.6	23.9	3.1
2	Mitral	Acute	49.8	43.1	6.9	43.1	58.7	34.3	1.9
	Aortic	Acute	52.7	51.0	3.9	38.1	65.9	26.5	2.3
3	Mitral	Acute	63.9	42.0	5.5	52.4	75.4	18.9	4.0
4	Aortic	Acute	68.1	56.0	7.4	33.7	71.6	22.0	3.3
Chronic valvulitis									
4	Mitral	Chronic active	49.4	47.4	7.4	44.3	53.7	38.8	1.4
5	Mitral	Chronic active	48.8	39.1	1.4	53.9	45.2	51.5	0.9
	Aortic	Chronic active	67.8	35.0	4.0	36.8	47.5	49.1	1.0
6	Mitral	Chronic active	41.8	23.4	8.0	65.9	57.3	33.3	1.7
	Aortic	Chronic active	69.6	48.7	6.2	30.1	58.2	32.6	1.8
7	Mitral	Chronic active	55.4	24.2	8.1	59.8	64.9	24.7	2.6
8	Mitral	Chronic active	80.4	34.1	13.4	44.4	44.8	50.9	0.9
9	Mitral	Chronic active	46.1	29.6	0.8	65.6	61.6	33.3	1.8

[a]Determined in the frozen valve samples studied.
[b](63D3) Monocytes/macrophages.
[c](Leu 16) B cells.
[d]Pan T cells.
[e]Helper T cells.
[f]Suppressor cells.

infiltrating mononuclear cells express DR antigens. A potentially important finding has been the observation that macrophage-like fibroblasts present in the diseased valves also express DR antigens (53) and might function as the antigen-presenting cells for the CD4$^+$ positive lymphocytes.

Increased cellular reactivity to streptococcal antigens has also been noted among the peripheral blood mononuclear cell preparations of ARF patients when compared to these cells isolated from nephritis patients (54). This abnormal reactivity peaks at 6 months after the attack, but may persist for as long as 2 years after the initial episode. Once again the reactivity was specific only for those strains associated with ARF, suggesting an abnormal humoral and cellular response to streptococcal antigens unique to ARF-associated streptococci.

Support for the potential pathologic importance of streptococcal antigen-reactive T cells is further strengthened by the observation that lymphocytes obtained from experimental animals sensitized to cell membranes, but not cell walls, are specifically cytotoxic for syngeneic embryonic cardiac myofibers *in vitro* (55). In humans, mononuclear cells obtained from healthy individuals and primed *in vitro* by M protein molecules from an ARF-associated strain are also cytotoxic for myofibers, but specificity solely for cardiac cells was lacking in the human studies (56). Similar studies have not yet been performed using lymphocytes from patients with active ARF.

CLINICAL FEATURES OF ACUTE RHEUMATIC FEVER

The clinical presentation of ARF is quite variable, and the lack of a single pathognomonic feature has resulted in the

TABLE 86.5. REVISED JONES CRITERIA FOR DIAGNOSIS OF ACUTE RHEUMATIC FEVER (ARF)

Major Criteria	Minor Criteria
Carditis	Fever
Polyarthritis	Arthralgias
Chorea	Previous ARF or RHD
Erythema marginatum	
Subcutaneous nodules	

Laboratory Findings
Elevated acute phase reactants
C-reactive protein
Erythrocyte sedimentation rate
Prolonged P-R interval
Supporting evidence of preceding streptococcal infection
Increased ASO or other streptococcal antibodies
Positive throat culture for group A–hemolytic streptococci
Recent scarlet fever

From Jones Criteria Update 1992. Guidelines for diagnosis of rheumatic fever. *JAMA* 1992;268:2069–2070.
ASO, anti-streptolysm O.

development of the revised Jones criteria, as illustrated in Table 86.5 (57), which are used to help establish a diagnosis. It should be noted that these criteria were established only as guidelines for the diagnosis and were never intended to be etched in stone. Thus, depending on the age, geographic location, or ethnic population, one criterion for the diagnosis of acute ARF may be more important than others. Manifestations of ARF that are not clearly expressed pose a dilemma because of the importance of identifying a first rheumatic attack clearly in order to establish the need for prophylaxis of recurrences. Some of the isolated manifestations, particularly polyarthritis, may be difficult or impossible to distinguish from other diseases, especially at their onset. The diagnosis can be made, however, when "pure" chorea is the sole manifestation because of the rarity with which this presentation is due to any other cause.

Arthritis

In the classic, untreated case, the arthritis of ARF affects several joints in quick succession, each for a short time. The legs are usually affected first and later the arms. The terms *migrating* and *migratory* are often used to describe the polyarthritis of ARF, but these designations are not meant to signify that the inflammation necessarily disappears in one joint when it appears in another. Rather, the various localizations usually overlap in time, and the onset, as opposed to the full course of the arthritis, "migrates" from joint to joint.

Joint involvement is more common, and also more severe, in teenagers and young adults than in children. Arthritis is usually the earliest symptomatic manifestation of the disease, although asymptomatic carditis may precede it. Rheumatic polyarthritis may be excruciatingly painful, but is almost always transient. The pain is usually more prominent than the objective signs of inflammation.

When the disease is allowed to express itself fully, unmodified by antiinflammatory treatment, over one-half of patients studied show a true polyarthritis, with inflammation in anywhere from 6 to 16 joints. Classically, each joint is maximally inflamed for only a few days, or a week at the most; the inflammation decreases, perhaps lingering for another week or so, and then disappears completely. Radiographs at this point may show a slight effusion but, most likely, will be unremarkable.

In routine practice, however, many patients with arthritis or arthralgias are treated empirically with salicylates or other nonsteroidal antiinflammatory drugs (NSAIDs). Accordingly, arthritis subsides quickly in the joint(s) already affected and does not migrate to new joints. Thus, therapy may deprive the diagnostician of a useful sign. In a large series of patients with ARF and associated arthritis, most of whom had been treated, involvement of only a single large joint was common (25%). One or both knees were affected in 76%, and one or both ankles in 50%. Elbows, wrists, hips, or small joints of the feet were involved in 12% to 15% of patients, and shoulder or small joints of the hand were affected in 7% to 8%. Joints rarely affected were the lumbosacral (2%), cervical (1%), sternoclavicular (0.5%), and temporomandibular (0.5%). Involvement of the small joints of the hands or feet alone occurred in only 1% of these patients (58).

Analysis of the synovial fluid in well-documented cases of ARF with arthritis generally reveals a sterile, inflammatory fluid. There may be a decrease of complement components C1q, C3, and C4, indicating local consumption, presumably by immune complexes in the joint fluid and tissue (59).

Poststreptococcal Reactive Arthritis

A number of investigators (60–62) have suggested that poststreptococcal migratory arthritis (both in adults and children) in the absence of carditis might be an entity distinct from ARF for these reasons:

1. The latent period between the antecedent streptococcal infection and the onset of poststreptococcal reactive arthritis is shorter (1 to 2 weeks) than the 3 to 4 weeks usually seen in classic ARF.
2. The response of the poststreptococcal reactive arthritis to aspirin and other nonsteroidal medications is poor in comparison to the dramatic response seen in classic ARF.
3. Evidence of carditis is not usually seen in these patients; further, the severity of the arthritis is quite marked.
4. Extraarticular manifestations (such as tenosynovitis and renal abnormalities) are often seen in these patients.

While these features may be seen (admittedly rare), migratory arthritis in the absence of other major Jones criteria, if supported by two minor manifestations (Table 86.5), must still be considered ARF, especially in children. Variations in the response to aspirin in these children often are not documented with serum salicylate levels and an unusual clinical course is not sufficient to exclude the diagnosis of ARF. Thus, appropriate prophylactic measures should be taken (reviewed in ref. 63). Support for this concept may be found in the work of Crea and Mortimer (64). In their series of patients with ARF, 50% of the children who presented solely with signs of migratory arthritis went on to develop significant valvular damage.

ARF in adults also occurs. Although migratory arthritis is a common presenting symptom, an outbreak in San Diego Naval Training Camp (65) revealed a 30% incidence of valvular damage in these patients.

The importance of clearly defining this reactive arthritis as an ARF variant has obvious implications for secondary prophylactic treatment. It has been suggested by some investigators, that poststreptococcal reactive arthritis is a benign condition without need for prophylaxis. Yet, as these patients generally do fulfill the Jones criteria (one major, two minor), they should be considered as having ARF and, in our opinion, treated as such.

Carditis

Cardiac valvular and muscle damage can manifest in a variety of signs and symptoms. These manifestations include organic heart murmurs, cardiomegaly, congestive heart failure, or pericarditis. Mild-to-moderate chest discomfort, pleuritic chest pain, or a pericardial friction rub are indications of pericarditis. On clinical examination, the patient may have new or changing organic murmurs, most commonly mitral regurgitant murmurs, and, occasionally, aortic regurgitant murmurs and systolic ejection murmurs, caused by acute valvular inflammation and deformity. Rarely, a Carey-Coombs mid-diastolic murmur caused by rapid flow over the mitral valve is heard. If the valvular damage is severe and there is concurrent cardiac dysfunction, congestive heart failure can occur. Congestive heart failure is the most life-threatening clinical syndrome of ARF, and must be treated aggressively and early with a combination of antiinflammatory drugs, diuretics, and, occasionally, steroids to acutely decrease cardiac inflammation. EKG abnormalities may include all degrees of heart block, including atrioventricular (A-V) dissociation, but first-degree heart block is not associated with a poor prognosis. Second- or third-degree heart block can occasionally be symptomatic. If heart block is associated with congestive heart failure, temporary pacemaker placement may be required. The most common manifestation of carditis is cardiomegaly, as seen on x-ray.

Among patients at the Rockefeller University Hospital who were diagnosed with acute ARF between 1950 and 1970 (average of 20 years of follow-up), 90% had evidence of carditis at diagnosis (Table 86.6). In Bland and Jones's (66) classic review of 1,000 patients with ARF, only 65% of the patients were diagnosed with carditis. However, when Doppler sonography was employed in the clinical evaluation of patients during the outbreak in Utah, 91% of patients had carditis (1) indicating that, with more sensitive measurements of cardiac dysfunction, almost all patients with ARF exhibit signs of acute carditis.

TABLE 86.6. PHYSICAL SIGNS AND SYMPTOMS OF ACUTE RHEUMATIC FEVER: ROCKEFELLER UNIVERSITY HOSPITAL 1950–1970

	RHD $n = 40$	No RHD $n = 47$	Total $n = 87$	Bland and Jones (67)
Carditis	100%	83.0%	90.1%	65.3%
Arthritis	67.5%	68.1%	67.8%	41.0%
Epistaxis	0	10.6%	5.7%	27.4%
Chorea	5.0%	2.1%	3.4%	51.8%
Pericarditis	2.5%	4.3%	3.4%	13.0%
Nodules	7.5%	0	3.4%	8.8%
Erythema marginatum	0	4.3%	2.3%	7.1%

Rheumatic Heart Disease

Rheumatic heart disease is the most severe sequela of ARF. Usually occurring 10 to 20 years after the original attack, it is the major cause of acquired valvular disease in the world. The mitral valve is mainly involved and aortic valve involvement occurs less often. Mitral stenosis is a classic rheumatic heart disease finding and can manifest as a combination of mitral insufficiency and stenosis, secondary to severe calcification of the mitral valve. When symptoms of left atrial enlargement are present, mitral valve replacement may become necessary.

In various studies, the incidence of rheumatic heart disease in patients with a history of ARF has varied. In Bland and Jones's (66) classic follow-up study of patients with ARF, after 20 years one-third of patients had no murmur, another one-third had died, and the remaining one-third were alive with rheumatic heart disease. A majority of the patients who died had rheumatic heart disease. While the classic dogma is that patients with rheumatic heart disease invariably had more than one attack of ARF, recent analysis of our patients at the Rockefeller University Hospital disproves this notion. The population studied was 87 patients who had only one documented attack of ARF, without any evidence (clinical or laboratory) of a recurrence during a 20-year follow-up under close supervision. Over 80% had carditis at admission, and approximately 50% now have organic murmurs (Table 86.6). Thus, valvular damage manifesting as organic murmurs later in life is still likely to occur in 50% of patients with ARF, particularly if they presented with evidence of carditis at initial diagnosis. All of the patients in our population who ended up with rheumatic heart disease had carditis at diagnosis.

Chorea

Sydenham's chorea, chorea minor, or "St. Vitus' dance" is a neurologic disorder consisting of abrupt, purposeless, nonrhythmic involuntary movements, muscular weakness, and emotional disturbances. Involuntary movements disappear during sleep, but may occur at rest and interfere with voluntary activity. Initially, it may be possible to suppress these movements, which may affect all voluntary muscles, with the hands and face usually the most obvious. Grimaces and inappropriate smiles are common. Handwriting usually becomes clumsy and provides a convenient way of following the patient's course. Speech is often slurred. The movements are commonly more marked on one side and are occasionally completely unilateral (hemichorea).

The muscular weakness is best revealed by asking the patient to squeeze the examiner's hands: the pressure of the patient's grip increases and decreases continuously and capriciously, a phenomenon known as relapsing grip, or milking sign.

The emotional changes manifest themselves in outbursts of inappropriate behavior, including crying and restlessness. In rare cases, the psychologic manifestations may be severe and may result in transient psychosis.

The neurologic examination fails to reveal sensory losses or pyramidal tract involvement. Diffuse hypotonia may be present. Chorea may follow streptococcal infections after a latent period, which is longer, on the average, than the latent period of other rheumatic manifestations. Some patients with chorea have no other symptoms, but other patients develop chorea weeks or months after arthritis. In both cases, examination of the heart may reveal murmurs.

Subcutaneous Nodules

The subcutaneous nodules of ARF are firm and painless. The overlying skin is not inflamed and can usually be moved over the nodules. The diameter of these round lesions varies from a few millimeters to 1 or even 2 cm. They are located over bony surfaces or prominences, or near tendons. Their number varies from a single nodule to a few dozen and averages three or four; when numerous, they are usually symmetric. Nodules are rarely present for more than a month. They are smaller and more short-lived than the nodules of RA. Although in both diseases the elbows are most frequently involved, the rheumatic nodules are more common on the olecranon, whereas nodules of RA are usually found 3 or 4 cm distal to it. Rheumatic subcutaneous nodules generally appear only after the first few weeks of illness, and usually only in patients with carditis.

Erythema Marginatum

Erythema marginatum is an evanescent, nonpruritic skin rash, pink or faintly red, usually affecting the trunk, sometimes the proximal parts or the limbs, but not the face. Lesions extend centrifugally while the skin in the center returns gradually to normal, hence the term *erythema marginatum.* The outer edge of the lesion is sharp, whereas the inner edge is diffuse. Because the margin of the lesion is usually continuous, making a ring, it is also known as "erythema annulare."

The individual lesions may appear and disappear in a matter of hours, usually to return. A hot bath or shower may make them more evident or may even reveal them for the first time.

Erythema marginatum usually occurs in the early phase of the disease. It often persists or recurs, even when all other manifestations of disease have disappeared. Occasionally, the lesions appear for the first time or, more likely, are *noticed* for the first time, late in the course of the illness or even during convalescence. This disorder usually occurs only in patients with carditis.

MINOR MANIFESTATIONS

Fever

Temperature is increased in almost all ARF attacks and ranges from 38.4°C to 40°C. Usually fever decreases in approximately 1 week without antipyretic treatment and may become low grade for another week or two. Fever rarely lasts for more than 3 to 4 weeks.

Abdominal Pain

The abdominal pain of RF resembles that of other conditions associated with acute microvascular mesenteric inflammation and is nonspecific. It usually occurs at or near the onset of the rheumatic fever attack so that other manifestations may not yet be present to clarify the diagnosis. In many cases, it may mimic acute appendicitis.

Epistaxis

In the past, epistaxis occurred most prominently and severely in patients with severe and protracted rheumatic carditis. Early clinical studies reported a frequency as high as 48%, but it probably occurs less frequently now (Table 86.6). Although epistaxis has been correlated in the past with the severity of rheumatic inflammation, it is difficult to assess retrospectively the possible thrombasthenic effect of large doses of salicylates, administered for prolonged periods in protracted attacks.

Rheumatic Pneumonia

Pneumonia may appear during the course of severe rheumatic carditis. This inflammatory process is difficult or impossible to distinguish from pulmonary edema or the alveolitis associated with respiratory distress syndromes due to a variety of pathophysiologic states.

LABORATORY FINDINGS

The diagnosis of ARF cannot readily be established by laboratory tests. Nevertheless, such tests may be helpful in two ways: first, in demonstrating that an antecedent streptococcal infection has occurred, and, second, in documenting the presence or persistence of an inflammatory process. Serial chest x-rays may be helpful in following the course of carditis, and the electrocardiogram may reflect the course of inflammatory involvement of the conduction system.

Throat cultures are usually negative by the time ARF appears, but an attempt should be made to isolate the organism. It is our practice to take three throat cultures during the first 24 hours, prior to administration of antibiotics. Streptococcal antibodies are more useful because (a) they reach a peak titer at about the time of onset of ARF; (b) they indicate true infection rather than transient carriage; and (c) by performing several tests for different antibodies, any significant recent streptococcal infection can be detected. To demonstrate a rising titer, it is useful to take a serum specimen when the patient is first seen and another 2 weeks later for comparison.

The specific antibody tests that have been used to diagnose streptococcal infections most frequently are those directed against extracellular products including antistreptolysin O, anti-DNase B, antihyaluronidase [anti–diphosphopyridine nucleotide (anti-DPNase)], and antistreptokinase. Antistreptolysin O has been the most widely used test and is generally available in hospitals in the United States.

Antistreptolysin O titers vary with age, season, and geography. They reach peak levels in the young school-age population. Titers of 200 to 300 Todd units per milliliter are common, therefore, in healthy children of elementary school age. After a streptococcal pharyngitis, the antibody response peaks at about 4 to 5 weeks, which is usually during the second or third week of ARF (depending on how early it is detected). Thereafter, antibody titers fall off rapidly in the next several months and, after 6 months, decline more slowly. Since only 80% of patients with acute ARF exhibit a rise in the antistreptolysin O titer, it is recommended that other antistreptococcal antibody tests be performed in the absence of a positive antistreptolysin O titer. These include anti-DNase B, antihyaluronidase, or antistreptozyme (which is a combination of various streptococcal antigens).

Streptococcal antibodies, when increased, support, but do not prove, the diagnosis of ARF, nor are they a measure of disease activity. Even in the absence of intercurrent streptococcal infection, titers decline during the attack despite the persistence or severity of disease activity.

Acute-Phase Reactants

Acute-phase reactants are elevated during ARF, just as they are during other inflammatory conditions. Both the C-reactive protein and erythrocyte sedimentation rate are almost invariably elevated during the active rheumatic process, if they are not suppressed by antirheumatic drugs. These may be normal, however, during episodes of pure chorea or persistent erythema marginatum. Particularly when treatment has been discontinued or is being tapered, the C-reactive protein or erythrocyte sedimentation rate are useful in monitoring "rebounds" of inflammation, which indicate that the rheumatic process is still active. If either the C-reactive protein or erythrocyte sedimentation rate remain normal a few weeks after discontinuing antirheumatic therapy, the attack may be considered ended unless chorea appears. Usually, there will be no exacerbation of the systemic inflammation, and chorea will be present as an isolated manifestation.

Anemia

A mild, normochromic, normocytic anemia of chronic infection or inflammation may be seen during ARF. Suppressing the inflammation usually improves the anemia; thus, hematinic therapy is usually not indicated.

Other Supporting Tests

As noted in Fig. 86.3 and Table 86.2, two other tests have, in our experience, been helpful in confirming the diagnosis of ARF especially when the diagnosis is in doubt.

First, one can detect elevated titers of heart-reactive antibodies directed against sarcolemmal antigens in the vast majority of patients with ARF. Elevated levels of these antibodies are not seen in either uncomplicated streptococcal infections or acute poststreptococcal glomerulonephritis. Using enzyme-linked immunosorbent assay (ELISA), antibodies directed against cytoskeletal constituents such as myosin and tropomyosin are also elevated in patients with ARF and might be helpful in determining whether or not cross-reactive antibodies unique to ARF exist (50).

Second, the use of the D8/17 monoclonal antibody mentioned earlier has also proved helpful in the differentiation of ARF from other disorders. In our hands, all patients with ARF express abnormal levels of D8/17$^+$ B cells, especially during the acute attack. In those cases where the diagnosis of ARF has been doubtful, the presence of elevated levels of D8/17$^+$ B cells has proven to be very helpful in establishing the correct diagnosis (41).

CLINICAL COURSE AND TREATMENT OF ACUTE RHEUMATIC FEVER

The mainstay of treatment for ARF has always been antiinflammatory agents, most commonly aspirin. Dramatic improvement in symptoms is usually seen after the initiation of therapy. Usually 80 to 100 mg/kg/day in children and 4 to 8 g/day in adults is required for an effect to be seen. Aspirin levels can be measured, and 20 to 30 mg/dL is the therapeutic range. Duration of antiinflammatory therapy can vary but needs to be maintained until all symptoms are absent and laboratory values are normal. If severe carditis is also present (as indicated by significant cardiomegaly, congestive heart failure, or third-degree heart block), steroid therapy can be instituted. The usual dosage is 2 mg/kg/day of oral prednisone during the first 1 to 2 weeks. Depending on clinical and laboratory improvement, the dosage is then tapered over the next 2 weeks, and during the last week aspirin may be added in the dosage recommended above, sufficient to achieve the 20 to 30 mg/dL level.

Whether or not signs of pharyngitis are present at the time of diagnosis, antibiotic therapy with penicillin should be started and maintained for at least 10 days, in doses recommended for the eradication of streptococcal pharyngitis. Additionally, all family contacts should be cultured and treated for streptococcal infection, if positive. If compliance is an issue, depot penicillin, i.e., benzathine penicillin G 600,000 units in children, 1.2 million units in adults, should be given. Recurrences of ARF are most common within 2 years of the original attack but can occur at any time. The risk of recurrence decreases with age. Recurrence rates have been decreasing, from 20% to 2–4% in recent outbreaks. This might be due to better surveillance and treatment.

PROPHYLAXIS

Antibiotic prophylaxis with penicillin should be started immediately following resolution of the acute episode. The optimal regimen consists of oral penicillin VK 250,000 twice a day or parenteral penicillin G, 1.2 million units i.m., every 4 weeks. One study suggests, however, that injections every 3 weeks are more effective than every 4 weeks at preventing acute RF recurrences (67). If the patient is allergic to penicillin, erythromycin 250 mg per day can be substituted.

The end point of prophylaxis is unclear; most believe it should continue at least until the patient is a young adult, which is usually 10 years from an acute attack with no recurrence. In our opinion, individuals with documented evidence of rheumatic heart disease should be on continuous prophylaxis indefinitely since our experience has been that ARF recurrences can occur even in the fifth or sixth decade. A potential source of ARF recurrences are young children in a household who may transmit new group A streptococcal infections to rheumatic susceptible individuals.

The alternative to long-term prophylaxis in an individual with ARF will be the introduction of streptococcal vaccines designed not only to prevent recurrent infections in susceptible individuals with previous ARF, but also to prevent streptococcal disease in general.

STREPTOCOCCAL VACCINE PROSPECTS

At present, the main approach to primary prevention of ARF is to treat all documented streptococcal pharyngitis with adequate doses of penicillin. Unfortunately, as emphasized by Veasy et al.'s (1) studies, the signs and symptoms of streptococcal pharyngitis can be so mild (especially in children) that the child is often not seen by the health care worker. Thus, no discussion of this disease would be complete without some mention of the current efforts toward developing an effective streptococcal vaccine that would protect against all streptococcal infections.

The classic observations by Lancefield (68) clearly demonstrated the importance of the M protein as a significant virulence factor. Antibodies to the M protein conferred type-specific immunity to that serotype but not to other type-specific M protein strains. Until 1970, few human trials of M protein vaccines were undertaken, mainly as a result of hypersensitivity reactions to the acid extracted M protein material (reviewed in ref. 20).

A breakthrough in this area was achieved by Beachey et al. (69), who used a purified M 24 protein devoid of hypersensitivity reactions to achieve type-specific opsonizing antibodies in humans. Encouraged by these studies and using the sequence data from the type-specific epitope of each M protein, they were able to synthesize hybrid peptides that were protective against two M proteins: namely, type 5 and 24 (70). Finally Dale et al. (71) extended these studies to produce a tetravalent antigen that induced opsonizing antibodies to four different M protein strains. While these results are promising, there are at least 30 known different types of M protein group A streptococci that can cause pharyngitis. Thus, the ability to protect against all group A streptococcal strains may not be possible.

The second approach is based on the observation by Bessen and Fischetti (72) that the C-repeat region of the M protein moiety is highly conserved in many group A streptococcal strains, and antibodies raised against this region might be protective. Using a group A streptococcal intranasal challenge mouse model, they were able to show protection against both homologous and heterologous type-specific strains immunized with C-repeat units of the M protein (73). While antibodies raised against these peptides are not opsonic, they do appear to protect against nasal invasion of the organism, thereby preventing attachment of the organism to the pharynx. These promising results in the mice will soon be evaluated in humans.

Although type-specific antibodies in human sera were clearly demonstrated by Lancefield, rarely did any given human serum contain multiple type-specific antibodies. In search of other antigens that might offer a more broadly based protection, Salvadori et al. (27) described the presence of anticarbohydrate antibodies in human sera that also are opsonic. These antibodies are effective against multiple M protein serotypes and the opsonic properties of these sera were directed against the *N*-acetylglucosamine moiety of the group A streptococci. Whether or not these antibodies are protective in active and passive protection challenge tests remains to be seen.

CONCLUSION

Despite its disappearance in many areas of the world, ARF continues to be a serious problem in geographic areas inhabited by two-thirds of the population. Even in developed countries with full access to medical care and better nutrition and housing, recent resurgence of the disease in these areas emphasizes the need for continued vigilance of physicians and other health officials in both diagnosing and treating ARF. Whether this resurgence represents a change in the virulence of the organism or failure to recognize the importance and adequate treatment of an antecedent streptococcal infection remains an area of intense debate and will therefore require careful and controlled epidemiologic surveillance. The importance of early diagnosis and therapy cannot be overemphasized. Although the joint manifestations are transient and self-limiting, the cardiac sequelae are chronic and life-threatening.

Nevertheless, ARF remains one of the few autoimmune disorders known to occur as a result of infection with a specific organism. The confirmed observation of an increased frequency of a B-cell alloantigen in several populations of rheumatics suggests that it might be possible to identify individuals susceptible to ARF at birth. If so, then from a public health standpoint (a) these individuals would be prime candidates for immunization with any streptococcal vaccine that might be developed in the future; (b) careful monitoring of streptococcal disease in the susceptible population could lead to early and effective antibiotic strategies, resulting in disease prevention; and (c) in individuals with previous ARF who later present with subtle or nonspecific manifestations of the disease, the presence or absence of the marker could be of value in arriving at a diagnosis.

The continued study of ARF as a paradigm for microbial-host interactions also has important implications for the study of autoimmune diseases in general and rheumatic diseases in particular. Further insights into this intriguing host parasite relationship may shed additional light into those diseases where an infection is presumed but not yet identified.

REFERENCES

1. Veasy LG, Wiedmeier SE, Orsmond GS, et al. Resurgence of acute rheumatic fever in the intermountain area of the United States. *N Engl J Med* 1987;316:421–427.
2. Gordis L. The virtual disappearance of rheumatic fever in the United States: lessons in the rise and fall of disease. *Circulation* 1985;72:1155–1162.
3. Pope RM. Rheumatic fever in the 1980s. *Bull Rheum Dis* 1989; 38:1–8.
4. Markowitz M. Rheumatic fever: recent outbreaks of an old disease. *Conn Med* 1987;51:229–233.
5. Kaplan EL, Johnson DR, Cleary PP. Group A streptococcal serotypes isolated from patients and sibling contacts during the resurgence of rheumatic fever in the United States in the mid-1980's. *J Infect Dis* 1989;159:101–103.
6. Whitnack E, Bisno AL. Rheumatic fever and other immunologically mediated cardiac diseases. In: Parker C, ed. *Clinical immunology,* vol 2. Philadelphia: WB Saunders, 1980:894–929.
7. Denny FW Jr, Wannamaker LW, Brink WR, et al. Prevention of rheumatic fever: treatment of the preceding streptococcal infection. *JAMA* 1950;143:151–153.
8. Markowitz M, Gordis L. *Rheumatic fever,* 2nd ed. Philadelphia: WB Saunders, 1972.
9. Stollerman GH, Lewis AJ, Schultz I, et al. Relationship of the immune response to group A streptococci to the cause of acute, chronic and recurrent rheumatic fever. *Am J Med* 1956;20: 163–169.
10. Potter EV, Svartman M, Mohammed I, et al. Tropical acute rheumatic fever and associated streptococcal infections compared with concurrent acute glomerulonephritis. *J Pediatr* 1978;92: 325–33.
11. Bessen D, Jones KF, Fischetti VA. Evidence for the distinct classes of streptococcal M protein and their relationship to rheumatic fever. *J Exp Med* 1989;169:269–283.
12. Kaplan EL, Anthony BF, Chapman SS, et al. The influence of the site of infection on the immune response to group A streptococci. *J Clin Invest* 1970;49:1405–1414.
13. Bisno AL, Nelson KE. Type-specific opsonic antibodies in streptococcal pyoderma. *Infect Immun* 1975;10:1356–1361.
14. Kendall F, Heidelberger M, Dawson M. A serologically inactive polysaccharide elaborated by mucoid strains of group A hemolytic streptococcus. *J Biol Chem* 1937;118:61–82.
15. Seastone CV. The virulence of group C hemolytic streptococci of animal origin. *J Exp Med* 1939;70:361–378.
16. Quinn RW, Singh KP. Antigenicity of hyaluronic acid. *Biochem J* 1957;95:290–301.
17. Fillit HM, McCarty M, Blake M. Induction of antibodies to hyaluronic acid by immunization of rabbits with encapsulated streptococci. *J Exp Med* 1986;164:762–776.
18. Faarber P, Capel PJ, Rigke PM, et al. Cross reactivity of anti DNA antibodies with proteoglycans. *Clin Exp Immunol* 1984;55: 402–412.
19. Stollerman GH. *Rheumatic fever and streptococcal infection*, vol 4. Orlando, FL: Grune & Stratton, 1975:70.
20. Fischetti VA. Streptococcal M protein: molecular design and biological behavior. *Clin Microbiol Rev* 1989;2:285–314.
21. Dale JB, Beachey EH. Multiple cross reactive epitopes of streptococcal M proteins. *J Exp Med* 1985;161:113–122.
22. Sargent SJ, Beachey EH, Corbett CE, et al. Sequence of protective epitopes of streptococcal M proteins shared with cardiac sarcolemmal membranes. *J Immunol* 1987;139:1285–1290.
23. Cunningham MW, McCormack JM, Talaber LR, et al. Human monoclonal antibodies reactive with antigens of the group A streptococcus and human heart. *J Immunol* 1988;141:2760–2766.
24. McCarty M. The streptococcal cell wall. *Harvey Lect* 1970;65: 73–96.
25. Goldstein I, Rebeyrotte P, Parlebas J, et al. Isolation from heart valves of glycopeptides which share immunological properties with streptococcus haemolyticus group A polysaccharides. *Nature* 1968;219:866–868.
26. Goldstein I, Caravano R. Determination of anti-group A streptococcal polysaccharide antibodies in human sera by an hemagglutination technique. *Proc Soc Exp Biol Med* 1967;124: 1209–1212.
27. Salvadori LG, Blake MS, McCarty M, et al. Group A streptococcus-liposome ELISA antibody titers to group A polysaccharide and opsonophagocytic capabilities of the antibodies. *J Infect Dis* 1995;171:593–600.

28. Chetty C, Schwab JH. Chemistry of endotoxins. In: Rietschel Elsenier ET, ed. *Handbook of endotoxin,* vol 1. Science Publishers BV, 1984;376–410.
29. Cromartie WJ, Craddock JB, Schwab JH, et al. Arthritis in rats after systemic injection of streptococcal cells or cell walls. *J Exp Med* 1877;146:1585–1602.
30. Cromartie WJ, Craddock JB. Rheumatic-like cardiac lesions in mice. *Science* 1966;154:285–287.
31. Heymer B, Schleifer KH, Read SE, et al. Detection of antibodies to bacterial cell wall peptidoglycan in human sera. *J Immunol* 1976;117:23–26.
32. Zabriskie JB. Rheumatic fever: the interplay between host genetics and microbe. *Circulation* 1985;71:1077–1086.
33. Kingston D, Glynn LE. A cross-reaction between *Streptococcus pyogenes* and human fibroblasts, endothelial cells and astrocytes. *Immunology* 1971;21:1003–1016.
34. Husby G, van de Rijn I, Zabriskie JB, et al. Antibodies reacting with cytoplasm of subthalmic and caudate nuclei neurons in chorea and acute rheumatic fever. *J Exp Med* 1976;144:1094–1110.
35. Froude J, Gibofsky A, Buskirk DR, et al. Cross reactivity between streptococcus and human tissue: a model of molecular mimicry and autoimmunity. *Curr Top Microbiol Immunol* 1989;145:5–26.
36. Cheadle WB. Harvean lectures on the various manifestations of the rheumatic state as exemplified in childhood and early life. *Lancet* 1889;1:821–832.
37. Wilson MG, Schweitzr MD, Lubschez R. The familial epidemiology of rheumatic fever. *J Pediatr* 1943;22:468–482.
38. Taranta A, Torosdag S, Metrakos JD, et al. Rheumatic fever in monozygotic and dizygotic twins. *Circulation* 1959;20:778–792.
39. Glynn LE, Halborrow EJ. Relationship between blood groups, secretion status and susceptibility to rheumatic fever. *Arthritis Rheum* 1961;4:203–208.
40. Patarroyo ME, Winchester RJ, Vejerano A, et al. Association of a B cell alloantigen with susceptibility to rheumatic fever. *Nature* 1979;278:173–174.
41. Khanna AK, Buskirk DR, Williams RC Jr, et al. Presence of a non-HLA B cell antigen in rheumatic fever patients and their families as defined by a monoclonal antibody. *J Clin Invest* 1989; 83:1710–1716.
42. Ayoub EA, Barrett DJ, Maclaren NK, et al. Association of class II human histocompatibility leucocyte antigens with rheumatic fever. *J Clin Invest* 1986;77:2019–2026.
43. Maharaj B, Hammond MG, Appadoo B, et al. HLA-A, B, DR and DQ antigens in black patients with severe chronic rheumatic heart disease. *Circulation* 1987;765:259–261.
44. Guilherme L, Weidenbach W, Kiss MH, et al. Association of human leucocyte class II antigens with rheumatic fever or rheumatic heart disease in a Brazilian population. *Circulation* 1991;83:1995–1998.
45. Watson RF, Hirst GK, Lancefield RC. Bacteriological studies of cardiac tissues obtained at autopsy from eleven patients dying with rheumatic fever. *Arthritis Rheum* 1961;4:74–85.
46. Halbert SP, Bircher R, Dahle E. The analysis of streptococcal infections. V. Cardiotoxicity of streptolysin O for rabbits in vivo. *J Exp Med* 1961;113:759–784.
47. Wagner BM. Studies in rheumatic fever. III. Histochemical reactivity of the Aschoff body. *Ann NY Acad Sci* 1960;86:992–1008.
48. Schlievert PM, Johnson LP, Tomai MA, et al. Characterization and genetics of group A streptococcal pyrogenic exotoxins. In: Ferretti J, Curtis R, eds. *Streptococcal genetics.* Washington, DC: ASM, 1987:136–142.
49. Paliard X, West SG, Lafferty JA, et al. Evidence for the effects of superantigen in rheumatoid arthritis. *Science* 1991;253:325–329.
50. Zabriskie JB, Hsu KC, Seegal BC. Heart-reactive antibody associated with rheumatic fever: characterization and diagnostic significance. *Clin Exp Immunol* 1970;7:147–159.
51. van de Rijn I, Fillit H, Brandeis WE, et al. Serial studies on circulating immune complexes in post-streptococcal sequelae. *Clin Exp Immunol* 1978;34:318–325.
52. Kemeny E, Grieve T, Marcus R, Sareli P, et al. Identification of mononuclear cells and T cell subsets in rheumatic valvulitis. *Clin Immunol Immunopathol* 1989;52:225–237.
53. Amoils B, Morrison RC, Wadee AA, et al. Aberrant expression of HLA-DR antigen on valvular fibroblasts from patients with acute rheumatic carditis. *Clin Exp Immunol* 1986;66:84–94.
54. Read SE, Reid HF, Fischetti VA, et al. Serial studies on the cellular immune response to streptococcal antigens in acute and convalescent rheumatic fever patients in Trinidad. *J Clin Immunol* 1986;6:433–441.
55. Yang LC, Soprey PR, Wittner MK, et al. Streptococcal induced cell mediated immune destruction of cardiac myofibers in vitro. *J Exp Med* 1977;146:344–360.
56. Dale JB, Beachey EH. Human cytotoxic T lymphocytes evoked by group A streptococcal M proteins. *J Exp Med* 1987;166: 1825–1835.
57. Jones Criteria 1992 update. Guidelines for diagnosis of rheumatic fever. *JAMA* 1992;268:2069–2070.
58. Feinstein AR, Spagnulo M. The clinical patterns of rheumatic fever: a reappraisal. *Medicine* 1962;41:279–305.
59. Svartman M, Potter EV, Poon-King T. Immunoglobulin components in synovial fluids of patients with acute rheumatic fever. *J Clin Invest* 1975;56:111–117.
60. Goldsmith DP, Long SS. Poststreptococcal disease of childhood—a changing syndrome. *Arthritis Rheum* 1982;25:S18 (abst).
61. Arnold MH, Tyndall A. Post-streptococcal reactive arthritis. *Ann Rheum Dis* 1989;48:681–688.
62. Fink CW. The role of streptococcus in post streptococcal reactive arthritis and childhood polyarteritis nodosa. *J Rheumatol* 1991; 18:14–20.
63. Gibofsky A, Zabriskie JB. Rheumatic fever: new insights into an old disease. *Bull Rheum Dis* 1994;42:5–7.
64. Crea MA, Mortimer EA. The nature of scarlatinal arthritis. *Pediatrics* 1959;23:879–884.
65. Wallace MR, Garst PD, Papadimos TJ, et al. The return of acute rheumatic fever in young adults. *JAMA* 1989;262:2557–2561.
66. Bland EF, Jones TD. Rheumatic fever and rheumatic heart disease: a twenty year report on 1,000 patients followed since childhood. *Circulation* 1951;4:836–843.
67. Lue HC, Mil-Wham W, Hsieh KH, et al. Rheumatic fever recurrences: controlled study of 3 week versus 4 week benzathnic penicillin prevention programs. *J Pediatr* 1986;108: 299–304.
68. Lancefield RC. Current knowledge of the type specific M antigens of group A streptococci. *J Immunol* 1962;89:307–313.
69. Beachey EH, Stollerman GH, Johnson RH, et al. Human immune response to immunization with a structurally defined polypeptide fragment of streptococcal M protein. *J Exp Med* 1979;150:862–877.
70. Beachey EH, Gras-Masse H, Tarter A, et al. Opsonic antibodies evoked by hybrid peptide copies of types 5 and 24 streptococcal M proteins synthesized in tandem. *J Exp Med* 1986;163: 1451–1458.
71. Dale JB, Chiang EY, Lederer JW. Recombinant tetravalent group A streptococcal M protein vaccine. *J Immunol* 1993;151: 2188–2194.
72. Bessen D, Fischetti VA. Role of nonopsonic antibody in protection against group A streptococcal infection. In: Lasky L, ed. *Technological advances in vaccine development.* New York: Alan R. Liss, 1988:493–502.
73. Bessen D, Fischetti VA. Influence of intranasal immunization with synthetic peptides corresponding to conserved epitopes of M protein on mucosal colonization by group A streptococci. *Infect Immun* 1988;56:2666–2672.

87

RELAPSING POLYCHONDRITIS

CLEMENT J. MICHET

Relapsing polychondritis is a rare disease of unknown etiology characterized by episodic attacks of inflammation of hyaline and elastic cartilaginous structures including the ears, nose, laryngotracheal, and articular cartilages, as well as the organs of special sense. It is thought to be an autoimmune disease based on these cardinal features, the observed association with other conditions such as vasculitis, the presence of cartilage inflammation on biopsy, anticollagen antibodies, and a therapeutic response to corticosteroid therapy.

HISTORICAL OVERVIEW AND DIAGNOSTIC CRITERIA

Relapsing polychondritis was first described in 1923 by Jaksch-Wartenhorst (1) as "polychondropathia" in a young man with fever, inflammatory arthritis, and nasal and auricular chondritis with hearing loss. Subsequent cases were reported and termed systemic chondromalacia or chronic chondromalacia. Carl Pearson and associates (2) in 1960 suggested the diagnostic term *relapsing polychondritis*, highlighting the episodic nature of the syndrome. They also emphasized the associated inflammatory manifestations occurring in noncartilaginous structures such as the middle and inner ear, sclera, and uveal tract, as well as the association of relapsing polychondritis with other rheumatic diseases.

Subsequently, McAdam et al. (3) suggested preliminary diagnostic criteria for relapsing polychondritis including (a) recurrent chondritis of both auricles; (b) nonerosive inflammatory polyarthritis; (c) nasal chondritis; (d) ocular inflammation including conjunctivitis, keratitis, scleritis/episcleritis, and/or uveitis; (e) respiratory tract chondritis involving laryngeal and/or tracheal cartilage; and (f) cochlear and/or vestibular damage resulting in neurosensory hearing loss, tinnitus, and/or vertigo. The authors suggested using the presence of at least three of the six criteria and a biopsy confirmation from either ear, nasal, or respiratory tract cartilage to make a diagnosis. Damiani and Levine (4) suggested modification of these criteria, providing three options to include one or more of McAdams's criteria with histologic confirmation; involvement of two or more separate cartilaginous sites with a therapeutic response to corticosteroids or dapsone; or, lastly, three or more cartilage sites without biopsy confirmation. Although these diagnostic criteria have not been independently tested in other patient groups, the characteristic clinical findings in relapsing polychondritis and the limited differential diagnostic possibilities have led to their adoption in clinical practice. Currently, most individuals afflicted with this syndrome do not require biopsy confirmation of their illness.

EPIDEMIOLOGY, DISEASE ASSOCIATIONS, AND PROGNOSIS

Polychondritis is rare and the annual incidence is uncertain. An estimate from the predominately Caucasian population of Rochester, Minnesota, revealed an incidence of 3.5 cases per million (author's personal observation). Cases are observed equally between the sexes and in all racial groups. Relapsing polychondritis occurs at all ages but is most frequently diagnosed in persons between 40 and 50 years of age. Disease manifestations may vary based on the age and sex of the patient. Nasal and subglottic chondritis are more common among younger patients, especially females. Approximately 40% of cases are associated with another rheumatic, inflammatory, or hematologic disorder (Table 87.1). Systemic vasculitis is the most commonly associated inflammatory syndrome, followed by rheumatoid arthritis, the spondyloarthropathies, and connective tissue disease disorders. Nonrheumatologic disease associations have included myelodysplastic syndromes and inflammatory bowel diseases. Usually relapsing polychondritis occurs after the onset of the other disease; often auricular chondritis is the only manifestation of relapsing polychondritis observed in this setting, although all of the major manifestations of the syndrome have been observed in some of these secondary cases. The life expectancy of persons with relapsing polychondritis is reduced. In one large series of referral cases, the overall 5-year survival was 74%, but only 45% among those with systemic vasculitis (5). Infection related either to immunosuppression or pneumonia complicating laryngotracheal obstruction is the leading cause of death directly attributable to relapsing

TABLE 87.1. CONDITIONS ASSOCIATED WITH POLYCHONDRITIS

Systemic vasculitis syndromes
Rheumatoid arthritis
Systemic lupus erythematosus
Sjögren's syndrome
Ankylosing spondylitis
Psoriasis and psoriatic arthritis
Reiter's syndrome
Inflammatory bowel disease
Behçet's syndrome
Myelodysplastic syndrome
Dermatitis herpetiformis
Hodgkin's disease
Panniculitis
Primary biliary cirrhosis
Retroperitoneal fibrosis
Thymoma

polychondritis, followed by inflammatory aneurysmal rupture or airway collapse. Complications from systemic vasculitis and glomerulonephritis are an important cause of death among cases associated with other rheumatic syndromes. Persons with an associated myelodysplastic syndrome usually die from that disorder (6).

CLINICAL MANIFESTATIONS

Relapsing polychondritis presents in varied patterns but with usually one or two areas of cartilaginous inflammation (Table 87.2). The mechanisms that determine the specific regions and combinations of site involvement in individual cases remain a complete mystery. Occasionally a prolonged fever with signs of systemic inflammation will precede any obvious signs of relapsing polychondritis; it is not clear whether vasculitis always underlies this presentation. Symptomatic recurrences are unique for each patient. Some always relapse at the same site, whereas others add new areas of cartilaginous involvement. The number of recurrences over time varies greatly. Attacks may occur frequently over several months or be limited to only one episode. A minority of patients have continuous inflammatory lesions despite ongoing treatment.

TABLE 87.2. CLINICAL MANIFESTATIONS OF RELAPSING POLYCHONDRITIS

Manifestation	Presenting (%)	Cumulative (Median 6-yr Follow-up) (%)
Auricular chondritis	39	85
Hearing loss	9	26
Vertigo	4	13
Nasal chondritis	24	54
Saddle nose	18	29
Laryngotracheal symptoms	26	48
Laryngotracheal stricture	15	23
Inflammatory arthritis	36	52
Valvular regurgitation	0	4
Aneurysm	0	4
Microhematuria	15	26
Elevated creatinine	7	13
Cutaneous	7	28

From Michel CJ, McKenna CH, Luthra HS, et al. Relapsing polychondritis. Survival and prediction role of early disease manifestation. *Ann Intern Med* 1986;104:74–78, with permission.

The herald sign of relapsing polychondritis is auricular chondritis, a manifestation of the illness in over 85% of patients. Unilateral, or bilateral in a simultaneous or sequential pattern, inflammation occurs in remitting and exacerbating attacks lasting for days to weeks. Characteristic findings include violaceous or erythematous tender swelling of the cartilaginous pinna with sparing of the soft lobule (Fig. 87.1). The external auditory canal may be involved, leading to narrowing. In patients who have suffered severe episodes, the ear may be left in a softened cauliflower deformity that may harden over time due to ossification of the damaged tissues (Fig. 87.2). In 30% of patients, hearing loss may occur coincident with auricular chondritis or even years after the attack. A variety of etiologies and patterns of hearing loss are encountered (7). A conductive loss related to serous otitis media and eustachian tube chondritis alone or in combination with a vestibular component presumed to be related to vasculitis of the vestibular branch of the internal auditory artery is observed. A second pattern of sensorineural loss with or without vestibular symptoms is hypothesized to result from vasculitis of the internal auditory artery. This latter pattern of hearing loss may progress suddenly, leading to unilateral or bilateral nerve deafness and may not respond as reliably to corticosteroids as does the hearing loss variant associated with serous otitis. Pure vestibular symptoms of vertigo and unsteadiness without auditory symptoms have not been observed in relapsing polychondritis.

Nasal chondritis may lead to collapse and a saddle nose deformity. Sudden, rapid progression has been described, but recurrent episodes, sometimes misdiagnosed as infection, are more common before the characteristic deformity appears.

Pulmonary involvement in the form of laryngotracheal or bronchial chondritis is one of the most feared complications of this disease; symptoms develop in nearly one-half of cases and anatomic narrowings are identified clinically in over 20% of cases. Airway chondritis may be encountered in patients of all ages; it is often associated with saddle nose deformity in younger individuals. Symptoms include sore throat, hoarseness, cough, inspiratory stridor (exertional or recumbent), choking, and dyspnea. As a presenting complaint, it has been misdiagnosed as refractory asthma, with the true situation only clarified when auricular or nasal chondritis develops. A superimposed infectious bronchitis

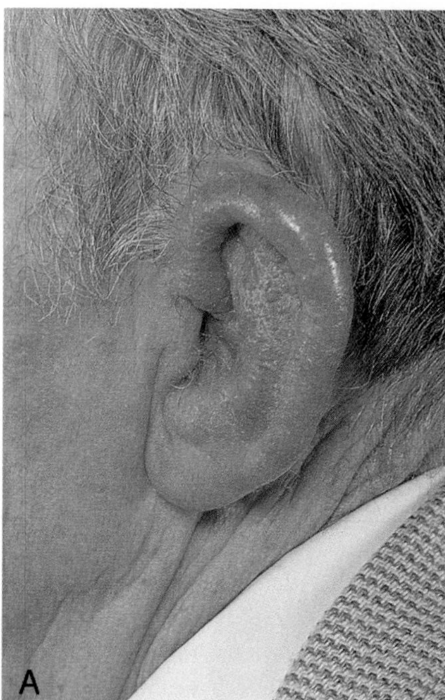

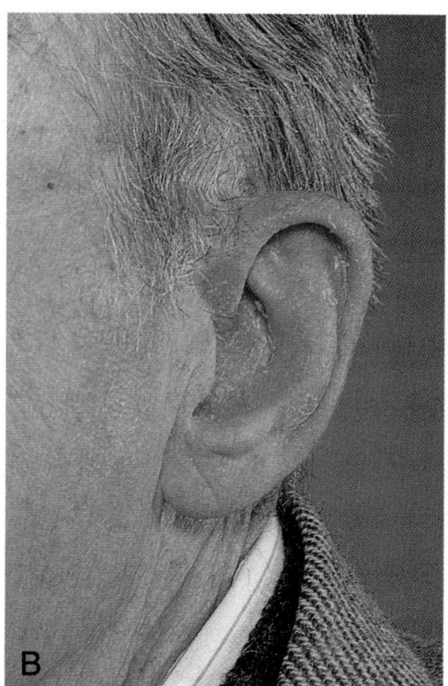

FIGURE 87.1. A: Acute auricular chondritis in an elderly man with an associated myelodysplastic syndrome. **B:** Inflammation has receded after 1 week of prednisone.

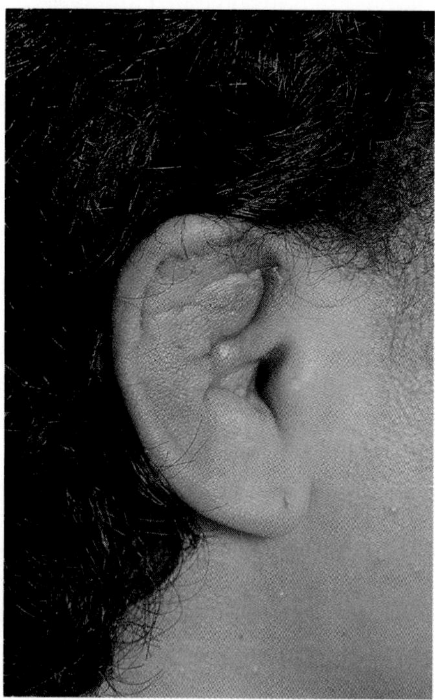

FIGURE 87.2. Chronic auricular deformity following several bouts of acute chondritis in a young woman with associated nasal and tracheal disease.

or pneumonia can seriously exacerbate the established symptoms or at times lead to the diagnosis of a previously unrecognized subglottic stenosis. This complication may lead rapidly to acute respiratory insufficiency.

The pulmonary problems resulting from airway chondritis are determined by the type and location of the lesion. Acutely, the airway may be obstructed by inflammatory edema (Fig. 87.3). Rarely, vocal cord paralysis may further compromise an extrathoracic tracheal obstruction (8). Later, a fixed fibrotic subglottic stenosis or a diffusely flaccid, dynamically collapsing tracheobronchial tree to the level of the segmental bronchi may be encountered. Bronchiectasis complicating the distal lesions has been observed (9). Airway collapse leads to tracheal narrowing as small as a few millimeters. Combinations of extrathoracic and intrathoracic fixed and flaccid lesions lead to mixed patterns of inspiratory and expiratory obstructive lung disease (10). While most subglottic lesions are symptomatic, loss of tracheobronchial cartilage rings may be clinically

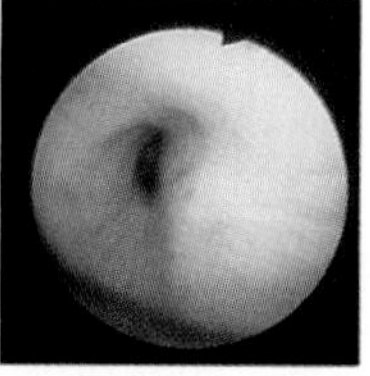

FIGURE 87.3. Bronchoscopic view of a man with acute laryngotracheal disease resulting in a flaccid airway.

inapparent in up to a third of the patients, with the lesions identified only by imaging and pulmonary function test examinations.

Synovitis occurs in up to 75% of patients with primary relapsing polychondritis and may be the presenting problem in 30%. Manifestations range from polyarthralgias or tendinitis to an oligoarticular arthritis. Joints most frequently affected include the knees, ankles, proximal interphalangeal and metacarpophalangeal joints, elbows, and forefeet. Parasternal articulations may be involved to such a degree that the resulting inflammation may mimic an infection (3). The peripheral arthritis is characteristically migratory and intermittent, and, in acute attacks, lasts for weeks (11). The episodes of synovitis may not temporally coincide with other inflammatory manifestations of relapsing polychondritis. Although usually subsiding, some cases of large joint synovitis in the knee or hip may persist despite resolution of other signs of active chondritis, leading to eventual cartilage damage and loss of joint space. Initially described as a nonerosive arthropathy, the small joint hand and foot involvement may progress to loss of joint space followed eventually by erosive changes over many years (12,13). It is not certain whether these cases represent a primary relapsing polychondritis arthropathy or an associated seronegative rheumatoid or spondyloarthropathy syndrome.

Cardiovascular manifestations occur throughout the course of polychondritis in about 10% of patients. Valvulitis leading to cusp rupture and aortic or mitral regurgitation has been noted to occur within months of disease onset (14). These lesions may also progress slowly and may occur in patients in whom there are no other signs of clinical disease activity. Later, aortitis may lead to annular dilatation and aortic valvular leak. Complete heart block due to inflammatory and fibrotic involvement of the membranous interventricular conduction system may further complicate the status of the patient (15). Inflammatory aneurysms of the ascending thoracic aorta occur more commonly than at the abdominal or iliac level and are identified months to years after disease onset (16). Multiple aneurysms may be present (17). A variety of clinical syndromes result, ranging from "pulseless disease," or subclavian steal, to sudden fatal ruptures of unrecognized silent aneurysmal lesions. Among patients with aortitis, other manifestations attributable to overlapping small vessel vasculitis such as scleritis and cutaneous vasculitis are observed simultaneously in some patients. Systemic polyarteritis is the most frequently reported vascular syndrome in patients without large vessel or valvular disease. Rarely an arterial thrombosis of a large vessel is encountered. One case was documented to be related to a circulating lupus anticoagulant (18). Antiphospholipid antibodies are also observed in relapsing polychondritis and may be related to an accompanying lupus syndrome (19).

At least 50% of patients with relapsing polychondritis have ocular involvement over the course of their illness, but most do not present with eye symptoms (20). Episcleritis and scleritis are the most prevalent problems. The scleritis may be anterior, diffuse, bilateral, and necrotizing, or rarely posterior. Scleritis is complicated by uveitis, keratitis, or corneal melt. The course of scleritis can become chronic with either recurrent attacks or episodes refractory to treatment, leading to scleromalacia. Painful proptosis with chemosis, "pseudotumor," is less common. Associated with extraocular muscle paresis, proptosis is likely related to inflammatory infiltration of the extraocular muscles. Lid edema without proptosis is also observed and is related to inflammation of the cartilaginous tarsal plate. Uncommon ocular manifestations include retinopathy, central retinal vein occlusion, chorioretinitis, and optic neuritis. Keratoconjunctivitis sicca is observed in up to 10% of cases. Rarely a conjunctival mass, a "salmon patch" of lymphoid hyperplasia, is observed (21).

As defined by microscopic hematuria and proteinuria, renal involvement in relapsing polychondritis occurs in approximately one-quarter of all patients seen in a referral practice. The usual problem is a glomerulonephritis, which occasionally develops in a patient who has only primary features of relapsing polychondritis, but more frequently occurs in the setting of an illness associated with other features of extrarenal microscopic polyangiitis. In this setting, the renal lesion is a segmental necrotizing cresenteric glomerulonephritis. This can be an aggressive process, constituting the major management problem in some cases. In the setting of relapsing polychondritis associated with Sjögren's syndrome or systemic lupus erythematosus, a diffuse proliferative glomerulonephritis may be encountered (22,23). Rarely, immunoglobulin A (IgA) nephropathy has been observed in relapsing polychondritis (24). Interstitial nephritis has also been observed on some biopsies and has been attributed to either nonsteroidal antiinflammatory drug (NSAID) toxicity or an associated Sjögren's syndrome (22).

Neurologic syndromes observed in relapsing polychondritis are attributable to vasculitis and are generally observed during the acute phase of the illness. The most common lesions consist of cranial second, third, sixth, seventh, or eighth cranial nerve mononeuropathies, mononeuritis multiplex, or diffuse peripheral sensorimotor neuropathies. Cerebrospinal fluid examination is normal in cases with isolated cranial neuropathies. Rare cases of central nervous system involvement presenting as encephalopathy or aseptic meningitis have been described (25). Lymphocytic pleocytosis, elevated cerebrospinal fluid proteins, and lymphocytic infiltration of the meninges accompanied by medium and small vessel cerebral vasculitis occur in this unusual setting (25–27). Contrast magnetic resonance imaging (MRI) scanning demonstrating leptomeningeal enhancement has been reported in one recent case (26).

Dermatologic manifestations are variable and may reflect vasculitis in the majority of cases. Up to 5% of patients will have cutaneous leukocytoclastic vasculitis. Other lesions include urticaria, angioedema, erythema multiforme, livedo reticularis, panniculitis, erythema nodosa, and migratory superficial thrombophlebitis (5). Transient mastitis, erythema elevatum diutinum, and oral and genital ulcers of Behçet's syndrome have been observed in association with relapsing polychondritis (28–30).

LABORATORY INVESTIGATION

There are no pathognomonic laboratory abnormalities in relapsing polychondritis. During the acute phase of the illness, the erythrocyte sedimentation rate and C-reactive protein are usually elevated. Thrombocytosis, mild leukocytosis, anemia, and hypergammaglobulinemia related to inflammation are also observed. A macrocytic anemia may be the first sign that there is an associated evolving myelodysplastic syndrome (31). Urinalyses should be obtained in all cases to screen for an accompanying glomerulonephritis.

Autoantibodies, including antinuclear antibodies and rheumatoid factor, are found in cases of relapsing polychondritis associated with connective tissue disease syndromes or rheumatoid arthritis. Hypocomplementemia is not observed unless it is related to an associated disease. Cryoglobulinemia is not found except in cases of related vasculitis. Antineutrophil cytoplasmic antibodies (ANCAs) occur in up to one-quarter of relapsing polychondritis cases during active flares (32). Both cytoplasmic ANCA (c-ANCA) and perinuclear ANCA (p-ANCA) antibodies with antimyeloperoxidase specifically have been reported. Not all of the c-ANCA–positive cases present with a clinically identifiable Wegener's granulomatosis nor have all the p-ANCA–positive cases been associated with glomerulonephritis or microscopic polyarteritis (32,33). Anticollagen antibodies are not routinely measured, are of uncertain sensitivity and specificity, and do not have a defined clinical utility in the management of relapsing polychondritis.

Evaluation of the airway in all patients with relapsing polychondritis is important because asymptomatic involvement, especially in the tracheobronchial region, may be present. Ideally, both pulmonary function testing and radiographic assessment should be performed since they are complementary. For example, radiographic or bronchoscopic evaluation of the laryngeal area may be unrevealing, yet pulmonary flow studies may demonstrate a grossly abnormal extrathoracic obstruction (10). Additionally, computed tomography (CT) scanning alone may underestimate the extent of dynamic collapse of the trachea (34). Pulmonary function testing should include both inspiratory and expiratory flow volume curves. Dyspnea may not be significant until the forced expiratory volume in 1 second (FEV_1) drops below 50% to 60% of expected (35). CT is best suited for imaging the laryngotracheal cartilage, because unlike conventional tomography, both airway narrowing and tracheal wall edema and fibrosis can be demonstrated (36). CT scanning should be performed in both routine inspiration as well as expiration or by cine CT to demonstrate abnormal variation in the tracheal diameter (Fig. 87.4). Sequential imaging may also be useful for monitoring the response to therapy by following tracheal wall thickness. However, these findings may be inaccurate for discriminating active inflammation from scarring. Gallium scintigraphy has been reported in one case to be a more sensitive indicator of tracheal inflammation. This observation requires confirmation in additional patients (37). Experience with MRI is not sufficient to evaluate its role in radiologic assessment of the airway. With the outlined approach, bronchoscopy is not routinely indicated in patients with laryngotracheal involvement. As there is some risk of precipitating an acute deterioration in respiratory status, the procedure should be reserved for cases in which the diagnosis is in question or a therapeutic stent placement is needed (35).

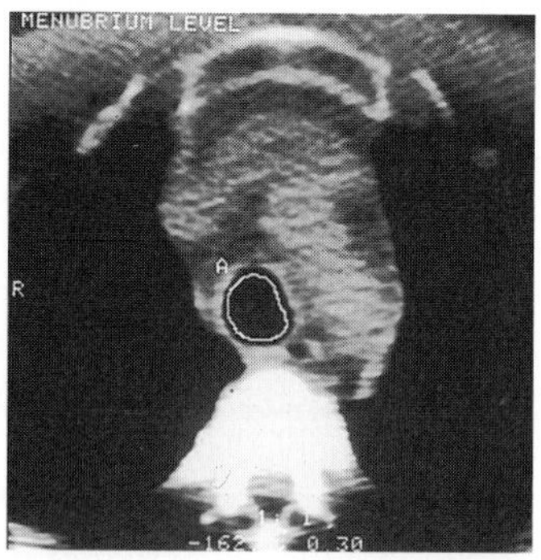

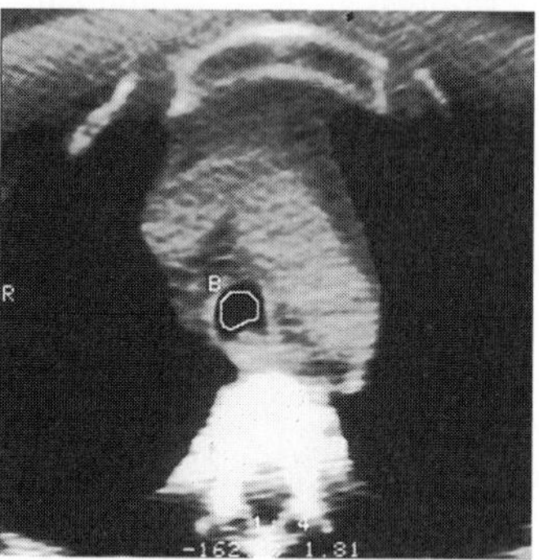

FIGURE 87.4. Cine computed tomography (CT) images of a flaccid trachea demonstrating a 66% variation in the airway diameter during respiration.

Echocardiography and angiography are indicated in selective cases to evaluate cardiovascular complications. Although echocardiography has been suggested as a routine procedure for the follow-up of patients with relapsing polychondritis, the incremental benefit provided by this procedure beyond auscultation has not been determined (38).

To date, there are no other proven laboratory methods for following relapsing polychondritis disease activity. Cytokine assays for indicators of active inflammation in relapsing polychondritis have not been evaluated. A report of elevated serum levels of a 148-kd tracheal, noncollagenous cartilage protein as a marker of disease activity has not been evaluated in a sufficient number of patients to evaluate its utility (39).

DIFFERENTIAL DIAGNOSIS

The multisite cartilaginous inflammation of relapsing polychondritis is unique, and when fully expressed the correct diagnosis is obvious. However, at initial presentation, patients will often have more limited syndromes and other conditions need to be considered. Unilateral auricular chondritis is confused with infection and frequently the correct diagnosis is only suspected when the contralateral ear becomes involved, repeated episodes occur, or there is a failure of empiric antibiotic treatment. Erysipelas may involve the ear. Fever, chills, and cellulitis spreading beyond the anatomic boundaries of the auricle are clues to the diagnosis.

Perichondritis related to *Pseudomonas aeruginosa* also mimics chondritis. A biopsy for culture to assist proper management is necessary in the setting of unilateral chondritis if no other manifestations of relapsing polychondritis are present. Chondrodermatitis helices is characterized by the appearance of a painful, tender, scaling, firm nodule on the helix of the ear and is usually easily distinguished from auricular chondritis. Rarely, other infiltrative lesions such as cutaneous lymphoma may involve the auricle and require biopsy for diagnosis.

Isolated nontraumatic subglottic stenosis may be related to prior endotracheal intubation, but is also observed in other inflammatory syndromes including amyloidosis, sarcoidosis, and Wegener's granulomatosis (40). The latter disease is complicated by features shared in common with relapsing polychondritis including saddle nose deformity, serous otitis, and proptosis. Mucosal ulcerations, pulmonary involvement, and a positive c-ANCA support a diagnosis of Wegener's granulomatosis. In the presence of auricular and costochondritis, overlapping syndromes of relapsing polychondritis and Wegener's granulomatosis can occur (41). A rare, inherited, pediatric disorder of hyaline cartilage has been described in an Indian family (42). This leads to saddle nose and noninflammatory subglottic cartilage degeneration and calcification. Other forms of tracheal disease, such as saber sheath trachea in chronic obstructive lung disease or tracheopathia osteoplastica in elderly patients, can be distinguished from relapsing polychondritis by the lack of other disease manifestations or characteristic CT scan appearance (43).

Cogan's syndrome is another inflammatory illness leading to nerve deafness and keratitis; however, the lack of cartilaginous involvement differentiates it from relapsing polychondritis. Systemic vasculitis syndromes with glomerulonephritis and either scleritis or serous otitis have been described. It is not clear whether these illnesses might represent variants of Wegener's granulomatosis or relapsing polychondritis.

PATHOGENESIS

The pathophysiologic mechanisms in relapsing polychondritis are incompletely understood. Factors initiating the cartilage inflammation are entirely unknown, but, once triggered, the evidence supports an immunologically mediated mechanism. Genetic susceptibility plays a role. Human leukocyte antigen HLA-DQ6/8 double transgenic mice developed polychondritis on immunization with type II collagen, whereas the parenteral strains do not (44). Immunogenetic analysis of a small number of patients with relapsing polychondritis confirmed an association with HLA-DR4 in 60% of cases compared to 25.5% of controls (19). Genotyping did not demonstrate a predominate DRB1*04 subtype allele as is seen in rheumatoid arthritis. Cell-mediated immunity to cartilage extracts, as well as collagen types II, IX, and XI, during active disease has been demonstrated (45,46). Histochemical staining of involved tissue reveals a predominance of HLA-DR$^+$ antigen-presenting cells and CD4$^+$ lymphocytes (47). Further evidence for cell-mediated immunity includes therapeutic observations of response in some refractory cases to cyclosporin A or anti-CD4 monoclonal antibodies (47–49).

A humoral immune response has been identified as part of the inflammatory process in relapsing polychondritis, but whether antibodies to collagen reflect a primary event or a secondary phenomenon resulting from an immune response to antigens released during cartilage destruction is not known. Neonatal polychondritis has been described in one infant who suffered a transient syndrome suggesting a primary role for transplacental anticollagen (or other unknown specificities) antibodies in causing the illness. Positive immunofluorescent assays for antibodies to cartilage matrix are observed (50). Analysis of the inflammatory reaction at the fibrocartilaginous junction of involved ear cartilage has revealed granular deposition of IgG, IgA, and C3, suggesting immune complex deposition (51). Circulating antibodies to native type II collagen during the acute stages of illness have been identified in some patients (52), and antibodies to minor collagens IX and XI have also been detected (53). One patient with relapsing polychondritis associated with microscopic polyarteritis expressed antibodies to native collagens II and IX. Several rheumatic diseases may lead to the production of anticollagen antibodies and a related secondary relapsing polychondritis syndrome. However, anticollagen antibodies in rheumatoid arthritis and relapsing polychondritis demonstrate different reactivities with cyanogen bromide digested peptides (54). This preliminary observation suggests that the clinical manifestations of anticollagen autoimmunity may be determined by the specific collagen epitope being targeted. Whether $DR4^+$ patients selectively produce anticollagen antibodies in relapsing polychondritis has not been clarified.

Animal models of type II collagen-induced chondritis have demonstrated the potential for an immunologic mechanism in relapsing polychondritis. Auricular chondritis occurs in outbred Wistar and Sprague-Dawley rats (55–57). Despite the appearance of antibodies to type II collagen coincident with the onset of arthritis in these animals, the extra-articular chondritis develops late in the course, suggesting a different pathogenic mechanism. The lack of a synovial membrane, and the thicker perichondrium impeding the ready deposition of IgG and complement and recruitment of neutrophils has been proposed as one mechanism for the late temporal evolution of auricular chondritis (55). Alternatively, a quantitative difference in IgG subclasses, a shift to immunity against minor collagen epitopes, or evolving immunity to proteoglycan antigens may explain this observation.

PATHOLOGY

The primary histopathology finding in relapsing polychondritis is destruction and loss of hyaline and elastic cartilage with an accompanying inflammatory cell infiltration of predominantly lymphocytes, plasma cells, and a few neutrophils. The fibrocartilaginous junction becomes indistinct, and damaged cartilage is fragmented into islands containing degenerating chondrocytes, surrounded by phagocytic macrophages and giant cells. Fibroblastic proliferation leads to replacement of cartilage with fibrous granulation tissue. Histochemical staining of involved cartilage reveals a characteristic loss of basophilic staining with hematoxylin and eosin and weak staining with Alcian blue compatible with matrix loss of glycosaminoglycans (58).

Electron microscopic examination of ear cartilage reveals that the superficial cartilage surface areas contain large amounts of electron-dense material lying in the matrix between scattered collagen fibers and on the surface of elastic fibers (59). Subsequent studies have suggested that there are a large number of extracellular small matrix granules of medium electron density, which are thought to be proteoglycans. Larger, dense membrane-bound vesicles of variable size are also observed. These appear to be released from chondrocytes into the extracellular space following budding from the tips of chondrocyte villi. It has been suggested that these lysosomal granules may contribute to the loss of cartilage matrix (60).

The synovium from an involved joint in relapsing polychondritis-associated arthritis reveals a chronic synovitis with a predominance of lymphocytes and plasma cells. Hyperplasia of type A synovial lining cells is also observed.

Cardiovascular pathology consists of valvulitis and aortic inflammation. The valvular tissue reveals neovascularization with foci of lymphocytes, plasma cells, and macrophages. The aortitis involves the media with increased neovascularization, perivascular mononuclear cellular infiltration, degeneration of collagen, and destruction of media elastic fibers, with replacement by fibrotic tissue.

In patients with scleritis, biopsies have demonstrated neutrophilic vasculitis, mononuclear cell infiltrates with mast cells, plasma cells, and lymphocytes in the conjunctiva and sclera. Immunofluorescent staining reveals immunoglobulin and C3 deposition in the vessel walls (61). Antibodies to corneal epithelium have been identified in a patient with corneal melt associated with scleritis (62). A biopsy of a patient with proptosis was described as showing a lymphocytic infiltrate in the region of the extraocular muscle (63).

TREATMENT

The treatment of relapsing polychondritis is based entirely on empiric clinical observations. Because of the rarity of the disease, no clinical trials have been performed. The mainstay of therapy is oral corticosteroids, which generally have a beneficial effect on the acute manifestations of chondritis. Initial doses of prednisone range from 0.5 to 1.0 mg/kg depending on the specific problems at presentation. Mild to moderate auricular and nasal chondritis may respond to lower doses, whereas scleritis, audiovestibular nerve involvement, laryngotracheal chondritis, or aortitis warrant initial high-dose treatment. NSAIDs can be utilized to manage mild auricular, nasal, and costochondral chondritis, or synovitis. Case reports have suggested the utility of dapsone (100 mg twice daily) or colchicine (0.6 mg twice daily) as alternatives to corticosteroids for managing auricular or nasal chondritis (64–66). If tolerated, an effective drug response should be seen within 1 to 2 weeks, hence longer trials of these agents are probably not warranted.

Unfortunately, there is a subset of patients with relapsing polychondritis that is resistant to corticosteroid treatment. This group often includes patients with necrotizing scleritis, progressive tracheal involvement, or vasculitis that progresses despite high-dose prednisone. Successful responses to azathioprine and oral or intravenous cyclophosphamide have been observed, but when these agents fail, cyclosporin A in a dose range of 3 to 5 mg/kg/day has been reported to be effective (47,67). The appropriate strategy of choice for second drug therapy for refractory patients is not clear. The increasing number of successful reports of cyclosporin A use suggests that it may be the best tolerated and most reliable drug for the corticosteroid-resistant patient. In individuals with an underlying systemic vasculitis, cyclosporin A may fail as a steroid-sparing agent. Limited successful experience with anti-CD4 monoclonal antibodies has been reported (48,49).

When relapsing polychondritis is associated with a systemic vasculitis, treatment should be tailored to the underlying arteritis. Cyclophosphamide should be considered using therapeutic approaches commonly employed for the treatment of systemic vasculitis. For the majority of patients with other forms of secondary relapsing polychondritis, corticosteroids alone are usually sufficient to manage the chondritis manifestations. Experience with using disease modifying antirheumatic drugs (DMARDs) such as hydroxychloroquine, methotrexate, or azulfidine for the management of relapsing polychondritis is limited. Methotrexate has not been effective in managing refractory scleritis in the setting of relapsing polychondritis (61); however, this drug has been found to be useful as a steroid-sparing agent by others (6,68).

Treatment of laryngotracheal relapsing polychondritis requires consideration of other issues beyond the choice of an immunosuppressant drug. A difficult problem is determining whether a flare of symptoms represents progression of the underlying disease or a superimposed bronchitis. Indirect laryngoscopy and CT scanning can be helpful in the assessment. Acute flares may be primarily related to airway edema leading to severe narrowing. Along with pulsed intravenous methylprednisolone, inhaled racemic ephedrine, a potent vasoconstrictor, has been reported to be effective (69,70). In cases with exclusively subglottic involvement, emergency tracheostomy may be necessary. For patients with diffuse airway damage and flaccid collapse, treatment options are very limited. Chronic pulmonary care with adequate hydration and prompt treatment of bronchitis is essential. Some patients may benefit from support with continuous positive airway pressure masks to allow improved pulmonary hygiene during bronchitis as well as relief from severe dyspneic symptoms during recumbency (71). Once the disease is quiescent, patients with fibrotic subglottic narrowing or segmental tracheobronchial damage only may be candidates for plastic repairs. For more extensive airway collapse or obstruction, stenting the involved bronchus with a silicon endoprosthesis can be attempted; however, these stents can be difficult to manage with mucous plugging, atelectasis, and pneumonia observed in some recipients. Neodymium:yttrium-aluminum-garnet (Nd:YAG) laser therapy has also been successfully used to treat localized inflammatory fibrotic narrowing of a main stem bronchus (72). Use of general anesthesia in a patient with relapsing polychondritis requires preoperative assessment of the airway with possible modification of usual intubation techniques (73).

Management of cardiovascular complications may require valvular replacement and aneurysmal repair in rare patients. Once corrected, long-term follow-up of these patients is mandatory, as they are at risk for ongoing inflammation. Postsurgical problems have included paravalvular prosthetic leaks and aneurysmal deterioration of vessels adjacent to graft repair sites. Because of the high prevalence of associated silent progressive aortitis, some surgeons have recommended considering replacement of the ascending aorta and reimplantation of the coronary arteries at the time of aortic valve replacement (74).

Relapsing polychondritis occurring during pregnancy has been rarely reported. Successful pregnancy without neonatal disease has been achieved in women treated with corticosteroids (75–77).

Long-term care of the patient with relapsing polychondritis requires periodic reassessment of the cardiovascular, pulmonary, and renal systems. A dilemma in managing the asymptomatic patient is the potential for progression of cardiac valvular, aortic, tracheobronchial, or renal lesions. Periodic reexamination, pulmonary function testing with serial flow volume loops, and assessment of renal function are necessary. This approach may be supplemented by selective application of CT scanning, vascular ultrasonography, and echocardiography in appropriate situations. Not all patients require continuous antiinflammatory treatment and many patients eventually "burn out" with no evidence of disease activity, sometimes after a very stormy initial illness.

REFERENCES

1. Jaksch-Wartenhorst R. Polychondropathia. *Med Klin* 1921;17: 93–100.
2. Pearson CM, Kline HM, Newcomer VD. Relapsing polychondritis. *N Engl J Med* 1960;263:51–58.
3. McAdam LP, O'Hanlan MA, Bluestone R, et al. Relapsing polychondritis. Prospective study of 23 patients and a review of the literature. *Medicine* 1976;55:193–215.
4. Damiani JM, Levine HL. Relapsing polychondritis—report of ten cases. *Laryngoscope* 1979;89:929–946.
5. Michet CJ, McKenna CH, Luthra HS, et al. Relapsing polychondritis. Survival and predictive role of early disease manifestations. *Ann Intern Med* 1986;104:74–78.
6. Trentham D, Le C. Relapsing polychondritis. *Ann Intern Med* 1998;129:114–122.
7. Cody DTR, Sones DA. Relapsing polychondritis; audiovestibular manifestations. *Laryngoscope* 1971;81:1208–1222.
8. Hussain SSM. Relapsing polychondritis presenting with stridor from bilateral vocal cord palsy. *J Laryngol Otol* 1991;105: 961–964.
9. Davis SD, Berkmen YM, King T. Peripheral bronchial involvement in relapsing polychondritis: demonstration by thin-section CT. *AJR* 1989;153:953–954.
10. Krell WS, Staats BA, Hyatt RE. Pulmonary function in relapsing polychondritis. *Am Rev Respir Dis* 1986;133:1120–1123.
11. O'Hanlan M, McAdam LP, Bluestone R, et al. The arthropathy of relapsing polychondritis. *Arthritis Rheum* 1976;19:191–194.
12. Booth A, Dieppe PA, Goddard PL, et al. The radiological manifestations of relapsing polychondritis. *Clin Radiol* 1989;40: 147–149.
13. Jawad ASM, Burrel M, Lim KL, et al. Erosive arthritis in relapsing polychondritis. *Postgrad Med J* 1990;66:768–770.
14. Marshall DAS, Jackson R, Rae AP, et al. Early aortic valve cusp rupture in relapsing polychondritis. *Ann Rheum Dis* 1992;51: 413–415.
15. Bowness P, Hawley IC, Morris T, et al. Complete heart block and severe aortic incompetence in relapsing polychondritis: clinicopathologic findings. *Arthritis Rheum* 1991;34:97–100.
16. Cipriano PR, Alonso DR, Baltaxe HA, et al. Multiple aortic

aneurysms in relapsing polychondritis. *Am J Cardiol* 1976;37: 1097–1102.

17. Giordano M, Valentini G, Sodano A. Relapsing polychondritis with aortic arch aneurysm and aortic arch syndrome. *Rheumatol Int* 1984;4:191–193.
18. Balsa-Criado A, Cuesta GHT, Aguado P, et al. Lupus anticoagulant in relapsing polychondritis. *J Rheumatol* 1990;17: 1426–1427.
19. Zeuner M, Straub RH, Schlosser U, et al. Antiphospholipid-antibodies in patients with relapsing polychondritis. *Lupus* 1998; 1:12–14.
20. Isaak BL, Liesegang TJ, Michet CJ Jr. Ocular and systemic findings in relapsing polychondritis. *Ophthalmology* 1986;93: 681–689.
21. Tucker SM, Linberg JV, Doshi HM. Relapsing polychondritis, another cause for a "salmon patch." *Ann Ophthalmol* 1993;25: 389–391.
22. Chang-Miller A, Okamura M, Torres VE, et al. Renal involvement in relapsing polychondritis. *Medicine* 1987;66:202–217.
23. Rodrigues MA, Tapanes FJ, Stekman IL, et al. Auricular chondritis and diffuse proliferative glomerulonephritis in primary Sjögren's syndrome. *Ann Rheum Dis* 1989;48:683–685.
24. Dalal BI, Wallace AC, Slinger RP. IgA neuropathy in relapsing polychondritis. *Pathology* 1988;20:85–89.
25. Stewart SS, Ashizawa T, Dudley AW Jr, et al. Cerebral vasculitis in relapsing polychondritis. *Neurology* 1988;38:150–151.
26. Kothare S, Chu C, VanLandingham K, et al. Migratory leptomeningeal inflammation with relapsing polychondritis. *Am Acad Neurol* 1998;51:614–617.
27. Brod S, Booss J. Idiopathic CSF pleocytosis in relapsing polychondritis. *Neurology* 1988;38:322–323.
28. Haigh R, Scott-Coombes D, Seckl JR. Acute mastitis; a novel presentation of relapsing polychondritis. *Postgrad Med J* 1987; 63:983–984.
29. Benard P, Bedane C, Delrous JL, et al. Erythema elevatum diutinum in a patient with relapsing polychondritis. *J Am Acad Dermatol* 1992;26:312–315.
30. Orme RL, Nordlund JJ, Barich L, et al. The MAGIC syndrome (mouth and genital ulcers with inflamed cartilage). *Arch Dermatol* 1990;126:940–944.
31. Van Besien K, Tricot G, Hoffman R. Relapsing polychondritis: a paraneoplastic syndrome associated with myelodysplastic syndromes. *Am J Hematol* 1992;40:47–50.
32. Papo T, Piette JC, Huong Du LT, et al. Antineutrophil cytoplasmic antibodies in polychondritis. *Ann Rheum Dis* 1993;52:384–385.
33. Handrock K, Gross WL. Relapsing polychondritis as a secondary phenomenon of primary systemic vasculitis. *Ann Rheum Dis* 1993;52:895–897.
34. Dunn WF, Hubmayr RD, Pairolero PC, et al. The assessment of major airway function in a ventilator-dependent patient with tracheomalacia. *Chest* 1990;97:939–942.
35. Tillie-LeBlond I, Wallaert B, LeBlond D, et al. Respiratory involvement in relapsing polychondritis. *Medicine* 1998;77:168–176.
36. Port JL, Khan A, Barbu RR. Computed tomography of relapsing polychondritis. *Comput Med Imaging Graph* 1993;17:119–123.
37. Okuyama C, Ushijima Y, Sugihara H, et al. Increased subglottic gallium uptake in relapsing polychondritis. *J Nucl Med* 1998;39: 1977–1979.
38. Buckley LM, Ades PA. Progressive aortic valve inflammation occurring despite apparent remission of relapsing polychondritis. *Arthritis Rheum* 1992;35:812–814.
39. Saxne T, Heingrd D. Involvement of non-articular cartilage, as demonstrated by release of a cartilage-specific protein, in rheumatoid arthritis. *Arthritis Rheum* 1989;32:1080–1086.
40. McDonald TJ, Devine KD, Weiland LH. Nontraumatic, nonneoplastic subglottic stenosis. *Ann Otol* 1975;84:757–763.
41. Cauhape P, Aumaitre O, Papo T, et al. A diagnostic dilemma: Wegener's granulomatosis, relapsing polychondritis or both? *Eur J Med* 1993;2:497–498.
42. Kurien M, Seshadri MS, Raman R, et al. Inherited nasal and laryngeal degenerative chondropathy. *Arch Otolaryngol Head Neck Surg* 1989;115:746–748.
43. Müeller NL, Miller RA, Ostrow DN, et al. Clinico-radiologic conference: diffuse thickening of the tracheal wall. *J Can Assoc Radiol* 1989;40:213–215.
44. Bradley D, Das P, Griffiths M, et al. HLA-DQ6/8 double transgenic mice develop auricular chondritis following type-II collagen immunization: a model for human relapsing polychondritis. *J Immunol* 1998;161:5046–5053.
45. Herman JH, Dennis MV. Immunopathologic studies in relapsing polychondritis. *J Clin Invest* 1973;52:549–558.
46. Rajapakse DA, Bywaters EGL. Cell-mediated immunity to cartilage proteoglycan in relapsing polychondritis. *Clin Exp Immunol* 1974;16:497–502.
47. Svenson KLG, Holmdahl R, Klareskog L, et al. Cyclosporin A treating in a case of relapsing polychondritis. *Scand J Rheumatol* 1984;13:329–333.
48. Choy EH, Chikanza IC, Kingsley GH, et al. Chimaeric anti-CD4 monoclonal antibody for relapsing polychondritis. *Lancet* 1991;338:450.
49. van der Lubbe PA, Miltenburg AM, Breedveld FO. Anti-CD4 monoclonal antibody for relapsing polychondritis. *Lancet* 1991; 337:1349.
50. Meyer O, Cyna J, Dryll A. Relapsing polychondritis-pathogenic role of anti-native collagen type II antibodies. A case report with immunological and pathological studies. *J Rheumatol* 1981;8: 820–824.
51. Valenzuela R, Cooperrider PA, Gogate P, et al. Relapsing polychondritis. *Hum Pathol* 1980;11:19–22.
52. Foidart JM, Abe S, Martin GR, et al. Antibodies to type II collagen in relapsing polychondritis. *N Engl J Med* 1978;299: 1203–1207.
53. Yang CL, Brinckmann J, Rui HF, et al. Autoantibodies to cartilage collagens in relapsing polychondritis. *Arch Dermatol Res* 1993;285:245–249.
54. Terato K, Shimozuru Y, Katayama K, et al. Specificity of antibodies to type II collagen in rheumatoid arthritis. *Arthritis Rheum* 1990;33:1493–1500.
55. Cremer MA, Pitcock JA, Stuart JM, et al. Auricular chondritis in rats. An experimental model of relapsing polychondritis induced with type II collagen. *J Exp Med* 1981;154:535–540.
56. McCune WJ, Schiller AL, Dynesius-Trantham RA, et al. Type II collagen-induced auricular chondritis. *Arthritis Rheum* 1982;25:266–273.
57. Prieur DJ, Young DM, Counts DF. Auricular chondritis in fawn-hooded rats. A spontaneous disorder resembling that induced by immunization with Type II collagen. *Am J Pathol* 1984;116: 69–76.
58. Verity MA, Larson WM, Madden SC. Relapsing polychondritis. *Am J Pathol* 1963;42:251–269.
59. Shaul SR, Schumacher HR. Relapsing polychondritis. Electron microscopic study of ear cartilage. *Arthritis Rheum* 1975;18: 617–625.
60. Hashimoto K, Arkin CR, Kang AH. Relapsing polychondritis. An ultrastructural study. *Arthritis Rheum* 1977;20:91–99.
61. Hoang-Xuan T, Foster CS, Rice BA. Scleritis in relapsing polychondritis. *Ophthalmology* 1990;97:892–898.
62. Albers FWJ, Majoor HJM, Van derGaag R. Corneal autoimmunity in a patient with relapsing polychondritis. *Eur Arch Otorhinolaryngol* 1992;249:296–299.
63. McKay DAR, Watson PG, Lyne AJ. Relapsing polychondritis and eye disease. *Br J Ophthamol* 1974;58:600–605.

64. Barranco VP, Minor DB, Solomon H. Treatment of relapsing polychondritis with dapsone. *Arch Dermatol* 1976;112:1286–1288.
65. Martin J, Roenigk HH Jr, Lynch W, et al. Relapsing polychondritis with dapsone. *Arch Dermatol* 1976;112:1272–1274.
66. Askari AD. Colchicine for treatment of relapsing polychondritis. *J Am Acad Dermatol* 1984;10:507–510.
67. Anstey A, Mayou S, Morgan K, et al. Relapsing polychondritis: autoimmunity to type II collagen and treatment with cyclosporin A. *Br J Dermatol* 1991;125:588–591.
68. Park J, Gowin K, Schumacher H. Steroid sparing effect of Methotrexate in relapsing polychondritis. *J Rheumatol* 1996;23: 937–938.
69. Gaffney RJ, Harrison M, Path FRC, et al. Nebulized racemic ephedrine in the treatment of acute exacerbations of laryngeal relapsing polychondritis. *J Laryngol Otol* 1992;106:63–64.
70. Lipnick RN, Fink CW. Acute airway obstruction in relapsing polychondritis: treatment with pulse methylprednisolone. *J Rheumatol* 1991;18:98–99.
71. Adliff M, Nagto D, Keshavjee S, et al. Treatment of diffuse tracheomalacia secondary to relapsing polychondritis with continuous positive airway pressure. *Chest* 1997;112:1701–1704.
72. Sacco O, Fregonese B, Oddone M, et al. Severe endobronchial obstruction in a girl with relapsing polychondritis: treatment with Nd YAG laser and endobronchial silicon stent. *Eur Respir J* 1997:10:494–496.
73. Burgess FW, Whitlock W, Davis MJ, et al. Anesthetic implications of relapsing polychondritis: a case report. *Anesthesiology* 1990;73:570–572.
74. Lang-Lazdunski L, Pansard Y, Hvass U. Aortic valve replacement in relapsing polychondritis. *J Thoracic Cardiovasc Surg* 1997;114: 131–132.
75. Arundell FW, Haserick JR. Familial chronic atrophic polychondritis. *Arch Dermatol* 1960;82:439.
76. Gimovsky ML, Nishiyama M. Relapsing polychondritis in pregnancy: a case report and review. *Am J Obstet Gynecol* 1989;161: 332–334.
77. Bellamy N, Dewar CL. Relapsing polychondritis in pregnancy. *J Rheumatol* 1990;17:1525–1526.

88

POLYMYALGIA RHEUMATICA AND GIANT CELL ARTERITIS

CORNELIA M. WEYAND
JÖRG J. GORONZY

Giant cell (temporal) arteritis is an inflammatory disease of medium-sized and large blood vessels in which injury to the arteries is caused by an immune-mediated mechanism. It is characterized by a wide spectrum of clinical signs and symptoms, only some of which are related to the vascular damage. Polymyalgia rheumatica is a closely related entity that affects the same patient population and has overlapping clinical and pathogenetic features.

Giant cell arteritis appears to be an old disease that may have already existed in the 15th century. At the end of the last century, several case reports described a new entity of temporal artery disease in combination with systemic symptoms. In 1932, Horton and co-workers (1) established the term *giant cell arteritis.* In 1957, Barber (2) defined polymyalgia rheumatica as a syndrome and introduced the name. During the past four decades, significant progress has been made in defining the spectrum of clinical manifestations, in optimizing diagnostic and therapeutic approaches, and in dissecting pathogenetic mechanisms.

DEFINITION

Giant cell arteritis is a chronic panarteritis that preferentially targets medium-sized and large arteries. Patients have involvement of the 2nd to 5th order branches of the proximal aorta, which possess well-defined internal and external elastic laminae. Often the inflammatory infiltrate is granulomatous and includes multinucleated giant cells. Because of the distribution of vessel involvement and the histomorphology, the disease also has been referred to as granulomatous arteritis, temporal arteritis, or cranial arteritis. Giant cell arteritis is the most frequent form of vasculitis in the Northern Hemisphere. It occurs almost exclusively in persons older than 50 years. Criteria for the classification of vasculitides have been published by the American College of Rheumatology (3). The criteria were developed to distinguish seven vasculitic syndromes and are useful for differentiating the various vasculitic diseases (Table 88.1). A patient with vasculitis is considered to have giant cell arteritis if three of the five criteria are present. Polymyalgia rheumatica is characterized by pain and stiffness in the muscles of the neck, the shoulder girdle, and the pelvic girdle of at least 4 weeks in duration (Table 88.2). Some, but not all, authors require an elevation of the erythrocyte sedimentation rate (ESR) above 40 mm/hour as a diagnostic criterion (4). The clinical signs and symptoms promptly respond to corticosteroid therapy (5). The diagnosis should be made only if other diseases, such as rheumatoid arthritis (RA), myositis, infection, and malignancy, have been excluded. Polymyalgia

TABLE 88.1. AMERICAN COLLEGE OF RHEUMATOLOGY 1990 CRITERIA FOR THE CLASSIFICATION OF GIANT CELL ARTERITIS (TRADITIONAL FORMAT)

Age at disease onset greater or equal to 50 years
Headache of new onset or new type
Tenderness or decreased pulsation of temporal artery
Elevated erythrocyte sedimentation rate
  (greater than or equal to 50 mm/hour)
Histologic changes of arteritis
  (either granulomatous lesions, usually with multinucleated giant cells, or diffuse mononuclear cell infiltration)

From Hunder GG, Bloch DA, Michel BA, et al. The American College of Rheumatology 1990 Criteria for the Classification of Giant Cell Arteritis. *Arthritis Rheum* 1990;33:1122–1128, with permission.

TABLE 88.2. CLINICAL FEATURES OF POLYMYALGIA RHEUMATICA

Pain in the muscles of the shoulder girdle, pelvic girdle,
  and neck (commonly bilateral and symmetrical,
  of at least 4 weeks in duration)
Stiffness after rest
Elevation of the erythrocyte sedimentation rate
  (greater than or equal to 40 mm/hour)
Frequent constitutional features including anemia, weight loss,
  fever, and general malaise
Prompt clinical response to corticosteroid treatment

rheumatica is diagnosed in patients without vasculitis; the documentation of inflammatory vascular lesions overrules the diagnosis of polymyalgia rheumatica and establishes the diagnosis of giant cell arteritis.

RELATIONSHIP BETWEEN POLYMYALGIA RHEUMATICA AND GIANT CELL ARTERITIS

The overlapping clinical features of polymyalgia rheumatica and giant cell arteritis and the occurrence of typical myalgias in patients with biopsy-proven giant cell vasculitis of the temporal artery suggest a close relationship between these two clinical syndromes. As long as an inciting agent has not been identified and as long as pathognomonic findings in polymyalgia rheumatica have not been clearly defined, the issue of whether polymyalgia rheumatica and giant cell arteritis are the same disease or are distinct diseases will remain controversial. Even before polymyalgia rheumatica was defined as a syndrome, it was observed that patients with giant cell arteritis and patients with "arthritis of the elderly" had common presenting features. In 1960, Paulley and Hughes (6) examined 67 patients who had giant cell arteritis and described the frequent occurrence of shoulder girdle and pelvic girdle pain in combination with morning stiffness. Subsequent studies established that patients with polymyalgia rheumatica may have positive temporal artery biopsy results despite a lack of evidence of cranial arteritis (7,8). Fauchald and co-workers (9) did not find any characteristic clinical features, except for symptoms directly related to arteritic involvement of cranial arteries, to distinguish patients with polymyalgia rheumatica and positive biopsy results from those with negative results.

Pathogenetic studies suggest that giant cell arteritis and polymyalgia rheumatica are variants of the same disease entity. Genetic studies demonstrated the preferential expression of certain human leukocyte antigen HLA-DRB1 alleles in both diseases (10–12). Molecular analyses have been used to identify the source of proinflammatory cytokines. Characteristically, both diseases have a high number of activated peripheral blood monocytes that are producing proinflammatory cytokines, distinguishing them from other chronic inflammatory diseases such as RA (13). The best evidence that polymyalgia rheumatica is indeed a variant of giant cell arteritis comes from studies analyzing the tissue expression of messenger RNA (mRNA) for inflammatory cytokines in temporal artery biopsy specimens (14). Temporal artery tissue from patients with polymyalgia rheumatica that was morphologically negative for inflammation contained locally produced transcripts of macrophage-derived and T-cell–derived cytokines. These studies established that polymyalgia rheumatica can have vascular involvement despite the lack of a microscopically detectable infiltrate.

EPIDEMIOLOGY

Giant cell arteritis is the most frequent vasculitis in North America and Western Europe. Its prevalence is highest in Scandinavian whites and lowest in Hispanics, blacks, and Orientals. Machado et al. (15) surveyed the incidence and prevalence of giant cell arteritis in Olmsted County, Minnesota, a population of mainly Northern European descent. Incidence rates averaged 17 per 100,000 persons, and prevalence rates averaged 223 per 100,000 in persons older than 50 years. There was an age-specific increase in incidence. Incidence increased from 2.6 per 100,000 persons in the age group 50 to 59 years to 44.7 per 100,000 in the population older than 80 years. Incidence and prevalence rates very similar to those in the Minnesotan population have been reported by several Scandinavian groups. A prospective study in Denmark found an incidence rate of 23.3 per 100,000 (16). In a 10-year survey of 284 cases of biopsy-proven giant cell arteritis in Göteborg, Sweden, the average annual incidence was 18.3 per 100,000 persons (17). The Scandinavian studies confirmed the observation of an increase in incidence with age, supporting the view that age is an important risk factor.

One autopsy study suggested that the true incidence of giant cell arteritis might be tenfold higher than indicated by epidemiologic surveys and that many cases might escape medical attention and take a benign, self-limited course (18). Striking differences in the prevalence in different racial groups, particularly in blacks and Hispanics, have been suggested by studies in Shelby County, Tennessee (19), and on the Texas Gulf Coast (20). The average annual incidence of biopsy-proven and probable temporal arteritis in Tennessee was 1.58 per 100,000. Epidemiologic studies in different regions of the world have supported the concept that ethnic and environmental differences influence the risk of development of giant cell arteritis. These differences might have been overemphasized in the earlier studies. Studies in Italy (21) and Israel (22) have reported incidence rates of 6.9 and 10.2 per 100,000, respectively, in a population older than 50 years. A follow-up study in Olmsted County suggested a nearly cyclical fluctuation in the incidence. Such fluctuations, which probably explain the increased frequencies observed in the mid-1980s in Minnesota and Sweden (15,17), add further complexity to investigations of the geographical distribution of the disease (23).

Differences in diagnostic criteria and lack of pathognomonic findings have complicated estimates of the prevalence and incidence of polymyalgia rheumatica. Generally, prevalence and incidence rates have paralleled those for giant cell arteritis in the different populations and are about two to three times higher. In a 10-year survey of the Olmsted County population, the average annual incidence was 53.7 per 100,000 persons and the prevalence was 500 per 100,000 (4), whereas Scandinavian studies estimated the annual incidence was 20.4 per 100,000 in persons 50 years or older (24). The disease is less common in Italy, where an average of 12.7 per 100,000 persons a year were diagnosed as having polymyalgia rheumatica (21). Kyle and co-workers (25) surveyed by questionnaire 656 persons older than 65 years of age and found higher estimates of prevalence rates in England (prevalence rate of 3,300 per 100,000). Further support for a role of inherited factors has come from several anecdotal reports of familial clustering of polymyalgia rheumatica and giant cell arteritis, although these data are limited. Familial aggregation was observed at a higher than expected frequency, with ten pairs of affected first-degree relatives in an estimated total patient population of about 500 (26). It is tempting to correlate annual or seasonal fluctuations in disease incidence rates or clustering of cases in space and time with environmental agents; however, these associations have remained hypothetical. Hepatitis B, contact with pet birds, respiratory syncytial virus, and adenovirus have been implicated, but these reports either have not been confirmed or await confirmation (27). In a more recent study, patients with giant cell arteritis and polymyalgia rheumatica were found to have elevated IgM titers to parainfluenza type I virus, indicating recent reinfection (28). Parvovirus-specific DNA sequences have been detected in arterial specimens from some giant cell arteritis patients (29).

PATHOLOGY

The diagnosis of giant cell arteritis is proven when typical histologic changes in arteries are noted (30). The histologic abnormalities vary, but the inflammatory infiltrates are generally centered in the arterial media with extension into the adventitia and intima (Fig. 88.1). Infiltrating cells include lymphocytes, macrophages, histiocytes, plasma cells, and some neutrophils and eosinophils. B cells are explicitly rare. Multinucleated giant cells are not always present and, although characteristic, are not required to establish the diagnosis. The arrangement of the inflammatory lesions has led to the distinction of two patterns of microscopic changes: (a) focal granulomatous lesions frequently including multinucleated giant cells, and (b) diffuse lymphomononuclear infiltrates giving the appearance of panarteritis. The clinical presentation does not appear to correlate with the pattern of vascular infiltration. If present, multinucleated giant cells are often close to a fragmented internal elastic lamina and may be located circumferentially along the degenerated elastic membrane. Occasionally, adventitial mononuclear infiltrates with perivascular cuffing of the vasa vasorum are found. Fibrinoid necrosis is rare. Intimal proliferation commonly occurs. The inflammatory response in giant cell arteritis is characterized by discontinuous lesions (skip lesions) leading to patchy damage of the elastic membrane and smooth muscle layer (31). Identification of inflammatory abnormalities may also be complicated by the coexistence of healed and fresh lesions. Healed vasculitis is diagnosed if neoangiogenesis, intimal fibrosis, and local medial scarring are present. However, these changes can be difficult to distinguish from age-related arterial changes.

In 90% of patients, histomorphologic changes occur in extracranial medium-sized branches of the aorta. The distribution pattern of involved arteries was established through an autopsy study by Wilkinson and Russell (32), who examined patients who died with active giant cell arteritis. Superficial temporal, vertebral, ophthalmic, and posterior ciliary arteries were involved most frequently. Vasculitic lesions also were detected in the internal and the external carotid and central retinal arteries. The infrequent involvement of intracranial vessels, which lack the external

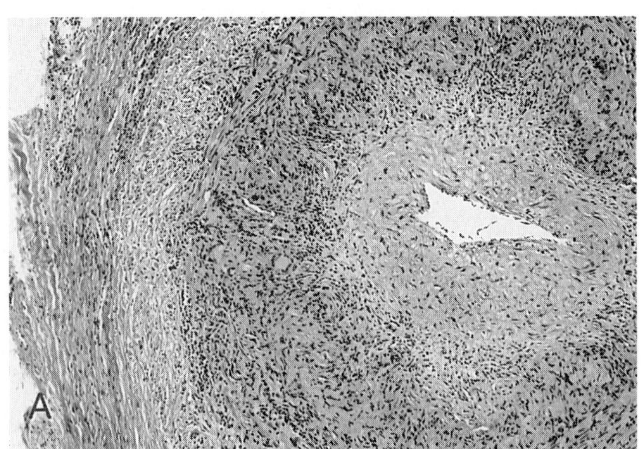

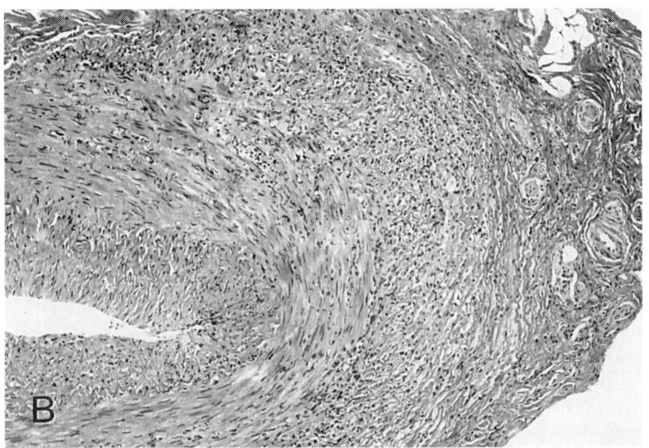

FIGURE 88.1. Histopathologic findings in giant cell arteritis. **A:** Granulomatous inflammation involving the media of the temporal artery with giant cell formation, predominantly at the intima/media junction. Concentric fibrosis of the media has caused intimal narrowing. **B:** Diffuse mononuclear infiltrate involving all three layers of the vessel wall, especially the expanded adventitia. No granulomas are identified. (H&E stain, ×100.) (Courtesy of Dr. J. Bjornsson, Mayo Clinic.)

elastic lamina, provided the basis for the hypothesis that a strict correlation exists between the presence of elastic laminae and inflammation.

In 10% to 15% of patients, inflammatory changes are found in large elastic arteries, including the aorta and its major branches and large pulmonary arteries (33). Infrequently, the process extends to other arteries, including small muscular arteries. Aside from the vasculature, inflammatory changes have been reported in synovial and hepatic tissue (34,35). Muscle biopsy specimens obtained from patients with polymyalgia rheumatica and giant cell arteritis have shown nonspecific type II muscle atrophy but no myositis.

CLINICAL FEATURES OF GIANT CELL ARTERITIS

Giant cell arteritis occurs almost exclusively in individuals older than 50 years; 70% to 80% of the patients are female. The mean age at disease onset is about 70 years. The disease causes a wide spectrum of symptoms (Table 88.3) (36). The vast majority of patients, 80% to 90%, have clinical findings related to involvement of extracranial branches of the proximal aorta. Systemic and local symptoms may be present only temporarily and do not necessarily persist despite continuous disease activity. The onset of the disease is often abrupt but also may be insidious. Giant cell arteritis is usually diagnosed within 2 to 6 months after symptom onset (37). Unusual manifestations may cause a delay in diagnosis. Increased awareness by physicians of the existence of this vasculitic entity causing constitutional symptoms in the elderly probably has expedited the diagnosis and led to the detection of giant cell vasculitis with unusual clinical manifestations.

TABLE 88.3. CLINICAL FEATURES OF GIANT CELL ARTERITIS

Symptoms directly related to vascular involvement
Frequent
Headaches
Abnormalities of temporal arteritis
Common
Ocular symptoms
Jaw claudication
Infrequent
Tongue claudication
Respiratory symptoms
Vision loss
Limb circulation
Circulatory insufficiency of central nervous system
Peripheral neuropathic syndromes
Aortic arch syndrome
Symptoms related to systemic illness
Frequent
Laboratory evidence for acute-phase response (elevated erythrocyte sedimentation rate, anemia, elevated C-reactive protein, elevated interleukin-6)
Common
Malaise, fever, anorexia, weight loss, night sweats, polymyalgia rheumatica
Infrequent
Arthralgias/arthritis

Headaches

The most common symptom is headache, which is present in 70% to 80% of patients at the initial examination. Although variable, it is usually severe. The patient describes throbbing, sharp, or dull pain that often is localized to one area of the head. The headache can be accompanied by scalp tenderness, but it can be severe even without tenderness of scalp arteries. Patients notice tenderness of the scalp, particularly in the temporal region, when wearing glasses, combing the hair, or touching the pillow with the head at night. The headache may improve despite ongoing disease activity. Abnormalities of the cranial arteries, including temporal, occipital, and superficial vessels, are frequent, particularly when carefully sought. However, in one-third of patients, temporal arteries are normal to palpation despite inflammatory involvement. Physical findings of significance are thickened vessels, tenderness, nodularity, and absent or reduced pulses.

Nonspecific Systemic Symptoms

Constitutional symptoms such as malaise, anorexia, weight loss, low-grade fever, fatigue, and depression are common, occurring in 40% to 50% of all cases. Symptoms of polymyalgia rheumatica are present in 40% to 60% of patients. Occasionally, fever of unknown origin with spiking temperatures and chills can be attributed to giant cell arteritis. Many of these manifestations are probably related to the increased production of proinflammatory cytokines and are closely associated with the induction of acute-phase reactants.

Visual Symptoms

Giant cell arteritis causes visual symptoms in 25% to 50% of all cases. The spectrum of ocular manifestations includes diplopia, amaurosis fugax, scotomata, ptosis, and partial or complete blindness. Symptoms can be transient or permanent. Visual loss is usually caused by anterior ischemic optic neuritis due to inflammation of posterior ciliary arteries. Infrequently, the central artery of the optic nerve or the retinal artery (both of which possess only an internal elastic lamina) is affected. Clinical features vary with the extent of optic nerve damage and include decreased acuity, field defects, impaired color vision, and defective pupil reactions. Funduscopic findings are normal or show pallor and edema of the optic disc, cotton-wool patches, and small hemorrhages.

Blindness due to retinal infarction or infarction of the occipital cortex is uncommon. Visual symptoms may also be caused by malfunctioning ocular muscles. Sudden blindness resulting from ischemic optic neuritis is a well-recognized and feared complication. It may be the presenting symptom of a patient lacking other manifestations of the disease, but it is most often preceded by other symptoms. Transient visual loss is a preceding symptom in only a minority of patients in whom permanent blindness develops. Visual defects in one eye often are followed by optic nerve damage of the other eye within days. Because visual loss is usually irreversible, ophthalmic symptoms are an emergency requiring prompt diagnosis and treatment. The risk of developing permanent visual defects after initiation of appropriate corticosteroid treatment is low (38). Ischemic optic neuritis, however, may complicate polymyalgia rheumatica treated with low-dose corticosteroids, particularly when the doses are tapered and signs of frank vasculitis develop.

Intermittent Claudication

Reduced blood flow in extracranial branches of the aorta, supplying the masseter and temporalis muscles, causes clinical manifestations that are relatively disease-specific. About 50% of patients complain of pain induced by chewing or prolonged talking. Jaw claudication is most evident with chewing meat and, rarely, can express as trismus. Other manifestations include claudication of the tongue and painful dysphagia related to ischemia of involved muscles. In contrast to Takayasu's arteritis, giant cell arteritis rarely produces neck, throat, or facial pain.

Large-Vessel Arteritis

Involvement of large arteries is appreciated in 10% to 15% of patients (33). Aortic arch syndrome is a serious complication of the disease and produces upper extremity claudication, decreased or absent peripheral pulses, paresthesias, and Raynaud's phenomenon. Vascular bruits can be heard over the carotid, subclavian, and axillary arteries. A recent case-control study has demonstrated that the clinical presentation of patients with large-vessel giant cell arteritis is different from patients with primarily cranial involvement (39). Specifically, headaches and jaw claudication are infrequent in patients with large-vessel arteritis. Signs of vascular insufficiency, particularly arm claudication, are the lead symptoms of the large-vessel variant of giant cell arteritis. Polymyalgia rheumatica is equally frequent in patients with classic large-vessel disease. Consistent with the absence of cranial symptoms, temporal artery biopsies are negative in 40% of patients with large-vessel involvement, emphasizing the need to consider the diagnosis of giant cell arteritis despite the absence of vascular lesions in the temporal artery. Aortic arch syndrome in giant cell arteritis is diagnosed by angiography that classically demonstrates lumen-compromising vascular lesions of the axillary and proximal brachial arteries. Abdominal aortic involvement, either independent or coexisting with arch disease, is rare.

Late complications of aortic involvement are more common than previously thought. In a population-based study cohort of giant cell arteritis in Olmsted County, Minnesota, thoracic aortic aneurysm developed in 11 of 96 patients. In eight patients, thoracic aortic aneurysm developed several years after the initial diagnosis. It has been estimated that patients with giant cell arteritis have a 17.3-fold increased risk for development of thoracic aortic aneurysm (40).

Clinical Features Manifesting in a Minority of Cases

Respiratory symptoms are probably referable to inflammatory lesions in pulmonary artery branches (41). They usually present as cough, hoarseness, and chest pain. Interstitial pulmonary infiltrates are rare. Soreness of the throat likely reflects ischemia of neck arteries. If respiratory symptoms dominate the clinical picture, they may be misleading and can cause undue delay in proper diagnosis.

Neurologic manifestations have probably been underestimated in frequency. Caselli and Hunder (42) described a diverse spectrum of neurologic problems occurring in 20% to 30% of patients. Narrowing and occlusion of carotid and vertebrobasilar arteries result in transient ischemic attacks or infarcts. Manifestations in the peripheral nervous system presenting as either mononeuritis or polyneuropathies are not uncommon, with 14% of cases affected.

Cardiac disease is rare. Clinical symptoms resemble those seen in Takayasu's arteritis and most often are related to coronary arteritis.

In recent years, an increasing number of case reports have emphasized that giant cell arteritis can produce very unusual clinical syndromes. On rare occasions, localized forms of the disease exist with vasculitic lesions in the female breast, ovaries, and uterus.

Clinical Features of Polymyalgia Rheumatica

Polymyalgia rheumatica is a syndrome that accompanies, precedes, or follows giant cell arteritis in 40% to 60% of cases, but it also occurs independently. Characteristic symptoms are aching and pain in the muscles of the neck, shoulders, lower back, hips, and thighs. The onset is often abrupt, and initial involvement of shoulder girdle muscles is frequent. Severe stiffness after periods of inactivity is a typical feature. Night pain is common, and patients frequently complain that they have difficulties getting up. Asymmetric patterns of involvement are unusual but do occur. Constitutional symptoms such as low-grade fever, weight loss, anorexia, malaise, and depression occur in more than 50% of patients. Pyrexia and chills are not considered part of the clinical spectrum. Synovitis of large joints probably contributes to the myalgic symptoms. Clinically appreciated synovitis involving knees and sternoclavicular joints was described by O'Duffy and associates (43). Joint inflammation has been documented by arthroscopic synovial biopsy and synovial fluid analysis (34,44,45). The issue of arthritis as a component of polymyalgia rheumatica, however, has remained controversial. Kyle and co-workers (46), using radiography, thermography, and isotope scanning, found synovitis in only 1 of 56 patients. The absence of florid arthritis and the benign course of the arthritis (when present) allow the distinction of polymyalgia rheumatica from other inflammatory arthropathies.

DIAGNOSTIC STUDIES

Histologic proof of vasculitis should be sought in a patient with suspected giant cell arteritis. In patients with findings suggestive of cranial arteritis, a clinically abnormal artery should be chosen, usually the temporal artery, infrequently the occipital artery. A normal physical examination of extracranial arteries does not exclude inflammatory involvement. Giant cell arteritis is characterized by discontinuous lesions, and the diagnosis can be missed if the biopsy specimen does not include one of the patchy infiltrates. Therefore, arterial segments of several centimeters should be removed, and multiple histologic sections should be examined routinely.

To minimize the rate of false-negative biopsy results, contralateral temporal artery biopsies have been recommended for cases in which cryosections of the first artery were negative. This approach has been shown to increase the rate of detecting vasculitic infiltrates by approximately 15% (47). Temporal artery biopsy is a highly sensitive diagnostic tool. Only 7% to 9% of patients who had a negative biopsy result of both temporal arteries presented with or developed unequivocal clinical evidence for vasculitis (48,49).

Whether patients with clear clinical evidence for giant cell arteritis need a confirmatory biopsy has been an issue of debate. The high rate of side effects in an elderly population treated with appropriate doses of corticosteroids warrants confirmation of an underlying inflammatory disease. Most of the clinical findings and certainly the laboratory abnormalities are not pathognomonic. Another controversy has been whether patients with polymyalgia rheumatica should undergo temporal artery biopsy. A subset of patients will have evidence for vasculitis on biopsy while lacking clinical signs of cranial arteritis. Depending on the population studied, 10% to 50% of patients with polymyalgia rheumatica may have giant cell arteritis at presentation or it will develop it during follow-up (4,50,51). Arterial biopsy is probably not necessary in patients with polymyalgia rheumatica if there is no clinical evidence of arteritis and if symptoms are mild and of recent onset or have remained stable over a long duration. Patients with a polymyalgic syndrome should be carefully evaluated clinically and should be monitored for signs of arteritis after initiation of treatment. Low-dose corticosteroid treatment does not prevent the progression of polymyalgia rheumatica to giant cell arteritis, and patients are particularly at risk for developing arteritis during periods of reduction or withdrawal of this treatment. If clinical signs of vasculitis develop, histologic proof should be sought.

Several studies have provided indirect evidence that corticosteroids given for a short period before the biopsy may not increase the rate of false-negative results (52,53). These studies have to be interpreted with some caution because the corticosteroid-treated patient cohort may have been biased for more severe disease, and the effect of corticosteroids may differ depending on the extent of inflammatory infiltrates. However, studies of temporal artery specimens that were engrafted into severe combined immunodeficiency mice have also shown that the inflammatory infiltrate persists in spite of corticosteroid treatment (54). Corticosteroids should therefore not be withheld if pertinent clinical evidence of arteritis is found and the biopsy cannot be done immediately.

Clinical findings indicating large-vessel involvement should prompt angiographic examination to document arteritic changes (33). Angiography of the aortic arch and its branches has been used successfully to establish the diagnosis of giant cell arteritis even in cases with negative results of temporal artery biopsy (39). Angiographically detected lesions have a typical distribution and are found in the carotid artery, in the subclavian artery, and often at the subclavian axillary junction (Fig. 88.2). Findings include segments of smooth wall stenosis, alternating with a normal or

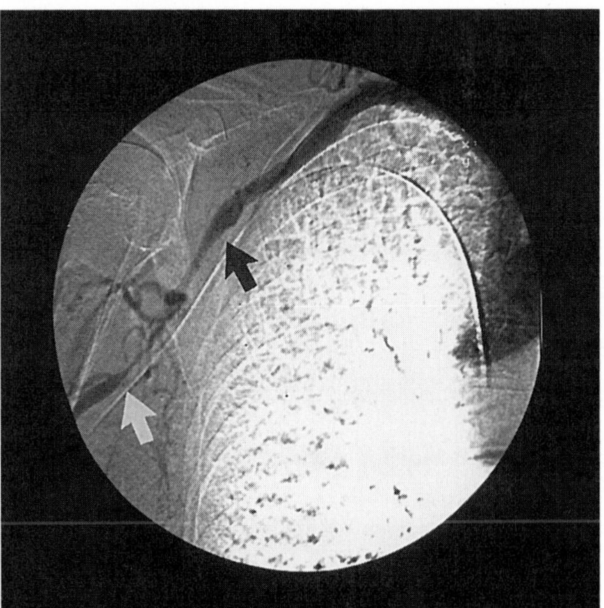

FIGURE 88.2. Intravenous digital subtraction angiogram showing typical findings of giant cell arteritis. The vasculitis has caused a tapered long segmental stenosis of the right distal axillary artery *(black arrow)* continuing to the proximal brachial artery *(white arrow)*.

an increased caliber, or smooth, tapered occlusions of large arteries. Irregular plaques and ulcerations should raise the suspicion of atherosclerosis causing narrowing or stenosis. Noninvasive vascular studies, including fluorescein angiography, transcranial Doppler flow studies, and Doppler ultrasonography to identify biopsy sites, may be helpful in some patients to detect vascular involvement (55). However, their general usefulness has not been established, and patients with unusual distribution patterns of vasculitis and patients with less pronounced arteritis may be missed (56).

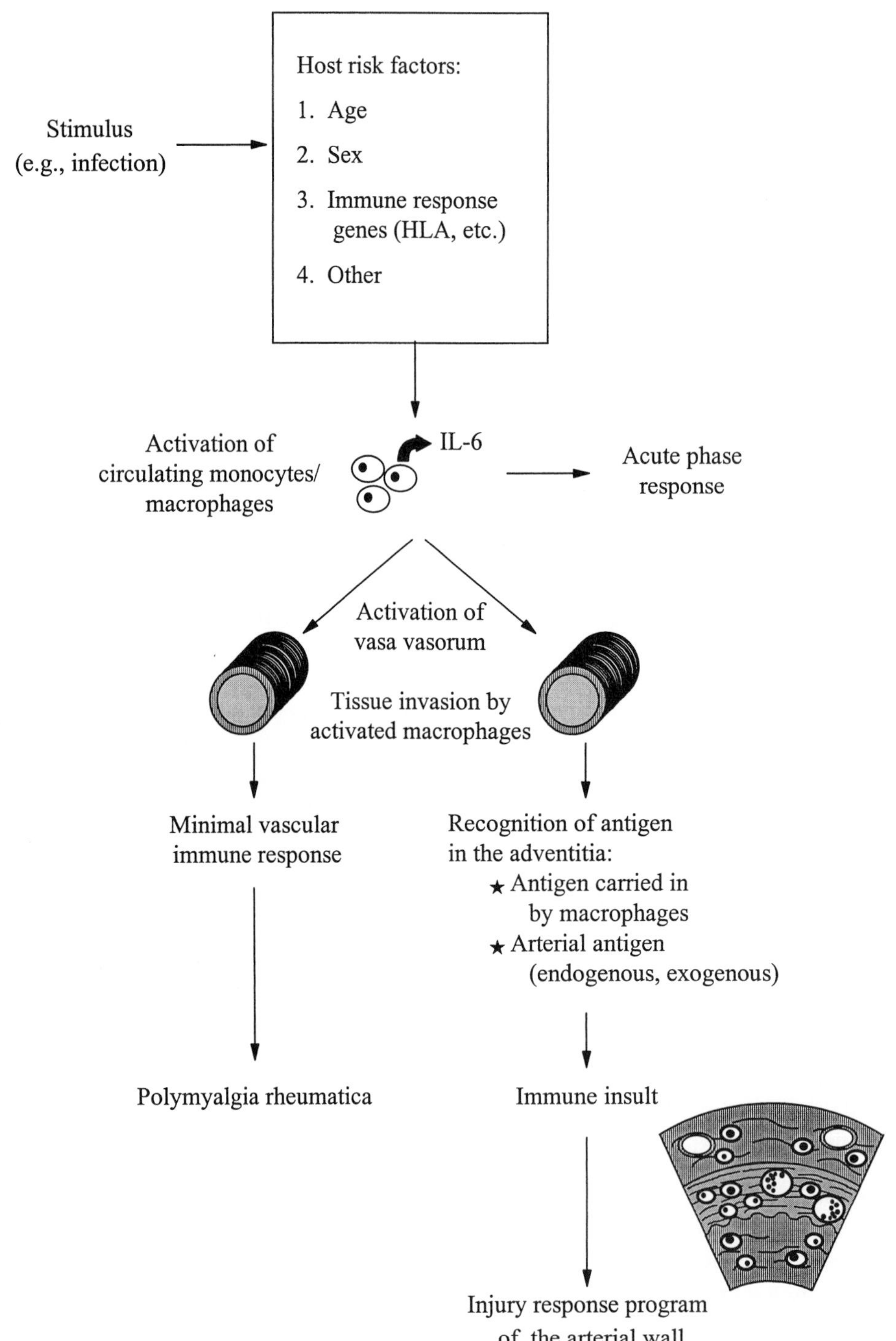

FIGURE 88.3. Schematic diagram of pathogenetic mechanisms in giant cell arteritis (From Hoffman G, Weyand C, eds. *Inflammatory diseases of blood vessels.* New York: Marcel Dekker, 1999, with permission.)

ROLE OF LABORATORY STUDIES

Giant cell arteritis and polymyalgia rheumatica cannot be diagnosed with a pathognomonic laboratory test. Laboratory abnormalities, however, are almost always present and are helpful for directing diagnostic decisions. Both diseases are characterized by an intense acute-phase reaction. The ESR is almost consistently elevated, often to more than 100 mm/hour. However, low or normal sedimentation rates in patients with positive biopsy results may be more frequent than previously appreciated. A mild-to-moderate normochromic or hypochromic anemia and elevated platelet counts are common. Peripheral eosinophilia occasionally occurs. Consistent with an acute-phase response, C-reactive protein and other acute-phase reactants are increased, and protein electrophoresis may show an elevated α_2-globulin level. C-reactive protein is probably no more useful for monitoring disease activity than sedimentation rates (57), although some reports have claimed a higher sensitivity. The level of interleukin-6 (IL-6), a proinflammatory cytokine with a major role in the induction of acute-phase proteins, is markedly increased (58,59). Elevated IL-6 concentrations are exquisitely sensitive to corticosteroid treatment, and withdrawal is associated with a prompt increase in IL-6 plasma levels even after several months of successful corticosteroid treatment. A recent study suggests that IL-6 plasma concentrations could be useful as a biomarker in monitoring disease activity in patients with polymyalgia rheumatica (60).

Contrary to many other chronic inflammatory diseases, polymyalgia rheumatica and giant cell arteritis are not characterized by autoantibody production. Antineutrophil cytoplasmic antibodies are rarely positive. Antinuclear antibodies and rheumatoid factors are not found more frequently than in an age-matched normal population. Anticardiolipin antibodies have been described in 31% of giant cell arteritis patients; however, they are also present in biopsy-negative patients with polymyalgia rheumatica (61), suggesting that they do not have a major role in vascular complications. Complement and immunoglobulin concentrations are usually normal.

In one-third of patients, liver function tests are mildly abnormal; usually alkaline phosphatase and, occasionally, aspartate aminotransferase activity are increased. Serum creatinine levels and urinary sediments are normal. Diagnostic tests evaluating muscle function such as determination of muscle enzymes, electromyographic studies, and muscle histology yield normal results. Proteins of endothelial origin, such as factor VIII/von Willebrand factor, have been found to be increased in patients with giant cell arteritis and polymyalgia rheumatica (62). Longitudinal studies have shown that plasma concentrations of von Willebrand factor have a tendency to eventually decrease but do not correlate with inflammatory activity (63,64).

ETIOLOGY AND PATHOGENESIS

The nonrandomness of incidence rates in different geographic regions and different ethnic or racial groups is highly suggestive of the contribution of genetic elements to disease pathogenesis (Fig 88.3). Female dominance, age restriction at onset of the disease, and the tissue tropism may also be surrogates for genetic risk factors. Thus far, convincing experimental data have been obtained only for one genetic system, the HLA-DR alleles. Whether uneven distribution of HLA genes is sufficient to explain the differences in disease incidence in different geographic regions of the world remains to be determined.

MAJOR HISTOCOMPATIBILITY COMPLEX (MHC) GENES IN GIANT CELL ARTERITIS AND POLYMYALGIA RHEUMATICA

In most studies analyzing an MHC association with giant cell arteritis, an overrepresentation of the HLA-DR4 haplotype has been found (10,11,65). This association is incomplete, and only 50% to 60% of patients with biopsy-proven disease express an HLA-DR4 haplotype. It has been suggested that MHC class II genes expressed in patients with giant cell arteritis share a sequence motif that is common to all different HLA-DRB1*04 variants but also expressed by several other HLA-DRB1 alleles. The sequence motif (amino acid positions 29 to 32) can be mapped to the antigen-binding site of the HLA-DR molecule, suggesting that the selective binding of a disease-inducing antigen by the HLA-DR molecule is a crucial event in the pathogenesis. Similarly, polymyalgia rheumatica has been found to have an HLA-DR4 association (10–12,66,67). The distributions of HLA-DRB1 alleles in these two diseases are indistinguishable, indicating that HLA-DR polymorphisms are not a genetic factor that determines the progression of polymyalgia rheumatica to vasculitis (12). In particular, a gene dosage effect of HLA-DRB1 polymorphisms, which has been described as an important progression factor in RA (68), cannot be demonstrated in giant cell arteritis.

HLA-DRB1*04 is not only a risk factor in giant cell arteritis but is also the most prominent allele associated with RA. HLA-DRB1*04 individuals, therefore, should have an increased risk for developing RA and, subsequently, also giant cell arteritis. This hypothesis was tested in a case series study of 835 patients with biopsy-proven giant cell arteritis (65). Only one patient with seropositive RA, instead of 22 expected cases, was identified, suggesting that these patients may be protected from developing giant cell arteritis. The mechanism of this protective effect is unclear, but these data provide interesting insights into the contrasting pathogenetic aspects.

Polymyalgia Rheumatica—An Incomplete Form of Giant Cell Arteritis

In addition to the shared HLA-DRB1 association of giant cell arteritis and polymyalgia rheumatica, multiple lines of evidence support the model that polymyalgia rheumatica is a forme fruste of giant cell arteritis. In essence, the polymyalgic syndrome exhibits the systemic component of disease while the vascular component often remains subclinical and can only be detected by molecular techniques (Fig 88.3) (14).

Patients with giant cell arteritis/polymyalgia rheumatica consistently have signs of pronounced systemic inflammation. The site of this inflammatory response has not been unequivocally identified. The inflammatory syndromes in polymyalgia rheumatica argue against the vascular tree as the sole location of the disease process. Systemic inflammation is closely linked to the laboratory abnormalities, reflecting a strongly upregulated acute-phase response that produces clinical manifestations of a wasting syndrome and that is explicitly sensitive to steroid-mediated immunosuppression. Pathogenic studies have demonstrated that circulating monocytes in both giant cell arteritis and polymyalgia rheumatica are constitutively activated and synthesize proinflammatory cytokines, such as IL-6 (13). Treatment with corticosteroids is followed by an abrupt decline in serum IL-6 levels, paralleled closely by an improvement of the clinical symptoms of myalgias and stiffness (59). Systemic monocyte activation is equally developed in giant cell arteritis and polymyalgia rheumatica, suggesting that it precedes the establishment of vascular lesions.

In patients with polymyalgia rheumatica, however, the arteries are not free of disease. Molecular analysis of tissue extracts from temporal arteries classified as negative pathologically have demonstrated that the monocyte-derived cytokines IL-1 and IL-6 are produced in the arterial wall (14). Local activation of macrophages is accompanied by the stimulation of T cells, demonstrated by the T-cell product IL-2 in the arterial tissue. Arteries from patients with polymyalgia rheumatica do not contain interferon-γ (IFN-γ), a T-cell cytokine released by differentiated, antigen-specific T cells. In contrast, IFN-γ is the dominant T-cell cytokine in artery specimens with classical arteritis.

The Nature of the Immune Response in the Arterial Wall

There is overwhelming evidence that vascular lesions in giant cell arteritis represent the consequence of a T-cell–dependent immune response (69). While the identification of the antigen driving T-cell activation in the arterial wall has not yet been achieved, accumulating data strongly support the concept that the vascular inflammation results from antigen-specific activation of T cells.

Vascular infiltrates are composed of T cells, mostly CD4$^+$ T cells, and macrophages; B cells are explicitly rare (70). IL-2 and IFN-γ are the dominant T-cell mediators produced *in situ* while IL-4 and IL-5 are absent (14). Attempts to study the relationship between the pathologic changes in the artery and the immune activation of T cells have led to the surprising finding that the adventitia is the site of the immunologic injury (71). Inflammation-related arterial wall destruction is focused on the medial layer where granulomas are formed, smooth muscle cells are damaged, and the bordering elastic laminae are fragmented. IFN-γ–producing CD4$^+$ T cells accumulate in the adventitia, raising the interesting question of how these cells are involved in regulating the media-based inflammation. Tissue-infiltrating T cells in temporal arteries undergo clonal proliferation, and T cells with identical T-cell receptors are concentrated in distinct regions of the arterial wall (72). Clonally expanded T cells proliferate in response to extracts from temporal artery tissue, suggesting a common antigen in different patients. Arteries from patients with polymyalgia rheumatica also contain the T-cell stimulatory material (73). The clonality, the clustering of IFN-γ–producing T cells in the adventitia, and the T-cell response to tissue extracts all support the role of antigen in driving this immune response. Studies in a human artery–mouse chimera model of giant cell arteritis provided direct evidence for this hypothesis. In this model, temporal arteries are engrafted into severe-combined immunodeficiency mice. Adoptive transfer of artery-derived T cells, but not of peripheral T cells from the same patient, amplifies cytokine production in the engrafted tissue (74).

Macrophages in the vascular lesions are highly specialized and display very distinct functional abilities, depending on their position in the arterial wall. Adventitial macrophages specialize in the production of IL-1β and IL-6, allowing them to interact with activated T cells in this arterial layer. Macrophages in the media are unable to release proinflammatory cytokines but are focused on the production of matrix metalloproteinases and growth factors. In several studies, medial macrophages were identified as cells with tissue-damaging potential (75–77). Matrix metalloproteinases have the potential to digest elastic fibers and are the likely cause of fragmentation of the elastic laminae (76,77). A novel mechanism of arterial wall damage has been attributed to the local production of toxic oxygen intermediates. Evidence of oxidative stress as an injurious mechanism in giant cell arteritis has been detected by demonstrating the presence of lipid peroxidation products in the media (75).

While histologic evaluation of inflamed temporal arteries has given rise to the speculation that giant cell formation results from the necessity to remove fragments of the internal elastic lamina, molecular studies have disputed this concept. Multinucleated giant cells, present in about 50% of all patients, represent a special form of media-based macrophages. Their product profile includes matrix metalloproteinase but they preferentially synthesize growth factors, such as platelet-derived growth factor and vascular endothelial growth factor (78,79), indicating that they have a role in tissue repair. There is evidence that the formation of giant cells in the lesions is under the control of IFN-γ, linking events in the media with the immune response in the adventitia (78).

Macrophages homing to the intimal layer are characterized by their ability to produce nitric oxide synthase 2 and they can thus elaborate nitric oxide in the inflamed artery (76). Whether nitric oxide has beneficial effects and regulates vasodilation or whether it contributes to inflammatory tissue damage is unresolved.

THE ARTERY'S INJURY-RESPONSE PROGRAM

The immunologic insult to the vascular wall is tissue-destructive, but the clinical manifestations and the pathology of giant cell arteritis are not that of aneurysm formation and hemorrhage. Rather, aneurysm formation is limited to the aorta and is not typical for arteries in the extracranial vascular bed. Clinical manifestations of giant cell arteritis result from tissue ischemia, a consequence of vascular occlusion. Luminal obstruction in giant cell arteritis is caused by a concentric growth of the intimal layer, similar to the intimal hyperplasia of atherosclerotic disease and the generation of neointima following angioplastic interventions. The outgrowth of hyperplastic intima is facilitated by the artery itself and represents attempted tissue repair. Recent pathogenic studies in giant cell arteritis have postulated that intimal hyperplasia, the underlying mechanism of giant cell arteritis–related morbidity, is a maladaptive response of the artery to the immunologic insult (Fig 88.3) (80). Conclusive evidence that this maladaptive reaction is under the control of the immune system comes from studies demonstrating that the growth factors necessary for tissue hyperplasia are supplied by tissue-infiltrating immune cells, specifically multinucleated giant cells producing an array of growth factors (78,79).

Upon injury, the resident cells of the arterial wall initiate an injury response program, including the mobilization of smooth muscle cells, their directed migration toward the lumen, and their proliferation in the intimal layer. Myofibroblast proliferation is combined with excessive production of extracellular matrix, producing the lumen-obstructive neotissue. Required molecular components for this process include matrix metalloproteinases, growth factors, such as platelet-derived growth factors, and mediators inducing matrix production. Clinical manifestations of cranial ischemia have been associated with the expression of platelet-derived growth factor and matrix metalloproteinases, produced by macrophages and multinucleated giant cells clustered in the media of inflamed arteries (78). Thus, the process of arterial occlusion is ultimately under the control of immune cells. Another pathway of the artery's response to inflammation involves the formation of new vasa vasorum. In normal arteries, microcapillaries are restricted to the adventitia. In inflamed arteries, new microvessels are generated throughout the media and intima. Vascular endothelial growth factor, identified as a critical mediator in the process, again originates from multinucleated giant cells and activated medial macrophages (79). Intimal hyperplasia and neoangiogenesis are both correlated with the production of IFN-γ by T cells in the adventitia (79,81). IFN-γ may induce the differentiation and activation of media macrophages and giant cells that regulate the artery's response (80). In summary, multiple pathways of the injury response program are counterproductive for the patient, exacerbate the consequences of vascular wall inflammation, and delay recovery. Molecular mediators controlling the maladapted injury response program of the arterial wall derive from tissue-invading inflammatory cells.

The artery's reaction to the immune insult is not exclusively tissue damaging. Analysis of genes induced by the vascular inflammation have indicated that protective mechanisms are also initiated. One of these potentially beneficial mechanisms ameliorating vascular injury is the induction of aldose reductase in temporal arteries from patients with giant cell arteritis. Aldose reductase is a reduced nicotinamide adenine dinucleotide phosphate (NADPH)-dependent oxidoreductase that metabolizes toxic aldehydes generated by reactive oxygen species, thereby protecting cellular membranes from destruction (82).

RELATIONSHIP TO OTHER DISEASES

Giant Cell Arteritis Versus Other Vasculitides

A vasculitic infiltration of the temporal arteries is sometimes found in other vasculitides; however, the histopathologic and clinical features are sufficiently distinct (83). There remains a small group of patients who, on clinical follow-up, have convincing signs of arteritis despite a negative biopsy result. Angiographic studies may document arteritis involving the large vessels, including the aortic arch and its proximal branches. This pattern of inflammatory vessel disease is considered unique for Takayasu's arteritis. In terms of pathology, clinical presentation, treatment response, and tissue tropism, giant cell arteritis and Takayasu's arteritis may be very similar, and only the age at onset may help to distinguish them.

Polymyalgia Rheumatica Versus Rheumatoid Arthritis

The diagnosis of polymyalgia rheumatica remains based on clinical presentation and, despite well-recognized laboratory abnormalities, no definite pathognomonic test exists. It is, therefore, likely that this diagnostic category includes a heterogeneous spectrum of disease processes (Table 88.4).

TABLE 88.4. DIFFERENTIAL DIAGNOSIS OF POLYMYALGIA RHEUMATICA

Arthropathies
Rheumatoid arthritis
Other inflammatory joint diseases in the elderly
Degenerative joint disease
Shoulder disorders
Inflammatory muscle disease
Malignant diseases
Infection
Hypothyroidism
Parkinson's disease
Functional myalgias

Frequently, the diagnosis has to be revised on follow-up. The distinction from inflammatory arthropathies is particularly difficult considering that synovitis of large joints is not uncommon in polymyalgia rheumatica and polymyalgic features are not uncommon in RA. Seronegative RA presenting with large joint disease may at times be indistinguishable from polymyalgia rheumatica. In a prospective study of 287 patients with polymyalgia rheumatica and giant cell arteritis, peripheral arthritis was found in 24% of the patients with polymyalgia rheumatica, while none of the patients with giant cell arteritis exhibited such manifestations (84). Diagnosis of polyarthritis exclusively in the patients with polymyalgia rheumatica may reflect the difficulties in separating polymyalgia rheumatica and seronegative RA. A prompt response to corticosteroids in doses of 10 to 20 mg daily is typical for polymyalgia rheumatica, whereas a partial response favors the diagnosis of seronegative RA. Increasing prominence of joint disease, involvement of small peripheral joints, and insufficient response to corticosteroid therapy should all prompt the physician to rethink the diagnosis of polymyalgia rheumatica and consider an inflammatory arthropathy of the elderly.

Polymyalgia Rheumatica Versus Other Inflammatory Diseases

Inflammatory myopathies that may present with muscle pain usually have objective signs of muscle weakness and laboratory and electromyographic evidence of myositis. Osteoarthritis of shoulders and hips can mimic a polymyalgic syndrome. Usually, radiographic studies and laboratory tests facilitate the diagnosis. Difficulties in diagnosis may arise in cases of bilateral capsulitis of the shoulders. The full range of passive motion of the shoulder joints in polymyalgia rheumatica should distinguish these cases. Diffuse myalgia is not infrequent in patients with infectious diseases; however, postviral syndromes usually do not persist for 2 months. Generally, patients with polymyalgia rheumatica do not have spiking fevers and chills, a feature that sets them apart from patients with chronic septicemia. Spiking fevers should always prompt a workup for underlying infectious diseases.

Polymyalgia Rheumatica Versus Malignant Diseases

It has been an issue of controversy whether polymyalgia rheumatica can represent a paraneoplastic syndrome. Diffuse myalgias, weight loss, anorexia, anemia, and elevated ESR, can be associated with a wide spectrum of malignant diseases. A careful clinical examination is appropriate, but invasive procedures are not recommended without additional clinical evidence for malignancy. An incomplete and delayed clinical response to corticosteroids should alert the physician to reevaluate the patient.

DISEASE COURSE, PROGNOSIS, AND THERAPEUTIC MANAGEMENT

Giant cell arteritis and polymyalgia rheumatica are chronic, but self-limiting, disorders. If diagnosed and treated promptly, patient prognosis is excellent. Managing these patients is gratifying for a physician. There is general agreement that corticosteroids are the treatment of choice. Controversy remains about the dose and the duration of therapy. Side effects of corticosteroid therapy are common in elderly patients (85). Corticosteroid-induced myopathy can complicate assessment of the clinical activity in polymyalgia rheumatica. Cataract formation can produce visual changes, raising the question of ophthalmic complications of giant cell arteritis. Osteoporosis and corticosteroid-induced glucose intolerance are feared complications. Corticosteroid-induced side effects, however, have to be weighed against disease-related morbidity. The therapeutic goal in patients with polymyalgia rheumatica is to control the very painful polymyalgias, the stiffness, and the constitutional features. It is very doubtful that the low-dose corticosteroids generally used in polymyalgia rheumatica are effective for preventing progression to vasculitis. Treatment with appropriate doses of corticosteroids is mandatory in giant cell arteritis to prevent vasculitic manifestations.

Several studies have addressed the question of what dose of corticosteroids should be used in polymyalgia rheumatica. Delecoeuillerie et al. (86) did not find an initial dose of 15 to 30 mg superior to 7 to 12 mg of prednisolone in a retrospective study. In contrast, Kyle and Hazleman (87) reported a high relapse rate when patients were treated with an initial dose of 10 mg daily. Dasgupta and co-workers (88) found 120 mg of intramuscular methylprednisolone acetate every 3 weeks equally effective to oral corticosteroids, but the cumulative dose and the number of osteopenic fractures were lower. Our current recommendation is to initiate treatment with 15 to 20 mg of prednisone per day. Prompt relief of myalgias can be expected within hours to days. However, a subset of patients has an incomplete response and daily doses of 30 mg of prednisone may be required for suppression of symptoms. Such patients can have persistent myalgias even after 4 weeks of treatment. Continuous elevation of IL-6 levels, despite therapy-induced normalization of ESRs, can be helpful in identifying them (60). Tapering of the corticosteroid dose should be guided by the clinical response. Generally, the daily dose of prednisone can be lowered by 2.5 mg every 2 weeks until a dose of 10 mg is reached. At that point, 1-mg decrements every 4 weeks are recommended.

A subset of patients can discontinue prednisone within 1 year. These patients are characterized by a less pronounced acute-phase response and may respond to smaller doses of corticosteroids initially (60). For the majority of patients, treatment for longer than 1 year is required, often with intermittent adjustment of the prednisone dose as directed by flares of clinical symptoms. Frequently, in these patients with relapsing disease, control of disease activity can be regained by increasing the daily dose of prednisone by just a few milligrams. ESR is only of limited value for diagnosing disease flares (60). Every patient with polymyalgia rheumatica should be considered to be at risk for giant cell arteritis and should be appropriately advised. Arteritic complications can develop in patients who do not have laboratory or clinical evidence of active disease. Patients with polymyalgia rheumatica should be monitored for the first 6 to 12 months after discontinuation of corticosteroids. Few patients can be effectively managed with nonsteroidal anti-inflammatory drugs. These agents can be tried in multiple-risk patients presenting with hypertension, diabetes, and ischemic heart disease.

Dose recommendations for giant cell arteritis vary but usually range from 40 to 60 mg prednisone per day. If the clinical response is inadequate, higher doses are necessary. Treatment studies in human artery–mouse chimeras have shown that corticosteroids function by repressing the transcription of proinflammatory cytokines and that standard doses of 1 mg/kg only achieve partial inhibition (54). Intravenous pulse methylprednisolone may therefore be given to patients with visual symptoms. The dose of 40 to 60 mg prednisone should be continued until remission of possibly reversible symptoms is reached and laboratory values are normal. Most patients are treated with the initial dose for 2 to 4 weeks before the dose can be reduced by 10% every 1 to 2 weeks. Few studies have addressed the issue of optimal dosing, but too rapid a tapering was associated with giant cell arteritis–related death in a cohort study of 284 patients (89) and with frequent relapses in a prospective treatment study (87). Not uncommonly, doses of 15 to 25 mg or more have to be given for several months before further dose reduction can be attempted. Alternate-day therapy is usually not sufficient to control disease activity (90). Monitoring of clinical symptoms and the ESR should guide the taper. The use of other acute-phase reactants has been suggested, but limited data are available to support their superiority over monitoring of the ESR. Significant, but inexplicable, increases in ESR are highly suspicious for disease flares, and corticosteroid doses should be adjusted accordingly. Once a dose of 10 mg per day is reached, 1-mg decrements every 4 weeks are usually tolerated. Exacerbations of the disease are unpredictable. They occur most frequently in the first 2 years after diagnosis.

Heterogeneity in patient cohorts and treatment responses may explain differences in disease duration observed by different investigators. In the epidemiologic studies in Minnesota, patients with polymyalgia rheumatica had a median disease duration of 11 months, and 75% were not receiving therapy 2 years after diagnosis (4). Most patients with giant cell arteritis had a disease course of less than 2 years (15). In European surveys, 30% to 50% of patients were able to discontinue use of corticosteroids after 2 years, but about one-half of all patients needed continuous management for longer than 2 years. There is a consensus that withdrawal from corticosteroids should be tried 2 years after initial diagnosis and that careful clinical monitoring is needed for 6 to 12 months after discontinuing treatment with corticosteroids. Better understanding of the heterogeneity of polymyalgia rheumatica and giant cell arteritis and more sensitive markers of disease activity will be necessary before corticosteroid dosing and treatment duration can be adapted to the needs of the individual patient. In some patients, the disease may smolder in the absence of clinical signs and laboratory abnormalities. Thoracic aorta aneurysm formation, which has been found more frequently than expected in patients with giant cell arteritis, occurred a median of 6 years after the initial diagnosis (36). Ongoing inflammation could be documented in selected cases.

In an attempt to minimize corticosteroid-related side effects, alternative types of corticosteroid therapy and corticosteroid-sparing agents have been explored. In contrast to other rheumatic diseases, alternate-day administration of corticosteroids has been unsuccessful (90). This clinical experience is in line with steroid-mediated suppression of cytokine gene transcription, which is transient in nature (54). Accordingly, IL-6 levels rebound to above normal within 24 hours after a single steroid dose (59). A controlled study with azathioprine has shown a modest corticosteroid-sparing effect (91). The efficacy and steroid-sparing potential of methotrexate in patients with polymyalgia rheumatica and giant cell arteritis has been explored in two studies. Both studies concluded that methotrexate was not beneficial (92,93).

CONCLUSION

The classic clinical presentation of giant cell arteritis is a combination of constitutional features associated with marked acute-phase reaction and symptoms related to the inflammation of extracranial branches of the proximal aorta. If treated promptly, mortality is low and feared consequences such as permanent vision loss and cerebral malperfusion can be prevented. Histologic confirmation should be sought in clinically suspected cases because the treatment of choice, high doses of corticosteroids given over several months, can cause serious side effects.

Molecular studies have profoundly improved the understanding of giant cell arteritis and polymyalgia rheumatica and will have impact on the diagnostic classification of patients and their management. Convincing evidence has been presented that polymyalgia rheumatica is an incomplete form of giant cell arteritis that shares genetic risk factors, excessive production of mediators inducing acute-phase responses, and system-wide activation of monocytes. Vascular lesions in polymyalgia rheumatica remain subclinical, escape detection by histomorphology, and are incompletely developed in terms of *in situ* production of inflammatory cytokines. The vascular lesions in full-blown giant cell arteritis include activated T cells with multiple features of antigen-reactive cells. They are localized in the adventitial layer, distant from the focus of arterial wall damage in the media, the intima, and the intima-media junction. Arterial wall damage is facilitated by tissue-injurious macrophages elaborating digestive enzymes and reactive oxygen intermediates. In response to the immunologic injury, the artery wall responds with an injury response program, which is intended to repair, but causes the formation of hyperplastic intima, leading to luminal occlusion and tissue ischemia. Mediators required in the process of intimal hyperplasia are provided by the invading immune cells, placing ultimate responsibility for the induction of clinical manifestations, such as ischemic optic neuropathy and cranial claudication, on the misled immune response occurring in the arterial wall. Progress in the management of patients can be expected with improved understanding of the pathomechanisms and with refined use of markers of disease activity such that the dosage and duration of corticosteroid therapy can be minimized, and undertreatment and potential long-term complications can be avoided.

REFERENCES

1. Horton BT, Magath TB, Brown GE. An undescribed form of arteritis of the temporal vessels. *Proc Staff Meet Mayo Clin* 1932; 7:700.
2. Barber HS. Myalgic syndrome with constitutional effects: polymyalgia rheumatica. *Ann Rheum Dis* 1957;16:230.
3. Hunder GG, Bloch DA, Michel BA, et al. The American College of Rheumatology 1990 criteria for the classification of giant cell arteritis. *Arthritis Rheum* 1990;33:1122–1128.
4. Chuang TY, Hunder GG, Ilstrup DM, et al. Polymyalgia rheumatica. A 10-year epidemiologic and clinical study. *Ann Intern Med* 1982;97:672–680.
5. Jones JG, Hazleman BL. Prognosis and management of polymyalgia rheumatica. *Ann Rheum Dis* 1981;40:1–5.
6. Paulley JW, Hughes JP. Giant cell arteritis or arthritis of the aged. *Br Med J* 1960;2:1562–1567.
7. Alestig K, Barr J. Giant cell arteritis: biopsy study of polymyalgia rheumatica, including one case of Takayasu's disease. *Lancet* 1963;1:1228–1230.
8. Hamrin B, Jonsson N, Landberg T. Involvement of large vessels in polymyalgia arteritica. *Lancet* 1965;1:1193–1196.
9. Fauchald P, Rygvold O, Oystese B. Temporal arteritis and polymyalgia rheumatica: clinical and biopsy findings. *Ann Intern Med* 1972;77:845–852.
10. Calamia KT, Moore SB, Elveback LR, et al. HLA-DR locus antigens in polymyalgia rheumatica and giant cell arteritis. *J Rheumatol* 1981;8:993–996.
11. Lowenstein MB, Bridgeford PH, Vasey FB, et al. Increased frequency of HLA-DR3 and DR4 in polymyalgia rheumatica-giant cell arteritis. *Arthritis Rheum* 1983;26:925–927.
12. Weyand CM, Hunder NNH, Hicok KC, et al. HLA-DRB1 alleles in polymyalgia rheumatica, giant cell arteritis, and rheumatoid arthritis. *Arthritis Rheum* 1994;37:514–520.
13. Wagner AD, Goronzy JJ, Weyand CM. Functional profile of tissue infiltrating and circulating CD68+ cells in giant cell arteritis. Evidence for two components of the disease. *J Clin Invest* 1994;94:1134–1140.
14. Weyand CM, Hicok KC, Hunder GG, et al. Tissue cytokine patterns in polymyalgia rheumatica and giant cell arteritis. *Ann Intern Med* 1994;121:484–491.
15. Machado EBV, Michet CJ, Ballard DJ, et al. Trends in incidence and clinical presentation of temporal arteritis in Olmsted County, Minnesota, 1950–1985. *Arthritis Rheum* 1988;31: 745–749.
16. Boesen P, Sorensen SF. Giant cell arteritis, temporal arteritis, and polymyalgia rheumatica in a Danish county. A prospective investigation, 1982–1985. *Arthritis Rheum* 1987;30:294–299.
17. Nordborg E, Bengtsson BA. Epidemiology of biopsy-proven giant cell arteritis (GCA). *J Intern Med* 1990;227:233–236.
18. Östberg G. An arteritis with special reference to polymyalgia arteritica. *Acta Pathol Microbiol Scand* 1973;237(suppl):1–59.
19. Smith CA, Fidler WJ, Pinals RS. The epidemiology of giant cell arteritis. Report of a ten-year study in Shelby County, Tennessee. *Arthritis Rheum* 1983;26:1214–1219.
20. Gonzalez EB, Varner WT, Lisse JR, et al. Giant-cell arteritis in the southern United States. An 11-year retrospective study from the Texas Gulf coast. *Arch Intern Med* 1989;149:1561–1565.
21. Salvarani C, Macchioni P, Zizzi F, et al. Epidemiologic and immunogenetic aspects of polymyalgia rheumatica and giant cell arteritis in northern Italy. *Arthritis Rheum* 1991;34:351–356.
22. Sonnenblick M, Nesher G, Friedlander Y, et al. Giant cell arteritis in Jerusalem: a 12-year epidemiological study. *Br J Rheumatol* 1994;33:938–941.
23. Salvarani C, Gabriel S, O'Fallon WM, et al. The incidence of giant cell arteritis in Olmsted County, Minnesota, apparent fluctuations in a cyclic pattern. *Ann Intern Med* 1995;123:192–194.
24. Bengtsson BA, Malmvall BE. Giant cell arteritis. *Acta Med Scand* 1982;658(suppl):1–102.
25. Kyle V, Silverman B, Silman A, et al. Polymyalgia rheumatica/giant cell arteritis in a Cambridge general practice. *Br Med J Clin Res* 1985;291:385–387.
26. Liang GC, Simkin PA, Hunder GG, et al. Familial aggregation of polymyalgia rheumatica and giant cell arteritis. *Arthritis Rheum* 1974;17:19–24.
27. Cimmino MA, Caporali R, Montecucco CM, et al. A seasonal pattern in the onset of polymyalgia rheumatica. *Ann Rheum Dis* 1990;49:521–523.
28. Duhaut P, Bosshard S, Calvet A, et al. Giant cell arteritis, polymyalgia rheumatica, and viral hypotheses: a multicenter, prospective case-control study. *J Rheumatol* 1999;26:361–369.

29. Gabriel SE, Espy M, Erdman DD, et al. The role of parvovirus B19 in the pathogenesis of giant cell arteritis: a preliminary evaluation. *Arthritis Rheum* 1999;42:1255–1258.
30. Lie JT. Illustrated histopathologic classification criteria for selected vasculitis syndromes. American College of Rheumatology Subcommittee on Classification of Vasculitis. *Arthritis Rheum* 1990;33:1074–1087.
31. Klein RG, Campbell RJ, Hunder GG, et al. Skip lesions in temporal arteritis. *Mayo Clin Proc* 1976;51:504–510.
32. Wilkinson IMS, Russell RWR. Arteries of the head and neck in giant cell arteritis. A pathological study to show the pattern of arterial involvement. *Arch Neurol* 1972;27:378–391.
33. Klein RG, Hunder GG, Stanson AW, et al. Large artery involvement in giant cell (temporal) arteritis. *Ann Intern Med* 1975; 83:806–812.
34. Chou CT, Schumacher HR Jr. Clinical and pathologic studies of synovitis in polymyalgia rheumatica. *Arthritis Rheum* 1984;27: 1107–1117.
35. Long R, James O. Polymyalgia rheumatica and liver disease. *Lancet* 1974;1:77–79.
36. Calamia KT, Hunder GG. Clinical manifestations of giant cell arteritis. *Clin Rheum Dis* 1980;6:389.
37. Hunder GG. Giant cell (temporal) arteritis. *Rheum Dis Clin North Am* 1990;16:399–409.
38. Aiello PD, Trautmann JC, McPhee TJ, et al. Visual prognosis in giant cell arteritis. *Ophthalmology* 1993;100:550–555.
39. Brack A, Martinez-Taboada V, Stanson A, et al. Disease pattern in cranial and large-vessel giant cell arteritis. *Arthritis Rheum* 1999;42:311–317.
40. Evans JM, O'Fallon WM, Hunder GG. Increased incidence of aortic aneurysm and dissection in giant cell (temporal) arteritis: a population-based study. *Ann Intern Med* 1995;122:502–507.
41. Larson TS, Hall S, Hepper NGG, et al. Respiratory tract symptoms as a clue to giant cell arteritis. *Ann Intern Med* 1984;101: 594–597.
42. Caselli RJ, Hunder GG. Neurologic aspects of giant cell (temporal) arteritis. *Rheum Dis Clin North Am* 1993;19:941–953.
43. O'Duffy JD, Hunder GG, Wahner HW. A follow-up study of polymyalgia rheumatica: evidence of chronic axial synovitis. *J Rheumatol* 1980;7:685–693.
44. Douglas WA, Martin BA, Morris JH. Polymyalgia rheumatica: an arthroscopic study of the shoulder joint. *Ann Rheum Dis* 1983;42:311–316.
45. Meliconi R, Pulsatelli L, Uguccioni M, et al. Leukocyte infiltration in synovial tissue from the shoulder of patients with polymyalgia rheumatica. Quantitative analysis and influence of corticosteroid treatment. *Arthritis Rheum* 1996;39:1199–1207.
46. Kyle V, Tudor J, Wraight EP, et al. Rarity of synovitis in polymyalgia rheumatica. *Ann Rheum Dis* 1990;49:155–157.
47. Hall S, Hunder GG. Is temporal artery biopsy prudent? *Mayo Clin Proc* 1984;59:793–796.
48. Hall S, Persellin S, Lie JT, et al. The therapeutic impact of temporal artery biopsy. *Lancet* 1983;2:1217–1220.
49. Vilaseca J, Gonzalez A, Cid MC, et al. Clinical usefulness of temporal artery biopsy. *Ann Rheum Dis* 1987;46:282–285.
50. Wilske KR, Healey LA. Polymyalgia rheumatica. A manifestation of systemic giant-cell arteritis. *Ann Intern Med* 1967;66:77–86.
51. Malmvall BE, Bengtsson BA. Giant cell arteritis. Clinical features and involvement of different organs. *Scand J Rheumatol* 1978;7: 154–158.
52. Cid MC, Campo E, Ercilla G, et al. Immunohistochemical analysis of lymphoid and macrophage cell subsets and their immunological activation markers in temporal arteritis. Influence of corticosteroid treatment. *Arthritis Rheum* 1989;32: 884–893.
53. Achkar AA, Lie JT, Hunder GG, et al. How does previous corticosteroid treatment affect the biopsy findings in giant cell (temporal) arteritis? *Ann Intern Med* 1994;120:987–992.
54. Brack A, Rittner HL, Younge BR, et al. Glucocorticoids mediated repression of cytokine gene transcription in human arteritis-SCID chimeras. *J Clin Invest* 1997;99:2842–2850.
55. Schmidt WA, Kraft HE, Vorpahl K, et al. Color duplex ultrasonography in the diagnosis of temporal arteritis. *N Engl J Med* 1997;337:1336–1342.
56. Hunder GG, Weyand CM. Sonography in giant-cell arteritis. *N Engl J Med* 1997;337:1385.
57. Kyle V, Cawston TE, Hazleman BL. Erythrocyte sedimentation rate and C-reactive protein in the assessment of polymyalgia rheumatica/giant cell arteritis on presentation and during follow up. *Ann Rheum Dis* 1989;48:667–671.
58. Dasgupta B, Panayi GS. Interleukin-6 in serum of patients with polymyalgia rheumatica and giant cell arteritis. *Br J Rheumatol* 1990;29:456–458.
59. Roche NE, Fulbright JW, Wagner AD, et al. Correlation of interleukin 6 production and disease activity in polymyalgia rheumatica and giant cell arteritis. *Arthritis Rheum* 1993;36:1286–1294.
60. Weyand CM, Fulbright JW, Evans JM, et al. Corticosteroid requirements in polymyalgia rheumatica. *Arch Intern Med* 1999; 159:577–584.
61. Duhaut P, Berruyer M, Pinede L, et al. Anticardiolipin antibodies and giant cell arteritis: a prospective, multicenter case-control study. *Arthritis Rheum* 1998;41:701–709.
62. Persellin ST, Daniels TM, Rings LJ, et al. Factor VIII–von Willebrand factor in giant cell arteritis and polymyalgia rheumatica. *Mayo Clin Proc* 1985;60:457–462.
63. Nordborg E, Andersson R, Tengborn L, et al. von Willebrand factor antigen and plasminogen activator inhibitor in giant cell arteritis. *Ann Rheum Dis* 1991;50:316–320.
64. Cid MC, Monteagudo J, Oristrell J, et al. Von Willebrand factor in the outcome of temporal arteritis. *Ann Rheum Dis* 1996;12: 927–930.
65. Weyand CM, Hicok KC, Hunder GG, et al. The HLA-DRB1 locus as a genetic component in giant cell arteritis. Mapping of a disease-linked sequence motif to the antigen binding site of the HLA-DR molecule. *J Clin Invest* 1992;90:2355–2361.
66. Richardson JE, Gladman DD, Fam A, et al. HLA-DR4 in giant cell arteritis: association with polymyalgia rheumatica syndrome. *Arthritis Rheum* 1987;30:1293–1297.
67. Sakkas LI, Loqueman N, Panayi GS, et al. Immunogenetics of polymyalgia rheumatica. *Br J Rheumatol* 1990;29:331–334.
68. Weyand CM, Hicok KC, Conn DL, et al. The influence of HLA-DRB1 genes on disease severity in rheumatoid arthritis. *Ann Intern Med* 1992;117:801–806.
69. Weyand CM, Goronzy JJ. Giant cell arteritis as an antigen driven disease. *Rheum Dis Clin North Am* 1995;21:1027–1039.
70. Martinez-Taboada V, Brack A, Hunder GG, et al. The inflammatory infiltrate in giant cell arteritis selects against B lymphocytes. *J Rheumatol* 1996;23:1011–1014.
71. Wagner AD, Björnsson J, Bartley GB, et al. Interferon gamma producing T cells in giant cell vasculitis represent a minority of tissue infiltrating cells and are located distant from the site of pathology. *Am J Pathol* 1996;148:1925–1933.
72. Weyand CM, Schönberger J, Oppitz U, et al. Distinct vascular lesions in giant cell arteritis share identical T cell clonotypes. *J Exp Med* 1994;179:951–960.
73. Martinez-Taboada V, Hunder NNH, Hunder GG, et al. Recognition of tissue residing antigen by T cells in vasculitic lesions of giant cell arteritis. *J Mol Med* 1996;74:695–703.
74. Brack A, Geisler A, Martinez-Taboada V, et al. Giant cell vasculitis is a T cell dependent disease. *Mol Med* 1997;81:29–55.
75. Rittner HL, Kaiser M, Brack A, et al. Tissue-destructive macrophages in giant cell arteritis. *Circ Res* 1999;84:1050–1058.

76. Weyand CM, Wagner AD, Björnsson J, et al. Correlation of topographical arrangement and the functional pattern of tissue-infiltrating macrophages in giant cell arteritis. *J Clin Invest* 1996;98:1642–1649.
77. Nikkari ST, Hoyhtya M, Isola J, et al. Macrophages contain 92-kd gelatinase (MMP-9) at the site of degenerated internal elastic lamina in temporal arteritis. *Am J Pathol* 1996;149: 1427–1433.
78. Kaiser M, Weyand CM, Björnsson J, et al. Platelet derived growth factor, intimal hyperplasia and ischemic complications in giant cell vasculitis. *Arthritis Rheum* 1998;41:623–633.
79. Kaiser M, Younge B, Björnsson J, et al. Formation of new vasa vasorum in vasculitis: Production of angiogenic cytokines by multinucleated giant cells. *Am J Pathol* 1999;155:765–774.
80. Weyand CM, Goronzy JJ. Arterial wall injury in giant cell arteritis. *Arthritis Rheum* 1999;42:844–853.
81. Weyand CM, Tetzlaff N, Björnsson J, et al. Disease patterns and tissue cytokine profiles in giant cell arteritis. *Arthritis Rheum* 1997;40:19–26.
82. Rittner HL, Hafner V, Klimiuk PA, et al. Aldose reductase functions as a detoxification system for lipid peroxidation products in vasculitis. *J Clin Invest* 1999;103:1007–1013.
83. Lie JT. When is arteritis of the temporal arteries not temporal arteritis? *J Rheumatol* 1994;21:186–189.
84. Myklebust G, Gran JT. A prospective study of 287 patients with polymyalgia rheumatica and temporal arteritis: clinical and laboratory manifestations at onset of disease and at the time of diagnosis. *Br J Rheumatol* 1996;35:1161–1168.
85. Gabriel SE, Sunku J, Salvarani C, et al. Adverse outcomes of anti-inflammatory therapy among patients with polymyalgia rheumatica. *Arthritis Rheum* 1997;40:1873–1878.
86. Delecoeuillerie G, Joly P, Cohen de Lara A, et al. Polymyalgia rheumatica and temporal arteritis: a retrospective analysis of prognostic features and different corticosteroid regimens (11 year survey of 210 patients). *Ann Rheum Dis* 1988;47:733–739.
87. Kyle V, Hazleman BL. Treatment of polymyalgia rheumatica and giant cell arteritis. II. Relation between steroid dose and steroid associated side effects. *Ann Rheum Dis* 1989;48:662–666.
88. Dasgupta B, Dolan AL, Panayi GS, et al. An initially double-blind controlled 96 week trial of depot methylprednisolone against oral prednisolone in the treatment of polymyalgia rheumatica. *Br J Rheumatol* 1998;37:189–195.
89. Nordborg E, Bengtsson BA. Death rates and causes of death in 284 consecutive patients with giant cell arteritis confirmed by biopsy. *Br Med J* 1989;299:549–550.
90. Hunder GG, Sheps SG, Allen GL, et al. Daily and alternate-day corticosteroid regimens in treatment of giant cell arteritis: comparison in a prospective study. *Ann Intern Med* 1975;82:613–618.
91. De Silva M, Hazleman BL. Azathioprine in giant cell arteritis/polymyalgia rheumatica: a double-blind study. *Ann Rheum Dis* 1986;45:136–138.
92. van der Veen MJ, Dinant HJ, van Booma-Frankfort C, et al. Can methotrexate be used as a steroid sparing agent in the treatment of polymyalgia rheumatica and giant cell arteritis? *Ann Rheum Dis* 1996;55:218–223.
93. Feinberg HL, Sherman JD, Schrepferman CG, et al. The use of methotrexate in polymyalgia rheumatica. *J Rheumatol* 1996;23: 1550–1552.

89

PREGNANCY AND RHEUMATIC DISEASES

MICHAEL D. LOCKSHIN

Pregnancy in women with rheumatic disease presents unique management problems. In the order of pregnancy frequency, the rheumatic diagnoses of pregnant women are systemic lupus erythematosus (SLE), antiphospholipid antibody syndrome, rheumatoid arthritis (RA), scleroderma, juvenile chronic arthritis, dermatomyositis/polymyositis, spondyloarthropathy, Takayasu's arteritis, polyarteritis nodosa, Wegener's granulomatosis, and relapsing polychondritis. Patients with genetic errors of connective tissue synthesis or metabolism (e.g., Ehlers-Danlos and Marfan syndromes) and local musculoskeletal conditions (hip replacement, tendinitis, and disc disease and low back pain) present a different set of management issues. Table 89.1 lists pregnancy-related maternal and fetal complications for the common illnesses.

TABLE 89.1. COMMON RHEUMATIC ILLNESS AND THEIR MAJOR PREGNANCY COMPLICATIONS

Disease	Maternal Complications	Fetal Complications	Comments
SLE	Flare, worsening renal function, low platelets	Prematurity, neonatal lupus	Anti-SSA/Ro, anti-SSB/La, antiphospholipid antibody common; renal flare, preeclampsia difficult to distinguish
APS	Phlebitis, stroke postpartum	IUGR, prematurity, death	Some patients have SLE
MCTD	Similar to SLE	Similar to SLE	Manage like SLE
UCTD	Similar to SLE	Similar to SLE	Manage like SLE
RA	Remission during pregnancy, flare after	None	Patient positioning difficult
Sjögren's	Similar to RA	Neonatal lupus	Anti-SSA/Ro, anti-SSB/La antibody common
JRA	Worsening during pregnancy	Insufficient data	Patient positioning difficult
SSc	Fluid volume a problem	Prematurity	Renal crisis life-threatening, difficult to distinguish from preeclampsia
AS, Reiter's syndrome	Worsens during, better after pregnancy	Probably none	Hip involvement common
Psoriatic arthritis	Improves during pregnancy, worsens after	Probably none	—
Dermatomyositis/ polymyositis	Respiratory insufficiency	Probably none	Maternal strength a problem
Takayasu's disease	Cardiac failure, hypertension hard to measure	Probably none	Hypertension hard to measure
Polyarteritis nodosa	Hypertension	Insufficient data	Very few cases known, high maternal morbidity
Wegener's granulomatosis	Worsens	Insufficient data	Very few cases known
Relapsing polychondritis	No change	Insufficient data	Normal delivery usual
Ehlers-Danlos syndrome	Uterine rupture	May be affected	—
Marfan syndrome	Aortic dissection	May be affected	—
Total hip replacement	Loosens	Insufficient data	Antibiotic coverage for delivery; positioning for vaginal delivery

SLE, systemic lupus erythematosus; APS, antiphospholipid antibody syndrome; aSSA/Ro, antibodies to Sjögren's syndrome A; aSSB/La, antibodies to Sjögren's syndrome B; MCTD, mixed connective tissue disease; UCTD, undifferentiated connective tissue disease; RA, rheumatoid arthritis; JRA, juvenile rheumatoid arthritis; SSc, systemic sclerosis (scleroderma); AS, ankylosing spondylitis; IUGR, intrauterine growth retardation.

NORMAL PREGNANCY

Definitions

Pregnancy begins when a fertilized ovum implants, either orthotopically or ectopically. The first laboratory marker of pregnancy is a rise in blood or urine (human) chorionic gonadotropin (hCG), usually by the time of the first missed menses. Proteinuria may cause a false-positive urine test. A fetus can be identified by ultrasound at 4 weeks and a fetal heartbeat can be seen at 8 to 10 weeks. Pregnancy loss before fetal heartbeat is spontaneous abortion, after fetal heartbeat fetal death, and after birth neonatal death. Although the end of pregnancy is delivery, physiologic changes of pregnancy require months to return to the nonpregnant state: maternal hormones take three or more months to return to baseline, bone recovery and ligament recovery may take a year, and fetal cells circulate in the mother's bloodstream for decades (1).

Organ System Changes

Blood volume and cardiac output increase by 45% during pregnancy. Glomerular filtration rate increases by 50%: a normal creatinine clearance in late pregnancy is 150 mL/minute. Patients with preexisting cardiac and renal insufficiency are at risk for hypertension and fluid overload as blood volume rises. Estradiol increases 100-fold and estriol 1,000-fold in pregnancy, and progesterone and prolactin excretion also rise by orders of magnitude. *In vitro,* estrogens upregulate and androgens downregulate T-cell responses, immunoglobulin synthesis, interleukin-1 (IL-1), IL-2, IL-6 and tumor necrosis factor-α (TNF-α), but changes in these cytokines are relatively small. In pregnancy, cell-mediated immunity is depressed, as reflected by abnormal lymphocyte stimulation, decreased T-cell/B-cell ratios, increased suppressor/helper T-cell ratios, and decreased lymphocyte/monocyte ratios, all of which vary with the stage of pregnancy. The pregnancy-specific proteins α-fetoprotein, β_1-glycoprotein, and β_2-macroglobulin suppress *in vitro* lymphocyte function (2,3). Cutaneous and humoral immune responses to specific microbial antigens are selectively depressed, as are leukocyte chemotaxis and adhesion. Polyspecific autoantibodies unaccompanied by symptoms occur in otherwise normal young women who have pregnancy complications. IL-1 and IL-3, TNF-α, interferon-γ, and granulocyte-macrophage colony-stimulating factor are critical in sustaining pregnancy (4). IL-3 levels are low in women with repeated pregnancy loss. Although in normal pregnancy total C3, C4, and hemolytic (CH_{50}) complement levels are usually unchanged or raised relative to nonpregnant levels, increases in classic pathway complement activation products (C3a, C4a, C5a, but not C1s-C1 inhibitor complex) suggest that low-grade classic pathway activation is a normal phenomenon in pregnant women. Platelet survival decreases and fibrinogen and coagulation factors VII, VIII, IX and X increase, while factors XI and XIII decrease. Thrombocytopenia is common in uncomplicated late pregnancy (5). Low-grade activation of intravascular coagulation occurs, particularly in patients with toxemia or ischemia, praevia, or abruption of the placenta. The normal anemia of late pregnancy may be exaggerated when it coexists with the anemia of chronic illness. Lordotic posture and ligament loosening of late pregnancy exacerbate preexisting musculoskeletal pain. Small noninflammatory knee effusions are

TABLE 89.2. COMMON PREGNANCY CHANGES THAT MAY INFLUENCE THE INTERPRETATION OR MANAGEMENT OF RHEUMATIC ILLNESS

Normal Pregnancy Change	Effect on Rheumatic Disease
Cardiovascular	
Increased intravascular volume	May cause heart failure, hypertension
Hematologic	
Hemodilutional anemia	Mimics disease exacerbation
Increased platelet activation	May worsen disease-induced thrombocytopenia
Increased fibrinogen	Suggests inflammation
Increased factor VIII, IX, X	Indicates endothelial activation or injury, suggesting vasculitis; lowers prothrombin time, thromboplastin time
Immunologic	
Immune complexes present	Mimics disease exacerbation
Increased complement	Modifies interpretation of disease-induced hypocomplementemia
Complement activation	Mimics disease exacerbation
Endocrine	
Increased cortisol	Induces remission during pregnancy? Decrease postpartum results in flare?
Increased estrogen	Worsens SLE?
Renal	
Increased clearance	If clearance does not increase, fluid overload occurs
Proteinuria/hypertension	Preeclampsia vs. disease exacerbation may be hard to distinguish
Joints	
Ligament loosening	Joint effusions mimic active arthritis; C1–2 subluxation may worsen in rheumatoid arthritis

frequent, and calcium supplements are required to prevent osteoporosis. Carpal tunnel syndrome occurs in late pregnancy. Drug metabolism increases during pregnancy, necessitating dose adjustments for some medications, such as anticonvulsants. Fatty liver of pregnancy, jaundice of pregnancy, and hepatic injury due to toxemia are potential threats to all pregnant women, independent of preexisting illness. Ovulation induction with exogenous hormones may induce ovarian cyst formation, ovarian hyperstimulation syndrome, and multiple gestation. Table 89.2 outlines the potential effects on rheumatic illness of normal physiologic changes of pregnancy.

Antirheumatic Drug Therapy During Pregnancy

Nonsteroidal antiinflammatory drugs may injure fetal kidneys or induce premature closure of the ductus arteriosus,

TABLE 89.3. DRUGS COMMONLY USED IN RHEUMATIC DISEASES

Drug	FDA Risk Category[a]	Safety	Comments
Aspirin[b]	C/D[c]	Variable: depends on dose and time of use	May be protective against fetal death in antiphospholipid antibody syndrome; may cause maternal and fetal bleeding if administered near term; high dose, uncertain safety
Naproxen, ibuprofen, ketoprofen, nabumetone, and similar drugs[b]	B/D[c]	Variable, depends on dose and time of use	Experience largely accumulated through treatment of headache or dysmenorrhea; no major teratogenicity noted; use at term not advised
Ketorolac[b]	C	Causes dystocia and neonatal death in animals	Insufficient human experience
Indomethacin[b]	B/D[c]	Variable, depends on dose and time of use	Rare cases of fetal pulmonary hypertension if used at term
Prednisone	B	Generally safe	Trivial passage across placenta; safe in lactation, but may suppress milk production
Methylprednisolone	B	Probably safe	Similar to prednisone, but fewer data available
Dexamethasone, betamethasone	C	Probably safe in late pregnancy	Important transfer across placenta; used to induce fetal lung maturation
Hydroxychloroquine	Unclassified	Questionable safety	Small published experience indicating safety
Azathioprine	D	Safety uncertain	Large experience with renal transplant patients indicates no immediate danger to offspring if maternal dose is <2 mg/kg/d; rare reports of congenital anomalies, including immunodeficiency
Cyclosporine	C	Probably safe	Little experience, none suggesting high fetal risk
Cyclophosphamide, methotrexate, chlorambucil	D	Dangerous	Abortifacient, teratogenic
Leflunomide	X	Dangerous	Abortifacient, teratogenic, no data available
Heparin	B	Appears to be safe	Anticoagulant of choice; usually given subcutaneously twice daily; dose control essential for safety; causes osteoporosis
Low molecular weight heparin	B[d]		
Warfarin	X	Teratogenic and possibly fetotoxic	Fetal warfarin syndrome when given in first trimester; may cause central nervous system defects in second and third trimesters; risk of severe neonatal hemorrhage when given near term
Etanercept	Unknown	Unknown	Unknown
Intravenous immunoglobulin	B[d]		

[a]Food and Drug Administration (FDA) pregnancy risk classification: A, controlled trials show no risk in humans; B, animal studies show no risk, no definitive studies in humans; C, animal studies show risk *or* no studies in humans *or* no information; D, positive evidence of risk, risk/benefit ratio may be acceptable in some circumstances; X, fetal risk, risk/benefit ratio always unacceptable.
[b]All inhibitors of prostaglandin synthesis activity may inhibit labor and prolong gestation. There is also a risk of in utero closure of the ductus arteriosus, particularly when used after the 34th gestational week.
[c]Risk category D when used in the third trimester.
[d]Assigned by author.

but such events are rare. Prednisone and methylprednisolone are inactivated by a placental hydroxylase and do not reach the fetus; fluorinated corticosteroids (dexamethasone and betamethasone) are not inactivated and should be used only with intent to treat the fetus. There is no published experience verifying safety of "pulse" bolus corticosteroid in pregnancy. Hydroxychloroquine is probably safe, though published experience is scant (6). Azathioprine, widely used in renal transplant patients, is relatively safe, but fetal cytopenias and malformations have occurred. It is considered Food and Drug Administration (FDA) risk category D (Table 89.3). Cyclosporine, which is fetotoxic at maternal toxic doses, is category C. Cyclophosphamide, methotrexate, and leflunomide are contraindicated in early pregnancy because of their teratogenic and abortifacient properties. Although listed as category D, they are clearly more dangerous than azathioprine. A few infants of women given cyclophosphamide late in pregnancy have been normal (7). Table 89.3 provides guidelines to commonly used antirheumatic drugs (8).

Methyldopa is the preferred antihypertensive agent in pregnant women. Hydralazine, labetalol, nifedipine, and diazoxide can also be used. Angiotensin-converting enzyme inhibitors and receptor inhibitors are not generally used, nor are diuretics. For gastric protection, antacids, sulcralfate, cimetidine, and ranitidine are considered safe (category B). Omeprazol and cisapride are category C. Misoprostol is an abortifacient and is contraindicated.

Fertility, Oral Contraception, and Paternity

Patients with SLE, antiphospholipid antibody syndrome, or spondyloarthropathy have normal fertility, and those with RA and scleroderma probably have slight reductions in fertility. A fear that oral contraceptives induce exacerbation of SLE is not supported by the literature; they have only small effect, if any, on disease incidence (9). Ovulation induction for purposes of *in vitro* fertilization likely does not induce flares of lupus; the effect of hormonal abortifacients such as RU-486 in rheumatic disease patients is unknown. Except for imparting genetic susceptibility, paternal rheumatic illness does not affect the child.

SPECIFIC RHEUMATIC DISEASES

Systemic Lupus Erythematosus

Although both men and women with SLE share increased plasma estrogen and decreased androgen levels that render patients feminized by biochemical but not by clinical criteria, these abnormalities have no discernible effect on pregnancy outcome. Whether pregnancy induces lupus flare remains controversial; flares, if they do occur, are generally mild (10). Diagnosing flare during pregnancy is difficult because pregnancy-induced thrombocytopenia, preeclamptic proteinuria, and erythemas all resemble SLE flare. Flare is most confidently diagnosed when a patient has new or increasing rash (not erythema alone), lymphadenopathy, arthritis, fever, or anti–double-stranded DNA (dsDNA) antibody.

Maternal Complications

Approximately one-fourth of all SLE patients develop thrombocytopenia during pregnancy. Patients with antiphospholipid antibody often have asymptomatic thrombocytopenia, which occurs before 15 weeks, does not fall lower than 50×10^9/L, stays constant throughout pregnancy, remits after delivery, and tends to recur with subsequent pregnancies. Thrombocytopenia due to preeclampsia appears after 25 weeks, worsens as pregnancy progresses, is associated with deteriorating maternal and fetal health, and remits after delivery. A similar type of thrombocytopenia occurs with the HELLP (hemolysis, elevated liver enzymes, low platelet count) syndrome, a virulent form of preeclampsia with liver failure. Modest (average 130×10^9/L) benign thrombocytopenia of late pregnancy is unrelated to SLE. Abrupt, severe thrombocytopenia of the immune thrombocytopenia (ITP) type and lupus-related low-grade chronic thrombocytopenia also occur. No specific test clearly differentiates among types of thrombocytopenia in pregnant patients with SLE, in whom thrombocytopenia is equally often due to antiphospholipid antibody, active SLE, and preeclampsia. Severe anemia (hematocrit <25%) due to chronic illness or to hemolysis indicates a need to use (higher doses of) corticosteroid or erythropoietin for protection of the fetus, even if the mother tolerates the anemia well.

Clinical signs of active SLE, rising anti-dsDNA antibody, and erythrocyte casts favor on a diagnosis of lupus nephritis as opposed to preeclampsia. Rapid worsening over days suggests preeclampsia. Hypertension, thrombocytopenia, hyperuricemia, and hypocomplementemia occur in both lupus nephritis and preeclampsia; low levels of alternate pathway complement components, when measurable, are more indicative of active SLE than are low levels of classic pathway components. Normal complement levels suggest preeclampsia. Two-thirds of pregnant lupus patients who enter pregnancy with prior renal disease develop preeclampsia, compared to less than 20% of those without prior kidney disease. In women with preexisting renal disease who develop preeclampsia, renal function may not return to its prepregnancy baseline.

Pregnancy erythemas of the face and hands resemble the rash of active SLE. Because skin blood flow increases in pregnancy, existing rash may become more prominent as pregnancy progresses. Patients who discontinue hydroxychloroquine for pregnancy often have recurrence of rash.

Joints previously damaged by lupus arthritis may develop noninflammatory effusions when ligament loosening occurs in late pregnancy. Neurologic lupus during pregnancy is rare. Chorea and transverse myelitis have been induced or exacerbated by pregnancy; the former occurs in pregnancy independent of SLE (chorea gravidarum). Seizures late in pregnancy, when accompanied by hypertension and renal failure, may require therapeutic trial to distinguish between cerebral SLE and eclampsia. Treatment for both is usually indicated. Pulmonary hypertension may develop or worsen during pregnancy.

Fetal Complications

The fetus may be injured by maternal fever, severe anemia, uremia, hypertension, or preeclampsia, but active SLE itself, in the absence of these abnormalities, does not compromise pregnancy. Maternal immunoglobulin G (IgG) (and hence autoantibody) is transmitted to the fetus; nonetheless, infants born of SLE mothers with IgG-induced thrombocytopenia usually have normal platelet counts. Occasionally, Coombs' hemolytic antibody causes hemolysis in the fetus, but anti-dsDNA antibody has no apparent pathologic effect. Infants are not leukopenic and usually do not have antiphospholipid antibody-associated clotting. With the exception of neonatal lupus, there are no congenital abnormalities associated with SLE.

The syndrome of *neonatal lupus* includes photosensitive rash, thrombocytopenia, hepatitis, and hemolytic anemia, all of which are transient, and congenital complete heart block, which is not (11). Mothers with anti-SSA/Ro and anti-SSB/La antibodies, whether or not they have a clinical diagnosis of SLE, are at risk to deliver a child with neonatal lupus. Approximately one-third of all SLE patients have one or both of these antibodies, as do a minority of patients with discoid lupus and a majority of those with subacute cutaneous lupus and with Sjögren's syndrome. Many infants with neonatal lupus are born of mothers who are clinically well, a small proportion of whom later develop SLE or Sjögren's syndrome. Congenital heart block is first diagnosable *in utero* by fetal electrocardiography, ultrasound, or cardiac rate monitoring between 18 and 25 weeks' gestation (average 23 weeks). Among SLE patients with anti-SSA/Ro antibody, the risk that a liveborn child will have neonatal lupus rash is 25%, and congenital complete heart block is less than 3%. However, the risk of recurrent congenital heart block is 18% and of recurrent neonatal lupus rash 25%. Heart block occurs most often in infants of mothers who have enzyme-linked immunosorbent assay (ELISA)-determined antibodies to both SSA/Ro and SSB/La antigens, or immunoblot-identified antibody to both 48-kd SSB/La and 52-kD SSA/Ro, but not to the 60-kd SSA/Ro, bands (12). Cardiac injury may be related to expression of the cardiac 52β Ro antigen during fetal development (13). No specific antibody pattern predicts neonatal lupus rash. Although animal models indicate that anti-Ro and La antibodies are directly toxic to fetal heart (14), several dizygotic twins and at least one monozygotic twin pair have been discordant for neonatal lupus, suggesting fetal contribution to illness.

Dexamethasone and plasmapheresis of the mother have been used, with variable success, to treat fetal incomplete heart block, myocarditis, heart failure, and hydrops fetalis (15). If fetal heart function deteriorates, early delivery is necessary. Complete heart block in a newborn usually requires a permanent pacemaker. Even with a pacemaker, cardiac failure and sudden death may occur before age 5.

Antiphospholipid Antibody Syndrome

Patients with antiphospholipid antibody syndrome and anticardiolipin antibody have a high frequency of midpregnancy intrauterine growth restriction or fetal death. High titer and IgG isotype suggest poor prognosis and are the only antibody characteristics that predict pregnancy outcome. Maternal history of prior fetal death markedly increases the risk of new fetal death. The combination of lupus anticoagulant and anticardiolipin antibody does not give a worse prognosis than either alone. Low-titer IgM and IgG anticardiolipin antibody are generally not associated with poor fetal outcome, nor is an isolated positive test for syphilis. Anti-β_2-glycoprotein I antibodies predict fetal death in the occasional patient who tests negative for both anticardiolipin and lupus anticoagulant. Fetal loss is not specific for the antiphospholipid antibody syndrome, since protein C, protein S, and antithrombin III deficiencies and factor V_{Leiden} and prothrombin mutations also predispose to fetal death (16).

Few antiphospholipid antibody patients suffer thromboses during pregnancy, possibly because most are prophylactically treated with heparin (17). Risk of stroke and thrombophlebitis is increased postpartum, especially after discontinuation of anticoagulant therapy. Ischemic cardiomyopathy and myocardial infarction may also occur postpartum. Thrombocytopenia, if present during pregnancy, usually remits after delivery.

An antiphospholipid antibody-compromised pregnancy is uniform: early pregnancy is uneventful except for thrombocytopenia. After 15 weeks, fetal growth rate slows. Over the next several weeks monitoring studies show nonreactive fetal heart rate pattern, spontaneous bradycardia, diminished fetal motion, decreased amniotic fluid, reduced placental size, and, if delivery is not accomplished, fetal death. The mother may show no evidence of illness other than thrombocytopenia or may develop severe preeclampsia or HELLP syndrome. Untreated women with secondary antiphospholipid antibody syndrome, anticardiolipin antibody of >80 GPL (IgG phospholipid) units/mL, and prior fetal deaths have fetal survival rates as low as 20%. With treatment, fetal survival rates of over 80% are possible. The goal of treatment is a liveborn child, not correction of the antibody. Pregnancy prognosis does not improve if lupus anticoagulant activity is corrected or if anticardiolipin antibody titer falls.

Placentae of SLE patients without antiphospholipid antibody exhibit ischemic-hypoxic change and chronic villitis, while those of patients with antiphospholipid antibody have decidual vasculopathy and extensive infarction, due to placental intraluminal thrombosis, to endothelial cell proliferation, or to other placental vasculopathy (18). Antiphospholipid antibody competes with placental anticoagulant protein I (PAP-I, also known as annexin V), possibly interdicting its anticoagulant function and permitting *in situ* coagulation to occur (19,20). Antiphospholipid antibody, β_2-glycoprotein-I, and PAP-I deposit together in placentas of mothers with antiphospholipid antibody syndrome (21). Laminin and collagen IV are present in excess amounts in the antiphospholipid antibody placenta.

Monitoring of antiphospholipid antibody pregnancies consists of ultrasound evaluation of fetal growth rate and placental volume and appearance. Weekly antepartum fetal heart rate testing may begin as early as 25 weeks (22). In the 25- to 28-week period occasional nonreactive tests (no increase in heart rate with fetal movement) are relatively common. After 28 weeks, any nonreactive test is abnormal. Spontaneous fetal sinus bradycardia indicates a need to deliver. The role of umbilical artery waveform determinations is not yet known, but it assists in timing delivery. Guidelines for pregnancy monitoring are given in Table 89.4. Choice of route of delivery is determined by obstetric criteria, including maternal and fetal platelet count. Antiphospholipid antibody is primarily IgG_2, which does not cross the placenta. Thus, many but not all infants of mothers with antiphospholipid antibody are antiphospholipid antibody negative. Even those who test positive rarely have pathologic clotting. Short-term follow-up studies of infant survivors of antiphospholipid antibody syndrome indicate that these children develop normally compared to children of equivalent prematurity.

Autoantibodies in general, and antiphospholipid antibody in particular, characterize patients with failed *in vitro* fertilization-embryo transfer, but the relationship of these antibodies to the failure is unknown. Murine models of antiphospholipid antibody syndrome show abnormal blastocyst development and impairment of embryo implantation (23). In animal models, fetal death is complement and adhesion molecule dependent; treatment with anticoagulation or IL-3, or immunization with peptides derived from β_2-glycoprotein I prevents fetal death (24).

Treatment recommendations for antiphospholipid antibody pregnancy are presented in Table 89.5. Controlled treatment trials of women with two or more pregnancy losses demonstrate that low-dose aspirin (81 mg/day) plus subcutaneous heparin, 5,000 to 12,000 units twice daily, begun after ultrasonographic confirmation of a viable pregnancy results in more than 80% live (not necessarily term) births (25,26). The lower heparin dose is as effective as higher doses. Full anticoagulant doses are necessary if a woman has had a prior thrombosis. Low molecular weight heparin has been used successfully but has not been tested in controlled trials. Intravenous immunoglobulin has not

TABLE 89.4. MONITORING OF THE PREGNANT RHEUMATIC DISEASE PATIENT[a]

Recommended Frequency	Monitoring Test
First visit	Complete blood count, including platelets
	Urinalysis
	Creatinine clearance
	Anticardiolipin antibody
	Lupus anticoagulant
	Anti-SSA/Ro and anti-SSB/La antibodies
	Anti-dsDNA antibody (SLE patients)
	Complement (C3 and C4 or CH_{50}) (SLE patients)
Monthly	Platelet count[b]
Each trimester	Creatinine clearance[b]
	24-hour urine protein if screening urinalysis abnormal[b]
	Anticardiolipin antibody
	Complement[b]
	Anti-dsDNA antibody[b]
Weekly (last trimester, mothers with antiphospholipid antibody)	Antenatal fetal heart rate testing ("nonstress test"), periodic biophysical profile[c]
Between 18 and 25 weeks (mothers with anti-SSA/Ro and anti-SSB/La antibodies)	Fetal echocardiogram, ?fetal electrocardiogram

[a]Note: The erythrocyte sedimentation rate is often abnormal in uncomplicated pregnancy.
[b]More frequently if abnormal.
[c]Measure of fetal size, activity, and amniotic fluid volume.
dsDNA, double-stranded DNA.

TABLE 89.5. TREATMENT RECOMMENDATIONS FOR PREGNANT WOMEN WITH ANTIPHOSPHOLIPID ANTIBODY

Patient Characteristic	Recommendation
High-titer IgG or IgM aPL antibody[a]	
Primipara	Consider aspirin, 81 mg/d, or no therapy initially; if modest (>50 × 10^9/L) thrombocytopenia occurs, add aspirin[b]
Multipara, most recent pregnancy liveborn	Consider aspirin, 81 mg/d, or no therapy initially; if modest (>50 × 10^9/L) thrombocytopenia occurs, add aspirin[a]
Multipara, most recent pregnancy failure <15 weeks (one loss)	Aspirin
Multipara, most recent pregnancy failure ≥15 weeks without other explanation, or >1 loss	Aspirin while trying to conceive; add heparin, 5,000 units b.i.d. at confirmation of fetal heartbeat, continue for duration of pregnancy
Low-titer IgG or IgM aPL antibody	
Primipara	No therapy
Multipara, no prior fetal loss	No therapy
Multipara, most recent pregnancy failure <15 weeks (one loss)	Aspirin
Multipara, most recent pregnancy failure ≥15 weeks without other explanation, or >1 loss	Aspirin while trying to conceive; add heparin, 5,000 units b.i.d. at confirmation of fetal heartbeat, continue for duration of pregnancy
Multipara, most recent pregnancy failure ≥15 weeks without other explanation	Aspirin while trying to conceive; add heparin, 5,000 units b.i.d. at confirmation of fetal heartbeat, continue for duration of pregnancy
Multipara, prior preeclampsia, IUGR, hypertension or renal disease	Aspirin, beginning after first trimester
Normal aPL antibody	
Primipara	No therapy
Multipara, prior preeclampsia, IUGR, hypertension, or renal disease	Aspirin, beginning after first trimester
Multipara, all others	No therapy indicated by antiphospholipid antibody

[a]At our institution normal IgG <16 GPL U/mL; low positive 16–40, high positive >40; normal IgM <8 MPL U/mL; low positive 8–40, high positive >40.
[b]For thrombocytopenia <50 × 10^9/L, consider intravenous immunoglobulin and/or prednisone.
aPL, antiphospholipid antibody; Ig, immunoglobulin; IUGR, intrauterine growth retardation.

shown benefit. Warfarin cannot be used because it is teratogenic.

For women who have received heparin, the drug should continue postpartum, or be changed to warfarin, for up to 3 months. Aspirin (if used during pregnancy) should also continue for at least 3 months. Absolute points at which anticoagulation might end have not been established.

Sjögren's Syndrome

Management of pregnancy of patients with secondary Sjögren's syndrome is that of the accompanying connective tissue disease. Treatment of the ocular and mucosal manifestations of primary Sjögren's syndrome is not altered by pregnancy. Patients with primary Sjögren's syndrome have an increased risk of fetal loss and of neonatal lupus in their offspring (27), the latter due to the high prevalence of anti-SSA/Ro and anti-SSB/La antibodies in this illness. Sjögren's pregnancies are otherwise similar to those of SLE patients.

Rheumatoid Arthritis

Whether a high frequency of pregnancy loss occurs in women before the clinical appearance of RA is controversial. Patients with established RA frequently experience amelioration of illness during pregnancy. Proposed reasons include endogenous corticosteroid, pregnancy-associated plasma protein A, and maternal-fetal human leukocyte antigen HLA-DQ and -DR disparity (28). Flare of RA often follows delivery, and the postpartum period is a time of increased risk for the new development of RA as well. Maternal exposure during pregnancy to fetally inherited paternal HLA-DR1 and DR4 genes, or to paternal DR genes similar to those of the mother, does not contribute to postpartum susceptibility to new disease (29).

Pregnancy is usually uneventful in rheumatoid patients. Rheumatoid joints may become unstable in late pregnancy as physiologic joint loosening occurs and as the patient's weight distribution changes. Undiagnosed cervical spine subluxation is a particular concern. Bacteremia occurring during labor, although rare, may seed involved joints. Anticardiolipin and anti-SSA/Ro and anti-SSB/La antibodies, hence neonatal lupus, are rarely present. High-risk pregnancy monitoring is not generally necessary. Gold, hydroxychloroquine, cyclosporine, and azathioprine have been used during pregnancy without apparent effect on the fetus, though the number of subjects is small. Cyclophosphamide, methotrexate, and leflunomide are contraindicated during early pregnancy and should be used in late pregnancy only in extreme circumstances. Moderate-dose aspirin and low-dose prednisone are the safest options. There are no specific hazards known regarding antirheumatic doses of other nonsteroidal antiinflammatory drugs, but little experience has accumulated regarding their use in pregnancy. Etanercept, infliximab, and other biologics have unknown effects in pregnancy and should not be used.

Before delivery, the team managing the patient must take special care to identify the patient's disabilities to prepare for labor. Points for special emphasis are hip, knee, and neck arthritis, and the potential risks of forcing motion beyond disease-imposed constraints, causing fracture or other injury. Elective cesarean section may be necessary. If intubation is planned, an anesthesiologist familiar with temporomandibular arthritis and rheumatoid cervical spine disease should be available.

There are no special risks to the fetus other than those related to maternal therapy.

Scleroderma

Patients with scleroderma may tolerate pregnancy well or poorly. Problems derive from nondistensible vascular beds and from preexisting renal, cardiac, and pulmonary insufficiency. Gastroesophageal reflux, common during pregnancy even in women with normal esophageal motility, can be disabling. Treatment is standard: small meals, elevating the head of the bed, histamine-2 blockers, and proton pump inhibitors, but not the prostaglandin E_1 analogue misoprostol. Maternal preeclampsia, congestive heart failure, pulmonary hypertension, pulmonary insufficiency, and renal insufficiency may occur. Renal scleroderma may be indistinguishable from preeclampsia; it may justify termination of pregnancy (30). Angiotensin-converting enzyme inhibitors are relatively contraindicated in pregnancy, except if renal hypertensive crisis occurs. Patients with severe atonic small bowel disease can carry a pregnancy to term with the use of parenteral nutritional support. Prematurity or intrauterine growth restriction are the greatest risks to the infant; otherwise pregnancy success rate is normal. A high and persistent degree of transplacental transfer of fetal cells occurs in scleroderma patients, but the relationship of this finding to disease pathogenesis is unknown (31). Years after pregnancy is over fetal cells can still be found in affected maternal skin sites (32).

Spondyloarthropathy

Female patients with ankylosing spondylitis have normal fertility. Most patients experience either no change or modest worsening of complaints during pregnancy; those who worsen return to baseline postpartum (33). Patients with psoriatic arthritis may improve during pregnancy. Other than the specific anatomic problems of spondyloarthropathy (restricted motion of the hips and lower back that might impede vaginal delivery), patients have no unusual problems with pregnancy.

Vasculitis

Patients with Takayasu's disease may do well, but renovascular occlusive disease, pulmonary hypertension, and cardiac insufficiency remain as important potential problems (34). Preeclampsia is common. Management during pregnancy involves careful monitoring and treatment of hypertension (which is difficult to measure when arteries are constricted) and aggressive hemodynamic and pharmacologic management in the peripartum period. Sixty percent of infants have intrauterine growth restriction, related to aortic involvement, hypertension, and preeclampsia. Pregnancy associated with polyarteritis nodosa (PAN) is rare. Onset of PAN during pregnancy results in high maternal morbidity, possibly because confusion of PAN with preeclampsia delays diagnosis. Maternal and fetal outcome for patients in clinical remission with stable established disease is good. Rarely, PAN occurs simultaneously in mother and neonate. Pregnancies in patients with leukocytoclastic vasculitis are uneventful. Some pregnant patients with Wegener's granulomatosis experience exacerbation and even death, but others do well (35). There are no data regarding the effect of Wegener's granulomatosis on the child. Because of the frequent need to use cyclophosphamide and the potential for rapidly progressive renal failure, pregnancy in this illness should be discouraged. Erythema nodosum may be triggered by pregnancy (erythema nodosum gravidarum), but it does not harm the fetus. The course of relapsing polychondritis does not change during pregnancy, and full-term pregnancy is probable (36).

Dermatomyositis/Polymyositis

Muscle fatigue and respiratory impairment are the greatest dangers for the pregnant patient with inflammatory myositis. Pulmonary fibrosis may compromise maternal respiratory reserve, especially in late pregnancy. Muscle strength and pulmonary function must be repeatedly monitored during pregnancy and delivery. Uterine muscle contraction in labor proceeds normally, but maternal weakness may be a limiting factor. Autoantibodies in dermatomyositis/polymyositis are not known to cause illness in the fetus. The risk to the fetus is that of the mother's therapy and of the complications she suffers during pregnancy. Because the disease is rare and variable in severity, management, counseling, and breast-feeding decisions must be individualized.

Heritable Disorders of Connective Tissue

Management during pregnancy in *Marfan syndrome* consists of extremely tight control of blood pressure and avoidance of strenuous Valsalva maneuvers to protect against aortic dissection. Antibiotic prophylaxis for cardiac valvular disease is appropriate. Elective cesarean section may also be appropriate. Patients with *Ehlers-Danlos syndrome* may develop cervical incompetence. Risks in pregnancy are those of joint dislocation and, very rarely, uterine rupture. Patients with *benign familial joint hyperlaxity,* possibly a mild variant of Ehlers-Danlos, are prone to unexplained antepartum hemorrhage.

Miscellaneous

Hip disease of any kind may interfere with normal vaginal delivery, because abduction may be severely limited. Forcing a patient's joint motion beyond the point at which she feels pain or at which resistance is encountered is not only painful, it also risks fracture, dislocation, or other permanent harm. Antibiotic coverage (a cephalosporin plus gentamicin, or vancomycin plus gentamicin) may be indicated in women with artificial joint replacements undergoing vaginal delivery. Pelvic and back pain may be caused by laxity of the pubic symphysis and sacroiliac joints, associated with increased levels of serum relaxin. Labor and delivery are occasionally complicated postpartum by infectious sacroiliitis or osteitis pubis. For diagnosis of back pain in pregnant patients, magnetic resonance imaging is preferable to computed tomography. Ultrasound, infrared therapy, and warm water therapeutic pool therapy may potentially injure the fetus.

PREGNANCY MANAGEMENT

Monitoring recommendations for rheumatic disease patients are presented in Table 89.4. Unexplained elevations of maternal α-fetoprotein and hCG (with estriol, the "triple screen" for Down syndrome) occurs in patients with lupus and with antiphospholipid antibody. It correlates with antiphospholipid antibody, preterm delivery, high prednisone dose, and fetal death (37). Because intervention with dexamethasone at the earliest sign of cardiac dysfunction may reverse myocarditis and possibly heart block, women with high titer anti-Ro and anti-La antibodies and those who have previously given birth to a child with any form of neonatal lupus should undergo fetal cardiac monitoring weekly during the vulnerable period, 18 to 25 weeks. In women known to have strongly positive *lupus anticoagulant* and anticardiolipin antibody, serial testing during pregnancy is unnecessary, since decrease in titer does not improve prognosis. In women with low titer or negative tests, repetition at least once each trimester is useful, since overall prognosis is that of the highest titer seen during the *pregnancy.* Platelet count should be repeated monthly. Women *both* positive for antiphospholipid antibody and having prior fetal losses should be treated with heparin.

Decisions regarding timing and route of delivery are dictated by the status of the fetus but may be influenced by maternal illness and its complications. Approximately one-third of SLE patients undergo operative delivery. The usual indications for cesarean section are fetal distress, prior cesarean section, prolonged ruptured membranes, failure to progress at labor and other obstetrical reasons, thrombocytopenia, and severe maternal illness.

There is little information about the use of tocolytics or stimulators of labor in rheumatic disease pregnancy. Ritodrine, magnesium sulfate, and prostaglandin suppositories have been used without incident. At delivery, "stress" corticosteroid doses (usually 100 mg hydrocortisone every 8 hours from onset of labor until 24 hours postdelivery) are administered to patients currently or recently taking corticosteroids. Asymptomatic bacteremia occurs during vaginal delivery in 3.6% of deliveries. Because of limited hip joint movement or risk of bacterial seeding, osteonecrosis of the hip may justify a decision for operative rather than vaginal delivery. Mode of delivery for patients with total hip replacements need not be surgical; patients have been delivered vaginally with appropriate attention paid to the positioning of the patient.

FETAL OUTCOME

Preliminary data suggest that boys of SLE mothers have developmental difficulties, the cause of which is unknown (38). In comparisons of such infants with sex- and gestational age-matched controls, intelligence is normal, but there is a high frequency of learning disabilities. Children with complete congenital heart block remain at risk for cardiac death. Although case reports have described survivors of neonatal lupus who developed systemic lupus when they became adults, such events are very rare. Other than the genetic risks, there are no other known risks to children of other rheumatic disease mothers.

REFERENCES

1. Maloney S, Smith A, Furst DE, et al. Microchimerism of maternal origin persists into adult life. *J Clin Invest* 1999;104:41–47.
2. Clark DA. T cells in pregnancy: illusion and reality. *Am J Reprod Immunol* 1999;41:233–238.
3. Austgulen R, Arntzen KJ, Ødegaard R. Circulating levels of cytokines and cytokine receptors in normal human pregnancy. *Scand J Rheumatol* 1998;suppl 107:18.
4. Hill JA. Cytokines considered critical in pregnancy. *Am J Reprod Immunol* 1992;28:123–126.
5. Crowther MA, Kelton, JG, Ginsberg J, et al. Thrombocytopenia in pregnancy: diagnosis, pathogenesis and management. *Blood* Rev 1996;10:8–16.
6. Parke AL. Antimalarial drugs in pregnancy. *Scand J Rheumatol* 1998;suppl 107:125–127.
7. Bermas BL, Hill JA. Effects of immunosuppressive drugs during pregnancy. *Arthritis Rheum* 1995;38:722–732.
8. Koren G, Pastuszak A, Ito S. Drugs in pregnancy. *N Engl J Med* 1998;338:1128–1137.
9. Petri M, Robinson C. Oral contraceptives and systemic lupus erythematosus. *Arthritis Rheum* 1997;40:797–803.

10. Ruiz-Irastorza G, Lima F, Alves J, et al. Increased rate of lupus flare during pregnancy and the puerperium: a prospective study of 78 pregnancies. *Br J Rheumatol* 1996;35:133–138.
11. Buyon JP, Hiebert R, Copel J, et al. Autoimmune-associated congenital heart block: demographics, mortality, morbidity and recurrence rates obtained from a national neonatal lupus registry. *J Am Coll Cardiol* 1998;31:1658–1666.
12. Buyon JP, Roubey R, Swersky S, et al. Complete congenital heart block: risk of occurrence and therapeutic approach to prevention. *J Rheumatol* 1988;15:1104.
13. Buyon JP, Tseng C-E, DiDonato F, et al. Cardiac expression of 52β, an alternative transcript of the congenital heart block-associated 52-kd SS-A/Ro autoantigen, is maximal during fetal development. *Arthritis Rheum* 1997;40:655–660.
14. Viana VS, Garcia S, Nascimento JT, et al. Induction of in vitro heart block is not restricted to affinity purified anti-52 kDa Ro/SSA antibody from mothers of children with neonatal lupus. *Lupus* 1998;7:141–147.
15. Rosenthal, D, Druzin M, Chin C, et al. A new therapeutic approach to the fetus with congenital complete heart block: preemptive targeted therapy with dexamethasone. *Obstet Gynecol* 1998;92:689–691.
16. Kupferminc MJ, Eldor A, Steinman N, et al. Increased frequency of genetic thrombophilia in women with complications of pregnancy. *N Engl J* Med 1999;340:9–13.
17. Lima F, Khamashta MA, Buchanan NM, et al. A study of sixty pregnancies in patients with antiphospholipid syndrome. *Clin Exp Rheumatol* 1996;14:131–136.
18. Magid MS, Kaplan C, Sammaritano LR, et al. Placental pathology in systemic lupus erythematosus: a prospective study. *Am J Obstet Gynecol* 1998;179:226–234.
19. Sammaritano LR, Gharavi AE, Soberano C, et al. Phospholipid binding of antiphospholipid antibodies and placental anticoagulant protein. *J Clin Immunol* 1992;12:27–35.
20. Rand JH, Wu XX, Andree HAM, et al. Pregnancy loss in the antiphospholipid-antibody syndrome—a possible thrombogenic mechanism. *N Engl J Med* 1997;337:154–160.
21. La Rosa L, Meroni PL, Tincani A, et al. Beta-2-glycoprotein I and placental anticoagulant protein I in placentae from patients with antiphospholipid antibody syndrome. *J Rheumatol* 1994; 21:1684–1693.
22. Adams D, Druzin ML, Edersheim T, et al. Antepartum testing-systemic lupus erythematosus and associated serologic abnormalities. *Am J Reprod Immunol* 1992;28:159–164.
23. Sthoeger ZM, Mozes E, Tartakovsky B. Anti-cardiolipin antibodies induce pregnancy failure by impairing embryonic implantation. *Proc Natl Acad Sci U S A* 1993;90:6464–6467.
24. Shoenfeld Y, Ziporen L. Lessons from experimental APS models. *Lupus* 1998;7:s158–s161.
25. Kutteh, WH, Ermel LD. A clinical trial for the treatment of aPL associated recurrent pregnancy loss with lower dose heparin and aspirin. *Am J Reprod Immunol* 1996;35:402–407.
26. Rai R, Cohen H, Dave M, et al. Randomized controlled trial of aspirin and aspirin plus heparin in pregnant women with recurrent miscarriage associated with phospholipid antibodies (or antiphospholipid antibodies). *Br Med J* 1997;314:253–257.
27. Julkunen H, Kaaja R, Kurki P, et al. Fetal outcome in women with primary Sjögren's syndrome: a retrospective case-control study. *Clin Exp Rheum* 1995;13:65–71.
28. Nelson JL, Hughes KA, Smith AG, et al. Maternal-fetal disparity in HLA class ll alloantigens and the pregnancy-induced amelioration of rheumatoid arthritis. *N Engl J Med* 1993;329:466–471.
29. Brennan P, Payton T, Ollier B, et al. Maternal exposure to paternal HLA does not explain the postpartum increase in rheumatoid arthritis. *Genet Epidemiol* 1996;13:411–418.
30. Steen VD, Medsger TA Jr. Fertility and pregnancy outcome in women with systemic sclerosis. *Arthritis Rheum* 1999;42: 763–768.
31. Nelson JL, Furst DE, Maloney S, et al. Microchimerism and HLA-compatible relationships of pregnancy in SSc. *Lancet* 1998; 351:559–562.
32. Artlett CM, Smith JB, Jimenez SA. Identification of fetal DNA and cells in skin lesions from women with systemic sclerosis. *N Engl J Med* 1998;338:1186–1191.
33. Gran JT, Östensen M. Spondylarthritides in females. *Baillieres Clin Rheumatol* 1998;12:695–715.
34. Bassa A, Desai DK, Moodley J. Takayasu's disease and pregnancy: three case studies and a review of the literature. *S Afr Med J* 1995;85:107–112.
35. Luisiri P, Lance NJ, Curran JJ. Wegener's granulomatosis in pregnancy. *Arthritis Rheum* 1997;40:1354–1360.
36. Papo T, Wechsler B, Bletry O, et al. Pregnancy in relapsing polychondritis: twenty-five pregnancies in eleven patients. *Arthritis Rheum* 1997;40:1245–1249.
37. Petri M, Ho AC, Patel J, et al. Elevation of maternal alpha-fetoprotein in systemic lupus erythematosus: a controlled study. *J Rheum* 1995;22:1365–1368.
38. McAllister DL, Kaplan BJ, Manzi S, et al. The influence of systemic lupus erythematosus on fetal development: cognitive, behavior and health trends. *J Int Neuropsych Soc* 1997;3:370–376.

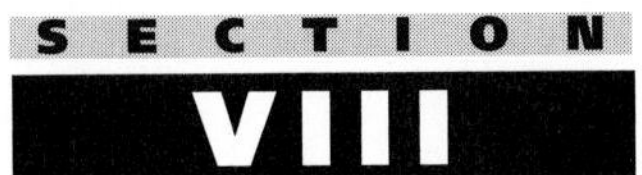

MISCELLANEOUS RHEUMATIC DISEASES

90

FIBROMYALGIA

LAURENCE A. BRADLEY
GRACIELA S. ALARCÓN

Fibromyalgia is a chronic musculoskeletal disorder characterized by widespread pain, exquisite tenderness at specific anatomic sites (i.e., tender points), and other clinical manifestations such as fatigue, sleep disturbance, and irritable bowel syndrome (1–10). Although fibromyalgia has been recognized for decades with descriptive terms such as *nonarticular rheumatism, psychogenic rheumatism,* and *fibrositis,* it was not until 1990 that reliable criteria for classifying patients with this disorder were developed and published by a multicenter committee of the American College of Rheumatology (ACR) (11). These criteria include widespread pain that persists for at least 3 months and tenderness in at least 11 of 18 specific anatomic sites. The publication of these criteria has contributed to a great increase in high-quality research on the epidemiology, etiopathogenesis, and consequences of fibromyalgia since 1990. Nevertheless, considerable controversy and debate about this condition exists. At one extreme of this controversy are those who deny its mere existence and consider fibromyalgia the result of the "medicalization" of unrelated symptoms; at the other extreme are those who consider fibromyalgia a defined disorder (12–15). A healthy middle ground has recently been proposed by Masi (16), who favors the designation of fibromyalgia as a syndrome (17).

Another alternative is to consider fibromyalgia a functional somatic disorder in which symptoms are magnified and perpetuated as a result of the belief that they are due to a serious disease or condition that may eventually have a catastrophic outcome (18). Cognizant of the fact that fibromyalgia may occur in the context of other well-defined diseases, such as systemic lupus erythematosus (SLE) or rheumatoid arthritis (RA), to cite but a few (19–21), the authors favor the designation of fibromyalgia syndrome when this disorder occurs in such circumstances and fibromyalgia per se, if no other well-defined rheumatic disorder is present.

CLINICAL FEATURES AND DIAGNOSIS

The ACR has defined widespread pain as (a) pain in the right and left sides of the body, (b) pain above and below the waist, and (c) axial skeletal pain (i.e., pain of the cervical spine, anterior chest, thoracic spine, or low back). The majority of patients with fibromyalgia report that they do not experience significant diurnal variation in the intensity or other characteristics of their pain. Moreover, they indicate that the most severe pain tends to localize to the axial skeleton, either in the upper back (paracervical and trapezius muscles) or the lower back (paralumbar and gluteus muscles). Some patients complain of pain in their hips and shoulders, whereas others indicate that pain is most severe in the peripheral skeleton (elbows, wrists, hands, knees, ankles, and feet) and often refer to this as "joint pain." Patients presenting for the first time to a general rheumatology clinic often report a peripheral onset of pain (22).

In addition to the widespread nature of pain associated with fibromyalgia, patients tend to experience pain or tenderness in response to relatively modest levels of pressure stimulation at multiple anatomic sites. The ACR multicenter committee identified 18 anatomic sites or tender points that best distinguish patients with fibromyalgia from patients with various other chronic pain syndromes, specifically, low back pain, RA, and SLE. These 18 tender points are the left and right (a) occiput, at the insertion of the suboccipital muscles; (b) lower cervical spine, at the anterior aspect of the intertransverse spaces between C5 and C7; (c) trapezius, at the midpoint of the upper border; (d) supraspinatus, at the origin of the muscle, above the scapula spine near the medial border; (e) second rib, at the second costochondral junction; (f) gluteal area, at the upper outer quadrant of buttocks; (g) epicondyle (lateral), 2 cm distal to the epicondyle; (h) greater trochanter, posterior to the trochanteric prominence; and (i) knee, at the medial fat pad, proximal to the articular line. The locations of these tender points are indicated in Fig. 90.1. During the evaluation of patients for fibromyalgia, pressure is applied with a force of approximately 4 kg with either the thumb (in the clinical setting) or a calibrated dolorimeter (in the research setting). Tenderness is defined by a verbal report of faint pain in response to the pressure stimulus. It has not been possible to establish normative values for the responses to

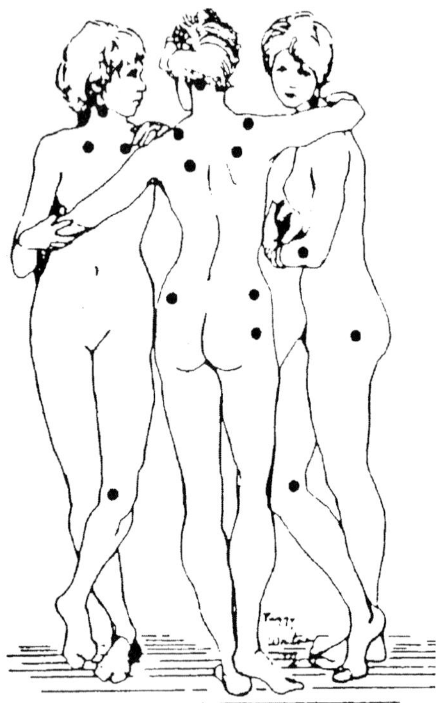

FIGURE 90.1. Tender point locations for the 1990 American College of Rheumatology classification criteria for fibromyalgia. (Adapted from Wolfe F, Smythe HA, Yunus MB, et al. The American College of Rheumatology 1990 criteria for the classification of fibromyalgia: report of the multicenter criteria committee. *Arthritis Rheum* 1990;33:160–172, with permission.)

tender point examinations of patients with fibromyalgia and healthy individuals. Independent laboratories have published different values, probably due to variations in evaluation procedures and dolorimeters (23,24). The authors have reported that the average Chatillon dolorimeter (Chatillon Instruments, Kew Gardens, NY) pressure required to elicit faint pain at the tender points is around 1.9 kg in patients who meet ACR criteria for fibromyalgia, compared to about 5.4 kg for healthy controls (25). Interestingly, for persons who meet ACR criteria for fibromyalgia but have not sought medical care for their symptoms *(vide infra)*, the pressure required is about 2.6 kg (25,26).

The ACR multicenter committee found that the criteria described above differentiated 293 patients with fibromyalgia from 265 control patients with other painful disorders (e.g., RA, low back pain) with a sensitivity of 88.4% and a specificity of 81.1% (11). The committee also assessed the responses of patients and control subjects to pressure stimulation at several anatomic sites in addition to the tender points. These "control points" were (a) the forearm, at the distal dorsal third of the forearm; (b) the midfoot, at the dorsal third metatarsal; and (c) the thumbnail. It was found that patients showed significantly greater tenderness at these points than the control subjects. However, responses to the control points differentiated patients from control subjects with less accuracy than the tender point responses. Other investigators, including our research group, have performed similar studies of responses to control point stimulation (25,27,28). Patients do report pain when relatively low levels of pressure are applied to various control points including those identified by the ACR committee; however, the pressure levels required to evoke pain at these control points tend to be greater than those needed to produce pain at the tender points (25,27). Wolfe (29) has recently proposed calling these anatomic sites "high threshold" points (rather than control points), but such terminology awaits acceptance.

SECONDARY CLINICAL MANIFESTATIONS

Musculoskeletal Symptoms

Individuals with fibromyalgia may report other musculoskeletal symptoms in addition to those in the ACR criteria. These symptoms include morning stiffness (lasting less than 1 hour), and diffuse arthralgias and myalgias, as well as subjective, but not demonstrable, joint and soft tissue swelling, mainly of the hands and feet. Indeed, patients often indicate that they have had to remove their rings or change shoe sizes because of swelling of the metacarpophalangeal and proximal and/or distal interphalangeal joints as well as the dorsal aspect of hands and fingers, feet, and toes (1,8,9). Some patients may also have carpal tunnel syndrome (30), whereas others may describe joint hypermobility that can be detected by physical examination (31,32). In fact, hypermobility has been identified as a contributing factor to exacerbations of fibromyalgia symptoms in both children and young adults (33,34). Patients frequently indicate that their symptoms vary with changes in weather, with some individuals being sensitive to high and others to low temperatures; still others report worsening of their symptoms with changes in barometric pressure (35,36). Of interest, Hagglund and colleagues (35) reported higher functional impairment in weather-sensitive patients with fibromyalgia than in those who were not sensitive to changes in weather.

Nonmusculoskeletal Symptoms

The most prominent nonmusculoskeletal manifestations associated with fibromyalgia are fatigue and sleep disturbances (1–4,8–11,37–40). It is very difficult to interpret reports of fatigue since they lack a physical examination correlate. The intensity of the fatigue described by patients with fibromyalgia tends to be variable. Only rarely is fatigue the primary symptom that limits activities of daily life; this differs from the reports of patients with chronic fatigue syndrome for whom fatigue is the dominant and truly incapacitating feature of the disorder (38,39,41). There are, however, patients who present both significant fatigue and pain; in fact, these patients may meet criteria for both fibromyalgia and chronic fatigue syndromes (42,43).

Sleep disturbances have been recognized for decades in patients with fibromyalgia. Regardless of the intensity of their pain, the large majority of patients suffer from insomnia or light and unrefreshing sleep. It is common for these patients to report that upon awakening they are more tired than when they went to bed the night before (37,41,44,45). Two factors have been associated with sleep disturbance in patients with fibromyalgia. Moldofsky and colleagues (30) have observed an abnormal pattern in the electroencephalographic (EEG) recordings of patients with fibromyalgia during deep sleep. This abnormal EEG pattern is described in greater detail in the section on the etiopathogenesis of fibromyalgia. Additionally, May and colleagues (46) have reported frequent occurrence of sleep apnea in men with fibromyalgia and have suggested that fibromyalgia should be regarded as a marker for sleep apnea. These authors have emphasized the need to elicit other symptoms of sleep apnea from patients, particularly, but not limited to obese men; these symptoms include restless sleep, daytime somnolence, morning fatigue, morning headaches, snoring, and observed breathing abnormalities. They also have indicated that the spouse/bed partner frequently is better able to provide this information than the patient is. The findings of May and associates differ from those reported by Alvarez-Lario and colleagues (47), however, who found that only 1 of 30 study patients with sleep apnea met criteria for the diagnosis of fibromyalgia. This frequency is comparable to that of fibromyalgia observed in the general population. These authors concluded that there is no association between sleep apnea and fibromyalgia.

Patients with fibromyalgia tend to report numerous other nonmusculoskeletal manifestations affecting almost every organ system (1–3,6,7,9,10,48–54). The ACR multicenter committee (11) noted the following: migraine and tension headaches; irritable bowel syndrome; dysmenorrhea and urinary frequency (i.e., female urethral or irritable bladder syndrome); paresthesias or dysesthesias (in the absence of neuropathy); Raynaud's phenomenon; and sicca symptoms. Other manifestations commonly described by patients with fibromyalgia include photosensitivity, skin rashes, and mucosal ulcerations (49,55–57). With the possible exception of Raynaud's phenomenon, these manifestations cannot be corroborated by physical examination (55). Granges and Littlejohn (4), however, found that reactive hyperemia and skin-fold tenderness can be objectively demonstrated in most patients with fibromyalgia. Similarly, cold-induced vasospasm, an infrequent event in normal adults, can be demonstrated in nearly 40% of patients with fibromyalgia (58).

It can be difficult to differentiate fibromyalgia from other rheumatic conditions. For example, Bonafede and colleagues (59) have reported that some patients with Sjögren's syndrome may be misdiagnosed with fibromyalgia. Conversely, patients with fibromyalgia who are antinuclear antibody (ANA)-positive with a history of photosensitivity, oral ulcerations, arthralgias, and joint swelling, may be erroneously diagnosed as having an undifferentiated connective tissue disease, or incomplete or latent lupus (60). We identified such a subset of patients among those referred, diagnosed, or followed with SLE at our institution (61), and are convinced many patients with fibromyalgia are indeed erroneously diagnosed as having SLE (62,63). Our data and those of Yunus and colleagues (64) show that the frequencies of ANA positivity and symptoms of connective tissue disease do not differ between patients with fibromyalgia and healthy controls. Indeed, in a longitudinal study of patients with early manifestations suggestive of a connective tissue disorder, but not diagnostic of any, very few patients evolved into lupus or other connective tissue disease, further questioning the wisdom of diagnosing such patients as having early SLE (65,66). Nevertheless, some of the ANA-positive patients in Yunus's study exhibited autoantibodies such as anti-Sm, anti-SSA, or anti-SSB, suggesting that they indeed may evolve into a more diffuse connective tissue disease (64).

Due to symptoms involving multiple organ systems, patients with fibromyalgia may present to a variety of specialists; it is not uncommon for them to undergo unnecessary and oftentimes invasive diagnostic or treatment procedures. For example, patients with undiagnosed fibromyalgia commonly are subjected to magnetic resonance or computed tomography of the head, chest, abdomen, or pelvis; echocardiograms; upper and lower gastrointestinal tract endoscopies; and cystoscopies. Even after the diagnosis of fibromyalgia is made, patients undergo an average of nearly 1 radiographic examination and 2.5 laboratory evaluations per year (67). Moreover, fibromyalgia patients may undergo more surgical procedures than nonfibromyalgia rheumatology patients (back and neck surgery, abdominal surgery, gynecologic surgery) (68,69). Table 90.1 lists some of the manifestations that may prompt fibromyalgia patients to consult different specialists, and tests commonly ordered in an effort to sort out the nature of their complaints. It should be clearly understood that patients with fibromyalgia are not malingerers with feigned manifestations. However, some patients may have difficulty accepting the diagnosis of fibromyalgia and of fibromyalgia-related conditions that cannot be cured with medications or surgical procedures (e.g., irritable bowel syndrome). This difficulty is especially likely to occur if patients receive little or no education regarding fibromyalgia. In fact, in a small study conducted by Hellstrom and colleagues (70) in Sweden, patients were interviewed and asked to describe the nature of their illness; they were found to be intensively involved in efforts to get their self-images of ill persons confirmed (70). As physicians learn more about the spectrum of clinical manifestations that characterize fibromyalgia and devote greater effort to patient education, it should be possible to

TABLE 90.1. SYMPTOMS, DIAGNOSTIC TESTS/PROCEDURES, AND DIAGNOSES IN PATIENTS WITH FIBROMYALGIA SEEKING HEALTH CARE

Specialist	Symptoms	Diagnostic Tests/Procedures	Possible Diagnoses[a]
Internist	Malaise, fatigue, weakness	Various	Various
Cardiologist	Palpitations, chest pain, syncope, hypotension	EKG, exercise tests, echocardiogram, conventional and MR-angiogram, heart catheterization, tilt table evaluations	Mitral valve prolapse Atypical angina Dysautonomia
Pulmonologist	Dyspnea, snoring	Pulmonary function tests, arterial blood gases, polysomnography	Asthma, sleep apnea Noncardiac chest pain
Gastroenterologist	Dysphagia, dyspepsia, abdominal pain, bloating, constipation, diarrhea	Upper and lower GI tract endoscopies, radiographs and/or biopsies, abdominal CT and/or ultrasound, abdominal angiogram	Irritable bowel syndrome Gastroesophageal reflux
Endocrinologist	Weakness, faintness	Fasting blood sugars, serum hormonal levels	Hypoglycemia
Rheumatologist	Myalgias, arthralgias, Raynaud's phenomenon, weakness, neck and/or back pain	Serologic tests, electrophysiologic studies	Latent or variant lupus Costochondritis Polymyalgia rheumatica Undifferentiated connective tissue disease
Dermatologist	Pruritus, hives, skin rashes, photosensitivity	Skin biopsies	Dermatitis
Allergologist	Allergies	Skin tests, suppression tests	Allergies Multiple chemical sensitivities
Neurologist	Dizziness, dysesthesias, vertigo, headache, syncope, seizures	CT scans and/or MRIs, MR-angiogram, electrophysiologic studies, lumbar puncture, biopsies	Headaches Restless leg syndrome Dysautonomia Anxiety
Gynecologist	Polyuria, dysuria, dyspareunia, vaginitis, pelvic pain	Cystoscopies, colposcopies	Urinary tract infection Cystitis Vaginitis Endometriosis
Otorhinolaringologist	Tinnitus, cough, headache, hoarseness, snoring, vertigo, dizziness	Audiograms, CT scans or MRIs, polysommography	Rhinitis Sinusitis Meniere's disease Sleep apnea
Orthopedist	Neck and/or back pain	Radiographs, MRIs and/or CT scans	Arthritis
Neurosurgeon	Headache, neck and/or back pain, dysesthesias	CT scans and/or MRIs, electrophysiologic studies	Spinal stenosis Radiculopathy
Ophthalmologist	Dry eyes, blurred vision, double vision	Shirmer's test, fluorescein test	Sicca syndrome
Psychiatrist	Anxiety, depression, insomnia, decreased memory, sexual and/or physical abuse	Neurocognitive evaluation, psychological tests	Anxiety Depression Abuse (sexual and/or physical)
Dentist	Dry mouth	Salivary gland biopsy	Sicca syndrome

[a]Some of these diagnoses represent true associations. Others, unfortunately, are given to patients in an effort to explain their symptoms, but lack organic bases.
CT, computed tomography; MRI, magnetic resonance imaging.

reduce the high frequencies of consultations and treatment-seeking behaviors exhibited by fibromyalgia patients.

Patient Subgroups

It is common practice to classify patients with fibromyalgia according to whether other medical conditions are associated with their fibromyalgia symptoms *(vide supra)*. Patients who meet ACR criteria for fibromyalgia for whom an underlying or concomitant medical condition cannot be identified are classified as having *primary fibromyalgia* or fibromyalgia per se. Patients who develop fibromyalgia also may have suffered for a period of time from other medical illnesses such as RA or osteoarthritis. Indeed, the symptoms of fibromyalgia may have greater importance to these patients than those of the underlying medical condition.

These patients are classified as having *secondary fibromyalgia* (11). The ACR multicenter committee recommended abolishing the use of the distinction between primary and secondary fibromyalgia for diagnostic purposes (11). Nevertheless, we believe the distinction is justifiable both in research and in clinical settings. With regard to the former, it is desirable to enter only patients with primary fibromyalgia in studies of etiopathogenesis so that any differences between patients and controls may be attributed to fibromyalgia per se and not to concomitant medical disorders. In addition, failure to differentiate primary fibromyalgia from secondary fibromyalgia may prevent investigators from identifying important biologic abnormalities associated only with primary fibromyalgia, e.g., elevated cerebrospinal fluid (CSF) levels of nerve growth factor (71).

It also is important in clinical settings to differentiate secondary fibromyalgia and fibromyalgia-related symptoms from preexisting rheumatic disorders or connective tissue diseases. For example, optimal management of patients with RA and secondary fibromyalgia requires efforts to reduce the inflammatory disease activity and joint pain of RA, as well as the sleep disturbance, fatigue, and generalized pain of fibromyalgia. Indeed, the secondary fibromyalgia symptoms may, in some patients, require greater attention than those associated with RA (72).

Patients with fibromyalgia also can be classified according to whether the onset of symptoms is acute or insidious. Patients who report an acute onset often attribute their symptoms to the occurrence of a precipitating event such as a defined infectious process (e.g., Lyme disease, or infection with parvovirus B19, coxsackievirus, hepatitis C, Epstein-Barr virus) (73–77), physical and/or emotional trauma (e.g., surgery, motor vehicle accident) (78–81), or stressful life events (e.g., divorce) (82,83). It also should be noted that the precipitating events identified by patients are not necessarily recent. For example, fibromyalgia has been found in a sizable proportion of women with the postparalytic polio syndrome (84). There is considerable controversy, however, regarding the extent to which some distal events such as sexual or physical abuse may be related to fibromyalgia symptoms (85–88). There also is conflicting evidence regarding whether physical trauma prior to pain onset is associated with higher levels of pain and disability than those observed in patients with insidious pain onset (82,89). Patients in whom a clear precipitating event is recognized are said to have "reactive" fibromyalgia (80).

Another clinical variable that may be used to classify patients with fibromyalgia is the presence or absence of familial aggregation (6,90). Familial aggregation may represent the influence of a genetic predisposition to neuroendocrine dysfunction, abnormal pain sensitivity, or muscle microtrauma; exposure to noxious environmental stimuli; or simply learned behavior (91). To the extent that this, and the other classifications described earlier, are used to advance our knowledge concerning fibromyalgia, they may be regarded as useful. For example, geographic clustering will be expected if environmental factors contribute significantly to the occurrence of fibromyalgia, but familial clustering will be expected if genetic features are important contributors to its occurrence. Registries of multiplex families and affected twins are being constituted at the present time; indeed a weak association (linkage) between fibromyalgia and the human leukocyte antigen (HLA) system has been reported by Yunus et al. (92), but these data await confirmation by other groups of investigators (see Etiopathogenesis, below).

Finally, there is some evidence that it is useful to classify patients with fibromyalgia on the basis of their psychosocial and behavioral responses to pain. A series of investigations using the Multidimensional Pain Inventory (93) suggest that 87% of tertiary care clinic patients with this disorder may be classified into one of three groups using a set of empirically derived rules (94,95). These groups were labeled as (a) dysfunctional (23%), (b) interpersonally distressed (33%), and (c) adaptive copers (31%). Patients in the dysfunctional and interpersonally distressed subgroups report higher levels of disability and depression than the adaptive copers (94). Moreover, an uncontrolled evaluation of a standard, interdisciplinary pain treatment program indicated that the patients classified as dysfunctional or as adaptive copers experienced significant improvements in pain; only the dysfunctional patients reported significant improvements in affective distress and disability (95). It may be useful, then, to tailor pain treatment plans based on patients' psychosocial and behavioral responses to the experience of chronic pain (95).

EPIDEMIOLOGY

Fibromyalgia is diagnosed mainly in middle-aged Caucasian women, although it has been observed in children and the elderly. Fibromyalgia is recognized primarily in persons from the middle and upper socioeconomic strata (96–101), although one Canadian population-based study suggests that relatively low levels of education are associated with increased risk for fibromyalgia (102). We have long suspected that fibromyalgia occurs less frequently in individuals from non-Caucasian ethnic groups, but information validating this assertion is just emerging (from Mexico, the India subcontinent, and Israel) (103–105). Population-based studies in North America have not carefully evaluated ethnic group differences in prevalence of fibromyalgia (98,102). However, one study performed in Wichita, Kansas, revealed that nonwhites composed 11% of the persons identified as fibromyalgia cases (98).

The incidence of fibromyalgia is unknown, but its prevalence has been estimated using population-based, primary care–based, or referral-based data (1,97,98,106–114). As noted by Raspe and Baumgartner (106), the prevalence estimates from various population-based studies are difficult to compare since different criteria have been used to define cases. Studies performed since 1989 have used either the ACR criteria (11) or earlier classification schemes such as the Yunus criteria (115). In some of these studies, primary and secondary fibromyalgia cases have been included, whereas in others only primary fibromyalgia has been considered. Recently, White and colleagues (116) have developed a questionnaire to screen for fibromyalgia in the general population. This questionnaire has six items, four related to pain and two related to fatigue. The instrument was tested in 31 patients with fibromyalgia, 30 patients with RA, and 30 healthy controls. For the pain criteria alone, the sensitivity was 100% and the specificity 100% when examined in comparison to healthy controls, but only 53% when the fibromyalgia patients were compared with the RA patients. For pain and fatigue, the sensitivity was 94% and the specificity 100% for the healthy controls, but 80% when tested against the RA patients. The authors emphasize that this questionnaire needs to be followed by a personal evaluation to confirm the distribution and duration of pain, as well as a tender point examination. Needless to say, persons performing these assessments should receive adequate training (117) to ensure reliability of tender point measurement (118,119).

The ages of the subjects have varied across the epidemiologic studies with some including only young adults and others including adults across the life span. The denominator also has varied, with some studies surveying only women, whereas others have included both men and women. Therefore, it is not surprising that population-based studies provide prevalence rates that vary between 0.7% and 13% in adult women and 0.2% and 3.9% in adult men. Population-based studies in Wichita, Kansas and London, Ontario have found overall prevalence rates of 2% and 3%, respectively (98,102). The prevalence rates for women in these studies were 3.4% and 4.9%, respectively (98,102); the prevalence rates for men were 0.5% and 1.6%. Both of these studies revealed that nearly 90% of the identified fibromyalgia cases were women.

Primary care–based studies have confirmed that fibromyalgia is a disorder that predominantly affects women. The frequency of fibromyalgia among men and women in the primary care setting varies between 1.9% and 3.7% (120,121). It is important to recognize, however, that not all patients with fibromyalgia are correctly identified in primary care settings. Indeed, some patients may be diagnosed as having myalgias, arthralgias, soft tissue rheumatism, regional pain syndromes, and/or panniculitis, or they may be ultimately diagnosed with disorders such as SLE, RA, polymyositis, polymyalgia rheumatica, or Sjögren's syndrome.

Fibromyalgia constitutes one of the most common diagnoses in referral-based rheumatology practices. The frequency of fibromyalgia, which varies from 3% to 20% in these practices, likely depends on interest in the disorder among rheumatologists, the degree of medical sophistication among patients, and the awareness of the condition among the referral sources (2,5,97,122).

ETIOPATHOGENESIS

A large number of studies have examined biologic and psychologic variables associated with fibromyalgia. However, relatively little attention has been devoted to the development of testable models of this disorder. Nevertheless, evidence is accumulating that suggests that genetic factors, in combination with abnormal peripheral and/or central pain mechanisms, are involved in the development of the widespread and chronic pain experienced by patients with fibromyalgia (3,123–126).

Genetic Factors

Several studies have examined the relationship between family history and pain experiences in community-based samples (127–129). All have shown that a family history of pain is associated with increased pain complaints among the respondents. Indeed, one of these studies revealed that the relationship is stronger for women than men (128). Similar findings recently have been produced in a small number of studies of persons with fibromyalgia.

Pellegrino and colleagues (124) performed the first study of familial aggregation in fibromyalgia. They reported that 52% of a group of fibromyalgia patients' first-degree relatives (71% of women and 35% of men) had findings consistent with fibromyalgia. Buskila and associates (130,131) reported similar findings. Moreover, these investigators reported that only the female relatives showed significantly lower pain threshold levels than male and female controls at both a subset of the ACR tender points and at a group of control points (131). In addition, female relatives of the fibromyalgia patients reported poorer health status than did the male relatives of the patients and the controls (132).

These findings suggest that a family history of pain may be a risk factor for the development of fibromyalgia. Most investigators have interpreted the data as indicating that there are strong environmental and behavioral contributors to the etiopathogenesis of fibromyalgia (91). However, both Pellegrino et al. (124) and Buskila et al. (131) have proposed that their findings indicate an autosomal-dominant genetic transmission of fibromyalgia. Indeed, Buskila and colleagues have suggested that this genetic factor may be sex-related, such that males show lower penetrance or milder expressivity. In response to these findings, Yunus and associates (92) recently studied 39 women with fibromyalgia who had at least one first-degree relative diagnosed with the same disorder. HLA typing revealed that the estimated HLA-specific risk to a female sibling of a woman with fibromyalgia was 1.22. While this value was statistically significant, the strength of the genetic linkage of fibromyalgia to the HLA region actually was quite modest. Thus, at present, it is premature to propose a substantial linkage of a fibromyalgia susceptibility gene to HLA in first-degree relatives of women with fibromyalgia.

Nevertheless, animal research suggests that there are important genetic influences on pain transmission and modulation that may be relevant to the familial aggregation of fibromyalgia among women (133). For example, several investigations have revealed a striking dependence of sex differences in pain sensitivity and pain modulation on the genetic background of the animal subjects (e.g., 134,135). A linkage mapping study revealed the presence of a sex-specific quantitative trait locus for nonopioid pain modulation produced by swim stress in two progenitor mouse strains (136). That is, a broad region of mouse chromosome 8 was identified that contains a gene(s) of major relevance to strain variability in this trait in female mice; the as yet unknown gene, however, was entirely irrelevant to that variability in male mice.

To summarize, then, both animal and human studies suggest that familial factors can significantly influence pain sensitivity, and this may be due in part to sex-related familial influences on pain transmission or pain modulation. No relationships have yet been identified between sex-related genetic influences on pain transmission or modulation and the higher prevalence of fibromyalgia in women compared to men. However, we believe it is quite likely that these relationships will be documented in the future.

Peripheral Mechanisms

Both patients and their health care providers tend to describe the pain of fibromyalgia as muscular in origin. It is not surprising, then, that a large number of investigators have attempted to identify abnormalities in the muscle tissue of patients with fibromyalgia that might account for their pain. For example, Bengtsson and colleagues (137,138) reported reductions in the levels of adenosine triphosphate (ATP) and phosphocreatine, as well as the appearance of ragged red fibers, in the tender areas of the trapezius muscle of patients with fibromyalgia. This may reflect the sequelae of continuous muscle microtrauma, which might contribute to the postexertional pain and other painful symptoms experienced by these patients (3). Other investigators have suggested that prolonged muscle tension and ischemia may account for the painful symptoms of fibromyalgia. For example, Lund et al. (139) found low levels of oxygenation in the tender points of the trapezius and brachioradial muscles of patients with fibromyalgia. Similarly, Bennett and colleagues (140) observed low blood flow in the muscles of patients with fibromyalgia during exercise compared to that of controls.

Despite these positive findings, no relationships have been found between muscle tension levels and pain in patients with fibromyalgia; moreover, electron microscopic evaluation of muscle biopsies has failed to reveal significant differences between tissue obtained from patients with fibromyalgia and healthy controls (141). One study of muscle tissue using immunohistochemical and molecular biologic methods revealed no differences between fibromyalgia patients and controls in neurochemicals involved in pain transmission and pain modulation such as substance P and serotonin (142).

Studies using ^{31}P nuclear magnetic resonance (NMR) spectroscopy have produced conflicting results. Initial investigations indicated that, although patients with fibromyalgia display reduced voluntary capacity for work, their biochemical response to work and recovery is normal (143–147). In contrast, Park and colleagues (148) recently showed that fibromyalgia patients, compared to controls, show significantly lower phosphorylation potential and total oxidative capacity in the quadriceps muscle during rest and exercise. Patients also display significantly lower levels of phosphocreatine and ATP, as well as a lower phosphocreatine/inorganic phosphate ratio in this muscle at rest. This represents the first strong evidence of metabolic abnormalities in muscle tissue that may contribute to the fatigue and weakness associated with fibromyalgia.

In summary, there is conflicting evidence regarding the role of muscle tissue abnormalities in the development of painful fibromyalgia symptoms. Nevertheless, investigators are continuing to examine the possibility that such abnormalities are involved in the etiopathogenesis of fibromyalgia.

Central Mechanisms

Numerous studies have shown that patients with fibromyalgia display generalized tenderness in response to pressure stimulation of both tender points in muscle tissue and a wide array of control points such as the mid-ulna, mid-tibia, and the thumb nail (4,9–11,27,28,149,150). These patients also show relatively low pain thresholds and tolerance levels in response to thermal and electrocutaneous stimulation, respectively (151,152). Moreover, counterstimulation produces pain inhibition among pain-free controls but not in patients with fibromyalgia (153,154). These findings suggest that the abnormalities in muscle tissue alone cannot account for the painful symptoms of fibromyalgia. Thus, attention has been directed to the identification of central mechanisms that distinguish patients with fibromyalgia from healthy persons.

NONRESTORATIVE SLEEP

Moldofsky and his colleagues (30) were the first to observe an abnormal pattern in the electroencephalographic (EEG) recordings of patients with fibromyalgia during deep sleep. This abnormal pattern, termed the alpha EEG nonrapid eye movement (NREM) anomaly, is characterized by a relatively fast frequency alpha EEG wave superimposed on a slower frequency delta EEG (30). The same investigators also demonstrated that when the alpha EEG NREM sleep anomaly was induced by slow wave sleep deprivation among healthy male volunteers, they exhibited increased tenderness in response to dolorimeter stimulation.

Although these investigators have replicated their finding, they also have found that it is not specific for patients with fibromyalgia (155,156). Moreover, an independent study of 22 patients with fibromyalgia found that only 36% exhibited the alpha EEG NREM sleep anomaly (157). Independent laboratory studies have not consistently shown that it is possible to induce muscle tenderness in healthy persons through slow wave sleep deprivation (158,159). However, it should be noted that the successful replication study (159) used middle-aged women, rather than the young men employed in studies with negative findings (158). Following three nights of slow wave sleep deprivation, these women reported increased fatigue and discomfort and displayed lower pain thresholds as well as increased flare response to mechanical stimulation (159). These findings suggest that slow wave sleep disruption may contribute to the development of fibromyalgia symptoms, although the sleep disturbance is not necessary for the syndrome to occur.

Regardless of the exact role of slow wave sleep disruption in the etiopathogenesis of fibromyalgia, studies indicate that there are important clinical sequelae associated with the sleep disturbance. For example, there is evidence that disordered sleep in patients with fibromyalgia is associated with slowed speed of performance on complex cognitive tasks as well as fatigue and negative mood (160). In addition, an intensive longitudinal investigation revealed that, among fibromyalgia patients, a night of poor sleep is followed by increased pain ratings and increased attention to pain on the following day (161).

Thus, poor sleep among fibromyalgia patients may contribute to the hypervigilance for abnormal somatic perceptions that has been documented in this population (162).

NEUROENDOCRINE ABNORMALITIES

Several laboratories have reported evidence that fibromyalgia is associated with a neuroendocrine disorder characterized by abnormal function of the hypothalamic-pituitary-adrenal (HPA) axis (163–166). McCain and Tilbe (163) first reported that patients with fibromyalgia showed reduced 24-hour, urinary free cortisol excretion as well as a loss of circadian fluctuation of glucocorticoid levels. Subsequently, two independent groups led by Crofford (164) and Griep (165) found that, following challenge with corticotropin-releasing hormone (CRH), fibromyalgia patients display exaggerated release of adrenocorticotropic hormone (ACTH) as well as a blunted cortisol response. The most recent study of HPA axis function showed normal, 24-hour, urinary free cortisol levels and normal cortisol response to ACTH infusion in patients with fibromyalgia (166). However, these patients, compared to controls, exhibited impairments in hypothalamic-pituitary and sympathoadrenal responses to stepped hypoglycemic challenge. Abnormalities in autonomic nervous system function also have been documented in studies of 24-hour heart rate variability (167) and response to orthostatic stress (168) in fibromyalgia patients.

In addition to the abnormalities described above, there is evidence of dysregulation of the hypothalamic-pituitary-thyroid (HPT) axis and the growth hormone axis in patients with fibromyalgia. For example, it has been shown that these patients display blunted secretion of thyroid-stimulating hormone and thyroid hormones in response to thyrotropin-releasing hormone, suggestive of a blunted pituitary response (169). Several investigators have documented changes in the growth hormone axis among fibromyalgia patients. Growth hormone, which is involved in muscle homeostasis, is maximally secreted during stage 4 of REM sleep. Bennett et al. (170) hypothesized that slow wave sleep abnormalities could disrupt the secretion of growth hormone and indirectly confirmed this by documenting low levels of insulin-like growth factor I (IGF-I) in patients with fibromyalgia (170). Moreover, growth hormone injections, compared to placebo, produce significant improvements among fibromyalgia patients in tender point scores and functional ability ratings, as well as sustained increases in IGF-I levels (171). The clinical significance of growth hormone deficiency is that it may contribute to poor healing of muscle microtrauma and thereby to prolonged nociceptive transmission by its influence on muscle metabolism (172,173). These findings, taken together with those described earlier regarding the HPA axis, suggest that in fibromyalgia, the pituitary release patterns of ACTH, thyroid-stimulating hormone, and growth hormone are altered substantially. The subsequent abnormalities in hormone levels (e.g., cortisol, IGF-I) may contribute to the pain, weakness, and fatigue experienced by patients with fibromyalgia. This evidence and that produced by the other studies reviewed above suggest that patients with fibromyalgia are characterized by multiple abnormalities of the neuroendocrine axes and the autonomic nervous system.

NEUROPEPTIDE ABNORMALITIES

Studies of neuropeptide levels in fibromyalgia patients and controls produced the earliest evidence of abnormal pain modulation functions. Russell and colleagues (174,175) performed a series of studies in which they found that, relative to healthy controls, patients with fibromyalgia are characterized by low blood serum levels of serotonin (174,175) and low CSF levels of the serotonin metabolite 5-hydroxyindole acetic acid (5-HIAA) (176). Similar findings have been reported by

Yunus and his associates (177). One report documented significantly higher binding of ^{3}H-imipramine among patients with fibromyalgia compared to controls (174). Moreover, the difference in ^{3}H-imipramine binding was eliminated following treatment of patients with alprazolam and ibuprofen. The reduction in ^{3}H-imipramine binding among the patients with fibromyalgia was significantly associated with reductions in their tender point index scores and in physician ratings of the patients' disease severity (174). The finding of high levels of ^{3}H-imipramine binding among patients with fibromyalgia has not been replicated consistently (178). Nevertheless, deficiencies of serotonin in blood plasma and low CSF levels of 5-HIAA may contribute to the sleep disturbance and abnormal pain sensitivity exhibited by patients with fibromyalgia.

Vaerøy and his associates (179) were the first to demonstrate that patients with fibromyalgia are characterized by significantly higher CSF levels of substance P than healthy controls. This finding has been replicated in independent samples of patients with fibromyalgia (180,181) and in a sample of community residents with fibromyalgia who had not sought medical care for their pain (181). Moreover, there is preliminary evidence that, unlike patients with fibromyalgia, patients with chronic fatigue syndrome exhibit CSF levels of substance P within the normal range (182). Thus, abnormal substance P levels may represent a biologic marker that distinguishes persons with fibromyalgia from those with chronic fatigue syndrome despite the symptoms shared by these disorders.

Recent data suggest that stress may perturbate the nociceptive effects of substance P release in persons with fibromyalgia. It has been shown that activation of the central nervous system (CNS) by stress stimulates mammotroph cells in the anterior pituitary to secrete prolactin and nerve growth factor (183). Consistent with these findings, patients with primary fibromyalgia are characterized by elevated CSF levels of nerve growth factor (71). Given that nerve growth factor regulates substance P expression in sensory nerves and may inhibit the antinociceptive effects of substance P metabolites (184), it is possible that stress may contribute in part to enhanced pain sensitivity in persons with fibromyalgia through its effects on nerve growth factor as well as its effects on HPA axis function.

There also is evidence that patients with fibromyalgia exhibit elevated CSF levels of dynorphin A (185) and calcitonin gene-related peptide (186), although the latter finding has not been replicated (187). Elevated levels of these neuropeptides and substance P are consistent with changes in CNS function that have been observed after tissue injury. Under these circumstances, a series of events can occur that produce allodynia, a phenomenon by which formerly innocuous stimuli such as light touch or mild heat are perceived as painful (188). One event is that new axon sprouts that are sensitive to stimulation often develop in the injured area of tissue. Spontaneous firings of these damaged nerves, as well as from the dorsal horn ganglion, increase the neuronal barrage into the CNS and contribute to the perception of pain. Similarly, spinal dorsal horn neurons also show increased excitability after injury, which is characterized by an enlargement of their peripheral receptive fields and greater responsiveness to mechanical, thermal, and chemical stimuli. This process of *central sensitization*, which also leads to increased neuronal input, is mediated by the activation of neurons through *N*-methyl-D-aspartate (NMDA) receptor sites by excitatory amino acids and is enhanced by neuropeptides such as dynorphin, substance P, and calcitonin gene-related peptide (188). There currently is no direct evidence of functional changes in peripheral or spinal dorsal horn neurons in patients with fibromyalgia. However, several laboratory studies of behavioral responses to noxious stimulation have shown that these patients display abnormal pain sensitivity consistent with the neuronal changes described above (189,190).

FUNCTIONAL BRAIN ACTIVITY ABNORMALITIES

Our laboratory has produced evidence that abnormalities occur in the functional activity of brain structures involved in pain perception as well as in neuropeptide levels among persons with fibromyalgia. We initially used single photo emission computed tomography (SPECT) imaging of resting state levels of regional cerebral blood flow (rCBF) in ten patients with fibromyalgia and seven healthy controls (149) (Fig 90.2). Our semiquantitated measures of rCBF reflect

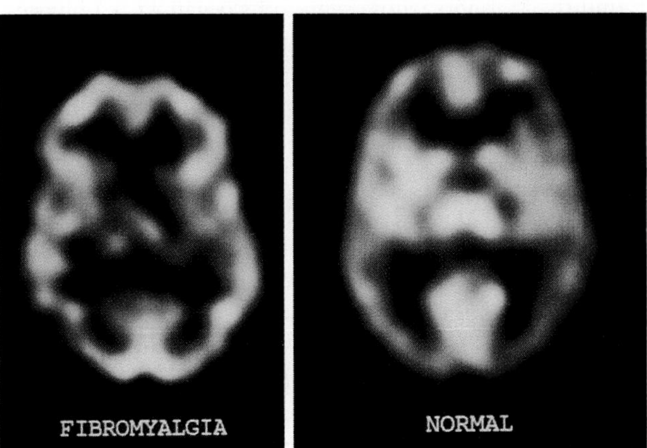

FIGURE 90.2. Single sections from single photon emission computed tomography (SPECT) brain scans, using ^{99m}technetium-hexamethylpropylene-amine oxime (^{99m}Tc-HMPAO), of a normal control subject and a patient with fibromyalgia. The section from the control subject shows normal cerebral perfusion, with clear visualization of the caudate head nuclei and thalami. This is contrasted to the regional cerebral blood flow seen in the scan of the fibromyalgia patient, which shows decreased tracer uptake in the caudate head nuclei and thalami. (From Mountz JM, Bradley LA, Modell JG, et al. Fibromyalgia in women: abnormalities of regional cerebral blood flow in the thalamus and caudate nucleus are associated with low pain threshold levels. *Arthritis Rheum* 1995;38:926–938, with permission.)

TABLE 90.2. MEAN (± SEM) REGIONAL CEREBRAL BLOOD FLOW (rCBF) IN THE THALAMUS AND CAUDATE NUCLEUS OF PATIENTS WITH FIBROMYALGIA (FM) AND HEALTHY CONTROLS

Location of rCBF Measurement	FM Patients (n = 10)	Healthy Controls (n = 7)	P Value
Right thalamus*	0.84 ± 0.04	1.05 ± 0.03	0.003
Left thalamus†	0.87 ± 0.05	1.04 ± 0.03	0.01
Right caudate‡	0.77 ± 0.03	0.88 ± 0.02	0.02
Left caudate**	0.77 ± 0.04	0.90 ± 0.02	0.01

*t = 3.76; †t = 3.04; ‡t = 2.60; **t = 2.97.
From Mountz JM, Bradley LA, Modell JG, et al. Fibromyalgia in women: abnormalities of regional cerebral blood flow in the thalamus and caudate nucleus are associated with low pain threshold levels. *Arthritis Rheum* 1995;38:926–938, with permission.

synaptic activity levels in specific brain structures. We found that patients, compared to controls, are characterized by significantly lower rCBF levels in the thalamus and caudate nucleus (Table 90.2). The thalamus is known to play an important role in the integration of pain signals as well as in the generation of signals that regulate HPA axis activity, whereas the caudate nucleus contains a large number of nociceptive-specific and wide-dynamic-range neurons that are involved in signaling the occurrence of noxious events (191–194). Additionally, electrical stimulation of the caudate nucleus produces analgesic effects (195,196).

Our finding of diminished rCBF in the thalamus and caudate nucleus have been replicated by two independent groups of investigators in Australia and Finland (197,198). We also replicated the finding in an independent group of fibromyalgia patients in our laboratory (181). However, we found that patients whose symptoms began with a physical trauma showed abnormal rCBF only in the thalamus, while those whose symptoms had an insidious onset were characterized by thalamic and caudate abnormalities (181). It should be noted that these abnormalities in resting state blood flow are not specific to fibromyalgia. Low thalamic rCBF levels also have been found in patients with posttraumatic neuropathic pain (199) and metastatic cancer pain (200). Abnormally low rCBF levels in the caudate nucleus have been documented in patients with pain related to spinal cord injury (201) and restless leg syndrome (202). Although the cause of thalamic and caudate abnormalities in rCBF is not known, it has been suggested that inhibition of thalamic activity may occur as a response to prolonged, excitatory nociceptive input (199). Indeed, we have proposed that the thalamic and caudate abnormalities in persons with fibromyalgia may be a marker for the presence of central sensitization (188,203). Over time, the modulatory actions of these structures in nociceptive transmission become compromised, thereby contributing to the abnormal pain sensitivity exhibited by persons with fibromyalgia.

If these premises were valid, one would expect that persons with fibromyalgia would show abnormal changes in rCBF in the thalamus and other structures involved in pain processing during exposure to acute, painful stimuli. It should be noted that normal individuals respond to painful phasic stimulation with increases in rCBF in the contralateral thalamus, anterior cingulate (AC) cortex, primary and secondary somatosensory (SS) cortices, and the insula (204–207). Moreover, as stimulus and perceived pain intensity increases, bilateral activation occurs in the thalamus, AC cortex, secondary SS cortex, and insula, as well as in the putamen and cerebellum (208). However, preliminary findings in our laboratory indicate that fibromyalgia patients with an insidious onset of pain show a different pattern of brain activation than healthy controls during exposure to phasic, right-side, painful stimulation that was calibrated to subjects' pain threshold levels. That is, controls showed significant increases in rCBF in the left SS cortex and left thalamus, whereas patients displayed significant activation of the left and right SS cortices and the right AC cortex. In addition, the patients' intensity ratings of the stimulation were twice as great as those of the controls, despite the fact that patients received significantly lower levels of stimulation than did the controls (209). None of the differences between patients and controls could be attributed to the confounding influence of depression, as the patients had been screened prior to study with structured psychiatric interviews to rule out the presence of depressive disorders.

We have not yet attempted to replicate these findings in fibromyalgia patients with histories of physical trauma prior to pain onset. Nevertheless, our studies of functional brain activity suggest that abnormal pain sensitivity in fibromyalgia is associated with abnormal brain rCBF during resting conditions as well as during exposure to acute pain in the laboratory. The rCBF abnormalities during acute pain are particularly interesting as they indicate that patients show bilateral activation of the SS cortices and produce high pain ratings during exposure to relatively low levels of noxious stimulation. In addition, the activation of the right SS cortex and AC cortex shown by the patients in response to right-sided stimulation is similar to the brain activation abnormalities displayed by patients with neuropathic pain and cluster headaches (210,211). Moreover, this finding is consistent with recent evidence that increased right frontal brain activity might be a biologic marker for abnormal pain sensitivity (210–212). It is necessary to determine, however, whether patients with fibromyalgia also show activation in the ipsilateral SS cortex and AC cortex during exposure to left-sided, painful stimulation.

PSYCHOLOGIC DISTRESS AND PSYCHIATRIC MORBIDITY

It is generally agreed that a large number of patients with fibromyalgia who obtain treatment at tertiary care centers or rheumatology specialty clinics display high levels of psychologic distress. This observation and the absence of a specific pathophysiologic mechanism underlying the symptoms of fibromyalgia have led some investigators to regard the disorder as psychologic in origin (88,213). A large number of studies have been performed in an attempt to better understand the relationship between psychologic distress and fibromyalgia.

Early studies of psychologic distress in fibromyalgia patients relied upon self-report measures such as the Minnesota Multiphasic Personality Inventory (MMPI). Wolfe and colleagues (214) found that the frequency of normal MMPI profiles among patients with primary fibromyalgia and patients with RA was 28% and 60%, respectively. Additionally, fibromyalgia patients exhibited significant elevations on the anxiety and depression scales of the Arthritis Impact Measurement Scales (AIMS). Similar findings were reported in MMPI studies of patients with fibromyalgia and RA conducted by Ahles and associates (215) and by Payne and associates (216).

It is possible, however, that the high levels of psychologic distress among fibromyalgia patients might be attributable to some unique characteristic of the MMPI. It has been shown, for example, that three MMPI scales (hypochondriasis, depression, and hysteria) are contaminated by items that focus on somatic symptoms (217,218). Additionally, it has been shown that patients with chronic pain may record elevated scores on the MMPI schizophrenia scale because several of its items refer to unusual somatic symptoms without an apparent underlying cause (219). Thus, patients with fibromyalgia might produce significantly higher MMPI scores than patients with RA due to a tendency to report a greater number of somatic symptoms than RA patients. It has been shown, however, that patients with fibromyalgia also record significantly higher scores than patients with RA on the Basic Personality Inventory (220) and the Hamilton Rating Scale for depression (213). In contrast, Ahles et al. (221) found that patients with fibromyalgia and those with RA did not differ from one another on the Zung Self-Rating Depression scale. Birnie and associates (222) also reported that patients with fibromyalgia and those with other chronic pain syndromes could not be distinguished on the hostility, anxiety, and depression scales of the Symptom Checklist-90 Revised (SCL-90-R) Scales. These studies suggest that, relative to patients with RA, patients with fibromyalgia generally report higher levels of psychologic distress, but this apparent difference in psychologic distress may, in part, reflect differences in reports of somatic symptoms.

It has been suggested that structured psychiatric interviews are superior to self-report measures in the psychologic evaluation of medical patients because these interviews may identify specific psychiatric illnesses that can be effectively treated with medication (223). Reductions in the symptoms of psychiatric disorders may then produce improvements in pain and disability. Hudson and colleagues have performed two studies in which patients with fibromyalgia were administered either the Diagnostic Interview Schedule (DIS) (213) or the Structured Clinical Interview (SCID-III-R) for the *Diagnostic and Statistical Manual of Mental Disorders*, third edition, revised (DSM-III-R) (224). In the former study, patients with fibromyalgia more frequently met DIS criteria for lifetime diagnoses of major depression and anxiety disorders than patients with RA. The patients with fibromyalgia also were characterized by high familial prevalence of major affective disorders. It was suggested that fibromyalgia might be a form of major affective disorder or that this psychiatric illness may predispose some individuals to develop fibromyalgia. The latter investigation involving the SCID-III-R also found high rates of lifetime psychiatric diagnoses of major depression and panic disorder as well as high familial rates of major affective disorders in an independent group of patients with fibromyalgia. Additionally, the patients were characterized by high frequencies of migraine headaches, irritable bowel syndrome, and chronic fatigue. It was suggested that fibromyalgia, major affective disorders, panic disorder, and irritable bowel syndrome might represent a family of related conditions, i.e., affective spectrum disorder, that share a common pathophysiology (224,225).

It should be noted that there are two groups of studies that do not support the findings described above. With regard to the responses of fibromyalgia patients to self-report measures, it has been shown that perceptions of environmental stress, as assessed by the Daily Hassles Scale, are significantly correlated with reports of psychologic distress on the AIMS (226) and on the SCL-90-R Scales (227). Indeed, Uveges and colleagues (227) demonstrated that the differences between patients with fibromyalgia and RA on the anxiety and paranoid ideation scales of the SCL-90-R were eliminated after controlling for group differences in daily hassles scores. Similarly, Aaron and colleagues (26) have shown that differences between patients with fibromyalgia and healthy controls on the Trait Anxiety Inventory and the Center for Epidemiological Studies–Depression Scale were eliminated after controlling for group differences in pain threshold levels and fatigue. Thus, the high levels of psychologic distress reported by fibromyalgia patients on questionnaires and inventories are associated with their physical symptoms and perceptions of environmental stress.

The findings described above cannot account for the high frequencies of psychiatric diagnoses found among patients with fibromyalgia. Two groups of investigators have produced evidence that psychologic distress and psychiatric diagnoses are found primarily among persons with fibromyalgia who seek medical care at tertiary care centers. Clark and colleagues (228) administered the SCL-90-R, Beck Depression Inventory, and the State-Trait Anxiety Inventory to individuals attending a general medical clinic who met research criteria for fibromyalgia but who were not seeking treatment for their pain. There were no differences on these measures between those individuals with fibromyalgia and a group of healthy controls that were administered the same self-report measures of psychologic distress.

Our research group evaluated the frequencies of lifetime psychiatric diagnoses in three groups of individuals using a computerized version of the DIS (26). These groups were (a) patients who met the ACR criteria for fibromyalgia, recruited from our university-based rheumatology clinics; (b) community residents (nonpatients) who also met ACR criteria for fibromyalgia but who had not sought treatment for their pain within the past 10 years; and (c) healthy community residents without any pain (controls). We found that patients with fibromyalgia met criteria for a significantly greater number of lifetime psychiatric diagnoses than either the nonpatients or the healthy controls (Fig. 90.3). Similar to the findings of Hudson and colleagues (213,225), patients with fibromyalgia reported very high rates of major mood disorders, such as major depressive episodes, and anxiety disorders, such as panic disorder with agoraphobia. Moreover, we found no difference in psychiatric morbidity between subjects with fibromyalgia who had not sought treatment and healthy controls. These findings strongly suggest that high levels of psychologic distress and psychiatric morbidity are found chiefly among individuals who seek health care for their fibromyalgia symptoms at tertiary care centers. Psychologic factors, therefore, may contribute to the decision of individuals to seek specialized health care for their fibromyalgia symptoms, but not to the etiopathogenesis of fibromyalgia. This conclusion is consistent with previous studies of persons with irritable bowel syndrome, which indicate that, after controlling for symptom severity, psychologic distress differentiates tertiary care patients from individuals with irritable bowel syndrome who do not seek treatment (229,230).

In addition to the evidence reviewed earlier, we have reported preliminary findings regarding the factors associated with health care seeking in a 30-month longitudinal study of 40 individuals with fibromyalgia who had not previously sought health care (231). We found that ten of these individuals eventually sought and obtained medical care (i.e., became patients) for their fibromyalgia symptoms during the 30-month study period. Those who became patients, relative to those who remained nonpatients, were more likely at baseline to report work-related stress, a psychiatric history of mood or substance abuse disorders, and use of prescription medication or medication for gastrointestinal disorders. However, the strongest predictor of seeking health care among these persons was the number of lifetime psychiatric diagnoses at baseline evaluation (232). The probability of not seeking care was 95% for individuals with no more than one psychiatric diagnosis, but 50% for those individuals with more than one diagnosis (Fig. 90.4).

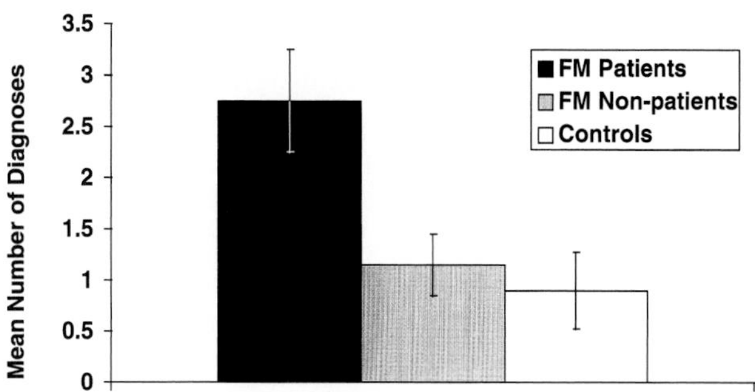

FIGURE 90.3. Mean [and standard error of the mean (SEM)] number of lifetime psychiatric diagnoses among patients with fibromyalgia (FM), community residents with fibromyalgia who had not sought treatment for their pain within the past 10 years (nonpatients), and healthy community residents without pain (controls). Patients met diagnostic criteria for a significantly greater number of psychiatric diagnoses than nonpatients and controls. Nonpatients did not differ from controls in psychiatric morbidity. (From Aaron LA, Bradley LA, Alarcón GS, et al. Psychiatric diagnoses are related to health care seeking behavior rather than illness in fibromyalgia. *Arthritis Rheum* 1996;39:436–445, with permission.)

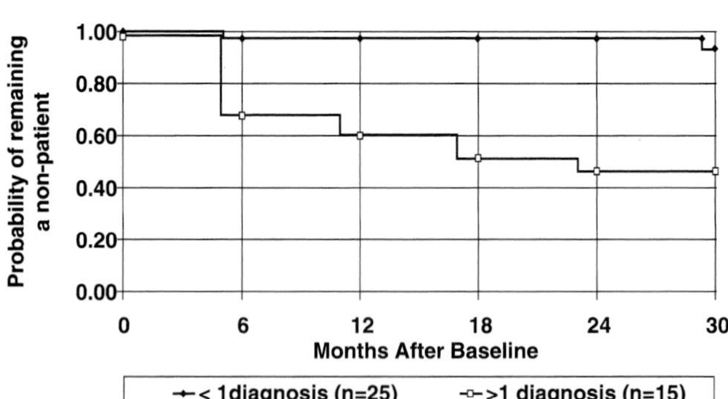

FIGURE 90.4. Probability of not seeking medical care for fibromyalgia symptoms (i.e., remaining a nonpatient) from baseline to 30-month follow-up evaluation as a function of baseline number of lifetime psychiatric diagnoses. Using a group of 40 persons with fibromyalgia, the probability of remaining a nonpatient was 95% for persons with no more than one psychiatric diagnosis. However, the probability was only 50% for persons with more than one diagnosis.

It should be noted that MacFarlane and colleagues (233) recently examined the relationship between psychiatric disorders, as measured by the General Health Questionnaire, and medical consultation in 88 men and 164 women community residents in the United Kingdom with chronic widespread pain and high levels of psychologic distress. Across all residents, there was no difference in the risk for psychiatric illness between those who sought medical consultation and those who did not. Among women, however, the risk of psychiatric illness among the consulters was more than twice that of the nonconsulters.

In summary, patients with fibromyalgia who are seen at tertiary care centers tend to display high levels of psychologic distress and histories of multiple psychiatric disorders during their lifetimes. Successful management of these patients may require a multidisciplinary approach involving psychologists, psychiatrists, and other health care professionals who are experienced in the management of persons with chronic pain (234). The abnormal pain perceptions and other symptoms of fibromyalgia cannot be attributed solely to psychiatric illness (26). However, we acknowledge that psychiatric illness and psychologic distress may enhance perceptions of pain intensity (88,162) and motivate persons with fibromyalgia to consult physicians for treatment.

FACTORS ASSOCIATED WITH SYMPTOM ONSET

Infectious Illness

As many as 55% of patients with fibromyalgia report that their symptoms began suddenly during or after a flu-like febrile illness (235). Additionally, fibromyalgia has been reported to occur after infection with coxsackievirus and parvovirus (75,236), as well as with human immunodeficiency virus (HIV) (237,238). Some patients may be diagnosed with fibromyalgia following the development of Lyme disease, suggesting an ongoing infection. However, many of these patients do not display improvement in their symptoms after appropriate antibiotic treatment for Lyme disease (73,74,239).

Several investigators have attempted to determine whether one or more immunologic abnormalities might be associated with fibromyalgia. However, the literature regarding these abnormalities consists primarily of exploratory studies rather than systematic series of investigations. Caro (240), for example, reported that 76% of patients with fibromyalgia had deposits of immunoglobulin G (IgG) at the dermoepidermal junction. Studies of other immunologic parameters in patients with fibromyalgia, such as the prevalence of ANA, generally have produced unreliable or inconclusive results (62,241,242). Other investigators have reported that patients with fibromyalgia, compared to healthy controls, are characterized by lower natural killer cell activity (243) and a decrease in T cells expressing activation markers (244). These findings may be due to the dependence of natural killer and T-cell activation on adequate levels of serotonin (245). Sprott and colleagues (246) observed collagen cuffs around the preterminal nerve fibers in skin samples obtained from the trapezius region in fibromyalgia patients. They suggested that these collagen cuffs, which might lower the firing thresholds of the nerves, may have been produced by remodeling of the extracellular matrix by injury-related stimulation of local nociceptors that, in turn, stimulated the release of proinflammatory cytokines [e.g., interleukin-1 (IL-I), IL-6] by macrophages. However, no investigators have attempted to test the validity of this hypothesis. In summary, there currently is not consistent evidence that fibromyalgia is directly related to a specific immunologic abnormality or infectious trigger.

Finally, Goldenberg (247) has suggested that infection may be one of several events that promote a maladaptive behavior pattern leading to the development of fibromyalgia. For example, highly anxious individuals with chronic infections such as Lyme disease may experience sleep disturbance and increased muscle tension levels and avoid physical activity. The stress associated with the chronically high levels of anxiety, in combination with sleep disturbance and physical reconditioning, may then lead to the neuroendocrine abnormalities described earlier in this chapter and thus contribute to the development of fibromyalgia.

Physical Trauma

Between 14% and 23% of patients with fibromyalgia report that their symptoms began following a physical injury or trauma such as surgery (79,80,247,248). It has been shown that physical injury may lead to alterations in C-fiber substance P levels and to the development of centrally mediated pain syndromes (249,250). However, a direct link between injury and chronic pain has not yet been demonstrated in patients with fibromyalgia.

Goldenberg (247) has posited that, similar to the association of fibromyalgia with infectious illness, physical injury or trauma among highly anxious persons may lead to development of fibromyalgia symptoms as a consequence of maladaptive behavior patterns. Indeed, it has been shown consistently that patients who develop fibromyalgia following physical injury are characterized by significantly higher levels of disability, inactivity, or financial compensation than patients without reactive fibromyalgia (80,82,89). For some patients, financial compensation actually may reinforce physical inactivity and other maladaptive behaviors and contribute to high levels of disability. For example, a meta-analytic study has shown that patients with chronic pain receiving financial compensation exhibit significantly poorer functional outcomes after treatment than patients without compensation (251). These data suggest that financial compensation may diminish the motivation of patients to change their behaviors or continue to reinforce pain complaints and maladaptive behaviors in spite of treatment. It is possible therefore, that physical injury contributes to the development of fibromyalgia both directly by means of changes in C-fiber substance P levels and, indirectly, through its association with financial compensation (249,251,252).

Emotional Trauma and Stress

It has been suggested that fibromyalgia is a stress-related disorder, similar to irritable bowel syndrome and chronic fatigue syndrome, because its symptoms are intensified by physical and emotional stress (253). Indeed, about 14% of patients who attend specialized rheumatology practices experience fibromyalgia symptoms after an emotionally traumatic event (247). We have shown that fibromyalgia patients with a history of sexual or physical abuse, compared to nonabused patients, report significantly higher levels of environmental stress, pain, fatigue, and functional disability (254). In addition, abused patients with fibromyalgia display a response bias toward perceiving a wide range of mechanical pressure stimuli as painful, regardless of their actual intensities (254). Studies from independent laboratories have suggested that the effects of abuse on pain and other physical symptoms are mediated by abnormalities in function of the HPA axis (255).

McBeth and colleagues (88) recently showed that reports of adverse childhood experiences, such as abuse, are associated with high tender point counts in community residents with high levels of psychologic distress. These investigators suggested, then, that adverse childhood experiences may contribute to the development of fibromyalgia. We acknowledge that this is possible in some individuals. However, we have found that community residents with fibromyalgia who have not sought medical care for pain do not differ from healthy controls in frequency of sexual or physical abuse histories (254). Thus, adverse childhood experiences do not appear to be necessary for the development of fibromyalgia.

ETIOPATHOGENETIC MODELS OF FIBROMYALGIA

A few investigators have proposed theoretic models for the etiopathogenesis of fibromyalgia on the basis of the studies reviewed earlier. Yunus (123) suggested that a complex interaction between central and peripheral factors was responsible for the high levels of pain and fatigue that characterize fibromyalgia (Fig. 90.5). Specifically, he suggested that genetically predisposed individuals who are exposed to viral infection or other stressors display neurohormonal dysfunction such as perturbed HPA axis activity. This neurohormonal dysfunction might lead to an aberrant central pain mechanism characterized by a functional deficiency of

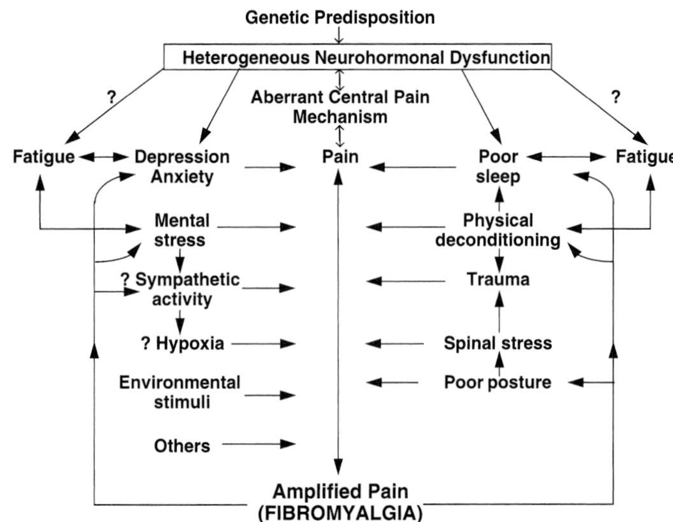

FIGURE 90.5. M. B. Yunus's model of central and peripheral mechanisms that may interact in persons with fibromyalgia leading to abnormal pain perception. Central factors are considered to be more important than peripheral factors in the development of pain and other symptoms of fibromyalgia. (From Yunus MB. Towards a model of pathophysiology of fibromyalgia: aberrant central pain mechanisms with peripheral modulation. *J Rheumatol* 1992;19:846–850, with permission.)

inhibitory neurotransmitters at the spinal or supraspinal levels (e.g., serotonin) or overactivity of excitatory neurotransmitters (e.g., substance P). A deficiency of serotonin and increased activity of substance P could account, in part, for abnormally low pain thresholds in persons with fibromyalgia (174,180). Another dimension of this aberrant central pain mechanism is the phenomenon of central sensitization described earlier (249).

Yunus's model also includes several other central and peripheral factors that may contribute to the pain and related symptoms of patients with fibromyalgia. Central factors include the alpha EEG NREM sleep anomaly described by Moldofsky et al. (30) and psychologic distress. The peripheral factors may include sympathetic overactivity, mechanical stress or trauma, physical deconditioning, and muscle microtrauma. Yunus, however, strongly suggests that central factors are most important in the development of fibromyalgia symptoms.

Bennett (3) also has proposed that fibromyalgia results from a complex interaction of central and peripheral factors. His model, however, suggests that pain in fibromyalgia is initiated by muscle microtrauma that occur at unusually low levels of physical exertion and do not heal normally. This muscle microtrauma may be attributed to genetic predisposition as well as to disruption of growth hormone secretion, blunted HPA axis function (163–166), the alpha

EEG NREM anomaly (30), or a regional pain syndrome (256). Bennett also posited a feedback loop in which the fatigue associated with the NREM sleep anomaly interacts with muscle pain; these factors together lead to physical inactivity and deconditioning, which also promote muscle microtrauma. The contribution of abnormalities in serotonin and substance P to enhanced perceptions of pain is also recognized. Indeed, Bennett (257) recently has emphasized the importance of central sensitization and other central nervous symptom abnormalities in the development of abnormal pain sensitivity in fibromyalgia (Fig. 90.6).

The authors' research group also has developed a model for the etiopathogenesis of abnormal pain sensitivity in fibromyalgia (Fig. 90.7) (203). This model, which includes elements of both the Yunus and Bennett proposals, emphasizes the role of central factors in fibromyalgia pain, including abnormal function of brain structures such as the thalamus and caudate nucleus. It posits that there is a genetic susceptibility to the development of abnormal pain sensitivity that involves the neuroendocrine axes, including the HPA axis, as well as specific structural defects in the musculoskeletal system and the CNS. Abnormal neuroendocrine and structural defects (e.g., following whiplash injury) (258) may produce enhanced nociceptive transmission from the peripheral nociceptors to the dorsal horns of the spinal cord. In addition, several environmental factors, such as physical trauma, stressful events, and infectious agents, may lead to high levels of nociceptive transmission to the dorsal horns by production of muscle microtrauma or release of nerve growth factor (NGF), which, in turn, regulates substance P expression in sensory nerves. However, we also proposed that the final common pathway for the actions of all of these precipitating factors is the process of central sensitization. Activation of neurons with NMDA receptor sites by excitatory amino acids and the release of substance P, calcitonin gene-related peptide, and dynorphin (259) lead to functional alterations in the dorsal horn spinal neurons that greatly increase nociceptive transmission to the brain. Based on our functional brain imaging studies and those of other investigators (e.g., 199), we suggested that increased nociceptive transmission eventually leads to functional alterations in the brain structures that are involved in modulating or processing the nociceptive input (e.g., thalamus, AC cortex). Moreover, there is a reciprocal interaction between brain limbic system structures (e.g., AC cortex) and the HPA axis such that alterations in the functioning of each of these systems may influence one another. Thus, the high level of perceived aversiveness of fibromyalgia pain, which is largely processed by brain limbic system functioning (260), may represent an emotional stressor that might contribute to and be influenced by the maintenance of HPA axis and related neuroendocrine abnormalities. The end points of all of these processes are the abnormal pain sensitivity and widespread persistent pain that characterize fibromyalgia. Moreover, even after these abnormalities in pain processing have been established, exposure to environmental stressors may heighten perceptions of pain-related affect due to increases in limbic system activity that alters functional activity in the AC cortex, prefrontal cortex, and the thalamus.

It should be noted that this model is consistent with Melzack's (125,126) revision of the gate control theory of pain transmission and modulation. The revised theory suggests that brain pathways linking the thalamus, cortex, and limbic system form a neuromatrix that generates patterns of neural activity. This pattern-generating mechanism underlies the awareness that one's body is distinct from the environment as well as perceptions of pain and pain behavior. Figure 90.8 shows that the function of the neuromatrix is influenced by multiple inputs including (a) endocrine,

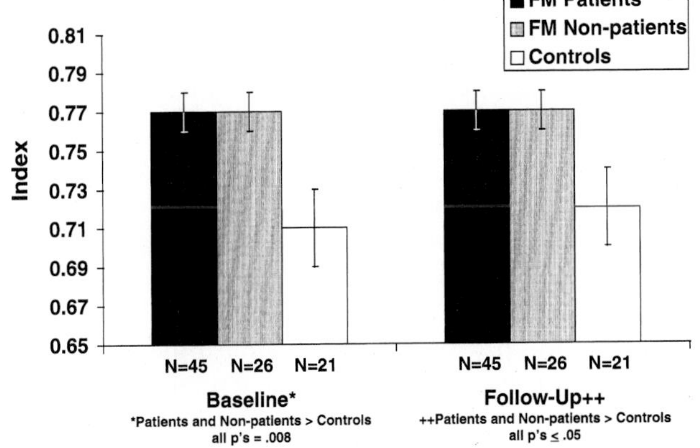

FIGURE 90.6. R. M. Bennett's model of central and peripheral mechanisms that may interact in persons with fibromyalgia leading to enhanced perceptions of pain. Muscle microtrauma is considered to be a key factor in the pain of fibromyalgia. (From Bennett RM. Fibromyalgia and the facts: sense or nonsense. *Rheum Dis Clin North Am* 1993;19: 45–59, with permission.)

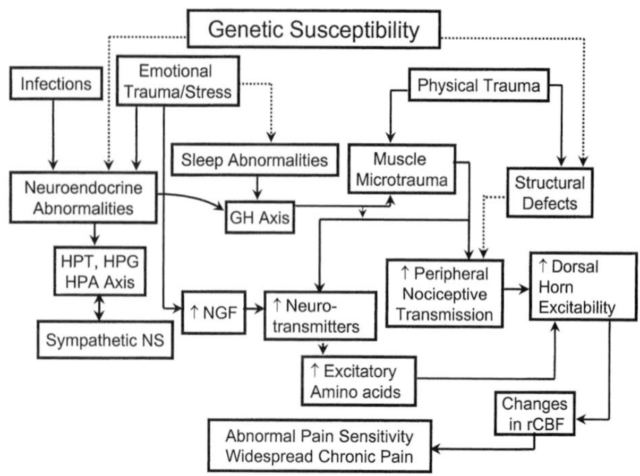

FIGURE 90.7. Authors' model of the etiopathogenesis of fibromyalgia. This model proposes that there may be a genetic susceptibility to the development of abnormal pain sensitivity that involves the neuroendocrine axes, as well as possible structural defects in the musculoskeletal system. Abnormal neuroendocrine activity and structural defects may produce enhanced nociceptive transmission from the peripheral nociceptors to the dorsal horns of the spinal cord. In addition, several environmental factors, such as physical trauma, stressful events, and infectious agents, may lead to high levels of nociceptive transmission to the dorsal horns by production of muscle microtrauma or release of nerve growth factor (NGF), which in turn regulates substance P expression in sensory nerves. However, the final common pathway for the actions of all of these precipitating factors is the process of central sensitization. Activation of neurons via *N*-methyl-D-aspartate (NMDA) receptor sites by excitatory amino acids, and the release of substance P, calcitonin gene-related peptide, and dynorphin leads to functional alterations in the dorsal horn spinal neurons that greatly increase nociceptive transmission to the brain. We posit that increased nociceptive transmission eventually leads to alterations in regional cerebral blood flow (rCBF) in the brain structures that are involved in modulating or processing the nociceptive input. The end points of all of these processes are the abnormal pain sensitivity and the widespread chronic pain that characterize fibromyalgia. *Solid lines* in this model represent established relationships and *dotted lines* represent relationships that are not yet well established. HPT, hypothalamic-pituitary-thyroid axis; HPG, hypothalamic-pituitary-gonadal axis; HPA, hypothalamic-pituitary-adrenal axis; GH, growth hormone; NS, nervous system; NGF, nerve growth factor.

immune, and autonomic system activity; (b) sources of afferent input (somatosensory, viscerosensory); (c) medullary descending inhibition; (d) pathologic input (e.g., from musculoskeletal defects; (e) CNS plasticity; (f) attention; and (g) psychosocial and health status factors (e.g., depression, anxiety). In addition, pain perception and pain behavior may influence one another through their effects on the inputs noted above. For example, coping strategies may influence attention and thus alter pain perception through effects on limbic system activity. Moreover, any factor (e.g., change in sex-related hormones, treatment interventions) that alter the function of the pain transmission or pain modulation pathways shown in our model and in the neuromatrix model may influence pain sensitivity.

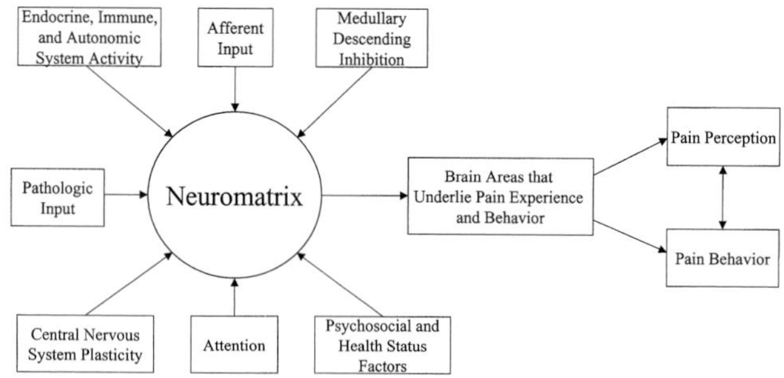

FIGURE 90.8. Model of the neuromatrix, which is a widespread network of brain neurons that generates patterns of activity responsible for perceptions of pain as well as reflexive and complex pain behaviors. The neuromatrix is influenced by multiple endogenous and exogenous factors. Pain perception and pain behavior may influence one another by altering the inputs to the neuromatrix. We propose that chronic pain syndromes, such as fibromyalgia, are produced by pathologic alterations in the nervous system and neuromatrix that cannot be restored to normal functioning.

NATURAL HISTORY OF FIBROMYALGIA

Although fibromyalgia often is considered to be a relatively benign disorder, this view is not supported by the few longitudinal studies that have been performed. For example, in a 5-year study of 56 Swedish patients with fibromyalgia, Henriksson (261) found that about one-half of the patients reported worsening of their symptoms, 20% reported improvement, and 30% experienced no change. Nørregaard and colleagues (262) performed a 4-year follow-up study of 91 Danish patients with fibromyalgia. Approximately 75% of the patients reported worsening of their symptoms, 10% reported improvement, and 15% reported their symptoms to be unchanged. Forseth and colleagues (263) from Norway studied a group of 214 women with self-reported musculoskeletal pain. Among them, there were 57 with chronic widespread pain (39 of whom met ACR criteria for fibromyalgia); 5½ years later 81 women had chronic widespread pain (71 of whom met ACR criteria for fibromyalgia). Eleven of the original 39 patients no longer fulfilled ACR criteria for fibromyalgia; based on these data, the authors concluded that chronic widespread pain and fibromyalgia portend a poor prognosis.

Three studies of the natural history of fibromyalgia have been performed in the United States (79,264,265). Each found that most patients' symptoms remained stable over periods ranging from 1 to 2 years. However, Granges and colleagues (266) reported conflicting findings in a group of 44 patients with fibromyalgia treated by community rheumatologists in Australia (266). Over a 2-year study, many of these patients no longer fulfilled the ACR criteria for fibromyalgia and 25% experienced a remission of their symptoms. With the exception of this study, the longitudinal studies indicate that the chronic pain and other symptoms of fibromyalgia change little over periods of 1 to 2 years.

Only a few investigators have examined the natural history of fibromyalgia in children (99,267,268). For example, Buskila and colleagues (99) followed 15 children with fibromyalgia over a 30-month period and found that 11 of the 15 no longer met criteria for fibromyalgia at the end of the study. Mikkelsson (268) in Finland reported similar data; he identified 22 children with fibromyalgia in a population-based study of 1,756 Finnish preadolescents. One year later, only 4 of the 16 children available for reexamination met criteria for the diagnosis of fibromyalgia (268).

In still another longitudinal study of children with fibromyalgia, a telephone interview was conducted at a mean of 2.6 years from the date of diagnosis in 33 of a total of 45 children initially diagnosed with fibromyalgia (267); improvement had occurred in the majority of these children. These three studies involved children who were not receiving medical care for their fibromyalgia symptoms; rather, they were identified as having fibromyalgia in a survey conducted among school-age children. Thus, these children were much like the adult nonpatients studied by both our research group (25,26) and Clark's group (120) who tend to suffer less severe symptoms than persons with fibromyalgia who are treated in tertiary care centers.

IMPACT OF FIBROMYALGIA

Despite the fact that patients with fibromyalgia do not experience any overt physical sequelae from this disorder, studies performed in different population groups have demonstrated that self-reported levels of pain and physical incapacitation in subjects afflicted with fibromyalgia are comparable to those reported by patients with RA (265,269,270). As a consequence, important functional losses (leisure/personal activities) as well as work disability are very likely to occur (98). In addition, and as already noted, patients with fibromyalgia tend to overutilize health care facilities with the corresponding cost (to themselves and to third party payers) (67). In fact, economic data for fibromyalgia are just emerging. White and colleagues (271) have reported data from the London Fibromyalgia Epidemiological Study (Ontario, Canada). Three subject groups were studied: subjects without pain, subjects with widespread pain not meeting ACR criteria for fibromyalgia, and a group of patients with fibromyalgia. A fourth healthy control group drawn from the Ontario Health Insurance Plan was also studied. Patients with fibromyalgia used outpatient health services and medications the most, and incurred twice the cost compared to both community and database health control groups (271). The economic burden of fibromyalgia has also been documented by other investigators around the world (67).

TREATMENT

The development of treatment interventions for patients with fibromyalgia has been hindered by the small amount of reliable data regarding the etiopathogenesis of this disorder. Nevertheless, several well-designed studies of treatment outcomes among patients with fibromyalgia have been published since 1986. These studies, which are reviewed next, may be classified into two broad categories: those that involve pharmacologic treatments and those that evaluate behavioral interventions.

Pharmacologic Interventions

Amitriptyline and Cyclobenzaprine

The first studies of pharmacologic interventions for fibromyalgia focused on the efficacy of amitriptyline and cyclobenzaprine. The use of these medications was based on the evidence that they tend to increase NREM stage IV sleep and the availability of brain serotonin as well as decrease muscle spasm (272). Amitriptyline is superior to placebo in decreasing patients' reports of pain intensity, sleep quality, and global symptom severity (Table 90.3) (273–275). Additionally, two of the three studies of amitriptyline show that this medication is associated with improvements in pain threshold or tender point counts (274,275).

Despite these promising results, some concerns have been raised regarding the long-term efficacy of amitriptyline. Goldenberg (272) surveyed each of the patients who participated in his study (275) 1 year after study termination. He reported that 69% of those patients who originally received amitriptyline were still taking this medication. However, as a group they showed substantial increases in their ratings of pain intensity, fatigue, sleep difficulty, and global symptom severity from posttreatment to the time of the survey. Thus, it appears that the efficacy of amitriptyline diminishes over time. This may be due to the tendency of tricyclic agents to suppress HPA axis function with long-term use (276).

The outcomes produced by cyclobenzaprine are similar to those produced by amitriptyline (Table 90.3) (277–280). Cyclobenzaprine appears to induce more consistent improvements in patients' ratings of sleep than in pain intensity, however. The findings reported by Carette and associates (279) raise some troubling issues concerning the efficacy of both cyclobenzaprine and amitriptyline. These investigators performed a large multicenter trial involving 208 patients with fibromyalgia that featured two methodologic advances. First, they evaluated outcome using measures of clinical improvement developed by Simms and colleagues (281) as well as conventional tests of statistical significance. Clinically significant improvement was recorded if at least four of the following criteria were met: (a) increase of 1 kg in total myalgic

TABLE 90.3. SUMMARY OF OUTCOMES PRODUCED BY AMITRIPTYLINE AND CYCLOBENZAPRINE

Study	Medication	Design	Number of Subjects	Significant Treatment Outcomes
Carette et al., 1986 (273)	50 mg amitriptyline vs. placebo	RCT	70	Improvements in patient ratings of pain, morning stiffness, sleep quality, and disease severity
Scudds et al., 1989 (274)	50 mg amitriptyline vs. placebo	Crossover	36	Improvements in patient ratings of pain and tender point pain thresholds
Goldenberg et al., 1986 (275)	25 mg amitriptyline, 1,000 mg naproxen vs. placebo	RCT	62	Only amitriptyline produced improvements in tender point count and patient ratings of pain, fatigue, morning tiredness, and global symptoms severity
Bennett et al., 1988 (277)	10–40 mg cyclobenzaprine vs. placebo	RCT	120	Improvements in patient ratings of pain and sleep quality as well as physician ratings of therapeutic response
Quimby et al., 1989 (278)	10–40 mg cyclobenzaprine vs. placebo	RCT	40	Improvements in patient ratings of sleep, stiffness, and aching as well as in physician global ratings
Carette et al., 1994 (279)	50 mg amitriptyline, 30 mg cyclobenzaprine vs. placebo	RCT	208	Both drugs superior to placebo at 1 month in producing clinically meaningful improvements; no group differences at posttreatment or 3-month follow-up due to improvements in all treatment conditions
Reynolds et al., 1991 (280)	20–40 mg cyclobenzaprine vs. placebo	Crossover	12	Improvements in patient ratings of evening fatigue and total sleep time; no effects on pain, mood, or tender point count

RCT, randomized controlled trial.

score; 50% change from baseline in patients' ratings of (b) sleep, (c) pain, (d) fatigue, and (e) global assessment; and (f) physician ratings of global assessment. The investigators also assessed outcomes at posttreatment and after a 3-month follow-up period. Both amitriptyline and cyclobenzaprine were significantly more effective in producing clinically meaningful outcomes than placebo after 1 month of treatment. Twenty-one percent of the amitriptyline-treated patients had improved compared to 12% of the patients treated with cyclobenzaprine and none of the patients who received placebo. However, patients in each group showed further improvements by the time of the 3-month follow-up assessment. At that time, 38% had improved with amitriptyline, 33% had improved with cyclobenzaprine, and 13% had improved with placebo.

In summary, the results of the outcome studies generally indicate that both amitriptyline and cyclobenzaprine are superior to placebo in producing subjective improvement in pain, sleep quality, and fatigue. These effects may appear within the first 4 weeks of treatment but they may diminish over extended periods of time. Only amitriptyline has been shown to reduce patients' tender point counts; no other directly observable measures of outcome have been assessed.

Other Psychotropic Medications

Anxiety and depression tend to amplify pain perception (125,126). Therefore, a number of antidepressants, anxiolytics, and psychotropic medications have been tried in patients with fibromyalgia in an effort to modify their symptoms. They include alprazolan, the selective serotonin reuptake inhibitors (SSRIs), and others (282–290). These drugs may moderate pain in patients with fibromyalgia who typically exhibit high levels of emotional distress (26). Alprazolam and ibuprofen together produce significantly greater reductions than placebo in the tender point index and patients' ratings of disease severity (Table 90.4) (282). Neither of these medications alone affected patients' responses on the outcome measures. It previously was shown that ibuprofen is not superior to placebo in reducing pain and tender point counts in patients with fibromyalgia (291). Thus, it appears that the coadministration of ibuprofen and alprazolam may have a synergistic effect on patient improvement. The effects of these medications have not been assessed longitudinally, however.

A great deal of interest has been generated in the use of SSRIs (283,285,288,292). This might be related to the central role that serotonin deficiency might play in the etiopathogenesis of fibromyalgia. It is surprising, then, that although fluoxetine and citalopram are associated with some positive effects on patients' ratings of depression and fatigue (283,288), they are not superior to placebo. It should be noted, however, that the citalopram study was confounded by the fact that patients were allowed to take medications such as codeine and acetaminophen during the trial (288). Additionally, there were a large number of dropouts in the fluoxetine trial (283).

TABLE 90.4. SUMMARY OF OUTCOMES PRODUCED BY ALPRAZOLAM AND SELECTIVE SEROTONIN REUPTAKE INHIBITORS

Study	Medication	Design	Number of Subjects	Significant Treatment Outcomes
Russell et al., 1991 (282)	0.5–3.0 mg alprazolam, and 2,400 mg ibuprofen vs. placebo	RCT	78	Alprazolam and ibuprofen together produced greater improvements than placebo in tender point index and patient ratings of disease severity
Wolfe et al., 1994 (283)	20 mg fluoxetine vs. placebo	RCT	42	No differences between fluoxetine and placebo; fluoxetine produced improvements in patient ratings of depression, fatigue, and sleep quality relative to baseline
Hannonen et al., 1998 (284)	450–600 mg moclobenide vs. 25–375 mg amitriptyline vs. placebo	RCT	130	54% of patients in moclobenide were responders vs. 49% in placebo and 74% in amitriptyline
Dwight et al., 1998 (285)	37.5 mg venlafaxine initially increased to a maximum of 375 mg	Open trial	15	Of 11 completers, six had ≥50% reduction in symptoms
Scharf et al., 1998 (286)	4.5 g (or slightly more) mg gamma-hydroxy-butyrate	Open trial	11	Improvement in pain, fatigue and in slow wave sleep; decrease in the severity of α sleep anomaly
Olin et al., 1998 (287)	10 mg ritanserin vs. placebo	RCT	51	Ritanserin-treated patience felt more refreshed and had less headaches; there were no differences between groups in pain, fatigue, sleep, morning stiffness, anxiety, and tender point count
Norregaard et al., 1995 (288)	20–40 mg citalopram vs. placebo	RCT	22	No differences between groups
Tavoni et al., 1987 (289)	200 mg SAMe vs. placebo	Crossover	17	Improvements in number of tender points and patient reports of depression in same group
Jacobsen et al., 1991 (290)	800 mg SAMe vs. placebo	RCT	44	Improvements in patient ratings of disease activity, pain, fatigue, morning stiffness, and mood; no effects on tender point score
Alberts et al., 1998 (292)	20 mg sertraline vs. placebo	RCT	14	Sertraline-treated patients showed increased pain thresholds at tender and control points and increased rCBF to the frontal regions relative to the placebo-treated patients

RCT, randomized controlled trial; SAMe, S-adenosylmethionene; rCBF, regional cerebral blood flow.

We have also conducted a small therapeutic blinded trial with sertraline hydrochloride (292). Patients received either sertraline hydrochloride or placebo for 3 months; they were evaluated prior to receiving treatment and at treatment termination, using self-report diaries of pain and mood as well as brain SPECT imaging of resting state rCBF levels. Patients in both the active drug and placebo conditions reported significant improvement from baseline to post-treatment in pain and mood. However, only the patients who received sertraline showed significant increases in pain thresholds at tender and control points as well as in rCBF in the right and left frontal cortices.

Another SSRI, venlafaxine (285), has been recently evaluated during an 8-week period in 15 patients with fibromyalgia who also had depression as determined by the structured clinical interview for axis 1 diagnoses from the DSM-IV. Of 11 completers, six had experienced a 50% or greater reduction of their fibromyalgia symptoms; the authors concluded that these patients improved because of the coexistence of depression. Whether or not this compound would benefit nondepressed patients with fibromyalgia was not investigated. Thus, it must be concluded that the effects of the SSRIs on fibromyalgia symptoms have not yet been adequately evaluated in clinical trials to date. SSRIs are, however, extensively used in the clinical setting, sometimes with very gratifying results.

Another antidepressant, moclobemide, a monoamine oxidase inhibitor, has recently been compared with amitriptyline in a 12-week study involving 130 women with fibromyalgia; no benefits from this compound were documented (284).

Another psychotropic, γ-hydroxybutyrate, has recently been investigated in a very small number of patients (286); it appears promising, but a double-blind study has not been done yet.

A different psychotropic, a long acting 5-hydroxytryptamine 2 (5-HT_2) receptor blocker (ritanserin) has been evaluated in a 16-week, double-blind study involving 51 women with fibromyalgia (287); 24 of the patients received ritanserin and 27 received placebo. At the end of the study, there were no differences between the study groups regarding pain, fatigue, anxiety, sleep, morning stiffness, and tender points; those patients receiving ritanserin, however, did significantly better in terms of feeling refreshed in the morning and in experiencing less severe headaches.

Two controlled trials performed in Europe have evaluated the effectiveness of S adenosylmethionine (SAMe) in patients with fibromyalgia (289,290). SAMe is a methyl donor that exerts antidepressant, antiinflammatory, and analgesic effects (290). This agent is available only by prescription in Europe, but it is not regulated in the United States. These two investigations demonstrated that SAMe is superior to placebo in producing improvement. The randomized controlled trial performed by Jacobsen and colleagues (290) suggested, however, that these effects are found only on patients' ratings of disease activity, pain, fatigue, and mood. The effect of SAMe on the tender point score was positive, but not superior to that of placebo. Moreover, it is not known whether the effects of SAMe are maintained during follow-up.

In summary, alprazolam, the SSRIs, other antidepressants, and other psychotropic agents have not been studied as intensively as amitriptyline and cyclobenzaprine. Nevertheless, regimens of SAMe as well as alprazolam combined with ibuprofen appear to be useful in the treatment of patients with fibromyalgia. It should be noted, however, that only the alprazolam and ibuprofen regimen reduces both the tender point index and patients' ratings of disease activity. Moreover, the long-term effects of these pharmacologic treatments have not been evaluated. Finally, limited studies of the SSRI medications, citalopram, fluoxetine, sertraline hydrochloride, and venlafaxine have produced variable results.

Other Pharmacologic Compounds

Generalists and specialists alike use numerous other agents for the treatment of patients with fibromyalgia (67). For the most part these compounds are used in an effort to modify the musculoskeletal manifestations of pain and stiffness, which can be quite devastating in some patients. These compounds can be divided into nonsteroidal antiinflammatory agents, nonnarcotic and narcotic analgesics, muscle relaxants, and miscellaneous.

Nonsteroidal Antiinflammatory Agents

These agents are prescribed for patients with fibromyalgia by a large proportion of practitioners as documented by Wolfe et al. (67). At antiinflammatory doses, these compounds are probably unnecessary since there is not a demonstrable component of inflammation in the painful musculoskeletal structures. They may be indicated for their antiinflammatory effect in specific situations such as in children and young adults with joint hypermobility who are likely to traumatize their muscles, joints, and tendons or when a superimposed regional pain syndrome (e.g., bicipital tendinitis) is present; in both situations these compounds should be used for a limited time rather than indefinitely.

Nonnarcotic Analgesics

The use of nonsteroidal antiinflammatory agents at analgesic doses may be supported by the study of the concomitant use of alprazolam and ibuprofen, as described. It should be remembered, however, that even at relatively small doses, the traditional nonsteroidal antiinflammatory agents [nonselective COX inhibitors] might produce significant renal and gastrointestinal side effects. The newer nonsteroidal compounds (primarily COX-2 specific inhibitors) have been approved for the treatment of acute, but not chronic, painful disorders; in theory at least, they are less likely to produce severe gastrointestinal side effects (renal side effects may still occur, however). Nevertheless, these compounds are being used at both antiinflammatory and analgesic doses in fibromyalgia, although there are no clinical trial data supporting such practice. Cost should be an important consideration when prescribing nonnarcotic analgesics. The currently available COX-2 inhibitors (celecoxobid and roxicobid in the United States) are much more expensive than plain analgesics such as acetaminophen.

Narcotic Analgesics

In our view and that of others, these compounds do not have a significant role in the treatment of patients with fibromyalgia (293). We are cognizant that some practitioners may advocate their use. Our clinical experience suggests, however, that patients with fibromyalgia do not significantly benefit from them. Moreover, once these compounds are started, they may be needed for life. Very few patients who are started on narcotics are able to discontinue them; although frank dose-escalation or class-progression may not be common, it does occur. Narcotic-like compounds such as tramadol have been proposed for the treatment of fibromyalgia (294); in fact, tramadol is being used by a significant proportion of fibromyalgia patients (257). These compounds' benefit may be quite limited, and their cost too high for them to be used other than on a short-term basis.

Muscle Relaxants

A number of compounds including carisoprodol, metaxalone, cyclobenzaprine, and others are approved for their short-term use as muscle relaxants. As already noted, only cyclobenzaprine has been formally tested in patients with fibromyalgia, with not very impressive long-term results. Nevertheless, fibromyalgia patients commonly receive these compounds for long periods of time with questionable beneficial effects.

Hormones

Two hormones, growth hormone (171) and calcitonin (295), have been tested in fibromyalgia. Whereas the preliminary data regarding growth hormone appears promising (but very expensive), the calcitonin trial produced negative data.

Gabapentin

Data on gabapentin have yet to be generated in patients with fibromyalgia, although the compound appears efficacious in some painful, difficult to treat, chronic conditions such as postherpetic neuralgia (296).

META-ANALYSIS OF PHARMACOLOGIC INTERVENTIONS

Rossy and colleagues (297) recently performed a literature meta-analysis regarding treatment interventions for patients with fibromyalgia. They evaluated 16 studies containing separate active drug and placebo groups and 17 trials with designs that included either (a) one-group, active drug or (b) crossover designs. It was found that, overall, antidepressant medications produced significant reductions in measures of fibromyalgia symptoms (e.g., self-reports of pain), and muscle relaxants produced significant reductions in measures of symptoms and physical status (e.g., tender point counts). However, only 4 of the 16 studies with separate active drug and placebo groups reported significant effects on outcome measures, whereas 13 of 17 studies with crossover or one-group designs produced significant improvements in these measures. Thus, the positive effects of pharmacologic interventions were observed primarily in studies with relatively weak experimental designs.

NONTRADITIONAL THERAPIES

Patients with fibromyalgia frequently seek treatments other than those provided by traditional health care providers. Indeed, one survey performed in Canada revealed that 91% of patients attending a university-based rheumatology clinic or a community-based private rheumatology practice reported using alternative treatments (298). Patients most frequently used over-the-counter products such as creams and rubs (50%) and vitamins (35%), spiritual practices such as prayers (41%) and meditation (38%), nonmedical practitioners such as chiropractors (19%) and massage therapists (10%), and dietary modifications (26%). The potential benefits of these and multiple other therapies are broadly proclaimed on the World Wide Web. However, these claims, which often are made by the treatment providers or manufacturers, should be viewed with great caution since the peer-review process usually has not been used to evaluate such information; in fact, very few data on alternative therapies have been published to date in conventional scientific sources. Dykman and colleagues (299), for example, have reported the beneficial effects of nutritional supplemental therapies (aloe vera gel extracts, plant-derived saccharides, freeze-dried fruits and vegetables); these data have been generated by the company producing these supplements and gathered by interviewing consumers of these products who had a physician diagnosis of fibromyalgia. Thus, the benefits of most alternative therapies have not been shown to be greater than those produce by credible placebos.

Behavioral Interventions

Aerobic Exercise

Interest in the therapeutic efficacy of aerobic exercise in patients with fibromyalgia began with the report by Bennett and colleagues (140) that 80% to 84% of a group of fibromyalgia patients fell below the average level of physical fitness established by the American Heart Association (300) and the Cooper Clinic Profiles (301). McCain and associates (302) compared the outcomes produced by a 20-week cardiovascular fitness training program with those produced by training in flexibility exercises (Table 90.5). It was found that cardiovascular fitness is superior to flexibility training in producing improvements in cardiovascular fitness indices, pain threshold, and subjective ratings of disease activity. Three subsequent investigations have reported similar findings for programs that provided cardiovascular fitness training (303), education and pool-based exercise training (304), and education with physical fitness training (305). Two of these studies documented that improvements in measures of cardiovascular fitness or physical function were maintained for periods ranging from 4 to 8 months following treatment (304,305). Only one study has shown that aerobic exercise and fitness training did not produce improvements in the outcome measures noted above (306). The meta-analysis performed by Rossy and colleagues (297) showed that aerobic exercise and other physically based interventions produced significant improvements in measures of fibromyalgia symptoms and physical status. Thus, it appears that a structured exercise program that emphasizes aerobic fitness training produces significant and sustained improvements in patients with fibromyalgia.

Cognitive-Behavioral Therapy

Cognitive-behavioral therapy (CBT) encompasses a variety of therapeutic interventions including relaxation training, reinforcement of healthy behavior patterns, coping skills training, and restructuring of maladaptive beliefs about one's ability to control painful symptoms (307). Since 1990, several investigations have examined the effects of CBT interventions on pain in patients with fibromyalgia.

TABLE 90.5. SUMMARY OF OUTCOMES PRODUCED BY BEHAVIORAL INTERVENTIONS

Study	Intervention	Design	Number of Subjects	Significant Treatment Outcomes
McCain et al., 1988 (302)	Cardiovascular fitness training vs. flexibility exercises	Randomized pretest-posttest design	42	Improvements in cardiovascular fitness, pain threshold, as well as patient and physician ratings of disease activity relative to flexibility exercise
Martin et al., 1996 (303)	Aerobic exercise vs. relaxation	Randomized, pretest-posttest design	60	Exercise produced greater improvement in tender point count, total myalgia scores, and aerobic fitness
Gowans et al., 1999 (304)	Exercise and education vs. waiting list control	Randomized, pretest-posttest design	41	Exercise produced greater improvement in 6-minute walk distance, sense of well-being, and fatigue; at 3 to 6 month follow-up, improvements were maintained in walk distance and sense of well-being
Burckhardt et al., 1994 (305)	Aerobic exercise vs. no adjunct treatment	Randomized, pretest-posttest design	85	Exercise and no adjunct treatment both produced negative results: decreases in peak power output and peak heart rate
Verstappen et al., 1997 (306)	Education and physical training vs. no treatment	Randomized, pretest-posttest design	99	Education and physical therapy together produced improvements in patient ratings of physical function; control over disease; and self-efficacy for pain, function, and other problems; improvements in function were maintained at 4- to 8-month follow-up assessment
White KP and Nielson WR, 1995 (310)	Cognitive-behavioral therapy	One group, pretest-posttest design	25	Improvements relative to baseline in patient ratings of pain intensity, emotional distress, life interference, depression, anxiety, and pain behavior
Goldenberg et al., 1994 (309)	Cognitive-behavioral therapy vs. no treatment control	Pretest-posttest design; no random assignment	79	Improvements relative to no treatment in patient ratings of pain intensity, fatigue, functional impact, and severity of psychologic distress
Turk et al., 1998 (311)	Interdisciplinary pain treatment program	One-group, pretest-posttest design	67	Treatment produced clinically significant improvement, as measured by Reliable Change Index, in pain severity ratings in 42% of patients
Bennett et al., 1996 (312) and 1991 (313)	Behavior modification, stress management, fitness training	One-group, pretest-posttest design	104	70% of patients had <11 tender points and disability scores decreased 25%
Buckelew et al., 1998 (314)	Biofeedback/relaxation training, exercise training, biofeed-back/relaxation/ exercise, or attention-placebo	Randomized, pretest-posttest design	119	Attention-placebo patients showed increased tender point sensitivity compared to all active treatment groups; no effects of active treatments on tender point sensitivity or measures of pain or pain behavior
Nicassio et al., 1997 (315)	Cognitive-behavioral therapy vs. attention-placebo	Randomized, pretest-posttest design	71	No differences between active treatment and attention-placebo in pain behavior, myalgia scores, or depression ratings
Vlaeyen et al., 1996 (316)	Cognitive-behavioral therapy, attention-placebo control, waiting list control	Randomized, pretest-posttest design	131	Cognitive-behavioral therapy was not superior to attention-placebo in any outcome measure
Ferraccioli et al., 1987 (320)	Electromyographic (EMG) biofeedback vs. false feedback	Randomized, pretest-posttest design	12	Improvements relative to baseline in tender point count and patient ratings of pain and morning stiffness
Haanen et al., 1991 (321)	Hypnotherapy vs. physical therapy	Randomized, pretest-posttest design with 12-week follow-up	40	Improvements relative to physical therapy in patient ratings of pain, fatigue, sleep disturbance, and psychologic distress; no effects on total myalgia score; improvements were maintained at follow-up

Most of these studies have reported that CBT interventions produce significant reductions in patients' ratings of pain, other clinical symptoms, functional disability, and in pain thresholds or tender point counts (95,308–313). None of these studies, however, used attention-placebo comparison groups to control for the nonspecific effects of prolonged or frequent contact with concerned health professionals. Thus, it is not possible to attribute the treatment gains documented in these studies to the CBT interventions, although it is promising that three studies reported that improvements in pain behavior and ratings of pain or functional ability were maintained up to 30 months after treatment termination (310–312). In addition, one investigation showed that the effects of CBT were clinically as well as statistically significant (311).

Three groups of investigators have performed placebo-controlled studies of behavioral treatments for patients with fibromyalgia. Each group examined the effects of CBT interventions, which included electromyographic biofeedback training, relaxation training (or both), and training in pain coping strategies (314–316). The attention-placebo control conditions consisted primarily of education on fibromyalgia and related health topics. Two of these groups found that CBT was not more effective than attention-placebo (315,316). The third group compared the effects of the CBT intervention to an exercise intervention, a combination of CBT and exercise, and the attention-placebo (314). It was found that all three active treatments produced significantly better tender point index scores than the attention-placebo. However, this effect primarily resulted from increased pain sensitivity observed among the attention-placebo patients over time. There were no significant CBT treatment effects on measures of pain or pain behavior. Nevertheless, a follow-up analysis revealed that across all treatment conditions, increases in self-efficacy were significantly associated with improvements in the tender point index and ratings of pain intensity (317).

These findings indicate that, at present, CBT interventions cannot be considered to be superior to placebo for the treatment of fibromyalgia. These negative findings are in contrast to those reported in studies of CBT interventions for patients with RA and osteoarthritis (318,319). Indeed, CBT represents a well-validated adjunct therapy for these rheumatologic disorders (307). It may be especially difficult for CBT to modify the function of CNS structures involved in abnormal stress responses and pain sensitivity (307). In addition, the high level of psychiatric morbidity among patients with fibromyalgia may reduce compliance with treatment and thus limit the potential effectiveness of CBT (307). Nevertheless, we believe that investigators should continue to study the potential benefits of CBT intervention for fibromyalgia, using rigorous experimental methodology and innovative approaches such as identification of patient subgroups who may be most likely to respond to treatment (e.g., 95).

Other Behavioral Therapies

Two groups of investigators have examined the effects of electromyographic (EMG) biofeedback training (320) and hypnotherapy (321) among patients with fibromyalgia. Both of these approaches yielded significant reductions in patients' pain intensity ratings; the EMG biofeedback training also was associated with a reduction in the tender point count. It should be noted, however, that the EMG biofeedback study evaluated only a select group of 12 patients. Half of these patients received both EMG biofeedback and relaxation training, whereas the other half received no training in relaxation or any EMG feedback signal. Thus, the positive effect of the biofeedback training may have been due largely to the relaxation training rather than to the biofeedback signal per se. Similarly, the hypnotherapy study examined the efficacy of autohypnosis and relaxation instructions recorded on audiotape for home practice as well as face-to-face hypnotic inductions. The comparison treatment consisted of massage and muscle relaxation instruction. It is possible, then, that the hypnotherapy intervention was superior to the comparison condition because the former was more effective in teaching relaxation skills to patients. Finally, one study has suggested that neck support may be an important element of a comprehensive therapeutic plan for patients with fibromyalgia, but data from large scale trials are lacking (322).

In summary, the data regarding behavioral treatments for fibromyalgia suggest that aerobic exercise produces reliable improvements in patients' reports of symptoms and functional abilities. The CBT interventions have not been shown to be superior to attention-placebo conditions. However, these interventions require additional rigorous evaluation in controlled studies before their efficacy can be fully assessed. Hypnotherapy and EMG biofeedback may be helpful for patients with fibromyalgia primarily due to their relaxation training components. Indeed, it may be found in future studies that structured relaxation training with home practice is equally effective and less expensive than hypnotherapy and biofeedback.

Other Therapeutic Maneuvers

Topical Treatment

Liniments and other topical preparations (substance P antagonist, capsaicin) have been used successfully for the treatment of limited or regional musculoskeletal syndromes. The diffuse and chronic nature of pain in fibromyalgia make their use problematic. Likewise, it is unclear (in the absence of a defined musculoskeletal regional pain syndrome) whether the injection of local anesthetics and/or corticosteroids into tender areas produce any long-lasting effect in patients with fibromyalgia. Nevertheless, they have been used with variable success in the clinic setting; whether their beneficial effect is due to "needling" (acupuncture) or to the effect of the pharmacologic compounds administered has not been studied in a systemic manner. Acupuncture has also been used, and in fact it is a recognized treatment modality for this condition according to a recent National Institutes of Health Consensus Conference (323,324).

Surgery

The claims made on the World Wide Web of the successful treatment of fibromyalgia with cervical spine decompressive surgery (325) are predicated on the possible association of fibromyalgia and Chiari malformation and/or other conditions capable of producing cervical spine stenosis. As to the modest association of fibromyalgia with Chiari malformation (326), this was a serendipitous finding our research group encountered while performing brain magnetic resonance imaging studies in patients and nonpatients with fibromyalgia (as well as in control subjects) prior to performing lumbar punctures for an ongoing investigation (181). In the conduct of our research studies we have encountered Chiari malformation not in any of our fibromyalgia nonpatients but rather in one normal subject. In addition, we did not find any differences between fibromyalgia patients with Chiari malformation versus those without Chiari with respect to CSF levels of substance P or self-reports of pain and fatigue (326). On the other hand, fibromyalgia has been reported to occur with increased frequency in patients who have sustained a cervical spine injury (258). However, patients with Chiari malformation and other stenosing lesions of the cervical spinal canal should only be offered decompressive surgery if unequivocal evidence of compressive myelopathy exists, but not otherwise (327).

RECOMMENDATIONS FOR FUTURE RESEARCH

The evidence reviewed above indicates that several medications (e.g., amitriptyline, cyclobenzaprine, SAMe), and aerobic exercise produce improvements in patients' reports of pain and other symptoms of fibromyalgia. However, a substantial number of clinical trials of the efficacy of these treatments and those of CBT and other behavioral interventions have failed to adequately control for the effects of the placebo response. Carette and colleagues (279) attempted to address this problem by randomly assigning a large number of subjects to medication or placebo conditions and by assessing clinically meaningful improvements with specific criteria for response to treatment (281). We suggest that future investigations of fibromyalgia treatments adopt a similar approach. We also believe that additional variables should be evaluated, such as measures of functional ability, quantifiable recordings of behaviors that are indicative of pain (328), pain beliefs, cognitions such as self-efficacy beliefs (329), and psychologic distress. Several investigators have suggested a broad array of measures that should be included in future treatment outcome studies (8,330–332).

Investigators also should consider using statistical approaches to assessing clinically meaningful change (311). One approach proposes that meaningful change represent a return to normal functioning (333,334). Thus, improvement in a specific variable might be defined as (a) a posttreatment score at least 2 standard deviations above or below the mean pretreatment score for the patient group, (b) a posttreatment score that is within 2 standard deviations of the mean score produced by a normal or healthy population, or (c) a posttreatment score that is closer to the mean score of a normal or healthy population than it is to the pretreatment score of the patient group.

Another statistical approach to measuring clinically meaningful change is represented by the Reliable Change Index (RCI) (334). The RCI is designed to overcome the problems associated with the statistical method described earlier in which there is considerable overlap between the score distributions of the patient group and those of a normal or healthy population. The RCI is defined as the patient's posttreatment score minus the patient's pretreatment score divided by the standard error of the difference between the two scores for the entire patient group. By this definition, an RCI equal to or greater than 1.96 is both statistically and clinically meaningful.

TREATMENT RECOMMENDATIONS

There is no generally accepted critical care pathway for the treatment of patients with fibromyalgia. However, there is agreement that successful treatment plans should begin with patient education and reassurance that the disorder is neither life threatening nor imaginary, and is not associated with development of joint deformities (335,336). We have found that patients in our clinic frequently have been told that their symptoms are psychiatric in origin or feigned. Thus, our patients usually are relieved to learn that although many patients who come to our clinic have psychiatric or psychologic problems, these problems are not the cause of their pain, fatigue, or other symptoms associated with fibromyalgia.

There also is general agreement that, although pharmacologic therapies do not eliminate pain, they may help patients better manage their pain. We tend to emphasize the use of medications such as amitriptyline and cyclobenzaprine. If these are ineffective, we often institute trials of SSRIs such as fluoxetine and sertraline despite the inconclusive or negative results of currently available trials regarding their efficacy. Alternatively, we may use anxiolytic medications such as alprazolam in patients who are highly anxious. Overall, we tend to limit the use of antiinflammatory agents, narcotic analgesics, and muscle relaxants *(vide supra)*.

It should be noted that patients often exhibit symptoms of both anxiety and depression. These patients frequently are difficult to treat and we tend to obtain consultations for them with colleagues who are highly experienced in managing persons with complex psychiatric disorders and somatic symptoms. Finally, on very rare occasions, we have resorted in a totally empiric fashion to short courses of very small doses of corticosteroids (prednisone 1 to 5 mg/day on a prn basis), in those patients with joint hypermobility in whom pain flares appear to be clearly related to physical trauma and who cannot take either the classic (nonselective COX inhibitors) or the newer (COX-2 specific inhibitors) nonsteroidal antiinflammatory agents. Nevertheless, we are aware that one study of the effectiveness of prednisone in patients with fibromyalgia reported negative results (337).

Another key element in the treatment of fibromyalgia is physical exercise. Consistent with the approach of McCain (338), we encourage our patients to engage in graduated aerobic exercise regimens led by physical therapists who are skilled in using learning principles to reward patients for meeting daily exercise quotas (339). It is essential that therapists make realistic assessments of the patients' exercise tolerance levels at baseline and devise exercise programs (e.g., water aerobics) that will meet patients' specific needs. Careful baseline assessment and tailoring of treatments to individual needs are essential to prevent patients from experiencing failure early in treatment and thus losing motivation to change their exercise behavior. This approach to physical therapy may be supplemented by palliative interventions such as massage or tender point injections.

Finally, persons who are experienced in providing CBT interventions should administer these therapies to patients who require training in pain coping skills and who appear able to practice and incorporate these skills in their daily routines. We are aware that, overall, the efficacy of CBT training for fibromyalgia has not been established in placebo-controlled trials. However, our experience is consistent with that of Turk et al. (95), who found that there are subgroups of patients who respond well to CBT training.

In summary, the treatment of patients with fibromyalgia is a complex and difficult endeavor that requires the integrated efforts of a large number of health professionals from various disciplines. It frequently is not possible to develop an interdisciplinary treatment team in many health care settings. Thus, it may be necessary to obtain consultations from, or refer patients to, centers capable of such therapeutic programs (234).

RESEARCH ISSUES

It is clear that our understanding of fibromyalgia is limited. There is a critical need to devote greater effort to research concerning the etiopathogenesis of the disorder. Indeed, it will not be possible to improve the effectiveness of our treatment approaches until we better understand the factors that contribute to the development of fibromyalgia. It is especially critical to better understand the interactions between genetic factors and peripheral and central pain mechanisms that appear to be involved in fibromyalgia.

Therapeutic studies involving patients with fibromyalgia have been limited by inadequate placebo controls, excessive emphasis on short-term outcomes, and reliance on conventional tests of statistical significance. It is essential to determine the extent to which these treatments reliably produce both statistically and clinically meaningful effects over time.

Although self-report measures of pain, disability, and psychologic distress are valuable, it also is necessary to evaluate changes in pain behavior, pain-related beliefs, and coping strategies. It is critically important to assess pain behavior given the high levels of psychologic distress shown by patients with fibromyalgia. That is, it is well known that there are substantial relationships between patients' reports of pain and psychologic distress (340). Thus, it is often difficult to determine if changes in self-reports of pain are due primarily to changes in psychologic distress. The use of reliable and objective measures of pain behavior, which are relatively independent of psychologic distress (328), should help us better evaluate the efficacy of interventions intended to alleviate pain in our patients. Moreover, it also is well known that pain beliefs and coping strategies are important determinants of adaptation to chronic pain (341). Evaluation of these cognitions and coping behaviors should help us to better understand factors that mediate therapeutic improvements in patients with fibromyalgia.

It was noted earlier that some effort has been made to measure clinically significant outcomes as well as conventional levels of statistical significance. We encourage investigators to devote greater attention to measuring clinical improvement as it is important to demonstrate that the changes produced by fibromyalgia treatments are meaningful as well as independent of chance factors.

Finally, patients with fibromyalgia experience high levels of pain and psychologic distress that do not vary greatly over time. Some adult patients are so incapacitated by their symptoms they have difficulty working and thus apply for disability benefits (342–348). There is evidence that the disability levels reported by patients with fibromyalgia are consistent with or greater than those reported by patients with RA (349,350). However, there is great variation across venues with regard to the extent that fibromyalgia is considered to be a legitimate cause of compensable disability. An international working group has encouraged research on the medicolegal issues related to disability in fibromyalgia (351). We also encourage this work so that judicial decisions may be made that are grounded in current knowledge on the etiopathogenesis and clinical features of this disorder and that will be fair to litigants without incurring excessive costs.

REFERENCES

1. Yunus MB. Fibromyalgia syndrome: clinical features and spectrum. In: Pillemer SR, ed. *The fibromyalgia syndrome: current research and future directions in epidemiology, pathogenesis, and treatment.* New York: Haworth Medical, 1994:5–21.
2. Yunus MB, Masi AT, Calabro JJ, et al. Primary fibromyalgia

(fibrositis): clinical study of 50 patients with matched normal controls. *Semin Arthritis Rheum* 1981;11:151–171.
3. Bennett RM. Fibromyalgia and the facts. Sense or nonsense. *Rheum Dis Clin North Am* 1993;19:45–59.
4. Granges G, Littlejohn GO. A comparative study of clinical signs in fibromyalgia/fibrositis syndrome, healthy and exercising subjects. *J Rheumatol* 1993;20:344–351.
5. Powers R. Fibromyalgia: an age-old malady begging for respect. *J Gen Intern Med* 1993;8:93–105.
6. Waylonis GW, Heck W. Fibromyalgia syndrome. New associations. *Am J Phys Med Rehabil* 1992;71:343–348.
7. Veale D, Kavanagh G, Fielding JF, et al. Primary fibromyalgia and the irritable bowel syndrome: different expressions of a common pathogenetic process. *Br Med J* 1991;30:220–222.
8. Littlejohn GO. A database for fibromyalgia. *Rheum Dis Clin North Am* 1995;21:527–557.
9. Jacobsen S, Petersen IS, Danneskiold-Samsøe B. Clinical features in patients with chronic muscle pain—with special reference to fibromyalgia. *Scand J Rheumatol* 1993;22:69–76.
10. Yunus MB, Ma i AT, Aldag JC. A controlled study of primary fibromyalgia sy idrome: clinical features and association with other functional syndromes. *J Rheumatol* 1989;16:62–71.
11. Wolfe F, Smythe HA, Yunus MB, et al. The American College of Rheumatology 1990 criteria for the classification of fibromyalgia. Report of the multicenter criteria committee. *Arthritis Rheum* 1990;33:160–172.
12. Solomon D, Liang MH. Fibromyalgia: scourge of humankind or bane of a rheumatologist's existence? *Arthritis Rheum* 1997;40:1553–1555.
13. Winfield JB. Pain in fibromyalgia. *Rheum Dis Clin North Am* 1998;25:55–79.
14. Yunus MB. Fibromyalgia syndrome: clinical features and spectrum. In: Pillemer SR, ed. *The fibromyalgia syndrome: current research and future directions in epidemiology, pathogenesis, and treatment.* Binghamton, NY: Haworth Medical, 1994:5–21.
15. Hadler NM. Fibromyalgia: la maladie est morte. Vive le malade! *J Rheumatol* 1997;27:1250–1251.
16. Masi AT. Concepts of illness in populations as applied to fibromyalgia syndromes: a biopsychosocial perspective. *Z Rheumatol* 1998;2:31–35.
17. Wolfe F. The fibromyalgia syndrome: a consensus report on fibromyalgia and disability. *J Rheumatol* 1996;23:534–539.
18. Barsky AJ, Borus JF. Functional somatic syndromes. *Ann Intern Med* 1999;130:910–921.
19. Abu-Shakra M, Mader R, Langevitz P, et al. Quality of life in systemic lupus erythematosus: a controlled study. *J Rheumatol* 1999;26:306–309.
20. Wang B, Gladman DD, Urowitz MB. Fatigue in lupus is not correlated with disease activity. *J Rheumatol* 1998;25:892–895.
21. Grafe A, Wollina U, Tebbe B, et al. Fibromyalgia in systemic lupus erythematosus. *Acta Der Venereol* 1999;79:62–64.
22. Reilly PA, Littlejohn GO. Peripheral arthralgic presentation of fibrositis/fibromyalgia syndrome. *J Rheumatol* 1992;19:281–283.
23. Cott A, Parkinson W, Bell MJ, et al. Interrater reliability of the tender point criterion for fibromyalgia. *J Rheumatol* 1992;19:1955–1959.
24. Smythe HA, Gladman A, Dagenais P, et al. Relation between fibrositic and control site tenderness: effects of dolorimeter scale length and footplate size. *J Rheumatol* 1992;19:284–289.
25. Bradley LA, Alarcón GS, Triana M, et al. Health care seeking behavior in fibromyalgia: associations with pain thresholds, symptom severity, and psychiatric morbidity. *J Musculoskel Pain* 1994;2:79–87.
26. Aaron LA, Bradley LA, Alarcón GS, et al. Psychiatric diagnoses are related to health care seeking behavior rather than illness in fibromyalgia. *Arthritis Rheum* 1996;39:436–445.
27. Tunks E, Crook J, Norman G, et al. Tender points in fibromyalgia. *Pain* 1988;34:11–19.
28. Kosek E, Ekholm J, Hansson P. Increased pressure pain sensibility in fibromyalgia patients is located deep to the skin, but not restricted to muscle tissue. *Pain* 1995;63:33–39.
29. Wolfe F. What use are fibromyalgia control points? *J Rheumatol* 1998;25:546–550.
30. Moldofsky H, Scarisbrick P, England R, et al. Musculoskeletal symptoms and non-REM sleep disturbances in patients with "fibrositis" syndrome and healthy subjects. *Psychosom Med* 1975;37:341–351.
31. Gedalia A, Press J, Klein M, et al. Joint hypermobility and fibromyalgia in school children. *Ann Rheum Dis* 1993;52:494–496.
32. Goldman JA. Hypermobility and deconditioning: important links to fibromyalgia/fibrositis. *South Med J* 1991;84:1192–1196.
33. Hudson N, Fitzcharles MA, Cohen M, et al. The association of soft-tissue rheumatism and hypermobility. *Br J Rheumatol* 1998;37:382–386.
34. Acasuso-Diaz M, Collantes-Estevez E. Joint hypermobility in patients with fibromyalgia syndrome. *Arthritis Care Res* 1998;11:39–42.
35. Hagglund KJ, Deuser WE, Buckelew SP, et al. Weather, beliefs about weather, and disease severity among patients with fibromyalgia. *Arthritis Care Res* 1994;7:130–135.
36. De Blecourt ACE, Knipping AA, de Voogd N, et al. Weather conditions and complains in fibromyalgia. *J Rheumatol* 1993;20:1932–1934.
37. Schaefer KM. Sleep disturbances and fatigue in women with fibromyalgia and chronic fatigue syndrome. *J Obstet Gynecol Neonatal Nurs* 1995;24:229–233.
38. Goldenberg DL. Fibromyalgia, chronic fatigue syndrome, and myofascial pain syndrome. *Curr Opin Rheumatol* 1995;7;127–135.
39. Goldenberg DL. Fibromyalgia, chronic fatigue syndrome, and myofascial pain syndrome. *Curr Opin Rheumatol* 1993;5:199–208.
40. White KP, Speechley M, Harth M, et al. The London epidemiology study: comparing the demographic and clinical characteristics in 100 random community cases of fibromyalgia versus controls. *J Rheumatol* 1999;26:1577–1585.
41. Wysenbeek AJ, Shapira Y, Leibovici L. Primary fibromyalgia and the chronic fatigue syndrome. *Rheumatol Int* 1991;10:227–229.
42. Demitrack MA. Chronic fatigue syndrome and fibromyalgia. Dilemmas in diagnosis and clinical management. *Psychiatric Clin North Am* 1999;21:671–692.
43. Demitrack MA, Crofford LJ. Evidence for and pathophysiologic implications of hypothalamic-pituitary-adrenal axis dysregulation in fibromyalgia and chronic fatigue syndrome. *Ann NY Acad Sci* 1998;840:684–697.
44. Branco J, Atalaia A, Paiva T. Sleep cycles and alpha-delta sleep in fibromyalgia syndrome. *J Rheumatol* 1994;21:1113–1117.
45. Jennum P, Drewes AM, Andreasen A, et al. Sleep and other symptoms in primary fibromyalgia and in healthy controls. *J Rheumatol* 1993;20:1756–1759.
46. May KP, West SG, Baker MR, et al. Sleep apnea in male patients with the fibromyalgia syndrome. *Am J Med* 1993;94:505–508.
47. Alvarez-Lario B, Teran J, Alonso JL, et al. Lack of association between fibromyalgia and sleep apnoea syndrome. *Ann Rheum Dis* 1992;51:108–111.
48. Cleveland CH Jr, Fisher RH, Brestel EP, et al. Chronic rhinitis: an underrecognized association with fibromyalgia. *Allergy Proc* 1992;13:263–267.
49. Paira SO. Fibromyalgia associated with female urethral syndrome. *Clin Rheumatol* 1994;13:88–89.

50. Chang L. The association of functional gastrointestinal disorders and fibromyalgia. *Eur J Surg* 1998;583:32–36.
51. Chun A, Deasutels S, Slivka A, et al. Visceral algesia in irritable bowel syndrome, fibromyalgia, and sphincter of oddi dysfunction, type III. *Dig Dis Sci* 1999;44:631–636.
52. Buskila D, Odes LR, Neumann L, et al. Fibromyalgia in inflammatory bowel disease. *J Rheumatol* 1999;26:1167–1171.
53. Nicolodi M, Volpe AR, Sicuteri F. Fibromyalgia and headache. Failure of serotonergic analgesia and N-methyl-D-aspartate–mediated neuronal plasticity: their common clues. *Cephalalgia* 1999;21:41–44.
54. Weiss DJ, Kreck T, Albert RK. Dyspnea resulting from fibromyalgia. *Chest* 1998;113:246–249.
55. Dinerman H, Goldenberg DL, Felson DT. A prospective evaluation of 118 patients with the fibromyalgia syndrome: prevalence of Raynaud's phenomenon, sicca symptoms, ANA, low complement, and Ig deposition at the dermal-epidermal junction. *J Rheumatol* 1986;13:368–373.
56. Bennett RM, Clark SR, Campbell SM, et al. Symptoms of Raynaud's syndrome in patients with fibromyalgia. A study utilizing the Nielsen test, digital photoplethysmography, and measurements of platelet alpha 2-adrenergic receptors. *Arthritis Rheum* 1991;34:264–269.
57. Grassi W, Core P, Carlino G, et al. Capillary permeability in fibromyalgia. *J Rheumatol* 1994;21:1328–1331.
58. Lapossy E, Gasser P, Hrycaj P, et al. Cold-induced vasospasm in patients with fibromyalgia and chronic low back pain in comparison to healthy subjects. *Clin Rheumatol* 1994;13:442–445.
59. Bonafede RP, Downey DC, Bennett RM. An association of fibromyalgia with primary Sjögren's syndrome: a prospective study of 72 patients. *J Rheumatol* 1995;22:133–136.
60. Greer JM, Panush RS. Incomplete lupus erythematosus. *Arch Intern Med* 1989;149:2473–2476.
61. Calvo-Alén J, Bastian HM, Burgard SL, et al. Identification of patient subsets of patients among those presumptively diagnosed with, referred and/or followed up for systemic lupus erythematosus at a large tertiary care center. *Arthritis Rheum* 1995;38:1475–1484.
62. Zonana-Nacach A, Alarcón GS, Reveille JD, et al. Clinical features of ANA-positive and ANA-negative fibromyalgia patients. *J Clin Rheumatol* 1998;4:52–56.
63. Bastian HM, Alarcón GS. A response on the positive ANA in an asymptomatic young woman [letter]. *J Clin Rheumatol* 1998; 4:169–170.
64. Yunus MB, Hussey FX, Aldag JC. Antinuclear antibodies and connective tissue disease features in fibromyalgia syndrome: a controlled study. *J Rheumatol* 1993;20:1557–1560.
65. Williams HJ, Alarcón GS, Joks R, et al. Early undifferentiated connective tissue disease VI. An inception cohort after ten years: disease remissions and changes in diagnosis in well-established and undifferentiated CTD. *J Rheumatol* 1999;26:816–825.
66. Williams HJ, Alarcón GS, Neuner R, et al. Early undifferentiated connective tissue disease. V. An inception cohort five years later: disease remissions and changes in diagnosis in well established and undifferentiated connective tissue diseases. *J Rheumatol* 1998;25:261–268.
67. Wolfe F, Anderson J, Harkness P, et al. A prospective, longitudinal, multicenter study of service utilization and costs in fibromyalgia. *Arthritis Rheum* 1997;40:1560–1570.
68. Ter Borg EJ, Gerards-Rociu E, Hannen HC, et al. High frequency of hysterectomies and appendectomies in fibromyalgia compared with rheumatoid arthritis: a pilot study. *Clin Rheumatol* 1999;18:1–3.
69. Mukerji B, Mukerji V, Alpert MA, et al. The prevalence of rheumatolgic disorders in patients with chest pain and angiographically normal coronary arteries. *Angiology* 1995;46:425–430.
70. Hellstrom O, Bullington J, Karlsson G, et al. A phenomenological study of fibromyalgia. Patient perspectives. *Scand J Prim Health Care* 1999;17:11–16.
71. Giovengo SL, Russell IJ, Larson AA. Increased concentrations of nerve growth factor in cerebrospinal fluid of patients with fibromyalgia. *J Rheumatol* 1999; 26:1564–1569.
72. Borenstein D. Prevalence and treatment outcome of primary and secondary fibromyalgia in patients with spinal pain. *Spine* 1995;20:796–800.
73. Sigal LH. Persisting symptoms of Lyme disease—possible explanations and implications for treatment. *J Rheumatol* 1994; 21:593–595.
74. Dinerman H, Steere AC. Lyme disease associated with fibromyalgia. *Ann Intern Med* 1992;117:281–285.
75. Berg AM, Naides SJ, Simms RW. Established fibromyalgia and parvovirus B19 infection. *J Rheumatol* 1993;20:1941–1943.
76. Buskila D, Shnaider A, Newmann L, et al. Musculoskeletal manifestations and autoantibody profile in 90 hepatitis C virus infected Israeli patients. *Semin Arthritis Rheum* 1998;28:107–113.
77. Rea T, Russo J, Katon W, et al. A prospective study of tender points and fibromyalgia during and after an acute viral infection. *Arch Intern Med* 1999;159:865–870.
78. Wolfe F. Post-traumatic fibromyalgia: a case report narrated by the patient. *Arthritis Care Res* 1994;7:161–165.
79. Waylonis GW, Perkins RH. Post-traumatic fibromyalgia. A long-term follow-up. *Am J Phys Med Rehabil* 1994;73:403–412.
80. Greenfield S, Fitzcharles MA, Esdaile JM. Reactive fibromyalgia syndrome. *Arthritis Rheum* 1992;35:678–681.
81. Culclasure TF, Enzenauer RJ, West SG. Post-traumatic stress disorder presenting as fibromyalgia. *Am J Med* 1993;94:548–549.
82. Aaron LA, Bradley LA, Alarcón GS, et al. Perceived physical and emotional trauma as precipitating events in fibromyalgia: association with health care seeking and disability status but not pain severity. *Arthritis Rheum* 1997;40:453–460.
83. Goldberg RT, Pachas WN, Keith D. Relationship between traumatic events in childhood and chronic pain. *Disability Rehab* 1999;21:23–30.
84. Trojan DA, Cashman NR. Fibromyalgia is common in a postpoliomyelitis clinic. *Arch Neurol* 1995;52:620–624.
85. Boisset-Pioro MH, Esdaile JM, Fitzcharles MA. Sexual and physical abuse in women with fibromyalgia syndrome. *Arthritis Rheum* 1995;38:235–241.
86. Hudson JI, Pope HG Jr. Does childhood sexual abuse cause fibromyalgia? *Arthritis Rheum* 1995;38:161–163.
87. Taylor ML, Trotter DR, Csuka ME. The prevalence of sexual abuse in women with fibromyalgia. *Arthritis Rheum* 1995;38: 229–234.
88. McBeth J, MacFarlane GJ, Benjamin J, et al. The association between tender points, psychological distres, and adverse childhood experiences: a community-based study. *Arthritis Rheum* 1999;42:1397–1404.
89. Turk DC, Okifuji A, Starz TW, et al. Effects of type of symptom onset on psychological distress and disability on fibromyalgia syndrome patients. *Pain* 1996;68:423–430.
90. Stormorken H, Brosstad F. Fibromyalgia: family clustering and sensory urgency with early onset indicate genetic predisposition and thus a "true" disease. *Scand J Rheumatol* 1992;21:207.
91. Schanberg LE, Keefe FJ, Lefebvre JC, et al. Social context of pain in children with juvenile primary fibromyalgia syndrome: parental pain history and family environment. *Clin J Pain* 1999; 14:107–115.
92. Yunus MB, Khan MA, Rawlings KK, et al. Genetic linkage analysis of multicase families with fibromyalgia syndrome. *J Rheumatol* 1999;26:408–412.
93. Kerns RD, Turk DC, Audy TE. The West Haven–Yale Multidimensional Pain Inventory (WHYMPI). *Pain* 1985;23:345–356.

94. Turk DC, Okifuji A, Sinclair JD, et al. Pain, disability, and physical functioning in subgroups of patients with fibromyalgia. *J Rheumatol* 1996;23:1255–1262.
95. Turk DC, Okifuji A, Sinclair JD, et al. Differential responses by psychosocial subgroups of fibromyalgia syndrome patients to an interdisciplinary treatment. *Arthritis Care Res* 1998;11:397–404.
96. Nørregaard J, Bülow PM, Prescott E, et al. Preliminary results of a 4 year follow-up study in fibromyalgia. In: Jacobsen S, Danneskiold-Samsœ B, Lund B, eds. *Musculoskeletal pain, myofascial pain syndrome, and the fibromyalgia syndrome.* New York: Haworth Press, 1993;159–163.
97. Masi AT. Review of the epidemiology and criteria of fibromyalgia and myofascial pain syndromes: concepts of illness in populations as applied to dysfunctional syndromes. In: Jacobsen S, Danneskiold-Samsœ B, Lund B, eds. *Musculoskeletal pain, myofascial pain syndrome, and the fibromyalgia syndrome.* New York: The Haworth Medical Press Inc, 1993;113–136.
98. Wolfe F, Ross K, Anderson J, et al. The prevalence and characteristics of fibromyalgia in the general population. *Arthritis Rheum* 1995;38:19–28.
99. Buskila D, Neumann L, Hershman E, et al. Fibromyalgia syndrome in children—an outcome study. *J Rheumatol* 1995;22: 525–528.
100. Lawrence RC, Helmick CG, Arnett FC, et al. Estimates of the prevalence of arthritis and selected musculoskeletal disorders in the United States. *Arthritis Rheum* 1998;41:778–799.
101. Buskila D, Press J, Gedalia A, et al. Assessment of nonarticular tenderness and prevalence of fibromyalgia in children. *J Rheumatol* 1993;20:368–370.
102. White KC, Speechley M, Harth M, et al. The London fibromyalgia epidemiology study: the prevalence of fibromyalgia syndrome in London, Ontario. *J Rheumatol* 1999;26:1570–1576.
103. Clark P, Burgos-Vargas R, Medina-Palma C, et al. Prevalence of fibromyalgia in children: a clinical study of Mexican children. *J Rheumatol* 1998;25:2009–2014.
104. Handa R, Aggarwal P, Wali JP, et al. Fibromyalgia in Indian patients with SLE. *Lupus* 1998;7:475–478.
105. Neumann L, Buskila D. Ethnocultural and educational differences in Israeli women correlate with pain perception in fibromyalgia. *J Rheumatol* 1998;25:1369–1373.
106. Raspe H, Baumgartner C. The epidemiology of the fibromyalgia syndrome: different criteria—different results. In: Jacobsen S, Danneskiold-Samsøe B, Lund B, eds. *Musculoskeletal pain, myofascial pain syndrome, and the fibromyalgia syndrome.* New York: Haworth Medical, 1993:149–152.
107. Prescott E, Jacobsen S, Kjoller M, et al. Preliminary communication on the prevalence of fibromyalgia in the adult Danish population. In: Jacobsen S, Danneskiold-Samsœ B, Lund B, eds. *Musculoskeletal pain, myofacial pain syndrome, and the fibromyalgia syndrome.* New York: The Haworth Medical Press Inc, 1993;153–157.
108. Prescott E, Kjoller M, Jacobsen S, et al. Fibromyalgia in the adult Danish population: I. A prevalence study. *Scand J Rheumatol* 1993;22:233–237.
109. Harvey CK. Fibromyalgia. Part II. Prevalence in the podiatric patient population. *J Am Podiatric Med Assoc* 1993;83:416–417.
110. Forseth KO, Gran JT. The occurrence of fibromyalgia-like syndromes in a general female population. *Clin Rheumatol* 1993; 12:23–27.
111. de Girolamo G. Epidemiology and social costs of low back pain and fibromyalgia. *Clin J Pain* 1991;7(suppl 1):S1–S7.
112. Makela M, Heliovaara M. Prevalence of primary fibromyalgia in the Finnish population. *Br Med J* 1991;303:216–219.
113. Schochat T, Croft P, Raspe H. The epidemiology of fibromyalgia. Workshop of the Standing Committee on Epidemiology European League Against Rheumatism (EULAR), Bad Sackingen, 19–21 November 1992. *Br J Rheumatol* 1994;33: 783–786.
114. Croft P, Rigby AS, Boswell R, et al. The prevalence of chronic widespread pain in the general population. *J Rheumatol* 1993; 20:710–713.
115. Yunus MB, Masi AT, Aldag JC. Preliminary criteria for primary fibromyalgia syndrome (PFS): multivariate analysis of a consecutive series of PFS, other pain patients, and normal subjects. *Clin Exp Rheumatol* 1989;7:63–69.
116. White KP, Harth M, Speechley M, et al. Testing an instrument to screen for fibromyalgia syndrome in general population studies: the London Fibromyalgia Epidemiology Study Screening Questionnaire. *J Rheumatol* 1999;26:880–884.
117. McIntosh MJ, Hewett JE, Buckelew SP, et al. Protocol for verifying expertise in locating fibromyalgia tender points. *Arthritis Care Res* 1998;11:210–216.
118. Okifuji A, Turk DC, Sinclair JD, et al. A standardized manual tender point survey. I. Development and determination of a threshold point for the identification of positive tender points in fibromyalgia syndrome. *J Rheumatol* 1997;24:377–383.
119. Ohrbach R, Crow H, Kamer A. Examiner expectancy effects in the measurement of pressure pain thresholds. *Pain* 1998;74: 163–170.
120. Campbell SM, Clark S, Tindall EA, et al. Clinical characteristics of fibrositis: 1. A "blinded," controlled study of symptoms and tender points. *Arthritis Rheum* 1983;26:817–825.
121. Hartz A, Kirchodoerfer E. Undetected fibrositis in primary care practice. *J Family Pract* 1987;25:365–369.
122. Wolfe F, Cathey MA. Prevalence of primary and secondary fibrositis. *J Rheumatol* 1983;10:965–968.
123. Yunus MB. Towards a model of pathophysiology of fibromyalgia: aberrant central pain mechanisms with peripheral modulation. *J Rheumatol* 1992;19:846–850.
124. Pellegrino MJ, Waylonis GW, Sommer A. Familial occurrence of primary fibromyalgia. *Arch Phys Med Rehabil* 1989;70:61–63.
125. Melzack R. Gate control theory: on the evolution of pain concepts. *Pain Forum* 1996;5:125–128.
126. Loeser JD, Melzack R. Pain: an overview. *Lancet* 1999;353: 1607–1609.
127. Sternbach RA. Survey of pain in the United States: the Nuprin Pain Report. *Clin J Pain* 1986;2:49–53.
128. Edwards PW, Zeichner A, Kuczmierczyk AR, et al. Familial pain models: the relationship between family history of pain and current pain experience. *Pain* 1985;21:379–384.
129. Lester N, Lefebvre JC, Keefe FJ. Pain in young adults: I. Relationship to gender and family pain history. *Clin J Pain* 1994;10: 282–289.
130. Buskila D, Neumann L, Hozanov I, et al. Familial aggregation in the fibromyalgia syndrome. *Semin Arthritis Rheum* 1996;26: 605–611.
131. Buskila D, Neumann L. Fibromyalgia syndrome (FM) and nonarticular tenderness in relatives of patients with FM. *J Rheumatol* 1997;24:941–944.
132. Neumann L, Buskila D. Quality of life and physical functioning of relatives of fibromyalgia patients. *Semin Arthritis Rheum* 1997;26:834–839.
133. Mogil JS, Sternberg WF, Marek P, et al. The genetics of pain and pain inhibition. *Proc Natl Acad Sci U S A* 1996;7:3048–3055.
134. Mogil JS, Richards SP, O'Toole LA, et al. Genetic sensitivity to hot-plate nociception in DBA/2J and C57BL/6J inbred mouse strains: possible sex-specific mediation by delta 2-opioid receptors. *Pain* 1997;70:267–277.
135. Elmer GI, Peiper JO, Negus SS, et al. Genetic variation in nociception and its relationship to the potency of morphine-induced analgesia in thermal and chemical tests. *Pain* 1998;75: 129–140.

136. Mogil JS, Richards SP, O'Toole LA, et al. Identification of a sex-specific quantitative trait locus mediating nonopioid stress-induced analgesia in female mice. *J Neurosci* 1997;17:7995–8002.
137. Bengtsson A, Henriksson KG, Larsson J. Muscle biopsy in primary fibromyalgia: light-microscopical and histochemical findings. *Scand J Rheumatol* 1986;15:1–6.
138. Bengtsson A, Henriksson KG, Larsson J. Reduced high-energy phosphate levels in the painful muscles of patients with primary fibromyalgia. *Arthritis Rheum* 1986;29:817–821.
139. Lund N, Bengtsson A, Thorborg P. Muscle tissue oxygen pressure in primary fibromyalgia. *Scand J Rheumatol* 1986;15:165–173.
140. Bennett RM, Clark SR, Goldberg L, et al. Aerobic fitness in patients with fibrositis: a controlled study of respiratory gas exchange and 133-xenon clearance from exercising muscle. *Arthritis Rheum* 1989;32:454–460.
141. Yunus MB, Kalyan-Raman UP, Masi AT. Electron microscopic studies of muscle biopsy in primary fibromyalgia syndrome: a controlled and blinded study. *J Rheumatol* 1992;16:97–101.
142. Sprott H, Bradley LA, Oh JJ, et al. Immunohistochemical and molecular biological detection of serotonin, substance P, galanin, pacap, and secretoneurin in fibromyalgia muscle tissue. *Arthritis Rheum* 1998;41:1689–1694.
143. Jacobsen S, Jensen KE, Thomsen C, et al. ^{31}P magnetic resonance spectroscopy of skeletal muscle in patients with fibromyalgia. *J Rheumatol* 1992;19:1600–1603.
144. Jubrias SA, Bennett RM, Klug GA. Increased incidence of a resonance in the phosphodiester region of ^{31}P nuclear magnetic resonance spectra in the skeletal muscle of fibromyalgia patients. *Arthritis Rheum* 1994;37:801–807.
145. Mengshoel AM, Saugen E, Forre Ø, et al. Muscle fatigue in early fibromyalgia. *J Rheumatol* 1995;22:143–150.
146. Sietsema KE, Cooper DM, Caro X, et al. Oxygen uptake during exercise in patients with primary fibromyalgia syndrome. *J Rheumatol* 1993;20:860–865.
147. Simms RW, Roy SH, Hrovat M, et al. Lack of association between fibromyalgia syndrome and abnormalities in muscle energy metabolism. *Arthritis Rheum* 1994;37:794–799.
148. Park JH, Phothimat P, Oates C, et al. Use of p-31 magnetic resonance spectroscopy to detect metabolic abnormalities in muscles of patients with fibromyalgia. *Arthritis Rheum* 1998;41: 406–413.
149. Mountz JM, Bradley LA, Modell JG, et al. Fibromyalgia in women. Abnormalities of regional cerebral blood flow in the thalamus and the caudate nucleus are associated with low pain threshold levels. *Arthritis Rheum* 1995;38:926–938.
150. Granges G, Littlejohn G. Pressure pain threshold in pain-free subjects, in patients with chronic regional pain syndromes, and in patients with fibromyalgia syndrome. *Arthritis Rheum* 1993; 36:642–646.
151. Gibson JJ, Littlejohn GO, Gorman MM, et al. Altered heat pain thresholds and cerebral event-related potentials following painful CO_2 laser stimulation in subjects with fibromyalgia syndrome. *Pain* 1994;58:185–193.
152. Arroyo JF, Cohen ML. Abnormal responses to electrocutaneous stimulation in fibromyalgia. *J Rheumatol* 1993;20:1925–1931.
153. Kosek E, Hansson P. Modulatory influence on somatosensory perception from vibration and heterotopic noxious conditioning stimulation (HNCS) in fibromyalgia patients with healthy subjects. *Pain* 1997;70:41–51.
154. Lautenbacher S, Rollman GB. Possible deficiencies of pain modulation in fibromyalgia. *Clin J Pain* 1997;13:189–196.
155. Moldofsky H, Lue FA, Smythe HA. Alpha EEG sleep and morning symptoms in rheumatoid arthritis. *J Rheumatol* 1983; 10:373–379.
156. Moldofsky H, Saskin P, Lue FA. Sleep and symptoms in fibrositis syndrome after a febrile illness. *J Rheumatol* 1988;15:1701–1704.
157. Carette S, Oakson G, Guimont C, et al. Sleep electroencephalography and the clinical response to amitriptyline in patients with fibromyalgia. *Arthritis Rheum* 1995;38: 1211–1217.
158. Older S, Battafrano D, Danning C, et al. The effects of delta wave sleep interruption on pain thresholds and fibromyalgia-like symptoms in healthy subjects; correlations with insulin-like growth factor. I. *J Rheumatol* 998;25:1180–1186.
159. Lentz MJ, Landis CA, Rathermel J, et al. Effects of selective slow wave sleep disruption on musculoskeletal pain and fatigue in middle aged women. *J Rheumatol* 1999;26:1586–1592.
160. Cote KA, Moldofsky H. Sleep, daytime symptoms, cognitive performance in patients with fibromyalgia. *J Rheumatol* 1997; 24:2014–2023.
161. Affleck G, Urrows S, Tennen H, et al. Sequential daily relations of sleep, pain intensity, and attention to pain among women with fibromyalgia. *Pain* 1996;68:363–368.
162. McDermid AJ, Rollman GB, McCain GA. Generalized hypervigilance in fibromyalgia: evidence of perceptual amplification. *Pain* 1996;66:133–144.
163. McCain GA, Tilbe KS. Diurnal hormone variation in fibromyalgia syndrome. A comparison with rheumatoid arthritis. *J Rheumatol* 1989;16:154–157.
164. Crofford LJ, Pillemer SR, Kalogeras KT, et al. Hypothalamic-pituitary-adrenal axis perturbations in patients with fibromyalgia. *Arthritis Rheum* 1994;37:1583–1592.
165. Griep EN, Boersma JW, deKloet ER. Altered reactivity of the hypothalamic-pituitary-adrenal axis in the primary fibromyalgia syndrome. *J Rheumatol* 1993;20:469–474.
166. Adler GK, Kinsley BT, Hurwitz S, et al. Reduced hypothalamic-pituitary and sympathoadrenal responses to hypoglycemia in women with fibromyalgia syndrome. *Am J Med* 1999;106: 534–543.
167. Martinez-Lavin M, Hermosillo AG, Rasas M, et al. Circadian studies of autonomic nervous balance in patients with fibromyalgia: a heart rate variability analysis. *Arthritis Rheum* 1998;41:1966–1971.
168. Martinez-Lavin M, Hermosillo AG, Mendoza C, et al. Orthostatic sympathetic derangement in subjects with fibromyalgia. *J Rheumatol* 1997;24:714–718.
169. Neeck G, Riedel W. Thyroid function in patients with fibromyalgia syndrome. *J Rheumatol* 1992;18:1120–1122.
170. Bennett RM, Clark SR, Campbell SM, et al. Low levels of somatomedin C in patients with the fibromyalgia syndrome: a possible link between sleep and muscle pain. *Arthritis Rheum* 1992;35:1113–1116.
171. Bennett RM, Clark SR, Walczyk J. A randomized, double-blind, placebo-controlled study of growth hormone in the treatment of fibromyalgia. *Am J Med* 1998;104:227–231.
172. Bennett RM. The origin of myopain: an integrated hypothesis of focal muscle changes and sleep disturbances in patients with the fibromyalgia syndrome. *J Musculoskel Pain* 1993;1:95–112.
173. Jacobsen S, Jensen LT, Foldager M, et al. Primary fibromyalgia: clinical parameters in relation to serum procollagen type II aminoterminal peptide. *Br J Rheumatol* 1990;29:174–177.
174. Russell IJ, Michalek JE, Vipario GA, et al. Platelet ^{3}H-imipramine uptake receptor density and serum serotonin levels in patients with fibromyalgia/fibrositis syndrome. *J Rheumatol* 1992;19:104–109.
175. Wolfe F, Russell IJ, Vipraio G, et al. Serotonin levels, pain threshold, and fibromyalgia symptoms in the general population. *J Rheumatol* 1997;24:555–559.
176. Vaerøy H, Helle R, Forre Ø, et al. Cerebrospinal fluid levels of B-endorphin in patients with fibromyalgia (fibrositis syndrome). *J Rheumatol* 1988;15:1804–1806.
177. Yunus MB, Dailey JW, Aldag JC, et al. Plasma tryptophan and

other amino acids in primary fibromyalgia: a controlled study. *J Rheumatol* 1992;19:90–94.
178. Kravitz HM, Katz R, Kot E, et al. Biochemical clues to a fibromyalgia-depression link: imipramine binding in patients with fibromyalgia or depression and in healthy controls. *J Rheumatol* 1992;19:1428–1432.
179. Vaerøy H, Helle R, Forre Ø, et al. Elevated CSF levels of substance P and high incidence of Raynaud phenomenon in patients with fibromyalgia: new features for diagnosis. *Pain* 1988;32:21–26.
180. Russell IJ, Orr MD, Littman B, et al. Elevated cerebrospinal fluid levels of substance P in patients with the fibromyalgia syndrome. *Arthritis Rheum* 1994;37:1593–1601.
181. Bradley LA, Sotolongo A, Alberts KR, et al. Abnormal regional cerebral blood flow in the caudate nucleus among fibromyalgia patients and non-patients is associated with insidious symptom onset. *J Musculoskel Pain* 1999;7:285–292.
182. Evengard B, Nilsson CG, Lindh G, et al. Chronic fatigue syndrome differs from fibromyalgia. No evidence for elevated substance P levels in cerebrospinal fluid of patients with chronic fatigue syndrome. *Pain* 1998;78:153–155.
183. Missole C, Toroni F, Sigala S, et al. Nerve growth factor in the anterior pituitary: localization in mammotroph cells and cosecretion with prolactin by a dopamine-regulated mechanism. *Proc Natl Acad Sci U S A* 1996;93:4240–4245.
184. Lindsay RM, Lockett C, Sternberg J, et al. Neuropeptide expression in cultures of adult sensory neurons: modulation of substance P and calcitonin gene-related peptide levels by nerve growth factor. *Neuroscience* 1989;33:53–65.
185. Vaeroy H, Nyberg F, Terenius L. No evidence for endorphin deficiency in fibromyalgia following investigation of cerebrospinal fluid (CSF) dynorphin A and Met-enkephalin-Arg6-Phe7. *Pain* 1991;46:139–143.
186. Vaeroy H, Sakurda T, Forre O, et al. Modulation of pain in fibromyalgia (fibrositis syndrome): cerebrospinal fluid (CSF) investigation of pain-related neuropeptides with special reference to calcitonin gene-related peptide (CGRP). *J Rheumatol* 1989;19:94–97.
187. Russell IJ. Neurochemical pathogenesis of fibromyalgia syndrome. *J Musculoskel Pain* 1996;4:61–92.
188. Pillemer SR, Bradley LA, Crofford LJ, et al. The neuroscience and endocrinology of fibromyalgia. *Arthritis Rheum* 1997;40: 1928–1937.
189. Bendsten L, Norregaard J, Jensen R, et al. Evidence of qualitatively altered nociception in patients with fibromyalgia. *Arthritis Rheum* 1997;40:98–102.
190. Kosek E, Ekholm J, Hansson P. Sensory dysfunction in fibromyalgia patients with implications for pathogenic mechanisms. *Pain* 1996;68:375–383.
191. Guilbaud G. Central neurophysiological processing of joint pain on the basis of studies performed in normal animals and in models of experimental arthritis. *Can J Physiol Pharmacol* 1991; 69:637–646.
192. Sorkin LS, McAdoo DJ, Willis WD. Stimulation in the ventral posterior lateral nucleus of the primate thalamus leads to release of serotonin in the lumbar spinal cord. *Brain Res* 1992;581:307–310.
193. Chudler EH, Swigiyama K, Dong WK. Nociceptive responses in the neostriatum and globus pallidus of the anesthetized rat. *J Neurophysiol* 1993;69:1890–1903.
194. Diorio D, Viau V, Meaney MJ. The role of the medical prefrontal cortex (cingulate gyrus) in the regulation of hypothalamic-pituitary-adrenal response to stress. *J Neurosci* 1983;13:3839–3847.
195. Lineberry CG, Vierck CJ. Attenuation of pain reactivity by caudate nucleus stimulation in monkeys. *Brain Res* 1975;9:119–134.
196. Acupuncture Anesthesia Coordinating Group. Observations on electrical stimulation of the caudate nucleus of human brain and acupuncture in treatment of intractable pain. *Chin Med J* 1977;3:117–124.
197. Kwiatek R, Barnden L, Rowe S. Pontine tegmental regional cerebral blood flow is reduced in fibromyalgia. *Arthritis Rheum* 1997;40:S43.
198. Airaksinen O, Vanninen E, Herno A, et al. Decrease in regional cerebral perfusion in fibromyalgia. In: *Abstracts of the 9th World Congress on Pain.* Seattle: IASP Press, 1999:43.
199. Iadarola MJ, Max MD, Berman KF, et al. Unilateral decrease in thalamic activity observed with position emission tomography in patients with chronic neuropathic pain. *Pain* 1995;63:55–64.
200. Di Piero V, Jones AKP, Iannotti F, et al. Chronic pain: a PET study of the central effects of percutaneous high cervical cordotomy. *Pain* 1991;46:9–12.
201. Ness TJ, San Pedro EC, Richards JS, et al. A case of spinal cord injury-related pain with baseline rCBF brain SPECT imaging and beneficial response to gabapentin. *Pain* 1998;78:139–143.
202. San Pedro EC, Mountz JM, Liu HG, et al. Familial painful restless leg syndrome correlates with a pain-dependent variation of blood flow to the caudate nucleus, thalamus, and anterior cingulate gyrus. *J Rheumatol* 1998;25:2270–2275.
203. Weigent DA, Bradley LA, Blalock JE, et al. Current concepts in the pathophysiology of abnormal pain perception in fibromyalgia. *Am J Med Sci* 1998;315:405–412.
204. Casey KL, Minoshima S, Berger KL, et al. Positron emission tomographic analysis of cerebral structures activated specifically by repetitive noxious heat stimuli. *J Neurophysiol* 1994;71:802–807.
205. Coghill RC, Talbot JD, Evans AC, et al. Distributed processing of pain and vibration by the human brain. *J Neurosci* 1994;14: 4095–4108.
206. Talbot JD, Marrett S, Evans AC, et al. Multiple representations of pain in the human cerebral cortex. *Science* 1991;251:1355–1358.
207. Jones AKP, Brown WD, Friston KJ, et al. Cortical and subcortical localization of response to pain in man using positron emission tomography. *Proc R Soc Lond [B]* 1991;244:39–44.
208. Coghill RC, Sang CN, Maisog JM, et al. Pain intensity processing within the human brain: a bilateral, distributed mechanism. *J Neurophysiology* 1999;82:1934–1943.
209. Bradley LA, Sotolongo A, Alarcón GS, et al. Dolimeter stimulation elicits abnormal pain sensitivity and regional cerebral blood flow (rCBF) in the right cingulate cortex (CC) as well as passive coping strategies in non-depressed patients with fibromyalgia (FM). *Arthritis Rheum* 1999;42:S342.
210. Hsieh J-C, Hannerz J, Ingvar M. Right-lateralized central processing for pain of nitroglycerin-induced cluster headache. *Pain* 1996;67:59–68.
211. Hsieh JC, Belfrage M, Stone-Elander S, et al. Central representation of chronic ongoing neuropathic pain studied by position emission tomography. *Pain* 1995;63:225–236.
212. Pauli P, Wiedemann G, Nickola M. Pain sensitivity, cerebral laterality, and negative affect. *Pain* 1999;80:359–364.
213. Hudson JI, Hudson MS, Pliner LF, et al. Fibromyalgia and major affective disorder: a controlled phenomenology and family history study. *Am J Psychiatry* 1985;142:441–446.
214. Wolfe F, Cathey MA, Kleinheksel SM, et al. Psychological status in primary fibrositis and fibrositis associated with rheumatoid arthritis. *J Rheumatol* 1984;11:500–506.
215. Ahles TA, Yunus MB, Riley SD, et al. Psychological factors associated with primary fibromyalgia syndrome. *Arthritis Rheum* 1984;27:1101–1106.
216. Payne TC, Leavitt F, Garron DC, et al. Fibrositis and psychological disturbance. *Arthritis Rheum* 1982;25:213–217.
217. Pincus T, Callahan LF, Bradley LA, et al. Elevated MMPI scores for hypochondriasis, depression, and hysteria in patients with rheumatoid arthritis reflect disease rather than psychological status. *Arthritis Rheum* 1986;29:1456–1466.

218. Prokop CK. Hysteria scale elevations in low back pain patients: a risk factor for misdiagnosis? *J Consult Clin Psychol* 1986;54: 558–562.
219. Moore JE, McFall ME, Kivlahan DR, et al. Risk of misinterpretation of MMPI Schizophrenia scale elevations in chronic pain patients. *Pain* 1986;32:207–213.
220. Scudds RA, Rollman GB, Harth M, et al. Pain perception and personality measures as discriminators in the classification of fibrositis. *J Rheumatol* 1987;14:563–569.
221. Ahles TA, Yunus MB, Masi AT. Is chronic pain a variant of depressive disease? The case of primary fibromyalgia syndrome. *Pain* 1987;29:105–111.
222. Birnie DJ, Knipping AA, van Rijswijk MH, et al. Psychological aspects of fibromyalgia compared with chronic and nonchronic pain. *J Rheumatol* 1991;18:1845–1848.
223. Clouse R. Psychopharmacologic approaches to therapy for chest pain of presumed esophageal origin. *Am J Med* 1992;92(suppl 5a):106S–113S.
224. Hudson JI, Goldenberg DL, Pope HG, et al. Comorbidity of fibromyalgia with medical and psychiatric disorders. *Am J Med* 1992;92:363–367.
225. Hudson JI, Pope HG. Fibromyalgia and psychopathology: is fibromyalgia a form of "affective spectrum disorder." *J Rheumatol* 1989;16:15–22.
226. Dailey PA, Bishop GD, Russell IJ, et al. Psychological stress and the fibrositis/fibromyalgia syndrome. *J Rheumatol* 1990;17: 1380–1385.
227. Uveges JM, Parker JC, Smarr KL, et al. Psychological symptoms in primary fibromyalgia syndrome: relationship to pain, life stress, and sleep disturbance. *Arthritis Rheum* 1990;33:1279–1283.
228. Clark S, Campbell SM, Forehand ME, et al. Clinical characteristics of fibrositis. II. A "blinded" controlled study using standard psychological tests. *Arthritis Rheum* 1985;28:132–137.
229. Drossman DA, McKee DC, Sandler RS, et al. Psychosocial factors in the irritable bowel syndrome: a multivariate study of patients and non-patients with irritable bowel syndrome. *Gastroenterology* 1988;95:701–708.
230. Whitehead WE, Bosmajian L, Zonderman AB, et al. Symptoms of psychologic distress associated with irritable bowel syndrome: comparison of community and medical clinic samples. *Gastroenterology* 1988;95:709–714.
231. Aaron LA, Bradley LA, Alexander MT, et al. Work stress, psychiatric history, and medication usage predict initial use of medical treatment for fibromyalgia symptoms: a prospective analysis. In: Jensen TS, Turner JA, Wiesenfeld-Hallin Z, eds. *Proceedings of the 7th World Congress on Pain. Progress in pain research and management,* vol 8. Seattle: IASP Press, 1999:683–691.
232. Aaron LA, Bradley LA, Alexander MT, et al. Prediction of health-care seeking for fibromyalgia (FM) symptoms among community residents with FM. *Arthritis Rheum* 1995;38:S230(abst).
233. MacFarlane GJ, Morris S, Hunt IM, et al. Chronic widespread pain in the community: the influence of psychological symptoms and mental disorder on health care seeking behavior. *J Rheumatol* 1999;26:413–419.
234. Bradley LA. Behavioral interventions for the management of chronic pain. *Bull Rheum Dis* 1994;43:2–5.
235. Buchwald D, Goldenberg DL, Sullivan JL, et al. The "chronic, active Epstein-Barr virus infection" syndrome and primary fibromyalgia. *Arthritis Rheum* 1987;30:1132–1136.
236. Leventhal LJ, Naides SJ, Freundlich B. Fibromyalgia and parvovirus infection. *Arthritis Rheum* 1991;34:1319–1324.
237. Buskila D, Gladman D, Langevitz P, et al. Fibromyalgia in human immunodeficiency virus infection. *J Rheumatol* 1990; 17:1202–1206.
238. Simms RW, Zerbini CA, Ferrante N, et al. Fibromyalgia syndrome in patients infected with human immunodeficiency virus. The Boston City Hospital Clinical AIDS Team. *Am J Med* 1992;92:368–374.
239. Hsu VM, Patella SJ, Sigal LH. "Chronic Lyme disease" as the incorrect diagnosis in patients with fibromyalgia. *Arthritis Rheum* 1993;36:1493–1500.
240. Caro XJ. Immunofluorescent detection of IgG at the dermal-epidermal junction in patients with apparent primary fibrositis syndrome. *Arthritis Rheum* 1984;27:1174–1179.
241. Whelton CL, Salit I, Moldofsky H. Sleep, Epstein-Barr virus infection, musculoskeletal pain, and depressive symptoms in chronic fatigue syndrome. *J Rheumatol* 1992;19:939–943.
242. Romano TJ, Homberger HA. Presence of anticardiolipin antibodies in the fibromyalgia syndrome. *Pain Clin* 1991;4:147–153.
243. Caligiuri M, Murray C, Buchwald D, et al. Phenotypic and functional deficiency of natural killer cells in patients with chronic fatigue syndrome. *J Immunol* 1987;139:3306–3313.
244. Hernanz W, Valenzuela A, Quijada J, et al. Lymphocyte subpopulations in patients with primary fibromyalgia. *J Rheumatol* 1994;21:2122–2124.
245. Hellstrand K, Hermodsson S. Role of serotonin in the regulation of human natural killer cell cytotoxicity. *J Immunol* 1987;139:869–875.
246. Sprott H, Muller A, Heine H. Collagen crosslinks in fibromyalgia. *Arthritis Rheum* 1997;40:1950–1954.
247. Goldenberg DL. Do infections trigger fibromyalgia [editorial]? *Arthritis Rheum* 1993;36:1489–1492.
248. Wolfe F. The clinical syndrome of fibrositis. *Am J Med* 1986;81: 7–14.
249. Coderre TJ, Katz J, Vaccarino AL, et al. Contribution of central neuroplasticity to pathological pain: review of clinical experimental evidence. *Pain* 1993;52:259–285.
250. Gracely RH, Lynch SA, Bennett GJ. Painful neuropathy: altered central processing maintained dynamically by peripheral input. *Pain* 1993;52:251–253.
251. Rohling ML, Binder LM, Langhinrichsen-Rohling J. Money matters: a meta-analytic review of the association between financial compensation and the experience and treatment of chronic pain. *Health Psychol* 1995;14:537–547.
252. Straaton KV, Maisiak R, Wrigley JM, et al. Barriers to return to work among persons unemployed due to arthritis and musculoskeletal disorders. *Arthritis Rheum* 1996;39:101–109.
253. Crofford LJ. Neuroendocrine abnormalities in fibromyalgia and related disorders. *Am J Med Sci* 1998;315:359–366.
254. Alexander RW, Bradley LA, Alarcón GS, et al. Sexual and physical abuse in women with fibromyalgia: association with outpatient health care utilization and pain medication usage. *Arthritis Care Res* 1998;11:102–115.
255. Heiss C, Ehlert V, Hander JP, et al. Abuse-related posttraumatic stress disorder and alterations of the hypothalamic-pituitary-adrenal axis in women with chronic pelvic pains. *Psychsom Med* 1998;60:309–318.
256. Lapossy E, Maleitzke R, Hrycaj P, et al. The frequency of transition of chronic low back pain to fibromyalgia. *Scand J Rheumatol* 1995;24:29–33.
257. Bennett RM. Emerging concepts in the neurobiology of chronic pain: evidence of abnormal sensory processing in fibromyalgia. *Mayo Clin Proc* 1999;74:385–398.
258. Buskila D, Neumann L, Vaisberg G, et al. Increased rates of fibromyalgia following cervical spine injury: a controlled study of 161 cases of traumatic injury. *Arthritis Rheum* 1997;40; 446–452.
259. Russell IJ. Advances in fibromyalgia: possible role for central neurochemicals. *Am J Med Sci* 1998;315:377–384.
260. Rainville P, Duncan GH, Price DD, et al. Pain affect encoded in human anterior cingulate but not somatosensory cortex. *Science* 1997;277:968–971.

261. Henriksson CM. Longterm effects of fibromyalgia on everyday life. A study of 56 patients. *Scand J Rheumatol* 1994;23:36–41.
262. Nørregaard J, Bülow PM, Prescott E, et al. A four-year follow-up study in fibromyalgia. Relationship to chronic fatigue syndrome. *Scand J Rheumatol* 1993;22:35–38.
263. Forseth DO, Forre O, Gran JT. A 5.5 year prospective study of self-reported musculoskeletal pain and of fibromyalgia in a female population: significance and natural history. *Clin Rheumatol* 1999;18:114–121.
264. Felson DT, Goldenberg DL. The natural history of fibromyalgia. *Arthritis Rheum* 1994;29:1522–1526.
265. Hawley DJ, Wolfe F, Cathey MA. Pain, functional disability, and psychological status: a 12-month study of severity in fibromyalgia. *J Rheumatol* 1988;15:1551–1556.
266. Granges G, Zilko P, Littlejohn GO. Fibromyalgia syndrome: assessment of the severity of the condition 2 years after diagnosis. *J Rheumatol* 1994;21:523–529.
267. Siegel DM, Janeway D, Baum J. Fibromyalgia syndrome in children and adolescents: clinical features at presentation and status at follow-up. *Pediatrics* 1998;101:377–382.
268. Mikkelsson M. One year outcome of preadolescents with fibromyalgia. *J Rheumatol* 1999;26:674–682.
269. White KP, Speechley M, Harth M, et al. Comparing self-reported function and work disability in 100 community cases of fibromyalgia syndrome versus controls in London, Ontario: the London Fibromyalgia Epidemiology Study. *Arthritis Rheum* 1999;42:76–83.
270. Hawley DJ, Wolfe F. Pain, disability, and pain/disability relationships in seven rheumatic disorders: a study of 1,522 patients. *J Rheumatol* 1991;18:1552–1557.
271. White KP, Speechley M, Harth M, et al. The London fibromyalgia epidemiology study: direct health care cost of fibromyalgia syndrome in London, Canada. *J Rheumatol* 1999;26: 885–889.
272. Goldenberg DL. A review of the role of tricyclic medications in the treatment of fibromyalgia syndrome. *J Rheumatol* 1989;16: 137–139.
273. Carette S, McCain GA, Bell DA, et al. Evaluation of amitriptyline in primary fibrositis: a double-blind, placebo-controlled study. *Arthritis Rheum* 1986;29:655–659.
274. Scudds RA, McCain GA, Rollman GB, et al. Improvements in pain responsiveness in patients with fibrositis after successful treatment with amitriptyline. *J Rheumatol* 1989;16(suppl 19):98–103.
275. Goldenberg DL, Felson DT, Dinerman H. A randomized, controlled trial of amitriptyline and naproxen in the treatment of patients with fibromyalgia. *Arthritis Rheum* 1986;29: 1371–1377.
276. Dessein PH, Shipton EA, Stanwix AE, et al. Neuroendocrine deficiency-mediated development and persistence of pain in fibromyalgia: a promising paradigm? *Pain* 2000;86:213–215.
277. Bennett RM, Gatter RA, Campbell SM, et al. A comparison of cyclobenzaprine and placebo in the management of fibrositis. A double-blind controlled study. *Arthritis Rheum* 1988;31: 1535–1542.
278. Quimby LG, Gratwick GM, Whitney CD, et al. A randomized trial of cylobenzaprine for the treatment of fibromyalgia. *J Rheumatol* 1989;16(suppl 19):140–143.
279. Carette S, Bell MJ, Reynolds WJ, et al. Comparison of amitriptyline, cyclobenzaprine, and placebo in the treatment of fibromyalgia: a randomized, double-blind clinical trial. *Arthritis Rheum* 1994;37:32–40.
280. Reynolds WJ, Moldofsky H, Saskin P, et al. The effects of cyclobenzaprine on sleep physiology and symptoms in patients with fibromyalgia. *J Rheumatol* 1991;18:452–454.
281. Simms RW, Felson DT, Goldenberg DL. Development of preliminary criteria for response to treatment in fibromyalgia syndrome. *J Rheumatol* 1991;18:1558–1563.
282. Russell IJ, Fletcher EM, Michalek JE, et al. Treatment of primary fibrositis/fibromyalgia syndrome with ibuprofen and alprazolam: a double-blind, placebo-controlled study. *Arthritis Rheum* 1991;34:552–560.
283. Wolfe F, Cathey MA, Hawley DJ. A double-blind placebo controlled trial of fluoxetine in fibromyalgia. *Scand J Rheumatol* 1994;23:255–259.
284. Hannonen P, Malminiemi K, Yli-Kerttula U, et al. A randomized, double-blind, placebo-controlled study of moclobemide and amitriptyline in the treatment of fibromyalgia in females without psychiatric disorder. *Br J Rheumatol* 1998;37: 1279–1286.
285. Dwight MD, Arnold LM, O'Brien H, et al. An open clinical trial of venlafaxine treatment of fibromyalgia. *Psychosomatics* 1998;39:14–17.
286. Scharf MB, Hauck M, Stover R, et al. Effect of gamma-hydroxybutyrate on pain, fatigue, and the alpha sleep anomaly in patients with fibromyalgia. Preliminary report. *J Rheumatol* 1998;25: 1986–1990.
287. Olin R, Klein R, Berg PA. A randomised double-blind 16-week study of ritanserin in fibromyalgia syndrome: clinical outcome and analysis of autoantibodies to serotonin, gangliosides and phospholipids. *Clin Rheumatol* 1998;17:89–94.
288. Nørregaard J, Volkmann H, Danneskiold-Samsøe B. A randomized controlled trial of citalopram in the treatment of fibromyalgia. *Pain* 1995;61:445–449.
289. Tavoni A, Vitali C, Bombardieri S, et al. Evaluation of S-adenosylmethionine in primary fibromyalgia: a double-blind crossover study. *Am J Med* 1987;83(suppl 5A):107–110.
290. Jacobsen S, Danneskiold-Samsøe B, Andersen RB. Oral S-adenosylmethionine in primary fibromyalgia: double-blind clinical evaluation. *Scand J Rheumatol* 1991;20:294–302.
291. Yunus MB, Masi AT, Aldag JC. Short term effects of ibuprofen in primary fibromyalgia syndrome: a double-blind, placebo controlled trial. *J Rheumatol* 1989;16:527–532.
292. Alberts KR, Bradley LA, Alarcón GS, et al. Sertraline hydrochloride alters pain threshold, sensory discrimination ability, and functional brain activity in patients with fibromyalgia (FM): a randomized, controlled trial (RCT). *Arthritis Rheum* 1998;41:S259.
293. Wallace DJ, Shapiro S, Panush RS. Update on fibromyalgia syndrome. *Bull Rheum Dis* 1999;48:1–5.
294. Biasi G, Manca S, Maganelli S, et al. Tramadol in the fibromyalgia syndrome: a controlled clinical trial versus placebo. *Int J Clin Pharmacol Res* 1998;18:13–19.
295. Bessette L, Carette S, Fossel AH, et al. A placebo controlled crossover trial of subcutaneous salmon calcitonin in the treatment of patients with fibromyalgia. *Scand J Rheumatol* 1998;27: 112–116.
296. Rowbotham M, Harden N, Stacey B, et al. Gabapentin of the treatment of postherpetic neuralgia a randomized controlled trial. *JAMA* 1998;280:1837–1842.
297. Rossy LA, Buckelew SP, Dorr N, et al. A meta-analysis of fibromyalgia treatment interventions. *Ann Behav Med* 1999;21: 180–191.
298. Pioro-Boisset M, Esdaile JM, Fitzcharles MA. Alternative medicine use in fibromyalgia syndrome. *Arthritis Care Res* 1996; 9:13–17.
299. Dykman KD, Tone C, Ford C, et al. The effects of nutritional supplements on the symptoms of fibromyalgia and chronic fatigue syndrome. *Integ Physiol Behav Sci* 1998;33:61–71.
300. Anonymous. *Exercise testing on apparently healthy individuals:* a handbook for physicians. Dallas: American Heart Association, 1975.

301. Borg GV, Linderholm H. Perceived exertion and pulse rate during graded exercise in various age groups. *Acta Med Scand* 1967;472(suppl):194–199.
302. McCain GA, Bell DA, Mai FM, et al. A controlled study of the effects of a supervised cardiovascular fitness training program on the manifestations of primary fibromyalgia. *Arthritis Rheum* 1988;31:1135–1141.
303. Martin L, Nutking A, McIntosh BR, et al. An exercise program in the treatment of fibromyalgia. *J Rheumatol* 1996;23: 1050–1053.
304. Gowans SE, deHuerck A, Voss S, et al. A randomized, controlled trial of exercise and education for individuals with fibromyalgia. *Arthritis Care Res* 1999;12:120–128.
305. Burckhardt CS, Mannerkorpi K, Hendenberg L, et al. A randomized, controlled clinical trial of education and physical training for women with fibromyalgia. *J Rheumatol* 1994;21: 714–720.
306. Verstappen FTJ, van Santen-Hoeuftt HMS, Bobvjn PH, et al. Effects of a group activity program for fibromyalgia patients on physical fitness and well being. *J Musculoskel Pain* 1997;5: 17–28.
307. Bradley LA, Alberts KR. Psychological and behavioral approaches to pain management for patient with rheumatic disease. *Rheum Dis Clin North Am* 1999;25:215–232.
308. Nielson WR, Walker C, McCain GA. Cognitive behavioral treatment of fibromyalgia syndrome: preliminary findings. *J Rheumatol* 1992;19:98–103.
309. Goldenberg DL, Kaplan KH, Nadeau MG, et al. A controlled study of a stress-reduction, cognitive-behavioral treatment program in fibromyalgia. *J Musculoskel Pain* 1994;2:53–66.
310. White KP, Nielson WR. Cognitive-behavioral treatment of fibromyalgia syndrome: a follow-up assessment. *J Rheumatol* 1995;22:717–721.
311. Turk DC, Okifuji A, Sinclair JD, et al. Interdisciplinary treatment for fibromyalgia syndrome: clinical and statistical significance. *Arthritis Care Res* 1998;11:186–195.
312. Bennett RM, Burckhardt CS, Clark SR, et al. Group treatment of fibromyalgia: a 6 month outpatient program. *J Rheumatol* 1996;23:521–528.
313. Bennett RM, Campbell S, Burckhardt C, et al. Balanced approach provides small but significant gains. A multidisciplinary approach to fibromyalgia management. *J Musculoskel Med* 1991;8:21–32.
314. Buckelew SP, Conway R, Parker J, et al. Biofeedback/relaxation training and exercise interventions for fibromyalgia: a prospective trial. *Arthritis Care Res* 1998;11:196–209.
315. Nicassio PM, Radojevic V, Weisman MH, et al. A comparison of behavioral and educational interventions with fibromyalgia. *J Rheumatol* 1997;24:2000–2007.
316. Vlaeyen JWS, Teeken-Gruben NJG, Boosens MEJB, et al. Cognitive-educational treatment of fibromyalgia: a randomized clinical trail. I. Clinical effects. *J Rheumatol* 1996;23: 1237–1245.
317. Buckelew SP, Huyser B, Hewett JE, et al. Self-efficacy predicts outcome among fibromyalgia subjects. *Arthritis Care Res* 1996; 9:97–104.
318. Bradley LA, Young LD, Anderson KO, et al. Effects of psychological therapy on pain behavior of rheumatoid arthritis patients. Treatment outcome and six-month followup. *Arthritis Rheum* 1987;30:1105–1114.
319. Keefe FJ, Caldwell DS, Williams DA, et al. Pain coping skills training in the management of osteoarthritis knee pain: a comparative study. *Behav Ther* 1990;21:49–62.
320. Ferraccioli G, Ghirelli L, Scita F, et al. EMG-biofeedback training in fibromyalgia syndrome. *J Rheumatol* 1987;14:820–825.
321. Haanen HCM, Hoenderdos HTW, van Romunde LKJ, et al. Controlled trial of hypnotherapy in the treatment of refractory fibromyalgia. *J Rheumatol* 1991;18:72–75.
322. Ambrogio N, Cuttiford J, Lineker S, et al. A comparison of three types of neck support in fibromyalgia patients. *Arthritis Care Res* 1998;11:405–410.
323. Berman BM, Ezzo J, Hadhazy V, et al. Is acupuncture effective in the treatment of fibromyalgia? *J Fam Pract* 1999;48:213–218.
324. Anonymous. Acupuncture. NIH Consensus Conference. *JAMA* 1998;280:1518–1524.
325. Hoh D. Spine, skull surgery may help many with CFIDS, FMS: Chiari malformation or cervical stenosis may be common in CFIDS and fibromyalgia. *CFIDS Chronicle* 1999;10:2.
326. Alarcón GS, Bradley LA, Hadley MN, et al. Does Chiari malformation contribute to fibromyalgia symptoms? *Arthritis Rheum* 1997;40:S190.
327. Alarcón GS, Bradley LA. Frequency of Chiari malformation in patients with fibromyalgia. *Arthritis Rheum.* 1999;42:2731–2732.
328. Baumstark KE, Buckelew SP, Sher KJ, et al. Pain behavior predictors among fibromyalgia patients. *Pain* 1993;55:339–346.
329. Buckelew SP, Parker JC, Keefe FJ, et al. Self-efficacy and pain behavior among subjects with fibromyalgia. *Pain* 1994;59: 377–384.
330. Bradley LA. Cognitive-behavioral therapy for primary fibromyalgia. *J Rheumatol* 1989;16(suppl 19):131–136.
331. Hewett JE, Buckelew SP, Johnson JC, et al. Selection of measures suitable for evaluating change in fibromyalgia clinical trials. *J Rheumatol* 1995;22:2307–2312.
332. Goldenberg DL, Mossey CJ, Schmid CH. A model to assess severity and impact of fibromyalgia. *J Rheumatol* 1995;22:2313–2318.
333. Blanchard EB, Schwarz SP. Clinically significant changes in behavioral medicine. *Behav Assess* 1988;10:171–188.
334. Jacobson NS, Truax P. Clinical significance: a statistical approach to defining meaningful change in psychotherapy research. *J Consult Clin Psychol* 1991;59:12–19.
335. Goldenberg DL. Treatment of fibromyalgia syndrome. *Rheum Dis Clin North Am* 1989;15:61–71.
336. Buckelew SP. Fibromyalgia: a rehabilitation approach. *Am J Phys Med Rehabil* 1989;68:37–42.
337. Clark S, Tindall E, Bennett RM. A double blind crossover trial of prednisone versus placebo in the treatment of fibrositis. *J Rheumatol* 1985;12:980–983.
338. McCain GA. Role of physical fitness training in the fibrositis/fibromyalgia syndrome. *Am J Med* 1986;81(suppl 3A):73–77.
339. Fordyce WE. *Behavioral methods for chronic pain and illness.* St. Louis: CV Mosby, 1976.
340. Bradley LA, McDonald JE, Richter JE. Psychophysiological interactions in the esophageal diseases: implications for assessment and treatment. *Semin Gastrointest Dis* 1990;1:5–22.
341. Keefe FJ, Bonk V. Psychosocial assessment of pain in patients having rheumatic diseases. *Rheum Dis Clin North Am* 1999; 25:81–103.
342. Hawley DJ, Wolfe F. Pain, disability, and pain/disability relationships in seven rheumatic disorders: a study of 1,522 patients. *J Rheumatol* 1991;18:1552–1557.
343. Burckhardt CS, Archenholtz B, Mannerkorpi K, et al. Quality of life of Swedish women with fibromyalgia syndrome, rheumatoid arthritis or systemic lupus erythematosus. In: Jacobsen S, Danneskiold-Samsøe B, Lund B, eds. *Musculoskeletal pain, myofascial pain syndrome, and the fibromyalgia syndrome.* New York: Haworth Medical, 1993:199–207.
344. Bruusgaard D, Evensen AR, Bjerkedal T. Fibromyalgia—a new cause for disability pension. *Scand J Soc Med* 1993;21:116–119.
345. Anonymous. Does fibromyalgia qualify as a work-related illness or injury? *J Occup Med* 1992;34:968.

346. Bennett RM. Disabling fibromyalgia: appearance versus reality. *J Rheumatol* 1993;20:1821–1824.
347. Capen K. The courts, expert witnesses and fibromyalgia. *Can Med Assoc J* 1995;153:206–208.
348. Romano TJ. Fibromyalgia 20 years later: What have we really accomplished? *J Rheumatol* 1996;23:192.
349. Burckhardt CS, Clark SR, Bennett RM. Fibromyalgia and quality of life: a comparative analysis. *J Rheumatol* 1993;20:475–479.
350. Martinez JE, Ferraz MB, Sato EI, et al. Fibromyalgia versus rheumatoid arthritis: a longitudinal comparison of the quality of life. *J Rheumatol* 1995;22:270–274.
351. Wolfe F, Aarflot T, Bruusgaard D, et al. Fibromyalgia and disability. Report of the Moss International Working Group on medico-legal aspects of chronic widespread musculoskeletal pain complaints and fibromyalgia. *Scand J Rheumatol* 1995;24:112–118.

91

NEUROPATHIC JOINT DISEASE (CHARCOT JOINTS)

MICHAEL H. ELLMAN

Neuropathic joint disease is a progressive degenerative arthritis with characteristic clinical and radiographic features. Described by Jean-Martin Charcot (1) in 1868 in patients with "l'ataxie locomotrice progressive," or tabes dorsalis, it is now most commonly seen in the mid- and forefoot and ankle of patients with diabetes mellitus (Fig. 91.1). The arthritis develops after sensory loss in a joint, increased local blood flow, osteopenia, and continued weight bearing; for unknown reasons, however, not all patients who meet these criteria develop neuroarthropathy.

It seems fitting that the eponym *Charcot joint* be retained as synonymous with neuropathic joint disease. Charcot (1825–1893) was a master of medicine with virtuoso contributions in neurology, psychiatry, and rheumatology (2). He is considered a father of neurology, but he had an avid interest in arthritis and his writings included a thesis, published in 1853, entitled "Primary Progressive Chronic Articular Rheumatism" (3). His progressive attitude toward medicine was revealed in a lecture at the Hospital of the Salpetriere in Paris in 1867, when he stated that the essential difference between ancient and modern medicine was that in the latter, "physicians could profit by the errors of their predecessors, which roads ought to remain closed to speculation and which, on the contrary, they may traverse without fear of losing themselves" (2).

Charcot's description of neuropathic joint disease has remained the best. He emphasized the suddenness of the arthritis, "most commonly without any pain whatever, or any febrile reaction." Charcot described the swelling of the joint and the presence of a hydrarthrosis: "On puncture being made, a transparent lemon-colored liquid has been frequently drawn from the joint." He also mentioned cracking sounds at the articular surfaces, luxations developing, rapid wasting of the muscles, the presence of foreign bodies, and the etiology of this arthritis, "produced . . . by the more or less energetic movements to which the patient sometimes continues to subject the affected members." Charcot felt that the joint changes were subordinate to sclerotic changes in the spinal cord, a concept of a trophic injury to nerves that became known as the French theory of neuropathic joint disease (1,4,5). This view was vigorously disputed by Volkmann and Virchow, who espoused the German theory, that neuropathic arthritis had a mechanical origin produced by insensitive joints and repeated subclinical trauma (4–6). Charcot also described an hyperacute variant of the disease with swelling and other signs of inflammation of such severity that joint sepsis would now be suspected. Schultze and Kahler described the relationship between syringomyelia and neuropathic joint disease in 1888 (7). Dearborn (8) in 1932 described the disease in a patient with congenital insensitivity to pain who billed himself as the "human pin cushion." Jordan (9) in 1936 chronicled neuropathic joint disease in diabetic neuropathy. By 1964, Robillard and associates (10) reviewed 100 cases of diabetic neuropathic joint disease in the medical literature, and in 1974, Clouse and co-workers (11) reported 90 cases of neuropathic joint disease and diabetes mellitus seen at a single institution over a 13-year span. Neuropathic-like joint disease without neurologic deficits has been described in patients receiving intraarticular corticosteroids (12–17) and in some individuals with calcium pyrophosphate dihydrate (CPPD) crystal deposition disease (18–29). A current but brief historical review of neuropathic arthropathy was written in 1993 (30).

Neuropathic joint disease has been described in a host of other diseases as disparate as yaws (31) and meningomyelocele (32). It is now most frequently seen by diabetologists, podiatrists, foot and ankle surgeons, and rheumatologists in patients with diabetes mellitus complaining of foot pain or swelling (10,11,33–41). Medical centers that have a multidisciplinary foot and ankle program may be the optimal place for the care of the patient with neuropathic joint disease involving the foot and ankle. If the disease is diagnosed early and treatment instituted promptly, the outcome is often surprisingly successful (10,33,35–39,41–44).

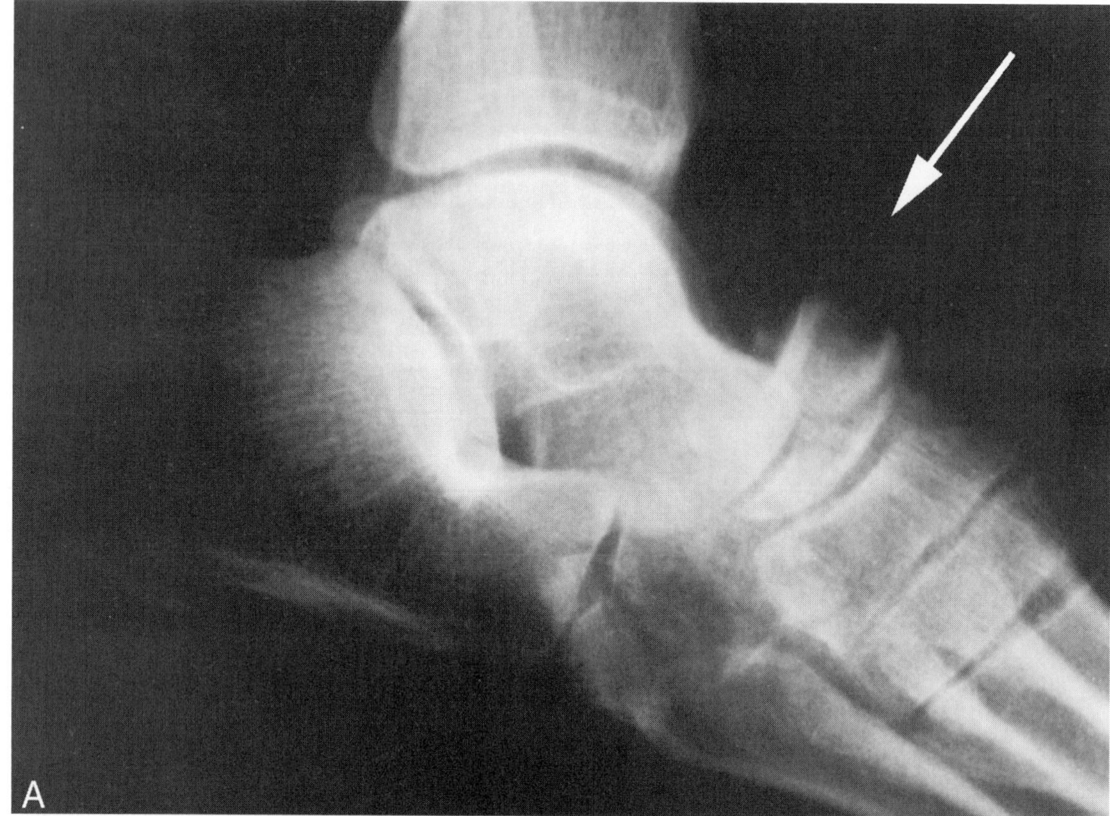

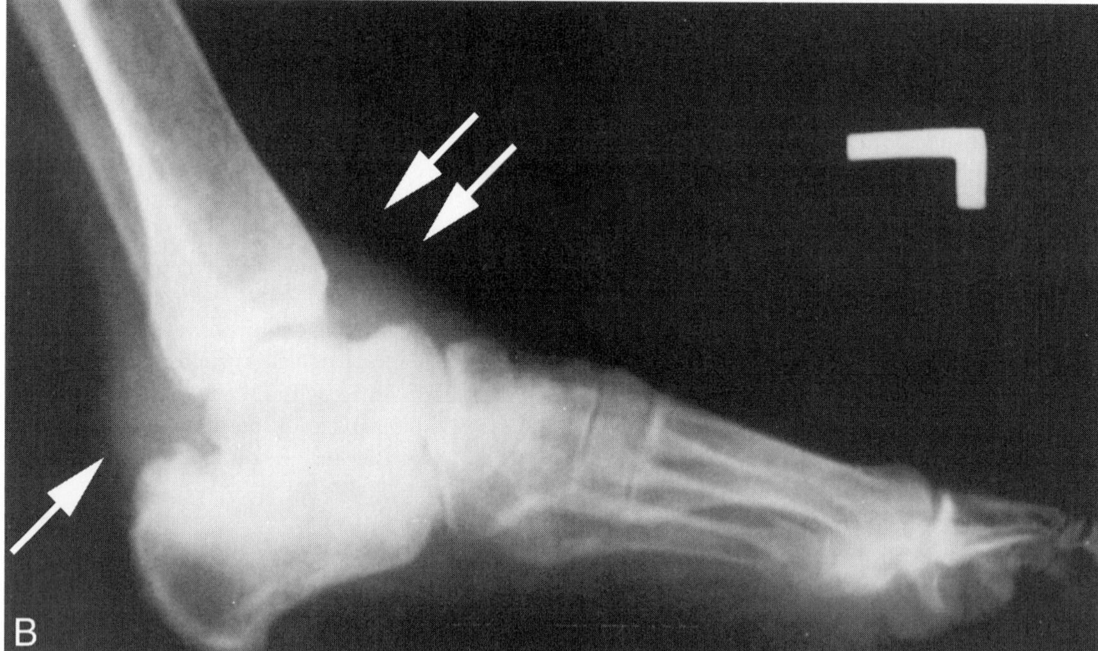

FIGURE 91.1. The radiographic appearance of neuropathic joint disease of the foot and ankle varies greatly. The foot is now the most common site of neuroarthropathy. **A:** This patient with diabetes mellitus had only moderate discomfort with the dislocation of the navicular bone *(arrow)*, which was the first indication of neuropathic joint disease. **B:** Massive soft tissue swelling surrounding the joint *(arrows)* is common in the neuropathic ankle and is frequently seen in neuroarthropathy accompanying diabetes mellitus, tabes dorsalis, congenital insensitivity to pain, or meningomyelocele.

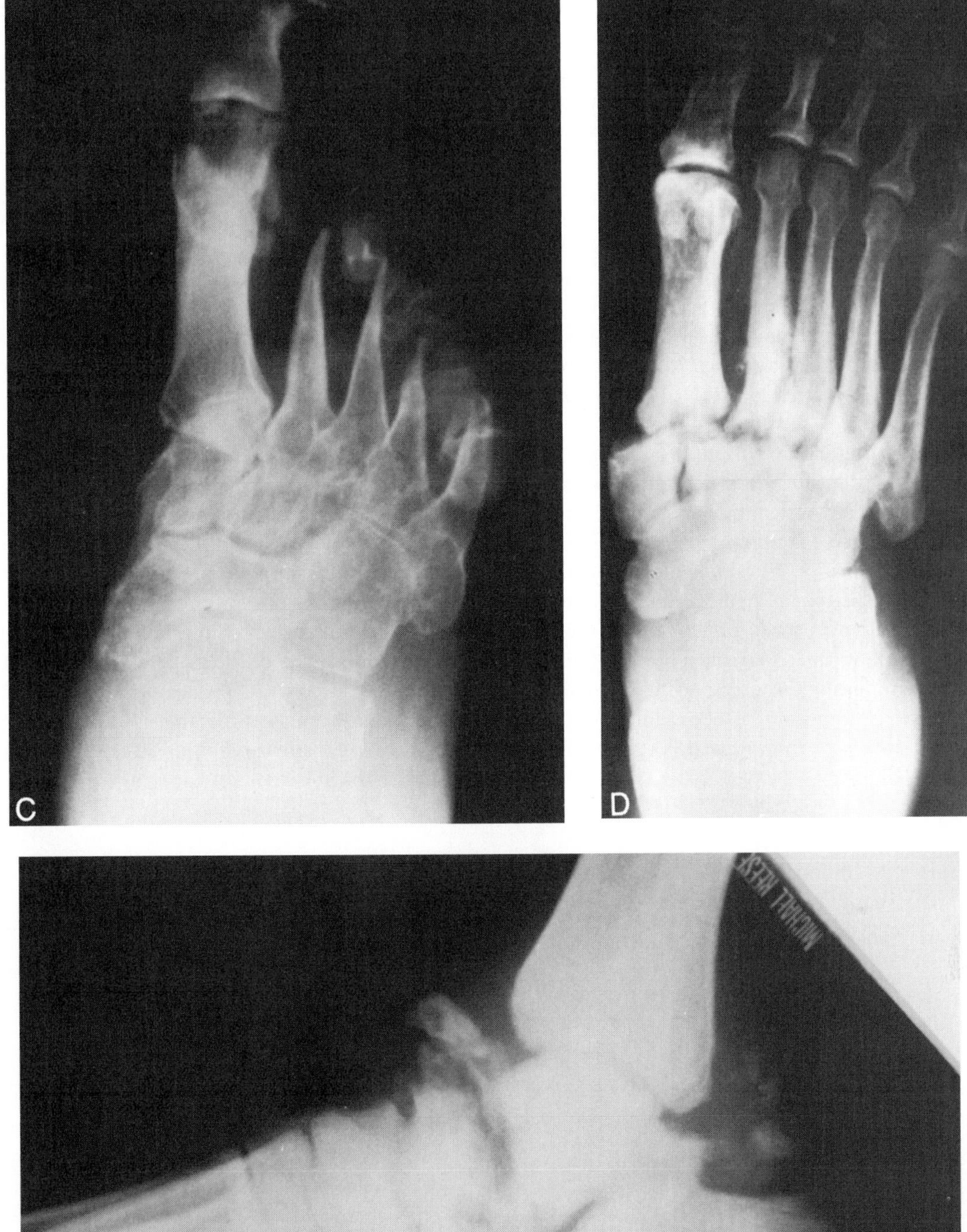

FIGURE 91.1. C: There is striking osteolysis of the metatarsals ("sucked candy" appearance) and the phalanges in this patient with chronic diabetes mellitus. **D:** This patient with diabetes mellitus exhibits destruction, fragmentation, and displacement of the tarsometatarsal joints, which are sometimes described as Lisfranc's fracture-dislocation (Lisfranc actually described amputation at that site) (38,103). **E:** Another patient with diabetes mellitus with typical soft tissue swelling and fragmentation of the navicular bone has sharply defined osseous debris at the dorsum and posterior foot and ankle.

CLINICAL FEATURES

The diseases giving rise to neuropathic joint disease have changed over the last several decades, as has the clinical picture. The decline in new cases of syphilis and the success of antibiotic treatment in curing existing cases has made tabetic neuropathic joint disease uncommon. These patients typically had monoarticular involvement, usually of the knee, with the hip, ankle, and lower axial skeleton less frequently involved (5,35,45–49). A painless lower extremity monoarticular arthritis in a patient with a neurologic deficit was usually ascribed to neurosyphilis (5,35, 46–50). Synovitis, progressive joint instability, bony overgrowth, and fragmentation led to the characteristic "bag of bones" sensation noted when the involved joint was palpated (5,35,47,51) (Figs. 91.2 and 91.3).

Pain is often the presenting symptom, although some patients have none, even after gross joint disintegration. Absent deep pain sensation, tested by squeezing the Achilles tendon, is the clinical sine qua non.

Most patients with neuropathic joint disease now have diabetes mellitus with peripheral neuropathy as the underlying cause. These patients usually present to the rheumatologist with a painful, warm, and swollen mid- or forefoot, ankle, or metatarsophalangeal joint with radiographic abnormalities demonstrating soft tissue swelling and demineralization suggestive of early infection (11,33,34,37,41, 52–54) (Fig. 91.1).

Upper extremity neuropathic joint disease usually is caused by syringomyelia (35,55–58). Proximal joints are most often involved, especially the shoulder (Fig. 91.4). The joints are swollen, warm, and often painful; subluxations may occur early in the course. In some patients, rapid dissolution of bone occurs (Fig. 91.4) (59,60).

Noninflammatory (group 1) joint fluid frequently is present when large joints are involved, although about half of the fluids obtained are grossly bloody or markedly xanthochromic (61). Inflammatory joint fluid containing CPPD crystals has been observed in some patients (18,21). Inflammatory fluid without the presence of CPPD crystals should raise the possibility of sepsis. Although uncommon, infection poses diagnostic difficulties because patients may complain of only mild increases in joint pain or swelling (62–65). Most of the reported cases of septic arthritis in large joint neuropathic disease have been caused by staphylococci, although tuberculous arthritis has been described (62–65). Perforating ulcerations of the foot in patients with neuropathic joint disease, described in 1818 as "plantaire mal perforant" (41,66,67), are distressingly common and often associated with infection (41,66,67).

The relative lack of pain makes a diagnosis of other complicating disorders difficult. For example, a traumatic false aneurysm developed after a hip fracture in a patient with tabes dorsalis and neuropathic joint disease. No pain was noted by the patient despite a large expanding hematoma, and the diagnosis was made only by the presence of an

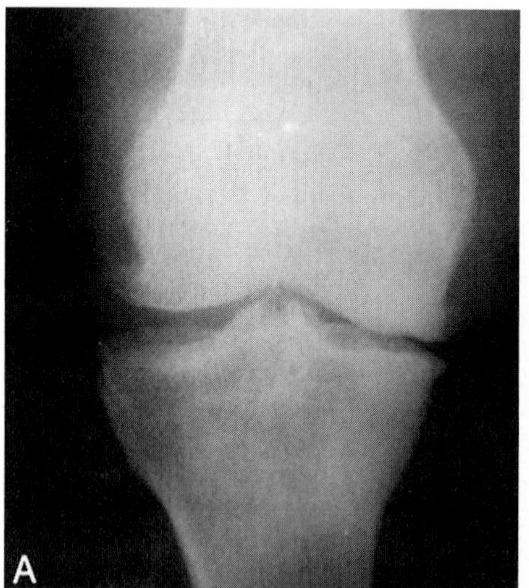

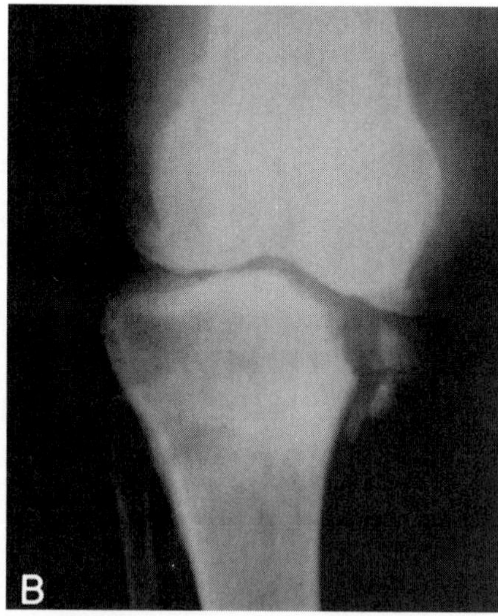

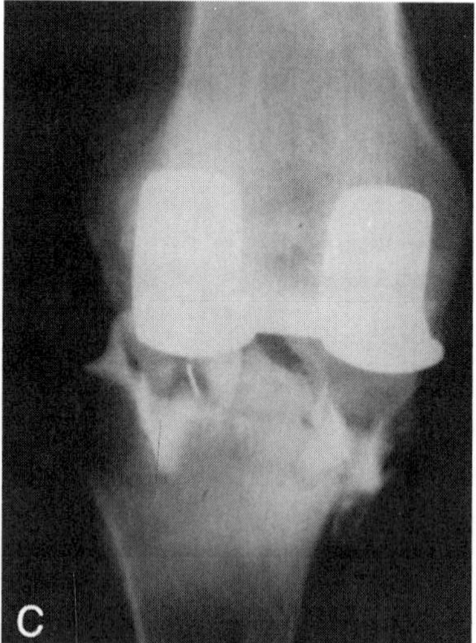

FIGURE 91.2. Neuroarthropathy of the knee joint in tabes dorsalis. **A:** This patient with tabes dorsalis was initially thought to have osteoarthritis and had been scheduled for total knee surgery, although there was minimal pain and the large joint effusion was atypical for primary osteoarthritis. **B:** A preoperative knee radiograph showed sharply defined fragmentation of bone at the medial tibial joint margin and a massive joint effusion, clues to the diagnosis of neuropathic joint disease that were, unfortunately, ignored by the surgeons. **C:** Two weeks after total knee surgery, the prosthesis had subluxed, and the knee was unstable. The patient had minimal knee pain but was not able to bear weight. Total joint replacement surgery is generally contraindicated in neuropathic joints.

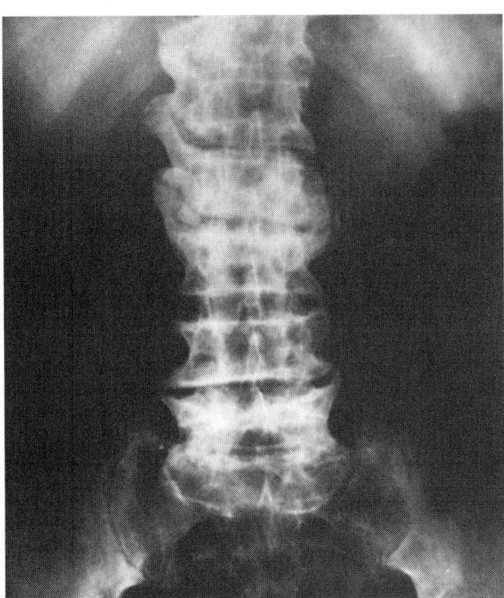

FIGURE 91.3. Neuropathic joint disease of the axial skeleton may mimic osteoarthritis or ankylosing hyperostosis. Irregular narrowing of the disc spaces, a vertebral fracture, subchondral sclerosis, and bulky-headed osteophytes resembling *les becs des parroquets* (parakeets' beaks) have developed in this 78-year-old man. (From Rodnan GP. Neuropathic joint disease (Charcot joints). In: McCarty DJ, ed. *Arthritis and allied conditions,* 10th ed. Philadelphia: Lea & Febiger, 1985:1101, with permission.)

ecchymosis in the flank accompanied by a falling hemoglobin (68).

Spontaneous fractures and dislocations are both very common in tabes dorsalis, diabetic neuropathy, congenital indifference to pain, and spinal dysraphism, and often call attention to the underlying disorder (45,53,69–77). Untreated fractures or dislocations may hasten the development and progression of the neuroarthropathy (72–78). The diagnosis of neuropathic joint disease is usually considered in a patient with arthritis accompanying a neurologic disorder. Most patients experience relatively less pain than expected, allowing continued use of the joint (5,47,79). The progression of the disease process varies widely (4,35). Many patients have sudden and dramatic symptoms with collapse of the joint because of intra- or juxtaarticular fractures (72,75). The use of pressure pattern analysis of the foot during gait may detect early abnormalities in the Charcot foot. The midtarsal area may sustain considerably more peak pressure with weight bearing and sustain this pressure for a longer period of time (80). The radiologic appearance is typical and nearly specific for the disease, although early in the course it may closely mimic the changes seen in osteoarthritis (3,11,26). Joint disease may also progress so slowly that review of serial radiographs correlated with the clinical features may be needed to confirm the diagnosis (26,51). In other patients, acute fractures, dislocations, subluxations, and gross disruption of the joint confirm the diagnosis on a single radiograph (26,28).

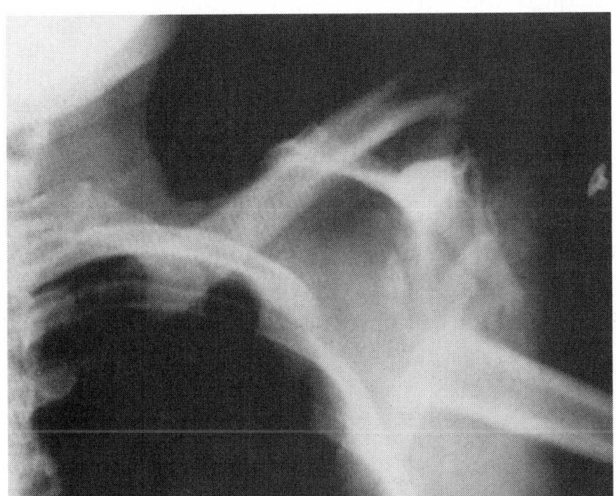

FIGURE 91.4. Shoulder neuroarthropathy is usually due to syringomyelia. Sterile inflammatory joint fluid was observed, and this patient experienced constant pain. The osteolysis of the proximal humerus and cloudy calcification of soft tissue are typical. Some patients have painless swelling; the progression of osteolysis may be exceedingly rapid.

RADIOLOGIC FEATURES

The radiographic appearance may be the first clue to the presence of neuroarthropathy. Joint effusion, soft tissue swelling, and osteophytes difficult to distinguish from primary osteoarthritis are early changes that are not diagnostic (26,50,51). Subluxation, paraarticular debris, and bony fragmentation strongly suggest the diagnosis of neuropathic joint disease (5,26,51).

More advanced radiographic changes include massive soft tissue enlargement, marked joint effusion, fractures, depression, and absorption of subchondral bone, and bony proliferation expressed as osteophytes and sclerosis (26, 35,50). Fragments of bone may accumulate in tissue distant from the joint. The focal disruption of bone and cartilage with collection of debris in synovial and paraarticular tissues may produce radiographic clues to the diagnosis before gross fragmentation becomes evident (26,50).

Malalignment with angular deformity and subluxation of the joint contribute to the fracturing. Pseudarthroses form at some joint surfaces as a result of fractures and deformities, leading to new bone approximations (11,26,50, 51,77).

In 1948, Hodgson and associates (81) directed attention to the difficulty in distinguishing the radiographic picture of neuroarthropathy from that of local infection. These authors found infection in the contiguous soft tissue in most of their patients with "neurotrophic" bone lesions and postulated that osteomyelitis contributed to the radiographic picture of neuropathic joint disease. Resnick and Niwayama (26) emphasized that the bony margins produced by osseous fragmentation in neuropathic joint disease are well defined and sharp; in contrast, fuzzy bony contours are atypical for neuroarthropathy and suggest infection or the presence of other inflammatory processes.

Bone scintigraphy with technetium ^{99m}Tc-labeled bisphosphonate revealed markedly abnormal uptake, even early in the disease (82–84). Radiopharmaceutical uptake was increased within 2 minutes after injection, indicating increased local blood flow (82). ^{67}Ga (radiogallium) uptake is an indicator of inflammation, and its accumulation in neuroarthropathy may be intense. Its distribution is less dependent on blood flow than is localization of ^{99m}Tc-labeled bisphosphonate (85,86). Of historic interest, six cases of neuropathic joint disease have been studied with angiography and three by lymphangiography (87,88). All showed increased local vascularity by angiography, whereas lymphangiography was normal. Computed tomography (CT) has been helpful in evaluating neuroarthropathy in the axial skeleton (89–93).

The diagnosis of infection in a Charcot joint remains difficult. The superimposition of the sometimes subtle clinical and radiographic findings of osteomyelitis on top of the neuroarthropathy is often diagnostically challenging. The sudden worsening of a previously stable neuropathic foot, increasing erythema without trauma, and systemic symptoms are clues to the possibility of infection. Osteomyelitis in the absence of chronic skin ulcers has been unusual in our experience. Positive blood, tissue, or bone cultures for a microorganism clarify the situation.

Indium-111 (^{111}In) leukocyte imaging has been studied in several series of patients with suspected osteomyelitis (Fig. 91.5). Maurer and co-workers (94), reported 13 patients with diabetic neuroarthropathy, four of whom had osteomyelitis. Three of the four patients with infection had a positive scintigram, but the negative results in eight of the nine patients without osteomyelitis were even more helpful. Seabold et al. (95) compared ^{111}In-leukocyte imaging with that obtained with ^{99m}Tc-bisphosphonate and magnetic resonance imaging (MRI) in patients with neuroarthropathy and suspected osteomyelitis. A negative ^{111}In–white blood cell (WBC) study indicated that osteomyelitis was unlikely, but positive imaging with any of the preceding techniques was compatible with infected neuroarthropathy. A technique that does not require leukocyte harvesting uses ^{111}In-labeled human nonspecific immunoglobulin G and may improve specificity for detecting infection in diabetic patients with foot ulcers, gangrene, or a Charcot joint when compared to conventional bone scans (96). Splittgerber and co-workers (97) and Kalen and co-workers (98)—the latter studying spinal neuroarthropathy—reported similar findings with the use of ^{111}In-WBC. Leukocyte imaging has the disadvantages of a long preparation time and low radionuclide count rates with poor spatial resolution. There also may be difficulty separating soft tissue from bony infection. Palestro and associates (99) found that the combination of indium-111 leukocyte and technetium-99m sulfur colloid scintigraphy was more specific for infected neuropathic joints than the combined use of triple-phase bone scans and leukocyte scintigraphy. The authors point out the nonspecificity of leukocyte scanning in neuroarthropathy and postulate that its increased radioactivity accumulation is related to marrow activity. Increased labeled leukocyte accumulation without corresponding activity on bone marrow images was felt to be typical of Charcot arthropathy and infection.

MRI has the ability to delineate soft tissue inflammation from bony structures (86) and is very helpful in diagnosing osteomyelitis (100), although in one study conventional radiography was comparable to MRI (101). It gives abnormal results in almost all patients with Charcot joints and is a sensitive tool for diagnosing the arthritis at the earliest

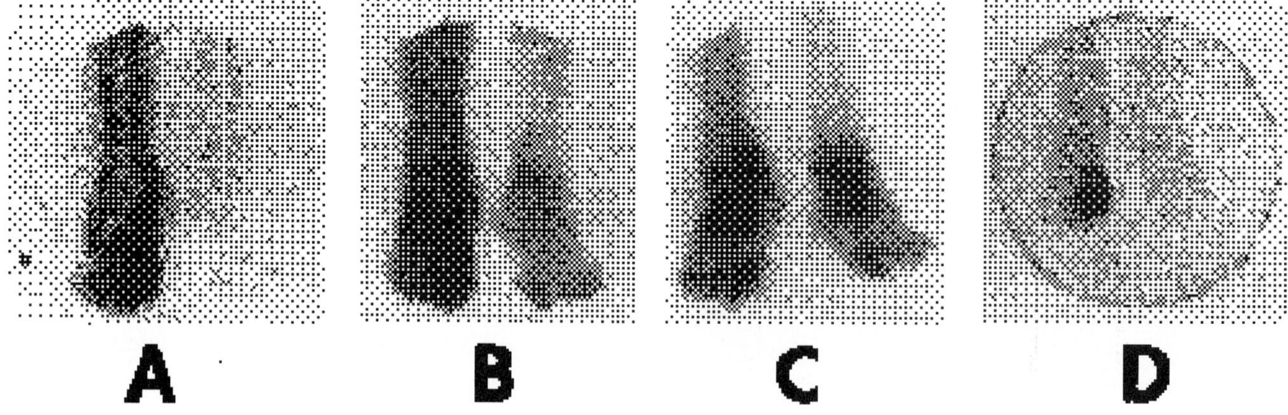

FIGURE 91.5. Selections from the three phases of a triple-phase technetium ^{99m}Tc-labeled bisphosphonate bone scintigram are shown. Radionuclide angiogram **(A)**, blood pool image **(B)**, and delayed bone image **(C)** in a patient with arthritis of the foot and ankle with suspected infection. **D:** The ^{111}In-labeled white blood count (WBC) scan demonstrates accumulation at the first toe. This site proved to be the only site of osteomyelitis.

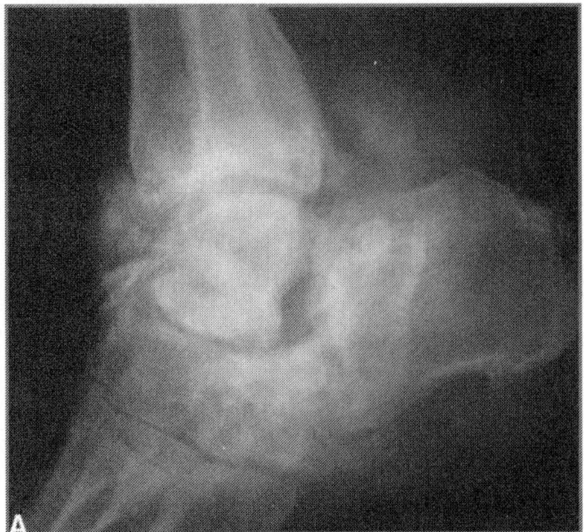
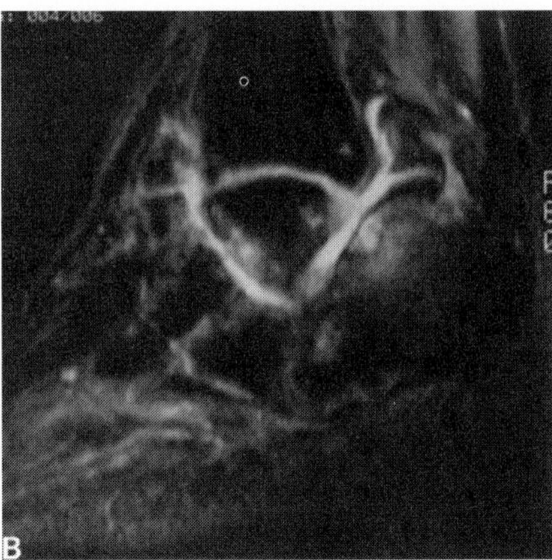
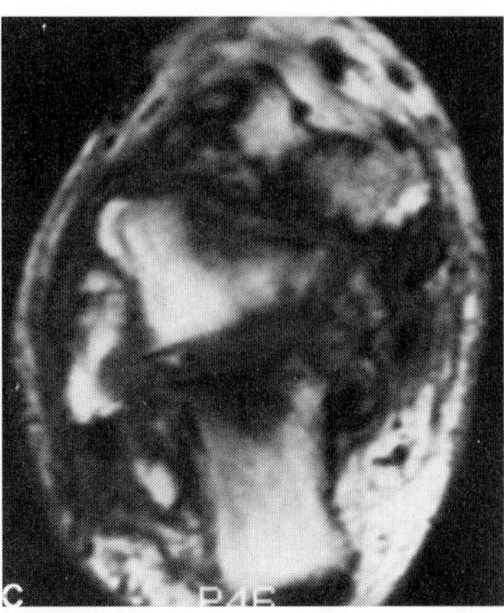

FIGURE 91.6. A: A lateral radiograph demonstrating neuroarthropathy involving the ankle with bony fragmentation, sclerosis, and soft tissue swelling. The appearance of this hypertrophic type of Charcot arthropathy has been described as "osteoarthritis with a vengeance." **B:** Sagittal view of the same ankle as in **A** with short T1 inversion recovery (STIR) (STIR–fat suppression technique) demonstrating foci (areas of high intensity) of bone marrow edema within the talus, which could represent either infection or fracture. **C:** Coronal view magnetic resonance imaging (MRI) of the same ankle (SE 600/20) demonstrating the bony fragmentation medial to the talus and calcaneus, soft tissue edema, tenosynovitis surrounding the peroneus longus and brevis tendons, and low signal focus in the calcaneus, probably representing sclerotic bone. (All photographs courtesy of Dr. Tom Grant.)

stage and for quantifying the extent of the abnormalities. Beltran and associates (102) found a distinctive pattern of low signal intensity on T1- and T2-weighted images within the bone marrow space adjacent to the involved joint in some Charcot patients. They also confirmed the helpfulness of MRI in differentiating neuropathy from osteomyelitis. Seabold and co-workers (95) found MRI abnormalities in all seven of the Charcot patients they studied, including decreased signal intensity on T1 images and increased signal on T2 and short T1 inversion recovery (STIR) images in joints and adjacent bone marrow (Figs. 91.6 and 91.7).

Resnick and Niwayama (26) stated, "The radiographic picture is that of a disorganized joint, characterized by simultaneously occurring bone resorption and formation.

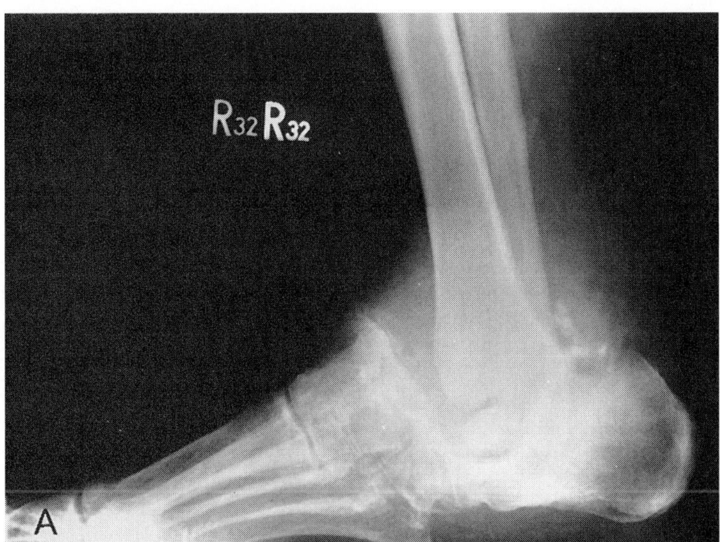

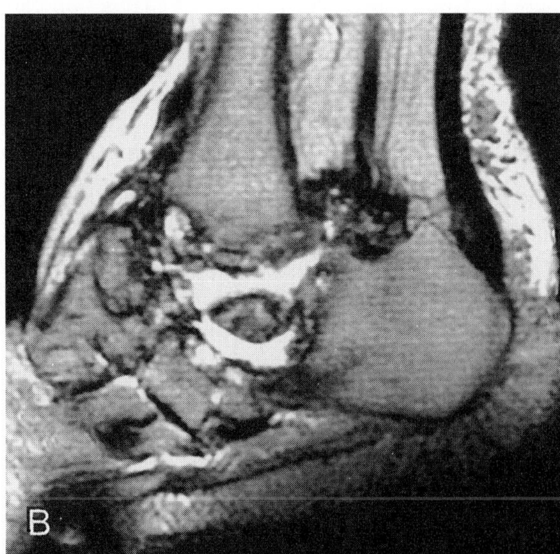

FIGURE 91.7. The patient is an elderly woman with diabetes mellitus and chronic Charcot arthropathy of the right ankle and foot manifested by persistent pain, swelling, and fever that prompted amputation of the ankle. **A:** Lateral radiograph revealed the extensive soft tissue swelling with destruction and collapse of the talus. **B:** MRI demonstrated fluid surrounding the remnant of the talus with destruction of the surrounding bones (T2-weighted image). The fluid was sterile at surgery. (Photographs courtesy of Dr. Larry Dixon.)

The degree of sclerosis, osteophytosis and fragmentation in this articular disorder is greater than that in any other process."

Diabetic Neuroarthropathy

The radiographic picture in diabetic neuroarthropathy has been divided into a destructive type affecting tarsal bones and an absorptive or mutilating type confined to the forefoot, with gradual disappearance of the epiphyseal ends with "pencil point" or "sucked candy" narrowing (Fig. 91.1C) (10,26,34,40,41,43,54). These types are not mutually exclusive. Destructive changes at the tarsometatarsal area are sometimes referred to as a Lisfranc fracture-dislocation (4,103) (Fig. 91.1D).

Forgacs (104) described the three radiographic stages of diabetic neuropathic joint disease, with stage I (initial findings) demonstrating only osteoporosis and cortical defects leading to stage II (progression) with osteolysis and fragmentation. In stage III (healing), there is deformity, ankylosis, refilling of cortical defects, and restitution (104).

The prevalence of neuroarthropathy in diabetes mellitus is not known. Clinically apparent peripheral neuropathy is present in more than 25% of diabetics and unrecognized foot fractures were found in 12 of 54 neuropathic patients (105). Cavanagh and co-workers (105) found that diabetes mellitus per se resulted in no excess of radiographic foot bony abnormalities compared with age-matched controls, but 16% of diabetics with neuropathy who had experienced foot ulcers exhibited radiographic changes characteristic of Charcot arthropathy. In a more recent study, 1.4% of 456 diabetic medicine clinic patients were found to have Charcot changes on plain foot radiographs. All of the patients had midfoot neuroarthropathy (106).

Tabes Dorsalis

The location of the joint involved may be the only differentiation between tabetic and diabetic neuropathic joint disease. Although nearly every joint has been involved in tabes dorsalis, the knee is most commonly affected, followed by the hip (5,35,49,50,69) (Fig. 91.2). Steindler (48) found genu varum deformity in 26 of 42 tabetic Charcot knees and free joint bodies in 24. Flattening of the tibial condyles was an early sign (46). In some cases, intramuscular and ligamentous ossifications formed a sheath of bone around the knee joint (48).

Axial neuroarthropathy is common in tabes dorsalis; 6% to 21% of tabetic neuropathic joints occur in the spine (42,45,90,92,107–115) (Fig. 91.3). Syringomyelia, paraplegia, and diabetes mellitus may also be associated with axial neuropathic joint disease, and rapid destruction of bone may occur (91,98,108,112,116,117). The axial neuroarthropathy of tabes dorsalis occurs most often in men in the sixth and seventh decades of life. Bone atrophy and hypertrophy often coexist, analogous to the peripheral arthropathy (113). Local bony outgrowths have been described as *les becs des parroquets* (parakeets' beaks) (112,113). Resnick and Niwayama (26) compared the radiographic features of axial arthropathy in tabes dorsalis with disorders that may mimic it such as infection, degenerative disc disease, and CPPD crystal deposition disease.

Syringomyelia

The neuroarthropathy in syringomyelia usually occurs in the shoulders, elbows, and cervical spine. The latter may be indistinguishable from ordinary cervical spondylosis (26,108,118,119). Large effusions and the loss of bone, especially involving the proximal humerus, are characteristic (57–60,118,120) (Fig. 91.4).

Calcium Pyrophosphate Dihydrate Crystal Deposition Disease

A destructive arthropathy resembling Charcot joints has been described in CPPD crystal deposition disease per se (18–20,22–29) (see Chapter 117). Jacobelli and co-workers (21) have suggested synergism between tabes dorsalis and CPPD arthropathy. Typical chondrocalcinosis with subsequent joint collapse and fragmentation, especially in the knee or hip, may suggest underlying CPPD crystal deposition (23–27) (Fig. 91.8).

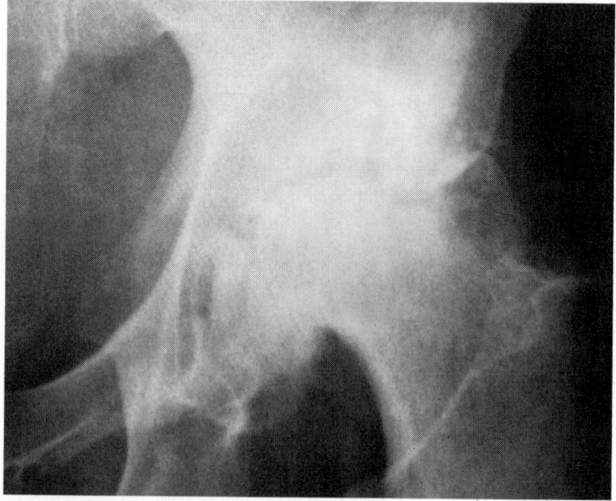

FIGURE 91.8. This elderly patient with no neurologic disease has calcium pyrophosphate dihydrate deposition disease with rapid, painful destruction of the hips, referred to as neuropathic-like or pseudoneuropathic joint. Joint replacement is not contraindicated if the patient is otherwise well.

PATHOPHYSIOLOGY

Charcot postulated a role for spinal cord lesions in the pathogenesis of neuropathic joint disease. Volkmann and Virchow felt that the striking joint destruction was primarily mechanical, caused by multiple episodes of trauma not perceived by the patient because of insensitivity of the affected joints (4–6,121).

Eloesser (122) studied a series of cats with posterior nerve root rhizotomy on one side; the contralateral side served as a control. Charcot joints developed only on the denervated side. Cats with posterior nerve root rhizotomy followed by induction of deforming arthritis with thermocautery developed accelerated neuropathic joint disease. Bone composition and strength under a given stress load was the same on both the rhizotomy side and the control side. Neuropathic joint disease resulting from nerve resection in healthy cats obviously could not be ascribed to syphilis or other infectious causes; trauma and lack of pain and proprioception appeared to be the cause of neuropathic joint disease. There was no osseous atrophy produced by disturbance in the nerve roots, making Charcot's trophic theory untenable (122).

Corbin and Hinsey (123) followed 13 cats with one hind limb completely denervated (lumbar sympathectomy and resection of L4-S3 dorsal roots) from 2 weeks to >3 years. No changes in the bones or joints were found as long as ambulation was restricted. In cats allowed to run free, hip arthritis developed. The authors concluded that activity was crucial to the development of arthritis and that nerves had no specific trophic function for joints.

Unilateral dorsal root ganglionectomy followed by transection of the ipsilateral anterior cruciate ligament in dogs produced remarkable gross and histologic lesions that resembled early neuroarthropathy (124). Dogs with transection of the anterior cruciate ligament only (no ganglionectomy) had more pain, as evidenced by limping, than did those with both cruciate ligament transection and ganglionectomy. Dogs subjected only to unilateral ganglionectomy, but no joint damage, developed no evidence of degenerative joint lesions. Investigators from the same university described three patients with diabetes mellitus and neuropathy who developed Charcot's arthropathy within weeks of minor trauma. The authors felt the neuropathy and minor trauma was the clinical counterpart of the dog model of transection of the cruciate ligament and ganglionectomy (125).

Finsterbush and Friedman (126), however, found that sensory denervation of the hind limb in rabbits produced chondrocyte degeneration even in rabbits in whom the affected limb was immobilized by a plaster cast. These cellular changes progressed over time in both rhizotomized immobilized and active rabbits. The authors postulated that the effects were mediated through altered nutrition produced by the nerve injury, not trauma, thus supporting Charcot's theory of nerve injury-mediated trophic changes in the joint.

Brower and Allman (127) also championed the Charcot trophic theory and nervous system control of bone and joint metabolism. They studied 91 radiographs of neuropathic joints. Approximately one-half of the patients had tabes dorsalis, syringomyelia, or diabetes mellitus, but fully one-third of the patients had no known underlying neurologic disease. Four patients were bedridden when the neuropathic joint disease developed, and the arthritis sometimes occurred with such rapidity that trauma could not be causal. They also noted striking bone resorption that also could not be adequately explained by trauma and suggested that increased bone blood flow with active bone resorption initiated by neurally controlled vascular reflex changes best explained their radiographic findings.

Evidence indicates that blood flow to Charcot joints is increased. Increased vascularity with increased venous draining and filling was shown by Kiss and co-workers (87) and Rabaiotti and co-workers (88). The latter authors commented that in some respects neuropathic joint vascularity was similar to that found in certain malignancies. Bone scintigraphy in neuropathic joint disease revealed diffuse and focal increases in joint uptake both at 2 minutes and 4 hours after injection (82,83). Scintigraphy demonstrated more extensive abnormalities than conventional radiographs, and these sometimes preceded radiographic changes (82,83). Although the increased blood flow to the neuropathic joints could be secondary to the arthritis, the disparity between the scintigrams and the radiographs was marked (83). A primary autonomic nerve defect, resulting in increased blood flow and increased osteoclastic activity, leading to bone damage after minor trauma, was postulated (82). Three diabetic patients developed neuroarthropathy of the ankle or foot after revascularization procedures restored blood flow to a neuropathic lower extremity, emphasizing that adequate blood flow plus neuropathy and trauma are necessary for the development of Charcot joints (128,129).

The increased blood flow to the feet of some patients with diabetes mellitus may lead to the development of local osteoporosis (105,130). Childs and co-workers (130) postulated that Charcot arthropathy is a late sequela of osteoporosis in combination with neuropathy. The authors suggest that Charcot arthropathy is in part a localized metabolic bone disorder. Shapiro and associates (131) found that diabetic Charcot arthropathy patients had a more normal response to high temperature stress by increasing foot peripheral blood flow then did diabetic patients without arthropathy. The authors further suggested that consequent osteopenia was a major risk factor for the development of the arthritis. Selby and co-workers (132) successfully used bisphosphonate treatment for six diabetic patients with neuroarthropathy (see Management, below).

The role of local anesthesia as a prerequisite for developing neuropathic joint disease remains controversial. The frequent development of neuropathic joints in patients insensitive to pain attests to the role of sensory nerves, yet many patients with neuropathic joint disease experience significant pain and near normal sensation (5,35). The majority of these patients have neurologic disease with diminished proprioception or diminished protective reflexes. Armstrong and Lavery (133) found that patients with diabetes mellitus and neuroarthropathy have significantly higher peak plantar pressures with ambulation than other diabetic patients (even those with neuropathy). The elevated plantar pressures were found in the forefoot, whereas the arthropathy was most often present in the midfoot, suggesting that the forefoot serves as a lever, forcing collapse of the midfoot.

The underlying neuropathy may be subtle. Dyck and coworkers (71) studied patients with neuropathic joint disease without overt neurologic signs; subclinical neuropathy and other factors such as trauma, obesity, and excessive activity were found. Sophisticated computer-assisted sensory examinations, nerve conduction velocities, and periosteal nociception testing were needed to detect the presence of the neurologic disorder in some of these patients.

The role of fractures was thoroughly studied by Johnson (73) when he reviewed 188 cases of neuropathic joint disease, 84 of which were tabetic. Fractures were of major importance in initiating or worsening the arthritis in the majority of patients (73,78). The serious prognostic significance of fractures was further documented by Clohisy and Thompson (134) in 18 juvenile-onset diabetes mellitus patients who had neuroarthropathy and fracture who were followed for a minimum of 1 year. Four of the patients became nonambulatory, and 14 depended on orthoses. Charcot (1), in his original article, called attention to the frequency of spontaneous fractures in tabes dorsalis. El-Khoury and Kathol (72) described unusual fractures in six diabetic patients, followed by the development of neuropathic joint disease. Even minor fractures may cause joint instability and increased susceptibility to abnormal stresses (70,73,77). When stress fractures or sprains occur in normal persons, pain stops further injurious activities. Such warning may not happen in patients with neurologic deficits. Trauma was identified as a precipitating cause in 13 of 55 cases of neuropathic joint disease (44). Poor vision in diabetes mellitus patients may lead to more frequent major and minor foot trauma including fracture (135). Bone mass is reduced in diabetes mellitus, increasing the risk of fracture (105). Newman (77) described spontaneous fractures of the foot and ankle in a patient with diabetic neuropathy that led to neuropathic joint disease. Neuropathic ankle joint disease developed in one patient after traumatic severance of the sciatic nerve (136). However, in another patient, denervation of the ankle joint, as treatment for unrelenting pain, did not cause neuropathic joint disease (137).

PATHOLOGY

The histologic findings in neuropathic joint disease are similar to those of osteoarthritis, with differences mainly of degree (5,50,79,138,139). Floyd and co-workers (140) stated that the essential pathologic difference between the two conditions is the presence of an active pannus in neuroarthropathy. Microscopic bone and cartilage fragments in the synovium are almost universal (50,138–141) (Fig. 91.9). Horwitz (139) stressed the importance of synovial debris in the early stages of neuropathic joint disease; in three of five patients, the finding of cartilage and bone detritus "ground" into the synovium first suggested the diagnosis. Few studies have been conducted of tissues from early neuropathic joints or the underlying nerve lesions.

In contrast, many authors have provided detailed descriptions of chronic neuropathic joints (5,47,48, 50,79,127). There is degeneration and disappearance of joint cartilage followed by eburnation of the bone ends that have been denuded of cartilage. In some areas, there is proliferation of cartilage resulting in new bone formation. The coincidental occurrence of massive bony disintegration and production of exuberant quantities of new bone is striking (5,44,48). Extraarticular bony fragments and periosteal bone production coexist with erosions and fractures and the devitalized bone. Intra- and extraarticular osteophytes and exostosis are found on gross examination (79).

Several authors describe hypertrophic and atrophic forms of neuropathic joint disease (48,50,142). Extra- and intraarticular exostoses, osteocytosis, and ossification of soft

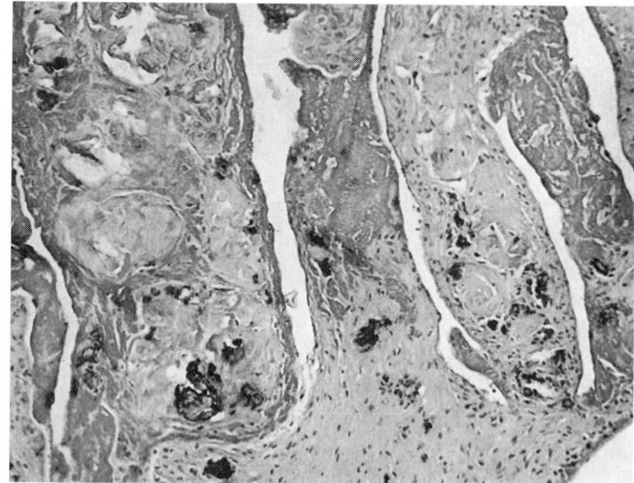

FIGURE 91.9. Photomicrograph of synovium from a neuropathic hip secondary to syphilitic tabes dorsalis. Note the surface hyalinization, dense fibrosis, and scattered areas of calcification. The presence of synovial proliferation and bone and cartilage detritus is very typical of neuropathic joint disease (hematoxylin and eosin stain). (From Rodnan GP. Neuropathic joint disease (Charcot joints). In: McCarty DJ, ed. *Arthritis and allied conditions,* 10th ed. Philadelphia: Lea & Febiger, 1985:1098, with permission.)

tissue are predominant in the former, whereas joint displacement and bone resorption characterize the latter. King (79) postulated that the hypertrophic changes are due to the stimulation of cellular proliferation by products of bone dissolution.

The microscopic changes depend on the stage and severity of the disease and the area of tissue examined. King (79) commented on the great variety of appearances presented by the diseased bone and cartilage. Steindler (48) described cartilage hyperplasia; some cartilage is invaded by pannus, leading to its destruction. A synovial cyst measuring 5 cm in diameter that presented as a slowly enlarging mass has been described (143). O'Connor and co-workers (124) found a variety of cartilage abnormalities in dogs subjected to anterior cruciate ligament transection after dorsal root ganglionectomy. Diminution of cartilage thickness, decreased cellularity, and staining with safranin O were common, although in other areas, hypercellularity and brood capsules were present.

Diabetic Neuropathic Joint Disease

It is not surprising that diabetes mellitus is the most common underlying condition associated with neuropathic joint disease. Perhaps 16 million Americans have diabetes mellitus, approximately 6% of the middle-aged population, and most diabetics have clinical or electromyographic evidence of neuropathy (66,144–147). Deaths from diabetes mellitus are declining, and diabetic patients are living longer, possibly increasing their risk of developing neuropathic joint disease (67).

Jordan (9) reviewed the neurologic manifestations of 226 diabetic patients at the Joslin Diabetic Center in 1936. The incidence of arthropathy was estimated to be between 0.1% and 0.5%, with an approximately equal sex ratio (67,104). The mean age at diagnosis of neuropathic joint disease is 55 years, and the mean duration of diabetes mellitus before the diagnosis of neuroarthropathy is 18 years, with a range of 8 months to 43 years (11,41). Esses and co-workers (53) described neuropathic arthritis in a 21-year-old diabetic patient. In one study of 90 diabetic patients with neuropathic joint disease, all had peripheral neuropathy (11). The preponderance of neuropathic joint disease occurring in diabetic rather than tabetic patients is a recent phenomenon. As late as 1964, tabes dorsalis accounted for 37 of a series of 52 cases of neuropathic joint disease, with diabetes mellitus only accounting for four (148).

The most common sites of neuropathic joints in diabetes are the tarsal and metatarsal joints with ankle involvement slightly less frequent (10,11,33,34,36,37, 142). The ankles were affected in 12% of 101 patients with neuropathic joint disease, while 24% had bilateral foot disease (41). Frykberg and Kozak (37) found bilateral foot disease in approximately 20% of their patients. Sinha and associates (41) reported that bony deformity was most common at the tarsometatarsal joints, skin ulceration at the metatarsophalangeal joints, and soft tissue swelling at the ankle. Metatarsophalangeal joint involvement may be more common than expected, and has been found in 15 of 21 patients with diabetic neuroarthropathy (149). Isolated great toe involvement can occur (150). Antecedent trauma was recalled most commonly in patients with tarsometatarsal joint disease. Neuropathic joint disease developing after fractures or dislocations in diabetic patients is common (39,53,70,72,78,129). Diabetic neuroarthropathy uncommonly occurs in joints above the ankle, but knee, spinal, and even upper extremity joint involvement have been reported (116,151,152). Wrist involvement was observed in a patient with diabetes mellitus and neuropathy relying on crutch walking to bear weight (153). Cauda equina syndrome has complicated diabetic neuropathic joint disease (91).

Schon and co-workers (154) in 1998 reviewed their experience and discussed management options in 221 patients culled over an 8-year period with Charcot arthropathy (presumably all or almost all with underlying diabetes mellitus). A total of 131 patients had midfoot involvement and 50 had ankle involvement.

Diabetic neuropathy was first described in 1798 (67,145). Distal, bilaterally symmetric polyneuropathy, predominantly sensory, is the most common finding. The distal portions of the longest nerves are affected first, explaining the inordinate degree of foot involvement (67,145). There is diminution of the nocifensor reflex, which is due to loss of small trophic fibers responsible for pain sensation, especially small unmyelinated C-fibers and thinly myelinated A-delta fibers (67,145,147). The sensory loss and recurrent daily trauma, combined with normal motor function and blood flow, allow the occurrence of abnormal joint hypermobility with development of external rotation and eversion of the foot. The stress of weight bearing leads to gradual, or at times sudden, breakdown of the foot (10,121,145).

The patient presents because of foot pain, although it is generally accepted that the pain in diabetic neuropathic joint disease is less than expected for the degree of deformity (36,37,41,55,155–158). Swelling almost always precedes pain and may be the only manifestation of early disease (38). Soft tissue ankle swelling is especially typical with ankle neuropathic joint disease (11,41) (Fig. 91.1B). Deep tendon reflexes of the ankle are diminished, with absent or diminished pain and vibration sensation and proprioception in most patients (67,145,147). The foot is erythematous, and the pulses are usually bounding (36,37). Increased mobility of the toes, especially in extension, with crepitation on palpation, may be present (41). Tarsometatarsal joint involvement may exhibit bony deformities with dorsal prominence or plantar protrusions. Downward collapse of the tarsal bones may produce convexity of the volar surface, forming a "rocker" foot or sole (11,36,37,41). Callus formation occurs over weight-bearing areas, especially the metatarsophalangeal joints, and is a frequent site of infection. Perforating ulcers of the foot associated with a neurologic deficit and arthritis are difficult to manage (66,158–161).

Tabes Dorsalis

The joint disorder that accompanied lesions of the central nervous system (CNS) described by Charcot was caused by tabes dorsalis; he emphasized the suddenness of the swelling and the lack of pain or fever. Swelling and hydrarthrosis occurred after a few days; and 1 to 2 weeks later "cracking sounds" developed, leaving a hypermobile joint with wearing away of the articular bones. "Besides the wearing down of the articular surfaces—you may notice the presence of foreign bodies, of bony stalactites, and in a word, all of the customary accompaniments of arthritis deformans" (1). Late tertiary syphilis includes cardiovascular, neurologic, and gummatous lesions. The neurologic lesions may be asymptomatic (abnormal cerebral spinal fluid only) or symptomatic, including tabes dorsalis (162). The posterior spinal column at the fasciculus gracilis is principally involved, but the fasciculus cuneatus also may be affected, accounting for the loss of proprioception (56,115). The proprioceptive loss generally is compensated for by intact visual pathways (56,115).

The Venereal Disease Research Laboratory (VDRL) or other nonspecific tests for syphilis, such as the rapid plasma reagin (RPR) test, are often negative in neurosyphilis because of prior treatment or the passage of time, but the specific tests, fluorescent treponemal antibody absorption (FTA-abs) and *Treponema pallidum* hemagglutination (TPHA) are positive in greater than 95% of patients with neurosyphilis. Testing of cerebrospinal fluid may be helpful; a positive cerebrospinal fluid VDRL usually indicates active syphilis, whereas a positive cerebrospinal fluid FTA usually indicates neurosyphilis (162).

The best single clinical criterion for diagnosing tabetic neuropathy is the absence of deep pain sensation (119). The Argyll-Robertson pupil may be absent or the irregularity in pupil size slight, although Koshino (84) found it to be the most important clinical finding in his cases (47,48,115, 140). A careful sensory examination is required. Knee reflexes are commonly absent (47,48,115,140). Neuropathic joint disease may be the first sign of tabes dorsalis. The classic picture of a large, firm, painless, and unstable joint is not always present, and the arthritis may remain undiagnosed for some time (46,140,148).

Neuropathic joint disease occurs in 4% to 10% of tabetics. Key (46) considered it rare in persons younger than 40 years of age. A history of syphilis is obtained in less than half the patients (46,140). The mean interval between the onset of the syphilis and the development of the neuropathic joint is 19 years. In Key's series of 69 cases, a total of 92 joints were involved; 18 patients had two joints and five had three joints affected. The knee was affected in 39; foot and ankle, 29; hip, 15; spine, 5; elbow, 2; and shoulder and wrist joint, 1 each. In another series, the knee was involved in 66% of the tabetic neuropathic joints and the ankle in 26%; 28% of patients had polyarticular involvement (49). Women composed one-third of these cases (49), but in most series men outnumbered women to an even greater extent (4,47,48,69). Beetham and co-workers (69) also described a patient with extensive polyarticular involvement.

The onset of joint disease in neurosyphilis is not always acute; the joint swelling may continue for months or years before disintegration occurs (46,49,69). Swelling is the most prominent sign of disease onset in the knee, ankle, and foot, but in the hip, a pathologic fracture is usually the presenting finding. In the spine, deformity is frequently the first finding (5,9,48,148).

Spinal neuroarthropathy is common (90,107–109,111, 112,114,115). As late as 1980, Wirth and associates (115) described 18 tabetic neuropathic spinal arthropathies culled from two institutions, and Campbell and Doyle (109) found eight cases within a 2-year period. The lesions were usually in the lumbar or lower dorsal vertebra with vertebral body destruction leading to posterior or lateral displacement, resulting in kyphotic and scoliotic deformity. Usually no bone tenderness occurred, but considerable discomfort was caused by compression of nerve roots (107,109,115). A "thud" on flexion-extension movement of the spine is said to be characteristic (111).

Syringomyelia

Syringomyelia frequently has been associated with neuropathic joint disease (4,55,57,59,118,120,163), since the original description by Schultze and Kahler in 1888 (7) (Fig. 91.10) Approximately 25% of syringomyelia patients have neuropathic arthritis, predominantly in the shoulders, elbows, and cervical spine, followed by the wrist, carpal, and small hand joints (26,118,120) (Fig. 91.11). Sternoclavicular joint involvement with massive swelling and destruction has been reported (164).

Syringomyelia (from the Greek *syrinx*—pipe or tube) is a chronic progressive, degenerative disorder of the spinal canal characterized clinically by weakness and atrophy of the hands and arms and segmental anesthesia of the dissociated type (loss of pain and temperature sensation but preservation of touch) especially at the neck, shoulders, and arms (56,120). There is cavitation of the central portion of the spinal canal, usually in the cervical region (56). The very high incidence of neuropathic joint disease in syringomyelia as compared to tabes dorsalis and diabetes mellitus is probably explained by the more profound sensory loss that occurs in syringomyelia (4,56). Amyotrophy and upper extremity areflexia are common in syringomyelia. Deep aching or boring pain is frequent (56). Neuropathic joint disease may occur early or late in the course of syringomyelia (56,58,113,118). Painful shoulder

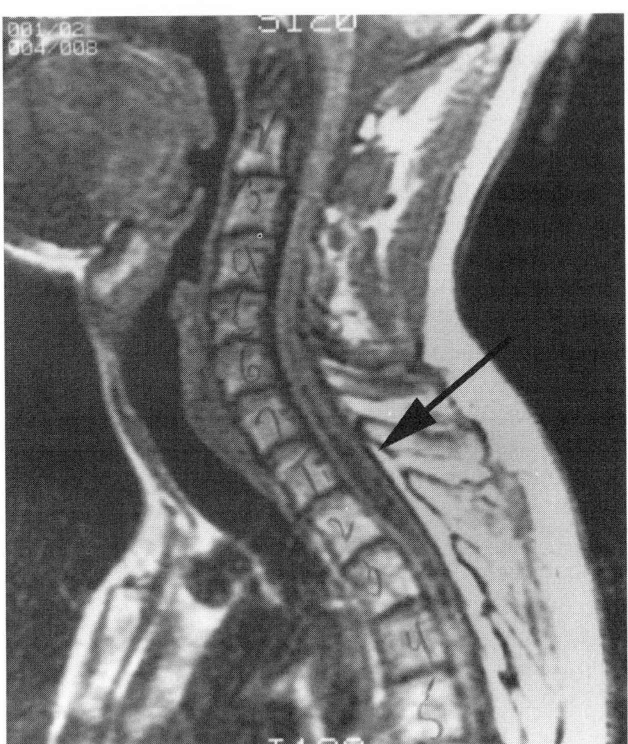

FIGURE 91.10. Sagittal section from an MRI study of the cervical spine in a patient with syringomyelia demonstrating a fluid-filled cavity *(arrow)* within the spinal canal.

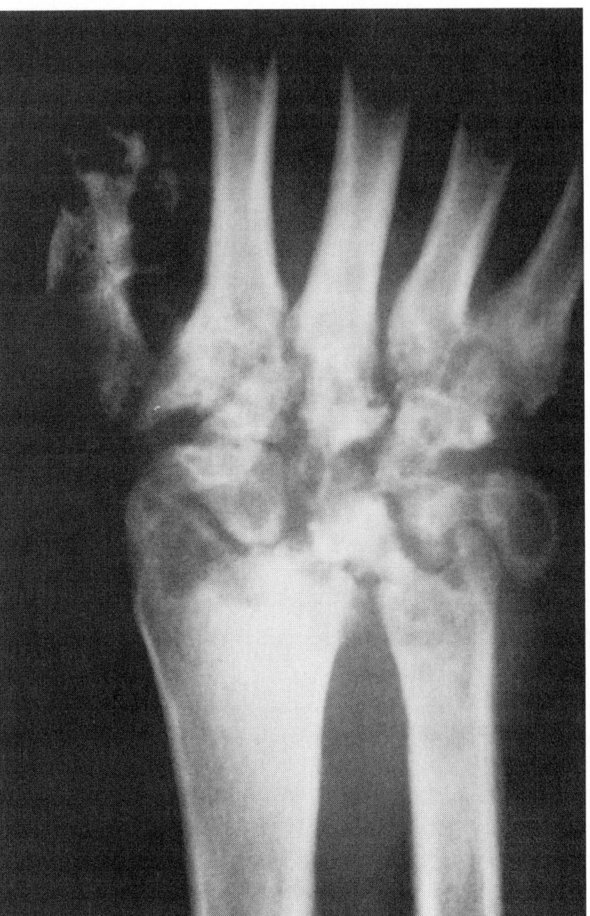

FIGURE 91.11. The wrist involvement in this patient with syringomyelia resembles the tarsometatarsal changes of the foot in diabetic neuroarthropathy. The combination of bony destruction and repair is frequently seen in neuropathic joint disease.

involvement was found in two patients as the first manifestation of syringomyelia (57) and rapid bone dissolution may occur (57). Multiple joints may be involved, even mimicking rheumatoid arthritis (165). In one series, three patients complained of pain, while in three others the condition was painless (58). Swelling was so pronounced that it limited arm motion in all patients (58). In two patients, no bony radiographic changes were found at the onset of the swelling, but, gradually, extensive joint destruction and calcification in the soft tissue developed, followed by slow resorption of bone (57). Cervical spine involvement is common in syringomyelia; early radiographic changes may be indistinguishable from cervical spondylosis (26,120).

When neuropathic joint disease occurs in the upper extremity, syringomyelia should be considered the most likely cause. The loss of deep tendon reflexes in the upper extremities, analgesia, and thermal anesthesia support the diagnosis (56). The diagnosis is confirmed by MRI detecting the syrinx (Fig. 91.10).

Calcium Pyrophosphate Dihydrate Crystal Deposition Disease

Jacobelli and co-workers (21) described the occurrence of CPPD crystal deposition and neuropathic joint disease (see Chapter 117) in four patients, three with tabes dorsalis, and one with no neurologic abnormalities but with a history of syphilis and positive VDRL and FTA-abs tests. All four patients had severe arthropathy of the knees, originally considered to be neuropathic joint disease only, until careful search revealed generalized CPPD crystal deposition. The patient without neurologic deficit developed an acute Charcot joint with collapse of the medial tibial plateau 24 hours after his first attack of pseudogout (18). As only 5% to 10% of tabetic patients develop neuropathic joints and the prevalence of CPPD deposition at age 70 years is about 5%, crystal deposition and neuropathic joint disease were postulated as analogous to the experimental findings of Eloesser (122) that were discussed above. Bennett and associates (18) suggested that the presence of CPPD crystals in joint fluid may explain some of the episodes of acute inflammation seen in some neuropathic joints.

CPPD crystal deposition and neuropathic joint disease were described in two patients without neurologic abnormalities or laboratory evidence of syphilis (20); the destructive arthropathy was described as neuropathic-like because of the presence of pain and lack of neurologic deficit.

Menkes and co-workers (25) described 15 cases of neuropathic-like destructive arthropathy in 125 patients with CPPD crystal deposition collected over a 3-year period. Knees, shoulders, hips, and wrists were most commonly involved. Resnick and co-workers (27) also described severe destructive arthropathy occurring frequently in their series of patients with CPPD crystal deposition. This variant has been called pseudoneuropathic joint disease (22). Fidler and associates (166) described a patient with cervical myelopathy due to a mass of CPPD crystal deposition contributing to compression of the spinal cord at the C2-C3 level. There was bilateral upper extremity neuroarthropathy as a result of the combination of true neuropathy plus the articular effects of crystal induced inflammation.

There is little doubt that CPPD crystal deposition alone can be associated with a destructive arthropathy (22), but it is important to separate neuropathic-like joint disease from true neuropathic joint disease because the former patients may be candidates for prosthetic joint surgery while the latter generally are not.

Intraarticular Corticosteroids

The possibility of iatrogenic neuropathic-like joint disease induced by intraarticular corticosteroids remains a concern (12–17,167). This form of local treatment of arthritis was popularized by Hollander and co-workers (168) in 1951. By 1961, they reported on more than 100,000 injections (articular and soft tissue) with careful observations on results and adverse effects (169). Instability of joints was noted in 0.7% of repeatedly injected weight-bearing joints. Proprioception or sensation loss was exhibited in the unstable joints, but in only four joints was the absorption of bone extensive. Kendall (170) noted an even lower incidence of untoward events in a series of 6,700 injections in 2,256 patients.

Chandler and associates (13) reported the rapid deterioration and development of a neuropathic-like hip joint in a patient with osteoarthritis injected at approximately monthly intervals (approximately 18 injections). Sweetnam and co-workers (16) described "steroid arthropathy" in four patients with rapid painless destruction of the hips; two had received intraarticular steroids and two had been treated with oral corticosteroids. Steinberg and co-workers (15) described neuropathic-like changes in a knee of a patient with rheumatoid arthritis treated locally with 22 corticosteroid injections over a period of 2 years. Alarcón-Segovia and Ward (12) described a similar case that developed after the patient received four to six yearly injections over a 6-year period.

Such neuropathic-like changes after local intraarticular steroid use are believed to result from the temporary suppression of pain induced by the medication, encouraging overuse of the damaged joint (14). Hollander and associates (169) advised protection from trauma and rest of weight-bearing joints after intraarticular corticosteroid therapy.

Neuropathic-like joint disease with intraarticular corticosteroid use must be uncommon. While reported cases of its occurrences may only represent a fraction of the actual number of cases, the widespread use of this technique by rheumatologists and orthopedic surgeons contrasted with the paucity of the reported neuroarthropathy is striking. However, caution must be used in patient selection and the frequency of the use of intraarticular corticosteroids in order to avoid this complication.

The early reports of neuropathic-like joint disease were associated with short-lived, relatively soluble corticosteroid preparations used repeatedly in weight-bearing joints. The deleterious effects of the newer, now more commonly used, less water soluble intraarticular corticosteroids are unclear, although there are few reports of the development of neuroarthropathy. Benefits from judicious intraarticular corticosteroids seem to greatly outweigh the risk of inducing joint instability and destruction (see Chapter 41). Corticosteroid injection into neuropathic joints is not recommended.

Congenital Insensitivity to Pain

Congenital insensitivity to pain, although rare, is so frequently associated with neuropathic joints that the diagnosis should be considered in children or young adults with atypical arthritis (8,12,171–180). Insensitivity to pain was first described in a sideshow participant advertised as the "human pin cushion" (8). "The patient cannot recall any pain except headache—and his memory is good." The diagnostic criteria are (a) pain sensation absent from birth, (b) the entire body affected, and (c) all other sensory modalities intact or only minimally impaired, with preservation of deep tendon reflexes (179). Subtle varieties of the condition include *congenital insensitivity to pain with anhidrosis* (181) and *congenital sensory neuropathy with neuropathic joint disease* (182). Feindel (183) described a patient with insensitivity to pain with histologically normal nerve endings around an affected joint.

Fractures of the metaphysis and diaphysis of long bones with epiphyseal separation and soft tissue ulcerations occur frequently and are often unrecognized (178). The radiographic appearance of injury (destruction) and repair (proliferation) of bone, occasionally complicated by infection, is similar to that seen in other causes of neuropathic joint disease (178). The ankle is most frequently involved, with joints of the feet, elbows, spine, and hip joints less commonly involved (184). In a patient with bilateral leg amputation because of complications of congenital insensitivity to pain, hand and wrist neuroarthropathy developed after use of the upper extremities for weight bearing (185). Truncal asymmetry developed in a pregnant 17-year-old with congenital insensitivity to pain that resulted in dense paraparesis requiring anterior decompression and stabilization of the spine (186). *Pain asymbolia,* an acquired equivalent of congenital insensitivity to pain, has not been reported in association with neuroarthropathy.

Spinal Dysraphism

The disorders of fusion of the dorsal midline structures at the primitive neural tube (especially meningomyelocele) are the most frequent cause of neuropathic joint disease in children (32,119,178,187). Evident at birth, the neurologic findings depend on the level of the lesion (32,56). Neuropathic joint disease most commonly affects the tarsal articulations and the ankle (32,178,187). Lower extremity long bone fractures are common in meningomyelocele because of osteoporosis that is due to immobility and sensory neuropathy (74,178,187,188). Children with myelomeningocele had less neuropathic joint disease and their fractures healed quicker than in children with congenital insensitivity to pain because children with the former walked less (178). The joints of children with meningomyelocele often are protected by braces at an early age, which may decrease the incidence of neuropathic joint disease (178).

Miscellaneous

Children with thalidomide-induced disease also may develop neuropathic joint disease (189). Because some adults treated with thalidomide also develop severe sensory peripheral neuropathy, McCredie (189) hypothesized that the embryo developed neuropathy at the time of thalidomide exposure, which later led to the neuropathic joint disease in childhood.

Neuropathic joint disease has been reported in familial amyloid neuropathy (190,191), nonfamilial amyloid neuropathy in a dialysis patient (192), amyloidosis associated with Waldenström's macroglobulinemia (193), the myelopathy of pernicious anemia (194), spinal cord trauma (148,195–197), neurofibromatosis (198), familial dysautonomia (199), multiple sclerosis (4), paraplegia (98,196), idiopathic neurogenic arthropathy (200–202), arachnoiditis secondary to tuberculosis (203), adhesive arachnoiditis (204), and neuropathy associated with leprosy (4,205). It has also been reported in acromegaly (206), yaws (31), juvenile rheumatoid arthritis (207), scleroderma (with cervical osteolysis) (89), the POEMS syndrome (polyneuropathy, organomegaly, endocrinopathy, M-protein, and skin changes) (208), and in patients undergoing chronic hemodialysis (209).

Neuropathic joint disease of the forefoot was described in 59 patients with severe alcoholism and polyneuropathy who were hospitalized at a single institution during a 3-year period (210). Patients were excluded if diseases usually associated with neuropathic joint disease, including diabetes mellitus, amyloidosis, or syphilis, were present. The patients were chronic heavy drinkers (mean age of 46.7 years) with painless foot ulcers, infections, and chronic venous insufficiency. Repeated bouts of cellulitis or lymphangitis were frequent. The association of alcohol and neuropathic joint disease had been described infrequently before this report (4,35,66).

A variety of other neurologic disorders may be associated with neuropathic joint disease. Because the common denominator of this arthritis is sensory loss and continued weight bearing, any disease with those features may be complicated by neuropathic joint disease. Hereditary sensory neuropathy (211–213), progressive hypertrophic polyneuritis (214), and peroneal muscular atrophy (Charcot-Marie-Tooth disease) (215) have all been associated with neuropathic joint disease. Bruckner and Kendall (215) described seven cases of neuropathic joint disease associated with the Charcot-Marie-Tooth disease. These patients had more severe muscle wasting and sensory loss than did patients with Charcot-Marie-Tooth disease without neuropathic joint disease (215). Neuroarthropathy of the shoulder developed in two patients with no underlying sensory abnormalities (216). Thus, Charcot arthropathy may develop before signs of an underlying neurologic disease become apparent. The patients described were followed for 14 and 2 years, respectively. In another patient, Charcot shoulder was an initial manifestation of Arnold-Chiari malformation (217).

MANAGEMENT

Most patients with neuropathic joint disease seen by a rheumatologist will have foot involvement resulting from diabetic neuropathy. Either painful or painless swelling in a diabetic foot should be considered possible neuropathic joint disease. An aggressive approach to diagnosis and treatment will help the patient. Molded or contour shoes, bracing, a course of non–weight bearing, patient education, and foot elevation may provide relief for most patients when treated early (36,37,39,43,79,121,154,173,218). Several authors have claimed that control of the diabetes mellitus improves the arthropathy (33,83). Dynamic measurements of plantar pressure may help design accommodative padding and shoes for individual patients (80). Schon and co-workers (154) described their management experience with both casting and surgery in 221 patients with Charcot foot with treatment depending on severity and locale of foot involvement.

Armstrong and co-workers (219) followed 55 diabetic patients with Charcot arthropathy of the feet, all of whom were treated with serial total contact casting for a mean of 18.5 weeks. They emphasized that acute neuroarthropathy requires "prompt, uncompromising reduction in weight bearing stress." The duration of total contact casting was based on clinical judgment combined with radiographic and thermometric assessments. Surgery was required in 25% of patients and that included plantar exostectomies and fusions of affected joints. A rigid orthotic with a custom insert designated the Charcot restraint orthotic walker (CROW) provides immobilization for prolonged periods of time. It was generally used after initial cast immobilization (220–222).

Sella and Barrette (221) described treatment consisting of limited weight bearing and observation for presumptive neuroarthropathy in the diabetic foot when there was warmth and swelling over the medial aspect of the foot but with normal radiographs. These patients had abnormal bone scanning results in spite of the normal radiographs.

Infection has to be excluded or treated before conservative treatment can begin. The intense inflammation of untreated, acute Charcot arthropathy, with its frequent exacerbations, can make differential diagnosis difficult. Help from radiologic studies, especially MRI and nuclear medicine diagnostic studies, has been described (see Radiologic Features, above). Osteomyelitis always must be considered in a patient with worsening neuroarthropathy.

A team approach is recommended to facilitate optimal treatment. The ideal team would consist of the attending physician, who treats the diabetes mellitus and other medical disorders if present and guides the patient through the slow recovery process, and the rheumatologist, orthopedist (now usually a foot and ankle specialist), and orthotist, who reworks and redesigns the orthotics so that the patient is always comfortable. The podiatrist consultation provides advice about the underlying arthropathy and ongoing treatment of the other foot disorders that diabetic patients so frequently experience.

Treatable conditions that may underlie neurologic disorders such as syphilis, yaws, and leprosy should always be kept in mind. Even when the underlying neurologic disease may be untreatable, prompt joint immobilization, cessation of weight bearing, accommodative footwear, and patient education often stabilize the neuropathic joint (39,75,121). Fractures and sprains heal with immobilization (38,73). Reduction of edema and treatment of infection and ulcerations are required for successful therapy of the diabetic foot (36,37,39). Refractory plantar ulcers can often be successfully treated with a wide plantar exposure, excision of the ulcer, and a generous saucerization of the convexity of the rocker bottom bony prominence (161). Immobilization or arthrodesis of the spine often is effective in axial skeleton neuroarthropathy (42,110,114,197). Crutch-walking is usually needed for hip joint neuropathic involvement. A patellar tendon-bearing orthosis has successfully reduced weight bearing in patients with neuropathic joint disease of the ankle or foot (34,223).

Arthrodesis of a neuropathic joint may fail because of nonunion or pin fracture (224,225), but successful fusion is possible and is often required for treatment of the neuropathic knee (44,171,224,226–228). Drennan and co-workers (226) in 1971 described successful knee arthrodesis in eight patients. The high rate of fusion was attributed to adequate bone resection and debridement, complete synovectomy, and firm interval fixation (bleeding bone to bleeding bone). Samilson and associates (44) emphasized the need for early arthrodesis. For example, arthrodesis of the spine is successful in achieving stability and relieving pain in most instances (42,110,115). Shibata and co-workers (229) successfully fused 19 of 26 ankles after intramedullary nailing with an average follow-up of 9 years.

Total joint replacement is generally contraindicated in neuropathic joint disease, although pain has been relieved with hip arthroplasty even though the joints have later subluxed or loosened (35,230–232). Charnley (233), the innovator of total hip joint surgery, warned against total joint replacement in neuropathic joint disease. Total glenohumeral joint replacement is contraindicated (234). The rapidity of loosening and subluxation of total joint prostheses in neuropathic joint disease attests to the importance of intact proprioception and deep pain sensation in stabilizing even carefully reconstructed joints. Sprenger and Foley (235) reviewed hip replacement surgery in neuropathic joint disease and described successful hip surgery in a patient with neurosyphilis. At 7-year follow-up, the patient was well and the hip prosthesis was stable. The authors ascribed the excellent result, contrary to the experience of other surgeons, to the lack of ataxia in their patient.

Soudry and co-workers (236) reported nine total knee arthroplasties in seven patients with neuropathic joint disease. Excellent results were obtained in eight and good results in one, with an average follow-up of 3 years. The histologic and radiologic findings were diagnostic of neuropathic joint disease, but four patients with clinically apparent neurologic abnormalities had no definable neurologic disease. Posterior stabilized components, ligamentous balancing, resection of adequate bone, bone grafting if required, or the use of a custom augmented prosthesis were considered the reasons for this unusual rate of success (236). Fullerton and Browngoehl (237) described the successful rehabilitation of a diabetic woman 61 years of age with bilateral knee neuroarthropathy who underwent arthrodesis of one knee and total arthroplasty of the other.

Lumbar sympathectomy was helpful in the diabetic neuropathic joint disease involving the foot in two patients with impaired circulation (238). Clinical healing occurred in three patients treated with non–weight bearing and the use of a pulsed electromagnetic field, inducing a weak electrical current in bone (239). Combined magnetic field bone growth stimulation was added to conventional treatment in 21 diabetic patients with foot neuroarthropathy (240). Significantly more rapid healing and less residual deformity was found in the treated patients compared to conventionally treated controls. The device was used for a half-hour daily. Magnetic fields have been extensively used as a treatment for fracture healing (241). This therapeutic modality appears to increase insulin-like growth factor II, which, in turn, may increase the rate of bone cell proliferation.

Amputation of the foot is occasionally required and often welcomed by patients with advanced neuroarthropathy, especially if infection complicates the arthritis. The improvements in amputation surgery and anesthesia and prompt use of orthotics and early weight bearing have made this treatment more acceptable. Exostectomies, when indicated, also have been reported to be helpful (218).

Selby and co-workers (132) studied the use of pamidronate in six diabetic patients with Charcot feet. Temperatures of the affected feet and serum alkaline phosphatase levels fell, which correlated with clinical improvement. Excess osteoclast activity is found in acute Charcot neuroarthropathy and the use of bisphosphonate treatment may be reasonable therapy, although controlled studies have not been performed (242,243). Guis and co-workers (244) describe the successful management with the use of pamidronate of a patient with Charcot foot secondary to hereditary sensory neuropathy. The patient refused foot immobilization, and treatment consisted only of pamidronate administered intravenously every 4 months for 2 years. That increased blood flow and subsequent osteopenia contribute to the fracturing of the Charcot joint is very likely, and attention to treatment of the localized bone disorder seems important.

REFERENCES

1. Charcot JM. Du Cerveau ou de la moelle epiniere. *Arch Physiol Nom Pathol* 1868;1:161–178,379–399.
2. Owen ARG. *Hysteria, hypnosis and healing:* the work of J-M Charcot. New York: Ganett, 1971.
3. Pemberton R, Osgood RB, eds. *The medical and orthopaedic management of chronic arthritis.* New York: Macmillan, 1934.
4. Bruckner FE, Howell A. Neuropathic joints. *Semin Arthritis Rheum* 1972;2:47–69.
5. Delano PJ. The pathogenesis of Charcot's joints. *AJR* 1946;56: 189–200.
6. Delano PJ (citing Volkmann R, Virchow R). The pathogenesis of Charcot's joints. *AJR* 1946;56:189–200.
7. Bruckner FE, Howell A (citing Schultze F, Kahler O). Neuropathic joints. *Semin Arthritis Rheum* 1972;2:47–69.
8. Dearborn GVN. A case of congenital general pure analgesia. *J Nerv Ment Dis* 1932;75:612–615.
9. Jordan WR. Neuritic manifestations in diabetes mellitus. *Arch Intern Med* 1936;57:307–366.
10. Robillard R, Gagnon PA, Alarie R. Diabetic neuroarthropathy: Report of four cases. *Can Med Assoc J* 1964;91:795–804.
11. Clouse ME, Gramm HF, Legg M, et al. Diabetic osteoarthropathy: clinical and roentgenographic observations in 90 cases. *AJR* 1974;121:22–34.
12. Alarcón-Segovia D, Ward LE. Charcot-like arthropathy in rheumatoid arthritis: consequence of overuse of a joint repeatedly injected with hydrocortisone. *JAMA* 1965;193:136–138.
13. Chandler GN, Jones PT, Wright V, et al. Charcot's arthropathy following intra-articular hydrocortisone. *Br Med J* 1959;1: 952–953.
14. Chandler GN, Wright V. Deleterious effect of intra-articular hydrocortisone. *Lancet* 1958;2:661–663.
15. Steinberg CL, Duthie RB, Piva AE. Charcot-like arthropathy following intra-articular hydrocortisone. *JAMA* 1962;181: 851–854.
16. Sweetnam DR, Mason RM, Murray RO. Steroid arthropathy of the hip. *Br Med J* 1960;1:1392–1394.
17. Parikh JR, Houpt JB, Jacobs S, et al. Charcot's arthropathy of the shoulder following intraarticular corticosteroid injections. *J Rheumatol* 1993;20:885–887.
18. Bennett RM, Mall JC, McCarty DJ. Pseudogout in acute neuropathic arthropathy. A clue to pathogenesis? *Ann Rheum Dis* 1974;33:563–567.
19. Genant HK. Roentgenographic aspects of calcium pyrophosphate dihydrate crystal deposition disease (pseudogout). *Arthritis Rheum* 1976;3:307–328.
20. Helms CA, Chapman GS, Wild JH. Charcot-like joints in calcium pyrophosphate dihydrate deposition disease. *Skeletal Radiol* 1981;7:55–58.
21. Jacobelli S, McCarty DJ, Silcox DC, et al. Calcium pyrophosphate dihydrate crystal deposition in neuropathic joints: four cases of polyarticular involvement. *Ann Intern Med* 1973;79: 340–347.
22. McCarty DJ Jr. *Arthritis and allied conditions,* 10th ed. Philadelphia: Lea & Febiger, 1985.
23. McCarty DJ Jr, Haskin ME. The roentgenographic aspects of pseudogout (articular chondrocalcinosis): an analysis of 20 cases. *Am J Roentgenol Radium Ther Nucl Med* 1963;90: 1248–1257.
24. Martel W, McCarter DK, Solsky MA, et al. Further observations on the arthropathy of calcium pyrophosphate crystal deposition disease. *Radiology* 1981;141:1–15.
25. Menkes CJ, Decraemere W, Postel M, et al. Destructive arthropathy in chondrocalcinosis articularis. *Arthritis Rheum* 1976;19:329–348.
26. Resnick D, Niwayama G. *Diagnosis of bone and joint disorders with emphasis on articular abnormalities.* Philadelphia: WB Saunders, 1981.
27. Resnick D, Niyama G, Georgen TG, et al. Clinical radiographic and pathologic abnormalities in calcium pyrophosphate dihydrate deposition disease (CPPD): pseudogout. *Radiology* 1977; 122:1–15.
28. Richards AJ, Hamilton EBD. Spinal changes in idiopathic chondrocalcinosis articularis. *Rheumatol Rehabil* 1976;15: 138–142.
29. Richardson BC, Genant HK. Destructive arthropathy in chondrocalcinosis: a case report. *Orthopedics* 1982;5:1482–1486.
30. Gupta R. A short history of neuropathic arthropathy. *Clin Orthop* 1993;296:43–49.
31. Smith FH. Charcot-like joints in yaws. *US Naval Med Bull* 1946;46:1832–1843.
32. Nellhaus G. Neurogenic arthropathies (Charcot's joints) in children. *Clin Pediatr* 1975;14:647–653.
33. Antes EH. Charcot joint in diabetes mellitus. *JAMA* 1954;156: 602–603.
34. Bailey CC, Root HF. Neuropathic foot lesions in diabetes mellitus. *N Engl J Med* 1947;236:397–401.
35. Eichenholtz SN. *Charcot joints.* Springfield, IL: Charles C Thomas, 1966.
36. Frykberg RG. Neuropathic arthropathy: the diabetic Charcot foot. *Diabetes Educator* 1984;9:17–20.
37. Frykberg RG, Kozak GP. Neuropathic arthropathy in the diabetic foot. *Am Fam Physician* 1978;5:105–113.

38. Herzwurm PJ, Barja RH. Charcot joints of the foot. *Contemp Orthop* 1987;14:17–22.
39. Jackson WPU, Louw JH. The diabetic foot. *S Afr Med J* 1979; 56:87–92.
40. Pogonowska MJ, Collins LC, Dobson HL. Diabetic osteopathy. *Radiology* 1967;89:265–271.
41. Sinha S, Munichoodappa CS, Kozak GP. Neuroarthropathy (Charcot joints) in diabetes mellitus. *Medicine* 1972;51:191–210.
42. Briggs JR, Freehafer AA. Fusion of the Charcot spine. *Clin Orthop* 1967;53:83–93.
43. Calabro JJ, Garg SL. Neuropathic joint disease. *Am Fam Physician* 1973;2:90–95.
44. Samilson RL, Sankaran B, Bersani FA, et al. Orthopedic management of neuropathic joints. *Arch Surg* 1959;78:115–121.
45. Charcot JM. Arthropathies, inxations et fractures spontanees chez une ataxique. *Bull Mem Soc Anat Paris* 1873;48:744–747.
46. Key JA. Clinical observations on tabetic arthropathies (Charcot joints). *Am J Syphilis* 1932;16:429–447.
47. Soto-Hall R, Haldeman KO. The diagnosis of neuropathic joint disease (Charcot joint). An analysis of 40 cases. *JAMA* 1940;114:2076–2078.
48. Steindler A. The tabetic arthropathies. *JAMA* 1931;96: 250–256.
49. Wile UJ, Butler MG. A critical survey of Charcot's arthropathy. Analysis of eighty-eight cases. *JAMA* 1930;94:1053–1055.
50. Potts WJ. The pathology of Charcot joints. *Ann Surg* 1927;86: 596–606.
51. Katz I, Rabinowitz JG, Dziadiw R. Early changes in Charcot's joints. *AJR* 1961;86:965–974.
52. Scartozzi G, Kanat IO. Diabetic neuroarthropathy of the foot and ankle. *J Am Podiatr Med Assoc* 1990;80:298–303.
53. Esses S, Langer F, Gross A. Charcot's joints: a case report in a young patient with diabetes. *Clin Orthop* 1981;156:183–186.
54. Kraft E, Spyropoulos E, Finby N. Neurogenic disorders of the foot in diabetes mellitus. *AJR* 1975;124:17–24.
55. Bhaskaran R, Suresh K, Iyer GV. Charcot's elbow—a case report. *J Postgrad Med* 1981;27:194–196.
56. Rowland LP, ed. *Merritt's textbook of neurology.* Philadelphia: Lea & Febiger, 1984.
57. Sackellares JC, Swift TR. Shoulder enlargement as the presenting sign of syringomyelia: report of two cases and review of the literature. *JAMA* 1976;236:2878–2879.
58. Skall-Jensen J. Osteoarthropathy in syringomyelia: analysis of seven cases. *Acta Radiol* 1952;38:382–388.
59. Meyer GA, Stein J, Poppel MH. Rapid osseous changes in syringomyelia. *Radiology* 1957;69:415–418.
60. Norman A, Robbins H, Milgram JE. The acute neuropathic arthropathy—a rapid, severely disorganizing form of arthritis. *Radiology* 1968;90:1159–1164.
61. Ropes MW, Bauer W. *Synovial fluid changes in joint disease.* Cambridge: Harvard University Press, 1953.
62. Bennet K, Hinricson H. A case of tuberculous infection of the knee with clinical and roentgenographic appearance of Charcot's disease. *J Bone Joint Surg* 1934;16:463–466.
63. Goodman MA, Swartz W. Infection in a Charcot joint: a case report. *J Bone Joint Surg* 1985;67A:642–643.
64. Martin JR, Root HS, Kim SO, et al. Staphylococcus suppurative arthritis occurring in neuropathic knee joints: a report of four cases with a discussion of the mechanisms involved. *Arthritis Rheum* 1965;8:389–402.
65. Rubinow A, Spark EC, Canoso JJ. Septic arthritis in a Charcot joint. *Clin Orthop* 1980;147:203–206.
66. Classen JN. Neurotrophic arthropathy with ulceration. *Ann Surg* 1964;6:891–894.
67. Marble A, Krall LP, Bradley RF, et al., eds. *Joslin's diabetes mellitus,* 12th ed. Philadelphia: Lea & Febiger, 1985.
68. Boynton EL, Paley D, Gross AE, et al. False aneurysm in a Charcot hip. *J Bone Joint Surg* 1986;68A:462–464.
69. Beetham WP Jr, Kaye RL, Polley HF. Charcot's joints: a case of extensive polyarticular involvement, and discussion of certain clinical and pathologic features. *Ann Intern Med* 1963;58: 1002–1012.
70. Coventry MB, Rothacker GW Jr. Bilateral calcaneal fracture in a diabetic patient. *J Bone Joint Surg* 1979;61A:462–464.
71. Dyck PJ, Stevens JC, O'Brien PC, et al. Neurogenic arthropathy and recurring fractures with subclinical inherited neuropathy. *Neurology* 1983;33:357–367.
72. El-Khoury GY, Kathol MH. Neuropathic fractures in patients with diabetes mellitus. *Radiology* 1980;134:313–316.
73. Johnson JTH. Neuropathic fractures and joint injuries: pathogenesis and rationale of prevention and treatment. *J Bone Joint Surg* 1967;49A:1–30.
74. Korhonen BJ. Fractures in myelodysplasia. *Clin Orthop* 1971; 79:145–155.
75. Kristiansen B. Ankle and foot fractures in diabetics provoking neuropathic joint changes. *Acta Orthop Scand* 1980;51:975–979.
76. Muggia FM. Neuropathic fracture: unusual complication in a patient with advanced diabetic neuropathy. *JAMA* 1965;191:336–338.
77. Newman JH. Spontaneous dislocation in diabetic neuropathy. A report of six cases. *J Bone Joint Surg* 1979;61B:484–488.
78. Slowman-Kovacs SD, Braunstein EM, Brandt KD. Rapidly progressive charcot arthropathy following minor joint trauma in patients with diabetic neuropathy. *Arthritis Rheum* 1990;33: 412–417.
79. King EJS. On some aspects of the pathology of hypertrophic Charcot's joints. *Br J Surg* 1930;18:113–124.
80. Wolfe L, Stess RM, Graf PM. Dynamic pressure analysis of the diabetic Charcot foot. *J Am Podiatr Med Assoc* 1991;81:281–287.
81. Hodgson JR, Pugh DG, Young HH. Roentgenologic aspects of certain lesions of bone: neurotrophic or infectious? *Radiology* 1948;50:65–71.
82. Edmonds ME, Clarke MB, Newton S, et al. Increased uptake of bone radiopharmaceutical in diabetic neuropathy. *Q J Med* 1985;224:843–855.
83. Eymontt MJ, Alavi A, Dalinka MK, et al. Bone scintigraphy in diabetic osteoarthropathy. *Radiology* 1981;140:475–477.
84. Koshino T. Stage classifications, types of joint destruction, and bone scintigraphy in Charcot joint disease. *Bull Hosp Joint Dis Orthop Inst* 1991;51:205–217.
85. Glynn TP Jr. Marked gallium accumulation in neurogenic arthropathy. *J Nucl Med* 1981;22:1016–1017.
86. Mack JM, Spencer RP. Role of radiopharmaceuticals in detection of osteomyelitis. In: Freeman LM, ed. *Nuclear medicine—annual 1990.* New York: Raven Press, 1990.
87. Kiss J, Martin JR, McConnell F, et al. Angiographic and lymphoangiographic examination of neuropathic knee joints. *J Can Assoc Radiol* 1968;19:19–24.
88. Rabaiotti A, Rossi L, Schittone N, et al. Vascular changes in tabetic arthropathy. *Ann Radiol Diag* 1960;3:115–121.
89. Clement GB, Grizzard K, Vasey FB, et al. Neuropathic arthropathy (Charcot joints) due to cervical osteolysis: a complication of progressive systemic sclerosis. *J Rheumatol* 1984;11:545–548.
90. Moran SM, Mohr JA. Syphilis and axial arthropathy. *South Med J* 1983;76:1032–1035.
91. Race MC, Keppler JP, Grant AE. Diabetic Charcot spine as cauda equina syndrome: an unusual presentation. *Arch Phys Med Rehabil* 1985;66:463–465.
92. Raynor RB. Charcot's spine with neurological deficit: computed tomography as an aid to treatment. *Neurosurgery* 1986; 19:108–110.

93. Kapila A, Lines M. Neuropathic spinal arthropathy: CT and MR findings. *J Comput Assist Tomogr* 1987;11:736–739.
94. Maurer AH, Millmond SH, Knight LC, et al. Infection in diabetic osteoarthropathy: use of indium-labelled leukocytes for diagnosis. *Radiology* 1986;161:221–225.
95. Seabold JE, Flickinger FW, Kao SCS, et al. Indium-111–leukocyte/technetium-99m-MDP bone and magnetic resonance imaging: difficulty of diagnosing osteomyelitis in patients with neuropathic osteoarthropathy. *J Nucl Med* 1990;31:569–556.
96. Oyen WJG, Netten PM, Lemmens JAM, et al. Evaluation of infectious diabetic foot complications with indium-111–labeled human nonspecific immunoglobulin G. *J Nucl Med* 1992;33: 1330–1336.
97. Splittgerber GF, Spiegelhoff DR, Buggy BP. Combined leukocyte and bone imaging used to evaluate diabetic osteoarthropathy and osteomyelitis. *Clin Nucl Med* 1989;14:156–159.
98. Kalen V, Isono SS, Cho CS, et al. Charcot arthropathy of the spine in longstanding paraplegia. *Spine* 1987;12:42–47.
99. Palestro CJ, Mehta HH, Patel M, et al. Marrow versus infection in the Charcot joint: indium-111 leukocyte and technetium-99m sulfur colloid scintigraphy. *J Nucl Med* 1998;39:346–350.
100. Meyers SP, Wiener SN. Diagnosis of hematogenous pyogenic vertebral osteomyelitis by magnetic resonance imaging. *Arch Intern Med* 1991;151:683–687.
101. Lipman BT, Collier BD, Carrera GF, et al. Detection of osteomyelitis in the neuropathic foot: nuclear medicine, MRI, and conventional radiography. *Clin Nucl Med* 1998;23:77–82.
102. Beltran J, Campanini DS, Knight C, et al. The diabetic foot: magnetic resonance imaging evaluation. *Skeletal Radiol* 1990; 19:37–41.
103. Giesecke SB, Dalinka MK, Kyle GC. Lisfranc's fracture-dislocation: a manifestation of peripheral neuropathy. *AJR* 1978; 131:139–141.
104. Forgacs S. Stages and roentgenological picture of diabetic osteoarthropathy. *Fortschr Rontgenstr* 1977;126:36–42.
105. Cavanagh PR, Vickers KL, Young MJ, et al. Radiographic abnormalities in the feet of patients with diabetic neuropathy. *Diabetes Care* 1994;17:201–209.
106. Smith DG, Barnes BC, Sands AK, et al. Prevalence of radiographic foot abnormalities in patients with diabetes mellitus. *Foot Ankle Int* 1997;18:342–346.
107. Alergant CD. Tabetic spinal arthropathy: two cases with motor symptoms due to root compression. Br J Venereol Dis 1960; 36:261–265.
108. Brain R, Wilkinson M. Cervical arthropathy in syringomyelia, tabes dorsalis and diabetes. *Brain* 1958;81:275–289.
109. Campbell DJ, Doyle JO. Tabetic Charcot's spine. Report of eight cases. *Br Med J* 1954;1:1018–1020.
110. Cleveland M, Wilson HJ Jr. Charcot disease of the spine: a report of two cases treated by spine fusion. *J Bone Joint Surg* 1959;41A:336–340.
111. Culling J. Charcot's disease of the spine. *Proc R Soc Med* 1974;67:1026–1027.
112. Feldman F, Johnson AM, Walter JF. Acute axial neuropathy. *Radiology* 1974;111:1–16.
113. Holland HW. Tabetic spinal arthropathy. *Proc R Soc Med* 1953;46:747–752.
114. Thomas DF. Vertebral osteoarthropathy of Charcot's disease of the spine. Review of the literature and report of two cases. *J Bone Joint Surg* 1952;34B:248–255.
115. Wirth CR, Jacobs RL, Rolander SD. Neuropathic spinal arthropathy: a review of the Charcot spine. *Spine* 1980;5:558–567.
116. Zucker G, Marder MJ. Charcot spine due to diabetic neuropathy. *Am J Med* 1952;12:118–124.
117. Crim JR, Bassett LW, Gold RH, et al. Spinal neuroarthropathy after traumatic paraplegia. *AJNR* 1988;9:359–362.
118. Rataj R. Artropatic w jamistorci rdzenia. *Neurol Neurochir Pol* 1964;14:439–445.
119. Rodnan GP. Neuropathic joint disease (Charcot joints). In: McCarty DJ, ed. *Arthritis and allied conditions,* 10th ed. Philadelphia: Lea & Febiger, 1985:1095–1107.
120. Williams B. Orthopaedic features in the presentation of syringomyelia. *J Bone Joint Surg* 1979;61B:314–323.
121. Lippmann HI, Perotto A, Farrar R. The neuropathic foot of the diabetic. *Bull NY Acad Med* 1976;52:1159–1178.
122. Eloesser L. On the nature of neuropathic affections of the joints. *Ann Surg* 1917;66:201–207.
123. Corbin KB, Hinsey JC. Influence of the nervous system on bone and joints. *Anat Rec* 1939;75:307–317.
124. O'Connor BL, Palmoski MJ, Brandt KD. Neurogenic acceleration of degenerative joint lesions. *J Bone Joint Surg* 1985;67A: 562–572.
125. Slowman-Kovacs SD, Braunstein EM, Brandt KD. Rapidly progressive Charcot arthropathy following minor joint trauma in patients with diabetic neuropathy. *Arthritis Rheum* 1990;33:412–417.
126. Finsterbush A, Friedman B. The effect of sensory denervation on rabbits' knee joints. *J Bone Joint Surg* 1975;57A:949–956.
127. Brower AC, Allman RM. Pathogenesis of the neurotropic joint: neurotraumatic vs neurovascular. *Radiology* 1981;139; 349–354.
128. Edelman SV, Kosofsky EM, Paul RA, et al. Neuro-osteopathy (Charcot's joint) in diabetes mellitus following revascularization surgery. Three case reports and a review of the literature. *Arch Intern Med* 1987;147:1504–1508.
129. Frykberg RG. Osteoarthropathy. *Clin Podiatr Med Surg* 1987;4: 351–359.
130. Childs M, Armstrong DG, Edelson GW. Is Charcot arthropathy a late sequela of osteoporosis in patients with diabetes mellitus? *J Foot Ankle Surg* 1998;37:437–439.
131. Shapiro SA, Stansberry KB, Hill MA, et al. Normal blood flow response and vasomotion in the diabetic Charcot foot. *J Diabetic Complications* 1998;12:147–153.
132. Selby PL, Young MJ, Boulton AJ. Bisphosphonates: a new treatment for diabetic Charcot neuroarthropathy? *Diabetic Med* 1994;11:28–23.
133. Armstrong DG, Lavery LA. Elevated peak pressures in patients who have Charcot arthropathy. *J Bone Joint Surg* 1998;80: 365–369.
134. Clohisy DR, Thompson RC Jr. Fractures associated with neuropathic arthropathy in adults who have juvenile onset diabetes. *J Bone Joint Surg* 1988;70A:1192–1200.
135. Shaw JE, Boulton AJ. Poor vision as a contributory factor in diabetic neuro-arthropathy. *Diabetes Res Clin Pract* 1997;38:21–23.
136. Kernwein G, Lyon WF. Neuropathic arthropathy of the ankle joint resulting from complete severance of the sciatic nerve. *Ann Surg* 1942;115:267–279.
137. Casagrande PA, Austin BP, Indeck W. Denervation of the ankle joint. *J Bone Joint Surg* 1951;33A:723–730.
138. Collins DH. *The pathology of articular and spinal diseases.* Baltimore: Williams & Wilkins, 1949.
139. Horwitz T. Bone and cartilage debris in the synovial membrane: its significance in the early diagnosis of neuroarthropathy. *J Bone Joint Surg* 1948;30A:579–588.
140. Floyd W, Lovell W, King RE. The neuropathic joint. *South Med J* 1959;52:563–569.
141. Rodnan GP, Yunis EJ, Totten RS. Experience with punch biopsy of synovium in the study of joint disease. *Ann Intern Med* 1960;53:319–331.
142. Raju UB, Fine G, Partamian JO. Neuropathic neuroarthropathy (Charcot's joints). *Arch Pathol Lab Med* 1982;106:349–351.
143. Brenner MA, Kalish SR, Lupo PJ, et al. The diabetic foot with synovial cyst. *Cutis* 1990;46:142–144.

144. Barrett-Connor E. The prevalence of diabetes mellitus in an adult community as determined by history or fasting hyperglycemia. *Am J Epidemiol* 1980;111:705–712.
145. Martin MM. Diabetic neuropathy: a clinical study of 150 cases. *Brain* 1953;76:594–624.
146. Ostrander LD Jr, Lamphiear DE, Block WD. Diabetes among men in a general population: prevalence and associated physiological findings. *Arch Intern Med* 1976;136:415–420.
147. Mulder DW, Lambert EH, Bastron JA, et al. The neuropathies associated with diabetes mellitus: a clinical and electromyographic study of 103 unselected diabetic patients. *Neurology* 1961;11:275–284.
148. Storey G. Charcot joint. *Br J Venereol Dis* 1964;40:109–117.
149. Scartozzi G, Kanat IO. Diabetic neuropathy of the foot and ankle. *J Am Podiatr Med Assoc* 1990;80:298–303.
150. Beals TC, Manoli A. Great toe neuroarthropathy: a report of two cases. *Foot Ankle Int* 1998;19:631–633.
151. Campbell WL, Feldman F. Bone and soft tissue abnormalities of the upper extremity in diabetes mellitus. *AJR* 1975;24:7–16.
152. Feldman MJ, Becker KL, Reefe WE, et al. Multiple neuropathic joints, including wrist, in a patient with diabetes mellitus. *JAMA* 1969;209:1690–1692.
153. Bayne O, Lu EJ. Diabetic Charcot's arthropathy of the wrist. *Clin Orthop* 1998;357:122–126.
154. Schon LC, Easley ME, Weinfeld SB. Charcot neuroarthropathy of the foot and ankle. *Clin Orthop* 1998;349:116–131.
155. Reiner M, Scurran BL, Karlin JM, et al. The neuropathic joint in diabetes mellitus. *Clin Podiatr Med Surg* 1988;5:421–437.
156. Brooks AP. The neuropathic foot in diabetes: part II. Charcot's neuropathy. *Diabetic Med* 1986;3:116–118.
157. Harrelson JM. Management of the diabetic foot. *Orthop Clin North Am* 1989;20:605–619.
158. Mizel MS. Diabetic foot infections. *Orthop Rev* 1989;18: 572–577.
159. Hart TJ, Healey K. Diabetic osteoarthropathy versus diabetic osteomyelitis. *J Foot Surg* 1986;25:464–468.
160. Subbarao J, Gratzer M, Pinzur MS, et al. Diabetic neuro-osteoarthropathy. Rehabilitation of a patient with both ankle joints involved and associated skin problems. *Orthop Rev* 1986; 15:85–92.
161. Leventen EO. Charcot foot—a technique for treatment of chronic plantar ulcer by saucerization and primary closure. *Foot Ankle* 1986;6:295–299.
162. Mandell GL, Douglas RG Jr, Bennett JE. *Principles and practice of infectious diseases,* 2nd ed. New York: Wiley, 1985.
163. Barber DB, Janus RB, Wade WH. Neuropathy: an overuse injury of the shoulder in quadriplegia. *J Spinal Cord Med* 1996;19:9–11.
164. Chidgey LK. Neuropathic sternoclavicular joint secondary to syringomyelia. A case report. *Orthopedics* 1988;11:1571–1573.
165. Steinberg VL. Clinical reports: syringomyelia with multiple neuropathic joints. *Ann Phys Med* 1956;3:103–104.
166. Fidler WK, Dewar CL, Fenton PV. Cervical spine pseudogout with myelopathy and Charcot joints. *J Rheumatol* 1996;23: 1445–1448.
167. Mankin HJ, Congler KA. The acute effects of intra-articular hydrocortisone on articular cartilage in rabbits. *J Bone Joint Surg* 1966;48A:1383–1388.
168. Hollander JL, Brown EM Jr, Jessar RA, et al. Hydrocortisone and cortisone injected into arthritis joints. Comparative effects of and use of hydrocortisone as a local antiarthritic agent. *JAMA* 1951;147:1629–1635.
169. Hollander JL, Jessar RA, Brown EM Jr. Intra-synovial corticosteroid therapy: a decade of use. *Bull Rheum Dis* 1961;11:239–240.
170. Kendall PH. Untoward effects following local hydrocortisone injection. *Ann Phys Med* 1958;4:170–175.
171. Abell JM Jr, Hayes JT. Charcot knee due to congenital insensitivity to pain. *J Bone Joint Surg* 1964;46A:1287–1291.
172. Drummond RP, Rose GK. A twenty-one year review of a case of congenital indifference to pain. *J Bone Joint Surg* 1975;57B: 241–243.
173. van der Houwen H. A case of neuropathic arthritis caused by indifference to pain. *J Bone Joint Surg* 1961;43B:314–317.
174. Mooney V, Mankin HJ. A case of congenital insensitivity to pain with neuropathic arthropathy. *Arthritis Rheum* 1966;9: 820–829.
175. Murray RO. Congenital indifference to pain with special reference to skeletal changes. *Br J Radiol* 1957;30:2–6.
176. Petrie JG. A case of progressive joint disorders caused by insensitivity to pain. *J Bone Joint Surg* 1953;35B:399–401.
177. Sandell LL. Congenital indifference to pain. *J Fac Radiol* 1958; 9:50–56.
178. Schneider R, Goldman AB, Bohne WHO. Neuropathic injuries to the lower extremities in children. *Radiology* 1978;128: 713–718.
179. Silverman FN, Gilden JJ. Congenital insensitivity to pain: a neurologic syndrome with bizarre skeletal lesions. *Radiology* 1959;72:176–189.
180. Thrush DC. Congenital insensitivity to pain: a clinical genetic and neurophysiological study of four children from the same family. *Brain* 1973;96:369–386.
181. Swanson AG, Buchan GC, Alvord EC Jr. Anatomic changes in congenital insensitivity to pain. *Arch Neurol* 1965;12:12–18.
182. Johnson RH, Spalding MK. Progressive sensory neuropathy in children. *J Neurol Neurosurg Psychiatry* 1964;27:125–130.
183. Feindel W. Note on the nerve endings in a subject with arthropathy and congenital absence of pain. *J Bone Joint Surg* 1953;35B:402–407.
184. Piazza MR, Bassett GS, Bunnell WP. Neuropathic spinal arthropathy in congenital insensitivity to pain. *Clin Orthop* 1988;236:175–179.
185. Parker RD, Froimson AI. Neurogenic arthropathy of the hand and wrist. *J Hand Surg* 1986;11A:709–710.
186. Heggeness MH. Charcot arthropathy of the spine with resulting paraparesis developing during pregnancy in a patient with congenital insensitivity to pain: a case report. *Spine* 1994;19:95–98.
187. Gyepes MT, Newbern DH, Neuhauser EBD. Metaphyseal and physeal injuries in children with spina bifida and meningomyelocele. *AJR* 1965;95:168–177.
188. Handelsman JE. Spontaneous fractures in spina bifida. *J Bone Joint Surg* 1972;54B:381.
189. McCredie J. Thalidomide and congenital Charcot's joints. *Lancet* 1973;2:1058–1061.
190. Pruzanski W, Baron M, Shupak R. Neuroarthropathy (Charcot joints) in familial amyloid polyneuropathy. *J Rheumatol* 1981;8:477–481.
191. Shiraishi M, Ando Y, Mizuto H, et al. Charcot knee arthropathy with articular amyloid deposition in familial amyloidotic polyneuropathy. *Scand J Rheumatol* 1997;26:61–64.
192. Peitzman SJ, Miller JL, Ortega L, et al. Charcot arthropathy secondary to amyloid neuropathy. *JAMA* 1976;235:1345–1347.
193. Scott RB, Elmore S McD, Brackett NC Jr, et al. Neuropathic joint disease (Charcot joints) in Waldenstrom's macroglobulinemia with amyloidosis. *Am J Med* 1973;54:535–538.
194. Halonen PI, Jarvinen KAJ. On the occurrence of neuropathic arthropathies in pernicious anemia. *Ann Rheum Dis* 1948;7: 151–155.
195. Kettunen KO. Neuropathic arthropathy caused by spinal cord trauma. *Ann Chir Gynaecol* 1957;46:95–100.
196. Slabaugh PB, Smith TK. Neuropathic spine after spinal cord injury. *J Bone Joint Surg* 1978;60A:1005–1006.
197. Sobel JW, Bohlman HH, Freehafer AA. Charcot's arthropathy

of the spine following spinal cord injury. *J Bone Joint Surg* 1985;67A:771–776.
198. Lokiec F, Arbel R, Isakov J et al. Neuropathic arthropathy of the knee associated with an intra-articular neurofibroma in a child. *J Bone Joint Surg* 1998;80B:468–470.
199. Brunt PW. Unusual cause of Charcot joints in early adolescence (Riley-Day Syndrome). *Br Med J* 1967;4:277–278.
200. Blanford AT, Keane SP, McCarty DJ, et al. Idiopathic Charcot joint of the elbow. *Arthritis Rheum* 1978;21:723–726.
201. Chillag KJ, Stevens DB. Idiopathic neurogenic arthropathy. *J Pediatr Orthop* 1985;5:597–600.
202. Meyn M Jr, Yablon IG. Idiopathic arthropathy of the elbow. *Clin Orthop* 1973;97:90–93.
203. Nissenbaum M. Neurotrophic arthropathy of the shoulder secondary to tuberculous arachnoiditis. A case report. *Clin Orthop* 1976;118:169–172.
204. Wolfgang GL. Neurotrophic arthropathy of the shoulder. A complication of progressive adhesive arachnoiditis. *Clin Orthop* 1972;87:217–221.
205. Horibe S, Tada K, Nagano J. Neuroarthropathy of the foot in leprosy. *J Bone Joint Surg* 1988;70B:481–485.
206. Daughaday WH. Extreme gigantism: analysis of growth velocity and occurrence of severe peripheral neuropathy and neuropathic arthropathy (Charcot joints). *N Engl J Med* 1977;23:1267–1270.
207. Rothschild BM, Hanissian AS. Severe generalized (Charcot-like) joint destruction in juvenile rheumatoid arthritis. *Clin Orthop* 1981;155:75–80.
208. Maurer M, Sommer C. POEMS-syndrom-ungewohnliche manifestation mit beidseitigem Charcot-Gelenk. *Dtsch Med Wochenschr* 1999;124:346–350.
209. Meneghello A, Bertoli M. Neuropathic (Charcot's) joints in dialysis patients. *Fortschr Rontgenstr* 1984;141:180–184.
210. Thornhill HL, Richter RW, Shelton ML, et al. Neuropathic arthropathic (Charcot forefoot) in alcoholics. *Orthop Clin North Am* 1973;4:7–20.
211. Heller IH, Robb P. Hereditary sensory neuropathy. *Neurology* 1955;5:15–29.
212. Murray TJ. Congenital sensory neuropathy. *Brain* 1973;96:387–394.
213. Pallis C, Schneeweiss J. Hereditary sensory radicular neuropathy. *Am J Med* 1962;32:110–118.
214. Russell WR, Garland HG. Progressive hypertrophic polyneuritis with case reports. *Brain* 1930;53:376–384.
215. Bruckner FE, Kendall BE. Neuroarthropathy in Charcot-Marie-Tooth disease. *Ann Rheum Dis* 1969;28:577–583.
216. Kuur E. Two cases of Charcot's shoulder arthropathy. *Acta Orthop Scand* 1987;58:581–583.
217. David RP, Ko KR, Sachdev VP, et al. Charcot shoulder as the initial symptom in Arnold-Chiari malformation with hydromyelia: case report. *Mt Sinai J Med (NY)* 1988;55:406–408.
218. Goldman F. Identification, treatment, and prognosis of Charcot joint in diabetes mellitus. *J Am Podiatry Assoc* 1982;10:485–490.
219. Armstrong DG, Todd WF, Lavery LA, et al. The natural history of acute Charcot's arthropathy in a diabetic foot specialty clinic. *Diabetic Med* 1997;14:357–363.
220. Morgan JM, Biehl WC 3d, Wagner FW Jr. Management of neuropathic arthropathy with the Charcot restraint orthotic walker. *Clin Orthop* 1993;296:58–63.
221. Sella EJ, Barrette C. Staging of Charcot neuroarthropathy along the medial column of the foot in the diabetic patient. *J Foot Ankle Surg* 1999;38:34–40.
222. Mehta JA, Brown C, Sargeant N. Charcot restraint orthotic walker. *Foot Ankle Int* 1998;19:619–623.
223. Gristina AG, Nicastro JF, Clippinger F, et al. Neuropathic foot and ankle patellar-tendon-bearing orthosis. As an adjunct to patient management. *Orthop Rev* 1977;6:53–59.
224. Brashear HR. The value of the intramedullary nail for knee fusion particularly for the Charcot joint. *Am J Surg* 1954;87:63–65.
225. Stack JK. Experiences with intramedullary fixation in knee fusion. *Am J Surg* 1952;83:291–299.
226. Drennan DB, Fahey JJ, Maylahn RJ. Important factors in achieving arthrodesis of the Charcot knee. *J Bone Joint Surg* 1971;53A:1180–1193.
227. Frymoyer JW, Hoaglund FT. The role of arthrodesis in reconstruction of the knee. *Clin Orthop* 1974;101:82–92.
228. Wiseman LW. Neurogenic arthritis and the problems of arthrodesis of the neurogenic knee. *Clin Orthop* 1956;8:218–226.
229. Shibata T, Tada K, Hashizume K, et al. The results of arthrodesis of the ankle for leprotic neuroarthropathy. *J Bone Joint Surg* 1990;72A:749–756.
230. Coventry MB, Upshaw JE, Riley LH, et al. Geometric total knee arthroplasty. II. Patient date and complications. *Clin Orthop* 1973;94:177–184.
231. Ritter MA, DeRosa GP. Total hip arthroplasty in a Charcot joint: a case with a six-year follow-up. *Orthop Rev* 1977;6:51–53.
232. Robb JE, Rymaszewski LA, Reeves BF, et al. Total hip replacement in a Charcot joint: brief report. *J Bone Joint Surg* 1988;70B:489.
233. Charnley J. Present status of total hip replacement. *Ann Rheum Dis* 1971;30:560–564.
234. Fenlin JM Jr. Total glenohumeral joint replacement. *Orthop Clin North Am* 1975;6:565–583.
235. Sprenger TR, Foley CJ. Hip replacement in a Charcot joint: a case report and historical review. *Clin Orthop* 1982;165:191–194.
236. Soudry M, Binazzi R, Johanson NA, et al. Total knee arthroplasty in Charcot and Charcot-like joints. *Clin Orthop* 1986;208:199–204.
237. Fullerton BD, Browngoehl LA. Total knee arthroplasty in a patient with bilateral Charcot knees. *Arch Phys Med Rehabil* 1997;78:780–782.
238. Parsons H, Norton WS II. The management of diabetic neuropathic joints. *N Engl J Med* 1951;244:935–938.
239. Hanft JR, Goggin JP, Landsman A, et al. The role of combined magnetic field bone growth stimulation as an adjunct in the treatment of neuroarthropathy/Charcot joint: an expanded pilot study. *J Foot Ankle Surg* 1998;37:510–515.
240. Bier RR, Estersohn HS. A new treatment for Charcot joint in a diabetic foot. *J Am Podiatry Med Assoc* 1987;77:63–69.
241. Ryaby JT. Clinical effects of electromagnetic and electric fields on fracture healing. *Clin Orthop* 1998;355S:S205–S215.
242. Gough A, Abraha H, Purewal TS, et al. Measurement of markers of osteoclast and osteoblast activity in patients with acute and chronic diabetic Charcot neuropathy. *Diabetic Med* 1997;14:527–531.
243. Frankart L, Nisolle JF, Ayoubi S, et al. Neuroarthropathy of the shoulder of unexpected origin. *Clin Rheumatol* 1997;16:413–416.
244. Guis S, Pellissier J-F, Arniaud D, et al. Healing of Charcot's joint by pamidronate infusion. *J Rheumatol* 1999;26:1843–1845.

92

AMYLOIDOSIS

MERRILL D. BENSON

The amyloidoses are a group of protein deposition diseases that are distinguished by the fibrillar nature and tinctorial properties of the tissue deposits. These deposits, called amyloid, are composed of fibrils having a diameter of 80 to 100 Å and specific tinctorial properties including the binding of Congo red in histologic sections, which gives a typical yellow/green birefringence when viewed by polarization microscopy (1). A current concept of amyloid formation is that specific proteins, which are normally soluble in physiologic systems, are transformed in such a way that they become insoluble and then aggregate along with other biologic substances to form proteolytically resistant tissue deposits. Since many proteins have a basic structure that can fulfill the requirements of a fibril subunit protein and are capable of undergoing the soluble to insoluble transformation, there are many different types of amyloid substance that can be formed. Therefore, there are many different types of amyloidosis and each type, characterized by a specific class of protein, must be considered a separate disease. These diseases have widely varying characteristics including pattern of organ system involvement, association with other disease conditions, rapidity of progression of the process, and prognosis. It is important for the physician to first recognize that a patient's illness is due to amyloidosis and then to determine which disease the patient has so that appropriate medical evaluation and intervention can be planned. This chapter discusses the major types of amyloidosis as separate diseases. After a brief review of classification and overall structural properties of amyloid substances, each of the major systemic forms of amyloidosis is discussed as a separate entity.

PHYSICAL PROPERTIES OF AMYLOID

The one factor common to all of the amyloidoses is the accumulation of fibrillar protein deposits in the extravascular space. The composition of these deposits (amyloid) may vary considerably from one disease to another, but the basic theme of all amyloid deposits is that there is a structurally unique subunit protein that is capable of aggregating to form fibril structures with diameter of 80 to 100 Å and indeterminate length (Fig. 92.1) (2). Varying amounts of glycosaminoglycans are also found in the deposits, but do not appear to be specific for any one type of amyloid substance. Amyloid P component, a pentagonal structured plasma protein (pentraxin), is also associated with amyloid deposits of all types. Additionally, there may be other constituents of amyloid deposits that have not yet been characterized but that may be important for stability of the fibril structure. Each of the amyloid constituents contributes to the physicochemical properties of the deposit, but it is the subunit protein that defines the basic structure of the fibril and gives the birefringent property to the deposits. The carbohydrate components probably confer stability and protection from proteolysis to the fibril. The carbohydrate moiety explains some of the tinctorial properties of amyloid deposits such as staining with periodic acid-Schiff (PAS) and the reaction with sulfuric acid and iodine, which led Virchow to coin the misnomer *amyloid* (starch-like) (3). Although amyloid P component may not be a significant structural component of the fibril, it may participate in resistance to proteolysis and is widely used as a marker for detection of amyloid deposits since all types of amyloid bind P component.

By light microscopy, amyloid deposits appear amorphous and eosinophilic (Fig. 92.2). The deposits are extracellular and, depending on the stage of the disease, give varying degrees of tissue distortion. Amyloid deposits may be limited to blood vessel walls where they may be difficult to appreciate on routine histology or be present as a massive accumulation along cell margins with displacement of cells and supporting structures. For example, in the liver it is not uncommon to see large collections of amyloid with no recognizable hepatocytes, and, in the heart, myocardial cells may be surrounded by rings of amyloid (Fig. 92.1). In the kidney, glomeruli may show complete replacement of normal structures by amorphous amyloid deposits (Fig. 92.2).

A number of histologic techniques have been used to identify deposits of amyloid. The metachromatic dyes, methyl violet and crystal violet, give specific staining reactions with amyloid. The fluorescent thioflavin dyes, although not as specific, are often used to localize amyloid deposits. At present, the alkaline Congo red stain is used most widely for the identification of amyloid. Congo red, a planar dye, has a particular affinity for amyloid fibril deposits. Tissue sections stained with alkaline Congo red

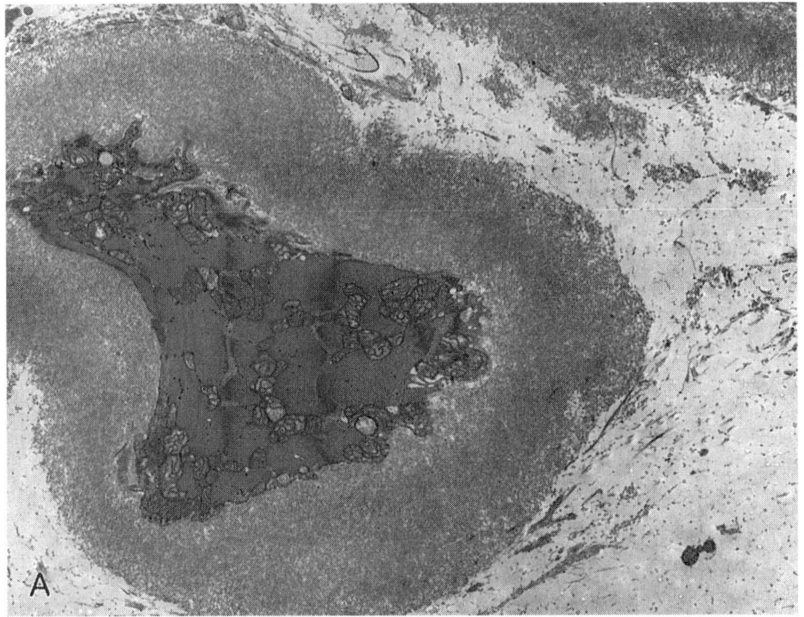

FIGURE 92.1. A: Electron micrograph of amyloid surrounding a cardiac myocyte (×20,125). **B:** High magnification showing typical fibrillar nature of amyloid deposit (×68,125).

show amyloid deposits as pink structures that, when viewed in the polarizing microscope, give a characteristic yellow/green color. This specific marker is due to the birefringent quality of the amyloid fibrils and their ability to bind Congo red. Unfortunately, the Congo red stain is not easily standardized and varying results can be obtained due to the thickness of the tissue section, the staining technique, and the availability of a suitable polarizing microscope.

By electron microscopy, amyloid deposits contain characteristic fibrillar structures, which are usually randomly arranged (Fig. 92.1). The fibrils are often in close contact with cytoplasmic membranes of cells, and occasionally reticuloendothelial cells may appear to contain inclusions of fibrils. The fibrils are nonbranching, of indeterminate length, and may consist of two or more parallel subunit filaments. Although there may be considerable structural variations from one fibril preparation to another, no ultrastructural features have been noted that differentiate the various chemical types of amyloid. Electron microscopy is often used for diagnosis of amyloidosis, but it probably should always be used in conjunction with light microscopy. It is not uncommon for other fibril structures in tissue preparations to be mistaken for amyloid fibrils, and this may lead to improper diagnosis.

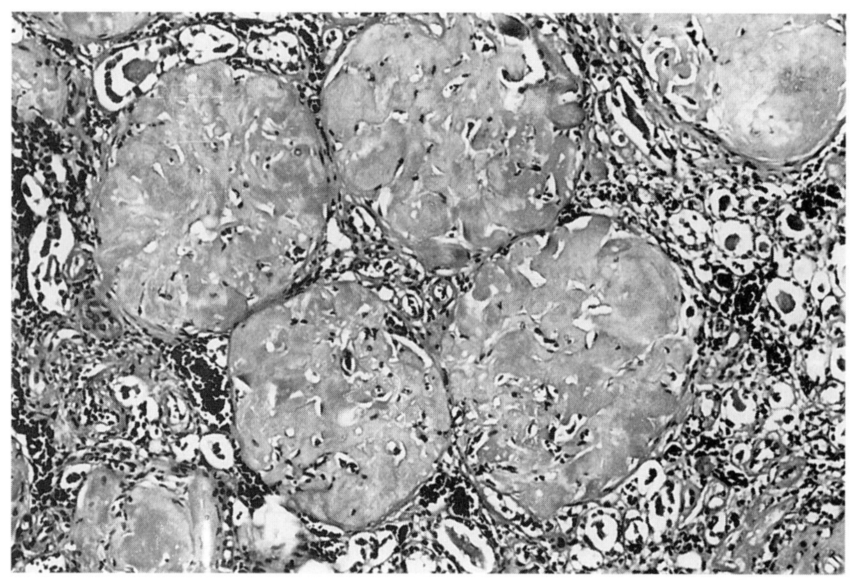

FIGURE 92.2. Renal biopsy showing obliteration of glomerular architecture by amorphous amyloid deposits.

The birefringence of amyloid fibril deposits is consistent with an ordered structure similar to that found in crystals. X-ray diffraction studies have shown that amyloid substances of diverse origins have predominantly β structure (4). This has been the basis for the antiparallel β-pleated sheet model of amyloid fibrils. Certainly, this is consistent with the finding that plasma proteins that are associated with amyloid fibril formation have significant amounts of β structure. This is true for the immunoglobulin light chain domains, which are the subunit proteins of immunoglobulin amyloidosis, and variant forms of transthyretin, which are the precursor proteins of amyloid fibrils in the most common form of hereditary amyloidosis.

CLASSIFICATION OF THE AMYLOIDOSES

There are four major types of systemic amyloidosis (Table 92.1):

1. Immunoglobulin light chain amyloidosis (AL) is always associated with a monoclonal plasma cell dyscrasia. The fibril subunit protein contains the variable segment of the light chain protein, either kappa or lambda. This may be the result of either a malignant plasma cell disease, such as multiple myeloma or Waldenström's macroglobulinemia, or a presumed benign monoclonal plasma cell dyscrasia (benign monoclonal gammopathy or monoclonal gammopathy of unknown significance).
2. Reactive amyloidosis (AA) is associated with chronic inflammatory disease. The amyloid fibril subunit protein is amyloid A (AA), a degradation product of the acute-phase plasma protein, serum amyloid A (SAA).
3. Hereditary amyloidosis includes a number of autosomal-dominant syndromes that are associated with mutations in specific plasma proteins including transthyretin, apolipoprotein A-I, gelsolin, fibrinogen, cystatin C, and lysozyme (5).

TABLE 92.1. SYSTEMIC AMYLOIDOSES

Type	Clinical Names	Subunit Protein	Distinguishing Feature
Immunoglobulin (AL)	Primary Myeloma-associated	Ig light chains (kappa or lambda)	Monoclonal Immunoglobulin
Reactive (AA)	Secondary	Amyloid A	Inflammatory disease
Hereditary	Familial Heredofamilial FAP	Transthyretin Apolipoprotein AI Gelsolin Fibrinogen Aα chain Lysozyme Cystatin C	Autosomal dominant
β_2-microglobulin (β_2M)	Dialysis	β_2-microglobulin	Renal dialysis

FAP, familial amyloid polyneuropathy.

4. β_2-Microglobulin amyloidosis is associated with chronic renal failure, and in almost all cases affected individuals have been treated with renal dialysis for a number of years. The amyloid fibril subunit protein is β_2-microglobulin, the light chain portion of the major histocompatibility complex (MHC) class I molecules.

Additionally, there are several forms of amyloidosis that are localized to specific tissues. These include Alzheimer's disease (central nervous system, CNS), prion disease (CNS), type II diabetes mellitus (islets of Langerhans), medullary carcinoma of the thyroid (thyroid), and isolated laryngeal, urinary tract, and cutaneous amyloid.

Nomenclature of Amyloid Syndromes

The International Amyloid Society has attempted to address the problem of standardizing nomenclature for the amyloid proteins and amyloidoses syndromes (6). The clinical terminology for various amyloid syndromes has generated considerable confusion in the past, mainly because of similarities at the clinical level of the different amyloid diseases and the fact that basic pathogenesis has not been defined for most of the syndromes. An example of this confusion is reflected in the description of many of the hereditary amyloidoses as *primary amyloidosis,* although this term was classically used to describe the sporadic disease with no obvious underlying cause. Amyloidosis occurring in individuals with chronic inflammatory disease, such as rheumatoid arthritis (RA), was appropriately called *secondary amyloidosis;* however, amyloidosis occurring in association with multiple myeloma was frequently called *amyloidosis secondary to multiple myeloma.* It is known now that amyloidosis associated with multiple myeloma is of the same chemical type as primary amyloidosis. With the identification of the various amyloid subunit proteins, attempts have been made to standardize the nomenclature using protein composition of the amyloid deposits rather than clinical parameters (Table 92.2). This has allowed clarification of the issue with immunoglobulin light chain amyloid (AL) representing primary and myeloma-associated amyloid, amyloid A (AA), representing the reactive secondary amyloidoses including those associated with familial Mediterranean fever and Muckle-Wells syndrome. The various hereditary forms of amyloidosis have now been named according to their subunit fibril protein (transthyretin, apolipoprotein A-I, etc.). Attempts to include all forms of localized amyloidosis have proved problematic since not all subunit proteins have been characterized. This is an ongoing project, how-

TABLE 92.2. STANDARDIZED NOMENCLATURE: THE 1990 GUIDELINES FOR NOMENCLATURE AND CLASSIFICATION OF AMYLOID AND AMYLOIDOSIS

Amyloid Protein[a]	Protein Precursor	Protein Type or Variant	Clinical
AA[b]	apoSAA		Reactive (secondary) Familial Mediterranean fever Familial amyloid nephropathy with urticaria and deafness (Muckle-Wells syndrome)
AL	kappa, lambda (e.g., κIII)	Aκ, A (e.g., AκIII)	Idiopathic (primary), myeloma or macroglobulinemia-associated
AH	(IgG I (λ1))	Aλ1	
ATTR	Transthyretin	e.g., Met30[c] e.g., Met111 TTR or Ile 122	Familial amyloid polyneuropathy (Portugese) Familial amyloid cardiomyopathy (Danish) Systemic senile amyloidosis
AApoAI	apoAI	Arg26	Familial amyloid polyneuropathy (Iowa)
AGel	Gelsolin	Asn187[d]	Familial amyloidosis (Finnish)
ACys	Cystatin C	G/n68	Hereditary cerebral hemorrhage with amyloidosis (Icelandic)
Aβ	β protein precursor (e.g., βPP)	G/n618	Alzheimer's disease Down's syndrome Hereditary cerebral hemorrhage with amyloidosis (Dutch)
$A\beta_2M$	β_2-microglobulin		Associated with chronic dialysis
AprP[e]	PrP[a]-cellular prion protein	PrP[Sc], PrP[CJD], e.g., P102L. A117V, F198S, Q217R	Scraple, Creutzfeldt-Jakob disease, kuru, Gerstmann-Sträussler-Scheinker syndrome
ACal	(Pro)calcitonin	(Pro)calcitonin	Medullary carcinoma of the thyroid
AANF	Atrial natriuretic factor		Isolated atrial amyloid
AIAPP	Islet amyloid polypeptide		Islets of Langerhans, diabetes type II, insulinoma

[a]Nonfibrillar proteins, e.g., protein AP (amyloid P-component) excluded
[b]Abbreviations not explained in table: AA, amyloid A protein; SAA, serum amyloid A protein; apo, apolipoprotein; L, immunoglobulin light chain; H, immunoglobulin heavy chain.
[c]ATTR Met30 when used in text
[d]Amino acid positions in the mature precursor protein. The position in the amyloid fibril protein is given in parentheses
[e]Modification suggested by editorial board.
From Natvig JB, Förre Ø, Husby G, et al., eds. *Amyloid amyloidosis.* Dordrecht: Kluwer Academic, 1990, with permission.

ever, and the current nomenclature is presented here to give some reference for understanding the scientific literature (7).

IMMUNOGLOBULIN, AL (PRIMARY) AMYLOIDOSIS

Immunoglobulin (primary) amyloidosis is the most common form of systemic amyloidosis. Although this disease is considered rare, the true incidence is not known. It is certainly more common than relapsing polychondritis and probably Wegener's granulomatosis. Several cases each year are seen in major academic medical centers, but because of the diverse clinical syndromes that AL amyloidosis generates, the cases are often spread over various divisions of medicine including cardiology, nephrology, rheumatology, and, unfortunately, sometimes just pathology. Recent canvassing of major medical centers that specialize in the treatment of patients with immunoglobulin amyloidosis revealed that the Mayo Clinic in Rochester, Minnesota, evaluates approximately 110 new patients per year (8), Boston University School of Medicine approximately 120 patients per year (9), and Indiana University School of Medicine approximately 20 patients per year. These numbers represent predominantly referred patients and are influenced by many factors including geographic location, socioeconomic status, age, sex, ethnicity, support groups, and the referring physician's knowledge of centers of research. There are three observations concerning these patients for which explanations are not completely clear: (a) males are more highly represented in referred groups than are females (60% to 65% males versus 35% to 40% females); (b) more patients with immunoglobulin amyloidosis are referred from physicians with no, or loose, affiliation with major academic centers than from physicians based at medical school centers; and (c) many patients refer themselves to centers specializing in amyloidosis after they are told that this is a rare disease for which there is no treatment. This latter factor may be related to a relative lack of information concerning amyloidosis in current medical texts. In any case, most investigators and students of amyloidosis would admit that the majority of individuals with amyloidosis are never seen in a major academic center, and many of them will never benefit from a definitive diagnosis.

Clinical Presentation

Immunoglobulin amyloidosis is associated with the most protean manifestations of all the systemic forms of amyloidosis. Pathology and, therefore, the clinical syndrome are directly related to the location and extent of amyloid deposition. Essentially every organ system in the body except for the CNS can be the site of amyloid deposits. The heart, kidneys, and liver are most prominently represented, with specific or overlapping syndromes. Other frequently involved organs include the gastrointestinal (GI) tract, spleen, thyroid, adrenals, lymph nodes, bone marrow, and lungs. This type of amyloid may occasionally infiltrate synovial structures (Fig. 92.3) and is the only major form of amyloidosis that involves skeletal muscle, skin (Fig. 92.4), and the tongue (Fig. 92.5). Although the CNS is spared amyloid deposition, presumably because of the blood–brain barrier that excludes immunoglobulin protein, the peripheral nervous system (PNS) enjoys no such protection. Sensory motor and autonomic neuropathy are frequent features of immunoglobulin amyloidosis.

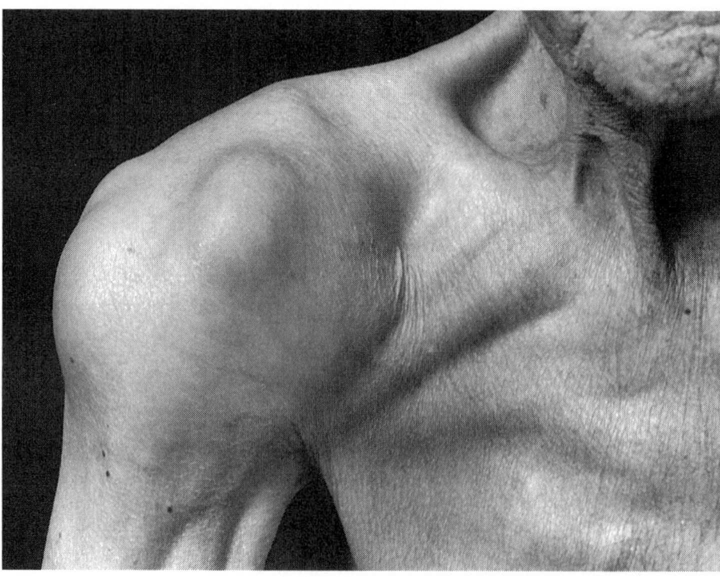

FIGURE 92.3. Articular amyloid infiltration in a 70-year-old man with AL amyloidosis. The subunit protein extracted from amyloid in the shoulder joint was a kappa III immunoglobulin light chain.

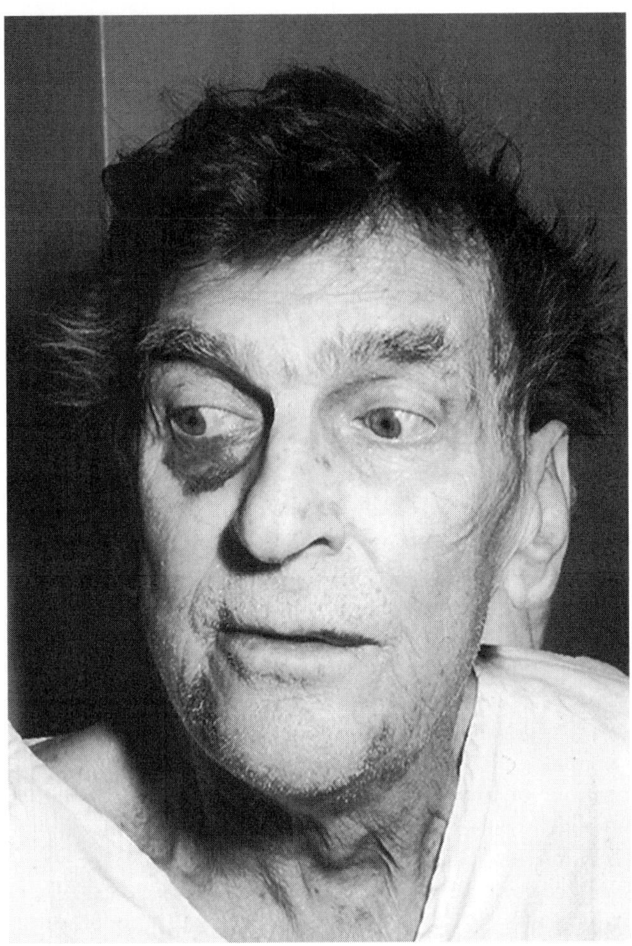

FIGURE 92.4. Periorbital purpura in AL amyloidosis. Frequently the patient gives no history of trauma to the areas of ecchymosis.

RENAL AMYLOID (AL)

Amyloid deposition in the kidney is usually glomerular, although varying degrees of interstitial fibril deposition may be seen. The nephrotic syndrome is the most frequent presentation and is the result of massive degrees of protein loss in the urine. Small amounts of urinary protein loss may be seen early in the course of immunoglobulin amyloidosis (i.e., 2 g/day); however, by the time a patient presents to the physician with persistent lower extremity edema, 24-hour urinary protein loss usually exceeds 5 g, is often in the 10- to 15-g range, and may exceed 25 g/day. Most of the urinary protein is albumin since this is the most abundant plasma protein and has a relatively low molecular weight. The basement membrane pathology of amyloidosis allows loss of the lower molecular weight proteins early in the course of the disease and, as the glomerular disease progresses, increasingly larger proteins are lost. Only immunoglobulin M (IgM) with molecular size of approximately 1,000,000 daltons and the lipoproteins, which are attached to high molecular weight lipoprotein particles, because of their size, are prevented from entering the urinary compartment. Presumably, the increased concentration of high molecular weight lipoproteins in the plasma is a direct result of the urinary protein loss in the nephrotic syndrome. It is not uncommon to find total plasma cholesterols that are well over 500 mg/dL and sometimes 1,000 mg/dL. Indeed, the finding of high cholesterol levels on routine blood chemistries should encourage an investigation of the urine for excessive amounts of protein loss. With or without treatment of primary amyloidosis, the nephrotic syndrome often persists for 1 or 2 years before the onset of renal failure, which is indicated by rising blood urea nitrogen and creatinine. Once the creatinine has started to

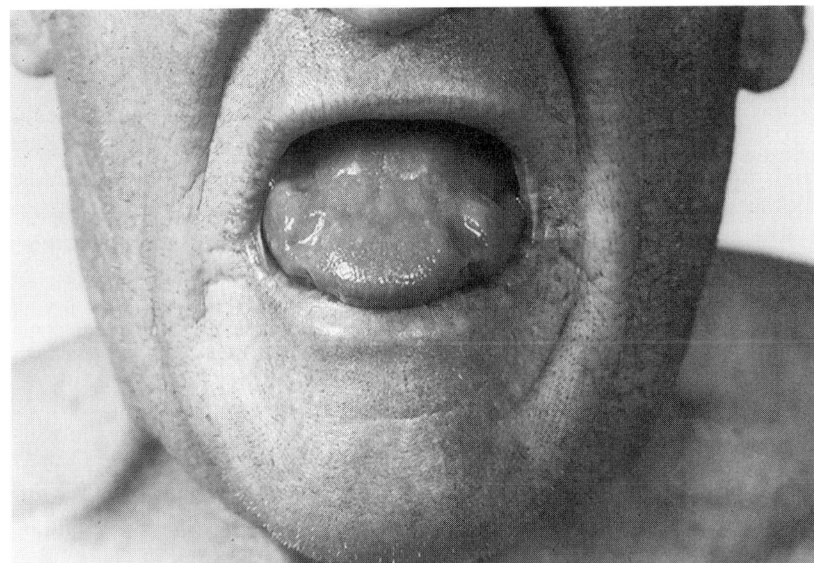

FIGURE 92.5. Macroglossia in AL amyloidosis. The tongue is firm to palpation. Note deep nonreducible impressions in the tongue caused by the teeth.

increase, the decline in renal function is precipitous. It is not uncommon for mild renal insufficiency with a serum creatinine of 2 to progress to complete renal failure with serum creatinine of 10 or greater within 6 to 12 months. The massive proteinuria, however, may not abate until almost complete anuria has occurred. This only serves to complicate the treatment of a patient who has volume depletion, orthostatic hypotension, and concomitant heart failure. Most published series of patients with immunoglobulin amyloidosis report kidney involvement as the most common presentation (10,11). This, in large part, is due to the fact that the nephrotic syndrome is relatively difficult to overlook, both by the patient and the physician. It demands diagnostic attention.

CARDIAC AMYLOID (AL)

Cardiac amyloidosis is a much more insidious process. By the time significant cardiac impairment is clinically apparent, the myocardium is usually severely damaged. Even in those cases in which a cardiac arrhythmia brings the patient to medical attention, cardiomegaly is usually present and significant decrease in cardiac reserve occurs (Fig. 92.6). Restrictive cardiomyopathy is the hallmark of myocardial amyloidosis. Systolic function usually is well maintained until late in the course of the disease; the problem is one of ventricular filling. Ejection fraction is usually well maintained, but stroke volume is decreased. The restrictive ventricular disease leads to atrial enlargement and very often supraventricular tachyarrhythmia. It is not uncommon for cardiac amyloidosis to present as florid congestive heart failure after the onset of a supraventricular tachycardia such as atrial fibrillation. Tachycardia further decreases diastolic filling time and severely compromises cardiac output. Successful treatment of the tachyarrhythmia can restore considerable cardiac function; however, many of the commonly used antiarrhythmic drugs have severe negative inotropic effects and, therefore, are contraindicated with amyloid cardiomyopathy. When the hemodynamics of restrictive cardiomyopathy are coupled with varying degrees of autonomic neuropathy, orthostatic hypotension is often the result. Individuals with amyloid cardiomyopathy have difficulty with adjustment of blood pressure on rising from the supine or sitting positions. This becomes even more pronounced when they are dehydrated by diuretic treatment of the congestive heart failure. While many patients with amyloidosis have either nephrotic syndrome or restrictive cardiomyopathy, a fair number have both organ systems involved, which adds significantly to the morbidity. If renal amyloidosis results in end-stage kidney failure, cardiac amyloidosis may preclude dialysis treatment of the azotemia.

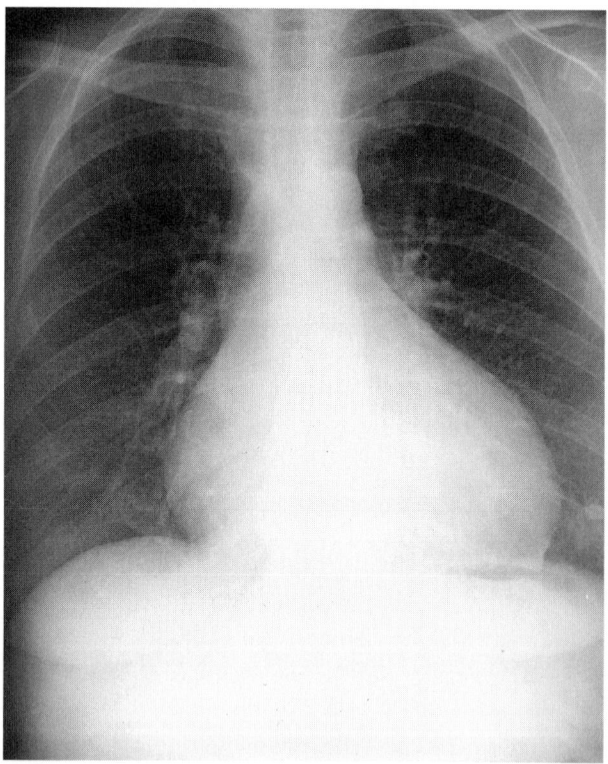

FIGURE 92.6. Chest radiograph showing massive cardiomegaly in a 45-year-old woman with AL amyloidosis. This patient's endocardial biopsy is featured in Fig. 92.1 and the two-dimensional echocardiogram in Fig. 92.16.

GASTROINTESTINAL TRACT (AL)

Clinically significant GI involvement in immunoglobulin amyloidosis is relatively common. It is usually manifest as one of two syndromes: motility disorders and bleeding.

Motility disturbances can be seen at all levels of the GI tract including the esophagus, stomach, small bowel, and large bowel. Most common, however, is delayed gastric emptying, noted by the patient as early satiety. Small bowel and large bowel involvement may cause alternating constipation and diarrhea, but measurement of transit times by standard tests is usually not of much diagnostic value. How much of the GI motility problem is due to actual infiltration of the bowel wall by amyloid versus autonomic nervous system impairment is usually difficult to gauge. In either case, bacteria overgrowth in the small bowel may occur and cause significant problems with absorption. This may result in low serum vitamin B_{12}, folic acid, and carotene levels. Occasionally, amyloid infiltration of the ileum leads to obstruction. This may present with the findings of an ileus, but may be mistaken for intestinal volvulus. In these patients, the small bowel wall is often very friable due to the amyloid infiltration and should be approached with care.

Bleeding may occur at any level of the GI tract. The stomach and small intestine are the most frequent sites of hemorrhage; however, occult bleeding may be the initial sign of AL amyloidosis and its origin often defies extensive investigation. GI bleeding may be severe and is frequently life-threatening.

Infiltration of the liver may occur as the major manifestation of immunoglobulin amyloidosis. It usually presents with moderate to massive hepatomegaly, usually without pain and often mistaken for metastatic neoplasia. Hepatic amyloidosis is often diagnosed by liver biopsy as the first diagnostic procedure (12). It is amazing how large the liver can become and the patient still not show evidence of hepatic decompensation. Serum alkaline phosphatase levels may be elevated and, in the end stages of hepatic amyloidosis, jaundice is common. When jaundice occurs, patients may inadvertently be referred for cholecystectomy and, if subjected to surgery, usually do not fare well. When hepatic amyloidosis occurs concurrently with either renal or cardiac amyloidosis, it is usually not the most life-threatening aspect of the disease. In patients suspected of having hepatic amyloidosis, a useful test for hepatic infiltration is the measurement of indocyanine green (ICG) extraction from the plasma (13). Less than 5% of ICG should remain in the serum 20 minutes after intravenous injection of 50 μg/kg body weight. Any elevation above this suggests that liver function is impaired. This test can be used as a serial monitor of amyloid progression or resolution. Liver spleen scan with technetium ^{99m}Tc sulfacolloid is useful to measure the size of the liver. Enlargement of the left lobe should raise the suspicion of amyloid since this lobe is less commonly the site of tumor metastases. Occasionally, defects in uptake can be mistaken for tumors, but usually the liver image is homogeneous. The spleen, on the other hand, very often shows decreased uptake of the radiotracer when heavily infiltrated with amyloid. This is evidence for functional asplenia and may correlate with hematologic findings (e.g., Howell-Jolly bodies). The amyloid-laden spleen may be enlarged, but in most autopsy series the organ is found to have only modest increase in weight, and is firm and relatively friable. The friable nature of the spleen will occasionally result in traumatic rupture of the organ.

NEUROPATHY (AL)

Peripheral neuropathy is a common feature of immunoglobulin amyloidosis, occurring in approximately 20% of affected individuals. It usually begins with paresthesias in lower extremities and progresses proximally. Sensory manifestations are most notable; however, motor involvement may lead to abnormalities of gait with bilateral foot drop. Demonstrable increase in nerve trunk size is not common. The neuropathy may occur months to years before visceral manifestations of AL amyloidosis and, indeed, patients with peripheral neuropathy are often considered to have better prognosis. These patients, however, do tend to progress to cardiac amyloidosis and die from heart failure or cardiac arrhythmia (14). Carpal tunnel syndrome unrelated to infiltration of nerves is frequently noted in the past medical history of patients and is the result of amyloid deposition in articular structures of the wrist resulting in compression of the median nerve. The carpal tunnel syndrome may occur one to several years prior to systemic disease manifestations and is usually relieved by surgical decompression of the median nerve. Unfortunately, tissue biopsy is rarely done at this stage of the disease because carpal tunnel syndrome is such a common entity and in only a small percentage of patients is it a result of amyloid deposition. Carpal tunnel syndrome is also a frequent manifestation of hereditary amyloidosis, and therefore complete evaluation for hereditary disease should be undertaken in patients with systemic amyloidosis and carpal tunnel syndrome. Autonomic neuropathy is common in AL amyloidosis. It may cause GI motility disorders and, frequently, impotence in males. The loss of ability in attaining an erection may precede signs of systemic disease such as weight loss, heart failure, or edema, by one or more years.

PULMONARY (AL)

Pulmonary amyloidosis may show two clinical presentations (15). The first is the development of tumoral masses of amyloid in the lung parenchyma, often with concomitant enlargement of hilar and peritracheal lymph nodes. The diagnosis of amyloid is usually made at the time of lung biopsy for suspected carcinoma (Fig. 92.7). The masses of amyloid tend to show progressive enlargement, but are not life-threatening unless accompanied by amyloid deposition in other organ systems. Patients may survive a number of years with these slowly enlarging tumors without any evidence of decreased pulmonary function. Frequent reevaluation of the patient for progression of the disease to other organ dysfunction (e.g., nephrotic syndrome) is recommended.

The second form of pulmonary amyloidosis manifests as diffuse interstitial infiltration of the entire lung parenchyma (Fig. 92.8). This results in "stiff" lungs with a restrictive pattern on pulmonary function testing and oxygen desaturation. This is often a rapidly progressing syndrome ending in severe air hunger that can only be temporarily assuaged by continuous oxygen therapy. Occasionally, more localized forms of amyloid deposition involve the respiratory tract with either laryngeal or tracheal/bronchial deposits. These may cause alterations in voice (hoarseness) or significant obstruction of the upper airways with pulmonary insufficiency. Local resection, usually by laser surgery, has become the standard treatment for this relatively localized form of AL amyloidosis.

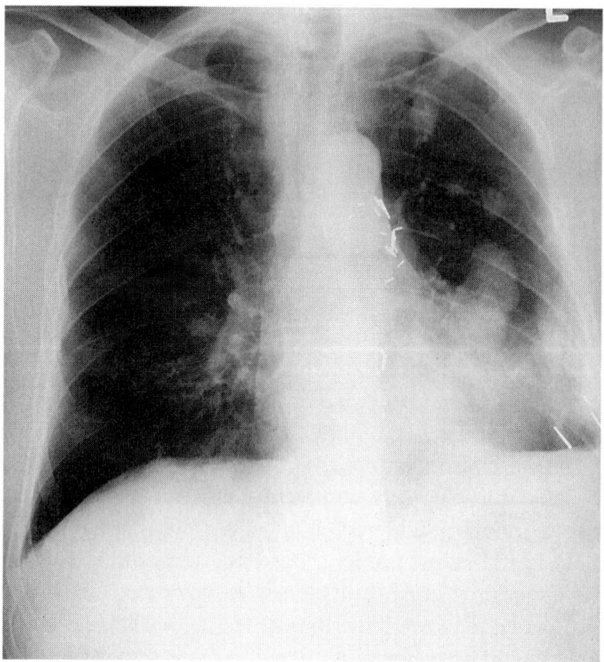

FIGURE 92.7. Chest radiograph of patient with tumoral amyloid in the pulmonary parenchyma. Diagnosis was by thoracotomy and biopsy.

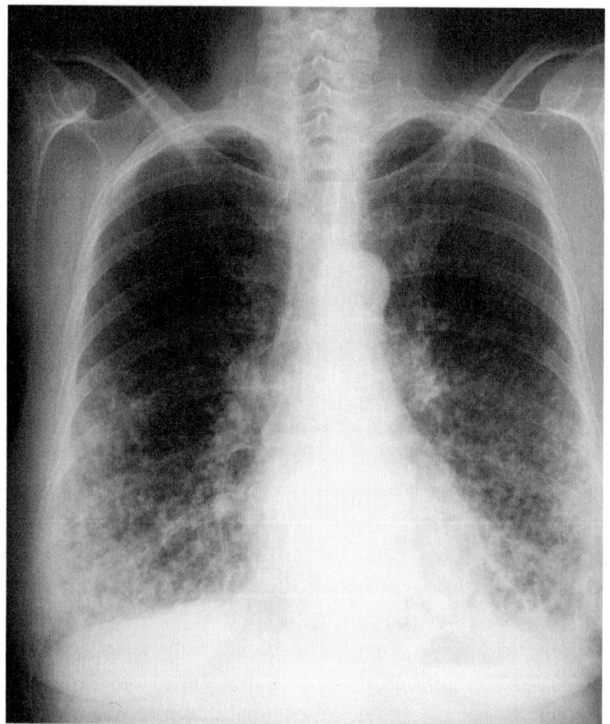

FIGURE 92.8. Chest radiograph of patient with diffuse pulmonary amyloid infiltration.

HEMATOLOGIC (AL)

Hematologic manifestations of AL amyloidosis include purpura, a result of infiltration of blood vessel walls by amyloid material that renders them friable (16). Purpura on the forearms, thorax, and around the eyes is the result of minor amounts of trauma causing extravasation of blood. Periorbital purpura may occur spontaneously after rubbing the eyes or even if the patient is in a head-down position for a prolonged period of time (Fig. 92.4). This manifestation may worsen when the patient is on small doses of aspirin, which is frequently used for its antiplatelet effect. Additionally, selective factor X deficiency, and, on occasion, factor IX, or even factor VIII, deficiency may occur in patients with AL amyloidosis (17). It has been hypothesized that factor X deficiency may be related to adsorption of the clotting factor by large splenic deposits of amyloid since amelioration of the syndrome has been seen after splenectomy (18). Another clotting abnormality caused by amyloid is increased coagulation with deep venous thrombosis, presumably a result of abnormalities in the plasminogen system that may occur in the presence of the nephrotic syndrome. Renal vein thrombosis is not uncommon in AL amyloidosis with the nephrotic syndrome.

ARTICULAR (AL)

Musculoskeletal and articular manifestations of AL amyloidosis include infiltration of skeletal muscle, which may result in pseudohypertrophy; this is relatively uncommon. Macroglossia is uncommon, occurring in no more than 10% of patients, but when it does occur it is essentially pathognomonic for AL amyloidosis. The organ is not only enlarged, but also firm to palpation and frequently shows persistent indentations from the teeth (Fig. 92.5). Macroglossia may be more real than apparent since enlargement at the base of the tongue may give a feeling of strangulation and problems with deglutition, although the tongue itself cannot be protruded for proper examination. Occasionally, macroglossia is so massive that a gastric feeding tube is necessary to sustain life.

The most striking articular involvement in AL amyloidosis is the "shoulder pad sign," a result of amyloid infiltration of tendons and capsular structures about the shoulders (Fig. 92.3). This process also occurs about the hip joints and may cause significant bony abnormalities. This articular involvement is often a source of considerable discomfort and severe limitation of motion. It may be accompanied by the carpal tunnel syndrome, which indicates that other articular regions of the body are also involved with this process. When coupled with the loss of the skeletal muscle mass frequently seen in AL amyloidosis, the shoulder pad sign may be very impressive.

Pathogenesis

The basic pathologic process in AL amyloidosis is a monoclonal plasma cell dyscrasia. The subunit protein of the AL fibril is derived from immunoglobulin light chain, which is the product of a single B-lymphocyte clone (19). Polyclonal light chain proteins do not form amyloid fibrils. The monoclonal light chain protein can be the product of either a malignant plasma cell clone, as seen in multiple myeloma or Waldenström's macroglobulinemia, or from an expanded clone that lacks malignant features. This latter condition is called benign monoclonal gammopathy or monoclonal gammopathy of unknown significance (MGUS). In either case, it is the immunoglobulin protein product of the clone that leads to the amyloid pathology and not the cellular proliferation itself. Monoclonal plasma cell expansion and protein synthesis, while necessary for AL amyloid, is not sufficient. The majority of individuals with multiple myeloma do not develop amyloidosis, indicating that there must be factors other than the production of monoclonal substrate that are important in fibrillogenesis. These factors may include the amount of protein synthesized, the structure of the protein, the metabolism of the protein, and the relative amounts of other fibril constituents. The amounts of monoclonal protein produced seem not to be a major factor in amyloid fibrillogenesis since individuals with large amounts of Bence-Jones protein very often do not form amyloid and others with very small amounts of monoclonal protein do form amyloid. Only 80% of patients with AL amyloidosis have detectable amounts of monoclonal protein in the serum or urine at the time of initial presentations (8). The other 20%, however, will be found to have monoclonal light chain as the constituent of their fibrils when they are examined biochemically after death. This suggests that despite the low plasma concentration of monoclonal protein, it can be selectively removed from the circulation and form the subunit of the amyloid fibrils.

Several factors suggest that the primary structure of the light chain protein is important in the generation of amyloid fibrils. Lambda light chains are represented in amyloid more frequently than kappa light chains, a reversal of the normal situation in plasma immunoglobulin proteins where the ratio is three kappa to two lambda. This suggests that lambda light chains have a greater propensity to form amyloid fibrils. Additionally, certain subtypes of light chain proteins are more frequently associated with amyloidosis. The lambda VI subtype is found only in patients with amyloidosis (20). In contrast, immunoglobulin light chain deposition disease, in which deposits of nonfibrillar light chain protein occur predominantly in the kidneys, is associated more frequently with kappa light chains than with lambda, suggesting that the kappa light chain structure is less capable of forming fibrils (21,22). Metabolism of the immunoglobulin light chain monoclonal protein is undoubtedly important in amyloid fibrillogenesis (23,24). The fibril subunit protein always involves the variable segment (VL) of the immunoglobulin light chain and may include the entire variable segment or only a part. Most frequently, the fibril protein represents the complete variable region and a portion of the constant region that is contiguous to the variable region (total mass is approximately 16,000 daltons). Occasionally the entire light chain protein (21,000 to 23,000 daltons) will be incorporated into fibrils, but this is uncommon. The immunoglobulin light chain domains, both VL and CL, have extensive β structures and it has been hypothesized that the VL domain plus one to three β strands of the CL domain constitute the amyloidogenic subunit for the fibrils (25). Proteoglycans found in amyloid fibril preparations may be an important constituent of the proteolytically resistant fibril. Proteoglycans also may play a role in the tissue tropism of amyloid fibrils. No good hypotheses have been put forth to explain why some patients have renal amyloid and others have cardiac amyloid or other organ involvement. This may be the result of local factors and other metabolic processes going on at the specific time of monoclonal protein availability. The role of amyloid P component never has been completely established. This protein is found in all forms of amyloid, but whether it is an integral part of the fibril, a stabilizing factor, and/or lends resistance to proteolysis, has not been determined.

It is commonly held that the pathology in AL amyloidosis is due to deposition of the fibrils themselves with displacement of normal structures. In the kidney, infiltration of the glomerular basement membrane clearly leads to early pathology. In the liver, large amounts of amyloid deposition can occur with expansion of the organ without severe derangement of liver function. A similar finding can occur in the heart where, in spite of cardiac weights of twice normal, muscle fibers continue to maintain respectable systolic contractility. In peripheral nerves, amyloid deposits either interfere with blood supply because of vascular wall infiltration, or deposits of amyloid actually result in demyelination and compressive neuropathy. Amyloid deposition can occur in practically any organ system of the body, although it is usually excluded from the CNS and probably from the eye. Previous reports of vitreous deposits in primary (AL) amyloidosis probably were misdiagnoses of the hereditary forms of amyloidosis. The location and the extent of amyloid dictates the severity of the condition, and this usually weighs heavily on the prognosis and survival. There is, however, considerable variation in the time frame of amyloid formation. We are frequently struck with the rapidity of the patient's decline after the diagnosis of amyloidosis, but often it is obvious that the process has been progressing for considerable time and normal organ reserves have delayed clinical expression of the disease. On the other hand, there are well-documented cases of AL amyloidosis in which the patient has gone from completely normal health status to severe incapacity within weeks.

Prognosis

AL amyloidosis is considered to be the most serious type of amyloidosis with regard to survival. Since it is a variable disease, it is difficult to be specific for any one patient. Relatively large clinical studies have shown that the median survival of patients with AL amyloidosis is presently between 18 and 24 months after tissue diagnosis (8). Attempts to date the onset of the disease retrospectively (prior to tissue diagnosis) do not give meaningful statistics for counseling patients. It is generally noted that individuals presenting with congestive heart failure have a shorter survival time. This is probably not due to a more rapid progression of the disease, but rather to the fact that the disease is fairly far advanced before congestive heart failure is appreciated. Patients who present with peripheral neuropathy or carpal tunnel syndrome, on the other hand, have a longer median survival. A more meaningful figure is the 5-year survival, which is approximately 20% in all series. AL amyloidosis is a very serious disease. In patients with multiple myeloma and amyloidosis, the morbidity of the malignant plasma cell disease and the protein deposition disease are additive and prognosis is even worse.

Treatment

The only specific treatment for AL amyloidosis is chemotherapy using chemical agents that alter the expanded plasma cell clone. The most common chemotherapy regimen is melphalan coupled with prednisone (26). This therapy has been used for multiple myeloma for many years and appears to be effective in AL amyloidosis in selected cases (13). Occasionally patients may be treated with cyclophosphamide and prednisone, and patients with Waldenström's macroglobulinemia and amyloidosis are often treated with chlorambucil. Although combination chemotherapy, as used for multiple myeloma, may be more effective in depleting the plasma cell clone, this may increase morbidity and mortality in amyloid patients. Patients with cardiac amyloidosis do not fair well when treated with Adriamycin, which has cardiotoxic effects, nor do they tolerate the use of vinca-alkaloids, which may aggravate their neuropathy. To date, the best survival rates continue to be seen with the older regimen of melphalan and prednisone. Colchicine in modest doses is sometimes added to the regimen, although it has not been definitely shown to be effective in AL amyloidosis. It does prevent amyloid in familial Mediterranean fever and the murine model of reactive amyloidosis, but these are two different disease conditions. In light of the variable nature of AL amyloidosis, no study has been done that shows significant changes in survival with chemotherapy versus no treatment. It is obvious, however, that certain individuals, particularly those with nephrotic syndrome, may have dramatic response to the chemotherapy (26). With the 5-year survival rate of only 20%, the patient certainly deserves consideration for this form of specific therapy.

High-dose intravenous melphalan (200 mg/per kg body weight) with autologous stem-cell rescue has become the preferred therapy for AL patients with acceptable medical status (27,28). Significant clinical improvement and disappearance of monoclonal proteins from serum and urine have been noted in 50% of patients, with more limited but significant improvement in patients in whom evidence of monoclonal disease persists. For patients with more advanced disease who may not tolerate the rigors of a bone marrow transplant, an intermediate dose of intravenous melphalan with stem-cell rescue may be effective. Advanced cardiac, renal, or hepatic amyloidosis is a relative contraindication to high-dose melphalan therapy. In general, cardiac and renal transplantations have not met with prolonged success due to recurrence of amyloid in the transplanted organ. If intravenous melphalan with stem-cell rescue proves to be a highly effective therapy for the plasma cell dyscrasia, selected patients with advanced disease may benefit from organ transplantation.

Nonspecific treatment of the patient with AL amyloidosis is very important. The use of potent diuretics can definitely prolong survival of patients with nephrotic syndrome and congestive heart failure. The correction of cardiac arrhythmias may increase cardiac hemodynamics and result in significantly prolonged survival. Either hemodialysis or peritoneal dialysis for renal failure can prolong the lives of some patients, although it is usually just a matter of time before another organ system fails. Renal transplants have been effective in some cases. Cardiac transplantation, however, is usually met with less than satisfactory results. Bleeding diathesis from factor X deficiency has been corrected in a few patients by splenectomy (18). Carpal tunnel release can give relief for patients with the carpal tunnel syndrome and should be done early in the course of the disease. Gastric emptying may be facilitated by use of metoclopramide, and intermittent courses of antibiotics may help relieve the diarrhea and malabsorption syndrome related to bacterial overgrowth in the gut.

One of the most important aspects of the treatment of patients with AL amyloidosis is performing a thorough evaluation of the organ systems involved and then informing the patient of what the process is and what to expect.

REACTIVE AA (SECONDARY) AMYLOIDOSIS

Reactive amyloidosis is usually associated with chronic inflammatory disease such as RA. This is undoubtedly the reason that practically all forms of amyloidosis have fallen into the realm of the rheumatologist. Fortunately, the incidence of reactive amyloidosis in patients with RA is low. The association of systemic amyloidosis and rheumatology, however, has persisted and the rheumatologist is called on to evaluate and treat the patient with primary (AL) amyloidosis (basically a disease of the immune system), and the systemic forms of hereditary amyloidosis (delayed-onset autosomal-dominant syndromes). Even so, the rheumatologist is probably the most qualified for dealing with these syndromes, which are multisystem diseases as are systemic lupus erythematosus and the vasculitides. Estimates of the prevalence of amyloidosis in patients with RA varied considerably in series of patients studied two to four decades ago (29,30). Recent studies that have been more scientifically rigorous suggest that biopsy evidence of amyloid can be found in approximately 6% to 8% of patients with long-standing RA. However, these data cannot be extrapolated directly to clinical practice situations where systemic amyloidosis will only be recognized in those individuals who have progressed to the point of having significant clinical pathology. In other words, not all individuals who have amyloid deposits demonstrated by biopsy of GI mucosa or other tissues will necessarily progress to having the nephrotic syndrome or liver function derangement from amyloid accumulation. The impression of most clinical rheumatologists is that reactive amyloidosis is quite rare in their patient populations with RA, certainly less than 5% and probably no more than 1% or 2%. Reactive amyloidosis, however, is associated with many types of chronic inflammatory disease including juvenile RA (31), psoriatic arthritis (32), and ankylosing spondylitis (33), and is even occasionally reported in association with systemic lupus erythematosus (34). It also has been reported in patients with cystic fibrosis, chronic bronchiectasis, granulomatous bowel disease, and osteomyelitis. In some parts of the world, it is a common complication of leprosy. Patients with quadriplegia or paraplegia who have recurrent infections have an increased incidence of reactive amyloidosis. There have also been several reports of reactive amyloidosis in intravenous drug users. Reactive amyloidosis also occurs in familial Mediterranean fever, an episodic inflammatory disease that is inherited as an autosomal-recessive trait (35). It is assumed that the amyloidosis is associated with the recurrent inflammatory episodes that are characterized by peritonitis and arthritis. A similar association of reactive amyloidosis and the hereditary Muckle-Wells syndrome (urticaria, deafness, amyloidosis) has been noted (36).

Clinical Presentation

The nephrotic syndrome is the most common presentation of reactive amyloidosis (Fig. 92.9). This often occurs in patients who have had inflammatory arthritis for at least 10, and often more than 20, years (37). In many cases, the inflammatory arthritis has become relatively quiescent, and the onset of peripheral edema is commonly mistaken as a manifestation of some other malady. In patients on prolonged treatment with gold salts or penicillamine, the persistence of proteinuria for more than 6 to 12 months after discontinuation of this therapy should raise the suspicion of renal amyloidosis. The degree of proteinuria is usually slowly progressive, but may reach levels in excess of 20 g of protein loss per day before renal insufficiency commences. The clinical course is then one of progressive renal insufficiency, which is the usual cause of death. Occasionally, patients present with azotemia without any history of the

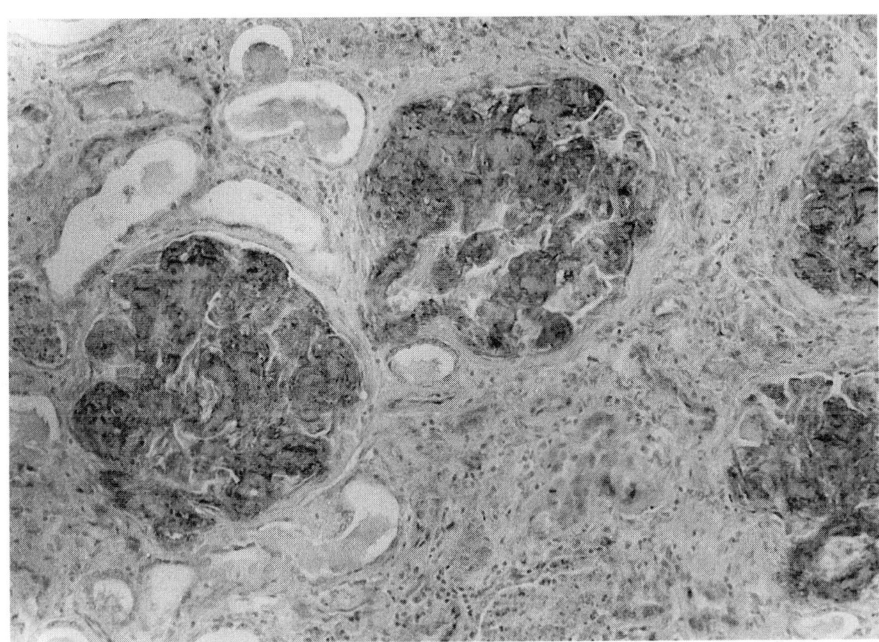

FIGURE 92.9. Immunohistochemical identification of reactive (secondary) glomerular amyloid with monoclonal antibody specific for protein AA.

nephrotic syndrome. In these individuals, the prognosis is extremely grave unless renal dialysis is instituted.

Gastrointestinal hemorrhage is relatively common in reactive amyloidosis and may be a presenting symptom. This presumably is due to amyloid infiltration of blood vessel walls throughout the entire length of the gut. GI motility disturbance is much less common in reactive amyloidosis than in immunoglobulin or hereditary amyloidosis (38). Hepatic amyloidosis is common, resulting in significant enlargement of the organ and eventually jaundice. However, liver function is usually relatively well maintained until late in the course of the disease. The spleen is practically always involved in patients with reactive amyloidosis. It rarely is more than modestly enlarged, but is usually firm and friable. Rare cases of splenic rupture due to relatively minor trauma have been reported. Although it has been reported, clinically significant cardiac amyloidosis is relatively uncommon in reactive disease and significant involvement of the tongue (macroglossia), skeletal muscle, and nerves is not seen. This helps to differentiate the disease from the immunoglobulin and hereditary forms of amyloidosis. Occasionally, an individual presents with reactive amyloidosis having no history or physical findings of inflammatory disease. This can occur in members of families with familial Mediterranean fever in which relatives have the complete syndrome and reactive amyloidosis. It also occasionally occurs in individuals with a history of neither familial Mediterranean fever nor any other inflammatory condition.

Pathogenesis

Serum amyloid A (SAA) is the precursor protein of reactive amyloid fibrils (39,40). There are a number of forms of SAA, each the product of a separate gene and expressed predominantly by hepatocytes. The family of SAA genes is localized to approximately 100 kilobase (kb) on the short arm of chromosome 11 (41). The SAA precursor of reactive amyloid fibril protein is an acute-phase reactant and is synthesized in response to an inflammatory stimulus (42). Under normal conditions, plasma levels of SAA are on the order of 1 to 3 μg/mL. Under acute-phase conditions, plasma levels of SAA may rise to 500 to 1,000 μg/mL, but usually fall back to normal levels within 2 to 3 days of resolution of the inflammatory stimulus (43,44). The inflammatory response is believed to be controlled by interleukin-1 (IL-1) and IL-6, which are produced predominantly by cells of the macrophage line (45,46). Other cytokines, such as tumor necrosis factor (TNF), may induce production of SAA proteins.

In humans, multiple forms of SAA have been identified. SAA1 and SAA2 proteins function as acute-phase reactants exhibiting elevated plasma levels in practically all instances of inflammatory disease (47,48). They are one of the most sensitive indicators of the acute-phase phenomenon. SAA plasma levels have been used to monitor organ graft rejection and myocardial infarction with significant elevation of plasma levels within 12 to 18 hours after an inflammatory stimulus. SAA4, on the other hand, is a constitutively produced protein with plasma concentration of 20 to 100 μg/mL without variation during the acute-phase response (49). This form of SAA has not been found as a constituent of amyloid fibrils, and its biologic function has not been delineated. The SAA3 gene, which has been shown to encode another form of SAA in mice and rabbits, is a pseudogene in the human and is not expressed (50,51). All of the SAA proteins are apolipoproteins (52). After synthesis by the liver and secretion into the plasma, they become part of the high-density lipoprotein (HDL) fraction of plasma and in times of high SAA production compete with the binding of apolipoprotein A-I for HDL. The subunit protein (AA) of amyloid fibrils in reactive amyloidosis is a degradation product of SAA. SAA1 and SAA2 are single polypeptide chains with 104 amino acid residues. In reactive amyloidosis, SAA undergoes enzymatic degradation, which usually results in the amino terminal 76 residues being incorporated into amyloid fibrils (53). The exact length of the AA protein does not seem to be a requirement for amyloid fibril formation since AA products representing residues 1–45, 1–54, 1–64, or even proteins longer than 76 residues have been found in selected cases (54,55). It would appear, however, that more of the SAA1 gene product is incorporated into amyloid fibrils than is the SAA2 protein, which is usually less than 20%. There is a more dramatic finding in the mouse model of amyloidosis, in which the product of only one gene (mouse SAA2) is found in the amyloid fibrils (56). These data suggest that some structural features of the SAA protein are important to fibril formation, but, as yet, no definite model for SAA fibril formation has been put forth. The fact that only a minority of individuals with chronic inflammatory disease ever develop reactive amyloidosis points out that there must be elements in reactive amyloid formation other than structure and production of SAA proteins.

Treatment and Prognosis

There is no specific treatment for reactive amyloidosis although control of chronic inflammation would seem logical, since presumably this would limit SAA production. Unfortunately, during the amyloid forming process, it would appear that relatively low levels of plasma SAA are sufficient to sustain fibril synthesis. Even so, resolution of reactive amyloidosis has been noted, particularly after control of systemic vasculitis and other relatively acute conditions such as Castleman's disease in which the lymphoid tumor has been removed. No such resolution has been reported for RA. Usually, patients with RA have received relatively maximum therapy to control their inflammatory disease, and, if reactive amyloidosis develops, there are limited remaining therapeutic options. Chemotherapy with drugs such as azathioprine, methotrexate, and chlorambucil has been reported to give favorable results, but no specific therapeutic protocol can be recommended. Colchicine is often given because it does prevent the occurrence of reactive amyloidosis in patients with familial Mediterranean fever (57), but, thus far, there is no definite evidence that it retards reactive amyloidosis related to other inflammatory diseases. Reactive amyloidosis is a slowly progressive condition. Patients often survive 5 or 10 years after the clinical onset of the disease. Supportive measures that may be effective in lengthening survival include renal dialysis, either hemodialysis or peritoneal dialysis, plus the use of diuretics, antibiotics, and measures used to treat the primary inflammatory disease.

β2-MICROGLOBULIN AMYLOIDOSIS

β_2-Microglobulin amyloidosis occurs predominantly in patients on hemodialysis. It is of particular interest to the rheumatologist since its principal manifestation is destruction of articular structures. The first manifestation is usually the carpal tunnel syndrome, although diffuse arthralgias, particularly involving the shoulders, are a common feature (58,59). This is a destructive disease with articular erosions and radiolucent cysts frequently in the shoulders, hips, and wrists (Fig. 92.10). Amyloid deposition can be seen in the synovium, subchondral bone, articular cartilage, and surrounding joint structures (60). Amyloid deposition in vertebral bodies is common and may cause vertebral collapse and consequent spinal cord impingement. Similar deposition in the hips may result in pathologic fracture.

The incidence of β_2-amyloidosis in patients on chronic hemodialysis is very high. Carpal tunnel syndrome is frequent in patients on dialysis for 7 years or longer and may be as high as 70% of patients on dialysis for 10 years. Most cases are associated with hemodialysis, but an increasing number of patients on chronic peritoneal dialysis are now being recognized as this form of dialysis has become more common.

Pathogenesis

The amyloid deposits in dialysis-related amyloidosis contain β_2-microglobulin, a part of human leukocyte antigen (HLA) class I molecules present on all nucleated cells (61,62). Under normal conditions, β_2-microglobulin (11.8 kd) is rapidly removed from the plasma by the kidney, where it is filtered and then reabsorbed by the proximal tubules and degraded. Plasma levels are approximately 2 mg/mL. Currently used kidney dialysis membranes fail to remove β_2-microglobulin from the plasma and levels as high as 60 times normal may be found in hemodialysis patients. Evidently, high levels of β_2-microglobulin lead to incorporation into amyloid fibrils and deposition in articular structures. The structure of β_2-microglobulin is analogous to a typical immunoglobulin domain with extensive β structure. There is no definite evidence that proteolytic cleavage is necessary for incorporation of β_2-microglobulin into fibrils, and it is not clear why this form of amyloid has a propensity for formation in articular structures. Some formation of β_2-microglobulin amyloid can occur in blood vessels throughout the body (e.g., intestines), and, therefore, this would appear to be a true systemic form of amyloidosis.

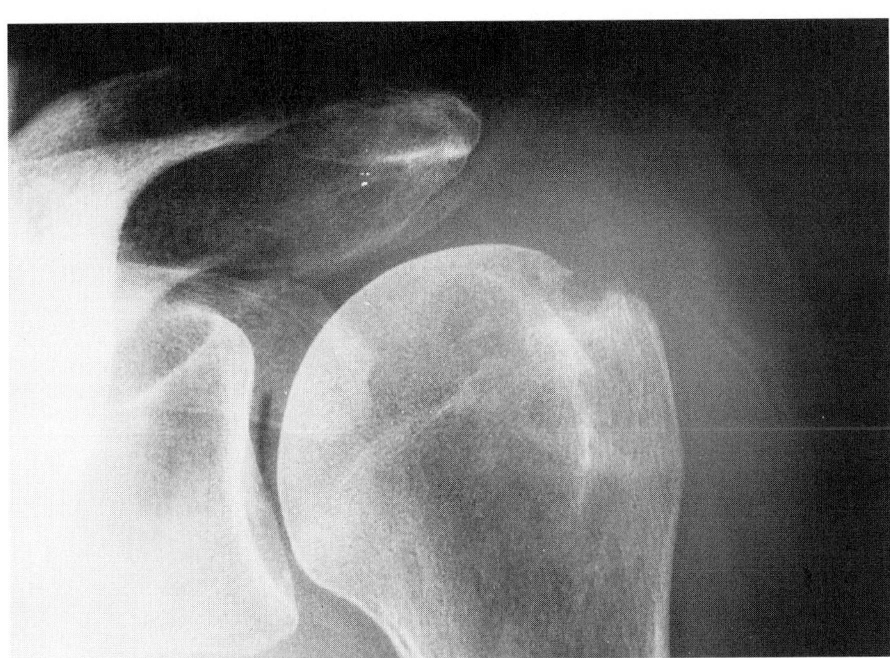

FIGURE 92.10. Cystic and erosive changes of the glenohumeral joint in β_2-microglobulin (dialysis) amyloidosis. The acromioclavicular joint is also involved.

Treatment and Prognosis

Specific treatment for dialysis-related amyloidosis is to remove the amyloid fibril forming substrate from the circulation. Unfortunately, no form of extracorporeal dialysis offers this treatment (63). When possible, renal transplantation will restore β_2-microglobulin levels to normal, and this presumably will ameliorate the syndrome. Unfortunately, many patients on chronic hemodialysis have already failed successful renal transplantation or are not suitable candidates for other reasons. Preliminary reports of removing β_2-microglobulin from the plasma by immunoabsorbent columns have not yet advanced to the stage of clinical application. In the meantime, nonspecific forms of therapy include surgery to relieve carpal tunnel syndrome. This may be very effective; however, articular pain, particularly in the shoulders, is usually not well controlled even with usually effective analgesics. Total hip arthroplasty may be used for destructive lesions of the femoral head. Stabilization of the spine may be necessary when β_2-microglobulin amyloidosis causes vertebral collapse.

HEREDITARY AMYLOIDOSIS

Hereditary amyloidosis is a heterogeneous disease (5). There are a number of mutated plasma proteins that are associated with amyloidosis. All are late-onset autosomal-dominant syndromes with varying degrees of cardiomyopathy, nephropathy, neuropathy, and other organ system involvement. They should be considered as separate disease entities rather than variations on a common theme, because each has unique features that may affect prognosis and treatment. The transthyretin amyloidoses are the most common form of systemic hereditary amyloidosis. However, similar syndromes may be caused by mutations in apolipoprotein A-I, plasma gelsolin, cystatin C, fibrinogen $A\alpha$ chain, lysozyme, and probably other proteins that have not yet been defined. Of particular concern is the tendency of the hereditary systemic amyloidoses to mimic the physical findings of immunoglobulin amyloidosis.

Transthyretin Amyloidoses

Pathogenesis

The majority of hereditary forms of amyloidosis are associated with variants of plasma transthyretin. There are more than 70 known mutations of transthyretin that are associated with systemic amyloidosis, plus another seven mutations that have not been associated with amyloid fibril formation (Table 92.3). Transthyretin is a normal plasma protein (64). It has two known plasma transport functions. It binds approximately 20% of the thyroxine in plasma, and also forms a noncovalent complex with retinol-binding protein and retinol (vitamin A) (65). The binding of retinol-binding protein–vitamin A to transthyretin prevents the loss of the lower molecular weight retinol-binding protein through the renal glomeruli. The actual biologic function of transthyretin is not completely clear since the knockout mouse model for transthyretin, while having very low levels of plasma vitamin A, shows no problems with development or maturation (66). Transthyretin is synthesized mainly by the liver as a single polypeptide chain of 127 amino acid residues (14,000 daltons) (64,67). In the plasma, transthyretin is a tetramer consisting of four identical monomers (55,000 daltons) (68). A central channel of the tetramer has a binding site for thyroxine, and retinol-binding protein forms a noncovalent association on the outside of the tetramer (Fig. 92.11) (69). Normal plasma concentrations of transthyretin are 20 to 40 mg/dL. Transthyretin is a negative acute-phase reactant, however, and during times of acute or chronic inflammation plasma levels are significantly depressed. Plasma levels are also modestly depressed in patients with transthyretin amyloidosis (70–72). This may represent increased metabolic turnover

TABLE 92.3. TRANSTHYRETIN AMYLOIDOSES

Mutation	Clinical Features	Geographic Kindreds
Cys10Arg	Heart, Eye, PN	United States (PA)
Leu12Pro	LM	United Kingdom
Asp18Glu	PN	South America
Asp18Gly	LM	Hungary
Val20Ile	Heart, CTS	Germany, United States
Ser23Asn	Heart, PN, Eye	United States
Pro24Ser	Heart, CTS, PN	United States
Val30Met	PN, AN, Eye, LM	Portugal, Japan, Sweden, United States (FAP I)
Val30Ala	Heart, AN	United States
Val30Leu	PN, Heart	Japan
Val30Gly	LM, Eye	United States
Phe33Ile	PN, Eye	Israel
Phe33Leu	PN, Heart	United States

TABLE 92.3. (continued)

Mutation	Clinical Features	Geographic Kindreds
Phe33Val	PN	United Kingdom, Japan
Arg34Thr	PN, Heart	Italy
Lys35Asn	PN, AN, Heart	France
Ala36Pro	Eye, CTS	United States
Asp38Ala	PN, Heart	Japan
Glu42Gly	PN, AN, Heart	Japan, United States, Russia
Glu42Asp	Heart	France
Phe44Ser	PN, AN, Heart	United States
Ala45Asp	Heart, PN	United States
Ala45Ser	Heart	Sweden
Ala45Thr	Heart	United States
Gly47Arg	PN, AN	Japan
Gly47Ala	Heart, AN	Italy, Germany
Gly47Val	CTS, PN, AN, Heart	Sri Lanka
Thr49Ala	Heart, CTS	France, Italy
Thr49Ile	PN, Heart	Japan
Ser50Arg	AN, PN	Japan, French/Italian
Ser50Ile	Heart, PN, AN	Japan
Glu51Gly	Heart	United States
Ser52Pro	PN, AN, Heart, Kidney	England
Gly53Glu	LM, Heart	Basque
Glu54Gly	PN, AN, Eye	England
Leu55Arg	LM	Germany
Leu55Pro	Heart, AN, Eye	United States, Taiwan
His56Arg	Heart	United States
Leu58His	CTS, Heart	United States (MD) (FAP II)
Leu58Arg	CTS, AN, Eye	Japan
Thr59Lys	Heart, PN, AN	Italy
Thr60Ala	Heart, CTS	United States (Appalachian)
Glu61Lys	PN	Japan
Phe64Leu	PN, CTS, Heart	United States, Italy
Phe64Ser	LM, PN, Eye	Canada, England
Ile68Leu	Heart	Germany
Tyr69His	Eye	United States
Lys70Asn	Eye, CTS, PN	United States
Val71Ala	PN, Eye, CTS	France, Spain
Ile73Val	PN, AN	Bangladesh
Ser77Phe		France
Ser77Tyr	Kidney	United States (IL, TX), France
Ile84Ser	Heart, CTS, Eye, LM	United States (IN), Hungary (FAP II)
Ile84Asn	Heart, Eye	United States
Ile84Thr		German, United Kingdom
Glu89Gln	PN, Heart	Italy
Glu89Lys	PN, Heart	United States
Ala91Ser	PN, CTS, Heart	France
Ala97Gly	Heart, PN	Japan
Ala97Ser	PN, Heart	Taiwan
Ile107Val	Heart, CTS, PN	United States
Ala109Ser		Japan
Leu111Met	Heart	Denmark
Ser112Ile	PN, Heart	Italy
Tyr114Cys	PN, AN, Eye, LM	Japan
Tyr114His	CTS	Japan
Tyr116Cys		France
Tyr116Ser		France
Ala120Ser	Heart	Afro-Caribbean
Val122Ile	Heart	United States
Val122	Heart, PN	United States (Ecuador)
Val122Ala	Heart, Eye, PN	United States

AN, autonomic neuropathy; CTS, carpal tunnel syndrome; Eye, vitreous deposits; LM, leptomeningeal; PN, peripheral neuropathy.

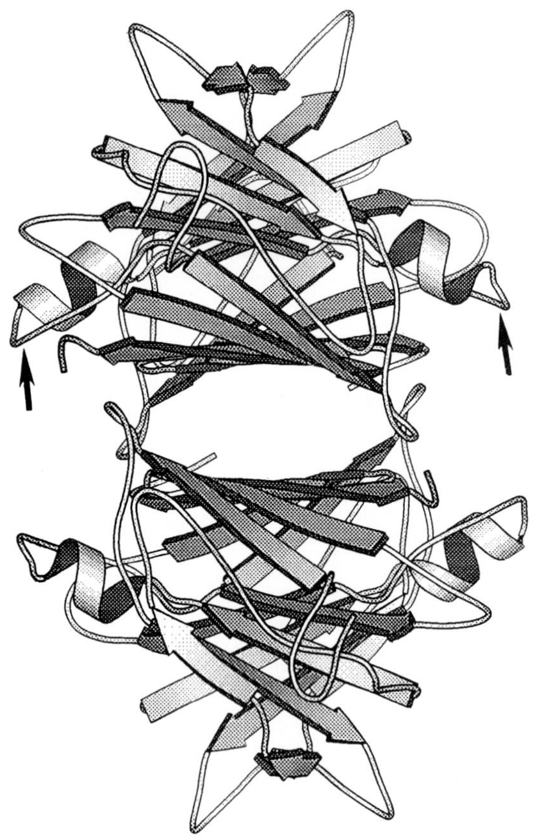

FIGURE 92.11. Computer graphic model of the transthyretin tetramer based on x-ray diffraction data. Thyroxine binds to the central cavity. Retinol-binding protein–vitamin A binds to the outside of the tetramer with amino acid Ile84 being central to the binding. Only two molecules of retinol-binding protein bind to one transthyretin tetramer since each molecule of retinol-binding protein (21,000 daltons) blocks the second potential binding site on that side of the tetramer.

of the variant molecules. Most individuals with transthyretin amyloidosis are heterozygous at the transthyretin gene locus on chromosome 18 (73). Expression of the two allelic protein products appears to be equal, and several reports have shown incorporation of both the normal gene product along with variant transthyretin into amyloid fibril deposits. Transthyretin has an extensive β structure, a property that most certainly is important in its tendency to form amyloid fibrils. It is hypothesized that single amino acid substitutions in transthyretin predispose to structural alterations that favor aggregation and fibril formation. There are also studies that suggest that normal transthyretin may be involved in amyloid formation as seen in senile systemic amyloidosis with cardiomyopathy (74). Although the principal site of synthesis for transthyretin is the liver, this protein is also synthesized in the choroid plexus of the brain and in the retinal pigment epithelium of the eye (75,76). Transthyretin produced in the choroid plexus may be important in the transport of thyroxine across the blood–brain barrier. Synthesis in the eye may be related to the vitreous amyloid deposits that are frequently seen in the transthyretin amyloid syndromes.

Clinical Syndromes

The first manifestation of most of the transthyretin amyloidoses is peripheral neuropathy (77,78). This may be a sensorimotor neuropathy starting in the lower extremities with progression proximally and subsequent upper extremity neuropathy. In some cases, however, the carpal tunnel syndrome, a compression neuropathy at the wrist, is the presenting symptom complex, and the sensory motor lower extremity neuropathy may follow. Symptoms of autonomic neuropathy may be the earliest and most pressing aspect of transthyretin amyloidosis with GI motility disturbances in most patients and frequently impotence in males. While the expression of the mutant transthyretin is present from birth, the formation of amyloid deposits and subsequent clinical disease usually start after the third decade of life and may not occur until advanced age. This variation in onset of clinical disease frequently clouds the autosomal-dominant genetics of transthyretin amyloidosis (Fig. 92.12) (5). This is of particular concern since the syndromes may be mistaken for immunoglobulin amyloidosis, which frequently presents with carpal tunnel syndrome or peripheral neuropathy. The motor neuropathy may progress to cause severe difficulty with ambulation and, with the sensory deficit, trophic ulcers of the lower extremities and traumatic injuries, including Charcot knee or ankle may occur. Chronic infections such as osteomyelitis are less common since the advent of antibiotics, but GI dysfunction often leads to severe cachexia. Delayed gastric emptying can be a particular problem. Cardiomyopathy is a leading cause of death in transthyretin amyloidosis. This is a restrictive cardiomyopathy with markedly thickened ventricular walls, a result of amyloid deposition. Diastolic filling is impaired and orthostatic symptoms are common. While systolic function is usually well maintained until the end stages of the disease, decreased cardiac filling and, therefore, low stroke volume leads to poor tissue perfusion. Renal failure often is a terminal event. Renal amyloid deposition may occur in the transthyretin syndromes, but is less frequent than cardiomyopathy. When this does occur, proteinuria is an initial feature followed by azotemia. Vitreous amyloid deposits are a common feature of transthyretin amyloidosis and explain the majority of cases that were previously thought to be related to primary amyloidosis. The amyloid deposits interfere with vision, and unless surgically removed, can lead to total blindness.

The incidence of transthyretin amyloidosis is not known. Attempts to determine accurate prevalence rates are confounded by the many mutations in transthyretin that are restricted to specific kindreds, and variations in the clinical syndromes (5). Table 92.3 lists the presently known mutations of transthyretin associated with amyloidosis,

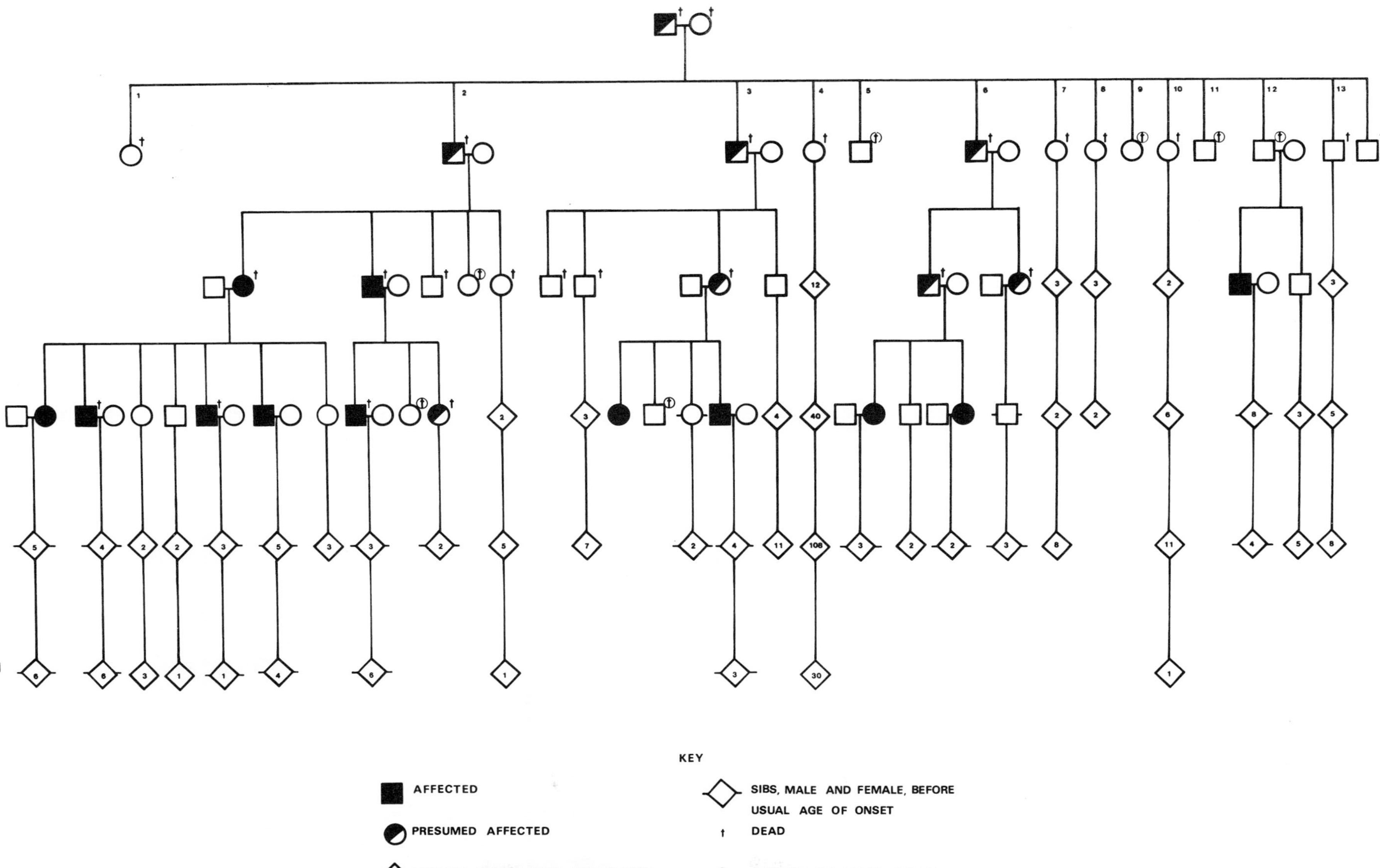

FIGURE 92.12. Pedigree of a typical family with autosomal-dominant transthyretin amyloidosis.

some of their prominent clinical features, and the geographic locations of many of these kindreds. The majority of transthyretin mutations that have been discovered in the United States have been in Caucasians of European origin. There is, however, one mutation (Val122I1e) that is restricted to the African American population with an allele frequency of 2% to 3% (79). This particular mutation is associated with late-onset restrictive cardiomyopathy and explains the majority of senile cardiac amyloidosis in African Americans. Several transthyretin mutations have been discovered in Japan, but none in mainland China, a finding most likely indicative of the level of sophistication of biomedical research.

DIAGNOSIS OF TRANSTHYRETIN-RELATED AMYLOIDOSIS

The transthyretin gene has four exons, with the amyloid-associated mutations dispersed over exons two, three, and four (80,81). Exon one, which encodes only the first three amino acid residues of the mature protein, has not been found to have an amyloid-associated mutation. Specific tests for each of the transthyretin mutations have been described. Most are based on polymerase chain reaction (PCR) amplification of the transthyretin exons coupled with restriction fragment length polymorphism (RFLP) analysis (Fig. 92.13) (82). DNA testing for only a fraction of the transthyretin mutations is commercially available, however, and consultation from a center for the study of amyloidosis is indicated when this diagnosis is suspected. Immunohistochemistry of biopsied nerve, carpal tunnel tissue, or GI mucosa with transthyretin specific antibodies can be used for diagnostic purposes, but this technique does not always give reliable results. Extensive documentation of family history with particular attention to ethnicity can be of great value in diagnosis.

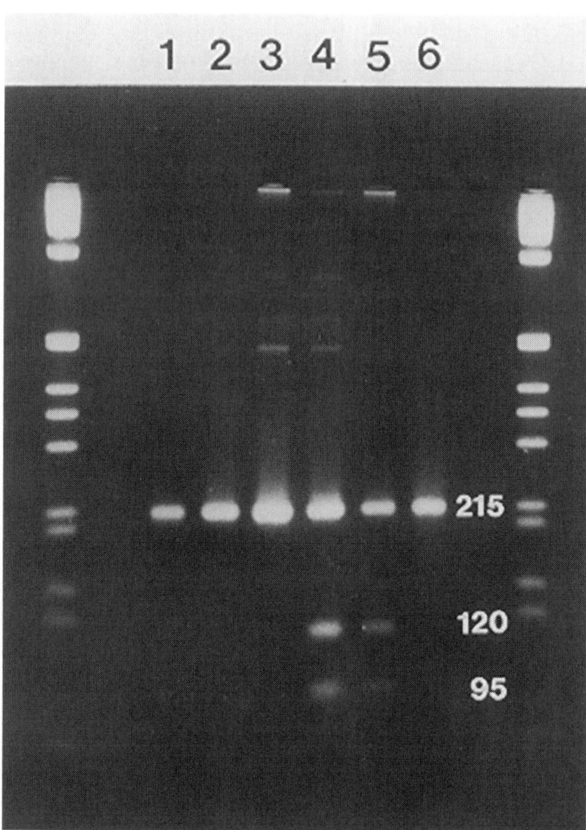

FIGURE 92.13. Diagnostic test for transthyretin Met30 amyloidosis. Genomic DNA from peripheral blood leukocytes is amplified by the polymerase chain reaction technique, in this case, exon 2 of transthyretin, to give a 215-nucleotide product. Digestion with the restriction enzyme NsiI identifies subjects 4 and 5 to be heterozygous for the transthyretin Met 30 mutation. Subjects 1, 2, 3, and 6 are normal.

TREATMENT OF TRANSTHYRETIN-RELATED AMYLOIDOSIS

The only specific treatment for transthyretin amyloidosis is liver transplantation (83). Since transthyretin is almost exclusively synthesized by hepatocytes, liver transplantation results in rapid disappearance of variant transthyretin from the circulation (84). This form of therapy is now being used for an increasing number of young individuals with transthyretin amyloidosis, although there are several problems. First, it has been found that there is increased surgical morbidity and mortality for patients who have progressed to a severe state of malnutrition before liver transplantation. Reversal of neuropathy is not to be expected, and therefore transplantation should be considered earlier in the course of clinical disease. However, graft rejection and risks from medication to prevent this must be factored into the equation for each patient. Cardiomyopathy related to transthyretin amyloidosis is often clinically significant only after age 60. Therefore, many individuals are not considered to be prime candidates for liver transplantation. There are, however, a number of nonspecific treatments that can significantly prolong life. Renal dialysis may be effective in patients with nephropathy. Cardiac pacemakers are often needed in individuals with sinus arrest or conduction abnormalities. The use of diuretics can improve quality of life for patients with restrictive cardiomyopathy, but relatively high central venous pressure is usually required to give adequate cardiac filling and tissue perfusion. GI dysfunction can be treated with medications to stimulate gastric emptying, antibiotics to alter bacterial overgrowth in the gut, and other agents to treat the persistent debilitating diarrhea. Colchicine is often given to patients with hereditary amyloidosis, but its efficacy has not been proven.

HEREDITARY AMYLOIDOSES OTHER THAN TRANSTHYRETIN AMYLOIDOSIS

Apolipoprotein A-I Amyloidosis

Seven mutations in apolipoprotein A-I (ApoAI) associated with hereditary systemic amyloidosis have been reported (Table 92.4). The first, in which glycine in position 26 of the mature protein is replaced by arginine, has been found in two American families and one Canadian family (85). The original American kindred, which originated in northern Britain, has peripheral neuropathy starting in the lower extremities associated with proteinuria and subsequent renal insufficiency. The second American family is of Italian origin. Amyloid deposits in spleen and liver are found in this syndrome, but renal amyloidosis is the most prominent feature. Age of onset is variable, ranging from the third to sixth decades. This disease is typical autosomal dominant but the degree of penetrance has not been determined. A second mutation in apolipoprotein (Leu60Arg) was described in an English family in which the propositus had splenic and hepatic amyloidosis at age 24 (86). Renal amyloidosis was found in other members of the kindred, but neuropathy was not reported in any of the affected individuals. A third ApoAI variant (Trp50Arg) was discovered in a family with hepatic and renal amyloidosis (87). Two deletion mutants of ApoAI have been reported in families with hepatic or renal amyloidosis (Table 92.4) (88,89). Recently, an unusual syndrome of cutaneous amyloid and cardiomyopathy has been reported in association with two different ApoAI single amino acid mutation variations (90,91). The first (Leu90Pro) is present in the amino terminal portion of the ApoAI that is found in the fibril deposits. The other (Arg173Pro) is present more in the C terminal and is not found in the fibrils.

The pathogenesis of ApoAI amyloidosis is not clear. It has been shown that plasma turnover of the variant Gly26Arg ApoAI protein is accelerated (92). This suggests involvement of metabolic processes. In all forms of ApoAI amyloidosis that have been studied biochemically including the C terminal Arg173Pro, the amyloid deposits contain only the amino terminal portion of the ApoAI molecule. This also indicates metabolic processing in the generation of amyloid fibrils. Additionally, while all individuals studied to date have been heterozygous, only the variant forms of ApoAI have been found in the amyloid deposits. This is different from the findings in transthyretin amyloidosis in which heterozygous individuals usually have a mixture of normal and variant transthyretin in the amyloid fibrils.

There is no specific treatment for this form of amyloidosis. Several patients have benefited from long-term renal dialysis. Although ApoAI is largely synthesized by the liver, significant synthesis by the intestine has also been demonstrated. Even so, liver transplantation has been suggested as a means of altering progression of the disease.

Gelsolin Amyloidosis

Lattice corneal dystrophy is the hallmark of gelsolin amyloidosis also known as Finnish familial amyloidosis (93,94). In addition to corneal deposits of amyloid derived from plasma gelsolin, progressive cranial neuropathy and cutis laxis are usually present. Amyloid deposition can also occur in visceral organs, with renal and cardiac amyloid being frequent. This is a relatively late-

TABLE 92.4. PLASMA PROTEINS (OTHER THAN TRANSTHYRETIN) ASSOCIATED WITH AUTOSOMAL DOMINANT SYSTEMIC AMYLOIDOSIS

Protein	Mutation	Clinical Features	Geographic Kindreds
Apolipoprotein AI	Gly26Arg	PN, nephropathy	United States
	Leu60Arg	Nephropathy	England
	Trp50Arg	Nephropathy	England
	del60-71 insVal/Thr	Hepatic	Spain
	del70-72	Nephropathy, hepatic	South Africa
	Leu90Pro	Cardiomyopathy, cutaneous	France
	Arg173Pro	Cardiomyopathy, cutaneous	United States
Gelsolin	Asp187Asn	PN, lattice corneal distrophy	Finland, United States, Japan
	Asp187Tyr	PN	Denmark, Czech
Cystatin C	Leu68Gln	Cerebral hemorrhage	Iceland
Fibrinogen	Arg554Leu	Nephropathy	Mexico
	Glu526Val	Nephropathy	United States
	4904delG	Nephropathy	United States
	4897delT	Nephropathy	France
Lysozyme	Ile56Thr	Nephropathy, petechiae	England
	Asp67His	Nephropathy	England

PN, peripheral neuropathy.

onset disease, although the corneal dystrophy can occur by age 20 to 30. Many affected individuals do not have a significantly shortened life span. The largest number of patients with this syndrome are in Finland, where the mutant gelsolin gene frequency is high and homozygous individuals have been identified. Homozygosity is associated with earlier onset and more aggressive disease. Individuals with this type of amyloidosis have been described also in the United States, Denmark, Canada, and Japan. The mutation in the gelsolin gene associated with this syndrome results in asparagine substitution for aspartic acid at position 187 of the mature gelsolin protein (95,96). Another mutation at this position, Asp187Tyr, has been reported and is associated with features similar to the Finnish amyloidosis, but this syndrome has not been investigated in any great detail (97). It was reported in two families, one from Denmark and the other from Czechoslovakia.

Pathogenesis

Gelsolin is an actin-binding plasma protein, which may play a role in the metabolic processing of actin. Only a fragment of the 93-kd plasma gelsolin is incorporated into amyloid fibrils. This suggests that, as with SAA and ApoAI, protein catabolism may play a significant role in amyloid fibril generation. The gelsolin gene, which is located on chromosome 9, spans approximately 70 kb of DNA and has at least 14 exons (98,99). Diagnostic DNA testing based on PCR coupled with RFLP is available and should be considered whenever amyloid is seen in a patient with lattice corneal dystrophy. It should be noted that there are a number of other corneal dystrophies with amyloid deposition that now have been proven not to be associated with gelsolin. There is no specific treatment for gelsolin amyloidosis. Even organ transplantation, such as with transthyretin, is not an option since gelsolin is synthesized in large part by skeletal muscle.

Fibrinogen-Associated Amyloidosis

Mutations in the fibrinogen A α chain are associated with familial amyloidosis characterized by renal pathology (100). The clinical syndrome typically starts with hypertension and proteinuria, leading subsequently to azotemia. While the liver and spleen also may have deposits, cardiac manifestations seem to be uncommon. The diagnosis is usually made by renal biopsy, and this entity can easily be mistaken for primary amyloidosis since no neuropathy is involved. The family history is variable, and clinical disease onset may range from age 30 to greater than 60 years. There are four known mutations in the fibrinogen A α chain that are associated with amyloidosis. All are in the carboxyl terminal portion of the fibrinogen A α chain (Glu526Val, Arg554Leu, 4904delG, 4897delT) (100–103).

Pathogenesis of this form of amyloidosis involves degradation of the protease sensitive carboxyl terminal portion of the fibrinogen A α chain protein (104). This suggests a significant role for proteolysis in generation of the amyloid fibrils. Fibrinogen, which is encoded by a gene on chromosome 4, is one of the most abundant plasma proteins and is one of the minor acute-phase proteins. Whether modulation of the plasma level with inflammation is relevant in patients with mutations of fibrinogen A α chain is not clear.

Treatment

Renal transplantation has been performed for patients affected with this type of amyloidosis. Amyloid deposition in the renal allograft, has occurred as early as 1 year after transplantation, but renal function may be adequate for as long as 8 to 10 years (101,103). Since fibrinogen is synthesized predominantly in the liver, liver transplantation may be a specific treatment for this disease. One patient with the Glu526Val mutation has undergone combined liver and kidney transplantation and is without progression of disease after 4 years.

Lysozyme-Associated Amyloidosis

Mutations in human lysozyme have been found to be associated with systemic amyloidosis with prominent renal failure (105). One mutation, Ile56Thr, is associated with a petechial skin rash from childhood and subsequent renal failure. Another mutation, Asp71His, is also associated with renal amyloidosis. Pathogenesis of this form of amyloidosis is not clear. The entire lysozyme molecule is incorporated into the amyloid deposits with only the variant protein being present in the fibrils. It might be assumed that the β structure of lysozyme predisposes the mutated forms of this protein to form amyloid fibrils. Lysozyme is produced by polymorphonuclear leukocytes and macrophages. No specific therapy for this form of amyloidosis is known.

Cystatin C Amyloidosis

Cystatin C, a cysteine protease inhibitor, is synthesized by many tissues including kidney, liver, gut, pancreas, and heart. A mutation in cystatin C (Leu68Gln) is associated with this autosomal-dominant form of amyloidosis (106). Clinically, the disease presents in young adulthood with recurrent hemorrhagic strokes (107). Amyloid deposition in leptomeningeal vessels results in frequent intracranial hemorrhage. Families with this disease are mainly in Iceland, but the disease has been reported in other geographic locations. Although the disease is largely localized to intracranial vessels, some systemic involvement with splenic deposits has been noted. Therefore, this syndrome may be considered one of the systemic forms of amyloidosis. Pathogenesis of cystatin C amyloidosis involves degradation of the cystatin C molecule with loss of the first 10 amino acid residues. Significantly lowered levels of cystatin C in the cerebrospinal fluid of affected individuals can be used as a diagnostic test as well as the standard DNA analysis based on PCR technology (108,109). There is no specific therapy for this form of amyloidosis, although control of blood pressure would seem important in decreasing the likelihood of hemorrhagic strokes.

Localized Amyloidosis

There are a number of types of amyloidosis that are localized to specific tissues or organs and these may be either sporadic or genetically determined. Tumoral deposits of amyloid frequently occur in the urinary tract (110). Clinical manifestations include obstruction if the amyloid deposit is in either the ureters or urethra, or hemorrhage if the deposits are in the urinary bladder. There are many anecdotal case reports in the literature, but no true incidence figures have been published. Amyloid deposits in the larynx or tracheal-bronchial tree may also occur in a sporadic fashion (111). Symptomatology will include hoarseness if the amyloid deposits involve the larynx, or respiratory obstruction if the trachea or bronchi have significant amounts of amyloid deposition. Amino acid sequence studies of both laryngeal and urinary tract amyloid have shown that the amyloid fibrils are derived from amyloid immunoglobulin light chain (112). Diagnosis of laryngeal amyloid can be suspected from the typical pale yellow appearance of the subepithelial deposits (Fig. 92.14). Similarly, urinary bladder amyloid is usually recognized as blue discoloration of the mucosa. Definitive diagnosis is made by tissue biopsy. Treatment is usually accomplished by laser excision of the deposits to relieve obstruction in the respiratory tract or to treat hemorrhage from the urinary bladder.

Sporadic occurrence of amyloid in the subcutaneous tissues, usually of the lower extremities, can occur, but this is very rare. Preliminary studies have shown immunoglobulin light chain subunit protein in these deposits. Again, diagnosis is by biopsy of these subcutaneous masses. There is no effective therapy. Cutaneous amyloidosis has also been reported as a hereditary condition with either autosomal-dominant or X-linked inheritance (113,114).

Hereditary forms of localized amyloidosis include multiple endocrine adenomatosis type II (MEA-II) in which the medullary carcinoma of the thyroid contains amyloid derived from procalcitonin (115,116). The genetics of several forms of late-onset localized amyloidosis are less clear. Alzheimer's disease, a form of amyloidosis localized to the CNS, is inherited as an autosomal-dominant trait in some kindreds. The cortical plaques and leptomeningeal vascular deposits of amyloid contain a subunit protein, amyloid β-peptide or βA4, with molecular weight of approximately 4,000 daltons (117). This amyloid subunit protein is a degradation product derived from the carboxyl terminal portion of a much larger protein, β protein precursor (βPP) (118). Several mutations in the βPP gene localized to chromosome 21 have been

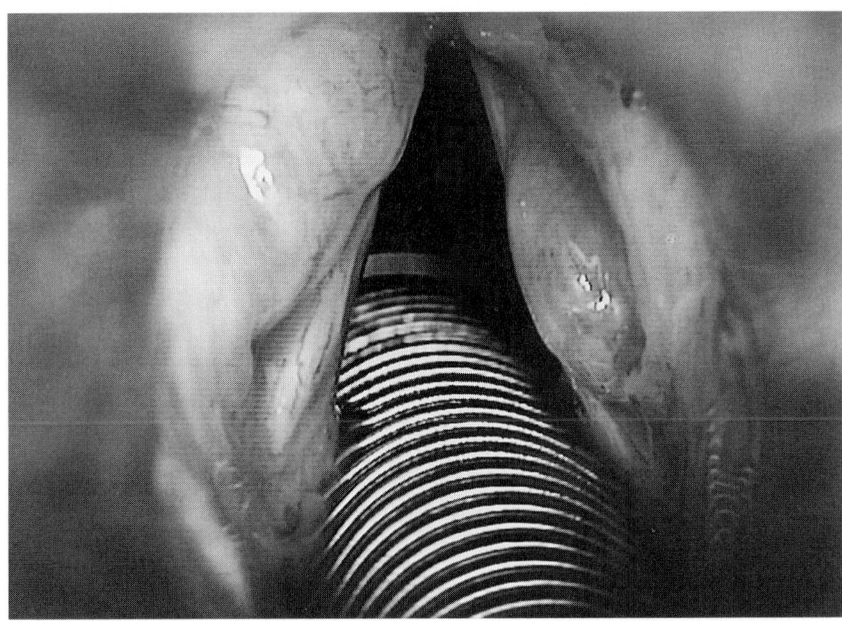

FIGURE 92.14. Enlargement of false vocal cord caused by amyloid deposition. This patient also had constriction of the tracheal airway due to subepithelial amyloid deposits.

shown to be associated with early-onset familial Alzheimer's disease (119–121). These βPP mutations, however, explain a very small percentage of familial Alzheimer disease. The majority of familial Alzheimer disease are associated with a gene localized to chromosome 14 that encodes a protein that may be a membrane receptor or ion channel (122). Apolipoprotein E (encoded on chromosome 19) has been shown to play a role in later-onset familial Alzheimer disease (123). Hereditary cerebral hemorrhage with amyloidosis of the Dutch type is also associated with a mutation in the βPP protein, but affected individuals in these kindreds die of cerebral hemorrhage without obvious clinical dementia (124). Whether the majority of Alzheimer disease in the elderly is genetically predetermined has not yet been answered.

Adult-onset diabetes mellitus is another form of localized amyloidosis. The islets of Langerhans contain hyalinized deposits that meet the criteria for amyloid. The subunit protein is a 37 amino acid peptide that is called either islet amyloid polypeptide (IAPP) or amylin (125,126). This peptide is synthesized by the β cells of the pancreas and is co-secreted with insulin. Its complete function is not known, and its relationship to the development of glucose intolerance also is not clear. There is an obvious genetic predisposition to type II diabetes, but the involvement of genetic factors in this form of localized amyloidosis is not clear. The same is true for isolated atrial amyloidosis in which a 28 amino acid residue carboxyl terminal degradation product of atrial natriuretic peptide is deposited in the walls of the cardiac atria (127,128). Long-standing congestive heart failure has been suggested to be a factor in pathogenesis. There is also a familial form of atrial standstill related to similar amyloid deposition (129). Isolated amyloid deposits in articular cartilage are frequently seen in elderly individuals with or without the presence of calcium pyrophosphate deposition disease (130). The chemical nature of this amyloid has not been determined.

Other forms of localized amyloidosis include the prion diseases. Creutzfeldt-Jakob disease may be either a sporadic infectious syndrome or inherited (131). Gerstmann-Sträussler-Scheinker disease is an inherited form of prion disease (132). Dementia is the clinical hallmark of these syndromes with progressive loss of cognitive functions and subsequent death from neural degeneration. The deposits in the CNS contain the prion protein and meet the criteria for amyloid deposits.

DIAGNOSIS OF AMYLOIDOSIS

The definitive diagnosis of amyloidosis depends on the histologic examination of tissue infiltrated with amyloid (Fig. 92.2). For the localized forms of amyloidosis, the diagnosis is usually straightforward. Localized amyloid deposition causes derangement of tissue structure or interference with function. This is true for urethral or ureteral obstruction, with bladder hemorrhage from mucosal amyloid deposits, and laryngeal amyloidosis that results in hoarseness. The abnormal tissue can be directly visualized, biopsied, and amyloid deposition recognized by appropriate pathologic examination. Diagnosis of localized forms of amyloidosis in organs less accessible for biopsy can be problematic, however. This is true for Alzheimer's disease and isolated cardiac atrial amyloidosis. The finding of amyloid deposition in medullary carcinoma of the thyroid is incidental to surgical resection of the primary tumor. There is no clinical need to demonstrate the amyloid in islets of Langerhans in diabetes mellitus type II. The main concern when tissue biopsy of a localized lesion demonstrates amyloid deposition is whether the process may be systemic.

Systemic amyloidosis should be suspected whenever there are functional abnormalities in more than one organ system. This may be as simple as congestive heart failure, angina with cardiomegaly, or cardiac arrhythmia in a patient who has symptoms of carpal tunnel syndrome, purpura, or GI hemorrhage. A more blatant, but not uncommon, presentation is the nephrotic syndrome in a patient who also has evidence of cardiac disease as well as hepatomegaly, macroglossia, and some degree of peripheral neuropathy. The individual with systemic amyloidosis usually seeks medical advice because of problems with one organ system. By the time of such presentation, however, the patient with systemic amyloidosis will often have evidence of other organ abnormalities that are apparent on careful examination. These multisystem abnormalities should always raise the suspicion of systemic amyloidosis.

Once the diagnosis of systemic amyloidosis is suspected or proven, it is necessary to determine which disease the patient has—immunoglobulin amyloidosis (AL), reactive amyloidosis (AA), or one of the forms of hereditary amyloidosis. There are a number of clues that may help in the diagnosis of each of the forms of systemic amyloidosis. For example, macroglossia (Fig. 92.5) and the shoulder pad sign (Fig. 92.3) due to amyloid infiltration of articular structures are signs of AL amyloidosis. Neither hereditary amyloidosis nor reactive (secondary) amyloidosis leads to macroglossia, nor do they cause infiltration of the joints. Carpal tunnel syndrome and peripheral neuropathy can be present in both AL amyloidosis and hereditary amyloidosis, but do not occur in reactive amyloidosis. The finding of monoclonal immunoglobulin protein on serum or urine electrophoresis is strongly indicative of AL amyloidosis since approximately 80% of AL patients will have a demonstrable M component (Fig. 92.15). Overt multiple myeloma in the patient with amyloidosis is strongly indica-

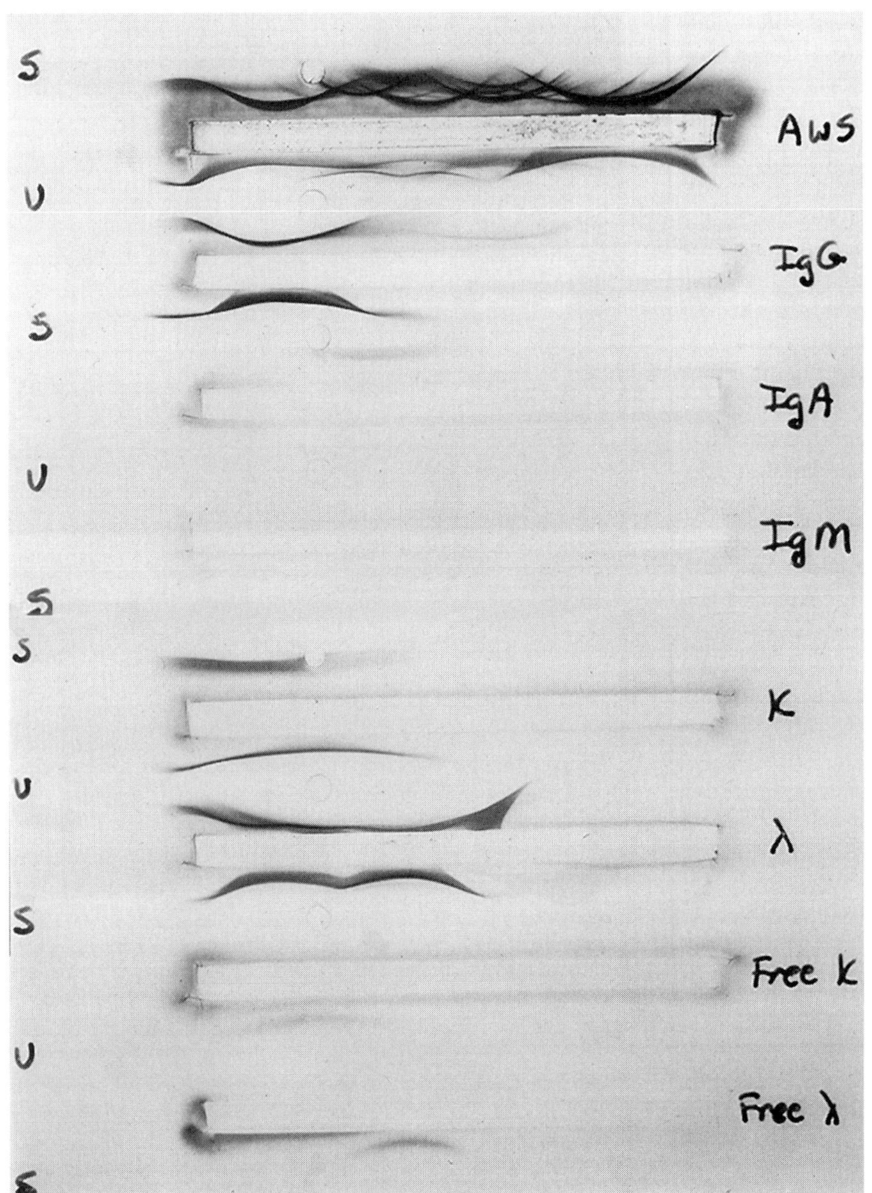

FIGURE 92.15. Immunoelectrophoresis of serum (S) and urine (U) from a patient with AL amyloidosis. The "gull-wing" pattern versus antilambda (λ) antiserum indicates a monoclonal (M) immunoglobulin in the serum and urine. In this case it is immunoglobulin Gλ (IgGλ).

tive of AL amyloidosis. All three forms of systemic amyloidosis may lead to the nephrotic syndrome. Restrictive cardiomyopathy is relatively uncommon in reactive amyloidosis, but it is very common in hereditary amyloidosis and AL amyloidosis. Hepatomegaly due to amyloid infiltration can be seen in AL amyloidosis and reactive amyloidosis, but is not to be expected in transthyretin amyloidosis. Reactive (secondary) amyloidosis usually occurs in association with a chronic inflammatory disease. These diseases include RA, granulomatous bowel disease, osteomyelitis, ankylosing spondylitis, psoriatic arthritis, and familial Mediterranean fever. History or physical findings of any such chronic inflammatory disease strongly support the diagnosis of reactive amyloidosis.

Peripheral neuropathy with or without the carpal tunnel syndrome is the hallmark of the transthyretin amyloidoses. Such findings should encourage pursuit of a thorough family history since the hereditary syndromes tend to have similar clinical presentation in subsequent generations. This often allows differentiation of hereditary amyloidosis from primary amyloidosis in which peripheral neuropathy may also occur. Vitreous amyloidosis probably only occurs in the hereditary transthyretin syndromes. Although hepatic amyloidosis is not a feature of the transthyretin amyloidoses, other hereditary types such as ApoAI, fibrinogen, and lysozyme may lead to hepatosplenomegaly.

Appropriate examination of biopsy specimens may be useful in diagnosing the correct form of amyloidosis. The Congo red stain, which is most commonly used to demonstrate amyloid deposits, gives a typical green birefringence to the amyloid deposits when viewed by polarization microscopy. Protein AA and transthyretin deposits usually stain better than AL amyloid deposits. This staining will disappear if unstained sections with AA amyloid are treated with potassium permanganate prior to staining with Congo red (133). On the other hand, AL amyloid proteins retain their positive Congo red staining after this treatment. An immunohistochemical test for AA amyloidosis using specific anti-AA antiserum is reliable (Fig. 92.9). Antiserum to transthyretin may be used to differentiate this form of hereditary amyloidosis, but this is not as reliable as anti-AA staining. Antisera to kappa or lambda light chain proteins tend to be less reliable for differentiating amyloid on paraffin fixed tissues. It is reported that they are more reliable when applied to frozen sections. Antiserum specific for the carboxyl terminal portion of the fibrinogen A α chain will identify that form of amyloid, but the antiserum is not readily available at this time.

For the diagnosis of systemic amyloidosis a number of different tissues may be biopsied. The most innocuous is the abdominal wall fat pad aspirate, which is then stained with Congo red (134). This method has proved successful in some laboratories, but not in others. A more time proven diagnostic method has been rectal biopsy in which approximately 70% of individuals with systemic amyloidosis of all forms will be proven positive. More recently, with the advent of upper endoscopy, both gastric and duodenal biopsies have been performed with favorable results. It is reported that duodenal biopsy has a somewhat higher yield than gastric biopsy. Skin biopsies are positive in only about 20% of patients and bone marrow biopsies in about 30% of patients with AL amyloidosis. If the less invasive types of tissue biopsy are not successful and the diagnosis of amyloidosis is strongly suspected, the organ with abnormal function can be biopsied with the highest yield. Renal, hepatic, and cardiac biopsy are all very informative for amyloid deposition in these organs if the proper histochemical evaluation is performed. Recently, an increase in use of endomyocardial biopsy has resulted in the more frequent diagnosis of amyloid restrictive cardiomyopathy.

Less invasive studies include echocardiography in which left ventricular wall thickness and cavity size can be indicative of amyloid deposition (Fig. 92.16). Notably, in patients with amyloid cardiomyopathy, systolic function of the left ventricle is usually well preserved despite advanced evidence of heart failure. Additionally, left atrial enlargement is suggestive of amyloid restrictive cardiomyopathy. The echocardiographic "sparkling" appearance of the myocardial texture, which has been reported, is more typical of hereditary transthyretin amyloidosis than it is of AL amyloidosis. The lack of this sparkling appearance should not preclude the diagnosis of cardiac amyloidosis. Electrocardiography is perhaps more sensitive with the typical amyloid pattern showing evidence for anteroseptal myocardial infarction with septal Q waves and decreased voltage in the precordial leads (Fig. 92.17). Prolongation of the PR interval is less common, but the presence of both atrial and ventricular extra systoles is very common. Nuclear scanning with ^{99m}Tc-labeled pyrophosphate may give specific uptake in the heart and is usually more prominent with transthyretin amyloidosis than with immunoglobulin amyloidosis (Fig. 92.18) (135).

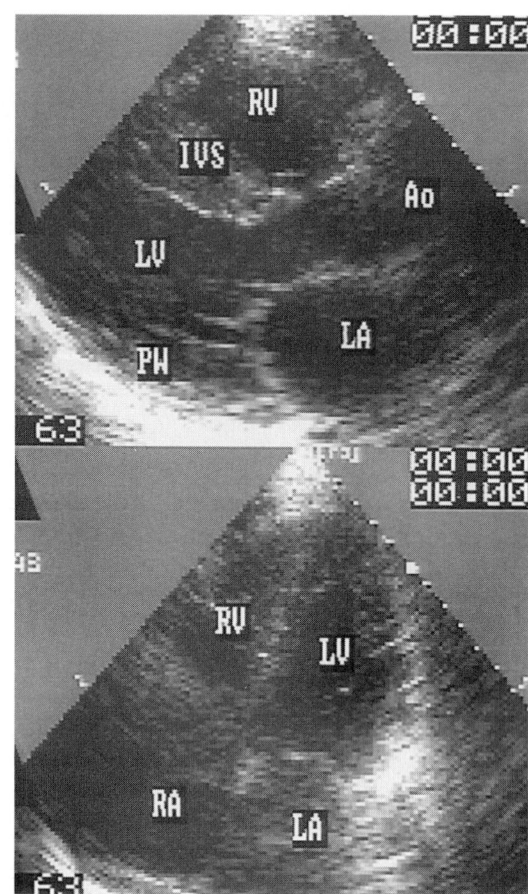

FIGURE 92.16. Two-dimensional echocardiogram for the same subject as depicted in Fig. 92.6. Classic features of amyloid cardiomyopathy are thickened intraventricular septum (IVS), left ventricular posterior wall (PW), and enlarged left atrium (LA).

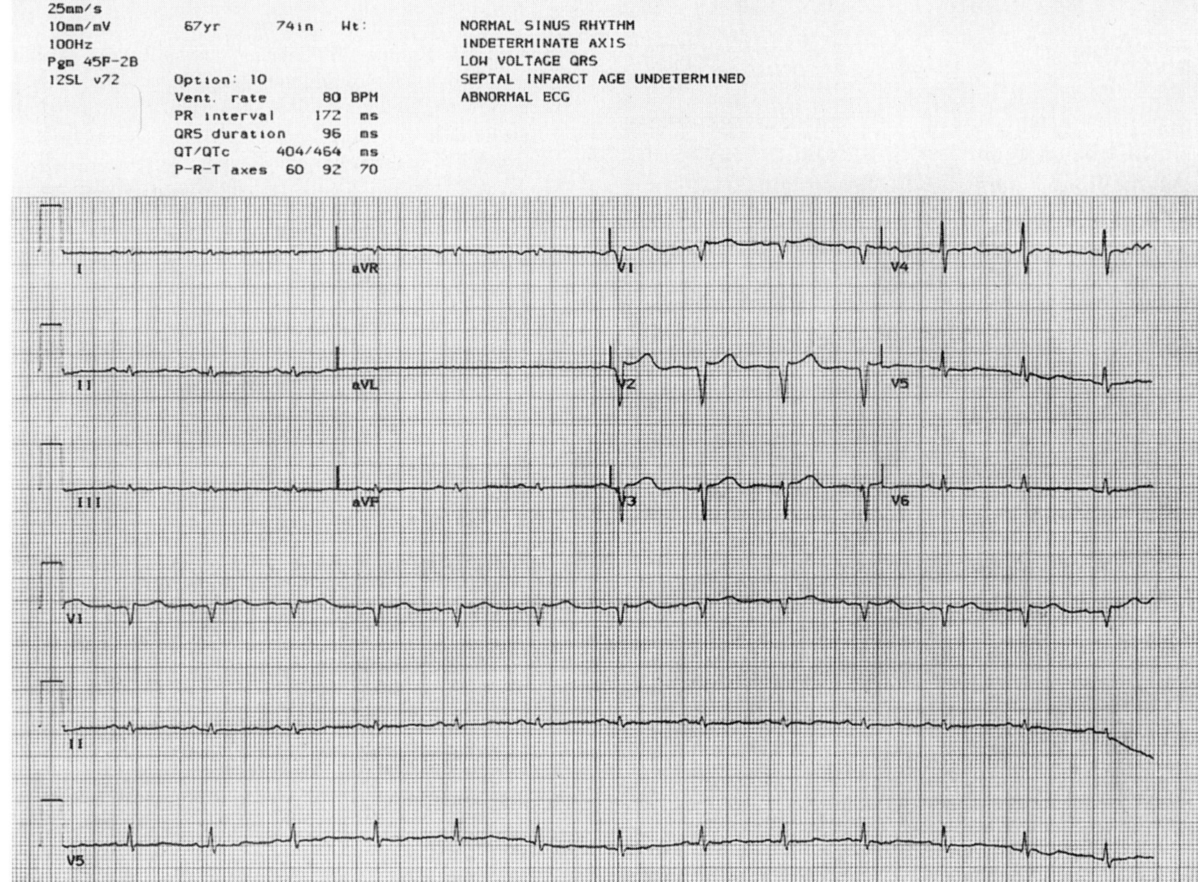

FIGURE 92.17. Electrocardiogram of patient with amyloid cardiomyopathy. Low voltage is a prominent feature and the standard, but erroneous, interpretation as "septal infarct, age indeterminate" is common.

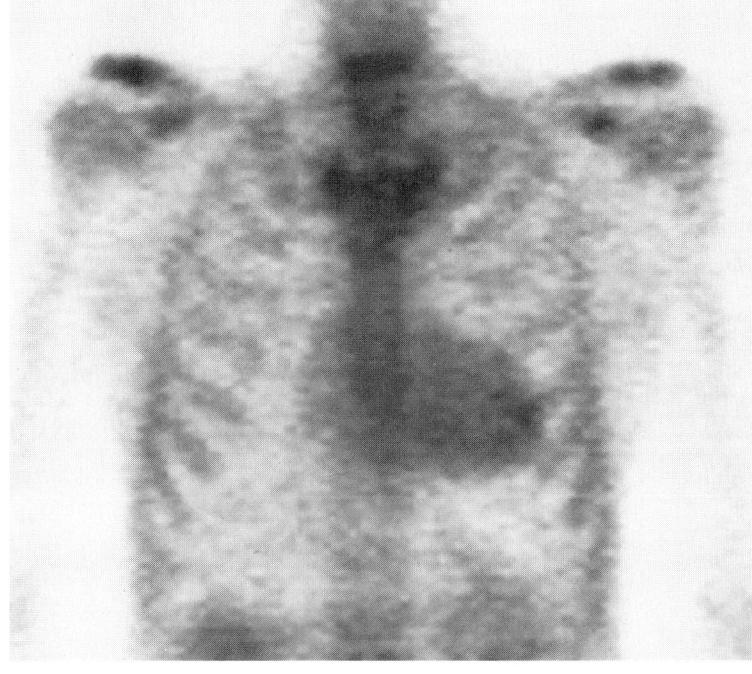

FIGURE 92.18. Myocardial uptake of technetium ^{99m}Tc pyrophosphate in a subject with transthyretin cardiomyopathy (radionuclide scan 3 hours after injection).

CONCLUSION

The diagnosis of systemic amyloidosis rests on a high index of suspicion whenever multisystem disease is present. In particular, the constellation of restrictive cardiomyopathy in a patient with or without the nephrotic syndrome and some degree of sensorimotor neuropathy should raise the possibility of amyloidosis. Definitive diagnosis is made by tissue biopsy.

ACKNOWLEDGMENTS

The research for this manuscript was supported by Veterans Affairs Medical Research (MRIS 583-0888), General Clinical Research Centers (GCRC), the United States Public Health Service (DK49596, DK42111, RR-00750), the Marion E. Jacobson Fund, and the Machado Family Research Fund.

REFERENCES

1. Glenner GG. Amyloid deposits and amyloidosis. The B-fibrilloses. *N Engl J Med* 1980;302:1283–1292,1333–1343.
2. Cohen AS, Calkins E. Electron microscopic observation on a fibrous component in amyloid of diverse origins. *Nature (Lond)* 1959;183:1202–1203.
3. Virchow VR. Ueber eineim Gehirn und Rueckenmark des Menschen aufgefundene Substanz mit der chemischen reaction der Cellulose. *Virchows Arch [A]* 1854;6:135–138.
4. Eanes ED, Glenner GG. X-ray diffraction studies of amyloid filaments. *J Histochem Cytochem* 1968;16:673–677.
5. Benson MD. Amyloidosis. In: Scriver CR, Beaudet AL, Sly WS, et al., eds. *The metabolic and molecular bases of inherited disease,* 7th ed, vol 3. New York: McGraw-Hill, 1995:4159–4191.
6. Husby G, Araki S, Benditt EP, et al. The 1990 guidelines for nomenclature and classification of amyloid and amyloidosis. In: Natvig JB, Förre Husby G, et al., eds. *Amyloid and amyloidosis.* VIth International Symposium on Amyloidosis. Norway. Dordrecht: Kluwer Academic, 1990:5–11.
7. Cohen AS. Guidelines for authors (Table III), amyloid. *Int J Exp Clin Invest* 1994;1.
8. Kyle RA, Gertz MA. Systemic amyloidosis. *Crit Rev Oncol Hematol* 1990;10:49–87.
9. Cohen AS, Rubinow A, Anderson JJ, et al. Survival of patients with primary (AL) amyloidosis. *Am J Med* 1987;82:1182–1190.
10. Brandt KD, Cathcart ES, Cohen AS. A clinical analysis of the course and prognosis of 42 patients with amyloidosis. *Am J Med* 1968;44:955–969.
11. Kyle RA, Greipp PR. Amyloidosis (AL): clinical and laboratory features in 229 cases. *Mayo Clin Proc* 1983;58:665–683.
12. Rubinow A, Koff RS, Cohen AS. Severe intrahepatic cholestasis in primary amyloidosis. A report of 4 cases and a review of the literature. *Am J Med* 1978;64:937–946.
13. Benson MD. Treatment of AL amyloidosis with melphalan, prednisone and colchicine. *Arthritis Rheum* 1986;29:683–687.
14. Kyle R, Bayrd E. Amyloidosis. Review of 236 cases. *Medicine* 1975;54:271–299.
15. Celli BR, Rubinow A, Cohen AS, et al. Patterns of pulmonary involvement in systemic amyloidosis. *Chest* 1978;74:543–547.
16. Yood RA, Skinner M, Rubinow A, et al. Bleeding and impaired hemostasis in 100 patients with amyloidosis. *JAMA* 1983;49:1322–1324.
17. Furie B, Greene E, Furie BC. Syndrome of acquired factor X deficiency and systemic amyloidosis: in vivo studies of the fate of factor X. *N Engl J Med* 1977;297:81–85.
18. Greipp PR, Kyle RA, Bowie WEJ. Factor-X deficiency in amyloidosis in a critical review. *Am J Hematol* 1981;11:443–550.
19. Glenner GG, Terry W, Harada M, et al. Amyloid fibril proteins: proof of homology with immunoglobulin light chains by sequence analysis. *Science* 1971;172:1150–1151.
20. Skinner M, Benson MD, Cohen AS. Amyloid fibril protein related to immunoglobulin lambda-chains. *J Immunol* 1975; 114:1433–1435.
21. Randall RE, Williamson WC Jr, Mullinax F, et al. Manifestations of light chain deposition. *Am J Med* 1976;60:293–299.
22. Preud'homme JL, Morel-Maroger L, Brovet JC, et al. Synthesis of abnormal immunoglobulin in lymphoplasmocytic disorders with visceral light chain deposition. *Am J Med* 1980;69:703–710.
23. Eulitz M, Linke RP. The precursor molecule of a Vλ immunoglobulin light chain-derived amyloid fibril protein circulates precleaved. *Biochem Biophys Res Commun* 1993;194: 1427–1434.
24. Myatt EA, Westholm FA, Weiss DT, et al. Pathogenic potential of human monoclonal immunoglobulin light chains: relationship of in vitro aggregation to in vivo organ deposition. *Proc Natl Acad Sci U S A* 1994;91:3034–3038.
25. Schormann N, Murrell JR, Liepnieks JJ, et al. Tertiary structure of an amyloid immunoglobulin light chain protein: a proposed model for amyloid fibril formation. *Proc Natl Acad Sci U S A* 1995;92:9490–9494.
26. Kyle RA, Wagoner RD, Holley KE. Primary systemic amyloidosis: resolution of the nephrotic syndrome with melphalan and prednisone. *Arch Intern Med* 1982;142:1445–1447.
27. Comenzo RL, Vosburgh E, Simms RW, et al. Dose-intensive melphalan with blood stem cell support for the treatment of AL amyloidosis: one-year follow-up in five patients. *Blood* 1996; 88:2801–2806.
28. Comenzo RL, Vosburgh E, Falk RH, et al. Dose-intensive melphalan with blood stem cell support for the treatment of AL (amyloid light-chain) amyloidosis: survival and responses in 25 patients. *Blood* 1998;91:3662–3670.
29. Laakso M, Mutru O, Isomaki H, et al. Mortality from amyloidosis and renal disease in patients with rheumatoid arthritis. *Ann Rheum Dis* 1986;45:663–667.
30. Boers M, Croonen AM, Kijkmans BAC, et al. Renal findings in rheumatoid arthritis: clinical aspects of necropsies. *Ann Rheum Dis* 1987;46:658–663.
31. Dhillon V, Woo P, Isenberg D. Amyloidosis in the rheumatic diseases. *Ann Rheum Dis* 1989;48:696–701.
32. David M, Abraham D, Weinberger A, et al. Generalized pustular psoriasis, psoriatic arthritis and nephrotic syndrome associated with systemic amyloidosis. *Dermatologica* 1982;165: 168–171.
33. Lehtinen K. Cause of death in 79 patients with ankylosing spondylitis. *Scand J Rheumatol* 1980;9:145–147.
34. Pettersson T, Tornroth T, Totterman KJ, et al. AA amyloidosis in systemic lupus erythematosus. *J Rheumatol* 1987;14: 835–838.
35. Sohar E, Gafni J, Pras M, et al. Familial Mediterranean fever. *Am J Med* 1967;43:227–253.
36. Muckle TJ, Wells M. Urticaria, deafness and amyloidosis: a new heredofamilial syndrome. *Q J Med* 1962;31:235–248.

37. Triger DR, Jockes AM. Renal amyloidosis—a fourteen year follow-up. *Q J Med* 1973;42:15–40.
38. Rubinow A, Burakoff RB, Cohen AS, et al. Esophageal manometry in systemic amyloidosis. *Am J Med* 1983;75:951–956.
39. Levin M, Pras M, Franklin EC. Immunologic studies of the major non-immunoglobulin protein of amyloid I. Identification and partial characterization of a related serum component. *J Exp Med* 1973;138:373–380.
40. Husby G, Natvig JB. A serum component related to immunoglobulin amyloid protein AS, a possible precursor of the fibrils. *J Clin Invest* 1974;53:1054–1061.
41. Kluve-Beckerman B, Naylor SL, Marshal A, et al. Localization of human SAA gene(s) to chromosome 11 and detection of DNA polymorphisms. *Biochem Biophys Res Commun* 1986;137: 1196–1204.
42. Rosenthal CJ, Franklin EC. Variation with age and disease of an amyloid A protein-related serum component. *J Clin Invest* 1975;55:746–753.
43. McAdam KPWJ, Sipe JD. Murine model for human secondary amyloidosis. Genetic variability of the acute-phase serum protein SAA response to endotoxins and casein. *J Exp Med* 1976; 144:1121–1127.
44. Benson MD, Scheinberg MA, Shirahama T, et al. Kinetics of serum amyloid protein A in casein-induced murine amyloidosis. *J Clin Invest* 1977;59:412–417.
45. Sipe JD, Vogel SN, Ryan JL, et al. Detection of a mediator derived from endotoxin-stimulated macrophages that induces the acute phase serum amyloid A response in mice. *J Exp Med* 1979;150:597–606.
46. Morrow JF, Stearman RS, Peltzman CG, et al. Induction of hepatic synthesis of serum amyloid A protein and actin. *Proc Natl Acad Sci U S A* 1981;78:4718–4722.
47. Dwulet FE, Wallace DK, Benson MD. Amino acid structures of multiple forms of amyloid-related serum protein SAA from a single individual. *Biochemistry* 1988;27:1677–1682.
48. Parmelee DC, Titani K, Ericsson LH, et al. Amino acid sequence of amyloid related apoprotein (apoSAA) from human high-density lipoproteins. *Biochemistry* 1982;21:3298–3303.
49. Whitehead AS, DeBeer MC, Steel DM, et al. Identification of novel members of the serum amyloid A protein superfamily as constitutive apolipoproteins of high density lipoprotein. *J Biol Chem* 1992;267:3862–3867.
50. Mitchell TI, Coon CI, Brinckerhoff CE. Serum amyloid A (SAA3) produced by rabbit synovial fibroblasts treated with phorbol esters or interleukin 1 induces synthesis of collagenase and is neutralized by specific antiserum. *J Clin Invest* 1991; 87:1177–1185.
51. Kluve-Beckerman B, Drumm ML, Benson MD. Nonexpression of the human serum amyloid A three (SAA3) gene. *DNA Cell Biol* 1991;10:651–661.
52. Benditt EP, Eriksen N. Amyloid protein SAA is associated with high density lipoproteins from human serum. *Proc Natl Acad Sci U S A* 1977;74:4025–4028.
53. Levin M, Franklin EC, Frangione B, et al. The amino acid sequence of a major nonimmunoglobulin component of some amyloid fibrils. *J Clin Invest* 1972;51:2773–2776.
54. Prelli F, Pras M, Frangione B. Degradation and deposition of amyloid AA fibrils are tissue specific. *Biochemistry* 1987;26: 8251–8256.
55. Liepnieks JJ, Kluve-Beckerman B, Benson MD. Characterization of amyloid A protein in human secondary amyloidosis. The predominant deposition of serum amyloid Al. *Biochim Biophys Acta* 1995;1270:81–86.
56. Hoffman JS, Ericsson LH, Eriksen N, et al. Murine tissue amyloid protein AA NH2-terminal sequence identity with only one or two serum amyloid protein (ApoSAA) gene products. *J Exp Med* 1984;159:641–646.
57. Zemer D, Pras M, Sohar E, et al. Colchicine in the prevention and treatment of the amyloidosis of familial Mediterranean fever. *N Engl J* Med 1986;314:1001–1005.
58. Assenat H, Calemard E, Charra B, et al. Hemodialyse, syndrome du canal carpien et substance amyloide. *Nouv Presse Med* 1980;9:1715.
59. Clanet M, Mansat M, Durroux R, et al. Syndrome du canal carpien, tenosynovite amyloide et hemodialyse periodique. *Rev Neurol (Paris)* 1981;137:613–624.
60. Bardin T, Kuntz D, Zingraff J, et al. Synovial amyloidosis in patients undergoing long-term hemodialysis. *Arthritis Rheum* 1985;28:1052–1058.
61. Gejyo F, Yamada T, Odani S, et al. A new form of amyloid protein associated with chronic hemodialysis was identified as β_2-microglobulin. *Biochem Biophys Res Commun* 1985;129:701–706.
62. Gorevic PD, Stone TT, Stone WJ, et al. β_2-Microglobulin is an amyloidogenic protein in man. *J Clin Invest* 1985;76: 2425–2429.
63. Floege J, Bartsch A, Schulze M, et al. Clearance and synthesis rates of β_2-microglobulin in patients undergoing hemodialysis and in normal subjects. *J Lab Clin Med* 1991;118:153–164.
64. Kanda Y, Goodman DS, Canfield RE, et al. The amino acid sequence of human plasma prealbumin. *J Biol Chem* 1974; 249:6796–6805.
65. Robbins J. Thyroxine-binding proteins. *Prog Clin Biol Res* 1976;5:331–355.
66. Episkopou V, Maeda S, Nishiguchi S, et al. Disruption of the transthyretin gene results in mice with depressed levels of plasma retinol and thyroid hormone. *Proc Natl Acad Sci U S A* 1993;90:2375–2379.
67. Costa RH, Lai E, Darnell JE. Transcriptional control of the mouse prealbumin (transthyretin) gene: both promotor sequences and a distinct enhancer are cell specific. *Mol Cell Biol* 1986;6:4697–4708.
68. Blake CCF, Geisow MJ, Swan IDA. Structure of human plasma prealbumin at 2.5 Å resolution. *J Mol Biol* 1974;88:1–12.
69. Monaco HL, Rizzi M, Coda A. Structure of a complex of two plasma proteins: transthyretin and retinol-binding protein. *Science* 1995;268:1039–1041.
70. Benson MD, Dwulet FE. Prealbumin and retinol binding protein serum concentrations in the Indiana type hereditary amyloidosis. *Arthritis Rheum* 1983;26:1493–1498.
71. Skinner M, Connors LH, Rubinow A, et al. Lowered prealbumin levels in patients with familial amyloid polyneuropathy (FAP) and their non-affected but at risk relatives. *Am J Med Sci* 1985;289:17–21.
72. Westermark P, Pitkanen P, Benson L, et al. Serum prealbumin and retinol-binding protein in the prealbumin-related senile and familial forms of systemic amyloidosis. *Lab Invest* 1985; 52:314–318.
73. Wallace MR, Naylor SL, Kluve-Beckerman B, et al. Localization of the human prealbumin gene to chromosome 18. *Biochem Biophys Res Commun* 1985;129:753–758.
74. Westermark P, Sletten K, Johansson B, et al. Fibril in senile systemic amyloidosis is derived from normal transthyretin. *Proc Natl Acad Sci U S A* 1990;87:2843–2845.
75. Stauder AJ, Dickson PW, Aldred AR, et al. Synthesis of transthyretin (prealbumin) mRNA in choroid plexus epithelial cells, localized by in situ hybridization in rat brain. *J Histochem Cytochem* 1986;34:949–952.
76. Soprano DR, Herbert J, Soprano KJ, et al. Demonstration of transthyretin mRNA in the brain and other extrahepatic tissues in the rat. *J Biol Chem* 1985;260:11793–11798.

77. Andrade C. A peculiar form of peripheral neuropathy. Familial atypical generalized amyloidosis with special involvement of the peripheral nerves. *Brain* 1952;75:408–427.
78. Andrade A, Araki S, Block WD, et al. Hereditary amyloidosis. *Arthritis Rheum* 1970;13:902–915.
79. Jacobson DR, Reveille JD, Buxbaum JN. Frequency and genetic background of the position 122 (Val-Ile) variant transthyretin gene in the black population. *Am J Hum Genet* 1991;49:192–198.
80. Tsuzuki T, Mita S, Maeda S, et al. Structure of the human prealbumin gene. *J Biol Chem* 1985;260:12224–12227.
81. Sasaki H, Yoshioka N, Takagi Y, et al. Structure of the chromosomal gene for human serum prealbumin. *Gene* 1985;37: 191–197.
82. Nichols WC, Benson MD. Hereditary amyloidosis: detection of variant prealbumin genes by restriction enzyme analysis of amplified genomic DNA sequences. *Clin Genet* 1990;37: 44–53.
83. Holmgren G, Ericzon B-G, Grotk C-G, et al. Clinical improvement and amyloid regression after liver transplantation in hereditary transthyretin amyloidosis. *Lancet* 1993;341: 1113–1116.
84. Holmgren G, Steen L, Ekstedt J, et al. Biochemical effect of liver transplantation in two Swedish patients with familial amyloidotic polyneuropathy (FAP-met30). *Clin Genet* 1991;40: 242–246.
85. Nichols WC, Gregg RE, Brewer HB Jr, et al. A mutation in apolipoprotein A-I in the Iowa type of familial amyloidotic polyneuropathy. *Genomics* 1990;8:318–323.
86. Soutar AK, Hawkins PN, Vigushin DM, et al. Apolipoprotein AI mutation Arg-60 causes autosomal dominant amyloidosis. *Proc Natl Acad Sci U S A* 1992;89:7389–7393.
87. Booth DR, Tan SY, Booth SE, et al. A new apolipoprotein AI variant, Trp50Arg, causes hereditary amyloidosis. *Q J Med* 1995;88:695–702.
88. Booth DR, Tan S-Y, Booth SE, et al. Hereditary hepatic and systemic amyloidosis caused by a new deletion/insertion mutation in the apolipoprotein AI gene. *J Clin Invest* 1996;97: 2714–2721.
89. Persey MR, Booth DR, Booth SE, et al. Hereditary nephropathic systemic amyloidosis caused by a novel variant apolipoprotein A-I. *Kidney Int* 1998;53:276–281.
90. Hamidi Asl L, Liepnieks JJ, et al. Hereditary amyloid cardiomyopathy caused by a variant apolipoprotein A1. *Am J Pathol* 1999;154:221–227.
91. Hamidi Asl K, Liepnieks JJ, Nakamura M, et al. A novel apolipoprotein A-1 variant, Arg173Pro, associated with cardiac and cutaneous amyloidosis. *Biochem Biophys Res Commun* 1999;257:584–588.
92. Rader DJ, Gregg RE, Meng MS, et al. In vivo metabolism of a mutant apolipoprotein, apoA-I_{Iowa} associated with hypoalphalipoproteinemia and hereditary systemic amyloidosis. *J Lipid Res* 1992;33:755–763.
93. Meretoja J. Familial systemic paramyloidosis with lattice dystrophy of the cornea, progressive cranial neuropathy, skin changes and various internal symptoms. *Ann Clin Res* 1969; 1:314–324.
94. Meretoja J. Genetic aspects of familial amyloidosis with corneal lattice dystrophy and cranial neuropathy. *Clin Genet* 1973; 4:173–185.
95. Maury CPJ, Kere J, Tolvanen R, et al. Finnish hereditary amyloidosis is caused by a single nucleotide substitution in the gelsolin gene. *FEBS Lett* 1990;276:75–77.
96. Levy E, Haltia M, Fernandez-Madrid I, et al. Mutation in gelsolin gene in Finnish hereditary amyloidosis. *J Exp Med* 1990; 172:1865–1867.
97. De La Chapelle A, Tolvanen R, Boysen G, et al. Gelsolin-derived familial amyloidosis caused by asparagine or tyrosine substitution for aspartic acid at residue 187. *Nature Genet* 1992;2:157–160.
98. Kwiatkowski DJ, Mehl R, Yin HL. Genomic organization and biosynthesis of secreted and cytoplasmic forms of gelsolin. *J Cell Biol* 1988;106:375–384.
99. Kwiatkowski DJ, Westbrook CA, Bruns GAP, et al. Localization of gelsolin proximal to ABL on chromosome 9. *Am J Hum Genet* 1988;42:565–572.
100. Uemichi T, Liepnieks JJ, Benson MD. Hereditary renal amyloidosis with a novel variant fibrinogen. *J Clin Invest* 1994; 93:731–736.
101. Benson MD, Liepnieks J, Uemichi T, et al. Hereditary renal amyloidosis associated with a mutant fibrinogen α-chain. *Nature Genet* 1993;3:252–255.
102. Uemichi T, Liepnieks JJ, Yamada T, et al. A frame shift mutation in the fibrinogen Aa-chain gene in a kindred with renal amyloidosis. *Blood* 1996;87:4197–4203.
103. Hamidi Asl L, Liepnieks JJ, Uemichi T, et al. Renal amyloidosis with a frame shift mutation in fibrinogen Aa-chain producing a novel amyloid protein. *Blood* 1997;90: 4799–4805.
104. Matsuda M, Yoshida N, Terukina S, et al. Molecular abnormalities of fibrinogen-the present status of structure elucidation. In: Matsuda M, Iwanage S, Takada A, et al., eds. *Fibrinogen 4:* current basic and clinical aspects. Amsterdam: Excerpta Medica, 1990:139–152.
105. Pepys MB, Hawkins PN, Booth DR, et al. Human lysozyme gene mutations cause hereditary systemic amyloidosis. *Nature* 1993;362:553–557.
106. Ghiso J, Pons-Estel B, Frangione B. Hereditary cerebral amyloid angiopathy: the amyloid fibrils contain a protein which is a variant of cystatin C, an inhibitor of lysosomal cysteine proteases. *Biochem Biophys Res Commun* 1986;136:548–554.
107. Gudmundsson G, Halgrimsson J, Jonasson TA, et al. Hereditary cerebral hemorrhage with amyloidosis. *Brain* 1972;95: 387–404.
108. Abrahamson M, Jonsdottir S, Olafsson I, et al. Hereditary cystatin C amyloid angiopathy: identification of the disease-causing mutation and specific diagnosis by polymerase chain reaction based analysis. *Hum Genet* 1992;89:377–380.
109. Jensson O, Luyendijk W, Pétursdóttir I, et al. Cystatin C values in the cerebrospinal fluid: comparison between the Icelandic and the Dutch type of hereditary central nervous system amyloid angiopathy. *Acta Neurol Scand* 1986;73:313.
110. Fujihara S, Glenner GG. Primary localized amyloidosis of the genitourinary tract: immunohistochemical study on eleven cases. *Lab Invest* 1981;44:55–59.
111. Thompson PJ, Citron KM. Amyloid and the lower respiratory tract. *Thorax* 1983;38:84–87.
112. Hamidi Asl K, Liepnieks JJ, Nakamura M, et al. Organ specific (localized) synthesis of Ig light chain amyloid. *J Immunol* 1999;162:5556–5560.
113. Sagher F, Shanon J. Amyloid cutis: familial occurrence in three generations. *Arch Dermatol* 1963;87:171–175.
114. Rajacopalan K, Tay CH. Familial lichen amyloidosis: report of 19 cases in 4 generations of a Chinese family in Malaysia. *Br J Dermatol* 1972;87:123–129.
115. Schimke RN, Hartmann WH. Familial amyloid-producing medullary thyroid carcinoma and pheochromocytoma: distinct genetic entity. *Ann Intern Med* 1965;63:1027–1039.
116. Sletten K, Westermark P, Natvig JB. Characterization of amyloid fibril proteins from medullary carcinoma of the thyroid. *J Exp Med* 1976;143:993–998.
117. Glenner GG, Wong CW. Alzheimer's disease: initial report of the purification and characterization of a novel cerebrovascular

amyloid protein. *Biochem Biophys Res Commun* 1984;120: 885–890.
118. Kang J, LeMaire H-G, Unterbeck A, et al. The precursor of Alzheimer's disease amyloid A4 protein resembles a cell-surface receptor. *Nature* 1987;325:733–736.
119. Goate A, Chartier-Harlin M-C, Mullan M, et al. Segregation of a missense mutation in the amyloid precursor protein gene with familial Alzheimer's disease. *Nature* 1991;349:704–706.
120. Murrell J, Farlow M, Ghetti B, et al. A mutation in the amyloid precursor protein associated with hereditary Alzheimer's disease. *Science* 1991;254:97–99.
121. Chartier-Harlin M-C, Crawford F, Houlden H, et al. Early-onset Alzheimer's disease caused by mutations at codon 717 of the β-amyloid precursor protein gene. *Nature* 1991;353: 844–846.
122. Sherrington R, Rogaev EI, Liang Y, et al. Cloning of a gene bearing missense mutations in early-onset familial Alzheimer's disease. *Nature* 1995;375:754–760.
123. Strittmatter WJ, Saunders AM, Schmechel D, et al. Apolipoprotein E. High-avidity binding to β-amyloid and increased frequency of type 4 allele in late-onset familial Alzheimer disease. *Proc Natl Acad Sci U S A* 1993;90: 1977–1981.
124. Levy E, Carman MD, Fernandez-Madrid IJ, et al. Mutation of the Alzheimer's disease amyloid gene in hereditary cerebral hemorrhage, Dutch type. *Science* 1990;248:1124–1126.
125. Westermark P, Wernstedt C, Wilander E, et al. Amyloid fibrils in human insulinoma and islets of Langerhans of the diabetic cat are derived from a neuropeptide-like protein also present in normal islet cells. *Proc Natl Acad Sci U S A* 1987;84: 3881–3885.
126. Roberts AN, Leighton B, Todd JA, et al. Molecular and functional characterization of amylin, a peptide associated with type 2 diabetes mellitus. *Proc Natl Acad Sci U S A* 1989;86: 9662–9666.
127. Johansson B, Wernstedt C, Westermark P. Atrial natriuretic peptide deposited as atrial amyloid fibrils. *Biochem Biophys Res Commun* 1987;148:1087–1092.
128. Linke RP, Voigt C, Storkel FS, et al. N-terminal amino acid sequence analysis indicates that isolated atrial amyloid is derived from atrial natriuretic peptide. *Virchows Arch [B]* 1988;55: 125–127.
129. Allensworth DC, Rice GJ, Lowe GW. Persistent atrial standstill in a family with myocardial disease. *Am J Med* 1969;47: 775–784.
130. Athanasou NA, Sallie B. Localized deposition of amyloid in articular cartilage. *Histopathology* 1992;20:41–46.
131. Prusiner SB, De Armond SJ. Prion protein amyloid and neurodegeneration. *Amyloid Int J Exp Clin Invest* 1995;2:39–65.
132. Ghetti B, Dlouhy SR, Giaccone G, et al. Gerstmann-Sträussler-Scheinker disease and the Indiana kindred. *Brain Pathol* 1995;5:61–75.
133. Wright JR, Calkins E, Humphrey RL. Potassium permanganate reaction in amyloidosis: a histologic method to assist in differentiating forms of the disease. *Lab Invest* 1977;36:274–281.
134. Libbey CA, Skinner M, Cohen AS. The abdominal fat tissue aspirate for the diagnosis of systemic amyloidosis. *Arch Intern Med* 1983;143:1549–1552.
135. Falk RH, Lee VW, Rubinow A, et al. Sensitivity of technetium-99m-pyrophosphate scintigraphy for the diagnosis of cardiac amyloidosis. *Am J Cardiol* 1983;51:826–830.

93

SARCOIDOSIS

H. RALPH SCHUMACHER, JR.

Sarcoidosis is a systemic disease characterized by a noncaseating granulomatous reaction of unknown origin. Our present concept of this syndrome has evolved from the early descriptions by Hutchinson, Besnier, and Boek (1), as well as by Schaumann (2). Symptoms and signs depend on the organs affected, most frequently the lymph nodes, lungs, liver, skin, and eyes. Muscle, spleen, bones, parotid glands, central nervous system, blood vessels, endocrine glands, and almost any other tissue, including the joints, may also be involved. Although generally a chronic disease, the onset of sarcoidosis can be acute, with hilar adenopathy, erythema nodosum, fever, and articular manifestations. This acute form is often termed Lofgren's syndrome (3).

PATHOLOGIC FEATURES

The characteristic histopathologic features of epithelioid tubercles with minimal necrosis and no true caseation, in contrast to the lesions of tuberculosis, are the hallmark of sarcoidosis (Figs. 93.1 and 93.2) (4). Studies on skin (Kveim reactions) and pulmonary lesions have identified large numbers of T lymphocytes around the epithelioid cells. At least in the lung lesions, these are usually enriched with $CD4^+$ helper T cells (5,6). Sarcoid granulomas often contain Langhans-type giant cells with three frequent types of cytoplasmic inclusions: (a) asteroid bodies, which appear to consist of criss-crossing bundles of collagen; (b) Schaumann bodies, which are round or oval laminated calcifications containing hydroxyapatite (Fig. 93.3); and (c) irregular, poorly stained, anisotropic, glass-like fragments (7). Such granulomas, even with the typical inclusions, are not pathognomonic for sarcoidosis. Similar granulomatous tissue reactions can be seen in histoplasmosis, coccidioidomycosis, tuberculosis, lymphoma, Hodgkin's disease, bronchogenic carcinoma, other tumors, foreign body granuloma, drug reactions, beryllium poisoning, syphilis, and leprosy. Functional impairment in sarcoidosis appears to result from both the active granulomatous disease and the secondary fibrosis.

CAUSE AND PREVALENCE

Many have speculated about the possible causes of sarcoidosis. The incidence of tuberculosis in sarcoidosis is 4%. An unusual reaction to *Mycobacterium tuberculosis* or to atypical mycobacteria is one suggested mechanism. High titers of antibody to a number of viruses and other organisms have been reported in sarcoidosis. Clustering of cases has raised suspicion of environmental factors (8). Circulating immune complexes can be identified in up to 50% of cases, but their pathogenic role is not clear. Alveolar macrophages may show increased receptor-mediated phagocytosis and express increased complement receptors (9). Despite cutaneous anergy and decreased circulating T lymphocytes, there is considerable evidence of cell-mediated immune reactivity in the pulmonary lesions (10). Patients who have inherited human leukocyte antigen (HLA) B8 may be more likely to express their sarcoidosis as

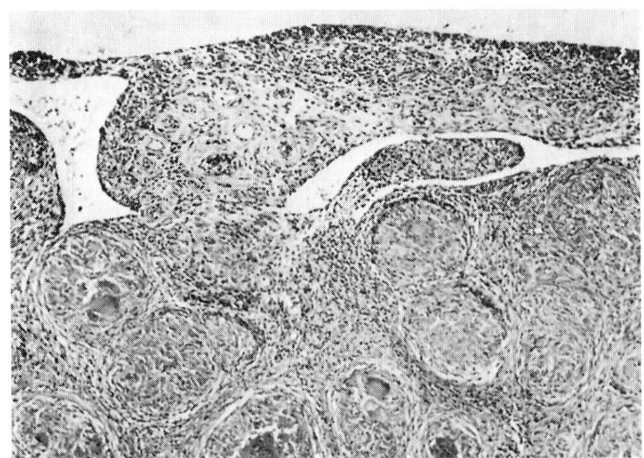

FIGURE 93.1. Granulomatous synovitis of the elbow in chronic sarcoid arthritis. (Hematoxylin and eosin stain, ×60.) The synovial tissue is crowded with discrete, noncaseating miliary tubercles. At the surface, the villi are hypertrophied and infiltrated with leukocytes and fibroblasts. The articular cartilage of this joint is intact, and the subchondral bone (olecranon and lateral condyle of humerus) is free of tubercles. (From Sokoloff L, Bunim JJ. Clinical and pathological studies of joint involvement in sarcoidosis. *N Engl J Med* 1959;260:842–847, with permission.)

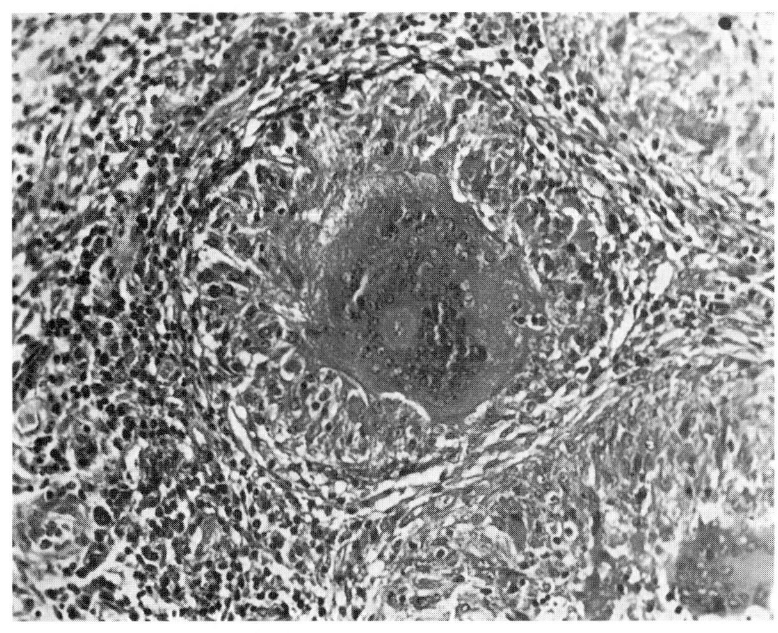

FIGURE 93.2. Multinucleated giant cell in the center of a tubercle of epithelioid cells. Surrounding the tubercle is a layer of fibroblasts and a cuff of lymphocytes, plasma cells, and mononuclear cells. This figure is an area from Fig. 93.1 under higher magnification (×175). (From Sokoloff L, Bunim JJ. Clinical and pathological studies of joint involvement in sarcoidosis. *N Engl J Med* 1959;260:842–847, with permission.)

erythema nodosum and acute arthritis (11). HLA-DR3 may predispose individuals to sarcoid arthritis (12). Several series in the United States show a higher incidence of sarcoidosis in black females than in the general population. The disease may begin at any age, including infancy, but it is most commonly diagnosed in the third and fourth decades. Females predominate slightly over males. Sarcoidosis has a worldwide distribution, with the estimated incidence of the disease reaching as high as 64/100,000 in Sweden. American veterans after World War II had an incidence of 11/100,000.

GENERAL MANIFESTATIONS AND PROGNOSIS

The severity of manifestations can vary from an asymptomatic chest roentgenogram to death in approximately 4% of patients. The most common symptoms and signs are fatigue (27%), malaise (15%), cough (30%), shortness of breath (28%), and chest pain (15%). Ninety-two percent of patients have abnormal chest roentgenograms. Pulmonary parenchymal involvement is more ominous than the more frequent hilar adenopathy. Restrictive lung disease and cor

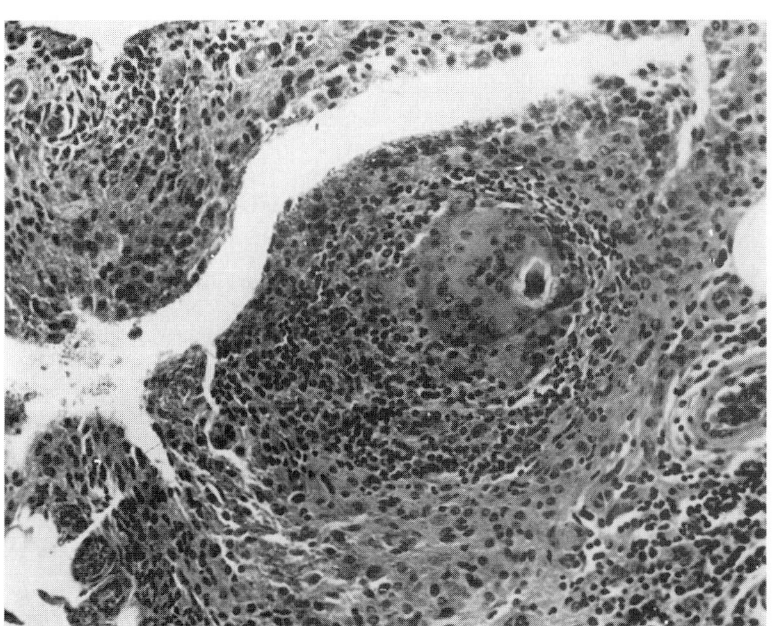

FIGURE 93.3. Section of synovial tissue from the knee of a 33-year-old African American woman with sarcoid polyarthritis of about 6 weeks' duration showing granulomatous synovitis and a Schaumann body. This Schaumann body appears in the cytoplasm of a giant cell as a circular clear space and consists of a colorless, crystalloid material that is doubly refractive. No bacteria or fungi were found with Brown-Brenn, Ziehl-Neelsen, or periodic acid-Schiff stains. (From Sokoloff L, Bunim JJ. Clinical and pathological studies of joint involvement in sarcoidosis. *N Engl J Med* 1959;260:842–847, with permission.)

pulmonale can develop. Granulomatous uveitis is the most frequent visual problem. Skin lesions occur in 30% of cases. They may be nondescript, but commonly are papular or nodular, erythematous, or violaceous lesions, which exhibit the typical granulomas on histologic examination. Erythema nodosum is common in sarcoidosis of acute onset. Liver involvement is almost always asymptomatic and is evidenced mainly by hepatomegaly. An elevated alkaline phosphatase level may suggest the presence of liver granulomas.

The acute form of sarcoidosis, accompanied by erythema nodosum, hilar adenopathy, and arthralgia, generally has the best prognosis. Despite the similar sarcoid tissue reaction, Truelove (13) has urged physicians to distinguish this syndrome from sarcoidosis. Certainly most patients with this acute syndrome have a full remission within 2 years, but up to 16% may have some chronic disease (14).

Vasculitis with vascular granulomas or nonspecific histology has been seen in sarcoidosis and occasionally can be life-threatening (15,16). Patients with vasculitis are easily confused with other rheumatic diseases. Parotid involvement and sicca features can also mimic Sjögren's syndrome (17).

DIAGNOSIS

The diagnosis of sarcoidosis is established by the demonstration of typical noncaseating granulomas in the absence of other identifiable causes of such granulomas (Table 93.1). Impaired delayed hypersensitivity on skin testing is characteristic but not invariable. Impaired tuberculin sensitivity after Bacille Calmette-Guérin (BCG) vaccination may persist even after apparent recovery from sarcoidosis. Antibody production is normal. The elevated immunoglobulins are of little help in the differential diagnosis. Leukopenia, anemia, eosinophilia, hypercalcemia, and elevated erythrocyte sedimentation rates may be seen. Hypercalciuria is found in most cases. The serum level of angiotensin-converting enzyme is typically elevated in active pulmonary or articular sarcoidosis (18). Angiotensin-converting enzyme is produced by the granulomas, which also secrete 1,25-dihydrocholecalciferol, responsible for the absorptive hypercalciuria. Although increased angiotensin-converting enzyme levels are seen in about 80% of patients, they are not unique to sarcoidosis and may also occur in inflammatory diseases of the liver (19), Gaucher's disease, leprosy silicosis, asbestosis, hyperthyroidism, and diabetes. Angiotensin-converting enzyme levels fall with successful therapy and may be useful in following treatment (20). These levels can also be followed, along with other findings, in patients with mild disease who are not treated, to look for early evidence of exacerbation.

TABLE 93.1. DIAGNOSTIC FEATURES OF SARCOIDOSIS

Noncaseating granulomas on biopsy: one must exclude other causes of granulomas
Hilar and right paratracheal adenopathy in 90%
Skin lesions, uveitis, or involvement of almost any tissue
Onset most often in third and fourth decades, but cases reported at all ages
Impaired delayed hypersensitivity in 85%
Frequent hyperglobulinemia
Increased angiotensin-converting enzyme levels in about 80%
Hypercalciuria in most: hypercalcemia in some

Tissue diagnosis is most expeditiously established by biopsy of a skin lesion or an accessible superficial lymph node. With such superficial material, additional evidence of generalized disease is also needed because foreign body reactions can be difficult to distinguish from sarcoidosis. Liver samples also can show granulomas, especially if the liver is palpably enlarged, but a granulomatous liver reaction is common in other liver diseases (21), and such granulomas are not as helpful in diagnosis as lymph node lesions. Mediastinoscopy in experienced hands is a safe and reliable method of obtaining lymph node tissue for diagnosis if hilar adenopathy is present. Transbronchial lung biopsy using the fiberoptic bronchoscope, is an attractive initial biopsy procedure yielding diagnoses in about 60% of cases in one series (22). In typical Lofgren's syndrome with asymptomatic hilar and right paratracheal adenopathy, one can sometimes observe the patient without performing a biopsy (23). Biopsies with serial sections often show granulomas in asymptomatic muscles (24). Israel and Sones (25) found muscle tissue positive in 89% of patients with erythema nodosum or arthralgias.

An intradermal injection of 0.2 mL of a 10% saline suspension of sarcoid tissue (the Kveim test) has previously been used for diagnosis. However, standardization of preparations has been difficult, and reliable material is not generally available (26).

Gallium scintigrams or bronchoalveolar lavage can assist in evaluating activity in alveolitis (20), and they may be abnormal even in patients with normal chest roentgenograms (27).

SPECIFIC MUSCULOSKELETAL MANIFESTATIONS

Muscle

Sarcoid granulomas in muscle are often asymptomatic, but they may be accompanied by local pain and tenderness, cramps, pseudohypertrophy, palpable nodules, and, occasionally, associated fasciitis. A symmetric proximal myopathy with weakness has also been described and reported to occur without evident sarcoidosis in other tissues (28,29). Any muscle including the diaphragm can be affected (30). Involved muscles often show noncaseating granulomas as well as lymphocytic infiltration, muscle necrosis, and regeneration. Creatine kinase levels may be elevated. Magnetic resonance imaging (MRI) can be used to identify nodular or myopathic patterns (31). Calcification of muscles and other soft tissues occasionally occurs in hypercalcemic patients. Neurosarcoidosis can produce a variety of musculoskeletal symptoms (32), as can vascular sarcoid.

Bone

Phalangeal cysts, often considered a helpful diagnostic clue in sarcoidosis (Fig. 93.4), were described in 14% of patients in one series (12). Although some of these cysts are due to sarcoid granulomas, others may be unrelated to sarcoidosis. Other bones, including the skull and vertebrae, may also develop cysts from sarcoid granulomas. Large lytic or sclerotic vertebral lesions can be seen (33). One report described a symptomatic tibial head cyst that was detected only by MRI as the presenting feature of sarcoidosis (34). MRI can also detect the extent of soft tissue involvement around bone lesions (35). Bone sarcoidosis is usually asymptomatic. The overlying cortex is typically intact, although cortical dissolution with scalloping or acro-osteolysis and fractures through large cysts have been described (36). The phalangeal lesions of sarcoidosis can also be associated with osteosclerosis (37). Cystic bone lesions only occasionally extend into the joint, in which case they may cause arthritis (4). Some destructive bony lesions are associated with overlying purplish red, nodular cutaneous masses, termed lupus pernio (7), or with a diffuse dactylitis (38).

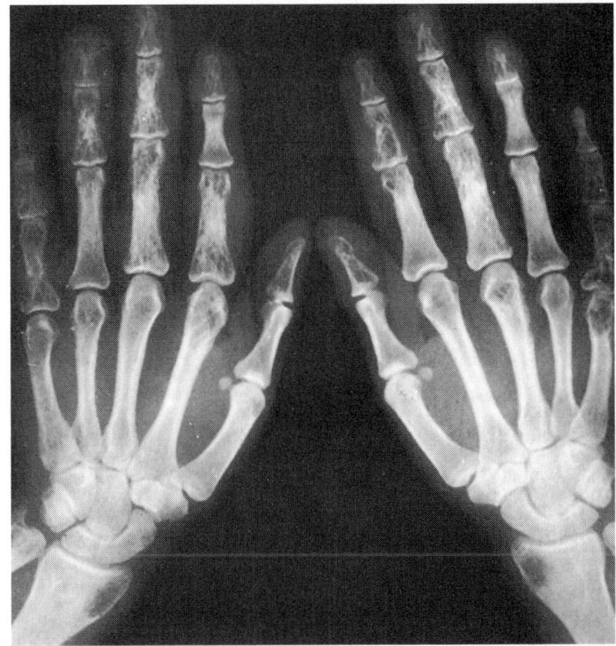

FIGURE 93.4. Radiographs of the hands showing unusually severe bone lesions of sarcoidosis. The bone cysts have not broken through the articular cortex. The hands shown in Fig. 93.5 have similar bone changes, but with extension into the distal interphalangeal joints.

Joints

Arthritis was first described with sarcoidosis in 1936. Since then, arthritis, periarthritis, or arthralgia has been reported in 2% to 38% of patients in various series (12,39–41). Chronic sarcoidosis is associated with fewer joint complaints than the acute form. Table 93.2 outlines the features of sarcoid arthropathy.

In acute sarcoidosis with hilar adenopathy, fever, and erythema nodosum, up to 89% of patients have articular symptoms, and 69% and 63% had articular or periarticular swelling, respectively, in the series of Lofgren (3) and James et al. (42). Ankle and knee joints are most frequently involved in acute sarcoidosis. Most other joints are occasionally involved. Heel pad pain is common; monarthritis is unusual (39). The patient generally has a dramatic, tender, warm, erythematous swelling that often is clearly periarticular rather than synovial. Such changes are occasionally difficult to distinguish from adjacent cutaneous erythema nodosum, and the histologic appearance of the lesions is identical. Joint motion is often painless; pain is much less than one would expect, considering the inflammatory signs. The frequency of severe, localized tenderness has been emphasized (43).

Roentgenograms show only soft tissue swelling. Such articular findings may antedate erythema nodosum by as much as 2 weeks and suggest a careful watch for the skin lesions. Both skin and joint lesions may antedate hilar adenopathy by several weeks. Ankle and knee involvement is often symmetric; joint involvement can be progressive. The acute inflammation often raises a suspicion of rheumatic fever, gonococcal or other infectious arthritis, and gout. Joint aspiration often yields no synovial fluid. When an effusion is aspirated, leukocyte counts can be as high as 42,500/mm^3, with 90% neutrophils (44). Most effusions are only mildly inflammatory, however, with leukocyte counts of less than 1,000/mm^3, predominantly lymphocytes and large mononuclear cells.

Cultures are negative and crystals cannot be identified by compensated, polarized light. Several patients with this syn-

TABLE 93.2. SARCOID ARTHROPATHY

Acute sarcoidosis (Lofgren's syndrome)
Often periarticular and tender, erythematous, warm swelling
Ankles and knees almost invariably involved
Joint involvement possibly the initial manifestation (chest film normal)
Joint motion possibly normal and pain absent or minimal
Synovial effusions infrequent and generally only mildly inflammatory
Usually nonspecific mild synovitis on synovial biopsy
Self-limited, lasting weeks to months
Chronic sarcoidosis
Arthritis possibly acute and evanescent, recurrent, or chronic
Noncaseating granulomas often demonstrable in synovium
Usually nondestructive, despite chronic or recurrent disease

drome, including an early case described by Hutchinson, were thought to have gout before the synovial fluid crystal identification was available to confirm the presence of gouty arthritis (45). That acute sarcoid arthritis may respond dramatically to colchicine further confuses the issue. Elevated uric acid levels have been noted in a small percentage of patients with sarcoidosis (41), but recent studies suggest that hyperuricemia should not be anticipated unless it is a result of drugs or renal failure. Needle synovial biopsy specimens in acute sarcoidosis most often show only mild nonspecific synovitis and some lining cell proliferation. Although much of the inflammation in acute sarcoidosis can be shown to be periarticular by ultrasonography (46), synovial granulomas are occasionally found during open surgical biopsy (4). Erythema nodosum occurred concomitantly with ankle periarthritis in one-third of 33 patients studied by Maña et al. (47) of Spain. Caplan et al. (48) have described an identical periarthritis in 19 patients with hilar adenopathy, none of whom had erythema nodosum. These workers found sarcoid granulomas in the subcutaneous tissue over three of seven inflamed ankles, but no granulomas in an open joint biopsy. Angiotensin-converting enzyme levels need not be elevated in patients with acute sarcoidosis without pulmonary parenchymal involvement (11).

The joint manifestations of acute sarcoidosis subside in 2 weeks to 4 months, although rare patients developing chronic sarcoid arthritis have been described (49). Erythema nodosum and a similar arthropathy can also be seen in lepromatous leprosy, ulcerative colitis, regional enteritis, tuberculosis, coccidioidomycosis, histoplasmosis, oral contraceptive and possibly other drug use, pregnancy, and psittacosis and other infections. Other cases are idiopathic.

In sarcoidosis of more insidious onset, joint manifestations are less common. In such cases, even with widespread systemic granulomatous disease, the arthritis may still be mild and evanescent, as in acute sarcoidosis. Arthritis can also be recurring or protracted with polysynovitis, however. Even in patients with chronic synovitis, joint destruction is infrequent, and most roentgenograms, show only soft tissue swelling. The destructive joint disease occasionally seen in sarcoidosis is illustrated in Fig. 93.5. Such severe arthritis is most common in patients with multisystemic granulomatous disease. Arthritis may occur as an initial manifestation or after years of systemic disease. Thus, such a variety of patterns can be seen that a high index of suspicion is needed to lead to biopsy and other diagnostic studies to differentiate this disorder from rheumatoid or other types of arthritis.

Reports of synovial fluid analysis are infrequent. We found joint fluid leukocyte counts of 250 to 6,250/mm^3 with predominantly mononuclear cells in six patients with arthritis associated with chronic sarcoidosis (50). Sokoloff and Bunim (4) found noncaseating granulomas in three of five surgical synovial biopsy specimens from patients with chronic arthritis. Additionally, the synovium showed diffuse chronic inflammation including plasma cells. None of their patients, and only 3.3% of those studied by Owen et al. (44), had any elevation of rheumatoid factor, but others have found rheumatoid factor in as many of 38% of patients with sarcoidosis (51). The presence of rheumatoid factor does not correlate with the presence or severity of joint disease. Tenosynovitis at the wrists and elsewhere can also be seen. Finger clubbing and hypertrophic osteoarthropathy (52) are occasional complications of pulmonary sarcoidosis.

Arthritis in early childhood sarcoidosis has been described, with especially large, painless, boggy synovial and tendon sheath effusions (53). The course of the disease is indolent, and constitutional symptoms are few. Despite prolonged synovitis, no erosive radiographic changes are seen. Synovial biopsy samples may show granulomas. Interestingly, the sarcoidosis reported in young children is associated with potentially devastating uveitis, but not with much lung disease or hilar adenopathy, so the relation of the syn-

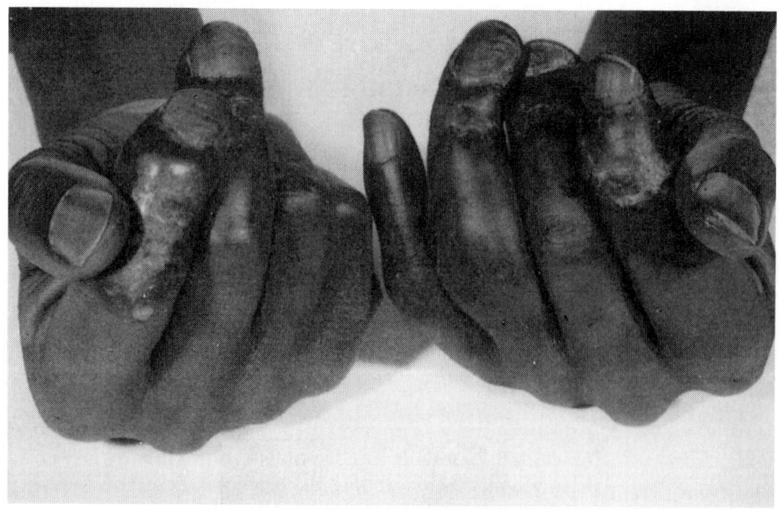

FIGURE 93.5. The hands of a 33-year-old African American man with sarcoidosis of 5 years' duration. Depigmented skin lesions are present on the dorsum of fingers, and the distal phalanx of the left fourth finger is displaced. Note the fusiform swelling of the proximal interphalangeal joint of the fourth and fifth fingers of the left hand (asymmetric). This patient does not have psoriasis. (From Sokoloff L, Bunim JJ. Clinical and pathological studies of joint involvement in sarcoidosis. *N Engl J Med* 1959;260:842–847, with permission.)

drome to adult sarcoidosis is not clear. Cases have been reported with vasculitis and one patient had premature aging (54). The term *juvenile systemic granulomatosis* has been suggested to distinguish this from adult sarcoidosis. A familial syndrome with granulomatous arthritis, uveitis, rash, and camptodactyly has also been described (55).

TREATMENT

Many patients with minimal symptoms require no treatment. No curative agent exists. Adrenal corticosteroids are commonly used to suppress potentially serious inflammatory reactions, such as ocular disease, pulmonary parenchymal disease, and central nervous system involvement, and are often effective. Corticosteroids can also lower persistently elevated serum calcium levels. Initial doses of 20 to 60 mg prednisone are tapered to the lowest effective maintenance dose. Alternate-day dosage seems effective for maintenance therapy. Objective long-term benefits from corticosteroids have often been difficult to demonstrate (56), but improved vital capacity even in severe disease has been shown in one series (57). Spontaneous remission can occur. Active articular disease almost always shows at least temporary improvement with corticosteroid therapy. When these agents are used, isoniazid coverage may be needed. Because joint disease is often self-limited, however, rest, salicylates, and other analgesics are often all that is required. Salicylates are often not as dramatically effective as in rheumatic fever. Colchicine shortens attacks of acute arthritis in some patients (43), but it is by no means invariably effective. Methotrexate at 7.5 to 15 mg/week has been effective in several open trials, although one review found 15% of patients develop hepatitis (58). Chloroquine or hydroxychloroquine have been reported to help cutaneous sarcoidosis (59) and may help some bone sarcoidosis (60). Uncontrolled reports of cyclosporine and azathioprine (61) use in sarcoidosis have suggested benefit in some patients.

REFERENCES

1. Boeck C. Multiple benign sarkoid of the skin. *J Cutan Genitourin Dis* 1899;17:543–550.
2. Schaumann JN. Etude sur le lupus pernio et ses rapports avec les sarcoides et la tuberculose. *Ann Dermatol Syph* 1916;6:357–373.
3. Lofgren S. Primary pulmonary sarcoidosis. I. Early signs and symptoms. *Acta Med Scand* 1953;145:424–431.
4. Sokoloff L, Bunim JJ. Clinical and pathological studies of joint involvement in sarcoidosis. *N Engl J Med* 1959;260:842–847.
5. Hunninghake GW, Crystal RG. Pulmonary sarcoidosis: a disorder mediated by excess helper T-lymphocyte activity at sites of disease activity. *N Engl J Med* 1981;305:429–434.
6. Konttinen YT, Tolvanen E, Visa-Tolvanen K, et al. Inflammatory cells of sarcoid granulomas detected by monoclonal antibodies and an esterase technique. *Clin Immunol Immunopathol* 1983;26: 380–389.
7. Longcope WT, Freiman DG. A study of sarcoidosis. *Medicine* 1952;31:1–32.
8. Veale D, Fitzgerald O. Acute sarcoid arthropathy—an infective cause? *Br J Rheumatol* 1990;29:158–159.
9. Petterson HB, Johnson E, Osen SS. Phagocytosis of agarose beads by receptors for C3b (CRI) and iC3b (CR3) on alveolar macrophages from patients with sarcoidosis. *Scand J Immunol* 1990;32:669–677.
10. Van Maarsseven ACM, Mullink H, Alons CL, et al. Distribution of T cell subsets in different portions of sarcoid granulomas. *Hum Pathol* 1986;17:493–500.
11. Fitzgerald AA, Davis P. Arthritis, hilar adenopathy, erythema nodosum complex. *J Rheumatol* 1982;9:935–938.
12. Krause A, Goebel KM. Class II MHC antigen (HLA DR3) predisposes to sarcoid arthritis. *J Clin Lab Immunol* 1987;24:25–27.
13. Truelove LH. Articular manifestations of erythema nodosum. *Ann Rheum Dis* 1960;19:174–180.
14. Neville E, Walker AN, James DG. Prognostic factors predicting the outcome of sarcoidosis: an analysis of 818 patients. *Q J Med* 1983;52:525–533.
15. Gran JT. Multiorgan sarciodosis presenting with symmetric polyarthralgia, cutaneous vasculitis and sicca symptoms. *Scand J Rheumatol* 1997;26:225–226.
16. Eld H, O'Connor CR, Catalano E, et al. Life-threatening vasculitis associated with sarcoidosis. *J Clin Rheumatol* 1998;4: 338–344.
17. Sack KE, Whitcher JP, Carteron NL, et al. Sarcoidosis mimicking Sjögren's syndrome: histopathologic observations. *J Clin Rheumatol* 1998;4:13–16.
18. Sequeira W, Stinar D. Serum angiotensin converting enzyme levels in sarcoid arthritis. *Arch Intern Med* 1986;146:125–127.
19. Matsuki K, Sakata T. Angiotensin-converting enzyme levels diseases of the liver. *Am J Med* 1982;73:549–551.
20. Lawrence EC, Teague RB, Gottlieb MS, et al. Serial changes in markers of disease activity with corticosteroid treatment in sarcoidosis. *Am J Med* 1983;74:747–756.
21. Fagan EA, Moore-Gillon JC, Turner-Warwick M. Multiorgan granulomas and mitochondrial antibodies. *N Engl J Med* 1983; 308:572–575.
22. Koontz CH, Joyner LR, Nelson RA. Transbronchial lung biopsy via the fiberoptic bronchoscope in sarcoidosis. *Ann Intern Med* 1976;85:64–66.
23. Winterbauer RH, Belic N, Moores KD. A clinical interpretation of bilateral hilar adenopathy. *Ann Intern Med* 1973;78:65–71.
24. Stjernberg N, Cajander S, Truedson H, et al. Muscle involvement in sarcoidosis. *Acta Med Scand* 1981;209:213–216.
25. Israel HL, Sones M. Selection of biopsy procedures for sarcoidosis diagnosis. *Arch Intern Med* 1964;113:255–260.
26. James DG. Kveim revisited, reassessed [editorial]. *N Engl J Med* 1975;292:859–860.
27. Nosal A, Schleissner LA, Mishkin FS, et al. Angiotensin-1-converting enzyme and gallium scan in non-invasive evaluation of sarcoidosis. *Ann Intern Med* 1979;90:328–331.
28. Wolfe SM, Pinals RS, Aelion JA, et al. Myopathy in sarcoidosis. *Semin Arthritis Rheum* 1987;16:300–306.
29. Janssen M, Dijkmans AC, Fulderink F. Muscle cramps in the calf as presenting symptom of sarcoidosis. *Ann Rheum Dis* 1991;50: 51–52.
30. Dewberry RG, Schneider BF, Cale WF, et al. Sarcoid myopathy presenting with diaphragm weakness. *Muscle Nerve* 1993;16: 832–835.
31. Otake S. Sarcoidosis involving skeletal muscle: imaging findings and relative value of imaging procedures. *AJR* 1994;162:369–375.
32. Chapelon C, Ziza JM, Piette JC, et al. Neurosarcoidosis: signs course and treatment in 35 confirmed cases. *Medicine* 1990;69: 261–276.

33. Perlman SG, Damergis J, Witorsch P, et al. Vertebral sarcoidosis with paravertebral ossification. *Arthritis Rheum* 1978;21: 271–277.
34. Blank NM, Steininger H, Kalden JR, et al. Symptomatic bone lesion of the tibial head as onset manifestation of sarcoidosis. *J Rheumatol* 1999;26:936–937.
35. Schorr AF, Murphy FT, Kelly WF, et al. Osseous sarcoidosis. Clinical, radiographic and therapeutic observations. *J Clin Rheumatol* 1998;4:186–192.
36. Sartoris DJ, Resnick D, Resnick C, et al. Musculoskeletal manifestations of sarcoidosis. *Semin Roentgenol* 1985;20: 376–386.
37. McBrine CS, Fisher MS. Acrosclerosis in sarcoidosis. *Radiology* 1975;115:279–281.
38. Liebowitz MR, Essop AR, Schamroth CL, et al. Sarcoid dactylitis in black South African patients. *Semin Arthritis Rheum* 1985; 14:232–237.
39. Gumpel JM, Johns CJ, Shulman LE. The joint disease of sarcoidosis. *Ann Rheum Dis* 1967;26:194–205.
40. Siltzbach LE, Duberstein JL. Arthritis in sarcoidosis. *Clin Orthop* 1968;57:31–50.
41. Spilberg I, Siltzbach LE, McEwen C. The arthritis of sarcoidosis. *Arthritis Rheum* 1969;12:126–137.
42. James DG, Thompson AD, Wilcox A. Erythema nodosum as a manifestation of sarcoidosis. *Lancet* 1956;2:218–221.
43. Kaplan H. Sarcoid arthritis with a response to colchicine. *N Engl J Med* 1960;268:778–781.
44. Owen DS, Waller M, Ray ES, et al. Musculoskeletal sarcoidosis and rheumatoid factor. *Med Coll VA Q* 1972;8:217–220.
45. Kaplan H, Klatskin G. Sarcoidosis, psoriasis, and gout: syndrome or coincidence? *Yale J Biol Med* 1960;32:335–352.
46. Kellner H, Spathling S, Herzer P. Ultrasound findings in Lofgren's syndrome: is ankle swelling caused by arthritis, tenosynovitis or periarthritis? *J Rheumatol* 1992;19:38–41.
47. Maña J, Gomez-Vaquero C, Salazar A, et al. Periarticular ankle sarcoidosis: a variant of Löfgren's syndrome. *J Rheumatol* 1996; 23:874–877.
48. Caplan HI, Katz WA, Rubenstein M. Periarticular inflammation, bilateral hilar adenopathy and a sarcoid reaction. *Arthritis Rheum* 1970;13:101–111.
49. Johard U, Eklund A. Recurrent Lofgren's syndrome in three patients with sarcoidosis. *Sarcoidosis* 1993;10:125–127.
50. Palmer DG, Schumacher HR. Synovitis with non-specific histologic changes in synovium in chronic sarcoidosis. *Ann Rheum Dis* 1984;43:778–782.
51. Oreskes I, Siltzbach LE. Changes in rheumatoid factor activity during the course of sarcoidosis. *Am J Med* 1968;55:60–67.
52. Rahbar M, Sharma OP. Hypertrophic osteoarthropathy in sarcoidosis. *Sarcoidosis* 1990;7:125–127.
53. North AF, Fink CW, Gibson WM, et al. Sarcoid arthritis in children. *Am J Med* 1970;48:449–455.
54. Umemoto M, Take H, Yamaguchi H, et al. Juvenile systemic granulomatosis manifesting as premature aging syndrome and renal failure. *J Rheumatol* 1997;24:393–395.
55. Raphael SA, Blau EB, Zhang WH, et al. Analysis of a large kindred with Blau syndrome for HLA, autoimmunity, and sarcoidosis. *Am J Dis Child* 1993;147:842–848.
56. Young RL, Harkleroad LE, Lordon RE, et al. Pulmonary sarcoidosis: a prospective evaluation of glucocorticoid therapy. *Ann Intern Med* 1970;73:207–212.
57. Emirgil C, Sobol BJ, Williams MH. Long-term study of pulmonary sarcoidosis. The effect of steroid therapy as evaluated by pulmonary function studies. *J Chronic Dis* 1969;22:69–86.
58. Newman LS, Rose CS, Maier LA. Sarcoidosis. *N Engl J Med* 1997;336:1224–1234.
59. Jones E, Callen JP. Hydroxychloroquine is effective therapy for control of cutaneous sarcoidal granulomas. *J Am Acad Dermatol* 1990;23:487–489.
60. De Simone DP, Brillant HL, Basile J, et al. Granulomatous infiltration of the talus and abnormal vitamin D metabolism in a patient with sarcoidosis; successful treatment with hydroxychloroquine. *Am J Med* 1989;87:694–696.
61. Krebs P, Abel H, Schonberger W. Behandling der boeckschan sarkoidose mit immunosuppressiven substanzen. Erfahrungen mit Azatioprin (Imurel). *Munchen Med Wochenschr* 1969;111: 2307–2311.

94

ARTHRITIS ASSOCIATED WITH HEMATOLOGIC DISORDERS, STORAGE DISEASES, DISORDERS OF LIPID METABOLISM, AND DYSPROTEINEMIAS

LOUIS W. HECK, JR.

Rheumatologists frequently are asked to evaluate patients of all ages who have undefined, vexing illnesses associated with regional or generalized pain, myalgias, arthralgias, and arthritis. Not infrequently, especially in large, tertiary-care medical centers, such illnesses reflect an underlying hematologic or lipid disorder, storage disease, or dysproteinemia. Some of the clinical aspects of these varied disorders, including diagnosis and treatment, which are of many etiologies and classes (neoplastic, inflammatory, and hereditary) are described in this chapter. The approach to such patients should include a thorough medical history, a careful physical examination, and judicious selection of laboratory and radiologic studies directed toward reaching a precise diagnosis, thereby facilitating optimal patient treatment and education. In hereditary disorders, testing, counseling, and education of family members should be done, all of which are critical to optimal patient care.

Current understanding of most of these disorders has evolved through laborious clinical-pathologic correlation studies. Treatments have improved but are not ideal. Precise understanding of these disorders will depend on new knowledge generated by efforts in molecular medicine. New information regarding fundamental genetic defects in hereditary disorders and the mechanisms of carcinogenesis is being generated at a blinding speed (1).

CHILDHOOD MALIGNANCIES

Acute lymphoid leukemia is the most common malignancy of children and accounts for approximately one-quarter of all new cases of neoplasms in children less than 15 years of age. It has a peak incidence between the ages of 3 and 5 years. Musculoskeletal manifestations of acute lymphoid leukemia are varied but may be either the presenting or dominant manifestation of this disorder. In a study of 584 children with acute lymphoid leukemia, 27% had bone or joint pain as the presenting symptom (2). The presenting symptom complex is diverse and may include intermittent or continuous fever, transient or persistent arthralgias and/or arthritis, and diffuse bone pain. The bone pain may be severe and incapacitating and is typically metaphyseal in location and out of proportion to the physical findings. The arthritis may be monarticular or polyarticular with a predilection for joints of the fingers, knees, and ankles (3,4). As the age of peak incidence of childhood acute lymphoid leukemia is identical to that of juvenile rheumatoid arthritis (JRA), the diagnosis of many children with acute lymphoid leukemia may be confused initially with any of the JRA onset types, most notably systemic-onset JRA, or other rheumatic illnesses such as systemic lupus erythematosus (SLE), acute rheumatic fever, or septic arthritis (5). Furthermore, the complete blood count (CBC) and platelet count may be normal and tests such as rheumatoid factor and antinuclear antibody (ANA) may be positive. Acute lymphoid leukemia should be considered in any young child presenting with musculoskeletal pain or JRA-like illnesses with an elevated erythrocyte sedimentation rate (ESR), normocytic anemia, low reticulocyte count, thrombocytopenia, or relative or absolute neutropenia. The blood smear should be carefully examined for circulating lymphoblasts, and if there is any question concerning acute lymphoid leukemia, a bone marrow aspiration and biopsy should be performed to exclude the diagnosis. In some cases, multiple bone marrow studies may have to be performed before establishing the diagnosis. The need for a correct diagnosis and prompt treatment is crucial since the emerging results of acute lymphoid leukemia outcome studies have shown that aggressive multidrug chemotherapy may produce long periods of disease-free remissions or even cure (2).

Neuroblastoma originates from sympathetic nerve tissue and is the most common solid tumor in children from ages

1 to 3 years. The presenting signs and symptoms of neuroblastoma are varied and may be caused by the primary tumor, metastatic disease, or paraneoplastic syndromes (6,7). Patients with metastatic neuroblastoma may have fever, cachexia, bone pain, subcutaneous nodules, hepatomegaly, lymphadenopathy, anemia, or pancytopenia, and mimic acute lymphoid leukemia or systemic-onset JRA. Unfortunately, this presentation is usually indicative of widespread metastatic neuroblastoma that responds poorly to treatment.

ADULT HEMATOLOGIC/LYMPHORETICULAR MALIGNANCIES

Adult leukemia may have prominent musculoskeletal manifestations with bone pain and arthralgias/arthritis. The true prevalence of joint involvement in adult leukemias is variable but it may be the presenting symptom complex in 13.5% of patients (8). Some patients may have symmetric arthralgias/arthritis involving the knees, ankles, shoulders, and hands, which resemble rheumatoid arthritis (RA), whereas others may have migratory asymmetric polyarthritis. Back pain presenting as a radiculopathy may be associated with meningeal infiltration by leukemia cells. Some patients with acute myelogenous leukemia may have symptomatic sternal tenderness. Synovial fluids have been studied in patients with leukemia-associated arthritis and the synovial fluid leukocyte counts have ranged from 50 to 50,000 cells/mm^3 (9). The mechanisms underlying the synovitis are not well understood. Studies of synovium obtained at autopsy and by biopsy have yielded negative results. However, two patients with lymphoblastic leukemia and one with T-cell leukemia have been reported with leukemic cells in synovial fluid using immunocytologic techniques (10,11).

Myelodysplastic syndromes (MDSs) are a collection of varied clonal hematologic disorders characterized by ineffective hematopoiesis (12). The French-American-British (FAB) classification of MDS includes refractory anemia, refractory anemia with ringed sideroblasts, refractory anemia with excess blasts, chronic myelomonocytic leukemia, and refractory anemia with excess blasts in transformation (12). These syndromes frequently present in men older than 70 years as isolated or multiple cytopenias. There is a significant association between these syndromes and rheumatic manifestations. In a prospective study of 162 patients with myelodysplastic syndromes, Castro et al. (13) found 10% with several rheumatic manifestations, which included cutaneous vasculitis, lupus-like manifestations, peripheral neuropathy, and rheumatic diseases, such as RA, Sjögren's syndrome, and mixed connective tissue disease (13). In another study, 8 of 28 patients had acute seronegative inflammatory arthritis at the time of discovery of the specific cytopenia (14). Illnesses such as cutaneous vasculitis and polymyalgia rheumatica–like syndromes have been described in patients with myelodysplastic syndromes (14,15). Besides occurring de novo in previously healthy individuals, MDS may develop in patients with rheumatic diseases treated with alkylating agents such as Cytoxan and chlorambucil (16). In a retrospective study of eight patients with MDS and rheumatic disease, seven had received a mean cumulative dose of 118 g of Cytoxan and one a cumulative dose of 6.5 g of chlorambucil. Six of the eight patients have died. Cytogenetic abnormalities included a deletion of all or part of chromosome 7 in five patients and a deletion of all or part of the long arm of chromosome 5 (16).

Hairy cell leukemia (HCL) is a rare, B lymphocyte, neoplastic disorder that occurs predominantly in young and middle-aged males and is characterized by splenomegaly, pancytopenia, and the presence of circulating mononuclear cells with hairy (cytoplasmic) projections. Sequential advances in treatment of this neoplastic disorder have included splenectomy, treatment with interferon-α, and, most recently, 2-chlorodeoxyadenosine. A recent report of a large multicenter trial involving 979 patients registered with HCL has shown 2-chlorodeoxyadenosine to be an excellent agent to treat this condition (17). Most of the patients were treated with a standard protocol of continuous intravenous infusion of this drug at a dose of 0.1 mg/kg/day for 7 consecutive days and followed for more than 4 years. An overall response rate of 87% was found in 861 assessable patients: 50% showed complete remission, 13% a good partial response, and 24% a partial response (17). Two rheumatic manifestations that have been described in association with HCL are a systemic vasculitis syndrome identical to polyarteritis nodosa and a symmetric arthritis similar to that of RA (18–24). Additionally, several patients with cutaneous small vessel vasculitis and erythema nodosum have been reported. Hairy cell infiltration of vessel walls and synovial fluid has been described, but the mechanism of inflammatory tissue injury has not been clarified (19). Treatment protocols utilizing prednisone and cyclophosphamide have been used with variable results. There is one report of autopsy-proven resolution of polyarteritis in a patient treated with interferon-α (22). Whether these rheumatic syndromes will occur in patients with HCL treated with 2-chlorodeoxyadenosine remains to be determined. Finally, bone involvement may occur in HCL and generally is responsive to radiation therapy (25).

T-cell large granular lymphocyte leukemia, which is a clonal expansion of CD3$^+$, CD8$^+$, CD16$^+$, and CD57$^+$ cells, may occur in patients with RA (26,27). Most of the patients present with neutropenia (<500/mm^3) which is associated with infections, and sometimes with splenomegaly, and may be misdiagnosed as having Felty's syndrome. In contrast to Felty's syndrome, however, patients with T-cell large granular lymphocyte leukemia present at an older age, and the neutropenia may appear within weeks to months of symptomatic joint disease and is usually associated with a normal or elevated blood leukocyte count. A characteristic finding on routine examination of the peripheral blood smear is the presence of increased numbers of large granular lymphocytes with abundant pale cytoplasm and prominent azurophilic granules. Treatment may consist of granulocyte-macrophage colony-stimulating factor (GM-CSF) to reverse neutropenia and a course of Cytoxan or continuous methotrexate (27). The successful treatment of refractory large granular lymphocytic leukemia with 2-chlorodeoxyadenosine has been reported (28).

Malignant lymphomas are a heterogeneous group of at least 15 neoplastic disorders defined broadly as either Hodgkin's disease (approximately 20%) or non-Hodgkin's lymphoma (approximately 80%). Bone involvement is common to all lymphomas, but the reported incidence varies depending on the method used to stage disease activity (29). For example, approximately 10% to 25% of patients with Hodgkin's disease have characteristic osseous changes by standard radiographic examination, but 50% have bone involvement at postmortem examination. Skeletal involvement in all lymphomas may involve the vertebrae, pelvis, ribs, long bones, and skull, and may include bone pain usually associated with active bone destruction involving the periosteum (29,30). Patients complain of pain that is deep, constant, and dull. The pain is typically worse at night and not relieved by rest. Sometimes the pain worsens on standing and walking in patients with vertebral or long bone involvement. Compressive nerve syndromes may arise from tumor infiltration of the spinal cord (myelopathy) or brachial/lumbosacral plexus roots (radiculopathy). A detailed description of specific pain syndromes in patients with lymphoma, cancer, or leukemia, which include permeative bone destruction or nerve involvement, is beyond the scope of this chapter but is given elsewhere (31,32). Bone destruction may manifest radiographically as osteolytic lesions, pathologic fractures of long bones and vertebrae, periostitis, or cortical destruction. As emphasized by Resnick (29), regional bone formation may occur in Burkitt's lymphoma (facial bones including maxilla and mandible), and solitary lesions with pathologic fractures in the femur and pelvic bones may be found in reticulum cell sarcoma.

Monarthritis or polyarthritis may be the presenting manifestations of *extranodal non-Hodgkin's lymphoma of the synovium.* In a review of six patients, four presented with knee monarthritis, one with sternoclavicular monarthritis, and one with polyarthritis; two had radiographic evidence of adjacent osteolysis, and one had a soft tissue mass (33). The precise diagnosis was made by synovial or bone biopsy. One patient had lymphoma presenting in bone (reticulum cell sarcoma) with extension into the synovium. In another series of 14 patients with reticulum cell sarcoma, four patients had complained of joint pain and three were evaluated without a rheumatologic diagnosis (34). All patients had persistent localized bone pain, swelling, or both, and had radiographic evidence of bone involvement.

Angioimmunoblastic lymphadenopathy with dysproteinemia is an uncommon peripheral T-cell (occasionally B-cell) lymphoma characterized by rash, constitutional symptoms, hepatosplenomegaly, lymphadenopathy, autoantibodies, thrombocytopenia, or hemolytic anemia (35–38). The diagnosis is made by lymph node biopsy and the characteristic histologic findings. Several patients have been reported with a symmetric, seronegative polyarthritis, which may occur transiently before or after the diagnosis is made (38–40). In one reported case, a lymphoid infiltrate in synovium resembled that found in a supraclavicular lymph node (39). No treatment protocol has been published, but there is a report of 2-chlorodeoxyadenosine in the treatment of two patients with refractory angioimmunoblastic lymphadenopathy with dysproteinemia (40).

Cutaneous T-cell lymphoma is a rare, cutaneous malignancy (mycosis fungoides) involving helper T cells, which may have a leukemic phase with abnormal circulating lymphocytes (Sezary syndrome). Two patients have been described with a symmetric seronegative arthritis (41,42), one of whom was initially seronegative but became rheumatoid factor positive and was refractory to conventional therapy but exhibited a partial response to anti-CD4 monoclonal antibody.

Lymphomatoid granulomatosis (LYG) is a rare disorder originally defined as a form of pulmonary angiitis and granulomatosis resembling Wegener's granulomatosis (43). This unique angiocentric and angiodestructive (necrotizing) infiltrative process involves the lungs predominantly, but also skin, central and peripheral nervous systems, liver, and spleen (43,44). Originally considered to be a systemic granulomatous vasculitis, LYG is an Epstein-Barr virus (EBV)-driven B-cell proliferation associated with an abundant T-cell infiltrate (45,46). Paradoxically, there is an associated immunodeficiency since there is evidence of defective T-cell function (45). In a longitudinal study of four patients with LYG followed for over a 5-year period, all biopsy specimens demonstrated medium to large B cells scattered in the background of a T-cell–rich infiltrate. Furthermore, double-labeling experiments showed localization of EBV sequences only to the B cells and not the T cells. Clonal immunoglobulin H (IgH) gene rearrangements were detected in two of three patients studied. The most common presenting symptoms were cough, dyspnea, and chest pain, which reflected the pulmonary involvement, and constitutional symptoms of fever, weight loss, and malaise. Arthralgias occurred in 6.3% of patients and myalgias in 2.8% in the extensive study of 152 patients reported by Katzenstein et al. (44). Several patients developed a symmetric seronegative polyarthritis (47). In this heterogeneous group of disorders, no standard treatment approach exists. However, responses to interferon-α_{2b} (45) and cyclosporin A (48) have been reported.

Although patients with RA exhibited an increased mortality, an excessive risk of lymphoma in this disorder, including those treated with methotrexate, has not been appreciated (49,50). However, a flurry of recent case reports have emphasized the increased occurrence of lymphoid neoplasms in RA patients (and a few in patients with dermatomyositis) receiving weekly, low-dose methotrexate (49–58) (see Chapter 35). Typically, these lymphoid neoplasms are non-Hodgkin's lymphomas, diffuse, large-cell type and of B-cell lineage. Exceptions include one reported case of T-cell lymphoma and two cases of Hodgkin's disease. One of the patients had sicca symptoms or Sjögren's syndrome. A remarkable feature in several cases has been the reversibility of the lymphomas; with cessation of methotrexate therapy, the lymphomas regressed completely. This suggests that methotrexate may be a cocarcinogen and may affect the metabolism of potentially carcinogenic compounds, impair the growth regulation of special immune cell types, or impair the ability of the immune system to eradicate tumors. The other remarkable feature was that the genomic DNA in most of these lymphomas harbored the EBV genome and the neoplastic cells were EBV latent membrane protein-1 positive, suggesting that EBV infection may be one of the triggering events in malignant lymphoproliferation. Regardless, all rheumatoid patients on low-dose methotrexate should be warned that there is a small chance of developing a malignancy and should be carefully examined for lymphadenopathy at each visit.

MULTIPLE MYELOMA AND AMYLOIDOSIS

Multiple myeloma (marrow tumor) is a common neoplastic disorder characterized by the uncontrolled growth of a single clone of plasma cells in the bone marrow. It may have varied musculoskeletal manifestations such as bone pain, resulting from pathologic bone resorption and osteoporosis, or joint pain. Malignant plasma cells infiltrate the bone marrow, demineralizing bone diffusely (diffuse osteoporosis) through a complex cascade mechanism involving the synthesis and secretion of bone-resorbing cytokines including tumor necrosis factor (TNF), interleukin-1, and interleukin-6 (59). Osteoclasts arise in the bone marrow from macrophage-granulocyte colony-forming units. The development of this bone resorbing cell is regulated under normal conditions by mesenchymal-osteoblast cells. Myeloma cells produce factors such as interleukin-6 and interleukin-11 that modulate the differentiation pathways of osteoclasts, leading to increased numbers of activated osteoclasts (59,60).

Skeletal pain may be the presenting and dominant symptom of myeloma (61,62). It may manifest initially as transient or mild pain, which begins insidiously or presents as severe, sudden pain of vertebrae, ribs, or extremities following minimal trauma usually due to fractures and sometimes associated with compression of the spinal cord or nerve roots. The radiographic bone survey remains the standard method to assess the extent of skeletal involvement, but newer imaging techniques such as computed tomography (CT) are superior to plain radiographs to delineate vertebral and long bone involvement (63). Furthermore, magnetic resonance imaging (MRI) can demonstrate the relationship between the vertebrae, spinal cord, and nerve roots, specifically defining exact sites of neural tissue compression (64).

Besides back pain, which is the most common rheumatic symptom in myeloma, arthralgias and arthritis have also been reported (61,62,65,66). Joint symptoms may occur at approximately the same time as symptomatic myeloma and include skeletal pain, joint stiffness and swelling, and carpal tunnel syndrome (67). These rheumatic manifestations are secondary to myeloma or an associated disorder called *primary amyloidosis* (68–72). Furthermore, patients with long-standing classic RA have subsequently developed myeloma, raising the possibility that this long-standing inflammatory disease triggered the onset of the neoplastic process (66).

Multiple myeloma and primary amyloidosis are characterized by the presence of a monoclonal (M) protein in serum or urine. Clinical consequences of an abundance of these abnormal proteins (paraproteins) include hyperviscosity with congestive heart failure, cryoglobulinemia with peripheral vascular insufficiency, deposition of light chains in the renal tubules (myeloma kidney), hypercalcemia from excessive bone resorption, and inactivation of plasma coagulation factors I, II, VIII, and IX by binding to the paraprotein. A rapid, sensitive, analytic technique to identify M proteins in these body fluids is immunofixation electrophoresis. Samples of diluted serum or concentrated urine are loaded into buffered agarose gel wells. After electrophoresis, each lane is incubated with antisera specific for IgG, IgM, or IgA heavy-chain polypeptides, κ and λ light-chain polypeptides, or with no antiserum. The antibodies diffuse into the gel matrix, bind to the specific antigen, and form an insoluble antigen-antibody immunofixation precipitin line. The extraneous soluble proteins are removed by gentle washing. The agarose gel is then dried and stained with a dye to reveal the M protein precipitin bands. The differential diagnoses of monoclonal gammopathies is extensive and usually requires further testing. The diagnoses in 851 patients with monoclonal gammopathies followed at the Mayo Clinic are shown in Table 94.1 (73). As shown, 66.9% of these patients had monoclonal gammopathies of undetermined significance (MGUS), which is considered a benign disorder, but some patients progressed to develop multiple myeloma, amyloidosis, macroglobulinemia, or other lymphoreticular malignancy. Representative immunofixation patterns are depicted in Fig. 94.1, including normal serum (A) and urine (B); serum (C) and urine (D) from a patient with a 13-year history of monoclonal gammopathy of unknown significance; and serum (E) and urine (F) from a patient with multiple myeloma.

Amyloidosis is not one clinical entity but rather a group of diverse structurally driven protein deposition diseases

TABLE 94.1. DIAGNOSIS IN 851 CASES OF MENOCLONAL GAMMOPATHY

Diagnosis	Frequency
Monoclonal gammopathy of unknown significance (MGUS)	66.9%
Plasma cell myeloma	13.5%
Primary amyloidosis	8.9%
Lymphoma	5.2%
Chronic lymphocytic leukemia	2.1%
Macroglobulinemia	2.0%
Indolent plasma cell myeloma	0.9%
Solitary plasmacytoma	0.5%

From Kyle RA, Lust JA. Monoclonal gammopathies of undetermined significance. *Semin Hematol* 1989;26:176–200, with permission.

that share some common properties but differ in biochemical composition (71,72). For example, they are similar in that protein deposition occurs extracellularly, and these deposits are eosinophilic with standard tissue histologic stains; bind Congo red dye, emitting an apple-green birefringence when using polarized light microscopy; exhibit metachromasia with crystal violet; have 100 Å nonbranching fibrils by electron microscopy; and exhibit a twisted β-pleated sheet antiparallel configuration by x-ray crystallography. They differ, however, in the biochemical nature of the proteinaceous deposits, the etiology of the associated diseases (neoplastic, inflammatory, degenerative, or hereditary), the tropism of protein deposition, and the spectrum of disease manifestations. By studying many different amyloid-laden tissues and using the aforementioned techniques, researchers have identified many different amyloid proteins and precursor proteins associated with clinical syndromes or specific diseases. There is no satisfactory clinical classification of the amyloidoses. One method is to consider three major systemic forms—AL (immunoglobulin light chain amyloid), AA (A protein amyloid), and ATTR (transthyretin amyloid); two major localized forms—Aβ_2 (β_2-microglobulin amyloid) and Aβ (β-protein amyloid); and several miscellaneous forms. Amyloidosis is discussed in greater detail in Chapter 92. Consideration of AL, AA,

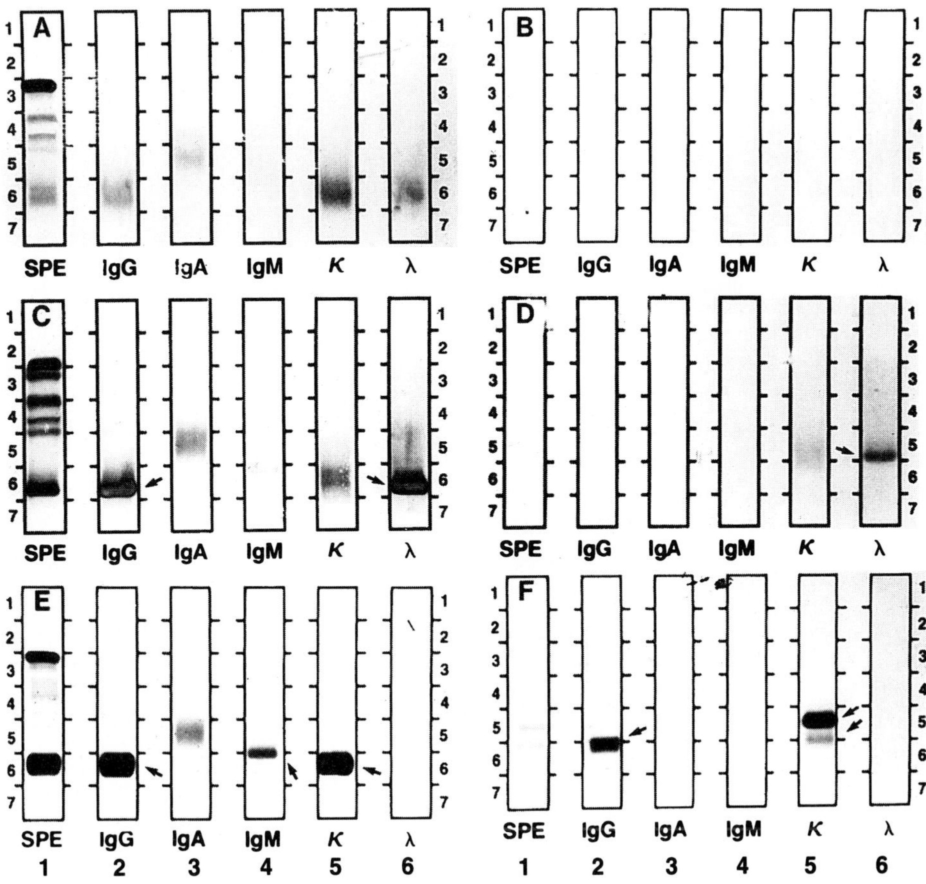

FIGURE 94.1. Immunofixation patterns of normal serum **(A)** and urine **(B)**; serum **(C)** and urine **(D)** from a 72-year-old man with a 12-year history of monoclonal gammopathy of undetermined significance; serum **(E)** and urine **(F)** from a 82-year-old man with multiple myeloma. In **A**, the prominent band in the SPE lane is albumin. No M protein is seen in the serum **(A)** or urine **(B)**. The following M proteins are noted: **C**—immunoglobulin G (IgG)λ; **D**—free λ light chains; **E**—IgGκ and a small amount of IgM (biclonal gammopathy); **F**—IgGκ and free κ light chains.

ATTR, and Aβ_2 forms of amyloid is of direct relevance in the evaluation of patients presenting with rheumatic symptoms.

Primary amyloidosis (AL) was the first amyloidosis to be defined biochemically. Solubilized purified amyloid protein was hydrolyzed and shown by amino acid sequence analysis to be identical to the variable region of immunoglobulin light chain (Bence Jones protein), thus proving the immunoglobulin origin of this protein. It is the most common of the systemic amyloidoses in the United States and is associated with plasma cell myeloma (20%) or plasma cell dyscrasias (80%) involving synovium, skin and subcutaneous tissue, nerve, liver, spleen, heart, kidney, and lung. In a large retrospective series of AL patients, approximately 50% had presenting symptoms of fatigue and weight loss; less frequent symptoms included peripheral edema, dyspnea, paresthesias, light-headedness, and hoarseness (74). Initial physical findings revealed a palpable liver and peripheral edema in one-third to one-half of the patients. Orthostatic hypotension, purpura, macroglossia, palpable spleen, skin papules, ecchymoses, and lymphadenopathy were less commonly present. Amyloid infiltration of synovial tissue may present as a symmetric polyarthritis resembling RA or with massive swelling of the periarticular structures of the shoulder producing the "shoulder pad" sign (68–70). Immunofixation studies showing an M component in the serum, but not urine, of a patient with primary amyloidosis are depicted in Fig. 94.2. Also depicted is a Congo-red stained fat aspirate demonstrating birefringence of the stained amyloid by polarized light microscopy. The immunofixation patterns of three patients with primary amyloidosis with different M proteins are shown in Fig. 94.3.

Examples of clinical syndromes associated with AL include those related to nerve tissue, such as carpal tunnel syndrome and peripheral neuropathy with paresthesias of the fingers and toes. Sympathetic dysfunction manifested by orthostatic hypotension, impotence, sweating abnormalities, and gastrointestinal disturbances due to autonomic nerve involvement may also occur. Congestive heart failure may appear with either predominant right-sided failure with restrictive cardiomyopathy due to stiff, noncompliant ventricles and thick intraventricular septum (multiple discrete 3- to 5-mm highly refractile echoes with a speckled pattern on two-dimensional echocardiogram) or, rarely, a dilated cardiomyopathy with biventricular failure. Both forms may be associated with conduction disturbances. Renal involvement with albuminuria, full-blown nephrotic syndrome, and slowly progressive renal failure may be seen.

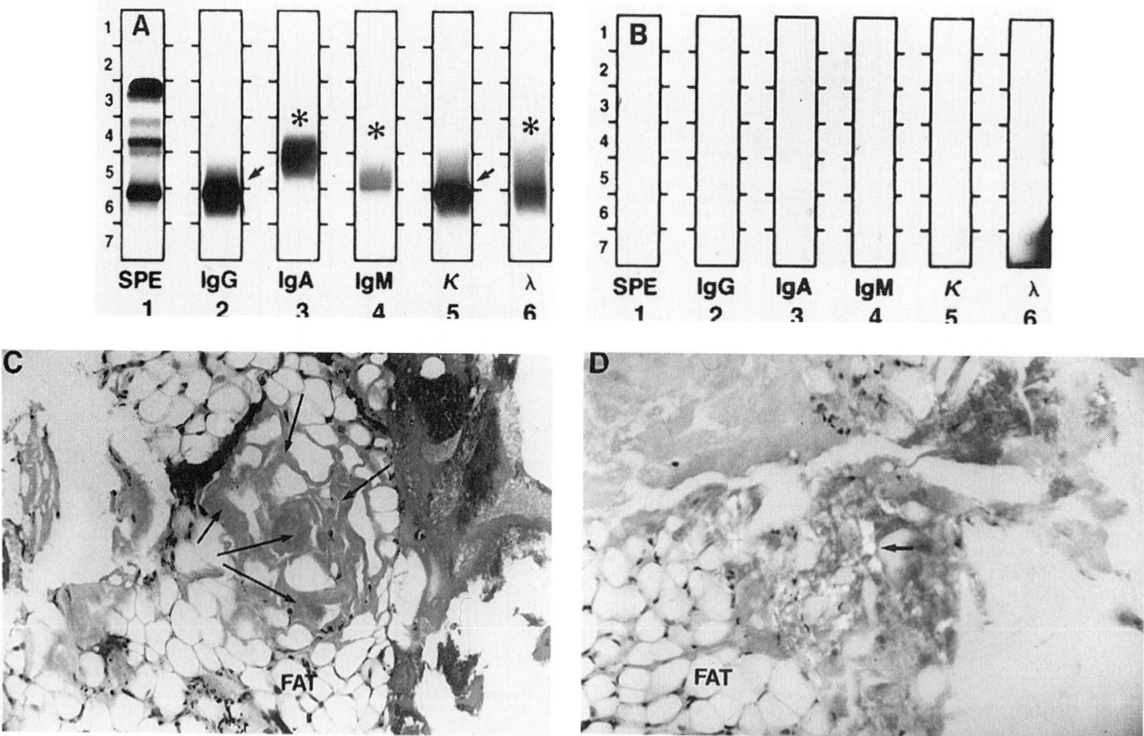

FIGURE 94.2. Immunofixation pattern of serum **(A)** and urine **(B)** and abdominal fat pad aspirate stained with Congo red **(C)** and examined by polarized light microscopy **(D)** from a 67-year-old man with primary amyloidosis. In **A**, the M protein is IgGκ; the asterisk above bands in lanes 3, 4, and 6 indicates artifacts that were confirmed by repeated studies using diluted serum and immunoelectrophoresis. No M protein was found in the urine. In **C**, the *arrows* point to congophilic material within the small arterioles and between fat cells. This congophilic material shows birefringence **(D)** by polarized light microscopy.

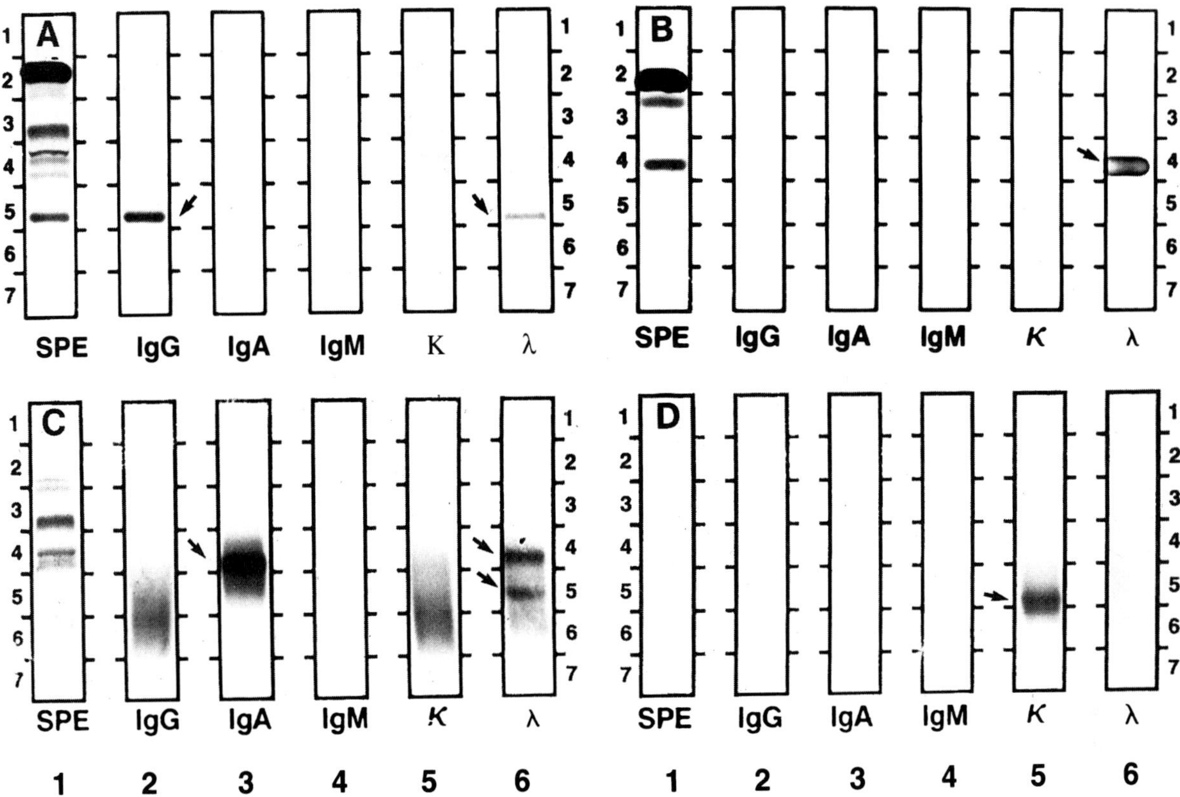

FIGURE 94.3. Immunofixation patterns from three patients with primary amyloidosis without multiple myeloma. Serum **(A)** and urine **(B)** from a 67-year-old woman with a history of carpal tunnel syndrome 27 years previous; serum **(C)** from a 62-year-old woman with sudden onset of congestive heart failure; and urine **(D)** from a 43-year-old woman with massive hepatomegaly. The following M proteins are noted: **A**—IgGλ; **B**—free λ light chains; **C**—IgAλ and free λ light chains (free λ light chains were also seen in urine; data not shown); **D**—free κ light chains in the urine (no M protein was found in the serum on several occasions).

Finally, ecchymoses and "pinch purpura" may result from minor skin trauma due to increased fragility of the small blood vessels from amyloid infiltration.

In a study of multiple myeloma patients with amyloid arthritis simulating RA, five patients were noted to have hand stiffness, swelling, and discomfort (68). Some patients had subcutaneous nodules, carpal tunnel syndrome, or proliferative synovitis with joint swelling, but no patient had metacarpophalangeal joint pain or swelling. Furthermore, there was no warmth over the swollen joints, and no rheumatoid factor, marginal erosions, or inflammatory effusions. Small fragments of amyloid-staining material were found in the synovial fluid of three patients. In some cases, amyloidosis infiltration of the synovial tissue may be extensive as shown in Fig. 94.4.

Primary amyloidosis is treated with mephalan, 0.15 mg/kg/day in two divided doses, and prednisone, 0.8 mg/kg/day in four divided doses. The duration of each treatment is 7 days with repeated cycles every 6 weeks (75). Trials from two major centers using slightly different treatment protocols have shown the efficacy of this cyclical chemotherapy as compared with no treatment or treatment with colchicine (reviewed in ref. 72). Disappointingly, the response rate is modest, with an increased median survival of 6 months between the untreated and treated patients. With some success in survival in treating multiple myeloma patients with combination high-dose chemotherapy and autologous stem cell transplantation, preliminary results have been reported regarding treatment of amyloidosis patients, but the role of this aggressive treatment approach remains indeterminate at the present time.

Secondary amyloidosis (AA) is the second systemic type of amyloidosis (72). In this disease, the precursor protein is a serum component (SAA), which is synthesized in the liver and may increase 100- to 200-fold with inflammatory stimuli. Certain monocyte/macrophage cytokines such as interleukin-1, TNF, and interleukin-6 may upregulate hepatic gene expression of this protein. Secondary amyloidosis usually involves the liver, spleen, and kidneys. Heart involvement is less frequently seen than in primary amyloidosis, and nerve involvement is rare. Some of the associated infectious diseases include osteomyelitis, tuberculosis, and bronchiectasis, and some of the noninfectious, chronic inflammatory states include RA, JRA, ankylosing spondyli-

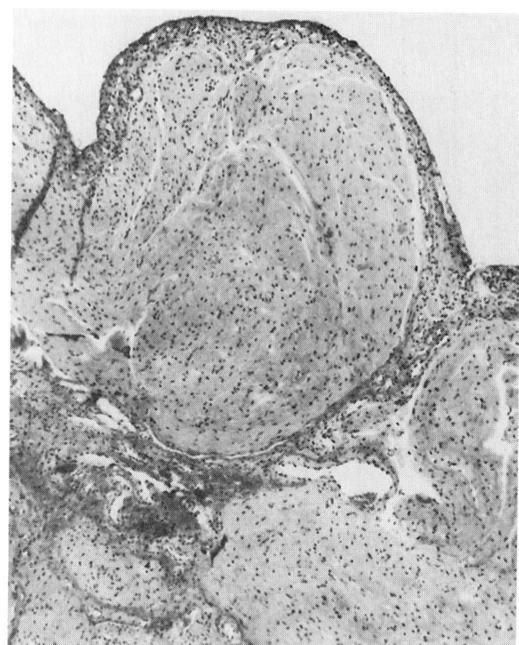

FIGURE 94.4. Photomicrograph of synovium obtained from the right shoulder of a 56-year-old woman with multiple myeloma who had developed pain in this shoulder and inability to use her arm 10 days earlier, following a fall. The humerus was dislocated. At the time of open reduction of this dislocation, large deposits of amyloid were found in the glenoid fossa. Note the mass of amyloid covered by a thin rim of synovium. The material in this nodule stained metachromatically with crystal violet.

tis, Crohn's disease, and familial Mediterranean fever. Curiously, the renal disease may be slow and indolent with progressive proteinuria evolving into nephrotic syndrome and persisting for 5 to 10 years before end-stage renal disease occurs. In Europe, renal amyloidosis has been reported as the major cause of death in patients with JRA, but this associated complication has not been seen in the United States. Another interesting observation is that amyloid deposits in AA disease may be resorbed *in vivo* as manifested by reduction in size of an enlarged liver or spleen or a reduction in proteinuria without defined treatment of the underlying disorder. Finally, the successful use of colchicine to reduce the attacks and development of amyloidosis in familial Mediterranean fever patients and to decrease proteinuria and improve renal function in some cases of AA disease mandates that AA disease be carefully considered and ruled out in all amyloid patients (76).

Familial amyloidosis (ATTR) is the third systemic amyloidosis to be defined and is associated with the deposition of an abnormal plasma prealbumin protein, designated transthyretin (72). This protein normally functions to transport thyroxine and retinol-binding protein. ATTR was defined originally as an autosomal-dominant, inherited, peripheral neuropathy occurring in mid-to-late life, progressing over the next several decades with the appearance of autonomic neuropathy and variable organ involvement, and occurring primarily in Portuguese patients. Subsequently, many clinical manifestations occurring in different kindred in Europe and the United States have been described that resulted from mutations in the gene for transthyretin, further resulting in amino acid substitutions in this transport molecule. These mutations have been associated with variable amyloid infiltration in heart, bowel, and kidney.

Dialysis-related amyloidosis, (AB_2M), a localized amyloidosis associated with arthropathy and carpal tunnel syndrome, occurs frequently in patients on maintenance hemodialysis or peritoneal dialysis of longer than 8 years' duration (77). It is due to the deposition of β_2-microglobulin amyloid in the periarticular, joint, bone, and carpal tunnel tissues (78). β_2-Microglobulin is the noncovalently associated β chain of class I human leukocyte antigen (HLA) molecules and is present on virtually all human nucleated cells. The catabolism of this small protein is dependent on normal kidney filtration and excretion. In dialysis patients and those with end-stage renal disease, plasma levels and tissue levels of β_2-microglobulin are elevated enhancing fibril formation. Although β_2-microglobulin may form amyloid fibrils *in vitro,* there is evidence that β_2-microglobulin within amyloid deposits may be modified by several post-translational modifications. For example, one study has shown that a more acidic β_2-microglobulin, modified with advanced glycation end products, was a major component of amyloid deposits in hemodialysis-associated amyloidosis and may be proinflammatory, acting to initiate and perpetuate inflammatory destruction of bone and joint tissues (79,80).

Some of the rheumatic complaints and findings associated with dialysis-related amyloidosis include chronic shoulder pain with tenderness over the subacromial bursae, pain and swelling of the wrist and finger joints, proliferative tenosynovitis involving the wrist extensor tendons, and intractable hand pain from carpal tunnel syndrome (77). The destructive nature of this arthropathy, unusual with other forms of amyloid, is evident from radiographic evidence of subchondral erosions of the carpal bones, femur, and humerus, sometimes associated with pathologic fractures of the femur and humerus. Involvement of the spine, unique to this amyloid type, may be associated with severe neurologic sequelae (81).

Management of dialysis-related amyloidosis is difficult. Efforts to effectively remove this protein using conventional dialysis membranes of cellulose acetate or cuprophane have not been successful due to poor protein clearance. Furthermore, these membranes induce complement activation and generation of interleukin-1, which may result in β_2-microglobulin accumulation and chemical modification. A new group of synthetic high-flux, highly permeable dialysis membranes (polycarbonate, polymethyl methacrylate, and polyacrylonitrile) is currently available but it is unknown if their use prevents β_2-microglobulin amyloid formation.

Although absorbent columns may remove β_2-microglobulin from blood, currently this is not a feasible approach to the problem (82). Endoscopic surgery to decompress the carpal tunnel and remove amyloid has been reported to be effective in dialysis patients (83). Finally, there has been a report of symptomatic improvement after renal transplantation (84).

The diagnosis of amyloidosis is made by detecting amyloid deposits in tissue preparations stained with Congo red, which emit an apple-green birefringence using polarized light microscopy. If a patient is suspected of having one of the systemic amyloidoses (AL, AA, ATTR), aspiration and staining of abdominal subcutaneous fat tissue should be performed. It can be done at the bedside quickly and safely. Fat tissue is obtained using a 16-gauge needle fixed to a 20- to 30-cc syringe. Repeated movements of the needle with gentle pulling of the syringe barrel to produce negative pressure should yield fragments of the fatty tissue (85). The fatty fluid and fragments are placed on alcohol-cleaned glass slides, air dried, and submitted for Congo red staining. There are reports of variable false-negative results, in which case a repeat biopsy of the subcutaneous tissue or of an alternative site such as the rectal mucosa is warranted. The redundant mucosal folds of the rectum (valves of Houston) may be directly visualized, tissue (including the vascular submucosa) obtained by pincer forceps, and bleeding controlled by cautery. Other biopsy sites include carpal tunnel tissue, kidney, sural nerve, heart (endomyocardial biopsy of right ventricle), bone, and synovium. Staining of amyloid deposits in synovial fluid of AL and Aβ_2-microglobulin patients has been described. In general, biopsy of the liver should be avoided due to the risk of bleeding. Attempts to define the chemical amyloid type should be undertaken. For example, specific antisera to κ and λ light chains, SAA, β_2-microglobulin, and transthyretin are commercially available for staining of the tissue using immunofluorescent or immunoperoxidase methods.

Immunotactoid glomerulonephritis and POEMS syndrome [polyneuropathy, organomegaly (splenomegaly, hepatomegaly, and lymphadenopathy), endocrinopathy (hypogonadism, hypothyroidism, and diabetes mellitus), monoclonal gammopathy, and skin changes (generalized hyperpigmentation, hypertrichosis, and skin thickening)] are included in the differential diagnoses of amyloidosis. Immunotactoid glomerulonephritis is a rare renal disorder characterized by the mesangial deposition of fibrillary material that does not stain with Congo red dye but is reactive with antipolyclonal immunoglobulin staining (immunotactoid) (86,87). POEMS syndrome is a rare multisystem disorder that may be a variant of myeloma (88,89).

In patients with suspected AL with or without myeloma, agarose gel electrophoresis of serum and concentrated urine may easily be performed (see above). Bone marrow aspiration and biopsy is usually performed to quantify the number of plasma cells and define myeloma. The bone marrow can then be stained for amyloid. Diagnosis by scintigraphy using radiolabeled P-component, which binds to all amyloid types, is considered an experimental procedure and its use cannot be justified currently as a screening or routine test.

HEMOGLOBINOPATHIES

Over 100 different hemoglobinopathies have been defined, but it is sickle cell anemia and its variants, in which the abnormal hemoglobin tends to crystallize or gel, the thalassemia syndromes, in which the hemoglobin chains are synthesized at unequal rates, or combinations of these two disorders that are associated with significant musculoskeletal pain and debility.

In the United States, *sickle cell anemia* (HbSS) occurs almost exclusively in African American patients who are homozygous for the sickle cell gene (approximately 0.2% of the African American population). In contrast, approximately 10% of those with sickle cell trait (HbSA) are symptomatic. All major clinical syndromes occur as a consequence of chronic hemolysis or acute intermittent crises related to vasocclusion, which may lead to end-organ failure (90,91). Local factors promoting red cell sickling include hypoxemia, acidosis, and red cell dehydration (92). Furthermore, sickled erythrocytes demonstrate an adhesiveness to endothelial cells, monocytes, and macrophages, and become aggregated and trapped leading to vessel occlusion (92,93). This vasocclusive process causes infarction of bone marrow and adjacent subchondral, trabecular, cortical bone, and muscle producing the various rheumatic disease syndromes (94).

Several hemoglobinopathies, clearly distinct from sickle cell anemia, but involving hemoglobin S, also feature musculoskeletal syndromes. The encompassing term *sickle cell disease* is used to describe these distinct entities that include sickle cell anemia (HbSS), sickle cell trait (HbSA), sickle cell–hemoglobin C disease (HbSC), sickle cell-α thalassemia (HbS-α (Thal), sickle cell-βE thalassemia (homozygote–no β-globin product) (HbS-βE Thal), and sickle cell-β^+ thalassemia (low synthesis of β-globin product) (HbS-β^+ Thal).

Musculoskeletal symptoms have been reported to occur in greater than 80% of patients with sickle cell anemia, and the distinction between the various clinical manifestations is often difficult but imperative since the treatments may differ considerably. True joint involvement, manifesting as a transient polyarthritis or monarthritis with warmth, swelling, or tenderness, is usually observed in association with sickle cell crises. In a survey of 70 patients with sickle cell disease followed over a period of 6 to 18 months, 32 developed a transient arthritis most commonly involving the knees but also elbows and hands, and they complained of pain in the lumbosacral spine, usually lasting 3 to 10 days (95). Synovial fluid analysis of 13 patients demonstrated both inflammatory (eight patients) and noninflammatory (five patients) characteristics, and sickled red cells were observed in 7 of 13 samples. No evidence of crystal deposition or infection was found. The pathogenesis of these effusions is unknown, but the occurrence of the effusions with painful crises, the radiographic evidence of adjacent bone infarctions, and synovial biopsies demonstrating microvascular thrombosis with thickening of the basement membrane with few infiltrating inflammatory cells all suggest ischemic injury to the joint, bone marrow, and adjacent bony structures as the most likely etiology (96).

In some cases, when the arthritis is migratory and the patient exhibits fever, leukocytosis, and flow murmurs with an enlarged heart, acute rheumatic fever must be considered. Typically, the arthritis is self-limited (1 to 2 weeks), responds to analgesic therapy, and leaves no permanent deformities. There have been reports of a severe disabling arthropathy in older patients with repeated bone infarcts near the knee joint resembling severe osteoarthritis (97). Septic arthritis, gout, and RA have all been reported in patients with sickle cell disease, and it is imperative to aspirate a warm swollen joint since the treatments of acute gout and septic arthritis differ considerably. Two patients with sickle cell anemia in whom destruction of hyaline articular cartilage occurred in association with chronic synovitis have been reported (98). Another patient has been reported with polyarticular chondrolysis with severe bilateral hip joint space narrowing (99). Light microscopy study of specimens from both hips demonstrated severe cartilage erosion, cartilage fibrillation, loss of chondrocytes with deep clones most prominent around the tidemark and no infarction of subchondral bone. Electron microscopy studies disclosed partially occluded blood vessels and phagocytic cells containing red cell debris and crystalline hemoglobin-like material. These studies suggest that the extracellular release of inflammatory mediators by phagocytic cells could lead to joint injury and destruction.

Localized bone marrow infarction of the carpal and tarsal bones and phalanges (sickle cell dactylitis or hand-foot syndrome) may be associated with excruciating painful swelling, erythema, and warmth of hands and feet in early childhood, most commonly at 6 months to 2 years of age, but occasionally also in adulthood (100). The reason cited for this preferential age range is that the presence of fetal hemoglobin protects the fetus and neonate from erythrocyte sickling. During the first year, hemoglobin F decreases, hemoglobin S increases, and erythrocyte sickling begins, and virtually never occurs in these bones after the age of 2 years due to the retreat of red marrow from these bones as a result of continuous asymptomatic bone marrow infarction with subsequent marrow fibrosis. This phenomenon occurs only in sickle cell anemia and not in other sickle cell diseases. The description by Diggs (94) of the clinical-radiologic features of sickle cell dactylitis cannot be improved upon:

> The infant is brought to the physician because there is swelling of the hands and/or the feet, pain, local elevation of temperature, limitation of movement and exquisite tenderness. The skin is tight and smooth, and the skin folds are effaced. The swelling is non-pitting and nonfluctuant. The lesions are often bilateral and in rare instances may involve both hands and both feet at the same time. There is fever and neutrophilic leukocytosis. Recurrences are frequent. Ischemic necrosis of marrow in the small bones of wrists, ankles or distal long bones may be coincident with infarcts of the bones of hands and feet. Roentgenograms taken during the first few days of pain reveal no abnormality other than soft-tissue swelling. After 10 to 14 days, when the symptoms are subsiding or have disappeared, roentgenologic changes appear. The lesions consist of periosteal elevation, subperiosteal new-bone formation and radiolucent areas intermingled with areas of increased density, giving a moth-eaten appearance. In rare instances, there may be a complete absence of visible calcific bone. In most instances, several tubular bones are affected at one time, with maximal involvement in the tarsal and the carpal bones and the proximal phalanges.

Long bone (diaphyseal) infarcts may be associated with recurrent attacks of excruciating pain and tenderness over bone with swelling/warmth mimicking soft tissue abscess or osteomyelitis (101). Infarction of trabecular bone is asymptomatic, but those involving a localized segment of the cortex may evoke a periosteal inflammatory reaction leading to the formation of an opacified thin line parallel to the shaft reflecting subperiosteal new bone formation (102). Diaphyseal infarction of larger tubular bones may lead to large areas of osteosclerosis simulating "bone-within-bone" appearance. In some cases, the osteosclerosis may be extensive and appear radiographically similar to Paget's disease or osteoblastic metastases. This occurs most commonly in HbSS but also in HbSC, HbS-α Thal, and least commonly in sickle cell trait. Typically, infarction of bone occurs in segments and does not involve the full circumferential thickness of the cortex.

Osteonecrosis of the femoral and humeral head is directly related to vascular occlusion of the cancellous and bony trabecula of the epiphysis of the proximal humerus and femur, usually in a symmetric manner, but occasionally occurs in other bones such as the distal humerus, distal femur, and talus (101–105). The patients usually report the insidious onset of aching while weight bearing or moving the involved joint. There may be an abrupt worsening of pain with any use or with rest. The pain may be severe and intractable but improves over time.

Osteonecrosis of the hip may be a difficult diagnostic and therapeutic problem (see Chapter 108). Arthrocentesis under fluoroscopy is indicated to rule out septic arthritis in the febrile patient presenting with acute hip pain and restricted hip flexion and internal rotation. Plain radiographs are unremarkable during the early stages of osteonecrosis until the repair process has changed the density of bone (cystic changes or osteosclerosis) (101). MRI may detect early osteonecrosis, but progressive changes are determined by radiologic staging (104). Most, but not all, patients with osteonecrosis have significant pain and debility. In a study of femoral head osteonecrosis as a complication of sickle cell disease, 2,590 patients age 5 or older were screened and followed for an average of 5.6 years (105). At study entry, 9.8% of patients were found to have osteonecrosis of one or both femoral heads. Over the follow-up period, the incidence of femoral head osteonecrosis, using age-adjusted rates for the sickle cell diseases, were HbSS-α Thal 4.46; HbS-βE 3.63; HBS-β^+ 2.35; HbSS 2.35; and HbSC 1.91. The frequency of painful crises and packed red cell volume were positively associated with osteonecrosis. While total hip arthroplasty is considered generally to be an effective treatment for femoral head osteonecrosis, some evidence suggests otherwise. In one study, 27 patients had total hip arthroplasties with 5 of the 27 requiring reoperation within 11 to 53 months of the initial surgery (105). Many continued to have significant pain with weight bearing. In another series of 22 total hip arthroplasties in 14 patients with sickle cell disease, there was a high perioperative complication rate ascribed to femoral intramedullary sclerosis and osteoporosis due to marrow hyperplasia (106).

Osteomyelitis is reported to occur approximately 100 times more frequently in patients with sickle cell disease than in normal individuals, with salmonella being the most common causative organism (107–113). Unfortunately, the onset of clinical osteomyelitis cannot be differentiated from diaphyseal infarctions since bone pain, fever, leukocytosis, and normal bone films are common to both. Over time, however, the presence of spiking fevers, persistent pain lasting more than 4 to 5 days, positive blood cultures, and changes on bone radiographs showing localized demineralization and periosteal elevation suggest osteomyelitis. Osteomyelitis may involve multiple bone sites (polyostotic), and both salmonella osteomyelitis and streptococcal soft tissue infections may mimic sickle cell dactylitis, but usually involve one hand or one foot. The definitive diagnosis of osteomyelitis can only be made by culture of material removed from beneath the periosteum before antibiotic treatment is initiated, however.

Hyperuricemia occurs in approximately 50% of adults with sickle cell disease, but gout is an uncommon finding (114). Likewise, septic arthritis is rarely seen in sickle cell disease patients in the United States. In a series of 600 children followed for 10 years, three cases of septic arthritis occurred and resulted from direct extension of osteomyelitis from adjacent bone (115). In contrast, in a total of 266 patients with sickle cell disease in Nigeria, 31 patients had 50 septic joints, most of which resulted from direct extension into the joint space from adjacent bone infection (116). Severe complications occurred in 76% of the cases due to delayed recognition and treatment and the high frequency of hip involvement.

Myonecrosis is a newly described complication of sickle cell disease. There have been reports describing myofascial pain with induration, tenderness, and swelling in adult patients (HbSS) during crises. In some cases, small painful swollen areas resembling furuncles were thought to occur at needle puncture sites. Drainage of purulent material from these sites and positive cultures for polymicrobial organisms suggested pyomyositis. Larger areas of symmetric induration and swelling over proximal muscle groups of the arms/legs remote from needle injections were observed subsequently. However, in four well-studied patients, muscle biopsy demonstrated acute myonecrosis with a minimal inflammatory response and occasional myofibrosis (117). No evidence suggesting pyomyositis was found. The clinical course of the four patients improved with symptomatic treatment. Some patients had recurrent symptoms and subsequent crises resulted in permanent sequelae of muscle atrophy, induration, and contractures.

These musculoskeletal complications of sickle cell disease result from local tissue thrombosis and infarction. Hyperplasia of bone marrow is also associated with skeletal abnormalities such as widening of medullary cavities, thinning of the trabeculae (osteoporosis), and depression of the upper and lower surfaces of the vertebral bodies (102).

Treatment protocols to prevent the vasocclusive, hemolytic and infectious complications of sickle cell disease are evolving and encouraging with regard to lengthening life span and also improving quality of life (93).

The *thalassemia syndromes* are characterized by an imbalanced synthesis of normal globin chains caused by mutations that impair either production or translation of globin messenger RNA. This reduction in globin chain production results in the formation of abnormally shaped erythroid precursor cells, which are short-lived, and die in the marrow or are prematurely destroyed in the circulation.

The β-thalassemias are characterized by diminished production of β-globin chains, which results in the accumulation and aggregation of excess α-globin chains. β-Thalassemia may exist in a homozygous form (Cooley's anemia), which is characterized by a severe anemia presenting within the first year of life with hepatosplenomegaly, jaundice, and marrow hyperplasia with skeletal changes. In β-thalassemia, the most severe form, no β-globin chains are synthesized. In β^+-thalassemia, which is less severe, small amounts of β chains and small quantities of hemoglobin A, in addition to hemoglobins A^2 and F, are found. Skeletal abnormalities, such as osteoporosis with/without pathologic fractures, delayed bone growth and short stature, and a lower extremity arthritis syndrome, are direct consequences of marrow hyperplasia (102).

Osteoporosis is common and usually severe, involving bones of the axial and appendicular skeleton. Bone expansion is associated with both marked trabecular and cortical thinning, cystic lesions, and associated osteopenia. Spontaneous recurrent fractures are not uncommon and most frequently involve the femur, tibia, forearm, and vertebrae (102). Growth disturbances with epiphyseal deformities related to premature closure of the epiphyses is a common finding in children with β-thalassemia. Erlenmeyer flask–shaped deformities with loss of normal concavity are seen in long bones. Bone reinforcement lines, which appear as transverse radiodense lines, also are seen frequently in long bones. Other radiographic fractures related directly to marrow hyperplasia include a "hair-on-end" appearance due to bony proliferation of the outer table of the vault, reduction of the air spaces of the paranasal sinuses due to bony expansion of the nasal and temporal bones, and maxillary alterations associated with hypertelorism and dental malocclusion, producing the "rodent-like" face (102).

A distinctive arthritis syndrome has been described in patients with β-thalassemia major (118). Twenty-four of 50 patients ranging from 5 to 23 years of age had tenderness to bone compression about the ankle joint over the malleoli, calcaneus, and midfoot. Two patients were wheelchair-bound because of ankle fractures. Eighteen patients had ankle pain that was precipitated by weight bearing and exertion but did not limit walking. Four patients could not ambulate without assistive devices because of incapacitating lower extremity pain. Two of these patients had effusions that were not inflammatory. Synovial biopsy demonstrated synovial lining cell hyperplasia and a heavy deposition of hemosiderin. Radiographic changes included marked reduction in trabecular and cortical bone consistent with severe osteoporosis and the presence of microfractures. Histologic studies of bone tissue revealed the presence of microfractures with increased resorptive and osteoid seams with iron deposition at the cement line and calcification front. Thus, thalassemic osteoarthropathy is considered to be due to juxtaarticular bone disease, but the role of iron overload in this disorder remains unknown.

Heterozygous β-thalassemia (thalassemia minor) is associated with milder clinical findings than thalassemia major, including a milder anemia, splenomegaly, and jaundice. Two arthritis forms have been reported in thalassemia minor (119–121). One type involves a chronic pauciarticular, asymmetric, seronegative arthropathy without detectable effusions with a predilection for the wrists, knees, and ankles (119). Juxtaarticular osteopenia without erosions or joint space narrowing of the involved joints was noted. An acute asymmetric arthritis lasting less than 10 days and described as "gout-like" also has been reported (120). Routine laboratory studies including ESR were normal. The synovial fluid white count ranged from 1,500 to 8,000 cells/mm^3 and consisted mostly of mononuclear cells. No crystals of monosodium urate or calcium pyrophosphate were observed. Synovial biopsy performed in two patients revealed nonspecific, mildly inflammatory synovitis. Radiographic studies were unremarkable. In another study of 80 patients with thalassemia minor, 52% complained of chronic pain (arthralgias) in the hands, wrists, and shoulders, and 4% had experienced arthritic attacks of short duration as described earlier (121). Finally, bilateral femoral head avascular necrosis has been reported in a 28-year-old woman with this condition (122).

HEMOPHILIA AND BLEEDING DISORDERS

Hemophilia is a group of disorders of blood coagulation due to a functional deficiency of a specific plasma clotting factor (123). Classic hemophilia (hemophilia A) and Christmas disease (hemophilia B) are deficiencies of factors VIII and IX, respectively. Approximately 80% of hemophiliac patients have hemophilia A. Both hemophilia A and B are X-linked recessive diseases and are associated with recurrent spontaneous and traumatic hemarthroses. The frequency and severity of the bleeding complications of hemophilia are related to the quantity of coagulation factor. For example, patients with 5% to 40% of normal activity (mild hemophilia) do well unless experiencing surgery or major trauma; those with 1% to 5% (moderate hemophilia) of normal activity have occasional spontaneous hemorrhage, but usually bleeding is provoked by trauma; and those with <1% (severe hemophilia) have frequent spontaneous hemarthroses and bleeding (123,124). There are several musculoskeletal manifestations of hemophilia; the most common are hemarthroses and muscle hemorrhage, with some patients developing a chronic arthritis and end-stage arthropathy (124,125). Some of these anatomic and radiographic changes are illustrated in Figs. 94.5 and 94.6.

Nearly all patients with severe hemophilia experience hemarthroses. Hemathroses first become manifest when the child begins to walk and run, between the ages of 12 and 24 months, and are a recurrent problem until adulthood. The most commonly affected joints are the knees, ankles, elbows, and shoulders. Bleeding into the joints of the fingers, wrists, feet, and axial spine is distinctly unusual. The patient can sense the hemarthroses developing with stiffness, fullness, and tingling, followed by pain and swelling of the joint. The patient often cannot tolerate any weight on the knee or ankle and must use crutches or a wheelchair. The joint is typically warm, swollen, and tender, and the patient will often have a low-grade fever.

The duration and severity of hemarthroses and subsequent joint deformity may be decreased substantially by prompt institution of factor replacement therapy. In practice, this should be started immediately during the prodromal symptoms while the patient is at home by infusing a dose of factor VIII concentrate to achieve a factor VIII activity of approximately 50% of normal and by immobilization of the joint for 3 to 4 days. Factor VIII infusions are

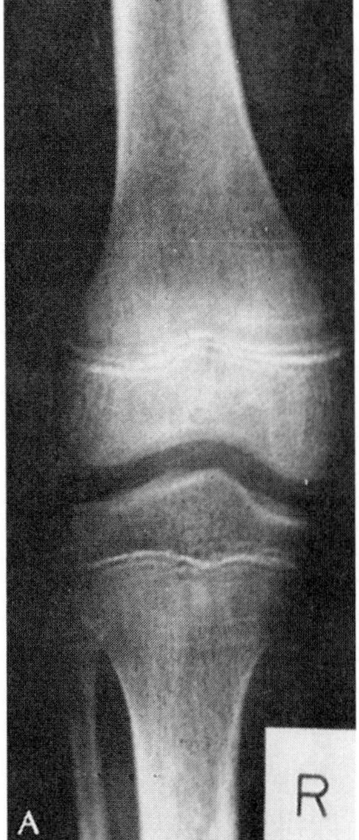

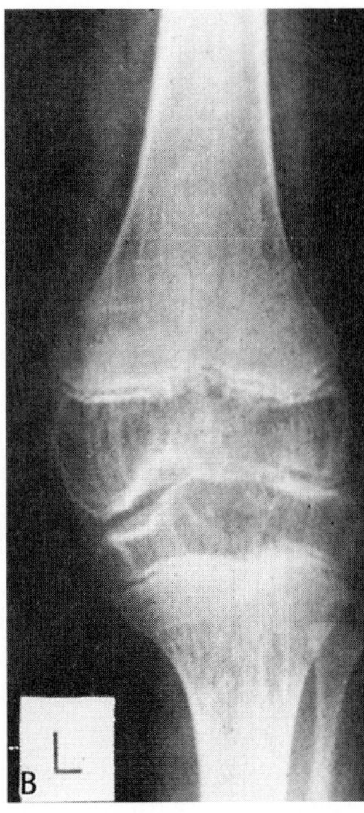

FIGURE 94.5. Radiographs of the knees of a 9-year-old boy with hemophilia and repeated hemarthroses involving the left knee. **A:** The right knee, which appears normal. **B:** The left knee. Note the loss of articular cartilage, the irregularity of bony surfaces, and the hypertrophy of the epiphyses of the femur and tibia.

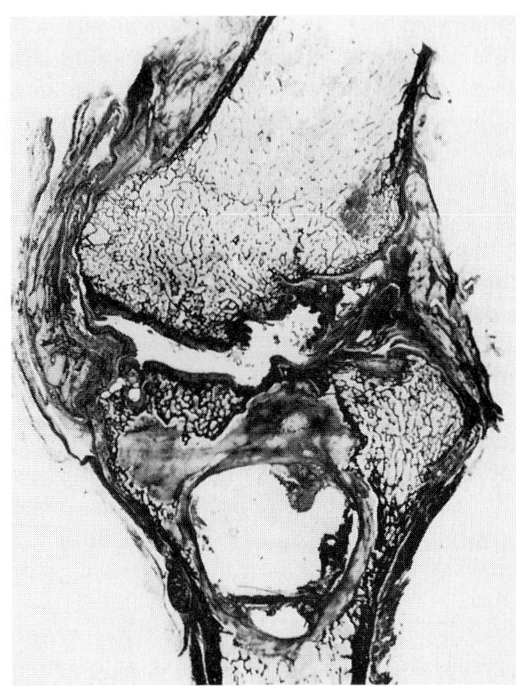

FIGURE 94.6. Sagittal section of the knee joint of a 49-year-old man with advanced hemophilic arthropathy. The femoral condyle appears flattened and the patella has virtually disappeared. The head of the tibia has undergone massive cystic resorption. The articular cartilage has disappeared from most of the joint surfaces, which have undergone partial fibrous ankylosis on the popliteal aspect on the right and have been replaced by fibrous tissue. The cyst in the tibia is lined by loose-textured fibrous tissue. The synovial and capsular tissues are thickened and infiltrated with many hemosiderin-laden mononuclear cells.

continued at one-half the initial dose every 8 hours for 2 days or until cessation of bleeding.

Unfortunately, many patients who received factor VIII cryoprecipitate in the late 1970s and 1980s became seropositive for HIV and hepatitis viruses B and C and died as a consequence of these illnesses (125,126). Infusions of recombinant factor VIII have been shown to be efficacious in the treatment of acute bleeding disorders and do not carry the risk of viral transmission, but, unfortunately, are expensive and thus are not routinely used (127). Currently, infusion of factor VIII concentrate is the preferred treatment for most patients with severe hemophilia A (126). Improved methods of screening donors, chemical and heat treatments of plasma concentrates, and immunoaffinity chromatography techniques have dramatically reduced (but not completely eliminated) the risks of viral transmission. After cessation of bleeding, physical therapy is then started to regain joint range of motion and to prevent contracture formation. Arthrocentesis is usually not indicated unless there is persistent fever, severe painful swollen joints, or neurovascular compromise, and it should never be performed unless the postinfusion factor deficiency is within the desired range (125).

Von Willebrand's disease is an autosomal-dominant disorder characterized by a variable decrease in factor VIII activity and prolonged bleeding time. It is not typically thought of as a disorder of recurrent hemarthroses and chronic arthritis (123). However, three reports have linked recurrent hemarthroses and chronic arthropathy with the degree of coagulation defect (factor VIII activity) (128–130). Two siblings with Glanzmann's thrombasthenia with recurrent hemarthroses and the occurrence of a chronic hemophiliac-like arthritis in the elbow of one sibling have been reported (131). A 47-year-old man with recurrent hemarthroses of the right ankle associated with factor XIII (fibrin stabilizing factor) deficiency has been reported, and 16 other cases were reviewed (132). Finally, hemarthroses and chronic arthritis have occurred in acquired hemorrhagic disorders associated with anticoagulant use (133–135).

Recurrent hemarthroses may lead to a chronic arthritis in which iron-containing, superficial lining cells of the synovium become hyperplastic. This hyperplastic synovial tissue, usually devoid of inflammatory cells, may form into an invasive pannus tissue, associated with marginal erosions of cortical bone and thinning of hyaline articular cartilage (124,125).

End-stage arthropathy is a result of chronic arthritis of one or more joints. Typically, there is bony enlargement, joint space narrowing with fibrous adhesions, restricted range of joint motion, marked flexion contractures, and muscle atrophy. Pain may be a prominent symptom, but usually it is not the major symptom. The chronic arthropathy affects only a few joints, most notably the knees and elbows, but the effective use of an extremity is severely compromised. Other joints such as shoulders, hips, and ankles are involved but to a lesser degree (125).

The chronic proliferative synovitis resulting from recurrent hemarthroses is associated with limitation of motion and radiographic progression of hemophiliac arthropathy. Open synovectomy has been demonstrated to reduce the number of hemarthroses and improve knee symptoms, but did not result in improved joint range of motion. Arthroscopic surgery is often effective in treating proliferative synovitis and is associated with minimal perioperative morbidity (136). With advanced joint disease, particularly of the knee associated with severe pain and limitation, total knee arthroplasty should be considered (137,138). The major contraindication is the presence of high titer factor VIII inhibitor.

Hemorrhage into muscles, bone, and soft tissues can present special problems (125). Bleeding into the thighs, calves, and forearms is common and may lead to myonecrosis, scarring, and flexion contracture. Bleeding into the gastrocnemius-soleus muscle may lead to a fixed talipes equinus deformity or to a compartment syndrome, which results when blood accumulates at a high-enough pressure within a closed muscle compartment, reducing capillary perfusion below that necessary to maintain tissue viability. In hemophilia, the most common compartment syndrome results from bleeding into the volar forearm muscles. If the pressure remains elevated for several hours, the normal function of muscles and nerves is compromised and, over time, muscle infarction and nerve injury lead to Volkmann's ischemic contracture. Prompt recognition and decompression with a fasciotomy is critical to restore adequate blood flow to ischemic tissues. Iliopsoas hemorrhage may compress the femoral nerve between the iliopectineal ligament and inguinal ligament, leading to muscle weakness and atrophy. Hemophiliac pseudotumors may result from subperiosteal or intraosseous hemorrhages. Retroperitoneal hemorrhage and bleeding about the tongue, mouth, or neck may impair respiration and may be life threatening (125).

Septic arthritis has been considered to be a rare complication of hemophilia. This view must be altered, however, due to the increasing number of reports detailing septic arthritis in predominantly HIV-positive hemophiliac patients (139).

LIPID STORAGE DISEASES

Clinically, there are three types of *Gaucher's disease*, an autosomal-recessive lysosomal glycolipid storage disease characterized by the accumulation of glucosylceramide in cells of the reticuloendothelial system (140). The three types are defined by the absence (type 1) or presence (types 2 and 3) and severity (type 2) of central nervous system involvement. All forms of Gaucher's disease are associated with hepatosplenomegaly and osteoporotic bone lesions and variable involvement of other organs. Type 1 Gaucher's disease, which accounts for more than 95% of the total cases, occurs most commonly as a familial disorder in Ashkenazi Jews. It is characterized by the lack of central nervous system involvement and variable degrees of severity and age of onset. For example, children up to age 10 may be diagnosed with massive hepatosplenomegaly associated with thrombocytopenia, hypersplenism, and skeletal abnormalities, or patients may be elderly at the time of diagnosis. Some patients may never come to medical attention. Type 2 (infantile form or neuronopathic form), which is seen in all ethnic groups, is usually apparent at 3 to 6 months of age and death occurs within the first 2 years of life. In patients with type 3 (juvenile form or Norrbottnian (Swedish) type), neurologic symptoms occur later and the course is more chronic and milder than type 2.

All the cells of the body are deficient in lysosomal β-glucosidase activity. In most cases, the enzyme is present but exhibits a decreased catalytic activity. A variety of mutations coding for β-glucosidase have been found to cause Gaucher's disease. Certain mutations cluster within a type, but there is varied phenotypic expression within all the genotypes.

It is the infiltrating glycosylceramide-laden macrophages that account for most, if not all, nonneurologic features of the disease. In general, musculoskeletal features may appear early in the course of Gaucher's disease, but are rarely the first symptom of the disease.

Skeletal manifestations may be extremely debilitating in types 1 and 3 disease (140). Approximately 20% to 40% of patients experience episodic, severe, bone pain in the hips, shoulders, and vertebrae. These attacks are more common within the first two decades but may also occur in later life. Typically, the attacks occur suddenly with a deep aching pain in the involved bone, which intensifies over the next 2 to 3 days and becomes excruciating in nature requiring narcotic medications. Within several days, the intense pain subsides to an aching pain, which persists for another 1 to 2 weeks. These bone crises, sometimes associated with fever, and reminiscent of sickle cell crises, have been termed "pseudo-osteomyelitis" (141). Microscopic examination of bony lesions demonstrates necrosis consistent with ischemic bone infarction and elevated intramedullary pressure due to resultant edema. An acute arthritis involving proximal interphalangeal joints, initially misdiagnosed as JRA, has been described in a 10-year-old boy with type 1 disease (142).

Radiographic bone abnormalities in Gaucher's disease are frequently seen even in those without skeletal pain. The Erlenmeyer-flask deformity of the distal femur is the most characteristic and common radiographic finding but is not invariably present. Generalized bone loss with pathologic fractures and vertebral body collapse with severe axial spine deformities may result. The vertebral collapse occurs most commonly in adolescent children during the pubertal growth spurt. Although children may complain of hip pain, avascular necrosis of the femur occurs later and pathologic fractures of the femoral neck occur more commonly in patients older than 30 (143). An example of avascular necrosis of the head of the femur is shown in Fig. 94.7.

In the past, the diagnosis of Gaucher's disease has been based on the presence of the glycosylceramide-laden cell (Gaucher cell) in various tissues. However, similar-appearing cells (pseudo-Gaucher cells) have been described in a variety of diseases associated with various cytopenias and hepatomegaly. Today, the most specific assays are biochemical quantitation of β-glucosidase activity in peripheral blood leukocytes and cultured skin fibroblasts. Furthermore, the DNA from these cells can be analyzed for mutations of the enzymes (140).

Enzyme replacement therapy using infusions of purified, modified human placental β-glucosidase (alglucerase) has been shown to be clinically effective but is extremely costly. Likewise, recombinant enzyme is anticipated to be very costly. Bone marrow transplantation can cure the disease but is currently considered a high-risk form of treatment. The feasibility of curing Gaucher's disease using gene therapy (transfer) is under consideration.

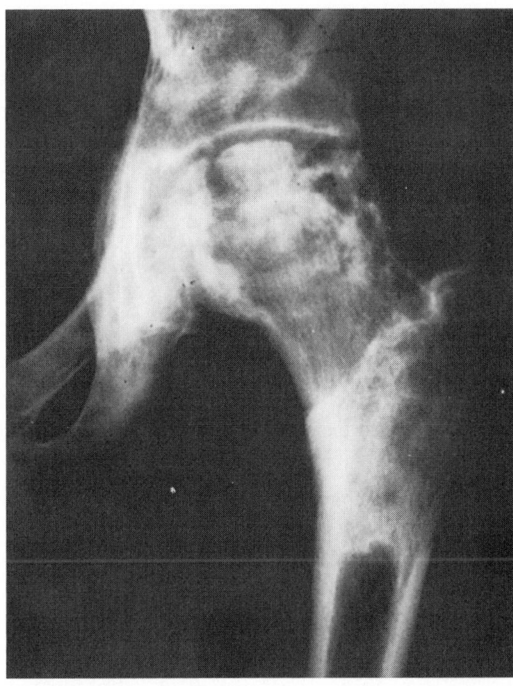

FIGURE 94.7. Radiograph of the left hip joint of a 22-year-old man with Gaucher's disease illustrating avascular necrosis of the head of the femur. This radiograph was obtained 2 years after the onset of pain in the hip.

Fabry's disease is an X-linked disorder of glycosphingolipid catabolism characterized by progressive systemic deposition of glycosphingolipids, predominantly globotriaosylceramide in lysosomes of endothelial, perithelial, and smooth-muscle cells of blood vessels (144). Pathologic storage may also occur in ganglion cells and in other cell types within the heart, eye, kidneys, bone marrow, and other tissues. Hemizygous males deficient in α-galactosidase A are affected; most heterozygous female carriers have an intermediate level of enzymatic activity and are asymptomatic. The clinical manifestations result directly from vascular glycolipid deposition (144–149). For example, the typical clusters of bluish to dark red angiokeratoma, which are more common in areas between the knees and buttocks and increase with age, are punctate telangiectasias, which may be flat or raised, do not blanch with applied pressure, and are venules with multiple layers of basement membrane within the vessel walls. These skin lesions are often missed, so the diagnosis is delayed. The usual clinical picture is that of an adolescent boy presenting with unexplained proteinuria and an abnormal urine sediment containing red cells, casts, and birefringent lipid globules detected by polarized light microscopy. There is gradual deterioration in renal function. Both cerebrovascular and cardiovascular insufficiency may result from multifocal small vessel occlusive disease and may be accentuated by hypertension from renal vascular disease. Death usually occurs after age 40 as a complication of vascular disease.

Pain may be a severe debilitating symptom of Fabry's disease and may be either intermittent or continuous (144–146). The severe intermittent crises may begin in childhood or adolescence and may herald the onset of the disease. Typically, the acral or solar areas are initially involved, but the pain may radiate to other areas of the body including the abdomen and back. In general, the periodic crises decrease with age. Many patients complain of daily intermittent paresthesias of the palmer and solar areas in the late afternoon. It is estimated that 10% to 20% of patients have no history of severe crises or acroparesthesias. Hypohidrosis is an early and constant finding, but some patients may have anhidrosis. The excruciating pain, acroparesthesias, and hypohidrosis are thought to result from glycolipid deposits in the ganglion cells of the autonomic nervous system.

Some patients develop a polyarthritis with swelling of the fingers, elbows, and knees. The most characteristic deformity, however, is in the distal interphalangeal joint causing limited extension (150). Avascular necrosis of the head of the femur or talus and multiple small opacities in the femoral head may be seen. Involvement of the temporomandibular joint, metacarpals, and metatarsal joints has been described. The mechanism of arthropathy is unclear. In one study, synovial biopsy of a proximal interphalangeal joint disclosed "foam" cells in the subsynovial and capsular capillaries without inflammation (150). Since the patient had prolonged distal latency but normal conduction velocities by nerve conduction studies, the authors suggested that the joint pain may have been related to neuroischemia.

The clinical diagnosis of Fabry's disease requires biochemical quantification of reduced α-galactosidase activity in plasma, leukocytes, or tears, or increased levels of globotriaosylceramide in plasma or urine sediment. Treatment has consisted of carbamazedine or diphenylhydantoin for agonizing pain, prophylactic oral anticoagulants for stroke-prone patients, and renal dialysis and kidney transplantation for end-stage renal disease. Therapeutic approaches involving replacement therapy and fetal liver transplantation have been reviewed (144).

Farber's disease (lipogranulomatosis) is a rare, autosomal-recessive disorder of infancy associated with tissue accumulation of ceramide due to a deficiency of lysosomal acid ceramidase (151). In studies of fewer than 50 patients, seven phenotypic subtypes have been defined with most patients fitting into types 1 and 2. Death usually occurs between 6 months and 2 years. This disease may be confused with systemic onset or polyarticular JRA (152) since the cardinal manifestations are painful swelling of proximal interphalangeal and metacarpophalangeal joints, wrists, elbows, knees, and ankles with a propensity to form severe flexion contractures. Other clinical features include subcutaneous nodules over pressure points and periarticular structures, and disturbances in respiration and swallowing due to involvement of the larynx and epiglottis involvement. Intermittent fever may be present. Other organs such as the heart, lungs, lymph nodes, and nervous system may be involved.

The mechanism of arthropathy appears to be the accumulation of macrophages and, in some instances, foam cells (granulomatosis infiltration) in synovial tissues and other organs with very little cellular reaction (153).

The diagnosis is based on demonstrating reduced functional activity of ceramidase in cultured skin fibroblasts or leukocytes. There is no specific therapy.

Lipochrome histiocytosis is an extremely rare familial lysosomal storage disease marked by pulmonary infiltrates, splenomegaly, polyarthritis, hypergammaglobulinemia, lipochrome pigmentation of histiocytes, and an increased susceptibility to infection (154,155). There is only one case report of arthritis associated with this disorder and this involved three sisters. One sister had intermittent polyarthritis and a biopsy-proven rheumatoid nodule; another had years of transient episodes of joint inflammation, then developed a symmetric polyarthritis, and the third had no rheumatic symptoms. All three had elevated titers of rheumatoid factor, hyperglobulinemia, and recurrent pulmonary infections. Metabolic and functional activity of peripheral blood leukocytes were studied in two of the sisters with lipochrome histiocytosis. A diminished capacity to reduce nitroblue tetrazolium dye with impaired respiration, hexose monophosphate shunt, and staphylococcal killing activity were found. This disorder is probably not a lipid storage disorder but rather a clinical variant of chronic granulomatous disease, even though a granulomatous response was not seen after examination of biopsy/autopsy tissues. Chronic granulomatous disease is reviewed elsewhere (156).

DISORDERS OF LIPID METABOLISM

Lipoprotein disorders, previously called hyperlipoproteinemias, result from a defect in either the synthesis or catabolism of lipoproteins. *Familial hypercholesterolemia* (previously called type IIa hyperlipoproteinemia) is an autosomal-dominant disorder caused by mutation in the gene encoding the low-density lipoprotein (LDL) receptor protein (157). In homozygotes with familial hypercholesterolemia, there is a functional or absolute LDL receptor deficiency resulting in high concentrations of LDL in connective tissue and arterial walls resulting in xanthomas and atherosclerosis. The prevalence is approximately one in 1 million people. Orange-yellow xanthomas develop usually before age 10 within the webbing of the fingers. Tendon xanthomas, typically within the extensor tendons of the hands and the Achilles tendon, subperiosteal olecranon and tibial tubercle nodules, and tuberous subcutaneous nodules are characteristically found. Coronary artery disease usually presents in the second decade of life. Homozygous familial hypercholesterolemia patients may have episodes of oligoarthritis or polyarthritis (158). Arthritis most commonly involves the knees or ankles, but also may involve the small joints of the hands or feet. These involved joints may be exquisitely tender, erythematous, and swollen. Attacks are self-limited, lasting several days to 10 to 14 days, thus resembling acute gout attacks. If the arthritis is a migratory polyarthritis, it may resemble acute rheumatic fever. No permanent joint damage has been reported. Recurrent acute tenosynovitis, with or without arthritis, may be a presenting symptom of familial hypercholesterolemia.

The heterozygous form of familial hypercholesterolemia is a common genetic disorder with a prevalence of about 1 in 500 people. In general, tendinous xanthomas usually appear in the second decade, and manifestations of coronary artery disease usually occur after the third decade (159–161). In the largest study of 73 patients with heterozygous familial hypercholesterolemia, 40% were reported to have had one episode of various rheumatic manifestations including Achilles tendon pain (18%), Achilles tendinitis (11%), oligoarticular arthritis (7%), and polyarticular or rheumatic fever-like arthritis (4%) (159).

Eruptive xanthomas over the back, shoulders, knees, and buttocks may be seen in types I, IV, and V hyperlipoproteinemias. Tendinous and tuberous xanthomas may occur in type III and IV hyperlipoproteinemias (162). Planar or palmer xanthomas occurring as yellow lipid deposits in the palmar creases are distinct for type III hyperlipoproteinemia (163).

Polyarthritis associated with elevated levels of very low density lipoprotein (VLDL) and triglyceride (previously called type IV hyperlipoproteinemia) has been reported (164,165). The arthritis typically presented as a persistent, bilateral, asymmetric oligoarthritis with minimal deformity. Synovial fluid analyses and synovial biopsies were performed in two patients. One synovial fluid analysis was inflammatory with a total white count of 8,050 of which 90% were mononuclear cells, whereas the other was reported as having 1,400 total white cells of which 60% were mononuclear cells. Both synovial biopsies demonstrated synovial cell layer hyperplasia, and only one demonstrated a mononuclear infiltrate. No crystals were seen by polarized light microscopy. Generalized osteoporosis was seen in five patients and bone cysts localized to the epiphyseal or metaphyseal regions were also observed in five patients. No joint space narrowing or periarticular erosions were noted. An example of paraarticular bone cysts in two patients with type IV hyperlipoproteinemia is shown in Fig. 94.8.

Eighty-eight consecutive patients with hyperlipidemia attending a lipid clinic [48 patients with adult familial hypercholesterolemia (ages 19 to 68); 16 patients with juvenile familial hypercholesterolemia (ages 5 to 16); and 24 patients with elevated cholesterol and triglycerides (mixed hyperlipidemia) (ages 19 to 69)] and 88 age/sex/race control patients with normal lipid levels were directly compared for rheumatic symptoms and physical findings (166). A significant association between the following were noted: tendon xanthomas (particularly the Achilles tendon) in patients with adult familial hypercholesterolemia and mixed hyperlipidemia; Achilles tendinitis in patients with adult familial hypercholesterolemia and mixed hyperlipidemia; and oligoarthritis in patients with mixed hyperlipidemia. Patients with juvenile familial hypercholesterolemia (38%) had rheumatic manifestations but did not significantly differ from that of the control group. The authors confirmed the findings from previous studies that rheumatic manifestations may predate the diagnosis of hyperlipidemia and that these manifestations may improve in patients treated with lipid-lowering agents (160,161, 164,165).

MULTICENTRIC RETICULOHISTIOCYTOSIS

Multicentric reticulohistiocytosis is a systemic disease of unknown etiology characterized by the infiltration of skin, synovia, and other tissues by lipid/periodic acid-Schiff

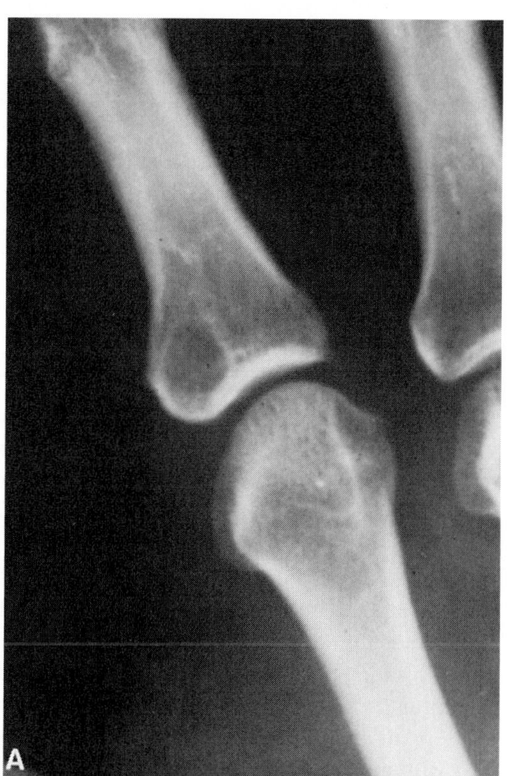

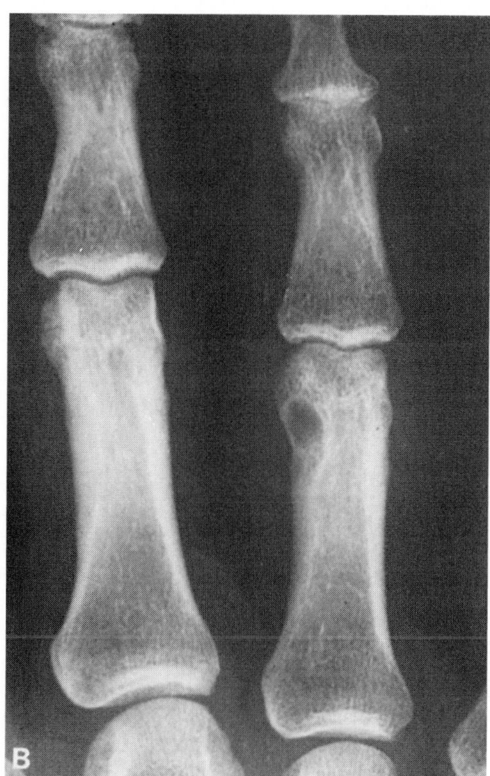

FIGURE 94.8. A and B: Radiographs showing prominent paraarticular bone cysts in the fingers of two patients with arthritis associated with type IV hyperlipoproteinemia. Both patients had polyarticular inflammatory disease.

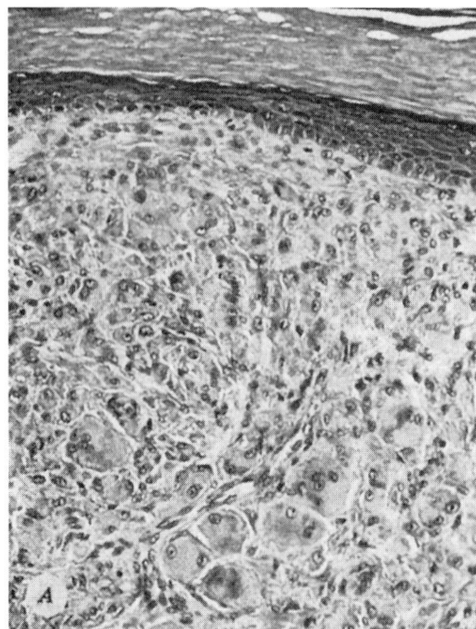

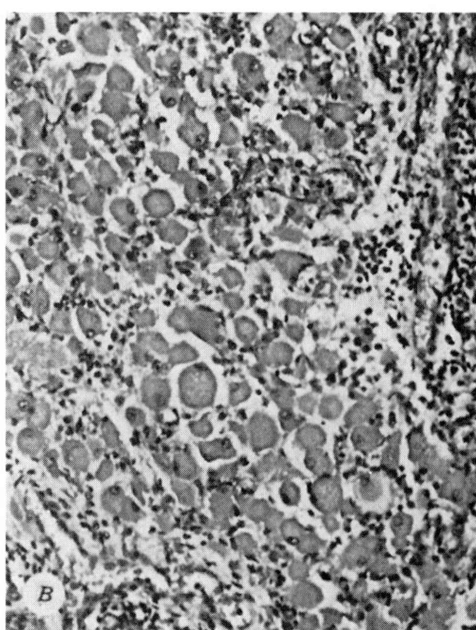

FIGURE 94.9. Photomicrograph of a skin nodule **(A)** and synovium (knee) **(B)** of a 54-year-old woman with multicentric reticulohistiocytosis. Numerous histiocytes and multinucleated giant cells contain large amounts of periodic acid-Schiff–positive material (×185).

(PAS)-laden histiocytes and multinucleated giant cells (167). A photograph illustrating the characteristic histologic features is shown in Fig. 94.9. At one time, multicentric reticulohistiocytosis was considered to represent a lipid storage disease, but no genetic association or consistent abnormality of serum lipoproteins or intracellular lipids has been defined. Other terms for this disorder have included *lipoid dermatoarthritis* and *normocholesterol xanthomatosis.* There is no known etiology.

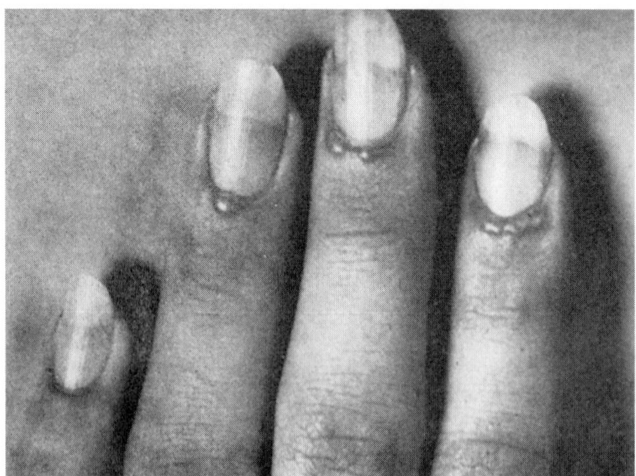

FIGURE 94.10. The fingers of a 16-year-old girl who had polyarthritis for 8 months and reddish brown "coral beads" around the nailfold for 5 months. Typical infiltrates of multicentric reticulohistiocytosis were found in biopsy specimens of both skin and synovium.

The natural course of this disease is variable. Systemic symptoms such as fever, weight loss, and generalized weakness may be prominent. Polyarthritis is the presenting sign in approximately 60% of cases followed by the appearance of nodular skin eruption months to years later. In the other 40% of cases, the skin nodules may accompany the arthritis or precede it. Typically, the arthritis resembles RA in that it is a symmetric inflammatory polyarthritis involving most commonly the distal interphalangeal joints but also other joints such as the proximal interphalangeal joints, metacarpophalangeal joints, metatarsophalangeal joints, knees, hips, shoulders, and elbows (167,168). Significant morning stiffness, warm, swollen joints, nodular lesions over the elbow extensor surfaces simulating rheumatoid nodules, and radiographic evidence of marginal erosions make this disorder difficult to distinguish from RA. Over time, the arthritis may worsen in approximately one-half of the patients leading to phalangeal resorption, marked shortening of the fingers, flail digits, and end-stage arthritis mutilans. Some patients may experience spontaneous remissions.

The skin nodules, which may vary from few to many hundred and measure from several millimeters to several centimeters, occur most frequently over the face, dorsum of the hands, ears, neck, forearms, and elbows. Small tumefactions around the nailfold termed "coral beads" are characteristic and are shown in Fig. 94.10. These cutaneous lesions may be discrete or coalesce into diffuse plaques. Furthermore, mucosal papules may occur over the lips, gingiva, tongue, buccal mucosa, and nasal septum. Less frequent complications include pericarditis, cardiac conduction abnormalities, pleuritis, pleural effusions, myositis, and paresthesias. Multicentric reticulohistiocytosis has been associated with various malignancies and may represent a paraneoplastic disorder in such cases (168). It is not clear from the current data whether the prevalence of malignancy is greater than that of an age-matched control group, however.

There is no standard treatment protocol for multicentric reticulohistiocytosis. In patients with mild arthritis, nonsteroidal antiinflammatory drugs and physical therapy should first be used. In more severe cases, treatment with either cyclophosphamide or chlorambucil for 6 to 24 months has induced complete remissions in five of six cases (169,170).

REFERENCES

1. Scriver CR, Beaudet AL, Sly WS, et al. *The metabolic and molecular bases of inherited disease,* 7th ed. New York: McGraw-Hill, 1995.
2. Crist WM, Pullen DJ, Rivera GK. Acute lymphoid leukemia. In: Fernbach DJ, Vietti TJ, eds. *Clinical pediatric oncology,* 4th ed. St. Louis: CV Mosby, 1991:305–335.
3. Fink CW, Windmiller J, Sartain P. Arthritis as the presenting feature of childhood leukemia. *Arthritis Rheum* 1972;15: 347–349.
4. Schaller J. Arthritis as a presenting manifestation of malignancy in children. *J Pediatr* 1972;81:793–797.
5. Brewer EJ. Differential diagnosis. In: Brewer EJ, Giannini EH, Person DA, eds. *Juvenile rheumatoid arthritis,* 2nd ed. Philadelphia: WB Saunders, 1982:78–100.
6. Aston JW Jr. Pediatric update #16. The orthopaedic presentation of neuroblastoma. *Orthop Rev* 1990;19:929–932.
7. Brodeur GM. Clinical and biological aspects on neuroblastoma. In: Scriver CR, Beaudet AL, Sly WS, et al., eds. *The metabolic and molecular bases of inherited disease,* 7th ed. New York: McGraw-Hill 1995:697–716.
8. Spilberg I, Meyer GJ. The arthritis of leukemia. *Arthritis Rheum* 1972;15:630–635.
9. Holdrinet RS, Corstens F, Van Horn JR, et al. Leukemic synovitis. *Am J Med* 1989;86:123–126.
10. Harden EA, Moore JO, Haynes BF. Leukemia associated arthritis: identification of leukemic cells in synovial fluid using monoclonal and polyclonal antibodies. *Arthritis Rheum* 1984; 27:1306–1308.
11. Fam AG, Voorneveld C, Robinson JB, et al. Synovial fluid immunocytology in the diagnosis of leukemic synovitis. *J Rheumatol* 1991;18:293–296.
12. Heaney ML, Golde DW. Myelodysplasia. *N Engl J Med* 1999; 340:1649–1660.
13. Castro M, Conn DL, Su WP, et al. Rheumatic manifestations in myelodysplastic syndrome. *J Rheumatol* 1991;18:721–727.
14. George SW, Newman ED. Seronegative inflammatory arthritis in the myelodysplastic syndromes. *Semin Arthritis Rheum* 1992; 21:345–354.
15. Kohli M, Bennett RM. The association of polymyalgia rheumatica with myeloplastic syndromes. *J Rheumatol* 1994;21: 1357–1359.
16. McCarthy CJ, Sheldon S, Ross CW, et al. Cytogenetic abnormalities and therapy-related myelodysplastic syndromes in rheumatic disease. *Arthritis Rheum* 1998;41:1493–1496.
17. Cheson BD, Sorensen JM, Vena DA, et al. Treatment of hairy cell leukemia with 2-chlorodeoxyadenosine via the Group C Protocol Mechanism of the National Cancer Institute: a report of 979 patients. *J Clin Oncol* 1998;16:3007–3015.
18. Elkon KB, Hughes GR, Catovsky D, et al. Hairy-cell leukaemia with polyarteritis nodosa. *Lancet* 1979;2:280–282.
19. Gabriel SE, Conn DL, Phyliky RL, et al. Vasculitis in hairy cell leukemia: review of literature and consideration of possible pathogenetic mechanisms. *J Rheumatol* 1986;13:1167–1172.
20. Gomez-Almaguer D, Herrera-Garza JL, Garcia-Guajardo BM, et al. Vasculitis in hairy-cell leukemia: rapid response to interferon alpha. *Am J Hematol* 1989;30:261–262.
21. Westbrook CA, Golde DW. Autoimmune disease in hairy cell leukemia: clinical syndromes and treatment. *Br J Haematol* 1985;61:349–356.
22. Carpenter MT, West SG. Polyarteritis nodosa in hairy cell leukemia: treatment with interferon-α. *J Rheumatol* 1994;21: 1150–1152.
23. Zervas J, Vayopoulos G, Kaklamanis PH, et al. Hairy-cell leukemia-associated polyarthritis: a report of two cases. *Br J Rheumatol* 1991;30:157–158.
24. Taylor HG, Davis MJ, Hothersall TE. Hairy cell leukaemia and rheumatoid arthritis. *Br J Rheumatol* 1991;30:391–192.
25. Demames DJ, Lane N, Beckstead JH. Bone involvement in hairy-cell leukemia. *Cancer* 1982;49:1697–1701.
26. Loughran TP Jr. Clonal diseases of large granular lymphocytes. *Blood* 1993;82:1–14.
27. Barton JC, Prasthofer EF, Egan ML, et al. Rheumatoid arthritis associated with expanded populations of granular lymphocytes. *Ann Intern Med* 1986;104:314–323.
28. Edelman MJ, O'Donnell RT, Meadows I. Treatment of refractory large granular lymphocytic leukemia with 2-chlorodeoxyadenosine. *Am J Hematol* 1997;54:329–331.
29. Resnick D. Myeloproliferative disorders in diagnosis of bone and joint disorders. In: Resnick D, ed. *Diagnosis of bone and joint disorders,* 2nd ed. Philadelphia: WB Saunders, 1988: 2459–2496.
30. VanSlyck EJ. The bony changes in malignant hematologic disease. *Orthop Clin North Am* 1972;3:733–744.
31. Foley KM. Advances in cancer pain. *Arch Neurol* 1999;56: 413–417.
32. Cherny NI, Portenoy RK. Cancer pain: principles of assessment and syndromes. In: Wall PD, Melzack R, eds. *Textbook of pain,* 3rd ed. Edinburgh: Churchill Livingstone, 1994:787–823.
33. Dorfman HD, Siegel HL, Perry MC, et al. Non-Hodgkin's lymphoma of the synovium simulating rheumatoid symptoms. *Arthritis Rheum* 1987;30:155–161.
34. Reimer RR, Chabner BA, Young RC, et al. Lymphoma presenting in bone: results of histopathology, staging, and therapy. *Ann Intern Med* 1977;87:50–55.
35. Steinberg AD, Seldin MF, Jaffe ES, et al. Angioimmunoblastic lymphadenopathy with dysproteinemia. *Ann Intern Med* 1988; 108:575–584.
36. Weiss LM, Strickler JG, Dorfman RF, et al. Clonal T cell populations in angioimmunoblastic lymphadenopathy and angioimmunoblastic lymphadenopathy-like lymphoma. *Am J Pathol* 1986;122:392–397.
37. Bignon YI, Janin-Mercier A, Dubost JJ, et al. Angioimmunoblastic lymphadenopathy with dysproteinaemia (AILD) and sicca syndrome. *Ann Rheum Dis* 1986;45:519–522.
38. McHugh NJ, Campbell GJ, Landreth JT. Polyarthritis and angioimmunoblastic lymphadenopathy. *Ann Rheum Dis* 1987; 46:555–558.
39. Boumpas DT, Wheby MS, Jaffe ES, et al. Synovitis in angioimmunoblastic lymphadenopathy with dysproteinemia simulating rheumatoid arthritis. *Arthritis Rheum* 1990;33:578–582.

40. Sallah S, Wehbie R, Lepera R, et al. The role of 2-chlorodeoxyadenosine in the treatment of patients with refractory angioimmunoblastic lymphadenopathy with dysproteinemia. *Br J Haematol* 1999;104:163–165.
41. Seleznick MJ, Aguilar JL, Rayhack J, et al. Polyarthritis associated with cutaneous T-cell lymphoma. *J Rheumatol* 1989;16: 1379–1382.
42. Berger RG, Knox SJ, Levy R, et al. Mycosis fungoides arthropathy. *Ann Intern Med* 1991;114:571–572.
43. Liebow AA, Carrington CR, Friedman PJ. Lymphomatoid granulomatosis. *Hum Pathol* 1972;3:457–558.
44. Katzenstein AL, Carrington CR, Liebow AA. Lymphomatoid granulomatosis: clinicopathological study of 152 cases. *Cancer* 1979;43:360–373.
45. Wilson WH, Kingsma DW, Raffeld M, et al. Association of lymphomatoid granulomatosis with Epstein-Barr viral infection of B lymphocytes and response to interferon-2b. *Blood* 1996;87: 4531–4537.
46. Jaffe ES, Wilson WH. Lymphomatoid granulomatosis: Pathogenesis, pathology, and clinical implications. *Cancer Surv* 1997; 30:233–248.
47. Clarke F, Crook P, McDonagh J. Lymphomatoid granulomatosis, an unusual cause of inflammatory arthritis. *J Rheumatol* 1994;21:774–775.
48. Raez LE, Temple JD, Saldana M. Successful treatment of lymphomatoid granulomatosis using cyclosporin A after failure of intensive chemotherapy. Am J Hematol 1996;53:192–195.
49. Reilly PA, Cosh JA, Maddison PJ, et al. Mortality and survival in rheumatoid arthritis: a 25-year prospective study of 100 patients. *Ann Rheum Dis* 1990;49:363–369.
50. Moder KG, Tefferi A, Cohen MD, et al. Hematologic malignancies and the use of methotrexate in rheumatoid arthritis: a retrospective study. *Am J Med* 1995;99:276–281.
51. Kingsmore SF, Hall BD, Allen NB, et al. Association of methotrexate, rheumatoid arthritis and lymphoma: report of 2 cases and literature review. *J Rheumatol* 1992;19:1462–1465.
52. Morris CR, Morris AJ. Localized lymphoma in a patient with rheumatoid arthritis treated with parenteral methotrexate. *J Rheumatol* 1993;20:2172–2173.
53. Taillan B, Garnier G, Castanet J, et al. Lymphoma developing in a patient with rheumatoid arthritis taking methotrexate. *Clin Rheumatol* 1993;12:93–94.
54. Kamel OW, van de Rijn M, Weiss LM, et al. Brief report: reversible lymphomas associated with Epstein-Barr virus occurring during methotrexate therapy for rheumatoid arthritis and dermatomyositis. *N Engl J Med* 1993;328:1317–1321.
55. Kamel OW, van de Rijn M, LeBrun DR, et al. Lymphoid neoplasms in patients with rheumatoid arthritis and dermatomyositis: frequency of Epstein-Barr virus and other features associated with immunosuppression. *Hum Pathol* 1994;25: 638–643.
56. Zimmer-Galler I, Lie JT. Choroidal infiltrates as the initial manifestation of lymphoma in rheumatoid arthritis after treatment with low-dose methotrexate. *Mayo Clin Proc* 1994;69: 258–261.
57. Liote F, Pertuiset E, Cochand-Priollet B, et al. Methotrexate related B lymphoproliferative disease in a patient with rheumatoid arthritis. Role of Epstein-Barr virus infection. *J Rheumatol* 1995;22:1174–1178.
58. Georgescu L, Quinn GC, Schwartzman S, et al. Lymphoma in patients with rheumatoid arthritis: association with the disease state or methotrexate treatment. *Semin Arthritis Rheum* 1997; 26:798–804.
59. Bataille R, Harousseau J-L. Multiple myeloma. *N Engl J Med* 1997;336:1657–1664.
60. Bataille R, Jourdan M, Zhang X-G, et al. Serum levels of interleukin 6, a potent myeloma cell growth factor, as a reflect of disease severity in plasma cell dyscrasias. *J Clin Invest* 1989;84: 2008–2011.
61. Kyle RA. Multiple myeloma. Review of 869 cases. *Mayo Clin Proc* 1975;50:29–40.
62. Hamilton EB, Bywaters EG. Joint symptoms in myelomatosis and similar conditions. *Ann Rheum Dis* 1961;20:353–362.
63. Solomon A, Rahamani R, Seligsohn U, et al. Multiple myeloma: early vertebral involvement assessed by computerised tomography. *Skeletal Radiol* 1984;11:258–261.
64. Ludwig H, Tscholakoff D, Neuhold A, et al. Magnetic resonance imaging of the spine in multiple myeloma. *Lancet* 1987; 2:364–366.
65. Hickling P, Wilkins M, Newman GR. A study of arthropathy in multiple myeloma. *Q J Med* 1981;50:417–433.
66. Wegelius O, Skrifvars B, Andersson L. Rheumatoid arthritis terminating in plasmacytoma. *Acta Med Scand* 1970;187: 133–138.
67. Zawadzki ZA, Benedek TG. Rheumatoid arthritis, dysproteinemic arthropathy and paraproteinemia. *Arthritis Rheum* 1969; 12:555–568.
68. Gordon DA, Pruzanski W, Ogryzlo MA, et al. Amyloid arthritis simulating rheumatoid disease in five patients with multiple myeloma. *Am J Med* 1973;55:142–154.
69. Goldenberg GJ, Paraskevas F, Israels LG. The association of rheumatoid arthritis with plasma cell and lymphocytic neoplasms. *Arthritis Rheum* 1969;12:569–579.
70. Wiernik PH. Amyloid joint disease. *Medicine* 1972;51: 465–479.
71. Glenner GG. Amyloid deposits and amyloidosis. *N Engl J Med* 1980;302:1283–1292,1333–1343.
72. Falk RH, Comenzo RL, Skinner M. The systemic amyloidoses. *N Engl J Med* 1997;337:898–909.
73. Kyle RA, Lust JA. Monoclonal gammopathies of undetermined significance. *Semin Hematol* 1989;26:176–200.
74. Kyle RA, Greipp PR. Amyloidosis (AL): clinical laboratory features in 229 cases. *Mayo Clin Proc* 1983;58:665–683.
75. Gertz MA, Kyle RA, Greipp PR. Response rates and survival in primary systemic amyloidosis. *Blood* 1991;77:257–262.
76. Zemer D, Pras M, Soher E, et al. Colchicine in the prevention and treatment of the amyloidosis of familial Mediterranean fever. *N Engl J Med* 1986;314:1001–1005.
77. Bardin T, Kuntz D, Zingraff J, et al. Synovial amyloidosis in patients undergoing longterm hemodialysis. *Arthritis Rheum* 1985;28:1052–1058.
78. Gejyo F, Yamada T, Odani S, et al. A new form of amyloid protein associated with hemodialysis was identified as beta-2 microglobulin. *Biochem Biophys Res Commun* 1985;129: 701–706.
79. Miyata T, Oda O, Inagi R, et al. Beta 2-microglobulin modified with advanced glycation end products is a major component of hemodialysis-associated amyloidosis. *J Clin Invest* 1993;92: 1242–1252.
80. Miyata T, Inagi R, Ida Y, et al. Involvement of Beta 2 microglobulin modified with advanced glycation end products in the pathogenesis of hemodialysis-associated amyloidosis. *J Clin Invest* 1994;93:521–528.
81. Davidson GS, Montanera WJ, Fleming JF. Amyloid destructive spondylarthropathy causing cord compression related to chronic renal failure and dialysis. *Neurosurgery* 1993;33: 519–522.
82. Gejyo F, Homma N, Hasegawa S, et al. A new therapeutic approach to dialysis amyloidosis: intensive removal of beta 2 microglobulin with adsorbent column. *Artif Organs* 1993;17: 240–243.
83. Okutsu I, Hamanaka J, Ninomiya S, et al. Results of endo-

scopic management of carpal tunnel syndrome in long-term haemodialysis versus idiopathic patients. *Nephrol Dial Transplant* 1993;8:1110–1114.
84. Nelson SR, Sharpston P, Kingswood JC. Dialysis-associated amyloidosis resolve after transplantation? *Nephrol Dial Transplant* 1993;8:369–370.
85. Libbey CA, Skinner M, Cohen AS. Use of abdominal fat tissue aspirate in the diagnosis of systemic amyloidosis. *Arch Intern Med* 1983;143:1549–1552.
86. Sturgill BC, Bolton WK, Griffith KM. Congo red-negative amyloidosis-like glomerulopathy. *Hum Pathol* 1985;16:220–224.
87. Korbet SM, Schwartz MM, Lewis FJ. Immunotactoid glomerulopathy. *Am J Kidney Dis* 1991;17:247–257.
88. Miralles GD, O'Fallon JR, Talley NJ. Plasma-cell dyscrasia with polyneuropathy: the spectrum of POEMS syndrome. *N Engl J Med* 1992;327:1919–1923.
89. Bardwick PA, Zvaifler NJ, Gill GN, et al. Plasma cell dyscrasia with polyneuropathy, organomegaly, endocrinopathy, M protein and skin changes: the POEMS syndrome. *Medicine* 1980; 59:311–322.
90. Powars DR. Natural history of disease: the first two decades. In: Embury SH, Hebbel RP, Mohandas N, et al., eds. *Sickle cell disease. Basic principles and clinical practice.* New York: Raven Press, 1994:395–412.
91. Charache S. Natural history of disease: adults in sickle cell disease. In: Embury SH, Hebbel RP, Mohandas N, et al., eds. *Sickle cell disease. Basic principles and clinical practice.* New York: Raven Press, 1994:413–422.
92. Hebbel RP, Mohandas N. Sickle cell adherence. In: Embury SH, Hebbel RP, Mohandas N, et al., eds. *Sickle cell disease. Basic principles and clinical practice.* New York: Raven Press, 1994: 217–230.
93. Steinberg MH. Management of sickle cell disease. *N Engl J Med* 1999;340:1021–1030.
94. Diggs LW. Bone and joint lesions in sickle-cell disease. *Clin Orthop* 1967;52:119–143.
95. Espinoza LR, Spilberg I, Osterland CK, et al. Joint manifestations of sickle cell disease. *Medicine* 1971;53:295–305.
96. Schumacher HR, Andrews R, McLaughlin G, et al. Arthropathy in sickle-cell disease. *Ann Intern Med* 1973;78:203–211.
97. Haberman ET, Grayzel AI. Bilateral total knee replacement in a patient with sickle cell disease. *Clin Orthop* 1974;100:211–215.
98. Schumacher HR, Dorwart BB, Bond J, et al. Chronic synovitis with early cartilage destruction in sickle cell disease. *Ann Rheum Dis* 1977;36:413–419.
99. Schumacher HR, van Linthoudt D, Manno CS, et al. Diffuse chondrolytic arthritis in sickle cell disease. *J Rheumatol* 1993; 20:385–389.
100. Weinberg AG, Curranino G. Sickle cell dactylitis: histopathologic observations. *Am J Clin Pathol* 1972;58:518–523.
101. Milner PF, Joe C, Burke GJ, et al. Bone and joint disease. In: Embury SH, Hebbel RP, Mohandas N, et al., eds. *Sickle cell disease. Basic principles and clinical practice.* New York: Raven Press, 1994:645–661.
102. Resnick D. Hemoglobinopathies and other anemias. In: Resnick D, ed. *Diagnosis of bone and joint disorders,* 2nd ed. Philadelphia: WB Saunders 1988:2320–2357.
103. Bennett OM, Namnyak SS. Bone and joint manifestations of sickle cell anemia. *J Bone Joint Surg* 1990;72A:494–499.
104. Steinberg ME, Steinberg DR. Evaluation and staging of avascular necrosis. *Semin Arthroplasty* 1991;2:175–181.
105. Milner PF, Kraus AP, Sebes JI, et al. Sickle cell disease as a cause of osteonecrosis of the femoral head. *N Engl J Med* 1991;325:1476–1481.
106. Moran MC, Huo MH, Garvin KL, et al. Total hip arthroplasty in sickle cell hemoglobinopathy. *Clin Orthop* 1993;294: 140–148.
107. Barrett-Conner E. Bacterial infection and sickle cell anemia. An analysis of 250 infections in 106 patients and a review of the literature. *Medicine* 1971;50:97–112.
108. Hook EW, Campbell CG, Weens HS, et al. Salmonella osteomyelitis in patients with sickle cell anemia. *N Engl J Med* 1957;257:403–407.
109. Silver HK, Simon JL, Clement DH. Salmonella osteomyelitis and abnormal hemoglobin disease. *Pediatrics* 1957;20: 439–447.
110. Syrogiannopoulos GA, McCracken GH, Nelson JD. Osteoarticular infections in children with sickle cell disease. *Pediatrics* 1986;78:1090–1096.
111. Ebong WW. Acute osteomyelitis in Nigerians with sickle cell disease. *Ann Rheum Dis* 1986;45:911–915.
112. Epps CH, Bryant DD, Coces MJM, et al. Osteomyelitis in patients who have sickle cell disease. *J Bone J Surg* 1991;73A: 1281–1294.
113. Piehl FC, Davis RJ, Prugh SI. Osteomyelitis is sickle cell disease. *J Pediatr Orthop* 1993;13:225–227.
114. Reynolds MD. Gout and hyperuricemia associated with sickle cell anemia. *Semin Arthritis Rheum* 1983;12:404–413.
115. Rao SP, Miller S, Solomon N. Acute bone and joint manifestations of sickle cell disease in children. *NY State J Med* 1986;86: 254–260.
116. Ebong WW. Septic arthritis in patients with sickle cell disease. *Br J Rheumatol* 1986;26:99–102.
117. Valeriano-Marcet J, Kerr LD. Myonecrosis and myofibrosis as complications of sickle cell anemia. *Ann Intern Med* 1991;115: 99–101.
118. Gratwick GM, Bullough PG, Bohne WHO, et al. Thalassemic osteoarthropathy. *Ann Intern Med* 1978;88:494–501.
119. Schlumph U, Gerber N, Bunzli H, et al. Arthritis in thalassemia minor. *Schweiz Med Wochenschr* 1977;107:1156–1162.
120. Gerster JC, Dardel R, Guggi S. Recurrent episodes of arthritis in thalassemia minor. *J Rheumatol* 1984;11:352–354.
121. Arman MI, Butun B, Doseyen A, et al. Frequency and features of rheumatic findings in thalassemia minor: a blind controlled study. *Br J Rheumatol* 1992;31:197–199.
122. Abou Rizk NN, Nasr FW, Frayha RA. Aseptic necrosis in thalassemia minor. *Arthritis Rheum* 1977;20:1147–1148.
123. Sadler JF, Davie EW. Hemophilia A, hemophilia B, and von Willebrand's disease. In: Stamatoyannopoulos K, Nienhuis AW, Majerus PW, et al., eds. *The molecular basis of blood diseases,* 2nd ed. Philadelphia: WB Saunders, 1994:657–675.
124. Madhok R, York R, Sturrock RD. Hemophiliac arthritis. *Ann Rheum Dis* 1991;50:588–591.
125. Duthie RB, Rizza CR, Giangrande PL, et al. *The management of musculoskeletal problems in the hemophilias.* Oxford: Oxford University Press, 1994.
126. Fricke WA, Lamb MA. Viral safety of clotting factor concentrates. *Semin Thromb Hemost* 1993;19:54–61.
127. Schwartz RS, Abildgaard CF, Aledort LM, et al. Human recombinant DNA-derived anti-hemophilic factor (factor VIII) in the treatment of hemophilia A. *N Engl J Med* 1990;323: 1800–1805.
128. Ahlberg A, Silwer JP. Arthropathy in von Willebrand's disease. *Acta Orthop Scand* 1970;41:539–544.
129. Sankarankutty M, Evans DI. Chronic arthropathy in von Willebrand's disease. *Clin Lab Haematol* 1983;5:149–156.
130. Macfarlane JD, Kroon HM, Caekebeke-Peerlinck KMJ, et al. Arthropathy in von Willebrand's disease. *Clin Rheumatol* 1989; 8:98–102.
131. Klofkorn RW, Lightsey AL. Hemarthrosis associated with Glanzmann's thrombasthenia. *Arthritis Rheum* 1979;22:1390– 1393.

132. Thakker S, McGehee W, Quismorio FP. Arthropathy associated with factor XIII deficiency. *Arthritis Rheum* 1986;29:808–811.
133. Katz AL, Alepa FP. Hemarthrosis secondary to heparin therapy. *Arthritis Rheum* 1976;19:996.
134. Wild JH, Zvaifler NJ. Hemarthrosis associated with sodium warfarin therapy. *Arthritis Rheum* 1976;19:98–102.
135. Andes WA, Edmunds JO. Hemarthroses and warfarin: joint destruction with anticoagulation. *Thromb Haemost* 1983;28: 187–189.
136. Triantafyllou SJ, Hanks GA, Handal JA, et al. Open and arthroscopic synovectomy in hemophilic arthropathy of the knee. *Clin Orthop* 1992;283:196–204.
137. Karthaus RP, Novakova IR. Total knee replacement in hemophilic arthropathy. *J Bone Joint Surg* 1988;70B:382–385.
138. Teigland JC, Tjonnfjord GE, Evensen SA, et al. Knee arthroplasty in hemophilia. *Acta Orthop Scand* 1993;64:153–156.
139. Gregg-Smith SJ, Pattison RM, Dodd CAF, et al. Septic arthritis in haemophilia. *J Bone Joint Surg* 1993;75B:368–370.
140. Buetler E, Grabowski G. Gaucher disease. In: Scriver CR, Beaudet AL, Sly WS, et al., eds. *The metabolic and molecular bases of inherited disease,* 7th ed. New York: McGraw-Hill, 1995: 2641–2670.
141. Schubiner H, Le Tourneau M, Murray DL. Pyogenic osteomelitis versus pseudo-osteomyelitis in Gaucher's disease. *Clin Pediatr* 1981;20:667–669.
142. Weizman Z, Tennenbaum A, Yatziv S. Interphalangeal joint involvement in Gaucher's disease, type 1, resembling juvenile rheumatoid arthritis. *Arthritis Rheum* 1982;25:706–707.
143. Lau MM, Lichtman DM, Hamati YI, et al. Hip arthroplasties in Gaucher's disease. *J Bone Joint Surg* 1981;63:591–601.
144. Desnick RJ, Ioannou YA, Eng C, et al. a Galactosidase A deficiency: Fabry disease. In: Scriver CR, Beaudet AL, Sly WS, et al., eds. *The metabolic and molecular bases of inherited disease,* 7th ed. New York: McGraw-Hill, 1995:2741–2784.
145. Wise D, Wallace HJ, Jellinck EH. Angiokeratoma corporis diffusum: a clinical study of eight affected families. *Q J Med* 1962; 31:177–206.
146. Lockman LA, Hunninghake DB, Krivit W, et al. Relief of pain of Fabry's disease by diphenylhydantoin. *Neurology* 1973;23: 871–875.
147. Pittelkow RB, Kierland RR, Montgomery H. Angiokeratoma corporis diffusum. *Arch Dermatol* 1955;72:556–561.
148. Fone D, King W. Angiokeratoma corporis diffusum. *Aust Ann Med* 1964;13:339–348.
149. Bethune JE, Landrigan PL, Chipman CD. Angiokeratoma corporis diffusum. *N Engl J Med* 1961;264:1280–1285.
150. Sheth KJ, Bernhard GC. The arthropathy of Fabry's disease. *Arthritis Rheum* 1979;22:781–783.
151. Moser HW. Ceramidase deficiency: Farber lipogranulomatosis. In: Scriver CR, Beaudet AL, Sly WS, et al., eds. *The metabolic and molecular bases of inherited disease,* 7th ed. New York: McGraw-Hill, 1995:2589–2601.
152. Jameson RA, Holt PJL, Keen JH. Farber's disease (lysosomal acid ceramidase deficiency). *Ann Rheum Dis* 1987;46:559–561.
153. Abul-Haj SK, Martz DG, Douglas WF, et al. Farber's disease: report of a case with observations on its histogenesis and notes on the nature of the stored material. *J Pediatr* 1962;61:221–232.
154. Ford DK, Price GE, Culling CFA, et al. Familial lipochrome pigmentation of histocytes with hyperglobulinemia, pulmonary infiltration, splenomegaly, arthritis and susceptibility to infection. *Am J Med* 1962;33:478–489.
155. Rodey GE, Park BH, Ford DK, et al. Defective bactericidal activity of peripheral blood leukocytes in lipochrome histiocytosis. *Am J Med* 1970;49:322–327.
156. Forehand JR, Nauseef WM, Curnutte JT, et al. Inherited disorders of phagocyte killing. In: Scriver CR, Beaudet AL, Sly WS, et al., eds. *The metabolic and molecular bases of inherited disease,* 7th ed. New York: McGraw-Hill, 1995:3995–4026.
157. Goldstein JL, Hobbs HH, Brown MS. Familial hypercholesterolemia. In: Scriver CR, Beaudet AL, Sly WS, et al., eds. *The metabolic and molecular bases of inherited disease,* 7th ed. New York: McGraw-Hill, 1995:1981–2030.
158. Khachadurian AK. Migratory polyarthritis in familial hypercholesterolemia (type II hyperlipoproteinemia). *Arthritis Rheum* 1968;11:385–393.
159. Rimon D, Cohen L. Hypercholesterolemic (type II hyperlipoproteinemic) arthritis. *J Rheumatol* 1989;16:703–705.
160. Shapiro JR, Fallat RW, Tsang RC, et al. Achilles tendinitis and tenosynovitis: a diagnostic manifestation of family type II hyperlipoproteinemia in children. *Am J Dis Child* 1974;128: 486–490.
161. Glueck CJ, Levy RI, Fredrickson DS. Acute tendinitis and arthritis. A presenting symptom of familial type II hyperlipoproteinemia. *JAMA* 1968;13:2895–2897.
162. Kane JP, Havel RJ. Disorders of the biogenesis and secretion of lipoproteins containing the B apolipoproteins. In: Scriver CR, Beaudet AL, Sly WS, et al., eds. *The metabolic and molecular bases of inherited disease,* 7th ed. New York: McGraw-Hill, 1995: 1853–1886.
163. Mahley RW, Rall SC. Type III hyperlipoproteinemia (dysbetapolipoprotenemia): the role of apolipoprotein E in normal and abnormal lipoprotein metabolism. In: Scriver CR, Beaudet AL, Sly WS, et al., eds. *The metabolic and molecular bases of inherited disease,* 7th ed. New York: McGraw-Hill, 1995: 1953–1980.
164. Goldman JA, Glueck CJ, Abrams NR, et al. Musculoskeletal disorders associated with type IV hyperlipoproteinaemia. *Lancet* 1972;2:449–452.
165. Buckingham RB, Bole GG, Bassett DR, et al. Polyarthritis associated with type IV hyperlipoproteinemia. *Arch Intern Med* 1975;135:289–290.
166. Klemp P, Halland AM, Majoos FL, et al. Musculoskeletal manifestations in hyperlipidaemia: a controlled study. *Ann Rheum Dis* 1983;42:519–523.
167. Barrow MV, Holubar K. Multicentric reticulohistiocytosis. *Medicine* 1969;48:287–307.
168. Catterall MD. Multicentric reticulohistiocytosis: a review of eight cases. *Clin Exp Dermatol* 1980;5:267–279.
169. Brandt F, Lipman M, Taylor JR, et al. Topical nitrogen mustard therapy in multicentric reticulohistiocytosis. *J Am Acad Dermatol* 1982;6:260–262.
170. Ginsburg WW, O'Duffy JD, Morris JL, et al. Multicentric reticulohistiocytosis: response to alkylating agents in six patients. *Ann Intern Med* 1989;111:384–388.

95

HERITABLE AND DEVELOPMENTAL DISORDERS OF CONNECTIVE TISSUE AND BONE

REED EDWIN PYERITZ

Any disorder can be described or studied by two fundamental approaches: etiology and pathogenesis. Either can be useful. An understanding of the causes of disease leads to reliable classification, diagnosis, and prevention, whereas an understanding of the mechanisms leads to effective prognosis and treatment. Unfortunately, the two approaches are often thought to be similar or even interchangeable—misconceptions that confuse nosology, management, and clinical investigation. Knowledge of etiology, no matter how refined, may shed no light on how the clinical manifestations (the phenotype) develop (1). For example, the "cause" of sickle cell disease is known at the highest level of resolution possible, the specific nucleotide mutation, whereas the mechanisms by which the diverse clinical features appear remain largely obscure. Conversely, the pathogenesis of acute gout is far better understood than is the etiology in most cases.

The role genetic factors play in the disorders of a given system has generally been considered etiology. The traditional approach has been to divide all disorders into nongenetic and genetic ones, and the latter into mendelian, chromosomal, and multifactorial categories. This scheme has increasingly outlived its utility (2,3). First, no disease is purely genetic or environmental in cause. Second, all diseases involve some interaction of genes and environment to produce the abnormal phenotype and to effect its resolution. Third, genes are important modifiers of pathogenesis; inheritance in a family of modifying genes, unlinked to a mutant gene that has a prime role in causing a disease, is one reason the phenotype can vary so widely among relatives. Finally, disorders due largely to single genes do not necessarily behave in families as Mendel would have predicted; this is especially true for genes on the mitochondrial chromosome, but imprinting, uniparental disomy, anticipation, and somatic and germinal mutation all introduce clinically important nuances to the principles of mendelian inheritance. These topics are discussed in a number of recent reviews and texts (2–8).

Virtually all diseases have genetic components in their causation and pathogenesis (1–3). The genetic factors in common diseases are increasingly being identified, and are discussed for osteoarthritis (OA), osteoporosis, and the rheumatic disorders in other chapters of this text (e.g., Chapters 29, 110, and 122). This chapter focuses on many of the conditions affecting the skeleton and other supporting elements in which a single mutant gene is of overriding causal importance, although its effect may be modulated by other genetic and environmental factors. These conditions occur in families in simple inheritance patterns, that is, autosomal dominant, autosomal recessive, X-linked, or maternal (mitochondrial). Nearly all these disorders are individually rare (prevalences of 1/104 to 1/106 in the general population), but because so many are now known [>10,844 in one tabulation as of late 1999 (9)], in the aggregate, they represent a substantial category of disease.

Chromosomal disorders are those in which an abnormal phenotype is associated with a chromosome aberration visible with the light microscope. For example, the Down syndrome is caused by the presence of three copies of chromosome 21 (trisomy 21), or by the patient having two normal chromosomes 21, and an additional copy of a short, critical segment of the long arm of chromosome 21, often attached to one of the other chromosomes. The number of syndromes known to be associated with chromosome aberrations continues to grow as improved cytogenetic techniques enhance resolution (10,11), resulting in a blurring of the distinctions between mendelian and cytogenetic disorders. Cytogenetic aberrations can provide crucial clues as to the genetic mapping of a disease-causing gene. For example, a number of patients with the Greig cephalopolysyndactyly syndrome had small deletions of the short arm of human chromosome 7 (involving band 7p13) (12). In one instructive family, the syndrome occurred only in relatives having an apparently balanced translocation between chromosomes 3 and 7, with one of the breakpoints in band 7p13. Disruption of the gene responsible for this rare condition by the deletions or the breakage and reunion of chromosome segments was the most likely causal explanation. This then led to an examination of genes already mapped to this band and the identification of the *GLI3* gene as the likely culprit (13).

The term *multifactorial* is often used to describe the important role that multiple genes and environmental factors have in determining a quantitative trait, such as stature or bone mass. Finding the genes that contribute to quantitative traits has become a major area of investigation (14). With regard to pathologic traits, multifactorial has a specific and a general meaning. Disorders such as pyloric stenosis, clubfoot, and idiopathic scoliosis, which conform to empiric predictions of recurrence, concordance in monozygotic twins, and differences in prevalence between sexes, are classified as multifactorial in the narrow sense (15,16). Conversely, any condition in which genes are a necessary but insufficient part of the cause and that are distributed in families in ways that do not fulfill any mendelian pattern can be described as multifactorial in the broad sense. The rheumatic disorders are examples.

The pace of discovery of new genes involved in extracellular matrix biology and pathobiology is accelerating, and both the investigator and the clinician must rely on interactive, on-line databases to stay current (9,15,16). The pace of description of new diseases involving the skeleton with a major genetic component, although not accelerating, continues rapidly enough that clinicians should be familiar with several useful databases (9,17–20), in addition to standard reference works (2,21,22). Table 95.1 lists mendelian disorders of the skeleton for which the cause is known at the genetic level; details about each condition can be found in reference 9. Some of the recent discoveries of mutations in previously unknown genes that cause rare disorders have had the additional benefit of identifying normal products that are crucial to skeletal development and bone mass (23,24).

A number of components of the extracellular matrix have not had human diseases associated with them. The genes specifying these components are "candidates" for linkage or mutation analysis whenever syndromes of unknown cause are investigated. One broad class of molecules under intense scrutiny is the metalloproteinases, including the cathepsins, which may underlie rare syndromes and play a role in common disorders such as rheumatoid arthritis (RA) and OA (25). Other categories of extracellular matrix components include receptors, such as for vitamin D (26); cytokines, such as interleukin-4 (IL-4) (27); and osteogenic proteins, such as bone morphogenic proteins (28). Osteogenic proteins have been associated with phenotypes as general as stature (29) and are being applied in clinical trials as exogenous adjuncts to bone remodeling and healing.

Increasingly, ideas about human disorders arise from targeted mutation, overexpression, or deletion ("knockout") of homologous genes in the mouse (30,31). Table 95.2 provides a partial list of mouse mutants that are models of human diseases.

The remainder of this chapter reviews some of the recent advances in the broad categories of heritable and developmental conditions that either affect the skeleton exclusively, or have important clinical manifestations in bone or cartilage.

HERITABLE DISORDERS OF CONNECTIVE TISSUE AND BONE

This category of human disease was defined in 1955 by McKusick (32), and in its first incarnation included only osteogenesis imperfecta, the Marfan syndrome, Ehlers–Danlos syndrome, pseudoxanthoma elasticum, and gargoylism (33). Over a period of more than three decades, more than 200 distinct mendelian disorders of connective tissue have been described and are now subject to periodic review by international committees charged with consensus development of diagnostic criteria and nosologic boundaries (34,35). Although much of their classification remains rooted in phenotypic distinctions, study of their causes at the biochemical and nucleic acid level is having increasing clinical utility.

The complexity of connective tissue is emphasized in Chapters 7 through 12. The heritable disorders of connective tissue are inborn errors of metabolism, as are the familial defects in amino acid and carbohydrate metabolism first investigated by Garrod at the turn of the century. With careful study, each of these disorders can serve as a window to understanding normal structure and function of the extracellular matrix. The disorders chosen for description in this chapter are relatively common and important in clinical rheumatology and orthopaedics, highly instructive about general principles, or both.

Marfan Syndrome

Patients with the Marfan syndrome have diverse abnormalities, especially in the skeletal, ocular, cardiovascular, and pulmonary systems (36,37). The diagnosis is based solely on the clinical features and the autosomal dominant inheritance pattern (38). This remains true despite the discovery of the basic defect, the gene specifying the large glycoprotein, fibrillin-1, which is the major constituent of the extracellular microfibril (32,33,39,40). More than 200 different mutations of the *FBN1* gene have been found in different patients with the Marfan syndrome, and there is no convincing evidence that any other gene is a primary cause of this autosomal dominant condition (41–43). Several issues limit the use of *FBN1* analysis in the many diagnostic dilemmas that commonly face clinicians trying to decide if tall, lanky people with myopia and mitral valve prolapse have the Marfan syndrome. First, *FBN1* is a large gene, and the mRNA contains about 10,000 nucleotides; routine

TABLE 95.1. MENDELIAN CONDITIONS THAT INVOLVE THE SKELETON WITH KNOWN GENETIC DEFECTS OF GENE MAPPING OF THE PHENOTYPE

Phenotype	Gene Symbol	OMIM no.*	Gene Map Locus
Developmental disorders			
Aarskog–Scott syndrome	*FGDI*	305400	Xp11.21
Acromesomelic dysplasia, Hunter–Thompson type	*GDF5*	601146	20q11.2
Apert syndrome	*FGFR2*	176943	10q26
Arthrogryposis congenita, distal, type I	*AMCD1*	108120	9p21–q21
Arthrogryposis congenita, distal, type II	*AMCD2B*	601680	11p15.5
Bardet–Biedl syndrome 1	*BBS1*	209901	11q13
Bardet–Biedl syndrome 2	*BBS2*	209900	16q21
Bardet–Biedl syndrome 3	*BBS3*	600151	3p13–p12
Bardet–Biedl syndrome 4	*BBS4*	600374	15q22.3–q23
Bardet–Biedl syndrome 5	*BBS5*	603650	2q31
Brachydactyly, type B1	*BDB1*	113000	9q33–q34
Brachydactyly, type C	*GDF5*	601146	20q11.2
Brachydactyly, type C	*BDC*	113100	12q24
Brachydactyly, type E (?)	*BDE*	113300	2q37
Brachydactyly–mental retardation syndrome	*BDMR*	600430	2q37
Cockayne syndrome	*CKN1*	216400	5
Coffin–Lowry syndrome	*RPS6KA3*	300075	Xp22.2–p22.1
Craniofacial-deafness-hand syndrome	*PAX3*	193500	2q35
Craniofrontonasal dysplasia	*CFNS*	304110	Xp22
Craniosynostosis, Adelaide type	*CRSA*	600593	4p16
Craniosynostosis, type 1	*CRS*	123100	7p21.3–p21.2
Craniosynostosis, type 2	*MSX2*	123101	5q34–q35
Crouzon syndrome	*FGFR2*	176943	10q26
Crouzon syndrome with acanthosis nigricans	*FGFR3*	134934	4p16.3
Ectrodactyly, ectodermal dysplasia, cleft lip/palate-1	*EEC1*	129900	17q11.2–q21.3
Ectrodactyly, ectodermal dysplasia, cleft lip/palate-2	*EEC2*	602077	19
Grieg cephalopolysyndactyly	*GLI3*	165240	7p13
Holt–Oram syndrome	*TBX5*	601620	12q24.1
Jackson–Weiss syndrome	*FGFR2*	176943	10q26
Jacobsen syndrome	*JBS*	147791	11q23
Klippel–Feil syndrome (?)	*KFS*	214300	5q11.2
Klippel–Feil syndrome with laryngeal malformation	*SGM1*	148900	8q22.2
Langer–Giedion syndrome	*LGCR*	150230	8q24.11–q24.13
Limb-mammary syndrome	*LMS*	603543	3q27
McKusick–Kaufman syndrome	*MKKS*	236700	20p12
Mulibrey nanism	*MUL*	253250	17q22–q23
Nail–patella syndrome	*LMX1B*	602575	9q34.1
Neurofibromatosis, type I	*NF1*	162200	17q11.2
Oculodentodigital dysplasia	*ODDD*	164200	6q22–q24
Pallister–Hall syndrome	*GLI3*	165240	7p13
Patella aplasia or hypoplasia	*PTHLAH*	168860	17q
Pfeiffer syndrome	*FGFR2*	176943	10q26
	FGFR1	136350	8p11.2–p11.1
Postaxial polydactyly, type A1	*GLI3*	165240	7p13
Postaxial polydactyly, type A2	*PAPA2*	602085	13q21–q32
Postaxial polydactyly, type A/B	*GLI3*	165240	7p13
Preaxial polydactyly type IV	*GLI3*	165240	7p13
Rothmund–Thompson syndrome	*RECOL4*	603780	8q24.3
Sacral agenesis syndrome	*HLXB9*	142994	7q36
Sacral agenesis-1	*SCRA1*	176450	7q36
Saethre–Chotzen syndrome	*TWIST*	601622	7p21
	FGFR2	176943	10q26
Schwartz–Jampel syndrome type 1	*SJS1*	255800	1p36.1–p34
Simpson dysmorphia syndrome	*GPC3*	300037	Xq26
Split hand/foot malformation, type 1	*SHFM1*	183600	7q21.2–q21.3
Split hand/foot malformation, type 2	*SHFM2*	313350	Xq26
Split hand/foot malformation, type 3	*SHFM3*	600095	10q24
Spondylocostal dysostosis	*SCDO1*	277300	19q13.1–q13.3
Symphalanagism, proximal	*NOG*	602991	17q22
Syndactyly, type III	*ODDD*	164200	6q22–q24

(continued)

TABLE 95.1. *(continued)*

Phenotype	Gene Symbol	OMIM no.*	Gene Map Locus
Developmental disorders *(continued)*			
Synostoses syndrome, multiple, 1	*NOG*	602991	17q22
Synpolydactyly, type II	*HOXD13*	142989	2q31–q32
Tetramelic mirror-image polydactyly (?)	*TMIP*	135750	14q13
Townes–Brocks syndrome	*SALL1*	602218	16q12.1
Treacher Collins mandibulofacial dysostosis	*TCOF1*	154500	5q32–q33.1
Triphalangela thumb-polysyndactyly	*TPTPS*	190605	7q36
Turner syndrome	*RPS4X*	312760	Xq13.1
Ulnar–mammary syndrome	*TBX3*	601621	12q24.1
Heritable disorders of connective tissue			
Albright hereditary osteodystrophy-2 (?)	*AHO2*	103581	15q11–q13
Bruck syndrome	*BRKX*	259450	17p12
Contractural arachnodactyly, congenital	*FBN2*	121050	5q23–q31
Cutis laxa	*ELN*	130160	7q11.2
Cutis laxa, marfanoid neonatal type (?)	*LAMB1*	150240	7q31.1–q31.3
Cutis laxa, neonatal	*ATP7A*	300011	Xq12–q13
Cutis laxa, recessive type I	*LOX*	153455	5q23.3–q31.2
Ehlers–Danlos syndrome, classic	*COL5A2*	120190	2q31
	COL5A1	120215	9q34.2–34.3
Ehlers–Danlos syndrome, hypermobility type	*COL3A1*	120180	2q31
Ehlers–Danlos syndrome, vascular type	*COL3A1*	120180	2q31
Ehlers–Danlos syndrome, kyphoscoliotic type	*PLOD*	153454	1p36.3–p36.2
Ehlers–Danlos syndrome, arthrochalasia type	*COL1A1*	120150	17q21,31-q22.05
	COL1A2	120160	7q22.1
Ehlers–Danlos syndrome, type X (?)	*FN1*	135600	2q34
Ehlers–Danlos–like syndrome	*TNXA*	600261	6p21.3
Fibrodysplasia ossificans progressiva (?)	*BMP2*	112261	20p12
	BMP4	112262	14q22–q23
Keutel syndrome	*MGP*	154870	12p13.1–p12.3
Marfan syndrome	*FBN1*	134797	15q21.1
MASS phenotype	*FBN1*	134797	15q21.1
Osteoarthritis, precocious	*COL2A1*	120140	12q13.11–q13.2
Osteogenesis imperfecta, four clinical forms	*COL1A1*	120150	17q21.31–q22.05
Osteogenesis imperfecta, three clinical forms	*COL1A2*	120160	7q22.1
Osteolysis, familial expansile	*OFE*	174810	18q21.1–q22
Osteopetrosis, type II	*OPTA2*	166660	1p21
Osteopetrosis, recessive	*OPTB1*	259700	11q12–q13
Osteoporosis	*CALCA*	114130	11p15.2p15.1
Osteoporosis, idiopathic	*COL1A1*	120150	17q21.31–q22.05
	COL1A2	120160	7q22.1
Osteoporosis, involutional (?)	*VDR*	601769	12q12–q14
Osteoporosis–pseudoglioma syn.	*OPPG*	259770	11q12–q13
Paget disease of bone (?)	*PDB*	167250	6p21.3
Paget disease of bone-2	*PDB2*	602080	18q21–q22
Sclerosteosis	*SOST*	269500	17q12–q21
Sclerosteolysis (?)	*TYS*	181600	4q28–q31
Shprintzen–Goldberg syndrome	*FBN1*	134797	15q21.1
Van Buchem disease	*VBCH*	239100	17q11.2
Metabolic disorders with secondary effect on connective tissue			
Alkaptonuria	*HGD*	203500	3q21–q23
Arthrocutaneouveal granulomatosis	*ACUG*	186580	16p12–q21
Aspartylglucosaminuria	*AGA*	208400	4q32–q33
Barth syndrome	*TAZ*	302060	Xq28
Fucosidosis	*FUCA1*	230000	1p34
Galactosialidosis	*PPGB*	256540	20q13.1
Gaucher disease	*GBA*	230800	1q21
Gigantism due to GHRF hypersecretion	*GHRH*	139190	20q11.2
GM_1 gangliosidosis	*GLB1*	230500	3p21.33
Hemochromatosis	*HFE*	235200	6p21.3
Homocystinuria	*CBS*	236200	21q22.3
Hyperparathyroidism, familial	*MEN1*	131100	11q13
Hyperparathyroidism, familial 1°	*HRPT2*	145001	1q21–q32
Hypocalcemia	*CASR*	601199	3q21–q24

TABLE 95.1. (continued)

Phenotype	Gene Symbol	OMIM no.*	Gene Map Locus
Hypocalciuric hypercalcemia, type I	*CASR*	601199	3q21–q24
Hypocalciuric hypercalcemia, type II	*HHC2*	145981	19p13.3
Hypoparathyroidism	*PTH*	168450	11p15.3–p15.1
Hypoparathyroidism, familial	*FIH*	146200	3q13
Hypoparathyroidism, X-linked	*HPT*	307700	Xq26–q27
Hypoparathyroidism–retardation–dysmorphisms syndrome	*HRD*	241410	1q42–q43
Hypophosphatasia, adult (?)	*ALPL*	171760	1p36.1–p34
Hypophosphatasia, childhood and infantile	ALPL	171760	1p36.1–p34
Hypophosphatemia, hereditary	*PHEX*	307800	Xp22.2–p22.1
Hypophosphatemia, type III	*CLCN5*	300008	Xp11.22
Hypophosphatemic rickets, dominant	*ADHR*	193100	12p13.3
Laron dwarfism	*GHR*	600946	5p13–p12
Mannosidosis, alpha, types I & II	*MANB*	248500	19cen-q12
Mannosidosis, beta	*MANBA*	248510	4q22–q25
Mucolipidosis II & III	*GNPTA*	252500	4q21–q23
Mucopolysaccharidosis IH, IS, IH/S	*IDUA*	252800	4p16.3
Mucopolysaccharidosis II	*IDS*	309900	Xq28
Mucopolysaccharidosis IIIA	*SGSH*	252900	17q25.3
Mucopolysaccharidosis IIIB	*NAGLU*	252920	17q21
Mucopolysaccharidosis IIIC	*MPS3C*	252930	14
Mucopolysaccharidosis IIID	*GNS*	252940	12q14
Mucopolysaccharidosis IVA	*GALNS*	253000	16q24.3
Mucopolysaccharidosis IVB	*GLB1*	230500	3p21.33
Mucopolysaccharidosis VI	*ARSB*	253200	5q11–q13
Mucopolysaccharidosis VII	*GUSB*	253220	7q21.11
Mucopolysaccharidosis IX	*HYAL1*	601492	3p21.3–p21.2
Neuraminidase deficiency	*NEU*	256550	6p21.3
Occipital horn syndrome	*ATP7A*	300011	Xq12–q13
Osteoporosis, postmenopausal susceptibility xxx	*CALCR*	114131	7q21.3
Pseudovitamin D deficiency rickets 1	*CYP27B1*	264700	12q14
Renal tubular acidosis–osteopetrosis	*CA2*	259730	8q22
Rickets, vitamin D-resistant	*VDR*	601769	12q12–q14
Scurvy	*GULOP*	240400	8p21.1
Neoplasia			
Chondrosarcoma	*EXT1*	133700	8q24.11–q24.13
Chondrosarcoma, extraskeletal myxoid	*CSMF*	600542	9q22
Diaphyseal medullary stenosis with malignant fibrous histiocytoma	*DMSFH*	112250	9p22–p21
Gardner syndrome	*APC*	175100	5q21–q22
Hereditary osteochondromas	*EXT1*	133700	8q24.11–q24.13
Hyperparathyroidism–jaw tumor syn.	*HRPT2*	145001	1q21–q32
Multiple endocrine neoplasia IIB	*RET*	164761	10q11.2
Osteosarcoma	*RB1*	180200	13q14.1–q14.2
	LOH18CR1	603045	18q21–q22
Neuromuscular disorders with secondary effect on joints			
Arthrogryposis congenita, neurogenic	*AMCN*	208100	5q35
Arthrogryposis, X-linked	*AMCX1*	301830	Xp11.3–q11.2
Osteochondrodysplasias			
Achondrogenesis Ib	*DTD*	222600	5q32–q33.1
Achondrogenesis–hypochondrogenesis, type II	*COL2A1*	120140	12q13.11–q13.2
Achondroplasia	*FGFR3*	134934	4p16.3
Acromesomelic dysplasia	*POMC*	176830	2p23.3
Atelosteogenesis II	*DTD*	222600	5q32–q33.1
Campomelic dysplasia	*SOX9*	114290	17q24.3–q25.1
Cartilage–hair hypoplasia	*CHH*	250250	9p13
Chondrocalcinosis, familial articular	*CCAL2*	118600	5p
Chondrocalcinosis with early-onset osteoarthritis	*CCAL1*	600668	8q
Chondrodysplasia, Grebe type	*GDF5*	601146	20q11.2
Chondrodysplasia punctata, brachytelephalangic	*ARSE*	300180	Xp22.3
Chondrodysplasia punctata, rhizomelic, type 1	*PEX7*	601757	6q22–q24
Chondrodysplasia punctata, rhizomelic, type 3	*AGPS*	603051	2q31
Chondrodysplasia, X-linked	*CDPX1*	300180	Xp22.3
Chondrodysplasia, X-linked	*CDPX2*	302960	Xq28
Cleidocranial dysplasia	*CBFA1*	600211	6p21

(continued)

TABLE 95.1. (continued)

Phenotype	Gene Symbol	OMIM no.*	Gene Map Locus
Osteochondrodysplasias *(continued)*			
Craniometaphyseal dysplasia	*CMGJ*	123000	5p15.2–p14.1
Diastrophic dysplasia	*DTD*	222600	5q32–q33.1
Ellis–van Creveld syndrome	*EVC*	225500	4p16
Hip dysplasia, Beukes type	*BHD*	142669	4q35
Hypochondroplasia	*FGFR3*	134934	4p16.3
Kniest dysplasia	*COL2A1*	120140	12q13.11–q13.2
Larsen syndrome	*LRS1*	150250	3p21.1–p14.1
Leri–Weill dyschondrosteosis	*SHOX*	312865	Xpter-p22.32
Marshall syndrome	*COL11A1*	120280	1p21
McCune–Albright polyostotic fibrous dysplasia	*GNAS1*	139320	20q13.2
Mesomelic dysplasia, Kantaputra type	*MMDK*	156232	2q24–q32
Metaphyseal chondrodysplasia, Murk Jansen type	*PTHR1*	168468	3p22–p21.1
Metaphyseal chondrodysplasia, Schmid type	*COL10A1*	120110	6p21–q22.3
Multiple epiphyseal dysplasia 1	*COMP*	600310	19p13.1
Multiple epiphyseal dysplasia 2	*COL9A2*	120260	1p33–p32.3
Multiple epiphyseal dysplasia 3	*COL9A3*	120270	20q13.3
Multiple exostoses, type 1	*EXT1*	133700	8q24.11–q24.13
Multiple exostoses, type 2	*EXT2*	133701	11p12–p11
Multiple exostoses, type 3	*EXT3*	600209	19p
OSMED syndrome	*COL11A1*	120290	6p21.3
Pseudoachondrydysplasia	*COMP*	600310	19p13.1
Pseudorheumatoid dysplasia	*WISP3*	208230	6q22
Pycnodysostosis	*CTSK*	601105	1q21
Spondyloepiphyseal dysplasia congenita	*COL2A1*	120140	12q13.11–q13.2
Spondyloepiphyseal dysplasia, tarda	*SEDL*	313400	Xp22.2–p22.1
Spondyloepimetaphyseal dysplasia, Pakistani type	*ATPSK2*	603005	10q23–q24
Spondyloepimetaphyseal dysplasia, Strudwick type	*COL2A1*	120140	12q13.11–q13.2
Stickler syndrome, type I	*COL2A1*	120140	12q13.11–q13.2
Stickler syndrome, type II	*COL11A2*	120290	6p21.3
Stickler syndrome, type III	*COL11A1*	120280	1p21
Thanatophoric dysplasia, types I and II	*FGFR3*	134934	4p16.3
Weissenbacher-Zweymuller syndrome	*COL11A2*	120290	6p21.3

Disorders may have been mapped by the phenotype, by the gene, or both; (?) after a disorder indicates the mapping data are still in limbo. An asterisk (*) refers to the entry for the locus in http://www.ncbi.nlm.nih.gov/htbin-post/Omim.

sequence analysis by any of a variety of techniques is time-consuming, costly, and not completely sensitive (44). Second, a number of conditions related to the Marfan syndrome, but with different clinical implications, also are due to diverse mutations in *FBN1*. Included are familial ectopia lentis, familial aortic aneurysm, and the MASS phenotype (Table 95.3). MASS is an acronym for *m*itral valve prolapse; mild, nonprogressive *a*ortic root dilatation; *s*triae atrophi-

TABLE 95.2. MOUSE MODELS OF HUMAN SKELETAL DISORDERS

Human Condition	Mouse Gene Name	Mouse Symbol	Mouse Chromosome
Acromesomelic chondrodysplasia	Growth differentiation factor 5	$Gdf5^{bp}$	2
Gaucher disease	Acid β-glucosidase	*Gba*	3
Growth hormone deficiency	Growth hormone–releasing hormone receptor	$Ghrhr^{lit}$	6
Homocystinuria	Cystathionine β-synthase	*Cbs*	17
Hypophosphatemic rickets, X-linked	Phosphate-regulating neutral endopeptidase	$Phex^{Hyp}$	X
Marfan syndrome	Fibrillin 1	$Fbn1^{Tsk}$	2
Menke disease	ATPase, Cu^{2+} transporting	$Atp7a^{Mo}$	X
MPS VII	β-Glucuronidase	gus^{mps}	5
Neurofibromatosis I	Neurofibromatosis	$Nf1^{tmiFcr}$	11
Osteogenesis imperfecta, EDS VII	$\alpha_2(1)$ Procollagen	$Cola2^{oim}$	6
Osteoporosis	Osteoprotegerin	Opg^{-}	
Pituitary hormone deficiency	Pituitary transcription factor	$Pit1^{dw}$	16
Pituitary hormone deficiency	Paired-box homeodomain transcription factor 1	$Prop1^{df}$	11

TABLE 95.3. FIBRILLINOPATHIES

Disorder	OMIM No. (18)
Confirmed	
Familial aortic aneurysm/dissection	132900
Familial ectopia lentis	129600
Familial tall stature	
Marfan syndrome	154700
MASS phenotype/familial mitral valve prolapse/familial myxomatous valvular disease	157700
Shprintzen–Goldberg syndrome	182212
Contractural arachnodactyly	121050
Possible	
Homocystinuria	236200
Bicuspid aortic valve/coarctation/ascending aortic aneurysm	109730
Weill–Marchesani syndrome	277600
Ectopia lentis et pupillae	225200
Marfanoid mental retardation syndrome	248770

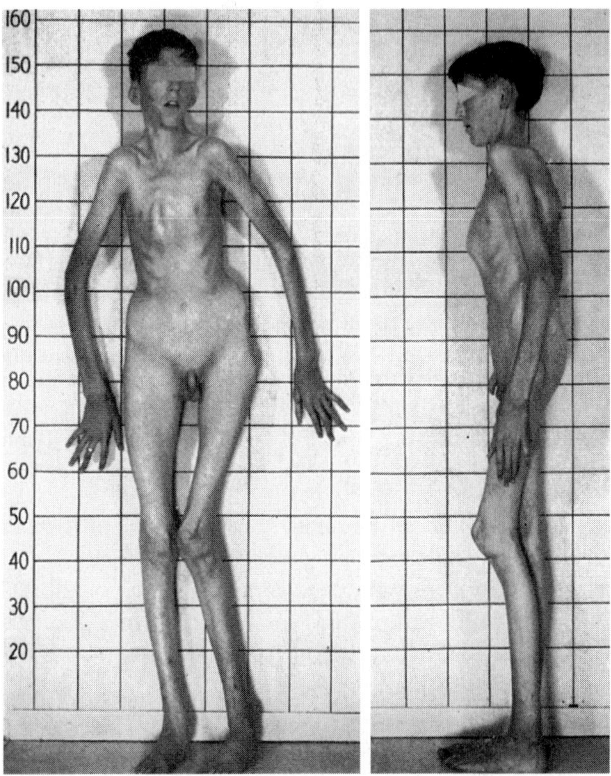

FIGURE 95.1. The Marfan syndrome in a 14-year-old boy. Note arachnodactyly, relatively long limbs (dolichostenomelia), pectus carinatum, sparse subcutaneous fat, unilateral genu valgum, and pes planus. Ectopia lentis and scoliosis also were present. This patient died of aortic rupture at age 15 years.

cae; and mild skeletal features, such as joint hypermobility, scoliosis, and anterior chest deformity. When a mutation in *FBN1* has been found in a patient, however, that change can be assayed relatively simply and inexpensively in relatives or in a fetus. Because the Marfan syndrome displays high penetrance (i.e., virtually never skips a generation), having a pathologic *FBN1* mutation ensures appearance of some features, although considerable intrafamilial variability confounds prognostication.

Skeletal Features

Patients with the Marfan syndrome (45) are excessively tall, or at least taller than unaffected relatives (Fig. 95.1). Body proportions show dolichostenomelia, with long arms (5% greater than height is unquestionably abnormal) and legs, the latter reflected in a low ratio of the upper segment to the lower segment (US/LS) for age. In practice, two measurements are made with the patient standing: height and lower segment (top of the pubic symphysis to floor). In normal, white adults, the mean ratio is about 0.92; in African-American adults, it is about 0.87. The US/LS varies with age, race, sex, and degree of vertebral column deformity in all persons, so that an isolated determination in a suspected patient must be interpreted with caution. The metacarpal index, the ratio of length to width of metacarpals, is said to be useful but requires a radiograph of the hands.

The ribs undergo excessive longitudinal growth as well. Depression of the sternum (pectus excavatum), protrusion (pectus carinatum; Fig. 95.1), or an asymmetric combination often results. The vertebral column is frequently deformed (46). The normal thoracic kyphos is often reduced, resulting in a "straight back" or an outright thoracic lordosis. Scoliosis may involve multiple segments and may progress rapidly, particularly during the adolescent growth spurt. Progression after skeletal maturity also is a possibility, and adults with curves of 30 degrees or more should be followed up regularly. Dural ectasia is usually an incidental finding on plain radiographs, computed tomography, or magnetic resonance imaging of the vertebral column (47). Back pain, so common in the general population, is even more frequent in the Marfan syndrome. The appearance of radicular pain in the buttocks or legs should suggest (in addition to the usual explanations), protrusion of dura through neural foramina. Occasional patients have problems with spinal fluid dynamics (resulting in headaches), abnormal response to spinal anesthesia, or pelvic masses as a consequence of anterior lumbosacral meningoceles.

Loose-jointedness is often striking in patients with the Marfan syndrome (48). Flat feet (pes planus) (49); hyperextensibility at the knees (genu recurvatum), elbows, and fingers; congenital dislocation of the hip (50); and recurrent dislocation of the patellae are manifestations of laxity of ligaments and joint capsules. A relatively narrow palm of the hand, long thumb, and longitudinal laxity of the hand are the bases for the *Steinberg thumb sign* (Fig. 95.2): the thumb apposed across the palm extends well beyond the ulnar margin of the hand. Another simple, but nonspecific, test is the wrist sign; the first and fifth digits, when wrapped around the contralateral wrist, overlap appreciably in the Marfan

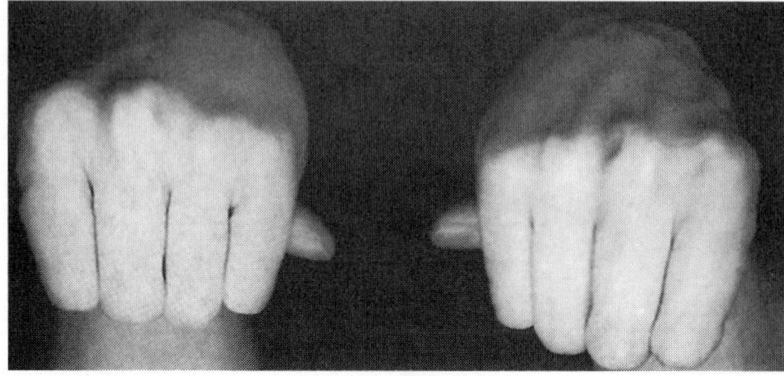

FIGURE 95.2. The Steinberg thumb sign in a patient with the Marfan syndrome. A positive test, such as this, consists of the distal phalanx of the thumb protruding beyond the ulnar border of the clenched fist and reflects both longitudinal laxity of the hand and a long thumb.

syndrome (Fig. 95.3). Acetabular protrusion is of increased prevalence but uncertain prognosis (51).

Joint laxity is so variable, even among relatives affected by the Marfan syndrome, that for a time, distinct disorders were suspected. About 10% of patients have some restriction of extension at one or more joints, usually of congenital onset; although a separate congenital contractual arachnodactyly syndrome exists (36,52), all patients with this signal feature should be evaluated as if they had the Marfan syndrome so that serious problems in other systems are not overlooked (53,54). The "Marfanoid hypermobility syndrome" (55) is not worth distinguishing as a separate entity.

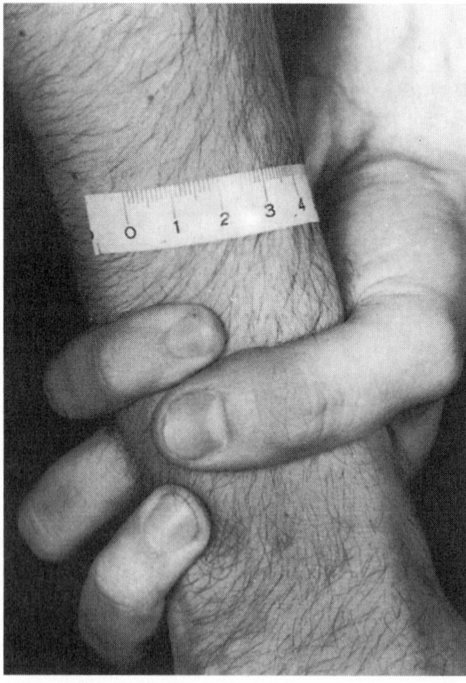

FIGURE 95.3. The wrist sign in a patient with the Marfan syndrome. In a positive test, the first phalanges of the thumb and fifth digit substantially overlap when wrapped around the opposite wrist.

Other Features

Most patients with the Marfan syndrome have myopia, and about one half have subluxation of the lenses (ectopia lentis). The ascending aorta bears the main stress of ventricular ejection, leading to progressive dilatation beginning in the sinuses of Valsalva. Aortic regurgitation and dissection are the main causes of death (36,37). Two decades ago, life expectancy was reduced, on average, by one third in patients with the Marfan syndrome. Subsequently, the development of reliable surgical procedures and their early application (56), and the widespread use of chronic β-adrenergic blockade to reduce stress on the aortic root (57), have greatly improved life expectancy (56,58). Mitral valve prolapse occurs in 80% of patients and leads to severe mitral regurgitation in about 10%; it is the most common cause of cardiovascular morbidity in children (53,59). Hernias are frequent (60), cystic changes in the lungs lead to pneumothorax (61), and striae distensae over the pectoral and deltoid areas and thighs are often first noticed in adolescence.

Management of the Skeletal Manifestations

The Marfan syndrome is compatible with a long and productive life; thus all patients deserve aggressive and prophylactic management of all organ systems at risk. For the skeletal system, management must begin in childhood because most problems are progressive during the years of growth.

Initial management of vertebral column deformity is by bracing. If abnormal curves can be stabilized, persistent bracing may be necessary until the skeleton matures. The presence of thoracic lordosis, common in the Marfan syndrome, unfortunately limits the effectiveness of most braces. Whenever scoliotic curves exceed 40 to 45 degrees, surgical stabilization and fusion are required (46).

Tall stature is usually not a problem in male patients. Girls, on the other hand, are more at risk for psychosocial difficulties as a result of their height. Analysis of growth shows that the average height for girls parallels the 95th percentile of the normal female growth curve; the average adult height is thus close to 6 feet. Early induction of puberty by administration of appropriate doses of sex hormones results in accelerated skeletal maturation. Beginning therapy well before the age of physiologic menarche lessens adult height (36). Furthermore, by acceleration of the "adolescent" growth spurt, there is less time for scoliosis to progress, and deformity is mitigated; this has never been tested in a controlled trial, however. Once the epiphyses are nearly fused or once the girl attains the age of physiologic menarche, hormonal therapy can be discontinued.

Deformity of the anterior chest progressively worsens as a result of rib growth. Repair of either pectus excavatum or pectus carinatum for cosmetic indications should thus be delayed until midadolescence, when the defect is not likely to recur (62). Occasionally, repair is needed earlier because of respiratory compromise.

Through young adulthood, disability resulting from hyperextensibility at other joints is uncommon, although complaints of joint pain are frequent (48). Dislocation of the patellae and the first metacarpal–phalangeal joints, severe pes planus, and metatarsus valgus are the most frequent problems. Physical therapy, muscular strengthening, and well-fitted shoes are useful (49). Surgery for these problems should be avoided if possible. As survival is now approaching the population average, an increased frequency of degenerative arthritis would be expected.

Other Disorders of the Microfibril

The microfibril, 10 to 12 nm in diameter, has a number of components (Table 95.4) that likely vary with organ, and serves several functions in the human extracellular matrix. First, microfibrils are formed early in tissues destined to become elastic. Tropoelastin is then deposited on the microfibrillar matrix, and the elastic fiber results. Microfibrils are ubiquitous, however, and occur in many organs or regions of tissues devoid of elastin. For example, the zonules of the eye are microfibrils, and autosomal dominant ectopia lentis is due to mutations of *FBN1*. Mutations in this locus also cause some cases of familial aortic aneurysm, familial aortic dissection, Shprintzen–Goldberg syndrome, and MASS phenotype (Table 95.3). This latter condition is much more common than the Marfan syndrome, and extends along the clinical continuum from mild Marfan syndrome to the fringes of the normal population (63). MASS has a generally excellent prognosis in the absence of aggressive treatment and is heritable as an autosomal dominant condition.

Fibrillin exists in two known isoforms, encoded by separate genes. *FBN2* encodes fibrillin-2, a glycoprotein deposited before fibrillin-1 in most tissues except those of the cardiovascular system. Thus fibrillin-2 plays a crucial role in embryonic extracellular matrices of the musculoskeletal system. Mutations in *FBN2* cause congenital contractural arachnodactyly, a relatively rare autosomal dominant condition (52,64,65). Patients have contractures of their digits, knees, and elbows at birth; these tend to improve with physical therapy started early in childhood. Scoliosis can be severe and progressive. Deformity ("crumpling") of the helix of the ear is common. A distinguishing feature from the Marfan syndrome should be the absence of aortic involvement. However, people with congenital contractural arachnodactyly have had severe mitral valve prolapse.

TABLE 95.4. CONSTITUENTS OF THE MICROFIBRIL

Protein	Gene	Map Locus
Confirmed		
Fibrillin-1	*FBN1*	15q21.1
Fibrillin-2	*FBN2*	5q23.q31
Latent transforming growth factor-β binding protein 1	*LTBP1*	2p12–q22
Latent transforming growth factor-β binding protein 2	*LTBP2*	14q24
Immunolocalized only		
Microfibril-associated protein-2 (formerly designated *MAGP1*)	*MFAP2*	1p36.1-p35
Microfibril-associated glycoprotein-2	*MAGP2*	12p13.1–p12.3
Microfibril-associated protein-3	*MAFP3*	5q32–q33.3
Lysyl oxidase (found in elastic fibers but not isolated microfibrils)	*LOX*	5q23.3–q31.2
Possible		
Microfibril-associated protein-1	*MFAP1*	15q15–q12
Latent transforming growth factor-β binding protein 2	*LTBP3*	11q12
Latent transforming growth factor-β binding protein 4	*LTBP4*	

Homocystinuria

Homocystinuria is an inborn error in the metabolism of methionine in which activity of the enzyme cystathionine β-synthase is deficient (66–69). Clinical features are superficially similar to those of the Marfan syndrome and include ectopia lentis, dolichostenomelia, arachnodactyly, and chest and spinal deformity (Fig. 95.4). Generalized osteoporosis, "tight" joints, arterial and venous thrombosis, malar flush, psychiatric disturbance, and mental retardation are features of homocystinuria usually not found in the Marfan syndrome (70). Aortic aneurysm and mitral prolapse are not features of homocystinuria. Homocystinuria is an autosomal recessive disorder, unlike the Marfan syndrome, which is a dominant trait. The hand in homocystinuria has none of the longitudinal laxity present in the Marfan syndrome, and the appendicular joints tend to have reduced mobility. Back pain resulting from osteoporosis occurs in some patients.

The pathogenesis of the three cardinal groups of manifestations—mental retardation, connective tissue disorder (ectopia lentis, osteoporosis, reduced joint mobility), and thrombosis—is not understood. Perhaps the reduced sulfhydryl groups of homocysteine or other substances that accumulate proximal to the block interfere with cross-linking of collagen, fibrillin, and other proteins of the extracellular matrix, thus accounting for the connective tissue manifestations. Such a mechanism occurs in the thiolism caused by prolonged administration of penicillamine, a compound structurally similar to homocysteine. An alternative, but not necessarily exclusive, hypothesis focuses on the deficiency of

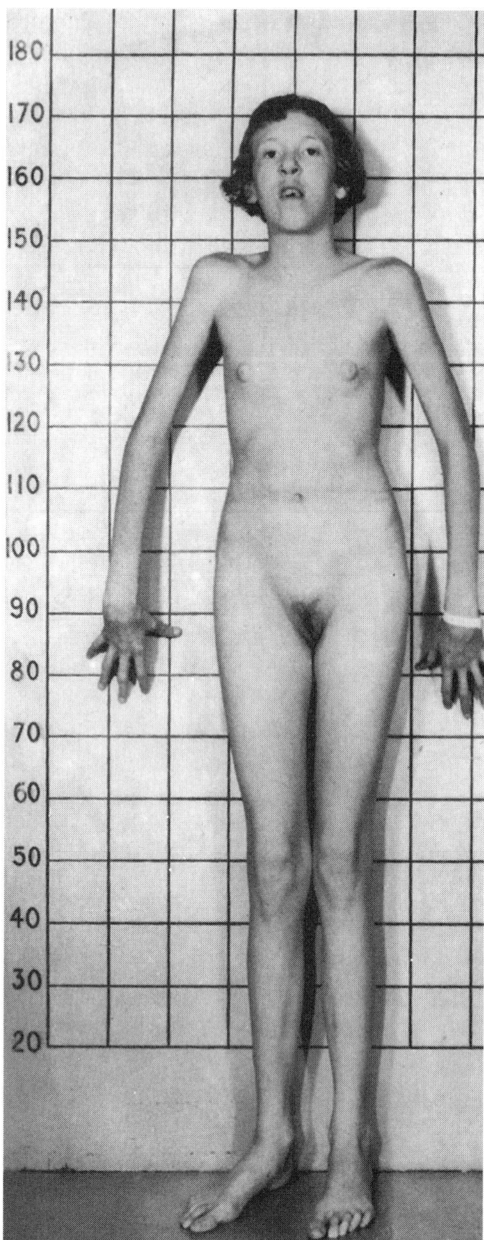

FIGURE 95.4. Homocystinuria in a 12-year-old girl. Note the excessive height, long, narrow feet, and mild anterior chest deformity. The teeth were crowded, ectopia lentis was present, and the joints showed moderate restriction of motion. Despite several episodes of pulmonary embolism and thrombophlebitis, she was active at age 40 years.

cysteine that results from the inability to join homocysteine with serine. Cysteine is one of the three amino acids that form glutathione; deficiency of this amino acid predisposes to damage from free radicals.

About one half of patients with homocystinuria respond to large doses of vitamin B_6 (pyridoxine) with clearing of homocysteine from the urine, lowering of plasma methionine and homocysteine, raising of cysteine to normal, and reducing the likelihood of developing clinical manifestations (66,67). Preexistent mental retardation and ectopia lentis are not improved by pyridoxine treatment in patients who show biochemical correction, emphasizing the need for early diagnosis and therapy. Because most states include testing for elevated blood methionine as part of the newborn screening program, early treatment is possible. Newborns with B_6-responsive cystathionine β-synthase deficiency may have sufficient pyridoxine from maternal sources to prevent hypermethioninemia during the first week of life, and thereby may escape detection. With supplementary folic acid (1 mg daily), as little as 20 mg of pyridoxine daily may be effective, although usually a dosage of 100 to 300 mg is required. In vitamin B_6 nonresponders, a low-methionine diet is the mainstay of management, although pyridoxine and folate should be included because of a tendency for deficiency of these cofactors. Because the low-methionine diet is relatively unpalatable, especially for people who begin protein restriction after infancy, alternative forms of therapy are being explored. The methyl donor betaine, when taken in pharmacologic doses of several grams per day, results in a lowering of plasma homocysteine concentrations and a concomitant increase in cysteine. Long-term clinical trials are needed. Additionally, sulfinpyrazone, dipyridamole, or aspirin, singly or in combination, may be useful in preventing thrombotic episodes in all homocystinurics, even though platelet survival is normal in most patients (71).

Weill–Marchesani Syndrome

Weill–Marchesani syndrome is another systemic disorder with ectopia lentis as a conspicuous feature (Fig. 95.5). The skeletal features are the antithesis of those in the Marfan syndrome: the patients are short, with particularly short hands and feet, and have stiff joints, especially in the hands. The hands sometimes show atrophy of the abductor pollicis brevis muscle consistent with carpal tunnel compression. Weill–Marchesani syndrome can be autosomal recessive or autosomal dominant (72). The basic defect remains unknown.

Ehlers–Danlos Syndromes

The Ehlers–Danlos syndromes (EDS) are a group of disorders of considerable diversity, largely caused by extensive genetic heterogeneity. The cardinal and unifying features relate to the joints and skin—hyperextensibility of skin, easy bruisability, dystrophic scarring, increased joint mobility, and abnormal tissue fragility (21,34,73–76). Internal manifestations, which include rupture of great vessels, hiatal hernia, diverticula of the gastrointestinal and genitourinary tracts, spontaneous rupture of the bowel, and spontaneous pneumothorax, tend to occur only in specific types of EDS.

The classification of EDS designates several general types on the basis of phenotypic and inheritance characteristics (Table 95.5) (74). Biochemical studies have demonstrated

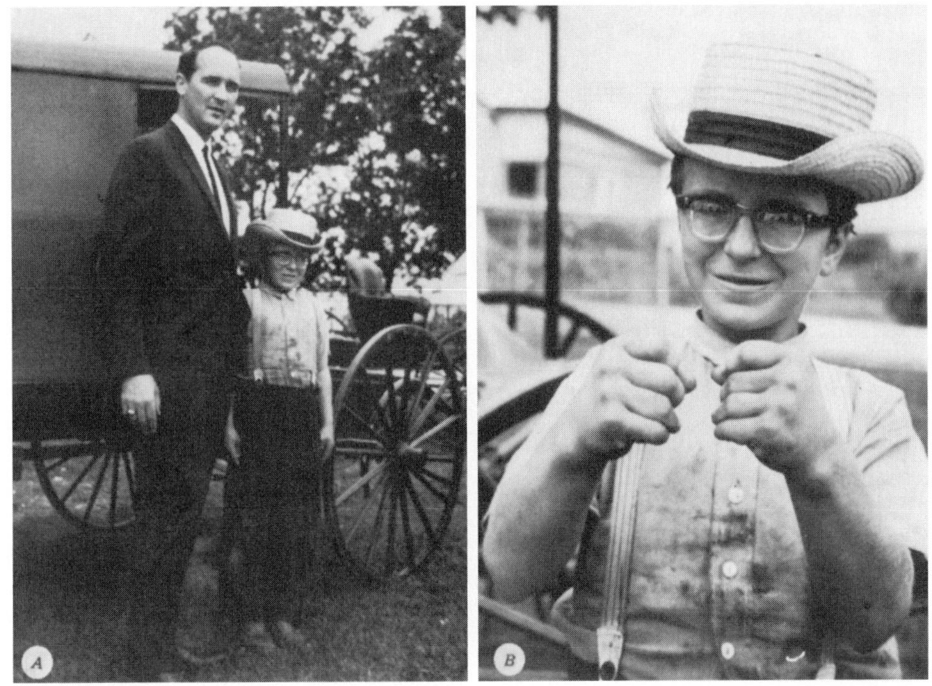

FIGURE 95.5. Weill–Marchesani syndrome in a 15-year-old Amish boy. **A:** Boy shown with normal adult male. Ectopia lentis was present, and attacks of acute glaucoma had occurred. **B:** The fingers were short with knobby joints and restricted flexion. Flattening of the thenar eminence was consistent with carpal tunnel compression.

TABLE 95.5. EHLERS–DANLOS SYNDROMES

Type	Former name	Clinical Features[a]	Inheritance	OMIM no.[b]	Molecular Defect
Classic	EDS I & II	Joint hypermobility; skin hyperextensibility; atrophic scars; smooth, velvety skin; subcutaneous spheroids	AD	130000 130010	Structure of type V collagen *COL5A1, COL5A2*
Hypermobility	EDS III	Joint hypermobility; some skin hyperextensibility, ± smooth and velvety	AD	130020	*COL3A1* in some
Vascular	EDS IV	Thin skin; easy bruising; pinched nose; acrogeria; rupture of large and medium-caliber arteries, uterus and large bowel	AD	130050 (225350) (225360)	Deficient type III collagen *COL3A1*
Kyphoscoliotic	EDS VI	Joint hypermobility; congenital, progressive scoliosis; scleral fragility with globe rupture; tissue fragility, aortic dilatation, mitral valve prolapse	AR	225400	Deficient procollagen-lysine, 2-oxoglutarate 5-dioxygenase *(PLOD)*
Arthrochalasia	EDS VII A & B	Joint hypermobility, severe, with subluxations; congenital hip dislocation; skin hyperextensibility; tissue fragility	AD	130060	No cleavage of N-terminus of type I procollagen 2° mutations in *COL1A1* or *COL1A2*
Dermatosparaxis	EDS VIIC	Severe skin fragility; decreased skin elasticity; easy brusing; hernias; premature rupture of fetal membranes	AR	225410	No cleavage of N-terminus of type I procollagen due to deficiency of peptidase
Unclassified types	EDS V	Classic features	XL	305200	?
	EDS VIII	Classic features and periodontal disease	AD	130080	?
	EDS X	Mild classic features, MVP	?	225310	? Deficient fibronectin
	EDS XI	Joint instability	AD	147900	?
	EDS IX	Classic features; occipital horns	XL	309400	Allelic to Menkes syndrome

AD, autosomal dominant; AR, autosomal recessive; MVP, mitral valve prolapse; XL, X-linked.
[a]Listed in order of diagnostic importance
[b]Entries in Online Mendelian Inheritance in Man (http://www.ncbi.nlm.nih.gov/htbin-post/Omin) for the phenotype; see Table 95.1 for OMIM entry no. for gene defect.

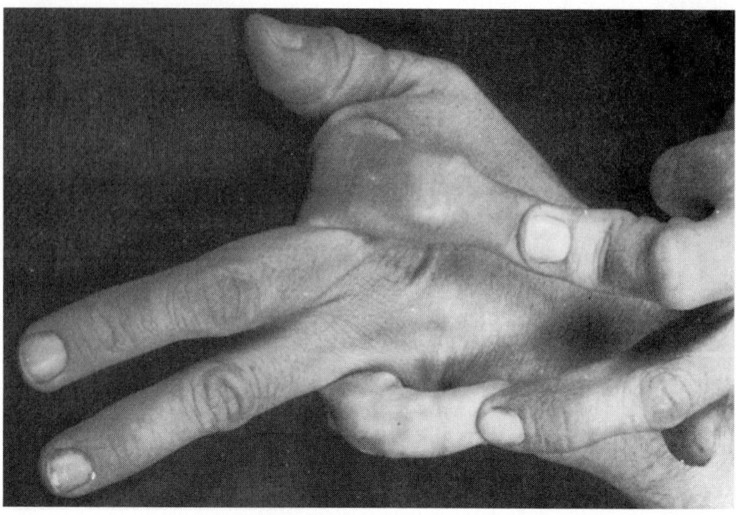

FIGURE 95.6. Joint hypermobility in the classic form of the Ehlers–Danlos syndrome.

considerable heterogeneity within individual types. This extensive phenotypic and biochemical characterization nonetheless fails the clinician as often as it helps; nearly one half of all patients who have at least one "cardinal" manifestation defy categorization.

Ehlers–Danlos Syndrome, Classic Type

Generalized hyperextensibility of joints (Fig. 95.6) and increased stretchability of skin are the hallmarks. Other features include bruising and fragility of the skin, with gaping wounds caused by minor trauma and with poor retention of sutures. Congenital dislocation of the hips in the newborn, habitual dislocation of selected joints in later life, joint effusions, clubfoot deformity of the feet, and spondylolisthesis are all consequences of the loose-jointedness. Hemarthroses and "hemarthritic disability" have been described and are analogous to bruising of the skin. Scoliosis is sometimes severe. Severe leg cramps occurring at rest and of unclear cause are troublesome to some patients. The fracture rate is increased modestly, and bone density is somewhat diminished (77) (Fig. 95.7).

This type is inherited as an autosomal dominant trait. A primary defect has been found in the genes that encode the α1 and 2 procollagen chains of type V collagen (*COL5A1* and *COL5A2*) (9). Type V collagen is a heterotrimer with three different chains; its distribution is similar to types I and III collagen, but in much smaller quantities.

Management of the classic type stresses prevention of trauma and great care in treating wounds. Young athletes benefit from wearing shin guards to protect their lower legs from the repeated minor injuries that lead to frequent hemorrhage, unsightly scars, and absence from school. Patients should be dissuaded from demonstrating their joint laxity as entertainment for their friends. Because the ligaments and joint capsules are lax, joint stability can be improved only by developing the muscles. Care must be used, however, in weight lifting and other forms of exercise because of the fragility of tendons.

Ehlers–Danlos Syndrome, Hypermobility Type

This condition has moderate dermal hyperextensibility and minimal fragility. The joint hyperextensibility ranges from extreme to bordering on normal. All too often, patients with mild joint laxity without joint instability or skin manifestations are labeled as this or some other form of EDS, particularly if relatives show a similar manifestation (78).

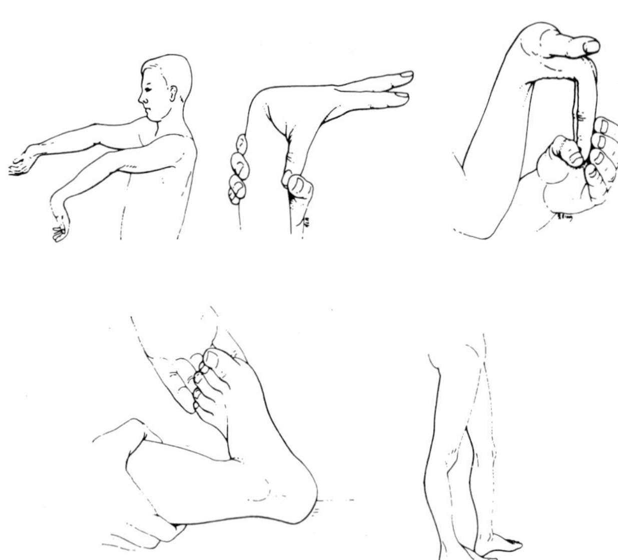

FIGURE 95.7. A method for evaluating joint mobility (73). Excessive joint laxity is judged to exist when at least three of the following five conditions are present: (a) elbows and (b) knees extend beyond 180 degrees; (c) thumb touches the forearm on flexing the wrist; (d) fingers are parallel to the forearm on extending the wrist and metacarpal joints; and (e) foot dorsiflexes to 45 degrees or more.

Such labeling may cause more harm than good, unless one makes it clear that little if any disability is likely to result. Indeed, hypermobility proves to be an asset in some senses, such as in repetitive motions required to play some musical instruments (79).

Ehlers–Danlos Syndrome, Vascular Type

This condition is by far the most serious type of EDS because of a propensity for spontaneous rupture of arteries and bowel (75,76). This type is particularly heterogeneous genetically, the unifying theme being abnormal production of type III collagen. Skin involvement is variable, with thin, nearly translucent skin present in some, and mildly hyperextensible skin the only feature in others. Joint laxity also is variable and may be limited to the digits. Affected women have a high risk of aortic rupture during pregnancy. Inheritance is usually autosomal dominant. Some patients without the classic vascular phenotype have been found to have mutations in *COL3A1,* so the biochemical phenotype does not necessarily predict the clinical (80).

Ehlers–Danlos Syndrome, Kyphoscoliotic Type

Fragility of the ocular globe and a propensity to severe scoliosis, in addition to the skin and joint involvement seen in EDS classic form, are the hallmarks of this autosomal recessive form of EDS. This is the first of the heritable disorders of connective tissue to have its basic defect elucidated, by Krane et al. in 1972 (81). Collagen in this condition contains little hydroxylysine because of deficiency of the enzyme that hydroxylates selected lysyl residues in the nascent collagen chains. Because hydroxylysine is normally involved, along with lysine, in cross-linking of collagen, the clinical features of this form of EDS are readily explained. Vitamin C is a necessary cofactor of lysyl hydroxylase and, in high doses, may be beneficial in some patients with EDS (82) (comparable to the benefit of vitamin B_6 in some cases of homocystinuria).

Ehlers–Danlos Syndrome, Arthrochalasia Type

Profound loose-jointedness with congenital dislocations dominates the clinical picture. The patients are moderately short of stature and the skin is variably, but usually mildly, involved (76). An inability to convert type I procollagen to mature collagen, by cleavage of the N-propeptide, has been found in all patients who have been studied (83). The genetic heterogeneity of this form of EDS is instructive. Deficiency of procollagen N-peptidase, the enzyme that cleaves the propeptide from the amino terminal end of type I procollagen, is deficient in fibroblasts from a minority of patients. Most have had normal N-peptidase activity and an amino acid sequence alteration around the site of the procollagen molecule where cleavage occurs. Two general types of mutations have been described thus far. In the first type, amino acids at the cleavage site in either the α1 (I) or the α2 (I) procollagen chain are mutated, disrupting the α-helix conformation requisite for peptidase activity. Alternatively, a deletion (or theoretically an insertion) of amino acids anywhere in either of the procollagen chains proximal to the N-peptidase cleavage site causes misregister of the three chains and disruption of the α-helix. Deficiency of peptidase activity would likely be an autosomal recessive trait. In distinction, the mutations causing amino acid alternations have all affected only one allele for either *COL1A1* or *COL1A2.* Because neither parent was affected in any of the cases examined biochemically so far, the mutation likely occurred in a parental gonad. The patients, however, should they choose to reproduce, will have a 50% chance of having an affected offspring, and their condition will readily be identified as an autosomal dominant trait.

Ehlers–Danlos Syndrome, Dermatosparaxis Type

This autosomal recessive enzymopathy is due functionally to the same defect in type I collagen as the previous type—an inability to cleave the N-propeptide from procollagen (84). Why the features are more severe in the skin and integument is unclear; perhaps the N-propeptidase has other molecules besides type I procollagen as substrate.

Ehlers–Danlos Syndrome, Unclassified Types

A rare, X-linked form most closely resembles the mild classic type (85). Although a deficiency of lysyl oxidase was claimed in one pedigree, this has not been confirmed or found in any other family.

A rare form is characterized by severe periodontal disease, with early loss of both primary and permanent teeth (86). The basic defect is unknown, and inheritance is autosomal dominant. Because the phenotypes of this type and the vascular type overlap, all such patients should be screened for deficiency of type III collagen.

One pedigree was reported with a phenotype inherited as an autosomal recessive, characterized by features of mild classic type EDS and associated with abnormal platelet aggregation (87). The platelet defect was corrected by exogenous plasma fibronectin.

Familial Articular Hypermobility Syndromes

This category of disorders includes generalized articular hypermobility with or without subluxation (34,81). Excluded are the skeletal dysplasias with joint hypermobility (e.g., Larsen syndrome) and the EDS (which all have some degree of skin involvement).

Familial Articular Hypermobility

This is a relatively common, autosomal dominant condition of unknown biochemical defect. Joint hypermobility is generalized, but rarely causes dislocation or disability (81,88). The incidence of congenital dislocation of the hip may be increased in families with his condition (89), which is also known as familial simple joint laxity.

Familial Articular Hypermobility, Dislocating Type

The cardinal feature of this autosomal dominant condition is instability of multiple appendicular joints; recurrent dislocation is the usual clinical finding. Joint hyperextensibility is variable but usually mild, and skin involvement is uncommon (90). This condition, which has been called both familial joint instability syndrome and EDS XI, may cause considerable disability. Clinical variability within a family is the rule, emphasizing the need for a comprehensive family history, including examination of close relatives if possible (Fig. 95.8).

This is an extremely difficult condition to manage successfully. For most patients, diagnosis is established only after multiple orthopedic surgical attempts (usually disappointing) to prevent recurrent dislocation of shoulders, knees, or elbows. As in the classic type of EDS, physical therapy of affected joints to increase periarticular muscle strength should be attempted first.

Cutis Laxa

The cardinal feature of these conditions is dermatologic: the skin is lax and loose, with none of the hyperelasticity seen in the EDS variants (91). Beyond childhood, the prominent skin folds and excessive wrinkling give a prematurely aged appearance. Both congenital (usually autosomal recessive) and late-onset (autosomal dominant) forms occur, and the basic defects, which presumably affect elastic fibers, are unclear. The skeletal system is largely unaffected, but the condition is of importance because of the phenocopy that rheumatologists may inadvertently cause in the offspring of their patients. A phenocopy is a disorder of nongenetic cause that mimics a hereditary disorder. Some fetuses exposed to D-penicillamine, as a result of maternal treatment of rheumatic disorders, Wilson disease, or cystinuria, develop a congenital syndrome indistinguishable from the severe, autosomal recessive form of cutis laxa (92). Neither the susceptible period of pregnancy nor the threshold dosage has been established.

Pseudoxanthoma Elasticum

The characteristic features occur in the skin, retina, and arteries (93,94). In areas of flexural stress, yellowish papules develop over time, giving the skin the appearance of that of a plucked chicken. As Bruch's membrane fragments, angioid streaks develop in the retina; hemorrhages lead to progressive visual loss. An arteriolar sclerosis, similar histopathologically to that of Mönckeberg, develops and leads to loss of peripheral pulses, myocardial infarction, and gastrointestinal hemorrhage. The skeleton is not involved in any obvious way. Both autosomal recessive (the most common) and autosomal dominant forms occur. The basic defect is unclear, but the pathognomonic dermatopathologic finding is calcification of elastic fibers. Restriction of nutritional calcium intake in early life may retard progression of the disease (95). Both the dominant and recessive forms have been mapped to 16p13.1 (96,97).

CONSTITUTIONAL DISEASES OF BONE

In addition to the disorders of connective tissue already discussed, a wide array of hereditary conditions affect the

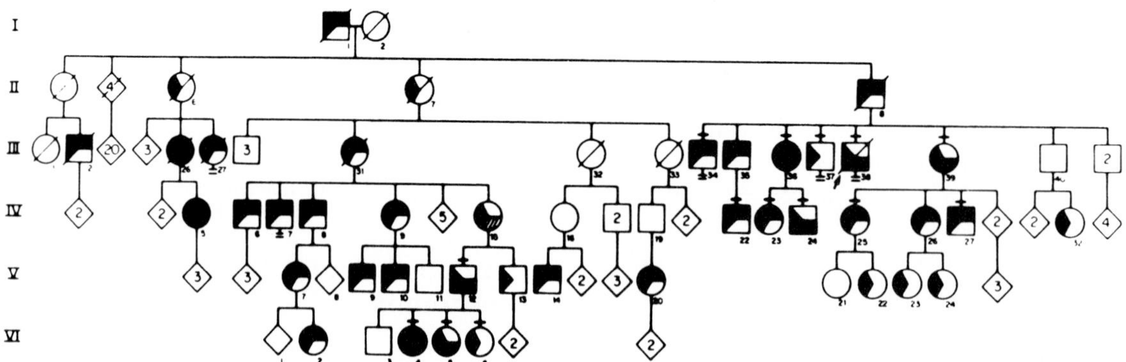

FIGURE 95.8. Pedigree of a family with familial articular hypermobility, dislocating type. The autosomal dominant transmission and variability of the phenotype are both well illustrated. Pedigree symbols: ◐, joint hypermobility; ◔, hip dislocation; ◓, patella dislocation; ●, possibly affected; ♂̄, examined by authors; ⌀, deceased. (Reproduced with permission from Horton WA, et al. Familial joint instability syndrome. *Am J Med Genet* 1980;6:221–228.)

skeleton. According to standard nomenclature, they are classified broadly as osteochondrodysplasia, dysostoses, idiopathic osteolyses, and primary metabolic abnormalities (35,98–100). The most common or instructive examples are presented here.

Osteogenesis Imperfecta Syndromes

Several phenotypically distinct osteogenesis imperfecta (OI) syndromes and even more classification schemes exist (34,101–103). The disorders share osseous, ocular, dental, aural, and cardiovascular involvement. The classification enjoying current application is based on clinical and inheritance pattern criteria (Table 95.6). Most but not all examples of OI are due to mutations in one of the genes encoding type I procollagen, *COL1A1* or *COL1A2* (104,105). Type I OI is the most common form and is associated with wide intrafamilial variability (106–108). One patient might be extremely short of stature, with frequent fractures and considerable disability, whereas an affected relative leads an unencumbered, vigorous life. Type II encompasses the class of "OI congenita" variants, most of which are lethal in infancy, if not *in utero* (105–110). Molecular characterization of type II is mature at both the collagen and the DNA level (73,111). Most cases arise as the result of a new mutation (the phenotype thus being transmissible as a dominant, if the patient could live and reproduce) in either *COL1A1* or *COL1A2.* A few patients have affected siblings and normal parents; rather than indicating autosomal recessive inheritance, some of these instances have been demonstrated to be due to germinal mosaicism. Specifically, fathers have had two populations of sperm, one with a mutation in procollagen type I and one without. Type III OI comprises miscellaneous phenotypes that cannot be classified better (112). Most cases include severe skeletal deformity and short stature as distinguishing features. Most occur sporadically. Some patients have mutations in type I collagen (113), but others do not (114). Type IV OI is similar to type I, only rarer and not associated with blue sclerae.

Accurate diagnosis is especially critical because of the not uncommon dilemma of distinguishing whether recurrent fractures in a young child represent brittle bones or child abuse (115).

Skeletal Features

"Brittle bones" are a familiar and dramatic feature of all the OI variants. Sometimes fractures occur *in utero,* particularly in type II, and permit radiographic antenatal diagnosis. In such cases, the limbs are likely to be short and bent at birth. Multiple rib fractures give a characteristic "beaded" appearance on radiographs. Some patients with types I or IV have few fractures or may escape them entirely, although blue sclerae, short stature, or deafness indicates the presence of the mutant gene. Brittleness and deformability result from a defect in the collagenous matrix of bone. The skeletal aspect of OI is, therefore, a hereditary form of osteoporosis. "Codfish vertebrae" (scalloping of the superior and inferior vertebral bodies by pressure from the expansible intervertebral disc) or flat vertebrae are observed, particularly in older patients in whom senile or postmenopausal changes exaggerate the change, or young patients immobilized after fracture or orthopedic

TABLE 95.6. OSTEOGENESIS IMPERFECTA SYNDROMES

Type	Clinical Features	Inheritance	OMIM No.[a]	Basic Defects
I	Fractures variable in number; little deformity; stature normal or nearly so; blue sclerae; hearing loss common but not always present; DI uncommon	AD	166200	Typically, one nonfunctional *COL1A1* allele
II	Lethal *in utero* or shortly after birth; many fractures at birth involving ribs (may appear "beaded") and other long bones; little mineralization of calvarium; pulmonary hypertension	AD AR	166210	*COL1A1* or *COL1A2:* typically substitution of glycyl residues; occasionally deletions of a portion of the triple-helical domain Deletion in *COL1A2* + nonfunctional allele
III	Fractures common, but long bones progressively deform starting *in utero;* stature markedly reduced; sclerae often blue, but become lighter with age; DI and hearing loss common	AD AR (rare)	259420	One (single amino acid substitution) or rarely two mutations in *COL1A1* and/or *COL1A2*
IV	Fractures common; stature usually reduced; bone deformity common but rarely severe; scleral hue normal to grayish; hearing loss variable; DI common	AD	166220	Point mutations in *COL1A1* or *COL1A2;* exon-skipping mutations in *COL1A2*

AD, autosomal dominant; AR, autosomal recessive; DI, dentinogenesis imperfecta.
[a]Entry in On-line Mendelian Inheritance in Man (http:/www.ncbi.nlm.nih.gov/htbin-post/Omim) for the phenotype; see Table 95.1 for OMIM entry no. for gene defect.

surgery. Usually the frequency of fractures decreases at puberty for patients with types I, III, and IV. Because of failure of union of fractures, pseudarthrosis (especially of the humerus or femur) occurs in some. Hypertrophic callous occurs frequently in patients with OI and is often difficult to distinguish from osteosarcoma. Debate continues as to whether the risk of true osteosarcoma is increased in any form of OI; regardless, the risk is not great, but worthy of consideration whenever skeletal pain occurs in the absence of fracture, particularly in an older patient. Loose-jointedness is sometimes striking in type I OI; dislocation of joints can result from deformity secondary to repeated fracture, ligamentous laxity, or rupture of tendons (especially the Achilles and patellar).

Ocular Features

Blue or bluish gray sclerae are present in types I, II, and III OI and are a valuable clue to the diagnosis. The cornea, like the sclera, is abnormally thin. The ocular features are usually not of great functional importance.

Aural Features

Hearing loss becomes detectable in many patients by the second or third decade of life. It was long assumed that deafness in OI was the result of precocious otosclerosis; alternatively, otosclerosis is such a common disorder in the general population that many OI patients are likely to develop it. A variety of aural abnormalities occurs in OI, and symptomatic hearing loss is nearly always multifactorial. The tympanic membrane may be thin, the pinna deformed, the ossicles disconnected, or the stapedial footplate thickened or degenerated. A surprisingly high percentage of patients have a sensorineural component, attributable in part to cochlear deformity, cochlear hair loss, and tectorial membrane distortion. Thus each patient must be evaluated in considerable detail to determine whether hearing impairment is present and whether it is conductive, sensorineural, or mixed.

Dental Features

The characteristic dental manifestation of OI is opalescent teeth caused by a defect in dentin morphogenesis (116). This finding is easily ascertained by direct observation of the blue or brown opalescent deciduous or permanent teeth or by the typical radiographic changes. This dental abnormality can be useful diagnostically because opalescent teeth, of all of the pleiotropic OI manifestations, tends to breed true in families, and forms the basis for subdividing types I and IV into disorders with and without opalescent teeth. Affected teeth wear poorly; enamel loss is secondary to fracture of the underlying dentin.

Other Features

Unusual bruising occurs in some patients, probably due to a defect in the connective tissue in the walls of small blood vessels or in the supporting connective tissues. Inconsistent defects of the coagulation mechanism or of platelet function have been demonstrated.

Mitral valve prolapse occurs in about 15% of patients with OI type I, several times more frequently than in the general population, and occasionally may progress to mitral regurgitation. Aortic dilatation and regurgitation also occur but are infrequent (117).

Differential Diagnosis

The differential diagnosis of OI includes idiopathic juvenile osteoporosis, juvenile osteoporosis with ocular and mental retardation, Cheney syndrome (osteoporosis, multiple wormian bones, acroosteolysis), pyknodysostosis (dwarfism, brittle bones, absent ramus of mandible, persistent cranial fontanels, acro-osteolysis), hypophosphatasia, and child abuse.

Management

The focus of management has largely been orthopaedic. Recent attempts at medical therapy have had encouraging results by addressing the increased bone resorption and decreased new bone formation that are both characteristic of severe OI. Bisphosphonates inhibit bone resorption, and the compound pamidronate administered intravenously produced increased bone density and decreased fracture frequency in children (118). A more permanent but highly experimental approach involves bone marrow transplantation, with the goal of repleting bone progenitors from the mesenchymal stem cells present in marrow. One trial in three patients with type III OI showed encouraging results (119).

OSTEOCHONDRODYSPLASIAS

These disorders affect development, growth, or both, of cartilage and bone. This category, often termed the skeletal dysplasias, has been divided into defects primarily of tubular bones, defects primarily of the spine, and defects of both the appendicular and axial skeleton. In some conditions, such as multiple epiphyseal dysplasia, only the skeleton is involved. In others, such as spondyloepiphyseal dysplasia congenita, other organs are affected as well. It also has been common practice to categorize conditions by age of onset and severity. Some do not become evident until a year or two of life, or even later. Others are so severe as to be lethal in the neonatal period.

Inborn Errors of Cartilage Collagen

Several groups of disorders, exceedingly diverse clinically, have long shared characteristic radiographic features, differing principally in severity (99). Some have been found to share defects in the principal collagen constituents of cartilage, specifically types II, IX, and XI. Some of the phenotypes in this category are described, beginning with the more severe.

Spondyloepiphyseal Dysplasia (SED) Congenita

As the name implies, short stature and gross skeletal deformity are obvious at birth (98–100). Platyspondyly contributes more to reduced height than does dysplasia of the limbs, which tends to be more severe proximally. Associated clinical features are cleft palate, pectus carinatum, kyphoscoliosis, vitreoretinal degeneration, myopia, and retinal detachment. The cervical spinal cord is vulnerable to subluxation of C1 on C2. The biochemical basis of SED congenita has been studied intensively (120,121). The phenotypes of patients with SED congenita comprise a clinical continuum, with severity positively correlated with how close the amino acid change is to the carboxyl end of the type II procollagen molecule, which determines the degree of posttranslational overmodification that occurs (122). Many cases of SED congenita are sporadic, with little likelihood that the affected women will reproduce because of the significant restriction in abdominal size. Pedigrees with autosomal dominant transmission and direct analysis of mutations suggest that most mutations that cause this disorder are heterozygous.

The radiographic features include a normal skull; platyspondyly; delayed ossification of a dysplastic odontoid; severe disorganization and delay in limb-ossification centers, more severe proximally and especially so at the femoral capital epiphyses; irregular, horizontal acetabula; mild involvement of the carpus; and minimal involvement of the digits. Whether two clinical subgroups can be distinguished based on the severity of coxa vara is unconfirmed.

Premature degenerative arthritis can be crippling. Early, aggressive realignment of the legs may have a clinical role, but long-term follow-up is still in progress.

Kniest Dysplasia

In this condition, the trunk is short because of both platyspondyly and kyphoscoliosis, limbs are generally short, myopia is severe with a predisposition to retinal detachment, and precocious deafness is common. Small deletions in the *COL2A1* gene account for some cases (123).

Spondyloepiphyseal Dysplasia Tarda

Although several types of late-onset SED exist, the majority are in male patients and occur in pedigrees consistent with X-linked recessive inheritance (124). The condition is often not diagnosed until degenerative arthritis develops in the shoulders and hips in late childhood or early adulthood. The radiographic findings in the femoral capital epiphyses and proximal humeral epiphyses are difficult to distinguish from multiple epiphyseal dysplasia. The spine, however, is not only more severely affected, but also characteristic (Fig. 95.9).

Stickler Syndrome

The cardinal features of this relatively common (at least 1 per 10,000 in the population) autosomal dominant condition are severe, progressive myopia; vitreal degeneration; retinal detachment; progressive sensorineural hearing loss; cleft palate; mandibular hypoplasia; hypermobility and hypomobility of joints; epiphyseal dysplasia; and variable disability resulting from joint pain, dislocation, or precocious osteoarthritis (125,126). In one large clinic for craniofacial anomalies, 6.6% of all patients with cleft palate but without cleft lip had Stickler syndrome (127). This condition, also called progressive arthroophthalmopathy, is clearly underdiagnosed, in part because patients often do not have the full syndrome and in part because the physician fails to obtain a detailed family history that might suggest a hereditary condition. The Stickler syndrome should be strongly considered in any infant with "swollen" wrists, knees, or ankles, the Robin triad (hypognathia, cleft palate, and glossoptosis), or flared (dumbbell-shaped) femoral metaphyses; in any adult with precocious degenerative arthritis of the hip, especially if relatives are similarly affected (128); and in any person with spontaneous retinal detachment.

Some nosologic confusion persists. The ocular features, first described in 1938, have been called the Wagner syndrome by ophthalmologists, but this is clearly a distinct condition. Some families with autosomal dominant severe myopia and hearing loss also have severe midfacial hypoplasia (not just flat malae), hypertelorism, a thick calvarium and abnormal frontal sinuses, and ectodermal dysplasia, findings termed Marshall syndrome (129). Patients with cleft palate, midfacial hypoplasia, small jaw, deafness, and SED who have normal eyes have been classified as having OSMED (oto-spondylo-megaepiphyseal dysplasia); this category subsumes those diagnosed as having Weissenbacher–Zweymüller syndrome.

The Stickler syndrome has been linked to the $\alpha 1$(II), $\alpha 1$(XI), and $\alpha 2$(XI) procollagen loci (130–133) and became the first human disease shown to be due to a heritable defect in the principal collagenous component of cartilage. Not all pedigrees with Stickler syndrome show linkage to these loci, and at least one other locus must be involved (131). The lack of eye involvement in patients with OSMED is explained by their defect in expression of *COL11A2*, a gene not normally expressed in the eye. Marshal syndrome is due to mutations in *COL11A1* that result in deletion of an entire exon (134).

"Generalized" Osteoarthritis

Some evidence exists for altered metabolism of type II collagen in cartilage from patients with OA (135). Further, mutations in *COL2A1* have been found in some patients with a family history of generalized OA (i.e., noninflammatory degenerative changes affecting multiple joints) (136). The patients with *COL2A1* mutations all had radiologic evidence of mild spinal chondrodysplasia. They were thus distinct from most patients in the population with OA in two respects: the spinal involvement and the family history. Sib-pair analysis of patients with generalized osteoarthritis from the population showed no linkage to *COL2A1* or to two other cartilage-specific genes, those for link protein and matrix protein (137). In a family with precocious OA with-

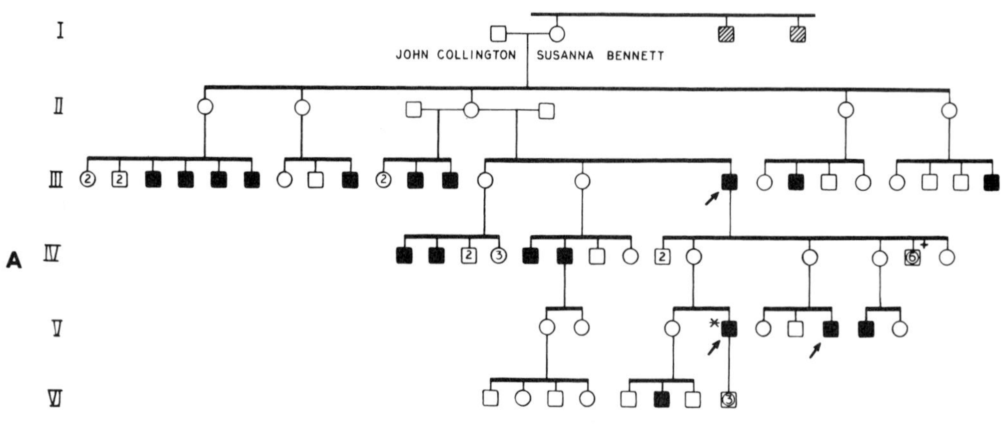

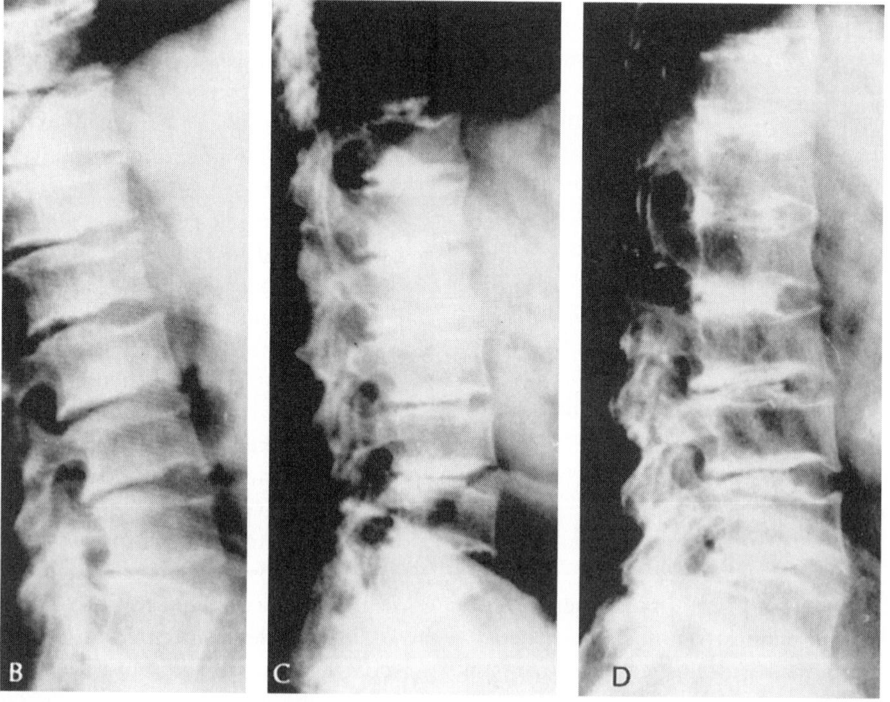

FIGURE 95.9. X-linked spondyloepiphyseal dysplasia tarda. **A:** Partially updated pedigree of family reported by Jacobsen. **B–D:** Radiographic changes in the spine are progressive; the heaping up of the posterior portion of the superior vertebral plate **(B)** is particularly distinctive. At first glance, the late changes **(D)** suggest those of alkaptonuria.

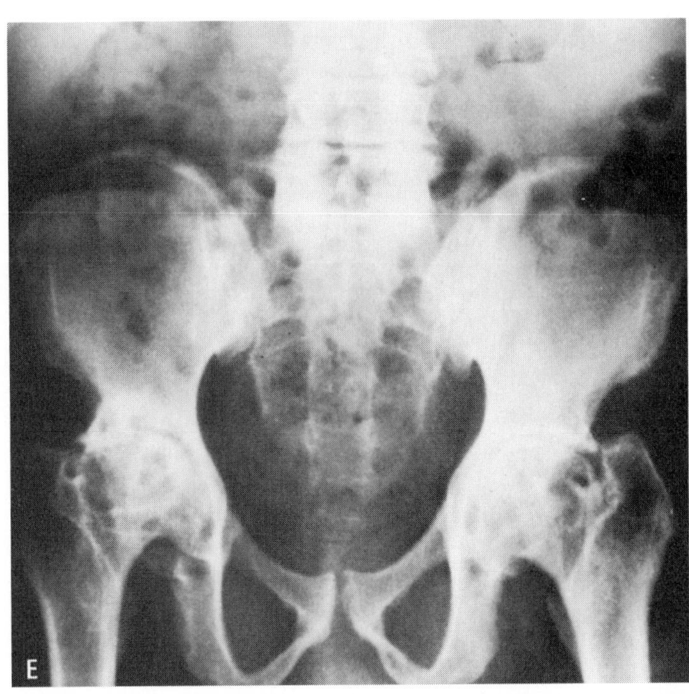

FIGURE 95.9. ***(continued)*** **E:** Late changes in the hips. Note the deep acetabula. (Radiographs courtesy of Dr. Leonard O. Langer, Jr., Minneapolis.)

out evidence of bone dysplasia, a variety of cartilage collagen and other candidate loci were excluded by linkage analysis (138). Thus mutations in *COL2A1* do account for a small percentage of cases of OA, but usually, and perhaps solely, with evidence of vertebral dysplasia (139). The search for a susceptibility locus for OA absent vertebral involvement and osteodysplasia continues; evidence from sib-pair analysis has suggested a locus on chromosome 11q (140).

Another component of cartilage, type IX collagen, is mutated in an autosomal dominant form of intervertebral disc disease. The defect occurred in the *COL9A2* locus (141).

Other Osteochondrodysplasias

Multiple Epiphyseal Dysplasias

This group of disorders is defined by disordered growth of the epiphyses of one or more pairs of joints that leads to a strong predisposition to early degenerative arthritis. Because of diversity in clinical phenotype and inheritance pattern among affected families, multiple epiphyseal dysplasia (MED) was long thought to be heterogenous. The most familiar form is autosomal dominant and comes to attention when a child is evaluated for short stature, abnormalities of gait, or hip pain. This condition is known by the eponym, Fairbanks type. Occasionally the diagnosis is not made until the third or fourth decade, when degenerative arthritis of the hips or occasionally of other joints occurs; this less severe condition has been called the Ribbing type of MED.

The most characteristic radiographic features occur in epiphyses of the limbs, with mild to no involvement of the spine and a normal skull. Joints are symmetrically involved. The appearance of ossification is delayed, and the centers then become irregular or even fragmented (98). Cone-shaped epiphyses of the metacarpals and phalanges may lead to brachydactyly and deformity of the interphalangeal joints, but surprisingly little pain or disability. The hips are nearly always affected, with abnormal ossification of the capital femoral epiphyses leading to a flattened femoral head (Fig. 95.10). The acetabulum is usually affected, and protrusio acetabuli is often seen.

The differential diagnosis includes Legg–Perthes disease, which is distinguished by being asymmetric, involving the metaphysis, sparing the acetabulum, and usually improving spontaneously; the spondyloepiphyseal dysplasias (especially in male patients, the tarda form), in which the spine is more severely affected than the limbs; and untreated hypothyroidism.

In some, but not all families with Fairbanks type, MED was linked to markers in chromosomal band 19p13.1 (142,143). Mutations in a Ca^{2+}-binding motif of the gene encoding cartilage oligomeric matrix protein (*COMP*), which maps to this region of chromosome 19, were subsequently discovered in some patients with MED (144,145). Interestingly, *COMP* is also the cause of some cases of pseudoachondroplasia. Other families with MED mapped to chromosome 1, and mutations in the *COL9A2* gene were found (146). Yet a third locus was identified on chromosome 20 at the site of the *COL9A3* locus (147). Rare cases of autosomal recessive MED have been found because of mutations in the *DTDST* gene, which also is responsible for diastrophic dysplasia (148).

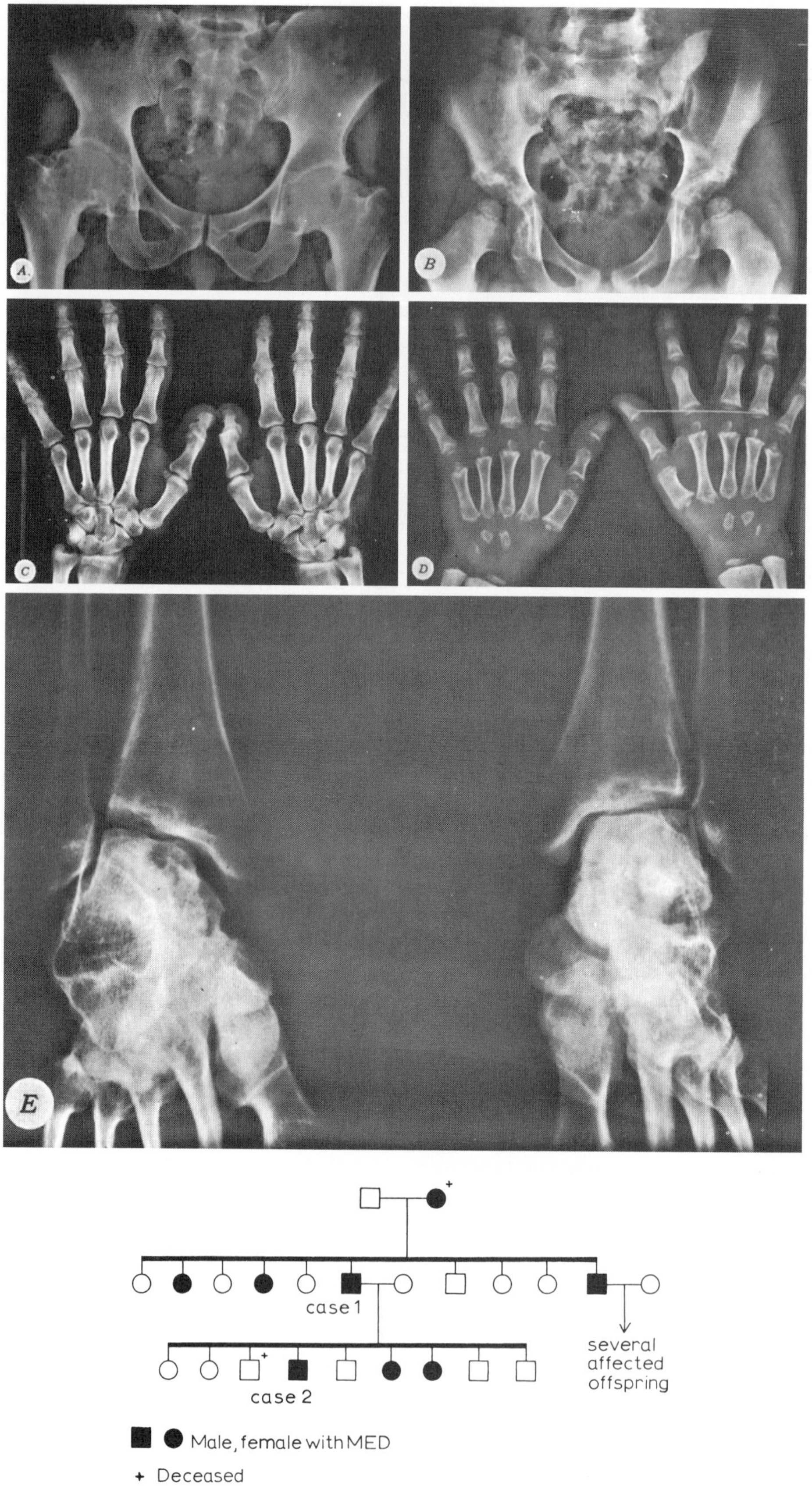

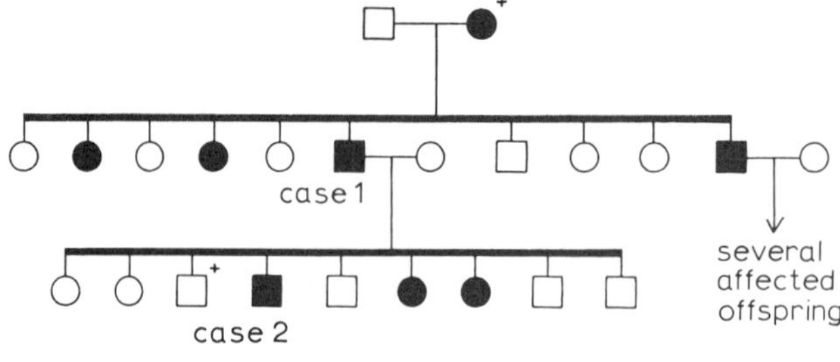

■ ● Male, female with MED

+ Deceased

F

Pseudoachondroplastic Dysplasia

This disorder affects the epiphyses, metaphyses, and the spine, and is therefore classified as a spondyloepimetaphyseal dysplasia (98). The skeletal changes, which can be severe and debilitating, are distinct from achondroplasia, despite the name. Short stature is not evident at birth, but growth falls off the standard curves by age 1 or 2 years (149). Typically the head and the face are spared. Generalized ligamentous laxity and early-onset OA are characteristic. Chondrocytes show accumulation of proteoglycan-like material in the endoplasmic reticulum. The basic defect resides in the same gene, *COMP,* that causes various forms of MED (144,150–153). Most families show autosomal dominant inheritance; suggestions of recessive inheritance were most likely due to germline mosaicism in a clinically unaffected parent (154).

Achondroplasia and Other Disorders of Fibroblast Growth Factor Receptors

This most common of the osteochondrodysplasias may occur as frequently as 1 per 50,000 births, and is the classic form of "short-limbed" dwarfism. In the medical literature before 1950, one has to view a diagnosis of "achondroplasia" with a healthy degree of skepticism because many conditions that affected the limbs more than the spine were so diagnosed. Achondroplasia is evident at birth (98,155,156), is heritable as an autosomal dominant trait, and affects other organ systems only secondarily (157). Midfacial hypoplasia produces a characteristic facies. General habitus and appearance are typified by rhizomelic (proximal) shortening of the limbs, flexion contractures of the elbows, bowed legs, hyperlordosis of the lumbosacral spine, and excessive body weight. Constriction of the craniocervical junction, particularly from a small foramen magnum (158), can produce quadriparesis, sleep apnea, and sudden death in infants (159). When to intervene with surgical decompression is a continuing matter of debate (160,161). The entire vertebral canal can be constricted, and in many patients, neurologic problems develop from impingement of the cord, roots, or cauda equina at ages ranging from early adolescence to late adulthood (162,163). The entire range of neurologic complications is only partly understood (164). Joint laxity of the shoulders and the knees can precipitate recurrent subluxation and predispose to degenerative arthritis.

The basic defect affects enchondral bone and produces diagnostic radiographic features (98). The skull base is short and the face small compared with the cranium; megalencephaly is part of the syndrome but may be accentuated by hydrocephalus (165). The posterior border of the vertebrae is scalloped, and the pedicles are short. In the lumbar spine, the interpedicular distance narrows caudally. In infants, a thoracolumbar gibbus is common; when it persists, anterior vertebral wedging results. The pelvis has square ilia with horizontal acetabular roofs and small sciatic notches. Appendicular metaphyses are widened.

Many patients benefit greatly from occupational and physical therapy, back braces, weight reduction, and various surgical procedures. Suboccipital craniectomy can be lifesaving in infancy (160). Straightening bowed legs can improve both gait and appearance (166). By using surgical techniques for lengthening limbs, pioneered by the Soviet orthopedist Ilizarov, the stature and arm span can be increased in achondroplasia, or indeed in many skeletal dysplasias. The incidence of vascular, neurologic, and infectious complications of the procedure has diminished with technical modifications and wider experience. Considerable debate continues, however, over whether the functional, cosmetic, and psychological benefits are worth the protracted disability, potential morbidity, and psychological and economic costs. Extended laminectomy for spinal stenosis, if performed early in the evolution of neurologic complications, can restore function (165).

The size of the head is increased in achondroplasia, not just in relation to stature. The cause is actual or arrested hydrocephalus. The head circumference must be monitored closely during infancy and childhood; a growth curve crossing percentiles for achondroplasia strongly suggests the need for shunting. Although cognitive skills are generally preserved, children with achondroplasia require careful follow-up and individual management (167).

The basic defect in achondroplasia is a mutation in the gene encoding fibroblast growth factor receptor 3 (*FGFR3*), which is located at chromosome 4p16.3 (168). More than 98% of mutations are identical, and involve substituting glycine for arginine at residue 280 in a transmembrane

FIGURE 95.10. Multiple epiphyseal dysplasia in father and son. Both were short in stature, the father being 153.7 cm (61.5 inches) tall. **A:** Hips in the father at age 44 years, showing advanced degenerative changes. **B:** Hips in the son at age 10 years, showing small femoral capital epiphyses and irregularities of the acetabula. **C:** Hands of the father showing brachydactyly, a short carpus, and degenerative joint disease. **D:** Hands of the son at age 10 years, showing dysplastic epiphyses and delayed development of the carpal bones. **E:** Sloping of the distal tibia is a clue to the diagnosis of multiple epiphyseal dysplasia in the adult. **F:** Family pedigree, in which cases 1 and 2 are the father and son illustrated here, demonstrates typical autosomal dominant inheritance of multiple epiphyseal dysplasia.

domain of the receptor (G380R). There is thus a simple DNA-based test for achondroplasia, which can be used in patients with equivocal diagnoses (an unusual occurrence) or prenatally. If one or both parents have achondroplasia, there is usually little interest in determining if a child is heterozygous for the mutation, but if both parents are affected, the risk is 25% that offspring will inherit both mutant alleles and have homozygous achondroplasia. This is a severe condition, and most patients do not survive infancy. Most cases of heterozygous achondroplasia are sporadic (i.e., neither parent is affected) and the result of a new mutation in one of the *FGFR3* alleles of the father (169).

A more severe condition, achondroplasia with developmental delay and acanthosis nigricans, is due to another distinct mutation in *FGFR3* (Lys650Met) (170).

Hypochondroplasia is a less severe condition, with milder radiologic features similar to those of achondroplasia (98), and is also due to mutations in *FGFR3,* but at a different codon. The common mutation causes substitution of an asparagine at residue 540 with lysine in a tyrosine kinase domain (N450K) (171). Individuals who inherit one G380R allele and one N450K allele have a condition more severe than either achondroplasia or hypochondroplasia, but not so severe as homozygous achondroplasia (172,173).

Thanatophoric dysplasia is one of the skeletal dysplasias considered a neonatal lethal; it also bears radiologic similarity to achondroplasia, albeit much more severe (98). Two types can be distinguished based on whether the femurs are short and curved (type I) or straight and relatively long (type II). Cloverleaf skull (kleblatschadel) is more common in type II. These conditions also are due to mutations in *FGFR3*: a glutamine-for-lysine change at codon 650 is typical of type I, whereas a cysteine-for-arginine substitution at codon 248 often occurs in type II (174).

Fibroblast growth factor receptors constitute a family of proteins of importance in diverse aspects of skeletal developmental (175). Thus far, mutations in *FGFR2* have been described in Crouzon syndrome and Jackson–Weiss syndrome (176,177), and mutations in *FGFR1* have been found in the Pfeiffer syndrome (178).

Metaphyseal Dysplasias

This is a heterogeneous grouping of disorders linked by primary radiographic abnormalities in the metaphyses of long bones (35,98). The Schmid form is characterized by short stature, bow legs, coxa vara, and autosomal dominance. Femoral and tibial osteotomies are common orthopaedic procedures. A defect in the gene encoding type X collagen, *COL10A1,* accounts for all patients studied thus far (179–181). This protein is a "short-chain" collagen and is expressed in hypertrophic chondrocytes; it has a prominent role in endochondral ossification.

The Jansen form of metaphyseal chondrodysplasia is associated with hypercalcemia and hypophosphatemia in the presence of normal levels of parathyroid hormone (PTH) and PTH-related protein (PTHrP). A defect in the PTH-PTHrP receptor was detected in a patient with this form of dwarfism (182).

The gene responsible for Ellis–van Creveld syndrome has been mapped to the short arm of chromosome 4 (183). This is a pleiotropic condition affecting bone, digital development, soft tissue of the mouth, and the interatrial septum.

Cartilage–hair hypoplasia (also known as metaphyseal chondrodysplasia, type McKusick) is particularly prevalent among the Finns and the Amish of Ohio. In addition to short-limbed dwarfism and thin hair that grows poorly, patients have deficient T-cell immunity, predisposition to hematopoietic malignancy, and decreased erythropoiesis (184). The gene maps to chromosome 9 (9p21-p31), and the same locus is involved in the disorder in diverse populations (185).

A number of spondylometaphyseal dysplasias (SMDs) exist, with metaphyseal changes indistinguishable from the Schmid form of metaphyseal dysplasia but with the added involvement of the spine (platyspondyly). One Japanese patient with SMD had a mutation in the *COL10A1* locus, but a number of other patients with SMD have had no detectable mutations in type X collagen (186).

Diastrophic Dysplasia

This autosomal recessive condition is evident at birth and prominently involves the spine, the feet, and the hands. Precocious calcification of cartilage leads to a "cauliflower" ear and symphalangism (the "hitchhiker's thumb"). Severe kyphoscoliosis, spinal stenosis, and C1–C2 subluxation pose threats to life. A defect of type IX collagen has been detected (187).

Cleidocranial Dysplasia

This autosomal dominant disorder is associated with abnormalities of both endochondral and membranous bone. Stature is mildly to moderately reduced, the clavicles are absent to hypoplastic, the anterior fontanel is large and patent, the midface is depressed, and dental abnormalities are prominent, including supernumerary and ectopic teeth (188). A gene for the condition was mapped to chromosome 6 (6p12) (189). One of the bone morphogenic proteins (BMP6) is a candidate.

Campomelic Dysplasia

This autosomal recessive disorder is unusual because although the sex ratio is 1:1 based on chromosome analysis (as would be expected), there is a preponderance of phenotypic female patients (190). The defect involves a gene encoding a transcription factor related to the product of the *SRY* gene, which induces testis development. The *SOX9* gene maps to 17q24.1-q25.1 and is mutated in patients with this extremely severe form of skeletal dysplasia associated with sex reversal (191).

Pycnodysostosis

This autosomal recessive condition, best known for affecting Henri de Toulouse-Lautrec, involves acroosteolysis, osteosclerosis, frequent fractures, delayed closure of cranial sutures (the hat often worn by the French artist presumably protected his persistent anterior fontanel), and short stature. The basic defect resides in a cathepsin K protein encoded at 1q21 (192).

Chondrodysplasia Punctata

This is a heterogeneous group of disorders that share abnormal calcification in developing endochondral bone. The physical features are similar to those of two other disorders, warfarin embryopathy and vitamin K epoxide reductase deficiency. The epiphyses of some bones appear stippled. One form is X-linked, and has been associated with deletions of the short arm. The defect involves mutation of one of the sulfatase genes located in band Xp22.3 (193).

Multiple Exostoses

This is a heterogeneous group of disorders, some associated with other features, such as in Langer–Gideon syndrome, due to contiguous gene deletions at 8q24.1. But isolated bony growths on long bones by themselves is heritable as an autosomal dominant trait (194). These protuberances can cause deformity and orthopaedic difficulties around joints. Males tend to be more severely affected, but penetrance is complete when radiography is used for diagnosis. Most families show linkage to either the *EXT1* gene on chromosome 8q23-q24 or the *EXT2* gene on 11p11-p12 (195). Both of these genes probably have tumor-suppressor functions.

Hyperostosis Corticalis Generalisata (Van Buchem Disease)

This autosomal recessive condition is characterized by osteosclerosis of the diaphyses of long bones, of the jaw, and of the skull. The changes become evident in childhood and do not predispose to fractures. Clinical sequelae result from encroachment on cranial foramina, leading to nerve palsy, deafness, and optic atrophy. The phenotype has been mapped to chromosome 17q12-q21 (196).

Skeletal Dysplasias with Prominent Joint Laxity

Many of the osteochondrodysplasias have variable degrees of joint laxity or instability as part of the overall phenotype. Several disorders, however, have such prominent joint hypermobility as to be the cardinal sign, and have been grouped in one category.

Larsen Syndrome

The Larsen syndrome is characterized by multiple congenital dislocations and characteristic facies: prominent forehead, depressed nasal bridge, and widely spaced eyes (197,198). Dislocation occurs at the knees (characteristically anterior displacement of the tibia on the femur), hips, and elbows. The metacarpals are short, with cylindric fingers lacking the usual tapering. Cleft palate, hydrocephalus, abnormalities of spinal segmentation, and moderate-to-severe short stature have occurred in some. Radiographic features that are helpful in diagnosis, in addition to congenital segmentation anomalies of the spine and congenital hip dislocation, are multiple ossification centers in the calcaneus and carpus. Several instances of multiple affected siblings with normal parents and one instance of consanguineous parents are known, suggesting autosomal recessive inheritance. But parent–child involvement also occurs, consistent with dominant inheritance; thus at least two clinically indistinguishable forms of the Larsen syndrome exist.

Dysostoses

This group of disorders involves malformations of individual bones, either singly or in combination. Some involve primarily the cranium and face [e.g., mandibulofacial dysostosis (199)], others the spine (e.g., Klippel–Feil deformities), and others the extremities [e.g., brachydactyly, symphalangism, polydactyly, and syndactyly (200)].

Symphalangism

Harvey Cushing (201) applied this term to a condition of hereditary ankylosis of the proximal interphalangeal joints. Fusion of carpal and tarsal bones also occurs in this autosomal dominant disorder.

Camptodactyly

Limited extension of the digits is a feature of more than 25 syndromes, including the Marfan syndrome, but occasionally is an isolated abnormality inherited as an autosomal dominant trait (200,202). Permanent flexion contractures are present at the proximal interphalangeal joints without limitation of flexion, typically accompanied by hyperextension at the metacarpophalangeal joints, and sometimes at the distal interphalangeal joints. Camptodactyly may be limited to the fifth finger or to other fingers. Rarely the thumb may be involved as well, with severity decreasing in the radial direction. A contracture band can often be felt on the volar surface of the affected proximal interphalangeal joint, and the transverse skin crease is invariably absent there. Camptodactyly is present from birth or early childhood and shows little tendency to progression. Because of compensatory hyperextension at the metacarpophalangeal joints, the contracture causes little disability. As was pointed out by Archibald Garrod, camptodactyly, when it involves multiple fingers, is often accompanied by knuckle pads, thickened skin on the dorsal aspect of the proximal interphalangeal joints. Camptodactyly is sometimes confused with Dupuytren's contracture, which is late in onset and has its primary site of contracture in the palm.

Hyperostosis Cranialis Interna

This autosomal dominant condition is limited to the calvaria and base of the skull (203). Patients have recurrent palsy of the facial nerve, and develop progressive impairment of balance, smell, taste, and vision.

Idiopathic Osteolyses

In the several, rare, heritable conditions that belong to this category, progressive dissolution of bone occurs, with predictable debilitating and disfiguring consequences. In no case, is either the cause or the pathogenesis understood (204,205).

Primary Metabolic Abnormalities

In each of the disorders in this category, an inborn error disrupts metabolism of a constituent of cartilage or bone. In many cases, the constituent also is present in the connective tissue of other organs, and associated features of each syndrome may be either primary or secondary to skeletal involvement. For example, homocystinuria (*vide supra*) represents a primary metabolic defect with secondary effect on the extracellular matrix and, hence, the skeleton.

Mucopolysaccharidoses

The conditions in this subgroup of the heteroglycanoses are the result of inborn errors of mucopolysaccharide metabolism. Although phenotypically diverse, the individual disorders share mucopolysacchariduria and deposition of mucopolysaccharides in various tissues. Numerous distinct types of mucopolysaccharidoses (MPSs) can be distinguished on the basis of combined clinical, genetic, and biochemical analysis (206). Table 95.7 summarizes the distinctive features of each. Additional biochemical and clinical variants undoubtedly remain to be described. All of these disorders are recessive, mucopolysaccharidosis II being X-linked, and the others autosomal.

Glycosaminoglycans (acid mucopolysaccharides) are the major constituents of the relatively amorphous part of the extracellular matrix that has been in the past referred to as "ground substance." The size, composition, and structure of proteoglycans vary widely in the human body (Chapter 10), but the hyaluronate backbone, core protein side chains, and link proteins that bind the glycosaminoglycan moieties are common to all. Proteoglycans, regardless of structural nuances and tissue distribution, share catabolic pathways; in particular, glycosaminoglycan degradation is largely catalyzed by lysosomal hydrolases. Thus a deficiency of one enzyme will affect the metabolism of a variety of glycosaminoglycans in a variety of tissues and is largely responsible for the pleiotropism of the MPS disorders, that is, the diversity of phenotypic features associated with a single mutant gene. All the MPS disorders are characterized by abnormal urinary excretion of glycosaminoglycans—"mucopolysacchariduria" of dermatan sulfate, heparan sulfate, and keratan sulfate—which is useful in screening and specific diagnosis.

Mucopolysacchariduria can be identified by several standard screening tests, at least one of which is part of the standard battery performed when a "metabolic screen" is ordered. Fractionation and characterization of the urinary mucopolysaccharides are useful in separating the several types of MPSs. For example, MPS III (Sanfilippo syndrome—the heparan sulfate excreters) and MPS IV (Morquio syndrome—the keratan sulfate excreters) in young subjects may be distinguished from the other types, especially MPS IH (Hurler syndrome—dermatan sulfate excreters), mainly by chemical analysis.

Studies with radioactive sulfate indicate accumulation of label in cultured fibroblasts and delayed washout, compatible with these disorders being due to a degradative defect. The specific lysosomal enzyme deficient in each is now known (Table 95.7). Like other lysosomal disorders, the MPSs have six distinctive characteristics: (a) intracellular storage of material occurs; (b) the storage materials are heterogeneous because the degradative enzymes are not strictly specific (e.g., in MPS IH, ganglioside is deposited in brain and predominantly mucopolysaccharide in the liver, and two glycosaminoglycans are excreted in the urine); (c) deposition is vacuolar (i.e., membrane bound) in the cytoplasm; (d) many tissues are affected; (e) the disorder is clinically progressive; and (f) replacement therapy is at least theoretically possible, through replacing the missing enzyme by the process of endocytosis, or by adding a functional copy of the relevant gene.

The possibility of replacement therapy in the MPSs is more than theoretic. Normal cells or the medium in which they have grown, when mixed with MPS fibroblasts, correct the metabolic defect (206). This finding indicates the production of a diffusible correction factor by normal cells, which is found also in normal urine. The correction factor is the enzyme deficient in the given disorder. Several trials of enzyme replacement therapy, using plasma exchange and fibroblast transplantation, have been attended by limited success, however, particularly in reversing established neurologic defects.

Bone marrow transplantation has been used in patients with MPSs that do and do not affect the brain (206,207). In either case, some improvement in somatic features (such as corneal clouding and joint stiffness) may occur, but mental retardation or other severe neurologic problems have been resistant to the presence of enzyme in the bloodstream. The complications of bone marrow transplantation now limit early intervention with this method when prevention of somatic features, rather than their reversal, might be possible. The differential features of the MPSs are summarized in Table 95.7, and the clinical features of MPS IH,

TABLE 95.7. GENETIC MUCOPOLYSACCHARIDOSES

Disorder OMIM[a] Eponym	Clinical Manifestations	Genetics	Urinary MPS	Enzyme Deficiency	Locus
MPS I 252800		AR	Dermatan sulfate Heparan sulfate	α-L-Iduronidase *IDUA*	4p16.3
MPS IH Hurler	Coarse facies, severe DM, clouding of cornea, progressive MR, death usually <10 y/o				
MPS IS Scheie	Stiff joints, cloudy cornea, aortic valve disease, normal intelligence and survival to adulthood				
MPS IH/S Hurler–Scheie	Intermediate phenotype				
MPS II 309900		XL	Dermatan sulfate Heparan sulfate	Iduronate sulfatase *IDS*	Xq28
Hunter, severe	No corneal clouding, otherwise similar to MPS IH, death before 15 years				
Hunter, mild	Stiff joints, survival to 30s to 60s, fair intelligence				
MPS IIIA 252900 Sanfilippo A	Mild physical features and DM, severe progressive MR	AR	Heparan sulfate	Heparan *N*-sulfatase (sulfamidase) *SGSH*	17q25.3
MPS IIIB 252920 Sanfilippo B	Indistinguishable from MPS IIIA	AR	Heparan sulfate	*N*-Acetyl-α-D-glucosaminidase *NAGLU*	17q21
MPS IIIC 252930 Sanfilippo C	Indistinguishable from MPS IIIA	AR	Heparan sulfate	Acetyl-CoA-α-glucosaminide *N*-acetyltransferase *MPS3C*	14
MPS III D 252940 Sanfilippo D	Indistinguishable from MPS IIIA	AR	Heparan sulfate	*N*-Acetylglucosamine-6-sulfate sulfatase *GNS*	12q14
MPS IV A 253000 Morquio A	Severe, distinctive bone changes, cloudy cornea, aortic regurgitation, thin enamel	AR	Keratan sulfate	Galactosamine-6-sulfate sulfatase *GALNS*	16q24.3
MPS IV B 253010 Morquio B (O'Brien–Arbisser)	Mild bone changes, cloudy cornea, hypoplastic odontoid, normal enamel	AR	Keratan sulfate	β-Galactosidase *GLB1*	3p21.33
MPS V	No longer used				
MPS VI 253200		AR	Dermatan sulfate	Arylsulfatase B (*N*-acetylgalactosamine 4-sulfatase) *ARSB*	5q11–q13
Maroteaux–Lamy Severe	Severe DM and corneal clouding, valvular heart disease, striking WBC inclusions, normal intellect, survival to 20s				
Intermediate	Same spectrum as severe, but milder				
Mild	Same spectrum as severe, but mild				
MPS VII 253230 Sly	DM, progressive MR, WBC inclusions, hepatosplenomegaly	AR	Dermatan sulfate Heparan sulfate	β-Glucuronidase *GUSB*	7q21.11
MPS VIII 253230	No longer used				
MPS IX 601492	Short stature, progressive soft tissue, and periarticular accumulations of hyaluronan	AR	Hyaluronic acid	Hyaluronidase *HYAL1*	3p21.3–p21.2

AD, autosomal dominant; AR, autosomal recessive; XL, X-linked; DM, dysostosis multiplex; MR, mental retardation.
Entry in On-line Mendelian Inheritance in Man (http://www.ncbi.nlm.nih.gov/htbin-post/Omim).

MPS IS, and MPS II are illustrated in Figs. 95.11, 95.12, and 95.13, respectively. The nosologic validity of this classification is supported by the results of cocultivation of fibroblasts. Mutual correction of their metabolic defects occurs when fibroblasts from MPS I and II, MPS I and III, and other combinations are studied. Failure of cross-correction between cultured fibroblasts of two patients indicates that they have the same enzyme deficiency, and that the mutations underlying them at a minimum are allelic, if not identical. Allelic variation at the loci responsible for MPS I, II, and VI accounts for the severe and milder forms of those disorders.

Skeletal Features

Relatively short stature is the rule in all patients with the MPS and can be profound in MPS IH, IV (the Morquio syndrome is the prototype "short trunk" form of dwarfism), and VI. Radiographically, the skeletal dysplasia is similar in character in all but MPS IV, differing among the others largely in severity (98). The term *dysostosis multiplex* has been applied, but is not specific for MPS, similar changes occurring in a variety of storage disorders. The chief radiographic features are a thick calvaria, an enlarged J-shaped sella turcica, a short and wide mandible, biconvex vertebral bodies, hypoplasia of the odontoid, broad ribs, short and thick clavicles, coxa valga, metacarpals with widened diaphyses and pointed proximal ends, and short phalanges.

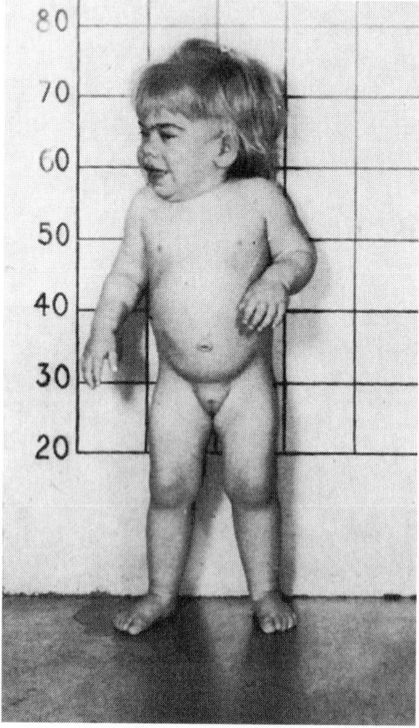

FIGURE 95.11. Mucopolysaccharidosis IH (Hurler syndrome) in a 2-year-old girl. Note the coarse facial features, prominent abdomen from hepatosplenomegaly, claw hands, and short stature. The joints generally had moderate restriction of motion. The patient died of congestive heart failure at age 12 years.

For the disorders compatible with survival to adulthood without severe retardation (MPS IS, II mild, IV, and VI), progressive arthropathy and transverse myelopathy secondary to C1–C2 subluxation account for considerable disability. Cervical fusion should be considered whenever upper motor neuron signs appear. Joint replacement, particularly of the hips, has been beneficial in MPS IS.

Stiff joints are a more or less striking feature of all forms except MPS IV. Like other somatic features, such as coarse facies, reduced joint mobility is less striking in MPS III. In the Scheie syndrome, stiff hands, together with clouding of the cornea, can lead to the main disability. In that condition, as in the others, carpal tunnel syndrome contributes to disability. Early decompression can be beneficial.

Other System Involvement

Regardless of the presence or severity of mental retardation or of the average life span, the major causes of death have as their pathogenesis the accumulation of glycosaminoglycan in soft tissues. The myocardium, cardiac valves, and coronary arteries are prime sites, and death of cardiac failure secondary to restrictive cardiopathy, severe valvular disease, or myocardial infarction is common (but often unrecognized) in MPS IH and IIA. Infiltration of the oropharynx and middle airways progresses to cause major clinical problems in most patients who survive cardiac disease (208). When attempting any procedure that requires sedation or anesthesia in a patient with an MPS, maximal precautions to protect the airway must be used. If possible, procedures should be performed under local anesthetic. Intubation of the airway should be attempted only after careful assessment of the anatomy, and with full respect for the possibility of atlantoaxial instability.

Phosphotransferase Deficiencies

Mucolipidosis II also is called I-cell disease (because of conspicuous inclusions in cultured cells). Mucolipidosis III also is called pseudo–Hurler polydystrophy. Neither shows mucopolysacchariduria despite lysosomal storage of mucopolysaccharide and a demonstrable defect in degradation of mucopolysaccharides. Both are inherited as autosomal recessive conditions, and some forms are likely allelic. The basic biochemical defect rests with an enzyme, UDP-*N*-acetylglucosamine:lysosomal enzyme, *N*-acetylglucosaminylphosphotransferase, responsible for post-translational modification of lysosomal enzymes (209). This defect results in multiple enzyme deficiencies and accumulation in tissues of both mucopolysaccharides and mucolipids.

Mucolipidosis II is a severe Hurler-like disorder. Survival rarely extends beyond the first decade. Mucolipidosis III is a distinctive disorder with stiff joints, cloudy cornea, carpal tunnel syndrome, short stature, coarse facies, and sometimes mild mental retardation, compatible with survival to adulthood (Fig. 95.14).

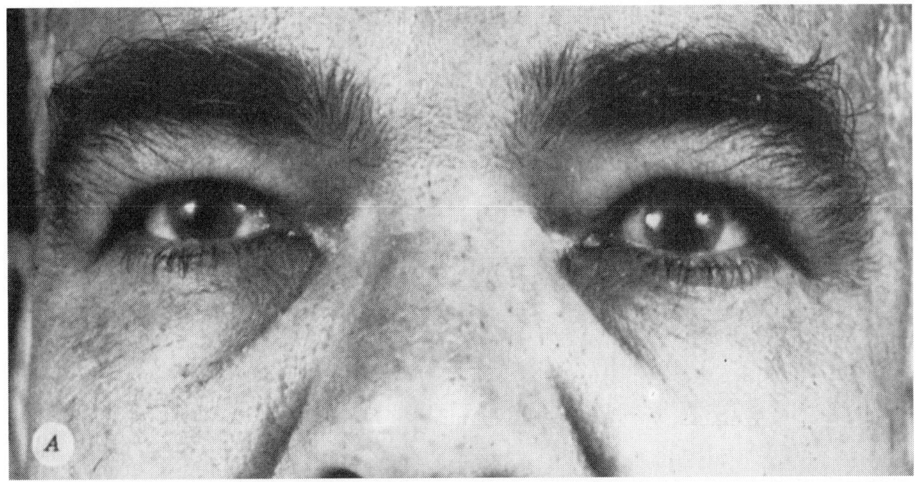

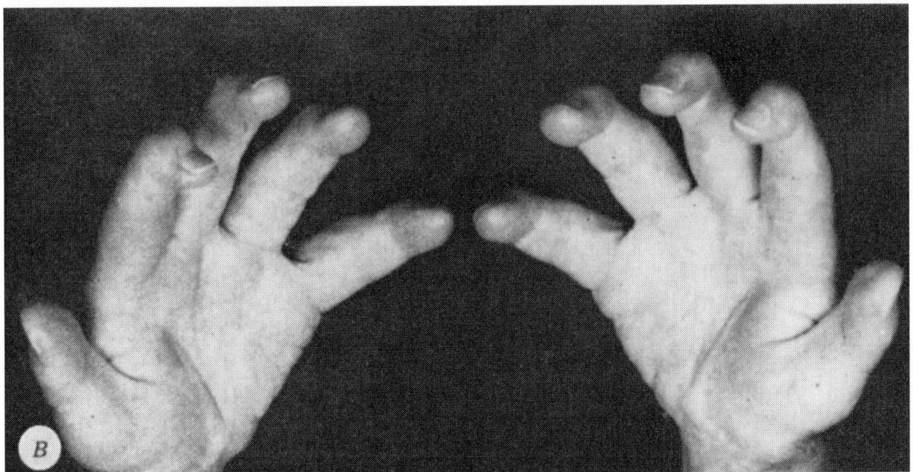

FIGURE 95.12. Mucopolysaccharidosis IS (Scheie syndrome) in a 54-year-old. **A:** Clouding of the cornea was densest peripherally. **B:** The hands were clawed; atrophy of the lateral aspect of the thenar eminences indicated carpal tunnel compression.

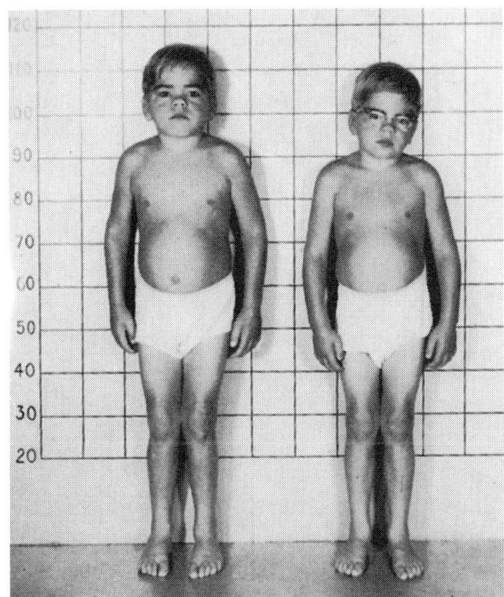

FIGURE 95.13. Mucopolysaccharidosis II, mild (Hunter syndrome, mild variant) in brothers, ages 7 and 6 years. Note the short stature, coarse facies, prominent abdomen, and clawed hands. Intellect was normal.

Mannosidosis

Deficiency of α-mannosidase, one of the many acid hydrolases found in lysosomes, causes phenotypic abnormalities of widely varying severity (210). Male and female subjects are affected with equal frequency, and symptomatic parents of patients have reduced levels of α-mannosidase, both features of autosomal recessive inheritance. Although the clinical conditions were initially thought to be limited to a severe and a mild form (designated types I and II), enough variation has been described to suggest a spectrum of phenotypes, presumably caused by an allelic series of mutations.

The most severe phenotype resembles the Hurler syndrome (MPS IH) in terms of coarse facial features, short stature, mental and motor retardation, hepatomegaly, and skeletal changes of dysostosis multiplex. Patients with severe mannosidosis have typical spoke-like posterior cataracts and lymphocytes with clear cytoplasmic vacuoles, and death in infancy of recurrent respiratory infections is common. At the other end of the phenotypic continuum, patients may

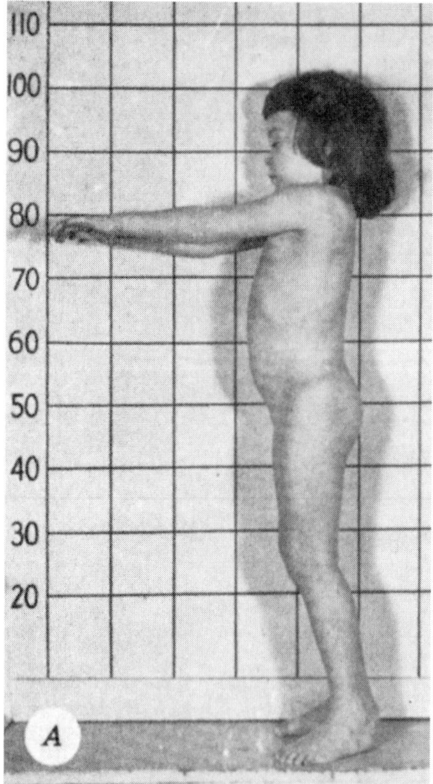

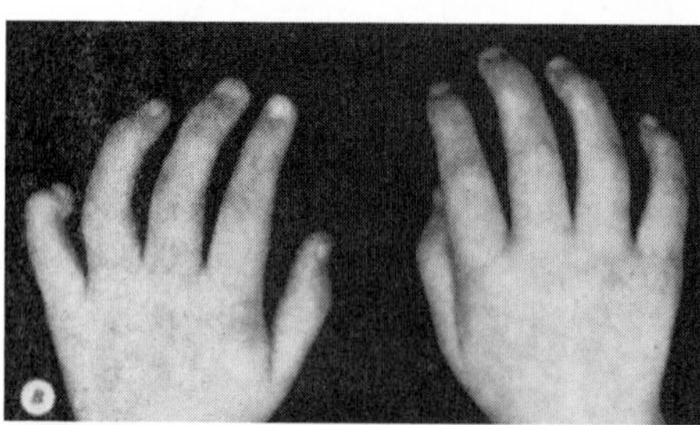

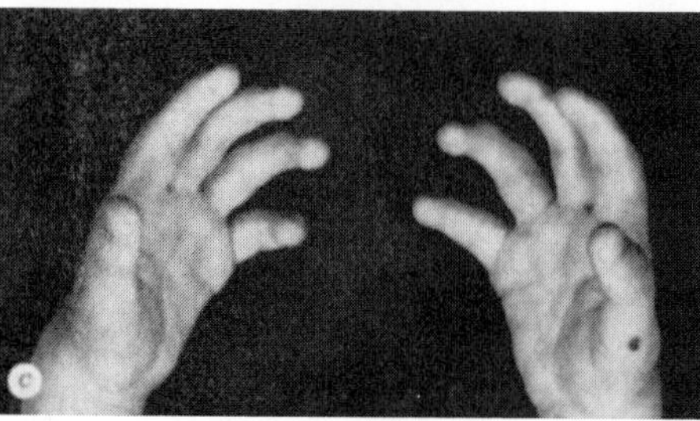

FIGURE 95.14. Mucolipidosis III (pseudo-Hurler polydystrophy) in a 6-year-old girl. **A:** Note the short stature and coarse facies. The corneas were clouded, motion of all joints was restricted, a murmur of aortic regurgitation was present, and intellect was mildly deficient. **B, C:** The hands were clawed, and atrophy of the thenar eminences indicated carpal tunnel compression, for which an operation was performed at age 13 years, with some benefit.

not be diagnosed until adulthood, have mild coarsening of facies, clear corneas, IQs in the borderline normal range, and joint hypermobility. They come to medical attention because of degenerative arthritis of the hips or cardiac problems similar to those described in the MPSs.

The diagnosis is suggested by screening urine for oligosaccharides and is confirmed by documenting decreased activity of α-mannosidase in cultured fibroblasts.

Alkaptonuria

This inborn error of amino acid metabolism was one of the original conditions studied by Archibald Garrod at the turn of the 20th century. A defect in tyrosine metabolism that results in accumulation of homogentisic acid in connective tissue, especially cartilage, has long been known (211). Degenerative arthropathy, especially of the knees and spine, develops at a relatively early age in adults. Accumulation also occurs in heart valves, and there may be a predisposition to atherosclerosis. The basic defect resides in the gene encoding the enzyme homogentisic acid oxidase (212,213).

Other Disorders That Simulate Arthritides

Hypophosphatemic and Vitamin D–resistant Bone Disease

Rickets of nutritional and environmental causes has largely been eliminated as a medical concern because of supplementation of the diet with vitamin D and exposure to sunlight. As a result, cases seen today are highly likely to have a genetic basis. In 1937, Albright et al. (214) described the first instance of a patient with rickets who responded only to supraphysiologic doses of vitamin D. This condition, now termed familial hypophosphatemic rickets or vitamin D–resistant rickets, is inherited as an X-linked dominant trait. Male and female patients both have reduced renal tubular reabsorption of phosphate that results in hypophosphatemia; however, serum calcium remains normal, and patients do not develop muscle weakness or tetany. The skeletal features, which are more severe in male patients (Fig. 95.15), are those of rickets and osteomalacia. In infancy and childhood, the epiphyses are broad and the metaphyses cupped; the epiphyses fuse early, the limbs bow, and the end plates of the vertebrae become sclerotic. Later in life, generalized bony sclerosis, scoliosis, protrusio acetabuli, and spinal stenosis from calcification of the ligamentum flavum develop. In adults, peripheral bone mass tends to be reduced, whereas axial bone mass is increased (215), consistent with degenerative arthritis of the legs rather than vertebral fractures being the most frequent late complication (216). The gene defect is expressed in teeth, resulting in abnormal secondary dentin, an effect apparently unrelated to hypophosphatemia. Therapy with both oral phosphate (four to five doses daily) and vitamin D can prevent skeletal changes. 1,25-Dihydroxyvitamin D (calcitriol) is preferable to vitamin D in producing optimal linear growth (217,218). The risks of nephrocalcinosis and secondary hyperparathyroidism increase with the dose of phosphate, so careful monitoring of children is necessary (218,219). Nephrocalcinosis is a complication of therapy, not an age-dependent feature. In the murine model for this disease (*Hyp* mouse; Table 95.2), transplantation of a normal kidney did not correct the serum phosphate or the fractional excretion of phosphate; transplantation of a kidney from a *Hyp* mouse to a normal mouse did not create abnormal phosphate balance (220), suggesting a humoral factor at work in the disorder. The gene for human hypophosphatemic rickets, *HYP*, maps to Xp22.1. A gene (*PHEX*) that encodes a neutral endopeptidase is mutated in patients (221,222).

Autosomal dominant and recessive forms of vitamin D–resistant rickets exist. The former is similar to the more common X-linked form except for the absence of overt rachitic changes. The condition is also more variable and may not be detected (usually on the basis of bone pain and dental abnormalities) until adolescence. Therapy usually requires calcitriol but not phosphate. A putative gene, *VWF*, of unknown function has been mapped to 12p13.3 (223).

In the hypocalcemic form of vitamin D–resistant rickets, an autosomal recessive disease, defects in the gene (*VDR*) for the cellular receptor for 1,25-dihydroxyvitamin D_3 occur (224). Alopecia is a prominent finding in some families. Resistance to exogenous vitamin D metabolites is often profound, but substantial benefit attends oral phosphate supplementation. Whether allelic variation at *VDR* plays an role in bone density, and osteoporosis in the general population continues to be an area of high activity and controversy (26,225).

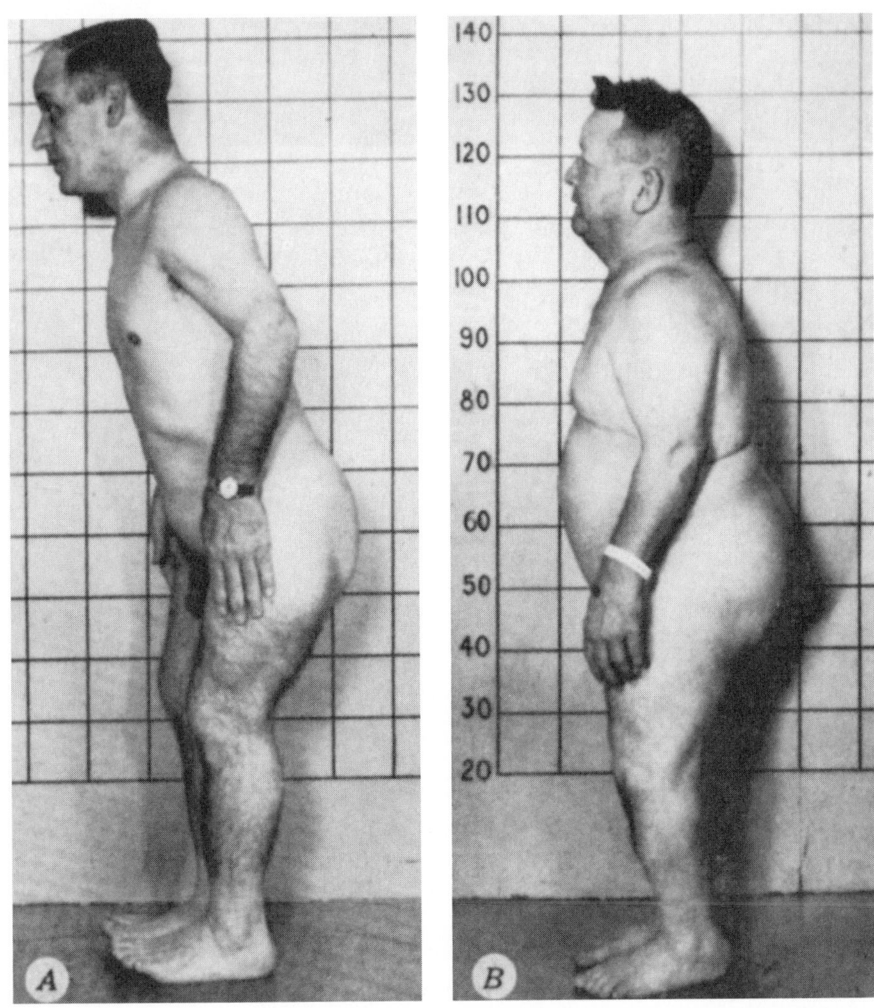

FIGURE 95.15. Ankylosing arthropathy in two men with vitamin D–resistant rickets. **A:** 41-year-old man. **B:** 61-year-old man. The younger man is the more severely affected, but both have almost complete ankylosis of the spine and similar changes in some peripheral joints. Note the short stature.

(continued on next page)

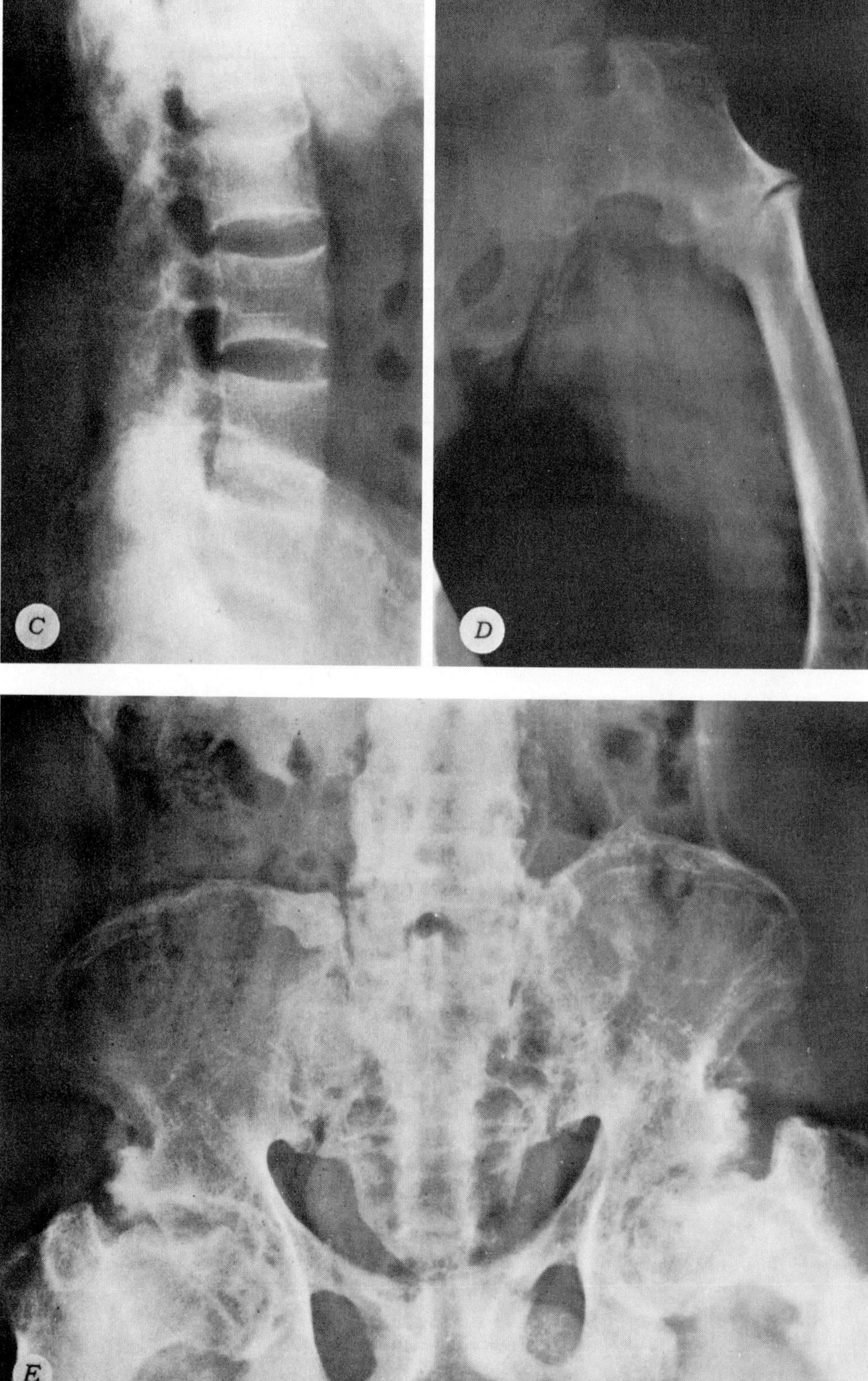

FIGURE 95.15. ***(continued)*** **C:** Lateral radiograph of the lower spine in the older patient. **D:** Left femur of the younger patient. Pseudofractures were situated symmetrically in the subtrochanteric area of both femurs. **E:** Pelvis of the 41-year-old patient.

Fibrodysplasia Ossificans Progressiva

This disorder, formerly called myositis ossificans progressiva, is uncommon and usually sporadic (226). Characterized by progressive ossification of ligaments, tendons, and aponeuroses, fibrodysplasia ossificans progressiva begins an inexorable, progressive course in the first year or so of life, usually with a seemingly inflammatory process and nodule formation on the back of the thorax, neck, or scalp. Local heat, leukocytosis, and elevated sedimentation rate are observed at this stage. Acute rheumatic fever is sometimes diagnosed. A valuable clue to the correct diagnosis is a short great toe with or without a short thumb; this is the leading cause of congenital hallux valgus (227). Life expectancy is considerably reduced, with progressive restriction in lung capacity contributing to respiratory insufficiency and terminal pneumonia (228,229).

From the few familial cases, autosomal dominant inheritance is likely, although most patients are the consequence of a new mutation. The finding of overexpression of bone morphogenic protein-4 in both lymphocytes and lesional cells from patients but not controls suggests that the basic defect may lie in the *BMP4* gene at 14q22-q23 (230).

Hypoparathyroidism

Hypocalcemia and its systemic consequences can be due to either inadequate or ineffective PTH. Both classes of defects have multiple genetic causes (Table 95.1). Aplasia of the parathyroid glands occurs as part of the DiGeorge sequence (third and fourth branchial arch syndrome), which is associated with an interstitial deletion of chromosome 22 (del22q11) (11).

The lack of effect of PTH leads to elevated hormone levels in the face of hypocalcemia and hyperphosphatemia. The phenotype termed Albright hereditary osteodystrophy (AHO; pseudohypoparathyroidism) shows, in addition to short stature and digits, variable mental retardation and ectopic calcification. Most patients with AHO exhibit an abnormal phosphaturic response to exogenous PTH; patients with type IA AHO also have a low output of cyclic adenosine monophosphate (cAMP) in response to PTH, whereas those with type IB have a normal or elevated cAMP excretion (231). Patients with the autosomal dominant type IA have ectopic calcification, especially of the basal ganglia and the paraspinal ligaments. A characteristic skeletal change is shortening of the metacarpals and metatarsals, especially the fourth. Failure to increase urinary cAMP in response to PTH is due to the basic defect, reduced function or synthesis of the α subunit of the stimulatory G protein of adenylate cyclase, encoded by the *GNAS1* locus (232). This defect in a second messenger accounts for the characteristic resistance to multiple hormones in AHO IA. Patients with pseudohypoparathyroidism can coexist in pedigrees with AHO IA, have the same skeletal phenotype, but not have endocrine abnormalities. Resistance to PTH and other hormones is imprinted, and the AHO IA phenotype occurs when the mutation is inherited from an affected mother (233).

The G proteins are normal in AHO IB, and patients with this form of PTH resistance have a normal appearance; whereas they have PTH-resistant hypocalcemia and hyperphosphatemia, responses to other hormones are normal. Interestingly, the condition maps to the same locus and shows the same dependence on parental imprinting as AHO IA (234).

A third condition, termed the AHO-like phenotype, includes short stature, sparse hair, short digits, a characteristic facies with deeply set eyes, bulbous nose, and thin upper lip, mental deficiency, and seizures. This disorder is associated with deletion of the end of the long arm of chromosome 2 (235).

Arthrogryposis Multiplex Congenita

The phenotype of congenital rigidity of multiple joints is of complex etiology, pathogenesis, and clinical presentation (236,237). In many instances, the disorder is a deformation of joints resulting from immobilization of the developing fetus, so that the proper stimulus for joint development is lacking. The cause of the immobilization may be a prenatal disorder of the brain, spinal cord, peripheral nerves, vasculature, or muscle. The affected baby is born with the arms and legs fixed in postures dictated by the position of the embryo and fetus in development. In addition to joint rigidity, dislocation of the hips and micrognathia are frequent findings. The Drachman theory of fetal immobilization as one cause of arthrogryposis multiplex congenita was developed from studies of the effects of neuromuscular blocking agents on chick embryos (238). His theory is supported by observation of arthrogryposis multiplex congenita in an infant born of a mother who received tubocurarine in early pregnancy for treatment of tetanus. The hereditary syndromes that include arthrogryposis multiplex congenita are exceedingly heterogeneous; at least three X-linked conditions affecting predominantly the distal joints have been described (239). A prenatally or neonatally lethal congenital contracture syndrome, inherited as an autosomal recessive trait, has been mapped to chromosome 9q34 (240). The pathologic hallmark is degeneration of motor neurons in the spinal cord.

Chondrocalcinosis

The deposition of calcium oxalate, phosphate, or pyrophosphate crystals (pseudogout) can lead to precocious osteoarthritis (cf. Chapters 117–119). Predispositions to each of these can be hereditary (Table 95.1).

Chondrocalcinosis is a classification of heterogeneous conditions associated by chronic arthritides with calcium salt crystals in synovial fluid and calcification of articular cartilage. Three broad categories exist: cases due to other metabolic disorders (e.g., hyperparathyroidism, hypothyroidism, Wilson disease, hemochromatosis); hereditary forms; and sporadic cases (at least some of which are likely genetic). Chondrocalcinosis 1 is an autosomal dominant condition associated with severe degenerative arthritis and linked to human chromosome 8q (241). Chondrocalcinosis 2 is also autosomal dominant with variable expression; it accounted for one fourth of chondrocalcinosis in one region of Spain (242). An unidentified gene maps to 5p15. Chondrocalcinosis is also a complication of Bartter syndrome, an autosomal recessive condition. In one family in which seven members had hypokalemic alkalosis with hypomagnesemia and hyperreninemic hyperaldosteronism, chondrocalcinosis was a prominent complication that improved with magnesium replacement (243).

Familial hypocalciuric hypercalcemia (FHH), which must be distinguished from familial multiple endocrine adenomatosis type I, is characterized by parathyroid hyperplasia, hypercalcemia, and no hypercalciuria (244). In some families, FHH mapped to 3q13, in the same location as the *CASR* gene, which encodes a calcium-sensing receptor (245). The range of expression is considerable, with some neonates suspected of having osteogenesis imperfecta (246). At least two other forms of FHH exist, one of which maps to 19q13 (247).

REFERENCES

1. Murphy EA, Pyeritz RE. Pathogenetics. In: Rimoin DL, Connor JM, Pyeritz RE, eds. *Principles and practice of medical genetics.* 3rd ed. New York: Churchill Livingstone, 1997:359–370.
2. Rimoin DL, Connor JM, Pyeritz RE. Nature and frequency of genetic disease. In: Rimoin DL, Connor JM, Pyeritz RE, eds. *Principles and practice of medical genetics.* 3rd ed. New York: Churchill Livingstone, 1997;31–34.
3. Childs B. *Genetic medicine.* Baltimore: Johns Hopkins University Press, 1999.
4. Rimoin DL, Connor JM, Pyeritz RE, eds. *Principles and practice of medical genetics.* 3rd ed. New York: Churchill Livingstone, 1997.
5. Wallace DC, Brown MD, Lott MT. Mitochondrial genetics. In: Rimoin DL, Connor JM, Pyeritz RE, eds. *Principles and practice of medical genetics.* 3rd ed. New York: Churchill Livingstone, 1997:277–332.
6. Pyeritz RE. Genetic approaches to cardiovascular disease. In: Chien KR, Breslow JL, Leiden JM, et al., eds. *Molecular basis of cardiovascular disease.* Philadelphia: WB Saunders, 1999:19–36.
7. Pyeritz RE. Genetics and cardiovascular disease. In: Braunwald E, ed. *Heart disease.* 6th ed. Philadelphia: WB Saunders (in press).
8. Pyeritz RE. Medical genetics. In: Tierney LM Jr, McPhee SJ, Papadakis MA, eds. *Current medical diagnosis and treatment 2000.* New York: Appleton & Lange, 2000:1574–1597.
9. McKusick VA. Online mendelian inheritance in man. www.ncbi.nlm.nih.gov/OMIM.
10. Ledbetter DH, Ballabio A. Molecular cytogenetics of contiguous gene syndrome: mechanisms and consequences of gene dosage imbalance. In: Scriver CR, Beaudet AL, Sly WS, et al., eds. *The metabolic and molecular bases of inherited disease.* New York: McGraw-Hill, 1995:811–842.
11. Spinner NB, Emanuel BS. Deletions and other structural abnormalities of autosomes. In: Rimoin DL, Connor JM, Pyeritz RE, eds. *Principles and practice of medical genetics.* 3rd ed. New York: Churchill Livingstone, 1997:999–1026.
12. Pettigrew AL, Greenberg F, Caskey CT, et al. Grieg syndrome associates with an interstitial deletion of 7p: confirmation of the localization of Grieg syndrome to 7p13. *Hum Genet* 1991;87: 452–456.
13. Vortkamp A, Gessler M, Le Paslier D, et al. Isolation of a yeast artificial chromosome contig spanning in Greig cephalopolysyndactyly syndrome (GCPS) gene region. *Genomics* 1994;22: 563–568.
14. Uitterlinden AG, Burger H, Huang Q, et al. Relation of alleles of the collagen type Iα1 gene to bone density and the risk of osteoporotic fractures in postmenopausal women. *N Engl J Med* 1998;338:1016–1021.
15. Holmes LB. Inborn errors of morphogenesis: a review of localized hereditary malformations. *N Engl J Med* 1983;291: 763–773.
16. Lathrop M, Terwilliger JD, Weeks DE. Multifactorial inheritance and genetic analysis of multifactorial disease. In: Rimoin DL, Connor JM, Pyeritz RE, eds. *Principles and practice of medical genetics.* 3rd ed. New York: Churchill Livingstone, 1997: 333–346.
17. *POSSUM 5.1.* Murdoch Institute for Research into Birth Defects. Melbourne: 1999:www.possum_support@cpgen.cpg.com.au.
18. Baraitser M, Winter R. *London dysmorphology database 2.1 and dysmorphology photo library 2.0.* London: Oxford University Press, 1999:www.oup.co.uk/isbn/0-19-268663-1.
19. *The genome data base.* www.gdb.org.
20. *A new gene map of the human genome.* www.ncbi.nlm.nih.gov/genemap99.
21. Royce PM, Steinmann B, eds. *Connective tissue and its heritable disorders.* New York: Wiley-Liss, 1993.
22. Scriver CR, Beaudet AL, Sly WS, et al., eds. *The metabolic and molecular bases of inherited disease.* New York: McGraw-Hill, 1995.
23. Beighton P. Sclerosteosis. *J Med Genet* 1988;25:200–203.
24. Balemans W, Van Den Ende J, Freire Paes-Alves A, et al. Localization of the gene for sclerosteosis to the van Buchem disease-gene region on chromosome 17q12-q21. *Am J Hum Genet* 1999;64:1661–1669.
25. Bryce SD, Lindsay S, Gladstone AJ, et al. A novel family of cathepsin L-like (CTSLL) sequences on human chromosome 10q and related transcripts. *Genomics* 1994;24:568–576.
26. Morrison NA, et al. Prediction of bone density from vitamin D receptor alleles. *Nature* 1994;367:284–286.
27. Lewis DB, et al. Osteoporosis induced in mice by overpopulation of interleukin 4. *Proc Natl Acad Sci U S A* 1993;90: 11618–11622.
28. Bonadio J, et al. A murine skeletal adaptation that significantly increases cortical bone mechanical properties. *J Clin Invest* 1993;92:1697–1705.
29. Thompson DB, Ossowski V, Janssen RC, et al. Linkage between stature and a region on chromosome 20 and analysis of the candidate gene encoding the bone morphogenetic protein 2. *Am J Med Genet* 1995;59:495–500.
30. Andrikopoulos K, et al. Targeted mutation in the *COL5A1* gene reveals a regulatory role for type V collagen during matrix assembly. *Nat Genet* 1995;9:31–36.
31. Erlebacher A, et al. Toward a molecular understanding of skeletal development. *Cell* 1995;80:371–378.
32. McKusick VA. The cardiovascular aspects of Marfan's syndrome: a heritable disorder of connective tissue. *Circulation* 1955;11:321–342.
33. McKusick VA. *Heritable disorders of connective tissue.* St. Louis: Mosby, 1956.

34. Beighton P, et al. International nosology of heritable disorders of connective tissue—Berlin, 1986. *Am J Med Genet* 1988;29: 581–594.
35. Rimoin DL. International nomenclature of constitutional diseases of bone with bibliography. *Birth Defects* 1979;15:30–55.
36. Pyeritz RE. Marfan syndrome and other disorders fibrillin. In: Rimoin DL, Connor JM, Pyeritz RE, eds. *Principles and practice of medical genetics.* 3rd ed. New York: Churchill Livingstone, 1997:1027–1066.
37. Pyeritz RE, Dietz HC. The Marfan syndrome and other fibrillinopathies. In: Royce PM, Steinmann B, eds. *Connective tissue and its heritable disorders:* molecular, *genetic and medical aspects.* 2nd ed. New York: Wiley-Liss (in press).
38. DePaepe A, Deitz HC, Devereux RB, et al. Revised diagnostic criteria for the Marfan syndrome. *Am J Med Genet* 1996;62: 417–426.
39. Sakai LY, Keene DR, Engvall E. Fibrillin, a new 350-kD glycoprotein, is a component of extracellular microfibrils. *J Cell Biol* 1986;103:2499–2509.
40. Maron BJ, Moller JH, Seidman CE, et al. Impact of laboratory molecular diagnosis on contemporary diagnostic criteria for genetically transmitted cardiovascular diseases: hypertrophic cardiomyopathy, long QT syndrome and Marfan syndrome. *Circulation* 1998;98:1460–1471.
41. Dietz HC, Cutting GR, Pyeritz RE, et al. Marfan syndrome caused by a recurrent de novo missense mutation in the fibrillin gene. *Nature* 1991;352:337–339.
42. Dietz HC, Pyeritz RE. Mutations in the human gene for fibrillin-1 (FBN1) in the Marfan syndrome and related disorders. *Hum Mutat* 1995;4:1799–1809.
43. Collod-Béroud G, Béroud C, Ades L, et al. Marfan database (3rd ed.): new mutations and new routines for the software. *Nucleic Acids Res* 1998;26:229–233.
44. Yuan B, Thomas JP, von Kodolitsch Y, et al. Comparison of heteroduplex analysis, direct sequencing and enzyme mismatch cleavage for detecting mutations in a large gene, *FBN1. Hum Mutat* 1999;14:440–446.
45. Magid D, Pyeritz RE, Fishman EK. Musculoskeletal manifestations of the Marfan syndrome. *Am J Radiol* 1990;155:99–104.
46. Sponseller PD, et al. The thoracolumbar spine in Marfan syndrome. *J Bone Joint Surg Am* 1995;77:867–876.
47. Pyeritz RE, et al. Dural ectasia is a common feature of the Marfan syndrome. *Am J Hum Genet* 1988;43:726–732.
48. Grahame R, Pyeritz RE. Marfan syndrome: joint and skin manifestations are prevalent and correlated. *Br J Rheumatol* 1995; 34:126–131.
49. Lindsey J, et al. The foot in Marfan syndrome: clinical findings and weight-distribution patterns. *J Pediatr Orthop* 1998;18: 755–759.
50. Sponseller PD, Tomek IM, Pyeritz RE. Developmental dysplasia of the hip in the Marfan syndrome. *Br J Paediatr Orthop* 1997;6:255–259.
51. Kuhlman JE, et al. Acetabular protrusion in the Marfan syndrome. *Radiology* 1987;164:415–417.
52. Viljoen D. Congenital contractural arachnodactyly (Beals syndrome). *J Med Genet* 1994;31:640–643.
53. Morse RP, et al. Diagnosis and management of Marfan syndrome in infants. *Pediatrics* 1990;86:888–895.
54. Desposito F, et al. Health supervision for children with Marfan syndrome. *Pediatrics* 1996;98:978–982.
55. Walker BA, Beighton PH, Murdoch JL. The marfanoid hypermobility syndrome. *Ann Intern Med* 1969;71:349–352.
56. Gott VL, et al. Surgery for ascending aortic disease in Marfan patients: a multi-center study. *N Engl J Med* 1999;340: 1307–1313.
57. Shores J, et al. Chronic β-adrenergic blockade protects the aorta in the Marfan syndrome: a prospective, randomized trial of propranolol. *N Engl J Med* 1994;330:1335–1341.
58. Silverman DI, et al. Life expectancy in the Marfan syndrome. *Am J Cardiol* 1995;75:157–160.
59. Sisk HE, Zahka KG, Pyeritz RE. The Marfan syndrome in early childhood: analysis of 15 patients diagnosed less than 4 years of age. *Am J Cardiol* 1983;52:353–358.
60. Parida SK, Kriss VM, Hall BD, Hiatus/paraesophageal hernias in neonatal Marfan syndrome. *Am J Med Genet* 1997;72: 156–158.
61. Hall J, et al. Pneumothorax in the Marfan syndrome: prevalence and therapy. *Ann Thorac Surg* 1984;37:500–504.
62. Arn PH, et al. Clinical outcome of pectus excavatum in the Marfan syndrome and in the general population. *J Pediatr* 1989;115:954–958.
63. Glesby MJ, Pyeritz RE. Association of mitral valve prolapse and systemic abnormalities of connective tissue: a phenotypic continuum. *JAMA* 1989;262:523–528.
64. Park ES, Putnam EA, Chitayat D, et al. Clustering of *FBN2* mutations in patients with congenital contractural arachnodactyly indicates an important role of the domains encoded by exons 24 through 34 during human development. *Am J Med Genet* 1998;78:350–355.
65. Babcock D, Gasner C, Francke U, et al. A single mutation that results in an Asp to His substitution and partial exon skipping in a family with congenital contractural arachnodactyly. *Hum Genet* 1998;103:22–28.
66. Mudd SH, et al. The natural history of homocystinuria due to cysthanthionine beta-synthase deficiency. *Am J Hum Genet* 1985;36:1–31.
67. Pyeritz RE. Homocystinuria. In: Beighton P, ed. *McKusick's heritable disorders of connective tissue.* St. Louis: CV Mosby, 1993:137–178.
68. Mudd SH, Levy HL, Skovby F. Disorders of transsulfuration. In: Scriver CR, Beaudet AL, Sly WS, et al., eds. *The metabolic and molecular bases of inherited disease.* New York: McGraw-Hill, 1995:1279–1328.
69. Kluijtmans LAJ, Boers GHJ, Kraus JP, et al. The molecular basis of cystathionine β-synthase deficiency in Dutch patients with homocystinuria: effect of CBS genotype on biochemical and clinical phenotype and on response to treatment. *Am J Hum Genet* 1999;65:59–67.
70. Abbott MH, Folstein SE, Abbey H, et al. Psychiatric manifestations of homocystinuria due to cystathionine beta-synthase deficiency. *Am J Med Genet* 1987;26:959–969.
71. Hill-Zobel RL, et al. Kinetics and biodistribution of ^{111}In-labeled platelets in homocystinuria. *N Engl J Med* 1982;307: 781–786.
72. Maumenee IH. The Weill-Marchesani syndrome. In: Beighton P, ed. *McKusick's heritable disorders of connective tissue.* St. Louis: CV Mosby, 1991:179–188.
73. Byers PH. Disorders of collagen biosynthesis and structure. In: Scriver CR, Beaudet AL, Sly WS, et al., eds. *The metabolic and molecular bases of inherited disease.* New York: McGraw-Hill, 1995:4029–4077.
74. Beighton P, et al. Ehlers-Danlos syndromes: revised nosology, Villefranche, 1997. *Am J Med Genet* 1998;77:31–37.
75. Byers PH. The Ehlers-Danlos syndromes. In: Rimoin DL, Connor JM, Pyeritz RE, eds. *Principles and practice of medical genetics.* 3rd ed. New York: Churchill Livingstone, 1997: 1067–1082.
76. Steinmann B, Royce PS, Superti-Furga A. The Ehlers-Danlos syndrome. In: Royce PM, Steinmann B, eds. *Connective tissue and its heritable disorders:* molecular, *genetic, and medical aspects.* New York: Wiley-Liss, 1993:351.
77. Dolan AL, Arden NK, Grahame R, Spector TD. Assessment of

bone in Ehlers-Danlos syndrome by ultrasound and densitometry. *Ann Rheum Dis* 1998;57:630–633.

78. Beighton P, Grahame R, Bird H. *Hypermobility of joints.* 2nd ed. New York: Springer-Verlag, 1989.
79. Larsson L-G, et al. Benefits and disadvantages of joint hypermobility among musicians. *N Engl J Med* 1993;329:1079–1082.
80. Hamel BC, Pals G, Engels CH, et al. Ehlers-Danlos syndrome and type III collagen abnormalities: a variable clinical spectrum. *Clin Genet* 1998;53:440–446.
81. Krane SM, Pinnell SR, Erbe RW. Lyso-protocollagen hydroxylase deficiency in fibroblasts from siblings with hydroxylysine deficient collagen. *Proc Natl Acad Sci U S A* 1972;69: 2899–2903.
82. Pasquali M, Still MJ, Vales T, et al. Abnormal formation of collagen cross-links in skin fibroblasts cultured from patients with Ehlers-Danlos syndrome type VI. *Proc Assoc Am Physicians* 1997;109:33–41.
83. Weil D, et al. Temperature-dependent expression of a collagen splicing defect in the fibroblasts of a patient with Ehlers-Danlos syndrome type VII. *J Biol Chem* 1989;264:16804–16809.
84. Colige A, Sieron AL, Li S-W, et al. Human Ehlers-Danlos syndrome type VII C and bovine dermatosparaxis are caused by mutations in the procollagen I N-proteinase gene. *Am J Hum Genet* 1999;65:308–317.
85. Beighton P, Curtis D. X-linked Ehlers-Danlos syndrome type V: the next generation. *Clin Genet* 1985;27:472–478.
86. Hartsfield JK Jr, Jousseff BG. Phenotypic overlap of Ehlers-Danlos syndrome types IV and VIII. *Am J Med Genet* 1990;37: 465–470.
87. Arneson MA, et al. A new form of Ehlers-Danlos syndrome: fibronectin corrects defective platelet function. *JAMA* 1980; 244:144–147.
88. Kirk JA, Ansell BM, Bywaters FGL. The hypermobility syndrome: musculoskeletal complaints associated with generalized joint hypermobility. *Ann Rheum Dis* 1967;26:419–425.
89. Wynne-Davies R. Acetabular dysplasia and familial joint laxity: two etiologic factors in congenital dislocation of the hip. *J Bone Joint Surg Br* 1970;52:704–716.
90. Horton WA, et al. Familial joint instability syndrome. *Am J Med Genet* 1980;6:221–228.
91. Uitto J, Fazio MJ, Christiano AM. Cutis laxa and premature aging syndromes. In: Royce PM, Steinmann B, eds. *Connective tissue and its heritable disorders.* New York: Wiley-Liss, 1993: 409–423.
92. Solomon I, et al. Neonatal abnormalities associated with D-penicillamine treatment during pregnancy. *N Engl J Med* 1977; 296:54–55.
93. Pope FM. Inherited abnormalities of elastic tissue. In: Rimoin DL, Connor JM, Pyeritz RE, eds. *Principles and practice of medical genetics.* 3rd ed. New York: Churchill Livingstone, 1997: 1083–1120.
94. Uitto J, Boyd CD, Lebwohl MG, et al. International centennial meeting on pseudoxanthoma elasticum: progress in PXE research. *J Invest Dermatol* 1998;110:840–842.
95. Renie WA, et al. Pseudoxanthoma elasticum: high calcium intake in early life correlates with severity. *Am J Med Genet* 1984;19:235–244.
96. Struk B, Neldner K, Rao V, et al. Mapping of both autosomal recessive and dominant variants of pseudoxanthoma elasticum to chromosome 16p13. *Hum Mol Genet* 1997;6:1823–1828.
97. Van Soest S, Swart S, Tijmes N, et al. A locus of autosomal recessive pseudoxanthoma elasticum, with penetrance of vascular symptoms in carriers, maps to chromosome 16p13.1. *Genome Res* 1997;7:830–834.
98. Wynne-Davies R, Hall CM, Apley AG. *Atlas of skeletal dysplasia.* Edinburgh: Churchill Livingstone, 1985.
99. Spranger J. Radiologic nosology of bone dysplasias. *Am J Med Genet* 1989;34:96–104.
100. Rimoin DL, Lachman RS. The chondrodysplasias. In: Rimoin DL, Connor JM, Pyeritz RE, eds. *Principles and practice of medical genetics.* 3rd ed. New York: Churchill Livingstone, 1997: 2779–2816.
101. Byers PH. Osteogenesis imperfecta. In: Royce PM, Steinmann B, eds. *Connective tissue and its heritable disorders: molecular, genetic, and medical aspects.* New York: Wiley-Liss, 1993:317.
102. Sillence DO. Disorders of bone density, volume, and mineralization. In: Rimoin DL, Connor JM, Pyeritz RE, eds. *Principles and practice of medical genetics.* 3rd ed. New York: Churchill Livingstone, 1997:2817–2836.
103. Sillence DO. Osteogenesis imperfecta: an expanding panorama of variants. *Clin Orthop* 1981;159:11–25.
104. Kuivaniemi H, Tromp G, Prockop DJ. Mutations in collagen genes: causes of rare and some common diseases in humans. *FASEB J* 1991;5:2052–2060.
105. Byers PH. Brittle bones-fragile molecules: disorders of collagen gene structure and expression. *Trends Genet* 1990;6:293–300.
106. Paterson CR, McAllion S, Miller R. Heterogeneity of osteogenesis imperfecta type I. *J Med Genet* 1983;20:203–205.
107. Constantinou CD, et al. Phenotypic heterogeneity in osteogenesis imperfecta: the mildly affected mother of a proband with a lethal variant has the same mutation substituting cysteine for a 1-glycine 904 in a type I procollagen gene (COL1A1). *Am J Hum Genet* 1990;47:670–679.
108. Cole WG, et al. The clinical features of three babies with osteogenesis imperfecta resulting from the substitution of glycine by arginine in the proa1(I) chain of type I procollagen. *J Med Genet* 1990;27:228–235.
109. Sillence DO, et al. Osteogenesis imperfecta type II: delineation of the phenotype with reference to genetic heterogeneity. *Am J Med Genet* 1984;17:407–423.
110. Cohn DH, et al. Lethal osteogenesis imperfecta resulting from a single nucleotide change in one human proa1(I) collagen allele. *Proc Natl Acad Sci U S A* 1986;83:6045–6057.
111. Khillan JS, Li S-W, Prockop DJ. Partial rescue of a lethal phenotype of fragile bones in transgenic mice with a chimeric antisense gene directed against a mutated collagen gene. *Proc Natl Acad Sci U S A* 1994;91:6298–6303.
112. Sillence DO, et al. Osteogenesis imperfecta type III: delineation of the phenotype with reference to genetic heterogeneity. *Am J Med Genet* 1986;23:821–832.
113. Rose NJ, et al. A Gly238Ser substitution in the $\alpha 2$ chain of type I collagen results in osteogenesis imperfecta type III. *Hum Genet* 1995;95:215–218.
114. Wallis GA, et al. Osteogenesis imperfecta type III: mutations in the type I collagen structural genes, COL1A1 and COL1A2, are not necessarily responsible. *J Med Genet* 1993;30:492–496.
115. Paterson CP, Burns J, McAllion SJ. Osteogenesis imperfecta variant vs child abuse: reply. *Am J Med Genet* 1995;56:117–118.
116. Levin LS. The dentition in the osteogenesis imperfecta syndromes. *Clin Orthop* 1981;159:64.
117. Hortop J, et al. Cardiovascular involvement in osteogenesis imperfecta. *Circulation* 1986;73:54–61.
118. Glorieux FH, Bishop NJ, Plotkin H, et al. Cyclic administration of pamidronate in children with severe osteogenesis imperfecta. *N Engl J Med* 1998;339:947–952.
119. Horowitz EM, et al. Bone marrow transplantation to correct the mesenchymal defect of children with osteogenesis imperfecta. *Nat Med* 1999;5:309–313.
120. Lee B, et al. Identification of the molecular defect in a family with spondyloepiphyseal dysplasia. *Science* 1989;244:978–980.
121. Tiller GE, et al. An RNA-splicing mutation ($G^{+}51VS20$) in the type II collagen gene (COL2A1) in a family with spondyloepi-

physeal dysplasia congenita. *Am J Hum Genet* 1995;56: 388–395.
122. Murray LW, et al. Type II collagen defects in the chondrodysplasia. I. Spondyloepiphyseal dysplasia. *Am J Hum Genet* 1989; 45:5–15.
123. Wilkin DJ, et al. Small deletions in the type II collagen triple helix produce Kniest dysplasia. *Am J Med Genet* 1999;85: 105–112.
124. Bannerman RM, Ingall GB, Mohn JF. X-linked spondyloepiphyseal dysplasia tarda: clinical and linkage data. *J Med Genet* 1971;8:291–301.
125. Herrmann J, et al. The Stickler syndrome (hereditary arthro-ophthalmology). *Birth Defects* 1975;11:76–103.
126. Liberfarb RM, Hirose T, Holmes LB. The Wagner-Stickler syndrome: a study of 22 families. *J Pediatr* 1981;99:394–399.
127. Shprintzen RJ, et al. Anomalies associated with cleft lip, cleft palate or both. *Am J Med Genet* 1985;20:585–595.
128. Rai A, et al. Hereditary arthro-ophthalmopathy (Stickler syndrome): a diagnosis to consider in familial premature osteoarthritis. *Br J Rheumatol* 1994;33:1175–1180.
129. Marshall D. Ectodermal dysplasia: report of kindred with ocular abnormalities and hearing defect. *Am J Ophthalmol* 1958;45: 143–156.
130. Knowlton RG, et al. Genetic linkage analysis of hereditary arthro-ophthalmopathy (Stickler syndrome) and the type II procollagen gene. *Am J Hum Genet* 1989;45:681–688.
131. Wilkin DJ, Mortier GR, Johnson CL, et al. Correlation of linkage data with phenotype in eight families with Stickler syndrome. *Am J Med Genet* 1998;80:121–127.
132. Körkkö J, Ritvaniemi P, Haataja L, et al. Mutation in type II procollagen (COL2A1) that substitutes aspartate for glycine (1-67 and that causes cataracts and retinal detachment: evidence for molecular heterogeneity in the Wagner syndrome and the Stickler syndrome (arthro-ophthalmopathy). *Am J Hum Genet* 1993;53:55–61.
133. Vikkula M, et al. Autosomal dominant and recessive osteochondrodysplasias associated with the COL11A2 locus. *Cell* 1995;80:431–437.
134. Griffith AJ, Sprunger LK, Sirko-Osadsa A, et al. Marshall syndrome associated with a splicing defect at the COL11A1 locus. *Am J Hum Genet* 1998;62:816–823.
135. Nelson F, Dahlberg L, Laverty S, et al. Evidence for altered synthesis of type II collagen in patients with osteoarthritis. *J Clin Invest* 1998;102:2115–2125.
136. Pun YL, et al. Clinical correlations of osteoarthritis associated with a single-base mutation (arginine[519] to cysteine) in type II procollagen gene. *Arthritis Rheum* 1994;37:264–269.
137. Loughlin J, et al. Sibling pair analysis shows no linkage of generalized osteoarthritis to the loci encoding type II collagen, cartilage link protein or cartilage matrix protein. *Br J Rheumatol* 1994;33:1103–1106.
138. Meulenbelt I, Bijkerk C, Breedveld FC, Slagboom PE. Genetic linkage analysis of 14 candidate gene loci in a family with autosomal dominant osteoarthritis without dysplasia. *J Med Genet* 1997;34:1024–1027.
139. Ala-Kokko L, et al. Single base mutation in the type II procollagen gene (COL2A1) as a cause of primary osteoarthritis associated with a mild chondrodysplasia. *Proc Natl Acad Sci U S A* 1990;87:6565–6568.
140. Chapman K, Mustafa Z, Irven C, et al. Osteoarthritis-susceptibility locus on chromosome 11q, detected by linkage. *Am J Hum Genet* 1999;65:167–174.
141. Annunen S, Paassilta P, Lohiniva J, et al. An allele of *COL9A2* associated with intervertebral disc disease. *Science* 1999;285: 409–412.
142. Oehlmann R, et al. Genetic linkage mapping of multiple epiphyseal dysplasia to the pericentromeric region of chromosome 19. *Am J Hum Genet* 1994;54:3–10.
143. Deere M, et al. Genetic heterogeneity in multiple epiphyseal dysplasia. *Am J Hum Genet* 1995;56:698–704.
144. Briggs MD, et al. Pseudoachondroplasia and multiple epiphyseal dysplasia due to mutations in the cartilage oligomeric matrix protein gene. *Nat Genet* 1995;10:330–336.
145. Deere M, Sanford T, Francomano CA, et al. Identification of nine novel mutations in cartilage oligomeric matrix protein in patients with pseudoachondroplasia and multiple epiphyseal dysplasia. *Am J Med Genet* 1999;85:486–490.
146. van Mourki JBA, Hamel BCJ, Mariman ECM. A large family with multiple epiphyseal dysplasia linked to the COL9A2 gene. *Am J Med Genet* 1998;77:234–240.
147. Paassilta P, Lohiniva J, Annunen S, et al. COL9A3: a third locus for multiple epiphyseal dysplasia. *Am J Hum Genet* 1999;64: 1036–1044.
148. Superti-Furga A, Neumann L, Riebel T, et al. Recessively inherited multiple epiphyseal dysplasia with normal stature, club foot, and double layered patella caused by a *DTDST* mutation. *J Med Genet* 1999;36:621–624.
149. Horton WA, et al. Growth curves for height for diastrophic dysplasia, spondyloepiphyseal dysplasia congenita, and pseudoachondroplasia. *Am J Dis Child* 1982;136:316–319.
150. Hecht JT, et al. Mutations in exon 17B of cartilage oligomeric matric protein (COMP) cause pseudoachondroplasia. *Nat Genet* 1995;10:325–329.
151. Deere M, Sanford T, Ferguson HL, et al. Identification of twelve mutations in cartilage oligomeric matrix protein (COMP) in patients with pseudoachondroplasia. *Am J Med Genet* 1998;80:510–513.
152. Ikegawa S, Ohashi H, Nishimura G, et al. Novel and recurrent COMP (cartilage oligomeric matrix protein) mutations in pseudoachondroplasia and multiple epiphyseal dysplasia. *Hum Genet* 1998;103:633–638.
153. Briggs MD, Mortier GR, Cole WG, et al. Diverse mutations in the gene for cartilage oligomeric protein in the pseudoachondroplasia-multiple epiphyseal dysplasia disease spectrum. *Am J Hum Genet* 1998;62:311–319.
154. Ferguson HL, Deere M, Evans R, et al. Mosaicism in pseudoachondroplasia. *Am J Med Genet* 1997;70:287–291.
155. Horton WA, et al. Standard growth curves for achondroplasia. *J Pediatr* 1978;93:435–438.
156. Hunter AGW, Hecht JT, Scott CI Jr. Standard weight for height curves in achondroplasia. *Am J Med Genet* 1996;62:255–261.
157. Nicoletti B, et al., eds. *Human achondroplasia.* New York: Plenum, 1988.
158. Hecht JT, et al. Growth of the foramen magnum in achondroplasia. *Am J Med Genet* 1989;32:528–535.
159. Reid CS, et al. Cervicomedullary compression in young patients with achondroplasia: value of comprehensive neurologic and respiratory evaluation. *J Pediatr* 1987;110:522–530.
160. Pauli RM, et al. Prospective assessment of risks for cervicomedullary-junction compression in infants with achondroplasia. *Am J Hum Genet* 1995;56:732–744.
161. Rimoin DL. Cervicomedullary junction compression in infants with achondroplasia: when to perform neurosurgical decompression. *Am J Hum Genet* 1995;56:824–827.
162. Pyeritz RE, Sack GH Jr, Udvarhelyi GB. Thoracolumbar laminectomy in achondroplasia: long-term results in 22 patients. *Am J Med Genet* 1987;28:433–444.
163. Hurko O, Uematsu S. Neurosurgical considerations in skeletal dysplasias. *Neurosurg Q* 1993;3:192–217.
164. Brinkmann G, et al. Cognitive skills in achrondroplasia. *Am J Med Genet* 1993;47:800–804.
165. Hurko O, Pyeritz RE, Uematsu S. Neurologic considerations in

achondroplasia. In: Nicoletti B, et al., eds. *Human achondroplasia.* New York: Plenum, 1988:153–162.
166. Kopits SE. Correction of bowleg deformity in achondroplasia. *Johns Hopkins Med J* 1980;146:206–209.
167. Thompson NM, Hecht JT, Bohan TP, et al. Neuroanatomic and neuropsychological outcome in school-age children with achondroplasia. *Am J Med Genet* 1999;88:145–153.
168. Shiang R, Thompson LM, Zhu Y-Z, et al. Mutations in the transmembrane domain of FGFR3 cause the most common genetic form of dwarfism, achondroplasia. *Cell* 1994;78: 335–342.
169. Wilkin DJ, Szabo JK, Cameron R, et al. Mutations in fibroblast growth-factor receptor 3 in sporadic cases of achondroplasia occur exclusively on the paternally derived chromosome. *Am J Hum Genet* 1998;63:711–716.
170. Bellus GA, Bamshad MJ, Przylepa KA, et al. Severe achondroplasia with developmental delay and acanthosis nigricans (SADDAN). *Am J Med Genet* 1999;85:53–65.
171. Bellus GA, et al. A recurrent mutation in the tyrosine kinase domain of fibroblast growth factor receptor 3 causes hypochondroplasia. *Nat Genet* 1995;10:357–359.
172. Huggins MJ, Smith JR, Chun K, et al. Achondroplasia-hypochondroplasia complex in a newborn infant. *Am J Med Genet* 1999;84:396–400.
173. Chitayat D, Fernandez B, Gardner A, et al. Compound heterozygosity for the achondroplasia-hypochondroplasia FGFR3 mutations: prenatal diagnosis and postnatal outcome. *Am J Med Genet* 1999;84:401–405.
174. Tavormina PL, et al. Thanatophoric dysplasia (types I and II) caused by distinct mutations in fibroblast growth factor receptor 3. *Nat Genet* 1995;9:321–328.
175. Mason IV. The ins and outs of fibroblast growth factors. *Cell* 1994;78:547–552.
176. Reardon W, et al. Mutations in the fibroblast growth factor receptor 2 gene cause Crouzon syndrome. *Nat Genet* 1994;8: 98–103.
177. Jabs EW, et al. Jackson-Weiss and Crouzon syndromes are allelic with mutations in fibroblast growth. *Nat Genet* 1994;8: 275–279.
178. Muenke M, et al. A common mutation in the fibroblast growth factor receptor 1 gene in Pfeiffer syndrome. *Nat Genet* 1994;8: 269–274.
179. Warman ML, et al. A type X collagen mutation causes Schmid metaphyseal chondrodysplasia. *Nat Genet* 1993;5:79–82.
180. Bonaventure J, Chaminade F, Maroteaux P. Mutations in three subdomains of the carboxy-terminal region of collagen type X account for most of the Schmid metaphyseal dysplasias. *Hum Genet* 1995;96:58–64.
181. McIntosh I, Abbott MH, Francomano CA. Concentration of mutations causing Schmid metaphyseal chondrodysplasia in the C-terminal noncollagenous domain of type X collagen. *Hum Mutat* 1995;5:121–125.
182. Schipani E, Kruse K, Jüppner H. A constitutively active mutant PTH-PTHrP receptor in Jansen-type metaphyseal chondrodysplasia. *Science* 1995;268:98–100.
183. Polymeropoulos MH, et al. The gene for the Ellis van Creveld syndrome is located on chromosome 4p16. *Genomics* 1996;35: 1–5.
184. Mäkitie O, et al. Cartilage-hair hypoplasia. *J Med Genet* 1995; 32:39–43.
185. Sulisalo T, et al. Genetic homogeneity of cartilage-hair hypoplasia. *Hum Genet* 1995;95:157–160.
186. Ikegawa S, Nishimura G, Nagai T, et al. Mutation of the type X collagen gene (*COL10A1*) causes spondylometaphyseal dysplasia. *Am J Hum Genet* 1998;63:1659–1662.
187. Diab M, Wu J-J, Shapiro F, Eyre D. Abnormality of type IX collagen in a patient with diastrophic dysplasia. *Am J Med Genet* 1994;49:402–409.
188. Mansour S, et al. A clinical and genetic study of campomelic dysplasia. *J Med Genet* 1995;32:415–420.
189. Feldman GJ, et al. A gene for cleidocranial dysplasia maps to the short arm of chromosome 6. *Am J Hum Genet* 1995;56: 928–943.
190. Foster JW, et al. Campomelic dysplasia and autosomal sex reversal caused by mutations in an SRY-related gene. *Nature* 1994;372:525–530.
191. Wagner T, et al. Autosomal sex reversal and campomelic dysplasia are caused by mutations in and around the SRY-related gene SOX9. *Cell* 1994;79:1111–1120.
192. Hou W-S, Brömme D, Zhao Y, et al. Characterization of novel cathepsin K mutations in the pro and mature polypeptide regions causing pycnodysostosis. *J Clin Invest* 1999;103: 731–738.
193. Franco B, et al. A cluster of sulfatase genes on Xp22.3: mutations in chondrodysplasia punctata (CDPX) and implications for warfarin embryopathy. *Cell* 1995;81:15–25.
194. Wicklund CL, Johnston PD, Hecht JT. Natural history study of hereditary multiple exostoses. *Am J Med Genet* 1995;55:43–46.
195. Wuyts W, Van Hul W, De Boulle K, et al. Mutations in the EXT1 and EXT2 genes in hereditary multiple exostoses. *Am J Hum Genet* 1998;62:346–354.
196. Van Hul W, Balemans W, Van Hul E, et al. Van Buchem disease (hyperostosis corticalis generalisata) maps to chromosome 17q12-q21. *Am J Hum Genet* 1998;62:391–399.
197. Laville JM, Lakermance P, Limouzy F. Larsen's syndrome: review of the literature and analysis of thirty-eight cases. *J Pediatr Orthop* 1994;14:63–73.
198. Latta RJ, et al. Larsen's syndrome: a skeletal dysplasia with multiple joint dislocations and unusual facies. *J Pediatr* 1971;78: 291–298.
199. Rovin S, et al. Mandibulofacial dysostosis, a familial study of five generations. *J Pediatr* 1964;65:215–221.
200. Temtamy S, McKusick VA. *The genetics of hand malformations.* New York: Alan R. Liss, 1978.
201. Strasburger AK, et al. Symphalangism: genetics and clinical aspects. *Bull Johns Hopkins Hosp* 1965;117:108–127.
202. Welch JP, Temtamy SA. Hereditary contractures of the fingers (camptodactyly). *J Med Genet* 1966;3:104–113.
203. Manni JJ, et al. Hyperostosis cranialis interna: a new hereditary syndrome with cranial-nerve entrapment. *N Engl J Med* 1990; 322:450–454.
204. Renie WA, Pyeritz RE. Idiopathic multicentric osteolysis in a 78-year-old woman. *Johns Hopkins Med J* 1981;148:165–171.
205. Carnevale A, et al. Idiopathic multicentric osteolysis with facial anomalies and nephropathy. *Am J Med Genet* 1987;26: 877–886.
206. Spranger J. Mucopolysaccharidoses. In: Rimoin DL, Connor JM, Pyeritz RE, eds. *Principles and practice of medical genetics.* 3rd ed. New York: Churchill Livingstone, 1997:2071–2080.
207. Hoogerbrugge PM, et al. Allogenic bone marrow transplantation for lysosomal storage diseases. *Lancet* 1995;345: 1398–1402.
208. Semenza GL, Pyeritz RE. Respiratory complications of the mucopolysaccharide storage disorders. *Medicine* 1988;67: 209–219.
209. Kornfield S, Sly WS. I-cell disease and pseudo-Hurler polydystrophy: disorders of lysosomal enzyme phosphorylation. In: Scriver CR, Beaudet AL, Sly WS, et al., eds. *The metabolic and molecular bases of inherited disease.* New York: McGraw-Hill, 1995:2495–2508.
210. Thomas GH, Beaudet AL. Disorders of glycoprotein degradation and structure: α-mannosidosis, β-mannosidosis, fucosido-

sis, sialidosis, aspartylglucosaminuria and carbohydrate-deficient glycoprotein syndrome. In: Scriver CR, Beaudet AL, Sly WS, et al., eds. *The metabolic and molecular bases of inherited disease.* New York: McGraw-Hill, 1995:2529–2562.
211. La Du BN. Alkaptonuria. In: Scriver CR, Beaudet AL, Sly WS, et al., eds. *The metabolic and molecular bases of inherited disease.* New York: McGraw-Hill, 1995:1371–1386.
212. McKusick VA. Alkaptonuria: tracked down to chromosome 3. *Genomics* 1994;19:3–4.
213. Gehrig A, Schmidt SR, Müller CR, et al. Molecular defects in alkaptonuria. *Cytogenet Cell Genet* 1997;76:14–16.
214. Albright F, Butler AM, Bloomberg E. Rickets resistant to vitamin D therapy. *Am J Dis Child* 1937;54:529–547.
215. Reid IR, et al. X-linked hypophosphatemia: skeletal mass in adults assessed by histomorphometry, computed tomography and absorptiometry. *Am J Med* 1991;90:63–69.
216. Reid IR, et al. X-linked hypophosphatemia: a clinical, biochemical and histopathologic assessment of morbidity in adults. *Medicine* 1989;68:336–352.
217. Balsan S, Tieder M. Linear growth in patients with hypophosphatemic vitamin D-resistant rickets: influence of treatment regimen and parental height. *J Pediatr* 1990;116:365–371.
218. Verge CF, et al. Effects of therapy in X-linked hypophosphatemic rickets. *N Engl J Med* 1991;325:1843–1848.
219. Glorieux FH, et al. Use of phosphate and vitamin D to prevent dwarfism and rickets in X-linked hypophosphatemia. *N Engl J Med* 1972;287:481–487.
220. Nesbitt T, et al. Crosstransplantation of kidneys in normal and *Hyp* mice: evidence that the *Hyp* mouse phenotype is unrelated to an intrinsic renal defect. *J Clin Invest* 1992;89:1453–1459.
221. The HYP Consortium. A gene (PEX) with homologies to endopeptidases is mutated in patients with X-linked hypophosphatemic rickets. *Nat Genet* 1995;11:130–136.
222. Filisetti D, et al. Non-random distribution of mutations in the *PHEX* gene, and under-detected missense mutations at non-conserved residues. *Eur J Hum Genet* 1999;7:615–619.
223. Econs MJ, et al. Autosomal dominant hypophosphatemic rickets is linked to chromosome 12p13. *J Clin Invest* 1997;100: 2653–2657.
224. Hughes MR, et al. Point mutations in the human vitamin D receptor gene associated with hypocalcemic rickets. *Science* 1988;242:1702–1705.
225. Gunnes M, et al. Lack of relationship between vitamin D receptor genotype and forearm bone gain in healthy children, adolescents and young adults. *J Clin Endocrinol Metab* 1997;82: 851–855.
226. Connor JM. Fibrodysplasia ossificans progressiva. In: Steinmann B, Royce PM, eds. *Connective tissue and its heritable disorders.* New York: Wiley-Liss, 1991:603–611.
227. Schroeber HW Jr, Zasloff M. The hand and foot malformations in fibrodysplasia ossificans progressiva. *Johns Hopkins Med J* 1980;147:73–78.
228. Conner JM, Evans DAP. Fibrodysplasia ossificans progressiva: the clinical features and natural history of 34 patients. *J Bone Joint Surg Br* 1982;64:766–783.
229. Smith R, Athanasou NA, Vipond SE. Fibrodysplasia (myositis) ossificans progressiva: clinicopathological features and natural history. *Q J Med* 1996;89:445–456.
230. Shafritz AB, et al. Overexpression of an osteogenic morphogen in fibrodysplasia ossificans progressiva. *N Engl J Med* 1996;335: 555–561.
231. Spiegel AM, Weinstein LS. Pseudohypoparathyroidism. In: Scriver CR, Beaudet AL, Sly WS, et al., eds. *The metabolic and molecular bases of inherited disease.* New York: McGraw-Hill, 1995:3073–3090.
232. Spiegel AM. Albright's hereditary osteodystrophy and defective G proteins. *N Engl J Med* 1990;322:1461–1462.
233. Wilson LC, et al. Parental origin of Gs-alpha gene mutations in Albright's hereditary osteodystrophy. *J Med Genet* 1994;31: 835–839.
234. Juppner H, et al. The gene responsible for pseudohypoparathyroidism type Ib is paternally imprinted and maps in four unrelated kindreds to chromosome 20q13.3. *Proc Natl Acad Sci U S A* 1998;95:11798–11803.
235. Bijlsma EK, Aalfs CM, Sluijter S, et al. Familial cryptic translocation between chromosomes 2qter and 8qter: further delineation of the Albright hereditary osteodystrophy-like phenotype. *J Med Genet* 1999;36:604–609.
236. Staheli LT, Hall JG, Jaffee KM, et al., eds. *Arthrogryposis.* Cambridge: Cambridge University Press, 1998.
237. Stevenson RE, Meyer LC. The limbs. In: Stevenson RE, Hall JL, Goodman RM, eds. *Human malformations and related anomalies.* New York: Oxford, 1993:699–803.
238. Drachman DB. The syndrome of arthogryposis multiplex congenita. *Birth Defects* 1971;7:90–97.
239. Hall JG, et al. Three distinct types of X-linked arthrogryposes seen in 6 families. *Clin Genet* 1982;21:81–97.
240. Makela-Bengs P, Jarvinen N, Vuopala K, et al. Assignment of the disease locus for lethal congenital contracture syndrome to a restricted region of chromosome 9q34, by genome scan using five affected individuals. *Am J Hum Genet* 1998;63:506–516.
241. Baldwin CT, et al. Linkage of early-onset osteoarthritis and chondrocalcinosis to human chromosome 8q. *Am J Hum Genet* 1995;56:692–697.
242. Balsa A, et al. Familial articular chondrocalcinosis in Spain. *Ann Rheum Dis* 1990;49:531–535.
243. Smilde TJ, et al. Familial hypokalemia/hypomagnesemia and chondrocalcinosis. *J Rheum* 1994;21:1515–1519.
244. Marx SJ, et al. Familial hypocalciuric hypercalcemia: recognition among patients referred after unsuccessful parathyroid exploration. *Ann Intern Med* 1980;92:351–356.
245. Chou Y-H, et al. Mutations in the human Ca(2+)-sensing-receptor gene that cause familial hypocalciuric hypercalcemia. *Am J Hum Genet* 1995;56:1075–1079.
246. Bai M, et al. Markedly reduced activity of mutant calcium-sensing receptor with an inserted Alu element from a kindred with familial hypocalciuric hypercalcemia and neonatal severe hyperthyroidism. *J Clin Invest* 1997;99:1917–1925.
247. Trump D, et al. Linkage studies in a kindred from Oklahoma, with familial benign (hypocalciuric) hypercalcaemia (FBH) and developmental elevations in serum parathyroid hormone levels, indicate a third locus for FBH. *Hum Genet* 1995;96:183–187.

96

HYPERTROPHIC OSTEOARTHROPATHY

ROY D. ALTMAN

Historically, clubbing was first recorded circa 400 BC by Hippocrates (1). Hypertrophic osteoarthropathy includes (a) clubbing of fingers and toes, (b) periostitis with new subperiosteal bone formation of long bones, and (c) arthritis. Synonyms have included familial idiopathic hypertrophic osteoarthropathy, Marie–Bamberger syndrome, osteoarthropathic hypertrophiante and pneumique, and secondary hypertrophic osteoarthropathy.

Hypertrophic osteoarthropathy is classified as either primary (hereditary) or secondary. The primary form usually appears in children or young adults. The secondary form can appear at any age and is often associated with neoplasms or infectious diseases. In the secondary form, associated diseases are more often intrathoracic rather than extrathoracic. Hypertrophic osteoarthropathy associated with infectious diseases is often characterized by an insidious development of mild rheumatic complaints over a period of months or years. In contrast, rapid onset and progression of hypertrophic osteoarthropathy with prominent joint pain is often associated with malignant diseases.

CLINICAL FEATURES

Clubbing

Clubbing is often discovered by a physician rather than by the patient. Although clubbing may be unsightly, it is rarely symptomatic. When symptoms do occur, they include clumsiness, stiffness, and burning or warmth of the finger tips. Clubbing is the most consistent feature of hypertrophic osteoarthropathy and is not invariably accompanied by periostitis or synovitis (2,3). It is unclear whether clubbing without the other features of hypertrophic osteoarthropathy is a separate disease or a *forme fruste* of hypertrophic osteoarthropathy (2,4). Clubbing itself does not distinguish primary from secondary disease, except that clubbing without periostitis generally occurs without associated disease. Increased digital blood flow is a constant feature of all forms of hypertrophic osteoarthropathy.

The first sign of clubbing is a softening of the nail bed that results in a fluctuant, "rocking" sensation on palpation of the proximal nail. Subsequently, there is periungual erythema with telangiectasia, local warmth, and sweating. The nail develops increased convexity in the sagittal and cross-sectional planes with loss of the normal 15 degree angle between the proximal nail and dorsal surface of the phalanx (Fig. 96.1). Excessive distal phalangeal resorption can lead to shortening of fingers and toes (5).

Associated changes may include excessive sweating or warmth of the fingertips, eponychia, paronychia, breaking or loosening of the nail, hangnails, and accelerated nail or cuticle growth. Advanced stages are associated with "drumstick" fingers (Fig. 96.2) and hyperextensibility of the distal interphalangeal joints (Fig. 96.1). Similar, but less clinically apparent changes occur in the toes. Spade-like enlargement of the hands and feet can occur as clubbing evolves over months or years.

Clubbing, when present, is usually clinically apparent. A qualitative measurement involves placing the dorsal surfaces of the contralateral ring (fourth) fingers together (6); the normal gap between the fingers at the nail bed disappears. Semiquantitative techniques include measuring the diameter of the thumbs and fingers at the base of the nails and at the distal interphalangeal joints; a sum of the 10 ratios (digital index) greater than 10 indicates clubbing (7). A "shadowgram" can be used to measure the hyponychial angle (8). A modified digital cast technique has been used to calculate a ratio of distal phalangeal and interphalangeal depth measured with calipers (9); one third of lung cancer patients had a ratio of more than 1.05.

Sporadic reports of unilateral clubbing (2) associated with arterial aneurysms (aorta, subclavian, or innominate), axillary tumors, subluxations of the shoulder, apical lung cancer, brachial arteriovenous aneurysm, and hemiplegia have appeared (10). Although uncommon, unidigital clubbing has been observed in sarcoidosis (11), tophaceous gout, and after injury to the median nerve. "Paddle fingers" occasionally develop in bass violin players. Unidigital clubbing is most often related to trauma (2). Clubbing of the toes alone has accompanied an infected abdominal aortic aneurysm.

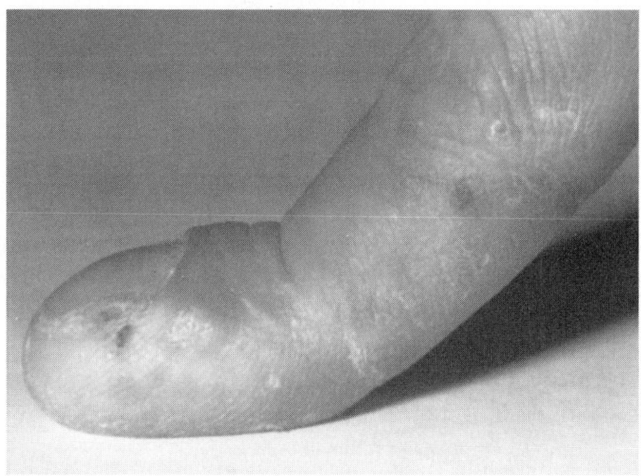

FIGURE 96.1. Lateral view of a distal digit with clubbing demonstrating loss of the normal 15 degree angle at the nail–nail bed junction and hyperextensibility of the distal interphalangeal joint.

Periostitis

Periostitis may be asymptomatic or may produce mild, deep-seated aching pain, burning pain, and tenderness over long bones. A unique feature of hypertrophic osteoarthropathy is aggravation of bone pain on dependency of the limbs, often relieved by elevation of the limbs. This phenomenon suggests that local vascular stasis plays a role in production of pain. The extent of periostitis depends on duration and not on primary or secondary disease. The patient also might complain of heat and swelling over the feet and legs. The distal extremities often appear broadened, with a palpable, firm, mildly pitting edema. Tenderness to pressure and warmth over the distal tibia, feet, radius, and ulna is usually present even in the absence of the complaint of pain.

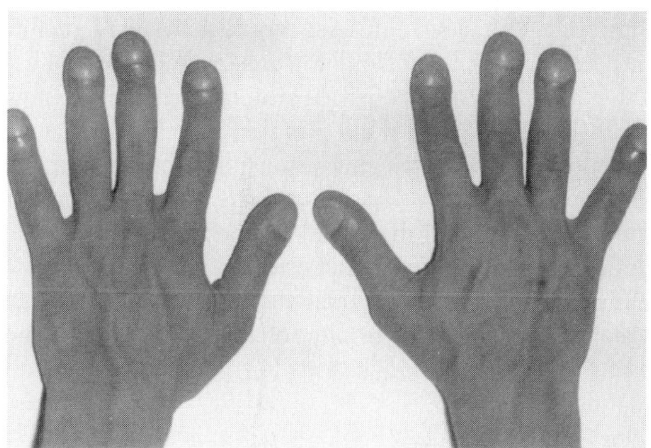

FIGURE 96.2. Clubbed digits of "Hippocratic" fingers show the drumstick appearance.

Arthritis

Patients may have oligoarthritis or polyarthritis with symptoms ranging from fleeting arthralgias to severe constant joint pain. Pain is most often symmetric and involves the knees, metacarpophalangeal joints, wrists, elbows, and ankles. Local warmth and erythema of the overlying skin, restricted joint motion, and swelling accompany pain. Ingestion of alcohol may worsen joint pain and swelling (12). Hypopigmentation of the skin and induration of the subcutaneous tissue around an affected joint suggest scleroderma. Effusions are usually mild but can be massive, particularly in hypertrophic osteoarthropathy associated with cyanotic congenital heart disease.

Additional Findings

Hypertrophic osteoarthropathy can be accompanied by signs of autonomic dysfunction including flushing, blanching, and profuse sweating, particularly in the hands and feet. Coarsening of the facial features and thickened furrowed skin of the face (leonine facies) and scalp might develop. Occasionally, patients develop gynecomastia, often associated with elevated levels of urinary estrogens (13).

CLINICAL SUBSETS

Pachydermoperiostosis

Primary hypertrophic osteoarthropathy also is referred to as pachydermoperiostosis or the Touraine–Solente–Golé syndrome. It has a bimodal onset with peaks at ages 1 and 15 years (14). The disease occurs within families, apparently transmitted by an autosomal dominant gene with variable penetrance. Currarino's disease is a variant in which there is delayed closure of the fontanelles and absence of skin involvement (15).

Symptoms most often occur in individuals before age 30 years (12,16,17). The onset of clubbing is insidious with "spade-like" enlargement of hands and feet. Signs and symptoms include cosmetic unsightliness, reduced dexterity, and awkwardness of the hands. There might be vague joint pain, bone pain, or both (16). Pain might be exacerbated by alcohol ingestion (12).

Cylindrical thickening of forearms and legs due to both bony and soft tissue proliferation accompanies clubbing (16). Recurrent, mildly symptomatic joint effusions and acrolysis involving the distal phalanges of hands and feet might occur (17). There is often excessive sweating, particularly of the hands and feet. Thickening and furrowing of facial skin with deep nasolabial folds and a corrugated scalp produce leonine features. The thickened skin is often "greasy" to the touch. These facial features, greasy skin, and sweating are uncommon in secondary hypertrophic osteoarthropathy. Although rare, gynecomastia, female hair distribution, striae, acne vulgaris, and cranial suture defects can occur. Nailfold capillary microscopy may reveal dilated, irregular, serpiginous capillary loops (17).

Secondary Hypertrophic Osteoarthropathy

Hypertrophic osteoarthropathy may accompany other illnesses, most commonly pulmonary neoplasms or infection of the lungs, mediastinum, or pleura.

Hypertrophic osteoarthropathy has been observed in 5% to 29% of patients with intrathoracic neoplasms (9,18,19), particularly bronchogenic carcinoma (20) and pleural tumors (21). Hypertrophic osteoarthropathy also may complicate lung abscess, bronchiectasis, chronic bronchitis, empyema, and acquired immunodeficiency syndrome (AIDS) (22). With improved therapy for chronic infections, hypertrophic osteoarthropathy is now often associated with chronic pneumonitis, pneumoconiosis, pulmonary tuberculosis, mediastinal Hodgkin's disease, sarcoidosis, immunodeficient children with recurrent pneumonitis, and cystic fibrosis (23,24). Hypertrophic osteoarthropathy with arthralgias can be the initial manifestation of interstitial pulmonary fibrosis (25). Numerous neoplasms have been reported with hypertrophic osteoarthropathy, many in association with intrathoracic metastases. Metastatic lesions *per se*, however, are not commonly associated with hypertrophic osteoarthropathy. Digital clubbing may be less common in small cell carcinoma than in non–small cell carcinoma of the lung as well as less common in men than in women (19).

Congenital heart malformations with cyanosis can cause clubbing (26). Hypertrophic osteoarthropathy is seldom seen in uncomplicated congenital heart disease without cyanosis. In up to 31% of patients with cyanotic congenital heart disease, hypertrophic osteoarthropathy develops, a fact that relates to the degree of right to left shunt (27). Other cardiac diseases that can be associated with hypertrophic osteoarthropathy include patent ductus arteriosus (28) and cardiac rhabdomyosarcoma (29). Clubbing in bacterial endocarditis might indicate embolization.

Gastrointestinal diseases associated with hypertrophic osteoarthropathy include ulcerative colitis, Crohn's disease, amebic colitis, subphrenic abscess, cirrhosis, idiopathic steatorrhea, sprue, neoplasms of the small intestine, multiple colonic polyposis, and carcinoma of the colon, esophagus, or liver (30). Hypertrophic osteoarthropathy also may accompany less common diseases such as primary cholangiolitic cirrhosis (31), secondary hepatic amyloidosis (perhaps related to infection), and biliary atresia (2,32). Hypertrophic osteoarthropathy of one or both lower extremities can be associated with an infected abdominal aneurysm or graft (33).

Less commonly, hypertrophic osteoarthropathy occurs after thyroidectomy for Graves' disease, and in hyperthyroidism, pregnancy, purgative abuse, connective tissue diseases, and hyperparathyroidism (2,18,34–36). Although uncommon, hypertrophic osteoarthropathy can occur with malignancy in childhood (37).

Thyroid Acropachy

This uncommon condition is characterized by clubbing of the fingers and asymptomatic periosteal proliferation of the bones of the hands and feet (38). It is associated with prior or active hyperthyroidism (Graves' disease), and most often is accompanied by exophthalmos and localized nonpitting soft tissue swelling of the extremities or pretibial myxedema. Long-acting thyroid stimulator (LATS) has been found in these cases (39).

LABORATORY AND ROENTGENOGRAPHIC FINDINGS

There is no test for hypertrophic osteoarthropathy. Antinuclear antibody and rheumatoid factor are not associated with hypertrophic osteoarthropathy. Acute phase reactants such as the erythrocyte sedimentation rate are often elevated. In the case of joint effusions, synovial fluids are group I (noninflammatory), clear, of high viscosity, and they usually have total leukocyte counts less than 2,000/mm^3 with fewer than 50% polymorphonuclear leukocytes (40,41). Serum and synovial fluid complement levels are normal in secondary hypertrophic osteoarthropathy (41).

The roentgenogram in periostitis is characteristic. There is subperiosteal new bone that appears symmetrically in the distal diaphyseal regions of long bones. This is present mostly in the legs and forearms, and less commonly in the phalanges (Fig. 96.3). Symptomatic disease in the absence of radiologic changes is rare (42). Subperiosteal new bone may be deposited in multiple layers, producing an "onion skin" appearance. The digital tuft hypertrophies in older patients, whereas there is acroosteolysis in younger patients.

Skeletal imaging using the ^{99m}Tc-bisphosphonate bone scanning agent may reveal a distinctive pattern (43). There is a pericortical linear accumulation of radiotracer along the long bones (Fig. 96.4). This pericortical accumulation of the nuclide also may occur along the proximal phalanges. There also may be increased periarticular uptake, reflecting synovitis. Involvement of the skull, scapulae, clavicles, and patellae is common. Asymmetric and irregular distribution is present in fewer than 20% of patients. Differentiation from the spotty localization of the nuclide of metastatic cancer is not difficult because hypertrophic osteoarthropathy produces a diffuse distribution of the radionuclide. Although the bone scan may suggest hypertrophic osteoarthropathy, it is not useful for staging of lung cancers (44).

PATHOLOGY

Histopathologic changes are similar in the primary (hereditary) and secondary forms of hypertrophic osteoarthropa-

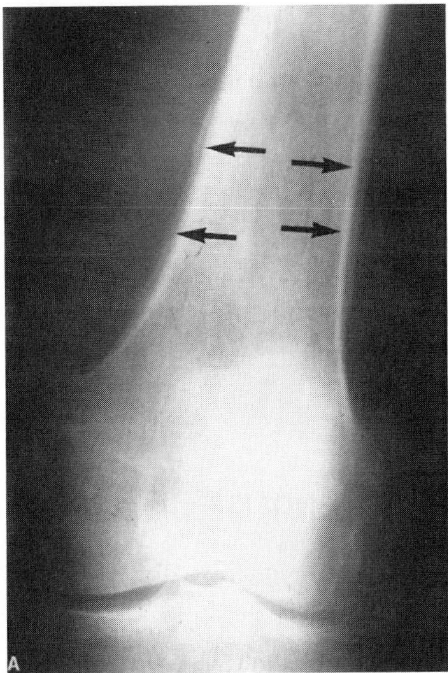

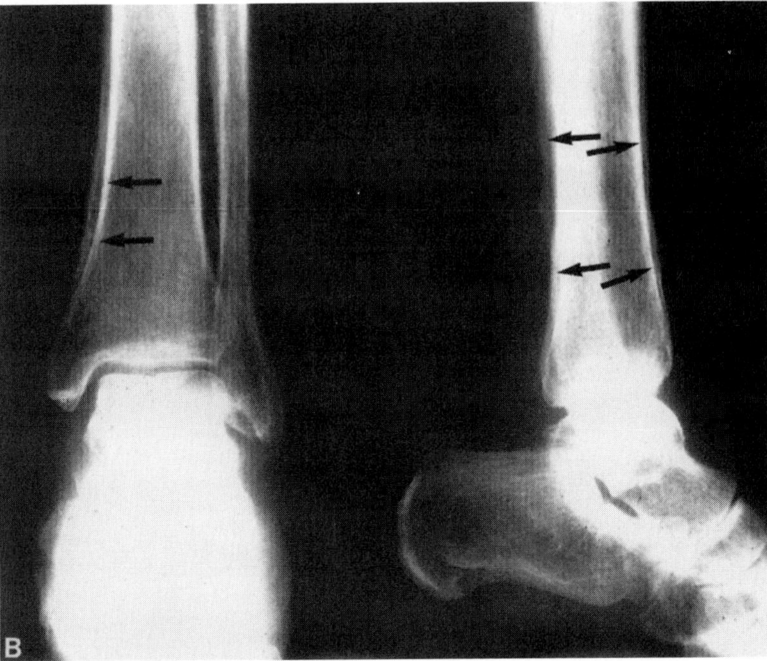

FIGURE 96.3. Hypertrophic osteoarthropathy. Radiodense bands along a margin of the shaft (*arrows*) indicate new osseous formation beneath the elevated periosteum. The appearance of these typical lesions is similar in the distal femur **(A)** to that of the distal tibia **(B)**.

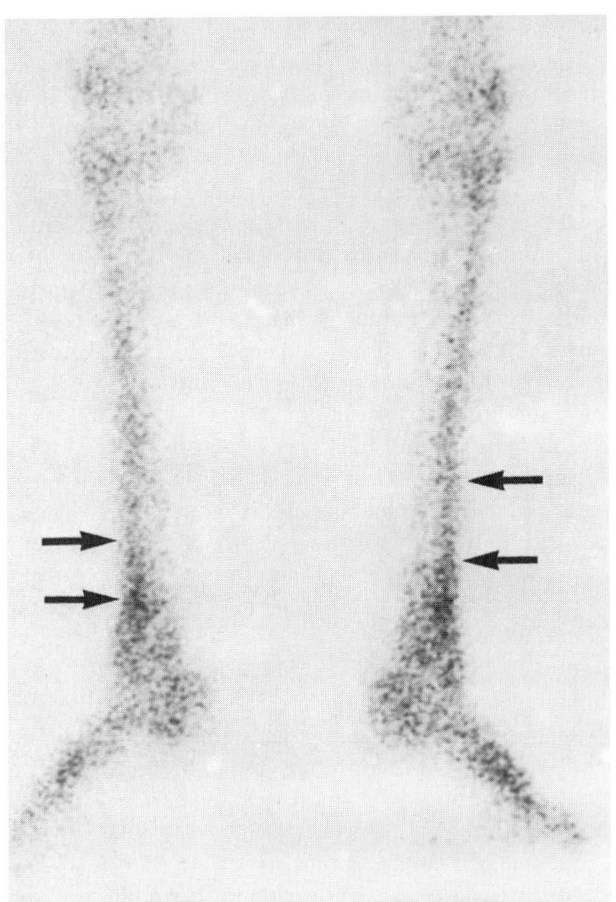

FIGURE 96.4. Bone scan using ^{99m}Tc-labeled methylene bisphosphonate demonstrating periosteal localization of the nuclide to the anterior tibiae (*arrows*).

thy. In clubbed phalanges, there is edema of the distal digital soft tissues, thickening of the blood vessel walls, cellular infiltration, fibroblastic proliferation, and deposition of new collagenous matrix, resulting in the uniform enlargement of terminal segments. Nail-bed and finger-pulp mast cell counts have been found to be lower in clubbed fingers as compared with control fingers (45).

Periostitis initially involves the distal end of metacarpals, metatarsals, long bones of the forearms, and legs. In severe disease, periostitis involving the ribs, clavicles, scapulae, pelvis, and malar bones is accompanied by round cell infiltration and edema of the periosteum, synovial membrane, articular capsule, and neighboring subcutaneous tissues. These changes are followed by periosteal elevation, deposition of subperiosteal osteoid, and subsequent mineralization. The distal long bones eventually become ensheathed with a cuff of new bone (Fig. 96.5). Concurrent with thickening, there is accelerated resorption of endosteal and haversian bone. The bony structure is weakened, and pathologic fractures sometimes occur. With advancing disease, these changes spread proximally along the bony shafts.

Synovial membranes adjoining the involved bones are often edematous and infiltrated with lymphocytes, plasma cells, and a few neutrophils. Advancing, proliferative, fibrous tissue at joint margins is sometimes associated with cartilage degeneration. Electron-microscopic studies of synovial membranes reveal alterations of the microcirculation, with dilatation of capillaries and venules, endothelial cell gaps, and multilamination of small vessel basement membranes (40). The significance of subendothelial electron-dense deposits in synovial membranes of patients with sec-

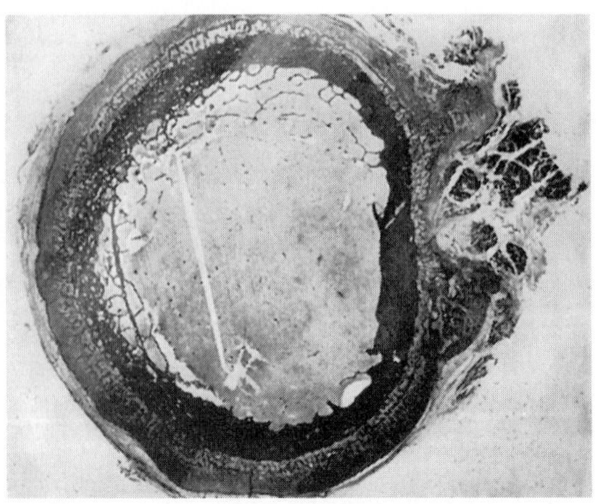

FIGURE 96.5. Cross section through a metatarsal of a patient with hypertrophic osteoarthropathy. The periosteum shows thickening, with an irregular cuff of new bone deposited over the cortex. (Reproduced with permission from Bartter FC, Bauer W. In: Cecil R, Loeb J, eds. *Textbook of medicine.* Philadelphia: WB Saunders, 1965.)

ondary hypertrophic osteoarthropathy is unclear (40). Negative immunofluorescent staining for gamma globulins and complement has been reported (46).

ETIOLOGY AND PATHOGENESIS

The nature of the genetic factors operative in the hereditary form of hypertrophic osteoarthropathy is unknown.

One theory implicates the development of pulmonary arteriovenous shunts, allowing a hormone or toxin that is normally inactivated in the lungs to escape into the systemic circulation and cause the pathologic changes. One suspected vasoactive substance is reduced ferritin. Some evidence suggests that the etiopathogenesis of hypertrophic osteoarthropathy may be related to platelet-derived vascular thrombi (46) or antiphospholipid antibodies (47).

Factors underlying development of hypertrophic osteoarthropathy in the setting of intrathoracic disease are unknown, but there is evidence for a local circulatory disorder (2,48). A locally acting circulating vasodilator has been demonstrated in some patients (49). Increased vascularity of clubbed fingers in secondary hypertrophic osteoarthropathy has been demonstrated by measurement of skin temperature, infrared photography, nailfold capillarioscopy, and postmortem arteriography (50). Elevated digital pulse pressure and blood flow have been shown to return to normal after removal of pulmonary lesions (2). Perhaps anomalous vascular control leads to such altered blood-flow patterns (51).

Plasma growth factors such as growth hormone, transforming growth factor-β, and hepatocyte growth factor were elevated in patients with lung cancers and clubbing (52–54). Elevated excretion of urinary estrogens also has been reported (13). A polypeptide substance differing from immunoreactive growth hormone, but related to somatotropins, might be a mediator in hypertrophic osteoarthropathy (55). A more recent report suggests an important role for platelet activation of endothelial cells with release of fibroblast growth factors (56,57).

Circulating tumor antigen–antibody complexes have been described in patients with a variety of tumors, including lung carcinomas. The electron-microscopic findings have been equivocal, but not inconsistent with the possibility that the synovitis seen in hypertrophic osteoarthropathy associated with bronchogenic carcinoma might be immune complex mediated.

DIFFERENTIAL DIAGNOSIS

The presence of clubbing simplifies diagnosis, and an underlying disease must be suspected. If acute polyarthritis precedes clubbing, the initial impression might be rheumatoid arthritis (RA) (58). In most instances, roentgenograms reveal subperiosteal new bone, which must be differentiated from that resulting from local tumors, lymphangitis, syphilis, or the hemorrhages of trauma or scurvy. Swelling and tenderness of the lower legs might falsely suggest thrombophlebitis, and bone pain might be misinterpreted as peripheral neuritis. The spoon-shaped nails of hypochromic anemia are easily distinguishable. Hypertrophic osteoarthropathy sometimes superficially suggests scleroderma.

Associated diseases should be excluded before assigning a patient to the ill-defined hereditary or idiopathic group. This point is emphasized because of the danger of overlooking infection, a resectable tumor, or another treatable condition. Separation of primary and secondary hypertrophic osteoarthropathy should not be difficult because the hereditary or idiopathic syndrome begins after puberty, follows a self-limited course of one to two decades, and occurs in other family members.

Florid, reactive periostitis occurring in young adults is not associated with clubbing and is more painful than the periostitis of hypertrophic osteoarthropathy (59).

TREATMENT

Clubbing is most often asymptomatic and usually requires no treatment *per se.* Disabling symptoms relating to periostitis, synovitis, or both often respond dramatically to removal of the primary pulmonary lesion or to intrathoracic vagotomy (60).

Nonsteroidal antiinflammatory drugs (NSAIDs) have been beneficial in reducing discomfort, but not in reversing the condition. Aspirin in modest doses or another NSAID, particularly indomethacin, is frequently effective (42,43).

Chemical vagotomy by atropine (61) or propantheline bromide has reportedly relieved symptoms (62). A variety of agents that cause vasodilation may prove of value, including calcium channel–blocking drugs as well as α-methyl dopa. Analgesics are appropriate. Adrenocortical steroid derivatives can be useful (63). Radiotherapy to the primary tumor site (64) or to the metastatic lesion (65,66), as well as chemotherapy (67), have relieved joint symptoms. Complete disappearance of hypertrophic osteoarthropathy is described after liver transplantation and after appropriate therapy for empyema, lung abscess, bronchiectasis, pneumonia, and bacterial endocarditis (30,68). Resolution of symptoms and signs has been shown to follow simple denervation of the hilum or vagotomy on the same side as the lesion. Thoracotomy without denervation in these studies was ineffective.

Intravenous pamidronate or subcutaneous octreotide have been helpful in controlling the pain of hypertrophic osteoarthropathy in lung cancer (69,70).

Treatment of idiopathic hypertrophic osteoarthropathy is symptomatic.

REFERENCES

1. Hippocrates (c. 400 BC). In: Adams F, trans. *The genuine works of Hippocrates.* Vol I. London: Syndenham Society, 1849:249.
2. Mendlowitz M. Clubbing and hypertrophic osteoarthropathy. *Medicine* 1942;21:269–306.
3. Fischer DS, Singer DH, Feldman SM. Clubbing: a review, with emphasis on hereditary acropachy. *Medicine* 1965;43:459–479.
4. Seaton DR. Familial clubbing of fingers and toes. *Br Med J* 1938;1:614–615.
5. Hedayati H, Barmada R, Skosey JL. Acrolysis in pachydermoperiostosis. *Arch Intern Med* 1980;140:1087–1088.
6. Schamroth L. Personal experience. *S Afr Med J* 1976;50: 297–300.
7. Vazquez-Abad D, Pineda C, Martinez-Lavin M. Digital clubbing: a numerical assessment of the deformity. *J Rheumatol* 1989;16:518–520.
8. Sinniah D, Omar A. Quantitation of digital clubbing by shadowgram technique. *Arch Dis Child* 1979;54:145–146.
9. Baughman RP, Gunther KL, Buchsbaur JA, et al. Prevalence of digital clubbing in bronchogenic carcinoma by a new digital index. *Clin Exp Rheumatol* 1998;16:21–26.
10. Denham MJ, Hodkinson HM, Wright BM. Unilateral clubbing in hemiplegia. *Gerontol Clin* 1975;17:7–12.
11. Hashmi S, Kaplan D. Asymmetric clubbing as a manifestation of sarcoid bone disease. *Am J Med* 1992;93:471.
12. Mueller M, Trevarthen D. Pachydermoperiostosis: arthropathy aggravated by episode alcohol abuse. *J Rheumatol* 1981;8: 862–864.
13. Jao JY, Barlow JJ, Krant MJ. Pulmonary hypertrophic osteoarthropathy, spider angiomata and estrogen hyperexcretion. *Ann Intern Med* 1969;70:581–584.
14. Martinez-Lavin M, Martucci-Cernic MM, Jajic I, et al. Hypertrophic osteoarthropathy: consensus on its definition, classification, assessment and diagnostic criteria. *J Rheumatol* 1993;20: 1386–1387.
15. Gaston-Garrette F, Porteau-Cassard L, Marc V, et al. A case of primary hypertrophic osteoarthropathy without skin involvement (Currarino's disease). *Rev Rhum Eng Ed* 1998;65: 591–593.
16. Vogl A, Goldfischer S. Pachydermoperiostosis: primary or idiopathic hypertrophic osteoarthropathy. *Am J Med* 1962;33: 166–187.
17. Fam AG, Chin-Sang H, Ramsay CA. Pachydermoperiostosis: scintigraphic, plethysmographic, and capillarscopic observations. *Ann Rheum Dis* 1983;42:98–102.
18. Wierman WJ, Clagett OT, McDonald JR. Articular manifestations in pulmonary diseases: an analysis of their occurrence in 1,024 cases in which pulmonary resection was performed. *JAMA* 1954;155:1459–1463.
19. Sridhar KS, Lobo CF, Altman RD. Digital clubbing and lung cancer. *Chest* 1998;114:1535–1537.
20. Freeman MH, Tonkin AK. Manifestations of hypertrophic pulmonary osteoarthropathy in patients with carcinoma of the lung: demonstration by ^{99m}Tc-pyrophosphate bone scans. *Radiology* 1976;120:363–365.
21. Briselli M, Mark J, Dickersin GR. Solitary fibrous tumors of the pleura: eight new cases and review of 360 cases in the literature. *Cancer* 1981;1:2678–2689.
22. Boonen A, Schrey G, Van der Linden S. Clubbing in human immunodeficiency virus infection. *Br J Rheumatol* 1996;35: 292–294.
23. West SG, Gilbreath RE, Lawless OJ. Painful clubbing and sarcoidosis. *JAMA* 1981;246:1338–1339.
24. Rush PJ, Gladman DD, Shore A, et al. Absence of an association between HLA typing in cystic fibrosis arthritis and hypertrophic osteoarthropathy. *Ann Rheum Dis* 1991;50:763–764.
25. Kupfer Y, Groopman JE, Aswini Lenora R, et al. Pulmonary hypertrophic osteoarthropathy as the initial manifestation of interstitial fibrosis. *N Y State J Med* 1989;89:234–235.
26. McLaughlin GE, McCarty DJ Jr, Downing DF. Hypertrophic osteoarthropathy associated with cyanotic congenital heart disease. *Ann Intern Med* 1967;67:579–587.
27. Martinez-Lavin M, Bobadilla M, Casanova J, et al. Hypertrophic osteoarthropathy in cyanotic congenital heart disease: its prevalence and relationship to bypass of the lung. *Arthritis Rheum* 1982;25:1186–1192.
28. Martinez-Lavin M, Pineda C, Navarro C, et al. Primary hypertrophic osteoarthropathy: another heritable disorder associated with patent ductus arteriosus. *Pediatr Cardiol* 1993;14:181–182.
29. Pascuzzi CA, Parkin TW, Bruwer AJ, et al. Hypertrophic osteoarthropathy associated with primary rhabdomyosarcoma of the heart. *Mayo Clin Proc* 1957;32:30–41.
30. Taillandier J, Alemanni M, Samuel D, et al. Hepatic hypertrophic osteoarthropathy: the value of liver transplantation. *Clin Exp Rheumatol* 1998;16:80–81.
31. Kieff ED, McCarty DJ. Hypertrophic osteoarthropathy with arthritis and synovial calcification in a patient with alcoholic cirrhosis. *Arthritis Rheum* 1969;12:261–268.
32. Epstein O, Dick R, Sherlock S. Prospective study of periostitis and finger clubbing in primary biliary cirrhosis and other forms of chronic liver disease. *Gut* 1981;22:203–206.
33. Sorin SB, Askari A, Rhodes RS. Hypertrophic osteoarthropathy of the lower extremities as a manifestation of arterial graft sepsis. *Arthritis Rheum* 1980;23:768–770.
34. Souders CR, Manuell JL. Skeletal deformities in hyperparathyroidism. *N Engl J Med* 1954;250:594–597.
35. Lovell RRH, Scott GBD. Hypertrophic osteoarthropathy in polyarteritis. *Ann Rheum Dis* 1956;15:46–50.
36. Borden EC, Holling HE. Hypertrophic osteoarthropathy and pregnancy. *Ann Intern Med* 1969;71:577–580.
37. Staaziman CR, Umans U. Hypertrophic osteoarthropathy in childhood malignancy. *Med Pediatr Oncol* 1993;21:676–679.
38. Curti LG, Siccardi M, Santienelo EB, et al. Full-blown hypothy-

roidism associated with vitiligo and acropachy: report of one case. *Thyroidol Clin Exp* 1992;4:111–117.
39. Lynch PJ, Maize JC, Sisson JC. Pretibial myxedema and nonthyrotoxic thyroid disease. *Arch Dermatol* 1973;107:107–111.
40. Schumacher HR. Articular manifestations of HPO in bronchogenic carcinoma: a clinical and pathologic study. *Arthritis Rheum* 1976;19:629–636.
41. Vidal AF, Altman RD, Pardo V, et al. Structural and immunologic changes of synovium of hypertrophic osteoarthropathy (HPO) [Abstract]. *Arthritis Rheum* 1977;20:139.
42. Pineda C, Fonseca C, Martinez-Lavin M. The spectrum of soft tissue and skeletal abnormalities of hypertrophic osteoarthropathy. *J Rheumatol* 1990;17:626–632.
43. Bomanji J, Nagaraj M, Jewkes R, et al. Pachydermoperiostosis: technetium-99m-methylene diphosphonate scintigraphic pattern. *J Nucl Med* 1991;32:1907–1909.
44. Morgan B, Coakley F, Finlay DB, et al. Hypertrophic osteoarthropathy in staging skeletal scintigraphy for lung cancer. *Clin Radiol* 1996;51:694–697.
45. Marshall R. Observations of the pathology of clubbed fingers with special reference to mast cells. *Am Rev Respir Dis* 1976;113:395–397.
46. Martucci-Cernic M, Martinez-Lavin M, Rojo F, et al. Von Willebrand factor antigen in hypertrophic osteoarthropathy. *J Rheumatol* 1992;19:765–767.
47. Harris AW, Harding TAC, Gaitonde MD, et al. Is clubbing a feature of the anti-phospholipid antibody syndrome? *Postgrad Med J* 1993;69:748–750.
48. Mendlowitz M, Leslie A. Experimental simulation in dogs of cyanosis and hypertrophic osteoarthropathy which are associated with congenital heart disease. *Am Heart J* 1942;24:141–152.
49. Shneerson JM. Digital clubbing and hypertrophic osteoarthropathy: the underlying mechanisms. *Br J Dis Chest* 1981;75:113–131.
50. Matucci-Cerinic M, Cinti S, Morroni M, et al. Pachydermoperiostosis (primary hypertrophic osteoarthropathy): report of a case with evidence of endothelial and connective tissue involvement. *Ann Rheum Dis* 1989;48:240–246.
51. Doyle L. Pathogenesis of secondary hypertrophic osteoarthropathy: a hypothesis. *Eur Respir J* 1989;2:105–106.
52. Goshney MA, Gosney JR, Lye M. Plasma growth hormone and digital clubbing in carcinoma of the bronchus. *Thorax* 1990;45: 545–547.
53. Hirakata Y, Kitamura S. Elevated serum transforming growth factor beta 1 level in primary lung cancer patients with finger clubbing. *Eur J Clin Invest* 1996;26:820–823.
54. Hojo S, Fujita J, Yamadori I, et al. Hepatocyte growth factor and digital clubbing. *Intern Med* 1997;36:44–46.
55. Audebert AA, Aubriot A, Krulik M, et al. Osteoarthropathie hypertrophiante pneumique associee a une quadruple secretion hormonale paraneoplasique. *Sem Hop Paris* 1982;158:529–530.
56. Martinez-Lavin M. Hypertrophic osteoarthropathy. *Curr Opin Rheumatol* 1997;9:83–86.
57. Silveri F, De Angelis R, Argentati F, et al. Hypertrophic osteoarthropathy: endothelium and platelet function. *Clin Rheumatol* 1996;15:435–439.
58. Polley HF, Clagett OT, McDonald JR, et al. Articular reactions with localized fibrous mesothelioma of the pleura. *Ann Rheum Dis* 1952;11:314.
59. Nance KV, Renner JB, Brashear HR, et al. Massive florid reactive periostitis. *Pediatr Radiol* 1990;20:186–189.
60. LeRoux BT. Bronchial carcinoma with hypertrophic pulmonary osteoarthropathy. *S Afr Med J* 1968;42:1074–1075.
61. Lopez-Enriquez E, Morales AR, Robert F. Effect of atropine sulfate in pulmonary hypertrophic osteoarthropathy. *Arthritis Rheum* 1980;23:822–824.
62. Schwartz HA. Pro-banthine for hypertrophic osteoarthropathy. *Arthritis Rheum* 1981;24:1588.
63. Holling HE, Brodey RS. Pulmonary hypertrophic osteoarthropathy. *JAMA* 1961;178:977–982.
64. Steinfeld AD, Munzenrider JE. The response of hypertrophic pulmonary osteoarthropathy to radiotherapy. *Radiology* 1974; 113:709–711.
65. Rao GM, Guruprakash GH, Poulose KP, et al. Improvement in hypertrophic pulmonary osteoarthropathy after radiotherapy to metastasis. *Am J Radiol* 1979;133:944–946.
66. Yeo W, Leung SF, Chan AT, et al. Radiotherapy for extreme hypertrophic pulmonary osteoarthropathy associated with malignancy. *Clin Oncol (R Coll Radiol)* 1996;8:195–197.
67. Evans WK. Reversal of hypertrophic osteoarthropathy after chemotherapy for bronchogenic carcinoma. *J Rheumatol* 1980;7: 93–97.
68. Shapiro CM, Mackinnon J. The resolution of hypertrophic pulmonary osteoarthropathy following treatment of subacute bacterial endocarditis. *Postgrad Med J* 1980;56:513–515.
69. Speden D, Nicklason F, Francis H, et al. The use of pamidronate in hypertrophic pulmonary osteoarthropathy (HPOA). *Aust N Z J Med* 1997;27:307–310.
70. Johnson SA, Spiller PA, Faull CM. Treatment of resistant pain in hypertrophic pulmonary osteoarthropathy with subcutaneous octreotide. *Thorax* 1997;52:298–299.

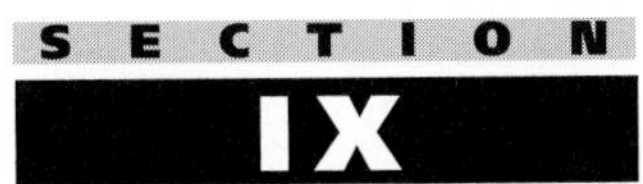

REGIONAL DISORDERS OF JOINTS AND RELATED STRUCTURES

97

TRAUMATIC ARTHRITIS AND ALLIED CONDITIONS

ROBERT S. PINALS

In its broadest sense, the term *traumatic arthritis* circumscribes a diverse collection of pathologic and clinical states that develop after single or repetitive episodes of trauma (Table 97.1). Although these conditions are frequently encountered by the rheumatologist, interest in the area has been casual, and studies of basic mechanisms of disease have been few as compared with those in the other rheumatic diseases. Because surgeons are more likely to deal with the sequelae of trauma, it is not surprising that the most significant contributions are to be found in the orthopedic literature. The credulous assignment of etiologic roles to trauma in early writings stands in sharp contrast to modern attitudes on the subject. Rheumatoid arthritis (RA), tuberculous arthritis, gout, and other rheumatic diseases were formerly attributed to trauma, which might alter the structural integrity of joints, predisposing them to inflammation. As other pathogenetic mechanisms have been revealed, it has become less necessary to invoke "unrecognized trauma," which was previously such a convenient explanation for poorly understood disorders. Even in osteoarthritis (OA), once the bellwether of traumatic disorders, considered by some to be synonymous with traumatic arthritis, increasing emphasis is being placed on altered cartilage metabolism, leaving an even smaller role for "multiple microtraumata."

TABLE 97.1. CLASSIFICATION OF TRAUMATIC ARTHRITIS AND ALLIED CONDITIONS

I. Articular trauma, single episode
   A. Traumatic synovitis, without disturbance of articular cartilage or disruption of major supporting structures. This type includes acute synovitis, with or without hemarthrosis, and most sprains. Healing is expected within several weeks, without permanent tissue damage
   B. Disruptive trauma, with infraction of the articular cartilage or complete rupture of major supporting structures. This type includes intraarticular fractures, meniscal tears, and severe sprains
   C. Posttraumatic osteoarthritis. This type includes cases of disruptive trauma in which major residual damage is present. Patients may have deformity, limited motion, or instability of joints.
II. Repetitive articular trauma. This type includes a variety of conditions related to occupation or sports and results in localized chronic arthritis
III. Induction or aggravation of another specific rheumatic disease by acute or repetitive trauma
IV. Conditions in which trauma may be one of several etiologic factors, or in which a relation has been suggested but not established: osteochondritis dissecans, osteitis pubis, Tietze's syndrome, and hypermobility syndrome
V. Disorders of extraarticular structures, such as tendons, bursae, and muscles, in which trauma commonly plays an etiologic role
VI. Nonmechanical types of trauma, such as arthropathy after frostbite, radiation, and decompression

ACUTE TRAUMATIC SYNOVITIS

After a direct blow or forced inappropriate motion to a joint, swelling and pain may develop. Because the knee is most commonly affected, the following discussion is directed at that joint, but one might follow a similar approach for a traumatic synovitis of the elbow, shoulder, or ankle. If the patient is able to walk without limping and has no effusion on examination, knee radiographs are probably unnecessary because fracture is highly unlikely (1). If an effusion is evident, it should be aspirated to determine whether hemarthrosis is present and to aid in further examination of the joint. Hemarthrosis is usually present if fluid appears within 2 hours after the injury. In about half the cases, swelling occurs within 15 minutes. Conversely, nonbloody effusions generally appear 12 to 24 hours after injury. With hemarthrosis, there is usually more pain, and at times a low-grade fever. Fractures, internal derangements, or major ligamentous tears must be ruled out by examination and radiographs, which suggest a cause for the bleeding in up to 75% of hemarthrosis cases. Arthroscopy and more sophisticated imaging techniques reveal a broader range of pathology (2,3). In a prospective series of 100 cases of traumatic hemarthrosis in nonathletes, magnetic resonance imaging (MRI) and arthroscopy, with ligament testing under anesthesia, demonstrated significant lesions in 99 cases even though routine roentgenograms were negative (2). Anterior cruciate ligament tears were found most frequently (67%), particularly with recreational injuries. Other causes included collateral and posterior cruciate ligament tears, meniscal and capsular tears, and chondral fractures. Although not indicated routinely, MRI permits identification of occult fractures and "bone bruises" (multiple impaction fractures), which can result in hemarthrosis (4). However, MRI does not add information on the status of the anterior cruciate ligament compared with a careful clinical examination (4). The presence of fat globules floating on the surface of bloody fluid usually indicates a fracture. At times, sufficient fat may be present to be detectable on a lateral knee radiograph as a radiolucent layer in the suprapatellar pouch (Fig. 97.1) (5). A similar appearance has been described in the elbow and hip. Among patients with hip trauma and negative roentgenograms, lipohemarthrosis on computed tomography is usually associated with an intraarticular fracture (6). Hemorrhagic fluid usually does not clot; coagulation may indicate more profound tissue damage and a poorer prognosis. Rarely, a chylous effusion may occur, either with or without an intraarticular fracture or hemarthrosis (7,8).

In the absence of gross bleeding, examination of the fluid reveals a variable number of red blood cells and 50 to 2,000 white blood cells, of which only a few are neutrophils. The protein content, mostly albumin, is two or three times that of normal fluid. Viscosity is slightly reduced, but the mucin clot is good. Synovial biopsy reveals some vasodilatation, edema, and an occasional small focus of synovial cell proliferation with mild lymphocytic infiltration (9).

A high leukocyte count in traumatic synovial effusions is rarely accompanied by intracellular and extracellular lipid globules, suggesting that lipid droplet phagocytosis might have provoked an inflammatory reaction (10). This hypothesis was supported by studies of dog knees subjected to blunt trauma, which resulted in clear effusions containing fat globules. Intraarticular injection of autologous fat was shown to induce phagocytosis and mild inflammation (see Chapter 119) (11).

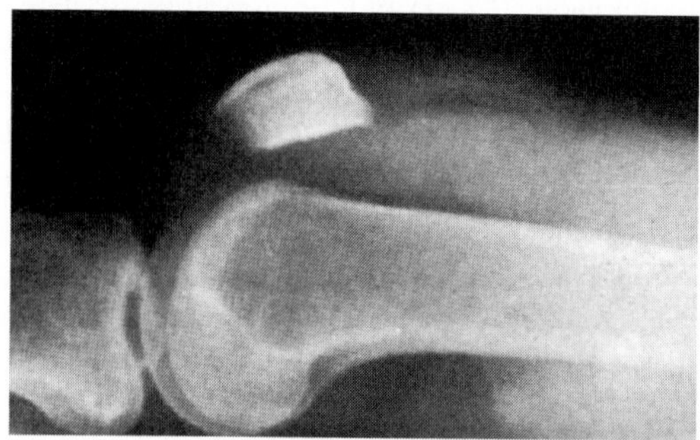

FIGURE 97.1. Traumatic hemarthrosis. Liquid fat and a fat–blood level are visible in the joint. (Reproduced with permission from Berk RN. Liquid fat in the knee joint after trauma. *N Engl J Med* 1967;277:1411–1412.)

Treatment may include such measures as cold packs initially and heat later, compression dressings, splinting with a brace that permits limited motion, graded quadriceps exercises, repeated aspiration if significant volumes of fluid reaccumulate, and a period of bed rest or partial weight bearing, depending on the severity of the injury. Early arthroscopic surgery is being advocated with increasing frequency, particularly in athletes. Partial cruciate ligament or meniscal disruptions may be recognized and repaired before progressing to complete tears (3). Short-term outcomes are excellent in the absence of improper treatment, such as cylinder cast immobilization, which may result in muscle atrophy and loss of motion, or premature weight bearing, which may in turn lead to an extended duration of synovitis.

SPRAINS

A sprain may be defined as a stretching or tearing of a supporting ligament of a joint by forced movement beyond its normal range. In its simplest form, there is minimal disruption of fibers, swelling, pain, and dysfunction. Severe sprains may cause total rupture of ligaments, marked swelling and hemorrhage, and joint instability, which may be permanent if untreated. Sprains occur most frequently in the ankle, but also are common in the knee, low back, and neck.

Ankle Sprains

Most ankle sprains result from unintentional weight bearing on the inverted, plantar-flexed foot. There is partial or total disruption of one or more of the three main lateral supporting structures that unite the fibula above with the calcaneus and talus below. Rupture of the anterior talofibular ligament is most common; this structure prevents anterior displacement of the talus out of the ankle joint mortise. With additional force, the calcaneofibular ligament, which prevents excessive inversion, also may rupture. The third ligament, the posterior talofibular ligament, is seldom torn with the usual type of injury. If it also tears, a completely unstable ankle results. Stretching of the medial supporting structures usually results in fracture and avulsion of the medial malleolus rather than a sprain.

The patient presents with severe pain and swelling on the outer aspect of the foot and ankle (12,13). Much of the early swelling is due to hemorrhage, resulting in ecchymosis several hours later. A history of something snapping, giving away, or slipping out of place may suggest a complete ligament rupture. The nature of the treatment largely depends on assessment of the integrity of these ligaments. This is most easily accomplished soon after the injury, before swelling and pain make forced motion difficult. Local anesthesia may be required for proper examination. The anterior drawer and talar tilt tests are manual stress tests to evaluate the anterior talofibular ligament and calcaneofibular ligament, respectively. Some orthopedists insist on stress roentgenograms after all severe sprains.

Early treatment of simple sprains may include elevation, ice packs, and compression dressing to prevent swelling, and early weight bearing. A lift on the outer border of the heel will maintain eversion and prevent strain on the injured ligament. Severe sprains may demand additional treatment, including casting and early or late surgical repair for marked instability. A follow-up study of patients with long-standing lateral ligament instability demonstrated a high incidence of degenerative changes in the articular cartilage of the medial joint surface (14).

Other Sprains

Knee sprains are considered in Chapter 98, and low back sprains in Chapter 102. Shoulder "sprain" is actually a subluxation of the acromioclavicular joint, commonly seen in body-contact sports. Wrist "sprain" may be a fractured navicular bone, often missed on initial roentgenograms. Traumatic torticollis may be called a neck sprain. Before a sudden twist or wrenching of the neck, pain and muscle spasm may result in involuntary assumption of a "wry neck" position. Spontaneous remission occurs after 1 to 2 weeks. Measures such as a cervical collar, traction, and heat may be helpful. The actual structures involved in neck sprain have not been well defined.

PERIARTICULAR OSSIFICATION

Heterotopic ossification, or bone formation outside the skeleton, is an unusual consequence of trauma. For instance, a linear ossification may develop in the area of the medial collateral ligament after acute knee trauma (Pellegrini–Stieda syndrome). A hematoma may be the initial event, but little is known about pathogenesis. Calcification is noted on roentgenograms obtained as early as 3 or 4 weeks after the injury. Few biopsies have been obtained in the early stages; those performed later show bone rather than a calcific deposit. The initial injury may be minor or may produce a fracture, torn meniscus, or ligamentous rupture. Initial signs and symptoms, as well as subsequent disability, are related more to this associated trauma than to the heterotopic bone itself. Fractures in the vicinity of the hip, elbow, and other joints may result in heterotopic bone formation, particularly if surgical intervention is delayed. A similar problem may occur after total hip replacement (15,16) (see Chapter 52). This is more likely to limit motion than to cause pain. Risk factors include underlying conditions such as ankylosing spondylitis and diffuse idiopathic skeletal hyperostosis.

Paraplegic and quadriplegic patients may develop ossification in soft tissues adjacent to joints that are located below the level of the neurologic lesion (17). The hips and knees are most commonly involved. This complication occurs in about 20% of patients with spinal cord injury and occasionally in other neurologic conditions. Although some of the milder cases may not be detected by physical examination, many patients have swelling, warmth, and erythema in the affected area, suggesting alternative diagnoses, such as cellulitis and thrombophlebitis. These signs may appear as early as 3 weeks after the injury, when radiographic findings are minimal or absent. At this stage, serum alkaline phosphatase may be elevated, and soft tissue uptake of radionuclide may be increased on a bone scan. After about 2 months, a firm mass of trabeculated bone may be detected on physical examination and demonstrated radiologically. This finding is often accompanied by loss of joint motion and occasionally by complete ankylosis. Serious functional impairment may result; for instance, the patient may be unable to sit because hip flexion is lost.

Heterotopic ossification also has been reported in critically ill patients requiring prolonged mechanical ventilation (18).

There is evidence to suggest that early treatment with indomethacin, diphosphonates, or radiotherapy inhibits the formation of heterotopic bone, regardless of its underlying cause (15,16). The osseous deposit may be excised when it reaches maturity, but it recurs in most patients.

Patients with spinal cord injury also may develop hydrarthrosis or hemarthrosis of the knee, presumed to be of traumatic origin (17,19). The effusion, which may precede the ossification, has a normal cell count but a discordantly high protein concentration (19).

DISRUPTIVE ARTICULAR TRAUMA: POSTTRAUMATIC OSTEOARTHRITIS

Permanent joint damage may be the result of various types of trauma, including fractures through the articular surface, dislocations, internal derangements, major ligamentous ruptures, and wounds, often with sepsis and foreign body implantation (Fig. 97.2). There may be permanent or progressive structural alterations [e.g., deterioration of articular cartilage, limitation of joint motion, instability, or angular deviation (20)]. Arthritis is more likely to develop in the legs than in the arms because of greater weight-bearing loads. Pathologically and radiographically, the condition has most of the characteristics of OA. However, a specific traumatic episode should not be definitely accepted as etiologically related to OA unless there is evidence establishing these points: (a) the joint was normal before injury; (b) records document either an effusion or structural damage shortly after the injury; and (c) similar disease has not occurred in nontraumatized joints. Other points favoring a

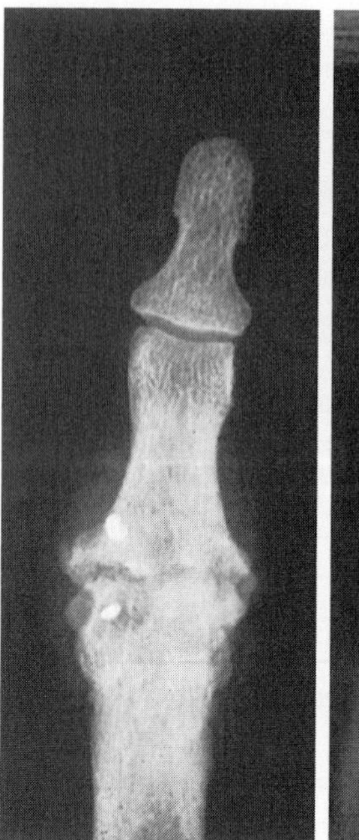
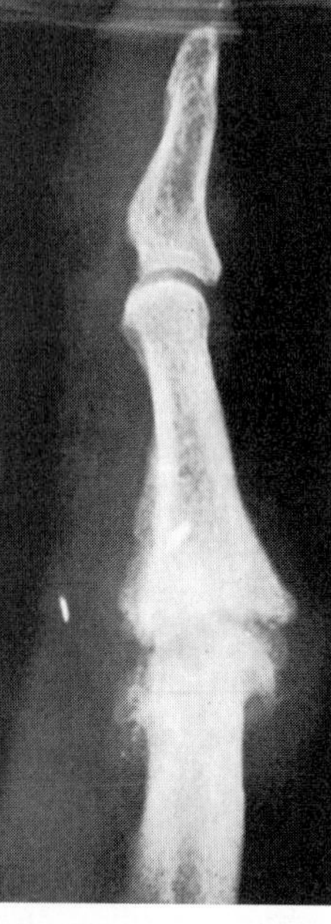

FIGURE 97.2. Arthritis due to foreign body. A piece of steel lodged in this index finger of the patient 4 years earlier. Swelling of the finger began about 2 years later and has continued to date. Radiograph shows marked deformity of the proximal interphalangeal joint of the right index finger. This consists of marked hypertrophic changes with possible ankylosis of the joint. There are two small opaque foreign bodies in relation to the palmar and radial aspects of the joint.

traumatic origin are the occurrence of significant isolated OA in a joint not usually involved by the idiopathic variety (such as ankle, wrist, elbow, or metacarpophalangeal joint) and radiologic demonstration of foreign bodies and healed fractures near the joint in question.

Soon after knee trauma, increased levels of metalloproteinases, proteoglycan fragments, and cartilage matrix proteins may be measured in joint fluid (21,22). These decrease over time, but elevations persist for several years after the injury. It is not yet clear whether these findings correlate with the development of posttraumatic OA.

REPETITIVE ARTICULAR TRAUMA

Osteoarthritis may develop in joints that are repeatedly traumatized as a result of certain occupations and sports. Radiographic abnormalities, such as joint-space narrowing, subcortical cysts, and marginal osteophytes, are common in some groups studied, but many of the affected individuals are asymptomatic. These changes occur in the hands and wrists of boxers and stone workers using pneumatic hammers, in the ankles of soccer players, in the first metatarsophalangeal joints of ballet dancers, and in the elbows of foundry workers.

ROLE OF TRAUMA IN OTHER TYPES OF ARTHRITIS

Trauma plays an important role in the development of neuropathic joint disease (see Chapter 91). Attacks of gouty arthritis and pseudogout often develop in recently injured joints. RA occasionally begins in a joint that has been injured or subjected to a surgical procedure. Posttraumatic onsets of seronegative spondyloarthropathy (23), as well as septic and tuberculous arthritis, have been described. A history of recent or old trauma to the affected joint is sometimes obtained from patients with septic or tuberculous arthritis. The evidence in these situations is anecdotal and difficult to evaluate. Data have not been gathered in an organized fashion, and the mechanisms involved are not well understood. In many instances, the trauma has been minimal, perhaps representing an unrelated antecedent to the joint disease.

In the absence of appropriate studies, the putative etiologic or precipitating role of trauma in chronic inflammatory arthritis remains speculative, but cannot be dismissed.

Preexisting arthritis may certainly be aggravated by trauma, but the magnitude and duration of exacerbation reasonably attributable to trauma are unknown, and each case must be considered on its own merits. Only minor force would be required to cause rupture of a frayed wrist-extensor tendon or collateral ligament in a patient with RA. Other acute episodes, such as abrupt increase in joint swelling or rupture of the posterior knee joint capsule, are commonly associated with unusual resistive exercise. Sanguineous joint fluid is sometimes aspirated from a knee or shoulder in patients with RA who report sudden increase in pain and swelling after relatively minor trauma. It is presumed that pinching or compressing the hypertrophied synovium may result in bleeding. In such cases, the synovial fluid hematocrit is fairly low, usually less than 10%.

Increased rates of fibromyalgia have been reported after cervical spine injury (24).

BENIGN HYPERMOBILITY SYNDROME

Generalized joint hypermobility due to ligamentous laxity occurs in about 5% to 12% of the population. The condition is regarded by some as a familial disorder that predisposes the affected individual to articular injuries, leading to chronic or recurrent arthralgia. However, all studies do not show an association between hypermobility and musculoskeletal pain (25). The term *hypermobility syndrome* refers to healthy subjects with joint laxity in the absence of major features of the Marfan or Ehlers–Danlos syndromes, and arthralgias and soft tissue rheumatism (26) for which no other explanation could be found. The syndrome has a marked female preponderance (26). Symptoms first appear in children or young adults (27,28). Hypermobile individuals are often able to hyperextend the knee and elbow beyond 10 degrees, to achieve sufficient lumbar flexion to place both palms on the floor without bending the knees, and to oppose the thumb passively to the flexor aspect of the forearm. Hypermobility may provide an advantage in the performance of certain activities, such as gymnastics, ballet, dancing, and playing musical instruments (29). Lacking the stability afforded by normal ligaments, hypermobile subjects may be more vulnerable to the adverse effects of injury and overuse, including sprains, traumatic synovitis, recurrent dislocations, tendinitis, and temporomandibular joint dysfunction (29,30). An association with mitral valve prolapse has been suggested but not confirmed in a recent study (31). A marfanoid habitus, thin skin (31), and uterine prolapse (32) also may be associated with hypermobility.

REFLEX SYMPATHETIC DYSTROPHY

After trauma to an extremity, severe pain, edema, vasomotor abnormalities, and atrophy of bone, muscle, and skin develop in a few patients (see Chapter 107). Many labels have been applied to this syndrome, depending on the feature of particular interest to the describer: *Sudeck's atrophy, Leriche's posttraumatic osteoporosis, Weir Mitchell's causalgia, algodystrophy,* and *chronic traumatic edema.* The term *causalgia* should probably be reserved for cases in which there has been injury to a major nerve trunk, but the resulting intense burning pain is not confined to the distribution of the nerve and may not differ from that which occurs in reflex dystrophy without nerve injury (33–35). Most patients are adults, but the condition also can occur in children. Another variant, the shoulder–hand syndrome, is usually not related to trauma and is described in detail in Chapter 107.

The antecedent injury may be a fracture, but it is often fairly trivial, such as a sprain or laceration, and it may occur with about equal frequency in an upper or lower extremity (33). Pain, of a quality and degree inappropriate for the injury, may begin immediately or not until several weeks after the trauma. Disinclination to move the extremity also is an early feature that is closely linked to the pain. The limb is painful on motion and may have striking cutaneous hyperalgesia and cold sensitivity. An early hyperemic stage may be noted in some cases, but a cold, moist, cyanotic, edematous hand or foot is more typical after 2 or 3 months. Roentgenograms, usually normal during the first month, later show patchy osteopenia, often periarticular in distribution initially, but diffuse later. Radionuclide bone scans show increased uptake in most adults (36), but normal or reduced uptake is more often characteristic in children. With continued immobility, muscle and skin atrophy occur, and joint motion is lost.

Pathogenesis and management are discussed in Chapter 107. It should be emphasized that early identification of patients and restoration of active motion are the keys to successful treatment. Early treatment with simple, conservative measures, including graded active exercises, heat, and elevation, may produce good results. Long-standing disease, with advanced atrophy of skin, muscle, and bone, may be largely irreversible. To obviate this irreversibility, more aggressive therapies have been proposed, but few have been studied in controlled trials. These measures include oral corticosteroids, sympathetic nerve blocks, transcutaneous nerve stimulation, and regional intravenous injection of corticosteroids, analgesics, or sympatholytic agents (34,35, 37). Most recently, intravenous biphosphonates (38) and gabapentin (39) have been advocated.

Another syndrome characterized by pain and osteopenia has been described as *migratory osteolysis, regional migratory osteoporosis,* and *transient osteoporosis.* The condition was first described during pregnancy, but subsequently has been noticed most often in middle-aged men, who develop a painful swelling in one region of a lower extremity, rarely with preceding trauma (40–42). Either the hip, knee, or foot may be involved. Pain is often severe, especially on motion and weight bearing. Although radiographs may be normal during the first 2 or 3 weeks of symptoms, severe osteoporosis in the painful region is readily apparent thereafter. This condition is unlikely to be related to disuse because uptake of a bone-seeking radioisotope is increased in the affected area during the first week, before immobilization of the extremity. The disorder is self-limited, with resolution of signs and symptoms in several months and eventual return of bone density to normal. Subsequent attacks may occur in other areas but not in previously involved joints. Nothing is known of the pathogenesis of this syndrome, but its resemblance to reflex sympathetic dystrophy has been noted (41,42). In both conditions, bone marrow edema may be an early finding on MRI.

OSTEOCHONDRITIS DISSECANS

This local disorder of subchondral bone is most commonly present in the knees of adolescents and young adults (43). A devitalized fragment of bone, with its articular cartilage still present, demarcates from its original site, usually on the lateral portion of the medial femoral condyle. Partial or complete detachment may occur eventually, with resulting signs and symptoms of a "loose body" in the joint; less frequently, the fragment may lodge in the intercondylar notch and may remain clinically silent.

Antecedent trauma, although common, seems to be only one of several etiologic factors. Anomalous ossification centers, locally deficient blood supply, and genetic factors are particularly important in the younger age group, whereas trauma plays a greater role in adults. The trauma involved may be endogenous, such as repeated contact between an unusually prominent tibial spine or aberrantly situated cruciate ligament and the femoral condyle. Osteochondritis has a different arthroscopic appearance from osteochondral fracture, and only the latter results in hemarthrosis.

The clinical picture in patients with knee involvement consists of mild discomfort rather than pain. This discomfort is aggravated by exercise, but there also may be some aching at rest. With separation of the fragment, the patient may complain of instability or "giving way." Often an unusual stance, due to external rotation of the tibia, may be noted. This stance diminishes contact between the tibial spine and the usual site of osteochondritis on the medial condyle, near the intercondylar notch. A sign that correlates with this may be demonstrated by forcing the tibia into internal rotation while slowly extending the knee from 90 degrees of flexion. At about 30 degrees, the patient complains of pain, which is relieved immediately by external rotation of the tibia.

Roentgenograms may be normal for as long as 6 months after the injury; the typical picture is that of a bony sequestrum lodged in a sharply defined cavity (Fig. 97.3). Recently MRI has been advocated as a useful tool in determining prognosis and assessing the need for surgical intervention. The lesion has a similar appearance when it occurs in other locations, such as the elbow (capitellum), ankle (talus), hip, and metatarsal head. Occasionally multiple sites are involved, particularly in individuals from predisposed families.

Treatment is conservative if the fragment remains in place. Loose fragments may be treated surgically, with either removal or fixation. Osteochondral grafts have been advocated by some surgeons, with variable success. The immediate prognosis is good, but OA may develop in some patients later in life.

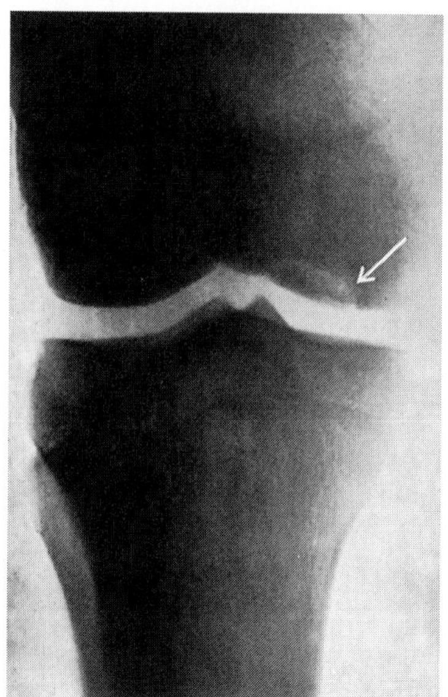

FIGURE 97.3. Osteochondritis dissecans. *Arrow,* Osseous fragment.

Epiphyseal Osteochondroses

Necrosis of an entire epiphysis is a common localized disorder in childhood (44,45). Vascular insufficiency is thought to be the most significant etiologic factor; trauma often is mentioned, but seldom established as a primary cause. Experimental evidence suggests that compression fractures may lead to disorderly epiphyseal ossification characteristic of osteochondroses. In the hip (*Legg–Calvé–Perthes disease*), osteochondroses occurs in younger children (age 2–10 years), usually seen with a limp rather than with pain (44). In the knee (*Osgood–Schlatter disease*) in older children (age 9–15 years) pain and swelling develop in the tibial tubercle; this condition may result from a traction injury. Osteochondritis of the vertebrae (*Scheuermann's disease*) is seen with juvenile kyphosis (45).

TIETZE'S SYNDROME: COSTOCHONDRITIS

Tietze's syndrome is a benign condition in which painful enlargement develops in the upper costal cartilages (46,47). The syndrome occurs with the same frequency in both sexes and on both sides of the chest. Involvement of only a single costal cartilage is found in 80% of patients, the second and third costal cartilages being most often affected. Onset of pain is either acute or insidious, usually without prior injury, with the exception of trauma, which may have occurred during vigorous coughing in a minority of cases. Pain is sometimes severe, is aggravated by motion of the rib cage, and may radiate to the shoulder and arm. Palpation of a firm tender fusiform swelling of the costal cartilage confirms the diagnosis. Biopsy usually shows normal cartilage, occasionally some edema of the perichondrium, and, rarely, nonspecific chronic inflammation in the surrounding tissues. The duration is variable, from a week to several years. Some patients have multiple episodes, but spontaneous remission is the rule. The swelling has been attributed to cartilaginous hypertrophy by some and to abnormal angulation by others, but nothing is known of the pathogenesis. Treatment may include analgesics, heat, local infiltration with corticosteroid (48), intercostal nerve block, and reassurance that symptoms are not due to heart disease.

Other disorders may produce pain, tenderness, or evidence of inflammation in the costochondral joints, but not a hard swelling as in Tietze's syndrome (Table 97.2). The

TABLE 97.2. CAUSES OF COSTOCHONDRAL PAIN

Isolated	Generalized
Tietze's syndrome	Fibromyalgia
Costochondritis	Rheumatoid arthritis
Xiphoidalgia	Seronegative spondyloarthropathies
Slipping rib syndrome	Crystal-induced arthropathies
Bacterial infection	

most common cause of chest wall pain in individuals who do not have a generalized rheumatic disease is an ill-defined condition usually called *costochondritis* or *perichondritis* (49,50). The pain may be severe, radiating widely, but is often worse on the left side. In some cases, it is aggravated by coughing, deep respiration, and motion of the thorax. Anxiety and hyperventilation are common accompaniments. Some episodes are brief and self-limited, but others are chronic, recurrent, and disabling. Tenderness over the costal cartilages, simulating or accentuating the spontaneous pain, is the main physical finding. The xiphoid may be tender in patients with generalized costochondritis, but there is also a syndrome of isolated xiphoidalgia, which may result in epigastric pain suggestive of various intraabdominal disorders. Reproduction of the pain by pressing over the xiphoid is the essential diagnostic maneuver. Little is known of the etiology and pathology of these conditions. In most cases there is no evidence for a traumatic cause, but emotional factors are frequently involved. Care must be taken to rule out coronary artery disease, which may occasionally be associated with chest wall hyperalgesia.

Sudden episodes of sharp pain at the costal margin may be caused by the *slipping rib* or *rib-tip syndrome* (51). This condition is due to hypermobility of the anterior end of a costal cartilage, usually that of the tenth rib, as a result of past trauma. The patients, usually middle-aged of either sex, complain of upper abdominal pain, precipitated by movement and by certain postures. A snapping sensation and point tenderness at the rib tip, relieved by a local anesthetic injection, will confirm the diagnosis.

A rare inflammatory condition, sternoclavicular hyperostosis, also can cause widespread pain, tenderness, and swelling in the anterior chest wall. This can be associated with palmoplantar pustulosis, severe acne, and spondyloarthropathy (52,53).

Painless enlargement of all the costochondral junctions (the acromegalic rosary) is a common clinical sign of previous or current growth hormone excess (54).

OSTEITIS PUBIS

Surgical trauma in the retropubic area may occasionally provoke an inflammatory process in the pubic symphysis and adjacent bone (55). Osteitis pubis may occur after prostate or bladder surgery and, more rarely, after herniorrhaphy or childbirth. Several weeks after surgery, pain develops over the symphysis, radiating down the inner aspects of the thighs, often aggravated by coughing and straining. Physical findings include an antalgic gait, point tenderness over the symphysis, spasm in the abdominal and hip adductor muscle groups, and a low-grade fever. Radiographs may be normal initially, but rarefaction and osteolysis develop around the symphysis within 2 to 4 weeks. A sterile chronic inflammatory process is usually noted on biopsy, but a true osteomyelitis may be discovered in a minority of patients, generally those with more marked bone destruction and fever (56). Tuberculosis and metastatic disease also must be considered in the differential diagnosis. Similar radiographic findings may be observed in ankylosing spondylitis and occasionally in chondrocalcinosis or in other types of polyarthritis, but pain is minimal or absent. Although spontaneous remission may be expected in osteitis pubis, disabling symptoms may persist for many months. The gamut of antiinflammatory drugs has been used with varying success. Other measures, such as immobilization, steroid injections (57), wearing a tight pelvic belt, and surgical debridement have been advocated. The pathogenesis is uncertain, but there is general agreement that one or more factors, in addition to trauma, may contribute.

Traumatic osteitis pubis in athletes, particularly soccer players, may be a result of an avulsion stress fracture at the origin of the gracilis muscle near the symphysis (58). A similar lesion may occur in osteoporotic patients with minimal trauma (59).

SYNOVIAL CYSTS OF THE POPLITEAL SPACE

Six primary bursae are associated with muscles and tendons on the posteromedial aspect of the knee. Communications between two bursae and between a bursa and the knee joint are common. Popliteal cysts may arise in three ways: (a) accumulation of fluid in a noncommunicating bursa; (b) distention of a bursa by fluid originating as a result of a lesion in the knee joint; and (c) posterior herniation of the joint capsule in response to increased intraarticular pressure. The communication between joint and cyst is generally narrow and the anatomy such that a flap-valve mechanism may be operative, allowing free passage of fluid from knee to cyst, but not in the opposite direction (60).

Popliteal cysts may be seen at all ages. Those in children are usually unassociated with joint disease and are often bilateral (61). Many disappear spontaneously. In most adult cases, some abnormality is evident in the knee joint, including OA, RA, internal derangements (62), and a variety of other conditions, and a connection between the cyst and joint can be demonstrated with arthrography. The cyst itself usually causes only mild discomfort; other symptoms may be related to the associated joint lesions. A fluctuant swelling is present in the popliteal area, occasionally extending well into the calf and seen superficially at the medial border of the gastrocnemius. The differential diagnosis, which includes aneurysms, benign neoplasms, abscesses, varicosities, and thrombophlebitis, is greatly facilitated by modern imaging techniques (61,63). The histopathologic characteristics of the cysts are varied and do not particularly correspond to the presumed origin, bursal or hernial. Most have a thin fibrous wall, lined by a single layer of flat cells. Others have structural characteristics of a synovial membrane, particularly those occurring in patients with RA. A few have a thickened, inflamed wall coated with fibrin, but no villus formation.

Definitive treatment is essentially surgical. In some cases, correction of knee joint pathology (such as synovectomy in a patient with RA) may result in spontaneous disappearance. Aspiration of the cyst and corticosteroid injections are often palliative.

A sudden increase of pressure within the popliteal cyst may result in rupture (64). The clinical picture simulates acute deep venous thrombosis, with calf swelling and tenderness, a positive Homans' sign, and pedal edema. Within a few days, a crescent-shaped ecchymosis may appear below one or both malleoli. A knee effusion or popliteal swelling present before the rupture may be less prominent or undetectable after the onset of acute calf pain. A popliteal cyst may still be demonstrable by sonography, but the rupture is best seen with arthrography or MRI. Imaging studies to rule out deep venous thrombosis also should be considered; in some patients, this may occur simultaneous with popliteal cyst rupture (64).

Synovial cysts in RA are seen in many other joints. Occasionally, a communicating cyst of traumatic or nonspecific origin may be seen elsewhere. For instance, a cyst connecting with the hip joint may be seen anteriorly as a mass in the groin or posteriorly with sciatic pain.

GANGLION

A ganglion is a cystic swelling that may be found near, and often attached to, a tendon sheath or joint capsule, and is believed to be derived from these structures (65). The cystic nature of the swelling is usually evident on physical examination, but some are firm; in these instances, a solid lesion may be ruled out by transillumination or ultrasonography (66). A slender connection may be demonstrated histologically and radiographically (67). The thick mucoid material within the ganglion contains hyaluronic acid, although no true synovial membrane lines the cavity. The most common location is on the dorsum of the wrist (Fig. 97.4), but ganglia also are frequently noted on the volar aspect of the wrist, the fingers, and the dorsum of the foot. Ganglia of the flexor tendon sheaths, at the base of the fingers, are common in typists. Ganglia are less common in the lower extremity, and most are in the foot and ankle (68). In most instances, there has been no definite relation to trauma. Small ganglia are more likely to be painful than are larger ones, probably because they are in the process of expanding. Most patients have few symptoms other than unsightly swelling and slight discomfort on motion.

Ganglia frequently disappear spontaneously (69). Treatment is not necessarily required, but is often demanded by the patient for cosmetic reasons. Most cases may be treated successfully with multiple punctures of the cyst wall with a large-bore needle and aspiration of the contents (70). If the ganglion recurs after this procedure, surgical excision may be performed.

TENOSYNOVITIS AND STENOSING TENOSYNOVITIS

Tenosynovitis is an inflammation of the cellular lining membrane of the fibrous tube through which a tendon moves. It may be produced by various diseases (e.g., RA, gout, gonococcal arthritis), but even more commonly by trauma. Such trauma may occur from a direct blow, from abnormal pressure on a tendon (such as from the stiff counter of a new shoe on the Achilles tendon) or, most often, from unusual activity involving a certain muscle–tendon unit. In industrial settings, the wrist and thumb extensors are frequently involved, often related to a new type of repetitive work or to resumption of work after vacation. The condition is identified by tenderness, swelling, and palpable crepitus over the tendon as it is moved (peritendinitis crepitans). Remission usually occurs if the affected part is rested for a few days.

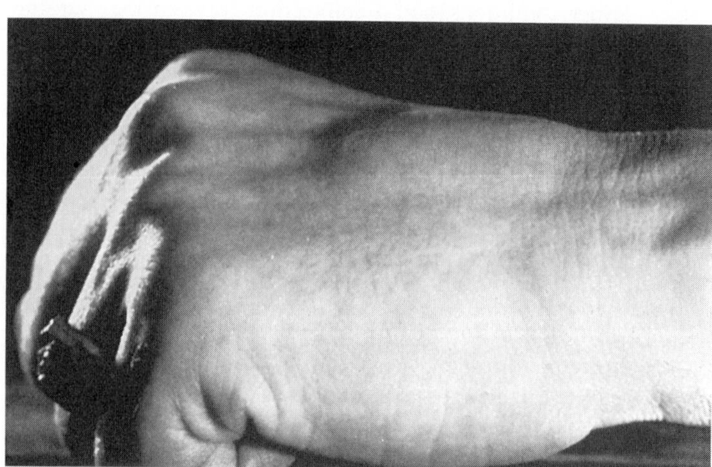

FIGURE 97.4. Ganglion arising from extensor tendon sheaths. An oval and flattened cystic mass is on the dorsum of the hand.

Stenosing tenosynovitis is primarily a disorder of the fibrous wall of the tendon sheath, particularly at locations where the tendon passes through a fibrous ring or pulley. Generally, an osseous groove is part of the ring, which is completed by a thickening of the tendon sheath. Such arrangements are found over bony prominences, such as the radial styloid and the flexor surfaces of the metacarpal and metatarsal heads. With prolonged mechanical stress from either tendon motion under an excessive load or external pressure, such as from the handles of pruning shears, abnormal proliferation of fibrous tissue in the ring constricts the lumen of the tendon sheath. Secondary degenerative changes may then occur in the tendon, usually with enlargement near the constriction ("tendinosis"). There may be a snapping sensation with movement of the enlarged segment of tendon through the narrowed ring ("trigger finger" and "snapping thumb"). Further progression may produce locking in flexion; the tendon may be pulled through the constriction by its own flexor muscle but not by its weaker extensor antagonist. When extension is forced, the bulbous portion suddenly pops back through the constriction, and the digit "unlocks." Tenosynovitis due to mechanical stress also may contribute to pain and loss of motion.

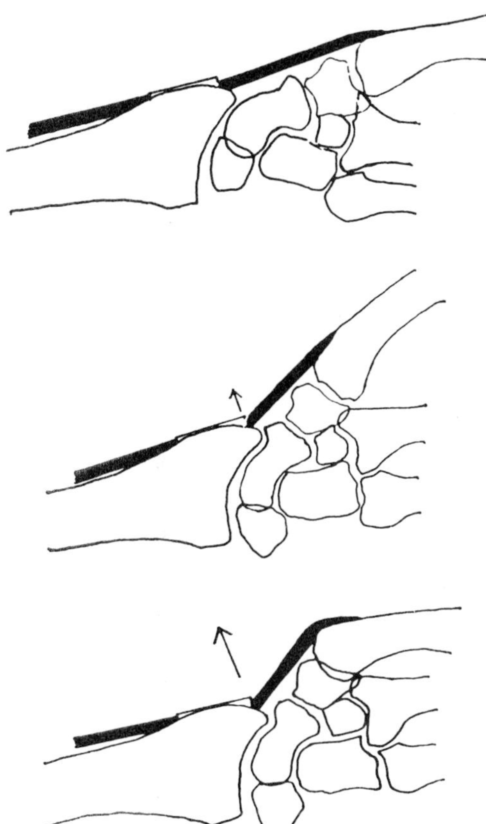

FIGURE 97.5. Top: Wrist and thumb in neutral position, tendons relaxed. **Center:** Radial deviation of wrist and thumb relaxed, minor tearing stress applied to retinaculum. **Bottom:** Radial deviation of wrist while gripping, strong tearing stress applied to retinaculum. (Reproduced with permission from Muckart RD. Stenosing tendovaginitis of abductor pollicis longus and extensor pollicis brevis at the radial styloid (de Quervain's disease). *Clin Orthop* 1964;33:201–207.)

Stenosing tenosynovitis of the abductor pollicis longus and extensor pollicis brevis at the radial styloid is known as *de Quervain's disease* (71). It is a common disorder among individuals who perform repetitive manual tasks involving grasping with the thumb accompanied by movement of the hand in a radial direction (Fig. 97.5). Occurrence during pregnancy, followed by spontaneous resolution, also has been reported (72). Symptoms include pain in the area of the radial styloid and weakness of grip. Examination reveals tenderness and thickening over the involved tendons and limited excursion of the thumb; locking and snapping seldom occur. The classic test is the demonstration of *Finkelstein's sign*. The thumb is placed in the palm of the hand and grasped by the fingers; ulnar deviation of the wrist elicits a sharp pain if inflammation of the tendon sheath is present.

The most common locations for stenosing tenosynovitis are the thumb flexor and extensor tendons and the finger flexors, but occasionally other sites are involved (73). These sites include the flexor carpi radialis tendon, resulting in pain at the base of the thenar eminence, the common peroneal sheath, causing pain on the lateral aspect of the ankle, and the tibialis posterior tendon, with pain below and behind the medial malleolus after prolonged standing and walking.

Treatment of Stenosing Tenosynovitis

Conservative measures such as (a) cessation of the repetitive activity thought to have provoked the condition, (b) immobilization with splints, and (c) local corticosteroid injections usually result in improvement (74), but recurrences are common. Tenosynovitis may subside, but the area of fibrous constriction is unlikely to be greatly altered by this approach, particularly when the duration of symptoms exceeds 4 months. It is sometimes necessary to resort to surgical excision of this portion of the sheath (75). In all the locations, the operation is simple and results in permanent remission, even allowing resumption of full activity in most cases. Trigger finger and snapping thumb may be treated successfully without surgery, with resolution of symptoms in nearly 90% of cases after one or two local corticosteroid injections (76).

Carpal and Tarsal Tunnel Syndromes

Tenosynovitis in the flexor compartment of the wrist, where the tendons are enclosed in a bony canal, roofed by a rigid transverse carpal ligament, may result in compression and degeneration of the median nerve that shares this space.

An entrapment neuropathy of the posterior tibial nerve behind and below the medial malleolus may be caused by tenosynovitis of the tendons that accompany the nerve through an osseofibrous tunnel. These and other nerve-entrapment syndromes are described in Chapter 105.

OTHER FORMS OF TENDINITIS AND BURSITIS

Painful conditions attributed to strain or injury of tendons and their attachments to bone are often loosely described by the term *tendinitis.* The supraspinatus and bicipital tendons of the shoulder, which are commonly affected, are discussed in Chapter 107. Frequently tendinitis is related to a particular occupation or sport. For instance, baseball pitchers, at the end of their delivery, stretch the attachment of the long head of the triceps to the inferior glenoid rim. This movement results in pain in the posterior axillary fold. It is presumed that inflammatory changes occur in the tendon attachment. A similar condition also may develop in baseball pitchers and golfers at the medial epicondyle of the elbow. Jumper's knee refers to tendinitis of the patellar tendon, at its attachment to the lower pole of the patella (77), or the quadriceps attachment to the upper pole (78). Semimembranosus tendinitis can cause posteromedial knee pain aggravated by weight-bearing exercise (79).

TENNIS ELBOW (EPICONDYLITIS)

This is a common condition, most often found in middle-aged persons of either sex, in which pain derives from the origin of the wrist and finger extensors at the lateral epicondyle. Although first described in tennis players, most cases are not related to that sport, but may be provoked by any exercise or occupation that involves repeated and forcible wrist extension or pronation–supination. The right elbow is involved more often than the left; the condition is seldom bilateral. Pain is usually gradual in onset, but is sometimes related to a specific traumatic incident. It often radiates to the forearm and dorsum of the hand. Physical examination reveals point tenderness at or near the lateral epicondyle, with little or no swelling. Elbow joint motion is unrestricted and painless, but resisted wrist extension results in accentuation of pain. Many possibilities have been suggested for its pathogenesis (80), including tendon rupture, radiohumeral synovitis, periostitis, neuritis, aseptic necrosis, and displacement of the orbicular ligament. The majority of cases are believed to be due to an injury to the common extensor tendon at or near its attachment to the lateral epicondyle. Specimens for histologic study are obtained only in chronic cases and show evidence of a failed healing process, leading to vascular and fibroblastic hyperplasia, and abnormal collagen production (80,81).

Management should be directed toward modifying the provocative activity. Many treatments have been proposed, including massage, ultrasonography, and other physical modalities, antiinflammatory drugs, wrist splinting in extension, and several surgical procedures (82–84). The most common approach, local corticosteroid injection, is usually successful (85). An attempted meta-analysis of 18 controlled trials of various therapies came to no conclusions favoring any single treatment (86).

BURSITIS

Bursae are closed sacs, lined with a cellular membrane resembling synovium (87). They serve to facilitate motion of tendons and muscles over bony prominences. There are over 80 bursae on each side of the body. Many are nameless, and additional ones may form at almost any point subjected to frequent irritation. Excessive frictional forces or, at times, direct trauma may result in an inflammatory process in the bursal wall, with excessive vascularity, exudation of increased amounts of viscous bursal fluid, and fibrin coating of the lining membrane. Only small numbers of inflammatory cells are found in bursal fluid in traumatic bursitis, but there may be a greater leukocyte response in bursitis secondary to other rheumatic diseases, such as RA or gout. Septic bursitis is usually caused by organisms introduced through punctures, wounds, or cellulitis in the overlying skin. Traumatic bursitis may be complicated by infection or hemorrhage (88). "Beat knee" and "beat shoulder" in miners are examples of this condition. Continuous abrasion of the skin with stone dust results in cellulitis, and repeated scraping of the bursa against rough stone surfaces leads to hemorrhage. After modification of occupations and habits, many of the classic forms of bursitis are encountered less frequently (e.g., "housemaid's knee," "weaver's bottom," and "policeman's heel"). Sports-related bursitis (e.g., "wrestler's knee," a prepatellar bursitis found in 10% of college wrestlers) is receiving greater emphasis (89).

Subdeltoid bursitis, which is described in detail in Chapter 107, is a very common bursitis. The following other types also are frequently seen.

TROCHANTERIC BURSITIS

Trochanteric bursitis is an inflammation of one or more of the bursae about the gluteal insertion on the femoral trochanter. This condition is most common in female patients and usually has insidious onset, preceded by apparent trauma in only about one fourth of the cases (90,91). Aching pain on the lateral aspect of the hip and thigh is aggravated by lying on the affected side. The patient experiences tenderness posterior to the trochanter, and pain with external rotation of the hip and with active abduction against resistance, but not with flexion and extension. Lumbar radiculopathy and entrapment of the lateral femoral cutaneous nerve must be considered in the differential diagnosis (92).

OLECRANON BURSITIS

An inflammation with effusion at the point of the elbow occurs frequently with RA and gout, as well as after trauma (93). Pain is usually minimal, except when pressure is applied to the swollen bursa. Elbow motion is unimpaired and usually painless. Fluid from the bursa is often serosanguineous with a low leukocyte concentration, consisting mainly of monocytes and T lymphocytes (94). Septic bursitis here is common and must be suspected even when cell counts are only moderately elevated. A controlled study has shown improved outcomes with an intrabursal steroid injection compared with naproxen or placebo (95). However, the swelling often subsides if additional trauma is prevented with a sponge ring.

ACHILLES BURSITIS

In this condition, an inflammation of the retrocalcaneal bursa occurs just above and anterior to the attachment of the Achilles tendon to the os calcis. However, most heel pain is related to a disorder of the Achilles tendon or plantar fascia (96) (see Chapter 99).

BUNION

A painful bursitis occurs over the medial surface of the first metatarsophalangeal joint, usually with a hallux valgus (see Chapter 99).

ISCHIAL BURSITIS

An inflammation of the bursa separating the gluteus maximus from the underlying ischial tuberosity is usually produced by prolonged sitting on hard surfaces ("weaver's bottom"). Weight loss, with reduction of protective padding in the buttock, also may be an etiologic factor (97). Buttock pain radiates down the posterior leg and may be aggravated by rectal examination.

PREPATELLAR BURSITIS

This type of bursitis is a swelling between the skin and lower patella or patellar tendon, resulting from frequent kneeling. Pain is usually slight unless there is direct pressure on the swollen area (Fig. 97.6).

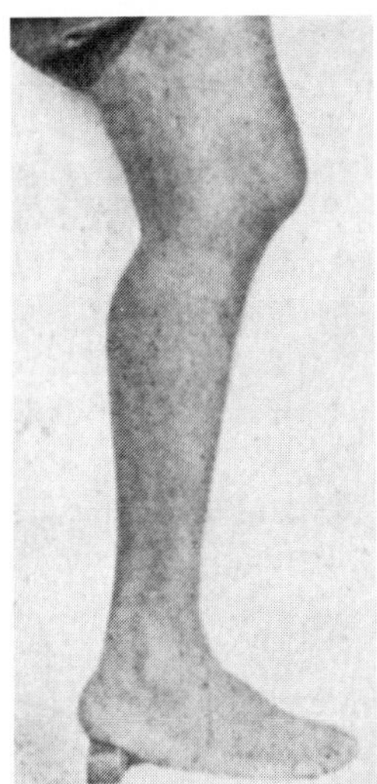

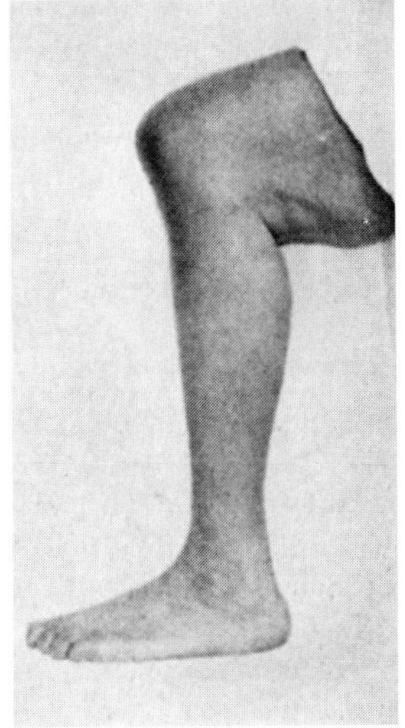

FIGURE 97.6. Bilateral prepatellar bursitis (housemaid's knee). (From Lewin P. *Orthopedic surgery for nurses.* Philadelphia: WB Saunders, 1947, with permission.)

ANSERINE BURSITIS

This inflammation of the sartorius bursa on the medial aspect of the knee about 4 cm below the joint line is seen most often in overweight women. Diabetes also may be a risk factor (98). The characteristic complaint is pain with stair climbing. In one series of bursitis in various locations, anserine bursitis was found to be the most common (90). Inflammation in another, nameless bursa located at the anterior edge of the medial collateral ligament also gives pain on the inner aspect of the knee, but with point tenderness in a different area.

ILIOPECTINEAL OR ILIOPSOAS BURSITIS

With this inflammation of a bursa between the iliopsoas and inguinal ligament, the patient complains of groin pain radiating to the knee, and often adopts a shortened stride to prevent hyperextension of the hip while walking (99). Examination reveals tenderness just below the inguinal ligament, lateral to the femoral pulse, and pain on hyperextension of the hip. Iliopsoas bursitis can also be a secondary manifestation of RA or OA of the hip, with an inguinal mass and leg swelling (99).

OBTURATOR INTERNUS BURSITIS

This may result in low back pain (100). There is local buttock tenderness just below the posterior inferior iliac spine; pain is reproduced by straight leg raising with maximal adduction and internal rotation.

Treatment

In general, therapy includes protection from irritation and trauma, either by modifying the patient's activities or by using appropriate padding. Antiinflammatory drugs, heat, and ultrasound also are commonly used. Local corticosteroid injections are usually successful, but there are occasional local complications such as infection and skin atrophy, particularly with olecranon bursitis (93). Surgical excision is reserved for refractory cases.

CALCIFIC TENDINITIS AND PERIARTHRITIS

Some cases of tendinitis and bursitis are associated with calcific deposits, most commonly with subdeltoid bursitis and trochanteric bursitis, but occasionally with tendinitis, bursitis, or periarthritis around the wrist, knee, or elbow (101). In these instances, the attacks are less likely to be preceded by recognized trauma. The attacks tend to be abrupt in onset, with intense local inflammatory signs resembling an attack of gout. These episodes, which may be examples of crystal-induced inflammation, are described further in Chapter 118.

INJURIES TO MUSCLES AND TENDONS

Rupture of tendons or muscles may occur during vigorous effort, accompanied by a sharp pain and a snapping sensation. After this, certain movements may be difficult to perform; before ecchymosis and swelling occur, a defect in the belly of the muscle may be apparent. Local anesthetic injection reduces pain and permits testing of muscular function. When diagnosis is difficult, soft tissue imaging may be useful (102,103). The supraspinatus muscle or tendon is the most likely to be torn in the upper extremity. The calf muscles, hamstrings, and the quadriceps are the most vulnerable in the lower extremity.

Because of their great tensile strength, rupture seldom occurs in the tendons, but rather at the muscle–tendon junction or at the bony insertion. Attrition of the musculotendinous cuff, secondary to local trauma by pulley systems and bony prominences, may lead to necrobiotic changes that predispose to rupture. Trauma is the immediate and direct cause of rupture; sudden application of a stretching force on a strongly contracting muscle results in tearing of muscle fibers, followed by hemorrhage, edema, and localized spasm (muscle strain) (103). In some cases, the primary mechanism is extreme passive stretching of a tendon attachment, such as the avulsion of the abductor insertion in the groin in a water skier falling with widely abducted hips. Muscle fatigue results in incomplete relaxation and predisposes to stretch injuries. Therefore, these injuries are more likely to occur in poorly conditioned athletes.

Tendon rupture, common in RA, is caused by the lytic effect of tenosynovial inflammation and, in addition, mechanical abrasion of tendons due to disruption of the contiguous bone. Injection of corticosteroids for tendinitis also has been said to predispose to tendon rupture, especially in the Achilles tendon.

Tears in the supraspinatus tendon occur in older individuals. It is presumed that attrition and trauma both contribute to the rupture (see Chapter 107).

Rupture of the long head of the biceps may be the final result of chronic frictional attrition of the tendon within the bicipital groove (see Chapter 107). The rupture may be accompanied by transient pain over the anterior aspect of the shoulder. The belly of the muscle assumes a spherical shape and lies closer to the elbow than normal. Surgical repair is often possible, but not mandatory, because disability is generally mild.

The greater or lesser rhomboid muscles may be strained by a sudden uncoordinated movement of the shoulder. This injury occurs frequently in industrial practice. These muscles arise from the ligamentum nuchae and the spinous processes of the seventh cervical through the fifth thoracic vertebrae, and they insert into the vertebral border of the scapula. Contraction of these muscles draws this border of the scapula upward.

After injury to the rhomboid muscles, there is a localized tenderness between the middorsal spine and the scapula. Pain occurs at this point if the shoulder is passively flexed forward or if it is extended against resistance. Other muscles arising from the spinous processes and inserting on the scapula or humerus include the levator scapulae, latissimus dorsi, and trapezius muscles. Strains of these muscles give a clinical picture somewhat similar to that for injury to the rhomboids.

Rupture of the pectoralis major muscle may occur in weight lifters during bench pressing (104), or may be caused by an abrupt traction injury, with sudden sharp pain in the shoulder and a snapping sensation. A tender mass is felt in the muscle, and there is ecchymosis of the overlying skin. Evacuation of the hematoma and surgical repair are the treatments of choice.

Rupture of the rectus abdominis muscle may at times be mistaken for intraperitoneal disease (such as appendicitis). Rupture of this muscle may occur after a severe bout of coughing or sneezing, during pregnancy or labor, or after influenza or typhoid fever (with degeneration of the muscle fibers). A large hematoma may form as a result of tears of branches of the epigastric vessels. The hematoma may require evacuation surgically.

Rupture of the quadriceps muscle or tendon is relatively common. This injury occurs at the point of attachment of the tendon to the patella or at the musculotendinous junction; occasionally, a tear may occur through the purely tendinous or muscular portions. The usual cause of this condition is a violent contraction of the muscle, such as falling on a flexed knee. The patient is unable to extend the knee actively, and a hiatus is seen in the tendon or muscle.

When the patellar tendon is ruptured, the patella lies higher than usual, a gap is noted, active knee extension is lost, and joint effusion is usually present. A roentgenogram will confirm the diagnosis.

Partial rupture of one of the calf muscles, termed *tennis leg,* usually involves a belly of the gastrocnemius muscle. Symptoms include a snap with sudden burning pain in the calf during a strong muscular contraction. The pain may extend to the popliteal space; it is aggravated by passive dorsiflexion of the ankle and may be confused with thrombophlebitis (105). Conservative treatment includes immobilization of the ankle in plantar flexion for several weeks, followed by heat, massage, and exercises.

Spontaneous rupture of the posterior tibial tendon results in pain, tenderness, and swelling behind and below the medial malleolus with loss of stability of the foot (106). Weakness of plantar flexion may be demonstrated by observing the patient's unsuccessful attempt at raising the heel of the involved foot, while the uninvolved foot is off the ground. This injury is usually preceded by chronic symptoms suggestive of tenosynovitis and is often associated with planovalgus feet. Treatment is either surgical repair, in cases diagnosed early, or an orthotic device.

Injury to the Achilles tendon may occur in runners or in middle-aged men unaccustomed to exertion who indulge in weekend athletics involving jumping (such as basketball and volleyball). There may be rupture at the musculotendinous junction or avulsion at the attachment to the calcaneus. Examination reveals a depression over the tendon and inability to flex the ankle against resistance. In partial rupture, the pain may be mild. Swelling and ecchymosis may conceal the depression usually noted with complete tears. Partial rupture may be treated conservatively with immobilization of the foot in plantar flexion; complete tears usually require surgical intervention (96). Sonography has been suggested as an inexpensive imaging technique that differentiates between conditions requiring surgery and those that will respond to conservative therapy (107). MRI allows more precise preoperative assessment (108). Prior local corticosteroid injections (109) and treatment with fluoroquinolone antibiotics (110) may play an etiologic role in some cases.

The *anterior tibial compartment syndrome* is an ischemic necrosis of muscle caused by swelling after unaccustomed exercise. The muscles in this compartment are confined by a tight fascial sheath, resulting in a compromised blood supply when swelling occurs. Examination shows a marked weakness of the involved muscle and local swelling and erythema. Sensation in the first two toes is often lost because of compression of the deep peroneal nerve. Immediate fasciotomy must be performed to prevent irreversible destruction of the muscle. Less frequently, similar problems may arise from high pressure in other muscle compartments of the lower leg and thigh.

FIBROTIC INDURATION AND CONTRACTURE OWING TO REPEATED INTRAMUSCULAR INJECTIONS

Certain drugs may cause local destruction of muscle tissue at injection sites, leading to fibrosis and contracture. Self-administration of pentazocine (Talwin) by patients with chronic pain has resulted in the most striking examples of this condition (111). The characteristic features are woody induration of the quadriceps, deltoids, and other muscles, needle marks and ulcerations in the overlying skin, and marked muscle shortening.

RUNNING INJURIES

The extraordinary popularity of running has engendered special interest in associated injuries and increased awareness of biomechanical aspects, including running techniques, conditioning, and equipment. These activities are often centered in special runners' clinics, in which the therapeutic goals may differ from those of conventional medicine. Emphasis is placed on continued participation and enhanced performance, in addition to the traditional aims of symptomatic relief and prevention of permanent tissue damage. The spectrum of running injuries encompasses virtually all the categories of musculoskeletal trauma (Table 97.3). About one third of running injuries involve the knee; heel pain is next in frequency. Certain preexisting conditions may predispose the runner to injury. For instance, a high-arched foot (pes cavus) does not pronate sufficiently to absorb shock during running, leading to Achilles tendinitis or plantar fasciitis. Running on a hyperpronated or flat foot may result in lateral ankle pain. Incongruity, faulty tracking, or laxity in the patellofemoral joint may predispose to patellar pain or chondromalacia. Recrudescent symptoms from virtually any previous articular derangement may develop when the individual begins to run regularly. Ill-fitting or poorly constructed footwear, hard or irregular running surfaces, poor running posture or technique, and inadequate warm-up or tendon stretching also increase the likelihood of injury. Detailed discussion of these matters is available elsewhere (112–114).

Stress fractures, also called fatigue fractures, are partial, cortical fractures related to prolonged, repetitive mechanical loading. A complete fracture may eventually result if the activity is continued. The presenting symptom is pain, which is generally aggravated by weight bearing and relieved by rest. In some areas, such as the tibia and fibula,

TABLE 97.3. COMMON DISORDERS IN RUNNERS

Disorder	Sites of Involvement
Stress fracture	Tibia, fibula, metatarsus, femur
Compartmental syndromes	
Sprains	
Bursitis	Retrocalcaneus, anserine, ischium, trochanter
Fasciitis	Plantar area, iliotibial band
Tendinitis	Achilles, anterior and posterior tibial, peroneal, quadriceps, patella
Tendon and muscle rupture	Achilles, hamstrings
Intraarticular disorders	Chondromalacia, meniscal tears, plica, "overuse" synovitis, ostearthritis
Cervical and lumbar disc degeneration	

tenderness, warmth, and swelling may occur over the fracture. The diagnosis is usually made radiographically, but typical findings of a linear cortical radiolucency or a localized area of periosteal new bone formation may not be present during the first week or two of symptoms. Therefore negative radiographs should be repeated if a stress fracture is strongly suspected. A bone scan or MRI demonstrates the stress fracture site at this early stage (112), but these expensive procedures are seldom justified in typical cases. The treatment of stress fractures depends on their location and severity. If the fibula is involved, continuation of running at a reduced level may be possible. At the other extreme, femoral fractures occasionally require surgical intervention.

Knee problems represent about one third of running injuries. They most frequently involve tracking abnormalities of the patella, often in relation to underlying anatomic and biomechanical factors (see Chapter 98). Internal derangements are seldom caused by running, but in patients with preexisting, asymptomatic lesions, pain and swelling are likely to develop under the stress of running. "*Overuse*" *synovitis* in the apparent absence of intra-articular pathology is noted occasionally with rapid increases in mileage. This condition should be managed with temporary cessation until the effusion resolves, with gradual resumption of the running program later. Lateral knee pain may result from the iliotibial band friction syndrome. A thick strip of fascia lata, which inserts into the lateral tibial condyle, may impinge on the femoral condyle during repeated flexion and extension of the knee, particularly in individuals with tibia vara and hyperpronated feet.

Heel pain, the second most frequent complaint among runners, results from various conditions that can usually be distinguished by physical examination and radiographs. These conditions include plantar fasciitis, calcaneal bursitis, Achilles tendinitis or rupture, and calcaneal stress fractures. Treatment includes instruction in running technique to avoid excessive heel strike, heel pads and orthotic devices, stretching exercises, temporary cessation or reduction in running, and antiinflammatory drugs.

Degenerative arthritis and disc disease may produce pain and limited activity among older runners, but there is little evidence that running causes OA in previously normal hips and knees (114). Substitution of an alternative exercise program with less impact loading, such as swimming or walking, may be recommended in such cases.

REPETITION STRAIN INJURY

Vague regional symptoms that are difficult to ascribe to a specific musculoskeletal injury may be encountered in patients whose occupations require fixed positions and repetitive movements, such as musicians (115), assembly-line workers, or accounting machine and computer operators (116). The complaints include muscular fatigue, stiffness and aching, weakness, paresthesia, and incoordination. Mental stress, various environmental factors, and adverse working conditions may influence the symptoms. Multiple pathogenetic factors may be involved, including muscle fatigue, tenosynovitis, nerve entrapments, compartment syndromes, synovitis, ligamentous strain, and referred pain from the cervical spine (117,118). Treatment usually depends on careful analysis and modification of performing techniques and may include rest, antiinflammatory drugs, and local injections.

RADIATION ARTHROPATHY AFTER NONMECHANICAL TRAUMA

Because articular cartilage is relatively radioresistant, the effects of radiation on joints are usually secondary to destruction of osteoblasts. Vascular damage (endarteritis) also may contribute to osteonecrosis. Because the field of radiotherapy is more likely to include the axial skeleton than the extremities, radiation arthropathy is usually seen in the hips, shoulder, spine, and sacroiliac and temporomandibular joints. Radiation changes are dose related; the threshold is 3,000 rads, with cell death occurring at 5,000 rads. Their occurrence depends not only on dosage, but on age, various technical factors, and superimposed trauma or infection. The time of onset of clinical manifestations is generally greater than 1 year, and is often several years after irradiation. Adults may have aseptic necrosis, fracture, or protrusio acetabuli (119,120). In children, slipped capital femoral epiphysis and scoliosis or kyphosis resulting from injury to the epiphyseal plates may develop, leading subsequently to wedge deformities of the vertebral bodies.

Changes resembling degenerative arthritis are occasionally found only in joints that had been included in the field of radiation many years previously. Radiographic findings include narrowing of the joint space, marginal new bone formation, and periarticular osteoporosis. Occasionally chondrocalcinosis and ankylosis may occur. A few examples of "rheumatoid-like" arthritis with soft tissue swelling have been noted. The spine may be involved, showing narrowing and calcification of intervertebral discs.

Irradiation of the rib cage may result in osteochondritis, with pain and swelling in the costal cartilages. These symptoms may suggest cancer or Tietze's syndrome, but, in contrast to these conditions, erythema exists in the tender area. High-dose ultrasound and diathermy have been reported to cause exacerbations of synovitis in RA.

FROSTBITE ARTHROPATHY

Frostbite injury to the distal extremities may occasionally involve the joints in addition to overlying soft tissues. Skeletal changes are not apparent until several months after frostbite, and include demineralization, juxtaarticular cysts, and joint-space narrowing. The late development of osteophytes results in a clinical picture closely resembling that of OA, with Heberden's and Bouchard's nodes (121). In children, destruction of the phalangeal epiphyses may lead to premature closure and digital growth impairment (122). These changes may be the result of direct chondrocyte injury during cold exposure.

REFERENCES

1. Weber JE, Jackson RE, Peacock WF, et al. Clinical decision rules discriminate between fractures and nonfractures in acute isolated knee trauma. *Ann Emerg Med* 1995;26:429–433.
2. Casteleyn PP, Handelberg F, Opdecam P. Traumatic haemarthrosis of the knee. *J Bone Joint Surg Br* 1988;70:404–406.
3. Maffulli N, Binfield PM, King JB, et al. Acute haemarthrosis of the knee in athletes. *J Bone Joint Surg Br* 1993;75:945–949.
4. Adalberth T, Roos H, Lauren M, et al. Magnetic resonance imaging, scintigraphy, and arthroscopic evaluation of traumatic hemarthrosis of the knee. *Am J Sports Med* 1997;25:231–237.
5. Berk RN. Liquid fat in the knee joint after trauma. *N Engl J Med* 1967;277:1411–1412.
6. Egund N, Nilsson CT, Wingstrand H, et al. CT scans and lipohaemarthrosis in hip fractures. *J Bone Joint Surg Br* 1990;72:379–382.
7. Reginato AJ, Feldman E, Rabinowitz JL. Traumatic chylous knee effusion. *Ann Rheum Dis* 1985;44:793–797.
8. White RE, Wise CM, Agudelo CA. Post-traumatic chylous joint effusion. *Arthritis Rheum* 1985;28:1303–1306.
9. Lindblad S, Wredmark T. Traumatic synovitis analysed by arthroscopy and immunohistopathology. *Br J Rheumatol* 1990;29:422–425.
10. Graham J, Goldman JA. Fat droplets and synovial fluid leukocytosis in traumatic arthritis. *Arthritis Rheum* 1978;21:76–80.
11. Weinberger A, Schumacher HR. Experimental joint trauma: synovial response to blunt trauma and inflammatory reaction to intra-articular injection of fat. *J Rheumatol* 1981;8:380–389.
12. Liu SH, Nguyen TM. Ankle sprains and other soft tissue injuries. *Curr Opin Rheumatol* 1999;11:132–137.
13. Klenerman L. The management of sprained ankle. *J Bone Joint Surg Br* 1998;80:11–12.
14. Harrington KD. Degenerative arthritis of the ankle secondary to longstanding lateral ligament instability. *J Bone Joint Surg Am* 1979;61:354–361.
15. Nilsson OS, Persson P-E. Heterotopic bone formation after joint replacement. *Curr Opin Rheumatol* 1999;11:127–131.
16. Knelles D. Prevention of heterotopic ossification after total hip replacement. *J Bone Joint Surg Br* 1997;79:596–602.
17. Rush PJ. The rheumatic manifestations of traumatic spinal cord injury. *Semin Arthritis Rheum* 1989;19:77–89.
18. Goodman TA, Merkel PA, Perlmutter G, et al. Heterotopic ossification in the setting of neuromuscular blockade. *Arthritis Rheum* 1997;40:1619–1627.
19. Yue CC, Regier A, Kushner I. Heterotopic ossification presenting as arthritis. *J Rheumatol* 1985;12:769–772.
20. Wright V. Post-traumatic osteoarthritis: a medicolegal minefield. *Br J Rheumatol* 1990;29:4744–4478.
21. Lohmander LS, Hoerrner LA, Dahlberg L, et al. Stromelysin, tissue inhibitor of metalloproteinases and proteoglycan fragments in human knee joint fluid after injury. *J Rheumatol* 1993;20:1362–1368.
22. Lohmander LS, Saxne T, Heinegard DK. Release of cartilage oligomeric matrix protein (COMP) into joint fluid after knee injury and in osteoarthritis. *Ann Rheum Dis* 1994;53:8–13.
23. Sandorfi N, Freundlich B. Psoriatic and seronegative inflammatory arthropathy associated with a traumatic onset: 4 cases and a review of the literature. *J Rheumatol* 1997;24:187–192.
24. Buskila D, Neumann L, Vaisberg G, et al. Increased rates of fibromyalgia following cervical spine injury: a controlled study of 161 cases of traumatic injury. *Arthritis Rheum* 1997;40:446–452.
25. Mikkelson M, Salminen JJ, Kautianen H. Joint hypermobility is not a contributing factor to musculoskeletal pain in pre-adolescents. *J Rheumatol* 1996;23:1963–1967.
26. Hudson N, Starr MR, Esdaile JM, et al.. Diagnostic associations with hypermobility in rheumatology patients. *Br J Rheumatol* 1995;34:1157–1161.
27. Gedalia A, Press J. Articular symptoms in hypermobile school children: a prospective study. *J Pediatr* 1991;119:944–946.
28. Arroyo IL, Brewer EJ, Giannini EH. Arthritis/arthralgia and hypermobility of the joints in schoolchildren. *J Rheumatol* 1988;15:978–980.
29. Larsson L-G, Baum J, Mudholkar GS, et al. Benefits and disadvantages of joint hypermobility among musicians. *N Engl J Med* 1993;329:1079–1082.
30. Harinstein D, Buckingham RB, Braun T, et al. Systemic joint laxity (the hypermobile joint syndrome) is associated with temporomandibular joint dysfunction. *Arthritis Rheum* 1988;31:1259–1264.
31. Mishra MB, Ryan P, Atkinson P, et al. Extra-articular features of benign joint hypermobility syndrome. *Br J Rheumatol* 1996;35:861–866.
32. Norton PA, Baker JE, Sharp HC, et al. Genitourinary prolapse and joint hypermobility in women. *Obstet Gynecol* 1995;85:225–228.
33. Bickerstaff DR, Kanes JA. Algodystrophy: an under-recognized complication of minor trauma. *Br J Rheumatol* 1994;33:240–248.
34. Chard MD. Diagnosis and management of algodystrophy. *Ann Rheum Dis* 1991;50:727–730.
35. Kozin F. Reflex sympathetic dystrophy syndrome: a review. *Clin Exp Rheumatol* 1992;10:401–409.
36. Holder LE, Cole LA, Myerson MS. Reflex sympathetic dystrophy in the foot: clinical and scintigraphic criteria. *Radiology* 1992;184:531–535.
37. Katz MM, Hungerford DS. Reflex sympathetic dystrophy affecting the knee. *J Bone Joint Surg Br* 1987;69:797–803.
38. Adami S, Fossaluzza V, Gatti D, et al. Biphosphonate therapy of reflex sympathetic dystrophy syndrome. *Ann Rheum Dis* 1997;56:201–204.
39. Mellick GA, Mellick LB. Reflex sympathetic dystrophy treated with gabapentin. *Arch Phys Med Rehabil* 1997;78:98–105.
40. Naides SJ, Resnick D, Zvaifler NJ. Idiopathic regional osteoporosis: a clinical spectrum. *J Rheumatol* 1985;12:763–768.
41. Guerra JJ, Steinberg ME. Distinguishing transient osteoporosis from avascular necrosis of the hip. *J Bone Joint Surg Am* 1995;77:616–624.
42. Froberg PK, Braunstein EM, Buckwalter KA. Osteonecrosis, transient osteoporosis and transient bone marrow edema. *Radiol Clin North Am* 1996;34:273–291.
43. Schenck RC Jr, Goodnight JM. Osteochondritis dissecans. *J Bone Joint Surg Am* 1996;78:439–456.
44. Herring JA. The treatment of Legg-Calvé-Perthes disease. *J Bone Joint Surg Am* 1994;76:448–458.
45. Lowe TG. Scheuermann disease. *J Bone Joint Surg Am* 1990;72:940–945.
46. Aeschlimann A, Kahn MF. Tietze's syndrome: a critical review. *Clin Exp Rheumatol* 1990;8:407–412.

47. Wise CM, Semble EL, Dalton CB. Musculoskeletal chest wall syndromes in patients with noncardiac chest pain: a study of 100 patients. *Arch Phys Med Rehabil* 1992;73:147–149.
48. Kamel M, Kotob H. Ultrasonographic assessment of local steroid injection in Tietze's syndrome. *Br J Rheumatol* 1997; 36:547–550.
49. Disla E, Rhim HR, Reddy A, et al. Costochondritis: a prospective analysis in an emergency department setting. *Arch Intern Med* 1994;154:2466–2469.
50. Kadzombe EA, Robson WJ. Perichondritis. *Lancet* 1988;2: 1010–1011.
51. Wright JT. Slipping-rib syndrome. *Lancet* 1980;2:632–634.
52. Kahn M-F, Chamot A-M. SAPHO syndrome. *Rheum Dis Clin North Am* 1992;18:225–246.
53. Benhamou CL, Chamot A-M, Kahn M-F. Synovitis-acne-pustulosis-hyperostosis-osteomyelitis syndrome (SAPHO): a new syndrome among spondyloarthropathies? *Clin Exp Rheumatol* 1988;6:109–112.
54. Ibbertson HK, Manning PJ, Holdaway IW, et al. The acromegalic rosary. *Lancet* 1991;1:154–156.
55. Lentz SS. Osteitis pubis: a review. *Obstet Gynecol Surv* 1995;50: 310–315.
56. Rosenthal RE, Spickard WA, Markham RD, et al. Osteomyelitis of the symphysis pubis: a separate disease from osteitis pubis. *J Bone Joint Surg Am* 1982;64:123–128.
57. Holt MA, Keene JS, Graf BK, Helwig DC. Treatment of osteitis pubis in athletes: results of corticosteroid injections. *Am J Sports Med* 1995;23:601–606.
58. Wiley JJ. Traumatic osteitis pubis: the gracilis syndrome. *Am J Sports Med* 1983;11:360–363.
59. Albertsen AM, Egund N, Jurik AG, Jacobsen E. Posttraumatic osteolysis of the pubic bone simulating malignancy. *Acta Radiol* 1994;35:40–44.
60. Rauschning W. Anatomy and function of the communication between knee joint and popliteal bursae. *Ann Rheum Dis* 1980;39:354–358.
61. Fielding JR, Franklin PD, Kustan J. Popliteal cysts: a reassessment using magnetic resonance imaging. *Skeletal Radiol* 1991; 20:433–435.
62. Stone KR, Stoller D, DeCarli A, et al. The frequency of Baker's cysts associated with meniscal tears. *Am J Sports Med* 1996;24: 670–671.
63. Szer IS, Klein-Gitelman M, DeNardo BA, et al. Ultrasonography in the study of prevalence and clinical evolution of popliteal cysts in children with knee effusions. *J Rheumatol* 1992;19:458–462.
64. Simpson FG, Robinson PJ, Bark M, et al. Prospective study of thrombophlebitis and "pseudothrombophlebitis." *Lancet* 1980; 1:331–333.
65. Young L, Bartell T, Logan SE. Ganglions of the hand and wrist. *South Med J* 1988;81:751–760.
66. Höglund M, Tordai P, Muren C. Diagnosis of ganglions in the hand and wrist by sonography. *Acta Radiol* 1994;35:35–39.
67. Greendyke SD, Wilson M, Shepler TR. Anterior wrist ganglia from the scaphotrapezial joint. *J Hand Surg (Am)* 1992;17: 487–490.
68. Rozbruch SR, Chang V, Bohne WHO, et al. Ganglion cysts of the lower extremity: an analysis of 54 cases and review of the literature. *Orthopedics* 1998;21:141–148.
69. Rosson JW, Walker G. The natural history of ganglion in children. *J Bone Joint Surg Br* 1989;71:707–708.
70. Korman J, Pearl R, Hentz VR. Efficacy of immobilization following aspiration of carpal and digital ganglions. *J Hand Surg (Am)* 1992;17:1097–1099.
71. Moore JS. De Quervain's tenosynovitis: stenosing tenosynovitis of the first dorsal compartment. *J Occup Environ Med* 1997;39: 990–1002.
72. Schumacher HR Jr, Dorwart BB, Korzeniowski OM. Occurrence of de Quervain's tendinitis during pregnancy. *Arch Intern Med* 1985;145:2083–2084.
73. Thorson E, Szabo RM. Common tendinitis problems in the hand and forearm. *Orthop Clin North Am* 1992;23:65–74.
74. Rankin ME, Rankin EA. Injection therapy for management of stenosing tenosynovitis (de Quervain's disease) of the wrist. *J Natl Med Assoc* 1998;90:474–476.
75. Sampson SP, Wisch D, Badalamente MA. Complications of conservative and surgical treatment of de Quervain's disease and trigger fingers. *Hand Clin* 1994;10:73–82.
76. Anderson B, Kaye S. Treatment of flexor tenosynovitis of the hand ("trigger finger") with corticosteroids. *Arch Intern Med* 1991;151:153–156.
77. Martens M, Wouters P, Burssens A, et al. Patellar tendinitis: pathology and results of treatment. *Acta Orthop Scand* 1982;53: 445–450.
78. Bodne D, Quinn SF, Murray WT, et al. Magnetic resonance images of chronic patellar tendinitis. *Skeletal Radiol* 1988;17: 24–28.
79. Ray JM, Clancy WG, Lemon RA. Semimembranosus tendinitis: an overlooked cause of medial knee pain. *Am J Sports Med* 1988;16:347–351.
80. Chard MD, Hazleman BL. Tennis elbow: a reappraisal. *Br J Rheumatol* 1989;28:186–190.
81. Chard MD, Cawston TE, Riley GP, et al. Rotator cuff degeneration and lateral epicondylitis: a comparative histologic study. *Ann Rheum Dis* 1994;53:30–34.
82. Gellman H. Tennis elbow (lateral epicondylitis). *Orthop Clin North Am* 1992;23:75–82.
83. Bennett JB. Lateral and medial epicondylitis. *Hand Clin* 1994;10:157–163.
84. Ernst E. Conservative therapy for tennis elbow. *Br J Clin Pract* 1992;46:55–57.
85. Stahl S, Kaufman T. The efficacy of an injection of steroids for medial epicondylitis. *J Bone Joint Surg Am* 1997;79:1648–1649.
86. LaBelle H, Guibert R, Joncas J, et al. Lack of scientific evidence for the treatment of lateral epicondylitis of the elbow: an attempted meta-analysis. *J Bone Joint Surg Br* 1992;74:646–651.
87. Bywaters EGL. Lesions of bursae, tendons and tendon sheaths. *Clin Rheum Dis* 1979;5:883–925.
88. Strickland RW, Vukelja SJ, Wohlgethan JR, et al. Hemorrhagic subcutaneous bursitis. *J Rheumatol* 1991;18:112–114.
89. Mysnyk MC, Wroble RR, Foster DT, et al. Prepatellar bursitis in wrestlers. *Am J Sports Med* 1986;14:46–54.
90. Larsson L-G, Baum J. The syndromes of bursitis. *Bull Rheum Dis* 1986;36:1–8.
91. Shbeeb MI, Matteeson EL. Trochanteric bursitis. *Mayo Clin Proc* 1996;71:565–569.
92. Traycoff RB. "Pseudotrochanteric bursitis": the differential diagnosis of lateral hip pain. *J Rheumatol* 1991;18:1810–1812.
93. Weinstein PS, Canoso JJ, Wohlgethan JR. Long-term follow-up of corticosteroid injection for traumatic olecranon bursitis. *Ann Rheum Dis* 1984;43:44–46.
94. Smith DL, Bakke AC, Campbell SM, et al. Immunocytologic characteristics of mononuclear cell populations found in nonseptic olecranon bursitis. *J Rheumatol* 1994;21:209–214.
95. Smith DL, McAfee JH, Lucas LM, et al. Treatment of nonseptic olecranon bursitis: a controlled, blinded prospective trial. *Arch Intern Med* 1989;149:2527–2530.
96. Myerson MS, McGarvey W. Disorders of the insertion of the Achilles tendon and Achilles tendinitis. *J Bone Joint Surg Am* 1998;80:1814–1824.
97. Mills GM, Baethge BA. Ischiogluteal bursitis in cancer patients: an infrequently recognized cause of pain. *Am J Clin Oncol* 1993; 16:229–231.

98. Cohen SE, Mahul O, Meir R, et al. Anserine bursitis and non-insulin dependent diabetes mellitus. *J Rheumatol* 1997;24:2152–2165.
99. Toohey AK, LaSalle TL, Martinez S, Polisson RP. Iliopsoas bursitis: clinical features, radiographic findings, and disease associations. *Semin Arthritis Rheum* 1990;20:41–47.
100. Swezey RL. Obturator internus bursitis: a common factor in low back pain. *Orthopedics* 1993;16:783–786.
101. Holt PD, Keats TE. Calcific tendinitis: a review of the usual and unusual. *Skeletal Radiol* 1993;22:1–9.
102. Deutsch AL, Mink JH. Magnetic resonance imaging of musculoskeletal injuries. *Radiol Clin North Am* 1989;27:983–1002.
103. Garrett WE Jr. Muscle strain injuries. *Am J Sports Med* 1996;24 (suppl):2–8.
104. Kretzler HH Jr, Richardson AB. Rupture of the pectoralis major muscle. *Am J Sports Med* 1989;17:453–458.
105. Agha A, DiMarcangelo MT, Reginato AJ. Calf pain and swelling (pseudothrombophlebitis) caused by rupture of the plantaris muscle/tendon: report of two cases with magnetic resonance imaging findings. *J Clin Rheumatol* 1996;2:147–151.
106. Conti SF. Posterior tibial tendon problems in athletes. *Orthop Clin North Am* 1994;25:109–121.
107. Mathieson JR, Connell DG, Cooperberg PL, et al. Sonography of the Achilles tendon and adjacent bursae. *AJR Am J Roentgenol* 1988;151:127–131.
108. Keene JS, Lash EG, Fisher DR, et al. Magnetic resonance imaging of Achilles tendon ruptures. *Am J Sports Med* 1989;17:333–337.
109. Mahler F. Partial and complete ruptures of the Achilles tendon and local corticosteroid injections. *Br J Sports Med* 1992;26:7–14.
110. Ribard P, Audisio F, Kahn M-F, et al. Seven Achilles tendinitis including 3 complicated by rupture during fluoroquinolone therapy. *J Rheumatol* 1992;19:1479–1481.
111. Oh SJ, Rollins JI, Lewis I. Pentazocine-induced fibrous myopathy. *JAMA* 1975;231:271–273.
112. Paty JG Jr. Running injuries. *Curr Opin Rheumatol* 1994;6:203–209.
113. Macera CA, Pate RR, Powell KE, et al. Predicting lower-extremity injuries among habitual runners. *Arch Intern Med* 1989;149:2565–2568.
114. Lane NE, Bloch DA, Wood PD, et al. Aging, long-distance running, and the development of musculoskeletal disability. *Am J Med* 1987;82:772–780.
115. Hoppmann RA, Patrone NA. A review of musculoskeletal problems in instrumental musicians. *Semin Arthritis Rheum* 1989;19:117–126.
116. McDermott FT. Repetition strain injury: a review of current understanding. *Med J Aust* 1986;144:196–200.
117. Bird HA, Hill J. Repetitive strain disorder: towards diagnostic criteria. *Ann Rheum Dis* 1992;51:974–977.
118. Smythe H. The "repetitive strain injury syndrome" is referred pain from the neck. *J Rheumatol* 1988;15:1604–1608.
119. Csuka ME, Brewer BJ, Lynch KL, et al. Osteonecrosis, fractures, and protrusio acetabuli secondary to x-irradiation therapy for prostatic carcinoma. *J Rheumatol* 1987;4:165–170.
120. Fu AL, Greven KM, Maruyama Y. Radiation osteitis and insufficiency fractures after pelvic irradiation for gynecologic malignancies. *Am J Clin Oncol* 1994;17:248–254.
121. Glick R, Parhami N. Frostbite arthritis. *J Rheumatol* 1979;6:456–460.
122. Carrera GF, Kozin G, McCarty DJ. Arthritis after frostbite injury in children. *Arthritis Rheum* 1979;22:1082–1087.

98

MECHANICAL DISORDERS OF THE KNEE

DENNIS W. BOULWARE

Mechanical disorders of the knee include clinical conditions caused by malfunction, trauma, or degeneration of a specific component of the knee, interfering with normal knee function. Normal knee operation is dependent on proper function of various intraarticular and extraarticular components. *Internal derangement of the knee* commonly refers to a disorder of the intraarticular components such as the articular cartilage, meniscus fibrocartilage, collateral ligaments, and/or cruciate ligaments. Disorders of extraarticular components of the knee joint include patellofemoral malalignment and insufficiency of the quadriceps or hamstring muscle groups and are also considered as mechanical disorders.

Mechanical disorders of the knee, if they continue unabated, eventually lead to osteoarthritis (OA). Several experimental animal models of OA (1–9) involve an initiating internal derangement of the joint. The most common models of experimental OA include partial medial meniscectomy (1,2) or transection of the anterior cruciate ligament (3,4) in canines and lapins. After the internal derangement is induced, the animal is required to exercise the limb and over time develops clinical OA. Other animal models of OA in guinea pigs (5,6), mice (7), and sheep (8), also require experimental disruption of the integrity of a variety of joints followed by use of the limb. As our population ages and becomes more engaged in recreational and sports-related activities, mechanical disorders of the knee will become more prevalent and, if not recognized early, will likely result in an increased prevalence of OA of the knee.

ANATOMY

Articular Hyaline Cartilage

The structure and function of cartilage in health and disease is covered in detail in Chapters 10 and 11. In brief, articular cartilage is a firm, resilient tissue capable of absorbing impact, transmitting load, and sustaining tremendous sheer forces. Changes in the macroscopic structure or proteoglycan content result in a diminished ability to function and remain resilient. Cartilage is an avascular structure, receiving its nutrients from synovial fluid during compressive loading and unloading. Any condition that affects the anatomic or biochemical integrity of hyaline cartilage of the knee predisposes an individual to a greater potential for a future mechanical disorder and places the knee at greater risk for eventual OA.

Meniscal Fibrocartilage

The structure and function of fibrocartilage are covered in detail in Chapter 7. In brief, the medial and lateral menisci are crescents of fibrocartilage, triangular in cross section, that modify the flat tibial plateau, creating a concave surface for the convex femoral condyles (Fig. 98.1). The menisci function by stabilizing the knee and limiting mobility to simple flexion and extension. The composition of fibrocartilaginous menisci differs biochemically from hyaline articular cartilage, with collagen composing 60% to 90% of the dry weight of fibrocartilage (10–12), whereas proteoglycans constitute less than 10% (13). In adulthood, the menisci are predominantly avascular structures with most of their nutrients being acquired from synovial fluid during loading and unloading. There is a vascular zone in the menisci adjacent to the bone, which accounts for their ability to undergo repair more readily than articular cartilage.

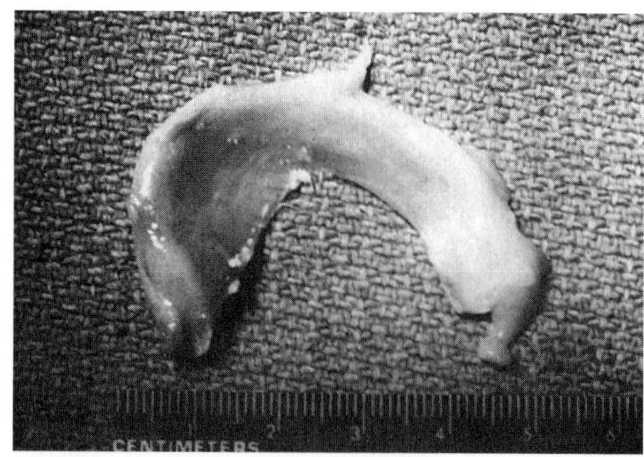

FIGURE 98.1. A normal human medial meniscus. Note the semilunar shape with a thin free edge and considerably thickened marginal attachment site. Menisci increase the stability of the joint and serve as weight-bearing structures in the knee.

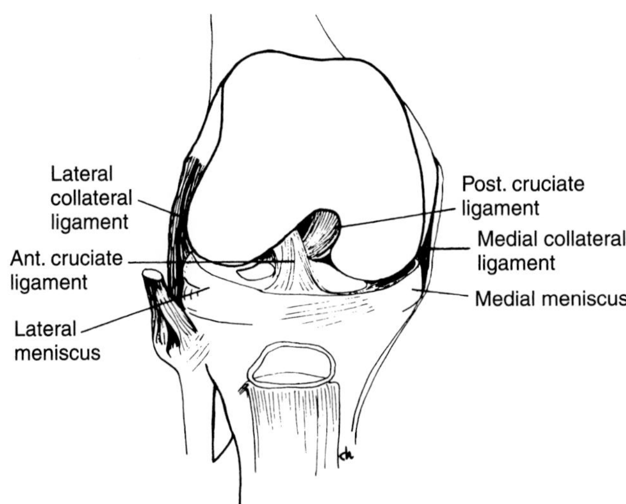

FIGURE 98.2. Diagram of the human knee joint. The patella and capsule have been removed. Note that the distal femur and proximal tibia are covered by hyaline articular cartilage. Affixed to the surface of the tibia are the medial and lateral collateral ligaments, stout collagenous bands, which provide stability in the coronal plane. The cruciate ligaments control stability in the sagittal plane.

Ligaments

Ligaments are composed nearly entirely of collagen and elastin in dense parallel organized bundles. They function to constrain knee mobility into desired flexion and extension (Fig. 98.2). The collateral ligaments prevent varus or valgus deviation, and the cruciate ligaments prevent anterior or posterior displacement of the tibial plateau as it pivots about the distal femoral condyles.

Patellofemoral Alignment

During flexion and extension of the knee, the patella glides superiorly and inferiorly along the femoral intercondylar groove. Patellar-tracking malalignment can occur with an imbalance of the vector forces of the quadriceps on the patellar tendon or in severe varus and valgus deformities. Similarly, the patella will exhibit abnormal tracking when there is significant subluxation of the patella secondary to patellar tendon laxity. Each of these anatomic aberrations can lead to a mechanical disorder of the knee with a major impact on the patellofemoral compartment.

MENISCAL DISORDERS

The medial and lateral menisci are crescent-shaped structures that appear triangular in configuration on cross-sectional examination. Their structure allows the knee to function with greater stability and improved joint congruity and to transmit 50% to 70% of the load across the knee during axial loading (14). Disorders of the menisci account for about two thirds of all derangements of the knee joint (15–20). Lesions of the menisci can be divided into *acute tears* and *chronic or degenerative tears*. The majority of acute tears occur after trauma, such as an athletic injury, in which there is abnormal excursion of the articular surfaces under conditions of loading, which entrap the menisci. Usually an acute tear will consist of a vertical and longitudinal tear. A chronic or degenerative tear often will not have a recognizable precipitating event. Symptoms are usually less severe in chronic tears, and the lesions often result in a horizontal cleavage, particularly in the posterior third of the meniscus.

In a large arthroscopic study (21) of symptomatic meniscal lesions, 81% of the patients were men, with medial meniscal lesions predominating. Approximately 75% of the medial meniscal tears were vertical, with the remainder being horizontal tears. Similarly, vertical tears were the more common pattern seen in lateral meniscal injuries.

Clinical Features

Historic Features

Acute meniscal injuries generally involve easily identifiable precipitating events, often followed by an associated limited range of motion with the pain. If the acute injury results in a displacement of the torn meniscus, patients will often complain of a painful "catching" or "popping" sensation in the knee. Although "buckling" sensations are often associated with meniscal tears, they are more common with anterior cruciate ligament injuries, but can be seen in any painful condition of the knee. They are caused by a reflexive muscle relaxation followed by "giving way."

A chronic tear of the meniscus is usually less painful than an acute tear, and there is frequently lack of any recognizable precipitating event. Usually associated with OA, a precipitating cause may be as simple as a squatting and twisting maneuver or a simple misstep. Complaints usually include chronic pain with use of the knee and occasional swelling. Limitation in range of motion is less a prominent feature than that with acute displaced tears.

Physical Examination

Joint effusions usually correlate with the severity of inflammation within the knee joint. Obviously, acute injuries generally have a greater associated effusion than do chronic degenerative tears. A limitation in passive range of motion will be seen if there is a displaced tear of the meniscus with entrapment of the meniscus. The entrapped fragment of the meniscus is frequently the culprit in limiting full flexion or full extension. The *McMurray test* is a specific test to induce entrapment of a meniscal tear. With the patient supine, the examiner grasps the affected leg and passively flexes the knee and hip maximally. At the point of maximal flexion, the knee is forcibly internally and externally rotated to attempt impingement of the torn lateral or medial meniscus. With the knee held in passive internal rotation in flexion, the knee is then extended to detect a palpable or audible snap in the joint. The maneuver is then repeated with the flexed knee held in full, passive, external rotation. Pain is not always present, particularly in an older degenerative tear. The *Apley grind test* also is used to detect possible meniscal derangement. This test is performed with the patient in a prone position and the knee flexed at 90 degrees. The examiner then manually loads the knee joint while rotating the knee in internal and external rotation. Tenderness elicited during this procedure is not specific for a meniscal injury, as an articular cartilage lesion also will produce tenderness. The combined presence of a "snap" and an abnormal Apley grind test is consistent with a torn meniscus.

Because of the anatomic location of the menisci near the medial and lateral joint lines, *joint-line tenderness* is the hallmark of a meniscal injury. The menisci are in close congruity with the peripheral joint capsule, which has a rich nerve supply, accounting for the localized tenderness. A combination of joint-line tenderness with a positive McMurray and/or Apley sign correlates well with a clinically torn meniscus.

Imaging Studies

Confirmation of a clinically suspected torn meniscus is usually achieved by using an imaging study, either noninvasive or invasive. Noninvasive studies include plain radiography, computerized tomography (CT), or magnetic resonance imaging (MRI; Fig. 98.3). Invasive imaging, including arthroscopy and arthrography, carries a higher accuracy. *Plain radiography* is a poor diagnostic modality for soft tissue injury. The only utility of plain radiography is to assess the severity of coexisting OA, a common comorbid feature of a degenerative or chronic tear. *MRI* has a diagnostic accuracy approaching 70% to 95% (22–27) (see Chapter 6). An excellent modality for evaluating soft tissue injuries, MRI is limited by the difficulty in differentiating a degenerative intact meniscus from a chronic or degenerative meniscal tear. The greatest utility of MRI is in a negative study because of its high negative predictive value. *CT* is of limited value in evaluating meniscal injuries when compared with the ability of MRI to differentiate soft tissue lesions.

Double-contrast *arthrography* previously had been the gold standard for meniscal tears (28). Its accuracy, however, is highly dependent on the experience of the interpreter and the severity of the lesion. *Arthroscopy* is a minor surgical procedure (Fig. 98.4), and at present should be considered the gold standard for the diagnosis of a meniscal tear (see Chapter 5) (29,30). There is still difficulty in visualizing the posterior horn of the medial meniscus, and the test is limited by the experience and efficiency of the operator. With a proper physical examination and the diagnostic utility of MRI, there is little need for diagnostic arthroscopy. This technique should be reserved for cases in which surgical intervention is deemed essential for treatment.

Treatment

A conservative versus surgical treatment approach is determined by the displacement of a meniscal tear. A dis-

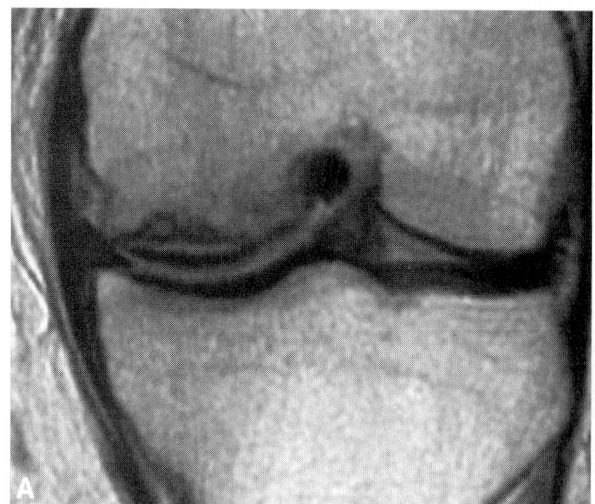

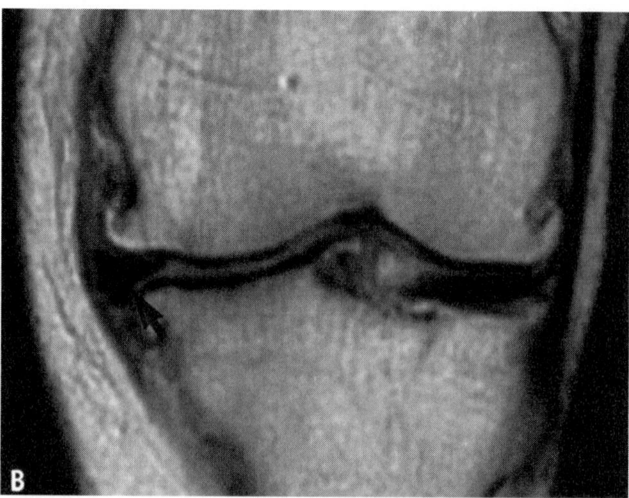

FIGURE 98.3. A: Magnetic resonance image of the knee of a 74-year-old man demonstrating concomitant spontaneous osteonecrosis of the medial femoral condyle. **B:** Complex degenerative horizontal cleavage tear of medial meniscus (*arrow*).

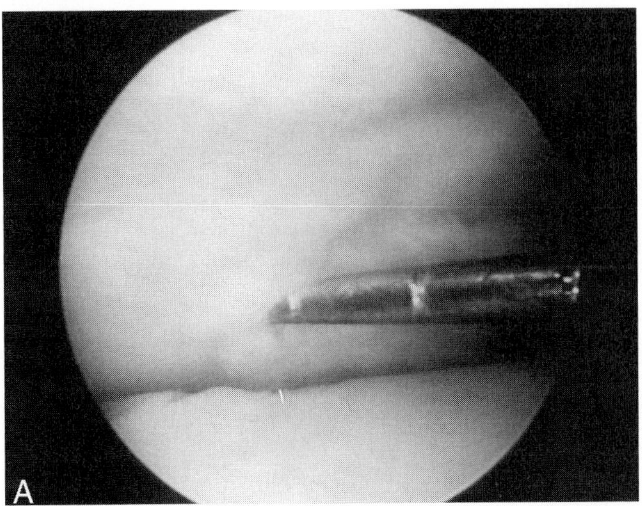

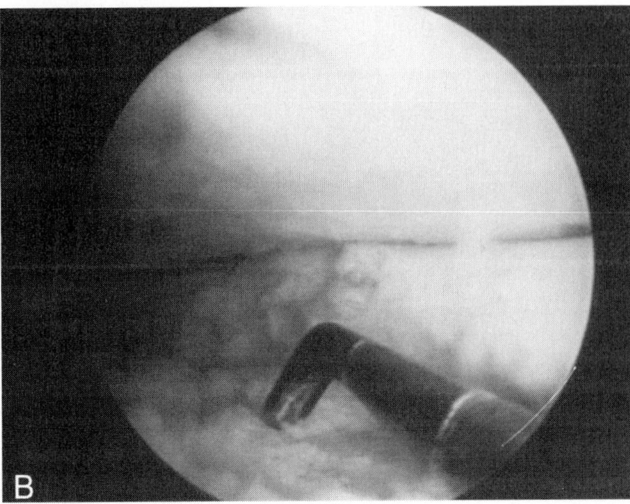

FIGURE 98.4. A: Arthroscopic appearance of the degenerative medial meniscus with probe in substance of tear. **B:** Associated chondral lesion with exposed subchondral bone.

placed meniscal tear resulting in entrapment and limitation of range of motion warrants surgical intervention. Tears that are nondisplaced or do not result in entrapment can be treated conservatively, including nonsteroidal antiinflammatory drugs for analgesic effect and supervised physical therapy to maintain passive range of motion and muscle strength. If a displaced meniscal tear requires surgical intervention, arthroscopic partial meniscectomy is preferable to open meniscectomy because of the advantage of more rapid recovery. The fraction of meniscus removed during meniscectomy should be minimized to maintain as much meniscal function as possible. Experimental models have found that postmeniscectomy OA changes vary directly with the fraction of meniscus removed during meniscectomy (31). Nonsteroidal antiinflammatory drugs and vigorous supervised physical therapy also are indicated for patients undergoing arthroscopic synovectomy.

LIGAMENTOUS DISORDERS

Normal knee stability and range of motion are dependent on intact ligaments. Four major ligaments restrict primary knee motion to flexion and extension: medial collateral ligament, lateral collateral ligament, anterior cruciate ligament, and posterior cruciate ligament. The *collateral ligaments* reside along the medial and lateral aspect of the knee and restrict the knee from varus or valgus angulation. The medial collateral ligament is firmly attached to the medial meniscus, and disruption of one structure often leads to injuries to the other structure in the medial compartment. The anterior and posterior *cruciate ligaments* function to retard anterior and posterior displacement of the tibia relative to the femoral condyles during flexion and extension. Acute injuries to the ligaments of the knee, particularly the anterior cruciate ligament, often result in a brisk hemarthrosis because of the vascularity of the ligaments. Acute injuries to the ligaments often have easily identifiable precipitating injuries.

Clinical Features

Historic Features

Injuries of the ligaments occur during activity and usually involve jumping or rapid changes in direction while running. Painful swelling of the joint, usually due to hemarthrosis, occurs precipitately within the first 2 to 6 hours after injury.

Physical Examination

Most ligamentous disorders can be easily detected by simple physical examination. *Medial and lateral collateral ligament injury* is best tested by passively placing the knee in 30 degrees of flexion. Applying passive stress that results in a valgus deviation of the knee would indicate a medial collateral ligament tear. Incomplete medial collateral ligament tears often result in tenderness over the medial compartment of the knee during this maneuver in the absence of valgus deviation. Conversely, a varus force applied to the knee still held in this position can be used to detect similar signs in the lateral compartment, implicating a lateral collateral ligament injury. Caution should be exercised in interpreting this maneuver, because "relative" laxity of the collateral ligaments is often seen in knees with loss of full articular cartilage thickness due to chronic OA.

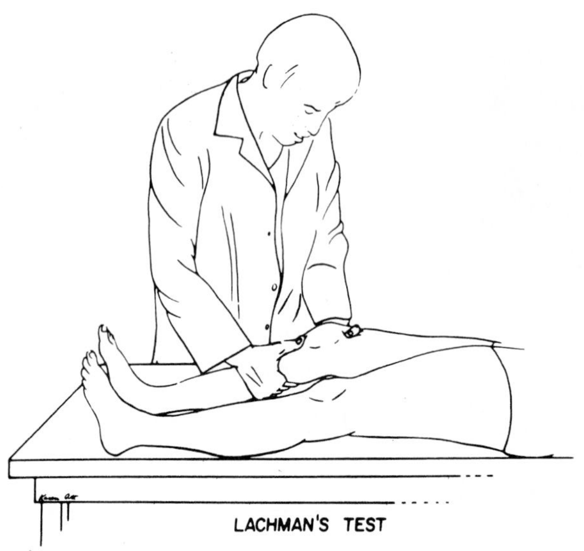

FIGURE 98.5. Lachman's test for anterior cruciate stability done with the knee at 25 degrees of flexion.

A torn *anterior cruciate ligament* is best tested by the anterior *drawer sign* or *Lachman's test* (Fig. 98.5). This maneuver is performed with the knee passively flexed to 25 degrees with an anterior force placed on the tibia relative to the femoral condyles. Anterior displacement of the tibia plateau relative to the femoral condyle indicates a torn or lax anterior cruciate ligament. Tenderness elicited by this maneuver in the absence of displacement suggests an incomplete tear of the anterior cruciate ligament. The *posterior cruciate ligament* is best tested by the posterior drawer sign, performed with the knee in 90 degrees of flexion. A posterior force is then placed on the tibia while looking for posterior displacement of the tibia relative to the femoral condyles. Again, caution should be exercised in interpreting these tests in patients with chronic OA and relative laxity of the ligaments due to articular cartilaginous loss.

Most ligamentous disruptions can be quantified by the degree of laxity or displacement. By using the normal contralateral knee as a reference point, a grade I laxity would represent up to 5 mm of additional motion; grade II, 6 to 10 mm; grade III, 11 to 15 mm; and grade IV, greater than 15 mm of additional displacement.

Imaging Studies

Diagnostic imaging, including plain radiography, CT, and MRI, offers little more to the diagnostic accuracy of the physical examination. Invasive arthroscopy should be considered in cases with a suspected associated torn meniscus or osteochondral fracture, requiring arthroscopic repair (32–35).

Treatment

The treatment of most ligamentous injuries is based on the severity or grade of the injury and anticipated or desired future functional capacity of the individual (36–40). For injuries to the *anterior cruciate ligament*, patients with grade I or II severity remain functionally stable after rehabilitation and modification of their activities. The decision to pursue a surgical reconstruction for grade III injuries is often dependent on the patient's desire to pursue future functional activities that will be demanding of the knee. Individuals with acute injuries resulting in grade IV laxity require surgical reconstruction to remain functional. Nonsteroidal antiinflammatory drugs for analgesia and vigorous supervised physical therapy are warranted for all individuals whether surgical candidates or not.

The treatment of a *medial collateral ligament* injury is similar to that of the anterior cruciate ligament (41,42). Injuries up to and including grade II can often be treated conservatively without surgery, including supervised physical therapy, nonsteroidal antiinflammatory drugs for analgesia, and the use of a hinged cast or brace for 3 to 6 weeks. Injuries with severity of grade III or greater often require surgical intervention for repair because of the likelihood of later problems with OA. *Lateral collateral ligament tears* of grade II or greater severity often require surgical reconstruction.

An isolated disruption of the *posterior cruciate ligament* is a rare event (43), but can result from an exaggerated pull of the quadriceps tendon on the patella to stabilize the knee in flexion, or with hyperextension injuries of the knee. Most patients are only modestly impaired from this injury, although the incidence of future OA remains high. Surgical repair is usually reserved for those cases in which there has been avulsion of a bone fragment. Midligamentous tears are usually not successfully repaired.

Combined injuries such as a medial collateral ligament disruption combined with an anterior cruciate ligament tear often require surgical repair (42).

Supervised rehabilitation is an important modality of treatment for all knee injuries, but particularly with ligamentous injuries. The goal of strengthening the hamstring muscle relative to the quadriceps is dependent on the type of ligamentous injury. After anterior cruciate ligament injuries, physical therapy should be directed toward achieving hamstring and quadriceps muscles of relative equal strength. This is unlike the normal situation in which the quadriceps muscle is roughly 50% stronger than the hamstring. In posterior cruciate ligament injuries, the quadriceps muscles are strengthened maximally to ensure knee stability. Each patient must have a physical strengthening regimen specifically tailored to the injury (see also Chapter 46).

PATELLOFEMORAL MALALIGNMENT

Malalignment of the patella as it tracks superiorly and inferiorly in the intercondylar groove of the femur is one of the most common causes of knee pain. Previously called *chondromalacia patella*, the associated degenerative process of the patellar cartilage is usually secondary to a malalignment of the patella within the intercondylar groove. Unlike the previously described disorders of the meniscus and ligament, patellofemoral malalignment is not associated with an injury. Problems with patellofemoral pain usually correlate with severity of abnormal patellar tilt, alignment, and/or subluxation.

Clinical Features

Historic Features

The most common complaint of patients with patellofemoral malalignment is exertional knee pain, particularly with activities involving active weight-bearing knee extension or flexion, such as stair climbing, running, jumping, and squatting. Interestingly, in patellofemoral disease, difficulty in descending stairs is often more symptomatic than is difficulty in ascending stairs. Prolonged periods of immobility with the knee in flexed positions such as sitting at a desk or riding in an automobile will often cause pain on resuming a standing position.

Physical Examination

Joint effusions are not commonly seen, but correlate with the degree of inflammation and histopathology of the patellar articular cartilage. Passive range of motion is frequently preserved. Crepitus is a common feature of patellofemoral malalignment and usually confined to the patellofemoral compartment. The patellofemoral compartment as a source of knee pain can be confirmed by reproducing the complaints by patellofemoral compression or patellar inhibition. There is often concomitant tenderness of the peripatellar muscles and iliotibial band.

An abnormal degree of *patellar tilt* or *patellar laxity* can be a cause of patellofemoral malalignment and subsequently a mechanical disorder of the knee (Fig. 98.6). The *passive patellar tilt* test measures patellar laxity. The tilting of the lateral patellar edge relative to the lateral femoral condyle tests the degree of lateral retinacular tightness. A zero-degree or a negative-angle tilt usually reflects excessive retinacular tightness. The *passive patellar glide test* allows the examiner to estimate the degree of lateral patellar deviation. The examiner passively displaces the patella laterally with the knee in passive full extension. The ability to displace the patellar more than one half of its total width suggests laxity of the medial retinacular restraints. Either medial retinacular laxity or lateral retinacular tightness will result in an abnormal tilt and malalignment of the patella.

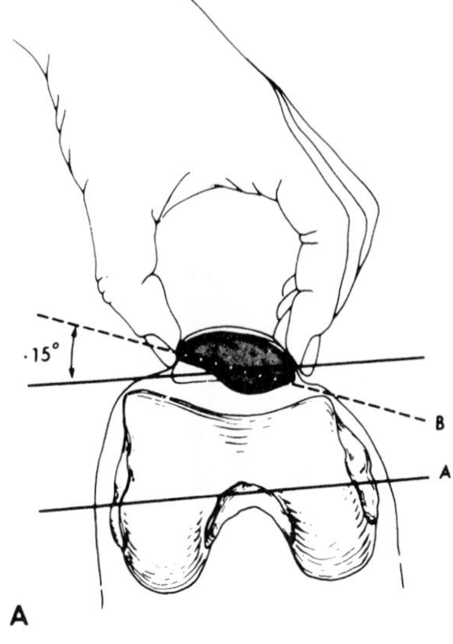

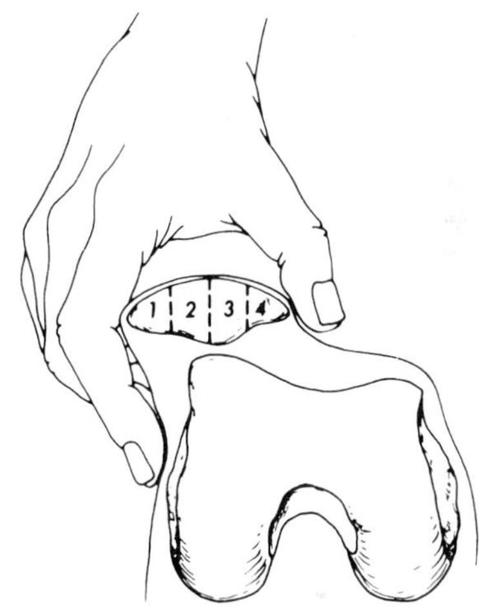

FIGURE 98.6. A: Passive patellar tilt indicates laxity of lateral ligamentous restraints. A patellar tilt of 0 degrees or less indicates tight lateral retinacular ligaments. **B:** Passive lateral glide test demonstrates the ability to displace the patella laterally with the knee in full extension; subluxation beyond one half of its width indicates laxity of medial retinacular restraints.

Overall *malalignment of the lower extremity*, particularly angulation of the knee, should be assessed with the patient standing. An increase in the Q angle (Fig. 98.7) results in abnormal patellar tracking. Similarly, vastus medialis muscle atrophy, valgus deformities of the knee, or forefoot pronation problems for any reason will result in patellofemoral malalignment (44).

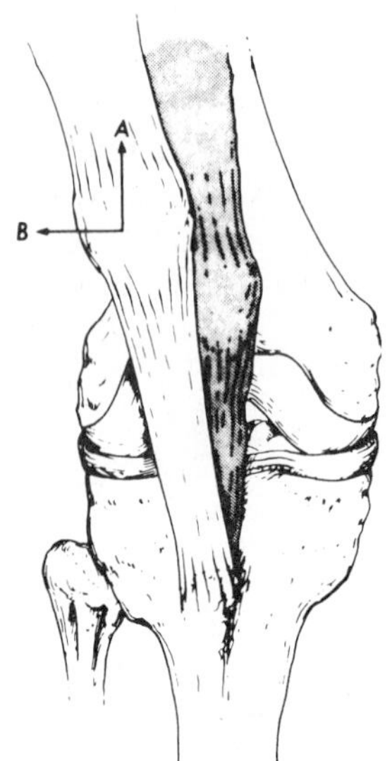

FIGURE 98.7. Increased "functional" Q angle is present if lateral excursion **(B)** exceeds proximal excursion **(A)**.

Imaging Studies

The clinical suspicion of a patellar tilt can usually be confirmed by *plain radiography* measuring the angle of Laurin. With the knee in 20 degrees of flexion, the lateral patellofemoral angle is measured (Fig. 98.8). In the normal patellofemoral compartment, the angle will open laterally when the angle of Laurin is positive. In the case of an abnormal patellar tilt, the angle of Laurin is negative and suggests an abnormal medial opening of the compartment (45,46).

CT and *MRI* are alternatives to plain radiography in confirming patellofemoral alignment and tilting problems (47,48). Although they offer a better view of the soft tissue of the knee compartment, their expense offers little justification for these imaging techniques.

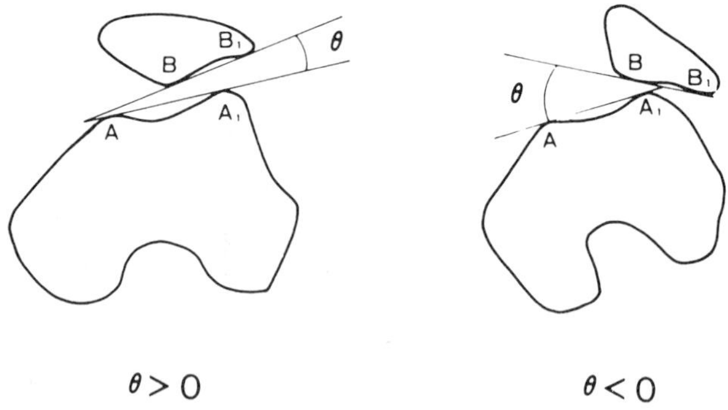

FIGURE 98.8. Angle of Laurin measures the lateral patellofemoral angle, where line *A–A1* passes through the femoral condyles and *B–B1* passes through the lateral patellar facet. The angle is positive if it opens laterally, and abnormal if it opens medially.

Arthroscopy is invaluable in grading the severity of patellar cartilage pathology, but offers little more in confirming the clinical suspicion than do the physical examination and plain radiography.

Treatment

Conservative management should be instituted for all degrees of severity of patellar malalignment (49). *Supervised physical therapy* is indicated to stretch the lateral retinaculum, hamstring, and iliotibial band in concert with strengthening exercises of the quadriceps muscles, particularly the vastus medialis. The use of external support such as elastic knee supports and orthotics also is helpful. Quadriceps-strengthening exercises using the last 30 degrees of extension to strengthen the vastus medialis muscle are an important modality. Heavily loaded isotonic exercises with full range of motion (i.e., full squats with weights) are to be avoided. Nonsteroidal antiinflammatory drugs are useful, not only for their analgesic properties but also in cases with large effusions.

Surgical management is occasionally required for severe malalignments. In the case of a chronic patellar subluxation, a lateral retinacular release may be helpful, although previous studies have been inconsistently successful when a lateral release is performed alone. Other surgical modalities including transposition of the vastus medialis insertion have similarly had equivocal outcomes (50).

CONCLUSIONS

Mechanical disorders of the knee can eventually lead to the final clinical pathway of OA. A severe derangement of any of the intraarticular or extraarticular components required for a normal functioning knee joint can result in OA. Early recognition, appropriate treatment, and modification of body habitus and lifestyle may retard the progression of mechanical disorders of the knee to clinical OA.

REFERENCES

1. Mehraban F, Kuo SY, Riera H, et al. Prostromelysin and procollagenase genes are differentially up-regulated in chondrocytes from the knees of rabbits with experimental osteoarthritis. *Arthritis Rheum* 1994;37:1189–1197.
2. Elmer RH, Moskowitz RW, Frankel VH. Meniscal regeneration and postmeniscectomy degenerative joint disease. *Clin Orthop* 1977;124:304–310.
3. Guilak F, Ratcliffe A, Lane N, et al. Mechanical and biochemical changes in the superficial zone of articular cartilage in canine experimental osteoarthritis. *J Orthop Res* 1994;12:474–484.
4. Pelletier JP, Mineau F, Raynauld JP, et al. Intra-articular injections with methylprednisolone acetate reduce osteoarthritic lesions in parallel with chondrocyte stromelysin synthesis in experimental osteoarthritis. *Arthritis Rheum* 1994;37:414–423.

5. Dedrick DK, Goulet R, Huston L, et al. Early bone changes in experimental osteoarthritis using microscopic computed tomography. *J Rheumatol* 1991;27(suppl):44–45.
6. Meacock SC, Bodmer JL, Billingham WE. Experimental osteoarthritis in guinea pigs. *J Exp Pathol (Oxford)* 1990; 71:279–293.
7. van der Kraan PM, Vitters EL, van Beuningen HM, et al. Degenerative knee joint lesions in mice after a single intra-articular collagenase injection: a new model of osteoarthritis. *J Exp Pathol (Oxford)* 1990;71:19–31.
8. Ishimaru J, Handa Y, Kurita K, et al. The effect of occlusal loss on normal and pathological temporomandibular joints: an animal study. *J Craniomaxillofac Surg* 1994;22:95–102.
9. Inerot S, Heinegard D, Olsson SE, et al. Proteoglycan alterations during developing experimental osteoarthritis in a novel hip model. *J Orthop Res* 1991;9:658–673.
10. Peters TJ, Smillie IS. Studies on the chemical composition of the menisci of the knee joint with special reference to the horizontal cleavage lesion. *Clin Orthop* 1972;86:245–252.
11. Ghosh P, Taylor TK. The knee joint meniscus: a fibrocartilage of some distinction. *Clin Orthop* 1987;224:52–63.
12. Aspden RM, Yarker YE, Hukins DW. Collagen orientations in the meniscus of the knee joint. *J Anat* 1985;140:371–380.
13. McDevitt CA, Webber RJ. The ultrastructure and biochemistry of meniscal cartilage. *Clin Orthop* 1990;252:8–18.
14. Walker PS, Erkman MJ. The role of the menisci in force transmission across the knee. *Clin Orthop* 1975;109:184–192.
15. Daniel D, Daniels E, Aronson D. The diagnosis of meniscus pathology. *Clin Orthop* 1982;163:218–224.
16. Hamberg P, Gillquist J, Lysholm J. Suture of new and old peripheral meniscus tears. *J Bone Joint Surg Am* 1983;65:193–197.
17. Jones RE, Smith EC, Resich JS. Effects of medial meniscectomy in patients older than forty years. *J Bone Joint Surg Am* 1978; 60:783–786.
18. Noble J, Erat K. In defense of the meniscus. *J Bone Joint Surg Br* 1980;62:7–11.
19. Sonne-Holm S, Fledelius I, Ahn N. Results after meniscectomy in 147 athletes. *Acta Orthop Scand* 1980;51:303–309.
20. Hough AJ, Webber RJ. Pathology of the meniscus. *Clin Orthop* 1990;252:32–40.
21. Dandy DJ. The arthroscopic anatomy of symptomatic meniscal lesions. *J Bone Joint Surg Br* 1990;72:628–633.
22. Polly DW, Callaghan JJ, Sikes RA, et al. The accuracy of selective magnetic resonance imaging compared with the findings of arthroscopy of the knee. *J Bone Joint Surg Am* 1988;70J: 192–198.
23. Watanabe AT, Carter BC, Teitelbaum GP, et al. Common pitfalls in magnetic resonance imaging of the knee. *J Bone Joint Surg Am* 1989;71:857–861.
24. Auge WK, Kaeding CC. Bilateral discoid medial menisci with extensive intra-substance cleavage tears: MRI and arthroscopic correlation. *Arthroscopy* 1994;10:313–318.
25. Mink JH, Deutsch AL. Magnetic resonance imaging of the knee. *Clin Orthop* 1989;244:29–47.
26. Raunest J, Oberle K, Lochnert J, Hoetzinger H. The clinical value of magnetic resonance imaging in the evaluation of meniscal disorders. *J Bone Joint Surg Am* 1991;73:11–29.
27. Glashow JL, Katz R, Schneider M, Scott WN. Double-blind assessment of the value of magnetic resonance imaging in the diagnosis of anterior cruciate and meniscal lesions. *J Bone Joint Surg Am* 1989;71:113–119.
28. Freiberger RH, Kaye JJ. *Arthrography.* New York: Appleton-Century-Crofts, 1979.
29. Casscells SW. The place of arthroscopy in the diagnosis and treatment of internal derangement of the knee: an analysis of 1000 cases. *Clin Orthop* 1980;151:135–142.
30. Curran WP, Woodward EP. Arthroscopy: its role in diagnosis and treatment of athletic knee injuries. *Am J Sports Med* 1980;8: 415–418.
31. Aglietti P, Zaccherotti G, De Biase P, et al. A comparison between medial meniscus repair, partial meniscectomy, and normal meniscus in anterior cruciate ligament reconstructed knees. *Clin Orthop* 1994;307:165–173.
32. Butler JC, Andrews JR. The role of arthroscopic surgery in the evaluation of acute traumatic hemarthrosis of the knee. *Clin Orthop* 1988;228:150–152.
33. Bumberg BC, McGinty JB. Acute hemarthrosis of the knee: indications for diagnostic arthroscopy. *J Arthrosc* 1990;6:221–225.
34. Kannus P, Jarvinen M. Long-term prognosis of nonoperatively treated acute knee distortions having primary hemarthrosis without clinical instability. *Am J Sports Med* 1987;15:138–148.
35. Casteleyn PP, Handelberg F, Opdecan P. Traumatic hemarthrosis of the knee. *J Bone Joint Surg Br* 1988;70:404–406.
36. Barrack RL, Buckley SL, Brucknes JD, et al. Partial versus complete acute anterior cruciate ligament tears. *J Bone Joint Surg Br* 1990;72J:622–627.
37. Noyes FR, Barber SD, Mangine RE. Bone-patellar ligament-bone and fascia latas allografts for reconstruction of the anterior cruciate ligament. *J Bone Joint Surg Am* 1990;72:1125–1136.
38. Noyes FR, Bassett RW, Grood ES, et al. Arthroscopy in acute traumatic hemarthrosis of the knee. *J Bone Joint Surg Am* 1980;62:687–695.
39. Kannus P, Jarvinen M. Conservatively treated tears of the anterior cruciate ligament. *J Bone Joint Surg Am* 1989;71:975–987.
40. Pattee GA, Fox JM, DelPizzo W, et al. Four to ten year followup of unreconstructed anterior cruciate ligament tears. *Am J Sports Med* 1989;17:430–435.
41. Belzer JP, Cannon D. Meniscus tears: treatment in the stable and unstable knee. *J Am Acad Orthop Surg* 1993;1:41–47.
42. Rubman MH, Noyes FR, Barber-Westin SD. Arthroscopic repair of meniscal tears that extend into the avascular zone: a review of 198 simple and complex tears. *Am J Sports Med* 1998;26:87–95.
43. Harner CD, Hoher J. Evaluation and treatment of posterior cruciate ligament injuries. *Am J Sports Med* 1998;26:471–482.
44. American Academy of Orthopaedic Surgery. *American Academy of Orthopaedic Surgery knowledge update.* Vol 2. Park Ridge, IL: American Academy of Orthopaedic Surgery, 1985.
45. Aglietti P, Insall JN, Cerulli G. Patella pain and incongruence. I. Measurements of incongruence. *Clin Orthop* 1983;176: 217–224.
46. Laurin CA, Lévesque HP, Dussault R, et al. The abnormal lateral patellofemoral angle: a diagnostic roentgenographic sign of recurrent patellar subluxation. *J Bone Joint Surg Am* 1978;60: 55–60.
47. Inoue M, Shino K, Hirose H, et al. Subluxation of the patella, computed tomography analysis of patellofemoral congruence. *J Bone Joint Surg Am* 1988;70:1331–1337.
48. Schutzer SF, Ramsby GR, Fulkerson JP. Computed tomographic classification of patellofemoral pain patients. *Orthop Clin North Am* 1986;17:235–248.
49. Arroll B, Ellis-Pegler E, Edwards A, et al. Patellofemoral pain syndrome: a critical review of nonoperative therapy. *Am J Sports Med* 1997;25:207–212.
50. Boden BP, Pearsall AW, Garrett WE, et al. Patellofemoral instability: evaluation and management. *J Am Acad Orthop Surg* 1997; 5:47–57.

99

PAINFUL FEET

JOSEPH J. BIUNDO
PERRY J. RUSH

Foot pain and loss of function may be caused by a multitude of maladies. As with other regions of the musculoskeletal system, the foot can manifest a large number of defined clinical entities. "Foot pain" is a symptom, not a diagnosis. A precise diagnosis should be made to ensure proper treatment, which is specific for that particular problem. Possible treatment may include medications, strategically placed local injections, thoughtfully chosen orthoses, exercise programs, and corrective surgery. Thus, if the physician perceives the problem simply as foot pain, it is unlikely that a successful outcome will ensue. The complaint of foot pain must be evaluated through a knowledgeable history taking, a hands-on physical examination, and selected imaging studies. The differential diagnosis takes place cognitively during this active process. Even though foot problems are extremely common, the foot is largely an ignored area. In chronic rheumatoid arthritis (RA), foot deformities occur in approximately 90% of patients (1). Typically, in general medicine, the foot is examined only for the presence of edema and the quality of pedal pulses. Even among rheumatologists, the foot often is not examined. A reluctance to ask the patient with impaired hand function to remove the shoes and socks may exist because of time constraints. The aesthetics of examining feet also may play a role. The biggest obstacle to a proper foot examination may, however, simply be the lack of expertise in this area.

Foot abnormalities may be clinically significant at any age. The infant can have clubfeet and other developmental defects, the young child can have one of the several osteochondroses, the adolescent can have tarsal coalition, and the young adult could have a spondyloarthritis involving the feet. Mechanical and degenerative problems become more prevalent with age, however, including such problems as hallux valgus, hallux rigidus, Morton's neuroma, and posterior tibial tendinitis and rupture. The anatomy of the foot is depicted in Fig. 99.1).

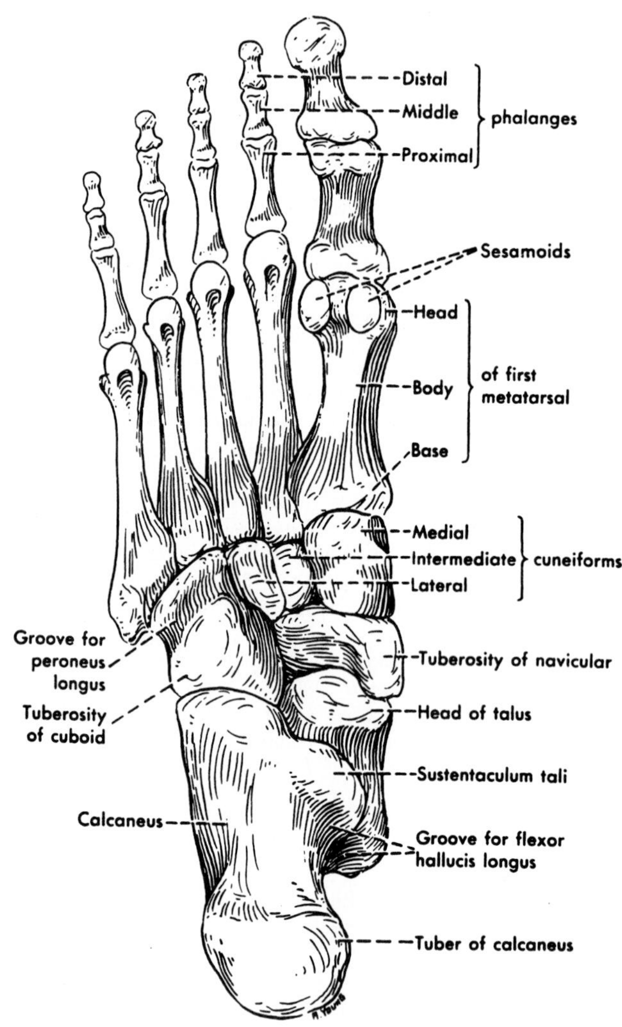

FIGURE 99.1. Plantar view of the bones of the foot. (Reproduced with permission from Hollinshead WH, Jenkins DB. *Functional anatomy of the limbs and back.* 5th ed. Philadelphia: WB Saunders, 1981:317.)

GAIT CYCLE AND BIOMECHANICS OF GAIT

To understand foot disorders and the prescription of appropriate foot orthoses, a basic comprehension of the normal gait cycle and the biomechanics of gait is essential (2,3). The normal gait cycle is divided into two main components, the stance phase which comprises 60% of the cycle, and the swing phase which comprises the remaining 40% (Fig. 99.2). The stance phase refers to contact of a limb with the floor. Five divisions of the stance phase exist: (a) heel strike, which is the initial contact of the heel with the floor; (b) foot-flat, which is the initial contact of the forefoot with the floor; (c) midstance, which occurs when the greater trochanter is in vertical alignment with the vertical bisector of the foot; (d) heel-off, which begins with plantar flexion and elevation of the heel; and (e) toe-off, the phase that begins with the elevation of the forefoot and ends at the point when the toes have left the floor. Other relevant terms include single support, which occurs when only one limb is in contact with the floor; double support, which occurs when both feet are simultaneously in contact with the floor; and push-off, which is a combination of the phases of heel-off and toe-off.

The swing phase of gait, which comprises 40% of the cycle, is divided into three phases: (a) acceleration, which occurs just as toe-off ends and the leg is posterior to the pelvis but moving anteriorly; (b) midswing, which occurs when the swinging limb passes the opposite limb in the stance phase, and the dorsiflexors of the ankle and foot contract to shorten the limb; and (c) deceleration, which occurs with eccentric contraction of the dorsiflexors to slow the movement of the limb, initiating heel strike.

The normal biomechanics of the foot and ankle are designed to absorb and direct the force occurring as a result of heel strike, foot plant, and toe push-off. The foot is unique in that it is flexible and rigid during different parts of the gait cycle. It becomes supple during the early part of stance and becomes rigid during the latter part of stance phase (4). As the foot is loaded, internal rotation of the tibia, eversion of the subtalar joint, dorsiflexion of the ankle (pronation), and abduction of the foot occur (5). Pronation is the flexible phase of heel strike in the gait cycle, allowing partial dissipation of the initial contact force. Supination is the stable configuration of the foot in which the subtalar joint is inverted and locked.

The key to understanding the foot is to start an evaluation from what is commonly known as the neutral position in which the talus and navicular bones and their related joint are congruous. In pes planus and hyperpronation, the longitudinal arch is depressed in midstance, and the foot does not supinate with toe-off. In pes cavus and limited subtalar motion, a decrease in ability of the foot to pronate and thereby dissipate the contact forces occurs. A tight Achilles tendon will limit ankle dorsiflexion, which leads to excessive pronation and abnormal stretching of the plantar fascia. Biomechanical stressors include running, sudden increase in activity, obesity, inadequate shoes, or prolonged standing or walking.

PHYSICAL EXAMINATION

A proper physical examination of the foot leads to the anatomic localization of the source of the pain symptoms, helps to identify the static and mechanical abnormalities of the foot, and aids in detecting an underlying disease (6–8). Look at the shoes for excessive wear on the heels and soles. Extreme lateral heel wear can signify hindfoot (calcaneal) varus. An examination of gait is valuable in diagnosing and treating many foot problems. The patient walks barefooted with the feet and ankles exposed, and the hindfoot, midfoot, and forefoot are separately viewed.

Observe the foot for swelling, deformity, and erythema or other skin changes. Palpation to detect tenderness is important for diagnosis. Palpate the subtalar joint in the neutral position for tenderness and alignment (9). Look for forefoot varus or forefoot valgus (Fig. 99.3). Examine the midtarsal area for tenderness and mobility. Examine for range of motion and tenderness or swelling of the metatarsophalangeal (MTP) joints. Check for hammer toes, cocked-up toes, and tenderness or swelling of toes. Observe the toenails for abnormalities. Check the calcaneus on the plantar surface for tenderness. Examine the Achilles tendon,

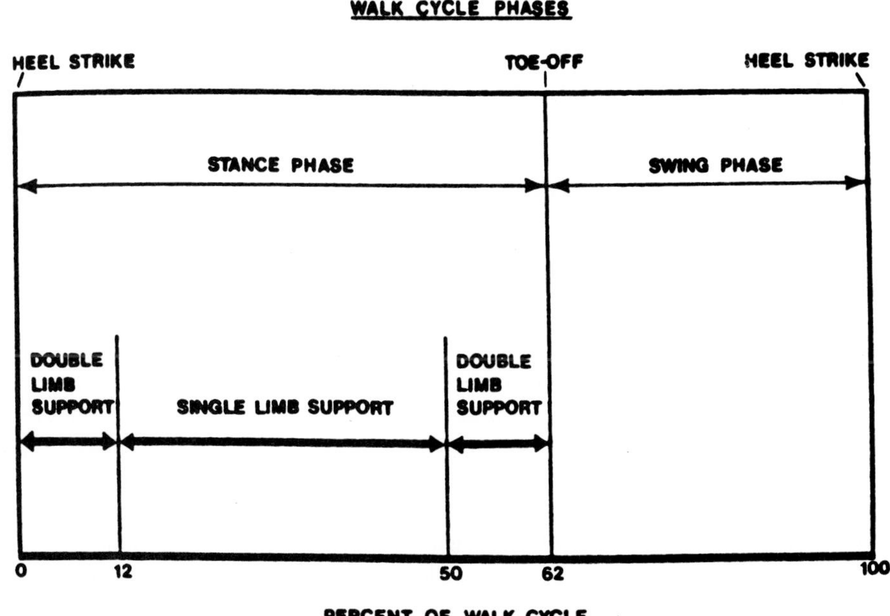

FIGURE 99.2. Gait cycle. (Reproduced with permission from Mann RA. Biomechanics of the foot and ankle. *Orthop Rev* 1978;7:43.)

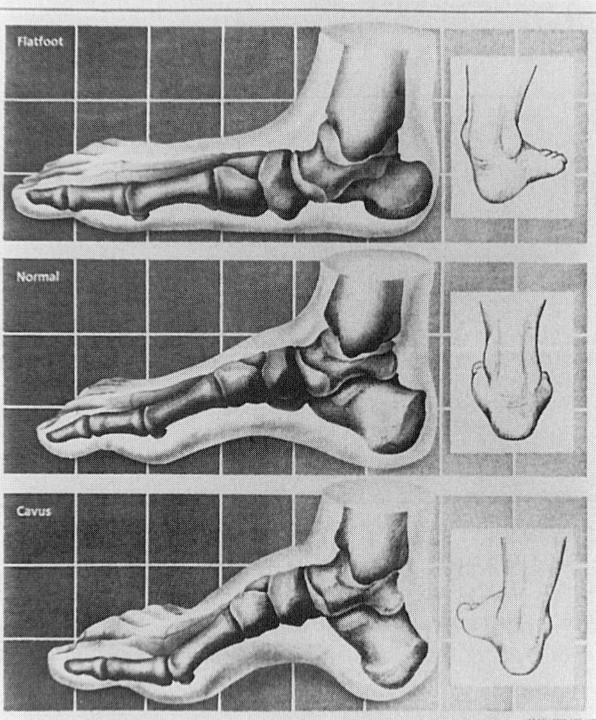

FIGURE 99.3. Feet are grouped into three types according to the way they function. The normal foot is supple on early weight-bearing and converts to a rigid structure for push-off. The flatfoot is supple and does not reconvert to form a rigid lever for push-off. In a flatfoot, the forefoot is typically abducted and in varus, and the heel is in valgus. The cavus foot is rigid and does not evert to become supple. In the cavus foot, the forefoot is adducted and in valgus. The heel in the cavus foot is in varus, and the first metatarsal is generally plantar flexed. (Reproduced with permission from Bordelon RL. Practical guide to foot orthoses. *J Musculoskeletal Med* 1989;6:73.)

retrocalcaneal bursa, posterior tibial tendon, and peroneal tendon for swelling, tenderness, subluxation, or rupture.

Identify calluses to reveal areas of excessive stresses on the foot. Describe the location of calluses. Identify corns, which are hyperkeratotic lesions secondary to pressure. Hard corns occur over bony prominences and typically are found on the lateral aspect of the fifth toe. Soft corns occur between the toes. Make note of the pulses. Check the spine for scoliosis and spinal mobility. Examine for hamstring and calf tightness, leg-length discrepancy, genu varus, genu valgus, patella position, and Q angle.

IMAGING OF THE FOOT

The standard plain radiograph views include the standing anteroposterior, standing lateral, and the oblique (pronated), depicting the medial aspect of the foot. It is important to obtain the anteroposterior and lateral radiographs in the standing position to demonstrate the anatomic relations of the foot in their functional position. In the lateral view, the x-ray

TABLE 99.1. INDICATIONS FOR SONOGRAPHY OF THE ANKLE AND FOOT

1. Tendon pathology: tenosynovitis, tendinosis, tendon tears, subluxation, or dislocation
2. Joint and bursal pathology: joint effusion, intraarticular loose bodies, or bursitis
3. Soft tissue pathology: foreign bodies, plantar fasciitis, Morton neuroma, ganglions, cellulites, or abscesses
4. Assessment when metallic artifact would limit imaging with MRI or CT
5. Guidance for intervention: joint aspiration, synovial or soft tissue biopsy, or joint or tendon sheath injection

Adapted from Fessell DP, Vanderschueten GM, Jacobson JA, et al. Ankle ultrasound: technique, anatomy and pathology. *Radiographics* 1998;18:325–340, with permission.
MRI, magnetic resonance imaging; CT, computed tomography.

beam passes from lateral to medial. Other special views are the lateral oblique (supinated) to visualize an accessory navicular bone; sesamoid view, which is an axial, oblique position (tilted lateral of sesamoids); and axial view of the heel (Harris) for calcaneal fractures and talocalcaneal coalition (10).

Computed tomography (CT) scanning is helpful in imaging the hindfoot, especially for subtalar joint pathology and fractures of the calcaneus. CT is beneficial in the diagnosis of fibrous and cartilaginous coalition, calcaneonavicular bony coalition, and talocalcaneal coalition. Magnetic resonance imaging (MRI) may be used to help diagnose tarsal coalition, osteomyelitis, osteonecrosis, tendinitis, tendon rupture, ligamentous injury, and osteochondral injuries of the talar dome (11). MRI is helpful in identifying soft tissue masses, such as ganglia, fibromatosis, Morton neuroma, and pigmented villonodular synovitis of the tendon sheath (12). Technetium bone scans can be used to determine stress fractures, especially of the metatarsals or calcaneus. Bone scans also are useful to detect inflammation in sites such as the plantar fascia (13). Diagnostic ultrasonography can help identify tendinitis and partial or complete tears of tendons of the foot, especially the Achilles tendon and the posterior tibial tendon. (14). Indications for the use of diagnostic ultrasonography are listed in Table 99.1.

MECHANICAL PROBLEMS

Forefoot Varus

This is an abnormality of the foot in which the forefoot is inverted in relation to the hindfoot when the subtalar joint is in the neutral position. The head of the first metatarsal is more dorsal than the head of the fifth metatarsal. The subtalar joint is in neutral position when the talonavicular joint is congruous. Forefoot varus is a major cause of compensatory subtalar pronation of an abnormal degree during the stance phase of gait. A foot orthosis with a medial wedge (post) may be needed to correct the biomechanical abnormality (Fig. 99.4) (15).

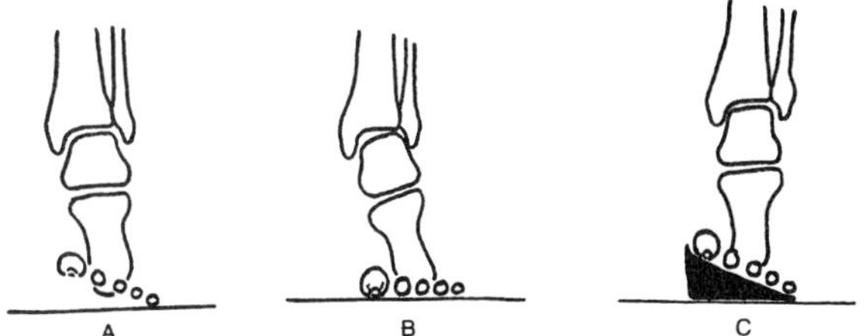

FIGURE 99.4. Demonstration of effect of biomechanical posting for abnormal forefoot and normal hindfoot. **A:** Foot in neutral position, showing the hindfoot in normal position and the forefoot in varus position. **B:** Demonstration of what happens when the foot hits the ground, with the foot collapsing so that the hindfoot is everted and the entire foot collapses. **C:** Correction of abnormality by placing a "post" beneath the medial side of the foot so that when the foot hits the ground, the hindfoot does not collapse, and normal function of the subtalar joint complex occurs. (Reproduced with permission from Bordelon RL. Orthotics, shoes, and braces. *Orthop Clin North Am* 1989;20:754.)

Forefoot Valgus

In this abnormality, the forefoot is everted in relation to the hindfoot when the subtalar joint is in neutral position. The fifth metatarsal head is more dorsal than the head of the first metatarsal head (15). A lateral wedge (post) orthosis may be needed to correct forefoot valgus (Fig. 99.5).

Hindfoot Valgus (Calcaneal Valgus, Rearfoot Valgus, Subtalar Valgus)

A lateral shift of the calcaneus occurs with medial rotation of the talus and a plantar drop of the talar head and navicular. This results in pronation of the foot and is seen in pes planus, RA, and posterior tibialis tendon rupture.

Hindfoot Varus

A medial shift of the calcaneus occurs. It is usually congenital and may be associated with pes cavus.

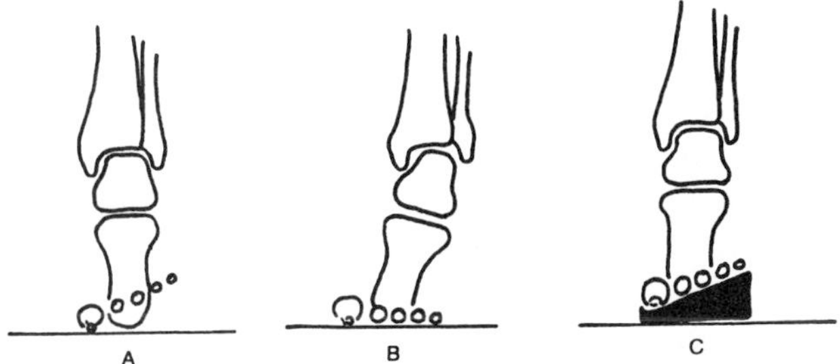

FIGURE 99.5. Demonstration of effect of lateral post. **A:** Examination of foot with foot in neutral position, showing valgus deformity of the forefoot. **B:** With weight bearing, the foot collapses and twists inward, producing an unstable foot with gait. **C:** Posting of lateral side of forefoot so that the subtalar joint complex remains in neutral during weight bearing, and the foot does not twist. (Reproduced with permission from Bordelon RL. Orthotics, shoes, and braces. *Orthop Clin North Am* 1989;20:755.)

Pes Planus

Pes planus, or flat feet, is often asymptomatic but may cause fatigue of the foot muscles and aching, with intolerance to prolonged walking or standing (16). The most common type is the flexible flatfoot (Fig. 99.3). Other causes of flatfoot are tarsal coalition, congenital vertical talus, and rupture of the tibialis posterior tendon, which causes the typical unilateral, acquired flatfoot. In pes planus, there is loss of the longitudinal arch on the medial side and prominence of the navicular bone and head of the talus. The calcaneus is everted (valgus), and on ambulation, out-toeing can be seen. The tendency for this condition is largely inherited and is seen with generalized hypermobility. A Thomas heel, firm shoes, grasping exercises to strengthen the intrinsic muscles, and toe walking to strengthen the tibialis posterior are helpful. A shoe orthosis may be needed for more severe cases. The asymptomatic flatfoot is left untreated.

Pes Cavus

An unusually high medial arch characterizes pes cavus, or claw foot, and in severe cases, a high longitudinal arch, resulting in shortening of the foot (Fig. 99.3) (16). These abnormally high arches result in some shortening of the extensor ligaments, causing dorsiflexion (extension) of the MTP joints and plantar flexion of the proximal interphalangeal and distal interphalangeal joints, thus giving the clawing appearance of the toes. The plantar fascia also may be contracted. The calcaneus is usually in a varus (inverted) position. Generally, a tendency to pes cavus is inherited, and in a high percentage of cases, an underlying neurologic disorder, such as myelomeningocele, Charcot-Marie-Tooth's disease, or Friedreich's ataxia, is present (17). Although pes cavus can cause foot fatigue and pain and tenderness over the metatarsal heads with callus formation, it also may be asymptomatic in the milder cases. Calluses also may be present over the dorsum of the toes. Use of metatarsal pads or bar is helpful, and stretching of the toe extensors is usually prescribed. In severe cases, surgical correction may be needed.

CLINICAL ENTITIES

Forefoot

Hallux Valgus

In hallux valgus, deviation of the large toe lateral to the midline and deviation of the first metatarsal medially occurs. A bunion (adventitious bursa) of the head of the first MTP joint may be present, often causing pain, tenderness, and swelling. Hallux valgus is more common in women and may be caused by a genetic tendency, wearing pointed shoes, or it can be secondary to RA or osteoarthritis (OA) (18). Stretching of shoes, use of bunion pads, or a surgical procedure may be indicated (19). Metatarsus primus varus, a condition in which the first metatarsal is angulated medially, is seen in association with, or secondary to, the hallux valgus deformity.

Hallux Rigidus

In hallux rigidus, immobility, especially on extension, of the first MTP joint is present. Limitation of plantar flexion also can occur. Pain is often present at the base of the big toe and is aggravated by walking, especially in high heels. A primary type of hallux rigidus is seen in younger persons, and the acquired form may be secondary to trauma, OA, RA, or gout. Osteophytes and sclerosis of the first MTP joint may be seen on radiographs. The term hallux limitus is sometimes used to denote a milder degree of immobility of the first MTP joint. The treatment of hallux rigidus generally consists of wearing shoes with a wide toe box and a rocker sole, because push-off during gait is limited. Surgery may be needed in some cases.

Bunionette

A bunionette, or tailor's bunion, is a prominence of the fifth metatarsal head resulting from the overlying bursa and a localized callus. The fifth metatarsal has a lateral (valgus) deviation (20). Pressure from shoewear can cause pain and tenderness may be present over the swollen bursa. Treatment consists of a wearing a shoe with a wide toe box, stretching of the shoe over the involved area, and use of a pad. In chronic, painful cases, surgical excision of the lateral eminence of the fifth metatarsal can be performed.

Hammer Toe

In hammer toe, the proximal interphalangeal joint is flexed, and the tip of the toe points downward (21). The second toe is most commonly involved. Calluses may form at the tip of the toe and over the dorsum of the interphalangeal joint, resulting from pressure against the shoe. Hammer toe may be congenital or acquired secondary to hallux valgus or improper footwear. When hammer toes are associated with hyperextension of the MTP joints, the deformity is known as "cocked-up toes." This may be seen in RA.

Metatarsalgia

Pain arising from the metatarsal heads, known as metatarsalgia, is a symptom resulting from a variety of conditions. Pain on standing and tenderness on palpation of the metatarsal heads are present. Calluses over the metatarsal heads are usually seen. The causes of metatarsalgia are many, including foot strain, use of high-heel shoes, everted foot, trauma, sesamoiditis, hallux valgus, arthritis, foot surgery, or a foot with a high longitudinal arch. Flattening of the transverse arch and weakness of the intrinsic muscles occur, resulting in a maldistribution of weight on the forefoot. Treatment is directed at elevating the middle portion of the transverse arch with an orthotic device, strengthening of the intrinsic muscles, weight reduction, and use of metatarsal pads or a metatarsal bar.

Metatarsal Stress Fracture

Stress fracture also is known as march fracture or fatigue fracture, because it was associated with a spontaneous fracture after long marches in army recruits. Pain, swelling, tenderness, and occasional erythema develop over the metatarsal area, usually without any clear history of trauma. On questioning, however, the episode of spontaneous pain related to the onset of the fracture can be identified in some cases. The neck of the second metatarsal bone is most frequently involved, but the other metatarsals also are sites of fracture. Athletic events, including jogging, or other activities stressful to the feet are common causes. Stress fractures may be seen in RA, generalized osteoporosis, or the elderly. The key to diagnosis of stress fractures of the foot is to have a high index of suspicion. The difficulty in making the diagnosis is that initial radiographs usually show no abnormalities or, at most, show only a faint fracture line (22). A repeated radiograph several weeks later may show healing with callus formation. Bone scans are essential to the early diagnosis and show an increase in uptake over the fracture site (Fig. 99.6) (23). Usually these fractures heal spontaneously, and rest and strapping of the foot or use of a postoperative shoe are helpful. Occasionally a cast may be needed.

Flexor Hallucis Longus Tendinitis

This tendon is the most posterior of the three tendons running posterior to the medial malleolus and passes through a fibroosseous tunnel. Inflammation can occur at this site, and triggering or snapping may develop as the tunnel becomes stenotic. In stenosing tenosynovitis, pain occurs during active plantar flexion of the big toe and on passive dorsiflexion. A snapping sensation may occur at the posteromedial aspect of the ankle. Occasionally, flexion of the big toe is impaired. A contracture of the flexor hallucis longus tendon is seen, and the big toe cannot be extended beyond neutral with the foot and ankle in neutral position or be passively extended with the ankle in plantar flexion. Rupture of the tendon can occur. Treatment of the tendinitis is usually conservative. Surgery may be used in severe cases.

Sesamoid Injuries

Lesions of the sesamoid bones of the big toe may exhibit local pain and tenderness under either the medial or lateral sesamoid (24). Pain may begin gradually or may be more abrupt after acute trauma, and usually increases with dorsiflexion of the digit or on weight bearing. Recognized causes of sesamoid pain, which has loosely been called sesamoidi-

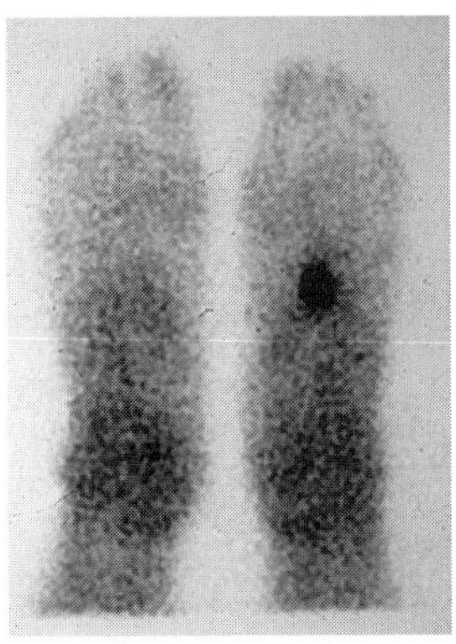

FIGURE 99.6. A plantar view on bone scan shows an intense uptake in metatarsal area of right foot, indicating a stress fracture.

tis, are repetitive strain from activities such as dancing or long-distance running, stress fracture, traumatic fracture, bipartite sesamoid, and osteochondritis (25). Treatment consists of eliminating the offending activity, avoidance of high heels, an orthosis that decreases weight bearing on the area, nonsteroidal antiinflammatory drugs (NSAIDs), and a local steroid injection. Surgery may be indicated to remove a painful, nonunited fractured sesamoid.

Freiberg's Disease

This condition is an osteochondrosis of the second metatarsal head, primarily affecting girls around age 12 years (26). Pain, tenderness, and swelling of the metatarsal are present. Fragmentation, sclerosis, and deformity of the metatarsal head are seen on radiographs. Treatment is aimed at reducing stress on the metatarsal joint with a metatarsal pad or metatarsal bar. Occasionally, a residual deformity with subsequent degenerative changes of the involved MTP joint occurs.

Midfoot

Sinus Tarsi Syndrome

Lateral foot pain and a feeling of instability of the ankle (27) characterize this syndrome. Marked tenderness is present on pressure over the sinus tarsi area. Prolonged standing, walking on uneven surfaces, or supination or adduction of the foot may initiate the pain. Rest usually alleviates the pain. Most patients with sinus tarsi syndrome have sustained either a single or repeated ankle sprain with an inversion injury (28). Other factors associated with the acquisition of this syndrome are inflammation from RA or gout and foot abnormalities such as pes cavus, pes planus with instability of the hindfoot, or forefoot valgus.

Usually, plain radiographs are negative. Subtalar arthrograms have revealed complete disappearance of the microrecesses along the interosseous ligament. MRI is helpful in identifying abnormalities of the interosseous talocalcaneal ligament, which fills the sinus tarsi (29).

Initial treatment often consists of a lidocaine and steroid injection into the sinus tarsi. If a biomechanical abnormality, such as forefoot valgus, is found, a foot orthosis is of benefit (30). In persistent cases, surgical excision of fatty tissue and part of the ligaments in the sinus tarsi may be performed. A triple arthrodesis has been successfully performed in a few reported cases.

Tarsal Coalition

Tarsal coalition is a fusion of two or more tarsal bones, and the connection may be fibrous (syndesmosis), cartilaginous (synchondrosis), or osseous (synostosis). The cause of coalition is congenital, but occasionally may be acquired because of trauma, prior foot surgery, inflammatory arthritis, degenerative arthritis, or infection.

The clinical manifestations consist of a dull pain of gradual onset that is perceived as foot fatigue or stiffness. Vigorous activities or prolonged standing may intensify the discomfort. The initial symptoms may follow such activity or begin after an injury such as an ankle sprain. On examination, limited or absent subtalar motion is usually present. Pes planus, tenderness of the medial aspect of the calcaneus (sustentaculum tali), and, occasionally, peroneal spasm may be found.

The most common site of involvement is a calcaneonavicular coalition, with 49% of cases in one study occurring at this location, whereas 37% were reported to have a talocalcaneal coalition (31). Talonavicular and calcaneocuboid coalitions were the next most frequent, and together totaled just under 10%.

On plain radiographs, the anteroposterior and lateral views usually fail to identify any bony union of the calcaneus and navicular or of the talus and calcaneus. A medial–oblique view of the foot, however, may reveal calcaneonavicular coalition, whereas an axial view (Harris–Beath view) of the foot can identify talocalcaneal coalition (32). A talar beak or large bony spur of the distal, dorsal surface of the talus may be seen in tarsal coalition. The subtalar joint may appear narrowed or tilted. CT is very helpful in diagnosis of fibrous and cartilaginous coalition, confirms calcaneonavicular bony coalition, and is excellent in diagnosing talocalcaneal coalition. MRI also can successfully identify tarsal coalition and is the most accurate technique to image fibrous coalitions (33).

Tarsal coalition may not cause symptoms. When present, however, symptoms are initially treated with NSAIDs, steroid injections, and shoeware modifications aimed at reducing stress on the talus, including heel wedges and closed-cell thermoplastic, polyethylene foam (Plastizote) inserts. Persistent symptoms may be treated with a walking cast for 3 to 6 weeks. A number of surgical procedures have been used in chronic cases, including resection of the coalition with interposition grafting or triple arthrodesis.

Kohler's Disease

This condition is an osteochondrosis of the navicular bone (26). The onset is gradual, beginning at about age 5 or 6 years and affecting boys more frequently. Occasionally, it is bilateral. Trauma is not thought to be the primary cause, but the initial pathology is that of avascular necrosis. The symptoms are discomfort over the dorsum of the foot and a limp. Tenderness and a mild swelling may be palpable over the affected navicular. A plain radiograph reveals a small, dense irregular navicular. Treatment is directed toward the pain, and a temporary medial arch support may be used. When more severe symptoms are present, immobilization with a splint may be used for a few weeks. The involved bone usually remodels to a correct form within 2 years.

Hindfoot

A complaint of heel pain is usually quite broad, and because heel pain can emanate from a number of different anatomic sites and from a number of different causes, it is essential to identify the specific location. The potential sites include the plantar surface (subcalcaneal), or posterior, medial, or lateral aspect of the heel.

Achilles Tendinitis

Achilles tendinitis usually results from trauma, athletic overactivity, or improperly fitting shoes with a stiff heel counter, but also can arise from inflammatory conditions such as ankylosing spondylitis, Reiter's syndrome, gout, RA, and calcium pyrophosphate deposition disease. Pain, swelling, and tenderness occur over the Achilles tendon at its attachment and in the area proximal to the attachment. Crepitus on motion and pain on dorsiflexion may be present. Management includes NSAIDs, rest, shoe corrections, heel lift, gentle stretching, and sometimes a splint with slight plantar flexion. The Achilles tendon is vulnerable to rupture, and the tendon itself must not be injected with a corticosteroid. However, peritendinous steroid injections for achillodynia have been reported (34).

Achilles Tendon Rupture

Spontaneous rupture of the Achilles tendon is well known and occurs with a sudden onset of pain during forced dorsiflexion (35). An audible snap may be heard, followed by difficulty in walking and standing on toes. Swelling and edema over the area usually develops. Diagnosis can be made with the Thompson test, in which the patient kneels on the chair with the feet extending over the edge, and the examiner squeezes the calf and pushes toward the knee. Normally this produces plantar flexion, but in a ruptured tendon, no plantar flexion occurs. Achilles tendon rupture is generally due to athletic events or trauma from jumps or falls. MRI can aid in the diagnosis and can distinguish a complete rupture from a partial one (36). The tendon is more prone to tear in persons having preexisting Achilles tendon disease or in those taking corticosteroids (37). Immobilization or surgery may be selected, depending on the situation (38).

Retrocalcaneal Bursitis

The retrocalcaneal bursa is located between the inside surface of the Achilles tendon and the calcaneus. The bursa's anterior wall is fibrocartilage where it attaches to the calcaneus, whereas its posterior wall blends with the epitenon of the Achilles tendon. Manifestations are pain at the back of the heel, tenderness of the area anterior to the Achilles tendon, and pain on dorsiflexion. Local swelling is present, with bulging on the medial and lateral aspects of the tendon. Retrocalcaneal bursitis, also called sub-Achilles bursitis, may coexist with Achilles tendinitis, and distinguishing the two is sometimes difficult. This condition may be secondary to RA, spondylitis, Reiter's syndrome, gout, and trauma. The treatment consists of NSAIDs, rest, and a local injection of a corticosteroid carefully directed into the bursa (39).

Subcutaneous Achilles Bursitis

A subcutaneous bursa posterior to the Achilles tendon may become swollen in the absence of systemic disease. This bursitis, known as "pump-bumps," is seen predominantly in women and results from pressure of shoes, although it also can result from bony exostoses. Other than relief from shoe pressure, no treatment is indicated.

Sever's Disease

This condition occurs especially in boys between the ages of 8 and 15 years and is characterized by pain, tenderness, and mild swelling involving the posterior heel (26). The pathology is a chronic sprain or partial avulsion of the calcaneal apophysis, which is the site where the Achilles tendon attaches to the calcaneus. Radiographs show the epiphyses to be irregular or segmented with areas of increased density. Somewhat problematic, however, is that such changes are seen in asymptomatic children and may be part of the normal ossification. The disorder is self-limiting, with improvement occurring in less than a year. Treatment includes prescription of a heel pad, reduction in activities, and use of a heel lift to reduce the traction of the Achilles tendon at its attachment during walking.

Plantar Fasciitis (Subcalcaneal Pain Syndrome)

Plantar fasciitis occurs primarily between 40 and 60 years of age. A gradual onset of pain in the plantar area of the heel usually occurs, but it may occur after trauma or from overuse after activities such as athletics, prolonged walking, wearing of improper shoes, or striking the heel with some force (40–43). The pain characteristically occurs in the

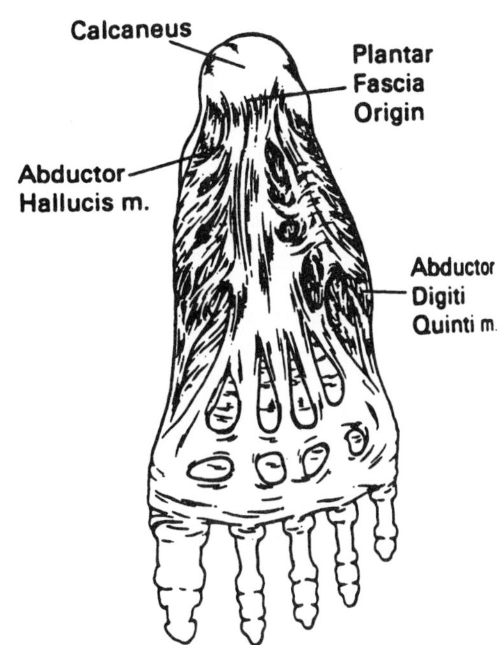

FIGURE 99.7. Anatomy of plantar fascia. (Reproduced with permission from Schepsis AA, Leach RE, Gorzyca J. Plantar fasciitis: etiology, treatment, surgical results, and review of the literature. *Clin Orthop* 1991;266:186.)

morning on arising. It is most severe for the first few steps. After an initial improvement, the pain may get worse later in the day, especially after prolonged standing or walking. The pain is burning, aching, and occasionally lancinating. Palpation typically reveals tenderness anteromedially on the medial calcaneal tubercle at the origin of the plantar fascia (Fig. 99.7). Less common is central heel tenderness. Passive stretching of the plantar fascia and eversion of the foot may exacerbate symptoms.

The pain is the result of degenerative changes in the origin of the plantar fascia and traction periostitis of the medial calcaneal tubercle resulting from overload. Over time and with repetitive stress, microtears can occur in the origin of the plantar fascia, generating an inflammatory response consisting of collagen necrosis, angiofibroblastic hyperplasia, mucinoid degeneration, chondroid metaplasia, and matrix calcification (41).

Most patients with heel pain have calcaneal spurs, but some do not. The spur itself is not likely to cause pain unless it is directed vertically downward. Calcaneal spurs are commonly seen in patients with spondyloarthropathies, and plantar fasciitis may be the presenting problem in such patients (44). Less common than plantar fasciitis, subcalcaneal pain also may occur from entrapment of the nerve to the abductor digiti quinti muscle, fat atrophy of the heel pad, or calcaneal stress fracture (42).

Treatment includes relative rest with a reduction in stressful activities, NSAIDs, and use of a heel pad or heel cup orthosis (45). A night splint with 5 degrees of dorsiflexion may help (43,46). Stretching of the calf muscles and plantar fascia is very important in the treatment. In some cases, physical therapy with strengthening, modalities with contrast baths, or ultrasound may be prescribed along with the stretching. A local injection, with a 25-gauge needle, with a corticosteroid is often of help. Ionotophoresis of dexamethasone also has been used to treat plantar fasciitis (47). Surgery may be indicated in chronic cases.

Posterior Tibial Tendinitis

Pain, swelling, and localized tenderness just posterior to the medial malleolus occurs in posterior tibial tendinitis (48). Extension and flexion may be normal, but pain is present on resisted inversion or passive eversion. The discomfort is usually worse after athletic events. Treatment is usually rest, NSAIDs, and possibly a local injection of a corticosteroid (49). Immobilization with a splint is sometimes needed.

Posterior Tibialis Tendon Rupture

Rupture of the posterior tibialis tendon, which is not commonly recognized, is a cause of progressive flatfoot (50–53). It may be caused by trauma, chronic tendon degeneration, or RA (54). An insidious onset of pain, swelling, and tenderness occurs along the course of the tendon just distal to the medial malleolus. The unilateral deformity of hindfoot valgus and forefoot abduction is an important finding. The forefoot abduction can best be seen from behind; more toes are seen from this position than would be seen normally. The result of the single heel rise test is positive when the patient is unable to rise onto the ball of the affected foot while the contralateral foot is off the floor. CT and MRI are helpful in the diagnosis of tendon rupture (52). Orthopedic consultation may help to determine whether the rupture should be treated conservatively with NSAIDs and casting or with a surgical repair.

Peroneal Tendon Dislocation and Peroneal Tendinitis

Dislocation of the peroneal tendon may occur from a direct blow, repetitive trauma, or sudden dorsiflexion with eversion (55,56). Sometimes a painless snapping noise is heard at the time of dislocation. Other patients report more severe pain and tenderness of the tendon area where it lies over the lateral malleolus. The condition may be confused with an acute ankle sprain. Conservative treatment with immobilization is often satisfactory because the peroneal tendon usually reduces spontaneously. If the retinaculum supporting the tendon is ruptured, however, surgical correction may be required. Peroneal tendinitis is manifested as localized tenderness and swelling over the lateral malleolus (56,57). Conservative treatment is usually indicated.

Neurologic Lesions

The foot is a frequent site of neurologic symptoms, some of which are common, whereas others are rare. The usual symptom is numbness of some portion of the foot, but this complaint is often ignored as being nonspecific. The symptoms are often not well described by the patient. Moreover, the patient is often not questioned by the physician in a manner specific enough to elicit a proper description of the problem. As with the upper extremity, numbness is often misinterpreted by the patient, and sometimes by the physician, as being due to "poor circulation." The symptoms of numbness, tingling, paresthesias, burning pain, or pins-and-needle sensation should first point to a possible neurologic lesion. The most common cause of numbness of the feet is peripheral neuropathy. If suspected, this can be confirmed by electrodiagnostic studies. A number of other local entities causing numbness of the foot, however, also should be considered.

Morton's Neuroma

Middle-aged women are most frequently affected by Morton's neuroma, an entrapment neuropathy of the interdigital nerve occurring most often between the third and fourth toe (58). Paresthesias and a burning, aching type of pain are usually experienced in the fourth toe. The symptoms are made worse by walking on hard surfaces or wearing tight shoes or high-heel shoes. Tenderness may be elicited by palpation between the third and fourth metatarsal heads. Occasionally a neuroma is seen between the second and third toes. Compression of the interdigital nerve by the transverse metatarsal ligament and possibly by an intermetatarsophalangeal bursa or synovial cyst may be responsible for the entrapment (59). Zanetti et al. (60) illustrated with excellent images the difficulty of diagnosing Morton neuroma only by clinical examination and the value of MRI in influencing diagnostic and therapeutic decisions.

Treatment of Morton's neuroma is usually with a metatarsal bar or pad or a local steroid injection into the web space (61). Ultimately, surgical excision of the neuroma and a portion of the nerve may be needed.

Tarsal Tunnel Syndrome

In tarsal tunnel syndrome, the posterior tibial nerve is compressed at or near the flexor retinaculum, which is located posterior and inferior to the medial malleolus. Just distal to the retinaculum, the nerve divides into the medial plantar, lateral plantar, and posterior calcaneal branches. Numbness, burning pain, and paresthesias of the toes and sole extend proximally to the area over the medial malleolus (62,63). Nocturnal exacerbation may be reported. The patient usually gets some relief by leg, foot, and ankle movements. A positive Tinel's sign is elicited on percussion posterior to the medial malleolus, and loss of pin-prick and two-point discrimination may be present. Women are more often affected. Trauma to the foot, especially fracture, valgus foot deformity, hypermobility, occupational factors, and synovitis may contribute to development of the tarsal tunnel syndrome (64). An electrodiagnostic test may show prolonged motor and sensory latencies and slowing of the nerve-conduction velocities (62,63,65). Additionally, a tourniquet test and pressure over the flexor retinaculum can induce symptoms. Shoe corrections and steroid injection into the tarsal tunnel may be of benefit, but often surgical decompression is needed (63).

Anterior Tarsal Tunnel Syndrome (Deep Peroneal Nerve Entrapment)

This is an entrapment neuropathy of the deep peroneal nerve at the inferior extensor retinaculum on the dorsum of the foot. The symptoms consist of numbness and paresthesias over the dorsum of the foot, especially at the web space (66). A tight feeling may be described over the anterior aspect of the ankle. The symptoms may arise after the wearing of tight shoes or high heels. Other causes include contusion of the dorsum of the foot, metatarsal fracture, talonavicular osteophytosis, and ganglion (67). Symptoms also tend to occur in bed at night and are relieved by standing or walking. Hypesthesia and hypalgesia may be present in the first dorsal web space, and a Tinel's sign may be elicited on percussion just anterosuperior to the medial malleolus. The extensor digitorum brevis may be atrophied and weak.

A diagnosis of anterior tarsal tunnel syndrome may be confirmed by electrodiagnostic studies (68). Conservative measures include avoiding shoes that might stretch or compress the nerve. Steroid injections have been used. In persistent cases, the deep peroneal nerve can be decompressed at the retinaculum (66).

Superficial Peroneal Nerve Entrapment (Intermediate and Medial Dorsal Cutaneous Nerves)

The superficial peroneal nerve bifurcates into the intermediate dorsal cutaneous and the medial dorsal cutaneous terminal nerves. The lateral aspect of the foot is usually innervated by a branch of the sural nerve, the lateral dorsal cutaneous nerve. When this branch is absent, then the intermediate branch of the superficial peroneal nerve supplies the innervation to the lateral foot.

The symptoms are pain, numbness, or tingling over the lateral aspect of the dorsum of the foot, worsened by exercise and often becoming more severe at night (69). The intermediate dorsal cutaneous branch, being very superficial, can be observed and palpated on plantar-flexing and inverting the foot. If this branch of the nerve is entrapped, then compression at this site will reproduce symptoms. A Tinel's sign is usually present. A decrease in sensation to light touch and pin prick may be present in the cutaneous distribution of the nerve.

The most common cause of this neuropathy is acute and chronic ankle sprains. Other causes include OA of tarsal bones and muscle herniation in the anterior compartment. Because the intermediate branch is so superficial, it is very susceptible to trauma, and may be the source of chronic posttrauma ankle and foot pain. Electrodiagnostic studies with abnormal sensory conduction velocity and prolonged distal latency help confirm the diagnosis. The treatment is a local steroid injection or, if persistent, surgical decompression.

Sural Nerve Entrapment

Entrapment of the sural nerve, although uncommon, may be overlooked because of its limited cutaneous distribution. This nerve, which is formed from branches of the posterior tibial and common peroneal nerves, descends lateral to the Achilles tendon, and after passing the lateral malleolus, the nerve turns anteriorly and continues as the lateral dorsal cutaneous nerve along the lateral side of the foot and the fifth toe.

The manifestations are numbness and a burning pain along the lateral side of the dorsum of the foot, which may be worse at night (70). A decrease in sensation and a Tinel's sign may be present. Trauma, scar tissue, and ganglia have been reported as causes of entrapment (71). Local decompression can relieve the symptoms.

FOOT REHABILITATION

Orthoses

Orthotics is the field of correcting foot deformities by means of external support; the name was coined by Nickel in 1953 (72). The devices used for this task are known as orthoses and not orthotics. These orthoses (orthotic devices) are used to relieve and/or cushion an area of pressure, support an area of collapse, or convert a biomechanically abnormal foot into a biomechanically functional foot during the stance phase of gait (15,16,73). In short, these mechanical devices help restore lost function or help maintain optimal function by altering biomechanics. Orthoses may provide pain relief and compensate for muscle and ligament weakness by decreasing forces passing through painful weight-bearing areas, stabilizing or immobilizing subluxing joints, and repositioning toes.

The range of these orthotic devices varies from simple inexpensive pads available in drug stores to complex, expensive, custom-made orthoses. The importance and value of foot orthoses in the treatment of foot disorders is often underrecognized. The physician should establish a relationship with a pedorthotist (an orthotist who is trained in foot devices), an orthotist, or a trained therapist who can fabricate orthoses that are specific for the problem (74).

Foot orthoses can be divided into three types: devices that relieve pressure on various parts of the foot; those that cushion the foot and decrease impact; and those that are custom made to correct abnormal biomechanics and restore better functioning foot (9,16). Orthoses that relieve pressure on specific areas of the foot are generally foam or felt with an adhesive backing. These can be shaped specifically for pressure areas such as under the first, second, or fifth metatarsal heads. The pad is placed just proximal to the area of pressure.

The second type of orthosis, which reduces impact and cushions the foot, is constructed of material such as Spenco, which is composed of microcellular rubber. These are transferable to different shoes and are used in mild cases. Spenco is available in most sporting goods and foot-care product stores. Additional materials used in orthoses that reduce impact and cushion the foot are Plastizote, Pelite, and Aliplast, which are closed-cell thermoplastic, polyethylene foam devices, and Sorbothane, a viscoelastic material. The material can be molded to the contour of the foot.

The third type of orthosis is the biomechanical custom-fabricated type, which attempts to restore the subtalar joint to a neutral position. These may be rigid, semiflexible, or soft, depending on the need. The thermoplastic materials are the semiflexible types. The rigid type is usually composed of an acrylic, rigid polyurethane foam, or polypropylene (74,75). As part of this type of orthosis, a "post," which is a wedge, can be incorporated to support the foot and correct the abnormality (Figs. 99.4 and 99.5) (15,16,73). If forefoot varus is present, then a medial post is used; and if forefoot valgus is present, then a lateral post is devised. Likewise, a medial post is used to correct pronation (eversion) of the hindfoot, whereas a lateral post is used to correct hindfoot supination (inversion). Typically, a custom-made orthosis may incorporate several features to address the foot problems, and if needed, all three types of foot orthoses can be combined into one orthosis (74). A depression can be made in the orthosis to relieve pressure in a specific area. Larger than normal or extra-depth shoes are needed for the orthosis to fit comfortably.

Ligament laxity is common in many inflammatory rheumatic diseases, often resulting in subluxation of joints. Subluxation of the MTP joint results in broadening of the forefoot, clawing of toes, and painful weight bearing on MTP heads. Callus, a protective reaction of the skin to stress, may be seen on the bottom of the foot. An internal or external metatarsal bar or pad can be placed in, or on, the shoes just behind the metatarsal heads to redistribute the weight away from this area to the metatarsal shafts. Alternatively, a metatarsal corset (a metatarsal pad attached directly to a toe with a strap, inside the sock) may be used in any shoe. Joint subluxation also results in loss of foot arches, uneven weight distribution, and pain. Arch supports such as a medial longitudinal arch support placed in the shoe can reform these arches. Spacers can be placed between toes to prevent overlapping and secondary calluses.

Shoe Modification

It is important to have a general understanding of shoe construction and available shoe modifications to help treat foot problems (76,77). As a start, one can simply examine shoe bottoms for wear and tear to determine the abnormal forces involved. A variety of modifications can be made. Extra-depth shoes with a large toebox should be used to accommodate fixed deformities such as clawed toes and to provide room for foot and ankle–foot orthoses (AFOs). Otherwise, corns may develop where the proximal interphalangeal joints of the toes or other parts of the foot rub on the superior part of the shoe. For patients with toe deformities, shoe closures can be modified. Traditional shoelaces can be changed to Velcro closures. Elastic laces can replace regular laces, effectively turning the shoe into a loafer type. Shoes with proper closures are generally preferred to loafers, however, as loafers maintain their place on the foot by tension.

A Thomas heel, which is a medial extension of the heel, may be added to support the longitudinal arch (78). Replacing the regular shoe heel with a "solid ankle cushion heel" may be helpful for heel pain or a fused ankle, as this heel can simulate ankle plantar flexion while walking (78). A rocker-bottom sole may be helpful for a fused ankle, hallux rigidus, or other toe deformities by substituting for the push-off and heel-strike phases of walking.

Lighter shoes are easier to wear, but have less stability and durability. Heavier shoes may have greater stability and durability, but are more difficult to carry. Ultimately, the shoe must be comfortable, have a good fit, and be aesthetically appealing. Otherwise, it will not be used. One can always advise patients to wear their special shoes at home and on the way to work and change when they get there.

In a leg-length discrepancy, a lift can be attached to the outside of the whole shoe of the short leg, and not just to the sole or heel. The shoe raise should be half to three fourths of the leg-length discrepancy. The difference should probably be greater than 1 cm to consider correcting. However, if the leg-length discrepancy is not a recent event, and especially if it is asymptomatic, it is probably best left untreated, because changing walking biomechanics after years of compensation may result in new symptoms.

Braces

A patellar tendon–bearing orthosis is helpful for the problem of pain and limitation in ambulation due to destructive changes of the ankle or subtalar joint subsequent to RA or other inflammatory arthritis (79). This patellar tendon–bearing brace, which provides weight bearing on the patellar tendon and tibial condyles through a molded upper-calf band, has a fixed ankle and a rocker-bottom sole. Thus, weight of the upper body can be directly transmitted from the knee region and calf to the floor, bypassing the ankle (Fig. 99.8) (80). This patellar tendon–bearing brace also is used to decrease stress on the ankle or subtalar joints in other conditions such as severe OA, Charcot joint, and nonunited fractures of the lower limb (81).

Other Modalities

The most commonly used modalities are heat and cold. Methods of superficial heating for the feet include hot packs, heating pads, hydrocollator packs, hot-water bottles, heated whirlpools, and infrared lamps. Hydrotherapy in a whirlpool can provide superficial heat to the whole foot. At home, hot baths and foot soaks, especially in the morning, can be used for relief. Ultrasound may be used to heat tendons and deeper structures.

Cooling of tissues can be obtained with coolant sprays, ice packs, basins of ice water, and frozen-food packages. Cooling also causes vasoconstriction with a reduction of blood flow and a decrease in metabolic activity in the region treated. Generally patients seem to prefer heat, however. Both heat and cold may be used alternatively as a contrast bath.

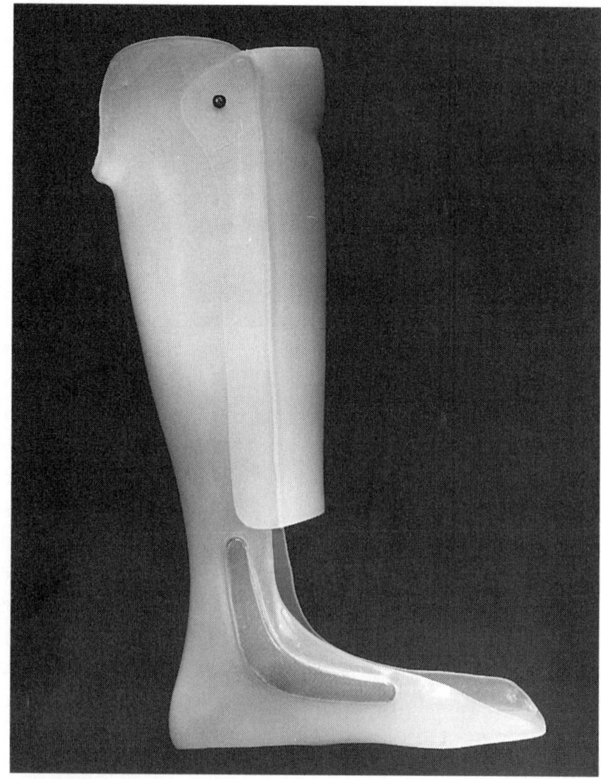

FIGURE 99.8. Patellar tendon– bearing orthosis used to decrease weight on ankle or subtalar joints.

Therapeutic Exercises

Therapeutic exercises may be broadly classified into three groups: (a) range of motion or stretching, (b) strengthening (resistive), and (c) aerobic (endurance). In many cases, a simple home exercise program is adequate and may be taught to the patient by the physician. Other cases require the prescription of a more formal physical therapy program. An exercise prescription should include the exercise frequency, intensity, type, and duration (timing), with the acronym FITT.

Range-of-motion exercises are important during the active phase of an inflammatory arthritis to maintain mobility of the ankle, subtalar, tarsal, and MTP joints. Ankle exercises include foot circles, active dorsiflexion, and plantar flexion. Writing the alphabet with the toes and cloth tugs with the toes and foot provide range of motion to the joints of the foot (82). After the acute phase has resolved, strengthening exercises against a resistance can be used (82). The ankle may be stretched with a rubber tubing. Patients can be asked to push their feet against a board attached to the bed. Bicycle riding, swimming, and a rowing machine are non–weight-bearing exercises that can help maintain cardiovascular conditioning.

REFERENCES

1. Calabro JJ. A critical evaluation of the diagnostic features of the feet in rheumatoid arthritis. *Arthritis Rheum* 1962;5:19–29.
2. Mann RA. Biomechanics of the foot and ankle. *Orthop Rev* 1978; 7:43–48.
3. Morris JM. Biomechanics of the foot and ankle. *Clin Orthop* 1977;122:10–17.
4. Mann RA. Biomechanics of the foot and ankle. In: Sammarco GJ, ed. *Foot and ankle manual.* Philadelphia: Lea & Febiger, 1991:32–41.
5. Perry J. Anatomy and biomechanics of the hindfoot. *Clin Orthop* 1983;177:9–15.
6. Shereff MJ. Clinical evaluation of the foot and ankle. In: Sammarco GJ, ed. *Foot and ankle manual.* Philadelphia: Lea & Febiger, 1991:42–53.
7. Smith RW. Evaluation of the adult forefoot. *Clin Orthop* 1979;142:19–23.
8. Polly HF, Hunder GG. The ankle and foot. In: *Physical examination of the joints.* 2nd ed. Philadelphia: WB Saunders, 1978: 239–274.
9. Riegler HF. Orthotic devices for the foot. *Orthop Rev* 1987;16: 293–303.
10. Brodsky JW. Radiology of the foot and ankle. In: Sammarco GJ, ed. *Foot and ankle manual.* Philadelphia: Lea & Febiger, 1991:54–67.
11. Beltran J. Magnetic resonance imaging of the ankle and foot. *Orthopedics* 1994;17:1075–1082.
12. Llauger J, Palmer J, Monill JM, et al. MR imaging of benign soft-tissue masses of the foot and ankle. *Radiographics* 1998;18: 1481–1498.
13. Graham CE. Painful heel syndrome: rationale of diagnosis and treatment. *Foot Ankle* 1983;3:261–267.
14. Klebo P, Allenmark C, Peterson L, Sward L. Diagnostic value of ultrasonography in partial ruptures of the Achilles tendon. *Am J Sports Med* 1992;20:378–381.
15. Bordelon RL. Orthotics, shoes, and braces. *Orthop Clin North Am* 1989;20:751–751.
16. Bordelon RL. Practical guide to foot orthoses. *J Musculoskeletal Med* 1989;6:71–87.
17. Ritterbusch JF, Drennan JC. The cavus foot: a review. *Contemp Orthop* 1992;24:525–532.
18. Inman VT. Hallux valgus: a review of etiologic factors. *Orthop Clin North Am* 1974;5:59–66.
19. Mann RA. Bunion surgery: decision making. *Orthopedics* 1990; 13:951–957.
20. Nestor BJ, Kitaoka HB, Illstrup DM, et al. Radiologic anatomy of the painful bunionette. *Foot Ankle* 1990;11:6–11.
21. Coughlin MJ. Lesser toe deformities. *Orthopedics* 1987;10:63–75.
22. Santi M, Sarttoris DJ, Resnick D. Diagnostic imaging of tarsal and metatarsal stress fractures. *Orthop Rev* 1989;18:178–185.
23. Prather JL, Nusynowitz ML, Snowdy HA, et al. Scintigraphic findings in stress fractures. *J Bone Joint Surg Am* 1977;59: 869–874.
24. Jahss MH. The sesamoids of the hallux. *Clin Orthop* 1981;157: 88–97.
25. Dietzen CJ. Great toe sesamoid injuries in the athlete. *Orthop Rev* 1990;19:966–972.
26. Brower AC. The osteochondroses. *Orthop Clin North Am* 1983; 14:99–117.
27. Kjaersgaard-Andersen P, Andersen K, Soballe K, et al. Sinus tarsi syndrome: presentation of seven cases and review of the literature. *J Foot Surg* 1989;28:3–6.
28. Taillard W, Meyer J-M, Garcia J, et al. The sinus tarsi syndrome. *Int Orthop* 1981;5:117–130.
29. Klein MA, Spreitzer AM. MR imaging of the tarsal sinus and canal: normal anatomy, pathologic findings, and features of the sinus tarsi syndrome. *Radiology* 1993;186:233–240.
30. Shear MS, Baitch SP, Shear DB. Sinus tarsi syndrome: the importance of biomechanically based evaluation and treatment. *Arch Phys Med Rehabil* 1993;74:777–781.
31. Carson CW, Ginsburg WW, Cohen MD, et al. Tarsal coalition: an unusual cause of foot pain: clinical spectrum and treatment in 129 patients. *Semin Arthritis Rheum* 1991;20:367–377.
32. Sartoris DJ, Resnick DL. Tarsal coalition. *Arthritis Rheum* 1985; 28:331–338.
33. Wechsler RJ, Schweitzer ME, Deely DM. Tarsal coalition: depiction and characterization with CT and MR imaging. *Radiology* 1994;193:447–452.
34. Reed MT. Safe relief of rest pain that eases with activity in achillodynia by intrabursal or peritendinous steroid injection: the rupture rate was not increased by these steroid injections. *Br J Sports Med* 1999;33:134–135.
35. Wills CA, Washburn MD, Caiozzo V, et al. Achilles tendon rupture: a review of the literature comparing surgical versus nonsurgical treatment. *Clin Orthop* 1986;207:156–163.
36. Panageas E, Greenberg S, Franklin PD, et al. Magnetic resonance imaging of pathologic conditions of the Achilles tendon. *Orthop Rev* 1990;19:975–980.
37. Holmes GB, Mann RA, Wells L. Epidemiologic factors associated with rupture of the Achilles tendon. *Contemp Orthop* 1991; 23:327–331.
38. Maffulli N. Rupture of the Achilles tendon. *J Bone Joint Surg* 1999;81:1019–1036.
39. Canoso JJ, Wohgethan JR, Newberg AH, et al. Aspiration of the retrocalcaneal bursa. *Ann Rheum Dis* 1984;43:308–312.
40. Baxter DE, Pfeffer GB, Thigpen M. Chronic heel pain: treatment rationale. *Orthop Clin North Am* 1989;20:563–569.
41. DeMaio M, Paine R, Mangine RE, et al. Plantar fasciitis. *Orthopedics* 1993;16:1153–1163.
42. Karr SD. Subcalcaneal heel pain. *Orthop Clin North Am* 1994; 25:161–175.

43. Michelson JD. Heel pain: when is it plantar fasciitis? *J Musculoskeletal Med* 1995;12:22–29.
44. Sebes JI. the significance of calcaneal spurs in rheumatic diseases. *Arthritis Rheum* 1989;32:338–340.
45. Martin RL, Irrgang JJ, Conti SF. Outcome study of subjects with insertional plantar fasciitis. *Foot Ankle Int* 1998;19:803–811.
46. Powell M, Post WR, Keener J, et al. Effective treatment of chronic plantar fasciitis with dorsiflexion night splints: a crossover prospective randomized outcome study. *Foot Ankle Int* 19998;19:10–18.
47. Gudeman SD, Eisele SA, Heidt RS, et al. Treatment of plantar fasciitis by iontophoresis of 0.45 dexamethasone: a randomized, double-blind, placebo-controlled study. *Am J Sports Med* 1998; 25:312–316.
48. Conti SF. Posterior tibial tendon problems in athletes. *Orthop Clin North Am* 1994;25:109–121.
49. Cozen L. Posterior tibial tenosynovitis secondary to foot strain. *Clin Orthop* 1965;42:101–102.
50. Mann RA, Thompson FA. Rupture of the posterior tibial tendon causing flat foot. *J Bone Joint Surg Am* 1985;67:556–561.
51. Supple KM, Hanft JR, Murphy BJ, et al. Posterior tibial tendon dysfunction. *Semin Arthritis Rheum* 1992;22:106–113.
52. Rosenberg ZS, Cheung Y, Jahss MH, et al. Rupture of posterior tibial tendon: CT and MR imaging with surgical correlation. *Radiology* 1988;169:229–235.
53. Churchill RS, Sferra JJ. Posterior tibial tendon insufficiency: its diagnosis, management, and treatment. *Am J Orthop* 1998;27: 339–347.
54. Downey DJ, Simkin PA, Mack LA, et al. Tibialis posterior tendon rupture: a cause of rheumatoid flat foot. *Arthritis Rheum* 1988;31:441–446.
55. Arrowsmith SR, Fleming LL, Allman FL. Traumatic dislocations of the peroneal tendons. *Am J Sports Med* 1983;11:142–146.
56. Sammarco GJ. Peroneal tendon injuries. *Orthop Clin North Am* 1994;25:135–145.
57. Parvin RW, Ford LT. Stenosing tenosynovitis of the common peroneal tendon sheath. *J Bone Joint Surg Am* 1956;38:1352–1357.
58. Alexander IJ, Johnson KA, Parr JW. Morton's neuroma: a review of recent concepts. *Orthopedics* 1987;10:103–106.
59. Bossley CJ, Cairney PC. The intermetatarsophalangeal bursa: its significance in Morton's metatarsalgia. *J Bone Joint Surg Br* 1980; 62:184–187.
60. Zanetti M, Strehle JK, Kundert HP, et al. Morton neuroma: effect of MR imaging findings on diagnostic thinking and therapeutic decisions. *Radiology* 1999;213:583–588.
61. Strong G, Thomas PS. Conservative treatment of Morton's neuroma. *Orthop Rev* 1987;16:343–345.
62. DeLisa JA, Saeed MA. The tarsal tunnel syndrome. *Muscle Nerve* 1983;6:664–670.
63. Wilemon WK. Tarsal tunnel syndrome: a 50-year survey of the world literature and a report of two new cases. *Orthop Rev* 1979; 8:111–118.
64. Grabois M, Puentes J, Lidsky M. Tarsal tunnel syndrome in rheumatoid arthritis. *Arch Phys Med Rehabil* 1981;62:401–403.
65. Galardi G, Amadio S, Maderna L, et al. Electrophysiologic studies in tarsal tunnel syndrome. *Am J Phys Med Rehabil* 1994;73: 193–198.
66. Dellon AL. Deep peroneal nerve entrapment on the dorsum of the foot. *Foot Ankle* 1990;11:73–80.
67. Gessini L, Jandolo B, Pietrangeli A. The anterior tarsal syndrome: report of four cases. *J Bone Joint Surg Am* 1984;66: 786–787.
68. Andressen BL, Wertsch JJ, Stewart WA. Anterior tarsal tunnel syndrome. *Arch Phys Med Rehabil* 1992;73:1112–1117.
69. Sridhara CR, Izzo KL. Terminal sensory branches of the superficial peroneal nerve: an entrapment syndrome. *Arch Phys Med Rehabil* 1985;68:789–791.
70. Pringle RM, Protheroe K, Mukherjee SK. Entrapment neuropathy of the sural nerve. *J Bone Joint Surg Br* 1974;56:465–468.
71. Bryan BM. Sural nerve entrapment after injury to the gastrocnemius: a case report. *Arch Phys Med Rehabil* 1999;80: 604–606.
72. Nickel VL. Orthotics in America: past, present and future. *Clin Orthop* 1974;102:10–17.
73. Donatelli R, Hurlbert C, Conaway D, et al. Biomechanical foot orthotics: a retrospective study. *J Orthop Sports Phys Ther* 1988; 10:205–212.
74. Janisse DJ. Indications and prescriptions for orthoses in sports. *Orthop Clin North Am* 1994;25:95–107.
75. Yates G. Molded plastics in bracing. *Clin Orthop* 1974;102: 46–57.
76. Bistevins R. Footwear and footwear modifications. In: Kottke FJ, Lehmann JF, eds. *Handbook of physical medicine and rehabilitation.* 4th ed. Philadelphia: WB Saunders, 1990:967–975.
77. Cowell HR. Shoes and shoe corrections. *Pediatr Clin North Am* 1977;24:791–797.
78. Milgram JE, Jacobson MA. Footgear: therapeutic modifications of sole and heel. *Orthop Rev* 1978;7:57–62.
79. Swezey RL. Below-knee weight-bearing brace for the arthritic foot. *Arch Phys Med Rehabil* 1975;56:176–179.
80. Lehmann JF, Warren CG, Pemberton DR, et al. Load-bearing function of patellar tendon bearing braces of various designs. *Arch Phys Med Rehabil* 1971;52:366–370.
81. Gristina AG, Nicastro JF, Clippinger F, et al. Neuropathic foot and ankle patellar-tendon-bearing orthosis as an adjunct to patient management. *Orthop Rev* 1977;6:53–59.
82. Kisner C, Colby LA. *Therapeutic exercise:* foundations and techniques. 2nd ed. Philadelphia: FA Davis, 1990.

100

CERVICAL SPINE SYNDROMES

JOE G. HARDIN, JR.
JAMES T. HALLA

Neck pain is a common problem in the general population whether or not a well-defined rheumatic disorder exists. It occurs at some time in one third or more of the population (1). Typically, the pain is perceived not only in the neck itself, but also in other regions, such as the back of the head, shoulder girdle, arm, and anterior chest. Pain originating from neck structures might be perceived exclusively in extracervical areas. In patients with unequivocal cervical trauma, cervical degenerative disc, and joint disease, including inflammatory arthropathies, the origin of the pain in the neck might be easy to establish, at least by inference. In individuals with pain but with none of these conditions, the cause is often impossible to establish with certainty. Fortunately, many of these pain syndromes are transient. The neck is an extraordinarily complex anatomic structure with many components that lend themselves poorly to diagnostic investigation.

It can be assumed that pain derived from the cervical spine originates in one or more of a limited number of structures: joints (either synovial or cartilaginous), ligaments, neural tissue (especially nerve roots), muscles, and tendons. Disease in one structure (i.e., a joint) often leads to symptoms in another (i.e., a nerve). Available diagnostic modalities can identify joints or neural tissue as a probable source of pain with relative ease; however, some of these techniques have been shown to be overly sensitive. Recognition of pathology in muscle or ligament is much more difficult, a fact that accounts for the difficulty in precise identification of the origin of cervical pain in individuals with no underlying rheumatic disorders.

In this chapter, the functional anatomy of the cervical spine and structures related to it is addressed first, followed by a review of cervical spine syndromes commonly encountered in otherwise normal individuals: syndromes associated with trauma, syndromes associated with degenerative disc and joint disease, and finally syndromes resulting from inflammatory arthropathies.

FUNCTIONAL ANATOMY

Emphasis in this section is on the spine, its articulations, and their relation to neural structures. Individual cervical vertebrae and their components are illustrated in Fig. 100.1. The atlas (C1) (Fig. 100.1A) is a ring of bone modified by articular facets anterolaterally. The superior facets articulate with the skull, forming relatively stable joints that permit only flexion–extension. The inferior facets articulate with their counterparts on the axis (C2; Fig. 100.1B). A third C1–C2 articulation also plays an important role in the motion occurring between these two vertebrae. This is the joint formed between the odontoid process of C2 and the anterior chamber of C1—the atlantoodontoid articulation. This joint is stabilized by the transverse ligament of C1 behind the odontoid and by ligaments between the odontoid and the occiput. The head and C1 move as a unit on C2 during cervical flexion. This motion stresses the stability of the atlanto-odontoid articulation and tends to force the odontoid posteriorly into the area occupied by the spinal canal. The three C1 to C2 articulations contribute about 50% of the rotational motion of the cervical spine, and all three are synovium-lined joints.

Below the axis, the remaining five cervical vertebrae (Fig. 100.1C) are relatively constant; their articulations account for the remaining motions permitted by the cervical spine. Anteriorly, the vertebral body articulates with its counterpart through the cartilaginous intervertebral disc. During youth, the disc is typical of others elsewhere in the spine with a dense outer annulus fibrosus and a central nucleus pulposus. Laterally, near the intervertebral neural foramina, the vertebral bodies are modified by superior uncinate processes (neurocentral lips) that articulate with a region of the vertebral bodies above them, forming the so-called "joints" of Luschka. The adult cervical disc loses its nucleus pulposus, and clefts develop at the site of the uncinate processes. With increasing age, these clefts dissect medially, bisecting the disc but not forming a true synovial joint (2,3). According to this observation, Luschka's joints are mythic (2,3).

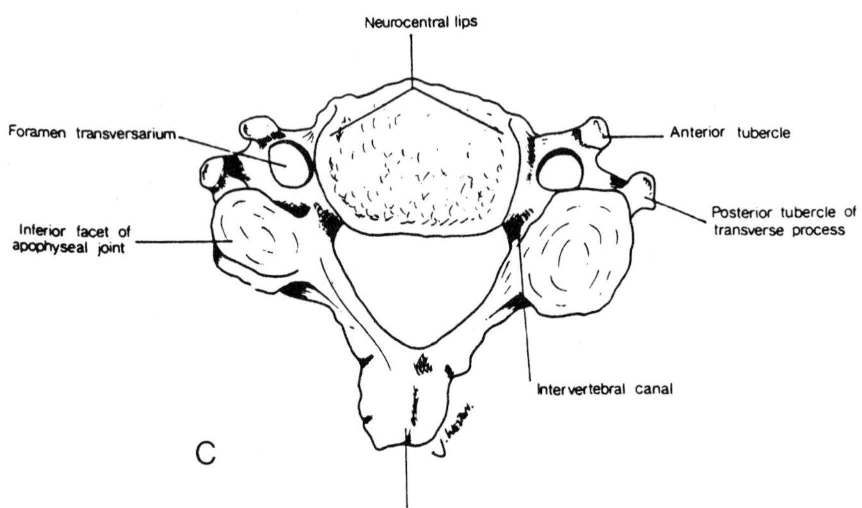

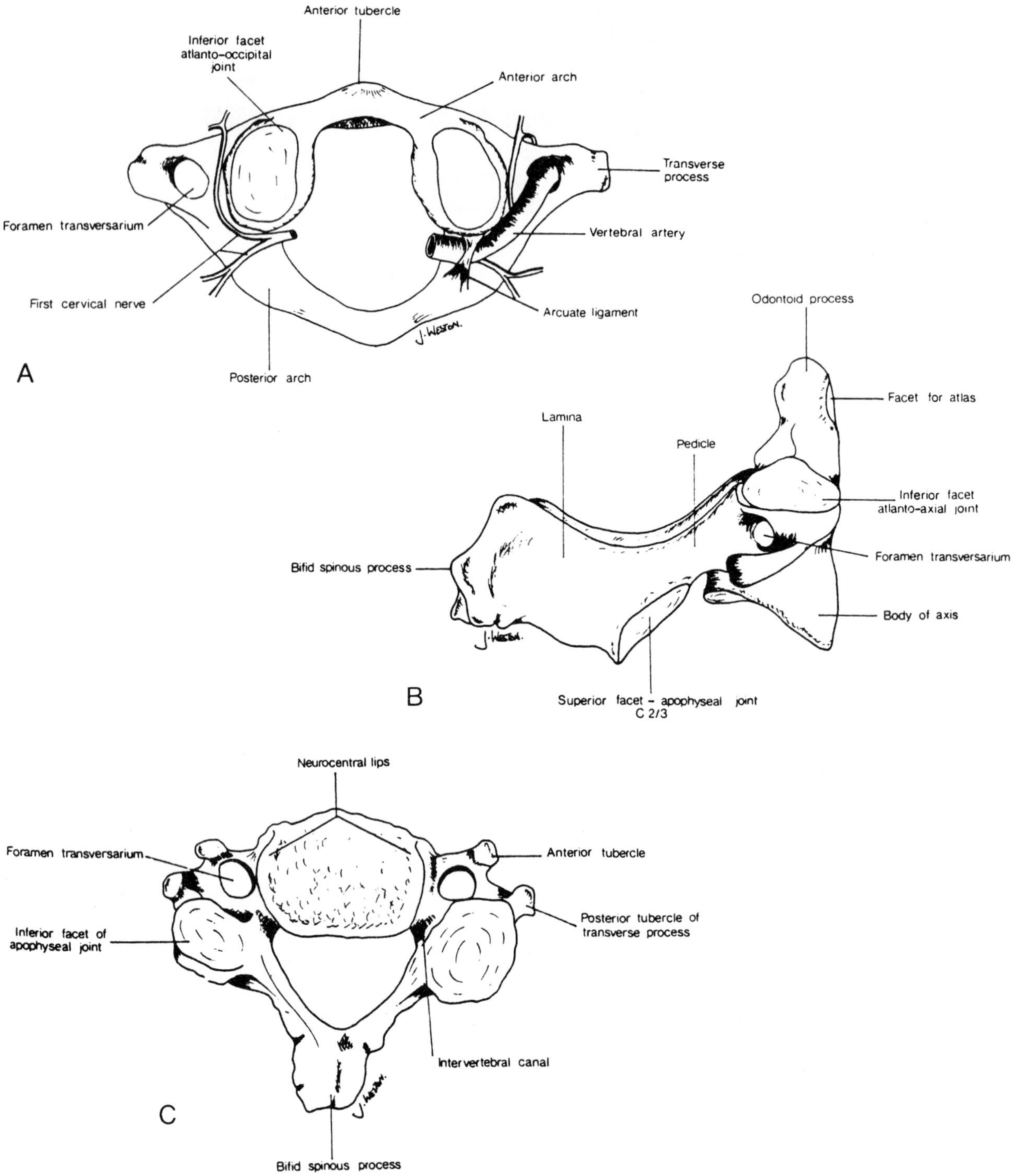

FIGURE 100.1. Atlas, axis, and typical lower cervical vertebra. **A:** Atlas, superior aspect. **B:** Axis, lateral view. **C:** Typical cervical vertebra, superior view. (Reproduced with permission from Jeffreys E. Disorders of the cervical *spine*. London: Butterworths, 1980:3.)

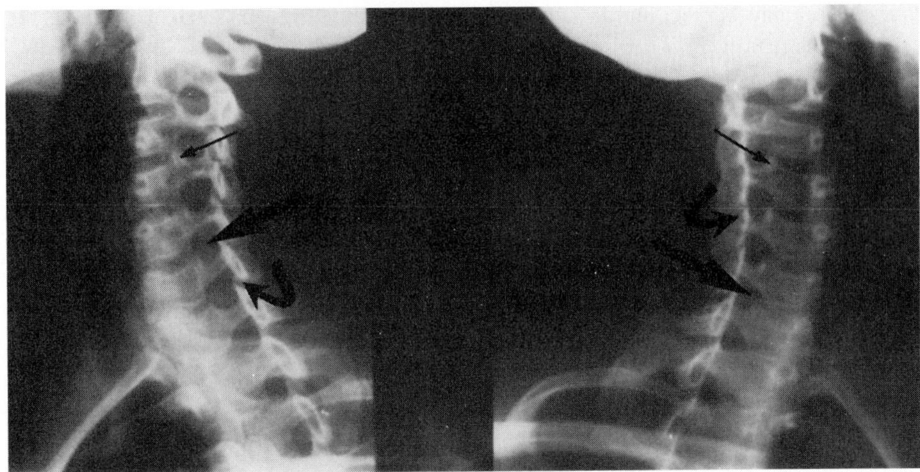

FIGURE 100.2. Right and left oblique views of the cervical spine demonstrating the intervertebral neural foramina (*large arrows*). Sites of the uncinate processes are indicated by *small arrows*, and the facet joints indicated by *curved arrows*.

The posterior elements of C2 and the lower five cervical vertebrae form the neural arch surrounding the spinal canal laterally and posteriorly. Laterally the narrow pedicles provide for the oval intervertebral neural foramina (Fig. 100.2), and the transverse processes, extending anterolaterally from the pedicles, form shelves or gutters for the exiting nerves. Except for that of C7, each transverse process, including those of C1 and C2, is perforated by a foramen for the vertebral artery (foramen transversum). The intervertebral neural foramina are best viewed obliquely in the anterolateral plane. Posterior to the pedicle, the neural arch flares inferiorly and superiorly to form the articular facets that lie considerably posterior to the articular facets of C1 and C2. The articulating surfaces of the facets face each other at an angle of about 45 degrees. The facet (apophyseal) joints are true synovial joints. The posterior elements (lamina) of the neural arch complete the spinal canal. Motions permitted by the cervical articulations vary with age, sex, and the observer measuring them. Average ranges are as follows: flexion–extension, 106 degrees; lateral flexion or bending, 178 degrees; and rotation, 131 degrees. Ranges in all directions decrease significantly with increasing age (4,5).

The first cervical nerve exits superior to C1 and posterior to the articular facet, and the second cervical nerve exits similarly superior and posterior to the superior articular facet of C2. All other cervical nerves pass anterolaterally through their respective gutters and posterior to the vertebral artery. After exiting the spinal canal, the posterior and anterior nerve roots join within their dural sleeve in the gutter to form the cervical nerve, with the posterior root lying superior to the anterior root. Their position in the foramina and the uncinate processes serves to protect the roots from protrusion or herniation of disc material.

Important ligaments add support to the cervical spine below the C1–C2 articulations. The anterior longitudinal ligament is bound to the front of the vertebral bodies, its fibers blending loosely with the annulus fibrosus as it crosses the disc spaces. The reverse is true for the posterior longitudinal ligament, which is loosely bound to the posterior aspects of the vertebral bodies but more firmly attached to the discs. The posterior longitudinal ligament is much thicker in the cervical area than in the thoracolumbar regions. The lamina or posterior aspects of the neural arch are bound to their inferior and superior counterparts by the tough elastic ligamenta flava, which extend anteriorly to blend in with the capsules of the facet joints.

A large muscle mass occupies the posterolateral cervical area. For the most part, these muscles are attached to the spine and to the skull, especially the occiput. In concert with the sternomastoid and the anterior neck muscles, they move the head and neck, support and stabilize the head and neck, and balance the head on the spine.

GENERAL APPROACHES TO CERVICAL SYMPTOMS

Most symptoms perceived in the neck are transient and of uncertain cause. Many probably qualify as myofascial (6). Symptoms are typically rapid in onset, are associated with limited or painful mobility of the neck and shoulder girdle, and seldom last longer than a week. The neurologic examination is normal; other physical findings are nonspecific, and diagnostic imaging is not helpful. This syndrome is often referred to by patients as a "crick." Persistent myofascial pain (in the presence or absence of an accompanying fibromyalgia syndrome) also may be a common cause of chronic symptoms in the neck region (7). The use of appropriate cervical contour pillows may be useful for this more persistent myofascial pain.

Symptoms persisting beyond 1 or 2 weeks or associated with certain other features must be taken more seriously. Other features suggesting a potentially serious or diagnosable cause include pain in other parts of the body, neurologic symptoms, abnormal neurologic findings, fever, and palpable or audible cervical crepitus. Polymyalgia rheumatica, fibromyalgia, and some of the inflammatory arthropathies might begin or predominate in the cervical region, as outlined in Table 100.1 (8). Symptoms or signs in other areas of the body might suggest one of these conditions. Cervical injuries also might trigger or precipitate a fibromyalgia syndrome; in a survey of patients with recent neck or lower extremity injuries, fibromyalgia was 13 times more frequent in those with the neck injury (9).

TABLE 100.1. DISORDERS THAT MAY INITIALLY HAVE SYMPTOMS IN THE NECK REGION

- Rheumatic diseases
  - Fibromyalgia
  - Polymyalgia rheumatica
  - Rheumatoid arthritis
  - Juvenile rheumatoid arthritis
  - Ankylosing spondylitis
  - Peripheral spondyloarthropathies
  - Crystal-deposition diseases
  - Degenerative disc and joint diseases
  - Diffuse idiopathic skeletal hyperostosis
- Trauma
  - Fractures–dislocations
  - Soft tissue injuries
- Regional cervical disorders
  - Myofascial pain
  - Osteomyelitis
  - Septic discitis
  - Septic arthritis
  - Congenital and acquired torticollis syndromes
  - Other congenital disorders of the cervical spine
  - Cervical lymphadenitis
  - Hyoid bone syndrome
  - Neck–tongue syndrome
  - Longus colli muscle tendinitis
  - Facet joint synovial cyst
  - Thyroiditis
  - Thoracic outlet syndrome
- Bone diseases
  - Paget's disease
  - Osteomalacia
  - Osteoporosis
  - Metastatic tumor
- Neuromuscular disorders
  - Meningitis
  - Cerebral palsy and other spastic conditions
  - Paralysis of cervical muscles from any cause

TABLE 100.2. USEFUL DIAGNOSTIC MANEUVERS IN PATIENTS WITH SYMPTOMS IN THE NECK REGION

- History
  - Duration
  - Trauma
  - Pain or similar symptoms elsewhere
  - Pain related to head–neck motion or position
  - Referral pattern and nature of referred pain
  - Neurologic symptoms
- Physical examination
  - Abnormal head position
  - Neck motion and pain on motion
  - Spine tenderness
  - Tender or trigger points in neck area
  - Motor or sensory deficits or reflex abnormalities, especially in the arms
- Diagnostic imaging
  - Routine radiographs (with oblique views)
  - Radioisotope scanning
  - Conventional tomography
  - Computed tomography
  - Magnetic resonance imaging
  - Myelography
- Electrodiagnostic studies
  - Nerve conduction studies
  - Electromyography

When the diagnosis is not apparent and the symptoms persist or seem potentially serious, further diagnostic efforts are indicated, as listed in Table 100.2. The history and physical examination maneuvers are routine, but very important. Cervical spine radiographs—anteroposterior, lateral, right and left oblique, and flexion and extension views in the lateral projection—are usually indicated. The facets between C1 and C2 are generally visualized by a view taken through the open mouth. Conventional tomography can be helpful if a bony defect or spinal derangement is suspected but not well defined by routine radiography or radioisotopic scintigraphy. Electrodiagnostic studies might confirm or better define a suspected neurologic deficit. Computed tomography (CT), magnetic resonance imaging (MRI), and myelography are used to define the source of a neurologic sign or symptom. Neural compression syndromes may be best defined by MRI (10,11); however, care must be taken not to overinterpret normal and age-related changes (12).

NECK PAIN ASSOCIATED WITH TRAUMA

Fractures and dislocations of the cervical spine must be excluded in symptomatic patients with a recent history of cervical trauma; however, blunt trauma elsewhere does not necessarily require cervical spine evaluation (13). A number of terms are used interchangeably to refer to the typical soft tissue injury syndrome including whiplash, cervical sprain or strain, and posttraumatic cervical syndrome. Although industrial or sports injuries might cause the problem, in the United States, most such injuries result from automobile collisions from the rear, most often with the victim using a seat belt (14). Medicolegal considerations can complicate and confound the clinical picture. The typical injury occurs as the head is first flexed and then forcibly hyperextended beyond its normal range of motion. Presumably the affected tissues include muscles, tendons, joints, ligaments, and perhaps nerve roots. The pathogenesis of the injury is not well understood. Usually the onset of pain begins within hours of the accident, and it predominates in the neck and medial aspects of the shoulder girdle. Headaches are common, and posttraumatic audiologic and vestibular dysfunction have been reported (15). Cervical radiographs can show loss of lordosis secondary to cervical muscle spasm; however, the significance of this finding may have been overinterpreted (16).

In one series, the syndrome had resolved in 52% of patients at 8 weeks and in 87% of patients at 5 months (17), but the natural history continues to be highly variable. In recent reviews, psychologic and medicolegal factors appear to have the major influence on the cause and severity of the problem (18,19). The cervical zygapophyseal joints have long been implicated as a source of persisting pain after cervical flexion–extension injuries, and provocation and blocking maneuvers have been used to support this notion (20). A recent controlled study failed to demonstrate any benefits of intraarticular corticosteroid injections in the implicated zygapophyseal joints in subjects with chronic whiplash pain (21). Collars, traction, other physical therapies, and analgesic agents can help symptomatically, although they do not seem to affect the course of the syndrome. A conservative approach is generally recommended (22,23).

DEGENERATIVE DISC AND JOINT DISEASES (INCLUDING DIFFUSE IDIOPATHIC SKELETAL HYPEROSTOSIS)

Although diffuse idiopathic skeletal hyperostosis (DISH) is usually readily identifiable from plain radiographs and typically produces few neck symptoms, degenerative disease of the spinal articulations can result in a confusing array of symptoms that are often difficult to explain. Confounding observations that can account for this difficulty are summarized in Table 100.3. Despite these difficulties, diagnoses continue to be made, and the conditions often are treated successfully. In few cases, however, is the precise pathogenesis clearly understood. Four syndromes will be addressed: presumed herniation of the nucleus pulposus, presumed osteophytic neural and vascular encroachment, facet joint osteoarthritis (OA), and DISH.

TABLE 100.3. FEATURES ASSOCIATED WITH DEGENERATIVE CERVICAL SPINE DISEASE THAT LEND DIFFICULTY TO PRECISE DIAGNOSES

Symptoms may arise from the facet joints or anulus fibrosus
Radiographic abnormalities are almost universal in the elderly population, most of whom are asymptomatic
Diagnostic imaging abnormalities may correlate poorly with symptoms. Distribution of diagnostic imaging abnormalities may correlate poorly with location of symptoms
Neurologic physical findings most often are absent
With age, the ligamenta flava become inelastic and may buckle into the spinal canal, causing symptoms
With age, the posterior longitudinal ligament may further thicken, encroaching on the spinal canal and causing symptoms
Even lesions that appear to encroach on neural structures (by diagnostic imaging) may not cause symptoms
By age 40 years, the nucleus pulposus appears to be no longer present in the cervical discs (suggesting that it cannot herniate) (3,24)
The posterior longitudinal ligament and the uncinate processes provide formidable barriers to disc herniation (3,24)
The lower cervical nerve roots appear to exit below the disc level, apparently protecting them from herniation in any event (3,24)
The anterior nerve roots appear to be set too low in the intervertebral foramina to be vulnerable to osteophytic encroachment (3,24)

Herniation of the Nucleus Pulposus

Disc ruptures, protrusions, and extrusions are used synonymously with herniation of the nucleus pulposus. Much of the literature concerning cervical disc disease fails to distinguish between herniation of the nucleus pulposus and osteophytic encroachment on neural structures, apparently because they often occur together. A distinctive clinical syndrome might be apparent, however. The herniation of the nucleus pulposus syndrome occurs at a younger age than the osteophytic one and more often affects men. Protrusion tends to occur acutely on one side and at one level (most often C6–7), dorsolaterally (compressing intrameningeal nerve roots) or intraforaminally (compressing the exiting nerve roots). Most often there is no history of trauma sufficient to account for the event. Symptoms often begin with neck pain that progresses to involve the scapular area, anterior chest, or arm, depending on which root is affected. Hyperextension of the neck or deviation of the head toward the side of the herniation of the nucleus pulposus can aggravate the pain. Neurologic findings and other signs often are present, depending on the site of the lesion (25,26).

The diagnosis may be supported by electromyography and confirmed by myelography, MRI, or CT. The procedure of choice is a matter of opinion, but most current experience favors MRI (27). Therapy is also a matter of opinion. Progressive neurologic deficits, signs of myelopathy, and intractable pain usually indicate surgery, however (see Chapter 51). Conservative therapy consists of intermittent or continuous cervical traction, bed rest, analgesics, and cervical collars for comfort (28).

Osteophytic Disease (Spondylosis)

Anterior osteophytes arising at the disc margins might imply more posterior disease, but of themselves are typically asymptomatic. The uncinate processes enlarge with age, so that what appear to be osteophytes in that area radiographically might not be, but foraminal bony encroachment from that region is seen commonly, as is similar encroachment from facet joint osteophytes posteriorly. Only the facet osteophytes are in a position to impinge on a nerve root, and only the posterior root is vulnerable (3,23). Posterior osteophytes from the vertebral bodies at the disc margins are common and can be sufficiently large to compress the spinal cord, although they, too, are most often asymptomatic. In general, the lower cervical spine, especially C5 through C6, is most prominently involved. Three overlapping syndromes can result from spondylitic osteophytic neural or vascular encroachment: nerve root compression (radiculopathy), spinal cord compression (myelopathy), and vertebral artery compression.

It might not be possible, even at surgery, to distinguish clearly between a radiculopathy due to a herniation of the nucleus pulposus and one due to osteophytic encroachment, and the reported clinical syndromes resulting from these events are similar, except as already mentioned. Herniation of the nucleus pulposus tends to occur in younger patients, affecting a single root. Approaches to diagnosis and therapy also are similar (29). A less dramatic and more ill-defined syndrome is more common than the classic one usually reported in textbooks. Older patients commonly experience neck, shoulder area, and arm pain, often aggravated by neck motion, and sometimes associated with intermittent paresthesias. Sometimes tests listed in Table 100.4 are positive, but neurologic deficits are absent. Plain cervical radiographs document neural foraminal osteophytic encroachment, often at several levels. More expensive diagnostic studies are seldom indicated. Symptoms tend to respond to conservative therapy, perhaps improving with time alone. Intermittent cervical traction is frequently helpful. It is seldom possible to document clearly an association between a given osteophytic encroachment and the symptoms.

Bland and Boushey (2) suggested that spondylitic myelopathy is more common than radiculopathy. The syndrome is seen more often in older men and is typically gradual in onset. Leg symptoms predominate, and spasticity is common. Radicular symptoms frequently accompany the myelopathy. A congenitally narrow spinal canal and posterior longitudinal ligament thickening or ossification may contribute to the compression. Myelography or MRI confirms the diagnosis, and surgical therapy is often indicated (30–33) (see Chapter 103).

Many symptoms can result from osteophytic compression of the vertebral artery, especially in the upper cervical region. These include autonomic symptoms, transient ischemic attacks, dizziness, vertigo, and headaches; symptoms are often related to cervical motion. The association of cervical spondylosis with headache has been questioned, however (34). The diagnosis of vertebral artery compression is usually made by angiography, and the treatment often involves surgical decompression.

Facet Joint Osteoarthritis

It is widely assumed, although difficult to prove, that neck discomfort in the older population is related to the radiographic findings of facet joint osteoarthritis (OA). In one follow-up study of 205 patients, such an association could not be documented (35). A few patients with cervical OA have symptoms arising primarily from the C1 through C2 facet joints, however. Patients with this syndrome tend to be older women complaining primarily of occipital pain. Crepitus in the upper cervical spine, occipital tender points, and a rotational head tilt deformity are common. These patients usually respond to conservative therapy, but surgical fusion is occasionally indicated for intractable pain (36).

TABLE 100.4. CLINICAL TESTS FOR CERVICAL NERVE ROOT COMPRESSION

Test	Technique
Neck compression test	With the patient sitting, examiner laterally flexes, slightly rotates, and then compresses the patient's head with a force of 7 kg; positive result is pain or paresthesias in distribution of affected root
Axial manual traction test	With the patient supine, examiner applies manual traction to neck with a force of 10–15 kg; positive result is relief of radicular symptoms
Shoulder abduction test	With patient sitting, the arm is actively abducted above the head; positive result is relief of radicular symptoms

Based on the results of myelography or magnetic resonance imaging, these tests are highly specific, but together have a sensitivity only in the range of 50% (25).

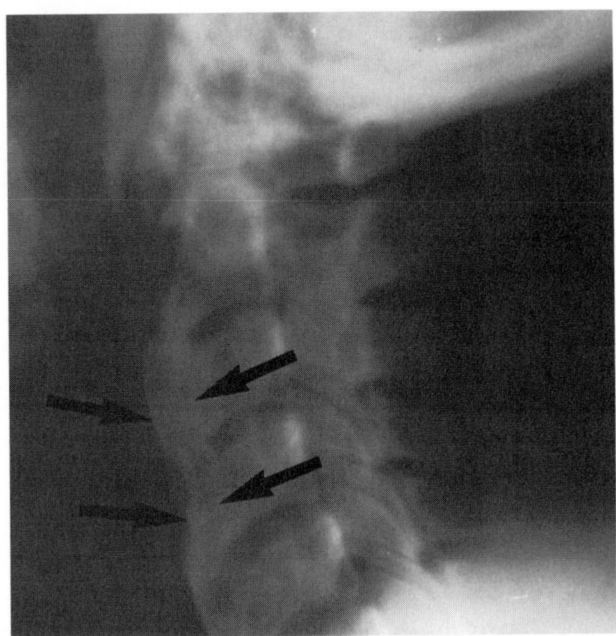

FIGURE 100.3. Cervical diffuse idiopathic skeletal hyperostosis (DISH). *Arrows,* Extent of the anterior longitudinal ligament ossification.

Diffuse Idiopathic Skeletal Hyperostosis

The anterior longitudinal ligament of the cervical spine is commonly ossified in patients with DISH, and sometimes the ossification is luxuriant (Fig. 100.3) Although most often asymptomatic, extensive ossification can be associated with limited neck mobility, anterior cervical masses, and dysphagia from esophageal compression (37). DISH also has been associated with ossification of the posterior longitudinal ligament, sometimes resulting in myelopathy with quadriplegia (38).

INFLAMMATORY ARTHROPATHIES

Neck syndromes are common in the inflammatory arthropathies (Table 100.1), especially rheumatoid arthritis (RA).

Rheumatoid Arthritis

Neck pain occurs in half of the patients with RA, but half of these symptomatic patients have normal cervical spine radiographs. Abnormalities of the rheumatoid cervical spine and its supporting structures occur in three patterns: (a) atlantoaxial (C1–C2) complex involvement with subluxation anteriorly or posteriorly with or without odontoid erosion; (b) C1 to C2 lateral facet joint and/or atlantooccipital joint involvement with lateral or rotatory subluxations; and (c) subaxial involvement with subluxation and/or spondylodiscitis (39).

More than one pattern might be seen in any individual patient, and each pattern might be associated with a distinctive clinical profile. For example, involvement of the C1 to C2 lateral facet joints, either unilaterally or bilaterally, is characterized by pain that parallels the degree of radiographic involvement, restricted neck motion, and a nonreducible rotational head tilt to the side of collapse and paralleling the degree of lateral mass collapse (Fig. 100.4). Neurologic symptoms are uncommon unless cranial settling is present (40,41).

Neck symptoms resulting from anteroposterior subluxations at the C1-to-C2 complex are less distinctive (Fig. 100.5). Anterior C1-to-C2 subluxation is the most frequent radiographic abnormality. The correlation is poor between the degree of subluxation demonstrated radiographically and symptoms, especially neurologic symptoms (42). However, patients with the following abnormalities are at the greatest risk for irreversible paralysis: (a) atlantoaxial subluxation and a posterior atlanto-odontoid interval of 14 mm or less; (b) atlantoaxial subluxation and at least 5 mm of cephalad migration of the odontoid tip due to cranial settling; and (c) subaxial subluxation and a sagittal diameter of the spinal canal of 14 mm or less (43).

Subaxial involvement includes vertebral end plate erosions, disc space narrowing without osteophytes, spondylodiscitis, and subluxation. Subluxation, either at single or multiple levels, is not uncommon, but rarely causes symptoms unless accompanied by discitis (39).

Treatment of neck pain in patients with RA should be guided by the radiographic pattern and by the nature of

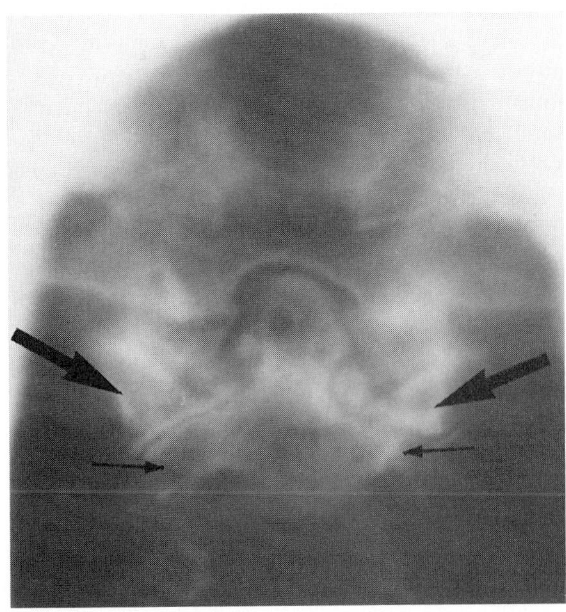

FIGURE 100.4. Conventional anteroposterior tomography of C1–C2 in a patient with severe rheumatoid arthritis. *Large arrows,* C1 lateral mass collapse; *small arrows,* C2 lateral mass collapse.

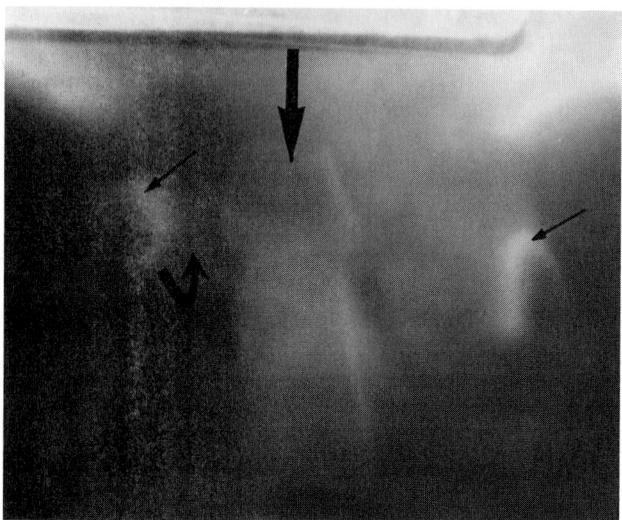

FIGURE 100.5. Conventional lateral tomography of C1–C2 area in a patient with severe rheumatoid arthritis. *Small arrows,* C1; *large arrow,* the odontoid process. The spinal canal is to the left (*curved arrow*). This patient had severe C1–C2 anterior subluxation with no symptoms!

symptoms. Sometimes no therapy is necessary, and conservative measures including physical therapy and drugs usually suffice. If pain is intractable, surgical fusion (occiput to C2 or C3) might give dramatic pain relief; this is especially true if the pain is due to C1 to C2 lateral facet joint disease (40,41,44,45).

Juvenile Rheumatoid Arthritis

Cervical spine involvement occurs in up to 50% of patients with juvenile rheumatoid arthritis (JRA), and is most prominently associated with polyarticular disease, a positive rheumatoid factor, or both. Manifestations include loss of cervical lordosis, apophyseal joint erosions and ankylosis, especially in the upper cervical spine, failure of vertebral body growth, C1-to-C2 anterior subluxation, and lateral facet joint disease with nonreducible rotational head tilt (46–48).

Neck pain can be either the presenting feature or a later manifestation of adult-onset Still's disease. Because the childhood and adult forms of Still's disease are similar in presentation and course, radiographic similarities are not unexpected. Unlike the childhood form, the adult disease tends to involve both the upper and lower cervical segments (49).

Ankylosing Spondylitis

Neck pain in ankylosing spondylitis is common. As many as 5% to 10% of patients have neck pain in the absence of back pain (50). Neck pain usually correlates with radiographic changes, but can occur in their absence. Conversely, radiographic abnormalities without neck pain are sometimes seen. Cervical spine involvement usually accompanies disease in the thoracolumbar spine, although women may have a higher frequency of isolated cervical spine disease (51).

Involvement of the C1–C2 complex occurs uncommonly; subluxation, usually anterior, and odontoid erosions are its usual manifestations (52). However, in one series, 22 of 103 ankylosing spondylitis patients had anterior subluxations, and they progressed over a 2-year period in about one third, five of whom required cervical fusion (53). The C1–C2 lateral facet joints might be the commonest source of severe neck pain in ankylosing spondylitis (47).

Cervical spine fracture, usually with minor trauma, is another cause of neck pain in patients with ankylosing spondylitis and is easily overlooked. These patients tend to be older men (mean age, 55 years) with advanced disease (average duration, 25 years). Neurologic deficits are common, and mortality is as high as 35% (54).

Spondylodiscitis is another source of neck pain in patients with ankylosing spondylitis. This radiographic finding occurs in 1% to 28% of patients, usually during the first 10 years of disease. The more destructive the lesion, the more likely there is to be widespread spinal ankylosis (55). Infectious spondylitis must be excluded.

Ossification of the posterior longitudinal ligament of the cervical spine occurs commonly in ankylosing spondylitis and other spondyloarthropathies; it generally correlates with disease severity and may cause or contribute to myelopathy (56).

Reiter's Syndrome

Cervical spine involvement in Reiter's syndrome is uncommon; fewer than 6% of patients demonstrate radiographic abnormalities. Manifestations include C1–C2 subluxations, C1–C2 lateral facet joint disease including nonreducible rotational head tilt, atlantooccipital joint involvement, anterior longitudinal ligamentous ossification, and spondylitis (57,58). All of these can be a source of neck pain.

Psoriatic Arthritis

Involvement of the cervical spine in psoriatic arthritis occurs in two patterns: a pattern similar to RA and a pattern similar to ankylosing spondylitis (59). Neck pain is common, and neurologic complications occur, especially in those patients with an RA-like pattern (60). The duration of psoriatic arthritis and the number of peripheral joints involved appear to be the major factors in determining cervical spine involvement (61).

Crystallopathies

As a group, the crystallopathies rarely affect the cervical spine. Gout can produce neck symptoms in a variety of ways, however, including intradural deposition of urate, discitis, and subluxations (62). In a group of 85 patients with calcium pyrophosphate deposition disease, ten had neck symptoms (63). Radiographic abnormalities included disc-space loss with vertebral sclerosis and osteophyte formation, facet joint abnormalities, and crystal deposition in synovial and ligamentous structures, including the ligamenta flava.

Crystal deposition, usually in the form of hydroxyapatite, also can occur in periarticular locations in the spine. Calcification within the longus colli muscle and tendon can be responsible for acute neck and occipital pain with or without dysphagia (64). Hydroxyapatite crystal deposition also has been reported in the infraoccipital region, interspinous bursae, and ligamenta flava, and has been associated with neck pain and neurologic manifestations (65).

REFERENCES

1. Bovin G, Schrader H, Sand T. Neck pain in the general population. *Spine* 1994;19:1307–1309.
2. Bland JG, Boushey DR. Anatomy and physiology of the cervical spine. *Semin Arthritis Rheum* 1990;20:1–20.
3. Bland JH. Basic anatomy. In: Bland JH, ed. *Disorders of the cervical spine.* 2nd ed. Philadelphia: WB Saunders, 1994:41–70.
4. O'Driscoll SL, Tomenson J. The cervical spine. In: Wright V, ed. *Clinics in rheumatic diseases.* Philadelphia: WB Saunders, 1982: 617–630.
5. Kuhlman KA. Cervical range of motion in the elderly. *Arch Phys Med Rehabil* 1993;74:1071–1079.
6. Rachlin ES. History and physical examination for regional myofascial pain syndrome. In: Rachlin ES, ed. *Myofascial pain and fibromyalgia.* St. Louis: CV Mosby, 1994:159–172.
7. Smythe HA. The C6-7 syndrome: clinical features and treatment response. *J Rheumatol* 1994;21:1520–1526.
8. Bland JH. Differential diagnosis and specific treatment. In: Bland JH, ed. *Disorders of the cervical spine.* 2nd ed. Philadelphia: WB Saunders, 1994:223–270.
9. Buskila D, Neumann L, Vaisberg G, et al. Increased rates of fibromyalgia following cervical spine injury. *Arthritis Rheum* 1997;40:446–452.
10. Kuroki T, Kumano K, Hirabayashi S. Usefulness of MRI in the preoperative diagnosis of cervical disk herniation. *Arch Orthop Trauma Surg* 1993;112:180–184.
11. Goto S, Mochizuki M, Watanabe T, et al. Long-term follow-up study of anterior surgery for cervical spondylotic myelopathy with special reference to the magnetic resonance imaging findings in 52 cases. *Clin Orthop* 1993;291:142–153.
12. Lehto IJ, Tertti MO, Komu ME, et al. Age-related MRI changes at 0.1 T in cervical discs in asymptomatic subjects. *Neuroradiology* 1994;36:49–53.
13. Roth BJ, Martin RR, Foley K, et al. Roentgenographic evaluation of the cervical spine. *Arch Surg* 1994;129:643–645.
14. Bauer W. Neck pain. In: Weisel SW, Feffer HL, Rothman RH, eds. *Neck pain.* Charlottesville: Michie Co., 1986:1–17.
15. Hildingsson C, Wenngren BI, Toolanen G. Eye motility dysfunction after soft-tissue injury of the cervical spine. *Acta Orthop Scand* 1993;64:129–132.
16. Helliwell PS, Evans PF, Wright V. The straight cervical spine: does it indicate muscle spasm? *J Bone Joint Surg Br* 1994;76: 103–106.
17. Pennie BH, Agambar LJ. Whiplash injuries. *J Bone Joint Surg Br* 1990;72:277–279.
18. Ferrari R, Russell AS. The whiplash syndrome: common sense revisited. *J Rheumatol* 1997;24:618–623.
19. Radanov BP. Common whiplash: research findings revisited. *J Rheumatol* 1997;24:623–625.
20. Bogduk N, Aprill C. On the nature of neck pain, discography and cervical zygapophysial joint blocks. *Pain* 1993;54:213–217.
21. Barnsley L, Lord SM, Wallis BJ, Bogduk N. Lack of effect of intraarticular corticosteroids for chronic pain in the cervical zygapophyseal joints. *N Engl J Med* 1994;330:1047–1050.
22. Carette S. Whiplash injury and chronic neck pain. *N Engl J Med* 1994;330:1083–1084.
23. Bogduk N, Lord SM. Cervical spine disorders. *Curr Opin Rheumatol* 1998;10:110–115.
24. Bland JH. New anatomy and physiology with clinical and historical implications. In: Bland JH, ed. *Disorders of the cervical spine.* 2nd ed. Philadelphia: WB Saunders, 1994:71–91.
25. Viikari-Juntura E, Porras M, Laasonen EM. Validity of clinical tests in the diagnosis of root compression in cervical disc disease. *Spine* 1989;14:253–257.
26. Dubuisson A, Lenelle J, Stevenaert A. Soft cervical disc herniation: a retrospective study of 100 cases. *Acta Neurochir* 1993;125: 115–119.
27. Van de Kelft E, Van Vyve M. Diagnostic imaging algorithm for cervical soft disc herniation. *J Neurol Neurosurg Psychiatry* 1994; 57:724–728.
28. Maigne JY, Deligne L. Computed tomographic follow-up study of 21 cases of nonoperatively treated cervical intervertebral soft disc herniation. *Spine* 1994;19:189–191.
29. Yu YL, Woo E, Huang CY. Cervical spondylotic myelopathy and radiculopathy. *Acta Neurol Scand* 1987;75:367–373.
30. Bernhardt M, Hynes RA, Blume HW, et al. Current contents review: cervical spondylotic myelopathy. *J Bone Joint Surg Am* 1993;75:119–128.
31. Sadsivan KK, Reed RP, Albright JA. The natural history of cervical spondylotic myelopathy. *Yale J Biol Med* 1993;66:235–242.
32. Law MD Jr, Bernhardt M, White AA. Cervical spondylotic myelopathy: a review of surgical indications and decision making. *Yale J Biol Med* 1993;66:165–177.
33. Houser OW, Onofrio BM, Miller GM, Folger WN, Smith PL. Cervical spondylotic stenosis and myelopathy: evaluation with computed tomographic myelography. *Mayo Clin Proc* 1994; 69:557–563.
34. Appenzeller O. The autonomic nervous system in cervical spine disorders. In: Bland JH, ed. *Disorders of the cervical spine.* 2nd ed. Philadelphia: WB Saunders, 1994:313–327.
35. Gore DR, Sepic SB, Gardner GM, et al. Neck pain: a long-term follow-up of 205 patients. *Spine* 1987;12:1–5.
36. Halla JT, Hardin JG. Atlantoaxial (C1-C2) facet joint osteoarthritis: a distinctive clinical syndrome. *Arthritis Rheum* 1987;30:577–582.
37. Kritzer RO, Rose JE. Diffuse idiopathic skeletal hyperostosis presenting with thoracic outlet syndrome and dysphagia. *Neurosurgery* 1988;22:1072–1074.
38. Pouchot J, Watts CS, Esdaile JM, et al. Sudden quadriplegia complicating ossification of the posterior longitudinal ligament and diffuse idiopathic skeletal hyperostosis. *Arthritis Rheum* 1987;30:1069–1072.
39. Halla JT, Hardin JG, Vitek J, et al. Involvement of the cervical spine in rheumatoid arthritis. *Arthritis Rheum* 1989;32:652–659.
40. Halla JT, Fallahi S, Hardin JG. Nonreducible rotational head tilt and lateral mass collapse: a prospective study of frequency, radiographic findings, and clinical features in patients with rheumatoid arthritis. *Arthritis Rheum* 1982;25:1316–1324.
41. Halla JT, Hardin JG. The spectrum of atlantoaxial (C1-C2) facet joint involvement in rheumatoid arthritis. *Arthritis Rheum* 1990; 33:325–329.

42. Weissman B, Aliabadi P, Weinfeld M, et al. Prognostic features of atlantoaxial subluxation in rheumatoid arthritis patients. *Radiology* 1982;144:745–751.
43. Boden SC, Dodge LD, Bohlman HH, Rechtine GR. Rheumatoid arthritis of the cervical spine. *J Bone Joint Surg Am* 1993;75:1282–1297.
44. Oostveen JCM, van de Laar MAFJ, Geelen JAG, et al. Successful conservative treatment of rheumatoid subaxial subluxation resulting in improvement of myelopathy, reduction of subluxation, and stabilisation of the cervical spine: a report of two cases. *Ann Rheum Dis* 1999;58:126–129.
45. Rawlins BA, Girardi FP, Boachie-Adjei O. Rheumatoid arthritis of the cervical spine. *Rheum Dis Clin North Am* 1998;24:55–65.
46. Ansell B, Kent P. Radiological changes in juvenile chronic polyarthritis. *Skeletal Radiol* 1977;1:129–144.
47. Halla JT, Fallahi S, Hardin JG. Nonreducible rotational head tilt and atlantoaxial lateral mass collapse. *Arch Intern Med* 1983;143:471–474.
48. Uziel Y, Rathaus V, Pomeranz A, et al. Torticollis as the sole initial presenting sign of systemic onset juvenile rheumatoid arthritis. *J Rheumatol* 1998;25:166–168.
49. Elkon K, Hughes G, Bywaters E, et al. Adult onset Still's disease: twenty-five year follow-up and further studies of patients with active disease. *Arthritis Rheum* 1982;25:647–654.
50. Hochberg M, Borenstein D, Arnett F. The absence of back pain in classic ankylosing spondylitis. *Johns Hopkins Med J* 1978;143:181–183.
51. Wiesner K, Bryan B. Clinical and radiographic abnormalities in ankylosing spondylitis: a comparison of men and women. *Radiology* 1976;119:293–297.
52. Sorin S, Askari A, Moskowitz R. Atlantoaxial subluxation as a complication of early ankylosing spondylitis. *Arthritis Rheum* 1979;22:273–276.
53. Ramos-Remus C, Gomez-Vargas A, Hernandez-Chavez A, et al. Two year followup of anterior and vertical atlantoaxial subluxation in ankylosing spondylitis. *J Rheumatol* 1997;24:507–510.
54. Murray G, Persellin R. Cervical fracture complicating ankylosing spondylitis. *Am J Med* 1981;70:1033–1041.
55. Dihlmann W. Current radiodiagnostic concept of ankylosing spondylitis. *Skeletal Radiol* 1979;4:179–188.
56. Ramos-Remus C, Russell AS, Gomez-Vargas A, et al. Ossification of the posterior longitudinal ligament in three geographically and genetically different populations of ankylosing spondylitis and other spondyloarthropathies. *Ann Rheum Dis* 1998;57:429–433.
57. Melsom R, Benjamin J, Barnes C. Spontaneous atlantoaxial subluxation: an unusual presenting manifestation of Reiter's syndrome. *Ann Rheum Dis* 1989;48:170–172.
58. Halla JT, Bliznak J, Hardin JG. Involvement of the craniocervical junction in Reiter's syndrome. *J Rheumatol* 1988;15:1722–1725.
59. Blau R, Kaufman R. Erosive and subluxing cervical spine disease in patients with psoriatic arthritis. *J Rheumatol* 1987;14:111–117.
60. Fam A, Cruickshank B. Subaxial cervical subluxation and cord compression in psoriatic spondylitis. *Arthritis Rheum* 1982;25:101–106.
61. Jenkinson T, Armas J, Evison G, Cohen M, Lovell C, McHugh NJ. The cervical spine in psoriatic arthritis: a clinical and radiological study. *Br J Rheumatol* 1994;33:255–259.
62. Resnick D, Niwayama G. Gouty arthritis. In: *Diagnosis of bone and joint disorders.* 2nd ed. Philadelphia: WB Saunders, 1988:1618–1671.
63. Haselwood D, Wiesner K. Clinical, radiographic and pathologic abnormalities in calcium pyrophosphate dihydrate deposition disease. *Pseudogout Radiol* 1977;122:1–15.
64. Resnick D, Niwayama G. Calcium hydroxyapatite crystal deposition disease. In: *Diagnosis of bone and joint disorders.* 2nd ed. Philadelphia: WB Saunders, 1988:1733–1764.
65. Nakajima K, Miyaoka M, Sumie H, et al. Cervical radiculomyelopathy due to calcification of the ligamenta flava. *Surg Neurol* 1984;21:479–488.

101

TEMPOROMANDIBULAR DISORDERS

M. FRANKLIN DOLWICK

Temporomandibular pain and dysfunction are common problems that occur in about 33% of the general population (1). It has been estimated that 75% of the population have symptoms and 33% have signs of temporomandibular disorders. Approximately 5% of the population will require treatment for temporomandibular disorders (2). Interestingly, the majority of patients seeking treatment are young women (age 20–40 years).

Typically, patients have complaints of orofacial pain, joint noise, and limitations of mandibular movement. Other symptoms such as headache, neckache, earache, dizziness, and tinnitus also have been associated with this condition. Despite extensive research during the past two decades, the etiology of the majority of cases remains elusive. Proposed etiologies include malocclusion (bad bite), bruxism (clenching or grinding the teeth), and trauma (3).

Because of the nonspecific nature of patient's symptoms, temporomandibular disorders have been difficult to classify. As a result, confusing terminologies have appeared in the literature. These include *temporomandibular joint* (TMJ), *Costen's syndrome, temporomandibular joint syndrome* (TMJS), *myofascial pain and dysfunction* (MPD), and *craniomandibular disorders* (CMDs). Currently, these complaints are broadly classified as *temporomandibular disorders* (TMDs). Collectively, temporomandibular disorders seem to represent an assemblage of disorders that can be divided into subcategories. It has been recognized finally that TMD complaints represent not a single disease entity, but a family of clinical conditions similar to those involving other joints (4). TMDs have, for the most part, been managed by dentists. Dentists became the primary care providers because the etiology was believed to be associated with abnormalities of occlusion, and therefore treatment was directed at modifying the dentition. In recent years, it has been recognized that the etiology is multifaceted and that malocclusion does not play a central role. It is important that physicians become informed about TMDs to facilitate diagnosis and treatment. Although no statistics exist, it is apparent that many patients undergo inappropriate and expensive diagnostic procedures because physicians do not consider TMDs in their differential diagnosis.

Physicians should plan an orderly evaluation of the patient with temporomandibular pain and dysfunction. A differential diagnosis should be established by medical history, physical examination, diagnostic imaging, and laboratory analysis. At the most basic level, the physician should determine whether the patient's complaints are caused by a musculoskeletal condition or some other condition. It is important that complaints such as headache, neckache, and ear pain be thoroughly evaluated.

Once a diagnosis has been made, a logical treatment plan can then be developed. The most common TMJ problems are self-limiting and rarely progress to more serious conditions. Therefore, initial treatment should be simple and reversible. Escalation toward nonreversible treatments should be made with caution.

ANATOMY

The TMJ is located anterior to the tragus of the ear and is the articulation between the base of the skull and the condyle of the mandible. The articular surface of the skull is the squamous part of the temporal bone. The bone has a concavity, the articular (glenoid) fossa, and a convexity, the articular eminence. The condyle is convex on surfaces that are load bearing. It is widest in the mediolateral direction.

The articular surfaces of the TMJ are covered with dense fibrous connective tissue instead of hyaline cartilage. Occasionally, cartilage cells occur within this tissue, in which case the surface is termed fibrocartilage. The surfaces are nonvascularized and noninnervated.

An articular capsule surrounds the joint. Laterally, the capsule is thickened to form the lateral (temporomandibular) ligament, which reinforces the joint. Capsular tissues are highly vascular and richly innervated.

The TMJ is a synovial joint. The articular space is divided into two synovial compartments by an articular disc (meniscus) (Fig. 101.1). The articular disc consists of dense, fibroelastic connective tissue and encloses the superior surface of the condyle. It attaches to the capsule and lateral pterygoid muscle anteriorly, joins the capsule mediolaterally, and

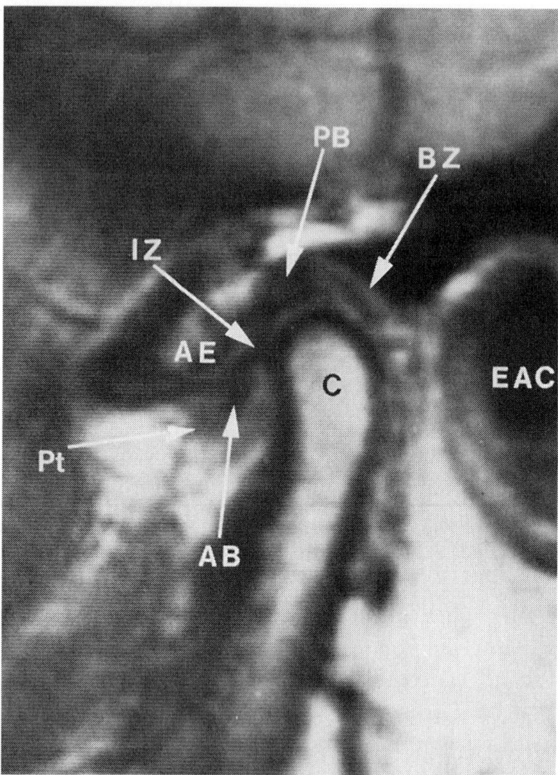

FIGURE 101.1. Magnetic resonance image of the left temporomandibular joint in closed position. *C*, Condyle; *AE*, articular eminence; *EAC*, external auditory canal; *BZ*, bilaminar zone; *PB*, posterior band of disc; *IZ*, intermediate zone; *AB*, anterior band of disc; *PT*, lateral pterygoid muscle.

attaches to loose, vascular connective tissue posteriorly. The superior compartment is largest and contiguous with the fossa. The inferior compartment is smallest and is reinforced by disc attachments. The condyle articulates with the disc with rotational movement occurring in the lower compartment between the condyle and disc. Sliding (translation) movement occurs in the upper compartment between the temporal bone and the disc–condyle complex. The disc maintains contact of the joint surfaces at rest and during function, serving important functions of load distribution and lubrication.

The main blood supply to the TMJ is derived from the terminal branches of the external carotid artery (the maxillary and superficial temporal arteries). The TMJ is innervated primarily by the auriculotemporal nerve.

Movement of the TMJ is produced by the muscles of mastication acting with the suprahyoid and infrahyoid muscle groups. Three large muscles, the masseter, medial pterygoid, and temporalis, function during closing movements of the mandible. The lateral pterygoid muscle functions during opening and excursive (protrusion and lateral) movements, whereas the suprahyoids act during opening of the mandible or with elevation of the hyoid bone. The infrahyoids function during depression of the hyoid bone or elevation of the larynx.

DIFFERENTIAL DIAGNOSIS

The evaluation of the patient with temporomandibular pain and dysfunction is like that of any other diagnostic workup (5). The evaluation should include a thorough history, physical examination of the masticatory system, and some type of plain TMP radiography. Special diagnostic studies such as laboratory tests or advanced imaging techniques should be performed only as indicated and not as routine studies.

HISTORY

The patient's history may be the most important part of the evaluation. It begins with the chief complaint; a statement of the patient's reason for seeking consultation or treatment. The history of the present illness should be comprehensive, including an accurate description of the patient's symptoms, chronology of the symptoms, determination of palliative and aggravating factors, description of how the problem affects the patient, and information about any previous treatments. Patients having TMD usually have complaints of orofacial pain that is worse during jaw function such as mastication and mandibular movement. Frequently patients also have complaints related to decreased mandibular range of motion.

PHYSICAL EXAMINATION

The physical examination consists of an evaluation of the entire masticatory system. The TMJs are examined for tenderness and noise. The most common forms of joint noise are clicking (a distinct sound) and crepitus (multiple, scraping sounds). Joint sounds occur in 33% to 50% of the population and are not necessarily significant, especially in the absence of pain or dysfunction. The mandibular range of motion is determined, with the normal range of movement of the adult's mandible being about 50 mm opening and 10 mm protrusively and laterally. The normal movement is straight and symmetric.

The masticatory muscles should be systematically examined. The head and neck should be inspected for soft tissue asymmetry and evidence of muscle hypertrophy. The patient should be observed for signs of jaw clenching or other habits. The muscles should be palpated for the presence of tenderness, fasciculations, spasm, or trigger points.

The dental examination is important. Odontogenic sources of pain should be eliminated. The teeth should be examined for wear facets, soreness, and mobility, which may be evidence of bruxism. Although the significance of occlusal (bite) abnormalities is controversial, the occlusion should be evaluated. Missing teeth should be noted, and dental and skeletal classification should be determined.

Finally, examination should be directed to specific areas of complaints. For example, patients complaining of ear symptoms should have an ear examination; patients complaining of neckache, a cervical examination.

ROUTINE IMAGING

Routine radiography of the TMJ is essential for the diagnosis of intraarticular osseous pathology. Lateral and anteroposterior views are recommended to evaluate the joint structures. A variety of lateral techniques exist, including transcranial, lateral pharyngeal, and panographic studies. Anteroposterior techniques include transorbital and modified Towne views. Currently, no single technique can be recommended as the best screening examination.

SPECIAL IMAGING STUDIES

Special imaging studies such as computerized tomography (CT), arthrography, magnetic resonance imaging (MRI), and scintigraphy should be used only when specifically indicated (6). Although TMJ arthrography and MRI have proven to be of value in identifying disc displacement, the clinical symptoms have often failed to correlate with the findings (7,8). Overreliance on the diagnostic value of imaging may lead to overdiagnosis and, hence, to overtreatment.

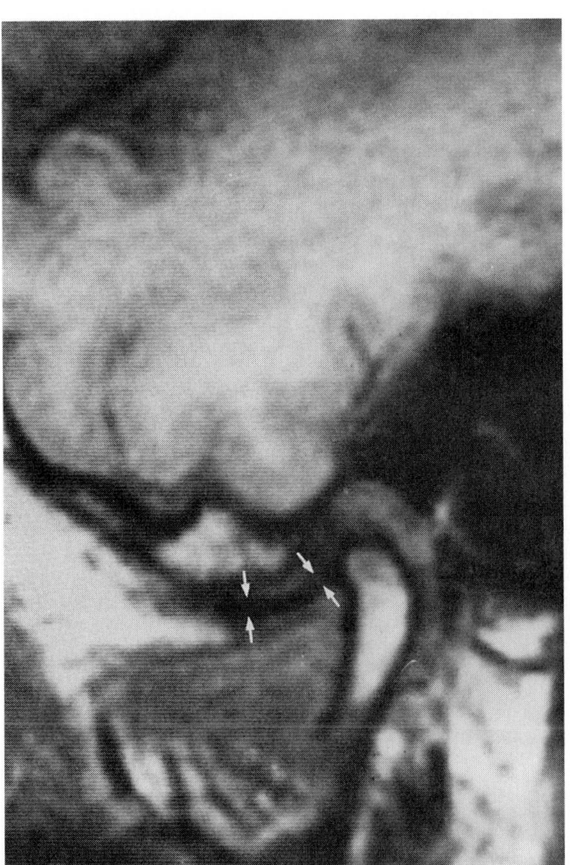

FIGURE 101.2. Magnetic resonance image of the left temporomandibular joint in closed position, showing an anteriorly displaced disc (*arrows*).

CT is indicated for the evaluation of osseous pathology. Condylar erosion, osteophytes, heterotopic bone, and osseous tumors can be seen with more detail than with plain radiography. CT has little role in the evaluation of disc displacement.

TMJ arthrography involves the injection of contrast medium into the synovial joint compartments followed by radiography of the joint. It is used to determine the position and shape of the disc. Arthrography is an invasive procedure and has been replaced for the most part by TMJ MRI.

TMJ MRI is the technique of choice for imaging the articular disc. It has been shown to reliably image the disc and its posterior attachment tissues; however, the clinical symptoms often do not correlate with the imaging findings (Figs. 101.1 and 101.2). Therefore, MRI should be used prudently. MRI also may identify joint effusions as well as avascular necrosis.

Although scintigraphy is rarely indicated, it may be helpful in the evaluation of osseous pathology such as cysts, tumors, or metastatic disease. It also can be useful in evaluating growth disturbances of the mandibular condyles such as condylar hyperplasia.

MYOFASCIAL PAIN AND DYSFUNCTION

MPD is the most common cause of masticatory pain and dysfunction for which patients seek evaluation and treatment (9). This subject is complex, involving several muscular disorders, which, for simplicity, are grouped together as MPD. Generally, the source of pain and dysfunction is muscular. The masticatory muscles become tender and painful as a result of abnormal muscular function. This abnormal muscular function is frequently, but not always, associated with bruxism.

The cause of MPD is controversial, although it is generally considered multifaceted. The most commonly accepted cause is bruxism secondary to stress and anxiety.

Clinical Findings

Patients with MPD generally complain of diffuse, poorly localized, preauricular and temporal pain, which may be cyclic in nature (Fig. 101.3). Patients frequently report that they have difficulty sleeping and that their pain is most severe in the morning on awakening. The patient also may complain of sore teeth. Generally, patients describe decreased and painful mandibular opening as well as pain associated with chewing. Headaches, usually bitemporal in location, also occur. Many patients are conscious of bruxing, although others are unaware of it. The pain most often exists or worsens during periods of stress and anxiety.

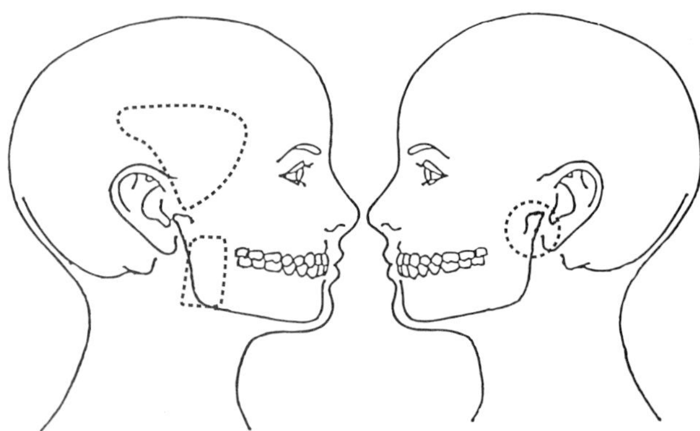

FIGURE 101.3. Facial pain diagram showing diffuse muscular pain associated with myofascial pain and dysfunction (**right**) and localized temporomandibular joint pain associated with internal derangement and osteoarthritis (**left**).

Examination of the patient reveals diffuse tenderness of the masticatory muscles. The TMJs are either nontender or mildly tender to palpation. Joint noise may be present, but is not usually associated with pain or mandibular dysfunction (catching or locking). The range of mandibular movement may be decreased and associated with deviation toward the most affected side. The teeth frequently have wear facets, particularly on the anterior teeth. However, the absence of wear facets does not eliminate bruxism as a cause of the problem.

Radiographic Findings

Radiographs of the TMJ are usually normal. Some patients may have evidence of degenerative joint changes including altered surface contours, erosion, or osteophytes. These changes, however, may be secondary to or unrelated to the MPD problem.

Treatment

The treatment of MPD should initially use reversible, noninvasive forms of therapy (10). Escalation of treatment to irreversible forms of therapy should be done slowly and only after failure to obtain satisfactory results with reversible methods. Initially, treatment involves a careful explanation of the problem to the patient. It is important to reassure the patient that the condition usually resolves with simple treatment and to alleviate concerns about more serious conditions such as tumors or cancer. Home care should include a soft diet, moist heat or cold treatments, muscle massage, and simple exercises consisting of opening and closing, protrusion, and right and left lateral movements of the mandible. Medical therapy should include some type of nonnarcotic analgesic, usually a nonsteroidal antiinflammatory medication, and, if sleep disturbance exists, a low-dose tricyclic antidepressant. The tricyclic antidepressants, particularly amitriptyline, have analgesic properties independent of an antidepressant effect and may be useful for chronic pain patients who have pain and sleep disturbance (11). They decrease the number of awakenings, increase stage IV (delta) sleep, and decrease time in rapid eye movement (REM) sleep. For these reasons, they have potential for the treatment of nocturnal bruxism. Dental treatment involves the use of an occlusal appliance (Fig. 101.4). The reduction of painful symptoms with occlusal appliance therapy has been well documented. Clark (12) reviewed the design, theory, and effectiveness of occlusal appliances and found a 70% to 90% rate of clinical success. Although the treat-

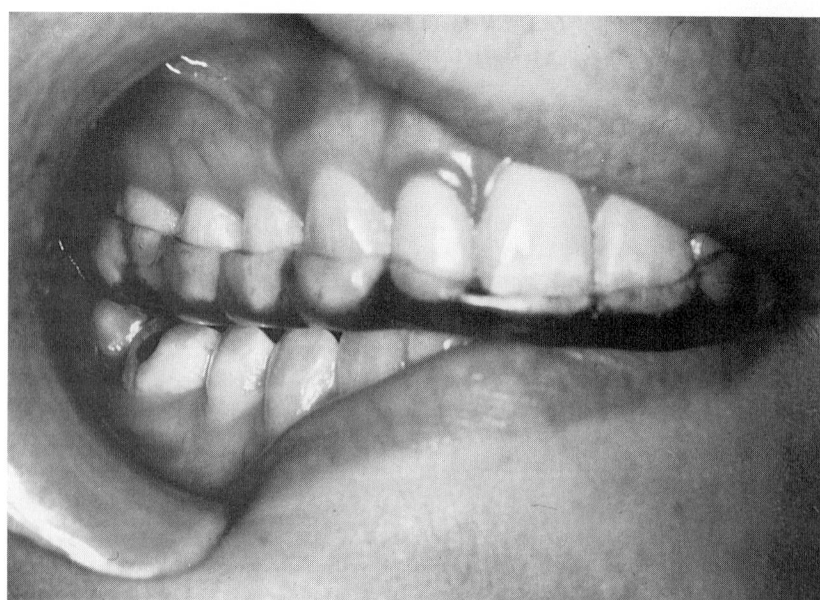

FIGURE 101.4. Maxillary occlusal appliance used for dental treatment of temporomandibular disorders.

ment effects are predictable, the physiologic basis of the treatment response has not been well understood. Patients who initially obtain relief of symptoms with occlusal appliance therapy may benefit from occlusal treatment, including occlusal adjustment, restorative dentistry, or orthodontics. Patients who have significant behavioral problems or who are refractory to treatment may benefit from psychologic evaluation and treatment (13).

It is important to recognize that MPD is usually a chronic problem associated with a behavioral etiology, and the treatment goal should be to manage the pain and dysfunction and not necessarily eliminate them totally. With the exception of dental treatments, MPD is managed similar to tension headaches and fibromyalgia. Surgery is not indicated in the treatment of MPD.

INTERNAL DERANGEMENT AND OSTEOARTHRITIS

Internal derangements and osteoarthritis (OA) are the most common joint causes of masticatory pain and dysfunction for which patients seek evaluation and treatment. This problem involves both disc derangement and OA, which, for simplicity, are grouped together. During the past two decades, disc position has been the focus of classification, diagnosis, and treatment of TMJ internal derangement (14). Recent observations have provided new insights into the pathology of TMJ internal derangement, and the evidence indicates that TMJ internal derangement is a complicated pathology involving disc displacement and deformity, synovitis, changes in articular cartilage, alteration in joint pressures and synovial fluid, and probably several yet-to-be-defined factors (15). The pathologic processes are probably similar to those seen in OA of other joints.

The cause of TMJ internal derangement is not well understood. The most commonly proposed etiologies are adverse joint loading secondary to bruxism and traumatic injuries.

Clinical Findings

Patients with internal derangement and OA often complain of well-localized pain, predominantly in front of the ear and over the joint structures (5) (Fig. 101.3). The pain is usually constant and increases in severity with jaw movements, particularly chewing. The patients also frequently complain of ear problems and headaches. Joint noise commonly exists and consists of either clicking or crepitus, and is usually associated with pain and interference with mandibular movement. Patients also may experience intermittent or permanent locking.

Examination of the patient reveals localized tenderness over the TMJ. However, diffuse muscle tenderness also may exist. Joint noise is commonly present. Patients with limited opening of less than 30 mm usually do not have joint noise. Crepitus may indicate disc perforation and advanced degenerative changes of the joint components. Mandibular movement is typically decreased and painful. The patient experiences increased joint pain when biting on the opposite side.

Radiographic Findings

Radiographs of the TMJ are normal in early cases and will demonstrate degenerative changes (irregularity of the articular surfaces and osteophytes) in more advanced cases. MRI is the preferred diagnostic procedure to demonstrate disc derangement (6) (Fig. 101.2); however, the correlation of the anatomic findings with symptoms is weak. Disc derangement is commonly observed with arthrography or MRI in individuals without pain (8).

Treatment

Clinical experience shows that the majority of patients will have a resolution of the symptoms with simple, reversible treatments (16,17). Toller (18) reported that 51% of patients with TMJ OA were pain free after 1 year, 76% after 2 years, and 98% after 5 years. The treatment of internal derangement and OA initially is similar to that for myofascial pain. A careful explanation of the problem, emphasizing the self-limiting nature, should be given to the patient. Home care should include a soft diet, jaw rest, and application of moist heat. Medical therapy is directed toward pain relief and reduction of inflammation by the use of nonsteroidal antiinflammatory medications. Narcotic analgesics should be avoided. Low-dose tricyclic antidepressants may be helpful if the patient is experiencing sleep disturbance. Dental treatment involves the use of occlusal appliances (Fig. 101.4). Whereas the physiologic basis for the effectiveness of occlusal appliances is poorly understood, they seem to reduce pain in 70% to 80% of the patients.

TMJ surgery plays an important but limited role in the treatment of patients whose symptoms are severe and refractory to conservative treatment (19). TMJ arthrocentesis and joint lavage has been shown to be effective in the management of acute cases with severe limitation of opening (20). The procedure is simple to perform and has no associated significant morbidity. TMJ arthroscopy has revolutionized the surgical approach to the treatment of internal derangement and osteoarthritis of the TMJ (21,22). Arthroscopic lavage and lysis of adhesions has proven effective in reducing pain and increasing range of motion in approximately 80% of the patients treated. Complications with TMJ arthroscopy are less common than with open surgery (23). Advanced arthroscopic operative techniques using rotary instruments, electrocautery, and lasers are being developed, but their effectiveness compared with simple lavage and lysis of adhesions has not been proven. TMJ arthrotomy procedures, including disc repositioning and arthroplasty or discectomy (meniscectomy), have been used for the treatment of severe symptoms for many years and are successful in the reduction of symptoms in about 80% of the patients (24). TMJ arthrotomy procedures are indicated for patients who have severe mechanical problems such as intermittent locking or patients who previously have undergone surgery. Complications associated with TMJ arthrotomy include facial nerve injury, malocclusion, and continued or increased symptoms (23). In past years, the use of alloplastic implants in the TMJ was popular; however, experience has shown that most of these patients developed particulation of the implant and foreign-body reactions. Therefore, the use of alloplastic implants in the TMJ is not recommended. In summary, TMJ surgical procedures benefit about 80% of the patients treated. Unfortunately, about 5% of patients who undergo surgery experience a worsening of their symptoms. The decision to proceed with surgery, therefore, must be carefully considered and made by both the patient and surgeon.

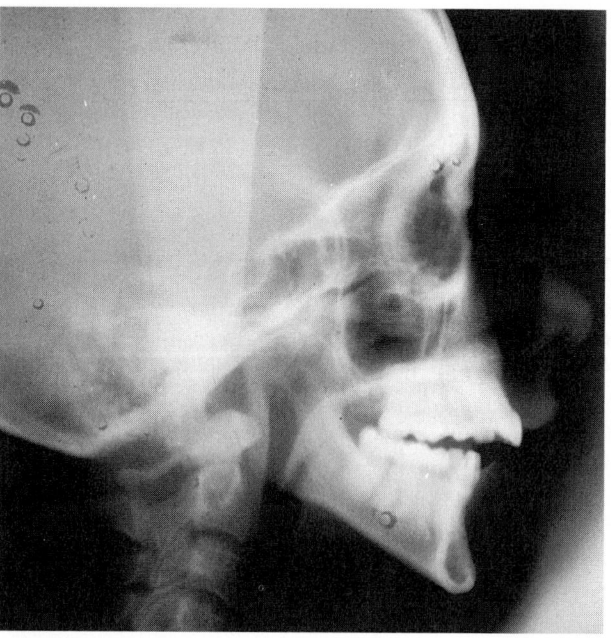

FIGURE 101.5. Lateral head radiograph showing posterior rotation of mandible associated with temporomandibular joint rheumatoid arthritis.

RHEUMATOID ARTHRITIS

Approximately 50% of patients with rheumatoid arthritis (RA) have involvement of the TMJ (25). Affected women outnumber affected men 3:1. TMJ involvement usually occurs late during the disease process and is more likely to occur in severe cases. The disease affects both TMJs. RA causes destruction of the mandibular condyles, frequently resulting in the development of a recessive mandible and open bite malocclusion.

Clinical Findings

Patients with RA with TMJ involvement may experience deep, dull, preauricular pain with exacerbation during function. TMJ tenderness, crepitation, and occasionally swelling over the joint also occur. Decreased range of motion, which is usually worse in the morning, may be noted by the patient. In patients with juvenile rheumatoid arthritis or with severe disease that has caused extensive resorption of the mandibular condyles, a recessive mandible and open-bite malocclusion may develop (Figs. 101.5 and 101.6). Hypomobility from fibrous or bony ankylosis also may occur.

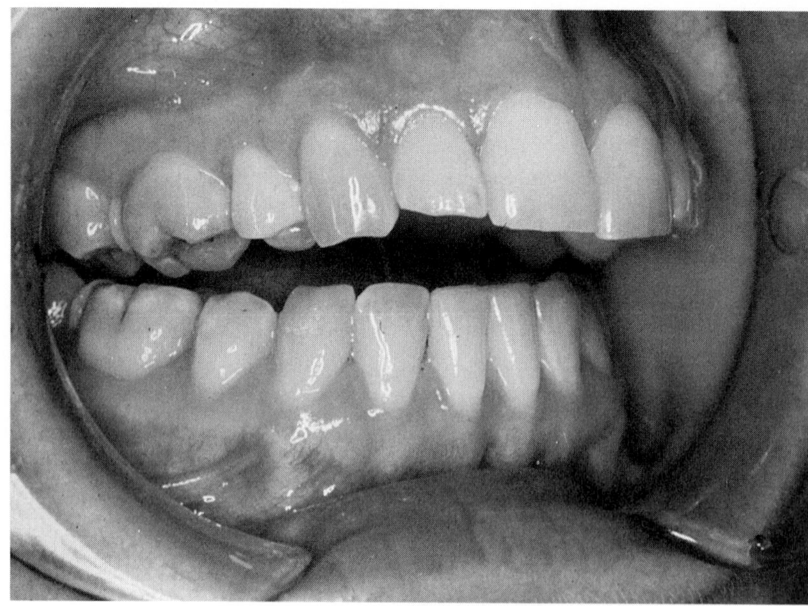

FIGURE 101.6. Open-bite malocclusion secondary to condylar resorption in patient with rheumatoid arthritis.

Radiographic Findings

TMJ radiographs may show flattening of the condylar heads. In advanced cases, a spiked appearance of the condyle is observed.

Treatment

Management of the TMJ affected by RA is directed toward management of the systemic disease (see Chapter 62). This includes medical management of symptoms and physical therapy designed to maintain functional range of motion. Dental therapy is directed at establishing and maintaining stable occlusal relations. Special oral hygiene programs may have to be developed for the patient who has a decreased ability to brush and floss.

Surgical intervention should be considered when persistent pain or significantly altered function is manifested by either severe hypomobility or the development of an openbite malocclusion. Generally, the surgical alternatives are either orthognathic surgery or total joint replacement.

OTHER DISEASES

The TMJ can be affected by any disease that involves synovial joints. Ankylosing spondylitis, psoriatic arthritis, and crystallopathies rarely affect the TMJs. Other conditions affecting the TMJ include hypermobility manifested by subluxation or dislocation of the condyles, fibrous or osseous ankylosis, and growth disturbances such as condylar hyperplasia or hypoplasia. Tumors are rare but do occur and must always be considered in the differential diagnosis. The most common benign tumor seen in the TMJ is osteochondroma, and the most common malignant tumor is osteo- or chondrosarcoma. Metastatic disease also may occur, especially with breast malignancies.

REFERENCES

1. Rugh JD, Solberg WK. Oral health status in the United States: temporomandibular disorders. *J Dent Educ* 1985;49:398–404.
2. Solberg WK, Woo MW, Houston JB. Prevalence of mandibular dysfunction in young adults. *J Am Dent Assoc* 1979;98:25–34.
3. McNeill C. Craniomandibular (TMJ) disorders: the state of the art: Part II. accepted diagnosis and treatment and modalities. *J Prosthet Dent* 1983;49:393–397.
4. McNeill C. Diagnostic classification. In: McNeill C, ed. *Temporomandibular disorders, guidelines for classification, assessment and management.* Chicago: Quintessence Publishing, 1993: 19–20.
5. Dolwick MF. Clinical diagnosis of temporomandibular joint internal derangement and myofascial pain and dysfunction. *Oral Maxillofac Surg Clin North Am* 1989;1:1–6.
6. Katzberg RW. Temporomandibular joint imaging. *Radiology* 1989;170:297–307.
7. Kaplan PA, Tu HK, Sleder PR, et al. Inferior joint space arthrography of normal TMJ: reassessment of diagnostic criteria. *Radiology* 1986;159:585–589.
8. Kiros LT, Ortendahl DA, Mark AS, et al. Magnetic resonance of the TMJ disc in asymptomatic volunteers. *J Oral Maxillofac Surg* 1987;45:852–854.
9. Laskin DM. Etiology of pain dysfunction syndrome. *J Am Dent Assoc* 1969;79:147–153.
10. Green CS, Laskin DM. Long-term evaluation of treatment for myofascial pain dysfunction syndrome: a comparative analysis. *J Am Dent Assoc* 1983;108:235–238.
11. Kreisberg MK. Tricyclic antidepressants: analgesic effect and indications in orofacial pain. *J Craniomandib Disord Facial Oral Pain* 1988;1:171–177.
12. Clark GT. A critical evaluation of orthopedic interocclusal appliance therapy: design, theory and overall effectiveness. *J Am Dent Assoc* 1984;108:359–364.
13. Rugh JD. Psychological components of pain. *Dent Clin North Am* 1987;31:579–594.
14. Dolwick MF, Katzberg RW, Helms CA. Internal derangements of the temporomandibular joint: fact or fiction? *J Prosthet Dent* 1983;49:415–418.
15. Stegenga B, DeBont LGM, Boering G, et al. Tissue responses to degenerative changes in the temporomandibular joint. *J Oral Maxillofac Surg* 1991;49:1079–1088.
16. Boering G. *Temporomandibular joint arthrosis:* an analysis of 400 cases. Leiden: Stafleu, 1966.
17. DeLeeuw R, Boering G, Stengenga B, et al. Clinical signs of TMJ osteoarthrosis and internal derangement 30 years after nonsurgical treatment. *J Orofac Pain* 1994;8:18–24.
18. Toller PA. Osteoarthrosis of the mandibular condyle. *Br Dent J* 1973;7:47.
19. Dolwick MF, Dimitroulis G. Is there a role for temporomandibular joint surgery? *Br J Oral Maxillofac Surg* 1994;32: 307–313.
20. Nitzan DW, Dolwick MF, Martinez A. Temporomandibular joint arthrocentesis: a simplified treatment for severe, limited mouth opening. *J Oral Maxillofac Surg* 1991;49:1163–1169.
21. Sanders B. Arthroscopic surgery of the temporomandibular joint: treatment of internal derangement with persistent closed lock. *Oral Surg* 1986;62:361–364.
22. McCain JP. Arthroscopy of the human temporomandibular joint. *J Oral Maxillofac Surg* 1988;46:648–652.
23. Vallerand WP, Dolwick MF. Complications of temporomandibular joint surgery. *Oral Maxillofac Surg Clin North Am* 1990;2:481–488.
24. Dolwick MF, Nitzan DW. The role of disc-repositioning surgery for internal derangement of the temporomandibular joint. *Oral Maxillofac Surg Clin North Am* 1994;6:271–275.
25. Ogus H. Rheumatoid arthritis of the temporomandibular joint. *Br J Oral Surg* 1975;12:275–284.

102

LOW BACK PAIN

NORTIN M. HADLER

Backache has bedeviled humans always. The quest to cope leaves in its wake a legacy of ingenuity, false starts, conceptions and misconceptions, illusion and disillusion that spans the globe and the ages. This history is a window on the vagaries of common sense. Medicine has always been a player, although not always a major player and not without its share of ignobility.

The dawn of medical interest in back pain was auspicious. The relevant hieroglyphics of the Edwin Smith Papyrus, the famous clinical document written around 1,500 BC and unearthed in Thebes in 1862, are translated as follows (1):

> If thou examinest a man having a sprain of the vertebra of his spinal column, Thou should say to him: Extend your legs and contract them both. He contracts them both immediately because of the pain he causes in the vertebra of the spinal column. Thou should say to him: One having a sprain in the vertebra of his spinal column, an ailment I shall treat. Thou should place him prostrate on his back. . . .

Medicine in Egypt in that day was preeminent. Practitioners were men of learning. Specialization flourished, and back pain commanded attention in a fashion that has returned to vogue today. The pain was thought to emanate from the vertebral body itself. The scribe was recording a description of a diagnostic maneuver of some form of Lesègue's sign. If only the next phrases of the papyrus had survived, perhaps the Egyptian physicians of old could have provided the therapeutic insight that we still lack. More likely, the next phrases were unfounded therapeutic assertions, because in the ensuing 3,500 years, those afflicted have gravitated to other remedies more often than to those offered by physicians.

Backache sufferers still do so today. The choice to be your patient for a backache is—nearly always—just that, a choice. Other options have been considered and discarded or tried and found to be lacking. The volitional aspect of seeking a physician's care must be appreciated to do justice to the choice; often the choice is driven by life's issues that confound the backache and that must be addressed if therapy is to succeed (2). This truth, which seldom finds its way into medical textbooks on any topic, is the secret to diagnosing and to managing low back pain. It is the subliminal force that has driven sufferers to seek cures high and low for millennia. This chapter dispels all that seems counterintuitive about this aphorism.

SYSTEMIC BACKACHE

Most patients with low back pain have a regional backache (i.e., one that is not caused by systemic disease). They have experienced no overtly traumatic precipitating event, and they would be well were it not for their use-related pain (3). Their plight is the focus of this chapter. On rare occasion, however, low back pain is a symptom of a systemic disorder, notably a primary or metastatic neoplastic or infectious disease, or idiopathic inflammatory disease for which specific therapy or special palliation is available. Modern medicine has the sensitive and specific means to diagnose each of these conditions safely and expeditiously. Expense aside, what do physicians have to lose if all backache patients are screened to assure ourselves and them that they are in the great majority who have a regional backache?

Plenty! Any prolonged diagnostic algorithm entails anxiety, some discomfort, and the potential for specious results. It also recruits the patient's active and intimate participation; symptoms grow in importance, rendering less pressing the development of coping skills that facilitate returning a patient with regional backache to function and then to healthfulness. By the time the patient has completed a laboratory battery, undergone imaging procedures, and been confronted with equivocal or misleading findings, the experience of illness is perturbed in a fashion that can be useful only if specific and effective therapy results. Even in the elderly presenting to a primary care physician, the likelihood of a neoplasm mimicking regional backache is less than 1:1,000 and, at any age, the likelihood of a mimicking infection is less than 1:10,000 (4). Therefore for nearly all patients with back pain, the diagnostic exercise, to varying degrees, is iatrogenic (5). The only defensible categoric screening must be completed during the course of the initial interaction.

TABLE 102.1. INDICATORS OF SYSTEMIC BACKACHE

Clinical Feature	Diagnostic Possibility
Weight loss	Metastatic neoplasia, chronic infection
Fever	Septic discitis, epidural abscess
Night pain causing fidgeting, pacing	Neoplasia
Night pain is less intense sitting	Cauda equina tumor
Paraparesis	Spinal infarct, neoplasia
Writhing pain	Vascular catastrophe, kidney stone
Cauda equina syndrome	Intrathecal tumors

Thus the burden is placed on the clinician's diagnostic acumen. Fortunately, most systemic diseases provoke back pain with distinctive qualities (Table 102.1). The presence of any such feature mandates appropriate laboratory and imaging studies. For many of these systemic diseases, sentinel clues can emerge during the expert physical examination that these patients deserve. It is to this end that the rheumatologist must be highly competent in all aspects of the physical examination. To confirm a clinical suspicion, or if serious doubt remains, most of the systemic processes that cause back pain can be readily detected by magnetic resonance imaging (MRI). If pathologic confirmation is necessary, appropriate tissue is accessible to imaging-guided needle biopsy. Unfortunately, in most series of patients whose backache had a systemic pathogenesis, as many as 50% lacked any clinical clue at presentation and for some time into their course. This holds for primary neoplasms (6), septic discitis (7), and epidural abscess (8). Even cord infarcts can produce weeks of low back pain before catastrophic paraparesis (9). So for the vast majority of backache patients who lack any hint of systemic pathogenesis, some small degree of uncertainty remains. That uncertainty, and the anxiety it provokes, is the purview of the treating physician. Some physicians seek reassurance in an erythrocyte sedimentation rate, accepting the limitations inherent in both the positive and negative predictive values of the test. In the course of managing putative regional backache, it behooves all physicians to introduce some forewarning regarding symptoms that should be brought to their attention (Table 102.1), while emphasizing the need to cope with all other symptoms. This is the conundrum of uncertainty for which society needs a physician.

REGIONAL LOW BACK PAIN

Back pain is a recurrent (10) nemesis: in adolescence (11), in the last decades of life (12,13), and in all decades in between (14). Based on telephone surveys, household interviews, questionnaires, and longitudinal diary studies (15) in many countries over many decades, back pain is a universal human predicament. As many as 50% of us recall such a challenge occurring in the past year. As many as 10% to 20% recall the challenge as daunting regardless of age, nationality, sex, or station in life. Low back pain is a predicament with which many individuals must cope, but they often must do so repeatedly and not always successfully. Telephone interviews with 4,437 randomly selected North Carolina adults unearthed the disturbing fact that 3.9% had chronic back pain during the course of a single year (16). "Chronic" meant they were in pain for more than 3 months that year, or experienced more than 25 episodes (Table 102.2).

Low back pain is a morbidity without human boundaries. It also is a morbidity that scorns the reductionism that contemporary Western medicine upholds with single-minded zeal; it is not simply a symptom of an underlying disease that needs to be caged by the power of diagnostics and then brought to heel by incisive treatment. Adherence to such an algorithm guarantees disservice for the patient

TABLE 102.2. CHARACTERISTICS OF 3.9% OF THE ADULT RESIDENTS OF NORTH CAROLINA WHO HAVE "CHRONIC" LOW BACK PAIN

Demographics		Clinical Features	
Mean age (yr)	52	Assessed health as fair or poor (%)	53
Female (%)	66	Permanently disabled from back pain (%)	34
Years since initial backache (mean)	14	Leg pain (%)	76
White race (%)	81	Days in bed past year (mean)	26
Currently employed (%)	42	Days off work in past year (mean)	21
Limited health insurance (%)	33	Sought care in past year (%)	73
Annual household income <$20,000 (%)	55	Ever hospitalized for back pain (%)	41
		Ever had surgery for back pain (%)	22

Reproduced with permission from Carey TS, Evans A, Hadler NM, Kalsbeek W, McLaughlin C, Freyer J. Care-seeking among individuals with chronic low back pain. *Spine* 1995,20:312–317.

with regional back pain. Similarly, structuring this chapter to serve such an algorithm would not serve the reader well. This topic (and many others in rheumatology and other fields) must be approached from the perspective of the individual who is having pain and who is considering options in recourse (17).

Processing the Predicament

Mobility and function that had been taken for granted become challenging in the predicament of regional back pain. The biomechanics of the lumbosacral spine are such that even leaning forward 20 degrees entails an impressive increment in force (Fig. 102.1). If writing at a desk can exacerbate the pain, lifting or assuming awkward postures can be prohibitive. Recumbency helps, but affected individuals have to be fully recumbent and persist in that posture in spite of boredom and uselessness. The pain always seems diabolic, no matter how sophisticated the person. Most individuals have learned to envision specters of disability, a ruptured disc, a "bad back," and back surgery. Each is forced to think about the pain, the predicament it is posing, and the options that are available. There are three (Fig. 102.2): one can persist somehow in remaining a person, in mobilizing personal resources in the hopes of steady improvement. If persevering presents an insurmountable challenge, one can choose to seek the ministrations of a doctor. If you find that you cannot perform in your workplace, most work settings in most industrial countries offer workplace health and safety programs.

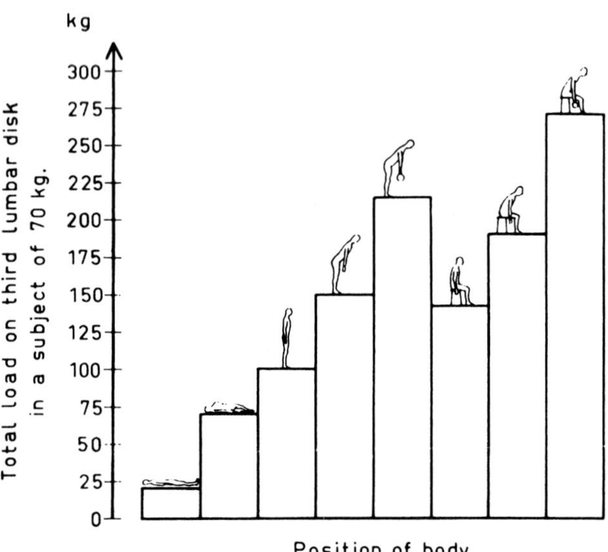

FIGURE 102.1. Total load on the L3 disk in different positions in a subject weighing 70 kg. Positions shown are **(a)** reclining (relaxed, supine), **(b)** reclining (lateral decubitus), **(c)** standing upright, **(d)** standing and 20 degree forward leaning without and **(e)** with a 20-kg load in arms, **(f)** sitting upright, arms and back unsupported, **(g)** sitting and 20 degree forward leaning without and **(h)** with a 20-kg load in arms. (Reproduced with permission from Nachemson A. In vivo discometry in lumbar discs with irregular nucleograms. Some differences in stress distribution between normal and moderately degenerated discs. *Acta Orthop Scand* 1965;36:426.)

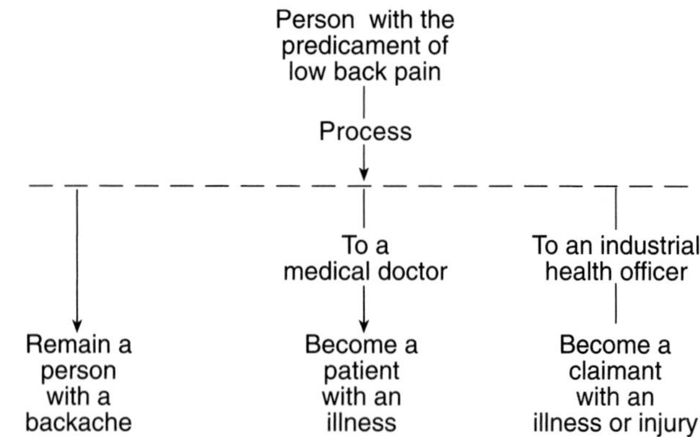

FIGURE 102.2. Processing the predicament of backache. Three options are available, each of which involves a choice between stations in life and each of which represents a very different contract. One can persevere. One can seek the assistance of a medical doctor. This figure is chauvinistic by intent. It should have been drawn to offer a number of alternatives that would involve choosing some person with certification or a degree, even a doctorate, in any number of disciplines purporting to offer expert assistance. However, the existence of these options is encompassed in the option of trying to "remain a person." However, the moment one talks to a medical doctor, that person is no longer a person with a predicament; he or she becomes a patient with the illness, backache. The third option is to tell someone in the context of the workplace that you are having a backache. Again you are no longer a person with a predicament. You instantly become a claimant, and your backache will be considered an illness or an injury, depending on the language heard when you describe the experience. If the language suggests you "injured your back," you are a claimant under workers' compensation insurance. Otherwise, if you simply started to hurt or the precipitant you perceive was not related to work or working, you are in a quest for whatever benefits are provided by your health insurance.

It has long been assumed that processing the predicament of backache is driven by the intensity of the illness and the autonomy one has in structuring daily physical demands. This assumption may indeed hold at the extremes. Sometimes the pain is so excruciating or is accompanied by neurologic symptoms so frightening that nothing short of medical care makes sense. Sometimes extraordinary physical demands cannot be avoided if one is to perform at all—a professional athlete, for example. But for most people faced with nearly all episodes of regional backache, processing is driven neither by the intensity of pain nor tasks that simply can not be circumvented. Rather, it is driven by personal psychosocial confounders. The pain is rendered far less tolerable when other aspects of our life are not in order. Then it can become the "straw that broke the camel's back"; any approach to the symptoms that ignores psychosocial confounders runs the risk of magnifying the predicament. This is readily demonstrable in the context of the workplace (18), but also holds for coping with regional musculoskeletal symptoms regardless of the setting (19).

An understanding of the reasoning behind and choices involved in "processing" is difficult to come by; there are important vagaries of recall that compromise interview surveys (20), although too close observation can perturb coping behavior. Asking people to keep a diary, as was done with a probability sample of 589 households in the 1977 Health in Detroit study (15), may be the closest we can come. This survey documented that 51% of adults can record musculoskeletal discomfort an average of 8 days of a 6-week period. More than 90% of this morbidity was low back pain. Most were otherwise asymptomatic and thought their symptoms were "not very serious." Most talked to their spouses about their predicament and ingested over-the-counter analgesics. Only 3% considered going to a doctor; 0.3% actually saw a doctor. There was one lost work day per two households over the course of these 6 weeks, but backache paled next to upper respiratory symptoms as the rationale. This survey is a glimpse of processing (Fig. 102.2) in one small universe, at one time. There is every reason to predict that this form of processing will not generalize. After all, it reflects common sense. Common sense is not common, either geographically or temporally, and it is relatively easy to perturb. Perturbing common sense is a fact of life and a goal of marketing.

Perhaps the best way to make this point is to contrast the Health in Detroit longitudinal survey with several other interview surveys in various populations including cross-sectional surveys conducted in Iowa (21) and Sweden (13) on elderly populations, probability samples of the entire population of the United States (14) and Finland (22), and another longitudinal interview survey of a probability sample of Glostrup, a suburb of Copenhagen (23). The magnitude of the differences in recall of the experience of backache and the perceived need to be a patient reflected across these surveys cannot simply be attributed to methodologic differences. Furthermore, these and other surveys provide documentation of the dramatic differences in the quantity and quality of the recourse sought by people whose most obvious differences relate to acculturation. If such differences can develop transnationally, just as they develop across sociologic strata (24), they can evolve. Medicine must be aware of its role in the dialectic, but first medicine must be aware of the dialectic itself. Processing the predicament of backache is one of life's ubiquitous challenges (Fig. 102.2). Perturbing processing has a history dating back millennia. The challenge is to gain certainty that any perturbation benefits the sufferer more than its provider or purveyor (25).

Coping with Back Pain

Attempting to cope with back pain is not a lonely exercise in any society. Everyone has advice to offer, mostly unsolicited. In advanced industrialized societies, inventive marketing offers everything from mattresses to automobile seats as solutions. There are people willing to push, pull, prod, and soak the sufferer. There are others to orchestrate exercise programs, offer education, or alter your lifestyle—all with unsubstantiated zeal (26). But everyone has a theory to explain the benefit that justifies their charges. This cacophony permeates our society; it always has and always will. It has a plasticity for which science is no match. Because of the natural history of low back pain, this marketplace enjoys a self-fulfilling prophecy that overwhelms *caveat emptor.* Low back pain is a chronic predicament characterized by intermittency and remittency. Nearly all episodes regress within a fortnight. What human being can purchase a modality, and then experience regression of symptoms, and not assume causality?

The pharmaceutical industry has long been a participant in this marketplace (27). In the 1960s, Americans consumed more than 40 tons of aspirin each day. That has fallen some 50% to be supplanted by prescription nonsteroidal antiinflammatory agents, approaching 100 million prescriptions annually through the 1980s (28). The pharmaceutical marketing strategy in the 1990s is to switch more and more of these drugs to the over-the-counter (OTC) market. Why? So that when Americans try to cope with their next episode of back pain or other regional musculoskeletal illness, their common sense will drive them toward OTC remedies before they need to consider a recourse other than their own devices. The ramifications for the American lifestyle boggle the mind. According to the Health in Detroit survey (15), 20 years ago the majority of people having the predicament of back pain sought relief in OTC remedies (often containing salicylates or phenacetin). More than half of the elderly in the Iowa 65+ Rural Health Study (21) were similarly inclined in the mid-1980s. Indubitably, this inclination can be encouraged so that more and more Americans of all ages learn to tolerate less and less regional musculoskeletal discomfort without consuming OTC analgesics. To whose benefit? At what risk?

Purchasing a pill, a mattress, or a membership in a health club entails little personal exposure. Not so, going to a healer. And healers abound outside of orthodox medicine today as they have for centuries. There are groups of healers whose practices are founded on principles, doctrines, and dogmas that are anathema to the orthodox medicine of the day. Some groups are outcasts from orthodox medicine, some are religious or quasireligious, and some evolve their doctrine from the teachings of a single eccentric proponent. These groups constitute "sectarian medicine" (29), and they flourish in America as elsewhere. Two of the sects that were founded in America a century ago thrive today in large part by offering themselves as a logical and ready option for any person faced with the predicament of low back pain. One, osteopathy, has abandoned most of its doctrines that orthodox medicine would consider deviant and has come to represent a different form of orthodox medicine that includes the application of mobilization and manipulative techniques to the plight of the sufferer with regional muscu-

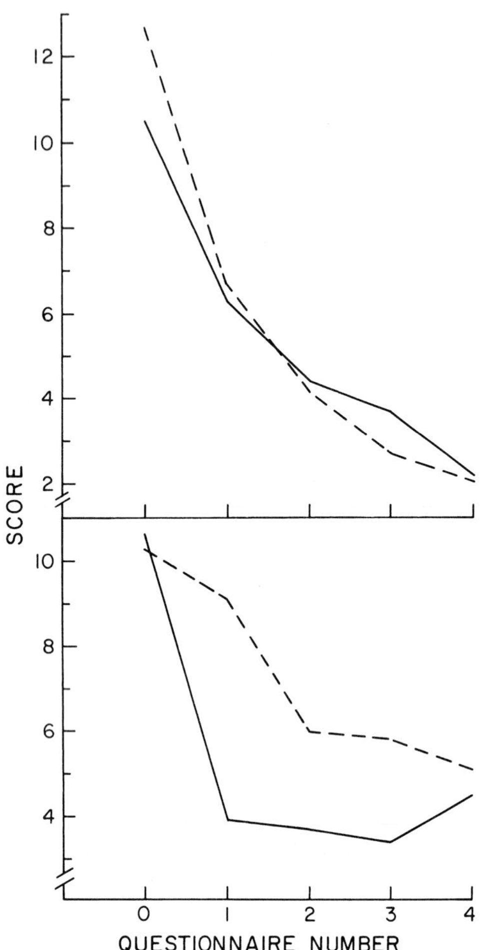

FIGURE 102.3. The University of North Carolina Trial of Spinal Manipulation. These plots show mean scores on a questionnaire that quantified the magnitude of illness from acute low back pain experienced by subjects in the University of North Carolina study of spinal manipulation. The questionnaire was administered just before entry into the study and at the time of telephone follow-up every 3 (±1) days after treatment. *Broken lines*, results from subjects randomized to be treated by mobilization entailing passive gentle motion of the spine; *solid lines*, those randomized to receive, in addition to mobilization, spinal manipulation using single, long lever-arm, high-velocity technique. All four groups were indistinguishable at entry and at 2 weeks after treatment. **Top:** Results for the stratum wherein all subjects had backache for <2 weeks at the time of entry into the protocol. **Bottom:** The stratum for subjects that had backaches for 2 to 4 weeks. Treatment effect was discernible only in the latter stratum ($p = 0.009$). In that stratum, those who underwent manipulation achieved a 50% reduction in score more rapidly than did those who underwent mobilization alone, although the latter caught up by 2 weeks. (Reproduced with permission from Hadler NM, Curtis P, Gillings DB, et al. A benefit of spinal manipulation as adjunctive therapy for acute low-back pain: a stratified controlled trial. *Spine* 1987;12:703–706.)

loskeletal illness (30). However, the other, the chiropractic, persists in staunch advocacy of many of its peculiar doctrines (31), is thriving in numbers of practitioners and patients, and has a growing presence in Canada (32) and elsewhere. Theories aside, it is clear that spinal manipulation can offer benefit to individuals faced with the predicament of low back pain (33). However, that benefit is most readily observed after a single treatment in individuals with uncomplicated low back pain of 2 to 4 weeks' duration (34), and it is hardly dramatic (Fig. 102.3). One can easily argue for including this maneuver among the options for medical management. However, there is no scientific support for manipulative therapy for any condition other than for this particular subset with low back pain, and no reason for multiple treatments (35).

Choosing to be a Patient with Regional Back Pain

Why would anyone abandon coping on their own, the benefit of nonprescription preparations, and the ministrations of those who push and pull and soak to see the advice of someone with a doctorate in medicine? Because the pain is intolerable? Never is the answer that straightforward. Remember we are considering a regional musculoskeletal illness; by definition, there are postures and positions that provide relief. The reason persons with regional low back pain assumes the vulnerability of becoming a patient is that they cannot cope on their own. If the response of the treating physician is to squelch pain with the prescription of analgesic and by the proscription of function, the result will be a costly compromise in the patient's satisfaction with care, understanding of the illness, and function (36). If the response to the treating physician is contingent on defining the cause of the pain, nearly always a diabolic fool's errand is enjoined. If the response of the treating physician is to seek to cure, the only ally in the exercise is natural history. American physicians, and all Americans, must be disabused of any notion to the contrary. The only patient–doctor contract that can be successfully enjoined relates to coping. The data disabusing all parties of any other preconceived notion are overwhelming.

In fact, the data addressing myriad issues that relate to the management of acute low back pain are rich and informative. They also are readily accessible, thanks to the work product, a "Clinical Practice Guideline," of a panel sponsored by the Agency for Health Care Policy and Research of the United States Department of Health and Human Services (37). The panel relied on a structured review of 360 clinical articles to derive an assessment of the substantive nature of current diagnostic and therapeutic inferences. Because I served as one of five formal consultants to this panel, the consonance of this text with the panel's conclusions is not surprising. The panel's conclusions reflect inferences I have drawn for nearly two decades (38,39). That does not make these Guidelines truth; they are heavily reflective of the values that dominate the interactions of the panel (40). Only occasionally is the science itself compelling. Even then, realize that to design a clinical experiment of the highest quality, one must focus the question, thereby reducing confidence that the result will generalize and *vice versa.* In other words, any panel is forced to weigh the value of "bad clinical science" performed on a

TABLE 102.3. EVIDENCE-BASED MANAGEMENT OF A PATIENT WITH A REGIONAL BACKACHE SEEKING THE MINISTRATIONS OF A RHEUMATOLOGIST

1. An elicitation of the history of the present illness that circumvents psychosocial confounders is inadequate. The impact of the back pain on coping at work and in the home—and vice versa—are more important features of the present illness than the quality of the pain
2. The elicitation of the history of the present illness is an instructional event for the patient as well as the physician. In the asking of questions, one communicates meaningfulness that may be not valid. The physician must be prepared to disabuse the patient of any resulting false inferences, including false inferences regarding causation, pathophysiology, and prognosis
3. The physical examination can assuage clinical uncertainty, to some degree, regarding the regional nature of the illness. It can exclude neurologic catastrophe, particularly overt leg weakness or cauda equina syndrome, in which case, surgical consultation is advisable. But it offers little else in terms of pathophysiologic insight. Focal neurologic signs are modestly useful in localization of pathology, but limited in specificity otherwise and in prognostic implications. Overinterpretation of such findings will inflame anxiety and thereby compromise palliation
4. Imaging modalities offer the potential for great anatomic definition. However, degenerative changes of the lumbosacral spine, even dramatic degenerative changes, are common in the asymptomatic and will persist in your patient long after symptoms have subsided. Given the lack of specificity, there is no justification for any imaging in this setting if the hypothesis one is testing is a regional disease
5. Do not invalid your patient either by your attitude or by your prescription. Urge coping and advise neutral postures, but do not prescribe bed rest
6. Do not prescribe an analgesic for impaired coping; doing so clouds the issues further and promulgates prolonged illness. Likewise, eschew agents that cloud the sensorium; coping requires one's wits. Seldom is any prescription analgesic mandatory. Attention to posture and to psychosocial confounders are the front line of therapy
7. Regional low back pain is not a surgical disease! There is no demonstrable benefit of any invasive, even "minimally invasive," technique. At best, the patient is "unharmed," but even this end is elusive. Submitting to aggressive, heroic, unfounded remedies fosters a sense of desperation that harbors the downfall of palliation
8. An array of widgets, physical therapies, and the like can be prescribed or suggested. At best, they are harmless. Always they instruct your patient in unfounded therapeutic and pathogenetic theories. To what end? Wouldn't enlightenment be preferable?

patient population representative of the vagaries of practice versus "good science" on a highly selected subset. It is no surprise that the "consensus" of any one panel need not generalize to another. Nonetheless, I urge rheumatologists to review this information in all its well-referenced breadth as a basis for personal conviction regarding the quality of evidence on which the Guidelines is based, if for no other reason than to be able to offer informed counsel to any patient who has sampled or wishes to sample alternatives to rheumatologic advice. I share the misgiving of many internists whenever "guidelines" are offered as a substitute for independent consideration by a physician faced with the idiosyncratic nature of any present illness (41).

Table 102.3 summarizes my version of defensible rheumatologic advice. Because this advice represents a radical departure from the tone and substance of previous chapters in this text, the readership is due some explanation.

Symptoms and Signs

Quantification of reproducibility (42), sensitivity, and specificity (43) places in perspective the physical signs long held to be useful in the diagnosis of regional backache. Short of cauda equina syndrome, none can offer substantial insights when it comes to the diagnosis or management of low back pain. Short of overt weakness, no finding, not even stretch signs or focal neurologic abnormalities, can alter the diagnostic synthesis or restructure therapeutic options for sciatica or other leg pain syndromes. The fact that the pain radiates into the leg already speaks to the presence of radiculopathy from the ipsilateral caudad lumbosacral roots; neither the presence nor absence of a stretch sign, nor a depressed tendon reflex, adds substantially to that insight, in terms of either localization or pathogenesis (44). The reason I still seek these signs is that I am tradition bound. However, I treat the findings or lack thereof with some diffidence. I also do not ascribe special importance to the presence of radiating pain. Sciatica is no more ominous a presentation than regional low back pain alone (45). The patient who is coping with leg pain should be afforded the same reasoned approach that is appropriate for the patient with regional low back pain without radiation.

TABLE 102.4. PRINCIPAL RESULTS AT 6 MONTHS OF THE REVEL RANDOMIZED CONTROLLED STUDY OF TREATING SCIATICA THAT HAD PERSISTED MORE THAN A MONTH BEFORE INTERVENTION

Patient's Global Assessment	Chemonucleolysis (*n* = 72)	Automated Percutaneous Discectomy (*n* = 69)
Very good and good	44	30
None and moderate	21	14
Subsequent surgery	5	23
Lost to follow-up	2	0
Technical failure	0	2

Reproduced with permission from Revel M, Payan C, Vallee C, et al. Automated percutaneous lumbar discectomy versus chemonucleolysis in the treatment of sciatica: a randomized multicenter trial. *Spine* 1993;18:1–7.

Imaging Modalities

If you actually pinpoint the cause of regional low back pain, you are extraordinarily lucky. After all, even the clue inherent in leg pain barely improves your odds. That is not to impugn the elegance of contemporary imaging modalities in defining anatomy and pathoanatomy. The conundrum rises from the fact that pathoanatomy is so ubiquitous in the adult as to be "normal" [i.e., a minority of adults have the pristine lumbosacral anatomy they were born with (46)]. The clinically meaningful question is not whether there is pathoanatomy. Rather, it is, "Which of the anatomic aberrations likely to be present at the lumbosacral spine accounts for this episode of regional low back pain, or of regional sciatica?" In this context, discal protrusions should be discounted as normal, and even discal extrusions should lead to tenuous inferences at best. That is not to say that these are examples of pathoanatomy without clinical correlate. Rather, even if they occur acutely and persist, they are associated with transient symptoms. A discal herniation may never hurt, may be responsible for a backache in the past, or may account for today's back pain—there is no rational basis for discerning among these possibilities.

Surgery and Other Invasive Interventions

In spite of 50 years of zeal, which appears to know no bounds (47) for particular American peer groups (48), the surgeon has little if anything to offer the patient with regional low back pain or regional sciatica. In other words, regional back disease is no more a surgical disease than is lupus, or even rheumatoid arthritis (RA). There are occasional patients for whom elective surgery is sensible, but they are exceptional. There are no substantive data whatsoever that invasive procedures of any kind afford palliation for regional low back pain beyond that of the natural history; for acupuncture (49) and facet injections (50), benefit proved elusive in well-designed studies with sufficient statistical power to detect even minor salutary effect. For sciatica, the jury is still out on epidural steroid injections, thanks to two decades of conflicting trials (51—53), but not on percutaneous discectomy, which proved more disappointing even than chemonucleolysis in an elegant study, the principal results of which are presented in Table 102.4 (54). Although there is no substantive scientific evidence that open surgery has anything to offer the patient with regional back pain, there is a suggestion—barely a suggestion—that surgery can help some patients with sciatica whose illness persists for a month or two. This suggestion drives the Guideline offered by the panel discussed earlier (37), appears in structured scholarly reviews (55), and threatens to become entrenched in clinical lore. However, it is based on a single trial (56), a single, barely interpretable trial that represents the underpinnings of one of the most frequently performed surgical procedures in the United States. It is worth close inspection (Table 102.5),

TABLE 102.5. THE WEBER EXPERIENCE (54) AS JUSTIFICATION FOR SURGERY IN PATIENTS WITH SCIATICA

	Conservative Group			Operative Group		
Result	No Surgery	Surgery	Total	No Surgery	Surgery	Total
Good	16	8	24	39	0	39
Fair	24	4	28	15	1	16
Poor	9	4	13	5	0	5
Bad	0	1	1	0	0	0
Total	49	17	66	59	1	60

and after close inspection, it provokes bewilderment at best. Table 102.5 summarizes the experience of H. Weber, a Norwegian orthopedist. In 1970, he admitted 281 patients with sciatica to his service. Of these, 87 seemed to be improving too rapidly to justify surgery, and 67, he thought, had unequivocal surgical indications. There remained 126 patients between 25 and 55 years of age who were still ill at 14 days but only to such a degree that Weber deemed surgery to be elective. He randomized these patients to laminectomy or continued conservative care. All had "definite herniation" demonstrable on myelography. The outcome at 1 year is tabulated in Table 102.5. By 4 years, no discernible difference remained between those subjected to surgery and those spared. This putative minor benefit of discectomy is not easily reproducible (57) or readily justifiable (58). Why should it hold sway? Even the author of this hortatory study now urges caution (59).

CLAIMANT WITH A BACKACHE

Few *patients* have chronic back pain. There are *people* with chronic back pain (16), but very few patients. Individuals who interact with the healthcare paradigm of the United States (and nearly all other advanced countries) for chronic low back pain are nearly always *claimants*; they are seeking redress, or seeking to prolong redress, to which they claim entitlement by virtue of indemnification for the illness of work incapacity consequent to their backache. Claimants with disabling backache are increasingly coming to the attention of rheumatologists. In part, this is because their absolute numbers continue to escalate, but in greater part, this is because insurers are seeking an approach other than that traditionally promulgated by orthopedic surgeons and neurosurgeons. Some of these claimants are the patients of the rheumatologist, but a growing number are referred by the insurer to the rheumatologist for expert advice as required under some disability insurance schemes. The rheumatologist is expected to opine whether further healing, with or without further intervention, is to be expected and whether the claimant with backache is really as disabled as he or she asserts.

One might imagine that the increase in numbers of claimants with disabling backache who are seeking and finding recourse in indemnity schemes reflects progressive growth in social conscience; the individual with chronic disabling back pain is thereby afforded solace in a time of need. However, I argue that for regional back pain, this is seldom the case. In seeking recourse, the individual with persistent back pain is poorly served by the existing paradigm. To understand such a counterintuitive assertion, one first needs a grasp of the paradigm itself.

European Roots of the American Scheme for Indemnifying Disabling Back Pain

Before the industrial revolution, the identification of and care of those who could not fend for themselves fell on the gentry. With industrialization, the inadequacies of *noblesse oblige* became obvious. The streets of western cities became home to thousands—all downtrodden, whether they were unemployed, unemployable, or unwilling to seek gainful employment (60). These "street people" were without voice and without champion. The mandate for change came from the work force itself, for whom the specters of unemployment and of ekeing out a living on the streets were inseparable. The English "Friendly Societies" and German "Krankenkassen" developed, usually trade based, so that artisans and more advantaged workers could purchase insurance that would provide some "sick pay," not medical treatment, should illness force them out of work. Workers often went into debt attempting to pay medical bills, and medical practice was plagued by receivable accounts. Although all workers lived in dread of losing income as a consequence of illness, that was not their greatest fear. Death loomed large. The industrial revolution was hazardous. As late as 1907, 7,000 American workers were killed in just two industries: railroading and bituminous coal mining (61). What became of their survivors? Most workers purchased insurance that provided for a decent burial; survivor benefits were beyond reach. Along with death, dismemberment, blindness, and other catastrophic events haunted the work force. Was there no recourse for the maimed other than to join the widows and children on the street? Was the employer or the state not responsible at some level? The answer was a resounding "No." "Common law" was fashioned by the ruling class to place the worker at an unsurmountable disadvantage in gaining any redress (62,63).

Reform first took hold in Germany—no testimony to the social conscience of the government of the day (64). Rather, Bismarck introduced social rights to avoid granting wider political rights. Workmens' Accident Insurance and Sickness Benefits, the first of the Prussian social legislation, passed into law in 1884. The Prussian statutes to follow were the fountainhead for all the social reform that swept across Europe around the turn of the century.

The Prussian precedent evolved over the course of nearly three decades. In 1911, a comprehensive program was enacted, the National Insurance Act, which included an administrative algorithm for redress for work incapacity that has dominated thinking ever since (Table 102.6). The dialectic that drove Prussian reform demanded that the injured worker be singled out for special consideration. A special fund was established to provide more than just reassurance that the worker would never again live in fear of being put out on the streets; it was to guarantee that everything possible would be done to return him to

TABLE 102.6. SALIENT FEATURES OF THE PRUSSIAN PARADIGM FOR REDRESS FOR THE ILLNESS OF WORK INCAPACITY

Level of Worthiness	Insurance Fund	Indemnification
Work incapacity is a consequence of work-related injury	Workmen's accident insurance	1. Wage replacement until the individual is able to return to prior work 2. Medical care and rehabilitation 3. Permanent partial awards
Work incapacity is a consequence of illness in a wage earner	Public pension insurance	1. Wage replacement for a finite period while under treatment and unable to return to the same job 2. Medical care and rehabilitation 3. Some level of monetary transfer if global disability persists
Work incapacity in one who was never a substantial wage earner	Public Aid	1. Sustenance 2. Medical care

full health. Short of that, he would not have a compromise in his wages even if he had a compromise in his wage-earning capacity.

Almost as worthy as the injured worker, in the social conscience of the day, was the working man who was forced out of work by blindness or other infirmity that was not work related. Redress for the ill worker was sought by the labor movement under a banner of compassion; workmen's compensation was demanded under the banner of righteousness. In response, legislation saw to it that the ill worker's job and wages were not at risk if he could not work, but only for a short period during which return to health might be anticipated with adequate medical care and efforts at rehabilitation. If the worker was not so fortunate as to regain sufficient health to return to his prior work, he was expected to seek less demanding employment. If he was not up to any employment, then he would receive money, usually called an "invalid pension," which would ward off the specter of life on the street. However, if one had seldom, if ever, worked, and was deemed incapable of any employment, then Public Aid provided shelter and sustenance.

This stratification must have seemed equitable at the time, judging from the way it was embraced across Europe. It was particularly seductive because it was grounded in medical science held to be incontrovertible (Table 102.7). Prussian medicine dominated the medical thinking of its day. It subjugated the French tradition of artfulness at the bedside and the British tradition of inferential reasoning at the bedside to dispassionate, distant, scientific reductionism (65). By 1911, Prussian tenets of scientific reductionism were the thrust of medical education across the industrial world, from America (66) to Japan (67), and remain so today. It was held that only if the "basic" principles underlying medical issues were dissected out and analyzed individually would valid constructs emerge that would generalize back to the bedside. The idea was that by studying the trees, one would understand the forest. Studying the forest itself was fraught with the phenomenologic and therefore unworthy.

Because of such reasoning, no one could imagine that defining an injury would prove difficult. After all, everyone envisioned a violent event with damage as outcome. No one could imagine that healing was an indistinct end point, and none could imagine that disability determination would prove so quarrelsome; after all, could it not be grounded in the medical determination of pathoanatomy (i.e., of impairment)? If you are not sufficiently impaired, you cannot be disabled.

TABLE 102.7. CLINICAL DECISION NODES THAT ARE THE UNDERPINNINGS FOR THE PRUSSIAN PARADIGM FOR PROVIDING REDRESS FOR THE ILLNESS OF WORK INCAPACITY

Clinical Decision Node	Criterion
Determine causation	Injured? In the course of employment?
Determine consolidation	Can anything more be done to cure, treat, or rehabilitate?
Determine disability	Based on the magnitude of pathoanatomic abnormality (impairment), can disability be inferred?

Such naiveté. Each of the three nodes for clinical decision-making (Table 102.7) are no match for reductionist thinking; they are multivariate, value-laden processes. The Prussian paradigm was doomed from the outset. There is no more astute a witness to this truth than Franz Kafka, who worked in the Workmen's Accident Insurance Institute for the Kingdom of Bohemia in Prague (68). Two years after the fully developed and vaunted Prussian response to the plight of the street people was in place, we learned that it is ponderous and kafkaesque. Rather than a hue and cry, rather than questioning if not abandoning the scheme, Europe took it to its bosom. Why? Certainly the political machinations in Berlin set the precedent for labor–management compromise elsewhere. But even more certainly, the fact that Germany offered the world the clinical reasoning (Table 102.7) on which to base the decisions of worthiness squelched debate. There seemed no better solution. For many countries, there still seems no better solution and no room for debate. Others have probed for options, but most of the probing commenced in the 1950s. For the first half of the century, the plight of the disabled was far from public conscience and seemed adequately met by the Prussian paradigm. During two World Wars, there was either too much to do to discard anyone who could contribute at all, or so much tragedy that survival was at stake. During the Great Depression, the plight of "those who can work" took primacy. Since the 1950s, the disabled are again recognized; redress has been offered, revised, and offered again. The Prussian precedent has been tampered with, particularly the clinical tenets (Table 102.7). Still the number of people on the rolls of the disabled grows, so that the number and the cost are an issue throughout the industrial world.

Scheme for Redress for Disabling Back Pain in the United States

America did not roil with social reform at the turn of the century. That was not for lack of street people, almshouses, and vestiges of the colonial Poor Laws. The Socialist Party was not a political threat, and the union movement was far less developed than that in Europe. Reform was spearheaded by "social progressive" academicians such as the economists John Commons of the University of Wisconsin and Henry Seager of Columbia University, who founded the American Association for Labor Legislation (AALL) in 1906. AALL sought to enlighten capitalism, not to abolish it.

The impact of AALL was limited. Only Workers' Compensation Insurance legislation survived the politics of the day, and not easily (69). Congress would not abide a national program; bills were drawn up painstakingly, one state at a time. The worker could ill afford any insurance. Management stepped up if the program included "tort immunity" and the ability to pass the cost on to the consumer. Was this taxation without representation? The New York statute survived this challenge before the U.S. Supreme Court in 1911. By 1949, all states independently administered Workers' Compensation Insurance programs. Today, the states are joined by the District of Columbia, the territories, federal employees, and railway workers; 58 independent jurisdictions administer insurance schemes, some of which are exclusively underwritten and managed by governmental agencies; others allow the employer to self-insure; and most are a marketplace for the private insurance industry. All are true to the Prussian paradigm except that they are "exclusive remedies." In other words, in accepting indemnification under Workers' Compensation, the American worker agrees to eschew any other form of redress. In particular, the worker agrees not to sue the employer (the employer has tort immunity), except in very special circumstances.

A central tenet of all Workers' Compensation programs is the provision of medical care aimed at returning the injured worker to the job. To this day, Workers' Compensation is the only health insurance mandated in America. Physicians and hospitals were ill prepared for this challenge early in the century (70) and remain ill prepared today. Workers' Compensation claimants became the special purview of the trauma surgeon. Early on the injuries that qualified were violent. However, the definition of "injury" became more expansive. This may be because Workers' Compensation was the only health insurance afforded the worker; if the illness was not considered compensable, the cost of medical care was out of pocket. Thus inguinal herniation could be considered an injury once it was termed a "rupture," and back pain qualified once the concept of the "ruptured disc" gained general credence in the 1930s (71,72). After World War II, most of the growth in compensation claims can be ascribed to expanding the definition of injury in this fashion. Workers' Compensation in America underwrites extraordinary surgical zeal aimed at the hurting back and more recently the aching arm (see Chapter 105). The American worker, in fact all Americans, have come to speak and think about musculoskeletal discomfort in an injury context. Seduced by the promise of diagnosis leading to cure, and the largesse of wage replacement or more, the American worker has been urged on by surgeons, lawyers, and, ultimately, common sense to confront the contest of causation with escalating vigor. The results are not always happy, judging from the proliferation of rehabilitation and pain-treatment facilities underwritten by Workers' Compensation insurers to reestablish a sense of future for all those who seem not to have benefited from their assault on the contest of causation. We shall return to this observation.

In 1911, when the first Workers' Compensation statute was implemented, the social progressives called for America to come to grips with the breadth of the illness of work incapacity as had Europe, and then move on to health insurance and the like. The members of AALL and men of similar mind had banded together to form the Progressive Party, and in 1912, recruited former President Theodore Roosevelt as their standard bearer. The American Medical Association (AMA), in a lucid and altruistic moment, came into the fold. I.M. Rubinow, a physician, actuary, socialist, and leading authority on social insurance, called for health insurance as the means to break the "vicious cycle" of disease and destitution (73). Theodore Roosevelt's defeat by Woodrow Wilson postponed for two decades further social reform.

The principal advance in social reform during Franklin Roosevelt's terms in office was the Social Security Act of 1935 providing an Old Age Pension for workers and their dependents. Health insurance and disability insurance schemes were squelched by political exigencies. The consensus of committee after committee for the next two decades (74) was that disability insurance was desirable, but management would be difficult and the cost, prohibitive unless some "safeguard" against unjustified claims, some "strict test," could be devised. By 1948, the Social Security Advisory Council was suggesting that disability could be "objectively determined by medical examination or tests," thereby avoiding the "danger of malingering." The idea that physicians could determine disability appealed to the congressional mind far more than that of the physicians who testified before Congressional Committees (74). Congress won out. The Prussian reductionist model of disease held sway; Congress decided that "real" disease can be reliably identified by physicians through clinical techniques that quantify impairment. Social Security Disability Insurance (SSDI) came into being to insure the workers of an adequate income if they no longer could earn such. The basis of an award was the magnitude of medically determinable disease, of impairment (75); the workers had to be sufficiently impaired so that one could infer with confidence that they could not "maintain substantial gainful employment," a shibboleth that translates to inability to earn even the minimum wage. A handbook was developed listing examples of the magnitude of impairment that would be a prerequisite. Once SSDI was in place, the strident objections of physicians to impairment rating schemes were superseded by acquiescence and remunerative participation. The AMA was quick to leap onto the impairment-rating bandwagon by publishing the "Guides to the Evaluation of Permanent Impairment." All editions of this popular and profitable guide contain the disclaimer that impairment need not correlate with disability. If that disclaimer were heeded, the Guides would have limited utility. However, they are widely used, particularly in disability determination for Workers' Compensation insurance, in which some jurisdictions require they be followed. This is in the face of overwhelming evidence that impairment, short of catastrophe, is a minor determinant of disability (76).

SSDI was developed to insure the worker who became globally disabled by disease; the disabled who never worked or hardly ever worked still had to turn to the welfare systems of the states, each of which, in its fashion, carried on the paternalistic tradition of the Elizabethan Poor Laws. Title XVI of the Social Security Act was passed into law in 1972, and by 1974 had imposed the rules and bureaucracy for administering SSDI on the state welfare programs. This Supplemental Security Income (SSI) program overwhelmed the agency, leading to a dramatic surge of individuals on the rolls and a dramatic surge in the cost of the federal disability insurance program. By 1977, nearly 3 million disabled Americans received benefits, nearly three-fold the number in 1967. In 1980, President Carter signed PL 96:265, requiring that the Social Security Administration commence periodic reviews of the validity of the disability claimed by all recipients. The intent was to purge the rolls of the unworthy, of those who could work. PL 96:265, enacted a century after the birth of social reform, produced one of the bleakest chapters in the annals of the disabled. Many did not meet impairment criteria. These claimants ascribed their disability to symptoms, particularly the symptom of pain, and were infuriated by a process that discounted the veracity of their symptoms in favor of the dearth of impairment. Nonetheless they were disallowed. That means that a person who survived on a meager SSDI/SSI pension (monthly payments averaged nearly $600 for the disabled and $165 for a dependent spouse or child) had to find work or plead poverty. Nonsense. Even claimants who perceive themselves disabled and are turned down by SSDI/SSI cannot find a niche in the labor force (77). Before the process was halted by class action suits before the federal judiciary, one of the more Kafkaesque sagas had played out (78). This was the saga that led Congress to charge the Institute of Medicine with finding a solution. How can the symptoms of pain be validated and quantified so that they will serve as a criterion for a disability award? A committee deliberated and produced a document (79) that concluded, in essence, that more research was needed. Neither this committee nor any other formal body is willing to replace the impairment rating for disability determination; they seem afraid of alternatives and seem no match for the sizable establishment that makes a living adhering to this sophism.

Today the U.S. has in place an unwieldy, inefficient, heavily bureaucratized version of the Prussian paradigm (Table 102.8). Conspicuously missing is health insurance for the working-age population. In the absence of health insurance, these disability schemes may be the only short-term or long-term medical recourse for anyone who cannot work, for anyone who will not work, and even for anyone who can work but is displaced or redundant. About 1% of Americans are on the rolls of SSDI/SSI; another 1% are denied each year.

TABLE 102.8. THE AMERICAN SCHEME

Level of Worthiness	Insurance Fund	Indemnification
Work incapacity is a consequence of work-related injury	Workers' Compensation Insurance	1. Wage replacement until the individual is able to return to prior work. 2. Medical care and rehabilitation 3. Permanent partial awards
Global work incapacity is a consequence of illness for >12 mo in a wage earner	Social Security Disability Insurance (SSDI)	1. No pension, medical care or rehabilitation before qualifying 2. Medical care (rehabilitation) 3. Some pension if disability persists
Global work incapacity for >12 mo in one who was never a substantial wage earner	Supplemental Security Income (SSI)	1. Sustenance 2. Medical care

Clinical Decision Node	Criterion
Determine causation	Injured? Often contested
Determine consolidation	Has everything been tried to cure, treat, or rehabilitate *only the injured worker?* The ill worker qualifies based on persistence alone
Determine disability	Impairment-based disability determination. *For SSDI/SSI, the residual functional capacity must preclude all substantial gainful employment*

The American Scheme evolved in a patchwork from 1910 to 1974. It incorporates most of the original Prussian paradigm. However, because there is no integral health insurance for those of working age, these programs with their various levels of largesse may be the only recourse for the redundant and the displaced, as well as the disabled worker

PHYSICIAN'S ROLE IN AMERICA'S SCHEME FOR INDEMNIFYING THE DISABLED

Many physicians, including a growing number of rheumatologists, find themselves participating in the gauntlet that awaits any American with disabling backache who seeks redress in Workers' Compensation or Social Security Disability insurance. If you are the treating physician, you have a privileged role and major responsibility. You can take advantage of the trust inherent in the patient–physician relationship to explain the process to your patient without eliciting distance or anger. If nothing else, the process is predictable. Although you cannot spare your patient any of its diabolic inconsistencies, by explaining what will happen, you can offer your patients a chance to preserve autonomy in making decisions that relate to their medical care, and a hope that they might preserve some equanimity, even some perspective. However, physicians are often recruited to serve the process as objective purveyors of expertise regarding their own or another physician's patient. This is tantamount to sitting in judgment in the eyes of the patient and often in the eyes of the contracted physician. If you serve in this capacity for your own patient, or even are perceived to do so, the trust inherent in the patient–physician contact is at great risk. In fact, to serve in this capacity at all, in obeisance to the Prussian paradigm (Table 102.8), is to test one's ethic.

Causation

Whenever a physician accepts payment from a workers' compensation carrier for service to a worker with regional back pain, the physician, *de facto,* is certifying that the worker has had a personal injury that "arose out of or in the course of employment." Providing service under such a contract is seductive; generous recompense fosters conviction that the injured worker is entitled to whatever care money can buy to attempt to heal the injury. Defense of the contract commences with the argument that there is no one more worthy than an individual whose work incapacity derived from the work itself. The test of the assertion is whether the worker is better off for the distinction. The answer is no. If a backache is considered compensable, that fact alone is associated with a delay in recovery not only when the back pain is chronic (80), but also from the initiation of the medical care (81).

Webster and Snook (82) have updated their analysis of the experience of Liberty Mutual Insurance Company in indemnifying Workers' Compensation claims for backache. The analysis is a reproach to the Workers' Compensation concept. This insurer, and presumably others in the industry, finds itself forced to raise premiums to underwrite an escalating likelihood that American workers with back injuries will find themselves facing temporary total disability if not permanent partial disability. Furthermore, this fate has not been thwarted by underwriting the increasingly costly ministrations of medical, chiropractic, osteopathic, and various other practitioners. Based on these descriptive statistics, Webster and Snook called for a concerted effort to identify responsible, remedial factors. Based on the same descriptive statistics, I would suggest that one such factor already stands out—the algorithm for recourse for low back pain promulgated by the Workers' Compensation system is dangerous, if not iatrogenic. It follows that the enormously costly enterprise of Workers' Compensation insurance benefits those who are involved in its execution far more than the unfortunate claimant with a regional backache (83).

Thus it behooves the treating physician to consider the human ramifications of accepting remuneration from Workers' Compensation for ministering to a patient/claimant with a regional backache. Realize that the injury concept, as applied to regional back pain, is a sophism kept alive by a century of tradition and bureaucratic expedience. Regional back pain arises "out of employment" far less predictably than the common cold, and we do not consider the common cold compensable. Based on many retrospective analyses, systematic reviews of the literature (18,84), and longitudinal observations (85,86), it is clear that psychosocial challenges at the workplace outstrip psychometrics, ergonomic challenges, or the quality of the illness to explain why a worker with a backache chooses to be a claimant. Once the choice to be a claimant is made, such variables as the magnitude of award, paucity of wages, and litigation are readily demonstrable direct correlates of the likelihood of a claim eventuating in either temporary or permanent disability (87).

It behooves the treating physician to reflect always on whether the complaint of back pain is a surrogate for the inability to cope with backache. The patient/claimant at the outset is better served by a physician who is aware of the sociopolitical complexity of the illness and who is far more ready to provide a wise ear, and an emotional port in the storm, than one who is seduced to become a functionary in the compensation paradigm. Society will be better served when regional backache is considered a challenge of ordinary life and not a work-related injury.

Consolidation

Seeking recourse for job dissatisfaction by claiming a compensable backache is dangerous. Physicians and surgeons are contracted to define the injury and put it right. However, when the pain is a surrogate for inability to cope with the pain—perhaps because the job provides so little that is satisfying and offers so little of the flexibility necessary to cope successfully—then the treating physician and the claimant are at cross purposes. The interventionalist is handsomely recompensed for applying any and all of the armamentarium of worthless and unproven remedies to the surrogate complaint. Predictably the claimant does not improve, is accused of "symptom magnification," impugned for not responding, and finally branded with the imprecation, "failed back." No wonder "caring" for the injured worker has promulgated even more unconscionable empiricisms (19,88) on the part of the "providers" than that which plagues society at large (89,90).

Disability Determination

Disability determination is based on the precept that "disability" is an outcome and not a process. Nonsense. As Mechanic (91) pointed out 35 years ago: "Illness and disability vary independently." Getting well, or as well as possible, from the reductionist perspective of biomedical science, does not mean that one can return to the prior job or even to the work force. There may be overriding personal needs. Or there may be much in the workplace that is unappealing, so that the disability label, earned by submitting to medical intervention or to a role of social deviance (92), is less demeaning. Do not for one moment assume that substantial gainful employment is preferable to being on the disability rolls! It is only if the employment leads to some degree of self-respect, even self-fulfillment. If it does not, the rolls may be the only way out (2).

Physicians are often recruited to participate in impairment rating for chronic regional backache by administrators of both Social Security and of Workers' Compensation paradigms (93). In the former, they do so by performing a "contracted examination," and in the latter, an "independent medical examination (IME)." In this role, the physician is expected to consider the claimant's symptoms, his or her illness, as too unreliable a basis for judging disability; only objective data are to be trusted (94). However, objective data, including those called for by the AMA Guides (95) or those generated by performance monitoring (96), are inadequate to the task. The upshot for Social Security is that awards for chronic back pain are nearly always based on more global illness than regional back pain alone (97). For Workers' Compensation schemes, disability determination is best described as idiosyncratic (98).

Furthermore, rather than a return to health, the fate of these Workers' Compensation claimants is a convoluted process of interventions and contests, which all too often leave them in a vortex of disability determination, visiting America's pain, work-hardening, and rehabilitation clinics trying to prove they hurt as much as they claim (99). These and others are the pressures brought to bear on any Workers' Compensation claimant with a regional backache. No wonder that more and more, they are increasingly rendered disabled in spite of more and more putatively effective clinical or ergonomic interventions.

Although several countries have subliminally moved away from impairment rating as a basis for disability determination (100), few have decried it. I will. It is a fantasy that supports an industry whose efforts are iatrogenic. Anyone who has to prove that he or she is ill cannot get better. In fact, they only can get more disabled; any other option will compromise their veracity.

QUO VADIS?

Regional backache is a nemesis for each of us as people, or it will be, or it will be again. Such is the human condition. A future edition of this text may educate the physician in a scientific approach to management based on a reliable and valid diagnostic algorithm. Perhaps. But I do not expect to live to see it. Nor do I consider that realization a pessimism. Life, lived fully, presents challenges including those consequent to the vicissitudes of morbidity. Not all morbidities cry out for the "scientific" solution. Regional backache, even prolonged regional backache, can be tolerable if personal resources are not compromised. We need to demedicalize the American population; we are in a position to expunge the myths and fears and counterproductive common sense (101). America must construct a workplace that is comfortable when we are well and accommodating when we are sick. There is no better solution lurking in the annals of disability determination (75).

REFERENCES

1. Breasted JH. *The Edwin Smith surgical papyrus.* Chicago: University of Chicago Press, 1930.
2. Hadler NM. The injured worker and the internist. *Ann Intern Med* 1994;120:163–164.
3. Hadler NM. Regional back pain. *N Engl J Med* 1986;315:1090–1092.
4. Liang M, Komaroff AL. Roentgenograms in primary care patients with acute low back pain. *Arch Intern Med* 1982;142:1108–1112.
5. Hadler NM. The dangers of the diagnostic process. In: *Occupational musculoskeletal disorders.* 2nd ed. Philadelphia: Lippincott Williams & Wilkins, 1999:18–45.
6. Delamarter RB, Sachs BL, Thompson GH, et al. Primary neoplasms of the thoracic and lumbar spine. *Clin Orthop* 1990;256:87–100.
7. Osenbach RK, Hitchon PW, Menezes AH. Diagnosis and management of pyogenic vertebral osteomyelitis in adults. *Surg Neurol* 1990;33:266–275.
8. Del Curling O, Gower DJ, McWhorter JM. Changing concepts in spinal epidural abscess: a report of 29 cases. *Neurosurgery* 1990;27:185–192.
9. Case records of the Massachusetts General Hospital. Case 5–1991. *N Engl J Med* 1991;324:322–332.
10. Carey TS, Garrett JM, Jackman A, et al. Recurrence and care seeking after acute back pain. *Med Care* 1999;37:157–164.
11. Brattberg G, Wickman V. Prevalence of back pain and headache in Swedish school children: a questionnaire survey. *Pain Clinic* 1992;5:211–220.
12. Hadler NM. Back pain in elderly people. In: Evans JG, Williams TF, eds. *Oxford textbook of geriatric medicine.* Oxford: Oxford University Press, 2000:558–565.
13. Bergstrom G, Bjelle A, Sundh V, Svanborg A. Joint disorders at ages 70, 75, and 79 years: a cross-sectional analysis. *Br J Rheumatol* 1986;25:333–341.
14. Deyo RA, Tsui-Wu Y-J. Descriptive epidemiology of low-back pain and its related medical care in the United States. *Spine* 1987;12:265–268.
15. Verbrugge LM, Ascione FJ. Exploring the iceberg: common symptoms and how people care for them. *Med Care* 1987;25:481–486.
16. Carey TS, Evans A, Hadler NM, et al. Care-seeking among individuals with chronic low back pain. *Spine* 1995;20:312–317.
17. Hadler NM. *Occupational musculoskeletal disorders.* 2nd ed. Philadelphia: Lippincott Williams & Wilkins, 1999.
18. Hadler NM. Back pain in the workplace: what you lift or how you lift matters far less than whether you lift or when. *Spine* 1997;22:935–940.
19. Hadler NM. Regional back pain: predicament at home, nemesis at work. *J Occup Environ Med* 1996;38:973–978.
20. Biering-Sørensen F, Hilden J. Reproducibility of the history of low-back trouble. *Spine* 1984;9:280–286.
21. Lavksy-Shulan M, Wallace RV, Kohout FJ, et al. Prevalence and functional correlates of low back pain in the elderly: the Iowa 65+ rural health study. *J Am Geriatr Soc* 1985;33:23–28.
22. Heliövaara M, Sievers K, Impivaara O, et al. Descriptive epidemiology and public health aspects of low back pain. *Ann Med* 1989;21:237–333.
23. Biering-Sørensen F. A prospective study of low back pain in a general population. *Scand J Rehabil Med* 1983;15:89–96.
24. Reisbord LS, Greenland S. Factors associated with self-reported back-pain prevalence: a population based study. *J Chronic Dis* 1985;38:691–702.
25. Hadler NM. Conservative, empirical, aggressive, alternative and complementary therapies. In: *Occupational musculoskeletal disorders.* 2nd ed. Philadelphia: Lippincott Williams & Wilkins, 1999:65–96.
26. Lahad A, Malter AD, Berg AO, et al. The effectiveness of four interventions for the prevention of low back pain. *JAMA* 1994;272:1286–1291.
27. Hadler NM. Daubert and the imperious p-value. In: *Occupational musculoskeletal disorders.* 2nd ed. Philadelphia: Lippincott Williams & Wilkins, 1999:46–64.
28. Brooks PM, Day RO. Nonsteroidal antiinflammatory drugs: differences and similarities. *N Engl J Med* 1991;324:1716–1725.
29. Gevitz N. Sectarian medicine. *JAMA* 1987;257:1636–1640.
30. Gevitz N. Osteopathic medicine: from deviance to difference. In: Gevitz N, ed. *Other healers:* unorthodox medicine in America. Baltimore: The Johns Hopkins University Press, 1988:124–156.
31. Wardwell WI. Chiropractors: evolution to acceptance. In: Gevitz N, ed. *Other healers:* unorthodox medicine in America. Baltimore: The Johns Hopkins University Press, 1988:157–191.
32. Manga P, Angus D, Papadopoulos C, et al. *The effectiveness and cost-effectiveness of chiropractic management of low-back pain: a*

report funded by the Ontario Ministry of Health. Ottawa: Pran Manga and Associates, 1993:1–104.
33. Shekelle PG, Adams AH, Chassin MR, et al. Spinal manipulation for low-back pain. *Ann Intern Med* 1992;117:590–598.
34. Hadler NM, Curtis P, Gillings DB, et al. A benefit of spinal manipulation as adjunctive therapy for acute low-back pain: a stratified controlled trial. *Spine* 1987;12:703–706.
35. Cherkin DC, Deyo RA, Battie M, et al. A comparison of physical therapy, chiropractic manipulation, and provision of an educational booklet for the treatment of patients with low back pain. *N Engl J Med* 1998;339:1021–1029.
36. Von Korff M, Barlow W, Chrekin D, Deyo RA. Effects of practice style in managing back pain. *Ann Intern Med* 1994;121:187–195.
37. Bigos S, Bowyer O, Braen G, et al. *Acute low back problems in adults:* clinical practice guideline No. *14. AHCPR Publication No. 95-0642.* Rockville, MD: Agency for Health Care Policy and Research, Public Health Service, U.S. Department of Health and Human Services, December 1994.
38. Quinet RJ, Hadler NM. Diagnosis and treatment of backache. *Semin Arthritis Rheum* 1979;8:261–287.
39. Hadler NM. *Medical management of the regional musculoskeletal diseases.* New York: Grune & Stratton, 1984:1–323.
40. Sox HC. Practice guidelines: *Am J Med* 1994;97:205–207.
41. Dans PE. Credibility, cookbook medicine, and common sense: guidelines and the college. *Ann Intern Med* 1994;120:966–968.
42. McCombe PF, Fairbank JCT, Cockersole BC, et al. Reproducibility of physical signs in low-back pain. *Spine* 1989;14: 908–918.
43. Deyo RA, Rainville J, Kent DL. What can the history and physical examination tell us about low back pain? *JAMA* 1992;268: 760–765.
44. van den Hoogen HMM, Koes BW, van Eijk JTHM, et al. On the accuracy of history, physical examination, and erythrocyte sedimentation rate in diagnosing low back pain in general practice: a criteria-based review of the literature. *Spine* 1995;20:318–327.
45. Weber H. The natural history of disc herniation and the influence of intervention. *Spine* 1994;19:2234–2238.
46. Jensen MC, Brant-Zawadski MN, Obuchowski N, et al. Magnetic resonance imaging of the lumbar spine in people without back pain. *N Engl J Med* 1994;331:69–73.
47. Davis H. Increasing rates of cervical and lumbar spine surgery in the United States, 1979-1990. *Spine* 1994;19:1117–1124.
48. McGuire SM, Phillips KT, Weinstein JN. Factors that affect surgical rates in Iowa. *Spine* 1994;19:2038–2040.
49. Mendelson G, Selwood TS, Kranz H, et al. Acupuncture treatment of chronic back pain: a double-blind placebo-controlled trial. *Am J Med* 1983;74:49–55.
50. Carette S, Marcoux S, Truchon R, et al. A controlled trial of corticosteroid injections into facet joints for chronic low back pain. *N Engl J Med* 1991;325:1002–1007.
51. Rogers P, Nash T, Schiller D, et al. Epidural steroids for sciatica. *Pain Clin* 1992;5:67–72.
52. Cuckler JM, Bernini PA, Wiesel SW, et al. The use of epidural steroids in the treatment of lumbar radicular pain. *J Bone J Surg Am* 1985;67:63–66.
53. Dilke TFW, Burry HC, Grahame R. Extradural corticosteroid injection in management of lumbar nerve root compression. *Br Med J* 1973;2:635–637.
54. Revel M, Payan C, Vallee C, et al. Automated percutaneous lumbar discectomy versus chemonucleolysis in the treatment of sciatica: a randomized multicenter trial. *Spine* 1993;18:1–7.
55. Hoffman RM, Wheeler KJ, Deyo RA. Surgery for the herniated lumbar discs: a literature synthesis. *J Gen Intern Med* 1993;8: 487–498.
56. Weber H. Lumbar disc herniation: a controlled, prospective study with ten years of observation. *Spine* 1983;8:131–140.
57. Alaranta H, Hurme M, Einola S, et al. A prospective study of patients with sciatica: a comparison between conservatively treated patients and patients who have undergone operation. Part II: Results after one year follow-up. *Spine* 1990;15:1345–1349.
58. Shvartzman L, Weingerten E, Sherry H, et al. Cost-effectiveness analysis of extended conservative therapy versus surgical intervention in the management of herniated lumbar intervertebral disc. *Spine* 1992;17:176–182.
59. Weber H. The natural history of disc herniation and the influence of intervention. *Spine* 1994;19:2234–2238.
60. Mayhew H. *London labour and the London poor.* Vol I–IV. New York: Dover Publications, 1968.
61. Berkowitz M, Burton JF. *Permanent disability benefits in workers' compensation.* Kalamazoo: WE Upjohn Institute, 1987:17.
62. Somers HM, Somers AR. *Workmen's compensation.* New York: John Wiley and Sons, 1954:18.
63. Rimlinger GV. *Welfare policy and industrialization in Europe, America and Russia.* New York: John Wiley and Sons, 1971.
64. Hadler NM. Disability determination and the social conscience. *Arthritis Care Res* 1996;9:163–169.
65. Altschule MD. *Essays on the rise and decline of bedside medicine.* Philadelphia: Lea & Febiger, 1989:375–421.
66. Ludmerer KM. *Learning to heal.* New York: Basic Books, 1985:93.
67. Hadler NM. Reflections of an American educator at the Japanese bedside. *Pharos* 1994;57:9–13.
68. Brod M. *Franz Kafka:* a biography. New York: Schockian, 1947:84.
69. Bohlen FH. A problem in the drafting of workmen's compensation acts. *Harv Law Rev* 1912;25:328–348.
70. Stevens R. *In sickness and in wealth.* New York: Basic Books, 1989:84–89.
71. Hadler NM. Regional musculoskeletal diseases of the low back: cumulative trauma versus single incident. *Clin Orthop* 1987; 221:33–41.
72. Hadler NM. Workers' compensation and chronic regional musculoskeletal pain. *Br J Rheumatol* 1998;37:815–818.
73. Kreader JL. Isaac Max Rubinow: pioneering specialist in social insurance. *Soc Serv Rev* 1976;50:402–425.
74. Osterweis M, Kleinman A, Mechanic D, eds. *Pain and disability.* Washington: National Academy Press, 1987:21–36.
75. Hadler NM. The disabled, the disallowed, the disaffected and the disavowed. *J Occup Environ Med* 1996;38:247–251.
76. Hadler N. *Occupational musculoskeletal disorders.* 2nd ed. Sect 3. Philadelphia: Lippincott Williams & Wilkins, 1999:221–416.
77. U.S. General Accounting Office Report to Congressional Requesters. *Social security disability:* denied applicants' health and financial status compared with beneficiaries'. Washington, DC: General Accounting Office, 1989:GAO/HRD-90-2: 1–78.
78. Mezey SG. *No longer disabled:* the federal courts and the politics of social security disability. New York: Greenwood Press, 1988: 1–195.
79. Osterweis M, Kleinman A, Mechanic D, eds. *Pain and disability.* Washington: National Academy Press, 1987:1–306.
80. Greenough CG, Fraser RD. The effects of compensation on recovery from low-back pain. *Spine* 1989;14:947–995.
81. Hadler NM, Carey TS, Garrett J. The influence of indemnification by workers' compensation insurance on recovery from acute backache. *Spine* 1995;20:2710–2715.
82. Webster BS, Snook SH. The cost of 1989 workers' compensation low back pain claims. *Spine* 1994;19:1111–1116.
83. Hadler NM. Workers with disabling back pain. *N Engl J Med* 1997;337:341–343.
84. Burton AK. Back injury and work loss: biomechanical and psychosocial influences. *Spine* 1997;22:2575–2580.

85. Papageorgiou AC, Croft PR, Thomas E, et al. Psychosocial risks for low back pain: are these related to work? *Ann Rheum Dis* 1998;57:500–502.
86. Bigos SJ, Battié MC, Spengler DM, et al. A prospective study of work perceptions and psychosocial factors affecting the report of back injury. *Spine* 1991;17:177–182.
87. Worrall JD, Appel D. The impact of workers' compensation benefits on low-back claims. In: Hadler NM, ed. *Clinical concepts in regional musculoskeletal illness.* Orlando: Grune & Stratton, 1987:281–297.
88. Hadler NM. Arm pain in the workplace: a small area analysis. *J Occup Med* 1992;32:113–119.
89. Greenwood J, Taricco A, eds. *Workers' compensation health care cost containment.* Horsham PA: LRP Publications, 1992:1–374.
90. Burton JF. Workers' compensation costs, 1960-1992: the increases, the causes and the consequences. *John Burton's Workers' Compensation Monitor* 1993:6–15.
91. Mechanic D. Illness and social disability: some problems in analysis. *Pac Sociol Rev* 1959;37–41.
92. Freidson E. Disability as social deviance. In: Sussman M, ed. *Sociology and rehabilitation.* Washington: American Sociological Association, 1965:1–99.
93. Carey TS, Hadler NM. The role of the primary physician in disability determination for social security insurance and workers' compensation. *Ann Intern Med* 1986;104:706–710.
94. Carey TS, Hadler NM, Gillings D, et al. Medical disability assessment of the back pain patient for the Social Security Administration: the weighting of presenting clinical features. *J Clin Epidemiol* 1988;41:691–697.
95. Boline PD, Keating JC, Haas M, et al. Interexaminer reliability and discriminant validity of inclinometric measurement of lumbar rotation in chronic low-back pain patients and subjects without low-back pain. *Spine* 1992;17: 335–338.
96. Estlander A-M, Venharanta H, Moneta GB, et al. Anthropometric variables, self-efficacy beliefs, and pain and disability ratings on the isokinetic performance of low back pain patients. *Spine* 1994;19:941–947.
97. Hadler NM. Work disability and musculoskeletal disease. *Arthritis Rheum* 1986;29:1410–1411.
98. Clark WL, Haldeman S, Hohnson P, et al. Back impairment and disability determination: another attempt at objective, reliable rating. *Spine* 1988;13:332–341.
99. Hadler NM. *Disability determination.* In: *Occupational musculoskeletal disorders.* 2nd ed. Philadelphia: Lippincott Williams & Williams, 1999:350–390.
100. Hadler NM. The disabling backache: an international perspective. *Spine* 1995;20:640–649.
101. Hadler NM, Carey TS. Low back pain: an intermittent and remittent predicament of life. *Ann Rheum Dis* 1998;57:1–2.

103

SPINAL STENOSIS

J. D. BARTLESON
J. DESMOND O'DUFFY

Spinal stenosis is a term that implies narrowing of the spinal canal by processes other than tumor or disk protrusion (1–10). This most commonly occurs in the cervical and lumbar regions, causing compression of the spinal cord and nerve roots of the cauda equina, respectively. Patients with such compression are typically older than 50 years. The two clinical syndromes of spinal stenosis are cervical myeloradiculopathy caused by cervical spondylosis (7–10) and neurogenic claudication (pseudoclaudication) caused by lumbar root compression from lumbar stenosis (1–6). In each case, the most common symptomatic presentation is a disturbance of gait. Both syndromes are manifestations of regional osteoarthritis (OA).

HISTORICAL OVERVIEW

In 1838, Key may have given the first account of spondylotic myelopathy, and in 1892, Horsley performed a cervical laminectomy in a patient with progressive lower limb weakness after trauma and found a transverse ridge of bone compressing the cervical spinal cord (11). Subsequent authors such as Stookey in 1928 (12) focused on the effects of acute cervical disc herniation but misidentified the disc material as tumorous chondromas. Brain et al. in 1948 (7) described the current concept of cervical spondylosis with cervical canal stenosis and the gradual onset of myelopathy with or without cervical radiculopathy and differentiated this from acute cervical disc rupture, which was more likely to be accompanied by pain and radiculopathy. In 1957, Payne and Spillane (13) identified the significance of a congenitally small cervical spinal canal in the pathogenesis of spondylotic myelopathy.

In 1893, Lane (14) described a 35-year-old woman with progressive lower limb weakness and reduced sensation due to degenerative spondylolisthesis, a concept that was further advanced by Junghanns (15), McNab (16), and Stewart (17). In 1945, Sarpyener (18) reported 12 children with various severe neurologic deficits due to a congenital narrowing of the lower spinal canal. Van Gelderen (19) described lumbar spinal canal stenosis and proposed that a hypertrophied ligamentum flavum was responsible. Verbiest, in 1954 (1,20), emphasized the contribution of congenital narrowing of the lumbar spinal canal to the development of stenosis. Debate persists over the relative contributions of congenital narrowing and hypertrophic changes for both cervical and lumbar canal stenoses.

CERVICAL SPINAL STENOSIS WITH MYELORADICULOPATHY

Definition and Incidence

Cervical spinal stenosis is a narrowing of usually the lower cervical spinal canal with compression of the spinal cord with or without additional compression of the exiting cervical nerve roots. The condition is associated with degenerative and hypertrophic changes in the cervical spine, and symptomatic myelopathy is more likely to occur if these changes are superimposed on a congenitally small spinal canal (7–10,13,21–24). Although significant cervical disc degeneration is present in 50% of persons at age 45 and in more than 90% after age 60, in only a minority does cervical myelopathy develop (25,26). The peak age at onset of symptoms is in the range of 40 to 60 years (24,25,27). Men predominate in a ratio of 3:2 and to an even greater extent beyond age 60. The precise incidence of symptomatic myeloradiculopathy due to cervical stenosis is uncertain; in a general adult practice, cervical stenosis will be the most common cause in patients with a slowly progressive myelopathy (10,11).

Etiology and Pathology

The myelopathy is caused by constricting degenerative and hypertrophic changes in the cervical spinal canal, with an added contribution from dynamic mechanical factors, chiefly flexion and extension (8–10,21–24). The cervical discs, especially C5–6, C6–7, and C4–5, degenerate. The degenerating annulus fibrosis and disc protrude and stimulate the growth of exostotic bone at the posterior margins of

TABLE 103.1. NONMALIGNANT CAUSES OF CERVICAL STENOSIS WITH MYELOPATHY

Acquired	Cervical spondylosis
	Paget's disease
	Fluorosis
	Ossification of posterior longitudinal ligament
	Diffuse idiopathic skeletal hyperostosis
	Gout
Congenital	Multiple hereditary exostoses
	Maroteaux–Lamy syndrome
	Achondroplasia

the adjacent vertebral bodies. These osteophytes form "spondylotic bars" that compress the anterior aspect of the spinal cord. Thickening of the ligamentum flavum encroaches on the spinal cord from behind (8). There can be contributions from osteoarthritic uncovertebral (Luschka) joints (23) and occasionally from a hypertrophied posterior longitudinal ligament (28). Acquired and congenital causes of cervical canal stenosis are listed in Table 103.1.

The corticospinal tracts are demyelinated at and below the level(s) of compression, whereas the ascending sensory dorsal columns are demyelinated above it (8). Postmortem specimens of the spinal cord show deep indentations by spondylotic bars (Fig. 103.1). When the bars extend into the intervertebral foramina, the nerve roots may become compressed and the dural sleeves fibrosed. The posterior and lateral white matter tracts are degenerated, whereas the anterior columns of white matter are relatively spared (8,23). At times, there is cord myelomalacia at and below the obstruction. The anterior horn cells within the spinal cord can be affected. A congenitally small cervical spinal canal no doubt predisposes to cord compression. Subluxation of one vertebra on another also can contribute. Most neuropathologists attribute the pathologic changes to static and dynamic (promoted by neck extension) compression of the spinal cord between the spondylotic bars anteriorly and the ligamentum flavum posteriorly, with a possible added vascular–ischemic contribution (9–11,21–23).

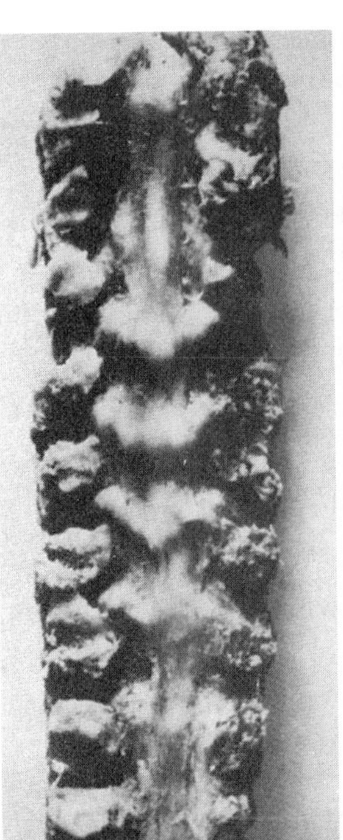

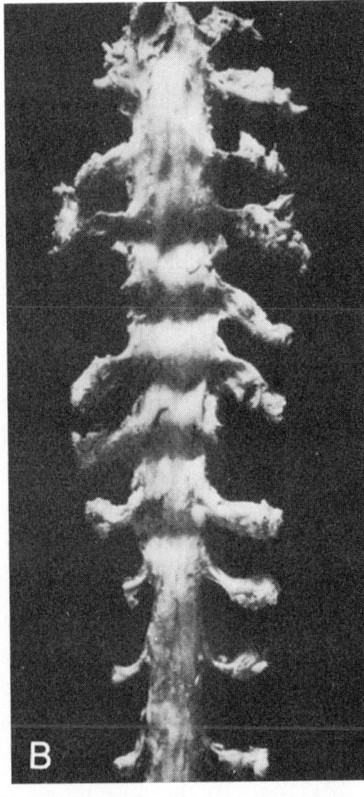

FIGURE 103.1. A: Posterior aspect of bodies of cervical vertebrae showing transverse spondylotic bars. **B:** Same patient showing indentations on anterior cervical cord and nerve roots corresponding to the spondylotic bars. (Reproduced with permission from Wilkinson M. Pathology: cervical myelopathy. In: Wilkinson M, ed. *Cervical spondylosis.* Philadelphia: WB Saunders, 1971:49–51.)

Signs and Symptoms

Patients with cervical spondylotic myelopathy typically have combinations of a spastic ataxic gait, upper extremity numbness, loss of hand dexterity, hyperreflexia in the lower limbs, and Babinski signs with variable degrees of neck and/or upper limb pain (9–11,26,29–31) (Table 103.2). Frequency and urgency of urination are common, whereas urinary incontinence and rectal sphincter dysfunction are uncommon.

TABLE 103.2. SYMPTOMS AND SIGNS IN 37 CASES OF CERVICAL SPONDYLOTIC MYELOPATHY

Type	Percentage of Patients
Abnormal reflexes	
Hyperreflexia	87
Babinski signs	54
Hoffman signs	13
Spasticity	54
Gait disturbance	49
Sphincter disturbance	49
Motor deficits	
Total with motor weakness	58
Upper limb weakness	31
Paraparesis	21
Hemiparesis	18
Quadriparesis	10
Brown–Séquard	10
Atrophy	13
Fasciculations	13
Sensory deficits	
Vague sensory level	41
Proprioceptive loss	39
Dermatomal upper limb	33
Paresthesias	21
Positive Romberg sign	15
Pain	
Radicular upper limb	41
Radicular lower limb	13
Cervical	8

Reproduced with permission from Lunsford LD, Bissonette DJ, Zorub DS. Anterior surgery for cervical disc disease. Part 2: Treatment of cervical spondylotic myelopathy in 32 cases. *J Neurosurg* 1980;53:12–19.

Depending on the site(s) of compression, there may be upper and/or lower motor neuron signs in the upper extremities. Thus the upper extremity reflexes can be decreased or increased (especially the triceps reflex). Hoffmann and Trömner signs may be present. Weakness and wasting in the hand and forearm muscles are common, and fasciculations can be seen. Patients may report Lhermitte's phenomenon, electric-like sensations or tingling down the back or limbs with neck flexion more often than extension (10,23). The effects on sensation may be complex. Pain and temperature reduction, loss of vibration and joint position sense, and dermatomal distribution deficits will depend on whether the spinothalamic tracts, posterior columns, or cervical nerve roots, respectively, are affected (9–11,23,26,30). If present, the upper limb pain can be sharp, aching, or even burning in nature and affect one or both sides. Neck range of motion is frequently restricted, whereas severe neck pain is uncommon (30,31). Sudden worsening of neurologic signs and symptoms may follow a mild neck injury with abrupt flexion and/or extension, as might occur in a simple fall. Symmetry in the symptoms and signs of myelopathy is not always present, and a partial Brown–Séquard's syndrome can be seen (7,30).

Diagnosis

Late-onset multiple sclerosis, subacute combined degeneration due to vitamin B_{12} deficiency, spinal cord tumor, amyotrophic lateral sclerosis, syringomyelia, arteriovenous malformation, neurosyphilis, human T-cell lymphotropic virus type 1 (HTLV-1) infection, human immunodeficiency virus (HIV) infection, and hereditary spastic paraparesis can be confused with spondylotic myeloradiculopathy (Table 103.3). Plain radiographs of the cervical spine usually show narrowed cervical disc spaces and osteophytes, especially at C5–6, and C6–7 (Fig. 103.2A) in adults who have reached middle age, and thus the radiographs are of limited diagnostic utility. Magnetic resonance imaging (MRI) of the cervical spine is the screening study of choice (10,32–34). The corkscrew shape of the cervical cord compressed at several levels is best seen on sagittal T2-weighted images (Fig. 103.2B). Axial MRI and postmyelogram computed tomography (CT) images demonstrate the compression and distortion of the spinal cord (Fig. 103.2C). Increased T2 signal within the cervical spinal cord at the level(s) of compression is thought to increase the likelihood that the impingement is responsible for accompanying signs and symptoms (Fig. 103.2D) (9). MRI can rule out mimics such as tumors, arteriovenous malformations, syringomyelia, and multiple sclerosis. Because intracranial processes can cause gait and limb dysfunction similar to those of cervical myelopathy, MRI of the brain is often obtained with imaging of the cervical spine. Myelography, and especially myelography with postmyelogram CT of the cervical spinal canal, also can demonstrate cervical stenosis with cord and nerve root compression and is complementary to MRI. Myelography has the advantage of allowing images to be obtained with the neck extended, which may show significantly more cord compression than imaging obtained with the neck in a neutral position. Cerebrospinal fluid (CSF) analysis may be helpful in excluding inflammatory myelopathies such as multiple sclerosis. In cervical spondylotic myelopathy associated with a block in the flow of CSF, the protein level can be significantly elevated if the fluid is obtained from below the level of compression. Electromyography and nerve-conduction velocity testing (EMG) can help to confirm the presence of cervical nerve root involvement and exclude other neurologic problems such as amyotrophic lateral sclerosis, peripheral neuropathy, and peripheral nerve entrapment.

TABLE 103.3. DIFFERENTIAL DIAGNOSIS OF CERVICAL SPONDYLOTIC MYELOPATHY

Cervical cord tumor
Syringomyelia
Cervical disc herniation
Arteriovenous malformation
Multiple sclerosis
Amyotrophic lateral sclerosis
Subacute combined degeneration (B_{12} deficiency)
Neurosyphilis
Rheumatoid arthritis or ankylosing spondylitis with subluxation
Hereditary spastic paraparesis
HTLV-1 or HIV infection
Adrenoleukodystrophy
Parasagittal cerebral lesion such as tumor

HTLV, human T-cell lymphotropic virus; HIV, human immunodeficiency virus.

Natural History and Treatment

Controversy surrounds the natural history of the myelopathy (23,25,27). Lees and Turner (25) followed up a cohort of 44 among 51 well-documented, and mostly not operated on, patients for 5 or more years. An injury often preceded the onset of symptoms. An indolent course was punctuated at long intervals by one or more neurologic exacerbations, but disability, often rated severe, did not change appreciably during observation. Conversely, Nurick (27), although extolling the virtue of nonoperative measures, found that 20% of the patients worsened. In favor of intervention is the fact that sudden deteriorations are unpredictable and that spontaneous improvement in myelopathy is rare.

Conservative therapy consists of use of a cervical collar, with the neck in a neutral or slightly flexed position, and physical therapy for weakness, gait difficulty, and neck pain (10,11,24). In the absence of controlled studies comparing operated on versus nonsurgical patients, there is a consensus that decompression is indicated for patients with moderate or severe deficits and for progressive neurologic worsening (9–11,25). Experience at our clinic with 84 patients operated on either through posterior laminectomy or anterior decompression and fusion, suggested a low morbidity, initial

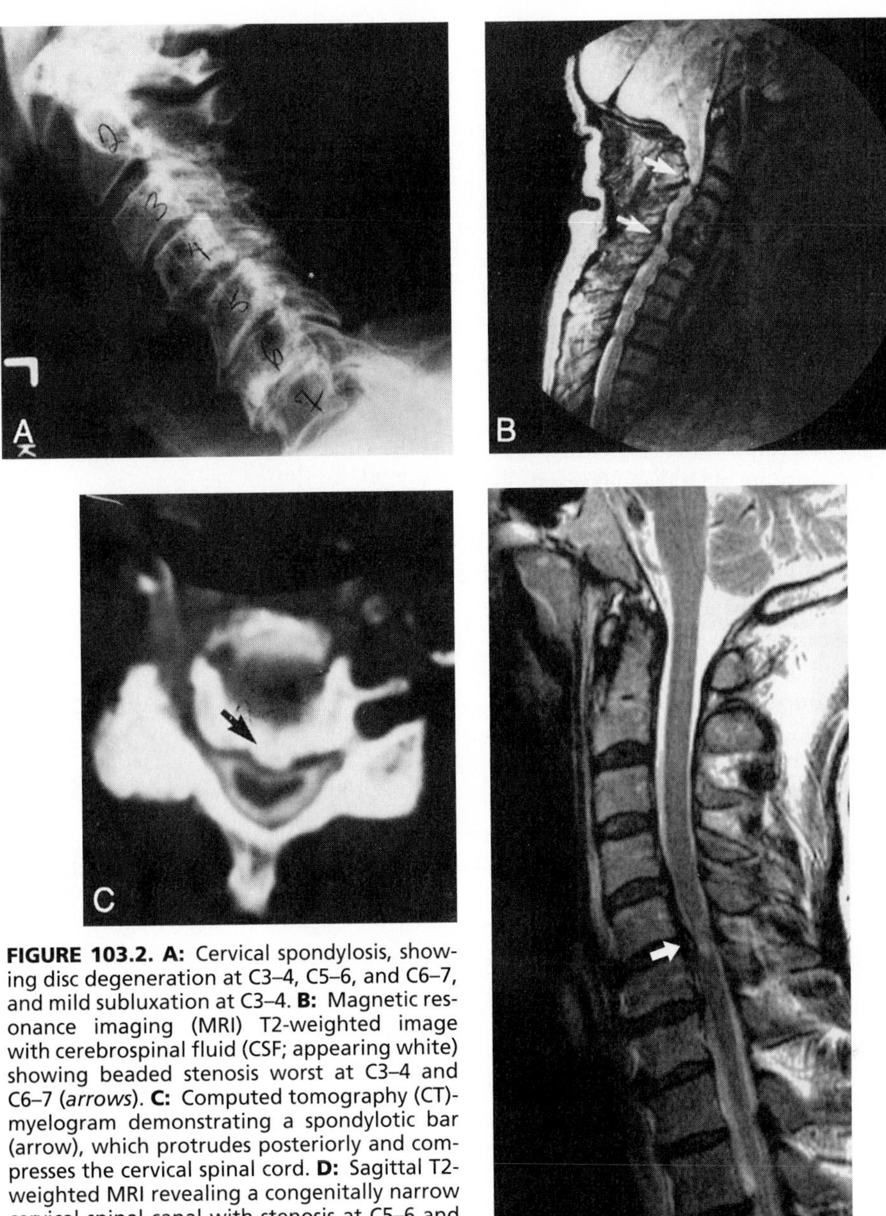

FIGURE 103.2. A: Cervical spondylosis, showing disc degeneration at C3–4, C5–6, and C6–7, and mild subluxation at C3–4. **B:** Magnetic resonance imaging (MRI) T2-weighted image with cerebrospinal fluid (CSF; appearing white) showing beaded stenosis worst at C3–4 and C6–7 (*arrows*). **C:** Computed tomography (CT)-myelogram demonstrating a spondylotic bar (arrow), which protrudes posteriorly and compresses the cervical spinal cord. **D:** Sagittal T2-weighted MRI revealing a congenitally narrow cervical spinal canal with stenosis at C5–6 and compression-related increased T2 signal within the spinal cord (arrow).

improvement in 70%, and then a tendency to deteriorate over many years, and a worse outcome in those with a longer preoperative duration of symptoms (31). When stenosis is multilevel, laminectomy is favored (9,31), and this resulted in improvement in 56% to 69% of patients in several series (27,31,35). Anterior decompression and fusion are favored in patients with an unstable spine or stenosis confined to one or two levels (10,24), and this approach is reported to benefit 50% to 72% of patients (30,31). Some patients may require combined anterior and posterior decompression for optimal results. Complications of surgery on the cervical spine include instability, infection, pain, and rarely acute quadriplegia. Surgical results are less influenced by the age of the patient than by preoperative duration of signs and symptoms (10,31). Patients who maintain a stable cervical spine fare better than those left with an increased range of motion (24,29). Strength and gait difficulty improve more than sensory symptoms. For patients who do not improve, it is thought that surgery helps to prevent progression of their myelopathy (9–11).

LUMBAR STENOSIS

Definition and Incidence

Lumbar spinal stenosis can be defined as narrowing of the spinal canal, its lateral recesses, and neural foramina, with associated compression of lumbosacral nerve roots (5,36). The stenosis can be symptomatic or asymptomatic, in which case, it is based on imaging studies alone. The narrowing can be single level or multilevel and can be decidedly asymmetric. Because of differences in the levels, symmetry, and severity of stenosis, the clinical syndrome is variable. The characteristic symptoms are a combination of pain, weakness and/or sensory symptoms in the lower limbs brought on by standing and/or walking and relieved by sitting or lying down (1,3,5,6,20,37–42). The constellation of symptoms is termed neurogenic claudication or pseudoclaudication because it can mimic the symptoms of vascular ischemic claudication of the lower limbs. The diagnosis is established through the use of MRI, CT scanning, and/or myelography with or without a postmyelogram CT scan.

The occurrence of lumbar spinal stenosis increases with advancing age, and the majority are older than 50 years. The precise incidence is not known. Probably because of aging of the population and increased recognition of the clinical syndrome, there has been a marked increase over time in the number of operations performed for lumbar spinal stenosis (43). An eight-fold increase in surgery rates for spinal stenosis for patients 65 years and older between 1979 and 1992 has been noted (43). The rate of surgery for lumbar spinal stenosis in 1989 for the National Hospital Discharge Survey was nearly 60 per 100,000 (43). In a meta-analysis of the literature, 56% of the patients undergoing surgery for lumbar spinal stenosis were men (44), whereas in the Medicare Cohort, 59% of the patients were women (43).

Etiology and Pathology

The lumbar spinal canal is bounded anteriorly by the vertebral bodies, intervertebral discs, and posterior longitudinal ligament; laterally by the vertebral body pedicles; and posteriorly by the facet joints, laminae, and ligamentum flavum (45–47). Narrowing can affect the spinal canal centrally or laterally and also can affect the intervertebral foramen, which extends from the medial to the lateral border of the pedicle at each vertebral level. Hypertrophy of any of the structures that border the canal can lead to stenosis, as shown diagrammatically in Fig. 103.3. Lumbar spinal stenosis can be due to congenital (primary, developmental) or acquired (secondary, degenerative) causes. Often degenerative changes are superimposed on a congenitally, relatively narrowed canal (36,46–48). Factors contributing to lumbar spinal stenosis are shown in Table 103.4.

Facet joint hypertrophy is the leading cause of lumbar stenosis (6,49). Examinations of the facet joints of resected specimens, compared with controls, showed that the hypertrophic changes are osteoarthritic, with type II collagen overgrowth and hyaline degeneration in the ligamentum flavum and bony hypertrophy at its attachment to the facet joints, at times with calcium pyrophosphate deposition, resulting in a greater than one-third reduction in cross-sectional area (by CT scan) of the canal (46,50). Synovial cysts may arise from the facet joints and further compromise the

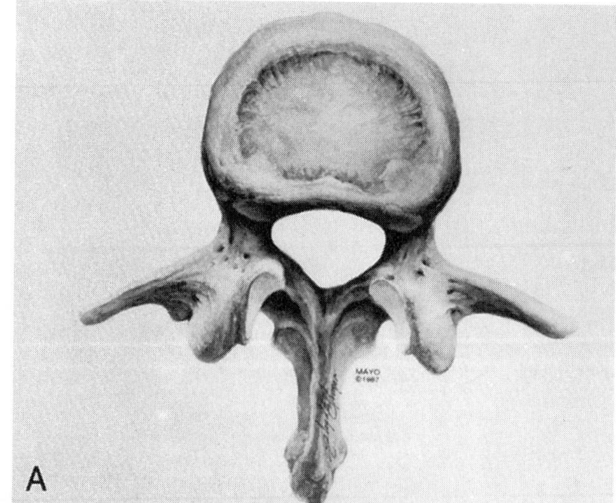

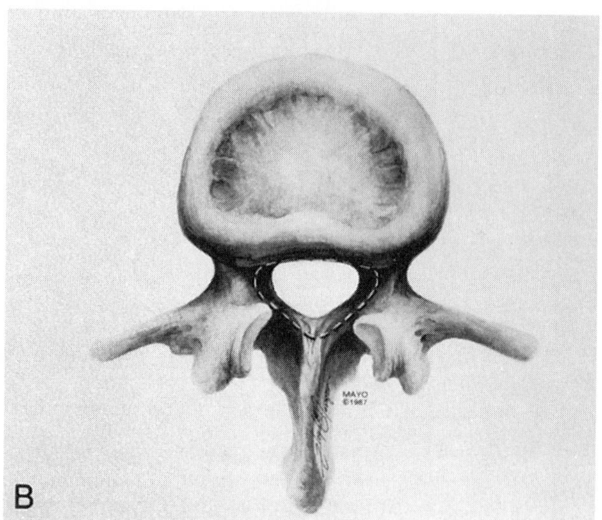

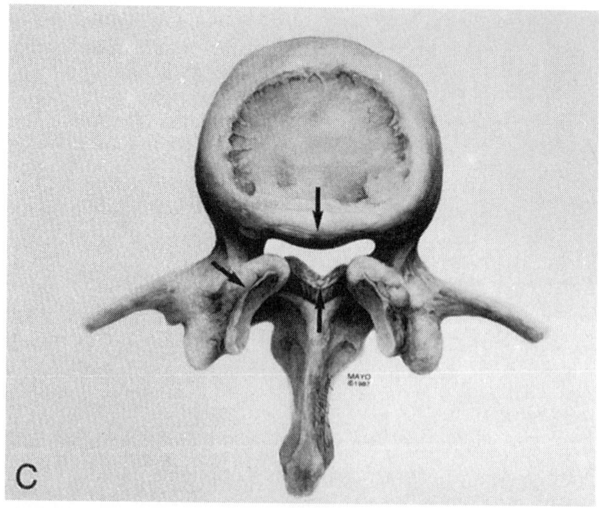

FIGURE 103.3. Types of lumbar spinal canal. **A:** Normal. **B:** Congenital narrowing. *Stippled line*, normal dimensions. **C:** Narrow lumbar canal due to hypertrophy of ligamentum flavum, enlargement of facet joints, and spondylotic hyperostosis of the vertebral body adjacent to the intervertebral disc (arrows). Floyd Hosmer, artist.

TABLE 103.4. FACTORS CONTRIBUTING TO LUMBAR STENOSIS

Degenerative changes
Hypertrophy of facet joints
Ligamentum flavum hypertrophy
Degenerative spondylolisthesis
Calcium salt deposition
Synovial cysts
Scoliosis
Congenital narrowing
Idiopathic
Achondroplasia
Less common causes
Paget's disease
Diffuse idiopathic skeletal hyperostosis
Fluorosis

canal. Degeneration of discs contributes to the syndrome (5,39,45,46). The ligamentum flavum, which normally should not exceed 3 to 4 mm in thickness, may be 7 to 8 mm thick (3,39,50). In descending order, the most commonly affected levels are L4–L5, L3–L4, L2–L3, L5–S1, and L1–L2; the majority of patients have narrowing at more than one level (41,44). Degenerative spondylolisthesis is present in one third of patients, often at L4–L5, and is due to facet joint instability (5,41,46,51). Lumbar stenosis has been described in achondroplasia (52), Paget's disease of bone, diffuse idiopathic skeletal hyperostosis (53), and rheumatoid arthritis (RA) (54). Calcium pyrophosphate crystals have been encountered in operated-on and nonsurgical cases (50,55). Lumbar scoliosis, especially in older women, appears to predispose to stenosis (56). In addition to the static narrowing produced by these factors, a dynamic component helps to account for the postural symptoms. When seated or recumbent, the lumbosacral spine is relatively straight, but when persons stand or walk, they develop lumbar lordosis and extension of the lumbosacral spine. The superior articular facets slide backward and downward on the inferior articular facets; the lumbar discs and posterior longitudinal ligaments may bulge posteriorly into the canal; and the ligamentum flavum may buckle forward into the canal, all of which further narrow the lumbar spinal canal and the intervertebral foramina and compress the lumbosacral nerve roots.

Through the years, there has been some controversy surrounding the mechanism of symptom production; does the stenosis compromise circulation to the nerve roots of the cauda equina or are the symptoms due to mechanical compression? In a patient of ours who died 12 hours after multilevel decompressive laminectomy for classic pseudoclaudication due to lumbar spinal stenosis, examination of the cauda equina roots showed evidence of chronic segmental compression at regular intervals corresponding to the levels of compression seen on preoperative myelography (41). This observation, the presence of abnormal EMG findings at rest, and the absence of a history of sudden loss of nerve root function, as might be seen in infarction, all suggest that direct pressure on the nerve roots rather than ischemia is the chief mechanism of symptom production.

Signs and Symptoms

The cardinal symptom is neurogenic claudication (pseudoclaudication) (1,3,5,6,20,37–42). Pseudoclaudication is usually bilateral and consists of painful discomfort mixed with weakness and/or sensory symptoms in the buttocks, thighs, and legs brought on by standing or walking and relieved by sitting or lying down. The symptoms are listed in Table 103.5. Patients describe pain, numbness, tingling, and/or weakness in the lower limbs, typically relieved or prevented by flexing forward at the waist. To alleviate symptoms, patients will rest against a wall or lean forward on a shopping cart or church pew. A history of increased tolerance for standing and walking behind a cart, walker, or lawn mower, which allows them to flex at the waist, is highly characteristic of pseudoclaudication. Pseudoclaudication is aggravated by factors that increase lumbar lordosis when upright, such as wearing higher-heeled shoes or walking down an incline. In advanced cases, not only is the pain provoked by standing and walking a short distance, but it may persist when recumbent, especially if lying prone. Lying on one side curled in a fetal position helps to relieve the discomfort. Occasional symptoms include restless legs and sexual and bladder dysfunction. In contrast to other types of cauda equina compression, sphincter disturbances are relatively rare. In our series, about 70% of patients reported a remote history of low back pain, and 19% had had sciatica in the past (41).

With vascular claudication, lower limb pain is provoked by walking and relieved by standing as well as sitting or

TABLE 103.5. SYMPTOMS OF LUMBAR STENOSIS IN 68 PATIENTS

Symptom	Percentage of Patients
Pseudoclaudication	94
Standing discomfort	94
Description	
Pain	93
Numbness	63
Weakness	43
Bilateral lower limb symptoms	69
Low back pain	65
Site	
Whole limb	78
Above knee only	15
Below knee only	7
Radicular pain only	6

Reproduced with permission from Hall S, Bartleson JD, Onofrio BM, et al. Lumbar spinal stenosis: clinical features, diagnostic procedures, and results of surgical treatment in 68 patients. *Ann Intern Med* 1985;103:271–275.

TABLE 103.6. NEUROLOGIC SIGNS OF LUMBAR STENOSIS IN 68 PATIENTS

Ankle reflex decreased or absent	43%
Knee reflex decreased or absent	18%
Objective weakness	37%
Positive straight leg–raising sign	10%
Electromyogram abnormal	92%

Reproduced with permission from Hall S, Bartleson JD, Onofrio BM, et al. Lumbar spinal stenosis: clinical features, diagnostic procedures, and results of surgical treatment in 68 patients. *Ann Intern Med* 1985;103:271–275.

lying down. In neurogenic claudication, the symptoms are typically provoked by standing as readily as by walking. Patients with neurogenic but not vascular claudication can ride a bicycle, stationary or otherwise, without experiencing discomfort. In general, the symptoms of vascular claudication clear a bit more quickly than those of neurogenic claudication. Nonetheless, it is not uncommon to encounter a patient who has undergone a vascular procedure before the neurogenic claudication is discovered. Patients often describe their symptoms with a sweeping downward motion of the hands indicating a buttock-to-heel distribution. Because the lower lumbar nerve roots are most likely to be affected, the pain usually affects the buttocks and posterior aspects of the lower limbs. The symptoms can be confined to above or below the knee. If the stenosis is asymmetric or affects only the lateral recess or intervertebral foramen, the symptoms will be unilateral. Patients seldom report aggravation of pain by Valsalva maneuver, or night wakening with pain; if they do or if straight-leg raising is prominently positive, they are more likely experiencing discogenic sciatica. Hip stiffness is absent, but lumbar spinal stenosis has been confused with hip disease (40). In most patients, the lumbar component of pain is mechanical and mild (38,39,41,57), but occasional patients report fairly significant low back pain, which has the same postural link as their lower extremity symptoms.

On examination, few physical signs are present (41,57) (Table 103.6). Pedal pulses are normal unless there is coexistent atherosclerosis, which is the case in about 9% of cases (41). Deep tendon reflexes were reduced at the ankle in 43% and at the knee in 18% of our series (41). Mild, often unilateral weakness, usually in an L5 and/or S1 distribution, is found in about one third of patients. The weakness is best demonstrated by asking the patient to walk on the heels and toes. Vibration sense is often reduced in the feet, but this is a common finding in older patients. Straight-leg raising should not evoke back pain (37,41). The patient may walk flexed forward at the waist, and the family or the patient may report that this is a new tendency. The normal degree of lumbar lordosis present when the patient is standing may be reduced. Range of motion of the lumbar spine can be normal or reduced, especially for extension (3,41). It is helpful to reproduce the patient's symptoms by having the patient walk 100 to 200 m or stand erect for 5 or 10 minutes. Characteristically, the patient will want to sit down or lean on the nearest support to reduce lower limb distress. New neurologic findings such as depressed deep tendon reflexes and L5 and/or S1 weakness may accompany the provoked symptoms (37), whereas the peripheral pulses are not reduced. Improvement in the provoked pseudoclaudication symptoms with forward flexion at the waist also is helpful diagnostically.

The prevalence of OA in the lower limb joints has not been studied in patients with lumbar stenosis, but successful joint arthroplasty may free the patient to walk distances that allow pseudoclaudication to emerge (58).

Diagnosis

The differential diagnosis of pseudoclaudication is (a) vascular claudication, (b) OA of the hips and/or knees, (c) lumbar disc protrusion with radiculopathy, and (d) other neurologic conditions including intraspinal tumor, arteriovenous malformation of the lower spinal cord, multiple sclerosis, and peripheral neuropathy (Table 103.7) (6,36,40,42).

Vascular laboratory evaluation can help to confirm or exclude lower extremity atherosclerotic occlusive disease. EMG can help to exclude peripheral neuropathy and frequently shows chronic neurogenic changes in the distribution of one or more lumbosacral nerve roots, usually bilaterally (41). In our series of patients with severe stenosis, 92% of patients studied with EMG had neurogenic changes compatible with nerve root injury (41). The muscles supplied by the L5 and S1 nerve roots are most commonly affected. A normal EMG does not exclude the possibility of lumbar spinal stenosis. CSF examination may show an ele-

TABLE 103.7. DIFFERENTIAL DIAGNOSIS OF LUMBAR STENOSIS

Vascular claudication: atherosclerotic	
Osteoarthritis of hips or knees	
Lumbar disc protrusion	
Unrecognized neurologic disease	Multiple sclerosis
	Intraspinal tumor
	Arteriovenous malformation of spinal cord
	Peripheral neuropathy

vated protein level, especially if the lumbar puncture is performed below a level of high-grade stenosis. When arthritis of a major lower limb joint such as the hip also is present, intraarticular injection of a local anesthetic can help determine the hip joint's contribution to the patient's symptoms.

Plain radiographs of the lumbar spine are nondiagnostic but characteristically show dense bony structures and one or more degenerated discs (5,36,41). The facet joints tend to show narrowing and bony sclerosis. If the facet joints are readily seen on anteroposterior views of the lumbar spine, this is suggestive of lumbar spinal stenosis. About one third of patients have degenerative spondylolisthesis, typically L4 on L5 (1,41).

Although some previous comparisons rated the accuracy of plain CT scan, MRI, and myelography as roughly equivalent in the accuracy of diagnosis of lumbar spinal stenosis (59), plain CT scanning does not reliably show the soft tissues surrounding the thecal sac and is now chiefly used as a screening test for patients unable to undergo MRI (5,6). Although myelography with CT, plain myelography, and MRI are roughly equivalent in diagnosing lumbar spinal stenosis (60), MRI is the screening examination of choice (Fig. 103.4A–C) (5,6). MRI provides superior delineation of the soft tissue elements of the spinal canal, including the intervertebral discs, and use of the contrast agent gadolinium can help identify tumors and differentiate between disc and scar (5,6,36). CT scanning with or without myelography better demonstrates bony pathology, including fractures, and can show whether calcification of discs or ligaments is present. Myelography with or without CT can

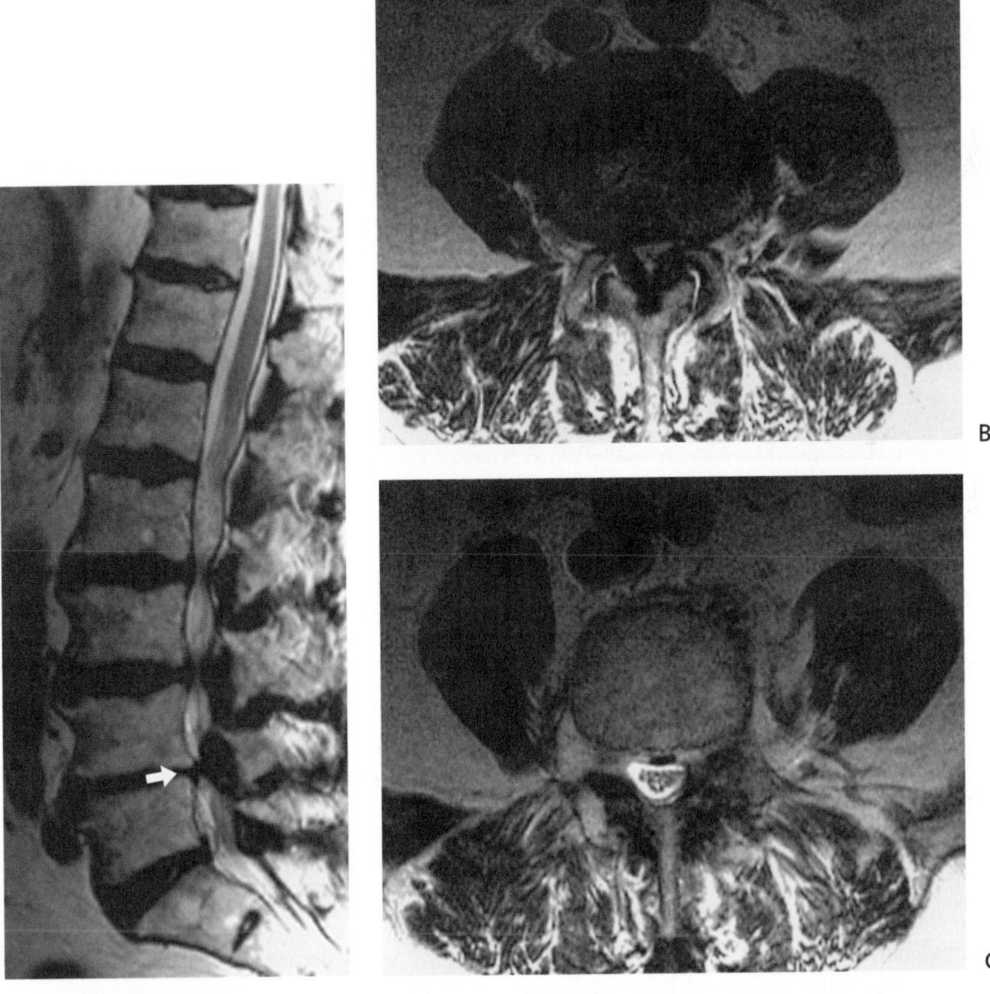

FIGURE 103.4. A: Sagittal T2-weighted magnetic resonance imaging of lumbar spine showing severe canal narrowing at L4–5 (*arrow*) and lesser stenosis at L3–4 more than L2–3. This patient has a congenitally narrow lumbar spinal canal. **B:** Axial T2-weighted image demonstrating marked central canal narrowing. **C:** Axial T2-weighted view at a slightly lower level shows mild to moderate stenosis with white-appearing cerebrospinal fluid surrounding the dark lumbosacral nerve roots of the cauda equina.

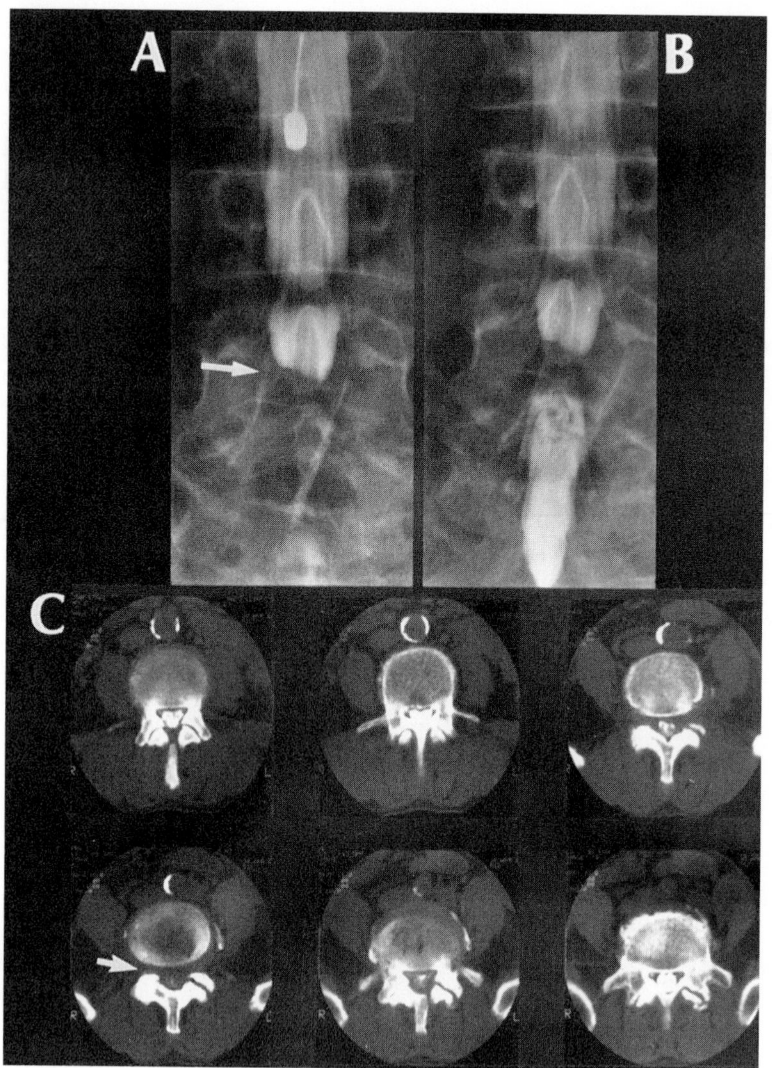

FIGURE 103.5. A: Myelogram done through a needle introduced at L2. Spine is in extension. There is complete block at L4–L5 (arrow). **B:** Needle is removed, and patient is allowed to flex his spine. Contrast now flows below the block. **C:** Postmyelographic computed tomography sequence from L3 to L4 (**top left**) through L5 (**bottom right**). Note the hypertrophic facet joints and the absence of contrast at L4–L5, the level of severe stenosis (*arrow*, **bottom left**).

demonstrate blockage in flow of contrast material because the films can be taken with the lumbar spine in partial extension (Fig. 103.5A) (1,41,45). Flexion of the lumbar spine will often allow the contrast material to flow through the stenotic region (Fig. 103.5B and C) (1,39,41,49). An hour-glass deformity shows the dual contribution from the facet joints and yellow ligament behind and from spondylosis in front of the cauda equina (Fig. 103.5A and B) (50). Lumbar spinal stenosis is frequently multilevel, and about 30% have multilevel block (41,45). Up to 10% of patients with lumbar stenosis may have coexisting cervical stenosis (6). Myelography has an advantage in that the thoracic and cervical spinal canal can be imaged at the same time as the lumbar canal. Of course, MRI also could be extended to include the entire spinal canal. Myelography with CT scanning and MRI are best viewed as complementary studies. In our practice, myelography with CT is usually reserved for patients who will be undergoing surgery and those in whom MRI leaves doubt about the presence, location, and severity of nerve root compression. Surgery can be performed on the basis of MRI alone. Because lumbar stenosis can be present on imaging studies without clinical accompaniment (61–63), surgery should be considered only in patients with a compatible clinical history.

Natural History and Treatment

There is no randomized study of patients treated conservatively versus surgically. In a retrospective, nonrandomized, admittedly biased study of 19 untreated versus 44 operated-on patients followed up for 2 to 3 years, it appeared that the group who declined surgery had a stable course (64,65). In a nonrandomized, 1-year outcome study of surgical versus nonsurgical treatment of severe lumbar spinal stenosis, greater improvement was reported by the surgically treated patients who had more severe preoperative stenosis and more severe symptoms; nonsurgical patients were unchanged (66). In another study of a matched pair of operated-on and nonsurgical patients, the overall results showed no statistical difference, but operated-on men had less pain 4 years after surgery than did their matched pairs (67). In these studies and in others, there appears to be a minority of patients with lumbar spinal stenosis, perhaps 10% to 20%, who improve partially without operative intervention (47,64–67).

Conservative treatment measures are characteristically unhelpful and include corsets and braces, exercises, nonsteroidal antiinflammatory drugs, and use of a short cane or walker. Substantial weight loss can occasionally be helpful by reducing the degree of lumbar lordosis needed to stand erect and reducing the axial load on the lumbar spine. Epidural steroid injections do not provide lasting benefit but may provide temporary pain relief (5,57,68,69).

The mainstay of effective therapy for lumbar spinal stenosis is surgical decompression, which may need to be coupled with fusion. Surgical intervention is completely elective. According to the Agency for Health Care Policy and Research Practice Guidelines, surgery for spinal stenosis should not be considered in the first 3 months of symptoms, and the decision to operate must take into account the patient's lifestyle, preferences, pseudoclaudication symptoms and associated limitations, other medical problems, and risks of surgery (70). Only patients with severely restricted activities who are otherwise in good health should be considered for an operation. Surgery sometimes needs to be extensive (4,41,44); many patients require laminectomy at two or three levels. Foraminotomies for lateral recess stenosis or intervertebral foramen stenosis may be needed. Part or all of one or more facet joints may need to be removed. A few patients have large discs or disc fragments that require removal. The thickness and density of the bones and ligaments add to the difficulty of operating (3,4,36,38,39).

A variety of surgical procedures for decompression of the stenotic lumbar canal have been described (36,46,47). Adequate decompression is essential. If spondylolisthesis is present preoperatively or is likely to occur as a result of the surgical intervention, simultaneous fusion is considered to prevent postoperative instability. One study showed little difference in clinical outcomes in patients with lumbar spinal stenosis undergoing laminectomy alone versus instrumented or noninstrumented fusion, but costs were significantly greater for the patients undergoing fusion (71). The majority of patients require decompression at more than one spinal level (41,44,72–78). Complications include infection, CSF leak, facet fracture, deep vein thrombophlebitis, nerve root damage, and segmental instability (5,36,41,44).

Decompressive laminectomy for lumbar spinal stenosis is not an unqualified success. In several reported groups of patients followed up for 1 to several years after surgery, about two thirds reported good to excellent relief of lower limb symptoms (41,44,72–77). The benefit from decompression is not sustained, and 5 to 10 years after the initial surgery, 10% to 20% of patients have undergone reoperation (6,44,72,75,78). Lower back pain, even if it is postural and accompanies the lower limb pseudoclaudication symptoms, may or may not improve after surgery. Factors associated with disappointing results include re-stenosis at the same or another level (6,75,78), absence of appropriate indications (79), inadequate decompression or an increase in mechanical back pain from further instability (6,75,78,79), a preceding low back operation (80), and comorbidities. In a 7-year to 10-year follow-up study of patients having undergone decompressive surgery for lumbar spinal stenosis, Katz et al. (78) found that 23% had undergone reoperation, and 33% had severe back pain, but 75% were satisfied with the results of the initial surgery. OA of major joints may require surgical attention either before or after spinal stenosis surgery (58).

ACKNOWLEDGMENT

We are deeply appreciative of the superior assistance provided by Ms. Linda A. Schmidt in the preparation of this manuscript.

REFERENCES

1. Verbiest H. A radicular syndrome from developmental narrowing of the lumbar vertebral canal. *J Bone Joint Surg Br* 1954;36: 230–237.
2. Jones RAC, Thomson JLG. The narrow lumbar canal. *J Bone Joint Surg Br* 1960;50:595–605.
3. Kirkaldy-Willis WJ, Paine KWE, Cauchoix J, et al. Lumbar spinal stenosis. *Clin Orthop* 1974;99:30–50.
4. Epstein JA, Epstein BS, Lavine L. Nerve root compression associated with narrowing of the lumbar spinal canal. *J Neurol Neurosurg Psychiatry* 1962;25:165–176.
5. Spivak JM. Degenerative lumbar spinal stenosis. *J Bone Joint Surg Am* 1998;80:1053–1066.
6. Epstein NE, Maldonado VC, Cusick JF. Symptomatic lumbar spinal stenosis. *Surg Neurol* 1998;50:3–10.
7. Brain WR, Knight GC, Bull JWD. Discussion on rupture of the intervertebral disc in the cervical region. *Proc R Soc Med* 1948; 41:509–516.
8. Wilkinson M. Pathology: cervical myelopathy. In: Wilkinson M, ed. *Cervical spondylosis:* its early diagnosis and treatment. Philadelphia: WB Saunders, 1971:49–55.
9. Braakman R. Management of cervical spondylotic myelopathy and radiculopathy [Editorial]. *J Neurol Neurosurg Psychiatry* 1994;57:257–263.
10. McCormack BM, Weinstein PR. Cervical spondylosis: an update. *West J Med* 1996;165:43–51.
11. Adams RD, Victor M. Cervical spondylosis with myelopathy. In: Adams RD, Victor M, eds. *Principles of neurology.* 5th ed. New York: McGraw-Hill, 1993:1100–1103.
12. Stookey B. Compression of the spinal cord due to ventral extradural cervical chondromas. *Arch Neurol Psychiatry* 1928;20: 275–291.
13. Payne EE, Spillane JD. The cervical spine: an anatomico-pathological study of 70 specimens (using a special technique) with particular reference to the problem of cervical spondylosis. *Brain* 1957;80:571–596.

14. Lane WA. Case of spondylolisthesis associated with progressive paraplegia: laminectomy. *Lancet* 1893;1:991.
15. Junghanns H. Spondylolisthesen ohne spalt im 3 weischengelenkstuck (pseudospondylolisthesen). *Arch Orthop Trauma Surg* 1930;29:118–127.
16. MacNab I. Spondylolisthesis with an intact neural arch: the so-called pseudo-spondylolisthesis. *J Bone Joint Surg Br* 1950;32: 325–333.
17. Stewart TD. Spondylolisthesis without separate neural arch (pseudospondylolisthesis of Junghanns). *J Bone Joint Surg* 1935; 17:640–648.
18. Sarpyener MA. Congenital stricture of the spinal canal. *J Bone Joint Surg* 1945;27:70–79.
19. Van Gelderen C. Ein orthotisches (lurdotisches) kaudasyndrom. *Acta Psychiatr Neurol* 1948;23:57–68.
20. Verbiest H. Further experiences on the pathological influence of a developmental narrowness of the bony lumbar vertebral canal. *J Bone Joint Surg Br* 1955;37:576–583.
21. Nurick S. The pathogenesis of the spinal cord disorder associated with cervical spondylosis. *Brain* 1972;95:87–100.
22. Dunsker SB. Cervical spondylotic myelopathy: pathogenesis and pathophysiology. In: Dunsker SB, ed. *Seminars in neurological surgery:* cervical spondylosis. New York: Raven Press, 1980: 119–134.
23. Bernhardt M, Hynes RA, Blume HW, et al. Current concepts review: cervical spondylotic myelopathy. *J Bone Joint Surg Am* 1993;75:119–128.
24. Fukui K, Kataoka O, Sho T, et al. Pathomechanism, pathogenesis, and results of treatment in cervical spondylotic myelopathy caused by dynamic canal stenosis. *Spine* 1990;15:1148–1152.
25. Lees F, Turner JWA. Natural history and prognosis of cervical spondylosis. *Br Med J* 1963;2:1607–1610.
26. Rowland LP. Myelopathy caused by cervical spondylosis. In: Rowland LP, ed. *Merritt's textbook of neurology.* 8th ed. Philadelphia: Lea & Febiger, 1989:409–412.
27. Nurick S. The natural history and the results of surgical treatment of the spinal cord disorder associated with cervical spondylosis. *Brain* 1972;95:101–108.
28. Hase H, Hirasawa Y, Ogura S, et al. Severe cervical myelopathy due to diffuse hypertrophy of the cervical posterior longitudinal ligament. *Spine* 1992;17:1417–1421.
29. Adams CBT, Logue V. Studies in cervical spondylotic myelopathy, Parts I, II, and III. *Brain* 1971;94:557–594.
30. Lunsford LD, Bissonette DJ, Zorub DS. Anterior surgery for cervical disc disease. Part 2: treatment of cervical spondylotic myelopathy in 32 cases. *J Neurosurg* 1980;53:12–19.
31. Ebersold MJ, Pare MC, Quast LM. Surgical treatment for cervical spondylotic myelopathy. *J Neurosurg* 1995;82:745–751.
32. Masaryk TJ, Modic MT, Geisinger MA, et al. Cervical myelopathy: a comparison of magnetic resonance and myelography. *J Comput Assist Tomogr* 1986;10:184–194.
33. Brown BM, Schwartz RH, Frank E, et al. Preoperative evaluation of cervical radiculopathy and myelopathy by surface coil MR imaging. *AJR Am J Roentgenol* 1988;151:1205–1212.
34. Houser OW, Onofrio BM, Miller GM, et al. Cervical spondylotic stenosis and myelopathy: evaluation with computed tomographic myelography. *Mayo Clin Proc* 1994;69:557–563.
35. Epstein JA. The surgical management of cervical spine stenosis, spondylosis, and myeloradiculopathy by means of the posterior approach. *Spine* 1988;13:864–869.
36. Epstein NE, Epstein JE. Lumbar decompression for spinal stenosis: surgical indications and techniques with or without fusion. In: Frymoyer JW, ed. *Adult spine:* principles and practice. 2nd ed. Philadelphia: Lippincott-Raven, 1997:2055–2088.
37. Blau JN, Logue V. Intermittent claudication of the cauda equina. *Lancet* 1961;1:1081–1086.
38. Pennal GF, Schatzker J. Stenosis of the lumbar spinal canal. *Clin Neurosurg* 1971;18:86–105.
39. Yamada H, Ohya M, Okada T, et al. Intermittent cauda equina compression due to narrow spinal canal. *J Neurosurg* 1972;37: 83–88.
40. Bohl WR, Steffee AD. Lumbar spinal stenosis: a cause of continued pain and disability in patients after total hip arthroplasty. *Spine* 1979;4:168–173.
41. Hall S, Bartleson JD, Onofrio BM, et al. Lumbar spinal stenosis: clinical features, diagnostic procedures, and results of surgical treatment in 68 patients. *Ann Intern Med* 1985;103:271–275.
42. Fritz JM, Delitto A, Welch WC, et al. Lumbar spinal stenosis: a review of current concepts in evaluation, management, and outcome measurements. *Arch Phys Med Rehabil* 1998;79:700–708.
43. Ciol MA, Deyo RA, Howell E, et al. An assessment of surgery for spinal stenosis: time trends, geographic variations, complications, and reoperations. *J Am Geriatr Soc* 1996;44:285–290.
44. Turner JA, Ersek M, Herron L, et al. Surgery for lumbar spinal stenosis: attempted meta-analysis of the literature. *Spine* 1992; 17:1–8.
45. Ehni G. Significance of the small lumbar canal: cauda equina compression syndromes due to spondylosis. Part 1. *J Neurosurg* 1969;31:490–494.
46. Jane JA Sr, Jane JA Jr, Helm GA, et al. Acquired lumbar spinal stenosis. *Clin Neurosurg* 1996;43:275–299.
47. Postacchini F. Management of lumbar spinal stenosis. *J Bone Joint Surg Br* 1996;78:154–164.
48. Arnoldi CC, Brodsky AE, Cauchoix J, et al. Lumbar spinal stenosis and nerve root entrapment syndromes: definition and classification. *Clin Orthop* 1976;115:4–5.
49. Penning L, Wilmink JT. Posture dependent bilateral compression of L4 or L5 nerve roots in facet hypertrophy: a dynamic CT myelographic study. *Spine* 1987;12:488–500.
50. Yoshida M, Shima K, Taniguchi Y, et al. Hypertrophied ligamentum flavum in lumbar spinal canal stenosis: pathogenesis and morphologic and immunohistochemical observation. *Spine* 1992;17:1353–1360.
51. Grobler LJ, Robertson PA, Novotny JE, et al. Etiology of spondylolisthesis: assessment of the role played by lumbar facet joint morphology. *Spine* 1993;18:80–91.
52. Pyeritz RE, Sack GH, Udvarhelyi GB. Cervical and lumbar laminectomy for spinal stenosis in achondroplasia. *Johns Hopkins Med J* 1980;146:203–209.
53. Karpman RR, Weinstein PR, Gall EP, et al. Lumbar spinal stenosis in a patient with diffuse idiopathic skeletal hypertrophy syndrome. *Spine* 1982;7:598–603.
54. Magnaes B, Hauge T. Rheumatoid arthritis contributing to lumbar spinal stenosis: neurogenic intermittent claudication. *Scand J Rheumatol* 1978;7:215–218.
55. Delamarter RB, Sherman JE, Carr J. Lumbar spinal stenosis secondary to calcium pyrophosphate crystal deposition (pseudogout). *Clin Orthop* 1993;289:127–130.
56. Simmons ED, Simmons EH. Spinal stenosis with scoliosis. *Spine* 1992;17(suppl):S117–S120.
57. Radu AS, Menkes CJ. Update on lumbar spinal stenosis: retrospective study of 62 patients and review of the literature. *Rev Rhum Engl Ed* 1998;65:337–345.
58. McNamara MJ, Barrett KG, Christie MJ, et al. Lumbar spinal stenosis and lower extremity arthroplasty. *J Arthritis* 1993;8: 273–277.
59. Kent DL, Haynor DR, Larson EB, et al. Diagnosis of lumbar spinal stenosis in adults: a meta-analysis of the accuracy of CT, MR, and myelography. *AJR Am J Roentgenol* 1992;158: 1135–1144.
60. Bischoff RJ, Rodriguez RP, Gupta K, et al. A comparison of computed tomography-myelography, magnetic resonance imaging,

and myelography in the diagnosis of herniated nucleus pulposus and spinal stenosis. *J Spinal Disord* 1993;6:289–295.
61. Boden SD, Davis DO, Dina TS, et al. Abnormal magnetic-resonance scans of the lumbar spine in asymptomatic subjects. *J Bone Joint Surg Am* 1990;72:403–408.
62. Jensen MC, Brant-Zawadzki MN, Obuchowski N, et al. Magnetic resonance imaging of the lumbar spine in people without back pain. *N Engl J Med* 1994;331:69–73.
63. Modic MT, Masaryk T, Boumphrey F, et al. Lumbar herniated disc disease and canal stenosis: prospective evaluation by surface coil MR, CT and myelography. *Am J Neuroradiol* 1986;7: 709–717.
64. Johnsson KE, Uden A, Rosen I. The effect of decompression on the natural course of spinal stenosis: a comparison of surgically treated and untreated patients. *Spine* 1991;16:615–619.
65. Johnsson KE, Rosen I, Uden A. The natural course of lumbar spinal stenosis. *Clin Orthop* 1992;279:82–86.
66. Atlas SJ, Deyo RA, Keller RB, et al. The Maine lumbar spine study, Part III. *Spine* 1996;21:1787–1795.
67. Herno A, Airaksinen O, Saari T, et al. Lumbar spinal stenosis: a matched-pair study of operated and non-operated patients. *Br J Neurosurg* 1996;10:461–465.
68. Rydevik BL, Cohen DB, Kostuik JP. Spine epidural steroids for patients with lumbar spinal stenosis. *Spine* 1997;22:2313–2317.
69. Fukusaki M, Kobayashi I, Hara T, et al. Symptoms of spinal stenosis do not improve after epidural steroid injection. *Clin J Pain* 1998;14:148–151.
70. Bigos S, Bowyer O, Braen G, et al. *Acute low back problems in adults:* Clinical Practice Guideline No. *14.* AHCPR Publication No. 95-0642. Rockville, MD: Agency for Health Care Policy and Research, Public Health Service, U.S. Department of Health and Human Services. December, 1994.
71. Katz JN, Lipson SJ, Lew RA, et al. Lumbar laminectomy alone or with instrumented or non-instrumented arthrodesis in degenerative lumbar spinal stenosis: patient selection, costs, and surgical outcomes. *Spine* 1997;22:1123–1131.
72. Tuite GF, Stern JD, Doran SE, et al. Outcome after laminectomy for lumbar spinal stenosis. Part I: Clinical correlations. *J Neurosurg* 1994;81:699–706.
73. Scholz M, Firsching R, Lanksch WR. Long-term follow-up in lumbar spinal stenosis. *Spinal Cord* 1998;36:200–204.
74. Javid MJ, Hadar EJ. Long-term follow-up review of patients who underwent laminectomy for lumbar stenosis: a prospective study. *J Neurosurg* 1998;89:1–7.
75. Jönsson B, Annertz M, Sjöberg C, et al. A prospective and consecutive study of surgically-treated lumbar spinal stenosis. Part II: Five-year follow-up by an independent observer. *Spine* 1997;22: 2938–2944.
76. Airaksinen O, Herno A, Turunen V, et al. Surgical outcome of 438 patients treated surgically for lumbar spinal stenosis. *Spine* 1997;22:2278–2282.
77. Hurri H, Slätis P, Soini J, et al. Lumbar spinal stenosis: assessment of long-term outcome 12 years after operative and conservative treatment. *J Spinal Disord* 1998;11:110–115.
78. Katz JN, Lipson SJ, Chang LC, et al. Seven- to ten-year outcome of decompressive surgery for degenerative lumbar spinal stenosis. *Spine* 1996;21:92–98.
79. Deen HG, Zimmerman RS, Lyons MK, et al. Analysis of early failures after lumbar decompressive laminectomy for spinal stenosis. *Mayo Clin Proc* 1995;70:33–36.
80. Herno A, Airaksinen O, Saari T, et al. The effect of prior back surgery on surgical outcome in patients operated on for lumbar spinal stenosis: a matched-pair study. *Acta Neurochir* 1996;138: 357–363.

104

FIBROSING SYNDROMES: DUPUYTREN'S CONTRACTURE, DIABETIC STIFF HAND SYNDROME, PLANTAR FASCIITIS, AND RETROPERITONEAL FIBROSIS

WILMER L. SIBBITT, JR.
RANDY R. SIBBITT

Fibrosis is the end stage of a reactive, usually inflammatory, process resulting in the invasion and replacement of normal tissue by connective tissue cells, collagen, and matrix proteins. Fibrosis interferes with the normal functioning of affected tissues by distorting anatomy, increasing rigidity, and entrapping critical neurovascular and musculotendinous structures (1–4). A fibrosing or sclerosing disease is characterized primarily by fibrosis that interferes with function. Representative diseases characterized by fibrosis are shown in Table 104.1.

PATHOGENESIS OF FIBROSIS

Fibrosis is mediated by the same processes that are responsible for normal tissue repair, but in fibrosis, these processes are exaggerated and detrimental (5,6). The normal healing process is characterized by four distinct phases: (a) initial tissue injury, (b) secondary inflammation, (c) tissue proliferation, and (d) tissue remodeling (Table 104.2). During the initial injury, type I and type III collagens are exposed, resulting in platelet adhesion and aggregation. Platelets release cytokines, which enhance fibroblast proliferation, promote leukocyte chemotaxis, and increase capillary permeability. During this phase, increased expression of chemotactic and adhesion molecules is prominent, resulting in the migration and adhesion of inflammatory cells to the region of injury. Neutrophils appear first, and then cells associated with chronic inflammation. Of the cells participating in the inflammatory phase of both wound healing and fibrosis, macrophages, eosinophils, mast cells, and fibroblasts play especially important roles, particularly because these are cells that can release or induce many cytokines implicated in fibrosis (5–8). If the injury is inflammatory or immunologic, then lymphocytes also contribute cytokines that influence both healing and fibrosis (6–9).

Many cytokines and adhesion molecules are released in the inflammatory phase of wound healing, including interleukin-1α (IL-1α) and IL-1β, IL-6, interferon (IFN-α, IFN-β, and IFN-γ), transforming growth factor-β (TGF-β), platelet-derived growth factor (PDGF), basic fibroblast growth factor (BFGF), leukotriene-B4 (LTB_4), monocyte chemotactic protein-1 (MCP-1), and tumor necrosis factor-α (TNF-α), as well as the neutrophil adhesion factor intercellular adhesion molecule-1 (ICAM-1) (9). Macrophages produce many factors with potential capacity to modulate local immune cells, fibroblasts, and/or extracellular matrix, including O_2^-, H_2O_2, NO, fibroblast chemoattractants (e.g., TGF-β, PDGF, and fibronectin), and factors that have been shown to stimulate or inhibit fibroblast growth or collagen production such as TNF-α, TGF-β, PDGF, insulin-like growth factor, and prostaglandin-E_2 (10).

These secreted cytokines and cell-surface adhesion molecules are essential for cell–cell and cell–matrix interactions, and regulate matrix turnover, procollagen gene expression, and protein synthesis (5). Activation of oncogenes in connective tissue by cytokines and production of specific growth or inhibitory proteins are critical steps in both the inflammatory reaction to injury and to the subsequent tissue and matrix remodeling (11). Cytokines particularly implicated in the fibrotic process are TNF-α, TGF-β, and endothelin-1 (12). Indeed, increased expression of TNF-α in resident connective tissue cells and elevated levels of circulating TNF-α and TNF-α receptor have been associated with the development of fibrosis, indicating the importance of the inflammatory phase in this process (13–16).

TABLE 104.1. FIBROSING DISEASES

Skin and musculoskeletal system	Sclerosing cholangitis
Progressive systemic sclerosis	Esophageal stricture
Morphea	Collagenous colitis
Graft–host reaction	Mesenteric fibrosis
Diabetic stiff-hand syndrome	Oral submucous fibrosis
Dupuytren's contracture	Diffuse pancreatic fibrosis
Aponeurotic plantar fibrosis	Inflammatory fibroid polyp of the gastrointestinal tract
Knuckle pads (Garrod's nodules)	Sclerosing peritonitis
Plantar fasciitis	Genitourinary
Keloids	Nephritis
Idiopathic fibrosing cervicitis (neck)	Nephrosclerosis
Focal myositis	Interstitial cystitis
Lungs	Peyronie's disease
Pulmonary fibrosis	Renal inflammatory pseudotumor
Chronic pleural reaction	Other
Peribronchial fibrosis	Pseudotumor
Cardiovascular	Calcifying fibrous pseudotumor
Constrictive pericarditis	Retroperitoneal fibrosis
Atherosclerotic plaques	Riedel's struma
Intimal proliferation	Cancer, especially sclerosing large cell lymphoma
Inflammatory abdominal aneurysm	Sjögren's syndrome
Chronic fibrosing periaortitis	Systemic idiopathic fibrosis
Gastrointestinal	Multifocal idiopathic fibrosclerosis
Chronic active hepatitis	Polyfibromatosis
Primary biliary cirrhosis	Inflammatory myofibroblastic tumor

Although many cytokines, including TNF-α, may be involved in both the initial injury to tissue and the subsequent inflammatory processes, TGF-β is especially important to the inflammatory and noninflammatory phases of wound healing and fibrosis (4,17–19). Elevated levels of TGF have been found in the circulation, extracellular matrix, and connective tissues of patients and animals with fibrosing diseases (4), and injection of TGF into animals induces fibrosis (20,21), whereas injection of inhibitors of TGF markedly reduces fibrosis (22–25). These data strongly support the critical role of TGF in wound healing and fibrosing diseases.

During tissue injury, TGF is released directly from platelets and by activation of latent TGF stored at the cell surface and in the extracellular matrix. Of the various isoforms of TGF, TGF-β_1 is particularly implicated in the development of fibrosis. Manipulation of the ratios of TGF-β superfamily members, particularly decreasing the ratio of TGF-β_1 relative to TGF-β_3, reduces scarring and fibrosis, whereas exogenous addition of TGF-β superfamily members accelerates the healing process (26). TGF-β1 is stored in platelets, at cell surfaces, and in the extracellular matrix in an inactive (latent) form, which must be converted to active TGF-β1 during inflammation (4). TGF-β1 is both an ago-

TABLE 104.2. THE NORMAL HEALING PROCESS

	Events in Progress	Time after Injury (Days)
Phase 1		
Tissue injury	Exposure of hidden proteins	0
Platelet activation	Release of mediators	0
Coagulation	Release of chemoattractants	0–2
Phase 2		
Secondary inflammation	Neutrophils and eosinophils	1–4
	Monocytes and macrophages	2–6
Phase 3		
Tissue proliferation	Fibroblast migration	1–7
	Vascular ingrowth	2–10
	Collagen secretion	2–21
	Myofibroblast differentiation	7–72
Phase 4		
Tissue remodeling	Modification by proteases	3–21
	Collagen cross-linking	7–72
	Contraction	21–72

nist and antagonist of inflammation and regulates PDGF, BFGF, TNF, and IL-1 by inhibiting and stimulating the production of these cytokines. TGF-β is a potent chemotactic factor and induces influx of neutrophils, T cells, fibroblasts, monocytes, and basophils (4,27).

TGF-β stimulates both infiltrating cells and resident fibroblasts to produce more TGF-β, resulting in a cascade of amplification that accelerates the fibrotic process. The increasing amounts of TGF-β stimulate resident connective tissue cells to produce massive amounts of matrix, which is critical to the development of fibrosis. Extracellular matrix is a dynamic noncellular structure composed of interrelated and self-aggregating molecules including collagen, proteoglycans, and fibronectin, to which cells are anchored by adhesion molecules including the integrins (28). Migrating fibroblasts exude extracellular strand-like arrays which include both collagen and adhesion proteins that firmly anchor the fibroblast to surrounding tissues, sense the direction of external stresses, bind and present cytokines, and regulate cell migration, growth, and activation. The extracellular matrix is not a passive structure, but rather, is itself continually remodeled by the secretion of new matrix and the action of proteases that digest matrix (29). TGF-β increases matrix by stimulating the production and secretion of matrix, decreasing the production of proteases, increasing the secretion of protease inhibitors, and accentuating the expression of integrins to enhance the adhesion of cells to the new matrix (4,22).

Chronic inflammatory processes repeatedly injure tissue, often producing vascular ablation, hypoxia, release of TNF-α and the generation of free radicals, which along with TGF-β, may stimulate fibroblasts to produce collagen (30). Central to this chronic inflammatory process is the expression and release of TNF-α, which is crucial to the maintenance of a sustained inflammatory reaction (31). Repeated injury and release of TNF-α does not permit the normal termination signals for TGF-β production, creating a chronic oversecretion of TGF-β_1, resulting in progressive fibrosis. Even brief exposure of fibroblasts to TGF-β may result in a persistent alteration of the biosynthetic phenotype, resulting in hypersecretion of collagen and disturbed regulation of collagen turnover by TGF-β, connective tissue growth factor (CTGF) and collagen receptors ($\alpha_1\beta_1$ and $\alpha_2\beta_1$ integrins) (32). Activation of fibroblasts by this process also may be responsible for perpetuating the inflammatory process by modulating the inflammatory cells that initially stimulated them or released TGF-β from matrix (33). CTGF, which has PDGF-like activities, is produced by fibroblasts after activation with TGF-β. CTGF expression is markedly increased in fibroblasts, contributing to the development of fibrosis (34).

Disordered apoptosis by both immune cells and fibroblasts may be important for perpetuation of inflammation and persistent connective tissue expansion (35). Fibroblasts with exaggerated activation and synthetic capabilities are preferentially recruited by TGF-β in certain susceptible individuals, and TGF-β may actually induce the phenotypic transformation of fibroblasts into myofibroblasts (36,37). Myofibroblasts are fibroblast-derived, contractile cells that participate in the inflammatory process, contain large amounts of the protein actin, and are crucial for scar formation (38). Myofibroblasts are very active metabolically and locally secrete matrix containing collagen types IV and VI, laminin, and fibronectin (39).

Contraction of healing tissue is mediated by myofibroblasts, fibroblasts, and epithelial cells. The contractures and distorted anatomy of fibrosing diseases are largely mediated by the powerful contraction of myofibroblasts in the maturing granulation tissue. The severity of the initial injury, the presence of repeated injury, overproduction of TGF-β, exaggerated responses of fibroblasts to TGF-β, and overexcretion of collagen and matrix are all important to the development of fibrosis. Under the influence of TNF-α, the myofibroblasts eventually undergo apoptosis (programmed cell death), and the resultant connective tissue is largely acellular (40).

From the earlier discussion, it is apparent that TGF, TNF-α, and their respective receptor proteins are critical to the processes leading to fibrosis. Therapeutic interventions focusing specifically on either the inflammatory or reactive fibrotic processes, especially blocking or modulating the effects of TNF-α and TGF-β, hold great promise for the prevention and treatment of fibrosing diseases (22–24,40–43).

DUPUYTREN'S CONTRACTURE

Pathology and Biochemistry

Dupuytren's contracture is characterized by nodular fibrosis of the palmar fascia and flexion contracture of the digits (1–3,44). This disorder was first described by Felix Plater in 1614, and later was given a full and accurate description by the French surgeon Baron Guillaume Dupuytren (45–47). Although usually an incidental finding, Dupuytren's contracture can be both deforming and disabling. Plantar fibromatosis is less common, but has identical histology, and is probably the same disorder (48). Dupuytren's diathesis consists of Dupuytren's contracture, nodules in the plantar fascia (Ledderhose disease), Peyronie's disease, and pads in the popliteal fossa, shoulder, knuckles, and other areas (Garrod's nodules) (49). Individuals with Dupuytren's diathesis usually have more severe fibrosis with increased postsurgical recurrences. Related, but more extensive fibrotic syndromes that can be associated with palmar fibromatosis include systemic idiopathic fibrosis, multifocal idiopathic fibrosclerosis, and polyfibromatosis (50).

Dupuytren's contracture is arbitrarily classified into three stages that resemble the phases of normal wound healing; and, as in most fibrosing diseases, overexpression of TGF-β has been implicated (51,52). The early or proliferative stage begins with the clinical appearance of a palmar nodule without contracture. Endothelial cell swelling, proliferation of the layers of basal laminae, microvascular occlusion, release of oxygen free radicals, and fibroblast proliferation are prominent.

The active phase is characterized by dimpling of the overlying skin, continued growth of existing nodules, and the development of thickened cords and bands in the fascia. Nodules and fibrotic cords contain fibroblast-like cells, type I and III collagen, fibronectin, and proteoglycans (53). Dermal dendrocytes, contractile myofibroblasts, and T lymphocytes are present throughout the lesion, and dense connective tissue accumulates in the nodules and cords. The cells in a Dupuytren's lesion are typical of a fibrosing disease and produce more cytokines and are more sensitive to cytokines (including IL-1, BFGF, PDGF, and TGF-β) than cells from normal palmar fascia. The contractile myofibroblasts are metabolically active and produce fibronectin, laminin, collagen type IV, and tenascin (54). Vascular elements are increasingly confined to the periphery of the lesions.

The advanced or residual stage of Dupuytren's disease is characterized by rigid, disabling contractures, thickened cords and nodules, and atrophy of the muscles of the hand and forearm. The tissue is largely acellular, presumably due to programmed cell death of the myofibroblasts, and consists overwhelmingly of matrix proteins, especially type I collagen (55).

Etiology

Heredity and preexisting disease are strongly associated with the development of Dupuytren's contracture (Table 104.3). Northern Europeans, especially Celts, have a prevalence of 25% to 30% among individuals in populations older than 60 years, and 40% of those aged 80 and older (56). However, despite an age dependence, Dupuytren's contracture does occur in both children and adolescents (57). In adult populations, an autosomal dominant inheritance pattern may be recognized, with 68% of first-degree relatives affected. Dupuytren's disease has been increasingly recognized in African and Asian populations, although with a lesser prevalence (1–3). Dupuytren's contracture is more common in men than in women (male/female ratio, 2:1), but the disease becomes increasingly common in women after age 75 years. Chromosomal abnormalities and mosaicism have been described, further implicating a genetic basis for this disorder, although this remains controversial (58,59).

TABLE 104.3. ASSOCIATIONS WITH DUPUYTREN'S CONTRACTURE

Intrinsic associations
Male gender
Northern European descent
Increasing age
Family history
Chromosomal abnormalities
HLA-DR3
Disease associations
Diabetes mellitus
Epilepsy
Plantar fasciitis
Peyronie's disease
Plantar fibrosis (Ledderhose's disease)
Knuckle pads (Garrod's nodules)
Carpal tunnel syndrome
Trigger finger
Rheumatoid arthritis
Eosinophilic fasciitis
Hyperlipidemia
Human immunodeficiency virus
Extrinsic associations
Palmar injury
Vibration injury (white-finger disease)
Alcoholism
Cigarette smoking
Anticonvulsant therapy

Dupuytren's contracture is often associated with chronic inflammatory and metabolic diseases (60). Increased prevalence of human leukocyte antigen (HLA)-DR3, autoantibodies to elastin and collagen subtypes, and immune activation are present in patients with Dupuytren's disease, indicating a possible autoimmune etiology (1–3). Circulating lymphocyte subpopulations are altered, strongly suggesting that the initial injury to tissue is immunologic (61). Dupuytren's contracture occurs in 20% to 42% of diabetic patients, although it is unknown whether metabolic derangements or genetic patterns create this association (62,63). Injury to the palmar structures, epilepsy, osteoarthritis (OA), peripheral vascular disease, anticonvulsant therapy, hepatic disease, carpal tunnel syndrome, trigger finger, alcoholism, cigarette smoking, chronic pulmonary tuberculosis, human immunodeficiency virus, eosinophilic fasciitis, rheumatoid arthritis (RA), and hyperlipidemia have all been associated with Dupuytren's disease (1–3,64). Age, total alcohol consumption, gender, and previous hand injuries, but not chronic liver disease are the most closely associated extrinsic associations with Dupuytren's disease. Occupation, except for repeated exposure to vibrating machinery or other recurrent trauma, does not appear to be closely related to the development of this disorder (65).

Clinical Findings

Patients note decreased mobility in the affected fingers and may complain of pain in the palm or digits. Both hands are often affected, and identical lesions may occur on the palmar surface of the feet. The ring finger is most commonly involved, but the fifth, third, and second digits in decreasing frequency also can be affected. Clinically, a nodular thickening is present in the palmar fascia. Unlike nodules associated with flexor tenosynovitis, the nodule of Dupuytren's is less discrete, does not move in the exact track of the tendon, and dimples the overlying skin (skin tethering; Fig. 104.1). Nodules are usually confined to the palmar aponeurosis, whereas bands and cords (long, fibrotic structures) extend into the digital fascia. Typically, the palmar aponeurosis, the flexor tendons, the neurovascular bundles, the skin, and the periarticular structures are entrapped by the active fibrotic process, resulting in pain, deformity, and progressive loss of function. Spiral nerves (distortion of the neurovascular bundle by fibrosis) are a particular hazard during fasciectomy.

Congenital flexion deformity, posttraumatic scar, immobilization contracture, Volkmann's ischemic contracture [wrist and proximal interphalangeal (PIP) flexed], primary joint contracture, tenosynovitis, fibrosarcoma (no contracture), and plantar fasciitis should be excluded by appropriate history and physical findings. In Dupuytren's contracture, the restriction of the flexor tendons is not altered by flexing the wrist (as in congenital or spastic contractures) or by flexing the metacarpophalangeal joints (as in contracture of the intrinsic muscles). If any question remains concerning the identity of the process, magnetic resonance imaging (MRI) is accurate in delineating the presence and stage of the Dupuytren's fibrotic mass (Fig. 104.2).

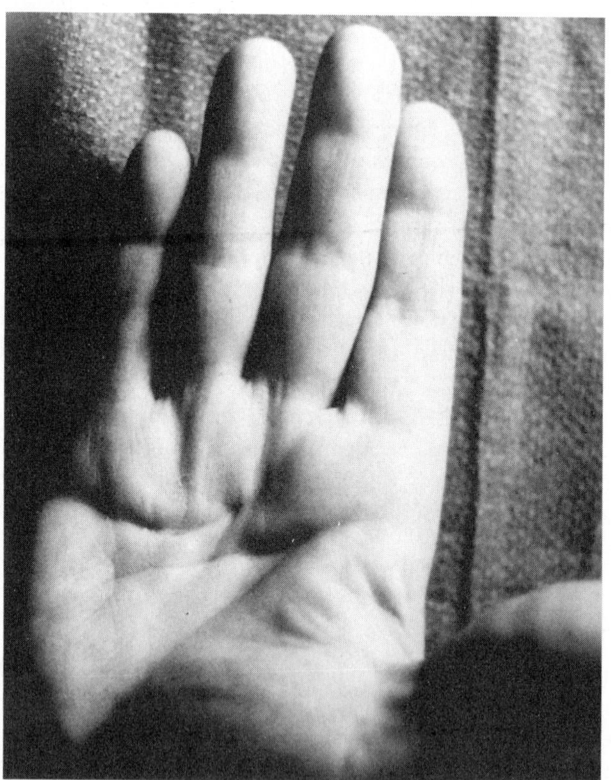

FIGURE 104.1. Dupuytren's Contracture. This is an early stage of Dupuytren's contracture characterized by a puckering of the skin and the presence of a nodular thickening of the palmar fascia. The contracture of the fourth metacarpophalangeal joint is in an incipient stage, but should progress with time. Similar lesions may be present in the plantar fascia (plantar fibromatosis).

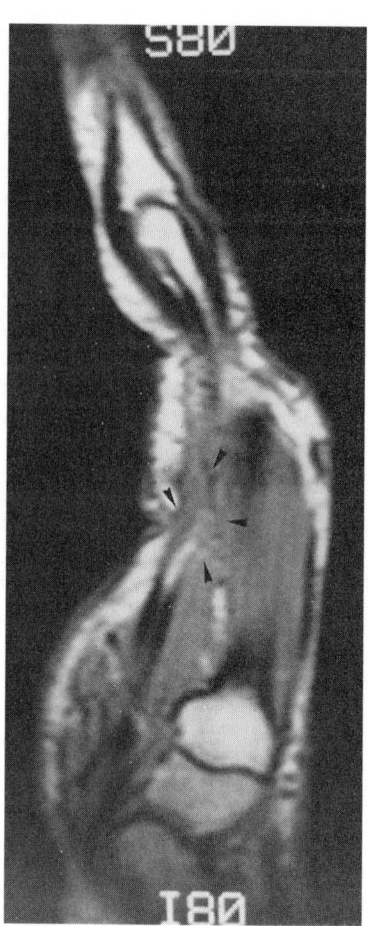

FIGURE 104.2. Dupuytren's contracture. This magnetic resonance imaging (MRI) scan of the same patient as in FIGURE 104.1 demonstrates the invading mass of connective tissue extending along the palmar fascia into the adjoining structures. The contractile mass of tissue has enmeshed itself around the flexor digitorum profundus and superficialis tendons and exerts traction, resulting in an angular deformity of the tendon and a clinical contracture.

Therapy

Reassurance, local heat, range-of-motion exercises, splinting, and an intralesional, long-acting corticosteroid injection may alleviate the symptoms and improve function for patients with an early, painful lesion without significant contracture. A new trend in therapy for more advanced Dupuytren's contracture has been the forced reduction of digital flexion contractures by using skeletal traction, continuous extension, or elongation techniques, resulting in considerable clinical regression (66). Forced, gradual reduction of flexion contractures results in complete remodeling and softening of the palmar fascial tissues, decreases anatomic distortions, and simplifies any subsequent surgery. Promising experimental medical therapies include injection of the palmar fascia with interferon-γ, the use of collagenase and other proteolytic enzymes, and oral colchicine (3,67,68).

Surgical approaches to the treatment of Dupuytren's contracture must necessarily be cautious, as the fibrotic tissue often affects the neurovascular bundles as well as the fascia and tendons (1–3). Complications associated with the surgical treatment of Dupuytren's contracture approach 20% and include flexion contractures, hematoma, skin necrosis, infection, reflex sympathetic dystrophy, and nodule recurrence. In patients with disabling contractures, surgery may be necessary to remove the mass of hypertrophied connective tissue from the flexor tendon and affected digits. Surgical procedures include nodule excision, limited fasciotomy, and dermatofasciectomy (radical fasciectomy) with skin grafting. The results of traditional surgical procedures at 10 years have been rather unsatisfactory, with high recurrence and extension rates (47% and 79%, respectively). Amputation of the affected digit remains a common surgical treatment for advanced Dupuytren's contracture.

THE SYNDROME OF LIMITED JOINT MOBILITY

Definition

The syndrome of limited joint mobility (SLJM) is characterized by decreased range of motion of the joints of the hands and wrists in a patient with diabetes mellitus without an apparent underlying inflammatory joint disease (1–3,69). Synonyms include cheiroarthropathy, diabetic stiff hand syndrome, and waxy contractures of diabetes. SLJM should be considered in the context of other diabetes-associated lesions of the hand and upper extremity (Table 104.4). These musculoskeletal disorders constitute a spectrum of pathology resulting from active fibrosis (Dupuytren's contracture, tenosynovitis), passive fibrosis (nonenzymatic glycosylation), motor neuropathy (neuropathic contractures), and autonomic disturbance (reflex sympathetic dystrophy) (69,70).

By definition, the SLJM is a complication of diabetes mellitus and must be distinguished from other diabetic and nondiabetic contractures. In normal populations, the range of motion of the small joints of the hands varies considerably, but decreases with aging. Because of these normal age-related changes, decreased range of motion of the joints in a younger individual with diabetes has far greater significance than do similar changes in an older individual. SLJM is most common in patients with type I diabetes, but is also frequent in type II patients. From 32% to 40% of all insulin-dependent diabetics may eventually be affected. SLJM is associated with increasing age, duration of diabetes, Dupuytren's contracture, palmar flexor tenosynovitis, retinopathy, neuropathy, and cigarette smoking.

TABLE 104.4. DIABETIC COMPLICATIONS INVOLVING THE UPPER EXTREMITY

Condition	Typical Joints Involved	Comments
Syndrome of limited joint mobility	MCP, PIP, wrists, other joints	Decreased range of motion of the small joints. Often associated with slecrodactyly
Diabetic sclerodactyly	Distal digits, but may extend to entire hand	Thickened, waxy skin
Reflex sympathetic dystrophy (RSD)	Contracture and edema of the entire hand, occasionally entire arm	More often bilateral (42%) than in other conditions (5%) Bone scan is positive
Adhesive capsulitis	Contracture of shoulder	Often associated with RSD or bicipital or supraspinatus tenosynovitis
Dupuytren's contracture	3rd, 4th, and 5th MCP and PIP contractures	Palpably thickened palmar fascia, dimpling of skin, associated with plantar fibromatosis
Flexor tenosynovitis	Any digit, but especially 2nd, 3rd, and 4th digits	Presence of painful trigger finger, thickened tendon sheath, nodule on tendon in area of pulley
Carpal tunnel syndrome	MCP and PIP contractures	Prominent pain, wasting of thenar musculature, positive Tinel's and Phelan's sign. Slowed nerve conduction
Diabetic neuropathy	Variable contractures	Dysesthesias, pain, loss of proprioception and fine touch. Abnormal nerve conduction.
Aseptic necrosis of humoral head	Shoulder contractures	Pain, loss of motion, radiographic changes delayed

MCP, Metacarpophalangeal joint; PIP, proximal interphalangeal joint; RSD, reflex sympathetic dystrophy.

Clinical Findings

SLJM is characterized by the presence of contractures involving the small joints of the hands, including the proximal and distal interphalangeal joints and the metacarpophalangeal joints (Fig. 104.3). The early stages of SLJM are usually asymptomatic, although accompanying aching, neuropathy, or vascular phenomena can occur. Later, when the contractures become more severe, the patient may complain of difficulty using the hands. When the contractures are severe, SLJM can be disabling because of decreased grip and impaired digital agility. The "prayer sign" is usually present, indicating the presence of contractures of the interphalangeal and metacarpophalangeal joints. Decreased extension at the wrists and metacarpophalangeal joints is the most reliable prognostic measure of disability in SLJM patients. Some patients also may have decreased range of motion in the shoulders and other large joints.

SLJM is often accompanied by diabetic sclerodactyly, a thickening and rigidity of the digital skin that resembles scleroderma (71). Conditions that can be confused with SLJM and diabetic sclerodactyly include true scleroderma, scleredema, reflex sympathetic dystrophy, diabetic neuropathy, Dupuytren's contracture, and flexor tenosynovitis with or without trigger finger.

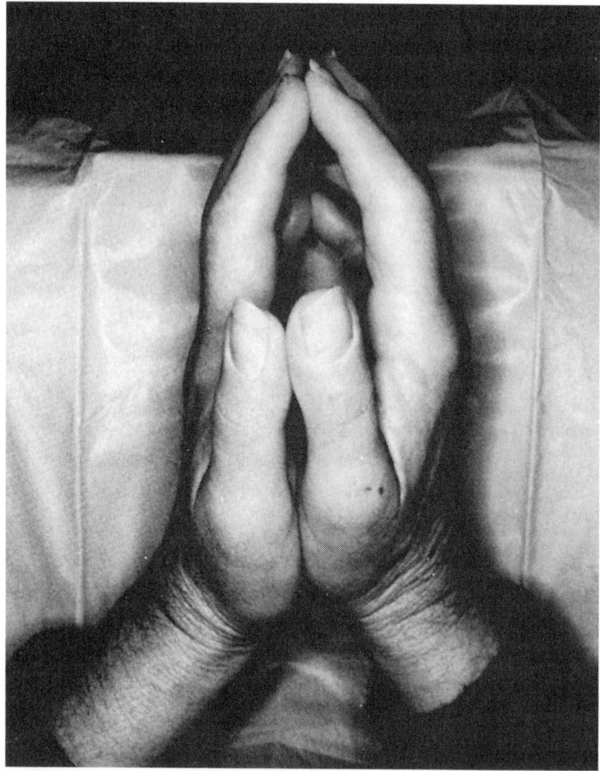

FIGURE 104.3. Syndrome of limited joint mobility (SLJM). This diabetic patient has contractures of the metacarpophalangeal, proximal interphalangeal, and distal interphalangeal joints, resulting in a prominent "prayer sign." The skin also is thickened and has lost most of the fine wrinkles, simulating true sclerodactyly.

Because SLJM is closely associated with the presence of retinopathy, nephropathy, and neuropathy, patients with classic diabetic complications should be carefully examined for a limitation of joint movement. Antinuclear antibodies and rheumatoid factor are negative in true SLJM, but may be positive in diabetes associated with scleroderma or lupus-like autoimmune syndromes. SLJM may be associated with restrictive pulmonary disease consistent with a generalized alteration of collagen (69).

Pathology

The etiology of SLJM and diabetic sclerodactyly is unknown, but is probably related to the same underlying mechanisms that induce other diabetic complications. Biopsies from patients with SLJM have demonstrated extensive fibrosis with markedly increased amounts of collagen in the dermis. This collagen has increased cross-linking and glycosylation, both of which may result in resistance to normal collagenase-mediated collagen turnover, with subsequent passive accumulation. The basement membranes of microvessels are thickened, endothelial cells demonstrate degenerative changes, binuclear fibroblasts are present, and muscle fibers reveal vacuolization and mitochondrial degeneration. These changes may be related to increased hydration of connective tissue associated with polyol accumulation and its metabolic consequences. There is very strong evidence that the primary cause of contracture in SLJM is involvement of the musculotendinous apparatus, causing tenosynovitis (72,73). Diabetic microvasculopathy of the digits is closely associated with both SLJM and diabetic sclerodactyly, and could promote fibrosis through chronic ischemia, analogous to that which occurs in progressive systemic sclerosis. More recently, fibrosis in diabetes has been linked to the more classic mechanisms of fibrosis discussed earlier, including the cascade of effects induced by TGF-β (74,75).

Treatment

Treatment of SLJM is controversial and unsatisfactory at this time. As with other diabetic complications, strict control of blood glucose is indicated (76). Range-of-motion exercises are essential to maintain strength and flexibility, but do not appear to reverse established contractures. Forced progressive extension has been effective in other digital contractures and could be considered in SLJM (66). Aldose reductase inhibitor agents may be effective, but remain experimental (77–79). Penicillamine and aminoguanidine, which may inhibit cross-linking of collagen, are possible therapies, but possess considerable toxicities and cannot be recommended at this time (69). Injection of the affected flexor tendon sheaths with a long-acting corticosteroid may be the safest and most effective therapy for symptomatic patients with fibrosing diabetic hand conditions at the present (73).

Plantar Fasciitis

The painful heel is one of the most common musculoskeletal complaints (1–3,80). Plantar fasciitis refers specifically to the clinical syndrome of pain, inflammation, and fibrosis of the plantar fascia and its calcaneal insertion. Plantar fasciitis is induced by excessive repetitive stresses applied to the foot, resulting in torsion and tension of the plantar fascia. Stress along the plantar fascia is increased with obesity, overuse, inappropriate footwear, and structural instability (the flexible flat foot), which has a tendency to pronate (evert) at the talonavicular and naviculocuneiform joints. These factors increase tension across the plantar fascia after heel strike and before toe-off, resulting in microavulsion, microtears, and inflammation of the plantar fascia and calcaneal periosteum.

Pathology

Histopathology of plantar fasciitis is characterized by collagen degeneration, angiofibroblastic hyperplasia, chondroid metaplasia, and calcification of degenerated matrix. Periosteal inflammation is ubiquitous, frequently inducing an anterior calcaneal spur (ostosis) at the insertion of the fascia. The anterior calcaneal ostosis remains after symptoms of pain have resolved, indicating that inflammation and injury, not the ostosis itself, is the usual etiology of pain.

Diagnosis

Plantar fasciitis is diagnosed with the following findings: (a) pain and morning stiffness involving the heel and plantar surface of the foot; and (b) maximal tenderness to palpation localized at the insertion of the plantar fascia on the calcaneal tuberosity. Inflammatory conditions, particularly the seronegative spondyloarthropathies, should be excluded by a careful history, physical examination, appropriate radiologic studies, and laboratory testing as indicated. Other causes of heel pain also should be excluded, as noted in Tables 104.5 and 104.6. The patient should be questioned about overuse, particularly long-distance running. The foot and heel should be deeply palpated to determine the site of pain. The structure and motion of the foot, ankle, knee, and hip should be carefully examined with weight bearing and walking for a tendency to pronate (evert).

Neurologic dysfunction as an etiology for heel pain should be considered, and tarsal tunnel syndrome in particular should be excluded. The patient's footwear should be examined for appropriate heel and midfoot support and for signs of excessive wear, instability, or loss of integrity. Radiologic

TABLE 104.5. INTRINSIC CAUSES OF HEEL PAIN

Disorder	Complaints	Diagnostic Sign
Plantar fasciitis	Plantar foot; anterior heel	Tenderness over calcaneal tuberosity. Anterior osteophyte
Achilles tendon		
Tenosynovitis	Tendon; posterior heel	Diffuse pain and swelling along tendon
Tendinitis	Tendon	Diffuse pain along tendon and calcaneal insertion
Subtendinous bursitis	Tendon; posterior heel	Pain, swelling superior posterior calcaneus
Subcutaneous bursitis	Tendon; posterior heel	Pain, swelling inferior posterior calcaneus
Rupture	Weakness; pain variable	Absence of tendon in area of rupture
Flexor hallucis longus		
Tendinitis or tenosynovitis	Ant. sup. heel Post. med. malleolus	Pain and swelling posterior to medial malleolus into plantar-foot
Tibialis posterior		
Tendinitis or tenosynovitis	Same as above	Same as above
Calcaneus		
Apophysitis	Posterior heel	Tenderness insertion of Achilles tendon, radiograph
Fracture	Heel	Stress fracture, radiograph
Periostitis	Heel	Tenderness, radiograph, systemic arthritis
Erosion	Heel	Same as above
Osteomyelitis	Heel	Radiograph, bone scan
Ostosis	Heel	Nonanterior calcaneal ostosis pain directly over ostosis
Tarsal tunnel syndrome	Heel or midfoot	Neurologic abnormalities in heel and plantar foot

TABLE 104.6. CONDITIONS ASSOCIATED WITH PLANTAR FASCIITIS

Inflammatory conditions
Reiter's syndrome
Ankylosing spondylitis
Psoriatic arthritis
Intestinal arthropathies
Behçet's disease
Rheumatoid arthritis
Systemic lupus erythematosus
Structural Abnormality
Pes valgus
Increased pronation
Flexible "flat foot"
Overuse
Long-distance running
Prolonged walking or standing
Aerobic dance
Other endurance exercise
Other
Poor footwear
Diabetes mellitus
Gout
Obesity
Calcaneal spurs
Dupuytren's contracture
Achilles tendinitis
Metabolic bone disease

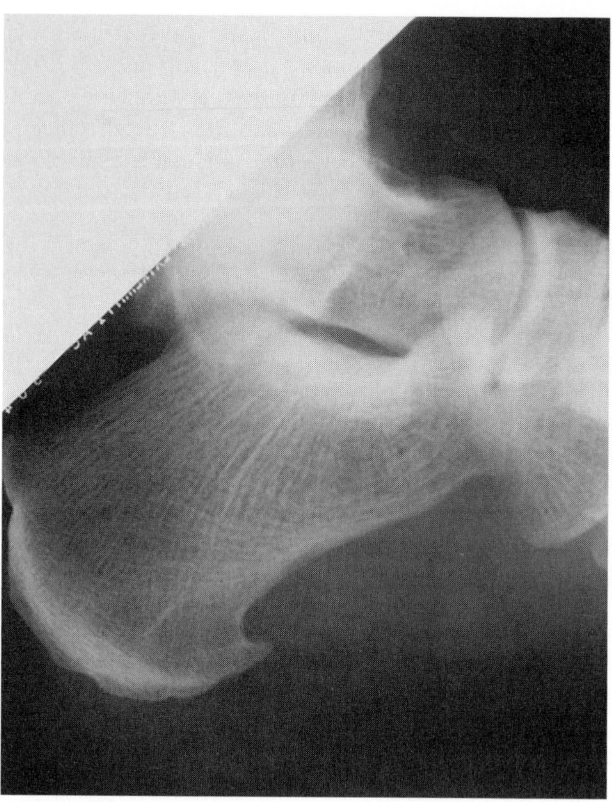

FIGURE 104.4. Plantar fasciitis. This patient was a long-distance runner who continued to run despite severe calcaneal pain secondary to plantar fasciitis. A large calcaneal hyperostosis extends anteriorly, following the plantar fascia. The patient responded to 8 months of abstinence from long-distance running and eventually was able to resume running at reduced distances with the use of antipronator running shoes.

studies may reveal small calcifications anterior to the calcaneal tuberosity or the presence of an exuberant anterior calcaneal ostosis (spur) (Fig. 104.4). The presence of an anterior heel spur is not necessary for the diagnosis of plantar fasciitis, but is confirmatory and implies that the process is chronic.

Therapy

Conservative therapy is very effective if the patient complies with the treatment plan. Torsion and injury to the plantar fascia should be reduced by resting, unloading, and stabilizing the foot. Obesity should be reduced, nonsupportive footwear should be discarded, and stable, comfortable footwear with excellent heel control and padding should be substituted. If greater stability is required, orthotic devices may be useful, including the varus wedge, plastic heel cup, medial arch support, night splint, or orthotics customized from plaster foot moldings and adjusted to the appropriate degree of correction (81,82).

There is some evidence that mechanical correction, including splinting, casting, and orthotics, is more effective that symptomatic therapy with antiinflammatory drugs (83). Long-distance running and other activities contributing to overuse should be suspended until the symptoms have completely resolved, a process that typically requires months. Substitution of exercise with less foot trauma such as bicycling or swimming is advised during this period of healing. Continued abuse of the foot will result in chronic, intractable pain and the development of a hyperostosis on the calcaneus.

Nonsteroidal antiinflammatory drugs diminish the pain and stiffness of plantar fasciitis, but are not curative. If 3 to 6 months of rest, nonsteroidal drugs, and foot stabilization with appropriate shoes or orthotics have not been effective, injection of the plantar fascia with corticosteroids may be considered. Before this is undertaken, an erythrocyte sedimentation rate and imaging consisting of radiographs, and in some instances MRI or radionuclide bone scan, should be considered to exclude confounding conditions including osteomyelitis, inflammatory joint disease, and stress fracture (84).

Corticosteroid injection of the plantar fascia should not be undertaken lightly because of potential complications including infection, plantar fascia rupture, chronic midfoot pain, and foot weakness (85). Injection of the plantar fascia is best accomplished through a lateral or medial approach, not through the plantar surface of the foot. If corticosteroid flows back along the needle track, atrophy of the plantar skin and calcaneal fat pad may occur, resulting in bone-on-skin in the critical weight-bearing pressure point of the heel.

For cases resistant to a minimum of 12 months of conservative therapy, surgical intervention may be considered. Fasciectomy, fasciotomy (fascial release), and exostectomy have been successful, although these procedures may increase the instability in the foot (86). The symptomatic effectiveness of surgical therapy may be related to hyperesthesia of the heel secondary to ablation of the lateral plantar nerve (87). Surgical therapy does not alter the forces that induced the fasciitis originally, except at the point of fascial insertion. Recurrence of foot pain is common.

RETROPERITONEAL FIBROSIS

Retroperitoneal fibrosis should be considered a member of the idiopathic fibrosclerotic disorders resulting in inflammatory pseudotumors (3,50,88,89) (Fig. 104.5). Specifically, retroperitoneal fibrosis is a fibrosing disease of the retroperitoneum that entraps and distorts retroperitoneal structures including the great vessels, ureters, nerves, kidneys, and biliary tree (90). Retroperitoneal fibrosis also may be a component of certain systemic fibrosing syndromes: (a) retroperitoneal, mesenteric, pulmonary, and periarticular fibrosis accompanied by subcutaneous panniculitis; or (b) a triad of sclerosing cholangitis, retroperitoneal fibrosis, and Riedel's thyroiditis, among other combinations (50,88–91). This syndrome is called multifocal idiopathic fibrosclerosis and also can be complicated by mediastinal fibrosis, orbital pseudotumor, Dupuytren's contractures, lymphoid hyperplasia, Peyronie's disease, vasculitis, testicular fibrosis, and pachymeningitis (92). Secondary retroperitoneal fibrosis can be caused by drugs and toxins (methylsergide, methyldopa, levodopa, ergot, bromocriptine, pergolide, asbestos), aortic aneurysm, malignant tumors (metastatic carcinomas, carcinoid, lymphoma), retroperitoneal injury (hemorrhage, infection, radiation, surgery, stenting, angioplasty), autoimmune disease, tuberculosis, sarcoidosis, biliary tract disease, gonorrhea, and ascending lymphangitis (3,93–95).

Clinical Signs and Symptoms

Pain in the lower abdomen, lumbosacral region, or flank is the most common presenting symptom. Signs of visceral obstruction may be present, including vomiting, diarrhea, or dehydration, and are the hallmark of retroperitoneal fibrosis. Hydronephrosis, renal insufficiency, severe peripheral edema, varicosities, or claudication may occur. Nerve entrapment and epidural cord compression may result in pain, dysesthesias, weakness, or spasticity. Pulmonary emboli, deep venous thrombosis, and obstruction of the bowel, bladder, or bronchi can occur. Mediastinal fibrosis may result in a lymphoma-like mass and superior vena caval syndrome with edema and venous dilatation of the arms, neck, and head. Extrahepatic portal vein obstruction, portal hypertension, esophageal varices, and uveitis may occur. A definitive diagnosis should be undertaken rapidly, and therapy seriously considered.

Pathology

Biopsies typically demonstrate fibrosis, granulation tissue, B cells, T-helper cells, large numbers of spindle-shaped cells expressing macrophage markers, and activated fibroblasts (96–98). T cell–receptor gene rearrangements have been reported as well as a 40% association with HLA-B27, but

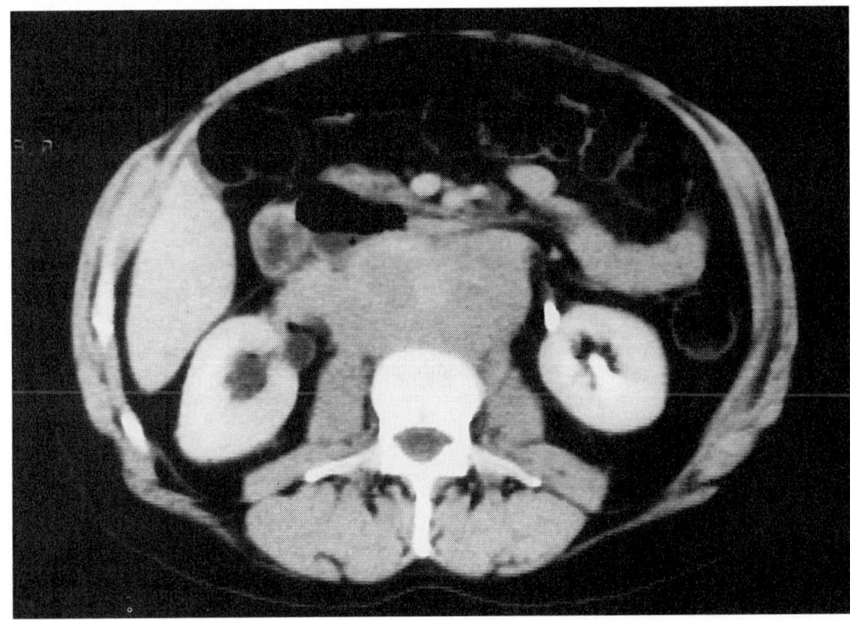

FIGURE 104.5. Retroperitoneal fibrosis. A tumor-like periaortic mass of homogeneous reactive fibrosis pulls the ureters medially in this contrasted computed tomography scan of the abdomen and retroperitoneum in a patient with retroperitoneal fibrosis.

these associations have not been proven (99,100). There is some evidence that degenerative and inflammatory diseases of the aorta resulting in aortic aneurysm (atherosclerosis, aortitis, inherited diseases of collagen, trauma, infection) shed inflammatory lipids and oxidized lipoproteins through the aortic adventitia, which trigger the retroperitoneal inflammatory process. Thus subclinical primary aortic disease must be suspected in all patients with idiopathic retroperitoneal fibrosis. Lymphoma, crystal-storing histiocytosis, immunocytoma, diffuse retroperitoneal carcinoma (pancreatic, scirrhous gastric, prostate, ovarian, renal, uterine cervix, carcinoid), Wegener's granulomatosis, xanthogranulomatous pyelonephritis, chronic pyelonephritis, tuberculosis, sarcoidosis, or aortic graft infection should be excluded by using appropriate imaging or by biopsy or aspiration of the retroperitoneal tissues or by careful examination of affected nonretroperitoneal tissues (101–103).

Diagnosis

A computed tomography (CT) or MRI scan with intravenous contrast or an intravenous urogram will demonstrate a retroperitoneal inflammatory reaction, obstruction of ureters, great vessels, biliary tree, or pancreatic ducts or the presence of diffuse or discrete unifocal or multifocal retroperitoneal masses (104,105). On occasion fibrosis may extend into the root of the mesentery, the bladder, and peribronchial areas, resulting in traction, distortion, and obstruction of the gut, urethra, and bronchi. Indium 111–labeled leukocyte or gallium radionuclide scans are useful to exclude abscess and other intensely inflammatory retroperitoneal processes and have been used to monitor disease activity (106,107). Autoimmune diseases should be excluded by careful examination and serologic testing. Drug use and toxin exposure should be carefully queried, and potentially offending drugs removed. After suggestive masses are identified, CT or ultrasound-guided percutaneous needle biopsy, laparoscopy, or retroperitoneal exploration can be undertaken to confirm the diagnosis and exclude confounding conditions, especially neoplasia and infection (108,109).

Treatment

Treatment for retroperitoneal fibrosis is unproven, but should seriously be considered because the disease is often progressive and fatal. Conventional treatment for obstructive retroperitoneal fibrosis consists of surgery to relieve ureteral and vascular entrapment and subsequent administration of long-term corticosteroids. An alternative approach is the use of ureteral stents to relieve obstruction, followed by pulse methylprednisolone therapy and long-term penicillamine, azathioprine, or cyclophosphamide (110,111). Tamoxifen has been used as primary therapy on a limited basis with some success and very little toxicity (107). Life-long anticoagulation is required for those patients with large vein involvement. Surgical repair of an abdominal aortic aneurysm may be either an exacerbating or an ameliorating factor for associated retroperitoneal fibrosis; thus therapy for these patients must be individualized.

REFERENCES

1. Sibbitt WL Jr. Fibrosing syndromes: diabetic stiff hand syndrome, Dupuytren's contracture, and plantar fasciitis. In: McCarty DJ, ed. *Arthritis and allied conditions.* Philadelphia: Lea & Febiger, 1989:1473–1485.
2. Sibbitt WL Jr. Fibrosing syndromes: diabetic stiff hand syndrome, Dupuytren's contracture, and plantar fasciitis. In: McCarty DJ, ed. *Arthritis and allied conditions.* Philadelphia: Lea & Febiger, 1993:1609–1618.
3. Sibbitt WL Jr. Fibrosing syndromes: diabetic stiff hand syndrome, Dupuytren's contracture, plantar fasciitis, and retroperitoneal fibrosis. In: Koopman W, ed. *Arthritis and allied conditions.* Lippincott Williams & Wilkins, 1997:1609–1618.
4. Border WA, Ruoslahti E. Transforming growth factor-beta in disease: the dark side of tissue repair. *J Clin Invest* 1992;90:1–7.
5. Mutsaers SE, Bishop JE, McGrouther G, Laurent GJ. Mechanisms of tissue repair: from wound healing to fibrosis. *Int J Biochem Cell Biol* 1997;29:5–17.
6. Trojanowska M, LeRoy EC, Eckes B, Krieg T. Pathogenesis of fibrosis: type 1 collagen and the skin. *J Mol Med* 1998;76: 266–274.
7. Gharaee-Kermani M, Phan SH. The role of eosinophils in pulmonary fibrosis. *Int J Mol Med* 1998;1:43–53.
8. Metcalfe DD, Baram D, Mekori YA. Mast cells. *Physiol Rev* 1997;77:1033–1079.
9. Haque MF, Harris M, Meghji S, Barrett AW. Immunolocalization of cytokines and growth factors in oral submucous fibrosis. *Cytokine* 1998;10:713–719.
10. Schins RP, Borm PJ. Mechanisms and mediators in coal dust induced toxicity: a review. *Ann Occup Hygiene* 1999;43:7–33.
11. Robledo R, Mossman B. Cellular and molecular mechanisms of asbestos-induced fibrosis. *J Cell Physiol* 1999;180:158–166.
12. Coker RK, Laurent GJ. Pulmonary fibrosis: cytokines in the balance. *Eur Respir J* 1998;11:1218–1221.
13. Miyazaki Y, Araki K, Vesin C, et al. Expression of a tumor necrosis factor-alpha transgene in murine lung causes lymphocytic and fibrosing alveolitis: a mouse model of progressive pulmonary fibrosis. *J Clin Invest* 1995;96:250–259.
14. Hasegawa M, Fujimoto M, Kikuchi K, Takehara K. Elevated serum tumor necrosis factor-alpha levels in patients with systemic sclerosis: association with pulmonary fibrosis. *J Rheumatol* 1997;24:663–665.
15. Majewski S, Wojas-Pelc A, Malejczyk M, Szymanska E, Jablonska S. Serum levels of soluble TNF alpha receptor type I and the severity of systemic sclerosis. *Acta Derm Venereol* 1999;79: 207–210.
16. Gruschwitz MS, Albrecht M, Vieth G, Haustein UF. In situ expression and serum levels of tumor necrosis factor-alpha receptors in patients with early stages of systemic sclerosis. *J Rheumatol* 1997;24:1936–1943.
17. Wahl SM. Transforming growth factor beta (TGF-beta) in inflammation: a case and a cure. *J Clin Immunol* 1992;12: 61–74.
18. Roulot D, Sevcsik AM, Coste T, Strosberg AD, Marullo S. Role of transforming growth factor beta type II receptor in hepatic

fibrosis: studies of human chronic hepatitis C and experimental fibrosis in rats. *Hepatology* 1999;29:1730–1738.
19. Clark DA, Coker R. Transforming growth factor-beta (TGF-beta). *Int J Biochem Cell Biol* 1998;30:293–298.
20. Terrell TG, Working PK, Chow CP, Green JD. Pathology of recombinant human transforming growth factor-beta1 in rats and rabbits. *Int Rev Exp Pathol* 1993;34:S43–S47.
21. Zugmaier G, Paik S, Wilding G, et al. Transforming growth factor beta1 induces cachexia and systemic fibrosis without an antitumor effect in nude mice. *Cancer Res* 1991;51:3590–3594.
22. Border WA, Okuda S, Languino LR, et al. Suppression of experimental glomerulonephritis by antiserum against transforming growth factor beta1. *Nature* 1990;346:371–374.
23. Shah M, Foreman DM, Ferguson MW. Control of scarring in adult wounds by neutralizing antibody to transforming growth factor beta. *Lancet* 1992;339:213–214.
24. Giri SN, Hyde DM, Hollinger MA. Effect of antibody to transforming growth factor beta on bleomycin induced accumulation of lung collagen in mice. *Thorax* 1993;48:959–966.
25. Border WA, Noble, NA, Yamamoto T, et al. Natural inhibitors of transforming growth factor-beta protects against scarring in experimental kidney disease. *Nature* 1992;360:361–364.
26. O'Kane S, Ferguson MW. Transforming growth factor betas and wound healing. *Int J Biochem Cell Biol* 1997;29:63–78.
27. Gruber BL, Marchese MJ, Kew RR. Transforming growth factor-beta1 mediates mast cell chemotaxis. *J Immunol* 1994;152: 5860–5867.
28. Kupper TS. Adhesion molecules in scleroderma: collagen binding integrins. *Int Rev Immunol* 1995;12:217–225.
29. Bissell DM. Hepatic fibrosis as wound repair: a progress report. *J Gastroenterol* 1998;33:295–302.
30. Wardle EN. Modulatory proteins and processes in alliance with immune cells, mediators, and extracellular proteins in renal interstitial fibrosis. *Renal Fail* 1999;21:121–133.
31. Feldmann M, Brennan FM, Maini R. Cytokines in autoimmune disorders. *Int Rev Immunol* 1998;17:217–228.
32. Haustein UF, Anderegg U. Pathophysiology of scleroderma: an update. *J Eur Acad Dermatol Venereol* 1998;11:1–8.
33. Hogaboam CM, Steinhauser ML, Chensue SW, et al. Novel roles for chemokines and fibroblasts in interstitial fibrosis. *Kidney Int* 1998;54:2152–2159.
34. Igarashi A, Nashiro K, Kikuchi K, et al. Connective tissue growth factor gene expression in tissue sections from localized scleroderma, keloid, and other fibrotic skin disorders. *J Invest Dermatol* 1996;106:729–733.
35. Greenhalgh DG. The role of apoptosis in wound healing. *J Biochem Cell Biol* 1998;30:1019–1030.
36. Gauldie J, Sime PJ, Xing Z, et al. Transforming growth factor-beta gene transfer to the lung induces myofibroblast presence and pulmonary fibrosis. *Curr Top Pathol* 1999;93:35–45.
37. Low RB. Modulation of myofibroblast and smooth-muscle phenotypes in the lung. *Curr Top Pathol* 1999;93:19–26.
38. Greenhalgh DG. The role of apoptosis in wound healing. *J Biochem Cell Biol* 1998;30:1019–1030.
39. Gauldie J, Sime PJ, Xing Z, et al. Transforming growth factor-beta gene transfer to the l nodular palmar fibromatosis (morbus Dupuytren). *Histol Histopathol* 1998;13:67–72.
40. Kapanci Y, Desmouliere A, Pache JC, et al. Cytoskeletal protein modulation in pulmonary alveolar myofibroblasts during idiopathic pulmonary fibrosis: possible role of transforming growth factor beta and tumor necrosis factor alpha. *Am J Respir Crit Care Med* 1995;152:2163–2169.
41. Maish GO III, Shumate ML, Ehrlich HP, Cooney RN. Tumor necrosis factor binding protein improves incisional wound healing in sepsis. *J Surg Res* 1998;78:108–117.
42. Cooney R, Iocono J, Maish G, et al. In vivo effects of tumor necrosis factor-alpha on incised wound and gunshot wound healing. *J Trauma* 1996;40(suppl 3):S140–S143.
43. Thrall RS, Vogel SN, Evans R, Shultz LD. Role of tumor necrosis factor-alpha in the spontaneous development of pulmonary fibrosis in viable motheaten mutant mice. *Am J Pathol* 1997; 151:1303–1310.
44. Benson LS, Williams CS, Kahle M. Dupuytren's contracture. *J Am Acad Orthop Surg* 1998;6:24–35.
45. Elliot D. The early history of contracture of the palmar fascia. Part 1: the origin of the disease; the curse of the MacCrimmons; the hand of benediction; Cline's contracture. Part 2: The revolution in Paris: Guillaume Dupuytren: Dupuytren's disease. *J Hand Surg Br* 1988;13:246–253, 371–378.
46. Elliot D. The early history of contracture of the palmar fascia. Part 3: the controversy in Paris and the spread of surgical treatment of the disease throughout Europe. *J Hand Surg* 1989;14: 25–31.
47. Elliot D. Pre-1900 literature on Dupuytren's disease. *Hand Clin* 1999;15:35–42.
48. de Palma L, Santucci A, Gigante A, et al. Plantar fibromatosis: an immunohistochemical and ultrastructural study. *Foot Ankle Int* 1999;20:253–257.
49. Classen DA, Hurst LN. Plantar fibromatosis and bilateral flexion contractures: a review of the literature. *Ann Plast Surg* 1992; 28:475–478.
50. Lee YC, Chan HH, Black MM. Aggressive polyfibromatosis: a 10 year follow-up. *Australas J Dermatol* 1996;37:205–207.
51. Badalamente MA, Sampson SP, Hurst LC, et al. The role of transforming growth factor beta in Dupuytren's disease. *J Hand Surg Am* 1996;21:210–215.
52. Badalamente MA, Hurst LC. The biochemistry of Dupuytren's disease. *Hand Clin* 1999;15:97–107.
53. Pasquali-Ronchetti I, Guerra D, Baccarani-Contri M, et al. A clinical, ultrastructural and immunochemical study of Dupuytren's disease. *J Hand Surg Br* 1993;18:262–269.
54. Berndt A, Kosmehyl H, Katenkamp D, et al. Appearance of the myofibroblastic phenotype in Dupuytren's disease is associated with a fibronectin, laminin, collagen type IV and tenascin extracellular matrix. *Pathobiology* 1994;62:55–58.
55. Wilutzky B, Berndt A, Katenkamp D, et al. Programmed cell death in nodular palmar fibromatosis (morbus Dupuytren). *Histol Histopathol* 1998;13:67–72.
56. Burge P. Genetics of Dupuytren's disease. *Hand Clin* 1999;15: 63–71.
57. Urban M, Feldberg L, Janssen A, et al. Dupuytren's disease in children. *J Hand Surg Br* 1996;21:112–116.
58. Chansky HA, Trumble TE, Conrad EU III, et al. Evidence for a polyclonal etiology of palmar fibromatosis. *J Hand Surg Am* 1999;24:339–344.
59. Dal Cin P, De Smet L, Sciot R, et al. Trisomy 7 and trisomy 8 in dividing and non-dividing tumor cells in Dupuytren's disease. *Cancer Genet Cytogenet* 1999;108:137–140.
60. Ross DC. Epidemiology of Dupuytren's disease. *Hand Clin* 1999;15:53–62.
61. Gudmundsson KG, Arngrimsson R, Arinbjarnarson S, et al. T- and B-lymphocyte subsets in patients with Dupuytren's disease: correlations with disease severity. *J Hand Surg Br* 1998;23: 724–727.
62. Yi IS, Johnson G, Moneim MS. Etiology of Dupuytren's disease. *Hand Clin* 1999;15:43–51.
63. Arkkila PE, Kantola IM, Viikari JS. Dupuytren's disease: association with chronic diabetic complications. *J Rheumatol* 1997; 24:153–159.
64. Burge P, Hoy G, Regan P, et al. Smoking, alcohol and the risk

of Dupuytren's contracture. *J Bone Joint Surg Br* 1997;79: 206–210.
65. Liss GM, Stock SR. Can Dupuytren's contracture be work-related? review of the evidence. *Am J Ind Med* 1996;29: 521–532.
66. Citron N, Messina JC. The use of skeletal traction in the treatment of severe primary Dupuytren's disease. *J Bone Joint Surg Br* 1998;80:126–129.
67. McCarthy DM. The long-term results of enzymic fasciotomy. *J Hand Surg Br* 1992;17:356.
68. Dominguez-Malagon HR, Alfeiran-Ruiz A, Chavarria-Xicotencatl P, et al. Clinical and cellular effects of colchicine in fibromatosis. *Cancer* 1992;69:2478–2483.
69. Kapoor A, Sibbitt WL Jr. Diabetic contractures: the syndrome of limited joint mobility. *Semin Arthritis Rheum* 1889;18: 168–174.
70. Chammas M, Bousquet P, Renard E, et al. Dupuytren's disease, carpal tunnel syndrome, trigger finger, and diabetes mellitus. *J Hand Surg Am* 1995;20:109–114.
71. Tuzun B, Tuzun Y, Dinccag N, et al. Diabetic sclerodactyly. *Diabetes Res Clin Pract* 1995;27:153–157.
72. Ismail AA, Dasgupta B, Tanqueray AB, et al. Ultrasonographic features of diabetic cheiroarthropathy. *Br J Rheumatol* 1996;35: 676–679.
73. Sibbitt WL Jr, Eaton RP. Corticosteroid responsive tenosynovitis is a common pathway for limited joint mobility in the diabetic hand. *J Rheumatol* 1997;24:931–936.
74. Border WA, Noble NA. Evidence that TGF-beta should be a therapeutic target in diabetic nephropathy. *Kidney Int* 1998; 54:1390–1391.
75. Phillips AO. Diabetic nephropathy: the modulating influence of glucose on transforming factor beta production. *Histol Histopathol* 1998;13:565–574.
76. Rosenbloom AL, Silverstein JH. Connective tissue and joint disease in diabetes mellitus. *Endocrinol Metab Clin North Am* 1996;25:473–483.
77. Eaton RP. Aldose reductase inhibition and the diabetic syndrome of limited joint mobility: implications for altered collagen hydration. *Metabolism* 1986;35:119–121.
78. Eaton RP, Sibbitt WL Jr, Harsh A. The effect of an aldose reductase inhibiting agent on limited joint mobility in diabetes mellitus. *JAMA* 1985;253:1437–1471.
79. Eaton RP, Sibbitt WL Jr, Shah VO, et al. A commentary on 10 years of aldose reductase inhibition for limited joint mobility in diabetes. *J Diabetes Complications* 1998;12:34–38.
80. Karr SD. Subcalcaneal heel pain. *Orthop Clin North Am* 1994; 25:S161–S175.
81. Sobel E, Levitz SJ, Caselli MA. Orthoses in the treatment of rearfoot problems. *J Am Podiatr Med Assoc* 1999;89:220–223.
82. Powell M, Post WR, Keener J, Wearden S. Effective treatment of chronic plantar fasciitis with dorsiflexion night splints: a crossover prospective randomized outcome study. *Foot Ankle Int* 1998;19:10–18.
83. Lynch DM, Goforth WP, Martin JE, et al. Conservative treatment of plantar fasciitis: a prospective study. *J Am Podiatr Med Assoc* 1998;88:375–380.
84. DiMarcangelo MT, Yu TC. Diagnostic imaging of heel pain and plantar fasciitis. *Clin Podiatr Med Surg* 1997;14:281–301.
85. Acevedo JI, Beskin JL. Complications of plantar fascia rupture associated with corticosteroid injection. *Foot Ankle Int* 1998;19: 91–97.
86. Benton-Weil W, Borrelli AH, Weil LS Jr, et al. Percutaneous plantar fasciotomy: a minimally invasive procedure for recalcitrant plantar fasciitis. *J Foot Ankle Surg* 1998;37:269–272.
87. Sammarco GJ, Helfrey RB. Surgical treatment of recalcitrant plantar fasciitis. *Foot Ankle Int* 1996;17:520–526.
88. Dehner LP, Coffin CM. Idiopathic fibrosclerotic disorders and other inflammatory pseudotumors. *Semin Diagn Pathol* 1998; 15:161–173.
89. Johal SS, Manjunath S, Allen C, et al. Systemic multifocal fibrosclerosis. *Postgrad Med J* 1998;74:608–609.
90. Kaipiainen-Seppanen O, Jantunen E, Kuusisto J, et al. Retroperitoneal fibrosis with antineutrophil cytoplasmic antibodies. *J Rheumatol* 1996;23:779–781.
91. Dehner LP, Moroni G, Farricciotti A, et al. Retroperitoneal fibrosis and membranous nephropathy: improvement of both diseases after treatment with steroids and immunosuppressive agents. *Nephrol Dial Transplant* 1999;14:1303–1305.
92. Levey JM, Mathai J. Diffuse pancreatic fibrosis: an uncommon feature of multifocal idiopathic fibrosclerosis. *Am J Gastroenterol* 1998;93:640–642.
93. Shaunak S, Wilkins A, Pilling JB, et al. Pericardial, retroperitoneal, and pleural fibrosis induced by pergolide. *J Neurol Neurosurg Psychiatry* 1999;66:79–81.
94. Sakr G, Cynk M, Cowie AG. Retroperitoneal fibrosis: an unusual complication of intra-arterial stents and angioplasty. *Br J Urol* 1998;81:768–769.
95. Sauni R, Oksa P, Jarvenpaa R, et al. Asbestos exposure: a potential cause of retroperitoneal fibrosis. *Am J Ind Med* 1998;33: 418–421.
96. Hughes D, Buckley PJ. Idiopathic retroperitoneal fibrosis is a macrophage-rich process. *Am J Surg Pathol* 1993;17:482–490.
97. Lee I. Human fibroblasts in idiopathic retroperitoneal fibrosis express HLA-DR antigens. *J Korean Med Sci* 1991;6:279–283.
98. Parums DV, Choudhury RP, Shields SA, et al. Characterization of inflammatory cells associated with idiopathic retroperitoneal fibrosis. *Br J Urol* 1991;67:564–568.
99. Dent GA, Baird DB, Ros DW. Systemic idiopathic fibrosis with T-cell receptor gene rearrangement. *Arch Pathol Lab Med* 1991; 115:80–83.
100. De Luca S, Terrone C, Manassero A, et al. Aetiopathogenesis and treatment of idiopathic retroperitoneal fibrosis. *Ann Urol (Paris)* 1998;32:153–159.
101. Garcia JF, Sanchez E, Lloret E, et al. Crystal-storing histiocytosis and immunocytoma associated with multifocal fibrosclerosis. *Histopathology* 1998;33:459–464.
102. Cuny C, Chauffert B, Lorcerie B, et al. Retroperitoneal fibrosis and infection of an aortic graft prosthesis: diagnosis and therapeutic problems. *Clin Cardiol* 1997;20:810–812.
103. Kaipiainen-Seppanen O, Jantunen E, Kuusisto J, et al. Retroperitoneal fibrosis with antineutrophil cytoplasmic antibodies. *J Rheumatol* 1996;23:779–781.
104. Engelken JD, Ros PR. Retroperitoneal MR imaging. *Magn Reson Imaging Clin North Am* 1997;5:165–178.
105. Kottra JJ, Dunnick NR. Retroperitoneal fibrosis. *Radiol Clin North Am* 1996;34:1259–1275.
106. Fink AM, Miles KA, Wraight EP. Indium-111 labelled leucocyte uptake in aortitis. *Clin Radiol* 1994;49:863–866.
107. Oosterlinck W, Derie A. New data on diagnosis and medical treatment of retroperitoneal fibrosis. *Acta Urol Belg* 1997;65: 3–6.
108. Stein AL, Bardawil RG, Silverman SG, et al. Fine needle aspiration biopsy of idiopathic retroperitoneal fibrosis. *Acta Cytol* 1997;41:461–466.
109. Kava BR, Russo P, Conlon KC. Laparoscopic diagnosis of malignant retroperitoneal fibrosis. *J Endourol* 1996;10:535–538.
110. Harreby M, Bilde T, Helin P, et al. Retroperitoneal fibrosis treated with methylprednisolone pulse and disease-modifying antirheumatic drugs. *Scand J Urol Nephrol* 1994;28:237–242.
111. Netzer P, Binek J, Hammer B. Diffuse abdominal pain, nausea and vomiting due to retroperitoneal fibrosis: a rare but often missed diagnosis. *Eur J Gastroenterol Hepatol* 1997;9:1005–1008.

105

NERVE ENTRAPMENT SYNDROMES

NORTIN M. HADLER

The major peripheral nerves of healthy individuals, with the few exceptions discussed later, withstand compromise in spite of their length and soft tissue shielding. Blunt trauma, fractures, and lacerations are the usual culprits and are the purview of trauma surgeons. Rheumatologists, however, traditionally care for the systemically ill patient in whom the soft tissue shielding of the peripheral nerves and the nerves themselves are often involved by synovitis and vasculitis, respectively. The challenge is to discern the symptoms and signs of peripheral neuropathy in a more general inflammatory disease setting.

Recently rheumatologists have been faced with ministering to individuals who would be well were it not for their arm discomfort which they and worker's compensation insurers consider work related. The diagnosis of entrapment neuropathy is often entertained. However, this is a population of individuals with arm pain unlike any other with which the rheumatologist is familiar. The diagnostic challenge merits separate treatment.

CLINICAL PRESENTATION

This chapter considers entrapment neuropathies of the major peripheral nerves as they course through the upper and lower extremities, focusing on those lesions likely to be seen by the rheumatologist; rare and exceptional sites of compression neuropathy require a more encyclopedic treatment (1). The differential diagnosis of peripheral compression neuropathies includes more proximal neurologic disease. Cervical and lumbar radiculopathies are discussed in Chapters 100, 102, and 103, and thoracic outlet syndrome and diseases of the brachial plexus in Chapter 107. Complementary essays are readily available (2,3). Rather than reemphasize the hallmarks of these confounding diagnoses, the distinctive features of peripheral entrapment neuropathies are emphasized here. Several of these features are common to all peripheral entrapment neuropathies and are discussed in the following paragraphs.

1. Dysesthesias are characteristic; they are often localized to the sensory distribution of the involved nerve.
2. The discomfort is variously described as burning, tingling, "pins and needles," or even "itchy" skin. Sometimes an aching pain is noted in the muscles, even the proximal muscles, innervated by the involved nerve.
3. The discomfort is not prominently use related. Tenderness in the distribution of the dysesthesias is not a feature; on the contrary, dysesthesias occurring at night and at rest plague these patients. The response is to attempt to rub or move the distal extremity, leading to further dismay if the patient has coincident inflammatory arthritis.
4. *Tinel's sign* is elicited by tapping the nerve at the site of entrapment. Focal tenderness is usually present but nonspecific, particularly in the setting of synovitis. The more specific response is to elicit pain and dysesthesias radiating into the sensory distribution of the nerve distal to the point of damage. The sign is useful both in the clinical diagnosis of entrapment neuropathy and in the localization of the compression in patients with systemic rheumatic disorders. Its utility pales when applied to any population other than that traditionally referred to rheumatologists. In particular, it is no match for the challenge of discerning entrapment as the cause of any pain in the work force.
5. The dysesthesias and associated symptoms reflect the greater vulnerability of the sensory fibers in the peripheral nerve to compressive damage. The process, however, rarely progresses to severe hypesthesia such that traditional testing with a pin is clearly abnormal. More subtle tests of tactile compromise, such as sensory thresholds, are unreliable in the hands of many experienced investigators. Regardless, a normal sensory examination does not militate against the diagnosis of an entrapment neuropathy.
6. With severe and prolonged compression, the motor function of the nerve is compromised as well. In instances of insidiously progressive compression, such as in some patients with rheumatoid arthritis (RA), motor compromise may be present with insignificant dysesthesias. In the upper extremity, motor compromise is manifest as clumsiness and decreased hand

function. In the lower extremity, a gait disorder may eventuate. Atrophy and weakness become evident in muscles innervated by the compressed nerve.
7. Discerning entrapment neuropathies in the setting of RA or other inflammatory arthritis is particularly difficult. With many idiopathic entrapments, particularly those occurring after subtle trauma, the involvement is often unilateral. Idiopathic carpal tunnel syndrome is an important exception. Symmetry of proliferative synovitis, however, can lead to symmetric entrapment neuropathies. Discerning the historic features of entrapment neuropathy among the more familiar inflammatory complaints is crucial. Inspecting the distal musculature is important, seeking asymmetry in the typical pattern of periarticular muscle atrophy, both between and within hands and feet, that might provide a clue to a peripheral neuropathy.
8. Although the patient may perceive that the involved distal extremity is "swollen," objective swelling or vasomotor phenomena are unusual in entrapment neuropathies, and their presence should lead to a restructuring of the differential diagnosis.
9. Entrapment neuropathies should be treated conservatively, unless symptoms become recalcitrant or weakness or atrophy supervenes. Atrophy is often obscured in the setting of inflammatory synovitis. Before considering surgical decompression, the physician should attempt to confirm the clinical diagnosis of entrapment and localize the compression by electroneurography. The sensitivity of these techniques varies depending on the lesion; for carpal tunnel syndrome in patients with or without systemic disease, it can approach 90% (4). However, the validity and reliability of electrodiagnosis, even for carpal tunnel syndrome, is critically dependent on the fastidiousness of the laboratory and the use of appropriate normal controls (5).

ENTRAPMENT NEUROPATHIES OF THE UPPER EXTREMITY

The three major nerves of the upper extremity course through the arm, protected from external compression short of that consequent to a humeral fracture or similar trauma. At the elbow, all three are at risk. Their course is more superficial at the elbow, even subcutaneous; they traverse synovial reflections that can proliferate in RA, and are sandwiched at points between long bones and muscles. At the wrist, they again are at risk for all of the preceding reasons except that the sandwich is between bony prominences and tendons. Each nerve is considered separately in the following sections.

Median Nerve

The median nerve approaches the antecubital fossa lying medial to the brachial artery and separates from the artery at the artery's bifurcation. The nerve passes between the two heads of the pronator teres (the ulnar artery is deep to this muscle) and courses through the forearm, lying between the flexors digitorum superficialis and profundus. It then passes through the carpal tunnel just beneath the transverse carpal ligament deep to the tendon of the palmaris longus. The median nerve supplies all the superficial and deep muscles of the volar forearm except the flexor carpi ulnaris. It also supplies nearly all the muscles of the thenar eminence: the abductor pollices brevis, the opponens pollices, and the superficial head of the flexor pollices brevis. The sensory distribution is illustrated in Fig. 105.1A.

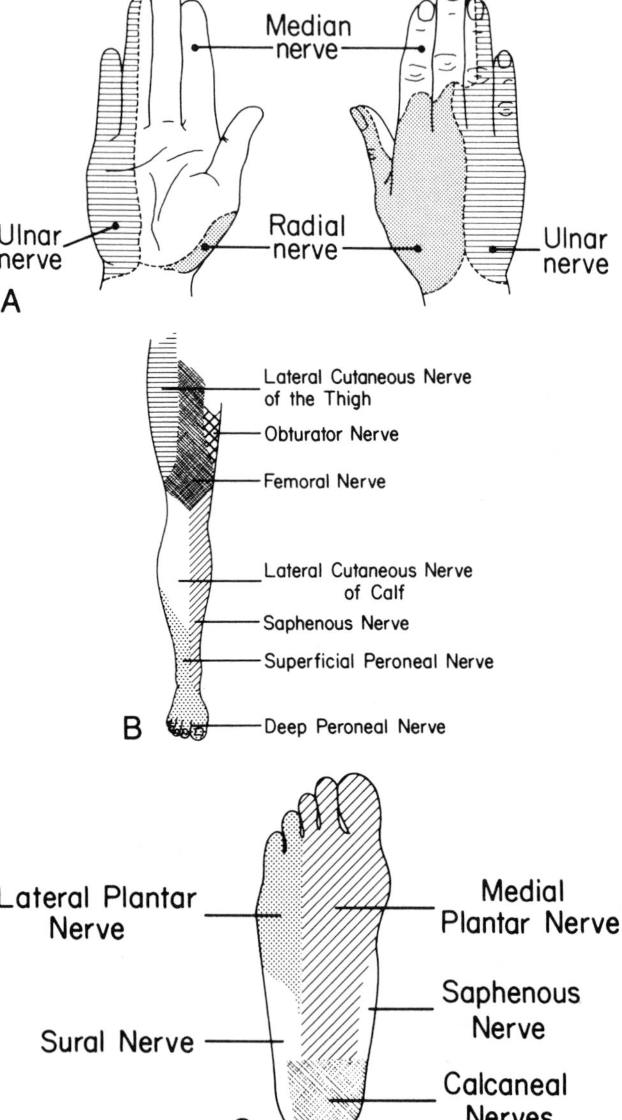

FIGURE 105.1. Distribution of the cutaneous nerves to the extremities. **A:** Sensory innervation of the palm and dorsum of the hand. **B:** Sensory innervation of the anterior aspect of the leg. **C:** Cutaneous innervation of the sole.

Entrapment neuropathy of the median nerve is the most common of the entrapment neuropathies. In fact, it is the most common peripheral neuropathy. Regardless of the clinical setting, the most common site of compression is within the carpal tunnel. Thus the carpal tunnel syndrome is the prototype entrapment neuropathy most likely to exhibit all of the preceding clinical features. Motor compromise involves the thenar eminence, with weakness and atrophy best detected by inspecting the contour of the abductor pollices brevis (Fig. 105.2). There is less uniformity of opinion regarding the sensitivity of provocative tests and the sensory examination. Some clinicians find the Tinel's and Phalen's signs useful (symptoms reproduced on flexion at the wrist), whereas most clinicians find sensory examinations very insensitive and provocative tests with a blood pressure cuff useless. When systematically assessed in patients with arm pain of various etiologies referred for electrodiagnostic tests, none of the classic signs has sufficient predictive value to be clinically useful in screening unless referral bias is so powerful that the patient has a very high *a priori* likelihood of having carpal tunnel syndrome (6–8).

Management of idiopathic carpal tunnel syndrome begins with splinting the wrist in the neutral position, particularly at night. In those with persistent symptoms in spite of splinting, steroid injection into the carpal tunnel provides complete relief in the majority, although many will relapse within 18 months. In cases severe enough to undergo carpal tunnel release, the pressure to which the nerve is subjected is increased. Thenar atrophy is a consensus indication for surgical intervention; recalcitrant symptoms, particularly atypical symptoms, call for perspicacity, judgment, and unequivocal electroneurographic confirmation of the diagnosis. It is important to emphasize that carpal tunnel syndrome is not prevalent; its incidence approximates 1/1,000 per year (9). Furthermore, it is not a consequence of performing repetitive motions if the elements of use are comfortable, and it does not occur in epidemics or even clusters (*vide infra*).

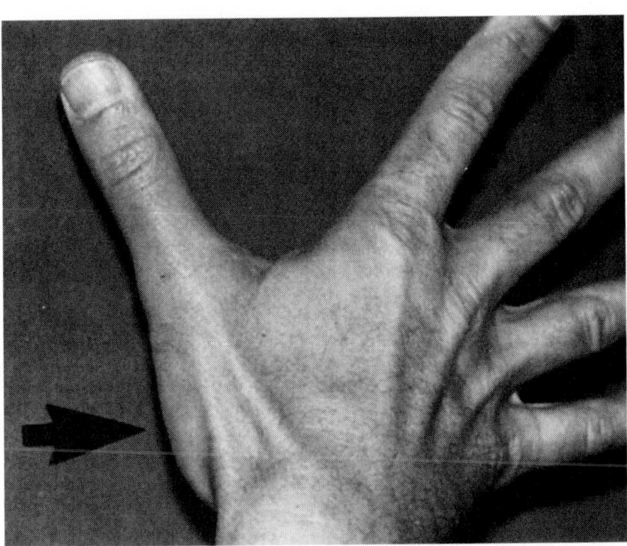

FIGURE 105.2. The lateral contour of the thenar eminence is the abductor pollicis brevis. Abduction against resistance allows one to assess the power of this muscle and inspect its bulk as a bulge (*arrow*). Because the innervation of this muscle is exclusively the median nerve, weakness and atrophy are specific signs of median neuropathy.

Carpal tunnel syndrome can complicate RA, even early in the course, and with bilateral involvement. Here, too, steroid injection can prove palliative with two provisos: first, thenar muscle atrophy secondary to median nerve compression can be obscured by that caused by articular inflammation, mandating close observation and ready recourse to surgical consultation. Second, injection therapy by the usual volar route carries greater risk of nerve infiltration and damage because of anatomic distortion secondary to articular destruction. Injecting the proximal radiocarpal joint by the dorsal approach carries no such risk and may produce the same result.

The differential diagnosis of carpal tunnel syndrome is broad and lengthy, but aside from pregnancy, most associated entities are exceedingly rare. Nonetheless, consideration and, on occasion, appropriate laboratory tests are germane because interventions vary considerably. Myxedema, tuberculous wrist, and gout are examples of medically treatable entities. Amyloid, multiple myeloma, and perhaps, diabetic or uremic involvement may not respond even to carpal tunnel release.

The median nerve is only rarely subjected to compression at sites other than the carpal tunnel. Compression between the heads of the pronator teres is suspected by a localizing Tinel's sign, confirmed by electrodiagnosis, and can be treated by constraining forceful pronation. Such a proximal median neuropathy may compromise the long flexors to the digits; the patient may be unable to flex distal interphalangeal joints, as confirmed in the clinical test of opposing the tips of the first and second digits to the thumb to form a circle.

Ulnar Nerve

The ulnar nerve parts from the brachial artery in the middle of the arm. It courses dorsally, piercing the medial intermuscular septum, and it lies in the condylar groove behind the medial epicondyle at the elbow. The nerve then courses in a volar direction, and 2 cm into the forearm, it enters the "cubital tunnel," the floor of which is the medial ligament of the elbow joint; the roof is the aponeurosis of the flexor carpi ulnaris muscle. It courses beneath this muscle and lies subcutaneous and lateral to the ulnar artery in the distal half of the forearm. The ulnar nerve enters the wrist superficial to the flexor retinaculum (here called the *pisohamate ligament*) between the pisiform and the hook of the hamate and deep to the superficial volar carpal ligament in a conduit called *Guyon's canal.* The ulnar nerve supplies the flexor carpi ulnaris and, with the median, the profundus in the forearm. In the palm it supplies the muscles of the hypothenar eminence, all the interossei, the third and fourth lumbricals, the adductor pollices, and part of the flexor pollices brevis. Its cutaneous distribution is shown in Fig. 105.1.

The ulnar nerve is at risk of compression at the condylar groove, in the cubital tunnel, and in Guyon's canal. Furthermore, all three sites are potential targets of proliferative synovitis in RA. The presentation can have all the features of compression neuropathy, but it is notoriously variable. Insidiously progressive atrophy can occur with little discomfort and even little sensory loss, the so-called "tardy ulnar palsy." Discerning early motor compromise is difficult and particularly challenging in the setting of RA. Weakness in apposition of the fourth and fifth digits and *Froment's* sign (Fig. 105.3) can be helpful, along with inspection of the hypothenar eminence for atrophy. Localization of the site of the compressive lesion can be challenging, particularly because the sensitivity of electrodiagnostic testing for ulnar neuropathy does not equal that for median neuropathies.

Ulnar neuropathies must be distinguished from lesions that involve the lower trunk of the brachial plexus. In these cases, the symptoms often extend proximal to the elbow. Pancoast tumors must be sought; a Horner syndrome may offer a clue. "Thoracic outlet syndrome" is an often abused and often tenuous concept (3). In an undisputed *axonopathic* form of neurogenic thoracic outlet syndrome, there is weakness and atrophy of median and ulnar innervated muscles of the hand and forearm with sensory disturbance in the ulnar, but not the median, distribution.

In the setting of RA, treatment of ulnar neuropathies includes injections of corticosteroids into the elbow or wrist joints to decrease the synovitis. Such maneuvers are of unproven benefit, however, in idiopathic ulnar neuropathies. In the absence of joint deformities, conservative management focuses on preventing trauma to the nerve at the elbow with padding and by restricting flexion. The decision to attempt "decompression" or nerve transposition will tax the judgment of any surgeon.

Radial Nerve

The radial nerve leaves the axilla, passes posterior to the humerus, through the lateral intermuscular septum just distal to the deltoid insertion to lie superficially in the lateral arm. The nerve then passes between the brachialis and brachioradialis to the front of the lateral epicondyle, near where it divides into two branches. The deep branch, the posterior interosseous nerve, passes into the supinator muscle through the arcade of Frohse and courses within the muscle in the supinator canal, from which it emerges to supply the extensor muscles of the digits and some of the wrist. The superficial radial nerve passes over the supinator and pronator teres muscles and descends along the lateral border of the forearm to provide the sensory distribution of the radial nerve (Fig. 105.1).

The radial nerve is at risk of compression on the humerus as it courses through the radial groove. Generally,

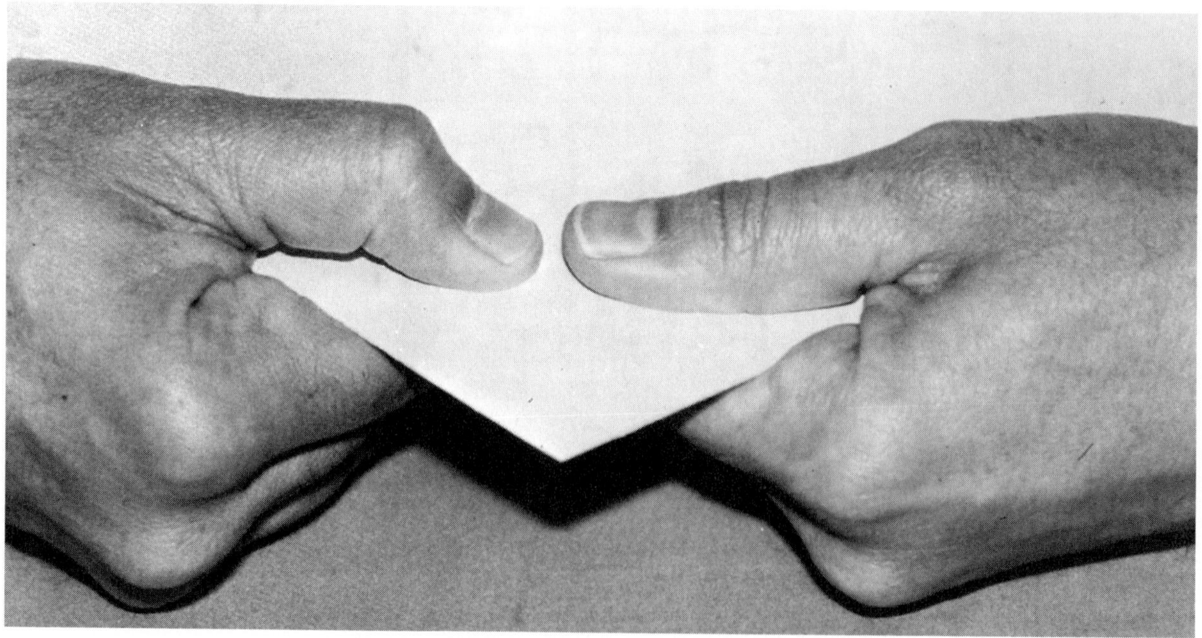

FIGURE 105.3. Froment's sign is the inability to maintain flexion of the interphalangeal joint of the thumb during forceful pinching. It is a subtle sign of intrinsic muscle compromise in ulnar palsy.

compression is the result of prolonged improper positioning during anesthesia or sleeping on the arm, often when inebriated or sedated ("Saturday night palsy") and results in wristdrop; sensory involvement is variable.

The posterior interosseous nerve is at risk of entrapment at the elbow by the proliferative synovitis of RA. Entrapment is manifest by weakness in the finger extensors more than in the wrist extensors and must be distinguished from compromise in the integrity of extensor tendons by dorsal synovitis at the wrist. Neither lesion produces a sensory deficit. It has been argued, although not convincingly, that entrapment of the posterior interosseus nerve in the arcade of Frohse or in the supinator canal is common and mimics lateral epicondylitis ("tennis elbow"). The superficial radial nerve is subject to external trauma, often resulting in distressing dysesthesias. Rarely, rupture of a rheumatoid elbow effusion can similarly compromise the nerve.

ENTRAPMENT NEUROPATHIES OF THE LOWER EXTREMITY

Compression or entrapment of the peripheral nerves in the absence of external force occurs less frequently in the lower extremity than in the upper. Lower extremity entrapment neuropathy is seldom recognized in RA. Nonetheless, a few examples are themselves important and enter into a differential diagnosis relevant to rheumatologic practice.

Femoral Nerve

The femoral nerve exits the pelvis beneath the medial aspect of the inguinal ligament to supply the quadriceps and the skin of the anterior thigh (Fig. 105.1B). It terminates at the saphenous nerve, which courses through the subsartorial canal before emerging through the fascia above the knee to supply the cutaneous innervation of the medial leg (Fig. 105.1). Aside from trauma and hematomas, femoral or saphenous entrapment is exceedingly rare. Saphenous entrapment is seen occasionally as a consequence of scarring from surgery on the venous system.

Lateral Cutaneous Nerve of the Thigh

The lateral cutaneous nerve of the thigh exits the pelvis either through or beneath the lateral inguinal ligament. The nerve is purely sensory (Fig. 105.1). Compression causes burning paresthesias and hyperpathia along the lateral aspect of the thigh, the syndrome of *meralgia paresthetica,* or *Bernhardt's disease* (*meralgia* derives from the Greek for pain in the thigh). The symptoms are worsened by standing and walking or by prolonged adduction or extension of the leg. The pathogenesis is thought to be entrapment of the nerve either at the inguinal ligament or when it pierces the fascia to reach the skin. The differential diagnosis includes an L3 radiculopathy or a femoral neuropathy, although both of these cause more anterior symptoms and rarely hyperesthesia. Rarely, retroperitoneal compression of the lumbar plexus by lymphoma or other neoplasms can provoke meralgia paresthetica. The diagnosis is based on the clinical features because there is no reliable electrodiagnostic test. Treatment is conservative because spontaneous regression of symptoms is the rule. Attempts should be made to eliminate compression by tight garments; weight loss often is advised. Surgical decompression has been disappointing (10).

Sciatic Nerve

The sciatic nerve exits the pelvis through the sciatic notch and lies between the greater trochanter and the ischial tuberosity deep to the gluteus maximus muscle. It courses deep to the hamstrings and supplies the posterior thigh muscles. In the pelvis, it is at risk for compression by neoplasms and inflammatory lesions such as a tuboovarian abscess. It is at some risk at the pyriform fossa, particularly with prolonged sitting on a hard surface or in a wheelchair. The "pyriformis syndrome" is a tenuous and controversial explanation for sciatica that invokes entrapment by the pyriformis muscle (11). Aside from overt trauma, the nerve is well cushioned throughout its course once it exits the pelvis, and compression from a gluteal abscess, for example, is exceedingly rare. Sciatic neuropathy as a manifestation of trochanteric bursitis has seldom been convincingly demonstrated (12). In the upper popliteal fossa, the sciatic nerve divides into the common peroneal nerve and the tibial nerve.

COMMON PERONEAL NERVE

The common peroneal nerve courses obliquely around the lateral aspect of the proximal fibula to pass through the superficial head of the peroneus longus muscle in the "fibular tunnel." On emerging, it divides into the superficial (musculocutaneous) and deep (anterior tibial) peroneal nerves. The former courses beside and supplies the peroneal muscles and supplies cutaneous innervation to the lateral and distal portion of the leg and dorsum of the foot (Fig. 105.1B). The deep peroneal nerve runs in the anterior compartment of the leg between the tibialis anterior and extensor hallucis longus muscles and tendons. It passes beneath the extensor retinaculum at the ankle and supplies most of the ankle and toes and the skin between the first and second toes.

The common peroneal nerve is particularly susceptible to compression in its superficial course around the fibula. Plaster casts and leg braces are frequent culprits, although prolonged pressure, prolonged squatting, and even habitual leg crossing have been implicated when no other explanation is patent. The syndrome includes footdrop and sensory compromise. The deep peroneal nerve can be compressed in the very rare anterior tibial syndrome. After trauma, or even excessive exercise, this compartment can become inflamed to the point at which timely surgical decompression is mandatory.

TIBIAL NERVE

The tibial nerve branches in the popliteal fossa to give off the sural nerve, which descends in the midline of the calf and passes behind the lateral malleolus to supply the skin over the lateral ankle and foot (Fig. 105.1C). The tibial nerve continues through the popliteal fossa and deep to the gastrocnemius to emerge at the medial aspect of the Achilles tendon. It then passes deep to the flexor retinaculum at the medial malleolus to enter the sole. This retinaculum forms the roof of the tarsal tunnel, which also contains the tendons of the tibialis posterior, flexor digitorum longus, and flexor hallucis longus muscles, as well as the posterior tibial artery and veins. The tibial nerve branches from the tarsal tunnel into two plantar nerves and calcaneal sensory branches. The tibial nerve supplies the flexors of the ankle and toes and provides cutaneous innervation (Fig. 105.1C).

The tibial nerve is at risk of entrapment beneath the flexor retinaculum, the tarsal tunnel syndrome. Although this syndrome is most often described after trauma, rheumatoid synovitis and focal lesions also are frequent settings (13). Paresthesias and, to a lesser extent, pain are the presenting complaints with the features previously listed. Occasionally, specific muscular atrophy can be discerned, although this is usually obscured by rheumatoid foot deformities. The distribution of paresthesias and a Tinel's sign suggest the diagnosis, which can be confirmed electrodiagnostically. The plantar and digital nerves also are subject to compression neuropathy, but specific diagnosis and differentiation from the tarsal tunnel syndrome is difficult if not elusive. Initial treatment is conservative, with systemic and local antiinflammatory agents and orthotic devices. Surgical decompression is technically demanding and reserved for the rare patient with recalcitrant symptoms or compromised muscle strength (14).

PUTATIVE CARPAL TUNNEL SYNDROME IN THE WORKPLACE

In the absence of trauma and systemic disease, most individuals have a month of neck or upper extremity morbidity every few years. Diabolical pain impedes function and assaults one's sense of invincibility. Can these regional musculoskeletal symptoms be ignored, even if they are familiar? With difficulty and with recourse to "common sense," but common sense varies temporally and geographically, and need not make "sense." To wit:

1. In the presence of pain, it is hard to imagine that nearly all regional musculoskeletal symptoms are self-limited. It can take months and the severity can be daunting, but patience is nearly always rewarded.
2. By definition, regional pain increases with use of the region that hurts, but that does not prove that the musculoskeletal use that causes the pain to worsen also caused the pain in the first place. Such thinking is inescapable; thus the vernacular tennis elbow and the like. However, it may be that these regional disorders spontaneously come and go; use makes us aware. Altering an imputable *pattern of use* can lead to palliation even if the cause is indeterminate. "Cause" is critical only if culpability must be assigned.
3. Over-the-counter potions are at-the-ready to provide relief. Prescription nonsteroidal antiinflammatory medications are ubiquitous. A multibillion dollar enterprise thrives on the diagnostic and prognostic uncertainties that are the regional musculoskeletal disorders.
4. Not only do pills and powders stand ready to help, but providers of physical and other alternative interventions also abound. This too is testimony to the empirical. *Caveat emptor: in the mind of the patient, benefits should clearly outweigh discomfort, inconvenience, stigmatization, or enforced disability.*

As difficult as it has become to cope with arm pain in modern life in general, it is even more difficult if the regional musculoskeletal symptoms interfere at all with function in the workplace (3).

Medicalization of the American Worker with Arm Pain

Individuals have three options in coping with regional musculoskeletal symptoms: rely on personal resources, seek care in the community, or turn to a "provider" in the context of the workplace. With the last choice, the individual assumes the role of claimant either for health benefits or for Worker's Compensation insurance. Workers' Compensation offers the greater largesse, but to qualify, the regional symptom must have arisen out of and in the course of employment and must be a (the) manifestation of injury. Recourse to Worker's Compensation has long seemed appropriate for low back pain (see Chapter 102), but not regional arm pain. Now there is new "common sense" in this country; tens of thousands of workers with arm pain access care under Worker's Compensation.

In the mid 1980s, the rubric "cumulative trauma disorders" was coined by the Occupational Safety and Health Administration (OSHA) and the National Institute of Occupational Safety and Health. The rationale harkens to metal fatigue; using the upper extremity in a repetitive fashion, even when performing tasks with comfortable and customary elements, will eventuate in damage. Promulgation of this hypothesis as policy has altered common sense in the work force; arm pain is now considered a consequence of task, signifies damage, requires medical intervention, and is compensable. The worker with arm pain has been instructed that anything short of immediate medical attention is a mistake. This view is scientifically insupportable: task relatedness is unproven, damage is elusive, and the empiric remedies are just that, empiric (15).

Furthermore, this algorithm holds great potential for iatrogenicity (3,16). In the absence of impressive pathoanatomy, the worker must prove persistence of symptoms to qualify for indemnification under Workers' Compensation insurance. Therein reside the seeds of a contest that encourages persistent illness; if you have to prove you are ill, it is very hard to perceive improvement, let alone to achieve healthfulness. It also is hard to maintain autonomy and perspective when considering therapeutic options. After all, if the claimant eschews an "indicated" intervention, veracity of symptoms rather than advisability for the intervention is called into question.

"Cumulative Trauma Disorders"—So-called

Nearly all these workers manifest no more than localized tenderness and pain with some motions; inflammation, dystrophy, atrophy, and unequivocal neurologic signs are exceptional. Because medical intervention pivots on diagnosis, what is the best label? Cumulative trauma disorder has no home in the clinical lexicon. Throughout the country, two diagnoses predominate: the entrapment neuropathy, carpal tunnel syndrome, or a soft tissue disorder such as "tendinitis." Neither designation is valid.

Putative Carpal Tunnel Syndrome

If one follows up 1,000 adults for 1 year, one expects one case of carpal tunnel syndrome to be diagnosed (9). Of these 1/1,000, an associated condition will be recognized in half; diabetes, RA, myxedema, and pregnancy lead the list. Thus idiopathic carpal tunnel syndrome afflicts 1/2,000 per year. There are no convincing examples of clustering or increased incidence (15,17). Therefore, most Americans who think they have carpal tunnel syndrome, or are told they have carpal tunnel syndrome, need to be disabused of this misdiagnosis.

The classic description of the clinical manifestations of carpal tunnel syndrome permeates the medical and the lay literature. This classic description has served experts well and maybe still serves some well. However, it serves primary care physicians and nurses poorly and renders patients a disservice. The traditional process of referral selected the patients that came to be so described. What happens if the same symptoms and signs are sought for in a far less selected population (18)? The answer is daunting. Assume that ten of 100 workers who report arm symptoms actually have carpal tunnel syndrome. How distinctive are these from the 90 with arm pain for whom the diagnosis of carpal tunnel syndrome is not justifiable? They can not be distinguished by any aspect of history or of physical examination; both groups are as likely to have Tinel's sign, Phalen's sign, or hypesthesia! We are all being led astray by the textbook descriptions.

How can it be determined whether the ten in the example actually have carpal tunnel syndrome? For most studies, authors rely on electrodiagnostic tests. Such a "gold standard" is useful for epidemiologic studies, but leaves much to be desired as a clinical tool. First, nerve conduction studies are technically demanding, uncomfortable, and expensive. Vasoconstriction from cold or anxiety will prolong conduction and must be avoided. Normal values must be established for each laboratory on populations appropriate to the work force being studied. That is critical because we know that "normal" for women, particularly the obese, the elderly, and even those with "square" wrists, is prolonged (5). It is also important to realize that "normal" is designed to encompass some 95% of the normal population; 5% of normal subjects are beyond the normal range. Therefore, one must be circumspect in interpreting mild conduction delays. Expert electrodiagnosticians are aware of these confounders and we hope are not blinded by zeal for their procedure. Nonetheless, physicians must bear responsibility for the interpretation of such studies.

From the earlier discussions, one might predict that finding people in the community that have symptomatic carpal tunnel syndrome but have not chosen to be patients is an exercise in futility. That prediction has been borne out in a recent British community-based survey of the point prevalence of hand symptoms and their correlation with median conductivity (19,20). The point prevalence of abnormal nerve conductions varied between 7% and 16% depending on how "abnormal" was defined. Regardless, the vast majority of people with abnormal tests had no symptoms. Of those with classic symptoms of carpal tunnel syndrome, only 18% had abnormal nerve conductions. Yes, this is circular reasoning.

So what is the solution? Vigilance regarding carpal tunnel syndrome has become a national policy, yet symptoms and signs are nonspecific and the gold standard is patently limited. Furthermore, mislabeling arm pain as carpal tunnel syndrome places the patient at risk for unnecessary, costly, and often damaging diagnostic and therapeutic interventions. Mislabeling arm pain as carpal tunnel syndrome and ascribing the disorder to hand use at work is a sophism that portends iatrogenicity (21). In my view, there is no choice but to err on the side of reassurance, knowing that a rare case of early carpal tunnel syndrome might be missed, but taking solace in the fact that such an oversight places the patient at little risk. At most, night splints and work modification should be offered as options, not mandates, to supplement a reassuring explanation. These patients should be followed up expectantly for thenar atrophy. Unbridled surgery cannot be justified to spare the occasional patient in whom atrophy will develop, and there is little evidence that atrophy is "too late" for surgical intervention.

There is no doubt that people, many of whom are workers, are increasingly likely to turn to physicians for assistance with regional musculoskeletal symptoms of the upper extremity, and there is no reason to doubt the veracity of these individuals when they describe their experience. But the treatment act needs to be informed by a compelling literature that decries both the application of diagnostic labels that are merely putative and the invalidated assignment of pathogenesis to use at work (22,23). The treatment act should be informed by a rich and growing literature that suggests that physical demands at work, or at home, are far less likely to render regional disorders of the upper extremity intolerable than is the psychosocial context in which the symptoms are experienced. The arm hurts, but the pain is rendered far less tolerable when coping is compromised by organizational, interpersonal, and financial confounders (24).

There is every reason to assert that these patients/claimants and society at large would be better served by empathetic physicians who understand the potential for disability insurance schemes and institutionalized medicine to do harm (3).

REFERENCES

1. Gelberman RH, ed. *Operative nerve repair and reconstruction.* Vols I and II. Philadelphia: JB Lippincott, 1991:1–1625.
2. Frymoyer JW, Ducker TB, Hadler NM, et al. eds. *The adult spine:* principles and practice. 2nd ed. Vols I and II. Philadelphia: Lippincott-Raven Press, 1997:1–2443.
3. Hadler NM. *Occupational musculoskeletal disorders.* 2nd ed. Philadelphia: Lippincott Williams & Wilkins, 1999:1–433.
4. Committee Report. Practice parameters for electrodiagnostic studies in carpal tunnel syndrome. *Muscle Nerve* 1993;16: 1390–1414.
5. Radecki P. Variability in the median and ulnar nerve latencies: implications for diagnosing entrapment. *J Occup Environ Med* 1995;37:1293–1299.
6. Kuhlman KA, Hennessey WJ. Sensitivity and specificity of carpal tunnel syndrome signs. *Am J Phys Med Rehabil* 1997;76: 451–457.
7. Heller L, Ring H, Costeff H, Solzi P. Evaluation of Tinel's and Phalen's signs in the diagnosis of the carpal tunnel syndrome. *Eur Neurol* 1986;25:40–42.
8. Katz JN, Larson MG, Sabra A, et al. The carpal tunnel syndrome: diagnostic utility of the history and physical examination findings. *Ann Intern Med* 1990;112:321–327.
9. Stevens JC, Sun S, Beard CM, et al. Carpal tunnel syndrome in Rochester, Minnesota, 1961-1980. *Neurology* 1988;38:134–138.
10. Macnicol MF, Thompson WJ. Idiopathic meralgia paresthetica. *Clin Orthop* 1990;254:270–274.
11. Jankiewicz JJ, Hennrikus WL, Houkom JA. The appearance of the pyriformis muscle syndrome in computed tomography and magnetic resonance imaging: a case report and review of the literature. *Clin Orthop* 1991;262;205–209.
12. Crisci C, Baker MK, Wood WJ, et al. Trochanteric sciatic neuropathy. *Neurology* 1989;39:1539–1541.
13. Erickson SJ, Quinn SF, Kneeland JB, et al. MR imaging of the tarsal tunnel and related spaces: normal and abnormal findings with anatomic correlation. *AJR Am J Roentgenol* 1990;155: 323–328.
14. Mackinnan SE, Dellon AL. Homologies between the tarsal and carpal tunnels: implications for treatment of the tarsal tunnel syndrome. *Contemp Orthop* 1987;14:75–84.
15. Hadler NM. Repetitive upper-extremity motions in the workplace are not hazardous. *J Hand Surg Am* 1997;22:19–29.
16. Hadler NM. Arm pain in the workplace: a small area analysis. *J Occup Med* 1992;34:113–119.
17. Hadler NM. A keyboard for "Daubert." *J Occup Environ Med* 1996;21:469–476.
18. Hadler NM. Carpal tunnel syndrome: diagnostic conundrum. *J Rheumatol* 1997;24:417–419.
19. Ferry S, Pritchard T, Keenan J, et al. Estimating the prevalence of delayed median nerve conduction in the general population. *Br J Rheumatol* 1998;37:630–635.
20. Ferry S, Silman AJ, Pritchard T, et al. The association between different patterns of hand symptoms and objective evidence of median nerve compression. *Arthritis Rheum* 1998;41:720–724.
21. Carmona L, Faucett J, Blanc PD, et al. Predictors of rate of return to work after surgery for carpal tunnel syndrome. *Arthritis Care Res* 1998;11:298–305.
22. Vender MI, Kasdan ML, Truppa KL. Upper extremity disorders: a literature review to determine work-relatedness. *J Hand Surg Am* 1995;20:534–541.
23. Barton NJ, Hooper G, Noble J, et al. Occupational causes of disorders in the upper limb. *Br Med J* 1992;304:309–311.
24. Hadler NM. Coping with arm pain in the workplace. *Clin Orthop* 1998;351:57–62.

106

TUMORS OF JOINTS AND RELATED STRUCTURES

JUAN J. CANOSO

Every practicing rheumatologist is bound to encounter, sooner or later, benign or malignant tumors that lie in, or adjacent to, articular tissues. The challenge is to distinguish these lesions from the overwhelmingly more common inflammatory or degenerative diseases. Prototypic situations exist in which knowledge of pathology, proficiency in physical examination, and expertise in the use of imaging techniques may lead to early diagnosis. A few examples follow:

1. A chronically swollen joint in a patient with normal laboratory tests including erythrocyte sedimentation rate (ESR) and C-reactive protein (CRP): Although this clinical presentation suggests the late effects of mechanical damage, psoriatic arthritis, thorn synovitis, and rarely chronic infection, it is also characteristic of pigmented villonodular synovitis, synovial chondromatosis, synovial hemangiomas, and lipoma arborescens.
2. Popliteal "cysts" that do not soften with knee flexion: The differential diagnosis here includes tense-packed cysts (knee disease should be apparent in these patients), ganglia, juxtaarticular myxomas, popliteal artery aneurysms, popliteal artery wall cysts, and, unfortunately, sarcomas.
3. Eccentric swellings that do not conform to the anatomic location of bursal, tenosynovial, or meniscal structures: These are a red flag, because a sarcomatous growth may be present. Two examples: (a) A young man was referred with a refractory tennis elbow. Surprisingly, full passive elbow extension could not be achieved, and a questionable bulge was palpable between the olecranon process and the lateral epicondyle. The eventual diagnosis was clear cell sarcoma. (b) A middle-age man presented with a slow-growing swelling in his hand; a fleshy mass was palpable deep in the first interosseal space. An initial consideration had been a proliferative type of flexor tenosynovitis. A sarcomatous growth was suspected, however. Pulmonary metastases were present. The diagnosis was synovial sarcoma.
4. Knee hemarthrosis in an older patient in the absence of trauma, anticoagulation, or crystals in the synovial fluid: The possibility of metastatic tumor synovitis should be considered in this patient. In a young adult or a child, especially if the hemarthrosis is recurrent, a synovial hemangioma should be suspected.
5. A finger lump: In addition to a ganglion, one must consider nodular pigmented synovitis and a fibroma of the tendon sheath. A 50-year-old man noted the slow growth of a lump in the palmar aspect of the right fifth digit. Flexion was limited by the bulk of the lesion. Pigmented nodular synovitis was suspected, and the diagnosis was confirmed at surgery. There was no recurrence.
6. An expanding nodule attached to fascia or tendon: Clear cell sarcoma and epithelioid sarcoma should be considered in the differential diagnosis.

Fortunately, the diagnosis of these lesions has been facilitated by techniques such as arthroscopy, computed tomography (CT), and especially magnetic resonance imaging (MRI).

BENIGN TUMORAL CONDITIONS

Benign tumoral conditions compose a heterogeneous group of disorders of joints, bursae, and tendon sheaths. They include pigmented villonodular synovitis (PVS), which is a chronic inflammatory lesion of unknown origin, synovial chondromatosis and other cartilaginous metaplasias of the subsynovial tissue, vascular malformations, fatty growths, fibromas, ganglia, and juxtaarticular myxomas.

Pigmented Villonodular Synovitis

The term *pigmented villonodular synovitis* denotes a group of interrelated tumorous disorders that involve the lining of joints, bursae, and tendon sheaths (1–9). These lesions, often locally aggressive but only exceptionally metastatic, consist of villous or nodular growths covered by a thin layer of synovial lining cells. The connective tissue stroma

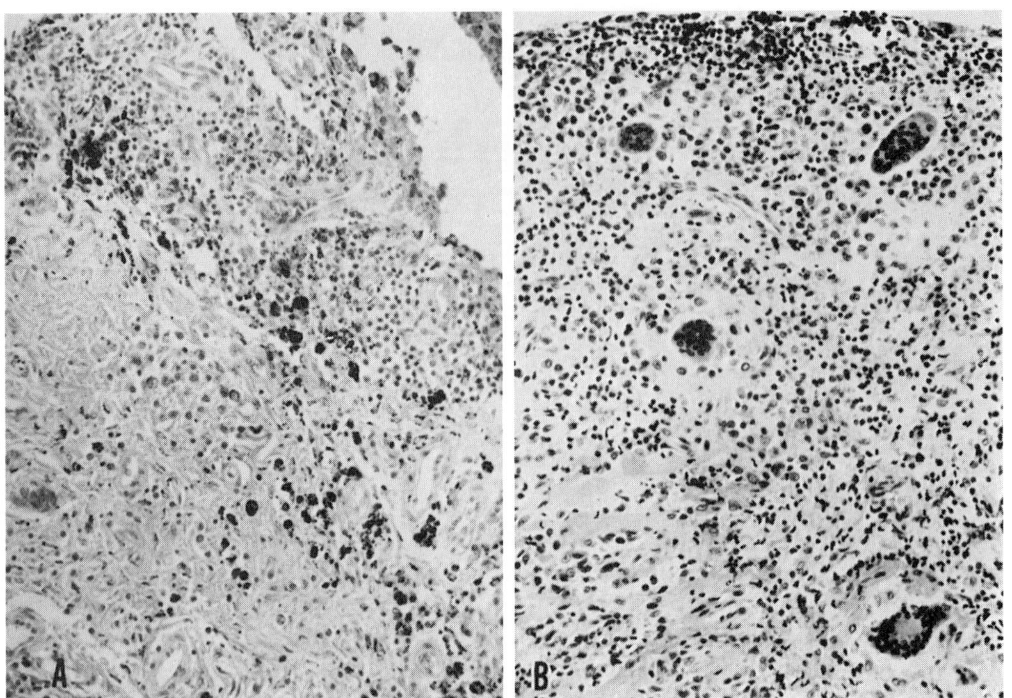

FIGURE 106.1. Circumscribed nodular synovitis; photomicrographs of a nodular lesion. **A:** Large deposits of hemosiderin pigment in richly cellular connective tissue stroma. **B:** Multinucleated giant cells amid a dense infiltrate of small round cells and large cells with pale, spindle-shaped nuclei (×175).

contains a heterogeneous, variably dense collection of cells, collagen bundles, and blood vessels. The cellular infiltrate consists of polyhedral, histiocytic-like cells; lipid-laden cells appearing as foam cells on routine histologic preparations; hemosiderin-laden cells; and multinucleated giant cells (Fig. 106.1). Electron-microscopic studies of both villous and nodular forms usually have revealed a predominance of cells resembling fibroblasts (synovial type-B cells) and a lesser number of cells resembling both macrophages (synovial type-A cells) and intermediate cells, consistent with derivation from normal synovium (10–13) (see Chapter 12). The iron tends to be deposited within lysosomal bodies (siderosomes) in deep type-B cells. Early lesions are highly vascular; old lesions are less vascular, exhibit more fibrosis and hyalinization, and may contain cholesterol crystals (1,14). The color of the lesion, ranging from yellow to dark brown, depends on the proportion of lipids and hemosiderin. In several cases involving the soft tissues of the hand (15) or the temporomandibular joint, PVS has coexisted with synovial chondromatosis (16). Bony invasion may result from direct penetration through vascular foramina and the chondro-osseous junction at the articular margin. The invading tissue carries its own blood supply, so there appears to be no attachment of the diseased tissue to the walls of the invasion cavity (17). There are several explanations for the erosive nature of PVS. On the one hand, there is pressure erosion (18). Also, collagenase and stromelysin produced by cells in the synovial lining and deep mononuclear infiltrates may play a major role in inducing osteolysis and formation of bone cysts (19). Finally, giant cells in PVS express features of osteoclasts and, following isolation, are able to form lacunar resorption pits on bone slices in short-term culture (20,21).

Clinical Findings

Involvement of the affected joint, tendon sheath, or bursa may be either diffuse or localized. The condition is typically monarticular and lacks systemic symptoms or findings. Rarely, two or more joints are affected (22–25). Several cases have been observed in association with rheumatoid arthritis (RA) (5,6,18,23,26) or psoriatic arthritis (27). It is unclear whether this is a true association or a detection bias. The ESR is usually normal (4,5,28), except in cases associated with RA or other systemic diseases.

Pigmented villonodular synovitis is classified according to location (articular, tenosynovial, or bursal) and lesional type (diffuse or nodular). These types may be difficult to distinguish in some cases. Confusion also occurs because some experts diagnose tenosynovial giant cell tumor, diffuse type, when a large extraarticular mass is present, with or without intraarticular involvement or actual tendon sheath involvement (29,30).

Articular, Diffuse

This condition occurs chiefly in young adults, equally in both sexes (3–5). The joint usually affected is the knee; much less commonly involved are the hip, ankle, shoulder, elbow, carpal joints, other joints of the hand, wrist, and tarsal joints. Rare locations include the temporomandibular joint (12,13,31,32) and the vertebral facet joint (33). The predominant symptom is pain, which may be mild and intermittent for a long period, and the principal sign is gradual swelling of the joint that is due to synovial proliferation and effusion. In the knee, focal masses are usually palpable, the joint is in slight flexion (25), and a popliteal cyst often develops (12,34). The joint fluid is usually sanguineous or dark brown, not viscous, and does not usually clot. One report noted an average of 26% neutrophils. Red blood cell counts have varied from 43,000 to 1,780,000/mm^3. Mucin clot tests varied from fair to good (35). The glucose content was normal. Intra- and extracellular lipid droplets producing Maltese crosses on polarizing microscopy have been reported (36). The frequency of this finding is unknown.

Radiographic examination shows capsular distention from increased joint fluid and sometimes lobulation and thickening of the synovial tissues. Lack of osteopenia, absence of heterotopic calcification, and mild spur formation are characteristic. Bony erosions in PVS occur as subchondral or paraarticular cysts, each surrounded by a well-defined sclerotic line. These may be multilocular and may involve both sides of the joint (Fig. 106.2). The differential diagnosis (37) of cystic lesions affecting both sides of a joint includes osteoarthritis, RA, hemophilia, gout, and calcium pyrophosphate dihydrate (CPPD) crystal deposition disease. Intraosseous ganglia, chondroblastoma, and metastatic carcinoma will generally affect only one side of the joint. In capacious joints such as the knee, erosions are uncommon (25% of cases), and when they occur, usually involve the patella (23). In tighter joints, such as the hip (90% of cases), elbow, and shoulder, as well as on occasion the wrist, finger, and temporomandibular joint, cyst formation is pronounced and one may see considerable concentric joint space narrowing (28,38). Many PVS lesions have been erroneously considered malignant, based on the extent of bone destruction (39–42). Although the findings are not pathognomonic, MRI is very useful in the diagnosis of PVS. Many previously misdiagnosed cases are being correctly identified as MRI is used in the evaluation of patients with protracted monarticular disease. MRI findings in PVS include synovial proliferation with focal decreases of signal intensity in both T1- and T2-weighted pulse sequences due to the paramagnetic effect of hemosiderin, joint effusion, and a full spectrum of articular, bursal, and osseous involvement (34,43,44). A similar focal decrease in signal intensity may occur as a result of blood flow and calcification. In isolation, MRI findings are insufficient to distinguish PVS from other forms of hemosideric synovitis such as chronic trauma, hemophilia, and some cases of RA. These and other conditions must be excluded on clinical, laboratory, and roentgenographic grounds. *A diagnosis of PVS requires demonstration of characteristic pathologic changes on tissue obtained arthroscopically or by open biopsy, plus the exclusion of mycobacterial and fungal infection* by the use of appropriate tissue stains and cultures.

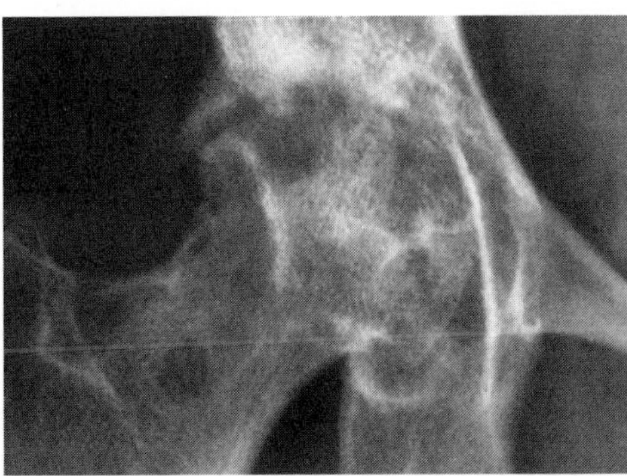

FIGURE 106.2. Cartilage narrowing and cystic erosive changes in the acetabulum and femoral head and neck from pigmented villonodular synovitis.

Articular, Circumscribed (Nodular)

Localized involvement of the synovium occurs less frequently than the diffuse form of the disease, with a ratio of 1:4 (5,45,46). Again, the knee is most commonly affected, and the patient is usually an adult with symptoms for many months or years. Symptoms are often episodic and consist of pain, swelling, locking, and "giving way" of the joint, mimicking a meniscal lesion (8,9). Acute symptoms may follow torsion and infarction of tissue (47). Small-to-moderate effusions and occasionally limited range of motion are found. The synovial fluid is less likely to be sanguineous. Roentgenograms usually show no abnormalities. The true nature of the process is not suspected until one or more nodular growths are found on an MRI study, arthroscopy, or at operation.

Tenosynovial, Circumscribed (Nodular)

This type constitutes by far the most common form of this disorder. It is ten times more common than circumscribed nodular synovitis (5,21). It is the second most common soft tissue tumor of the hand, outnumbered only by ganglia (48). The majority of patients are mature adults. Women are affected more often than men and the incidence is higher in the dominant hand. The fingers are most frequently involved, particularly the index or middle, on the volar (60%), dorsal, or lateral aspect where a firm, slow-growing, painless nodular mass develops. Less often, the lesion is found near a metacarpophalangeal joint, wrist, ankle, or toe. Radiographic examination shows only a soft tissue mass in 50% of cases, extensive pressure erosion of adjacent bone in larger lesions, or normal findings (49).

The origin of lesions arising in sites devoid of tendon sheaths, such as the lateral or dorsal aspect of fingers, is controversial. The differential diagnosis includes ganglia, foreign body granulomas, tendinous xanthomas, necrobiotic granulomas, and fibromas of the tendon sheath (7).

Tenosynovial, Diffuse

Diffuse involvement of tendon sheaths and other soft tissues may occur with or without evidence of intraarticular disease. Such lesions become quite large, pursue an aggressive course, and are locally destructive, resulting in erosion of neighboring bone (1,29,50–52).

Bursal

This uncommon lesion, usually diffuse, may be found in a deep bursa such as the subacromial (53), iliopsoas (54), gastrocnemius-semimembranosus with (12,34) or without (1) concomitant disease in the knee joint, suprapatellar (in unusual cases in which this bursa is separate from the joint) (55), anserine (1,56), and an unspecified ankle region bursa (1). No instances have been described involving subcutaneous bursae.

Pathogenesis

Whether PVS represents a true neoplasm of synovial tissue, a proliferative reaction to recurrent hemarthrosis, or an inflammatory reaction to an as yet unidentified microbial agent is not clear. The nodular growth pattern, the relative lack of inflammatory cells, the frequent erosion of adjacent bone by these lesions, and their recurrence after synovectomy have been thought to favor the theory of a neoplasm. Based on karyotypic abnormalities, in particular trisomy of chromosomes 5 and/or 7 in diffuse forms and rearrangement of the short arm of chromosome 1 in over 50% of both the localized and the diffuse forms, a neoplastic origin of PVS has been suggested (51,57). Indeed, there are a few cases reported in which late metastatic disease occurred in otherwise routine cases of PVS (30).

Similarities in pathology between PVS, hemophilia, and intraarticular hemangioma have led many to consider that the lesion might result from recurrent hemarthrosis (58). In support of this view, changes resembling those of the human disease have been experimentally produced in dogs and in rhesus monkeys by repeated intraarticular injection of blood and colloidal iron (59,60). Moreover, multiple lesions in children have been associated with cutaneous or synovial hemangiomas (61,62), suggesting a pathogenetic role for recurrent hemarthrosis. No evidence of vascular malformation, however, exists in most instances of PVS, and giant cells and foam cells do not occur in hemosideric synovitis induced experimentally (60,63) or in hemophilic joints (64). A related hypothesis is that recurrent lipohemarthrosis could explain the deposition of both hemosiderin and lipids. This view is supported by the finding that, in over 50% of patients, acute or repetitive local trauma preceded the appearance of the lesion (5). In contrast to hemophilic synovitis, in which the siderosomes occur in type-A cells and are surrounded by damaged organelles, iron deposits are found in type-B cells in PVS, without evidence of intracellular damage (65).

Finally, a microbial cause of the lesion has been sought but not found. Cultures have been routinely negative. There is an obvious need to reinvestigate a possible microbial cause with newer molecular techniques, using synovial fluid or tissue samples. Although the possibility remains that the lesion may result from more than one causative mechanism (12), the pendulum of opinion is currently moving toward a neoplastic origin of PVS.

Treatment

Although PVS is considered to be a benign lesion, usually confined to a single joint or soft tissue structure, the results of surgical treatment are often disappointing. Resection of nodular synovitis of tendon sheaths has a recurrence rate of approximately 20%, presumably owing to incomplete removal of the lesion. A follow-up study of 11 patients with diffuse PVS affecting the knee, treated with total knee arthroplasty, documented recurrence in only two patients at an average follow-up of 10.3 years (66). A similar rate of recurrence was seen in a comparable series of patients who had arthroscopic total synovectomy (67–69). In the hip, complete synovectomy (achieved by dislocating the joint) may be effective in early lesions in which the joint space is preserved and no erosions are present (70). Because bone erosion is present in most cases, however, the usual treatment consists of total hip replacement. The treatment of recurrent PVS is unsatisfactory. Arthroscopic surgical procedures (8,67–69) have the advantage of low morbidity, and they can be repeated easily if necessary. Another approach is the use of total joint replacement or arthrodesis, if the initial failed procedure was a synovectomy. Finally, intraarticular administration of the radioisotope yttrium-90 silicate, which may be effective in early cases as an alternative to synovectomy, had disappointing results in patients with failed synovectomy (71–73). Despite residual or recurrent disease in some cases, functional results of treatment of PVS are good (3,66,67).

Synovial Chondromatosis

Synovial chondromatosis is characterized by multiple cartilaginous nodules within the joint space. A similar disorder may occur in the joint capsule, tendon sheath, bursa, or paraarticular connective tissue (2,74–79). The nodules may be buried in the synovial membrane (Fig. 106.3), may be pedunculated, or may lie free within the synovial cavity (80-82). These cartilage nodules may calcify or even ossify,

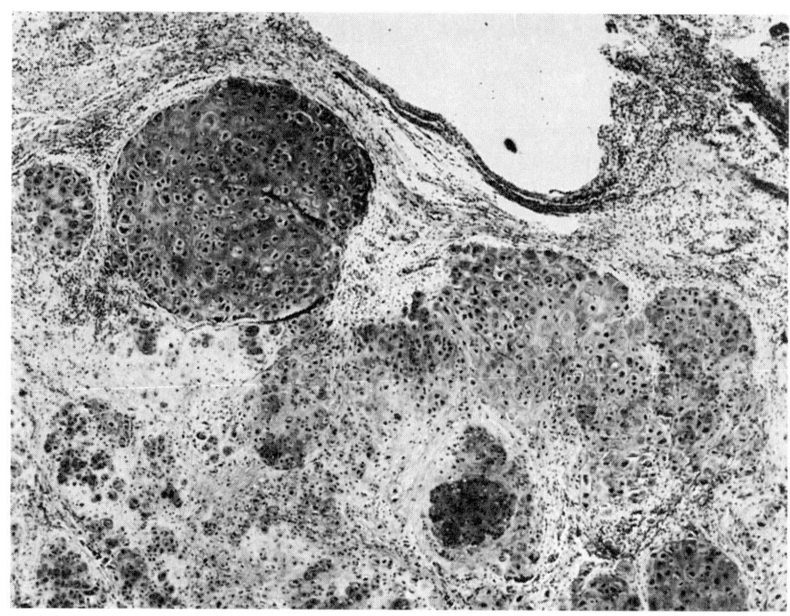

FIGURE 106.3. Synovial chondromatosis; photomicrograph of synovium showing several small islands of cellular cartilage lying just beneath the surface of the membrane (×25).

leading to the term *osteochondromatosis.* The origin of the disorder is unknown. The lesion undergoes malignant change in up to 5% of cases (79,83).

Synovial chondromatosis occurs most often as a monarticular disturbance in young or middle-aged adults and is about as common in men as in women. Pediatric cases are rare (84,85). There is a report of familial chondromatosis (86) in which calcium CPPD crystal deposition disease was not excluded as a predisposing factor.

Clinical Findings

Articular

The joint most frequently involved is the knee, followed by hip, elbow, ankle, shoulder, and wrist (74,75,78,79). Osteochondromatosis of the temporomandibular joint, sometimes in association with PVS (15,16), has also been reported (16,87,88). In uncommon cases of multiple joint involvement, both knees or both hips are usually affected (89).

Patients may have pain, swelling, and limited joint motion, or they may be asymptomatic, with the lesion discovered by accident. Even in patients with free intracavitary nodules, locking of the joint is uncommon (76,77). Examination often reveals the presence of loose bodies and increased amounts of normal synovial fluid. Compression neuropathies may occur (90).

The diagnosis, usually established by radiographic examination, discloses multiple stippled calcifications within the confines of the joint capsule in approximately 90% of patients (Fig. 106.4). Single, large lesions reminiscent of chondrosarcoma or parosteal osteosarcoma may occur (91). Pressure erosions are frequent, particularly in the femoral neck and proximal humerus, and may lead to a pathologic fracture (89,92). The joint otherwise appears normal.

The differential diagnosis of synovial chondromatosis includes several other conditions associated with loose joint bodies, such as severe osteoarthritis with intraarticular osteophytic fragments, osteochondritis dissecans, neuropathic arthropathy, and the Milwaukee shoulder (93). Synovial calcification, mimicking osteochondromatosis, can also occur in CPPD crystal deposition disease (94).

Extraarticular

Synovial chondromatosis may occur in tendon sheaths (95–97) and bursae such as the ischial (98), iliopsoas (76,91), anserine (76), gastrocnemius-semimembranosus (75,76,99), an adventitious deep bursa (100), retrocalcaneal (101), and prepatellar (102) in patients with or without concurrent articular disease. Moreover, chondromatosis may involve the soft tissue of the extremities without an apparent connection with synovial structures (97).

Pathogenesis

Gross examination of the affected joint reveals variably large and compact clusters of flat or pedunculated cartilaginous nodules protruding from the thickened synovial membrane, as well as loose bodies within the joint cavity. Microscopic study reveals cartilaginous masses with chondrocytes arranged in small clusters within the masses, separated into lobules by acellular septa (Fig. 106.3). Subtle transition between subsynovial fibrocytes and fully developed chondrocytes has been shown by electron microscopy (103). Early calcification occurs in the perilacunar matrix. In extensively calcified masses, a fatty marrow is frequently found in the center. Pedunculated or free bodies exhibit similar findings.

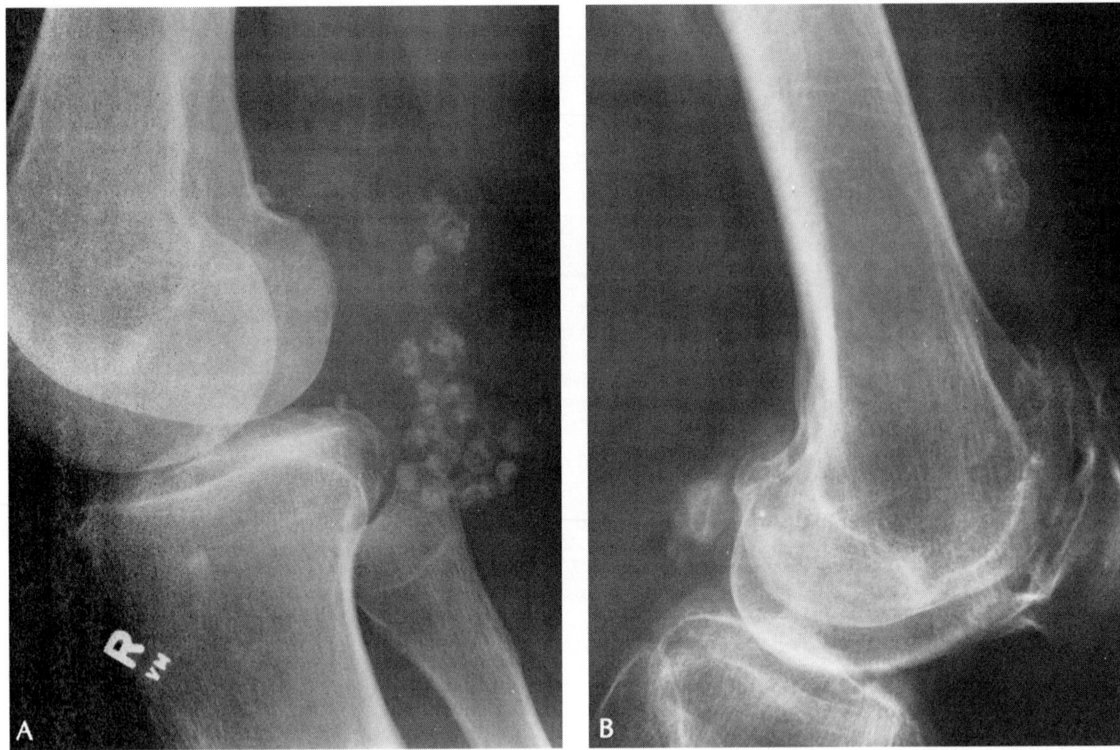

FIGURE 106.4. A: Primary synovial osteochondromatosis with multiple loose bodies extruded into a Baker's cyst. **B:** Advanced degenerative joint disease with effusion and secondary osteochondromatosis.

The differentiation from chondrosarcoma may be difficult. In malignancy, the cloning pattern of chondrocytes, which are arranged in sheaths, is lost; there are myxoid changes in the matrix and crowding of cells with spindling of the nuclei at the periphery. Necrosis may be present, and bone erosion is not by pressure but by permeation with filling of marrow spaces (83).

Detailed analysis of histologic findings in loose bodies and the synovial membrane has permitted a reconstruction of the natural history of the disease (80). At first, cartilage metaplasia occurs in the subsynovial tissue in a multifocal fashion (phase I). In a later stage, some of the growing nodules become pedunculated and are finally released as loose joint bodies, whereas others remain buried in the membrane (phase II). Finally, the synovial membrane resumes its normal morphologic features, probably by resorption of residual foci of cartilaginous metaplasia, while the loose bodies undergo further remodeling (phase III). Calcification and ossification of the nodules can occur either before or after their release into the joint cavity. It is clear now that there are chondroprogenitor cells in synovial tissue (104). Histologically, the cartilage in synovial chondromatosis is usually cellular with binucleate forms, suggesting that the disease is not merely a metaplasia, but implies a proliferative component. An absence of mitotic figures and the lack of the proliferating nuclear antigen Ki-67 in cartilaginous nodules of synovial chondromatosis are in keeping with a metaplastic, rather than proliferative, origin of the condition. However, image cytometry suggests a proliferative process, in at least some of the cases of synovial chondromatosis. Thus, synovial chondromatosis appears to occupy an intermediate point between benign enchondromas and malignant chondrosarcomas (105).

Treatment

When synovial chondromatosis is suspected, arthroscopy or arthrotomy should be undertaken to remove the loose bodies, to determine the condition of the synovial membrane and remove the involved tissue, and to assess the integrity of the articular cartilage (78,106). Open synovectomy, however, involves major operative trauma and is often followed by considerable stiffness that may require prolonged physiotherapy or even manipulation under anesthesia. As arthroscopic experience has accrued (99,107), it has become evident that the results of arthroscopic surgery are at least equal to surgical synovectomy, but with far less morbidity. Although some authors have advocated for the removal of loose bodies only, the additional removal of any abnormal synovial tissue appears prudent. Arthroscopic surgery is emerging as the treatment of choice for any stage of the disease (99). More than one arthroscopic procedure may be needed. Provided that no significant osteoarthritis is present, an asymptomatic joint can be expected in almost all patients.

Intracapsular, Extrasynovial Chondroma

Intracapsular, extrasynovial chondroma is an unusual lesion that occurs most frequently in the knee (46,77,108,109). The patient has discomfort and a firm mass distal to the patella and deep to the patellar tendon. Lateral radiographs reveal a calcified lesion within the infrapatellar fat pad. Treatment is surgical excision.

Hemangioma

Joint and tendon sheath hemangiomas represent an unusual location of the most common type of benign soft tissue tumors in infancy and childhood (7,63,110,111). Synovial hemangiomas occur most often in adolescents or in young adults, many of whom have had symptoms since childhood; this characteristic suggests that the lesion may represent a congenital vascular malformation. The knee joint is most commonly affected (60%), followed by the elbow (30%) (2,63,112). The lesion, which may grow as a pedunculated nodule or as a diffuse process, in most cases corresponds histologically to a cavernous (massively engorged capillary vessels) hemangioma. Other histologic types include lobular capillary hemangiomas in which "feeder vessels" can be identified, arteriovenous hemangiomas formed by thick-walled arterial and venous vessels, and, rarely, venous hemangiomas (63). Nodular lesions often originate in the infrapatellar fat pad (46,113). The usual history is one of recurrent pain and swelling. Documentation of hemarthrosis is uncommon, probably reflecting incomplete ascertainment. Chronic limb pain (113) and bland, nonhemorrhagic effusions may also occur. In some cases, a doughy mass decreases in size with compression or elevation of the limb. There is no association with cutaneous hemangiomas.

When marked arteriovenous shunting is present, the leg may be hypertrophic, including increased length, and a high cardiac output state may be present. The *Klippel-Trenaunay syndrome* is characterized by port-wine cutaneous angiomatous nevi, varicose veins, and an hypertrophic leg (114). In the *Parkes Weber syndrome*, the same findings are associated with arteriovenous fistulas. Large vascular tumors may be complicated by thrombocytopenia and a consumption coagulopathy known as the *Kasabach-Merritt syndrome* (115,116). In this condition, the thrombocytopenia appears to be caused by platelet trapping by the abnormal endothelium of the tumor (116).

Radiographic examination is usually normal in nodular angiomas. Phleboliths, often present in larger angiomas, are helpful in the differential diagnosis of articular masses and paraarticular masses with muscle involvement (112,117). Recurrent hemangiomatous bleeding may lead to enlarged epiphyses, joint-space narrowing, and enlargement of the intercondylar notch resembling hemophilic arthropathy (118). MRI findings include high signal intensity in both T1- and T2-pulse sequences, a striated-septal configuration, and fluid-fluid levels (117,119). In patients with a large limb and varicosities, when a doughy compressible mass is present, or if physical examination reveals a bruit, arteriography is extremely helpful to reveal the nature, anatomic distribution, and feeding vessels of the lesion (117). Intramuscular lesions should be differentiated from alveolar soft-part sarcoma, a highly vascularized sarcoma that may be pulsatile and has angiographic and MRI findings resembling hemangioma (120,121). When hemangioma is suspected in a patient with recurrent hemarthrosis, arthroscopy without the use of a tourniquet usually reveals the nature of the lesion. It may be difficult macroscopically to distinguish synovial hemangiomas with heavy hemosiderin deposits from PVS. Histologically, however, sheet-like histiocytic infiltrates and giant cells, which are routine findings in PVS, are absent in hemangioma. Several reports have documented the concurrence of the two lesions (61,62).

Surgical excision, usually simple and effective in patients with synovial hemangioma, is often unsatisfactory in patients with extensive angiomatosis. In these cases, parts of the lesion may be missed, or the process may be so extensive as to render full resection unrealistic. Arteriography followed by embolotherapy should be considered in these patients (63).

Hemangiomas may also occur in tendon sheaths, involving both the tendon itself and the surrounding structures. A soft compressive swelling, which decreases when the limb is elevated and increases when a tourniquet is placed proximal to the mass, is usually noted. Radiographic examination frequently reveals many phleboliths. In contrast with synovial hemangiomas, the hand, forearm, and ankle are the sites favored by this lesion, which is treated by surgical excision (63).

Fat Tumors

Lipomas, tumors composed of mature fat, occur rarely in joints and tendon sheaths. Articular lipomas have been found predominantly in the knee joint in relation to the subsynovial fat on either side of the patellar ligament or the anterior surface of the femur (2). Tendon sheath lipomas may occur in the hand, wrist, feet, and ankles (122). Extensor tendons are affected more often than flexor tendons, but involvement may be bilateral.

Additional examples of lipomatous growths include synovial hyperplasia (including subsynovial fat) seen near affected articular surfaces in osteoarthritis (123,124), called *lipoma arborescens* and *Hoffa's disease*. Lipoma arborescens (2,123–127) is a rare condition of unknown origin in which villous proliferation involves the entire synovial lining of a joint, most prominently in cases affecting the knee in the suprapatellar pouch. Each villus consists of mature stromal fat lined by flattened synovium. Lipoma arborescens occurs predominantly in males. It is usually found in the knee and is bilateral in approximately 20% of cases. Rarely, it involves the wrist, hip, or occurs in multiple joints. If osteoarthritis coexists, it is usually mild, suggesting a fortuitous association. In a typical case, a knee has been swollen for years with episodic inflammation after trauma. Laboratory studies are normal including the ESR. The diagnosis may be suggested by a lobulated, low-density mass seen in the suprapatellar pouch on lateral roentgenograms of the knee. MRI findings include a villous mass with a high signal similar to that of fat on T1-weighted and T2-weighted images. The lesion may appear as multiple villous lipomatous synovial proliferations, isolated frond-like subsynovial fat, or as a mixed pattern. Cases associated with trauma or chronic inflammatory conditions have a multiple villous pattern or a mixed pattern (125). Synovectomy is curative. The term *Hoffa's disease* (128) designates traumatic inflammation of the infrapatellar fat pad. Patients are in pain, and the usual finding is swelling in the infrapatellar region, deep to the patellar tendon. The differential diagnosis includes pretendinous bursitis, deep infrapatellar bursitis, and intracapsular, extrasynovial chondroma (46).

Fibroma

Intraarticular fibroma is rare (129), but fibroma of a tendon sheath is frequent (7,130,131). The great majority of fibromas occurs in the fingers, hand, and wrist, and consists of a firm, lobulated, painless nodule, usually measuring 1 to 2 cm in diameter, firmly attached to tendon or tendon sheath. Flexion may be limited. Carpal tunnel syndrome is a rare manifestation of the condition (132). The nodules, which consist of myofibroblasts, fibroblasts, and dense collagen, are frequently divided by narrow clefts. The lesion is benign, but recurrences have been noted in 24% of cases after local excision.

Juxtaarticular Myxoma

These tumors usually occur in the vicinity of the knee. Rarely, the acromioclavicular and other joints may be involved (133). A history of trauma and findings of meniscal degeneration and osteoarthritis are often present. This lesion, which predominantly involves the subcutaneous tissue, may impinge on the joint capsule or extend to neighboring bursae. Growth occurs over years, but sudden enlargement may bring the patient for evaluation. A malignant lesion may be suspected. On gross pathology, the mass is mucoid or myxoid and often has cystic spaces. Histologically, the cellular component consists of fibroblast-like cells in an abundant glycosaminoglycan matrix (Fig. 106.5). There is a resemblance to intramuscular myxomas (which tend to involve large muscles, and ganglion cysts), which occur predominantly around the wrist. In contrast to the latter, a synovial connection does not occur in juxtaarticular myxoma. Recommended treatment includes excision of the mass and meniscectomy if the adjacent meniscus is degenerated. Recurrences are frequent. They also are treated conservatively.

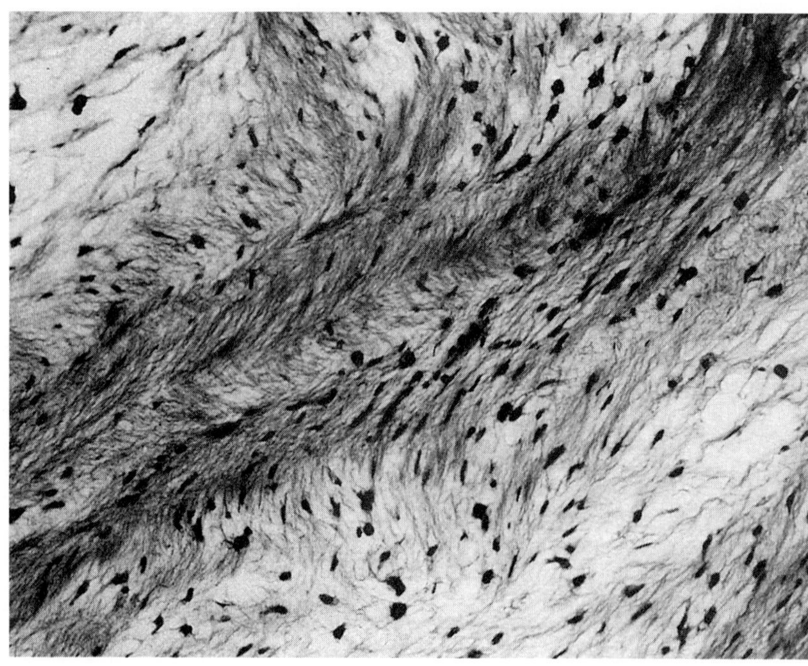

FIGURE 106.5. Juxtaarticular myxoma composed of fibroblast-like cells with small hyperchromatic nuclei and delicate cytoplasmic processes within a myxoid matrix (×150). (From Meis JM, Enzinger FM. Juxtaarticular myxomas. *Hum Pathol* 1992;23:639–646, with permission.)

MALIGNANT NEOPLASMS OF JOINTS

Malignant neoplasms of joints may be either primary or secondary. Primary intraarticular tumors are very rare and are represented by synovial sarcomas, cases of malignant PVS, and chondrosarcomas, which originate in synovial chondromatosis (30,79,83,134). Far more frequently, synovial sarcomas arise in the vicinity of large joints, particularly the knee (7). Other malignant tumors with an origin in the fascial tissues of the extremities include clear cell sarcomas of tendons and aponeuroses (135) and epithelioid sarcoma (136). Secondary involvement of joints occurs as a complication of the contiguous spread of malignant bone tumors, metastases of carcinoma, leukemia, or lymphoma. Rheumatologic manifestations of malignant hematologic diseases are discussed in Chapter 94.

Synovial Sarcoma

Clinical Findings

Synovial sarcoma is a malignant and histologically complex neoplasm generally found near a large joint (7,137–142). The tumor, which seldom originates within the joint itself (144) (Table 106.1), represents 10% of all soft tissue sarcomas and is preceded in frequency only by malignant fibrous histiocytoma, leiomyosarcoma, and liposarcoma. Synovial sarcoma occurs most often in young adults, although it has been observed at all ages from birth to 80 years. A slight preponderance is seen in men. The lower limb is more commonly the site of primary involvement than the upper limb. Other primary sites have included the buttocks, penis, abdominal wall, retroperitoneum, chest, neck, face, orbit, mouth, larynx, pharynx, esophagus, pericardium, heart, mediastinum, nerves such as the median, and veins such as the femoral and inferior vena cava (7,143–146). The characteristic history is that of a slowly growing, often painless mass that, in the case of a deeply situated lesion, may reach a considerable size before detection. Infrequently, pain or tenderness is the first manifestation of the disease.

The typical radiographic appearance of synovial sarcoma is that of a nonspecific paraarticular soft tissue mass of homogeneous water density, possibly lobulated, with a sharp, discrete border. Less often, the mass is irregular in outline and is not clearly separable from the surrounding tissues. In 30% of patients, the tumor contains small (rarely large) foci of amorphous calcification (7,138,147). In 10% to 20% of patients, secondary involvement of contiguous bone produces periosteal reaction, surface erosion, or bone invasion.

Although the rate of growth and the rapidity of metastatic spread vary, the disease characteristically follows a

TABLE 106.1. CHARACTERISTICS OF MALIGNANT SYNOVIAL TUMORS (7,136,139,141,169,173,177)

	Synovial Sarcoma	Clear Cell Sarcoma of Tendons and Aponeuroses	Epithelioid Sarcoma
Age			
Median	34	25	30
Greatest prevalence	20–40	10–40	10–35
Sex, male/female	1.5:1	1:1.2	2:1
Clinical features	Deep mass related to joints; most frequent in lower extremities	Deep-seated nodule adherent to tendon or aponeurosis; most frequent in foot and ankle	Slow-growing nodule in finger, hand, forearm, knee, lower leg; rare in other locations; central necrosis common; ulceration
Radiologic calcification	30%	Occasional	Rare
Histology	Biphasic (epithelial cells, spindle cell stroma); monophasic; undifferentiated[a]	Nests or fascicles of fusiform or rounded cells with clear cytoplasm	Large ovoid to plumb spindle cells arranged in a nodular pattern
Immunohistochemistry	Cytokeratin	S-100 protein	Cytokeratin
Electron microscopy	Basal lamina, zonulae adherens, desmosomes	Melanosomes or premelanosomes	Zonulae adherens, desmosomes, watertight junctions
Histologic grade[b]	2 or 3	2 or 3	2 or 3
Metastases	Lung, lymph nodes, bone	Lung, lymph nodes, bone	Lymph nodes, lungs, skin
Recurrence rate	25%	15–20%	70%
5-year survival	50–60%	40%	NA

[a]In all types, a biphasic cellular pattern is required in at least one portion of the neoplasm.
[b]Grade is determined by a combined assessment of cellularity, cellular anaplasia or pleomorphism, mitotic activity, expansive or infiltrative growth, and necrosis
NA, not available; S-100 protein, a neuroectodermal marker.

malignant course. The mass grows centrifugally, and compression of the surrounding tissues forms a pseudocapsule that is often perforated by fingers of tumor cells, leading to satellite lesions. As is true for other soft tissue sarcomas, synovial sarcoma spreads by direct extension along tissue planes, muscle bundles, nerves, and by way of the vascular system. Invasion of regional lymph nodes occurs in approximately 20% of cases. The most common site of visceral metastasis is the lung, in which the lesions appear as multiple large densities or as a diffuse infiltrate; cavitary metastases are rare (148). The pleura, diaphragm, pericardium, and skin also may be involved. Bone marrow lesions are seen in approximately 20% of cases. Osteolytic lesions are more common than sclerotic changes radiographically.

Histopathologic Findings

The gross appearance of synovial sarcoma depends on its origin, duration, rapidity of its growth, and cellular composition. The color of the tumor varies from a pale gray-yellow to a deep red, usually the result of hemorrhage. The tumor may feel uniformly firm when spindle cell elements predominate, or it may be soft and contain cystic spaces filled with mucoid secretions when epithelial cells predominate.

Synovial sarcomas are pleomorphic tumors (137–141). The classic type is characterized by a biphasic cellular pattern that includes epithelial cells arranged in nests, tubules, and acini, and a mesenchymal-appearing stroma of spindle cells and abundant reticulin fibers (Fig. 106.6). Other tumors are monophasic, most commonly of the spindle-cell type and less commonly of the epithelial-cell type. Finally, an undifferentiated type is also recognized. Calcification may occur in any of the four types of synovial sarcoma; it may consist of small elements, usually in the periphery of the tumor, or it may occupy large areas. Synovial sarcomas exhibit prominent vascularity, and vascular invasion is often apparent.

Regardless of the type, the diagnosis of synovial sarcoma requires the presence of a biphasic cellular pattern in at least one portion of the primary or recurrent tumor. The most distinctive histologic feature of synovial sarcoma is the presence of clefts and cystic spaces, lined by cuboidal or columnar cells, and containing a mucin-rich secretion that is resistant to hyaluronidase. A second type of mucinous material, present in the spindle cell areas, is sensitive to hyaluronidase.

Immunocytochemical studies have proven helpful in differentiating synovial sarcoma from other soft tissue tumors and have provided intriguing information regarding histogenesis (141,142). Biphasic and most monophasic synovial

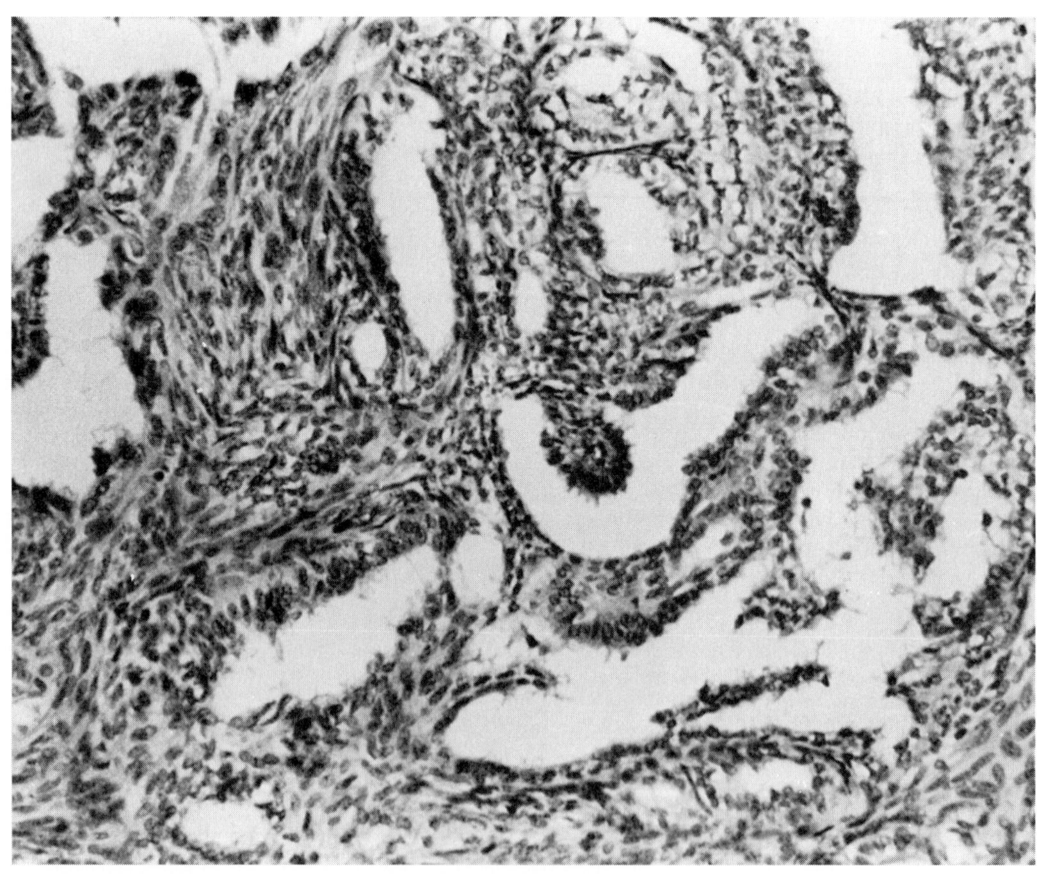

FIGURE 106.6. Biphasic synovial sarcoma. Note the irregular spaces lined with columnar cells in addition to the spindle-cell stroma (×100).

sarcomas are reactive for cytokeratin, epithelial membrane antigen, and Bcl 2 protein, and negative for CD34. Many express S-100 protein and CD99 allowing the exclusion of fibrosarcoma, malignant schwannoma, and hemangiopericytoma. Vimentin, an intermediate filament associated with mesenchymal cells and mesenchymal cell tumors, is present in the spindle cells of both biphasic and monophasic tumors. The epithelial structures are surrounded by laminin and type IV collagen basement membrane, whereas the extracellular matrix of the spindle cell areas is positive for types I and III collagen and fibronectin. Tenascin is restricted to the mesenchymal tissue that surrounds the epithelial structures (149).

The ultrastructural characteristics of these tumors are unique and intriguing in terms of histogenesis (150,151). The epithelial cells have a well-defined ovoid nucleus and abundant mitochondria, a prominent Golgi complex, and smooth and rough endoplasmic reticulum. Cellular arrangements in clusters and gland-like structures are frequent, and microvilli are present on the apical cell surfaces facing pseudoglandular spaces. Epithelial cells enclosing gland-like lumina are connected by junctional complexes, desmosomes, and zonulae adherens, which are not present in normal synovial tissue. Furthermore, most observations have revealed the presence of a continuous basal lamina at the epithelial-stromal junction, a structure also absent from normal synovial tissue. The spindle cells generally resemble fibroblasts, but have less cytoplasm and a less-developed endoplasmic reticulum than do fibroblasts.

The random location of synovial sarcoma in relation to joints, the lack of effect of hyaluronidase on the tinctorial characteristics of the mucinous material, and the presence of cytokeratin and ultrastructural findings that do not occur in synovial tissue clearly show that, despite its name, synovial sarcoma is unrelated to synovium. Synovial sarcomas probably arise from primitive mesenchymal cells (the arthrogenic mesenchyma) with an inherent or acquired ability to undergo epithelial cellular differentiation (7,150). A reciprocal translocation involving the chromosomes X and 18, t(X; 18) (p11.2; q11.2) has been demonstrated by chromosomal analysis to occur in 90% of synovial sarcomas (141,142,152).

Diagnosis

Synovial sarcoma should be suspected when a deep-seated swelling or a palpable mass develops in the vicinity of a joint in a young patient. Plain roentgenograms of the region are useful to determine the general characteristics of the mass and the possible presence of phleboliths, amorphous calcification, or bone abnormalities. Sonography is important to exclude cystic lesions such as a Baker's cyst, meniscal cyst, or ganglion. If the mass is solid, the next question is to determine if one is dealing with a benign or malignant lesion (153). Patients in whom a soft tissue sarcoma is suspected should be referred to an experienced surgical oncologist prior to biopsy (154). Solid masses more than 5 cm in diameter deep to the fascia are likely to be a sarcoma. MRI is the most efficient means of defining the exact location of the tumor and the possible involvement of neighboring structures in transverse and sagittal views (155,156). Synovial sarcoma is suggested by a relatively well-defined, nonhomogeneous hemorrhagic lesion near a joint with bone contact. CT may be required if the integrity of cortical bone is in question. A chest radiograph and CT, and a bone scan are obtained routinely to detect metastatic disease, which if present may alter the treatment of the primary tumor. Because no clinical or imaging procedures can reliably distinguish benign from malignant lesions, however, a biopsy is always necessary (155). A primary diagnosis requires an open procedure involving excision or incision of the tumor mass, or a closed procedure performed with needles or trephines. Excisional biopsies imply the "shelling out" of the entire tumor and are used exclusively for small lesions. Incisional biopsies, in which only part of the tumor is removed, are used for masses greater than 3 cm in diameter and should be obtained at a site that can be excised en bloc with the tumor when the definitive procedure is performed. The biopsy, performed with open or closed procedures, should be done in such a way as to (a) avoid unnecessary tissue manipulation; (b) excise the track en bloc with the tumor; (c) avoid violation of additional compartments or neurovascular structures; and (d) obtain the tissue from a soft tissue mass rather than bone, to prevent a fracture. Because frozen sections (which are useful to determine adequacy of the sample) are suboptimal to distinguish the various types of soft tissue sarcoma, a definitive diagnosis rests on the interpretation of permanent sections. Closed biopsies are particularly helpful to document local or distant metastases, or in suspected recurrence.

Prognosis and Treatment

Adverse prognostic factors in synovial sarcoma include older age, male sex, proximal tumors, deep tumors, absence of extensive calcification, evidence of nodal involvement, invasion of neurovascular structures or bone, a high mitotic rate of the tumor, and, in particular, a tumor size greater than 5 cm in diameter (142,157–162).

Because of the pattern of tumor spread, en bloc excision of the tumor and the entire muscle compartment, or radical amputation in which the joint proximal to the involved compartment is disarticulated, is often required. With these procedures, the rate of local recurrence should be less than 20%; however, a 31% recurrence rate was observed after inadequate initial surgery (161). Alternatively, one of several limb-sparing procedures may be considered. A frequently used approach (163) is wide local excision in which the tumor is removed along with several centimeters of normal tissue in all directions, along with lymphadenectomy, given the frequent nodal involvement in synovial sarcoma. The procedure may be preceded by, or (usually) followed by, radiotherapy, often in association with adjuvant chemotherapy. Microscopic involvement of the surgical margins has a dire effect on prognosis. In a randomized trial of amputation compared with limb-sparing surgery in which all patients received postoperative radiotherapy and chemotherapy, the rate of local recurrence was extremely low (0/16 in amputated patients and 4/27 in patients treated with limb-sparing surgery), and the survival at 5 years was 83% and 88%, respectively (164). Although various drugs have been used in adjuvant chemotherapy, the most promising include doxorubicin, ifosfamide, and cisplatin (165,166). Local recurrences and isolated pulmonary metastases may be treated surgically (167).

Clear Cell Sarcoma of Tendons and Aponeuroses

Clear cell sarcoma (7,135,168,169) is a peculiar neoplasm that affects children and young adults, more frequently women (Table 106.1). Clinically, it presents as a deep, painless, slow-growing mass intimately associated with tendons or aponeuroses. In approximately 75% of cases, the site of the lesion is in the lower extremity, predominantly the foot or ankle, and less frequently the knee or thigh. Most of the remaining lesions occur in the upper extremity.

The tumor consists of peculiar compact nests and fascicles of round or fusiform, pale (glycogen)-staining cells with vesicular nuclei and prominent nucleoli (Fig. 106.7). Because intracellular melanin is found in nearly half the cases, and because melanosomes and the neuroectodermal S-100 protein are virtually always present, a neuroectodermal origin for clear cell sarcoma appears certain (7,170). At the genetic level, however, 60% to 75% of cases of clear cell sarcomas have a translocation (12;26) while a broad range of genetic alterations are found in malignant melanoma, most commonly involving chromosomes 1, 5, and 6 (171). Prognosis is generally poor, particularly when the tumor mass is 5 cm or larger in diameter. Local recurrences are common, and lymph node, lung, and bone metastases occur in most cases (7,172,173). Treatment of this lesion includes radical excision or amputation, combined with radiotherapy and adjuvant chemotherapy. Lymph node excision should be included, because regional node involvement occurs in about 30% of cases.

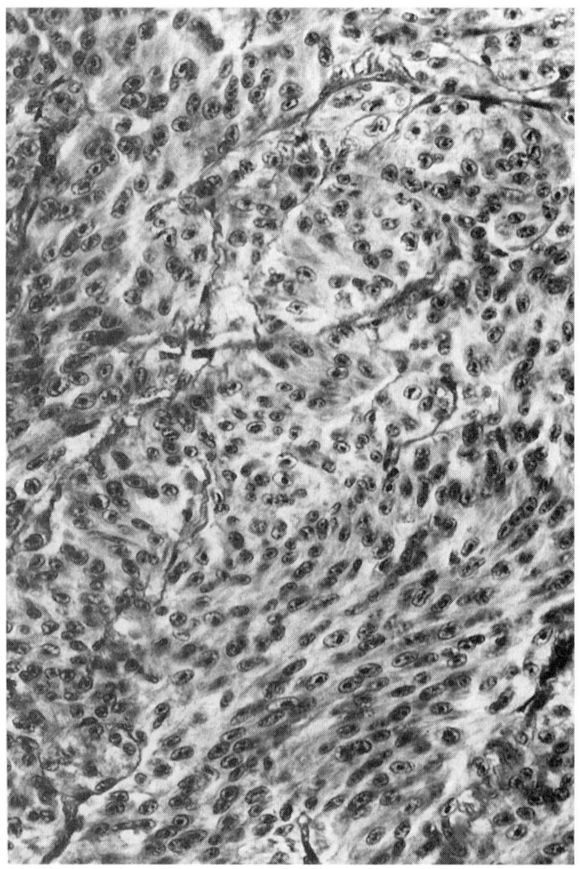

FIGURE 106.7. Classic architectural pattern of clear-cell sarcoma: clusters of tumor cells separated by delicate fibroconnective tissue septa. (From Lucas DR, Nascimento AG, Sim FH. Clear cell sarcoma of soft tissues. *Am J Surg Pathol* 1992;16:1197–1204, with permission.)

Epithelioid Sarcoma

This distinctive sarcoma occurs predominantly in young adults (Table 106.1) (136), usually in the hand, wrist, forearm, or lower leg. The lesion may arise in the subcutis or deeper tissues such as tendon, tendon sheaths, and deep fascia. Superficial lesions, which have a predilection for the fingers, forearms, and tibial regions, develop as raised, slow-growing, woody nodules that become ulcerated weeks or months later. Understandably, these lesions tend to be confused with necrotizing infectious granulomas, ulcerating squamous cell carcinomas, necrobiosis lipoidica, granuloma annulare, and rheumatoid nodules. Deep lesions tend to be larger and are firmly attached to the fibrous structure on which they grow. Although initially they may be interpreted as nodular tendinitises, subsequent growth suggests a sarcomatous origin. Microscopically, the tumor includes large, acidophilic polygonal cells and spindle cells arranged in irregular nodules in which central necrosis is frequent (Fig. 106.8) (7,136). Immunohistochemical stains are positive for cytokeratin, usually for vimentin, and negative for the S-100 protein (174–176). Electron microscopy reveals polygonal and spindle-shaped cells with interdigitating cellular processes. Maculae adherens and desmosomes are present, but a basal lamina is absent (7). Epithelioid sarcoma is a tumor with a tendency to recur, sometimes repeatedly, over many years. Metastases develop in 45% of cases, predominantly to regional lymph nodes and lung. Treatment of this lesion requires wide or radical resection (177) plus adjuvant therapy similar to synovial sarcoma.

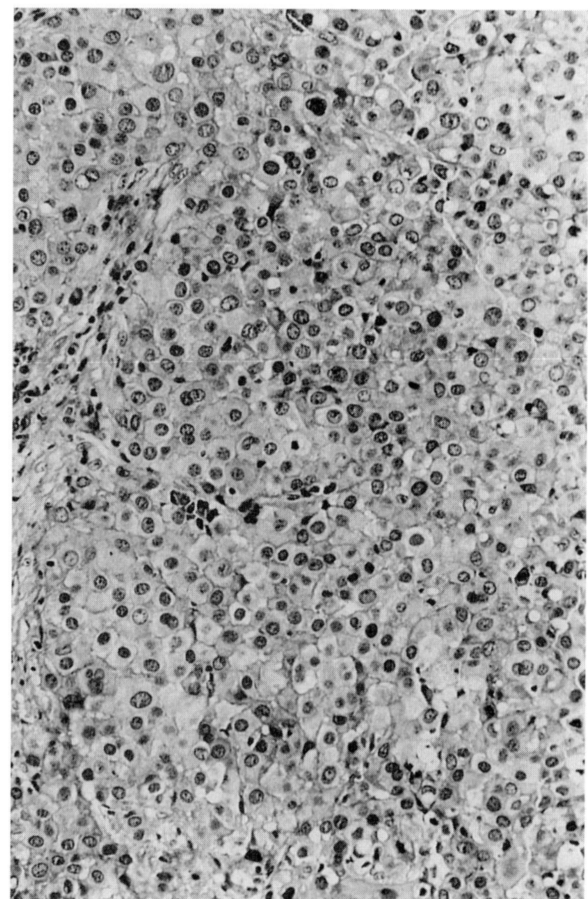

FIGURE 106.8. Epithelioid sarcoma composed of sheets of tumor cells with abundant eosinophilic cytoplasm. (From Arber DA, Kandalaft PL, Mehta P, Battifora H. Vimentin-negative epithelioid sarcoma. *Am J Surg Pathol* 1993;17:302–307, with permission.)

Synovial Angiosarcoma

Angiosarcomas usually involve skin, soft tissues, the heart, or the liver. Primary synovial angiosarcoma is truly exceptional (178).

Involvement of Joints by Primary Bone Tumors

Metaphyseal bone tumors, chiefly osteosarcoma, fibrosarcoma, and chondrosarcoma, often invade joints (179). Ewing's sarcoma usually involves the diaphysis, but cases that originate in the epiphysis may involve a joint (180). Articular (hyaline) cartilage is thought to act as a barrier to local tumor angiogenesis (181). Tumor penetration eventually occurs, however, whether peripherally beneath the joint capsule, at the bone attachment of intracapsular ligaments such as the cruciate ligaments of the knee, or across cartilage itself. Bland synovial effusions may indicate early invasion of the joint (182). The transarticular extension of sarcomas that originated in the iliac bone has been studied: 11 of 47 sarcomas invaded the sacrum through the sacroiliac joint (183).

Carcinomatous Synovitis

That metastases to synovium are clinically rare is surprising given the high frequency of disseminated carcinomas and the rich vascular supply of synovial tissue. Knees are most commonly affected (184–189). Other evidence of disseminated tumor is usually present, but, rarely, joint metastases are the first indications of malignant disease or of tumor dissemination (184,185,187). Radiographic studies of such joints demonstrate lytic lesions of the patella, femur, or tibia, but patients with early cases may lack abnormal findings (184,187).

Bone scanning may reveal increased local radionuclide uptake. Multiple focal lesions of increased activity throughout the skeleton provide further evidence of metastatic disease. Synovial fluid is hemorrhagic, with 100 to 8,000 white blood cells (WBCs)/mm^3, predominantly mononuclear cells. The fluid of one patient exhibited eosinophilia (184). Tumor cells are found in synovial fluid in about 80% of patients. Arthroscopy is valuable in the diagnosis of synovial metastases when the results of other tests are inconclusive (189).

Metastases to Bones of the Hands and Feet

Bone metastasis of the hands and feet is an unusual form of arthritis that occurs in patients with disseminated carcinoma. Metastases occur in small bones, particularly the distal phalanges, and the tarsal bones. Clinically, these resemble paronychia or gout. Lytic lesions, sometimes with pathologic fractures, are usually present (190–194).

Metastases to Shoulders

Bone metastases in renal cell carcinoma exhibit a curious predilection for the clavicle, acromion, and proximal humeral head (195). Painful lytic lesions in these areas should direct attention to the kidney. An instance of nasopharyngeal carcinoma, metastatic to both acromioclavicular joints, has been reported (196).

Lymphoma

Musculoskeletal manifestations of lymphoma (197–202), both Hodgkin's and non-Hodgkin's, include pain caused by bone metastasis or primary involvement of bone, anterior chest wall pain (203), hypertrophic osteoarthropathy in patients with intrathoracic lesions, and, very rarely, arthritis caused by lymphomatous synovial infiltration. The latter is usually monarticular (204), but polyarticular cases may resemble RA (200,205,206).

NONMETASTATIC (PARANEOPLASTIC) SYNDROMES

The nonmetastatic syndromes comprise a variety of conditions (Table 106.2) (207,208).

Hypertrophic Osteoarthropathy

The well-known association of intrathoracic tumors and hypertrophic osteoarthropathy is discussed in Chapter 96. It can be considered the prototype of a tumor-associated paraneoplastic process; its onset often leads to the discovery of an unsuspected intrathoracic malignant process (209,210).

Pancreatic Cancer with Arthropathy and Fat Necrosis

Panniculitis resembling erythema nodosum accompanied by synovitis and serositis is a well-known accompaniment of pancreatic carcinoma, particularly of the acinar-cell type, as well as of pancreatitis. The pancreatitis is often silent. Its pathogenesis includes fat necrosis in subcutaneous tissue, bone marrow, and subsynovial fat, as a result of high levels of circulating pancreatic lipase (211–216).

TABLE 106.2. RHEUMATOLOGIC SYNDROMES ASSOCIATED WITH NONHEMATOLOGIC MALIGNANT DISEASES

- By direct extension or metastasis
  - Primary bone tumors
  - Carcinomatous (metastatic) synovitis
  - Metastases to small bones
- Nonmetastatic (paraneoplastic)
  - Articular
    - Hypertrophic osteoarthropathy
    - Subcutaneous nodules, arthritis, and serositis (fat necrosis) in pancreatic cancer (or pancreatitis)
  - Cancer arthritis
  - Tumor-induced osteomalacia
  - Hyperuricemia and gout, hypouricemia
  - Carcinoid arthropathy
  - Multicentric reticulohistiocytosis
  - Palmar fasciitis and polyarthritis associated with carcinoma
  - Coincidental arthritis of any type
- Muscular
  - Type II muscle fiber atrophy
  - Dermatomyositis
  - Eaton-Lambert syndrome
  - Hypophosphatemic myopathy
  - Carcinoid myopathy
  - Coincidental myopathy of any type
- Cutaneous
  - Carcinoid "scleroderma"
- As complications of therapy
  - Aseptic necrosis of bone
  - Septic arthritis
  - Corticosteroid myopathy
  - Chemotherapy-induced fibrotic syndromes
  - Interleukin-2–induced polyarthritis
  - α-Interferon–induced polyarthritis
  - BCG immunotherapy–induced polyarthritis

Cancer Arthritis

Several observers have described a syndrome resembling RA with typical or atypical features (217–219), having its onset a few months before the discovery of a tumor. The atypical form is characterized by explosive onset, asymmetry of joint involvement, sparing of wrists and small joints of the hand, absence of subcutaneous nodules, and seronegativity. All patients in one series were in their fifth decade or older. Removal or successful treatment of the tumor was associated with remission of the arthritis in approximately half of these patients. Remission was more frequent in the atypical than in the typical RA-like pattern. The validity of these associations has not been definitely established by epidemiologic data.

Supporting evidence of a causal association between carcinoma and rheumatic disease has been provided by anecdotal observations, in which removal of carcinoma has been followed by complete clinical and serologic remission of the syndrome. The tumors involved included lung (220,221), esophageal (222,223), gastric (224), colonic (225), and breast carcinoma (226), and ovarian dysgerminoma (227,228).

Tumor-Induced Osteomalacia

Osteomalacia, including generalized osteopenia, multiple fractures, Looser's zones, hypophosphatemia, hyperphosphaturia, and low serum levels of 1,25-hydroxyvitamin D may be caused by a variety of benign and malignant tumors, most commonly mesenchymal tumors and hemangiopericytomas (229–231). Clinically, ankylosing spondylitis may be suggested (including bilateral "sacroiliitis"), but coexistent hypophosphatemic myopathy should lead to the correct diagnosis. Removal of the tumor results in regression of biochemical findings, resolution of myopathy, and improvement of skeletal lesions.

Hyperuricemia and Gout

The degree of hyperuricemia in patients with carcinoma correlates with the extent of the disease, involvement of the liver, and the presence of hypercalcemia. Gout occurred in only five of 70 patients studied. In two of these patients, gout preceded the tumor (232). The frequency of hyperuricemia and gout in a cancer patient population remains to be elucidated. Hyperuricemia has been noted in association with cisplatin therapy (233). Interestingly, hypouricemia has also been described in association with disseminated carcinoma (234).

Carcinoid Arthropathy

This peculiar form of arthropathy characterized by arthralgias, juxtaarticular demineralization, erosions, and subchondral cysts were observed in four of five consecutive patients with the carcinoid syndrome (235, 236).

Angiocentric T-Cell Lymphoma

Arthralgia, polyarthritis (237), and cutaneous pseudovasculitis (238) may be associated with this peculiar T-cell lymphoproliferative disorder, which is characterized by angiodestructive lymphoreticular proliferative granulomata.

Multicentric Reticulohistiocytosis

An association may well be present between multicentric reticulohistiocytosis and cancer; 28% of the 82 cases in one review had an associated neoplasm (239).

Palmar Fasciitis and Polyarthritis Associated with Carcinoma

Medsger and co-workers (240) have described a unique syndrome, including palmar fasciitis and polyarthritis, in six patients with ovarian carcinoma, predominantly of the endometrioid type. Other tumors also produce this syndrome (241). The palmar changes ranged from diffuse, globular swelling with warmth and erythema to typical Dupuytren's contractures, including plantar nodular fasciitis. The shoulders and the metacarpophalangeal and proximal interphalangeal joints were most frequently involved and exhibited painful limitations of motion and flexor contractures. Morning stiffness was prominent. Although two of these patients had carpal tunnel syndrome, none had Raynaud's phenomenon, dermal or pulmonary fibrosis, or evidence of myositis. In five patients, the articular symptoms preceded the diagnosis of malignant disease by several months to 2 years. In the remaining patient, the articular symptoms preceded tumor recurrence. In all patients, the ovarian tumor was extensive and gave evidence of intra- and extraperitoneal spread. The median survival time after diagnosis of the tumor was 6 months. The syndrome may be limited to polyarthritis and severe joint contractures (242). The pathogenesis of this syndrome, which resembles reflex sympathetic dystrophy but tends to be more disseminated, remains unexplained.

Other Rheumatologic Syndromes

Polymyositis (dermatomyositis) and other muscle syndromes associated with tumors are discussed in Chapter 78.

COMPLICATIONS OF CANCER TREATMENT

When a patient with underlying malignant disease is receiving corticosteroid or immunosuppressive therapy, secondary joint manifestations related to these drugs may occur (Table 106.2). These manifestations include aseptic necrosis of bone (see Chapters 40 and 108), septic arthritis (see Chapters 126 and 128), and steroid myopathy (see Chapter 40). Additionally, chemotherapy with bleomycin can give rise to a fibrotic syndrome resembling systemic sclerosis (see Chapter 80), and cases of polyarthritis have followed interleukin-2 infusions (243), and possibly α-interferon (244), and intravesical Bacille Calmette-Guérin (BCG) immunotherapy (245).

REFERENCES

1. Jaffe HL, Lichtenstein L, Sutro CJ. Pigmented villonodular synovitis, bursitis and tenosynovitis. *Arch Pathol* 1941;31:731–765.
2. Jaffe HL. *Tumors and tumorous conditions of the bones and joints.* Philadelphia: Lea and Febiger, 1958.
3. de Visser E, Veth RP, Pruszczynski M, et al. Diffuse and localized pigmented villonodular synovitis: evaluation and treatment of 38 patients. *Arch Orthop Trauma Surg* 1999;119:401–404.
4. Docken WP. Pigmented villonodular synovitis: a review with illustrative case reports. *Semin Arthritis Rheum* 1979;9:1–22.
5. Myers BW, Masi AT, Feigenbaum SL. Pigmented villonodular synovitis and tenosynovitis: a clinical epidemiology study of 166 cases and literature review. *Medicine* 1980;59:223–238.
6. Rao AS, Vigorita VJ. Pigmented villonodular synovitis (giant-cell tumor of the tendon sheath and synovial membrane). *J Bone Joint Surg* 1984;66A:76–94.
7. Enzinger FM, Weiss SW. *Soft tissue tumors,* 2nd ed. St. Louis: CV Mosby, 1988.
8. Bentley G, McAuliffe T. Pigmented villonodular synovitis. *Ann Rheum Dis* 1990;49:210–211.
9. Klompmaker J, Veth RPH, Robinson PH, et al. Pigmented villonodular synovitis. *Arch Orthop Trauma Surg* 1990;109: 205–210.
10. Reginato A, Martinez V, Schumacher HR, et al. Giant cell tumor associated with rheumatoid arthritis. *Ann Rheum Dis* 1974;33:333–341.
11. Ghadially FN, Lalonde JM, Dick CE. Ultrastructure of pigmented villonodular synovitis. *J Pathol* 1979;127:19–26.
12. Schumacher HR, Lotke P, Athreya B, et al. Pigmented villonodular synovitis: light and electron microscopic studies. *Semin Arthritis Rheum* 1982;12:32–43.
13. Ushijima M, Hashimoto H, Tsuneyoshi M, et al. Pigmented villonodular synovitis. A clinicopathologic study of 52 cases. *Acta Pathol Jpn* 1986;36:317–326.
14. Rosenthal DI, Coleman PK, Schiller AL. Pigmented villonodular synovitis: correlation of angiographic and histologic findings. *AJR* 1980;135:581–583.

15. Dahlin DC, Salvador AD. Cartilaginous tumors of the soft tissues of the hands and feet. *Mayo Clin Proc* 1974;49:721–726.
16. Takagi M, Ishikawa G. Simultaneous villonodular synovitis and synovial chondromatosis of the temporomandibular joint. Report of a case. *J Oral Surg* 1981;39:699–701.
17. Scott PM. Bone lesions in pigmented villonodular synovitis. *J Bone Joint Surg* 1968;50B:306–311.
18. Dorwart RH, Genant HK, Johnston WH, et al. Pigmented villonodular synovitis of synovial joints: clinical, pathologic and radiologic features. *AJR* 1984;143:877–885.
19. Darling JM, Glimcher LH, Shortkroff S, et al. Expression of metalloproteinases in pigmented villonodular synovitis. *Hum Pathol* 1994;25:825–830.
20. Darling JM, Goldring SR, Harada Y, et al. Multinucleated cells in pigmented villonodular synovitis and giant cell tumor of tendon sheath express features of osteoclasts. *Am J Pathol* 1997;150:1383–1393.
21. Neale SD, Kristelly R, Gundle R, et al. Giant cells in pigmented villonodular synovitis express and osteoclast phenotype. *J Clin Pathol* 1997;50:605–608.
22. Wendt RG, Wolfe F, McQueen D, et al. Polyarticular pigmented villonodular synovitis in children: evidence for a genetic contribution. *J Rheumatol* 1986;13:921–926.
23. Flandry F, McCann SB, Hughston JC, et al. Roentgenographic findings in pigmented villonodular synovitis of the knee. *Clin Orthop* 1989;247:208–219.
24. Vedantam R, Strecker WB, Schoenecker PL, et al. Polyarticular pigmented villonodular synovitis in a child. *Clin Orthop* 1998;348:208–211.
25. Flandry F, Hughston JC, McCann SB, et al. Diagnostic features of diffuse pigmented villonodular synovitis of the knee. *Clin Orthop* 1994;298:212–220.
26. Torisu T, Watanabe H. Pigmented villonodular synovitis occurred in a rheumatoid patient. *Clin Orthop* 1973;91:134–140.
27. Archer-Harvey JM, Henderson DW, Papadimitriou JM, et al. Pigmented villonodular synovitis associated with psoriatic polyarthropathy: an electron microscopic and immunocytochemical study. *J Pathol* 1984;144:57–68.
28. Flipo RM, Desvigne-Noulet MC, Cotten A, et al. La synovite villo-nodulaire pigmentee de la hanche. *Rev Rheumatol* 1994;61:85–95.
29. Abdul-Karim FW, El-Naggar AK, Joyce MJ, et al. Diffuse and localized tenosynovial giant cell tumor and pigmented villonodular synovitis. A clinicopathologic and flow cytometric DNA analysis. *Hum Pathol* 1992;23:729–735.
30. Bertoni F, Unni KK, Beabout JW, et al. Malignant giant cell tumor of the tendon sheaths and joints (malignant pigmented villonodular synovitis). *Am J Surg Pathol* 1997;21:153–163.
31. Curtin HD, Williams R, Gailla L, et al. Pigmented villonodular synovitis of the temporomandibular joint. *Comput Radiol* 1983;7:257–260.
32. Dawiskiba S, Eriksson L, Elner A, et al. Diffuse pigmented villonodular synovitis of the temporomandibular joint demonstrated by fine-needle aspiration cytology. *Diagn Cytopathol* 1989;5:301–304.
33. Karnezis TA, McMillan RD, Ciric I. Pigmented villonodular synovitis in a vertebra. A case report. *J Bone Joint Surg* 1990;72A:927–930.
34. Steinbach LS, Neumann CH, Stoller DW, et al. MRI of the knee in diffuse pigmented villonodular synovitis. *Clin Imaging* 1989;13:305–316.
35. Ropes MW, Bauer W. *Synovial fluid changes in joint disease.* Cambridge: Harvard University Press, 1953.
36. Ugai K, Kurosaka M, Hirohata K. Lipid microspherules in synovial fluid of patients with pigmented villonodular synovitis. *Arthritis Rheum* 1988;31:1442–1446.
37. Bullough PG, Bansal M. The differential diagnosis of geodes. *Radiol Clin North Am* 1988;26:1165–1184.
38. Abrahams TG, Pavlov H, Bansal M, et al. Concentric joint space narrowing of the hip associated with hemosiderotic synovitis (HS) including pigmented villonodular synovitis. *Skeletal Radiol* 1988;17:37–45.
39. Nilsonne U, Moberger G. Pigmented villonodular synovitis of joints. Histological and clinical problems in diagnosis. *Acta Orthop Scand* 1969;40:448–460.
40. Jergesen HE, Mankin HJ. Diffuse pigmented villonodular synovitis of the knee mimicking primary bone neoplasm. A report of two cases. *J Bone Joint Surg* 1978;60A:825–829.
41. Andersen JA, Ladefoged C. A case of aggressive pigmented villonodular synovitis. *Acta Orthop Scand* 1988;59:467–470.
42. Nielsen AL, Kiaer T. Malignant giant cell tumor of synovium and locally destructive pigmented villonodular synovitis. Ultrastructural and immunohistochemical study and review of the literature. *Hum Pathol* 1989;20:765–771.
43. McKenzie AF. The role of magnetic resonance imaging. When to use it and what to look for. *Acta Orthop Scand Suppl* 1997;273:21–24.
44. Miller TT, Potter HG, McCormack RR. Benign soft tissue masses of the wrist and hand: MRI appearances. *Skeletal Radiol* 1994;23:327–332.
45. Mancini GB, Lazzeri S, Bruno G, et al. Localized pigmented villonodular synovitis of the knee. *Arthroscopy* 1998;14:532–536.
46. Jacobson JA, Lenchik L, Ruhoy MK, et al. MR imaging of the infrapatellar fat pad of Hoffa. *Radiographics* 1997;17:675–691.
47. Howie CR, Smith GD, Christie J, et al. Torsion of localized pigmented villonodular synovitis of the knee. *J Bone Joint Surg* 1985;67B:564–566.
48. Shenaq SM. Benign skin and soft-tissue tumors of the hand. *Clin Plast Surg* 1987;14:403–412.
49. Karasick D, Karasick S. Giant cell tumor of tendon sheath: spectrum of radiologic findings. *Skeletal Radiol* 1992;21:219–224.
50. Schajowicz F, Blumenfeld I. Pigmented villonodular synovitis of the wrist with penetration into bone. *J Bone Joint Surg* 1968;50B:312–317.
51. Sciot R, Rosai J, Dal Cin P, et al. Analysis of 35 cases of localized and diffuse tenosynovial giant cell tumor: a report from the Chromosomes and Morphology (CHAMP) study grou. *Mod Pathol* 1999;12:576–579.
52. De Beuckeleer L, De Schepper A, De Belder F, et al. Magnetic resonance imaging of localized giant cell tumour of the tendon sheath (MRI of localized GCTTS). *Eur Radiol* 1997;7:198–201.
53. Konrath GA, Nahigian K, Kolowich P. Pigmented villonodular synovitis of the subacromial bursa. *J Shoulder Elbow Surg* 1997;6:400–404.
54. Weisser JR, Robinson DW. Pigmented villonodular synovitis of the iliopectineal bursa. *J Bone Joint Surg* 1951;33A:988–992.
55. Katz DS, Levinsohn EM. Pigmented villonodular synovitis of the sequestered suprapatellar bursa. *Clin Orthop* 1994;306:204–208.
56. Present DA, Bertoni F, Enneking WF. Case report 384. *Skeletal Radiol* 1986;15:236–240.
57. Ray RA, Morton CC, Lipinski KK, et al. Cytogenetic evidence of clonality in a case of pigmented villonodular synovitis. *Cancer* 1991;67:121–125.
58. Hawley WL, Ansell BM. Synovial hemangioma presenting as monoarticular arthritis of the knee. *Arch Dis Child* 1981;56:558–560.
59. Roy S, Ghadially FN. Synovial membrane in experimentally produced chronic hemarthrosis. *Ann Rheum Dis* 1969;28:402–414.

60. Singh R, Grewal DS, Chakravarti RN. Experimental production of pigmented villonodular synovitis in the knee and ankle joints of Rhesus monkeys. *J Pathol* 1969;98:137–142.
61. Bobechko WP, Kostuik JP. Childhood villonodular synovitis. *Can J Surg* 1968;11:480–486.
62. Juhl M, Krebs B. Arthroscopy and synovial hemangioma or giant cell tumour of the knee. *Arch Orthop Traum Surg* 1989;108:250–252.
63. Devaney K, Vinh TN, Sweet DE. Synovial hemangioma: a report of 20 cases with differential diagnostic considerations. *Hum Pathol* 1993;24:737–745.
64. Duthie RB, Rizza CR. Rheumatological manifestations of the hemophilias. *Clin Rheum Dis* 1975;1:53–93.
65. Morris CJ, Blake DR, Wainwright AC, et al. Relationship between iron deposits and tissue damage in the synovium: an ultrastructural study. *Ann Rheum Dis* 1986;45:21–26.
66. Hamlin BR, Duffy GP, Trousdale RT, et al. Total knee arthroplasty in patients who have pigmented villonodular synovitis. *J Bone Joint Surg* 1998;80A:76–82.
67. Zvijac JE, Lau AC, Hechtman KS, et al. Arthroscopic treatment of pigmented villonodular synovitis of the knee. *Arthroscopy* 1999;15:613–617.
68. Ogilvie-Harris DJ, McLean J, Zarnett ME. Pigmented villonodular synovitis of the knee. Results of total arthroscopic synovectomy, partial arthroscopic synovectomy, and arthroscopic local resection. *J Bone Joint Surg* 1992;74A:119–123.
69. Flandry F, Hughston JC, Jacobson KE, et al. Surgical treatment of pigmented villonodular synovitis of the knee. *Clin Orthop* 1994;300:189–194.
70. Gitelis S, Heligman D, Morton T. The treatment of pigmented villonodular synovitis of the hip. A case report and review of the literature. *Clin Orthop* 1989;239:154–160.
71. Robert D'Eshoughes J, Delcambre B, Delbart P. Pigmented villonodular synovitis and radioisotopic synoviorthesis. *Lille Med* 1975;20:438–446.
72. O'Sullivan MM, Yates DB, Pritchard MH. Yttrium 90 synovectomy. A new treatment for pigmented villonodular synovitis. *Br J Rheumatol* 1987;26:71–72.
73. Franssen MJAM, Boerbooms AMTh, Karthaus RP, et al. Treatment of pigmented villonodular synovitis of the knee with yttrium-90 silicate: prospective evaluations by arthroscopy, histology, and 99mTc pertechnetate uptake measurements. *Ann Rheum Dis* 1989;48:1007–1013.
74. Murphy FP, Dahlin DC, Sullivan CR. Articular synovial chondromatosis. *J Bone Joint Surg* 1962;44A:77–86.
75. Milgram JW. Synovial osteochondromatosis. A histopathological study of thirty cases. *J Bone Joint Surg* 1977;59A: 792–801.
76. Sim FH, Dahlin DC, Ivins JC. Extra-articular synovial chondromatosis. *J Bone Joint Surg* 1977;59A:492–495.
77. Karlin CA, De Smet AA, Neff J, et al. The variable manifestations of extraarticular synovial chondromatosis. *AJR* 1981;137: 731–735.
78. Maurice H, Crone M, Watt I. Synovial chondromatosis. *J Bone Joint Surg* 1988;70B:807–811.
79. Davis RI, Hamilton A, Biggart JD. Primary synovial chondromatosis: a clinicopathological review and assessment of malignant potential. *Hum Pathol* 1998;29:683–688.
80. Milgram JW. The classification of loose bodies in human joints. *Clin Orthop* 1977;124:282–291.
81. Milgram JW. The development of loose bodies in human joints. *Clin Orthop* 1977;124:292–303.
82. Saotome K, Tamai K, Koguchi Y, et al. Growth potential of loose bodies: an immunohistochemical examination of primary and secondary synovial osteochondromatosis. *J Orthop Res* 1999;17:73–79.
83. Bertoni F, Unni KK, Beabout JW, et al. Chondrosarcomas of the synovium. *Cancer* 1991;67:155–162.
84. Carey RPL. Synovial chondromatosis of the knee in childhood. A report of two cases. *J Bone Joint Surg* 1983;59A:444–447.
85. Pelker RR, Drennan JC, Ozonoff MB. Juvenile synovial chondromatosis of the hip. *J Bone Joint Surg* 1983;65A:552–554.
86. Steinberg GG, Desai SS, Malhorta R, et al. Familial synovial chondromatosis. *J Bone Joint Surg* 1989;71B:144–145.
87. Dolan EA, Vogler JB, Angelillo JC. Synovial chondromatosis of the temporomandibular joint diagnosed by magnetic resonance imaging: report of a case. *J Oral Maxillofac Surg* 1989;47: 411–413.
88. Rosati LA, Stevens C. Synovial chondromatosis of the temporomandibular joint presenting as an intracranial mass. *Arch Otolaryngol Head Neck Surg* 1990;116:1334–1337.
89. Norman A, Steiner GC. Bone erosion in synovial chondromatosis. *Radiology* 1986;161:749–752.
90. Jones JR, Evans DM, Kaushik A. Synovial chondromatosis presenting with peripheral nerve compression. Report of two cases. *J Bone Joint Surg* 1987;12B:25–27.
91. Eideken J, Eideken BS, Ayala AG, et al. Giant synovial chondromatosis. *Skeletal Radiol* 1994;23:23–29.
92. Szypryt P, Twining P, Preston BJ, et al. Synovial chondromatosis of the hip joint presenting as a pathologic fracture. *Br J Radiol* 1986;59:399–401.
93. McCarty DJ, Halverson PB, Carrera GF, et al. "Milwaukee shoulder"—association of microspheroids containing hydroxyapatite crystals, active collagenase, and neutral protease with rotator cuff defects. I. Clinical aspects. *Arthritis Rheum* 1981; 24:464–473.
94. Ellman MH, Krieger MI, Brown N. Pseudogout mimicking synovial chondromatosis. *J Bone Joint Surg* 1975;57A:863–865.
95. DeBenedetti MJ, Schwinn CP. Tenosynovial chondromatosis of the hand. *J Bone Joint Surg* 1979;61A:899–903.
96. Cremone JC, Wolff TW, Wolfort FG. Synovial chondromatosis of the hand. *Plast Reconst Surg* 1982;69:871–874.
97. Roulot E, Le Viet D. Primary synovial osteochondromatosis of the hand and wrist. *Rev Rhum* (English edition) 1999;66: 256–266.
98. Pope TL Jr, Keats TE, de Lange EE, et al. Idiopathic synovial chondromatosis in two unusual sites: inferior radioulnar joint and ischial bursa. *Skeletal Radiol* 1987;16:205–208.
99. Coolican MR, Dandy DJ. Arthroscopic management of synovial chondromatosis of the knee. Findings and results in 18 cases. *J Bone Joint Surg* 1989;71B:498–500.
100. Milgram JW, Keagy RD. Bursal osteochondromatosis: a case report. *Clin Orthop* 1979;144:269–271.
101. Giordano V, Giordano M, Knackfuss IG, et al. Synovial osteochondromatosis of the retrocalcaneal bursa: a case study. *Foot Ankle Int* 1999;20:534–537.
102. Wilner D. *Radiology of bone tumors and allied disorders*, vol 4. Philadelphia: WB Saunders, 1982:3941.
103. McCarthy EF, Dorfman HD. Primary synovial chondromatosis. An ultrastructural study. *Clin Orthop* 1982;168:178–186.
104. Nishimura K, Solchaga LA, Caplan AI, et al. Chondroprogenitor cells of synovial tissue. *Arthritis Rheum* 1999;42:2631–2637.
105. Davis RI, Foster H, Arthur K, et al. Cell proliferation studies in primary synovial chondromatosis. *J Pathol* 1998;184:18–23.
106. Shpitzer T, Ganel A, Engelberg S. Surgery for synovial chondromatosis: 26 cases followed up for 6 years. *Acta Orthop Scand* 1990;61:567–569.
107. Okada Y, Awaya G, Ikeda T, et al. Arthroscopic surgery for synovial chondromatosis of the hip. *J Bone Joint Surg* 1989; 71B:198–199.
108. Nuovo MA, Desai P, Shankman S, et al. Intracapsular paraarticular chondroma of the knee. *Bull Hosp Jt Dis* 1990;50:189–194.

109. Steiner GC, Meushar N, Norman A, et al. Intracapsular and paraarticular chondromas. *Clin Orthop* 1994;303:231–236.
110. Watson WL, McCarthy WD. Blood and lymph vessel tumors. A report of 1056 cases. *Surg Gynecol Obstet* 1940;71:569–585.
111. Drolet BA, Esterly NB, Frieden IJ. Hemangiomas in children. *N Engl J Med* 1999;341:173–181.
112. Greenspan A, Azouz EM, Matthews J 2nd, et al. Synovial hemangioma: imaging features in eight histologically proven cases, review of the literature, and differential diagnosis. *Skeletal Radiol* 1995;24:583–590.
113. Ryd L, Stenstrom A. Hemangioma mimicking meniscal injury. A report of 10 years of knee pain. *Acta Orthop Scand* 1989; 60:230–231.
114. Berry SA, Peterson C, Mize W, et al. Klippel-Trenaunay syndrome. *Am J Med Genet* 1998;79:319–326.
115. El-Dessouky M, Azmy AF, Raine PAM, et al. Kasabach-Merritt syndrome. *J Pediatr Surg* 1988;23:109–111.
116. Seo SK, Suh JC, Na GY, et al. Kasabach-Merritt syndrome: identification of platelet trapping in a tufted angioma by immunohistochemistry technique using monoclonal antibody to CD61. *Pediatr Dermatol* 1999;16:392–394.
117. Greenspan A, McGahan JP, Vogelsang P, et al. Imaging strategies in the evaluation of soft-tissue hemangiomas of the extremities: correlation of the findings of plain radiography, angiography, CT, MRI, and ultrasonography in 12 histologically proven cases. *Skeletal Radiol* 1992;21:11–18.
118. Resnick D, Oliphant M. Hemophilia-like arthropathy of the knee associated with cutaneous and synovial hemangiomas. *Radiology* 1975;114:323–326.
119. Ehara S, Sone M, Tamakawa Y, et al. Fluid-fluid levels in cavernous hemangioma of soft tissue. *Skeletal Radiol* 1994;23: 107–109.
120. Nakashima Y, Kotoura Y, Kasakura K, et al. Alveolar soft-part sarcoma. *Clin Orthop* 1993;294:259–266.
121. Temple HT, Scully SP, O'Keefe RJ, et al. Clinical presentation of alveolar soft-part sarcoma. *Clin Orthop* 1994;300:213–218.
122. Sullivan CR, Dahlin DC, Bryan RS. Lipoma of the tendon sheath. *J Bone Joint Surg* 1956;38A:1275–1280.
123. Placeo F, Tassi D. Clinical considerations regarding 62 cases of posttraumatic lipoma arborescens of the knee, with or without a meniscal lesion. *Minerva Chir* 1953;8:316–322.
124. Hubscher O, Costanza E, Elsner B. Chronic monoarthritis due to lipoma arborescens. *J Rheumatol* 1990;17:861–862.
125. Soler T, Rodriguez E, Bargiela A, et al. Lipoma arborescens of the knee: MR characteristics in 13 joints. *J Comput Assist Tomogr* 1998;22:605–609.
126. Kloen P, Keel SB, Chandler HP, et al. Lipoma arborescens of the knee. *J Bone Joint Surg* 1998;80B:298–301.
127. Narváez J, Narváez JA, Ortega R, et al. Lipoma arborescens of the knee. *Rev Rhum* (English edition) 1999;66:351–353.
128. Hoffa A. The influence of the adipose tissue with regard to the pathology of the knee joint. *JAMA* 1904;43:795–796.
129. Ogata K, Ushijima M. Tendosynovial fibroma arising from the posterior cruciate ligament. *Clin Orthop* 1987;215:153–155.
130. Chung EB, Enzinger FM. Fibroma of tendon sheath. *Cancer* 1979;44:1945–1954.
131. Millon SJ, Bush DC, Garbes AD. Fibroma of tendon sheath in the hand. *J Hand Surg* 1994;19A:788–793.
132. Evangelisti S, Reale V. Fibroma of tendon sheath as a cause of carpal tunnel syndrome. *J Hand Surg* 1992;17A:1026–1027.
133. Meis JM, Enzinger FM. Juxta-articular myxoma: a clinical and pathologic study of 65 cases. *Hum Pathol* 1992;23:639–646.
134. McKinney CD, Mills SE, Fechner R. Intraarticular synovial sarcoma. *Am J Surg Pathol* 1992;16:1017–1020.
135. Enzinger FM. Clear-cell sarcoma of tendons and aponeuroses. An analysis of 21 cases. *Cancer* 1965;18:1163–1174.
136. Enzinger FM. Epithelioid sarcoma. A sarcoma simulating a granuloma or a carcinoma. *Cancer* 1970;26:1029–1041.
137. Haagensen CD, Stout AP. Synovial sarcoma. *Ann Surg* 1944;120:826–842.
138. Cadman NL, Soule EH, Kelly P. Synovial sarcoma. An analysis of 134 tumors. *Cancer* 1965;18:613–627.
139. Soule EH. Synovial sarcoma. *Am J Surg Pathol* 1986;10(suppl 1):78–82.
140. Brodsky JT, Burt ME, Hajdu SI, et al. Tendosynovial sarcoma. Clinicopathologic features, treatment and prognosis. *Cancer* 1992;70:484–489.
141. Fisher C. Synovial sarcoma. *Ann Diagn Pathol* 1998;2:401–421.
142. Skytting BT, Bauer HCF, Larsson O. Diagnosis, treatment and prognosis of patients with synovial sarcoma. *Acta Orthop Scand* 1999;70(suppl 285):47–49.
143. Witkin GB, Miettinen M, Rosai J. A biphasic tumor of the mediastinum with features of synovial sarcoma. A report of four cases. *Am J Surg Pathol* 1989;13:490–499.
144. Pai S, Chinoi RF, Pradhan SA, et al. Head and neck synovial sarcomas. *J Surg Clin Oncol* 1993;54:82–86.
145. Al-Rikabi AC, Diab AR, Buckai A, et al. Primary synovial sarcoma of the penis- case report and literature review. *Scand J Urol Nephrol* 1999;33:413–415.
146. Chesser TJ, Geraghty JM, Clarke AM. Intraneural synovial sarcoma of the median nerve. *J Hand Surg* 1999;24B:373–375.
147. Milchgrub S, Ghandur-Mnaymneh L, Dorfman HD, et al. Synovial sarcoma with extensive osteoid and bone formation. *Am J Surg Pathol* 1993;17:357–363.
148. Traweek ST, Rotter AJ, Swartz W, et al. Cystic pulmonary metastatic sarcoma. *Cancer* 1990;65:1805–1811.
149. Guarino M, Christensen L. Immunohistochemical analysis of extracellular matrix components in synovial sarcoma. *J Pathol* 1994;172:279–286.
150. Ghadially FN. Is synovial sarcoma a carcinosarcoma of connective tissue? *Ultrastruct Pathol* 1987;11:147–151.
151. Lopes JM, Bjerkehagen B, Sobrinho-Simoes M, et al. The ultrastructural spectrum of synovial sarcomas: a study of the epithelial type differentiation of primary tumors, recurrences, and metastases. *Ultrastruct Pathol* 1993;17:137–151.
152. Sreekantaiah C, Ladanyi M, Rodriguez E, et al. Chromosomal aberrations in soft tissue tumors. Relevance to diagnosis, classification, and molecular mechanisms. *Am J Pathol* 1994;144: 1121–1134.
153. Toolanen G, Lorentzen R, Friberg S, et al. Sonography of popliteal masses. *Acta Orthop Scand* 1988;59:294–296.
154. Gustafson P, Dreinhofer KE, Rydholm A. Soft tissue sarcoma should be treated at a tumor center. A comparison of the quality of surgery in 375 patients. *Acta Orthop Scand* 1994;65: 47–50.
155. Peabody TD, Gibbs CP Jr, Simon MA. Evaluation and staging of musculoskeletal neoplasms. *J Bone Joint Surg* 1998;80A: 1204–1218.
156. Jones BC, Sundaram M, Kransdorf MJ. Synovial sarcoma: MR imaging findings in 34 patients. *AJR* 1993;161:827–830.
157. Varela-Durán J, Enzinger FM. Calcifying synovial sarcoma. *Cancer* 1982;50:345–352.
158. Jensen OM, Hogh J, Ostgaard SE, et al. Histopathological grading of soft tissue tumours. Prognostic significance in a prospective study of 278 consecutive cases. *J Pathol* 1991;163:19–24.
159. Saddegh MK, Lindholm J, Lundberg A, et al. Staging of soft-tissue sarcomas. Prognostic analysis of clinical and pathologic features. *J Bone Joint Surg* 1992;74B:495–500.
160. Peabody TD, Monson D, Montag A, et al. A comparison of the prognoses for deep and subcutaneous sarcomas of the extremities. *J Bone Joint Surg* 1994;76A:1167–1173.
161. Bergh P, Meis-Kindblom JM, Gherlinzoni F, et al. Synovial sar-

comas: identification of low and high risk groups. *Cancer* 1999; 15:2596–2607.
162. Machen SK, Easley KA, Goldblum JR. Synovial sarcoma of the extremities: a clinicopathological study of 34 cases, including semi-quantitative analysis of spindled, epithelial, and poorly differentiated areas. *Am J Surg Pathol* 1999;23: 268–275.
163. Herbert SH, Corn BW, Solin LJ, et al. Limb-preserving treatment for soft tissue sarcomas of the extremities. *Cancer* 1993;72:1230–1238.
164. Rosenberg SA, Tepper J, Glatstein E, et al. The treatment of soft tissue sarcomas of the extremities. *Ann Surg* 1982;196:305–315.
165. Kampe CE, Rosen G, Eilber F, et al. Synovial sarcoma. A study of intensive chemotherapy in 14 patients with localized disease. *Cancer* 1993;72:2161–2169.
166. Rosen G, Forscher C, Lowenbraun S, et al. Synovial sarcoma. Uniform response of metastases to high dose ifosfamide. *Cancer* 1994;73:2506–2511.
167. van Geel AN, van Coevorden F, Blankensteijn JD, et al. Surgical treatment of pulmonary metastases from soft tissue sarcomas: a retrospective study in the Netherlands. *J Surg Oncol* 1994;56:172–177.
168. Chung EB, Enzinger FM. Malignant melanoma of soft parts. A reassessment of clear cell sarcoma. *Am J Surg Pathol* 1983;7: 405–413.
169. Lucas DR, Nascimento AG, Sim FH. Clear cell sarcoma of soft tissues. Mayo Clinic experience with 35 cases. *Am J Surg Pathol* 1992;16:1197–1204.
170. Mii Y, Miyauchi Y, Hohnoki K, et al. Neural crest origin of clear cell sarcoma of tendons and aponeuroses. *Virchows Arch [A]* 1989;415:51–60.
171. Graadt van Roggen JF, Mooi WJ, Hogendoorn PC. Clear cell sarcoma of tendons and aponeuroses (malignant melanoma of soft parts). And cutaneous melanoma: exploring the histogenetic relationship between these two clinicopathological entities. *J Pathol* 1998;186:3–7.
172. Chinoi RF, Jadav J. Clear cell sarcomas of the tendon sheath. An experience of 22 cases seen over 16 years. *Indian J Cancer* 1989;26:164–174.
173. Sara AS, Evans HL, Benjamin RS. Malignant melanoma of soft parts (clear cell sarcoma). A study of 17 cases, with emphasis on prognostic factors. *Cancer* 1990;65:367–374.
174. Chase DR, Weiss SW, Enzinger FM, et al. Keratin in epithelioid sarcoma. An immunohistochemical study. *Am J Surg Pathol* 1984;8:435–441.
175. Daimaru Y, Hashimoto H, Tsuneyoshi M, et al. Epithelial profile of epithelioid sarcoma. Immunohistochemical analysis of eight cases. *Cancer* 1987;59:134–141.
176. Arber DA, Kandalaft PL, Mehta P, et al. Vimentin-negative epithelioid sarcoma. *Am J Surg Pathol* 1993;17:302–307.
177. Steinberg BD, Gelberman RH, Mankin HJ, et al. Epithelioid sarcoma in the upper extremity. *J Bone Joint Surg* 1992;74A:28–35.
178. Case 43-1983. *N Engl J Med* 1983;309:1042–1049.
179. Simon MA, Hecht JD. Invasion of joints by primary bone sarcomas in adults. *Cancer* 1982;50:1649–1655.
180. McGirr EE, Edmonds JP. Ewing's sarcoma presenting as monoarthritis. *J Rheumatol* 1984;11:534–536.
181. Folkman J, Klagsburn M. Angiogenic factors. *Science* 1987;235: 442–447.
182. Lagier R. Synovial reaction caused by adjacent malignant tumors: anatomopathological study of three cases. *J Rheumatol* 1977;4:65–72.
183. Ozaki T, Lindner N, Hillmann A, et al. Transarticular invasion of iliopelvic sarcomas into the sacrum. Radiological analysis of 47 cases. *Acta Orthop Scand* 1997;68:381–383.
184. Goldenberg DL, Kelley W, Gibbons RB. Metastatic adenocarcinoma of synovium presenting as acute arthritis: diagnosis by closed synovial biopsy. *Arthritis Rheum* 1975;18:107–110.
185. Fam AG, Kolin A, Lewis AJ. Metastatic carcinomatous arthritis and carcinoma in the lung: a report of two cases diagnosed by synovial fluid cytology. *J Rheumatol* 1980;7:98–104.
186. Murray GC, Persellin RH. Metastatic carcinoma presenting as monoarticular arthritis: a case report and review of the literature. *Arthritis Rheum* 1980;23:95–100.
187. Weinblatt ME, Karp GI. Monoarticular arthritis: early manifestations of a rhabdomyosarcoma. *J Rheumatol* 1981;8:685–688.
188. Thompson KS, Reyes CV, Jensen J, et al. Synovial metastasis: diagnosis by fine-needle aspiration cytologic investigation. *Diagn Cytopathol* 1996;15:334–337.
189. Tandogan RN, Aydogan U, Demirhan B, et al. Intra-articular metastatic melanoma of the right knee. *Arthroscopy* 1999; 15:98–102.
190. Colson GM, Willcox A. Phalangeal metastases in bronchogenic carcinoma. *Lancet* 1948;1:100–102.
191. Vaezy A, Budson DC. Phalangeal metastases from bronchogenic carcinoma. *JAMA* 1978;239:226–227.
192. Amadio PC, Lombardi RM. Metastatic tumors of the hand. *J Hand Surg* 1987;12A:311–316.
193. Zindrick MR. Metastatic tumors of the foot. *Clin Orthop* 1982;170:219–225.
194. Besser E, Roessner A, Brug E, et al. Bone tumors of the hand. A review of 300 cases documented in the Westphalian Bone Tumor Register. *Arch Orthop Trauma Surg* 1987;106: 241–247.
195. Ritch PS, Hansen RM, Collier D. Metastatic renal cell carcinoma presenting as shoulder arthritis. *Cancer* 1983;51:968–972.
196. Rozboril MB, Good AE, Zarbo RJ, et al. Sternoclavicular joint arthritis: an unusual presentation of metastatic carcinoma. *J Rheumatol* 1983;10:499–502.
197. Newcomer LN, Silverstein MB, Cadman EC, et al. Bone involvement in Hodgkin's disease. *Cancer* 1982;49:338–342.
198. Rice DM, Semble E, Ahl ET, et al. Primary lymphoma of bone presenting as monoarthritis. *J Rheumatol* 1984;11:851–854.
199. Barton A, Hickling P. Synovial involvement in Hodgkin's disease. *Br J Rheumatol* 1986;25:391–392.
200. Dorfman HD, Siegel HL, Perry MC, et al. Non-Hodgkin's lymphoma of the synovium simulating rheumatoid arthritis. *Arthritis Rheum* 1987;30:155–161.
201. Hicks DG, Gokan T, O'Keefe RJ, et al. Primary lymphoma of bone. *Cancer* 1995;75:973–980.
202. Mulligan ME, McRae GA, Murphey MD. Imaging features of primary lymphoma of bone. *AJR* 1999;173:1691–1697.
203. Toussirot E, Gallinet E, Auge B, et al. Anterior chest wall malignancies. A review of ten cases. *Rev Rhum* (English edition) 1998;65:397–405.
204. Mariette X, de Roquancourt A, d'Agay M-F, et al. Monoarthritis revealing non-Hodgkin's T cell lymphoma of the synovium. *Arthritis Rheum* 1988;31:571–572.
205. Savin H, Zimmermann B III, Aaron RK, et al. Seronegative symmetric polyarthritis in Sezary syndrome. *J Rheumatol* 1991; 18:464–467.
206. Peeva E, Davidson A, Keiser HD. Synovial non-Hodgkin lymphoma in a human immunodeficiency virus infected patient J Rheumatol 1999;26:696–698.
207. Campanella N, Moraca A, Pergolini M, et al. Paraneoplastic syndromes in 68 cases of resectable non-small cell lung carcinoma: can they help in early detection? *Med Oncol* 1999;16: 129–133.
208. Naschitz JE, Rosner I, Rozenbaum M, et al. Rheumatic syndromes: clues to occult neoplasia. *Semin Arthritis Rheum* 1999; 29:43–55.
209. Schumacher HR Jr. Articular manifestations of hypertrophic

pulmonary osteoarthropathy in bronchogenic carcinoma. *Arthritis Rheum* 1976;19:629–636.

210. Martínez-Lavín M. Hypertrophic osteoarthropathy. In: Klippel JH, Dieppe PA. *Rheumatology*, 2nd ed. London: CV Mosby, 1998:8.46.1–4.
211. Good AE, Schnitzer B, Kawanishi H, et al. Acinar pancreatic tumor with metastatic fat necrosis: report of a case review of rheumatic manifestations. *Am J Dig Dis* 1976;21:978–987.
212. Mullin GT, Caperton E, Crespin S, et al. Arthritis and skin lesions resembling erythema nodosum in pancreatic disease. *Ann Intern Med* 1968;68:75–87.
213. Simkin PA, Brunzell JD, Wisner D, et al. Free fatty acids in the pancreatic arthritis syndrome. *Arthritis Rheum* 1983;26: 127–132.
214. van Klaveren RJ, de Mulder PH, Boerbooms AM, et al. Pancreatic carcinoma with polyarthritis, fat necrosis, and high serum lipase and trypsin activity. *Gut* 1990;31:953–955.
215. Agarwal N, Pitchumoni CS. Acute pancreatitis: a multisystem disease. *Gastroenterologist* 1993;115–128.
216. Dahl PR, Su WP, Cullimore KC, et al. Pancreatic panniculitis. *J Am Acad Dermatol* 1995;33:413–417.
217. Mackenzie AH, Sherbel AL. Connective tissue syndromes associated with carcinoma. *Geriatrics* 1963;18:745–753.
218. Sheon RP, Kirsner AB, Tangsintanapas P, et al. Malignancy in rheumatic disease: inter-relationships. *J Am Geriatr Soc* 1977; 25:20–27.
219. Strandberg B. Rheumatoid arthritis and cancer arthritis. *Scand J Rheumatol* 1974;5(suppl):1–14.
220. Litwin SD, Allen JC, Kunkel HG. Disappearance of the clinical and serological manifestations of rheumatoid arthritis following a thoracotomy for a lung tumor. *Arthritis Rheum* 1966; 9:865.
221. Bradley JD, Pinals RS. Carcinoma polyarthritis: role of immune complexes in pathogenesis. *J Rheumatol* 1983;10:826–828.
222. Cayla J, Rondier J, Leger JM, et al. Esophageal carcinoma revealed by acute polyarthritis. *Rev Rhum Mal Osteoartic* 1981;48:595–600.
223. Burki F, Treves R. Polyarthritis and esophageal carcinoma. *Rev Rhum Mal Osteoartic* 1986;53:547–549.
224. Chaun H, Robinson CE, Sutherland WH, et al. Polyarthritis associated with gastric carcinoma. *Can Med Assoc J* 1984;131: 909–911.
225. Simon RD, Ford LE. Rheumatoid-like arthritis associated with colonic carcinoma. *Arch Intern Med* 1980;140:698–700.
226. Chan MK, Hendrickson CS, Taylor KE. Polyarthritis associated with breast carcinoma. *West J Med* 1982;137:132–133.
227. Kahn MF, Ryckewaert A, Cannat A, et al. Systemic lupus erythematosus and ovarian dysgerminoma: remission of the systemic lupus erythematosus after extirpation of the tumor. *Clin Exp Immunol* 1966;1:355–359.
228. Bennett RM, Ginsberg MH, Thomsen S. Carcinomatous polyarthritis: the presenting symptoms of an ovarian tumor and association with a platelet activating factor. *Arthritis Rheum* 1976;19:953–958.
229. Cai Q, Hodgson SF, Kao PC, et al. Inhibition of renal phosphate transport by a tumor product in a patient with oncogenic osteomalacia. *N Engl J Med* 1994;330:1645–1649.
230. Nelson AE, Robinson BG, Mason RS. Oncogenic osteomalacia: is there a new phosphate regulating hormone? *Clin Endocrinol* 1997;47:635–642.
231. Zura RD, Minasi JS, Kahler DM. Tumor-induced osteomalacia and symptomatic Looser zones secondary to mesenchymal chondrosarcoma. *J Surg Oncol* 1999;71:58–62.
232. Ultman JE. Hyperuricemia in disseminated neoplastic disease other than lymphomas and leukemias. *Cancer* 1962;15: 122–129.
233. Nanji AA, Mikhael NZ, Stewart DJ. Increase in serum uric acid level associated with cisplatin therapy. *Arch Intern Med* 1985; 145:2013–2014.
234. Morales M, García-Nieto V. Hypouricemia and cancer. A study of the mechanisms of renal urate wasting in two cases. *Oncology* 1996;53:345–348..
235. Plonk JW, Feldman JM. Carcinoid arthropathy. *Arch Intern Med* 1974;134:651–654.
236. Crisp AJ. Carcinoid arthropathy [letter]. *Br J Radiol* 1983;56: 782.
237. Bergin C, Stein HB, Boyko W, et al. Lymphomatoid granulomatosis presenting as polyarthritis. *J Rheumatol* 1984;11: 537–539.
238. Thomas R, Vuitch F, Lakhanpal S. Angiocentric T cell lymphoma maskerading as cutaneous vasculitis. *J Rheumatol* 1994; 21:760–762.
239. Nunnink JC, Krusinski PA, Yates JW. Multicentric reticulohistiocytosis and cancer: a case report and review of the literature. *Med Pediatr Oncol* 1985;13:273–279.
240. Medsger TA Jr, Dixon JA, Garwood VF. Palmar fasciitis and polyarthritis associated with ovarian carcinoma. *Ann Intern Med* 1982;96:424–431.
241. Pfinsgraff J, Buckingham RB, Killian PJ, et al. Palmar fasciitis and arthritis with malignant neoplasms: a paraneoplastic syndrome. *Semin Arthritis Rheum* 1986;16:118–125.
242. Eekhoff EM, van der Lubbe PA, Breedveld FC. Flexion contractures associated with a malignant neoplasm: "a paraneoplastic syndrome?" *Clin Rheumatol* 1998;17:157–159.
243. Massarotti EM, Liu NY, Mier J, et al. Chronic inflammatory arthritis after treatment with high-dose interleukin-2 for malignancy. *Am J Med* 1992;92:693–697.
244. Ueno Y, Sohma T. Alfa-interferon-induced nodular rheumatoid arthritis in renal cell carcinoma. *Ann Intern Med* 1992;117: 266–267.
245. Clavel G, Grados F, Cayrolle G, et al. Polyarthritis following intravesical BCG immunotherapy. Report of a case and review of 26 cases in the literature. *Rev Rhum* (English edition) 1999; 66:115–118.

107

PAINFUL SHOULDER AND THE REFLEX SYMPATHETIC DYSTROPHY SYNDROME

JEAN G. GISPEN

The main function of the shoulder is to place the hand in a functional position for grasping and seizing (1). As the upper extremity became prehensile and manipulative rather than weight bearing, humans and other primates evolved highly mobile shoulders (2). All primates have clavicles, which serve as struts to hold the shoulder girdle away from the body, slightly forward, thereby allowing the hand to be used efficiently in front of the body. The scapula is long and narrow, the acromion is large, and the deltoid is more powerful than in most animals, with a more distal insertion on the humerus. The humerus twisted as primates became erect, so that the bicipital groove is anterior, the scapula more dorsal than lateral, and the hand in a more useful position relative to the trunk (2,3). These evolutionary changes in the muscles and bones of the shoulder girdle gave humans a marvelously complex, enormously mobile, and fairly unstable shoulder.

ANATOMY

"The shoulder" refers to the glenohumeral joint, but in fact the four joints of the shoulder girdle move synchronously to allow effective hand placement, and all four joints are potential sites of pain or dysfunction. These joints are the sternoclavicular, the acromioclavicular, the glenohumeral, and the scapulothoracic.

The sternoclavicular joint is the shoulder girdle's only bony attachment to the axial skeleton. It can be thought of as the apex of an imaginary cone. The lateral clavicle sweeps in a circular arc at the base of the cone, while the medial clavicle glides in its socket at the sternoclavicular joint. It is an incongruous joint, formed by a sternal articular surface that is concave from above downward and slightly convex front to back, a fairly flat clavicular articular surface, and the cartilage of the first rib. An articular disc between the sternum and clavicle improves the fit of the joint. The disc is attached to the clavicle above and to the first costal cartilage below, making the sternoclavicular joint very stable (4,5).

The costoclavicular ligament is just lateral to the sternoclavicular joint, and prevents excessive elevation or protraction of the clavicle. The subclavius muscle is just lateral to the ligament, and performs the same functions.

The acromioclavicular joint lies at the lateral end of the clavicle and allows the acromion (and scapula) to rotate on the clavicle. It often contains an articular disc. Medial to the acromioclavicular joint, where the lateral third of the clavicle begins, is the coracoclavicular ligament. This broad ligament transmits force applied to the scapula to the medial two-thirds of the clavicle, and ensures that the clavicle and scapula move together as a unit in all large motions.

The sternoclavicular joint and acromioclavicular joint permit shrugging (elevation and depression of the shoulder girdle) as well as the leaning-forward posture of a seamstress and the exaggerated shoulders-back posture of military personnel (protraction and retraction of the shoulder girdle, respectively). In elevation of the arm above the head, movement at the sternoclavicular joint is seen in the first 90 degrees, with 4-degree elevation of the clavicle for every 10-degree elevation of the humerus. Movement at the acromioclavicular joint is important in the latter phase of abduction, above 135 degrees (6).

The acromion lies at the lateral end of the scapular spine and projects over the glenohumeral joint, protecting it posteriorly and superiorly from trauma. It and the coracoacromial ligament form a rigid arch overlying the glenohumeral joint (Fig. 107.1), and restricting upward motion of the humerus. There is just barely enough room beneath this arch for the joint capsule, the muscles of the rotator cuff, and the subacromial bursa. For abduction above 90 degrees, the humerus must rotate externally, so that the greater tuberosity can slip beneath the acromion. If this external rotation is impaired, the greater tuberosity hits the acromion, blocking further abduction. Full flexion of the arm requires internal rotation of the humerus, so that the lesser tuberosity of the humerus can slide beneath the coracoacromial ligament without abutting (7). The distance from the top of the humerus to the inferior surface of the acromion measures 9 to 10 mm on a standard anteroposterior radiograph of a normal shoulder. The space is slightly larger in men than in women, and in men decreases slightly with age (8).

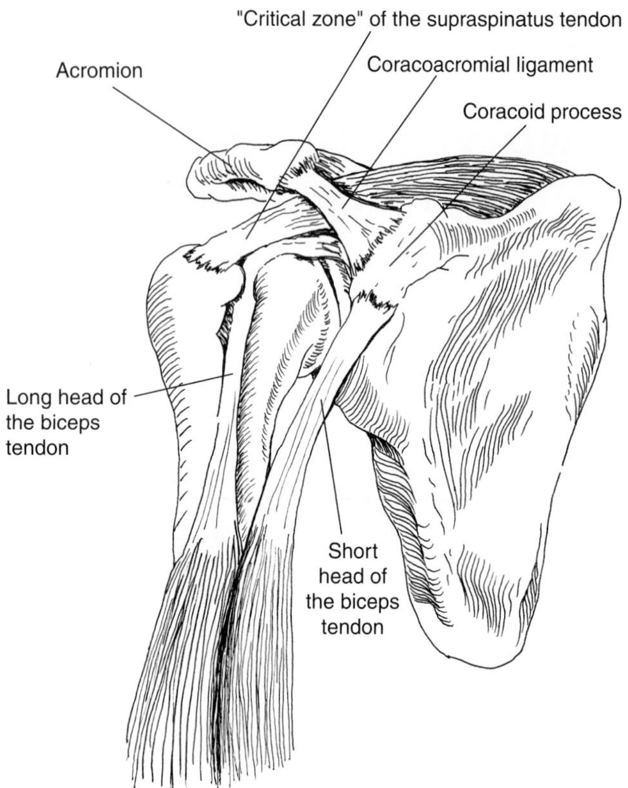

FIGURE 107.1. The glenohumeral joint, illustrating the relationships of the acromion, biceps tendon long and short heads, coracoacromial ligament, and the supraspinatus tendon.

The glenoid fossa is a very shallow, concave space, narrow superiorly and broader inferiorly. It tilts further anteriorly in humans than in other primates, hence predisposing to greater anterior instability (9). The humeral head is more convex than the glenoid is concave, which makes the glenohumeral joint incongruous (1). The humerus is not deeply seated in the glenoid fossa as the femoral head is seated within the acetabulum (10), but is held in place in its socket by the stabilizing rotator cuff muscles. The humeral head both rotates and glides (translates) within the glenoid fossa. As a multiaxial ball-and-socket joint, the glenohumeral joint rotates around many different centers with no static fulcrum. Only a small fraction of the humeral articular surface is in contact with the glenoid at a given time (9), and these contact points change with movement (11).

The glenoid fossa is surrounded by a fibrocartilaginous labrum, which effectively deepens the glenoid. The glenohumeral joint capsule arises from the labrum and inserts upon the anatomic neck of the humerus. Its volume, twice that of the humeral head (3,9), allows for the great mobility of the glenohumeral joint. Anteriorly the capsule thickens into three pleats, or folds, called the superior, middle, and inferior glenohumeral ligaments. These reinforce the capsule, and, together with the subscapularis muscle, protect against anterior dislocation of the humeral head (10,12).

The capsule is lined by synovium. The biceps tendon's long head, which runs within the bicipital groove between the greater and lesser tuberosities of the humerus and inserts on the superior glenoid fossa, is intracapsular but extrasynovial (1).

The muscles of greatest importance to the glenohumeral joint are the four muscles of the rotator cuff: supraspinatus, infraspinatus, teres minor, and subscapularis (Fig. 107.2), as well as the deltoid, the pectoral muscles, latissimus dorsi, and teres major. The supraspinatus originates above the spine of the scapula, runs beneath the coracoacromial ligament and directly above the glenohumeral joint to insert high on the greater tuberosity. It is innervated by the suprascapular nerve, from cervical roots C4, C5, and C6. The infraspinatus originates below the spine of the scapula, runs behind the glenohumeral joint, and inserts on the lateral tubercle. It also is innervated by the suprascapular nerve. The teres minor arises from the lateral border of the scapula and runs beside the infraspinatus to insert lower down on the lateral tubercle. These two muscles are external rotators of the humerus. Their tendons join with the supraspinatus tendon to form the rotator cuff. The fourth muscle of the rotator cuff, subscapularis, arises from the thoracic surface of the scapula and runs laterally to insert on the lesser tuberosity of the humerus. It has the most anterior and most medial insertion of the rotator cuff muscles, and it functions as an internal rotator of the humerus.

The rotator cuff muscles are even more important as stabilizers of the humeral head than they are as rotators of the glenohumeral joint. During abduction, they work together with the deltoid muscle in what is called a *force couple mechanism* (10). The infraspinatus, teres minor, and subscapularis hold the humeral head tightly compressed into the glenoid fossa and pull down on the humeral head, preventing upward subluxation by the deltoid muscle (13). The deltoid and supraspinatus work together throughout abduction (14), with maximal deltoid activity by electromyography (EMG) at 120-degree abduction and peak supraspinatus activity by EMG near 100-degree abduction (10). The del-

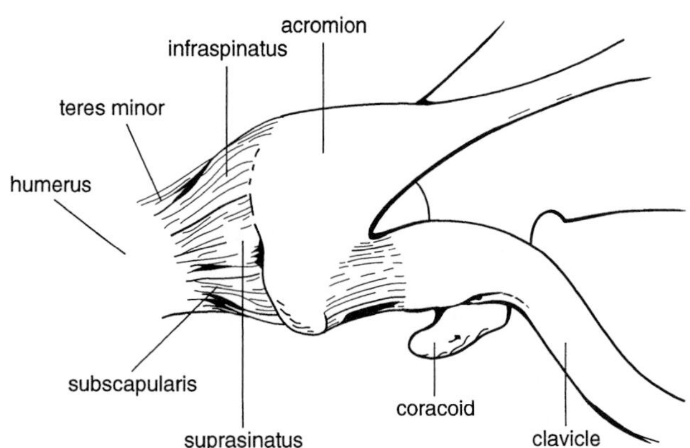

FIGURE 107.2. The rotator cuff viewed from above. (Courtesy of Dr. Franklin Kozin.)

toid can initiate abduction in a shoulder whose supraspinatus muscle is paralyzed (14).

The glenohumeral joint and the scapulothoracic joint move synchronously in what is termed scapulohumeral rhythm. In the plane of the scapula (a plane tilted 30 degrees anterior from the coronal plane), glenohumeral abduction accounts for 103 degrees and scapular movement 65 degrees during full abduction. The glenohumeral joint moves approximately 3 degrees (2.5 to 4 degrees) for every 2 degrees of scapular motion (6,9,15). If the scapulohumeral rhythm is abnormal and this ratio does not apply, usually the shoulder girdle has been injured (15).

The subacromial bursa allows the rotator cuff tendons to glide freely beneath the coracoacromial arch, without friction. The subdeltoid bursa, subcoracoid bursa, and supraspinatus bursa are extensions of the subacromial bursa, which serves as a secondary scapulohumeral joint or suprahumeral joint, separating the humerus from the fibroosseous coracoacromial arch (3). The bursa does not communicate with the glenohumeral joint unless there is a full-thickness rotator cuff tear.

Six major arteries supply the shoulder. The suprascapular, anterior circumflex humeral, and posterior circumflex humeral arteries are always present, while the thoracoacromial, suprahumeral, and subscapular arteries are more variable (3,9). The supraspinatus tendon has a critical zone of hypovascularity about 1 cm proximal to its insertion on the humerus (9,16). This is a zone where small collaterals anastomose, but in the anatomic position of adduction, neutral rotation, and a dependent arm, the anastomoses are compressed by the stretching of the tendon over the underlying humeral head, and this area becomes ischemic (16). Contraction of the supraspinatus muscle (whose tendon is flat and whose blood supply runs longitudinally primarily) also compresses the anastomotic area (1,16). The critical zone is hyperemic when the arm is passively supported and the rotator cuff muscles relaxed (1). The zone is mechanically squeezed between the humerus and the coracoacromial arch during glenohumeral abduction. This area of repeated mechanical impingement and recurring ischemia is the site of initial degenerative changes in the supraspinatus tendon and the most common site of rotator cuff tear.

EPIDEMIOLOGY

Shoulder pain is a common musculoskeletal complaint, roughly equal in incidence to neck pain (17). It could be anticipated in those athletes or laborers who perform repetitive overarm movements. Shipyard welders, for example, have an 18.3% prevalence of rotator cuff tendinitis, and steel plate workers a 16.2% prevalence (18). What is perhaps unanticipated and not generally recognized is the high frequency of shoulder pain and resultant disability in the general population.

Of 400 randomly selected adults in Great Britain, 135 reported shoulder pain at that moment or during the preceding month (19). Twenty-one of 100 hospitalized patients over age 70 described shoulder pain, though only 3 of the 21 (14%) had ever sought medical treatment for the pain (20); 170 (26%) of 644 nonhospitalized elderly reported shoulder symptoms, with 136 (21%) having identifiable shoulder disorders, mostly related to the rotator cuff. Fewer than 40% of the 136 persons with shoulder disease had consulted their primary care physicians, and of these, only 40% received any treatment for the pain, despite high levels of disability; 93 of the 136 had pain at night, 65 had pain at rest, 83 had difficulty with washing or personal care, 73 had difficulties with housework, and 108 had problems with lifting or with working above shoulder height (21).

Chakravarty and Webley (22) studied 100 apparently healthy adults over age 64; 24 had symptoms involving the shoulder girdle, and 10 more had clinical signs of shoulder disease. Clinical diagnoses included glenohumeral osteoarthritis, rotator cuff tendinitis or tear, and acromioclavicular osteoarthritis; 16 of the 34 with shoulder disorders had consulted their general practitioners more than twice. Treatments offered included nonsteroidal antiinflammatory drugs (NSAIDs) and physical therapy, but no one received intraarticular steroids. Ten of the 16 were told that their symptoms were incurable because of age.

Winters and co-workers (23) studied 101 patients seeing general practitioners in Groningen, the Netherlands, with shoulder pain; 51% of patients still had complaints at 26 weeks, though 80% felt cured (that is, there were no symptoms or the symptoms were so mild that they didn't interfere with normal work activities, the symptoms were no longer inconvenient, and the patients felt no treatment was needed); 41% of patients still had complaints at 12 to 18 months, but again 80% felt cured. That so many patients who still had complaints felt cured is very consistent with the known fact that many patients have shoulder pain for which they never seek medical care.

In another study, 544 people who sought orthopedic care for one of five common shoulder conditions (anterior glenohumeral instability, complete reparable rotator cuff tear, frozen shoulder, glenohumeral osteoarthritis, or impingement) filled out the SF-36 Health Survey, which measures the impact of disease on a person's perception of his own health. Compared with the United States norms for the general population, these patients had significant decreases in physical functioning, role–physical (which measures problems with work or other activities of daily living because of physical health), bodily pain, social functioning, and role–emotional (which measures problems with work or other daily activities because of emotional problems) (24). These results emphasize the effect chronic musculoskeletal pain or the inability to put on a shirt easily has on one's sense of physical and emotional well-being.

EXAMINATION

Appropriate therapy of shoulder disease rests upon an accurate diagnosis. This is not always easily achieved clinically. Winter and co-workers (25) reported only a 60% diagnostic agreement between two carefully trained, experienced physiotherapists who independently examined 201 patients with shoulder pain after taking the history jointly. They found it especially difficult to define the anatomic site of the problem in patients with severe pain, chronic complaints, and bilateral involvement. In a study by Bamji and colleagues (26), three consultant rheumatologists agreed on the diagnosis of shoulder disease in fewer than 50% of the cases. An accurate clinical diagnosis of shoulder pain (without the help of imaging) can be difficult and is not always possible, but the effort is aided by a thorough examination and an awareness by the examiner of the potential pathologic entities and their ramifications for the patient.

Examination of the shoulder begins with a careful, detailed history. Where is the pain precisely? When did the pain begin? Was the onset sudden or gradual and insidious? Was trauma involved or is there a history of chronic (over)use? What exacerbates the pain, and what alleviates the pain? Does it occur with motion, at rest, or at night? What movements are involved in work, hobbies, or sports? Can the patient reproduce the motion or motions that cause or aggravate the pain? Is the shoulder stiff, unstable, or weak? Are there underlying systemic illnesses? Are other joints involved?

TABLE 107.1. DISEASES AFFECTING THE SHOULDER AND SHOULDER GIRDLE

- Rotator cuff disease
  - Subacromial impingement
  - Rotator cuff tendinitis
  - Rotator cuff tear
  - Cuff-tear arthropathy
  - Calcific tendinitis
- Subacromial bursitis
- Biceps disease
  - Tendinitis associated with impingement
  - Primary bicipital tendinitis
  - Dislocation, subluxation of tendon
  - Rupture of the biceps tendon
  - SLAP lesions
- Disorders of the shoulder capsule
  - Frozen shoulder (adhesive capsulitis)
  - Glenohumeral instability
- Disorders of the labrum
  - Labral tears, including SLAP lesions
  - Posterosuperior glenoid impingement
- Disorders of the glenohumeral joint
  - Osteoarthritis
    - Dislocation arthropathy
    - Capsulorrhaphy arthropathy
  - Rheumatoid arthritis
  - Crystal-induced arthritis
  - Spondyloarthropathies
  - Septic arthritis
  - Polymyalgia rheumatica
  - Cuff-tear arthropathy
    - Milwaukee shoulder
    - Idiopathic destructive arthritis
  - Avascular necrosis
- Disorders of the sternoclavicular joint
  - Septic arthritis
  - Sternocostoclavicular hyperostosis, SAPHO
  - Dislocations, subluxations
  - Systemic arthritides
- Disorders of the acromioclavicular joint
  - Osteoarthritis
  - Osteolysis of the distal clavicle
  - Systemic arthritides
- Disorders of soft tissue pain
  - Postural shoulder pain
  - Fibromyalgia
- Congenital anomalies
- Snapping scapula
- Disorders of muscles
  - Deltoid muscle contractures
  - Muscular dystrophy
  - Polymyositis
- Problems with bones
  - Fractures
  - Infections
- Shoulder pain of neurologic etiology
  - Neuralgic amyotrophy
  - Cervical radiculopathy
  - Brachial plexus lesions
  - Nerve palsies
  - Suprascapular nerve entrapment
  - Myelopathy or syringomyelia
    - Neuroarthropathy
  - Shoulder pain in quadriplegia, paraplegia
  - Shoulder pain in hemiplegia
- Shoulder pain of neurovascular etiology
  - Thoracic outlet syndrome
  - Reflex sympathetic dystrophy
- Neoplasm involving the shoulder girdle
- Referred pain from visceral disease
- Shoulder involvement in systemic disease
  - Amyloidosis
    - Hemodialysis arthropathy
  - Diabetes mellitus
  - Hyperparathyroidism
  - Ochronosis
  - Wilson's disease
  - Hemochromatosis
  - Alkaptonuria

SAPHO, synovitis acne pustulosis hyperostosis osteomyelitis syndrome; SLAP, superior labrum anterior posterior tears.

What adjectives describe the pain? Is it sharp, dull, knifelike, burning, constant, or intermittent? Burning, electric pain, or other paresthesias often indicate a neuropathic etiology.

It is helpful to think of possible etiologies of the shoulder pain during the patient interview and examination (Table 107.1). First, is the shoulder pain intrinsic or extrinsic? Extrinsic causes of pain generally are associated with painless full range of motion, and a shoulder girdle that is normal on inspection and palpation. Potential extrinsic etiologies include myocardial infarction, gallbladder disease, subphrenic abscess, splenic trauma, and neuropathies such as cervical radiculopathies or thoracic outlet syndrome. Intrinsic etiologies can be divided according to anatomic location. Does the pain arise in the glenohumeral capsule (too loose in the unstable shoulder or too tight in the frozen shoulder), in the rotator cuff tendons (tear, tendinitis, or impingement), in the biceps tendon (tendinitis, subluxation, or rupture), or in one of the four shoulder girdle joints (osteoarthritis, rheumatoid arthritis, infectious arthritis, or other arthritides)? Is the problem in the humerus (avascular necrosis, fracture, infection, or neoplasm) or in the soft tissues (postural or fibromyalgia)?

The patient should be examined sitting or standing, with both shoulders exposed and the shoulder girdle inspected. Are the glenohumeral, acromioclavicular, and sternoclavicular joints symmetrical? The physician should (a) look for swelling, erythema, abnormal deltoid contours, or bony enlargement; (b) look above and below the spine of the scapula for supraspinatus or infraspinatus atrophy, as one might see with a long-standing rotator cuff tear; (c) ask the patient to shrug; and (d) look for scapular winging as the patient does a pushup against the wall or in a corner; this suggests serratus anterior weakness.

Also, the biceps tendon should be palpated. When the arm is rotated 10 degrees internally, the bicipital groove lies anteriorly over the proximal humerus. The biceps tendon normally is somewhat tender to palpation, but check for asymmetry between the two arms as a possible indication of bicipital tendinitis. Check for pain over the biceps tendon when the muscle contracts against resistance, which might indicate bicipital tendinitis (Table 107.2).

Since shoulder pain can be referred from the neck, the cervical range of motion should be ascertained. Perform a careful neurologic exam of the upper extremities, particularly in the patient with weakness or paresthesias. Cervical radicular pain may radiate below the elbow to the hand, and may be completely relieved by elevating the arm above 120 degrees (2).

Examination for crepitus about the shoulder should be done. The sensation is one of fine gravel moving beneath the examining fingertips. Subacromial crepitus can be felt by putting the hand over the superior shoulder and rotating the slightly abducted arm internally and externally. Glenohumeral crepitus is felt about the glenoid as the adducted arm is rotated. Scapulothoracic crepitus is felt over the superomedial scapula as the arm is elevated or shoulder protracted.

Passive range of motion at the glenohumeral joint often exceeds the active range of motion in the patient with rotator cuff tendinitis or tear. Both passive and active range of motion are diminished in patients with adhesive capsulitis. To evaluate active range of motion, the examiner must observe the patient anteriorly, laterally, and posteriorly. Does the shoulder shrug with abduction? Patients do this to try to compensate for decreased glenohumeral movement of adhesive capsulitis, for the weakness associated with a rotator cuff tear, or for the painful arc associated with rotator cuff tendinitis or tear. The scapula elevates and rotates, but the humerus doesn't abduct or externally rotate normally. In general, intrinsic shoulder pain will disturb normal scapulohumeral rhythm, and this can be seen on active range of motion.

Shoulder range of motion should be assessed with the patient sitting, to eliminate compensatory and potentially confusing leg and lumbar spine movements. The patient (a) raises both arms sideways until the hands touch overhead to test abduction, (b) crosses straight arms in front of his chest to test adduction, (c) swings the arms forward and backward to test flexion and extension, (d) clasps the hands behind his neck to check both external rotation and abduction, and (e) should attempt to bring a thumb up the center of his back as high as he can as a convenient way to check internal rotation. Rotation also can be measured with the patient supine and the adducted arm and elbow close to the body, rotating the forearm toward the stomach (internal rotation) or away from the body (external rotation). Young patients should have a rotary arc of at least 70 degrees (2).

When testing abduction of the shoulder passively, the scapula should be fixed with one hand while moving the arm with the other hand. Normal abduction is 90 to 120 degrees. This normal range decreases with age. Changes in abduction and rotation at the glenohumeral joint are the best early indicators of glenohumeral joint pathology.

Specific provocative tests for impingement, for glenohumeral instability, for SLAP lesions (tears in the superior labrum extending anterior and posterior), for rotator cuff tears, and for bicipital tendinitis (Table 107.2) should be performed as indicated.

In the young patient with shoulder pain, look carefully for signs of instability, particularly if the pain is atraumatic. The older the patient is, the less likely the shoulder problem is caused by instability. Any patient over age 40 with prolonged shoulder pain and no obvious arthritis has rotator cuff tendinitis or tear until proven otherwise.

TABLE 107.2. PHYSICAL EXAMINATION PROVOCATIVE TESTS

Sign or Test	Suspected Diagnosis	Description
Impingement sign	Rotator cuff impingement	Pain with forced forward flexion to 180 degrees or further (Neer); pain with arm flexed to 90 degrees and internally rotated (Hawkins-Kennedy)
Impingement test	Rotator cuff impingement	Inject 10 mL 1% lidocaine in the subacromial space; repeat the impingement signs; if the pain is significantly lessened, this indicates impingement of the rotator cuff tendons between the humerus and the coracoacromial arch
Drop arm test	Rotator cuff tear	Arm is placed in maximum forward flexion, or above 90 degrees elevation in the plane midway between frontal and coronal planes; thumb is down; lower the arm slowly; if the arm drops suddenly, this suggests a rotator cuff tear (it is not pathognomonic); this test may be repeated after subacromial Xylocaine; in the setting of a rotator cuff tear, the arm still drops suddenly
Supraspinatus test	Supraspinatus tendinitis	Pain when the arm is held at 90-degree elevation in a plane between flexion and abduction against resistance
Yergason's test	Bicipital tendinitis	Arm flexed at the elbow, with forearm pronated; pain over the anterior, medial shoulder when the forearm is then supinated against resistance
Speed's test	Bicipital tendinitis	Arm is held with the forearm supinated and elbow extended; flexion of the arm against resistance causes pain
Painful arc	Rotator cuff impingement, tendinitis	Arm abducted (in the coronal plane); patient feels pain from 60 to 100 or 120 degrees, perhaps maximal about 90 degrees, as the inflamed rotator cuff tendons slide under the coracoacromial arch; slumped-shoulder posture causes the painful arc at lesser degrees of abduction
SLAPrehension test	Superior glenoid labral lesion	Arm flexed to 90 degrees and adducted across the chest, with elbow extended and forearm pronated; a positive test is one of apprehension, pain in the bicipital groove, and an audible or palpable clink; repeated test with the arm in supination is less painful (27)
Clunk test	Labral tear	Patient lies supine; arm externally rotated and extended; examiner moves shoulder into forward flexion and internal rotation; a clunking sensation suggests a free labral fragment caught between the glenoid and the humeral head, as does a "click" on manipulation of the glenohumeral joint (28)
Anterior slide test	Labral tear	Patient sits or stands; hands on hips, thumbs posterior; examiner puts one hand over shoulder, one behind elbow, then pushes anteriorly and superiorly against the flexed elbow; patient resists; pain/pop/click localized to the anterosuperior shoulder suggests superior glenoid labral tear (28)
Push-pull test	Glenohumeral instability	Patient sits; one hand of the examiner stabilizes the scapula; other hand pushes the proximal humerus forward and backward; normally the humeral head will move up to 50% of its diameter backward, but will not come forward
Posterior stability check	Glenohumeral instability	Examiner pushes posteriorly on proximal humerus when shoulder is relaxed, flexed, and abducted; translation of up to 50% of the humeral head diameter can be normal

(continued)

TABLE 107.2. (continued)

Sign or Test	Symptom	Description
Apprehension shoulder	Anterior glenohumeral stability	Patient is supine; one of the examiner's hands is under the shoulder; the arm is abducted, extended, and externally rotated; this is done *slowly* (this is the position of the arm in a swimmer's backstroke flip turn, the old way); is the patient apprehensive that the shoulder will "go out"?; if there is pain that is relieved by pushing backward on the anterior shoulder, the patient has a positive "relocation test" for anterior instability
Sulcus sign	Inferior glenohumeral instability	Examiner holds the seated patient's elbow and pulls inferiorly; if the skin dimples next to the acromion, it may indicate excessive inferior translation of the humeral head

ROTATOR CUFF DISEASE

Impingement

Impingement refers to the trapping of the rotator cuff tendons (and the long head of the biceps) between the underlying humeral head and the overlying coracoacromial arch as the arm is raised to an overhead position. Because use of the arm occurs primarily in front of the body, rather than to the side, impingement occurs against the anterior edge and the underside of the anterior third of the acromion, the coracoacromial ligament, and at times the acromioclavicular joint (29). Cadaver studies prove this, with osteophytes, roughness, and erosions found on the anteroinferior surface of the acromion, where the greater tuberosity has hit repeatedly during life. There is a finite space beneath the bony arch. Impingement may be caused by an increase in the volume of the tendons and subacromial bursa that run beneath the arch or by a diminution of the enclosed space, secondary to acromial shape, osteophytes, or superior migration of the humeral head in a patient with a rotator cuff tear (30). An acromion that is hooked or has a prominent anterior edge (Fig. 107.3), or an acromion that is less sloped is more prone to cause impingement, and impingement causes 95% of rotator cuff tears (29). Bigliani and Morrison (31,32) found that 70% of patients with surgically confirmed full-thickness rotator cuff tears and 70% of cadavers with rotator cuff tears had hooked acromions. Rounded, sloped-shoulder posture causes impingement at an earlier angle of abduction (1). Inflammation or edema of the rotator cuff tendons (which can be caused by impingement in the first place) worsens impingement by increasing the volume of the structures that must fit under the coracoacromial arch. Rheumatoid synovitis, synovial osteochondromatosis (33), or iatrogenic postsurgical thickening of the subacromial bursa can lead to impingement.

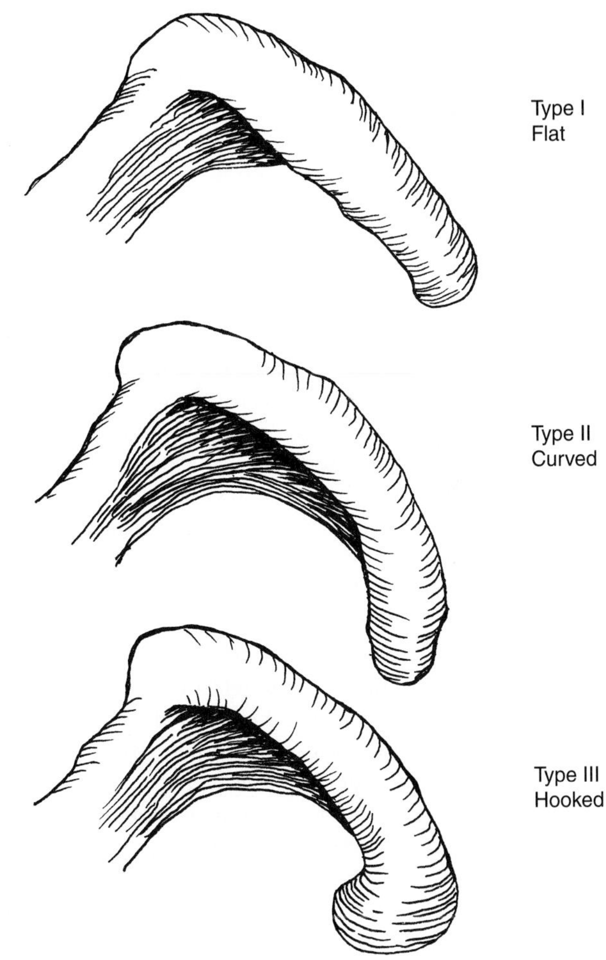

FIGURE 107.3. Potential shapes of the acromion. The lateral view demonstrates a flat, curved, or hooked anterior prominence. The hooked acromion is associated with a higher risk of impingement and rotator cuff tear.

The first clue to shoulder impingement is an insidious development of shoulder pain with overhead activity. A patient will often describe pain at a certain point in abduction or flexion of the arm, beyond which the pain disappears again. This "painful arc of motion" occurs between 60 and 120 degrees, when an inflamed rotator cuff or subacromial bursa tries to squeeze beneath the coracoacromial arch, as the arm is raised or lowered (34). Once the inflamed structure fully passes beneath the arch, the pain disappears, until the arm is brought back to its prior position and the inflamed tendons or bursa must pass beneath the coracoacromial arch again.

Two physical signs suggest impingement (Table 107.2). In the Neer maneuver, the patient's scapula is immobilized and the painful arm is passively flexed as far as it will go. This pinches the critical zone of the supraspinatus tendon between the anterior acromion and the greater tuberosity of the humerus. The patient grimaces or complains (29). (This maneuver can be done actively also, with the patient flexing the arm to 180 degrees, and the scapula free.) Hawkins and Kennedy (30) described pain when the arm is flexed to 90 degrees, then internally rotated. This pinches the critical zone against the coracoacromial ligament.

In the "impingement test," the examiner injects 10 cc of 1% Xylocaine subacromially. The local anesthesia relieves or dramatically decreases the painful arc of motion and the pain of the Neer and Hawkins-Kennedy maneuvers in the patient with impingement. Subacromial Xylocaine does not relieve the pain in patients with anterior subluxation, arthritis, calcific tendinitis, or shoulder stiffness.

Neer divided the impingement syndrome into three clinical stages. The separation into stages is somewhat artificial, as pathologic changes occur in a continuum, but the separation is useful in terms of thinking about treatment. Stage I is rotator cuff tendinitis. Histologically the changes are of edema and hemorrhage in the supraspinatus tendon. Typically these patients are younger than 25 years of age, but this stage can occur at any age. It is reversible, with time and conservative management. Pain occurs after exercise, but then resolves. Stage II is fibrosis and more severe tendinitis. The bursa becomes thickened and fibrotic. Some of this scarring may be irreversible. This is typical in laborers or athletes ages 25 to 40. The shoulder hurts during and after activity, and there may be night pain. Stage III lesions are partial or complete rotator cuff tears due to degenerative changes in the supraspinatus tendon resulting from many years of overarm use and impingement. The bony and tendinous changes are irreversible. The shoulder is stiff, weak, and continuously painful. Bicipital ruptures commonly accompany rotator cuff ruptures, as the biceps long head tendon also is squeezed, at the proximal end of the bicipital groove.

Rotator Cuff Tendinitis

Rotator cuff tendinitis is common, and is clinically defined as shoulder pain exacerbated by movement against resistance when the shoulder is abducted (supraspinatus tendinitis), externally rotated (infraspinatus tendinitis), or internally rotated (subscapularis tendinitis) (35). Active range of motion may be limited by pain, but passive range of motion is full.

One can divide the causes of rotator cuff tendinitis (or tendinopathy) into those extrinsic and intrinsic to the tendons themselves. The primary and most obvious extrinsic cause is impingement. Muscle imbalance about the shoulder due to glenohumeral instability or laxity or due to biceps or labral tears leads to an increased dependence on the rotator cuff muscles for stability. This can result in muscle fatigue and overuse tendinopathy. Trauma, either as a single event or as repeated microtraumas, can cause rotator cuff tendinitis. Intrinsic causes of tendinitis include the poor vascular supply of the critical zone, degenerative changes in the tendons associated with aging, and local calcium deposits worsening mechanical impingement and fanning inflammation (calcific tendinitis).

Rotator cuff tendinitis can develop in teenage athletes who overuse their arms in overhead positions, or in older athletes and laborers in response to overuse. It can occur spontaneously in persons aged 40 or above, with edema and inflammation superimposed on an aging tendon. Initially pain is felt only during active use of the shoulder, but the tendinitis can progress to cause pain during and after movement, and finally to cause continuous pain.

Chard and co-workers (36) studied the long-term course of 137 patients with rotator cuff tendinitis, finding more than 25% with persistent symptoms at 19-month follow-up, despite treatment. In this retrospective study, early treatment led to a better outcome.

The initial therapy is avoidance of aggravating activities and attention to good posture. Relief of pain is essential in order to restore normal motion and scapulohumeral rhythm, and to lessen the likelihood of a secondary adhesive capsulitis. NSAIDs are given commonly, and are effective in some patients (37,38), but often give no significant relief (36,38). Subacromial steroid injections should be given to those who do not respond to rest, physical therapy, and NSAIDs within several weeks (37,38). The effectiveness of this treatment, however, also is controversial (39). In one study, patients' pretreatment clinical status in terms of pain, function, and degrees of active abduction possible meant more in determining treatment outcome than did the type of therapy given (37). This argues strongly for early treatment of rotator cuff tendinitis.

In addition to rest of the shoulder, avoidance of painful movements, ice, heat, and possibly ultrasound, treatment must include physical therapy. This should begin with Codman pendular exercises (Fig. 107.4), in which the patient's active body movements result in passive shoulder range of motion exercises (1,40). The consequent motion at the glenohumeral joint prevents adhesion between adjacent inflamed structures and protects against frozen shoulder. Active range of

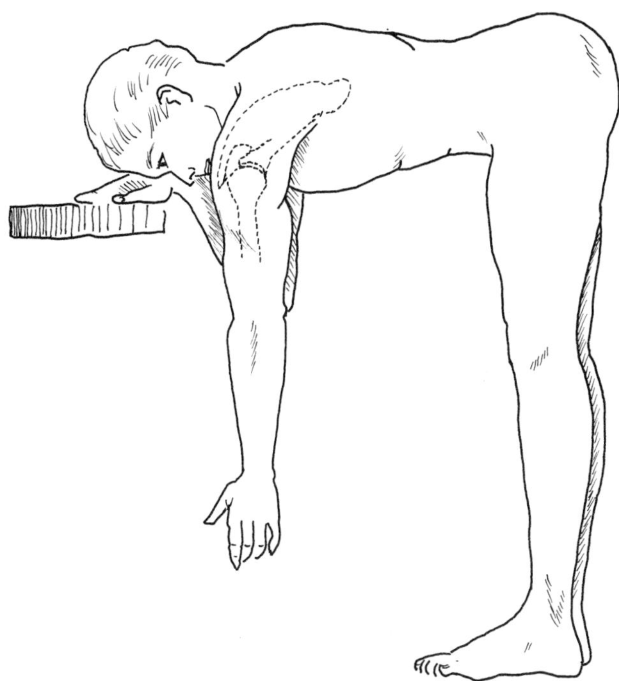

FIGURE 107.4. The position for Codman pendular exercises. The principle of the bent-forward position is that the arm is flexed by gravity, without the need for supraspinatus or deltoid contraction.

motion is avoided at first to minimize muscle contraction and impingement, which could worsen the tendinitis. The shoulder should be warmed immediately prior to the exercises. The patient must bend forward at the waist, with the affected arm dangling vertically. Knees are flexed. No weight is held in the hand. This puts the arm at almost 90-degree forward flexion, without any muscle contractions in the deltoid or rotator cuff. Gravity elongates the glenohumeral joint capsule slightly and pulls the humeral head slightly away from the glenoid. The body is then moved forward, backward, sideways, and in a circular motion, with the arm hanging passively. Because of the body's motions, the glenohumeral joint is extended, flexed, abducted, adducted, and rotated.

When the shoulder pain has subsided, the patient can begin active pendular exercises. These again should be done bending forward from the waist, with the involved arm hanging freely. The arm is swung front to back, side to side, and in circles, both clockwise and counterclockwise. "Walking the wall," both facing the wall and sideways to the wall, is another active stretching maneuver to help maintain or restore range of motion.

Rotator cuff strengthening exercises are added next, once the shoulder is pain-free, or almost pain-free (Table 107.3, Fig. 107.5). These should be done two to four times a day, keeping the arm below shoulder height to minimize impingement. The theory underlying rotator cuff exercises

TABLE 107.3. ROTATOR CUFF STRENGTHENING EXERCISES

1. Stand with your back and heels against the wall, arms hanging at the sides, palms in. Slowly bring the arm forward, as if you were goose-stepping. Take the arm up to just below shoulder height, hold briefly at the top, then lower slowly. Repeat ten times. A resistive flexion exercise is performed by standing on one end of a long length of tubing or Theraband. The injured arm holds the other end. The arm is slowly raised, with the elbow straight and the palm facing in, to just below shoulder level. Lower. Repeat.
2. Stand sideways to the wall, with the uninjured shoulder next to the wall. The palm of the free outside arm faces in. This arm is slowly abducted, held for an instant just below shoulder level, then lowered. Repeat ten times. This exercise, particularly if done in a plane 20 to 30 degrees anterior to the coronal plane, stresses the supraspinatus muscle. Be careful, especially if using resistive tubing, not to put too much stress on the supraspinatus, exacerbating tendinitis.
3. Lie on your side, and exercise the upper arm as follows. Bend the elbow to 90 degrees and keep the elbow tucked tightly against your waist. Begin with your arm across your chest, like Napoleon Bonaparte, then raise your forearm and hand off your chest until they are parallel to the floor. Hold briefly, lower. Repeat ten times. A resistive exercise to strengthen the infraspinatus (for external rotation) is done standing at right angles to a closed door, with the injured shoulder away from the door. Surgical tubing or Theraband is attached to the door handle. Reach across the front of the body to grasp the tubing with the outside hand. Pull the tubing back across the body, holding the upper arm tight against the lateral chest and the elbow bent, externally rotating against resistance, then passively internally rotating as the stretched tubing pulls the arm back to the starting position. Repeat.
4. Lie on your side as in exercise 3, but it is the underneath arm that exercises, internally rotating, then externally rotating back to the starting position. Again, do ten. To strengthen the subscapularis (for internal rotation) with resistive tubing, stand at right angles to the closed door, but this time the injured shoulder is near the door. Slowly pull the tubing across the body (actively internally rotating against resistance), then return to the beginning position (passively externally rotating). Repeat.

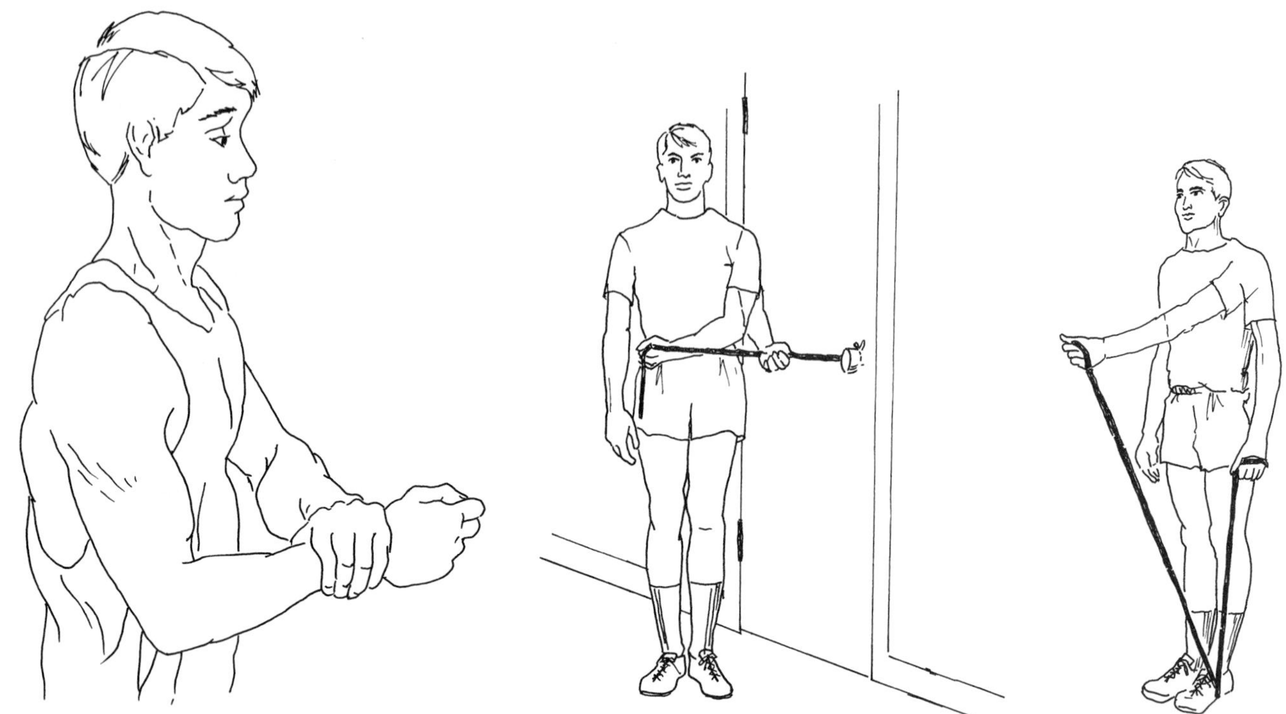

FIGURE 107.5. Strengthening exercises for the rotator cuff. Initially, the exercises are done isometrically. The patient tries to rotate the injured right arm against the resistance of the normal left hand and arm **(A)**. The injured left arm rotates internally **(B)** and flexes **(C)** against resistance provided by tubing.

is twofold: stronger muscles have a better blood supply and therefore can repair microtears quicker, and stronger rotator cuff muscles can better stabilize the glenohumeral joint.

If pain from rotator cuff tendinitis persists after 12 to 18 months' treatment, the physician must consider surgical options such as bursectomy, splitting of the coracoacromial ligament, or anterior acromioplasty.

Rotator Cuff Tear

Partial or complete rotator cuff tears represent Neer's stage III impingement lesions. Most commonly occurring in the critical zone of the supraspinatus tendon, rotator cuff tears disrupt the ability of these muscles to hold the humeral head firmly against the glenoid, leading to abnormal scapulohumeral rhythm, worsened impingement, and pain. Complete rotator cuff tears in cadavers are seen with a frequency of 5% overall (29) to 32% in cadavers above age 40 (41). Generally, tears are the culmination of years of degenerative changes, beginning with rotator cuff tendinitis and fibrosis. Tears seldom occur before age 40 in the absence of significant acute trauma, such as a fall on an outstretched arm. Typically, patients have a prolonged history of shoulder pain that interferes with overhead movements. Sometimes, but not always, they recall an acute traumatic episode that markedly worsened shoulder function. Associated bicipital findings and acromioclavicular tenderness are common. Clinically, one often finds supraspinatus and infraspinatus atrophy, with painful, limited abduction and external rotation. Passive range of motion exceeds active range of motion and can be full. Occasionally, a patient with a rotator cuff tear presents with a frozen shoulder, because the shoulder was so painful that the patient avoided movement. Acute rotator cuff tears in the absence of preceding shoulder symptoms are rare, accounting for only 8% in a Mayo Clinic series of 510 patients with tears (41).

A positive drop arm test strongly suggests a rotator cuff tear (Table 107.2). In this maneuver the arm is passively abducted to 90 degrees, then released. Persons with rotator cuff tears cannot hold the arm up, and it drops. No clinical sign is pathognomonic for rotator cuff tear. The classic picture of a person with a rotator cuff tear is someone over the age of 40 who feels a snap in the shoulder after a fall or a lifting strain and then develops severe pain and weakness or inability to move the joint. Some patients with rotator cuff tears, however, have pain but negative drop arm tests, no muscle atrophy, full range of motion without a painful arc, and no significant weakness (42).

Radiology

Radiographic findings on plain films are those of chronic impingement. They can include subacromial calcification, sclerosis or irregularity of the greater tuberosity, cystic changes in the upper two-thirds of the anatomic neck of the humerus, a concave acromion, subacromial osteophytes, and degenerative changes at the acromioclavicular joint (43). Narrowing of the acromiohumeral gap to 5 mm or less is highly suggestive of a (large) rotator cuff tear. This narrowing is partly due to the decreased thickness of rotator cuff tissues, but also may be due to an impaired balance between the deltoid and the rotator cuff forces, so that the deltoid overwhelms the rotator cuff and pulls the humeral head proximally (44).

Ultrasound is a good screening tool for rotator cuff tears, with favorable sensitivities and specificities compared with operative findings and arthrograms (45). If the ultrasound is negative but clinical symptoms imply a tear, an arthrogram or magnetic resonance imaging (MRI) should be performed. Positive arthrography shows escape of the contrast material outside the glenohumeral capsule, usually into the subacromial bursa. An arthrogram is cheaper than an MRI, but obviously painful and invasive. MRIs are very helpful in the diagnosis of rotator cuff tears, demonstrating the size of a tear, the amount of retraction, and even atrophy or scarring in the rotator cuff muscles (28), although it is at times difficult to distinguish partial tears from tendinitis. An MRI with the arm abducted can document impingement (46).

Treatment

Whether surgical or nonsurgical treatment of rotator cuff tear is optimal depends on the patient's age, function, pain, and treatment goals.

Pathologic specimens of partial supraspinatus tears show avascularity in the proximal stumps and hypervascularity distally with areas of granulation tissue. No histologic evidence of active repair is seen in the proximal stumps or in the space between the stumps (47). An experimentally notched tendon experiences increased tensile stress at the notch (48), which implies that partial tears inexorably will tear further. The hope underlying conservative, nonoperative treatment of rotator cuff tears is that rest and avoidance of impingement will allow tendons to heal, but the foregoing data indicate that the possibility of spontaneous healing is extremely low. It may be that when conservative treatment is successful, the patient simply has learned to compensate for the torn tendon through strengthening of other muscles.

The natural history of unrepaired rotator cuff tears is not known. Some patients have minimal difficulties with shoulder pain, weakness, or loss of function. Other patients, estimated at 4% of those with complete rotator cuff tears, progress to the debilitating cuff-tear arthropathy (49). Persons with massive tears perhaps are more likely to progress to the arthropathy, but other prognostic factors are not known.

Conservative treatment of a rotator cuff tear is as described for rotator cuff tendinitis with rest, avoidance of aggravating motions, NSAIDs, range of motion exercises, and rotator cuff strengthening exercises. The use of subacromial or intraarticular steroids is debated, with some authors claiming benefit and others no benefit (50). If success is defined as slight or no pain, even though the shoulder may be weak, conservative treatment of rotator cuff tears is successful in 44% to 74% (51–53). For an elderly person who has a high surgical or anesthetic risk, these chances and this definition of success may be enough. An athlete or a laborer who desires not only pain relief but also maximal function and strength is better served surgically.

Those unusual patients with a massive acute tear and sudden shoulder weakness (in the absence of prior shoulder symptoms) are offered early surgical repair, in hopes that there are few degenerative changes in the tendon and that a primary repair of the tendon is possible. Strength and return of motion are better if the repair is done within 3 to 6 weeks of the injury (41).

In patients with chronic shoulder pain culminating in a rotator cuff tear, conservative treatment is given for 6 to 12 months (29,42) before surgical treatment is offered. Anterior (54) or anteroinferior acromioplasty (55) with excision of the coracoacromial ligament is the standard surgical procedure. Routine distal clavicular resection and biceps tenodesis (56) generally are not performed, though the biceps tendon and the acromioclavicular joint should be inspected at surgery. Unaddressed acromioclavicular arthritis can lead to a poor surgical result. Complete bicipital tendon ruptures are not repaired, but many surgeons will perform a tenodesis for patients with such inflammation beneath the transverse humeral ligament and attenuation of the biceps tendon that rupture seems imminent. A hypertrophied bicipital tendon (to two or three times normal size), seen in some patients with rotator cuff tears, is left alone, for it reinforces the anterior shoulder capsule and functions as a depressor of the humeral head.

Patients under the age of 40 who fail conservative treatment for impingement may respond to excision of the coracoacromial ligament alone. Persons with rotator cuff tears or those over the age of 40 who fail conservative treatment require more extensive surgical relief of impingement. Open surgical procedures give good to excellent relief of pain in 80% to 90% of patients (29,41,52,57), with patient satisfaction averaging in the upper 70th percentiles (41). Postoperative function and strength are dependent on the size of the tear (58,59).

Arthroscopic acromioplasty seems to give equivalent results when compared to the open acromioplasties (60–62). A greater return-to-sports percentage for athletes with rotator cuff lesions is seen with arthroscopic acromioplasties (61,63), perhaps because of avoidance of deltoid detachment and a quicker surgical recovery following the arthroscopic procedure.

A new technique for repair of large rotator cuff lesions and relief of impingement, the lift-up osteotomy of the acromion (64), allows a clear view of the rotator cuff and as much subacromial space as needed, and has given good results in more than 100 patients.

Surgical treatment of chronic shoulder impingement does not necessarily prevent the progression of rotator cuff tendinitis to rotator cuff tear. Of 93 patients (96 shoulders) with intact rotator cuff tendons at the time of open acromioplasties for impingement, 12 shoulders had complete tears and 7 had partial tears by MRI or arthrogram 9 years later (65). Such a progression to rotator cuff tear despite acromioplasty might be predicted in light of previous chronic damage sustained by the tendons.

Cuff Tear Arthropathy

Cuff-tear arthropathy (49) is probably the same entity as Milwaukee shoulder (66–68) and idiopathic destructive arthritis (69). It occurs in the elderly, often women, in the dominant or both shoulders. The glenohumeral joint is markedly degenerated and disorganized; the rotator cuff is massively torn or absent (49,66,70,71). Voluminous joint effusions often are bloody, but contain low cell counts with a paucity of neutrophils. McCarty's group (66,67,71) described microspheroids containing hydroxyapatite crystals and particulate collagen within the synovial fluid. Activated collagenase and neutral proteases are found in the synovial fluids of some patients, but not all.

There is a vicious cycle of damage in these shoulders, but what the initiating event (or events) is (or are) is unclear (72). Neer et al. (49) emphasized the pathologic findings of atrophic articular cartilage of the humeral head, sclerotic subchondral bone in areas denuded of articular cartilage, and fragmented articular cartilage found in subsynovial layers. They hypothesized that a massive rotator cuff tear exposed a large portion of articular cartilage, impaired normal glenohumeral movements, and caused the joint to become unstable. They further postulated that the loss of a closed joint space led to decreased perfusion of nutrients to the articular cartilage, and thereby to atrophy of the articular cartilage. Instability of the joint, atrophic articular cartilage, and disuse osteoporosis of subchondral bone all combined to cause collapse of subchondral bone and marked glenohumeral osteoarthritis.

McCarty et al. (66,67) theorized that crystal deposition in degenerated tissues came first, rather than the rotator cuff tear. These basic calcium phosphate crystals in synovial fluid, when phagocytosed by macrophage-like synovial cells, stimulated the release of collagenase and neutral proteases. The enzymes then attacked periarticular tissues, causing the "strip mining" of more crystals, which perpetuated the cycle. The rotator cuff tears and instability resulted from damage done by the activated enzymes.

It may be that either scenario can lead to the same final arthritis.

Treatment of Milwaukee shoulder or cuff-tear arthropathy is difficult. Rest, NSAIDs, and repeated aspirations with corticosteroid injections generally give only transient benefit (70). Tidal irrigation followed by intraarticular methylprednisolone and tranexamic acid benefited two patients with Milwaukee shoulder syndrome (73). Patel and co-workers (70) reported good results in a patient using colchicine b.i.d. (chosen because of its usefulness in pseudogout) and choline magnesium trisalicylate (chosen because magnesium enhances the solubility of calcium and inorganic pyrophosphate and increases the enzymatic dissolution of inorganic pyrophosphate by alkaline phosphatase). Humeral hemiarthroplasty is a surgical option, recognizing that postoperative strength and active mobility are limited by the rotator cuff deficiency (74) and poor bone stock.

Calcific Tendinitis

Calcium deposits are seen about the shoulder on routine radiographs in 2.7% (75) to 8% (76) of adult shoulders. Codman (40) estimated that all calcium deposits larger than 1.5 cm became symptomatic, and that 34.6% of all calcium deposits in the rotator cuff structures would be symptomatic at some time. Mavrikakis and co-workers (78) saw calcifications on standard anteroposterior films of the shoulders in 25.7% of hospitalized adults over age 33—in 31.8% of 824 diabetics and 10.3% of 320 nondiabetics; 32% of the 262 diabetics with shoulder calcifications had experienced shoulder pain or loss of motion during or before the study. Calcium deposits are less common and less often symptomatic in the elderly (79,80).

Calcific deposits in the rotator cuff structures were thought initially to represent a degenerative process (80). The proposed sequence of events included hyaline degeneration in the collagen of the tendon due to aging or microtrauma, then fibrillation of these degenerated strands. The fibrillated strands broke with motion, then formed a small rice-like body in a cavity within the tendon. Continued motion pulverized the bodies into necrotic debris, which then calcified. Uhthoff et al. (81) conceptualized a different process, based not on degenerative changes within the tendon, but on a poor vascular supply and lowered oxygen tensions within the tissues triggering metaplasia of tendon to fibrocartilage, with a tendency to mineralize. Diminished blood flow facilitates calcium deposition into tendons (48). The hypothesis of poor oxygen supply can explain both the increased incidence of calcific tendinitis in adults with diabetic vasculopathy (78) and the location of most calcium deposits in the critical zone of the supraspinatus. Patients with uremia or hypervitaminosis D have an increased prevalence of tendon calcification, without any underlying degenerative changes being necessary (2).

The calcium deposits that cause clinical calcific tendinitis are intratendinous, often bilateral and multifocal (77). The supraspinatus tendon is affected more than 50% of the time, followed in frequency by infraspinatus, teres minor, and subscapularis. The clinical syndromes are illnesses of middle age, peaking in the fifth decade. Sexes appear to be equally affected (2); however, there may be a female predominance (82). When unilateral, the dominant shoulder is more likely to be affected (78,82).

Four histologic patterns can be seen in calcific tendinitis, and all patterns often coexist in the patient: (a) Precalcific changes are those of focal fibrocartilaginous transformation within the tendon. (b) The calcific phase is one of intratendinous calcium deposits without any inflammatory response. (c) The resorptive phase is that associated clinically with acute excruciating pain. Phagocytic cells, some of them multinucleated, surround the calcium deposit, along with multiple vascular channels. (d) The repair pattern is one of reconstitution of tendinous tissue (82).

Three clinical pictures occur. The first actually "exists," rather than "occurs," for the calcifications are clinically silent, are discovered incidentally, and never cause symptoms. The second picture, chronic calcific tendinitis, has varying symptoms, dependent on the tendon or tendons involved. Generally the patient complains of chronic anterior aching about the shoulder, with increased pain on flexion and abduction. In the patient with posterior infraspinatus or teres minor calcifications, pain is felt posteriorly as a sudden catching on specific movements such as putting the arm into a sleeve. Subscapularis calcifications usually are asymptomatic (1). Chronic calcifications appear homogeneous and smooth-bordered on radiographs (Fig. 107.6A). Their consistency is that of dry, granular chalk. Chronic calcifications increase the volume of the tendon, thereby increasing the risk of painful mechanical impingement.

Acute calcific tendinitis causes sudden excruciating shoulder pain. The patient guards the afflicted arm, supporting it with his good hand, unable to move the arm or to find a comfortable position. He cannot sleep at night. The pain radiates from the suprahumeral space toward the deltoid insertion on the upper humerus and at times proximally to the base of the neck. The dried chalky material within the tendon has become a milky emulsion, with the consistency of toothpaste. On x-ray films, it looks fluffy or fuzzy. Chemically, the material is still hydroxyapatite; scanning electron microscopic and x-ray diffraction studies show no difference between the crystal lattice structures of chronic and acute calcium deposits (83).

The pathologic sequence in acute tendinitis begins with toothpaste-like calcium under pressure forming a "calcium boil" within the tendon, pushing up against the floor of the subacromial bursa. This calcium boil irritates all contiguous tissues, including the supraspinatus tendon, the subacromial bursa, the synovial joint capsule, and even the biceps tendon (1). Examination of the shoulder is difficult because of pain, but there is an area of maximal tenderness, fullness, and erythema, corresponding to the site of the calcium boil. The boil ruptures spontaneously into the subacromial bursa (Fig. 107.6B) in 4 to 7 days. The pressure is relieved, and the crystals are dispersed throughout the subacromial bursa and locally phagocytosed. The pain diminishes markedly, generally disappearing fully within 48 more hours.

The acute pain corresponds to an increase in resorptive changes histologically (81,82) and to a change in the calcium deposit from dense and homogeneous to flocculent radiologically. Precisely what precipitates the spontaneous resorption of calcium deposits is not known. Often minor trauma or strain precedes acute calcific tendinitis by several hours, perhaps affecting the tendons that overlie the intratendinous calcium deposit and allowing the calcium to come into contact with the subacromial bursa where it incites inflammation, becomes hydrated, and swells into a calcium boil.

Acute calcific tendinitis is self-limited, but it is a rare person who can wait out the pain. Colchicine often helps with the pain, just as in acute gout or pseudogout (2). Needling of the calcium deposit with a large-bore needle and barbotage (using two needles to irrigate the deposit with saline and aspirate calcium flecks) give good results by decreasing the pressure within the calcium boil (1,84). Local steroid

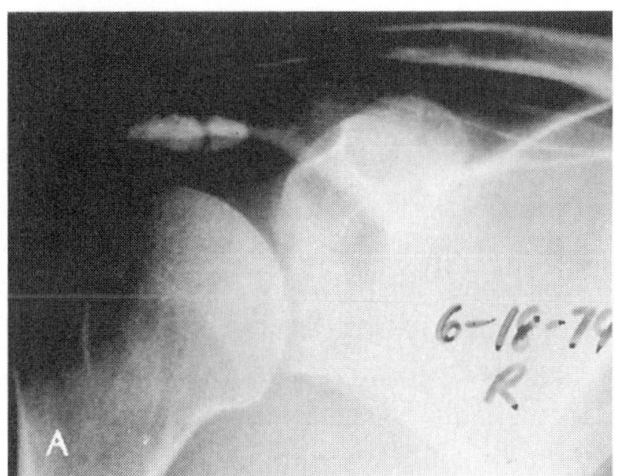

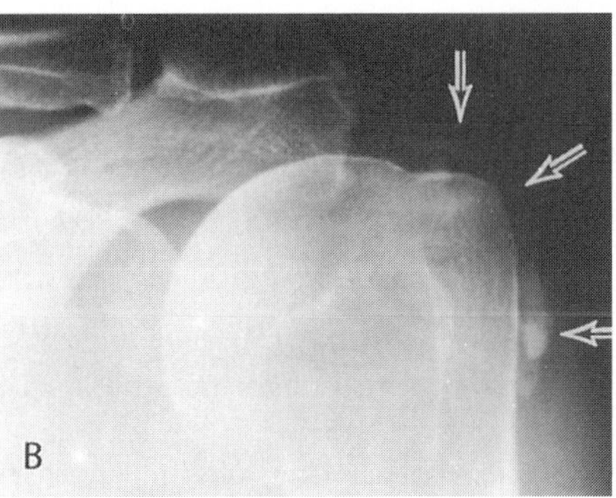

FIGURE 107.6. Plain radiographs of the shoulder in a patient with calcification in the supraspinatus tendon **(A)** and in the subacromial bursa **(B)**. Note the calcium extending into the subdeltoid area in **B** (*arrows*). (Courtesy of Dr. Franklin Kozin.)

injections are avoided, for they abort the natural resorptive process and promote recurrences (84). There is also the fear of local tissue necrosis and lessened tendon strength after steroid injections (81). Surgical removal of an acutely inflamed calcific deposit is not a commonly offered option. Lithotripsy for symptomatic chronic calcific tendinitis (unresponsive to conservative treatment for impingement) is safe and effective (85,86).

SUBACROMIAL BURSITIS

The subacromial bursa caps the rotator cuff, buffering these muscles from the overlying acromion and deltoid. The inferior synovial wall of the subacromial bursa is the outer synovial lining of the supraspinatus tendon (1). The roof of the bursa is attached to the underside of the acromion and the coracoacromial ligament. The bursa extends medially and inferiorly to the coracoid process and laterally to the greater tuberosity. It extends distally superficial to the bicipital groove and under the deltoid for variable distances (87). The subdeltoid and subacromial bursae are contiguous in 78% to 95% of patients (87,88); 11% to 20% of patients have communications between the subcoracoid and subacromial bursae.

Prior to the development of MRI and ultrasound, subacromial bursography was used to differentiate subtle instability from coracoacromial arch impingement syndromes and to document bursal side rotator cuff tears. The normal subacromial bursa holds 5 to 10 mL of contrast medium easily. The chronically inflamed or irritated bursa accepts only a few milliliters of contrast or cannot be demonstrated radiographically by this technique. Strizak and co-workers (87) studied 31 athletes with symptoms of subacromial impingement, and found that those with abnormal subacromial bursograms responded well to decompressive surgery, and that those with normal bursograms received little benefit from decompressive procedures.

Primary subacromial bursitis is rare. Typically subacromial bursitis accompanies inflammation of the glenohumeral joint or supraspinatus tendon. It occurs with subacromial impingement, rotator cuff tear, crystal deposition disease, inflammatory arthritis, polymyalgia rheumatica (89,90), calcific tendinitis, or septic bursitis (particularly in intravenous drug users). Rarely, direct trauma to the top of the shoulder causes an acute hemorrhagic subacromial bursitis (1,91). Prolonged hyperabduction of the shoulder, as during a breast cancer operation, can precipitate subacromial bursitis due to the prolonged compression of the bursa (40).

Subacromial steroid injections, placing Xylocaine and a long-acting steroid preparation into the subacromial bursa, often are helpful in the treatment of rotator cuff tendinitis and impingement syndrome (Fig. 107.7).

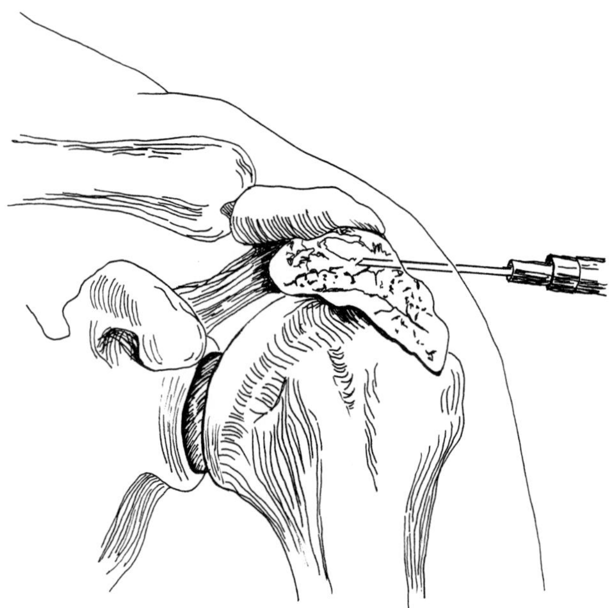

FIGURE 107.7. Subacromial injection. A 25-gauge 1 1/2 inch needle is inserted beneath the acromion, approximately halfway between the anterior and posterior lateral acromial borders. The needle is directed from posterior to anterior to enter the subacromial bursa.

BICIPITAL SYNDROMES

The long head of the biceps originates from the supraglenoid tubercle and the most superior part of the glenoid labrum. The tendon runs across the humeral head, intraarticularly but extrasynovially, then bends to run in the bicipital groove on the ventral aspect of the humerus. The groove is roofed by fibrous tissue, and is reinforced anteriorly by the coracohumeral ligament proximally and the transverse humeral ligament distally. A synovial sheath that extends from the glenohumeral joint to surround the biceps tendon lines the groove. The humeral head slides on the biceps tendon, resulting in a shorter intraarticular portion when the arm is abducted. The tendon is stabilized by the supraspinatus, the subscapularis, the coracohumeral and the superior glenohumeral ligaments. If the rotator cuff is intact, the bicipital tendon cannot be displaced from its groove, even if the transverse humeral ligament is transected (92).

The biceps muscle flexes the elbow, supinates the forearm, and contracts eccentrically to decelerate the arm during throwing. It is a weak static depressor of the humeral head, and normally only a weak dynamic depressor. If there is a rotator cuff tear, however, the biceps can partially compensate, assuming a greater role in abduction and flexion, depression of the humeral head, and stabilization of the anterior joint capsule (92–95). In this case, the tendon of the long head often hypertrophies (55,95).

The biceps tendon is at risk for degenerative changes because of the angle it makes as it courses over the humeral head (which tends to "wring out" its blood supply) and because of its close proximity to the coracoacromial ligament during forward flexion of the shoulder (which predisposes to impingement) (57). Because the tendon's synovial sheath is continuous with the shoulder joint, bicipital tendinitis accompanies rheumatoid synovitis of the shoulder, septic arthritis, gout or pseudogout of the shoulder, hemodialysis arthropathy, and other inflammatory processes involving the glenohumeral joint.

Bicipital Tendinitis

Ninety-five percent of bicipital tendinitis is associated with rotator cuff disease and impingement (54). The patient has anterior shoulder pain, which may extend to the biceps muscle belly, but does not radiate to the neck or past the biceps insertion distally. Usually, there is no history of trauma, but rather a history of repetitive use, often overhead. The pain worsens with lifting, carrying, or any use of the biceps. It is chronic and may worsen at night. On exam, the patient has point tenderness over the biceps tendon (felt directly anterior and about 2 to 3 inches below the acromion when the arm is internally rotated 10 degrees) (92). The area of point tenderness moves as the arm rotates, which distinguishes it from tenderness arising from the underlying bone. Flexion against resistance with the elbow extended and the forearm supinated causes pain over the biceps tendon (Speed's test). Supination of the forearm against resistance when the elbow is flexed also causes pain over the proximal anteromedial arm (Yergason's sign). Maneuvers that stretch the inflamed biceps tendon (such as backward extension and external rotation with an extended elbow) cause pain (96). Impingement testing generally is positive.

Primary bicipital tendinitis, not associated with impingement or with inflammatory processes in the glenohumeral joint, is rare. The tendon narrows within the bicipital groove beneath a thickened stenotic synovial sheath. The tendon may become adherent to the underlying joint capsule and then rupture, with acute relief of pain and improved joint motion (96), or the tendon may elongate due to chronic friction and secondary tendon attrition (2).

Subluxation or Dislocation

Bicipital subluxation is the slipping of the biceps tendon in and out of the intertubercular groove as the arm is internally and externally rotated, respectively. Dislocation means that the tendon has slipped out and stayed out. This happens in older individuals with elongated tendons (and/or rotator cuff tears) or in younger throwing athletes. Those persons with shallow bicipital grooves or grooves with medial wall angles that are more oblique are predisposed to displacement of the tendon. Clinically, the patient complains of anterior upper arm or shoulder pain with popping, clicking, or snapping when the arm reaches a certain position in the rotation arc.

Rupture of the Biceps Tendon

The biceps tendon can rupture when the muscle contracts forcefully unexpectedly (as in catching an object that is surprisingly heavy) or with minimal exertion in the middle-aged or elderly with a history of chronic shoulder pain. In young people, biceps ruptures are uncommon, but may occur at the distal musculotendinous junction. These ruptures should be surgically repaired at the time of injury.

Ruptures occurred after lifting, pushing, pulling, or falling in just over half of 42 middle-aged patients with proximal tendon ruptures, in one series. Five of the seven patients who ruptured after minimal exertion (such as pulling up a stocking) had received a steroid injection within the preceding 3 weeks. At follow-up almost 8 years later, there was no significant functional difference between the patients treated conservatively and those treated surgically (97).

The Ludington test is the easiest way to pick up a biceps rupture because subtle changes in the biceps contours are more apparent. The patient puts both hands behind his head and flexes the biceps. A proximal biceps tendon rupture causes a distal bulge of bunched-up muscle.

The importance of proximal bicipital rupture is that it is a clue to possible impingement and impending rotator cuff tear. Neer (29) estimated that the pinched biceps tendon ruptures before the pinched supraspinatus tendon one time out of eight.

Superior Labrum Anterior and Posterior (SLAP) Lesions

SLAP lesions are uncommon injuries to the glenoid labrum near the biceps insertion, with tears beginning posteriorly and extending anteriorly (98). In a Belgian series of 530 arthroscopies, a 6% incidence of SLAP lesions was found (99). The injury was due to compression in 28% of the 32 patients. A fall on an outstretched arm, an automobile accident where the driver braces against the steering wheel as he is hit from behind (100), or a direct blow on the lateral shoulder can compress the humeral head against the labrum. An inferior traction pull (lifting a weight) caused 22% of the injuries in this series. Deceleration forces tugging on the biceps anchor during overhead sports activities or throwing caused 25% of the lesions. Dislocation or subluxation accounted for 22% of the lesions (99).

Cordasco and co-workers (101) found instability on examination under anesthesia in 70% of 27 patients with SLAP lesions, and suggested that occult instability might underlie labral tears. In a cadaver model by Bey and colleagues (102) that produced traction on the biceps tendon, inferior subluxation of the humeral head did facilitate the creation of SLAP lesions.

Patient complaints are vague and inconsistent, including pain while lifting weights or clicking and an unstable feeling. The SLAP prehension test, which is 87.5% sensitive for unstable SLAP lesions, entails adducting the affected shoulder with the shoulder flexed to 90 degrees, the elbow extended, and the forearm pronated (27). A positive test causes apprehension, pain felt at the bicipital groove, or a click that is heard or felt. The test causes less pain if repeated with the forearm supinated (which decreases traction on the biceps tendon).

MRI (103), MRI arthrography (104), and computed tomography (CT) arthrography (105) can demonstrate SLAP lesions. Arthroscopy allows not only diagnosis, but also classification as to type, and treatment of the unstable lesions by reanchoring the torn labrum and biceps anchor to the glenoid.

Radiology

Plain radiographs of the shoulder usually are normal in patients with bicipital disease, though a special bicipital groove view (106) might show bony intertubercular spurs. Radiographic signs of impingement may be present. Arthrography can outline the bicipital groove, but in patients with associated rotator cuff tears the synovial sheath does not fill reliably. Ultrasonography gives as good a picture of the bony anatomy of the bicipital groove and a better look at the biceps tendon itself (107). Dynamic sonography allows documentation of biceps tendon subluxations and assessment of the three-dimensional relationships between the biceps tendon, the rotator cuff, and the coracoacromial arch. Ultrasonography is limited by calcifications about the shoulder that interfere with imaging of the biceps and by poor visualization of the intraarticular portion of the tendon (108). MRI gives a clear picture of the intraarticular and extraarticular biceps tendon, as does CT arthrography, and both demonstrate any associated rotator-cuff or intraarticular pathology, but both are expensive. Arthroscopy allows direct visualization of the intraarticular portion of the biceps tendon and is the best method for evaluation of SLAP lesions.

Treatment

Treatment of bicipital tendinitis begins with rest of the arm and discontinuation of activities that cause pain. Antiinflammatory drugs are used. If the patient doesn't respond, a subacromial steroid/Xylocaine injection may treat impingement-associated tendinitis, and a steroid/Xylocaine injection into the bicipital sheath may help the rare patient with primary bicipital tendinitis. This should be repeated no more than once (or twice in rare cases) at an interval of not less than 4 to 6 weeks. Kennedy and Willis (109) documented disorganization and loss of the normal parallel collagen arrangement in tendons experimentally injected with steroids. Failure strength was decreased by 35% 48 hours after the injection and only returned to normal 2 weeks after the injection. Ultrastructural changes persisted for 6 weeks. These findings and the frequent ruptures after steroid injections in Phillip's et al.'s (97) study suggest that the patient should baby the biceps tendon for 3 weeks or longer after a steroid injection.

When acute symptoms resolve, physical therapy is used to maintain strength and range of motion. Rotation is emphasized in an effort to strengthen the rotator cuff muscles, while abduction is avoided initially. If the patient doesn't respond to conservative care after 6 to 12 months, further evaluation for impingement or other joint pathology is indicated, and surgical treatment is considered.

Conservative care for the subluxating or dislocating tendon also begins with rest of the biceps and avoidance of aggravating activities. NSAIDs are used. If conservative care fails, exploration of the biceps groove with replacement of the biceps tendon is indicated in young patients. Tears in the supraspinatus, the subscapularis, and the coracohumeral ligament are sought and repaired (92,93). The older patient may respond to tenodesis and subacromial decompression.

Proximal bicipital ruptures in older sedentary patients are treated conservatively with NSAIDs and biceps rest, with a resultant mild cosmetic deformity but ample elbow flexion and forearm supination for activities of daily living. Younger patients who require maximal supination strength benefit from subacromial decompression and biceps tenodesis (94).

CAPSULAR DISEASE

Frozen Shoulder

Frozen shoulder is the name given to a painful stiff shoulder, whose glenohumeral motion is globally limited by a contracted, poorly compliant joint capsule (110). Its cause is unknown, though it is quite common, estimated to occur in 2% to 3% of the general population and 11% to 19% of diabetics (111,112). Frozen shoulder is also called adhesive capsulitis, based on Neviaser's (113) pathologic studies, in which he felt the capsule peeled off the humeral head at surgery the way an adhesive plaster peels off skin. Adhesive capsulitis has been reported in the wrist, the ankle, and the hip, though in much lower incidences than in the shoulder (114–116). Other synonyms for frozen shoulder include check-rein shoulder, periarthritis of the shoulder, and scapulohumeral periarthritis.

Frozen shoulder is rare before age 40, and generally involves persons aged 50 to 70. Women are affected slightly more than men (117). The disease is bilateral 5% to 25% of the time (112,118), sequentially or simultaneously. It is thought that frozen shoulder will not recur in a shoulder that has been affected previously.

The patient with a frozen shoulder experiences diffuse shoulder pain, often night pain, and a gradual loss of mobility. Fastening a bra behind the back, putting on a shirt or coat, reaching for a wallet in the back hip pocket, or combing the back of the hair becomes difficult. Active and passive mobility of the shoulder is limited, even if the examiner uses Xylocaine injections to eliminate pain during the exam. External rotation, abduction, and internal rotation are the motions most affected, but all motions of the glenohumeral joint are involved. The patient may have pain-free motion within the confines of his decreased range, with pain only at the extremes of his range. Scapulothoracic motion remains normal, and is used by the patient to try to compensate for lost glenohumeral mobility.

Frozen shoulder is a diagnosis of exclusion, and must be differentiated from chronic posterior dislocations, rotator cuff disease, septic arthritis, avascular necrosis, fracture, bony or pulmonary neoplasm, osteoarthritis of the shoulder or cervical spine, or other shoulder arthropathies. The shoulder with a torn or inflamed rotator cuff generally has limited motion in only one or two directions, and has full passive motion once Xylocaine is used to eliminate pain and muscle spasm.

The cause of frozen shoulder is unknown, but it has been associated with a number of other diseases (Table 107.4). The association with diabetes is strong: it occurs in 11% to 19% of diabetics, and the incidence increases with both duration (111) and severity (112) of the diabetes. Patients with frozen shoulder should be screened for diabetes, particularly if the illness is bilateral (119). Some authors have suggested an association with a depressive personality (120), but others have disputed this (112,118). One study suggested an association with human leukocyte antigen HLA-B27 (121) and another an association with decreased serum immunoglobulin A (IgA) levels (122), but other studies did not confirm these findings (117,119). One factor that many associated conditions have in common is immobility of the shoulder, for whatever reason.

TABLE 107.4. CONDITIONS ASSOCIATED WITH FROZEN SHOULDER

Trauma
Immobility of the shoulder
Diabetes mellitus
Thyroid disease
Cervical spine disease
Hemiparesis
Myocardial infarction, coronary artery disease, or cardiac catheterization
Parkinson's disease
Impairment of consciousness
Prolonged intravenous therapy
Pancoast tumors, other lung or chest wall neoplasms
Tuberculosis, emphysema, or chronic bronchitis
Breast, chest, or shoulder surgery
Hypoadrenalism
Other intrinsic shoulder disease
Reflex sympathetic dystrophy
Isoniazid
Scleroderma
Phenobarbital?

Pathologic studies in frozen shoulder show increased fibrosis in the glenohumeral joint capsule. The capsule is thickened, contracted, and adherent to the underlying humeral head (113). The normal axillary pouch is missing, and synovial fluid is conspicuously absent. Biochemical changes of increased glycosaminoglycans, decreased glycoproteins, and decreased hyaluronic acid reflect fibroplasia, much as is seen in patients with Dupuytren's contracture (123). [In Bridgman's (112) series, 2.3% of the 600 nondiabetics, 2.75% of the 800 diabetics, and 2.38% of the 714 diabetics without frozen shoulder had Dupuytren's contractures, but 5.8% of the 86 diabetics with frozen shoulder had Dupuytren's contractures.]

The natural history of frozen shoulder has been divided into three phases: freezing, frozen, and thawing (124). The freezing phase may last 10 to 36 weeks, with generalized pain and growing stiffness. The second phase of marked stiffness typically lasts 4 to 12 months, and is less painful. The thawing phase generally lasts 5 to 26 months, and is characterized by gradual return of glenohumeral motion and function. Spontaneous recovery is the usual course of frozen shoulder. The total duration of the illness in Reeves's (124) 49 patients averaged 30.1 months. More than 50% were left with some limitation of movement, although only three patients had significant functional disabilities. Other authors have found limited motion in 30% to 42% of patients at 6- to 7-year follow-up (125,126), but few patients with functional loss. The cause of the spontaneous recovery from frozen shoulder is unknown but perhaps is due to an inadvertent, unrecognized tear of the joint capsule or to mechanical attrition of the tightened capsule (117).

Plain radiographs typically are normal in patients with frozen shoulder, or show disuse osteopenia. Periarticular calcifications are seen in 7% to 9%, which is the frequency in the general population. An axillary view of the shoulder should be done in addition to standard anteroposterior views, to rule out unrecognized dislocations, fractures, or osteophytes. An arthrogram showing a significant loss of joint capsule volume and obliteration of the normal axillary pouch (Fig. 107.8) fully confirms the diagnosis of frozen shoulder. The normal glenohumeral joint capsule accepts 20 to 30 mL of contrast, as opposed to 5 to 10 mL contrast in the frozen shoulder.

Exercises form the basis of every treatment proposed for frozen shoulder. Prophylaxis is important in situations that might predispose to frozen shoulder, and includes such active and passive range of motion programs as the Reach to Recovery program used after mastectomies and the range of motion exercises done by physical therapists for comatose patients.

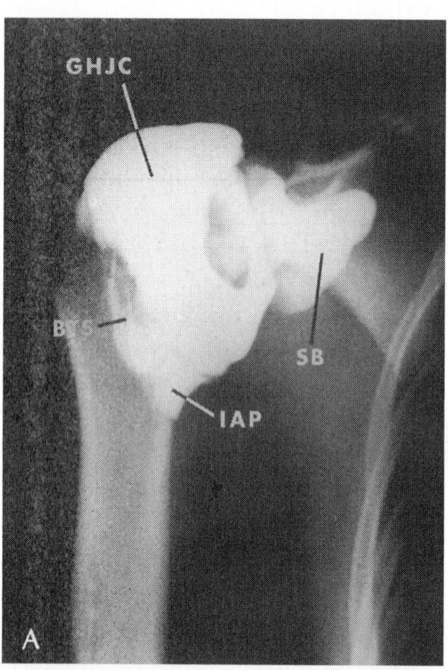

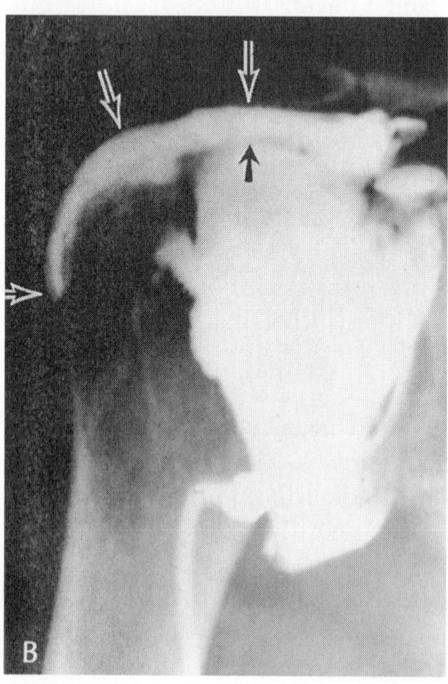

FIGURE 107.8. A: Arthrogram of the normal shoulder, showing the glenohumeral joint capsule (GHJC), the subscapular bursa (SB), the inferior axillary pouch (IAP), and the bicipital tendon sheath (BTS). **B:** Arthrogram of the shoulder in a patient with a complete rotator cuff rupture, demonstrating contrast in the subacromial bursa *(arrows)*. (Courtesy of Dr. Franklin Kozin.)

During the freezing phase, the emphasis is on pain relief. This can be accomplished with a sling, moist heat, NSAIDs, analgesics, oral steroids (2), and/or local steroids. Ultrasound and nerve stimulation also can be used. Gentle range of motion exercises may help maintain mobility. During the frozen stage, exercises should be done four to five times a day if possible (Fig. 107.9). They should not be so aggressive as to aggravate the pain and lead to further guarding of the shoulder. If performed after the shoulder is warmed with a shower, sweater, or moist heat, stretching exercises are easier for the patient. The underlying concept is to stretch the shoulder capsule using a mechanical advantage rather than with active muscular contraction. First, the patient is taught Codman's pendular exercises. The shoulder can be stretched passively using the contralateral arm. For example, the unaffected arm can push the affected arm up the back when the involved arm is internally rotated, with the thumb against the spinal column. This stretches the anterior capsule. A 3-foot length of broom handle or stiff tubing can be used to stretch the involved shoulder. The unaffected side powers the stick, while the affected side is moved passively, in all directions. A pulley system is another way to passively move the frozen shoulder by actively pulling with the contralateral arm. Hooking the hand of the frozen shoulder on the top of a door, then bending the knees while trying to press the axilla against the door uses the weight of the entire body to stretch the shoulder (110,127,128).

Treating the patient "patiently" with such exercises and no referral for more formal physical therapy returned functional motion to 50 patients at an average of 14 months (with a range from 3 to greater than 36 months), with no treatment complications in one series (127).

Local steroid injections benefit pain more than they increase range of motion. Intraarticular and subacromial injections seem more effective than trigger point injections (129). Koppel and Thompson (130) proposed the use of suprascapular nerve blocks, postulating that frozen shoulder might arise as a complication of suprascapular neuropathy. Electrophysiologic studies do not support this etiologic theory, but a suprascapular nerve block during the freezing stage might give enough pain relief to allow better maintenance of motion (117).

Joint brisement is the act of placing fluid into the contracted capsule under pressure, making the capsule expand and eventually rupture. It can be accomplished by distention arthrography, by injection of bacteriostatic saline and local anesthetic (with or without a small amount of steroids), or arthroscopically (131–133). It must be followed by a careful regimen of passive stretching exercises.

Manipulation under anesthesia is reserved for recalcitrant cases of frozen shoulder, as potential complications

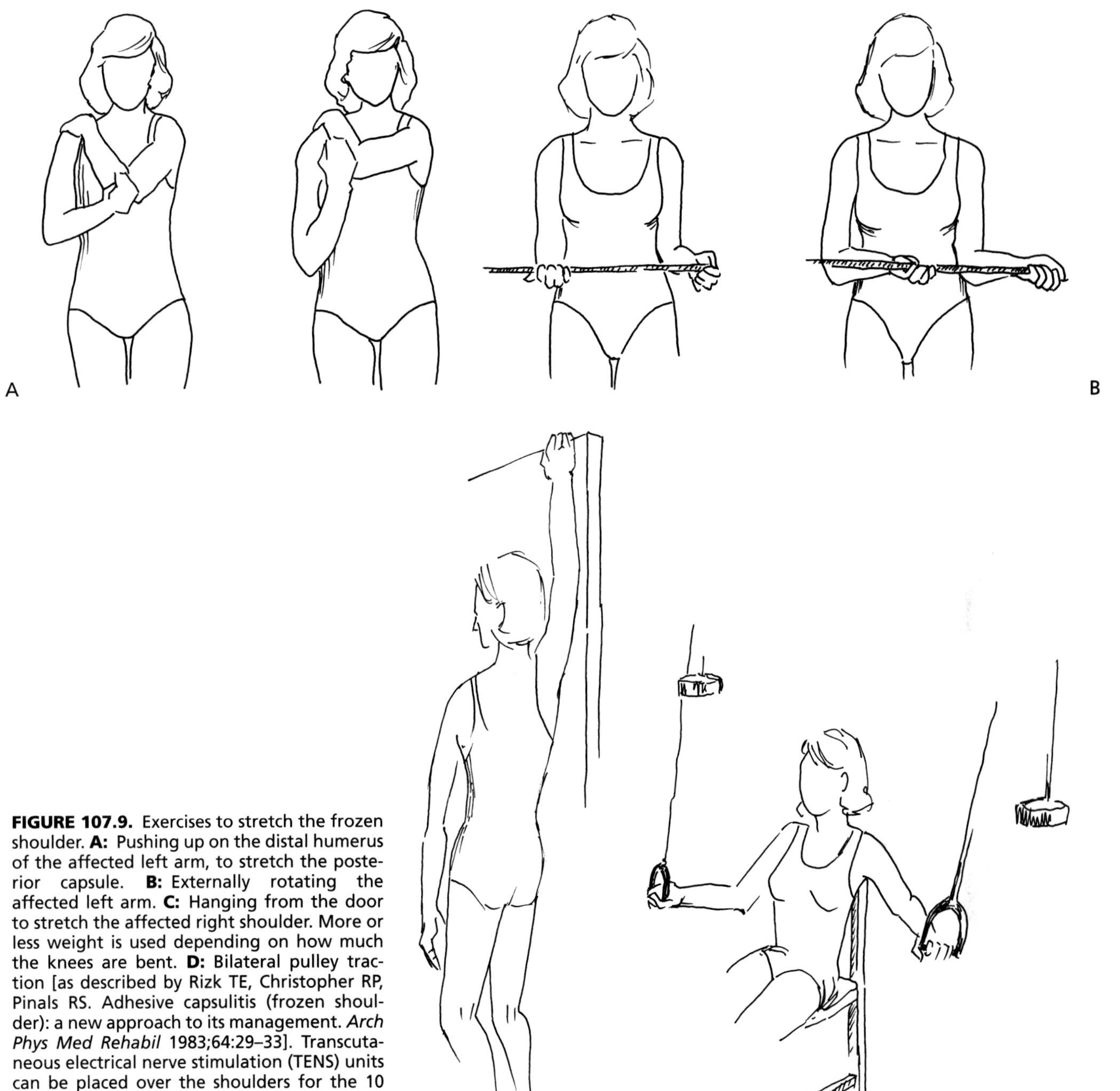

FIGURE 107.9. Exercises to stretch the frozen shoulder. **A:** Pushing up on the distal humerus of the affected left arm, to stretch the posterior capsule. **B:** Externally rotating the affected left arm. **C:** Hanging from the door to stretch the affected right shoulder. More or less weight is used depending on how much the knees are bent. **D:** Bilateral pulley traction [as described by Rizk TE, Christopher RP, Pinals RS. Adhesive capsulitis (frozen shoulder): a new approach to its management. *Arch Phys Med Rehabil* 1983;64:29–33]. Transcutaneous electrical nerve stimulation (TENS) units can be placed over the shoulders for the 10 minutes prior to traction and the entire traction time to reduce patient discomfort.

include fracture, glenohumeral dislocation, rotator cuff tear, traction injuries of the brachial plexus, and hemarthrosis (128). Manipulation is contraindicated in the osteoporotic patient or anyone whose frozen shoulder resulted from a proximal humeral fracture or dislocation. A second option for the patient who has not improved after prolonged conservative therapy is open or arthroscopic release of contracted tissues, followed by faithful performance of passive stretching exercises. Recalcitrant diabetic frozen shoulders have been successfully treated with a regimen of manipulation under anesthesia, arthroscopic capsular releases, and postoperative passive mobilization under interscalene block anesthesia via an indwelling catheter (128).

Glenohumeral Instability

Glenohumeral instability is increasingly recognized as a cause of shoulder pain or dysfunction. The glenohumeral joint depends on the joint capsule, the labrum, glenohumeral ligaments, and negative intraarticular pressure

(134) for static support. These static constraints are most important at extremes of the range of motion. In the midpoints of the ranges of motion, the dynamic support provided by the rotator cuff and the long head of the biceps is crucial. Because the glenohumeral joint is so highly mobile, it is the most frequently dislocated joint in the body. Dislocations occur with a bimodal pattern, peaking in the twenties because of athletic injuries and in the sixties to eighties because of falls (135). "Dislocation" means that the articular surfaces lose contact with each other, without spontaneous relocation. Subluxation is a transient symptomatic excessive translation of the humeral head on the glenoid without complete disassociation of the articular surfaces (136). Subtle subluxations are thought to underlie many of the impingement symptoms in younger throwing athletes.

The dead-arm syndrome in patients with recurring anterior subluxations of the shoulder is a sudden severe pain or paralysis when the abducted, extended arm is externally rotated (137). The pain subsides quickly, but the arm remains sore or weak for several hours. Some patients are aware that the shoulder is slipping out of joint, but others are unaware of the subluxation, recognizing only pain and an inability to use the arm forcefully overhead. Patients with dead-arm syndrome have positive apprehension tests, and shoulder radiographs may show Hill-Sachs lesions of the humeral head (posterior and lateral indentations or compression fractures in the humeral head that indicate a prior anterior subluxation or dislocation has occurred). Dead arms resulting from injuries or excessive throwing maneuvers must be differentiated from thoracic outlet syndromes, cervical disc syndromes, brachial plexus stretching, acromioclavicular disease, rotator cuff tears, and biceps lesions.

Acute traumatic dislocations usually are unmistakable; 95% are anterior, occurring after forceful abduction and external rotation. The normal deltoid contour is lost, and the humeral head can be palpated anteriorly in a subcoracoid, subglenoid, or subclavicular position. The arm often is held abducted in external rotation or at the side, for the patient is unwilling or unable to internally rotate the arm (136). The main prognostic factor in anterior dislocations is the age of the patient at the time of the first dislocation. Patients younger than 35 have a higher rate of redislocation than those over 40 (138,139), although older patients have a greater incidence of associated rotator cuff tears (140). Most second dislocations occur within 2 years of the first dislocation (139,141). Aggressive physical therapy to strengthen the rotator cuff muscles, the deltoid, and the scapula stabilizers can lessen the redislocation rate to as low as 17.3% to 25% in young males, a rate much lower than the 33% to 50% rates of redislocation initially reported in young age groups (142).

Posterior dislocations are far less common, accounting for 4% of traumatic glenohumeral dislocations and resulting from a direct blow to the anterior shoulder, a seizure or electrical shock, or an indirect blow to the adducted, flexed, internally rotated arm. Posterior dislocations can mimic frozen shoulders, because of the pain and diminished external rotation. Physical examination shows asymmetric shoulders, a prominent coracoid process, and an inability to externally rotate the arm when the elbow is flexed at 90 degrees. An axillary radiograph will often demonstrate the displaced humeral head behind the glenoid fossa (136).

Thomas and Matsen (143) introduced the acronym TUBS to describe *t*raumatic *u*nilateral instability, with *B*ankhart lesions (detachment of the anterior capsule and labrum from the glenoid); *s*urgery often is needed to remedy this instability.

Some patients have atraumatic dislocations of the glenohumeral joint. Usually, they have generalized ligamentous laxity [hyperextensible elbows and knees, ability to touch the thumb to the volar forearm, ability to extend the metacarpophalangeals (MCPs) past 90 degrees] and multidirectional instability at the glenohumeral joint. They have inferior instability with a positive sulcus sign, and either anterior or posterior instability, often with positive apprehension signs. Thomas and Matsen (143) described such persons with the acronym AMBRI: *a*traumatic, *m*ultidirectional instability, often *b*ilateral, responds to *r*ehabilitation, may have a redundant *i*nferior capsule requiring surgery to tighten it. Burkhead and Rockwood (144) found a good or excellent response to rehabilitative exercises in 80% of 66 shoulders with atraumatic subluxation, and felt that most patients with multidirectional instability did best without any surgery.

A torn labral fragment can catch between the humeral head and the glenoid, causing a catching, slipping, locking sensation of unreliability that is called functional glenohumeral instability (145). These patients have no anatomic dislocation or subluxation, merely a situation in the shoulder analogous to that occurring in a knee with a torn medial meniscus.

Instability should be sought in young patients with shoulder pain, especially as instability is more common than subacromial impingement and rotator cuff disease in this age group. Anterior instability is diagnosed by the feeling of apprehension and impending joint slippage when the extended, abducted arm is externally rotated (Table 107.2). Posterior instability can be felt as too great a translation of the humeral head posteriorly on the glenoid, when the patient is lying supine and the humerus is displaced posteriorly. Inferior instability is manifest as a sulcus that appears below the acromion laterally as the humerus is distracted downward.

The exercise program used to treat instability is essentially the same program used to treat subacromial impingement (144,146). Exercises to strengthen the rotator cuff and deltoid initially are isometric, and then are done with Theraband or resistive surgical tubing. External rotation to 45 degrees, abduction to 45 degrees, extension to 45 degrees, internal rotation to 45 degrees, and flexion to 45 degrees are all performed with the elbow bent at a 90-degree angle, and the tubing attached to a door handle (Table 107.3, Fig. 107.5). The resistance is very slowly increased, over a matter of weeks to months. Shoulder-shrug exercises strengthen the trapezius and levator scapulae. Wall pushups, knee pushups, and then regular pushups are done to strengthen the serratus anterior and the rhomboids. After the shoulder has been rehabilitated, the exercises must be continued two to three times a week indefinitely to best maintain shoulder stability (144).

Articular mechanoreceptors, specialized neurons that transform mechanical deformation into electrical signals to give the brain information about joint position and motion, are found in the glenoid labrum and glenohumeral ligaments. Muscle spindle receptors work as well to provide proprioceptive feedback to the brain. Unstable shoulders have small deficits in the threshold for detection of passive motion and in the reproduction of passive positioning (147). These deficits may contribute to ongoing instability via altered reflex muscle contractions about the joint in response to (abnormal) joint movements. Proprioception in shoulders whose anterior instability has been surgically repaired is normal, perhaps because the tighter capsules allow better functioning of the mechanoreceptors or perhaps because proprioception has been relearned during rehabilitative exercises (147). If proprioception can indeed be learned through exercises, these exercises should join the traditional rotator cuff strengthening exercises as part of the standard rehabilitative effort.

Shoulder dislocations and subluxations are relatively common and glenohumeral osteoarthritis is relatively rare. Nonetheless, Samilson and Prieto (148) described "dislocation arthropathy" in 74 shoulders with prior single or multiple dislocations. The number of dislocations was not related to the severity of the arthritis, but age at the time of the first dislocation correlated positively with the severity of arthritis. Unrecognized posterior dislocations that were reduced late were prone to osteoarthritis. Shoulders with posterior instability were more prone to moderate or severe arthritis than shoulders with anterior or multidirectional instability. Shoulders that have undergone instability surgery with internal hardware or with excessive tightening of the anterior capsule are more prone to glenohumeral osteoarthritis than are virgin shoulders (149). The arthritis of dislocation and capsulorrhaphy arthritis can be so painful and disabling that shoulder arthroplasty is often the best treatment, despite the youth of affected patients (150).

SHOULDER PAIN IN ATHLETES

Athletic endeavors often involve repetitive shoulder motions, at extremes of the range of motion and at near-maximal tolerance. Nicholas et al. (151) broke down the inherent movements of various sports into six different categories: throw, stance, jump, kick, run, and walk. The frequency of use of these different movements followed the order in which they are listed, with throwing being the most commonly used. Throwing was defined as a ballistic motion of the upper extremity whereby the center of mass of the arm or an external object was propelled away from or around the body's center of mass. The shoulder is at risk in all throwing sports.

The forces of throwing can be divided into three types: explosive, dynamic, and static (152). Professional baseball pitchers generate explosive forces, experiencing maximal forces about the shoulder for short periods of time. The forces about a swimmer's shoulder are dynamic. The shoulder and arm move continuously and repetitively throughout workouts lasting 1 to 2 hours, with rest breaks of minutes or seconds. Static forces occur when gymnasts and weight lifters sustain isometric contractions in the rotator cuff and scapular muscles. The injuries of a given sport vary with the type of force used in that sport.

The shoulder joint is anatomically balanced between mobility and stability, with much of the stability due to soft tissues. Optimal athletic performance requires a balance between the looseness needed for the extreme external rotation of pitching or of backstroking and the tightness needed to prevent subluxations or secondary impingement. Joint laxity may contribute to athletic success, but a stretched glenohumeral capsule also predisposes to instability and recurrent subluxations (153).

Falls onto the shoulder or outstretched arm contribute to the 10% to 14% incidence of shoulder injuries in football players, which include acromioclavicular separations, glenohumeral dislocations, and muscle strains. Wrestling, with its twisting and falling motions, has a 12.5% to 18% incidence of shoulder injuries (152). Acute traumatic subacromial bursitis, common in contact sports or sports such as skiing where hard falls occur, can result when the humerus is driven against the acromion in a fall (91).

Microtrauma results from the chronic overuse of the shoulder in overarm sports. No single catastrophic injury occurs; rather, damage is cumulative, from small repeated insults that do not have time to heal before the next practice or the next game.

Baseball

The pitching motion has been broken down into sequential movements: windup, cocking, acceleration, deceleration, and follow-through (154–157). In late cocking, the shoulder is abducted to 90 degrees, hyperextended, and in extreme external rotation. Both the biceps and the triceps are taut, as are the forearm flexors and extensors. The humeral head translates anteriorly on the glenoid, stressing the anterior joint capsule, the inferior glenohumeral ligament, and the subscapularis. The greater tuberosity of the humerus abuts the posterosuperior glenoid rim, sometimes catching the labrum between the underside of the rotator cuff and the humeral head. This is called *internal impingement* or *posterosuperior glenoid impingement.*

Subacromial impingement of the rotator cuff or biceps tendon can occur during acceleration when the shoulder is whipped from extreme external rotation to internal rotation, as the forearm, hand, and ball come forward. During deceleration, the biceps contracts eccentrically to slow elbow extension, tugging on its origin in so doing, and at times causing SLAP lesions.

Internal impingement is thought to be the most common cause of rotator cuff pathology in the young throwing athlete (158). It often is associated with glenohumeral instability, for if the humerus subluxates anteriorly during abduction and external rotation, the impingement of the posterosuperior glenoid labrum is increased. This causes labral fraying or tears, tears on the undersurface (not the subacromial side) of the supraspinatus and infraspinatus tendons, and cystic changes in the greater tuberosity beneath the insertions of the supraspinatus and infraspinatus. Clinically, the thrower experiences posterior pain, worst during the late cocking phase. Internal impingement was not recognized until arthroscopy (159) and MRI came into being. Treatment of posterosuperior glenoid impingement rests largely on ensuring anterior stability of the glenohumeral joint: the less the humeral head translates anteriorly on the glenoid, the less the posterosuperior humeral head contacts the glenoid during abduction and external rotation. The rotator cuff muscles are strengthened to try to stabilize the joint, with special attention given to the subscapularis muscle, which stabilizes the anterior joint dynamically during extreme external rotation. The muscles about the scapula are strengthened, as a greater scapulothoracic range of motion decreases the stress on the glenohumeral joint during throwing. If the athlete has unilateral anterior instability and has failed rehabilitative exercises, surgical reconstruction of the anterior capsule and inferior glenohumeral ligament may be appropriate.

Little Leaguer's shoulder was described by Carson and Gasser (160) as pain localizing to the proximal humerus during throwing. Widening of the proximal humeral physis was seen on radiographs of the throwing arm. After 3 months of rest from throwing, 21 of 23 children could throw again without pain.

Primary subacromial anterior impingement in young athletes occurs mainly in those who have hooked acromions, which result in smaller subacromial spaces. Secondary subacromial impingement can follow anterior humeral subluxation. The anterior capsule, labrum, and inferior glenohumeral ligament experience microtrauma during late cocking, and can stretch and become attenuated. The rotator cuff muscles, biceps, and scapular rotators try to compensate, to hold the humeral head tight into the glenoid, but when they fatigue, the humeral head tends to subluxate anteriorly and superiorly, increasing the likelihood of subacromial impingement as well as posterosuperior glenoid impingement. The appropriate treatment in this scenario is not to approach the (secondary) impingement per se, but to treat the instability (156).

Swimming and Water Polo

Swimmers have generalized joint laxity, perform a high number of revolutions about the shoulder with each practice session, and function at extremes of shoulder range of motion (161). The incidence of swimmer's shoulder increases with the ability of the swimmer and with the number of years of competitive swimming. In one study, 58% of the 40 swimmers on a world championship team had shoulder pain, as did 53% of the 38 elite swimmers at an Olympic training camp, and 27% of the nonelite swimmers at the training camp (162). Fifty percent of competitive swimmers have shoulder pain severe enough to make them stop swimming for 3 weeks or longer at least once in their careers (161).

The pathophysiology is subacromial impingement of the supraspinatus and biceps tendons, occurring as the internally rotated, adducted arm enters the water at the beginning of the freestyle and butterfly pulls. The microtrauma caused by the impingement is exacerbated by the avascularity in the supraspinatus tendon at the end of the pull when the adducted internally rotated arm is at the swimmer's side and the tendon is "wrung out" over the humeral head (163,164). The cycle repeats as long as the stroke is continued, and microtrauma accumulates.

The breaststroke does not predispose to shoulder pain. The pull begins similarly, with the arms above the head, adducted and internally rotated, but the pull ends at shoulder level (except for the first pull after the start or after a turn), and so the supraspinatus is rarely wrung out over the humeral head. The shoulders are flexed throughout the entire breaststroke race, because the stroke recovery is underwater rather than through the air.

Women are more prone to shoulder pain than men, because they take more strokes per lap. Hand paddles predispose to shoulder pain. Middle-distance and sprint swimmers are more likely to have pain than distance swimmers. Butterfliers can develop bilateral pain; freestylers more often have pain on the breathing side.

Treatment of swimmer's shoulder is treatment of anterior impingement, including ice, rest, massage, ultrasound, oral NSAIDs, transcutaneous electrical nerve stimulation (TENS) unit, and judicious use of subacromial steroid injections. Yardage is decreased, hand paddles are avoided, and the stroke technique is reviewed. Conditioning is maintained with strokes that don't hurt and with kicking. Swimmers unresponsive to conservative treatment may benefit from resection of the coracoacromial ligament.

Apprehension shoulder is now an uncommon problem, for most competitive backstrokers turn by flipping onto their stomachs and doing a front-flip turn, pushing off from the wall on their backs. Previously, the back-flip turn entailed pushing upward against the wall with the extended, externally rotated, abducted arm, ducking the head and flipping backward. This is the position of the "apprehension sign" for anterior subluxation, and caused pain in loose-jointed backstrokers with anterior instability (171). The back-flip turn remains legal in competitive swimming but is used rarely.

Giombini and co-workers (165) described 11 male and female national-caliber water polo players with shoulder pain. Plain radiographs in four cases showed erosions of the posterosuperior glenoid, and in five cases showed osteochondral defects of the posterior aspect of the humeral head. All 11 subjects had posterosuperior labral damage, partial tears of the undersurface of the rotator cuff, and posterosuperior glenoid impingement, seen by MRI and confirmed by arthroscopy.

Tennis

Tennis shoulder refers to a postural droop in the dominant shoulder of tennis players and overhand throwers. The suspensory muscles of the shoulder (trapezius, levator scapulae, and rhomboids) are repeatedly stretched during the tennis serve, in the overhead reach for the ball, the acceleration phase, and the follow-through. The racket arm has a greater mass than the free arm, due to hypertrophy of muscles and bone from repeated exercise. These two facts combine to pull the dominant shoulder down, causing an apparent scoliosis in the tennis player (166). Often this postural change is asymptomatic, but thoracic outlet syndrome has been described in a player with a depressed tennis shoulder. Tennis shoulder can be treated by conscious elevation of the dominant shoulder, or prevented by exercises to strengthen the nonplaying arm and to stretch its shoulder elevators, to maintain a symmetrical physique.

Gymnastics

Caraffa and co-workers (167) studied elite male gymnasts, finding a surprising number with labral damage, particularly SLAP lesions, though the gymnasts had no history of dislocations or shoulder instability. Five of five elite and one of eight intermediate gymnasts surveyed had shoulder pain, most often acute in onset. Rings were the apparatus that caused pain, particularly just before the gymnast hung vertically from the rings after coming down from a handstand. EMG studies of this maneuver showed that the activity of the pectoralis major, biceps, deltoid, triceps, trapezius, and latissimus dorsi approximated only 10% of maximal activity at this point, even though the forces across the shoulder were high. It is possible that the pull of the body on the shoulder when the large muscles are not fully protecting the joint causes the labral damage. SLAP lesions result if the tendon of the long head of the biceps pulls on its attachment to the glenoid labrum with too great a force. Female gymnasts who do not perform on the rings have a much lower incidence of shoulder pain that is largely due to impingement (168).

GLENOHUMERAL OSTEOARTHRITIS

Primary glenohumeral osteoarthritis is uncommon, perhaps because the joint is non–weight-bearing and not a target joint for generalized osteoarthritis. The joint is subject to high forces across it (96), largely related to the weight of the arm and the forces needed to hold the humeral head against the glenoid during abduction. Degenerative changes in the articular cartilage are more common and more severe on the glenoid side of the joint posteriorly. Fibrillation, softening, and fraying of articular cartilage are seen, with cartilage loss, subchondral bone sclerosis, and subchondral cyst formation. The humeral head loses articular cartilage in a central baldness pattern. Anterior glenoid articular cartilage and a rim of humeral head articular cartilage are relatively spared. Marginal osteophytes appear, inferiorly and anteriorly about the glenoid and all around the rim of the humeral head (Fig. 107.10), due to traction of the joint capsule on these areas (96,169,170). Anterior capsular contractures and posterior humeral subluxation are common.

Clinically, primary glenohumeral arthritis causes decreased motion, particularly decreased rotation and abduction. Crepitus is felt with joint motion. Severe pain is unusual, and if it is present, an alternative explanation for the pain should be sought in the tendons and ligaments

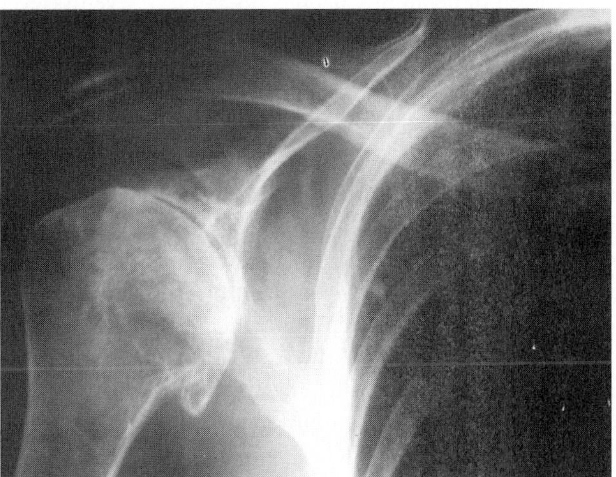

FIGURE 107.10. Glenohumeral osteoarthritis in an 87-year-old woman. The joint space is narrowed. Subchondral sclerosis of the humeral head and the glenoid and large inferior osteophytes are present.

(rotator cuff tendinitis or tear, calcific tendinitis) or neighboring joints (referred pain from the acromioclavicular joint or the neck) (96). Treatment of glenohumeral osteoarthritis includes NSAIDs, analgesics, and avoidance of painful movements. Occasionally, joint arthroplasty or arthrodesis is indicated, depending on the functional demands on the shoulder.

Secondary glenohumeral osteoarthritis occurs in the setting of chronic unreduced dislocation, fracture with malunion or a healed incongruous joint surface, avascular necrosis, and recurrent subluxations or dislocations (dislocation arthropathy) especially if the patient has had surgery for instability with internal fixation devices. Capsulorrhaphy arthropathy is an arthritis following an instability procedure wherein the capsule has been overtightened, usually anteriorly. The humeral head undergoes obligatory posterior translation, which causes eccentric glenohumeral contact and excessive wear of the posterior glenoid and central humeral articular cartilage. Patients are young, with an average age of 46, as opposed to an average age in the 60s for primary osteoarthritis (169).

The rotator cuff is almost always intact in patients with primary glenohumeral osteoarthritis, which, combined with the relative lack of pain and the wear on the central humeral articular cartilage distinguish primary osteoarthritis from the Milwaukee shoulder (cuff-tear arthropathy).

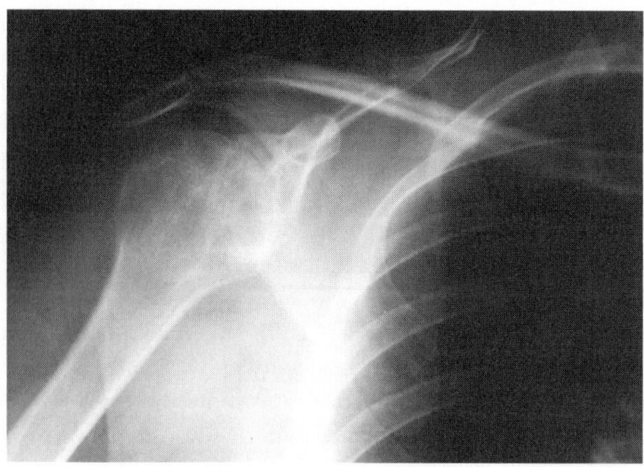

FIGURE 107.11. Rheumatoid arthritis of 10 years' duration in a 38-year-old woman. The joint space is diffusely and symmetrically narrowed. The humeral head shows cystic changes due to synovial invasion.

SHOULDER INVOLVEMENT IN SYSTEMIC DISEASE

Any of the systemic arthritides can affect the shoulder joints and bursae, as can many metabolic diseases. *Osteoarthritis* has been discussed in this chapter and is covered in Chapters 111 and 112. *Rheumatoid arthritis* (RA) (Fig. 107.11) is discussed in detail in Chapters 58 and 62. Seventy-seven percent of 105 patients with a mean duration of RA of 17 years had constant or intermittent shoulder pain (171). With increasing duration of RA, destructive joint changes in the shoulder progress and mobility lessens; 68% of 74 patients with seropositive erosive RA followed for 15 years from disease onset had definite rheumatoid involvement of the acromioclavicular joint radiographically (172). Thirty to forty percent of rheumatoid patients develop sternoclavicular erosions, generally by the end of the first year of illness (173). A sonographic study demonstrated that RA afflicts the shoulder diffusely, involving the glenohumeral and acromioclavicular joints and the biceps tendon sheath often, and the subacromial bursa and rotator cuff tendons occasionally (174).

Sternoclavicular tomograms (175), scintigraphy (176), arthroscopy, and synovial biopsy (177,178) have proven the existence of proximal synovitis in *polymyalgia rheumatica* (PMR). Shoulder MRI performed on 13 patients with untreated PMR and an average erythrocyte sedimentation rate (ESR) of 79 mm/hour revealed subacromial bursitis in all, glenohumeral joint synovitis in 77%, and biceps tenosynovitis in 54% (89). The widespread inflammation of the shoulder girdle seen in the MRI study may explain the diffuse proximal aching of patients with PMR that seems so out of proportion to the mild synovitis found on biopsy. Salvarani et al. (90) postulate that bursitis and tenosynovitis, rather than synovitis, may be the dominant features of the illness.

Crystal-induced arthritis can affect the sternoclavicular, acromioclavicular, or glenohumeral joints. *Gout* in the shoulder is unusual, though one series among alcohol users in Zimbabwe reported shoulder involvement in 5 of 23 patients (179). *Pseudogout* of the shoulders is common, though it is less frequent than pseudogout of the knees, wrists, and hips. *Tophaceous pseudogout* is rare, but when involving the sternoclavicular joint, may present as a mass effect on underlying nerves or blood vessels (180).

Shoulder arthropathy appears in approximately 50% of persons on *hemodialysis* for more than 10 years, usually attributable to articular and periarticular *amyloid* deposition. The amyloid-thickened rotator cuff and subacromial bursa may cause impingement symptoms, which can be relieved via arthroscopic or open resection of the coracoacromial ligament and acromial arthroplasty (181,182).

Hyperparathyroidism can cause pseudogout or inferior resorption of the distal third of the clavicles. Erosions about the humeral head and adjacent to the acromioclavicular joints may occur (183).

Avascular necrosis of the humeral head, like that of the femoral head, may follow steroid use, barotrauma, chronic alcohol use, sickle cell infarctions of bone (Fig. 107.12), trauma, or other causes. Pain precedes the collapse of the

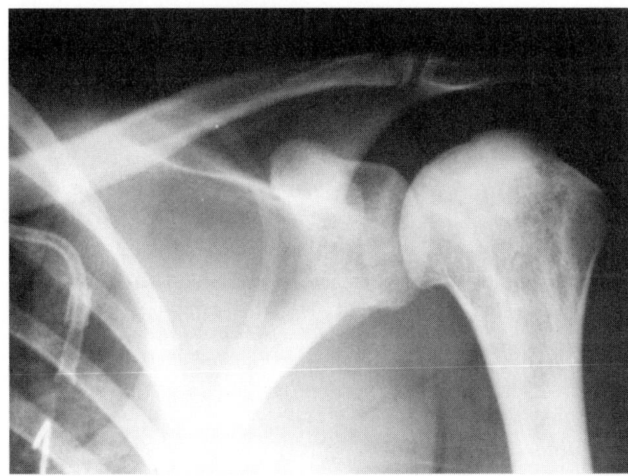

FIGURE 107.12. Avascular necrosis in a 24-year-old man with sickle cell disease. A crescent sign is seen beneath a small area of cortical collapse (lines).

humeral head. The irregular, collapsed head causes joint incongruity, and secondary osteoarthritis results.

Diabetes mellitus has numerous rheumatologic consequences in addition to its metabolic effects. Diabetics have an increased frequency of soft tissue calcifications about the shoulder (184), an increased risk of frozen shoulder (112), and a poorer prognosis for regaining mobility after frozen shoulder; 42% of 48 unselected insulin-dependent diabetics had restricted shoulder movements on exam in one study (185).

Shoulder pain may be the sole presenting complaint in *Parkinson's disease, cerebral tumor*, or *progressive focal encephalopathy* (186). The common physical finding in these patients is hypertonicity of the shoulder girdle muscles. Muscle disease such as *polymyositis* or *muscular dystrophy* may cause pain about the shoulder via changes in muscle tone or via weakness and altered scapulohumeral mechanics.

Shoulder arthropathy may also occur in the metabolic diseases *ochronosis, Wilson's disease, hemochromatosis, alkaptonuria*, and *amyloidosis*.

Sternoclavicular Disease

Primary osteoarthritis of the sternoclavicular (SC) joint is uncommon, for the intraarticular disc is massive and functions effectively as a buffer within the joint through the seventh decade (96). Posttraumatic osteoarthritis of the SC joint is more common, occurring after subluxations or dislocations or after a fracture of the medial clavicle. Anterior dislocations of the SC joint may result from athletic injuries or automobile accidents. Generally, no treatment is needed, though the clavicle may subluxate in and out of position, moving forward when the shoulder is braced back, and returning to its anatomic position when the shoulder is brought forward. Posterior dislocations are rare, but potentially disastrous, as the dislocated clavicle can disrupt the brachial plexus, pleura, esophagus, trachea, or major vessels, which lie behind the joint (96).

Involvement of the sternoclavicular joint in RA is frequent. Paice and co-workers (175) reported sternoclavicular erosions in 11 of 25 consecutive patients with PMR, as evaluated by sternoclavicular tomography. There was a strong correlation with the length of disease: six of seven patients with PMR for longer than 12 months had erosions (175).

Bacterial arthritis of the sternoclavicular joint represents 5% to 10% of all septic arthritis cases. Intravenous drug users, hemodialysis patients, and persons with indwelling intravenous catheters are especially susceptible (187).

Sternocostoclavicular hyperostosis (188,189) is an uncommon syndrome characterized by bony lesions of the anterior chest wall, and sometimes associated with rashes. It is felt to be a seronegative spondyloarthropathy (190) or a subset of psoriatic arthritis (191), and has been described under various names, including pustulotic arthro-osteitis (192), chronic recurrent multifocal osteomyelitis (the pediatric form of the syndrome), and SAPHO (synovitis-acne-pustulosis-hyperostosis-osteomyelitis) (193). Patients with Tietze's syndrome may in fact have SAPHO (194). The syndrome is seen primarily in children and young and middle-aged adults. Most reported cases are from Japan or northwestern Europe. The anterior chest wall is affected in all cases, with pain, tenderness, and swelling of gradual onset. Enlargement of the medial ends of the clavicles, upper ribs, and sternum; bony sclerosis or lytic lesions; and soft tissue ossification between the upper ribs and the clavicle are the characteristic radiographic findings (195). The technetium bone scan is positive, but typical findings on plain films make the diagnosis. The bony lesions are frequently associated with palmoplantar pustulosis, or with other skin diseases including psoriasis vulgaris (190,191), acne fulminans, hidradenitis suppurativa, and acne conglobata. Sacroiliitis occurs in up to 33% of patients (194), diffuse idiopathic skeletal hyperostosis (DISH) in up to 23% (188), and peripheral inflammatory arthritis in up to a third (188). The etiology is unknown, and biopsies of the bony lesions show only chronic nonspecific inflammation. Rarely, cultures of a bony lesion have grown *Proprionibacterium acnes* (194), but usually cultures are negative. Several Japanese authors have suggested that the syndrome is an allergic or inflammatory response to a focal infection, and they cite cases of palmoplantar pustulosis that have improved after tonsillectomy (189).

The clinical course is one of exacerbations and remissions of the painful chest wall lesions. The illness tends to remit spontaneously in patients over age 60 (189). Treatment with antibacterials is effective in some patients (189), but ineffective in most (194). NSAIDs are the mainstay of treatment. Colchicine has been used, as has sulfasalazine

(194). Intraarticular steroid injections may give some relief (2). Intravenous pamidronate has been used successfully for sternal pain in a patient (195); calcitonin also has helped with painful bone lesions (196).

ACROMIOCLAVICULAR DISEASE

The acromioclavicular (AC) joint is a common source of shoulder pain. The articular surfaces are small, usually incongruous, and variable. The intraarticular disc is rarely complete, deteriorates with aging, and does not protect the articular surfaces well. Most people have advanced degenerative arthritis of the AC joint by mid-life (96). The AC joint is subject to frequent direct or indirect trauma, because of its exposed location. AC strains, subluxations, and complete dislocations (shoulder separations) all predispose to osteoarthritis. Osteophytes extending inferiorly from an arthritic AC joint compromise the subacromial space and can cause rotator cuff impingement symptoms.

Clinically, the patient with AC osteoarthritis experiences a diffuse shoulder pain, radiating down into the lateral deltoid or up into the neck. Pain is worsened by overhead activities or by lying on the shoulder. The patient may describe a painful arc of motion, which at 120 to 180 degrees is higher than the painful arc of rotator cuff disease. The joint is tender to palpation. Pushups and horizontal cross-chest adduction with the arm at 90-degree elevation stress the AC joint. Grasping the unaffected shoulder with the hand and pulling toward the affected side is painful. Trying to pull apart the interlocked hands when the arms are held at shoulder height also causes pain from compression of the arthritic joint (197). A lidocaine injection into the AC joint can be used diagnostically to determine whether a joint that is arthritic by radiographic examination is in fact the cause of the shoulder pain.

Treatment of AC arthritis begins with avoidance of activities above 120-degree abduction. NSAIDs are used orally; an intraarticular steroid injection can be tried. Shoulder range of motion exercises and scapular stabilizer strengthening exercises are used. Open or arthroscopic resection of the distal 1 to 2 cm of the clavicle is consistently quite successful in relieving osteoarthritic pain that has not responded to conservative treatment (197).

Edelson (198) examined 300 cadaveric bony specimens, finding no arthritis in AC joints that were adjacent to healed clavicular fractures. He speculated that the clavicular shortening served as a "physiologic arthroplasty" to protect the AC joint from compressive forces and the subsequent development of osteoarthritis.

A less common cause of AC pain and tenderness is osteolysis of the distal clavicle. This can occur several weeks to years after direct trauma (199) or can occur atraumatically in weight lifters, gymnasts, and laborers whose AC joints experience repeated stresses (200,201). Patients typically are in their teens to thirties, and insidiously develop pain with overhead activities. Radiographs show osteoporosis, cystic changes, and loss of subchondral bony detail in the distal clavicle and sometimes in the acromion. The AC joint space widens. Bone scintigraphy is positive during this lytic process. The causes of posttraumatic and atraumatic osteolysis of the distal clavicle are unknown. Proposed etiologies include autonomic nervous system dysfunction with secondary ischemia, stress fractures, avascular necrosis, and synovial hyperplasia. Treatment is cessation of any provoking activities and rest of the AC joint. This in itself can relieve pain and lead to partial or complete reossification of the clavicle. Oral NSAIDs and steroid injections generally are not helpful, but the nonsteroidals should be tried. Patients who do not improve with conservative treatment, or who cannot or will not change their activities, respond to excision of the distal clavicle.

NEOPLASM INVOLVING THE SHOULDER GIRDLE

Primary bone tumors involving the shoulder are infrequent (202). Metastatic cancer to the highly vascular upper humerus is not uncommon, occurring in breast, lung, kidney, prostate, and thyroid cancers. Multiple myeloma can cause shoulder pain via involvement of the ribs, spine, scapula, clavicle, or proximal humerus.

REFERRED PAIN FROM VISCERAL DISEASE

Shoulder pain may be the sole or presenting symptom of underlying distant visceral disease. When this extrinsic cause of shoulder pain exists, physical examination of the shoulder is normal. Active and passive ranges of motion are full, there is no point tenderness, and there is no crepitus or muscle atrophy. Referred pain may arise from thoracic or abdominal illnesses that irritate the phrenic nerve or the diaphragm. Potential thoracic causes of referred pain include myocardial ischemia or infarction, lung neoplasm (especially Pancoast tumors) or infarction, esophageal spasm, and dissecting aortic aneurysm. Potential abdominal causes of referred pain include gallbladder disease, subphrenic abscess, splenic trauma, and perforated peptic ulcers or diverticulae.

POSTURE

Persons whose work demands a head-forward position and those with a dorsal kyphosis due to skeletal abnormalities or habitual posture are particularly susceptible to postural shoulder pain. Muscle tightness secondary to psychological or physical stress and poor muscle tone due to chronic illness or deconditioning exacerbate this susceptibility. When the head and arms are held in front of the body's center of gravity for a prolonged time, active muscle contractions are needed to maintain balance. Muscle fatigue can lead to a dull aching pain about the neck and shoulders, particularly in the trapezius, rhomboids, and latissimus dorsi. Acutely, massage or ultrasound of the affected muscles is helpful. Long-term relief entails postural retraining, workstation modification, and strengthening exercises for the scapular stabilizers.

CONGENITAL ANOMALIES

The most common congenital abnormality of the shoulder is Sprengel's deformity, or congenital elevation of the scapula. Although Eulenberg first described the condition in 1863, Sprengel in 1891 was the first to theorize that it resulted from failure of the scapula to descend during intrauterine development. The scapula is hypoplastic and retains the fetal shape of an equilateral triangle (203). Sprengel's deformity is highly associated with other skeletal and soft tissue abnormalities: scoliosis in 47%, rib abnormalities in 38%, and Klippel-Feil syndrome (brevicollis) in 29%. Missing or ectopic kidneys occur in up to 6% of patients (204).

Congenital fibrotic bands within the deltoid muscles are far less common than acquired fibrosis from repeated intramuscular injections, but have the same clinical picture.

DELTOID CONTRACTURES

Fibrotic contractures can develop in the quadriceps, the gluteus muscles, the deltoid, or the triceps in children or adults, typically after repeated intramuscular injections. No particular drug has been implicated more than any other (though several reports in adults involved pentazocine). The common factor in reported cases has been frequent intramuscular injection of fairly high volumes of fluid into the involved muscle (205). As the deltoid muscle develops fibrous bands, the patient develops an abduction contracture, with extension of the shoulder and scapular winging. Scapular winging disappears when the arm is abducted above 90 degrees.

The major consequences of deltoid contractures in adults are pain in the neck and shoulder girdle and inconveniences associated with activities of daily living. Untreated deltoid contractures in children are less frequently painful, but can have more serious consequences. The fibrous band in the deltoid acts as the fulcrum of a lever, and the weight of the abducted arm tends to push the humeral head superiorly. Compressive forces lead to flattening of the humeral head. Scoliosis or narrowing of the thoracic cage may develop in response to the weight of the abducted arm (206). Treatment of the contractures includes cessation of intramuscular injections and surgical resection of the fibrous bands. The arm then can be adducted, the scapular winging resolves, and if a child is still young enough to remodel bones, the humeral head regains its normal contour.

SNAPPING SCAPULA

Snapping scapula refers to crepitus felt or heard beneath the scapula as it moves over the thorax. Scapulothoracic crepitus is present physiologically in some people (207), but in others the sounds are louder or the grating coarser, and the scapulothoracic motion is painful. These persons may have chronic shoulder girdle or neck pain, with tenderness along the medial scapular border. If a person with a snapping scapula puts the ipsilateral hand on the contralateral shoulder, thereby moving the medial scapula away from the underlying chest wall, the crepitus and pain are lessened.

The etiology of snapping scapula is not always known. Occasionally a specific bony abnormality is found, which diminishes the normal separation between the scapula and the chest wall. Examples include scapular exostoses, osteochondromas, healed scapular fractures, a tubercle of Luschka (a prominent bony or fibrocartilaginous nodule at the superomedial angle of the scapula), anterior angulation of the superior angle of the scapula, or underlying rib abnormalities (208). At times snapping occurs in association with Sprengel's deformity (congenital undescended scapula), probably because of the unusual scapular shape.

Soft tissue pathology can cause snapping. Percy et al. (209) thought that the levator scapulae and rhomboids could, through repeated overhead motions, develop tendinitis at the insertions into the medial scapula. They likened the process to tennis elbow, resulting from repeated microtraumas and overuse. Snapping can occur in the setting of serratus anterior atrophy or subscapularis atrophy, perhaps from altered scapulothoracic mechanics or perhaps from a lessening of the muscle cushion between the scapula and the ribs. Snapping scapula has been described in people who have undergone a first rib resection for thoracic outlet syndrome, probably because of altered muscle mechanics postoperatively (208).

Acquired, or adventitious, bursae may be present beneath the scapula (40). Bursitis due to frictional scapulothoracic forces can cause crepitus.

The differential diagnosis of snapping scapula is basically the differential diagnosis of posterior shoulder pain, and includes referred pain from the glenohumeral joint, from the subacromial space, or from the neck. Thoracic outlet syndrome should be considered. Fibromyalgia can cause very similar pain and tenderness, but generally these patients have widespread trigger points.

The conservative treatment of snapping scapula may include NSAIDs, ultrasound, transcutaneous nerve stimulation, or a local subscapular injection of steroid and anesthetic. These often help pain, though they may not relieve the snapping. Postural exercises and strengthening exercises for the scapular stabilizers are the primary treatment, helping both pain and the crepitus. Many physicians believe that only conservative treatment should be offered (209). Others perform open or arthroscopic (210) resection of the superomedial or medial scapula in patients with recalcitrant pain, particularly if a bony abnormality is demonstrated by oblique radiographs, CT scans, or fluoroscopy. Postoperatively, strengthening of scapular adduction and postural shoulder-shrug exercises are reemphasized (207).

NEUROLOGIC CAUSES OF SHOULDER PAIN

Brachial Plexus Injuries

The brachial plexus is most commonly injured via a traction mechanism, wherein the head is forcefully tilted away from the shoulder in a fall (211), a blow to the shoulder, or a motorcycle or automobile accident. Which portion of the brachial plexus is injured depends to a great extent on the position of the arm in relation to the body at the time of injury. If the arm is adducted, the upper plexus (formed from cervical roots C5, C6, and C7) is injured. Clinical signs include weakness of abduction and external rotation of the shoulder due to deltoid and spinatus paresis. Elbow flexion is affected because of bicipital weakness. If the arm is abducted at the time of injury, the lower plexus (formed from C8 and T1 roots) is involved. The resultant paresis of the intrinsic muscles of the hand diminishes grip strength.

Penetrating wounds due to knives or bullets can damage the brachial plexus. Compression injuries from backpacks (212), figure-of-eight splints for clavicular fractures, or excessive callus formation after clavicular fractures are less common than traction injuries, but generally resolve fully with time. Postoperative brachial palsies can be avoided by limiting abduction of the arm during anesthesia to 90 degrees, and by preventing posterior displacement of the arm. Most postoperative brachial palsies are neurapraxias, which means that there is physiologic disturbance of nerve function, but no anatomic damage to the nerve. They resolve completely, usually within 6 weeks (211).

Burners or stingers are brachial plexus injuries common in contact sports such as football or rugby. They are brief episodes of burning dysesthesias, often of the entire arm, after a blow to the shoulder or head during a tackle or a fall. Weakness of the deltoid, biceps, and spinatus muscles can follow the severe dysesthesias and pain, moments or even days later. The burners result most often from a stretching of the upper brachial plexus as the shoulder is forced downward and the head tilted in the opposite direction. In the person who has an underlying congenital anomaly or spinal stenosis, burners may result from extension of the neck with rotation or tilting toward the affected side. Treatment is conservative, including avoidance of contact until the neurologic symptoms fully resolve and exercises to maintain strength and flexibility about the shoulder (213).

The differential diagnosis of brachial plexus injuries includes neuralgic amyotrophy, cervical radiculopathy, dead arm syndrome caused by occult glenohumeral subluxation, cervical fracture, and transient quadriplegia from a spinal cord contusion (213). The prognosis for brachial plexus lesions depends on the exact site of the lesion and its severity. Severe burning pain is a poor prognostic sign for recovery.

Neuralgic Amyotrophy (Parsonage-Turner Syndrome, Paralytic Brachial Neuritis, Acute Brachial Plexitis)

Neuralgic amyotrophy is an illness of unknown etiology, characterized by the sudden onset of severe pain about the shoulder girdle that lasts a few hours to several weeks, followed by variable degrees of motor loss in the affected shoulder and/or forearm, then eventual spontaneous recovery (214–216). The annual incidence has been estimated at 1.64/100,000 (217). It can affect any age, but most nonfamilial cases occur between ages 20 and 60, with a predilection for males. Neuralgic amyotrophy may follow an infection, surgery in a remote site, or immunization, or may occur in a totally healthy individual. The rare familial cases are indistinguishable from nonfamilial cases clinically, except for an earlier age of onset, a tendency to recurrence, and a positive family history (218). Epidemics of brachial plexus neuritis have been reported (219,220).

Fever and constitutional signs are lacking. The pain often begins in the scapular region, or can involve the top of the shoulder, the side of the neck, or the upper arm. Movement of the shoulder or elbow exacerbates the pain, but coughing, sneezing, and neck motions do not. Patients often appear with the arm held in a position of shoulder adduction and elbow flexion.

The pain lasts from several hours to several weeks generally, and paresis appears within 14 days of the onset of pain. The motor loss is in the area of one or more peripheral nerves, or one or more nerve roots, or some combination of nerves and cervical roots. Profound atrophy appears rapidly. Because the upper brachial plexus is involved more frequently than the lower plexus, the shoulder musculature is affected more than that of the elbow or the wrist. Sensory loss is variable, and is mild in comparison to the motor findings. The most common sensory finding is a small area of hypoesthesia over the deltoid muscle, in the distribution of the axillary nerve.

Electromyographic studies document muscle denervation, and may demonstrate subclinical involvement of the opposite brachial plexus. (Clinical bilateral involvement does occur, but is uncommon.) Nerve biopsies show profound axonal degeneration. Analysis of the blood and cerebrospinal fluid is generally normal. Radiographs are normal or nonspecific.

The prognosis of neuralgic amyotrophy is good. Tsairis et al. (221) reported 80% functional recovery by 2 years and 90% functional recovery by 3 years in a series of 99 patients. Treatment is supportive, with analgesics during the painful phase, passive range of motion exercises during the atrophic phase, then active exercises during recovery.

Cervical Radiculopathies

The most common causes of cervical radiculopathies are a herniated cervical disc and cervical degenerative arthritis. When the C5 or C6 nerve root is involved pain is often felt in the shoulder or posterior neck. Clues to cervical radiculopathy are a dermatomal pattern to the pain and motor or sensory loss, pain that extends distally past the elbow, normal passive shoulder range of motion, and worsening of the pain or dysesthesias with coughing or sneezing.

Axillary Nerve Palsy

Axillary nerve palsy is most common after shoulder dislocation or fracture of the surgical neck of the humerus, but it also can follow blunt trauma to the shoulder without fracture or dislocation. Deltoid function is lost, but adjacent muscles that originate from the C5 nerve root are unaffected. Sensory loss may or may not be present. Patients with incomplete paralysis have a better outcome than those with complete paralysis. If the palsy is complete, the patient should be examined monthly for evidence of neurologic recovery. If no recovery is seen clinically or by electromyography by 3 to 4 months, surgery should be considered to see if the nerve is in discontinuity and if so, to attempt a nerve graft (222).

Spinal Accessory Nerve Palsy

Paralysis of the trapezius can result from trauma to or postviral inflammation of the spinal accessory nerve. The patient experiences a persistent dull ache in the shoulder, with weak abduction, drooping, and loss of shoulder shrugging. On active abduction, the scapula moves down and outward away from the spine; abduction is limited to 180 degrees. Recovery may occur over 3 to 12 months (96).

Long Thoracic Nerve Palsy

The long thoracic nerve arises from the ventral rami of C5, C6, and C7 nerve roots and supplies the serratus anterior, a major scapular stabilizer that holds the scapula closely applied to the posterior chest wall. Long thoracic nerve palsy causes winging of the scapula, which means that the scapula is not held in its proper position against the chest wall. It may follow infections, ingestion of toxins, trauma, breast cancer surgery, transaxillary first rib resection for thoracic outlet syndrome, transaxillary breast augmentation, anesthesia, or participation in sports such as wrestling, weight lifting, tennis, or ballet (223). It may be idiopathic. Abduction is weak and limited, because the scapula shifts upward and inward when it is attempted. The inferior angle of the scapula moves toward the spine and, with the vertebral scapular border, juts out from the chest wall. Winging is particularly apparent when the patient pushes against a wall with his arms in front of him. Long thoracic nerve palsies are usually due to stretching injuries, and may resolve over a 3- to 12-month period (96).

Suprascapular Nerve Palsy

Suprascapular nerve entrapment is an underrecognized cause of posterolateral shoulder pain. The suprascapular nerve is a mixed sensorimotor nerve that arises from the ventral fibers of C5 and C6, with contributions from C4 about half the time. It runs beneath the omohyoid and trapezius muscles, then enters the supraspinous fossa at the suprascapular notch (Fig. 107.13), ducking beneath the (superior) transverse scapular ligament (224). It runs deep to the supraspinatus muscle, giving off motor branches to the supraspinatus and sensory branches to the glenohumeral and AC joints. At the lateral border of the scapular spine, it runs through the spinoglenoid notch to enter the infraspinous fossa. The nerve is relatively fixed at the suprascapular notch, though the notch itself moves with excursions of the scapula during arm movements (225). Suprascapular nerve entrapment most commonly occurs here, at the suprascapular notch.

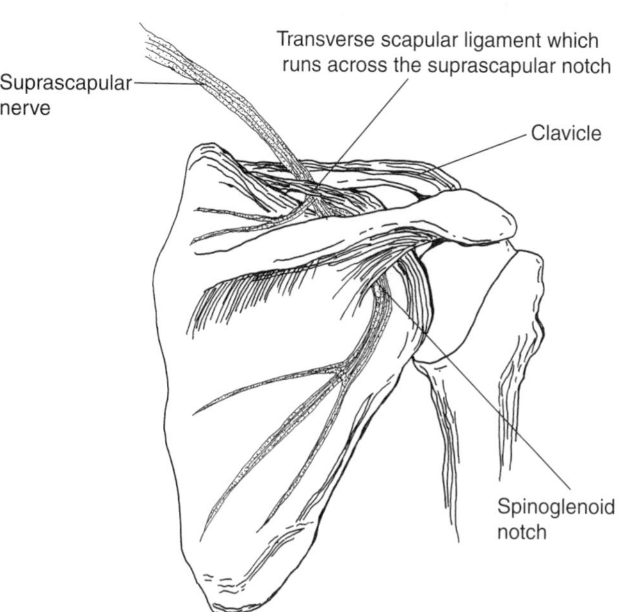

FIGURE 107.13. Course of the suprascapular nerve.

The patient experiences a deep aching or burning posterolateral shoulder pain. It may radiate medially up into the neck, or medially to the interscapular region, or laterally down the arm (225). Both spinatus muscles atrophy if the nerve is compressed at the suprascapular notch. The infraspinatus alone atrophies if the nerve lesion is more distal, at the spinoglenoid notch. External rotation and abduction are weak, external rotation slightly more so (226).

The nerve can be compressed at the suprascapular notch by ganglia, tumors, scapular fractures, lipomas, anterior glenohumeral dislocation, or direct trauma. Occasionally the transverse scapular ligament is partially or completely ossified, which makes it more rigid and more likely to inflame the tethered underlying suprascapular nerve in the setting of heavy shoulder use. The suprascapular notch may be small and V-shaped, rather than U-shaped, which may predispose to traction injuries of the nerve (227). The nerve is also prone to traction injuries if the supraspinatus muscle is advanced laterally during repair of a massive rotator cuff tear (228).

Compression at the spinoglenoid notch can result from ganglia arising from the posterior glenohumeral joint capsule and underlying labral tears (229) or from the mass lesions listed above. The nerve is prone to traction injuries as the nerve is stretched around the lateral scapular spine with cross-body adduction and internal rotation of the shoulder, or with other motions that cause wide scapular excursions. The nerve can be compressed under a hypertrophied inferior transverse scapular ligament (spinoglenoid ligament), though this ligament is not present in all shoulders (230). Sandow and Ilic (231) proposed that the suprascapular nerve is subject to direct compression between the lateral scapular spine and the aponeurotic connection between the supraspinatus and infraspinatus components of the rotator cuff. When the shoulder is abducted and externally rotated, as in the cocking movement of the baseball pitcher or the volleyball server, the rotator cuff seems to impinge on the lateral scapular spine, trapping the suprascapular nerve. This can explain the infraspinatus atrophy and weakness of external rotation seen in a significant number of world-class volleyball players (231,232).

Diagnosis of suprascapular neuropathy rests first upon the awareness of the syndrome, then upon the typical clinical picture of deep posterior shoulder pain with atrophy of the spinatus muscles and weakness of external rotation. Electromyography confirms the diagnosis by demonstrating denervation in the spinatus muscles (or infraspinatus alone), and localizes the problem to the suprascapular notch or the spinoglenoid notch. Nerve conduction velocities are often but not always slowed (226). MRI is used to look for mass lesions impinging upon the nerve, and to document atrophic muscle.

The initial treatment is conservative, and includes NSAIDs for their antiinflammatory and analgesic properties, and Neurontin or amitriptyline for the neuropathic pain. Exercises are done to strengthen the rotator cuff muscles, the deltoid, and the scapular stabilizers. Steroid injections at the suprascapular notch have been used successfully in some cases (233). The patient with a discrete anatomic lesion or with no response to conservative treatment should undergo surgery to remove mass lesions, drain ganglia, or resect overlying ligaments. Patients who undergo surgery within 6 months of the onset of symptoms do better than those who wait a longer time (234).

Syringomyelia and Neuroarthropathy (Charcot Joint)

Syringomyelia is a rare condition characterized by a liquid-filled cavity occupying the central part of the spinal cord in the cervical region, at times extending up into the medulla oblongata or down into the thoracic or lumbar regions. Sensitivity to pain and sensitivity to temperature are lost in the affected regions of the arms, shoulders, and neck; sensitivity to touch and position sense remain intact. Muscle atrophy (amyotrophy) develops in patients with syringomyelia, as does thoracic kyphoscoliosis (thought to be secondary to asymmetric weakness of the paravertebral muscles). Syringomyelia is congenital or idiopathic or posttraumatic (occurring in approximately 1.3% of patients with spinal cord injuries) (235). Neuroarthropathy develops in 10% to 25% of patients with syringomyelia (235,236), most commonly in the shoulder, followed in frequency by the elbow and then the wrist.

Two theories of pathogenesis of Charcot joints exist. The neurotraumatic theory states that when a joint is insensate, cumulative microtrauma leads to joint destruction. The neurovascular theory postulates an alteration in sympathetic nervous activity, leading to joint hyperemia and accelerated osteolysis by osteoclasts. Joint destruction is secondary and occurs with weight bearing. The glenohumeral joint is highly mobile, and it is easy to imagine that microtrauma in such a mobile joint would be frequent when abnormal movements are not felt as being painful.

Shoulder neuroarthropathy can be the presenting sign of syringomyelia (235–237). The shoulder swells and can be hot, but remains relatively painless. Radiographs show marked destruction of the humeral head and glenoid cavity. The joint is disorganized, with a large effusion and periarticular soft tissue edema and bony debris. The proximal humerus may subluxate. Destructive changes occur as rapidly as 8 to 21 days after the onset of symptoms (237).

Bisphosphonates have been used successfully to treat diabetic Charcot joints in the feet (238,239), and should be evaluated in the treatment of shoulder neuroarthropathy (236). Parenteral pamidronate 90 mg intravenously every 4 months is a potential regimen (238).

Shoulder Pain in Quadriplegia, Paraplegia, and Hemiplegia

Patients with spinal cord injuries at level C5 or lower have the potential to use their shoulders in a weight-bearing fashion for independent transfers and decompression raises. The shoulder is needed for wheelchair propulsion and for hand positioning in the performance of activities of daily living. Shoulder pain can make the difference between independence and dependence in these paraplegic or quadriplegic patients.

Shoulder pain occurs in 75% of quadriplegic patients during the first 6 months after the spinal cord injury. Rotator cuff pathology and frozen shoulder are the dominant causes. Thirty to sixty percent of patients have shoulder pain chronically. Instability is the major problem in this group. When the spinal cord level is C5 or higher, some rotator cuff function is lost, and thus dynamic stability of the shoulder is lessened. Static instability arises from the stretching of the capsuloligamentous structures over time (240). Among wheelchair-bound paraplegics who transfer independently, the most common cause of shoulder pain is subacromial impingement (241).

Lal (242) examined 33 quadriplegic and 20 paraplegic patients prospectively, finding 72% with radiographic changes of osteoarthritis, primarily at the AC joint. Patients with a higher level of wheelchair activity, those above age 30, and women were more likely to have these changes. Only 11% complained of shoulder pain (242).

The patient with hemiplegia from a completed stroke may be left with a painful nonfunctioning shoulder, a partially functioning shoulder, a frozen shoulder, or reflex sympathetic dystrophy. The first stage is a flaccid shoulder. The humeral head subluxates down and out because of loss of tone in the supraspinatus muscle. The angle of the glenoid fossa changes because loss of tone in the trapezius and serratus anterior muscles leads to scapular depression and outward rotation. The vertical spine bends toward the side of the hemiparesis. Treatment during the flaccid stage revolves around careful positioning of the spine, the scapula, and the glenohumeral joint. The scapula is kept protracted, and the scapula is held during transfers, not the upper arm.

Most patients with stroke will progress to a spastic phase, in which the scapula remains depressed and retracted, the glenohumeral joint is subluxated, the humerus is adducted and internally rotated, the elbow flexed, the forearm pronated, and the wrists and fingers flexed. The patient may progress further to the synergy stage, wherein any movement to the patient or attempted by the patient reflexly initiates the above flexor pattern. Treatment during these phases involves intensive muscle reeducation by physicians and therapists trained in rehabilitation (1).

NEUROVASCULAR CAUSES OF SHOULDER PAIN

Thoracic Outlet Syndrome

The thoracic outlet syndrome is defined as neurovascular compression of the subclavian artery and vein and the brachial plexus as they run through a narrow canal of bones and soft tissues from the apex of the thorax and base of the neck toward the axilla. Three areas in this canal are potential sites of compression: (a) the scalene triangle, bounded by the scalenus anterior and scalenus medius and by the first rib inferiorly; (b) the costoclavicular space, bounded by the clavicle and subclavius muscle superiorly and laterally, the first rib inferiorly, and the scapula posteriorly; and (c) the pectoralis minor muscle where it inserts on the coracoid process. The existence of thoracic outlet syndrome is unquestioned, but its incidence is unknown and controversial.

Neurologic symptoms predominate. Ninety percent of cases of thoracic outlet syndrome are due to nerve compression, with only 10% being solely or dominantly due to vascular compression; 90% to 95% of patients have pain and paresthesias in the shoulder, neck, arm, and hand, and 10% have motor weakness. The inferior portion of the brachial plexus is most vulnerable to compression and angulation as it runs through the thoracic outlet; thus, neurologic symptoms and signs are often in the C8-T1 distribution. Paresthesias are frequently segmental, in the distribution of the ulnar nerve. The arm becomes intolerant of cold and fatigues easily. Overhead use of the arms or downward traction on the arms worsens the symptoms.

Pain begins insidiously, but occasionally it begins so suddenly and so severely in the anterior chest and periscapular region that it mimics angina (243). Other atypical presentations of pain include occipital or orbital headaches, syncope with dizziness, and tinnitus initiated or exacerbated by hyperabduction of the arm (244).

Patients with the proximal nerve compression of thoracic outlet syndrome are more vulnerable to peripheral nerve compression as well, in a double-crush phenomenon. Up to 44% of patients with thoracic outlet syndrome have an associated distal compressive neuropathy (245).

Vascular compressive symptoms are less common than neurologic symptoms, and arterial compression is less likely than venous compression, in a ratio of 1:4 (246). Venous stasis, swelling of the arm, a heavy sensation, cyanosis (puffy blue hands), and distention of venous collaterals about the shoulder and anterior chest may all occur. Thrombosis of the subclavian/axillary vein in an active healthy individual who overuses the arm (baseball player or tennis player, for example) is called effort thrombosis or Paget-Schroetter syndrome. It usually indicates compression in the costoclavicular space.

Arterial compression causes weakness and coldness of the arm, occasionally with Raynaud's phenomenon or even ischemic ulceration in the fingers. Pain results from an ischemic neuritis. Arterial compression often occurs when there is a cervical rib, and a poststenotic aneurysm of the subclavian artery may result.

Osseous abnormalities are seen in 30% of the patients with thoracic outlet syndrome (247), most commonly a cervical rib or a clavicular deformity. Cervical ribs occur in 0.5% to 1.0% of the population, but are symptomatic only 5% to 10% of the time (248). In roughly half to two-thirds of the cases, cervical ribs are bilateral, but symptoms usually are unilateral and right-sided (249).

The age of onset of thoracic outlet symptoms is most often between 20 and 40. Women are affected more often than men. Poor posture predisposes to thoracic outlet syndrome, for the clavicle is depressed and the scapula is pushed forward when shoulders sag; space within the thoracic outlet shrinks. Heavy-breasted women can experience compression in the costoclavicular region, for the bra strap pulls the clavicle down with the weight of the breasts (250). Climbers, soldiers, or students who wear heavy backpacks are at risk via the same mechanism. Persons who sleep or work with the arms abducted to 180 degrees over the head are prone to compression in the pectoralis minor region as the neurovascular bundle is slung around the pectoralis minor insertion on the coracoid and trapped between the pectoralis minor and the subscapular muscles. Women with long swan necks and low-set shoulders can experience pain and dysesthesias in the arms due to stretching of the brachial plexus (251).

Diagnosis of thoracic outlet syndrome is difficult, and it is here that controversy arises. Cases of venous or arterial compression are easily diagnosed with the aid of Dopplers or venograms and noninvasive arterial studies or arteriograms, in the setting of an appropriate history and clinical exam, but vascular thoracic outlet syndrome is uncommon. Neurologic compression infrequently has objective physical findings. Some investigators find ulnar nerve conduction velocity testing across the clavicle to be helpful (247); others find that nerve conduction velocities and EMGs rarely are abnormal (252). Somatosensory evoked potentials recorded from the brachial plexus and cervical spine, after median and ulnar nerve stimulation in one study, were more sensitive than nerve conduction velocity testing in the diagnosis of thoracic outlet syndrome (253).

Four provocative physical maneuvers are used in the diagnosis of thoracic outlet syndrome. The scalenus maneuver or Adson's test constricts the scalene outlet. The patient takes a deep breath (to raise the first rib), extends his neck, and turns the head toward the arm that is being examined. The examiner looks for a diminution or obliteration of the radial pulse in the tested arm and asks the patient if neurologic symptoms are reproduced. In the costoclavicular test, the patient sits or stands at attention, in an exaggerated military posture, with the shoulders pressed down and back. Again, he takes a deep breath, the radial pulse is monitored and the presence or absence of paresthesias is noted. The hyperabduction test or Wright's test involves abducting the arm to 180 degrees while the pulse is monitored and paresthesias asked about. The Roos test is one in which the arm is abducted to 90 degrees and externally rotated, and the patient repeatedly clenches and unclenches his fist. This test is performed for 3 minutes and is positive if the patient experiences paresthesias in the arm at any point during the 3 minutes. The latter two procedures evaluate the pectoralis minor space. It is important to realize that in 50% to 87% of normal people (245,254), the radial pulse is diminished or obliterated (and infraclavicular or supraclavicular bruits may be produced) by at least one of these provocative tests. A neurologic response to at least one provocative maneuver occurs in 41% of normals (245). The high percentage of positive tests in normal people obviously lessens the usefulness of these maneuvers.

For many clinicians thoracic outlet syndrome is a diagnosis of exclusion. Mimickers of neurologic thoracic outlet syndrome include cervical spine disease or herniated cervical discs, amyotrophic lateral sclerosis, syringomyelia, multiple sclerosis, brachial plexitis, postural palsies, peripheral neuropathies, and distal compressive neuropathies including cumulative trauma disorder (255). Malignancies of the lung apex, the mediastinum, or neck can affect the brachial plexus. Takayasu's arteritis and other vasculitides, angina, arterial embolism, thromboangiitis obliterans, Raynaud's disease or phenomenon, and reflex sympathetic dystrophy should be considered in the differential diagnosis, as well as thrombophlebitis associated with malignancy, birth control pills, or anticardiolipin antibody syndrome.

Treatment of thoracic outlet syndrome begins with attention to posture and strengthening exercises for the rhomboids, the levator scapulae, and the trapezius muscles. Heavy-breasted women should wear underwire bras with broad shoulder straps. Neurologic symptoms alone rarely mandate surgery (255), but vascular compression frequently does. Transaxillary resection of the first rib is a favored surgical approach, though some surgeons prefer an anterior approach if arterial compression exists (249).

Reflex Sympathetic Dystrophy

Reflex sympathetic dystrophy (RSD) is a syndrome of extremity pain, swelling, stiffness, and discoloration often leading to disability, usually occurring after trauma or in association with a disease or a drug. Mitchell et al. (256), during the American Civil War, described "causalgia" as a burning pain in the extremity after a gunshot wound. Numerous investigators have described causalgia and RSD since, each emphasizing various signs and symptoms within the syndromes. Different names are used for RSD, including algodystrophy (in Europe), Sudeck's atrophy, shoulder-hand syndrome, postinfarction sclerodactyly, sympathetic trophoneurosis, and complex regional pain syndrome type I. The International Association for the Study of Pain (IASP) coined the last term at a consensus meeting in 1993. Complex regional pain syndrome type II was defined as causalgia, a painful dystophy following injury of a peripheral nerve. RSD was renamed complex regional pain syndrome (CRPS) type I. The IASP's definition of CRPS type I was "a syndrome that usually develops after an initiating noxious event, is not limited to the distribution of a single peripheral nerve, and is apparently disproportionate to the inciting event. It is associated at some point with evidence of edema, changes in skin blood flow, abnormal sudomotor activity in the region of the pain, or allodynia or hyperalgesia" (257). CRPS type I is felt to be a spectrum of entities, with pain as the primary characteristic of the illness. "Complex" refers to its variability over time and from person to person. It also refers to the plethora of inflammatory, autonomic, motor, cutaneous, and dystrophic signs that can accompany the neuropathic pain. "Regional" reflects the involvement of an area beyond the area initially injured. The area involved does not represent the distribution of any single peripheral nerve (258). This name does not imply any particular pathophysiology. It is well known that RSD does not necessarily involve nervous reflexes, may or may not include sympathetically maintained pain in a given patient, and may lead to dystrophy or may resolve fully with no sequelae. Nevertheless, for historical reasons, this chapter uses the term *reflex sympathetic dystrophy.*

The prevalence of RSD is not known. It can be associated with one of a number of diseases, drugs, or injuries (Table 107.5). More than 25% of the time, no associated precipitant is found (2). Trauma is the most common inciting factor, but the trauma can be very minor. Reported incidences of RSD range from 5% to 20% of patients with myocardial infarctions (2), 12% to 21% of patients with hemiplegia (2), 0.2% to 35% after Colles' fracture (2,259,260), and 2% to 5% after peripheral nerve injury (261). Some investigators have suggested that certain personality types predispose to RSD or that stressful life events increase the risk of RSD (262,263), but others feel that depression, anxiety, and other psychological disturbances are the result of the RSD rather than a cause (264,265).

TABLE 107.5. CONDITIONS ASSOCIATED WITH REFLEX SYMPATHETIC DYSTROPHY

Trauma: major, minor, or surgical
Ischemic heart disease
Cerebrovascular disease with hemiplegia; hemiplegia from other causes
Cervical osteoarthritis with neural foraminal encroachment or cervical herniated disc[a]
Fractures, especially Colles' fracture
Herpes zoster
Epilepsy
Brain tumors
Spinal cord lesions: syringomyelia, polio, myelopathy
Lumbar herniated disk
Barbiturates or other anticonvulsants
Antituberculous therapy, especially isoniazid
Peripheral neuropathy
Carpal tunnel release
Rotator cuff tendinitis
Arthroscopy
Ergotamine
Cyclosporin A
Arteriovenous shunt

[a]May be an innocent bystander, rather than a causal association.

Clinical Features

The diagnosis of RSD is made clinically. Various diagnostic criteria have been proposed (Table 107.6) (2,266). Not all symptoms and signs are present simultaneously, and one or another may dominate the presentation. Generally, severe pain is the paramount symptom, considerably worse than one would expect from the initial injury or the underlying illness. The pain is often described as burning, constant, or intense. Pain, swelling, color, and temperature changes are aggravated by any motion of the extremity or by dependency. Patients often will consult the physician with the extremity held protectively, wrapped in a moist towel or wet dressing, as the moisture seems to them to lessen the burning. The extremity is diffusely tender, perhaps slightly more so periarticularly. *Allodynia* is pain felt in response to stimuli that normally are not noxious stimuli. Allodynia can result from light touch, pressure, changes in temperature, or joint movement. *Hyperpathia* is an abnormally exaggerated response to painful stimuli, such as persistent pain after mild pressure to the affected area. In 829 patients with RSD, Veldman and co-workers (260) found hyperpathia in 75% during the first 2 months of illness. Blumberg and Jänig (267) found no hyperpathia in a series of 203 patients, and mechanical allodynia in only 8%, but generally these symptoms are thought to occur more frequently in RSD.

TABLE 107.6. KOZIN'S DIAGNOSTIC CRITERIA FOR REFLEX SYMPATHETIC DYSTROPHY

Definite reflex sympathetic dystrophy
Pain with allodynia or hyperpathia
Tenderness
Vasomotor and sudomotor changes: cool, pallid extremity (vasospasm) or warm, erythematous extremity (hyperemia); hyperhidrosis; hypertrichosis
Dystrophic skin changes: shiny, with loss or wrinkling; atrophy; scaling; nail changes; thickened palmar or plantar fascia
Swelling
Probable reflex sympathetic dystrophy
Pain and allodynia
Vasomotor or sudomotor changes
Swelling
Possible reflex sympathetic dystrophy
Vasomotor or sudomotor changes
Swelling

In the upper extremity, the shoulder motion typically is limited, the elbow is spared, and the hand is swollen and painful, thus the term *shoulder-hand syndrome* (Fig. 107.14). Frozen shoulder is considered by some to be a forme fruste of RSD.

Swelling is the first physical sign of RSD, and may be pitting or nonpitting. Early in the disease it is soft, but as the illness progresses the edema becomes hard and brawny. Stiffness of the extremity increases over time, initially due to the edema, and later due to fibrotic changes in the soft tissues. Discoloration of the extremity is related to vasomotor instability. In warm-onset RSD, the extremity is red and warm, and both arteries and veins within the extremity are dilated. In cold-onset RSD, the extremity is pale or cyanotic, and the vessels to the extremity have constricted.

Sudomotor changes in the extremity are common, with increased sweating early in the disease, and sometimes a dry extremity later in the illness. Temperature changes reflect the spasm or dilatation of the underlying blood vessels. Trophic changes appear in the skin, the hair, and the nails.

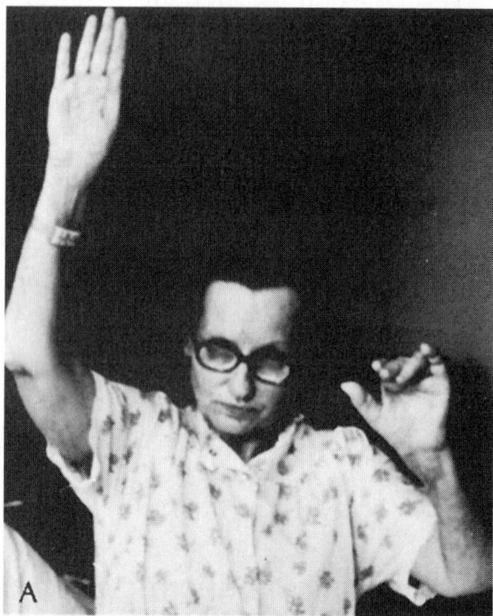

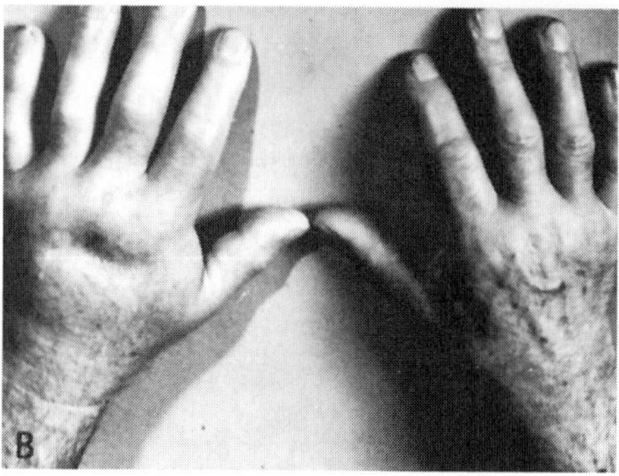

FIGURE 107.14. A: A patient with shoulder-hand syndrome who has limited shoulder motion and diffuse swelling of the hand. **B:** Note the shiny skin, flexion contractures of the hand, and the presence of pitting edema. (Courtesy of Dr. Franklin Kozin.)

The skin is shiny with fewer wrinkles when the extremity is edematous. When subcutaneous tissues and the skin atrophy, the skin is smooth and glossy. Hypertrichosis of the extremity can be a prominent complaint. Thickening of the palmar or plantar fascia occurs, and nodules can be felt through the skin. Other skin lesions may also occur, including nonimmune bullous lesions (268), hyperpigmentation (260), pustular lesions, telangiectasias, ulcers (269), and cellulitis (270).

Motor abnormalities are also part of RSD, though they have been less emphasized than the sensory and pseudoinflammatory changes. They may precede pain, may appear suddenly, and may occur in the affected extremity or on the contralateral side of the body (271). Veldman et al. (260) reported a tremor of the affected limb in 49% of patients, muscular incoordination in 54%, and weakness in 95%. Severe muscle spasms appeared in 25% of patients with RSD of longer duration. The tremor, most commonly a flexion-extension tremor of the fingers brought on by an attempt to move the hand (271), should be considered an enhanced physiologic tremor (272). Sympathetic blockade in early RSD or recovery from RSD makes the tremor disappear (271). Van der Laan et al. (270) found dystonia in 50 extremities (19 upper and 31 lower) of 1,006 patients with RSD. In the arm this appeared as a clenched fist with a flexed wrist, flexed elbow, and adducted shoulder, and in the leg as an inverted equinus position of the foot. Myoclonus occurred in 21 limbs, 9 of which also had dystonia.

Steinbrocker and co-workers (273,274) described three clinical stages of RSD in discussing the shoulder-hand syndrome. The first, the acute stage, was characterized by soft edema, pain, paresthesias, decreased motion because of pain, vasodilation with erythema, increased warmth, increased sweating, and the beginning of patchy osteoporosis. The second, the dystrophic stage, from 3 to 9 or 12 months after the initial symptoms, was marked by continued pain, stiffening and brawny edema, and vasospasm with cooling of the hand and pallor or cyanosis. Other features were early palmar fasciitis, polar demineralization, and skin glossiness because of atrophy rather than because of edema. The third, the atrophic stage, began at 9 to 12 months and was characterized by stiffness and flexion contractures in the hand, muscle atrophy and weakness, profound osteoporosis, pallor, coolness, and somewhat diminished pain at rest with continued pain with attempted motion. It is not clear that separation of RSD into such clinical stages is accurate or helpful, as there is no clear progression from one stage to the next, some patients begin with the cold second stage, and some patients fluctuate between the first two stages. RSD may spontaneously resolve at any time before the development of contractures (2). Dividing RSD into warm onset and cold onset based on the observed or remembered temperature in the extremity at the onset of illness (266,270) is useful prognostically.

Severe complications such as infection, ulcers, chronic edema, dystonia, and myoclonus are more likely to occur in patients with cold-onset disease than in patients with an afflicted extremity that is red and warm, initially (270).

Among adults, women are slightly more prone to RSD than men (260,275,276), unless the underlying illness (such as myocardial infarction) is male-linked (2,275). RSD in children differs from RSD in adults in that girls exceed boys by 2–6:1 and lower extremity involvement far exceeds upper extremity involvement (266,277). Trauma is a common precipitant in children. The typical child with RSD is a preteen girl. Allodynia occurs in a high percentage of patients, and vasomotor changes in 83% (278). Bone scans are not useful diagnostically, as uptake may be increased, decreased, or normal (278,279). Noninvasive, nonpharmacologic treatment (physical therapy, psychologic support for the child and her family, TENS unit) is often, but not always successful in treatment (278).

Reflex sympathetic dystrophy is bilateral in at least 25% of cases clinically (280); bone scanning and dolorimeter testing indicate some degree of bilaterality in a far higher percentage (280,281). RSD involving three or four limbs has been reported (260). Different limbs may be involved in multiple episodes (282,283). Typically the entire foot or hand is affected, but RSD also appears in segmental forms: involving one or more digits (radial form) (284,285), involving a single joint such as the knee or the hip (286–288), or involving part of the femoral head or the patella (zonal form).

Transient osteoporosis or migratory osteolysis may be an incomplete form of RSD. This is a syndrome of pregnant women or middle-aged men, who develop unprovoked painful osteoporosis in a foot, ankle, knee, or hip. It is characterized by intense homogeneous increased uptake in the affected area on bone scans (289). It is a self-limited condition, with resolution of pain and swelling within several months, and eventual return of the bone density in the affected region to normal (290–292).

Laboratory Testing

Complete blood counts; sedimentation rate, C-reactive protein, and other acute-phase reactants; chemistries; populations of T and B lymphocytes, natural killer cells, and activated T cells (293); and autoimmune profiles are normal the vast majority of the time. When abnormal they may reflect an underlying associated illness. Nerve conduction velocities and somatosensory evoked potentials also are normal. EMGs are normal or show minimal nonspecific neuropathic and myopathic changes (294).

The resting sweat output, if elevated in a patient with extremity pain and edema, has a 94% specificity for RSD. If the patient also has a decreased sweat output elicited by the axon reflex, he has a 98% likelihood of having RSD. Unfortunately, these tests have a poor sensitivity, so they are only useful if positive and meaningless in terms of diagnosing RSD when negative (295).

Radiology

Radiographs of affected limbs typically show patchy or spotty osteopenia, as early as 4 to 8 weeks from the onset of symptoms (296,297). This represents irregular resorption of trabecular bone (281,298). Such osteopenia does not occur in all patients, and is not pathognomonic for RSD, as a similar picture is seen in persons with prolonged immobilization in casts. The osteoporosis of RSD tends to be more severe and to develop more rapidly than disuse osteoporosis (298) or postmenopausal osteoporosis (299). Subchondral, intracortical, subperiosteal, and endosteal bone resorption also takes place. Fine-detail radiographs with optical magnification can document subtle surface erosions like those of early RA, with loss of the cortical margin. These are most common in the metacarpophalangeal or metatarsophalangeal joints. "Crumbling" erosions of marginal bones with superimposed new bone formation may be seen in distal or proximal interphalangeal joints. These resemble changes seen in hyperparathyroidism, Wilson's disease, or degenerative joint disease (281,298). Joint space is normal. Later in the illness the affected bones may exhibit a ground-glass appearance on radiographs, reflecting diffuse osteoporosis.

Bone scanning with technetium has diagnostic and predictive value in RSD. Scintigraphy is more specific in the diagnosis of RSD than plain films, with no loss of sensitivity (281). The three-phase bone scan is typically used (Fig. 107.15). A positive flow study shows flow to be diffusely increased to all parts of the wrist and hand (or foot, for lower limb RSD). The blood pool (or tissue phase) image, which immediately follows the flow studies, is positive if activity is diffusely increased on the affected side. The delayed image, done 2.5 to 3 hours later, again demonstrates diffusely increased activity on the affected side, with juxtaarticular accentuation of the uptake. An abnormality in all three phases is seen in less than half the patients with RSD. The delayed images seem to be the most sensitive in diagnosing RSD (300). In the upper extremity, delayed uptake alone may be a sufficient test, but in the lower extremity blood flow and blood pool phases help in making the diagnosis (301). In clinical studies, the sensitivity of scintigraphy in the diagnosis of RSD ranges from 54% to 100% and the specificity ranges from 85% to 98% (300). These values depend on the duration of illness, the age of the patients, the location of the disease, and the specific clinical criteria for diagnosis.

Positive bone scans may predict the development of RSD in asymptomatic patients with strokes and hemiparesis (302) and in patients with lumbar radiculopathy (303). Bone scans help in the diagnosis of segmental forms of RSD (284,288) as well. Bone scans (296) and vascular scans with

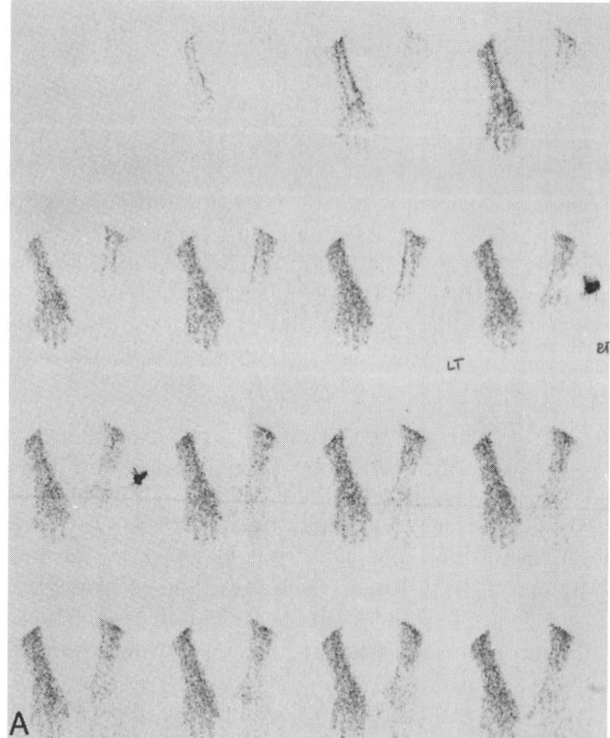

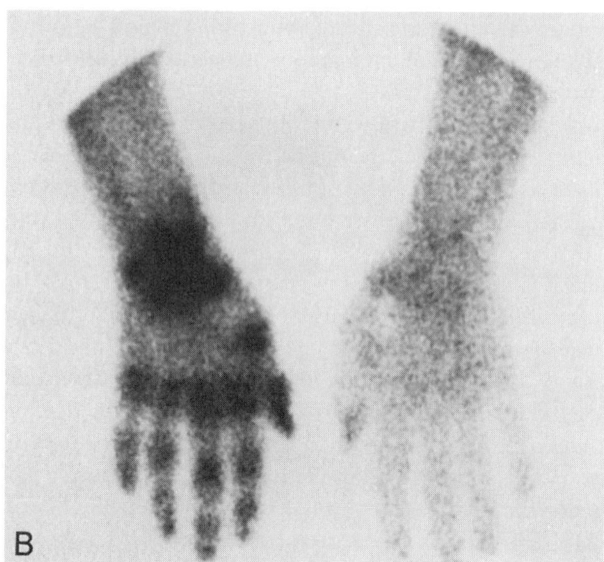

FIGURE 107.15. A three-phase bone scintigram in a patient with reflex sympathetic dystrophy affecting the left hand is illustrated. The characteristic changes are shown in the flow study **(A)** in which there is more rapid accumulation of radionuclide in the left hand, and in the 2.5-hour delayed bone scan **(B)** in which increased radionuclide is present in the periarticular tissues. (Courtesy of Dr. Franklin Kozin.)

technetium-labeled human serum albumin (304,305) can be used to monitor treatment.

Approximately one-third of the bone mineral content and cortical thickness is lost in bones affected by RSD (298). Dual-energy x-ray absorptiometry documents loss of bone mineral content and bone mineral density in patients with RSD (306–308), but clearly cannot distinguish RSD from other potential causes of unilateral demineralization. Chapurlat and co-workers (306), measuring whole body bone mineral density, found (a) no difference in bone mineral density between the affected and unaffected legs within the first 100 days of disease, (b) a significant difference in bone mineral density between the affected and unaffected legs when measured 55 weeks after disease onset, and (c) no increase in bone mineral density of the affected or unaffected leg 1 year after treatment of the RSD with calcitonin and then intravenous pamidronate. Laroche and co-workers (308) described pretreatment losses of bone mineral content and bone mineral density of 8.8% and 9.6% compared to the unaffected limb in RSD of 8 months' duration, but saw increases in bone mass 9 to 12 months later in those patients whose RSD had improved clinically. Persistent osteoporosis after RSD may predispose a patient to insufficiency fractures in the affected area (309).

MRIs in patients with warm-onset RSD show bone marrow edema (hyperemia). When the limb is cold, the MRI is normal, or rarely has a "Swiss-cheese" appearance (294).

Differential Diagnosis

Localized infection or fracture should be sought in the patient with extremity edema, warmth, and pain. Crystal-induced arthritis, early RA, and spondyloarthropathy must be entertained as possible diagnoses. If neuropathic pain dominates the clinical picture, radiculopathy, peripheral nerve impingement (310), or actual nerve injury should be considered. A severe thoracic oulet syndrome, particularly one with subclavian vein stenosis (311), resembles RSD. Scleroderma is mimicked by the puffy fingers and stiffness of early RSD and by the flexion contractures and stiffness of late RSD. Factitious edema, as a part of Münchausen's syndrome, can simulate RSD (312).

Palmar fasciitis and polyarthritis associated with ovarian carcinoma is a paraneoplastic syndrome that closely resembles RSD. Bilateral pain and limitation of shoulder and hand motion, palmar fasciitis, and arthritis of other joints including elbows may predate the diagnosis of ovarian malignancy by 5 to 25 months. There is no response to steroid treatment (313). Other malignancies also have been associated with palmar fasciitis and with RSD (314).

Pathology

The affected bone in patients with RSD is hyperemic. Some authors report prominent osteoclastic activity in the areas of patchy osteoporosis (315–317), while others do not see the hyperosteoclastic activity one might expect given the rapidity of the bone loss (294). Synovial biopsies show proliferation and disarray of synovial lining cells, synovial and subsynovial edema, capillary proliferation, and subsynovial fibrosis. Very few inflammatory cells are seen (280).

In eight patients with spontaneous pain, hyperpathia, paresis, allodynia, and anesthesia dolorosa (no sensibility to touch, but severe pain present in the anesthetic area) who underwent amputation for chronic RSD, myelinated nerve fibers were normal, but axonal degeneration of small afferent C fibers was seen in four. Skeletal muscle abnormalities included a decrease in type I fibers, an increase in lipofuscin pigment, atrophic fibers, and markedly thickened capillary basement membranes. These changes were similar to those seen in muscle biopsies of patients with diabetes mellitus, though none of the eight patients had diabetes (318).

Pathophysiology

The pathogenesis of RSD remains an enigma. An alteration in the sympathetic nervous system is the basis of one pathogenetic theory. The other main etiologic theory invokes an uncontrolled regional inflammatory response.

Roberts (319) developed a scheme for sympathetically maintained pain in RSD that began with trauma in a peripheral tissue activating unmyelinated C nociceptors. This activity led to long-term sensitization of wide dynamic range (WDR) neurons in the spinal cord, making them more responsive to all subsequent afferent signals. He then proposed that stimulation of A-fiber mechanoreceptors by touch or via peripheral sympathetic efferents could excite the WDR neurons further, and that a high rate of firing from WDR neurons would result in the sensation of pain. This theory would explain allodynia, but it would predict that TENS units would exacerbate RSD pain, whereas clinically they often diminish pain.

Arguments in support of sympathetic nervous system involvement in RSD rest on patient responses to sympathetic blockade, to intravenous α-adrenergic antagonists such as phentolamine, and to oral phenoxybenzamine. Controlled double-blind studies of regional intravenous sympatholytics, however, suggest these agents are little better than placebo (320–322). The blood flow in RSD hands typically is increased, with normal autoregulation and vasoconstrictor responses (323,324). This argues for decreased basal sympathetic tone in the extremity, but a functioning sympathetic nervous system. Venous norepinephrine levels are lower in the affected extremity than in the unaffected extremity (325,326), which is also consistent with decreased sympathetic activity in the affected limb. Arnold and co-workers (327) have demonstrated increased responsiveness of α-adrenoceptors to norepinephrine in blood vessels of the affected limb. If the α-adrenoceptors of nociceptor and mechanoreceptor neurons also are hyperresponsive, this could explain hyperalgesia and allodynia, respectively.

Schwartzman and Kerrigan (271) suggested that an interaction between substance P and the sympathetic nervous system might underlie the dystonia of RSD. Schott (328) postulated a role for substance P and calcitonin gene-related peptide in the pathogenesis of RSD.

Investigators in Nijmegen, the Netherlands, have again focused attention on Sudeck's (329) theory of an exaggerated peripheral inflammatory response as the cause of RSD. Oxygen consumption studies in eight patients with acute warm RSD of a hand found increased arterial blood flow, but a high venous oxygen saturation. This implied poor oxygen extraction, which suggested that there was tissue hypoxia despite a high oxygen supply (330). Phosphocreatine levels measured by phosphorus 31-nuclear magnetic resonance spectroscopy are low in skeletal muscle of patients with chronic RSD. Phosphocreatine is needed for the resynthesis of adenosine triphosphate (ATP) after exercise, but its own synthesis is oxygen dependent. Because RSD tissues are hypoxic, they cannot synthesize adequate phosphocreatine or ATP, and the patient is physically unable to exercise (331).

Patients with acute RSD have extravasation of macromolecules in the affected hand as indicated by indium 111–immunoglobulin G scintigraphy, suggesting regional inflammation that damages vascular endothelium and increases vascular permeability (332). The lipofuscin seen in RSD skeletal muscle biopsies is thought to represent oxidative stress (318). Infusion of free radicals into the hindlimb of unanesthetized rats leads to increased skin temperature, edema, erythema, dysfunction of the limb, spontaneous pain behavior, and increased sensitivity to mechanical and thermal stimuli, in a syndrome resembling RSD (333). The therapeutic effectiveness of corticosteroids (280,334,335) and free-radical scavengers (336) provide further suggestive evidence that inflammation is involved in the pathogenesis of RSD.

Treatment

An *awareness* of RSD and the injuries, illnesses, and drugs that can provoke it is the first step in the treatment of RSD. It is thought that early mobilization after myocardial infarctions, trauma, and strokes can lessen the likelihood of developing RSD.

The severity of RSD, its duration, and prognosis are unrelated to the severity of the underlying injury or provocation. *Early treatment* of RSD leads to a better outcome. Rosen and Graham (337) found a good or excellent response to treatment in 43% of patients with symptoms less than 6 months, but only 20% of patients with a longer duration of disease did as well. Elevated resting skin temperature, edema, and disease duration of less than 6 months are the best predictors of a good response to sympathetic block (especially in upper extremity RSD) (295). Patients with disease of less than 1 year seem to respond better to intravenous pamidronate (338).

Other prognostic factors exist. Children seem to do better, and may need less aggressive treatment, though not all children recover fully by any means (277). Patients whose RSD is primarily cold at the onset of disease have a worse functional outcome; a higher incidence of recurrence or development of RSD in a second limb; a greater likelihood of developing severe complications such as infection, ulcers, chronic edema, dystonia, or myoclonus (270); and a greater chance of needing eventual amputation (339). These patients are slightly younger than adults with warm-onset RSD and are more likely to have lower-extremity involvement (270).

Treated or untreated RSD can disable. In a late 1970s study of upper-extremity RSD, only 10 patients of 77 queried had no residual pain or stiffness in the shoulder or the hand; 19 of these 77 patients were working full-time and performed 100% of normal daily activities without the use of medications, but only one of these 19 was pain-free. Another five patients were free of all symptoms, but had retired (340). In Geertzen et al.'s (341) study of 65 patients with RSD of the upper extremities 5.5 years after the onset of disease, pain was found to be the most disabling effect of the RSD. Weakness of grip strength also caused difficulties with activities of daily living; 26% of patients changed professions because of RSD, and almost 30% had to stop work for more than a year because of RSD (342). Patients with atrophy and flexion contractures, patients with chronically infected or ulcerated extremities, and patients with dystonia or myoclonus clearly have limited function socially and professionally.

After the recognition of RSD, treatment begins with pain control. Nonsteroidals and narcotics give poor pain control in RSD. Corticosteroids do help with pain, as might sympathetic blockade. Gabapentin can relieve the burning pain in some patients. When the pain is controlled, a physical therapist can work with the patient to mobilize the extremity and to relieve edema. Contrast baths are helpful in some patients. Ice reduces swelling and stiffness, but not every patient can tolerate the temperature changes. The extremity should be elevated as much as possible to *minimize edema.* The patient should only *exercise* the extremity actively *within his pain-free ranges,* even if the amplitude of joint movement is small. If he exceeds these ranges, he may perpetuate local inflammation, free radical generation, and pain cycling. A program of stress loading can be used to exercise the hand without active joint motion (343). *Psychological support* is necessary for all patients and families, as anxiety and depression always accompany the other clinical signs of RSD.

Treatment must be *multimodal* and coordinated temporally. For example, the best time for a patient to work with the physical therapist may be immediately after a sympathetic block, when he is experiencing less pain or is painfree. The preferred treatment for RSD varies a great deal with the specialty of the treating physician and his geographic location. In Europe, calcitonin has been the initial treatment for years, though sympathetic blockade is also used. Recently, Dutch investigators have used primarily free radical scavengers. In the United States, corticosteroids or sympathetic blocks have been the standard interventions.

Though widely used, the value of *sympathetic blockade* remains controversial (344,345). Kozin (2) estimated long-lasting diminution of clinical symptoms or lessening of disability with sympathetic blockade in 14% to 25% of patients so treated. Clinical response to a limited number of blocks may occur (346–348); but Kozin has found that one or two blocks often are inadequate for diagnosis or treatment, that a minimum of three blocks in a 7- to 10-day period should be used for diagnostic purposes, and that up to 6 to 12 blocks may be needed for treatment. Wang et al. (347), using repeated lumbar sympathetic blocks, and Cortet et al. (348), using regional intravenous buflomedil, both reported better response rates when the duration of RSD was less than 6 months. Malik et al. (349), in a study of five patients treated with regional intravenous phenoxybenzamine, reported good long-term relief (months) in three patients with short-duration RSD, but also in two patients who had been symptomatic for 60 and 18 months.

Ganglion blockade of the stellate ganglion or lumbar ganglia is usually done intermittently, but may be performed continuously. Morphine injected about the stellate ganglion does not modulate the sympathetic nervous system or give pain relief (350).

Brachial plexus blockade, performed intermittently or continuously, has been used to block C- and A-fibers in addition to sympathetic efferents. The C- and A-fibers not only initiate afferent sensory signals, but also release neuropeptides that can cause local inflammation, possibly perpetuating the RSD (351). Because these blocks give sensory and motor deficits, physical therapy postblock must be passive.

Continuous or intermittent *epidural blocks* may be used. Cooper et al. (352) used indwelling lumbar epidural catheters for 2 to 7 days, to instill first bupivacaine, then narcotic anesthesia, in patients with RSD of the knee. This regimen allowed aggressive physical therapy, including continuous passive motion, manipulation, muscle stimulation, and contrast baths; 11 of 14 patients recovered fully. Rauck and colleagues (353) gave continuous epidural clonidine to 19 patients with chronic RSD who had responded to intermittent epidural clonidine. Infusion of clonidine for a mean of 43 days did give pain relief, but also an unacceptable infection rate of 6 out of 19.

Regional intravenous sympathetic blockade, using a Bier block, has been widely used since Hannington-Kiff (354) reported success with regional intravenous guanethidine in 1977. This method is comparable to stellate ganglion block (355) and is technically easier. Many drugs have been used, including guanethidine (unavailable in the United States and France) (320–322,356,357), reserpine (320,357), droperidol (358), atropine (359), bretylium (360), ketanserin (361), buflomedil (348,362), and phenoxybenzamine (349). Several studies have shown regional intravenous guanethidine to be no better than intravenous saline placebo or no treatment (320,322,357,363), but only Ramamurthy and Hoffman's (322) study used more than one regional intravenous block, and clinically multiple blocks are given (364). Regional intravenous block with saline in one study gave 83% of patients pain relief lasting more than 24 hours (320), which implies a strong placebo effect or benefit from the local anesthetic or the tourniquet. Bupivacaine can decrease adrenergic transmission experimentally (365), and intravenous lidocaine can lessen allodynia in neuropathic rats (366). If an Esmarch bandage or equivalent is wrapped around an affected limb from distal to proximal to reduce the volume of the extremity, and then a proximal cuff is inflated to a pressure above systolic blood pressure, the diffuse deep pain in the extremity is abolished or reduced after 1 to 2 minutes. Blumberg and Hoffman (367) have used this finding as a supplemental test in the diagnosis of RSD, and Blumberg and Jänig (267) have suggested that pain relief in the ischemia test predicts pain relief with sympatholytic interventions.

Intravenous phentolamine infused over 5 to 20 minutes may give relief of spontaneous and evoked pain in an affected extremity. A positive response to intravenous phentolamine is a strong predictor of response to regional sympatholytic treatment (368).

Open *sympathectomy*, endoscopic sympathectomy, and percutaneous radiofrequency lesioning of the sympathetic trunk (345) are not widely used, but are potential treatments for those patients with good, but temporary, responses to sympathetic blocks. Sympathectomy is not a panacea, even in this select group, as patients can develop sympathalgia, and Kozin (2) estimates fewer than 25% of patients get lasting pain relief from sympathectomy. Sympathectomy may be more likely to succeed if done early in the disease (369).

Oral α_1-receptor antagonists such as *phenoxybenzamine* (370,371), *terazosin* (372), and *prazosin* (362) have been used with variable success. Their chronic use is limited primarily by orthostatic hypotension. *Clonidine*, an α_2-adrenergic agonist, has been used in RSD topically (373) and epidurally (353).

Corticosteroids give good pain relief and reduction of heat, erythema, and edema in a number of patients (280,334,335,374). They seem to be most helpful in the upper extremity in "warm" disease (2). They have no role in the atrophic phase of RSD. Kozin (2) has recommended a 28-day course of prednisone (or its equivalent) beginning at 15 mg q.i.d. for 4 days, then 10 mg q.i.d. for 4 days, then 10 mg t.i.d. for 4 days, then 10 mg b.i.d for 4 days, then 15 mg qd for 4 days, 10 mg qd for 4 days, and finally 5 mg qd for 4 days. Patients may flare transiently (lasting 3 to 7 days) after the steroids have ended. Occasionally a second course of steroids is helpful, this time with 8 days at each level, and some patients need low-dose maintenance steroids at 5 to 10 mg per day. Obviously, the longer a patient uses steroids and the higher the doses used, the greater the risk of steroid side effects including glucose intolerance, hypertension, visual changes, worsening of osteoporosis, and avascular necrosis.

Approximately 50% of RSD patients have a *trigger point* within the affected extremity (330). This term, as used by van der Laan and Goris (330), refers to a point that is a source of pain (and potentially inflammation), not caused by the RSD. Examples are tendinitis of the patellar tendon, lateral/medial epicondylitis, carpal tunnel syndrome, trigger finger, or a painful neuroma. *Removal of a neuroma*, an *orthotic*, or a *local steroid/anesthetic* injection may give significant pain relief.

Calcitonin, given intramuscularly, subcutaneously (375), or intranasally (376,377) daily over a 15- to 20-day course helps in about 60% of patients (266). The injected dose is 100 to 150 IU daily. When calcitonin helps, its effect is seen within a few days.

Bisphosphonates seem to be a promising treatment (338,378,379). Adami and co-workers (378) treated 20 patients with either *alendronate* or a placebo intravenously daily for 3 days in a blinded fashion. Two weeks later, all patients received 3 days of alendronate. At 4 weeks, spontaneous pain had decreased by more than 75% in five patients and by more than 50% in eight patients. At 12 months, nine patients (seven of whom received two courses of alendronate) were in full remission, four patients were lost to follow-up, and seven patients (four of whom received only one course of alendronate) had relapsed (378). Maillefert and colleagues (338) reported pooled results from two open trials of pamidronate in 35 patients who had failed calcitonin. Disease duration was greater than 3 months. Patients received 30 mg *pamidronate* intravenously daily for 3 consecutive days or 1 mg/kg per day for 1, 2, or 3 days, as tolerated. Overall, pain by visual analogue scale decreased at 1 and 3 months, and physician global assessment increased at 1 and 3 months. The decrease in pain was greater in patients with non-posttraumatic RSD. Improvement in physician global assessment was higher in patients with disease duration less than a year and in patients with non-posttraumatic RSD. Double-blind controlled studies are needed.

Dutch investigators have promoted the use of *free-radical scavengers* in the treatment of acute RSD. The most severe cases are given continuous *intravenous mannitol* (10%, 1 L/24 hours) for a week, watching carefully for hyperosmolality in patients with renal insufficiency. This treatment is followed by *dimethylsulfoxide (DMSO) cream* (50% in a fatty base) to the skin of the affected area five times daily for 2 to 3 months. Less severe cases are treated with DMSO from the beginning (330,380). Geertzen et al. (262) found DMSO was more effective than six twice-weekly regional intravenous guanethidine blocks in 26 patients with early RSD. DMSO causes an oniony-garlic taste and smell, but is low in cost and can be self-applied.

Several French investigators reported good results with *beta blockers*, especially *propranolol* and *pindolol* (381), though these drugs should be avoided in cold-onset RSD. Every effort should be made to increase perfusion to the affected limb in cold-onset RSD. *Verapamil, nifedipine* (371), or other calcium channel blockers, *ketanserin*, or *pentoxifylline* can be used. If the extremity remains cold despite vasodilators, Dutch investigators proceed to sympathetic block (330).

Gabapentin, an anticonvulsant, is very helpful in the treatment of peripheral neuropathy, postherpetic neuralgia, and radicular neuropathic pain. Mellick and Mellick (382) reported a 60% to 100% reduction in pain in six patients with RSD using gabapentin. One patient was cured of early disease with 800 mg gabapentin t.i.d. as her only treatment. Mellick and Mellick began at a dose of 300 mg the first day, 300 mg b.i.d. the second day, and then 300 mg t.i.d. thereafter, with dose increases as needed and as tolerated. (Side effects include somnolence, dizziness, ataxia, and confusion.) Some patients required doses as high as 600 to 900 mg q.i.d., but the authors remarked that they had yet to see a gabapentin treatment failure in the management of RSD. I have used gabapentin in three patients with RSD, beginning at 100 mg qhs and allowing the patients to self-adjust very quickly up to 300 to 400 mg t.i.d. One woman with atrophic RSD of an upper extremity experienced marked improvement of ipsilateral lower extremity dystonia. One woman with acute RSD of a lower extremity and a man with acute upper extremity RSD had rapid relief of edema and allodynia. Gabapentin's mechanism of action in RSD is unknown. Double-blind placebo-controlled trials are needed.

Lioresal helps the muscle spasms of late RSD (271).

Generally one medication at a time is tested in clinical trials, but it seems reasonable to use a many-barreled approach in RSD, just as the oncologists use a multiple drug approach to chemotherapy. A combination regimen using medications with different potential sites of action and different side effect profiles should be tested. Two such regimens (for acute warm-onset RSD) might be (a) DMSO locally, calcitonin or a bisphosphonate, and gabapentin; or (b) corticosteroids, calcitonin or a bisphosphonate, and gabapentin.

Phenytoin (383), *griseofulvin* (384), and *topical capsaicin* (385) are other medications that have been tried in RSD. TENS is helpful in some patients with acute RSD. Though it tends to become less effective over time, some patients with chronic RSD also benefit from its use (386) or from neuroaugmentation with implanted spinal cord stimulators or implanted peripheral nerve stimulators (387–390).

Amputation is an extreme therapy when all other treatments for RSD have failed, and the patient has intractable pain, recurrent infection, or a useless limb that gets in the way. Of 28 patients with RSD who underwent amputations, only two patients were relieved of pain, but 10 of 14 were cured of infection and 9 of 15 patients could function better. RSD recurred in the stump of 28 of the 34 amputations, generally when the amputation was done at a level that was not free of symptoms (339). Phantom sensation is very common after amputation (339,391).

ACKNOWLEDGMENTS

I am grateful to Kim Allen of Baptist Memorial Hospital–North Mississippi and to the Interlibrary Loan staff of the University of Mississippi for their help in obtaining books and articles.

REFERENCES

1. Cailliet R. *Shoulder pain,* 3rd ed. Philadelphia: FA Davis, 1991.
2. Kozin F. Painful shoulder and the reflex sympathetic dystrophy syndrome. In: Koopman WJ, ed. *Arthritis and allied conditions,* 13th ed. Baltimore: Williams & Wilkins, 1997:1887–1922.
3. Bland JH, Merrit JA, Boushey DR. The painful shoulder. *Semin Arthritis Rheum* 1977;7:21–47.
4. Basmajian JV. *Primary anatomy,* 6th ed. Baltimore: Williams & Wilkins, 1970.
5. Warwick R, Williams PL. *Gray's anatomy,* 35th British ed. Philadelphia: WB Saunders, 1973.
6. Inman VT, Saunders M, Abbott LC. Observations on the function of the shoulder joint. *J Bone Joint Surg* 1944;26:1–30.
7. McGregor L. Rotation at the shoulder. A critical inquiry. *Br J Surg* 1937;24:425–438.
8. Petersson CJ, Redlund-Johnell I. The subacromial space in normal shoulder radiographs. *Acta Orthop Scand* 1984;55:57–58.
9. Rothman RH, Marvel JP, Heppenstall RB. Anatomic considerations in the glenohumeral joint. *Orthop Clin North Am* 1975;6:341–352.
10. Lucas DB. Biomechanics of the shoulder joint. *Arch Surg* 1973;107:425–432.
11. Saha AK. Dynamic stability of the glenohumeral joint. *Acta Orthop Scand* 1971;42:491–505.
12. Turkel SJ, Panio MW, Marshall JL, et al. Stabilizing mechanisms preventing anterior dislocation of the glenohumeral joint. *J Bone Joint Surg* 1981;63A:1208–1217.
13. Poppen NK, Walker PS. Forces at the glenohumeral joint in abduction. *Clin Orthop* 1978;135:165–170.
14. Howell SM, Imobersteg AM, Seger DH, et al. Clarification of the role of the supraspinatus muscle in shoulder function. *J Bone Joint Surg* 1986;68A:398–404.
15. Poppen NK, Walker PS. Normal and abnormal motion of the shoulder. *J Bone Joint Surg* 1976;58A:195–201.
16. Rathbun JB, MacNab I. The microvascular pattern of the rotator cuff. *J Bone Joint Surg* 1970;52B:540–553.
17. Jacobsson L, Lindgarde F, Manthorpe R. The commonest rheumatic complaints of over six weeks' duration in a twelve-month period in a defined Swedish population. *Scand J Rheumatol* 1989;18:353–360.
18. Herberts P, Kadefors R, Hogfors C, et al. Shoulder pain and heavy manual labor. *Clin Orthop* 1984;191:166–178.
19. MacFarlane GJ, Hunt IM, Silman AJ. Predictors of chronic shoulder pain: a population based prospective study. *J Rheumatol* 1998;25:1612–1615.
20. Chard MD, Hazleman BL. Shoulder disorders in the elderly (a hospital study). *Ann Rheum Dis* 1987;46:684–687.

21. Chard MD, Hazleman R, Hazleman BL, et al. Shoulder disorders in the elderly: a community survey. *Arthritis Rheum* 1991;34:766–769.
22. Chakravarty KK, Webley M. Disorders of the shoulder: an often unrecognized cause of disability in elderly people. *Br Med J* 1990;300:848–849.
23. Winters JC, Sobel JS, Groenier KH, et al. The long-term course of shoulder complaints: a prospective study in general practice. *Rheumatology* 1999;38:160–163.
24. Gartsman GM, Brinker MR, Khan M, et al. Self-assessment of general health status in patients with five common shoulder conditions. *J Shoulder Elbow Surg* 1998;7:228–237.
25. Winter AF de, Jans MP, Scholten RJPM, et al. Diagnostic classification of shoulder disorders: interobserver agreement and determinants of disagreement. *Ann Rheum Dis* 1999;58: 272–277.
26. Bamji AN, Erhardt CC, Price TR, et al. The painful shoulder: can consultants agree? *Br J Rheumatol* 1996;35:1172–1174.
27. Berg EE, Ciullo JV. A clinical test for superior glenoid labral or "SLAP' lesions. *Clin J Sport Med* 1998;8:121–123.
28. Evans PJ, Miniaci A. Rotator cuff tendinopathy. Many causes, many solutions. *J Musculoskel Med* 1997;14:47–61.
29. Neer CS. Impingement lesions. *Clin Orthop* 1983;173:70–77.
30. Hawkins RJ, Kennedy JC. Impingement syndrome in athletes. *Am J Sports Med* 1980;8:151-158.
31. Bigliani LU, Morrison DS. The morphology of the acromion and its relationship to rotator cuff tears. *Orthop Trans* 1986; 10:228.
32. Morrison DS, Bigliani LU. The clinical significance of variations in acromial morphology. *Orthop Trans* 1987;11:234.
33. DeFerm A, Lagac K, Bunker T. Synovial osteochondromatosis: an unusual cause for subacromial impingement. *Acta Orthop Belg* 1997;63:218–220.
34. Kessel L, Watson M. The painful arc syndrome. Clinical classification as a guide to management. *J Bone Joint Surg* 1977;59B: 166–172.
35. Cyriax J. *Textbook of orthopaedic medicine. Vol I:* Diagnosis of soft tissue lesions, 7th ed. London: Ballière Tindall, 1978.
36. Chard MD, Sattelle LM, Hazleman BL. The long-term outcome of rotator cuff tendinitis—a review study. *Br J Rheumatol* 1988;27:385–389.
37. Petri M, Dobrow R, Neiman R, et al. Randomized, double-blind, placebo-controlled study of the treatment of the painful shoulder. *Arthritis Rheum* 1987;30:1040–1045.
38. Adebajo AO, Nash P, Hazleman BL. A prospective double blind dummy placebo controlled study comparing triamcinolone hexacetonide injection with oral diclofenac 50 mg TDS in patients with rotator cuff tendinitis. *J Rheumatol* 1990;17: 1207–1210.
39. Vecchio PC, Hazleman BL, King RH. A double-blind trial comparing subacromial methylprednisolone and lignocaine in acute rotator cuff tendinitis. *Br J Rheumatol* 1993;32:743–745.
40. Codman EA. *The shoulder. Rupture of the supraspinatus tendon and other lesions in or about the subacromial bursa.* Brooklyn, NY: G. Miller, 1934.
41. Cofield RH. Rotator cuff disease of the shoulder. *J Bone Joint Surg* 1985;67A:974–979.
42. Neviaser JS. Ruptures of the rotator cuff of the shoulder. New concepts in the diagnosis and operative treatment of chronic ruptures. *Arch Surg* 1971;102:483–485.
43. Norwood LA, Barrack R, Jacobson KE. Clinical presentation of complete tears of the rotator cuff. *J Bone Joint Surg* 1989;71A: 499–505.
44. Weiner DS, MacNab I. Superior migration of the humeral head. A radiological aid in the diagnosis of tears of the rotator cuff. *J Bone Joint Surg* 1970:52B:524–527.
45. Mack L, Matsen FA, Kilcoyne RF, et al. US evaluation of the rotator cuff. *Radiology* 1985;157:205–209.
46. Shibuta H, Tamai K, Tabuchi K. Magnetic resonance imaging of the shoulder in abduction. *Clin Orthop* 1998;348:107–113.
47. Fukuda H, Hamada K, Yamanaka K. Pathology and pathogenesis of bursal-side rotator cuff tears viewed from en bloc histologic sections. *Clin Orthop* 1990;254:75–80.
48. MacNab I. Rotator cuff tendinitis. *Ann R Coll Surg Engl* 1973;53:271–287.
49. Neer CS, Craig EV, Fukuda H. Cuff-tear arthropathy. *J Bone Joint Surg* 1983;65A:1232–1244.
50. Weiss JJ. Intra-articular steroids in the treatment of rotator cuff tear: reappraisal by arthrography. *Arch Phys Med Rehabil* 1981; 62:555–557.
51. Takagishi N. Conservative treatment of ruptures of the rotator cuff. *J Japanese Orthop Assoc* 1978;52:781–787.
52. Samilson RL, Binder WF. Symptomatic full thickness tears of the rotator cuff. An analysis of 292 shoulders in 276 patients. *Orthop Clin North Am* 1975;6:449–466.
53. Bokor DJ, Hawkins RJ, Huckle G, et al. Long-term follow-up of full thickness tears of the rotator cuff treated non-operatively. *J Bone Joint Surg* 1989;71B:880–881.
54. Neer CS. Anterior acromioplasty for the chronic impingement syndrome in the shoulder. *J Bone Joint Surg* 1972;54A:41–50.
55. Rockwood CA, Lyons FR. Shoulder impingement syndrome: Diagnosis, radiographic evaluation, and treatment with a modified Neer acromioplasty. *J Bone Joint Surg* 1993;75A: 409–424.
56. Neviaser TJ, Neviaser RJ, Neviaser JS, et al. The four-in-one arthroplasty for the painful arc syndrome. *Clin Orthop* 1982; 163:107–112.
57. Penny JN, Welsh RP. Shoulder impingement syndromes in athletes and their surgical management. *Am J Sports Med* 1981;9: 11–15.
58. Gore DR, Murray MP, Sepic SB, et al. Shoulder-muscle strength and range of motion following surgical repair of full-thickness rotator-cuff tears. *J Bone Joint Surg* 1986;68A: 266–272.
59. Hawkins RJ, Misamore GW, Hobeika PE. Surgery for full-thickness rotator-cuff tears. *J Bone Joint Surg* 1985;67A:1349–1355.
60. Lindh M, Norlin R. Arthroscopic subacromial decompression versus open acromioplasty. A two-year follow-up study. *Clin Orthop* 1993;290:174–176.
61. Altchek DW, Warren RF, Wickiewicz TL, et al. Arthroscopic acromioplasty. Technique and results. *J Bone Joint Surg* 1990; 72A:1198–1207.
62. Gartsman GM, Khan M, Hammerman SM. Arthroscopic repair of full-thickness tears of the rotator cuff. *J Bone Joint Surg* 1998;80A:832–840.
63. Tibone JE, Elrod B, Jobe FW, et al. Surgical treatment of tears of the rotator cuff in athletes. *J Bone Joint Surg* 1986;68A: 887–891.
64. Thür C, Jülke M, Bircher HP. Die Aufrichteosteotomie des Akromions (AAO) als neue Prinzip in der Behandlung des Impingementsyndroms, inbesonders im Zummenhang mit der Rekonstruktion von grossen Rotatorenmanschettenläsionen. *Unfallchirurg* 1998;101:176–183.
65. Hyvönen P, Lohi S, Jalovaara P. Open acromioplasty does not prevent the progression of an impingement syndrome to a tear. Nine-year follow-up of 96 cases. *J Bone Joint Surg* 1998;80B: 813–816.
66. McCarty DJ, Halverson PB, Carrera GF, et al. "Milwaukee shoulder"—association of microspheroids containing hydroxyapatite crystals, active collagenase, and neutral protease with rotator cuff defects. I. Clinical aspects. *Arthritis Rheum* 1981; 24:464–473.

67. Halverson PB, Cheung HS, McCarty DJ, et al. "Milwaukee shoulder"—association of microspheroids containing hydroxyapatite crystals, active collagenase, and neutral protease with rotator cuff defects. II. Synovial fluid studies. *Arthritis Rheum* 1981;24:474–483.
68. Garancis JC, Cheung HD, Halverson PB, et al. "Milwaukee shoulder"—association of microspheroids containing hydroxyapatite crystals, active collagenase, and neutral protease with rotator cuff defects. III. Morphologic and biochemical studies of an excised synovium showing chondromatosis. *Arthritis Rheum* 1981;24:484–491.
69. Campion GV, McCrae F, Alwan W, et al. Idiopathic destructive arthritis of the shoulder. *Semin Arthritis Rheum* 1988;17: 232–245.
70. Patel KJ, Weidensaul D, Palma C, et al. Milwaukee shoulder with massive bilateral cysts: effective therapy for hydrops of the shoulder. *J Rheumatol* 1997;24:2479–2483.
71. Halverson PB, Carrera GF, McCarty DJ. Milwaukee shoulder syndrome. Fifteen additional cases and a description of contributing factors. *Arch Intern Med* 1990;150:677–682.
72. Dieppe PA. Milwaukee shoulder. *Br Med J* 1981;283:1488–1489.
73. Caporali R, Rossi S, Montecucco C. Tidal irrigation in Milwaukee shoulder syndrome. *J Rheumatol* 1994;21:1781–1782.
74. Zeman CA, Arcand MA, Cantrell JS, et al. The rotator cuff-deficient arthritic shoulder: diagnosis and surgical management. *J Am Acad Orthop Surg* 1998;6:337–348.
75. Bosworth BM. Calcium deposits in the shoulder and subacromial bursitis. A survey of 12,122 shoulders. *JAMA* 1941; 116:2477–2482.
76. Boyle AC. Joints and their disease; disorders of the shoulder joint. *Br Med J* 1969;3:283–285.
77. Simon WH. Soft tissue disorders of the shoulder. *Orthop Clin North Am* 1975;6:521–539.
78. Mavrikakis ME, Drimis S, Kontoyannis DA, et al. Calcific shoulder periarthritis (tendinitis) in adult onset diabetes mellitus: a controlled study. *Ann Rheum Dis* 1989;48:211–214.
79. Kernwein GA. Roentgenographic diagnosis of shoulder dysfunction. *JAMA* 1965;194:179–183.
80. McLaughlin HL. Lesions of the musculotendinous cuff of the shoulder. III. Observation on the pathology, course, and treatment of calcific deposits. *Ann Surg* 1946;124:354–362.
81. Uhthoff HK, Sarkar K, Maynard JA. Calcifying tendinitis. A new concept of its pathogenesis. *Clin Orthop* 1976;118: 164–168.
82. McKendry RJR, Uhthoff HK, Sarkar K, et al. Calcifying tendinitis of the shoulder: prognostic value of clinical, histologic, and radiologic features in 57 surgically treated cases. *J Rheumatol* 1982;9:75–80.
83. Gartner J, Simons B. Analysis of calcific deposits in calcifying tendinitis. *Clin Orthop* 1990;254:111–120.
84. Comfort TH, Arafiles RP. Barbotage of the shoulder with image-intensified fluoroscopic control of needle placement for calcific tendinitis. *Clin Orthop* 1978;135:171–178.
85. Rompe JD, Rumler F, Hopf C, et al. Extracorporeal shock wave therapy for calcifying tendinitis of the shoulder. *Clin Orthop* 1995;321:196–201.
86. Ebenbichler GR, Erdogmus CB, Resch KL, et al. Ultrasound therapy for calcific tendinitis of the shoulder. *N Engl J Med* 1999;340:1533–1538.
87. Strizak AM, Torrance LD, Jackson DW, et al. Subacromial bursography. An anatomical and clinical study. *J Bone Joint Surg* 1982;64A:196–201.
88. Bureau NJ, Dussault RG, Keats TE. Imaging of bursae around the shoulder joint. *Skeletal Radiol* 1996;25:513–517.
89. Salvarani C, Cantini F, Olivieri I, et al. Proximal bursitis in active polymyalgia rheumatica. *Ann Intern Med* 1997;127:27–31.
90. Salvarani C, Cantini F, Olivieri I, et al. Polymyalgia rheumatica: a disorder of extraarticular synovial structures? [Editorial]. *J Rheumatol* 1999;26:517–521.
91. Neer CS, Welsh RP. The shoulder in sports. *Orthop Clin North Am* 1977;8:583–591.
92. Burkhead WZ, Arcand MA, Zeman C, et al. The biceps tendon. In: Rockwood CA, Matsen FA, eds. *The shoulder,* 2nd ed. Philadelphia: WB Saunders, 1998:1009–1063.
93. Nove-Josserand L, Levigne CH, Boileau P, et al. Resultats preliminaires des recentrages du tendon long biceps. *Rev Chir Orthop* 1994:80(suppl 1):195.
94. Curtis AS, Snyder SJ. Evaluation and treatment of biceps tendon pathology. *Orthop Clin North Am* 1993;24:33–43.
95. Sakurai G, Ozaki J, Tomita Y, et al. Morphologic changes in long head of biceps brachii in rotator cuff dysfunction. *J Orthop Sci* 1998;3:137–142.
96. DePalma AF. *Surgery of the shoulder,* 3rd ed. Philadelphia: JB Lippincott, 1983.
97. Phillips BB, Canale ST, Sisk TD, et al. Ruptures of the proximal biceps tendon in middle-aged patients. *Orthop Rev* 1993;22:349–353.
98. Snyder SJ, Karzel RP, Del Pizzo W, et al. SLAP lesions of the shoulder. *Arthoscopy* 1990;6:274–279.
99. Handelberg F, Willems S, Shahabpour M, et al. SLAP lesions: a retrospective multicenter study. *Arthroscopy* 1998;14:856–862.
100. Morgan CD, Burkhart SS, Palmeri M, et al. Type II SLAP lesions: three subtypes and their relationships to superior instability and rotator cuff tears. *Arthroscopy* 1998;14: 553–565.
101. Cordasco FA, Steinmann S, Flatow EL, et al. Arthroscopic treatment of glenoid labral tears. *Am J Sports Med* 1993;21:425–431.
102. Bey MJ, Elders GJ, Huston LJ, et al. The mechanism of creation of superior labrum, anterior, and posterior lesions in a dynamic biomechanical model of the shoulder: the role of inferior subluxation. *J Shoulder Elbow Surg* 1998;7:397–401.
103. Monu JUV, Pope TL, Chabon SJ, et al. MR diagnosis of superior labral anterior posterior (SLAP) injuries of the glenoid labrum: value of routine imaging without intraarticular injection of contrast material. *AJR* 1994;163:1425–1429.
104. Bresler F, Blum A, Braun M, et al. Assessment of the superior labrum of the shoulder joint with CT-arthrography and MR-arthrography: correlation with anatomical dissection. *Surg Radiol Anat* 1998;19:57–62.
105. Hunter JC, Blatz DJ, Escobedo EM. SLAP lesions of the glenoid labrum: CT arthrographic and arthroscopic correlation. *Radiology* 1992;184:513–518.
106. Cone RO, Danzig L, Resnick D, et al. The bicipital groove:radiographic, anatomic and pathologic study. *AJR* 1983;141: 781–783.
107. Middleton WD, Reinus WR, Totty WG, et al. US of the biceps tendon apparatus. *Radiology* 1985;157:211–215.
108. Farin PU. Sonography of the biceps tendon of the shoulder: normal and pathologic findings. *J Clin Ultrasound* 1996;24: 309–316.
109. Kennedy JC, Willis RB. The effects of local steroid injections on tendons: a biomechanical and microscopic correlative study. *Am J Sports Med* 1976;4:11–21.
110. Harryman DT, Lazarus MD, Rozencwaig R. The stiff shoulder. In: Rockwood CA, Matsen FA, eds. *The shoulder,* 2nd ed. Philadelphia: WB Saunders, 1998:1064–1112.
111. Friedman NA, LaBan MM. Periarthrosis of the shoulder associated with diabetes mellitus. *Am J Phys Med Rehabil* 1989; 68:12–14.
112. Bridgman JF. Periarthritis of the shoulder and diabetes mellitus. *Ann Rheum Dis* 1972;31:69–71.
113. Neviaser JS. Adhesive capsulitis of the shoulder. A study of the

pathological findings in periarthritis of the shoulder. *J Bone Joint Surg* 1945;27:211–222.

114. Brandser EA, Renfrew DL, Schenck RR. Adhesive capsulitis of the wrist. *Can Assoc Radiol J* 1995;46:137–138.
115. Gusman DN, Dockery GL. Adhesive lesions of the talocrural joint. *Clin Podiatr Med Surg* 1994;11:385–394.
116. Mont MA, Lindsey JM, Hungerford DS. Adhesive capsulitis of the hip. *Orthopedics* 1999;22:343–345.
117. Rizk TE, Pinals RS. Frozen shoulder. *Semin Arthritis Rheum* 1982;11:440–452.
118. Wright V, Haq AMMM. Periarthritis of the shoulder. I. Aetiological considerations with particular reference to personality factors. *Ann Rheum Dis* 1976;35:213–219.
119. Withrington RH, Girgis FL, Seifert MH. A comparative study of the aetiological factors in shoulder pain. *Br J Rheumatol* 1985;24:24–26.
120. Bruckner FE, Nye CJS. A prospective study of adhesive capsulitis of the shoulder ("frozen shoulder") in a high risk population. *Q J Med* 1981;198:191–204.
121. Bulgen DY, Hazleman BL, Voak D. HLA B-27 and frozen shoulder. *Lancet* 1976;1:1042–1044.
122. Bulgen DY, Hazleman BL, Ward M, et al. Immunological studies in frozen shoulder. *Ann Rheum Dis* 1978;37:135–138.
123. Lundberg BJ. Glycosaminoglycans of the normal and frozen shoulder-joint capsule. *Clin Orthop* 1970;69:279–284.
124. Reeves B. The natural history of frozen shoulder syndrome. *Scand J Rheumatol* 1975;4:193–196.
125. Shaffer B, Tibone JE, Kerlan RK. Frozen shoulder, a long-term follow-up. *J Bone Joint Surg* 1992;74A:738–746.
126. Clarke GR, Willis LA, Fish WW, et al. Preliminary studies in measuring range of motion in normal and painful stiff shoulders. *Rheum Rehabil* 1975;14:39–46.
127. Miller MD, Wirth MA, Rockwood CA. Thawing the frozen shoulder: the "patient" patient. *Orthopedics* 1996;19:849–853.
128. Duralde XA, Pollock RG, Flatow EL, et al. Frozen shoulder: prevention, diagnosis, and management. *J Musculoskel Med* 1993;10:64–72.
129. Zuckerman JD, Cuomo F. Frozen shoulder. In: Matsen FA, Fu FH, Hawkins RJ, eds. *The shoulder:* a balance of mobility and stability. Rosemont, IL: American Academy Orthopaedic Surgeons, 1993:253–267.
130. Koppel HP, Thompson WAL. Pain and the frozen shoulder. *Surg Gynecol Obstet* 1959;109:92–96.
131. Rizk TE, Gavant ML, Pinals RS. Treatment of adhesive capsulitis (frozen shoulder) with artherographic capsular distention and rupture. *Arch Phys Med Rehabil* 1994;75:803–807.
132. Fareed DO, Gallivan WR. Office management of frozen shoulder syndrome: treatment with hydraulic distension under local anesthesia. *Clin Orthop* 1989;242:177–183.
133. Older MW, McIntyre JL, Lloyd GJ. Distention arthrography of the shoulder joint. *Can J Surg* 1976;19:203–207.
134. Woo SL-Y, McMahon PJ, Debski RE, et al. Factors limiting and defining shoulder motion: what keeps it from going farther? In: Matsen FA, Fu FH, Hawkins RJ, eds. *The shoulder:* a balance of mobility and stability. Rosemont, IL: American Academy Orthopaedic Surgeons, 1993:141–158.
135. Chan KM, Maffulli N, Nobuhara M, et al. Shoulder instability in athletes: the Asian perspective. *Clin Orthop* 1996;323:106–112.
136. Itamura JM, Burkhead WZ, Shankwiler JA. Decision making in shoulder dislocation and instability. *J Musculoskel Med* 1995;12:48–57.
137. Rowe CR, Zarins B. Recurrent transient subluxation of the shoulder. *J Bone Joint Surg* 1981;63A:863–872.
138. Hovelius L, Gaevle KE, Falun HF, et al. Recurrences after initial dislocation of the shoulder. Results of a prospective study of treatment. *J Bone Joint Surg* 1983;65A:343–349.
139. Simonet WT, Cofield RH. Prognosis in anterior shoulder dislocation. *Am J Sports Med* 1984;12:19–24.
140. Pevny T, Hunter RE, Freeman JR. Primary traumatic anterior shoulder dislocation in patients 40 years of age and older. *Arthroscopy* 1998;14:289–294.
141. Protzman RR. Anterior instability of the shoulder. *J Bone Joint Surg* 1980;62A:909–918.
142. Aronen JG, Regan K. Decreasing the incidence of recurrence of first time anterior shoulder dislocations with rehabilitation. *Am J Sports Med* 1984;12:283–291.
143. Thomas SC, Matsen FA. An approach to the repair of glenohumeral ligament avulsion in the management of traumatic anterior glenohumeral instability. *J Bone Joint Surg* 1989;71A: 506–514.
144. Burkhead WZ, Rockwood CA. Treatment of instability of the shoulder with an exercise program. *J Bone Joint Surg* 1992; 74A:890–896.
145. Pappas AM, Goss TP, Kleinman PK. Symptomatic shoulder instability due to lesions of the glenoid labrum. *Am J Sports Med* 1983;11:279–288.
146. Garth WP, Allman FL, Armstrong WS. Occult anterior subluxations of the shoulder in noncontact sports. *Am J Sports Med* 1987;15:579–585.
147. Lephart SM, Warner JJP, Borsa PA, et al. Proprioception of the shoulder joint in healthy, unstable, and surgically repaired shoulders. *J Shoulder Elbow Surg* 1994;3:371–380.
148. Samilson RI, Prieto V. Dislocation arthropathy of the shoulder. *J Bone Joint Surg* 1983;65A:456–460.
149. Matsen FA, Thomas SC, Rockwood CA, et al. Glenohumeral instability. In: Rockwood CA, Matsen FA, eds. *The shoulder,* 2nd ed. Philadelphia: WB Saunders, 1998:611–754.
150. Brems JJ. Arthritis of dislocation. *Orthop Clin North Am* 1998; 29:453–466.
151. Nicholas JA, Grossman RB, Hershman EB. The importance of a simplified classification of motion in sports in relation to performance. *Orthop Clin North Am* 1977;8:499–532.
152. Hill JA. Epidemiologic perspective on shoulder injuries. *Clin Sports Med* 1983;2:241–246.
153. Jobe FW, Jobe CM. Painful athletic injuries of the shoulder. *Clin Orthop Rel Res* 1983;173:117–124.
154. Tullos HS, King JW. Throwing mechanism in sports. *Orthop Clin North Am* 1973;4:709–720.
155. Craig EV. Shoulder arthroscopy in the throwing athlete. *Clin Sports Med* 1996;15:673–700.
156. Arroyo JS, Hershon SJ, Bigliani LU. Special considerations in the athletic throwing shoulder. *Orthop Clin North Am* 1997; 28:69–78.
157. Roger B, Skaf A, Hooper AW, et al. Imaging findings in the dominant shoulder of throwing athletes: comparison of radiography, arthrography, CT arthrography, and MR arthrography with arthroscopic correlation. *AJR* 1999;172:1371–1380.
158. Jobe CM. Superior glenoid impingement. *Orthop Clin North Am* 1997;28:137–143.
159. Walch G, Boileau P, Noel E, et al. Impingement of the deep surface of the supraspinatus tendon on the posterosuperior glenoid rim: an arthroscopic study. *J Shoulder Elbow Surg* 1992;1: 238–245.
160. Carson WG Jr, Gasser SI. Little Leaguer's shoulder. A report of 23 cases. *Am J Sports Med* 1998;26:575–580.
161. Pink M, Perry J, Browne A, et al. The normal shoulder during freestyle swimming: an electromyographic and cinematographic analysis of 12 muscles. *Am J Sports Med* 1991;19:569–576.
162. Richardson AB, Jobe FW, Collins HR. The shoulder in competitive swimming. *Am J Sports Med* 1980;8:159–163.
163. Kennedy JC, Hawkins R, Krissoff WB. Orthopaedic manifestations of swimming. *Am J Sports Med* 1978;6:309–322.

164. Fowler P. Swimmer problems. *Am J Sports Med* 1979;7: 141–142.
165. Giombini A, Rossi F, Pettrone FA, et al. Posterosuperior glenoid rim impingement as a cause of shoulder pain in top level water polo players. *J Sports Med Phys Fitness* 1997;37:273–278.
166. Priest JD, Nagel DA. Tennis shoulder. *Am J Sports Med* 1976;4: 28–42.
167. Caraffa A, Cerulli G, Rizzo A, et al. An arthroscopic and electromyographic study of painful shoulders in elite gymnasts. *Knee Surg Sports Traumatol Arthrosc* 1996;4:39–42.
168. Wadley GH, Albright JP. Women's intercollegiate gymnastics. Injury patterns and "permanent" medical disability. *Am J Sports Med* 1993;21:314–320.
169. Matsen FA, Rockwood CA, Wirth MA, et al. Glenohumeral arthritis and its management. In: Rockwood CA, Matsen FA, eds. *The shoulder,* 2nd ed. Philadelphia: WB Saunders, 1998: 840–964.
170. Bullough PG. Pathology and pathogenesis of osteoarthritis. In: Matsen FA, Fu FH, Hawkins RJ, eds. *The shoulder:* a balance of mobility and stability. Rosemont, IL: American Academy Orthopaedic Surgeons, 1993:229–237.
171. Petersson CJ. Painful shoulders in patients with rheumatoid arthritis. *Scand J Rheumatol* 1986;15:275–279.
172. Lehtinen JT, Kaarela K, Belt EA, et al. Incidence of acromioclavicular joint involvement in rheumatoid arthritis: a 15 year endpoint study. *J Rheumatol* 1999;26:1239–1241.
173. Kalliomäki JL, Viitanen S-M, Virtama P. Radiological findings of sternoclavicular joints in rheumatoid arthritis. *Acta Rheum Scand* 1968;14:233–240.
174. Coari G, Paoletti F, Iagnocco A. Shoulder involvement in rheumatic diseases. Sonographic findings. *J Rheumatol* 1999;26: 668–673.
175. Paice EW, Wright FW, Hill AGS. Sternoclavicular erosions in polymyalgia rheumatica. *Ann Rheum Dis* 1983;42:379–383.
176. O'Duffy JD, Wahner HW, Humder GG. Joint imaging in polymyalgia rheumatica. *Mayo Clin Proc* 1976;51:519–524.
177. Douglas WA, Martin BA, Morris JH. Polymyalgia rheumatica: an arthroscopic study of the shoulder joint. *Ann Rheum Dis* 1983;42:311–316.
178. Meliconi R, Pulsatelli L, Uguccioni MG, et al. Leukocyte infiltration in synovial tissue from the shoulder of patients with polymyalgia rheumatica. Quantitative analysis and influence of corticosteroid treatment. *Arthritis Rheum* 1996;39:1199–1207.
179. Lutalo SK. Gout: an experience from Zimbabwe. *Cent Afr J Med* 1993;39:60–62.
180. Richman KM, Boutin RD, Vaughan LM, et al. Tophaceous pseudogout of the sternoclavicular joint. *AJR* 1999;172: 1587–1589.
181. Bernageau J, Bardin T, Goutallier D, et al. Magnetic resonance imaging findings in shoulders of hemodialyzed patients. *Clin Orthop* 1984;304:91–96.
182. Nagoshi M, Hashizume H, Masaoka S, et al. Surgical treatment for shoulder arthropathy induced by dialysis-related amyloidosis. *J Shoulder Elbow Surg* 1998;7:337.
183. Nussbaum AJ, Doppman JL. Shoulder arthropathy in primary hyperparathyroidism. *Skeletal Radiol* 1982;9:98–102.
184. Kaklamanis Ph, Rigas A, Giannatos J, et al. Calcification of the shoulders and diabetes mellitus [letter]. *N Engl J Med* 1975; 293:1266–1267.
185. Trapp RG, Soler NG. Musculoskeletal abnormalities of the upper extremities and neck in insulin dependent diabetics: symptomatology and physical findings. *Arthritis Rheum* 1983; 26(suppl):S47.
186. Wallace TW. Shoulder pain and occult disease of the central nervous system [letter]. *JAMA* 1970;212:1709.
187. Ike, RW. Bacterial arthritis. In: Koopman WJ, ed. *Arthritis and allied conditions,* 13th ed. Baltimore: Williams & Wilkins, 1997:2267–2295.
188. Sartoris DJ, Schreiman JS, Kerr R, et al. Sternoclavicular hyperostosis: a review and report of 11 cases. *Radiology* 1986;158: 125–128.
189. Chigira M, Maehara S, Nagase M, et al. Sternocostoclavicular hyperostosis. A report of nineteen cases, with special reference to etiology and treatment. *J Bone Joint Surg* 1986;68A:103–112.
190. Hayem G, Bouchaud-Chabot A, Palazzo E, et al. Psoriasis vulgaris, as palmoplantar pustulosis and severe acne, can be associated with bone involvement (SAPHO syndrome). *Arthritis Rheum* 1994;37:S205.
191. Helliwell PS, Marchessoni A, Peters M, et al. A revaluation of the osteoarticular manifestations of psoriasis. *Br J Rheumatol* 1991;30:339–345.
192. Sonozaki H, Mitsui H, Miyanaga Y, et al. Clinical features of 53 cases with pustulotic arthro-osteitis. *Ann Rheum Dis* 1981;40: 547–553.
193. Benhamou CL, Chamot AM, Kahn MF. Synovitis acne pustulosis hyperostosis osteomyelitis syndrome (SAPHO). A new syndrome among the spondylo-arthropathies? *Clin Exp Rheumatol* 1988;6:109–112.
194. Kahn MF, Chamot AM. SAPHO syndrome. *Rheum Dis Clin North Am* 1992;18:225–246.
195. Watts RA, Crisp AJ, Hazleman BL, et al. Arthro-osteitis—a clinical spectrum. *Br J Rheumatol* 1993;32:403–407.
196. Misaki T, Doksh S, Mori E. Calcitonin treatment for intersternocostoclavicular ossification. Clinical experience in two cases. *Ann Rheum Dis* 1991;50:813–816.
197. Corso SJ, Furie E. Arthroscopy of the acromioclavicular joint. *Orthop Clin North Am* 1995;26:661–670.
198. Edelson JG. Clavicular fractures and ipsilateral acromioclavicular arthrosis. *J Shoulder Elbow Surg* 1996;5:181–185.
199. Quinn SF, Glass TA. Posttraumatic osteolysis of the clavicle. *S Med J* 1983;76:307–308.
200. Kaplan PA, Resnick D. Stress-induced osteolysis of the clavicle. *Radiology* 1986;158:139–140.
201. Slawski DP, Cahill BR. Atraumatic osteolysis of the distal clavicle. Results of open surgical excision. *Am J Sports Med* 1994;22: 267–271.
202. Matsen FA, Bonica JJ, Franklin J. Pain in the shoulder, arm, and elbow. In: Bonica JJ, ed. *The management of pain,* 2nd ed. Philadelphia: Lea and Febiger, 1990:906–923.
203. Chung SMK, Nissenbaum MM. Congenital and developmental defects of the shoulder. *Orthop Clin North Am* 1975;6: 381–392.
204. Wood VE, Marchinski L. Congenital anomalies of the shoulder. In: Rockwood CA, Matsen FA, eds. *The shoulder,* 2nd ed. Philadelphia: WB Saunders, 1998:99–163.
205. Groves RJ, Goldner JL. Contracture of the deltoid muscle in the adult after intramuscular injections. Report of three cases. *J Bone Joint Surg* 1974;56A:817–820.
206. Ogawa K, Yoshida A, Inokuchi W. Deltoid contracture: a radiographic survey of bone and joint abnormalities. *J Shoulder Elbow Surg* 1999;8:22–25.
207. Butters KP. The scapula. In: Rockwood CA, Matsen FA, eds. *The shoulder.* Philadelphia: WB Saunders, 1998:391–427.
208. Carlson HL, Haig AJ, Stewart DC. Snapping scapula syndrome: three case reports and an analysis of the literature. *Arch Phys Med Rehabil* 1997;78:506–511.
209. Percy EC, Birbrager D, Pitt MJ. Snapping scapula: a review of the literature and presentation of 14 patients. *Can J Surg* 1988; 31:248–250.
210. Harper GD, McIlroy S, Bayley JIL, et al. Arthroscopic partial resection of the scapula for snapping scapula: a new technique. *J Shoulder Elbow Surg* 1999;8:53–57.

211. Leffert RD. Brachial-plexus injuries. *N Engl J Med* 1974;291: 1059–1067.
212. Hirasawa Y, Sakakida K. Sports and peripheral nerve injury. *Am J Sports Med* 1983;11:420–426.
213. Garth WP. Evaluating and treating brachial plexus injuries. *J Musculoskel Med* 1994;11:55–67.
214. Parsonage MJ, Turner JWA. Neuralgic amyotrophy: shoulder-girdle syndrome. *Lancet* 1948;1:973–978.
215. Magee KR, DeJong RN. Paralytic brachial neuritis. Discussion of clinical features with review of 23 cases. *JAMA* 1960;174: 1258–1262.
216. Aymond JK, Goldner JL, Hardaker WT. Neuralgic amyotrophy. *Orthop Rev* 1989;18:1275–1279.
217. Beghi E, Kurland LT, Mulder DW, et al. Brachial plexus neuropathy in the population of Rochester, Minnesota, 1970–1981. *Ann Neurol* 1985;18:320–323.
218. Wiederholt WC. Hereditary brachial neuropathy. Report of two families. *Arch Neurol* 1974;30:252–254.
219. Spillane JD. Localized neuritis of shoulder girdle: report of 46 cases in MEF. *Lancet* 1943;2:532–535.
220. Bardos V, Somadsha V. Epidemiologic study of a brachial plexus neuritis outbreak in Northeastern Czechoslovakia. *World Neurol* 1961;2:973–979.
221. Tsairis P, Dyek PJ, Mulder DW. Natural history of brachial plexus neuropathy: report on 99 patients. *Arch Neurol* 1972; 27:109–117.
222. Berry H, Bril V. Axillary nerve palsy following blunt trauma to the shoulder region: a clinical and electrophysiological review. *J Neurol Neurosurg Psychiatry* 1982;45:1027–1032.
223. Ebraheim NA, Lu J, Porshinsky B, et al. Vulnerability of long thoracic nerve: an anatomic study. *J Shoulder Elbow Surg* 1998; 133:458–461.
224. Rengachary SS, Burr D, Lucas S, et al. Suprascapular entrapment neuropathy: a clinical, anatomical, and comparative study. Part 2: Anatomical study. *Neurosurgery* 1979;5:447–451.
225. Clein LJ. Suprascapular entrapment neuropathy. *J Neurosurg* 1975;43:337–342.
226. Martin SD, Warren RF, Martin TL, et al. Suprascapular neuropathy. Results of nonoperative treatment. *J Bone Joint Surg* 1997;79A:1159–1165.
227. Ticker JB, Djurasovic M, Strauch RJ, et al. The incidence of ganglion cysts and other variations in anatomy along the course of the suprascapular nerve. *J Shoulder Elbow Surg* 1998;7: 472–478.
228. Warner JJP, Krushell RJ, Masquelet AL, et al. Anatomy and relationships of the suprascapular nerve: anatomical constraints to mobilization of the supraspinatus and infraspinatus muscles in the management of massive rotator-cuff tears. *J Bone Joint Surg* 1992;74A:36–45.
229. Ferrick MR, Marzo JM. Suprascapular entrapment neuropathy and ganglion cysts about the shoulder. *Orthopedics* 1999;22: 430–435.
230. Demirhan M, Imhoff AB, Debski RE, et al. The spinoglenoid ligament and its relationship to the suprascapular nerve. *J Shoulder Elbow Surg* 1998;7:238–243.
231. Sandow MJ, Ilic J. Suprascapular nerve rotator cuff compression syndrome in volleyball players. *J Shoulder Elbow Surg* 1998; 7:516–521.
232. Ferretti A, Cerullo G, Russo G. Suprascapular neuropathy in volleyball players. *J Bone Joint Surg* 1987;69A:260–263.
233. Torres-Ramos FM, Biundo JJ. Suprascapular neuropathy during progressive resistive exercises in a cardiac rehabilitation program. *Arch Phys Med Rehabil* 1992;73:1107–1111.
234. Fabre TH, Piton C, Leclouerec G, et al. Entrapment of the suprascapular nerve. *J Bone Joint Surg* 1999;81B:414–419.
235. Barber DB, Janus RB, Wade WH. Neuroarthropathy: an overuse of the shoulder in quadriplegia. *J Spinal Cord Med* 1996;19:9–11.
236. Frankart L, Nisolle J-F, Ayoubi S, et al. Neuroarthropathy of the shoulder of unexpected origin. *Clin Rheumatol* 1997;16:413–416.
237. Rockwood CA, Wirth MA, Hatzis N. Neuropathic arthropathy of the shoulder. *J Shoulder Elbow Surg* 1998;7:307.
238. Guis S, Pellissier J-F, Arniaud D, et al. Healing of Charcot's joint by pamidronate infusion. *J Rheumatol* 1999;26: 1843–1845.
239. Selby PL, Young MJ, Boulton AJM. Bisphosphonates: a new treatment for diabetic Charcot neuroarthropathy? *Diabetic Med* 1994;11:28–31.
240. Campbell CC, Koris MJ. Etiologies of shoulder pain in cervical spinal cord injury. *Clin Orthop* 1996;322:140–145.
241. Bayley JC, Cochran TP, Sledge CB. The weight-bearing shoulder. The impingement syndrome in paraplegics. *J Bone Joint Surg* 1987;69A:676–678.
242. Lal S. Premature degenerative shoulder changes in spinal cord injury patients. *Spinal Cord* 1998;36:186–189.
243. Urschel HC, Razzuk MA, Hyland JW, et al. Thoracic outlet syndrome masquerading as coronary artery disease (pseudoangina). *Ann Thorac Surg* 1973;16:239–248.
244. Timmis HH. Comment on: Dale WA, Lewis MR. Management of thoracic outlet syndrome. *Ann Surg* 1975;181:575–585.
245. Rayan GM. Thoracic outlet syndrome. *J Shoulder Elbow Surg* 1998;7:440–451.
246. Atasoy E. Thoracic outlet compression syndrome. *Orthop Clin North Am* 1996;27:265–303.
247. Urschel HC, Razzuk MA. Management of the thoracic-outlet syndrome. *N Engl J Med* 1972;286:1140–1143.
248. Bertelsen S. Neurovascular compression syndromes of the neck and shoulder. *Acta Chir Scand* 1969;135:137–148.
249. Tyson RR, Kaplan GF. Modern concepts of diagnosis and treatment of the thoracic outlet syndrome. *Orthop Clin North Am* 1975;6:507–519.
250. DeSilva M. The costoclavicular syndrome: a "new cause." *Ann Rheum Dis* 1986;45:916–920.
251. Swift TR, Nichols FT. The droopy shoulder syndrome. *Neurology* 1984;34:212–215.
252. Wilbourn AJ, Lederman RJ. Evidence for conduction delay in thoracic-outlet syndrome is challenged [letter]. *N Engl J Med* 1984;310:1052–1053.
253. Yiannikas C, Walsh JC. Somatosensory evoked responses in the diagnosis of thoracic outlet syndrome. *J Neurol Neurosurg Psychiatry* 1983;46:234–240.
254. Gergoudis R, Barnes RW. Thoracic outlet arterial compression: prevalence in normal persons. *Angiology* 1980;31:538–541.
255. Mackinnon SE. Thoracic outlet syndrome [editorial]. *Ann Thorac Surg* 1994;58:287–289.
256. Mitchell SW, Morehouse GR, Keen WW. *Gunshot wounds and other injuries of nerves.* New York: JB Lippincott, 1864.
257. Wilson PR. Post-traumatic upper extremity reflex sympathetic dystrophy. Clinical course, staging, and classification of clinical forms. *Hand Clin* 1997;13:367–372.
258. Wong GY, Wilson PR. Classification of complex regional pain syndromes. New concepts. *Hand Clin* 1997;13:319–325.
259. Atkins RM, Duckworth T, Kanis JA. Features of algodystrophy after Colles' fracture. *J Bone Joint Surg* 1990;72:105–110.
260. Veldman PHJM, Reynen HM, Arntz IE, et al. Signs and symptoms of reflex sympathetic dystrophy: prospective study of 829 patients. *Lancet* 1993;342:1012–1016.
261. Omer GC, Thomas MS. Treatment of causalgia. *Tex Med* 1971;67:93–96.
262. Geertzen JHB, de Bruijn H, de Bruijn-Kofman AT, et al. Reflex sympathetic dystrophy: early treatment and psychological aspects. *Arch Phys Med Rehabil* 1994;75:442–446.

263. Geertzen JHB, de Bruijn-Kofman AT, de Bruijn HP, et al. Stressful life events and psychological dysfunction in complex regional pain syndrome type I. *Clin J Pain* 1998;14:143–147.
264. Lynch ME. Psychological aspects of reflex sympathetic dystrophy: a review of the adult and paediatric literature. *Pain* 1992;49:337–347.
265. Didierjean A. Psychological aspects of algodystrophy. *Hand Clin* 1997;363–366.
266. Doury PCC. Algodystrophy. A spectrum of disease, historical perspectives, criteria of diagnosis, and principles of treatment. *Hand Clin* 1997;13:327–337.
267. Blumberg H, Jänig W. Clinical manifestations of reflex sympathetic dystrophy and sympathetically maintained pain. In: Wall PD, Melzack R, eds. *Textbook of pain,* 3rd ed. Edinburgh: Churchill Livingstone, 1994:685–698.
268. Webster GF, Iozzo RV, Schwartzman RJ, et al. Reflex sympathetic dystrophy: occurrence of chronic edema and nonimmune bullous skin lesions. *J Am Acad Dermatol* 1993;28:29–32.
269. Greipp ME, Thomas AF. Skin lesions occurring in clients with reflex sympathetic dystrophy syndrome. *J Neurosci Nurs* 1994;26:342–346.
270. Van der Laan L, Veldman PHJM, Goris RJA. Severe complications of reflex sympathetic dystrophy: infection, ulcers, chronic edema, dystonia, and myoclonus. *Arch Phys Med Rehabil* 1998;79:424–429.
271. Schwartzman RJ, Kerrigan J. The movement disorder of reflex sympathetic dystrophy. *Neurology* 1990;40:57–61.
272. Deuschl G, Blumberg H, Lücking CH. Tremor in reflex sympathetic dystrophy. *Arch Neurol* 1991;48:1247–1252.
273. Steinbrocker O, Friedman HH, Lapin L. The shoulder-hand syndrome. (Reflex neurovascular dystrophy of the upper extremity.) *Postgrad Med* 1954;16:46–57.
274. Steinbrocker O, Argyros TG. The shoulder-hand syndrome: present status as a diagnostic and therapeutic entity. *Med Clin North Am* 1958;42:1533–1553.
275. Bremer C. Shoulder-hand syndrome. A case of unusual aetiology. *Ann Phys Med* 1968;9:168–171.
276. Pak TJ, Martin GM, Magness JL, et al. Reflex sympathetic dystrophy. Review of 140 cases. *Minn Med* 1970;53:507–512.
277. Wilder RT, Berde CB, Wolohan M, et al. Reflex sympathetic dystrophy in children. *J Bone Joint Surg* 1992;74A:910–919.
278. Dietz FR, Mathews KD, Montgomery WJ. Reflex sympathetic dystrophy in children. *Clin Orthop* 1990;258:225–231.
279. Stanton RP, Malcolm JR, Wesdock KA, et al. Reflex sympathetic dystrophy in children: an orthopedic perspective. *Orthopedics* 1993;16:773–780.
280. Kozin F, McCarty DJ, Sims J, et al. The reflex sympathetic dystrophy syndrome. I. Clinical and histologic studies: evidence for bilaterality, response to corticosteroids and articular involvement. *Am J Med* 1976;60:321–331.
281. Kozin F, Genant HK, Bekerman C, et al. The reflex sympathetic dystrophy syndrome. II. Roentgenographic and scintigraphic evidence of bilaterality and of periarticular accentuation. *Am J Med* 1976;60:332–338.
282. Schiffenbauer J, Fagien M. Reflex sympathetic dystrophy involving multiple extremities. *J Rheumatol* 1993;20:165–169.
283. Barrera P, van Riel PLCM, De Jong AJL, et al. Recurrent and migratory reflex sympathetic dystrophy syndrome. *Clin Rheumatol* 1992;11:416–421.
284. Laukaitis JP, Varma VM, Borenstein DG. Reflex sympathetic dystrophy localized to a single digit. *J Rheumatol* 1989:16:402–405.
285. Helms CA, O'Brien ET, Katzberg RW. Segmental reflex sympathetic dystrophy syndrome. *Radiology* 1980;135:67–68.
286. Corbett M, Colston JR, Tucker AK. Pain in the knee associated with osteoporosis of the patella. *Ann Rheum Dis* 1977;36:188–191.
287. Kim HJ, Kozin F, Johnson RP, et al. Reflex sympathetic dystrophy of the knee following menisectomy. Report of three cases. *Arthritis Rheum* 1979;22:177–181.
288. Tietjen R. Reflex sympathetic dystrophy of the knee. *Clin Orthop* 1986;209:234–243.
289. Gaucher A, Colomb J-N, Naoun AR, et al. The diagnostic value of 99m Tc-diphosphonate bone imaging in transient osteoporosis of the hip. *J Rheumatol* 1979;6:574–583.
290. Curtiss PH, Kincaid WE. Transitory demineralization of the hip in pregnancy: a report of three cases. *J Bone Joint Surg* 1959;41A:1327–1333.
291. Langloh ND, Hunder GG, Riggs BL, et al. Transient painful osteoporosis of the lower extremities. *J Bone Joint Surg* 1973;55A:1188–1196.
292. Mailis A, Inman R, Pham D. Transient migratory osteoporosis: a variant of reflex sympathetic dystrophy? Report of 3 cases and literature review. *J Rheumatol* 1992;19:758–764.
293. Ribbers GM, Oosterhuis WP, van Limbeek J, et al. Reflex sympathetic dystrophy: is the immune system involved? *Arch Phys Med Rehabil* 1998;79:1549–1552.
294. Masson C, Audran M, Pascaretti C, et al. Further vascular, bone and autonomic investigations in algodystrophy. *Acta Orthop Belg* 1998;64:77–87.
295. Chelimsky TC, Low PA, Naessens JM, et al. Value of autonomic testing in reflex sympathetic dystrophy. *Mayo Clin Proc* 1995;70:1029–1040.
296. Kozin F, Ryan LM, Carerra G, et al. The reflex sympathetic dystrophy syndrome (RSDS). III. Scintigraphic studies, further evidence for the therapeutic efficacy of systemic corticosteroids, and proposed diagnostic criteria. *Am J Med* 1981;70:23–30.
297. Kozin F, Soin JS, Ryan LM, et al. Bone scintigraphy in the reflex sympathetic dystrophy syndrome. *Radiology* 1981;138:437–443.
298. Genant HK, Kozin F, Bekerman C, et al. The reflex sympathetic dystrophy syndrome. A comprehensive analysis using fine-detail radiography, photon absorptiometry, and bone and joint scintigraphy. *Radiology* 1975;117:21–32.
299. Bickerstaff DR, Charlesworth D, Kanis JA. Changes in cortical and trabecular bone in algodystrophy. *Br J Rheumatol* 1993;32:46–51.
300. Fournier RS, Holder LE. Reflex sympathetic dystrophy: diagnostic controversies. *Semin Nucl Med* 1998;28:116–123.
301. Davidoff G, Werner R, Cremer S, et al. Predictive value of the three-phase technetium bone scan in diagnosis of reflex sympathetic dystrophy syndrome. *Arch Phys Med Rehabil* 1989;70:135–137.
302. Weiss L, Alfano A, Bardfeld P, et al. Prognostic value of triple phase bone scanning for reflex sympathetic dystrophy in hemiplegia. *Arch Phys Med Rehabil* 1993;74:716–719.
303. Carlson DH, Simon H, Wegner W. Bone scanning and diagnosis of reflex sympathetic dystrophy secondary to herniated lumbar discs. *Neurology* 1977;27:791–793.
304. Blockx P, Driessens MF. The use of Tc-99m HAS dynamic vascular examination in the staging and therapy monitoring of reflex sympathetic dystrophy. *Nucl Med Commun* 1991;12:725–731.
305. Schiepers C. Clinical value of dynamic bone and vascular scintigraphy in diagnosing reflex sympathetic dystrophy of the upper extremity. *Hand Clin* 1997;13:423–429.
306. Chapurlat RD, Duboeuf FP, Liens D, et al. Dual energy x-ray absorptiometry in patients with lower limb reflex sympathetic dystrophy syndrome. *J Rheumatol* 1996;23:1557–1559.
307. Lovy MR, Goodman R. Dual energy x-ray absorptiometry in reflex sympathetic dystrophy [letter]. *J Rheumatol* 1997;24:812–814.

308. Laroche M, Redon Dumolard A, Mazieres B, et al. An x-ray absorptiometry study of reflex sympathetic dystrophy syndrome. *Rev Rhum* (English edition) 1997;64:106–111.
309. Sarangi PP, Ward AJ, Smith EJ, et al. Algodystrophy and osteoporosis after tibial fractures. *J Bone Joint Surg* 1993;75B: 450–452.
310. Parano E, Pavone V, Greco F, et al. Reflex sympathetic dystrophy associated with deep peroneal nerve entrapment. *Brain Dev* 1998;20:80–82.
311. Wilhelm A. Stenosis of the subclavian vein. An unknown cause of resistant reflex sympathetic dystrophy. *Hand Clin* 1997;13: 387–411.
312. Chevalier X, Claudepierre P, Larget-Piet B, et al. Münchausen's syndrome simulating reflex sympathetic dystrophy. *J Rheumatol* 1996;23:1111–1112.
313. Medsger TA, Dixon JA, Garwood VF. Palmar fasciitis and polyarthritis associated with ovarian carcinoma. *Ann Intern Med* 1982;96:424–431.
314. Michaels RM, Sorber JA. Reflex sympathetic dystrophy as a probable paraneoplastic syndrome: case report and literature review. *Arthritis Rheum* 1984;27:1183–1185.
315. DeTakats G. Reflex dystrophy of the extremities. *Arch Surg* 1937;34:939–956.
316. Sudeck P. Über die akute entzündliche Knochenatrophie. *Arch Klin Chir* 1900;62:147–156.
317. Miller DS, deTakats G. Posttraumatic dystrophy of the extremities. Sudeck's atrophy. *Surg Gynecol Obstet* 1941;125:558–582.
318. Van der Laan L, ter Laak HJ, Gabreëls-Festen A, et al. Complex regional pain syndrome type I (RSD). Pathology of skeletal muscle and peripheral nerve. *Neurology* 1998;51:20–25.
319. Roberts WJ. A hypothesis on the physiological basis for causalgia and related pains. *Pain* 1986;24:297–311.
320. Blanchard J, Ramamurthy S, Walsh N, et al. Intravenous regional sympatholysis: a double-blind comparison of guanethidine, reserpine, and normal saline. *J Pain Symptom Manage* 1990;5:357–361.
321. Jadad AR, Caroll D, Glynn CJ, et al. Intravenous regional sympathetic block for pain relief in reflex sympathetic dystrophy: a systemic review and a randomized double blind crossover study. *J Pain Manage* 1995;10:13–20.
322. Ramamurthy S, Hoffman J. Intravenous regional guanethidine in the treatment of reflex sympathetic dystrophy/causalgia: a double blind study. Guanethidine Study Group. *Anesth Analg* 1995;81:718–723.
323. Christensen K, Henriksen O. The reflex sympathetic dystrophy syndrome-an experimental study of blood flow and autoregulation in subcutaneous tissue. *Arthritis Rheum* 1982; 25:S145(abst).
324. Ide J, Yamaga M, Kitamura T, et al. Quantitative evaluation of sympathetic nervous system dysfunction in patients with reflex sympathetic dystrophy. *J Hand Surg* 1997;22B:102–106.
325. Drummond PD, Finch PM, Smythe GA. Reflex sympathetic dystrophy: the significance of differing plasma catecholamine concentrations in affected and unaffected limbs. *Brain* 1991;114:2025–2036.
326. Harden RN, Duc TA, Williams TR, et al. Norepinephrine and epinephrine levels in affected versus unaffected limbs in sympathetically maintained pain. *Clin J Pain* 1994;10:324–330.
327. Arnold JMO, Teasell RW, MacLeod AP, et al. Increased venous alpha-adrenoceptor responsiveness in patients with reflex sympathetic dystrophy. *Ann Intern Med* 1993;118:619–621.
328. Schott GD. An unsympathetic view of pain. *Lancet* 1995;345:634–636.
329. Sudeck P. Die sogenannte akute Knochenatrophie als Entzündungsvorgang. *Chirurg* 1942;15:449–458.
330. Van der Laan L, Goris RJA. Reflex sympathetic dystrophy. An exaggerated regional inflammatory response? *Hand Clin* 1997; 13:373–385.
331. Heerschap A, den Hollander JA, Reynen H, et al. Metabolic changes in reflex sympathetic dystrophy: a 31P NMR spectroscopy study. *Muscle Nerve* 1993;16:367–373.
332. Oyen WJG, Arntz IE, Claessens RAMJ, et al. Reflex sympathetic dystrophy of the hand; an excessive inflammatory response? *Pain* 1993;55:151–157.
333. Van der Laan L, Kapitein PJC, Oyen WJG, et al. A novel animal model to evaluate oxygen derived free radical damage in soft tissue. *Free Radic Res* 1997;26:363–372.
334. Christensen K, Jensen EM, Noer I. The reflex sympathetic dystrophy syndrome response to treatment with systemic corticosteroids. *Acta Chir Scand* 1982;148:653–655.
335. Mowat AG. Treatment of the shoulder-hand syndrome with corticosteroids. *Ann Rheum Dis* 1974;33:120–123.
336. Zuurmond WWA, Langendijk PNJ, Bezemer PD, et al. Treatment of acute reflex sympathetic dystrophy with DMSO 50% in a fatty cream. *Acta Anaesthesiol Scand* 1996;40:364–367.
337. Rosen PS, Graham W. The shoulder-hand syndrome: historical review with observations on 73 patients. *Can Med Assoc J* 1957; 77:86–91.
338. Maillefert JF, Cortet B, Aho S. Pooled results from 2 trials evaluating bisphosphonates in reflex sympathetic dystrophy [letter]. *J Rheumatol* 1999;26:1856–1857.
339. Dielissen PW, Claassen ATPM, Veldman PHJM, et al. Amputation for reflex sympathetic dystrophy. *J Bone Joint Surg* 1995: 77B:270–273.
340. Subbarao J, Stillwell GK. Reflex sympathetic dystrophy syndrome of the upper extremity: analysis of total outcome of management of 125 cases. *Arch Phys Med Rehabil* 1981;62:549–554.
341. Geertzen JHB, Dijkstra PU, Groothoff JW, et al. Reflex sympathetic dystrophy of the upper extremity—a 5.5-year follow-up. Part I. Impairments and perceived disability. *Acta Orthop Scand* 1998;69(suppl 279):12–18.
342. Geertzen JHB, Dijkstra PU, Groothoff JW, et al. Reflex sympathetic dystrophy of the upper extremity—a 5.5 year follow-up. Part II. Social life events, general health and changes in occupation. *Acta Orthop Scand* 1998;69(suppl 279):19–23.
343. Watson HK, Carlson L. Treatment of reflex sympathetic dystrophy of the hand with an active "stress loading" program. *J Hand Surg* 1987;12A:779–785.
344. Farcot JM, Gautherie M, Foucher G. Regional intravenous sympathetic nerve blocks. *Hand Clin* 1997;13:499–517.
345. Schott GD. Interrupting the sympathetic outflow in causalgia and reflex sympathetic dystrophy. A futile procedure for many patients. *Br Med J* 1998;316:792–793.
346. Steinbrocker O, Neustadt D, Lapin L. Sympathetic block compared with corticotropin and cortisone therapy. *JAMA* 1953; 153:788–791.
347. Wang JK, Johnson KA, Ilstrup DM. Sympathetic blocks for reflex sympathetic dystrophy. *Pain* 1985;13–17.
348. Cortet B, Guyot M-H, Dabouz R, et al. Evaluation de l'efficacité des blocs intra-veineux au buflomedil au cours de l'algodystrophie. A propos de 213 cas chez 81 patients. *Rhumatologie* 1997;49:230–234.
349. Malik VK, Inchiosa MA, Mustafa K, et al. Intravenous regional phenoxybenzamine in the treatment of reflex sympathetic dystrophy. *Anesthesiology* 1998;88:823–827.
350. Glynn C, Casale R. Morphine injected around the stellate ganglion does not modulate the sympathetic nervous system nor does it provide pain relief. *Pain* 1993;53:33–37.
351. Ribbers GM, Geurts AC, Rijken RA, et al. Axillary brachial plexus blockade for the reflex sympathetic dystrophy syndrome. *Int J Rehabil Res* 1997;20:371–380.
352. Cooper DE, DeLee JC, Ramamurthy S. Reflex sympathetic

dystrophy of the knee. Treatment using continuous epidural anesthesia. *J Bone Joint Surg* 1989;365–369.

353. Rauck RL, Eisenach JC, Jackson, et al. Epidural clonidine treatment for refractory reflex sympathetic dystrophy. *Anesthesiology* 1993;79:1163–1169.
354. Hannington-Kiff JG. Relief of Sudeck's atrophy by regional intravenous guanethidine. *Lancet* 1977;1:1132–1133.
355. Bonelli S, Conoscente F, Movilia PG, et al. Regional intravenous guanethidine vs. stellate ganglion block in reflex sympathetic dystrophies; a randomized trial. *Pain* 1083;16:297–307.
356. Glynn CJ, Basedow RW, Walsh JA. Pain relief following post-ganglionic sympathetic blockade with i.v. guanethidine. *Br J Anesth* 1981;53:1297–1301.
357. Rocco AG, Kaul AF, Reisman RM, et al. A comparison of regional intravenous guanethidine and reserpine in reflex sympathetic dystrophy: a controlled, randomized, double-blind cross-over study. *Clin J Pain* 1989;5:205–209.
358. Kettler RE, Abram SE. Intravenous regional droperidol in the management of reflex sympathetic dystrophy: a double-blind, placebo-controlled, crossover study. *Anesthesiology* 1988;69: 933–936.
359. Glynn CJ, Stannard C, Collins PA, et al. The role of peripheral sudomotor blockade in the treatment of patients with sympathetically maintained pain. *Pain* 1993;53:39–42.
360. Hord AH, Rooks MD, Steohens BO, et al. Intravenous regional bretylium and lidocaine for treatment of reflex sympathetic dystrophy: a randomized double-blind study. *Anesth Analg* 1992; 74:818–821.
361. Hanna MH, Peat SJ. Ketanserin in reflex sympathetic dystrophy. A double-blind placebo controlled cross-over trial. *Pain* 1989;38:145–150.
362. Farcot JM, Grasser C, Foucher G, et al. Traitements locaux intra-veineux des algodystrophies de la main: Buflomédil versus guanéthidine, suivi à long terme. *Ann Chir Main Membr Super* 1990;9:296–304.
363. Field J, Atkins RM. Effect of guanethidine on the natural history of post-traumatic algodystrophy. *Ann Rheum Dis* 1993;52: 467–469.
364. Kingery WS. A critical review of controlled clinical trials for peripheral neuropathic pain and complex regional pain syndromes. *Pain* 1997;73:123–139.
365. Szocik JF, Gardner CA, Webb RC. Inhibitory effects of bupivacaine and lidocaine on adrenergic neuroeffector junctions in rat tail artery. *Anesthesiology* 1993;78:911–917.
366. Chaplan SR, Bach FW, Shafer SL, et al. Prolonged alleviation of tactile allodynia by intravenous lidocaine in neuropathic rats. *Anesthesiology* 1995;83:775–785.
367. Blumberg H, Hoffmann U. Der "Ischämie-Test"-ein neues Verfahren in der klinischen Diagnostik der sympathischen Reflexdystrophie (Kausalgie, M Sudeck). *Der Schermz* 1992;6: 196–198.
368. Arnér S. Intravenous phentolamine test: diagnostic and prognostic use in reflex sympathetic dystrophy. *Pain* 1991;46: 17–22.
369. Aburahma AF, Robinson PA, Powell M, et al. Sympathectomy for reflex sympathetic dystrophy: factors affecting outcome. *Ann Vasc Surg* 1994;8:372–379.
370. Ghostine SY, Comair YG, Turner DM, et al. Phenoxybenzamine in the treatment of causalgia. A report of 40 cases. *J Neurosurg* 1984;60:1263–1268.
371. Muizelaar JP, Kleyer M, Hertogs IAM, et al. Complex regional pain syndrome (reflex sympathetic dystrophy and causalgia): management with the calcium channel blocker nifedipine and/or the alpha-sympathetic blocker phenoxybenzamine in 59 patients. *Clin Neurol Neurosurg* 1997;99:26–30.
372. Stevens DS, Robins VF, Price HM. Treatment of sympathetically maintained pain with terazocin. *Reg Anesth* 1993;18: 318–321.
373. Davis KD, Treede RD, Raja SN, et al. Topical application of clonidine relieves hyperalgesia in patients with sympathetically maintained pain. *Pain* 1991;47:309–317.
374. Braus DF, Krauss JK, Strobel J. The shoulder-hand syndrome after stroke: a prospective clinical trial. *Ann Neurol* 1994;36: 728–733.
375. Gobelet C, Meier JL, Schaffner W, et al. Calcitonin and reflex sympathetic dystrophy syndrome. *Clin Rheumatol* 1986;5: 382–388.
376. Bickerstaff DR, Kanis JA. The use of nasal calcitonin in the treatment of post-traumatic algodystrophy. *Br J Rheumatol* 1991;30:291–294.
377. Gobelet C, Waldburger M, Meier JL. The effect of adding calcitonin to physical therapy on reflex sympathetic dystrophy. *Pain* 1992;48:171–175.
378. Adami S, Fossaluzza V, Gatti D, et al. Bisphosphonate therapy of reflex sympathetic dystrophy. *Ann Rheum Dis* 1997;56: 201–204.
379. Cortet B, Flipo R-M, Coquerelle P, et al. Treatment of severe recalcitrant reflex sympathetic dystrophy: assessment of efficacy and safety of the second generation bisphosphonate pamidronate. *Clin Rheumatol* 1997;16:51–56.
380. Goris RJA. Treatment of reflex sympathetic dystrophy with hydroxyl radical scavengers. *Unfallchirurg* 1985;88:330–332.
381. Arlet J, Mazières B. Medical treatment of reflex sympathetic dystrophy. *Hand Clin* 1997;13:477–483.
382. Mellick GA, Mellick LB. Reflex sympathetic dystrophy treated with gabapentin. *Arch Phys Med Rehabil* 1997;78:98–105.
383. Chaturvedi SK. Phenytoin in reflex sympathetic dystrophy. *Pain* 1989;36:379–380.
384. Cohen A, Goldman J, Daniels R. Treatment of shoulder-hand syndrome with griseofulvine (preliminary communication). *JAMA* 1960;173:542–543.
385. Cheshire WP, Snyder CR. Treatment of reflex sympathetic dystrophy with topical capsaicin. Case report. *Pain* 1990;42: 307–311.
386. Johnson MI, Ashton CH, Thompson JW. An in-depth study of long-term users of transcutaneous electrical nerve stimulation (TENS). Implications for clinical use of TENS. *Pain* 1991;44: 221–229.
387. Hassenbusch SJ, Stanton-Hicks M, Schoppa D. Long-term results of peripheral nerve stimulation for reflex sympathetic dystrophy. *J Neurosurg* 1996;84:415–423.
388. Kumar K, Nath RK, Toth C. Spinal cord stimulation is effective in the management of reflex sympathetic dystrophy. *Neurosurgery* 1997;40:503–509.
389. Calvillo O, Racz G, Didie J, et al. Neuroaugmentation in the treatment of complex regional pain syndrome of the upper extremity. *Acta Orthop Belg* 1998;64:57–63.
390. Kemler MA, Barendse GAM, Van Kleef M, et al. Electrical spinal cord stimulation in reflex sympathetic dystrophy: retrospective analysis of 23 patients. *J Neurosurg* (Spine 1) 1999;90: 79–83.
391. Jensen TS, Krebs B, Nielsen J. Immediate and long-term phantom limb pain in amputees: incidence, clinical characteristics and relationship to pre-amputation pain. *Pain* 1985;21:267–278.

108

OSTEONECROSIS

JOHN PAUL JONES, JR.

The terms *osteonecrosis, avascular (aseptic) necrosis, bone infarction,* and *osseous ischemia* indicate death of the cellular constituents of both bone and bone marrow. A minimum of 2 hours of complete ischemia and total anoxia is required to cause irreversible osteocytic necrosis (1). Although the etiology is multifactorial, intravascular coagulation (2) appears to be the final common pathway in the early pathogenesis of osteonecrosis.

PATHOPHYSIOLOGIC FEATURES

Traumatic (Macrovascular) Damage

Posttraumatic osteonecrosis is caused by disruption of the *arterial* blood supply to bone. Thus, the likelihood of developing osteonecrosis is directly proportional to the amount of initial displacement of the fracture fragments (3). It usually involves those vulnerable bones covered extensively by cartilage, with few vascular foramina and limited collateral circulation. For example, since blood to the superolateral two-thirds of the femoral head comes almost entirely from the lateral epiphyseal branches of the medial femoral circumflex artery, this area is particularly susceptible to osteonecrosis. The only other blood available to the femoral head flows through the ligamentum teres (medial epiphyseal artery), which has limited anastomoses with these lateral epiphyseal vessels. Intracapsular fractures of the hip interrupt most blood flow through the subsynovial retinacular vessels (4), including these important lateral epiphyseal arteries. About 80% of postfracture femoral head specimens were partially or totally avascular (2). Late segmental collapse of the articular surface occurs in about 30% of displaced fractures and 10% of hip dislocations without fractures, since dislocations usually rupture the ligamentum teres. Four-part fractures of the proximal humerus may impair humeral head circulation (5), primarily arising from the ascending branch of the anterior circumflex artery (6), which often results in osteonecrosis. The carpal scaphoid and body of the talus are also vulnerable to osteonecrosis, in addition to several other bones with precarious vascularity.

Nontraumatic (Microvascular) Damage

Intravascular Coagulation (Thrombosis)

Although thermal injuries and irradiation (7) can cause localized osteonecrosis, other patients may have multifocal involvement of additional and often contiguous bones, suggesting systemic osseous devascularization from an underlying disease process (8). For example, in one patient magnetic resonance imaging (MRI) revealed osteonecrosis in 19 sites (9). These patients often have bilaterally symmetrical involvement of their femoral heads, knees, and humeral heads (10). Osteonecrosis is due to a single ischemic event rather than repetitive episodes (reinfarction), since no extension of the necrotic lesion was found in 604 of 606 (99.7%) affected femoral heads studied histopathologically (11). Furthermore, sequential MRI studies have not shown the presence of recurrent osteonecrosis (12).

Intravascular coagulation with fibrin thrombus propagation appears to be the intermediary pathophysiology and final common pathway producing osteonecrosis in several different conditions (Table 108.1) (13–15). Direct histologic evidence of intravascular coagulation has been discovered in humans with intraosseous fibrin-platelet thromboses within prenecrotic femoral and humeral head segments, both 70 minutes (16) and 18 hours (17) after a known ischemic event, and prior to complete autolytic reduction of the avascular zone. These femoral head lesions appeared similar to very early osteonecrosis, which was discovered in the femoral heads of a horse (18). In both the horse (19) and the human (13), aortoiliac thrombosis can result from disseminated intravascular coagulation. Intraosseous arterial and arteriolar thromboses have also been observed histologically within later lesions (13,20–22). For example, intravascular coagulation would explain the coexistent osteonecrosis involvement of bones contiguous to the talus (23), including the distal tibia, calcaneus, and navicular (24), as well as combined osteonecrosis of the femoral head and the acetabular region (25).

Thrombosis of the microcirculation of susceptible intraosseous end-organs appears to be the genesis of nontraumatic osteonecrosis, and it results from a combination of at least three factors: (a) stasis, (b) hypercoagulability, and (c)

TABLE 108.1. RISK FACTORS POTENTIALLY ACTIVATING INTRAVASCULAR COAGULATION AND CAUSING OSTEONECROSIS

- Familial thrombophilia
  - Activated protein C resistance
- Prothrombin mutation 20210 GA
- Heparin cofactor II deficiency
- Platelet glycoprotein III a gene A1/A2 polymorphism
  - Protein C deficiency
  - Protein S deficiency
  - Antithrombin III deficiency
  - Factor VIII elevation
  - Hyperhomocysteinemia
- Hyperlipemia and embolic lipid
  - Alcoholism
  - Carbon tetrachloride poisoning
  - Diabetes mellitus
  - Fat emulsion therapy
  - Hypercortisonism (or Cushing's disease)
  - Hyperlipemia (Types II and IV)
    - C-reactive protein increased
  - Obesity
  - Pregnancy (fatty liver)
  - Disrupted adipocytes
    - Dysbaric phenomena
    - Hemoglobinopathies
    - Pancreatitis (lipase)
    - Severe burns
    - Unrelated fractures
- Hypersensitivity reactions
  - Allograft organ rejection
    - Kidney, heart, liver, marrow
  - Anaphylactic shock
  - Antiphospholipid antibodies
  - Immune complexes
  - Immune globulin therapy
  - Serum sickness
  - Systemic lupus erythematosus
    - Anticardiolipin antibodies
    - Lupus anticoagulant
  - Transfusion reactions
- Hypofibrinolysis
  - Lipoprotein(a)
  - Plasminogen deficiency
  - Tissue plasminogen activator (TPA) decreased
  - Plasminogen activator inhibitor type 1 (PAI 1) increased (gene 4G 4G)
- Infections
  - Bacterial endotoxic reactions
    - *Neisseria meningitidis*
    - *Haemophilus influenzae*
    - *Escherichia coli*
    - Others
  - Bacterial lipopolysaccharides
  - Bacterial mucopolysaccharides
  - Corticosteroid suppression
    - Prepares Shwartzman reaction
  - Intravenous drug abuse
  - Septic abortion
  - Toxic shock
    - *Staphylococcus* exotoxin
  - Viruses
    - *Cytomegalovirus*
    - Hepatitis
    - Human immunodeficiency (HIV)
    - *Rubella*
    - *Varicella*
    - Others
- Proteolytic enzymes
  - Pancreatitis (trypsin)
  - Snake venom
- Tissue factor release
  - Inflammatory bowel disease
    - Crohn's disease
    - Ulcerative colitis
  - Malignancies
    - Acute leukemias
    - Hodgkin's disease
    - Metastatic carcinoma
    - Others
    - Chemotherapy
      - L-asparaginase
  - Neurodamage
    - Brain injury/surgery
    - Spinal injury/surgery
  - Pregnancy
    - Abortion (hypertonic saline)
    - Amniotic fluid embolism
    - Normal pregnancy
      - Prepares Shwartzman reaction
    - Retained fetus in utero
    - Toxemia
- Other prethrombotic conditions
  - Acidosis
  - Anorexia nervosa
  - Anovulatory agents (estrogens)
  - Cigarette smoking
  - Decompression sickness
  - Dehydration
  - Diabetic angiopathy
  - Gaucher crisis
  - Hemolysis
  - Hemolytic-uremic syndrome
  - Hepatic failure
  - Hyperfibrinogenemia
  - Hypertension
  - Hypertrophy fatty marrow
  - Hyperviscosity
  - Hypotension (shock)
  - Immobilization
  - Nephrotic syndrome
  - Patent foramen ovale
  - Polycythemia
  - Postoperative states
  - Raynaud's phenomenon
  - Sickle-cell crisis
  - Storage diseases
    - Fabry-Anderson disease
    - Gaucher disease
  - Polyvinylpyrrolidone (PVP)
  - Thrombocytosis
  - Thrombocytopenic purpura
  - Vasoconstriction
    - Catecholamines
    - Endothelin-1
  - Vascular disorders
    - Aneurysms
    - Arteriosclerosis
    - Coarctation
    - Giant hemangiomas
    - Vasculitis
  - von Willebrand factor (VWF)

endothelial damage. The initial lesion is localized to the subchondral bone, which has a vulnerable microanatomy, facilitating stasis. Terminal arteries with few collaterals supply subchondral areas, which favors embolic occlusion and thrombosis, especially with localized vasoconstriction, or possibly, vasospasm (Raynaud's phenomenon). Endothelins are potent vasoconstrictor peptides that may be stimulated by thrombin, endotoxin, or hypoxia, and they are also associated with the no-reflow phenomenon following reperfusion (26). Intramedullary pressure and blood flow are reduced in the fatty subchondral bone of epiphyseal regions with long, narrow arcades of subchondral end-capillaries (27). Relative stasis also occurs in sinusoids and the central veins.

Hypercoagulability (28) occurs under local conditions of increased concentration and potency of procoagulant activities, decreased anticoagulant activities, vasoconstriction (neural, metabolic, and humoral) of the subchondral arteriolar bed, and, especially, decreased fibrinolysis (29). For example, protein C and S deficiencies, resistance to activated protein C (factor V Leiden mutation), antithrombin III (AT III) deficiency, hyperviscosity, hyperlipemia, hyperfibrinogemia, polycythemia, lupus anticoagulant, thrombocytosis, elevated plasminogen activator inhibitor type 1 (PAI-1) (30,31), and other platelet activating factors (Table 108.1) most likely produce a decreased threshold resistance to thrombogenesis and osteonecrosis.

The surface/volume ratio of the subchondral capillary bed results in a marked increase of endothelial cells in direct contact with blood. In the perturbed state, subchondral cells can be thrombogenic through the synthesis of von Willebrand factor antigen (vWF:Ag, factor VIIIa), PAI-1, and especially tissue factor (TF) (thromboplastin), a high-affinity, cell-surface receptor for factor VII. This functional bimolecular complex mediates the initial proteolytic activation of the extrinsic coagulation cascade. Endothelial damage of subchondral capillaries and sinusoids, with release of TF, is the most likely event triggering platelet aggregation and fibrin thrombosis, with progressive involvement of venules, veins, arterioles, and occasionally extraosseous arteries (13).

Intravascular Coagulation (Edema and Hemorrhage)

The duration of ischemia and reperfusion injury determines the extent of tissue damage. Subchondral fibrin-platelet thrombosis is usually followed by some degree of secondary, endogenous fibrinolysis. Reperfusion of these necrotic vessels subsequently results in peripheral marrow hemorrhage (Fig. 108.1) adjacent to the anemic infarction (13). Ischemia-reperfusion injuries (32) also cause lipid peroxidation of endothelial cell membranes by toxic oxygen free radicals, which increase capillary permeability that contributes to tissue edema, and also potentiates microfocal bleeding. Ischemia-reperfusion injury was recently detected by intravital microscopy through a bone chamber window implanted in

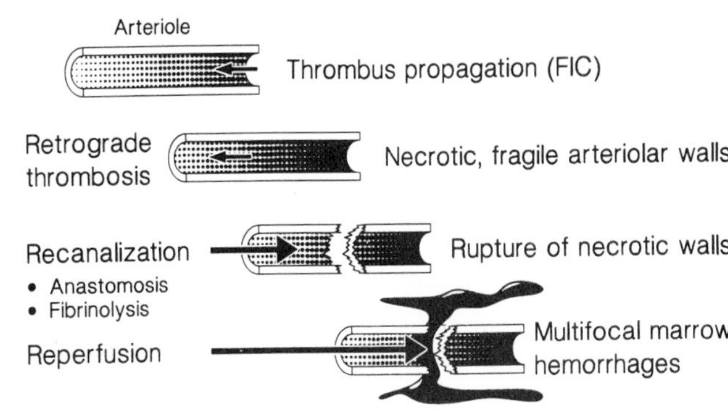

FIGURE 108.1. Probable mechanism for the development of focal intramedullary hemorrhages resulting from focal intravascular coagulation (FIC) of marrow veins, sinusoids, and capillaries, and retrograde fibrin-platelet thrombosis with fibrinolysis and rupture of necrotic arteriolar walls with reperfusion.

rabbit tibias (33). Reperfusion injury occurred after ischemia doses as short as 4 hours, and included leukocyte adherence, abnormal vessel leakage (edema), and secondary ischemia (no-reflow). It is conceivable that there is an ischemic threshold between reversible intraosseous hypoxia (bone marrow edema syndrome) and irreversible intraosseous anoxia (osteonecrosis) and that borderline necrosis occurs in the transition zone of this ischemic threshold (34).

Hemorrhage also occurs in very early osteonecrosis with extravasation of erythrocytes between marrow adipocytes (Fig. 108.2), hemosiderin deposition, and deposition of eosinophilic amorphous material and fibrin between

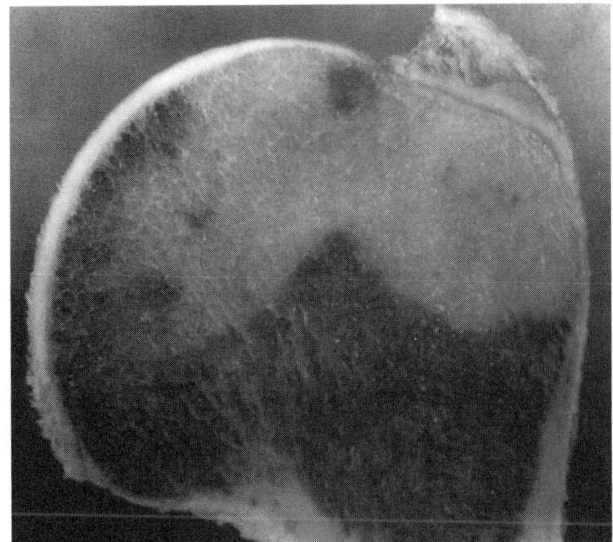

FIGURE 108.2. Coronal section of left humeral head in a patient who expired 18 hours after developing anaphylactic shock. Disseminated intravascular coagulation (DIC) had resulted in fibrin thromboses of vessels, with infarction of adipocytic marrow tissue *(nonviable light areas)* and secondary fibrinolysis and interadipocytic hemorrhage of adjacent marrow *(viable dark areas)*. This classic distribution of osteonecrosis was also seen in this patient's right humeral head and both femoral heads.

adipocytes (2,16,21). Furthermore, biopsies of precollapse femoral heads in steroid-treated patients showed multifocal marrow hemorrhages with damaged or ruptured blood vessels in the hemorrhagic areas (35,36). After a few days the affected capillaries and sinusoids may disappear altogether. However, focal or disseminated intravascular coagulation is not the cause of osteonecrosis but is always an intermediary event trigger-activated by some other underlying etiologic factor (37).

Risk Factors

Risk factors may be reversible or irreversible, subthreshold or suprathreshold, as well as additive or multiplicative, so that individuals with several suprathreshold factors may be at a substantially increased relative risk for subsequently developing osteonecrosis (8,38).

Dysbaric Phenomena

Evidence of osteonecrosis has been discovered in the fossilized (64 to 100 million years) humeral heads and vertebral bodies of deep-diving mosasaur lizards and turtles (39). Virtually identical lesions have been found in those humans exposed to changes in atmospheric pressure in the course of their occupations, principally divers and compressed-air (tunnel or caisson) workers. Using conventional radiographic examinations, osteonecrosis was found in 1% to 13% of compressed-air workers using current engineering technology (40,41). Generally, the risk of decompression sickness (DCS) is minimal if working pressures are kept below 11 pounds per square inch gauge (psig), but pressures greater than 17 psig increase DCS and the risk of osteonecrosis (42). Also, the presence of a patent foramen ovale (PFO) occurs in about 30% of the normal population. The presence of a PFO increases the odds ratio for developing serious (type II) DCS by about 2.5 times (43).

Advances in diving research now permit safe and effective underwater operations in depths to 1,600 feet. Four groups of divers are considered: (a) breath-hold divers, in whom osteonecrosis is nonexistent, and sport scuba divers, in whom it is virtually nonexistent; (b) navy divers, who have a 1% to 3% incidence of osteonecrosis, using standard tables; (c) commercial divers who have a 4% incidence overall and 1% juxtaarticular incidence; and (d) diving fishermen, who may have a 50% or higher incidence of osteonecrosis lesions (10). For example, in Korean diving fishermen, the incidence of DCS was 89%, and 171 of 256 (67%) divers were found with osteonecrosis (44).

There is no direct evidence that dysbaric osteonecrosis results from the primary embolic or compressive effects of nitrogen bubbles alone on the osseous vasculature (16). However, secondary injury to the marrow adipose tissue may result from rapidly expanding nitrogen gas that triggers focal intravascular coagulation, and probably disseminated intravascular coagulation. Following a single hyperbaric air exposure with inadequate decompression, osteonecrosis can appear in humans and sheep (45). Dysbaric osteonecrosis has also been produced in obese mice subjected to multiple hyperbaric exposures (2). Intravascular fat and TF accelerate disseminated intravascular coagulation after decompression sickness. Fibrinogen, lipid, and platelet aggregation at the blood–bubble interface are associated with disseminated intravascular coagulation and postdive red blood cell (RBC) aggregation, thrombocytopenia, accelerated platelet and fibrinogen turnover, decreased AT III activity, prolongation of the prothrombin time, and increased fibrin degradation products (13).

Autopsy of a diver who expired 70 minutes after surfacing with DCS revealed gas bubbles in the fatty marrow of his femoral and humeral heads (16). Lipid and platelet aggregates were found on the surface of marrow bubbles. Fibrin thrombi occluded dilated sinusoids adjacent to the bubbles, as well as veins, capillaries, and arterioles. Since pulmonary, renal, and intraosseous (subchondral) fat embolism and fibrin thromboses were also observed, it was suggested that injured marrow adipocytes can release liquid fat (46), TF, and other vasoactive substances, which appear to play a systemic procoagulant role in triggering disseminated intravascular coagulation and additional osteonecrosis.

Hypersensitivity Reactions

Intravascular coagulation can be induced in several human and animal models, producing osteonecrosis. The earliest case of osteonecrosis, affecting both humeral (Fig. 108.2) and femoral heads, with subchondral fat embolism (Fig. 108.3A) and disseminated intravascular coagulation, occurred 18 hours after anaphylactic shock (17). Subchondral fibrin thrombosis (Fig. 108.3B) and peripheral interadipocytic hemorrhage resulting from secondary fibrinolysis and reperfusion of necrotic vessels were found (Fig. 108.1). Moreover, subclinical transfusion reactions may induce disseminated intravascular coagulation and cause osteonecrosis, which potentially also can occur in hemophilia, aplastic anemia (47), and thalassemia (48).

Circulating immune complexes are associated with marrow necrosis (49). An animal model (type III hypersensitivity, immune-complex mediated) likewise suggests intravascular coagulation to be the final common pathway (50,51). Serum sickness, with and without corticosteroid treatment, produced microthrombi in the marrow as a result of immune complex deposition, leading to necrotic femoral lesions with erythrocyte extravasation. These early necrotic lesions could be detected by gadolinium-enhanced and fat suppression T1-weighted MRI at 1 week after the final injection of horse serum (52).

Osteonecrosis often develops in systemic lupus erythematosus (SLE) patients, but lesions may spontaneously repair without progression (53). The high incidence and polyarticular involvement of osteonecrosis in SLE suggests that there are several risk factors for disseminated intravascular coagulation (54–57). Maximal prednisone doses, cushingoid appearance,

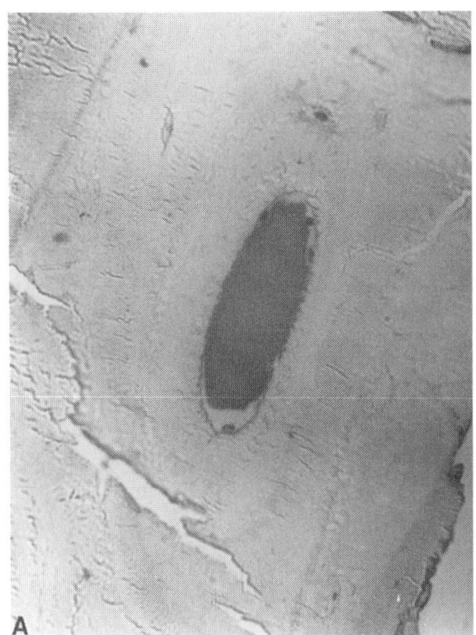

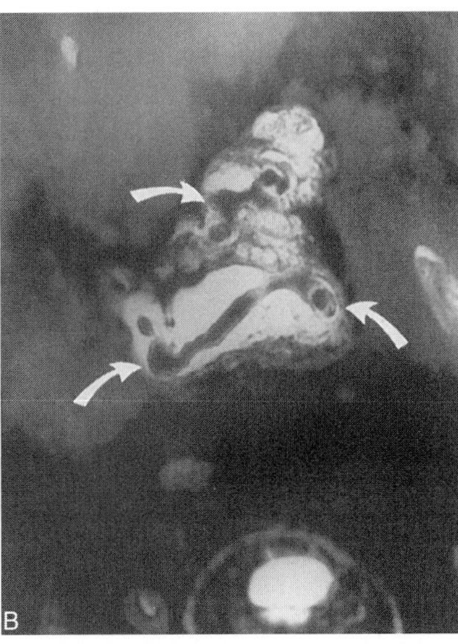

FIGURE 108.3. A: Photomicrograph of subchondral bone from humeral head showing pyknotic-appearing endothelial cell within a haversian canal that is completely occluded by a deformed fat embolus (S. B. Doty modification of osmium-potassium dichromate technique stain, ×400). **B:** Photomicrograph of humeral head at the tidemark revealing subchondral capillaries occluded with multiple fibrin thrombi *(arrows)* (phosphotungstic acid-hematoxylin stain, ×200).

immunoglobulin G (IgG) anticardiolipin levels, venous thrombosis, and vasculitis were found to be associated with osteonecrosis in SLE patients (58). Osteonecrosis was associated with elevated levels of PAI-1 (59). Precipitating autoantibodies may also be predictive of osteonecrosis (60). Although thrombosed vessels have been found adjacent to areas of necrotic bone in SLE (13,24), usually local activation of the coagulation system in SLE remains subclinical.

Antiphospholipid Antibody Syndrome

Although extensive bone infarctions probably result from a consumptive coagulopathy in SLE (54), it has been observed that osteonecrosis can occur in SLE patients who have never received corticosteroids. Antiphospholipid antibodies can cause a coagulopathy with venous and arterial thromboses, as well as osteonecrosis of the femoral heads (61,62). Osteonecrosis in the antiphospholipid antibody syndrome has been observed in patients without SLE who have never received corticosteroids, the so-called primary antiphospholipid antibody syndrome (63,64). Protein C deficiency with lupus anticoagulants can also result in arterial occlusions. Thrombocytopenia is associated with antiphospholipid antibody, suggesting platelet aggregation, and it is now considered that these antibodies initiate thrombosis by activating platelets. Disseminated intravascular coagulation has been observed in 14 of 50 (28%) patients with this syndrome (65).

Endotoxic (Shwartzman) Reactions

Rabbits administered bacterial endotoxins not only develop disseminated intravascular coagulation, but also hyperlipemia, fatty liver, systemic fat embolism, and fibrin thrombosis during the generalized Shwartzman phenomenon (13). Depletion of extrinsic pathway inhibitor (66) also sensitizes rabbits to disseminated intravascular coagulation and the Shwartzman reaction, or focal intravascular coagulation, which can involve a single target organ almost exclusively (67). Widespread osteonecrosis can complicate postmeningococcal (52,68) or posthemophilus disseminated intravascular coagulation (Fig. 108.4) (13, 69, 70)

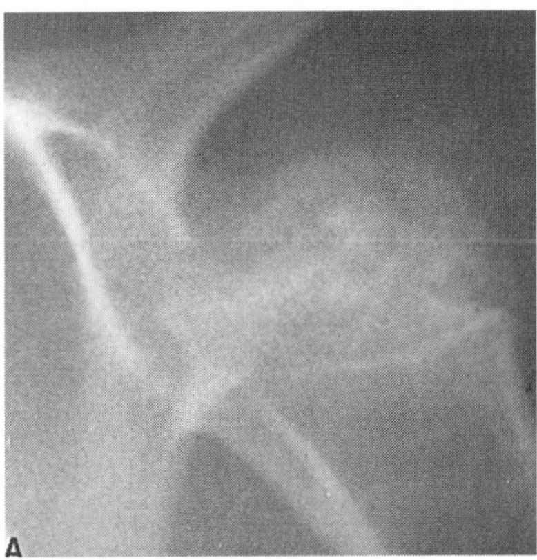

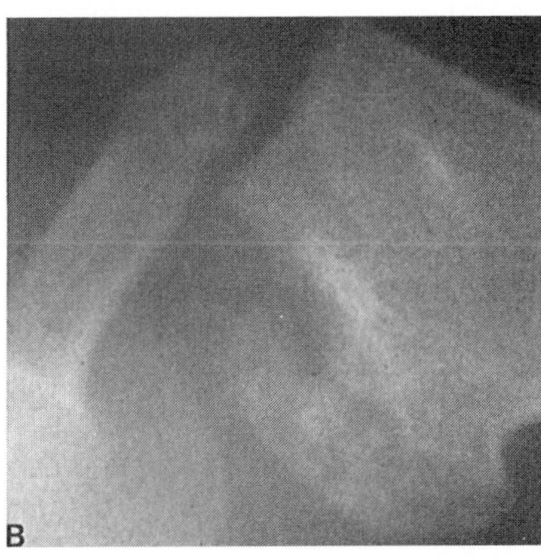

FIGURE 108.4. A and B: Radiographic views of left shoulder demonstrating osteonecrosis with hypoplasia, irregularity, and fragmentation of the capital humeral epiphysis. This 22-month-old girl had recovered from disseminated intravascular coagulation following infection with *Haemophilus influenzae* at age 2 months. (Courtesy of Louise S. Acheson, M.D.)

Endotoxin (lipopolysaccharide) may be the single most potent activator of disseminated intravascular coagulation resulting in osteonecrosis. Fifty-one osteonecrosis lesions, including the humeral (Fig. 108.4) and femoral heads, complicated disseminated intravascular coagulation in eight children (Shwartzman phenomenon) (2). Patellar osteonecrosis was found in four additional children (2). Another child developed postmeningococcal disseminated intravascular coagulation with gangrene, requiring amputations of her left fingers and right hand, and was found to have nine osteonecrosis lesions (71), including both distal tibias and tali. Histologic studies (72) reveal ischemia and fibrin thrombi within the microvasculature adjacent to the necrotic bone, as was observed in a partially necrotic talus from a postmeningococcal patient with disseminated intravascular coagulation and osteonecrosis. These clinical studies have been confirmed in rabbits in which *Escherichia coli* endotoxin-induced Shwartzman reactions cause disseminated intravascular coagulation with hepatic necrosis, thrombosis, and osteonecrosis (73). This ischemic process is enhanced by corticosteroid treatment.

Various viral illnesses can also induce disseminated intravascular coagulation, including cytomegalovirus, hepatitis, rubella, rubeola, and varicella. Human immunodeficiency virus (HIV) disease is associated with disseminated intravascular coagulation (37) and osteonecrosis (74), as well as hypertriglyceridemia and anticardiolipin antibodies. A Shwartzman reaction also occurs after human renal homotransplantation. Disseminated intravascular coagulation can also be triggered by hyperacute rejection of other organ allografts (75). Corticosteroid immunosuppression also enhances the Shwartzman reaction and facilitates sepsis and endotoxemia in patients with SLE and inflammatory bowel disease.

Alcoholism

There appears to be a dose-related cumulative alcohol-induced osteonecrosis response (76). In 164 patients with alcohol-induced osteonecrosis, the average duration of alcohol abuse was 9.5 years, ranging form 8 to 20 years, and hyperlipemia was found in 38% of cases (77). In this author's experience, the exposure threshold for alcohol-associated osteonecrosis (at a consumption of 400 mL or more of absolute ethanol a week) is about 150 L of 100% ethanol. However, the early detection of necrotic lesions by dynamic contrast-enhanced MRI (78,79) and the prothrombotic and hypofibrinolytic effects of multiple coexistent factors (Table 108.1) will decrease this exposure threshold.

Of 38 alcoholics with osteonecrosis, 24 (63%) had type II or type IV hyperlipemia and biopsy-proven fatty livers (2). The alcohol-induced fatty liver is conceivably the most common source of continuous, low-grade, and relatively asymptomatic showers of systemic fat emboli (27). In one study, 80% of alcohol-associated osteonecrosis cases had increased levels of serum γ-glutamyltransferase (GGT) (64). Alcohol-induced osteonecrosis usually affects patients under age 50 (80), and younger alcoholics with hyperlipemia, hypofibrinolysis, and liver disease may have a greater susceptibility to developing disseminated intravascular coagulation (81).

Hypercortisonism

Endogenous (Cushing's syndrome) (82) and exogenous hypercortisonism can cause osteonecrosis (83,84). In my experience, the at-risk cumulative dose threshold for the adult is about 2,000 mg of continuously administered prednisone, unless other prothrombotic or hypofibrinolytic factors are present (Table 108.1). Up to 30% of adults with SLE treated with steroids may develop osteonecrosis. The metacarpal heads, carpal bones, elbow, mandible, humeral and femoral heads, distal femoral condyles, tibial plateaus, patella, distal tibia, and talus and other foot bones may be involved. Osteonecrosis occurs in about 8% of bone marrow transplant recipients (85,86) and 3% of cardiac transplant patients (87). In combining previous studies, 299 of 2,285 (13%) renal transplant recipients developed osteonecrosis (2), but recent MRI screening of asymptomatic renal transplant recipients reveals a prevalence of femoral head osteonecrosis of about 6% to 8% (88,89).

Exogenous glucocorticoids contribute to the occurrence, localization, and persistence of fibrin thrombi in disseminated intravascular coagulation by (a) preparing the microcirculation for the generalized endotoxin-induced Shwartzman reaction by stimulating α-adrenergic receptors; (b) potentiating the effects of catecholamines on vessels (90); (c) facilitating hypofibrinolysis by decreasing tissue plasminogen activator synthesis and by increasing PAI-1 activity (91); (d) impairing phagocytic activity of endotoxin-producing bacteria and reducing reticuloendothelial clearance of fibrinogen degradation products, circulating soluble fibrin monomer, or activated coagulation factors; (e) increasing marrow fat content (92) with loss of venous capacity and reduced blood flow (93); and (f) causing hyperlipemia and fatty liver with intraosseous fat embolism (27).

Hyperlipemia and Embolic Lipid

Hyperlipemia (types II and IV) is associated with intravascular coagulation (94). In histologic studies of osteonecrosis patients with alcoholism and hypercortisonism, intravascular lipid (95,96) and thrombosis of the femoral heads were observed. These fat emboli may arise from fatty liver (mechanism A), destabilization and coalescence of chylomicrons and very low density lipoproteins (mechanism B), which may undergo calcium-dependent agglutination and binding by C-reactive protein resulting in the generation of fat emboli (97), and disruption of fatty bone marrow or other adipose tissue depots (mechanism C). Platelet aggregation occurs *in vivo* over the surface of intravascular fat globules, which is followed within 2 hours by the appearance of fibrin-platelet microthrombi (2,13,16). Subchondral osteonecrosis may be precipitated by an absolute overload (98,99) of intraosseous fat emboli, generating unbound free fatty acids that can produce rapid endothelial sloughing and release of TF (17), with platelet aggregation and fibrin thrombosis of intravascular coagulation (27).

EXPERIMENTAL CONFIRMATION

Studies of the induction of osteonecrosis have been conducted in corticosteroid-treated rabbits in several laboratories (2). In summary, hyperlipemia, fatty liver, pulmonary fat embolism, systemic fat embolism, and subchondral fat embolism of the femoral (and humeral) heads were uniformly observed. Focal osteocyte death in the femoral heads occurred in six of the eight studies. Corticosteroids caused hyperlipemia, particularly very low density, pre-B lipoproteins, after 4 to 7 days. Fatty liver and significant systemic fat embolism to the subchondral arterioles and capillaries of the femoral heads occurred after 2 to 3 weeks. Marrow necrosis occurred as early as 3 weeks. Increased intrafemoral head pressure, with decreased blood flow, occurred after 6 to 8 weeks.

EXTRAVASCULAR LIPID MIGRATION

There is rapid centrifugal movement of intravascular macromolecules into the peripheral osteocytic lacunae of the osteon. Prelabeled intravascular fat also extends circumferentially through canaliculi to become deposited within individual osteocytic lacunae (27). This lipid most likely reaches osteocytes by traversing the space of Neumann between the cell-process membrane and the lacunar-canalicular collagen matrix wall. There is an accumulation of lipid in subchondral osteocytes that subsequently become necrotic, both experimentally (100) and clinically (101), in both alcoholism and hypercortisonism. The sequence of intraosseous fat embolism, endothelial cell necrosis, extravascular lipid migration, reduced osteoblastic activity, and fatty osteocytic necrosis has been observed in space-flight rats (102).

Pregnancy

Pregnancy is accompanied by the physiologic activation of intravascular coagulation. Osteonecrosis can develop in pregnancy (103), usually in the third trimester or early postpartum period, and often in association with hypercoagulability. Hypercoagulability is often first manifested when venous thrombosis, usually of the lower extremities, develops during oral contraceptive use, during pregnancy, or in the postpartum period. However, most persons with hypercoagulability do not develop overt thrombosis unless an additional risk factor is present, i.e., the two-hit phenomenon. For example, young women who smoke heavily and are heterozygous for factor V Leiden or prothrombin gene mutation may conceivably be at increased risk for not only myocardial infarction (104) but also bone infarction. When the thrombophilic effects of exogenous estrogens were superimposed on the factor V Leiden mutation, thrombophilia was augmented, and the risk of osteonecrosis was increased (105).

Massive marrow necrosis can occur with disseminated intravascular coagulation as a complication of pregnancy (106). In the bone marrow edema syndrome (BMES), rapid and complete fibrinolysis might result in transient hypervascularity, postischemic inflammatory marrow edema, and transient demineralization, rather than persistent thrombosis and osteonecrosis (107). Plasma lipid levels increase after the third month of gestation when adrenocortical activity is elevated. Either exogenous corticosteroids (90) or pregnancy may be preparatory for the Shwartzman reaction. For example, pregnant animals require only one injection of bacterial endotoxin to precipitate disseminated intravascular coagulation, rather than the two (preparatory and trigger) injections that are usually required. Hypercoagulability also occurs during late pregnancy with hyperlipemia, depression of the fibrinolytic system with increased PAI-1 (108), and occasionally, decreased AT III. Although osteonecrosis can follow normal deliveries, it is also related to fatty liver of pregnancy (27,109), retained fetus *in utero* (13), toxemia (preeclampsia or eclampsia), and several other obstetric problems. These disorders can induce disseminated intravascular coagulation because of the rich content of TF in human placental tissues, which may gain access to the maternal circulation (37).

Inherited thrombophilia is usually transmitted in an autosomal-dominant fashion. These patients frequently present with deep venous thrombosis, usually of the lower extremities. It is recommended that women who develop osteonecrosis should be tested for factor V Leiden, the prothrombin gene mutation, deficiencies of AT III or proteins C and S, PAI-1, antiphospholipid syndrome, and hyper-homocysteinemia, which may be either inherited or acquired as a result of dietary folate deficiency. Hyperhomocysteinemia is an independent risk factor for thrombosis (110); it is also a recently discovered risk factor for osteonecrosis.

Malignancies

TF produced by various neoplastic cells, especially metastatic carcinoma, lymphoma, and acute promyelocytic or lymphoid leukemias, can activate disseminated intravascular coagulation (37) and cause acute marrow necrosis and bone pain (111,112). Osteonecrosis can also occur in chemotherapy patients who have not received corticosteroids (113,114). Steroid therapy for malignant lymphoma may further increase the incidence of osteonecrosis (115). For example, 9 of 24 (38%) steroid-treated patients with acute lymphoblastic leukemia developed osteonecrosis (116). Osteonecrosis occurred in 6 of 53 (11%) patients with Hodgkin's disease (117), where TF is also associated with intravascular thrombosis (118). Systemic L-asparaginase chemotherapy with a reduction in AT III can also cause thrombosis and bone infarction (7). Additionally, the proteolytic enzyme, trypsin, may be systemically released in pancreatic carcinoma and trigger disseminated intravascular coagulation. Osteonecrosis in pancreatitis, without coexistent alcoholism, may also result from trypsin-induced disseminated intravascular coagulation.

Neurotrauma

In addition to the placenta, brain and spinal cord tissue are also rich in TF (119) and may gain access to the systemic circulation following trauma or surgery and activate the extrinsic clotting cascade. Postmortem examination found that head injury has been complicated by disseminated intravascular coagulation, as well as the formation of fibrin microthrombi within bone marrow (120). Coagulopathies resulting from TF, fat embolism, and elevated PAI-1 activity are also associated with spinal surgery (121,122) and other postoperative states (123,124). Increased catecholamines and corticosteroids may aggravate this process. Osteonecrosis is likely to occur when short-term, high-dose glucocorticoids are used for their antiinflammatory effects (13).

Inflammatory Bowel Disease

Episodes of thrombosis in ulcerative colitis and regional enteritis (Crohn's disease) most often occur during the active stage of disease. Disseminated intravascular coagulation is probably enhanced by chronic thromboplastin release (37), circulating immune complexes, thrombocytosis, hyperfibrinogenemia, anticardiolipin antibodies, increased PAI-1 and factor VIII, decreased AT III, protein C and S deficiency (125), decreased tissue plasminogen activator, intravenous fat emulsion therapy (99) with increased C-reactive protein (97), hypercortisonism, and bacterial endotoxemia (Shwartzman reactions) resulting from superimposed sepsis. Moreover, C-reactive protein induces blood monocytes to synthesize tissue factor, which may contribute to the development of disseminated intravascular coagulation in these inflammatory conditions (126). Multifocal lower extremity lesions are usually found, but the wrist and elbow may rarely be involved (127). In one study (128), 7 of 161 (4%) of steroid-treated patients with inflammatory bowel disease developed osteonecrosis. Bilateral osteonecrosis of the femoral heads may also occur in patients with inflammatory bowel disease who have not received any corticosteroid therapy (129).

Hemoglobinopathies

Osteonecrosis in sickle cell anemia and its variants has previously been considered to be due solely to plugging of intraosseous vessels by sickled erythrocytes. However, disseminated intravascular coagulation can also occur during sickle cell crises (130,131). Infarctions of the phalanges and metacarpals in infancy (sickle dactylitis) appear similar to postmeningococcal-disseminated intravascular coagulation lesions in children (132). Osteonecrosis also complicates sickle cell trait. Patients with the hemoglobin SS genotype, especially when associated with α-thalassemia (133,134), have the highest risk of osteonecrosis.

Normally, the erythroid hyperplasia of the sickle hemoglobinopathies results in increased marrow blood flow. However, a hypercoagulable state (135) with increased platelet activation, enhanced thrombin generation, fibrin deposition, and impaired fibrinolysis occurs at the same time as erythrocyte sequestration (136–138). Thrombosis with increased levels of serum fibrinogen degradation products most likely results from activation of the coagulation system in the sickle hemoglobinopathies by a combination of fat and marrow embolism, thrombocytosis, hyperfibrinogenemia, hyperviscosity, increased factor VIII, plasma B-thromboglobulin, platelet factor 4, thromboxane B_2, decreased clotting factors V and XIII, plasminogen, tissue plasminogen activator, and proteins C and S (137).

An increase in circulating endothelial cells in sickle cell crisis is compatible with local vascular damage. Necrotic marrow can be aspirated from the site of the acutely painful bone crisis. The source of the pain is presumed to be an increased intramedullary pressure from the secondary inflammatory response, since MRI studies indicate acute infarction with edema in the majority of patients with painful crisis (139,140).

Gaucher's Disease

Gaucher's disease is associated with thrombocytopenia, hyperviscosity, and decreased levels of a wide spectrum of coagulation factors, including factor IX (hemophilia B) and protein C (2). Disintegrating Gaucher cells can enter hepatic sinusoids and perhaps trigger disseminated intravascular coagulation. Bone crises have been reported in 23% to 37% of patients with type I Gaucher's disease. At the onset of a crisis, scintigraphy reveals decreased radionuclide uptake at the site of pain providing evidence of ischemia (141). Four initially photopenic femoral heads showed radiographic evidence of osteonecrosis 6 months after the onset of acute pain (142). MRI during a painful crisis reveals increased marrow and subperiosteal signal, presumably related to edema and hemorrhage following an avascular incident (143).

Obesity

Obesity is an independent risk factor not only for osteonecrosis (27), but also for primary osteoarthritis (144), suggesting a systemic mechanism. Fatty liver occurs in obesity (145), and obesity precedes osteoarthritis of the hand

(146). Moreover, the arthropathy of frostbite (147) may be caused by osteonecrosis and be similar to primary osteoarthritis, since Heberden's and Bouchard's nodes may develop in both conditions. Conceivably, chronic low-grade showers of the subchondral (articular and vertebral) end plates with fat emboli (146) (or other coactivating risk factors for intravascular coagulation and fibrin thrombosis) results in ischemic necrosis of primarily the calcified chondrocytes and subjacent osteocytes (2,148), largely sparing the subjacent adipocytes.

Recent studies of spontaneous osteoarthritis in the macaque monkey and guinea pig indicate that subchondral bone changes precede cartilage changes. Focal subchondral osteonecrosis might also be related to osteoarthritis in mice (149). In obesity there is a decrease in fibrinolytic activity (108), which may prolong the ischemic effect of subchondral fibrin thrombi. Decreased fibrinolysis also occurs in primary osteoarthritis, in addition to increased fibrinogenesis and hypercoagulability with hyperlipidemia (95). Subchondral hypoxia and histologic evidence of necrosis have been observed as early manifestations of both primary osteoarthritis and osteonecrosis (150). Intraosseous fat emboli (17,95) and fibrin thrombi (151) have been observed in both osteonecrosis and, to a lesser extent, in primary osteoarthritis, where hyperlipidemia, hypercoagulability, and hypofibrinolysis have also been detected (152).

Organic substances can diffuse through cartilage of intact articular joints. For example, lipid readily enters cartilage and rapidly appears in chondrocytes, which may become necrotic (2). With advancing age there is an increase in the intra- and extracellular lipids of human articular cartilage, hypofibrinolysis (95), and an association between lesion severity, total lipid content, and fatty acid levels (153). Perhaps subchondral hypoxia (150) stimulates osteoblastic new bone formation in subchondral regions with fractional osteocytic necrosis.

Articular (noncalcifying) cartilage normally inhibits capillary invasion. Although plasminogen activator activity is elevated during vascular invasion (154), the cartilage synthesizes the serine protease inhibitor PAI-1 (155). In a primate model of naturally occurring osteoarthritis, tidemark vascular invasion and osteophytes were present before any evidence of damage to articular cartilage (156). If the reparative revascularization process targets fractional necrosis of the subchondral plate, there may be chondroclastic resorption with abnormal capillary penetration through the (reduplicating and advancing) tidemark. For example, repetitive subchondral ischemia (13 decompressions) was shown in sheep to produce 13 reduplicated tidemarks (45). Acute DCS is known to produce fat embolism in sheep and humans. Embolic lipid and fibrin thrombi have been observed within subchondral capillaries of the femoral and humeral heads of a human diving fatality with DCS (16).

As this calcification front slowly extends toward the joint surface there is reciprocal thinning and secondary degradation of the existing hyaline cartilage. Chondroclastic resorption with hypervascularity of the deep cartilage layer may release metabolites and inflammatory mediators that cause further cartilage destruction. Accelerated subchondral remodeling may also cause marginal capillary penetration of cartilage and endochondral new bone formation, which extends beyond the original subchondral end plate as central sclerosis and peripheral osteophytes, appearing in osteoarthritis associated with aging and obesity (157).

Other Prethrombotic and Hypofibrinolytic Conditions

Thrombophilia and hypofibrinolysis are risk factors for osteonecrosis (158). These factors include decreased endogenous anticoagulants (AT III, protein C, protein S, and especially heterozygosity for factor V Leiden) (13,14). Nineteen patients with protein C deficiency and four patients with protein S deficiency have been reported with Legg-Perthes disease (159). Seven additional children had a high level of lipoprotein (a), a thrombogenic lipoprotein associated with osteonecrosis in adults. Perhaps children with thrombophilia or hypofibrinolysis (160) may be more susceptible to developing disseminated intravascular coagulation and osteonecrosis (Legg-Perthes disease) following certain viral or bacterial (endotoxic) infections, since increases in immunoglobulins (IgG and IgM) are also found in this disease (2). Recently, Legg-Perthes disease was discovered in three siblings, two heterozygous and one homozygous for the factor V Leiden mutation (161).

Disseminated intravascular coagulation with end-organ damage is enhanced by the inhibition or impairment of secondary endogenous fibrinolysis (13). To exceed the ischemic threshold and produce a bone infarction, it is likely that significant fibrin microthrombi must remain within the intraosseous vasculature for a minimum of 2 to 6 hours, and not be immediately dissolved by endogenous fibrinolysis. Hypofibrinolysis results from increased PAI-1 in the nephrotic syndrome, hemolytic-uremic syndrome, thrombotic thrombocytopenic purpura, smoking, and hypertriglyceridemic syndromes II and IV, which are all associated with osteonecrosis. Although the most dramatic elevations of serum triglycerides occur in types I and V, osteonecrosis is most common in types II and IV where elevated soluble fibrin complexes are found. Eight family members had type IV hyperlipidemia and osteonecrosis of the femoral heads (27). In addition to hyperlipidemia and diabetes, obese patients may also have increased PAI-1, factor VII coagulant activity, and fibrinogen. The coagulation and fibrinolysis systems are also involved in diabetes (162) and atherosclerosis (163). Lipemia inhibits fibrinolysis (108), and very low density lipoprotein (VLDL) causes the release of PAI-1 from cultured endothelial cells. Increased

PAI-1 has been reported in several patients with idiopathic osteonecrosis (30,31).

Moreover, hyperviscosity, hyperfibrinogemia, polycythemia, thrombocytosis, and other unknown factors could also facilitate thrombogenesis, including decreased tissue plasminogen activator. Disseminated intravascular coagulation and osteonecrosis have also been observed in anorexia nervosa (2). Moreover, the nephrotic syndrome is associated with several other coagulation abnormalities (164), including thrombocytosis and platelet hyperaggregability, increased factors V and VIII, increased fibrinogen with hyperviscosity, and decreased protein S and AT III. The hyperlipemia of the nephrotic syndrome may also be exacerbated by corticoid therapy, further increasing osteonecrosis susceptibility. Similarly, the coagulation pathway is activated in the hemolytic uremic syndrome.

Hyperviscosity and the gradual obliteration of vascular lumina by progressive lipid (or polyvinylpyrrolidone) (165) storage within marrow histiocytes or endothelial cells could conceivably cause osteonecrosis in Gaucher's disease and Fabry-Anderson disease. However, the acutely painful crises in Gaucher's disease, acute leukemia, sickle hemoglobinopathies, and DCS result from sudden ischemia and acute infarction; scintigraphy shows decreased uptake shortly after symptoms appear, consistent with acute thrombosis of intravascular coagulation.

DIAGNOSIS AND MANAGEMENT OF OSTEONECROSIS

This discussion focuses on management of lesions affecting the juxtaarticular regions because metadiaphyseal lesions are not disabling.

In 1993, the Committee on Terminology and Staging of the Association Research Circulation Osseous (ARCO) proposed a five-stage (0–IV) international classification of osteonecrosis (Fig. 108.5), which was in large part derived from the Japanese system (based on lesion location) and the Philadelphia system (based on lesion size).

STAGE	0	1	2	3	4
FINDINGS	All present techniques normal or non-diagnostic	X-ray and CT are normal. At least ONE of the below is positive	NO CRESCENT SIGN: X-RAY ABNORMAL: sclerosis, lysis, focal porosis	CRESCENT SIGN on the X-ray and/or flattening of articular surface of femoral head	OSTEOARTHRITIS joint space narrowing, acetabular changes, joint destruction
TECHNIQUES	X-ray CT Scintigraph MRI	Scintigraph MRI *QUANTITATE on MRI	X-ray, CT Scintigraph MRI *QUANTITATE MRI & X-ray	X-ray, CT ONLY *QUANTITATE on X-ray	X-ray ONLY
LOCATION	NO	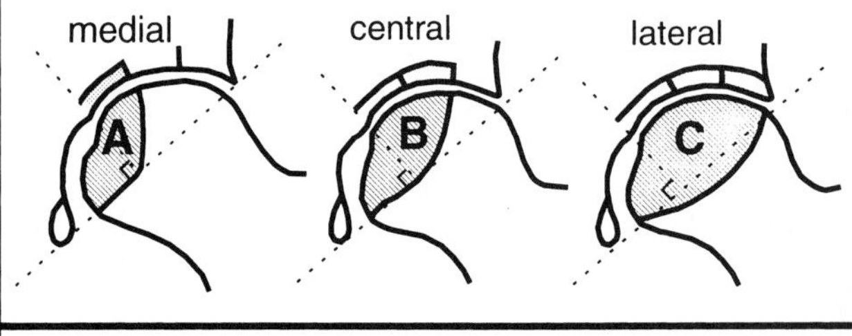 medial A	central B	lateral C	NO
SIZE	NO	**QUANTITATION** % AREA INVOLVEMENT: minimal A < 15%; moderate B 15-30%; extensive C > 30% LENGTH of CRESCENT: A < 15%; B 15-30%; C > 30% % SURFACE COLLAPSE & DOME DEPRESSION: 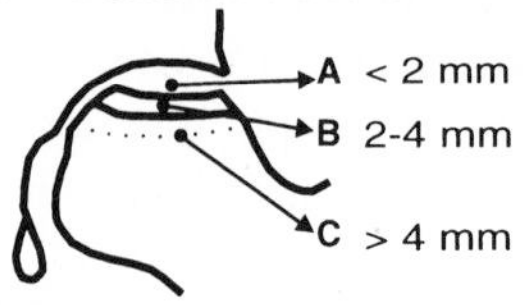 A < 2 mm; B 2-4 mm; C > 4 mm			NO

FIGURE 108.5. Schematic modified outline of the five-stage Association Research Circulation Osseous (ARCO) international classification for osteonecrosis of the femoral head.

Stage 0

Stage 0 is the etiology and early pathogenesis of osteonecrosis. Traumatic osteonecrosis results from a sudden ischemic event (arterial severance). Etiologic risk factors potentially capable of triggering intravascular coagulation and nontraumatic osteonecrosis are listed in Table 108.1. Prevention of osteonecrosis requires avoidance of the risk factors.

Stage I Lesion

The generalized stage I lesion (dead bone without repair) occurs with physiologic death of the skeleton and appears in dehydrated and nonpermineralized paleopathologic specimens (Fig. 108.6) (2). The living patient with very early osteonecrosis is usually asymptomatic (except during the acute pain of decompression sickness, or sickle cell and Gaucher's disease crises) with no physical or radiographic findings. However, in some cases of suspected disseminated intravascular coagulation there may be a transient episode of painful swelling of the knees and ankles, as a nonspecific arthritis.

Pathologic Features

Histologically, localized stage I lesions in the living patient will initially appear normal without evidence of repair. Within 2 weeks of the ischemic event there will be evidence of necrotic marrow, and usually by 3 weeks there will be some absent osteocytes in dead trabeculae. Marrow changes occur before alterations in the trabeculae. If a biopsy is performed too soon after the infarction, there may not be any obvious changes on routine light microscopy, except for marginal hemorrhage (Fig. 108.2) or edema.

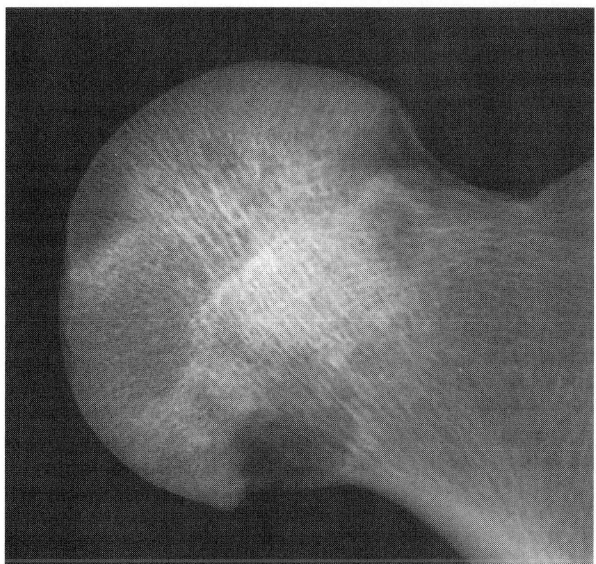

FIGURE 108.6. Radiograph of the 60,000-year-old left femoral head from a Neanderthal man, ordinally identified in 1856 by Fuhlrott, showing excellent preservation of the three main trabecular patterns and demonstrating that prehistoric bone that dies and undergoes natural mummification (dehydration without permineralization), without repair, does not spontaneously collapse. (Courtesy of Paul Dann, M.D.)

The hematopoietic marrow cells and capillary endothelial cells will be the first to appear necrotic, followed by adipocytic necrosis. More than 200 biopsy specimens of early lesions indicated interstitial edema and necrosis of fatty and hematopoietic marrow and rupture of lipocytes, producing large, fatty cysts and liquefaction necrosis, amorphous debris, sinusoidal distention, and arteriolar thrombosis (21). The presence or absence (empty lacunae) of osteocyte nuclei was variable, because of wide variations in autolytic rates after functional death. At the margin of the necrotic sequestrum in early osteonecrosis, sinusoids may be enlarged and contain lipid droplets, and there may be hemorrhagic marrow lesions (Fig. 108.2) with macrophages filled with hemosiderin (2). With thrombosis of the subchondral capillary and venous sinusoidal bed, there is venous congestion and increased venous-outlet resistance. Perinecrotic inflammatory marrow edema progresses within the rigid bony compartment, further aggravating the preexisting ischemic perfusion damage.

Postischemic interstitial edema probably occurs very rapidly after intraosseous intravascular coagulation. Cytokine mediators such as interleukin-1 and tumor necrosis factor may cause a nonspecific secondary inflammatory response to a severe ischemic insult. Neutrophil activation and release of proteases induces vascular damage, cellular destruction, increased vascular permeability, and further intraosseous edema. Cytokines also increase TF exposure and decrease thrombomodulin expression and increase secretion of PAI-1, which further contributes to microvascular thrombosis. With progressive venous thrombosis, marrow venous drainage is decreased, intraosseous pressure is increased, and marrow perfusion is further decreased.

Laboratory Tests

Since the duration of the stage I lesion is only about 1 to 2 weeks, asymptomatic lesions are rarely discovered. Certain tests may be useful for persons suspected of having an associated condition (discussed previously). Elevated plasma fibrinopeptide A was found in two stage I patients with evidence of systemic fat embolism and arterial interruptions detected by superselective angiography (27). Another stage I patient had elevated D-dimer fibrin fragments and decreased AT III (17).

Because osteonecrosis is selective, radiographs should concentrate on the shoulder, hip, and knee joints with two rotational views of each shoulder, and an anteroposterior and lateral projection of each hip and knee. Conventional radiography and computed tomography (CT) are not suitable for the early diagnosis of osteonecrosis because death of bone and marrow, without repair, produces no radiologic abnormality.

Scintigraphy

A photon-deficient "cold" lesion provides the best noninvasive evidence for a stage I lesion (2,166). Cold lesions commonly occur immediately after sickle cell and Gaucher's disease crises or decompression sickness (167), and represent acute bone infarctions (168). Interpretations of technetium ^{99m}Tc-methylene diphosphonate scintigrams are generally based on asymmetric radioisotope uptake, so diagnosis becomes more difficult in patients with bilateral involvement. Osteonecrosis on the less affected side is often overlooked. Single photon emission computed tomography (SPECT) more sensitively defines photon-deficient areas during the early avascular phase (166,169).

Magnetic Resonance Imaging

Because of false-negative studies, conventional MRI is not useful for stage I lesions (166,170). MRI studies can appear normal for at least 12 to 14 days after a known ischemic event (170,171). However, animal studies indicate that very early detection of acute osteonecrosis can be obtained by dynamic contrast-enhanced MRI (78,79). Probably the earliest positive findings in conventional MRI of osteonecrosis is an edema pattern with indistinct areas of intermediate signal intensity on T1-weighted images that increase on T2-weighted, fat saturation, and short tau inversion recovery (STIR) sequences. This pattern suggests increased perinecrotic free water, which may be located either in capillaries and sinusoids in the form of vascular congestion or hyperemia, in the interstitial space in the form of perinecrotic edema or hemorrhage (172), or within ischemic and swollen cells (hydropic degeneration).

This nonspecific marrow edema pattern also occurs in transient osteoporosis of the hip (2), acute marrow infarction in sickle cell crisis (139), trauma, tumors, osteomyelitis, reflex sympathetic osteodystrophy, and other conditions. It is likely that some patients experience complete endogenous fibrinolysis of thrombi with only transient postischemic inflammatory marrow edema rather than irreversible osteonecrosis. In MRI images obtained with a T1-weighted, spin echo pulse, the normal marrow is characterized by a signal of high intensity, resulting from the high content of hydrogen-rich marrow fat (173).

Normally, high signal intensity (white) appears on coronal images of the humeral and femoral heads. In stage I the necrotic zone will retain high signal intensity (isointense with viable marrow fat) if the nonviable fat cells and fatty cysts have not yet saponified. However, the necrotic zone will exhibit homogeneous low signal intensity on T1-weighting if liquefaction necrosis and saponification have resulted in degradation of the preexisting fat into amorphous granular debris. Heterogeneous hypointensity most likely occurs when only a portion of the nonviable fat undergoes saponification.

Intraosseous Pressure and Venography

Peripheral hemorrhage (Fig. 108.2) and perinecrotic inflammatory edema consistently cause elevation of intraosseous pressure in very early osteonecrosis (21,166). This appears to be a very early secondary, but nonspecific, effect within the postischemic marrow cavity. Venous obstruction with intramedullary stasis has also been consistently observed by intraosseous venography in early osteonecrosis (21). Even if the major extraosseous arterial and venous circulation appears normal, the capillary and sinusoidal microcirculation may be thrombosed and destroyed, and the contrast media is not absorbed but diffuses slowly through the medullary space.

Increased levels of circulating free fatty acids may lead directly to increased production of prostaglandins, which may cause intramedullary edema and increased intraosseous pressure. Twofold elevations in both unbound free fatty acids and plasma prostaglandins occur 1 to 2 weeks after initiation of corticosteroids in rabbits (2). Elevated serum total lipids and free fatty acids, as well as intraosseous fat emboli and increased prostaglandins, were found in the necrotic femoral heads of steroid-treated rabbits. The prostaglandin E_2 (PGE_2)-like activity increased eightfold and 16-fold after 30 and 90 days, respectively, of prednisolone administration (174).

Digital Subtraction and Superselective Angiography

If the scintigram or MRI is abnormal, superselective angiographic studies may reveal an abrupt interruption of the medial femoral circumflex (27), or absence of its lateral epiphyseal (superior retinacular) branches (166,175).

Stage II Lesion

The patient with a stage II lesion is usually asymptomatic and still has no physical findings. The bony lesion shows repair without collapse (Fig. 108.5).

Pathologic Features

A lag period occurs before the repair response is activated. Collateral circulation is stimulated and endogenous fibrinolysis with reperfusion rapidly occurs through existing vessels. Beyond the ischemic margin, the slow process of neovascularization begins. Angiogenesis of postischemic marrow may be initiated by endothelin-1 (176) or platelet-derived growth factor (Fig. 108.7), and osteoclast migration may be stimulated by necrotic collagen degradation products. Spontaneous

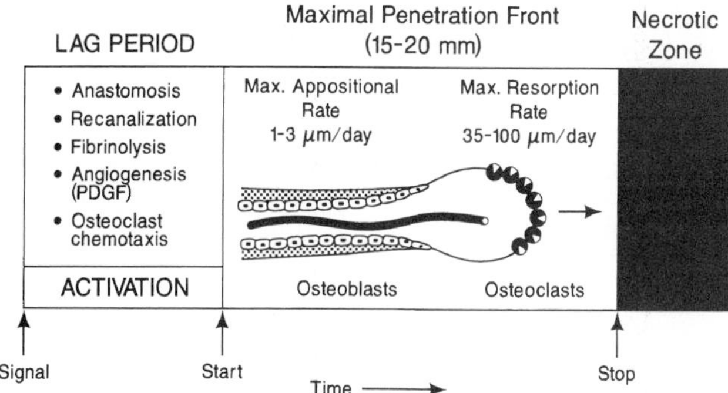

FIGURE 108.7. Chronologic concept of various components causing an activation lag period, which is followed by generation and penetration of a revascularization front *(cutting cone)* into the necrotic bone. Maximal penetration of the overall front is finite in cancellous, and especially in cortical (subchondral) bone. A subchondral zone of residual necrosis usually remains if the trabecular lesion is over 15 to 20 mm in diameter. PDGF, platelet-derived growth factor.

revascularization of segmental necrotic lesions of the femoral head from the cancellous region is possible, within certain limits (15–20 mm). Because the osteonecrotic segment is avascular, repair can begin only along its outer perimeter, at the junction of the ischemic zone surrounding the dead area, and the viable area with intact circulation (the hyperemic zone). Primitive, undifferentiated mesenchymal cells and capillary buds, containing endothelial cells, proliferate, and differentiate to fibroblasts, which begin synthesizing collagen. Subsequently, these mesenchymal cells differentiate to osteoblasts. The dead trabeculae are partially or completely resorbed by osteoclasts and are replaced or covered with new appositional bone, resulting in thickened, reinforced trabeculae. Reossification usually occurs distal to the revascularization and resorption front. The revascularization front includes osteoclasts, fibroblasts, and capillaries. Intimal thickening and myointimal cell proliferation with subendothelial fibrosis following endothelial cell injury or recanalization can result in narrowing of the arterial lumen.

Radiographic Features

Radiographic changes produced by infarcted bone marrow vary according to location. Areas of focal demineralization beneath an intact articular surface first appear on conventional radiographic examination as less dense areas, the result of subchondral bone resorption (radiolucency) and surrounding appositional new bone formation (radiosclerosis). Metaphyseal lesions often appear as irregular lucencies or linear or mottled densities. Shaft or diaphyseal lesions often show serpentine calcification. No evidence of secondary subchondral fracture exists; the radiolucent "crescent" sign is not yet seen (Fig. 108.5).

Magnetic Resonance Imaging

MRI is the most sensitive, specific, low-risk, noninvasive test for determining the size and location of osteonecrosis in stage II. Eventual bilaterality occurs in the majority of nontraumatic lesions. The presence of a sealed-off epiphyseal scar may be associated with increased risk of femoral head osteonecrosis (177).

In general, stage II lesions show either rings (focal smaller lesions) (Fig. 108.8) or bands (larger lesions) (Fig. 108.9) or subchondral crescents of low signal intensity, representing the combined revascularization and reossification front surrounding the necrotic zone. Once an enlarging revascularization (repair) front begins penetrating into the necrotic zone,

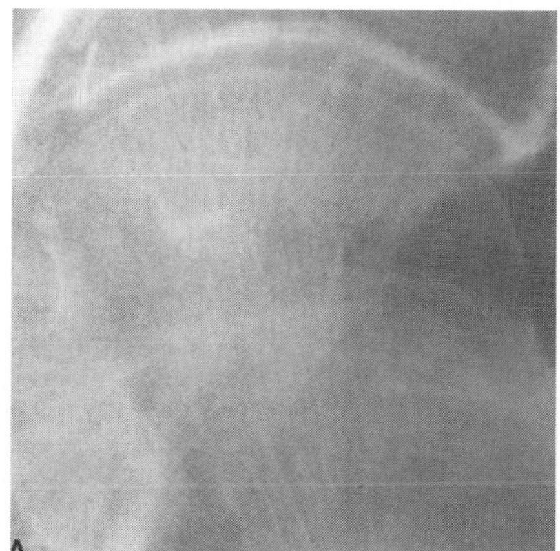

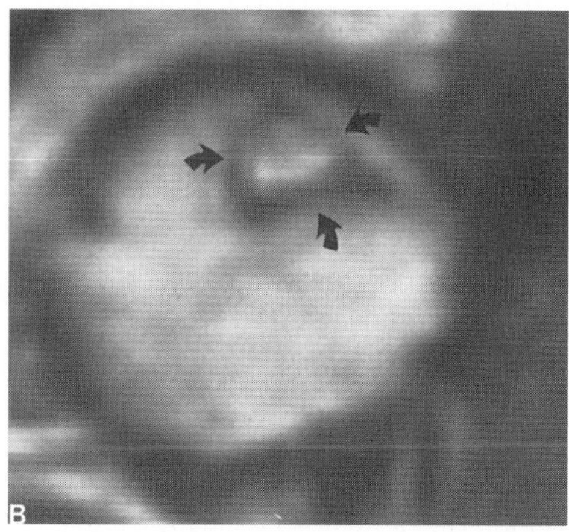

FIGURE 108.8. A focal stage II lesion is silently undergoing repair without collapse. **A:** It is not visualized in a normal-appearing plain radiograph of the femoral head. **B:** Magnetic resonance imaging (MRI) with T1 weighting demonstrated a single reparative ring of low-intensity signal *(arrows)* in the superolateral femoral head. The central, residual necrotic nidus is isointense with the normal high-intensity, perinecrotic region.

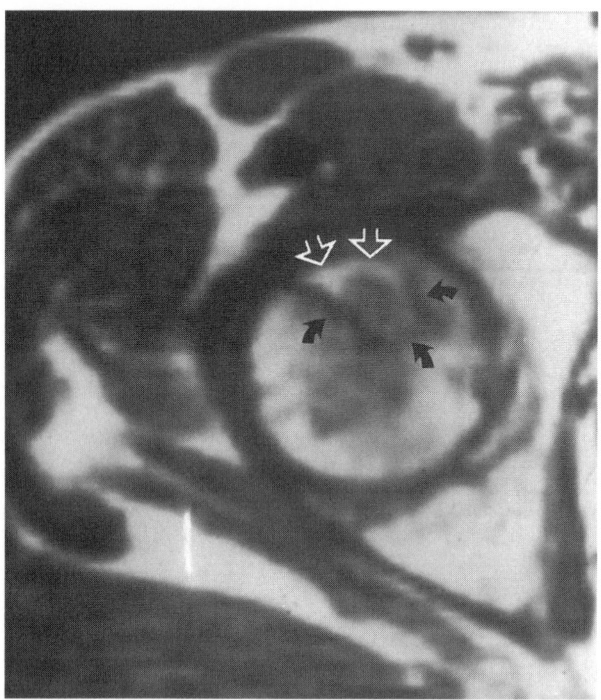

FIGURE 108.9. MRI (T1-weighted) of femoral head in axial plane showing a classic, reparative lesion without collapse (stage II) that is surrounded by a dark band *(black arrows)*, the revascularization front. Heterogeneous signal intensity in the necrotic segment results from residual, dead, unsaponified adipocytes in the anterior third of the lesion *(white arrows)*. This patient was an alcoholic with pancreatitis and diabetes.

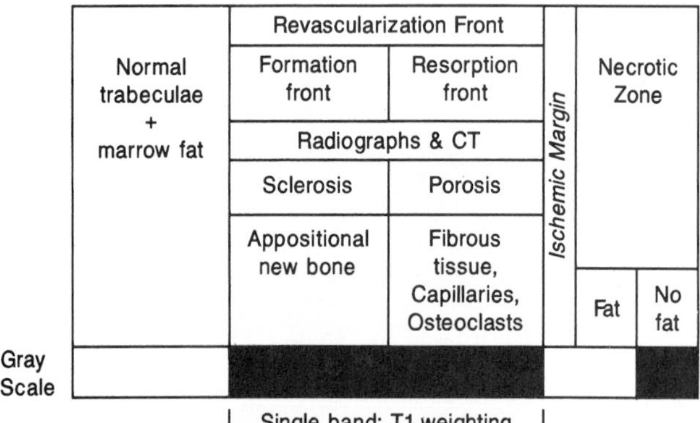

Normal trabeculae + marrow fat
Revascularization Front
Formation front
Resorption front
Radiographs & CT
Sclerosis
Porosis
Appositional new bone
Fibrous tissue, Capillaries, Osteoclasts
Ischemic Margin
Necrotic Zone
Fat
No fat
Gray Scale
Single band: T1 weighting

FIGURE 108.10. Gray-scale analysis of various components of stage II lesion using MRI with T1 weighting (short TR/TE). The single band (or ring) usually represents the combined revascularization (resorption and formation) front, appearing as porosis and sclerosis on radiographs and computed tomography (CT). The necrotic zone will have high signal intensity and erroneously will appear normal if the dead fat had not yet saponified, and low intensity if it had already undergone liquefaction and coagulation necrosis and become amorphous debris. The stage I lesion has no discernible revascularization front (no single band).

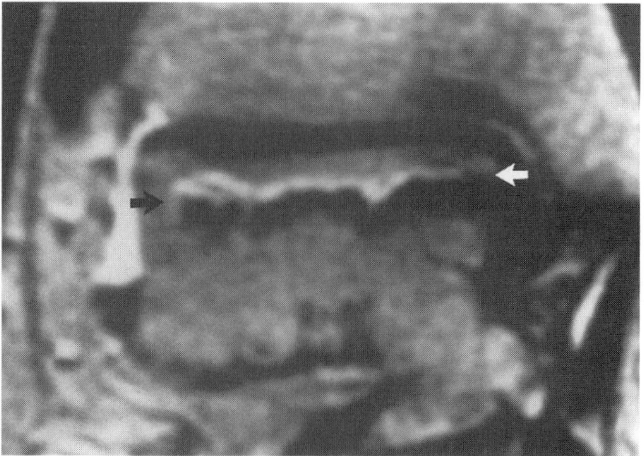

FIGURE 108.11. The double-line sign *(arrows)* is obvious on the T2-weighted (TR/TE, 2400/20) MRI appearing as a transverse double band (compare with Fig. 108.13) across the dome of the body of the right talus, immediately beneath the ankle mortise. This patient had morbid obesity, diabetes, and hyperlipemia.

there is a further delay before a discrete band is obvious on MRI. In stage II, a repair (revascularization) front appears as a single band or ring of decreased signal intensity on T1 weighting (Fig. 108.10). This band is composed of viable tissue without fat cells and includes two parts: a resorption front, which is usually proximal, and a formation front, which is usually more distal. These two parts may be visualized with T2 weighting as the double-line sign (Fig. 108.11). This appearance may represent chemical shift artifact (178), or the high-intensity proximal part of the sign may represent granulation tissue with inflammatory edema and hyperemia (the resorption front), and the low-intensity distal band may represent thickened trabeculae (Fig. 108.12). A prospective MRI study found that 14 of 31 (45%) femoral head lesions

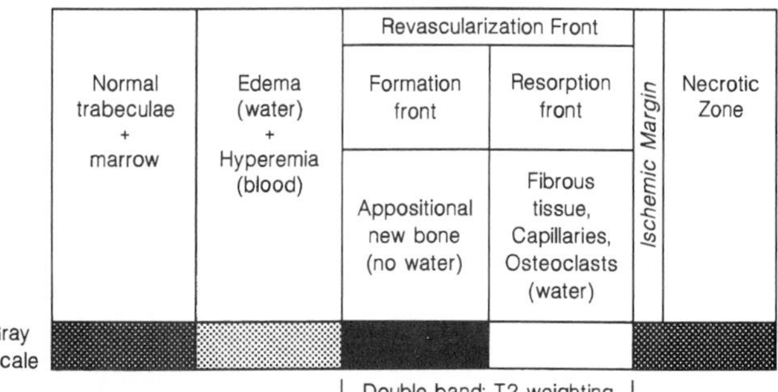

Normal trabeculae + marrow
Edema (water) + Hyperemia (blood)
Revascularization Front
Formation front
Resorption front
Appositional new bone (no water)
Fibrous tissue, Capillaries, Osteoclasts (water)
Ischemic Margin
Necrotic Zone
Gray Scale
Double band: T2 weighting

FIGURE 108.12. Gray-scale analysis of various components of stage II lesions using MRI with T2 weighting (long TR/TE). The double band usually represents the revascularization front with a proximal (*white* = high signal intensity) resorption front with hyperemia (blood and edema), and distal (*black* = low intensity signal) formation front. Marrow edema (water) often appears distal to the revascularization front in the form of intermediate-to-high signal intensity. The stage I lesion often shows an edema pattern (high intensity, T2 weighting) but has no discernible revascularization front (no double-line sign).

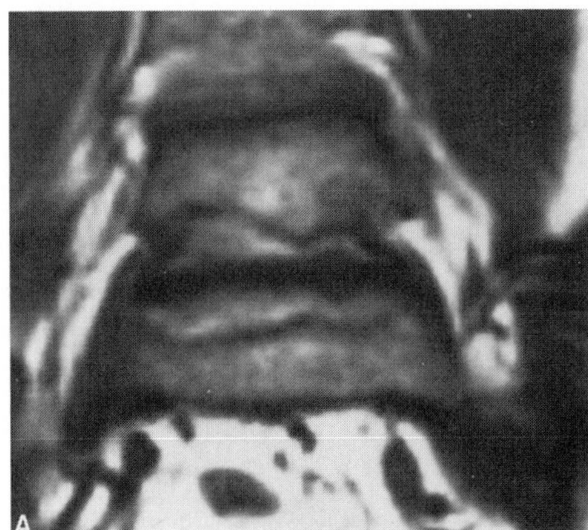

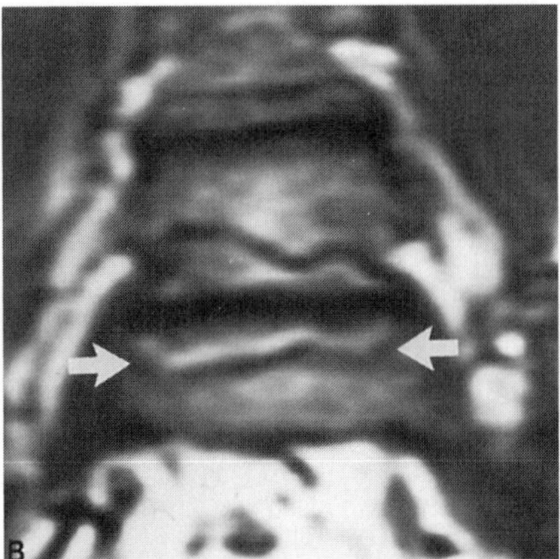

FIGURE 108.13. A: T1-weighted (TR/TE, 600/20) MRI of the lumbosacral spine demonstrating transverse single-banded revascularization fronts involving the inferior L5 and superior S1 vertebral bodies. **B:** T2-weighted (TR/TE, 2000/20) MRI reveals an obvious double-banded (resorption/formation) front *(arrows)* within the superior aspect of S1 (compare with Fig. 108.11). This vertebral end-plate necrosis perhaps caused degenerative disc disease at L5-S1 by creating diffusion barriers to hydration of the nucleus pulposus. This former United States Navy diver also had a focal stage II lesion in his left femoral head and stage IV postcollapse osteonecrosis involving his right hip. (Courtesy of Paul Swenson, M.D.)

underwent a spontaneous reduction in size (179). Lesions either stay the same size or become slightly smaller; they do not enlarge (11).

Adjacent vertebral bodies can be similarly affected with precollapse (stage II) lesions (Figs. 108.1, 108.2, and 108.13) and be associated with both degenerative disc disease and osteonecrosis of the femoral heads (13). Other patients with degenerative disc disease have MRI alterations in the vertebral end plates and marrow with bands of decreased intensity on T1 weighting (180) and increased intensity on T2 weighting, similar to the MRI findings in osteonecrosis of the hip. Abnormalities in the cartilaginous end plates may precede histologic changes in the nucleus pulposis and anulus fibrosus. Conceivably, necrotic vertebral end plates, caused by various risk factors (Table 108.1), may provide a diffusion barrier to normal hydration of the nucleus pulposus resulting in degenerative disc disease and spinal osteoarthritis (157).

Scintigraphy

With revascularization, ^{99m}Tc-MDP (methylene diphosphonate) is localized along mineralization fronts of newly formed bone on the 2-hour delayed images. Stage II lesions show increased radionuclide uptake. In the transition from a stage I "cold" lesion to a stage II "hot" lesion is an intermediate stage II "cold and hot" lesion, in which revascularization surrounds the necrotic zone.

Single Photon Emission Computed Tomography

The advantage of triple-head SPECT over planar imaging is that it allows more accurate localization of photopenic defects with greater contrast and anatomic clarity than with a conventional scan by eliminating superimposed activity (169). In stage II lesions, osteonecrosis is suspected by SPECT when an area of no uptake or an area of diminished uptake is surrounded by an area of increased uptake (Fig. 108.14).

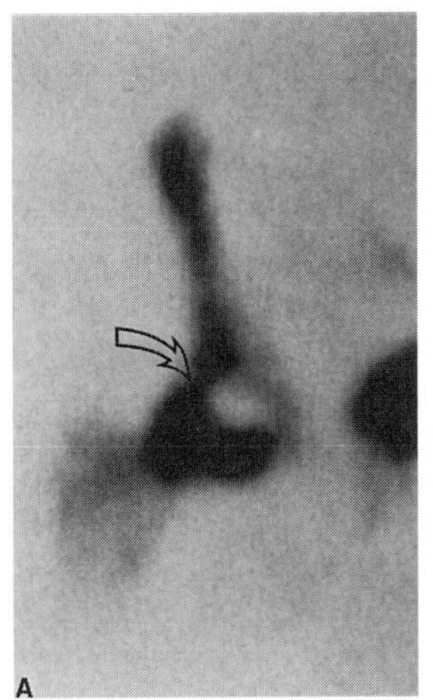

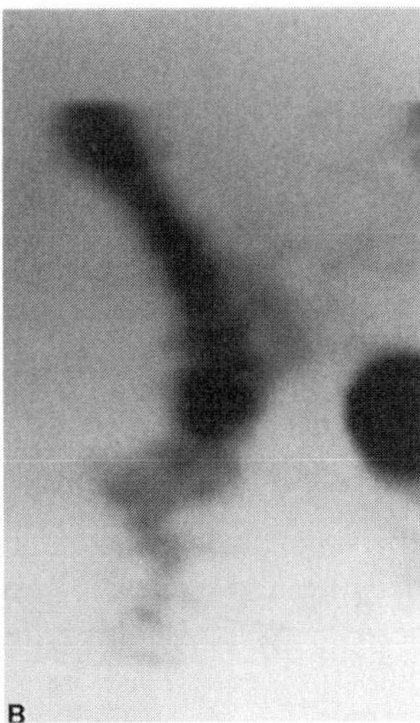

FIGURE 108.14. Single photon emission computed tomography (SPECT) image of a partially revascularized precollapse femoral head lesion (stage II) with a photopenic superomedial necrotic zone surrounded by a hyperemic (resorptive) margin with increased radionuclide uptake. **A:** A transitional cold/hot lesion of this magnitude has a poor prognosis, since it is especially vulnerable to collapse near the superolateral chondro-osseous junction (arrow). **B:** SPECT image of a diffusely hot, but much smaller, femoral head lesion (stage II), which has a much better prognosis, because it has repaired without collapsing.

Computed Tomography with Multiplanar Reconstructions

Although the possibility of articular collapse (stage III lesion) can be directly evaluated by arthroscopy of the shoulder, hip, or knee, CT with multiplanar reconstructions (CT/MPR) is noninvasive and is also sensitive to small changes of contour (subchondral collapse) and differences in radiographic density. Necrosis of the contralateral hip was found by CT/MPR in 16% (9/55 patients), most of whom had stage II lesions (2).

Superselective Angiography

When performed in hips with stage II to III lesions, superselective angiography indicates hypervascularity of the femoral head by probable recanalized lateral epiphyseal vessels with neovascularization about a subchondral zone of devascularization. Ultimately, there may also be some collateral circulation of the lateral epiphyseal vessels derived from the uninvolved lateral femoral circumflex arterial tributaries, the inferior gluteal vessels, and the obturator artery and its medial epiphyseal branches traversing the ligamentum teres. These are known to anastomose with lateral epiphyseal (superior retinacular) vessels to a limited extent.

Treatment

The risk of collapse (stage II to III conversion) is related to several variables, including the size and location of the stage II lesion. Although certain stage II lesions that are small or medium size may spontaneously heal and not collapse (88,181–183); it has not yet been shown that improved diagnostic accuracy of the large lesion has resulted in treatment strategies that can consistently prevent their ultimate collapse (184). In one study of stage II femoral head lesions treated with electrical stimulation (pulsed electromagnetic fields) and followed for 6 years, 71% exhibited stability with no radiographic progression (185).

Although core decompression provides immediate pain relief, it remains a controversial treatment modality and may possibly facilitate the collapse of large nonsclerotic lesions due to increased structural weakness of the femoral head. The success rate of this procedure has varied widely in different studies (186), with an overall rate, in 24 reports, of clinical success of 64% (187). More clinical trials with long-term follow-up are necessary to determine if core decompression can significantly modify the natural course of osteonecrosis and prevent collapse of large lesions in vulnerable locations (188). Free vascularized fibular bone grafts have been successfully performed for femoral head osteonecrosis (189,190). A total of 1,303 procedures were reported from seven centers. In the precollapse stage the survival rate ranged from 76 to 100% (mean, 88%).

Stage III Lesions

Often the patient remains asymptomatic until the articular surface undergoes late segmental collapse. When a stage II lesion converts to a stage III lesion (Fig. 108.5), the patient reports symptoms of acute joint pain and occasionally, spasm, usually aggravated by weight bearing and relieved by rest. Joint tenderness and slight limitation of motion are often present, especially on internal rotation of the hip in flexion.

Pathologic Features

Late segmental collapse is a result of the repair process. If repair were prevented entirely, the necrotic femoral head would not collapse because dead bone (stage I) is essentially as strong as living bone (Fig. 108.6). In stage III lesions, however, the radiolucent revascularization front has resorbed subchondral bone and uncalcified articular cartilage. Intracapital fractures begin in a focal area of osteoclastic resorption at the chondro-osseous junction (Fig. 108.15). Stress risers are created by focal resorption of the subchondral plate. The low elastic modulus of this region may reduce its ability to resist deformation.

Impulse loading leads to shear-induced microfractures of the preexisting necrotic trabeculae, beginning at the stress risers, which propagate into the femoral head. Finally, the anterosuperior portion of the femoral head or the central portion of the humeral head buckles and collapses. Fibrocartilaginous metaplasia often occurs beneath the subchondral fracture, blocking further revascularization. This metaplasia probably develops as a result of micromotion or

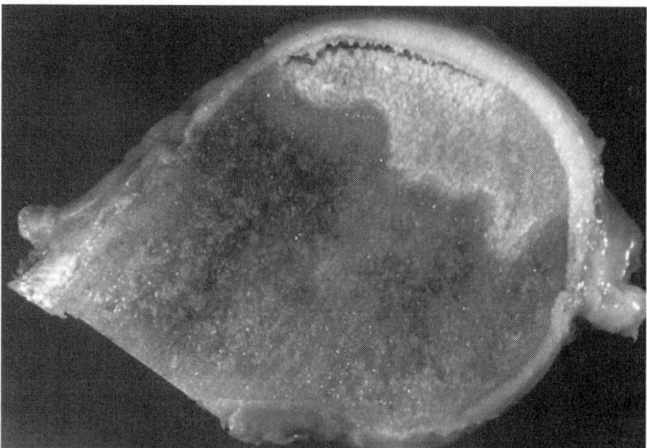

FIGURE 108.15. Gross sagittal section of right femoral head showing a stage III postcollapse lesion with an extensive subchondral fracture (radiolucent crescent) with incomplete detachment of the overlying cartilage, and a dark zone of revascularization, especially in the region of the lateral epiphyseal vessels. This patient had morbid obesity, diabetes, fatty liver, arterial fat embolism, increased free fatty acids, and intravascular coagulation.

terminal hypoxia at the revascularization front. Perinecrotic arteries may show concentric intimal proliferation and thickening with narrowed lumina, probably resulting from endothelial denudation and recanalization (2). Microangiography of postcollapse specimens may reveal extraosseous interruption of superior retinacular arteries with newly formed branches arising from their stumps (175).

Radiographic Features

Radiographic examination, particularly external rotation views of the shoulder and lateral views of the hip, indicate architectural failure and structural collapse. A unipolar subchondral fracture is often apparent. A positive, radiolucent, crescent (meniscus) sign indicates a stage III lesion. Once a break has occurred in the smooth, spherical, articular cartilage and in subchondral bone, the necrotic lesion is irreversible, inevitably progressing to further collapse, with articular incongruity and secondary degenerative changes. Vertebral collapse is especially common in sickle cell and Gaucher's disease (191,192). The presence on plain radiographs of an intravertebral vacuum cleft in a partially collapsed vertebra is considered virtually pathognomonic of osteonecrosis.

Treatment

Using an angulatory intertrochanteric osteotomy (193) or a rotational transtrochanteric osteotomy (194), smaller necrotic areas can be moved so that maximal stress may fall on the uninvolved surface of the femoral head. Surface hemiarthroplasty may also provide symptomatic relief and defer the need for total hip replacement (195). However, total replacement is often indicated when there is extensive involvement of the femoral head.

Stage IV Lesions

These patients have continuous joint pain, limpness, stiffness, and weakness. Physical findings include tenderness, deformity, crepitation, contracture, and limited motion.

Pathologic Features

As subchondral collapse continues, joint destruction occurs with advanced changes typical of secondary osteoarthritis, including a narrowed, incongruous joint space, diffuse hypertrophy with extensive marginal osteophytic proliferation, and degenerative cyst formation.

Treatment

Total joint replacement is recommended for stage IV lesions (196).

REFERENCES

1. James J, Steijn-Myagkaya GL. Death of osteocytes. Electron microscopy after in vitro ischemia. *J Bone Joint Surg* 1986;68B:620–624.
2. Jones JP. Osteonecrosis. In: Koopman WJ, ed. *Arthritis and allied conditions:* a textbook of rheumatology, 13th ed. Baltimore: Williams & Wilkins, 1997:1923–1942.
3. Hughes LO, Beaty JH. Fractures of the head and neck of the femur in children. *J Bone Joint Surg* 1994;76A:283–292.
4. Swiontkowski MF. Intracapsular fractures of the hip. *J Bone Joint Surg* 1994;76A:129–138.
5. Brooks CH, Revell WJ, Heatley FW. Vascularity of the humeral head after proximal humeral fractures. *J Bone Joint Surg* 1993;75B:132–136.
6. Gerber C, Schneeberger AG, Vinh TS. The arterial vascularization of the humeral head. *J Bone Joint Surg* 1990;72A:1486–1494.
7. Takahashi S, Sugimoto M, Kotoura Y, et al. Long-term changes in the haversian systems following high-dose irradiation. *J Bone Joint Surg* 1994;76A;722–738.
8. Jones JP. Risk factors potentially activating intravascular coagulation and causing nontraumatic osteonecrosis. In: Urbaniak JR, Jones JP, eds. *Osteonecrosis: etiology, diagnosis, and treatment.* Rosemont, IL: American Academy of Orthopedic Surgeons, 1997:89–96.
9. Nishii T, Sugano N, Ohzono K, et al. Multiple lesions of osteonecrosis depicted by magnetic resonance imaging. *Am J Knee Surg* 1995;8:137–140.
10. LaPorte DM, Mont MA, Mohan V, et al. Multifocal osteonecrosis. *J Rheumatol* 1998;25:1968–1974.
11. Yamamoto T, DiCarlo EF, Bullough PG. The prevalence and clinicopathological appearance of extension of osteonecrosis in the femoral head. *J Bone Joint Surg* 1999;81B:328–332.
12. Shimizu K, Moriya H, Akita T, et al. Prediction of collapse with magnetic resonance imaging of avascular necrosis of the femoral head. *J Bone Joint Surg* 1994;76A:215–223.
13. Jones JP. Intravascular coagulation and osteonecrosis. *Clin Orthop* 1992;277:41–53.
14. Glueck CJ, Freiberg R, Gruppo R, et al. Thrombophilia and hypofibrinolysis: reversible pathogenetic etiologies of osteonecrosis. In: Urbaniak JR, Jones JP, eds. *Osteonecrosis: etiology, diagnosis, and treatment.* Rosemont, IL: American Academy of Orthopedic Surgeons, 1997:105–110.
15. Arruda VR, Belangero WD, Ozelo MC, et al. Inherited risk factors for thrombophilia among children with Legg-Calve-Perthes disease. *J Pediatr Orthop* 1999;19:84–87.
16. Jones JP, Ramirez S, Doty SB. The pathophysiologic role of fat in dysbaric osteonecrosis. *Clin Orthop* 1993;296:256–264.
17. Jones JP. Fat embolism, intravascular coagulation, and osteonecrosis. *Clin Orthop* 1993;292:294–308.
18. Welch RD, Hogan PM, Groom LJ, et al. Osteonecrosis of the femoral head associated with colitis in a horse. In: Urbaniak JR, Jones JP, eds. *Osteonecrosis: etiology, diagnosis, and treatment.* Rosemont, IL: American Academy of Orthopedic Surgeons, 1997:181–187.
19. Moore LA, Johnson PJ, Bailey KL. Aorto-iliac thrombosis in a foal. *Vet Rec* 1998;142:459–462.
20. Arlet J, Laroche M, Soler R, et al. Histopathology of the vessels of the femoral heads in specimens of osteonecrosis, osteoarthritis and algodystrophy. *Clin Rheumatol* 1993;12:162–165.
21. Ficat RP, Arlet J. *Ischemia and necrosis of bone.* Baltimore: Williams & Wilkins, 1980.
22. Spencer JD, Brookes M. Avascular necrosis and the blood supply of the femoral head. *Clin Orthop* 1988;235:127–140.

23. Delanois RE, Mont MA, Yoon TR, et al. Atraumatic osteonecrosis of the talus. *J Bone Joint Surg* 1998;80:529–536.
24. Resnick D, Pineda C, Trudell D. Widespread osteonecrosis of the foot in systemic lupus erythematosus: radiographic and gross pathologic correlation. *Skeletal Radiol* 1985;13:33–38.
25. Fink B, Assheuer J, Enderle A, et al. Avascular osteonecrosis of the acetabulum. *Skeletal Radiol* 1997;26:509–516.
26. Briggs PJ, Moran CG, Wood MB. Actions of endothelin-1, 2, and 3 in the microvasculature of bone. *J Orthop Res* 1998; 16:340–347.
27. Jones JP. Fat embolism and osteonecrosis. *Orthop Clin North Am* 1985;16:595–633.
28. Korompilias AV, Ortel TL, Gilkeson GS, et al. Hypercoagulability and osteonecrosis. In: Urbaniak JR, Jones JP, eds. *Osteonecrosis: etiology, diagnosis, and treatment.* Rosemont, IL: American Academy of Orthopedic Surgeons, 1997:111–116.
29. Muller-Berghaus G. Pathophysiologic and biochemical events in disseminated intravascular coagulation: dysregulation of procoagulant and anticoagulant pathways. *Semin Thromb Hemostasis* 1989;15:58–87.
30. Glueck CJ, Freiberg R, Glueck HI, et al. Hypofibrinolysis: a common, major cause of osteonecrosis. *Am J Hematol* 1994;45: 156–166.
31. Van Veldhuizen PJ, Neff J, Murphey MD, et al. Decreased fibrinolytic potential in patients with idiopathic avascular necrosis and transient osteoporosis of the hip. *Am J Hematol* 1993; 44:243–248.
32. Pollock FE, Smith TL, Koman LA, et al. Decreased microvascular perfusion in the rabbit ear after six hours of ischemia. *J Orthop Res* 1994;12:48–57.
33. Winet H, Hsieh A, Bao JY. Approaches to study of ischemia in bone. *J Biomed Mater Res* 1998;43:410–421.
34. Koo KH, Jeong ST, Jones JP. Borderline necrosis of the femoral head. *Clin Orthop* 1999;358:158–165.
35. Saito S, Inoue A, Ono K. Intramedullary hemorrhage as a possible cause of avascular necrosis of the femoral head. *J Bone Joint Surg* 1987;69B:346–351.
36. Saito S, Ohzono K, Ono K. Early arteriopathy and postulated pathogenesis of osteonecrosis of the femoral head. *Clin Orthop* 1992;277:98–110.
37. Bick RL. Disseminated intravascular coagulation. *Clin Lab Med* 1994;14:729–768.
38. Swales JD, de Bono DP. *Cardiovascular risk factors.* London: Gower, 1993.
39. Martin LD, Rothschild BM. Paleopathology and diving mosasaurs. *Am Sci* 1989;77:460–467.
40. Lam TH, Yau KP. Dysbaric osteonecrosis in a compressed air tunneling project in Hong Kong. *Occup Med* 1992;42: 23–29.
41. Zhang LD, Kang JF, Xue HL. Distribution of lesions in the head and neck of the humerus and the femur in dysbaric osteonecrosis. *Undersea Biomed Res* 1990;17:353–358.
42. Jones JP, Behnke AR. Prevention of dysbaric osteonecrosis in compressed-air workers. *Clin Orthop* 1978;130:118–128.
43. Bove AA. Risk of decompression sickness with patent foramen ovale. *Undersea Hyper Med* 1998;25:175–178.
44. Yoo MC, Cho YJ, Lee SG. Bony lesions of professional divers in Korea. *J Korean Orthop Assoc* 1992;27:331–340.
45. Lehner CE, Wilson MA, Dueland RT, et al. Sheep model of dysbaric osteonecrosis in divers and caisson workers. In: Urbaniak JR, Jones JP, eds. *Osteonecrosis: etiology, diagnosis, and treatment.* Rosemont, IL: American Academy of Orthopedic Surgeons, 1997:145–152.
46. Kitano M, Hayashi K. Acute decompression sickness—report of an autopsy case with widespread fat embolism. *Acta Pathol Jpn* 1981;31:269–276.
47. Murayama S, Borne JA, Robinson AE, et al. MR imaging of pediatric hematologic disorders. *Acta Radiol* 1991;32:267–270.
48. Katz K, Horev G, Goshen J, et al. The pattern of bone disease in transfusion-dependent thalassemia major patients. *Isr J Med Sc* 1994;30:577–580.
49. Bernard C, Sick H, Boilletot A, et al. Bone marrow necrosis. Acute microcirculation failure in myelomonocytic leukemia. *Arch Intern Med* 1978;138:1567–1569.
50. Matsui M, Saito S, Ohzono K, et al. Experimental steroid-induced osteonecrosis in adult rabbits with hypersensitivity vasculitis. *Clin Orthop* 1992;277:61–72.
51. Nakata K, Masuhara K, Nakamural N, et al. Inducible osteonecrosis in a rabbit serum sickness model: deposition of immune complexes in bone marrow. *Bone* 1996;18:609–615.
52. Sakai T, Sugano N, Tsuji T, et al. Early magnetic resonance imaging in a rabbit osteonecrosis model. *Trans Orthop Res Soc* 1999;24:584.
53. Nagasawa K, Tsukamoto H, Tada Y, et al. Imaging study on the mode of development and changes in avascular necrosis of the femoral head in systemic lupus erythematosus. *Br J Rheumatol* 1994;33;343–347.
54. Nagasawa K, Ishii Y, Mayumi T, et al. Avascular necrosis of bone in systemic lupus erythematosus: possible role of hemostatic abnormalities. *Ann Rheum Dis* 1989;48:672–676.
55. Leong KH, Koh ET, Feng PH, et al. Lipid profiles in patients with systemic lupus erythematosus. *J Rheumatol* 1994;21: 1264–1267.
56. Ono K, Tohjima T, Komazawa T. Risk factors of avascular necrosis of the femoral head in patients with systemic lupus erythematosus under high-dose corticosteroid therapy. *Clin Orthop* 1992;277:89–97.
57. Shimamoto Y, Ohta A, Sano M, et al. Improved or fatal acute disseminated intravascular coagulation in systemic lupus erythematosus. *Am J Hematol* 1993;42:191–195.
58. Mont MA, Glueck CJ, Pacheco IH, et al. Risk factors for osteonecrosis in systemic lupus erythematosus. *J Rheumatol* 1997;24:654–662.
59. Sheikh JS, Retzinger GS, Hess EV. Association of osteonecrosis in systemic lupus erythematosus with abnormalities of fibrinolysis. *Lupus* 1998;7:42–48.
60. Watanabe T, Tsuchida T, Kanda N, et al. Avascular necrosis of bone in systemic lupus erythematosus. The predictive role of precipitating autoantibodies. *Scand J Rheumatol* 1997;26: 184–187.
61. Asherson RA, Khamashta MA, Ordi-Ros J, et al. The "primary" antiphospholipid syndrome: major clinical and serological features. *Medicine* 1989;68:366–374.
62. Asherson RA, Liote F, Page B, et al. Avascular necrosis of bone and antiphospholipid antibodies in systemic lupus erythematosus. *J Rheumatol* 1993;20:284–288.
63. Seleznick MJ, Silveira LH, Espinoza LR. Avascular necrosis associated with anticardiolipid antibodies. *J Rheumatol* 1991; 18:1416–1417.
64. Vela P, Salas E, Batlle E, et al. Primary antiphospholipid syndrome and osteonecrosis. *Clin Exp Rheumatol* 1991;9:545–546.
65. Asherson RA, Cervera R, Piette JC. Catastrophic antiphospholipid syndrome. Clinical and laboratory features of 50 patients. *Medicine* 1998;77:195–207.
66. Sandset PM, Warn-Cramer BJ, Maki SL, et al. Immunodepletion of extrinsic pathway inhibitor sensitizes rabbits to endotoxin-induced intravascular coagulation and the generalized Shwartzman reaction. *Blood* 1991;78:1496–1502.
67. Ohno Y, Shiga J, Mori W. Selective segmental hepatic necrosis produced by the Shwartzman mechanism in rabbits. *Virchows Arch [A]* 1989;416:75–80.
68. Damry N, Schurmans T, Perlmutter N. MRI evaluation and

follow-up of bone necrosis after meningococcal infection and disseminated intravascular coagulation. *Pediatr Radiol* 1993;23:429–431.

69. Acheson LS. Disturbances of bone growth in a child who survived septic shock. *J Fam Pract* 1986;23:321–329.
70. Duncan JS, Ramsey LE. Widespread bone infarction complicating meningococcal septicaemia and disseminated intravascular coagulation. *Br Med J* 1984;288:111–112.
71. Santos E, Boavida JE, Barroso A, et al. Late osteoarticular lesions following meningococcemia with disseminated intravascular coagulation. *Pediatr Radiol* 1989;19:199–202.
72. Grogan DP, Love SM, Ogden JA, et al. Chondroosseous growth abnormalities after meningococcemia. *J Bone Joint Surg* 1989;71A:920–928.
73. Yamamoto T, Hirano K, Tsutsui H, et al. Corticosteroid enhances the experimental induction of osteonecrosis in rabbits with Shwartzman reaction. *Clin Orthop* 1995;316:235–243.
74. Chevalier X, Larget-Piet B, Hernigou P, et al. Avascular necrosis of the femoral head in HIV-infected patients. *J Bone Joint Surg* 1993;75B:160–161.
75. Pardo-Mindan FJ, Salinas-Madrigal L, Idoate M, et al. Pathology of renal transplantation. *Semin Diagn Pathol* 1992;9:185–199.
76. Matsuo K, Hirohata T, Sugioka Y, et al. Influence of alcohol intake, cigarette smoking and occupational status on idiopathic osteonecrosis of the femoral head. *Clin Orthop* 1988;234:115–123.
77. Jacobs B. Alcoholism-induced bone necrosis. *NY State J Med* 1992;92:334–338.
78. Lang P, Mauz M, Schorner W, et al. Acute fracture of the femoral neck: assessment of femoral head perfusion with gadopentetate dimeglumine-enhanced MR imaging. *AJR* 1993;160:335–341.
79. Nadel SN, Debatin JF, Richardson WJ, et al. Detection of acute avascular necrosis of the femoral head in dogs: dynamic contrast-enhanced MR imaging vs spin-echo and STIR sequences. *AJR* 1992;159:1255–1261.
80. Antti-Poika I, Karaharju E, Vankka E, et al. Alcohol-associated femoral head necrosis. *Ann Chir Gynaecol* 1987;76:318–322.
81. Carr JM. Disseminated intravascular coagulation in cirrhosis. *Hepatology* 1989;10:103–110.
82. Alexakis PG, Wallack M. Idiopathic osteonecrosis of the femoral head associated with a pituitary tumor. *J Bone Joint Surg* 1989;71A:1412–1414.
83. Felson DT, Anderson JJ. Across-study evaluation of association between steroid dose and bolus steroids and avascular necrosis of bone. *Lancet* 1987;8538:902–905.
84. Mirzai R, Chang C, Greenspan A, et al. The pathogenesis of osteonecrosis and the relationships to corticosteroids. *J Asthma* 1999;36:77–95.
85. Socie G, Selimi F, Sedel L, et al. Avascular necrosis of bone after allogeneic bone marrow transplantation: clinical findings, incidence and risk factors. *Br J Haematol* 1994;86:624–628.
86. Bizot P, Nizard R, Socie G, et al. Femoral head osteonecrosis after bone marrow transplantation. *Clin Orthop* 1998;357:127–134.
87. Bradbury G, Benjamin J, Thompson J, et al. Avascular necrosis of bone after cardiac transplantation. *J Bone Joint Surg* 1994;76A:1385–1388.
88. Mulliken BD, Renfrew DL, Brand RA, et al. Prevalence of previously undetected osteonecrosis of the femoral head in renal transplant recipients. *Radiology* 1994;192:831–834.
89. Tervonen O, Mueller DM, Matteson EL, et al. Clinically occult avascular necrosis of the hip: prevalence in an asymptomatic population at risk. *Radiology* 1992;182:845–847.
90. Lopez-Garrido J, Galera-Davidson H, Medina IO, et al. Dexamethasone-prepared *Escherichia coli*–induced disseminated intravascular coagulation. *Lab Invest* 1987;56:534–543.
91. Schneiderman J, Adar R, Sawdey M. Chronic glucocorticosteroid administration modulates the response of the fibrinolytic system to bacterial lipoplysaccharide. *Fibrinolysis* 1994;8:238–244.
92. Koo KH, Daussault RG, Kaplan PA, et al. Fatty marrow conversion of the proximal femoral metaphysis in osteonecrotic hips. *Clin Orthop* 1999;361:159–167.
93. Wang GJ, Hubbard SL, Reger SI, et al. Femoral head blood flow in long-term steroid treatment (study of rabbit model). In: Arlet J, Ficat RP, Hungerford DS, eds. *Bone circulation.* Baltimore: Williams & Wilkins, 1984:35–37.
94. Carvalho AC, Lees RS, Vaillancourt RA, et al. Intravascular coagulation in hyperlipidemia. *Thromb Res* 1976;8:843–857.
95. Cheras PA, Freemont AJ, Sikorski JM. Intraosseous thrombosis in ischemic necrosis of bone and osteoarthritis. *Osteoarth Cartilage* 1993;1:219–232.
96. Tsai CL, Liu TK. Evidence for eicosanoids within the reparative front in avascular necrosis of human femoral head. *Clin Orthop* 1992;281:305–312.
97. Hulman G. The pathogenesis of fat embolism. *J Pathol* 1995;176:3–9.
98. Haber LM, Hawkins EP, Seilheimer DK, et al. Fat overload syndrome. An autopsy study with evaluation of the coagulopathy. *Am J Clin Pathol* 1988;90:223–227.
99. Shapiro SC, Rothstein FC, Newman AJ, et al. Multifocal osteonecrosis in adolescents with Crohn's disease: a complication of therapy? *J Pediatr Gastroenterol Nutr* 1985;4:502–506.
100. Kawai K, Tamaki A, Hirohata K. Steroid-induced accumulation of lipid in the osteocytes of the rabbit femoral head. *J Bone Joint Surg* 1985;67A:755–763.
101. Muratsu H, Shimizu T, Kawai K, et al. Alcohol-induced accumulations of lipids in the osteocytes of the rabbit femoral head. *Trans Ortho Res Soc* 1990;15:402(abst).
102. Doty SB, Morey-Holton ER, Durnova GN, et al. Cosmos 1887: morphology, histochemistry, and vasculature of the growing rat tibia. *FASEB* 1990;4:16–23.
103. Montella BJ, Nunley JA, Urbaniak JR. Osteonecrosis of the femoral head associated with pregnancy. In: Urbaniak JR, Jones JP, eds. *Osteonecrosis: etiology, diagnosis, and treatment.* Rosemont, IL: American Academy of Orthopedic Surgeons, 1997:125–130.
104. Rosendaal FR, Siscovick DS, Schwartz SM, et al. A common prothrombin variant (20210 G to A) increases the risk of myocardial infarction in young women. *Blood* 1997;90:1747–1750.
105. Glueck CJ, McMahon RE, Bouguot JE, et al. Heterozygosity for the Leiden mutation of the factor V gene, a common pathoetiology for osteonecrosis of the jaw, with thrombophilia augmented by exogenous estrogens. *J Lab Clin Med* 1997;130:540–543.
106. Szasz I, Morrison RT, Lyster DM, et al. Bone scintigraphy in massive disseminated bone necrosis. *Clin Nucl Med* 1981;97–100.
107. Jones JP Jr. Osteonecrosis and bone marrow edema syndrome: Similar etiology but a different pathogenesis. In: Urbaniak JR, Jones JP, eds. *Osteonecrosis: etiology, diagnosis, and treatment.* Rosemont, IL: American Academy of Orthopedic Surgeons, 1997:181–187.
108. Takada A, Takada Y, Urano T. The physiological aspects of fibrinolysis. *Thromb Res* 1994;76:1–31.
109. Jones MB. Pulmonary fat emboli associated with acute fatty liver of pregnancy. *Am J Gastroenterol* 1993;88:791–792.
110. den Heijer M, Koster T, Blom HJ, et al. Hyperhomocysteinemia as a risk factor for deep-vein thrombosis. *N Engl J Med* 1996;334:759–762.

111. Dunn P, Shih LY, Liaw SJ, et al. Bone marrow necrosis in 38 adult cancer patients. *J Formosan Med Assoc* 1993;92: 1107–1110.
112. Limentani SA, Pretell JO, Potter D, et al. Bone marrow necrosis in two patients with acute promyelocyte leukemia during treatment with all-trans retinoic acid. *Am J Hematol* 1994;47: 50–55.
113. Marymont J, Kauffman E. Osteonecrosis of bone associated with combination chemotherapy without corticosteroids. *Clin Orthop* 1986;204:150–153.
114. Harper G, Trask C, Souhami RL. Avascular necrosis of bone caused by combination chemotherapy without corticosteroids. *Br Med J* 1984;288:267–268.
115. Chan-Lam D, Prentice AG, Copplestone JA, et al. Avascular necrosis of bone following intensified steroid therapy for acute lymphoblastic leukemia and high-grade malignant lymphoma. *Br J Haematol* 1994;86:227–230.
116. Ojala AE, Paakko E, Lanning FB, et al. Osteonecrosis during the treatment of childhood acute lymphoblastic leukemia: a prospective MRI study. *Med Pediatr Oncol* 1999;32:11–17.
117. Ellis J, MacLeod U, Sammon D, et al. Osteonecrosis following treatment for Hodgkin's disease. *Clin Lab Haematol* 1994;16: 3–8.
118. Ruco LP, Pittiglio M, Dejana E, et al. Vascular activation in the histopathogenesis of Hodgkin's disease: potential role of endothelial tissue factor in intravascular thrombosis and necrosis. *J Pathol* 1993;171:131–136.
119. Pattisapu JV, Miller JD, Bell WN, et al. Spinal cord thromboplastin-induced coagulopathy in a rabbit model. *Neurosurgery* 1990;27:549–553.
120. Fujii Y, Mammen EF, Farag A, et al. Thrombosis in spinal cord injury. *Thromb Res* 1992;68:357–368.
121. Mayer PJ, Gehlsen JA. Coagulopathies associated with major spinal surgery. *Clin Orthop* 1989;245:83–88.
122. Miller JD, Pattisapu JV. Disseminated intravascular coagulation associated with spinal cord laceration. *J Trauma* 1989;29: 1178–1179.
123. Eriksson BI, Eriksson E, Risberg B. Impaired fibrinolysis and post-operative thromboembolism in orthopedic patients. *Thromb Res* 1991;62:55–64.
124. Pugh SC. Disseminated intravascular coagulation complicating bilateral cemented total hip arthroplasty. *Anaesth Intensive Care* 1991;19:106–108.
125. Jorens PG, Hermans CR, Haber I, et al. Acquired protein C and S deficiency, inflammatory bowel disease and cerebral arterial thrombosis. *Blut* 1990;61:307–310.
126. Cermak J, Key NS, Bach RR, et al. C-reactive protein induces human peripheral blood monocytes to synthesize tissue factor. *Blood* 1993;82:513–520.
127. Madsen PV, Andersen G. Multifocal osteonecrosis related to steroid treatment in a patient with ulcerative colitis. *Gut* 1994;35:132–134.
128. Vakil N, Sparberg M. Steroid-related osteonecrosis in inflammatory bowel disease. *Gastroenterology* 1989;96:62–67.
129. Freeman HJ, Kwan WCP. Non-corticosteroid-associated osteonecrosis of the femoral heads in two patients with inflammatory bowel disease. *N Engl J Med* 1993;329:1314–1316.
130. Devine DV, Kinney TR, Thomas PF, et al. Fragment D-dimer levels: an objective marker of vasoocclusive crisis and other complications of sickle cell disease. *Blood* 1986;68:317–319.
131. Garza JA. Massive fat and necrotic bone marrow embolization in a previously undiagnosed patient with sickle cell disease. *Am J Forensic Med Pathol* 1990;11:83–88.
132. Tochen ML. Bone lesions in a child with meningococcal meningitis and disseminated intravascular coagulation. *J Pediatr* 1977;91:342–343.
133. Milner PF, Kraus AP, Sebes JI, et al. Sickle cell disease as a cause of osteonecrosis of the femoral head. *N Engl J Med* 1991; 325:1476–1481.
134. Milner PF, Kraus AP, Sebes JI, et al. Osteonecrosis of the humeral head in sickle cell disease. *Clin Orthop* 1993;289: 136–143.
135. Francis RB. Platelets, coagulation, and fibrinolysis in sickle cell disease: their possible role in vascular occlusion. *Blood Coagulation Fibrinolysis* 1991;2:341–353.
136. Beurling-Harbury C, Schade SG. Platelet activation during pain crisis in sickle cell anemia patients. *Am J Hematol* 1989; 31:237–241.
137. Peters M, Plaat BEC, Ten Cate H, et al. Enhanced thrombin generation in children with sickle cell disease. *Thromb Haemost* 1994;71:169–172.
138. Rickles FR, O'Leary DS. Role of coagulation system in pathophysiology of sickle cell disease. *Arch Intern Med* 1986;133: 635–641.
139. Rao VM, Fishman M, Mitchell DG, et al. Painful sickle cell crises: bone marrow patterns observed with MR imaging. *Radiology* 1986:161:21–215.
140. Van Zanten TEG, Statius van Eps LW, Golding RP, et al. Imaging the bone marrow with magnetic resonance during a crisis and in chronic forms of sickle cell disease. *Clin Radiol* 1989; 40:486–489.
141. Israel O, Jerushalmi J, Gront D. Scintigraphic findings in Gaucher disease. *J Nucl Med* 1986;27:1557–1563.
142. Katz K, Mechlis-Frish S, Cohen IG, et al. Bone scans in the diagnosis of bone crisis in patients who have Gaucher disease. *J Bone Joint Surg* 1991;73A:513–517.
143. Lanir A, Hadar H, Cohen I, et al. Gaucher disease: assessment with MR imaging. *Radiology* 1986;161:239–244.
144. Van Saase JLCM, Vandenbroucke JP, van Romunde LKJ, et al. Osteoarthritis and obesity in the general population. A relationship calling for an explanation. *J Rheumatol* 1988;15: 1152–1158.
145. Clain DJ, Lefkowitch JH. Fatty liver disease in morbid obesity. *Gastroenterol Clin North Am* 1987;16:239–252.
146. Carmen WJ, Sowers M, Hawthorne V, et al. Obesity as a risk factor for osteoarthritis of the hand and wrist: a prospective study. *Am J Epidemiol* 1994;139:119–129.
147. Solomon SD. Frostbite arthritis. *Arthritis Rheum* 1980:23: 1332.
148. Wong SYP, Evans RA, Needs C, et al. The pathogenesis of osteoarthritis of the hip. Evidence for primary osteocyte death. *Clin Orthop* 1987;214:305–312.
149. Yamasaki K, Itakura C. Aseptic necrosis of bone in ICR mice. *Lab Anim* 1988;22:51–53.
150. Kiaer T. Bone perfusion and oxygenation. Animal experiments and clinical observations. *Acta Orthop Scand* 1994;65(suppl 257):1–40.
151. Arnoldi CC. Vascular aspects of degenerative joint disorders. *Acta Orthop Scand* 1994;65(suppl 261):1–82.
152. Cheras PA. Role of hyperlipidemia, hypercoagulability, and hypofibrinolysis in osteonecrosis and osteoarthritis. In: Urbaniak JR, Jones JP, eds. *Osteonecrosis: etiology, diagnosis, and treatment.* Rosemont, IL: American Academy of Orthopedic Surgeons, 1997:97–104.
153. Lippiello L, Walsh T, Feinhold M. The association of lipid abnormalities with tissue pathology in human osteoarthritic articular cartilage. *Metabolism* 1991;40:571–576.
154. DeSimone DP, Reddi AH. Vascularization and endochondral bone development: changes in plasminogen activator activity. *J Orthop Res* 1992;10:320–324.
155. Treadwell BV, Pavia M, Towle CA, et al. Cartilage synthesizes the serine protease inhibitor PAI-1: support for the involvement

of serine proteases in cartilage remodeling. *J Orthop Res* 1991; 9:309–316.
156. Carlson CS, Loeser RF, Jayo MJ, et al. Osteoarthritis in cynomolgus macaques: a primate model of naturally occurring disease. *J Orthop Res* 1994;12:331–339.
157. Jones JP Jr. Subchondral osteonecrosis can conceivably cause disk degeneration and "primary" osteoarthritis. In: Urbaniak JR, Jones JP, eds. *Osteonecrosis: etiology, diagnosis, and treatment.* Rosemont, IL: American Academy of Orthopedic Surgeons, 1997:135–142.
158. Glueck CJ, Glueck HI, Welch M, et al. Thrombophilia and hypofibrinolysis: pathophysiologies of osteonecrosis. *Clin Orthop* 1997;334:43–56.
159. Glueck CJ, Crawford A, Roy D, et al. Association of antithrombotic factor deficiencies and hypofibrinolysis with Legg-Perthes disease. *J Bone Joint Surg* 1996;78A;3–13.
160. Gregosiewicz A, Okonski M, Stolecka D, et al. Ischemia of the femoral head in Perthes' disease: is the cause intra- or extravascular. *Pediatr Orthop* 1989;9:160–162.
161. Gruppo R, Glueck CJ, Wall E, et al. Legg-Perthes disease in three siblings, two heterozygous and one homozygous for the factor V Leiden mutation. *J Pediatr* 1998;132:885–888.
162. Van Wersch JWJ, Westerhuis LWJJM, Venekamp WJRR. Coagulation activation in diabetes mellitus. *Hemostasis* 1990; 20:263–269.
163. Tanaka K, Sueishi K. The coagulation and fibrinolysis systems and atherosclerosis. *Lab Invest* 1993;69:5–18.
164. Kanfer A. Coagulation factors in nephrotic syndrome. *Am J Nephrol* 1990;10(suppl 1):63–68.
165. Kim YY, Bae DK, Suh DS, et al. Osteonecrosis of the femoral head associated with polyvinylpyrrolidone storage. *Korean J Orthop Surg* 1982;598–606.
166. Koo KH, Kim R, Cho SH, et al. Angiography, scintigraphy, intraosseous pressure, and histologic findings in high-risk osteonecrotic femoral heads with negative magnetic resonance images. *Clin Orthop* 1994;308:127–138.
167. Macleod MA, McEwan AJB, Pearson RR, et al. Functional imaging in the early diagnosis of dysbaric osteonecrosis. *Br J Radiol* 1982;55:497–500.
168. Sebes AJ. Diagnostic imaging of bone and joint abnormalities associated with sickle cell hemoglobinopathies. *AJR* 1989;152: 1153–1159.
169. Kim KY, Lee SH, Moon DH, et al. The diagnostic value of triple head single photon emission computed tomography (3H-SPECT) in avascular necrosis of the femoral head. *Int Orthop* 1993;17:132–138.
170. Asnis SE, Gould ES, Bansal M, et al. Magnetic resonance imaging of the hip after displaced femoral neck fractures. *Clin Orthop* 1994;298:191–198.
171. Ruland LJ, Wang GJ, Teates CD, et al. A comparison of magnetic resonance imaging to bone scintigraphy in early traumatic ischemia of the femoral head. *Clin Orthop* 1992;285:30–34.
172. Horev G, Kornreich L, Hadar H, et al. Hemorrhage associated with "bone crisis" in Gaucher's disease identified by magnetic resonance imaging. *Skeletal Radiol* 1991;20:479–482.
173. Lang P, Jergesen HE, Genant HK. The hip. In: Chan WP, Lang P, Genant HK, eds. *MRI of the musculoskeletal system.* Philadelphia: WB Saunders, 1994:233–262.
174. Surat A. Isolation of prostaglandin E2-like material from osteonecrosis induced by steroids and its prevention by kallikrein inhibitor, aprotinin. *Prostaglandins Leukotrienes Med* 1984;13:159–167.
175. Atsumi T, Kuroki Y. Role of impairment of blood supply of the femoral head in the pathogenesis of idiopathic osteonecrosis. *Clin Orthop* 1992;277:22–30.
176. Battistini B, Chailler P, D'Orleans-Juste P, et al. Growth regulatory properties of endothelins. *Peptides* 1993;14:385–399.
177. Jiang CC, Shih TT. Epiphyseal scar of the femoral head: risk factor of osteonecrosis. *Radiology* 1994;191:409–412.
178. Vande Berg BE, Malghem JJ, Labaisse MA, et al. MR imaging of avascular necrosis and transient marrow edema of the femoral head. *Radiographics* 1993;13:501–520.
179. Sakamoto M, Shizu K, Iida S, et al. Osteonecrosis of the femoral head. A prospective study with MRI. *J Bone Joint Surg* 1997;79B:213–219.
180. Toyone T. Takahashi K, Kitahara H, et al. Vertebral bone-marrow changes in degenerative lumbar disc disease. *J Bone Joint Surg* 1994;76B:757–764.
181. Berg BCV, Malghem J, Goffin EJ, et al. Transient epiphyseal lesions in renal transplant recipients: presumed insufficiency stress fractures. *Radiology* 1994;191:403–407.
182. Fordyce MJF, Solomon L. Early detection of avascular necrosis of the femoral head by MRI. *J Bone Joint Surg* 1993;75B: 365–367.
183. Kopechy KK, Boudysova M, Zanotti F, et al. Apparent avascular necrosis of the hip; appearance and spontaneous resolution of MR findings in renal allograft recipients. *Radiology* 1991; 179:523–527.
184. Lafforgue P, Dahan E, Chagnaud C, et al. Early-stage avascular necrosis of the femoral head: MR imaging for prognosis in 31 with at least 2 years of follow-up. *Radiology* 1993;187:199–204.
185. Aaron, RK. Treatment of osteonecrosis of the femoral head with electrical stimulation. In: Schafer M, ed. *Instructional course lectures.* Chicago: American Academy of Orthopedic Surgeons, 1994:495–498.
186. Bozic KJ, Zurakowski D, Thornhill TS, et al. Survivorship analysis of hips treated with core decompression for nontraumatic osteonecrosis of the femoral head. *J Bone Joint Surg* 1999;81A:200–209.
187. Mont MA, Carbone JJ, Fairbank AC. Core decompression versus nonoperative management for osteonecrosis of the hip. *Clin Orthop* 1996;324:169–178.
188. Koo KH, Song HR, Jeong ST, et al. Preventing collapse in early osteonecrosis of the femoral head. A randomized clinical trial of cone decompression. *J Bone Joint Surg* 1995;77B:870–874.
189. Coogan PG, Urbaniak JR. Multicenter experience with free vascularized fibular grafts for osteonecrosis of the femoral head. In: Urbaniak JR, Jones JP, eds. *Osteonecrosis: etiology, diagnosis, and treatment.* Rosemont, IL: American Academy of Orthopedic Surgeons, 1997:327–346.
190. Yoo MC, Chung DW, Hahn CS. Free vascularized fibula grafting for the treatment of osteonecrosis of the femoral head. *Clin Orthop* 1992;277:128–138.
191. Katz K, Sabato S, Horev G, et al. Spinal involvement in children and adolescents with Gaucher's disease. *Spine* 1993;18: 332–335.
192. Sadat-Ali M, Ammar A, Corea JR, et al. The spine in sickle cell disease. *Int Orthop* 1994;18:154–156.
193. Scher MA, Jakim I. Intertrochanteric osteotomy and autogenous bone-grafting for avascular necrosis of the femoral head. *J Bone Joint Surg* 1993;75A:1119–1133.
194. Sugioka Y, Hotokebuchi T, Tsutsui H. Transtrochanteric anterior rotational osteotomy for idiopathic and steroid-induced necrosis of the femoral head. *Clin Orthop* 1992;277:111–120.
195. Amstutz HC, Grigoris P, Safran MR, et al. Precision-fit surface hemiarthroplasty for femoral head osteonecrosis. *J Bone Joint Surg* 1994;76B:423–427.
196. Ortiguera CJ, Pulliam IT, Cabanela ME. Total hip arthroplasty for osteonecrosis: matched-pair analysis of 188 hips with long-term followup. *J Arthroplasty* 1999;14:21–28.

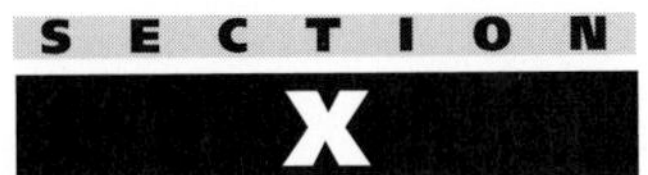

OSTEOARTHRITIS

109

PATHOLOGY OF OSTEOARTHRITIS

AUBREY J. HOUGH, JR.

One purpose of studying a disease is to gain insight concerning its causation. Osteoarthritis (OA), despite widespread occurrence in the adult population, offers formidable obstacles to the acquisition of such understanding. The very term *osteoarthritis* is a misnomer, because it implies an inflammatory process. The original usage of the term by John Spender in 1886 was as a synonym for rheumatoid arthritis (RA) and not as the disorder we recognize today (1). The term, however, has been used in the English-speaking world for several generations, and neither the pathologically more accurate term *degenerative joint disease* nor the European term *osteoarthrosis* have displaced it. Osteoarthritis has also suffered from a lack of consensus regarding its definition.

Different classification schemes for OA have emerged based on putative mechanical and biologic factors culminating in the disorder. The current working definition of OA incorporates these into a working formulation stating "morphologic, biochemical, molecular, and biomechanical changes of both cells and matrix which lead to softening, fibrillation, ulceration, and loss of articular cartilage, sclerosis, and eburnation of subchondral bone, osteophytes, and subchondral cysts" (2). In less comprehensive terms, OA is thus characterized by a deterioration of articular cartilage and formation of new bone at the joint surfaces (Fig. 109.1). The relationship between cartilaginous and bony changes has long been a source of contention. The nature of this relationship is central to the explanation of the pathologic changes seen in OA.

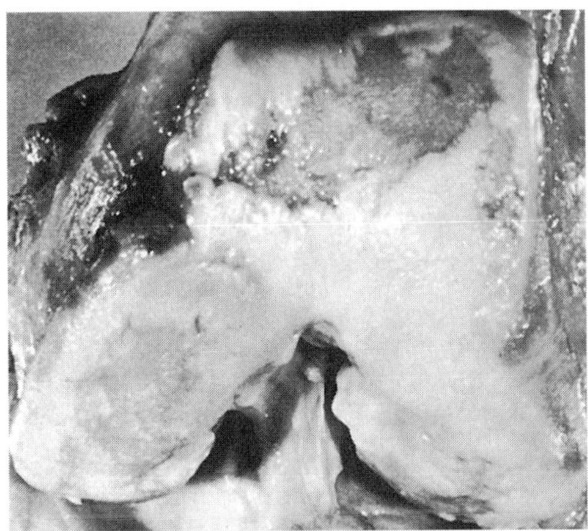

FIGURE 109.1. Degenerative joint disease of the knee. Large areas of erosion of articular cartilage are present on the patellar facet and on the condyles of the femur. These erosions occupy principally the central portions of the joint surfaces and spare the marginal regions. The cartilage at the eroded edges is fibrillated. The irregular elevations at the periphery of the surfaces are osteophytes.

OSTEOARTHRITIS AND REMODELING

Remodeling is defined as the gradual alteration of the internal architecture of the skeleton in response to mechanical loading (3). The removal of bone from certain sites coincides with the simultaneous formation of new bone elsewhere (4). Remodeling of bone explains changes in the shape of the joints both with age and in OA. In experimental models, these forces can produce resorption of calcified cartilage in areas of decreased pressure and necrobiosis of chondrocytes in areas of increased pressure (3). Similar changes occur in human OA (5). Likewise, rapidly destructive variants of OA that are associated with accelerated subchondral remodeling and osteocyte death also have been described (6,7).

Accounts of early OA usually maintain that fibrillation of articular cartilage precedes the development of other lesions. Biopsies of cartilage in early OA show that fibrillation is the earliest gross pathologic change observed (8). Similar changes are seen in early OA induced by partial meniscectomy in rabbits (9) and anterior cruciate transection in dogs (10). Cartilaginous changes, however, may not occur first, as changes in adjacent bony structures may precede them. The relationships between the cartilaginous and bony changes are complex, and the hypotheses relating them have been summarized by Sokoloff (11). OA can be viewed as a degeneration of articular cartilage progressively leading to denudation of the joint surface. If this chondrogenic theory were valid, little or no concomitant remodeling of bone would occur. This pattern does occur, most commonly in the hip joint, but is rather uncommon (3) and usually results from inflammatory lysis of cartilage rather than from mechanical overloading. In keeping with this hypothesis, the extent of remodeling in surgically resected femoral heads is generally greater in OA (coxa magna) than in RA (4). Similar lack of remodeling is seen in ochronotic arthropathy, perhaps due to the cartilage lysis that characterizes the disorder.

A second hypothesis is that cartilage fibrillation (Fig. 109.2A) sets in motion a cascade of events leading to secondary bony remodeling of the joint (4). This concept is very difficult to substantiate from the cartilaginous pathology alone because other morphologic events often occur in cartilage and subchondral bone simultaneously. For instance, age-related remodeling (12–14) in the osteochondral junction may coexist with surface fibrillation, albeit at different sites. Remodeling of the basal calcified cartilage is usually more apparent in non–weight-bearing areas of the joint (13), in contrast to fibrillation, which is more prominent in the weight-bearing areas. Thus, direct causal relationships between these two early changes are difficult to establish. Microfractures of the calcified cartilage, however, may presage the development of later cartilage degeneration by penetrating into the underlying bone marrow (14–16).

A third hypothesis proposed that OA is a consequence of increased stiffness of subchondral bone (4). Radin and Rose (17) postulated that microfractures of subchondral bone precede cartilage damage, because bone, rather than cartilage, absorbs most of the energy of impact loading transmitted through the extremities. Repair of these microfractures results in a net increase in bone stiffness, causing the overlying cartilage to absorb a greater proportion of the transmitted energy. This repartition of forces is postulated to result eventually in degeneration of the articular cartilage. Although this hypothesis has a distinct biomechanical logic, there are, as with the previous two hypotheses, certain limitations. The first is that the microfractures of the subchondral bony trabeculae may actually be a protective mechanism to maintain normal joint function because their numbers are decreased in OA, as compared to normal joints (18,19). This view holds that the remodeling of the subchondral trabeculae into thicker structures is the primary event rather than the microfractures. Bone morphometric studies of several types have confirmed that subchondral bone remodeling is consistently seen in OA (20,21). Another source of the confusion is the failure to distinguish between microfractures of the subchondral bony plate itself and those occurring at some distance in the underlying trabecular bone. The former are clearly involved in the formation of subchondral pseudocysts (Fig. 109.3). The latter are variously influenced by the systemic state of the skeleton, aging, and the extent of remodeling activities (22). Studies indicate that, in OA, trabecular histomorphometric changes of the iliac crest bone may not accurately reflect those occurring in subchondral bone in femoral heads (23). This may be due to the existence of distinct subpopulations of patients with atrophic and hypertrophic OA of the hip, the former being more likely to have thin bone trabeculae (24).

These degenerative and remodeling events are intertwined to the extent that identification of a unique initial event in the process of OA, if one exists, has not been possible. The same processes that culminate in destruction of the osteoarticular junction and the abrasion of the cartilage surface also result in proliferation of new cartilage and bone at or near the joint surface (Fig. 109.4). Although the exact cause of this proliferation has not been established, the generation of the new cartilage in defects in the joint surface that penetrate into the subjacent bone marrow has been documented in experimental models (4). In humans, this abortive repair process produces islands of cartilaginous

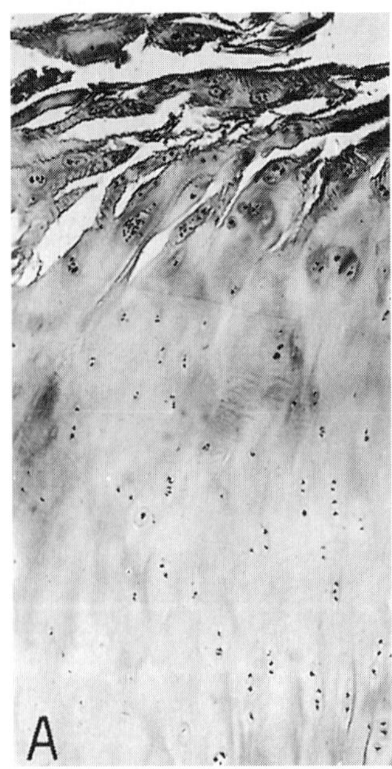

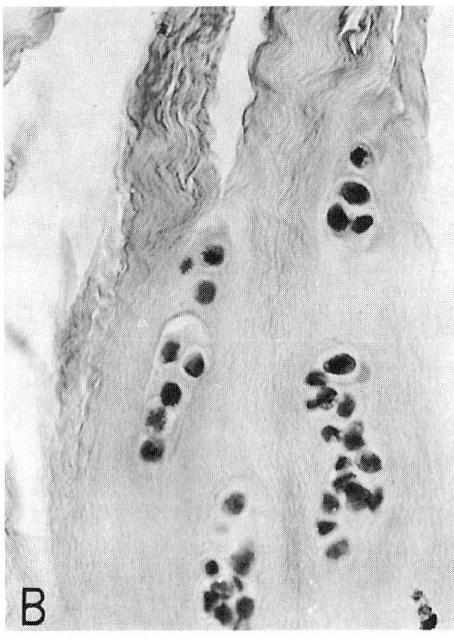

FIGURE 109.2. Fibrillation of articular cartilage. **A:** The most superficial dehiscences are oriented parallel to the surface and then arch downward in a more vertical direction. This pattern corresponds to the fibrous planes of the cartilage. (Hematoxylin and eosin stain, ×40.) **B:** Higher magnification (×240) of the fibrillated edge. The collagen fibrils at the surface have been "unmasked" from the hyaline matrix and appear frayed. Clusters of chondrocytes have proliferated to form so-called brood capsules.

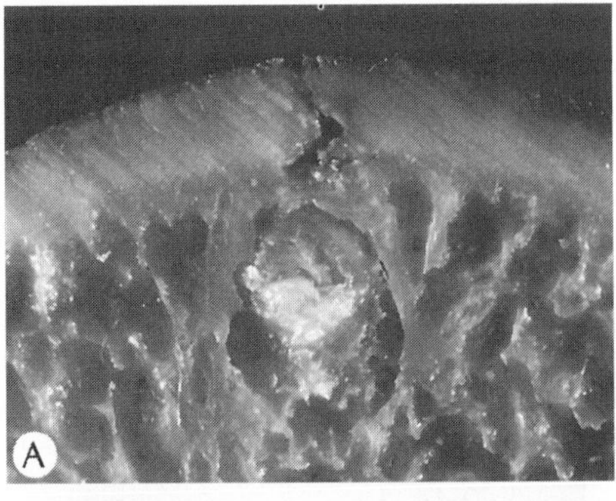

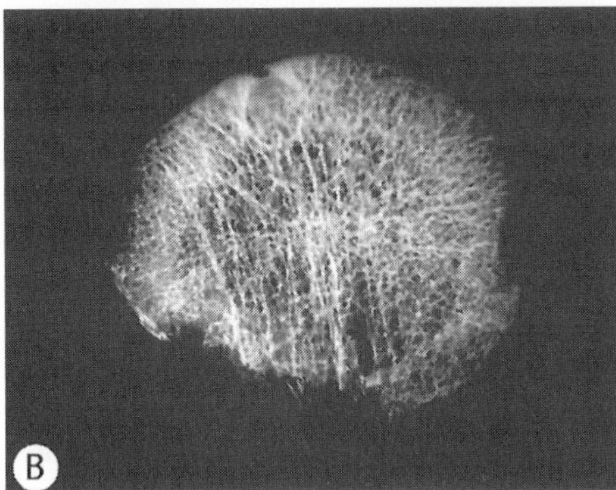

FIGURE 109.3. Relationship between a pseudocyst and a microfracture of the subchondral plate. This fortuitous slab section is from a recently fractured femoral head of a 77-year-old woman. Although moderate fibrillation is present elsewhere in the cartilage surface, the sole pseudocyst is located immediately beneath the minute discontinuity in the otherwise intact cartilage and osteochrondral junction. **A:** Gross appearance (approximately ×4). **B:** Roentgenogram, showing the gap in the subchondral plate and the sclerotic wall of the cyst.

proliferation interspersed with foci of new bone formation in the subchondral bone marrow. Using this attribute of cartilage to advantage, autografts of cultured articular chondrocytes have been employed to repair full-thickness cartilage defects in the knee joints (25).

Among the most prominent features of remodeling in OA are osteophytes (Fig. 109.4). Although they are a conspicuous feature of advanced OA, it would be erroneous to conclude that they represent merely a late change in the evolution of the joint lesions. Periarticular bone remodeling appears early in the course of experimental canine OA (26,27) parallel to changes in the composition of articular cartilage. In this regard, OA represents not so much the inability of the joint surface to initiate repair but rather the failure of repair to restore function (3).

ARTICULAR CARTILAGE

Microscopic Changes

Microscopic changes in articular cartilage are a consistent feature in early OA of both human and experimen-

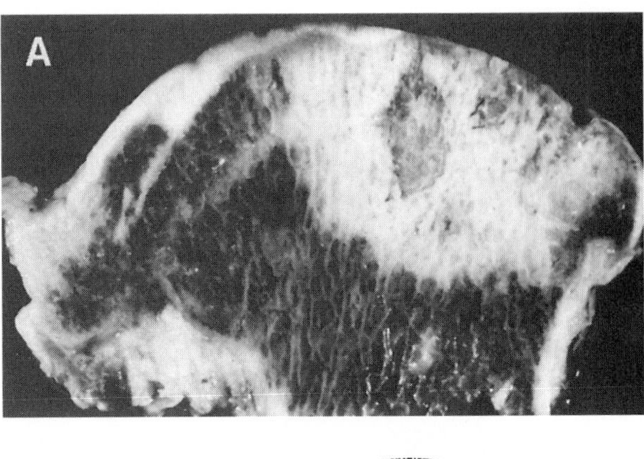

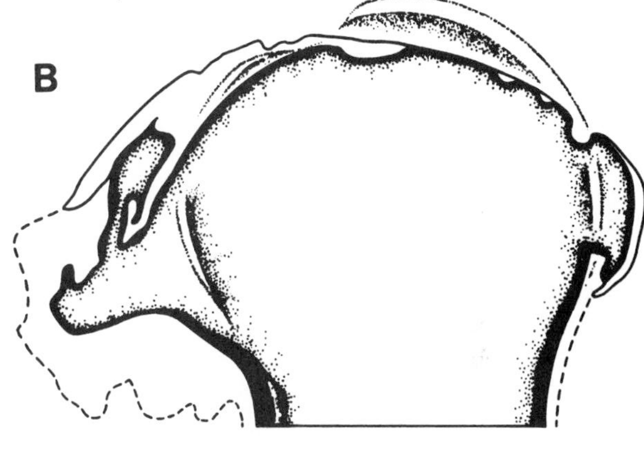

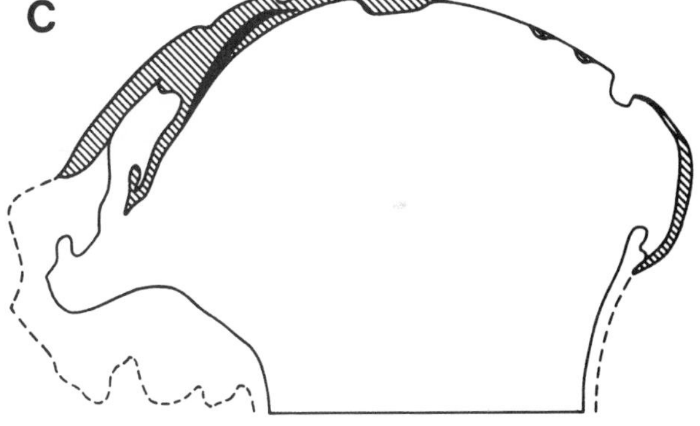

FIGURE 109.4. Advanced osteoarthritis of the head of the femur. **A:** The contour has been deformed both by abrasion of the bearing surface and by formation of marginal osteophytes. The large inferomedial spur at the left has grown not only to the side, but also into the original joint cartilage. Subchondral pseudocysts approach the eroded surface through slender crevices. The pallor of the eburnated zone reflects the condensation of bony trabeculae and compact fibrous tissue, in contrast to the darker, vascular hematopoietic marrow. **B:** Schematic representation of the remodeling. The outline of the gross specimen is superimposed on a best-fit contour of a normal femoral head of corresponding size. Bone appears *black;* cartilage, *white* outlined by a *solid line.* The *broken line* demarcates retinacular synovium. The loss of substance affects both articular cartilage and the immediately subjacent bone. **C:** Newly formed cartilage as deduced from the difference in the corresponding outlines in B. Only a minute residue of the original cartilage *(black)* persists at the base of the inferomedial osteophyte. The bulk of the cartilage must have therefore formed in the retinaculum or the subchondral bone marrow.

tal animal subjects (4). However, opinions differ as to the relative importance of individual lesions in the overall pathogenetic schema. Correlation of these early changes with biochemical and molecular changes is hampered by regional variations in the types of response to injury. As an example, repair cartilage, often of the fibrocartilaginous type, frequently overlies or is juxtaposed to degenerating hyaline cartilage in OA (Fig. 109.5F). Nevertheless, numerous specific lesions are described below.

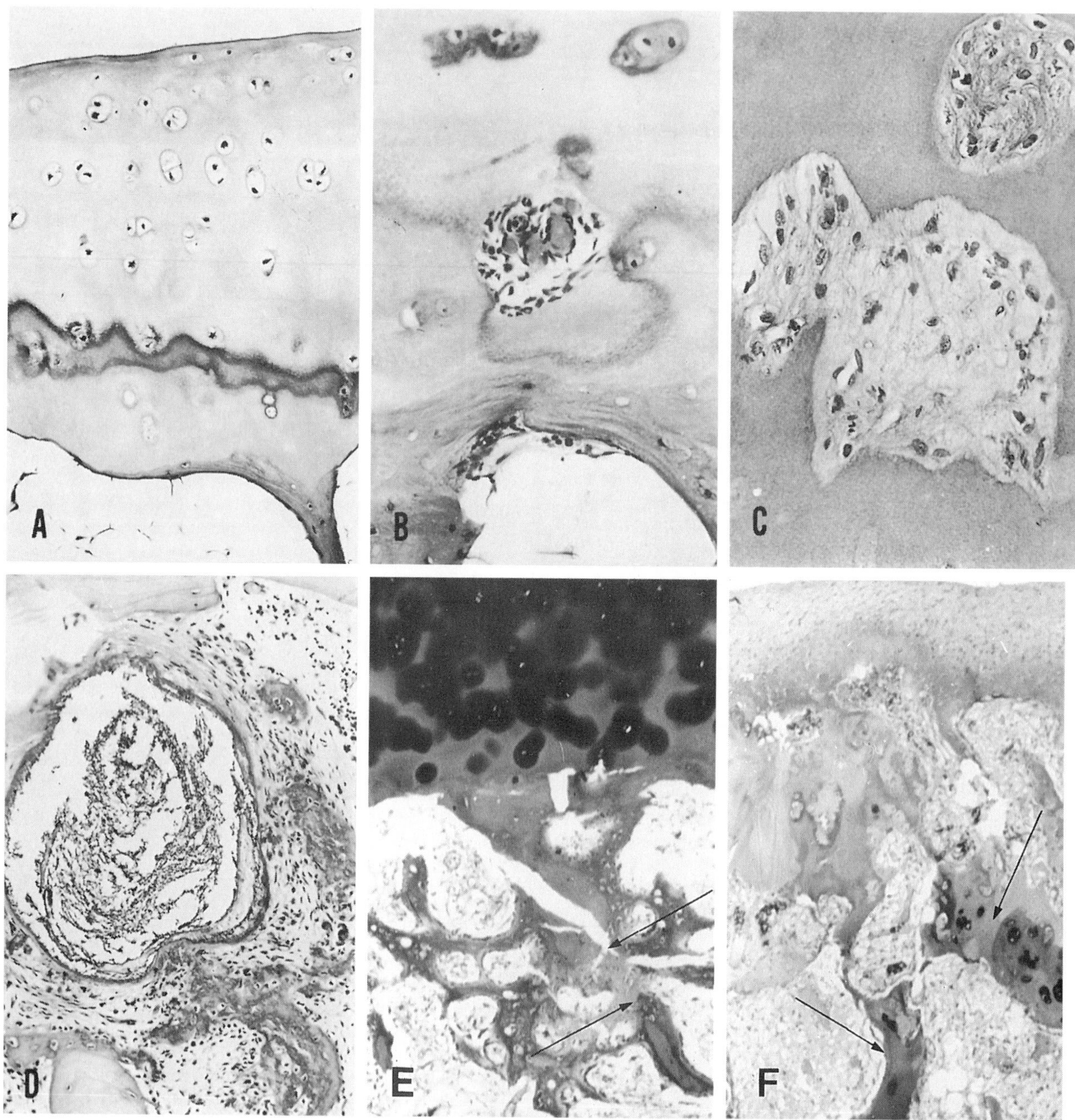

FIGURE 109.5. Miscellaneous remodeling and degenerative changes; all sections are stained with hematoxylin and eosin. **A:** Reduplication of calcification tidemark (×95). **B:** Vascularization of base of articular cartilage; the dark-stained material in the capsules of the chondrocytes is calcific (×183). **C:** Weichselbaum's lacunar resorption; small, geographic areas of hyaline cartilage are replaced by loose-textured, cellular fibrous tissue (×210). **D:** Early subchondral cystic degeneration; a small true cyst, filled with mucoid material, has a fibrous border. New bone formation is seen in the adjacent marrow (×90). **E:** Subchondral microfractures (arrows) of the femoral head in early osteoarthritis. Note proliferative callus (×70). **F:** Advancing ossification front has obliterated all but remnants of original articular cartilage (arrows). Reparative fibrocartilage occupies joint surface (×70).

Focal Chondromucoid Degeneration

Bennett et al. (28) concluded that focal swelling of the cartilage matrix associated with increased affinity for hematoxylin constituted the initial event in the process of OA. This superficial mucoid transformation is associated with an increased number of chondrocytes adjacent to the alteration (29). This change is prominent in the precocious OA variant of the patellofemoral joint (chondromalacia patellae).

Some differences have been described between the histology of chondromalacia and progressive OA of older adults (30). Some authors have gone as far as suggesting that chondromalacia patellae without malalignment does not ordinarily progress to clinical OA (31).

FOCAL LOSS OF METACHROMASIA

Loss of metachromatic staining material, presumably chondroitin sulfate, from all but the deepest portion of the radial zone of articular cartilage has been proposed as a histologic counterpart of chondromalacia leading to OA (4). Decreased metachromasia is accompanied by a loss of affinity for hematoxylin, in contrast to the view of Bennett et al. (28). Quantitative and qualitative changes in matrix protein polysaccharides accompany the loss of metachromasia (32). Furthermore, severity of histologic change in cartilage correlates with proteoglycanase activity in human OA (33,34) and increased amounts of proteoglycan fragments circulate in plasma in OA (35–37).

PROLIFERATION OF CHONDROCYTES

Small clusters of chondrocytes are common at the margin of minute fissures in the surface of the cartilage. These chondrocytes have apparently proliferated in response to the dehiscence of the tissue (Fig. 109.2). The preponderance of evidence supports focal mitotic activity as the source of the increased cellularity in these so-called chondrons (38,39). Tetraploidy and unstable DNA have been described also in chondrocytes associated with osteoarthritic erosions (40), as have somatic mutations, particularly involving chromosome 7 (41,42). Whether these changes in DNA are involved in the pathogenesis of OA is unclear.

WEICHSELBAUM'S LACUNAR RESORPTION

Focal dissolution of matrix by chondroclastic cells in cartilage lacunae was once regarded as a specific feature of OA (Fig. 109.5C) but is more characteristic of RA (see Chapter 56). Evidence that cytokines, particularly interleukin-1 (IL-1), can stimulate chondrocytes to release matrix-destroying proteases (33,43) supports the observation that lacunar resorption is a significant pathologic process in cartilage destruction, regardless of disease specificity. Also, evidence has been presented that chondrocytes in OA are more sensitive to IL-1 action (43) due to increased receptor density (44).

DIMINUTION OF CHONDROCYTES

Once adulthood is reached, the unit number of chondrocytes changes little in articular cartilage with simple aging uncomplicated by disease (4). In contrast to chondrocyte proliferation associated with fibrillation, diffuse chondrocyte loss is frequently found in all layers of articular cartilage in OA. Relics of disintegrated cells are often seen associated with microscars. Similar changes have been described in experimental OA (4). Other experimental and clinical studies have suggested that chondrocyte necrosis is associated with areas of increased pressure (3). More recently, increased numbers of apoptotic chondrocytes have been demonstrated in OA (45).

FATTY DEGENERATION

Fine fat deposits in the interterritorial matrix represent an early degenerative change in cartilage; these may become larger, forming coarse droplets at the "capsule" of the chondrocyte. The content of triglyceride and complex lipids increases with age in the cells and in cartilage matrix even before fibrillation. Similar lipid degeneration has been described in osteoarthritic joint capsular tissues that have undergone nodular chondroid metaplasia (46). Increased arachidonic acid, the precursor of prostaglandins, is confined to the tangential layer (4). Prostaglandin release from osteoarthritic cartilage has been described (47), as well as qualitative and quantitative changes in gangliosides (48).

ALTERATION OF COLLAGEN FIBRILS

In aging articular cartilage, the general architecture and appearance of the collagen fibrils are preserved, although looser packing and occasional fragmentation are sometimes seen in the superficial layers. The aforementioned microscars increase in number as OA evolves. Some of the fragmented fibrils in these areas have a larger diameter. A progressive radial reorientation of the collagen fibrils has been noted by electron microscopy and by x-ray diffraction. Although amianthoid (asbestos-like) degeneration of the matrix has been described as a late feature of OA (49), this process typically occurs in costal and other extraarticular cartilage rather than in joint cartilage. In progressive OA, unraveling and disaggregation of collagen fibrils is usually apparent (50), although this may be secondary to changes in matrix protein polysaccharides.

GROSS CHANGES

Localized areas of softening of the cartilage are associated with a fine, velvety disruption of the surface. In these areas, one sees dehiscence of the cartilage along the axes of the matrix collagen fibers. In disruption confined to the surface tangential layer, the process is referred to as flaking; when the process extends to the deeper radial layer, it is described as fibrillation (Fig. 109.2). Because these minute discontinuities in the surface are readily stained grossly by India ink (4), they lend themselves to quantitative study. Abrasion of the fibrillated cartilage results in progressive erosion that may expose the underlying bony cortex (Fig. 109.1). The sites of predilection for destruction of the joint surface are those subject to greatest load bearing or shearing stress. Earliest fibrillation, however, is often present in regions with presumably low compressive stress, such as the infrafoveal portion of the femoral head. In the patella, the central facets are the sites most prone to erosion (4). Although not a weight-bearing joint, the patella is subjected to enormous loads by leverage when the knee is flexed, such as in stair-climbing or squatting. Repair cartilage, often of fibrocartilaginous type, is demonstrable grossly due to its bosselated, knobby appearance. As OA progresses, little original hyaline cartilage may remain. If osteophytes are present, these will be covered by a mixture of fibrocartilage and fibrous tissue. Hence, the translucent qualities of healthy hyaline cartilage will be absent.

LATE HISTOLOGIC CHANGES

In fibrillated regions, continuity of the surface of the articular cartilage is disrupted. The height of the fronds is in the range of 20 to 150 μm (4). Ground-substance metachromasia is reduced, and the matrix has a fibrillary, disheveled appearance. Birefringence of collagen fibrils is increased. Clusters of chondrocytes, long known as brood capsules, are located close to the margins of the clefts (Fig. 109.2B). The proliferative and proteoglycan-producing activities of these cells have been amply documented both *in vivo* and *in vitro* (38,39,51). Little or no collagen is seen within the clones, and it must be presumed that chondrolytic enzymes, including collagenases (33,34,52–54), have been generated to remove matrix to make room for the new cells (see Chapter 110).

The ultimate fate of these cellular clusters has been the subject of debate. Although small areas of necrobiosis are seen, these are not necessarily limited to the cell clusters. Focal proliferation of chondrocytes is also seen in deeper areas when severe lesions have disrupted the surrounding matrix. The matrix in these areas has a pale, myxoid appearance. Evidence indicates that type II collagen degradation products are present in osteoarthritic cartilage (4), along with enhanced synthesis of type II collagen (55). A class switch to production of types I and III collagens may occur as osteoarthritic changes progress, however (56–58). These collagens are predominantly deposited in the pericellular matrix (56,57). In these proliferative clusters, type X collagen has been identified and provides further evidence of chondrocyte hypertrophy (59,60) in osteoarthritic cartilage.

Suppression of matrix protein synthesis has been identified in the superficial zones of osteoarthritic cartilage (61). However, increases in biosynthetic activity of articular chondrocytes, even at some distance from the sites of overt damage to the cartilage, also have been described (4). Part of the confusion relates to the stage of OA from which cartilage has been obtained for study. In advanced lesions, the bulk of the cartilage is of a new and immature type. Thus, reparative cartilage typically is composed of a mixed hyaline and fibrocartilaginous tissue with more conspicuous fibrillary collagen and less intense staining for proteoglycan. Osteophytes are covered by a combination of a fibrocartilaginous surface with areas of overt fibrous tissue. In many cases, secondary degenerative change and fibrillation are then superimposed on the reparative cartilage, further complicating the histologic appearance. As a result, the histochemical and immunocytochemical features of the matrix are heterogeneous (4).

Degenerative changes in the basal calcified zone of articular cartilage are a consistent feature of OA. The junction of this calcified zone with the deep radial zone of articular cartilage is demarcated by an undulating hematoxyphlic line known as the tidemark. Reduplication of the tidemark (Fig. 109.5A) is exaggerated in the vicinity of the fibrillated cartilage and, more remotely, at the margin of the joint (4). Several types of degenerative change in the calcified zone have been described (12,62,63). Calcium-containing crystals are deposited in the territorial matrix of the adjacent chondrocytes as forward remodeling occurs. These crystals appear as basophilic granules in demineralized sections (Fig.109.5B) and within or around matrix vesicles in electron micrographs (12). The numbers and calcium-precipitating activities of matrix vesicle enzymes are increased in osteoarthritic cartilage compared to normal control articular cartilage (4,64). Osteonectin, a protein identified with early stages of calcification, was detected in chondrocytes above the calcified zone in osteoarthritic, but not in normal, cartilage (65). The process of pathologic advancement of the calcified zone contributes to bone production that consumes the articular cartilage from the subchondral aspect (Fig. 109.5F) and is an important aspect in the development of exposed bone (eburnation) at the joint surface.

BONE

New bone formation occurs in two separate locations in relation to the joint surface: in exophytic growths at the margins of the articular cartilage and in the immediately subjacent bone marrow (Fig. 109.4). Marginal osteophytes have two patterns of growth. One consists of a protuberance into the joint space, whereas the other develops within capsular and ligamentous attachments to the joint margins. In each circumstance the direction of the osteophyte is governed by the lines of mechanical force exerted on the area of growth, generally corresponding to the contour of the joint surface from which the osteophyte protrudes. The osteophyte consists in large part of bone that merges imperceptibly with the other cortical and cancellous tissue of the subchondral bone. The osteophyte is capped by a layer of hyaline and fibrocartilage continuous with the adjacent synovial lining. In advanced lesions, the landmarks are obliterated because the osteophytic surface itself undergoes degeneration, and fibrous tissue may cover the marginal portions of the osteophyte.

On the femoral head, proliferative tissue frequently occupies the fovea of the ligamentum teres and extends down along the femoral neck to form buttress osteophytes. These buttress osteophytes may obscure the normal boundary between the femoral head and the femoral neck. In most surgical specimens of the femoral head removed for OA, the combination of degenerative and proliferative activity has destroyed virtually all of the native articular cartilage.

The proliferation of bone in the subchondral tissue is most marked in areas denuded of their cartilaginous covering (4). In these regions, the articulating surface consists of bone that has been rubbed smooth. The glistening appearance of this polished sclerotic surface suggests ivory, hence the name eburnation. Nubbins of newly proliferated cartilage usually protrude through minute gaps in the eburnated bone. Proliferation of new bone at these sites is an integral part of eburnation (14,66). Dense bone at the articular surface is accompanied by marked sclerosis of the underlying subchondral bone (67).

"Cystic" areas of rarefaction of bone are commonly seen immediately beneath eburnated surfaces in the hip (Fig. 109.4A). Such structures are much less frequent in other joints. The cystic areas occur on both femoral and acetabular sides of the joint. The lesions are most frequently present on the superolateral weight-bearing surface. In severe instances, they may involve other regions of the hip as well (4). In a few cases, these lesions appear roentgenographically before narrowing of the joint space has given evidence of cartilage destruction. The lesions only infrequently contain pockets of mucoid fluid, and thus are not truly cystic (Fig. 109.5). The trabeculae in the affected areas disappear, and the bone marrow undergoes fibromyxoid degeneration. Fragments of dead bone, cartilage, and amorphous debris are often interspersed within them. In time, the entire area is encircled by a rim of reactive new bone and compact fibrous tissue (Fig. 109.3B). Minute gaps in the overlying articular cortex, resulting from microfractures, are commonly seen at the apex of the pseudocysts (Fig. 109.3). These findings are consistent with an intrusion of pressure, if not of synovial fluid, from the joint cavity through a defect in the articular cortex into the subchondral bone marrow. Intraarticular pressures exceeding 1,000 mm Hg occur in hip joints with effusions (4). The increased pressure is dissipated radially into the adjacent bone marrow, compressing the medullary blood vessels, and thereby leading to the retrogressive changes. This mechanism is not contradicted by observations that the intraosseous pressure is normal in osteoarthritic femoral heads at the time of arthroplasty. In these specimens, bulk pressures, rather than localized gradients, are measured. Furthermore, remodeling has compensated so that cysts are much less prominent in advanced lesions subjected to total hip arthroplasty. The "punched out" lesions observed radiographically in gout and the bone "cysts" in hemophilic arthropathy correspond pathologically to the pseudocysts in OA, except that they have specific exudates within the pseudocysts that are absent in OA.

New bone formation also occurs in the form of focal enchondral ossification at the base of the articular cartilage (62,63). Such metaplasia is a component of the remodeling process through which bone is added to a portion of the articular cortex while other areas of the joint undergo resorption of bone. The osteochondral junction is juxtaposed to a zone of calcified cartilage. During the period of active skeletal growth, this osteochondral junction has an epiphysis-like function that permits actual enlargement of the bone through sequential ossification of the calcified cartilage. In adults, the interface between calcified and noncalcified hyaline articular cartilage is demarcated by a thin, undulating, hematoxyphilic line known as the tidemark (Fig. 109.5A). In older persons, this line is usually transformed into several parallel discontinuous ones whose presence is clear evidence of the progression of calcification front into the articular cartilage (12). The possibility that the progression of the basilar calcification might lead to thinning of the articular cartilage (senile atrophy) in the absence of pathologic new bone formation in OA has not been substantiated (4).

The role of osteonecrosis in the generation of OA has been the subject of considerable discussion. Much of the deformity in symptomatic OA results from collapse of the joint surface. Localized areas of necrosis are seen frequently in this location, and occlusion of minute intramedullary arteries has been demonstrated in the past by angiography (4).

Furthermore, distinctive histologic differences have been noted between subchondral vessels of resected femoral heads in osteonecrosis and OA (68). Small secondary infarcts of eburnated bone are seen in approximately 6% to 14% of surgically resected femoral heads (69–71). Histochemical staining for lactate dehydrogenase has been used to show that the osteocytes of many bone trabeculae in OA are nonviable (72). Extensive morphologic studies have led to past suggestions that osteonecrosis might be involved in all cases of OA of the hip, but this clearly exceeds the evidence (4). Hypercoagulability demonstrated in patients with primary OA might also be operative in this complication (73). Nevertheless, rapidly destructive variants of OA are frequently accompanied by subchondral bone necrosis (74). Some patients with progressive OA have demonstrated sterile subchondral inflammatory foci histologically distinct from both pseudocyts and secondary osteonecrosis (75). These may also contribute to collapse of the articular surface.

CHONDROCALCINOSIS

The frequency of chondrocalcinosis, especially in the older age group (see also Chapters 117 and 118), has generated divergent opinions regarding the relationship of this condition to OA. Confusion over the exact role of chondrocalcinosis in OA is enhanced by the fact that calcium pyrophosphate dehydrate (CPPD) deposition disease, the most common form of chondrocalcinosis, occurs in both primary and secondary variants. The latter form of the disorder is associated with a wide range of conditions including hemochromatosis, ochronosis, hepatolenticular degeneration, hyperparathyroidism, acromegaly, and hemophilic arthropathy. The primary form of CPPD is frequently found in association with OA, especially in older patients (76). However, chondrocalcinosis is also exceptionally common as an asymptomatic phenomenon in the knee joints of elderly persons (77). The experience of Sokoloff and Varma (78) indicates that meniscal chondrocalcinosis is present in roughly half of knees treated surgically for OA after age 68. The risk for meniscal calcinosis in surgically removed knees was sixfold that of an age- and sex-adjusted postmortem population. Felson and co-workers (79) found a lower but significant association between OA of the knee and chondrocalcinosis using radiographic assessment in an epidemiologic study. By contrast, CPPD crystals are rarely found in femoral heads removed for OA. Chondrocalcinosis also is relatively infrequent in fractured hips before the age of 85 (4). Why the meniscus is the predominant site of involvement in OA of the knee, while the hyaline articular cartilages are largely spared, remains a matter of conjecture (80). Ordinarily, the deposition of CPPD in the osteoarthritic knee engenders no inflammatory reaction. Deposits of lipid are associated with CPPD deposits and are also present in the adjacent chondrocytes (81). The role of this lipid material in the deposition of crystals is unclear. Early CPPD deposition has also been associated with intracellular proteoglycan deposits in adjacent chondrocytes, suggesting an abnormal secretion pattern (4). In contrast to the articular chondrocytes that degenerate at sites of CPPD crystal deposition (82), meniscal fibrochondrocytes apparently remain metabolically active in the presence of these crystals (4). Several observers have noted that joint mice are more frequent in OA specimens with chondrocalcinosis than in those without crystal deposition.

In a recent study, serum nucleotide pyrophosphohydrolase activity was increased in patients with OA whether or not CPPD crystals were present in joints (83). To further complicate the situation, some cases of OA harbor CPPD crystals that are too small to be resolved by conventional polarizing microscopy (84). This leads to the possibility that the role of CPPD crystals in the pathogenesis of OA might be underestimated. Since apoptotic chondrocytes produced pyrophosphate in one study (85), a common basic mechanism of chondrocyte injury may be operative whether or not CPPD crystals are produced as the end result.

Another form of radiologic chondrocalcinosis is associated with deposition of basic calcium phosphate (BCP) (apatite) crystals. The observation that BCP crystals are quantitatively associated with more severe cases of OA of the knee has promoted the theory that BCP crystals might be released from abraded eburnated surfaces (4), but this has not been established. However, BCP crystal deposition is characteristically associated with more severe arthropathy and occasional Charcot-like breakdown of joints (see Chapter 118). Unlike CPPD crystals, most of which can be seen with conventional polarizing microscopy, BCP crystals are too small (84) and require specialized techniques such as alizarin red staining of centrifuged synovial fluid for detection (see Chapter 118). Thus, it is difficult to establish the presence of BCP crystals in severe OA unless a specific search is employed.

SOFT TISSUE

During recent years, the inflammatory manifestations of OA have stimulated considerable discussion. By definition, OA is inherently a noninflammatory condition, but some degree of synovial villous hypertrophy and fibrosis are seen in the majority of symptomatic cases (Fig. 109.6). A moderate focal chronic synovitis has been described in about one-fifth of surgically resected specimens (4). This synovitis is characterized by hyperplasia and enlargement of synovial lining cells and by the presence of lymphocytes and mononuclear cells (86,87). The infiltrate is generally mild and heterogeneous with respect to immunopathology (4). Polyclonal B lymphocytes compose part of the infiltrate, and extracellular deposits of complement component C3 also have been described (4). Fibronectin is deposited in exudative foci (4). Other tissue changes such as hemosiderin deposition, foreign body reaction to joint detritus, and xanthoma-like changes around fat necrosis may be seen. The stage of any particular case may be important, as the synovial response has been visualized as evolving from an early exudative to a late fibrotic stage (88). In a few cases the synovial inflammation may be so pronounced as to resemble RA. Immunopathologic studies, however, show significant qualitative differences in the infiltrates charac-

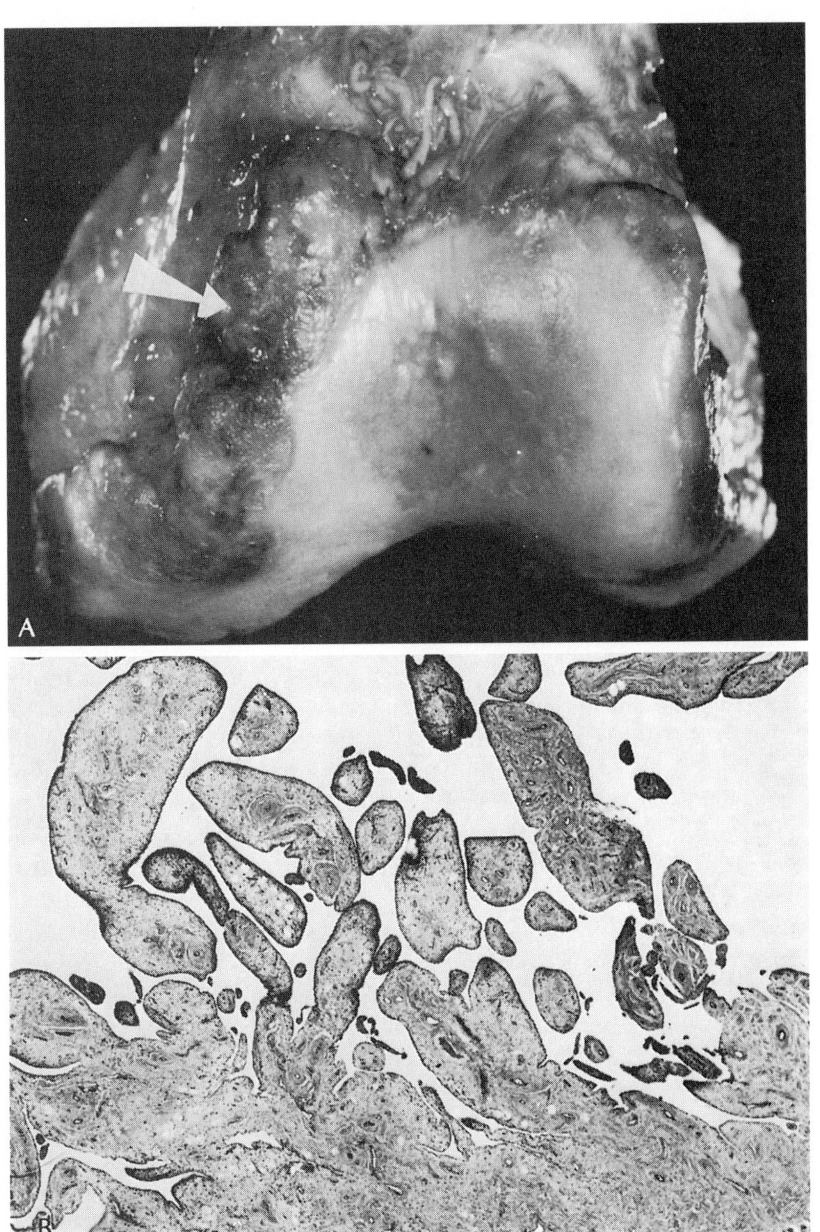

FIGURE 109.6. Synovial hypertrophy in severe osteoarthritis. The patient is a 63-year-old man whose left knee had been enlarged for 23 years following an automobile accident. **A:** A massive osteophyte *(arrow)* is seen at the medial border of the articular surface. The adjacent synovial tissue has undergone prominent papillary thickening. **B:** Histologically, the villous processes are made up of compact tissue not infiltrated by inflammatory cells. (H&E ×16.)

terizing the two diseases. Synovial macrophages are more frequent in RA (89,90), as are cells bearing activation antigens (89). The mean nuclear density of cellularity is higher in RA, and immunoglobulin-producing plasma cells, common in RA, are rare in osteoarthritic synovia (86). Immunoblasts are not seen in the synovial fluid in OA (4). Helper/suppressor (CD4/CD8) ratios vary between upper and lower synovial regions in RA but are uniform throughout the synovium in OA (86). Although $CD4^+$ T cells are more numerous in RA synovium (91), natural killer (NK) cells with $CD16/56^+$ phenotype are more frequent in OA (92). In line with this latter observation, NK cell–associated granzyme expression is also increased in osteoarthritic synovial specimens (93). Mast cells are also found in increased numbers in the synovium of patients (94) with OA and in one recent report were actually more numerous than in synovium from RA patients (95). Their actual participation in joint damage in OA has not been established.

Taken as a whole, these findings clearly differentiate the cellular inflammatory responses in OA from those in RA. However, the presence of inflammation in many cases of OA is undeniable. Epidemiologic studies have linked progression of early radiologic OA of the knee to higher serum levels of the inflammatory marker C-reactive protein (96). Similar low-grade inflammatory responses occur in other joint diseases of nonphlogistic origin such as those accompanying acromegaly, ochronosis, and neuropathic arthropathies.

Autosensitization to joint detritus is an attractive consideration in the genesis of the inflammatory reaction. A so-called detritic synovitis is observed in many cases of severe OA requiring joint replacement, but is much less common in early cases treated with arthroscopic surgery (97). The resulting reaction to osteocartilaginous fragments not only results in inflammation, but may result in generation of cytokines by synovial macrophages. Such cytokines are associated with synovial inflammation in OA (98). Detritic synovitis also produces a possible mechanism for autosensitization to cartilage structural proteins. In fact, cartilage-derived molecules are present in sera of patients with OA (99,100), as well as other diseases (101).

Additional supportive evidence for autosensitization is the finding of autoantibodies directed against both native and denatured type II collagen in 50% of OA cartilage extracts (4). Analysis of DNA restriction enzyme patterns of T lymphocytes from osteoarthritic synovia show an oligoclonal pattern of T-cell receptor β chain gene rearrangements, suggesting a response by a limited number of T-cell clones (102), as might occur in a response to released indigenous articular cartilage molecules. Peripheral blood lymphocytes from OA patients are highly reactive in proliferation assays against human cartilage link protein (103). Evidence for an immune response in certain types of OA also includes the finding of immunoglobulin-complement complexes deposited in the superficial zones of osteoarthritic articular cartilage (104). Whether the deposits in OA are a primary phenomenon or merely a response to matrix damage is not known, but autoantibodies associated with deposition in articular cartilage are a recognized finding in generalized, nodal OA (105).

As previously discussed, another possible mechanism for the inflammatory changes in the synovium involves responses to CPPD or BCP crystals (106,107). Both species occur in the synovium in cartilage and in the synovial fluid (see Chapters 117 and 118). Crystals have been proposed as one mechanism for induction of cytokine release, particularly IL-1. IL-1 stimulates synovial cells and articular chondrocytes to release neutral proteases capable of destroying cartilage matrix (44). Studies have also implicated tumor necrosis factor (TNF) in the process (108). Human osteoarthritic cartilage is enriched with partially degraded type II collagen (109), indicating that this mechanism may be of significance in perpetuating articular destruction.

Other soft tissues also participate in OA. Minute tears in capsular tissue appear as slender, fibrovascular seams disrupting the principal axes of the collagen bundles. Secondary osteochondromatosis occurs at times, but is much more characteristic of neuropathic arthropathy than of OA. In the hip joints, the ligamentum teres commonly disintegrates. In the knee joint, the cruciate ligaments and menisci also become frayed. Substantial clinical (110) and experimental (4) evidence suggests that meniscectomy leads to OA, but no correlation has been found in autopsy material between tears or other lesions of the semilunar cartilages and OA (4). Furthermore, postmeniscectomy OA of the knee shows a strong association with OA of the hands and opposite knee (111). Degeneration was more severe, however, on the operated side and was independent of age and sex. This study suggests that a predisposition to primary OA influences the development of secondary degeneration and makes a clear distinction between these two subsets of the disease more difficult. Others have found evidence of increased prevalence of generalized OA in individuals with severe knee (4) or hip OA (112). Although meniscectomy resulted in OA, underlying or systemic factors may thus have contributed to its severity.

Among other soft tissue changes, fibrillation and fibrosis of the synovial surface and even mild cartilaginous metaplasia of the patellar tendon have been described. Lipochondral degeneration is seen in hip capsular tissues that have previously undergone nodular chondroid metaplasia (46). Amyloid deposits have been reported in the joint capsule in OA (113), but they also occur in joint capsules and articular cartilage of normal joints and in the intraarticular discs of older individuals (4,114). An association with CPPD crystals has been described (4). Amyloid or amyloid-like materials, however, have been described in several different tissues of aged individuals (4). Any claim for specificity for amyloid in cartilage requires a considerably more discriminatory technique than screening by green birefringence after Congo red staining, the usual histochemical method. Destructive amyloid arthropathy is characteristic not of OA, but of dialysis-associated osteoarthropathy due to β_2-microglobulin retention (114) (see Chapters 92 and 94).

A progressive increase in the amount of fibrous tissue separating the synovial capillaries from the joint space has been described as an age-related finding, but it is unlikely that this condition interferes with the nourishment of the cartilage. Focal hyaline sclerosis of minute vessels is a common finding even in joint tissues of young individuals (4). It is unlikely that this finding is directly related to OA. Periarticular muscle undergoes atrophy with type 2 myofibers being affected primarily (4).

BIOCHEMICAL PATHOLOGY OF OSTEOARTHRITIS

Understanding of the biochemical changes in OA has been rapidly advanced in recent years, as discussed in Chapter 110. The principal pitfalls in interpreting biochemical data are the problems of sampling variability and of discriminating changes associated with OA from those associated with aging (see Chapter 11). When living tissue is required for metabolic studies, the source is frequently surgically resected femoral heads. Sampling of reparative rather than degenerated native cartilage from such specimens probably accounts for the major discrepancies noted between biochemical data from articular cartilage obtained from necropsy (4) and that from surgically resected specimens (see Chapter 110). Similar variability can be introduced by using fractured femoral heads as a source of control cartilage because such tissue undergoes secondary changes following injury (4). The knee joint is recommended for study by some authors for this reason. Although the destructive process commonly is unicompartmental, the other condyle is not immune from the complex processes that are in part proliferative. Finally, biochemical properties in nonarticular cartilages show significant differences in some parameters (4). Thus, such findings are difficult to extrapolate to the pathobiology of articular cartilage.

The cell and molecular biology of cartilage collagens also provides insight into the changes in structural proteins occurring in OA. Type II collagen accumulates in the matrix in early OA (4), accompanied by increased synthesis of the molecule (55). Although type II collagen continues to be produced by osteoarthritic repair cartilage, types I and III collagens are also demonstrated in more advanced cases of OA (56–58). Evidence is accumulating that changes in the distribution of minor collagens found in articular cartilage (types VI, IX, and XI) may predispose to breakdown of the principal collagen, type II (116). Type VI collagen is normally found in very small amounts in the pericellular domains (4) of normal cartilage, but increases markedly in early experimental OA (4). Type X collagen, normally associated with hypertrophic epiphyseal chondrocytes, also appears in osteoarthritic cartilage (59,60). Cartilage matrix protein synthesis is suppressed in the more superficial zones of cartilage in OA as well (61). Immunohistochemical techniques are necessary to localize collagens and other proteins to specific areas because biochemical findings from fibrillated articular cartilage may differ considerably from those in nondegenerated areas.

COMPARATIVE PATHOLOGY OF OSTEOARTHRITIS

Osteoarthritis occurs widely in the vertebrae kingdom, regardless of the position of the species in the taxonomic scale. Osteophytic lesions, sometimes leading to ankylosis, were common in certain giant dinosaurs 100 million years ago. The disorder has been observed in large and small mammals, in animals that swim (cetaceans) rather than bear their weight on their extremities, and also, to a mild degree, in birds (117). It is of considerable economic importance in livestock commerce, the horse-racing industry, and veterinary practice.

In small laboratory animals, it has been possible to study a number of pathogenetic concepts of OA. The importance of genetic factors has been established in mice (4) The inheritance appears to be polygenic and the overall behavior recessive. No evidence suggests major sex linkage, although male mice consistently develop more severe OA than do females. Obesity is not an important factor (4). In laboratory rodents, the knee and elbow joints are commonly affected severely, but the hips rarely. That inheritable biochemical defects are major factors in the development of OA is suggested by the frequency of osteoarthritic lesions in blotchy (BLO) mice, in which a mutant gene leads to inadequate cross-linking of collagen (118). In the STR/ORT mouse, widely studied for its predisposition to OA (119–121), Walton (122) attributed knee joint changes to spontaneous patellar subluxation. Surgical containment of the subluxation prevented the development of OA. Susceptibility to OA in these animals seems attributable to abnormal mechanical loading rather than to a cartilage metabolic abnormality. Although impressive, these data are difficult to reconcile with Sokoloff's (3) observations that lesions in STR/IN mice were not confined to the knee but were more generalized. One study suggested that synovial acute and chronic inflammatory infiltrates of the patellofemoral joints in STR/ORT mice are so prominent that the use of this strain as a model of human OA should be questioned (119). More generalized cartilage degeneration has been observed in guinea pigs as well (123), especially in the Dunkin-Hartley strain (124). Genetic factors influencing the development of OA may be exerted at many levels—local and generalized, mechanical and metabolic.

The genetic aspects of OA are also manifested by variable susceptibility of different species to its development. Rats, for example, are generally resistant, whereas another rodent, *Mastomys natalensis,* develops a severe generalized OA by the age of 2 years. Another desert rodent, the Mediterranean sand rat *(Psammomys obesus)* develops a severe degenerative spondylosis with disc thinning and anterior vertebral hyperostosis reminiscent of human hyperostotic spondylosis (125). Genetic contributions to OA are also seen in certain breeds of cattle and swine. The fundamental pathogenetic problem is whether these genetic factors are local and articular, related to the configuration and mechanical forces exerted on the joint, as in the dysplastic hips of German shepherd dogs (126,127), or whether they are more generalized metabolic properties of the articular tissues. Such concerns complicate the use of spontaneous animal models of OA as paradigms of the human disease, as well as influence the choice of various species and strains as subjects for experimental induction of OA.

EXPERIMENTAL INDUCTION

Numerous animal models of OA have been developed (128). Some directly damage articular cartilage. Small surgically induced defects do not usually produce OA. Larger defects deforming the joint contour, however, may result in OA, and direct damage to cartilage by heat, freezing (4), or other physical agents may also cause OA. Synovitis induced by intrasynovial instillation of irritants may eventuate in osteoarthritic changes, but these may have acted on the cartilage as well (4). Subluxation of the patella and hip dislocation have produced early remodeling and later OA. Surgical interruption of the cruciate ligaments, usually the anterior, are frequently used to induce OA in a relatively short time in both dogs (10,129,130) and rabbits (131,132). Partial meniscectomy is used in a similar way in rabbits (9,133) and valgus tibial osteotomy in dogs (134,135). Prolonged compression of the articular cartilages for even a few days causes death of chondrocytes, which may be followed by OA. This sequence is presumably due to prevention of percolation of interstitial fluids into the cartilage (4). Restriction of joint motion was found in older studies to lead to degeneration resembling OA, but one problem with such studies is that it is difficult to restrict joint mobility without altering joint loading (136). Others have found that motion in the absence of weight-bearing does not maintain normal articular cartilage (4). In humans immobilized for long periods, contracture and fibrous ankylosis develop rather than OA (4). A similar pattern is seen in immature spastic cerebral palsy (137).

Repetitive impact loading has been used to induce degenerative changes resembling early OA in animal models (138). Intraarticular instillation of abrasive particles such as Carborundum induces superficial degeneration of articular cartilage and a foreign body reaction in the synovium. The similarity to the pattern of synovitis induced by cartilage detritus is apparent (6). Enzymes, such as bacterial collagenase, induce degenerative changes and osteophyte formation when injected into mouse joints (139). A variety of experimental manipulations that directly affect the viability of articular chondrocytes or the integrity of the surrounding matrix can result in OA-like disease. Other procedures placing abnormal mechanical stresses on joints can induce remodeling of articular contours (140). The application of any of these models to human disease requires discretion.

DEGENERATIVE DISEASE OF THE SPINAL COLUMN

Degenerative changes in the spine affect two discrete, but interrelated, articular systems: the amphiarthroses (discs) and the diarthrodial (zygapophyseal or facet) joints. The former develop qualitative and quantitative changes (141) with increasing age, characterized by loss of ground substance metachromasia (4) and matrix water content, increased vascularization of the hyaline cartilage end plates, and disorderly and attenuated collagen fibrils (4). In many individuals, such degeneration leads to annulus fibrosis tears (142), disc herniation, and to the breakdown of the cartilaginous end plates with the development of spinal osteochondrosis (143). The prominent osteochondral osteophytes (144) that develop in this condition have led to the wide use of the term *spondylosis deformans* (see Chapters 102 and 103). Osteophytes are most commonly found at the T9-10 and L3 interspaces (145). However, the cervical spine is very susceptible to the clinical manifestations of this condition (146).

The spinal diarthrodial joints develop osteoarthritic changes similar to those in peripheral joints. This distinction in terms should not lead to the conclusion that the two processes are unrelated, because the pathologic findings in the joints are similar. The nucleus pulposus becomes fissured and deformed, and similar cracks appear in the annulus fibrosus (142). Fibrillary disintegration of the hyaline cartilage plates, through which the disc is attached to the vertebral bodies, cannot be distinguished histologically from the changes in diarthrodial OA. Eburnation of the subchondral bony plate develops in like manner. Marginal osteophytes arise under the mechanical stimulus of horizontal pulsion of the annulus fibrosus and its periosteal attachments as a result of collapse and spreading out of the nucleus pulposus. Traction forces by spinal muscles on the tendinous insertions in this region also have been implicated in this disorder. Furthermore, intervertebral disc disease shifts a greater proportion of the compressive and torsional loads on the apophyseal facet joints (4), contributing to further degenerative changes.

Another feature of spinal osteochondrosis is the development of nodules of cartilaginous and fibrous tissue beneath the subchondral plate of the vertebral bodies called Schmorl's nodes, which are usually attributed to the displacement of a nucleus pulposus into a vertebral body (4). These islands are often surrounded by a shell of bone and, except for their greater content of cartilage, are reminiscent of the subchondral cysts in osteoarthritic peripheral joints. Schmorl's nodes are not a pathognomonic feature of vertebral osteoporosis, because they occur commonly in degenerative disc disease not associated with osteopenia. Several studies have confirmed that degenerative disc disease and osteochondrosis are positively associated with increased bone mass (147–149). A similar relationship has been described for OA of the hands (150).

Although the marginal osteophytes develop most often on the anterolateral aspects of the vertebral bodies, posterior osteophytic protrusions occur and may affect the spinal cord and its roots. In the cervical region, spondylosis constitutes a hazard among older patients because of the resultant spinal stenosis (see Chapter 103). In the lumbar region, spinal stenosis develops with encroachment of osteophytes on the spinal canal and is frequently due to degenerative spondylolisthesis associated with OA of the apophyseal joints (143). Osteophytes in the Luschka (uncovertebral, neurocentral) joints have been shown by anatomic and angiographic means to compromise the neighboring vertebral arteries (see Chapter 100). The narrowing of the vascular lumen is most marked during rotation of the head and provides the basis for the posterior cervical sympathetic or Barre-Lieou syndrome.

OA does not characteristically lead to ankylosis; however, in at least three forms of segmental disease of the senescent spine, bony bridges unite the vertebral bodies. The proclivity for ankylosis may be related to the inherent limited mobility of the intervertebral disc.

HYPEROSTOTIC SPONDYLOSIS

Of the vertebral ankylosing disorders, the best known entity goes by several names: hyperostotic spondylosis, senile ankylosing hyperostosis of Forestier and Rotes-Querol, and spondylorrheostosis. Hyperostotic spondylosis nominally is distinguished from ordinary spondylosis by the absence of disc degeneration (4,151). The distal thoracic spine is the site of predilection (143). The ankylotic bridges are located on the anterolateral portions of the vertebral bodies and extend into the anterior longitudinal ligaments (Fig. 109.7). This appearance has often led to confusion with ankylosing spondylitis. However, ankylosing hyperostosis is not an inflammatory disorder, unlike the spondyloarthropathies. Ossification of the posterior longitudinal ligament is also frequently associated with vertebral hyperostosis (152) as is ossification of the stylohyoid ligament (153). In some instances the vertebral lesion is accompanied by excessive osteophyte formation in peripheral joints. From this feature comes still another term for this condition, *diffuse idiopathic skeletal hyperostosis* (DISH) (154–156). Currently, no consensus exists as to the definition of the DISH syndrome. Hyperglycemia is a common clinical finding in these patients (see Chapter 111). A possible relationship to relative excess of growth hormone has been postulated (157).

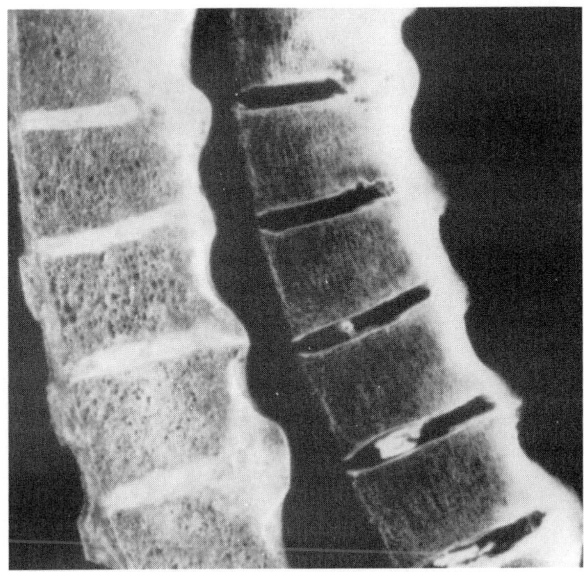

FIGURE 109.7. Hyperostotic spondylosis in the thoracic spine of an elderly male. Unlike the lesions of ankylosing spondylitis (Marie-Strumpell arthritis), the vertebral bodies do not manifest a "squared" appearance. Ossification has developed in the intervertebral discs, and the disc space is also narrowed anteriorly. Ossification in the anterior longitudinal ligament has blended with a hyperostotic response of the anterior vertebral bodies forming a continuous bony bridge (×0.5). (Courtesy of Professor W. A. Gardner, M.D., University of South Alabama.)

ANKYLOSIS

Ankylosis, distinct from that of hyperostotic spondylosis, may accompany severe spondylosis in humans and other species. The disc space is narrowed. Destructive changes are present in the cortex of the anterior portion of the vertebral bodies (143,146). Dense new bone formation is seen in the anterior longitudinal ligament. The appearance suggests that the ligament is first avulsed from the osteophyte and then repaired.

OTHER SEGMENTAL DISEASE

Several patterns of dorsal protrusion and bridging of cervical vertebrae (posterior spondylotic osteophytes) may cause life-threatening cervical myelopathy (146). The relation of physiologic vertebral ligamentous ossification to the preceding disorder and to hyperostotic spondylosis is uncertain (152). It occurs in 7% of Japanese (158) and 0.3% of United States adults (4). These lesions are asymptomatic in individuals with large spinal canals, but they require surgical decompression when spinal canals are small and myelopathy has developed (159).

Baastrup's syndrome, an OA-like change that is due to bursitis between the distal portions of "kissing" lumbar dorsal spinous processes (143), is usually associated with severe spondylosis.

SPECIAL FORMS OF OSTEOARTHRITIS

Heberden's Nodes

Despite the relative antiquity of the description of Heberden's nodes and their frequency, comparatively little information is available on their histopathology. They are usually manifested as marginal osteophytes of the distal interphalangeal joints. In more advanced cases, these lesions are indistinguishable from those arising in osteoarthritic remodeling in other sites (Fig. 109.8). Ossific transformation of the tendinous insertion into the joint capsule creates the osteophytosis. In other instances, mucoid transformation of the periarticular fibroadipose tissue is associated with proliferation of myxoid fibroblasts and cyst formation.

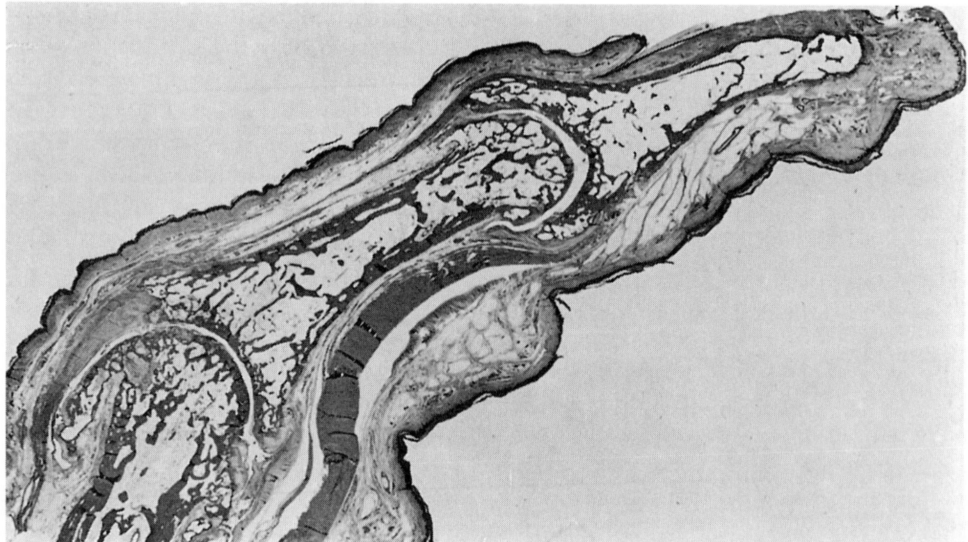

FIGURE 109.8. Heberden node. The articular cartilage has completely disappeared from the surfaces of the distal interphalangeal joint. Bony osteophytes, directed toward the base of the finger, are present on the dorsal and palmer aspects of both articulating surfaces. Advanced osteoarthritic changes also are present in the proximal interphalangeal joint and form a so-called Bouchard node. (H&E ×20.)

These types of Heberden's nodes are usually associated with radiographically demonstrable distal interphalangeal osteophytes but not invariably so (160). These cysts, like the osteophytes, are not unique anatomic features of Heberden's nodes. Indistinguishable changes may be present in other osteoarthritic joints and in other species. The process has certain morphologic similarities to ganglion formation or to cystic degeneration of the semilunar cartilages and to the subchondral pseudocysts of OA. Unilateral sparing from Heberden nodes after hemiplegia has been reported (161). This observation suggests the possibility of neurovascular contributions to the development of the lesion, but does not exclude a biomechanical explanation since one study comparing groups of women with qualitatively similar manual tasks definitely related Heberden node formation to the quantitative use of the hands (162). The association of the paraarticular mucous cysts of the distal interphalangeal joints with osteophytes has been emphasized because they are likely to recur following excision unless the osteophytes are also removed (see Chapter 48).

The term *erosive osteoarthritis* (see Chapter 111) has been applied to a disorder resembling OA in its predilection for the distal and proximal interphalangeal joints, but in which a distinct inflammatory component exists (163). A nonspecific, chronic synovial lymphocytic and mononuclear cell infiltrate is present. The nosologic status of the disorder is uncertain. One possibility is that this entity simply represents OA with a prominent, detritic synovitis. In a few cases, the lesion disseminates (4) to other joints and has been reported to evolve into RA. Such RA patients, however, are generally seronegative and show a much greater tendency toward osteophyte formation than patients with seropositive RA. Variants of nodal OA associated with chronic sialadenitis have also been described (164) whose relationships to erosive arthritis and seronegative RA are unclear. Bony ankylosis may occasionally occur in the finger joints in association with Heberden's nodes, especially of the inflammatory type.

GENERALIZED FORMS OF OSTEOARTHRITIS

The generalized forms of OA are variants having in common a marked tendency to polyarticular involvement. With the exception of most endemic arthritis, all have degrees of heritability and some are now linked to specific molecular defects in structural or regulatory proteins.

Primary Generalized Osteoarthritis

Primary generalized OA was first defined as an entity by Kellgren et al. (165). Conspicuous features of the disorder included a preponderance in middle-aged women, Heberden node formation, and involvement of the first carpometacarpal and knee joints. Hip joints were affected less commonly. Key features of the syndrome included signs of articular inflammation and radiologic evidence that proliferation of adjacent bone, rather than erosion of articular cartilage, was the primary event in the genesis of the lesions. The description of the syndrome was based on limited anatomic material, a situation not entirely corrected by succeeding studies (160,163).

The status of generalized OA remains controversial. Most patients with this pattern of disease do not present for surgical intervention. Thus, the condition is far more common in rheumatologic than in orthopedic practice. Some studies have confirmed an association of generalized OA with OA of the hips (166), whereas others have denied this relationship. The association of OA of the hands and knees has been established by radiologic studies (167). From the obverse viewpoint (4), patients requiring hip and knee surgery for localized OA are significantly more likely to have generalized disease as well. When hip disease is associated with Heberden's nodes, particularly in patients with inflammatory features, it is of the concentric type (4) rather than the more common deforming type. Some authors maintain that this pattern is only a part of the generalized OA syndrome (4). The genetic predisposition to the development of generalized OA has been related to several types of markers. These include increased frequency of human leukocyte antigens HLA-A1 and HLA-B8 (168), certain hereditary polymorphisms of the estrogen receptor gene (169), and abnormalities on chromosome 2q (170). Using radiographic hand and knee OA as the index condition, segregation analyses suggest a significant contribution from a major recessive gene together with possible environmental factors (171). This supports the observations made a generation previously (165).

Osteoarthritis Caused by Heritable Collagen Defects

Other forms of polyarticular OA associated with mutant type II collagens have been described in several unrelated families (172–175) (see Chapters 9, 110, and 111). These disorders produce precocious generalized OA with accentuated involvement of weight-bearing joints. In one family, a mild spondylodysplasia with truncal shortening was present (172), and in two others more severe manifestations of spondyloepiphyseal dysplasia were noted (173,176). In the mildly spondylodysplastic family, a single point mutation at residue 519 in the triple helical domain substituted cysteine for arginine, producing abnormal posttranslational overmodification (174). The abnormal collagen has been isolated from cartilage remaining on a surgically excised femoral head from an affected family member (177) in which about one-quarter of the α1(II) chains contained the substitution. This was associated with severe precocious ulceration of articular cartilage. In a more severely dysplastic family, an entire exon coding for 36 amino acids was deleted from the type II triple helical domain (176) with a calculated effect that 90% of the type II collagen homotrimers would be abnormal in the heterozygous state. Electron microscopy of articular cartilage in one kindred demonstrated parallel lamellar arrays of collagen fibrils rather than the normal structure (175). Affected families showed definite or probable autosomal-dominant inheritance (172–175) with an age-dependent penetrance approaching 100%. Some other family studies suggest an inherited defect in one of the introns or promoters for the procollagen II gene (178).

Evidence to link defects in the type II procollagen gene to the common type of generalized nodal OA has not as yet been readily forthcoming. Molecular analysis of DNA from cases of generalized erosive nodal OA failed to disclose evidence of a single point mutation in collagen II α1(II) chain residue 519 (174). Sibling pair analysis in generalized nodal OA also fails to suggest linkage to loci encoding type II collagen (179). Some studies have suggested differential allelic expression from sequence dimorphisms of the type II collagen gene in osteoarthritic cartilage, but this could be a manifestation of somatic mutation (180). Furthermore, the usual pattern in generalized OA does not include a clinically detectable spondyloarthropathy (see Chapter 111).

OCHRONOTIC ARTHROPATHY

Alkaptonuria is caused by a deficiency in homogentisic acid oxidase caused by a mutation on chromosome 3q (181) that eventually results in a generalized degeneration of joints similar to OA (see Chapter 121). Several differences are notable, however. External remodeling is less prominent than in idiopathic OA (4). Destructive spinal changes are marked. This includes a calcification or ossification of the nucleus pulposus of the intervertebral discs and breakdown of the vertebral end plates. Osteophyte production is not a conspicuous feature of the spondylopathy either. In many cases, the spinal disease is so severe as to imitate that of a mucopolysaccharidosis (see Chapter 94) or ankylosing spondylitis (182). The pigmented cartilage is extremely brittle, so that comminution with a resultant detritic synovitis is prominent. Pigmented cartilage fragments are found in the synovial fluid (183). Reactive polyps of the synovium containing these fragments are common and may be mistaken for loose bodies on radiographs. Fibrosis near ulcerated zones of the articular surface along with wavy alterations of the cartilage collagenous fibrillar ultrastructure has been noted (184). A complicating feature is that both calcium pyrophosphate and BCP crystals have been identified in ochronotic cartilage (4). Homogentisic acid, the substance that accumulates in cartilage in ochronosis, has been shown to inhibit chondrocyte metabolism *in vitro* (185), possibly by producing oxidative DNA damage (186).

GOUT

The arthropathy of gout develops as a consequence of the deposition of monosodium urate monohydrate crystals in and around joint tissues (see Chapter 114). Mono-, oligo-, and polyarticular forms occur. The character of the lesions depends on the amount, location, and duration of the deposits. Acute inflammatory episodes are a hallmark of the disease. These are likely to affect the small joints of the feet, particularly the first metatarsophalangeal joint, but large weight-bearing joints also can be involved.

Although tophaceous deposits can cause massive disorganization of articular structures, most cases with recurrent acute gout result in secondary OA of the postinflammatory type. Even in the absence of clinical acute inflammation, urate crystals may still be detected by polarized light microscopy of synovial fluid (187). Pathologically, the urate crystals are deposited not only in and on the surface of the articular cartilage, but also in the subchondral marrow. Chondrocytes are characteristically necrotic and often surrounded by an oxyphilic matrix in areas of urate crystal deposition. Urate crystals are quite soluble in neutral buffered 4% formaldehyde, the routine histologic fixative. If tissue confirmation of gout is required, fixation in 95% alcohol should be employed (188).

ENDEMIC OSTEOARTHRITIS

The term *endemic osteoarthritis* encompasses special types of noninflammatory deforming joint disease occurring frequently in certain geographically confined areas (4). Although these disorders have certain features in common with generalized OA, they differ from the latter in affecting younger individuals and in producing stunted growth. Although evidence of pathogenesis is accumulating in several different countries, workers continue to speculate on the cause of these disorders. Three types currently receiving attention are discussed here.

Kashin-Beck Disease

Kashin-Beck disease, formerly known as *endemic osteoarthrosis deformans*, affects at least 2 million individuals in northern China, North Korea, Siberia (189), and Tibet (190). The changes first appear during childhood and develop with variable severity in different affected individuals. The early changes consist of a zonal necrosis of the articular and epiphyseal chondrocytes (191). Profound deformity is the result in many affected individuals (192). Several theories as to the cause of the disorder have emerged. The most evidence favors the soil and water in the region being deficient in selenium and iodine (193,194), and the combination of these two factors results in the disorder. Although earlier studies failed to demonstrate inhibitory effects of selenium deficiency on short-term chondrocyte monolayer cultures (195), intact selenium-deficient mice develop a Kashin-Beck type osteoarthropathy when supplemented with dietary fulvic acid, a product of mold growth (196). Interestingly, mycotoxins, particularly those of *Fusarium* sp. have long been suspected as having some role in the disorder (4). Fulvic acid, a complex contaminant of water derived from decay of moldy soil, inhibits processing of type II procollagen in chicken articular cartilage (197). Related mold-derived compounds known as the humic acid solvent extraction fraction induce oxidative stress in cultured rabbit articular chondrocytes (198). Thus, a synergism between selenium deficiency and mold toxins may be the basis of the disorder.

Mseleni Disease

Mseleni disease, common in northern Zululand, has been described more recently than Kashin-Beck disease. The disorder is polyarticular and noninflammatory, and the hip is particularly susceptible. In surgically resected femoral heads, eburnation was absent. The joint surface was instead covered by a combination of regenerated and degenerated cartilage (199). Some investigators have proposed that the disorder is heterogeneous, in part being hereditary spondyloepiphyseal dysplasia (200). With regard to spondyloepiphyseal dysplasia, localized occurrences of a dwarfing variant have been described (201), and some studies have suggested mutation in the type II collagen gene (202). Patients with Mseleni joint disease are also more likely to show histologic evidence of osteopenia, osteomalacia, and osteoclast failure, but abnormalities in calcium metabolism have not been identified (203). Generalized OA of the usual sort seen in predominantly European populations occurs less frequently in black Africans (204). Handigodu disease is another form of proliferative OA seen in a geographically confined region of South India. The disorder is polyarticular, affects both genders, and can lead to severe deformity. Many similarities to Mseleni osteoarthropathy exist. However, Handigodu disease demonstrates an autosomal-dominant pattern of inheritance (205). Heredity dwarfing variants of Mseleni disease have been previously discussed (201).

HEMOPHILIC ARTHROPATHY

Joint disease following recurrent hemarthroses in the hemophilias has many features in common with OA (206). Like ordinary OA, erosion of articular cartilage occurs early accompanied by eburnation of bone and marginal osteophyte formation. Unlike the subchondral pseudocysts of OA, those in hemophilic arthropathy are filled with hemorrhagic material. The synovium usually contains such immense quantities of hemosiderin that it appears reddish-brown grossly, but only minute quantities can be detected in articular chondrocytes (4). How the iron reaches the chondrocytes is unknown because excessive iron is not detectable in the matrix (4). In advanced lesions, the destruction of the joint is more profound than that seen in OA, with disintegration and fibrous ankylosis being the end result. Although hemophilic arthropathy may affect any combination of joints, the larger peripheral joints are particularly prone to severe involvement, especially the knee and elbow joints.

The pathogenesis of the cartilage destruction is not completely understood, although it is somehow related to recurrent articular hemorrhage (see Chapter 94). Two general hypotheses are entertained. One is that chondrolytic enzymes are released from hemosiderin-laden synovial macrophages (4). A second is that cartilage damage is due to toxic products of hemoglobin degradation such as free radicals created by ionic iron from degraded hemoglobin. Iron may also chelate proteoglycans and alter the elastic properties of the matrix (4).

OSTEOARTHRITIS ASSOCIATED WITH OTHER HERITABLE OSTEOARTICULAR DISEASES

A number of types of multiple epiphyseal dysplasia have been described (207). In these rare conditions, epiphyseal growth and maturation of variable portions of the axial and appendicular skeleton are defective. Some are known to be associated with abnormalities of the type II procollagen gene (172,177), as described previously. Many affected persons die in infancy (206), but precocious OA develops with great frequency in those who survive childhood. In many instances, the OA has supervened in joints where the contiguous bone is markedly deformed. In some instances, the anatomic changes are indistinguishable from those of common OA; in others, eburnation is absent, and the articular surface is covered by a shaggy reparative cartilage (4). The femoral heads of such patients are small and flattened. Similar changes are seen on the surface of femoral heads removed from children with spastic cerebral palsy, although many of these children are afflicted with hip dislocations as well (208). OA has been reported in patients with a rare form of heritable osteochondrosis of the digits known as the nail-patella syndrome (hereditary osteo-onychodysplasia, Turner-Kieser syndrome, iliac horn syndrome). Heritable causes of joint laxity such as osteogenesis imperfecti (209), Ehlers-Danlos syndrome (210,211), and Larsen syndrome (212) are also associated with precocious OA.

Osteoarthritis commonly follows congenital hip dysplasia in humans, possibly caused by elevated pressure resulting from the distribution of forces over the reduced contact area of the dysplastic femoral head (213). The disorder is relatively common, occurring approximately in 1.5 per 1,000 live births (214), and more frequently in females. The disorder is usually clinically manifest at birth with hip dislocation (215). The existence of unrecognized forme fruste variants causing localized hip OA in a greater number of individuals in adult life is controversial (4). The hereditary contribution to the prevalence of this condition is also the subject of debate. Its frequency is increased in conditions with oligohydramnios (4), pointing toward an acquired defect *in utero.* The disorder is definitely more common in offspring of diabetic mothers (216). Other studies suggest a more generalized connective tissue defect in some cases (215,217). In dogs, however, the evidence supports a strong genetic contribution (218). Certain breeds, such as German shepherds, commonly develop it, whereas others, such as American greyhounds, do not. Shepherd dogs are also prone to dysplasia and secondary OA of the elbow. The condition is of considerable economic importance in work dogs of other types as well.

LOCALIZED FORMS OF OSTEOARTHRITIS

Malum Coxae Senilis

Several childhood hip abnormalities lead to premature osteoarthritic degeneration in adult life. Such disorders include congenital hip dysplasia (213–215), Legg-Calvé-Perthes disease (219), slipped capital femoral epiphysis (220), and congenital coxa vara. At times there is such a clear history that a pathogenetic sequence seems certain. In other patients, however, no precursor state is evident. These patients are sometimes considered to have a forme fruste of congenital hip dysplasia (4). This retrospective view may be questioned because subluxation has been documented only as a late manifestation of the joint deformity. Earlier views that subclinical hip dysplasia is frequently responsible for isolated OA of the hip have not been substantiated (221,222). Legg-Calvé-Perthes disease results from necrosis of the growth center of the femoral head in childhood. A severe secondary OA characterized by a flattened femoral head with bilateral beak-like osteophytes results. Because synovitis is a feature of early stages in the disorder (223), increased intraarticular pressure has been implicated. Hypercoagulability due to increased prevalence of inherited factor V (Leiden) mutations also has been implicated (224). Slipped capital femoral epiphysis occurs in older boys of endomorphic habitus and results from a fracture through the physeal growth plate. Complete or total detachment is characterized by secondary osteonecrosis and severe precocious OA (220). Between 25% and 40% of cases are bilateral (225). The disorder is associated with acromegaly and conditions treated with synthetic growth hormone such as renal failure (226). Studies of archived human skeletons suggested that 8% were involved by slipped capital femoral epiphyses, and that the condition was associated with severe OA (227).

Chondromalacia Patellae

The term *chondromalacia patellae* is used loosely to describe a clinically distinctive, posttraumatic softening of the articular cartilage of the patella in young persons (see Chapter 98). The anatomic lesions resemble those of early OA, although subtle differences have been described by some authors (29,30). Changes involve the cartilage and the subchondral bone (4). Softening, swelling, and increased water content of cartilage have all been reported in the early stages of chondromalacia. In a minority of patients, a significant inflammatory component may be present secondary to irritation of synovium from detachment of cartilage fragments (detritic synovitis). Some studies have suggested that many cases of chondromalacia patellae do not progress to OA of the type seen in older individuals (31). Some evidence favors hypermobility of the knee joint as an evocative factor (228).

Neuropathic Arthropathies

Neuropathic arthropathies comprise articular degenerations with varying morphologies according to the duration and type of the underlying sensory defects (229). Collectively, these are called Charcot joints owing to their description by J. M. Charcot in 1868. The changes resemble those of severe OA but are more profoundly destructive. Extensive detritic synovitis is characteristic and is frequently accompanied by secondary osteochondromatosis. The pathogenesis of these lesions is complex, with damaged neurovascular reflexes, sensory denervation, and metabolic factors all having advocates (see Chapter 91). In the diabetic foot, the most frequent site of Charcot joints in the United States (230), the landmarks of the tarsal bones are often obliterated by fusion (4), indicating extensive remodeling. Some authors have proposed that subtle sensory deprivation contributes to the acceleration of some cases of idiopathic OA (231). The clinical and pathologic similarity between Charcot joints and severe examples of CPDD crystal arthropathy is described in Chapter 117.

Associated Osteonecrosis

Osteoarthritis as a late sequela of previous bone infarction (osteonecrosis) has been the subject of a large body of literature (see Chapter 108). The epiphyseal ends of the bones are involved primarily in osteonecrosis because they receive a discrete arterial supply distinct from that to the remainder of the bone (232). The femoral and humeral heads are the most frequent sites of osteonecrosis (233). Articular cartilage derives nutrition from synovial fluid, so infarction is limited to the subchondral bone and marrow, which fractures and collapses, leading to loss of the normal congruency of the joint surface. Proliferative remodeling leads to osteophyte formation. As the disorder progresses, the articular cartilage may slough, leading to exposure of bone and further remodeling. Osteonecrosis principally begins in only one articular member of a joint, but in later stages secondary degeneration involves the mating articular surfaces (234). Although overt OA may ensue, eburnation is usually not a conspicuous feature. Ordinary OA of the hip may be associated with areas in which the osteocytes of underlying subchondral bone are necrotic (70–72). The preponderance of evidence, however, suggests that such necrosis is a secondary event (70) that may contribute to rapid progression of deformity (6). Primary osteonecrosis is associated with a number of conditions that enhance thrombosis of the osseous microcirculation (235). The possible role, if any, of hypercoagulability and venous occlusive disease observed in some cases of OA (73) secondary to osteonecrosis has not been established.

A special form of osteonecrosis of the medial femoral condyle develops in elderly persons (4) leading to gonarthrosis. The sudden onset of symptoms (pain) may have been precipitated by a segmental fracture with depression of the articular cortex. Others have associated the disorder with medial meniscus tears (4) and with meniscectomy (236). OA has been described as a late consequence of meniscal disease as well. Thus, when segmental infarction occurs in OA of the knee (237), it probably is a secondary phenomenon, as in the hip.

ROLE OF ARTICULAR CARTILAGE REPAIR

The persistent erosion of articular cartilage in OA has long aroused interest in the limited ability of this tissue to grow (4). By all measures, the metabolic activity of hyaline cartilage is low. Experimentally induced gaps in articular cartilage show little tendency to repair if they do not penetrate into the vascularized bone marrow, leading to a common view that failure of cartilage repair is responsible for the irreversible development of OA (4).

Such dogma warrants serious reconsideration. Chondrocytes are capable of brisk mitotic and metabolic activities *in vitro* (4). Their release from surrounding matrix by enzymes provides a stimulus to cell division *in vivo,* as illustrated by proliferating cell clones near areas of matrix fibrillation (Fig. 109.2). Thymidine incorporation (39) and biosynthetic activities of chondrocytes (32,55–57) are increased in OA. Although their rate of repair is low, it may be significant over the extended periods required for the development of OA. Cartilage defects may be reconstituted by autologous chondrocyte transplants, further indicating a capacity for repair (25) under the right conditions.

The more obvious mechanism of cartilage repair lies in the proliferation and differentiation from pluripotential cells in the subchondral bone marrow. The fibrocartilaginous covering of osteophytes illustrates repair by this mechanism (58). Foci of hyaline and fibrocartilage also develop in the fibro-osseous granulation tissue forming beneath metallic joint prostheses (4). Wedge osteotomies designed to redistribute forces in hips with OA have resulted in radiologic widening of the joint space and, in a few instances, in fibrocartilaginous recovering of joint spaces. Thus, despite evidence of both increased apoptosis (5,238) and somatic mutations (41) in chondrocytes in OA, there is ample evidence of proliferation and repair *in vivo.*

CONCEPTS OF PATHOGENESIS

The clinical and experimental pathology of OA suggests certain concepts about pathogenesis. These should be viewed as subject to modification as our knowledge of the molecular events underlying the morphologic lesions is enhanced.

Primary Versus Secondary Osteoarthritis

Osteoarthritis frequently develops in joints with clear-cut preexisting structural abnormalities. These cases are classified as secondary OA. In primary OA, no trauma or other predisposition can be identified, and intrinsic alterations of the articular tissues, or response to normal cumulative stresses, are presumed to be responsible. Differences in the conformation of OA joints in ochronotic or postinflammatory arthropathies suggest that intrinsic cartilage damage is also responsible for concentric (nonhypertrophic) OA, whereas mechanical overloading is responsible for the much more common varieties in which overt joint remodeling is conspicuous. In the hip joint, the patterns of cartilage loss and osteophyte development have been proposed as representative of the original causal abnormalities (4). Use of surgically resected femoral heads to support such causal explanations is quite difficult, owing to the advanced nature of the changes in such specimens. One school of thought proposes that a preexisting structural basis for OA of the hip can be identified in most cases (239). The entire issue is controversial, because others report a much lower percentage of preexisting conditions (4,221,222,227,240) and recognize primary OA of the hip as the dominant entity (241,242), presenting evidence that generalized OA is common in individuals requiring hip surgery for localized disease (166). Similar frequency of polyarticular disease is found in patients who present with OA of the knee (167). Since the possibility exists that a genetic predisposition to generalized OA (171) might predispose to secondary OA (111), the entire issue is far from resolved.

Origin in Bone or in Cartilage

If the earliest events in the progression to OA occur in articular cartilage (5,8,15,32,34,38), then the bone remodeling results from the loss of energy-absorbing function of the cartilage. The osteophytes in primary OA can thus be viewed as an attempt to redistribute the increased transmitted forces over a greater surface area. If the primary alteration is in the subchondral bone (13,17–20,23,24) or in the basal layer of calcified cartilage (12,14,15,16), then the cartilage changes represent a failure of cartilage repair to compensate for the remodeling, including that of calcified cartilage (12,14). Evidence that bony changes underlie the deterioration of cartilage includes the following: (a) articular cartilage has little measurable impact-absorbing function; (b) microfractures and subchondral trabecular sclerosis precede measurable changes in the cartilage; and (c) cartilage is mechanically more susceptible to impact loading that produces deformation of subchondral bone than to shearing stresses (17,138). Osteophytes, the most conspicuous features of established OA of the hip, develop very early, concomitant with the first radiologic evidence of joint space narrowing (4). Similar early remodeling changes are present in experimental OA in rabbits (9) and dogs (10). The pathogenesis of OA likely involves an interaction between intrinsic deranged cartilage metabolism and extrinsic potentiating mechanical factors. Their relative contribution may vary in different joints and in different forms of OA. This subject is considered in further detail in Chapter 110.

Systemic Contributions to Osteoarthritis

Several systemic factors have been previously considered in relation to OA, including age, metabolic and genetic influences, obesity, and exercise. A salient feature of OA is a strong association with advancing age (11). This may suggest either that a series of cumulative insults is required to produce disease or that time-dependent molecular alterations engendered by genetic defects occur independently of environmental insults. Some degree of deterioration of the articular surface occurs linearly with increasing age, but the rate is greater in some joints than others (242). The changes in surgically resected osteoarthritic hip and knee specimens are far outside the normal distribution of changes seen in natural aging, suggesting that other local or systemic factors are necessary for progressive OA to occur (240–242).

Metabolic Factors

The increased prevalence of OA in patients with several different types of metabolic disease (e.g., ochronosis and acromegaly) has suggested that systemic factors are important (see Chapter 111). Likewise, CPDD deposition disease with secondary OA is common in hemochromatosis (243) and hyperparathyroidism (76) and may eventuate in a pattern of secondary OA. The contribution of the most common of all metabolic disorders (244), diabetes mellitus, to OA is more difficult to demonstrate. Some authors have associated hyperglycemia on clinical and epidemiologic grounds with symptomatic OA (245), but others have not (246). Diabetes is associated with several other joint disorders including neuropathic arthropathy (230), ankylosing hyperostosis (157), and other manifestations of the DISH syndrome, as well as the syndrome of fibrositis with limited joint mobility (244). The contribution of maternal diabetes mellitus to congenital hip dysplasia has been discussed elsewhere (215,216). It is more difficult to demonstrate molecular and biochemical pathology directly linking diabetes to primary OA. The relationship is complicated by the association of obesity to both type II diabetes mellitus and OA (241,242).

Other systemic factors may influence OA as well. Important sex differences in human OA exist, and multiple joint involvement is far more frequent in women (166,167,247). In men, OA of hips, wrist, and spine (248) is more frequent. The influence of endocrinopathies on the development of rheumatic disease is discussed in Chapter 124.

Osteoporosis

Although both osteoporosis and OA are diseases that appear in older individuals, they do not frequently coexist. The age-corrected incidence of OA is decreased in individuals with osteoporosis (24,145,249,250). Conversely, the existence of OA may retard the development of osteoporosis (147,251,252). Increased tissue concentrations of insulin-like growth factors I and II (253) and osteocalcin (254) in bone have been identified in association with OA. This raises the possibility that local accumulation might be the mechanism of increased bone density in some cases of OA. The subject is complex due to differences in types of OA used to assess patient status. Furthermore, osteoblastogenesis is inhibited by glucocorticoids, which also promote osteocyte apoptosis (255). Inhibition of the role of subchondral bone formation in the genesis of OA could be a possible mechanism explaining the inverse relationship between OA and osteoporosis in some cases.

Genetic Factors

Genetic factors contributing to OA in humans (166,167) and other species may have systemic, metabolic, or, as in the dysplasias, local effects (see Chapter 110). Data regarding inheritance of Heberden's nodes have been interpreted as reflecting involvement of a single gene, which is dominant in females and recessive in males (165). In other studies, mendelian recessive inheritance for OA in hand and knee joints with a multifactorial additional component has been advanced (171). Increased frequency of certain HLA antigens in patients with generalized OA suggests a genetic component (168), as does association with estrogen gene polymorphisms (169) and chromosomal 2q abnormalities (170). Likewise, vitamin D receptor gene polymorphism (256) has been associated with early OA of the knee, and specific genotypes of the cartilage matrix protein genes are significantly associated with polyarticular OA in men (257). Likewise, twin studies have shown an increased likelihood of OA in identical as opposed to fraternal twins, leading to the conclusion that the genetic influence on hand and knee involvement ranges up to 65% (258).

The contribution of inherited abnormalities in type II collagens to the overall incidence of primary OA remains uncertain. Due to the number of exons in the gene (178), large-scale screening of patients with generalized OA is conceptually difficult. However, the available evidence does not indicate genetic linkage of generalized OA of the usual sort to the loci encoding type II collagen (179). Genetic linkage of a multiple epiphyseal dysplasia phenotype to a specific defect of the $\alpha 2$ chain of type IX collagen has been demonstrated (259), but a role in common varieties of OA for so-called minor collagen constituents of cartilage is problematic.

Obesity

Obesity is accepted as a definite contributory factor. It seems self-evident that excessive weight imposes a mechanical burden on the joints undergoing impulse loading, but several studies indicate that the situation is not so simple. In mice, obesity itself does not have an important effect on OA (4). However, epidemiologic data support an association of human OA of the knee with obesity (247,260,261), especially in women. The association with OA of the hip is weaker, perhaps due to confounding variables such as the local factors discussed previously (240–242,262). Heberden's nodes are apparently not associated with obesity (4), although OA of the hand and wrist are more common in obese patients (263). The caveat that patients with OA are likely to exercise less and thus become obese is worthy of consideration (248). This may be one factor in the observation that survival is reduced in women with increasing prevalence of full-body radiographically defined OA (264). Spondylosis is also more common in obese persons than in those of normal weight (4). Because joints involved in such studies are often not weight bearing, constitutional effects of obesity may be as important as biomechanical considerations. One plausible explanation is the increase in generalized bone density (150) seen in obese as opposed to nonobese individuals (4).

Ligamentous Laxity

A variety of postural abnormalities of joints associated with laxity of the ligamentous structures (207) also predispose patients to OA. Severe joint hypermobility occurring in states such as the Marfan and Ehlers-Danlos syndromes is associated with OA (210,265). Joint degeneration in patients with osteogenesis imperfecti is due not only to structural abnormality of underlying bone, but also to ligamentous laxity as well (207,209). Some other states, such as the Larsen syndrome, combine multiple congenital joint dislocations and epiphyseal dysplasias (207,212). Other studies have implicated an increased frequency of OA, especially of the knee and shoulder, occurring with idiopathic joint hypermobility (4). In particular, chondromalacia patellae is associated with hypermobility of the knee in young, active individuals (228).

Mechanical Factors in OA

Mechanical factors have been proposed to evoke OA in specific joints. Elbow OA of foundry workers using long tongs to lift hot metals and "coal miner's back" are two such examples. Vibratory trauma has been implicated in the cause of OA of the hands and feet in some studies, but not others (248). OA of the knee was more common in a study in individuals whose occupations involve heavy labor (265). OA of the hip has been correlated with heavy physical workload in women (240) and men (266). Heavy use of the hands is linked with interphalangeal OA (162) as well.

In numerous studies, the occurrence of OA in runners was not increased over control populations. Other types of athletic activity may not be as uninfluential. Retired soccer players, for example, had more OA of the hips than age- and weight-matched control group athletes in one study, but not in another (4). Nevertheless, competitive sports have been considered a major risk factor for OA of the hips (268). The possibility that repetitive trauma induces OA more commonly in genetically predisposed susceptible individuals cannot be excluded (112,162). Single injuries probably do not cause OA unless they are severe enough to disorganize the joint surface or its major stabilizing structures (Fig. 109.6).

Direct evidence for the mechanical abrasion of cartilage from the joint surface is provided by the shards of cartilage found in the synovial fluid and synovium in OA (97). In ochronosis, such joint detritus is a dominant feature of the disease and incites significant immune and inflammatory response in the synovium (183). The actual mechanical basis of the abrasion injuries in common OA is less obvious but their presence is undeniable.

One cause of increased cartilage abrasion could be decreased or disordered joint lubrication (4). The articular cartilage of animal joints oscillated *in vitro* in the absence of synovial fluid undergoes rapid frictional destruction. Instillation of testicular hyaluronidase also leads to *in vitro* scoring of joint surfaces. Although the depolymerization of synovial mucin could account for the friction, it is possible that the hyaluronidase may also have acted directly on the cartilage matrix. The subject of joint lubrication has attracted much interest in recent years. Hyaluronidase abolishes the viscosity of synovial fluid but not its lubricating ability (4). Under conditions reproducing the joint loading occurring during walking, the friction on human femoral heads increased after hyaluronidase digestion of synovial fluid (4). These studies reflect the different characteristics of boundary and fluid film lubrication processes operating in joint function (269).

The volume, hyaluronate content, and relative viscosity of synovial fluid are usually normal in OA, although other studies have shown diminished polymerization of synovial mucin and a reduction of the hyaluronate content (4). The contradictory data arise in part because truly normal synovial fluids are not readily obtained for comparison. In the absence of joint disease, the amount of synovial fluid within joints is small, and many joints aspirated have low-grade synovitis (4). The synovial fluid also contains a lubricating glycoprotein called lubricin (269) and a surface active phospholipid (270) produced by synovial cells (271). The latter is bound to the surface of cartilage, probably transported to that site by the former (272). Lubricin thus functions in lubrication as a carrier for the phospholipid (273). Studies of femoral heads and knees removed for severe OA showed decreased surface active phospholipid recoverable from the surface of worn as opposed to unworn areas (274). Whether this is a primary or secondary phenomenon is unclear. In a synthetic bearing test system, no deficiency in the boundary-lubricating ability of synovial fluid was found in OA in previous studies (4).

The forces applied over the hip, knee, and ankle joints are characterized by being intermittent and are often several multiples of the body weight (4), even in simple apparently nonstressful movements such as walking on level ground. The resistance to wear under such conditions is a complex function involving lubrication, the elastic properties of the articular cartilage, and the deformation of the underlying bone. This subject is discussed in detail in Chapter 7. The elastic properties of cartilage, as measured by either stiffness or recovery from deformation, are not altered by aging unless fibrillation is also present (4).

The stiffness of the underlying bone has been increasingly considered as a factor in the development of OA (17,18,20), and the decreased stiffness of osteoporotic bone may explain why OA is less common in osteoporotic patients (24,249,252). However, some evidence from studies of comparative pathology of OA suggests that deficiency of mineralized bone may adversely affect cartilage (4). Such deficiency of mechanical support may contribute to the arthropathy seen in hyperparathyroidism (76). Conversely, osteopetrosis, a rare condition characterized by markedly increased stiffness of bone, favors the development of premature OA (4). The cause-and-effect relationship, however, is still unclear because fractures with deformity also characterize this disorder.

Paget's disease (osteitis deformans) produces significant bone deformation that may extend into the subchondral osteoarticular junction and produce irregularities at the joint surface. The hip is frequently the site of mixed patterns of Paget's disease and OA, and protrusio acetabuli develops in approximately 25% of such patients, a far higher frequency than in OA without Paget's disease (275).

CONCLUSION

Understanding the pathogenesis of OA requires reconciliation of apparently divergent biomechanical and biochemical concepts about the initial events in its evolution. The nature of the lesions and numerous lines of experimental work seem to reaffirm an interdependence between mechanical wear-and-tear processes and an altered metabolic state of articular tissues (4). The pathologic findings in OA do not establish that the disease is an inevitable concomitant of aging (11) or that the lesions, once developed, have no biologic potential for repair. Furthermore, secondary variants of OA develop commonly in association with a number of systemic or localized conditions. In some cases, such as ochronosis, hemophilia, and osteonecrosis, specific pathology gives evidence of a preexisting disease state. In others such information is lacking. In secondary OA following long-standing RA of the hip, the stigmata of previous inflammatory insult to the cartilage and subchondral bone may be minimally, if at all, evident. Such scenarios serve to confound attempts to distinguish between primary and secondary OA on pathologic grounds in many cases. In other cases, coexistence of OA and other states, such as chondrocalcinosis, makes establishment of causality difficult. This phenomenon contributes to continuing disputes on the contributions of systemic factors to localized OA, especially of the hip joint. Inasmuch as OA is a pathologic final common pathway for a number of predisposing disease conditions, a relative degree of uncertainty about the primacy of local versus systemic factors will persist pending availability and application of more discriminatory molecular pathologic techniques to augment traditional pathologic methodology.

REFERENCES

1. Parish LC. An historical approach to the nomenclature of rheumatoid arthritis. *Arthritis Rheum* 1963;6:138–158.
2. Keuttner KE, Goldberg V, eds. *Osteoarthritic disorders.* Rosemont, IL: American Academy of Orthopedic Surgeons 1995:21–25.
3. Sokoloff L. Osteoarthritis as a remodeling process. *J Rheumatol* 1987;14 (suppl 14):7–10.
4. Hough AJ. Pathology of osteoarthritis. In: Koopman WJ, ed. *Arthritis and allied conditions,* 13th ed. Philadelphia: Lea and Febiger, 1996:1945–1968.
5. Blanco FJ, Guitian R, Vasquez-Martul E, et al. Osteoarthritis chondrocytes die by apoptosis. A possible pathway for osteoarthritis. *Arthritis Rheum* 1998;441:284–289.
6. Mitrovic DR, Riera H. Synovial, articular cartilage and bone changes in rapidly destructive arthropathy (osteoarthritis) of the hip. *Rheumatol Int* 1992;12:17–22.
7. Rosenberg ZS, Shankman S, Steiner GC, et al. Rapidly destructive osteoarthritis: clinical, radiographic, and pathologic features. *Radiology* 1992;182:213–216.
8. Soren A, Cooper NS, Waugh TR. The nature and designation of osteoarthritis determined by its histopathology. *Clin Exp Rheumatol* 1988;6:41–46.
9. Malemud CJ, Goldberg VM, Moskowitz RW. Pathological, biochemical, and experimental therapeutic studies in meniscectomy models of osteoarthritis in the rabbits relationship to human joint pathology. *Br J Clin Pract* 1986;43 (suppl):21–31.
10. Dedrick DK, Goldstein SA, Brandt KD, et al. A longitudinal study of subchondral plate and trabecular bone in cruciate-deficient dogs with osteoarthritis followed up to 54 months. *Arthritis Rheum* 1993;36:1460–1467.
11. Sokoloff L. Aging and degenerative diseases affecting cartilage. In: Hall BK, ed. *Cartilage,* vol 3. New York: Academic Press, 1987:110–141.
12. Bullough PG, Jagannath A. The morphology of the calcification front in articular cartilage. *J Bone Joint Surg* 1983;65B:72–78.
13. Clark JM, Huber JD. The structure of the human subchondral plate. *J Bone Joint Surg* 1990;72B:866–873.
14. Oegema TR, Carpenter RJ, Hofmeister F, et al. The interaction of the zone of calcified cartilage and subchondral bone in osteoarthritis. *Microsc Res Tech* 1997;37:324–332.
15. Mori S, Haruff R, Burr DB. Microcracks in the articular cartilage of human femoral heads. *Arch Pathol Lab Med* 1993;117: 196–198.
16. Sokoloff L. Microcracks in the calcified layer of articular cartilage. *Arch Pathol Lab Med* 1993;117:191–195.
17. Radin EL, Rose RM. Role of subchondral bone in the initiation and progression of cartilage damage. *Clin Orthop* 1986;213: 34–40.
18. Fazzalari NL, Vernon-Roberts B, Darracott J. Osteoarthritis of the hip. Possible protective and causative roles of trabecular microfractures in the head of the femur. *Clin Orthop* 1987; 216:224–233.
19. Koszyca B, Fazzalari NL, Vernon-Roberts B. Microfractures in coxarthrosis. *Acta Orthop Scand* 1990;61:307–310.
20. Fazzalari NL, Parkinson IH. Fractal properties of subchondral cancellous bone in severe osteoarthritis of the hip. *J Bone Miner Res* 1997;12:632–640.
21. Moore RJ, Fazzalari NL, Manthey BA, et al. The relationship between head-neck-shaft angle, calcar width, articular cartilage thickness and bone volume in arthrosis of the hip. *Br J Rheumatol* 1994;33:432–436.
22. Koszyca B, Fazzalari NL, Vernon-Roberts B. Trabecular microfractures. Nature and distribution in the proximal femur. *Clin Orthop* 1989;244:208–216.
23. Fazzalari NL, Moore RJ, Manthey BA, et al. Comparative study of iliac crest and subchondral bone in osteoarthritic patients. *Bone* 1992;13:331–335.
24. Schnitzler CM, Mesquita JM, Wane L. Bone histomorphometry of the iliac crest and spinal fracture prevalence in atrophic and hypertrophic osteoarthritis of the hip. *Osteoporosis Int* 1992;2:186–194.
25. Brittberg M, Lindahl A, Nilsson A, et al. Treatment of deep cartilage defects in the knee with autologous chondrocyte transplantation. *N Engl J Med* 1994;331:889–895.
26. Oettmeier R, Arokoski J, Roth AJ, et al. Quantitative study of articular cartilage after strenuous running training. *Bone Miner Res* 1992;7 (suppl 12):S419–424.
27. Brandt KD, Myers SL, Burr D, et al. Osteoarthritic changes in canine articular cartilage, subchondral bone, and synovium fifty-four months after transection of the anterior cruciate ligament. *Arthritis Rheum* 1991;34:1560–1570.
28. Bennett GA, Waine H, Bauer W. *Changes in the knee joint at various ages.* New York: Commonwealth Fund, 1942.
29. Ohno O, Naito J, Iguchi T, et al. An electron microscopic study of early pathology in chondromalacia of the patella. *J Bone Joint Surg* 1988;70A:883–899.
30. Mori Y, Kubo M, Okumo H, et al. Histological comparison of patellar cartilage degeneration between chondromalacia in youth and osteoarthritis in aging. *Knee Surg Sports Traumatol Arthrosc* 1995;3:167–172.
31. Jensen DB, Albrektsen SB. The natural history of chondromalacia patellae. A 12-year follow-up. *Acta Orthop Belg* 1990;56:503–506.
32. Cs-Szabo G, Melching LI, Rhoughley PJ, et al. Changes in mes-

senger RNA and protein levels of proteoglycans and link protein in human osteoarthritic cartilage samples. *Arthritis Rheum* 1997;40:1037–1045.

33. Testa V, Capasso G, Maffulli N, et al. Proteases and antiproteases in cartilage homeostasis. *Clin Orthop* 1994;308:79–84.
34. Walter H, Kawashima A, Nebelung W, et al. Immunohistochemical analysis of several proteolytic enzymes as parameters of cartilage degradation. *Pathol Res Pract* 1998;194:73–81.
35. Lohmander LS, Lark MW, Dahlberg L, et al. Cartilage matrix metabolism in osteoarthritis: markers in synovial fluid, serum, and urine. *Clin Biochem* 1992;25:167–174.
36. Goldberg RL, Huff JP, Lenz ME, et al. Elevated plasma levels of hyaluronate in patients with osteoarthritis and rheumatoid arthritis. *Arthritis Rheum* 1991;34:799–807.
37. Pitsillides AA, Will RK, Bayliss MT, et al. Circulating and synovial fluid hyaluronan levels. *Arthritis Rheum* 1994;37: 1030–1038.
38. Poole CA, Matsuoka A, Schofield JR. Chondrons from articular cartilage III. Morphologic changes in the cellular microenvironment of chondrons isolated from osteoarthritic cartilage. *Arthritis Rheum* 1991;34:22–35.
39. Rotzer A, Mohr W. [^{3}H-thymidine incorporation into chondrocytes of arthritic cartilage]. *Z Rheumatol* 1992;51:172–176.
40. Macha N, Older J, Bitensky L, et al. Abnormalities of DNA in human osteoarthritic articular cartilage. *Cell Biochem Funct* 1993;11:63–69.
41. Mertens F, Palsson E, Lindstrand A, et al. Evidence of somatic mutations in osteoarthritis. *Hum Genet* 1996;98:651–656.
42. Broberg K, Limon J, Palsson E, et al. Clonal chromosome aberrations are present in vivo in synovia and osteophytes from patients with osteoarthritis. *Hum Genet* 1997;101:295–298.
43. Ismaiel S, Atkins RM, Pearse MF, et al. Susceptibility of normal and arthritic human cartilage to degradative stimuli. *Br J Rheumatol* 1992;31:369–373.
44. Martel-Pelletier J, McCollum R, DiBattista J, et al. The interleukin-I receptor in normal and osteoarthritic human articular chondrocytes. Identification as the type I receptor and analysis of binding kinetics and biologic function. *Arthritis Rheum* 1992;35:530–540.
45. Hashimoto S, Ochs RL, Komiya S, et al. Linkage of chondrocyte apoptosis and cartilage degradation in human osteoarthritis. *Arthritis Rheum* 1998;41:1632–1638.
46. Sokoloff L, DiFrancesco L. Lipochondral degeneration of capsular tissue in osteoarthritic hips. *Am J Surg Pathol* 1995;19: 278–283.
47. Wittenberg RH, Willburger RE, Kleemeyer KS, et al. In vitro release of prostaglandins and leukotrienes from synovial tissue, cartilage, and bone in degenerative joint diseases. *Arthritis Rheum* 1993;36:1444–1450.
48. David MJ, Portoukalian J, Rebbaa A, et al. Characterization of gangliosides from normal and osteoarthritic human articular cartilage. *Arthritis Rheum* 1993;36:938–942.
49. Ghadially FN, Lalonde JM, Yong NK. Ultrastructure of amianthoid fibers in osteoarthritic cartilage. *Virchows Arch [B]* 1979;31:81–86.
50. Curtin WA, Reville WJ. Ultrastructural observations on fibril profiles in normal and degenerative human articular cartilage. *Clin Orthop* 1995;313:224–230.
51. Lafeber FP, Van der Kraan PM, Van Roy HL, et al. Local changes in proteoglycan synthesis during culture are different for normal and osteoarthritic cartilage. *Am J Pathol* 1992;140: 1421–1429.
52. Tsuchiya K, Maloney WJ, Vu T, et al. Osteoarthritis: differential expression of matrix metalloproteinase-9 mRNA in nonfibrillated and fibrillated cartilage. *J Orthop Res* 1997;15:94–100.
53. Shlopov BV, Lie WR, Mainard CL, et al. Osteoarthritic lesions:involvement of three different collagenases. *Arthritis Rheum* 1997;40:2065–2074.
54. Imai K, Ohta S, Matsumoto T, et al. Expression of matrix metallo-proteinase and activation of progelatinase A in human osteoarthritic cartilage. *Am J Pathol* 1997;151:245–256.
55. Aigner T, Stoss H, Weseloh G, et al. Activation of collagen type II expression in osteoarthritic and rheumatoid cartilage. *Virchows Arch B* 1992;62:337–345.
56. Nerlich AG, Wiest I, Von der Mark K. Immunohistochemical analysis of interstitial collagens in cartilage of different stages of osteoarthrosis. *Virchows Arch B* 1993;63:249–255.
57. Aigner T, Bertling W, Stoss H, et al. Independent expression of fibril-forming collagens I, II, and III in chondrocytes of human osteoarthritic cartilage. *J Clin Invest* 1993;91:829–837.
58. Misoge N, Waletzko K, Bode C, et al. Light and electron microscopic in situ hydridization of collagen type I and type II mRNA in the fibrocartilaginous tissue of late-stage osteoarthritis. *Osteoarthritis Cartilage* 1998;6:278–285.
59. Girkontaite I, Frischholz S, Lammi P, et al. Immunolocalization of type X collagen in normal fetal and adult osteoarthritic cartilage with monoclonal antibodies. *Matrix Biol* 1996;15: 231–238.
60. Walker GD, Fischer M, Gannon J, et al. Expression of type-X collagen in osteoarthritis. *J Orthop Res* 1995;13:4–12.
61. Aigner T, Vornehm SI, Zeiler G, et al. Suppression of cartilage matrix gene expression in upper zone chondrocytes of osteoarthritic cartilage. *Arthritis Rheum* 1997;40:562–569.
62. Revell PA, Pirie C, Amir G, et al. Metabolic activity in the calcified zone of cartilage: observations on tetracycline labeled articular cartilage in human osteoarthritic hips. *Rheumatol Int* 1990;10:143–147.
63. Amir G, Pirie CJ, Rashad S, et al. Remodelling of subchondral bone in osteoarthritis: a histomorphometric study. *J Clin Pathol* 1992;45:990–992.
64. Derfus B, Kranendonk S, Camacho N, et al. Human osteoarthritic cartilage matrix vesicles generate both calcium pyrophosphate dihydrate and apatite in vitro. *Calcif Tissue Int* 1998;63:258–262.
65. Nanba Y, Nishida K, Yoshikawa T, et al. Expression of osteonectin in articular cartilage of osteoarthritic knees. *Acta Med Okayama* 1997;51:239–243.
66. Burr DB, Schaffler MB. The involvement of subchondral mineralized tissues in osteoarthrosis: quantitative microscopic evidence. *Microsc Res Tech* 1997;37:343–351.
67. Kamibayashi L, Wyss UP, Cooke TD, et al. Trabecular microstructure in the medial condyle of the proximal tibia of patients with knee osteoarthritis. *Bone* 1995;17:27–35.
68. Arlet J, Laroche M, Soler R, et al. Histopathology of the vessels of the femoral heads in specimens of osteonecrosis, osteoarthritis, and algodystrophy. *Clin Rheumatol* 1993;12:162–165.
69. Milgram JW. Morphologic alterations in the subchondral bone in advanced degenerative arthritis. *Clin Orthop* 1983;173: 293–312.
70. Ilardi CF, Sokoloff L. Secondary osteonecrosis in osteoarthritis of the femoral head: a pathological study. *Hum Pathol* 1984;15: 79–83.
71. Franchi A, Bullough PG. Secondary avascular necrosis in coxarthrosis: a morphologic study. *J Rheumatol* 1992;19: 1263–1268.
72. Wong SYP, Evans RA, Needs C, et al. The pathogenesis of osteoarthritis of the hip. Evidence for primary osteocyte death. *Clin Orthop* 1987;214:305–312.
73. Cheras PA, Whitaker AN, Blackwell EA, et al. Hypercoagulability and hypofibrinolysis in primary osteoarthritis. *Clin Orthop* 1997;334:57–67.
74. Ryu KN, Kim EJ, Yoo MC, et al. Ischemic necrosis of the entire

femoral head and rapidly destructive hip disease: potential causative relationship. *Skeletal Radiol* 1997;26:143–149.
75. O'Connell JT, Nielsen GP, Rosenberg AE. Subchondral acute inflammation in severe arthritis: a sterile osteomyelitis? *Am J Surg Pathol* 1999;23:192–197.
76. Pritzker KPH. Articular-skeletal system: muscle, fat, and other connective tissues. In: Kovacs K, Asa SL, eds. *Functional endocrine pathology,* 2nd ed. Oxford: Blackwell, 1998:766–769.
77. Pereira ER, Brown RR, Resnick D. Prevalence and patterns of tendon calcifications in patients with chondrocalcinosis of the knee: radiographic study of 156 patients. *Clin Imaging* 1998; 22:371–375.
78. Sokoloff L, Varma AA. Chondrocalcinosis in surgically resected joints. *Arthritis Rheum* 1988:750–756.
79. Felson OT, Anderson JJ, Naimark A, et al. The prevalence of chondrocalcinosis in the elderly and its association with knee osteoarthritis: the Framingham study. *J Rheumatol* 1989;16: 1241–1245.
80. Hough AJ, Webber RJ. The pathology of the meniscus. *Clin Orthop* 1990;252:32–40.
81. Ohira T, Ishikawa K, Masuda T, et al. Histologic localization of lipid in the articular tissues in calcium pyrophosphate dihydrate crystal deposition disease. *Arthritis Rheum* 1988;31:1057–1062.
82. Pritzker KP, Cheng PT, Renlund RC. Calcium pyrophosphate crystal deposition in hyaline cartilage: ultrastructural analysis and implications for pathogenesis. *J Rheumatol* 1988;15: 828–835.
83. Cardenal A, Masuda I, Ono W, et al. Serum nucleotide pyrophosphatase activity; elevated levels in osteoarthritis, calcium pyrophosphate crystal deposition disease, scleroderma, and fibromyalgia. *J Rheumatol* 1998;25:2175–2180.
84. Swan A, Chapman B, Heap P, et al. Submicroscopic crystals in osteoarthritic synovial fluids. *Ann Rheum Dis* 1994;53: 467–470.
85. Hashimoto S, Ochs RL, Rosen F, et al. Chondrocyte-derived apoptotic bodies and calcification of articular cartilage. *Proc Natl Acad Sci U S A* 1998;95:3094–3099.
86. Kennedy TD, Plater-Zyberk C, Partridge TA, et al. Morphometric comparison of synovium from patients with osteoarthritis and rheumatoid arthritis. *J Clin Pathol* 1988; 41:847–852.
87. Schulte E, Fisseler-Eckhoff A, Muller KM. [Differential diagnosis of synovitis. Correlation of arthroscopic-biopsy to clinical findings]. *Pathologie* 1994;15:22–27.
88. Dijkgraaf LC, Liem RS, de Bont LG. Ultrastructural characteristics of the synovial membrane in osteoarthritic temporomandibular joints. *J Oral Maxillofac Surg* 1997;55:1269–1279.
89. Helbig B, Gross WL, Borisch B, et al. Characterization of synovial macrophages by monoclonal antibodies in rheumatoid arthritis and osteoarthritis. *Scand J Rheumatol* 1988;76 (suppl): 61–66.
90. Demaziere A. Macrophages in rheumatoid synovial membrane: an update. *Rev Rhum* 1993:60:568–579.
91. Ezawa K, Yamamura M, Matsui H, et al. Comparative analysis of CD45RA-and CD45RO-positive CD4+T cells in peripheral blood, synovial fluid and synovial tissue in patients with rheumatoid arthritis and osteoarthritis. *Acta Med Okayama* 1997; 51:25–31.
92. Fort JG, Flanigan M, Smith JB. Mononuclear cell (MNC) subtypes in osteoarthritis synovial fluid. *J Rheumatol* 1995;22: 1335–1337.
93. Kummer JA, Tak PP, Brinkman BM, et al. Expression of granzymes A and B in synovial tissue from patients with rheumatoid arthritis and osteoarthritis. *Clin Immunol Immunopathol* 1994;73:88–95.
94. Dean G, Hoyland JA, Denton J, et al. Mast cells in the synovium and synovial fluid in osteoarthritis. *Br J Rheumatol* 1993;32:671–675.
95. Pu J, Nishida K, Inoue H, et al. Mast cells in osteoarthritic and rheumatoid arthritic synovial tissues of the human knee. *Acta Med Okayama* 1998;52:35–39.
96. Spector TD, Hart DJ, Nandra D, et al. Low-level increases in serum C-reactive protein are present in early osteoarthritis of the knee and predict progressive disease. *Arthritis Rheum* 1997; 40:723–733.
97. Myers SL, Flusser D, Brandt KD, et al. Prevalence of cartilage shards in synovium and their association with synovitis in patients with early and endstage osteoarthritis. *J Rheumatol* 1992;19:1247–1251.
98. Smith MD, Triantafillou S, Parker A, et al. Synovial membrane inflammation and cytokine production in patients with early osteoarthritis. *J Rheumatol* 1997;24:365–371.
99. Lohmander LS, Lark MW, Dahlberg L, et al. Cartilage matrix metabolism in osteoarthritis: markers in synovial fluid, serum, and urine. *Clin Biochem* 1992;25:167–174.
100. Pitsillides AA, Will RK, Bayliss MT, et al. Circulating and synovial fluid hyaluronan levels. Effects of intraarticular corticosteroid on the concentration and the rate of turnover. *Arthritis Rheum* 1994;37:1030–1038.
101. Anderson-Gare B, Fasth A. Serum concentration of hyaluronan, IgM and IgA rheumatoid factors in a population-based study of juvenile chronic arthritis. *Scand J Rheumatol* 1994;23:183–190.
102. Stamenkovic I, Stegagno M, Wright KA, et al. Clonal dominance among T-lymphocyte infiltrates in arthritis. *Proc Natl Acad Sci U S A* 1988;85:1179–1183.
103. Guerassimov A, Zhang Y, Cartman A, et al. Immune responses to cartilage link protein and the G1 domain of proteoglycan aggrecan in patients with osteoarthritis. *Arthritis Rheum* 1999; 42:527–533.
104. Vetto AA, Mannik M, Zatarain-Rios E, et al. Immune deposits in articular cartilage of patients with rheumatoid arthritis have a granular pattern not seen in osteoarthritis. *Rheumatol Int* 1990;10:13–20.
105. Hopkinson ND, Powell RJ, Doherty M. Autoantibodies, immunoglobulins, and Gm allotypes in nodal generalized osteoarthritis. *Br J Rheumatol* 1992;31:605–608.
106. Ali SY, Rees JA. Microcrystal deposition in cartilage and in osteoarthritis. *Bone Miner* 1992;17:115–118.
107. Schumacher HR. Synovial inflammation, crystals, and osteoarthritis. *J Rheumatol* 1995;43 (suppl):101–103.
108. Webb GR, Westacott CI, Elson CJ. Chondrocyte tumor necrosis factor receptors and focal loss of cartilage in osteoarthritis. *Osteoarthritis Cartilage* 1997;5:427–437.
109. Dodge GR, Poole AR. Immunohistochemical detection and immunohistochemical analysis of type II collagen degradation in human normal, rheumatoid, and osteoarthritic articular cartilages and in explants of bovine articular cartilage cultured with Interleukin 1. *J Clin Invest* 1989;83:647–661.
110. Lanzer WL, Komenda G. Changes in articular cartilage after meniscectomy. *Clin Orthop* 1990;252:41–48.
111. Doherty M, Watt I, Dieppe PA. Influence of primary generalized osteoarthritis on development of secondary osteoarthritis. *Lancet* 1983;2:8–11.
112. Croft P, Cooper C, Wickham C, et al. Is the hip involved in generalized osteoarthritis? *Br J Rheumatol* 1992;31:325–328.
113. Ladefoged C, Merrild V, Jorgensen B. Amyloid deposits in surgically removed articular and periarticular tissue. *Histopathology* 1989;15:289–296.
114. Maury CP. Beta 2-microglobulin amyloidosis. A systemic amyloid disease affecting primarily synovium and bone in long-term dialysis patients. *Rheumatol Int* 1990;10:1–8.
115. Nelson F, Dahlberg L, Laverty S, et al. Evidence for altered syn-

thesis of type II collagen in patients with osteoarthritis. *J Clin Invest* 1998;102:2115–2125.
116. Kuettner KE. Biochemistry of articular cartilage in health and disease. *Clin Biochem* 1992;25:155–163.
117. Anderson-Mackenzie JM, Hulmes DJ, Thorp BH. Degenerative joint disease in poultry-differences in composition and morphology of articular cartilage are associated with strain susceptibility. *Res Vet Sci* 1997;63:29–33.
118. Glasson SS, Trubetskoy OV, Harlan PM, et al. Blotchy mice: a model of osteoarthritis associated with a metabolic defect. *Osteoarthritis Cartilage* 1996;4:209–212.
119. Das-Gupta EP, Lyons TJ, Hoyland JA, et al. New histological observations in spontaneously developing osteoarthritis in the STR/ORT mouse questioning its acceptability. *Int J Exp Pathol* 1993;74:627–634.
120. Munasinghe JP, Tyler JA, Hodgson RJ, et al. Magnetic resonance imaging, histology, and X-ray of three stages of damage to the knees of STR/ORT mice. *Invest Radiol* 1996;31: 630–638.
121. Brewster M, Lewis EJ, Wilson KL, et al. Ro 32-3555, an orally active collagenase selective inhibitor, prevents structural damage in the STR/ORT mouse model of osteoarthritis. *Arthritis Rheum* 1998;41:1639–1644.
122. Walton M. Patella displacement and osteoarthrosis of the knee joint in mice. *J Pathol* 1979;127:165–172.
123. Bendele AM, Hulman JF. Spontaneous cartilage degeneration in guinea pigs. *Arthritis Rheum* 1988;31:561–565.
124. Jimenez PA, Glasson SS, Truketskoy OV, et al. Spontaneous osteoarthritis in Dunkin-Hartley guinea pigs: histologic, radiologic, and biochemical changes. *Lab Anim Sci* 1997;47:598–601.
125. Moskowitz RW, Ziv I, Denko CW, et al. Spondylosis in sand rats: a model of intervertebral disc degeneration and hyperostosis. *J Orthop Res* 1990;8:401–411.
126. Ohlerth S, Busato A, Gaillard C, et al. [Epidemiologic and genetic studies of canine hip dysplasia in a population of labrador retrievers: a study over 25 years]. *Dtsch Tierarztl Wochenschr* 1998;105:378–383.
127. Lust G. An overview of the pathogenesis of canine hip dysplasia. *J Am Vet Med Assoc* 1997;210:1443–1445.
128. Moskowitz RW. Experimental models of osteoarthritis. In: Moskowitz RW, Howell DS, Goldberg VM, et al., eds. *Osteoarthritis: diagnosis and medical/surgical management*, 2nd ed. Philadelphia: WB Saunders, 1992:213–232.
129. Pidd JG, Gardner DL, Adams ME. Ultrastructural changes in the femoral condylar cartilage of mature American foxhounds following transection of the anterior cruciate ligament. *J Rheumatol* 1988;15:663–669.
130. Fernandes JC, Jovanovic D, Dehnade F, et al. [Resection of the anterior cruciate ligament of the knee using arthroscopy induces arthrosis in dogs. Validity of the Pond-Nuki model]. *Ann Chir* 1998;52:768–775.
131. Chang DG, Iverson EP, Schinagl RM, et al. Quantitation and localization of cartilage degeneration following the induction of osteoarthritis in the rabbit knee. *Osteoarthritis Cartilage* 1997; 5:357–372.
132. Hashimoto S, Takahashi K, Amiel D, et al. Chondrocyte apoptosis and nitric oxide production during experimentally induced osteoarthritis. *Arthritis Rheum* 1998;41:1266–1274.
133. Fernandes J, Tardif G, Martel-Pelletier J, et al. In vivo transfer of interleukin-1 receptor antagonist gene in osteoarthritic rabbit knee joints: prevention of osteoarthritis progression. *Am J Pathol* 1999;154:1159–1169.
134. Panula HE, Lohmander LS, Ronkko S, et al. Elevated levels of synovial fluid PLA 2, stromelysin (MMP-3) and TIMP in early osteoarthrosis after tibial valgus osteotomy in young beagle dogs. *Acta Orthop Scand* 1998;69:152–158.
135. Panula HE, Hyttinen MM, Arokoshi JP, et al. Articular cartilage superficial zone collagen birefringence reduced and cartilage thickness increased before surface fibrillation in experimental osteoarthritis. *Ann Rheum Dis* 1998;57:237–245.
136. Buckwalter JA. Osteoarthritis and articular cartilage use, disuse, and abuse: experimental studies. *J Rheumatol* 1995;43 (suppl): 13–15.
137. Gamble JG, Rinsky LA, Bleck EE. Established hip dislocations in cerebral palsy. *Clin Orthop* 1990;253:90–99.
138. Farquhar T, Xia Y, Mann K, et al. Swelling and fibronectin accumulation in articular cartilage explants after cyclical impact. *J Orthop Res* 1996;14:417–423.
139. Van Osch GJ, van der Kraan PM, van Valburg AA, et al. The relation between cartilage damage and osteophyte size in a murine model for osteoarthritis in the knee. *Rheumatol Int* 1996;16:115–119.
140. Panula HE, Helminen HJ, Kiviranta I. Slowly progressive osteoarthritis after tibial valgus osteotomy in young beagle dogs. *Clin Orthop* 1997;343:192–202.
141. Bishop PB, Pearce RH. The proteoglycans of the cartilaginous end-plate of the human intervertebral disc change after maturity. *J Orthop Res* 1993;11:324–331.
142. Vernon-Roberts B, Fazzalari NL, Manathey BA. Pathogenesis of tears of the anulus investigated by multiple-level transaxial analysis of the T12-L1 disc. *Spine* 1997;22:2641–2646.
143. Bullough PG, Boachie-Adjei O. *Atlas of spinal diseases.* Philadelphia: JB Lippincott, 1988:77–97.
144. Heggeness MH, Doherty BJ. Morphologic study of lumbar vertebral osteophytes. *South Med J* 1998;91:187–189.
145. O'Neill TW, McCloskey EV, Kanis JA, et al. The distribution, determinants, and clinical correlates of vertebral osteophytosis: population based survey. *J Rheumatol* 1999;26:842–848.
146. Boushey DR, Bland JH. Pathology. In: Bland JH, ed. *Disorders of the cervical spine.* Philadelphia: WB Saunders, 1987:64–73.
147. Jones G, Nguyen T, Sambrook PN, et al. A longitudinal study of the effect of spinal degenerative disease on bone density in the elderly. *J Rheumatol* 1995;22:932–936.
148. Liu G, Peacock M, Eilam O, et al. Effect of osteoarthritis in the lumbar spine and hip on bone mineral density and diagnosis of osteoporosis in elderly men and women. *Osteoporos Int* 1997;7: 564–569.
149. von der Recke P, Hansen MA, Overgaard K, et al. The impact of degenerative conditions in the spine on bone mineral density and fracture prediction. *Osteoporos Int* 1996;6:43–49.
150. Marcelli C, Favier F, Kotzki PO, et al. The relationship between osteoarthritis of the hands, bone mineral density, and osteoporotic fractures in elderly women. *Osteoporos Int* 1995;5:382–388.
151. Tanaka N, Tsuchiya T, Shiokawa A, et al. [Histopathological studies of the osteophytes and ossification of the posterior longitudinal ligament (OPLL) in the cervical spine]. *Nippon Seikeigeka Gakkai Zasshi* 1996;60:323–336.
152. Ono K, Yonenobu K, Miyamoto S, et al. Pathology of ossification of the posterior longitudinal ligament and ligamentum flavum. *Clin Orthop* 1999;359:18–26.
153. Guo B, Jaovisidha S, Sartoris DJ, et al. Correlation between ossification of the stylohyoid ligament and osteophytes of the cervical spine. *J Rheumatol* 1997;24:1575–1581.
154. Cammisa M, De Serio A, Guglielmi G. Diffuse idiopathic skeletal hyperostosis. *Eur J Radiol* 1998;27 (suppl 1):S7–S11.
155. Pappone N, Di Girolamo C, Del Puente A, et al. Diffuse idiopathic skeletal hyperostosis (DISH): a retrospective analysis. *Clin Rheumatol* 1996;15:121–124.
156. Resnick D, Niwayama G. Diffuse idiopathic hyperostosis (DISH) (ankylosing hyperostosis of Forestier and Rotes-Querol). In: Resnick D, ed. *Diagnosis of bone and joint disorders,* 3rd ed. Philadelphia: WB Saunders, 1995:1463–1495.

157. Denko CW, Boja B, Moskowitz RW. Growth promoting peptides in osteoarthritis and diffuse idiopathic skeletal hyperostosis-insulin, insulin-like growth factor I, growth hormone. *J Rheumatol* 1994;21:1725–1730.
158. Tsuyama N. Ossification of the posterior longitudinal ligament of the spoine. *Clin Orthop* 1984;184:71–84.
159. Miyasaka K, Kaneda K, Sato S, et al. Myelopathy due to ossification or calcification of the ligamentum flavum: radiologic and histologic evaluations. *Am J Neurol Radiol* 1983;4:629–632.
160. Cicuttini FM, Baker J, Hart DJ, et al. Relation between Heberden's nodes and distal interphalangeal joint osteophytes and their role as markers of generalized disease. *Ann Rheum Dis* 1998;57:246–248.
161. Segal R, Avrahami E, Lebdinski E, et al. The impact of hemiparalysis on the expression of osteoarthritis. *Arthritis Rheum* 1998;41:2249–2256.
162. Nakamura R, Ono Y, Horii E, et al. The aetiological significance of workload in the development of osteoarthritis of the distal interphalangeal joint. *J Hand Surg [Br]* 1993;18: 540–542.
163. Smith D, Braunstein EM, Brandt KD, et al. A radiographic comparison of erosive osteoarthritis and idiopathic nodal osteoarthritis. *J Rheumatol* 1992;19:896–904.
164. Kassimos DG, Shirlaw PJ, Choy H, et al. Chronic sialadenitis in patients with nodal osteoarthritis. *Br J Rheumatol* 1997;36: 1312–1317.
165. Kellgren JH, Lawrence JS, Bier F. Genetic factors in generalized osteoarthritis. *Ann Rheum Dis* 1963;22:237–255.
166. Hirsch R, Lethbridge-Cejku M, Hanson R, et al. Familial aggregation of osteoarthritis: data from the Baltimore Longitudinal Study on Aging. *Arthritis Rheum* 1998;41:1227–1232.
167. Hirsch R, Lethbridge-Cejku M, Scott WW, et al. Association of hand and knee osteoarthritis: evidence for a polyarticular disease subset. *Ann Rheum* Dis 1996;55:25–29.
168. Pattrick M, Manhire A, Ward AM, et al. HLA-A, B antigens and alpha 1-antitrypsin phenotypes in nodal generalized osteoarthritis and erosive osteoarthritis. *Ann Rheum Dis* 1989; 48:470–475.
169. Ushiyama T, Ueyama H, Inoue K, et al. Estrogen receptor gene polymorphism and generalized osteoarthritis. *J Rheumatol* 1998;25:134–137.
170. Wright GD, Hughes AE, Regan M, et al. Association of two loci on chromosome 2q with nodal osteoarthritis. *Ann Rheum Dis* 1996;55:317–319.
171. Felson DT, Couropmitree NN, Chaisson CE, et al. Evidence for a Mendelian gene in segregation analysis of generalized radiographic osteoarthritis: The Framingham Study. *Arthritis Rheum* 1998;41:1064–1071.
172. Knowlton RG, Katzenstein PL, Moskowitz RW, et al. Genetic linkage of a polymorphism in the type II procollagen gene (COL2A1) to primary osteoarthritis associated with mild chondrodysplasia. *N Engl J Med* 1990;332:526–530.
173. Reginato AJ, Passano GM, Neumann G, et al. Familial spondyloepiphyseal dysplasia tarda, brachydactyly, and precocious osteoarthritis associated with an arginine T5 cysteine mutation in the procollagen type II gene in a kindred of chiloe islanders. *Arthritis Rheum* 1994;37:1078–1086.
174. Pun YL, Moskowitz RW, Lie S, et al. Clinical correlations of osteoarthritis associated with a single-base mutation (arginine 519 to cysteine in type II procollagen gene. A newly defined pathogenesis. *Arthritis Rheum* 1994;37:264–269.
175. Bleasel JF, Bisagni-Faure A, Holderbaum D, et al. Type II procollagen gene (COL2A1) mutation in exon II associated with spondyloepiphyseal dysplasia, tall stature, and precocious osteoarthritis. *J Rheumatol* 1995;22:255–261.
176. Lee B, Vissing H, Ramirez F, et al. Identification of the molecular defect in a family with spondyloepiphyseal dysplasia. *Science* 1989;244:978–980.
177. Eyre DR, Weis MA, Moskowitz RW. Cartilage expression of a type II collagen mutation in an inherited form of osteoarthritis associated with a mild chondrodysplasia. *J Clin Invest* 1991;87: 357–361.
178. Vikkula M, Palotie A, Ritvaniemi P, et al. Early onset osteoarthritis linked to the type II procollagen gene. Detailed clinical phenotype and further analyses of the gene. *Arthritis Rheum* 1993;36:401–409.
179. Loughlin J, Irven C, Fergusson C, et al. Sibling pair analysis shows no linkage of generalized osteoarthritis to the loci encoding type II collagen, cartilage link protein or cartilage matrix protein. *Br J Rheumatol* 1994;33:1103–1106.
180. Loughlin J, Irven C, Athanasou N, et al. Differential allelic expression of the type II collagen gene (COL2A1) in osteoarthritic cartilage. *Am J Hum Genet* 1995;56:1186–1193.
181. Janocha S, Wolz W, Srsen S, et al. The human gene for alkaptonuria (AKU) maps to chromosome 3q. *Genomics* 1994;19: 5–8.
182. Kabasakal Y, Kiyici I, Ozmen D, et al. Spinal abnormalities similar to ankylosing spondylitis in a 58-year-old woman with ochronosis. *Clin Rheumatol* 1995;14:355–357.
183. Stiehl P, Kluger KM. [Joint effusion findings in alkaptonuric arthropathy]. *Z Rheumatol* 1994;53:150–154.
184. Melis M, Onori P, Aliberti G, et al. Ochronotic arthropathy: structural and ultrastructural features. *Ultrastruct Pathol* 1994; 18:467–471.
185. Angeles AP, Badger R, Gruber H, et al. Chondrocyte growth inhibition induced by homogentensic acid and its partial prevention with ascorbic acid. *J Rheumatol* 1989;16:512–517.
186. Hiraku Y, Yamasaki M, Kawanishi S. Oxidative DNA damage included by homogentisic acid, a tyrosine metabolite. *FEBS Lett* 1998;432:13–16.
187. Pascual E. Persistence of monosodium urate crystals and low grade inflammation in the synovial fluid of patients with untreated gout. *Arthritis Rheum* 1991;34:141–145.
188. Bancroft JD, Stevens A. *Theory and practice of histological techniques,* 3rd ed. Edinburgh: Churchill-Livingstone, 1990:262–263.
189. Sokoloff L. The history of Kashin-Beck disease. *NY State J Med* 1989;89:343–351.
190. Mathieu F, Begaux F, Lan ZY, et al. Clinical manifestations of Kashin-Beck disease in Nyemo Valley, Tibet. *Int Orthop* 1997; 21:151–156.
191. Sokoloff L. Endemic forms of osteoarthritis. *Clin Rheum Dis* 1985;11:187–202.
192. Wang Y, Yang Z, Gilula LA, et al. Kashin-Beck disease: radiographic appearance in the hands and wrists. *Radiology* 1996; 201:265–270.
193. Yang GQ, Xia YM. Studies on human dietary requirements and safe range of dietary intakes of selenium in China and their application in the prevention of related endemic diseases. *Biomed Environ Sci* 1995;8:187–201.
194. Moreno-Reyes R, Suetens C, Mathieu F, et al. Kashin-Beck osteoarthropathy in rural Tibet in relation to selenium and iodine status. *N Engl J Med* 1998;339:1112–1120.
195. Wei XQ, Wright GC, Sokoloff L. The effect of sodium selenite in chondrocytes in monolayer culture. *Arthritis Rheum* 1986; 29:660–664.
196. Yang C, Niu C, Bodo M, et al. Fulvic acid supplementation and selenium deficiency disturb the structural integrity of mouse skeletal tissue. An animal model to study the molecular effects of Kashin-Beck disease. *Biochem J* 1993;289: 829–835.
197. Yang C, Bodo M, Holger N, et al. Fulvic acid disturbs processing of procollagen II in articular cartilage of embryonic chicken

and may also cause Kashin-Beck disease. *Eur J Biochem* 1991; 202:1141–1146.
198. Liang HJ, Tsai CL, Lu FJ. Oxidative stress induced by humic acid solvent extraction fraction in cultured rabbit articular chondrocytes. *J Toxicol Environ Health* 1998;54:477–489.
199. Sokoloff L, Fincham JE, du Toit GT. Pathological features of the femoral head in Mseleni disease. *Hum Pathol* 1985;16: 117–120.
200. Solomon L. Distinct types of hip disorder in Mseleni joint disease. *S Afr Med J* 1986:69:15–17.
201. Viljoen D, Fredlund V, Ramesar R, et al. Brachydactylous dwarfs of Mseleni. *Am J Med Genet* 1993;46:636–640.
202. Ballo R, Viljoen D, Machadu M, et al. Mseleni joint disease—a molecular genetic approach to defining the aetiology. *S Afr Med J* 1996;86:956–958.
203. Schnitzler CM, Pieczkowski WM, Fredlund V, et al. Histomorphometric analysis of osteopenia associated with endemic osteoarthritis (Mseleni joint disease). *Bone* 1988;9:21–27.
204. Adebajo AO. Pattern of osteoarthritis in a west African teaching hospital. *Ann Rheum Dis* 1991;50:20–22.
205. Agarwal SS, Phadke SR, Fredlund V, et al. Mseleni and Handigodu familial osteoarthropathies. Syndromic identity? *Am J Med Genet* 1997;72:435–439.
206. Roosendaal G, van Rinsum AC, Vianen ME, et al. Hemophilic arthropathy resembles degenerative rather than inflammatory joint disease. *Histopathology* 1999;34:144–153.
207. Yang SS. The skeletal system. In: Wigglesworth JS, Singer DB, eds. *Textbook of fetal and perinatal pathology,* 2nd ed. London: Blackwell, 1998:1039–1068.
208. Gamble JG, Rinsky LA, Bleck EE. Established hip dislocations in cerebral palsy. *Clin Orthop* 1990;253:90–99.
209. Beighton PM, DePaepe A, Hall JG, et al. Molecular nosology of the heritable disorders of connective tissue. *Am J Med Genet* 1992;42:431–448.
210. Giunta C, Superti-Furga A, Spranger S, et al. Ehlers-Danlos syndrome type VII: clinical features and molecular defects. *J Bone Joint Surg* 1999;81A:225–238.
211. Badelon O, Bensahel H, Csukonyi Z, et al. Congenital dislocation of the hip in Ehlers-Danlos syndrome. *Clin Orthop* 1990; 255:138–143.
212. Vujic M, Hallstensson, Wahlstrom J, et al. Localization of a gene for autosomal dominant Larsen syndrome to chromosome region 3 p21.1-14.1 in the proximity of, but distinct from the COL 7A1 locus. *Am J Hum Genet* 1995;57:1104–1113.
213. Hadley NA, Brown TD, Weinstein SL. The effects of contact pressure elevations and aseptic necrosis on the longterm outcome of congenital hip dislocation. *J Orthop Res* 1990;8: 504–513.
214. Tredwell SJ. Neonatal screening for hip joint instability. *Clin Orthop* 1992;281:63–68.
215. Wilkinson JA. Etiological factors in congenital displacement of the hip and myelodysplasia. *Clin Orthop* 1992;281:75–83.
216. Hod M, Merlob P, Friedman S, et al. Prevalence of congenital anomalies and neonatal complications in the offspring of diabetic mothers in Israel. *Isr J Med Sci* 1991;27:498–502.
217. Uden A, Lindhagen T. Inguinal hernia in patients with congenital hip dislocation. *Acta Orthop Scand* 1988;59:667–668.
218. Todhunter RJ, Acland GM, Olivier M, et al. An outcrossed canine pedigree for linkage analysis of hip dysplasia. *J Hered* 1999;90:83–92.
219. Guille JT, Lipton GE, Szoke G, et al. Legg-Calve-Perthes disease in girls. A comparison of the results with those seen in boys. *J Bone Joint Surg* 1998;80A:1256–1263.
220. Weinstein SL. Natural history and treatment outcomes of childhood hip disorders. *Clin Orthop* 1997;344:227–242.
221. Lane WE, Neuitt MC, Cooper C, et al. Acetabular dysplasia and osteoarthritis of the hip in elderly white women. *Ann Rheum Dis* 1997;56:627–630.
222. Smith RW, Egger P, Coggon D, et al. Osteoarthritis of the hip joint and acetabular dysplasia in women. *Ann Rheum Dis* 1995; 54:179–181.
223. Hochbergs P, Eckerwall G, Egund N, et al. Synovitis in Legg-Calvé-Perthes disease. Evaluation with MR imaging in 84 hips. *Acta Radiol* 1998;39:532–537.
224. Arruda VR, Belangero WD, Ozelo MC, et al. Inherited risk factors for thrombophilia among children with Legg-Calvé-Perthes disease. *J Pediatr Orthop* 1999;19:84–87.
225. Stasikelis PJ, Sullivan CM, Phillips WA, et al. Slipped capital femoral epiphysis. Prediction of contralateral involvement. *J Bone Joint Surg* 1996;78A:1149–1155.
226. Fine RN. Growth hormone treatment of children with chronic renal insufficiency, end-state renal disease and following renal transplantation—update 1997. *J Pediatr Endocrinol Metab* 1997;10:361–370.
227. Goodman DA, Feighan JE, Smith AD, et al. Subclinical slipped capital femoral epiphysis. Relationship to osteoarthrosis of the hip. *J Bone Joint Surg* 1997;79A:1489–1497.
228. al-Rawi Z, Nessan AH. Joint hypermobility in patients with chondromalacia patellae. *Br J Rheumatol* 1997;36:1324–1327.
229. Gupta R. A short history of neuropathic arthropathy. *Clin Orthop* 1993;296:43–49.
230. Squeira W. The neuropathic joint. *Clin Exp Rheumatol* 1994; 12:325–327.
231. Sharma L, Pai Y-C, Holtkamp K, et al. Is knee joint proprioception worse in the arthritic knee versus the unaffected knee in unilateral knee osteoarthritis. *Arthritis Rheum* 1997;40: 1518–1525.
232. Brighton CT. Morphology and biochemistry of the growth plate. *Rheum Dis Clin North Am* 1987;13:75–100.
233. Koo KH, Kim R, Cho S-H, et al. Angiography, scintigraphy, intraosseous pressure, and histologic findings in high-risk osteonecrotic femoral heads with negative magnetic resonance images. *Clin Orthop* 1994;308:127–138.
234. Steinberg ME, Corces A, Fallon M. Acetabular involvement in osteonecrosis of femoral head. *J Bone Joint Surg* 1999;81A: 60–65.
235. Jones JP. Coagulopathies and osteonecrosis. *Acta Orthop Belg* 1999;65 (suppl 1):5–8.
236. Muscolo DL, Costa-Paz M, Makino A, et al. Osteonecrosis of the knee following arthroscopic meniscectomy in patients over 50 years old. *Arthroscopy* 1996;12:273–279.
237. Ahuja SA, Bullough PG. Osteonecrosis of the knee: a clinicopathological study in twenty-eight patients. *J Bone Joint Surg* 1978;60A:191–197.
238. Hashimoto S, Ochs RL, Komiya S, et al. Linkage of chondrocyte apoptosis and cartilage degradation in human osteoarthritis. *Arthritis Rheum* 1998;41:1632–1638.
239. Harris WH. Etiology of osteoarthritis of the hip. *Clin Orthop* 1986;213:20–33.
240. Vingard E, Alfredsson L, Malchau H. Osteoarthritis of the hip in women and its relation to physical load at work and in the home. *Ann Rheum Dis* 1997;56:293–298.
241. Cooper C, Inship H, Croft P, et al. Individual risk factors for hip osteoarthritis: obesity, hip injury, and physical activity. *Am J Epidemiol* 1998;147:516–522.
242. Felson DT, Zhang Y. An update on the epidemiology of knee and hip osteoarthritis with a view to prevention. *Arthritis Rheum* 1998;41:1343–1355.
243. Axford JS, Bomford A, Revell P, et al. Hip arthropathy in genetic hemochromatosis. Radiographic and histologic features. *Arthritis Rheum* 1991;34:357–361.
244. Rosenbloom AL, Silverstein JH. Connective tissue and joint

disease in diabetes mellitus. *Endocrinol Metab Clin North Am* 1996;25:473–483.

245. Cimmino MA, Cutolo M. Plasma glucose concentration in symptomatic osteoarthritis. A clinical and epidemiological survey. *Clin Exp Rheumatol* 1990;8:251–257.
246. Frey MI, Barrett-Connor E, Sledge PA, et al. The effect of noninsulin dependent diabetes mellitus on the prevalence of clinical osteoarthritis. A population based study. *J Rheumatol* 1996; 23:716–722.
247. Davis M, Ettinger WH, Neuhaus JM, et al. Sex differences in osteoarthritis of the knee. The role of obesity. *Am J Epidemiol* 1988;127:1019–1030.
248. Peyron JG, Altman RD. The epidemiology of osteoarthritis. In: Moskowitz RW, Howell DS, Goldberg VM, et al., eds. *Osteoarthritis: diagnosis, and medical/surgical management*, 2nd ed. Philadelphia: WB Saunders 1992:15–37.
249. Belmonte-Serrano MA, Block DA, Lane NE, et al. The relationship between spinal and peripheral osteoarthritis and bone density measurements. *J Rheumatol* 1993;20:1005–1013.
250. Verstraeten A, Van Ermen H, Haghebaert G, et al. Osteoarthritis retards the development of osteoporosis. *Clin Orthop* 1991;264:169–177.
251. Hannan MT, Anderson JJ, Zhang Y, et al. Bone mineral density and knee osteoarthritis in elderly men and women. *Arthritis Rheum* 1993;36:1671–1680.
252. Ito M, Hayashi K, Yamada M, et al. Relationship of osteophytes to bone mineral density and spinal fracture in men. *Radiology* 1993;189:497–502.
253. Dequeker J, Mohan S, Finkelman RD, et al. Generalized osteoarthritis associated with increased insulin-like growth factor types I and II and transforming growth factor β in cortical bone from iliac crest. *Arthritis Rheum* 1993;36:1702–1708.
254. Raymackers G, Aerssens J, Van der Eynde R, et al. Alterations of the mineralization profile and osteocalcin concentrations in osteoarthritic cortical iliac crest bone. *Calcif Tissue Int* 1992; 51:269–275.
255. Weinstein RS, Jilka RL, Parfitt AM, et al. Inhibition of osteoblastogenesis and promotion of apoptosis of osteoblasts and osteocytes by glucocorticoids. Potential mechanisms of their deleterious effects on bone. *J Clin Invest* 1998;102: 274–282
256. Keen RW, Hart DJ, Lanchbury JS, et al. Association of early osteoarthritis of the knee with a Taq I polymorphism of the vitamin D receptor gene. *Arthritis Rheum* 1997;40:1444–1449.
257. Meulenbelt I, Bijerk C, de Wildt SC, et al. Investigation of the association of the CRTM and CRTL1 genes with radiographically evident osteoarthritis in subjects from the Rotterdam study. *Arthritis Rheum* 1997;40:1760–1765.
258. Spector TD, Cicuttini F, Baker J, et al. Genetic influences on osteoarthritis in women: a twin study. *Br Med J* 1996;312: 940–943.
259. Muragaki Y, Mariman ECM, van Beersum SEC, et al. A mutation in the gene encoding the α2 chain of the fibril-associated collagen IX, COL9A2 causes multiple epiphyseal dysplasia (EDM2). *Nat Genet* 1996;12:103–105.
260. Davis MA, Neuhaus JM, Ettinger WH. Body fat distribution and osteoarthritis. *Am J Epidemiol* 1990;132:701–707.
261. Spector TD, Hart DJ, Doyle DV. Incidence and progression of osteoarthritis in women with unilateral knee disease in the general population: the effect of obesity. *Ann Rheum Dis* 1994; 53: 565–568.
262. Tepper S, Hochberg MC. Factors associated with hip osteoarthritis: data from the First National Health and Nutrition Examination Survey (NHANES-1). *Am J Epidemiol* 1993; 127:1081–1088.
263. Sowers M, Zobel D, Weissfeld L, et al. Progression of osteoarthritis of the hand and metacarpal bone loss. *Arthritis Rheum* 1991;34:36–42.
264. Cerhan JR, Wallace RB, el-Khoury GY, et al. Decreased survival with increasing prevalence of full-body radiographically defined osteoarthritis in women. *Am J Epidemiol* 1995;141:225–234.
265. Lindberg H, Montgomery F. Heavy labor and the occurrence of gonarthrosis. *Clin Orthop* 1987;214:235–236.
266. Roach KE, Persky V, Miles T, et al. Biomechanical aspects of occupation and osteoarthritis of the hip: a case-control study. *J Rheumatol* 1994;21:2334–2340.
267. Lane NE, Michel B, Bjorkengren A, et al. The risk of osteoarthritis with running and aging: a five-year longitudinal study. *J Rheumatol* 1993;20:461–468.
268. Olsen O, Vingard E, Koster M, et al. Etiologic fractions for work load, sports and overweight in the occurrence of coxarthrosis. *Scand J Work Environ Health* 1994;20:184–188.
269. Swann DA, Silver FH, Slayter HS, et al. The molecular structure and lubricating activity of lubricin isolated from bovine and human synovial fluids. *Biochem J* 1985;25:195–201.
270. Woo S L-Y, Kwan MK, Coutts RD, et al. Biomechanical considerations. In: Moskowitz RW, Howell DS, Goldberg VM, et al., eds. *Osteoarthritis: diagnosis and medical/surgical management*, 2nd ed. Philadelphia: WB Saunders, 1992:191–211.
271. Hills BA, Monds MK. Enzymatic identification of the load-bearing boundary lubricant in the joint. *Br J Rheumatol* 1998;37:137–142.
272. Schwarz IM, Hills BA. Synovial surfactant: lamellar bodies in type B synoviocytes and proteolipid in synovial fluid and the articular lining. *Br J Rheumatol* 1996;35:821–827.
273. Schwarz IM, Hills BA. Surface-active phospholipid as the lubricating component of lubricin. *Br J Rheumatol* 1998;37:21–26.
274. Hills BA, Monds MK. Deficiency of lubricating surfactant lining the articular surfaces of replaced hips and knees. *Br J Rheumatol* 1998;37:143–147.
275. Ludkowski P, Wilson-MacDonald J. Total arthroplasty in Paget's disease of the hip. *Clin Orthop* 1990;255:160–167.

110

ETIOPATHOGENESIS OF OSTEOARTHRITIS

JEAN-PIERRE PELLETIER
JOHANNE MARTEL-PELLETIER
DAVID S. HOWELL

Osteoarthritis (OA) results from a complex of biologic processes, both degradative and reparative, with involvement of all tissues of the joint. Inflammatory components to a variable degree afflict the majority of patients. The secondary form of OA, for the most part, may be divided into two categories: the imposition of a structurally or biomechanically faulty joint, and superimposed risk factors that affect the intensity and distribution of loading forces across the joint surfaces. This chapter focuses on research advances in the understanding of pathogenesis, emphasizing cellular and molecular biology and the biochemistry of the joint tissues, as well as inflammation and relevant growth factors. A brief clinical sketch of the etiologic categories is given before the main review on pathogenesis.

PHYSICAL INSULTS IN ETIOLOGY

Neuromuscular control of the limbs is impaired in diseases such as tabes dorsalis and syringomyelia (Table 110.1). Also, there is evidence that such control may be subtly impaired in aging patients with OA where digging of the heels on force plate analysis has been shown (1). Loss of muscle strength in the quadriceps and other muscle groups retards smooth attenuation of loading forces (2). Obesity is an important risk factor that causes joint overload and is associated with radiographically dense bones (3). Joint location and cartilage matrix vulnerability to chemical and mechanical injury are highly correlated with risk of developing OA (4,5). Theoretically, the evolutionary adaptations by humans to upright posture, involving redistribution of loading forces across the hips, knees, bunion joints, and low back, as well as changes in the hand could be considered OA risk factors (6).

Overexercise, macrotrauma, and microtrauma have been studied in detail in relation to human occupations and sports (7), and the cartilage cell mechanics (8) and matrix responses to trauma have been examined (9). Her-

TABLE 110.1. CLASSIFICATION OF OSTEOARTHRITIS

Primary idiopathic
Peripheral joints (single versus multiple joints)
  Interphalangeal joints (nodal) (e.g., DIP PIP)
  Other small joints (e.g., CMC, first MTP)
  Large joints (e.g., hip, knee)
Spine
  Apophyseal joints
  Intervertebral joints
Variant subsets
  Erosive inflammatory osteoarthritis (EOA)
  Generalized osteoarthritis (GOA)
  Chondromalacia patellae
  Diffuse idiopathic skeletal hyperostosis (DISH, ankylosing hyperostosis)
Secondary
  Trauma
    Acute
    Chronic (occupational, sports, obesity)
  Other joint disorders
    Local (fracture, avascular necrosis, infection)
    Diffuse (rheumatoid arthritis, hypermobility syndrome, hemorrhagic diatheses)
  Systemic metabolic disease
    Ochronosis (alkaptonuria)
    Hemochromatosis
    Wilson's disease
    Kashin-Beck disease
  Endocrine disorders
    Acromegaly
    Hyperparathyroidism
    Diabetes mellitus
  Calcium crystal deposition diseases
    Calcium pyrophosphate dihydrate
    Calcium apatite
  Neuropathic disorders (Charcot joints) (e.g., tabes dorsalis, diabetes mellitus, intraarticular steroid overuse)
  Bone dysplasias (multiple epiphyseal dysplasia, spondyloepiphyseal dysplasia)
  Miscellaneous
    Frostbite
    Long-leg arthropathy

DIP, distal interphalangeal joint; PIP, proximal interphalangeal joint; CMC, carpometacarpal joint; MTP, metatarsal phalangeal joint.

itable collagen hyperelasticity seen in Ehlers-Danlos syndrome causes joint hypermobility, increasing the risk of OA in several joints. Premature onset of primary OA has been studied in different generations of nonconsanguineous families (10), and radiographic and clinical changes of OA were identified in multiple joints in the second and third decades of life. Pedigree studies revealed an autosomal-dominant trait mapped to alleles of type II procollagen gene located on chromosome 12. Specifically, a mutation introducing cysteine (in place of arginine) into the triple helix domain of type II procollagen chains at position 519 was associated with the disease phenotype (10). OA is caused predominantly by weakening of the cartilage matrix due to the above faulty collagen structure in joint cartilage in adults. New research on these and other hereditary disorders relevant to OA development has been reviewed recently (10,11). Chronic inflammatory diseases either by direct injury of joints or through induction of abnormalities of growth plate function and/or bone growth can render joints vulnerable to the development of OA.

Most developmental abnormalities predisposing to OA are idiopathic. Examples include "pistol grip" deformities of the hip (12), shallowness or bony ridge formation of the acetabulum (13), tilted position of the femoral head on the femoral neck (13), and genu varus or genus valgus, as well as unequal limb length. Differences in OA prevalence according to joint location (e.g., knee vs. ankle sites) have led to biochemical and biomechanical studies comparing the two sites.

Osteoarthritis also develops in patients with injury of cartilage cells related to exposure to unique deposits or infiltrates in the cartilage matrix found in metabolic diseases such as hemochromatosis, ochronosis (alkaptonuria), Wilson's disease, and Gaucher's disease, as well as cartilage disturbed by endocrine disorders, such as acromegaly (Table 110.1).

The role of nutritional factors in the etiopathology of OA has been reexamined in epidemiologic studies (14). Evidence suggesting an increased risk of OA in the knees related to low vitamin D status was obtained, and protection against OA progression was associated with a high intake of the antioxidants ascorbic acid and β-carotene (14). In Asia, Kashin-Beck disease, a form of OA, has been related to dietary exposure to an endemic fungus (15). Of interest, hypothyroidism afflicts many of these patients due to the presence of dietary selenium deficiency (16). A chick model with dietary vitamin B_6 deficiency exhibited articular cartilage fissuring, joint effusion, and loss of decorin from cartilage surfaces (17).

Elucidation of pathogenic pathways involved in OA has come from biochemical and biomechanical studies of various animal models of OA (18). Interestingly, disuse immobilization followed by overexercise can lead to cartilage injury associated with altered biochemical composition (19–21) and elevated metalloproteases in the cartilage (22,23). Following cruciate ligament transection in dogs, a predictable chronology of changes in cartilage, bone, ligaments, and synovia occurs. The earliest changes in the knee articular cartilage reflect a hypertrophic biochemical repair reaction, with enhanced synthesis of matrix components and increase in matrix content (24,25). The hypertrophic stage clearly precedes the occurrence of the deep lesional stage with its characteristic focal loss of cartilage. In this model, the biomechanical properties correlated well with the significantly reduced distribution and size of the large and small proteoglycan aggregates measured by transport ultracentrifugation, concurrent loss of hyaluronan and link protein from cartilage, as well as upregulated collagenase (21,26–28). Degradation was shown by upregulation of link protein and aggrecan ligands in synovial fluid indicative of proteolysis (29).

MINERAL DEPOSITION AND OSTEOARTHRITIS

In many patients, crystal deposition of calcium pyrophosphate dihydrate (CPPD) or basic calcium phosphate (BCP) precedes development of clinical or radiographic evidence of OA (30,31). However, because chondrocalcinosis and OA are both common in the elderly, correlations must be interpreted cautiously. In a large autopsy series, articular cartilage staining for calcium salts was positive in over 90% of the subjects (32). A high frequency of calcium-containing crystals on OA cartilage surfaces was shown in another study (33). Such calcium minerals have been detected in 60% of synovial fluids in one study of osteoarthritic patients (34). These cases include idiopathic OA with the usual distribution of joint pathology (30). Mineral deposition in CPPD has a different pattern of involved joints than idiopathic OA with localization in the former typically involving the shoulders, wrists, and metacarpophalangeal joints (30).

Although under certain conditions CPPD crystals and hydroxyapatite crystal aggregates are dramatically phlogistic in both animal models and cell culture systems, there is equivocal evidence in cartilage that crystals are taken up by or injure chondrocytes directly (31,35,36). Phlogistic secondary effects on cartilage cells of such crystals through their induction of synovial cell factors have been comprehensively reviewed (37). As is the case in growth cartilage, matrix vesicle fractions from articular cartilages have been detected in osteoarthritic joints that generate CPPD crystals and BCP crystals (38,39). In recent years, chondrocytic production of large amounts of nitric oxide in articular cartilage, together with the demonstration that nitric oxide induces programmed cell death in chondrocytes, has stimulated studies of traumatized human tissue and of animal models of traumatic responses for the presence of nitric oxide production, apoptosis, and prostaglandin E_2 (PGE_2) release. The similarity of apoptotic cell particles to matrix vesicles was recently demonstrated regarding several parameters, including their capability of generating minerals in the presence of adenosine triphosphate (ATP) *in vitro* (40). The severity of experimental OA was reduced by treatment with a specific inhibitor of inducible nitric oxide synthase (41). Phosphocitrate, a potent blocker of CPPD and BCP crystal formation, arrested nitric oxide–induced calcification of cartilage, as well as calcification of apoptotic bodies, probably through its effects on crystal surfaces but not inhibition of the critical enzyme NTP pyrophoshydrolase (NTPPPH) (42). In aging human cartilage, increased apoptotic cells and apoptotic particles have been observed using histologic techniques, particularly in the surface cartilage layers (43). Several reports have suggested loss of cellularity at the articular cartilage surface and empty lucunae (44). Certainly, this is seen in OA. These cell modulations have been compared to those of growth plates because of similarities in the pattern of terminal differentiation, as exemplified by the expression of growth plate type markers [e.g., collagen type X (45) and parathyroid hormone (PTH)-related peptide (PTHrP)] (46). This interesting theory relating chondrocyte apoptosis to the pathogenesis of OA has become the subject of an expanding research field (see below).

ETIOPATHOLOGY OF OSTEOARTHRITIS

In osteoarthritis (OA), articular cartilage, subchondral bone, and synovial membrane are the major sites of change in the course of the disease process. OA is characterized by degradation and loss of articular cartilage, hypertrophic bone changes with osteophyte formation, subchondral bone remodeling, and, at the clinical stage of the disease, chronic inflammation of the synovial membrane.

Prior to the onset of proteoglycan depletion and loss of cartilage, biosynthetic activity of the chondrocytes may lead to an increase in proteoglycan concentration of the cartilage, resulting in thickening of the tissue during the earlier stages of OA. These new proteoglycan molecules appear abnormal as their structure is significantly altered. Nevertheless, the repair process appears to keep pace with the disease, and this response may be sufficient to maintain joint function for many years. As the disease progresses, however, the degradative process eventually exceeds the anabolic, leading to a progressive loss of cartilage and eburnation of bone. This appears to occur when the physiologic balance between the synthesis and degradation of the extracellular matrix favors catabolism. At the clinical stage of the disease, an inflammatory reaction involving the synovial membrane is often present. This process favors the synthesis of inflammatory mediators, which impact on cartilage matrix homeostasis by altering chondrocyte metabolism to enhance catabolism while reducing the anabolism.

Cartilage

The alterations in OA cartilage are numerous and involve morphologic and synthetic changes of chondrocytes as well as biochemical and structural alterations of the extracellular matrix macromolecules. Evidence has accumulated favoring an important role for metabolic changes in these pathologic chondrocytes, with elaboration of pathologic factors causing matrix degradation (47).

In the normal joint, there is a balance between the continuous processes of cartilage matrix degradation and repair. These functions are performed almost solely by resident chondrocytes dispersed in their lacunae throughout the matrix, lasting a lifetime under normal conditions. Chondrocytes function in response to cytokines and growth factor signals, and to direct physical stimuli, which interact in a complex manner. The end result is a change in the rate of synthesis versus that of enzymatic breakdown of the cartilage matrix, occurring both around the cells and at some distance. Both autocrine and paracrine actions have been demonstrated in chondrocytes as well as in synovial lining cells. In OA, there is a disruption of this homeostatic state. In most sites of OA change, the anabolic processes of these cells become deficient relative to their catabolic influences (Fig. 110.1, stage I). Focal repair responses are inadequate to maintain normal matrix integrity. At the time of histologic appearance of OA lesions, the matrix has reached the critical point where its viscoelastic properties become insufficient to withstand normal joint loads, and progressive cartilage loss may follow. Biomechanical factors then assume a more prominent role.

Synovial Membrane

As is well known, even if articular tissue destruction characterizes the OA condition, synovial membrane inflammation is also of importance in the progression of cartilage lesions in this disease. In most patients with OA, focal or scattered sites of synovial inflammation are detected (48–50). OA patients who have undergone either total knee or total hip replacement are often found to have a prominent inflammatory synovitis that may resemble the inflammatory changes seen in rheumatoid arthritis (RA). Osteoarthritic synovial membrane histology is quite heterogeneous. At one end of the spectrum there is marked hyperplasia of the synovial lining layer, with a dense cellular infiltrate composed mainly of lymphocytes and monocytes. At the opposite end, the synovial membrane is thickened by fibrotic tissue, with a very sparse cellular infiltrate. Cytokines in the synovial fluid are believed to

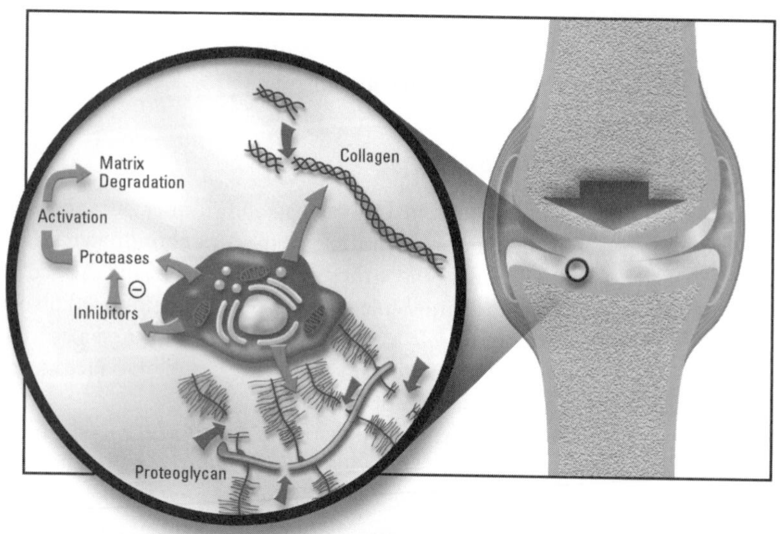

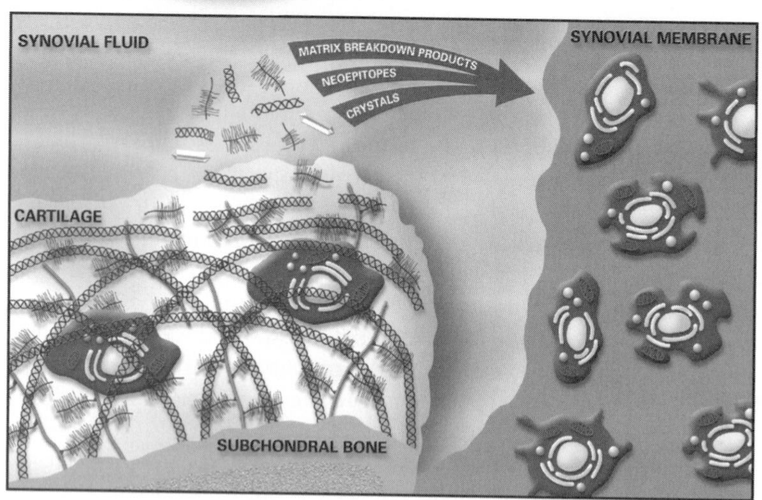

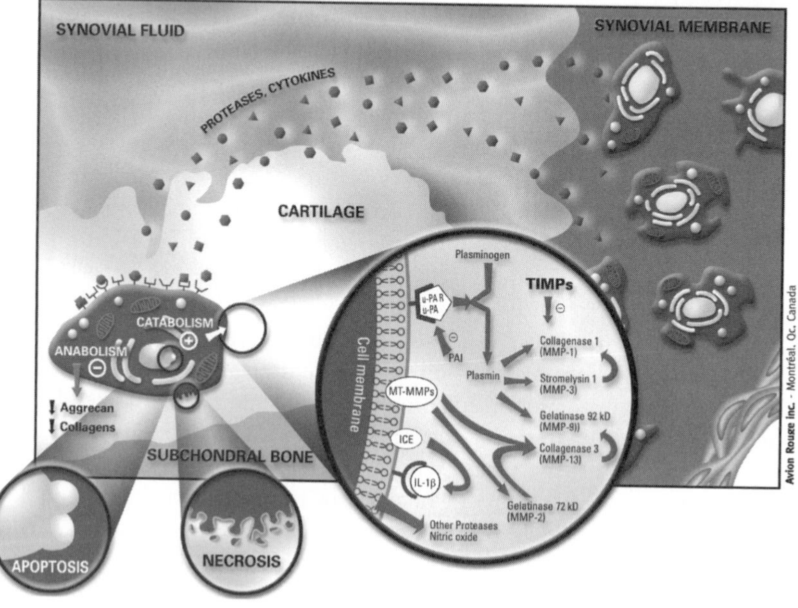

FIGURE 110.1. The evolution of the osteoarthritis disease process is arbitrarily divided into three stages. **Stage I (top)**: proteolytic breakdown of cartilage matrix. **Stage II (middle)**: fibrillation and erosion of cartilage surface with release of matrix molecule breakdown products into the synovial fluid. **Stage III (bottom)**: the phagocytosis of cartilage matrix breakdown products and other materials by synovial macrophages induces a chronic inflammatory reaction of the synovium, thereby producing local synthesis of proteases and proinflammatory cytokines. The proteases and cytokines released by the synovium diffuse through the synovial fluid and into the cartilage, induce additional cartilage breakdown by direct macromolecule proteolysis and by stimulation of cytokine secretion by chondrocytes to increase the synthesis of proteases. At this stage the chondrocytes are hypersensitive to cytokine stimulation because of an increased level of cytokine receptors on the cell membrane. Stage III modified from Amershan Pharmacia Biotech, hc.

originate from increased synthesis by the membrane, but this is certainly not the primary cause of the synovitis. Synovial inflammation in OA is almost certainly secondary and is related to multiple factors, including microcrystals, mechanical stress, and enzymatic breakdown of OA cartilage, producing wear particles and soluble cartilage-specific degradation of macromolecules (Fig. 110.1, stage II). Cartilage matrix components are released into the synovial fluid, then taken up by synovial lining macrophages or, like keratan sulfate, escape into the blood (51). Proteolytic enzymes release increased amounts of cartilage matrix fragments into synovial fluid, which can promote inflammation in the synovial membrane. The inflammation, through the synthesis of mediators, creates a vicious circle, with increased cartilage degradation and subsequent provocation of more inflammation (Fig. 110.1, stage III).

Articular Joint Tissue Catabolism

Biochemical changes in OA affect several cartilage components, including its major matrix constituents—proteoglycan aggregates (aggrecan) and collagens. Aggrecans are probably the first cartilage constitutent to be affected, because they are progressively depleted in parallel with the severity of the disease. At a certain stage of evolution of OA, the chondrocytes appear unable to compensate fully for proteoglycan loss by increased synthesis, resulting in a net loss of matrix. The structure of the proteoglycan remaining in the cartilage is altered in different ways (52–55). Generally, the presence of aggregates appears to reduce the vulnerability of proteoglycans to enzymatic attack. In OA, proteases able to attack the proteoglycan monomer, particularly at the hyaluronic acid (HA)-binding region, have been demonstrated (56–61). Such degraded fragments can rapidly diffuse from cartilage, leaving behind normal proteoglycan still capable of aggregation. This important finding may explain why few breakdown products of proteoglycans have been found in OA cartilage. As soon as the degradation occurs, the products are either further degraded by chondrocyte enzymes or rapidly diffuse into the synovial fluid. Alternatively, but not excluding the latter, the reduction in the HA content of OA cartilage, causing a diminution in the size of the aggrecans as a result of facilitated diffusion of linear polymers, could favor a loss of proteoglycan breakdown products from cartilage. Proteoglycan degradation products have been identified in synovial fluid of patients with OA (62–65). Cleavage at the interglobular domain between G1 and G2 has been demonstrated and seems to be of particular importance in the pathophysiology of OA (59,63). The decreased proteoglycan content of the matrix in association with damaged collagen structure (28) leads to functional loss of normal matrix physiologic properties. Epitopes near the collagenase cleavage site of type II collagen fibers have been detected in OA cartilage with the use of antibodies (66). Moreover, the first damage to type II collagen is seen in pericellular sites around chondrocytes, directly implicating the chondrocyte in this collagen alteration.

In addition to mechanical factors, evidence suggests a role for enzymatic pathways in OA cartilage matrix degradation (67) (Fig. 110.2, top panel). Enzymatic processes resemble a cascade similar to that of the coagulation or complement systems. In RA, the synovium is the most abundant source of degradative enzymes, but in OA, chondrocytes seem to be the prime source of enzymes responsible for cartilage matrix catabolism. The enzyme family identified as playing a major role in OA pathophysiology is the metalloprotease. Other enzymes belonging to the serine proteases and thiol proteases also appear to be important during this disease process. However, a role for still other enzymes cannot be ruled out.

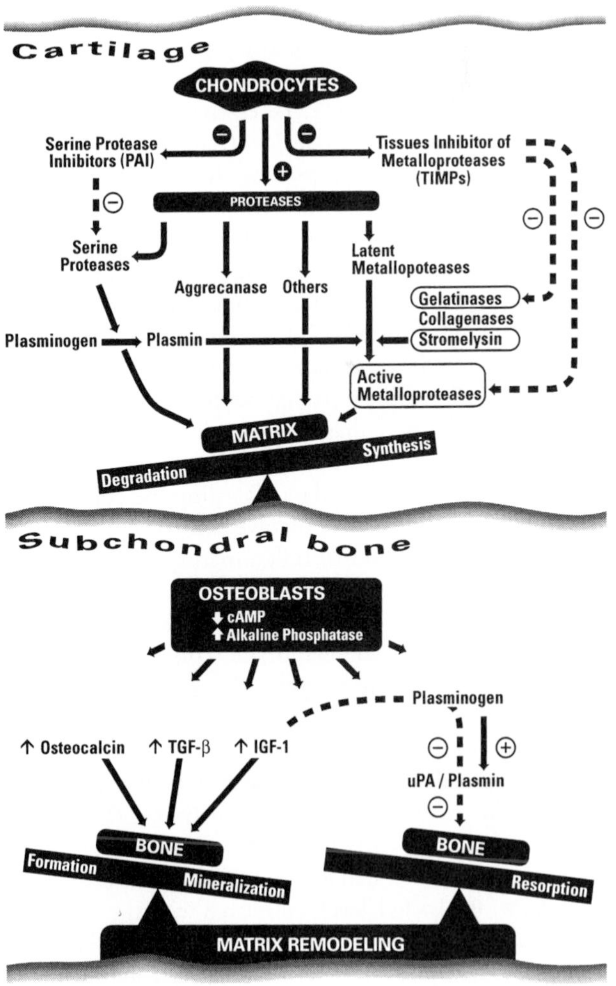

FIGURE 110.2. Schematic representation of the local enzymes or factors regulating articular cartilage catabolism and subchondral bone remodeling. (–), inhibition; (+), stimulation.

Metalloproteases

Matrix metalloproteases (MMPs) are broadly divided into groups based on substrate specificity and cellular location: collagenases, stromelysins, gelatinases, and membrane-type MMP (MT-MMP) (Fig. 110.2, top panel). In the last few years, another subgroup of MMPs, consisting of zinc-binding MMPs (designated adamalysin), has also been identified.

In OA, collagenase is responsible for the breakdown of collagen type II scaffolding in cartilage. Three collagenases have been identified in human cartilage—collagenase-1 (MMP-1), collagenase-2 (MMP-8), and collagenase-3 (MMP-13)—and their levels of expression and synthesis are clearly elevated in OA (68–74). Although all three collagenases are active on collagen fibrils, they are biochemically different. The coexistence of different types of collagenases in articular tissue, and their elevation during the OA process, point to distinct roles and regulation for each (70). All three collagenases cleave type II collagen. Collagenase-3 is at least five times more active on this substrate than collagenase-1; collagenase-2 has a higher specificity for type I collagen, and collagenase-1 for type III collagen. Within OA cartilage, it has also been demonstrated that a different topographical distribution exists among collagenase-1, collagenase-2, and collagenase-3, suggesting a selective involvement of each collagenase during the disease process. In this OA cartilage, collagenase-1 and -2 are located predominantly in the superficial and upper layers, whereas collagenase-3 is found mostly in the lower intermediate and deep layers (72,75–77). Moreover, in an immunohistochemical study using an OA animal model, it has been shown that the collagenase-1 chondrocyte score increased steadily in the superficial zone of the cartilage with progression of the lesions, whereas the collagenase-3 cell score in the deep zone reached a plateau at the moderate stage of the disease (76). Taken together, data regarding the collagenases in OA cartilage suggest an involvement of collagenase-1 during the catabolic and/or inflammatory phase, and collagenase-3 in the remodeling phase. The specific role of collagenase-2 in OA cartilage still remains to be determined. In OA synovial membrane, collagenase-1 is the predominant form. This enzyme, along with stromelysin-1, has been demonstrated in lining cells of OA synovia by immunolocalization (78–80).

Three stromelysins have also been described in human tissues: stromelysin-1 (MMP-3), stromelysin-2 (MMP-10), and stromelysin-3 (MMP-11). Of these, only stromelysin-1 has been found in elevated levels in OA tissues. As with collagenase, stromelysin-1 levels correlated with the histologic severity of OA lesions in both cartilage and synovial membrane (68,81). Stromelysin-1 has also been found in OA synovial fluid (64,82). Histochemical studies suggest a relationship between the level of stromelysin and the severity of degradation of pericellular proteoglycan. Degradation of type IX collagen—a glycoprotein with both collagenous and noncollagenous domains that plays an important role in cartilage matrix stability by linking type II collagen and proteoglycan—also occurred through the action of stromelysin (83). Interestingly, stromelysin-1 is also implicated in the enzymatic cascade responsible for the activation of procollagenase (84). Thus, this enzyme may have a dual role in OA pathophysiology.

Two gelatinases have been found in articular tissues: gelatinase 92 kd (gelatinase B or MMP-9) and gelatinase 72 kd (gelatinase A or MMP-2) (85). Further, gelatinase 92 kd was reported to be expressed and synthesized in OA, but not in normal cartilage (86). The fact that gelatinase 92 kd was found to be selectively expressed in OA fibrillated cartilage is consistent with the possibility that this enzyme could be responsible for progressive articular cartilage degradation in OA. Gelatinase 72 kd expression was also recently shown to be elevated in OA synovial membrane (87). This, however, contrasts with an earlier report in which only a few OA synovia demonstrated gelatinase 72 kd (88).

To date, four members of the MT-MMP subgroup have been identified and designated MT1-MMP through MT4-MMP. MT1-MMP is expressed in human articular cartilage and possesses collagenolytic activity (89). Both MT1-MMP and MT2-MMP activate gelatinase 72 kd and collagenase-3 (90,91). However, the relevance of these enzymes in the pathogenesis of OA has yet to be determined.

Analysis of aggrecan fragments in different catabolic systems indicates that cleavage of the Glu373-Ala374 bond of the interglobular domain, between the G1 and G2 domains of aggrecan, plays a central role in destroying the function of the molecule (59,63,65). An increased level of aggrecan fragments exhibiting this specific cleavage pattern was found in OA synovial fluid (65), indicating that a specific enzyme is involved in OA cartilage aggrecan degradation. This proteolytic activity is believed to be related to the action of a novel protease termed aggrecanase (63). This enzyme has recently been identified and belongs to the adamalysin family (61). It exhibits a zinc-binding domain similar to that found in several MMPs, and an aspartic acid residue following the third conserved histidine similar to that found in the adamalysin family. Interestingly, it contains a probable cysteine switch and a potential furin cleavage site, suggesting that this enzyme is synthesized in the inactive pro-form and requires a proteolytic cleavage to generate the mature active enzyme. The level of aggrecanase appeared to be increased by interleukin-1 (IL-1) (64).

Metalloprotease Regulation

The synthesis, activation, and inhibition of MMPs are tightly regulated at several levels in order to maintain a proper balance between the anabolism and catabolism of the articular joint tissue, since excessive amounts of MMPs would result in the overall destruction of the extracellular matrix. Regulatory pathways are found at the transcriptional [stimulation or inhibition of messenger RNA (mRNA)] and posttranslational levels (activation of the secreted latent enzymes and inhibition of activated MMPs.

In normal articular joint tissues, metalloprotease genes are generally expressed at low levels, and their transcription is induced by factors such as proinflammatory cytokines [IL-1β, tumor necrosis factor-α (TNF-α)] and some growth factors [epidermal growth factor (EGF), platelet-derived growth factor (PDGF), basic fibroblast growth factor (bFGF), transforming growth factor-β (TGF-β)]. For most of these factors, transcription activation of the MMP genes depends, at least in part, on the presence of an activator protein-1 (AP-1) site (92). Proteins of the Jun and Fos families of transcription factors bind the AP-1 site as dimers (Jun/Jun or Jun/Fos) and contribute to both basal and induced MMP transcription. Although important, this factor is not the only regulator of transcription but rather, seems to act in concert with other *cis*-acting sequences. For example, in the collagenase-1 promoter, the AP-1 and PEA3 (polyomavirus enhancer A) sites have been found to act as a transcriptional unit to achieve maximal induction. Metalloprotease gene transcription can be suppressed by various factors, and those of physiologically interest for articular tissues are the growth factor TGF-β (depending on the cell type, the state of the cell, and the isoforms), vitamin A analogues (retinoids), and glucocorticoids. Although each of these agents has its own pathway for inhibiting metalloprotease gene transcription, the presence of an AP-1 site in the promoter of MMP genes appears to be a key element in the inhibitory effect.

Metalloprotease activity is controlled by physiologic inhibitors and activators. Tissue inhibitors of MMPs (TIMPs) are the specific physiologic inhibitors of MMPs, and bind the active site of the MMPs and inhibit their catalytic activity. These molecules are synthesized by the same cells that produce MMPs. Although four TIMP molecules have been identified (TIMP-1 to -4) (93), at present, only the first three have been identified in human joint tissues, and are synthesized by chondrocytes (68,87,88,94,95). TIMP-3 is found exclusively in the extracellular matrix and not in conditioned medium (96). Although elevated levels of TIMP-1 and TIMP-3, but not TIMP-2, have been found in OA tissues (68,87,94), the presence of an imbalance between the amount of TIMPs and MMPs was demonstrated in these diseased tissues, resulting in a relative inhibitor deficiency (68,97). This finding could explain the increased level of active MMPs found in OA cartilage. All active MMPs are inhibited by TIMP with a stoichiometric ratio of 1:1. MMP inhibition by TIMPs is the result of their specific noncovalent binding to the active site of MMPs, and to the proforms of gelatinase 72 kd (TIMP-2, -3, -4) and 92 kd (TIMP-1 and -3). These latter complexes can still be activated, but show lower specific activities than the noncomplexed gelatinases. Moreover, TIMPs also inhibited MT1-MMP, and TIMP-3 and TIMP-2 appear to be better inhibitors of this enzyme than TIMP-1 (98).

There are at least two activation processes for MMPs. Extracellular activation occurs in the tissue for most of the MMPs and at the cell surface for collagenase-3 and gelatinase 72 kd, and some are intracellularly activated (99). Extracellular activation is a stepwise process in which an activator generates an intermediate and the intermediate or partially activated MMPs then fully activate the MMPs. This process allows for very fine regulation of the enzyme activity. Several enzyme families have been proposed as activators of MMPs. Enzymes from the serine protease and thiol-dependent protease families, such as plasminogen activator (PA)/plasmin system and cathepsin B, have been suggested as possible activators of MMPs. Activation of latent collagenase involves a cascade of events starting with cleavage of the amino terminal end by a protease such as plasmin and an additional proteolytic cleavage by stromelysin-1 at the carboxyl terminal end for full activation (99,100). Moreover, the collagenases and gelatinases can also be activated by other active MMPs (99–101). MT1-MMP activates collagenase-3, and gelatinase 72 kd potentiates the latter activation; MT1-MMP also activates gelatinase 72 kd. Collagenase-3 is itself capable of activating progelatinase 92 kd. Stromelysin-1 has been shown to cleave the proforms of both collagenase-1 and collagenase-3 and gelatinase 92 kd. In addition, some MMPs such as the MT-MMP and stromelysin-3 are activated intracellularly by a Golgi-associated protease, the furin.

Serine Proteases

The urokinase-type (uPA) and tissue-type (tPA) plasminogen activators are proteases that convert plasminogen to plasmin. In articular tissue, uPA appears to play the predominant role. The PA/plasmin proteases have a broad spectrum of activity. Their increased levels in OA joints, as well as their stimulation by IL-1, suggest a role in this disease (102,103). Although their role in cartilage metabolism is still not fully understood, they may directly digest connective tissue glycoprotein (104). Moreover, plasmin has the potential to degrade cartilage proteoglycans (105) as well as to activate latent MMPs, hence likely playing an important role in cartilage degradation. This enzyme system also appears to be involved in subchondral bone remodeling (see below).

In OA cartilage a direct, positive correlation was found between the level of plasmin and active collagenase (103). Several physiologic serine protease inhibitors also have been found in cartilage (103,106,107). In particular, the specific

PA inhibitor PAI, and more particularly PAI-1, exhibited decreased levels in OA cartilage (103). This, combined with the increased level of PA, may contribute, at least in part, to the increased level of biologically active MMPs found in OA tissue.

Thiol Proteases

The degradation of cartilage extracellular matrix macromolecules, as demonstrated by ultrastructural and microscopic examination, often occurs in the perilacunar area where the matrix pH is in the acid range. Cathepsins are lysosomal enzymes with a maximal activity at acid pH and require thiol as an activator. In cartilage, it is believed that cathepsin B plays a role in tissue degradation. This enzyme, in addition to having a direct degradation effect on both collagen and proteoglycans, may also be an MMP activator (108). Only *in vitro* studies support this notion so far. The maximal activity of cathepsin B is at pH 6.0, but it can exert proteolytic activity for a limited time at neutral pH (109).

As in several human enzyme systems, the proteolytic effect of cathepsin B is regulated by specific inhibitors. Two such inhibitors of high (67 kd) and low (16 kd) molecular weights (MWs) have been found in articular cartilage (107,110), which appear to be kininogen (high MW) (111) and a cystatin (low MW) (112), respectively. In diseased cartilage such as in OA, cathepsin B levels are increased, with a concomitant decrease in cysteine protease inhibitory activity (110). This imbalance may also be an important contributing factor in OA cartilage degradation.

Other Proteases

Although lysosomes of cultured chondrocytes contain exo-B-n-D-hexosaminidase and exo-B-d-glucuronidases capable of degrading oligosaccharides, no enzyme capable of cleaving the chains of chondroitin sulfate and releasing sulfated oligosaccharides has been found in adult cartilage. A hyaluronidase has been isolated from adult articular cartilage, but it was not active at the physiologic pH of cartilage matrix. The cationic protein lysozyme is abundant in cartilage, where it can regulate the size of proteoglycan aggregates (113).

PROINFLAMMATORY CYTOKINES

Enzymatic alterations in articular cartilage may explain the exhaustive degradation of this tissue but do not provide an explanation for the increased synthesis and expression of proteolytic enzymes, particularly MMPs. There is compelling evidence suggesting that secreted inflammatory mediators including cytokines impact cartilage matrix homeostasis by altering chondrocyte metabolism. Existing data suggest that in OA, it is the synovial lining cells that play a major role as proinflammatory effector cells (114,115). Evidence points to the importance of the cytokines IL-1β and TNF-α in the catabolic process in OA. It is still unclear whether IL-1β and TNF-α act independently or in concert in the pathogenesis of OA, or if a functional hierarchy exists between these proinflammatory cytokines. Studies performed on human OA tissues showed that IL-1β appears to be the major cytokine involved in articular cartilage destruction, and that TNF-α drives the inflammatory process (116–118). Both these cytokines have been found in enhanced amounts in OA synovial membrane, synovial fluid, and cartilage (114,115, 119–121). The association of these cytokines with tissue damage arises from their propensity to stimulate the proteolytic pathways of extracellular matrix degradation and, at the same time, suppress the synthetic pathways leading to new matrix formation.

IL-1 and TNF-α can increase the synthesis of proteases, including MMPs and PA, and these cytokines are probably responsible for increasing protease synthesis in OA synovium. Metalloproteases such as stromelysin and collagenase have been identified in these synovia (78,79,114). Their production correlated with the severity of inflammation, which in turn correlated positively with the level of synovial fluid IL-1 (121). In this tissue, protease inhibitors, such as PAI-1 or TIMP-1, are either suppressed or unaffected by these proinflammatory cytokines. Some mediators of the inflammatory process, such as PGE_2, are also stimulated (122,123), which could, in turn, be responsible for several symptoms observed in patients with OA. Because synoviocytes can secrete IL-1β, it is tempting to speculate that autocrine stimulation may also play a role in the regulation of synoviocyte enzyme synthesis. IL-1 may also contribute to the fibrosis observed in arthritic synovium, since it increases the synthesis of type I and III collagens by synovial fibroblasts (124,125).

Interleukin-1β

There is increasing evidence supporting the involvement of proinflammatory cytokines in OA cartilage degradation. Messenger RNA coding for IL-1α and IL-1β, has been demonstrated in chondrocytes (114,120,126,127). Immunohistochemical studies of cartilage showed the presence of IL-1β in OA chondrocytes, predominantly in the superficial layer. A major question arises as to how and in what manner chondrocytes are induced to produce cytokines. Whether this represents an autocrine or a paracrine stimulation is still undetermined. Evidence supports their involvement in modulating chondrocyte synthetic pathways, including matrix macromolecules (128,129). The increase of minor types of collagen in OA cartilage strongly suggests an influence of IL-1β. In fact, this cytokine stimulated chondrocyte collagen type I and III synthesis and decreased the synthesis of collagen types II and IX (129). Such changes could result in inappropriate matrix repair and lead to further cartilage erosion. Similarly, the decreased proteoglycan synthesis found in OA cartilage lesions may be attributable to IL-1β. It has been shown *in vivo* in an animal model of OA that blocking IL-1 activity with the specific IL-1 receptor antagonist (IL-1Ra) markedly reduced the progression of the tissue structural changes of OA (116,130,131).

The balance between inhibition and activation of MMPs in OA tissue could also very well be modulated by cytokines. For instance, the imbalance in TIMP-1 and MMP levels found in OA (68,78,97,132) could be mediated by IL-1β, because this cytokine decreased TIMP-1 synthesis *in vitro* in parallel with increased MMP synthesis in articular chondrocytes (68,133). The PA system is similarly modulated by IL-1β. The *in vitro* effect of IL-1 on articular cartilage showed a dose-dependent increase in PA synthesis, and a decrease in PAI-1 levels (102,133). These *in vitro* effects of IL-1 on cartilage complement the *ex vivo* findings in OA cartilage and stress the likely role of this cytokine in the pathophysiology of OA. Furthermore, the profound effect of IL-1 on PAI-1, in combination with the PA enhancement, is a powerful mechanism boosting the generation of both plasmin and MMP activation. In addition, IL-1β may be involved in proliferative events in OA, such as osteophyte formation, by stimulating the proliferation of human osteoblast-like cells, leading to increased periarticular bone formation (134).

IL-1β is primarily synthesized as a 31-kd precursor (pro-IL-1β) devoid of a conventional signal sequence, and subsequently released in the active form of 17.5 kd. In articular joint tissue, including synovial membrane, synovial fluid, and cartilage, IL-1β has been found in the active form. Some proteases can process pro-IL-1β to bioactive forms, but only one belonging to the cystein-dependent protease family and named IL-1β converting enzyme (ICE or caspase-1) can specifically generate the mature cytokine (135,136). ICE is a proenzyme polypeptide of 45 kd located in the cellular membrane. Active ICE is produced following proteolytic cleavage of the proenzyme, generating two subunits known as p10 and p20, both of which are essential for enzymatic activity. Recently, the presence of active ICE was demonstrated in both synovial membrane and cartilage, with a marked increase in OA tissues (127). In OA cartilage, ICE is located throughout the tissue, with a significant increase in the superficial zone. In synovial membrane, ICE was identified in the lining cells, mononuclear cell infiltrate, and the endothelial blood vessel cells. In these disease tissues, this enzyme was also found to be intimately involved in the IL-1β maturation, as incubation of tissue explants with a specific ICE inhibitor (YVAD) completely abrogated the production of the mature form of IL-1β (127).

The biologic activation by IL-1 of cells such as chondrocytes and synovial cells is mediated through association with a specific cell-surface protein, IL-1 receptor (IL-1R). Two types of IL-1R have been identified, type I and type II, with type I being responsible for signal transduction (137). It has been shown that the elevated expression of type I IL-1R in chondrocytes and synovial fibroblasts in OA may render these cells more sensitive to stimulation by IL-1 (138,139), thereby increasing their potential to secrete MMP and mediate joint destruction. The action of IL-1 can be inhibited by IL-1Ra, a natural competitive inhibitor of IL-1 (137). IL-1Ra inhibits the action of IL-1 by specifically binding to IL-1R without eliciting a biologic response. It is believed that IL-1Ra has a pivotal role in homeostasis in the joint. Its production in OA synovium may not be in sufficient amounts to inhibit the effects of locally produced IL-1 (116,130, 131,140). This may be another factor favoring the catabolism of cartilage in this disease.

Both types of IL-1R can also be shed from the cell surface, and exist extracellularly in truncated forms; they are named IL-1 soluble receptors (IL-1sR). For IL-1, the shed receptor may function as a receptor antagonist because the ligand-binding region is preserved, and thus is capable of competing with the membrane-associated receptors of the target cells. As well, shedding of surface receptors may decrease the responsiveness of target cells to the ligand. Type II IL-1R appears to serve as the main precursor for shed soluble receptors. The binding affinity of IL-1sR to both IL-1 isoforms and IL-1Ra differs. Type II IL-1sR binds IL-1β more readily than IL-1Ra; in contrast, type I IL-1sR binds IL-1Ra with high affinity (141,142). Therefore, when IL-1Ra and type I IL-1sR are present concurrently, their individual inhibitory effects are abrogated; however, when type II IL-1sR and IL-1Ra are combined, the resulting effect appears to be beneficial.

Tumor Necrosis Factor-α

In OA, TNF-α also appears to be an important mediator of matrix degradation and a pivotal cytokine in synovial membrane inflammation, although this cytokine is detected in OA articular tissue at low levels. TNF-α is synthesized as a precursor protein with amino-terminal extensions that are cleaved from the mature sequence prior to secretion. The proteolytic cleavage takes place at the cellular surface, via a TNF-α converting enzyme named TACE belonging to the adamalysin subfamily (143). This enzyme is also required for shedding of TNF receptors (TNF-R). Upregulation of TACE mRNA in human OA cartilage has recently been reported (144).

TNF-α also acts by binding to two specific receptors on the cell membrane, named according to their molecular weight: TNF-R55 and TNF-R75. In articular tissue cells, TNF-R55 seems to be the dominant receptor responsible for mediating TNF-α activity. In osteoarthritic chondrocytes and synovial fibroblasts, enhanced expression of TNF-R55 has been reported (145,146). Although it is accepted that TNF-R55 is biologically relevant for several cell types, including chondrocytes and synoviocytes, both receptor types appear to be actively involved in signal transduction (145,147,148). It is suggested that both membrane receptors, TNF-R55 and TNF-R75, are linked to distinct intracellular second-messengers. Moreover, it has been reported that TNF-R75 may regulate the rate of TNF-α association with TNF-R55 (149). As is the case for IL-1R, both TNF-R55 and -R75 can also be shed from chondrocyte and fibroblast synovial membranes (119,145,150). In OA, an upregulation in the release of TNF-R75 has been found (145). However, the exact role of these TNF soluble receptors (TNF-sRs) in the control of TNF-α action remains under debate, and may depend on their relative free abundance. It has been reported that TNF-sR acts as a receptor antagonist, mediates TNF-α activity, and/or stabilizes TNF-α.

Other Proinflammatory Cytokines

Other proinflammatory cytokines such IL-6, leukemia inhibitory factor (LIF), and IL-17 have also been considered potential contributing factors in the pathogenesis of this disease. In OA, it has been shown that IL-1β, IL-6, and TNF-α coexist in synovial fluid.

Several studies have reported the presence of IL-6 in arthritic tissues; this cytokine was detected in the synovial fluid of patients with various arthropathies, including OA and RA (151). In OA, the exact role of IL-6 has not yet been clearly defined. The ability of IL-1β and TNF-α to induce IL-6 protein and mRNA in synovial fibroblasts (152) suggests that this cytokine may be an important intermediate signal in the induction of other cellular responses to these cytokines. IL-6 has no direct effect on the synthesis of proteases, prostaglandins, or matrix proteins, but stimulates synthesis of TIMP-1 (153). It is suggested that IL-6, by its in vivo activation of synovial type B cells (synovial lining cells, macrophage type), may contribute to the immunologic phenomenon; its role in inflammation may be via regulation of changes in the concentrations of acute-phase proteins.

LIF is another cytokine of the IL-6 family that is upregulated in OA synovial membrane and fluid, and produced by chondrocytes in response to the proinflammatory cytokines IL-1β and TNF-α (154–156). This cytokine stimulates cartilage proteoglycan degradation, as well as MMP synthesis and nitric oxide cellular production. In OA, however, its role has not yet been clearly defined.

IL-17 is a newly discovered cytokine present as a homodimer, and variably glycosylated. This cytokine upregulates a number of gene products involved in cell activation, including proinflammatory cytokines IL-1β, TNF-α, and IL-6, as well as MMPs, in target cells such as human macrophages (157). IL-17 also increases the production of nitric oxide by chondrocytes, and appears to signal through nuclear factor NFκB with MAPKAP-K acting as a transactivating factor (158–160).

Recently, another cytokine, IL-18, also known as the interferon-γ–inducing factor (IGIF), has also been found to be expressed and produced within articular cartilage (127,161). In OA, a significantly higher frequency of chondrocytes producing this cytokine was found compared to normal (127). IL-18 is synthesized as an inactive precursor protein, and activation cleavage is catalyzed by ICE/caspase-1. To date, very few studies have been conducted on IL-18 in cartilage. However, it has recently been suggested that IL-18 might be involved in the release of glycosaminoglycans (161).

Antiinflammatory Cytokines

Natural inhibitors of proinflammatory cytokines, IL-4, IL-10, and IL-13, have also been identified in articular joint tissues. These cytokines are able to modulate various inflammatory processes, including a decreased production of proinflammatory cytokines such IL-1β, TNF-α, as well as some proteases. Moreover, they are also able to upregulate IL-1Ra and TIMP production (162–166). The antiinflammatory potential of these factors depends greatly on the target cell, which appears to be related to different individual cell-binding properties. For example, IL-13 and IL-4 receptors consist of several chains; as a result, the type of the receptor complex expressed depends on the cell and which of the possible receptor components are present. Finally, individual effects on cellular signaling pathways may also vary greatly (167).

OTHER INFLAMMATORY AGENTS

Nitric Oxide

Nitric oxide (NO), an inorganic free radical, has been implicated in the regulation of cartilage catabolism in OA. NO is synthesized from L-arginine by the action of an NO synthase (NOS). At present, the major isoforms of NOS include the constitutive type (cNOS) and an inducible type (iNOS). The latter is generally expressed after activation of cells by cytokines. Compared to normal, OA cartilage produces a large amount of NO, both under spontaneous and proinflammatory cytokine-stimulated conditions (168,169). Clinical evidence of NO production in OA joints has been documented from measurement of nitrites and nitrates in patients' synovial fluid (170). Cytokines such as IL-1β, TNF-α, and some inflammatory factors, such as lipopolysaccharides, were shown to stimulate NO production by human cartilage explants and chondrocytes, but not (or very little) by synoviocytes (169,171–173). NO appears to contribute to IL-1–induced degradation of cartilage, mainly by affecting

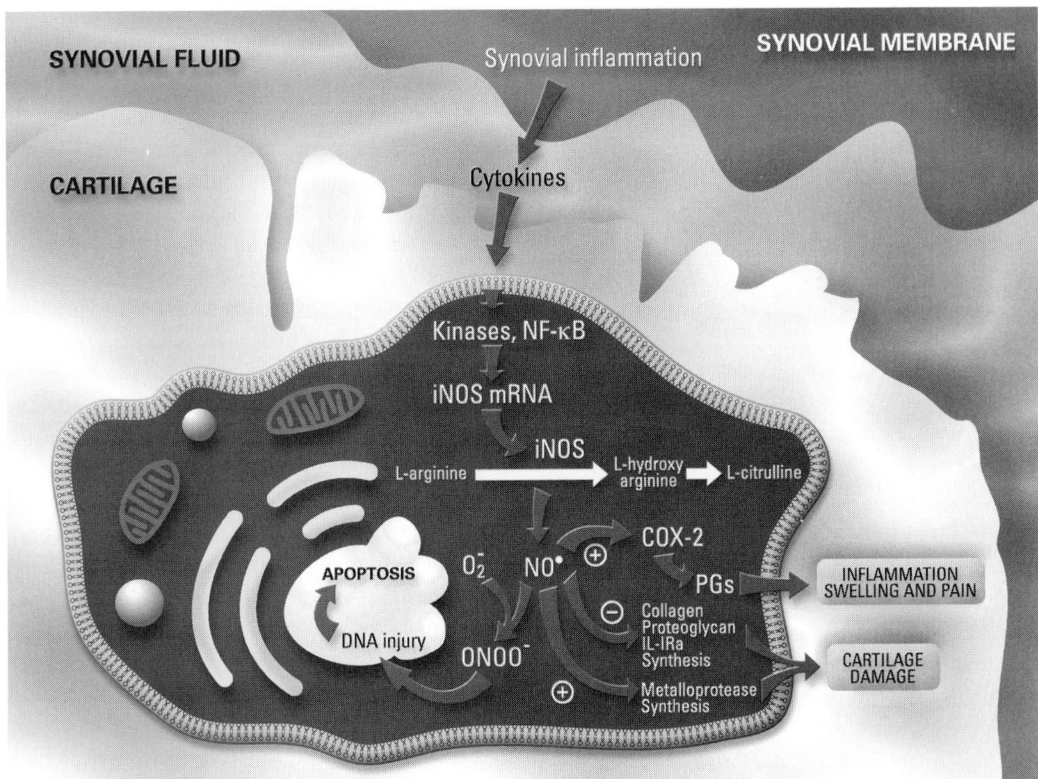

FIGURE 110.3. Pathways of nitric oxide (NO) formation and effects on articular chondrocytes –, inhibition; +, stimulation.

biosynthesis of aggrecan and collagen, and by enhancing MMP activity (174–177) *(Fig. 110.3).* Other effects have also been noted and include the reduction of IL-1Ra synthesis by chondrocytes (168). *In vivo,* therapeutic effects of a selective inhibitor of iNOS on the progression of lesions in experimental arthritis and OA models have been reported (178–180).

Prostaglandins and Cyclooxygenase

Prostaglandins (PGs) are biologically active metabolites of arachidonic acid. The biosynthesis of PGs is initiated by cyclooxygenase (COX). PGE_2 is a well-characterized mediator of inflammation and has multiple effects on connective tissue cell functions. It may affect cartilage remodeling directly or function indirectly as an autocrine regulatory factor (181). Many of the effects of PGE_2 are due to activation of adenylate synthase through binding to specific membrane receptors. It is believed that several of the effects of IL-1 are associated with the stimulation of PGE_2 production. In addition to exerting inflammatory actions of their own, PGE_2 can potentiate the effects of other mediators of inflammation.

COX enzyme exists as two isoforms, COX-1 and COX-2. COX-1 is a constitutive protein and is responsible for physiologic production of PGs. COX-2 is synthesized only after induction by mediators such as IL-1 and TNF-α. Although both COX isoforms have a similar affinity for arachidonic acid, they have a 60% homology between them, show different substrate specificities, and are found in different locations. There are also differences in the genes encoding the two enzymes. In particular, there are substantial differences in the promoter sites and, in contrast with COX-1, the COX-2 promoter contains binding sites for many regulators, including cytokines and glucocorticoids. In the inflammatory response of OA articular cells, the changes in COX-2 expression and/or activity seems to be one of the major determinants of PGE_2 production (182). In human articular cartilage, COX-1 appears at a very low level. However, although the COX-2 enzyme is not present in normal articular tissues, it is detected in OA tissues.

Interestingly, while the induction of COX-2 and iNOS appears to be through separate processes, interaction in some target cells between these two systems was reported (183) (Fig. 110.3). It has been shown that peroxynitrite, a product of the interaction of NO with superoxide, directly activates the PG endoperoxide synthases (184). Moreover, both IL-1β–induced NO and TNF-α–induced COX-2 expressions were suggested as being mediated by cyclic guanosine monophosphate (cGMP). Surprisingly, it was shown that inhibition of NO production by chondrocytes enhanced PGE_2 production (185).

Substance P

Emerging evidence also points to the involvement of substance P in the pathogenesis of OA. This neuropeptide has been detected in the synovial membrane and fluid obtained from patients with OA (186,187). Its secretion is believed to originate from the nonmyelinated sensory neurons in the synovium in response to the inflammatory changes occurring in this tissue. Substance P has been shown to activate both inflammatory cells and synoviocytes (186,188–191), to stimulate the secretion of IL-1 (192), and to potentiate the action of this cytokine (193).

APOPTOSIS

Chondrocyte death may represent an important component in the pathogenesis of OA as hypocellularity is often observed. Apoptosis, or programmed cell death, is a naturally occurring process for cell removal, and has been proposed to be, at least in part, involved in OA cartilage hypocellularity. This process can be distinguished morphologically and biologically from necrosis. The characteristic morphologic features of apoptosis include DNA fragmentation, chromatin condensation, membrane blebbing, cell shrinkage, and disassembly into membrane-enclosed vesicles. *In vivo* this process culminates with the engulfment of apoptotic bodies by other cells, preventing complications that would result from release of intracellular contents. Phagocytes are not believed to be activated on ingestion, and apoptosis usually occurs without the inflammatory changes that accompany necrosis.

Apoptosis has been observed in freshly isolated chondrocytes and in cartilage from OA patients (43). However, the pathways linked to the occurrence of chondrocyte apoptosis are unknown. A relationship between chondrocyte apoptosis and the extent of matrix degradation, however, was reported (194), and generally apoptotic chondrocytes from OA cartilage were prominent in the superficial zone of cartilage. It has been suggested that apoptosis is a consequence of an inflammatory process associated with OA, rather than a typical feature of this disease. Indeed, in OA, some cells from the articular joints are known to produce several mediators having the potential to induce chondrocyte death through apoptosis. These mediators include IL-1, TNF-α, IL-17, Fas ligand, the oxygen radicals, etc. In addition, *in vitro* stimulation with NO was reported to induce apoptosis in chondrocytes (194,195). However, this can also occur as an attempted repair process.

CARTILAGE REPAIR AND GROWTH FACTORS

Cartilage extracellular matrix structure plays an integral role in the function of this tissue. Matrix homeostasis is controlled by chondrocytes through a balanced regulation of synthesis and degradative events, with the rate of new matrix synthesis being equal to the rate of matrix degradation. Both processes are controlled by a variety of extracellular messenger proteins, termed growth factors and cytokines. Disturbance or alteration in the net effects of multiple growth factors and cytokines may compromise the macromolecule synthesis and degradation pattern, therefore being responsible for the development of pathologic conditions.

Using experimental models, two types of repair reactions have been identified in cartilage. On the one hand, the reparative process of osteochondral defects involves the migration of mesenchymal cells from subchondral bone. On the other hand, attempted repair of more superficial chondral defects occurs during the early period following a cartilage lesion. This reparative process is characterized by chondrocyte clustering, cartilage hypertrophy, and an increase in fibronectin and water content, and in glycosaminoglycan synthesis (196,197). Unfortunately, this reparative phase ultimately falters as cartilage destruction becomes chronic. Several factors could be involved in the aborted repair reaction, including alteration in the macromolecule structure, chondrocyte phenotypic change, overproduction of proinflammatory cytokines, increased susceptibility of chondrocytes to cytokine-induced degradation, overexpression of IL-1β and TNF-α receptors, growth factor synthesis and bioactivity downregulation, reduction of chondrocyte sensitivity to growth factors, chondrocyte apoptosis, etc. (43, 198,199).

The cartilage repair reaction is regulated by factors locally produced by chondrocytes and neighboring tissues, mainly synovial membrane and subchondral bone. Growth factors such as insulin-like growth factor-1 (IGF-1), TGF-β, and bFGF are generally associated with the stimulation of connective tissue synthesis, whereas cytokines such as IL-1β and TNF-α are usually associated with the stimulation of molecules leading to matrix degradation. Factors including PDGF and bone morphogenic protein (BMP) could also have important regulatory functions.

TGF-β is the prototypic member of the large TGF superfamily, sharing functional and signaling homology with the BMPs. This growth factor enhances aggrecan production, but also stimulates the production of the smaller proteoglycans, which are found in OA cartilage (53,200). In OA, significant levels of TGF-β are found in the synovial fluid as well as in the synovial membrane, in cartilage and in subchondral bone (198,201,202). In synovial membrane, coexpression of TGF-β with TNF-α and IL-1 is seen at sites of inflammation, whereas exclusive of TGF-β expression is noted in fibrotic areas (203). TGF-β can counteract the effect of IL-1β. The mechanism involved was thought to be through a downregulation of IL-1 receptor by TGF-β (204,205). TGF-β stimulates collagen and proteoglycan core protein transcription. Furthermore, and depending on the cell type, TGF-β isoforms, and physiologic state of the cells, it can stimulate some MMP synthesis and inhibit others. TGF-β also induces the synthesis of TIMP-1 and PAI-1 by connective tissue cells (206). This growth factor, however, was also shown to induce osteophyte formation (207). Some BMPs (BMP-2, BMP-7, and BMP-9) also strongly stimulate chondrocyte proteoglycan synthesis (208–210).

IGF-1 is another candidate to regulate the anabolism of cartilage matrix molecules. The parallel between serum and skeletal IGF-1 levels may not be readily explained since hormones and factors regulating the synthesis of IGF-1 in the liver, which determines levels of systemic IGF-1, and in the skeleton are different. Several investigations of the relationship between serum levels of IGF-1 and the presence and severity of OA have been performed over the years, but have yielded conflicting results (211–216). One study showed no association between serum IGF-1 concentrations and OA (214), and the earlier data may have been skewed by the confounding effects of age. The observations that focus on serum levels of IGF-1 do not exclude a role for local production of IGF-1 in articular tissues. In fact, levels of IGF-1 were found to be increased in human OA synovial fluid, cartilage, synovial membrane, and subchondral bone (217–223). Despite an increased IGF-1 mRNA level in OA articular tissue (217) and IGF-1 protein production by OA chondrocytes (217,218), the latter cells are hyporesponsive to IGF-1 stimulation (224). This phenomenon is not related to a downregulation of the type I IGF receptor but, at least in part, to an increased amount of the IGF-binding proteins (IGF-BPs) in this pathologic tissue (224,225). This hyporesponsiveness may well account for the decrease in cartilage reparative capacity found at the advanced stages of the disease, and may explain the progressive nature of OA. Proinflammatory cytokines such as IL-1β and TNF-α could also be implicated in the hyporesponsiveness of pathologic chondrocytes to IGF-1. While these cytokines activate the release of IGF-1 from chondrocytes, they also trigger the release of IGF-BPs (226–229). Alternatively, and not exclusively of the latter, IL-1 may participate in this process via activation of proteases. Proteases such as the PA/plasmin system as well as other cell surface proteases, including cathepsin G and γ-glutamyl transpeptidase, can cleave IGF-1 in other cell systems. One of the most important modulating agents of IGF-1 is the growth hormone. In adult chondrocytes, it has been shown that elevated synthesis of IGF-1 did not occur through a growth hormone (GH) GHF receptor mechanism (218). This suggests that other factors are capable of controlling local IGF-1 production in osteoarthritic chondrocytes, including TGF-β and other pituitary growth factors.

Fibroblast growth factor (FGF) has been identified in synovial fluid of patients with different forms of arthritis (230). FGF stimulated mitotic activity in articular cartilage chondrocytes (231), but did not stimulate the synthesis of glycoaminoglycans (232). Although the role of FGF in the etiopathogenesis of OA is still under debate, it is of potential therapeutic interest because, administered intraarticularly, it promoted the healing of articular cartilage in a rabbit knee model (233).

Imbalance between anabolic growth factors and catabolic cytokine synthesis and/or bioactivity could be the key of cartilage repair failure. Several mechanisms can control growth factors and cytokine bioactivity during OA development. Interactions of binding proteins, soluble receptors, and matrix components with growth factors or cytokines may modulate their effects on chondrocyte metabolism. A synergy between growth factors or a coordinate regulation of cytokines and growth factors in articular cartilage is becoming accepted as contributing to the overall tissue response governing repair. For example, proliferation of chondrocytes was found to be amplified by the combination of FGF and IGF (234,235). Moreover, it was demonstrated that IL-6 and TGF-β function synergistically to stimulate the chondrocyte proliferative response (236). A marked synergy was also shown in normal cartilage with IGF-1 and a number of growth factors in activation of chondrocyte proteoglycan synthesis (237).

SUBCHONDRAL BONE AND OSTEOARTHRITIS

Osteoarthritis is a disease that involves all tissues of the joint. Subchondral bone sclerosis and osteophyte formation are well-recognized manifestations of human OA, although their exact roles in the disease process remain largely unknown. It is suggested that osteophyte formation may play a compensatory role in the redistribution of biochemical forces to provide articular cartilage protection. The mechanisms responsible for osteophyte formation in OA have not yet been elucidated; however, it was shown in the murine knee joint that TGF-β and IL-1β, among other factors, might be implicated (207) (Fig. 110.4). The data also

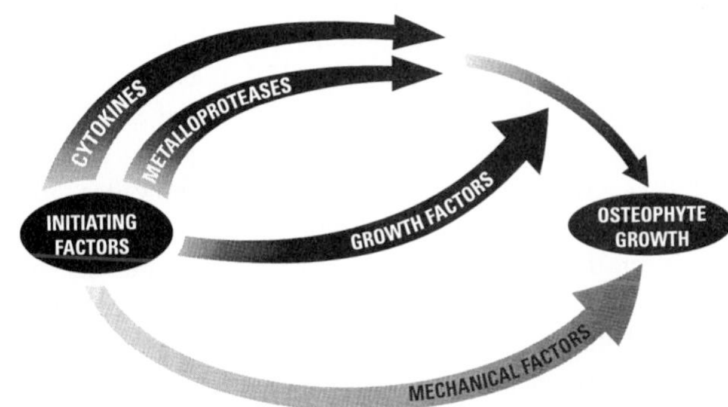

FIGURE 110.4. Suggestive scheme for events in osteophyte formation. (Modified from Moskowitz RW. Bone remodeling in osteoarthritis: subchondral and osteophytic responses. *Osteoarthritis Cartilage* 1999;7:323–324.)

suggest that the vitamin D receptor genotype is involved in osteophyte formation (238).

Subchondral bone appears to be the structural element of most importance in this disease. Indeed, one of the most powerful known predictors of structural change in established knee OA is a positive bone scintigraphy, which reflects subchondral bone turnover. Scintigraphic evidence of increased activity of bone appears to switch on and off in a phasic manner, and to precede episodes of progression of radiographic changes (239).

It is currently suggested that subchondral bone alterations may be more intimately related to the OA process rather than merely be a consequence of this disease (240). However, the question that still remains to be answered is whether changes in subchondral bone induce or participate in the disease progression. Two theories are currently proposed. Mechanical stress on weight-bearing joints may contribute to increased microfractures in the bone plate and overlying cartilage. As articular cartilage slowly erodes, sclerosis of the subchondral bone plate also progresses and bone stiffness increases in this tissue, possibly contributing to further mechanical disturbances of the cartilage. On the other hand, changes in the subchondral bone such as sclerosis may precede cartilage damage in OA. A steep stiffness gradient in the underlying subchondral bone may therefore be an initiating mechanism of OA since the integrity of the overlying articular cartilage depends on the mechanical properties of its bony bed.

Evidence suggests that the subchondral bone sclerosis in OA results from an increased stiffness, and not an increase in bone mineral density (241) (Fig. 110.2, bottom panel). Association of thickening of subchondral bone with an abnormally low mineralization pattern has been identified in OA patients (242,243), indicating that dysregulation of bone remodeling may be an integral part of OA. These findings suggest that this might be due to a subchondral bone osteoblast defect.

Bone resorption and formation do not occur randomly but follow a precise remodeling schedule regulated by hormones and local growth factors and cytokines. It was recently reported that osteoblasts from subchondral bone in OA exhibited altered metabolism as assessed by specific bone biomarkers (223,244) (Fig. 110.2, bottom panel). Indeed, these cells had a lower production of 3′,5′-cyclic adenosine monophosphate (cAMP) in response to PTH and PGE_2 than normal osteoblasts; they showed a 50% blunted response to PTH; and no response to PGE_2 (223). Moreover, they released more osteocalcin than normal cells in response to vitamin D_3 stimulation and exhibited increased alkaline phosphatase activity (223). An imbalance between collagen and noncollagen protein production, such as osteocalcin, can lead to an increase in bone volume without a concomitant increase in the bone mineralization pattern. Evidence that osteocalcin knockout mice had an increased mineralization pattern without significant effects on bone resorption (245) suggests that the elevated osteocalcin levels in OA could be responsible for the abnormal mineralization pattern in these patients. Moreover, in the cancellous bone compartment in the hip of OA patients, a combination of increased gelatinase 72 kd and alkaline phosphatase activity, indicating increased collagen turnover, has been observed (246). Bone sclerosis noted in OA subchondral bone may be linked to an abnormal regulation of the uPA/plasmin system, IGF-1/IGF-BP and TGF-β (223,247,248). They may all influence the production of collagenases and other proteolytic pathways, ultimately promoting matrix remodeling/degradation. An example of this was recently described (Fig. 110.2, bottom panel). In OA subchondral bone osteoblasts, uPA was found to regulate its own activity via a positive feedback loop whereby plasmin generated by uPA-dependent plasminogen hydrolysis can stimulate uPA activity directly (248). Interestingly, in these OA cells, IGF-1 can block this positive feedback loop, with no effect on normal cells. If this *in vitro* data reflects the *in vivo* situation, then this mechanism could retard bone remodeling in OA, ultimately favoring the development of bone sclerosis.

Taking into account all the observations on the OA subchondral bone, the following hypothesis has been proposed (47). At onset or early in the OA process, a thickening of the underlying subchondral bone is noted. This could result from repetitive loading, microfracture, and/or the activity of the IGF/IGF-BP system, leading to abnormal response of the subchondral bone. This, in turn, creates local microfractures in the cartilage, inducing cartilage matrix damage. This cartilage damage is normally repaired by either local synthesis, or the release of IGF-1/IGF-BP that stimulates matrix formation in the cartilage. At a certain point, however, chondrocytes from OA patients seem unresponsive to IGF-1 challenge (224). At the same time, the elevated IGF-1 in OA bone osteoblasts could promote bone formation, but could also prevent normal bone remodeling by inhibiting the uPA/plasmin activity, explaining abnormal bone mineralization and tissue sclerosis. On the other hand, the local activation of the PA/plasmin system in cartilage promotes local cartilage alteration. Thus, the local induction in bone and cartilage of IGF-1 and other protease regulatory systems promotes both cartilage damage and subchondral bone plate thickening; this last pathway leads to further cartilage damage. The imbalance in the repair capacity and damage of cartilage due to subchondral plate thickening subsequently leads to a progressively abnormal cartilage matrix, and eventually to OA, hence explaining the slow progression of the disease.

CONCLUSION

Expanded research in biomechanics and cell and molecular biology has led to an increased understanding of the etiopathology of OA. Although some of the factors bearing on this disorder are becoming clearer, certainly many additional etiologic variables remain to be discovered. Nevertheless, these very important findings are paving the way for breakthrough discoveries that should lead to the development of curative treatment for this disease.

REFERENCES

1. Radin EL, Yang KH, Riegger C, et al. Relationship between lower limb dynamics and knee joint pain. *J Orthop Res* 1991; 9:398–405.
2. Yang KH, Riegger CL, Rodgers MM, et al. Diminished lower limb deceleration as a factor in early stage osteoarthritis. *Trans Orthop Res Soc* 1989;14:52(abst).
3. Felson DT. Epidemiology of osteoarthritis. In: Brandt KD, Doherty M, Lohmander LS, eds. *Osteoarthritis.* Oxford: Oxford University Press, 1998:13–22.
4. Huch K, Kuettner KE, Dieppe P. Osteoarthritis in ankle and knee joints. *Semin Arthritis Rheum* 1997;26:667–674.
5. Kang Y, Koepp H, Cole AA, et al. Cultured human ankle and knee cartilage differ in susceptibility to damage mediated by fibronectin fragments. *J Orthop Res* 1998;16:551–556.
6. Hutton CW. Generalised osteoarthritis: an evolutionary problem? *Lancet* 1987;1:1463–1465.
7. Buckwalter JA. Osteoarthritis and articular cartilage use, disuse, and abuse: experimental studies. *J Rheumatol Suppl* 1995;43: 13–15.
8. Grodzinsky AJ, Kim YJ, Buschmann MD. Response of the chondrocyte to mechanical stimuli. In: Brandt KD, Doherty M, Lohmander LS, eds. *Osteoarthritis.* Oxford: Oxford University Press, 1998:123–136.
9. Setton LA, Elliott DM, Mow VC. Altered mechanics of cartilage with osteoarthritis: human osteoarthritis and an experimental model of joint degeneration. *Osteoarthritis Cartilage* 1999;7:2–14.
10. Holderbaum D, Haqqi TM, Moskowitz RW. Genetics and osteoarthritis: exposing the iceberg. *Arthritis Rheum* 1999;42: 397–405.
11. Olsen BR. Role of cartilage collagens in formation of the skeleton. In: de Crombrugghe B, Horton WA, Olsen BR, eds. *Molecular and developmental biology of cartilage.* New York: New York Academy of Sciences, 1996:124–130.
12. Harris WH. Idiopathic osteoarthritis of the hip. A twentieth century myth? Proceedings, 6th combined meeting. *J Bone Joint Surg* 1977;59B:121.
13. Murray RO. The aetiology of primary osteoarthritis of the hip. *Br J Radiol* 1965;38:810–824.
14. McAlindon T, Felson DT. Nutrition: risk factors for osteoarthritis. *Ann Rheum Dis* 1997;56:397–400.
15. Sokoloff L. The history of Kashin-Beck disease. *NY State J Med* 1989;89:343–351.
16. Utiger RD. Kashin-Beck disease—expanding the spectrum of iodine-deficiency disorders. *N Engl J Med* 1998;339:1156–1158.
17. Masse PG, Carrino DA, Morris N, et al. Loss of decorin from the surface zone of articular cartilage in a chick model of osteoarthritis. *Acta Histochem* 1997;99:431–444.
18. Moskowitz RW. Experimental models of osteoarthritis. In: Moskowitz RW, Howell DS, Goldberg VM, et al., eds. *Osteoarthritis. diagnosis and medical/surgical management,* 2nd ed. Philadelphia: WB Saunders, 1992:213–232.
19. Palmoski MJ, Brandt KD. Running inhibits the reversal of atrophic changes in canine knee cartilage after removal of a leg cast. *Arthritis Rheum* 1981;24:1329–1337.
20. Kiviranta I, Tammi M, Jurvelin J, et al. Articular cartilage thickness and glycosaminoglycan distribution in the young canine knee joint after remobilization of the immobilized limb. *J Orthop Res* 1994;12:161–167.
21. Muller FJ, Setton LA, Manicourt DH, et al. Centrifugal and biochemical comparison of proteoglycan aggregates from articular cartilage in experimental joint disuse and joint instability. *J Orthop Res* 1994;12:498–508.
22. Grumbles RM, Howell DS, Howard GA, et al. Cartilage metalloproteases in disuse atrophy. *J Rheumatol Suppl* 1995;43: 146–148.
23. Cheung HS, Setton LA, Guilak F, et al. Metalloproteinase levels in articular cartilage resultant from disuse immobilization, as well as subsequent vigorous exercise. *Trans Orthop Res Soc* 1999;24:40(abst).
24. Adams ME, Brandt KD. Hypertrophic repair of canine articular cartilage in osteoarthritis after anterior cruciate ligament transection. *J Rheumatol* 1991;18:428–435.
25. Brandt KD, Braunstein EM, Visco DM, et al. Anterior (cranial) cruciate ligament transection in the dog: a bona fide model of osteoarthritis, not merely of cartilage injury and repair. *J Rheumatol* 1991;18:436–446.
26. Manicourt DH, Pita JC, Thonar EJ, et al. Proteoglycans nondissociatively extracted from different zones of canine normal articular cartilage: variations in the sedimentation profile of aggregates with degree of physiological stress. *Connect Tissue Res* 1991;26:231–246.
27. Manicourt DH, Thonar EJ, Pita JC, et al. Changes in the sedimentation profile of proteoglycan aggregates in early experimental canine osteoarthritis. *Connect Tissue Res* 1989;23:33–50.
28. Pelletier JP, Martel-Pelletier J, Altman RD, et al. Collagenolytic activity and collagen matrix breakdown of the articular cartilage in the Pond-Nuki dog model of osteoarthritis. *Arthritis Rheum* 1983;26:866–874.
29. Ratcliffe A, Beauvais PJ, Saed-Nejad F. Differential levels of synovial fluid aggrecan aggregate components in experimental osteoarthritis and joint disuse. *J Orthop Res* 1994;12:464–473.
30. McCarty DJ. Calcium pyrophosphate dihydrate crystals deposition disease (pseudogout syndrome)—clinical aspects. *Clin Rheum Dis* 1977;3:61–89.
31. Schumacher HR Jr. Synovial inflammation, crystals, and osteoarthritis. *J Rheumatol* 1995;43:101–103.
32. Gordon GV, Villanueva T, Schumacher HR, et al. Autopsy study correlating degree of osteoarthritis, synovitis and evidence of articular calcification. *J Rheumatol* 1984;11:681–686.
33. Ali SY, Rees JA, Scotchford CA. Microcrystal deposition in cartilage and in osteoarthritis. *Bone Miner* 1992;17:115–118.
34. Swan A, Chapman B, Heap P, et al. Submicroscopic crystals in osteoarthritic synovial fluids. *Ann Rheum Dis* 1994;53: 467–470.
35. Watanabe W, Baker DG, Schumacher HR Jr. Comparison of the acute inflammation induced by calcium pyrophosphate dihydrate, apatite and mixed crystals in the rat air pouch model of a synovial space. *J Rheumatol* 1992;19:1453–1457.
36. Fam AG, Morava-Protzner I, Purcell C, et al. Acceleration of experimental lapine osteoarthritis by calcium pyrophosphate microcrystalline synovitis. *Arthritis Rheum* 1995;38:201–210.
37. Ryan LM, Cheung HS. The role of crystals in osteoarthritis. In: Brandt KD, ed. *Osteoarthritis, rheumatic diseases of America,* vol 25. Philadelphia: WB Saunders, 1999:257–267.
38. Derfus B, Kranendonk S, Camacho N, et al. Human osteoarthritic cartilage matrix vesicles generate both calcium pyrophosphate dihydrate and apatite crystals in-vitro. *Calcif Tissue Int* 1998;163:258–262.
39. Derfus B, Steinberg M, Mandel N, et al. Characterization of an additional articular cartilage vesicle fraction that generates cal-

cium pyrophosphate dihydrate crystals in vitro. *J Rheumatol* 1995;22:1514–1519.

40. Hashimoto S, Ochs RL, Rosen F, et al. Chondrocyte-derived apoptotic bodies and calcification of articular cartilage. *Proc Natl Acad Sci U S A* 1998;95:3094–3099.
41. Pelletier JP, Jovanovic D, Fernandes JC, et al. Reduced progression of experimental osteoarthritis in vivo by selective inhibition of inducible nitric oxide synthase. *Arthritis Rheum* 1998;41: 1275–1286.
42. Cheung HS, Ryan LM. Phosphocitrate blocks nitric oxide induced mineralization in cartilage and chondrocyte-derived apoptotic bodies. *Osteoarthritis Cartilage* 1999;7:409–412.
43. Blanco FJ, Guitian R, Vazquez-Martul E, et al. Osteoarthritis chondrocytes die by apoptosis. A possible pathway for osteoarthritis pathology. *Arthritis Rheum* 1998;41:284–289.
44. Vignon E, Arlot M, Patricot LM, et al. The cell density of human femoral head cartilage. *Clin Orthop* 1976;303–308.
45. von der Mark K, Kirsch T, Nerlich A, et al. Type X collagen synthesis in human osteoarthritic cartilage. Indication of chondrocyte hypertrophy. *Arthritis Rheum* 1992;35:806–811.
46. Terkeltaub R, Lotz M, Johnson K, et al. Parathyroid hormone-related proteins is abundant in osteoarthritic cartilage, and the parathyroid hormone-related protein 1–173 isoform is selectively induced by transforming growth factor beta in articular chondrocytes and suppresses generation of extracellular inorganic pyrophosphate. *Arthritis Rheum* 1998;41:2152–2164.
47. Martel-Pelletier J, Di Battista JA, Lajeunesse D. Biochemical factors in joint articular tissue degradation in osteoarthritis. In: Reginster JY, Pelletier JP, Martel-Pelletier J, et al, eds. *Osteoarthritis:* clinical and experimental aspects. Berlin: Springer-Verlag, 1999:156–187.
48. Goldenberg DL, Egan MS, Cohen AS. Inflammatory synovitis in degenerative joint disease. *J Rheumatol* 1982;9:204–209.
49. Lindblad S, Hedfors E. Arthroscopic and immunohistologic characterization of knee joint synovitis in osteoarthritis. *Arthritis Rheum* 1987;30:1081–1088.
50. Haraoui B, Pelletier JP, Cloutier JM, et al. Synovial membrane histology and immunopathology in rheumatoid arthritis and osteoarthritis. In vivo effects of anti-rheumatic drugs. *Arthritis Rheum* 1991;34:153–163.
51. Lohmander LS. The role of molecular markers to monitor breakdown and repair. In: Reginster JY, Pelletier JP, Martel-Pelletier J, et al., eds. *Osteoarthritis:* clinical and experimental aspects. Berlin: Springer-Verlag, 1999:296–311.
52. Rizkalla G, Reiner A, Bogoch E, et al. Studies of the articular cartilage proteoglycan aggrecan in health and osteoarthritis. Evidence for molecular heterogeneity and extensive molecular changes in disease. *J Clin Invest* 1992;90:2268–2277.
53. Cs-Szabo G, Roughley PJ, Plaas AH, et al. Large and small proteoglycans of osteoarthritic and rheumatoid articular cartilage. *Arthritis Rheum* 1995;38:660–668.
54. Malemud CJ, Papay RS, Hering TM, et al. Phenotypic modulation of newly synthesized proteoglycans in human cartilage and chondrocytes. *Osteoarthritis Cartilage* 1995;3:227–238.
55. Cs-Szabo G, Melching LI, Roughley PJ, et al. Changes in messenger RNA and protein levels of proteoglycans and link protein in human osteoarthritic cartilage samples. *Arthritis Rheum* 1997;40:1037–1045.
56. Tyler JA. Chondrocyte-mediated depletion of articular cartilage proteoglycans in vitro. *Biochem J* 1985;225:493–507.
57. Campbell IK, Roughley PJ, Mort JS. The action of human articular-cartilage metalloproteinase on proteoglycan and link protein. Similarities between products of degradation in situ and in vitro. *Biochem J* 1986;237:117–122.
58. Martel-Pelletier J, Pelletier JP, Malemud CJ. Activation of neutral metalloprotease in human osteoarthritic knee cartilage: evidence for degradation in the core protein of sulphated proteoglycan. *Ann Rheum Dis* 1988;47:801–808.
59. Sandy JD, Neame PJ, Boynton RE, et al. Catabolism of aggrecan in cartilage explants. Identification of a major cleavage site within the interglobular domain. *J Biol Chem* 1991;266: 8683–8685.
60. Lark MW, Bayne EK, Flanagan J, et al. Aggrecan degradation in human cartilage: evidence for both matrix metalloproteinase and aggrecanase activity in normal, osteoarthritic, and rheumatoid joints. *J Clin Invest* 1997;100:93–106.
61. Arner EC, Pratta MA, Trzaskos JM, et al. Generation and characterization of aggrecanase. A soluble, cartilage-derived aggrecan-degrading activity. *J Biol Chem* 1999;274:6594–6601.
62. Saxne T, Heinegard D. Synovial fluid analysis of two groups of proteoglycan epitopes distinguishes early and late cartilage lesions. *Arthritis Rheum* 1992;35:385–390.
63. Sandy JD, Flannery CR, Neame PJ, et al. The structure of aggrecan fragments in human synovial fluid. Evidence for the involvement in osteoarthritis of a novel proteinase which cleaves the Glu 373-Ala 374 bond of the interglobular domain. *J Clin Invest* 1992;89:1512–1516.
64. Lohmander LS, Hoerrner LA, Lark MW. Metalloproteinases, tissue inhibitor and proteoglycan fragments in knee synovial fluid in human osteoarthritis. *Arthritis Rheum* 1993;36: 181–189.
65. Lohmander LS, Neame PJ, Sandy JD. The structure of aggrecan fragments in human synovial fluid: evidence that aggrecanase mediates cartilage degradation in inflammatory joint disease, joint injury, and osteoarthritis. *Arthritis Rheum* 1993;36: 1214–1222.
66. Hollander AP, Heathfield TF, Webber C, et al. Increased damage to type II collagen in osteoarthritic articular cartilage detected by a new immunoassay. *J Clin Invest* 1994;93: 1722–1732.
67. Martel-Pelletier J, Tardif G, Fernandes JC, et al. Metalloproteases and their modulation as treatment in osteoarthritis. In: Tsokos GC, ed. *Molecular rheumatology.* Totowa, NJ: Humana Press, 1999 *(in press).*
68. Martel-Pelletier J, McCollum R, Fujimoto N, et al. Excess of metalloproteases over tissue inhibitor of metalloprotease may contribute to cartilage degradation in osteoarthritis and rheumatoid arthritis. *Lab Invest* 1994;70:807–815.
69. Reboul P, Pelletier JP, Tardif G, et al. The new collagenase, collagenase-3, is expressed and synthesized by human chondrocytes but not by synoviocytes: a role in osteoarthritis. *J Clin Invest* 1996;97:2011–2019.
70. Martel-Pelletier J, Pelletier JP. Wanted—the collagenase responsible for the destruction of the collagen network in human cartilage! *Br J Rheumatol* 1996;35:818–820.
71. Mitchell PG, Magna HA, Reeves LM, et al. Cloning, expression, and type II collagenolytic activity of matrix metalloproteinase-13 from human osteoarthritic cartilage. *J Clin Invest* 1996;97:761–768.
72. Chubinskaya S, Huch K, Mikecz K, et al. Chondrocyte matrix metalloproteinase-8: up-regulation of neutrophil collagenase by interleukin-1β in human cartilage from knee and ankle joints. Lab Invest 1996;74:232–240.
73. Cole AA, Chubinskaya S, Schumacher BL, et al. Chondrocyte matrix metalloproteinase-8. Human articular chondroctyes express neutrophil collagenase. *J Biol Chem* 1996;271: 11023–11026.
74. Shlopov BV, Lie WR, Mainardi CL, et al. Osteoarthritic lesions: involvement of three different collagenases. *Arthritis Rheum* 1997;40:2065–2074.
75. Moldovan F, Pelletier JP, Hambor J, et al. Collagenase-3 (matrix metalloprotease 13) is preferentially localized in the deep layer

of human arthritic cartilage in situ: in vitro mimicking effect by transforming growth factor beta. *Arthritis Rheum* 1997;40: 1653–1661.

76. Fernandes JC, Martel-Pelletier J, Lascau-Coman V, et al. Collagenase-1 and collagenase-3 synthesis in early experimental osteoarthritic canine cartilage. An immunohistochemical study. *J Rheumatol* 1998;8:1585–1594.
77. Nguyen Q, Mort JS, Roughley PJ. Preferential mRNA expression of prostromelysin relative to procollagenase and in situ localization in human articular cartilage. *J Clin Invest* 1992;89: 1189–1197.
78. Firestein GS, Paine M, Littman BH. Gene expression (collagenase, tissue inhibitor of metalloproteinases, complement, and HLA-DR) in rheumatoid arthritis and osteoarthritis synovium: quantitative analysis and effect of intra-articular corticosteroids. *Arthritis Rheum* 1991;34:1094–1105.
79. McCachren SS. Expression of metalloproteinases and metalloproteinase inhibitor in human arthritic synovium. *Arthritis Rheum* 1991;34:1085–1093.
80. Zafarullah M, Pelletier JP, Cloutier JM, et al. Elevated metalloproteinase and tissue inhibitor of metalloproteinase mRNA in human osteoarthritic synovia. *J Rheumatol* 1993;20:693–697.
81. Pelletier JP, Martel-Pelletier J, Cloutier JM, et al. Proteoglycan-degrading acid metalloprotease activity in human osteoarthritic cartilage, and the effect of intraarticular steroid injections. *Arthritis Rheum* 1987;30:541–548.
82. Walakovits LA, Moore VL, Bhardwaj N, et al. Detection of stromelysin and collagenase in synovial fluid from patients with rheumatoid arthritis and posttraumatic knee injury. *Arthritis Rheum* 1992;35:35–42.
83. Okada Y, Konomi H, Yada T, et al. Degradation of type IX collagen by matrix metalloproteinase 3 (stromelysin) from human rheumatoid synovial cells. *FEBS Lett* 1989;244:473–476.
84. Murphy G, Cockett MI, Stephens PE, et al. Stromelysin is an activator of procollagenase. A study with natural and recombinant enzymes. *Biochem J* 1987;248:265–268.
85. Murphy G, Crabbe T. Gelatinases A and B. *Methods Enzymol* 1995;248:470–484.
86. Mohtai M, Smith RL, Schurman DJ, et al. Expression of 92-kD type IV collagenase/gelatinase (gelatinase B) in osteoarthritic cartilage and its induction in normal human articular cartilage by interleukin-1. *J Clin Invest* 1993;92:179–185.
87. Su S, Grover J, Roughley PJ, et al. Expression of the tissue inhibitors of metalloproteinases (TIMPs) gene family in normal and osteoarthritic joints. *Rheumatol Int* 1999;18:183–191.
88. Hembry RM, Bagga MR, Reynolds JJ, et al. Immunolocalisation studies on six matrix metalloproteinases and their inhibitors, TIMP-1 and TIMP-2, in synovia from patients with osteo- and rheumatoid arthritis. *Ann Rheum Dis* 1995;54:25–32.
89. Ohuchi E, Imai K, Fujii Y, et al. Membrane type 1 matrix metalloproteinase digests interstitial collagens and other extracellular matrix macromolecules. *J Biol Chem* 1997;272:2446–2451.
90. Imai K, Ohuchi E, Aoki T, et al. Membrane-type matrix metalloproteinase 1 is a gelatinolytic enzyme and is secreted in a complex with tissue inhibitor of metalloproteinases 2. *Cancer Res* 1996;56:2707–2710.
91. Buttner FH, Chubinskaya S, Margerie D, et al. Expression of membrane type 1 matrix metalloproteinase in human articular cartilage. *Arthritis Rheum* 1997;40:704–709.
92. Benbow U, Brinckerhoff CE. The AP-1 site and MMP gene regulation: what is all the fuss about? *Matrix Biol* 1997;15: 519–526.
93. Gomez DE, Alonso DF, Yoshiji H, et al. Tissue inhibitors of metalloproteinases: structure, regulation and biological functions. *Eur J Cell Biol* 1997;74:111–122.
94. Zafarullah M, Su S, Martel-Pelletier J, et al. Tissue inhibitor of metalloproteinase-2 (TIMP-2) mRNA is constitutively expressed in bovine, human normal, and osteoarthritic articular chondrocytes. *J Cell Biochem* 1996;60:211–217.
95. Su S, Dehnade F, Zafarullah M. Regulation of tissue inhibitor of metalloproteinases-3 gene expression by transforming growth factor-beta and dexamethasone in bovine and human articular chondrocytes. *DNA Cell Biol* 1996;15:1039–1048.
96. Apte SS, Mattei M-G, Olsen BR. Cloning of the cDNA encoding human tissue inhibitor of metalloproteinases-3 (TIMP-3) and mapping of the TIMP3 gene to chromosome 22. *Genomics* 1994;19:86–90.
97. Dean DD, Martel-Pelletier J, Pelletier JP, et al. Evidence for metalloproteinase and metalloproteinase inhibitor imbalance in human osteoarthritic cartilage. *J Clin Invest* 1989;84:678–685.
98. Will H, Atkinson SJ, Butler GS, et al. The soluble catalytic domain of membrane type 1 matrix metalloproteinase cleaves the propeptide of progelatinase A and initiates autoproteolytic activation. Regulation by TIMP-2 and TIMP-3. *J Biol Chem* 1996;271:17119–17123.
99. Nagase H. Activation mechanisms of matrix metalloproteinases. *Biol Chem* 1997;378:151–160.
100. Nagase H, Enghild JJ, Suzuki K, et al. Stepwise activation mechanisms of the precursor of matrix metalloproteinase 3 (stromelysin) by proteinases and (4-aminophenyl) mercuric acetate. *Biochemistry* 1990;29:5783–5789.
101. Knauper V, Will H, Lopez-Otin C, et al. Cellular mechanisms for human procollagenase-3 (MMP-13) activation. Evidence that MT1-MMP (MMP-14) and gelatinase a (MMP-2) are able to generate active enzyme. *J Biol Chem* 1996;271:17124–17131.
102. Campbell IK, Piccoli DS, Butler DM, et al. Recombinant human interleukin-1 stimulates human articular cartilage to undergo resorption and human chondrocytes to produce both tissue- and urokinase-type plasminogen activator. *Biochim Biophys Acta* 1988;967:183–194.
103. Martel-Pelletier J, Faure MP, McCollum R, et al. Plasmin, plasminogen activators and inhibitor in human osteoarthritic cartilage. *J Rheumatol* 1991;18:1863–1871.
104. Quigley JP. Phorbol ester-induced morphological changes in transformed chick fibroblasts: evidence for direct catalytic involvement of plasminogen activator. *Cell* 1979;17:131–141.
105. Mochan E, Keler T. Plasmin degradation of cartilage proteoglycan. *Biochim Biophys Acta* 1984;800:312–315.
106. Andrews JL, Ghosh P. Low molecular weight serine proteinase inhibitors of human articular cartilage. Isolation, characterization, and biosynthesis. *Arthritis Rheum* 1990;33:1384–1393.
107. Killackey JJ, Roughley PJ, Mort JS. Proteinase inhibitors of human articular cartilage. *Coll Relat Res* 1983;3:419–430.
108. Eeckhout Y, Vaes G. Further studies on the activation of procollagenase, the latent precursor of bone collagenase. Effects of lysosomal cathepsin B, plasmin and kallikrein, and spontaneous activation. *Biochem J* 1977;166:21–31.
109. Mort JS, Recklies AD, Poole AR. Extracellular presence of the lysosomal proteinase cathepsin B in rheumatoid synovium and its activity at neutral pH. *Arthritis Rheum* 1984;27:509–515.
110. Martel-Pelletier J, Cloutier JM, Pelletier JP. Cathepsin B and cysteine protease inhibitors in human OA: effect of intra-articular steroid injections. *J Orthop Res* 1990;8:336–344.
111. Legris F, Martel-Pelletier J, Pelletier JP, et al. An ultrasensitive chemiluminoenzyme immunoassay for the quantification of human tissue kininogens: application to synovial membrane and cartilage. *J Immunol Methods* 1994;168:111–121.
112. Werb Z, Alexander CM. Proteinases and matrix degradation. In: Kelley WN, Harris ED Jr, Ruddy S, et al., eds. *Textbook of rheumatology,* 4th ed. Philadelphia: WB Saunders, 1992: 248–268.
113. Woessner JF Jr, Howell DS. Hydrolytic enzymes in cartilage. In:

Maroudas A, Holborow EJ, eds. *Studies in joint disease,* vol 2. Tunbridge Wells, England: Pitman Medical, 1981:4–152.
114. Pelletier JP, Faure MP, Di Battista JA, et al. Coordinate synthesis of stromelysin, interleukin-1, and oncogene proteins in experimental osteoarthritis. An immunohistochemical study. *Am J Pathol* 1993;142:95–105.
115. Farahat MN, Yanni G, Poston R, et al. Cytokine expression in synovial membranes of patients with rheumatoid arthritis and osteoarthritis. *Ann Rheum Dis* 1993;52:870–875.
116. Caron JP, Fernandes JC, Martel-Pelletier J, et al. Chondroprotective effect of intraarticular injections of interleukin-1 receptor antagonist in experimental osteoarthritis: suppression of collagenase-1 expression. *Arthritis Rheum* 1996;39:1535–1544.
117. Van de Loo FAJ, Joosten LA, van Lent PL, et al. Role of interleukin-1, tumor necrosis factor alpha, and interleukin-6 in cartilage proteoglycan metabolism and destruction. Effect of in situ blocking in murine antigen- and zymosan-induced arthritis. *Arthritis Rheum* 1995;38:164–172.
118. Plows D, Probert L, Georgopoulos S, et al. The role of tumour necrosis factor (TNF) in arthritis: studies in transgenic mice. *Rheumatol Eur* 1995;suppl 2:51–54.
119. Chikanza IC, Roux-Lombard P, Dayer JM, et al. Tumour necrosis factor soluble receptors behave as acute phase reactants following surgery in patients with rheumatoid arthritis, chronic osteomyelitis and osteoarthritis. *Clin Exp Immunol* 1993;92:19–22.
120. Pelletier JP, Martel-Pelletier J. Evidence for the involvement of interleukin 1 in human osteoarthritic cartilage degradation: protective effect of NSAID. *J Rheumatol* 1989;16:19–27.
121. Wood DD, Ihrie EJ, Dinarello CA, et al. Isolation of an interleukin 1 like factor from human joint effusions. *Arthritis Rheum* 1983;26:975–983.
122. Dayer JM, Beutler B, Cerami A. Cachectin/tumor necrosis factor stimulates collagenase and prostaglandin E2 production by human synovial cells and dermal fibroblasts. *J Exp Med* 1985;162:2163–2168.
123. Dayer JM, de Rochemonteix B, Burrus B, et al. Human recombinant interleukin 1 stimulates collagenase and prostaglandin E2 production by human synovial cells. *J Clin Invest* 1986; 77:645–648.
124. Krane SM, Dayer JM, Simon LS, et al. Mononuclear cell-conditioned medium containing mononuclear cell factor (MCF), homologous with interleukin 1, stimulates collagen and fibronectin synthesis by adherent rheumatoid synovial cells: effects of prostaglandin E2 and indomethacin. *Coll Relat Res* 1985;5:99–117.
125. Postlethwaite AE, Raghow R, Stricklin GP, et al. Modulation of fibroblast functions by interleukin 1: increased steady-state accumulation of type I procollagen messenger RNAs and stimulation of other functions but not chemotaxis by human recombinant interleukin 1 alpha and beta. *J Cell Biol* 1988;106:311–318.
126. Ollivierre F, Gubler U, Towle CA, et al. Expression of IL-1 genes in human and bovine chondrocytes: a mechanism for autocrine control of cartilage matrix degradation. *Biochem Biophys Res Commun* 1986;141:904–911.
127. Saha N, Moldovan F, Tardif G, et al. Interleukin -1β-converting enzyme/caspase-1 in human osteoarthritic tissues: localization and role in the maturation of IL-1β and IL-18. *Arthritis Rheum* 1999;42:1577–1587.
128. Tyler JA. Articular cartilage cultured with catabolin (pig interleukin 1) synthesizes a decreased number of normal proteoglycan molecules. *Biochem J* 1985;227:869–878.
129. Goldring MB, Birkhead J, Sandell LJ, et al. Interleukin 1 suppresses expression of cartilage-specific types II and IX collagens and increases types I and III collagens in human chondrocytes. *J Clin Invest* 1988;82:2026–2037.
130. Pelletier JP, Caron JP, Evans CH, et al. In vivo suppression of early experimental osteoarthritis by IL-Ra using gene therapy. *Arthritis Rheum* 1997;40:1012–1019.
131. Fernandes JC, Tardif G, Martel-Pelletier J, et al. In vivo transfer of interleukin-1 receptor antagonist gene in osteoarthritic rabbit knee joints: prevention of osteoarthritis progression. *Am J Pathol* 1999;154:1159–1169.
132. Clark IM, Powell LK, Ramsey S, et al. The measurement of collagenase, tissue inhibitor of metalloproteinases (TIMP), and collagenase-TIMP complex in synovial fluids from patients with osteoarthritis and rheumatoid arthritis. *Arthritis Rheum* 1993;36:372–379.
133. Martel-Pelletier J, Zafarullah M, Kodama S, et al. In vitro effects of interleukin 1 on the synthesis of metalloproteases, TIMP, plasminogen activators and inhibitors in human articular cartilage. *J Rheumatol* 1991;18(suppl 27):80–84.
134. Bunning RA, Richardson HJ, Crawford A, et al. The effect of interleukin-1 on connective tissue metabolism and its relevance to arthritis. *Agents Actions Suppl* 1986;18:131–152.
135. Black RA, Kronheim SR, Cantrell M, et al. Generation of biologically active interleukin-1 beta by proteolytic cleavage of the inactive precursor. *J Biol Chem* 1988;263:9437–9442.
136. Kronheim SR, Mumma A, Greenstreet T, et al. Purification of interleukin-1 beta converting enzyme, the protease that cleaves the interleukin-1 beta precursor. *Arch Biochem Biophys* 1992; 296:698–703.
137. Arend WP. Interleukin-1 receptor antagonist. *Adv Immunol* 1993;54:167–227.
138. Martel-Pelletier J, McCollum R, Di Battista JA, et al. The interleukin-1 receptor in normal and osteoarthritic human articular chondrocytes. Identification as the type I receptor and analysis of binding kinetics and biologic function. *Arthritis Rheum* 1992;35:530–540.
139. Sadouk M, Pelletier JP, Tardif G, et al. Human synovial fibroblasts coexpress interleukin-1 receptor type I and type II mRNA: the increased level of the interleukin-1 receptor in osteoarthritic cells is related to an increased level of the type 1 receptor. *Lab Invest* 1995;73:347–355.
140. Pelletier JP, McCollum R, Cloutier JM, et al. Synthesis of metalloproteases and interleukin 6 (IL-6) in human osteoarthritic synovial membrane is an IL-1 mediated process. *J Rheumatol* 1995;22:109–114.
141. Svenson M, Hansen MB, Heegaard P, et al. Specific binding of interleukin-1 (IL-1) and IL-1 receptor antagonist (IL-1ra) to human serum. High-affinity binding of IL-1ra to soluble IL-1 receptor type I. *Cytokine* 1993;5:427–435.
142. Dinarello CA. Biologic basis for interleukin-1 in disease. *Blood* 1996;87:2095–2147.
143. Black RA, Rauch CT, Kozlosky CJ, et al. A metalloproteinase disintegrin that releases tumour-necrosis factor-alpha from cells. *Nature* 1997;385:729–733.
144. Patel IR, Attur MG, Patel RN, et al. TNF-alpha convertase enzyme from human arthritis-affected cartilage: isolation of cDNA by differential display, expression of the active enzyme, and regulation of TNF-alpha. *J Immunol* 1998;160: 4570–4579.
145. Alaaeddine N, Di Battista JA, Pelletier JP, et al. Osteoarthritic synovial fibroblasts possess an increased level of tumor necrosis factor-receptor 55 (TNF-R55) that mediates biological activation by TNF-alpha. *J Rheumatol* 1997;24:1985–1994.
146. Westacott CI, Atkins RM, Dieppe PA, et al. Tumour necrosis factor-alpha receptor expression on chondrocytes isolated from human articular cartilage. *J Rheumatol* 1994;21: 1710–1715.
147. Naume B, Shalaby R, Lesslauer W, et al. Involvement of the 55- and 75-kDa tumor necrosis factor receptors in the generation of

lymphokine-activated killer cell activity and proliferation of natural killer cells. *J Immunol* 1991;146:3045–3048.
148. Hohmann HP, Brockhaus M, Baeuerle PA, et al. Expression of the types A and B tumor necrosis factor (TNF) receptors is independently regulated, and both receptors mediate activation of the transcription factor NF-kappa B. TNF alpha is not needed for induction of a biological effect via TNF receptors. *J Biol Chem* 1990;265:22409–22417.
149. Tartaglia LA, Pennica D, Goeddel DV. Ligand passing: the 75-kDa tumor necrosis factor (TNF) receptor recruits TNF for signaling by the 55-kDa TNF receptor. *J Biol Chem* 1993;268: 18542–18548.
150. Roux-Lombard P, Punzi L, Hasler F, et al. Soluble tumor necrosis factor receptors in human inflammatory synovial fluids. *Arthritis Rheum* 1993;36:485–489.
151. Guerne PA, Zuraw BL, Vaughan JH, et al. Synovium as a source as interleukin-6 in vitro: contribution to local and systemic manifestations of arthritis. *J Clin Invest* 1989;83:585–592.
152. Kohase M, Henriksen-DeStefano D, May LT, et al. Induction of beta 2-interferon by tumor necrosis factor: a homeostatic mechanism in the control of cell proliferation. *Cell* 1986; 45:659–666.
153. Lotz M, Guerne PA. Interleukin-6 induces the synthesis of tissue inhibitor of metalloproteinases-1/erythroid potentiating activity. *J Biol Chem* 1991;266:2017–2020.
154. Lotz M, Moats T, Villiger PM. Leukemia inhibitory factor is expressed in cartilage and synovium and can contribute to the pathogenesis of arthritis. *J Clin Invest* 1992;90:888–896.
155. Hamilton JA, Waring PM, Filonzi EL. Induction of leukemia inhibitory factor in human synovial fibroblasts by IL-1 and tumor necrosis factor-alpha. *J Immunol* 1993;150:1496–1502.
156. Campbell IK, Waring P, Novak U, et al. Production of leukemia inhibitory factor by human articular chondrocytes and cartilage in response to interleukin-1 and tumor necrosis factor alpha. *Arthritis Rheum* 1993;36:790–794.
157. Jovanovic D, Di Battista JA, Martel-Pelletier J, et al. Interleukin-17 (IL-17) stimulates the production and expression of proinflammatory cytokines, IL-beta and TNF-alpha, by human macrophages. *J Immunol* 1998;160:3513–3521.
158. Attur MG, Patel RN, Abramson SB, et al. Interleukin-17 up-regulation of nitric oxide production in human osteoarthritis cartilage. *Arthritis Rheum* 1997;40:1050–1053.
159. Shalom-Barak T, Quach J, Lotz M. Interleukin-17–induced gene expression in articular chondrocytes is associated with activation of mitogen-activated protein kinases and NF-κB. *J Biol Chem* 1998;273:27467–27473.
160. Martel-Pelletier J, Mineau F, Jovanovic D, et al. Mitogen-activated protein kinase and nuclear factor-κB together regulate interleukin-17–induced nitric oxide production in human osteoarthritic chondrocytes: possible role of transactivating factor mitogen-activated protein kinase-activated protein kinase (MAPKAPK). *Arthritis Rheum* 1999;42:2399–2409.
161. Olee T, Hashimoto S, Quach J, et al. IL-18 is produced by articular chondrocytes and induces proinflammatory and catabolic responses. *J Immunol* 1999;162:1096–1100.
162. Hart PH, Vitti GF, Burgess DR, et al. Potential antiinflammatory effects of interleukin 4: suppression of human monocyte tumor necrosis factor alpha, interleukin 1, and prostaglandin E2. *Proc Natl Acad Sci U S A* 1989;86:3803–3807.
163. Lacraz S, Nicod L, Galve-de Rochemonteix B, et al. Suppression of metalloproteinase biosynthesis in human alveolar macrophages by interleukin-4. *J Clin Invest* 1992;90:382–388.
164. Jenkins JK, Malyak M, Arend WP. The effects of interleukin-10 on interleukin-1 receptor antagonist and interleukin-1β production in human monocytes and neutrophils. *Lymphokine Cytokine Res* 1994;13:47–54.
165. de Waal Malefyt R, Figdor CG, Huijbens R, et al. Effects of IL-13 on phenotype, cytokine production, and cytotoxic function of human monocytes. Comparison with IL-4 and modulation by IFN-gamma or IL-10. *J Immunol* 1993;151: 6370–6381.
166. Jovanovic D, Pelletier JP, Alaaeddine N, et al. Effect of IL-13 on cytokines, cytokine receptors and inhibitors on human osteoarthritic synovium and synovial fibroblasts. *Osteoarthritis Cartilage* 1998;6:40–49.
167. Alaaeddine N, Di Battista JA, Pelletier JP, et al. Inhibition of tumor necrosis factor alpha-induced prostaglandin E2 production by the antiinflammatory cytokines interleukin-4, interleukin-10, and interleukin-13 in osteoarthritic synovial fibroblasts: distinct targeting in the signaling pathways. *Arthritis Rheum* 1999;42:710–718.
168. Pelletier JP, Mineau F, Ranger P, et al. The increased synthesis of inducible nitric oxide inhibits IL-1Ra synthesis by human articular chondrocytes: possible role in osteoarthritic cartilage degradation. *Osteoarthritis Cartilage* 1996;4:77–84.
169. Rediske J, Koehne CF, Zhang B, et al. The inducible production of nitric oxide by articular cell types. *Osteoarthritis Cartilage* 1994;2:199–206.
170. Farrell AJ, Blake DR, Palmer RM, et al. Increased concentrations of nitrite in synovial fluid and serum samples suggest increased nitric oxide synthesis in rheumatic diseases. *Ann Rheum Dis* 1992;51:1219–1222.
171. Stadler J, Stefanovic-Racic M, Billiar TR, et al. Articular chondrocytes synthesize nitric oxide in response to cytokines and lipopolysaccharide. *J Immunol* 1991;147:3915–3920.
172. Palmer RM, Hickery MS, Charles IG, et al. Induction of nitric oxide synthase in human chondrocytes. *Biochem Biophys Res Commun* 1993;193:398–405.
173. Stefanovic-Racic M, Stadler J, Georgescu HI, et al. Nitric oxide and energy production in articular chondrocytes. *J Cell Physiol* 1994;159:274–280.
174. Evans CH, Watkins SC, Stefanovic-Racic M. Nitric oxide and cartilage metabolism. *Methods Enzymol* 1996;269:75–88.
175. Murrell GAC, Jang D, Williams RJ. Nitric oxide activates metalloprotease enzymes in articular cartilage. *Biochem Biophys Res Commun* 1995;206:15–21.
176. Hauselmann HJ, Oppliger L, Michel BA, et al. Nitric oxide and proteoglycan biosynthesis by human articular chondrocytes in alginate culture. *FEBS Lett* 1994;352:361–364.
177. Taskiran D, Stefanovic-Racic M, Georgescu HI, et al. Nitric oxide mediates suppression of cartilage proteoglycan synthesis by interleukin-1. *Biochem Biophys Res Commun* 1994;200: 142–148.
178. Pelletier JP, Lascau-Coman V, Jovanovic D, et al. Selective inhibition of inducible nitric oxide synthase in experimental osteoarthritis is associated with a reduction of tissular levels of catabolic factors. *J Rheumatol* 1999;26:2002-2014.
179. Connor JA, Manning PT, Settle SL, et al. Suppression of adjuvant-induced arthritis by selective inhibition of inducible nitric oxide synthase. *Eur J Pharmacol* 1995;273:15–24.
180. Stefanovic-Racic M, Meyers K, Meschter C, et al. N-monomethyl arginine, an inhibitor of nitric oxide synthase, suppresses the development of adjuvant arthritis in rats. *Arthritis Rheum* 1994;37:1062–1069.
181. Goldring MB, Suen L-F, Yamin R, et al. Regulation of collagen gene expression by prostaglandins and interleukin-1β in cultured chondrocytes and fibroblasts. *Am J Ther* 1996;3:301–308.
182. Berenbaum F, Jacques C, Thomas G, et al. Synergistic effect of interleukin-1 beta and tumor necrosis factor alpha on PGE2 production by articular chondrocytes does not involve PLA2 stimulation. *Exp Cell Res* 1996;222:379–384.
183. Tetsuka T, Daphna-Iken D, Miller BW, et al. Nitric oxide

amplifies interleukin 1–induced cyclooxygenase-2 expression in rat mesangial cells. *J Clin Invest* 1996;97:2051–2056.

184. Landino LM, Crews BC, Timmons MD, et al. Peroxynitrite, the coupling product of nitric oxide and superoxide, activates prostaglandin biosynthesis. *Proc Natl Acad Sci U S A* 1996; 93:15069–15074.
185. Amin AR, Attur MG, Patel RN, et al. Superinduction of cyclooxygenase-2 activity in human osteoarthritis-affected cartilage. Influence of nitric oxide. *J Clin Invest* 1997;99:1231–1237.
186. Matucci-Cerinic M, Lombardi A, Leoncini G, et al. Neutral endopeptidase (3.4.24.11) in plasma and synovial fluid of patients with rheumatoid arthritis. A marker of disease activity or a regulator of pain and inflammation? *Rheumatol Int* 1993;13:1–4.
187. Menkes CJ, Renoux M, Laoussadi S, et al. Substance P levels in the synovium and synovial fluid from patients with rheumatoid arthritis and osteoarthritis. *J Rheumatol* 1993;20:714–717.
188. Koff WC, Dunegan MA. Modulation of macrophage-mediated tumoricidal activity by neuropeptides and neurohormones. *J Immunol* 1985;135:350–354.
189. Lotz M, Carson DA, Vaughan JH. Substance P activation of rheumatoid synoviocytes: neural pathway in pathogenesis of arthritis. *Science* 1987;235:893–895.
190. Laurenzi MA, Persson MA, Dalsgaard CJ, et al. Stimulation of human B lymphocyte differentiation by the neuropeptides substance P and neurokinin A. *Scand J Immunol* 1989;30:695–701.
191. Matsuda H, Kawakita K, Kiso Y, et al. Substance P induces granulocyte infiltration through degranulation of mast cells. *J Immunol* 1989;142:927–931.
192. Kimball ES, Persico FJ, Vaught JL. Substance P, neurokinin A, and neurokinin B induce generation of IL-1–like activity in P388D1 cells. Possible relevance to arthritic disease. *J Immunol* 1988;141:3564–3569.
193. Kimball ES, Fisher MC. Potentiation of IL-1–induced BALB/3T3 fibroblast proliferation by neuropeptides. *J Immunol* 1988;141:4203–4208.
194. Hashimoto S, Takahashi K, Amiel D, et al. Chondrocyte apoptosis and nitric oxide production during experimentally induced osteoarthritis. *Arthritis Rheum* 1998;41:1266–1274.
195. Blanco FJ, Ochs RL, Schwarz H, et al. Chondrocyte apoptosis induced by nitric oxide. *Am J Pathol* 1995;146:75–85.
196. Kouri JB, Jimenez SA, Quintero M, et al. Ultrastructural study of chondrocytes from fibrillated and non-fibrillated human osteoarthritic cartilage. *Osteoarthritis Cartilage* 1996;4: 111–125.
197. Aigner T, Gluckert K, von der Mark K. Activation of fibrillar collagen synthesis and phenotypic modulation of chondrocytes in early human osteoarthritic cartilage lesions. *Osteoarthritis Cartilage* 1997;5:183–189.
198. Chambers MG, Bayliss MT, Mason RM. Chondrocyte cytokine and growth factor expression in murine osteoarthritis. *Osteoarthritis Cartilage* 1997;5:301–308.
199. Towle CA, Hung HH, Bonassar LJ, et al. Detection of interleukin-1 in the cartilage of patients with osteoarthritis: a possible autocrine/paracrine role in pathogenesis. *Osteoarthritis Cartilage* 1997;5:293–300.
200. Roughley PJ, Melching LI, Recklies AD. Changes in the expression of decorin and biglycan in human articular cartilage with age and regulation by TGF-β. *Matrix* 1994;14:51–59.
201. Fava R, Olsen N, Keski-Oja J, et al. Active and latent forms of transforming growth factor β activity in synovial effusions. *J Exp Med* 1989;169:291–296.
202. Schlaak JF, Pfers I, Meyer Zum Buschenfelde KH, et al. Different cytokine profiles in the synovial fluid of patients with osteoarthritis, rheumatoid arthritis and seronegative spondylarthropathies. *Clin Exp Rheumatol* 1996;14:155–162.
203. Chu CQ, Field M, Abney E, et al. Transforming growth factor-beta 1 in rheumatoid synovial membrane and cartilage/pannus junction. *Clin Exp Immunol* 1991;86:380–306.
204. Dubois CM, Ruscetti FW, Palaszynski EW, et al. Transforming growth factor beta is a potent inhibitor of interleukin 1 (IL-1) receptor expression: proposed mechanism of inhibition of IL-1 action. *J Exp Med* 1990;172:737–744.
205. Harvey AK, Hrubey PS, Chandrasekhar S. Transforming growth factor-beta inhibition of interleukin-1 activity involves down-regulation of interleukin-1 receptors on chondrocytes. *Exp Cell Res* 1991;195:376–385.
206. Campbell IK, Wojta J, Novak U, et al. Cytokine modulation of plasminogen activator inhibitor-1 (PAI-1) production by human articular cartilage and chondrocytes. Down-regulation by tumor necrosis factor alpha and up-regulation by transforming growth factor-β basic fibroblast growth factor. *Biochim Biophys Acta* 1994;1226:277–285.
207. van Beuningen HM, Van der Kraan PM, Arntz OJ, et al. Transforming growth factor-beta 1 stimulates articular chondrocyte proteoglycan synthesis and induces osteophyte formation in the murine knee joint. *Lab Invest* 1994;71:279–290.
208. Luyten FP, Yu YM, Yanagishita M, et al. Natural bovine osteogenin and recombinant human bone morphogenetic protein-2B are equipotent in the maintenance of proteoglycans in bovine articular cartilage explant cultures. *J Biol Chem* 1992; 267:3691–3695.
209. Lietman SA, Yanagishita M, Sampath TK, et al. Stimulation of proteoglycan synthesis in explants of porcine articular cartilage by recombinant osteogenic protein-1 (bone morphogenetic protein-7). *J Bone Joint Surg* 1997;79A:1132–1137.
210. van Beuningen HM, Glansbeek HL, van der Kraan PM, et al. Differential effects of local application of BMP-2 or TGF-beta 1 on both articular cartilage composition and osteophyte formation. *Osteoarthritis Cartilage* 1998;6:306–317.
211. Schouten JS, Van den Ouweland FA, Valkenburg HA, et al. Insulin-like growth factor-1: a prognostic factor of knee osteoarthritis. *Br J Rheumatol* 1993;32:274–280.
212. McAlindon TE, Teale D, Dieppe PA. Insulin-like growth factor 1: effect of age accounts for apparent correlation with sclerosis and osteophytosis in osteoarthritis of the knee. *Br J Rheumatol* 1992;31(suppl 2):213.
213. Denko CW, Boja B, Moskowitz RW. Growth promoting peptides in osteoarthritis: insulin, insulin-like growth factor-I, growth hormone. *J Rheumatol* 1990;17:1217–1221.
214. Hochberg MC, Lethbridge-Cejku M, Scott WW Jr, et al. Serum levels of insulin-like growth factor I in subjects with osteoarthritis of the knee. Data from the Baltimore Longitudinal Study of Aging. *Arthritis Rheum* 1994;37:1177–1180.
215. Lloyd ME, Hart DJ, Nandra D, et al. Relation between insulin-like growth factor-1 concentrations, osteoarthritis, bone density, and fractures in the general population: the Chingford study. *Ann Rheum Dis* 1996;55:870–874.
216. Denko CW, Boja B. Growth factors in asymptomatic osteoarthritis—insulin, insulin-like growth factor-1, growth hormone. *Immunopharmacology* 1993;2:71–76.
217. Middleton JF, Tyler JA. Upregulation of insulin-like growth factor-1 gene expression in the lesions of osteoarthritic human articular cartilage. *Ann Rheum Dis* 1992;51:440–447.
218. Doré S, Abribat T, Rousseau N, et al. Increased insulin-like growth factor 1 production by human osteoarthritic chondrocytes is not dependent on growth hormone action. *Arthritis Rheum* 1995;38:413–419.
219. Schneiderman R, Rosenberg N, Hiss J, et al. Concentration and size distribution of insulin-like growth factor-I in human normal and osteoarthritic synovial fluid and cartilage. *Arch Biochem Biophys* 1995;1:173–188.

220. Tavera C, Abribat T, Reboul P, et al. IGF and IGF-binding protein system in the synovial fluid of osteoarthritic and rheumatoid arthritic patients. *Osteoarthritis Cartilage* 1996; 4:263–274.
221. Fernihough JK, Billingham ME, Cwyfan-Hughes S, et al. Local disruption of the insulin-like growth factor system in the arthritic joint. *Arthritis Rheum* 1996;39:1556–1565.
222. Olney RC, Tsuchiya K, Wilson DM, et al. Chondrocytes from osteoarthritic cartilage have increased expression of insulin-like growth factor 1 (IGF-1) and IGF-binding protein-3 (IGFBP-3) and -5, but not IGF-II or IGFBP-4. *J Clin Endocrinol Metab* 1996;81:1096–1103.
223. Hilal G, Martel-Pelletier J, Pelletier JP, et al. Osteoblast-like cells from human subchondral ostoearthritic bone demonstrate an altered phenotype in vitro: possible role in subchondral bone sclerosis. *Arthritis Rheum* 1998;41:891–899.
224. Doré S, Pelletier JP, Di Battista JA, et al. Human osteoarthritic chondrocytes possess an increased number of insulin-like growth factor 1 binding sites but are unresponsive to its stimulation. Possible role of IGF-1–Binding Proteins. *Arthritis Rheum* 1994;37:253–263.
225. Martel-Pelletier J, Tardif G, Reboul P, et al. Human osteoarthritic chondrocytes expressed a normal level of type I IGF-receptor but an increased expression and synthesis of IGF binding proteins. *Trans Orthop Res Soc* 1995;20:372(abst).
226. Yateman ME, Claffey DC, Cwyfan Hughes SC, et al. Cytokines modulate the sensitivity of human fibroblasts to stimulation with insulin-like growth factor-1 (IGF-1) by altering endogenous IGF-binding protein production. *J Endocrinol* 1993;137: 151–159.
227. Matsumoto T, Tsukazaki T, Enomoto H, et al. Effects of interleukin-1 beta on insulin-like growth factor-1 autocrine/ paracrine axis in cultured rat articular chondrocytes. *Ann Rheum Dis* 1994;53:128–133.
228. Scharla SH, Strong DD, Mohan S, et al. Effect of tumor necrosis factor-alpha on the expression of insulin-like growth factor 1 and insulin-like growth factor binding protein 4 in mouse osteoblasts. *Eur J Endocrinol* 1994;131:293–301.
229. Olney RC, Wilson DM, Mohtai M, et al. Interleukin-1 and tumor necrosis factor-alpha increase insulin-like growth factor-binding protein-3 (IGFBP-3) production and IGFBP-3 protease activity in human articular chondrocytes. *J Endocrinol* 1995;146:279–286.
230. Hamerman D, Taylor S, Kirschenbaum I, et al. Growth factors with heparin binding affinity in human synovial fluid. *Proc Soc Exp Biol Med* 1987;186:384–389.
231. Sachs BL, Goldberg VM, Moskowitz RW, et al. Response of articular chondrocytes to pituitary fibroblast growth factor (FGF). *J Cell Physiol* 1982;112:51–59.
232. Kato Y, Gospodarowicz D. Sulfated proteoglycan synthesis by confluent cultures of rabbit costal chondrocytes grown in the presence of fibroblast growth factor. *J Cell Biol* 1985;100: 477–485.
233. Cuevas P, Burgos J, Baird A. Basic fibroblast growth factor (FGF) promotes cartilage repair in vivo. *Biochem Biophys Res Commun* 1988;156:611–618.
234. Kato Y, Hiraki Y, Inoue H, et al. Differential and synergistic actions of somatomedin-like growth factors, fibroblast growth factor and epidermal growth factor in rabbit costal chondrocytes. *Eur J Biochem* 1983;129:685–690.
235. Trippel SB, Wroblewski J, Makower AM, et al. Regulation of growth-plate chondrocytes by insulin-like growth-factor I and basic fibroblast growth factor. *J Bone Joint Surg* 1993;75A: 177–189.
236. Guerne PA, Lotz M. Interleukin-6 and transforming growth factor-beta synergistically stimulate chondrosarcoma cell proliferation. *J Cell Physiol* 1991;149:117–124.
237. Verschure PJ, Joosten LA, van der Kraan PM, et al. Responsiveness of articular cartilage from normal and inflamed mouse knee joints to various growth factors. *Ann Rheum Dis* 1994;53:455–460.
238. Uitterlinden AG, Burger H, Huang Q, et al. Vitamin D receptor genotype is associated with radiographic osteoarthritis at the knee. *J Clin Invest* 1997;100:259–263.
239. Dieppe P, Cushnaghan J, Young P, et al. Prediction of the progression of joint space narrowing in osteoarthritis of the knee by bone scintigraphy. *Ann Rheum Dis* 1993;52:557–563.
240. Moskowitz RW. Bone remodeling in osteoarthritis: subchondral and osteophytic responses. *Osteoarthritis Cartilage* 1999;7: 323–324.
241. Li B, Aspden RM. Composition and mechanical properties of cancellous bone from the femoral head of patients with osteoporosis or osteoarthritis. *J Bone Miner Res* 1997;12:614–651.
242. Grynpas MD, Alpert B, Katz I, et al. Subchondral bone in osteoarthritis. *Calcif Tissue Int* 1991;49:20–26.
243. Puzas JE, ed. *Primer on the metabolic bone diseases and disorders of mineral metabolism,* 2nd ed. New York: Raven Press, 1993.
244. Westacott CI, Webb GR, Warnock MG, et al. Alteration of cartilage metabolism by cells from osteoarthritic bone. *Arthritis Rheum* 1997;40:1282–1291.
245. Ducy P, Desbois C, Boyce B, et al. Increased bone formation in osteocalcin-deficient mice. *Nature* 1996;382:448–452.
246. Mansell JP, Tarlton JF, Bailey AJ. Biochemical evidence for altered subchondral bone collagen metabolism in osteoarthritis of the hip. *Br J Rheumatol* 1997;36:16–19.
247. Martel-Pelletier J, Hilal G, Pelletier JP, et al. Evidence for increased metabolic activity in human osteoarthritic subchondral bone explants. *Arthritis Rheum* 1997;40:S182(abst).
248. Hilal G, Martel-Pelletier J, Pelletier JP, et al. Abnormal regulation of urokinase plasminogen activator by insulin-like growth factor-1 in human osteoarthritic subchondral osteoblasts. *Arthritis Rheum* 1999;42:2112–2122.

111

CLINICAL AND LABORATORY FINDINGS IN OSTEOARTHRITIS

ROLAND W. MOSKOWITZ
DANIEL HOLDERBAUM

Osteoarthritis (OA) is a slowly evolving articular disease characterized by the gradual development of joint pain, stiffness, and limitation of motion. The terms degenerative joint disease or OA may be more precise because degeneration of cartilage is the most prominent pathologic change. Both experimental (1) and clinical (2) studies have shown mild-to-moderate synovitis, although inflammatory changes may be absent early (3). Some favor a particular form of nomenclature, but at present, the terms OA, osteoarthrosis, and degenerative joint disease are used interchangeably. Although OA is often benign, severe degenerative changes may cause serious disability. Newer concepts of pathogenesis suggest that OA is not an inevitable sequence of aging itself and raise the possibility of rational preventive and therapeutic approaches in the future.

CLASSIFICATION

Classification of OA is difficult because of its variable presentation. It has been suggested that OA may represent several disease subsets leading to similar clinical and pathologic alterations, rather than being one specific disorder. The disease is classified as primary or idiopathic when it occurs in the absence of any known underlying predisposing factor. In contrast, secondary OA is that form of the disease after an identifiable underlying local or systemic pathogenetic factor. The distinctions on which this simple classification is based may be artificial, however. Studies on OA of the hip, for example, show that many cases of primary OA are actually secondary to anatomic abnormalities that result in articular incongruity and premature cartilage degeneration, such as congenital hip dysplasia and slipped capital femoral epiphysis of childhood (4).

Classification criteria for OA of the knee (5), hand (6), and hip (7) have been developed by the American College of Rheumatology (ACR). Development of such criteria is important for various purposes, including epidemiologic and case–control studies, studies of disease natural history and prognosis, and therapeutic responses. Although classification criteria should not be used as diagnostic criteria, because sensitivity and specificity are not 100%, they are valuable in standardization for reporting of series of cases, in performing investigational studies, and in improving consistency in communication. Alternative sets of criteria may be used under different circumstances. For example, criteria not involving radiographs can be used for screening purposes in an office practice. Clinical trials in which radiographs are obtained routinely and in which other parameters are frequently quantified, allow use of criteria based on clinical examination, laboratory tests, and radiographs. Criteria based on clinical examination alone are useful for population surveys and other epidemiologic studies. Difficulties inherent in development of classification criteria of clinical OA are related to imprecisely defined clinical symptoms, disparity between pathologic and clinical findings, absence of specific diagnostic tests, and differences in criteria related to different joints involved. Although algorithms using surrogate variables have been developed for use when primary variables are not available, their complexity makes them less practical for everyday use (5–7).

Various forms of the disease, such as primary generalized OA, erosive inflammatory OA, and chondromalacia patellae, have different clinical, pathologic, and radiographic findings, and are generally considered distinct syndromes. A working classification of OA based on known anatomic and etiologic mechanisms is presented in Table 111.1.

PRIMARY OSTEOARTHRITIS

Interpretation of data regarding the natural history of primary OA is complicated by the different case-finding techniques, whether clinical, radiographic, or pathologic, used in many of the reported studies. Moreover, studies focused on different joints cannot be compared, even when similar

TABLE 111.1. CLASSIFICATION OF OSTEOARTHRITIS

Primary (Idiopathic)
- Peripheral joints
- Spine
  - Apophyseal joints
  - Intervertebral joints
- Subsets
  - Generalized osteoarthritis
  - Erosive inflammatory osteoarthritis
  - Diffuse idiopathic skeletal hyperostosis
  - Chondromalacia patellae
- Hereditary (type II collagen gene mutations)

Secondary
- Trauma
  - Acute
  - Chronic (occupational, sports)
- Underlying joint disorders
  - Local (fracture, infection)
  - Diffuse (rheumatoid arthritis)
- Systemic metabolic or endocrine disorders
  - Ochronosis (alkaptonuria)
  - Wilson's disease
  - Hemochromatosis
  - Kashin–Beck disease
  - Acromegaly
  - Hyperparathyroidism
- Crystal-deposition disease
  - Calcium pyrophosphate dihydrate (pseudogout)
  - Basic calcium phosphate (hydroxyapatite–octacalcium phosphate–tricalcium phosphate)
  - Monosodium urate monohydrate (gout)
- Neuropathic disorders (Charcot joints)
  - Tabes dorsalis
  - Diabetes mellitus
- Intraarticular corticosteroid overuse
- Miscellaneous
  - Bone dysplasia (multiple epiphyseal dysplasia; achondroplasia)
  - Frostbite

case-finding methods are used. Nevertheless, sufficient data permit a reasonable approximation of the natural course of the disease.

Epidemiologic Features

A comparison of epidemiologic surveys undertaken to characterize the prevalence and clinical characteristics of OA requires close attention to variations in analytic techniques and populations studied (8) (see Chapters 1 and 3). Such variations may have a major impact on the data obtained. Studies derived from autopsy analyses, for example, define earlier disease manifestations than do clinical studies based on symptoms that develop later. In clinical surveys, disease definitions must be clear, and the use of prospective or retrospective techniques must be taken into account. Data obtained from radiographic studies depend on the number and location of joints studied (9). Surveys of hospitalized patients, in contrast to those in the general population, are narrow in scope, but they may be useful in identifying certain disease subsets.

Prevalence

Autopsy studies show that degenerative joint changes begin in the second decade (10). By age 40 years, 90% of all persons have such changes in their weight-bearing joints, even though clinical symptoms are generally absent. Radiographic manifestations of the disease increase progressively with age. Studies in a Dutch population demonstrated that, by age 40 years, 10% of the population had distal interphalangeal OA, and 20% had metatarsophalangeal disease (11). Knee OA alone leads to disability as often as heart disease and chronic obstructive lung disease (12).

Signs and symptoms suggestive of OA of the knee were evaluated in 682 elderly people (13). The frequency of signs and symptoms and their degree of severity remained constant in the seventh, eighth, and ninth decades, suggesting that OA of the knee was indeed common in the elderly but not inevitably progressive. In a study performed in a large health maintenance organization (HMO) in New England, OA occurred more frequently in women than in men (ratio, 2:1); the incidence increased until age 80 years, after which there was a leveling off or decline in the rates for OA for all joints observed (14). In contrast to these observations, however, OA of the knee increased in both prevalence and incidence with age (15). In a study of hand OA, it was observed that radiologic progression of OA increased most rapidly in the most elderly members studied (16). In another study of patients with OA of the knee followed up over a period of 12 years, individuals older than 60 years had an almost fourfold higher rate of joint space loss than those aged 45 to 49 years (17). Increased risk with age appeared to be statistically independent of gender and weight. Hip OA was observed to be more prevalent at older ages (18). In a study of subjects aged 55 to 74 years, the risk of hip OA increased with age, adjusting for gender, race, marital status, education, and family income.

These and other studies emphasize the high frequency of OA in the general population. It has been estimated that approximately 21 million Americans between ages 25 and 75 years have clinical signs and symptoms of OA, and it is estimated that by the year 2020, with an aging population, millions more will be afflicted with this disease.

Gender, Race, and Heredity

Evaluations of the relations of gender to OA involve considerations of the influence of sex hormones, job, sports-related effects, and heavy physical activity. In a longitudinal study carried out as a component of the Framingham investigation, OA of the knee was seen to occur more frequently in women than in men; analyses were adjusted for age, body mass index, smoking, injury, chondrocalcinosis, and physical activity (19). Studies by Anderson and Felson (20) demonstrated an increased frequency of radiographic OA with age in both sexes; beginning with individuals in the age decade 45 to 54 years, however, OA was greater in women than in men. Van Sasse et al. (11), in studies of a Dutch population, also noted an increased prevalence in women versus men; hand OA appeared to be significantly more common in women. Studies suggest that hip OA is more common in men, particularly at older ages; the female preponderance of OA in the knee and hand is not seen with hip OA (11,18,21,22).

Differences in the prevalence of OA in black and white races have been noted, particularly when patterns of joint involvement are analyzed (23,24). African-American women had higher rates of knee OA than did white American women, even after adjustment for age and weight (20). Differences in certain predisposing genetic factors, such as congenital subluxation of the hip, may play a role.

Southern Chinese (25), South African blacks (24), and East Indians (26) have a lower incidence of OA of the hip than do European or American whites. In the Chinese, the hip joint may be protected by the extreme range of motion required for frequent squatting. A decreased frequency of predisposing factors such as rheumatoid arthritis (RA), congenital dysplasia of the hip, and slipped femoral capital epiphysis, all believed to be uncommon in the Chinese, may also explain some of the differences (25). In contrast, Japanese have a high incidence of secondary OA of the hip, related to antecedent congenital hip disease, especially dislocation or acetabular dysplasia (27). Marked variations in racial rates of total hip arthroplasty for primary hip OA were noted in a population-based study in San Francisco; total hip replacement rates were much lower for Asians, Hispanics, and black subjects than for the white population (28). The racial distribution of primary OA of the hip among patients who underwent total hip replacement appeared consistent with distribution patterns observed in international studies. Painful arthropathy of the hips described in the black population around Mseleni in southern Africa appears to be the result of two distinct abnormalities: protrusio acetabuli, affecting mainly women and increasing in frequency with age; and hip dysplasia, which does not increase in frequency with age (29). Degenerative joint disease was more prevalent in Native Americans than in the general population (30).

A role for genetic factors in OA has been suggested for more than half a century, based on clinical findings demonstrating that Heberden's nodes were 10 times more likely to occur in women than in men, and that mothers and sisters of affected women were two to three times more likely to be affected than was the general population (31–33). Subsequent studies demonstrated an increased frequency of human leukocyte antigens HLA-A1 and HLA-B8 in patients with OA as compared with reference populations (34,35). More recently, a cross-sectional study of patients undergoing total hip or total knee replacement in Britain suggested that siblings had an increased risk for both hip and knee replacement compared with spouses, suggesting that genetics may play a more important role than environment in predicting risk of severe degenerative joint disease (36).

Investigation of relative disease incidence in monozygotic and dizygotic twins is a powerful means of determining whether certain conditions that appear to "run in families" have a heritable basis. Spector et al. (37) have shown an increased correlation of radiographic OA of hands and knees among identical twins when compared with fraternal twins. They concluded that the genetic influence on hand and knee OA ranged from 39% to 65%. Wright et al. (38) applied affected sib-pair analysis to siblings with nodal OA and found a significant association with two loci on the long arm of chromosome 2. Candidate genes (genes possibly affecting cartilage structure or metabolism) in the vicinity of the two markers associated with OA include COL5A2 (the α_2-chain of type V collagen), COL6A3 (the α_3-chain of type VI collagen), FN1 (fibronectin) and IL-8R (the interleukin-8 receptor). Felson et al. (39) recently examined hand and knee OA in parents and adult children, with OA assessment by hand and knee radiographs. Their genetic modeling demonstrated a best fit of the data for a mendelian recessive trait with significant polygenic or environmental factors. Studies of primary generalized OA using the sib-pair approach showed no linkage to type II collagen, cartilage matrix protein, or link protein, although strong evidence of a heritable pattern was evident (40).

A linkage between generalized OA accompanied by mild spondyloepiphyseal dysplasia and mutations in the type II collagen gene has been described (41–44). The presence of a single base mutation in exon 31 in the COL2A1 gene was associated with precocious generalized OA in affected family members. This single base substitution converted the codon for arginine at position 519 in the α_1(II) chain to a codon for cysteine, an amino acid normally not found in the triple helical region of type II collagen. Subsequently, nine additional families with precocious generalized OA cosegregating with the same mutation at position 519 have been identified. Other mutations of the COL2A1 gene in the setting of accelerated OA and spondyloepiphyseal dysplasia have been identified, including mutations in exons 11 (44; D. Holderbaum and R.W. Moskowitz, unpublished data) and 41 (45). The occurrence of multiple unrelated families with the same mutation in the COL2A1 gene raises the question of mutational sites of susceptibility, so-called "hot spots." Defects in collagen related to collagen gene mutations appear to translate into a failure of cartilage matrix leading to OA changes, representing a defined cause of primary OA. No specific mutations have been found that result in a phenotype that includes OA without some underlying chondrodysplasia. Several reports have, however, suggested genetic linkage of primary OA to several different chromosomal loci. Vikkula et al. (46) demonstrated linkage of OA to type II collagen in two Finnish families. The radiographic findings in these Finnish kindreds were negative for chondrodysplasia or other underlying anatomic abnormality. The families had symptoms affecting primarily knees, hips, and hands. Sequence data from the 54 exons of COL2A1 failed to show any amino acid substitutions, suggesting that the defect was either in a non–protein coding region of the gene (i.e., an intronic or regulatory region), or perhaps in another gene tightly linked to the COL2A1 gene. Loughlin et al. (47) in the U.K. found differential expression of a rare, polymorphic allele of COL2A1 in patients with generalized OA without dysplasia. As in the previous studies, mutation of protein-coding DNA was not detected, suggesting the possibility of a mutated regulatory region.

Several recent investigations have suggested association of OA with certain candidate gene loci. A vitamin D–receptor haplotype was shown to be associated with higher risk of knee OA in both men and women, in a population-based study conducted in The Netherlands (48). These investigators concluded that the approximately 2.27-fold increase in OA associated with this haplotype was due to increased osteophytosis rather than to joint-space narrowing, suggesting that radiologic changes indicative of cartilage degeneration were not associated with this haplotype. At nearly the same time, a study based on a vitamin D–receptor genotype in British women was reported (49). This study used a single polymorphic marker [Taq I restriction fragment length polymorphism (RFLP)] and determined that women who had either one or two alleles in which the restriction site was absent had an approximate threefold increase in risk of knee OA. It is interesting to note that the vitamin D–receptor locus is genetically very close (<1 million base pairs) to the gene for type II collagen (COL2A1) on chromosome 12q. Further analysis will be required to determine whether the vitamin D receptor is itself the causal locus or is in linkage disequilibrium with a neighboring disease-causing gene.

Climate

Geographic studies in Northern Europe and America suggest that OA is less frequent farther north (23). The prevalence of OA may be lower in Alaskan Eskimos (50) and less prevalent in Finland than in the Netherlands (51). Studies comparing populations in Jamaica and Great Britain, however, revealed an equal frequency in the two climates (23). Factors such as race, culture, and environment complicate comparisons of climatic effects on disease prevalence. Symptoms may be less severe in a warmer climate, related perhaps to higher temperatures, greater amounts of sunshine, and lighter-weight clothes.

Obesity, Body Somatotype, and Bone Density

Although the role of obesity in the etiology of OA requires further definition, a positive relation with knee OA has been demonstrated in multiple studies (52,53). Higher baseline body mass index increases the risk of OA, and weight change was directly correlated with OA risk (19). Weight loss was associated with a lower risk of OA. Similar findings were observed in a longitudinal study of women in an English population; women in the top tertile of body mass index were observed to have an increased risk of knee OA (54). In addition to a relation of obesity to disease prevalence in certain joints, several studies have reported that obese patients are more likely to experience progressive disease (17,55,56). Clinical studies demonstrated that joint symptoms in patients with OA improve with weight loss (52,57). It has been suggested that obesity in OA patients may be secondary to the relative inactivity brought on by joint pain and limitation of motion; although this may pertain to some of the relation, it is more likely that obesity plays a direct role in onset and progression of OA of the knee. In contrast to the knee, studies suggest only a limited association, if any, between body weight and hip OA (18,58).

After controlling for metabolic factors such as serum cholesterol, serum uric acid, diabetes, and blood pressure, no significant reduction in the association between obesity and knee OA was observed, thereby failing to support a metabolic link between obesity and knee OA (53).

In addition to the possible biomechanical effects of obesity on the origin of OA, a metabolic role for fat in disease pathogenesis has been suggested (59). Studies in strains of mice that develop OA showed that diets enriched with lard, a saturated fat, increased the frequency and severity of the degenerative lesions. When unsaturated fat was fed to achieve the same body weight, however, no adverse effect was noted. Perhaps obesity in humans is related to OA not only through its biomechanical effects, but also as a result of still obscure metabolic changes in cartilage. Such a mechanism might explain the increased incidence of OA in non–weight-bearing joints, such as sternoclavicular and distal interphalangeal joints (60).

Hormonal factors have been implicated in the etiology of OA with particular attention on growth hormone, insulin-like growth factor-1 (IGF-1), and sex hormones, including estrogens and testosterone. In one study, patients with OA were observed to have elevated levels of serum insulin and diminished levels of IGF-1 as compared with age-, sex-, and race-matched controls (61). In other studies, no correlations were reported between radiographic changes in knee OA and serum IGF-1 values (62); other investigations noted a relation between IGF-1 concentrations and osteophyte growth but not joint-space narrowing (63). OA has been observed as a significant clinical finding in patients with acromegaly; conversely, the prevalence of radiographic OA was noted to be low in older patients with a deficiency of growth hormone (64).

The interrelations of estrogenic hormones and OA have shown inconsistent results. Some studies have demonstrated an increased relative risk among women who had received estrogen replacement therapy in the postmenopausal period (65). Other investigations, however, have demonstrated a possible inverse relation between the intake of estrogen and knee OA (66–69). Spector et al. (70) noted that current use of estrogen was associated with a protective effect on knee OA. A moderate protective effect of estrogen on hip OA was observed in studies by Vingärd et al. (71). Animal studies have demonstrated differing effects of estrogens on the OA process, depending on such factors as differences in species and the animal model studied (72).

OA has been associated with specific somatotypes; its prevalence is greater in stout individuals than in thin ones (73). Patients with OA of the hip or femoral neck fractures were compared; 94% of the former were endomorphic mesomorphs, whereas the majority of patients with fractures were ectomorphic (74).

Bone density is associated with OA. In studies of the femoral head, a diminished bone mass was associated with femoral neck fracture; increased bone mass, on the other hand, showed a positive correlation with OA (75).

Patients with OA have higher bone marrow density and bone volume than do age-matched controls, even at sites distant from the arthritis (76,77). Additional studies suggested that osteophyte formation was linked to high bone mass, whereas loss of joint space in cartilage was not (78). It has been suggested that stiffer, denser subchondral bone alters the amount and distribution of mechanical forces acting through cartilage, with resultant predisposition to degenerative change (80).

Increased ligamentous laxity correlated positively with joint degeneration. Patients with joint hypermobility had an increased prevalence of generalized OA compared with age- and sex-matched control subjects (80). Conversely, when patients with OA were evaluated, the prevalence of generalized joint hypermobility was higher than that in matched control subjects. Synovial effusions and chondrocalcinosis were common in patients with hypermobility syndrome.

Occupation and Sports

Mechanical stress related to occupation or sports activities has been implicated in the induction of OA in a number of investigations. OA of the hips, knees, and shoulders was more common in miners than in porters or clerks (81); dock workers showed a higher prevalence of OA of the fingers, elbows, and knees than did age-matched civil servants (83); farmers had a high risk of developing hip OA (58); and prolonged or repeated heavy overuse of joints has been related to an increased frequency of OA in bus drivers (32).

Occupational knee bending appears to play a significant role in the development of OA in various occupations (20). Radiographic evidence of knee OA was higher in individuals aged 55 to 64 years whose jobs required knee bending than in those whose jobs required no knee bending; no similar association was noted in younger workers. Similar analyses (83) revealed an association between knee bending and knee OA related to duration of knee-bending activities in male carpenters, floor layers, and painters. An increased risk of knee OA was observed in individuals whose main job entailed more than 30 minutes per day of squatting or kneeling, or climbing more than 10 flights of stairs (84). Kneeling, squatting, or climbing stairs, as well as regularly lifting more than 25 kg, led to a risk of knee OA five times that of individuals with no exposure to these same activities. With respect to hip OA, a positive but weak relation between work-related exposure, such as farming, has been reported (86). In another study, individuals in intermediate or heavy work categories had increased frequency of hip OA (86). Longitudinal studies have defined a relation between level of current physical activity and knee OA (19). The odds of developing OA of the knee were increased by heavy, but not by moderate or light physical activity, adjusting for other factors such as age, gender, and body mass index.

The relation of occupational activity to OA was demonstrated in a study of repetitive manual work performed by women in a weaving factory. Subjects confirmed that the right hand was more severely involved, and it was noted that the pattern of hand and finger lesions could be directly related to the type of work done by each group, with OA being most severe in joints used most repetitively (87). Severe OA of the metacarpophalangeal joints, so-called Missouri metacarpal syndrome, was associated with heavy manual labor involving sustained gripping motions of both hands for 30 years or more (88).

Involvement of millions of individuals in aerobic exercise of various sorts, especially running, has intensified interest in the possible relation of joint overuse to OA. An older study showed no increase in OA of the hip in Finnish running champions as compared with age- and sex-matched controls (89). A later study comparing knee radiographs of long-distance runners aged 50 to 72 years with those of community controls revealed a statistically significant increase in knee sclerosis in women but not in men and no differences in joint-space narrowing, crepitus, joint stability, or symptomatic OA (91). Follow-up studies of these individuals over an additional 5-year period revealed a similar age-related increase in OA in both the runners and controls (91). A study of men who ran many miles per week over many years showed no evidence of premature OA in the lower extremities (92). The effects of habitual running on development of premature OA were studied in Danes who had been running for an average of 40 years at mileage levels comparable to recreational runners of today (93); no differences in OA between runners and nonrunners were noted.

In studies of former elite female athletes including runners and tennis players, increased rates of knee OA were observed when compared with age-matched nonathletes. In studies of male former elite athletes, soccer players had an increased prevalence of knee OA (94). These findings in elite runners are in contrast to the lack of increased rates of OA associated with recreational running.

In contrast to the absence of an association between knee OA and recreational running, increased nonoccupational physical activity may be associated with increased hip OA (95). These investigations revealed that increased sports activities of all kinds were associated with an increased risk of hip OA, depending on the number of years of exposure. Increased risk was associated with sports of all types including track and field, as well as racket sports (95). Lane et al. (96) noted a modest increased risk of hip OA in elderly women who had engaged in weight-bearing physical activities earlier in life.

Accordingly, data thus far suggest that runners are not at increased risk for knee OA. Unfortunately, these studies represent retrospective investigations of the prevalence of OA in self-selected individuals with a demonstrated ability to maintain active running. Selective bias cannot be excluded in any of these studies; that is, individuals with a predisposition to OA (because of obesity, habitus, or metabolic or structural connective tissue abnormalities) may not have chosen this particular form of exercise. Additionally, individuals who developed OA early may have discontinued running.

In contrast to studies of the relation of running to knee OA, an increased risk of hip OA in runners has been suggested in recent epidemiologic reports (95,97).

Increased OA may be associated with sports other than running. An increased incidence of OA changes related to sports injuries has been described in American football players, baseball pitchers, and competitive soccer players (98–101).

Symptoms and Signs

The symptoms of OA are localized to the affected joints (Table 111.2). Involvement of many joints may suggest a systemic form of arthritis. Frequently, little or no correlation exists between the joint symptoms and the extent or degree of pathologic or radiographic change. Only about 30% of persons with radiographic evidence of OA complained of pain at the relevant sites (102). Except for lumbar apophyseal joints, persons with radiographic OA were predisposed to develop related symptoms. Similarly, a positive correlation between clinical symptoms and radiographic evidence of OA of the knee was noted (103). Some of the apparent disparity between symptoms and radiographic abnormalities may relate to the radiographic definition of OA. For example, the use of osteophytes alone as a diagnostic feature has been questioned. Long-term radiographic studies of the hip and knee suggest that the presence of osteophytes does not imply later development of other structural changes of OA, such as joint-space narrowing, subchondral bone cysts, and eburnation (104). Correlation of symptoms with these more definitive structural abnormalities might well provide evidence of a positive interrelation.

TABLE 111.2. CLINICAL PROFILES OF OSTEOARTHRITIS

Factor	Characteristics and Occurrence
Age	Usually advanced; symptoms uncommon before age 40, unless due to secondary cause
Joint involvement	Commonly, distal interphalangeal, proximal interphalangeal, first carpometacarpal, hip, knee, first metatarsophalangeal joints, and lower lumbar and cervical vertebrae. Rarely, metacarpophalangeal, wrist, elbow, or shoulder joints, except after trauma
Joint effusion	Little or none
Onset	Usually insidious
Systemic manifestations	Rare
True bony ankylosis	Uncommon
Symptoms	Pain on motion (early); pain at rest (later); pain aggravated by prolonged activity, relieved by rest; localized stiffness of short duration ("gelling") relieved by exercise; possibly painful muscle spasm; limitation of motion; "flares" associated with crystal-induced synovitis
Signs	Localized tenderness; crepitus and cracking on motion; mild joint enlargement with firm consistency from proliferation of bone and cartilage; synovitis (less common), gross deformity (later)

The cardinal symptom of OA is pain, which at first occurs after joint use and is relieved by rest. The pain is usually aching in character and is poorly localized. As the disease progresses, pain may occur with minimal motion or even at rest. In advanced cases, pain may awaken the patient from sleep because of the loss of protective muscular joint splinting, which during the waking hours limits (103) painful motion. Because cartilage has no nerve supply and is insensitive to pain, the pain in OA must arise from noncartilaginous intraarticular and periarticular structures. The pain is usually multifactorial and may result from elevation of the periosteum accompanying marginal bony proliferation, pressure on exposed subchondral bone, venous engorgement with intramedullary hypertension, trabecular microfractures, involvement of intraarticular ligaments, capsular distention, and pinching or abrasion of synovial villi. Additional contributory factors include synovitis and capsulitis. Although prostaglandins released from synovial tissues and chondrocytes may theoretically contribute to the pain response, a parallel between the inflammatory response and joint fluid prostaglandin concentrations has not been described (105). Periarticular tissues, such as tendons and fascia, are supplied with sensory nerves and are an important source of pain. Muscle spasms around the joint or pressure on contiguous nerves may be more painful than the pain of articular origin. Frequently, as with other types of joint disease, the pain is intensified just before weather changes.

OA is sometimes associated with acute or subacute inflammation. This response is most common in erosive (inflammatory) OA of the hands, but it may occur in other peripheral joints. When seen in peripheral joints other than the hands, such inflammatory "acute flares" have been attributed to various degrees of trauma or to crystal-induced synovitis in response to calcium pyrophosphate or other crystals (106).

Stiffness on awakening in the morning and after periods of inactivity during the day is a common complaint. Such stiffness is of short duration, rarely lasting for more than 15 minutes. Articular gelling, a transient stiffness lasting only for several flexion–extension cycles, is extremely common, especially in the lower extremity joints of elderly patients. This occurs often in the absence of other symptoms of OA and follows prolonged inactivity. Limitation of motion develops as the disease progresses, owing to joint-surface incongruity, muscle spasm and contracture, capsular contracture, and mechanical block from osteophytes or loose bodies. In weight-bearing joints, abrupt giving way may occur. Objectively, joints may show localized tenderness, especially if synovitis is present. Pain on passive motion may be a prominent finding even without local tenderness. Crepitus, a crackling or grating sound as the joint is moved, may result from cartilage loss and joint-surface irregularity. Compartment-directed (patellofemoral, medial and lateral tibiofemoral) evidence of crepitus has a high degree of diagnostic specificity and sensitivity (107). Enlargement of the joint may be caused by secondary synovitis, an increase in synovial fluid, or marginal proliferative changes in cartilage or bone (osteophytes). Osteophytes can be readily palpated along the margins of the affected joint. Late stages of the disease are associated with gross deformity and subluxation resulting from cartilage loss, collapse of subchondral bone, formation of bone cysts, and gross bony overgrowth. Although these symptoms and signs are common to OA in general, the clinical picture and course depend on the particular joint(s) involved.

Specific Joint Involvement

Heberden's Nodes

One of the most common manifestations of primary OA, Heberden's nodes (108) (Figs. 111.1 and 111.2), represents cartilaginous and bony enlargement of the dorsolateral and dorsomedial aspects of the distal interphalangeal joints of the fingers, often associated with flexion and lateral deviation of the distal phalanx. Similar nodes may be seen in the proximal interphalangeal joints, and are called Bouchard's nodes (Fig. 111.3). Heberden's nodes may be single, but they usually are multiple. They begin most often after age 45 years, but can begin in the third decade of life. Women are affected much more frequently than men, at a ratio of approximately 10:1 (109). Heredity plays a large part in the origin of these lesions, particularly in the female side of the family (i.e., in mothers, daughters, and sisters) (110). Heberden's nodes were twice as common in mothers and three times as common in sisters of affected women than in the general population (33). Stecher (110) postulated a single autosomal gene, sex-influenced, dominant in females and recessive in males, with complete penetrance by age 70 years, because all who had this gene developed the lesions. Although idiopathic Heberden's nodes undoubtedly have a genetic origin, the exact mode of transmission remains open to question because

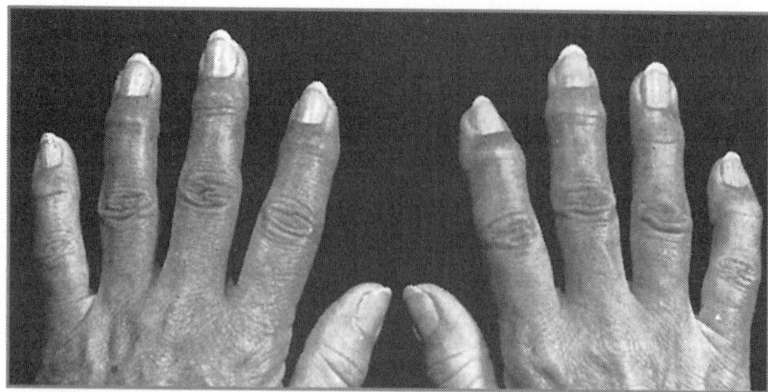

FIGURE 111.1. Typical Heberden's nodes, the cardinal sign of primary osteoarthritis. Note their characteristic position at the distal interphalangeal joints. The proximal interphalangeal joints may be involved later.

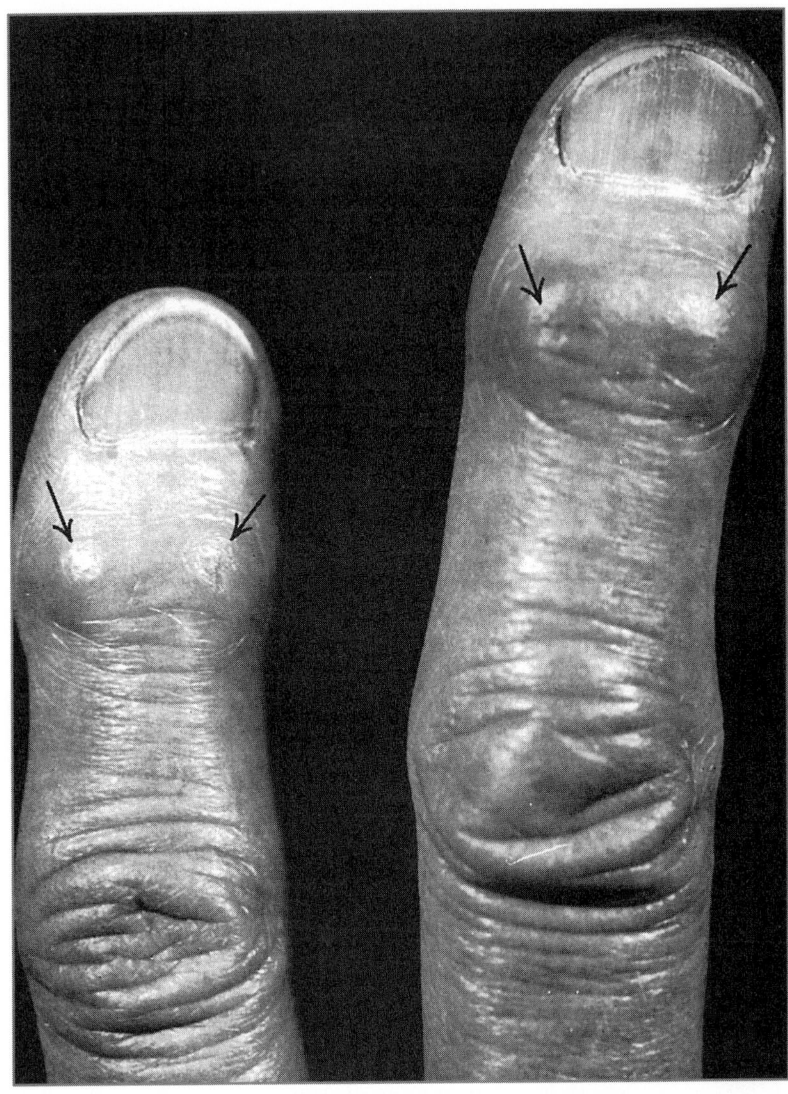

FIGURE 111.2. Close-up view of Heberden's nodes (*arrows*) affecting the index and middle fingers.

several genetic patterns fit the available data (36–39,111). As noted earlier, the demonstration of gene-related abnormalities for type II collagen in OA (41–44) promises further clarification of inheritance patterns.

Clinically, Heberden's nodes may develop gradually with little or no pain and may progress essentially unnoticed for months or years. In other cases, they appear rapidly, with redness, swelling, tenderness, and aching, particularly after use. Afflicted individuals may complain of paresthesias and loss of dexterity. Many joints may be involved almost simultaneously, or one or two joints may be involved for a long time before others develop similar changes. The swollen joints may feel either soft and fluctuant or hard. Small, gelatinous cysts may appear, generally on the dorsal aspects of the joint or just proximal to it. These cysts, which are often attached to tendon sheaths and resemble ganglia, may recede spontaneously or may persist indefinitely. At times, they precede the appearance of Heberden's nodes themselves. The cause of the cysts is uncertain. Studies have demonstrated communication of the cysts with the distal interphalangeal joint space (112). This communication may later be pinched off, but at some stage in development, the cysts are in direct communication with the joint space. As noted previously, the proximal interphalangeal joints of the fingers also may be involved, usually after several distal joints are affected. Horizontal deviation of the distal and proximal interphalangeal joints may lead to a snake-like configuration of the fingers. Metacarpophalangeal joint involvement is rare; when it does occur, it involves the joints of the second and third fingers. It should be noted that the ACR classification criteria for reporting a diagnosis of OA of the hands requires the presence of bony enlargement in two of ten selected joints, swelling of fewer than three metacarpophalangeal joints, and bony enlargement of at least two distal interphalangeal joints (6).

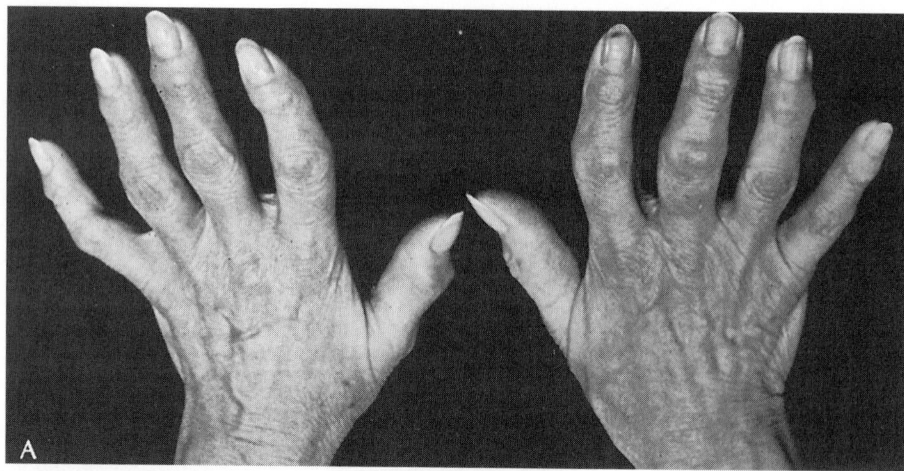

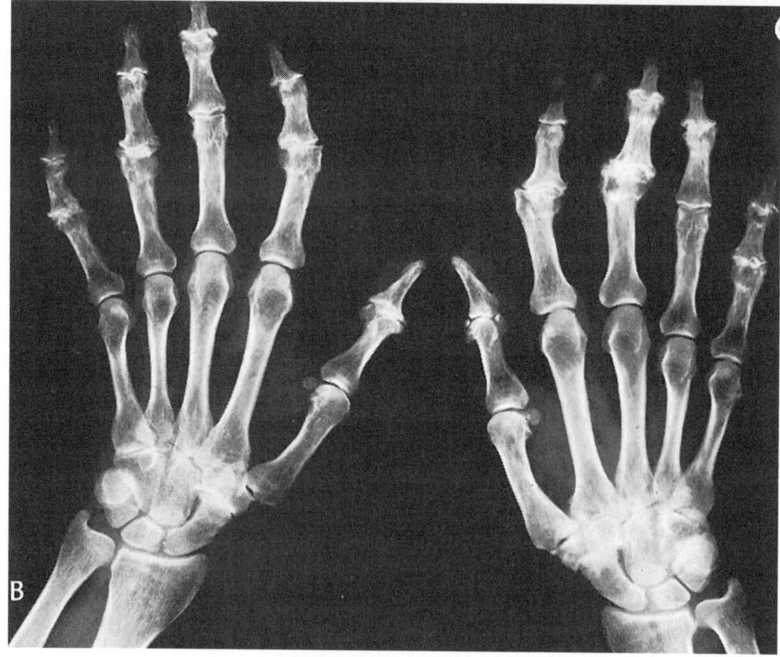

FIGURE 111.3. A: Primary osteoarthritis of the hands with marked proximal interphalangeal joint involvement (Bouchard's nodes), as well as distal interphalangeal joint involvement (Heberden's nodes). **B:** Radiographic appearance of the same hands.

Carpometacarpal and Trapezioscaphoid Joints

Degenerative changes involving the first carpometacarpal joint are often present. Pain and localized tenderness may suggest a stenosing tenosynovitis. The patient often has a tender prominence at the base of the first metacarpal bone, and the joint in this area may have a squared appearance (shelf sign) (Fig. 111.4). Motion is often limited and painful. Radiographic examination may reveal subluxation of the base of the first metacarpal bone in addition to joint-space narrowing and osteophyte formation.

OA changes in the trapezioscaphoid joint of the wrist are common (113). Such changes may occur in association with OA of the first carpometacarpal and distal interphalangeal joints, or they may be an isolated finding. Symptoms and signs include pain in the wrist and thumb

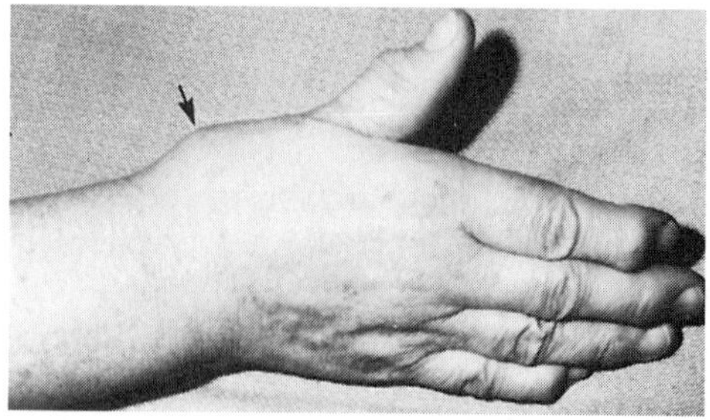

FIGURE 111.4. Severe osteoarthritis of the carpometacarpal joint leads to a prominent squaring (shelf sign) at the base of the thumb (*arrow*). Heberden's nodes also are seen.

base, radial and volar swelling, and tenderness over the scaphoid bone.

Metatarsophalangeal Joints

One of the most common sites of primary OA is the first metatarsophalangeal joint of the foot; OA of the other metatarsophalangeal joints occurs to a lesser degree. The onset is usually insidious, with gradual progression of swelling and pain. Symptoms may be aggravated by wearing tight shoes. A sudden increase in swelling and pain may accompany inflammation of the bursa at the medial aspect of the joint (bunion). The irregular contour of the involved joint can be felt. Foot symptoms also may result from OA of the subtalar and other tarsal joints. Pain of subtalar origin is aggravated by inversion and eversion of the foot, and symptoms may make walking difficult.

Acromioclavicular and Manubriosternal Joints

OA of the acromioclavicular joint is common and frequently overlooked as a cause of shoulder pain and disability. Symptoms are usually poorly localized to the joint, and shoulder motion is nearly normal, although painful. Tenderness localized to the joint is the key finding. Radiographic changes of degeneration are often minimal. OA of the manubriosternal joint is rare, but it may result in chest pain and tenderness.

Temporomandibular Joints

OA produces symptoms of crepitus, stiffness, and pain on chewing. Similar symptoms may be caused by disturbances in temporomandibular joint dynamics (temporomandibular dysfunction syndrome), rather than by structural degenerative change. The patient may complain of joint noise and pain, masticatory muscle tenderness, limited motion, and deviation of the jaw to the affected side. The distinction between OA and other causes of jaw pain are discussed in detail in Chapter 101.

Knee

The knee joint is frequently affected by primary OA, with involvement of one or more of its three compartments (medial femorotibial, lateral femorotibial, and patellofemoral; Fig. 111.5). Symptoms consist of pain on motion, relieved by rest, stiffness, particularly after sitting or rising in the morning, and crepitus on motion. Little objective change might be found on examination. At times, the patient has localized tenderness over various aspects of the joint and pain on passive motion. Marginal osteophytes may be seen and felt. These are often more prominent on physical examination than they are on radiography. Mild synovitis and joint effusion may be present. Crepitus can often be detected when the examiner's hand is held over the patella as the knee is flexed. Pain may be elicited by the examiner by holding the patella tight against the femur with the quadriceps relaxed and then requesting that the

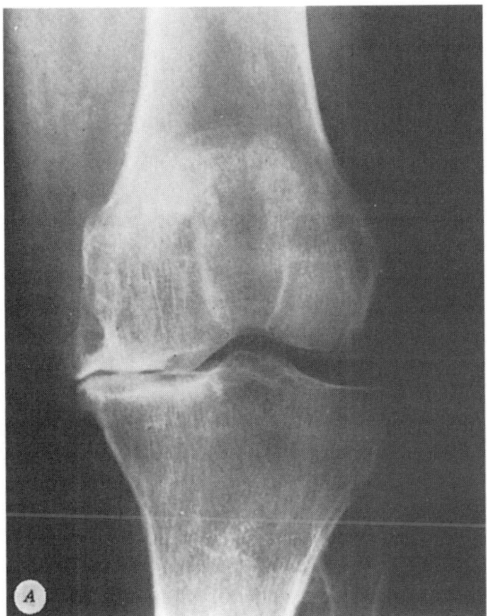

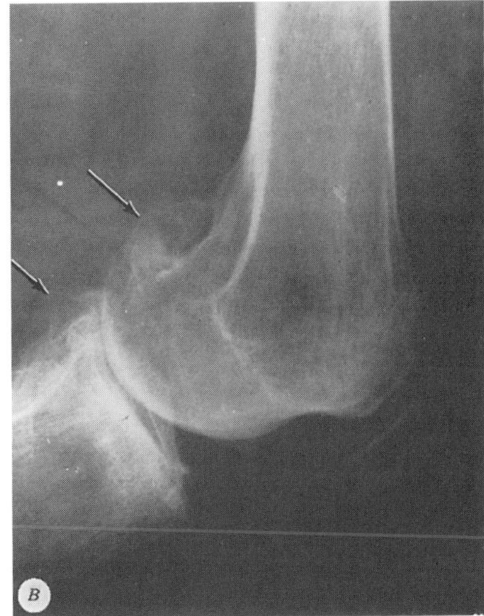

FIGURE 111.5. A: Osteoarthritis of the knee; medial joint-space narrowing is prominent and is associated with subchondral bony sclerosis (eburnation) and osteophyte formation. **B:** Lateral view of the same knee; large osteophytes can be seen at the posterior aspects of the femur and tibia (*arrows*).

patient contract this muscle. Limitation of joint motion, usually extension, on both active or passive motion may be noted. Muscle atrophy about the knee may occur rapidly, especially with disuse. Disproportionate degenerative changes localized to the medial or lateral compartment of the knee may lead to secondary genu varus or, much less commonly, to genu valgus with joint instability and subluxation. Instability is further aggravated by laxity of the collateral ligaments. Isolated patellofemoral compartment or tricompartmental involvement should alert the clinician to underlying calcium pyrophosphate dihydrate (CPPD) crystal deposition. Joint fluid basic calcium phosphate crystals were associated with lateral tibiofemoral disease in patients with concomitant (Milwaukee) shoulder joint disease (114). Ike et al. (115) found erosions of the articular cartilage of the lateral compartment arthroscopically in all patients with lateral tibiofemoral joint space narrowing by radiographic examination, and all had CPPD deposits. They also found medial meniscal degeneration and cartilage erosions in all patients with medial tibiofemoral compartment narrowing. Although chondrocalcinosis was significantly associated with OA after controlling for age, both OA and chondrocalcinosis increased independently with age as well (116).

Individuals with OA of one knee have an increased likelihood of involvement of the contralateral knee (117,118). Among patients studied in Chingford, England, in 34% of individuals with OA of one knee, OA developed in the contralateral knee within a 2-year period. In an investigation of 63 patients with knee OA, 12 of 13 patients with unilateral OA of the knee at baseline developed bilateral knee OA over the subsequent 11 years of follow-up (119). Accordingly, individuals with unilateral and bilateral knee OA appear to represent similar subsets.

Hip

OA of the hip, also known as malum coxae senilis or morbus coxae senilis, may be disabling (Fig. 111.6). Symptoms usually first appear in older individuals. This condition occurs more frequently in men than in women and may be unilateral or bilateral. In a study of the natural history of hip OA, Evarts (120) noted that over an 8-year period, in 10% of patients with unilateral hip degeneration, bilateral disease developed.

Data on the frequency of right and left hip involvement in unilateral disease are conflicting. One study of 54 patients with idiopathic OA of the hip noted that the two sides were affected with equal frequency when disease was unilateral (121). Another study of 175 patients found that 13% of men and 29% of women had unilateral disease (122). The latter patients had a significant predilection for a particular side; 20 right and 10 left hips were involved, a 2:1 ratio. In those with the onset of symptoms after age 60 years, the ratio of right to left hip involvement was even

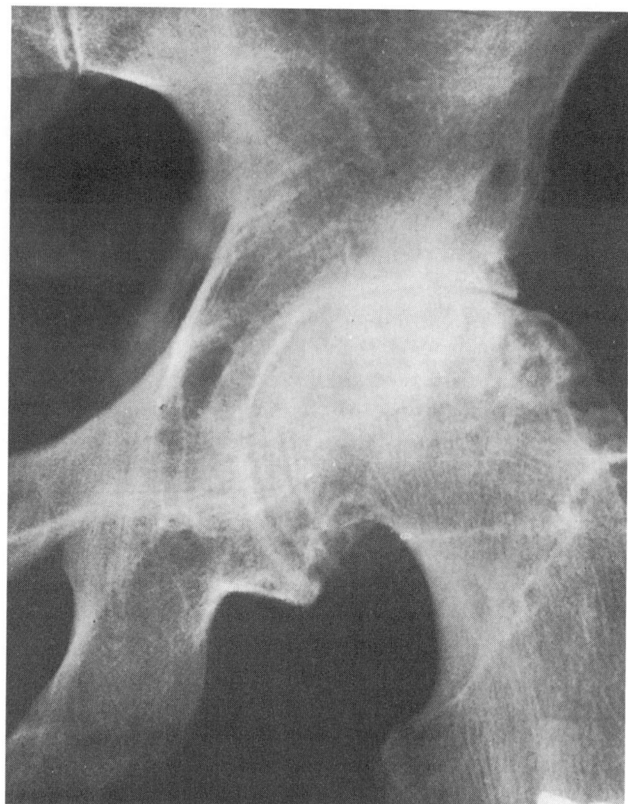

FIGURE 111.6. Osteoarthritis of the hip. Note the almost complete loss of articular cartilage, flattening of the femoral head, and small cystic areas in the head and neck of the femur. Subchondral bone is sclerotic.

more marked, 7:1. In another study (22), bilateral involvement of the hip was reported in up to 42% of individuals. As with knee OA, involvement of one hip increases the likelihood of involvement of the contralateral joint (118). Superior or lateral involvement of the hip is more common than medial involvement (22,123). Superomedial and medial/axial patterns were more common in women; superolateral patterns were seen more commonly in men (22).

The main symptom of OA of the hip is insidious pain followed by a characteristic limp (antalgic gait). Pain in the "hip" may often not originate there, and pain actually arising in the hip joint may be referred to other areas. True hip pain is usually felt on its outer aspect, the groin, or along the inner aspect of the thigh. It may be referred to the buttocks or sciatic region and is often referred down the obturator nerve to the knee. Occasionally, most of the pain is in the knee, and its true origin is overlooked. The degree of pain varies widely and does not always correlate with the extent of cartilaginous and osseous changes. Weakness of the hip muscles may be demonstrated by the Trendelenburg sign whereby standing on the involved extremity causes the contralateral hip to drop due to weakening of the ipsilateral hip abductors. Trochanteric bursitis, caused by inflammation of the bursa over the greater trochanter, produces pain and tenderness at the lateral aspect of the hip; symptoms and physical findings may simulate those seen in patients with OA of the hip. Pain is exaggerated by weight bearing, and a mild limp is common; however, hip motion is normal, in contrast to the invariable limitation of motion seen in OA of the hip joint. Localized tenderness over the bursa is characteristic. Rapid relief of symptoms after bursal injection with local corticosteroids and lidocaine is diagnostically helpful.

Stiffness is common and increases after inactivity. Examination reveals varying degrees of limited motion. The leg is often held in external rotation with the hip flexed and adducted. Severe backache may result from the compensatory lordosis accompanying flexion contracture. Functional shortening of the extremity may occur. The gait is frequently awkward with shuffling or waddling. Sitting is difficult, as is rising from this position, owing to limitation of motion.

Other Peripheral Joints

In addition to characteristic involvement of joints noted previously, primary OA was opined to occur in sites generally considered "protected." Sixteen patients with elbow OA not associated with nodal- or crystal-related degenerative changes were reported (124). Elbow OA appeared to affect primarily middle-aged men and was commonly associated with metacarpophalangeal OA. In another report, the unrecognized association of nodal OA of the fingers with OA of interphalangeal joints of the toes was emphasized (125).

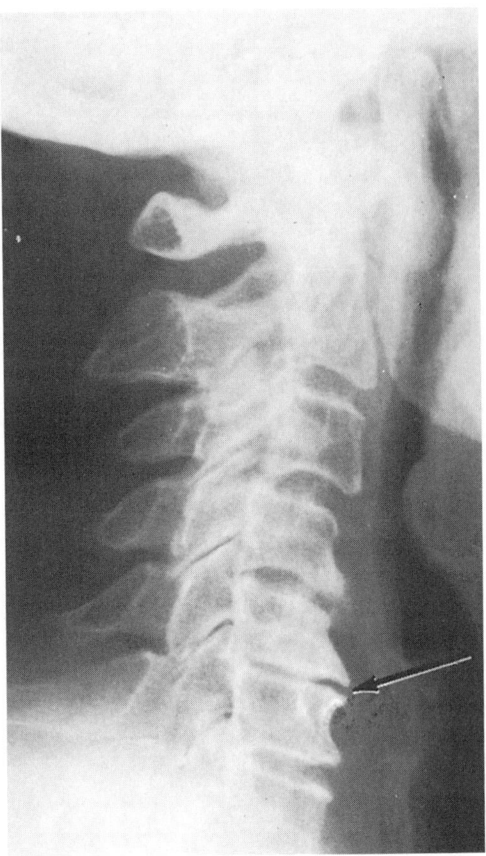

FIGURE 111.7. Osteoarthritis changes in the lower cervical spine. Spur formation is prominent. Note the marked narrowing of the intervertebral disc between C-5 and C-6 vertebrae (*arrow*) and subluxation of C-3–C-4.

Spine

OA of the spinal joints is common (Fig. 111.7; see Chapters 100, 102, and 103). It often results from degenerative changes in the intervertebral fibrocartilaginous discs, from damage to vertebral bodies, or from degeneration in the posterior apophyseal articulations themselves. Disc narrowing may cause subluxation of the posterior apophyseal joints (see Chapter 100). Lipping or spur formation (osteophytosis) on the vertebral bodies is a prominent finding (Fig. 111.8). Anterior spurs are most prevalent. Although usually asymptomatic, large anterior osteophytes in the cervical spine may give rise to symptoms of dysphagia (126). Respiratory symptoms such as hoarseness, coughing, and aspiration may be noted. Joint-space narrowing, bony sclerosis, and spur formation often are seen in apophyseal joints. Some authors make a distinction between degenerative changes involving the discs and vertebral bodies, for which they use the term spondylosis, and degenerative changes of the apophyseal joints, which are classified as true OA, because radiologic abnormalities more closely resemble those seen in other diarthrodial joints.

Degenerative changes of all types are most frequent in the areas of the lordotic and kyphotic apices, C-5, T-8, and L-3 to L-4, and correlate in general with the areas of maximal spine motion. In some older individuals, however, osteophytes may extend along the entire length of the spine, with prominent involvement of the thoracic region (Fig. 111.9). These osteophytes may be striking, and coalescence with fusion may occur (Fig. 111.10). Forestier et al. (127) have suggested the name ankylosing hyperostosis for these severe cases, which may be associated with moderate-to-severe spinal limitation. The frequent extraspinal manifestations of "Forestier's disease" have led to the term diffuse idiopathic skeletal hyperostosis (DISH) (128,129), discussed later in this chapter.

Symptoms of spinal OA include localized pain and stiffness and radicular pain. Localized pain has been assumed to originate in paraspinal ligaments, joint capsules, and periosteum. Such changes may explain spontaneous fluctuations of symptoms in the presence of persistent or progressive cartilage degeneration and spur formation. Spasm of paraspinal muscles is common and may be a major cause of pain. Radicular pain may be due to compression of nerve roots, or it may represent pain referred along dermatomes related to the primary local lesion. Nerve root compression

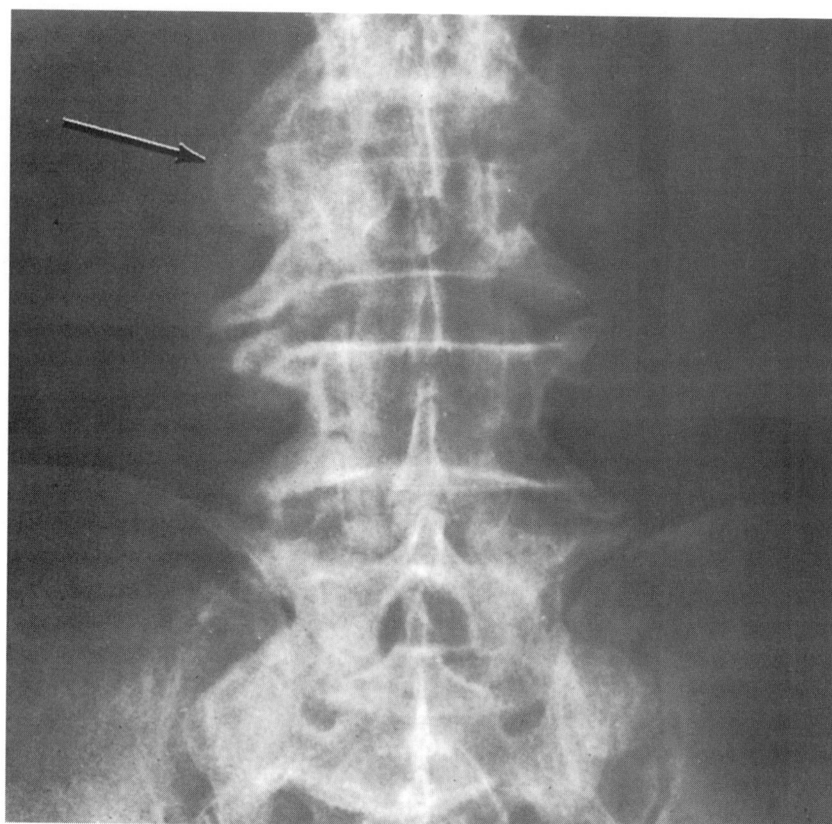

FIGURE 111.8. Osteoarthritis of the lumbar spine. Note the marked osteophyte formation with bridging of spurs between L-2 and L-3 on the right (*arrow*).

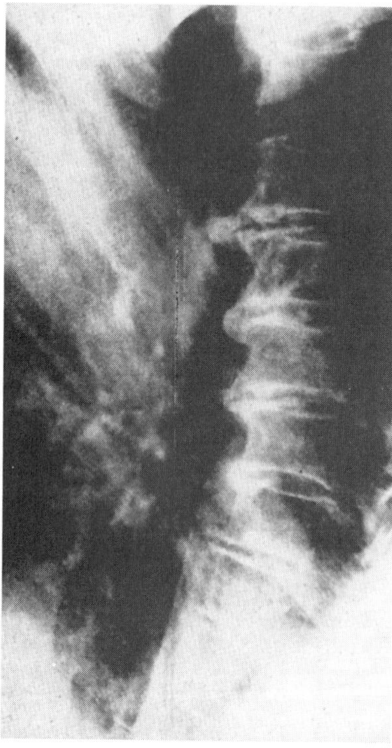

FIGURE 111.9. Osteoarthritis of the thoracic spine. Note the pronounced exostoses at the anterior vertebral margins and the narrowed intervertebral disc spaces.

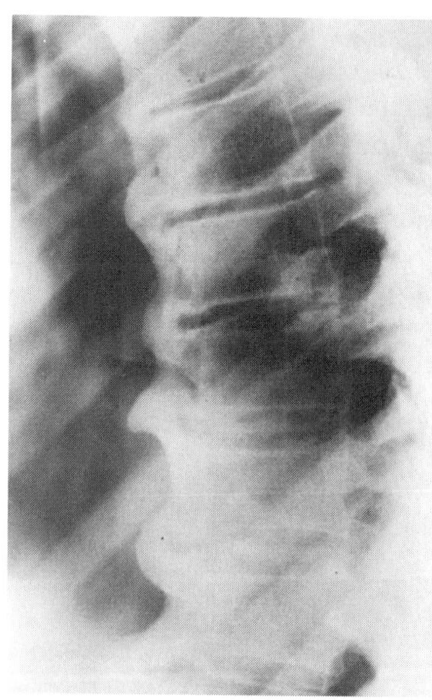

FIGURE 111.10. Florid hyperostosis of the spine in a patient with Forestier's disease (diffuse idiopathic skeletal hyperostosis). A flowing mantle of ossification from ligamentous calcification and coalescence of osteophytes is seen at the anterior aspect of the spine. (Courtesy of Dr. Donald Resnick.)

causing neuropathy is common. This disorder may result from impingement on the nerve root by spurs that compromise the foraminal space (Fig. 111.11), by lateral prolapse of a degenerated disc, or by foraminal narrowing from apophyseal joint subluxation. Pressure on nerve roots may cause radicular pain, paresthesias, and reflex and motor changes in the distribution of the involved root. Neurologic complications of this type occur most frequently in the neck because of its small spinal canal and intervertebral foramina, but they can occur in other areas of the spine. Nerve root compression in the dorsal spine may result in radicular pain radiating around the chest wall in a girdle distribution. This must be differentiated from symptoms caused by other disorders. Involvement of nerve roots in the lumbosacral area is associated with low back pain and neurologic signs and symptoms, which frequently allow localization of specific nerve root compression. Involvement of the L-3 or L-4 nerve roots is associated with a diminished or absent patellar reflex; an absent ankle jerk indicates involvement of the S-1 nerve root. Sensory loss over the anteromedial aspect of the leg is consistent with L-4 nerve root compression. A lesion at L-5 causes sensory changes at the anterolateral aspect of the leg and the medial aspect of the foot and weakness of dorsiflexion of the foot and great toe. S-1 nerve root compression results in sensory changes at the posterolateral aspect of the calf and the lateral foot. Gastrocnemius muscle weakness may be evident.

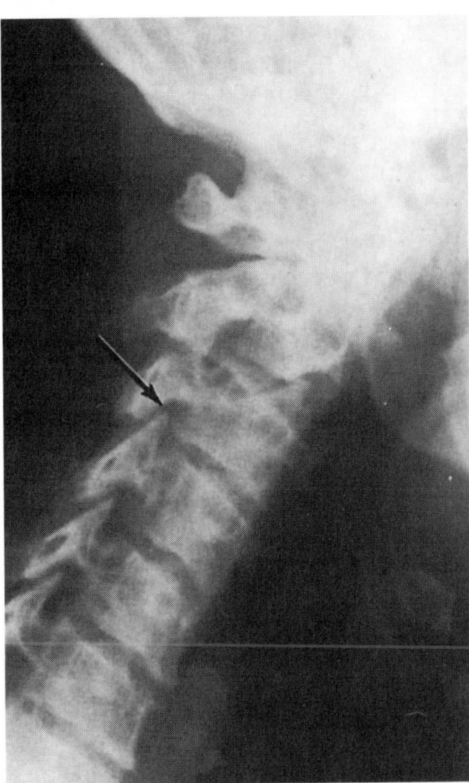

FIGURE 111.11. Osteoarthritis of cervical spine, oblique radiographic view. The foraminal space between C-3 and C-4 (*arrow*) is compromised by marked posterior spur formation.

Neurologic symptoms also may be associated with cervical OA if large posterior spurs or protruded discs compress the spinal cord. In these cases, upper-motor-neuron and other long-tract signs may be observed. Compression of the anterior spinal artery may produce a central cord syndrome. The blood supply to the brain may be compromised if large spurs compress the vertebral arteries. The spectrum of clinical signs and symptoms is similar to that in basilar artery insufficiency. Exacerbations are often associated with postural neck changes, resulting in compression of vertebral arteries by osteophytes. Angiographic studies of carotid and vertebral arteries are diagnostically helpful.

OA of the atlantoaxial joint has been described (130). Radiographic signs consisted of joint-space narrowing, marginal cortical thickening, and osteophyte formation. Involvement of the lateral atlantoaxial joint, the articulation of the atlas with the odontoid, or mixed involvement were found. Patients complained of occipital pain, stiffness of the shoulder, and paresthesias of the fingers. Conservative treatment provided satisfactory relief of symptoms, except in one patient who required a transoral atlantoaxial fusion.

Spinal cord lesions as a result of OA of the dorsal spine are rare. Spinal cord compression is not seen in patients with lumbosacral lesions because the spinal cord ends at the level of L-1, but cauda equina syndrome with sphincter dysfunction may develop.

Spinal stenosis (Chapter 103) may produce symptoms in the lower back and the lower extremities. Pain may be constant or intermittent. It is often worsened by exercise, simulating intermittent claudication. Hyperextension of the spine often exacerbates symptoms; relief is noted with flexion. The patient may stand with knees, hips, and lumbar spine flexed (simian stance). Sensory change may be present, and motor power in the legs may be diminished. As noted, ambulation usually aggravates symptoms; there appears to be a "resting urgency," with a need to stop immediately after walking variable distances. The patient is usually able to resume walking for a short while until pain requires stopping once again. Characteristic features of lumbar spinal stenosis include age older than 65 years; severe pain in the lower extremities, absent on being seated at rest; a wide-based gait; an abnormal Romberg test; pain in the thighs after 30 seconds of lumbar extension; and neuromuscular defects. Neurologic examination, however, may often be normal (131). Symptoms of lumbar spinal stenosis may be confused with symptoms related to hip OA, and the two entities often coexist.

Stenosis is usually caused by combined anatomic abnormalities because congenital narrowing alone is generally asymptomatic (132). Commonly associated causes include degenerative spurs, disc herniation, ligamentous hypertrophy, and spondylolisthesis. Trauma, postoperative fibrosis, Paget's disease, and fluorosis are less commonly associated.

Stenosis of the cervical spinal canal may be associated with similar symptoms involving the upper extremities. The patient may complain of radicular symptoms, exacerbated by hyperextension and relieved by flexion of the cervical spine.

Radiographic evidence of degenerative disease in the spine may be extensive but may still bear little relation to the patient's symptoms. Conversely, severe symptoms may develop with minor spur formation if the spur is located in a critical area. Radiographic changes of marginal lipping, sclerosis of the articular margins, and narrowing have been found in sacroiliac joints with increasing age, but it is unlikely that such changes lead to symptoms.

Laboratory Findings

No specific diagnostic laboratory abnormalities exist in primary OA (Table 111.3). The erythrocyte sedimentation rate, routine blood counts, urinalyses, and blood chemical determinations are normal in patients with primary disease but are important in excluding other forms of arthritis considered in the differential diagnosis, and they may identify systemic metabolic disorders associated with secondary OA. For example, patients with associated CPPD crystal deposition disease may have evidence of underlying primary hyperparathyroidism with elevation of serum calcium and an increase in serum parathyroid hormone level (see Chapter 124). Patients with Paget's disease exhibit elevated serum alkaline phosphatase levels and increased urinary hydroxyproline excretion (see Chapter 123). In patients with joint disease associated with ochronosis, the presence of homogentisic acid metabolites in the urine darkens the urine on standing or causes a false-positive Benedict's test result for glycosuria (see Chapter 121).

Much interest has been directed toward the study of cartilage matrix components in synovial fluid, serum, or urine as a measure of cartilage degradation (133–154). The search for such markers has been advanced by the availability of monoclonal or polyclonal antibodies raised against various cartilage and bone macromolecules. Study of synovial fluid, serum, or urine markers is complicated by the fact that levels of such markers in various body fluids represent an interplay of synthesis and degradation as well as effects related to transit of markers from synovial fluid through the lymphatic and vascular systems, hepatic metabolism, and urinary excretion.

Joint fluid has a number of advantages as a source for measuring response markers because the concentration of such markers is usually higher in joint fluid than in other body fluids. Joint fluid is, however, more difficult to obtain than urine or blood. Measurement of cartilage-related markers in serum, on the other hand, may represent a more balanced measure of overall metabolic activities occurring in total body cartilage content. Serum is easier to obtain, and measurement is independent of local joint volume flux. Urine markers are limited by the low concentrations of macromolecules that are generally present.

Among potential markers, keratan sulfate has been most extensively studied in experimental models and in humans (133,135–137,141,147). Serum keratan sulfate concentrations were shown to be increased in patients with OA or RA as compared with normal subjects or patients with fibromyalgia syndrome (133); but no correlation between the level of keratan sulfate and the joint score or the duration of disease

TABLE 111.3. LABORATORY AND RADIOGRAPHIC FINDINGS IN PRIMARY OSTEOARTHRITIS

Laboratory Tests	Results
Erythrocyte sedimentation rate	Usually normal
Routine blood counts	Normal
Rheumatoid factor	Negative
Antinuclear antibody	Negative
Serum calcium, phosphorus, alkaline phosphatase, serum protein electrophoresis	Normal
Synovial fluid analysis	Good viscosity with normal mucin clot; modest increase in leukocyte number. Presence of fibrils and debris (wear particles)
Radiographic Findings	**Causes**
Narrowing of joint space	Articular cartilage ulceration
Subchondral bony sclerosis (eburnation)	New bone formation
Marginal osteophyte formation	Proliferation of cartilage and bone
Bone cysts and bony collapse	Subchondral microfractures
Gross deformity with subluxation and loose studies	Ligamentous laxity as a result of mechanical forces

was found, in either OA or RA. Other studies demonstrated an increase in the serum level of antigenic keratan sulfate in the presence of knee injury in humans (139). The concentration and total amount of proteoglycan-related fragments were found to be increased in the joint fluid of patients with OA (137,154). Similarly, concentrations of catabolic enzymes such as stromelysin and collagenase and of tissue inhibitor of metalloproteinase (TIMP) were higher in the joint fluid of patients with traumatic or primary OA (140,148,149,155). Cartilage oligomeric protein appears to reflect proteoglycan degradation (142), and has been shown to be elevated in progressive OA (151,156). Antibody to 846, which binds to an epitope on the chondroitin sulfate moiety of the proteoglycan aggrecan, is thought to identify the most recently synthesized molecules, thereby representing a putative marker of aggrecan synthesis (157). This epitope has recently been found to be elevated in the synovial fluid of patients with either progressive OA or traumatic injury of the knee (153). The level of C-propeptide of type II collagen (CPII) reflects collagen synthesis (145).

Serum hyaluronate concentrations are elevated in the presence of OA (138). Hyaluronate levels were elevated in patients with OA and were even higher in patients with RA (138). In a study of knee OA by Sharif et al. (158), hyaluronate levels at study entry correlated with disease duration, minimal joint space, and previous surgery. Radiographic progression was greater in those individuals found retrospectively to have higher hyaluronate levels at baseline. In another investigation, however, no correlation was observed between hyaluronate levels and the Lequesne algofunctional index, duration of symptoms, C-reactive protein (CRP), or severity of radiographic changes (159). Inflamed synovium is probably the main source of these elevated concentrations.

Recent studies have linked CRP elevations but not erythrocyte sedimentation rate with clinical severity of OA of the hip and knee (160). CRP was significantly associated with disability, joint tenderness, pain, fatigue, global severity, and depression. In a study of 845 women in the Chingford study group, CRP levels were initially elevated in women with radiographic evidence of knee OA of Kellgren–Lawrence grade II or greater, as compared with 740 women without OA. In addition, these investigators found that CRP levels were elevated in individuals whose knee OA progressed by at least one grade during the 4-year study when compared with women whose OA did not progress (161). Because levels of CRP were monitored at the beginning of the study, a potential prognostic value for this evaluation is suggested.

Measurements of urinary pyridinium cross-links were suggested as an indicator of cartilage and bone collagen degradation in both OA and RA (144).

Although the literature relative to investigations on serum markers has increased extensively over the past decade, difficulties in interpretation as outlined earlier dictate that the use of serum markers for diagnostic and prognostic purposes remains investigational (162).

Synovial fluid in primary OA is "noninflammatory," with no abnormalities other than a slight increase in white cells. Viscosity is good, and the mucin clot formed after addition of glacial acetic acid is normal. Synovial fluid fibrils, morphologically indistinguishable from sloughed collagen fibers, are often seen. The collagen fibers seen in synovial fluid in OA appear to be type II, derived from articular hyaline cartilage (163). CPPD or basic calcium phosphate crystals may be present. Cholesterol crystals have been identified by light microscopy in synovial fluids of patients with OA with recurrent knee effusions (164). Although evidence of altered cellular and humoral immune mechanisms has been described, its significance remains to be determined.

Histologic examination of the synovium in primary OA reveals nonspecific changes of chronic mild inflammation, particularly in more advanced disease.

Scintigraphy

Bone and joint scintigraphy using ^{99m}Tc as the pertechnetate has been of limited diagnostic value, but studies using 4-hour ^{99m}Tc coupled with bone-seeking diphosphonates correlated with radiographic abnormalities in OA of hand joints (165). Abnormalities predicted the development of radiographic signs, and joints abnormal on scintigraphy showed the greatest progression in follow-up studies (166,167). Some joints were abnormal on either radiograph or scan alone, and others showed a marked disparity in the degree of abnormality on radiographic evaluation compared with isotopic evaluation. These discrepancies suggested that scintigraphy offers a different way of assessing OA changes, perhaps useful in evaluating response to therapeutic strategies. Further studies demonstrated that scintigraphy using technetium-labeled diphosphonates was similarly highly predictive of subsequent radiographic progression in OA of the knee (167). In contrast to these studies, however, correlations of radiographs of the hand and bone scans in patients with symptomatic hand OA, including level of initial isotope retention and changes in scintigraphy score, were of no predictive value with respect to radiographic progression of the OA (168). Expanded studies will further define the role of scintigraphy in evaluation of OA with respect to diagnosis and prognosis. Scintigraphy may prove especially useful in the diagnosis of preclinical OA. Positive correlation of scintigraphy and disease progression would be of value in studies of disease-modifying agents in clinical trials.

Although intraosseous phlebography and thermography have been used in studies of OA, the role of these techniques in the routine diagnosis of OA remains limited and poorly defined; they usually add little to observations evident on routine physical examination.

Radiographic Appearance

The radiographic appearance may be normal if the pathologic changes leading to clinical symptoms are sufficiently mild. Many gradations of abnormality may be noted as the disease progresses (Table 111.3). Joint-space narrowing occurs as a result of degeneration and disappearance of articular cartilage.

Studies have demonstrated a disparity between radiographic findings and arthroscopically defined changes (169). Significant pathologic abnormalities in the form of cartilage loss were observed arthroscopically in the presence of essentially normal radiographic findings; further, the presence of joint-space narrowing indicative of OA on radiologic study was often associated with more advanced disease by intraarticular study. The converse of this discordance whereby apparent joint-space narrowing seen on radiographs was not corroborated on intraarticular study was a less common finding.

Subchondral bony sclerosis (eburnation) is noted as increased bone density. Marginal osteophyte formation takes place as a result of proliferation of cartilage and bone. Cysts, varying in size from several millimeters to several centimeters, are seen as translucent areas in periarticular bone. Gross deformity, subluxation, and loose bodies may occur in advanced cases.

Although osteophytes are usually regarded as a manifestation of OA, the use of this feature alone in diagnosis has been questioned, as noted earlier in this chapter. Osteophytes correlate with aging and are not necessarily an early sign of OA (104,170). The diagnosis of OA of the peripheral joints may be more validly based on radiographic findings of structural abnormalities in cartilage (decreased joint space) or in subchondral bone (cysts and eburnation) or in both.

The origin of the subchondral "detritus" cysts has been explained as follows: (a) a failure in the bone-remodeling process, in which local osteoclastic activity outstrips that of osteoblasts; or (b) the result of pressure transmitted from the joint surface to subarticular bone through cracks in the subchondral plate (trabecular microfractures). The cysts may contain fluid, nonspecific detritus, or a primitive mesenchymal tissue that undergoes fibrosis. These cysts may be prominent even in joints with adequately preserved joint space when seen radiographically.

Ankylosis in OA is uncommon. It is seen occasionally in OA of the hands, especially in its erosive inflammatory form.

Osteophytes are usually located on the anterior and anterolateral borders of the vertebral bodies and are best visualized on lateral radiographs. The amount of bony overgrowth varies. Spurs arising from the posterior margins of the vertebral bodies or from the margins of the articular facets are less common but are of greater clinical importance, owing to their proximity to neural structures. Narrowing of intervertebral joint spaces results from disc degeneration; this is most frequent and usually most marked in the lower cervical and lower lumbar regions. Sclerosis of adjacent bone is common, and one sometimes sees wedging of the anterior borders of the vertebral bodies. Apophyseal joints may show joint-space narrowing, sclerosis, and associated spur formation. Osteoporosis is not a component of OA.

Many of the previously mentioned radiographic abnormalities may be visualized on routine posteroanterior and lateral views. Oblique views of the cervical and lumbar spine should be performed routinely, if degenerative changes involving intervertebral foramina and apophyseal joints are to be accurately delineated. Myelography may be of help when symptoms are severe and a surgical procedure is contemplated. Although computed tomography (CT) scanning has been useful diagnostically in patients with OA of the spine, especially when the procedure is combined with myelography, the use of this technique for noninvasive imaging has been generally superseded by magnetic resonance imaging (MRI). Advances in MRI technology have allowed its use as a satisfactory alternative to CT scans and myelography for most patients with suspected disease both for general diagnostic purposes and for preoperative evaluation. In contrast to its functional advantages in studies of degenerative disease of the spine, MRI offers little benefit in the routine study of peripheral OA. It is particularly helpful in differentiating lesions such as internal joint derangements, avascular necrosis, and pigmented villonodular synovitis from OA. MRI is finding increased application as an investigational tool in defining cartilage responses to therapeutic agents and in epidemiologic studies.

Radiographic study of Heberden's and Bouchard's nodes reveals joint-space narrowing, bony sclerosis, and cyst formation. Spur formation, best seen radiologically on routine posteroanterior views, is prominent and appears to develop at the attachments of the flexor and extensor tendons to the distal phalanx. In some patients, however, spurs may be directed anteroposteriorly rather than mediolaterally, and lateral views with the fingers spread may be necessary to demonstrate changes. Although the nodes may feel hard, only minimal spur formation may be visible radiographically, and the enlargement may consist of soft tissue and cartilage. OA of metacarpophalangeal joints is uncommon, but hook-like osteophytes were noted on the radial side of the head of the metacarpal bones in seven of 100 patients with nodal OA (171). These changes, seen primarily in patients older than 65 years, may result from tension on capsular ligaments caused by contraction of interosseous muscles at the radial side of the metacarpal head.

Anteroposterior views of the pelvis should be obtained routinely when OA of the hip is suspected. This view is especially informative in that the hips, sacroiliac joints, symphysis pubis, and pelvic bones are visualized. Special views of the hips, including lateral views and tomograms, may be of value when pathologic changes are suspected but not seen with routine techniques. Advanced disease may demonstrate striking abnormalities such as protrusio acetabuli (arthrokatadysis), a condition in which the floor of the acetabulum is displaced medially by the head of the femur, so that the femoral head may bulge into the pelvis ("Otto's pelvis").

Although OA changes of the knee are usually readily seen on routine anteroposterior and lateral views, special views are often helpful. Tunnel views taken with the knee in flexion expose the intercondylar notch and enable one to identify loose bodies, intraarticular spurs, and changes in the tibial spines. Tunnel views may best reveal loss of the joint space. Their effectiveness in delineating cartilage loss may relate to the visualization of a more posterior portion of the femoral condyles, where cartilage loss may be significant. "Skyline" (Hughston) views taken from above allow more detailed study of the patellofemoral compartment. Films obtained when the patient is bearing weight allow optimal demonstration of genu varus or genu valgus and medial or lateral compartment narrowing. Radiographs of the contralateral joint are helpful in evaluating observed changes.

Additional imaging modalities such as ultrasonographic techniques and macroradiographic examination of joints with quantitative microfocal assessments are of interest, but are costly techniques that provide little additional information for routine OA diagnosis (172–176). It is of interest that ultrasound studies may prove to be of value in detecting not only changes in cartilage depth, but also qualitative changes in cartilage occurring as a result of the degenerative process (177).

Variant Forms

The clinical, radiographic, and pathologic findings in certain patients with primary OA are sufficiently different from those usually seen to warrant consideration of these cases as distinct symptom complexes (128,129,178–181). One such group, characterized by diffuse polyarticular involvement, has been termed primary generalized OA (180). A second group demonstrating similar features has been given the name ankylosing hyperostosis or diffuse idiopathic skeletal hyperostosis (128,129,181). It should be noted that although diffuse idiopathic skeletal hyperostosis is frequently included in discussions of degenerative joint disease of the spine, this entity differs from classic intervertebral disc disease and spondylosis, with respect to both etiopathogenesis and clinical presentation. A third group, characterized by inflammatory synovitis of interphalangeal joints of the hands in association with juxtaarticular bone erosions, has been termed erosive inflammatory OA (129,180). Finally, a fourth group of patients may exhibit evidence of chondromalacia patellae with variable degrees of progression to full forms of OA change (182).

Primary Generalized Osteoarthritis

This pattern of "nodal" OA occurs predominantly in middle-aged women (180). Distal and proximal interphalangeal joints and first carpometacarpal joints are sites of predilection and are often affected in succession. Other peripheral joints including knees, hips, and metatarsophalangeal joints are frequently involved, as are joints of the spine. An acute inflammatory phase commonly precedes chronic articular symptoms. The erythrocyte sedimentation rate is normal or slightly elevated; serum rheumatoid factor is absent. Although the overall pattern of radiologic changes is similar to that usually seen in localized OA, certain differences are notable. Articular facets, neural arches, and spinous processes of the vertebral column are often enlarged, leading to the radiographic designation of "kissing spines." Knee films show marked joint-space narrowing with "molten wax" osteophytes as opposed to ordinary, sharply pointed osteophytes. Patients with advanced cases show radiographic changes in excess of the clinical findings. Joint function is often only mildly affected despite severe anatomic changes.

The concept of primary generalized OA as a distinct subset is still controversial. This form may simply reflect more severe disease differentiated only by polyarticular involvement.

In some patients with generalized OA, chondrocalcinosis has been noted (106,183). Studies have demonstrated the presence of diffuse deposits of CPPD crystals (184). A familial form of chondrocalcinosis associated with "apatite" crystal deposition has been described in patients exhibiting symptoms indistinguishable from those seen in generalized OA alone (185). Synovial fluid basic calcium phosphate crystals (apatite-type) correlated well with the severity of radiographic joint degeneration, and synovial fluid CPPD crystals correlated with patient age but not with degeneration (186).

Calcium pyrophosphate–deposition disease (chondrocalcinosis, pseudogout) and associated OA has been linked to chromosome 8q by Baldwin et al. (187). It is likely that multiple pathways contribute deposition of calcium pyrophosphate crystals in articular cartilage because other kindreds with familial chondrocalcinosis have been shown to have the phenotype genetically linked to a region of chromosome 5p (188,189). Further refinement of the genetic linkage of calcium pyrophosphate–deposition disease to chromosome 5p indicates that the gene responsible lies in an area of less than 1 cM in this area of chromosome 5p (190).

Erosive Inflammatory Osteoarthritis

Erosive inflammatory (180) OA is another variant of "nodal" disease and involves primarily the distal and proximal interphalangeal joints. The metacarpophalangeal joints also may be involved. The disease is usually hereditary.

Painful inflammatory episodes eventually lead to joint deformity and sometimes to ankylosis. Postmenopausal women are most frequently affected. Acute flares may occur for years, but eventually, the affected joints often become asymptomatic. Gelatinous cysts, variably painful and tender, may develop over the involved joints. Inflammation and swelling may be sufficiently severe to suggest a diagnosis of RA. Radiographic examination reveals loss of joint cartilage, spur formation, and subchondral bony sclerosis. Bony erosions are prominent. Bony ankylosis, commonly seen, may be the result of synovial inflammation and pannus formation, healing of denuded cartilage surfaces, or coalescence of adjacent osteophytes. Studies of synovium may reveal an intense proliferative synovitis, often indistinguishable from that of RA. The erythrocyte sedimentation rate is usually normal or only slightly elevated.

Rheumatoid factor and antinuclear antibodies are absent. The presence of abnormal immune mechanisms has been suggested, however, by the demonstration of immune complexes in involved synovium (191). Synovial fluid and synovial specimens from patients with erosive OA have increased numbers of T lymphocytes expressing major histocompatibility complex (MHC) class II antigens, similar to those seen in specimens from patients with RA (192). These findings are not present in patients with OA of other types. Evidence of sicca syndrome in patients with erosive OA suggests the presence of some immunologic abnormality (193). Such individuals may well represent a subset of erosive inflammatory OA with an autoimmune background.

Diffuse Idiopathic Skeletal Hyperostosis; Ankylosing Hyperostosis

As noted earlier, DISH likely represents a disease state different from OA, based on etiopathogenic and clinical considerations. Given many similarities to intervertebral disc disease, however, it is frequently discussed as an OA variant. The disease is characterized by an unusual type of florid hyperostosis of the spine, with large spurs or marginal bony proliferations in the form of anterior osseous ridges (128,129,181). Fusion of these ridges often has a flowing appearance (Fig. 111.10). Ossification occurs in the connective tissue surrounding the spine, such as the anterior longitudinal ligament and peripheral disc margins. A predilection exists for involvement of the dorsal spine, although all levels of the spine may be affected. Lesions are most marked at the anterior and right lateral aspects of the vertebral column. The observation of left-sided vertebral bridging in patients with situs inversus suggests that the descending thoracic aorta plays a role in the location of vertebral calcification. Although most common in older patients, the disease has been noted in younger persons. Despite extensive anatomic abnormalities, pain is often minimal or absent, and spinal motion is only moderately limited.

Subsequent studies have further defined the clinical and pathologic features of this syndrome and have demonstrated extraspinal manifestations (128). An increased frequency of clinically palpable OA of the distal and proximal interphalangeal joints of the hands was documented in a study of patients with DISH syndrome as compared with matched DISH-negative controls (194). Resnick et al. (195) defined specific criteria for vertebral involvement, to allow differentiation of this disorder from degenerative disc disease or ankylosing spondylitis. The criteria include flowing ossification along the anterolateral aspect of at least four contiguous vertebral bodies, preservation of disc height, absence of vacuum phenomena or vertebral body marginal sclerosis, and absence of apophyseal joint ankylosis or sacroiliac joint erosions, sclerosis, or fusion. Frequently, radiolucency is apparent between the abnormal calcification and the underlying vertebral body. Extraspinal manifestations include irregular new bone formation or "whiskering," large bony spurs, seen particularly on the olecranon process and the calcaneus (Fig. 111.12), and severe ligamentous calcification, seen mainly in the sacrotuberous, iliolumbar (Fig. 111.13), and patellar ligaments. Periarticular osteophytes are conspicuous.

Spinal stiffness is a prominent clinical complaint despite surprising maintenance of spinal motion with minimal pain. Involvement of the cervical spine may lead to a number of specific associated symptoms including dysphagia (196), cervical myelopathy (197), and distortion of the airway, leading to unexpected difficulties during intubation for surgery (198). Peripheral joint symptoms include pain in involved elbows, ilia, shoulders, hips, knees, and ankles. Heel pain related to a calcaneal spur is common. The diffuse radiographic findings involving both spinal and extraspinal structures have led to the suggestion that this disorder represents an "ossifying diathesis," rather than merely a localized disorder of the spine. Coexistence of DISH and ankylosing spondylitis in the same patient has been described (199).

Hyperglycemia is the most common laboratory abnormality noted in patients with this syndrome, with an incidence of abnormal glucose tolerance tests about twice that

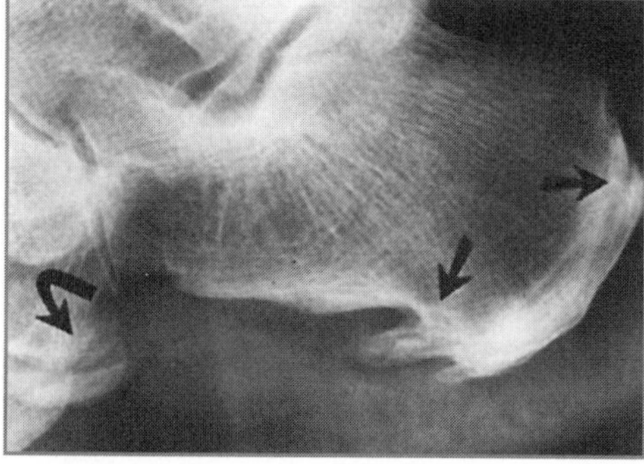

FIGURE 111.12. Diffuse idiopathic skeletal hyperostosis. The calcaneus demonstrates large, irregular spurs at its posterior and plantar aspects (*straight arrows*). Associated irregularity at the area of the cuboid and fifth metatarsal bones is seen (*curved arrow*). (Courtesy of Dr. Donald Resnick.)

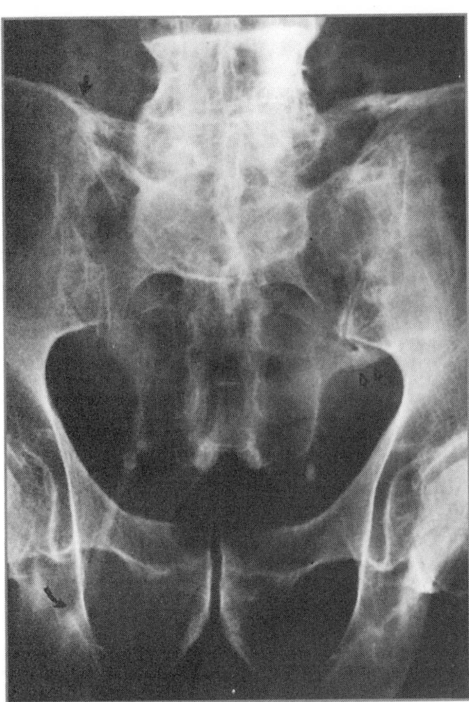

FIGURE 111.13. Radiogram of the pelvis in a patient with diffuse idiopathic skeletal hyperostosis reveals iliolumbar (*straight arrow*) and sacrotuberous (*curved arrow*) ligament ossification and paraarticular sacroiliac osteophyte formation (*open arrows*). (From Resnick D, Shaul SR, Robins JM. Diffuse idiopathic skeletal hyperostosis (DISH): Forestier's disease with extraspinal manifestations. *Radiology* 1975;115:513–524, with permission.)

seen in an age-, sex-, and weight-matched population. In a recent study, diabetes mellitus was present in 40% of these patients (200). Growth hormone and somatomedin (insulin-like growth factor) levels are normal in DISH, but insulin levels have been shown to be elevated (201,202). In patients with DISH syndrome, a significant increase in the concentration of growth hormone was noted at 30 and 45 minutes after an intravenous insulin tolerance test as compared with controls (203).

The etiopathogenesis of DISH is unknown. In one report, 16 of 47 patients with this syndrome were HLA-B27$^+$ (204). In other studies, however, a statistically significant increase in HLA-B27 has not been confirmed. Studies of Pima Indians have shown this syndrome to be present in 50% of all individuals, with a 20% frequency of HLA-B27 (205). No significant association was seen, however, with HLA-B locus antigens when Pima Indians with the syndrome were compared with age-matched control subjects. Patients with DISH have increased levels of serum vitamin A (206). Of special interest in this regard is the observation that patients receiving high doses of synthetic vitamin A derivatives, retinoids, develop an ossification disorder resembling DISH (207). Radiographic features may simulate vertebral and extravertebral manifestations of DISH syndrome, or may be limited to extraspinal tendon and ligament calcification with minimal or absent vertebral involvement. Biochemical studies also have demonstrated increased concentrations of endogenous 13-*cis*- and all-*trans*-retinoic acids in DISH, as demonstrated by high-pressure liquid chromatography (HPLC) (208). Five patients with DISH syndrome were noted to have elevated plasma and urine fluoride levels (209). Abnormal levels of fluoride were, however, not noted in other studies (129).

A syndrome characterized by ossification of the posterior longitudinal ligament has been described, occurring mainly in Japanese (210). It has been estimated that more than 4,000 patients in Japan are afflicted with this disorder. Radiographic study of the spine reveals lumpy or linear bony masses across one or more disc spaces, sometimes extending from the superior cervical spine to the thoracic region. Ankylosing hyperostosis of the type seen in DISH may be associated. Clinical manifestations may be severe because of spinal cord compression.

Chondromalacia Patellae

This disorder is characterized by degenerative changes of the cartilage of the patella and is included in those conditions associated with OA changes in the knee (see Chapter 98). Although previously identified as a specific entity, chondromalacia patellae is now thought to result from many conditions affecting the knee that lead to cartilage degeneration (182). The malacic changes are considered to be simply the final common pathway through which articular cartilage of the patella degenerates. The specific conditions effecting these changes—such as primary meniscal disease, knee laxity, or abnormal patellar positions such as patella alta—may lead to a similar end-stage complex of symptoms. The syndrome is often associated with repeated trauma, as occurs in recurrent lateral subluxation of the patella. Pain is present about the patella and is aggravated by activity such as ascending or, particularly, descending stairs. Paradoxically, vague knee pain may occur after periods of inactivity in the flexed position, such as watching a movie. The disease is typically seen in young adults, especially women, and may be a precursor to the development of patellofemoral compartment OA. On routine radiologic study, changes of chondromalacia may be limited or absent. Detailed studies evaluating the relative efficacies of conventional MRI, magnetic resonance arthrography, and CT arthrography demonstrated that all imaging techniques were insensitive to grade I lesions, and highly sensitive to grade IV lesions, so that no significant difference among the techniques could be shown; all imaging techniques studied had a high specificity and accuracy in the detection and grading of chondromalacia patellae overall (211).

Although the findings described in the foregoing discussion support the existence of various forms of OA, the validity of classifying these as distinct symptom complexes or entities remains open to question. OA may affect many joints in any given patient, so generalized involvement may merely reflect one end of the spectrum of clinical severity. Inflammation may occur in early OA, whether localized or generalized, and its use as a differentiating characteristic is not definitive. In some patients, it is difficult to rule out the coexistence of seronegative RA and OA. Ankylosing hyperostosis has many characteristics that distinguish it from the more common forms of OA. The pathologic changes may be indistinguishable, however, especially in early disease.

Prognosis

The outlook for patients with primary OA is variable, depending on the extent and site of the disease. Involvement of the distal interphalangeal joints, for example, may be associated with a moderate amount of pain, but usually causes little limitation of function unless fine-finger motion is required occupationally, such as in typing or in playing musical instruments. Involvement of weight-bearing joints, on the other hand, may lead to marked disability. Similarly, OA of the cervical spine may not only give rise to distressing symptoms but may also lead to severe objective neurologic deficits and disability.

Studies of disease progression in specific joints suggest that not all cases of OA inevitably deteriorate (212,213). As noted earlier, joint deterioration is more likely to occur in association with aging and obesity. Spector et al. (56) demonstrated a high frequency of involvement of the previously uninvolved contralateral knee within a 2-year period in obese patients. Patients with a larger number of joints affected by OA throughout the body experienced a more rapid progression of knee OA than did those with lesser numbers of joint involvement (56). Presence of bilateral knee OA, as contrasted to unilateral involvement, is associated with a higher rate of joint deterioration (119). Other similar studies noted that a diagnosis of generalized OA increased the likelihood of progressive cartilage loss in the knee by threefold (17).

Occasional patients may develop a rapidly progressive, destructive OA of the hip (214). Severe changes are seen both in the acetabulum and in the femoral head. Degenerative pseudocysts and lack of osteophyte formation are characteristic findings. Synovitis noted at operation is of a low grade. Such rapid deterioration of hip joints may be associated with use of nonsteroidal antiinflammatory drugs (NSAIDs) (215). Such an association, if real, might be related to increased joint use permitted by the analgesic action of these drugs, to a direct effect of these drugs on cartilage with inhibition of proteoglycan synthesis, or both. As noted, similar rapid destructive changes have been described, unrelated to the use of analgesic agents, and the overall clinical experience with these agents over many years in the treatment of various forms of arthritis is reassuring.

The incidence and progression of various radiographic features were examined in a study of the natural history of hand OA (16). These features increased with age, although their rate of progression slowed as disease severity increased. The earliest radiographic signs of OA were joint-space narrowing and possible osteophytes regardless of age. Approximately 10 to 20 years elapsed before any of the radiographic features progressed one grade and even longer before OA progressed from intermediate to late stages. Slowing of OA progression at higher levels of severity has important implications when assessing outcome variables in clinical trials.

Treatment may retard the progression of the disease and is of further value in protecting the contralateral joints exposed to increased stress. Patients should be reassured that the general outlook is favorable and disability is uncommon, in contrast to the threat of crippling seen in patients with RA. Patients should be told that involvement of certain joints may be associated with localized pain, stiffness, and limitation of motion. OA is certainly not always benign.

Differential Diagnosis

The differentiation of primary OA from other disorders of the musculoskeletal system depends on a correlation of clinical, laboratory, and radiographic findings. OA may be confused with other forms of arthritic disease because pain, stiffness, and limitation of motion are common features in all these disorders. Differential diagnosis is further complicated by the high radiographic prevalence of OA in the general population that often bears no relation to the musculoskeletal complaints of a given patient.

In most patients, the diagnosis is simple. In others, however, atypical disease presentation and behavior may require extensive differential diagnostic considerations. Examples of such presentations include OA occurring in an atypical site such as the shoulder, association with a significant inflammatory element, coexistence with other entities such as CPPD crystal deposition, precocious occurrence in young individuals, and OA of the spine with neurologic findings that simulate other underlying neurologic disorders.

RA can usually be differentiated on the basis of its more inflammatory nature and the characteristic pattern of joint involvement. If RA begins as monoarticular disease of the knee or hip, however, differentiation from OA may be difficult without prolonged follow-up study. An increase in the erythrocyte sedimentation rate, a positive test for rheumatoid factor, and synovial fluid analysis are helpful (see Chapter 60). RA may be particularly difficult to differentiate from erosive OA. The pattern of joint involvement is of diagnostic value because the latter is limited mainly to the distal and proximal interphalangeal joints of the hands; RA usually affects the metacarpophalangeal and the wrist and carpal joints and peripheral joints elsewhere. Joints afflicted with active seropositive RA rarely develop osteophytes. Some patients with Heberden's nodes or erosive OA may later develop RA, in which case osteophytes precede rheumatoid involvement, and a careful clinical history is necessary to identify the presence of a "mixed" arthritis. Mixed disease also may be present when RA leads to secondary degenerative change, but bony overgrowth occurs only in "burned out" disease, and even then, osteophyte formation is abortive. Proximal or distal interphalangeal joint involvement in juvenile rheumatoid arthritis (JRA) or psoriatic arthritis is frequently accompanied by nodal formation in these joints.

Rheumatic syndromes characterized by involvement of the distal interphalangeal joints of the hands, such as psoriatic arthritis, Reiter's syndrome, and the arthritis of chronic ulcerative colitis, may be confused with OA of the nodal type. The associated clinical findings of the underlying disease in these patients usually suffice to clarify the diagnosis. Pseudogout syndrome, or chondrocalcinosis articularis, may simulate OA when low-grade arthralgias result from the presence of CPPD crystals in synovial fluid. The pattern of arthritis is clearly different in these patients; the metacarpophalangeal joints, wrists, elbows, shoulders, knees, hips, and ankles are often affected (see Chapter 117). Symptoms related to early manifestations of localized joint disorders such as osteonecrosis, pigmented villonodular synovitis, and chronic infectious arthritis may be mistakenly attributed to degenerative changes seen as coincidental radiographic findings. Neurologic symptoms secondary to spinal OA must be differentiated from those that result from other neurologic disorders. The symptoms of OA of the cervical spine may simulate those of multiple sclerosis, syringomyelia, amyotrophic lateral sclerosis, progressive spinal atrophy, and spinal cord tumors (see Chapter 100).

SECONDARY OSTEOARTHRITIS

The term secondary OA describes those cases that follow a recognizable underlying local or systemic factor, some of which are noted in Table 111.1. A diagnosis of secondary OA should be considered, particularly when the disease develops at an early age.

Acute Trauma

Joint degeneration may follow acute injury. The history includes the injurious event followed by redness, soft tissue swelling, and pain over the involved joint. In several months, the inflammatory changes subside and are replaced by a hard, painless enlargement. The deformity is localized to the injured joint. The anatomic changes are similar to those seen in primary OA. Injury of this nature involving the distal interphalangeal joints of the hands may lead to traumatic Heberden's nodes (109). Acute trauma to any of the interphalangeal joints of the hands may lead to the common "baseball finger" (Fig. 111.14).

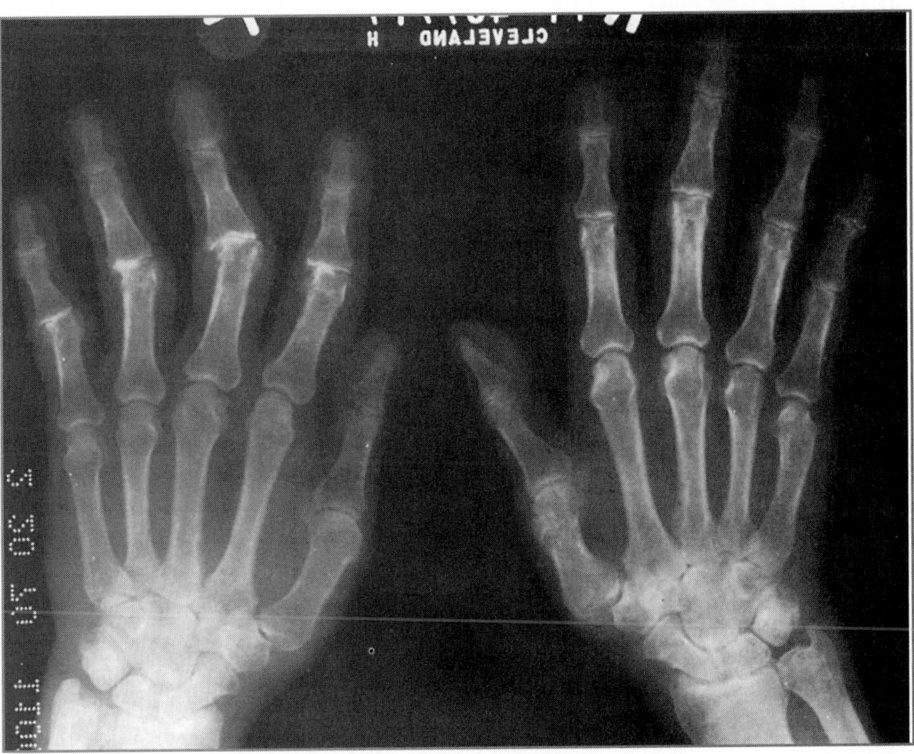

FIGURE 111.14. Secondary osteoarthritis of the second, third, fourth, and fifth proximal interphalangeal joints of the left hand ("baseball fingers") in a patient with recurrent episodes of acute trauma while a semiprofessional baseball player.

Chronic Trauma

An increased prevalence of OA is associated with chronic trauma related to certain occupations. Although exposure of a joint to subtle chronic trauma, or microtrauma, has been suggested as an etiologic factor in the development of primary OA, the relation between trauma and joint changes, as described previously, seems more clear cut and supports the classification of such lesions as secondary.

Other Joint Disorders

Such disorders may be either local or diffuse. Secondary localized OA may follow local joint disorders of other causes such as fractures, aseptic necrosis, or acute or chronic infection. Early-age OA in the knee may be the result of torn menisci, patellar dislocation, stress resulting from obesity, poor mechanics as a result of genu varus, or tibial torsion. Localized OA of the hip may follow childhood disorders such as congenital dysplasia of the hip, slipped capital epiphysis, and Legg–Calvé–Perthes disease. OA of the midfoot or hindfoot may result in patients with congenital calcaneonavicular and talocalcaneal coalition.

Diffuse secondary degenerative changes may supervene in patients with RA, in patients with bleeding dyscrasias in whom repeated hemarthroses may occur, or in dwarfs with achondroplasia.

Systemic Metabolic or Endocrine Disorders

Osteoarthritis changes may follow several metabolic or endocrine disorders (see Chapters 121 and 124).

Alkaptonuria (Ochronosis)

This inherited metabolic disease, associated with absence of homogentisic acid oxidase and characterized by the excretion of homogentisic acid in the urine and by the binding of its metabolic products to connective tissue components, is associated with generalized OA (216). The disease appears to be the result of a mutation mapped to chromosome 3q (217). Tissue deposition of brown–black pigment, or ochronosis, is seen primarily in cartilage, skin, and sclera. Degenerative disease of the spine occurs frequently; calcification of numerous intervertebral discs is a characteristic finding. Arthritis of peripheral joints such as hips, knees, and shoulders is less common and develops later. Tissue damage may involve an inhibitory effect of homogentisic acid on chondrocyte growth (see Chapter 121).

Wilson's Disease

Hepatolenticular degeneration, or Wilson's disease, is an inherited disorder associated with a variety of mutations in a gene (ATP7B) on chromosome 13q14.3 (218). It is characterized by excessive retention of copper, with degenerative changes in the brain and hepatic cirrhosis. Premature OA has been described as one component of associated articular manifestations of this disorder (219). In a small series of patients, copper was demonstrated in cartilage (219). Copper also has been observed in synovial tissue, where it might alter production of cytokines and proteases (220) (see Chapter 121).

Hemochromatosis

This chronic disease is associated with excessive deposition of iron and fibrosis in a variety of tissues. Although it can result from long-term overingestion of iron and from multiple transfusions, the disease is most often idiopathic. OA changes occur in 20% to 50% of patients (221). Hands, knees, and hips are most commonly involved, although virtually any joint, including those in the feet, can be affected. Involvement of the second and third metacarpophalangeal joints of the hands is particularly characteristic. Synovial tissue shows a striking deposition of iron, most prominently in the synovial lining cells. Radiographs reveal joint-space narrowing and irregularity, subchondral sclerosis, cystic erosions, bony proliferation, and, at times, subluxation. Chondrocalcinosis with deposits of CPPD is seen in up to 60% of patients.

Kashin–Beck Disease

This disorder, characterized by disturbances in growth and maturation in children, is endemic in eastern Siberia, northern China, and northern Korea (222). Abnormalities in enchondral bone growth lead to dystrophic changes in epiphyseal and metaphyseal areas. Severe secondary OA involves the peripheral joints and the spine. Various causes have been suggested, including a relation to a fungus ingested with cereal grains, iron excess, or selenium deficiency (223).

Acromegaly

Hypersecretion of growth hormone by the anterior pituitary gland in adults leads to a slowly progressive overgrowth of soft tissue, bone, and cartilage. Peripheral and spinal OA is common. Peripheral joint symptoms occur in about 60% of patients (224). Most commonly involved are the knees, hips, shoulders, and elbows. Carpal tunnel syndrome is frequently seen. Backache is common, but back motion is often normal or increased because of the thickened intervertebral discs and the laxity of acromegalic ligaments. Early, increased cartilage thickness results in wide joint spaces on radiographs. Later, joint-space narrowing, osteophyte formation, and subchondral sclerosis occur. Prominent new bone formation is similar to that seen in DISH syndrome and may bear a relation to increased levels of serum growth hormone (225). A relation of growth hormone and insulin-like growth factors also has been suggested in studies of patients with OA not associated with acromegaly (62–64) (see Chapter 124).

Hyperparathyroidism

Increased levels of parathyroid hormone, whether primary or secondary, can produce many rheumatic problems. It has been postulated that degenerative changes result from damage to cartilage related either to CPPD crystal deposition or to subchondral bony erosion from the resorptive effects of parathyroid hormone. Radiographs classically show subperiosteal bone resorption, cystic or sclerotic changes in bones, and chondrocalcinosis (see Chapter 124).

Crystal Deposition Disease

Generalized OA has been reported in patients with idiopathic articular chondrocalcinosis (226). Large joints of the lower limbs and intervertebral joints of the lumbar spine are especially involved. Although a destructive arthropathy has been described in patients with articular chondrocalcinosis, these changes appear to be much more common when generalized OA and chondrocalcinosis coexist (227). Weight-bearing joints are frequently affected, but involvement of non–weight-bearing joints such as the elbows, shoulders, wrists, and metacarpophalangeal joints also occurs. Several mechanisms have been postulated to explain the association of calcium pyrophosphate crystal deposition with OA (226). In certain patients, obvious crystal deposition antedates significant OA; alterations in cartilage matrix in these patients may predispose them to degenerative changes. In other patients, OA is present for a prolonged period, and crystal deposition disease occurs later in the disorder. Whether changes in cartilage matrix as a result of OA may favor the deposition of these crystals is still unclear.

An association between basic calcium phosphate (apatite-type) crystal deposition and OA has been described (186,228). The disease in patients with identifiable basic calcium phosphate crystals in synovial fluid is similar to other forms of OA, except the presence of crystals correlates with more severe radiographic change. Whether apatite crystals are a result of or a cause of OA is unknown. Severe degenerative changes of the shoulder in association with basic calcium phosphate crystal deposition have been described by Halverson et al. (229), and termed Milwaukee shoulder. Similar changes have been observed in other joints, such as the knee (186,228). Injection of CPPD crystals in a lapine model of OA accelerated the OA disease process (229) (see Chapters 117 and 118).

Neuropathic Disorders

Severe OA occurs in association with neuropathic disorders, as first described by Charcot (230). The loss of proprioceptive or pain sensation, or both, relaxes the normal protective mechanisms of the joint and leads to articular instability and an exaggerated response to normal daily stresses. Although first described in patients with tabes dorsalis, similar lesions may be seen in other diseases associated with neuropathy including diabetes mellitus, syringomyelia, meningomyelocele, and peripheral nerve section (see Chapter 91).

Overuse of Intraarticular Corticosteroid Therapy

The development of localized OA has been ascribed to the repeated use of intraarticular injections of corticosteroids (231). In these patients, pain relief may allow overuse of already damaged joints and may thereby promote degenerative change. A direct, deleterious effect of corticosteroids on cartilage may represent a second mechanism for the development of those degenerative changes.

Symptoms and signs, laboratory findings, and radiographic abnormalities of secondary OA are generally similar to those seen in the primary form of the disease. Additional findings related to the associated underlying disease state also are present. The management of secondary OA is similar to that of the primary form of the disease (see Chapter 112).

REFERENCES

1. Moskowitz RW, Goldberg VM, Berman L. Synovitis as a manifestation of degenerative joint disease: an experimental study. *Arthritis Rheum* 1976;19:813(abst).
2. Goldenberg DL, Egan MS, Cohen AS. Inflammatory synovitis in degenerative joint disease. *J Rheumatol* 1982;9:204–209.
3. Myers SL, Brandt KD, Ehrlich JW, et al. Synovial inflammation in patients with early osteoarthritis of the knee. *J Rheumatol* 1990;17:1662–1669.
4. Murray RO. The aetiology of primary osteoarthritis of the hip. *Br J Radiol* 1965;50:81–83.
5. Altman R, Asch E, Bloch D, et al. Development of criteria for the classification and reporting of osteoarthritis: classification of osteoarthritis of the knee. *Arthritis Rheum* 1986;29:1039–1049.
6. Altman R, Alarcón G, Appelrouth D, et al. Criteria for classification and reporting of osteoarthritis of the hand. *Arthritis Rheum* 1990;33:1601–1610.
7. Altman R, Alarcon G, Bloch ADD, et al. Criteria for classification and reporting of osteoarthritis of the hip. *Arthritis Rheum* 1991;34:505–514.
8. Peyron J. Epidemiologic and etiologic approach of osteoarthritis. *Semin Arthritis Rheum* 1979;8:288–306.
9. Bland JH, Soule AB, Van Buskirk FW, et al. A study of inter- and intra observer error in reading plain radiographs of the hands: "to err is human." *Am J Radiol* 1969;105:853–859.
10. Lowman EW. Osteoarthritis. *JAMA* 1955;157:487–488.
11. Van Saase JLCM, Van Romunde K, Cats A, et al. Epidemiology of osteoarthritis: Zoetermeer survey: comparison of radiological osteoarthritis in a Dutch population with that in 10 other countries. *Ann Rheum Dis* 1989;48:271–280.

12. Guccione AA, Felson DT, Anderson JJ, et al. The effects of specific medical conditions on the functional limitations of elders in the Framingham Study. *Am J Public Health* 1994;84: 351–357.
13. Forman M, Malamet R, Kaplan D. A survey of osteoarthritis of the knee in the elderly. *J Rheumatol* 1983;10:283–287.
14. Oliveria SA, Felson DT, Reed JI, et al. Incidence of symptomatic hand, hip, and knee osteoarthritis among patients in a health maintenance organization. *Arthritis Rheum* 1995;38: 1134–1141.
15. Felson D, Naimark A, Anderson J, et al. The prevalence of knee osteoarthritis (OA) in the elderly: the Framingham study. *Arthritis Rheum* 1987;30:914–915.
16. Kallman DA, Wigley FM, Scott WW, et al. The longitudinal course of hand osteoarthritis in a male population. *Arthritis Rheum* 1990;33:1323–1332.
17. Schouten JSAG, van den Ouweland FA, Valkenburg HA. A 12 year follow up study in the general population on prognostic factors of cartilage loss in osteoarthritis of the knee. *Ann Rheum Dis* 1992;51:932–937.
18. Tepper S, Hochberg MC. Factors associated with hip osteoarthritis: data from the First National Health and Nutrition Examination Survey (NHANES-I). *Am J Epidemiol* 1993; 137:1081–1088.
19. Felson DT, Zhang Y, Hannan MT, et al. Risk factors for incident radiographic knee osteoarthritis in the elderly. *Arthritis Rheum* 1997;40:728–733.
20. Anderson J, Felson DT. Factors associated with knee osteoarthritis (OA) in the HANES I survey; evidence for an association with overweight, race and physical demands of work. *Am J Epidemiol* 1988;128:179–189.
21. Danielsson L, Lindberg H, Nilsson B. Prevalence of coxarthrosis. *Clin Orthop* 1984;191:110–115.
22. Ledingham L, Dawson S, Preston B, et al. Radiographic patterns and associations of osteoarthritis of the hip. *Ann Rheum Dis* 1992;51:1111–1116.
23. Bremner JM, Lawrence JS, Miall WE. Degenerative joint disease in a Jamaican rural population. *Ann Rheum Dis* 1968; 27:326–332.
24. Solomon L, Beighton P, Lawrence JS. Rheumatic disorders in the South African Negro. Part II. Osteoarthrosis. *South Afr Med J* 1975;49:1737–1740.
25. Hoaglund FT, Yau ACMC, Wong WL. Osteoarthritis of the hip and other joints in Southern Chinese in Hong Kong. *J Bone Joint Surg Am* 1973;55:645–657.
26. Mukhopadhaya B, Barooah B. Osteoarthritis of hip in Indians: an anatomical and clinical study. *Indian J Orthop* 1967;1:55–62.
27. Hoaglund FT, Shiba R, Newberg AH, et al. Diseases of the hip: a comparative study of Japanese oriental and American white patients. *J Bone Joint Surg* 1985;67:1376–1383.
28. Hoaglund FT, Oishi CS, Gialamas GG. Extreme variations in racial rates of total hip arthroplasty for primary coxarthrosis: a population-based study in San Francisco. *Ann Rheum Dis* 1995;54:107–110.
29. Solomon L, Beighton P, Lawrence JS. Distinct types of hip disorder in Mseleni joint disease. *South Afr Med J* 1986;69:15–17.
30. Roberts J, Burch TA. *Prevalence of osteoarthritis in adults by age, sex, race, and geographic area: United States, 1960-1962:* National Center for Health Statistics: *data from the National Health Survey.* Washington: United States Government Printing Office: Publ. 1000, Series 11, No 15, 1966.
31. Lawrence JS. Hypertension in relation to musculoskeletal disorders. *Ann Rheum Dis* 1975;34:451–456.
32. Lawrence JS. Generalized osteoarthrosis in a population sample. *Am J Epidemiol* 1969;90:381–389.
33. Stecher RM, Hersh AH, Hauser H. Heberden's nodes: family history and radiographic appearance of large family. *Am J Hum Genet* 1953;5:46–60.
34. Doherty M, Pattrick M, Powell R. Nodal generalized osteoarthritis is an autoimmune disease. *Ann Rheum Dis* 1990;49:1017–1020.
35. Pattrick M, Manhire M, Milford-Ward A, et al. HLA-A, B antigens alpha-1-antitrypsin phenotypes in nodal generalized osteoarthritis. *Ann Rheum Dis* 1989;48:470–475.
36. Chitnavis J, Sinsheimer JS, Clipsham K, et al. Genetic influences in end-stage osteoarthritis: sibling risks of hip and knee replacement for idiopathic osteoarthritis. *J Bone Joint Surg Br* 1997;79:660–664.
37. Spector TD, Cicuttini F, Baker J, et al. Genetic influences on osteoarthritis in women: a twin study. *Br Med J* 1996;312: 940–943.
38. Wright G, Hughes AE, Regan M, et al. Association of two loci on chromosome 2q with nodal osteoarthritis. *Ann Rheum Dis* 1996;55:317–319.
39. Felson DT, Couropmitree NN, Chaisson CE, et al. Evidence for a mendelian gene in a segregation analysis of generalized radiographic osteoarthritis: the Framingham Study. *Arthritis Rheum* 1998;41:1064–1071.
40. Loughlin L, Irven C, Fergusson C, et al. Sibling pair analysis shows no linkage of generalized osteoarthritis to the loci encoding type II collagen, cartilage link protein or cartilage matrix protein. *Br J Rheumatol* 1994;33:1103–1106.
41. Ala-Kokko L, Baldwin CT, Moskowitz RW, et al. Single base mutation in the type II procollagen gene (COL2A1) as a cause of primary osteoarthritis associated with a mild chondrodysplasia. *Proc Natl Acad Sci U S A* 1990;87:6565–6568.
42. Pun YL, Moskowitz RW, Lie S, et al. Clinical correlations of osteoarthritis associated with a single-base mutation (arginine^{519} to cysteine) in type II procollagen gene, a newly defined pathogenesis. *Arthritis Rheum* 1994;37:264–269.
43. Eyre DR, Weis MA, Moskowitz RW. Cartilage expression of a type II collagen mutation in an inherited form of osteoarthritis associated with a mild chondrodysplasia. *J Clin Invest* 1991; 87:357–361.
44. Bleasel JF, Bisagni-Faure A, Holderbaum D, et al. Type II procollagen gene (COL2A1) mutation in exon 11 associated with spondyloepiphyseal dysplasia, tall stature and precocious osteoarthritis. *J Rheumatol* 1995;22:255–261.
45. Chan D, Taylor TKF, Cole WG. Characterization of an arginine^{789} to cysteine substitution in α_1(II) collagen chains of a patient with spondyloepiphyseal dysplasia. *J Biol Chem* 1993; 268:15238–15245.
46. Vikkula M, Palotie A, Ritvaniemi P, et al. Early-onset osteoarthritis linked to the type II procollagen gene. *Arthritis Rheum* 1993;36:401–409.
47. Loughlin J, Irven C, Athanasou N, et al. Differential allelic expression of the type II collagen gene (COL2A1) in osteoarthritic cartilage. *Am J Hum Genet* 1995;56:1186–1193.
48. Uitterlinden AG, Burger H, Huang QJ, et al. Vitamin D receptor genotype is associated with radiographic osteoarthritis at the knee. *J Clin Invest* 1997;100:259–263.
49. Keen RW, Hart DJ, Lanchbury JS, et al. Association of early osteoarthritis of the knee with a Taq I polymorphism of the vitamin D receptor gene. *Arthritis Rheum* 1997;40:1444–1449.
50. Blumberg BS, Bloch K, Black RL, et al. A study of the prevalence of arthritis in Alaskan Eskimos. *Arthritis Rheum* 1961;4: 325–341.
51. Lawrence JS, DeGraff R, Laine VAI. Degenerative joint disease in random samples and occupational groups. In: Kellgren JH, Jeffrey MR, Ball J, eds. *The epidemiology of chronic rheumatism.* Vol 1. Oxford: Blackwell, 1963.
52. Felson DT. Epidemiology of hip and knee osteoarthritis. *Epidemiol Rev* 1988;10:1–18.

53. Davis MA, Ettinger WM, Neuhaus JM. The role of metabolic factors and blood pressure in the association of obesity with osteoarthritis of the knee. *J Rheumatol* 1988;5:1827–1832.
54. Hart DJ, Doyle DV, Spector TD. Incidence and risk factors for radiographic knee osteoarthritis in middle-aged women: the Chingford Study. *Arthritis Rheum* 1999;42:17–24.
55. Altman RD, Fried JF, Bloch DA, et al. Radiographic assessment of progression in osteoarthritis. *Arthritis Rheum* 1987;30: 1214–1225.
56. Dougados M, Gueguen A, Nguyen M, et al. Longitudinal radiologic evaluation of osteoarthritis of the knee. *J Rheumatol* 1992;19:378–383.
57. McGoey BV, Deitel N, Saplys RJF, et al. Effect of weight loss on musculoskeletal pain in the morbidly obese. *J Bone Joint Surg Br* 1990;72:322–323.
58. Croft P, Coggon D, Cruddas M, et al. Osteoarthritis of the hip: an occupational disease in farmers. *Br Med J* 1992;304: 1269–1272.
59. Silberberg M, Silberberg R. Osteoarthritis in mice fed diets enriched with animal or vegetable fat. *Arch Pathol* 1960;70: 385–390.
60. Kellgren JH, Lawrence JS. Osteo-arthrosis and disk degeneration in an urban population. *Ann Rheum Dis* 1958;17: 388–397.
61. Denko CW, Boja B, Moskowitz RW. Growth promoting peptides in osteoarthritis: insulin, insulin-like growth factor-I, growth hormone. *J Rheumatol* 1990;17:1217–1221.
62. McAlindon RE, Teale JD, Dieppe P. Levels of insulin related growth factor 1 in osteoarthritis of the knee. *Ann Rheum Dis* 1993;52:229–231.
63. Schouten JSAG, van den Ouweland FA, Valkenburg HA, et al. Insulin-like growth factor-1: a prognostic factor of knee osteoarthritis. *Br J Rheumatol* 1993;32:274–280.
64. Bagge E, Eden S, Rosen T, et al. The prevalence of radiographic osteoarthritis is low in elderly patients with growth hormone deficiency. *Acta Endocrinol* 1993;129:296–300.
65. Sandmark H, Hogstedt C, Lewold S, et al. Osteoarthrosis of the knee in men and women in association with overweight, smoking and hormone therapy. *Ann Rheum Dis* 1999;58:151–155.
66. Samanta A, Jones A, Regan M, et al. Is osteoarthritis in women affected by hormonal changes or smoking? *Br J Rheumatol* 1993;32:366–370.
67. Hannan MT, Felson DF, Anderson JJ, et al. Estrogen use and radiographic osteoarthritis of the knee in women. *Arthritis Rheum* 1990;33:525–532.
68. Wolfe F, Altman R, Hochberg M, et al. Postmenopausal estrogen therapy is associated with improved radiographic scores in osteoarthritis and rheumatoid arthritis. *Arthritis Rheum* 1994; 37(suppl):S231.
69. Zhang YZ, McAlindon T, Hannan MT, et al. A longitudinal study of the relation of estrogen replacement therapy (ERT) to the risk of radiographic knee osteoarthrosis (OA). *Arthritis Rheum* 1995;38:S269.
70. Spector TD, Nandra D, Hart DJ, et al. Is hormone replacement protective for hand and knee osteoarthritis in women? The Chingford Study. *Ann Rheum Dis* 1997;56:432–434.
71. Vingård E, Alfredsson L, Malchau H. Lifestyle factors and hip arthrosis: a case referent study of body mass index, smoking and hormone therapy. *Acta Orthop Scand* 1997;68:216–220.
72. Rosner IA, Malemud CJ, Goldberg VM, et al. Pathologic and metabolic responses of experimental osteoarthritis to estradiol and an estradiol antagonist. *Clin Orthop* 1982;171:280–286.
73. Acheson RM, Collart AN. New Haven survey of joint diseases XIII: relationship between some systemic characteristics and osteoarthrosis in a general population. *Ann Rheum Dis* 1975;34:379–387.
74. Solomon L, Schnitzler CN, Browett JP. Osteoarthritis of the hip: the patient behind the disease. *Ann Rheum Dis* 1982;41:118–125.
75. Weintroub S, Papo J, Ashkenazi M, et al. Osteoarthritis of the hip and fractures of the proximal end of the femur. *Acta Orthop Scand* 1982;53:261–264.
76. Gevers G, Dequeker J, Geusens P, et al. Physical and histomorphological characteristics of iliac crest bone differ according to the grade of osteoarthritis at the hand. *Bone* 1989;10:173–177.
77. Dequeker J Goris P, Utterhoeven R. Osteoporosis and osteoarthritis (osteoarthrosis): anthropometric distinctions. *JAMA* 1983;249:1448–1451.
78. Hannan MT, Anderson JJ, Zhang Y, et al. Bone mineral density and knee osteoarthritis in elderly men and women. *Arthritis Rheum* 1993;36:1671–1680.
79. Radin EL, Martin BR, Burr DB, et al. Effects of mechanical loading on the tissues of the rabbit knee. *J Orthop Res* 1984;2: 221–234.
80. Bird HA, Tribe CR, Bacon PA. Joint hypermobility leading to osteoarthrosis and chondrocalcinosis. *Ann Rheum Dis* 1978; 37:203–211.
81. Schlomka G, Schroter G, Ocherwal A. Über der bedeutung der beruflischer Belastung für die entsehung der degenerativen Gelenkleiden. *Z Gesamte Inn Med* 1955;10:993–999.
82. Partridge REH, Duthie JJR. Rheumatism in dockers and civil servants: a comparison of heavy manual and sedentary workers. *Ann Rheum Dis* 1968;27:559–568.
83. Kivimaki J, Riihimake H, Hanninen K. Knee disorders in carpet and floor layers and painters. *Scand J Work Environ Health* 1992;18:310–316.
84. Cooper C, McAlindon T, Coggon D, et al. Occupational activity and osteoarthritis of the knee. *Ann Rheum Dis* 1994;53:90–93.
85. Maetzel A, Makela M, Hawker G, et al. Osteoarthritis of the hip and knee and mechanical occupational exposure: a systematic overview of the evidence. *J Rheumatol* 1997;24:1599–1607.
86. Roach KE, Persky V, Miles T, et al. Biomechanical aspects of occupation and osteoarthritis of the hip: a case-control study. *J Rheumatol* 1994;21:2334–2340.
87. Hadler NM, Gillings DB, Imbus HR, et al. Hand structure and function in an industrial setting: influence of three patterns of stereotyped repetitive usage. *Arthritis Rheum* 1978;21:210–220.
88. Williams WV, Cope R, Gaunt WD, et al. Metacarpophalangeal arthropathy associated with manual labor (Missouri metacarpal syndrome). *Arthritis Rheum* 1987;30:1362–1381.
89. Puranen J, Ala-Ketola L, Peltokallio P, et al. Running and primary osteoarthrosis of the hip. *Br Med J* 1975;2:424–425.
90. Lane NE, Bloch DA, Jones HH, et al. Long distance running, bone density, and osteoarthritis. *JAMA* 1986;255:1147–1151.
91. Lane NE, Michel B, Bjorkengren A, et al. The risk of osteoarthritis with running and aging: a five year longitudinal study. *J Rheumatol* 1993;20:461–468.
92. Panush RS, Schmidt C, Caldwell JR, et al. Is running associated with degenerative joint disease? *JAMA* 1986;255:1152–1154.
93. Konradsen L, Hansen E-M, Sondergaard L. Long distance running and osteoarthrosis. *Am J Sports Med* 1990;18:379–381.
94. Kujala UM, Kettunen H, Paananen H, et al. Knee osteoarthritis in former runners, soccer players, weight lifters and shooters. *Arthritis Rheum* 1995;38:539–546.
95. Vingård E, Alfredsson L, Goldie I, et al. Sports and osteoarthrosis of the hip: an epidemiologic study. *Am J Sports Med* 1993; 21:195–200.
96. Lane NE, Hochberg MC, Pressman A, et al. Recreational physical activity and the risk of osteoarthritis of the hip in elderly women. *J Rheumatol* 1999;26:849–854.
97. Marti B, Knobloch M, Tschopp A, et al. Is excessive running predictive of degenerative hip disease? Controlled study of former athletes. *Br Med J* 1989;229:91–93.

98. Linberg H, Roos H, Gardsell P. Prevalence of coxarthrosis in former soccer players. *Acta Orthop Scand* 1993;64:165–167.
99. Adams JE. Injury to the throwing arm: a study of traumatic changes in the elbow joints of boy baseball players. *Calif Med* 1965;102:127–129.
100. Bennet GE. Shoulder and elbow lesions of the professional baseball pitcher. *JAMA* 1941;117:510–514.
101. Rall K, McElroy G, Keats TE. A study of the long term effects of football injury in the knee. *Mo Med* 1964;61:435–438.
102. Cobb S, Merchant WR, Rubin T. The relation of symptoms to osteoarthritis. *J Chronic Dis* 1957;5:197–204.
103. Gresham GE, Rathey UK. Osteoarthritis in knees of aged persons: relationship between roentgenographic and clinical manifestations. *JAMA* 1975;233:168–170.
104. Hernborg J, Nilsson BE. The relationship between osteophytes in the knee joint, osteoarthritis and aging. *Acta Orthop Scand* 1973;44:69–74.
105. Tokunaga M, Ohuchi K, Yoshizawa S, et al. Change of prostaglandin E level in joint fluids after treatment with flurbiprofen in patients with rheumatoid arthritis and osteoarthritis. *Ann Rheum Dis* 1981;40:462–465.
106. Schumacher HR, Gordon G, Paul H, et al. Osteoarthritis, crystal deposition, and inflammation. *Semin Arthritis Rheum* 1981;11(suppl):116–119.
107. Ike RW, O'Rourke KS. Compartment-directed physical examination of the knee can predict articular cartilage abnormalities disclosed by needle arthroscopy. *Arthritis Rheum* 1995;38: 917–925.
108. Heberden W. *Commentaries on the history and cure of diseases.* London: T Payne, 1803.
109. Stecher RM, Hauser H. Heberden's nodes: roentgenological and clinical appearance of degenerative joint disease of fingers. *Am J Radiol* 1948;59:326–327.
110. Stecher RM. Heberden's nodes: heredity in hypertrophic arthritis of finger joints. *Am J Med Sci* 1941;201:801–809.
111. Horton WE, Lethbridge-Çejku M, Hochberg MC. An association between an aggrecan polymorphic allele and bilateral hand osteoarthritis in elderly white men: data from the Baltimore Longitudinal Study for Aging (BLSA). *Osteoarthritis Cartilage* 1998;6:245–251.
112. Eaton RG, Dobranski AI, Littler JW. Marginal osteophyte excision in treatment of mucous cysts. *J Bone Joint Surg Am* 1973; 55:570–574.
113. Patterson AC. Osteoarthritis of the trapezioscaphoid joint. *Arthritis Rheum* 1975;18:375–379.
114. Halverson BP, Cheung HS, McCarty DJ. Milwaukee shoulder syndrome (MSS): description of predisposing factors. *Arthritis Rheum* 1987;30:S131.
115. Ike RW, Arnold WJ, Simon C. Correlations between radiographic (XR) changes, meniscal chondrocalcinosis and other intra-articular (IA) abnormalities (ABN) in patients (PT) with osteoarthritis of the knee (OAK) undergoing arthroscopy (AR). *Arthritis Rheum* 1987;30:S131(abst).
116. Felson DT, Anderson JJ, Naimark A, et al. The prevalence of chondrocalcinosis in the elderly and its association with knee osteoarthritis: the Framingham study. *J Rheumatol* 1989;16: 1241–1245.
117. Felson DT, Zhang Y, Hannan MT, et al. The incidence and natural history of knee osteoarthritis in the elderly: the Framingham osteoarthritis study. *Arthritis Rheum* 1995;38: 1500–1505.
118. Cooper C, Egger P, Coggon D, et al. Generalized osteoarthritis in women: pattern of joint involvement and approaches to definition for epidemiological studies. *J Rheumatol* 1996;23:1938–1942.
119. Spector TD, Dacre JE, Harris PA, et al. Radiological progression of osteoarthritis: an 11 year follow-up study of the knee. *Ann Rheum Dis* 1992;51:1107–1110.
120. Evarts CM. Challenge of the aging hip. *Geriatrics* 1969;24: 112–119.
121. Meachim G, Whitehouse GH, Pedley RB, et al. An investigation of radiological, clinical and pathological correlations in osteoarthrosis of the hip. *Clin Radiol* 1980;31:565–574.
122. Macys JR, Bullough PG, Wilson PDJ. Coxarthrosis: a study of the natural history based on a correlation of clinical, radiographic, and pathologic findings. *Semin Arthritis Rheum* 1980; 10:66–80.
123. Jorring K. Osteoarthritis of the hip, epidemiology and clinical role. *Acta Orthop Scand* 1980;51:523–530.
124. Doherty M, Preston B. Primary osteoarthritis of the elbow. *Ann Rheum Dis* 1989;48:743–747.
125. McKendry RJR. Nodal osteoarthritis of the toes. *Arthritis Rheum* 1986;16:126–134.
126. Prince DS, Luna RF, Cohn MN, et al. Osteophyte-induced dysphagia: occurrence in ankylosing hyperostosis. *JAMA* 1975; 234:77–78.
127. Forestier J, Jaqueline F, Rotes-Querol J. *Ankylosing spondylitis: clinical considerations, roentgenology, pathologic anatomy, treatment.* Springfield, IL: Charles C Thomas, 1956.
128. Resnick D, Shaul SR, Robins JM. Diffuse idiopathic skeletal hyper-ostosis (DISH): Forestier's disease with extraspinal manifestations. *Radiology* 1975;115:513–524.
129. Utzinger PD, Resnick D, Shapiro R. Diffuse skeletal abnormalities in Forestier disease. *Arch Intern Med* 1976;136:763–768.
130. Harata S, Tohno S, Kawagishi T. Osteoarthritis of the atlanto-axial joint. *Int Orthop* 1981;5:277–282.
131. Katz JN, Dalgas M, Stucki G, et al. Degenerative lumbar spinal stenosis: diagnostic value of the history and physical examination. *Arthritis Rheum* 1995;38:1236–1241.
132. Arnoldi CC, Brodsky AE, Cauchoix J. Lumbar spinal stenosis and nerve root entrapment syndromes: definition and classification. *Clin Orthop* 1976;115:4–5.
133. Mehraban F, Finegan CK, Moskowitz RW. Serum keratan sulfate: quantitative and qualitative comparisons in inflammatory arthritides. *Arthritis Rheum* 1991;34:1435–1441.
134. Lohmander LS, Dahlberg L, Ryd L, et al. Increased levels of proteoglycan fragments in the knee joint after injury. *Arthritis Rheum* 1989;32:1434–1442.
135. Thonar EA-MA, Shinmei M, Lohmander L. Body fluid markers of cartilage changes in osteoarthritis. *Rheum Dis Clin North Am* 1993;19:635–657.
136. Campion GV, McCrae F, Schnitzer TJ, et al. Levels of keratan sulfate in the serum and synovial fluid of patients with osteoarthritis of the knee,. *Arthritis Rheum* 1991;34:1254–1259.
137. Carroll GJ, Bell MC, Laing BA, et al. Reduction of the concentrations and total amount of keratan sulphate in synovial fluid from patients with osteoarthritis during treatment with piroxicam. *Ann Rheum Dis* 1992;51:850–854.
138. Goldberg RL, Huff JP, Lenz ME, et al. Elevated plasma levels of hyaluronate in patients with osteoarthritis and rheumatoid arthritis. *Arthritis Rheum* 1991;34:799–807.
139. Lohmander LS. Markers of cartilage metabolism in arthrosis. *Acta Orthop Scand* 1991;62:623–632.
140. Lohmander LS, Hoerrner LA, Lark MW. Metalloproteinases, tissue inhibitor, and proteoglycan fragments in knee synovial fluid in human osteoarthritis. *Arthritis Rheum* 1993;36: 181–189.
141. Ratcliffe A, Israel HA, Saed-Nejad F, et al. Keratan sulfate epitope levels are elevated in synovial fluids from joints with arthroscopically diagnosed early osteoarthritis. *Orthop Res Soc Trans* 1991;16:228.

142. Saxne T, Heinegard D. Cartilage oligomeric matrix protein: a novel marker of cartilage turnover detectable in synovial fluid and blood. *Br J Rheumatol* 1992;31:583–591.
143. Saxne T, Heinegard D, Synovial fluid analysis of two groups of proteoglycan epitopes distinguishes early and late cartilage lesions. *Arthritis Rheum* 1992;35:385–390.
144. Siebel MJ, Duncan A, Robins SP. Urinary hydroxypyridinium crosslinks provide indices of cartilage and bone involvement in arthritic diseases. *J Rheumatol* 1989;16:964–970.
145. Shinmei N, Nagaya I, Miyanaga J, et al. Clinical usefulness of type II procollagen carboxypeptide (C-II propeptide, pColl-II-C) in synovial fluid as a marker of collagen metabolism in cartilage. *Ryumachki* 1992;32:453–460.
146. Thompson PW, Spector TD, James IT, et al. Urinary collagen crosslinks reflect the radiographic severity of knee osteoarthritis. *Br J Rheumatol* 1992;31:759–761.
147. Thonar EJ, Glant T. Serum keratan sulfate—a marker of predisposition to polyarticular osteoarthritis. *Clin Biochem* 1992; 25:175–180.
148. Walkovits LA, Bhardwaj N, Gallick GS, lMW. Detection of high levels of stromelysin and collagenase in synovial fluid from patients with rheumatoid arthritis and post-traumatic knee injury. *Arthritis Rheum* 1992;35:35–42.
149. Shinmei M, Inamori Y, Yoshihara Y, et al. The potential of cartilage markers in joint fluid for drug evaluation. In: Kuettner KE, Schleyerback R, Peyron JG, et al., eds. *Articular cartilage and osteoarthritis.* New York: Raven Press, 1992:597.
150. Manicourt DH, Lenz ME, Druetz-Van Egeren A, et al. Rapid and sustained rise in the serum level of hyaluronan following anterior cruciate ligament transection in the dog knee joint. *J Rheumatol* 1995;22:262–269.
151. Bleasel JF, Poole AR, Heinegård D, et al. Changes in serum cartilage marker levels indicate altered cartilage metabolism in families with osteoarthritis-related type II collagen (COL2A1) mutation. *Arthritis Rheum* 1999;42:39–45.
152. Ishiguro N, Ito T, Ito H, et al. Relationship of matrix metalloproteinases and their inhibitors to cartilage proteoglycan and collagen turnover: analyses of synovial fluid from patients with osteoarthritis. *Arthritis Rheum* 1999;42:129–136.
153. Lohmander LS, Ionescu M, Jugessur H, et al. Changes in joint cartilage aggrecan after knee injury and in osteoarthritis. *Arthritis Rheum* 1999;42:534–544.
154. Carroll GJ. Spectrophotometric measurement of proteoglycans in osteoarthritic synovial fluid. *Ann Rheum Dis* 1987;46:375–379.
155. Lohmander LS, Hoerrner LA, Dahlberg L, et al. Tissue inhibitor of metalloproteinases and proteoglycan fragments in human knee joint fluid after injury. *J Rheumatol* 1993;20: 1362–1368.
156. Conrozier T, Saxne T, Fan CS, et al. Serum concentrations of cartilage oligomeric matrix protein and bone sialoprotein in hip osteoarthritis: a one year prospective study. *Ann Rheum Dis* 1998;57:527–532.
157. Poole A, Ionescu M, Swan A, et al. Changes in cartilage metabolism in arthritis are reflected by altered serum and synovial fluid levels of the cartilage proteoglycan aggrecan. *J Clin Invest* 1994;94:25–33.
158. Sharif M, George E, Shepstone L, et al. Serum hyaluronic acid level as a predictor of disease progression in osteoarthritis of the knee. *Arthritis Rheum* 1995;38:760–767.
159. Balblanc JC, Hartmann D, Noyer D, et al. L'acide hyaluronique serique dans l'arthrose. *Rev Rheum Ed Fr* 1993;60:194–202.
160. Wolfe F. The C-reactive protein but not the erythrocyte sedimentation rate is associated with clinical severity in patients with osteoarthritis of the knee or hip. *J Rheumatol* 1997;24: 1486–1488.
161. Spector TD, Hart DJ, Nandra D, et al. Low-level increases in serum C-reactive protein are present in early osteoarthritis of the knee and predict progressive disease. *Arthritis Rheum* 1997; 40:723–727.
162. Brandt KD. A pessimistic view of serologic markers for diagnosis and management of osteoarthritis: biochemical, immunologic and clinicopathologic barriers. *J Rheumatol* 1989;16(suppl 18):39–42.
163. Cheung HS, Ryan LM, Kozin F, et al. Identification of collagen subtypes in synovial fluid sediments from arthritic patients. *Am J Med* 1980;68:73–79.
164. Fam AG, Pritzker KPH, Cheng P-T, et al. Cholesterol crystals in osteoarthritic joint effusions. *J Rheumatol* 1981;8:273–280.
165. Hutton CW, Watt I, Dieppe PA. Technetium-99m HMDP bone scanning in osteoarthritis: a predictor of joint progression. *Br J Radiol* 1986;59:807–808.
166. McCrae F, Shouls J, Dieppe P, et al. Scintigraphic assessment of osteoarthritis of the knee joint. *Ann Rheum Dis* 1992;51: 938–942.
167. Dieppe P, Cushnaghan J, Young P, et al. Prediction of the progression of joint space narrowing in osteoarthritis of the knee by bone scintigraphy. *Ann Rheum Dis* 1993;52:557–563.
168. Balblanc JC, Mathieu P, Mathieu L, et al. Second scintigraphy and radiographic progression of digital osteoarthritis. *Osteoarthritis Cartilage* 1994;2:38.
169. Fife RS, Brandt KD, Braunstein EM, et al. Relationship between arthroscopic evidence of cartilage damage and radiographic evidence of joint space narrowing in early osteoarthritis of the knee. *Arthritis Rheum* 1991;34:377–382.
170. Hernborg JS, Nilsson BE. The natural course of untreated osteoarthritis of the knee. *Clin Orthop* 1977;123:130–137.
171. Swezey RL, Peter JB, Evans PL. Osteoarthritis of the metacarpophalangeal joint: hook-like osteophytes. *Arthritis Rheum* 1969;12:405–410.
172. Martel W, Adler RS, Chan K, et al. Overview: new methods of imaging osteoarthritis. *J Rheumatol* 1991;18(suppl 27):32–37.
173. Li KC, Higgs J, Alsen AM, et al. MRI in osteoarthritis of the hip: gradations of severity: magnetic resonance imaging 1988;6: 229–236.
174. Bongartz G, Bock E, Horbach T, et al. Degenerative cartilage lesions of the hip: magnetic resonance evaluation. *Magn Reson Imaging* 1989;7:179–186.
175. Buckland-Wright JC, MacFarlane DG, Lynch JA, et al. Quantitative microfocal radiographic assessment of progression in osteoarthritis of the hand. *Arthritis Rheum* 1990;33:57–65.
176. Buckland-Wright JC, Bradshaw CR. Clinical applications of high definition microfocal radiography. *Br J Radiol* 1989;62: 209–217.
177. Myers SL, Dines K, Brandt DA, et al. Experimental assessment by high frequency ultrasound of articular cartilage thickness and OA changes. *J Rheumatol* 1995;22:109–116.
178. Kellgren JH, Moore R. Generalized osteoarthritis and Heberden's nodes. *Br Med J* 1952;1:181–187.
179. Crain DC. Interphalangeal osteoarthritis. *JAMA* 1961;175: 1049–1053.
180. Ehrlich GE. Inflammatory osteoarthritis. I. The clinical syndrome. *J Chronic Dis* 1972;25:317–328.
181. Forestier J, Lagier R. Ankylosing hyperostosis of the spine. *Clin Orthop* 1971;74:65–83.
182. DeHaven KE, Dolan WA, Mayer PJ. Chondromalacia patellae in athletes. *Am J Sports Med* 1979;7:1–5.
183. Dieppe PA, Doyle DV, Huskisson EC, et al. Mixed crystal deposition disease in osteoarthritis. *Br Med J* 1978;1: 150–152.
184. Dieppe PA, Alexander GJM, Jones HE, et al. Pyrophosphate

arthropathy: a clinical and radiological study of 105 cases. *Ann Rheum Dis* 1982;41:371–376.

185. Marcos JC, de Banyacar MA, Garcia-Morteo O, et al. Idiopathic familial chondrocalcinosis due to apatite crystal deposition. *Am J Med* 1981;71:557–564.
186. Halverson PB, McCarty DJ. Patterns of radiographic abnormalities associated with basic calcium phosphate and calcium pyrophosphate dihydrate crystal deposition in the knee. *Ann Rheum Dis* 1986;45:603–605.
187. Baldwin C, Farrer LA, Adair R, et al. Linkage of early-onset osteoarthritis and chondrocalcinosis to human chromosome 8q. *Am J Hum Genet* 1995;56:692–697.
188. Hughes AE, McGibbon D, Woodward E, et al. Localisation of a gene for chondrocalcinosis to chromosome 5p. *Hum Mol Genet* 1995;4:1225–1228.
189. Williams CJ, Hardwick LJ, Butcher S, et al. Linkage of chondrocalcinosis to chromosome 5p15.1-.2 in a large Argentinian pedigree. *Am J Hum Genet* 1996;S59:A242.
190. Andrew LJ, Brancolini V, delaPena L, et al. Refinement of the chromosome 5p locus for familial calcium pyrophosphate dihydrate deposition disease. *Am J Hum Genet* 1999;64:136–145.
191. Ohno O, Cooke TD. Electron microscopic morphology of immunoglobulin aggregates and their interaction in rheumatoid articular collagenous tissues. *Arthritis Rheum* 1978;21: 516–517.
192. Utzinger PD, Fite FL. Immunologic evidence for inflammation (I) in osteoarthritis (OA): high percentage of Ia+ T lymphocytes (L) in the synovial fluid (SL) and synovium (S) of patients with erosive osteo-arthritis (EOA). *Arthritis Rheum* 1982;25:S44(abst).
193. Shuckett R, Russell ML, Gladman DD. Atypical erosive osteoarthritis and Sjögren's syndrome. *Ann Rheum Dis* 1986;45:281–288.
194. Schlapbach P, Beyeler CH, Gerber NJ, et al. The prevalence of palpable finger joint nodules in diffuse idiopathic skeletal hyperostosis (DISH): a controlled study. *Br J Rheumatol* 1992; 31:531–534.
195. Resnick D, Shapiro RF, Wiesner KB, et al. Diffuse idiopathic skeletal hyperostosis (DISH) (ankylosing hyperostosis of Forestier and Rotes-Querol). *Semin Arthritis Rheum* 1978;7: 153–187.
196. Kmucha ST, Cravens RBJ. DISH syndrome and its role in dysphagia. *Otolaryngol Head Neck Surg* 1994;110:431–436.
197. Stechison MT, Tator CH. Cervical myelopathy in diffuse idiopathic skeletal hyperostosis: case report. *J Neurosurg* 1990;73: 279–282.
198. Crosby ET, Grahovac S. Diffuse idiopathic skeletal hyperostosis: an unusual cause of difficult intubation. *Can J Anesth* 1993; 40:54–58.
199. Maertens M, Mielants H, Verstraete K, et al. Simultaneous occurrence of diffuse idiopathic skeletal hyperostosis and ankylosing spondylitis in the same patient. *J Rheumatol* 1992;19: 1978–1982.
200. Robbes-Ruyn E, Rojo-Mejia, Harrison-Garcin Calderon J, et al. Diffuse idiopathic skeletal hyperostosis: clinical and radiologic manifestations in 50 patients. *Arthritis Rheum* 1982;25:S101(abst).
201. Littlejohn GO. Insulin and new bone formation in diffuse idiopathic skeletal hyperostosis. *Clin Rheum* 1985;4:294–300.
202. Denko CW, Boja B, Moskowitz RW. Growth-promoting peptides: insulin-like growth factor-1, insulin, growth hormone in diffuse idiopathic skeletal hyperostosis. *Arthritis Rheum* 1989;32(suppl):S84(abst).
203. Altomonte L, Zoli A, Mirone L, et al. Growth hormone secretion in diffuse idiopathic skeletal hyperostosis. *Ann Ital Med Int* 1992;7:30–33.
204. Shapiro R, Utsinger PD, Wiesner KB. The association of HLA-B27 with Forestier's disease (vertebral ankylosing hyperostosis). *J Rheumatol* 1976;3:4–8.
205. Spagnole A, Bennett P, Terasaki P. Vertebral ankylosing hyperostosis (Forestier's disease) and HLA antigens in Pima Indians. *Arthritis Rheum* 1978;21:467–472.
206. Abiteboul M, Mazieres B, Laffont F, et al. Hyperostose vertebral ankylosante et metabolisme de la vitamine A. *Rev Rhum* 1981; 9:8–9.
207. DiGiovanni JJ, Helfgott RK, Gerber HL, et al. Extraspinal tendon and ligament calcification associated with long-term therapy with etretinate. *N Engl J Med* 1986;315:1177–1182.
208. Periquet B, Lambert W, Garcia J, et al. Increased concentrations of endogenous 13-cis- and all-trans-retinoic acids in diffuse idiopathic skeletal hyperostosis, as demonstrated by HPLC. *Clin Chim Acta* 1991;203:57–65.
209. Mills DM, Taves DR, Pal DP, et al. Association of diffuse idiopathic spinal hyperostosis and fluorosis. *Arthritis Rheum* 1983; 26(suppl):511.
210. Ono K, Ota H, Tada K, et al. Ossified posterior longitudinal ligament: a clinicopathologic study. *Spine* 1977;2:126–138.
211. Gagliardi JA, Chung EM, Chandnani VP, et al. Detection and staging of chondromalacia patellae: relative efficacies of conventional MR imaging, MR arthrography, and CT arthrography. *Am J Radiol* 1994;163:629–636.
212. Nilsson BE, Danielsson LG, Hernborg SAJ. Clinical feature and natural course of coxarthrosis and gonarthrosis. *Scand J Rheumatol* 1982;43(suppl):13–21.
213. Felson DT. The course of osteoarthritis and factors that affect it. *Rheum Dis Clin North Am* 1993;19:607–615.
214. Rosenberg ZS, Shankman S, Steiner GC, et al. Rapid destructive osteoarthritis: clinical, radiographic and pathologic features. *Radiology* 1992;182:213–216.
215. Brandt KD. Should osteoarthritis be treated with nonsteroidal antiinflammatory drugs? *Rheum Dis Clin North Am* 1993;19: 697–712.
216. O'Brien WM, La Du BN, Bunim JJ. Biochemical, pathologic and clinical aspects of alcaptonuria, ochronosis and ochronotic arthropathy: review of world literature (1584-1962). *Am J Med* 1963;34:813–838.
217. Janocha S, Wolz W, Soren S, et al. The human gene for alkaptonuria maps to chromosome 3q. *Genomics* 1994;19:5–8.
218. Maier-Dobersberger T, Fererci P, Polli C, et al. Detection of the His 1069 Gln mutation in Wilson disease by rapid polymerase chain reaction. *Ann Intern Med* 1997;127:21–26.
219. Menerey KA, Eider W, Brewer GJ, et al. The arthropathy of Wilson's disease: clinical and pathologic features. *J Rheumatol* 1988;15:331–337.
220. Kramer U, Weinberger A, Yarom R, et al. Synovial copper distribution as a possible explanation for arthropathy in Wilson's disease. *Bull Hosp Joint Dis* 1993;52:46–49.
221. Schumacher RH. Articular cartilage in the degenerative arthropathy of hemochromatosis. *Arthritis Rheum* 1982;25: 1460–1468.
222. Nesterov AI. The clinical course of Kashin-Beck disease. *Arthritis Rheum* 1964;7:29–40.
223. Wei XW, Wright GC, Sokoloff L. The effect of sodium selenite on chondrocytes in monolayer culture. *Arthritis Rheum* 1986; 29:660–664.
224. Bluestone R, Bywaters EGL, Hartog M, et al. Acromegalic arthropathy. *Ann Rheum Dis* 1971;30:243–258.
225. Littlejohn GO, Hall S, Brand CA, et al. New bone formation in acromegaly. *Clin Exp Rheum* 1986;499–104.
226. Wilkins E, Dieppe P, Maddison P, et al. Osteoarthritis and articular chondrocalcinosis in the elderly. *Ann Rheum Dis* 1983;42: 280–284.

227. Gerster JC, Vischer TL, Fallet GH. Destructive arthropathy in generalized osteoarthritis with articular chondrocalcinosis. *J Rheumatol* 1975;2:265–269.
228. Halverson BP, McCarty DJ, Cheung HS, et al. Milwaukee shoulder syndrome: eleven additional cases with involvement of the knee in seven (basic calcium phosphate crystal deposition disease). *Semin Arthritis Rheum* 1984;14:36–44.
229. Fam AG, Protzner EM, Carrie P, et al. Acceleration of experimental osteoarthritis by calcium pyrophosphate microcrystalline synovitis. *Arthritis Rheum* 1995;38:201–210.
230. Charcot JM. Sur quelques arthropathies qui paraissent dépendre d'une lésion du cerveau ou de la moelle épinère: arthridited dans l'hémiplégie de cause cérébrale. *Arch Physiol Norm Pathol* 1868;2:379–400.
231. Gottlieb NL, Risken WG. Complications of local corticosteroid injections. *JAMA* 1980;243:1547–1548.

112

MANAGEMENT OF OSTEOARTHRITIS

CARLOS J. LOZADA
ROY D. ALTMAN

Osteoarthritis (OA) is the most common articular rheumatic disease, affecting approximately 12% of the United States population between the ages of 25 and 74 years (1). Although variable in its presentation, OA often carries significant morbidity. In addition to the effects on the individual, the economic impact of OA on society is significant. This cost is related to the high prevalence of OA, reduced avocational and vocational activities of patients with OA, the occasional loss of patient's ability at self-care, and the related drain on health care resources (2). With significant improvement in our understanding of the etiopathogenesis of OA, there have been changes in the conceptual approach to management, providing new emphasis on potential preventive measures and a more comprehensive approach to treatment (3). Guidelines for the management of OA at specific sites have been developed and reported (4,5). Guidelines for the conduct of clinical trials in OA have likewise been developed (6).

Therapeutic considerations must incorporate concepts that OA is no longer considered a "degenerative" or "wear and tear" arthritis, but rather involves dynamic biomechanical, biochemical, and cellular processes (7). The joint damage that occurs in OA occurs at least in part through active remodeling involving all the joint structures (8). Although articular cartilage continues to be at the center of change, OA is now viewed as a disease of the entire joint, and therefore failure of the joint as an organ.

Before considering a therapeutic regimen for OA, the correct diagnosis must be verified (9–11). The development of a therapeutic program also must consider that OA differs in symptoms, signs, and function in different joints, implying different therapeutic options. The most effective therapeutic program is prevention. Several factors may predispose to the development of OA, such as trauma, infection, and obesity. Specific preventive measures can be directed at altering these risk factors.

Presently most therapy is directed at symptoms. Although a variety of symptoms exist—such as "giving way," instability, weakness, limited function, and deformity—pain is the most common symptom that causes the patient to seek assistance.

With the advent of new approaches to therapy, medication-based interventions for the treatment of OA are now classified as follows; (12) (a) symptom-modifying agents. These may be directed at short-term benefit [e.g., nonsteroidal antiinflammatory drugs (NSAIDs)] or long-term benefit (e.g., intraarticular depocorticosteroids or hyaluronate); and (b) structure (disease)-modifying agents. These medications are intended to prevent, arrest, or reverse the process of OA. These agents are classified according to whether they directly affect symptoms or have no direct effects on symptoms.

There also has been an effort to subject therapies that have been generally considered "alternative" (13, 14) to appropriate clinical trials as both symptom modifying or structure modifying.

PAIN

Pain is most often the reason a patient with OA will seek the help of a physician (15). It is unclear why only 40% of patients with severe radiographic OA [Kellgren and Lawrence grade III and IV (16)] have pain (17). Even when it is present, the origin of the pain is often not clear, as pain in OA has many potential causes (18). Pain can be difficult to localize to an area within the joint. In knee OA, patients will most commonly describe their pain as involving the entire joint. In one study, medial knee pain was reported in 34% of patients with OA of the knee as compared with 52% reporting "generalized" knee pain (19). A thorough history and physical examination may help direct symptomatic therapy by revealing and hence allowing the physician to address the origin of the pain. We have elected to categorize the origin of pain by anatomic site (Table 112.1). Therapy is more effective when directed at the causes of pain.

Indirect Causes of Pain

Damage to *articular cartilage* is the hallmark of OA, yet articular cartilage does not generate a pain response because

TABLE 112.1. PAIN IN OSTEOARTHRITIS

Structure	Mechanism
Cartilage	"Char" fragments
	Crystal release
	Enzyme release
	Stimulation of inflammatory mediators
	Stress on subchondral bone
	Joint instability
Menisci	Tearing or degeneration/stretching at their insertion to the capsule
Synovium	Increased in fluid volume, which can carry cartilage products and inflammatory cells
	Infiltration with inflammatory cells
Subchondral bone	Ischemia and increased vascular pressure
	Repair of infarcted bone
Osteophytes	Periosteal elevation
	Neural impingement
Joint capsule	Stretch from joint distention
	Stress at insertion to periosteum and bone
Ligaments	Stretch at insertion to periosteum and bone
Bursae	Inflammation, with or without calcification
Muscle	Spasm
	Nocturnal myoclonus
	Contractures
Central nervous system	Psychologic stress/sleep deprivation

it lacks nerve endings (20,21). *Menisci* similarly do not contain nerves, except away from compressive forces on their outer third, and cannot directly account for pain. Teleologically, it makes evolutionary sense that compressive or shear forces on cartilage would not elicit pain, as pain would make locomotion burdensome. Nevertheless, *articular cartilage, menisci,* and even *synovial fluid* can indirectly cause pain in OA. Damaged *articular cartilage* causes symptoms as a result of structural damage, structural debris, and its loss. Structurally damaged cartilage no longer has the ability to allow the even gliding characteristic of smooth cartilage surfaces. This results in a grinding or clicking sensation to the patient and crepitus on examination. Some patients interpret these sensations as painful.

Damaged *cartilage "char" fragments* released into the synovial cavity are removed by the synovium, stimulating an inflammatory synovial response. Other microscopic and submicroscopic particulate material released from damaged articular cartilage—such as collagen, proteoglycans, crystals, proteolytic enzymes and cytokines—trigger a synovial inflammatory response of varying degrees. Although inflammation of the synovium in OA is most often less severe than in the "inflammatory" arthritides such as rheumatoid arthritis (RA) and gout, some degree of inflammation is almost always present in the joints affected by OA (justifying the terminology of osteoarthritis) (22,23).

Abnormal cartilage may contain a variety of basic calcium phosphate crystals, such as calcium pyrophosphate dihydrate. Surface disruption may lead to "crystal shedding" into the joint cavity, stimulating varying degrees of inflammation (24). In cases in which cartilage is fissured and the subchondral bone is exposed, hydroxyapatite crystals from bone or cartilage may leach out or be sheared into the synovial cavity. A role has been proposed for hydroxyapatite crystals in causing inflammation (25,26). The absence of articular cartilage allows loosening and instability of the joint with resultant changes in the paraarticular structures described later.

Other loose bodies in the joint (27) are potential indirect causes of pain. Torn *menisci* can be displaced and inserted between normally smooth, gliding articular surfaces, altering normal biomechanics and causing direct articular cartilage damage. Vertically fissured menisci such as "bucket-handle" and "parrot's beak" tears, do not provide the appropriate biomechanical support for the joint, altering mechanical loading, and promoting cartilage damage. Pain can sometimes be elicited on examination when the torn meniscus is stressed at its outer third or when partially torn menisci "catch" between cartilage surfaces. Horizontal fissures usually do not cause symptoms, but fragments of the defective menisci may elicit an inflammatory response or act as loose bodies in the joint cavity. Therapy, mostly arthroscopic, of torn menisci is directed at retention or restoration of normal anatomy.

Synovial fluid can indirectly cause pain by serving as a transport medium, distending the joint capsule and limiting joint function. The synovial fluid shuttles inflammatory mediators back and forth between the cartilage and synovium. Synovial fluid also serves as a reservoir for inflammatory products, cells, and crystals. Furthermore, synovial fluid distends the joint capsule, potentially compressing blood vessels, leading to the stimulation of pressure receptors in the capsule (28–30) and the nerves that innervate the compressed blood vessels. Joint distention also compromises the transport of nutrients and oxygen from the synovium to cartilage and waste products from cartilage to synovium. These waste products then linger in the synovial space, perpetuating inflammation. Thus, removal of excess synovial fluid volume with its inflammatory mediators is in itself an effective therapeutic modality, even in the absence of other interventions.

Direct Causes of Pain

Unmyelinated C fibers and partially myelinated A-delta fibers carry pain from the periphery to the central nervous system (31). These pain receptors may be activated through peripheral mechanical, thermal, and noxious stimuli. These noxious stimuli include bradykinin, histamine, prostaglandins, and leukotrienes (32).

The *synovium* contains nerve fibers, including A-beta large myelinated mechanoreceptors, A-delta small myelinated nociceptors, and C-small nonmyelinated nociceptors. These nociceptors can release both substance P and calcitonin gene–related peptide (CGRP). Substance P stimulates both the pain response and inflammation (33).

The *subchondral bone* might directly contribute to pain in OA by virtue of nociceptors such as substance P and CGRP (34). When subchondral ischemia or increased arterial pressures occur, these peptides are released from the nerve endings in bone (35). The pain of ischemic bone is aching and deep-seated. When bone death occurs (avascular necrosis), there is a pain-free period. Pain recurs with bone repair and remodeling. In OA, subchondral cysts and sclerosis are the eventual radiographic evidence that localized avascular necrosis has taken place. Relief of the pain of ischemic bone has not been specifically studied; analgesics, NSAIDs, and/or salmon calcitonin may be of value. It is uncertain whether there is a component of neurogenic pain to the bone pain for which a different set of medications might be considered.

Osteophytes are the most consistent clinical finding related to the presence of pain. The mechanisms are not clear, but osteophytes may cause pain directly by distending the periosteum; pain can sometimes be elicited by applying pressure over the osteophyte. Pain from osteophytes may be from concomitant inflammation, the latter potentially treatable with NSAIDs or local injection of lidocaine (with or without depocorticosteroids). Osteophytes in the spinal facets are often an indirect cause of pain and other symptoms by compressing nerves as they traverse the spinal foramina (e.g., cervical, lumbar lateral recess) or within the spinal canal (e.g., lumbar spinal stenosis).

The *joint capsule* and periarticular *ligaments* are stretched by synovial effusions (see earlier) or instability and may cause pain through mechanoreceptors and nociceptors. Stress at the ligamentous insertion on the *periosteum* stimulates nociceptors. When the joint periarticular tissues are distorted, the ligaments may be abnormally stressed or may be understressed (e.g., varus deformity of the knee stresses the lateral ligaments and fully relaxes the medial ligaments). These phenomena, labeled stress enhancement and stress deprivation (36), result in contractures of the capsule and ligaments. Contractures result in decreasing function and increasing pain. Under these conditions, range-of-motion exercises are needed to prevent/reverse contractures. NSAIDs are of value if inflammation is present, but otherwise have limited use.

Periarticular *bursae* may become inflamed and hence a source of pain. Often detected on physical examination, the associated inflammation tends to respond more effectively to local lidocaine injections containing depocorticosteroids than to NSAIDs. Bursal inflammation is sometimes associated with calcium formation (e.g., calcific bursitis). Aspiration of inflammatory fluid and calcium followed by injection of depocorticosteroids with lidocaine (as an anesthetic) is most often effective. It is uncommonly necessary to remove calcium deposits surgically from a bursa.

Muscle spasm is probably a common source of pain in OA, particularly in cervical and lumbar spine OA. Muscle spasm may occur in the form of nocturnal myoclonus, altering sleep patterns and resulting in fibromyalgia-like symptoms (37). Muscle spasm of the lower extremities must be differentiated from pain of vascular (e.g., night cramps) or spinal radicular origin. Muscle contractures in OA can cause pain on stretching.

Finally, joint pain is related to the individual's perception of that pain and to the individual's unique ethnic, cultural, and personal circumstances. Pain tends to be more severe in the evenings, on weekends, and early in the work week (38). Pain is complicated by the presence of dysthymia, other forms of depression, cyclothymia, and secondary gains. Psychologic intervention may be needed in the evaluation of the overlying psychologic influences on the pain response.

PREVENTIVE THERAPY

Although many of the presently established risk factors, such as age and genetics, cannot be modified, some risk factors can be altered. Based on emerging epidemiologic data, the single most important factor emerging from epidemiologic trials that can potentially be altered is obesity. Obesity in women has been linked to OA of the knees (39,40) and is probably a risk factor in both the hip and knee joints in both sexes (41). A link between weight and OA of the hands has been proposed as well (42,43). The mechanisms have not been clearly elaborated and may include increase in body mass, altered biodynamics of gait (44), genetic predisposition (genetically obese mice get more OA), and/or altered metabolism (e.g., estrogens).

Metabolic correlates of OA have been investigated as well. Data from 1,003 women between the ages of 45 and 64 years from the Chingford population study has suggested that, even after adjustment for age and body mass index, hypertension, hypercholesterolemia, and elevated blood glucose may be associated with unilateral and bilateral OA of the knee (45). The Baltimore Longitudinal Study of Aging cohort did not show these relations when adjustments for age and obesity were made (46).

Weight loss should be a goal in obese patients, as modest weight loss has been accompanied by a decrease in symptoms (47) and perhaps reduced radiographic progression. Other studies have shown that a reduction in percentage of body fat rather than weight may be significant in reducing pain from OA of the knee (48).

The role of occupational trauma in OA is not always clear. However, occupations involving considerable bending seem to be related to OA of the knees. Changes in certain repetitive motions, severe trauma, and bending may be indicated. Weakness of the quadriceps muscles, relative to body weight, has been reported as a possible risk factor for OA of the knees (49).

SYMPTOMATIC THERAPY

An individualized therapeutic program should be designed once the causes of pain have been assessed. The most effective symptomatic therapy combines several approaches and may be more effective if multidisciplinary (e.g., the rheumatologist, physiatrist, orthopedist, physical therapist, occupational therapist, psychologist, psychiatrist, nurse/nurse coordinator, dietitian, and social worker).

The physician-directed therapeutic program should include a combination of physical measures, medicinal measures, psychological approaches, and surgical interventions.

Physical Measures

A variety of physical modalities are of value for relieving pain, reducing stiffness, and limiting muscle spasm. These include strengthening the paraarticular structures to provide improved joint support. Physical measures make up an integral part of any successful therapeutic program for OA. Physical measures may be subdivided into exercise, supportive devices, alterations in activities of daily living, and thermal modalities (Table 112.2).

Exercise is the most commonly used physical measure and is most effective after some pain relief has been obtained. In patients with OA, exercise programs have been linked to reduced pain and improved function (50,51). Although professional guidance will be required in some patients, in most instances, exercises can be performed by the patient after minimal instruction. Range-of-motion exercises can be active or passive. Active exercises involve strengthening and can be isometric, isotonic, or isokinetic (52). Improved muscle tone reduces muscle spasm and prevents contractures. It is theorized that improved muscle support of the joint will retard the progression of OA. Exercises that improve muscle tone must be isometric and isotonic (which improve the function of the red "endurance" muscle fibers) as well as aerobic (53), perhaps even including progressive resistance exercises (which improve white "strength" fibers). Commonly used aerobic exercises include walking, swimming, and (stationary) bicycle riding. Selective atrophy of the type I "red" fibers occurs with immobilization (54).

TABLE 112.2. PHYSICAL MEASURES IN THE MANAGEMENT OF OSTEOARTHRITIS

- Exercise
  - Passive range of motion
  - Rest periods
  - Active: range of motion, isometric, isotonic, isokinetic
- Support devices and orthotics
  - Canes
  - Crutches
  - Collars
  - Shoe insoles
  - Medial taping of the patella
  - Knee braces
- Modified activities of daily living
  - Proper positioning and support when sitting, sleeping, or driving a car
  - Adjusting ways of performing such activities as getting dressed, etc.
  - Adjusting furnishings around the house or at work (e.g., raising the level of a chair or toilet seat)
- Thermal modalities
  - Superficial heat (e.g., hot packs, paraffin baths)
  - Deep heat (e.g., ultrasound)
  - Cold applications (e.g., cold packs, vapocoolant sprays)
- Miscellaneous
  - Pulsed electromagnetic fields
  - Transcutaneous electrical nerve stimulation (TENS)
  - Acupuncture
  - Chiropractic
  - Spa, massage, and yoga therapy

Improved strength of the paraarticular structures resulting from exercise adds stability and support to the joint and appears to reduce symptoms. A supervised program of fitness walking and education improves functional status without worsening OA of the knee (55). Patients with OA should be encouraged to exercise—the myth that any exercise worsens arthritis should be dispelled. The onset of the exercise program should be carefully graded. If the regimen is advanced too quickly, symptoms may worsen, and compliance is threatened. The patient should be advised that worsening pain is a warning sign that exercise tolerance has been reached.

It is proposed that lumbar spine exercises are effective in providing better function, decreased pain, and improved flexibility (56). Back schools teach an exercise program consisting of stretching of proximal thigh muscles, strengthening abdominal and paraspinal muscles, posture training, and an aerobic conditioning program. Among the specific exercises sometimes used in back pain patients are the Williams flexion exercises (56–58). These are indicated for musculoskeletal and mechanical low back pain and mild spinal stenosis. They are contraindicated in patients with osteoporosis or symptomatic herniated nucleus pulposus. In these patients, McKenzie exercises could be useful (56,58). There is no advantage to bed rest for patients with acute or chronic low back pain (59). The value of exercise for chronic low back pain should not be confused with the advantages of normal physical activities for acute low back pain (60).

Other muscle groups should be exercised. Strengthening of the quadriceps muscles in a patient with knee OA can improve function and decrease pain for up to 8 months (61). Indeed, there is some question as to whether the muscle weakness actually precedes the development of symptomatic OA. Care should be taken to choose exercises that maximize muscle strengthening while minimizing stress on the affected joints. Involvement in some particular sport or activity may need to be curtailed or replaced. Swimming is particularly effective in that it exercises multiple muscle groups and is useful in nearly all forms of OA. There are exceptions in which specific exercises may actually worsen symptoms: for instance, chondromalacia patella may be worsened by bicycle riding, and lumbar facet OA may be worsened by hyperextension of the spine such as in swimming.

Supportive devices are often of value as a supplement to the exercise program. Supportive devices partially unload the joint and may improve symptoms. Some of these devices include canes, crutches, walkers, corsets, collars, orthotics for shoes, and sometimes cervical traction. Canes, when properly used, can increase the base of support, and decrease loading and demands on the lower limb and its joints (62). As a consequence, devices such as canes, forearm crutches, crutches, and walkers can improve balance and decrease pain. The total length of a properly measured cane should be equal to the distance between the upper border of the greater trochanter of the femur and the bottom of the heel of the shoe. This should result in elbow flexion of about 20 degrees. The cane should be held in the hand contralateral to and moved together with the affected limb. The healthier limb should precede the affected limb when climbing up stairs; when climbing down stairs, the cane and the affected limb should be advanced first. The cane can unload the affected hip by 60% (63).

Proper footwear and orthotic shoes can be of great value. A short leg that accentuates lumbar scoliosis may be helped through a unilateral heel or sole lift. An orthotic device, or shoe insert, may help the patient with subluxed metatarsophalangeal joints (64). Walking ability and pain in early medial compartment OA of the knee can be improved by the use of a lateral heel-wedged insole (65,66). Athletic shoes with good mediolateral support, good medial arch, and calcaneal cushion can be of benefit.

Medial taping of the patella has been advocated for patients with OA of the patellofemoral compartment of the knee (67). Knee braces may be of use in some patients with tibiofemoral disease (68), especially those with lateral instability and those with a tendency for the knee to "give out."

All these various supports and orthotics will allow the patient to pursue more activities, improve compliance, and allow the patient to retain functional independence. The use of the devices should be frequently monitored to ensure proper use. Examples of this include use of cervical collars intermittently at the start, proper sizing of the collar, and proper orientation of the collar. Cane/crutch tips should be changed when worn, to avoid slipping on smooth or wet surfaces.

There may need to be some alteration in performance of *activities of daily living*. Simple instructions on adjusting daily activities may be very helpful in decreasing symptoms. For example, patients with back pain should be instructed not to sit on soft couches or recliners and not to lie in bed with a pillow under the knees. They should be advised to sit in straight-back chairs with good structural support (cushions allowed). Raising the level of a chair or toilet seat can be helpful because the hip and knee are subjected to the highest pressures during the initial phase of rising from the seated position (69). However, lift chairs are only rarely necessary. The patient should also be advised to use a firm bed, perhaps with a bed board, and not to slouch, even when driving. The car seat should be placed forward so that the knees are flexed during driving. Stress on low back structures from slouching or sitting in soft chairs/recliners often becomes manifest the next morning when the patient has pain on rising from bed.

Thermal modalities can be particularly effective. There is no advantage of superficial heat modalities over cold applications (70). The use of heat, cold, or alternating heat and cold are based on patient preference. Traditionally, the more acute the process, the more likely cold applications will be of benefit (71). The use of heat can be subdivided into superficial and deep, with no proven advantage of one over the other (72–74). Hot packs, paraffin baths, fluidotherapy, hydrotherapy, and radiant heat are vehicles for providing superficial heat. Deep heat can be provided by using ultrasound, usually for larger joints such as hips. The therapeutic value of applying heat includes decreasing joint stiffness, alleviating pain, relieving muscle spasm, and preventing contractures. Heat modalities should be used with caution in anesthetized, somnolent, or obtunded patients. The use of heat is contraindicated over tissues with inadequate vascular supply, bleeding, or cancer. Heat also should be avoided in areas close to the testicles or near developing fetuses (75). The range of temperatures used are from 40°C to 45°C (104°F–113°F) (76) for 3 to 30 minutes. Cold is used mostly in the form of cold packs or vapocoolant sprays to relieve muscle spasm, decrease swelling in acute trauma, and relieve pain from inflammation.

There are several *miscellaneous* physical modalities, such as massage, yoga therapy (77), acupressure, acupuncture (78), magnets, pulsed electromagnetic fields (79), transcutaneous neural stimulation (TENS) (80), and spa therapy. Many of these programs are of unproven value and work through unclear mechanisms. Chiropractic or other forms of manipulation will often transiently relieve the pain of muscle spasm; repeated manipulations are often needed because of the short-lived benefit. Some other physical measures have advocates. Spa therapy (mud packs, mineral baths) was superior to tap-water baths in the treatment of OA of the knee in one trial (81). TENS is cumbersome, expensive, and may be better suited to acute or subacute pain than to chronic pain of OA.

Medication-based Symptomatic Therapy

Medications used to treat symptoms in OA can be divided into categories of antiinflammatory agents, nonantiinflammatory analgesic agents, antispasmodics, and depocorticosteroids (Table 112.3).

TABLE 112.3. MEDICINAL MEASURES IN THE MANAGEMENT OF OSTEOARTHRITIS

- Symptomatic therapy
  - Short acting
    - Nonsteroidal antiinflammatory agents
    - COX-2 inhibitors
    - Nonantiinflammatory analgesics (opioids, nonopioids)
    - Antispasmodics
  - Long acting
    - Intraarticular depocorticosteroids
    - Intraarticular hyaluronic acid
    - *S*-adenosylmethionine (SAM)[a]
    - Chondroitin sulfate[a]
    - Glucosamine sulfate[a]
    - Intraarticular orgotein[a]
    - Diacerhein[a]
    - Estrogens[a]
    - Avocado/soy nonsaponifiables[a]
    - Pulse electromagnetic fields[a]
    - Ginger extracts[a]
    - "Popular culture" remedies[a]
- Disease-modifying agents
  - Tetracyclines[a]
  - Collagenase inhibitors[a]
  - Glycosaminoglycan polysulfuric acid (GAGPS)[a]
  - Glycosaminoglycan–peptide complexes[a]
  - Pentosan polysulfate[a]
  - Growth factors and cytokines (e.g., TGF-β)[a]
  - Genetic therapy[a]
  - Osteochondral grafts and stem cell transplantation[a]

COX, cyclooxygenase.
[a]Investigational therapy

Patients often inquire about the benefit of diets, vitamins, and minerals. At this time, there is no adequate evidence that any of these improve the symptoms or underlying disease. That is, they do not seem to affect the metabolism of cartilage or the natural history of OA. Therefore ingestion of special diets, vitamins, zinc, or copper, beyond the recommended daily requirements, is not encouraged.

Antiinflammatory Drugs

NSAIDs are the most commonly prescribed agents (82) for treatment of both pain and inflammation in OA. Discussions of the pharmacology and potential differences among these agents are included in Chapter 32 and published elsewhere (83).

Analgesia can be achieved at smaller doses of most NSAIDs than are needed for antiinflammatory effects (84). Indeed, for most NSAIDs, the greater the dose, the greater the antiinflammatory effect (also the greater risk of an adverse reaction). Because inflammation is usually not severe in OA, only smaller doses of NSAIDs may be required. In OA, the NSAID can be titrated to the lowest effective dose. Because the pain of OA is often intermittent, the use of NSAIDs in OA also can similarly be intermittent. There is some indication that analgesics lacking significant antiinflammatory effects may be of benefit in many patients with OA (85).

The major potential adverse effects of NSAIDs are gastrointestinal (peptic ulcer disease, gastritis) (86) and renal (interstitial nephritis, prostaglandin-inhibition–related renal insufficiency). These adverse effects are more prevalent in the elderly (87), the population with the highest prevalence of OA.

Effective strategies have been developed to mitigate the gastrointestinal toxicity of the NSAIDs: use of low-dose NSAID, use of a nonacetylated salicylate, concomitant use of misoprostol or a gastrointestinal proton pump inhibitor, use of a specific cyclooxygenase (COX)-2 inhibitor, topical analgesics, and/or intraarticular therapy with a depocorticosteroid or hyaluronate.

The timing of the dose of the NSAID may be important; indomethacin administered at 8 p.m. caused fewer adverse reactions than when administered at 8 a.m. (88). The effects of NSAIDs on articular cartilage and the outcome of OA are controversial (89,90). However, there is increasing evidence that indomethacin has long-term adverse effects on the outcome of OA (91).

Misoprostol, a synthetic prostaglandin E_1 analog, can be taken orally and reduces the incidence of gastric adverse events in patients receiving NSAIDs (92). In several clinical trials, the incidence of gastroduodenal ulceration in patients taking NSAIDs has been reduced by misoprostol in doses ranging from 200 μg b.i.d. to q.i.d (93). However, the incidence of diarrhea and abdominal pain is increased (94).

Misoprostol also is available as a combination product with diclofenac. The combination diclofenac/misoprostol (50 or 75 mg diclofenac/200 μg misoprostol) has comparable efficacy to diclofenac, with reduced gastric and duodenal ulceration. The incidence of diarrhea and flatulence was increased with diclofenac/misoprostol (95).

Proton-pump inhibitors such as omeprazole (20 mg p.o., q.d.) have also been shown to reduce the incidence of gastric and duodenal endoscopic ulceration when taken by patients taking NSAIDs (96). Their beneficial effect on gastric mucosa, as assessed endoscopically, has been equivalent to that of full doses of misoprostol (200 μg, q.i.d.) in some studies (97). Although effective for symptoms, other purported gastroprotective agents such as H_2 blockers have not been so effective (98).

Patients vary in their benefit from and adverse reactions to the various NSAIDs. Differences in half-lives of the NSAIDs may influence patient compliance and dosing.

In selected patients, the nonacetylated salicylates may be of value because they do not inhibit prostaglandins at the usual doses and have reduced effects on the gastric mucosa, renal function, and platelet adhesiveness.

The discovery of two forms of COX has quickly been transformed into clinical practice. The original NSAIDs work through nonspecific inhibition of COX isoforms 1 and 2 (COX-1 and COX-2), although alternative modes of action have been proposed (99). COX-1 is constitutively expressed in platelets, kidneys, and gastrointestinal tissues, among others. COX-2 is constitutive in the brain, ovaries, kidneys, and small and large bowel but is inducible at sites of inflammatory responses. Both pain and inflammation are only in the domains of COX-2. In contrast, the gastrointestinal (gastritis, peptic ulcer disease) adverse effects of NSAIDs are in the domain of COX-1 inhibition. Hence a specific COX-2 inhibitor would potentially avoid the gastrointestinal side effects.

In relation to other major effects of NSAIDs, platelet aggregation and bleeding time are not affected by specific COX-2 inhibition; however, localization studies in animals have shown expression of COX-2 in the macula densa and medulla of the kidney, raising concerns about the renal effects of COX-2 inhibition (100,101).

Several excellent reviews address the COX isoenzymes and their roles (102,103). The initially available COX-2 inhibitors are celecoxib and rofecoxib. A double-blind, placebo-controlled trial of rofecoxib in 672 patients with hip and knee OA showed superiority to placebo at 6 weeks as assessed by the Western Ontario and McMaster Universities Osteoarthritis Index (WOMAC) pain scale, patient global assessment of response to therapy, and physician assessment of disease status (104). Subsequent studies have shown clinical efficacy comparable to that of diclofenac and ibuprofen by using the WOMAC visual analog pain scale as the primary end point (105,106). A 2-week randomized, double-blind, placebo-controlled trial of celecoxib in OA of the knee showed it to be significantly better than placebo as judged by patient global assessment and OA severity index (107). A longer, 12-week study in 1,004 patients with OA of the knee showed superiority of celecoxib to placebo and no statistical difference with naproxen in arthritis assessments (108). Gastrointestinal adverse events and withdrawal rates were similar to those with placebo.

Celecoxib was compared with naproxen in a 1-week, double-blind, placebo-controlled endoscopic study. Thirty-two normal volunteers with negative baseline upper endoscopies were randomized to one of four arms (placebo; naproxen, 500 mg b.i.d.; celecoxib, 100 mg b.i.d.; and celecoxib, 200 mg b.i.d.). Endoscopy at day 7 revealed no ulcers in the placebo or either of the celecoxib groups. There were six (19%) patients with endoscopic gastric ulcers in the naproxen arm (109). Further studies have demonstrated that the clinical efficacy of celecoxib is comparable to that of diclofenac in RA (110) and showed no pharmacologic interaction with methotrexate (111). However, both celecoxib and rofecoxib have been shown to prolong the prothrombin time (PT) and PT-INR of patients on warfarin by about 10%.

Other NSAIDs are purportedly COX-2 selective, such as flosulide (112) and meloxicam. Meloxicam was tested versus diclofenac in a 6-month, multicenter, double-blind study of 336 patients. Severe adverse events, treatment discontinuation, and clinically significant laboratory abnormalities were numerically but not statistically more common with diclofenac than with meloxicam (113,114).

COX-2 inhibitors may have effects through modulation of nitric oxide pathways. Prostaglandin E_2 (PGE_2) levels have been found to be 50-fold higher than those in normal cartilage in *ex vivo* culture, and this coincides with local upregulation of COX-2. The addition of nitric oxide (NO) inhibited prostaglandin production, whereas the NO inhibitor N(G)-monomethyl-L-arginine (L-NMMA) augmented PGE_2 production (115). This may point to an anti-inflammatory role for NO and its derivatives in OA.

The *nonantiinflammatory* analgesic acetaminophen has a weak COX inhibitory effect and was as effective as ibuprofen for the treatment of pain in OA of the knee (85). In contrast, ibuprofen, 1,200 mg, was more effective than and as well tolerated as acetaminophen, 4,000 mg, in a 6-day study for those with more severe pain (116). Acetaminophen appears free of gastric adverse effects, but hepatotoxicity occurs when ingested at high doses; there is epidemiologic evidence of renal toxicity even when it is ingested at the recommended dose (117).

Topical agents can be useful adjuncts in the treatment of OA. The use of capsaicin has been supported in double-blind trials (118,119). Capsaicin is derived from capsicum, the common pepper plant (120). It is available as an over-the-counter nonprescription agent in two strengths. It is applied from 2 to 4 times daily. It also has been used in post-herpetic neuralgia and diabetic neuropathy (121). Capsaicin is absorbed topically and interferes with substance P–mediated pain transmission by reversibly depleting stores of substance P in unmyelinated C fiber afferent neurons (122). Over the first several days of administration, until the nerve endings are depleted of substance P, capsaicin applications are accompanied by a sensation of heat or burning in the area of the skin where it is applied. If it is not used continuously, the nerve endings will renew their supply of and sensitivity to substance P. Care should be taken to avoid the inadvertent application of capsaicin in the eyes.

A variety of other topical analgesics, menthol- and salicylate-based over-the-counter topical preparations, are available in the U. S., but despite their popularity, there are no published trials supporting their use in OA. Topical NSAIDs are in common use in many parts of the world (123,124).

Pain of OA is generally responsive to *narcotic analgesics.* Mildly potent and minimally addictive narcotic analgesics, such as codeine and propoxyphene, have been used effectively in patients with OA, especially in combination with nonnarcotic analgesics (e.g., acetaminophen).

Tramadol has mild suppressive effects on the μ opioid receptor and also inhibits the uptake of norepinephrine and serotonin (125). Tramadol does not have significant addictive tendencies (126) and is not a controlled schedule prescription in the U.S. However, there have been some reports of abuse by opioid-dependent patients. Seizures and allergic reactions also have been reported (127). Nevertheless, tramadol appears to have a place in the therapy of OA (128) and may have NSAID-sparing properties (129). Tramadol commonly produces nausea and central nervous system side effects that can be reduced by starting with 50 mg, twice daily for 3 days, and slowly escalating the dose to the maximum or until the desired pain relief is achieved.

The chronic nature of the pain in OA and the addictive potential of the stronger opiates and opioids test the skill of the physician in the use of these agents. With great care and judgment, narcotic analgesics have a place in the care of many chronic pain states, even OA. There is still uncertainty regarding how to block nonnarcotic central nervous system pain receptors. Guidelines for the use of narcotics in patients with nonmalignant pain have been published (130).

Any analgesic program can be supplemented with tricyclic antidepressants—these agents potentiate the analgesic effects of the other analgesics. In addition, they may exert part of their benefit in those patients having sleep disturbances due to nocturnal myoclonus and fibromyalgia-like complaints.

Antispasmodics are useful in the reduction of muscle pain and spasm in OA. Although the main treatment for muscle spasm is through the physical modalities noted earlier, pain associated with muscle spasm may be reduced with an injection of lidocaine with or without a depocorticosteroid. The value of oral medications in relieving the pain of muscle spasm is controversial—clinical trials have not convincingly demonstrated any medication to be superior to placebo. However, centrally acting agents may be helpful for their sedating qualities and potential for disrupting neurologic transmission of the pain sensation. Sedation is of value to improve sleep patterns, but is no longer proposed for the majority of patients with muscle spasm (particularly related to low back pain).

Oral corticosteroids are not indicated for the treatment of OA. In contrast, *intraarticular depocorticosteroids* are thought to be of value when there is evidence of synovial inflammation. Synovial effusions should be removed before injection. Infiltration of depocorticosteroids also may be helpful in treatment of periarticular soft tissue complications, such as anserine bursitis. They have not been consistently helpful in facet joints for treatment of chronic low back pain (131) but have been useful in many patients as epidural injections for symptomatic spinal stenosis (56). In spite of the impression of many clinicians that intraarticular depocorticosteroids are of benefit in OA, few published double-blind trials support their benefit over aspiration alone (132). Some trials have shown short-term benefit (133). Reduction in pain, as judged by a visual analogue scale, lasted up to 4 weeks when compared with a normal saline injection as a placebo (134). Despite the clinical impression that they are of value in the presence of inflammation, no consistent clinical predictors of response to intraarticular depocorticosteroids have been found to aid in patient selection for this therapy (135).

In general, depocorticosteroid injections should be limited to four injections into any single joint per year (136). Complications of intraarticular depocorticosteroids, such as septic arthritis, are rare if proper aseptic technique is used. Depocorticosteroids are crystalline and can induce a transient synovitis or "flare." A flare occurs within several hours of the injection. This is in contrast to infection, which most often occurs 24 to 72 hours after the procedure. The application of cold compresses often reduces the pain until the flare resolves within several hours (137). The suspicion of infection should prompt immediate reaspiration with subsequent Gram stain and cultures.

Psychosocial Measures

Pain and disability are not solely related to physical and mechanical impairment. Psychosocial factors are very much intertwined with the perception of pain and associated disability. Several factors have been linked to the propensity to be disabled in patients with musculoskeletal complaints. These include older age, lower educational level, lower income, unmarried status, and non-Caucasian race (138).

Reassurance, counseling, and education by the physician are important in trying to minimize the negative effects of psychosocial factors. Patients should be encouraged to participate in their care and to understand their disease. This should lead the patient to better acceptance, adaptation, and compliance. Periodic telephone support has been found to be beneficial and to promote self-care in patients with OA (139).

Another potential need for psychosocial intervention is with obese patients. Weight-loss groups and a stable social support system may be helpful in a concerted effort at weight reduction.

Patients can often have sexual problems secondary to the symptoms from their OA but may be reluctant to discuss these unless specifically queried (140). Psychosocial intervention and counseling can be effective in this area as well.

Depression must be recognized and treated.

Surgical Intervention

The primary reason for elective orthopedic surgery is intractable pain. A secondary reason for surgery is restoration of compromised function. Interventions include removal of loose bodies, stabilization of joints, redistribution of joint forces (e.g., osteotomy), relief of neural impingement (e.g., spinal stenosis, herniated disc), and joint replacement (e.g., total knee replacement).

Total hip and knee arthroplasties have improved the morbidity and probably the indirect mortality of OA. Most series report good to excellent long-term results in more than 90% of patients undergoing either hip or knee replacement (132), with 85% success rates at 20 years' follow-up of the Charnley total hip prosthesis. These procedures appear cost effective when the improved quality of life and the alternatives are considered. Osteotomies may serve as alternatives to arthroplasty in younger, overweight patients and in unicompartmental disease of the knee. This may delay progression of disease (hence the need for total joint replacement). However, only 50% of patients with knee osteotomies have satisfactory results at 10 years (141). Hip osteotomies have less certain long-term results.

Arthroscopic intervention should be limited to patients in whom an additional diagnosis is suspected. Surgical arthroscopy is useful for repair and for partial removal of damaged menisci, as described earlier. The value of synovectomy and debridement has not been established in OA. Abrasion chondroplasty leads to partial cartilage repair and provides the same symptomatic improvement as irrigation and debridement alone (142,143). This procedure should be avoided.

Arthroscopic lavage also has been tried, with some success. Large-bore needle lavage with saline may be of value in selected patients (144). It has been shown to be effective in the relief of pain in OA of the knees for up to 6 months (145).

LONG-ACTING SYMPTOMATIC THERAPY

Medications in this class have a variable onset of benefit with a prolonged effect on discontinuation (Table 112.3) Many of the medications in this group are considered investigational in the U.S. and are not approved for use. Some are being investigated as disease-modifying agents.

Intraarticular depocorticosteroids (discussed in earlier section) may have long-term effects. There is some evidence that depocorticosteroids may slow cartilage catabolism *in vitro* and in animal models (146). There is contradictory evidence that they may advance OA (147).

Synthetic and naturally occurring *hyaluronic acid (HA) derivatives* are administered intraarticularly. They are prepared in a variety of molecular weights (range, <100,000 to >1,000,000 Svedberg units). In general, they are reported to reduce pain for prolonged periods and potentially to improve mobility (148,149). The mechanism(s) of action are not known. However, there is evidence for an antiinflammatory effect (particularly at high molecular weight), a short-term lubricant effect, an analgesic effect by direct buffering of synovial nerve endings, and a stimulating effect on synovial lining cells on the production of normal HA, perhaps through binding to synovial cell CD44HA receptors.

Three weekly HA (Synvisc) intraarticular injections provided comparable pain relief to a single depocorticosteroid intraarticular injection at 1-week follow-up; at 45-day follow-up, HA was superior to the depocorticosteroid (150). An intraarticular HA (Hyalgan) derivative was compared with oral naproxen or placebo in a 14-week double-blind study (151). Pain relief was prolonged with the HA, and at 6 months, more than 60% of the completers had at least a 20% reduction of pain (pain free in half of that group). Even though 40% of the placebo group improved, there was significant improvement in the HA-injected group when compared with placebo. The benefit compared favorably with that of naproxen, with significantly fewer adverse effects (fewer gastrointestinal complaints). In another study, three weekly intraarticular injections of HA (Synvisc) were compared with their combination with an NSAID, and with the NSAID alone. At 12 weeks and a telephone 26-week follow-up, the groups receiving the HA were better in terms of rest pain and lateral joint tenderness (152). Other HA derivatives are under investigation (Artz, DHA, Orthovisc).

S-Adenosylmethionine (SAMe), a methyl group donor (153) and oxygen radical scavenger, has been used in intravenous loading and oral maintenance. In one study, the two centers reported differing results. One center reported reductions in overall pain and rest pain over placebo; the other showed no significant difference between the test group and placebo but treated patients with more severe OA (154).

Glucosamine sulfate, an intermediate in mucopolysaccharide synthesis, has been tested orally and intramuscularly. Glucosamine sulfate, 400 mg twice weekly intramuscularly for 6 weeks, reduced the severity of disease as judged by the

Lequesne Index when compared with placebo (155). Glucosamine sulfate, 500 mg 3 times daily orally, was compared with ibuprofen, 400 mg 3 times daily, in OA of the knee in a randomized, double-blind parallel-group, 4-week study. The response to ibuprofen was more rapid, but at 4 weeks, there was no statistically significant difference in the two agents (reduction of at least 2 points in the Lequesne Index) (156). A double-blind study in China tested 178 patients with OA of the knee on oral glucosamine sulfate, 1,500 mg daily, versus ibuprofen, 1,200 mg daily for 4 weeks. Knee pain at 4 weeks was numerically but not statistically superior with glucosamine sulfate. Adverse drug reactions were reported in 6% of the glucosamine group and 16% of the ibuprofen group, with no discontinuations in the glucosamine group and 10% discontinuations in the ibuprofen group (157).

The mechanism of action of glucosamine sulfate is uncertain. Some *in vitro* experiments have shown stimulation of the synthesis of cartilage glycosaminoglycans and proteoglycans (158,159). Enhanced synovial production of HA has been proposed as a mechanism in one study (160). There is evidence of structure/disease modification in animal studies showing decreased cartilage erosion (161).

Oral *chondroitin sulfate,* a glycosaminoglycan with a molecular mass of approximately 14,000 daltons, is composed of repeating units of *N*-acetyl galactosamine and glucuronic acid. A double-blind, placebo-controlled study investigating this agent included a 3-month treatment phase followed by a 2-month treatment-free phase. The major outcome parameter was NSAID consumption. Those receiving chondroitin sulfate consumed fewer NSAIDs than the controls at both the completion of the treatment and the treatment-free phase (162). Another study compared chondroitin sulfate, 1,200 mg daily for 3 months, with diclofenac sodium, 150 mg daily for 1 month, both followed by placebo to 6 months in a double-dummy protocol. The diclofenac group had quicker response to therapy, whereas the chondroitin group had a more prolonged improvement, as measured by the Lequesne Index, visual analogue scale for pain, 4-point scale for pain, and acetaminophen (Paracetamol) use (rescue medication) (163). A meta-analysis of four double-blind, randomized, placebo- or NSAID-controlled trials with chondroitin sulfate showed chondroitin sulfate to be superior to placebo regarding Lequesne Index visual analog scale for pain, and co-medication consumption (164). Most of the effects became evident after 60 days of chondroitin sulfate.

However, another meta-analysis and quality assessment of the studies of glucosamine and chondroitin in OA of hip or knee concluded that insufficient information about study design and conduct has generally been provided with these trials to allow a definitive evaluation of either agent (165). Larger studies with longer follow-up periods are needed.

One double-blind, placebo-controlled crossover trial evaluated men with pain and radiographic knee or low back pain OA on the combination of glucosamine HCl, 1,500 mg/day; chondroitin sulfate, 1,200 mg/day; and manganese ascorbate, 228 mg/day. Thirty-four patients were enrolled in this 16-week trial. Patients with knee OA reported improvement in visual analog scale for pain, patient assessment of treatment effect, and a summary disease score (pain questionnaire, functional questionnaire, physical examination score, and running time). No benefit was reported among patients with spinal OA (166). Another study reported benefit of the glucosamine/chondroitin combination in patients with OA of the temporomandibular joint (TMJ) (167).

Glucosamine and chondroitin sulfates are considered nutritional supplements in the U.S. and are not regulated by the strict rules of the U.S. Food and Drug Administration. Quality control of the products from health food stores is variable, and there is inadequate evidence that these agents individually, or in combination, are "cures" for OA.

Recombinant human superoxide dismutase (rH-SOD) has been tested in animal models (168). It catalyzes peroxide formation from free radicals, therefore limiting free radical concentrations and ability to inflict damage in the joint. Intraarticular orgotein, a metalloproteinase with superoxide dismutase activity, has been investigated as a therapeutic agent in OA (169). One trial suggested benefit as assessed by decreased pain for up to 6 months (170). Another group reported decreased pain and improved function and global assessment in OA of the knee (171). Trials were discontinued because of toxicity.

Radioactive synovectomy is still being performed with agents such as yttrium (172) or osmic acid. A recent trial reported benefit similar to that of joint lavage plus intraarticular depocorticosteroid injection at 6 months after treatment (173).

Diacerein is the acetylated form of the naturally occurring dihydroxyanthraquinone rhein, related to the senna compounds. Diacerein inhibits the synthesis of interleukin-1β (IL-1β) in human OA synovium *in vitro* as well as the expression of IL-1 receptors on chondrocytes (174). IL-1–dependent stromelysin-1 production was also diminished. No effects were observed on tumor necrosis factor (TNF) or its receptors. Other observed effects of rhein have included inhibition of superoxide anion production, chemotaxis, and phagocytosis by neutrophils and macrophages. Collagenase production also has been reduced, and articular damage has been reduced by diacerein in animal models (175–177). In human clinical trials, oral diacerein (50 mg twice daily) improved pain scores as compared with placebo. Both diacerein and tenoxicam were superior to placebo in OA of the hip (178). Diarrhea is the main side effect and can be observed in up to 30% of patients (179). The presence of diarrhea is inversely related to absorption; newer formulations of diacerein have improved absorption.

Estrogens have been studied in OA, although they are prescribed for reasons other than OA. Epidemiologic studies of women receiving estrogen replacement therapy (ERT), however, have reported that they have a lower prevalence of OA than those not receiving ERT (180). The Chingford data show an inverse association of current ERT use and radiologic OA of the knee. The effect was statistically significant for the presence of osteophytes or for Kellgren–Lawrence grade in knee OA, but not for distal interphalangeal OA (181). ERT has also been associated with a lower risk of hip OA in elderly white women (odds ratio, 0.62) (182). Results from another study did not support an association between endogenous estrogen levels and the severity of radiographic hand OA (183). Additionally, estrogen receptor gene polymorphisms have been confirmed as genetic markers for generalized OA. One particular gene polymorphism was associated with an odds ratio of 1.86 (184).

Avocado/soybean unsaponifiables (that part of the oil that does not hydrolyze and form soap and glycerin) may have potential as slow-acting symptom-relieving drugs for OA. Prior testing was in scleroderma (185). Avocado/soy nonsaponifiables have been found potentially to modulate chondrocyte synthetic and repair activity (186–188). In a 3-month prospective, multicenter, randomized, double-blind, placebo-controlled trial of 162 patients with OA of the hip or knee, one daily tablet of avocado/soybean unsaponifiables was compared with placebo. NSAID use was 43% in the avocado/soybean group versus 70% in the placebo group (189). Pain scores were similar in both groups, but the Lequesne functional index was significantly improved in the avocado/soy unsaponifiable group. Avocado/soy unsaponifiable was compared with placebo in a 6-month study of patients with OA of the hip or knee (190), with efficacy measured by the Lequesne functional index and visual analogue pain scale. Those taking avocado/soybean unsaponifiables had significant symptomatic improvement over placebo, with the effect appearing after the second month of therapy. There was also less NSAID use in the active treatment group.

Pulsed electromagnetic fields have been evaluated for healing of bone (191) and are being investigated for their effects on pain in OA. (192). One double-blind, placebo-controlled trial reported benefit in knee and cervical spine OA. Improvement was significant when compared with placebo as judged by patients and physician overall assessment, pain, and pain on motion.

Ginger-based products have been used for OA in some areas and are currently in clinical trials (193). Other "nutritional supplements" entrenched in popular culture such as "cat's claw" and shark cartilage are being used with increasing frequency and being sold over the counter in pharmacies and health food stores. There are no carefully performed trials to support their use.

Structure/Disease-modifying Agents

Structure/disease-modifying agents for OA refers to medications that are intended to retard the progression of OA and/or enhance the normal reparative process (Table 112.3). Because OA is a disease of the entire joint, the prior term "chondroprotection" is inappropriate. It appears most difficult to establish the value of a structure/disease-modifying drug in a disease process that progresses at variable rates and has no definable clinical or laboratory marker of activity/progression. Measures used to identify structure/disease modification include radiographic assessment of joint space, such as fluoroscopically positioned anteroposterior radiographs of the knee or magnetic resonance imaging (MRI) (194). Although several agents are being evaluated for these properties, none has been established as effective. Several of the agents discussed earlier have structure/disease-modifying potential. These agents may be listed as subsets as follows: (a) growth factors and cytokines; (b) sulfated and nonsulfated sugars; (c) hormones and other steroids; and (d) enzyme inhibitors.

Tetracyclines, apart from any antimicrobial effect, are inhibitors of tissue metalloproteinases. This could be due to their ability to chelate calcium and zinc ions. There also has been investigation into the potential role of nitric oxide in the mechanism of action of the tetracyclines (195). Doxycycline and, to a lesser extent, minocycline block spontaneous and IL-1β–induced OA cartilage nitric oxide synthase (NOS) activity in *in vitro* experiments. More recently, however, tetracyclines have been shown to be capable of upregulating COX-2 and PGE_2 production, independent of any effects on NO (196). The clinical significance of this, as human trials with tetracyclines in OA go forth, is unclear. Minocycline has been used in the management of RA (197). Doxycycline, another tetracycline derivative, has been shown to inhibit articular cartilage collagenase and activity (198,199).

Doxycycline also has reduced the severity of OA in canine models. In one study, there was preservation of medial femoral condyle cartilage in treated dogs compared with the untreated group. Other lesions such as medial trochlear ridge cartilage damage, superficial fibrillation of the medial tibial plateau, and osteophytosis were unaffected by treatment. Collagenolytic and gelatinolytic activity, however, were reduced to one fifth and one fourth, respectively, when compared with the untreated dogs. In an *in vitro* model, not only did doxycycline reduce collagenase and gelatinase activity in cartilage, but it also prevented proteoglycan loss, cell death, and deposition of type X collagen matrix (200).

A study of 21 human femoral heads from patients undergoing arthroplasty for end-stage hip OA measured the activities of collagenase and gelatinase in OA cartilage extracts from patients on doxycycline, 100 mg b.i.d. or q a.m. for 5 days before surgery, 200 mg as a single dose 3 days before surgery, or no doxycycline. The single dose of 200 mg was ineffective in inhibiting metalloproteases, whereas the dose of 100 mg b.i.d. inhibited both collagenase and gelatinase. The 100 mg q a.m. dose was statistically significant in inhibiting gelatinase but not collagenase (201).

Further animal and human studies are needed in this area. One study showed symptomatic benefit and decreased collagenase activity when doxycycline was used at 50 mg twice a day for 3 months in patients with OA of the TMJ (202). A multicenter, double-blind, placebo-controlled trial using doxycycline for "structure modification" in obese women with OA of the knee is ongoing. Other compounds with collagenase-inhibiting properties are being developed and investigated as structure/disease-modifying agents not only in OA, but also in RA (203).

A chemically modified tetracycline has been used to inhibit matrix metalloproteinases in the spontaneous OA model in guinea pigs. The oral compound, called CMT-7, was given prophylactically for 4 to 8 months to guinea pigs. Cartilage fibrillation and destruction in addition to subchondral bone sclerosis and cyst formation were decreased in the central compartment of the medial condyle (204). In the same study, the changes were not decreased in a group of guinea pigs taking doxycycline.

Glycosaminoglycan polysulfuric acid (GAGPS, Arteparon, Adequan) has been proposed to be a disease-modifying agent in OA and to work through a reduction in collagen degradation as a result of its effect on collagenase. It is a highly sulfated glycosaminoglycan, ranging from 2,000 to 16,000 in molecular weight (205) derived from bovine tracheal cartilage with some heparin-like properties. In a therapeutic canine model of OA, GAGPS was administered intraarticularly twice weekly for 4 weeks (206). Four weeks after completion of the GAGPS, gross and histologic medial femoral condylar lesions had developed to a lesser degree in the treated group than in saline-treated dogs. Uronic acid and hydroxyproline levels were significantly higher, and levels of active and latent collagenase were lower in the dogs receiving GAGPS. Furthermore, swelling, an indicator of collagen network integrity, remained near control levels in the treatment group. OA of the human knee was studied in a 5-year trial showing improvement in multiple measured parameters including less time lost from work (207). Adverse reactions were minimal, but potential allergy and heparin-like effects have caused the use of GAGPS to become controversial. GAGPS is still available for equine use.

Another extract, a *glycosaminoglycan–peptide complex (Rumalon),* is a highly sulfated polysaccharide with undefined peptides derived from bovine tracheal cartilage and bone marrow that is administered intramuscularly (208,209). It has been shown to increase the levels of tissue inhibitor of metalloproteinases (TIMP) (210). Long-term studies on hip and knee have shown the agent to improve most measured parameters (205). However, a 5-year prospective trial involving 400 patients with OA of the hip and knee has failed to demonstrate disease-modifying properties (K. Pavelka, personal communication, 1999). Adverse events are particularly uncommon. It has limited availability in parts of Europe and South America.

Pentosan polysulfate (Cartrofen) is a purified extract of beech hemicellulose administered intramuscularly, or orally as a calcium salt. It is an inhibitor of granulocyte elastase. Experimental studies in a variety of animal models suggest that it helps to preserve cartilage proteoglycan content and retards cartilage degradation (211,212).

Several peptides are being investigated that have inhibitory effects on metalloproteinase activity. In a rabbit model, an orally active metalloproteinase inhibitor blocked proteoglycan release (assessed through knee lavage) after injection of stromelysin into the knees (213).

Data from the Framingham study has indicated that *estrogen replacement therapy* may delay progression of radiographic OA of the knee. The analysis of the cohort prospective study revealed a moderate, but not statistically significant protective effect of estrogens on the progression of OA (214).

Growth factor and cytokine manipulation are areas of potential intervention (215). In an animal model, induction of repair in partial-thickness articular cartilage lesions by timed release of transforming growth factor-β (TGF-β) with liposomes has been attempted. The defects exhibited an increase in cellularity, being populated by cells of mesenchymal origin from the synovial membrane. The appearance of the repaired cartilage resembled hyaline cartilage, and its integrity persisted up to 1 year after surgery (216). Genetic therapy may also be in the future of OA. The control of genes such as the TIMP and the metalloproteinase (MMP) genes would, in theory, provide the opportunity to modulate the patients' disease. Expression of TGF-β has been achieved in chondrocytes and synoviocytes of guinea pigs using adenovirus as the vector (217). Using this same vector, temporary expression of the transduced β galactosidase gene has been seen in human chondrocytes (218). Reduction in the macroscopic and histologic severity of cartilage lesions was achieved in an anterior cruciate ligament model of dog OA by transfecting the IL-1 receptor–antagonist gene into synovial fibroblast-like cells (219).

In the future, better results and techniques may be achieved through the use of *osteochondral grafts.* Implantation of chondrocytes into cartilage defects has become possible in humans (220), and even implantation of stem cells into defects with eventual differentiation into bone and cartilage has been accomplished in a rabbit model (221). If these procedures become practical, they may radically alter the management of OA. They may lead not only to "chondroprotection" but also to the preservation of the entire joint organ.

It is suggested that combination therapy may be needed for joint repair. In a study of canine induced OA, sodium pentosan polysulfate, when combined with insulin-like growth factor 1 (IGF-1), reduced stromelysin activity with an added increase in TIMP (222).

Structure/disease modification has yet to be achieved in OA, and any claims are premature until well-designed, double-blind, placebo-controlled trials are conducted. Trials currently under way could provide an answer as to whether this is a realistic goal.

It also is possible that some of the drugs being now tested for structure/disease modification could provide symptom relief and could add to our armamentarium in that capacity, even if not successful as structure/disease-modifying agents.

CONCLUSIONS

Therapy for OA is potentially directed at symptomatic relief or structure/disease modification. Presently, therapy of OA is aimed at symptom relief. One must clinically attempt to define the cause of the symptoms, most often pain. This allows goal-directed therapy. Effective therapy combines many of the tools available, including physical measures, medications, psychologic approaches, and surgery. An algorithm for the therapy of OA is reflected in Fig. 112.1.

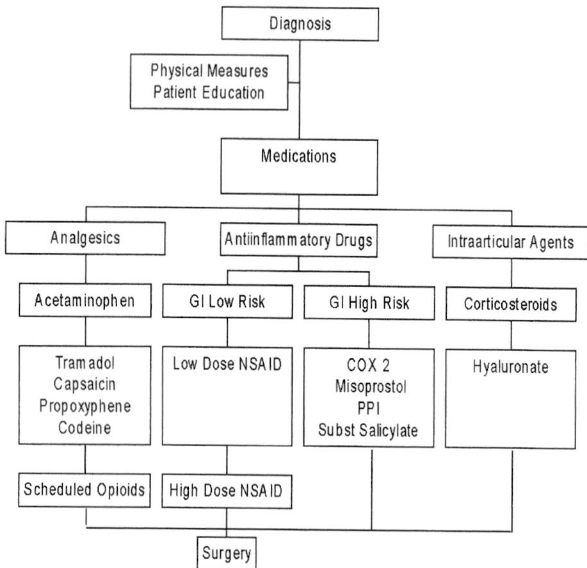

FIGURE 112.1. Flow chart for the therapy of osteoarthritis. Physical measures and patient education are the baseline of therapy and must be continued throughout the program. Medications are potentially used singly or in combination. Surgery is an option when the physical and medicinal programs fail to provide adequate symptomatic relief. *GI*, Risk of gastrointestinal adverse event; *NSAID*, nonsteroidal antiinflammatory drug; *COX-2*, cyclooxygenase 2 specific inhibitor; *PPI*, protein pump inhibitor; *Subst Salicylate*, substituted (nonacetylated) salicylate.

REFERENCES

1. Lawrence RC, Hochberg MC, Kelsey JL, et al. Estimates of the prevalence of selected arthritic and musculoskeletal diseases in the United States. *J Rheumatol* 1989;16:427–441.
2. Levy E, Ferme A, Perocheau D, et al. Socioeconomic costs of osteoarthritis in France. *Rev Rhum* 1993;60:63S–67S.
3. Lozada CJ, Altman RD. Osteoarthritis: a comprehensive approach to management. *J Musculoskeletal Med* 1997;14: 26–38.
4. Hochberg MC, Altman RD, Brandt KD, et al. Guidelines for the medical management of osteoarthritis. Part II: Osteoarthritis of the knee. *Arthritis Rheum* 1995;38:1541–1546.
5. Hochberg MC, Altman RD, Brandt RD, et al. Guidelines for the medical management of osteoarthritis. Part I: Osteoarthritis of the hip. *Arthritis Rheum* 1995;38:1535–1540.
6. Altman R, Brandt K, Hochberg M, et al. Design and conduct of clinical trials in patients with osteoarthritis: recommendations from a task force of the Osteoarthritis Research Society. *Osteoarthritis Cartilage* 1996;4:217–243.
7. Hutton CW. Osteoarthritis: the cause not result of joint failure? *Ann Rheum Dis* 1989;48:958–961.
8. Liang MH, Fortin P. Management of osteoarthritis of the hip and knee [Editorial]. *N Engl J Med* 1991;325:125–127.
9. Altman R, Appelrouth D, Asch E, et al. Criteria for classification and reporting of osteoarthritis of the hand. *Arthritis Rheum* 1990;33:1601–1610.
10. Altman R, Alarcón G, Appelrouth KD, et al. Criteria for classification and reporting of osteoarthritis of the hip. *Arthritis Rheum* 1991;34:505–514.
11. Altman R, Appelrouth D, Asch E, et al. Development of criteria for the classification and reporting of osteoarthritis: classification of osteoarthritis of the knee. *Arthritis Rheum* 1986;29: 1039–1049.
12. Lequesne M, Brandt K, Bellamy N, et al. Guidelines for testing slow acting drugs in osteoarthritis. *J Rheumatol* 1994;21(suppl): 4165–4173.
13. Trock DH, Bollet AJ, Dyer RH Jr, et al. A double-blind trial of the clinical effects of pulsed electromagnetic fields in osteoarthritis. *J Rheumatol* 1993;20:459–460.
14. Lewis D, Lewis B, Sturrock RD. Transcutaneous electrical nerve stimulation in osteoarthrosis: a therapeutic alternative? *Ann Rheum Dis* 1984;43:47–49.
15. Brandt KD. Pain, synovitis, and articular cartilage changes in osteoarthritis. *Semin Arthritis Rheum* 1989;18(suppl 2):77–80.
16. Kellgren JH, Lawrence RC. Radiological assessment of osteoarthrosis. *Ann Rheum Dis* 1957;16:494–501.
17. Hochberg MC, Lawrence RC, Everett DF, et al. Epidemiologic associations of pain in osteoarthritis of the knee: data from the National Health and Nutrition Examination-I epidemiologic follow-up survey. *Semin Arthritis Rheum* 1989;18(suppl 2):4–9.
18. Altman R, Dean D. Introduction and overview: pain in osteoarthritis. *Semin Arthritis Rheum* 1989;(suppl 2):1–3.
19. Creamer P, Lethbridge-Cejku M, Hochberg MC. Where does it hurt? Pain localization in osteoarthritis of the knee. *Osteoarthritis Cartilage* 1998;6:318–323.
20. Harkness IAL, Higgs ER, Dieppe PA. Osteoarthritis. In: Wall PD, Melzadk R, eds. *Textbook of pain.* London: Churchill Livingstone, 1984:215–224.
21. Wyke B. The neurology of joints: a review of general principles. *Clin Rheum Dis* 1981;7:223–239.
22. Lindblad S, Hedfors E. Arthroscopic and immunohistologic characterization of knee joint synovitis in osteoarthritis. *Arthritis Rheum* 1987;30:1081–1088.
23. Lindblad S, Hedfors E. Arthroscopic and synovial correlates of

pain in osteoarthritis. *Semin Arthritis Rheum* 1989;18(suppl 2):91–93.

24. Schumacher HR. The role of inflammation and crystals in the pain of osteoarthritis. *Semin Arthritis Rheum* 1989;18(suppl 2): 81–85.
25. Schumacher HR, Somyo AP, Tse RL, et al. Arthritis associated with apatite crystals. *Ann Intern Med* 1977;87:411–416.
26. Fam AG, Stein J. Hydroxyapatite pseudopodagra in young women. *J Rheumatol* 1992;19:662–664.
27. Evans CH, Mears DC, McKnight JL. A preliminary ferrographic survey of the wear particles in human synovial fluid. *Arthritis Rheum* 1981;24:912–918.
28. Schaible H-G, Schmidt RF. Effects of an experimental arthritis on the sensory properties of fine articular afferent units. *J Neurophysiol* 1985;54:1109–1122.
29. Grigg P, Schaible H-G, Schmidt RF. Mechanical sensitivity of group III and IV afferents from posterior articular nerve in normal and inflamed cat knee. *J Neurophysiol* 1986;55:635–643.
30. Schaible H-G, Neugebauer V, Schmidt RF. Osteoarthritis and pain. *Semin Arthritis Rheum* 1989;18:30–34.
31. Georgepoulos AP. Functional properties of primary afferent units probably related to pain mechanisms in primate glabrous skin. *J Neurophysiol* 1974;39:71–83.
32. Kantor TG. Concepts in pain control. *Semin Arthritis Rheum* 1989;18(suppl 2):94–99.
33. Kolasinski SL, Haines KA, Siegel EL, et al. Neuropeptides and inflammation: a somatostatin analog as a selective antagonist of neutrophil activation by substance P. *Arthritis Rheum* 1992;35:369–375.
34. Badalamente MA, Cherney SB. Periosteal and vascular innervation of the human patella in degenerative joint disease. *Semin Arthritis Rheum* 1989;18(suppl 2):61–66.
35. Kiaer T, Gronlund J, Sorensen KH. Intraosseous pressure and partial pressures of oxygen and carbon dioxide in osteoarthritis. *Semin Arthritis Rheum* 1989;18(suppl 2):57–60.
36. Akeson WH, Garfin S, Amiel D, et al. Para-articular connective tissue in osteoarthritis. *Semin Arthritis Rheum* 1989;18(suppl 2):41–50.
37. Moldofsky H. Sleep influences on regional and diffuse pain syndromes associated with osteoarthritis. *Semin Arthritis Rheum* 1989;18(suppl 2):18–21.
38. Bellamy N, Sothern RB, Campbell J, et al. Circadian and circaseptan variation in pain perception in osteoarthritis of the knee. *J Rheumatol* 1990;17:364–372.
39. Felson DT. The epidemiology of knee osteoarthritis: results from the Framingham Osteoarthritis Study. *Semin Arthritis Rheum* 1990;20:42–50.
40. Hubert HB, Bloch DA, Fries JF. Risk factors for physical disability in an aging cohort: the NHANES 1 epidemiologic follow-up study. *J Rheumatol* 1993;20:480–488.
41. Hochberg MC, Lethbridge-Cejku M, Scott WW Jr, et al. The association of body weight, body fatness and body fat distribution with osteoarthritis of the knee: data from the Baltimore Longitudinal Study of Aging. *J Rheumatol* 1995;22:488–493.
42. Oliveira SA, Felson DT, Cirillo PA, et al. Body weight, body mass index, and incident symptomatic osteoarthritis of the hand, hip, and knee. *Epidemiology* 1999;10:161–166.
43. Carman WJ, Sowers M, Hawthorne VM, et al. Obesity as a risk factor for osteoarthritis of the hand and wrist: a prospective study. *Am J Epidemiol* 1994;139:119–129.
44. Leach RE, Baumgard S, Broom J. Obesity: its relationship to osteoarthritis of the knee. *Clin Orthop* 1973;93:271–273.
45. Hart DJ, Doyle DV, Spector TD. Association between metabolic factors and knee osteoarthritis in women: the Chingford Study. *J Rheumatol* 1995;22:1118–1123.
46. Martin K, Lethbridge-Cejku M, Muller DC, et al. Metabolic correlates of obesity and radiographic features of knee osteoarthritis: data from the Baltimore Longitudinal Study of Aging. *J Rheumatol* 1997;24:702–707.
47. Felson DT, Zhang Y, Anthony JM, et al. Weight loss reduces the risk for symptomatic knee osteoarthritis in women. *Ann Intern Med* 1992;116:535–539.
48. Toda Y, Toda T, Takemura S, et al. Change in body fat, but not body weight or metabolic correlates of obesity, is related to symptomatic relief of obese patients with knee osteoarthritis after a weight control program. *J Rheumatol* 1998;25: 2181–2186.
49. Slemenda C, Heilman DK, Brandt KD, et al. Reduced quadriceps strength relative to body weight: a risk factor for knee osteoarthritis in women? *Arthritis Rheum* 1998;41:1951–1959.
50. Fisher NM, Pendergast DR, Gresham GE, et al. Muscle rehabilitation: its effect on muscular and functional performance of patients with knee osteoarthritis. *Arch Phys Med Rehabil* 1991; 72:367–374.
51. van Baar ME, Dekker J, Oostendorp RA, et al. The effectiveness of exercise therapy in patients with osteoarthritis of the hip or knee: a randomized clinical trial. *J Rheumatol* 1998;25: 2432–2439.
52. Joynt RL. Therapeutic exercise. In: DeLisa JA, et al., eds. *Rehabilitation medicine principles and practice.* Philadelphia: JB Lippincott, 1988:346–371.
53. Ytterberg SR, Mahowald ML, Krug HE. Exercise for arthritis [Review]. *Baillieres Clin Rheumatol* 1994;8:161–189.
54. Merritt JL. Soft tissue mechanisms of pain in osteoarthritis. *Semin Arthritis Rheum* 1989;18(suppl 2):51–56.
55. Kovar PA, Allegrante JP, MacKenzie R, et al. Supervised fitness walking in patients with osteoarthritis of the knee. *Ann Intern Med* 1992;116:529–534.
56. Fast A. Low back disorders: conservative management. *Arch Phys Med Rehabil* 1988;69:880–891.
57. Deyo RA. Conservative therapy for low back pain. *JAMA* 1982;250:1057–1062.
58. Ponte DJ, Jensen GJ, Kent BE. A preliminary report on the use of the McKenzie protocol versus Williams protocol in the treatment of low back pain. *J Orthop Sports Phys Ther* 1984;6:130–139.
59. Waddell G. A new clinical model for the treatment of low-back pain. *Spine* 1987;12:632–641.
60. Malmivaara A, Hakkinen V, Aro T, et al. The treatment of acute low back pain-bed rest: exercises, or ordinary activity? *N Engl J Med* 1995;332:351–355.
61. Fisher NM, Pendergast DR, Gresham GE, et al. Muscle rehabilitation: its effects on muscular and functional performance of patients with knee osteoarthritis. *Arch Phys Med* 1991;72: 367–374.
62. Blount WP. Don't throw away the cane. *J Bone Joint Surg Am* 1956;38:695–708.
63. Brand SA, Crowninshield RD. The effect of cane use on hip contact force. *Clin Orthop* 1980;147:181–184.
64. Thompson JA, Jennings MB, Hodge W. Orthotic therapy in the management of osteoarthritis. *J Am Podiatr Med Assoc* 1992;82:136–139.
65. Keating EM, Faris PM, Ritter MA, et al. Use of lateral heel and sole wedges in the treatment of medial osteoarthritis of the knee. *Orthop Rev* 1993;22:921–924.
66. Liang MH, Fortin P. Management of osteoarthritis of the hip and knee. *N Engl J Med* 1991;325:125–127.
67. Cushnagan J, McCarthy C, Dieppe PA. Taping the patella medially: a new treatment for osteoarthritis of the knee joint? *Br Med J* 1988;308:753–755.
68. Rubin G, Dixon M, Danisi M. prescription procedures for knee orthosis and knee-ankle-foot orthosis. *Orthot Prosthet* 1977;31: 15–25.

69. Kirk JA, Kersley GD. Heat and cold in the physical treatment of rheumatoid arthritis of the knee: a controlled clinical trial. *Ann Phys Med* 1967;9:270–274.
70. Felson DT, Zhang Y, Anthony JM, et al. Weight loss reduces the risk for symptomatic knee osteoarthritis in women. *Ann Intern Med* 1992;116:535–539.
71. Swezey RL. Essentials of physical management and rehabilitation in arthritis. *Semin Arthritis Rheum* 1974;3:349–368.
72. Fontain P, Gersten J, Sengir O. Decrease in muscle spasm produced by ultrasound, hot packs and infrared radiation. *Arch Phys Med Rehabil* 1960;41:293–298.
73. Cordray YM, Krusen EM. Use of hydrocollator packs in the treatment of neck and shoulder pains. *Arch Phys Med Rehabil* 1959;40:105.
74. Lehman JF, Brunner GD, Stow RW. Pain threshold measurements after therapeutic application of ultrasound, microwaves, and infrared. *Arch Phys Med Rehabil* 1958;39:560—565.
75. Lehman JF, DeLateur BJ. Diathermy and superficial heat, laser, and cold therapy. In: Kottke FJ, Lehman JF, eds. *Krusen's handbook of physical medicine and rehabilitation.* 4th ed. Philadelphia: WB Saunders, 1990:283–367.
76. Basford JR. Physical agents and biofeedback. In: DeLisa JA, eds. *Rehabilitation medicine: principles and practice.* Philadelphia: JB Lippincott, 1988:257–275.
77. Garfinkel MS, Shumacher HR Jr, Husain A, et al. Evaluation of a yoga based regimen for treatment of osteoarthritis of the hands. *J Rheumatol* 1994;21:2341–2343.
78. Christensen BV, Iuhl IU, Bulow H-H, et al. Acupuncture treatment of severe knee osteoarthrosis: a long-term study. *Acta Anaesthesiol Scand* 1992;36:519–525.
79. Trock DH, Bollet AJ, Dyer JR, et al. A double-blind trial of the clinical effects of pulsed electromagnetic fields in osteoarthritis. *J Rheumatol* 1993;20:456–460.
80. Lewis D, Lewis B, Sturrock RD. Transcutaneous electrical stimulation in osteoarthrosis: a therapeutic alternative? *Ann Rheum Dis* 1984;43:47–49.
81. Elkayam O, Wigler I, Tishler M, et al. Effect of spa therapy in Tiberias on patients with rheumatoid arthritis and osteoarthritis. *J Rheumatol* 1991;18:1799–1803.
82. McAlindon T, Dieppe P. The medical management of osteoarthritis of the knee: an inflammatory issue? *Br J Rheumatol* 1990;29:471–473.
83. Brooks PM, Day PO. Nonsteroidal antiinflammatory drugs: differences and similarities. *N Engl J Med* 1991;324:1716–1725.
84. Mazzuca SA, Brandt KD, Anderson SE, et al. The therapeutic approaches of community based primary care practitioners to osteoarthritis of the hip in an elderly patient. *J Rheumatol* 1991;18:1593–1600.
85. Bradley JD, Brandt KD, Katz BP, et al. Comparison of an antiinflammatory dose of ibuprofen, an analgesic dose of ibuprofen, and acetaminophen in the treatment of patients with osteoarthritis of the knee. *N Engl J Med* 1991;325:87–91.
86. Roth SH. Non-steroidal anti-inflammatory drugs: gastropathy, deaths, and medical practice. *Ann Intern Med* 1988;109:353–354.
87. Griffin MR, Ray WA, Schaffner W. Nonsteroidal anti-inflammatory drug use and death from peptic ulcer in elderly persons. *Ann Intern Med* 1988;109:359–363.
88. Levi F, Le Louran C, Reinberg A. Timing optimizes sustained-release indomethacin treatment of osteoarthritis. *Clin Pharmacol Ther* 1985;37:77–84.
89. Palmoski MJ, Brandt KD. Effects of some nonsteroidal antiinflammatory drugs on proteoglycan metabolism and organization in canine articular cartilage. *Arthritis Rheum* 1980;23:1010–1020.
90. Herman JH, Appel AM, Hess EV. Modulation of cartilage destruction by select non-steroidal anti-inflammatory drugs. *Arthritis Rheum* 1987;30:257–265.
91. Huskisson EC, Berry H, Geshen P, et al. On behalf of the LINK Study Group: effects of antiinflammatory drugs on the progression of osteoarthritis of the knee. *J Rheumatol* 1995;22:1941–1946.
92. Graham DY, Agrawal NM, Roth SH. Prevention of NSAID-induced gastric ulcer with misoprostol: multicenter, double-blind, placebo-controlled trial. *Lancet* 1988;2:1277–1280.
93. Agrawal NM, Van Kerckhove HE, Erhardt LJ, et al. Misoprostol coadministered with diclofenac for prevention of gastroduodenal ulcers: a one-year study. *Dig Dis Sci* 1995;40:1125–1131.
94. Melo Gomes JA, Roth SH, Zeeh J, et al. Double-blind comparison of efficacy and gastroduodenal safety of diclofenac/misoprostol, piroxicam, and naproxen in the treatment of osteoarthritis. *Ann Rheum Dis* 1993;52:881–885.
95. Bocanegra TS, Weaver AL, Tindall EA, et al. Diclofenac/misoprostol compared with diclofenac in the treatment of osteoarthritis of the knee or hip: a randomized, placebo controlled trial. *J Rheumatol* 1998;25:1602–1611.
96. Cullen D, Bardhan KD, Eisner M, et al. Primary gastroduodenal prophylaxis with omeprazole for non-steroidal anti-inflammatory drug users. *Aliment Pharmacol Ther* 1998;12:135–140.
97. Hawkey CJ, Karrasch JA, Szczepanski L, et al. Omeprazole compared with misoprostol for ulcers associated with nonsteroidal antiinflammatory drugs: Omeprazole versus Misoprostol for NSAID-induced Ulcer Management (OMINUM) Study Group. *N Engl J Med* 1998;338:727–734.
98. Yeomans ND, Tulassay Z, Juhasz L, et al. A comparison of omeprazole with ranitidine for ulcers associated with nonsteroidal antiinflammatory drugs: Acid Suppression Trial: Ranitidine versus Omeprazole for NSAID-Associated Ulcer Treatment (ASTRONAUT) Study Group. *N Engl J Med* 1998;338:719–726.
99. Abramson SB, Weissmann G. The mechanism of action of nonsteroidal antiinflammatory drugs. *Arthritis Rheum* 1989;32:1–9.
100. Harris RC, McKanna JA, Akai Y, et al. Cyclooxygenase-2 is associated with the macula densa in rat kidney and increases with salt restriction. *J Clin Invest* 1994;94:2504–2510.
101. Guan Y, Chang M, Cho W, et al. Cloning, expression, and regulation of rabbit cyclooxygenase-2 in renal medullary interstitial cells. *Am J Physiol* 1997;273:F18–F26.
102. Dubois RN, Abramson SB, Crofford L, et al. Cyclooxygenase in biology and disease. *FASEB J* 1998;12:1063–1073.
103. Vane JR, Botting RM. Mechanism of action of aspirin-like drugs. *Semin Arthritis Rheum* 1997;26:2–10.
104. Ehrich E, Schnitzer T, Kivitz A, et al. MK-966, a highly selective COX-2 inhibitor, was effective in the treatment of osteoarthritis (OA) of the knee and hip in a 6-week placebo controlled study. *Arthritis Rheum* 1997;40:S85(abst).
105. Cannon G, Caldwell J, Holt P, et al. MK-0966, a specific COX-2 inhibitor, has clinical efficacy comparable to diclofenac in the treatment of knee and hip osteoarthritis (OA) in a 26-week controlled clinical trial. *Arthritis Rheum* 1998;41(suppl):S196.
106. Saag K, Fisher C, McKay J, et al. MK-0966, a specific COX-2 inhibitor, has clinical efficacy comparable to ibuprofen in the treatment of knee and hip osteoarthritis (OA) in a 6-week controlled clinical trial. *Arthritis Rheum* 1998;41(suppl):S196.
107. Hubbard RC, Koepp RJ, Yu RS, et al. SC-58635, a novel COX-2 selective inhibitor, is effective as treatment for osteoarthritis (OA) in a short-term pilot study. *Arthritis Rheum* 1996;39(suppl):S226.
108. Hubbard R, Geis GS, Woods E, et al. Efficacy, tolerability and safety of celecoxib, a specific COX-2 inhibitor in osteoarthritis. *Arthritis Rheum* 1998;41(suppl):S196.

109. Lanza FL, Callison DA, Hubbard RC, et al. A pilot endoscopic study of the gastroduodenal effects of SC-58635, a COX-2 selective inhibitor. *Arthritis Rheum* 1997;40:S93(abst).
110. Geis GS, Stead H, Morant S, et al. Efficacy and safety of celecoxib, a specific COX-2 inhibitor, in patients with rheumatoid arthritis. *Arthritis Rheum* 1998;41(suppl):S316.
111. Karin A, Tolbert D, Piergies A, et al. Celecoxib, a specific COX-2 inhibitor, lacks significant drug-drug interactions with methotrexate or warfarin. *Arthritis Rheum* 1998;41(suppl): S315.
112. Bjarnason I, Macpherson A, Rotman H, et al. A randomized, double-blind, crossover comparative endoscopy study on the gastroduodenal tolerability of a highly specific cyclooxygenase-2 inhibitor, flosulide, and naproxen. *Scand J Gastroenterol* 1997; 32:126–130.
113. Hosie J, Distel M, Bluhmki E. Meloxicam in osteoarthritis: a 6-month, double-blind comparison with diclofenac sodium. *Br J Rheumatol* 1996;35(suppl 1):39–43.
114. Linden B, Distel M, Bluhmki E. A double-blind study to compare the efficacy and safety of meloxicam 15 mg with piroxicam 20 mg in patients with osteoarthritis of the hip. *Br J Rheumatol* 1996;35(suppl 1):35–38.
115. Amin AR, Attur M, Patel RN, et al. Superinduction of cyclooxygenase-2 activity in human osteoarthritis-affected cartilage: influence of nitric oxide. *J Clin Invest* 1997;99:1231–1237.
116. Altman RD, and the IAP Study Group. Ibuprofen, acetaminophen and placebo in osteoarthritis of the knee: a six-day double-blind study. *Arthritis Rheum* 1999;42(Suppl): S403(abst.).
117. Perneger TV, Whelton PK, Klag MJ. Risk of kidney failure associated with the use of acetaminophen, aspirin, and nonsteroidal antiinflammatory drugs. *N Engl J Med* 1994;331:1675–1679.
118. McCarthy GM, McCarthy DJ. Effect of topical capsaicin in the therapy of painful osteoarthritis of the hands. *J Rheumatol* 1992;19:604–607.
119. Deal CL, Schnitzer TJ, Lipstein E, et al. Treatment of arthritis with topical capsaicin: a double-blind trial. *Clin Ther* 1991; 13:383–389.
120. Virus RM, Gebhart GF. Pharmacologic actions of capsaicin: apparent involvement of substance P and serotonin. *Life Sci* 1979;25:1273–1284.
121. Zhang WY, Li Wan Po A. The effectiveness of topically applied capsaicin: a meta-analysis. *Eur J Clin Pharmacol* 1994;46: 517–522.
122. Rains C, Bryson HM. Topical capsaicin: a review of its pharmacological properties and therapeutic potential in post-herpetic neuralgia, diabetic neuropathy and osteoarthritis. *Drugs Aging* 1995;7:317–328.
123. Dreiser RL, Tisne-Camus M. DHEP plasters as a topical treatment of knee osteoarthritis: a double-blind placebo-controlled study. *Drugs Exp Clin Res* 1993;19:117–123.
124. Rolf C, Engstrom B, Beauchard C, et al. Intra-articular absorption and distribution of ketoprofen after topical plaster application and oral intake in 100 patients undergoing knee arthroscopy. *Rheumatology* 1999;38:564–567.
125. Raffa RB, Friederichs E, Reimann W, et al. Opioid and non-opioid components independently contribute to the mechanism of action of tramadol, an "atypical" opioid analgesic. *J Pharmacol Exp Ther* 1992;260:275–285.
126. Katz WA. Pharmacology and clinical experience with tramadol in osteoarthritis. *Drugs* 1996;52(suppl 3):39–47.
127. Goeringer KE, Logan BK, Christian GD. Identification of tramadol and its metabolites in blood from drug-related deaths and drug-impaired drivers. *J Anal Toxicol* 1997;21:529–537.
128. Roth SH. Efficacy and safety of tramadol HCl in breakthrough musculoskeletal pain attributed to osteoarthritis. *J Rheumatol* 1998;25:1358–1363.
129. Schnitzer TJ, Kamin M, Olson WH. Tramadol allows reduction of naproxen dose among patients with naproxen-responsive osteoarthritis pain: a randomized, double-blind, placebo-controlled study. *Arthritis Rheum* 1999;42:1370–1377.
130. AGS Panel on Chronic Pain in Older Persons. The management of chronic pain in older persons. *J Am Geriatr Soc* 1998;46: 635–651.
131. Carette S, Marcoux S, Truchon R, et al. A controlled trial of corticosteroid injections into facet joints for chronic low back pain. *N Engl J Med* 1991;325:1002–1007.
132. Miller JH, White J, Norton TH. The value of intra-articular injections in osteoarthritis of the knee. *J Bone Joint Surg Am* 1958;40:636–643.
133. Dieppe PA, Sathapatayavongs B, Jones HE, et al. Intra-articular corticosteroids in osteoarthritis. *Rheumatol Rehabil* 1980;19: 212–217.
134. Ravaud P, Moulinier L, Giraudeau B, et al. Effects of joint lavage and steroid injection in patients with osteoarthritis of the knee: results of a multicenter, randomized, controlled trial. *Arthritis Rheum* 1999;42:475–482.
135. Jones A, Doherty M. Intra-articular corticosteroids are effective in osteoarthritis but there are no clinical predictors of response. *Ann Rheum Dis* 1996;55:829–832.
136. Schnitzer TJ. Osteoarthritis treatment update. *Postgrad Med* 1993;93:89–93.
137. Altman RD. Osteoarthritis: aggravating factors and therapeutic measures. *Postgrad Med* 1986;80:150–163.
138. Cunningham LS, Kelsy JL. Epidemiology of musculoskeletal impairments and associated disability. *Am J Public Health* 1984;74:574–579.
139. Rene J, Weinberger M, Mazzuca SA, et al. Reduction of joint pain in patients with knee osteoarthritis who have received monthly telephone calls from lay personnel and whose medical treatment regimens have remained stable. *Arthritis Rheum* 1992;35:511–515.
140. Currey LF. Osteoarthrosis of the hip joint and sexual activity. *Ann Rheum Dis* 1970;29:488–491.
141. Oldenbring S, Egund N, Knutson K, et al. Revision after osteotomy for gonarthrosis: a 10-19 year follow-up of 314 cases. *Acta Orthop Scand* 1990;61:128–130.
142. Gibson JNA, White MD, Chapman VM, et al. Arthroscopic lavage and debridement for osteoarthritis of the knee. *J Bone Joint Surg Br* 1992;74:534–537.
143. Chang RW, Falconer J, Stulberg SD, et al. A randomized, controlled trial of arthroscopic surgery versus closed-needle joint lavage for patients with osteoarthritis of the knee. *Arthritis Rheum* 1993;36:289–296.
144. Liveseley PJ, Doherty M, Needoff M, et al. Arthroscopic lavage of osteoarthritic knees. *J Bone Joint Surg Br* 1991;73:922–926.
145. Ravaud P, Moulinier L, Giraudeau B, et al. Effects of joint lavage and steroid injection in patients with osteoarthritis of the knee. *Arthritis Rheum* 1999;42:475–482.
146. Pelletier JP, Martell-Pelletier J. Protective effects of corticosteroids on cartilage lesions and osteophyte formation in the Pond-Nuki dog model of osteoarthritis. *Arthritis Rheum* 1989; 32:181–193.
147. Wada J, Koshino T, Morii T, et al. Natural course of osteoarthritis of the knee treated with or without intraarticular corticosteroid injections: *Bull Hosp Joint Dis* 1993;53:45–48.
148. Peyron JG. Intraarticular hyaluronan injections in the treatment of osteoarthritis: state-of-the art review. *J Rheumatol* 1993;20(suppl 39):10–15.
149. Dougados M, Nguyen M, Listrat V. High molecular weight sodium hyaluronate (hyalectin) in osteoarthritis of the knee: a 1 year placebo-controlled trial. *Osteoarthritis Cartilage* 1993;1: 97–103.

150. Leardini G, Mattara L, Franceschini M, et al. Intra-articular treatment of knee osteoarthritis: a comparative study between hyaluronic acid and 6-methyl prednisolone acetate. *Clin Exp Rheumatol* 1991;9:375–381.
151. Altman RD, Moskowitz R. Intraarticular sodium hyaluronate (Hyalgan) in the treatment of osteoarthritis of the knee: a randomized clinical trial: Hyalgan Study Group. *J Rheumatol* 1998;25:2203–2212.
152. Adams MF, Atkinson M, Lussler AJ, et al. Comparison of intra-articular Hyalgan G-F (Synvisc): a viscoelastic derivative of hyaluronan and continuous NSAID therapy in patients with osteoarthritis of the knee. *Arthritis Rheum* 1993;37:S165.
153. McCarty MF. The neglect of glucosamine as a treatment for osteoarthritis: a personal perspective. *Med Hypotheses* 1994;42: 323–327.
154. Bradley JD, Flusser D, Katz BP, et al. A randomized, double blind, placebo controlled trial of intravenous loading with S-adenosylmethionine (SAM) followed by oral SAM therapy in patients with knee osteoarthritis. *J Rheumatol* 1994;21: 905–911.
155. Reichelt A, Forster KK, Fischer M, et al. Efficacy and safety of intramuscular glucosamine sulfate in osteoarthritis of the knee: a randomised, placebo-controlled, double-blind study. *Arzneimittelforschung* 1994;44:75–80.
156. Muller-Fabender H, Bach GL, Haase W, et al. Glucosamine sulfate compared to ibuprofen in osteoarthritis of the knee. *Osteoarthritis Cartilage* 1994;2:61–69.
157. Qiu GX, Gao SN, Giacovelli G, et al. Efficacy and safety of glucosamine sulfate versus ibuprofen in patients with knee osteoarthritis. *Arzneimittelforschung* 1998;48:469–474.
158. Karzel K, Domenjoz R. Effects of hexosamine derivatives and uronic acid derivatives on glycosaminoglycan metabolism of fibroblast cultures. *Pharmacology* 1971;5:337–345.
159. Bassleer C, Reginster JY, Franchimont P. Effects of glucosamine on differentiated human chondrocytes cultivated in clusters. *Rev Esp Reum* 1993;20(suppl 1):96(abst).
160. McCarty MF. Enhanced synovial production of hyaluronic acid may explain rapid clinical response to high-dose glucosamine in osteoarthritis. *Med Hypotheses* 1998;50:507–510.
161. Mathieu M, Piperno S, Annefeld M, et al. Glucosamine sulfate significantly reduced cartilage destruction in a rabbit model of osteoarthritis. *Arthritis Rheum* 1998;41(suppl):S147.
162. Mazieres B, Loyau G, Menkes CJ, et al. Chondroitin sulfate in the treatment of gonarthrosis and coxarthrosis: 5-month results of a multicenter double-blind controlled prospective study using placebo. *Rev Rhum* 1992;59:466–472.
163. Morreale P, Manopulo R, Galati M, et al. Comparison of the antiinflammatory efficacy of chondroitin sulfate and diclofenac sodium in patients with knee osteoarthritis. *J Rheumatol* 1996; 23:1385–1391.
164. Leeb BF, Schweitzer H, Montag K, et al. A meta-analysis of chondroitin sulfate in the treatment of osteoarthritis. *Arthritis Rheum* 1998;41(suppl):S198.
165. McAlindon TE, Gulin J, Felson DT. Glucosamine (GL) and chondroitin (CH) treatment for osteoarthritis (OA) of the knee or hip: meta-analysis and quality assessment of clinical trials. *Arthritis Rheum* 1998;41(suppl):S198.
166. Leffler CT, Philippi AF, Leffler SG, et al. Glucosamine, chondroitin and manganese ascorbate for degenerative joint disease of the knee or low back: a randomized, double-blind, placebo-controlled pilot study. *Mil Med* 1999;164:85–91.
167. Shankland WE II. The effects of glucosamine and chondroitin sulfate on osteoarthritis of the TMJ: a preliminary report of 50 patients. *Cranio* 1998;16:230–235.
168. Hoedt-Schmidt S, Schneider B, Kahlben DA. Histomorphological studies on the effect of recombinant human superoxide dismutase in biochemically induced osteoarthritis. *Pharmacology* 1993;47:252–260.
169. Mazieres B, Masquelier AM, Capron MH. A French controlled multicenter study of intraarticular orgotein versus intraarticular corticosteroids in the treatment of knee osteoarthritis. *J Rheumatol* 1991;27(suppl):134–137.
170. Gammer W, Broback L-G. Clinical comparison of orgotein and methylprednisolone acetate in the treatment of osteoarthritis of the knee joint. *Scand J Rheumatol* 1984;13:108–112.
171. McIlwain H, Silverfield JC, Cheatum DE, et al. Intra-articular orgotein in osteoarthritis of the knee: a placebo-controlled efficacy, safety, and dosage comparison. *Am J Med* 1989;87: 295–300.
172. Stucki G, Bozzone P, Treuer E, et al. Efficacy and safety of radiation synovectomy with yttrium-90: a retrospective long-term analysis of 164 applications in 82 patients. *Br J Rheumatol* 1993;32:383–386.
173. Hilliquin P, Le Devic P, Menkes CJ. Comparison of the efficacy of nonsurgical synovectomy (synoviorthosis) and joint lavage in knee osteoarthritis with effusions. *Rev Rhum Engl Ed* 1996;63: 93–102.
174. Martel-Pelletier J, Mineau F, Jolicoeur FC, et al. In vitro effects of diacerhein and rhein on interleukin 1 and tumor necrosis factor-alpha systems in human osteoarthritic synovium and chondrocytes. *J Rheumatol* 1998;25:753–762.
175. Carney SL, Hicks CA, Tree B, et al. An in vivo investigation of the effect of anthraquinones on the turnover of aggrecans in spontaneous osteoarthritis in the guinea pig. *Inflamm Res* 1995; 44:182–186.
176. Brun PH. Effect of diacetylrhein on the development of experimental osteoarthritis: a biochemical investigation [Letter]. *Osteoarthritis Cartilage* 1997;5:289–291.
177. Brandt K, Smith G, Kang SY, et al. Effects of diacerhein in an accelerated canine model of osteoarthritis. *Osteoarthritis Cartilage* 1997;5:438–449.
178. Nguyen M, Dougados M, Berdah L, et al. Diacerhein in the treatment of osteoarthritis of the hip. *Arthritis Rheum* 1994; 37:529–537.
179. Spencer CM, Wilde MI. Diacerein. *Drugs* 1997;53:98–108.
180. Felson DT, Nevitt MC. The effects of estrogen on osteoarthritis. *Curr Opin Rheumatol* 1998;10:269–272.
181. Spector TD, Nandra D, Hart DJ, et al. Is hormone replacement therapy protective for hand and knee osteoarthritis in women? The Chingford Study. *Ann Rheum Dis* 1997;56:432–434.
182. Nevitt MC, Cummings SR, Lane NE, et al. Association of estrogen replacement therapy with the risk of osteoarthritis of the hip in elderly white women: study of Osteoporotic Fractures Research Group. *Arch Intern Med* 1996;156:2073–2080.
183. Cauley JA, Kwoh CK, Egeland G, et al. Serum sec hormones and severity of osteoarthritis of the hand. *J Rheumatol* 1993;20: 1170–1175.
184. Ushiyama T, Ueyama H, Inoue K, et al. Estrogen receptor gene polymorphism and generalized osteoarthritis. *J Rheumatol* 1998;25:134–137.
185. Szczepanski A, Dabrowska H, Moskalewska K. An appraisal of the effect of Piascledine in the treatment of scleroderma. *Przeg Derm* 1975;LXII:4.
186. Harmand MF. Etude de l'action des insaponifiables d'avocat et de soja sur les cultures de chondrocytes articulaires. *Gazette Med France* 1985;92:No 29.
187. Loyau G, Pujol JP, Mauviel A. Effet des insaponifiables d'avocat/soja aur l'activite collagenolytique de cultures de synoviocytes rhumatoides humains et de chondrocytes articulaires de lapin traites par l'interleukine-1. *Rev Rhum* 1991;58:241–245.
188. Chevalier X, Feng XZ, Groult N, et al. Modulation of fibronectin biosynthesis, elastase activity, cell proliferation and

cell phenotype of rabbit chondrocytes by soja and avocado extracts: communication at the 12th European Congress on Rheumatology-Budapest 7/1991.

189. Blotman F, Maheu E, Wulwik A, et al. Efficacy and safety of avocado/soybean unsaponifiables in the treatment of symptomatic osteoarthritis of the knee and hip: a prospective, multicenter, three-month, randomized, double-blind, placebo-controlled trial. *Rev Rhum Engl Ed* 1997;64:825–834.
190. Maheu E, Mazieres B, Valat JP, et al. Symptomatic efficacy of avocado/soybean unsaponifiables in the treatment of the knee and hip: a prospective, randomized, double-blind, placebo-controlled, multicenter clinical trial with a six month treatment period and a two-month follow-up demonstrating a persistent effect. *Arthritis Rheum* 1998;41:81–91.
191. Mammi GI, Rocchi R, Cadossi R, et al. The electrical stimulation of tibial osteotomies: double-blind study. *Clin Orthop* 1993;288:246–253.
192. Trock DH, Bollet AJ, Markoll R. The effect of pulsed electromagnetic fields in the treatment of osteoarthritis of the knee and cervical spine: report of randomized, double blind, placebo controlled trials. *J Rheumatol* 1994;21:1903–1911.
193. Srivasta KC, Mustafa T. Ginger (*Zingiber officinale*) in rheumatism and musculoskeletal disorders. *Med Hypotheses* 1992;39:342–348.
194. Lozada CJ, Altman RD. Chondroprotection in osteoarthritis. *Bull Rheum Dis* 1997;46:5–7.
195. Amin AR, Attur MG, Thakker GD, et al. A novel mechanism of action of tetracyclines: effects on nitric oxide synthases. *Proc Natl Acad Sci U S A* 1996;93:14014–14019.
196. Amin AR, Patel RN, Attur MG, et al. Tetracyclines upregulate COX-2 expression and PGE_2 production independently from the inhibition of nitric oxide. *Arthritis Rheum* 1998;41 (suppl):S342.
197. Tilley BC, Alarcon GS, Heyse SP, et al. Minocycline in rheumatoid arthritis: a 48-week, double-blind, placebo-controlled trial. *Ann Intern Med* 1995;122:81–89.
198. Cole AD, Chubinskaya S, Luchene LJ, et al. Doxycycline disrupts chondrocyte differentiation and inhibits cartilage matrix degradation. *Arthritis Rheum* 1994;32:1727–1734.
199. Yu LP Jr, Smith GN Jr, Hasty KA, et al. Doxycycline inhibits type XI collagenolytic activity of extracts from human osteoarthritic cartilage and of gelatinase. *J Rheumatol* 1991; 18:1450–1452.
200. Brandt KD, Yu LP, Amith G, et al. Therapeutic effect of doxycycline (doxy) in canine osteoarthritis (OA). *Osteoarthritis Cartilage* 1993;1:14.
201. Smith GN Jr, Yu LP Jr, Brandt KD, et al. Oral administration of doxycycline reduces collagenase and gelatinase activities in extracts of human osteoarthritic cartilage. *J Rheumatol* 1998;25:532–535.
202. Israel HA, Ramamurthy NS, Greenwald R, et al. The potential role of doxycycline in the treatment of osteoarthritis of the temporomandibular joint. *Adv Dent Res* 1998;12:51–55.
203. Lewis EJ, Bishop J, Bottomley D, et al. Ro32-3555, an orally active collagenase inhibitor, prevents cartilage breakdown in vitro and in vivo. *Br J Pharmacol* 1997;121:540–546.
204. de Bri E, Lei W, Svensson O, et al. Effect of an inhibitor of matrix metalloproteinases on spontaneous osteoarthritis in guinea pigs. *Adv Dent Res* 1998;12:82–85.
205. Burkhardt D, Ghosh P. Laboratory evaluation of antiarthritic drugs as potential chondroprotective agents. *Semin Arthritis Rheum* 1987;17(suppl 1):3–34.
206. Altman RD, Dean DD, Muniz OE, et al. Prophylactic treatment of canine osteoarthritis with glycosaminoglycan polysulfuric acid ester. *Arthritis Rheum* 1989;32:759–766.
207. Rejholec V. Long-term studies of antiosteoarthritic drugs: an assessment. *Semin Arthritis Rheum* 1987;17(suppl 1):35–53.
208. Moskowitz RW, Reese JH, Young RG, et al. The effects of Rumalon, a glycosaminoglycan peptide complex, in a partial meniscectomy model of osteoarthritis in rabbits. *J Rheumatol* 1991;18:205–209.
209. Dean DD, Muniz OE, Rodriguez I, et al. Amelioration of lapine osteoarthritis by treatment with glycosaminoglycan-peptide association complex (Rumalon). *Arthritis Rheum* 1991;34:304–313.
210. Howell DS, Altman RD. Cartilage repair and conservation in osteoarthritis. *Rheum Dis Clin North Am* 1993;19:713–724.
211. Golding JC, Ghosh P. Drugs for osteoarthrosis I: the effects of pentosan polysulphate (SP54) on the degradation and loss of proteoglycans from articular cartilage in a model of osteoarthrosis induced in the rabbit knee joint by immobilization. *Curr Ther Res* 1983;32:173–184.
212. Smith MM, Ghosh P, Numata Y, et al. The effects of orally administered calcium pentosan polysulfide on inflammation and cartilage degradation produced in rabbit joints by intraarticular injection of a hyaluronate-polylysine complex. *Arthritis Rheum* 1994;37:125–136.
213. Doughty J, Spirito S, Ganu V, et al. An orally active metalloproteinase inhibitor blocks proteoglycan release in rabbit knees after injection of stromelysin but not interleukin-1. *Trans 41st Annu Meet Orthop Res Soc* 1995;20:414.
214. Zhang Y, McAlindon TE, Hannan MT, et al. Estrogen replacement therapy and worsening of radiographic knee osteoarthritis: The Framingham study. *Arthritis Rheum* 1998;41:1867–1873.
215. Pelletier JP, Roughley PJ, DiBattista JA, et al. Are cytokines involved in osteoarthritic pathophysiology? *Semin Arthritis Rheum* 1991;20(suppl 2):12–25.
216. Hunziker EB, Rosenberg L. Induction of repair in partial thickness articular cartilage lesions by timed release of TGF-beta. *Trans 40th Annu Meet Orthop Res Soc* 1994;19:236.
217. Ikeda T, Kubo T, Arai Y, et al. Adenovirus mediated gene delivery to the joints of guinea pigs. *J Rheumatol* 1998;25:1666–1673.
218. Doherty PJ, Zhang H, Tramblay L, et al. Resurfacing of articular cartilage explants with genetically-modified human chondrocytes in vitro. *Osteoarthritis Cartilage* 1998;6:153–159.
219. Pelletier JP, Caron JP, Evans C, et al. In vivo suppression of early experimental osteoarthritis by interleukin-1 receptor antagonist using gene therapy. *Arthritis Rheum* 1997;40:1012–1019.
220. Brittberg M, Lindahl A, Nilsson A, et al. Treatment of deep cartilage defect in the knee with autologous chondrocyte transplantation. *N Engl J Med* 1994;331:889–895.
221. Wakitani S, Goto T, Pineda SJ, et al. Mesenchymal cell-based repair of large, full-thickness defects of articular cartilage. *J Bone Joint Surg Am* 1994;76:579–592.
222. Rogachefsky RA, Dean DD, Howell DS, et al. Treatment of canine osteoarthritis with insulin-like growth factor-1 (IGF-1) and sodium pentosan polysulfate. *Osteoarthritis Cartilage* 1993; 1:105–114.

113

ARTICULAR CARTILAGE REPAIR

ROBERT L. SAH
ALBERT C. CHEN
SILVIA S. CHEN
KELVIN W. LI
MICHAEL A. DIMICCO
MELISSA S. KURTIS
LISA M. LOTTMAN
JOHN D. SANDY

Throughout adult life, the articular cartilage of diarthrodial joints experiences a high level of biomechanical stress (1). In many individuals and in most anatomic sites, cartilage can tolerate years of repetitive loading. However, with trauma and aging, cartilage damage occurs often in particular sites, for example, in the hip and knee. After even minor injuries, adult cartilage, as a tissue, has a highly limited intrinsic capacity to repair (2). Cartilage defects that currently appear to represent good candidates for surgical repair are those that are focal and occupy a surface area of several square centimeters on the femoral, tibial, or patellar surfaces of the knee. Such defects typically result from sports-related injury (3), occult osteochondral lesions after anterior cruciate ligament (ACL) rupture (4), or osteochondritis dissecans in the mature knee (5).

In practice, two distinct but related clinical problems must be addressed. In one case, a chondral defect, the damage is restricted to the cartilage layer; in the other case, an osteochondral defect, both the cartilage and the subchondral bone tissues are involved (Fig. 113.1). Repair strategies that include subchondral penetration may be applicable to both chondral and osteochondral defects, especially because it has been noted that attempts to debride damaged cartilage from a superficial lesion can sometimes result in penetration of the subchondral bone (6,7). However, repairs limited to the cartilage will be applicable only to chondral defects. As discussed in detail later, the biologic responses to cartilage injury are highly dependent on whether the defect penetrates through the calcified cartilage to expose the marrow elements (2,8).

The inability of adult articular cartilage to mount an effective wound-repair response, such as that commonly seen in an adult bone fracture or skin lesion, is a consequence of a number of unique properties of this tissue. Articular cartilage is composed primarily of cells (chondrocytes) embedded sparsely in a fiber-reinforced hydrated gel. The fibers consist of collagen, largely types II, IX, and XI. The gel is a highly electronegative composite of protein and sulfated glycosaminoglycans (chondroitin sulfate and keratan sulfate), the major structural element of which is the proteoglycan called *aggrecan.* Unlike bone or skin, mature cartilage is avascular and receives nutrients primarily from the synovial fluid that bathes the articular surface (9). This inability of blood vessels to penetrate the mature articular cartilage matrix results to some degree from an abundance of angiostatic molecular factors in the tissue (10,11). This fact essentially eliminates a central feature of normal wound repair, that of inflammation and resorption of the damaged tissue by inflammatory cells. Unlike the repair fibroblasts of skin or the osteoblasts of bone, chondrocytes within cartilage tissue are essentially immobilized within the dense extracellular matrix. These cells therefore exhibit little or no

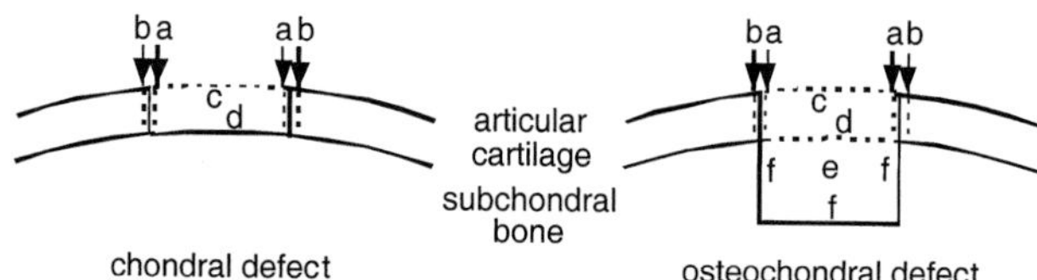

FIGURE 113.1. Schematic of two broad categories of cartilage defects seen clinically. The chondral defect (**left**) involves only the cartilage, and the repair strategy may or may not involve subchondral bone. The osteochondral defect (**right**) involves both cartilage and bone, and repair of both is required. Tissues and interface areas of particular importance are shown as *a*, interface of implant with host cartilage; *b*, interface of host cartilage with implant; *c*, implant providing repair cartilage; *d*, interface of repair cartilage with subchondral bone; *e*, repair bone; and *f*, interface of repair bone with host bone. (Adapted from Hjertquist SO, Lemperg R. Histological, autoradiographic, and microchemical studies of spontaneously healing osteochondral articular defects in adult rabbits. *Calcif Tissue Res* 1971;8: 54–72, with permission.)

intrinsic repair responses, such as proliferation and migration to the injury site (12,13). In addition, the matrix is metabolized rather slowly. Other major obstacles to effective repair and generation of a stable and functional composite are the filling of defect regions with cartilaginous tissue with the integration of the repair tissue with the surrounding tissue (14). Finally, the joint is a biomechanically complex environment, and mechanical activity or inactivity may alter the cellular and extracellular processes that are needed for effective repair.

In a recent review of the field (2), the authors summarized a possible *multistage clinical approach* to restoring a functional articular surface in a damaged joint. This included (a) analysis of the structural and functional abnormalities of the involved joint and the patient's expectations for future use, (b) mechanical correction for malalignment or instability, (c) debridement that may include penetration of subchondral bone to allow access of reparative mesenchymal stem cells, (d) implanting a construct that may contain a natural or synthetic matrix as well as growth factors and cells, and (e) a postoperative course of controlled loading and motion.

In this chapter, we summarize the available information primarily in the area of implant design and application (stage d, above). In particular, we focus on the application to the defect site of an implant composed of one or several of the following components: tissues, cells, natural or synthetic materials, and growth factors. A summary of some of the specific components currently in investigative and clinical use is provided in Fig. 113.2. Many issues arise regarding the choice of particular components and the production and delivery of the implant. These issues are central to the emerging discipline of tissue engineering. Tissue engineering of articular cartilage has received a great deal of interest, both in the scientific literature (15) and the popular press (16,17). Tissue engineering has been defined as *the application of principles and methods of engineering and life sciences toward fundamental understanding of structure–function relations in normal and pathologic mammalian tissues and the development of biologic substitutes to restore, maintain, or improve tissue functions* (18). The major factor that distinguishes cartilage tissue-engineering therapies from others,

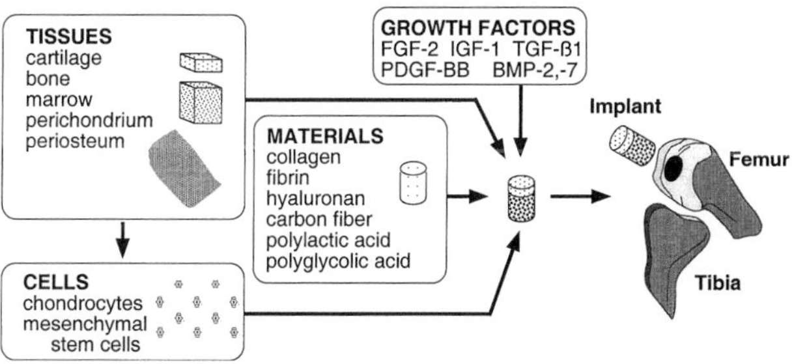

FIGURE 113.2. Tissue-engineering strategies to repair an articular cartilage defect in the femoral condyle.

such as joint replacement with metal and plastic prostheses, is the primary involvement of living cells; the engineered implant either includes living cells or is designed to modulate the function of endogenous cells (19–21).

INTRINSIC CARTILAGE REPAIR AFTER SUBCHONDRAL PENETRATION

Because of the long-standing realization that superficial adult cartilage lesions are essentially nonreparative (22), many of the current clinical procedures for repair of cartilage defects purposefully penetrate through the base of cartilage defects into the subchondral vasculature. These procedures include subchondral drilling (23), microfracture (3,24), abrasion (25,26), and spongiolization (27). Such penetrating defects elicit an exuberant repair response, in contrast to lacerations confined to the articular cartilage (8). Thus it is useful to first consider the natural repair processes that are triggered by the creation of an osteochondral defect. The exact details of the repair process may depend on a number of factors including the size, shape, and location of the defect, as well as the maturity (28) and species of the animal. Nevertheless, such repair generally exhibits a number of cellular and matrix remodeling processes that result in a characteristic evolution of structural, compositional, and functional features.

The process of tissue overgrowth after subchondral penetration has been studied extensively in adult rabbits (28,29) and has been described in detail as follows (30):

> In the first few days, fibrinous arcades were established across the defect, from surface edge to surface edge, and this served to orient mesenchymal cell ingrowth along the long axes. The first evidence of a cartilage matrix, as defined by safranin-O staining, appeared at 10 days. At 2 weeks, cartilage was present immediately beneath the surface of collagenous tissue that was rich in flattened fibrocartilaginous cells in virtually all specimens. At 3 weeks, the sites of almost all of the defects had a well-demarcated layer of cartilage containing chondrocytes. An essentially complete repopulation of the defects occurred at 6, 8, 10, and 12 weeks, with progressive differentiation of cells to chondroblasts, chondrocytes, and osteoblasts. Autoradiography, after labeling with ^{3}H-thymidine and ^{3}H-cytidine, demonstrated that chondrocytes from the residual adjacent articular cartilage did not participate in the repopulation of the defect. The repair was mediated wholly by the mesenchymal cells of the marrow. Thus the early stages of this repair response include the migration, adhesion, proliferation, and differentiation of cells extrinsic to cartilage.

Clinical experiences (3,23,24) suggest that, in some patients, repair after subchondral penetration can provide a significant improvement of joint function and pain relief for many years. However, it also is clear that, for many other patients, such approaches do not provide a long-term solution. Indeed, the unsuccessful patients in these studies appear to undergo matrix remodeling and degeneration processes that are clearly delineated at later times in animal studies. Poor healing at the cartilage–cartilage interface has been implicated as an important deficit. In studies on the long-term repair response to a laceration type of chondral injury in rabbits, local cell death and a limited local proliferation response without healing led to cartilage fissures both within and outside the original injury sites by 18 to 24 months (22). In studies of osteochondral defects in rabbits (29,30), the majority of the tissue formed at 12 weeks typically turned into fibrocartilage that initially filled the bulk of the defect but ultimately broke down. Early traces of degeneration of the cartilage matrix were seen in many defects at 12 to 20 weeks, with the prevalence and intensity of the degeneration increasing at 24, 36, and 48 weeks. Polarized light microscopy demonstrated failure of the newly synthesized repair matrix to become adherent to, and integrated with, the cartilage immediately adjacent to the drill-hole, even when light microscopy had shown apparent continuity of the tissue. In many instances, a clear gap was seen between repair and residual cartilage (30). These interface regions between repair and host cartilage were observed to be associated with the absence of live cells. In addition, complete restoration of the subchondral bone plate was inconsistent (28), although occasionally, by 24 weeks, both the tidemark and the compact lamellar subchondral bone plate were reestablished. The cancellous woven bone that had formed initially in the depths of the defect was replaced by lamellar, coarse cancellous bone (30).

These morphologic features of the intrinsic repair after subchondral bone penetration are associated with abnormal matrix constituents and biomechanical properties. Biochemically, the tissue has a proteoglycan content that does not reach that of normal articular cartilage, whereas the collagen component includes an abnormally high content of type I collagen. Type I collagen composes 70% of the total (types I and II) collagen at 3 weeks, and about 20% of the total at 24 to 48 weeks (31). With respect to interpreting biochemical data as a measure of the repair response and the degree of filling of cartilage defects, it should be emphasized that the way in which biochemical composition is described is critical. Because cartilaginous tissue contains both fluid and solid components with an overall tissue density close to unity (32), normalization of a chemical constituent to tissue wet weight (roughly equivalent to normalization to tissue volume) provides an index of the degree of filling of the defect. In contrast, normalization of a constituent to the sample dry weight typically does not provide a quantity that is directly comparable to that for normal cartilage, because the hydration of the repair tissue is typically greater than that of normal cartilage. The abnormal composition of fibrocartilaginous repair tissue is associated with load-bearing biomechanical properties that are inferior to those of normal articular cartilage (28,33–39).

This description of morphologic, biochemical, and biomechanical assessments provides detail on several possible undesirable outcomes for a repair process. These include a filling of the defect that is incomplete, fibrous, and not durable; an inadequate integration of the repair tissue with the surrounding cartilage; and an inconsistent restoration of subchondral bone (30,40). Each of these features may be a precipitating factor in the eventual degeneration of the repair tissue.

EXTRINSIC COMPONENTS FOR ENHANCING CARTILAGE REPAIR

A range of approaches is used currently to optimize the possibility of achieving fully functional and integrative cartilage repair. To evaluate the success of a particular repair strategy, a variety of outcomes can be measured (41). Ideally, successful repair would lead to a consistent restoration of functional joint tissues and long-term symptomatic relief and preservation of the surrounding cartilage. In a clinical situation, important end-point measures are restoration of joint function and attainment of pain relief. In studies on animals, all tissues can be harvested and analyzed at several time points and levels of detail. When extrinsic cells are implanted into a defect, the localization and adhesion of these cells can be assessed. At the tissue level, the composition, structure, metabolism, and function of the bulk of the repair tissue can be compared with those of normal tissues. This tissue-level comparison presumes that restoration of these parameters will lead to restoration of overall joint function. At the organ level, overall joint function and absence of deterioration can be analyzed directly. In this section we summarize the use of various extrinsic components for repairing cartilage defects in relation to the restoration of the normal structure, composition, and function of articulating joints.

Tissues

Transplantation of various tissues has been performed clinically for the repair of cartilage defects and also studied experimentally in animals. The choice of tissue may depend largely on the clinical picture (lesion area, depth, location, patient age, etc.), but tissue availability also will be a determinant. At one extreme are tissues, such as cartilage and osteochondral fragments, that contain normal articular cartilage and thus, at the time of implant, are fully formed, metabolically active, and mechanically functional. Alternatively, tissues such as periosteum and perichondrium are used with the intent of developing into biomechanically functional cartilage and bone. Tissue implants also have been used to contribute indirectly to repair, for example, by functioning to retain or modulate other reparative cells. Conversely, because intact tissues have a discrete structure, they may impede integration between the implant and the host tissues. The origin of the tissue to be transplanted also is a critical issue. Thus whereas fresh allogeneic tissue can be difficult to obtain and there is a need to screen for disease transmission, autogeneic tissue removal necessarily creates a defect at the donor site, which itself must heal or be repaired.

Once a tissue fragment or construct has been prepared *ex vivo,* it must be fixed to the cartilage defect site. Physical methods of fixing the implant include press-fit and the use of fastening devices. For implants containing extensive amounts of subchondral bone, such as osteochondral fragments, biodegradable pins (42–47) have been buried through the soft tissue substance into the bone. Alternatively, screws have been used to fix the subchondral bone portion of the implant to the host. Implants that are relatively soft have been fixed by using other methods. For defects that are relatively deep, press-fit methods have been used (48–50). For more shallow defects or for relatively thin tissue implants, sutures have been used. For example, to hold periosteal tissue in place at the base of an osteochondral defect, sutures are passed through drill holes, exiting laterally through subchondral bone (51). When periosteum is used as a covering flap, it is affixed by placing sutures into the surrounding tissues, including articular cartilage (52). Such application of a suture through the articular cartilage may have a mild detrimental effect (6,53). Adhesive chemicals and materials, described later, provide alternative methods of fixing an implant and may allow direct bonding of entire areas of the implant to the host.

Cartilage Implants

There have been a few studies examining the application of articular cartilage tissue to the repair of a chondral defect. Animal studies demonstrated the possibility of affixing such implants by using fibrin adhesive. In sheep, tissue retention was evident with bony union at 7 months (54). However, cartilage degeneration occurred in allogeneic cartilage grafts by 12 to 18 months (55). In rabbits, application of multiple cartilage slices did not lead to complete integration with the host cartilage at 40 weeks (56). In the limited clinical experiences in humans (57,58), the grafted cartilage, at 1 year, typically showed apposition with the surrounding cartilage and subchondral bone. However, some grafts showed evidence of degeneration, and, for allograft cartilage, a pannus-like tissue overgrowth, suggesting a possible immune response.

Osteochondral Implants

Osteochondral fragments have been used extensively as a clinical treatment for cartilage defects and also in experimental studies. Such fragments consist of normal full-thickness articular cartilage and a layer of attached subchondral bone. For the past several decades, transplantation of site-matched allogeneic osteochondral fragments has been performed for cartilage defects, especially those that are relatively large, and the clinical outcome has been reasonably good in long-term studies (43,44,46,59–65). Here, efforts are made to keep the indwelling chondrocytes alive by using the allografts soon after donor harvest and by incubating the fragment in a nutrient solution in the interim. Clinical studies report varied levels of apparent cartilage integration after osteochondral grafting (60,62,63). To minimize delivery of immunogenic marrow cells within the allogeneic donor bone, the bone portion of an osteochondral fragment can be prepared to be thin (several millimeters) and rinsed by pulsatile lavage before implantation (43,44).

The use of an autogeneic osteochondral graft (66–68) avoids problems associated with allogeneic tissue. However, other problems can arise with the use of autogeneic tissue. There is morbidity at the donor site and difficulty in creating a graft that is matched geometrically to the recipient site. The use of multiple osteochondral autografts, in the form of cylindrical cores (69–71), allows better fitting of the implant to the host site, while generating more interfaces between portions of the graft. Osteochondral autografts have been used for various joints (72–74), and the surgical procedure has been described in detail with encouraging short-term clinical data (an average follow-up of about 2 years) (75). In a modification of these osteochondral autograft approaches, a combination of microfracture and transplantation of a cartilage–bone paste has also been used; the paste is prepared from a full-depth cartilage bone plug removed from the intercondylar notch of the knee under treatment (76). The mixture of articular cartilage and cancellous bone appears to provide a supportive matrix for cartilage formation, and clinical evaluation indicated that the procedure provided pain relief and an increase in activity level. However, both hyaline cartilage and nonfibrous tissue were evident in biopsies.

Periosteal Implants

The use of periosteum for cartilage repair has been studied in animals and explored in humans, as described in a recent review (51). Periosteum is a tissue that covers bones and consists of an outer fibrous layer and an inner cambium layer. The cambium layer of periosteum contains stem cells that can differentiate into chondrocytes. Periosteum-derived cells form cartilage and bone during normal physiologic development and growth, as well as fracture healing. Such cells have the capacity to form cartilage exuberantly, as evidenced by the growth of periosteal explants during *in vitro* incubation and after *in vivo* implantation (77,78). Experimental studies in rabbits indicate that the source of repair cells in the cartilage defect after periosteal transplantation is largely from the implanted periosteum (78,79). The harvest technique is critical to the survival of the cells in the periosteum tissue (51). Clinically, autologous periosteum has been used as an exogenous source of cells for repairing relatively large cartilage defects in knee joints. The periosteum tissue has been placed against the subchondral bone of a defect with the cambium side facing either the articular surface (80–85) or the subchondral bone (51). Here, short-term clinical follow-up indicates that repair can be excellent in some patients, but unsatisfactory in others (51,80,81,83). Both in clinical and animal studies, periosteum has been used as a flap (with the cambium layer facing down toward the bone), overlying injected chondrocytes (see later).

Perichondrial Implants

Perichondrium, like periosteum, has been used for repair of cartilage defects both in animal experiments and in the clinic. Perichondrium is the transitional zone between connective tissue and cartilage (86), and consists of an outer fibrous layer, an intermediate proliferative layer, and an inner layer that transitions to attached cartilage (87). The outer fibrous layer contains a sparse population of fibrocyte cells, whereas the intermediate and transition layers contain cells that take on an increasingly round, chondrocyte-like morphology toward the transition layer. It was recognized that perichondrium from the ear has the capacity to form cartilage *in vivo,* and formation of cartilage from perichondrium may be responsible for "cauliflower ear," the common disfigurement afflicting wrestlers (88). When perichondrium is cultured *in vitro* (86,89) or transplanted into cartilage defects in animals, cartilage is formed (86,90). Although perichondrium from the ear was studied for repair of articular cartilage defects, it formed cartilage less consistently than perichondrium from ribs, and it also synthesized elastin, which is not normally found in articular cartilage (86,91). Thus for studies on cartilage repair, perichondrium tissue obtained from the ribs has been used most commonly. When placed in cartilage defects, the perichondrium appears to be the source of reparative cells that proliferate and differentiate into chondrocytes (92). Although the formation of repair tissue is somewhat inconsistent, the cartilaginous tissue that does form at 1 year exhibits a biochemical composition (indices of collagen type and proteoglycan content) and biomechanical properties approaching those of normal cartilage (90). Clinically, perichondrial transplants have been used mostly to repair cartilage defects in finger joints (93–97), but also for other small joints [temporomandibular, toe, elbow (94,98)] and the knee (99,100). The long-term results for small joints (94) appear to be better than those for the knee (100,101).

Cells

As already implied in the preceding section on cell-laden tissue implants for cartilage repair, it seems likely that a truly effective repair strategy for articular cartilage lesions will require, at a minimum, the implantation of cells. In this regard, it is important to appreciate that the donor "repair" cells may fulfill one or more of several possible roles in the repair process. In the common situation in which mature differentiated chondrocytes are used, the rationale is that the cells will maintain a stable phenotype and directly synthesize and organize a functional mature cartilage matrix. A second approach is to use a "precursor" cell population and, in this case, the rationale calls for the cells to differentiate into chondrocytes and then produce a stable matrix. In a third conceivable scenario, cells of a different phenotype might be added to condition the microenvironment, for example, to encourage the migration and stable differentiation of precursor cells from the host tissues.

Typically the cells are introduced by injection or by placement within a scaffold material (see later section) that serves as a carrier. In clinical chondrocyte transplantation protocols, a cell density of 25×10^6 cells/cm^3 (a cell pellet of 12 million cells and an additional 0.4 mL of medium) is used (102), and this is intermediate to the cell density of articular cartilage during growth and development and that in mature humans (103). Over time, the local cell density may be modulated by the cellular processes of adhesion, migration, proliferation, and death, and the activity of cells may be modulated by biochemical and biophysical factors that affect cell metabolism. Although the optimal number of cells for repair of a particular sized cartilage defect is not known, the development of methods to deliver a controlled number of cells consistently is likely to be a critical step in repair therapies.

Chondrocytes

As might be expected for cartilage repair, the majority of cell-implant studies have been done with chondrocytes, and these have either been allogeneic cells from immature or adolescent donors (in animal studies) or autogeneic cells from young adults (in human studies). In rabbits, chondrocytic cells have been harvested from various cartilage tissues (35,49,104–107) or rib perichondrium (37,108) and placed in carbon fiber pads or collagen materials for implantation. Articular chondrocytes have also been prepared for implantation in the horse (109–111), injected under a periosteal flap in the dog (6,53,112), and added with fibrin glue in the goat (113,114). In humans, the use of autologous, culture-expanded articular chondrocytes implanted under a sutured periosteal flap in the knee (52) is now in extended clinical use, and this is discussed later.

The success of chondrocyte transplantation appears to be very dependent on the nature of the vehicle used to retain the cells in the implant. A number of early studies concerning treatment of osteochondral defects examined the application of isolated chondrocytes (48,115–118). This approach appeared to result in an inconsistent adherence of the implanted cells to the repair site (115), and this variability may have led to the formation of isolated islands of cartilage tissue (48,116). To enhance retention of injected cells in the defect site, chondrocytes have been injected underneath an autologous periosteal patch that was sutured over the cartilage defect. This configuration has been used both in animal studies (6,53,112,119,120) and in humans (7,52,121,122), and more recently, the periosteum–cartilage interface has been sealed with fibrin glue (6,7,53,112,121,122). In animals, several studies have established that this treatment does lead to an increased filling of the defect with cartilaginous tissue at 6 weeks (119) and up to 1 year (120), whereas in another study (6), this was not achieved. The application of this procedure to humans, especially for defects of the femoral condyle, has often led to an improvement in joint function and a subsequent decrease in pain and swelling (52,121–123). Recommendations have been given for complications, including incomplete graft incorporation and delamination, as well as hypertrophy (7). How this procedure, commercialized as Carticel by Genzyme Tissue Repair in the United States, compares with others that are used clinically (and that do not involve the use of cultured cells) is unclear; the lack of a direct comparison has incited much controversy (124–128).

A number of other important questions have arisen about the chondrocyte transplantation procedure currently in clinical use. For example, the survival period of the transplanted cells and the periosteal flap within the cartilage defect, and the likely effect of a sealant on this process is unclear. After 6 weeks in rabbit and dog animal models, only a small and variable portion of the cells in the defect site were found to contain molecular markers that had been applied to the injected cells (53,119). This indicates several possibilities, including the loss of transplanted cells from the defect site, the influx of host cells into the repair site, or loss of the tag from the transplanted cells. The circumstances under which each applied component (i.e., injected chondrocytes, periosteal patch, sutures, fibrin sealant) contribute independently or interactively to repair remains to be established (126,129,130).

Mesenchymal Stem Cells

It has long been realized that bone marrow and certain other tissues, such as periosteum and perichondrium, contain stem cells that can differentiate into chondrocytes and osteoblasts. Isolation, expansion, purification, and genetic manipulation of these cells have therefore been considered as a realistic alternative to the use of mature chondrocytes in cell-based cartilage repair (131). Conversely, it is possible that a biomaterial could be designed that will alone be capable of inducing the invasion and retention of chondrogenic mesenchymal cells, for example, from the synovial membrane of the host (132). Attempts to translate the experience obtained from animal studies to the human clinical problem are also now under consideration (133–135).

Growth Factors

In addition to providing the appropriate cell and/or matrix to enable effective repair, a further consideration has been an exogenous supply of growth factor (136). This factor addition can be seen as either enhancing the proliferation/differentiation of prechondrogenic cells and/or maintaining the stable chondrocyte phenotype of a repair cell. Such modulating factors have been applied either as a natural tissue component or, more recently, in purified form.

Demineralized Bone Matrix

Demineralized bone matrix (DBM) has been used for many years to stimulate repair of bone (137). DBM can induce the differentiation of mesenchymal cells into cartilage and bone (138), and because osteoinduction by DBM is preceded by an intermediate cartilaginous stage, implantation of DBM has been considered as a possible cartilage repair treatment. When DBM was placed directly into osteochondral defects, however, there appeared to be only a slight enhancement, if any, of cartilage repair (139,140). Whether such DBM preparations release growth factors that modulate repair of cartilage defects remains to be established. Alternatively, DBM may serve as a temporary scaffold for cell ingrowth. In addition, DBM has been used with chondrocytes (118,141) and also with perichondrium (139) to form implants, and it may modulate the effects of co-implanted cells and materials through either biologic or physical mechanisms.

Purified Growth Factors

Because it was shown that a variety of growth factors, such as transforming growth factor-β (TGF-β) superfamily members purified from DBM, are capable of stimulating cartilage matrix synthesis and assembly *in vitro* (136,142), many studies have examined the effects of addition of purified or recombinant growth factor proteins to cartilage repair *in vivo.* For example, the intrinsic repair of osteochondral defects in rabbits was more effective in the presence of either hepatocyte growth factor (143), bone morphogenic protein-7 (BMP-7) (144) or fibroblast growth factor-2 (FGF-2) (145,146). In a similar type of study, a 3-mm defect filled with a collagen sponge was repaired more effectively if the sponge was impregnated with BMP-2 (147). Modulation of human chondrocytes isolated from elderly patients with a combination of TGF-β and FGF-2 produced an active chondroprogenitor population, which might be useful for autologous repair (148). The potential importance of TGF-β also has been emphasized in studies examining chondrogenesis from periosteal implants (51). The possibility of using insulin-like growth factor-1 (IGF-1)–laden fibrin composites to enhance intrinsic repair of full-thickness defects has also been studied in horses (149), and the potential importance of platelet-derived growth factor-BB (PDGF-BB) in promoting chondrogenesis *in vivo* is also now under investigation (150). Although an exogenous supply of growth factor may be important in repair initiation, it seems likely that the subtle interplay of factors required to achieve and maintain cartilage repair and homeostasis over an extended period will result from the activity of the implanted or host cells.

Matrices and Scaffolds

The use of materials, other than tissues, cells, and growth promoters, may well be required to form or deliver effective constructs for cartilage repair. Matrix or scaffold materials can provide mechanical support (for example, as a resilient load-bearing material), and they can serve as a carrier of a biologically active substance, such as growth factor. In addition, a matrix may be required for the transfer of cells into a defect or may act as a template to which cells can attach, migrate, and guide tissue growth. Such guided growth may occur either *in vivo* or *in vitro,* for example, during synthesis of a cell-laden tissue construct.

Biologic Materials

Gels and scaffolds, made primarily from type I collagen, have been used both to carry chondrocytes into cartilage defects and to encapsulate chondrocytes and thereby guide the *in vitro* formation of an implantable tissue construct. Soluble collagen can be induced to form a gel *in vitro,* and chondrocytes have been added during the gelling stage. When such gels were mixed with young allogeneic chondrocytes and placed soon afterward into osteochondral defects in rabbits, the repair was markedly improved compared with empty defects, defects treated with collagen alone, or chondrocytes alone (35,118,151). However, even with optimal cartilage formation, the restoration of the subchondral plate was inconsistent at 6 months and 1 year. The preparation of more mature tissue constructs with chondrocytes in type I collagen gels and scaffolds has been achieved after several weeks of culture (49,107,109,110,152,153). Cells in such constructs can maintain the chondrocyte phenotype for as long as 6 weeks (154–156). Implanting such constructs into osteochondral defects in rabbits has produced encouraging results out to 6 months (49,107,153). However, similar studies of large osteochondral defects in horses (109,110) have met with limited success at 4 or 8 months.

Another gelling substance that has been used for chondrocyte delivery into rabbit defects is the polysaccharide hyaluronan (157–159). Hyaluronan is abundant in normal adult articular cartilage and also in the developing mesenchyme of the embryo, where it mediates cell migration (160). Cell-laden hyaluronan constructs were more effective than hyaluronan alone, and the cellular effect also was seen when the hyaluronan was used in conjunction with carbon-fiber pads (161). In an extension of this, scaffolds formed from chemically derivatized hyaluronan have been used as a delivery vehicle for mesenchymal stem cells (162).

Fibrin glue, also called fibrin sealant, is another biomaterial that has been examined for use in a number of orthopedic procedures (163,164). This material is prepared by mixing the blood proteins fibrinogen and thrombin and allowing the thrombin to digest the fibrinogen to fibrin monomers that aggregate to form a clot. Thrombin also activates factor XIII, converting it to the transglutaminase, factor XIIIa, which in turn cross-links monomers to an alpha-polymer through peptide bridges. In general, covalent bonds may be formed between fibrin and fibrin, collagen, or other matrix molecules. The exact composition of fibrin sealant, as well as the method of fibrin preparation and delivery, may affect the biologic and biomechanical properties of the formed material. The fibrinogen component can be autologous, where it is typically prepared by cryoprecipitation. Alternatively, fibrinogen solutions are prepared from allogeneic blood; commercial preparations (e.g., Tisseel, Baxter Hyland Immuno) provide a high and defined concentration of fibrinogen. In addition, the degradation of an implanted fibrin clot can be modulated by inclusion of proteinase inhibitors, such as aprotinin, in the clot (165).

Fibrin glue has been used for several purposes in cartilage repair procedures. The adhesive properties of fibrin allow it to be used to affix a variety of tissues at the site of cartilage defects, including a periosteal patch overlying injected chondrocytes, as noted earlier. The adhesive strength of tissues attached with fibrin is modest, and factor XIIIa, transglutaminase, develops a somewhat similar adhesive strength (14,166). Alone, the application of commercial fibrin glue does not markedly enhance repair of osteochondral defects, and such a fibrin preparation appears to effectively form a seal and prevent migration or ingress of cells at early times after application (120). This is in contrast to the effects of a naturally formed endogenous fibrin clot (29,30,120) or that applied to an osteochondral defect (167). Fibrin sealant has been used as a delivery vehicle for transplanting cells into cartilage defects (111,168). Indeed, the injection of chondrocytes within gel-forming fibrin into the subcutaneous tissue of immunodeficient mice leads to development of cartilaginous tissue (169,170). Fibrin implants also can be loaded effectively with growth factors (149), and they also have been used to encapsulate cells to form a tissue construct *in vitro* (113,165,171–173).

Nonbiologic Matrices

Several types of matrices with low degradation rates have been used to provide a permanent scaffold within repairing cartilage defects. These matrices include felts of carbon fiber (174–177), polytetrafluoroethylene (Teflon™) (178–180), and polyester (Dacron™) (178–182). Clinical observations with carbon fiber pads and rods for articular resurfacing have been somewhat mixed (177,183–185). Whereas encouraging clinical results were initially found in 80% of patients after several years (177,183), a more recent clinical study (185) showed a low degree of patient satisfaction after several years. In the recent study, synovial biopsies often demonstrated the incorporation of carbon fibers and an associated foreign-body and low-grade inflammatory reaction, indicating disruption of the implant. This reaction may have a long-term detrimental effect on joint homeostasis.

Other matrices with relatively high degradation rates have been used to provide a temporary scaffold for repair cells (186). The materials commonly used include poly-lactic acid (PLA), poly-glycolic acid (PGA), and their copolymers (PLGA). PLA and PGA are degraded *in vivo* through (nonenzymatic) hydrolysis, with degradation times ranging from several weeks for PGA (187) to many months for PLA (188) and with intermediate times for copolymers (189–191). The degradation products appear to induce little or no host response (188,192), unless a large amount is present and local degradation rates are high (186,193,194). Cartilage-producing cells have been seeded into scaffolds of PGA (50,195–197) and PLA (37,198,199). Other materials have been designed so that cross-links can be formed by photoactivation and thus can be used to bridge between tissue surfaces (200) or encapsulate cells *in situ* (201).

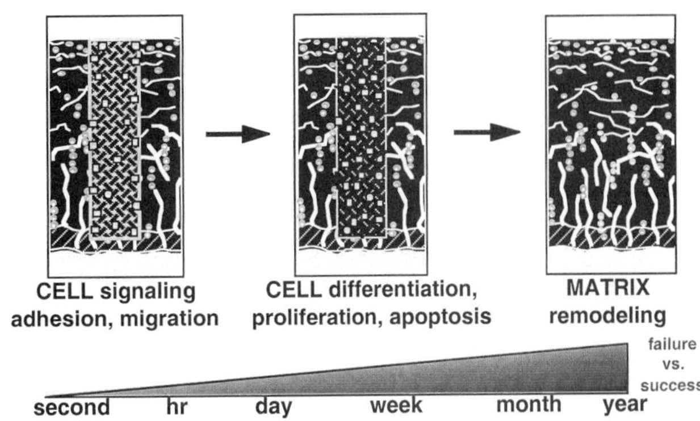

FIGURE 113.3. Time scale of processes occurring during repair of an articular cartilage defect confined to the body of the cartilage and involving the application of a cell-laden matrix (*shaded area*, **left**). In most cases, assessments regarding the "success" or "failure" of the repair strategy can be made only after extended periods of matrix remodeling and tissue integration.

DESIGN STRATEGIES FOR ENHANCING CARTILAGE REPAIR

For repair of both chondral and osteochondral defects, the attainment of a number of specific design goals is considered critical to development of a successful repair strategy. One goal is to deliver viable repair cells within and adjacent to the defect site. If this is attempted by placing cells in the defect, these cells will need to remain at the defect site long enough to contribute to the repair process. A second goal is that these cells be regulated to form repair tissue with the desired site-specific characteristics of functional articular cartilage and subchondral bone. For this to occur, the cells should become stable and ultimately attain the characteristics of the cells of the desired tissue. Thus, cells within the cartilage layer should be maintained as articular chondrocytes and not undergo dedifferentiation into fibroblasts or exhibit terminal differentiation and form bone. Particularly challenging is the maintenance and stabilization of the mature chondrocyte phenotype in which the cells produce a matrix composition without cell cloning or vascularization, as is seen in progressive osteoarthritis (OA). A further goal is that the repair tissue should integrate firmly with the surrounding tissue, not only to the bone below, but also to the adjacent host cartilage. Each of these goals is associated with particular locations within the repair site (Fig. 113.1) and characteristic time frames (Fig. 113.3). Finally, overall repair will occur under the influence of certain postoperative rehabilitation regimens and increasing postsurgical biomechanical demands, and so these regimens should be developed to optimize repair.

Cartilage repair strategies that have been used to address these goals are summarized in this section. A particular strategy may involve the implant or the host, and it may help achieve one or several of the mentioned goals. At the outset, it should be noted that the outcome of a particular design strategy under experimental conditions in animal studies is likely to be highly dependent on a number of factors that may or may not be present in clinical scenarios. For example, in many animals, the thickness of the articular cartilage and the size of the joint are severalfold less than those in humans (202). This makes application of implants technically difficult and raises questions about what size of defect is relevant for study (129) and how to scale the results from animals to humans. Nevertheless, *in vivo* animal studies are useful for providing insight into potential repair problems and potential solutions that ultimately can be tested and validated as efficacious in clinical studies.

Engineered Tissue Constructs

Many forms of cartilage repair constructs have been generated by combining cells and materials and then incubating the combination for various periods. Such constructs have not yet been evaluated clinically, but have been examined both *in vitro* and in animal studies. Much as was seen for intrinsic repair of osteochondral defects (see earlier), construct-initiated repair shows encouraging results at early times after implant (up to about 6 months in the rabbit) (49,107,153). However, as is also the case for intrinsic repair, longer term outcomes have been inconsistent and showed deterioration (37,50,106,109–111,113,114,199).

The extent of cell attachment and tissue cohesion may be critical factors for effective tissue implants. At one extreme, cells are seeded onto a carrier scaffold and incubated for an extended duration so that a substantial tissue forms (48,50,109,110,118,152,195,203–206). At the other end of the spectrum, cells are seeded for only a short time (e.g., hours) before implantation (34,35,37,108,111,151,157,

158,161,168,177,199). The latter constructs may allow proliferation and migration of implanted cells within the repair site, as well as the influx of host cells. Conversely, because the cells have not yet formed a cohesive tissue, they may have relatively weak attachments and be dislodged from the carrier and lost from the defect site. Indeed, in one study, with cells that had been cultured for 7 to 10 days in a collagen matrix and tagged with a molecular marker (203), there was a major loss (90%) of tagged cells from the defect site within the first day. Whether this was due to loss of implanted cells from the defect site or loss of marker expression from implanted cells is not clear. Constructs containing substantial matrix may be sufficiently cohesive to retain the donor cells while generally excluding host cells. Constructs formed after a moderate duration of incubation may integrate with the host tissue better than constructs incubated for a prolonged duration in which a more mature tissue is formed (50,197).

Most recently, multicompartment implants have been designed to enhance repair of specific regions of tissue within the cartilage defect. Some constructs consist of a bone-repair component topped with a cartilage-repair component, with the latter consisting of seeded cells or tissue (49,90,114,118,139,207–211). Implants forming a region of calcified cartilage also are under investigation (212–214).

Modifications to Enhance Cell Adhesion and Tissue Integration

A major consideration in cell-laden constructs is that repair cells are needed both in the body of the defect for matrix assembly and also near or at the interfaces to achieve integration with the host tissue. Thus for integrative repair, adhesion of the implanted cells or cell-laden construct to the host tissues would appear to be critical. One strategy to increase cell adhesion at the defect site is to treat host cartilage enzymatically to remove antiadhesive molecules at the tissue surface. It has been hypothesized that proteoglycans prevent cell adhesion to matrix-binding sites. *In vivo* studies suggest that treatment of host cartilage with the matrix-degrading enzymes chondroitinase ABC (132,215,216) or trypsin (131,217) enhance repair by increasing cell adhesion to the cartilage defect. Direct measurement of chondrocyte adhesive force to cartilage indicates that chondroitinase ABC treatment at a high concentration and/or long treatment duration significantly increases chondrocyte adhesion (218). An understanding of the way in which injected cells adhere to the surrounding tissue may allow rational cell manipulations or matrix treatments to enhance cell adhesion and retention in the defect site. In this regard, recent studies have implicated β_1-integrins as a mediator of the attachment of cultured chondrocytes to cartilage (219). Another strategy is to seed cells onto the implant (cartilage) surface (220), such as the vertical surfaces of osteochondral cores (221), in an attempt to enhance integration of the implanted tissue with the host cartilage (222,223). Pretreatment of the vertical cartilage surface of implantable osteochondral tissue cylinders with chondroitinase ABC enhances seeding of chondrocytes onto such tailored implants (221). It remains to be determined if any of these design strategies are effective in the clinic.

Modulation of the Biomechanical Environment

The effectiveness of a repair strategy is likely to be modulated by biomechanical regulators. It has been well established that chondrocytes are highly responsive to variation in their biomechanical environment and that both compression and shear forces can markedly modify biosynthetic processes (224,225). The biomechanical environment of tissue within and around an osteochondral defect has been examined experimentally (226) and theoretically (227–229). Qualitatively and quantitatively, the relatively soft repair tissue and the residual host cartilage would be predicted to be compressed more than normal cartilage under the same loading conditions; the interface between host cartilage and repair tissue also may undergo sizeable shear strain or stress (14,230). The mechanical environment of the implant and surrounding host tissue also would be expected to be sensitive to the tightness of the fit of an implant into a cartilage defect.

Certain mechanical factors that can be manipulated intraoperatively or postoperatively have been identified as affecting cartilage repair, and these factors would be expected also to regulate the postoperative remodeling of implanted constructs. The repair of cartilage after fracture of an osteochondral fragment extending into the joint space in the medial femoral condyle of rabbits was markedly enhanced by reduction of the surfaces with a large force such that the fracture was barely visible (231). Reduction with a small force allowed the formation of a fibrous repair tissue between the apposing surfaces, whereas application of a large force resulted in integrative repair, including electron-microscopic evidence of collagen fibril integrity across the repair site. Clinically, after an autologous chondrocyte transplantation procedure, specific postoperative rehabilitation protocols have been recommended to enhance repair of the defect while minimizing the development of adhesions (121,123). These protocols include continuous passive motion, largely based on the basic research studies of Salter et al. (232), who defined the role of continuous passive motion in enhancing repair of full-depth defects in rabbits. Clinical observations also suggest that perichondrial grafting is enhanced by continuous passive motion (80).

In this regard, it has been emphasized that the most suitable patients for the chondrocyte transplantation procedure are those in whom a physiologic biomechanical environment can be restored. Thus ideal patients are those with a single cartilage defect, without a defect on the apposing surface, and without clinical signs of OA (123). In keeping with the multistage and multidisciplinary approach to this problem advocated by Buckwalter and Mankin (2), any existing orthopedic problems (malalignment, incongruity, etc.) must be corrected before the use of the transplantation procedure to optimize results. Alternatively, it has been suggested that if stable fixation can be achieved after osteotomy, a chondrocyte transplantation procedure can be done concomitantly, and postoperative motion therapies can be initiated immediately (123).

THE FUTURE IN CARTILAGE REPAIR

It was noted by Hunter in 1743 that "it is universally allowed that ulcerated cartilage is a troublesome thing, and that once damaged, it is not repaired" (233). This view of the inability of articular cartilage to recover from injury is prevalent even today, because there remains no established treatment to reverse or even slow the progression of cartilage degradation once it has begun. Short of total joint replacement with a metal and plastic prosthesis, no suitable method currently exists for resurfacing degraded articular cartilage on a whole-joint scale. Conversely, focal chondral or osteochondral defects can be treated now by a number of surgical procedures, including subchondral penetration, osteochondral allografting and autografting, autologous chondrocyte transplantation, and, likely in the future, by transplantation of engineered cell-laden tissue constructs.

Although the tissue engineered constructs described earlier are suitable for defects of a focal nature, more widespread joint damage is present in many individuals. For such persons, an emerging concept currently at the very early experimental stages is that of replacing entire joints with a suitably engineered biologic construct. Whole-joint construction presents special challenges because of the complexity of the desired structure, including multiple tissues and cell types. The concept of synthesizing joint structures was demonstrated dramatically when mesenchymal tissue was transformed into cartilage and vascularized bone that formed the shape of a hip (234). More recently, composite tissues were formed into the shape of a human phalange and small joint (235). As such, an engineered biologic joint implant increases in size relative to the remaining host tissue, the implant increasingly will need to bear the functional biomechanical demands of the joint during postoperative rehabilitation. In principle, such a biologic joint has advantages over the current generation of metal and plastic prostheses, because application of the latter is limited by activity-induced formation of wear debris that leads to prosthesis failure. In contrast, biologic replacements could adapt metabolically to functional demands. Clearly at present, such constructs are far from the point of clinical applicability, but their potential promise is enormous.

REFERENCES

1. Hodge WA, Fijan RS, Carlson KL, et al. Contact pressures in the human hip joint measured in vivo. *Proc Natl Acad Sci U S A* 1986;83:2879–2883.
2. Buckwalter JA, Mankin HJ. Articular cartilage: degeneration and osteoarthritis, repair, regeneration, and transplantation. *Instr Course Lect* 1998;47:487–504.
3. Blevins FT, Steadman JR, Rodrigo JJ, et al. Treatment of articular cartilage defects in athletes: an analysis of functional outcome and lesion appearance. *Orthopedics* 1998;21:761–768.
4. Faber KJ, Dill JR, Amendola A, et al. Occult osteochondral lesions after anterior cruciate ligament rupture: six-year magnetic resonance imaging follow-up study. *Am J Sports Med* 1999;27:489–494.
5. Anderson AF, Lipscomb AB, Coulam C. Antegrade curettement, bone grafting and pinning of osteochondritis dissecans in the skeletally mature knee. *Am J Sports Med* 1990;18:254–261.
6. Breinan HA, Minas T, Hsu H-P, et al. Effect of cultured autologous chondrocytes on repair of chondral defects in a canine model. *J Bone Joint Surg Am* 1997;79:1439–1451.
7. Minas T, Peterson L. Advanced techniques in autologous chondrocyte transplantation. *Clin Sports Med* 1999;18:13–44, v–vi.
8. Mankin HJ. The response of articular cartilage to mechanical injury. *J Bone Joint Surg Am* 1982;64:460–466.
9. McKibbin B, Maroudas A. Nutrition and metabolism. In: Freeman MAR, ed. *Adult articular cartilage*. 2nd ed. Tunbridge Wells, England: Pitman Medical, 1979:461–486.
10. Kostoulas G, Lang A, Nagase H, et al. Stimulation of angiogenesis through cathepsin B inactivation of the tissue inhibitors of matrix metalloproteinases. *FEBS Lett* 1999;455:286–290.
11. Moses MA, Wiederschain D, Wu I, et al. Troponin I is present in human cartilage and inhibits angiogenesis. *Proc Natl Acad Sci U S A* 1999;96:2645–2650.
12. Saadeh PB, Brent B, Mehrara BJ, et al. Human cartilage engineering: chondrocyte extraction, proliferation, and characterization for construct development. *Ann Plast Surg* 1999;42:509–513.
13. Kieswetter K, Schwartz Z, Alderete M, et al. Platelet derived growth factor stimulates chondrocyte proliferation but prevents endochondral maturation. *Endocrine* 1997;6:257–264.
14. Ahsan T, Sah RL. Biomechanics of integrative cartilage repair. *Osteoarthritis Cartilage* 1999;7:29–40.
15. Mankin HJ. Chondrocyte transplantation: one answer to an old question. *N Engl J Med* 1994;331:940–941.
16. The promise of tissue engineering. *Sci Am* 1999;280:59.
17. Thomsen I. High-tech body shop: doctors are now using cartilage cultured in labs to repair injured knees. *Sports Illust* 1999;90:18–19.
18. Skalak R, Fox CF, eds. Tissue engineering: proceedings of a workshop held at Granlibakken, Lake Tahoe, California, February 26-29, 1988. In: *UCLA symposia on molecular and cellular biology*. Vol 107. New York: Liss, 1988.
19. Galletti PM. Let's do tissue engineering right: viewpoint. *IEEE Spectrum* 1996;33:94.
20. Langer R, Vacanti JP. Tissue engineering. *Science* 1993;260:920–926.
21. Nerem RM, Sambanis A. Tissue engineering: from biology to biological substitutes. *Tissue Eng* 1995;1:3–13.

22. Ghadially FN, Thomas I, Oryschak AF, et al. Long term results of superficial defects in articular cartilage: a scanning electron microscope study. *J Pathol* 1977;121:213–217.
23. Muller B, Kohn D. Indikation und durchführung der knorpel-knochen-anbohrung nach Pridie. *Orthopade* 1999;28:4–10.
24. Steadman JR, Rodkey WG, Briggs KK, et al. Die technik der mikrofrakturierung zur behandlung von kompletten knorpeldefekten im kniegelenk. *Orthopade* 1999;28:26–32.
25. Johnson LL. The sclerotic lesion: pathology and the clinical response to arthroscopic abrasion arthroplasty. In: Ewing JW, ed. *Articular cartilage and knee joint function:* basic science and arthroscopy. New York: Raven Press, 1990:319–933.
26. Friedman MJ, Berasi CC, Fox JM, et al. Preliminary results with abrasion arthroplasty in the osteoarthritic knee. *Clin Orthop* 1984;182:200–205.
27. Ficat RP, Ficat C, Gedeon P, et al. Spongiolization: a new treatment for diseased patellae. *Clin Orthop* 1979;144:74–83.
28. Wei X, Messner K. Maturation-dependent durability of spontaneous cartilage repair in rabbit knee joint. *J Biomed Mater Res* 1999;46:539–548.
29. Hjertquist SO, Lemperg R. Histological, autoradiographic and microchemical studies of spontaneously healing osteochondral articular defects in adult rabbits. *Calcif Tissue Res* 1971;8:54–72.
30. Shapiro F, Koido S, Glimcher MJ. Cell origin and differentiation in the repair of full-thickness defects of articular cartilage. *J Bone Joint Surg Am* 1993;75:532–553.
31. Furukawa T, Eyre DR, Koide S, et al. Biochemical studies on repair cartilage resurfacing experimental defects in the rabbit knee. *J Bone Joint Surg Am* 1980;62:79–89.
32. Maroudas A. Physico-chemical properties of articular cartilage. In: Freeman MAR, ed. *Adult articular cartilage.* 2nd ed. Tunbridge Wells, England: Pitman Medical, 1979:215–290.
33. Coletti JM, Akeson WH, Woo SL-Y. A comparison of the physical behavior of normal articular cartilage and the arthroplasty surface. *J Bone Joint Surg Am* 1972;54:147–160.
34. Wakitani S, Goto T, Pineda SJ, et al. Mesenchymal cell-based repair of large, full-thickness defects of articular cartilage. *J Bone Joint Surg Am* 1994;76:579–592.
35. Wakitani S, Goto T, Young RG, et al. Repair of large full-thickness articular cartilage defects with allograft articular chondrocytes embedded in a collagen gel. *Tissue Eng* 1998;4:429–444.
36. Mow VC, Ratcliffe A, Rosenwasser MP, et al. Experimental studies on repair of large osteochondral defects at a high weight bearing area of the knee joint: a tissue engineering study. *J Biomech Eng* 1991;113:198–207.
37. Dounchis J, Harwood FL, Chen AC, et al. Repair of osteochondral defects with perichondrocyte-polylactic acid scaffold grafts: autogenic vs. allogenic cells. *Clin Orthop* (in press).
38. Wei X, Gao J, Messner K. Maturation-dependent repair of untreated osteochondral defects in the rabbit knee joint. *J Biomed Mater Res* 1997;34:63–72.
39. Athanasiou KA, Fischer R, Niederauer GG, et al. Effects of excimer laser on healing of articular cartilage in rabbits. *J Orthop Res* 1995;13:483–494.
40. Hjertquist SO, Lemperg R. Transplantation of autologous costal cartilage to an osteochondral defect on the femoral head: histological and autoradiographical studies in adult rabbits after administration of ^{35}S-sulphate and ^{3}H-thymidine. *Virchows Arch Pathol Anat Physiol Klin Med* 1969;346:345–360.
41. Buckwalter JA. Evaluating methods of restoring cartilaginous articular surfaces. *Clin Orthop* 1999;367S:224–238.
42. Oates KM, Chen AC, Young EP, et al. Effect of tissue culture storage on the in vivo survival of canine osteochondral allografts. *J Orthop Res* 1995;13:562–569.
43. Bugbee WD, Convery FR. Osteochondral allograft transplantation. *Clin Sports Med* 1999;18:67–75.
44. Chu CR, Convery FR, Akeson WH, et al. Articular cartilage transplantation: clinical results in the knee. *Clin Orthop* 1999;360:159–168.
45. Garrett JC. Osteochondral allografts for reconstruction of articular defects of the knee. *Instr Course Lect* 1998;47:517–522.
46. Ghazavi MT, Pritzker KP, Davis AM, et al. Fresh osteochondral allografts for post-traumatic osteochondral defects of the knee. *J Bone Joint Surg Br* 1997;79:1008–1013.
47. Plaga BR, Royster RM, Donigian AM, et al. Fixation of osteochondral fractures in rabbit knees: a comparison of Kirschner wires, fibrin sealant, and polydioxanone pins. *J Bone Joint Surg Br* 1992;74:292–296.
48. Aston JE, Bentley G. Repair of articular surfaces by allografts of articular and growth-plate cartilage. *J Bone Joint Surg Br* 1986;68:29–35.
49. Frenkel SR, Toolan B, Menche D, et al. Chondrocyte transplantation using a collagen bilayer matrix for cartilage repair. *J Bone Joint Surg Br* 1997;79:831–836.
50. Schreiber RE, Ilten-Kirby BM, Dunkelman NS, et al. Repair of osteochondral defects with allogeneic tissue engineered cartilage implants. *Clin Orthop* 1999;367S:382–395.
51. O'Driscoll SW. Articular cartilage regeneration using periosteum. *Clin Orthop* 1999;367S:186–203.
52. Brittberg M, Lindahl A, Nilsson A, et al. Treatment of deep cartilage defects in the knee with autologous chondrocyte transplantation. *N Engl J Med* 1994;331:889–895.
53. Breinan HA, Minas T, Barone L, et al. Histological evaluation of the course of healing of canine articular cartilage defects treated with cultured autologous chondrocytes. *Tissue Eng* 1998;4:101–114.
54. Passl R, Plenk H Jr, Sauer G, et al. Die homologe reine gelenkknorpeltransplantation im tierexperiment: vorläufie experimentelle studien am schaf. *Arch Orthop Unfallchir* 1976;86:243–256.
55. Passl R, Plenk H, Sauer G, et al. Fibrinklebung von knorpelflächen: experimentelle studien und klinische ergebnisse. *Med Sport* 1979;19:23–28.
56. Albrecht F, Roessner A, Zimmermann E. Closure of osteochondral lesions using chondral fragments and fibrin adhesive. *Arch Orthop Trauma Surg* 1983;101:213–217.
57. Kaplonyi G, Zimmerman I, Frenyo AD, et al. The use of fibrin adhesive in the repair of chondral and osteochondral injuries. *Injury* 1988;19:267–272.
58. Passl R, Plenk H Jr. Die fibrinklebung von knorpelflächen. *Beitr Orthop Traumatol* 1989;36:503–507.
59. Bakay A, Csonge L, Papp G, et al. Osteochondral resurfacing of the knee joint with allograft: clinical analysis of 33 cases. *Int Orthop* 1998;22:277–281.
60. Fitzpatrick PL, Morgan DA. Fresh osteochondral allografts: a 6-10 year review. *Aust N Z J Surg* 1998;68:573–579.
61. Garrett JC. Fresh osteochondral allografts for treatment of articular defects in osteochondritis dissecans of the lateral femoral condyle in adults. *Clin Orthop* 1994;303:33–37.
62. McDermott AG, Langer F, Pritzker KP, et al. Fresh small-fragment osteochondral allografts: long-term follow-up study on first 100 cases. *Clin Orthop* 1985;Jul–Aug:96–102.
63. Oakeshott RD, Farine I, Pritzker KPH, et al. A clinical and histologic analysis of failed fresh osteochondral allografts. *Clin Orthop* 1988;233:283–294.
64. Johnson DL, Warner JJ. Osteochondritis dissecans of the humeral head: treatment with a matched osteochondral allograft. *J Shoulder Elbow Surg* 1997;6:160–163.
65. Marco F, Lopez-Oliva F, Fernandez-Arroyo JM, et al. Osteochondral allografts for osteochondritis dissecans and

osteonecrosis of the femoral condyles. *Int Orthop* 1993;17: 104–108.

66. Yamashita F, Sakakida K, Suzu F, et al. The transplantation of an autogeneic osteochondral fragment for osteochondritis dissecans of the knee. *Clin Orthop* 1985;201:43–50.
67. Outerbridge HK, Outerbridge AR, Outerbridge RE. The use of a lateral patellar autologous graft for the repair of a large osteochondral defect in the knee. *J Bone Joint Surg Am* 1995;77: 65–72.
68. Outerbridge HK, Outerbridge AR, Outerbridge RE, et al. The use of lateral patellar autologous grafts for the repair of large osteochondral defects in the knee. *Acta Orthop Belg* 1999; 65:129–135.
69. Matsusue Y, Yamamuro T, Hama H. Arthroscopic multiple osteochondral transplantation to the chondral defect in the knee associated with anterior cruciate ligament disruption. *Arthroscopy* 1993;9:318–321.
70. Bobic V. Arthroscopic osteochondral autograft transplantation in anterior cruciate ligament reconstruction: a preliminary clinical study. *Knee Surg Sports Traumatol Arthrosc* 1996;3:262–264.
71. Hangody L, Kish G, Karpati Z, et al. Treatment of osteochondritis dissecans of the talus: use of the mosaicplasty technique: a preliminary report. *Foot Ankle Int* 1997;18:628–634.
72. Berlet GC, Mascia A, Miniaci A. Treatment of unstable osteochondritis dissecans lesions of the knee using autogenous osteochondral grafts (mosaicplasty). *Arthroscopy* 1999;15:312–316.
73. Ishida O, Ikuta Y, Kuroki H. Ipsilateral osteochondral grafting for finger joint repair. *J Hand Surg [Am]* 1994;19:372–377.
74. Sandow MJ. Proximal scaphoid costo-osteochondral replacement arthroplasty. *J Hand Surg [Br]* 1998;23:201–208.
75. Kish G, Modis L, Hangody L. Osteochondral mosaicplasty for the treatment of focal cartilage and osteochondral lesions of the knee and talus in the athlete: rationale, indications, techniques, and results. *Clin Sports Med* 1999;18:45–66, vi.
76. Stone KR, Walgenbach A. Surgical technique for articular cartilage transplantation to full-thickness cartilage defects in the knee joint. *Oper Tech Orthop* 1997;7:305–311.
77. Rubak JM, Poussa M, Ritsilä V. Chondrogenesis in repair of articular cartilage defects by free periosteal grafts in rabbits. *Acta Orthop Scand* 1982;53:181–186.
78. Zarnett R, Delaney JP, Driscoll SWO, et al. Cellular origin and evolution of neochondrogenesis in major full-thickness defects of a joint surface treated by free autogenous periosteal grafts and subjected to continuous passive motion in rabbits. *Clin Orthop* 1987;222:267–274.
79. Zarnett R, Salter RB. Periosteal neochondrogenesis for biologically resurfacing joints: its cellular origin. *Can J Surg* 1985;32: 171–174.
80. Alfredson H, Lorentzon R. Superior results with continuous passive motion compared to active motion after periosteal transplantation: a retrospective study of human patella cartilage defect treatment. *Knee Surg Sports Traumatol Arthrosc* 1999;7:232–238.
81. Alfredson H, Thorsen K, Lorentzon R. Treatment of tear of the anterior cruciate ligament combined with localised deep cartilage defects in the knee with ligament reconstruction and autologous periosteum transplantation. *Knee Surg Sports Traumatol Arthrosc* 1999;7:69–74.
82. Lorentzon R, Alfredson H, Hildingsson CH. Treatment of deep cartilage defects of the patella with periosteal transplantation. *Knee Surg Sports Traumatol Arthrosc* 1998;6:202–208.
83. Hoikka VEJ, Jaroma HJ, Ritsila VA. Reconstruction of the patellar articulation with periosteal grafts. *Acta Orthop Scand* 1990;61:36–39.
84. Korkala OL, Kuokkanen HO. Autoarthroplasty of knee cartilage defects by osteoperiosteal grafts. *Arch Orthop Trauma Surg* 1995;114:253–256.
85. Niedermann B, Boe S, Lauritzen J, et al. Glued periosteal grafts in the knee. *Acta Orthop Scand* 1985;56:457–460.
86. Engkvist O, Skoog V, Pastacaldi P, et al. The cartilaginous potential of the perichondrium in rabbit ear and rib: a comparative study in vivo and in vitro. *Scand J Plast Reconstr Surg* 1979;13:275–280.
87. Bruns J, Meyer-Pannwitt U, Silbermann M. The rib perichondrium: an anatomical study in sheep of a tissue used as transplant in the treatment of hyaline-cartilage defects. *Acta Anat* 1992;144:258–266.
88. Skoog T, Ohlsen L, Sohn SA. Perichondrial potential for cartilaginous regeneration. *Scand J Plast Reconstr Surg* 1972;6: 123–125.
89. Bulstra SK, Homminga GN, Buurman WA, et al. The potential of adult human perichondrium to form hyalin cartilage in vitro. *J Orthop Res* 1990;8:328–335.
90. Coutts RD, Woo SL-Y, Amiel D, et al. Rib perichondrial autografts in full-thickness articular cartilage defects in rabbits. *Clin Orthop* 1992;275:263–273.
91. Upton J, Sohn SA, Glowacki J. Neocartilage derived from transplanted perichondrium: what is it? *Plast Reconstr Surg* 1981; 68:166–174.
92. Engkvist O, Wilander E. Formation of cartilage from rib perichondrium grafted to an articular defect in the femur condyle of the rabbit. *Scand J Plast Reconstr Surg* 1979;13:371–376.
93. Skoog T, Johansson SH. The formation of articular cartilage from free perichondrial grafts. *Scand J Plast Reconstr Surg* 1976; 57:1–6.
94. Engkvist O, Johansson SH. Perichondrial arthroplasty: a clinical study in twenty-six patients. *Scand J Plast Reconstr Surg* 1980;14:71–87.
95. Katsaros J, Milner R, Marshall NJ. Perichondrial arthroplasty incorporating costal cartilage. *J Hand Surg [Br]* 1995;20: 137–142.
96. Sully L, Jackson IT, Sommerlad BC. Perichondrial grafting in rheumatoid metacarpophalangeal joints. *Hand* 1980;12:137–148.
97. Jackson IT, Sully L, Tanner NS, et al. An interpositional elastomeric cap for metacarpophalangeal joint perichondroplasty in rheumatoid arthritis. *Hand* 1981;13:158–163.
98. Tajima S, Aoyagi F, Maruyama Y. Free perichondrial grafting in the treatment of temporomandibular joint ankylosis: preliminary report. *Plast Reconstr Surg* 1978;61:876–880.
99. Hvid I, Andersen LI. Perichondrial autograft in traumatic chondromalacia patellae: report of a case. *Acta Orthop Scand* 1981; 52:91–93.
100. Bouwmeester SJ, Beckers JM, Kuijer R, et al. Long-term results of rib perichondrial grafts for repair of cartilage defects in the human knee. *Int Orthop* 1997;21:313–317.
101. Bouwmeester P, Kuijer R, Terwindt-Rouwenhorst E, et al. Histological and biochemical evaluation of perichondrial transplants in human articular cartilage defects. *J Orthop Res* 1999; 17:843–849.
102. Carticel: autologous cultured chondrocytes for implantation. Cambridge, MA: Genzyme Tissue Repair, 1997.
103. Stockwell RA, Meachim G. The chondrocytes. In: Freeman MAR, ed. *Adult articular cartilage.* 2nd ed. Tunbridge Wells, England: Pitman Medical, 1979:69–144.
104. Grande DA, Singh IJ, Pugh J. Healing of experimentally produced lesions in articular cartilage following chondrocyte transplantation. *Anat Rec* 1987;218:142–148.
105. Brittberg M, Nilsson A, Lindahl A, et al. Rabbit articular cartilage defects treated with autologous cultured chondrocytes. *Clin Orthop* 1996;326:270–283.
106. Rahfoth B, Weisser J, Sternkopf F, et al. Transplantation of allograft chondrocytes embedded in agarose gel into cartilage defects of rabbits. *Osteoarthritis Cartilage* 1998;6:50–65.

107. Kawamura S, Wakitani S, Kimura T, et al. Articular cartilage repair: rabbit experiments with a collagen gel-biomatrix and chondrocytes cultured in it. *Acta Orthop Scand* 1998;69:56–62.
108. Chu CR, Coutts RD, Yoshioka M, et al. Articular cartilage repair using allogeneic perichondrocyte seeded biodegradable porous polylactic acid (PLA): a tissue engineering study. *J Biomed Mater Res* 1995;29:1147–1154.
109. Sams AE, Nixon AJ. Chondrocyte-laden collagen scaffolds for resurfacing extensive articular cartilage defects. *Osteoarthritis Cartilage* 1995;3:47–59.
110. Sams AE, Minor RR, Wootton JAM, et al. Local and remote matrix responses to chondrocyte-laden collagen scaffold implantation in extensive articular cartilage defects. *Osteoarthritis Cartilage* 1995;3:61–70.
111. Hendrickson DA, Nixon AJ, Grande DA, et al. Chondrocyte-fibrin matrix transplants for resurfacing extensive articular cartilage defects. *J Orthop Res* 1994;12:485–497.
112. Shortkroff S, Barone L, Hsu HP, et al. Healing of chondral and osteochondral defects in a canine model: the role of cultured chondrocytes in regeneration of articular cartilage. *Biomaterials* 1996;17:147—154.
113. van Susante JL, Buma P, Schuman L, et al. Resurfacing potential of heterologous chondrocytes suspended in fibrin glue in large full-thickness defects of femoral articular cartilage: an experimental study in the goat. *Biomaterials* 1999;20:1167–1175.
114. van Susante JL, Buma P, Homminga GN, et al. Chondrocyte-seeded hydroxyapatite for repair of large articular cartilage defects: a pilot study in the goat. *Biomaterials* 1998;19: 2367–2374.
115. Bentley G, Gree RB. Homotransplantation of isolated epiphyseal and articular cartilage chondrocytes into the joint surfaces of rabbits. *Nature* 1971;230:385–388.
116. Bentley G, Smith AU, Mukerhjee R. Isolated epiphyseal chondrocyte allografts into joint surfaces: an experimental study in rabbits. *Ann Rheum Dis* 1978;37:449–458.
117. Chesterman PJ, Smith AU. Homotransplantation of articular cartilage and isolated chondrocytes: an experimental study in rabbits. *J Bone Joint Surg Br* 1968;50:184–197.
118. Green WT. Articular cartilage repair: behavior of rabbit chondrocytes during tissue culture and subsequent allografting. *Clin Orthop* 1977;124:237–250.
119. Grande DA, Pitman MI, Peterson L, et al. The repair of experimentally produced defects in rabbit articular cartilage by autologous chondrocyte transplantation. *J Orthop Res* 1989;7:208–218.
120. Brittberg M, Sjogren-Jansson E, Lindahl A, et al. Influence of fibrin sealant (Tisseel) on osteochondral defect repair in the rabbit knee. *Biomaterials* 1997;18:235–242.
121. Gillogly SD, Voight M, Blackburn T. Treatment of articular cartilage defects of the knee with autologous chondrocyte implantation. *J Orthop Sports Phys Ther* 1998;28:241–251.
122. Cartilage repair registry: periodic report. Cambridge, MA: Genzyme Tissue Repair, 1999.
123. Minas T, Peterson L. Chondrocyte transplantation. *Oper Tech Orthop* 1997;7:323–333.
124. Jackson DW, Simon TS. Chondrocyte transplantation. *Arthroscopy* 1996;12:732–738.
125. McPherson JM, Tubo R, Barone L. Chondrocyte transplantation. *Arthroscopy* 1997;13:541–547.
126. Messner K, Gillquist J. Cartilage repair: a critical review. *Acta Orthop Scand* 1996;67:523–529.
127. Brittberg M, Lindahl A, Homminga G, et al. A critical analysis of cartilage repair. *Acta Orthop Scand* 1997;68:186–191.
128. Buckwalter JA. Cartilage researchers tell progress: technologies hold promise, but caution urged. *Am Acad Orthop Surg Bull* 1996;44:24–26.
129. Hunziker EB. Biologic repair of articular cartilage: defect models in experimental animals and matrix requirements. *Clin Orthop* 1999;367S:135–146.
130. O'Driscoll SW. The healing and regeneration of articular cartilage. *J Bone Joint Surg Am* 1998;80:1795–1813.
131. Caplan AI, Elyaderani M, Mochizuki Y, et al. Principles of cartilage repair and regeneration. *Clin Orthop* 1997;342:254–269.
132. Hunziker EB, Rosenberg LC. Repair of partial-thickness defects in articular cartilage: cell recruitment from the synovial membrane. *J Bone Joint Surg Am* 1996;78:721–733.
133. Johnstone B, Yoo JU. Autologous mesenchymal progenitor cells in articular cartilage repair. *Clin Orthop* 1999;367S:156–162.
134. Yoo JU, Barthel TS, Nishimura K, et al. The chondrogenic potential of human bone-marrow-derived mesenchymal progenitor cells. *J Bone Joint Surg Am* 1998;80:1745–1757.
135. Grande DA, Breitbart AS, Mason J, et al. Cartilage tissue engineering: current limitations and solutions. *Clin Orthop* 1999; 367S:176–185.
136. Coutts RD, Sah RL, Amiel D. Effect of growth factors on cartilage repair. *Instr Course Lect* 1997;46:487–494.
137. Glowacki J, Mulliken JB. Demineralized bone implants. *Clin Plast Surg* 1985;12:233–241.
138. Urist MR, Nogami H. Morphogenetic substratum for differentiation of cartilage in tissue culture. *Nature* 1970;225:1051–1052.
139. Billings E, von Schroeder HP, Mai MT, et al. Cartilage resurfacing of the rabbit knee: the use of an allogeneic demineralized bone matrix-autogeneic perichondrium composite implant. *Acta Orthop Scand* 1990;61:201–206.
140. Dahlberg L, Kreicbergs A. Demineralized allogeneic bone matrix for cartilage repair. *J Orthop Res* 1991;9:11–19.
141. van Susante JLC, Burma P, van Osch GJVM, et al. Culture of chondrocytes in alginate and collagen carrier gels. *Acta Orthop Scand* 1995;66:549–556.
142. Dounchis JS, Goomer RS, Harwood FL, et al. Chondrogenic phenotype of perichondrium-derived chondroprogenitor cells is influenced by transforming growth factor-beta 1. *J Orthop Res* 1997;15:803–807.
143. Wakitani S, Imoto K, Kimura T, et al. Hepatocyte growth factor facilitates cartilage repair: full thickness articular cartilage defect studied in rabbit knees. *Acta Orthop Scand* 1997;68: 474–480.
144. Grgic M, Jelic M, Basic V, et al. Regeneration of articular cartilage defects in rabbits by osteogenic protein-1 (bone morphogenetic protein-7). *Acta Med Croatica* 1997;51:23–27.
145. Fujimoto E, Ochi M, Kato Y, et al. Beneficial effect of basic fibroblast growth factor on the repair of full-thickness defects in rabbit articular cartilage. *Arch Orthop Trauma Surg* 1999;119: 139–145.
146. Otsuka Y, Mizuta H, Takagi K, et al. Requirement of fibroblast growth factor signaling for regeneration of epiphyseal morphology in rabbit full-thickness defects of articular cartilage. *Dev Growth Differ* 1997;39:143–156.
147. Sellers RS, Peluso D, Morris EA. The effect of recombinant human bone morphogenetic protein-2 (rhBMP-2) on the healing of full-thickness defects of articular cartilage. *J Bone Joint Surg Am* 1997;79:1452–1463.
148. Bradham DM, Horton WE. In vivo cartilage formation from growth factor modulated articular chondrocytes. *Clin Orthop* 1998;352:239–249.
149. Nixon AJ, Fortier LA, Williams J, et al. Enhanced repair of extensive articular defects by insulin-like growth factor-I-laden fibrin composites. *J Orthop Res* 1999;17:475–487.
150. Lohmann CH, Schwartz Z, Niederauer GG, et al. Pretreatment with platelet derived growth factor-BB modulates the ability of costochondral resting zone chondrocytes incorporated into PLA/PGA scaffolds to form new cartilage in vivo. *Biomaterials* 2000;21:49–61.

151. Wakitani S, Kimura T, Hirooka A, et al. Repair of rabbit articular surfaces with allograft chondrocytes embedded in collagen gel. *J Bone Joint Surg Br* 1989;71:74–80.
152. Noguchi T, Oka M, Fujino M, et al. Repair of osteochondral defects with grafts of cultured chondrocytes. *Clin Orthop* 1994; 302:251–258.
153. Ben-Yishay A, Grande DA, Schwartz RE, et al. Repair of articular cartilage defects with collagen-chondrocyte allografts. *Tissue Eng* 1995;1:119–133.
154. Nixon AJ, Sams AE, Lust G, et al. Temporal matrix synthesis and histologic features of a chondrocyte-laden porous collagen cartilage analogue. *Am J Vet Res* 1993;54:349–356.
155. Grande DA, Halberstadt C, Naughton G, et al. Evaluation of matrix scaffolds for tissue engineering of articular cartilage grafts. *J Biomed Mater Res* 1997;34:211–220.
156. Kimura T, Yasui N, Ohsawa S, et al. Chondrocytes embedded in collagen gels maintain cartilage phenotype during long-term cultures. *Clin Orthop* 1984;186:231–239.
157. Robinson D, Halperin N, Nevo Z. Regenerating hyaline cartilage in articular defects of old chickens using implants of embryonal chick chondrocytes embedded in a new natural delivery substance. *Calcif Tissue Int* 1990;46:246–253.
158. Robinson D, Halperin N, Nevo Z. Long-term follow-up of the fate of xenogeneic transplants of chondrocytes implanted into joint surfaces. *Transplantation* 1991;52:380–383.
159. Butnariu-Ephrat M, Robinson D, Mendes DG, et al. Resurfacing of goat articular cartilage by chondrocytes derived from bone marrow. *Clin Orthop* 1996;330:234–243.
160. Toole BP. Hyaluronan in morphogenesis. *J Intern Med* 1997; 242:35–40.
161. Robinson D, Efrat M, Mendes DG, et al. Implants composed of carbon fiber mesh and bone-marrow-derived, chondrocyte-enriched cultures for joint surface reconstruction. *Bull Hosp Joint Dis* 1993;53:75–82.
162. Solchaga LA, Dennis JE, Goldberg VM, et al. Hyaluronic acid-based polymers as cell carriers for tissue-engineered repair of bone and cartilage. *J Orthop Res* 1999;17:205–213.
163. Schlag G, Redl H. Fibrin sealant in orthopedic surgery. *Clin Orthop* 1988;227:269–285.
164. Weber SC, Chapman MW. Adhesives in orthopaedic surgery: a review of the literature and in vitro bonding strengths of bone-bonding agents. *Clin Orthop* 1984;191:249–261.
165. Meinhart J, Fussenegger M, Hobling W. Stabilization of fibrin-chondrocyte constructs for cartilage reconstruction. *Ann Plast Surg* 1999;42:673–678.
166. Jürgensen K, Aeschlimann D, Cavin V, et al. A new biological glue for cartilage-cartilage interfaces: tissue transglutaminase. *J Bone Joint Surg Br* 1997;79:185–193.
167. Paletta GA, Arnoczky SP, Warren RF. The repair of osteochondral defects using an exogenous fibrin clot: an experimental study in dogs. *Am J Sports Med* 1992;20:725–731.
168. Itay S, Abramovici A, Nevo Z. Use of cultured embryonal chick epiphyseal chondrocytes as grafts for defects in chick articular cartilage. *Clin Orthop* 1987;220:284–303.
169. Sims CD, Butler PE, Cao YL, et al. Tissue engineered neocartilage using plasma derived polymer substrates and chondrocytes. *Plast Reconstr Surg* 1998;101:1580–1585.
170. Silverman RP, Passaretti D, Huang W, et al. Injectable tissue-engineered cartilage using a fibrin glue polymer. *Plast Reconstr Surg* 1999;103:1809–1818.
171. Homminga GN, Buma P, Koot HW, et al. Chondrocyte behavior in fibrin glue in vitro. *Acta Orthop Scand* 1993;64:441–445.
172. Ting V, Sims CD, Brecht LE, et al. In vitro prefabrication of human cartilage shapes using fibrin glue and human chondrocytes. *Ann Plast Surg* 1998;40:413–420.
173. Hendrickson DA, Nixon AJ, Erb HN, et al. Phenotype and biological activity of neonatal equine chondrocytes cultured in a three-dimensional fibrin matrix. *Am J Vet Res* 1994;55:410–414.
174. Minns RJ, Muckle DS, Donkin JE. The repair of osteochondral defects in osteoarthritic rabbit knees by the use of carbon fibre. *Biomaterials* 1982;3:81–86.
175. Minns RJ, Muckle DS. Mechanical and histological response of carbon fibre pads implanted in the rabbit patella. *Biomaterials* 1989;10:273–276.
176. Kaar TK, Fraher JP, Brady MP. A quantitative study of articular repair in the guinea pig. *Clin Orthop* 1998;346:228–243.
177. Brittberg M, Faxen E, Peterson L. Carbon fiber scaffolds in the treatment of early knee osteoarthritis: a prospective 4-year followup of 37 patients. *Clin Orthop* 1994;307:155–164.
178. Messner K. Durability of artificial implants for repair of osteochondral defects of the medial femoral condyle in rabbits. *Biomaterials* 1994;15:657–664.
179. Messner K, Gillquist J. Synthetic implants for the repair of osteochondral defects of the medial femoral condyle: a biomechanical and histological evaluation in the rabbit knee. *Biomaterials* 1993;14:513–521.
180. Messner K, Lohmander LS, Gillquist J. Neocartilage after artificial cartilage repair in the rabbit: histology and proteoglycan fragments in joint fluid. *J Biomed Mater Res* 1993;27:949–954.
181. Messner K. Hydroxylapatite supported Dacron plugs for repair of isolated full-thickness osteochondral defects of the rabbit femoral condyle: mechanical and histological evaluations from 6-48 weeks. *J Biomed Mater Res* 1993;27:1527–1532.
182. Messner K, Gillquist J, Björnsson S, et al. Proteoglycan fragments in rabbit joint fluid correlated to arthrosis stage. *Acta Orthop Scand* 1993;64:312–316.
183. Pongor P, Betts J, Muckle DS, et al. Woven carbon surface replacement in the knee: independent clinical review. *Biomaterials* 1992;13:1070–1076.
184. Muckle DS, Minns RJ. Biological response to woven carbon fibre pads in the knee. *J Bone Joint Surg Br* 1989;71:60–62.
185. Meister K, Cobb A, Bentley G. Treatment of painful articular cartilage defects of the patella by carbon-fibre implants. *J Bone Joint Surg Br* 1998;80:965–970.
186. Bostman O. Absorbable implants for the fixation of fractures. *J Bone Joint Surg Am* 1991;73:148–153.
187. Chu CC, Browning A. The study of thermal and gross morphologic properties of polyglycolic acid upon annealing and degradation treatments. *J Biomed Mater Res* 1988;22:699–712.
188. Matsusue Y, Yamamuro T, Oka M, et al. In vitro and in vivo studies on bioabsorbable ultra-high-strength poly(L-lactide) rods. *J Biomed Mater Res* 1992;26:1553–1567.
189. Athanasiou KA, Schmitz JP, Agrawal CM. The effects of porosity on in vitro degradation of polylactic acid-polyglycolic acid implants used in repair of articular cartilage. *Tissue Eng* 1998; 4:53–63.
190. Therin M, Christel P, Li S, et al. In vitro degradation of massive poly(α-hydroxy acids): validation of in vitro findings. *Biomaterials* 1992;13:594–600.
191. Spain TL, Agrawal CM, Athanasiou KA. New technique to extend the useful life of a biodegradable cartilage implant. *Tissue Eng* 1998;4:343–352.
192. Athanasiou KA, Korvick D, Schenck RC. Biodegradable implants for the treatment of osteochondral defects in a goat model. *Tissue Eng* 1997;3:363–373.
193. Suganuma J, Alexander H. Biological response of intramedullary bone to poly-L-lactic acid. *J Appl Biomater* 1993;4:13–27.
194. Paivarinta U, Bostman O, Majola A, et al. Intraosseous cellular response to biodegradable fracture fixation screws made of polyglycolide or polylactide. *Arch Orthop Trauma Surg* 1993; 112:71–74.

195. Freed LE, Grande DA, Lingbin Z, et al. Joint resurfacing using allograft chondrocytes and synthetic biodegradable polymer scaffolds. *J Biomed Mater Res* 1994;28:891–899.
196. Freed LE, Martin I, Vunjak-Novakovic G. Frontiers in tissue engineering. In vitro modulation of chondrogenesis. *Clin Orthop* 1999;367S:46–58.
197. Vunjak-Novakovic G, Martin I, Obradovic B, et al. Bioreactor cultivation conditions modulate the composition and mechanical properties of tissue-engineered cartilage. *J Orthop Res* 1999; 17:130–139.
198. Chu CR, Monosov AZ, Amiel D. In situ assessment of cell viability within biodegradable polymer matrices. *Biomaterials* 1995;16:1381–1384.
199. Chu CR, Dounchis JS, Yoshioka M, et al. Osteochondral repair using perichondrial cells: a one year study in rabbits. *Clin Orthop* 1997;340:220–229.
200. Jackson RW, Judy MM, Matthews JL, et al. Photochemical tissue welding with 1,8 naphthalimide dyes: in vivo meniscal and cartilage welds. *Trans Orthop Res Soc* 1997;22:650.
201. Elisseeff J, Anseth K, Sims D, et al. Transdermal photopolymerization for minimally invasive implantation. *Proc Natl Acad Sci U S A* 1999;96:3104–3107.
202. Simon WH. Scale effects in animal joints. *Arthritis Rheum* 1971;14:493–502.
203. Baragi VM, Renkiewicz RR, Qiu L, et al. Transplantation of adenovirally transduced allogeneic chondrocytes into articular cartilage defects in vivo. *Osteoarthritis Cartilage* 1997;5:275–282.
204. Freed LE, Marquis JC, Nohria A, et al. Neocartilage formation in vitro and in vivo using cells cultured on synthetic biodegradable polymers. *J Biomed Mater Res* 1993;27:11–23.
205. Kawabe N, Yoshinao M. The repair of full-thickness articular cartilage defects. *Clin Orthop* 1991;268:279–293.
206. Kandel RA, Chen H, Clark J, et al. Transplantation of cartilaginous tissue generated in vitro into articular joint defects. *Artif Cells Blood Substit Immobil Biotechnol* 1995;23:565–577.
207. Amiel D, Coutts RD, Abel M, et al. Rib perichondrial grafts for the repair of full-thickness articular-cartilage defects. *J Bone Joint Surg Am* 1985;67:911–920.
208. Kreklau B, Sittinger M, Mensing MB, et al. Tissue engineering of biphasic joint cartilage transplants. *Biomaterials* 1999;20: 1743–1749.
209. Peel SAF, Chen H, Renlund R, et al. Formation of a SIS-cartilage composite graft in vitro and its use in the repair of articular cartilage defects. *Tissue Eng* 1998;4:143–155.
210. Toolan BC, Frenkel SR, Pereira DS, et al. Development of a novel osteochondral graft for cartilage repair. *J Biomed Mater Res* 1998;41:244–250.
211. von Schroeder HP, Kwan M, Amiel D, et al. The use of polylactic acid matrix and periosteal grafts for the reconstruction of rabbit knee articular defects. *J Biomed Mater Res* 1991;25:329–339.
212. Yu H, Grynpas M, Kandel RA. Composition of cartilaginous tissue with mineralized and non-mineralized zones formed in vitro. *Biomaterials* 1997;18:1425–1431.
213. Kandel RA, Boyle J, Gibson G, et al. In vitro formation of mineralized cartilaginous tissue by articular chondrocytes. *In Vitro Cell Dev Biol Anim* 1997;33:174–181.
214. Kandel R, Hurtig M, Grynpas M. Characterization of the mineral in calcified articular cartilaginous tissue formed in vitro. *Tissue Eng* 1999;5:25–34.
215. Rosenberg L, Hunziker EB. Cartilage repair in osteoarthritis: the role of dermatan sulfate proteoglycans. In: Kuettner KE, Goldberg VM, eds. *Osteoarthritic disorders*. Rosemont, IL: American Academy of Orthopaedic Surgeons, 1995:341–356.
216. Hunziker EB, Kapfinger E. Removal of proteoglycans from the surface of defects in articular cartilage transiently enhances coverage by repair cells. *J Bone Joint Surg Br* 1998;80: 144–150.
217. Mochizuki Y, Goldberg VM, Caplan AI. Enzymatical digestion for the repair of superficial articular cartilage lesions. *Trans Orthop Res Soc* 1993;18:728.
218. Lee MC, Sung K-LP, Kurtis MS, et al. Adhesive force of chondrocytes to cartilage: effects of chondroitinase ABC. *Clin Orthop* 2000;Jan:286–294.
219. Kurtis MS, Gaya OA, Tu BP, et al. Mechanisms of chondrocyte adhesion to cartilage: role of β1 integrins, CD44, and anchorin CII. *Trans Orthop Res Soc* 1999;24:105.
220. Chen AC, Nagrampa JP, Schinagl RM, et al. Chondrocyte transplantation to articular cartilage explants in vitro. *J Orthop Res* 1997;15:791–802.
221. Albrecht DR, Chen AC, Sah RL. Tailoring cartilage implants by targeted chondrocyte seeding: towards enhancement of integrative cartilage repair. *Tissue Eng* (in press).
222. Peretti GM, Randolph MA, Caruso EM, et al. Bonding of cartilage matrices with cultured chondrocytes: an experimental model. *J Orthop Res* 1998;16:89–95.
223. Peretti GM, Bonassar LJ, Caruso EM, et al. Biomechanical analysis of a chondrocyte-based repair model of articular cartilage. *Tissue Eng* 1999;5:317–326.
224. Sah RL, Grodzinsky AJ, Plaas AHK, et al. Effects of static and dynamic compression on matrix metabolism in cartilage explants. In: Kuettner KE, Schleyerbach R, Peyron JG, et al., eds. *Articular cartilage and osteoarthritis*. New York: Raven Press, 1992:373–392.
225. Guilak F, Sah RL, Setton LA. Physical regulation of cartilage metabolism. In: Mow VC, Hayes WC, eds. *Basic orthopaedic biomechanics*. 2nd ed. New York: Raven Press, 1997:179–207.
226. Brown TD, Pope DF, Hale JE, et al. Effects of osteochondral defect size on cartilage contact stress. *J Orthop Res* 1991; 9:559–567.
227. Hale JE, Rudert MJ, Brown TD. Indentation assessment of biphasic mechanical property deficits in size-dependent osteochondral defect repair. *J Biomech* 1993;26:1319–1325.
228. Mow VC, Bachrach NM, Ateshian GA. The effects of a subchondral bone perforation on the load support mechanism within articular cartilage. *Wear* 1994;175:167–175.
229. Athanasiou KA, Rosenwasser MP, Buckwalter JA, et al. Biomechanical modeling of repair articular cartilage: effects of passive motion on osteochondral defects in monkey knee joints. *Tissue Eng* 1998;4:185–195.
230. Wayne JS, Woo SLY, Kwan MK. Application of the u-p finite element method to the study of articular cartilage. *J Biomech Eng* 1991;113:397–403.
231. Mitchell N, Shepard N. Healing of articular cartilage in intra-articular fractures in rabbits. *J Bone Joint Surg Am* 1980;62: 628–634.
232. Salter RB. The biologic concept of continuous passive motion of synovial joints: the first 18 years of basic research and its clinical application. *Clin Orthop* 1989;242:12–25.
233. Hunter W. On the structure and diseases of articulating cartilage. *Trans R Soc Lond* 1743;42:514–521.
234. Khouri RK, Koudsi B, Reddi H. Tissue transformation into bone in vivo: a potential practical application. *JAMA* 1991;266: 1953–1955.
235. Isogai N, Landis W, Kim TH, et al. Formation of phalanges and small joints by tissue-engineering. *J Bone Joint Surg Am* 1999; 81:306–316.

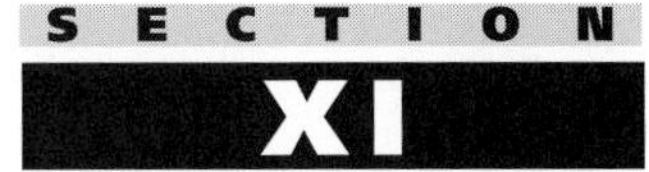

METABOLIC BONE AND JOINT DISEASES

114

CLINICAL GOUT AND THE PATHOGENESIS OF HYPERURICEMIA

MICHAEL A. BECKER

Gout is a heterogeneous group of diseases resulting from tissue deposition of monosodium urate or uric acid crystals from extracellular fluids supersaturated with respect to this end product of human purine metabolism. The limited range of clinical manifestations of urate deposition includes recurrent attacks of a unique type of acute inflammatory arthritis (acute gout); accumulation of potentially destructive crystalline aggregates (tophi), especially in connective tissue structures; uric acid urolithiasis; and infrequently, renal impairment (gouty nephropathy). *Hyperuricemia* (supersaturation for urate in serum) is the pathogenetic common denominator through which diverse etiologic influences predispose to crystal deposition and the potential for clinical events. Although hyperuricemia is a necessary underlying feature of gout, it is in the majority of instances insufficient for expression of the disorder. Thus the distinction between hyperuricemia, a biochemical aberration, and gout, a disease state, is essential. Recognition of this distinction, in conjunction with increasing evidence that hyperuricemia and gout are, at worst, only weak risk factors for the development of chronic renal insufficiency, has promoted conservatism in the use of drug therapy to treat asymptomatic hyperuricemia and even the early stages of gout.

HISTORICAL OVERVIEW

Gout is among the most illustrious and well-described human diseases, and it is likely not coincidental that contemporary understanding of the pathogenesis of hyperuricemia and gout is quite extensive (1). The distinctive clinical features of gouty arthritis were recognized by Hippocrates in the 5th century BC and were described in the oldest known medical text. The Roman physicians Galen (who was the first to describe gouty tophi) and Celsus recognized that gout afflicted the rich and powerful, especially those who were most overindulgent. An inherited tendency to gout (gouty diathesis) also was suspected by the Romans two millennia before the inclusion of gout among the first group of "inborn errors of metabolism" by Sir Archibald Garrod in 1909 (2). The medieval concept that gout arises as a consequence of poisonous "noxa" appears to be the basis for the term gout, derived from the Latin *guta,* meaning "a drop." In view of the contemporary understanding of gout as monosodium urate crystal deposition disease, the term reflects a certain prescience.

A relation between gout and uric acid has long been recognized. Van Leeuwenhoek (3), the Dutch microscopist, sketched needle-shaped crystals obtained from a gouty tophus in 1679, and, a century later, Scheele, a Swedish chemist, identified urolithic (uric) acid in a urinary calculus. In 1797, the British chemist Wollaston identified urate as the major constituent of a gouty tophus (1). The demonstration of excess uric acid in the acidified serum from patients with gout by using a "thread test" provided the basis for Alfred Baring Garrod's remarkably clear and accurate postulates concerning gouty pathogenesis (1859, 1863) and also was a pioneering achievement in the new science of clinical chemistry (4). Garrod described asymptomatic hyperuricemia, the relation of hyperuricemia to gout, the cause and effect relation between urate crystal deposition and gouty inflammation, and roles for increased uric acid formation and impaired renal uric acid excretion among patients with gout. Surprisingly, this work was largely forgotten until monosodium urate crystals were specifically identified in the synovial fluid of patients with acute gouty arthritis by McCarty and Hollander in 1961 (5).

Since the 1960s, sophisticated biochemical, isotopic, and cell biologic studies of the pathophysiology of hyperuricemia and gout have resulted in a unified concept of gout centering on the role of urate crystal deposition. Concomitantly, this period has witnessed development of highly successful management modalities based on rational therapeutics and the availability of multiple classes of agents to achieve the major aims of therapy in gout: treatment of acute inflammation, prevention of recurrent attacks of arthritis and urinary tract stones, and reversal of hyperuricemia. These therapeutic achievements are the culmination of nearly 1,000 years of medical intervention in gout, dating from the introduction of colchicine in the Middle Ages (1).

DEFINITION OF HYPERURICEMIA

Physicochemical and epidemiologic definitions of hyperuricemia have been proposed. Solubility product considerations dictate that at the sodium concentrations prevailing in extracellular fluids, serum at 37°C is supersaturated for monosodium urate at concentrations greater than about 6.8 mg/dL (6) (Fig. 114.1). Above this theoretic limit of solubility, increasing risks for gout and urinary tract stones have been documented (7,8). In most population groups tested, application of the specific uricase-spectrophotometric serum uric acid assay has established upper limits of normal (mean + 2 SD) of about 7.0 mg/dL in adult men and 6.0 mg/dL in premenopausal women (9). Nevertheless, hyperuricemia defined by the solubility of urate is preferable to population-defined hyperuricemia, because the distribution of serum urate values is not symmetric about the mean but is skewed so that the majority of values falling outside 2 SD from the mean are high (10).

Automated enzymatic methods rely on the production of H_2O_2 generated during the oxidation of urate by uricase and constitute the most common and convenient procedures now used for measurement of serum and urinary uric acid values (11). These methods are subject to minor nonspecific interference, but with proper standardization, they are sufficiently accurate for routine clinical practice and represent a considerable improvement on prior colorimetric methods, which have largely been abandoned.

Serum urate values in children are lower than those in adults, and, during male puberty, values increase into the adult male range (10,12). The lower serum urate values in women of reproductive age compared with their male counterparts have been ascribed to lower renal postsecretory uric acid reabsorption and thus increased urate clearance in women of childbearing age (12,13), but the suspected role of estrogenic compounds remains unclarified. With the onset of menopause, serum urate values in women approach or equal those of men of corresponding age, and this physiologic change is accompanied by an increase in the incidence of gout.

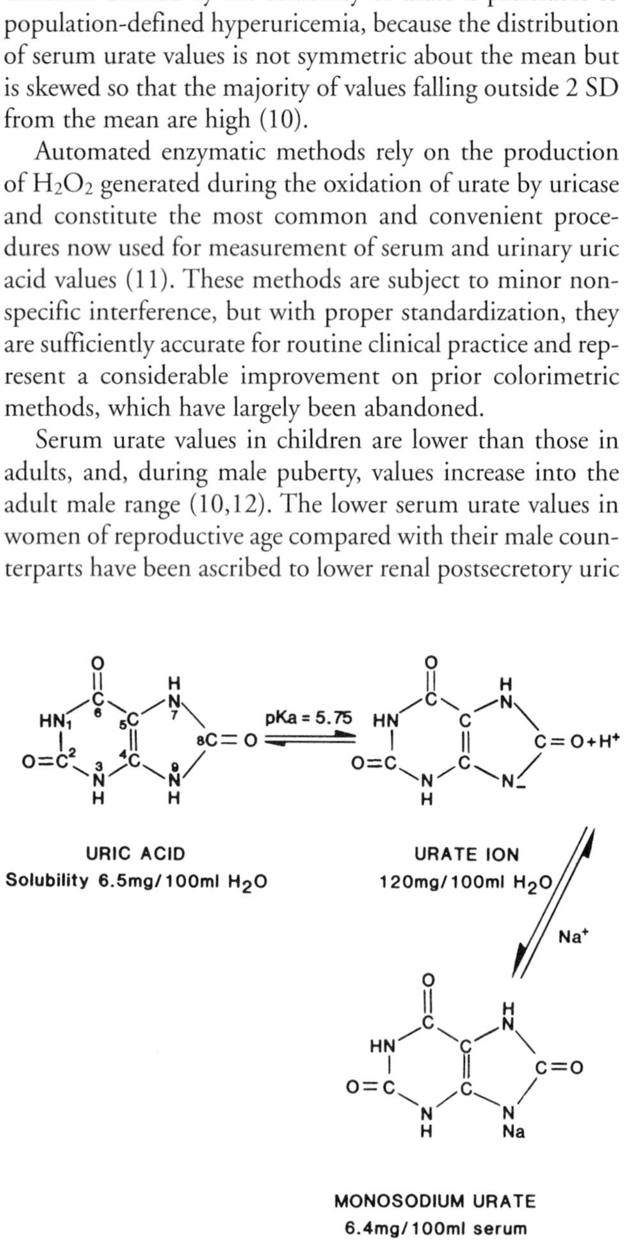

URIC ACID
Solubility 6.5mg/100ml H_2O

pKa = 5.75

URATE ION
120mg/100ml H_2O

Na^+

MONOSODIUM URATE
6.4mg/100ml serum

FIGURE 114.1. Solubility of uric acid species.

Asymptomatic Hyperuricemia

The term *asymptomatic hyperuricemia* is applied to the state in which the serum urate concentration is abnormally high, but symptoms have not occurred. In men, primary hyperuricemia frequently begins at puberty, whereas in women, it is usually delayed until menopause. Once developed, asymptomatic hyperuricemia frequently lasts a lifetime, but gout may develop in hyperuricemic individuals at any point. The prevalence of asymptomatic hyperuricemia among adult American men has been estimated at 5% to 8%, but even higher prevalence rates have been reported in Asian-Pacific populations (14,15). Management of hypertension and congestive heart failure with diuretics has expanded an already large population of individuals with asymptomatic hyperuricemia, particularly among elderly women.

Few studies have assessed the risks of asymptomatic hyperuricemia. In a cohort of 2,046 initially healthy men followed up for 15 years with serial measurements of serum urate concentrations, the annual incidence rate of gout was 4.9% for a serum urate of 9 mg/dL or more (7). In contrast, the incidence rate was only 0.5% for values between 7.0 and 8.9 mg/dL, and 0.1% for values below 7.0 mg/dL. Throughout this prospective study, there was no evidence of renal deterioration attributable to hyperuricemia. This finding was confirmed by a study of 3,693 subjects enrolled in a hypertension detection and follow-up program (16). Therapy with thiazide-type diuretics increased both serum urate and creatinine concentrations. However, reducing urate values with drug therapy did not influence creatinine values. Additionally, the incidence of gouty attacks in subjects at risk was only 2.7% over a 5-year period. Fessel (17) concluded that hyperuricemia is of no clinical importance with respect to renal outcomes until serum urate levels reach at least 13 mg/dL in men and 10 mg/dL in women, limits beyond which little information is available. Urolithiasis was rare among previously asymptomatic hyperuricemic individuals, with an annualized incidence rate of 0.4% compared with 0.9% in gouty patients. In the Framingham study, gout developed in only 12% of patients with urate levels between 7 and 7.9 mg/dL over a period of 14 years (8). Values greater than 9 mg/dL had a sixfold greater predictive value but represented only 20% of the gouty population.

The available data thus do not justify therapy for most patients with asymptomatic hyperuricemia. Nevertheless, hyperuricemia does predispose individuals to both articular gout and nephrolithiasis. Once a hyperuricemic individual experiences one of these complications, the asymptomatic phase is ended, and medical management of hyperuricemia may be indicated (see Chapter 115).

PATHOGENESIS OF HYPERURICEMIA AND GOUT

Among mammalian species, only humans and the great apes excrete uric acid as the end product of purine metabolism, reflecting the lack of the enzyme uricase, which catalyzes the degradation of uric acid to the readily excretable compound, allantoin (18). Uric acid is a weak organic acid (pK_{a1}, 5.75) that is sparingly soluble both in the unionized acid form prevalent in normal urine and in the ionized urate form at the pH and sodium concentration of other extracellular fluids (6) (Fig. 114.1). The combination of lack of uricase and the solubility properties of uric acid conditions humans to the deposition of urate from supersaturated (hyperuricemic) body fluids, with the consequent risk of clinical sequelae (gout). The magnitude of this problem is dramatized by the fact that, at least among normal adult white men, mean serum urate concentrations are within 1 mg/dL of the theoretic limit of urate solubility in serum. The factors determining who will develop hyperuricemia and, among this group, who will develop gout are diverse and are best understood in the context of how purine compounds are normally metabolized (Fig. 114.2) and the physiologic mechanisms maintaining uric acid homeostasis.

Purine Metabolism in Humans

Net contributions to body pools of purine compounds are provided by dietary purine ingestion and the endogenous pathway of *de novo* purine nucleotide synthesis. The latter is a sequence of ten enzymatic reactions by which small molecule precursors of uric acid are incorporated into a purine ring (Fig. 114.3), synthesized on a ribose phosphate backbone donated by 5-phosphoribosyl 1-pyrophosphate (PRPP) (19) (Fig. 114.4). This pathway requires 6 moles of adenosine triphosphate (ATP) for generation of each mole of inosinic acid, the first purine nucleotide product of the pathway. A complex network of purine interconversion

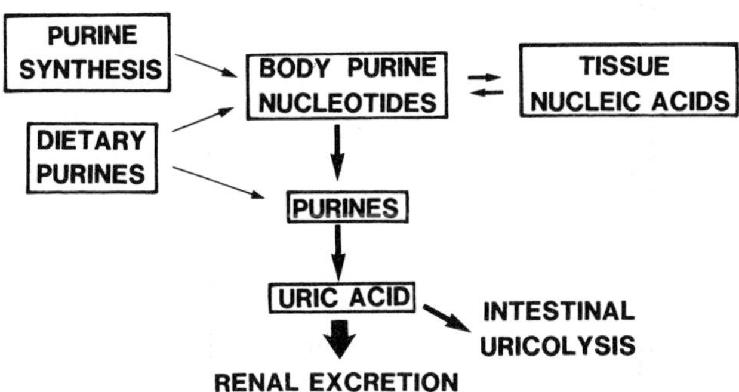

FIGURE 114.2. Human purine metabolism. (Courtesy of Dr. J. Edwin Seegmiller.)

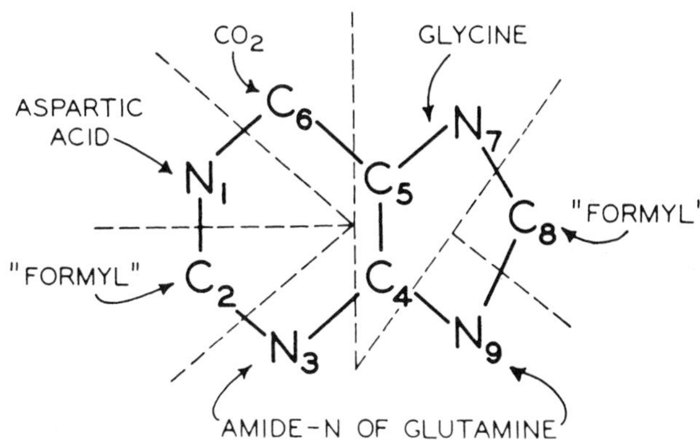

FIGURE 114.3. Precursors of the purine ring.

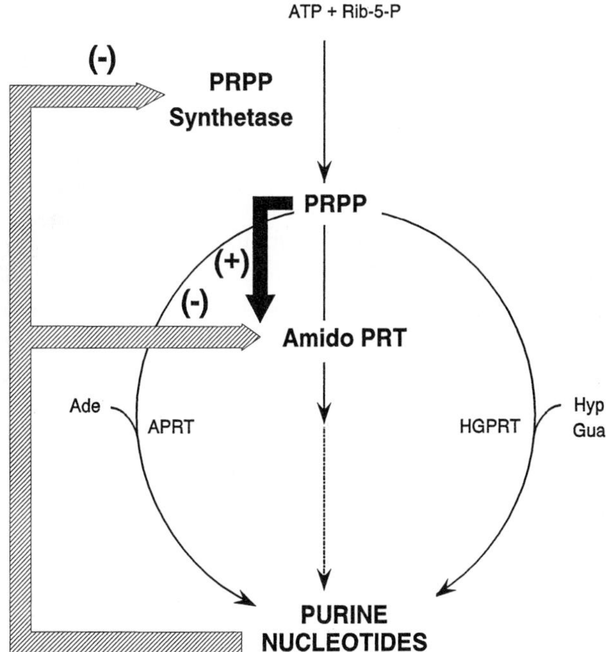

FIGURE 114.4. Pathways of phosphoribosylpyrophosphate (PRPP) and purine nucleotide synthesis and regulation of rates of purine synthesis *de novo* by PRPP and purine nucleotide end products. *Curved arrows,* Single-step purine base salvage pathways catalyzed by the phosphoribosyltransferase (PRT) enzymes APRT and HGPRT. Purine synthesis *de novo* is shown by a *thin solid arrow*, representing the initial and rate-limiting AmidoPRT reaction and a *dashed arrow* depicting the final nine steps in this reaction sequence. Purine nucleotide inhibition (–) of PRPP synthetase and AmidoPRT is indicated by the *heavy hatched arrow*, and allosteric activation (+) of AmidoPRT by PRPP is shown by the *heavy dark arrow. Rib-5-P*, ribose-5-phosphate; *Ade*, adenine; *Hyp*, hypoxanthine; *Gua*, guanine.

reactions ensures efficient reuse of preformed purines, so that much of the cellular energy that would otherwise be consumed in *de novo* synthesis of purines is conserved. Foremost among these are the single-step salvage reactions, involving the two enzymes adenine and hypoxanthine-guanine phosphoribosyltransferase (APRT and HGPRT), which catalyze conversion of the respective purine bases directly to the corresponding nucleotides by reaction with PRPP (20).

Together, purine base salvage and *de novo* purine synthesis pathways provide alternative, but concerted, means for adjusting the production of purine nucleotides to needs. The molecular mechanisms effecting this regulation have been defined (21,22). Control of purine synthesis *de novo* (Fig. 114.4) is exerted in large part in a regulatory domain encompassing the first reaction uniquely committed to the pathway, catalyzed by amidophosphoribosyltransferase (AmidoPRT) (21), and the preceding PRPP synthetase reaction in which PRPP is generated (22). The allosteric regulatory properties of AmidoPRT reflect an antagonistic interaction at the level of the enzyme between PRPP and pathway end products (21,23,24). AmidoPRT activity is inhibited by purine nucleotides, and this feedback inhibition is reversed by PRPP (23). Concentrations of PRPP in normal cells are below the apparent affinity constant of AmidoPRT for PRPP (23,25), suggesting that availability of this compound is the basis of rate limitation at the AmidoPRT reaction. AmidoPRT can assume two subunit conformations (21,24). The active 133-kd monomer can be reversibly converted into an inactive 270-kd dimer by addition of purine nucleotide inhibitors, and this effect is blocked by increasing concentrations of PRPP. This molecular mechanism provides a structural basis for control of AmidoPRT activity and has been demonstrated *in vivo* (25), as well as in purified preparations of the enzyme (21). Cloning of human AmidoPRT cDNA (26) and resolution of the crystal structure of the Bacillus protein by x-ray diffraction analysis (27) have recently helped shed further light on molecular mechanisms through which this critical enzyme is expressed.

A second level of inhibitory control of purine synthesis *de novo* is exerted by purine nucleotides on the activity of PRPP synthetase (Fig. 114.4), but this enzyme is less sensitive than AmidoPRT to nucleotide inhibition (22,28). Moreover, PRPP synthetase activity also is inhibited by pyrimidine and, perhaps, pyridine nucleotides, products of pathways that also require PRPP (25,29). Overall, the dual regulation of purine nucleotide production is admirably suited to maintain both fine and broad control over changes in end product availability—the former by alterations in AmidoPRT subunit structure and activity in response to small changes in purine concentrations (21,22,24,28), and the latter, by changes in the activity of PRPP synthetase in response to larger variations in concentrations of the nucleotide products of several metabolic pathways (22,28,30).

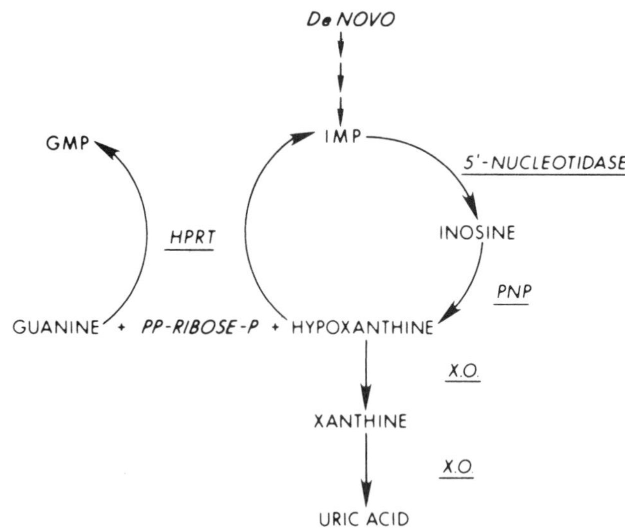

FIGURE 114.5. Schematic representation of purine nucleotide catabolism, purine base salvage, and purine base oxidation to uric acid. Reactions of adenylate metabolism are omitted. *HPRT*, hypoxanthine-guanine phosphoribosyltransferase; *IMP*, inosinic acid; *PNP*, purine nucleoside phosphorylase; *XO*, xanthine oxidase.

Adenine and guanine nucleotides are intracellular building blocks for RNA and DNA, and purine compounds also are essential in energy metabolism and intercellular signaling, including neural transmission. Balanced production of adenylates and guanylates is expedited by nucleotide interconversion pathways, which also appear to be regulated to ensure that the distribution of nucleotide classes meets both baseline requirements of all cells and the specific needs of specialized cells (31). On the catabolic side of purine metabolism (Fig. 114.2), purine nucleotides are degraded through purine nucleoside and purine base forms, with ultimate irreversible oxidation of unreclaimed hypoxanthine to xanthine and xanthine to uric acid, a reaction sequence catalyzed by xanthine oxidase (18) (Fig. 114.5).

Uric Acid Homeostasis in Normal and Gouty Individuals

Uric acid, synthesized mainly in the liver, is released into the circulation, where only a small percentage (less than 4% under physiologic conditions) (32) is bound nonspecifically to albumin or to a specific urate-binding globulin (9). The vast majority of circulating urate is thus readily available for filtration at the glomerulus and for participation in a complex series of renal uric acid–handling mechanisms, as discussed later. When tracer doses of isotopically labeled uric acid (e.g., [^{15}N] urate) are given intravenously to normal individuals at steady state, the size and dynamics of the miscible pool of uric acid can be quantitated, and the overall contribution of renal excretion to uric acid disposal can be estimated from the isotopic enrichment of urinary uric acid (9,33). The miscible urate pool in normal men averages about 1,200 mg, and mean turnover of this pool is approximately 0.6 pools/day (9,34). In women, the average urate pool size is about 600 mg, and the turnover rate of the pool is also about 0.6 pools/day. In both sexes, urinary uric acid excretion accounts for approximately two thirds of the uric acid turned over daily, with degradation by gut bacteria of uric acid secreted into the intestine (intestinal uricolysis) accounting for nearly all of the additional urate disposed of by extrarenal routes (9,33).

Uric acid pool size is enlarged in all untreated patients with gout regardless of the magnitude of urinary uric acid excretion (9,33). (Uric acid pools in gout patients are usually in the range of 2,000 to 4,000 mg in the absence of evident tophi but may reach 30,000 mg or more in tophaceous gout.) In hyperuricemic individuals or gouty patients, extrarenal uric acid disposal is invariably normal or increased (to as much as 50% of total daily excretion), excluding impaired intestinal uricolysis as a mechanism of hyperuricemia (33). Although many patients with gout have rates of turnover of the uric acid pool that overlap the normal range (34), increased rates of turnover are uniformly found in patients who show excessive rates of incorporation of radioactively labeled precursor molecules (such as [^{14}C] glycine) into urinary uric acid (a measure of purine nucleotide and uric acid synthesis) and daily urinary uric acid excretion clearly exceeding that of normal individuals (9,34,35).

These findings provided the first evidence of heterogeneity in the mechanisms accounting for uric acid accumulation, hyperuricemia, and the consequent predisposition to urate crystal deposition in gout (34,35). Additional study has confirmed that excessive production and diminished renal excretion of uric acid, operating singly or in combination, are the major abnormalities demonstrable among hyperuricemic individuals with or without gout (9). Whether the hyperuricemia occurs exclusive of a coexisting disease or aberrant physiologic state (primary hyperuricemia) or is a consequence of one of the conditions listed in Table 114.1 (secondary hyperuricemia), one or both of these mechanisms underlie the development of hyperuricemia.

Distinction in individual patients between uric acid overproduction and impaired renal uric acid excretion as the basis of hyperuricemia has therapeutic as well as investigative significance and is warranted in most patients with gout and perhaps all who have normal renal function (36). The most practical approach to achieving this distinction is measurement of daily urinary uric acid excretion. This determination is best made on 2 consecutive days, 5 days after initiation of an isocaloric purine-free diet and at least 10 days after medications affecting uric acid production or excretion have been discontinued. [Indomethacin and colchicine do not alter uric acid production or excretion and may be given during the study period, but radiologic contrast agents should be avoided because of their uricosuric effects (9).] Under these conditions of steady state with regard to uric acid metabolism, urinary excretion of uric acid represents a minimal esti-

TABLE 114.1. CAUSES OF HYPERURICEMIA IN MAN

Increased purine biosynthesis or urate production
Inherited enzyme defects
Hypoxanthine–guanine phosphoribosyltransferase deficiency
Phosphoribosylpyrophosphate synthetase overactivity
Glucose-6-phosphatase deficiency (glycogenosis I)
Clinical disorders leading to purine overproduction
Myeloproliferative disorders
Lymphoproliferative disorders
Polycythemia vera
Malignant diseases
Hemolytic disorders
Psoriasis
Obesity
Tissue hypoxia
Glycogenosis III, V, VII
Drugs or dietary habits
Ethanol
Diet rich in purines.
Pancreatic extract
Fructose
Nicotinic acid
Ethylamino-1,3,4-thiadiazole
4-Amino-5-imidazole carboxamide riboside
Vitamin B_{12} (patients with pernicious anemia)
Cytotoxic drugs
Warfarin
Decreased renal clearance of urate
Clinical disorders
Chronic renal failure
Lead nephropathy
Polycystic kidney disease
Hypertension
Dehydration
Salt restriction
Starvation
Diabetic ketoacidosis
Lactic acidosis
Obesity
Hyperparathyroidism
Hypothyroidism
Diabetes insipidus
Sarcoidosis
Toxemia of pregnancy
Bartter's syndrome
Chronic beryllium disease
Down syndrome
Drugs or dietary habits
Ethanol
Diuretics
Low doses of salicylates
Ethambutol
Pyrazinamide
Laxative abuse (alkalosis)
Levodopa
Methoxyflurane
Cyclosporine

mate of the rate of uric acid synthesis (uncorrected for extrarenal uric acid disposal), which, in groups of white men, averages about 425 mg/day with an SD of 75 to 80 mg/day (9,34). Excretion of urinary uric acid in excess of 600 mg/day (mean + 2 SD) indicates uric acid overproduction.

The strict dietary control necessary for the accuracy of this determination is difficult to achieve in ambulatory patients. Measurement of daily urinary uric acid excretion during normal dietary intake is an alternative approach frequently used. Excretion in excess of 1,000 mg/day is regarded as clearly excessive. Values between 800 and 1,000 mg/day are equivocal, requiring retesting under closer dietary control (9,37). Women, children, nonwhite men, and obese or very large individuals are groups for which normal values are not readily available. For such persons, daily urinary uric acid excretion exceeding about 12 mg/kg body weight most likely represents uric acid overproduction.

Overproduction of Uric Acid

Excessive daily urinary uric acid excretion is demonstrable in 10% to 15% of patients with gout and primary hyperuricemia and in most patients whose hyperuricemia reflects increased cell turnover (e.g., a myelo- or lymphoproliferative disease) or a toxic state or pharmacologic intervention resulting in increased uric acid production (9) (Table 114.1). *In vivo* isotopic labeling studies applied to such individuals almost invariably confirm the presence of increased purine nucleotide and uric acid synthesis (9,34). The consistency of this relation renders the highly accurate but cumbersome and expensive isotopic procedures unnecessary in this group.

In some circumstances, however, rates of uric acid synthesis are increased, as determined isotopically in patients with normal or even reduced daily urinary uric acid excretion values (34). These discrepancies usually reflect increased extrarenal contributions to uric acid disposal, such as with deposition of urate in the tophi of patients with extensive tophaceous gout or with increased intestinal uricolysis in patients with renal insufficiency. Failure to confirm a strong suspicion of uric acid overproduction by urinary uric acid excretion measurements in patients with tophi or renal insufficiency should prompt consideration for direct measurement of rates of purine nucleotide synthesis either by *in vivo* labeling or by measurement of rates of purine synthesis *de novo* in fibroblasts cultured from skin biopsy material (30). The latter method provides a sensitive and reliable means for detecting purine overproduction in patients with primary hyperuricemia (38). These alternatives to daily urinary uric acid excretion studies also are valuable in detecting the occasional patient whose cryptic uric acid overproduction is accompanied by impaired renal uric acid disposal but who has neither tophi nor overt reduction in glomerular filtration rate.

Persistent uric acid overproduction in patients with gout and primary hyperuricemia indicates excessive rates of purine synthesis *de novo.* In keeping with the proposed scheme for regulation of the rate of this pathway, involving antagonistic interaction of PRPP and purine nucleotides on AmidoPRT activity (21,22) (Fig. 114.4), altered balance in the availability of these small molecule effectors has been identified under several circumstances in which inherited or acquired hyperuricemia is associated with uric acid overproduction. In these instances, either increased PRPP availability or diminished purine nucleotide concentrations (or both) constitutes the immediate stimulus for excessive purine nucleotide and uric acid production. Although an AmidoPRT with decreased response to nucleotide inhibition or increased response to PRPP also could result in purine overproduction (9,38), defects in this enzyme have yet to be confirmed among gouty individuals.

Increased PRPP Availability

A wealth of biochemical, pharmacologic, and clinical data support the role of PRPP as a critical component in the regulation of purine synthesis and thus of uric acid production (9,21,22,25). Increased PRPP availability as the driving force for excessive rates of purine synthesis *de novo* is best exemplified in the two X chromosome–linked inborn errors of purine metabolism, HGPRT deficiency (39,40) and PRPP synthetase superactivity (41,42) (Figs. 114.4 and 114.6). In both of these disorders, uric acid overproduction, hyperuricemia, and hyperuricosuria occur in conjunction with increased PRPP levels but not with a decrease in purine nucleotide concentrations (9,22,30,42,43). A unique or contributing role for increased PRPP availability in uric acid overproduction also has been suggested in several other proposed or established enzymatic defects or metabolic states (Fig. 114.6), but the associations remain to be more fully delineated.

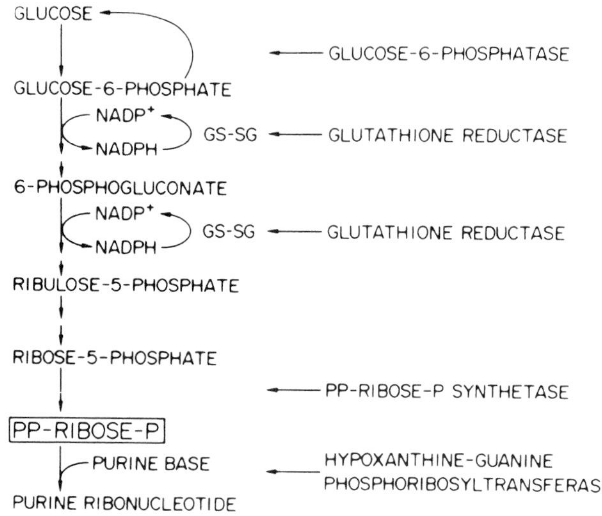

FIGURE 114.6. Enzymatic defects that may result in increased phosphoribosylpyrophosphate availability. *NADP,* Nicotinamide adenine dinucleotide phosphate; *NADPH,* reduced nicotinamide adenine dinucleotide phosphate.

HGPRT Deficiency

HGPRT catalyzes the salvage reactions of the purine bases hypoxanthine and guanine with PRPP (Figs. 114.4 and 114.5) to form the respective mononucleotides inosine monophosphate (IMP) and guanosine monophosphate (GMP) (19). The presence of HGPRT activity in all cells suggests a "housekeeping" function (44), although recent evidence suggests functionally significant regulation of the expression of the HGPRT gene in some cell types. Despite alternative routes of purine nucleotide synthesis, HGPRT function is clearly not redundant, as revealed by the consequences of inherited deficiency of the enzyme (45).

Deficiency of HGPRT is expressed in two clinical forms, only one of which appears among hemizygous affected male subjects in a single family. In general, those phenotypes correlate with the presence or absence of residual HGPRT activity. The Lesch–Nyhan syndrome (46) appears in infancy or early childhood in conjunction with complete HGPRT deficiency (39) (Fig. 114.7). This is a dramatic and devastating disorder in which the clinical consequences of hyperuricemia and hyperuricosuria (most frequently uric acid urolithiasis) are usually secondary in importance to a neurobehavioral constellation that includes most or all of the following features: choreoathetosis, spasticity, varying degrees of mental retardation, and compulsive self-mutilation. How the neurologic features of the syndrome relate to the inherited defect in purine metabolism is uncertain (45). Nevertheless, abnormalities in the dopaminergic neurotransmitter pathway from the substantia nigra to the putamen and caudate nucleus have been identified in brains of Lesch–Nyhan syndrome patients (47), implicating these regions of the brain despite the minimal histologic damage found at necropsy. Furthermore, aberrant dopaminergic brain function and behavior have been induced in HGPRT-deficient mice treated with amphetamine (48), providing the possibility of an animal model to assess this relation.

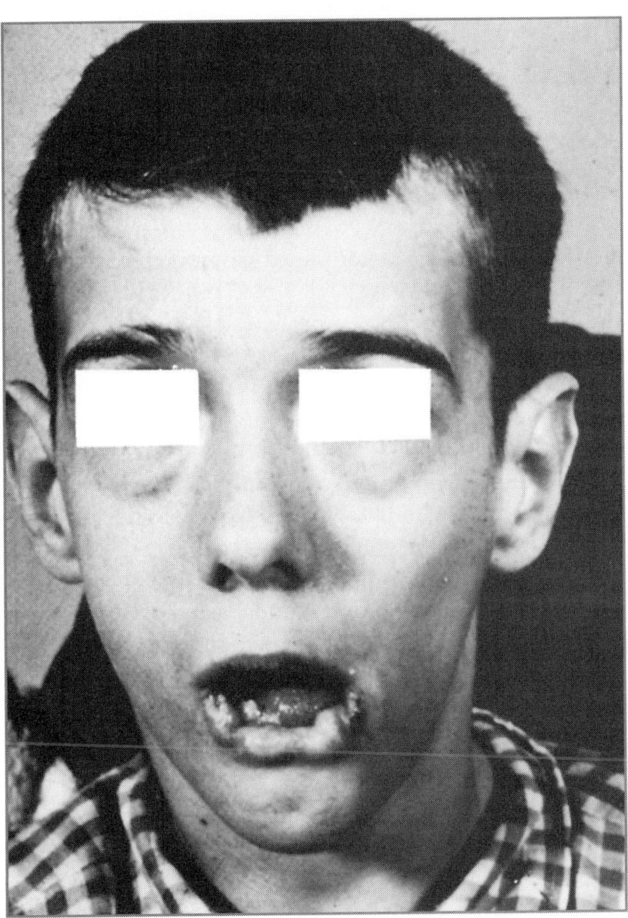

FIGURE 114.7. Patient with the Lesch–Nyhan syndrome. Note the mutilation of the lower lip. (Courtesy of Dr. J. Edwin Seegmiller.)

Partial deficiencies of HGPRT are associated with clinical manifestations directly correlated with severe uric acid overproduction, hyperuricemia, and hyperuricosuria: gouty arthritis and uric acid urolithiasis, appearing in male subjects in late adolescence or early adulthood (40,43). Neurobehavioral defects are not infrequent among patients with partial HGPRT deficiency, in which residual enzyme activity may be less than 1% that of normal. At the other end of the spectrum, residual HGPRT activities of up to 60% have been reported among affected male subjects in certain families, but closer examination has usually revealed kinetic defects in HGPRT, resulting in more severely reduced HGPRT function under conditions occurring in intact cells (9,49).

Expression of HGPRT deficiency is virtually restricted to male subjects, reflecting the fact that the HGPRT gene maps to a 44-kb DNA sequence (50) on the long arm of the X chromosome (Xq26) (51). Extensive analyses of normal and mutant human HGPRT genes, cDNAs, and enzymes have revealed marked heterogeneity in the precise structural defects associated with enzyme deficiencies and with the distinctive clinical phenotypes (45,49,52–54). HGPRT is undetectable both enzymatically and immunochemically in the cells of the majority of patients with Lesch–Nyhan syndrome (49). HGPRT gene transcripts (mRNAs) can, however, be detected at normal or reduced abundance in most instances, and a wide range of genetic defects characteristic of these families have been identified by direct sequencing of amplified mutant transcripts (53,54). Nucleotide deletions, additions, and, most frequently, base substitutions have been revealed by these studies. The identification of multiple sites of mutation leading to severe enzyme deficiency has shed some light on the relation of HGPRT primary structure and enzymatic function (45), a relation now more precisely defined as a result of x-ray diffraction resolution of crystals of human HGPRT protein (55). Recent technologic advances also have permitted development of oligonucleotide-specific hybridization analysis for detection of carriers and prenatal diagnosis of affected fetuses in individual families (45).

Partial deficiencies of HGPRT are most often accompanied by a residual HGPRT protein (45,49,52), allowing the possibility of characterization of mutations by protein analysis as well as by the cloning techniques necessary for analysis of severe enzyme deficiencies. Protein chemical analyses of HGPRT isolated from the cells of patients with partial enzyme deficiency (and even a few with Lesch–Nyhan syndrome) have been achieved by means of enzyme purification and peptide sequencing (52). These studies have revealed amino acid substitutions correlated with varying degrees of enzyme deficiency, providing further insight into enzyme structure–function relations (45,55).

The study of HGPRT deficiency has reached a high level of sophistication, particularly at the levels of basic cell biology, protein structure analysis (55), and molecular genetics (45). Current model systems designed to transfer human HGPRT DNA into the nervous systems of experimental animals may ultimately provide the basis for attempts at correcting the genetic and biochemical defects in the Lesch–Nyhan syndrome (47,48,56). Given the available analytic expertise, measurement of HGPRT activity should be undertaken in patients with demonstrated primary uric acid overproduction and is especially important in those families with infantile or childhood onset of symptoms and a neurologic syndrome.

Despite the structural heterogeneity underlying HGPRT deficiency and the consequent variability in the magnitude of the derangement in purine synthesis, the biochemical mechanism of purine nucleotide and uric acid overproduction is unitary (Fig. 114.4). PRPP availability is increased as a result of decreased use of this compound in the salvage of hypoxanthine and guanine (9,30). Overall synthesis of PRPP is not increased, and purine nucleotide concentrations are not diminished (9,30). Accumulation of PRPP activates AmidoPRT, the rate-determining reaction of purine synthesis *de novo,* and thus accelerates the pathway (24). Once the excessive purine nucleotide products of the pathway are converted into hypoxanthine or guanine, failure of purine base reutilization means that these purine bases are directed to formation of uric acid (30,57,58) (Fig. 114.5). The inability to salvage hypoxanthine and guanine not only contributes to hyperuricemia but also precludes the salvage synthesis of purine nucleotide feedback inhibitors of purine synthesis *de novo,* which would normally modulate the rate of the pathway (30,58) (Fig. 114.4).

Purine nucleoside phosphorylase (PNP) deficiency, an enzyme defect resulting in inherited immunodeficiency, also results in purine overproduction as a consequence of impaired PRPP use in purine base salvage (59). This disorder, however, is accompanied by hypouricemia because PNP is required for formation of hypoxanthine and guanine, without which only limited amounts of uric acid can be produced.

PRPP Synthetase Superactivity

This enzyme catalyzes synthesis of PRPP from ribose-5-phosphate and MgATP in a reaction dependent on inorganic phosphate (Pi) and Mg^{2+} as activators. The reaction is subject to inhibition by a variety of phosphorylated compounds, including purine and pyrimidine nucleotides (25,60) (Fig. 114.4). In common with HGPRT deficiency, PRPP synthetase superactivity is inherited as an X chromosome–linked trait (61,62), which is expressed in two clinical phenotypes. The more severe phenotype also involves infantile or early childhood neurodevelopmental impairment in association with more severe kinetic derangement in enzyme function and more aberrant PRPP and purine metabolism in the affected individuals and their cells in culture (63). The enzymatic alterations resulting in PRPP synthetase superactivity are heterogeneous, reflecting differences in molecular pathology. Kinetic abnormalities include (a) enzyme overactivity in which increased catalytic velocity results from an overabundance of normal enzyme (42,64,65); (b) defective allosteric regulation of PRPP synthetase activity by purine nucleotide inhibition and Pi activation (63,66–69); (c) combined catalytic and regulatory defects (70); and (d) increased affinity for the substrate ribose-5-phosphate (38).

In all affected individuals, purine and uric acid overproduction results from increased PRPP availability, which is, in turn, a consequence of increased PRPP synthesis (30,67). In this regard, PRPP synthetase superactivity differs from HGPRT deficiency, in which increased PRPP concentrations result from impaired use in purine base salvage, and rates of PRPP synthesis are normal. Families with regulatory or combined kinetic defects in PRPP synthetase generally have higher rates of PRPP production and, consequently, greater acceleration of purine nucleotide and uric acid synthesis (30). Affected hemizygous male members of such families are likely to show infantile or early childhood symptoms and signs of uric acid overproduction in conjunction with neurodevelopmental impairment, most frequently sensorineural deafness (63,64,68,70). Heterozygous female carriers in these families may develop gout during the reproductive period, sometimes in association with deafness (63,70). In contrast, in families with overabundance of normal PRPP synthetase alone, clinical presentation is almost always restricted to affected male members in whom gout and uric acid urolithiasis, without neurologic defects, become evident in early adulthood (42,64,71).

A family of at least three human PRPP synthetase genes has been identified and mapped (72–74), and genes for two PRPP synthetase–associated proteins have been demonstrated (75,76). PRPP synthetase genes code for structurally homologous but functionally distinctive proteins (74,77,78) that appear to be independently active isoforms (74,79). Two of the PRPP synthetase genes map to the X chromosome but to different regions (72,73).

Point mutations (single base substitutions) in the protein coding region of the PRPP synthetase 1 gene (which is located on the long arm of the X chromosome at Xq22-q24) (73) have been identified in the PRPP synthetase 1 cDNAs from affected male subjects in six unrelated families in whom aberrant allosteric regulation of PRPP synthetase activity results in enzyme overactivity (69,80). In each case, expression of the mutant PRPP synthetase 1 cDNA in bacterial cells results in a recombinant human PRPP synthetase with aberrant kinetic properties closely resembling those in cultured cells from the corresponding patient (69,80). Thus mutations in the PRPP synthetase 1 gene provide the basis for inherited PRPP synthetase superactivity associated with altered purine nucleotide and Pi responsiveness, a class of defects usually accompanied by a neurodevelopmental as well as metabolic clinical phenotype. Although the enzymatic basis of uric acid overproduction and gout in individuals with these mutations is clearly explained, the basis of the associated neurologic and developmental impairments remains undefined (69).

The functional basis of excessive expression of normal activity (65) in individuals with phenotypically less severe enzyme superactivity has recently been established as accelerated transcription of the *PRPS1* gene, which results in increased PRPP synthetase 1 isozyme concentration and activity (81). The genetic defect underlying this unusual form of inherited disease remains to be established.

PRPP Availability in Other States of Purine Overproduction and/or Gout

Together, HGPRT deficiency and PRPP synthetase superactivity account for only a small proportion (10–15%) of patients with primary uric acid overproduction (9). Other enzyme defects that may shed light on additional members of this group of individuals as a consequence of increased PRPP production have been studied (Fig. 114.6).

In patients with glucose-6-phosphatase deficiency (glycogen storage disease, type I; von Gierke's disease), hyperuricemia appears as early as infancy, and gout has been reported by the end of the first decade. Patients surviving into adulthood with this autosomal recessive disorder may then have tophaceous gout and gouty renal disease as major clinical problems unless effective management is instituted (82,83).

The pathophysiology of hyperuricemia in glucose-6-phosphatase–deficient patients is multifactorial, involving both purine nucleotide and uric acid overproduction, confirmed by *in vivo* isotopic labeling (9), and impaired renal uric acid excretion that is due to lacticacidemia and ketonemia (82,83). Dual mechanisms through which increased PRPP production may contribute to the hyperuricemia of this disease have been proposed (9,84). First, glucose-6-phosphate accumulation, resulting from the inherited enzyme deficiency, may provide increased hepatic substrate for and stimulation of the oxidative branch of the pentose phosphate pathway, which leads to increased ribose-5-phosphate and, ultimately, PRPP synthesis. Second, diminished concentrations of inhibitory purine nucleotides occurring in the livers of patients with this disease during recurrent episodes of hypoglycemia (84) may result in activation of AmidoPRT and PRPP synthetase by release of one or both of these enzymes from nucleotide feedback inhibition (24). The extent to which these possibly potentiating mechanisms play roles in purine nucleotide overproduction in glucose-6-phosphatase deficiency in humans is uncertain, but results with human and animal experimental models indicate that both are tenable (24,82,84).

Increased PRPP production as a consequence of enhanced oxidative pentose phosphate pathway production of ribose-5-phosphate also has been hypothesized to explain hyperuricemia in some gout patients without glucose-6-phosphatase deficiency. Increased concentrations and rates of production of ribose-5-phosphate and PRPP were shown in fibroblasts cultured from two patients with documented purine nucleotide and uric acid overproduction (38). A high frequency of overactive, electrophoretically variant forms of glutathione reductase also were reported in red blood cell lysates from patients with gout (9). Activity of glutathione reductase promotes reduction of glutathione and oxidation of reduced nicotinamide adenine dinucleotide phosphate (NADPH) to nicotinamide adenine dinucleotide phosphate (NADP), a cofactor in the first two reactions of the oxidative pathway. Because the rate of operation of the pathway depends at least in part on the regulation of glucose-6-phosphate dehydrogenase activity by the ratio [NADPH]/ [NADP], increased glutathione reductase activity could provide a tenable mechanism for excessive PRPP synthesis and purine nucleotide and uric acid overproduction.

Purine overproduction was, however, not demonstrated in the initial report of variant glutathione reductase activity (9), and several subsequent studies have failed to confirm either abnormal enzyme activity or electrophoretically altered glutathione reductase in hemolysates from gouty patients (85). Additionally, definitive experimental evidence linking rates of the oxidative and nonoxidative pathways of pentose phosphate generation to control of rates of PRPP and purine nucleotide synthesis under physiologic conditions has not been provided. Despite the absence of confirmatory data, a connection between accelerated carbohydrate metabolism and rates of PRPP production could provide a basis for the association of metabolic disorders, such as obesity and hypertriglyceridemia, with hyperuricemia. In states of carbohydrate excess or increased lipogenesis, a mechanism for accelerated production of PRPP would be provided by increased pentose phosphate shunt activity, resulting in increased ribose-5-phosphate and PRPP synthesis.

Decreases in Purine Nucleotide Concentrations

Although deficiency of HGPRT might be expected to result in reduced intracellular purine nucleotide concentrations, such reductions have not been found in extracts of HGPRT-deficient cells (30,58,86). Nevertheless, circumstances in which uric acid overproduction results from nucleotide depletion have been identified (Fig. 114.8). These circumstances have in common net degradation of ATP as a consequence of increased ATP consumption or impaired ATP regeneration (87). In conditions in which the availability of Pi, oxygen, glucose, or fatty acids is restricted, optimal rates of ATP synthesis may be impaired, and severe ATP depletion and accompanying hyperuricemia may ensue, especially if the demands for ATP consumption are increased. Net ATP degradation results in accumulation of adenosine diphosphate (ADP) and adenosine monophosphate (AMP), which are rapidly converted to uric acid through the intermediates adenosine, inosine, hypoxanthine, and xanthine. Thus increases in any or all of these intermediates accompanying excessive uric acid levels in serum or urine provide evidence in support of this mechanism of hyperuricemia (88–97).

The effects of rapid administration of fructose in humans provides an experimental model for this mechanism (87). Fructose phosphorylation in the liver uses ATP, and the accompanying Pi depletion limits regeneration of ATP from ADP, which, in turn, serves as substrate for the catabolic pathway to uric acid formation (87). Thus within minutes after fructose infusion, plasma (and later urinary) inosine, hypoxanthine, xanthine, and uric acid concentrations are increased (90). In conjunction with purine nucleotide depletion, rates of purine synthesis *de novo* are accelerated, thus potentiating uric acid production (91). Evidence from these studies and from fructose administration in rats confirms that the increased purine synthetic rate is accompanied by increased PRPP levels, presumably as a result of release of nucleotide inhibition of PRPP synthetase (24,91). Additionally, the distribution of AmidoPRT in hepatic tissue is shifted toward the active monomeric form, as might be predicted from the acceleration of purine synthesis *de novo* (24).

Among the clinical states associated with net ATP degradation and consequent hyperuricemia are glycogen storage diseases, type III (debranching enzyme deficiency), type V (myophosphorylase deficiency), and type VII (muscle phosphofructokinase deficiency), in which mild exercise provokes "myogenic hyperuricemia" and hyperuricosuria as a consequence of impaired glucose availability for regeneration of ATP from ADP in muscle (93). In affected individuals, even daily activities, as well as mild exercise not exceeding the anaerobic threshold, may produce persistent hyperuricemia (96). Strenuous exercise exceeding the anaerobic threshold (97) or prolonged training in otherwise normal individuals may result in muscle hypoxia, leading to muscle adenylate depletion and generation of hypoxanthine (87). This purine base is then transported to the liver for conversion to uric acid, ultimately contributing more to the ensuing hyperuricemia than the accompanying hyperlacticacidemia and dehydration. In glucose-6-phosphatase deficiency, hypoglycemia or glucagon administration result in reduced hepatic ATP concentrations and increased purine catabolism (91), contributing to the multifactorial hyperuricemia discussed earlier.

Hyperuricemia resulting at least in part from net ATP degradation is encountered quite commonly in two additional situations. First, in acutely ill patients with diseases such as adult respiratory distress syndrome (ARDS), myocardial infarction, or status epilepticus, tissue hypoxia may impair ATP synthesis from ADP in mitochondria, resulting in ADP catabolism and high plasma and urinary concentrations of inosine, hypoxanthine, xanthine, and uric

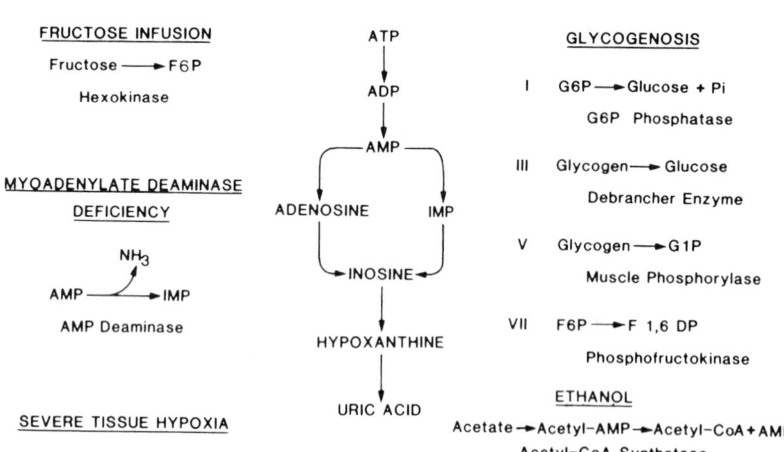

FIGURE 114.8. Conditions resulting in accelerated adenine nucleotide catabolism. *F6P*, Fructose-6-phosphate; *G6P*, glucose-6-phosphate; *G1P*, glucose-1-phosphate; *F 1,6 DP*, fructose-1,6-diphosphate; *ADP*, adenosine diphosphate; *IMP*, inosinic acid; *Pi*, inorganic phosphate.

acid (88,89). The fact that these findings are associated with a poor prognosis in such patients suggests that significant hypoxia is required for activation of the purine catabolic pathway. Second, alcohol consumption results in accelerated conversion of ATP to AMP and enhanced production of uric acid and its immediate precursors when the rate of ATP use in ethanol metabolism through acetate to form acetyl coenzyme A (CoA) exceeds the capacity for ATP regeneration (92,94). This mechanism can play a major role in the hyperuricemia associated with ethanol ingestion, along with renal uric acid retention in the course of dehydration and metabolic acidosis.

EXCRETION OF URIC ACID

In normal persons, approximately two thirds of the uric acid produced daily is excreted by the kidney, one third is eliminated by the gastrointestinal tract, and less than 1% is excreted in sweat (9,98). In gouty patients, decreased renal clearance commonly leads to hyperuricemia despite increased gastrointestinal urate excretion.

Control of Uric Acid Excretion by the Kidney

Renal excretion of uric acid is a complicated physiologic function (Fig. 114.9), the component mechanisms of which have been defined as a result of pharmacologic and physiologic studies in experimental animals and in humans. Despite essentially free filtration of urate at the glomerulus, renal clearance of uric acid in normal adult subjects is only 7% to 12% that of creatinine or inulin clearances (9). [The function ($C_{urate}/C_{creatinine} \times 100$) is referred to as fractional urate excretion or FE_{urate}, expressed as a percentage.] This discrepancy implies that about 90% of filtered urate is subjected to tubular reabsorption (99). Available animal studies indicate that the major site of uric acid reabsorption is in the proximal renal tubule and is facilitated by an active transport process independent of nonionic diffusion or passive forces (100,101).

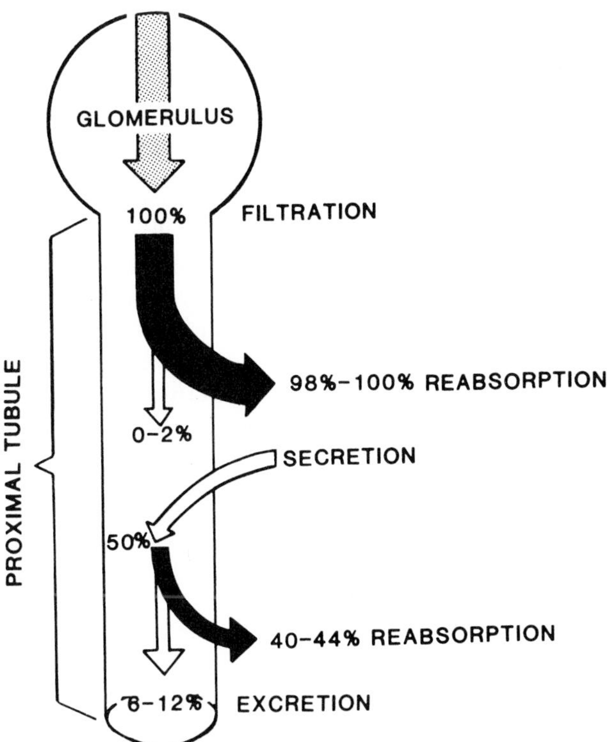

FIGURE 114.9. Four-component model illustrating bidirectional urate transport by the kidney. Tubular reabsorption and secretion are shown as a percentage of filtered urate.

Evidence that a two-component system, involving glomerular filtration and proximal tubular reabsorption, was insufficient to define renal urate handling completely came from two sources. First, an otherwise healthy man was identified in whom marked hypouricemia was accompanied by a urate clearance that was 146% that of inulin clearance (100). In this individual with an apparent selective defect in uric acid reabsorption, tubular urate secretion was postulated. The existence of this mechanism also appeared to explain a second experimental observation: the paradoxic effects of salicylates and probenecid on uric acid excretion (9). In low doses, these drugs decrease uric acid excretion, but high doses result in uricosuria (9,100). These phenomena were best explained by hypothesizing inhibition of tubular secretion at low doses and inhibition of both secretion and reabsorption at higher doses. Subsequently, tubular secretion as a third mechanism of renal uric acid handling was confirmed after urate loading, mannitol diuresis, and large doses of probenecid both in normal subjects and in animal studies using micropuncture techniques (100,102). The latter method has identified the proximal nephron as the major site of tubular secretion, and a study in humans has shown that the proximal but not the distal nephron can transport urate from plasma to tubular fluid (100). Finally, urate secretion in humans appears to be mediated by a transport system shared with other organic acids such as salicylates, acetoacetate, lactate, β-hydroxybutyrate, branched-chain ketoacids, and pyrazinoic acid, the major metabolite of pyrazinamide (100).

Even though tubular urate secretion may be the single most important mechanism determining renal uric acid excretion, there remains uncertainty regarding the relative contributions of reabsorption and secretion to this process in humans (103,104). A variety of paradoxic drug effects on human uric acid excretion and studies in Cebus monkeys and in individuals and families with defects in renal uric acid handling have caused the three-component model of renal urate handling to be reassessed (103,105). A four-component model incorporating extensive postsecretory reabsorption of secreted urate at a site either coextensive with or distal to the secretory site has been proposed (103–105) (Fig. 114.9). Hypouricemic individuals have been studied who have enhanced fractional excretion of urate, a normal response to pyrazinamide, and reduced uricosuric responses to benzbromarone or probenecid, findings most easily interpreted as reflecting an isolated defect in postsecretory reabsorption of uric acid (106–108). Nevertheless, validation of the four-component model of urate handling remains incomplete (99), and quantitation of the flux of uric acid by the individual transport mechanisms will require studies beyond the scope of *in vivo* pharmacologic manipulation. Whether or not postsecretory reabsorption of urate proves to be an operative mechanism in humans (99), the pyrazinamide suppression test, formerly used to distinguish the relative contributions to urinary uric acid excretion of secreted and filtered but nonreabsorbed uric acid appears to be invalid (103,105).

Decreased Uric Acid Excretion in Gout

A reduction of uric acid clearance may contribute to hyperuricemia in as many as 90% of patients with primary gout. Over a wide range of filtered urate loads, most gouty subjects have a lower FE_{urate} than do nongouty subjects (109) (Fig. 114.10). Simkin (109) has shown that gouty individuals excrete on average 41% less uric acid than normal subjects for any given plasma concentration of urate. Patients with primary hyperuricemia also have a greater increment in plasma urate concentrations in response to exogenous purines, a finding attributed to decreased urate clearances (110). Gouty subjects require urate levels 2 to 3 mg/dL higher than nongouty subjects to achieve equivalent uric acid excretion rates (109,111).

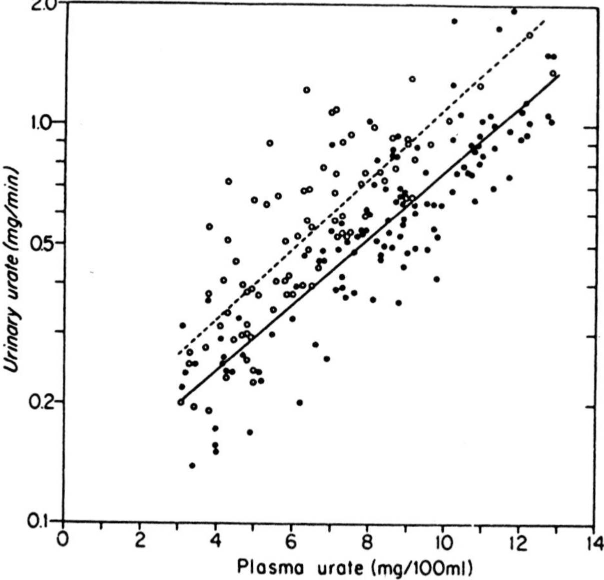

FIGURE 114.10. Urate excretion at various plasma urate concentrations in gouty (*solid symbols*) and nongouty (*open symbols*) subjects. (Reproduced from Simkin PA. Urate excretion in normal and gouty men. *Adv Exp Med Biol* 1977;76B:41–45, with permission.)

Decreased urate clearance in primary gout could be due to reduced urate filtration, enhanced uric acid reabsorption, or decreased urate secretion. The filtered load of urate could be decreased as a result of increased urate binding to plasma proteins. This defect has been proposed in the hyperuricemia of the Maoris of New Zealand (14) and in a few gouty subjects, but this requires confirmation. Both increased reabsorption and decreased secretion of uric acid have been proposed as the basis for the lower urate clearances observed in patients with primary gout. Overall, there is no compelling experimental evidence to affirm enhanced tubular reabsorption of uric acid as one mechanism. In contrast, diminished renal urate secretion per nephron has been implicated in the hyperuricemia of primary gout not associated with overproduction of uric acid (112). Studies using the uricosuric response to benzbromarone, a drug that selectively inhibits reabsorption of secreted urate, to measure minimum tubular secretory rate are reported to show decreased secretion of uric acid in such patients compared with controls or with gouty subjects with overproduction hyperuricemia (103). To date, no alteration in postsecretory reabsorption has been documented in patients with primary gout.

CLINICAL DESCRIPTION OF GOUT

Acute gouty arthritis, intercritical gout, and chronic tophaceous gout represent the three classic stages in the natural history of progressive urate crystal deposition disease. Contemporary management modalities are highly efficient in interrupting the progression of the disorder and in reducing the frequency of acute gouty arthritis, urolithiasis, and tophus formation. Thus gout only infrequently unfolds in the classic manner at present, and this is largely among noncompliant individuals and patients in whom the management scheme has not been appropriately communicated or the diagnosis of gout has not been made. Of special concern with regard to the latter circumstance is the recently noted increasing incidence of gout among elderly women, often with mild renal insufficiency, osteoarthritic nodes, atypical and mild joint inflammation, and tophaceous deposits resembling rheumatoid nodules (113–116).

Acute Gouty Arthritis

> The patient goes to bed and sleeps quietly till about two in the morning when he is awakened by a pain which usually seizes the great toe, but sometimes the heel, ankle, or instep. The pain resembles that of a dislocated bone . . . and is immediately preceded by a chillness and slight fever in proportion to the pain which is mild at first but grows gradually more violent every hour; sometimes resembling a laceration of ligaments, sometimes the gnawing of a dog, and sometimes a weight and constriction of the parts affected, which becomes so exquisitely painful as not to endure the weight of the clothes nor the shaking of the room from a person walking briskly there-in. [From Sydenham, quoted in Copeman (117).]

The acute gouty attack, so vividly described by Sydenham, lasts from a few days to several weeks in untreated patients. With multiple recurrences, shorter intervals, separate attacks, and polyarticular involvement are more frequent. Chronic inflammation with superimposed acute exacerbations may progress to a crippling arthritis. Various studies, heavily weighted to male patients, cite the peak age at onset of gouty arthritis to be between the fourth and sixth decades (9,118), but, in women, initial episodes often arise in the sixth to eighth decades (113,114). Onset before age 30 years or in a premenopausal woman should raise suspicion of an inherited enzyme defect, an inherited or toxic renal disease, or induction by a drug or toxic agent [such as ethanol or lead or even a prolonged ingestion of diuretic (119)].

In older series describing the natural history of gout in men, fully 90% of patients experienced acute attacks at the base of the great toe (podagra) at some time during the course of their disease, and the first metatarsophalangeal joint was involved in about 50% of first attacks (9,118). Reductions in these figures are the case now, given the truncated history of the joint disease under appropriate therapy and the recognition of atypical joint involvement in women (113–116). Although it is generally accepted that about 80% of initial attacks are monoarticular, polyarticular first attacks are more common in elderly women and in patients with gout accompanying myeloproliferative disorders or the use of cyclosporine (120–124). In a recent series of 92 women with gout, 70% had had polyarticular attacks, and 35% gave no history of preceding monoarthritis (114). Other common initial sites of involvement include the instep, ankle, heel, knee, wrist, fingers, and elbows (olecranon bursa). Rarely involved sites include the shoulders, sternoclavicular joints, hips, spine, and sacroiliac joints. Conceptually, acute gout remains predominantly a disease of the lower extremity, and the more distal the site of involvement, the more typical the attack. Although urate-induced inflammation in unusual joints and soft tissue sites is often preceded by typical attacks in the usual distal joints, initial appearance in the former locations can cause diagnostic confusion (125). The occurrence of gouty inflammation (and even tophus formation) in prior sites of osteoarthritic node involvement of distal and proximal interphalangeal finger joints warrants particular mention, both for its frequency and for the potential difficulty in recognizing the coexistence of these arthritic processes (126,127).

Trivial episodes of pain ("petite attacks") lasting only hours and sometimes recurrent over several years may precede the first dramatic gouty attack. The initial attack of gout often occurs with explosive suddenness, typically awakening the patient or becoming apparent as a foot is placed on the floor on arising. The skin over the affected joint soon becomes reddened and warm; extreme tenderness of the affected joint and periarticular tissues is noted (Fig. 114.11). The slightest pressure produces exquisite pain. Fever, leukocytosis, and elevation of the erythrocyte sedimentation rate often occur. The skin over the joint may desquamate as the episode subsides.

The course of untreated acute gout is variable. Mild attacks may subside in several hours or may persist for only a few days and not reach the intensity described by Sydenham. Severe attacks may last many days to several weeks. A

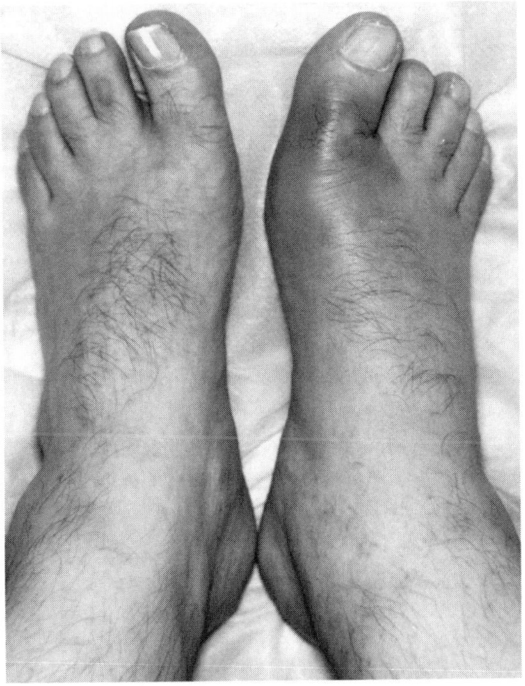

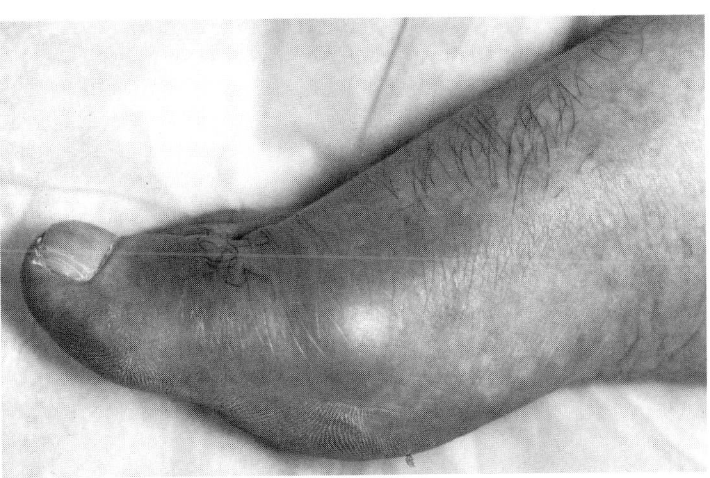

FIGURE 114.11. Acute gouty arthritis of the right first metatarsophalangeal joint. Note the swelling and hyperemia about the affected joint.

number of physiologic responses that contribute to the spontaneous and complete resolution of gouty arthritis have recently been reviewed (128,129) (see Chapter 116).

On recovery, the patient reenters an asymptomatic phase termed *the intercritical period.* Even though the attack may have been incapacitating, with excruciating pain and swelling, resolution is usually complete, and the patient is once again well. This freedom from symptoms during the intercritical period is an important feature in the diagnosis of acute arthritis as gout.

Provocative or Possible Etiologic Factors

Factors capable of provoking episodes of acute gouty arthritis include trauma, surgery, alcohol ingestion, starvation, overindulgence in foods with high purine content, and ingestion of drugs that cause changes in urate concentrations. The precise relation of these factors to the attacks remains speculative. For example, the first metatarsophalangeal joint as a primary weight-bearing area is subject to considerable microtrauma. It is tenable that degenerative changes of the bunion joint, perhaps in conjunction with locally elevated urate concentrations as proposed by Simkin, render this site unusually susceptible to urate crystal deposition (130). In a report of a patient with tophaceous gout and persistent normouricemia, McCarty (131) emphasized an additional local factor, reduced temperature in poorly perfused acral tissues, as a candidate to reduce regional urate solubility and promote crystal formation and deposition. Each of the other factors is capable of provoking more generalized disturbances in extracellular urate concentrations. Alcohol binges, acute overeating, or starvation can induce marked increases in serum urate and acute attacks. The administration of drugs—such as thiazide diuretics for the treatment of hypertension (120), cyclosporine for immunosuppression (121–124), or uricosuric agents or allopurinol for treatment of hyperuricemia (120)—can result in gout with either elevated or lowered urate concentrations. Intravenous hyperalimentation is capable of provoking attacks of gout in predisposed individuals despite the associated hypouricemia (132). Finally, surgery and acute trauma may predispose to gout as a consequence of the stress response and the attendant hyperuricosuria and hypouricemia (131).

Intercritical Gout and Recurrent Episodes

A clear and detailed history of an acute arthritic attack followed by a completely asymptomatic intercritical period before a recurrence is valuable in pointing toward the diagnosis of gout. During this period, aspiration of a previously inflamed joint can frequently corroborate the diagnosis of gout. For example, in an untreated gouty population, 36 of 37 synovial fluid aspirates obtained during intercritical periods yielded urate crystals if the knee aspirated had been subject to past gouty attacks (133). By comparison, the yield was only 22% if there was no history of prior acute involvement in the aspirated knee and was 50% in previously inflamed knees in patients taking urate-lowering medication. The presence of crystals deposited in joints during the intercritical period supports the view that the stages of clinical gout represent arbitrary designations reflecting only the state of inflammation and the size of urate accumulations at a specific time. That is, by the time of the first attack of gouty arthritis, clinically inapparent crystal aggregates are likely to be present in the great majority of gout patients. Nevertheless, the duration of the intercritical period is variable. Without therapy, most gouty patients will experience a second episode within 2 years. In one large series (9), 62% of patients had recurrences within the first year, and 78% within 2 years, with only 7% free of recurrences for 10 years or more (7).

As the disease progresses in the untreated patient, acute attacks occur with increasing frequency and are often polyarticular, more severe, longer lasting, and occasionally associated with a febrile course. Although affected joints may continue to recover completely, bony erosions may develop. As many as one third of patients with late polyarticular attacks reported that their initial attack was also polyarticular (134). Joints may flare in sequence, in a migratory pattern, or, as in pseudogout, several neighboring joints may be involved simultaneously in a cluster attack. Frequently periarticular sites such as bursae and tendons also are involved.

Eventually the patient may have chronic polyarticular gout without pain-free intercritical periods. Gout at this stage may be confused with rheumatoid arthritis (RA), especially if tophi are mistaken for rheumatoid nodules. On occasion, the disease may progress from initial podagra to an RA-like chronic deforming arthritis without remissions but with synovial thickening and the early development of nodules (tophi). Unlike RA, in which polyarticular inflammation is most often synchronous, inflamed gouty joints are frequently out of phase—a flare in one joint may coincide with subsidence of inflammation in another joint. Conversely, subcutaneous nodules in patients with "rheumatoid nodulosis" are easily confused with tophi (135). Up to 30% of patients with tophaceous gout have low serum titers of rheumatoid factor (136). In a study of 160 patients with RA, hyperuricemia was found in 7.5%, a finding that was correlated inversely with disease activity (137). Coexistence of gout and RA is rare, however, and the appropriate diagnosis is best established by demonstrating the presence or absence of urate crystals by aspiration of affected joints or tophaceous deposits.

Chronic Tophaceous Gout

Chronic tophaceous gout (Fig. 114.12) is characterized by the identifiable deposition of solid urate (tophi) in connec-

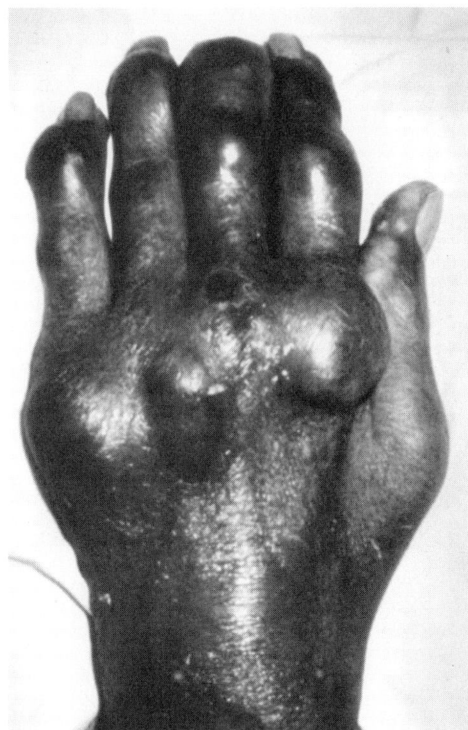

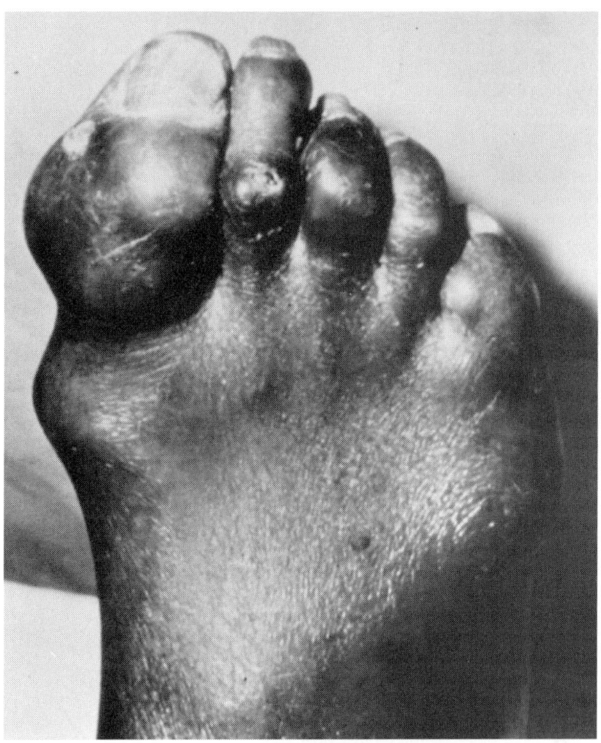

FIGURE 114.12. Chronic tophaceous gout manifested as multiple skin and joint deformities in a hand and foot.

tive tissues, including articular structures, with ultimate development of a destructive arthropathy, often with secondary degenerative changes. The identification of tophi with or before the initial gouty attack, once considered rare in primary gout (125), has been documented more frequently in recent years (138,139). This occurrence has also been observed in 0.5% of subjects with gout secondary to myeloproliferative disease (9), and in patients with type 1 glycogen storage disease (82) and the Lesch–Nyhan syndrome (9). In Gutman's series (140), the rate of urate deposition in joint tissue correlated with both the duration and degree of hyperuricemia. In patients without tophi, the mean serum urate concentration was 9.2 mg/dL. Values of 10 to 11 mg/dL were found in subjects with minimal-to-moderate deposits, and patients with extensive tophaceous deposits had urate concentrations in excess of 11 mg/dL. In untreated patients, the interval from the first gouty attack to the beginning of chronic arthritis or visible tophi is highly variable, ranging from 3 to 42 years with an average of 11.6 years (9). A retrospective analysis of 1,165 patients in the pretreatment era found that 70% were free of demonstrable tophi 5 years after the first gouty attack; at 10 years, only 50% remained without tophi; and by 20 years, this proportion had declined to 28% (140). The percentage of patients with severe tophaceous gout reached appreciable proportions (24%) 20 years after the first attack. In a population of 4,110 gouty Japanese subjects followed up for 19 years, only 9.2% had tophaceous deposits (141).

Tophaceous gout is often associated with an early age at onset, a long duration of active but untreated disease, frequent attacks, high serum urate values, and a predilection for upper extremity and polyarticular episodes (142). A prospective study of 106 consecutive gouty men in a Veterans Administration (VA) hospital substantiated these observations, including episodes of polyarticular gout in 40% of patients (143). Characteristics of the arthritis included asymmetric, ascending joint involvement in which chronic inflammation was typical. Although ethanol consumption and diuretic use were frequently associated with gout in this population, suboptimal management and patient compliance were considered to be major factors in the progression from monoarticular gout to polyarticular status.

A second group of more compliant elderly patients is also prone to develop polyarticular and tophaceous gout (113–116). Of 60 consecutive gouty patients seen in a rheumatology unit, 15% were elderly women (mean age, 82 years), all of whom were taking diuretic therapy, and most of whom had tophi in osteoarthritic interphalangeal joints (113) (Fig. 114.13). In another series of 149 gout patients, 17% were found to have gout in joints affected with nodal osteoarthritis (OA) (126). Mean age was 71 years, gender was evenly distributed, and the mean urate

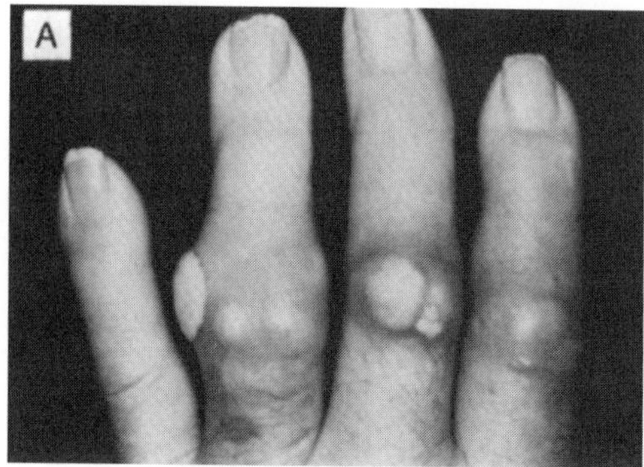

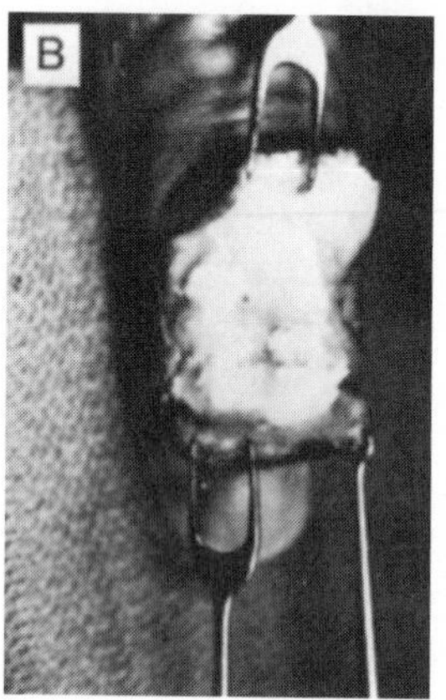

FIGURE 114.13. A: Impostumous gout involving osteoarthritic joints of an elderly woman receiving diuretic therapy for hypertension. **B:** Extensive urate deposits in periarticular tissue from a similar patient. (Courtesy of Dr. Michael Jablon.)

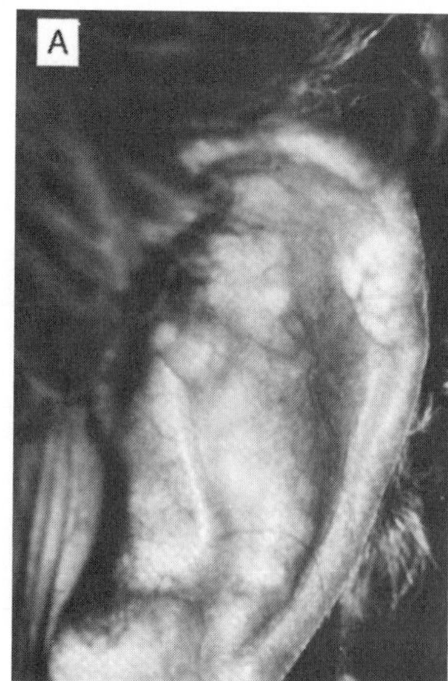

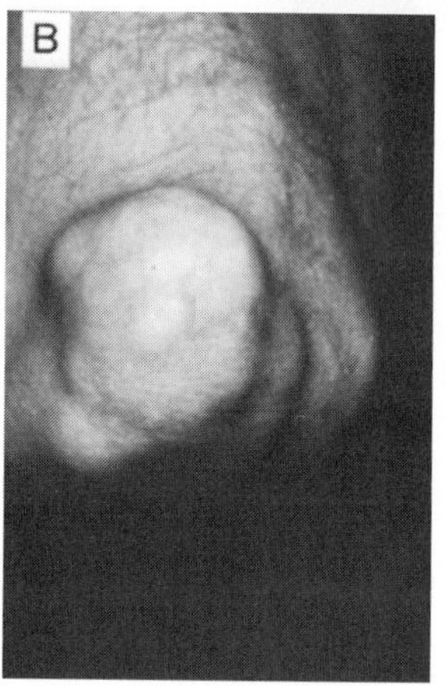

FIGURE 114.14. Tophi in **(A)** helix of ear and **(B)** olecranon bursa.

concentration was 11 mg/dL. Diuretics were being used by 72% of these patients, and impaired renal function was present in 60%. The combination of diuretic-induced hyperuricemia, renal insufficiency, and nodal OA appears to predispose the elderly to tophaceous gout arising in nodal tissue (127,144,145). The clinical features of this group of patients, in which women are clearly overrepresented (impostumous gout) (146), set it apart from the classically described group of middle-aged male patients with tophaceous gout who have a higher incidence of hypertension, obesity, and ethanol abuse.

Organ transplant recipients treated with cyclosporine (and often diuretics as well) compose another group at increased risk for the accelerated development of chronic tophaceous gout (120–124). Both renal and cardiac transplant patients, particularly those with compromised renal function, have developed severe and often difficult-to-manage complications of the effects of cyclosporine on renal urate clearance.

The helix of ear is a classic extraarticular location for tophaceous deposits, which take the form of small white excrescences (Fig. 114.14A). Other sites of predilection include the olecranon (Fig. 114.14B) and prepatellar bursae, ulnar surfaces of the forearm, Achilles tendons, and finger pads, where urate crystal deposits may be intradermal as well as subcutaneous (147,148). Deposits may produce irregular and often grotesque tumescences on the hands or feet with accompanying joint destruction and crippling (Figs. 114.12 and 114.13). The tense, shiny skin overlying the tophus may ulcerate and extrude white, chalky material composed of needle-shaped (acicular) urate crystals (Fig. 114.15). Ulcerated tophi rarely become secondarily infected. Bony ankylosis also is unusual (149).

The process of tophus formation advances insidiously, the patient often noting progressive stiffness and aching of affected joints. Tophi or a secondary degenerative process may limit joint mobility by mechanical destruction of the joints and adjacent structures. Likewise, the axial skeleton does not escape urate crystal deposition, which may mimic a tumor or protruded disc (150). Tophaceous involvement of the sacroiliac joint and aseptic necrosis of the hip have been reported as manifestations of gout. Monosodium urate crystals have been identified in avascular bone,

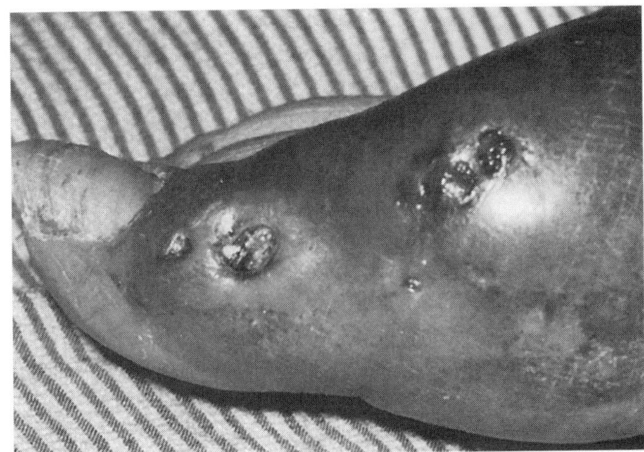

FIGURE 114.15. Ulcerated tophi. (Courtesy of Dr. Ira Melnicoff.)

although no cases of avascular necrosis of the femoral head were found in a systematic study of 138 gouty patients (151).

As tophi and often associated renal disease advance, acute attacks may recur less frequently and may be milder; late in the illness, they may disappear entirely or may be superimposed on indolently inflamed joints. Virtually all parenchymal organs except the brain have been sites of tophus formation in one or another report (152,153).

The availability of uricosuric agents and allopurinol has resulted in a significant decline in visible tophi and chronic gouty arthritis. Before the introduction of these drugs, tophaceous deposits were found in as many as 70% of gouty patients (9); more recent surveys report frequencies of less than 5% (154). In some population groups, however, residual frequencies of tophaceous gout approaching 50% have been reported (142,143). Factors such as noncompliance, poor physician–patient communication, misdiagnosis, aggressive management of hypertension with diuretics, especially in the elderly, and use of cyclosporine in transplant recipients make further reduction in the current low frequency of tophaceous gout unlikely in the future.

Urolithiasis and Gout

Uric acid stones account for 5% to 10% of all renal stones in the United States and Europe and 40% of renal stones in Israel (155). The overall prevalence of uric acid stones in the adult U.S. population is estimated to be 0.01%, but in a series of 1,258 patients with primary gout and 59 patients with secondary gout, the prevalence of renal lithiasis was 22% and 42%, respectively (156). Fourteen years later, when the primary gout population had increased to 2,038, the prevalence of uric acid stone disease was 23% (157). More than 80% of calculi in these gouty patients consisted entirely of uric acid, with the remainder containing calcium oxalate or calcium phosphate, often with a central nidus of uric acid. The several hundred–fold higher incidence of uric acid stones in gout patients is accompanied by a 10- to 30-fold increased incidence of calcium oxalate stones (158). Renal stones antedated arthritis in 40% of subjects with primary gout and occurred more frequently than arthritis as a first manifestation before the fourth decade (157). When the prevalence of urolithiasis was related to serum urate values in the Framingham study, 12.7% of male subjects with urate values between 7 and 7.9 mg/dL and 40% of subjects with urate values greater than 9 mg/dL gave a history of renal stones (8). The annual incidence of urolithiasis increased from 0.2% in normouricemic controls and 0.3% in asymptomatic hyperuricemic subjects to 0.9% in patients with gout (17). About one third of nongouty hyperuricemic patients in whom uric acid stones developed gave a family history of gout (156). In studies of gouty individuals, higher prevalence rates of uric acid urolithiasis are associated with increased uric acid excretion. In gouty patients with daily excretion of more than 1,100 mg of uric acid, the prevalence of stones was 50%, or 4.5-fold greater than in patients excreting less than 300 mg/day (156). Many clinical circumstances result in hyperuricosuria, including inherited enzymatic defects and hematologic disorders that lead to accelerated purine biosynthesis, diets high in purine content (110), and the administration of uricosuric drugs (which cause only a transient increase in uric acid excretion). The increase in uric acid excretion seen in patients ingesting large amounts of dietary purines may contribute to the development of calcium oxalate stones (158). Low urine volume as well as chronic excessive bicarbonate loss may be predisposing factors for the development of uric acid calculi in patients with ileostomies or colostomies (159), and reduced urine volumes contribute heavily to uric acid stone formation among people living in hot, arid climates (155).

Because the hydrogen ion concentration in urine is a critical determinant of uric acid solubility, the excretion of a persistently acid urine is another predisposing factor to the development of uric acid stones. For example, at pH 5.0, the limit of solubility of uric acid in urine is 15 mg/dL, but if the pH is increased to 7.0, solubility is increased to 200 mg/dL because 95% of uric acid is present as the more soluble urate ion (155). Low urinary pH is a well-documented characteristic of patients with primary gout, in general, and in gout patients with uric acid stones, in particular (155–157).

The low urinary pH of patients with uric acid calculi has been ascribed by some investigators to a defect in ammonium excretion (160) and by others to an increase in titratable acidity. These conflicting suggestions, reviewed by Yü (155), have not been thoroughly evaluated because other variables have not been adequately controlled. These include age, reduced nephron mass, and diets high in protein and purines. One hypothesis offered to explain the defect in ammonium excretion observed in gouty patients suggests that a deficiency of renal glutaminase activity results in reduced glutamine use for ammonium production by the kidney (160). In direct assays, however, renal glutaminase activity is normal in gouty subjects (161).

Substances that may affect both uric acid solubility and crystal growth are important additional factors to consider in the pathogenesis of uric acid and calcium oxalate stones in patients with idiopathic hyperuricosuria. Regarding uric acid solubility, the presence of a nondialyzable mucoprotein in urine, which retards uric acid precipitation, has been suggested (162). No difference was found, however, in the amount of this substance in urine from patients with urolithiasis and healthy controls. Heterogeneous nucleation of calcium oxalate crystals can occur either on monosodium urate or uric acid seed crystals in patients with hyperuricosuria (163,164). Additionally, a glycoprotein containing carboxyglutamic acid (nephrocalcin) has been isolated from kidney and urine (165). This protein and Tamm–Horsfall protein appear to inhibit calcium oxalate crystal growth and clearly warrant further study.

Kidney Disease in Gout

Apart from arthritis and tophus formation, renal disease is the most frequently reported clinical association of hyperuricemia (9). Hyperuricemia may affect the kidney through (a) deposition of urate crystals in the renal interstitium, referred to as *urate nephropathy,* (b) deposition of uric acid crystals in the collecting tubules, an entity referred to as *uric acid nephropathy,* and (c) *uric acid urolithiasis.* The distinction between the first two entities is often unclear, and the term gouty kidney has been used for both. Urate nephropathy is not uncommon, by pathologic criteria at least, in patients with gout, regardless of the accompanying excretion of uric acid. In contrast, both uric acid nephropathy and urolithiasis are more common in patients with excessive uric acid production and excretion. Acute uric acid nephropathy with accompanying acute renal tubular damage and an obstructive uropathic clinical picture is very uncommon except in patients with malignancy and hyperuricemia treated with radiation or chemotherapy, or with inherited enzyme defects resulting in markedly increased uric acid excretion. In addition to these direct effects of hyperuricemia, other causes of renal dysfunction such as hypertension, diabetes mellitus, alcohol abuse, nephrotoxic drug therapy, and lead nephropathy also are prevalent in the gouty population. The isolation of hyperuricemia or gout as primary risk factors for progressive renal disease is thus exceedingly difficult (7,17,166–168).

Urate nephropathy, if progressive at all, is only slowly progressive and does not materially reduce life expectancy (17,167). The incidence of proteinuria in gout patients varies from 15% to 20% (169). Hypertension is at least as common as proteinuria. It is not entirely clear whether hypertension is the result of hyperuricemia and urate nephropathy or whether it is a cause of renal dysfunction observed in gouty patients (170). Study of 273 gout patients provided evidence that uncontrolled hypertension was responsible for a significant amount of the observed renal dysfunction (169), and other studies support this view (17,166).

Significant impairment of renal function in up to 40% of patients with gout was reported in older series of patients (9,171), and renal failure was the eventual cause of death in 18% to 25% of patients in one of these series (171). Recent evaluations, however, have deemphasized a primary causal relation between hyperuricemia/gout and renal disease (17,166). The incidence of renal disease among gouty individuals is probably no greater than that in subjects of comparable age with similar degrees of hypertension, obesity, and primary renal disease.

Considerable interest has focused on an inherited disorder, transmitted in an autosomal dominant fashion, in which hyperuricemia (and frequently gout) is associated with early and progressive renal impairment and hypertension (172–174). The term familial juvenile hyperuricemic (or gouty) nephropathy has been used to describe this syndrome (172,173), the molecular basis for which is unclear (173). Although hyperuricemia clearly precedes renal insufficiency in most instances, there is no substantial evidence that renal deposition of urate is responsible for the observed interstitial and tubular nephropathy (173,174). The most characteristic features of the disorder in affected individuals include hyperuricemia disproportionate to the degree of renal dysfunction and severe uric acid hypoexcretion reflecting marked reduction of FE_{urate} at the earliest points studied (172–174). Reduced excretion of hypoxanthine and xanthine as well as uric acid, marked elevation of renal vascular resistance (174), and a similar clinical course in a family with identical renal histopathologic changes in the absence of hyperuricemia (175) support the view that hyperuricemia is not of pathogenetic relevance but may be a consequence of a primary disorder of renal hemodynamics (174). In this regard, a more descriptive term for this disorder may be hereditary nephropathy associated with hyperuricemia and gout (174). Long-term results of allopurinol in forestalling progression of the disorder are controversial (172–174).

PREVALENCE AND INCIDENCE OF PRIMARY GOUT

Although the prevalence of gout varies worldwide, it appears to be similar in Europe (0.3%) and North America (0.27%) (9), although a recent self-reported incidence estimate of 0.8% was obtained in the U.S. (176). A prevalence of 0.2% was found in Framingham, among 5,127 subjects (2,283 men and 2,844 women) with a mean age of 44 years (8). Fourteen years later, the prevalence had increased to 1.5% (mean age, 58 years): 2.8% in men and 0.4% in women. Among 4,663 Parisian men aged 35 to 44 years, the prevalence was 1.1% in the age group 35 to 39 and 2% in men aged 40 to 44 years (177). The prevalence of hyperuricemia and gout is much higher among Pacific Islanders and the Maori of New Zealand (14,15,178–180). In the latter group, the prevalence of gout is 10.3% in men and 4.3% in women (14,180).

More than 90% of patients with primary gout are men, and the age of peak incidence in men (118) is earlier than that of affected women, who rarely develop the disorder before menopause (113–116,181). In a prospectively studied cohort of 1,338 physicians (91% men), the cumulative incidence of gout was 8.6% over a period of 20 years (182). No gouty women were identified. Higher percentages of women have been reported in series that included patients with secondary gout complicated by renal disease or diuretic therapy (113–116). Gout is uncommon before the third decade. In the Framingham study, the cumulative incidence rate in men appeared to be approaching a plateau at about age 58 years, although only one third of patients with urate levels 8 mg/dL or more had developed gout (8). The proposed relation between the incidence of gout and the magnitude of hyperuricemia (8) has been confirmed in recent studies (7). Moreover, the fact that distinctive peak age incidences of gout in men and women occur about two to three decades after the respective sex-specific physiologic increments in serum urate suggests that on average hyperuricemia of many years' duration precedes the occurrence of symptomatic events.

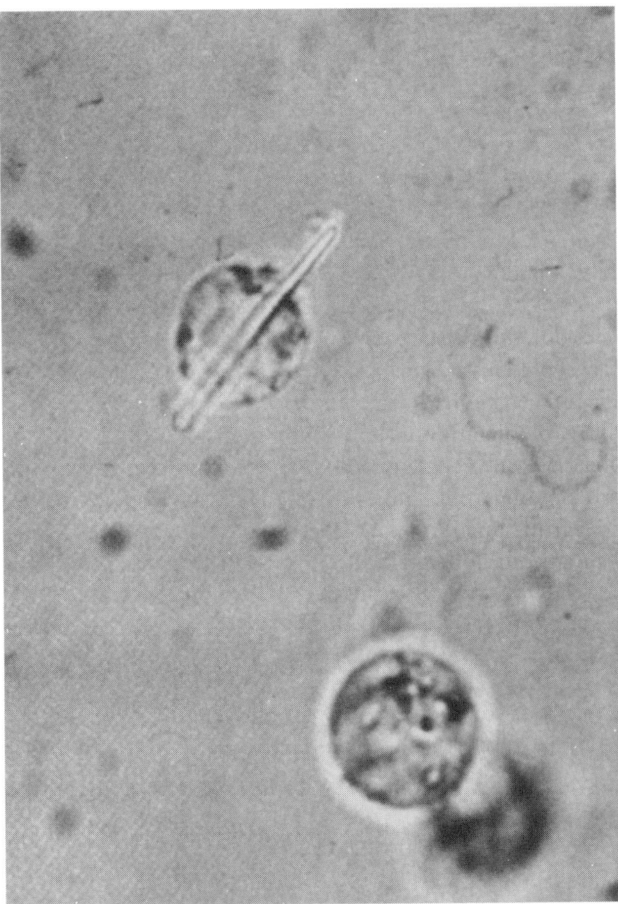

FIGURE 114.16. Polymorphonuclear leukocyte containing a phagocytized monosodium urate crystal.

DIAGNOSIS OF GOUTY ARTHRITIS

The diagnosis of gout should be established on firm criteria to ensure that expensive and toxic medications are not prescribed unnecessarily. Available data do not support therapeutic intervention for the great majority of patients with asymptomatic hyperuricemia (see Chapter 115). A definitive diagnosis of gout is established by demonstration of intracellular monosodium urate crystals in synovial fluid neutrophils by polarized compensated light microscopy (Fig. 114.16) (see Chapter 4). In a study conducted by the American College of Rheumatology Subcommittee on Diagnostic and Therapeutic Criteria, the sensitivity of this technique in patients with gouty arthritis and an acutely inflamed joint was 84.4%; the specificity for gout was absolute (100%) (183). It is, however, important to recall the occasional patient in whom acute gouty arthritis coexists with another type of joint disease such as septic arthritis, calcium pyrophosphate dihydrate (CPPD) crystal deposition disease (pseudogout), or even basic calcium phosphate crystal deposition disease (184,185).

Extracellular urate crystals also are identifiable in synovial fluid from previously affected joints in 70% to 97% of gouty patients during asymptomatic intervals (133,186). In one study documenting this point, only one of 19 asymptomatic hyperuricemic controls and two of nine patients with renal failure but no history of acute arthritis had demonstrable extracellular urate crystals (186). In another study, crystals were identified in only one of 31 subjects with asymptomatic hyperuricemia, and in none of six patients with renal failure (187). Thus extracellular urate crystals in synovial fluid are common during intercritical gout, but this finding is of lesser sensitivity and specificity for gout than is the case for intracellular urate crystal identification during episodes of acute arthritis.

Demonstration of urate crystals in tophi is nearly as specific for gout as is synovial fluid crystal identification. Because, however, tophi are found in only a minority of patients with gout, this diagnostic test is of limited sensitivity. In the absence of the means to identify urate crystals or a negative polarized light microscopic study, the following combination of findings may be useful in suggesting a diagnosis of gout: (a) a classic history of monoarticular arthritis followed by an intercritical period completely free of symptoms, (b) rapid resolution of synovitis after colchicine therapy, and (c) hyperuricemia (183).

Normouricemia does not preclude the diagnosis of gout, given that up to 40% of patients have normal serum urate levels at the time of acute attacks (188). Urate diuresis due to stress-related cortisol release; correction of risk factors such as alcoholism, obesity, or diuretic therapy; and management of hyperuricemia may result in normal serum urate values at the time of an acute gouty attack. Although hyperuricemia and gout are causally related, they should be regarded as separate phenomena. Criteria for improvement resulting from colchicine therapy include major subsidence of objective joint inflammation within 48 hours and no recurrence of inflammation in any joint for at least 7 days (189). Arthritis alone in a hyperuricemic patient is insufficient to establish a diagnosis of gout. Pseudogout (CPPD) and basic calcium phosphate crystal-induced inflammation are diseases difficult to differentiate clinically from acute gout. Self-limited attacks of acute inflammation in the first metatarsophalangeal joint (pseudopodagra), resulting from transient amorphous calcific deposits, have been described in premenopausal women (184). Septic arthritis, cellulitis, and fractures are additional processes that often need careful exclusion in the clinical setting, suggesting acute gouty arthritis. The resemblance of gouty inflammation to cellulitis points up the diffuse, periarticular nature of gouty arthritis, which differentiates this process from primary synovitic disorders such as RA.

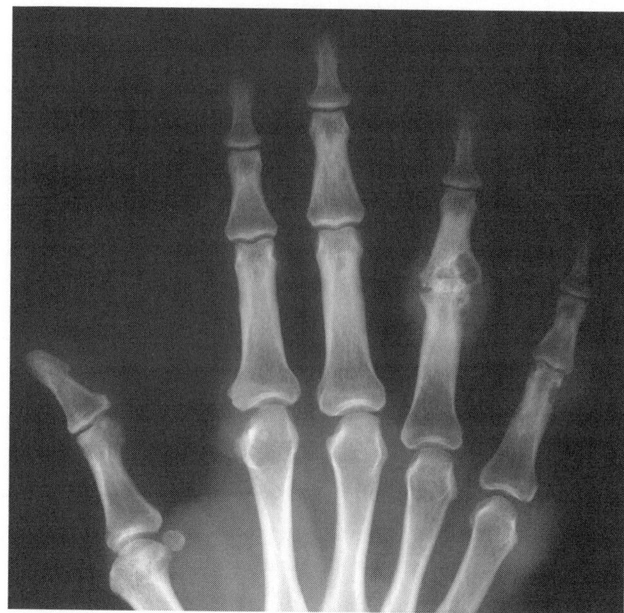

FIGURE 114.17. Radiographic features of gout are prominently displayed in the fourth and fifth proximal interphalangeal joints of the right hand of this individual. Soft tissue swellings (tophi) surround both joints, and there are marginal erosions with sclerotic borders and overhanging edges as well as osseous cysts. Bony mineralization is generally well maintained, and the joint space of the fifth proximal interphalangeal joint remains intact. (Courtesy of Dr. Larry B. Dixon.)

RADIOGRAPHIC FINDINGS IN GOUT

The major value of radiographic examination during the initial attack of gout is to exclude other types of arthritis. At this stage, the findings related to gout are nonspecific, usually in the form of soft tissue swelling. The radiographic hallmarks of long-standing gout are those of an asymmetric, inflammatory, erosive arthritis often accompanied by soft tissue nodules, but generally with retention of normal bone and periarticular density and joint spaces.

Sharply "punched-out," round, or oval defects situated in the marginal areas of the joint and surrounded by a sclerotic border suggest gout (Fig. 114.17). Bony (intraosseous) tophaceous lesions almost always antedate subcutaneous tophi and may be seen in joints that have never been clinically inflamed (142). In about 40% of patients with gouty erosions in bone, an elevated margin extends outward into the soft tissue covering the tophaceous nodule (190). This "overhanging margin" of bone, which may result from bony resorption beneath the enlarging tophus and periosteal apposition of the involved cortex, helps to distinguish gouty erosions from the "pocketed" erosions seen in RA. Bony erosions occur relatively late in gout, and many patients with repeated acute attacks show neither bone nor soft tissue lesions. Another feature useful in distinguishing gout from RA is the infrequency of periarticular osteopenia in the former.

Bony erosions caused by deposits of urate crystals are related to both the duration and severity of gout. In patients with advanced chronic tophaceous gout, joint destruction may be extensive. Bony ankylosis with obliteration of the joint space is rare except in the interphalangeal joints of the hands and feet and in the intercarpal region (149). The presence of a relatively normal joint space in a joint with extensive erosions is an important radiologic characteristic of gout.

Tophi in soft tissues are typically deposited in an asymmetric distribution, reflected radiographically as nodular swellings particularly frequent in the feet, hands, ankles, elbows, and knees. Soft tissue prominences about the dorsum of the foot and calcaneus are also characteristic. Calcification of tophi is unusual in the absence of renal impairment (Fig. 114.18). Soft tissue tophi are often accompanied by erosions in adjacent bone with typical overhanging margins, helping to distinguish urate crystal aggregates from nodular lesions associated with other types of arthritic and metabolic disorders. Osteolytic lesions (tophaceous pseudotumors) in the superolateral portion of the patella, often associated with peripatellar calcified soft tissue masses, have been described (191). Identification of such lesions as tophi may obviate invasive diagnostic procedures.

The identification of urate tophi in articular and organ structures has been attempted by means of magnetic resonance or computed tomographic imaging. The features of tophi revealed by these techniques do not provide the speci-

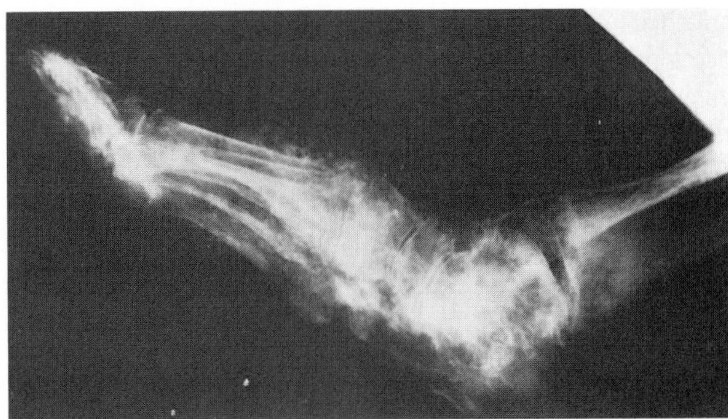

FIGURE 114.18. Calcified soft tissue prominence over the dorsum of the foot, and destruction of the talocalcaneus joint in a 63-year-old man with polyarticular tophaceous gout. (Courtesy of Dr. David Tartof.)

ficity needed for definitive diagnosis (192–194). Dodds and Steinbach (195) found that 10 of 31 patients with gout had meniscal calcification of the type usually associated with CPPD crystal deposits. In another study, calcification of one or more menisci was found in only two (5%) of 43 patients with gout, roughly the incidence of chondrocalcinosis observed in elderly populations (196). Because of the high incidence of gout in patients with pseudogout (5%) and vice versa, the presence of cartilage calcification in a patient with gout should suggest that pseudogout also may be present.

Subchondral lesions are occasionally observed near the sacroiliac joints in patients with chronic tophaceous gout (Fig. 114.19). Sclerotic punched-out lesions in the sacroiliac joints are usually found in advanced disease, associated with tophaceous deposits in the extremities (9). In a prospective radiologic survey of 143 gout patients, 24 individuals with tophi developed sacroiliac changes, which included sclerosis and irregularity of joint margins, focal osteoporosis, and cysts with sclerotic rims (197).

Uric acid stones are radiolucent and appear radiologically as "filling defects." Cysteine, xanthine, and 2,8-dihydroxyadenine stones also are radiolucent, but most radiolucent stones are composed of uric acid. Uric acid stones or gravel may be white or pink ("brick dust") as a result of absorption of a pigment that has not been identified. Patients with brick dust urine may present with what they believe to be hematuria. Radiopaque stones also occur with greatly increased frequency in gouty subjects and are composed largely of calcium oxalate. These stones often contain a small amount of uric acid, which probably serves as a nidus for the deposition of calcium oxalate by epitaxial overgrowth.

HEREDITY IN GOUT

Inherited influences have long been suspected in primary gout (1,2). English observers reported gout in family members of 38% to 81% of patients, and in series reported from the U.S., familial incidence figures have ranged from 6% to 18% (1,9). Among hyperuricemic relatives of gout patients, the incidence of gout averaged 20% in five series reviewed by Smyth (198). In family members of gouty probands, the incidence of asymptomatic hyperuricemia ranged from

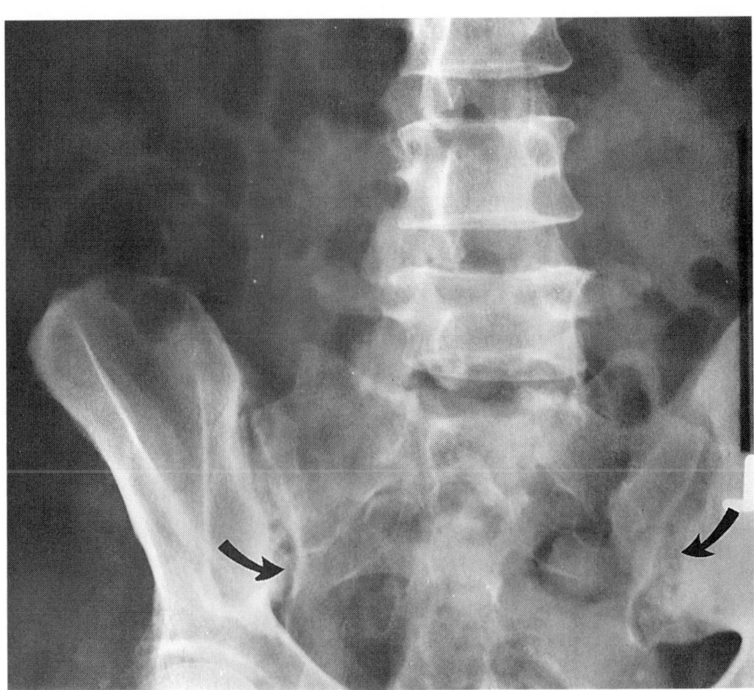

FIGURE 114.19. Sacroiliac joints showing scalloped erosions (*arrows*) and adjacent bony sclerosis. (Courtesy of Dr. Nancy Brown.)

25% to 27% (199). A convincing example of hereditary influence in the absence of a defined enzymatic defect is provided by consideration of patients with early-onset gout or hyperuricemia, often associated with nephropathy (172–174). In one study of 21 subjects of mean age 28 years, a family history of gout was noted in 71% (200).

Although some studies of restricted populations (i.e., racially selected, geographically isolated, or families of gouty probands) showed a bimodal distribution of serum urate values, supporting a single dominant gene hypothesis (201), abundant data indicate that serum urate concentration is continuously distributed in both male and female populations (10), although skewed toward higher values. Whether this finding is definitive evidence that multiple genes determine hyperuricemia in primary gout patients (9) remains controversial, as does the proposal of a major dominant gene hypothesis in primary gout (202). A study of Blackfeet and Pima Indians showed strong polygenic hereditary influences on serum urate and suggested both autosomal dominant and X-linked transmission patterns (203). Additional studies also have favored multifactorial inheritance, demonstrating a prevalence of high urate values without evidence of bimodality (8,199). In general, polygenic control is more prominent the greater the population heterogeneity (199). Thus within limited groups of individuals, a single gene may influence urate values to the relative exclusion of other influences that may reveal themselves in broader populations in the form of apparent multigenic expression.

PATHOLOGIC FEATURES OF GOUT

The most frequent sites of monosodium urate crystal deposition are cartilage, epiphyseal bone, periarticular structures, and the kidney. Although organs such as the liver, spleen, voluntary muscle, and nerve tissue are characteristically spared, crystal deposits have been described at one time or another in most organs other than the brain. Crystal aggregates produce local necrosis, and, unless the tissue is avascular, a foreign-body reaction ensues with proliferation of fibrous tissues. Tophi thus consist of a multicentric deposit of urate crystals and intercrystalline matrix, together with a foreign-body reaction. In the early stage of crystallization, needle-shaped urate crystals may be clustered radially in a sporulated form (resembling beach balls) embedded beneath the synovial lining cells (204,205). Affected joints may develop cartilaginous degeneration, synovial proliferation, erosion of marginal bone, or, rarely, ankylosis (Fig. 114.20). No joint is exempt, although those of the lower extremities are more commonly involved. The significance of the rich proteoglycan matrix of tophi is uncertain (206). It is important to recall that urate crystals are water soluble, and nonaqueous fixation (such as in absolute alcohol) is necessary to preserve urate deposits in histologic sections.

The only distinctive histologic feature of urate nephropathy is the presence of urate crystals and a surrounding giant cell reaction (Fig. 114.21). Crystal deposition in the kidney may be associated with interstitial or vascular changes or both. That some of the vascular changes may be related to concomitant hypertension emphasizes the difficulty of attributing pathologic changes to a single factor. In a review of 191 gout patients in whom clinical information and postmortem renal tissue permitted adequate evaluation, all but three showed either urate crystals or pyelonephritic or vascular changes (171). These features were present in variable proportion and severity. Vascular lesions included arterial and arteriolar sclerosis and, in 11 instances, findings of malignant hypertension. Kidneys from 30 patients revealed both well-developed vascular changes and pyelonephritis with extensive structural alterations and urate deposits.

Some exceptions were found related to the correlation of clinical severity and renal pathology. A few patients with severe tophaceous gout showed only minimal clinical evi-

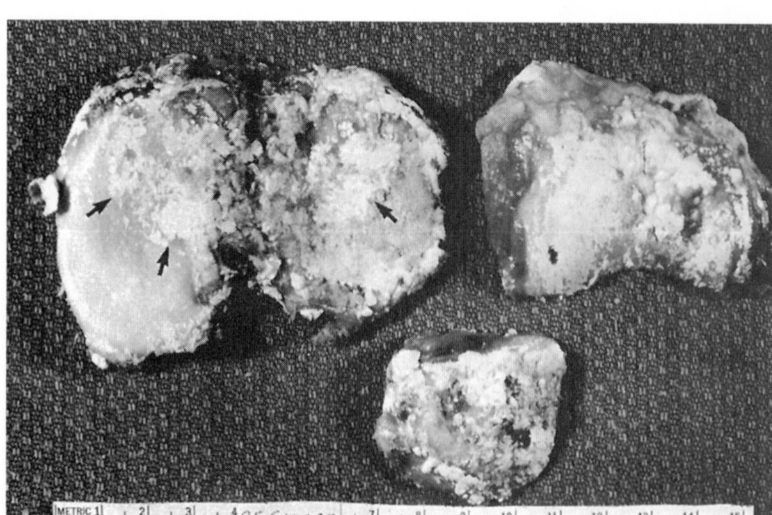

FIGURE 114.20. Encrusted urate deposits on eroded articular cartilage of the tibial plateau (**Upper Left**) and fragments of the femoral condyle. (Courtesy of Dr. Mitchell Krieger.)

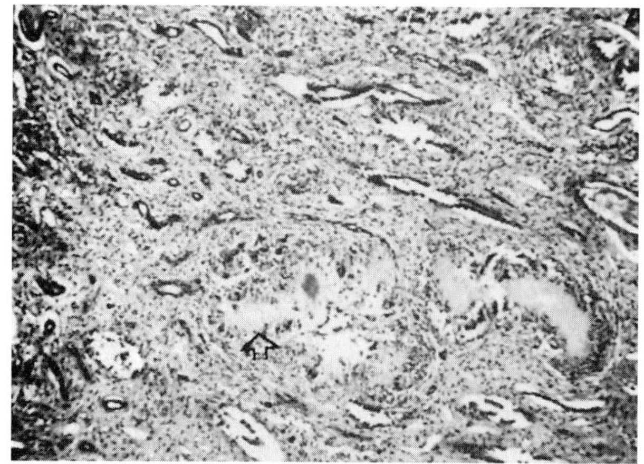

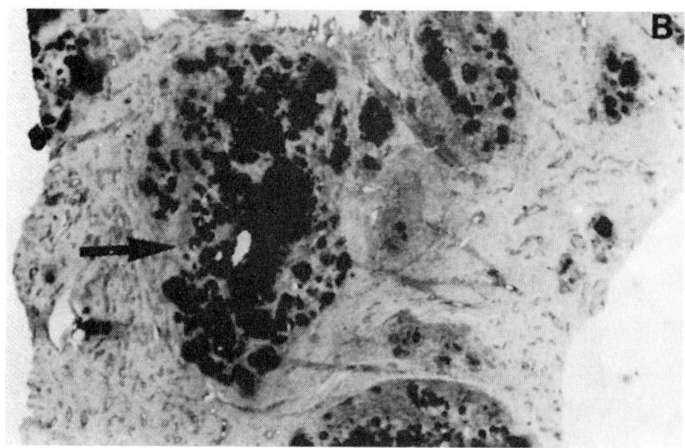

FIGURE 114.21. **A:** Urate deposit in the medulla of the kidney fixed in alcohol (hematoxylin & eosin stain: ×100). **B:** Same deposit stained with methenamine silver (×375). (Courtesy of Dr. Wellington Jao.)

dence of renal insufficiency, and other patients with severe renal disease had only minimal articular disease. In the latter patients, renal disease may have caused premature death, such as portrayed in a few reports of "gouty nephrosis" occurring without clinical evidence of gout (207). In the rare patients with this syndrome, however, serum urate concentrations have not been reported.

A number of mechanisms have been proposed to explain the various pathologic findings reported in urate nephropathy. The renal lesions may stem from deposition of uric acid in collecting tubules with resultant obstruction, atrophy of the more proximal tubules, and secondary necrosis and fibrosis (9). The associated interstitial inflammatory process has been attributed to complicating pyelonephritis. Other studies have shown that tubular damage is an early structural abnormality associated with an interstitial reaction; this finding suggests a relation between the interstitial and tubular changes (208). For example, studies of the interaction of urate crystals with a cultured renal collecting duct epithelium cell line support the notion that interstitial urate deposits are derived from intratubular crystals reacting with tubular epithelium (209). Within hours of exposure, crystals are found within intercellular spaces and also within intracellular vacuoles (phagolysosomes), leading to lysosomal enzyme release. This process could expedite passage of crystals into the interstitium *in vivo.*

HYPERURICEMIA AND GOUT AS CONSEQUENCES OF DRUGS, TOXINS, ABNORMAL PHYSIOLOGIC STATES, OR OTHER DISEASES

The mechanisms underlying secondary hyperuricemia are precisely those responsible for primary hyperuricemia, although in the former case, activation of the abnormal metabolism is associated with a drug therapy, environmental factor, or associated disease process. Gout arises in these contexts as a consequence of urate crystal deposition and the identical attendant consequences as in primary gout, although, in some instances, the pace of clinical manifestations may be accelerated.

Drugs

Diuretic therapy is one of the most frequent causes of secondary hyperuricemia. Diuretics were implicated in 20% of hyperuricemic men admitted to a VA hospital (210). Fifty percent of the new cases of gout in the Framingham study developed in subjects taking thiazides or ethacrynic acid (8). Surveillance of the Framingham study population years later showed that 20% of men and 25% of women reported taking antihypertensive medications, and the mean serum urate concentration was 0.8 mg/dL higher for this group than for the untreated subjects (211). Similar increments were observed in a short-term study of 358 mildly hypertensive subjects treated with very low doses of hydrochlorothiazide (212). Other series reported increments in urate concentrations of 1.3 to 1.8 mg/dL during prolonged thiazide administration (8).

The primary mechanism of urate retention among diuretic-treated patients appears to be enhanced tubular reabsorption of both sodium and uric acid, because urate excretion is unchanged when volume depletion is prevented with intravenous saline (213,214). Additionally, furosemide and diazoxide can induce hyperlacticacidemia sufficient to suppress tubular secretion of urate. Neither of these mechanisms represents a direct drug effect on bidirectional urate transport. Spironolactone may decrease the renal clearance of uric acid but has no consistent effect on urate values (215). The substantial prevalence of tophaceous gout among elderly women receiving long-term diuretic therapy (113–116) attests to the importance of recognizing this consequence of drug therapy in an increasingly elderly population. A recent study concluded that in contrast to the common occurrence of hyperuricemia, diuretic-induced gout occurs, with few exceptions, in patients with an additional cause of hyperuricemia, usually impaired renal function (216).

A wide variety of other drugs can induce hyperuricemia. Renal uric acid retention as a result of ingestion of low doses of salicylates (less than 2 g/day) has been discussed earlier (120). Suppression of tubular secretion of urate occurs at the resulting concentrations of free salicylate in tubular urine. Doses of aspirin exceeding about 3 g/day result in suppression of both reabsorption and secretion, and the consequent net effect is uricosuria. The antituberculous drugs pyrazinamide and ethambutol (120) decrease the renal clearance of uric acid, as does nicotinic acid (217), but the last of these drugs and warfarin may also stimulate purine synthesis *de novo* (218). Hyperuricemia and gout occur frequently in transplant patients receiving the immunosuppressive agent cyclosporine (120–124,219). The degree of hyperuricemia and the severity of gout associated with this drug is often unusual, with early progression to polyarticular attacks and tophaceous deposits. Impaired renal urate excretion is the basis of cyclosporine-induced hyperuricemia, but the mechanisms of this effect are complex. Acute cyclosporine nephrotoxicity is a prerenal process, altering filtration and promoting urate retention as a result of increased tubular reabsorption (122,220). Chronic cyclosporine-induced renal insufficiency is characterized primarily by interstitial fibrosis and arteriolar damage, leading to a decreased filtered load of urate and adaptive declines in urate tubular handling mechanisms. Additionally, a direct effect of cyclosporine on tubular urate transport remains a possibility, and the hyperuricemic effect appears to be potentiated by simultaneous administration of diuretics (122).

Toxins

As previously discussed, ethanol can result in hyperuricemia either as a consequence of enhanced nucleotide catabolism with excessive uric acid production or dehydration and lacticacidemia, leading to reduced renal uric acid excretion (92,94). Epidemiologic studies show a strong correlation between serum urate levels and habitual alcohol intake, and gouty individuals consume more alcohol than do nongouty counterparts (221). In most large series of gout patients, heavily weighted toward a predominance of men, the proportion of patients who abuse alcohol ranges from 30% to 50% (7,118).

Lead nephropathy is a chronic tubulointerstitial nephritis caused by chronic lead poisoning. An increased incidence of gout is found in patients with chronic lead nephropathy (saturnine gout); reduced renal clearance of uric acid is the primary mechanism of hyperuricemia (222). In Australia (223), leaded paint has provided the major source of lead exposure, in contrast to the southeastern U.S., where toxic exposure results from lead contamination during distillation or storage of unbonded alcohol, or "moonshine" (222,224).

Increased mobilizable lead also has been demonstrated in patients with gout and renal insufficiency but no known lead exposure (225,226), and a reciprocal relation between lead excretion after intravenous chelation with ethylenediamine tetraacetic acid (EDTA) and creatinine clearance was described in groups of such patients (225,226). These findings were the basis for the hypothesis that lead may be responsible for the decline in renal function observed in some gouty patients (225). However, a controlled study failed to confirm this relation and questioned the importance of lead intoxication as a primary factor for decreased creatinine clearance in gouty patients (227). In the latter study, nongouty moonshiners had lead stores comparable to those of gouty ingestors of moonshine, who, in turn, had no greater renal impairment than a group of patients with gout but no history of lead exposure. Moreover, chelation therapy, resulting in normalization of mobilizable lead in six gouty patients with renal insufficiency, altered neither creatinine clearances nor plasma and urinary concentrations of hypoxanthine, xanthine, and uric acid (228). Factors other than lead nephropathy, such as obesity, alcohol consumption, and hypertension thus appear to be the major factors contributing to decreased renal function in patients with gout, and increased mobilizable lead in gouty patients with renal impairment is likely to be an associated but *infrequently* pathogenetic factor.

Abnormal Physiologic States

Total caloric restriction results in hyperuricemia, largely attributed to reduced renal urate clearance (9). Urate retention correlates best with ketosis, especially concentrations of β-hydroxybutyrate and acetoacetate (229). Carbohydrate, protein, or purine refeeding causes a prompt increase in urinary uric acid excretion and return of serum urate to control values (221), but ketosis persists if a fat diet succeeds a fast. If starvation is attended by nucleotide depletion, excessive uric acid production may contribute to the associated hyperuricemia. Attacks of gout may occur during periods of starvation, usually in patients with a history of hyperuricemia or gout.

Hyperuricemia is common in uremic patients, but gouty arthritis is unusual and occurs in fewer than 1% of uremic individuals. Extremely high serum urate values are unusual in chronic renal failure, owing in part to increased fractional excretion of uric acid. This results from persistence of tubular secretory capacity, even as glomerular filtration rate decreases, and from reduced tubular uric acid reabsorptive capacity at glomerular filtration rates less than 10 mL/min (230). Additionally, extrarenal disposal of uric acid assumes a major role in urate homeostasis as renal function deteriorates, reaching up to 50% of total uric acid disposal (231). The rarity of gout associated with uremia has been attributed to a shortened life span and a decreased ability to respond to an inflammatory stimulus.

Recurrent attacks of acute inflammatory arthritis or periarthritis occur in patients with chronic renal failure treated with long-term hemodialysis. Although the clinical features of these episodes in the setting of hyperuricemia often suggest gouty arthritis (232), tissue and synovial fluid examination may show crystals of basic calcium phosphate (apatite), or of calcium oxalate (233), rather than urate crystals.

Other Diseases

In a series of patients with leukemia, myeloid metaplasia, polycythemia vera, and multiple myeloma, increased cell and nucleic acid turnover resulted in hyperuricemia in 66% of 113 men and 69% of 73 women (234). Gouty arthritis was noted in 10 patients, an incidence similar to the 3.7% and 4.5% incidence of gouty arthritis reported in other series of patients with myeloproliferative and lymphoproliferative diseases (9). In myeloid metaplasia, the incidence of gout, often complicated by early development of tophaceous deposits, may be as great as 27%, the longer survival of patients with this disorder perhaps accounting for the higher incidence.

Mean urate excretion of 634 mg/24 hours was found in a group of 27 patients with gout and hematoproliferative diseases in comparison with a value of 497 mg/24 hours in a control group. In these conditions, the miscible pool of uric acid is enlarged, and uric acid turnover accelerated (9). Peak incorporation of labeled precursors into uric acid and urinary purines occurs earlier than normal, indicating rapid turnover of newly synthesized nucleotides. A secondary peak of urinary uric acid labeling after 1 to 2 weeks reflects the rapid turnover of cells of the abnormal hematopoietic line.

Hyperuricemia also is a relatively common finding in secondary polycythemias (235,236), hemoglobinopathies (237), pernicious anemia (especially after vitamin B_{12} therapy), and chronic hemolytic states (238). Occasionally, disseminated carcinomas with rapid cell turnover are accompanied by hyperuricemia. Among patients with homozygous sickle cell disease, the frequency of hyperuricemia ranges from 26% to 39%, principally among patients in the third decade of life who have reduced renal urate secretory capacity (237). Excessive urinary uric acid excretion, increased precursor labeling of urinary uric acid, and increased fractional excretion of uric acid in younger patients with sickle cell anemia also suggest excessive production of uric acid in this population (239). Gouty arthritis is, however, unusual in patients with sickle cell anemia, probably because of shortened life span (240).

Hyperuricemia is frequent in patients with hyperparathyroidism (241). In most studies, however, hypertension, obesity, and renal disease have obscured the significance of elevated serum urate levels (241,242). Shelp et al. (243) infused 14 volunteers with parathyroid hormone and did not alter the renal excretion of uric acid. In a large series of patients with primary hyperparathyroidism, the incidence of gouty arthritis was reported to be 3% to 9% (9), but polarization of synovial fluid to detect and differentiate urate and calcium pyrophosphate crystals (pseudogout) was not performed in these earlier studies. An association between psoriasis and hyperuricemia is postulated to result from increased epidermal cell turnover, but not all studies confirm the association. The disparate prevalence rates (0–50%) (9,244) may reflect differences in disease severity or individual differences in bidirectional urate transport (245). The pattern of labeled glycine incorporation into urinary uric acid in psoriatic individuals is consistent with accelerated nucleic acid turnover, presumably in the cells of psoriatic plaques. An association of sarcoidosis, psoriasis, and gout is regarded by some authors as a syndrome, but may represent a chance occurrence. A study demonstrated an increased prevalence of hypothyroidism in urate crystal–proven gout (246).

Hyperuricemia also has been reported in patients with Down syndrome (9), cystinuria, primary oxaluria, Paget's disease of bone (247), and Bartter's syndrome (248), and episodes of gouty arthritis have been noted in the latter two of these conditions. Uric acid nephrolithiasis is described in cystinuria. Reduced renal uric acid clearance has been proposed in Bartter's syndrome (248), Down syndrome, and hyperoxaluria (233).

DISORDERS ASSOCIATED WITH HYPERURICEMIA AND GOUT

Gout and hyperuricemia occur with increased frequency in several important disorders in which no cause–effect relation has been established. Primary management of potentially serious disorders such as hypertension should not be withheld or delayed because of concern over the degree of hyperuricemia or the frequency of gouty attacks, issues that can most often be readily managed.

Obesity

A strong positive correlation between body weight and serum urate concentration has been documented, but the relation is both complex and multifactorial (249–254). In a study of 73,000 obese women, the crude relative risk for gout was 2.56, and women who were 85% above desirable body weight (255) had gout 1.56 times more frequently than women weighing within 10% of ideal body weight. In the Framingham study, the correlation between uric acid levels and weight was particularly marked in the age group from 35 to 44 years, with lower correlations seen in older age groups (256). In a group of male physicians studied prospectively, weight gain before age 35 appeared to be one determinant of the occurrence of gout. In another study, 52% of gouty patients were more than 20% over ideal body weight (228). The fact that 85% were hypertensive and

48% had abnormal glucose tolerance tests and hyperlipidemia points out the multiplicity of variables relating to obesity and its metabolic complications. An increased incidence of obesity and decreased fractional excretion of uric acid also have been reported among hyperuricemic Maori men (14). Obesity has several effects on urate metabolism including decreased renal urate clearance and increased uric acid production (257). Weight reduction is associated with a modest lowering of serum urate concentration and a decrease in the rate of *de novo* purine synthesis (257).

Hyperlipidemia

An association between hypertriglyceridemia and hyperuricemia is well established (258). Up to 80% of individuals with hypertriglyceridemia have hyperuricemia, and 50% to 75% of gouty patients have hypertriglyceridemia. Confounding the interpretation of these relations are other variables observed in this population, including obesity and excessive alcohol intake. In one study of 40 gouty subjects, a correlation was found between the ponderal index and serum triglycerides (259). Fasting triglyceride values were, however, not significantly higher than those of obese controls. The 17 gouty subjects in this study who drank excessive alcohol had higher triglyceride values than those who abstained. Another study reported a 1.6-fold increase in the frequency of hypertriglyceridemia independent of alcohol intake in a group of obese gouty patients whose hyperuricemia was normalized with either allopurinol or probenecid (260). In 108 gouty Japanese men, hyperlipoproteinemia was seen in 56% and appeared to be independent of both alcohol intake and obesity (261). Additional observations demonstrate a correlation between 24-hour urinary uric acid excretion and serum triglyceride levels (262). In another study of Japanese gout patients, elevated triglyceride levels were accompanied by reduced serum high-density lipoprotein C (HDL-C) and HDL2-C concentrations. By logistic regression analysis, serum triglyceride levels and alcohol consumption discriminated gout patients from controls, but HDL levels and body mass index did not, suggesting that increased triglyceride levels are intrinsic to gout and that reduced HDL levels are attributable to altered triglyceride metabolism (263). Finally, no change was found in levels of serum urate or uric acid excretion when triglycerides were acutely elevated in three gouty subjects receiving intravenous intralipid (264).

Evidence to support the view that the association of hypertriglyceridemia and hyperuricemia might, in many instances, be part of a more extensive metabolic syndrome has recently been reviewed by Emmerson (265). Both experimental and epidemiologic investigations are in accord with the concept that hyperuricemia resulting from reduced renal uric acid clearance (266,267) is an intrinsic component of the metabolic syndrome of hyperinsulinemia and resistance to insulin action (268). This syndrome is characterized, in addition, by increased body mass index, abdominal obesity (269), hypertriglyceridemia (270,271), increased apolipoprotein B and VLDL cholesterol, reduced HDL cholesterol, hypertension, and coronary artery disease (272). A corollary of these observations is that hyperuricemic individuals, particularly those with abdominal obesity, may be a high-risk group for the cardiovascular correlates of insulin resistance.

Hypertension

Hyperuricemia is reported in 22% to 38% of untreated hypertensive patients, and increases to 47% to 67% when therapy and renal disease are included (9). The prevalence of gout in the hypertensive population is between 2% and 12%. Although the prevalence of hyperuricemia in the general population increases with increasing blood pressure, no consistent relations emerge. In the Tecumseh study, no correlation was found between urate concentration and age, sex, anthropometric data, or level of blood pressure (273). Likewise, only 1% of blood pressure variation could be accounted for by serum urate values in the Israeli ischemic heart study of 10,000 men aged 40 years or older (274). Conversely, among patients with classic gout, 25% to 50% have hypertension that is unrelated to the duration of gout and is more common in obese patients (118,275).

Causal factors relating hyperuricemia and hypertension are unclear. Renal urate clearances, which depend on tubular secretory and postsecretory reabsorption rates, are reported to be inappropriately low relative to glomerular filtration rates in both adult and childhood essential hypertension (9,276). This process may be regulated in part, by renal blood flow. A recent study has documented reduced renal blood flow and increased renal vascular resistance and total peripheral resistance in subjects with essential hypertension and hyperuricemia (170). In contrast, glomerular filtration rates, cardiac output, and intravascular volume were not specifically affected in this group. The authors suggested that hyperuricemia in patients with essential hypertension reflects early nephrosclerosis. The importance of this relation should not be overlooked in the management of gout because untreated hypertension may contribute to renal morbidity in these patients.

Atherosclerosis

Since an early description of an increased frequency of hyperuricemia in a group of young patients with coronary heart disease, the issue of hyperuricemia as an independent risk factor for atherosclerosis has been a subject of controversy. Additional reports have noted a relation between hyperuricemia and atherosclerosis (9,277–279), but no clear association was found in the Tecumseh study when adjustments were made for age, sex, and relative weight (273). Serum urate values did not differ significantly in the coronary heart disease group from the mean value of the entire population. With multivariate analysis of risk factors at the 13th biennial evaluation of the original Framingham cohort, serum urate values did not add independently to the prediction of coronary heart disease (211). Analysis of this population, segregated by diuretic use, however, showed that among gouty men who had never received diuretics, a 60% excess of coronary artery disease was present (280). Alcohol intake, systolic blood pressure, and body mass index were higher in the gouty subjects. Among Polynesians, hypertension, diabetes mellitus, and atherosclerosis are correlates of obesity rather than of hyperuricemia (281). Thus in hyperuricemic patients, a tangled web of coronary risk factors such as obesity, hypertension, insulin resistance, and hypertriglyceridemia appears to contribute to the observed association between elevated urate values and atherosclerosis.

A recent extension of the Framingham study (282) supports the contention that it is these risk factors, each associated with hyperuricemia and cardiovascular disease and death, rather than hyperuricemia itself that are primary casual factors in atherosclerotic heart disease. In this study of 6,763 subjects whose baseline serum urate levels were established in 1971 to 1976, hyperuricemia was not associated (by 1994) with an increased risk for adverse outcome (coronary heart disease, death of cardiovascular disease, or death of all causes) in men or, after adjustment for other cardiovascular risk factors, in women.

ACKNOWLEDGMENT

This study was supported by National Institutes of Health Grant DK-25584. I thank Ms. Danette Shine for excellent preparation of the manuscript.

REFERENCES

1. Porter R. Gout: framing and fantasizing disease. *Bull Hist Med* 1994;68:1–28 and references therein.
2. Garrod AE. *The inborn factors in disease:* an essay. New York: Oxford University Press, 1931:106–111.
3. McCarty DJ. A historical note: Leeuwenhoek's description of crystals from a gouty tophus. *Arthritis Rheum* 1970;13: 414–418.
4. Garrod AB. *Treatise on gout and rheumatic gout.* 3rd ed. London: Longmans, Green, 1876.
5. McCarty DJ, Hollander JL. Identification of urate crystals in gouty synovial fluid. *Ann Intern Med* 1961;54:452–460.
6. Loeb J. The influence of temperature on the solubility of monosodium urate. *Arthritis Rheum* 1972;15:189–192.
7. Campion EW, Glynn RJ, DeLabry LO. Asymptomatic hyperuricemia: risks and consequences in the normative aging study. *Am J Med* 1987;82:421–426.
8. Hall AP, Barry PE, Dawber TR, et al. Epidemiology of gout and hyperuricemia: a long-term population study. *Am J Med* 1967; 42:27–37.
9. Wyngaarden JB, Kelley WN. *Gout and hyperuricemia.* New York: Grune & Stratton, 1976, and references therein.
10. Mikkelsen WM, Dodge HJ, Valkenburg H. The distribution of serum uric acid values in a population unselected as to gout or hyperuricemia: Tecumseh, Michigan 1959-60. *Am J Med* 1965;39:242–251.
11. Price CP, James DR. Analytical reviews in clinical biochemistry: the measurement of urate. *Ann Clin Biochem* 1988;25: 484–498.
12. Munan L, Kelley A, Petitclerc C. Serum urate levels between ages 10 and 14: changes in sex trends. *J Lab Clin Med* 1977;90: 990–996.
13. Mateos Anton F, Puig JG, Ramos T, et al. Sex differences in uric acid metabolism in adults: evidence for a lack of influence of estradiol 17β (E_2) on the renal handling of urate. *Metabolism* 1986;35:343–348.
14. Gibson T, Waterworth R, Hatfield P, et al. Hyperuricemia, gout and kidney function in New Zealand Maori men. *Br J Rheumatol* 1984;23:276–282.
15. Darmavan J, Valkenburg HA, Muirden KD, et al. The epidemiology of gout and hyperuricemia in a rural population of Java. *J Rheumatol* 1992;19:1595–1599.
16. Langford HG, Blaufox MD, Borhani NO, et al. Is thiazide-produced uric acid elevation harmful? Analysis of data from the hypertension detection and follow-up program. *Arch Intern Med* 1987;147:645–649.
17. Fessel JW. Renal outcomes of gout and hyperuricemia. *Am J Med* 1979;67:74–82.
18. Hitchings GH. Uric acid: chemistry and synthesis. In: Weiner IM, Kelley WN, eds. *Uric acid:* handbook of experimental pharmacology. Vol 51. New York: Springer-Verlag, 1978:1–20.
19. Holmes EW. Regulation of purine biosynthesis de novo. In: Weiner IM, Kelley WN, eds. *Uric acid:* handbook of experimental pharmacology. Vol 51. New York: Springer-Verlag, 1978:21–41.
20. Arnold WJ. Purine salvage enzymes. In: Weiner IM, Kelley WN, eds. *Uric acid:* handbook of experimental pharmacology. Vol 51. New York: Springer-Verlag, 1978:43–73.
21. Holmes EW, Wyngaarden JB, Kelley WN. Human glutamine phosphoribosylpyrophosphate amidotransferase: two molecular forms interconvertible by purine nucleotide and phosphoribosylpyrophosphate. *J Biol Chem* 1973;248:6035–6040.
22. Becker MA, Kim M. Regulation of purine synthesis de novo in human fibroblasts by purine nucleotides and phosphoribosylpyrophosphate. *J Biol Chem* 1987;262:14531–14537.
23. Holmes EW, McDonald JA, McCord JM, et al. Human glutamine phosphoribosylpyrophosphate amidotransferase: kinetic and regulatory properties. *J Biol Chem* 1973;248:144–150.
24. Itakura M, Sabina RL, Heald PW, et al. Basis for the control of purine biosynthesis by purine ribonucleotides. *J Clin Invest* 1981;67:994–1002.
25. Becker MA, Raivio KO Seegmiller JE. Synthesis of phosphoribosylpyrophosphate in mammalian cells. *Adv Enzymol* 1979;49:281–306.
26. Iwahana H, Oka J, Mizusawa N, et al. Molecular cloning of human amidophosphoribosyltransferase. *Biochem Biophys Res Commun* 1993;190:192–200.
27. Smith JL, Zaluzec EJ, Wery J-P, et al. Structure of the allosteric regulatory enzyme of purine biosynthesis. *Science* 1994;264: 1427–1433.
28. Yen RCK, Raivio KO, Becker MA. Inhibition of phosphoribosylpyrophosphate synthesis by 6-methylthioinosinate. *J Biol Chem* 1981;256:1839–1845.
29. Fox IH, Kelley WN. Human phosphoribosylpyrophosphate synthetase: distribution, purification, and properties. *J Biol Chem* 1971;246:5739–5748.

30. Becker MA, Losman MJ, Kim M. Mechanisms of accelerated purine nucleotide synthesis in human fibroblasts with superactive phosphoribosylpyrophosphate synthetases. *J Biol Chem* 1987;262:5596–5602.
31. Hershfield MS, Seegmiller JE. Regulation of de novo purine biosynthesis in human lymphoblasts: coordinate control of proximal (rate-determining) steps and the inosinic acid branch point. *J Biol Chem* 1976;251:7348–7354.
32. Kovarsky J, Holmes EW, Kelley WN. Absence of significant urate binding to human serum proteins. *J Lab Clin Med* 1979;93:85–91.
33. Sorensen LB. Degradation of uric acid in man. *Metabolism* 1959;68:687–703.
34. Seegmiller JE, Grayzel AI, Laster L, et al. Uric acid production in gout. *J Clin Invest* 1961;40:1304–1314.
35. Wyngaarden JB. Overproduction of uric acid as the cause of hyperuricemia in primary gout. *J Clin Invest* 1957;36: 1508–1515.
36. Becker MA. Clinical aspects of monosodium urate monohydrate crystal deposition disease (gout). *Rheum Dis Clin North Am* 1988;14:377–394.
37. Berger L, Yu T-F. Renal function in gout: an analysis of 524 gouty subjects including long-term follow-up studies. *Am J Med* 1975;59:605–613.
38. Becker MA. Patterns of phosphoribosylpyrophosphate and ribose-5-phosphate concentration and generation in fibroblasts from patients with gout and purine overproduction. *J Clin Invest* 1976;57:308–318.
39. Seegmiller JE, Rosenbloom FM, Kelley WN. Enzyme defect associated with sex linked human neurological disorder and excessive purine synthesis. *Science* 1967;155:1682–1684.
40. Kelley WN, Rosenbloom FM, Henderson JF, et al. A specific enzyme defect in gout associated with overproduction of uric acid. *Proc Natl Acad Sci U S A* 1967;57:1735–1739.
41. Sperling O, Boer P, Persky-Brosh S, et al. Altered kinetic property of erythrocyte phosphoribosylpyrophosphate synthetase in excessive purine production. *Rev Eur Etud Clin Biol* 1972;17: 703–706.
42. Becker MA, Meyer LJ, Wood AW, et al. Purine overproduction in man associated with increased phosphoribosylpyrophosphate synthetase activity. *Science* 1973;179:1123–1126.
43. Kelley WN, Greene ML, Rosenbloom FM, et al. Hypoxanthine-guanine phosphoribosyltransferase deficiency in gout. *Ann Intern Med* 1969;70:155–206.
44. Rincon-Limas DE, Krueger DA, Patel PI. Functional characterization of the human hypoxanthine phosphoribosyltransferase gene promoter: evidence for a negative regulatory element. *Mol Cell Biol* 1991;11:4157–4164.
45. Rossiter BJF, Caskey CT. Hypoxanthine-guanine phosphoribosyltransferase deficiency: Lesch-Nyhan syndrome and gout. In: Scriver CR, Beaudet AL, Sly WS, et al., eds. *The metabolic and molecular bases of inherited disease*. 7th ed. New York: McGraw-Hill 1995:1679–1706.
46. Lesch M, Nyhan WL. A familial disorder of uric acid metabolism and central nervous system function. *Am J Med* 1964; 36:561–570.
47. Lloyd KG, Hornykiewicz O, Davidson L, et al. Biochemical evidence of dysfunction of brain neurotransmitters in the Lesch-Nyhan syndrome. *N Engl J Med* 1981;305:1106–1111.
48. Jinnah HA, Gage FH, Friedmann T. Amphetamine-induced behavioral phenotype in a hypoxanthine-guanine phosphoribosyltransferase-deficient model of the Lesch-Nyhan syndrome. *Behav Neurosci* 1991;105:1004–1112.
49. Wilson JM, Stout JT, Palella TD, et al. A molecular survey of hypoxanthine-guanine phosphoribosyltransferase deficiency in man. *J Clin Invest* 1986;77:188–195.
50. Patel PI, Framson PE, Caskey CI, et al. Fine structure of the human hypoxanthine phosphoribosyltransferase gene. *Mol Cell Biol* 1986;6:393–403.
51. Seravelli E, DeBona P, Velisavakis M, et al. Further data on the cytologic mapping of the human X chromosome with man-mouse cell hybrids. *Cytogenet Cell Genet* 1976;16:219–222.
52. Wilson JM, Baugher BW, Landa L, et al. Human hypoxanthine-guanine phosphoribosyltransferase: purification and characterization of mutant forms of the enzyme. *J Biol Chem* 1981; 256:10306–10312.
53. Davidson BL, Tarle SA, Palella TD, et al. Molecular basis of hypoxanthine-guanine phosphoribosyltransferase deficiency in ten subjects determined by direct sequencing of amplified transcripts. *J Clin Invest* 1989;84:342–346.
54. Davidson BL, Tarle SA, Palella TD, et al. Identification of 17 independent mutations responsible for human hypoxanthine-guanine phosphoribosyltransferase (HPRT) deficiency. *Am J Hum Genet* 1991;49:951–958.
55. Eads JC, Scapin G, Xu Y, et al. The crystal structure of human hypoxanthine-guanine phosphoribosyltransferase with bound GMP. *Cell* 1994;78:325–334.
56. Palella TD, Silverman LJ, Schroll CT, et al. Herpes simplex virus-mediated human hypoxanthine-guanine phosphoribosyltransferase gene transfer into neuronal cells. *Mol Cell Biol* 1988; 8:457–460.
57. Edwards NL, Recker D, Fox IH. Overproduction of uric acid in hypoxanthine-guanine phosphoribosyltransferase deficiency: contribution by impaired purine salvage. *J Clin Invest* 1979;63:922–930.
58. Hershfield MS, Seegmiller JE. Regulation of de novo purine synthesis in human lymphoblasts: similar rates during growth by normal cells and mutants deficient in hypoxanthine-guanine phosphoribosyltransferase. *J Biol Chem* 1977;252:6002–6010.
59. Thompson LF, Willis RC, Stoop JW, et al. Purine metabolism in cultured fibroblasts from patients deficient in hypoxanthine phosphoribosyltransferase, purine nucleoside phosphorylase, or adenosine deaminase. *Proc Natl Acad Sci U S A* 1978;75: 3722–3736.
60. Fox IH, Kelley WN. Human phosphoribosylpyrophosphate synthetase: kinetic mechanism and end-product inhibition. *J Biol Chem* 1972;247:2126–2131.
61. Zoref E, deVries A, Sperling O. Metabolic cooperation between human fibroblasts with normal and with superactive phosphoribosylpyrophosphate synthetase. *Nature* 1976;260:786–788.
62. Yen RCK, Adams WB, Lazar C, et al. Evidence for X-linkage of human phosphoribosylpyrophosphate synthetase. *Proc Natl Acad Sci U S A* 1978;75:482–485.
63. Becker MA, Puig JG, Mateos FA, et al. Inherited superactivity of phosphoribosylpyrophosphate synthetase: association of uric acid overproduction and sensorineural deafness. *Am J Med* 1988;85:383–390.
64. Becker MA, Losman MJ, Rosenberg AL, et al. Phosphoribosylpyrophosphate synthetase superactivity: a study of five patients with catalytic defects in the enzyme. *Arthritis Rheum* 1986;29:880–888.
65. Becker MA, Taylor W, Smith PR, et al. Overexpression of the normal phosphoribosylpyrophosphate synthetase 1 isoform underlies catalytic superactivity of human phosphoribosylpyrophosphate synthetase. *J Biol Chem* 1996;271:19894–19899.
66. Sperling O, Persky-Brosh S, Boer P, et al. Human erythrocyte phosphoribosylpyrophosphate synthetase mutationally altered in regulatory properties. *Biochem Med* 1973;7:389–395.
67. Zoref E, deVries A, Sperling O. Mutant feedback resistant phosphoribosylpyrophosphate synthetase associated with purine overproduction and gout. *J Clin Invest* 1975;56:1093–1099.
68. Becker MA, Losman MJ, Wilson J, et al. Superactivity of phos-

phoribosylpyrophosphate synthetase due to altered regulation by nucleotide inhibition and inorganic phosphate. *Biochim Biophys Acta* 1986;882:168–176.
69. Becker MA, Smith PR, Taylor W, et al. The genetic and functional basis of purine nucleotide feedback-resistant phosphoribosylpyrophosphate synthetase superactivity. *J Clin Invest* 1995;96:2133–2141.
70. Becker MA, Raivio KO, Bakay B, et al. Variant human phosphoribosylpyrophosphate synthetase altered in regulatory and catalytic functions. *J Clin Invest* 1980;65:109–120.
71. Akaoka I, Fujimori S, Kamatani N, et al. A gouty family with increased phosphoribosylpyrophosphate synthetase activity: case reports, family studies, and kinetic studies of the abnormal enzyme. *J Rheumatol* 1981;8:563–574.
72. Taira M, Kudoh J, Minoshima S, et al. Localization of human phosphoribosylpyrophosphate synthetase subunit I and II genes (PRPS 1 and PRPS 2) to different regions of the X chromosome and assignment of two PRPS-related genes to autosomes. *Somat Cell Mol Genet* 1989;15:29–37.
73. Becker MA, Heidler SA, Bell GI, et al. Cloning of cDNAs for human phosphoribosylpyrophosphate synthetases 1 and 2 and X chromosome localization of PRPS 1 and PRPS 2 genes. *Genomics* 1990;8:555–561.
74. Taira M, Iizasa T, Shimada H, et al. A human testis-specific mRNA for phosphoribosylpyrophosphate synthetase that initiates from a non-AUG codon. *J Biol Chem* 1990;265: 16491–16495.
75. Ishizuka T, Kita K, Sonoda T, et al. Cloning and sequencing of human complementary DNA for the phosphoribosylpyrophosphate synthetase-associated protein 39. *Biochim Biophys Acta* 1996;1306:27–30.
76. Sonoda T, Ishizuka T, Kita K, et al. Cloning and sequencing of rat cDNA for the 41-kDa phosphoribosylpyrophosphate synthetase-associated protein has a high homology to the catalytic subunits and to 39 kDa associated protein. *Biochim Biophys Acta* 1997;1350:6–10.
77. Iizasa T, Taira M, Shimada H, et al. Molecular cloning and sequencing of human cDNA for phosphoribosylpyrophosphate synthetase subunit II. *FEBS Lett* 1989;244:47–50.
78. Sonoda T, Taira M, Ishijima S, et al. Complete nucleotide sequence of human phosphoribosylpyrophosphate synthetase subunit I (PRSI) cDNA and a comparison with human and rat PRPS gene families. *J Biochem* 1991;109:361–364.
79. Nosal JM, Switzer RL, Becker MA. Overexpression, purification, and characterization of recombinant human 5-phosphoribosyl-1-pyrophosphate synthetase isozymes I and II. *J Biol Chem* 1993;268:10168–10175.
80. Roessler BJ, Nosal, JM, Smith PR, et al. Human X-linked phosphoribosylpyrophosphate synthetase superactivity is associated with distinct point mutations in the PRPS1 gene. *J Biol Chem* 1993;268:26476–26481.
81. Ahmed M, Taylor W, Smith PR, et al. Accelerated transcription of PRPS1 in X-linked overactivity of normal human phosphoribosylpyrophosphate synthetase. *J Biol Chem* 1999;274: 7482–7488.
82. Chen Y-T, Burchell A. Glycogen storage diseases. In: Scriver CR, Beaudet AL, Sly WS, et al., eds. *The metabolic and molecular bases of inherited disease.* 7th ed. New York: McGraw-Hill, 1995:935–965.
83. Reitsma-Bierens WCC. Renal complications in glycogen storage disease type I. *Eur J Pediatr* 1993;152:S60–S62.
84. Greene HL, Wilson FA, Hefferan P, et al. ATP depletion, a possible role in the pathogenesis of hyperuricemia in glycogen storage disease, type I. *J Clin Invest* 1978;62:321–328.
85. Breven J, Hardwell TR, Hickling P, et al. Effect of treatment erythrocyte phosphoribosylpyrophosphate synthetase and glutathione reductase activity in patients with primary gout. *Ann Rheum Dis* 1986;45:941–944.
86. Rosenbloom FM, Henderson JF, Caldwell IC, et al. Biochemical bases of accelerated purine biosynthesis de novo in human fibroblasts lacking hypoxanthine-guanine phosphoribosyltransferase. *J Biol Chem* 1968;243:1166–1173.
87. Fox IH, Palella TD, Kelley WN. Hyperuricemia: a marker for cell energy crisis. *N Engl J Med* 1987;317:111–112.
88. Woolliscroft JO, Colfter H, Fox IH. Hyperuricemia in acute illness: a poor prognostic sign. *Am J Med* 1982;72:58–62.
89. Woolliscroft JO, Fox IH. Increased body fluid purine levels during hypotensive events: evidence for ATP degradation. *Am J Med* 1986;81:472–478.
90. Fox IH, Kelley WN. Studies on the mechanism of fructose-induced hyperuricemia in man. *Metabolism* 1972;21:713–721.
91. Raivio KO, Becker MA, Meyer LJ, et al. Stimulation of human purine synthesis de novo by fructose infusion. *Metabolism* 1975; 24:861–869.
92. Faller J, Fox IH. Ethanol-induced hyperuricemia: evidence for increased urate production by activation of adenine nucleotide turnover. *N Engl J Med* 1982;307:1598–1602.
93. Mineo I, Kono N, Hara N, et al. Myogenic hyperuricemia: a common pathophysiological feature of glycogenesis types III, V, and VII. *N Engl J Med* 1987;317:75–80.
94. Puig JG, Fox IH. Ethanol-induced activation of adenine nucleotide turnover: evidence for a role of acetate. *J Clin Invest* 1984;74:36–41.
95. Fox IH. Adenosine triphosphate degradation in specific disease. *J Lab Clin Med* 1985;106:101–110.
96. Jinnai K, Kono N, Yamamoto Y, et al. Glycogenosis V (McArdle's disease) with hyperuricemia: a case report and clinical investigation. *Eur Neurol* 1993;33:204–207.
97. Yamanaka H, Kawagoe Y, Taniguchi A, et al. Accelerated purine nucleotide degradation by anaerobic but not by aerobic ergometer muscle exercise. *Metabolism* 1992;41:364–369.
98. Sorensen LB. The elimination of uric acid in man studied by means of ^{14}C-labelled uric acid. *Scand J Clin Lab Invest* 1960;12 (suppl):1–214.
99. Roch-Ramel F, Diezi J. Renal transport of organic ions and uric acid. In: Schrier RW, Gottschalk CE, eds. *Diseases of the kidney* 6th ed. Boston: Little, Brown and Company, 1996: 231–249.
100. Steele TH. Urate excretion in man, normal and gouty. In: Weiner IM, Kelley WN, eds. *Uric acid:* handbook of experimental pharmacology. Vol 51. New York: Springer-Verlag, 1978:257–286 and references therein.
101. Roch-Ramel F, Weiner IM. Excretion of urate by the kidneys of Cebus monkeys: a micropuncture study. *Am J Physiol* 1973; 224:1369–1374.
102. Weiner IM, Fanelli GM Jr. Renal urate excretion in animal models. *Nephron* 1975;14:33–47.
103. Levinson DJ, Sorensen LB. Renal handling of uric acid in normal and gouty subjects: evidence for a 4-component system. *Ann Rheum Dis* 1980;39:173–179.
104. Puig GJ, Mateos Anton F, Jimenez ML, et al. Renal handling of uric acid in gout: impaired tubular transport of urate not dependent on serum urate levels. *Metabolism* 1996;35: 1147–1153.
105. Diamond HS, Paolino JS. Evidence for a post-secretory reabsorptive site for uric acid in man. *J Clin Invest* 1973;52: 1491–1499.
106. Sorensen LB, Levinson DJ. Isolated defect in postsecretory reabsorption of uric acid. *Ann Rheum Dis* 1980;39:180–183.
107. Smetana SS, Bar-Khayim Y. Hypouricemia due to renal tubular defect: a study with the probenecid-pyrazinamide test. *Arch Intern Med* 1985;145:1200–1203.

108. Tofuku Y, Kuroda M, Takeda R. Hypouricemia due to renal urate wasting. *Nephron* 1982;30:39–44.
109. Simkin PA. Urate excretion in normal and gouty men. *Adv Exp Med Biol* 1977;76B:41–45.
110. Zollner N, Griebsch A. Diet and gout. *Adv Exp Med Biol* 1974; 41B:435–442.
111. Levinson DJ, Decker DE, Sorensen LB. Renal handling of uric acid in man. *Ann Clin Lab Sci* 1982;12:73–77.
112. Rieselbach RE, Sorensen LB, Shelp WD, et al. Diminished renal urate secretion per nephron as a basis for primary gout. *Ann Intern Med* 1970;73:359–366.
113. Macfarlane DG, Dieppe PA. Diuretic-induced gout in elderly women. *Br J Rheumatol* 1985;24:155–157.
114. Meyers OL, Monteagudo FSE. Gout in females: an analysis of 92 patients. *Clin Exp Rheumatol* 1985;3:105–109.
115. Lally EW, Ho G Jr, Kaplan SR. The clinical spectrum of gouty arthritis in women. *Arch Intern Med* 1986;146:2221–2225.
116. Puig JG, Michan AD, Jimenez ML, et al. Female gout: clinical spectrum and uric acid metabolism. *Arch Intern Med* 1991; 151:726–732.
117. Copeman WSC. *A short history of the gout and the rheumatic diseases.* Berkeley: University of California Press, 1964:66–79.
118. Grahame R, Scott JT. Clinical survey of 354 patients with gout. *Ann Rheum Dis* 1970;29:461–468.
119. Hayem G, Delahousse M, Meyer O, et al. Female premenopausal tophaceous gout induced by long term diuretic abuse. *J Rheumatol* 1996;23:2166–2167.
120. Scott JT. Drug-induced gout. *Ballieres Clin Rheumatol* 1991;5: 39–60.
121. Kahl LE, Thompson ME, Griffith BP. Gout in the heart transplant recipient: physiologic puzzle and therapeutic challenge. *Am J Med* 1989;87:289–294.
122. Lin HY, Rocher LL, McQuillan MA, et al. Cyclosporine-induced hyperuricemia and gout. *N Engl J Med* 1989;321: 287–292.
123. Burack DA, Griffith BP, Thompson ME, et al. Hyperuricemia and gout among heart transplant recipients receiving cyclosporine. *Am J Med* 1992;92:141–146.
124. Baethge BA, Work J, Landreneau MD, et al. Tophaceous gout in patients with renal transplants treated with cyclosporine A. *J Rheumatol* 1993;20:718–720.
125. Wernick R, Winkler C, Campbell S. Tophi as the initial manifestation of gout: report of six cases and review of the literature. *Arch Intern Med* 1992;152:873–876.
126. Lally EV, Zimmerman B, Ho G Jr, et al. Urate-mediated inflammation in nodal osteoarthritis: clinical and roentgenographic correlations. *Arthritis Rheum* 1989;32:86–90.
127. Simkin PA, Campbell PM, Larson EB. Gout in Heberden's nodes. *Arthritis Rheum* 1983;26:94–97.
128. Terkeltaub RA, Dyer CA, Martin J, et al. Apolipoprotein (apo) E inhibits the capacity of monosodium urate crystals to stimulate neutrophils: characterization of intraarticular apo E and demonstration of apo E binding to urate crystals in vivo. *J Clin Invest* 1991;87:20–26.
129. Terkeltaub RA. What stops a gouty attack? *J Rheumatol* 1992; 19:8–10.
130. Simkin PA. The pathogenesis of podagra. *Ann Intern Med* 1977; 86:230–233.
131. McCarty DJ. Gout without hyperuricemia. *JAMA* 1994;271: 302–303.
132. Derus CL, Levinson DJ, Bowman B, et al. Altered fractional excretion of uric acid during total parenteral nutrition. *J Rheumatol* 1987;114:978–981.
133. Pascual E. Persistence of monosodium urate crystals and low-grade inflammation in the synovial fluid of patients with untreated gout. *Arthritis Rheum* 1991;34:141–145.
134. Raddatz DA, Mahowald ML, Bilka PJ. Acute polyarticular gout. *Ann Rheum Dis* 1983;42:117–122.
135. Ginsberg, MH, Genant HK, Yü T-F, et al. Rheumatoid nodulosis: an unusual variant of rheumatoid disease. *Arthritis Rheum* 1975;18:49–58.
136. Kozin F, McCarty DJ. Rheumatoid factors in the serum of gouty patients. *Arthritis Rheum* 1977;20:1559–1560.
137. Agudelo CA, Turner RA, Panetti M, et al. Does hyperuricemia protect from rheumatoid inflammation? *Arthritis Rheum* 1984; 27:443–448.
138. Iglesias A, Londono JC, Saaibi DL, et al. Gouty nodulosis: widespread subcutaneous deposits without gout. *Arthritis Care Res* 1996;9:74–77.
139. Liu K, Moffatt EJ, Hudson ER, et al. Gouty tophus presenting as a soft-tissue mass diagnosed by fine needle aspiration: a case report. *Diagn Cytopathy* 1996;15:246–249.
140. Gutman AB. The past four decades of progress in the knowledge of gout with an assessment of the present status. *Arthritis Rheum* 1973;16:431–445.
141. Nishioka N, Mikanagi K. Clinical features of 4,000 gouty subjects in Japan. *Adv Exp Med Biol* 1980;122A:47–54.
142. Nakayama DA, Barthelemy C, Carrera G, et al. Tophaceous gout: a clinical and radiographic assessment. *Arthritis Rheum* 1984;27:468–471.
143. Lawry GV II, Fan PT, Bluestone R. Polyarticular versus monoarticular gout: a prospective comparative analysis of clinical features. *Medicine* 1988;67:335–343.
144. Fam AG, Stein JG, Rubenstein J. Gouty arthritis in nodal osteoarthritis. *J Rheumatol* 1996;23:684–689.
145. Foldes K, Petersilge CA, Weisman MH, et al. Nodal osteoarthritis and gout. *Skeletal Radiol* 1996;25:421–424.
146. Doherty M, Dieppe PA. Crystal deposition disease in the elderly. *Clin Rheum Dis* 1986;12:97–116.
147. Holland NW, Jost D, Beutler A, et al. Finger pad tophi in gout. *J Rheumatol* 1996;23:690–692.
148. Fam AG, Assad D. Intradermal urate tophi. *J Rheumatol* 1997; 24:1126–1131.
149. Good AE, Rapp R. Bony ankylosis: a rare manifestation of gout. *J Rheumatol* 1978;5:335–337.
150. Varga J, Giampaola C, Goldenberg DL. Tophaceous gout of the spine in a patient with no peripheral tophi: case report and review of the literature. *Arthritis Rheum* 1985;28:1312–1315.
151. Stockman A, Darlington LG, Scott JT. Frequency of chondrocalcinosis in the knees and avascular necrosis of the femoral head in gout: a controlled study. *Ann Rheum Dis* 1980;39:7–11.
152. Lichtenstein L, Scott HW, Levin MH. Pathologic changes in gout: survey of 11 necropsied cases. *Am J Pathol* 1956;32: 871–895.
153. Stark TW, Hirokawa RH. Gout and its manifestations in the head and neck. *Otolaryngol Clin North Am* 1982;15:659–664.
154. O'Duffy JD, Hunder GG, Kelly PJ. Decreasing prevalence of tophaceous gout. *Mayo Clin Proc* 1975;50:227–228.
155. Yü T-F. Uric acid nephrolithiasis. In: Weiner IM, Kelley WN, eds. *Uric acid:* handbook of experimental pharmacology. Vol 51. New York: Springer-Verlag, 1978:397–422.
156. Yü T-F, Gutman AB. Uric acid nephrolithiasis in gout: predisposing factors. *Ann Intern Med* 1967;67:1133–1148.
157. Yü T-F. Urolithiasis in hyperuricemia and gout. *J Urol* 1981; 126:424–430.
158. Coe FL, Kavalach AG. Hypercalciuria and hyperuricosuria in patients with calcium nephrolithiasis. *N Engl J Med* 1974; 291:1344–1350.
159. Preminger GM. Renal calculi: pathogenesis, diagnosis, and medical therapy. *Semin Nephrol* 1992;12:200–216.
160. Gutman AB, Yü, T-F. An abnormality of glutamine metabolism in primary gout. *Am J Med* 1963;35:820–831.

161. Pollak VE, Mattenheimer H. Glutaminase activity in the kidney in gout. *J Lab Clin Med* 1965;66:564–570.
162. Sperling O, De Vries A, Kedem O. Studies on the etiology of uric acid lithiasis: 4. Urinary non-dialyzable substances in idiopathic uric acid lithiasis. *J Urol* 1965;94:286–292.
163. Coe FL, Lawton RL, Goldstein RB, et al. Sodium urate accelerates precipitation of calcium oxalate in vitro. *Proc Soc Exp Biol Med* 1975;149:926–929.
164. Ryall RL, Grover PK, Marshall VR. Urate and calcium stones—picking up a drop of mercury with one's fingers? *Am J Kidney Dis* 1991;17:426–430.
165. Nakagawa Y, Abram V, Coe FL. Isolation of calcium oxalate crystal growth inhibitor from rat kidney and urine. *Am J Physiol* 1984;247:F765–F772.
166. Berger L, Yü T-F. Renal function in gout: 4. An analysis of 524 gouty subjects including long-term follow-up studies. *Am J Med* 1975;59:605–613.
167. Reif MC, Constantiner A, Levitt MF. Chronic gouty nephropathy: a vanishing syndrome? *N Engl J Med* 1981;304:535–536.
168. Liang MH, Fries JF. Asymptomatic hyperuricemia: the case for conservative management. *Ann Intern Med* 1978;666–670.
169. Yü T-F, Berger L. Renal disease in primary gout: a study of 253 gout patients with proteinuria. *Semin Arthritis Rheum* 1975;4: 293–305.
170. Messerli FH, Frohlich ED, Dreslinski GR, et al. Serum uric acid in essential hypertension: an indicator of renal vascular involvement. *Ann Intern Med* 1980;93:817–821.
171. Talbott JH, Terplan KL. The kidney in gout. *Medicine* 1960;39:405–468.
172. Moro E, Ogg CS, Simmonds HA, et al. Familial juvenile gouty nephropathy with renal urate hypoexcretion preceding renal disease. *Clin Nephrol* 1991;35:263–269.
173. Cameron JS, Moro F, Simmonds HA. Gout, uric acid and purine metabolism in paediatric nephrology. *Pediatr Nephrol* 1993;7:105–118.
174. Puig JG, Miranda ME, Mateos FA, et al. Hereditary nephropathy associated with hyperuricemia and gout. *Arch Intern Med* 1993;153:357–365.
175. Stabellini N, Storari A, Aleotti A, et al. Familial interstitial nephropathy without hyperuricemia. *Nephron* 1994;66:215–218.
176. Lawrence RC, Helmick CG, Arnett FC, et al. Estimates of the prevalence of arthritis and selected musculoskeletal disorders in the United States. *Arthritis Rheum* 1998;41:778–799.
177. Zalokar J, Lellouch J, Claude JR. Goutte et uricemie dans une population de 4663 hommes jeunes actifs. *Sem Hop Paris* 1981; 57:664–670.
178. Prior IAM, Rose BS. Uric acid, gout and public health in the South Pacific. *N Z Med J* 1966;65:295–300.
179. Reed D, Labarthe D, Stallones R. Epidemiological studies of serum uric acid levels among Micronesians. *Arthritis Rheum* 1972;15:381–390.
180. Klemp P, Stansfield SA, Castle B, et al. Gout is on the increase in New Zealand Maori men. *Ann Rheum Dis* 1997;56:22–26.
181. Turner RE, Frank MJ, VanAusdal D, et al. Some aspects of the epidemiology of gout: sex and race incidence. *Arch Intern Med* 1960;106:400–406.
182. Roubenoff R, Klag MJ, Mead LA, et al. Incidence and risk factors for gout in white men. *JAMA* 1991;266:3004–3007.
183. Wallace SL, Robinson H, Masi AT, et al. Preliminary criteria for the classification of the acute arthritis of primary gout. *Arthritis Rheum* 1977;20:895–900.
184. Fam AG, Rubenstein J. Hydroxyapatite pseudopodagra: a syndrome of young women. *Arthritis Rheum* 1989;32:741–747.
185. Mines D, Abduhl SB. Hydroxyapatite pseudopodagra: acute calcific periarthritis of the first metatarsophalangeal joint. *Am J Emerg Med* 1996;14:180–182.
186. Rouault T, Caldwell DS, Holmes EW. Aspiration of the asymptomatic metatarsophalangeal joint in gout patients and hyperuricemic controls. *Arthritis Rheum* 1982;25:209–212.
187. Weinberger A, Agudelo CA, Schumacher HR, et al. Frequency of intra-articular monosodium urate (MSU) crystals in asymptomatic hyperuricemic subjects. *Adv Exp Med Biol* 1986;195A: 431–434.
188. Logan JA, Morrison E, McGill P. Serum uric acid in acute gout. *Ann Rheum Dis* 1997;56:696–697.
189. Wallace SL, Bernstein D, Diamond H. Diagnostic value of colchicine therapeutic trial. *JAMA* 1967;199:525–528.
190. Martel W. The overhanging margin of bone: a roentgenologic manifestation of gout. *Radiology* 1968;91:755–756.
191. Recht MP, Seragini F, Kramer J, et al. Isolated or dominant lesions of the patella in gout: a report of seven patients. *Skeletal Radiol* 1994;23:113–116.
192. Popp JD, Bidgood WD JR, Edwards NL. Magnetic resonance imaging of tophaceous gout in the hands and wrists. *Semin Arthritis Rheum* 1996;25:282–289.
193. Yu JS, Chung C, Recht M, et al. MRI imaging of tophaceous gout. *AJR Am J Roentgenol* 1997;168:523–527.
194. Gerster JC, Landry M, Duvoisin B, et al. Computed tomography of the knee joint as an indicator of intraarticular tophi in gout. *Arthritis Rheum* 1996;39:1406–1409.
195. Dodds WJ, Steinbach HL. Gout associated with calcification of cartilage. *N Engl J Med* 1966;275:745–749.
196. Good AE, Rapp R. Chondrocalcinosis of the knee with gout and rheumatoid arthritis. *N Engl J Med* 1967;277:286–290.
197. Alarcon-Segovia DA, Cetina JA, Diaz-Jouanen E. Sacroiliac joints in primary gout: clinical and roentgenographic study of 143 patients. *AJR Am J Roentgenol* 1973;118:438–443.
198. Smyth CJ. Hereditary factors in gout: a review of recent literature. *Metabolism* 1957;6:218–229.
199. Hauge M, Harvald B. Hereditary in gout and hyperuricemia. *Acta Med Scand* 1955;152:247–257.
200. Calabrese G, Simmonds HA, Cameron JS, et al. Precocious familial gout with reduced fractional urate clearance and normal purine enzymes. *Q J Med* 1990;78:441–445.
201. Laskarzewski PM, Khoury P, Morrison JA, et al. Familial hyper- and hypouricemia in random and hyperlipidemic recall cohorts: the Princeton School District Family Study. *Metabolism* 1983; 32:230–243.
202. Short EM. Hyperuricemia and gout. In: King RA, Rotter JI, Motulsky AG, eds. *Genetic basis of common diseases.* New York: Oxford University Press, 1992:482–506.
203. O'Brien WM, Burch TA, Bunim JJ. Genetics of hyperuricemia in Blackfeet and Pima Indians. *Ann Rheum Dis* 1966;25: 117–119.
204. Fiechtner JJ, Simkin PA. Urate spherulites in gouty synovia. *JAMA* 1981;245:1533–1536.
205. Weinberger A. Spherulite crystals in synovial tissue of a patient with recurrent monarthritis. *Clin Exp Rheumatol* 1984;2: 63–65.
206. Perricone E, Brandt KD. Enhancement of urate solubility by connective tissue: 1. Effect of proteoglycan aggregates and buffer cation. *Arthritis Rheum* 1978;21:453–460.
207. Brown J, Mallory GK. Renal changes in gout. *N Engl J Med* 1950;243:325–329.
208. Gonick HC, Rubini ME, Gleason IO, et al. The renal lesion in gout. *Ann Intern Med* 1965;62:667–674.
209. Emmerson BT, Cross M, Osborne JM, et al. Ultrastructural studies of the reaction of urate crystals with a cultured renal tubular cell line. *Nephron* 1991;59:403–408.
210. Paulus HE, Coutts A, Calabro JJ, et al. Clinical significance of hyperuricemia in routinely screened hospitalized men. *JAMA* 1970;211:277–281.

211. Brand FN, McGee DL, Kannel WB, et al. Hyperuricemia as a risk factor of coronary heart disease: the Framingham study. *Am J Epidemiol* 1985;121:11–18.
212. Maroko PR, McDevitt JT, Fox MJ, et al. Antihypertensive effectiveness of very low doses of hydrochlorothiazide: results of the PHICOG Trial. *Clin Ther* 1989;11:94–119.
213. Steele TH, Oppenheimer S. Factors affecting urate excretion following diuretic administration in man. *Am J Med* 1969;47:564–574.
214. Steele TH. Evidence for altered renal urate reabsorption during changes in volume of the extracellular fluid. *J Lab Clin Med* 1969;74:288–299.
215. Roos JC, Boer P, Peuker KH, et al. Changes in intrarenal uric acid handling during chronic spironolactone treatment in patients with essential hypertension. *Nephron* 1982;32: 209–213.
216. Scott JT, Higgens CS. Diuretic-induced gout: a multifactorial condition. *Ann Rheum Dis* 1992;51:259–261.
217. Gershon SL, Fox IH. Pharmacologic effects of nicotinic acid on human purine metabolism. *J Lab Clin Med* 1974;84:179–186.
218. Menon RK, Mikhailides BP, Bell JL, et al. Warfarin administration increases uric acid concentration in plasma. *Clin Chem* 1986;32:1557–1559.
219. Gores PF, Fryd DS, Sutherland DER, et al. Hyperuricemia after renal transplantation. *Am J Surg* 1988;156:397–400.
220. Gupta AK, Rocher LL, Schmaltz SP, et al. Short-term changes in renal function, blood pressure and electrolyte levels in patients receiving cyclosporine for dermatologic disorders. *Arch Intern Med* 1991;151:356–362.
221. MacLachlan MJ, Rodnan GP. Effects of food, fast and alcohol on serum uric acid and acute attacks of gout. *Am J Med* 1967; 42:38–57.
222. Ball GV, Sorensen LB. Pathogenesis of hyperuricemia in saturnine gout. *N Engl J Med* 1969;280:1199–1202.
223. Emmerson BT. Chronic lead nephropathy: the diagnostic use of calcium EDTA and the association with gout. *Aust Ann Med* 1963;12:310–324.
224. Halla JT, Ball GV. Saturnine gout: a review of 42 patients. *Semin Arthritis Rheum* 1982;11:307–314.
225. Batuman V, Moesaka JK, Haddad B, et al. The role of lead in gout nephropathy. *N Engl J Med* 1981;304:520–523.
226. Crosswell PW, Price J, Boyle PD, et al. Chronic renal failure with gout: a marker of chronic lead poisoning. *Kidney Int* 1984; 26:319–323.
227. Miranda ME, Puig JG, Mateos FA, et al. The role of lead in gout nephropathy reviewed: pathogenic or associated factor. *Adv Exp Med Biol Am* 1991;309:209–212.
228. Reynolds PP, Knapp MJ, Baraf HSB, et al. Moonshine and lead. Relationship to the pathogenesis and hyperuricemia in gout. *Arthritis Rheum* 1983;26:1057–1064.
229. Goldfinger S, Klinenberg JR, Seegmiller JE. Renal retention of uric acid induced by infusion of beta-hydroxybutyrate and acetoacetate. *N Engl J Med* 1965;272:351–355.
230. Steele TH, Rieselbach RE. The contribution of residual nephrons within the chronically diseased kidney to urate homeostasis in man. *Am J Med* 1967;43:876–886.
231. Sorensen LB, Levinson DJ. Origin and extrarenal elimination of uric acid in man. *Nephron* 1975;14:7–20.
232. Caner JEZ, Decker JL. Recurrent acute (gouty) arthritis in chronic renal failure treated with periodic hemodialysis. *Am J Med* 1964;36:571–582.
233. Reginato AJ, Ferreiro Seoane JL, Barbazan Alvarez, et al. Arthropathy and cutaneous calcinosis in hemodialysis oxalosis. *Arthritis Rheum* 1986;29:1387–1396.
234. Lynch EC. Uric acid metabolism in proliferative diseases of the marrow. *Arch Intern Med* 1962;109:639–653.
235. Martinez-Lavin M, Amigo M-C, Castillejos G, et al. Coexistent gout and hypertrophic osteoarthropathy in patients with cyanotic heart disease. *J Rheumatol* 1984;11:832–834.
236. Ross EA, Perloff JK, Danovitch GM, et al. Renal function and urate metabolism in late survivors with cyanotic congenital heart disease. *Circulation* 1986;73:396–400.
237. Diamond HS, Meisel A, Sharon E, et al. Hyperuricosuria and increased tubular secretion of urate in sickle cell disease. *Am J Med* 1975;59:796–802.
238. Paik CH, Alavi I, Dunea G, et al. Thalassemia and gouty arthritis. *JAMA* 1970;213:296–297.
239. Diamond HS, Meisel AD, Holden D. The natural history of urate overproduction in sickle cell anemia. *Ann Intern Med* 1979;90:752–757.
240. Espinoza LR, Spillberg I, Osterland CK. Joint manifestations of sickle cell disease. *Medicine* 1974;53:295–305.
241. Scott JT, Dixon A StJ, Bywaters EGL. Association of hyperuricemia and gout with hyperparathyroidism. *Br Med J* 1964; 1:1070–1073.
242. Castrillo JM, Diaz-Curiel M, Rapado A. Hyperuricemia in primary hyperparathyroidism: incidence and evolution after surgery. *Adv Exp Med Biol* 1984;165A:151–157.
243. Shelp WD, Steele TH, Rieselbach RE. Comparison of urinary phosphate, urate and magnesium excretion following parathyroid hormone administration to normal man. *Metabolism* 1969; 18:63–70.
244. Lambert JR, Wright V. Serum uric acid levels in psoriatic arthritis. *Ann Rheum Dis* 1977;36:264–267.
245. Puig JG, Mateos FA, Jimenez ML, et al. Uric acid metabolism in psoriasis. *Adv Exp Med Biol* 1986;195A:411–416.
246. Erickson AR, Enzenauer RJ, Nordstrom DM, et al. The prevalence of hypothyroidism in gout. *Am J Med* 1994;97:231–234.
247. Altman RD, Collins B. Musculoskeletal manifestations of Paget's disease of bone. *Arthritis Rheum* 1980;23:1121–1127.
248. Meyer WJ III, Gill JR Jr, Bartter FC. Gout as a complication of Bartter's syndrome: a possible role for alkalosis in the decreased clearance of uric acid. *Ann Intern Med* 1975; 83:56–59.
249. Brauer GW, Prior IAM. A prospective study of gout in New Zealand Maoris. *Ann Rheum Dis* 1978;37:466–472.
250. Fessel WJ, Bar GD. Uric acid, lean body weight and creatine interactions: results from regression analysis of 78 variables. *Semin Arthritis Rheum* 1977;7:115–121.
251. Glynn RJ, Campion EW, Silbert JE. Trends in serum uric acid levels 1961-1980. *Arthritis Rheum* 1983;26:87–93.
252. Scott JT. Obesity and hyperuricaemia. *Clin Rheum Dis* 1977; 3:25–35.
253. Sturge RA, Scott JT, Kennedy AC, et al. Serum uric acid in England and Scotland. *Ann Rheum Dis* 1977;36:420–427.
254. Seidell JC, Bakx KC, Deurenberg P, et al. Overweight and chronic illness: a retrospective cohort study with a follow-up of 6-17 years, in men and women of initially 20-50 years of age. *J Chronic Dis* 1986;39:585–593.
255. Bray GA. Complications of obesity. *Ann Intern Med* 1985;103: 1052–1062.
256. Kannel WB, Gordon T. Physiological and medical concomitant of obesity: the Framingham study. In: Bray GA, ed. *Obesity in America.* Bethesda: National Institutes of Health, DHEW No. (NIH), 1979:79–359.
257. Emmerson BT. Alteration of urate metabolism by weight reduction. *Aust N Z J Med* 1973;3:410–412.
258. Barlow KA. Hyperlipidemia in primary gout. *Metabolism* 1968; 17:289–299.
259. Gibson JT, Grahame R. Gout, hypertriglyceridemia, and alcohol consumption. *Ann Rheum Dis* 1974;33:109–110.
260. Naito HK, Mackenzie AH. Secondary hypertriglyceridemia and

hyperlipoproteinemia in patients with primary asymptomatic gout. *Clin Chem* 1979;25:371–375.

261. Jiao S, Kameda K, Matsuzawa Y, et al. Hyperlipoproteinemia in primary gout: hyperlipoproteinemic phenotype and influence of alcohol intake and obesity in Japan. *Ann Rheum Dis* 1986;45:308–313.
262. Matsubara K, Matsuzawa Y, Jiao S, et al. Relationship between hypertriglyceridemia and uric acid production in primary gout. *Metabolism* 1989;38:698–701.
263. Takahashi S, Yamamoto T, Moriwaki Y, et al. Impaired lipoprotein metabolism in patients with primary gout: influence of alcohol intake and body weight. *Br J Rheumatol* 1994;33: 731–734.
264. Fox IH, John D, DeBruyne S, et al. Hyperuricemia and hypertriglyceridemia: metabolic basis for the association. *Metabolism* 1985;34:741–746.
265. Emmerson B. Hyperlipidaemia in hyperuricaemia and gout. *Ann Rheum Dis* 1998;58:509–510.
266. Facchini F, Chen Y-D, Hollenbeck CB, et al. Relationship between resistance to insulin-mediated glucose uptake, urinary uric acid clearance, and plasma uric acid concentration. *JAMA* 1991;266:3008–3011.
267. Vuorin-Markkola H, Yki-Jarvonen H. Hyperuricemia and insulin-resistance. *J Clin Endocrinol Metab* 1994;78:25–29.
268. Reaven GM. Role of insulin-resistance in human disease. *Diabetes* 1988;37:1596–1607.
269. Carey GDP. Abdominal obesity. *Curr Opin Lipidol* 1998;9: 35–40.
270. Collantes Estevez E, Pineda Priego M, A-Non Barbudo J, et al. Hyperuricemia-hyperlipidemia association in the absence of obesity and alcohol abuse. *Clin Rheumatol* 1990;9:28–31.
271. Wiedemann E, Rose H, Schwartz E. Plasma lipoproteins, glucose tolerance and insulin response in primary gout. *Am J Med* 1972;53:299–307.
272. Lee J, Sparrow D, Vokonas PS, et al. Uric acid and coronary heart disease risk: evidence for a role of uric acid in the obesity-insulin resistance syndrome. *Am J Epidemiol* 1995;142: 288–294.
273. Myers AR, Epstein FH, Dodge HJ, et al. The relationship of serum uric acid to risk factors in coronary heart disease. *Am J Med* 1968;45:520–528.
274. Kahn HA, Medalie JH, Neufeld HN, et al. The incidence of hypertension and associated factors: the Israel ischemic heart disease study. *Am Heart J* 1972;84:171–182.
275. Rapado A. Relationship between gout and arterial hypertension. *Adv Exp Med Biol* 1974;41B:451–459.
276. Prebis JW, Gruskin AB, Polinsky MS, et al. Uric acid in childhood essential hypertension. *J Pediatr* 1981;98:702–707.
277. Freedman DS, Williamson DF, Gunter EW, et al. Relation of serum uric acid to mortality and ischemic heart disease: the NHANES I epidemologic follow-up study. *Am J Epidemiol* 1995;141:637–644.
278. Yano K, Reed DM, McGee DL. Ten year incidence of coronary heart disease in the Honolulu heart program: relationship to biologic and lifestyle characteristics. *Am J Epidemiol* 1984;119: 653–666.
279. Lehto S, Niskanen L, Ronnemaa T, et al. Serum uric acid is a strong predictor of stroke in patients with non-insulin dependent diabetes mellitus. *Stroke* 1998;29:635–639.
280. Abbott RD, Brand FN, Kannel WB, et al. Gout and coronary heart disease: the Framingham study. *J Clin Epidemiol* 1988;41: 237–242.
281. Prior IAM, Rose BS, Harvey HP, et al. Hyperuricemia, gout and diabetic abnormality in Polynesian people. *Lancet* 1966;1: 333–338.
282. Culleton BF, Larson M, Kannel WB, et al. Serum uric acid and risk for cardiovascular disease and death: the Framingham heart study. *Ann Intern Med* 1999;131:7–13.

115

MANAGEMENT OF HYPERURICEMIA

N. LAWRENCE EDWARDS

Hyperuricemia is a common biochemical abnormality that in the majority of affected individuals will not result in clinical disease state or tissue pathology. It is frequently associated with other metabolic perturbations such as increased body mass, hypertension, hypertriglyceridemia, and non–insulin-dependent diabetes mellitus (1,2). Large population studies in the United States have demonstrated an overall prevalence of approximately 5% (3,4). Studies of hyperuricemia in hospitalized populations reveal a much higher prevalence of 17% to 28% because of the combined effects of illnesses and medications (5,6). Aside from its classic clinical associations with gout and nephrolithiasis, hyperuricemia has recently come under intense scrutiny for its possible pathogenic role in the development of renal disease, coronary artery disease, and salt-dependent hypertension (7).

A rational approach to hyperuricemia requires the clinician to answer the following questions: (a) Is the individual truly hyperuricemic? (b) What is the basis of the hyperuricemia? and (c) Is it important to lower the serum urate concentration? (8).

DEFINITION OF HYPERURICEMIA

Hyperuricemia can be defined either physiologically or epidemiologically. The serum urate value is theoretically elevated when it exceeds 6.4 mg/dL, the limit of solubility of monosodium urate (MSU) in serum at 37°C. In most epidemiologic studies, the upper limit is 7.0 mg/dL in men and 6.0 mg/dL in women (9). Many clinical laboratories, however, will indicate that a serum urate value is elevated only when it is greater than two standard deviations above the mean value of the population served. With this mechanism for defining hyperuricemia, it is not uncommon for the upper limit of normal range to be as high as 8.0 to 8.5 mg/dL.

The serum urate concentration varies with both the sex and the age of the patient. Children of both sexes normally have a serum urate concentration of 3 to 4 mg/dL (9). At puberty, boys exhibit a further elevation in serum urate concentration of 1 to 2 mg/dL, which is generally sustained throughout life. In girls, there is little if any change in serum urate levels through adolescence and young adult life. At menopause, however, the serum urate concentration increases and approaches the value for adult men.

In the Normative Aging Study, subjects with serum urate levels of 9.0 mg/dL or more had a cumulative incidence of gouty arthritis of 22% at 5 years, whereas those with urate concentrations of 7.0 to 8.9 mg/dL had a 5-year cumulative incidence of 3% (10). The incidence of gout increases with age and with the degree of hyperuricemia, but it is important to distinguish hyperuricemia from gout. A sustained elevation in serum urate is essential in the pathogenesis of gout but by itself is insufficient to cause gout. The vast majority of patients with hyperuricemia will never develop symptoms associated with uric acid excess, such as gout, tophi, or kidney stones (11).

CAUSES OF HYPERURICEMIA

Hyperuricemia may be classified as either primary or secondary. Primary hyperuricemia refers to those cases that are not associated with other clinical disorders or medications. Whereas some cases of primary gout have a genetic basis, others do not. Secondary hyperuricemia refers to cases that develop in the course of another disease or as a consequence of drug intake. The relative frequency of primary versus secondary forms of hyperuricemia depends on the clinical setting. One study of hospitalized subjects reported a 30% and 70% incidence of primary and secondary hyperuricemia, respectively (5).

There are two major causes of hyperuricemia: increased production of uric acid and decreased excretion of uric acid. Overproduction of uric acid is, by far, less common and may account for as little as 5% of hyperuricemia in the gouty population (9).

Increased Uric Acid Production

Two inborn errors in purine metabolism account for virtually all the cases of primary uric acid overproduction (Table

TABLE 115.1. CAUSES OF HYPERURICEMIA: INCREASED URIC ACID PRODUCTION

Primary hyperuricemia
- HPRT deficiency
  - Complete: Lesch–Nyhan syndrome
  - Partial: Kelley–Seegmiller syndrome
- PP-ribose-P synthetase overactivity

Secondary hyperuricemia
- Increased ATP degradation
  - Glucose-6-phosphatase deficiency
  - Tissue hypoxia
  - Ethanol consumption
- Increased nucleic acid turnover
  - Blood dyscrasias
  - Malignancy
  - Infectious mononucleosis
  - Psoriasis
  - Tumor lysis syndrome

HPRT, hypoxanthine–guanine phosphoribosyl transferase; PP-ribose-P synthetase, 5-phosphoribosyl-1 pyrophosphate synthatase; ATP, adenosine triphosphate.

115.1). Intracellular 5-phosphoribosyl-1-pyrophosphate (PP-ribose-P) is a high-energy sugar that activates amidophosphoribosyltransferase, the rate-limiting enzyme of *de novo* purine biosynthesis. Patients with hypoxanthine-guanine phosphoribosyltransferase (HPRT) deficiency have a decreased consumption of PP-ribose-P (12). In these rare patients and the very rare subjects with phosphoribosylpyrophosphate synthetase overactivity, the accumulated PP-ribose-P accelerates purine biosynthesis and results in uric acid overproduction (13).

Multiple causes of secondary hyperuricemia are associated with increased production of uric acid (Table 115.1). In various disease states, accelerated consumption of adenosine triphosphate (ATP) results in increased uric acid synthesis. In glucose-6-phosphatase deficiency (von Gierke's disease), hypoglycemia-induced glycogen degradation results in depletion of the hepatic ATP pool. Hyperuricemia is observed in many acutely ill patients and may be related to accelerated ATP degradation (14,15). Patients in the intensive care unit with acute myocardial infarction, smoke inhalation, respiratory failure, and status epilepticus are in this category. Finally, excessive alcohol consumption is associated with increased synthesis of uric acid secondary to accelerated degradation of ATP (16).

Hyperuricemia also occurs as a result of an increased turnover of DNA and RNA (Table 115.1). A number of diseases including the myeloproliferative and lymphoproliferative disorders, multiple myeloma, secondary polycythemia, pernicious anemia, certain hemoglobinopathies, hemolytic anemias, infectious mononucleosis, psoriasis, and some carcinomas may be associated with increased marrow activity or increased cell turnover at other sites. Tumor lysis syndrome is a generalized metabolic disturbance associated with lymphoproliferative malignancies after spontaneous or chemotherapy-induced cytolysis (17). Hyperuricemia is frequently the most dramatic and damaging consequence of tumor lysis syndrome.

Decreased Uric Acid Excretion

Uric acid is the end product of purine metabolism in humans, and its excretion is by renal and extrarenal routes. Two thirds of daily urate turnover is accounted for in the urine. The other one third is excreted in intestinal secretions (saliva, gastric juice, bile, and pancreatic secretions). Bacteria degrade uric acid in these secretions to allantoin and carbon dioxide by a process called intestinal uricolysis (18). The rate of intestinal loss of uric acid is directly dependent on serum urate concentration.

The kidney's mechanisms of handling uric acid excretion are localized primarily in the glomerulus and in the proximal convoluted tubule (Fig. 115.1). This widely accepted four-component model of renal uric acid disposal consists of filtration, tubular reabsorption (early), tubular secretion, and postsecretory tubular reabsorption (late). Plasma urate is thought to be freely filterable at the glomerulus except for the very small fraction that is protein bound (1–4%). The filtered urate is then almost completely reabsorbed by an active transport system in the proximal tubule. Linkage between urate reabsorption and the reabsorption of other components of the glomerular filtrate such as sodium, glucose, calcium, and bicarbonate has been demonstrated (19,20). There continues to be debate as to whether urate is

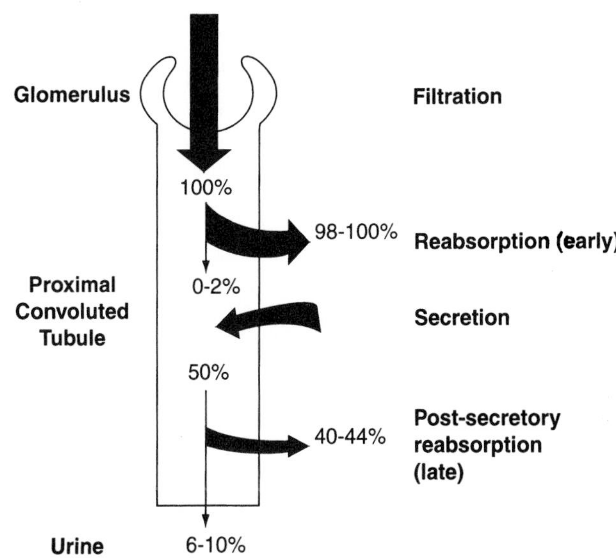

FIGURE 115.1. The four-component model of urate handling by the kidney. Uric acid is filtered at the glomerulus and then undergoes bidirectional transport within the proximal convoluted tubule. The percentages represent the fraction of urate filtered at the glomerulus that is subsequently transported.

secreted into the collecting system by a secretory pathway shared by many weak organic acids (like lactate, β-hydroxybutyrate, acetoacetate, and keto acids) or through a urate-specific secretory mechanism. A final adjustment in the amount of uric acid to be either retained or excreted is made by a postsecretory reabsorptive process. It is this latter mechanism in the proximal tubule that is influenced by our current uricosuric agents.

Most patients with primary hyperuricemia (85% to 90%) have a defect in renal handling of uric acid. Gouty subjects and nongouty controls have similar sigmoidal relations between plasma urate concentration and uric acid excretion rate (Fig. 115.2). However, subjects with primary gout excrete relatively less uric acid in the urine for any given plasma urate concentration. This "shift to the right" of excretory kinetics in subjects with primary gout (compared with nongouty subjects) may be caused by one or more perturbations of urate handling in the proximal convoluted tubule (Table 115.2). The favored hypotheses underlying this defect include enhanced postsecretory reabsorption and decreased secretory response for a given level of urate (21,22).

A decreased renal excretion of uric acid is the most common cause of secondary hyperuricemia. Virtually any form of renal disease that leads to functional impairment

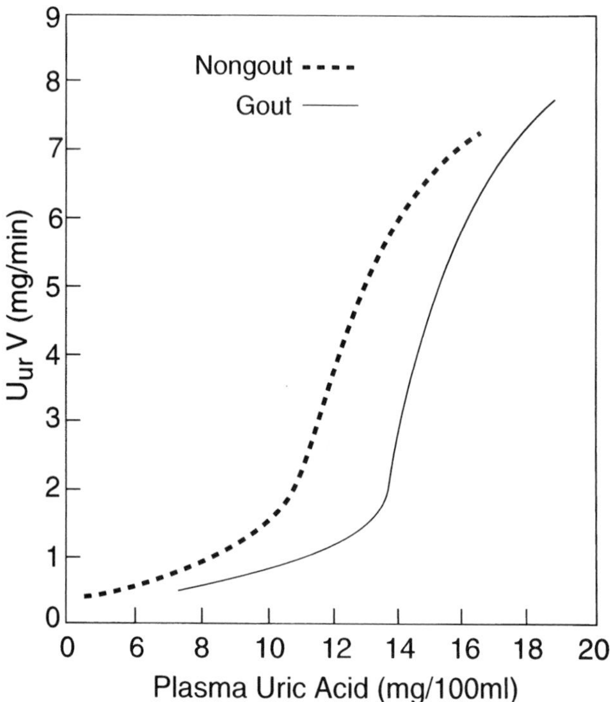

FIGURE 115.2. The relation between plasma urate concentration and the rate of urinary uric acid excretion in nongouty and gouty subjects. Patients with primary gout have less efficient excretion kinetics, resulting in greater retention of uric acid. (Adapted from Wyngaarden JB. Gout. *Adv Metab Dis* 1965;2:1–78, with permission).

TABLE 115.2. CAUSES OF HYPERURICEMIA: DECREASED URIC ACID EXCRETION

Primary hyperuricemia
- Decreased filtered load
- Increased tubular reabsorption
- Decreased tubular secretion

Secondary hyperuricemia
- Reduced renal functional mass
  - Chronic renal disease
- Increased tubular reabsorption: contraction of extracellular volume
  - Dehydration
  - Diabetes mellitus
  - Diuretics
- Decreased tubular secretion: associated with increased organic acidemia
  - Starvation
  - Diabetic ketoacidosis
  - Acute ethanol ingestion
  - Toxemia of pregnancy
- Decreased tubular secretion: associated with drug administration
  - Salicylates (<2 g/24 h)
  - Phenylbutazone (<200 mg/24 h)
  - Thiazide diuretics
  - Cyclosporine
  - Levodopa
  - Ethambutol
  - Nicotinic acid
- Mechanism not established
  - Chronic lead exposure
  - Berylliosis
  - Sarcoidosis

many result in hyperuricemia. In chronic renal insufficiency, urate excretion per unit of glomerular filtration rate tends to increase progressively with advancing severity of disease. However, this adaptation is incomplete, and hyperuricemia occurs. Other renal conditions that result in increased tubular reabsorption or decreased tubular secretion also will lead to hyperuricemia (Table 115.2). Chronic lead intoxication, beryllıosis, and sarcoidosis also affect kidneys in such a manner as to result in secondary hyperuricemia, although the exact mechanism(s) remains unclear.

COMPLICATIONS OF HYPERURICEMIA

Tissue damage associated with hyperuricemia is caused by the precipitation of urate crystals in soft tissues and organ parenchyma. Urate crystals are the classic needle-like crystals associated with gouty arthritis. Uric acid crystals also can form, but only at very low pH, as in the lumen of renal collecting tubules. These crystals are usually amorphous in shape. Regional factors that influence the precipitation of urate include urate concentration, temperature, ambient pH, and the presence of nucleation factors. The current list of physiologically important nucleators is short, with the leading contenders being type I collagen and a γ globulin subfraction (11,23).

Gouty Arthritis

The most widely recognized complications of hyperuricemia are the acute and chronic forms of arthritis associated with gout. Arthritis usually occurs after decades of "asymptomatic hyperuricemia," although the duration of this asymptomatic period will vary greatly depending on the degree of serum urate elevation and other factors. In cyclosporine-induced hyperuricemia, the asymptomatic interval may be as short as 6 to 12 months (24–26).

The period of acute intermittent gout may last for a decade or more. During this stage, the joints and bony structures generally remain free of significant destruction, as demonstrated by a lack of radiographic changes (other than transient soft tissue swelling), and a return to normal pain-free function of involved joint(s) during intercritical periods is characteristic.

Chronic tophaceous gout, on the other hand, is a disabling, erosive arthritis in which entire bones are occasionally replaced with deposits of MSU. Unfortunately, plain radiographs and physical examination tend to underestimate the amount of skeletal destruction associated with chronic gouty arthritis (27).

Nodules

The subcutaneous tophus is the most characteristic lesion of chronic gouty arthritis. Similar-appearing nodules are clinically observed in other rheumatic disorders such as rheumatoid arthritis (RA) (28) and multicentric reticulohistiocytosis (29) and may lead to diagnostic confusion. Parallels can be drawn between nodule formation in RA and tophus formation in gout. The nodular aspects of both diseases are generally observed in the most chronic and severe cases, but are not a universal consequence of the disease process and may appear in patients with clinically inapparent joint disease. However, a subcutaneous collection of MSU crystals is pathognomonic for gout. Subcutaneous gouty tophi may be found anywhere over the body but occur most commonly at pressure points. Tophi also may occur in and around articular structures as well as the connective tissues at other sites (e.g., tendons, renal pyramids, heart valves, and sclerae). As with the chronic destructive arthritis they are frequently associated with, tophi themselves may lead to physical disability and pain (30).

Nephrolithiasis

The renal collecting ducts are the only site in the body where local pH is low enough to allow the formation of amorphous uric acid crystals. At a pH of 7.4, 98% of uric acid is the form of the monosodium salt of the urate ion (MSU). At a pH of 5.7 or less, most of the urate ion is converted to nonionized uric acid. In water, uric acid is 20-fold less soluble than urate, and solubility declines with decreasing pH (31). Uric acid crystallization in urine is primarily influenced by urine pH and the concentration of uric acid being excreted. The presence or absence of natural inhibitors of crystallization, including citrate and glycosaminoglycan, also is an important factor (32).

In approximately 20% of individuals with gout, uric acid kidney stones will develop at some time in their disease course. Occasionally, symptomatic uric acid calculi will precede other complications of hyperuricemia such as gouty arthritis or tophi formation. Nearly 75% of all patients with uric acid stones will demonstrate no other manifestations of hyperuricemia (33). Whether this is because local renal factors other than hyperuricemia play a disproportionately large role in stone formation or because of therapeutic intervention is not clear.

Pure uric acid stones are radiolucent and therefore difficult to detect by routine radiographic studies. Although these compose only 10% of all kidney stones, a uric acid nidus may be at the core of many of the more common calcium-containing calculi (34). For this reason, hyperuricemic patients with calcium oxalate stones or normouricemic stone formers who have a daily uric acid excretion in excess of 750 mg are usually given allopurinol to prevent recurrent stone formation.

Renal Insufficiency

Two types of renal parenchymal pathology have been attributed to hyperuricemia. *Acute uric acid nephropathy* develops in the setting of sudden uricosuria associated with chemotherapy for hematologic malignancies. *Chronic urate nephropathy* is a more insidious condition in which microtophi of MSU crystals form in the tubulointerstitium of the renal medulla. Although both conditions are widely recognized, the etiopathogenesis and significance of the latter have been debated.

Acute uric acid nephropathy is a preventable complication of the tumor lysis syndrome (17,35). Patients undergoing chemotherapy or radiation therapy for leukemia or lymphoma can develop massive uricosuria. Crystallization of uric acid/urate within the collecting systems and tubules can be precipitate and result in acute renal failure. Whereas most patients will demonstrate marked increases in serum urate levels, the urinary uric acid concentration is of greater importance in establishing the diagnosis. A ratio of uric acid to creatinine of greater than 1.0 in the urine of a patient with acute renal failure is pathognomonic for this condition (36).

The role of hyperuricemia in chronic renal insufficiency has been debated for decades. The presence of MSU microtophi in the medullary tubulointerstitium is a common finding in chronic hyperuricemia. Whether these pathologic changes are responsible for the progressive and irreversible renal insufficiency observed in these individuals is not clear. This population of hyperuricemic patients is almost always hypertensive. Yu et al. (37) examined renal dysfunction in their large gouty population and assumed that hypertension and hyperuricemia were independent events. As a result, they excluded all hypertensive subjects (two thirds of total population) and concluded that hyperuricemia and gout were not directly injurious to the kidney. Recently, however, a direct connection between tubulointerstitial damage from urate microtophi and the development of salt-dependent hypertension has been postulated (38). According to this hypothesis, some forms of hypertension are the result of acquired structural injury to the kidney that leads to impaired salt excretion. The linkage of urate and sodium reabsorption in the proximal tubule further exacerbates this form of hypertension in hyperuricemic subjects. Although unproven, this scenario raises the cautionary point that in young gouty patients with no obvious renal disease, destructive and irreversible structural changes may be occurring in the kidney.

Hypertension and Cardiovascular Disease

Hyperuricemia is strongly associated with excess mortality from many forms of cardiovascular disease (39). If a patient is hyperuricemic and hypertensive, there is an increased risk for both coronary and cerebral vascular diseases compared with individuals that are hypertensive alone. Several studies have demonstrated a threefold to fivefold increase in coronary artery disease and cerebrovascular events in hyperuricemic compared with normouricemic individuals with hypertension (40,41). However, a direct effect of hyperuricemia on cardiovascular disease appears less likely since the release of The Framingham Study (42). Hyperuricemia is a component of a cluster of abnormalities associated with insulin resistance, termed syndrome X (43–45). This syndrome, which also includes hyperinsulinemia, hypertension, high plasma triglycerides, and low high-density lipoprotein cholesterol, is associated with coronary artery disease. This may explain the previously recognized association between hyperuricemia and heart disease. Although not a direct risk factor, hyperuricemia may be considered an indicator of heart disease, as well as other forms of global hypoxia including obstructive pulmonary disease and neonatal hypoxia (46,47). Hyperuricemia is predictive of high blood pressure in adolescent boys, but not in women (48). In patients with essential hypertension, hyperuricemia most likely reflects early renal vascular involvement (nephrosclerosis) (49). No study has demonstrated that reducing the serum urate concentration in either an asymptomatic hyperuricemic person or a patient with gout prevents cardiac disease or decreases hypertension.

EVALUATION OF HYPERURICEMIA

The significance of hyperuricemia in an individual is readily determined with a good history and physical examination and the use of several basic laboratory tests. The evaluation is directed at establishing that the hyperuricemia as either primary or secondary. A detailed history and physical examination will go a long way in making this distinction. The hyperuricemia can be further defined by evaluating the individual for reduced renal clearance of uric acid versus purine overproduction. This latter categorization will frequently require laboratory evaluation. A final aspect of the evaluation is to determine what damage, if any, is being caused by the hyperuricemia.

The main causes of secondary hyperuricemia are listed in Tables 115.1 and 115.2. They include diabetes mellitus, chronic renal insufficiency, alcohol consumption (especially beer), or the use of any medications that adversely affect serum urate concentration. When detailed history taking has excluded any of these secondary causes, then the hyperuricemia is said to be "primary." Although there is considerable overlap, serum urate concentration is generally higher with secondary causes (Fig. 115.3). A serum urate value of 11 mg/dL or higher is very suggestive of a secondary form of hyperuricemia (50).

Serum uric acid measurement with the uricase method is the accepted standard for detecting hyperuricemia. The

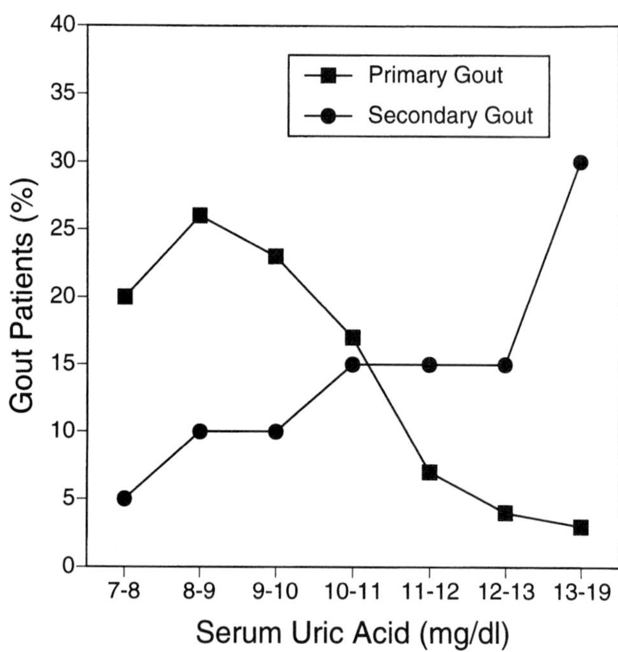

FIGURE 115.3. The distribution of serum urate levels in primary and secondary gout. Few subjects with primary gout have serum urate values >11 mg/dL. Only 25% of secondary gout is associated with urate levels <10 mg/dL. (Adapted from Talbott JH, Yu T-F. Secondary gout. In: *Gout and uric acid metabolism.* New York: Stratton Medical Book Co., 1976:191–204).

older colorimetric assays for uric acid were less reliable because of interference by several drugs. Two new methods for assessing uric acid levels have recently been reported. Salivary uric acid levels were tested in gouty and healthy controls. The assay appears to be a sensitive, reliable, and noninvasive surrogate for standard serum sampling (51). Another noninvasive approach for monitoring uric acid concentration is by scalp hair sampling (52). Hair from hyperuricemic patients and normouricemic volunteers was collected, and the portion 10 to 20 mm from the scalp was sampled for uric acid. This 10-mm sample represents 1 month of hair growth, and the urate concentration correlated well with serum values obtained 1 month before.

Single serum urate determinations are not adequate for documenting the presence and degree of hyperuricemia. Dietary changes, exercise, and medications cause considerable flux in urate concentration. The stress of severe pain has a uricosuric effect, and approximately 40% of patients with acute gouty attacks will have normal serum urate levels (53,54). The preattack hyperuricemia will again become evident as the pain of acute gout subsides.

A 24-hour urinary uric acid measurement is the standard used to determine whether hyperuricemia is caused by purine overproduction or uric acid underexcretion. The classic studies were conducted on men ingesting purine-free diets and suggested that a 24-hour urinary uric acid of greater that 600 mg was characteristic of purine overproduction states; less than 600 mg per day in the face of hyperuricemia suggested renal underexcretion as the causative mechanism (55). In the normal clinical setting, it is not practical to place patients on purine-free diets for 3 to 5 days before collecting a 24-hour urine sample. On a regular Western diet, a 24-hour urinary uric acid value in excess of 1,000 mg per day is clearly abnormal, whereas 800 to 1,000 mg per day is a borderline value.

Simplified methods have been sought for assessing uric acid overproduction. Proposed techniques included determining the ratio of uric acid to creatinine in a "spot urine" or the ratio of uric acid clearance to creatinine clearance (56). Comparison of these two ratios with the 24-hour urinary uric acid excretion, however, reveals a poor correlation, largely because of a striking diurnal variation in the excretion of uric acid (57).

Traditionally, the 24-hour urine collection for uric acid has been viewed as a valuable tool in assessing risk of stones, elucidating underlying factors, and determining which urate-lowering agent to use (58,59). How useful this time-honored measurement is to the clinical management of gout and hyperuricemia remains controversial (60).

TREATMENT TECHNIQUES

General Approach

The stereotype of the gouty patient as a corpulent, hypertensive, overimbibing, middle-aged man is an accurate characterization often enough that there is usually a role for lifestyle modification in the management of hyperuricemia and gout. Before the advent of effective uric acid–lowering agents, dietary purine restriction was a mainstay of therapeutic intervention (61). Unfortunately, even a severe reduction in purine intake will rarely reduce serum urate levels by more than 1 mg/dL unless the patient has an unusually high consumption of purine-rich foods on a long-term basis. It is worthwhile to quiz hyperuricemic subjects for a dietary pattern that may contain unusual quantities of purine-rich foods (Table 115.3). If an excessive pattern of purine consumption is identified, the subject should be counseled regarding moderation. With the availability of modern uric acid–reducing agents, there is little benefit from severe purine restriction in most patients.

TABLE 115.3. COMMON FOODS WITH HIGH PURINE CONTENT

Very High	High
Brewer's yeast	Bacon
Anchovies	Beer
Herring	Liver
Sardines	Lobster
Mussels	Salmon
Clams	Sweetbreads (pancreas)
	Turkey
	Veal

Other lifestyle modifications also can be helpful in the treatment of hyperuricemia. Dietary counseling for weight loss in obese and hypertensive patients will help reduce urate levels. Regular alcohol consumption should be discouraged because it can stimulate increased purine production (16). Episodic acute intoxication also can cause hyperuricemia on the basis of transient hyperlacticacidemia and interference with renal uric acid excretion (62). Beer drinking can be especially problematic because it not only exerts an ethanol effect on purine production and elimination but also is a purine-rich food.

Before initiating uric acid–reducing therapy, the physician should review the patient's current medications to determine if any might be contributing to the hyperuricemia (Table 115.2). Potential offending drugs (especially thiazide diuretics) should be replaced with alternatives. Several medications have a paradoxic effect on uric acid excretion (Table 115.4); that is, a low dose of these medications results in elevated serum urate levels, whereas a higher dose results in hypouricemia. The mechanism for

TABLE 115.4. DRUGS WITH PARADOXIC EFFECTS ON URATE EXCRETION

Salicylate	Ethacrinic acid
Probenicid	Acetazolamide
Phenylbutazone	Pyrazinamide

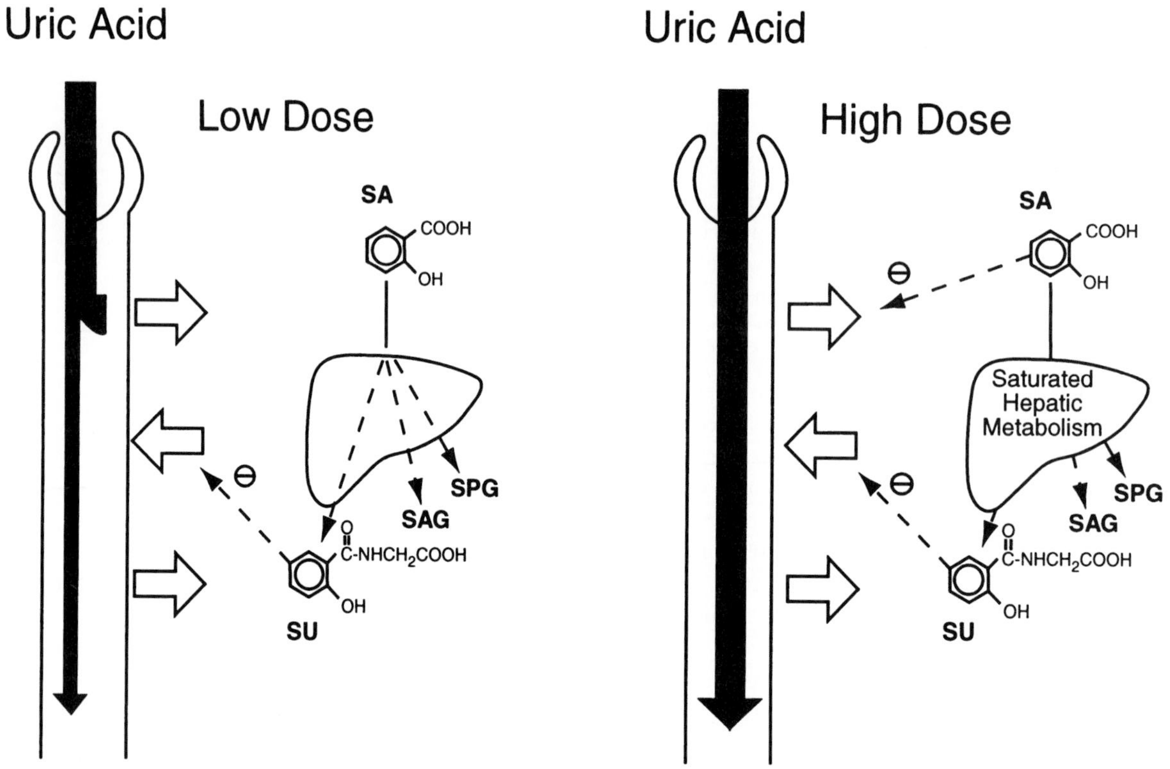

FIGURE 115.4. The proposed mechanism for the paradoxic effect of salicylate (*SA*) on serum urate levels. At low-dose aspirin, salicylurate (*SU*) is the main metabolite and is a competitive inhibitor of uric acid secretion in the proximal tubule, leading to hyperuricemia. At high-dose aspirin, serum SA levels increase and inhibit early reabsorption of uric acid. This results in hypouricemia.

this paradoxic effect has not been elucidated for all of these medications. For salicylate, a mechanism has been proposed that may, in general, be applicable to the other agents listed in Table 115.4. When aspirin is administered in low doses (<1.5 g/day), its metabolism and elimination are by hepatic conjugation to form salicylurate (SU) and, to a lesser extent, salicyl acyl glucuronide (SAG) and salicyl phenolic glucuronide (SPG) (Fig. 115.4). SU is a competitive inhibitor of the urate secretory system, resulting in hyperuricemia. When aspirin intake is increased to 4.8 g per day (approximately 14 tablets), hepatic metabolism of salicylate to SU becomes saturated. Salicylate concentration in the serum increases, and salicylate becomes a major excretory product along with SU. Salicylate inhibits tubular reabsorption of urate at the early and, possibly, late sites, resulting in uricosuria and hypouricemia (63).

Urate-lowering Drugs

Reduction of the serum urate concentration is achieved pharmacologically by (a) increasing the renal excretion of uric acid or (b) by decreasing uric acid synthesis. The urate-lowering drugs (ULDs) most widely used in the United States are the uricosuric agents, probenecid and sulfinpyrazone, and the uric acid synthesis inhibitor, allopurinol. Benzbromarone is a uricosuric drug not available in the U.S., but extensively used in other parts of the world. The antiinflammatory agent, diflunisal, and the angiotensin II receptor antagonist, losartan, both have uricosuric effects that may, in selected patients, have clinical utility.

Uricosuric Agents

Uricosuric agents are successful 70% to 80% of the time in achieving optimal serum urate levels. These drugs lose effectiveness as renal function deteriorates and are completely ineffective when the glomerular filtration rate reaches 30 mL per minute or less. Probenecid and sulfinpyrazone require multiple doses per day and may interfere with other medications being used by the patient. For these reasons, compliance becomes a problem in the long-term use of these agents. A reasonable candidate for treatment with uri-

TABLE 115.5. INDICATIONS FOR USE OF URICOSURIC AGENTS

Hyperuricemia with uric acid urinary excretion of less than 800 mg/24 h on a regular diet
Satisfactory renal function (creatinine clearance greater than 50 ml/min)
No history of renal calculi
Younger than 60 years
Lack of polypharmacy

cosuric agents might be a gouty subject with the features described in Table 115.5.

Probenecid

Probenecid was initially developed as a drug to help maintain higher serum levels of penicillin when penicillin was a rare and precious commodity after World War II (64). Probenecid is rapidly and completely absorbed by the gastrointestinal tract and is more than 70% eliminated from the circulation in 24 hours (65). The biologic half-life is between 6 and 12 hours and is dose dependent. The uricosuric activity of probenecid is due largely to inhibition of renal tubular reabsorption of uric acid at the postsecretory reabsorptive site (Fig. 115.1).

Therapy is begun at 250 mg twice each day and is increased as necessary up to 3 g per day. Optimal serum urate control can be achieved with 1 g day or less in 50% of gouty patients and in 85% with 2 g per day or less (66). Because of the serum half-life of 6 to 12 hours, probenecid should be taken in two or three evenly spaced doses.

Probenecid is generally well tolerated, with approximately 5% of patients developing complications such as rash, fever, gastric irritation, or precipitation of acute gout or nephrolithiasis. Acute gouty arthritis can usually be avoided by the concomitant use of colchicine or a nonsteroidal antiinflammatory drug (NSAID). Renal stones can be avoided by maintaining adequate urine volume and an alkaline urine pH, as well as a slow escalation of the probenecid dose. Gastric irritation is usually abated by taking the medication with meals. Other rare toxicities of probenecid include nephrotic syndrome (67) and hepatotoxicity (68). Probenecid influences the metabolism and elimination of multiple other medications (Table 115.6).

TABLE 115.6. DRUG–DRUG INTERACTIONS WITH PROBENECID

Ampicillin	Salicylates
Penicillin	Indomethacin
Nafcillin	Heparin
Cephradine	Dapsone
Cephaloridine	Rifampicin

Sulfinpyrazone

Sulfinpyrazone is an analogue of the antiinflammatory drug phenylbutazone. Sulfinpyrazone has no antiinflammatory activity, but is a potent uricosuric and also exerts an antiplatelet effect. Like probenecid, it is rapidly absorbed in the gastrointestinal tract, although its plasma half-life is much shorter at 1 to 3 hours (69). Renal insufficiency lessens the effectiveness of sulfinpyrazone, but not to the same extent as with probenecid. Its mechanism of action is the same as that of probenecid.

In the treatment of gout, sulfinpyrazone is initiated at a dose of 50 mg, twice a day, with incremental increases to 100 mg and then 200 mg twice daily as needed to achieve optimal urate control. This medication is generally well tolerated, with many of the same complications as probenecid. Gastrointestinal side effects are found in 10% to 15% of treated subjects. Bone marrow toxicity has been reported (70) and drug–drug interactions with oral hypoglycemic agents and sulfa drugs also have been described (71).

Benzbromarone

Benzbromarone is a very potent uricosuric drug that is widely used outside of the U.S. In animal studies it exhibits weak inhibitory effects on xanthine oxidase, although in humans, this effect is clinically insignificant (72,73). Its mechanism of action is similar to that of probenecid and sulfinpyrazone (74), but it is much more effective in renal insufficiency than is either of these other uricosurics. However, a creatinine clearance of less than 20 mg per minute renders this drug inactive as well. Only 21 of 780 subjects taking benzbromarone discontinued the drug because of side effects (75). The medication is administered in a once-a-day schedule, with doses ranging from 25 to 120 mg.

Diflunisal

Diflunisal (Dolobid) is a fluorinated salicylate that is commonly used as an NSAID. From the time of its release, diflunisal was known to have moderate uricosuric effects at all dose levels studied (76,77). Early studies suggested that diflunisal induced a competitive inhibition of xanthine oxidase *in vitro,* whereas *in vivo* studies in gouty subjects indicated a complex hypouricemic effect that depended on the uric acid excretory characteristics of the individual patients (78). Follow-up investigations showed no increase in plasma xanthine levels in subjects taking diflunisal, thus discounting any significant xanthine oxidase inhibition (79). This same study demonstrated a mean reduction in plasma urate of 33% with diflunisal compared with a 48% decrease with allopurinol. Dosing at 500 to 1,000 mg per day in divided doses is effective for both analgesic and uricosuric effects.

Losartan

Losartan is a member of a new class of antihypertensive agents: the angiotensin II receptor antagonists. It is as effective as angiotensin-converting enzyme (ACE) inhibitors, calcium channel blockers, or β-blockers in lowering blood pressure, but losartan also possesses uricosuric activity (80). Investigators have found this drug useful in treating cyclosporine-induced hyperuricemia in renal and heart transplant recipients (81). In patients with recalcitrant hyperuricemia because of dependency on diuretics, the addition of ACE inhibitors also is helpful in reducing serum urate levels (82).

Inhibitors of Urate Synthesis

Allopurinol

Allopurinol is the most commonly prescribed ULD because of its easy dosing regimen, its broad range of efficacy, and its generally good safety profile. Allpurinol is a structural analogue of hypoxanthine, in which a pyrazolo instead of an imidazole ring is attached to pyrimidine ring (Fig. 115.5). Although it was originally designed to be an antitumor agent, its primary biologic activity is to inhibit the uric acid–generating enzyme, xanthine oxidase (83). Allopurinol is both a substrate and competitive inhibitor of xanthine oxidase. The plasma half-life of allopurinol is only 1 to 3 hours, as it is extensively catabolized to oxypurinol, a structural analogue of xanthine (Fig. 115.5). Oxypurinol has a half-life of 17 to 40 hours, depending on renal function, and also is a potent inhibitor of xanthine oxidase (84). The formation of oxypurinol provides a more stable level of xanthine oxidase inhibition, as well as a once-a-day dosing schedule for the parent drug, allopurinol (85).

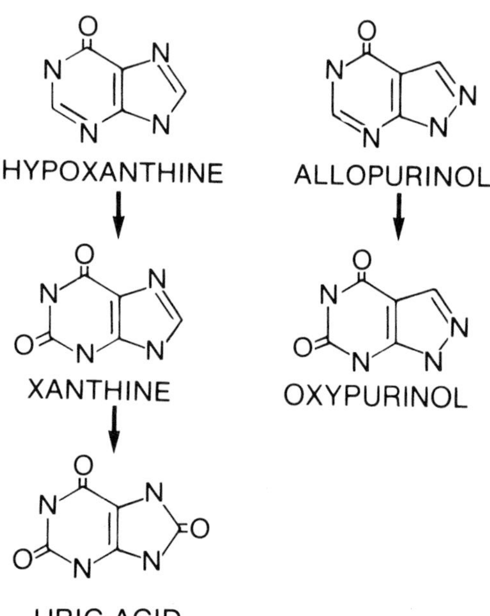

FIGURE 115.5. Xanthine oxidase catalyzes the conversion of hypoxanthine to xanthine, of xanthine to uric acid, and of allopurinol to oxypurinol.

Within 1 to 2 days of allopurinol administration, the serum urate concentration begins to decrease, reaching a nadir within 7 to 14 days. This decline in serum urate level is accompanied by a marked drop in urinary uric acid excretion. This is an important difference from the urate-lowering activities of the uricosuric agents. Hypoxanthine and xanthine levels increase in both serum and urine as a result of allopurinol therapy. Both of these compounds are more soluble and readily excretable than is uric acid. Total purine excretion also declines by 10% to 60% of pretreatment levels when allopurinol is taken. This decline results from increased salvage of hypoxanthine to inosine monophosphate (IMP) and from the concomitant reduction in the rate of *de novo* purine biosynthesis, an effect of feedback inhibition by allopurinol ribonucleotides (86) (Fig. 115.6).

Allopurinol is a potent ULD for virtually all causes of hyperuricemia, but it is particularly indicated for patients with the following conditions: (a) gout and either renal insufficiency and/or a 24-hour urinary uric acid excretion of greater than 1,000 mg/day; (b) noncompliance with uricosuric agents; (c) allergy or failure to respond to uricosuric agents; (d) a history of renal calculi of any type and a urinary uric acid excretion of greater than 600 mg per 24 hours; and (e) prophylaxis for or treatment of tumor lysis syndrome.

Caution should be exercised in the initiation of allopurinol in patients with renal failure or in patients taking azathioprine (Imuran), 6-mercaptopurinol (Purinethol), or other purine-based antimetabolites. There has been a widely accepted trend over the last decade to initiate allopurinol at a low dose in all patients and gradually increase the dose until the optimal serum urate level is achieved. The traditional approach had been to start all gouty subjects on 300 mg per day as a "standard" dose. At this dose of allopurinol, 85% of patients will normalize their serum urate levels, although some might require only 100 to 200 mg per day (87). Starting all patients at 100 mg per day and gradually increasing the dose every 4 weeks until a target serum urate level is reached greatly decreases the chances of precipitating an acute gouty attack or of triggering a severe hypersensitivity reaction. The exception to this scheme is the patient with a creatinine clearance of less than 20 mL per minute. In this case, a starting dose of 100 mg every other day or even every third day is recommended (88). Even in these more extreme cases of renal failure, the dose of allopurinol will frequently need to be escalated to achieve normouricemia. Even after allopurinol has been started, it is important to continue to look for and correct any secondary causes of hyperuricemia. This may include lifestyle modifications or changes in other medications.

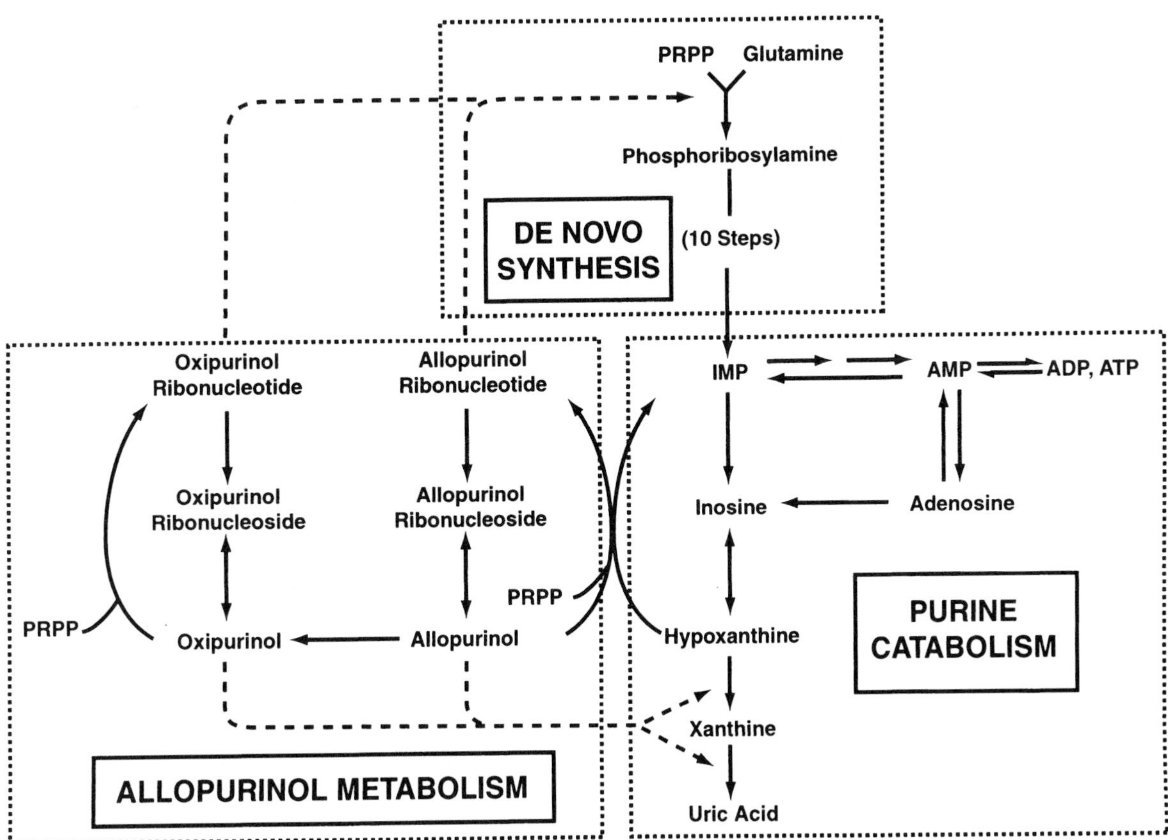

FIGURE 115.6. Parallels and interactions between the metabolic pathways of purines and allopurinol. *Dashed lines,* Sites of inhibition of allopurinol and oxypurinol on xanthine oxidase as well as inhibition of *de novo* purine synthesis by the ribonucleotide forms of allopurinol and oxypurinol.

Allopurinol may interfere with the metabolism of drugs other than the purine derivatives mentioned earlier. Increased levels of theophylline and warfarin may occur in patients taking allopurinol because of altered hepatic metabolism. Cyclophosphamide toxicity and bone marrow suppression is enhanced with allopurinol, although the mechanism for this is not clear (89). A 20% incidence of skin rash has been reported in patients taking allopurinol with either ampicillin or amoxicillin (90). Other drugs potentially affected by allopurinol therapy are listed in Table 115.7.

Side effects of allopurinol are infrequent and generally mild. The most frequently encountered problems include rashes, gastrointestinal distress, diarrhea, and headache. Mild rashes may occur in 2% of patients taking allopurinol. In most cases, a reduction in dose will allow the rash to clear. In subjects with more persistent rashes or other mild allergic responses to allopurinol, desensitizing by either oral or intravenous routes can be attempted (91,92).

A severe hypersensitivity reaction to allopurinol is rare but potentially life threatening. The true incidence of this immunologically mediated syndrome is not known, but estimates of 0.1% to 0.4% are reported (88,93). There is a characteristic setting for this hypersensitivity reaction, and special precautious may help avoid it. The allopurinol hypersensitivity syndrome (AHS) is characterized by fever, rash, hepatitis, leukocytosis with eosinophilia, and worsening renal function (94,95). Death is reported in 25% to 30% of these cases, even when allopurinol is quickly discontinued. Fever and rash are present acutely in 95% of AHS cases. The fever is usually in the range of 39.0°C to 39.5°C (102°F to 103°F). The skin involvement may include generalized exfoliative erythroderma, marked palmar/plantar hyperkeratosis, Stevens–Johnson syndrome, or toxic epidermal necrolysis ("scalded skin" syndrome). From 80% to 90% of patients with AHS will have elevated serum transaminase levels that may occasionally progress into

TABLE 115.7. DRUG–DRUG INTERACTIONS WITH ALLOPURINOL

Ampicillin/Amoxicillin	6-Mercaptopurine
Azathioprine	Probenecid
Chlorpropamide	Vidarabine
Cyclophosphamide	Warfarin
Dilantin	ACE inhibitors[a]

ACE, angiotensin-converting enzyme.
[a]Suspected.

hepatic failure. A leukocytosis is observed in 40% and is frequently associated with eosinophilia and lymphopenia (96). A peripheral eosinophilia is found in 75% of AHS cases. The causes of death in AHS include acute renal and hepatic failure, gastrointestinal bleeding, and sepsis associated with skin exfoliation.

The clinical setting for AHS is consistent in most published series. Eighty percent have mild renal dysfunction, and 50% are taking thiazide diuretics at the time allopurinol is initiated. The majority of AHS patients develop their symptoms soon after starting a "standard" dose (300 mg/day) of allopurinol. The mean duration from start of therapy to onset of symptoms is 3 weeks (88). Tragically, more than half of the patients in whom this life-threatening reaction develops have no clear indication for being started on allopurinol.

By recognizing the risk factors of mild renal dysfunction combined with the use of thiazide diuretics and by adopting the "go low, go slow" approach to initial allopurinol dosing, AHS can be prevented in many cases. Treatment of AHS consists of early recognition, discontinuation of allopurinol, and supportive measures. The benefit of using corticosteroids in treating AHS is controversial (94,97).

Oxypurinol

Oxypurinol is the active product of allopurinol oxidation and has pharmacologic effects similar to those of allopurinol. In direct comparative studies, allopurinol is more effective because of better gastrointestinal absorption (71). Although neither the oral nor intravenous forms of oxypurinol are commercially available in the U.S., it has been used on a compassionate basis for many years in individuals with severe allopurinol hypersensitivity who experience acute urate overload from tumor lysis syndrome. However, cross-reactivity between allopurinol and oxypurinol is reported at 30%.

Uricase

Unlike humans, in whom uric acid is the final product of purine catabolism, most other members of the animal kingdom have an additional purine catabolic enzyme, uricase or urate oxidase. Uricase further catabolizes uric acid by opening its ring structures and renders it quite soluble. Hence, with rare exceptions, gout and uric acid nephrolithiasis are diseases peculiar to humans. Because uricase is a foreign protein, some difficulty has been encountered in developing stable and active formulations for treating human disease. Uricase is available in Europe, but not in the U.S. The enzyme is extracted from several fungal species and given either intramuscularly or intravenously. Polyethylene glycol modification has helped reduce the risks of anaphylaxis and hemolytic anemia (98).

When to Start Urate-lowering Drugs

Asymptomatic Hyperuricemia

The majority of subjects with chronic hyperuricemia will never develop symptoms of urate deposition. It is, therefore, generally not advisable to begin ULDs on the basis of elevated serum urate alone. Many experts have published recommendations for treating asymptomatic hyperuricemia when the urate levels are very high (12 or 13 mg/dL or greater). The justification for this is the high likelihood of gouty symptoms or nephrolithiasis developing in the subsequent 6 to 12 months. This approach has not been validated by controlled clinical trials, and therefore each case must be considered individually. Regardless of whether UDLs are used, it is universally advised to evaluate patients with the markedly elevated urate levels thoroughly for the underlying diseases or medications listed in Tables 115.1 and 115.2.

Gout

ULDs are indicated in all patients with chronic gouty arthritis, with or without tophi. From the first episode of acute gout, however, it may take years or decades to reach this stage of chronic nonremitting arthritis. There has been considerable controversy as to when to initiate UDLs during this long period of "intermittent gout.' There is no evidence of bony destruction early in the course of intermittent gout. As episodes of acute gout recur in the same joint, bony destruction takes place. As many as 42% of subjects with intermittent gout will demonstrate radiographic evidence of joint deterioration before the development of subcutaneous tophi or chronic arthritis (99,100). If the goal of therapy in gout is to prevent destructive changes in bones and joints, then clearly ULDs must be started sometime between the stages of asymptomatic hyperuricemia and chronic tophaceous gout. Serial monitoring for radiographic changes has been proposed as a useful mechanism for determining when to begin ULDs (101). The cost-effectiveness of urate-lowering therapy has been analyzed by comparing treated and nontreated groups (102). Treatment of patients who had two or more gouty attacks per year resulted in an overall cost savings when compared with the costs avoided by not having to treat acute episodes or the complications of NSAID use.

The optimal target range for serum urate reduction is another area dominated by opinions rather than controlled studies. Preventing recurrent gouty attacks can usually be achieved by reducing the serum urate to between 5 and 6 mg/dL (300 μM and 360 μM), respectively (59,103). Resorption of subcutaneous tophi may require a serum urate reduction of less than 5 mg/dL (59,100).

The decision regarding which type of ULD to choose as the initial urate-lowering therapy is dictated by the indications and contraindications for uricosurics and allopurinol discussed earlier. In gouty subjects who excrete less than 800 mg of uric acid per day, reduction in serum urate can be achieved with either allopurinol or the uricosuric agents. They may rarely require both types of ULDs. Early studies found no clear advantage for allopurinol compared with uricosurics (104), whereas subsequent reports demonstrated better long-term treatment outcomes with allopurinol (105,106). In a recent study from Spain, benzbromarone was thought to be superior to allopurinol in achieving optimal serum urate levels (107,108). Despite a lack of compelling, well-controlled data on the long-term treatment of hyperuricemia in gout, a strong bias toward the initial use of allopurinol has emerged. Virtually all practicing rheumatologists in Ontario, Canada, chose allopurinol as the initial ULD in a published survey (109). Another study reported that 66% of rheumatologists use allopurinol first (110), and 30% of French rheumatologists claimed that they never use uricosurics (111).

Nephrolithiasis

Uric acid calculi occur frequently in patients with gout but can occur in subjects with no previous evidence of uric acid–related symptoms. The development of gout and tophi correlates closely with serum urate levels. Uric acid stone disease, conversely, is correlated with urinary uric acid concentration and urine pH. In urine, uric acid becomes insoluble at acid pH but has more than tenfold greater solubility with pH over 7.0. Regardless of serum urate concentration, patients with renal calculi should have a 24-hour urine examined for pH, volume, and uric acid excretion. Volume deficits and acidic pH should be corrected. Patients with renal calculi who have daily urinary uric acid excretion of greater than 800 mg should be given allopurinol regardless of the composition of the stone. Potassium citrate (30 to 80 mEq/day orally in divided doses) is a good approach for correcting a consistently acid urine. It can be used alone or in combination with allopurinol (112).

When to Stop Urate-lowering Drugs

For patients with chronic tophaceous gout who have experienced resolution of tophi and complete abatement of arthritis through the use of ULDs, the traditional approach is to continue the ULD indefinitely (59). Given the cost of medications and their monitoring, the possibilities of side effects, and the burden of taking drugs on a daily basis, alternatives to life-long use of ULDs have been investigated.

The effect of discontinuing ULDs in gouty subjects in remission has been studied on several occasions (113–115). Recurrent arthritis was observed in approximately 50% of patients within 2 to 3 years of ULD discontinuation. In one study that selectively enrolled patients who formerly had chronic tophaceous gouty arthritis, 81% had recurrent arthritis, and 43% redeveloped tophi within 3 years (115).

The effect of intermittent control of hyperuricemia in gouty patients who had stopped ULDs also was examined. Twenty-five patients were administered allopurinol 2 months per year and compared with 25 subjects who received continuous allopurinol (116). By the second year of observation, seven of the 25 patients receiving intermittent allopurinol had experienced ten episodes of arthritis compared with no episodes in the continuously treated group. Clinical factors that might predict early recurrence of arthritis and tophi after ULDs are discontinued include severity of basal hyperuricemia, duration of gouty symptoms, duration of ULD therapy, and obesity. These, however, have not been studied in a systematic fashion.

No intermittent ULD treatment regimen is now comparable to continuous life-long therapy.

Special Considerations

Transplantation Gout

Hyperuricemia and gout are common occurrences in subjects who have undergone solid organ transplantation and are receiving cyclosporine to prevent rejection (117). Allopurinol is the most frequently used ULD after renal or cardiac transplantation (26). Of concern, however, is the drug–drug interaction between allopurinol and azathioprine, a common co-therapy with cyclosporine. A general guideline for initiating allopurinol therapy in the presence of azathioprine has been published (26). Allopurinol is begun at 50 mg per day, and the dose of azathioprine is reduced by 50%. Serum urate, cyclosporine levels, and white blood cell count are monitored weekly. The dose of allopurinol is escalated in 50-mg increments every 2 to 3 weeks. As the serum urate level decreases toward the target range of 5 to 6 mg/dL, the azathioprine is reduced to about 25% of the initial dose. Markers of rejection must be monitored closely.

The uricosuric properties of the angiotensin II receptor antagonist, losartan, is a possible alternative to allopurinol, provided the urinary uric acid excretion does not exceed 800 mg per day and the patient can maintain good hydration (81). Consideration might also be given to benzbromarone for patients being treated outside the U.S. Similarly, uricase has been used successfully in cyclosporine-induced gout (118,119) but is not available in the U.S.

Tumor Lysis Syndrome

Tumor lysis syndrome describes a constellation of metabolic abnormalities associated with lymphoproliferative malignancies after spontaneous or chemotherapy-induced cytolysis (120). The biochemical aberrations include hyperphosphatemia, hyperkalemia, hypocalcemia, and azotemia, but the most clinically important is hyperuricemia. Early prophylactic measures can greatly reduce the frequency and severity of complications associated with tumor lysis syndrome. Allopurinol in full doses is given to prevent uric acid formation. Vigorous hydration to ensure good renal blood flow and urine volume are important in preventing acute renal failure. Alkalinization of the urine with sodium bicarbonate is important to improve uric acid solubility. The alkalinization should, however, not be overly zealous because massive phosphate crystalluria might occur (121). A target urine pH of 6.5 to 7.0 is adequate. In severe cases of tumor lysis syndrome, hemodialysis may be an important salvage technique because uric acid is readily dialyzable. Uricase also has been used experimentally in tumor lysis syndrome (122).

REFERENCES

1. Freedman DS, Williamson DF, Gunter EW, et al. Relation of serum uric acid to mortality and ischemic heart disease: the NHANES I Epidemiologic Follow-up Study. *Am J Epidemiol* 1995;141:637–644.
2. Goldbourt U, Medalie JH, Herman JB, et al. Serum uric acid: correlation with biochemical, anthropometric, clinical and behavioral parameters in 10,000 Israeli men. *J Chronic Dis* 1980;33:435–443.
3. Mikkelsen WM, Dodge HJ, Valkenburg H. The distribution of serum uric acid values in a population unselected as to gout or hyperuricemia: Tecumseh, Michigan 1959-1960. *Am J Med* 1965;39:242–251.
4. Hall AP, Barry PE, Dawber TR, et al. Epidemiology of gout and hyperuricemia: a long term population study. *Am J Med* 1967;42:27–37.
5. Paulus HE, Coutts A, Calabro JJ, et al. clinical significance of hyperuricemia in routinely screened hospitalized men. *JAMA* 1970;21:277–281.
6. Saggiani F, Pitati S, Targher G, et al. Serum uric acid and related factors in 500 hospitalized subjects. *Metabolism* 1996;45: 1557–1561.
7. Johnson RJ, Kivlighn SD, Kim Y-G, et al. Reappraisal of the pathogenesis and consequences of hyperuricemia in hypertension, cardiovascular disease, and renal disease. *Am J Kidney Dis* 1999;33:225–234.
8. Wortmann RL. Management of hyperuricemia. In: Koopman WJ, ed. *Arthritis and allied conditions.* 13th ed. Philadelphia: Lea & Febiger, 1997:2073–2081.
9. Edwards NL, Fox IH, Disorders Associated with purine and pyrimidine metabolism. In: Cohen MP, Foa PP, eds. *Special topics in endocrinology and metabolism.* Vol 6. New York: Alan R. Liss, 1984:95–140.
10. Campion EW, Glynn RJ, DeLabry LO. Asymptomatic hyperuricemia: risks and consequences in the Normative Aging Study. *Am J Med* 1987;82:421–426.
11. Popp JD, Edwards NL. New insights into gouty arthritis. *Contemp Intern Med* 1995;7:55–64.
12. Edwards NL, Recker D, Fox IH. Overproduction of uric acid in hypoxanthine-guanine phosphoribosyltransferase deficiency: contribution by impaired purine salvage. *J Clin Invest* 1979; 63:922–930.
13. Becker MA, Raivio KO, Bakay B, et al. Variant human phosphoribosylpyrophosphate synthetase altered regulatory and catalytic functions. *J Clin Invest* 1980;65:109–120.
14. Wooliscroft JO, Colfer H, Fox IH. Hyperuricemia in acute illness: a poor prognostic sign. *Am J Med* 1982;72:58–62.
15. Leyva F, Chua TP, Anker SD, et al. Uric acid in chronic heart failure: a measure of the anaerobic threshold. *Metabolism* 1998; 47:1156–1159.
16. Faller J, Fox IH. Ethanol-induced hyperuricemia: evidence for increased urate production by activation of adenine nucleotide turnover. *N Engl J Med* 1982;307:1598–1602.
17. Jones DP, Mahmoud H, Chesney RW. Tumor lysis syndrome: pathogenesis and management. *Pediatr Nephrol* 1995;9: 206–212.
18. Sorensen LB. Degradation of uric acid in man. *Metabolism* 1959;8:687–703.
19. Holmes EW, Kelley WN, Wyn Gaarden JB. The kidney and uric acid excretion in man. *Kidney Int* 1972;2:115–118.
20. Weinman EJ, Eknoyan G, Suki WN. The influence of the extracellular fluid volume on the tubular reabsorption of uric acid. *J Clin Invest* 1975;55:283–291.
21. Puig JG, Mateos FA, Jimenez ML, et al. Renal handling of uric acid in gout: impaired tubular transport of urate not dependent on serum urate levels. *Metabolism* 1986;35:1147–1153.
22. Puig JG, Mateos FA, Jimenez ML, et al. Renal excretion of hypoxanthine and xanthine in primary gout. *Am J Med* 1988; 85:533–537.
23. McGill NW, Dieppe PA. The role of serum and synovial fluid components in the promotion of urate crystal formation. *J Rheumatol* 1991;18:1042–1046.
24. Marcen R, Gallego N, Gamez C, et al. Hyperuricemia after kidney transplantation in patients treated with cyclosporine. *Am J Med* 1992;93:354–355.
25. West C, Carpenter BJ, Hakala TR. The incidence of gout in renal transplant recipients. *Am J Kidney Dis* 1987;10:369–371.
26. Howe S, Edwards NL. Controlling hyperuricemia and gout in cardiac transplant recipients. *J Musculoskeletal Med* 1995;12: 15–24.
27. Popp JD, Bidgood WD, Edwards NL. Magnetic resonance imaging of tophaceous gout in the hands and wrists. *Semin Arthritis Rheum* 1996;25:282–289.
28. Ziff M. The rheumatoid nodule. *Arthritis Rheum* 1990;33: 761–767.
29. Campbell DA, Edwards NL. Multicentric reticulohistiocytosis: systemic macrophage disorder. *Clin Rheumatol* 1991;5: 301–319.
30. Popp JD, Bidgood WD, Edwards NL. The gouty tophus. *Rheumatol Rev* 1993;2:163–168.
31. Wilcox WR, Khalaf A, Weinberger A, et al. The solubility of uric acid and monosodium urate. *Med Biol Eng* 1972;10: 522–531.
32. Emmerson BT. Gout and renal disease. In: Smyth CJ, Holers VM, eds. *Gout, hyperuricemia, and other crystal-associated arthropathies.* New York: Marcel Dekker, 1999:241–260.
33. Yu T. Urolithiasis in hyperuricemia and gout. *J Urol* 1981;126: 424–430.
34. Coe FL. Uric acid and calcium oxalate nephrolithiasis. *Kidney Int* 1983;24:392–403.
35. Conger ID. Acute uric acid nephropathy. *Med Clin North Am* 1990;74:859–871.
36. Kelton J, Kelley WN, Holmes EW. A rapid method for the diagnosis of acute uric acid nephropathy. *Arch Intern Med* 1978; 138:612.
37. Yu T, Berger L, Dorph DJ, et al. Renal function in gout. V. Factors influencing the renal hemodynamics. *Am J Med* 1979;67: 766–771.
38. Johnson RJ, Schreiner GF. Hypothesis: the role of acquired

tubulointerstitial disease in the pathogenesis of salt-dependent hypertension. *Kidney Int* 1997;52:1169–1179.
39. Levine W, Dyer AR, Shekelle RB, et al. Serum uric acid and 1.5 year mortality of middle-aged women of the Chicago Heart Association detection project in industry. *J Clin Epidemiol* 1989;42:257–267.
40. Breckenridge A. Hypertension and hyperuricemia. *Lancet* 1966;1:15–18.
41. Hiyamuta K, Toshima H, Koga Y, et al. Relationship between coronary risk factor and arteriographic feature of coronary atherosclerosis. *Jpn Circ J* 1990;59:442–447.
42. Brand FEN, McGee DL, Kannel WB, et al. Hyperuricemia as a risk factor of coronary artery disease: the Framingham study. *Am J Epidemiol* 1985;121:11–18.
43. Moller DE, Filer JS. Mechanisms of disease: insulin resistance-mechanisms, syndromes and implications. *N Engl J Med* 1991;325:938–948.
44. Cappuccio FP, Strazzullo P, Farinaro E, et al. Uric acid metabolism and tubular sodium handling: results from a population based study. *JAMA* 1993;270:354–359.
45. Zavaroni I, Mazza S, Fantuzzi M, et al. Changes in insulin and lipid metabolism in males with asymptomatic hyperuricemia. *J Intern Med* 1993;234:25–30.
46. Elsayed NM, Nakashima JM, Postlewait EM. Measurement of uric acid as a marker of oxygen tension in the lung. *Arch Biochem Biophys* 1993;302:228–232.
47. Porter KB, O'Brien WF, Benoit R. Comparison of cord purine metabolites to maternal and neonatal variables of hypoxia. *Obstet Gynecol* 1992;79:394–397.
48. Goldstein HS, Manowitz P. Relation between serum uric acid and blood pressure in adolescents. *Ann Hum Biol* 1993;20: 423–431.
49. Messerli FH, Frohlich ED, Dreslinski GR, et al. Serum uric acid in essential hypertension: an indicator of renal vascular involvement. *Ann Intern Med* 1980;93:817–821.
50. Talbott JH, Yu T-F. Secondary gout. In: *Gout and uric acid metabolism.* New York: Stratton Medical Book Co., 1976: 191–204.
51. Owen-Smith B, Quiney J, Read J. Salivary urate in gout, exercise and diurnal variation. *Lancet* 1998;351:1932.
52. Kobayashi K, Morioka Y, Esaka Y, et al. Determination of uric acid in scalp hair for non-invasive evaluation of uricemic controls in hyperuricemia. *Biol Pharm Bull* 1998;21:398–400.
53. Schlesinger N, Baker DG, Schumacher HR. Serum uric acid during bouts of acute gouty arthritis. *J Rheumatol* 1997;24: 2265–2266.
54. Logan JA, Morrison E, McGill PE. Serum uric acid in acute gout. *Ann Rheum Dis* 1997;56:696–697.
55. Coe FL, Kaualach AG. Hypercalcemia and hyperuricemia in patients with calcium nephrolithiasis. *N Engl J Med* 1976; 295:1449–1454.
56. Simkin PA, Hoover PL, Paxson CS, et al. Uric acid excretion: quantitative assessment from spot, midmorning serum and urine samples. *Ann Intern Med* 1979;91:44–47.
57. Wortmann RL Fox IH. Limited value of uric acid to creatinine ratios in estimating uric acid excretion. *Ann Intern Med* 1980; 93:822–825.
58. McDonald E, Marino C. Stopping progression to tophaceous gout: when and how to use urate-lowering therapy. *Postgrad Med* 1998;104:117–127.
59. Emmerson BT. The management of gout. *N Engl J Med* 1996;334:445–451.
60. Schlesinger N, Baker DG, Schumacker HR. How well have diagnostic tests and therapies for gout been evaluated? *Curr Opin Rheumatol* 1999;11:441–445.
61. Talbott JH. Solid and liquid nourishment in gout: selected historical excerpts, largely empiric or fashionable and current scientific (?) concepts in the management of gout and gouty arthritis. *Semin Arthritis Rheum* 1981;11:288–306.
62. MacLachlan MJ, Rodnan GP. Effect of food, fast, and alcohol on serum uric acid and acute attacks of gout. *Am J Med* 1967;42:38–57.
63. Diamond HS, Sterba G, Jayadeven K, et al. On the mechanism of the paradoxical effect of salicylate on urate excretion. *Adv Exp Med Biol Am* 1980;122:221–231.
64. Burnell JM, Kerby WMM. Effectiveness of a new compound, Benemid, in elevating serum penicillin concentrations. *J Clin Invest* 1951;109:346–353.
65. Dayton PG, Yu T-F, Chen W, et al. The physiological disposition of probenecid, including renal clearance in man, studied by an improved method for its estimation in biological material. *J Pharmacol Exp Ther* 1963;140:278–291.
66. Gutman AB, Yu T-F. Protracted uricosuric therapy in tophaceous gout. *Lancet* 1957;111:1258–1260.
67. Ferris TF, Morgan WS, Levitin H. Nephrotic syndrome caused by probenecid. *N Engl J Med* 1961;265:381–383.
68. Reynolds ES, Schlant RC, Gonick HC, et al. Fatal massive necrosis of the liver as a manifestation of hypersensitivity to probenecid. *N Engl J Med* 1957;265:592.
69. Emmerson BT. A comparison of uricosuric agents in gout with special reference to sulfinpyrazone. *Med J Aust* 1963;1: 839–844.
70. Gutman AB. Uricosuric drugs with special reference to probenecid and sulfinpyrazone. *Adv Pharmacol* 1966;4:91–142.
71. Khawaja AT, Diamond HS. Hypouricemic drugs. In: Smyth CV, Holers VM, eds. *Gout, hyperuricemia, and other crystal-associated arthropathies.* New York: Marcel Dekker, 1999:219–240.
72. Deltour G, Broekhuysen J, Ghislain M, et al. Research in the series of benfuranes XXI. Inhibition of phenoly derivatives of benzfuranes and various analogues of the liver xanthine oxidase of the rat. *Arch Int Pharmacodyn Ther* 1967;165:25–37.
73. Broekhuysen J, Pacco M, Sion R, et al. Metabolism of benzbromarone in man. *Eur J Clin Pharmacol* 1972;4:125–132.
74. Grantham JJ, Chonko AM. Renal handling of organic anions and cations, excretion of uric acid. In: Brenner BM, Rector FC, eds. *The kidney.* 4th ed. Philadelphia: WB Saunders, 1991:483–509.
75. Massbernard A, Guilbaud J, Droniou J. Clinical experiences with long term treatment of gout with iodine and bromide derivatives of benzofuranes. *Lyon Med* 1971;225:683–691.
76. Dresse A, Fischer P, Gerard MA, et al. Uricosuric properties of diflunisal in man. *Br J Clin Pharmacol* 1979;7:267–272.
77. van Loenhout JWA, van de Putte LBA, Gribnau FWJ, et al. Persistent hypouricemic effect of long-term diflunisal administration. *J Rheumatol* 1981;8:639–642.
78. Ferraccioli G, Spisni A, Ambanelli U. Hypouricemic action of diflunisal in gouty patients: in vitro and In vivo studies. *J Rheumatol* 1984;11:330–332.
79. Emmerson BT, Hazelton RA, Whyte IMacG. Comparison of the urate lowering effects of allopurinol and diflunisal. *J Rheumatol* 1987;14:335–337.
80. Burnier M, Rutschmann B, Nussberger J, et al. Salt dependent renal effects of an angiotensin II antagonist in healthy subjects. *Hypertension* 1993;22:339–347.
81. Minghelli G, Seydoux C, Goy J-J, et al. Uricosuric effect of the angiotensin II receptor antagonist losartan in heart transplant recipients. *Transplantation* 1998;66:268–271.
82. Leary WP, Reyes AJ. Angiotensin I converting enzyme inhibitors and the renal excretion of urate. *Cardiovasc Drugs Ther* 1987;1:29–38.
83. Elion GB, Callahan S, Nathan H, et al. Potentiation by inhibition of drug degradation: 6-substituted purines and xanthine oxidase. *Biochem Pharmacol* 1963;12:85–98.

84. Elion GB, Yu T-F, Gutman AB, et al. Renal clearance of oxypurinol, the chief metabolite of allopurinol. *Am J Med* 1968; 45:69–75.
85. Rodnan GP, Robin JA, Tolchin SF, et al. Allopurinol and gouty hyperuricemia: efficacy of a single daily dose. *JAMA* 1975; 231:1143–1149.
86. Edwards NL, Recker D, Airozo D, et al. Enhanced purine salvage during allopurinol therapy: an important pharmacologic property in humans. *J Lab Clin Med* 1981;98:673–683.
87. Day RO, Miners JO, Birkett DJ, et al. Allopurinol dosage selection: relationships between dose and plasma oxypurinol and urate concentrations and urinary urate excretion. *Br J Clin Pharmacol* 1988;26:423–428.
88. Hande KR, Noone RM, Stone WJ. Severe Allopurinol toxicity: description and guidelines for prevention in patients with renal insufficiency. *Am J Med* 1984;76:47–56.
89. Fox IH, Kelley WN. Management of gout. *JAMA* 1979;242: 361–364.
90. Boston Collaborative Drug Surveillance Program. Excess of ampicillin rashes associated with allopurinol therapy or hyperuricemia. *N Engl J Med* 1972;286:505–507.
91. Fam AG, Lewtas J, Stein J, et al. Desensitization to allopurinol in patients with gout and cutaneous reactions. *Am J Med* 1992; 93:299–302.
92. Walz-LeBlanc BAE, Reynolds WJ, MacFadden DK. Allopurinol sensitivity in a patient with chronic tophaceous gout: success of intravenous desensitization after failure of oral desensitization. *Arthritis Rheum* 1991;34:1329–1331.
93. McInnes GT, Lawson DH, Jick H. Acute adverse reactions attributed to allopurinol in hospitalized patients. *Ann Rheum Dis* 1981;40:245–249.
94. Arellano F, Sacristan JA. Allopurinol hypersensitivity syndrome: a review. *Ann Pharmacother* 1993;27:337–343.
95. Edwards NL. Allopurinol hypersensitivity. In: Klippel JH, Dieppe PA, eds. *Rheumatology.* 2nd ed. London: Mosby, 1998:8.19.11–19.12.
96. Lockard O, Harmon C, Nolph K, et al. Allergic reactions to allopurinol with cross-reactivity to oxypurinol. *Ann Intern Med* 1976;85:333–335.
97. Lang PG. Severe hypersensitivity reactions to allopurinol. *South Med J* 1979;72:1361–1368.
98. Chua CC, Greenberg MI, Viau AT, et al. Use of polyethylene glycol-modified uricase (PEG-uricase) to treat hyperuricemia in a patient with non-Hodgkin's lymphoma. *Ann Intern Med* 1988;109:114–117.
99. Nakayama DA, Barthelemy C, Carrera GF, et al. Tophaceous gout: a clinical and radiographic assessment. *Arthritis Rheum* 1984;27:468–471.
100. McCarthy GM, Barthelenay CR, Veum JA, et al. Influence of antihyperuricemic therapy on the clinical and radiographic progression of gout. *Arthritis Rheum* 1991;34:1489–1494.
101. Barthelemy CR, Nakayama DA, Carrera GF, et al. Gouty arthritis: a prospective radiographic evaluation of sixty patients. *Skeletal Radiol* 1984;11:1–8.
102. Ferraz MB, O'Brien B. A cost effectiveness analysis of urate lowering drugs in nontophaceous recurrent gouty arthritis. *J Rheumatol* 1995;22:908–914.
103. Howe S, Edwards NL. Hyperuricemia and gout. In: Rakel RE, ed. *Conn's current therapy*. Philadelphia: WB Saunders, 1995: 503–505.
104. Scott JT. Comparison of allopurinol to probenecid. *Ann Rheum Dis* 1966;25:623–626.
105. Weinberger A, Schreiber M, Sperling O, et al. Comparative evaluation of uricosuric and allopurinol treatment in a series of 183 patients. *Int Rev Rheum* 1975;5:681–692.
106. Rundles RW, Metz EN, Silberman HR. Allopurinol in the treatment of gout. *Ann Intern Med* 1966;64:229–258.
107. Perez-Ruiz F, Alonso-Ruiz A, Calaaboza M, et al. Efficacy of allopurinol and benzbromazone for control of hyperuricemia: a pathogenic approach to the treatment of primary chronic gout. *Ann Rheum Dis* 1998;57:545–549.
108. Perez-Ruiz F, Calaabozo M, Fernandez-Lopez J, et al. Treatment of chronic gout in patients with renal impairment: an open, randomized, actively controlled study. *J Clin Rheumatol* 1999; 5:49–55.
109. Bellamy N, Gilbert JR, Brooks PR, et al. A survey of current prescribing practices of anti-inflammatory and urate lowering drugs in gouty arthritis in the Province of Ontario. *J Rheumatol* 1988;15:1841–1871.
110. Medellin MV, Erickson AR, Enzenauer RJ. Variability of treatment for gouty arthritis between rheumatologists and primary care physicians. *J Clin Rheumatol* 1997;3:24–27.
111. Pawlotsky Y. What is the optimal treatment for acute crystal induced arthritis? *Rev Rheum* 1996;63:231–233.
112. Pak CYC, Sakhaee K, Fuller C. Successful management of uric acid nephrolithiasis with potassium citrate. *Kidney Int* 1986; 30:422–428.
113. Loebl WY, Scott JT. Withdrawal of allopurinol in patients with gout. *Ann Rheum Dis* 1974;33:304–307.
114. Gast LF. Withdrawal of long term antihyperuricemic therapy in tophaceous gout. *Clin Rheumatol* 1987;6:70–73.
115. van Lieshout-Zuidema MF, Breedveld FC. Withdrawal of long term antihyperuricemic therapy in tophaceous gout. *J Rheumatol* 1993;20:1383–1385.
116. Bull PW, Scott JT. Intermittent control of hyperuricemia in the treatment of gout. *J Rheumatol* 1989;16:1246–1248.
117. Lin H, Rocher LL, McQuillan MA, et al. Cyclosporine induced hyperuricemia and gout. *N Engl J Med* 1989;321:287–292.
118. Rosenberg S, Koeger AC, Bourgeois P. Urate-oxidase for gouty arthritis in cardiac transplant recipients. *J Rheumatol* 1993;20: 12–14.
119. Ippoliti G, Negri M, Campana C, et al. Urate oxidase in hyperuricemic heart transplant recipients treated with azathioprine. *Transplantation* 1997;63:1370–1371.
120. Jones DP, Mahmoud H, Chesney RW. Tumor lysis syndrome: pathogenesis and management. *Pediatr Nephrol* 1995;9: 206–212.
121. Stapleton FB, Strother DR, Roy S, et al. Acute renal failure at onset of therapy for advanced stage Burkitt lymphoma and B cell acute lymphoblastic leukemia. *Pediatrics* 1988;82: 863–869.
122. Masera G, Jankovic M, Zurlo MG, et al. Urate oxicase prophylaxis of uric acid-induced renal damage in childhood leukemia. *J Pediatr* 1982;100:152–155.

116

PATHOGENESIS AND TREATMENT OF CRYSTAL-INDUCED INFLAMMATION

ROBERT A. TERKELTAUB

The cellular and molecular pathogenetic mechanisms and treatment of the inflammatory host response to several microcrystals implicated in human rheumatic diseases are discussed in this chapter. Techniques used for identification of crystals in clinical practice and in experimental work are discussed in Chapters 4 and 115.

NUCLEATION, GROWTH, AND SHEDDING OF CRYSTALS

The nucleation and growth of monosodium urate monohydrate (MSU) and calcium pyrophosphate dihydrate (CPPD) crystals will serve as examples for this discussion.

Deposition of Monosodium Urate Crystals

Urate crystallizes as its monosodium salt in oversaturated tissue fluids (1). MSU crystals found in joint fluid at the time of an acute attack may derive from rupture of preformed synovial deposits (Fig. 116.1) or may precipitate *de novo,* as exemplified in certain instances by the recognition of urate spherulites (1) (see Chapter 4).

The onset of acute attacks of gout in patients correlates with the rate of change of levels of serum urate (either up or down) rather than with a steady-state level. Initial treatment with allopurinol commonly produces an abrupt decline in urate levels and precipitates an acute attack of gout. Additionally, heavy alcohol users with acute gout (e.g., "aldermanic gout") may have particularly large fluctuations in serum urate concentrations (1,2). Decreasing serum urate levels may promote the release of MSU crystals from packed tophaceous deposits through a slight decrease in the size of crystals, loosening them from their organic matrix (crystal "shedding").

Arthroscopically, the earliest urate crystal deposits are apparently most often in the synovium, rather than in cartilage; they appear as white furuncles with an erythematous base. Investigators have identified tophi in the synovial membrane at the time of the first gouty attack (1). Additionally, in some individuals with gout (or with asymptomatic hyperuricemia), urate crystals can be found in asymptomatic metatarsophalangeal and knee joints never previously involved with acute gout (1,3). Thus gout, like CPPD crystal deposition, can exist in an asymptomatic state.

Only a minority of individuals with sustained hyperuricemia develop tophi and gouty arthropathy (1). Furthermore, gout can occur, albeit rarely, in individuals without hyperuricemia (4). Although many factors are implicated in the tissue deposition of MSU crystals (Table 116.1), the reasons underlying the clinical selectivity of tophus formation are poorly understood at present (1,5–7).

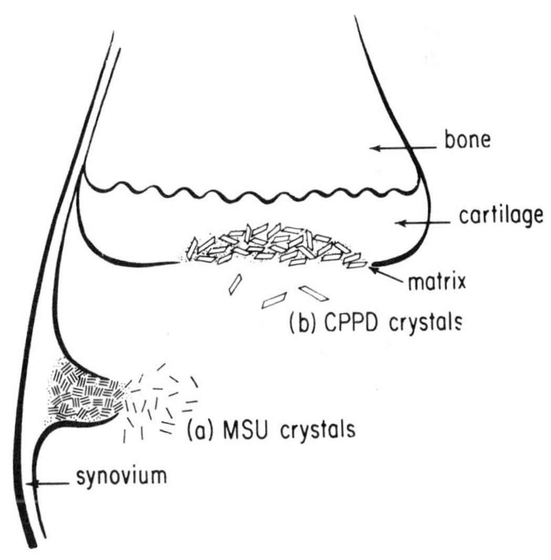

FIGURE 116.1. Autoinjection of monosodium urate (MSU) crystals **(a)** from preformed tophus in synovium into adjacent joint space. Autoinjection of calcium pyrophosphate dihydrate (CPPD) crystals **(b)** from preformed cartilaginous deposit into adjacent joint space, as a result of crystal shedding. Both concepts are still hypothetic and have only indirect supportive evidence. See text for details.

TABLE 116.1. FACTORS PROPOSED TO MODULATE TISSUE DEPOSITION OF MSU CRYSTALS

Temperature
pH
Trauma, tissue injury
Glycosaminoglycans and connective tissue turnover
Degenerative joint disease (e.g., tophi in Heberden's nodes)
Plasma proteins (e.g., IgG, albumin)
Concentrations of other solutes (e.g., lead, calcium, sodium)
Urate secretion and sequestration within macrophage acini
Unknown factors

MSU, monosodium urate; Ig; immunoglobulin.

ROLE OF TEMPERATURE, PH, AND SOLUTES

The decreased solubility of sodium urate at the lower temperatures of peripheral structures such as the toes and ears may help explain why MSU crystals deposit in these areas (1). The predilection for marked MSU crystal deposition in the first metatarsophalangeal joint also may relate to repetitive minor trauma at this site. Simkin (1) demonstrated that the rate of diffusion of urate molecules from the synovial space to plasma is only half that of water. Thus the urate concentration in a small effusion in a dependent joint, such as the great toe, could equilibrate with plasma urate during the day. Subsequently, as the effusion resorbed during recumbency, a localized increase in urate level would be expected. This phenomenon may explain the usual nocturnal onset of acute gouty symptoms in a dependent joint. Additionally, such a mechanism might also account for Schumacher's observation of rapid tophus formation at the site of a burn (1).

Acidification may enhance urate nucleation *in vitro* by the formation of protonated solid phases (1). However, the solubility of sodium urate, as opposed to that of uric acid, actually increases as pH decreases from 7.4 to 5.8, and measurements of both pH and buffering capacity in gouty joints have failed to demonstrate significant acidosis. Thus acute pH changes are unlikely to significantly influence articular MSU crystal formation.

Critical urate supersaturation levels can be altered *in vitro* by the concentrations of a number of other solutes, including sodium and calcium (1). Additionally, lead, at 100 mg/L, can effectively nucleate MSU from a normal saline solution containing 10 mg/dL urate (1). Such high levels are found only in acute lead poisoning, however, making it unlikely that lead acts as a nucleating agent, even in saturnine gout. Whether relative changes in solute concentrations contribute to the well-documented lack of tophi in gout secondary to the hyperuricemia of renal disease is unknown (1).

ROLE OF CONNECTIVE TISSUE MATRIX

Urate is more soluble in the presence of aggregated proteoglycans than of nonaggregated proteoglycans (1). Furthermore, the concentrations of insoluble collagen and chondroitin sulfate appear to influence urate crystal formation *in vitro* (6,7). Katz (1) observed threefold elevations of serum uronic acid in patients with articular gout, but not in patients with hyperuricemia or other inflammatory diseases, suggesting a possible specificity for MSU crystal deposition. The normalization of these elevated levels by the usual therapeutic doses of colchicine lends further credence to this finding and suggests that at least one of the prophylactic mechanisms of colchicine may be different from those operating in the treatment of established acute gouty arthritis, and might relate to effects of colchicine on matrix metabolism (1). The observations that hemiplegia appears to have a sparing effect on the development of tophi and acute gout on the paretic side (1) and that tophi and acute gout occur in distal interphalangeal joints at the location of Heberden's nodes (8) further emphasize the potential importance of focal connective tissue structure and turnover.

Variable amounts of lipid debris have been detected in the intercrystalline matrix of tophi (1). A similar physical association of lipids with cartilaginous deposits of CPPD crystals also has been described, but could represent the presence of phospholipids from membrane-derived cartilage matrix vesicles (see Chapter 11). Whether lipids are innocent bystanders, a causative factor, or consequence of urate crystal deposition remains unknown. Further studies are needed to ascertain whether the heightened frequency of hypothyroidism in gout (9) may predispose to crystal deposition (e.g., by alteration of matrix metabolism).

Mononuclear phagocytes in various stages of maturity encircle deposited urate in many small tophi but not always in larger urate deposits (10). Olecranon bursa tophi contain small acini of macrophages surrounding necrotic tissues that do not contain internal urate crystals. Palmer et al. (10) have hypothesized that macrophages may play an active role in urate deposition through their ability to transport (and perhaps centripetally sequester) organic anions (11).

EFFECTS OF PLASMA PROTEINS

The role of plasma proteins in MSU crystal nucleation and growth *in vivo* remains controversial. Several studies suggested that uric acid binding to plasma proteins is generally weak and reversible and that plasma proteins have minimal effects on the distribution of uric acid in equilibrium dialysis (12). Evidence for a role of plasma protein in binding to uric acid and maintaining its solubility has been suggested by the finding of a partial deficiency of a uric acid–binding α-globulin in one kindred with gout (1). Various plasma proteins have been reported to enhance MSU crystallization from supersaturated uric acid solutions *in vitro* (1,6,13); however, the effects have varied from laboratory to laboratory, and are dependent on the heat stability of the proteins and the ambient pH (1,6,13). For example, human albumin accelerates

MSU nucleation at a pH higher than 7.5, but the effects of albumin are minimal at pH 7.0, possibly because of a requirement for available albumin hydroxylate groups (13). Interestingly, albumin appears to interact selectively with one of the hydrophilic faces of urate crystals (13).

Immunoglobulin G (IgG) has been proposed to act as a nucleating factor for MSU crystals in patients with gout (6,14). In particular, IgG isolated from several gouty synovial fluids [but not from synovial fluids from patients with osteoarthritis (OA), rheumatoid arthritis (RA), or pseudogout] increased the rate of nucleation of MSU crystals from supersaturated fluid *in vitro* (14). Additionally, injection of rabbits with MSU crystals (once a week for 8 weeks) was associated with induction of serum IgG that was capable of increasing the rate of nucleation of MSU crystals (14). This effect gradually disappeared if no booster doses of crystals were given to the rabbits. Weekly injections with crystallized allopurinol, or MSU crystals in adjuvant failed to elicit detectable serum IgG that promoted crystallization of MSU (14). Thus it was suggested that microcrystals of MSU, under certain conditions, might act as "antigenic surfaces" promoting urate nucleation (14).

In several studies, joint fluid supernatants from gouty joints have enhanced MSU crystal formation *in vitro* (1,6). Whether such effects can be attributed to increased nucleation or an enhanced rate of crystal growth through the possible participation of ultramicrocrystals in the gouty fluids as "seeds" remains to be determined.

STUDIES IN URATE OXIDASE KNOCKOUT MICE

Mice in which the uric acid–degrading enzyme urate oxidase has been eliminated by homologous recombination (urate oxidase knockout mice) have a tenfold elevation in serum uric acid (mean serum urate of 11 mg/dL) and urinary uric acid, rapidly progressive urate nephropathy, a very high mortality rate in the first weeks of life, and therapeutic responsiveness to allopurinol (15). In this valuable small animal model of human hyperuricemia, subcutaneous tophi and articular urate deposition are not detected in the first 4 weeks of life. Additionally, the high mortality has made it difficult to ascertain whether tophi and joint disease can occur later in life in these animals. This model system provides a unique opportunity to determine experimentally the factors critical in regulating tophus formation.

Shedding of CPPD Crystals

The initial site of CPPD crystal formation is probably articular cartilage, but "crystal traffic" from cartilage to other articular sites can coexist with primary CPPD crystals deposition in synovium, extraarticular tendons, ligaments, and bursae. Cartilage inorganic phosphate (Pi) metabolism and the pathogenesis of CPPD crystal deposition are discussed at length in Chapter 117.

Assuming that the CPPD crystals residing in their cartilaginous mold of proteoglycan are in thermodynamic equilibrium with Ca^{2+} and $P_2O_7^{-4}$ (the ions from which they were formed), conditions that either reduce ionized calcium or reduce Ca^{2+} and $P_2O_7^{-4}$ should increase the solubility of these crystals and free them from their mold. This hypothetic phenomenon has been designated *crystal shedding* (1). The marked effect of even small changes in ionized calcium level on crystal solubility *in vitro,* the onset of acute pseudogout after lavage of joints with solubilizers of CPPD crystals such as ethylenediaminetetraacetic acid (EDTA) or Mg^{2+}-containing buffers (1), and the clinical correlation of acute arthritis with decreasing serum calcium concentrations (1) all support this hypothesis. Joint fluid Pi levels are lower during acute attacks of pseudogout, owing to a more rapid equilibration with the much lower plasma Pi level (2 m*M*). Thus once an acute attack begins, the decrease in ambient Pi that is due to increased synovial blood flow may further increase crystal solubility and shedding.

Other postulated mechanisms for the autoinjection of CPPD crystals presumed to precede acute pseudogout include mechanical disruption of cartilage accompanying subchondral microfracture (1). In this regard, trauma is a common antecedent of acute pseudogout. "Enzymatic strip mining" of crystals from preformed cartilaginous deposits can occur. Presumably, any significant intrasynovial discharge of inflammatory proteases might digest the components of the "mold," releasing crystals into the joint space (1). For example, CPPD crystals were readily released from cartilage incubated *in vitro* with synovial cell collagenase (1). *Thus, the mere presence of CPPD or MSU crystals in joint fluid must be interpreted in the clinical context because they might be a result, as well as a cause, of joint inflammation.*

PATHOGENESIS OF CRYSTAL-INDUCED INFLAMMATION

Gout will serve as a paradigm for the following discussion. Acute onset, severity, edema, and erythema extending beyond the joint margin, neutrophil influx, and systemic manifestations are the hallmarks of articular inflammation in a gouty paroxysm. These features reflect the ability of MSU crystals to activate a remarkable number of humoral and cellular inflammatory mediator systems. Human acute gouty synovial fluids contain a "broth" of cell-derived mediators [including interleukin-1 (IL-1), tumor necrosis factor-α (TNF-α), leukotriene B_4 (LTB_4), IL-6, and IL-8; Fig. 116.2]. MSU crystal–induced activation of cells and the induction of cytokine release by crystals appear to be the central events in the pathogenesis of gouty inflammation. Inflammatory crystals other than MSU have been less thoroughly studied but

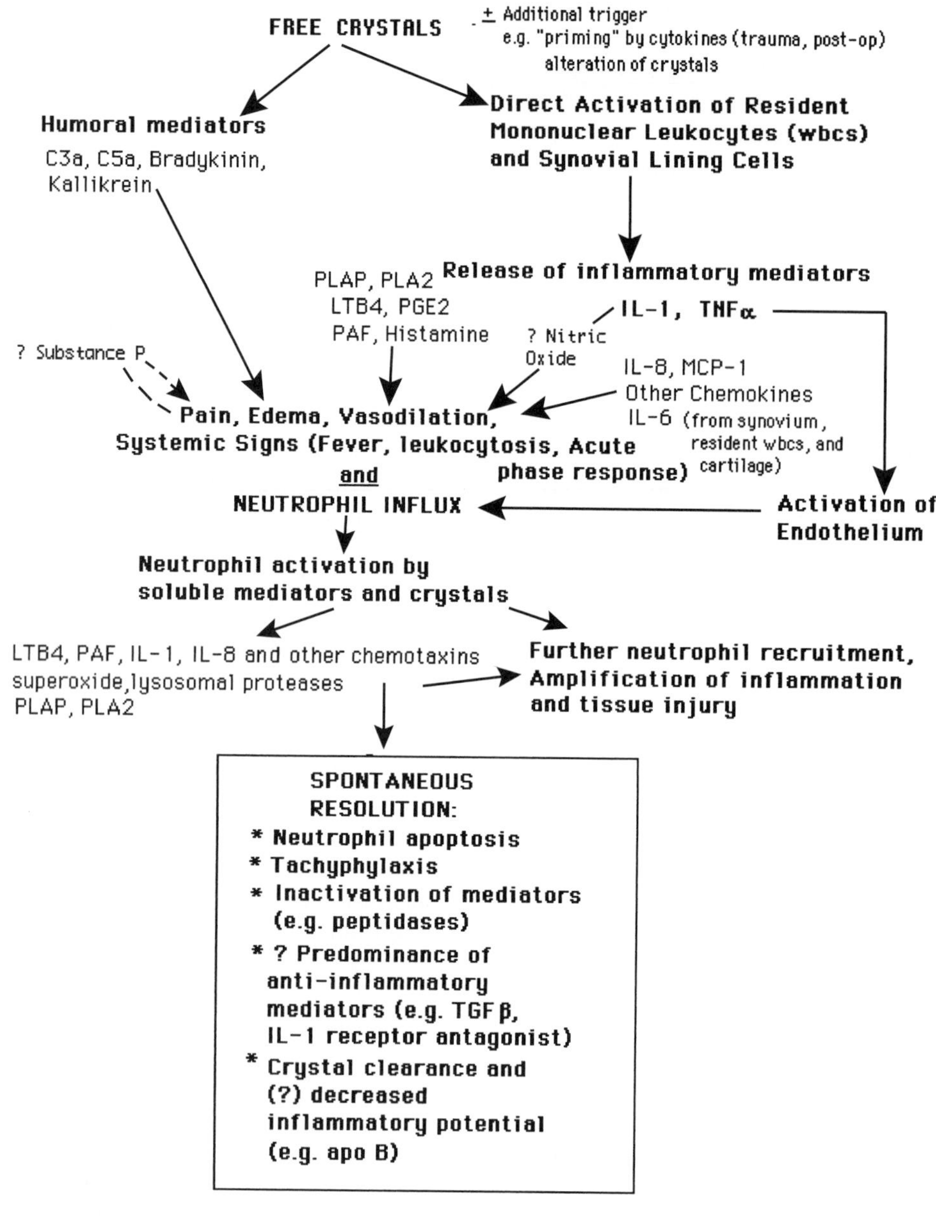

FIGURE 116.2. Hypothetic pathways involved in the triggering, amplification, and spontaneous resolution of acute gouty arthritis. *PLA2*, Phospholipase A2; *PLAP*, PLA2-activating protein; *MCP*, monocyte chemoattractant protein-1; *IL-8*, interleukin-8; *LTB4*, leukotriene B_4; *PAF*, platelet activating factor. See text for details.

share the ability of MSU crystals to activate multiple pathways that generate inflammatory mediators.

Generation and Release of Inflammatory Mediators

Complement and Coagulation System Activation

MSU crystals activate the classic complement pathway *in vitro* (1). They can bind and induce cleavage of purified macromolecular C1 in the absence of immunoglobulin (1,16). Additionally, classic pathway activation is amplified by bound IgG or C-reactive protein (1). Alternative pathway activation also occurs *in vitro* at higher crystal concentrations when classic pathway activation is inhibited (1). Direct cleavage of C5 to C5a and C5b also is effected by a stable C5 convertase formed on the crystal surface (1). Complement activation occurs in many human gouty synovial fluids (1). Although the amount of complement in normal joint fluid is low, C5a and C5a-des-arg are known to exert chemotactic effects at low concentrations (see Chapter 22).

MSU crystals activate Hageman factor and the contact coagulation system *in vitro,* resulting in generation of kallikrein, bradykinin, plasmin, and other inflammatory mediators (1). Joint fluids in acute gout (and in models of gout) contain elevated levels of kinins (1).

Monosodium Urate Crystal–induced Elaboration of Mediators from Cells

MSU crystals interact physically with synovial lining cells and mononuclear phagocytes in gouty joints (1). They also stimulate the transcription and elaboration of several proinflammatory cytokines (including IL-1, TNF-α, IL-6, and IL-8) (17–20) from cultured monocytes and synoviocytes. Additionally, the crystals are known to induce release of activated phospholipase A2 (PLA2) and a PLA2-activating protein (PLAP) (21), vasoactive prostaglandins, certain proteases from monocytes, and collagenase from fibroblasts *in vitro* (1).

MSU crystals induce neutrophils to elaborate lysosomal proteases (1), superoxide (1), activated PLA2 and PLAP (21), and lipoxygenase-derived products of arachidonic acid, including LTB_4 (1). Additionally, MSU crystals induce the production and release of IL-1 and IL-1β by neutrophils (22,23).

Certain low molecular weight polypeptides with neutrophil chemotactic activity also are transcriptionally activated and secreted in neutrophils after phagocytosis of MSU and certain other particulates (24). The grouping of these mediators under the term *crystal-induced chemotactic factor* (24) likely represented an early, seminal description of members of the chemokine family of low molecular weight polypeptide chemotactic cytokines (see Chapter 20). Several closely related chemokines of the C-X-C subfamily, including IL-8, GROβ, and GROγ, are potent neutrophil chemoattractants that share specific receptors, and are often released simultaneously in response to specific cytokines (e.g., IL-1) and other inflammatory stimuli (25). Substantial production of IL-8 by neutrophils can be induced by a variety of phagocytosable particles (including MSU crystals) as well as by certain soluble mediators (26).

The participation of synovial mast cells, platelets, or both in acute gout is theoretically possible; platelets are among the earliest cells to mediate inflammatory responses (see Chapter 19), and their interaction with urate crystals *in vitro* is well recognized (1). Mast cells (see Chapter 18) reside in the synovium, and stimulation of these cells *in vitro* by C3a, C5a, and IL-1 results in the release of a variety of inflammatory mediators, including histamine. Early articular swelling has been diminished by antihistamines in experimental MSU crystal–induced inflammation (1), and mast cell depletion inhibits experimental urate crystal–induced peritonitis (27).

Basic Mechanisms of Monosodium Urate Crystal–induced Cellular Activation

Crystal-induced Membrane Perturbation and Lysis

The considerable surface reactivity of the MSU crystal imparts to it a high capacity to induce perturbation and delayed lysis of plasma membranes and model liposomes (1,28,29). Furthermore, rapid cellular responses not mediated by membrane lysis are prominent, including secretion of platelet serotonin, neutrophil superoxide anion, and lysosomal proteases (1). Membrane cholesterol and MSU crystal–induced cross-linking of mobile membrane glycoproteins have been proposed to be important factors in MSU crystal–induced membrane lysis (1,28,29).

Phagocytosis of MSU crystals by neutrophils is followed by rapid dissolution of the phagolysosomal membrane. This process has been termed *suicide sac formation* by Weissmann et al. (1) because internal release of the lysosomal contents supervenes, and is followed by cellular swelling and death. Protein-coated MSU crystals are probably stripped of surface proteins by enzymatic digestion within phagolysosomes. Because the protein coat of MSU crystals inhibits membrane injury (1), its removal allows phagolysosome membrane lysis to occur. Cell death after phagocytosis of membranolytic crystals may also depend on influx of extracellular calcium into the damaged cell (1).

Signal Transduction

The ability of MSU crystals to induce functional responses [e.g., degranulation, reduced nicotinamide adenine dinucleotide phosphate (NADPH) oxidase activation] and gene expression in such a broad variety of cells indicates that heterogeneous mechanisms must be involved (Fig. 116.3). MSU crystals appear to activate membrane G proteins (including G_i α2) in neutrophils (30). Although MSU crystals can increase membrane permeability by lytic effects (1), MSU crystals also induce rapid cytosolic calcium mobilization modulated by phosphatidylinositol-4,5-bisphosphate (PIP_2) hydrolysis and inositol 1,4,5-trisphosphate (IP_3) generation in neutrophils (31). Unlike neutrophil activation induced by chemotactic factors, however, MSU crystal–induced PIP_2 hydrolysis and cytosolic calcium mobilization peak slowly, and these signals and subsequent functional responses do not require the activation of a pertussis toxin–sensitive G protein (30,31). PIP_2 hydrolysis is not the sole indication of plasma membrane phospholipase activation by MSU in leukocytes. For example, MSU crystals also induce cellular PLA2 and D activity in leukocytes (21,32).

MSU (and CPPD) crystals induce activation of certain tyrosine kinases in neutrophils (Fig. 116.3), generating a stimulus-specific array of phosphoproteins (33–36). Activation of the Src family tyrosine kinase *lyn* is an element of

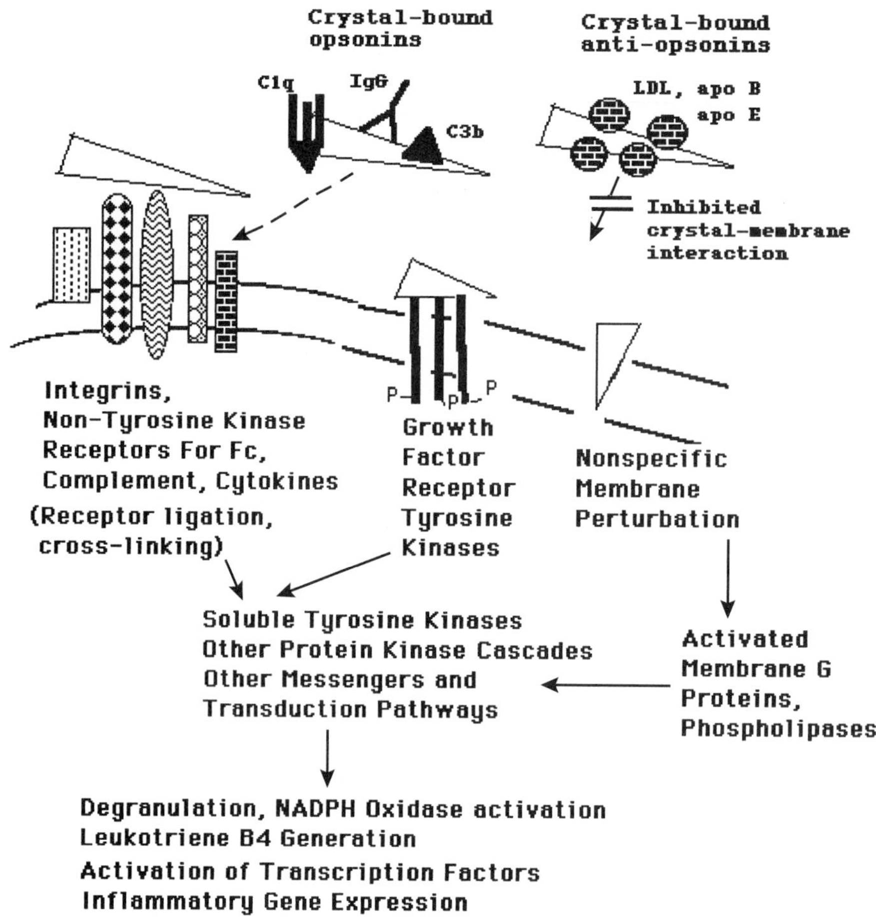

FIGURE 116.3. Hypothetic model for signal transduction in the activation of inflammatory cells by urate crystals. In this model, plasma membrane receptors that both nonspecifically bind naked urate crystals and specifically bind to crystal-bound opsonins [e.g., immunoglobulin G (IgG), C1q, C3b], are cross-linked and clustered, with the participation of the cytoskeleton (not shown). These events stimulate effector responses partly through attendant tyrosine kinases and other signals, including activation of membrane G proteins and phospholipases. Nonspecific membrane perturbation by urate crystals, and the capacity of crystal-bound proteins with antiopsonic activity [e.g., low-density lipoprotein (LDL) apoB] to diminish cell activation by inhibition of crystal–membrane binding also are indicated. See text for details.

this signal-transduction pathway (37). It is likely that Src family tyrosine kinase activation and the activation of certain other protein kinases (38,39) play a significant (and possibly central) role in several of the rapid responses to crystals (calcium mobilization, degranulation, and possibly NADPH oxidase activation) (36) as well as in proinflammatory gene expression (40).

MSU crystal–induced signal transduction is believed to be modulated by (a) membrane perturbation; (b) the previously mentioned surface reactivity of the MSU crystal, which gives it the ability to bind and potentially cross-link and cluster mobile membrane proteins (1), including integrins such as CD11b/CD18 and receptors including the Fc receptor CD16 on neutrophils (41); and (c) cytoskeletal interactions with such membrane proteins (34,35) (Fig. 116.3). In platelets, the membrane integrin Gp IIb/IIIa clearly binds to urate crystals, and partially mediates urate-induced platelet serotonin secretion (42).

Cross-linking and clustering of membrane proteins by multivalent ligands such as crystals (as depicted in Fig. 116.3) may be analogous to the effects on leukocytes of cross-linking certain membrane proteins [including Fc receptors (43)] or solid-phase bound CD44 and CD45 (44), which can result in pertussis toxin–insensitive cytosolic calcium mobilization (43) or cytokine induction (44). Tyrosine kinase activation plays a role in cell responses to many inflammatory ligands (e.g., cytokines) whose receptors possess no intrinsic tyrosine kinase activity, but can interact with attendant tyrosine kinases (see Chapter 22). Moreover, specific, ligand-induced dimerization is an important step in activation of growth factor receptors with intrinsic tyrosine kinase activity (45) (Fig. 116.3).

Fc receptor–mediated particle phagocytosis by macrophages (46) as well as unopsonized zymosan-induced arachidonate release in monocytes (47) can be mediated by activation of tyrosine kinases. In this light, opsonization of MSU crystals is not required for cell activation (Fig. 116.3). Whether cell adhesion to MSU is crystal face specific (48) remains to be determined.

Urate crystal–induced signal transduction culminating in proinflammatory cytokine gene expression has been studied in detail with IL-8 as a model (49). Urate crystals activate the mitogen-activated protein kinases p38, ERK1/ERK2, and JNK (49), and ERK1/ERK2 activation is critical for crystal-induced IL-8 expression in monocytic cells. Activation of the transcription factor AP-1 (mediated by JNK) also plays an essential role in IL-8 transcription in response to urate crystals (49). ERK1/ERK2, NF-κB, and AP-1 activation also have been observed to mediate inflammatory gene expression in response to CPPD and hydroxyapatite crystals in certain cells (including neutrophils, monocytes, and fibroblasts) (49–51).

Initiation, Propagation, and Spontaneous Resolution of Acute Gout

Hypothetic Sequence of Events

MSU crystals liberated from synovial microtophi, or precipitated *de novo,* are believed to activate humoral and cellular inflammatory mediator cascades and to upregulate neutrophil–endothelial adhesion (Fig. 116.2). For example, injection of free MSU crystals into the joint space of the knee in pigs induces marked upregulation of E-selectin in the synovial microvascular endothelium within hours (52). Triggering factors other than the new appearance of crystals must come into play in certain patients. These likely include changes in the surface, cell-activating properties of crystals, and "priming" effects on synovial inflammatory cells by cytokines (e.g., trauma, after surgery, intercurrent medical illness, or onset of gout in another joint; Fig. 116.2). Priming by cytokine release under such conditions may ignite a smoldering subclinical inflammatory response in otherwise asymptomatic joints (53) and help to explain the occurrence of polyarticular gouty attacks.

Early vasodilatation, enhanced vascular permeability, and pain in gouty arthritis are likely mediated by vasoactive prostaglandins, kinins (which also potentiate prostaglandin synthesis through release of membrane arachidonate), complement cleavage peptides, and histamine (1). The role of prostaglandins (54) as mediators of pain in gout is underlined by the strikingly complete suppression of tenderness (out of proportion to its effects on swelling, local heat, and volume of local effusion) in synovitis induced by MSU crystals in normal human volunteers pretreated with aspirin (1). Theoretically, pain signals also may mediate acute gout by the release from nociceptive afferent sensory nerve fibers of substance P, which has a number of proinflammatory functions (55,56). Surprisingly, the role of nitric oxide induction remains to be defined in crystal-induced arthritis (Fig. 116.2), although nitric oxide synthesis is triggered by IL-1 and other mediators (57) (see Chapter 20).

Neutrophil influx and activation appear to be the major effector arms in acute gouty arthritis. This is supported by the striking accumulation of these cells in both the joint fluid and synovial membrane, where they phagocytose crystals actively, and aggregate and degranulate in the microvasculature in areas remote from crystals (1). Phelps and McCarty (1) established that experimental urate crystal–induced synovitis is suppressed in neutrophil-depleted animals. Finally, a number of agents that suppress neutrophil inflammatory function are effective in preventing and terminating acute gouty inflammation.

Central Role of IL-8 and Related C-X-C Chemokines in Neutrophilic Gouty Inflammation

Neutrophils are virtually absent in normal joint fluid (see Chapter 4), and thus resident cell-derived humoral mediators must trigger initial neutrophil ingress into joints. MSU crystal–induced release of IL-1 and TNF-α from monocytes and synovial lining cells likely promotes neutrophil ingress through the induction of activation of the endothelial cells of postcapillary venules (see Chapters 16 and 21). IL-1 and TNF-α also induce the release of several chemotactic cytokines (chemokines; see Chapter 20) including IL-8, GROβ, GROγ, and monocyte chemoattractant protein-1 (MCP-1) from mononuclear phagocytes, fibroblasts, chondrocytes (58–62), and certain other cells (25,26). In this regard, IL-8 is the major neutrophil chemotactic factor released from monocytes activated by MSU crystals *in vitro,* and is particularly abundant in acute gout (and pseudogout) joint fluids (20,63).

Neutrophil chemotactic C-X-C subfamily chemokines other than IL-8 also are expressed at sites of gouty inflammation (25,64,65). There is expression in the joint space, and by the synovium or synovium-like lining, in rodent models of acute gout, of GROα, and the GROβ and GROγ homologue monocyte inhibition protein-2 (MIP-2; a much more potent neutrophil chemotaxin than GROα) (65). There are two IL-8 receptors in humans (CXCR1 and CXCR2), but CXCR2 is much more promiscuous than CXCR1 and binds the GRO chemokines and certain other C-X-C chemokines with the potential to be expressed in the joint (including ENA-78 and GCP-2) (25,65).

In the mouse, neutrophils express a homologue of CXCR2 but not CXCR1 (63), and mice do not express IL-8. We studied acute urate crystal–induced inflammation in CXCR2 knockout mice (65). The neutrophils of these mice respond normally to chemotaxins other than CXCR2 ligands. However, acute urate crystal–induced neutrophilic inflammation (4 hours after crystal injection into a subcutaneous air pouch) was completely dependent on CXCR2 ligands (65). Nevertheless, a proteinaceous exudate was induced in the pouch 4 hours after crystal injection in CXCR2 knockout mice, indicating a role, in this component of the inflammatory response, for mediators other than CXCR2 ligands (likely including arachidonate metabolites).

Study of urate crystal–induced joint inflammation in rabbits treated with antibody to IL-8 indicated that the early neutrophilic influx was suppressed but not abrogated, consistent with a likely role for synovium-derived GRO chemokines, and possibly other CXCR2 ligands distinct from IL-8 in initiating acute gouty arthritis (66). Neutrophil influx was inhibited by approximately two thirds at 24 hours after crystal injection in the rabbits treated with neutralizing antibody to IL-8 (66). Thus it is likely that IL-8 derived from not only synovial lining cells but also activated, infiltrating neutrophils, markedly amplifies early crystal-induced inflammation (Fig. 116.2). Specifically, the release of neutrophil-derived mediators [e.g., IL-1, chemokines, LTB_4, and platelet activating factor (PAF) (67)] in response to contact with both intraarticular MSU crystals and fluid-phase IL-8, and other CXCR1 and CXCR2 ligands, appears to play a major role in gouty inflammation by establishing a self-amplifying cycle of further neutrophil ingress and neutrophil activation (Fig. 116.2).

Direct crystal–neutrophil interaction detected by compensated polarized light microscopy is diagnostic in acute crystal arthritis (see Chapter 4). However, the findings discussed earlier indicate that direct crystal–neutrophil (as opposed to crystal–synovial lining cell interaction) may not be essential to the pathologic process in acute gout. This likely explains why crystals are not detected within synovial fluid neutrophils at all times in all cases.

Systemic Manifestations and Chronic Inflammation

The elaboration of MSU crystal–induced IL-1, TNF-α, IL-8, and IL-6 (17–20) into the circulation likely plays a critical role in the development of systemic manifestations (including low-grade fever, leukocytosis, and the hepatic acute phase protein response). MSU crystal deposition may be associated not only with episodic acute inflammation but also with chronic synovitis, articular erosions, and cartilage and subchondral osseous destruction. The MSU crystal–induced release from resident mononuclear phagocytes and synovial lining cells of the previously mentioned cytokines and of proteases and biologic oxidants likely fuels chronic inflammation and connective tissue degradation. Thus adequate and expeditious measures to reduce hyperuricemia and to lessen crystal deposition are imperative. Destructive articular changes and joint deformities can progress despite uric acid–reducing therapy that adequately diminishes further episodes of acute gout (68).

Regulation of the Inflammatory Potential of the Monosodium Urate Crystal

Self-limitation of Acute Gouty Inflammation

The self-limitation of acute gouty inflammation has been known since the time of Hippocrates. Additionally, the remarkable efficacy of short-term treatment for acute gout suggests the additional participation of significant natural mechanisms that limit gouty inflammation. Factors other than cell-mediated MSU crystal dissolution (1) or crystal sequestration must play a role in terminating attacks, as free MSU crystals are often found in synovial fluid for many weeks after subsidence of an acute gouty paroxysm. Several events might contribute (Table 116.2). In this regard, neutrophil apoptosis (see Chapter 16) is a fundamental mechanism in the resolution of acute tissue inflammation (69,70). Neutrophils in acute crystal synovitis joint fluids undergo apoptosis (71), a process that can be accelerated by TNF-α and other inflammatory agonists (72). Such effects (and the usual limitation by apoptosis of the maximal neutrophil functional life span to a few days) (72,73) likely mandate continued recruitment of new neutrophils to the gouty inflammatory locus to sustain acute inflammation (74).

Another mode of inflammatory autoregulation is inactivation of mediators (e.g., LTB_4 omega-oxidation and regulation of expression of related peptidases that can inactivate IL-1β, substance P, C5a, and other mediators) (75). IL-8 and other chemokines are particularly resistant to proteolytic inactivation (20,25,26). Thus tachyphylaxis to such mediators (76), and the cross-desensitization of leukocytes to chemotaxins (77) also may play a significant role.

Changes in the balance between molecules that exert pro- and antiinflammatory effects during the course of

TABLE 116.2. POTENTIAL MECHANISMS TO EXPLAIN SPONTANEOUS RESOLUTION IN ACUTE GOUT

1. Neutrophil apoptosis
2. Tachyphylaxis to inflammatory mediators
3. Inactivation of mediators (e.g., peptidases)
4. ? Change in the balance of antiinflammatory mediators
   IL-1 receptor antagonist
   TGF-β
   Soluble TNF and Fc receptors
   Peroxisome proliferator activated receptor (PPAR) subtypes (α,γ)
5. Crystal clearance and (? decreased crystal inflammatory potential secondary to bound apoB, apoE)

IL, interleukin; TGF, transforming growth factor; TNF, tumor necrosis factor; apo, apolipoprotein.

acute crystal-induced inflammation are likely to modulate the clinical features. Activated inflammatory cells can release a variety of substances that are capable of diminishing inflammation (78). In gouty inflammation, these would be expected to first include the E-series prostaglandins, which inhibit IL-1 and TNF-β production, suppress neutrophil function (see Chapter 16), and suppress MSU crystal–induced inflammation in rat air pouches (79). Second, IL-1–receptor antagonist activity is expressed physiologically (80) and also is present in acute crystal arthritis synovial fluids (81). Third, transforming growth factor-β (TGF-β), although it has a number of proinflammatory activities that could help ignite acute synovitis (82,83), is a potent inhibitor of IL-1–receptor expression and IL-1–driven cellular responses (83,84). TGF-β is known to be released from activated monocytes and from other cells and is abundant in some acute gouty synovial fluids (85). Administration of TGF-β into a rat air pouch 2 hours after MSU crystal substantially inhibited leukocyte accumulation (86). Fourth, IL-6 can inhibit TNF-β release under certain conditions (87), and can, along with IL-1, induce central adrenocorticotropin (ACTH) release with subsequent endogenous adrenal glucocorticoid release. Fifth, shedding of soluble Fc and TNF-β receptors by activated neutrophils (88,89) may inhibit phagocytosis, neutrophil priming, and other proinflammatory events. Recent work has demonstrated antiinflammatory negative-feedback loops involving peroxisome proliferator–activated receptor (PPAR) subtypes α and γ (90–92) and in some cases LTB_4 (90) (which is by itself not critical for neutrophil influx in experimental acute gouty inflammation) (65,93). Last, changes in crystal surface-bound proteins, which have been described during the evolution of the gouty paroxysm (94), also may modulate inflammation.

Crystals with and without Inflammation

The lack of direct correlation between the amount of urate crystal deposition and the severity of acute gouty inflammatory reactions is well documented (1,3). For example, large quantities of crystals (joint milk) may be aspirated from joints that show little or no sign of inflammation (95). In other patients, only a few crystals might be detected despite full-blown acute gouty arthritis. A striking absence of inflammation adjacent to subcutaneous deposits of urate crystals is the rule, and some patients with chronic tophaceous gout give no history of acute attacks (1).

Putative Regulatory Factors for Crystal-induced Inflammation

Host factors that may modulate MSU crystal–induced inflammation include renal failure and RA. Patients with chronic renal insufficiency have diminished inflammatory responses to the subcutaneous injection of MSU crystals (1), and it has been suggested that gouty attacks are less severe and less frequent in such individuals (1). The high incidence of gouty arthritis in association with lead nephropathy and cyclosporine use seem paradoxic.

The coexistence of RA and gout is much more rare than expected statistically (1), perhaps attributable to the hypouricemic and antiinflammatory effects of many therapeutic agents used routinely in RA, and the elevated intraarticular temperature of active RA joints.

Polymeric hyaluronic acid inhibits both neutrophil chemotactic mobility and phagocytosis of MSU crystals in a dose-dependent manner and thus may regulate crystal-induced inflammation (1). A decrease in hyaluronate concentration as a result of development of an effusion (e.g., after trauma) might dilute its inhibitory effect on crystal–cell interactions and render the crystals more inflammatory. Urate in solution suppresses protein adsorption by neutrophil plasma membranes and could result in increased crystal-induced membranolysis (1). No correlation exists between crystal size and the severity of MSU-induced inflammation (1). Fam's work (1) has suggested that urate spherulites may have a different inflammatory potential, however, and it is conceivable that subtle variations in the means by which MSU crystals are nucleated (13) can alter their inflammatory potential.

Alteration of Monosodium Urate Crystal–induced Cell Activation by Crystal-bound Proteins

Much attention has been focused on the possibility that protein adsorbed to MSU crystal surfaces (1,96,97) could be a critical determinant of their inflammatory potential. For example, removal or proteolytic digestion of proteins coating the surface of MSU crystals isolated from quiescent tophi can markedly alter their capacity to activate neutrophils *in vitro* (98,99). Additionally, binding of neutrophil lysosomal enzymes to MSU crystals can displace IgG from the crystal surface and render MSU crystals less able to stimulate neutrophils *in vitro* (100). The binding of fibronectin to MSU crystals (1) also could enhance integrin-mediated crystal binding to cells (101).

Synthetic MSU crystals (and monosodium urate crystals from tophi) preincubated with whole serum become markedly less stimulatory for leukocytes (96). The effects of serum are mainly due to the binding of apolipoprotein (apo) B–containing lipoproteins (96). Low density lipoprotein (LDL), the predominant apoB lipoprotein, suppresses cellular responses to MSU by binding to the crystal surface, thereby physically inhibiting particle–cell interaction, phagocytosis, and membrane activation (Fig. 116.3) (96,102). ApoB is both necessary and sufficient for this activity of LDL (96). MSU crystals in quiescent tophaceous synovial deposits are physically associated with various amounts of surface proteins and lipids (1). The lipids in tophi include cholesteryl esters, which are predominantly carried by plasma LDL. Furthermore, LDL binds to MSU crystals *in vivo* (94,97).

Apolipoprotein (apo) E also can be bound to MSU crystals *in vivo,* and at physiologic concentrations, MSU crystal–bound apoE blunts crystal-induced neutrophil activation *in vitro* (103). ApoE, unlike apoB, is synthesized within synovial joints by cells of the monocyte/macrophage lineage (103), and thus it exemplifies a locally produced factor capable of markedly altering the inflammatory potential of MSU crystals.

The proteins coating MSU crystals undergo dynamic changes during the evolution of acute gout and experimental gouty inflammation *in vivo* (94,97). Crystal-bound IgG, which enhances the intrinsic capacity of MSU to stimulate neutrophils and certain other cells (1) (Fig. 116.3) generally becomes less abundant with time (94). Conversely, little apoB is initially detected on MSU crystals, but crystal-bound apoB becomes substantially more abundant coincident with the resolution of intraarticular leukocytosis (94). LDL is capable of markedly inhibiting the inflammatory potential of MSU crystals injected into rat air pouches *in vivo* (E. Ortiz-Bravo et al., unpublished data, 1990). Further studies on the potential effects of MSU crystal–bound LDL *in vivo* in gout are indicated because oxidation of LDL lipids, which has been documented in inflammatory joint fluids, actually renders LDL capable of inducing the elaboration by monocytes of several proinflammatory cytokines, including IL-8 (104).

Gout Paradigm and Inflammation Caused by Other Crystals

The range in intensity of acute synovitis associated with intraarticular crystals other than MSU is broad. Similarly, the pathogenesis of inflammation induced by other microcrystals appears complex. In addition, acute synovitis associated with CPPD crystals is sometimes relatively long-lived and refractory to treatment. Ingested CPPD crystals (and basic calcium phosphate crystals) are relatively potent mitogens for synovial cells (105) compared with MSU crystals, and thus a heightened relative role of synovial proliferation in acute articular inflammation provoked by CPPD and other calcium-containing crystals is a possibility.

CPPD Crystal–induced Inflammation

Monoclinic versus Triclinic CPPD Crystals

Acute pseudogout is associated with neutrophil leukocytosis in synovial fluid and with intracellular crystals. CPPD crystals activate complement (1), trigger cytosolic calcium mobilization and tyrosine kinase activation in neutrophils (33,106) and the release of leukotrienes, IL-1, chemotactic cytokines, and PLAP from phagocytes (1,20,21). Several studies with CPPD crystals suggested, however, that their capacity to induce the release of a number of cytokines (including IL-1 and IL-6) from phagocytes is weaker than that of MSU crystals (18,107,108). The inflammatory potential of CPPD crystals appears to be markedly influenced by their structure. Specifically, the experimental injection of monoclinic CPPD crystals into rodent air pouches and pleural spaces produces substantially greater inflammation than did the injection of triclinic CPPD crystals (109,110). In a clinical study, the ratio of monoclinic to triclinic CPPD crystals was elevated in acute pseudogout synovial fluids in comparison to noninflamed CPPD deposition disease and osteoarthritic synovial fluids containing CPPD crystals (111). Monoclinic crystals are larger than triclinic crystals, and the increased surface area may be vital for increased adsorption of opsonizing serum proteins, as proposed by Burt and Jackson (112).

As described by Mandel (1), negativity of crystal surface charge and surface irregularity appear to be important determinants of the inflammatory potential of crystals; that is, the crystal surfaces of more inflammatory membranolytic crystals (MSU, CPPD, the α-quartz form of silicon dioxide) are irregular and possess a high density of charged groups, whereas the surfaces of nonhemolytic noninflammatory crystals (e.g., diamond dust and the stishovite and anatase forms of silicon dioxide) are smooth. Brushite and hydroxyapatite crystals present a less negatively charged surface atomic array than the more membranolytic CPPD crystals (1), which may explain why these crystals are less frequently associated with acute inflammation.

Basic Calcium Phosphate Crystals

Basic calcium phosphate crystals have a remarkable tendency to form aggregates, the larger of which (“too big to swallow”) may escape endocytosis. However, hydroxyapatite and their basic calcium phosphates directly stimulate both leukocytes and synoviocytes *in vitro.* These crystals are phlogistic when injected into animals and are sometimes associated with severe acute articular and periarticular inflammation in humans. They also are associated with widespread articular inflammation in *ank/ank* mice (113).

Thus definition of other factors that account for the remarkable lack of acute articular inflammation and leukocytosis generally associated with the presence of intraarticular basic calcium phosphate crystals in humans is required. Such factors may include the low complement-activating potential of basic calcium phosphate crystals relative to MSU (1); the diminished ability of basic calcium phosphate to induce release of cytokines (e.g., IL-1) from human monocyte/macrophages (17), and chemotactic factors from neutrophils (108); and the inability of hydroxyapatite crystals (unlike MSU and silica crystals) to activate neutrophil membrane G proteins directly (30). It is possible that hydroxyapatite crystals are less able than urate crystals to activate tyrosine kinase signaling in phagocytes (50). Additionally, adsorbed molecules may mediate the inflammatory potential of basic calcium phosphate crystals, as already demonstrated for MSU. Phosphocitrate, an inhibitor of calcium phosphate crystallization that is constitutively present in the mitochondria (the intracellular compartment containing by far the most Pi), also markedly inhibits several basic calcium phosphate and CPPD crystal–induced cell-activation events, including membranolysis, mitogen activated protein kinase (MAPK) activation, and mitogenesis (105). α2-HS-glycoprotein, a serum protein produced by the liver that localizes to mineralizing bone, is a major specific inhibitor of neutrophil responses to basic calcium phosphate crystals *in vitro* (114).

Advances in understanding how physical changes in the structure and surface coat of crystals could regulate crystal–membrane interaction and inflammation *in vitro* and *in vivo* should be facilitated by the advent of atomic force microscopy, which can be used to identify microcrystals readily and to resolve their surface constituents in exquisite detail in biologic samples (115,116).

Experimental Models of Crystal-induced Arthritis

Animal model systems have been useful in the dissection of some critical features of the host response to crystals. Such models have used dog, bird, porcine, and rabbit joints (66); rat paws; and rat pleural spaces (1,48). The rodent subcutaneous air pouch, which is lined by cells histologically similar to synoviocytes, and created by repeated injection of sterile air, is a useful model (65,110). Such artificial "joints," however, do not contain hyaluronate-rich fluid. Moreover, it has not been established that MSU crystal–induced inflammation is neutrophil dependent, and indomethacin treatment failed to suppress MSU crystal–induced neutrophil influx in this model system (117).

Experimental crystal-induced inflammation in humans can be successfully used for testing for drug effectiveness (1). For example, the intradermal injection of sterile MSU crystals in humans provokes a transient, self-limited local response, and a systemic response exemplified by leukocytosis and an increase in serum amyloid A protein, which peaks while the intradermal lesion is resolving (118).

TREATMENT OF CRYSTAL-INDUCED INFLAMMATION

Gout

The aims of therapy in gout are to alleviate pain, which is often excruciating, and to restore the inflamed joint to useful function. After protection of the joint by splinting and administration of analgesics, a wide choice of effective drugs is available.

Colchicine

Therapy of Acute Gout and Toxicities Observed

Under most circumstances, colchicine has the poorest therapeutic benefit/toxicity ratio of drugs available for the primary treatment of acute gout (1,119,120) (Table 116.3). For this reason, the use of colchicine as a primary treatment justifiably has been eclipsed by the use of other modalities. In particular, the standard oral colchicine regimen discussed later usually provokes diarrhea, which can be severe.

Colchicine is most effective as primary therapy in gout when administered in the first 24 hours after onset of the acute attack. The drug can be given orally; a standard regimen is 0.5 or 0.6 mg/hour until relief or side effects occur, or until a predetermined maximal total dose has been given (i.e., a maximal total of 6 mg over a total of 12 hours in normal individuals, but less than this amount of colchicine in those with renal insufficiency and in the elderly). Signs and symptoms of inflammation generally subside in 12 to 24 hours, and pain is gone in 90% of patients in 24 hours (1). A useful alternative approach is to add low doses of oral colchicine (e.g., 0.6 mg p.o., b.i.d.) as an adjunct to another, better-tolerated primary treatment approach [e.g., nonsteroidal antiinflammatory drugs (NSAIDs) or ACTH], particularly if the patient is a candidate to start uric acid–lowering therapy after resolution of the acute gouty attack.

A response to colchicine treatment has been reported in a number of articular conditions other than gout [including sarcoid arthritis, calcific tendinitis, and pseudogout (1)].

TABLE 116.3. MANIFESTATIONS OF COLCHICINE TOXICITY

Intravenous
Bone marrow depression producing peripheral thrombocytopenia and neutropenia (nadir of values about 3–6 days after drug is given; recovery in absence of additional drug in 4–7 days)
Cellulitis or thrombophlebitis at injection site
Alopecia
Gastrointestinal: Abdominal pain, nausea, vomiting, diarrhea (rare)
CNS dysfunction
Peripheral neuropathy
Myopathy (proximal weakness and elevated serum creatine kinase)
Shock: Delayed and associated with oliguria, hematuria, weakness, paralysis, delirium, convulsions, and (often) death
Oral
Gastrointestinal: Cramps, diarrhea (most common), nausea, vomiting
Neuropathy myopathy alopecia (uncommon)
Bone marrow depression (uncommon)
Shock (rare)
Effects on sperm production and function (controversial)

CNS, central nervous system.

Thus a response to colchicine alone is insufficient to confirm the diagnosis of acute gout.

Colchicine cannot be given orally in persons with postoperative acute gout. ACTH or intraarticular steroid injection is preferable in these circumstances. The use of intravenous colchicine under most circumstances is questionable (120,121). However, in the rare event that other treatments are contraindicated or ineffective, intravenous colchicine can be used as follows: intravenous colchicine, 1 mg, diluted in 20 mL of normal saline is administered slowly (not less than 10 minutes). Colchicine, 1 mg, given as a single dose is adequate for most attacks. Care is necessary to avoid extravasation because of the marked irritating properties of the drug. *No more than 2 mg of colchicine should be given in a single intravenous dose, and a total intravenous dose of greater than 4 mg and repeated intravenous administration time beyond 24 hours for one attack of gout are inadvisable.* Furthermore, it has been recommended that patients should receive no more colchicine by any route for the first 7 days after intravenous colchicine therapy (122,123).

Intravenous colchicine should be used only if strict precautions are followed (1,124). First, because colchicine is excreted in urine and bile, patients with oliguria, severe renal insufficiency (creatinine clearance <10 mL/min), significant hepatic dysfunction, and biliary tract obstruction should be treated with alternative agents. In patients with renal failure, severe marrow suppression is a particular risk (even with low doses of intravenous colchicine). Second, individuals with significant cardiac dysfunction, persons with depressed bone marrow function or receiving cytotoxic chemotherapy, and those with severe infection have an increased risk of colchicine toxicity, mandating a dose reduction and strong consideration of alternative therapy. Third, the maximal dose of intravenous colchicine should be decreased by 50% in the elderly. Fourth, intravenous colchicine should be avoided, or used only judiciously, in patients with a history of immediate prior use of therapeutic or daily, prophylactic oral colchicine.

Manifestations of intravenous and oral colchicine toxicity are listed in Table 116.3, and have been reviewed in more detail elsewhere (124,125). A reversible syndrome of gastrointestinal dysfunction, deterioration of hepatic and renal function, and neuromyopathy has been reported in some patients taking colchicine in conjunction with cyclosporine (126). Conversely, colchicine appeared to protect against experimental cyclosporine nephrotoxicity in rats (127).

Treatment of colchicine overdose with colchicine-specific antibodies holds considerable therapeutic promise (128,129). Furthermore, colchicine analogues have been described with comparable antiinflammatory activities *in vivo* but less toxicity (1,130). The possible therapeutic use of these compounds, and of liposomal formulations of colchicine for local delivery (131) remain to be explored.

Prophylactic Use

Because the total leukocyte and absolute neutrophil counts in asymptomatic gouty knee joints are significantly reduced by a prophylactic colchicine treatment regimen (53), it is conceivable that "prophylactic" colchicine actually works in part by diminishing subclinical inflammation.

Acute gouty attacks are effectively prevented by small daily doses of colchicine. Doses of 0.5 to 1.8 mg daily are given; the average patient requires about 1 mg. Such doses either completely prevented attacks or greatly reduced their frequency in 93% of a large series of gouty patients during many years of follow-up (1). Only 4% had gastrointestinal toxicity, and many of these patients had underlying intestinal disease. Even with a standard prophylactic dose of 1.2 mg/day, renal failure (particularly with concomitant hepatic disease or cytotoxic drug treatment) predisposes to more serious toxicity, including bone marrow depression (132) and a reversible polymyositis-like proximal myopathy (133), which can occur within weeks of initiating therapy (134). Colchicine-induced rhabdomyolysis also has been reported (135).

A dose-reduction schedule for patients with renal insufficiency is strongly advised (132,134). For example, patients with severe renal insufficiency can be maintained on as little as 0.6 mg oral colchicine q3–4 days with continuing therapeutic efficacy. Additionally, caution should be exercised when concurrently using drugs (e.g., cimetidine, tolbutamide, erythromycin) that can additively interfere with colchicine metabolism in the face of coexistent hepatic or renal disease (124,136–138). Transplacental passage of colchicine and entry into the breast milk of nursing mothers also have been documented (139). The overall effects of low-dose colchicine regimens on rates of miscarriages and congenital malformations and female and male fertility are unclear (138–140).

Acute attacks may be heralded by "twinges" in the target joint. If attacks are relatively infrequent (fewer than three per year), the patient not receiving daily prophylactic doses can often abort an attack by taking 1 mg of oral colchicine at the first symptom and 0.5 mg every 2 hours thereafter (to a maximal total of 6 mg) until symptoms are relieved.

Metabolism

After a single, 2-mg intravenous dose of colchicine, the drug is still detectable in plasma by radioimmunoassay days later (1). The mean plasma half-life has been estimated to be 58 ± 20 minutes with a peak plasma concentration of 2.9 ± 1.5 mg/dL (10^{-7} *M*) under these conditions. In volunteers given a single, 1-mg oral dose of colchicine, peak plasma levels of up to 0.6 mg/dL (10^{-8} *M*) have been measured. The drug is concentrated in leukocytes at tenfold or greater levels relative to plasma, however (141). In this regard, the absence of the multidrug resistance gene drug export channel (P glycoprotein) in neutrophils may allow even greater concentration (and efficacy) of the drug in neutrophils relative to mononuclear leukocytes (142). Although maximal urinary excretion occurs 2 hours after intravenous colchicine administration, the overall excretion of the drug is slow, and it has been detected in the urine 10 days after injection.

Mechanism of Action

Peak colchicine concentration in peripheral blood leukocytes after a standard intravenous dose can reach 1 to 2 × 10^{-5} *M*; at 72 hours after injection, leukocyte colchicine levels of 5 × 10^{-6} *M* have been reported, and detectable drug levels can still be found in cells isolated from the blood 10 days later (1). The ability of colchicine to concentrate in leukocytes appears central to its efficacy (Table 116.4). Colchicine binds irreversibly to tubulin dimers and prevents their assembly into microtubules (1,141). This property makes colchicine, like other tubulin-binding plant alkaloids (e.g., vinblastine), a potent, and potentially lethal, antimitotic cell toxin (111,128,138).

The broad spectrum of colchicine effects on neutrophils (Table 116.4) is consistent with its particularly rapid and consistent efficacy (measured in a few hours) in a predominantly neutrophil-mediated inflammatory process such as acute gout. The effects of colchicine on neutrophil–endothelial adhesion (see Chapters 16 and 21) are particularly potent and may be critical to its efficacy (143). Specifically, colchicine at nanomolar concentrations achievable with low-dose, oral, prophylactic colchicine regimens alters the distribution of E-selectin–mediated increase in endothelial adhesiveness for neutrophils in response to IL-1 and TNF-α (144,145). Colchicine at higher, therapeutic concentrations (300 n*M* or greater) diminishes the expression of L-selectin on neutrophils (but not lymphocytes) and diminishes the L-selectin–mediated rolling of leukocytes in the microvasculature (145).

TABLE 116.4. PROPOSED MECHANISMS FOR EFFICACY OF COLCHICINE IN ACUTE CRYSTAL-INDUCED ARTHRITIS

- Inhibits inflammatory neutrophil function
  - Inhibits upregulated neutrophil–endothelial adhesion (particularly potent effect)
  - Increases cAMP
  - Inhibits crystal-induced tyrosine kinase activation
  - Selectively inhibits mediator release (e.g., decreases IL-1 and chemotactic cytokine release, but not IL-1 receptor antagonist release)
  - Inhibits crystal-induced PLA2 activity, and PLAP and LTB_4 release
  - Inhibits migration
  - Inhibits phagocytosis
- Other inhibitory effects
  - TNF receptors/responses in macrophages and endothelium (not in neutrophils)
  - Histamine release from mast cells

cAMP, cyclic adenosine monophosphate; IL, interleukin; PLA2, phospholipase A2; PLAP, PLA2 activating protein; LT, leukotriene; TNF, tumor necrosis factor.

At higher concentrations that are achievable therapeutically, colchicine also suppresses many other neutrophil functions, including random motility, chemotaxis, PLA2 activation and the stimulated elaboration of PLAP, and certain chemotactic factors (e.g., LTB_4) (1,21–23). Neutrophil responses to a number of soluble chemotactic agonists (including LTB_4, IL-8, and other chemotactic cytokines) are markedly inhibited by colchicine (1). Production and secretion of cytokines and proteases, however, appear to be inhibited selectively and in a ligand-specific manner by colchicine (1,23,146–148). In this regard, the release of IL-1–receptor antagonist by activated neutrophils does not appear to be suppressed by colchicine (23). Colchicine inhibits IL-1 production by activated neutrophils (22,23), however, although the drug may have different effects on IL-1 production by other cells (1,107). Colchicine also inhibits phagocytosis of certain particulates, but these effects are relatively weak, and colchicine does not inhibit superoxide generation by neutrophils (1).

Colchicine also may act by directly downregulating TNF-α receptors (and TNF-α–driven responses) in macrophages and endothelial cells (149), whereas neutrophil TNF-α receptors are unaffected under identical conditions. Colchicine also can inhibit mast cell histamine release (1,141).

Colchicine appears to effect neutrophil inhibition by heterogeneous mechanisms. First, colchicine directly elevates cyclic adenosine monophosphate (AMP) levels, and potentiates prostaglandin E-induced and β-adrenergic–induced increases in neutrophil cyclic AMP, probably by stimulating the guanosine triphosphatase (GTPase) activity of tubulin (1,141). Some work suggests that the ability of colchicine to promote cAMP elevation in neutrophils can be enhanced by concomitant administration of the prostaglandin E analogue misoprostol (150). Elevation of cAMP can globally depress neutrophil function. Second, intact microtubule function clearly contributes to optimal expression of neutrophil 5- and 15-lipoxygenase activity, and colchicine markedly suppresses these activities in neutrophils (146). Third, colchicine (at levels of 10^{-5} *M*) inhibits MSU and CPPD crystal–induced tyrosine kinase activation in neutrophils (34). This effect is specific, as activation induced by several soluble agonists [including the chemotactic peptides *N*-formyl-methionyl-leucyl-phenylalanine (FMLP) and C5a] are not suppressed and may be mediated by effects on microtubule-modulated membrane protein clustering and movement (1,34). Fourth, colchicine may alter diacylglycerol generation (147) and thus modulate certain stimulus–response coupling mechanisms (1). Last, the stabilization by colchicine of labile microtubules normally required for leukocyte motility may inhibit chemotaxis, phagocytosis, and adhesiveness (1).

The effects of colchicine on microtubules may not be the only explanation for the drug's effectiveness. Colchicine also binds to leukocyte membrane proteins, which might be tubulin-like attachment points for microtubules (1,147). Furthermore, certain colchicine analogues that do not effectively bind to tubulin, and which are not metabolized to colchicine in humans, appear to have antiinflammatory effects in animal model systems and in gouty patients (1,130). Conversely, certain colchicine analogues that effectively bind tubulin have little antiinflammatory activity (1,130).

Nonsteroidal Antiinflammatory Agents

Many NSAIDs provide effective therapy for acute gout (1,122) and can also be used (at lower doses) for prophylaxis of gouty attacks. Caution must be exercised in the elderly and in other patient subsets (e.g., individuals with dehydration or renal insufficiency), as discussed in Chapter 32. The basis for the neutrophil-suppressive and antiinflammatory activities of NSAIDs are reviewed in Chapters 16 and 32. For example, NSAIDs diminish adhesion mediated by the integrin CD11b/CD18 (144).

Indomethacin is an effective agent for acute gout (an adequate dose is generally 150–200 mg/day for 2–3 days, and then 75–100 mg daily over the next week, or until pain and inflammation subside). Naproxen, 750 mg as a single dose followed by maintenance doses (375–500 mg b.i.d.), is a reasonable alternative (109). Tolmetin sodium has been claimed to be less effective for acute gout (151). There are no published data, at this time, to indicate whether the newer, selective cyclooxygenase-2 (COX-2) inhibitor NSAIDs are more or less effective than indomethacin or naproxen for acute (and chronic) crystal-induced arthritis.

Azapropazone (1) and other NSAIDs that possess uricosuric effects (e.g., the fluorinated salicylate diflunisal) (152) require further investigation for adequacy and safety in long-term gout prophylaxis and uric acid reduction.

Corticosteroids and ACTH

Thorough aspiration of the joint, often possible at the time of diagnostic arthrocentesis to obtain fluid for crystal identification, can be followed by local injection of microcrystalline adrenocorticosteroid esters. Such therapy is ideal in a single large joint; crystal-induced inflammation subsides predictably within 12 hours of treatment, regardless of the prior duration of the acute attack.

Therapy with ACTH (153–157) is a particularly useful approach for polyarticular gout refractory to NSAIDs, or for gout in settings in which NSAIDs are absolutely contraindicated (including renal failure, gastrointestinal bleeding, and certain postoperative states). ACTH may be conveniently administered by intramuscular and subcutaneous routes (153–156). The dose can be repeated (e.g., q12 hours for 1–3 days in incomplete responders) (157). A single dose of 25 to 40 IU i.m. of synthetic ACTH is often sufficient for early, monoarticular attacks. For example, in one therapeutic trial for monoarticular gout, ACTH, given as a single intramuscular injection (40 IU), was consistently and rapidly effective (relief of pain in 3 hours), and tolerance was excellent (154). Clinical rebound can be a problem, however (156,157), and may be reduced by timely initiation of prophylactic low-dose colchicine. Acute polyarticular gout attacks may require more prolonged ACTH treatment (155). In my experience, more severe polyarticular gout attacks usually are treated successfully with one dose of intravenous ACTH [prepared by suspending a lyophilized ACTH preparation (40 IU) in saline and administering it by slow intravenous infusion]. With this regimen, it is sometimes necessary to readminister 40 IU ACTH intravenously (e.g., 18–24 hours later) to patients who respond incompletely. Synthetic ACTH preparations are preferable to ACTH prepared from animal tissues, as the risk of anaphylaxis is decreased.

In my opinion, ACTH is generally more rapidly acting and preferable to oral prednisone, which is effective for gout only at initial doses of 30 mg/day (tapering to less than 20 mg per day by 1 week, followed by continuing therapy for 1 to 3 weeks) (153). Intravenous methylprednisolone (individual doses of 50–150 mg) can be used in place of prednisone where necessary.

Acute gout can be observed in transplant patients receiving maintenance doses of prednisone (158), underscoring the relatively low potency of systemic steroids in acute crystal-induced inflammation. Additionally, because rebound can be observed after cessation of therapy with systemic steroids (156), adjunctive low-dose daily colchicine (e.g., 0.6 mg p.o., b.i.d.) or an NSAID is often required.

Some patients receiving long-term, low-dose prednisone therapy for other conditions (and presumably manifesting a diminished capacity for adrenal stimulation by ACTH) exhibit therapeutic responsiveness to ACTH (155). In this regard, peripheral leukocytes can manufacture ACTH (56), and ACTH and certain related peptides have been suggested to have some direct antiinflammatory properties through antagonism of several cytokines (159). Thus antiinflammatory effects of ACTH in gout might be partially effected by direct action at the periphery.

Pseudogout

Supportive measures are useful in the treatment of pseudogout, as outlined previously. Thorough aspiration of a large joint often effectively controls acute inflammation even without local corticosteroid injection, presumably because of removal of sufficient crystals to control what may be a dose-related response. One study corroborated the clinical impression that in pseudogout, in comparison to gout, there is a clearer dose-dependence between inflammation and recoverable synovial fluid crystal load (111).

Concomitant use of local corticosteroid ester crystals is virtually 100% effective in control of acute pseudogout in a single large joint, although a postinjection flare has been implicated as precipitating acute pseudogout, possibly due to the enzymatic strip-mining mechanism previously discussed.

NSAIDs and ACTH (155,157) are usually effective in comparable doses as used for the treatment of acute gout. Colchicine effectiveness is less predictable for acute pseudogout when the drug is given orally. Intravenous colchicine (1–2 mg) more predictably controls acute pseudogout, probably because it produces much higher intracellular levels, as outlined previously. The frequency of acute attacks of pseudogout can be diminished by the use of small daily prophylactic doses of colchicine as used for gout (160).

REFERENCES

1. Terkeltaub R. Pathogenesis and treatment of crystal-induced inflammation. In: Koopman WJ, ed. *Arthritis and allied conditions.* 13th ed. Baltimore: Williams & Wilkins, 1997:2085–2102.
2. Vandenberg MK, Moxley G, Breitbach A, et al. Gout attacks in chronic alcoholics occur at lower serum urate levels than nonalcoholics. *J Rheumatol* 1994;21:700–704.
3. Bomalaski JA, Lluberas G, Schumacher HR Jr. Monosodium urate crystals in the knee joints of patients with asymptomatic nontophaceous gout. *Arthritis Rheum* 1986;39:1480–1484.
4. McCarty DJ. Gout without hyperuricemia. *JAMA* 1994;271: 302–303.
5. Pritzker KP. Gout and the gullible. *J Rheumatol* 1994;21: 2175–2176.
6. Burt HM, Dutt YC. Growth of monosodium urate monohydrate crystals: effect of cartilage and synovial fluid components on in vitro growth rates. *Ann Rheum Dis* 1986;45:858–864.
7. McGill NW, Dieppe PA. The role of serum and synovial fluid components in the promotion of urate crystal formation. *J Rheumatol* 1991;18:1042–1045.
8. Lally EV, Zimmerman B, Ho G Jr, et al. Urate-mediated inflammation in nodal osteoarthritis: clinical and roentgenographic correlations. *Arthritis Rheum* 1989;32:86–90.
9. Erickson AR, Enzenauer RJ, Nordstrom DM, et al. The prevalence of hypothyroidism in gout. *Am J Med* 1994;97:231–234.
10. Palmer DG, Highton J, Hessian PA. Development of the gouty tophus: an hypothesis. *Am J Clin Pathol* 1989;91:190–195.
11. Steinberg TH, Newman AS, Swanson JA, Silverstein SC. Macrophages possess probenecid-inhibitable organic anion transporters that remove fluorescent dyes from the cytoplasmic matrix. *J Cell Biol* 1987;105:2695–2702.
12. Hardwell TR, Manley G, Braven J, et al. The binding of urate plasma proteins determined by four different techniques. *Clin Chim Acta* 1983;133:75–83.
13. Perl-Treves D, Addadi L. A structural approach to pathological crystallizations: gout: the possible role of albumin in sodium urate crystallization. *Proc R Soc Lond* 1988;235:145–159.
14. Kam M, Perl-Treves D, Caspi D, et al. Antibodies against crystals. *FASEB J* 1992;6:2608–2613.
15. Wu X, Wakamiya M, Vaishnav S, et al. Hyperuricemia and urate nephropathy in urate oxidase-deficient mice. *Proc Natl Acad Sci U S A* 1994;91:742–746.
16. Terkeltaub R, Tenner AJ, Kozin F, et al. Plasma protein binding by monosodium urate crystals: analysis by two-dimensional gel electrophoresis. *Arthritis Rheum* 1983;26:775–783.
17. Di Giovine FS, Malawista SE, Nuki G, et al. Interleukin-1 (IL-1) as a mediator of crystal arthritis: stimulation of T cell and synovial fibroblast mitogenesis by urate crystal-induced IL-1. *J Immunol* 1987;138:3213–3218.
18. Guerne PA, Terkeltaub R, Zuraw B, et al. Stimulation of IL-6 production in human monocytes and synoviocytes by inflammatory microcrystals. *Arthritis Rheum* 1989;32: 1443–1452.
19. di Giovine FS, Malawista SE, Thornton E, et al. Urate crystals stimulate production of tumor necrosis factor alpha from human blood monocytes and synovial cells: cytokine mRNA and protein kinetics, and cellular distribution. *J Clin Invest* 1991;87:1375–1381.
20. Terkeltaub R, Zachariae C, Santoro D, et al. Monocyte-derived neutrophil chemotactic factor/IL-8 is a potential mediator of crystal-induced inflammation. *Arthritis Rheum* 1991;34: 894–903.
21. Bomalaski JS, Baker DG, Brophy LM, et al. Monosodium urate crystals stimulate phospholipase A2 enzyme activities and the synthesis of a phospholipase A2-activating protein. *J Immunol* 1990;145:3391–3397.
22. Roberge CJ, Grassi J, DeMedicis R, et al. Crystal-neutrophil interactions lead to interleukin-1 synthesis. *Agents Actions* 1991; 34:38–41.
23. Roberge C, de Medicis R, Dayer J-M, et al. Crystal-induced neutrophil activation. V. Differential production of biologically active IL-1 and IL-1 receptor antagonist. *J Immunol* 1994;152: 5485–5494.
24. Bhatt A, Spilberg I. Purification of crystal induced chemotactic factor from human neutrophils. *Clin Biochem* 1988;21: 341–345.
25. Ahuja SK, Gao J-L, Murphy PM. Chemokine receptors and molecular mimicry. *Immunol Today* 1994;15:281–287.
26. Bazzoni F, Cassatella MA, Rossi F, et al. Phagocytosing neutrophils produce and release high amounts of the neutrophil-activating peptide 1/interleukin 8. *J Exp Med* 1991;173: 771–774.
27. Getting SJ, Flower RJ, Parente L, et al. Molecular determinants of monosodium urate crystal-induced murine peritonitis: a role for endogenous mast cells and a distinct requirement for endothelial-derived selections. *J Pharmacol Exp Ther* 1997;283: 123–130.
28. Herring FG, Lam E, Burt HM. A spin label study of the membranolytic effects of crystalline monosodium urate monohydrate. *J Rheumatol* 1986;13:623–630.
29. Burt HM, Jackson JK. Role of membrane proteins in monosodium urate crystal-membrane interactions. II. Effect of pretreatments of erythrocyte membranes with membrane permeable and impermeable protein crosslinking agents. *J Rheumatol* 1990;17:1359–1363.
30. Terkeltaub R, Sklar LA, Mueller H. Neutrophil activation by inflammatory microcrystals of monosodium urate monohydrate utilizes pertussis toxin-insensitive and sensitive pathways. *J Immunol* 1990;144:2719–2724.
31. Onello E, Traynor-Kaplan A, Sklar L, et al. Mechanism of neutrophil activation by an unopsonized inflammatory particulate: monosodium urate crystals induce pertussis toxin-insensitive hydrolysis of phosphatidylinositol 4,5-bisphosphate. *J Immunol* 1991;146:4289–4299.
32. Marcil J, Harbour D, Houle MG, et al. Monosodium urate-crystal-stimulated phospholipase D in human neutrophils. *Biochem J* 1999;337:185–192.
33. Gaudry M, Roberge C, Medicis R, et al. Crystal-induced neutrophil activation III: inflammatory microcrystals induce a distinct pattern of tyrosine phosphorylation in human neutrophils. *J Clin Invest* 1993;91:1649–1655.
34. Roberge C, Gaudry M, Medicis R, et al. Crystal-induced neu-

trophil activation. IV. Specific inhibition of tyrosine phosphorylation by colchicine. *J Clin Invest* 1993;92:1722–1729.
35. Smallwood J, Malawista S. Colchicine, crystals, and neutrophil tyrosine phosphorylation. *J Clin Invest* 1993;92:1602–1603.
36. Burt H, Jackson J, Salari H. Inhibition of crystal-induced neutrophil activation by a protein tyrosine kinase inhibitor. *J Leukoc Biol* 1994;55:112–119.
37. Gaudry M, Gilbert C, Barabe F, et al. Activation of *lyn* is a common element of the stimulation of human neutrophils by soluble and particulate agonists. *Blood* 1995;86:3567–3574.
38. Jackson JK, Lauener R, Duronio V, et al. The involvement of phosphatidylinositol 3-kinase in crystal-induced human neutrophil activation. *J Rheumatol* 1997;24:341–348.
39. Naccache PH, Gilbert C, Barabe F, et al. Agonist-specific tyrosine phosphorylation of Cbl in human neutrophils. *J Leukoc Biol* 1997;2:901–910.
40. Geng Y, Zhang B, Lotz M. Protein tyrosine kinase activation is required for lipopolysaccharide induction of cytokines in human blood monocytes. *J Immunol* 1993;151:6692–6700.
41. Barabe F, Gilbert C, Liao N, et al. Crystal-induced neutrophil activation VI: involvement of FcgamaRIIIB (CD16) and CD11b in response to inflammatory microcrystals. *FASEB J* 1998;12:209–220.
42. Jaques BC, Ginsberg MH. The role of cell surface proteins in platelet stimulation by monosodium urate crystals. *Arthritis Rheum* 1982;25:508–521.
43. Kimberly RP, Ahlstrom JW, Click ME, et al. The glycosyl phosphatidylinositol-linked Fcgamma RIIIPMN mediates transmembrane signalling events distinct from Fcgamma RII. *J Exp Med* 1990;171:1239–1255.
44. Webb DS, Shimizu Y, Van Seventer GA, et al. LFA-3, CD44, and CD45: physiologic triggers of human monocyte TNF and IL-1 release. *Science* 1990;249:1295–1297.
45. Ohashi H, Maruyama K, Liu Y-C, et al. Ligand-induced activation of chimeric receptors between the erythropoietin receptor and receptor tyrosine kinases. *Proc Natl Acad Sci U S A* 1994; 91:158–162.
46. Greenberg S, Chang P, Silverstein C. Tyrosine phosphorylation is required for Fc receptor-mediated phagocytosis in mouse macrophages. *J Exp Med* 1993;177:529–534.
47. Sanguedolce M-V, Capo C, Bouhamdan M, et al. Zymosan-induced tyrosine phosphorylations in human monocytes. *J Immunol* 1993;151:405–414.
48. Hanein D, Geiger B, Addadi L. Differential adhesion of cells to enantiomorphous crystal surfaces. *Science* 1994;263:1413–1416.
49. Liu R, O'Connell M, Johnston K, et al. Monosodium urate and calcium pyrophosphate crystal-induced IL-8 expression requires activation of Erk1/Erk2 MAP kinase and activation of the NF-κB binding domain of the IL-8 promoter in monocytes. *Arthritis Rheum* 1998;41:S358.
50. McCarthy GM, Augustine JA, Baldwin AS, et al. Molecular mechanism of basic calcium phosphate crystal-induced activation of human fibroblasts. *J Biol Chem* 1998;273:35161–36169.
51. Tudan C, Jackson JK, Charlton L, et al. Activation of S6 kinase in human neutrophils by calcium pyrophosphate dihydrate crystals: protein kinase C-dependent and phosphatidylinositol-3-kinase-independent pathways. *Biochem J* 1998;331:531–537.
52. Chapman PT, Jamar F, Harrison AA, et al. Noninvasive imaging of E-selectin expression by activated endothelium in urate crystal-induced arthritis. *Arthritis Rheum* 1994;37:1752–1756.
53. Pascaul E, Castellano JA. Treatment with colchicine decreases white cell counts in synovial fluid asymptomatic knees that contain monosodium urate crystals. *J Rheumatol* 1992;19:600–603.
54. Pouliot M, James MJ, McColl SR, et al. Monosodium urate microcrystals induce cyclooxygenase-2 in human monocytes. *Blood* 1998;91:1769–1776.
55. Lotz M, Carson D, Vaughan JH. Substance P activation of rheumatoid synoviocytes: neural pathway in pathogenesis of arthritis. *Science* 1987;235:893–895.
56. Mantyh PW. Substance P and the inflammatory and immune response. *Ann N Y Acad Sci* 1991;632:263–271.
57. Nussler AK, Billiar TR. Inflammation, immunoregulation, and inducible nitric oxide synthase. *J Leukoc Biol* 1993;54:171–178.
58. Lotz M, Terkeltaub R, Villiger PM. Chondrocytes and joint inflammation: expression of IL-8 in response to peptide regulatory factors and proinflammatory agents. *J Immunol* 1992;148: 466–473.
59. Villiger PM, Terkeltaub R, Lotz M. Monocyte chemoattractant protein-1 (MCP-1) expression in human cartilage: induction by leukemia inhibitory factor (LIF) and differential regulation by dexamethasone and retinoic acid. *J Clin Invest* 1992;90: 488–496.
60. Tessier PA, Naccache PH, Clark-Lewis I, et al. Chemokine networks in-vivo. *J Immunol* 1997;159:3595–3602.
61. Matsukawa A, Miyazaki S, Maeda T, et al. Production and regulation of monocyte chemoattractant protein-1 in lipopolysaccharide- or monosodium urate crystal-induced arthritis in rabbits: roles of tumor necrosis factor α, interleukin-1, and interleukin-8. *Lab Invest* 1998;78:973–985.
62. Matsukawa A, Yoshimura T, Maeda T, et al. Analysis of the cytokine network among tumor necrosis factor, interleukin-1β, interleukin-8, and interleukin-1 receptor antagonist in monosodium urate crystal-induced rabbit arthritis. *Lab Invest* 1998;78:559–569.
63. Miller EJ, Brelsford WG. Interleukin 8: the major neutrophil chemotaxin in a case of pseudogout. *J Rheumatol* 1993;20: 1250–1251.
64. Koch AE, Kunkel SL, Harlow LA, et al. Epithelial neutrophil activating peptide-78: a novel chemotactic cytokine for neutrophils in arthritis. *J Clin Invest* 1994;94:1012–1018.
65. Terkeltaub R, Baird S, Sears P, et al. The murine homolog of the interleukin-8 receptor CXCR-2 is essential for the occurrence of neutrophilic inflammation in the air pouch model of acute urate crystal-induced gouty synovitis. *Arthritis Rheum* 1998;41: 900–909.
66. Nishimura A, Akahoshi T, Takahashi M, et al. Attenuation of monosodium urate crystal-induced arthritis in rabbits by a neutralizing antibody against interleukin-8. *J Leukoc Biol* 1997;62:444–449.
67. Miguelez R, Palacios I, Navarro F, et al. Anti-inflammatory effect of a PAF receptor antagonist and a new molecule with antiproteinase activity in an experimental model of acute urate crystal arthritis. *J Lipid Mediat Cell Signal* 1996;12:35–49.
68. McCarthy GM, Barthelemy CR, Veum JA, et al. Influence of antihyperuricemic therapy on the clinical and radiographic progression of gout. *Arthritis Rheum* 1991;34:1489–1494.
69. Jones J, Morgan BP. Apoptosis is associated with reduced expression of complement regulatory molecules, adhesion molecules and other receptors on polymorphonuclear leukocytes: functional relevance and role in inflammation. *Immunology* 1995;86:651–660.
70. Haslett C, Savill JS, Whyte MK, et al. Granulocyte apoptosis and the control of inflammation. *Trans R Soc Lond* 1994; 345:327–333.
71. Jones SM, Denton J, Holt PL, et al. Possible clearance of effete polymorphonuclear leucocytes from synovial fluid by cytophagocytic mononuclear cells: implications for pathogenesis and chronicity in inflammatory arthritis. *Ann Rheum Dis* 1993;52:121–126.
72. Takeda Y, Watanabe H, Yonehara S, et al. Rapid acceleration of neutrophil apoptosis by tumor necrosis factor-alpha. *Int Immunol* 1993;5:691–694.

73. Savill JS, Wyllie AH, Henson JE, et al. Macrophage phagocytosis of aging neutrophils in inflammation: programmed cell death in the neutrophil leads to its recognition by macrophages. *J Clin Invest* 1989;83:865–875.
74. Haslett C, Jose PJ, Giclas PC, et al. Cessation of neutrophil influx in C5a-induced acute experimental arthritis is associated with loss of chemoattractant activity from the joint space. *J Immunol* 1989;142:3510–3517.
75. VanHal PW, Hopstaken-Broos JM, Prins A, et al. Potential indirect anti-inflammatory effects of IL-4: stimulation of human monocytes, macrophages, and endothelial cells by IL-4 increases aminopeptidase-N (CD13; EC 3.4.11.2). *J Immunol* 1994;153:2718–2728.
76. Cybulsky MI, Colditz IG, Movat HZ. The role of interleukin-1 in neutrophil leukocyte emigration induced by endotoxin. *Am J Pathol* 1986;124:367–372.
77. Tomhave ED, Richardson RM, Didsbury JR, et al. Cross-desensitization of receptors for peptide chemoattractants: characterization of a new form of leukocyte regulation. *J Immunol* 1994;153:3267–3275.
78. Arend WP, Dayer JM. Cytokines and cytokine inhibitors or antagonists in rheumatoid arthritis. *Arthritis Rheum* 1990;33:305–315.
79. Tate GA, Mandell BF, Schumacher HR, et al. Suppression of acute inflammation by 15-methylprostaglandin E_1. *Lab Invest* 1988;59:192–199.
80. Matsukawa A, Fukumoto T, Maeda T, et al. Detection and characterization of IL-1 receptor antagonist in tissues from healthy rabbits: IL-1 receptor antagonist is probably involved in health. *Cytokine* 1997;9:307–315.
81. Malyak M, Swaney RE, Arend WP. Levels of synovial fluid interleukin-1 receptor antagonist in rheumatoid arthritis and other arthropathies. *Arthritis Rheum* 1993;36:781–789.
82. Fava RA, Olsen NJ, Postlethwaite AE, et al. Transforming growth factor beta 1 (TGF-β1) induced neutrophil recruitment to synovial tissues: implications for TGF-β-driven synovial inflammation and hyperplasia. *J Exp Med* 1991;173:1121–1132.
83. McCartney-Francis NL, Wahl SM. Transforming growth factor beta: a matter of life and death. *J Leukoc Biol* 1994;55:401–409.
84. Dubois CM, Ruscetti FW, Palasynski EW, et al. Transforming growth factor beta is a potent inhibitor of interleukin 1 (IL-1) receptor expression: proposed mechanism of inhibition of IL-1 action. *J Exp Med* 1990;172:737–744.
85. Fava RA, Olsen J, Keski-Oja HL, et al. Active and latent forms of transforming growth factor beta activity in synovial effusions. *J Exp Med* 1989;169:291–296.
86. Liote F, Ortiz-Bravo E, Bardin T. TGF-beta inhibits monosodium urate crystal-induced acute inflammation in vivo (rat air pouch, synovium-like model). *Arthritis Rheum* 1993;36:S109(abst).
87. Aderka D, Le J, Vilcek J. IL-6 inhibits lipopolysaccharide-induced tumor necrosis factor production in cultured human monocytes, U937 cells, and in mice. *J Immunol* 1989;143:3517–3523.
88. Huizinga TWJ, de Haas M, Kleijer M, et al. Soluble Fc gamma receptor III in human plasma originates from release by neutrophils. *J Clin Invest* 1990;86:416–423.
89. Porteau F, Nathan C. Shedding of tumor necrosis factor receptors by activated human neutrophils. *J Exp Med* 1990;172:599–607.
90. Devchand PR, Keller H, Peters JM, et al. The PPARalpha-leukotriene B_4 pathway to inflammation control. *Nature* 1996;384:39–43.
91. Ricote M, Li AC, Willson TM, et al. The peroxisome proliferator-activated receptor-gamma is a negative regulator of macrophage activation. *Nature* 1998;391:79–82.
92. Jiang C, Ting AT, Seed B. PPAR-gamma agonists inhibit production of monocyte inflammatory cytokines. *Nature* 1998;391:82–86.
93. Forrest MJ, Aammit V, Brooks PM. Inhibition of leukotriene B_4 synthesis by BW 755c does not reduce polymorphonuclear leucocyte accumulation induced by monosodium urate crystals. *Ann Rheum Dis* 1988;47:241–246.
94. Ortiz-Bravo E, Sieck M, Schumacher R. Changes in the proteins coating monosodium urate crystals during active and subsiding inflammation. *Arthritis Rheum* 1993;9:1274–1285.
95. Horowitz MD, Abbey L, Sirota DK, et al. Intraarticular noninflammatory free urate suspension (urate milk) in 3 patients with painful joints. *J Rheumatol* 1990;17:712–714.
96. Terkeltaub R, Martin J, Curtiss L, et al. Apolipoprotein B mediates the capacity of low density lipoprotein to suppress neutrophil stimulation by particulates. *J Biol Chem* 1986;261:15662–15667.
97. Ortiz-Bravo E, Schumacher HR. Components generated locally as well as serum alter the phlogistic effect of monosodium urate crystals in vivo. *J Rheumatol* 1993;20:1162–1166.
98. Gordon TP, Roberts-Thompson PJ. Preliminary evidence for the presence of an inhibitor on the surface of natural monosodium urate crystals. *Arthritis Rheum* 1986;29:1172–1173.
99. Stankovic A, Front P, Barbara A, et al. Tophus-derived monosodium urate monohydrate crystals are biologically much more active than synthetic counterpart. *Rheumatol Int* 1991;10:221–226.
100. Rosen MS, Baker DG, Schumacher HR Jr, et al. Products of polymorphonuclear cell injury inhibit IgG enhancement of monosodium urate-induced superoxide production. *Arthritis Rheum* 1986;29:1473–1479.
101. Kolb-Bachofen V. Uptake of toxic silica particles by isolated rat liver macrophages (Kupffer cells) is receptor mediated and can be blocked by competition. *J Clin Invest* 1992;90:1819–1824.
102. Terkeltaub R, Smeltzer D, Curtiss LK, et al. Low density lipoprotein inhibits the physical interaction of phlogistic crystals and inflammatory cells. *Arthritis Rheum* 1986;29:363–370.
103. Terkeltaub R, Dyer C, Martin J, et al. Apolipoprotein E (apo E) inhibits the capacity of monosodium urate crystals to stimulate neutrophils: characterization of intraarticular apo E and demonstration of apo E binding to urate crystals in vivo. *J Clin Invest* 1991;87:20–26.
104. Terkeltaub R, Banka C, Solan J, et al. Oxidized LDL induces the expression by monocytic cells of IL-8, a chemokine with T lymphocyte chemotactic activity. *Arterioscler Thromb* 1994;14:47–53.
105. Nair D, Misra RP, Sallis JD, et al. Phosphocitrate inhibits a basic calcium phosphate and calcium pyrophosphate dihydrate crystal-induced mitogen-activated protein kinase cascade signal transduction pathway. *J Biol Chem* 1997;272:18920–18925.
106. Burt HM, Jackson JK. Cytosolic Ca^{2+} concentration determinations in neutrophils stimulated by monosodium urate and calcium pyrophosphate crystals: effect of protein adsorption. *J Rheumatol* 1994;21:138–144.
107. Malawista SE, Duff G, Atkins E, et al. Crystal-induced endogenous pyrogen production: a further look at gouty inflammation. *Arthritis Rheum* 1985;28:1039–1046.
108. Swan A, Dularay B, Dieppe P. A comparison of the effects of urate, hydroxyapatite and diamond crystals on polymorphonuclear cells: relationship of mediator release to the surface area and adsorptive capacity of different particles. *J Rheumatol* 1990;17:1346–1352.
109. Roch-Arveiller M, Legros R, Chanaud B, et al. Inflammatory reactions induced by various calcium pyrophosphate crystals. *Biomed Pharmacother* 1990;44:467–474.
110. Watanabe W, Baker DG, Schumacher HR. Comparison of the

acute inflammation induced by calcium pyrophosphate dihydrate, apatite and mixed crystals in the rat air pouch model of a synovial space. *J Rheumatol* 1992;19:1453–1457.

111. Swan A, Heywood B, Chapman B, et al. Characterization of the crystals responsible for attacks of "pseudogout." *Arthritis Rheum* 1994;37:S427(abst).
112. Burt HM, Jackson JK. Enhancement of crystal induced neutrophil responses by opsonisation of calcium pyrophosphate dihydrate crystals. *Ann Rheum Dis* 1993;52:599–607.
113. Krug HE, Mahowald ML, Halverson JS, et al. Phosphocitrate prevents disease progression in murine progressive ankylosis. *Arthritis Rheum* 1993;11:1603–1611.
114. Terkeltaub R, Santoro D, Mandel G, et al. Serum and plasma inhibit neutrophil stimulation by hydroxyapatite crystals: evidence that serum alpha 2 HS-glycoprotein is a potent and specific crystal-bound inhibitor. *Arthritis Rheum* 1988;31:1081–1089.
115. Hansma H, Weisenhorn A, Edmundson A, et al. Atomic force microscopy: seeing molecules of lipid and immunoglobulin. *Clin Chem* 1991;37:1497–1501.
116. Blair JM, Sorensen LB, Arnsdorf MF, et al. The application of atomic force microscopy for the detection of microcrystals in synovial fluid from patients with recurrent synovitis. *Semin Arthritis Rheum* 1995;24:359–369.
117. Gordon TP, Kowasko IC, James M, et al. Monosodium urate crystal-induced prostaglandin synthesis in the rat subcutaneous air pouch. *Clin Exp Rheumatol* 1985;3:291–295.
118. Hutton CW, Collins AJ, Chambers RE, et al. Systemic response to local urate crystal induced inflammation in man: a possible model to study the acute phase response. *Ann Rheum Dis* 1985;44:533–536.
119. Neuss MN. Long-term colchicine administration leading to colchicine toxicity and death. *Arthritis Rheum* 1986;29:448–449.
120. Roberts WM, Liang MH, Stern SH. Colchicine in acute gout. *JAMA* 1987;257:1920–1921.
121. Moreland LW, Ball GV. Colchicine and gout [Editorial]. *Arthritis Rheum* 1991;34:782–786.
122. Wallace SW, Singer JZ. Therapy in gout. *Rheum Dis Clin North Am* 1988;14:441–458.
123. Wallace SL, Singer JZ. Review: systemic toxicity associated with the intravenous administration of colchicine—guidelines for use. *J Rheumatol* 1988;15:495–499.
124. Ben-Chetrit E, Levy M. Colchicine: 1998 update. *Semin Arthritis Rheum* 1998;28:48–59.
125. Milne ST, Meek PD. Fatal colchicine overdose: report of a case and review of the literature. *Am J Emerg Med* 1998;16:603–608.
126. Yussim A, Bar-Nathan N, Lustig S, et al. Gastrointestinal, hepatorenal and neuromuscular toxicity caused by cyclosporine-colchicine interaction in renal transplantation. *Transplant Proc* 1994;26:2825–2826.
127. Sobh M, Sabry A, Moustafa F, et al. Effect of colchicine on chronic cyclosporin nephrotoxicity in Sprague-Dawley rats. *Nephron* 1998;79:452–457.
128. Edmond-Rouan SKE, Otterness IG, Cunningham AC, et al. Reversal of colchicine-induced mitotic arrest in Chinese hamster cells with a colchicine-specific monoclonal antibody. *Am J Pathol* 1990;137:779–787.
129. Baud FJ, Sabouraud A, Vicaut E, et al. Brief report: treatment of severe colchicine overdose with colchicine-specific Fab fragments. *N Engl J Med* 1995;332:642–645.
130. Sugio K. Separation of tubulin-binding and anti-inflammatory activity in colchicine analogs and congeners. *Life Sci* 1987;40: 35–39.
131. Kulkarni SB, Singh M, Betageri GV. Encapsulation, stability and in-vitro release characteristics of liposomal formulations of colchicine. *J Pharm Pharmacol* 1997;49:491–495.
132. Wallace SL, Singer JZ, Duncan GJ, et al. Renal function predicts colchicine toxicity: guidelines for prophylactic use of colchicine in gout. *J Rheumatol* 1991;18:264–269.
133. Kuncl RW, Duncan GJ, Watson D, et al. Colchicine myopathy and neuropathy. *N Engl J Med* 1987;316:1562–1568.
134. Schiff D, Drislane FW. Rapid-onset colchicine myoneuropathy. *Arthritis Rheum* 1992;35:1535–1536.
135. Dawson TM, Starkebaum G. Colchicine induced rhabdomyolysis. *J Rheumatol* 1997;24:2045–2046.
136. Caraco Y, Putterman C, Rahamimov R, et al. Acute colchicine intoxication: possible role of erythromycin administration. *J Rheumatol* 1992;19:494–496.
137. Ben-Chetrit E, Scherrmann J-M, Zylber-Katz E, et al. Colchicine disposition in patients with familial Mediterranean fever with renal impairment. *J Rheumatol* 1994;24:710–713.
138. Putterman C, Ben-Chetrit E, Caraco Y, et al. Colchicine intoxication: clinical pharmacology, risk factors, features, and management. *Semin Arthritis Rheum* 1991;21:143–155.
139. Amoura Z, Schermann J-M, Wecisler B, et al. Transplacental passage of colchicine in familial Mediterranean fever. *J Rheumatol* 1994;21:383.
140. Haimov-Kochman R, Ben-Chetrit E. The effect of colchicine treatment on sperm production and function: a review. *Hum Reprod* 1998;13:360–362.
141. Famaey JD. Colchicine in therapy: state of the art and new perspectives for an old drug. *Clin Exp Rheumatol* 1988;6: 305–317.
142. Ben-Chetrit E, Levy M. Does the lack of the P-glycoprotein efflux pump in neutrophils explain the efficacy of colchicine in familial Mediterranean fever and other inflammatory diseases? *Med Hypotheses* 1998;51:377–380.
143. Cronstein BN, Molad Y, Reibman J, et al. Colchicine alters the quantitative and qualitative display of selectins on endothelial cells and neutrophils. *J Clin Invest* 1995;96:994–1002.
144. Cronstein BN, Weissmann, G. The adhesion molecules of inflammation. *Arthritis Rheum* 1993;36:147–157.
145. Asako H, Kubes P, Baethge BA, et al. Colchicine and methotrexate reduce leukocyte adherence and emigration in rat mesenteric venules. *Inflammation* 1992;16:45–56.
146. Reibman J, Weissmann G. Colchicine inhibits ionophore-induced formation of leukotriene B_4 of microtubules. *J Immunol* 1986;136:1027–1032.
147. Reibman J, Haines KA, Gude D, et al. Differences in signal transduction between Fc gamma receptors (Fc gamma R II, Fc gamma R 111) and FMLP receptors in neutrophils: effects of colchicine on pertussis toxin sensitivity and diacylglycerol formation. *J Immunol* 1991;146:988–996.
148. Djeu JY, Matsushima K, Oppenheim JJ, et al. Functional activation of neutrophils by recombinant monocyte-derived neutrophil chemotactic factor/IL-8. *J Immunol* 1990;144:2205–2210.
149. Ding AH, Porteau P, Sanchez F, et al. Downregulation of tumor necrosis factor receptors on macrophages and endothelial cells by microtubule depolymerizing agents. *J Exp Med* 1990;171: 715–727.
150. Smallwood JI, Malawista SE. Misoprostol stimulates leukocyte cyclic adenosine 3′, 5′ monophosphate production and synergizes with colchicine: novel combination of established drugs may boost anti-inflammatory potential. *J Pharmacol Exp Ther* 1994;269:1196–1204.
151. Furst DE. Are there differences among nonsteroidal antiinflammatory drugs? Comparing acetylated salicylates, nonacetylated salicylates, and nonacetylated nonsteroidal antiinflammatory drugs. *Arthritis Rheum* 1994;37:1–9.
152. Emmerson BT, Hazelton RA, Whyte IM. Comparison of the urate lowering effects of allopurinol and diflunisal. *J Rheumatol* 1987;14:335–337.
153. Groff GD, Frank WA, Raddatz DA. Systemic steroid therapy

for acute gout: a clinical trial and review of the literature. *Semin Arthritis Rheum* 1990;19:329–336.

154. Axelrod D, Preston S. Comparison of parenteral adrenocorticotrophic hormone with oral indomethacin in the treatment of acute gout. *Arthritis Rheum* 1988;31:803–805.
155. Ritter J, Kerr LD, Valeriano-Marcet J, et al. ACTH revisited: effective treatment for acute crystal induced synovitis in patients with multiple medical problems. *J Rheumatol* 1994;21:696–699.
156. Siegel LB, Alloway JA, Nashel DJ. Comparison of adrenocorticotrophic hormone and triamcinolone in the treatment of acute gouty arthritis. *J Rheumatol* 1994;21:1325–1327.
157. Rosenthal AK, Ryan LM. Treatment of refractory crystal-associated arthritis. *Rheum Dis Clin North Am* 1995;21:151–162.
158. Kahl LE, Thompson ME, Griffith BP. Gout in the heart transplant recipient: physiologic puzzle and therapeutic challenge. *Am J Med* 1989;87:289–294.
159. Hiltz ME, Catania A, Lipton JM. Alpha-MSH peptides inhibit acute inflammation induced in mice by rIL-1 beta, rIL-6, rTNF-alpha and endogenous pyrogen but not that caused by LTB_4, PAF and rIL-8. *Cytokine* 1992;4:320–328.
160. Alvarellos A, Spilberg I. Colchicine prophylaxis in pseudogout. *J Rheumatol* 1986;13:804–805.

117

CALCIUM PYROPHOSPHATE CRYSTAL DEPOSITION DISEASE, PSEUDOGOUT, AND ARTICULAR CHONDROCALCINOSIS

ANN K. ROSENTHAL
LAWRENCE M. RYAN

The application of polarized light microscopy to synovial fluid analysis led to the discovery of nonurate crystals in joint fluids from patients with acute gout-like arthritis (1,2). These crystals were identified as calcium pyrophosphate dihydrate ($Ca_2P_2O_7{\cdot}2H^2O$, or CPPD) crystals and the associated clinical syndrome was called pseudogout (3) (Fig. 117.1A). Injection of either monosodium urate or CPPD crystals into normal human and canine joints was followed by an acute inflammatory response, demonstrating the pathogenicity

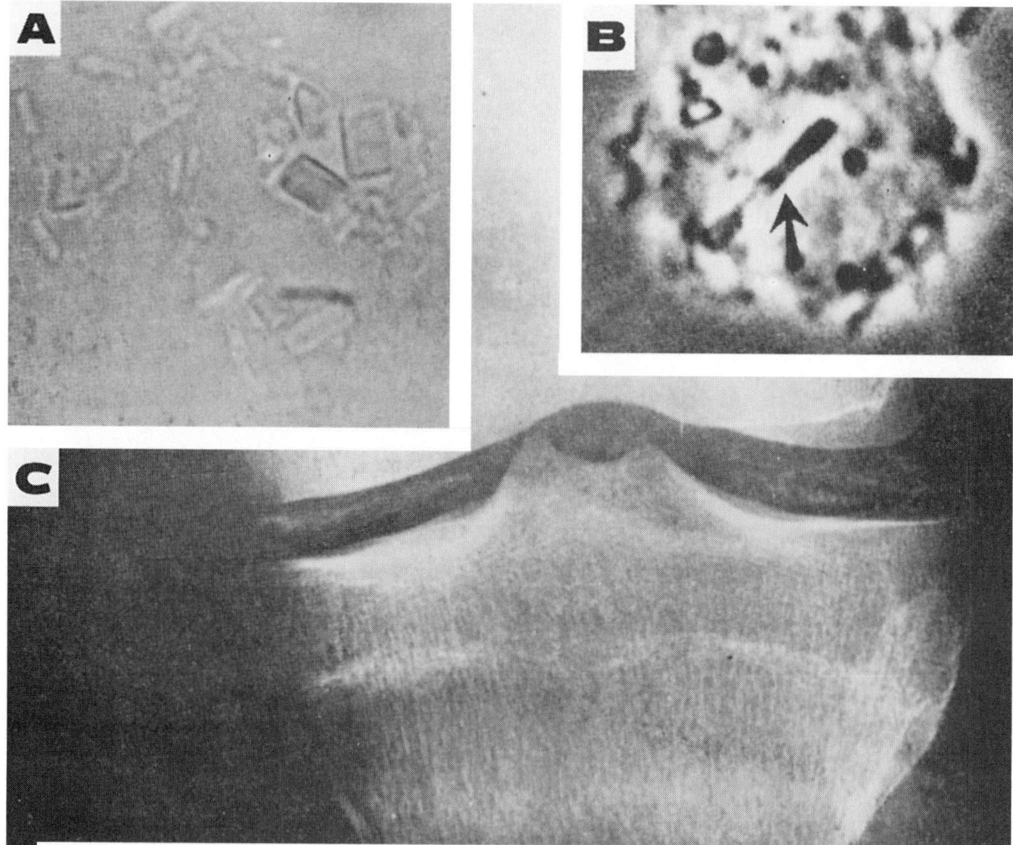

FIGURE 117.1. A: Weakly birefringent monoclinic and triclinic calcium pyrophosphate dihydrate (CPPD) microcrystals in synovial fluid removed from a chronically symptomatic knee (polarized light ×1,250). **B:** Phagocytosed crystal *(arrow)* in a polymorphonuclear leukocyte (phase contrast ×1,250). **C:** Anteroposterior radiograph of the knee showing typical punctate and linear deposits of CPPD in the menisci and articular hyaline cartilage.

of these crystals (4,5). In the 40 years since this initial observation, CPPD deposition disease has emerged as a complex and clinically heterogeneous disease, with distinct differences from gout. Although both urate and CPPD crystals can cause an acute arthritis, the clinical features of articular CPPD deposition, particularly the frequent occurrence of severe cartilage degeneration, suggest that CPPD crystals have far more complex biologic effects in the joint than do gout crystals. Likewise, the link between CPPD deposition, advanced age, and a handful of seemingly heterogeneous metabolic diseases suggests a similar complexity to the factors causing CPPD crystal formation. While a clear delineation of both cause and effect in urate gout resulted in effective therapies for this disease, no specific treatments for CPPD deposition disease yet exist.

NOMENCLATURE

The acute arthritis associated with CPPD crystal deposition was initially termed *pseudogout* because of the obvious parallel with true (urate) gout (2). Many patients with symptomatic arthritis, however, do not have acute attacks, so this term should be reserved for the acute episodes associated with articular CPPD crystals. The term *chondrocalcinosis* refers to the characteristic radiologic features of CPPD crystal deposition and is attributed to Zitnan and Sitaj (6). However, while chondrocalcinosis is highly suggestive of CPPD crystal deposition, crystals other than CPPD can rarely cause a similar radiographic appearance (7). Hence, this term should not be used synonymously with more specific terms for the clinical syndromes associated with CPPD crystals. The term *pyrophosphate arthropathy* was coined in 1969 by H. L. F. Currey, and is widely used in the United Kingdom (8). It has not achieved popularity in the United States, perhaps because it does not reflect the important role of the whole CPPD crystal in causing this disease. At present, the most widely accepted and accurate name for the clinical syndromes associated with articular CPPD crystals is *CPPD crystal deposition disease.*

EARLY REPORTS

Seven patients with acute arthritis and synovial fluid CPPD crystals were described by McCarty and co-workers (2) in 1962 (Fig. 117.1A,B). The radiographic appearance of calcification in fibroarticular and hyaline articular cartilage was noted (Fig. 117.1C). Analysis of such deposits showed CPPD crystals identical to those seen in joint fluid. X-ray diffraction powder patterns were obtained from at least one tissue deposit or from crystals harvested from synovial fluid in 51 of the first 80 cases reported by McCarty et al.; all were CPPD (9).

In addition to pseudogout attacks and a chronic degenerative arthropathy, other key findings in this initial group of patients have been confirmed by subsequent separate reports and suggested early on the clinical heterogeneity of this disorder. For example, a destructive arthropathy resembling Charcot arthropathy, radiologic lesions resembling osteochondromas, hemorrhagic joint fluids, prominent subchondral cysts, and the simultaneous presence of urate crystals were all documented at least once in this initial series.

When the clinical and radiographic findings in this group were analyzed, a review of the literature revealed a similarity to chondrocalcinosis polyarticularis (familiaris), as described in 1958 by Zitnan and Sitaj (6). These workers used the characteristic radiographic appearance as the unifying diagnostic feature. They pointed out that the menisci of the knee were most commonly involved (Fig. 117.1C). These authors later reported 27 cases, 21 from five Hungarian families living in a single village in Slovakia (10).

Perhaps the first report of CPPD deposition was made in 1903 by Bennett (11). He described an elderly man with mineral deposits in cartilage of the hips, shoulders, and sternoclavicular and temporomandibular joints at autopsy. Chemical analysis revealed the presence of calcium and carbonate in these deposit, and the murexide test for urate was negative. Morphologically, these crystals were smaller than urate crystals and were rhomboidal in shape under an ordinary light microscope. Other historic reports have been previously reviewed (12).

PREVALENCE

The incidence and prevalence of clinically important CPPD deposition disease are not known. Most studies have used radiologic or anatomically defined articular calcification as a marker for CPPD deposition disease (12). The study of elderly subjects by Ellman and Levin (13) is of particular interest (13). Fully 27.6% of their ambulatory volunteers showed calcific deposits on high-resolution radiographs. Assuming that all were CPPD deposits, this finding implicated age as a factor in the expression of the condition. These findings were confirmed by a report using standard radiographs of the knee in 108 women over 80 years of age (14). Meniscal calcification was found in 16% of the 55 women aged 80 to 89 and in 30% of 53 women aged 89 to 99; 22 of 25 with chondrocalcinosis of the knee had deposits in other joints as well. A radiographic survey of patients admitted to a geriatric unit disclosed a 44% prevalence of chondrocalcinosis in patients over 84 years of age when films of the hands and wrist, pelvis, and knees were examined (15). The prevalence was 15% in patients between 65 and 74 years of age and 36% in those between 75 and 84 years. Data from the Framingham study showed an overall prevalence of radiographic chondrocalcinosis of 8.1% in the population over the age of 63 (16).

Anatomic studies confirm the high prevalence of CPPD crystals in the elderly. A study of over 800 menisci from 215 cadavers (17) showed at least one small calcific deposit in the type-M radiograph in 22% of excised menisci. Most deposits were too small to permit dissection, much less identification, but 15 sets of mensici contained crystals that were amenable to further analysis. Of these, seven sets of menisci (3.2% of cadavers) showed linear and punctate deposits of CPPD. Mitrovic and associates (18) showed prevalence rates of 20% in knee joints of patients over the age of 60, and rates as high as 50% in patients over the age of 90.

JOINT FLUID FINDINGS

The presence of CPPD crystals in synovial fluid originally defined the clinical syndrome we know as CPPD crystal deposition disease. Like monosodium urate crystals, CPPD crystals exhibit monoclinic and triclinic dimorphism and frequently show twinning. In addition to their resistance to digestion by uricase, CPPD crystals differ from urate crystals in several ways. Under polarized light, they demonstrate weakly positive birefringence and inclined extinction. In contrast, urate crystals are negatively birefringent with axial extinction. Some CPPD crystals are isotropic (nonrefractile) under polarized light. Nearly all fluids aspirated from inflamed joints showed phagocytosed CPPD microcrystals (2) (Fig. 117.1B). CPPD crystals are much more difficult to see by polarized light microscopy than are monosodium urate crystals, and we routinely use phase contrast in addition to polarized light at 1,000-fold magnification for crystal identification. Even using these sensitive techniques, ultramicrocrystals cannot be detected (19,20). The number of crystals bears some relation to the acuteness of inflammation because pellets from joint fluid taken during acute attacks contain much more pyrophosphate on chemical analysis then do pellets from noninflamed joints (12). Exceptions occur, however. Some fluids from inflamed joints have few CPPD crystals, and some fluids from noninflamed joints are milky because of the large number of crystals present. This same phenomenon is described in true gout.

Other features of the synovial fluid may support the diagnosis of CPPD crystal deposition disease. The mean leukocyte concentration in acute attacks is exactly the same as in urate gout, about 20,000/mm^3, with over 90% polymorphonuclear cells. In the absence of active inflammation, white cell counts are typically in the noninflammatory range. As already noted, the fluid in pseudogout may be tinged with blood, especially early in the acute episode (12). In at least one case, such fluid was associated with subchondral bony fractures (21). Synovial fluids containing CPPD crystals more often than not also contain basic calcium phosphate. Of 30 CPPD-containing knee fluids in one study, 22 also contained showed basic calcium phosphate (BCP) crystals (22) (see Chapter 118).

DIAGNOSTIC CRITERIA

A diagnostic classification, based on the premise that CPPD crystals are the specific feature of the disease (5), has been modified to include radiographic findings as suggested by Resnick et al. (23) and Martel et al. (24) (Table 117.1). A case is considered definite if CPPD crystals are demonstrated in tissues or synovial fluid or if crystals compatible with CPPD are demonstrated by compensated polarized light microscopy and typical calcifications are seen on radiographs. If only one

TABLE 117.1. DIAGNOSTIC CRITERIA AND CATEGORIES FOR CALCIUM PYROPHOSPHATE DIHYDRATE CRYSTAL DEPOSITION DISEASE (PSEUDOGOUT)

Criteria

I. Demonstration of CPPD crystals, obtained by biopsy, necropsy, or aspirated synovial fluid, by definitive means; e.g., characteristic "fingerprint" by x-ray diffraction powder pattern or by chemical analysis.

II. A. Identification of monoclinic or triclinic crystals showing a weakly positive, or a lack of, birefringence by compensated polarized light microscopy.
  B. Presence of typical calcifications on radiographs.[a]

III. A. Acute arthritis, especially of knees or other large joints, with or without concomitant hyperuricemia.
  B. Chronic arthritis, especially of knee, hip, wrist, carpus, elbow, shoulder, and metacarpophalangeal joints, particularly if accompanied by acute exacerbations; the chronic arthritis shows the following features helpful in differentiating it from osteoarthritis (23).
    1. Uncommon site for primary osteoarthritis; e.g., wrist, metacarpophalangeal joints, elbow, or shoulder.
    2. Radiographic appearance; e.g., radiocarpal or patellofemoral joint space narrowing, especially if isolated (patella "wrapped around" the femur),[b] femoral cortical erosion superior to the patella on the lateral view of the knee.
    3. Subchondral cyst formation.
    4. Severe progressive degeneration, with subchondral bony collapse (microfractures), and fragmentation, with formation of intraarticular radiodense bodies.
    5. Variable and inconstant osteophyte formation.
    6. Tendon calcifications, especially of Achilles, triceps, and obturator tendons.
    7. Involvement of the axial skeleton with subchondral cysts of apophyseal and sacroiliac joints, multiple levels of disc calcification and vacuum phenomenon, and sacroiliac vacuum phenomenon.

Categories

A. Definite—criteria I or II(A) and II(B) must be fulfilled.
B. Probable—criteria IIA or IIB must be fulfilled.
C. Possible—criteria IIIA or IIIB should alert the clinician to the possibility of underlying CPPD deposition.

CPPD, calcium pyrophosphate dihydrate.
[a]Heavy punctate and linear calcifications in fibrocartilages, articular (hyaline) cartilages, and joint capsules, especially if bilaterally symmetric; faint or atypical calcifications may be due to dicalcium phosphate dihydrate (DCPD) ($CaHPO_4 \cdot 2H_2O$) deposits or to vascular calcifications; both are also often bilaterally symmetric.
[b]Also described as a feature of the arthritis of hyperparathyroidism.

of these criteria is found, a probable diagnosis is made. The clinical findings or the radiologic clues given in Table 117.1 should alert the clinician to the possible presence of underlying CPPD crystal deposition disease.

CLINICAL FEATURES

In a series of over 1,000 definite and probable cases of CPPD deposition disease, men predominated in a ratio of 1.5:1 (12). A similar sex ratio was recorded at the Mayo Clinic (25). In contrast, female predominance has been reported in three other surveys of patients with symptomatic CPPD deposition (16,26,27). Patients' ages averaged 72 years at the time of diagnosis (12).

The various patterns of arthritis encountered clinically are summarized in Fig. 117.2. We regard CPPD deposition as a great mimic because it not only can resemble gout, but may also mimic rheumatoid arthritis (RA), osteoarthritis (OA), and other types of joint disease (8,28).

Type A—Pseudogout

The pseudogout pattern is marked by acute or subacute arthritic attacks lasting from 1 day to 4 weeks. These episodes are self-limited and generally involve only one or a few appendicular joints. Such attacks can be as severe as those of true gout, but they usually take longer to reach peak intensity and are less painful and disabling. Inflammation may begin in a single "mother" joint with spread to involve other nearby "daughter" joints, the so-called cluster attack of the crystal deposition diseases. Mild "petite" attacks also occur, as in urate gout, and these may often outnumber full-blown attacks. Such attacks produce local effusions, joint stiffness, and warmth of the overlying skin, but they are not painful. Leukocytosis is noted in the synovial fluid. Injection of CPPD crystals into the joints of volunteers confirmed that the inflammatory response is dose related. Pain is the last symptom to appear and the first to disappear.

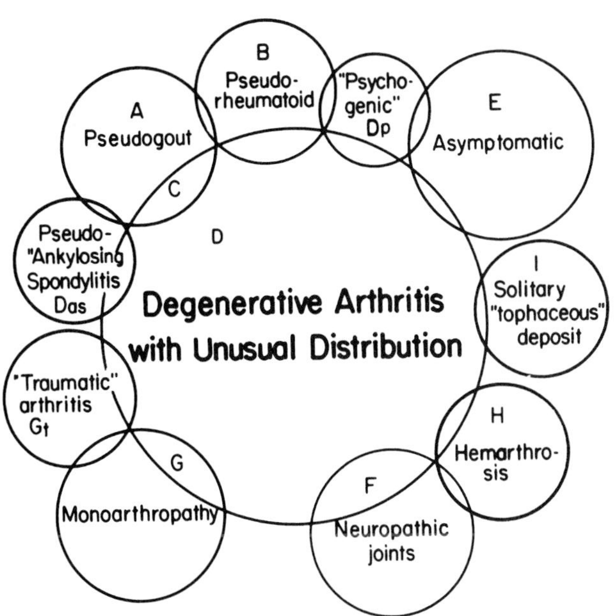

FIGURE 117.2. Diagrammatic representation of various clinical presentations of joint disease associated with calcium pyrophosphate dihydrate crystal deposition. (From McCarty D. The Heberden oration, 1982. Crystals, joints, and consternation. *Ann Rheum Dis* 1983;42:243–253, with permission.)

About 25% of patients show this gout-like, type A pattern. Men predominate. As in gout, the patients are usually completely asymptomatic between attacks. Radiographic evidence of CPPD deposits is found in most patients with this pattern of disease (Figs. 117.3A,B, 117.4, and 117.5). The knee joint is to pseudogout as the first metatarsal phalangeal joint is to gout, and it is the site of over half of all acute attacks. Conversely, CPPD-induced podagra of the first metatarsophalangeal joint has been reported, but is quite rare (12). Approximately 20% of patients with CPPD deposits have hyperuricemia, and about 5% have monosodium urate crystal deposits as well.

Provocation of acute episodes by a surgical procedure or by medical illness is common in both gout and pseudogout. The percentage of patients with either disease who had at least a single episode after operation was similar: 8.3% of 168 gouty patients and 9.4% of 106 patients with pseudogout (28). Parathyroidectomy is particularly likely to precipitate acute arthritis (25,29). Similarly, severe medical illness, particularly vascular occlusion such as stroke or myocardial infarction, provoked attacks in 20.3% of 167 gouty subjects, as opposed to 24% of 104 patients with pseudogout. Trauma may provoke acute arthritis in patients with either gout or pseudogout. Because both types of crystals are often found in the same subject and because either may cause self-limited attacks under identical clinical circumstances and may respond similarly to treatment, joint aspiration and specific crystal identification are essential for precise differential diagnosis.

Although not nearly as predictably effective as in gout, oral colchicine may provide dramatic relief in pseudogout. The release of a chemotactic factor by polymorphonuclear leukocytes after phagocytosis of either monosodium urate or CPPD crystals (30) (Chapter 116) is inhibited by colchicine in concentrations easily reached in serum by the usual therapeutic doses. The inhibition of urate crystal-induced release was more predictable than that induced by CPPD crystals, an *in vitro* result parallel to the clinical experience in patients. Spilberg and associates (31) found that colchicine, 1 to 2 mg, given intravenously predictably controls acute attacks of pseudogout.

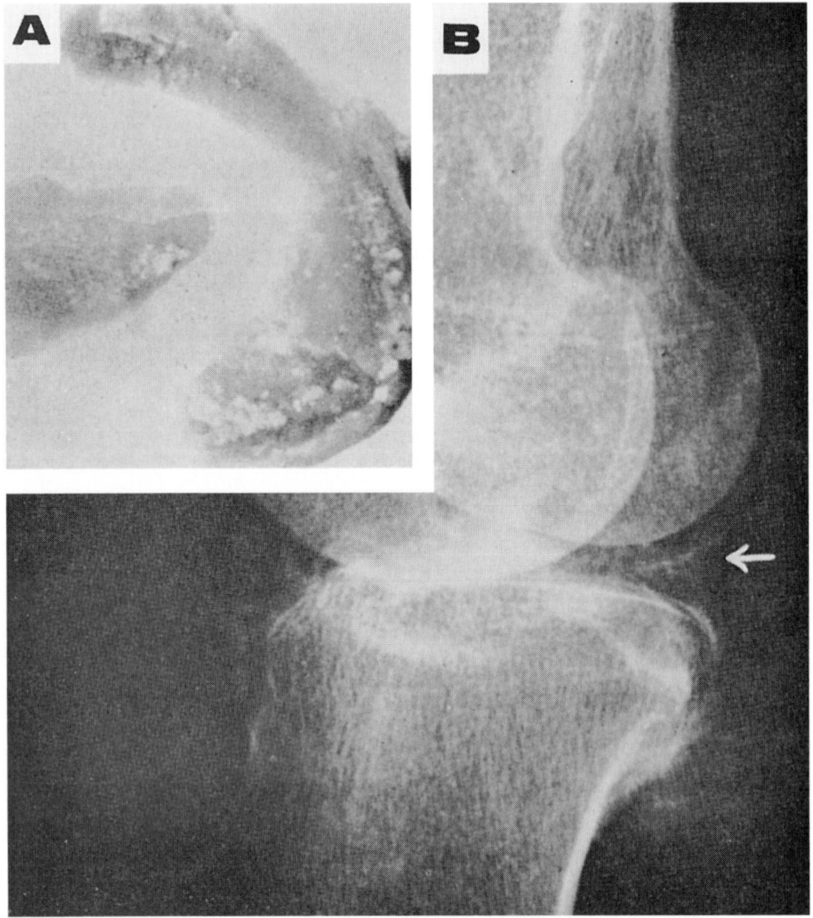

FIGURE 117.3. A: Meniscus excised at necropsy showing punctate and linear aggregates of calcium pyrophosphate dihydrate microcrystals; a wedge of articular cartilage from the tibial plateau shows similar deposits. **B:** Lateral radiograph of the knee showing the typical Y-shaped appearance of meniscal calcification *(arrow)*.

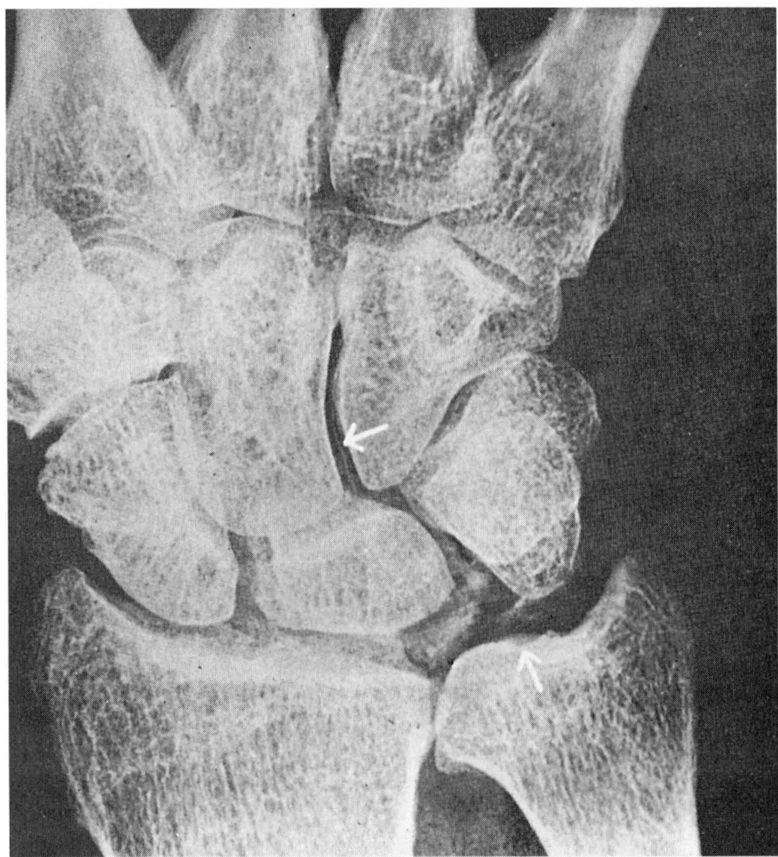

FIGURE 117.4. Anteroposterior radiograph of the wrist showing calcification of the fibrocartilaginous articular disc and a fine line of calcification parallel to the radiodensity of the underlying bone, indicative of articular cartilage calcification *(arrow)*.

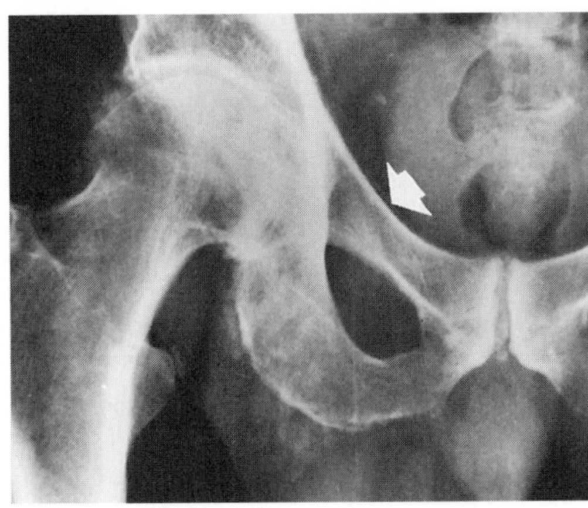

FIGURE 117.5. Calcific deposits in the symphysis pubis, the hyaline cartilage, and the acetabular labrum of the hip, the origin of the adductor tendons on the ischium and lesser trochanter, and Cooper's ligament *(arrow)*. (Courtesy of Dr. Harry K. Genant.)

Type B—Pseudorheumatoid Arthritis

Approximately 5% of patients have multiple joint involvement with subacute attacks lasting 4 weeks to several months. Nonspecific symptoms of inflammation, such as morning stiffness and fatigue, are common; signs such as synovial thickening, localized pitting edema, limitation of joint motion due to inflammation or to flexion contractures, and elevated erythrocyte sedimentation rates are found. Such patients are often thought to have RA (32). Additionally, because about 10% of patients with CPPD-related arthritis have positive tests for rheumatoid factor (RF) (28), albeit usually in low titer, the opportunities for confusion abound. The presence of high titers of RF and typical radiographic erosions favor a diagnosis of true RA (33). Interestingly, urate gout may also present with polyarticular involvement, RF in 10% of cases, and symptoms mimicking those of rheumatoid arthritis (34).

CPPD deposits have been described both histologically (35) and radiographically (36) in patients with presumably bona fide RA. By chance alone, at least 1% of patients with CPPD joint deposits would be expected to have RA. This figure agrees with the finding of nine cases of true RA in our series. A lower incidence (3%) of joint cartilage calcification in RA subjects was found in one study as compared to controls (14%), but the high incidence in the latter group, whose average age was 64.8 years, is greater than that usually observed in an asymptomatic population (37). This disparity may be due to the use as controls of patients presenting to the emergency unit with knee pain. Conversely, the coincidence of crystal-proven gout and RA is quite rare (12).

The type B pattern is intended to apply only to patients (a) whose joints are inflamed "out of phase" with one another, as in gout, rather than "in phase," as in RA; (b) who form osteophytes; (c) who have CPPD crystals in joint fluid leukocytes; and (d) who do not have typical radiographic erosive disease. When RA and CPPD crystal deposition coexist, the radiographic appearance of the former is said to be atypical for RA (37). Asymmetric disease, retained bone density, prominent osteophytes, well-corticated cysts, and paucity of erosions were found in seven of ten patients thought to have both diseases. It seems probable that those seven patients actually had the *pseudorheumatoid* pattern of CPPD crystal deposition.

A variant of pseudorheumatoid arthritis (type B) can cause confusion clinically. The patient, usually elderly, has multiple acutely inflamed joints, marked leukocytosis, fever of 102 to 104°F, and mental confusion or disorientation (38). Systemic sepsis is suspected by the attending physicians, and antibiotics have usually been prescribed despite negative cultures. The entire clinical picture reverses with antiinflammatory drug therapy.

Types C and D—Pseudo-Osteoarthritis

Approximately half the patients with CPPD deposition disease have progressive degeneration of multiple joints (Figs. 117.6, 117.7, and 117.8). Women predominate. The knees are most commonly affected, followed by the wrists, metacarpophalangeal joints, hips, spine, shoulder, elbows, and ankles. Involvement is generally symmetric, although the degenerative process may be much further advanced on one side, especially in joints that have been subjected to fracture or trauma. Flexion contractures of the involved joints are common. CPPD crystal deposition should be suspected in patients with bilateral or unilateral valgus deformity, or flexion contractures of the knees, especially if accompanied by osteophytes and flexion contractures of other joints not usually affected by primary OA, such as the wrists, elbows, shoulders, and metacarpophalangeal joints.

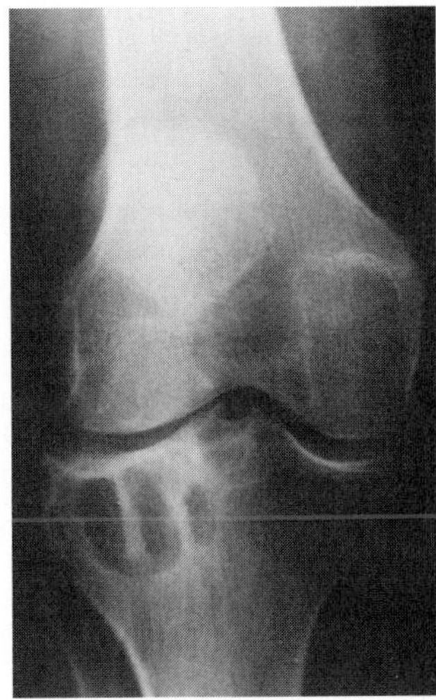

FIGURE 117.6. Subchondral bone cyst under the lateral tibial plateau in a patient with generalized calcium pyrophosphate dihydrate deposition and hyperparathyroidism.

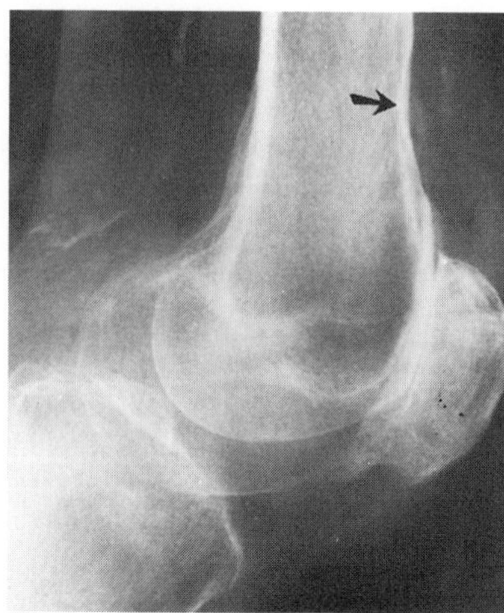

FIGURE 117.7. Lateral radiographs of the knee showing peculiar erosion of the femoral cortex superior to the patella *(arrow)*. Note the patella "wrapped around" the femur. (Courtesy of Dr. Harry K. Genant.)

About 25% of the total series, or about half of those with types C and D disease, have a history of episodic, superimposed acute attacks, and have been classified as type C. Those without an apparent inflammatory component have been classified as type D.

Characteristic CPPD crystal deposits may or may not be visible on radiographs of involved joints. CPPD crystals are often found in radiographically negative joints, especially those with extensive degenerative change. Serial radiographic studies by Zitnan and Sitaj (39) contain examples of joints with obvious calcific deposits at an early phase of the disease that may be difficult to discern when severe degeneration has supervened. Fine-detail radiographs are helpful in the detection of small or faint deposits (40).

Martel and co-workers (41), as well as Hamilton and his colleagues (42), described squaring of bone ends, subchondral cystic changes, and hook-like osteophytes, especially in the metacarpophalangeal joints associated with CPPD crystal deposition. Atkins and associates (43) compared the radiographic features of metacarpophalangeal degeneration in sporadic CPPD crystal deposition disease with that associated with hemochromatosis; they found more severe changes in a greater proportion of patients with hemochromatosis-associated CPPD.

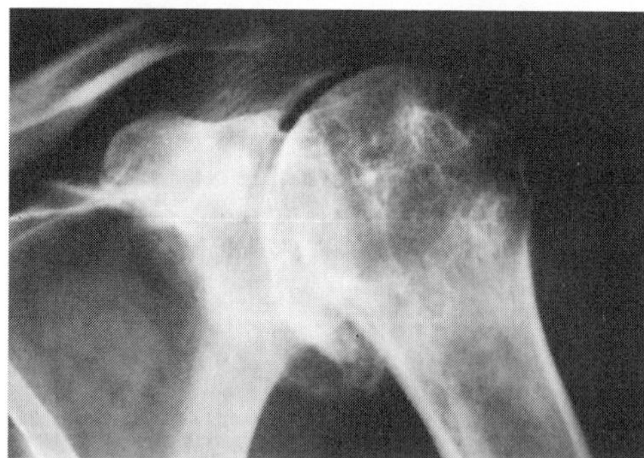

FIGURE 117.8. Anteroposterior radiograph of the shoulder showing neurotrophic joint appearance with extensive cystic bone lesions and powdered bony fragments in the synovial recesses inferiorly.

Resnick and his colleagues (23) have studied patients with CPPD deposition using age- and sex-matched control subjects. Useful diagnostic clues have been incorporated into the criteria outlined in Table 117.1. Axial skeleton involvement is frequent and is characterized by calcification of the annulus fibrosus, multiple levels of disc degeneration with vacuum phenomenon and subchondral erosions, and vacuum phenomena of the sacroiliac joints (23,24).

The pattern of joint degeneration in types C and D (e.g., wrists, metacarpophalangeal joints, elbow, and shoulder) is clearly different from that of primary OA (e.g., proximal and distal interphalangeal and first carpometacarpal joints). The knee is commonly affected in both conditions. Concomitant Heberden's and Bouchard's nodes, as well as other stigmata of primary OA, often coexist with the pattern of joint involvement peculiar to CPPD crystal deposition, probably a chance association of two common conditions in elderly persons.

Type E—Lanthanic (Asymptomatic) Calcium Pyrophosphate Dihydrate Crystal Deposition

Type E CPPD crystal deposition may be the most common clinical presentation of CPPD deposition disease. Most joints with CPPD deposits plainly visible on radiographs are not symptomatic, even in patients with acute or chronic symptoms in other joints. Wrist complaints and genu varus deformities, but not acute joint inflammation, were more common in patients with CPPD deposits than in control subjects from the same elderly population (13).

Type F—Pseudoneuropathic Joints

One of the patients in the original report of CPPD deposition disease had a Charcot-like arthropathy of a knee in the absence of neurologic abnormality (2). Subsequently, three of four cases of "neuropathic" arthritis of the knees associated with polyarticular CPPD deposition had mild tabes dorsalis; the fourth case also had late latent syphilis, but no neurologic abnormality (44). One of these patients later developed an acute Charcot joint with hemorrhagic joint fluid and acute pseudogout (21). Other reports of destructive arthropathy similar to neurotrophic arthropathy in patients with CPPD deposits and normal neurologic examinations underscore this association (45–48). Severe degeneration of the neuropathic type has even been reported in the temporomandibular joints (49).

Charcot knee joints develop in only 5% to 10% of patients with tabes dorsalis. Because CPPD deposition affects about 5% of the adult population, the two conditions might be expected to coexist by chance alone in only 1 of 20 tabetics with Charcot joints. Thus, it was postulated that neurotrophic joints actually develop in the 5% of tabetic patients who have underlying CPPD crystal deposition (44). That CPPD crystals alone can be associated with a destructive arthropathy, without the help of a neurologic deficit, reinforces this hypothesis (Fig. 117.8).

Other Patterns of Crystal Deposition

Multiple other patterns of disease have been described (8). Stiffening of the spine that mimics ankylosing spondylitis or diffuse idiopathic skeletal hyperostosis has been observed, particularly in familial CPPD deposition (10,48). True bony ankylosis was observed in Chilean familial cases; none of the affected individuals had the human leukocyte antigen HLA-B27 (50).

Neurologic presentations of CPPD crystal deposition are increasingly recognized. A syndrome of acute neck pain ascribed to CPPD or BCP deposits associated with a tomographic appearance of calcification surrounding the odontoid process has been termed the *crowned dens syndrome* (51). At times, neck pain has been accompanied by stiffness and fever so as to mimic meningitis (52). Other patients have developed long tract signs and symptoms related to deposits of CPPD crystals and adjacent tissue hypertrophy in the cervical spine (53–56). The ligamentum flavum has been the most regularly reported cervical site of CPPD crystal deposition (Fig. 117.9) (57). Crystal deposits, ligament hypertrophy, and chondroid metaplastic growths all contribute to encroachment on the cord. Less frequently, involvement of the posterior longitudinal ligament or facet joints has been reported (58,59). Surgical decompression has generally been effective. Lumbar spine involvement may manifest as acute radiculopathy or neurogenic claudication from central spinal stenosis (60). In one study, CPPD crystals occurred in the ligamentum flavum of 29% of unselected patients undergoing surgery for spinal stenosis (61).

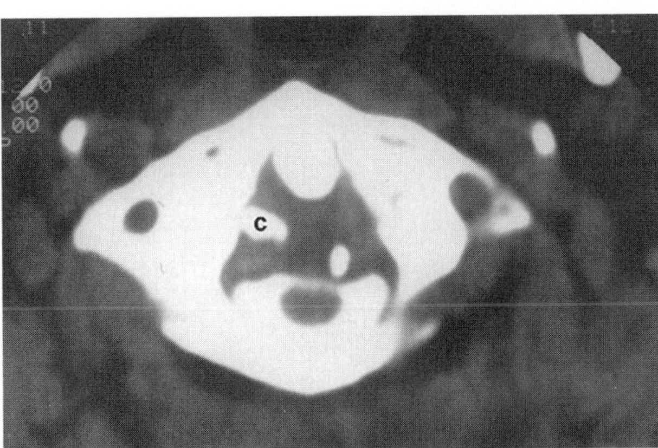

FIGURE 117.9. Excess calcification (C) at the C1-C2 level in a patient with chondrocalcinosis and long tract signs. Surgical specimen revealed crystal deposits in metaplastic fibrocartilage.

Monoarticular inflammation or degeneration may occur in CPPD secondary to trauma or attendant operations. This presentation is particularly common in the knee, years after meniscectomy (62), after operations to remove osteochondral fragments in osteochondritis dissecans (63), or in disc fibrocartilage after lumbar surgical procedures (64,65).

The frequent finding (8%) of polymyalgia rheumatica in a series from the United Kingdom suggests that CPPD deposition may mimic the proximal stiffness, pain, and elevated erythrocyte sedimentation rate of polymyalgia rheumatica (26). Rarely, a localized, progressively destructive, solitary, "tophaceous" mass of CPPD crystals occurs in synovial tissue with chondroid metaplasia (12).

It is clear from the long-term observations of the natural history of CPPD joint deposition in familial cases by Zitnan and Sitaj (39) that a given patient may show one pattern of arthritis early in the course of the disease and a different pattern later; many type A patients may eventually have pattern C, D, or F, for example.

Systemic findings during an acute attack are frequent but not invariable (2). These include a fever of 99 to 103°F, leukocytosis of 12,000 to 15,000/mm^3 with a "left shift," and an elevated erythrocyte sedimentation rate and serum acute-phase reactants. Interleukin-6 may mediate some of these systemic effects (66).

Acute attacks of pseudogout occurred during the second and third trimester of otherwise normal pregnancies (67). Each patient had a clearly identifiable cause for CPPD deposition at a young age. The release of crystals from cartilage may have been due to partial dissolution of deposits by alkaline phosphatase of placental origin, which may degrade CPPD crystal components under physiologic conditions (68).

Calcium Pyrophosphate Dihydrate Deposits in Animals

CPPD crystals have been identified in the cartilage of a Barbary ape, in elderly rhesus monkeys, and in dogs (12). Calcifications in old rabbits have also been found, but were composed of BCP rather than of CPPD.

ETIOLOGIC CLASSIFICATION

A tentative classification of CPPD deposition disease is given in Table 117.2. The genetic aberrations responsible for each of the ten largest reported series of hereditary

TABLE 117.2. ETIOLOGIC CLASSIFICATION OF CALCIUM PYROPHOSPHATE DIHYDRATE CRYSTAL DEPOSITION DISEASE

I. Hereditary (see Table 117.3)
II. Sporadic (idiopathic)
III. Associated with metabolic disease (see Table 117.4)
IV. Associated with trauma or surgical procedures

cases probably differ. Table 117.3 lists the evidence. Most families show disease transmission as an autosomal-dominant trait. The Hungarian group has an HLA association, no male-to-male transmission, and symptomatic heterozygotes. Five of the other series showed male-to-male transmission of disease, indicating autosomal inheritance. Because nearly half the offspring of a heterozygote in all series eventually developed radiographic evidence of CPPD crystal deposition, penetrance is nearly complete. Associated metabolic conditions, such as hyperparathyroidism, were rare in any of these kindreds. Phenotypic manifestations of the disease were severe in some kindreds and mild in others. The Hungarian homozygotes had severe disease, and the heterozygotes developed milder disease. In one of several English kindreds, childhood seizures presaged development of CPPD deposition in adulthood (69). Recently, the gene for some forms of familial CPPD deposition disease has been localized to the short arm of chromosome 5 (70).

The so-called sporadic or idiopathic cases of CPPD deposition disease warrant comment. Generally, no systematic search for the condition had been conducted among blood relatives, and none of the putative metabolic disease associations had been found. Such a study is difficult in the United States in view of the extreme mobility of the population and the widespread psychologic resistance to submit to study because of possible discovery of abnormality. When 12 families of patients suspected to have the sporadic form of CPPD crystal deposition disease were thoroughly studied, three were found to have more than one member with CPPD deposition disease (12). In Spain, a study of 46 apparently sporadic cases revealed a familial pattern in five (11%) (71). This finding could represent a coincidence of sporadic cases in aged subjects. Other surveys in Spain noted a 27% to 28% prevalence of familial CPPD deposition, defined as at least one other blood relative with evidence of CPPD deposits (72,73). It is likely that a thorough study of sporadic cases would result in reclassification of many as either hereditary or as associated with metabolic disease.

ASSOCIATED DISEASES

A number of metabolic diseases and physiologic stresses, such as aging and trauma, have been associated with CPPD crystal deposition. Only aging and previous joint surgery have been statistically proven to be associated with CPPD deposition. Nonetheless, strong circumstantial evidence suggests that many of these other associations are true, and the converse has often been proved, that is, that radiographically evident chondrocalcinosis occurred more frequently in patients with several of these conditions, notably gout (74), hemochromatosis (75), and hyperparathyroidism (76), than in age- and sex-matched control populations. Even when associations seem significant, however, a cause-and-effect relationship should not be inferred.

Reported associations must be interpreted with caution because CPPD deposits occur in about 5% of the adult population and are associated with nearly all diseases by chance alone. Pragmatically, the clinician is well advised to keep in mind the diseases listed in Table 117.4 when con-

TABLE 117.3. CHARACTERISTICS OF HEREDITARY CALCIUM PYROPHOSPHATE DIHYDRATE CRYSTAL DEPOSITION DISEASE

Series	Type	Male-to-Male Transmission	Associations		HLA Antigens
			Arthritis	Onset	
Slovakian (Hungarian gene)	AD	No	Severe	Early	Yes
Chilean (Spanish gene)	AD	Yes	Severe	Early	No
French	AD	Yes	Severe	Early	No
Japanese	AD	Yes	Severe	Early	NA
Swedish	AD	Yes	Severe	Early	No
Dutch	AD	Yes	Mild	Early	No
Mexican-American	AD	Yes	Mild	Early	No
French-Canadian	AD	Yes	Mild	Early	No
Spanish	AD	?	Mild	Late	
NA					
Jewish (77)	AD	No	Mild	Early	NA

AD, autosomal dominant; HLA, human leukocyte antigen; NA, not available.

TABLE 117.4. CONDITIONS PROBABLY ASSOCIATED WITH CALCIUM PYROPHOSPHATE DIHYDRATE CRYSTAL DEPOSITION

Aging
Trauma, including surgery
Hyperparathyroidism
Familial hypocalciuric hypercalcemia
Hemochromatosis
Hemosiderosis
Hypophosphatasia
Hypomagnesemia
Hypothyroidism
Gout
Neuropathic joints
Amyloidosis

fronted with a case of CPPD crystal deposition disease. Unsuspected hyperparathyroidism, hypothyroidism, and other metabolic abnormalities have been found repeatedly when appropriate laboratory studies were performed in such patients. Conversely, when arthritis supervenes in a patient with one of these metabolic conditions, the possibility of CPPD deposition disease should be considered in the differential diagnosis.

Hyperparathyroidism

Numerous reports of CPPD crystal deposition in patients with hyperparathyroidism have appeared (76,78–80), and most series of patients with CPPD deposition show an incidence of 2% to 15% (47,81,82). Conversely, 20% to 30% of patients with hyperparathyroidism have radiologic chondrocalcinosis (76,83). Of historic note, the first case of osteitis fibrosa cystica complicating hyperparathyroidism also displayed typical chondrocalcinosis when preserved humeri were radiographically examined over two centuries later (84). Hyperparathyroid patients with CPPD deposits are older than those without such deposits. In most surgically treated cases, parathyroid adenomas rather than hyperplasia have been found. Acute attacks of pseudogout are common after parathyroidectomy (25,29). A long-term postoperative follow-up study demonstrated persistence of the calcific deposits despite return of serum calcium levels to normal (83,85,86).

It has long been assumed that the persistent hypercalcemia associated with hyperparathyroidism contributes to the formation of CPPD crystals in the joint. This is reinforced by the reported associations of joint symptoms and radiologic chondrocalcinosis suggestive of CPPD crystal deposits in persons with a benign lifelong condition called hypocalciuric hypercalcemia (87,88). A better rheumatologic analysis of such patients is needed.

Hemochromatosis

The original report of arthritis in patients with hemochromatosis noted one example of articular cartilage calcification (89). Many subsequent reports have documented this association (90). Nearly half the patients with hemochromatosis have arthritis, and half of these have radiologic chondrocalcinosis (91,92). Again, these are the older patients in the series (92,93). CPPD deposition and related joint complaints are often present in patients with asymptomatic hemochromatosis. Involvement of metacarpophalangeal joints was more common in patients with hemochromatosis than in those with idiopathic chondrocalcinosis (43), but the appearance of "squared off" bone ends, joint space narrowing, and subchondral cysts in these joints was identical to that described by Martel and colleagues (41) in patients with idiopathic chondrocalcinosis. Adamson et al. (94) pointed out more prominent narrowing of the metacarpophalangeal joints, especially those in the second and third digits, peculiar hook-like osteophytes on the radial aspect of the metacarpal heads, and less scapholunate separation in CPPD crystal deposition. Appropriate treatment of the iron overload did not prevent the development of new calcifications over a 10-year period (75). Radiologic evidence of CPPD crystal deposition increased from 7 to 13 of the 18 patients followed.

That iron itself may be directly related to the calcific deposits is suggested by reports of CPPD deposition in patients with transfusion hemosiderosis (90) and hemophilia (12). *In vitro,* there is also some support for a role for iron in CPPD crystal deposition (95). Ferrous ions inhibit the pyrophosphatases responsible for degrading CPPD crystals (96). Synovial hemosiderosis slowed the metabolic clearance of radiolabeled CPPD crystals from rabbit joints by about 50% (97). However, other explanations for the link between hemochromatosis and CPPD deposition exist. For example, normocalcemic hyperparathyroidism may occur in up to 50% of patients with hemochromatosis (98). Pawlotsky et al. (99) recently demonstrated increased levels of specific parathyroid hormone (PTH) fragments in patients with hemochromatosis. They showed that levels of these specific fragments correlated with the presence of arthritis. Thus, common etiologic factors may be present in both hyperparathyroidism and hemochromatosis.

Other Disorders

O'Duffy (100) reported a patient with *hypophosphatasia* and CPPD deposits, and subsequently several others have been described (101,102). Inorganic pyrophosphate (PPi) is the anionic component of the CPPD crystal and is a natural substrate of alkaline phosphatase. As urinary and plasma PPi levels are elevated in hypophosphatasia (103,104), it is not surprising that hypophosphatasia may be associated with CPPD crystal deposition. BCP crystal deposition may also be common in this population (105). Attempts at replacing alkaline phosphatase by infusing plasma from patients with Paget's disease of bone into a patient with infantile hypophosphatasia had no appreciable effect on the urinary excretion of PPi but may have improved the bony abnormalities (106).

Hypomagnesemia associated with CPPD crystal deposition was first described in 1974 (107). At least ten cases have been reported since then (12). This association makes sense teleologically, because magnesium increases the solubility of CPPD crystals (108) and is also an important cofactor for alkaline phosphatase (109), as well as for many inorganic pyrophosphatases (96). In most reported instances, the defect appeared to be a failure of renal conservation of magnesium. In two cases, magnesium replacement therapy decreased radiologic calcification (110,111). A controlled study of oral magnesium therapy in patients with CPPD crystal deposits showed statistically significant beneficial effects on articular signs and symptoms but not on radiographic calcification (112). CPPD deposition has also been reported in *Bartter's syndrome* (12), perhaps secondary to the associated hypomagnesemia. Abnormalities in urinary or serum magnesium, however, are not present in most patients with CPPD crystal deposition (107).

Hypothyroidism has been associated with CPPD deposits but the association of these common conditions remains controversial. Deposits may remain asymptomatic until after treatment with thyroid hormone (113). One survey reported that 11% of 105 consecutive patients with CPPD deposition were hypothyroid (114), more than detected in comparable populations of patients with acute medical conditions or OA. A meta-analysis indicates a significant although small association of CPPD deposition with hypothyroidism (115). However, two studies of patients with hypothyroidism could not demonstrate an increased prevalence of radiographic knee chondrocalcinosis compared to a euthyroid control group (116,117).

Periarticular and intraarticular *amyloid deposits* have been noted in association with CPPD deposition since the first report in 1976 (118). Four of five elderly patients with amyloid arthropathy, most of whom had carpal tunnel syndrome and pitting edema of the hands, had chondrocalcinosis (119). Subsequent histologic studies have shown frequent amyloid deposits in cartilage and synovium, often in close proximity to the CPPD crystals (90). Because most such patients are elderly, this association may represent the chance concurrence of two age-related processes. Amyloid is known to bind PPi analogues (120), as well as calcium, however, and local sequestration could favor CPPD crystal formation. Amyloid has also been described in osteoarthritic cartilage (121,122) and in joints of senescent mice.

Hyperuricemia, often accompanying mild azotemia, hypertension, or diuretic use, is common in the elderly population. The coexistence of pseudogout and *urate gout* varies from 2% to 8% in most reported series (90,123). If the prevalence of monosodium urate crystal deposition were estimated at 2% of the adult male population, (17), then this association could be one of chance. Although 32% of a series of 31 gouty patients had radiologically evident chondrocalcinosis, only 5% of another series of 43 gouty patients showed such deposits, a percentage no greater than in control subjects (36). In carefully controlled prospective studies, the prevalence of chondrocalcinosis in patients with gout was 8 of 138; in age-matched normal control patients and in asymptomatic hyperuricemic patients, the prevalence was 0 of 142 and 1 of 84, respectively (77,124). These results imply an association of CPPD with gout but not with hyperuricemia.

An association of chondrocalcinosis and *spondyloepiphyseal dysplasia* has been postulated (125–127). This relationship has not been extensively investigated.

Ankylosing hyperostosis has been noted in serial studies of hereditary cases of CPPD deposition in Slovakia (39). It appeared in one-third of 18 Japanese patients (128) and was found in a number of hereditary cases studied in the Netherlands (129). Conversely, CPPD deposits were found in 6% of 34 patients with ankylosing hyperostosis.

The relationship between OA and CPPD deposition is complex. There are studies to support a correlation between CPPD crystals and severe radiographic joint degeneration. Swan and co-workers (130) showed that calcium containing crystals occur frequently in patients with apparent primary OA. They obtained synovial fluids from knee joints of 12 patients with large knee effusions, OA, no radiographic evidence of chondrocalcinosis, and no synovial fluid crystals detected by routine compensated polarized light microscopy. Eleven of these fluids demonstrated calcium containing crystals, three CPPD, six BCP, and two a mixture of both crystal types. The authors postulated that most synovial fluids from patients with OA may contain CPPD or BCP crystals too small or too infrequent to detect by routine microscopy. Sanmarti and associates (131) demonstrated that radiologic OA was positively associated with chondrocalcinosis in a population-based study in Spain. On the other hand, Felson and coworkers (132) showed that chondrocalcinosis was not an independent risk factor for incident OA in the elderly. Thus, CPPD crystals may initiate or worsen OA or may simply represent a separate entity altogether.

We suggest that *the routine examination of a newly diagnosed patient with CPPD deposition should include determinations of the following: serum calcium, magnesium, phosphorus, alkaline phosphatase, ferritin, iron and total iron-binding capacity, and thyroid-stimulating hormone,* with further metabolic study if abnormalities are found. However, hypomagnesemia and hypophosphatasia need not be considered in patients over 60 years of age.

Trauma/Surgery

Mounting evidence links CPPD deposition with antecedent joint trauma or surgical procedures. In 1942,

Weaver (133) discussed monarticular calcific deposition following trauma. Arthroscopic findings in such joints have been described (134). Radiographic chondrocalcinosis has been recognized in hypermobile joints (135), unstable joints (136), and neuropathic joints (44). The most compelling evidence was presented by Linden and Nilsson (63) and Doherty and co-workers (62). In the former study, 25 of 42 knees previously treated operatively for osteochondritis dissecans of the femoral condyle developed chondrocalcinosis in the operated, but not the contralateral, knee. A control group of meniscectomy patients developed chondrocalcinosis in 14 of 41 operated knees. In the latter study of postmeniscectomy patients, knee radiographs were obtained a mean of 25 years after operation; at that time, 20% of operated, but only 4% of contralateral, knees showed chondrocalcinosis. A case of monarticular chondrocalcinosis following local radiation therapy has also been reported (137).

Drugs

The administration of pamindronate, granulocyte-macrophage colony-stimulating factor, and intraarticular hyaluronan preparations have been associated with pseudogout attacks in isolated case reports (138–140).

RADIOGRAPHIC FEATURES

CPPD deposition disease has characteristic radiographic features, but radiographic changes should not be overly relied upon as a diagnostic test. Chondrocalcinosis may not always represent CPPD deposits. Conversely, Fisseler-Eckhoff and Muller (141) reported that radiographic chondrocalcinosis may only identify a minority (39%) of patients with pathologically demonstrable CPPD crystal deposits at the time of arthroscopy. Heavy CPPD crystal deposits in fibrocartilaginous structures, hyaline (articular) cartilage, ligaments, and joint capsules have a characteristic appearance that is diagnostically helpful. Punctate and linear radiodensities are most frequently seen in the fibrocartilaginous menisci of the knee and usually involve both menisci of both knees (Figs. 117.1C and 117.3B). Other fibrocartilaginous structures often calcified in this miliary fashion are the articular discs of the distal radioulnar joint (Fig. 117.4), the symphysis pubis (Fig. 117.5), the glenoid and acetabular labra, and the annulus fibrosus of the intervertebral discs. The articular discs of the sternoclavicular joints are often involved, but those of the temporomandibular joint are usually spared.

Calcification of the hyaline articular cartilage is common; the deposits in the midzonal layer appear as a radiopaque line paralleling the density of the underlying bone (Figs. 117.3B and 117.4). The larger joints show these deposits most frequently, although they have been observed in nearly every diarthrodial joint. On magnetic resonance imaging (MRI), hyaline articular CPPD deposits appear as hypointense foci best shown on two- and three-dimensional gradient-echo (GRE) sequences, while meniscal calcification is often missed (142). Calcifications of articular capsules or synovium, especially of the elbow, shoulder, hip, and knee, are frequently seen; the deposits appear as a faintly opaque line more diffuse than that seen in cartilage.

Calcification of bursae, tendons, and ligaments also occurs in CPPD deposition disease. This calcification may represent BCP crystal deposition in some patients, but crystal-proven CPPD deposits have been reported in all the aforementioned sites. Synovial deposits may be so large as to mimic synovial chondromatosis (143), and ligamentous or tendinous deposits may produce local compressive symptoms, such as carpal tunnel syndrome (144) or myelopathy, as already outlined.

Subchondral bone cysts are common and can attain a large size. Histologic examination of the walls of the lesion shown in Fig. 117.6 confirmed that it was only a bone cyst. How such lesions are related to CPPD deposition disease is unknown, but they occur frequently enough to be a diagnostic clue (23).

A number of distinct local radiographic abnormalities may suggest CPPD deposition. A peculiar erosion of the femoral cortex superior to the patella has been reported (145,146). This lesion appears to correlate with OA of the patellofemoral compartment (Fig. 117.7). Carpal instability reported in association with CPPD deposits resembles that of RA (147). A particular propensity for radiocarpal involvement has been observed. Navicular-lunate dissociation is thought to result from degeneration of the ligamentous structures. Axial involvement has been described (24). In the lumbar spine, multiple levels of annulus fibrosus calcification, vacuum disc phenomena, and disc narrowing are emphasized. A syndrome of acute neck pain associated with calcifications surrounding the odontoid process, the "crowned dens syndrome," has been described (51) (Fig. 117.9). It has occurred in patients who have either BCP or CPPD crystal deposition in peripheral joints. Sacroiliac joint abnormalities include subchondral erosions, reactive sclerosis, and bilateral vacuum phenomena. Axial involvement is particularly prominent in uremic patients with secondary hyperparathyroidism (83).

Features that may accompany CPPD crystal deposition include joint degeneration, tibial stress fractures, and avascular necrosis of the medial or lateral femoral condyle. Degenerative changes in joints not commonly involved in primary OA, such as the metacarpophalangeal, radiocarpal, elbow, and shoulder joints, may suggest underlying CPPD crystal deposition even in the absence of radiographic chondrocalcinosis. Subchondral cysts, bone and cartilage fragmentation, and variable osteophyte formation are characteristic (Fig. 117.8). The best serial studies are those of the familial Hungarian cases (39). CPPD deposits first appeared in radiographically normal cartilage, and degeneration inevitably followed. Tibial stress fractures were reported in five elderly patients with CPPD deposition and severe degenerative knee disease (148). Because their knees were usually painful before the fractures, the source of increased pain was not readily apparent. Interestingly, 4 of 14 patients with osteonecrosis of the medial femoral condyle had CPPD knee deposits (149), an association subsequently confirmed (150).

A patient may be screened for CPPD deposition with four suitably exposed radiographs: an anteroposterior view of each knee, an anteroposterior view of the pelvis, and a posteroanterior view of the wrists. If nothing diagnostic is seen on these films, a more extensive survey is unlikely to be helpful.

The chemical composition of the crystal deposits may be inferred with confidence when typical chondrocalcinosis is present on radiographs. Caution must be exercised when the calcifications are faint or atypical, however, because of the possibility that these represent dicalcium phosphate dihydrate, BCP, or calcium oxalate crystal deposits or vascular calcifications (17).

PATHOLOGIC FEATURES

The distribution of CPPD crystals in affected tissues has been extensively examined in seven cadavers (12), and generally parallels that seen on radiographs. Joint capsules, especially in the hip and shoulder, and the midzonal and superficial areas of hyaline articular cartilages were often affected, but the heaviest deposits were distributed diffusely in fibrocartilaginous structures (Fig. 117.10). The menisci of the knee were involved in all cases (Fig. 117.3A). Heavy deposits were often noted in tendons and in intraarticular ligaments, such as the cruciate ligaments in the knee. Microscopically, the deposits were composed of various-sized microcrystalline aggregates of CPPD (Fig. 117.11). Their diameters varied from 15 μm to 0.6 cm; the larger ones appeared grossly as white chalky deposits. It was difficult on gross inspection to distinguish these deposits (Fig. 117.3A) from the white chalky lesions of true gout.

CPPD crystals are far more common in cartilage than in other articular tissues. Periarticular deposits of CPPD, however, have been reported in tendons, dura mater, ligamenta flava, and the olecranon bursa, as well as in isolated tophi (12). A survey of a large number of pathologic nonarticular calcifications using crystallographic techniques showed no CPPD crystals and thus established their relative specificity for articular tissue (151). Identification of crystals in aortic plaques, costal cartilages, pancreas, and pineal glands obtained from pseudogout patients at necropsy showed only apatite deposits.

Histologic abnormalities in joint tissues during attacks of acute pseudogout have also been noted. Cartilage sections from these patients showed neutrophils migrating into the matrix (152). Intracellular CPPD crystals were observed within invading neutrophils. The superficial cartilage was eroded, and collagen fibers were degraded. Presumably, the neutrophils generated enzymes and free oxygen radical species harmful to adjacent matrix and cells.

The histologic appearance of CPPD crystal deposition in articular cartilage is well described. The smallest, and presumably the earliest, crystals appear at the lacunar margin

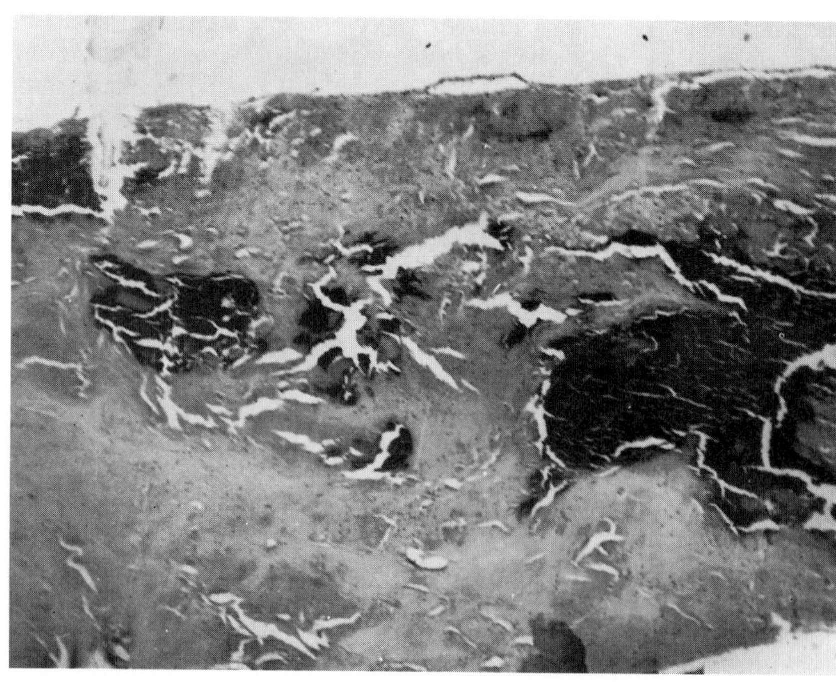

FIGURE 117.10. Photomicrograph of a section through the meniscus shown in Fig. 117.3A, various-sized aggregates of calcified material are distributed throughout (hematoxylin and eosin stain, ×26).

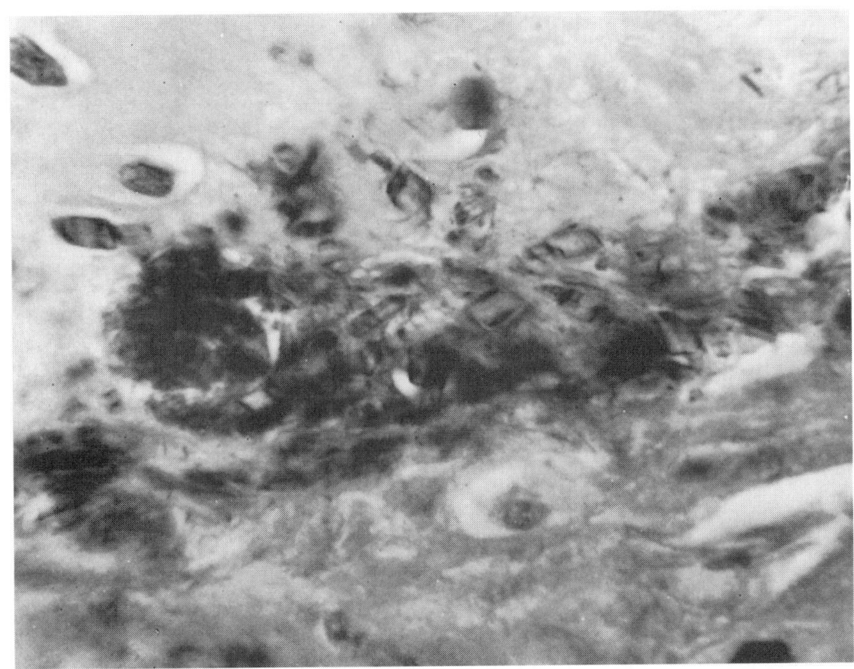

FIGURE 117.11. Photomicrograph of the smallest deposits found shows them surrounding the lacunae of the chondrocytes. This process begins in the midzonal layer of articular cartilage, more diffusely in fibrocartilage. Individual crystals of calcium pyrophosphate dihydrate are visible in this section (alazarin red, ×800; linear magnification ×3).

of chondrocytes. When adjacent chondrocytes are damaged, chondrocyte-derived membrane bound vesicles, known as *matrix vesicles*, are often seen pericellularly. Increased glycogen islands and rough endoplasmic reticulum are present in the chondrocytes (153). The surrounding matrix may appear normal or granular. Collagen fibril fragmentation in uncalcified areas of CPPD cartilage has been described in familial cases (154). Larger superficial deposits occur in degenerative cartilages, usually at sites of surface ulcerations and fissuring and are often associated with chondrocyte "cloning."

Chondrocytes from cartilage with CPPD deposits appear morphologically abnormal. Ishikawa and co-workers (155) have shown convincing evidence of abnormal proteoglycan deposition within chondrocytes in the immediate vicinity of early CPPD crystal deposits. These "red cells," stained with safranin-0, were not seen if the tissue was first exposed to either papain or chondroitinase ABC, which confirms their proteoglycan nature. Red cells were a constant feature of evolving, but not of mature, CPPD crystal deposits in fibrocartilage, hyaline cartilage, and synovium showing chondroid metaplasia (155). They were seen in tissue from both sporadic and familial cases. Ishikawa et al. also found the following: (a) absence of normal safranin-0 staining in the matrix in areas of early crystal deposition; (b) "packing" of the proteoglycan-denuded collagen fibers in these same areas; (c) hypertrophy and mitotic activity of the red cells; (d) the appearance of CPPD crystals in empty chondrocyte lacunae; and (e) mature deposits were ringed with dense, proteoglycan-free collagen, but the crystals were coated with a thin film of proteoglycan. No collagen or cells could be identified within these crystal masses by light or electron microscopy. The surrounding matrix now contained normal-appearing cells and stained normally. Ishikawa et al. speculated that the cell-associated proteoglycan may indicate faulty release from the chondrocytes after synthesis, or that it may enter these cells by endocytosis. Their findings warrant further exploration and, if confirmed, must be taken into account in any scheme of the pathogenesis of CPPD crystal deposition.

Ohira and co-workers (156) reported that articular hyaline and fibrocartilage as well as synovium from patients with CPPD deposits contain excess lipid. Sites of crystal deposits stained strongly with Sudan III. Adjacent metaplastic chondrocytes contained large Sudan III–positive granules. The lipid nature of this material was confirmed by extraction with chloroform/ethanol. The role of lipid in mineralization could not be elucidated, but lipid may bind calcium needed for CPPD formation. A calcium-binding protein, S-100, has also been immunolocalized to CPPD-containing articular tissues, but not CPPD-free tissues from patients with OA (157). Others, however, noted increased S-100 protein in degenerative joints without crystals (158).

In three patients, superficial amyloid deposits occurred adjacent to CPPD crystals (121). Isolated descriptions of CPPD crystals within chondrocytes have been reported (159–162), indicating that chondrocytes may phagocytose crystals with attendant biologic consequences (Chapter 116). A single case of temporomandibular joint CPPD deposition was found to contain numerous crystals within chondrocytes, possibly within mitochondria (163). A unique abnormality of mitochondrial PPi metabolism was postulated to result in intracellular CPPD crystal deposition.

Synovial biopsy material showed inflammatory and reparative changes consistent with the clinical state of the joint at the time of biopsy. Early in an acute attack, the edematous synovium was infiltrated with polymorphonuclear leukocytes; later, mononuclear infiltration and fibroblastic proliferation were seen. Synovial proliferation and infiltration with chronic inflammatory cells in chronically symptomatic joints can resemble rheumatoid pannus. Crystals have been identified in the superficial synovium under polarized light and by electron microscopy (161). In patients with pseudo-OA undergoing knee replacement, synovial deposits were focal and concentrated in avascular areas (162). In synovium, CPPD crystals appear to align along collagen fibers and in proximity to foci of chondroid metaplasia (164). Collagen fibers may be a nucleating site for CPPD crystals, constituent PPi being generated by the adjacent metaplastic chondroid tissue. Excised surgical samples from involved ligaments have shown chondroid metaplasia, occasional matrix vesicles, and CPPD crystals.

In six cases, CPPD deposits were identified in periarticular bone (165). High PPi levels in bone may foster deposition at this site, or PPi needed for crystal deposition could have been derived from synovial fluid enzymes acting on extracellular adenosine triphosphate (ATP) as described below.

PATHOGENESIS

The cause of CPPD crystal deposition is unknown. Conceptually, formation of CPPD crystals in cartilage may result from elevated levels of either calcium or PPi, from changes in the matrix that promote crystal formation, or from combinations of these factors. Because CPPD crystal deposition is a clinically heterogeneous disorder, different factors may predominate in individual cases, much as hyperuricemia preceding monosodium urate crystal deposition may have different causes.

Bjelle (154) favors the hypothesis that matrix changes antedate and facilitate CPPD crystal formation. In studies of Swedish patients with familial CPPD deposition, he found weakly staining midzonal matrix with decreased collagen content, some fragmentation of collagen fibers, and an abnormal hexosamine profile. The proportions of keratan sulfate and chondroitin 6-sulfate were increased, and those of chondroitin 4-sulfate were decreased. A decrease in mucin-like oligosaccharides was found. Because these changes were independent of the amount of crystal deposits and because morphologically abnormal crystal-free areas in midzonal cartilage were seen by electron microscopy, Bjelle postulated a primary role of a matrix abnormality in promoting CPPD mineral phase. Alterations of matrix collagen and proteoglycan were reported by Masuda et al. (157) in sporadic cases of CPPD crystal deposition disease.

The inorganic composition of matrix may also affect CPPD crystal formation. Ferrous ions inhibited some pyrophosphatases (96), and ferric ions lowered the formation product for CPPD crystals *in vitro* (95) and slowed the intracellular degradation of CPPD crystals injected into rabbit joints (97). Hypomagnesemia, both primary and secondary to Bartter's syndrome, has also been associated with chondrocalcinosis. Magnesium is a cofactor for many pyrophosphatases and increases the solubility of CPPD crystals (108). Therefore, its deficiency may decrease hydrolysis of PPi and may slow crystal dissolution. Profound hypomagnesemia induced by dietary magnesium deprivation did not change the rate of CPPD crystal clearance from rabbit joints, however (166). Elevations of inorganic phosphate have promoted CPPD crystal nucleation and growth *in vitro* and may act similarly *in vivo* (167). The effect of inorganic phosphate in aqueous solution on CPPD crystal formation is most prominent in the 0.01- to 1.0-mM range (168). That such an aberration may exist is suggested by the finding of elevated levels of inorganic phosphate in synovial fluid in pseudogout (169).

Studies of crystal formation in gels provide indirect evidence that organic matrix components may be nucleating agents in CPPD crystal formation. In aqueous solutions, CPPD crystal synthesis occurred at acid pH or at high ionic concentrations (4,168). In model collagen gels, however, crystals formed at neutral pH (170), and at PPi concentrations between 2 and 20 μM (171). Formation of amorphous calcium pyrophosphate and orthorhombic calcium pyrophosphate tetrahydrate preceded formation of monoclinic and triclinic CPPD crystals identical to those observed *in vivo* (172). These studies seem particularly relevant because cartilage is a gel. The modulatory effect of other organic matrix components, such as proteoglycans, on CPPD crystal formation has not been carefully studied.

No systematic study has been made of cartilage interstitial fluid calcium in patients with CPPD deposition. Clearly, some of these patients have hyperparathyroidism, usually due to adenoma, with associated hypercalcemia. CPPD deposition has also been noted in patients with familial hypocalciuric hypercalcemia (87,88), further supporting a role for elevated ionized calcium levels in promoting CPPD deposition.

In contrast to what is known about calcium, there is a large body of evidence suggesting that the metabolism of PPi, the anionic component of the CPPD crystal, is abnormal in CPPD deposition disease. PPi is produced by many biosynthetic reactions during macromolecular synthesis (103). The ubiquitous pyrophosphatases, hydrolyzing PPi into inorganic orthophosphate, drive these reactions in the direction of synthesis; but the intracellular enzymatic hydrolysis of PPi does not go to completion, and detectable amounts are measurable in cells, including fibroblasts and chondrocytes (173).

The amount of PPi produced in the body is immense. It has been calculated that 30 g are made daily in the human liver as a by-product of the synthesis of albumin alone (103). Only a small amount of that synthesized appears in the urine (approximately 10 to 100 μmol daily), where it acts as a powerful inhibitor of crystal nucleation and growth. The turnover rate of plasma PPi in dogs is only about 2 minutes, which further complicates the interpretation of plasma values. Neither the source nor the fate of plasma PPi is known.

Much PPi is adsorbed to bone mineral (174–176), where it is thought to act as a regulator of mineralization. In addition to its effect on crystal precipitation, it retards the conversion of amorphous calcium phosphate into crystalline hydroxyapatite, inhibits crystal aggregation, and slows the dissolution rate of hydroxyapatite crystals. The diphosphonates, which have P-C-P bonds, instead of P-O-P bonds, are nonhydrolyzable analogues of PPi. These compounds have similar biologic effects and are used as therapeutic agents in various diseases of mineral metabolism and, coupled with tin and technetium ^{99m}Tc, as bone-scanning agents.

Studies of PPi metabolism were stimulated by recognition of this substance as a constituent of the crystal deposits. Because urinary levels are much easier to quantify than those in plasma, these were measured earliest and were found to be normal in patients with CPPD deposition disease (176,177). Blood levels of PPi were later measured; serum contained two to three times the concentration of plasma (178). This increase resulted from the release of PPi by platelets during clotting. Plasma concentrations in sporadic cases of CPPD deposition were similar to those in osteoarthritic or normal control subjects (179). In patients with hypophosphatasia, a disease associated with CPPD deposition, both urinary and plasma levels of PPi were elevated (104,180), presumably as a result of decreased hydrolysis.

Abnormal local metabolism of PPi was suggested by reports of elevated levels in synovial fluids from patients with CPPD crystal deposition, although elevations were also observed in synovial fluids from patients with gout, OA, and even RA. The highest joint fluid levels were found in the most severely degenerated joints, as judged radiographically (169). PPi levels were lower during acute attacks and rose as the episode subsided (169,181), probably because of increased synovial blood flow during acute attacks with more rapid equilibration with plasma PPi. The elevated synovial fluid levels could not be explained by dissolution of crystals in the fluid. The gradient between synovial fluid and plasma implied a local origin of PPi (169). Even normal synovial fluid PPi concentrations exceed those in plasma (182). The site of the synovial fluid production was expected to be cartilage, based on the histologic observation that the smallest and presumably the earliest crystals are seen adjacent to chondrocytes. Subsequent studies indicated that articular hyaline and fibrocartilages in organ culture liberated PPi into the ambient media, whereas synovium, subchondral bone, and nonarticular (elastic) cartilages did not (183,184). Extrapolation of the amount produced by incubated slices to the estimated mass of cartilage in a whole knee joint yielded figures for local production of the same order of magnitude as estimated from *in vivo* kinetic experiments (183,185). Demonstration of a single PPi pool that included synovial fluid might suggest that both cartilage extracellular fluid and synovial fluid accumulate and dispose of PPi at similar rates. Thus, cartilage is the most likely source of locally elevated concentrations of PPi in CPPD deposition.

There is evidence for three pathways of extracellular PPi generation by chondrocytes: (a) extracellular generation by extracellular or ectoenzymes (ectoenzyme hypothesis); (b) "leakage" or transport from chondrocytes containing excess PPi (secretion hypothesis); and (c) release of PPi together with matrix-destined synthetic products (coexport hypothesis) (Fig. 117.12). Whether each pathway is important in all patients or whether abnormal PPi generation occurs via different pathways in different patients is unknown. As in

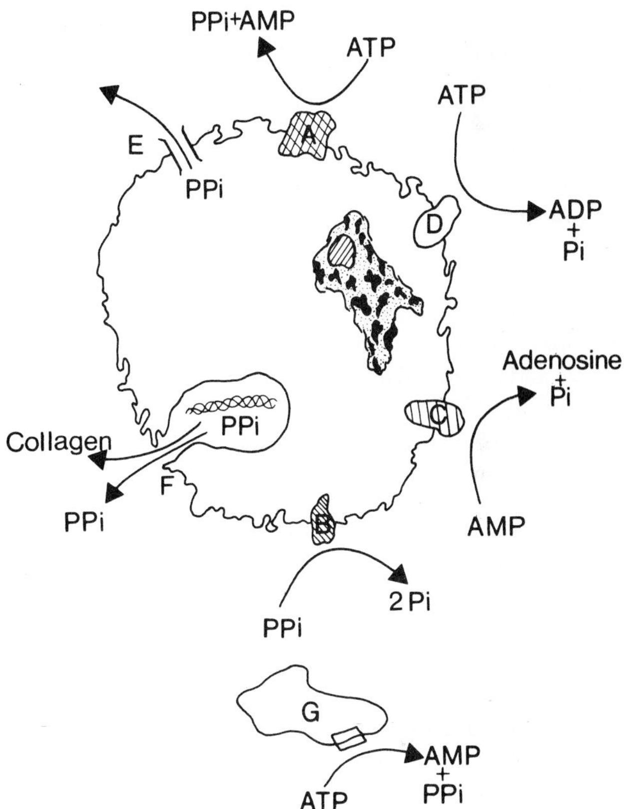

FIGURE 117.12. Putative factors in release of extracellular inorganic pyrophosphate (PPi) by chondrocytes. PPi generated from extracellular adenosine triphosphate (ATP) by ectonucleoside triphosphate pyrophosphohydrolase (ectoenzyme hypothesis) **(A)**. Degradation of extracellular PPi by ecto- or extracellular PPi-ase **(B)**. 5′-Nucleotidase degrades adenosine monophosphate (AMP), promoting reaction A **(C)**. Ecto-ATPase competes with reaction A for substrate **(D)**. PPi leak or secretion from chondrocyte cytoplasm **(E)**. Release of PPi together with matrix molecules (coexport hypothesis) **(F)**. Vesicles derived from chondrocytes contain nucleoside triphosphate pyrophosphohydrolase and other enzymes **(G)**.

gout, the crystals represent a final common pathway of anion accumulation. In contrast to systemic hyperuricemia in gout, the excess anion (PPi) concentration is purely local in CPPD deposition.

Several observations support the ectoenzyme hypothesis. Augmented PPi generation was found in the presence of ATP by extracts of cartilages from patients with CPPD deposition, as compared with extracts of osteoarthritic or normal cartilages (186). ATP was enzymatically hydrolyzed to adenosine monophosphate and PPi by ATP pyrophosphohydrolase. A similar activity had been described in calcifying sheep cartilage (187). Subsequent reports have verified the presence of this enzyme in matrix vesicle fractions of epiphyseal cartilage (188,189), where it may play a role in calcium phosphate precipitation (190,191). We have characterized this activity as a chondrocyte nucleoside triphosphate pyrophosphohydrolase (NTPPPH) with broad substrate reactivity and as an ectoenzyme (192). The cell surface location of this enzyme was confirmed by Howell et al. (193) and by Caswell and Russell (194).

There is now evidence for three enzymes with ectoNTPPPH activity. One, termed PC-1 (plasma cell glycoprotein), has been cloned and sequenced, and was originally isolated from a plasmacytoma (195). It is situated on the plasma membranes of various cells including osteoblasts, skin fibroblasts, and chondrocytes (196). A soluble form of PC-1 has been described. Transfection of PC-1 into simian fibroblasts increased their generation of ATP-induced extracellular PPi elaboration (197). A second enzyme, NTPPPH, a 127-kd molecule, appears to be specific for cartilage, ligament, and tendon (198,199). It is pelletable and is associated with 100-nm vesicles released from these tissues. The 127-kd molecule and enzymatically active split products have been identified in cartilage organ culture conditioned medium. A 61-kd porcine protein has now been cloned, and represents the carboxyl terminal portion of the 127-kd protein (200). Its human homologue has been recently cloned and designated cartilage intermediate layer protein (201). A 58-kd protein with NTPPPH activity has also been isolated. All three enzymes have been identified in human synovial fluids (202). NTPPPH activity in human serum or plasma samples from a given subject was identical and due to a 100-kd split product of the 127-kd enzyme (203).

Because CPPD crystals appear first extracellularly adjacent to chondrocytes and because PPi does not passively cross cell membranes (204), the external position of this enzyme might allow the generation of PPi at the site of crystal formation in the presence of suitable substrate. Levels of NTPPPH activity were higher in the synovial fluid of patients with CPPD deposition and OA than in fluids from patients with RA or gout (181). Activity was also elevated in synovial fluids containing BCP crystals, implying a broader connection between NTPPPH and mineralization in general (205). Enzyme activity correlated directly with the concentration of PPi in synovial fluid. In addition to elevated NTPPPH activity in detergent extracts of cartilages with CPPD deposition, Tenenbaum et al. (186) also described higher levels of 5′-nucleotidase activity and lower levels of alkaline phosphatase and PPiase activity than in osteoarthritic cartilages. All of these aberrations would favor the accumulation of PPi in the ectoenzyme system shown in Fig. 117.13.

ATP was found in both platelet-poor plasma (100–800 nM) and synovial fluid (206). Levels of extracellular ATP were higher in fluids from joints containing CPPD crystals than in fluids from patients with OA (200 nM in CPPD vs. 100 nM in OA). Alternatively, chondrocytes may discharge cellular nucleoside triphosphate (NTP) substrates for their own ectoenzyme without requiring synovial fluid ATP.

The rate of hydrolysis of ATP in cell-free synovial fluid incubated under physiologic conditions was rapid; the half-life averaged 72 seconds in OA fluids, 30 seconds in CPPD fluids, and 86 seconds in one normal fluid (207). When ATP was infused into such fluids at rates intended to mimic *in vivo* steady-state levels, it was converted predominantly to PPi (60–83%). Synovial fluid was as effective as whole cartilage in generating PPi from extracellular ATP. Total PPi production in a human knee would be 0.3 to 1.75 μmol per hour by extrapolation from synovial fluid production rates to the pool size determined earlier *in vivo* (185). This compares with quantitative estimates of PPi production using two other methods. Pool and turnover studies using radiolabeled PPi suggest 0.1 to 0.8 μmol of PPi production per hour in human arthritic knees (185), and production of PPi by organ culture of normal human hyaline articular knee cartilage is 0.08 μmol per hour (207). Taken together, the data suggest that much of PPi production in joint tissues derives from extracellular ATP via ectoNTPPPH (208).

Vesicles, derived by collagenase digestion of articular cartilage and resembling matrix vesicles, are also rich in NTPPPH. These structures promoted calcium mineral formation when incubated with ATP in defined media. The precipitates contained PPi derived from the ATP and posi-

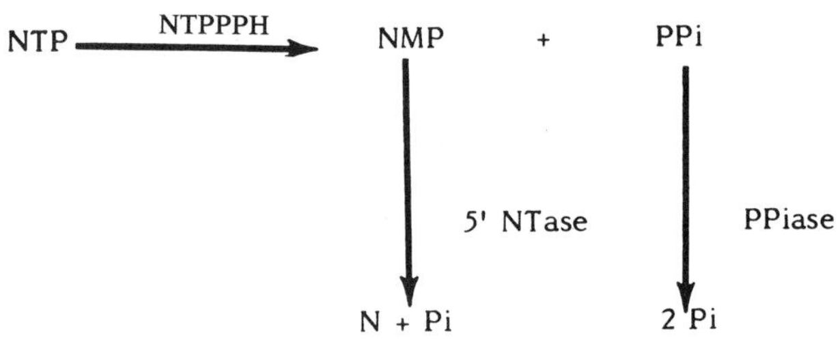

FIGURE 117.13. Postulated enzymatic cascade of inorganic pyrophosphate (PPi) production from nucleotide triphosphate (NTP). Elevated NTP pyrophosphohydrolase and 5′-nucleotidase activities and decreased inorganic pyrophosphatase activity in chondrocalcinosic cartilages all favor PPi accumulation. 5′-NTase, 5′-nucleotidase; PPiase, inorganic pyrophosphatase; Pi, inorganic phosphate; N, nucleotide; NMP, nucleotide monophosphate.

tively birefringent crystals resembling monoclinic CPPD. These dissolved when incubated with yeast inorganic pyrophosphatase (209). Fourier transform infrared spectroscopy identified peaks characteristic of P-P bonds in the mineral. EM diffraction confirmed spacings closely matching those of standard CPPD crystals in mineralized porcine cartilage vesicles (210). Thus, ectoenzyme associated with cell-derived membrane particles, as well as with intact cells, may promote CPPD crystal formation.

Alternatives to the ectoenzyme hypothesis are necessary, since rabbit chondrocytes stripped of their ectoNTPPPH activity by protease treatment still generate extracellular PPi (211). Support for the secretion hypothesis is derived from the work of Lust and associates (173,212), who found intracellular PPi levels twice those of control subjects in cultured skin fibroblasts and in lymphoblasts obtained from affected members of a French kindred with familial CPPD deposition. A generalized metabolic abnormality phenotypically expressed only in chondrocytes was postulated. The total and releasable PPi content of platelets in five patients with sporadic or familial CPPD deposition was similar to that of 17 control subjects (213), but a significant positive correlation was found between platelet PPi content and the age of the donor.

PPi levels in cultured skin fibroblasts from patients with both sporadic and familial CPPD crystal deposition were significantly elevated compared to those from normal persons or subjects with OA (214). Activity of ectoNTPPPH was elevated in fibroblasts from sporadic, but not familial, CPPD crystal deposition (214). Lastly, intracellular PPi levels and ectoNTPPPH activity were positively correlated in fibroblasts from each of the groups studied. This may be a result of transient expression of NTPPPH intracellularly prior to its translocation as suggested by PC-1 transfection experiments (197).

The export of chondrocyte PPi is greatly enhanced by transforming growth factor-β (TGF-β) (215). This enhanced export is inhibited by insulin-like growth factor-1 (IGF-1), interleukin-1 (IL-1), and tumor necrosis factor-α (TNF-α) (216). Thus, the physiologic decline in IGF-1 production with aging was postulated to promote age-related CPPD crystal formation. A mechanism of export is suggested by the finding that the TGFβ–induced rise in extracellular PPi around cultured chondrocytes is inhibited by the anion transport inhibitor probenecid (217).

Last, the coexport of PPi, formed during synthesis of matrix-destined macromolecules, and its metabolic coproducts was investigated. Liberation of PPi correlated with release of uronic acid in one study (184), but chondrocyte coexport of PPi and glycosaminoglycans was later disproved (211,218). However, incubation of adult articular hyaline cartilage with ascorbate, which stimulates collagen synthesis, markedly increased PPi elaboration. This effect was reversed when ascorbate oxidase was added (219). General protein synthesis inhibitors and more specific inhibitors of collagen production prevented ascorbate enhancement of PPi elaboration. Interestingly, cycloheximide, a nonspecific protein synthesis inhibitor, abrogated ascorbate-enhanced PPi production, but not basal PPi production by unstimulated cells. This implies at least two modes of extracellular PPi elaboration, one independent of protein synthesis and the other cycloheximide inhibitable, possibly co-secretion of collagen and PPi.

Although these biochemical changes cannot yet be directly related to the pathogenesis of CPPD crystal deposition, they represent the earliest biochemical correlates of this metabolic arthropathy.

THERAPY

Acute attacks of pseudogout are readily treated by several methods, including (a) thorough aspiration of the joint to remove crystals; (b) administration of nonsteroidal antiinflammatory drugs, such as indomethacin, (c) joint immobilization; and (d) local injection of microcrystalline corticosteroid esters. Intravenous colchicine is as effective in pseudogout as it is in gout (31). Oral colchicine reduced the number of acute attacks when given prophylactically (220). Use of adrenocorticotropic hormone (ACTH) or systemic corticosteroids has been advocated in special circumstances where conventional treatments may be contraindicated (221).

No known way exists to halt the progressive deposition of crystals or to remove those already deposited. Correction of associated metabolic disorders such as hyperparathyroidism, myxedema, and hemochromatosis has not resulted in the disappearance of radiographic cartilage calcification. New calcifications have developed in some such patients (75). Attempts at lavage of affected knee joints with magnesium chloride were unsuccessful in removing enough CPPD crystals to change the radiographic appearance, but acute attacks were precipitated (222). Several examples of spontaneous disappearance of calcific deposits have been reported. Wrist calcification disappeared in one case after immobilization and subsequent development of reflex sympathetic dystrophy (223). Radiologic evidence of decreased meniscal calcification in two cases with associated hypomagnesemia occurred after prolonged magnesium treatment (110,111). In a double-blinded, placebo-controlled trial of magnesium carbonate treatment for sporadic CPPD crystal deposition, radiographic calcification did not change over 6 months, although symptoms improved significantly (112). Repeated intraarticular injections of glycosaminoglycan polysulfate (Arteparon) in 12 patients with CPPD crystal deposition reduced pain and increased mobility compared to the contralateral, untreated knee joints (224) Radiographic calcification decreased after 2 to 7 weeks of treatment. However, several recent case reports describe precipitation of acute pseudogout attacks with hyaluronan preparations (140).

Treatment of the frequently associated degenerative disease is the same as for OA. Intraarticular injection with ^{90}Y ameliorated pain and stiffness and decreased the size of effusions in affected knee joints over a 6-month period (225). Joint deformity and radiographic changes were not improved, however.

Even if effective treatments were available, two problems remain. First, no biochemical marker identifies those patients who will develop crystal deposition. We must await radiographic evidence of cartilage calcification or identification of crystals in joint fluids, both of which probably signal long-standing disease. Therapeutic interventions at this stage may be much less effective. Second, although treatment of the crystal deposition would probably ameliorate or prevent acute pseudogout attacks, it might have no effect on the much more significant degenerative joint disease. Figure 117.14 illustrates three potential pathogenetic sequences relating degenerative disease to crystal deposition. Only in sequence 3, analogous to the pathogenesis of tophaceous gout, would removal or prevention of crystal formation affect cartilage degeneration. Doherty and coworkers (62) have postulated that the biologic effects of CPPD crystals may act as an amplification loop, as shown by the hatched lines in sequences 1 and 2, which envision crystal formation as an epiphenomenon and as a coincidental phenomenon, respectively. Radiographic evidence of chondrocalcinosis as a primary determinant of the rate of radiographic deterioration supports this thesis (226). If an amplification loop exists, then prevention of crystal formation and crystal removal would both have a salutary effect. Perhaps each of the paradigms shown here occurs in patients with CPPD crystal deposition, with varying sequences in different patients. Because the clinical importance of CPPD crystals will surely rise as the population ages, these therapeutic considerations are of more than theoretic interest.

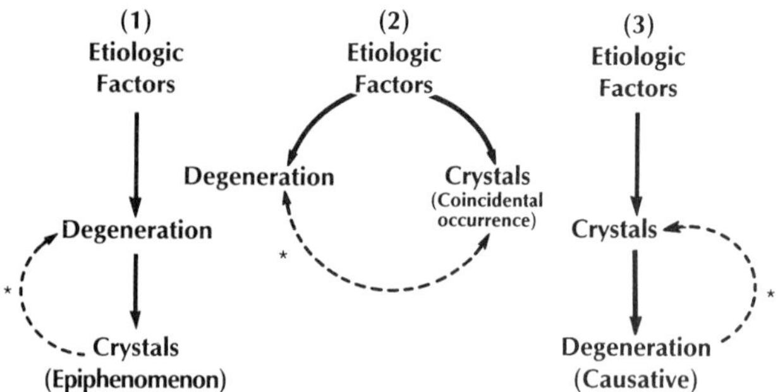

FIGURE 117.14. Prevention of crystal formation or dissolution of calcium pyrophosphate dihydrate crystals would have little effect on cartilage degeneration except in schema number 3 or if an amplification loop exists. *, amplification loop.

ACKNOWLEDGMENTS

This work was supported by National Institutes of Health (NIH) grants RO-AR38656 (L.M.R.) and RO-AG15337 (A.K.R), and a Veterans Affairs (VA) Merit Review (A.K.R.).

REFERENCES

1. McCarty DJ, Hollander JL. Identification of urate crystals in gouty synovial fluid. *Ann Intern Med* 1961;54:452–460.
2. McCarty DJ, Kohn NN, Faires JS. The significance of calcium phosphate crystals in the synovial fluid of arthritis patients: the "pseudogout syndrome." I. Clinical aspects. *Ann Intern Med* 1962;56:711–737.
3. Kohn NN, Hughes RE, McCarty DJ, et al. The significance of calcium phosphate crystals in the synovial fluid of arthritis patients: the "pseudogout syndrome." II. Identification of crystals. *Ann Intern Med* 1962;56:738–745.
4. Brown EH, Lehr JR, Smith JP, et al. Preparation and characterization of some calcium pyrophosphates. *J Agr Food Chem* 1963;11:214–222.
5. McCarty DJ. Crystal-induced inflammation: syndromes of gout and pseudogout. *Geriatrics* 1963;18:467–478.
6. Zitnan D, Sitaj S. Mnohopocentna familiarna kalcifikacin articularnych chrupiek. *Bratisl Lek Listy* 1958;38:217–228.
7. Uri DS, Martel W. Radiologic manifestations of the crystarelated arthropathies. *Semin Roentgenol* 1996;31:229–238.
8. McCarty DJ. The Heberden oration, 1982. Crystals, joints, and consternation. *Ann Rheum Dis* 1983;42:243–253.
9. McCarty DJ. Calcium pyrophosphate deposition disease. In: Hollander JL, ed. *Arthritis and allied conditions.* Philadelphia: Lea & Febiger, 1966:947–964.
10. Zitnan D, Sitaj S. Chondrocalcinosis articularis. Section I. Clinical and radiological study. *Ann Rheum Dis* 1963;22: 142–169.
11. Bennett EH. Abnormal deposits in joints. *Dublin J Med Sci* 1903;65:161–163.
12. Ryan L, McCarty D. Calcium pyrophosphate crystal deposition disease; pseudogout; articular chondrocalcinosis. In: McCarty DJ, ed. *Arthritis and allied conditions,* 11th ed. Philadelphia: Lea & Febiger, 1989:1711–1736.
13. Ellman MH, Levin B. Chondrocalcinosis in elderly persons. *Arthritis Rheum* 1975;18:43–47.
14. Memin Y, Monville C, Ryckewaert A. La chondrocalcinose articulaire apres 80 ans. *Rev Rheum Mal Osteoartic* 1978;45: 77–82.
15. Wilkins E, Dieppe P, Maddison P, et al. Osteoarthritis and articular chondrocalcinosis in the elderly. *Ann Rheum Dis* 1983;42: 280–284.
16. Felson DT, Anderson JJ, Naimark A, et al. The prevalence of chondrocalcinosis in the elderly and its association with knee osteoarthritis: the Framingham study. *J Rheumatol* 1989;16: 1241–1245.
17. McCarty DJ, Hogan JM, Gatter RA, et al. Studies on pathological calcifications in human cartilage. I. Prevalence and types of crystal deposits in the menisci of two hundred fifteen cadavera. *J Bone Joint Surg* 1966;48A:308–325.
18. Mitrovic DR, Stankovic A, Iriarte-Borde O, et al. The prevalence of chondrocalcinosis in the human knee joint. *J Rheumatol* 1988;15:633–641.
19. Bjelle A, Crocker P, Willoughby D. Ultra-microcrystals in pyrophosphate arthropathy. *Acta Med Scand* 1980;207:89–92.

20. Parel H, Reginato A, Schumacher HR. Alizarin red S staining as a screening test to detect calcium compounds in synovial fluid. *Arthritis Rheum* 1983;26:191–200.
21. Bennett RM, Mall JC, McCarty DJ. Pseudogout in acute neuropathic arthropathy: a clue to pathogenesis. *Arthritis Rheum Dis* 1974;33:563–567.
22. Rachow JW, Ryan LM, McCarty DJ, et al. Synovial fluid inorganic pyrophosphate concentration and nucleotide pyrophosphohydrolase activity in basic calcium phosphate deposition arthropathy and Milwaukee shoulder syndrome. *Arthritis Rheum* 1988;31:408–413.
23. Resnick D, Niwayama G, Goergen TG, et al. Clinical, radiographic and pathologic abnormalities in calcium pyrophosphate dihydrate deposition disease (CPPD) pseudogout. *Diagn Radiol* 1977;122:1–15.
24. Martel W, McCarter DK, Solsky MA, et al. Further observations on the arthropathy of calcium pyrophosphate crystal deposition disease. *Radiology* 1981;141:1–15.
25. O'Duffy JD. Clinical studies of acute pseudogout attacks. *Arthritis Rheum* 1976;19(suppl):349–353.
26. Dieppe PA, Alexander GJM, Jones HE, et al. Pyrophosphate arthropathy: a clinical and radiological study of 105 cases. *Ann Rheum Dis* 1982;41:371–376.
27. Fam AG, Topp JR, Stein HB, et al. Clinical and roentgenographic aspects of pseudogout: a study of 50 cases and review. *Can Med Assoc J* 1981;124:545–550.
28. McCarty DJ. Diagnostic mimicry in arthritis: patterns of joint involvement associated with calcium pyrophosphate dihydrate crystal deposits. *Bull Rheum Dis* 1975;25:804–809.
29. Bilezikian JP, Aurbach GD, Connor TB, et al. Pseudogout after parathyroidectomy. *Lancet* 1973;1:445–449.
30. Phelps P. Polymorphonuclear leukocyte motility in vitro. IV. Colchicine inhibition of chemotactic activity formation after phagocytosis of urate crystals. *Arthritis Rheum* 1970;13:1–9.
31. Spilberg I, McLain D, Simchowitz L, et al. Colchicine and pseudogout. *Arthritis Rheum* 1980;23:1062–1063.
32. Moskowitz RW, Harris BK, Schwartz A, et al. Chronic synovitis as a manifestation of calcium crystal deposition disease. *Arthritis Rheum* 1971;14:109–116.
33. Resnick D, Williams G, Weisman MH, et al. Rheumatoid arthritis and pseudorheumatoid arthritis in calcium pyrophosphate dihydrate crystal deposition disease. *Radiology* 1981;140: 615–621.
34. Wallace SL, Robinson H, Masi AT, et al. Preliminary criteria for the classification of the acute arthritis of primary gout. *Arthritis Rheum* 1977;20:895–900.
35. Bywaters EGL. Calcium pyrophosphate deposits in synovial membrane. *Ann Rheum Dis* 1972;31:219–220.
36. Good AE, Rapp R. Chondrocalcinosis of the knee with gout and rheumatoid arthritis. *N Engl J Med* 1967;277:286–290.
37. Doherty M, Dieppe P, Watt I. Low incidence of calcium pyrophosphate dihydrate crystal deposition in rheumatoid arthritis, with modification of radiographic features in coexistent disease. *Arthritis Rheum* 1984;27:1002–1009.
38. Bong D, Bennett R. Pseudogout mimicking systemic disease. *JAMA* 1981;246:1438–1440.
39. Zitnan D, Sitaj S. Natural course of articular chondrocalcinosis. *Arthritis Rheum* 1976;19(suppl):363–390.
40. Genant HK. Roentgenographic aspects of calcium pyrophosphate dihydrate crystal deposition disease (pseudogout). *Arthritis Rheum* 1976;19:307–328.
41. Martel W, Champion CK, Thompson GR, et al. A roentgenologically distinctive arthropathy in some patients with pseudogout syndrome. *Am J Roentgenol* 1970;109:587–605.
42. Hamilton EBD, Williams R, Barlow K, et al. The arthropathy of idiopathic haemochromatosis. *Q J Med* 1968;37:171–182.
43. Atkins CJ, McIvor J, Smith PM, et al. Chondrocalcinosis and arthropathy: studies in haemochromatosis and in idiopathic chondrocalcinosis. *Q J Med* 1970;39:71–79.
44. Jacobelli SG, McCarty DJ, Silcox DC, et al. Calcium pyrophosphate dihydrate crystal deposition in neuropathic joints: four cases of polyarticular involvement. *Ann Intern Med* 1973;79: 340–347.
45. Gerster JC, Vischer TL, Fallet GH. Destructive arthropathy in generalized osteoarthritis with articular chondrocalcinosis. *J Rheumatol* 1975;2:265–269.
46. Hamilton EBD, Richards AJ. Destructive arthropathy in chondrocalcinosis articularis. *Ann Rheum Dis* 1974;33:196–203.
47. Menkes CJ, Simon F, Chourki M. Les arthropathies destructrices de la chondrocalcinose. *Rev Rhum Mal Osteoartic* 1973;40: 115–123.
48. Reginato AJ, Valenzuela F, Martinez V, et al. Polyarticular and familial chondrocalcinosis. *Arthritis Rheum* 1970;13:197–213.
49. Pritzker KPH, Philips H, Luc SC, et al. Pseudotumor of temporomandibular joint: destructive calcium pyrophosphate dihydrate arthropathy. *J Rheumatol* 1976;3:70–81.
50. Reginato AJ, Schiapachasse V, Zmijewski CM, et al. HLA antigens in chondrocalcinosis and ankylosing chondrocalcinosis. *Arthritis Rheum* 1979;22:928–932.
51. Bouvet J, le Parc J-M, Michalski B, et al. Acute neck pain due to calcifications surrounding the odontoid process: the crowned dens syndrome. *Arthritis Rheum* 1985;28:1417–1420.
52. LeGoff P, Penunec Y, Youinou P. Signes cervicaux aigus pseudomeninge, relateurs de la chondrocalcinose articulaire. *Sem Hop Paris* 1980;56:1515–1518.
53. Kawano N, Matsuno T, Miyazawa S, et al. Calcium pyrophosphate dihydrate crystal deposition disease in the cervical ligamentum flavum. *J Neurosurg* 1988;68:613–620.
54. Berghausen EJ, Balogh K, Landis WJ, et al. Cervical myelopathy attributable to pseudogout. *Clin Orthop Rel Res* 1987;214: 217–221.
55. Gomez H, Chou SM. Myeloradiculopathy secondary to pseudogout in the cervical ligamentum flavum. *Neurosurgery* 1989;25:298–302.
56. Kawano N, Yoshida S, Ohwada T, et al. Cervical radiculomyelopathy caused by deposition of calcium pyrophosphate dihydrate crystals in the ligamenta flava. *J Neurosurg* 1980; 52:279–283.
57. Baba H, Maezawa Y, Kawahara N, et al. Calcium crystal deposition in the ligamentum flavum of the cervical spine. *Spine* 1993;18:2174–2181.
58. Parker PD, Jones NR, Scott G. Cervical myelopathy in CPPD deposition disease. *Australas Radiol* 1990;34:82–85.
59. Ciricillo SF, Weinstein PR. Foramen magnum syndrome from pseudogout of the atlanto-occipital ligament. *J Neurosurg* 1989; 71:141–143.
60. Sadique T, Bradley JG, Jackson AM. Central spinal stenosis due to pseudogout. *J Bone Joint Surg* 1994;76B:672–673.
61. Markiewitz AD, Boumphrey FR, Bauer TW et al. Calcium pyrophosphate dihydrate crystal deposition disease as a cause of lumbar canal stenosis. *Spine* 1996;21:506–511.
62. Doherty M, Watt I, Dieppe PA. Localised chondrocalcinosis in post-meniscectomy knees. *Lancet* 1982;1:1207–1210.
63. Linden B, Nilsson BE. Chondrocalcinosis following osteochondritis dissecans in the femur condyle. *Clin Orthop* 1978;130: 223–227.
64. Andres TL, Trainer TD. Intervertebral chondrocalcinosis: a coincidental finding possibly related to previous surgery. *Arch Pathol Lab Med* 1980;104:269–271.
65. Ellman MH, Vazquez LT, Brown NKL, et al. Calcium pyrophosphate dihydrate deposition in lumbar disc fibrocartilage. *J Rheumatol* 1981;8:955–958.

66. Guerne PA, Terkeltaub R, Zuraw B, et al. Inflammatory microcrystals stimulate interleukin-6 production and secretion by human monocytes and synoviocytes. *Arthritis Rheum* 1989;32:1443–1452.
67. Regan M, Clarke AK, Doherty MP. Pseudogout provoked by pregnancy. *Br J Rheumatol* 1993;32:245–247.
68. Whyte MP, Landt M, Ryan LM, et al. Alkaline phosphatase: placental and tissue-nonspecific isoenzymes hydrolyze phosphethanolamine, inorganic pyrophosphate, and pyridoxal 5′-phosphate. *J Clin Invest* 1995;95:1440–1445.
69. Doherty M, Hamilton E, Henderson J, et al. Familial chondrocalcinosis due to calcium pyrophosphate dihydrate crystal deposition in English families. *Br J* Rheumatol 1991;30:10–15.
70. Andrew LJ, Brancolini V, Serrano de la Pena L, et al. Refinement of the chromosome 5p locus for familial calcium pyrophosphate dihydrate deposition disease. *Am J Hum Genet* 1999;64:136–145.
71. Rodriguez-Valverde V, Zuniga M, Casanueva B, et al. Hereditary articular chondrocalcinosis. *Am J Med* 1988;84:101–106.
72. Fernandez Dapica M, Gomez-Reino J. Familial chondrocalcinosis in the Spanish population. *J Rheumatol* 1986;13:631–633.
73. Balsa A, Martin-Mola E, Gonzalez T, et al. Familial articular chondrocalcinosis in Spain. *Ann Rheum Dis* 1990;49:531–535.
74. Hollingworth P, Williams PL, Scott JT. Frequency of chondrocalcinosis of the knees in asymptomatic hyperuricemia and rheumatoid arthritis: a controlled study. *Ann Rheum Dis* 1982;41:344–346.
75. Hamilton EBD, Bomford AB, Laws JW, et al. The natural history of arthritis in idiopathic haemochromatosis: progression of the clinical and radiological features over ten years. *Q J Med* 1981;50:321–329.
76. Rynes RI, Merzig EG. Calcium pyrophosphate crystal deposition disease and hyperparathyroidism: a controlled prospective study. *J Rheumatol* 1978;5:460–468.
77. Eshel G, Gulik A, Halperin N, et al. Hereditary chondrocalcinosis in an Ashkenazi Jewish family. *Ann Rheum Dis* 1990;49:528–530.
78. Aitken RE, Kerr JL, Lloyd HM. Primary hyperparathyroidism with osteosclerosis with calcification in articular cartilage. *Am J Med* 1964;37:813–820.
79. Bywaters EGL, Dixon A St J, Scott JT. Joint lesions of hyperparathyroidism. *Ann Rheum Dis* 1963;22:171–187.
80. Zvaifler NJ, Reefe WE, Black RL. Articular manifestations in primary hyperparathyroidism. *Arthritis Rheum* 1962;5:237–249.
81. Currey HLF, Key JJ, Mason RM, et al. Significance of radiological calcification of joint cartilage. *Ann Rheum Dis* 1966;25:295–306.
82. Skinner M, Cohen AS. Calcium pyrophosphate dihydrate crystal deposition disease. *Arch Intern Med* 1969;123:636–644.
83. Van Geertruyden J, Kinnaert P, Frederic N, et al. Effect of parathyroid surgery on cartilage calcification. *World J Surg* 1986;10:111–115.
84. Buchanan WW, Kraag GR, Palmer DG, et al. The first recorded case of osteitis fibrosa cystica. *Can Med Assoc J* 1981;124:812–815.
85. Glass JS, Grahame R. Chondrocalcinosis after parathyroidectomy. *Ann Rheum Dis* 1976;35:521–525.
86. Pritchard MH, Jessop JD. Chondrocalcinosis in primary hyperparathyroidism. *Ann Rheum Dis* 1977;36:146–151.
87. Marx SJ, Attie MF, Levine MA, et al. The hypocalciuric or benign variant of familial hypercalcemia: clinical and biochemical features in fifteen kindreds. *Medicine* 1981;60:397–412.
88. Marx SJ, Spiegel AM, Levine MA, et al. An association between neonatal severe primary hyperparathyroidism and familial hypocalciuric hypercalcemia in three kindreds. *N Engl J Med* 1982;306:257–263.
89. Schumacher HR. Hemochromatosis and arthritis. *Arthritis Rheum* 1964;7:41–50.
90. Ryan L, McCarty DJ. Calcium pyrophosphate crystal deposition disease; pseudogout; articular chondrocalcinosis. In: McCarty DJ, ed. *Arthritis and allied conditions,* 10th ed. Philadelphia: Lea & Febiger, 1985:1515–1546.
91. Dorfmann H, Solonia J, DiMenza CL, et al. Les arthropathies des hemochromatoses: resultats d'une enquete prospective portant sur 54 malades. *Sem Hop Paris* 1969;45:416–523.
92. Dymock IW, Hamilton EBD, Laws JW, et al. Arthropathy of hemochromatosis. *Ann Rheum Dis* 1970;29:469–476.
93. Hamilton EBD. Diseases associated with CPPD deposition disease. *Arthritis Rheum* 1976;19(suppl):353–357.
94. Adamson TC, Resnik CS, Guerra J, et al. Hand and wrist arthropathies of hemochromatosis and calcium pyrophosphate deposition disease: distinct radiographic features. *Radiology* 1983;146:377–381.
95. Hearn PR, Russell RGG, Elliott JC. Formation product of calcium pyrophosphate crystals in vitro and the effect of iron salts. *Clin Sci Mol Med* 1978;54:29–33.
96. McCarty DJ, Pepe PF. Erythrocyte neutral inorganic pyrophosphatase in pseudogout. *J Lab Clin Med* 1972;79:277–284.
97. McCarty DJ, Palmer DW, Garancis JC. Clearance of calcium pyrophosphate dihydrate crystals in vivo. III. Effects of synovial hemosiderosis. *Arthritis Rheum* 1981;24:706–710.
98. Pawlotsky Y, Lancien Y, Roudier G, et al. Histomorphometrie osseuse et manifestations osteo-articulares de l'hemochromatose idiopathique. *Rev Rheum* 1979;46:91–99.
99. Pawlotsky Y, Le Dantec P, Moirand R, et al. Elevated parathyroid hormone 44–68 and osteoarticular changes in patients with genetic hemochromatosis. *Arthritis Rheum* 1999;42:799–805.
100. O'Duffy JD. Hypophosphatasia associated with calcium pyrophosphate dihydrate deposits in cartilage. *Arthritis Rheum* 1970;13:381–388.
101. Earde AW, Swannell AJ, Williamson NR. Pyrophosphate arthropathy in hypophosphatasia. *Ann Rheum Dis* 1981;40:164–170.
102. Whyte MP, Murphy WA, Fallon MD. Adult hypophosphatasia with chondrocalcinosis and arthropathy: variable penetrance of hypophosphatemia in a large Oklahoma kindred. *Am J Med* 1982;72:631–641.
103. Russell RGG. Metabolism of inorganic pyrophosphate (PPi). *Arthritis Rheum* 1976;19(suppl):463–478.
104. Russell RGG, Bisaz S, Donath A, et al. Inorganic pyrophosphate in plasma in normal persons and in patients with hypophosphatasia osteogenesis imperfecta and other disorders of bone. *J Clin Invest* 1971;50:961–969.
105. Chuck AJ, Pattrick MG, Hamilton E, et al. Crystal deposition in hypophosphatasia: a reappraisal. *Ann Rheum Dis* 1989;48:571–576.
106. Whyte MP, Valdes R, Ryan LM, et al. Infantile hypophosphatasia: enzyme replacement therapy by intravenous infusion of alkaline phosphatase-rich plasma from patients with Paget's bone disease. *J Pediatr* 1982;101:379–386.
107. McCarty DJ, Silcox DC, Coe F, et al. Diseases associated with calcium pyrophosphate dihydrate crystal deposition: a controlled study. *Am J Med* 1974;56:704–714.
108. Bennett RM, Lehr JR, McCarty DJ. Factors affecting the solubility of calcium pyrophosphate dihydrate crystals. *J Clin Invest* 1975;56:1571–1579.
109. McCarty DJ, Solomon SD, Warnock M, et al. Inorganic pyrophosphate concentrations in the synovial fluid of arthritis patients. *J Lab Clin Med* 1971;78:216–229.
110. Runeberg L, Collan Y, Jokinen EJ, et al. Hypomagnesemia due to renal disease of unknown etiology. *Am J Med* 1975;59:873–881.
111. Smilde TJ, Haverman JF, Schipper P, et al. Familial

hypokalemia/hypomagnesemia and chondrocalcinosis. *J Rheumatol* 1994;21:1515–1519.

112. Doherty M, Dieppe PA. Double blind, placebo controlled trial of magnesium carbonate in chronic pyrophosphate arthropathy. *Ann Rheum Dis* 1983;42(suppl):106–107(abst).
113. Dorwart BB, Schumacher HR. Joint effusions, chondrocalcinosis and other rheumatic manifestations in hypothyroidism. *Am J Med* 1975;59:780–789.
114. Alexander GM, Dieppe PA, Doherty M, et al. Pyrophosphate arthropathy: a study of metabolic associations and laboratory data. *Ann Rheum Dis* 1982;41:377–381.
115. Jones AC, Chuck AJ, Arie EA, et al. Diseases associated with calcium pyrophosphate deposition disease. *Semin Arthritis Rheum* 1992;22:188–202.
116. Komatireddy GR, Ellman MH, Brown NL. Lack of association between hypothyroidism and chondrocalcinosis. *J Rheumatol* 1989;16:807–808.
117. Chaisson CE, McAlindon TE, Felson DT, et al. Lack of association between thyroid status and chondrocalcinosis or osteoarthritis: the Framingham osteoarthritis study. *J Rheumatol* 1996;23:711–715.
118. Kaplinski N, Biran D, Frankl O. Pseudogout and amyloidosis. *Harefuah* 1976;91:59.
119. Ryan LM, Liang G, Kozin F. Amyloid arthropathy: possible association with chondrocalcinosis. *J Rheumatol* 1982;9:273–278.
120. Yood RA, Skinner M, Cohen AS, et al. Soft tissue uptake of bone seeking radionuclide in amyloidosis. *J Rheumatol* 1981;8:760–766.
121. Egan MS, Goldenberg DL, Cohen AS, et al. The association of amyloid deposits and osteoarthritis. *Arthritis Rheum* 1982;25:204–208.
122. Ladefoged C. Amyloid in osteoarthritic hip joints: a pathoanatomical and histological investigation of femoral head cartilage. *Acta Orthop Scand* 1982;53:581–586.
123. Jaccard YB, Gerster JC, Calame L. Mixed monosodium urate and calcium pyrophosphate crystal-induced arthropathy: a review of 17 cases. *Rev Rhum* (English Edition) 1996;63:331–315.
124. Stockman A, Darlington LG, Scott JT. Frequency of chondrocalcinosis of the knees and avascular necrosis of the femoral heads in gout: a controlled study. *Ann Rheum Dis* 1980;39:7–11.
125. Hamza M, Bardin T. Camptodactyly, polyepiphyseal dysplasia and mixed crystal deposition disease. *J Rheumatol* 1989;16:1153–1158.
126. Sambrook PN, de Jager JP, Champion GD, et al. Synovial complications of spondyloepiphyseal dysplasia of late onset. *Arthritis Rheum* 1988;31:282–287.
127. Kahn MF, Corvol MT, Jurmand SH, et al. Le rhumatisme chondrodyplasique. *Sem Hop Paris* 1970;46:1938–1953.
128. Okazaki T, Sato T, Mitomo T, et al. Pseudogout: clinical observations and chemical analyses of deposits. *Arthritis Rheum* 1976;19:293–305.
129. VanderKorst JK, Geerards J, Driessens FCM. A hereditary type of idiopathic articular chondrocalcinosis. *Am J Med* 1974;56:307–314.
130. Swan A, Chapman B, Heap P, et al. Submicroscopic crystals in osteoarthritic synovial fluids. *Ann Rheum Dis* 1994;53:467–470.
131. Sanmarti R, Kanterewicz E, Pladevall M, et al. Analysis of the association between chondrocalcinosis and osteoarthritis: a community based study. *Ann Rheum Dis* 1996;55:30–33.
132. Felson DT, Zhang Y, Hannan MT, et al. Risk factors for incident radiographic knee osteoarthritis in the elderly: the Framingham study. *Arthritis Rheum* 1997;40:718–733.
133. Weaver JB. Calcification and ossification of the menisci. *J Bone Joint Surg* 1942;24:873–882.
134. Altman RD. Arthroscopic findings of the knee in patients with pseudogout. *Arthritis Rheum* 1976;19:286–292.
135. Bird HA, Tribe CR, Bacon PA. Joint hypermobility leading to osteoarthrosis and chondrocalcinosis. *Ann Rheum Dis* 1978;37:203–211.
136. Settas L, Doherty M, Dieppe P. Localized chondrocalcinosis in unstable joints. *Br Med J* 1982;285:175–176.
137. Collis CH, Dieppe PA, Bullimore JA. Radiation-induced chondrocalcinosis of the knee articular cartilage. *Clin Radiol* 1989;39:450–451.
138. Malnick SD, Ariel-Ronen S, Evron E, et al. Acute pseudogout as a complication of pamidronate. *Ann Pharmacother* 1997;31:499–500.
139. Sandor V, Hassan R, Kohn E. Exacerbation of pseudogout by granulocyte colony-stimulating factor. *Ann Intern Med* 1996;125:781.
140. Luzar MJ, Altawil B. Pseudogout following intraarticular injection of sodium hyaluronate. *Arthritis Rheum* 1998;41:939–940.
141. Fisseler-Eckhoff A, Muller KM. Arthroscopy and chondrocalcinosis. *Arthroscopy* 1992;8:98–104.
142. Beltran J, Marty-Defaut E, Bencardino J, et al. Chondrocalcinosis of the hyaline cartilage of the knee: MRI manifestations. *Skeletal Radiol* 1998;27:369–374.
143. Ellman M, Krieger MI, Brown N. Pseudogout mimicking synovial chondromatosis. *J Bone Joint Surg* 1975;57A:863–865.
144. Gerster JC, Laiger R, Boivin G, et al. Carpal tunnel syndrome in chondrocalcinosis of the wrist. *Arthritis Rheum* 1980;23:926–931.
145. Ahlgren P. Chondrocalcinois og knogleusurer. *Nord Med* 1965;73:309–313.
146. Lagier R. Case report: rare femoral erosions and osteoarthritis of the knee associated with chondrocalcinosis. A histological study of this cortical remodeling. *Virchows Arch* 1974;364:215–223 (abst).
147. Resnick D, Niwyama G. Carpal instability in rheumatoid arthritis and calcium pyrophosphate deposition disease. *Ann Rheum Dis* 1977;36:311–318.
148. Ross DJ, Dieppe PA, Watt I, et al. Tibial stress fracture in pyrophosphate arthropathy. *J Bone Joint Surg* 1983;65B:474–477.
149. Houpt JB, Sinclair DS. Spontaneous osteonecrosis of the medial femoral condyle. *J Rheumatol* 1974;1(suppl):117(abst).
150. Watt I, Dieppe P. Medial femoral condyle necrosis and chondrocalcinosis: a causal relationship. *Br J Radiol* 1983;56:7–22.
151. Gatter RA, McCarty DJ. Pathological tissue calcification in man. *Arch Pathol* 1967;84:346–353.
152. Ishikawa H, Ueba Y, Isobe T, et al. Interaction of polymorphonuclear leukocytes with calcium pyrophosphate dihydrate crystals deposited in chondrocalcinosis cartilage. *Rheumatol Int* 1987;7:217–221.
153. Ali SY, Griffiths S, Bayliss MT, et al. Ultrastructural studies of pyrophosphate crystal deposition in articular cartilage. *Ann Rheum Dis* 1983;42(suppl):97–98.
154. Bjelle A. Cartilage matrix in hereditary pyrophosphate arthropathy. *J Rheumatol* 1981;8:959–964.
155. Ishikawa K, Masuda I, Ohira T, et al. A histological study of calcium pyrophosphate dihydrate crystal-deposition disease. *J Bone Joint Surg* 1989;71A:875–886.
156. Ohira T, Ishikawa K, Masuda I, et al. Histologic localization of lipid in the articular tissues in calcium pyrophosphate dihydrate crystal deposition disease. *Arthritis Rheum* 1988;31:1057–1062.
157. Masuda I, Ishikawa I, Usuku G. A histologic and immunohistochemical study of calcium pyrophosphate dihydrate crystal deposition disease. *Clin Orthop* 1991;263:272–287.
158. Chen F, Kerner MB, Dorfman HD, et al. The distribution of S-100 protein in articular cartilage from osteoarthritic joints. *J Rheumatol* 1990;17:1676–1681.

159. Boivin G, Lagier R. An ultrastructural study of articular chondrocalcinosis in cases of knee osteoarthritis. *Virchows Arch* 1983;400:13–29(abst).
160. Mitrovic D. Pathology of articular deposition of calcium salts and their relationship to osteoarthritis. *Ann Rheum Dis* 1983; 42(suppl):19–26.
161. Schumacher HR. The synovitis of pseudogout: electron microscopic observations. *Arthritis Rheum* 1968;11:426–435.
162. Schumacher HR. Articular cartilage in the degenerative arthropathy of hemochromatosis. *Arthritis Rheum* 1982;25: 1460–1468.
163. Dijkgraaf LC, Liem RS, de Bont GM, et al. Calcium pyrophosphate dihydrate crystal deposition disease: a review of the literature and a light and electron microscopic study of a case of the temporomandibular joint with numerous intracellular crystals in the chondrocytes. *Osteoarthritis Cartilage* 1995;3:35–45.
164. Beutler A, Rothfuss S, Clayburne G, et al. Calcium pyrophosphate dihydrate crystal deposition in synovium. *Arthritis Rheum* 1993;36:704–715.
165. Keen CE, Crocker PR, Brady K, et al. Calcium pyrophosphate dihydrate deposition disease: morphological and microanalytical features. *Histopathology* 1991;19:529–536.
166. McCarty DJ, Palmer DW, James C. Clearance of calcium pyrophosphate dihydrate crystals in vivo: II. Studies using triclinic crystals doubly labeled with 45Ca and 85Sr. *Arthritis Rheum* 1979;22:1122–1131.
167. Hearn PR, Guilland-Cumming DF, Russell RGG. Effect of orthophosphate and other factors on the crystal growth of calcium pyrophosphate. *Ann Rheum Dis* 1983;42(suppl):101.
168. Cheng PT, Pritzker K. Pyrophosphate, phosphate ion interaction: effects on calcium pyrophosphate and calcium hydroxyapatite crystal formation in aqueous solution. *J Rheumatol* 1983; 10:769–777.
169. Silcox DC, McCarty DJ. Elevated inorganic pyrophosphate concentrations in synovial fluid in osteoarthritis and pseudogout. *J Lab Clin Med* 1974;83:518–531.
170. Pritzker KPH, Cheng P-T, Adams ME, et al. Calcium pyrophosphate dihydrate crystal formation in model hydrogels. *J Rheumatol* 1978;5:469–473.
171. Mandel NS, Mandel GS. Nucleation and growth of CPPD crystals and related species in vitro. In: Rubin RP, Weiss G, Putner JW, eds. *Calcium in biological systems.* New York: Plenum Press, 1985:711–717.
172. Mandel N, Mandel G, Carroll D, et al. Calcium pyrophosphate crystal deposition. An in vitro study using a gelatin matrix model. *Arthritis Rheum* 1984;27:789–796.
173. Lust G, Faure G, Netter P, et al. Increased pyrophosphate in fibroblasts and lymphoblasts from patients with hereditary diffuse articular chondrocalcinosis. *Science* 1981;214:809–810.
174. Jung A, Bisaz S, Fleisch H. The binding of pyrophosphate and two diphosphonates by hydroxyapatite crystals. *Calcif Tiss Res* 1973;11:269–280.
175. McGaughey C. Binding of polyphosphates and phosphonates to hydroxyapatite, subsequent hydrolysis, phosphate exchange and effects on demineralization, mineralization, and microcrystal aggregation. *Caries Res* 1983;17:229–241.
176. Russell RGG, Bisaz S, Fleisch H. Inorganic pyrophosphate in plasma, urine and synovial fluid of patients with pyrophosphate arthropathy (chondrocalcinosis or pseudogout). *Lancet* 1970;2: 899–902.
177. Pflug M, McCarty DJ, Kawahara F. Basal urinary pyrophosphate excretion in pseudogout. *Arthritis Rheum* 1969;12: 228–231.
178. Silcox DC, Jacobelli SG, McCarty DJ. The identification of inorganic pyrophosphate in human platelets and its release on stimulation with thrombin. *J Clin Invest* 1973;52:1595–1600.
179. Ryan LM, Kozin F, McCarty DJ. Quantification of human plasma inorganic pyrophosphate: I. Normal values in osteoarthritis and calcium pyrophosphate dihydrate crystal deposition disease. *Arthritis Rheum* 1979;22:886–891.
180. Sorensen SA, Flodgaard H, Sorensen E. Serum alkaline phosphatase, serum pyrophosphatase, phosphoreylethanolamine, and inorganic pyrophosphate in plasma and urine: a genetic and clinical study of hypophosphatasia. *Monogr Hum Genet* 1978; 10:66–69.
181. Rachow J, Ryan L. Adenosine triphosphate pyrophosphohydrolase and neutral inorganic pyrophosphatase in pathologic joint fluids. *Arthritis Rheum* 1985;28:1283–1288.
182. Hamilton E, Pattrick M, Doherty M. Inorganic pyrophosphate, nucleoside triphosphate pyrophosphatase, and cartilage fragments in normal human synovial fluid. *Br J Rheumatol* 1991;30:260–264.
183. Howell DS, Muniz O, Pita JC, et al. Extrusion of pyrophosphate into extracellular media by osteoarthritic cartilage incubates. *J Clin Invest* 1975;56:1473–1480.
184. Ryan LM, Cheung HS, McCarty DJ. Release of pyrophosphate by normal mammalian articular hyaline and fibrocartilage in organ culture. *Arthritis Rheum* 1981;24:1522–1527.
185. Camerlain M, McCarty DJ, Silcox DC, et al. Inorganic pyrophosphate pool size and turnover rate in arthritic joints. *J Clin Invest* 1975;55:1373–1381.
186. Tenenbaum J, Muniz O, Schumacher HR, et al. Comparison of phosphohydrolase activities from articular cartilage in calcium pyrophosphate deposition disease and primary osteoarthritis. *Arthritis Rheum* 1981;24:492–500.
187. Cartier P, Picard J. La mineralisation du cartilage ossifiable: III. Le mechanisme de la reaction atpasique du cartilage. *Bull Soc Chim Biol* 1955;37:1159–1168.
188. Hsu H. Purification and partial characterization of ATP pyrophosphohydrolase from fetal bovine epiphyseal cartilage. *J Biol Chem* 1983;258:3463–3468.
189. Siegel SA, Hummel CF, McCarty RP. The role of nucleoside triphosphate pyrophosphohydrolase in vitro nucleoside triphosphate-dependent matrix vesicle calcification. *J Biol Chem* 1983;258:8601–8607.
190. Hsu H, Anderson H. The deposition of calcium pyrophosphate and phosphate by matrix vesicles isolated from fetal bovine epiphyseal cartilage. *Calcif Tiss Int* 1984;36:615–621.
191. Hsu H, Anderson H. The deposition of calcium pyrophosphate by NTP pyrophosphohydrolase of matrix vesicles from fetal bovine epiphyseal cartilage. *Int J Biochem* 1986;18:1141–1146.
192. Ryan LM, Wortmann RL, Karas B, et al. Cartilage nucleoside triphosphate (NTP) pyrophosphohydrolase: I. Identification as an ectoenzyme. *Arthritis Rheum* 1984;27:913–918.
193. Howell D, Martel-Pelletier J, Pelletier J-P, et al. NTP pyrophosphohydrolase in human chondrocalcinotic and osteoarthritic cartilage: II. Further studies on histologic and subcellular distribution. *Arthritis Rheum* 1984;27:193–199.
194. Caswell A, Russell RGG. Identification of ecto-nucleoside triphosphate pyrophosphatase in human articular chondrocytes in monolayer culture. *Biochim Biophys Acta* 1985;847:40–47.
195. Rebbe NF, Tong BD, Hickman S. Expression of nucleotide pyrophosphatase and alkaline phosphodiesterase. I. Activities of PC-1 the murine plasma cell antigen. *Mol Immunol* 1993; 30:87–93.
196. Huang R, Rosenbach M, Vaughn R, et al. Expression of the murine plasma cell nucleotide pyrophosphohydrolase PC-1 is shared by human liver, bone, and cartilage cells. *J Clin Invest* 1994;94:560–567.
197. Terkeltaub R, Rosenbach M, Fong F, et al. Causal link between nucleotide pyrophosphohydrolase overactivity and increased intracellular inorganic pyrophosphate generation demonstrated

by transfection of cultured fibroblasts and osteoblasts with plasma cell membrane glycoprotein. *Arthritis Rheum* 1994;37: 934–941.

198. Masuda I, Hamada J, Haas A, et al. A unique ectonucleotide pyrophosphohydrolase associated with porcine chondrocyte-derived vesicles. *J Clin Invest* 1995;95:699–704.
199. Cardenal A, Masuda I, Haas A, et al. Specificity of an ecto-nucleoside triphosphate pyrophosphohydrolase unique to chondrocyte-derived vesicles. *Arthritis Rheum* 1994;37:S412.
200. Masuda I, Halligan BD, Barbieri JT, et al. Molecular cloning and expression of a porcine chondrocyte nucleotide pyrophosphohydrolase. *Gene* 1997;197:277–287.
201. Lorenzo P, Bayliss MT, Heinegard D. A novel cartilage protein (CILP) present in the mid-zone of articular cartilage increases with age. *J Biol Chem* 1998;273:23463–23468.
202. Masuda I, Cardenal A, Ono W, et al. Nucleotide pyrophosphohydrolase in human synovial fluid. *J Rheumatol* 1997;24: 1588–1594.
203. Cardenal A, Masuda I, Ono W, et al. Serum nucleotide pyrophosphohydrolase activity: elevated levels in osteoarthritis, calcium pyrophosphate dihydrate deposition disease, scleroderma and fibromyalgia. *J Rheumatol* 1998;25; 2175–2180.
204. Felix R, Fleisch H. The effect of pyrophosphate and diphosphonates on calcium transport in red cells. *Experientia* 1977; 33:1003–1005.
205. Rachow JW, Ryan LM, McCarty DJ, et al. Synovial fluid inorganic pyrophosphate concentration and nucleotide pyrophosphohydrolase activity in basic calcium phosphate deposition arthropathy and Milwaukee shoulder syndrome. *Arthritis Rheum* 1988;31:408–413.
206. Ryan L, Rachow J, McCarty DJ. Synovial fluid ATP: a possible substrate for generation of inorganic pyrophosphate in calcium pyrophosphate dihydrate (CPPD) crystal deposition disease. *J Rheumatol* 1991;18:716–720.
207. Park W, McCarty DJ. Intraarticular inorganic pyrophosphate genesis in human synovial fluid is driven by extracellular adenosine triphosphate. *Arthritis Rheum* 1994;37:S427.
208. Ryan LM, McCarty DJ. Understanding inorganic pyrophosphate metabolism—toward prevention of calcium pyrophosphate dihydrate crystal deposition. *Ann Rheum Dis* 1995;54: 939–941.
209. Derfus BA, Rachow JW, Mandel NS, et al. Articular cartilage vesicles generatem calcium pyrophosphate dihydrate-like crystals in vitro. *Arthritis Rheum* 1992;35:231–240.
210. Derfus BA, Honari D, Ryan LM, et al. EM diffraction confirms calcium pyrophosphate dihydrate deposition by articular cartilage vesicles. *Arthritis Rheum* 1994;37:S412.
211. Prins APA, Kiljan E, van de Stadt RJ, et al. Inorganic pyrophosphate release by rabbit articular chondrocytes in vitro. *Arthritis Rheum* 1986;29:1485–1492.
212. Lust G, Fare G, Netter P, et al. Evidence of a generalized metabolic defect in patients with hereditary chondrocalcinosis. *Arthritis Rheum* 1981;24:1517–1521.
213. Ryan LM, Lynch MP, McCarty DJ. Inorganic pyrophosphate levels in blood platelets from normal donors and patients with calcium pyrophosphate dihydrate crystal deposition disease. *Arthritis Rheum* 1983;26:564–566.
214. Ryan L, Wortmann RL, Karas B, et al. Pyrophosphohydrolase activity with inorganic pyrophosphate content of cultured human skin fibroblasts. *J Clin Invest* 1986;77:1689–1693.
215. Rosenthal AK, Cheung HS, Ryan LM. Transforming growth factor β1 stimulates inorganic pyrophosphate elaboration by porcine cartilage. *Arthritis Rheum* 1991;34:904–911.
216. Olmez U, Ryan LM, Kurup IV, et al. Insulin-like growth factor-1 suppresses pyrophosphate elaboration by transforming growth factor β1-stimulated chondrocytes and cartilage. *Osteoarthritis Cartilage* 1994;2:149–154.
217. Rosenthal AK, Ryan LM. Probenecid inhibits transforming growth factor β1 induced pyrophosphate elaboration by chondrocytes. *J Rheumatol* 1994;21:896–900.
218. Ryan LM, Kurup I, McCarty DJ, et al. Cartilage inorganic pyrophosphate elaboration is independent of sulfated glycosaminoglycan synthesis. *Arthritis Rheum* 1990;33:235–240.
219. Ryan LM, Kurup I, Cheung HS. Stimulation of cartilage inorganic pyrophosphate elaboration by ascorbate. *Matrix* 1991; 11:276–281.
220. Alvarellos A, Spilberg I. Colchicine prophylaxis in pseudogout. *J Rheumatol* 1986;13:804–805.
221. Ritter J, Kerr LD, Valeriano-Marcet J, et al. ACTH revisited: effective treatment for acute crystal induced synovitis in patients with multiple medical problems. *J Rheumatol* 1994;21: 696–699.
222. Bennett RM, Lehr JR, McCarty DJ. Crystal shedding and acute pseudogout: a hypothesis based on a therapeutic failure. *Arthritis Rheum* 1976;19:93–97.
223. Fam AG, Stein G. Disappearance of chondrocalcinosis following reflex sympathetic dystrophy. *Arthritis Rheum* 1981;24: 747–749.
224. Sarkozi AM, Nemeth-Csoka M, Bartosiewicz G. Effect of glycosaminoglycan polysulphate in the treatment of chondrocalcinosis. *Clin Exp Rheumatol* 1988;6:3–8.
225. Doherty M, Dieppe PA. Effect of intra-articular yttrium-90 on chronic pyrophosphate arthropathy of the knee. *Lancet* 1981;1: 1243–1246.
226. Ledingham J, Regan M, Jones A, et al. Factors affecting radiographic progression of knee osteoarthritis. *Ann Rheum Dis* 1995;54:53–58.

118

BASIC CALCIUM PHOSPHATE (APATITE, OCTACALCIUM PHOSPHATE, TRICALCIUM PHOSPHATE) CRYSTAL DEPOSITION DISEASES AND CALCINOSIS

PAUL B. HALVERSON

There are innumerable reports of pathologic calcium phosphate mineral phase deposition in various human tissues. These reports are largely descriptive, and most present no clear pattern of disease. Basic calcium phosphate (BCP) crystals, formerly thought to be hydroxyapatite (HA), have long been associated with calcific periarthritis and tendinitis (1). BCP crystals were later found in synovial fluid by scanning electron microscopy (SEM) or transmission electron microscopy (TEM) (2,3).

CRYSTAL IDENTIFICATION

The study of BCP crystal-associated arthritis has been relatively difficult because of the lack of a simple, reliable diagnostic test (see also Chapter 4). Heterogeneity of crystal species in periarticular shoulder joint calcifications was first established by Faure et al. (4), who directly measured the interplanar spacings of individual apatite crystals using high-resolution TEM. These crystals were largely carbonate-substituted, and other nonapatitic calcium phosphates were found. Fourier transform infrared (FTIR) analysis of shoulder joint fluid crystals, of calcified rabbit synovium, and of subcutaneous calcifications from dermatomyositis showed that each contained partially carbonate-substituted HA, octacalcium phosphate (OCP), and particulate collagens (Table 118.1) (5). Samples from one patient had tricalcium phosphate instead of octacalcium phosphate. BCP is therefore used generically to designate these crystal mixtures. *Basic calcium phosphate crystal deposition disease* is proposed as the most appropriate term for the associated clinical syndromes.

Radiography

Basic calcium phosphate crystal deposits are rounded or fluffy calcifications varying from a few millimeters to several centimeters in diameter. They may occur either as solitary nodules or as multiple deposits. Occasionally, paradia-

TABLE 118.1. CHEMICAL FORMULAE AND MOLAR RATIOS OF CALCIUM (CA) TO PHOSPHORUS (P) OF CALCIUM-CONTAINING CRYSTALS FOUND IN HUMAN SYNOVIAL FLUID, CARTILAGE, OR SYNOVIUM

Crystal	Formula	Ca/P
Basic calcium phosphate (BCP)		
Hydroxyapatite (HA)	$Ca_5(PO_4)_3OH2H_2O$	1.67
Octacalcium phosphate (OCP)	$Ca_8H_2(PO_4)_65H_2O$	1.33
Tricalcium phosphate (TCP) (whitlockite)	$Ca_3(PO_4)_2$	1.5
Other		
Dicalcium phosphate dihydrate (brushite)	$CaHPO_42H_2O$	1.0
Calcium pyrophosphate dihydrate	$Ca_2P_2O_7H_2O$	1.0
Calcium oxalate	$CaC_2O_4H_2O$	

physeal tendon calcifications may cause cortical erosions in adjacent bone (6). Although radiography is a useful diagnostic tool, it is both relatively insensitive and nonspecific in the diagnosis of BCP crystal arthropathies (7). Asymptomatic periarticular calcific deposits are frequently observed as incidental findings.

Synovial Fluid

Phase-contrast polarized light microscopy, invaluable for the detection of the larger monosodium urate monohydrate and calcium pyrophosphate dihydrate (CPPD) crystals, provides little help with BCP crystals, because their size is below the limits of resolution of optical microscopy. Although these crystals tend to aggregate, their orientation within an aggregate is usually random, and they are not birefringent. Rarely, birefringence is noted because thousands of ultramicroscopic crystals are oriented along the same axis (8). Individual needle- or plate-shaped crystals are usually less than 0.1 μm long (Fig. 118.1). BCP crystal aggregates may be visible by light microscopy as shiny laminated "coins." Alizarin red S staining of synovial fluid pellets has been suggested as a screening technique for BCP crystals (9). The method is sensitive to 0.005 μg of HA standard per milliliter, but it is not specific for calcium phosphates and may provide many false-positive results (10,11). Another study using fresh and alcohol-fixed cytospin preparations found that alizarin red allowed confident identification of intracellular BCP crystals (12). Artifacts rendered the technique useless for extracellular BCP crystals, however.

A semiquantitative technique using the binding of (^{14}C) ethane-1-hydroxy-1, 1-diphosphonate (EHDP) to BCP crystals has proved useful as a screening test. It is sensitive to about 2 μg/mL HA standard (1,13). Synovial fluid binding of (^{14}C) EHDP correlated strongly with the radiographic grade of osteoarthritis (OA) present (Fig. 118.2) (1,14). Synovial fluid pellets that bound (^{14}C) EHDP were examined routinely by SEM. Microspheroidal aggregates approximately 1 to 19 μm in diameter were generally found (Fig. 118.3A). These aggregates were then further characterized by x-ray energy dispersive analysis (1,13). The spectrum was analyzed for calcium and phosphorus, and the relative molar amounts of each element were calculated using an on-line computer (Fig. 118.3B). Cherian and Schumacher (15) suggested the routine use of TEM, which has the advantage of better definition of crystal morphology and location (e.g., in cells). Arsenazo III has been used for quantitative analysis of calcium containing crystals (16).

X-ray diffraction of BCP mineral by the powder method is relatively insensitive. Such small, poorly crystallized material yields broad diffraction minima that cannot differentiate between closely related calcium phosphate compounds. Electron diffraction, high-resolution TEM, atomic force microscopy (17), and FTIR spectrophotometry are useful research tools but are not practical for everyday clinical use.

Direct chemical analysis for calcium and phosphorus of several pellets from joint fluid that bound (^{14}C) EHDP showed levels of 12 to 45 μg BCP mineral per milliliter (13).

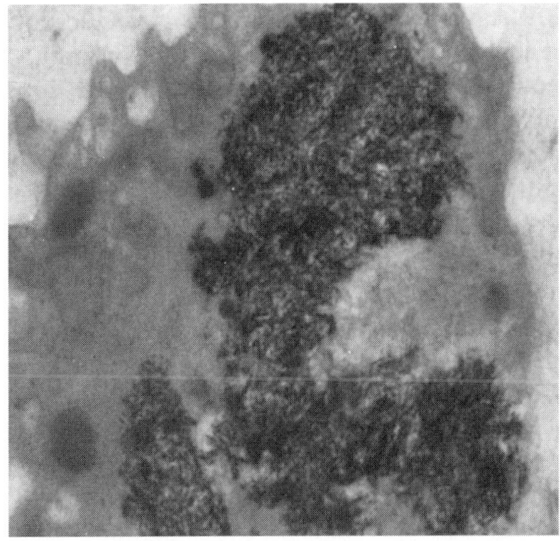

FIGURE 118.1. Aggregate of needle-shaped crystals within a synovial fibrocyte. No limiting membrane can be identified (×43,800).

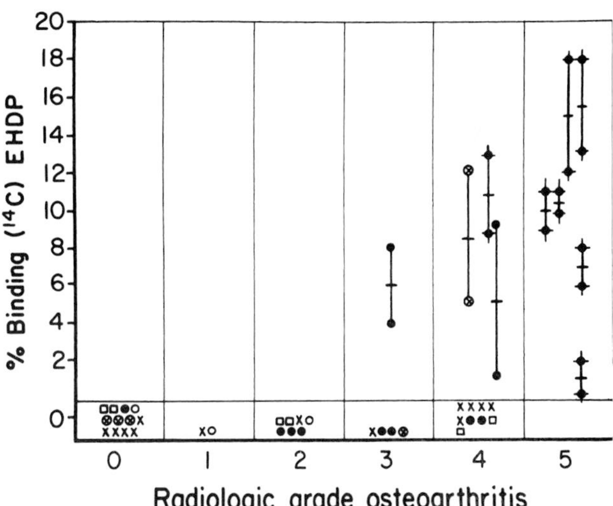

FIGURE 118.2. Fluids that bound (^{14}C) ethane-1-hydroxy-1, 1-diphosphonate (EHDP) generally were obtained from joints with advanced degenerative changes (radiologic grades 4 and 5). □, internal derangement of knee; ●, osteoarthritis; +, osteoarthritis with few calcium pyrophosphate deposition crystals in fluid; x, inflammatory arthritis with white blood cell (WBC) concentration >3,000 mm^3; ⊗, inflammatory arthritis with WBC concentration <3,000 mm^3; ○, miscellaneous arthritis. Positive results are shown in duplicate. (From Halverson PB, McCarty DJ. Identification of hydroxyapatite crystals in synovial fluid. *Arthritis Rheum* 1979;22:389–395, with permission.)

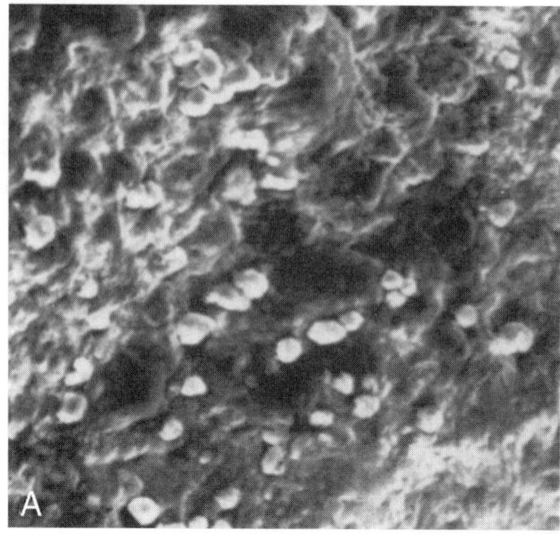

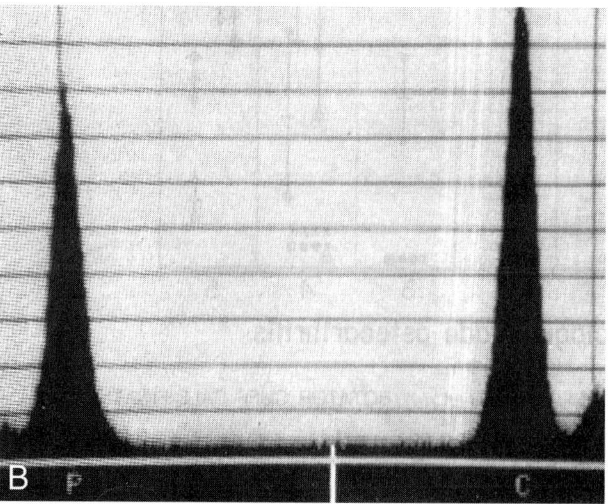

FIGURE 118.3. A: Scanning electron micrograph of synovial fluid sediment showing typical microspheroidal crystal aggregates (×525). (From Halverson PB, Cheung HS, McCarty DJ. "Milwaukee shoulder": association of microspheroids containing hydroxyapatite crystals, active collagenase and neutral protease with rotator cuff defects: II. Synovial fluid studies. Arthritis Rheum 1981;24:474–483, with permission.) **B:** Spectrograph from x-ray energy dispersive analysis showing peaks for phosphorus and calcium.

TABLE 118.2. BASIC CALCIUM PHOSPHATE CRYSTAL-ASSOCIATED JOINT DISEASE[a]

- Calcific periarthritis
  - Unifocal
    - Hydroxyapatite pseudopodagra (19)
  - Multifocal
  - Familial (19)
- Calcific tendinitis and bursitis (20)
- Intraarticular BCP arthropathies
  - Acute (gout-like) attacks
  - Milwaukee shoulder/knee syndrome (7) (idiopathic destructive arthritis; cuff tear arthropathy)
  - Erosive polyarticular disease
  - Mixed crystal deposition disease (BCP and CPPD)
- Tumoral calcinosis
  - Hyperphosphatemic
  - Nonhyperphosphatemic
- Secondary BCP crystal arthropathies/periarthropathies[b]
- Calcinosis
  - Metastatic
    - Hyperphosphatemia states: chronic renal failure, hypoparathyroidism, pseudohypoparathyroidism
    - Hypercalcemia states: primary hyperparathyroidism; hypervitaminosis D; milk-alkali syndrome; neoplasms, sarcoidosis
  - Dystrophic
    - Primary connective tissue disease (21,22); scleroderma, either diffuse or limited formed; dermatomyositis, polymyositis; Ehlers-Danlos syndrome; pseudoxanthoma elasticum
    - Metabolic diseases: gout; diabetes mellitus; alkaptonuria (ochronosis); porphyria cutanea tarda; pseudopseudohypoparathyroidism; Werner's syndrome; progeria; myositis ossificans progressiva
    - Parasitic infestation
    - Neurologic injury/paralysis paraarticular calcification

BCP, basic calcium phosphate; CPPD, calcium pyrophosphate dihydrate.
[a]See ref. 1 for references to older publications.
[b]Mineral deposits may also occur in fibrous tissues remote from joints in these conditions.

DISEASES

Several articular and periarticular conditions associated with BCP crystals have been described (Table 118.2). Calcific tendinitis and bursitis are discussed also in Chapters 97 and 107. The secondary BCP arthropathies occur in conditions known to predispose to such crystal deposition (Table 118.2).

Rotator Cuff Calcifications

In the shoulder, the location of rotator cuff calcifications has been related to etiopathogenesis, natural history, and prognosis (22). Sarkar and Uhthoff (22) found that calcifications at the tidemark of the rotator cuff insertion into the greater tuberosity of the humerus represented degenerative enthesopathy with *secondary calcification*. These and the secondary calcification of the torn ends of a rotator cuff are irreversible. On the other hand, *primary calcification* in the rotator cuff, approximately 1.5 cm away from the tidemark in Codman's critical area, occurred in metaplastic fibrocartilage. These deposits were associated with matrix vesicles and with crystal phagocytosis by macrophages and giant cells. *The natural history of such deposits is resorption.* Scalloping of the fluffy radiodense deposits on roentgenograms represents the radiologic correlate of cellular resorption of mineral (22). Others have not found chondroid metaplasia or matrix vesicles in calcific tenosynovitis but found instead psammoma bodies and calcification within necrotic cells (23).

Cartilage and Synovial Calcifications

Ali and Griffiths (24) presented electron microscopic evidence for pericellular matrix vesicles in normal articular cartilage, which they regard as a latent growth plate. Vesicles were present at all levels of the cartilage but were most numerous near the tidemark adjoining the subchondral bone. Microcrystals within mineral nodules (0.6 μm in diameter) were noted in various stages of formation. Both vesicles and mineral were greatly increased in osteoarthritic cartilage; quantitatively, this increase was reflected by a marked increase (up to 30-fold) in alkaline phosphatase activity. Three distinct types of calcification in osteoarthritic cartilage were seen. In addition to the mineral nodules just discussed, dense cuboidal-shaped crystals resembling whitlockite morphologically, but with a molar Ca/P of 1.72, were found in pericellular matrix around the surface chondrocytes. Fine needle-shaped crystal clusters were observed on the cartilage surface in the acellular amorphous zone (lamina splendens). These clusters had a molar Ca/P of 1.7 and resembled the crystals found in synovial fluid. Matrix vesicles and crystals were seen in rabbit fibrocartilage that had formed from autologous grafts of synovial tissue implanted into defects produced surgically in hyaline cartilage but not in sham-operated joints (25).

A systematic study of articular cartilage from 28 patients with advanced OA showed superficial HA-type needle-shaped crystals in 56%; calcified deposits were found in 36% in deeper repair-type fibrocartilage, and CPPD crystals were seen in 11% of cases (26). Overall, 75% of the cartilages had microcrystalline deposits of some kind. Synovium from the same joints all showed a patchy lining cell hyperplasia and giant cells, whether or not calcific deposits were present in the area. Calcific deposits were present in 70% of synovial specimens. All were of the HA type, but four specimens also showed CPPD deposits. The pathologic prevalence of 70% to 75% synovial calcification is in accord with a radiologic survey of osteoarthritic knee joints, wherein 72% showed periarticular or intraarticular calcification (27).

Calcific Periarthritis

Periarticular calcifications are found most commonly around the shoulder but have been described near many other joints. Calcific scapulohumeral periarthritis was first described in 1870 (1). Roentgenographic demonstration of periarticular shoulder calcifications was accomplished in 1907 (1), and a classic review of 329 cases of peritendinitis calcarea was presented in 1938 (1). Calcium deposits were found in one or both shoulders of 138 of 5,061 employees of a life insurance company (1). More than 70% of patients were under the age of 40 years, and many remained asymptomatic, although large deposits usually caused acute painful inflammation at some point in time. Spontaneous resorption of some deposits, especially the smaller ones, occurred. Nearly half of these subjects had bilateral deposits.

Most cases of acute calcific periarthritis consist of a single attack in a single area, frequently with localized warmth, erythema, swelling, and pain lasting a few days to a few weeks. Sepsis is frequently the initial diagnosis. The radiographic finding of periarticular calcification is useful as a confirmatory diagnostic aid.

Hydroxyapatite pseudopodagra is a term used by Fam and Rubenstein (19) to describe acute inflammation in the first metatarsal phalangeal joint, usually in young women. Radiographs show periarticular calcific deposits, which later disappear. Acute calcific periarthritis less commonly involves the small joints of the hand, wrist, and elbow and also occurs predominantly (80%) in women (28).

Recurrent attacks of calcific periarthritis occurring at multiple sites suggest a more generalized condition rather than a chance localized process with resultant calcification (1). Several reports describe familial occurrences of calcific arthritis and periarthritis (1,18).

Episodic attacks of calcific periarthritis have been treated successfully with a variety of nonsteroidal antiinflammatory drugs (NSAIDs) and colchicine (1). Needle aspiration of the paste-like calcific deposits with or without irrigation may be helpful (1). Mechanical disruption and dispersion of the deposits may speed their removal by increasing the surface available to phagocytic cells, as outlined by Sarkar and Uhthoff (22). Surgical removal of large calcific deposits may be needed for permanent symptomatic relief. Codman considered this procedure to be essential for relief of chronic shoulder symptoms (1). Ultrasound treatment may be a novel method for disruption and more rapid resolution of symptomatic tendon calcifications (29).

Basic Calcium Phosphate Crystal–Related Arthritis

Basic calcium phosphate crystals may be found within joint fluid as well as in cartilage and synovium. Schumacher and associates (3) have described both acute and chronic forms of arthritis. Acute attacks of arthritis in relatively young persons occurred with pain, swelling, and erythema resembling gout. Crystals resembling BCP were found by TEM in synovial fluid pellets with significantly elevated synovial fluid leukocyte counts and normal joint roentgenograms. Persons with chronic degenerative arthropathy and three patients with erosive arthritis were described. Recurrent episodes of pain and swelling were associated with gradual erosion and destructive changes in metacarpophalangeal, proximal interphalangeal, and wrist joints. One of the three patients had chronic renal failure. Although all had radiographic evidence of periarticular calcific deposits, no synovial fluid was obtained; therefore, it remains unclear whether intrasynovial crystals were present.

In 1976, Dieppe and co-workers (2) reported that synovial fluid from five patients with clinical evidence of OA contained 0.15 to 0.8 μm crystals, which, by x-ray energy dispersive analysis, were compatible with apatite (2). Others reported apatite crystals in approximately 30% to 60% of synovial fluid from patients with knee joint OA (14,30,31). Even synovial fluids from patients with OA, which appeared to contain no crystals by routine light microscopy, usually had BCP or CPPD crystals when subjected to enzymatic and hypochlorite extraction and examined by analytic electron microscopy (32,33). Leukocyte levels in synovial fluid from osteoarthritic joints were no different whether or not crystals were present (30). BCP and CPPD crystals were found more frequently together than separately in fluid from joints of patients with OA of the knee; the presence of BCP crystals correlated with joint deterioration, whereas the finding of CPPD crystals correlated with patient age (14). BCP and CPPD crystals were found together in soft tissues in association with carpal tunnel syndrome (34).

Milwaukee Shoulder/Knee Syndrome

The authors have studied 30 cases of a peculiar arthropathy, which we named *Milwaukee shoulder syndrome* (MSS) (7).

TABLE 118.3. FEATURES OF MILWAUKEE SHOULDER/KNEE SYNDROME

Clinical features
- Elderly, predominance in women
- Dominant shoulder usually affected but often bilateral
- Symptoms variable—asymptomatic to severe pain at rest; mostly painful after use and at night; glenohumeral joint stiffness or instability

Radiographic features
- Glenohumeral joint degeneration
- Soft tissue calcification
- Upward subluxation of the humeral head

Synovial fluid
- Low leukocyte counts; few to many erythrocytes
- Basic calcium phosphate crystal aggregates
- Particular collagens
- Elevated protease activities in some fluids

Robert Adams (35,36) of Dublin was the first to describe this entity as rheumatic arthritis of the shoulder in 1857 (37). Salient clinical, radiographic, and synovial fluid findings are listed in Table 118.3.

Adams and Smith described the regular disappearance of the rotator cuff and the intraarticular portion of the tendon of the long head of the biceps. Because the process was often bilateral and patients had no history of trauma, Adams and Smith attributed such massive loss of fibrous tissue to an intraarticular disease process and not to a traumatic cuff tear. They described upward subluxation of the humeral head with eburnation of its superior aspect as it formed a pseudoarticulation with the coracoacromial vault. Synovial hypertrophy with frequent formation of pedunculated loose bodies and separation of the acromion into two parts along the plane of the epiphysis was also clearly described.

Clinical Features

The primary findings of MSS include predominance in women (80%), greater or exclusive involvement on the dominant side, glenohumeral joint degeneration, and lysis of the rotator cuff. Others have described similar patients under a variety of descriptive terms. The reported studies are summarized in Table 118.4. The average age of patients was 72 years with range of 50 to 90 years. The average duration of symptoms, when ascertainable, was 3.8 years, but the range was variable (1 to 10 years). The exact time of onset could not be determined in some cases. The syndrome appeared to evolve slowly over a span of years in most patients. Symptoms also varied. Three patients with bilateral shoulder involvement had asymptomatic disease on the nondominant side. Most persons experienced mild to moderate

TABLE 118.4. SUMMARY OF REPORTS DESCRIBING 72 PATIENTS WITH SEVERE SHOULDER DEGENERATION

n	Male/Female	Mean Age (Years)	Age Range	Bilateral (%)
72	13/59	72	50–90	46 (64)

Data from refs. 1 and 7.

pain, especially after use, but one patient had severe pain even at rest. Other symptoms included limited motion, stiffness, and night pain. Examination showed reduced active range of motion in all affected shoulders, sometimes associated with pronounced joint instability. Crepitation and pain were often noted when the humerus was grated passively against the glenoid. Unusual features may include acromioclavicular joint cyst, acromial stress fracture, and formation of a sinus draining into the tissues of the anterior chest wall (38–40).

Aspiration of the affected shoulder joints routinely yielded 3 to 40 mL of synovial fluid that was frequently blood tinged. Occasionally, hydrops of the shoulder yielding 130 mL or more of synovial fluid was encountered (Fig. 118.4). In two instances, hydrops was associated with joint rupture and dissection of fluid into the anterior chest wall. This event can be precipitated by intraarticular bleeding and may be accompanied by subcutaneous ecchymosis covering the trunk and upper arm—the "quarter panel" sign (41).

Associated Factors

Several factors that may predispose to the development of Milwaukee shoulder syndrome have been identified (7). Trauma or overuse was observed in nine of our 30 cases. Four patients had fallen on an outstretched hand, and one was involved in a motor vehicle accident. Two men had "traumatic" professions (jackhammer operation and professional wrestling), and two other men had experienced recurrent shoulder dislocations. Recurrent dislocation has been identified as a predisposing cause of shoulder arthropathy (42). Two patients with paraparesis used their shoulders as weight-bearing joints while crutch-walking and later using wheelchairs—conditions described as the "impingement syndrome of paraplegia" (18). Another patient had a dysplastic left shoulder from birth and developed Milwaukee shoulder syndrome on the opposite side. Eight patients were found to have BCP and CPPD crystals simultaneously and all but one of them also had symptomatic knee involvement. Three

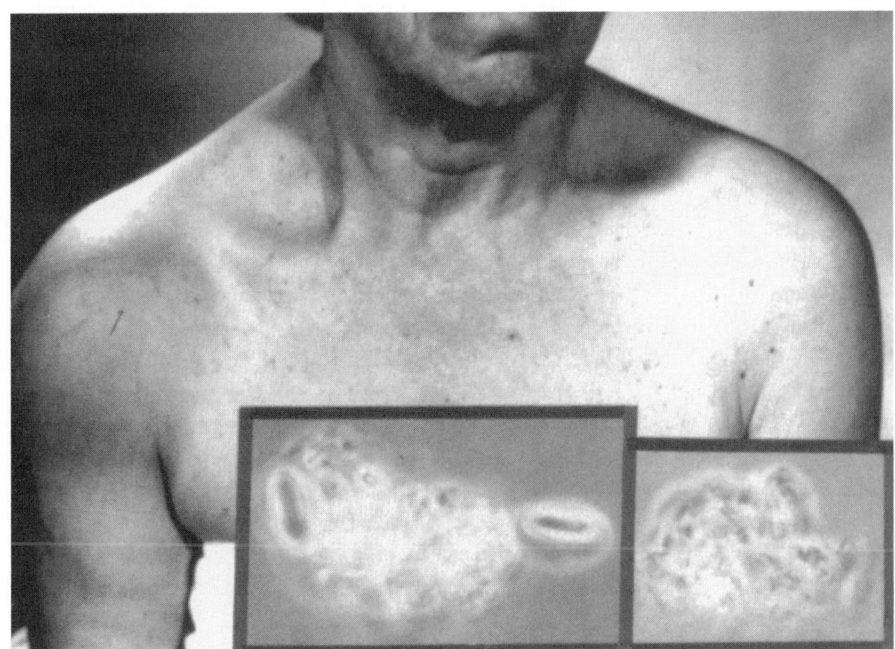

FIGURE 118.4. Photograph of a 62-year-old woman with grotesque swelling of the right shoulder. Inserts show two crystal masses found in a wet preparation of fresh joint fluid. Note the erythrocytes for size comparison (phase contrast ×1,000).

patients had severe neurologic disorders (syringomyelia in one and cervical radiculopathies in two). Thus, the shoulder disease was partially attributable to denervation resulting in neuropathic joints. One patient had chronic renal failure requiring hemodialysis. The remaining one-third of patients, all of them women, had no identifiable contributing factor. One patient with hyperparathyroidism had her shoulder effusion resolve following resection of her parathyroid adenoma (43).

Milwaukee shoulder/knee syndrome may represent the final common pathway of several conditions, although other factors must also be involved because these associated conditions do not always progress to such severe joint destruction.

Radiographic Features

Glenohumeral joint degeneration was noted in 49 of 55 shoulders examined in our series of 30 cases. Soft tissue calcifications were present in 55% of shoulders. Upward subluxation of the humeral head or arthrographic evidence of rotator cuff defects was evident in 46 of 55 shoulders (Fig. 118.5). The distance from the superior rim of the humeral head to the acromion, measured on routine roentgenograms with the patient erect, was reduced to 2 mm or less in all but three patients in the series of 26 patients reported by Neer et al. (1). Erosion of the coracoid process, of the undersurface of the anterior third of the acromion, and of the acromioclavicular joint was common (Figs. 118.6 and 118.7); in many instances, a rounding off of the greater tuberosity occurred with loss of the sulcus demarcating the anatomic neck of the humerus. Erosions, subchondral cysts, and roughening of the bony cortex over the greater tuberosity at the site of the insertion of the rotator cuff were also noted frequently.

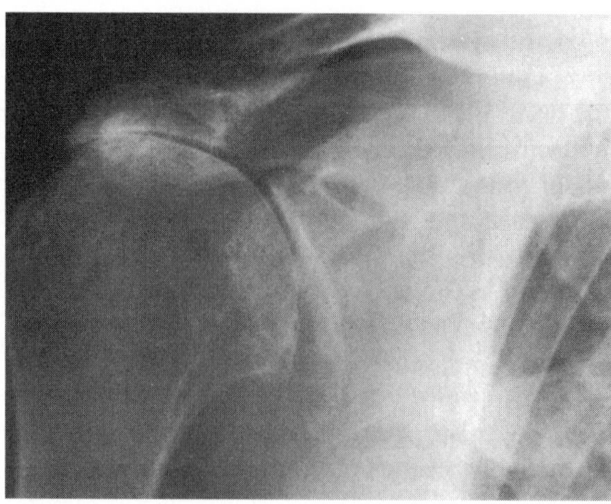

FIGURE 118.6. Anteroposterior radiograph of the right shoulder in a patient showing more advanced changes. Superior displacement of the humeral head has resulted in a pseudoarticulation with the acromion. Sclerosis, cystic changes, and irregularity of the humeral head are also present.

Arthrograms or bursagrams were performed in all 26 of the patients studied by Neer et al. (1). Each showed a grossly defective rotator cuff with communication between the glenohumeral and acromioclavicular joints in ten instances. Arthro-

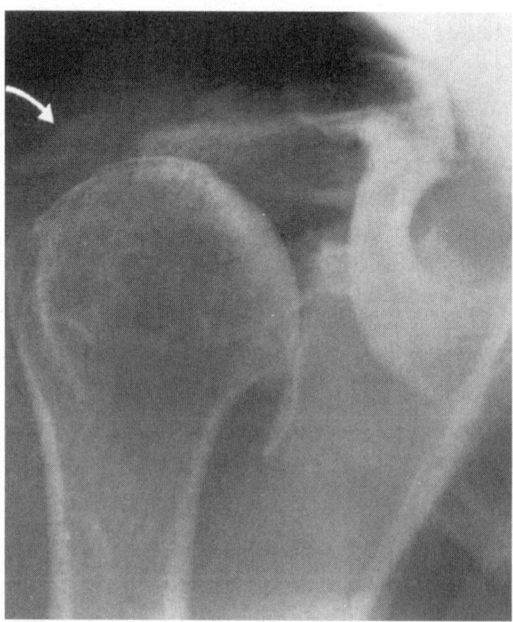

FIGURE 118.5. Anteroposterior radiograph of the right shoulder showing soft tissue calcifications *(arrow)* and superior subluxation and sclerosis of the humeral head.

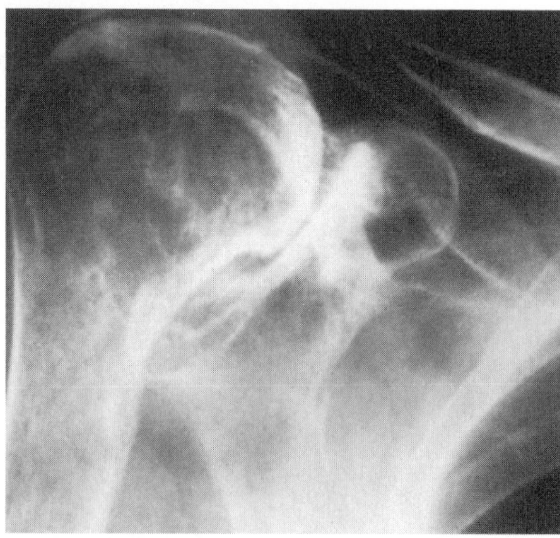

FIGURE 118.7. Anteroposterior radiograph of the right shoulder of another patient showing superior displacement of the humeral head and pseudoarticulation with the clavicle, acromion, and coracoid process. The humeral head is partly collapsed with eburnation only in its inferomedial articulating surface. Note the absence of osteophytes.

grams of the contralateral shoulder were performed in 11 of the 26 patients, and all showed a complete tear of the rotator cuff, although only five had typical radiographic changes in the glenohumeral joint. Pseudarthrosis formation between the humeral head and the acromion and clavicle was common (Fig. 118.6). Bony destruction of the humeral head was also common, whereas osteophyte formation was usually modest (1). An area of collapse of the proximal aspect of the humeral articular surface was present in all patients in the Neer series and was a requirement for the diagnosis. These changes are not those of OA of the shoulder where the rotator cuff remains intact with sclerosis of bone and prominent osteophytes.

Synovial Fluid Features

Synovial fluid leukocyte counts were usually less than 1,000 per mm^3 (76 of 78 fluids). When the fluids were assayed for BCP crystals by (^{14}C) diphosphonate binding as described previously, 73 of 78 fluids were positive. CPPD crystals were also seen in eight fluids. Crystal concentrations estimated serially in fluids from two shoulders were remarkably constant for nearly a year, suggesting that they were under homeostatic control. Microspheroidal aggregates were found by SEM in 33 of 46 fluids that bound (^{14}C) diphosphonate. The molar Ca/P of these aggregates ranged from 1.4 to 1.7 by x-ray energy dispersive analysis (7).

Low levels of collagenolytic activity, either active or latent, were found in at least one synovial fluid supernatant from half our patients. The total protein concentration in these fluids was 3 to 4 g/dL, mostly albumin. Low levels of α_2-macroglobulins, a natural inhibitor of collagenase, and α_1-antitrypsin were found. Synovial fluids also demonstrated types I, II, and III particulate collagens and elevated neutral protease activities (13). FTIR analyses showed collagen as a constant feature in these joint fluid pellets (6).

Knee Involvement

In our series of 30 patients with shoulder disease, 16 had symptomatic knee involvement. Lateral tibiofemoral compartment narrowing occurring in 14 of 36 patients (39%) (Figs. 118.8 and 118.9), as is often seen in CPPD crystal

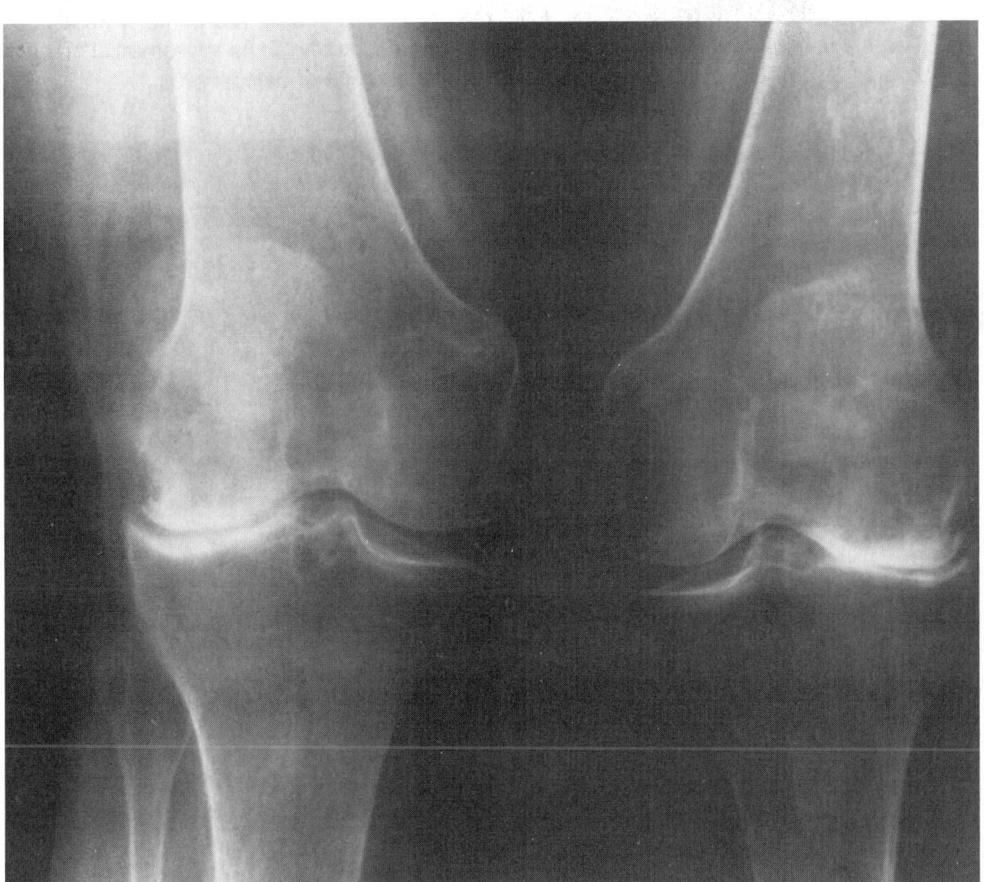

FIGURE 118.8. Standing anteroposterior roentgenogram of the knees from a patient with Milwaukee shoulder syndrome showing lateral tibiofemoral compartment narrowing and incongruity with subchondral bony sclerosis but minimal osteophyte formation.

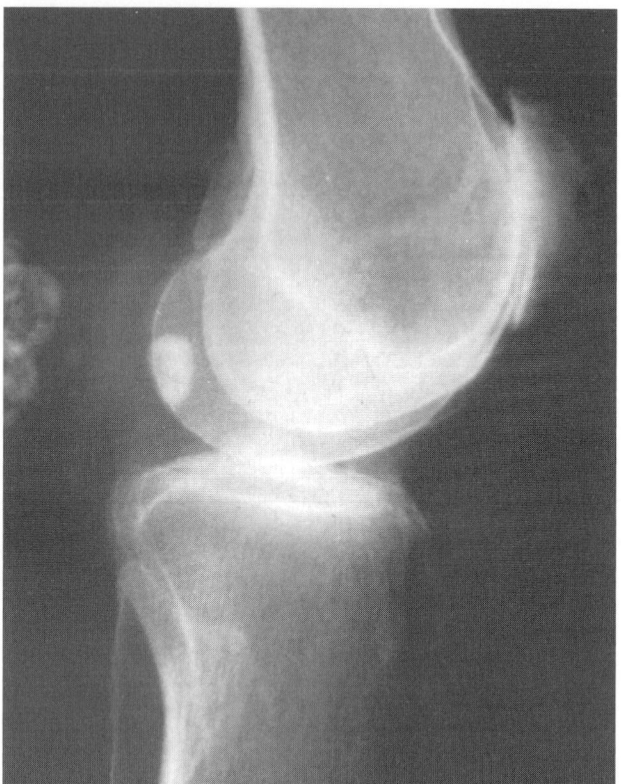

FIGURE 118.9. Lateral radiograph of the right knee of another patient showing isolated patellofemoral osteoarthritis (patella "wrapped around" the femur), femoral cortical defect, and chondrocalcinosis of the femoral articular cartilage. Osteochondromata can be seen in the posterior joint recess.

deposition disease (see Chapter 117), exceeded medial compartment narrowing in 11 of 36 patients (31%). This differed significantly from 56 patients (62 evaluable knees) with symptomatic OA of the knee without shoulder joint involvement ($p < .01$) (7). CPPD crystal deposition was detected either in synovial fluid or by radiographs in seven patients. One patient had osteochondromatosis, and another lateral femoral condylar osteonecrosis, both of which have also been associated with CPPD crystal deposition. Dieppe's patients also showed primarily hip and lateral compartment knee involvement (1). Thus, the pattern of knee joint degeneration in patients with shoulder joint disease appears to differ from that of primary OA of the knee, where medial tibiofemoral compartment disease predominates.

Other Joint Involvement

Two of our patients had severe degenerative arthritis of the hips, but because they already had prosthetic joint replacement, there was no fluid to study. Whether a similar process was involved in pathogenesis is unclear. We have also studied a man with bilateral elbow joint degeneration and synovial fluid findings consistent with those of Milwaukee shoulder syndrome. The erosive arthropathy of wrists and small hand joints associated with periarticular calcific deposits described by Schumacher et al. (1), may share some of these features, although again, no fluid had been obtained for analysis.

Pathology

Synovial biopsies obtained at the time of operation from the shoulders of four patients demonstrated increased numbers of villi, focal synovial lining cell hyperplasia, a few giant cells, fibrin, and BCP crystal deposits (Fig. 118.10) (Table 118.5) (44). Electron microscopy showed crystals being engulfed by synovial lining cells and histiocytes (Fig. 118.11). Calcific deposits in synovial microvilli appeared to have access to the joint space through areas denuded of synovial lining cells (Fig. 118.12).

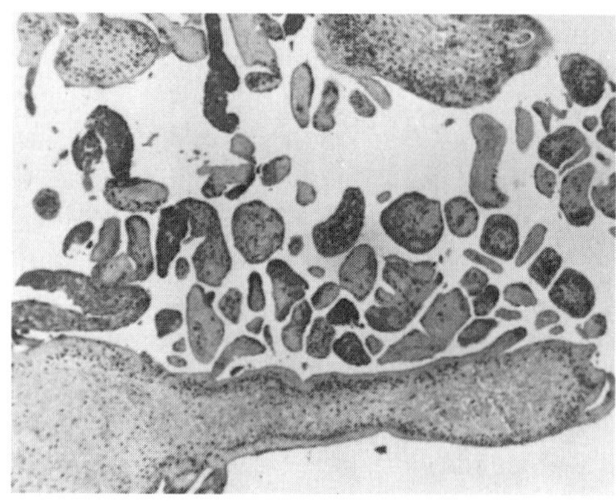

FIGURE 118.10. Light micrograph of synovium showing many villi and focal synovial cell hyperplasia. In cross section, the branching villi appear as free bodies. Some villi are partially covered with fibrin or contain fibrin in various stages of organization (×110).

TABLE 118.5. MICROSCOPIC FEATURES OF SYNOVIAL MEMBRANE IN MILWAUKEE SHOULDER/KNEE SYNDROME

Villous hyperplasia
Focal synovial lining cell hyperplasia
Basic calcium phosphate crystal deposition (extracellular, intracellular)[a]
Fibrin deposition
Giant cells
Fibrosis
Vascular congestion
No inflammatory cells

[a]The only specific feature.

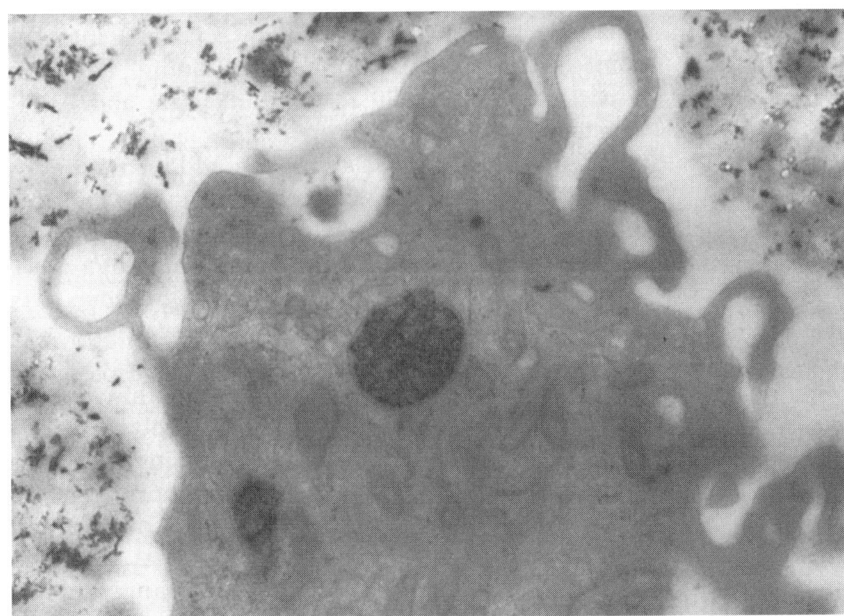

FIGURE 118.11. Electron micrograph of a hyperplastic synovial cell. Crystals within phagolysosomes are bounded by distinct limiting membranes. Many extracellular crystals are also present (×26,400).

In the series of Neer et al., a large, complete cuff tear was found in each patient at operation (1,42). The humeral head could be dislocated passively in 14 instances and was fixed in a dislocated position in the remaining 12 shoulders. The supraspinatus tendon was completely ruptured in all patients, and the infraspinatus tendon in all but one instance. The teres minor and subscapularis tendons were usually involved, but some vestiges remained in all patients. The tendon of the long head of the biceps was ruptured, dislocated, or frayed in 18, 3, and 5 patients, respectively. The subdeltoid bursa was thickened, forming a large loose pouch around the head of the biceps, and contained variable amounts of (often) sanguineous synovial fluid. The articular cartilage was pebble-like, and the collapsed articular surface, the major point of contact with the acromion, was eburnated and denuded of cartilage with small marginal osteophytes. The remainder of the humeral head was covered with degenerated cartilage and fibrous tissue. The subchondral bone could be indented easily with a finger. The anterior acromial epiphysis had failed to fuse in three patients, which may have contributed to subacromial impingement.

Histologically, the atrophic articular cartilage of the humeral head was covered to a variable degree with a fibrous membrane (pannus). In these areas, the adjacent bone was osteoporotic and hypervascularized with attempts at repair at points of bony collapse. At points of contact between the humeral head and scapula, the cartilage was completely denuded and the bone was sclerotic. Fragments of articular cartilage were found in the subsynovium. These fragments resembled those found in neuropathic joints, albeit less extensive.

In glenohumeral OA, the entire humeral head is sclerotic without large areas of softening (42), and is enlarged by

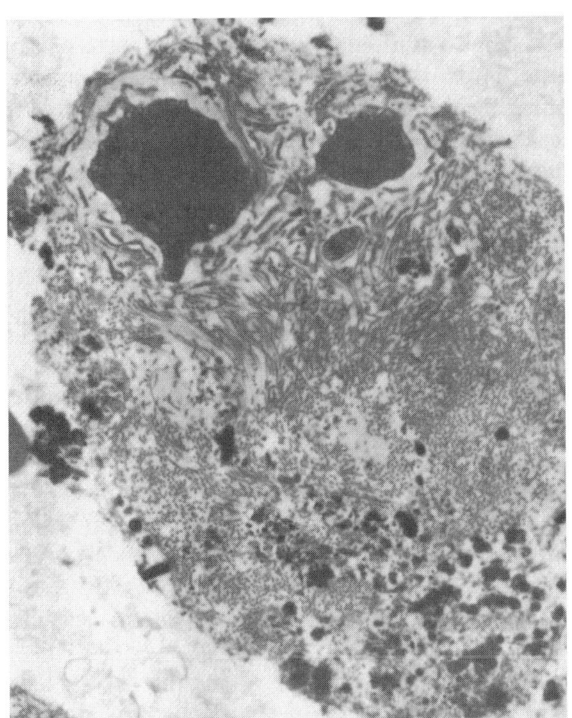

FIGURE 118.12. Electron micrograph showing a small villus in cross section. Synovial lining cells are absent. Crystal microaggregates are seen dispersed among collagen fibers, lying free on the surface and in the synovial space. Several fibrocytes are present

marginal osteophytes without collapse (1). The rotator cuff is nearly always intact (42).

Pathogenesis

A hypothesis was formulated (Fig. 118.13) in which BCP crystals, and possibly particulate collagens, are endocytosed by synovial lining cells. These cells are then stimulated to produce prostaglandin E_2 (PGE_2) and enzymes such as collagenase, stromelysin, and, perhaps, other proteases. Although collagenase is not a constant finding in synovial fluids and was not identified by Dieppe et al. (45) in any shoulder joint fluid, it has been identified in OA synovial fluids by others (46). The massive lysis of the rotator cuff and only the intrasynovial portion of the long head of the biceps tendon is difficult to explain without implicating this enzyme. Synovial lining cells metabolize BCP crystals in acidic phagolysosomes. The release of calcium within the cell (47) may contribute to synovial cell proliferation in which BCP crystals from eburnated bone, metaplastic synovium, and perhaps cartilage are probably continually released by mechanical forces, and possibly by enzymatic "strip" mining as previously postulated for sodium urate and CPPD crystal release (see Chapters 116 and 117).

Particulates such as latex beads, added to rabbit synovial cells in culture, are phagocytosed, stimulating increased secretion of proteases, including collagenase (42). This increased secretion continued until the ingested particles were biodegraded, at which time it returned to baseline. Collagen also stimulated collagenase release from cultured human skin fibroblasts (48), and synovial fluid "wear" particles released neutral proteases from cultured synovial cells (49).

This hypothesis was tested by adding natural or synthetic BCP, CPPD, and other crystals to cultured human or canine synovial cells (50). Neutral protease (stromelysin) and collagenase secretion were augmented in a dose-related fashion approximately five to eight times over control cultures incubated without crystals. Collagenase and stromelysin messenger RNA induction were shown by Northern blot analysis in chondrocytes in primary culture as well (18). Partially purified mammalian collagenase released BCP crystal microspheroidal aggregates from calcified synovial tissue *in vitro* (51). The mean diameter and size ranges of the released aggregates were identical to those observed in synovial fluids obtained from the same patient. Fluid obtained several weeks after synovectomy of the affected shoulder in this patient showed no mineral by (^{14}C) EHDP binding and greatly reduced protease activities (13).

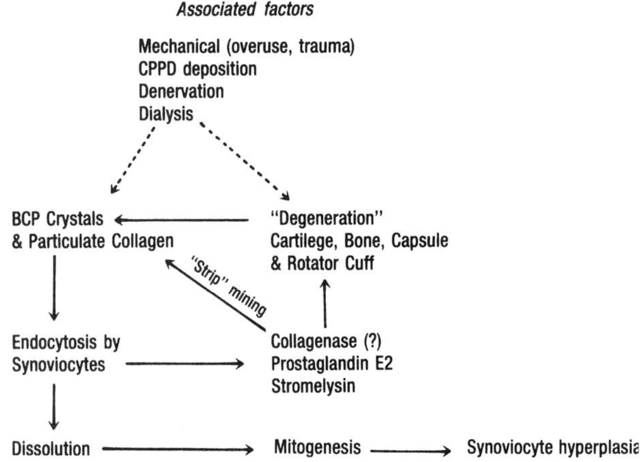

FIGURE 118.13. Hypothetical schema relating the various features of Milwaukee shoulder/knee syndrome.

In addition to the stimulation of relentless enzyme secretion, BCP or CPPD crystal endocytosis was associated with a massive genesis of prostaglandins, especially PGE_2 (52,53). PGE_2 release and collagenase release have been found after exposure of macrophages or synovial cells to sodium urate crystals also and have been related to the hard tissue destruction in gout (Chapter 116). PGE_2 was found in joint fluid from our patients (13) and was isolated from the periarticular calcium phosphate deposits from a patient with phalangeal osteolysis (53).

This hypothesis is consistent with the concept of "crystal traffic" derived from studies of the fate of radiolabeled CPPD or BCP crystals injected intrasynovially. One half of a dose of CPPD crystals was cleared from human joints in 30 to 90 days and from rabbit joints in 16 to 20 days (1). Clearance rates were inversely proportional to crystal size. Injected crystals were phagocytosed by synovial cells, where virtually all dissolution appeared to take place. This phenomenon was evidenced by localization of all nuclide in synovial tissue, the finding of all crystals inside cells by electron microscopy, the lack of effect on clearance rate of extracellular magnesium depletion by dietary deprivation, the failure of joint lavage to remove significant radionuclide, and reduction of clearance rate by 65% in the presence of synovial cell hemosiderosis induced by injection of autologous blood (1). Both CPPD crystals and hemosiderin were shown in the same cells by TEM and x-ray energy dispersive analysis. ^{85}Sr-labeled BCP crystals were cleared from rabbit joints with a half-life of about 6 days, about three times faster than CPPD crystals (54).

The focal cell hyperplasia found in the four synovial membranes we examined (43) was described by Doyle (26) as a constant feature of synovial membranes containing calcium crystals. This finding might be related to their mitogenic properties. BCP, CPPD, calcium urate, calcium diphosphonate, and calcium carbonate, but not crystals or particulates without calcium (such as sodium urate, diamond, silicon dioxide, or latex beads), were capable of substituting for serum growth factors in certain cell systems (18,55). Crystals must undergo endocytosis and dissolution by cells for mitogenesis to occur (18). Calcium-containing crystals act as a "competence" factor, because they can substitute for growth factors found in serum (platelet-derived growth factor, PDGF); like PDGF, calcium-containing crystals require a progression factor, such as insulin-like growth factor-1 (somatomedin C) for full expression of mitogenic potency (56). ^{45}Ca-BCP crystals added to cultured synovial cells, skin fibroblasts, or peripheral blood monocytes were phagocytosed and degraded, probably by the adenosine triphosphatase (ATPase)-driven lysosomal proton pump (18). Weak bases, such as chloroquine or $NH4^+$, inhibited BCP crystal solubilization in a dose-dependent fashion (18). Calcium crystal-induced mitogenesis was also reduced in a parallel dose-dependent fashion by these inhibitors, but serum-stimulated mitogenesis was unaffected (18).

Basic calcium phosphate crystal stimulation of fibroblasts includes activation of protein kinase C and the induction of the proto-oncogenes c-*fos,* c-*myc,* and c-*jun* (57). Messenger RNA for stromelysin, and probably gelatinase, is induced (58). Inhibitors of BCP crystal dissolution block mitogenesis but not collagenase induction or secretion.

The stimulation of cytokines by BCP crystals has not been thoroughly studied. Available data suggest a limited role if any. HA crystals induced tumor necrosis factor-α (TNF-α) expression in a mononuclear cell line (59). In a study of synovial fluids from OA patients, levels of TNF-α, but not interleukin-1 (IL-1), were increased relative to rheumatoid arthritis (60).

Although BCP crystals may elicit a major acute inflammatory response as in hydroxyapatite pseudopodagra (19), BCP crystals as found in OA synovial fluid do not stimulate a neutrophilic response very often. This may be related to a lesser phlogistic potential or to adsorbed surface proteins, which modulate crystal-cell interactions. BCP crystals generated reduced amounts of chemotactic factors from neutrophils, and these showed greater surface binding to BCP crystals in comparison to monosodium urate (MSU) crystals (61). Further, other proteins adsorbed onto the surface of BCP crystals, such as α_2-HS glycoprotein, inhibited superoxide generation and chemiluminescence (62).

Indirect evidence does suggest that BCP crystals contribute to low-grade joint inflammation. The severity of joint symptoms in OA correlated with the synovial fluid leukocyte count and with the presence of HA crystals and other particulates (63). In patients with OA of the knee, synovial effusions were larger when BCP crystals were present (64). Gerster (65) found that the presence of HA crystals in distal interphalangeal joints correlated with progression to erosive OA (65).

Neer and co-workers favor a pathogenesis based on disuse osteoporosis and mechanical instability (1). The greater severity of symptoms, radiologic evidence of destruction, the higher joint fluid levels of crystals and enzymes in the shoulder on the dominant side, and the frequent history of overuse or trauma support a pathogenetic role of movement. But the finding of destructive arthropathies of the knee and possibly other joints in the same patients suggests that systemic metabolic effects might be operative. Biomechanical factors probably play a major role in the pathogenetic scheme outlined in Figure 118.13.

Treatment

The treatment of Milwaukee shoulder syndrome is generally unsatisfactory. A conservative approach including NSAIDs, repeated shoulder aspirations, and decreased joint use has sometimes controlled symptoms satisfactorily. Treatment with oral colchicine and an NSAID containing magnesium was effective in one patient (66). Tidal irrigation therapy resulted in symptomatic improvement and resolution of joint effusions for up to 1 year in two patients (67). Several patients have responded to a series of three hylan g-f20 injections (personal observation). Surgical complete arthroplasty is usually successful for relief of pain and restoration of some function, as described in Chapter 49.

At the time of diagnosis, advanced destructive changes are usually present, and may even be asymptomatic. Thus, there is no a priori way to identify persons at risk for this condition.

Secondary Basic Calcium Phosphate Arthropathies

Several conditions, including chronic renal failure, the connective tissue diseases, and neurologic injury, have been associated with calcification that may occur in almost any tissue (Table 118.2). In these conditions, BCP crystals have been found in periarticular soft tissues, in bursae, and within joints and are often associated with symptoms.

Soft tissue calcifications involving the fibrous tissue in skin or muscle occur in the connective tissue diseases (1). Rare cases of intraarticular calcification have been reported in scleroderma, one case with a chalky joint effusion (1), and cases with polymyositis (18,68) and mixed connective tissue disease (21). Several patients with scleroderma have experienced episodes of acute calcific periarthritis with severe pain, swelling, and erythema (69). In contrast to patients with idiopathic calcific periarthritis, these patients had recurrent episodes of periarthritis, and the calcifications did not disappear.

Heterotopic ossification mimicking arthritis has been described following neurologic catastrophes (1). Such ossification tends to occur in periarticular tissues. The mechanisms are unknown. Low synovial fluid leukocyte counts and high protein concentrations have been found.

Several miscellaneous causes of BCP crystal deposition have been described (1). One patient had Laennec's cirrhosis, hypertrophic osteoarthropathy, and synovial calcifications in the knees probably related to vitamin D intoxication. A patient with "draft dodger's knee" developed calcifications around the knee many years after self-injection of olive oil.

The intraarticular injection of triamcinolone hexacetonide has been associated with the formation of periarticular calcifications along the injection tract, which may become apparent months after the injection (1,70,71). Such calcifications may gradually be resorbed over a period of months to years. A young woman developed a large periarticular calcification near her shoulder following three injections of paramethasone (72).

Arthropathy in Chronic Renal Failure

Although patients with chronic renal failure are susceptible to virtually any type of arthritis, uremia and hemodialysis predispose to osteodystrophy, tendinitis, tendon rupture (73), carpal tunnel syndrome, and several forms of arthritis and periarthritis (Table 118.6).

Musculoskeletal symptoms occur in 57% to 82% of patients on long-term dialysis (74–76). One study of 80 patients showed that arthralgias were the most common complaint (74%), but radiographic evaluation disclosed erosive arthropathy of the fingers (8%) and spine (9%), bone cysts of the carpus (10%), humeral head (9%), and hip (11%), cervical spondylolisthesis (5%), and multiple diaphyseal lacunae (1%) (74).

In the small joints of the hands, erosive arthropathy has been ascribed to secondary hyperparathyroidism (77). Erosive disease has also been observed in axial joints and large joints, especially the shoulder (78–80). "Erosive azotemic arthropathy" described a subset of patients with erosive changes in large and small joints, "noninflammatory" synovial fluids, and renal osteodystrophy (81). Histologic analysis of material found in bone cysts has shown amyloid composed of β_2-microglobulin (82) (see also Chapter 92). β_2-microglobulin modified with advanced glycation end products, but not the unmodified form, is chemotactic for human monocytes and increased secretion of TNF and IL-1 by macrophages (83). Cases with carpal tunnel syndrome have consistently demonstrated this type of amyloid as well (84). Amyloid has been detected in synovium, tenosynovium, capsule, and extraarticular locations (85). The term *dialysis myelopathy* has been used to describe a case of quadriparesis resulting from extradural amyloid deposition (86).

TABLE 118.6. ARTHROPATHIES AND PERIARTHROPATHIES ASSOCIATED WITH CHRONIC RENAL FAILURE

Periarthritis/tendinitis
  Tendon rupture
Erosive arthropathy
  Hands (secondary hyperparathyroidism)
  Large joints (especially shoulders)
  Axial skeleton
  "Erosive azotemic arthropathy" (large and small joints and renal osteodystrophy)
Crystal deposition
  Monosodium urate monohydrate
  Calcium pyrophosphate dihydrate
  Basic calcium phosphates
  Calcium oxalate
  Aluminum phosphate
β_2-microglobulin amyloid
  Carpal tunnel syndrome
  Bone cysts

Crystal-induced arthritis appears to be common in uremia (Table 118.6). Hyperuricemia predisposes to acute gout, although attacks are less common than might be expected. BCP crystals are likely to form in or around joints and in other tissues in the milieu of excess phosphorus or calcium and may cause acute episodes of articular and periarticular inflammation, although greater attention to control of calcium and phosphorus plasma levels has reduced this complication (87). CPPD crystal deposition has been associated with hyperparathyroidism (1). Calcium oxalate has been found in the synovial fluid from patients receiving chronic hemodialysis (88), especially in those receiving ascorbic acid supplementation (89). Worcester et al. (90) showed that uremic serum is supersaturated with respect to calcium oxalate. Calcium oxalate deposition may be associated with chondrocalcinosis and inflammatory bursitis, tenosynovitis, and acute, subacute, or chronic arthritis. Finally, aluminum phosphate has been demonstrated in the synovium of patients taking aluminum compounds by mouth to bind intestinal phosphate (91,92).

Synovial fluid leukocyte counts are generally not increased, although leukocytosis was found in two of three inflamed shoulders in dialysis patients (1), and BCP crystals were found in two of these.

Calciphylaxis is an unusual occlusive vascular disease usually associated with end-stage renal disease and hyperparathyroidism. Lesions are primarily cutaneous including ischemic skin necrosis and digital gangrene which may be confused with vasculitis (93,94). Visceral calcification has been reported following parenteral corticosteroid therapy (95). Vascular occlusion results from medial arterial calcification and endovascular fibrosis, which may be diagnosed by skin biopsy (96,97).

CALCINOSIS

Calcinosis, or pathologic calcification of the soft tissues, occurs in a variety of systemic and localized conditions (Table 118.2). Ectopic calcification is generally classified into two groups—those conditions that result from persistent hypercalcemia or hyperphosphatemia (metastatic calcification), and those conditions that follow a local metabolic or degenerative tissue abnormality (dystrophic calcification).

Metastatic Calcification

Calcareous deposits, common in hypercalcemic states, are found in the kidney (nephrocalcinosis), stomach, lung, brain, eyes (band keratopathy), skin, subcutaneous and periarticular tissues, and arterial walls. The milk-alkali syndrome and vitamin D intoxication are two such conditions that may affect rheumatic disease patients who become hypercalcemic because of overzealous treatment to prevent duodenal ulcer or osteoporosis (98,99). Pulmonary calcification was observed in 5% of cases following orthotopic liver transplantation (100). Affected patients had increased serum calcium and phosphate levels in comparison to nonaffected patients. Calcification of the articular cartilage and menisci (chondrocalcinosis) and joint capsules is a well-recognized feature of hyperparathyroidism. For some persons, an attack of CPPD crystal-induced synovitis (pseudogout) represents the first clinical manifestation of this disease. Accordingly, the possibility of primary hyperparathyroidism should be carefully considered in all patients with CPPD arthropathy. Immediately following resection of a parathyroid adenoma, patients are at high risk to develop attacks of pseudogout (42). Rarely, tumoral collections of CPPD crystals have been found in soft tissues (101).

Normocalcemic-hyperphosphatemic hyperparathyroidism secondary to renal insufficiency may cause soft tissue calcification, although it seldom affects the skin (102) and does not affect ocular structures. Calcinosis may also occur in hyperparathyroid renal transplant patients despite a normal calcium-phosphate product (103). Renal calculus formation is less frequent than in the hypercalcemic states. The removal of pyrophosphate, a physiologic inhibitor of calcification, may be responsible for this phenomenon (42). Treatment with phosphate-binding agents has resulted in a significant reduction of serum phosphorus levels, disappearance of cutaneous calcinosis, and relief from the articular attacks (92). Malabsorption of phosphate binders may be a problem (104). Reversal of uremic tumoral calcinosis was achieved by daily hemodialysis using a very low calcium dialysate (105).

In hypoparathyroidism, pseudohypoparathyroidism, and pseudopseudohypoparathyroidism, calcification may occur in the brain, particularly in the basal ganglia, as well as in subcutaneous tissue. Acute calcific periarthritis in hypoparathyroidism has been reported to occur in association with a fall in serum calcium (106), similar to the same phenomenon observed in surgically treated primary hyperparathyroidism (42) and gout.

Radiographically obvious biopsy-proved metastatic calcification has been detected by bone scanning [technetium (^{99m}Tc)-labeled methylene diphosphonate] in numerous areas, including the lung, gastric wall, heart, and kidney (42). Such uptake, caused by the affinity of the tracer for the surface of HA crystals, has also been shown in the subcutaneous tissues and skin (42).

Tumoral Calcinosis

Tumoral calcinosis is separable from other causes of metastatic calcification because visceral involvement is absent. This rare entity, also called *lipocalcinosis granulomatosis,* is characterized by the rapid development of large, multilobulated calcific masses in the subcutaneous tissue and muscles surrounding the hips, shoulders, elbows, hands, fingers (107), and chest wall in otherwise healthy young persons. Smaller tumors occur adjacent to the spine, wrists, feet, lower ribs, sacrum, and ischium. There is no sex predilection, but there is a considerably increased prevalence among African Americans and black Africans (108). These firm, nontender deposits may increase to a diameter of 20 cm or larger over a period of months to years. Little or no articular limitation occurs unless masses become very large or are complicated by the development of fistulous tracts caused by either infection or attempts at surgical drainage. Nerve root impingement (especially sciatica) may result. Curiously, several patients have had angioid streaks of the retina.

Most patients with tumoral calcinosis have normal serum calcium and alkaline phosphatase values, but hyperphosphatemia (109) and elevated levels of 1,25-dihydroxyvitamin D (42) have been noted in several cases. Rapid exchange of calcium between serum and calcific masses is evident, along with an increased intestinal absorption of dietary calcium, with no defect in the turnover of skeletal calcium (109). An intrinsic renal proximal tubular defect allowing enhanced phosphate reabsorption has been postulated. Elevated 1,25-dihydroxyvitamin D levels are present after phosphate depletion, suggesting dysregulation of its synthesis or metabolism or an as yet undiscovered stimulus for its production (110). Approximately half of the patients with tumoral calcinosis reported to date have had affected siblings. This observation, together with the occurrence of hyperphosphatemia, has led to the suggestion that there is a heritable disturbance in the metabolism of phosphorus (109). Although an autosomal-recessive mechanism has been considered, the report of this condition in four generations of one family, coupled with a unique dental lesion (teeth with short, bulbous roots and nearly total obliteration of pulp cavities) suggests the possibility of an autosomal-dominant heredity with variable expression (111). Early diagnosis was suggested in some patients by head and neck abnormalities including mucosal macules, gingivitis, and hoarseness (112). On sectioning, calcific deposits are found to be composed of multilocular cysts enclosing pockets of milky fluid or pasty microcrystalline calcareous matter. The tissue lining the walls of these cysts contains mononuclear cells, which are rich in alkaline phosphatase and believed to be responsible for local accumulation of calcium phosphate. Foreign body giant cells are also present (108). Local hemorrhage may initiate the lesions, followed by aggregation of histiocytes and eventual transformation into cystic cavities with some features of adventitious bursae (113). Calcification seems to occur on membrane fragments in large cytoplasmic vesicles inside osteoclastic appearing giant cells and mononuclear lining cells and also, extracellularly, in locules containing cellular debris. The masses contain pure calcium carbonate and phosphate, a mixture of the two salts, or HA crystals (114).

Treatment at present consists mainly of early surgical excision of the calcareous masses, which rarely recur at the same site. As a rule, the prognosis is good, although new deposits may appear in time around other joints and, in some instances, secondary infection of the deposits has led to multiple draining sinuses, cachexia, and amyloidosis. A low-calcium and low-phosphorus diet and large oral doses of antacids containing aluminum hydroxide have resulted in negative balances of both calcium and phosphorus with clinical improvement (42). Intravenous calcitonin infusion has been reported to cause phosphaturia and a significant fall in serum phosphorus level (115).

Dystrophic Calcification

Many investigators restrict the use of the term *calcinosis* to those patients in whom the deposition of calcium salts in the soft tissues occurs in the absence of any generalized disturbance in calcium or phosphorus metabolism.

Myositis (Fibrodysplasia) Ossificans Progressiva

Patients with this uncommon disorder have widespread ectopic calcification and ossification in fascia, aponeuroses, and other fibrous structures related to muscles. The initial symptoms usually appear in early childhood, often preceded by local trauma (Fig. 118.14). The disease occurs in families and appears to be transmitted as an autosomal-dominant trait with irregular penetrance. Associated congenital anomalies of the digits include microdactyly or total absence of the thumbs and great toes.

Onset usually consists of a very painful localized area of swelling, redness, and warmth in the neck or paravertebral area. After several days, the inflammation subsides, leaving an area of residual doughy firmness that appears fibromatous and gradually ossifies over the following weeks. Scanning with ^{99m}Tc-pyrophosphate may be useful in the detection of areas of ossification before roentgenographic changes become apparent (116). The replacement of the tendon and muscle by bone leads to characteristic contracture deformities. Once ossification occurs, further change is minimal. Recurring bouts of inflammation and ossification result in progressive damage to much of the striated musculature. Involvement of the muscles of the chest wall and back may lead to restrictive pulmonary disease (117). Death usually ensues from respiratory failure and/or pulmonary infection resulting from ossification of the muscles of the thorax or from inanition as a result of damage to the muscles of mastication.

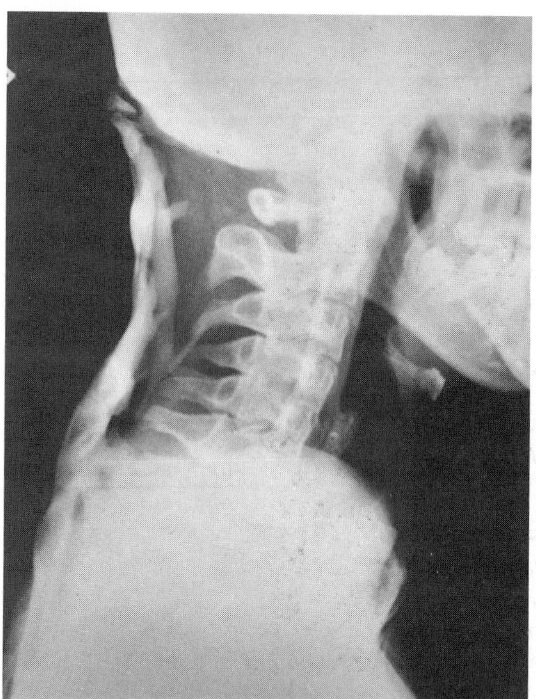

FIGURE 118.14. Radiograph illustrating new bone formation in the cervical area of a 17-year-old girl with myositis ossificans progressiva. She first noted pain, swelling, and limitation of motion in this area after trauma 10 years previously.

Diphosphonate treatment may suppress, at least temporarily, the development of new areas of mineralization following surgical excision of ectopic bone, but the ultimate value of these agents is uncertain (42). Corticosteroids may relieve the acute symptoms of inflammation and retard progression of the disease in some patients (42).

Calcinosis Associated with Connective Tissue Disease

In systemic sclerosis, the calcareous deposits are generally confined to the extremities and are particularly frequent on the flexor surfaces of the terminal phalanges, around joints, and near other bony eminences (calcinosis circumscripta) (Fig. 118.15). Cervical paraspinal calcification in patients with scleroderma appeared to be located in cervical synovial articulations and were associated with pain and radiculopathy (118). Constrictive pericarditis in a patient with CREST syndrome was attributed to pericardial calcification (119). Most of these patients suffer from the limited cutaneous (CREST syndrome) variant. In contrast, widespread encasing calcification of the skin, subcutaneous and periarticular tissues, as well as involvement of the deeper structures, occurs later in the course of polymyositis-dermatomyositis (calcinosis universalis). This process includes

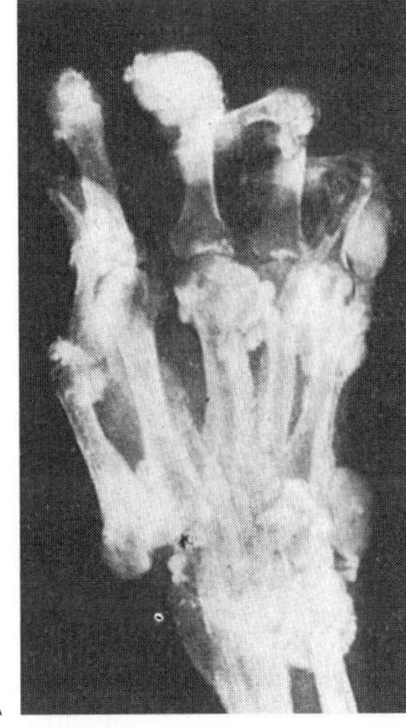

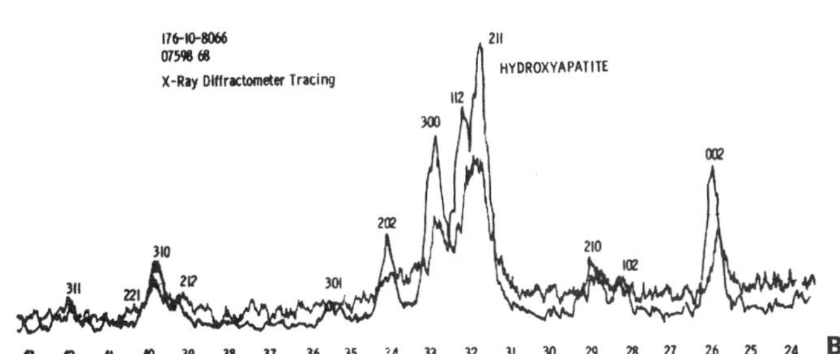

FIGURE 118.15. Dystrophic calcinosis. **A:** Radiograph of the hand of a woman with polymyositis showing extensive calcinosis involving both subcutaneous tissues and tendon sheaths. **B:** X-ray diffraction patterns. The labeled spectra are derived from a hydroxyapatite control, and the spectra with lower peak heights are from the patient. Correspondence of peak positions suggests the presence of hydroxyapatite. (See Chapter 117 for additional information on identification of calcium phosphate crystals.)

tendons, tendon plaques, and nodules and is often associated with erosive arthropathy, severe joint contractures, or ankylosis (120). Calcinosis most often complicates childhood dermatomyositis (40–74% of cases) and is associated with late treatment, suboptimal dosage of corticosteroids, or severe myopathy unresponsive to steroids (121). The latter patients more frequently demonstrate a linear, reticular pattern of calcification (122). In one patient with systemic lupus erythematosus receiving hemodialysis, calcinosis cutis was associated with pseudocyst formation around interphalangeal joints (123).

The standard method of detection of dystrophic calcification has been the roentgenogram. However, computed tomographic scanning can identify calcinosis in symptomatic but radiographically normal areas (124). The precipitates of calcium in the skin appear as pleomorphic crystals—needles and large plates—in the elastic fibers of the connective tissue (125). X-ray diffraction and electron microscopy identify these crystals as HA (126), although they undoubtedly include other members of the BCP crystal family (6).

Patients have normal concentrations of serum calcium, phosphorus, and alkaline phosphatase activity, but calcium balance studies have yielded conflicting data. In patients with calcinosis cutis, increased absorption and retention of calcium has been evident. Paradoxically, this is associated with a more rapid disappearance rate of radiolabeled calcium injected intradermally (42). When a woman with scleroderma and calcinosis was placed on a calcium-restricted diet, the bone resorption rate increased, and urinary excretion of calcium fell normally, but the net calcium accretion rate (which included extraosseous calcium deposition) remained constant (127). Urinary excretion of a vitamin K–dependent, calcium-binding protein called γ-carboxyglutamic acid, or Gla, is increased in dermatomyositis and scleroderma patients with calcinosis (42,128).

Animal Models of Basic Calcium Phosphate Crystal Deposition

The basis of the deposition of calcium salts in the tissues of patients with systemic connective tissue disorders and other forms of dystrophic calcification is unclear. Spontaneous periarticular calcinosis has been reported in dogs (129,130) and may be familial. Renal failure and associated hyperphosphatemia caused tumoral calcifications in a dog (131). In a canine model of OA, HA crystals were detected in synovial fluids early in the course of the arthritis (132). Several different forms of cutaneous, subcuticular, periarticular, and visceral calcification have been produced experimentally in the rat by calciphylaxis, but none serves as a model of human calcinosis. The initial precipitation of calcium salts in experimental cutaneous calcinosis in the rat occurs in areas rich in proteoglycan or, in some instances, in collagen fibers, which appear to act as a matrix for calcification. Reginato et al. (133) calcified rabbit synovium with vitamin D. These deposits were composed of BCP crystals identical to those found in the synovial fluid of patients (6). Calcification of porcine cardiac valve prostheses has been shown to occur on devitalized porcine connective tissue cells and collagen fibers, and abnormal collagen cross-links have been implicated in this process (42).

Treatment

Numerous drugs, hormones, and a host of nonspecific measures have been used unsuccessfully in the treatment of calcinosis (42). The identification of the calcium-binding amino acid Gla (γ-carboxyglutamic acid) in pathologic soft tissue calcification (128,134) provides a rationale for the use of warfarin therapy. Synthesis of Gla-containing proteins, such as prothrombin, is vitamin K–dependent. Reports of success (134,135), however, must be viewed in the light of the natural tendency for spontaneous resorption as already discussed. Probenecid and aluminum hydroxide have been used successfully to treat calcinosis in dermatomyositis, but the same caveat applies in the absence of suitable controls (136,137). Diltiazem has been reported to control calcinosis in limited scleroderma (138). Surgical excision of large calcareous masses may be helpful in selected instances (42,139). Resolution of calcinosis in juvenile dermatomyositis was accompanied by serious hypercalcemia in one case (140). Colchicine may be effective in reducing soft tissue inflammation surrounding such deposits (141). Ectopic calcification following paraplegia or hip surgery in animals was prevented by indomethacin and prednisone plus low-dose radiation therapy (142).

OTHER LOCALIZED CALCIFIC SYNDROMES

A variety of local and regional sites of calcification have been associated with rheumatic complaints. In addition to the common syndromes of the shoulder and hip, idiopathic calcific tendinitis and tenosynovitis have produced instances of carpal tunnel syndrome (143) and wrist and finger flexor tenosynovitis (144), all believed to be due to repeated minor trauma. A similar cause has been suggested for calcinosis cutis affecting the knee (42) and probably accounts for cases of penile (145) and scrotal calcification (146), and calcinosis cutis following electromyography (147). Milia-like calcinosis (and connective tissue nevi) were reported in a patient with Down syndrome (148). Synthetic retinoid therapy is associated with spinal hyperostosis, diffuse idiopathic skeletal hyperostosis (DISH), and extraspinal tendon and ligament calcification (149). DISH (150) and ligamentum flavum calcification (151) may cause cervical myelopathy. Nontraumatic causes of neck pain now include calcific tendinitis of the longus colli muscle (152) and retropharyngeal calcific tendinitis (153). Gastric mucosal calcinosis, consisting of calcified aluminum phosphate deposits, has been observed in some organ transplant patients ingesting antacids containing aluminum or sucralfate (154). A patient with multiple myeloma developed progressive respiratory failure from pulmonary calcinosis (155).

UNANSWERED QUESTIONS

Many questions about BCP crystal arthropathies and periarthropathies remain. Such crystals have been described in the synovial fluid of patients with many different types of joint disease. Whether BCP crystals participate in the inflammation or degeneration of OA and other diseases or merely represent an epiphenomenon is unknown (42).

Campion and co-workers (156) found a considerable overlap in the features of patients with destructive shoulder arthritis resulting from different primary etiologies. They refer to severe, destructive shoulder lesions unassociated with any other definable arthropathy as "idiopathic destructive arthritis of the shoulder," and suggest that crystals are not related to any specific type of arthropathy (156), a proposition with which the authors agree.

Perhaps the greatest mystery is the mechanism of pathologic calcification. Codman considered the formation of periarticular calcific deposits in the shoulder to be secondary to tissue necrosis (1), but Sarkar and Uhthoff (22) were unable to detect histologic evidence of necrosis. They hypothesized that hypoxia induces tendon metaplasia into fibrocartilage. BCP crystals then form in matrix vesicles generated by chondrocytes, subsequently coalescing into larger deposits (1). Vascular invasion and cellular resorption of the calcific deposits follow, leaving a reconstituted vascularized tendon.

Anderson has presented a unified concept of pathologic calcification encompassing both metastatic and dystrophic forms. Matrix vesicles or mitochondria may serve as repositories for calcium and, on exposure to sufficient phosphate, mineralization begins (157). The mechanism responsible for most pathologic calcifications occurring in the absence of hypercalcemia or hyperphosphatemia is unclear.

REFERENCES

1. Halverson PB, McCarty DJ. Basic calcium phosphate (apatite, octacalcium phosphate, tricalcium phosphate) crystal deposition diseases. In: McCarty DJ, ed. *Arthritis and allied conditions,* 11th ed. Philadelphia: Lea & Febiger, 1989:1737–1755.
2. Dieppe PA, Crocker P, Huskisson EC, et al. Apatite deposition disease. A new arthropathy. *Lancet* 1976;1:266–269.
3. Schumacher HR, Smolyo AP, Tse RL, et al. Arthritis associated with apatite crystals. *Ann Intern Med* 1977;87:411–416.
4. Faure G, Daculsi G, Netter P, et al. Apatites in heterotopic calcifications. *Scan Electron Microsc* 1982;4:1624–1634.
5. McCarty DJ, Lehr JR, Halverson PB. Crystal populations in human synovial fluid. Identification of apatite, octacalcium phosphate, tricalcium phosphate. *Arthritis Rheum* 1983;26:1220–1224.
6. Fritz P, Bardin T, Laredo, J-D, et al. Paradiaphyseal calcific tendinitis with cortical bone erosion. *Arthritis Rheum* 1994;37:718–723.
7. Halverson PB, Carrera GF, McCarty DJ. Milwaukee shoulder syndrome: fifteen additional cases and a description of contributing factors. *Arch Intern Med* 1990;150:677–682.
8. Schumacher HR, Rothfuss S, Bertken R, et al. Unusual laminated birefringent arrays of apatite crystals in inflammatory arthritis. *Arthritis Rheum* 1987;30:S106.
9. Paul H, Reginato AJ, Schumacher HR. Alizarin red S staining as a screening test to detect calcium compounds in synovial fluid. *Arthritis Rheum* 1983;26:191–200.

10. Bardin T, Bucki B, Lansaman J, et al. Coloration par le rouge alizarine des liquides articulaires. *Rev Rhum Mal Osteoartic* 1987;54:149–154.
11. Gordon C, Swan A, Dieppe P. Detection of crystals in synovial fluids by light microscopy: sensitivity and reliability. *Ann Rheum Dis* 1989;48:737–742.
12. Lazcano O, Li CY, Pierre RV, et al. Clinical utility of the alizarin red S stain on permanent preparations to detect calcium-containing compounds in synovial fluid. *Am J Clin Pathol* 1993; 99:90–96.
13. Halverson PB, Cheung HS, McCarty DJ. "Milwaukee shoulder": association of microspheroids containing hydroxyapatite crystals, active collagenase and neutral protease with rotator cuff defects: II. Synovial fluid studies. *Arthritis Rheum* 1981;24:474–483.
14. Halverson PB, McCarty DJ. Patterns of radiographic abnormalities associated with basic calcium phosphate and calcium pyrophosphate dihydrate crystal deposition in the knee. *Ann Rheum Dis* 1986;45:603–605.
15. Cherian PV, Schumacher HR. Diagnostic potential of rapid electron microscopic analysis of joint effusions. *Arthritis Rheum* 1982;25:98–100.
16. Fernandez-Dupica MP, Reginato AJ, Ramachandrula A. Quantitative analysis of BCP crystals in synovial fluid using Arsenazo III. *Arthritis Rheum* 1994;37:S413.
17. Blair JM, Sorenson LB, Arnsdorf MF, et al. The application of atomic force microscopy for the detection of microcrystals in synovial fluid from patients with recurrent synovitis. *Semin Arthritis Rheum* 1995;24:359–369.
18. Halverson PB. Basic calcium phosphate (apatite, octacalcium phosphate, tricalcium phosphate) crystal deposition diseases; Calcinosis. In: Koopman WJ, ed. *Arthritis and allied conditions,* 13th ed. Baltimore: Williams & Wilkins, 1997:2127–2146.
19. Fam AG, Rubenstein J. Hydroxyapatite pseudopodagra. *Arthritis Rheum* 1989;32:741–747.
20. Uhthoff HK, Sarkar K, Maynard JA. Calcifying tendinitis. *Clin Orthop Rel Res* 1976;118:164–168.
21. Hutton CW, Maddison PJ, Collins AJ, et al. Intra-articular apatite deposition in mixed connective tissue disease: crystallographic and technetium scanning characteristics. *Ann Rheum Dis* 1988;47:1027–1030.
22. Sarkar K, Uhthoff HK. Rotator cuff tendinopathies with calcification. In: Rubin RP, Weiss G, Putney JW, eds. *Calcium in biological systems.* New York: Plenum Press, 1984:725–730.
23. Gravanis MG, Gaffney EF. Idiopathic calcifying tenosynovitis. Histopathologic features and possible pathogenesis. *Am J Surg Pathol* 1983;7:359–361.
24. Ali SY, Griffiths S. New types of calcium phosphate crystals in arthritis cartilage. *Semin Arthritis Rheum* 1981;11:124–126.
25. Stein H, Bab IA, Sela J. The occurrence of hydroxyapatite crystals in extracellular matrix vesicles after surgical manipulation of the rabbit knee joint. *Cell Tissue Res* 1981;214:449–454.
26. Doyle DV. Tissue calcification and inflammation in osteoarthritis. *J Pathol* 1982;136:199–216.
27. Huskisson EC, Dieppe PA, Tucher AC, et al. Another look at osteoarthritis. *Ann Rheum Dis* 1979;38:423–428.
28. Yosipovitch G, Yosipovitch Z. Acute calcific periarthritis of the hand and elbows in women. *J Rheumatol* 1993;20:1533–1538.
29. Ebenbichler GR, Derdogmus CB, Resch KL, et al. Ultrasound therapy for calcific tendinitis of the shoulder. *N Engl J Med* 1999;340:1533–1538.
30. Dieppe PA, Crocker PR, Corke CF, et al. Synovial fluid crystals. *Q J Med* 1979;192:533–553.
31. Gibilisco PA, Schumacher HR, Hollander JL, et al. Synovial fluid crystals in osteoarthritis. *Arthritis Rheum* 1985;28: 511–515.
32. Swan A, Chapman B, Heap P, et al. Submicroscopic crystals in osteoarthritic synovial fluids. *Ann Rheum Dis* 1994;53: 467–470.
33. Swan AJ, Heywood BR, Dieppe PA. Extraction of calcium containing crystals from synovial fluids and articular cartilage. *J Rheumatol* 1992;19:1764–1773.
34. Lagier R, Boivin G, Gerster JC. Carpal tunnel syndrome associated with mixed calcium pyrophosphate dihydrate and apatite crystal deposition in tendon synovial sheath. *Arthritis Rheum* 1984;27:1190–1195.
35. Adams R. *A treatise on rheumatic gout or chronic rheumatic arthritis of all the joints,* 2nd ed. Dublin: Fannin, 1873.
36. Adams R. *Illustration of the effects of rheumatic joint in chronic rheumatic arthritis of all the articulations; with descriptive and explanatory statements.* London: John Churchill, 1857:1–31.
37. McCarty DJ. Robert Adams' rheumatic arthritis of the shoulder: Milwaukee shoulder revisited. *J Rheumatol* 1989;16: 668–670.
38. Craig EV. The acromioclavicular joint cyst. *Clin Orthop Rel Res* 1986;202:189–192.
39. Dennis DA, Ferlic DC, Clayton MD. Acromial stress fracture associated with cuff-tear arthropathy. *J Bone Joint Surg* 1986; 68A:937–940.
40. Klimaitis A, Carroll G, Owen E. Rapidly progressive destructive arthropathy of the shoulder—a viewpoint on pathogenesis. *J Rheumatol* 1988;15:1859–1862.
41. McCarty DJ, Swanson AB, Elihart RH. Hemorrhagic rupture of the shoulder. *J Rheumatol* 1994;21:1134–1137.
42. Halverson PB, McCarty DJ. Basic calcium phosphate (apatite, octacalcium phosphate, tricalcium phosphate) crystal deposition diseases. In: McCarty DJ, ed. *Arthritis and allied conditions,* 12th ed. Philadelphia: Lea & Febiger, 1993:1857–1872.
43. Ter Borg EJ, Eggelmijer F, Jaspers PJTM, et al. Milwaukee shoulder associated with primary hyperparathyroidism. *J Rheumatol* 1995;22:561–562.
44. Halverson PB, Garancis JC, McCarty DJ. Histopathologic and ultrastructural studies of Milwaukee shoulder syndrome—a basic calcium phosphate crystal arthropathy. *Ann Rheum Dis* 1984;43:734–741.
45. Dieppe PA, Cawston T, Mercer E, et al. Synovial fluid collagenase in patients with destructive arthritis of the elbow joint. *Arthritis Rheum* 1988;31:882–890.
46. Vignon E, Balblance JC, Mathieu P, et al. Metalloprotease activity, phospholipase A2 activity and cytokine concentration in osteoarthritis synovial fluids. *Osteoarthritis Cartilage* 1993;1: 115–120.
47. Halverson PB, Greene AS, Cheung HS. Intracellular calcium responses to basic calcium phosphate crystals in fibroblasts. *Osteoarthritis Cartilage* 1998;6:324–329.
48. Biswas C, Dayer J. Stimulation of collagenase production by collagen in mammalian cell cultures. *Cell* 1979;18:1035–1041.
49. Evans CH, Means DC, Cosgrove JR. Release of neutral proteinase from mononuclear phagocytes and synovial cells in response to cartilaginous wear particles in vitro. *Biochim Biophys Acta* 1981;677:287–294.
50. Cheung HS, Halverson PB, McCarty DJ. Release of collagenase, neutral protease and prostaglandins from cultured synovial cells by hydroxyapatite and calcium pyrophosphate dihydrate. *Arthritis Rheum* 1981;24:1338–1344.
51. Halverson PB, Cheung HS, McCarty DJ. Enzymatic release of microspheroids containing hydroxyapatite crystals from synovium and of calcium pyrophosphate dihydrate crystals from cartilage. *Ann Rheum Dis* 1982;41:527–531.
52. McCarty DJ, Cheung HS. Prostaglandin (PG)E2 generation by cultured synovial fibroblasts exposed to microcrystals containing calcium. *Ann Rheum Dis* 1985;44:316–320.
53. Caniggia A, Gennari C, Vattimo A, et al. Prostaglandin

(PGE2): a possible mechanism for bone destruction in calcinosis circumscripta. *Calcif Tissue Res* 1978;25:53–57.
54. Palmer DW, McCarty DJ. Clearance of 85Sr labelled calcium phosphate (CP) crystals from normal rabbit joints. *Arthritis Rheum* 1984;27:427–432.
55. Cheung HS, Ryan LM. Role of crystal deposition in matrix degradation. In: Woessner JF Jr, Howell DS, eds. *Joint cartilage degradation—basic and clinical aspects.* New York: Marcel Dekker, 1993:209–223.
56. Cheung HS, Van Wyk JJ, Russell WE, et al. Mitogenic activity of hydroxyapatite: requirement for somatomedin C. *J Cell Physiol* 1986;128:143–148.
57. Mitchell PG, Pledger WJ, Cheung HS. Molecular mechanisms of basic calcium phosphate crystal-induced mitogenesis: role of protein kinase. *J Biol Chem* 1989;264:14071–14077.
58. McCarthy GM, Mitchell PG, Cheung HS. The mitogenic response to stimulation with basic calcium phosphate crystals is accompanied by induction and secretion of collagenase in human fibroblasts. *Arthritis Rheum* 1991;34:1021–1030.
59. Meng ZH, Hudson AP, Schumacher HR Jr, et al. Monosodium urate, hydroxyapatite, and calcium pyrophosphate crystals induce tumor necrosis factor-α expression in a mononuclear cell line. *J Rheumatol* 1997;24:2385–2388.
60. Westacott CI, Whicher JT, Barnes IC, et al. Synovial fluid concentrations of five different cytokines in rheumatic diseases. *Ann Rheum Dis* 1990;49:676–681.
61. Swan A, Dularay B, Dieppe P. A comparison of the effects of urate, hydroxyapatite and diamond crystals on polymorphonuclear cells: relationship of mediator release to the surface area and adsorptive capacity of different particles. *J Rheumatol* 1990;17:1346–1352.
62. Terkeltaub RA, Santoro DA, Mandel G, et al. Serum and plasma inhibit neutrophil stimulation by hydroxyapatite crystals: evidence that serum α2-HS glycoprotein is a potent and specific crystal-bound inhibitor. *Arthritis Rheum* 1988;31: 1081–1089.
63. Schumacher HR Jr, Stineman M, Rahman M, et al. The relationship between clinical and synovial fluid findings and treatment response in osteoarthritis (OA) of the knee. *Arthritis Rheum* 1990;33:S92.
64. Carroll GJ, Stuart RA, Armstrong JA, et al. Hydroxyapatite crystals are a frequent finding in osteoarthritic synovial fluid, but are not related to increased concentrations of keratan sulfate or interleukin-1 beta. *J Rheumatol* 1991;18:861–865.
65. Gerster JC. Intraarticular apatite crystal deposition as a predictor of erosive osteoarthritis of the fingers. *J Rheumatol* 1994;21:2164–2165.
66. Patel KJ, Weidensaul D, Palma C, et al. Milwaukee shoulder with massive bilateral cysts: effective therapy for hydrops of the shoulder. *J Rheumatol* 1997;24:2479–2483.
67. Caporali R. Tidal irrigation in Milwaukee shoulder syndrome. *J Rheumatol* 1994;21:1781–1782.
68. Citera G, Lazaro MA, Maldonado Cocco JA, et al. Apatite deposition in polymyositis subluxing arthropathy. *J Rheumatol* 1996;23:22551–553.
69. Fam AG, Pritzker KPH. Acute calcific periarthritis in scleroderma. *J Rheumatol* 1992;19:1580–1585.
70. Gilsanz V, Bernstein BH. Joint calcification following intraarticular corticosteroid therapy. *Radiology* 1984;151:647–649.
71. Dalinka MK, Stewart V, Bomalski JS, et al. Periarticular calcifications in association with intra-articular corticosteroid injections. *Radiology* 1984;153:615–618.
72. Toussirot E, Kremer P, Benmansour A, et al. Giant calcification in soft tissue after shoulder corticosteroid injection. *J Rheumatol* 1996:23:181–182.
73. Lauerman WC, Smith BG, Kenmore PI. Spontaneous bilateral rupture of the extensor mechanism of the knee in two patients on chronic ambulatory peritoneal dialysis. *Orthopedics* 1987;10:589–591.
74. Brown EA, Arnold IR, Gower PE. Dialysis arthropathy: complication of long term hemodialysis. *Br Med J* 1986;292: 163–166.
75. Hardouin P, Flipo R-M, Foissac-Gegoux P, et al. Current aspects of osteoarticular pathology in patients undergoing hemodialysis: study of 80 patients: 1. Clinical and radiological analysis. *J Rheumatol* 1987;14:780–783.
76. Menery K, Braunstein E, Brown M, et al. Musculoskeletal symptoms related to arthropathy in patients receiving dialysis. *J Rheumatol* 1988;15:1848–1854.
77. Resnick DL. Erosive arthritis of the hand and wrist in hyperparathyroidism. *Radiology* 1974;110:263–269.
78. Kuntz D, et al. Destructive spondyloarthropathy in hemodialyzed patients: a new syndrome. *Arthritis Rheum* 1984;27: 369–375.
79. Goldstein S, et al. Chronic arthropathy in long-term hemodialysis. *Am J Med* 1985;78:82–86.
80. McCarthy JT, Dahlberg PJ, Krieghauser JS, et al. Erosive spondyloarthropathy in long-term dialysis patients: relationship to severe hyperparathyroidism. *Mayo Clin Proc* 1988;63: 446–452.
81. Rubin LA, Fam AG, Rubenstein J, et al. Erosive azotemic arthropathy. *Arthritis Rheum* 1984;27:1086–1094.
82. Huaux J, Noel H, Malghem J, et al. Erosive azotemic osteoarthropathy: possible role of amyloidosis. *Arthritis Rheum* 1985;28:1075–1076.
83. Miyata T, Inagi R, Iida Y, et al. Involvement of (beta) 2–microglobulin modified with advanced glycation end products in the pathogenesis of hemodialysis-associated amyloidosis. *J Clin Invest* 1994;93:521–528.
84. Bardin T, Kuntz D, Zingraff J, et al. Synovial amyloidosis in patients undergoing long-term hemodialysis. *Arthritis Rheum* 1985;28:1052–1058.
85. Bardin T, Zingraff J, Shirahama T, et al. Hemodialysis-associated amyloidosis and beta-2 microglobulin. *Am J Med* 1987; 83:419–424.
86. Allain TJ, Stevens PE, Bridges LR, et al. Dialysis myelopathy: quadriparesis due to extradural amyloid of α_2 microglobulin origin. *Br Med J* 1988;296:752–753.
87. Moskowitz RW, Vertes V, Schwartz A, et al. Crystal-induced inflammation associated with chronic renal failure treated with periodic hemodialysis. *Am J Med* 1969;47:450–460.
88. Hoffman GS, Schumacher HR, Paul H, et al. Calcium oxalate microcrystalline-associated arthritis in end-stage renal disease. *Ann Intern Med* 1982;97:36–42.
89. Reginato A, Seoane JLF, Alvarez CB, et al. Arthropathy and cutaneous calcinosis in hemodialysis oxalosis. *Arthritis Rheum* 1986;29:1387–1396.
90. Worcester E, Nakagawa Y, Bushinsky D, et al. Evidence that serum calcium oxalate supersaturation is a consequence of oxalate retention in patients with chronic renal failure. *J Clin Invest* 1986;77:1888–1896.
91. Netter P, Delongeas JL, Faure G, et al. Inflammatory effect of aluminum phosphate. *Ann Rheum Dis* 1983;42(suppl):114.
92. Netter P, Kessler M, Durnel D, et al. Aluminum in joint tissues of chronic renal failure patients treated with regular hemodialysis and aluminum compounds. *J Rheumatol* 1984;11:66–70.
93. Melikoglu M, Apaydin S, Hamuryudan V, et al. Calciphylaxis: a condition mimicking necrotizing vasculitis. *Clin Rheumatol* 1996;15:498–500.
94. Barri YM, Graves GS, Knochel JP. Calciphylaxis in a patient with Crohn's disease in the absence of end-stage renal disease. *Am J Kidney Dis* 1997;29:773–776.

95. Tamura M, Hiroshige K, Osajima A, et al. A dialysis patient with systemic calciphylaxis exhibiting rapidly progressive visceral ischemia and acral gangrene. *Internal Med* 1995;34:908–912.
96. Fischer AH, Morris DJ. Pathogenesis of calciphylaxis:study of three cases with literature review. *Hum Pathol* 1995;26:1055–1064.
97. Worth RL. Calciphylaxis: pathogenesis and therapy. *J Cutaneous Med Surg* 1998;2:245–248.
98. Butler RC, Dieppe PA, Keat ACS. Calcinosis of joints and periarticular tissues associated with vitamin D intoxication. *Ann Rheum Dis* 1985;44:494–498.
99. Duthie JS, Solanki HP, Krishnamurthy M, et al. Milk-alkali syndrome with metastatic calcification. *Am J Med* 1995;99:102–103.
100. Libson E, Wechsler RJ, Steiner RM. Pulmonary calcinosis following orthotopic liver transplantation. *J Thorac Imaging* 1993;8:305–308.
101. Yu SL, Li RZ, Bian ZH. Tumoral calcium pyrophosphate dihydrate deposition disease. Report of a case with a review of the literature. *Chin Med J* 1992;105:780–784.
102. deGraaf P, Ruiter DJ, Scheffer E, et al. Metastatic skin calcifications: a rare phenomenon in dialysis patients. *Dermatologica* 1980;161:28–32.
103. Wenzel-Seifert K, Harwig S, Keller F. Fulminant calcinosis in two patients after kidney transplantation. *Am J Nephrol* 1991;11:497–500.
104. Kovarik J, Frühwald F, Seidl G, et al. Tumorous paraarticular calcifications due to undigested phosphate-binders in a patient undergoing regular hemodialysis [letter]. *Clin Nephrol* 1984;21:141–142.
105. Fernandez E, Montoliu J. Successful treatment of massive uraemic tumoral calcinosis with daily haemodialysis and very low calcium dialysate. *Nephrol Dial Transplant* 1994;9:1207–1209.
106. Walton K, Swinson DR. Acute calcific periarthritis associated with transient hypocalcaemia secondary to hypoparathyroidism. *Br J Rheumatol* 1983;22:179–180.
107. Malik M, Acharya S. Tumoral calcinosis of the fingers. *Int Orthop* 1993;17:279–281.
108. McKee PH, Liomba NG, Hutt MSR. Tumoral calcinosis: a pathological study of fifty-six cases. *Br J Dermatol* 1982;107:669–674.
109. Zerwekh JE, Sanders LA, Townsend J, et al. Tumoral calcinosis: evidence for concurrent defects in renal tubular phosphorus transport and in 1α,25-dihydrocholecalciferol synthesis. *Calcif Tissue Int* 1980;32:1–6.
110. Lufkin EG, Kumar R, Heath H III. Hyperphosphatemic tumoral calcinosis: effects of phosphate depletion on vitamin D metabolism, and of acute hypocalcemia on parathyroid hormone secretion and action. *J Clin Endocrinol Metab* 1983;56:1319–1322.
111. Lyles KW, Burkes EJ, Ellis GJ, et al. Genetic transmission of tumoral calcinosis: autosomal dominant with variable clinical expressivity. *J Clin Endocrinol Metab* 1985;60:1093–1096.
112. Gal G, Metzker A, Garlick J, et al. Head and neck manifestations of tumoral calcinosis. *Oral Surg* 1994;77:158–166.
113. Slavin RE, Wen J, Kumar D, Evans EB. Familial tumoral calcinosis—a clinical, histopathologic, and ultrastructural study with an analysis of its calcifying process and pathogenesis. *Am J Surg Pathol* 1993;17:788–802.
114. Boskey AL, Vigorita VJ, Sencer O, et al. Chemical, microscopic, and ultrastructural characterization of the mineral deposits in tumoral calcinosis. *Clin Orthop Rel Res* 1983;178:258–269.
115. Salvi A, Cerudelli B, Cimino A, et al. Phosphaturic action of calcitonin in pseudotumoral calcinosis. *Horm Metab Res* 1983;15:260.
116. Suzuki Y, Bisada K, Takeda M. Demonstration of myositis ossificans by 99mTc pyrophosphate bone scanning. *Radiology* 1974;111:663–664.
117. Buhain WJ, Rammohan G, Berger HW. Pulmonary function in myositis ossificans progressiva. *Am Rev Respir Dis* 1974;110:333–337.
118. Schweitzer ME, Cervilla V, Manaster BJ, et al. Cervical paraspinal calcification in collagen vascular diseases. *AJR* 1991;157:523–525.
119. Pancal P, Adams E, Hsieh A. Calcific constrictive pericarditis. *Arthritis Rheum* 1996;39:347–350.
120. Kazmers IS, Scoville CD, Schumacher HR. Polymyositis associated apatite arthritis. *J Rheumatol* 1988;15:1019–1021.
121. Bowyer SL, Blane CE, Sullivan DB, et al. Childhood dermatomyositis: factors predicting functional outcome and development of dystrophic calcification. *J Pediatr* 1983;103:882–888.
122. Blane CE, White SJ, Braunstein EM, et al. Patterns of calcification in childhood dermatomyositis. *AJR* 1984;142:397–400.
123. Kumakiri M, Kokuba J, Tanaka H, et al. Pseudocysts around the interphalangeal joints as a manifestation of calcinosis cutis in a patient with lupus nephritis undergoing hemodialysis. *Arch Dermatol* 1992;128:120–121.
124. Randle HW, Sander HM, Howard K. Early diagnosis of calcinosis cutis in childhood dermatomyositis using computed tomography. *JAMA* 1986;256:1137–1138.
125. Leroux J-L, Pernot F, Fedou P, et al. Ultrastructural and crystallographic study of calcifications from a patient with CREST syndrome. *J Rheumatol* 1983;10:242–246.
126. Kawakami T, Nakamura C, Hasegawa H, et al. Ultrastructural study of calcinosis universalis with dermatomyositis. *J Cutan Pathol* 1986;13:135–143.
127. Kales AN, Phang JM. Dietary calcium perturbation in patients with abnormal calcium deposition. *J Clin Endocrinol Metab* 1970;31:204–212.
128. Moore SE, Jump AA, Smiley JD. Effect of warfarin sodium therapy on excretion of 4-carboxy-L-glutamic acid in scleroderma, dermatomyositis, and myositis ossificans progressiva. *Arthritis Rheum* 1986;29:344–351.
129. Ellison GW, Norrdin RW. Multicentric periarticular calcinosis in a pup. *J Am Vet Med Assoc* 1980;177:542–546.
130. Woodard JC, Shields RP, Aldrich HC, et al. Calcium phosphate deposition disease in Great Danes. *Vet Pathol* 1982;19:464–485.
131. Croom AL, Houston DM. Hyperphosphatemic tumoral calcinosis in a young dog with renal failure. *Can Vet J* 1994;35:438–440.
132. Schumacher HR, Rubinow A, Rothfuss S, et al. Apatite crystal clumps in synovial fluid (SF) are an early finding in experimental canine osteoarthritis (OA). *Arthritis Rheum* 1994;37:S346.
133. Reginato AJ, Schumacher HR, Brighton CT. Experimental hydroxyapatite synovial and articular cartilage calcification: light and electron microscopic studies. *Arthritis Rheum* 1982;25:1239–1249.
134. Berger RG, Hadler NM. Treatment of calcinosis universalis secondary to dermatomyositis or scleroderma with low dose warfarin. *Arthritis Rheum* 1983;26:S11.
135. Yoshida S, Torikai K. The effects of warfarin on calcinosis in a patient with systemic sclerosis. *J Rheumatol* 1993;20:1233–1235.
136. Skuterud E, Sydnes AO, Haavik TK. Calcinosis in dermatomyositis treated with probenecid. *Scand J Rheumatol* 1981;10:92–94.
137. Nakagawa T, Takaiwa T. Calcinosis cutis in juvenile dermato-

myositis responsive to aluminum hydroxide treatment. *J Dermatol* 1993;20:558–560.

138. Palmieri GMA, Sebes JI, Aelion JA, et al. Treatment of calcinosis with diltiazem. *Arthritis Rheum* 1995;38:1646–1654.
139. Jones NF, Imbriglia JE, Steen VD, et al. Surgery for scleroderma of the hand. *J Hand Surg* 1987;12A:391–400.
140. Wilsher ML, Holdaway IM, North JDK. Hypercalcaemia during resolution of calcinosis in juvenile dermatomyositis. *Br Med J* 1984;288:1345.
141. Fuchs D, Fruchter L, Fishel B, et al. Colchicine suppression of local inflammation due to calcinosis in dermatomyositis and progressive systemic sclerosis. *Clin Rheumatol* 1986;5:527–530.
142. Ahrengart L, Lindgren V, Reinholt EP. Comparative study of the effects of radiation, indomethacin, prednisolone and ethane-1-hydroxy-1′, 1-diphosphonate (EHDP) in the prevention of ectopic bone formation. *Clin Orthop Res* 1988;229: 265–273.
143. Edwards AJ, Sill BJ, Macfarlane I. Carpal tunnel syndrome due to dystrophic calcification. *Aust NZ J Surg* 1984;54:491–492.
144. Selby CL. Acute calcific tendinitis of the hand: an infrequently recognized and frequently misdiagnosed form of periarthritis. *Arthritis Rheum* 1984;27:337–340.
145. Katoh N, Okabayashi K, Wakabayashi S, et al. Dystrophic calcinosis of the penis. *J Dermatol* 1993;114:114–117.
146. Germiyanoglu C, Ozkardes H, Peskircioglu L, et al. Scrotal calcinosis. *Int Urol Nephrol* 1994;26:349–352.
147. Johnson RC, Fitzpatrick JE, Hahn DE. Calcinosis cutis following electromyographic examination. *Cutis* 1993;52:161–164.
148. Sais G, Jucgla A, Moreno A, et al. Milia-like idiopathic calcinosis cutis and multiple connective tissue nevi in a patient with Down syndrome. *J Am Acad Dermatol* 1995;32:129–130.
149. DiGiovanna JJ, Helfgott RK, Gerber LH, et al. Extraspinal tendon and ligament calcification associated with long-term therapy with etretinate. *N Engl J Med* 1986;315:1177–1182.
150. Sakkas L, Thouas B, Kotsou S, et al. Cervical myelopathy with ankylosing hyperostosis of the spine. *Surg Neurol* 1985;24:43–46.
151. Miyasaka K, Kaneda K, Sato S, et al. Myelopathy due to ossification or calcification of the ligamentum flavum: radiologic and histologic evaluations. *Am J Neurol Radiol* 1983;4:629–632.
152. Widlus DM. Calcific tendinitis of the longus colli muscle: a cause of a traumatic neck pain. *Ann Emerg Med* 1985;14: 1014–1017.
153. Benanti JC, Gramling P, Bulat PI, et al. Retropharyngeal calcific tendinitis: report of five cases and review of the literature. *J Emerg Med* 1986;4:15–24.
154. Greenson JK, Trinidad SB, Pfeil SA, et al. Gastric mucosal calcinosis: calcified aluminum phosphate deposits secondary to aluminum-containing antacids or sucralfate therapy in organ transplant patients. *Am J Surg Pathol* 1993;17:45–50.
155. Kaburgi T, Nagai H, Sasaki T, et al. Case report of multiple myeloma with diffuse pulmonary calcinosis. *Jpn J Thorac Dis* 1991;29:1479–1483.
156. Campion GV, McCrae F, Alwan W, et al. Idiopathic destructive arthritis of the shoulder. *Semin Arthritis Rheum* 1988;17: 232–245.
157. Anderson HC. Calcific diseases—a concept. *Arch Pathol Lab Med* 1983;107:341–348.

119

CALCIUM OXALATE AND OTHER CRYSTALS OR PARTICLES ASSOCIATED WITH ARTHRITIS

ANTONIO J. REGINATO

Besides monosodium urate monohydrate (MSU), calcium pyrophosphate dihydrate (CPPD), and basic calcium phosphates (BCP), other crystals have been found in synovial fluid of patients with arthritis (1–3) (Table 119.1). Sufficient information is available to describe the clinical manifestations associated with calcium oxalate (1–16), cholesterol (1,3,17–26), lipid liquid crystals (1–3,27–34), cryoglobulin crystals (1–3,35–44), Charcot-Leyden crystals (1–3,45–49), and synthetic corticosteroid crystals (3) (see also Chapter 4). Other crystals such as cystine (1–3,50–54), hypoxanthine and xanthine (1–3,55–57), aluminum phosphate (1–3,58–64), hemoglobin (1–3, 65–68), hematoidin (1–3,65), and other crystalline lipids, thought to be fatty acids (2,69,70) have been described in synovial fluid, synovium muscle, or bone only in single case reports.

Exogenous particles described in association with foreign-body synovitis also often have a crystalline structure (2,3,71–80). Sea urchin spines, for example, are formed from calcium carbonate crystals (2,73), and talcum powder consists of magnesium silicate crystals or starch granules (74). Also, other foreign bodies such as plant thorns (71,77–79) and polyethylene and polymethyl methacrylate (75) particles have a paracrystalline or crystalline structure (2,66,71).

TABLE 119.1. CRYSTALS AND BIREFRINGENT PARTICLES UNCOMMONLY FOUND IN JOINT, MUSCLE, OR BONE

Calcium oxalate
Cholesterol
Lipid liquid crystals
Other crystalline lipids
Synthetic corticosteroid
Cystine
Xanthine
Hypoxanthine
Cryoglobulins
Charcot-Leyden (lysophospholipase) crystals
Aluminum
Hemoglobin
Hematoidin
Foreign bodies
Plant thorns
Sea urchin spines (calcium carbonate)
Polyethylene polymer
Methylmethacrylate polymer

CALCIUM OXALATE CRYSTAL DEPOSITION

The articular manifestations of both primary oxalosis and secondary oxalosis occurring in uremic patients managed with long-term hemodialysis have been confused in the past with those of gout and pseudogout (Fig. 119.1). Such patients may present a variety of articular manifestations (Fig. 119.2), as well as life-threatening organ involvement, which includes devastating peripheral vascular insufficiency with gangrene (1,3,81), cardiomyopathy (1,3,82), complete heart block (83), peripheral neuropathy (1,2), and pancytopenia (84).

Primary Oxalosis

Three types of primary oxalosis have been recognized. Primary hyperoxaluria type 1 (PH1) is a rare, autosomal-recessive, inborn error of glyoxylate metabolism caused by a deficiency of the liver-specific peroxisomal enzyme alanine glyoxylate aminotransferase (AGT) (85–88) (Fig. 119.3). The disease is characterized biochemically by increased synthesis and excretion of oxalate and glyoxylate, as a result of blockage of glyoxylate alternate pathways (Fig. 119.3), and clinically by urolithiasis, nephrocalcinosis, and, in severe cases, renal failure and systemic oxalosis. The disease is strikingly heterogeneous, both clinically and biochemically (85–93). From the clinical point of view, the disease exhibits wide variation with regard to age at disease onset (1 to 57 years), severity of clinical manifestations, degree of hyperoxaluria and hyperglycolic aciduria, rate of progression to systemic oxalosis, pyridoxine response, and age at death (1 to 65 years). Also, these patients show wide variation in the enzymatic activity, subcellular distribution, and genetic coding sequence of AGT (89–91). A study of 116 PH1

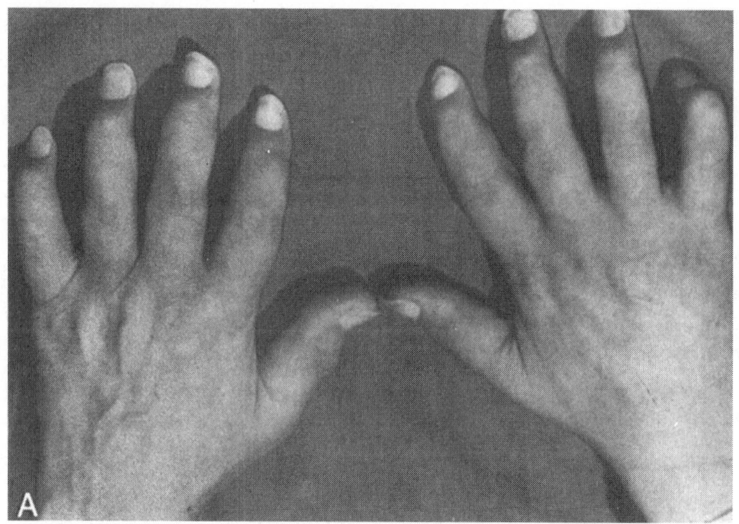

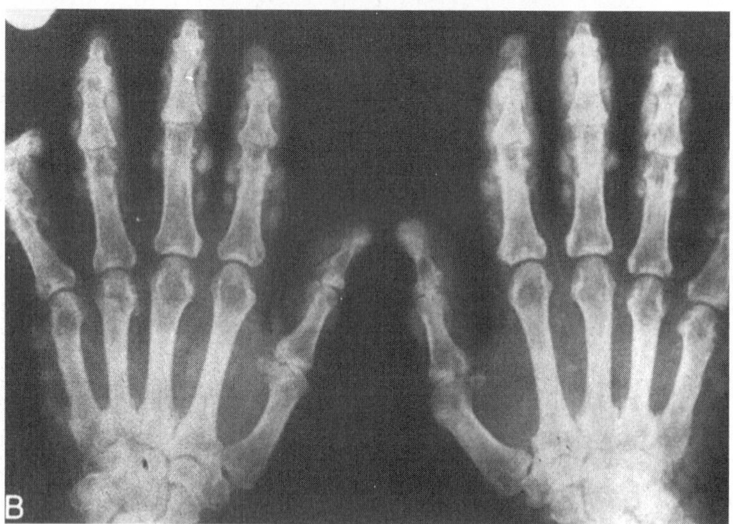

FIGURE 119.1. A: Hands of a patient with primary oxalosis mimicking gout or rheumatoid arthritis. **B:** Radiographs of the same hands, showing periarticular calcific deposits, bony erosions, and resorption of distal phalanges (From Schmidt KL, Leber HW, Schutterle G. Arthropathies bei primarer Oxalose-Krystallsynovitis oder Osteopathie. *Dtsch Med Wochenschr* 1981;106:19, with permission.)

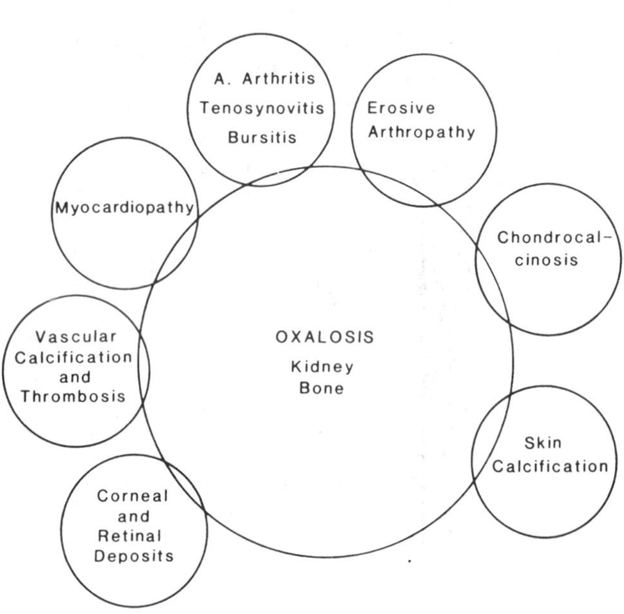

FIGURE 119.2. Clinical manifestations of oxalosis. A, acute.

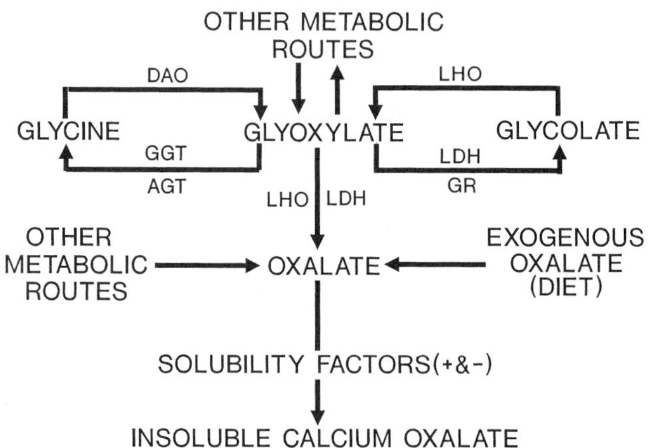

FIGURE 119.3. Genetic and environmental factors likely to affect oxalate metabolism. Peroxisomal enzymes: alanine: glyoxylate aminotransferase/serine: pyruvate aminotransferase (AGT) (deficient in PH1); D-amino acid oxidase/glycine oxidase (DAO); L-α-hydroxy acid oxidase/glycolate oxidase (LHO). Cytosolic enzymes: glutamate: glyoxylate aminotransferase/alanine; 2-oxiglutarate aminotransferase (GGT); glyoxyalate reductase/D-glycerate dehydrogenase (GR) (deficient in PH2); lactate dehydrogenase (LDH). (From Danpure CJ. Molecular clinical heterogeneity in primary hyperoxaluria type I. *Am J Kidney Dis* 1991;17:364–369, with permission.)

patients over the past 8 years has shown four main enzymatic phenotypes: (a) absence of both AGT catalytic activity and immunoreactive AGT protein (40% of patients); (b) absence of AGT catalytic activity but presence of immunoreactive protein (16% of patients); (c) presence of both AGT catalytic activity and immunoreactive protein (41% of patients) (in such cases, the AGT generally is mistargeted to the mitochondria instead of the peroxisome (91); and (d) a variation of the mistargeting phenotype in which AGT is equally distributed between peroxisomes and mitochondria, but is aggregated into matrical core-like structures in peroxisomes (3% of patients) (90–92). Several point mutations, each occurring at conserved positions in the coding region of the AGT gene, have been identified in these patients (85,92–95) (Fig. 119.4). The most common mutation leads to a Gly170 Arg amino acid substitution (85,94–97). The enzymic defect can be diagnosed using liver tissue obtained by needle biopsy (87), but cloning and sequencing of the human AGT gene will permit future screening for defects using genomic DNA from peripheral blood leukocytes (96,97).

Primary hyperoxaluria type 2 (PH2) is a recessive disorder that is the result of a defect in hydroxypyruvate metabolism due to deficiency of glyoxylate reductase (GR), which also has D-glycerate dehydrogenase activity (85,88,98,99) (Fig. 119.3). Both of these enzymic activities appear to reside in a single enzyme. Deficiency of D-glycerate dehydrogenase activity causes accumulation of its substrate, hydroxypyruvate, which is then converted to L-glycerate by the action of L-lactate dehydrogenase. Deficiency of glyoxylate reductase causes impaired conversion of glyoxylate to glycolate. Conversion of glyoxylate to oxalate by L-lactate dehydrogenase would explain the observed hyperoxaluria (Fig. 119.3). Decreased activity of D-glycerate acid dehydrogenase has been demonstrated in leukocytes of patients with PH2 (88). Sixteen of the 21 patients previously reported with type 2 hyperoxaluria initially had renal calculi between 6 months and 24 years of age (99–101). Five affected relatives seemed to have had no symptoms and were identified only because their siblings also had the disorder (100,101), thus suggesting that this subset of asymptomatic patients may be more common than originally suspected. PH2 may be a more benign disease with a better long-term prognosis for renal function than PH1 (101).

A third form of hyperoxaluria, PH3, is due to primary increased absorption of oxalate from the small bowel (85). In PH1 and PH2, the renal insufficiency is associated with rapid, progressive deposition of calcium oxalate crystals in kidney, myocardium, skin, bone, and blood vessels (88). Oxalate crystals have been described in synovium, tendon sheaths, articular cartilage, and bone (1). Several reports have described in detail the clinical and radiographic musculoskeletal manifestations of PH1 (10–12,15,16) (Table 119.2).

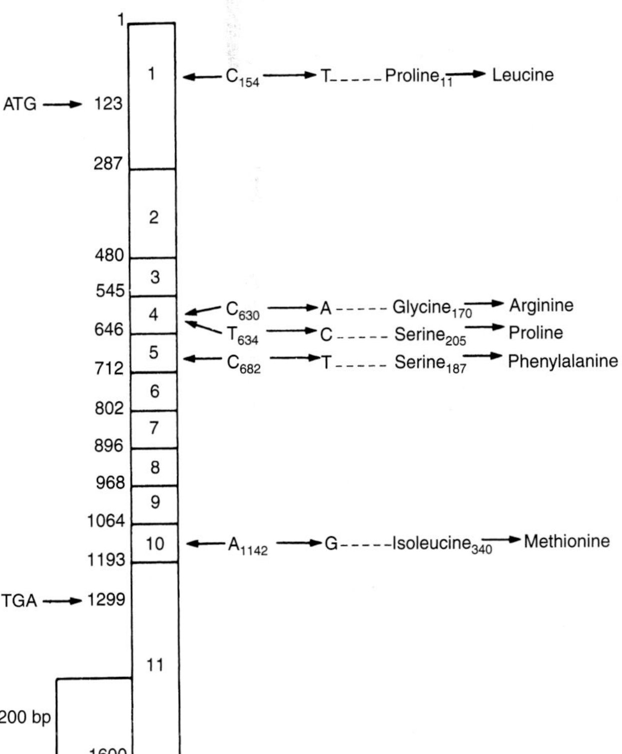

FIGURE 119.4. Diagram of full length AGT cDNA divided into numbered boxes representing 11 exons. Point mutations are shown to the **right** of the diagram. The coding region extends from nucleotide 123 to nucleotide 1299. (Data from Purdue PE, Lumb MJ, Fox M, et al. Characterization and chromosomal mapping of a genomic clone encoding human alanine: glyoxylate aminotransferase. *Genomics* 1991;10:34–42; from Watts RWE. Primary hyperoxaluria type I. *Q J Med* 1994;97:593–600, with permission.)

TABLE 119.2. SKELETAL MANIFESTATIONS OBSERVED IN 23 PATIENTS WITH PRIMARY HYPEROXALURIA TYPE 1 AND END-STAGE RENAL DISEASE[a]

Skeletal Manifestations	No. of Patients
Bone pain	22
Dense bones	18
Osteitis fibrosa	14
Osteomalacia	3
Fracture separation epiphysis[b]	3
Vertebral fractures	3
Multiple fractures	1
Joint pain	18
Polyarticular pain	10
Acute arthritis	8
Chronic arthritis	7
Destructive finger arthropathy[c]	8
Chondrocalcinosis	4
Chronic shoulder destructive arthropathy	1
Tendon/bursal pain	
Calcified flexor finger tendon sheaths	9
Calcified olecranon bursitis	2

[a]Managed with dialysis for 1–7.7 years, mean 6.7 years. Ages: 6–60 years, mean 24 years (10,12,15,16).
[b]Children only.
[c]Cutaneous calcinosis in three patients.

Acquired Oxalosis

Oxalic acid is the metabolic end product of glycine, serine (Fig. 119.3), tryptophan and ascorbic acid (1–3,88). Large amounts of oxalate are also found in certain foods such as spinach and rhubarb (102,103). Oxalate is readily absorbed after ingestion. It is removed from the body almost entirely by glomerular filtration and secretion in the proximal tubule. Hyperoxalemia, hyperoxaluria, oxalate kidney stones, and crystalline tissue deposits may be the result of several contributing factors that may affect oxalate metabolism (1,3,88) (Table 119.3). Excessive oxalate in the diet (102,103) or increased absorption in patients with chronic inflammatory bowel disease, small bowel resection, intestinal bypass (104), external biliary drainage (105), and intestinal lymphangiectasia (106) can lead to hyperoxalemia. Methoxyflurane (2), ethyleneglycol (2), ascorbic acid, and xylitol (102) are all metabolized to oxalate.

Thiamine and pyridoxine deficiencies may inhibit glyoxylate metabolism, thereby increasing oxalate production (88). *Aspergillus niger* can synthesize oxalic acid, which may crystallize in infected tissues and in aspergillomas (2,107). Chronic renal failure can lead to serum oxalate levels four- to eightfold greater than normal (88,108). Serum oxalate levels parallel those of creatinine, becoming saturated when levels of serum creatinine reach 8 to 9 mg/dL (4,108).

The formation of calcium oxalate crystals in biologic fluids and tissues occurs when the limits of solubility are exceeded. In the urine as well as in the serum, the degree of saturation of calcium oxalate expressed in terms of the ionic concentration of calcium and oxalic acid is the most important single factor in the formation of oxalate crystals (88,108). Similar mechanisms may operate in synovial fluid and other tissues (1,2). Some tissues, such as kidney, myocardium, and retina, and *A. niger* infections produce oxalic acid, so that local oxalic acid concentrations may exceed that of serum (108). This may account for the calcium oxalate crystal formation observed in idiopathic calcium urolithiasis (108), aspergillosis (107), granulomatous lymphadenitis (109), and dystrophic retinal damage (110), which are associated with normal serum oxalate.

TABLE 119.3. TYPES OF OXALOSIS

Familial
- Primary hyperoxaluria
  - Type 1: AGT deficiency
  - Type 2: GR deficiency
  - Type 3: Increased oxalate absorption

Acquired
- Diet rich in oxalate, e.g., rhubarb
- Increased ingestion or administration of oxalate precursors, e.g., ascorbic acid, ethyleneglycol, and xylitol
- Increased absorption, e.g., small bowel resection or bypass, inflammatory bowel disease, or external biliary drainage
- Increased production, e.g., deficiency of thiamine or pyridoxine, *Aspergillus niger* infection
- Decreased renal excretion: uremia
- Dystrophic: retinal damage

AGT, alanine: glyoxylate aminotransferase; GR, Glyoxylate reductase/D-glycerate dehydrogenase.

Radiographic Manifestations

The radiographic appearance of primary and secondary oxalosis is similar, characteristically involving the hands and feet, with skin (Figs. 119.1B and 119.5), vascular, periarticular, and intraarticular calcifications (1,4,10,15,16) (Figs. 119.1B, 119.6, and 119.7). Rosette-like areas of bony sclerosis in hands and feet, metaphyseal sclerotic bands, pathologic fractures, multiple bilateral fractures, separation of epiphyses (15), and pseudoarthrosis may be seen alone or in combination with the bony changes of renal osteodystrophy (4,10,15,16). Large shallow areas of subperiosteal resorption and bone erosions can be seen in the absence of secondary hyperparathyroidism (4,10,111–115). Chondrocalcinosis of larger joints and periarticular calcified masses have also been described (4,6,14) (Fig. 119.7).

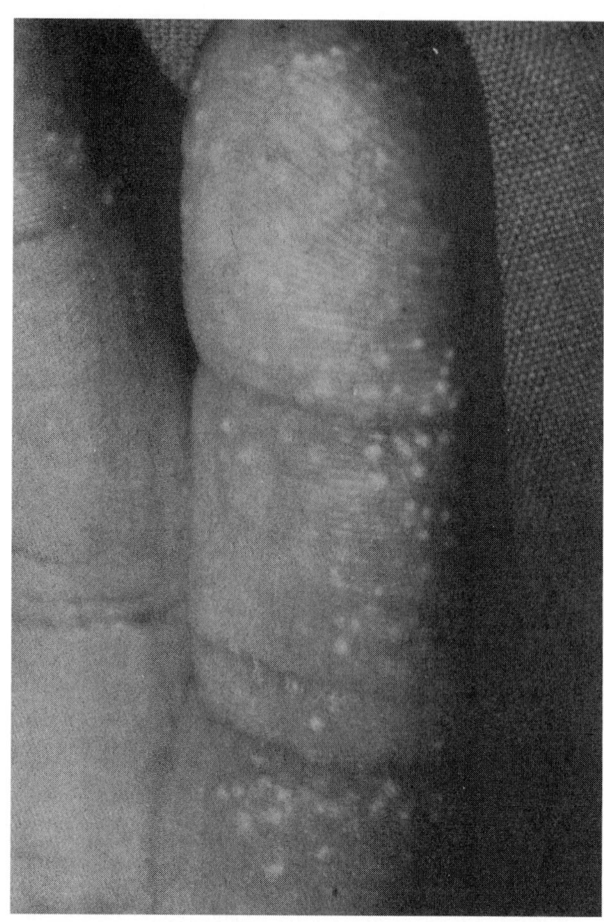

FIGURE 119.5. Miliary skin deposits in a patient with hemodialysis oxalosis. (From Reginato AJ, Ferreiro JL, Barbazan C, et al. Arthropathy and cutaneous calcinosis in hemodialysis oxalosis. *Arthritis Rheum* 1986:29:1387–1396, with permission.)

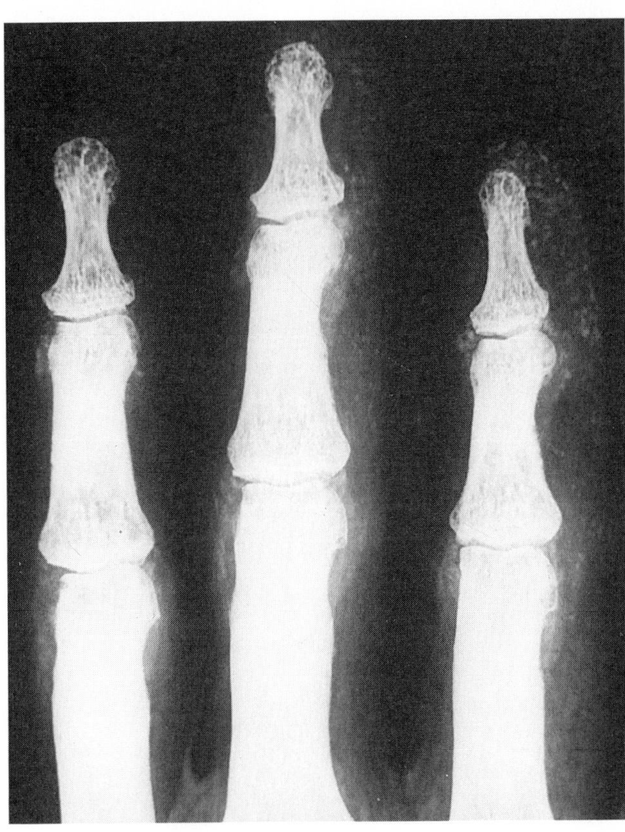

FIGURE 119.6. Radiograph of a patient with hemodialysis oxalosis, showing skin, vascular and periarticular calcifications. (From Reginato AJ, Ferreiro JL, Barbazan C, et al. Arthropathy and cutaneous calcinosis in hemodialysis oxalosis. *Arthritis Rheum* 1986;29:1387–1396, with permission.)

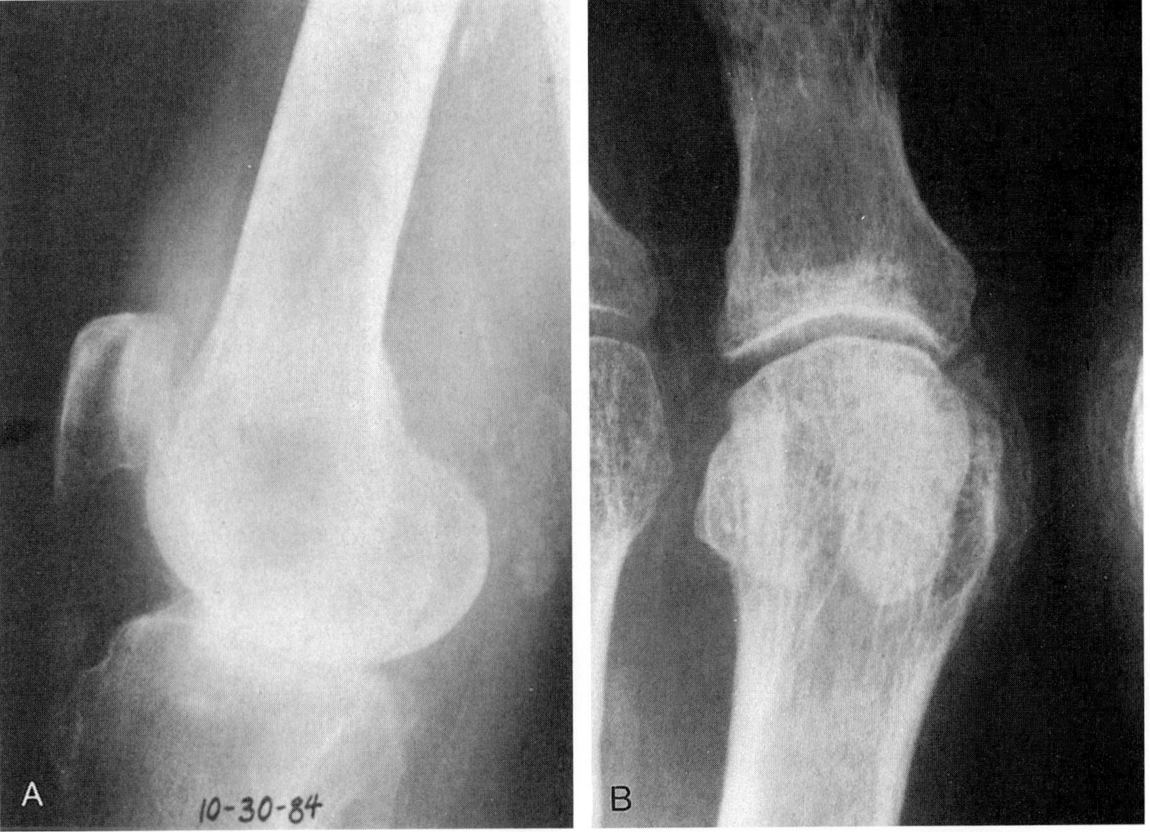

FIGURE 119.7. Radiographs of patient with secondary oxalosis due to end-stage renal disease. **A:** Large calcified masses observed in the popliteal space and infrapatellar tendon along with arterial calcifications. (From Schumacher HR, Reginato AJ, Pullman S. Synovial fluid oxalate deposition complicating rheumatoid arthritis with amyloidosis and renal failure: demonstration of intracellular oxalate crystals. *J Rheumatol* 1987;4:361–366.) **B:** First metatarsophalangeal joint showing synovial calcifications and chondrocalcinosis. (From Reginato AJ, Kurnik B. Calcium oxalate and other crystals associated with kidney diseases and arthritis. *Semin Arthritis Rheum* 1989;18:198–224, with permission.)

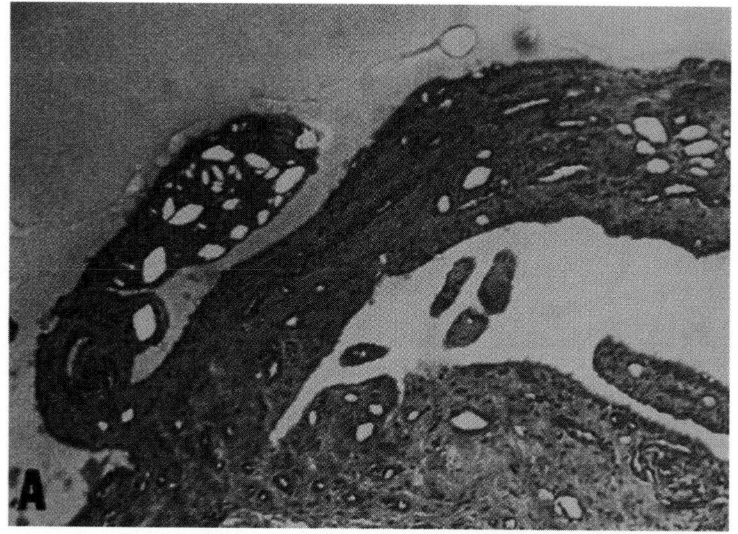

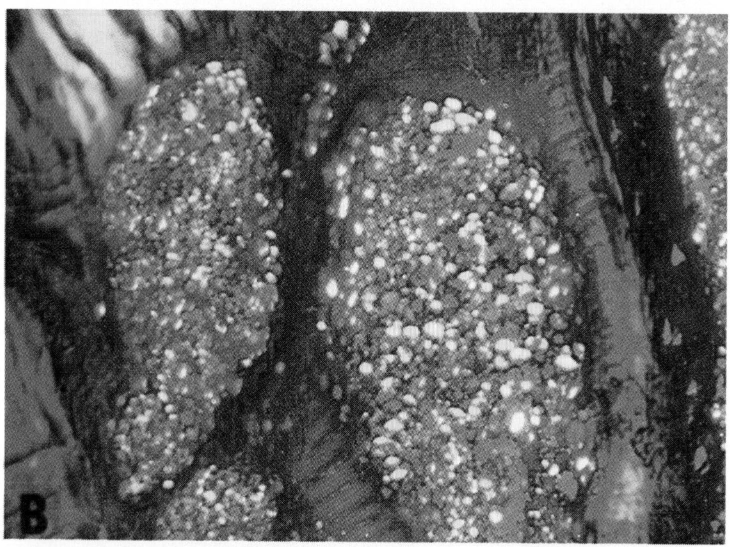

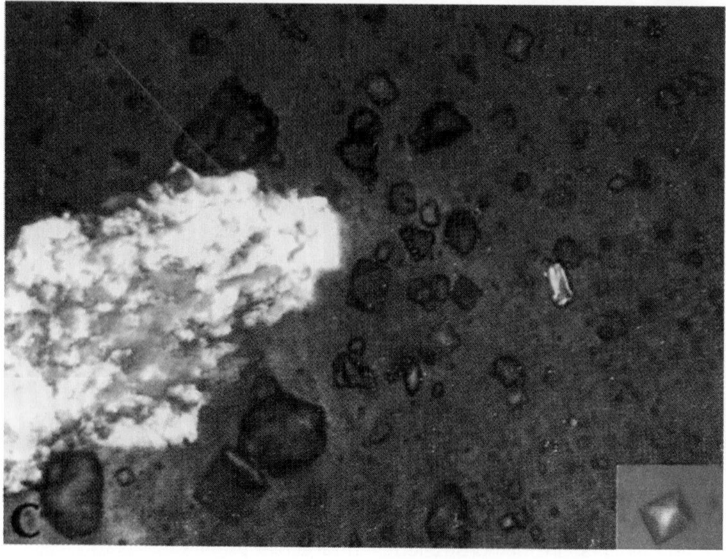

FIGURE 119.8. A: Calcium oxalate crystals in the synovium of the first metatarsophalangeal joint (hematoxylin and eosin stain, ×180). **B:** Tophaceous deposit of birefringent crystals observed in synovial membrane of the same joint. Compensated polarized microscopy (×180). **C:** Calcium oxalate crystals in synovial fluid. Pseudotophaceous deposits surrounded by abundant polymorphic and a few dipyramidal crystals showing no birefringence and weak or intense birefringence with positive elongation (**insert**). Compensated polarized microscopy (×400). (From Reginato AJ, Ferreiro JL, Barbazan C, et al. Arthropathy and cutaneous calcinosis in hemodialysis oxalosis. *Arthritis Rheum* 1986;29: 1387–1396, with permission.)

Pathologic Studies

Synovium

Synovium obtained from patients with chronic synovitis has exhibited mild synovial cell hyperplasia with hyperemia and pleomorphic calcium oxalate crystals lying in a mildly fibrotic interstitium with scarce mononuclear cells and a few giant cells (1,4,14) (Fig. 119.8A,B). Clumps of closely packed crystals with intensely and weakly positive birefringence may be seen in the subsynovium without an inflammatory reaction (Fig. 119.8A,B).

Cartilage, Meniscus, and Bone

Few studies of articular cartilage in oxalosis have been performed (1,4,14). Hoffman and co-workers (14) found oxalate crystals in a large cystic area of a meniscus of a patient with hemodialysis-associated oxalosis. Bone histology in most patients with oxalosis shows oxalate crystal deposits surrounded by giant cell granulomas and bone marrow fibrosis (2,4,10,12,114,115). These deposits correlate with radiologic areas of subperiosteal resorption, endosteal erosions, pseudofractures, or localized osteosclerosis resulting from deposits of radiopaque calcium oxalate crystals in the bone marrow (10,12,114,115).

Crystallographic Features

Calcium oxalate crystal deposits occur in bone, tendon, articular cartilage, menisci, and synovium (1,2) (Fig. 119.8A,B). These sites are probably the source of crystals found in joint fluid (Fig. 119.8C). Two types of oxalate crystals have been identified: (a) characteristic dipyramidal crystals formed by calcium oxalate dihydrate (weddellite), and (b) polymorphic crystals composed of calcium oxalate monohydrate (whewellite). The latter appear as irregular squares, chunks, short rods, stretched ovals, dumbbells, and even microspherules (1). Sizes range from 5 to 30 μm. Some calcium oxalate crystals show strong birefringence with positive elongation (for concepts of birefringence and elongation see Chapter 4 on synovial fluid analysis), but most exhibit weakly positive birefringence or none at all (Fig. 119.8C). Most fresh preparations of oxalate crystals stain with alizarin red S (4) and those in tissue deposits can also be recognized with Pizzolato's stain (4,10,14). Under transmission electron microscopy, they are electron dense with sharp margins and a foamy structure similar to that of CPPD crystals (3,4,14). As a result of their polymorphism and variable intensity of birefringence, calcium oxalate crystals can easily be confused with CPPD crystals or even with BCP crystal microspherules when synovial fluid is examined only by ordinary or compensated polarized light (2,66). The phlogistic potency of calcium oxalate crystals is similar to that of monosodium urate crystals or calcium phosphate crystals when assessed by injections of synthetic preparations into dog knees or rat paws (2,116). Crystalline calcium oxalate–induced formation of giant cell granulomas also stimulated synovial cells to synthesize and release latent collagenase and prostaglandins (116). Activation of synovial cells, fibroblasts, and osteoclasts by calcium oxalate crystals may induce bone erosions, bone cysts, and even pathologic fractures (10,12).

Biochemical Features

Serum oxalate levels have been measured in two of the five reports of articular oxalosis complicating long-term dialysis (4,6,7,9,14). The levels ranged from 168 to 204 mg/L^2, about eightfold higher than normal. Synovial fluid oxalate levels in these patients were considerably higher than those present in fluid of patients with rheumatoid arthritis (RA), osteoarthritis (OA), or pseudogout (14). Most patients with end-stage renal disease and oxalosis had a low serum calcium level, although a few were hypercalcemic in the absence of secondary hyperparathyroidism (1,111,114).

Hypercalcemia could be a contributory factor in precipitating calcium oxalate crystals in tissues, but parathyroidectomy, performed in a few patients with bone oxalosis and end-stage renal disease, was ineffective in correcting the elevated serum calcium or in decreasing crystal deposits (4,10). Another possible explanation for the hypercalcemia seen in these patients is increased osteoclastic bone resorption at the site of oxalate deposits in bone (2,4,10,12,114).

Oxalate is removed by both hemodialysis and peritoneal dialysis, but neither procedure induces a negative balance required for effective removal of oxalate from tissues of patients with either primary oxalosis or end-stage renal disease (1,88,117). Table 119.4 summarizes the clinical manifestations of 12 patients with oxalosis due to end-stage renal disease and dialysis. Autopsy series reveal that renal and bone oxalosis occur in about 90% of patients with end-stage renal disease managed with long-term hemodialysis (1,114). Several reports of articular oxalosis associated with renal failure have implicated ascorbic acid administration in aggravating oxalate

TABLE 119.4. CLINICAL MANIFESTATIONS IN 12 REPORTED PATIENTS WITH SECONDARY OXALOSIS DUE TO END-STAGE RENAL DISEASE AND DIALYSIS

Manifestations	No. of Patients
Bone pain	11
Joint pain	12
Arthritis	11
Acute	3
Chronic	11
Skin oxalate deposits	7
Myocardiopathy	2
Obliterative vascular disease	3
Periodontitis	1

From refs. 1, 4, 7, 9, and 13.

deposition (1,4,14,118–120). In the past, most patients with articular oxalosis and end-stage renal disease received 500 to 1,000 mg of ascorbic acid after each dialysis (4,14).

Clinical Manifestations

Diffuse bone pain; compression fractures; acute, symmetric, proximal interphalangeal and metacarpophalangeal joint arthritis (with or without flexor tenosynovitis); miliary calcific deposits of digits; and digital vascular calcifications are the most characteristic clinical presentations (4,11,13,14) (Figs. 119.1, 119.5 to 119.7) (Tables 119.2 and 119.4). Acute or chronic effusions of larger joints including knees, elbows, or ankles may develop (4–6). Podagra, Achilles tenosynovitis, and bursitis have been observed in single patients (2,4) (Fig. 119.7B). In most patients, the initial acute synovitis follows a chronic course, responding poorly to colchicine, nonsteroidal antiinflammatory drugs (NSAIDs), intraarticular injections of corticosteroids, or even increased frequency of dialysis (4,13,14). Synovial fluids from acute and chronic effusions have been clear or bloody with normal viscosity (3,4,14). Leukocyte counts have been low, ranging from 150 to 2,100 cells/µL with 60% to 90% polymorphonuclear cells in some samples (3). In others, a predominance of large mononuclear cells was observed (4,14). Abundant clumps of oxalate crystals are usually seen, most of which are extracellular (Fig. 119.8C), but intracellular crystals were found in fluid from several patients (6,7).

Therapy

The efficacy of the management of primary hyperoxaluria depends on early diagnosis (85,87). Before renal failure occurs, there are several medical interventions that may be effective in minimizing renal and extrarenal oxalate crystal deposition (85,88). These measures include maintenance of a high urine output of about 3 L per day and avoidance of foods that contain high levels of oxalate such as tea, chocolate, spinach, and rhubarb. The diet should provide only the minimum requirement of vitamins C and D (85). Nonspecific inhibitors of crystallization and subsequent crystal aggregation such as neutral orthophosphate (121), pyrophosphate, magnesium oxide, and potassium citrate (122) can be used to increase the solubility of calcium oxalate. Pharmacologic doses of pyridoxine are indicated in some patients with PH1 (121–124), as pyridoxine is a coenzyme for AGT that stimulates the conversion of glyoxylate to glycine (Fig. 119.3). In a report describing the pathway for glyoxylate synthesis, L-oxothiazolidine-4 carboxylate manifested potential as a drug that may inhibit oxalate synthesis (123). This drug is being evaluated in a phase II clinical trial. The ideal drug may be an antisense oligonucleotide that blocks the expression of glycolate oxidase, a key enzyme in hepatic oxalate synthesis.

Early transplantation preceded by aggressive preoperative hemodialysis and the use of a living, related graft donor have been tried to improve the outcome of renal transplantation. However, the kidney transplant experience has been disappointing due to graft oxalosis (125). Combined liver-kidney transplantation is the treatment of choice for children with PH1 and advanced renal failure. The liver provides sufficient enzyme to lower oxalate production to the normal range and induce resolution of life-threatening myocardiopathy, and oxalate osteopathy (126–128). The use of gene therapy in this inborn error of metabolism awaits further technical advances in the field.

Acute and chronic arthropathy due to oxalate crystals have been managed with NSAIDs, intraarticular corticosteroid, and colchicine with poor-to-mediocre improvement (4,14).

SYNDROMES ASSOCIATED WITH CHOLESTEROL CRYSTALS AND OTHER CRYSTALLINE LIPIDS

Cholesterol Crystals

Cholesterol crystals are occasionally identified in RA joint fluid (17,26), rheumatoid nodules (2), or bursal effusions (1–3,17,23,24). They are rarely observed in the synovial fluid from patients with OA (19), chronic tophaceous gout (2), systemic lupus erythematosus (3,17), tumoral calcinosis associated with dermatomyositis (129), and scleroderma (21), and a variety of other chronic effusions (2,17). Cholesterol crystal clefts are also found in xanthomas, and necrobiotic xanthogranulomas with paraproteinemia. Table 119.5 summarizes conditions associated with cholesterol crystal deposition.

TABLE 119.5. CONDITIONS ASSOCIATED WITH CHOLESTEROL CRYSTAL DEPOSITION

Skin
- Xanthomas (1,3)
- Necrotic xanthogranulomas with paraproteinemia (3)
- Cholesterol tophus (20,21)
- Monosodium urate tophus (1,3)
- Calcific exudate [scleroderma (21), dermatomyositis (3)]
- Rheumatoid nodules (3); rheumatoid nodulosis (3)

Joints, bursae, tendons
- Rheumatoid arthritis (1,2,17,23,24,26)
- Systemic lupus erythematosus (1,3)
- Ankylosing spondylitis (1,3)
- Degenerative joint disease (19)
- Chronic tophaceous gout (1,3)
- Hyperbetalipoproteinemia (3)

Bone
- Unicameral bone cyst (3)
- Bone granulomatosis (Erdhein Chester's disease) (3)

Pleural/pericardial effusions
- Rheumatoid arthritis (24)
- Malignancy (1,3)
- Tuberculosis (1)

Arteries
- Atheromas (1)
- Cholesterol emboli (130)

The few studies performed on synovial fluid of patients with arthritis associated with hyperlipoproteinemias have failed to show cholesterol or other crystalline lipids (1–3). Xanthomas often develop in the Achilles tendon and extensor tendon sheaths of the hands of patients with familial hypercholesterolemia (18). Incompletely characterized rod-like crystals have been identified in a single patient with hyperbetalipoproteinemia with Achilles tendinitis (18). The syndrome of multiple cholesterol emboli may present a constellation of systemic manifestations mimicking necrotizing vasculitis (130) (see also Chapter 84).

Crystallographic Features

Synovial fluid containing cholesterol crystals often has a golden-honey or yellow-brown color (1), but cholesterol crystals have also been observed in chalky calcific exudates obtained from the skin of patients with scleroderma or dermatomyositis (21,129). Cholesterol crystals in synovial fluid are extracellular but are often associated with intra- and extracellular birefringent "Maltese crosses" (1–3) (Fig. 119.9). Cholesterol crystals show two morphologic forms (1–3): (a) highly birefringent, large, flat, rectangular plates with one or more notched corners, ranging from 8 to 100 μm (Fig. 119.10), and (b) rod- or needle-shaped, strongly birefringent crystals with either positive or negative elongation, ranging from 2 to 20 μm long (Fig. 119.10). Needle-shaped crystals may be confused with monosodium urate, while short plates can be confused with CPPD crystals (1–3).

Many factors are probably involved in the formation of cholesterol crystals in inflamed tissues including increased cholesterol synthesis, *in situ* bleeding, lipid release from damaged cell membranes and organelles, and

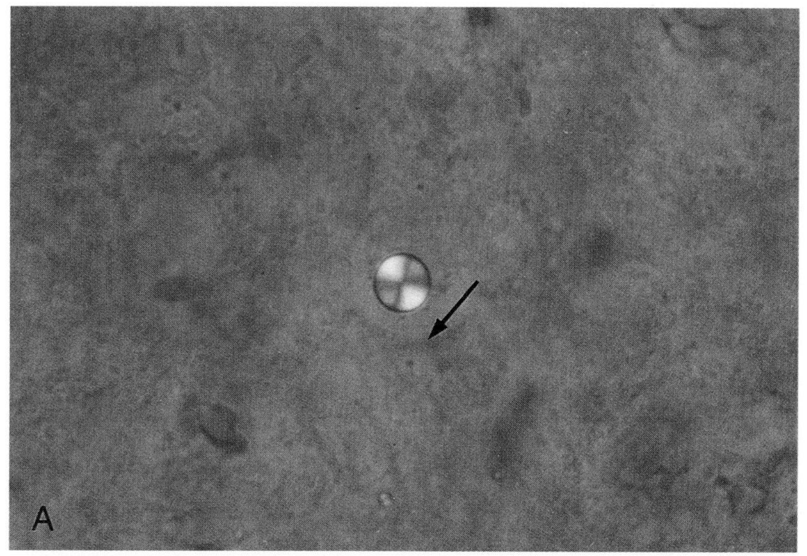

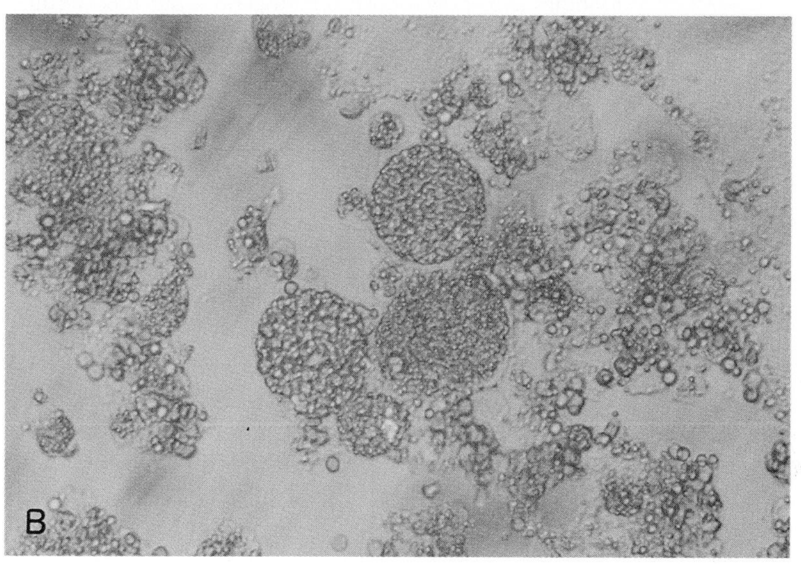

FIGURE 119.9. Lipid liquid crystals. **A:** Single, large, double-positive birefringent microspherule showing positive elongation. ***Arrow*** marks the orienting line of the compensator. **B:** Abundant, small, birefringent microspherules seen both inside and outside cells. Compensated polarized microscopy (×200).

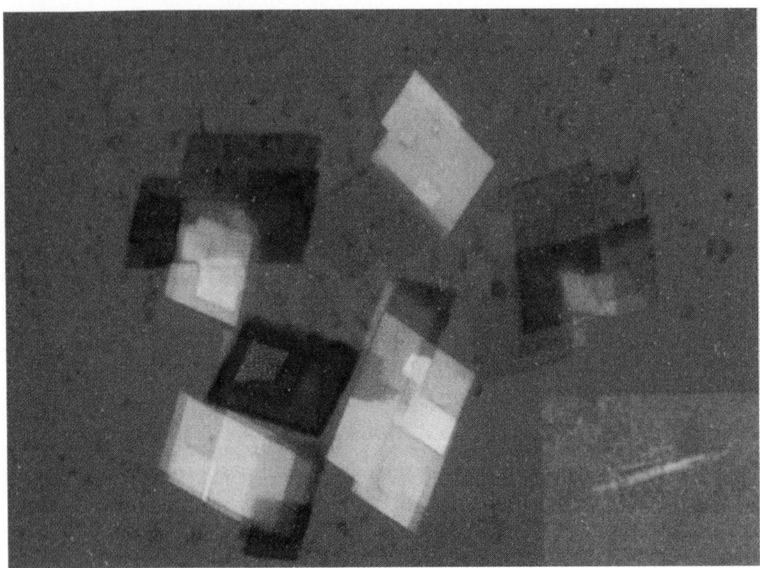

FIGURE 119.10. Characteristic highly birefringent plate-like cholesterol crystals. **Insert:** Needle-shaped cholesterol crystals showing a negative elongation. Compensated polarized light (×200).

abnormal intracellular transport of lipids resulting from chronic inflammation or infection (3,17,26). The capability of synthetic cholesterol crystals to induce moderate acute and chronic inflammation in skin, subcutaneous tissue, and knee joints of rabbits has been demonstrated in several studies (1,22). Cholesterol crystals have not been observed inside human phagocytes, as occurs with monosodium urate, CPPD, or BCP crystals. Because pyrogen contamination was not excluded and the similarity of crystal structure with that of natural cholesterol crystals was not shown in any of these studies, extrapolation of these observations to human disease states remains speculative. Although cholesterol crystals may activate serum complement, which might potentiate inflammation and aggravate joint destruction in RA and even OA, there is no clinical evidence to support this concept (1–3).

Lipid Liquid Crystals

Lipid liquid crystals represent states of matter having properties of both liquids and solids (27). These inclusions are formed by phospholipid or by other polar molecules that also be arranged as liquid crystals (1–3) (Fig. 119.9).

As previously noted, birefringent Maltese crosses occasionally have been found in synovial or bursal fluids of patients with RA (1–3). They have also been identified in synovial fluid of acute monarthritis (27–32), acute olecranon bursitis (2), pigmented villonodular synovitis (31), acute RA flare (32), and in one patient with chronic unexplained symmetric polyarthritis (29) and monoarthritis (28).

Crystallographic Features

Under compensated polarized light, these microspherules have an intense birefringence with positive elongation (Fig. 119.9). Sizes range from 2 to 8 µm. In atherosclerotic plaques, bile, and synovial fluid, these liquid lipid microspherules precede the formation of cholesterol crystals (2). They are commonly seen inside cells, stain with Sudan black B, and are dissolved completely in 1:1 alcohol-ether (3). Smaller microspherules may appear to be anisotropic (nonbirefringent) (Fig. 119.9B). These birefringent Maltese crosses with positive elongation must be differentiated from those with negative elongation such as monosodium urate microspherules, rarely seen in patients with gout, and from positive birefringent talcum powder crystals that may contaminate synovial fluids when gloves are used during arthrocentesis (1–3). The latter are magnesium silicate or starch granules and show a positive elongation, but their outlines are more irregular than the monosodium urate and lipid crystal microspherules (3).

Clinical Features

Acute Arthritis

All patients described have experienced acute onset of monarticular synovitis as often seen in other crystal-associated arthritis (1–3). The knee is most commonly involved, although wrist involvement was noted in one instance (27). Synovial fluid is inflammatory, with white cell counts ranging from 10,000 to 45,000/µL with 75% to 90% neutrophils. About 20% of these neutrophils contain doubly birefringent microspherules. Arthritis in all patients subsided completely within 1 week after NSAIDs were given.

Synovium has been obtained in only two patients with acute synovitis (1,29). Mild inflammatory changes with rare lymphocytic, mononuclear, or polymorphonuclear cell infiltrates were seen in both cases, and in one specimen, intracellular birefringent microspherules were seen within mononuclear cells (29).

Synthetic lipid liquid crystals injected into rabbit knees induced either acute or subacute synovitis (33). The origin of these microspherules in articular tissues is unknown. Injection of autologous blood into rabbit knee joints was associated with formation of similar Maltese crosses (34). Similar spherules seen in human joints may be formed by lipids derived from breakdown of membranes of platelets, erythrocytes, or leukocytes, and even from serum lipids (3).

Other Crystalline Lipids

Other crystalline lipids, thought to be fatty acids, have been described in skin fat necrosis of newborns (1). Identical structures have been observed in synovial fluid of patients with OA associated with large bone cysts, in hemarthrosis, and in synovial fluid examined several days after arthrocentesis (1–3). Such crystals may have either a strongly positive or negative elongation and may present with needle, plate, or rod shapes. Some may form clumps or rosettes (1–3,65,66). The rod- and needle-shaped crystals can be confused with CPPD or monosodium urate crystals (Fig. 119.11).

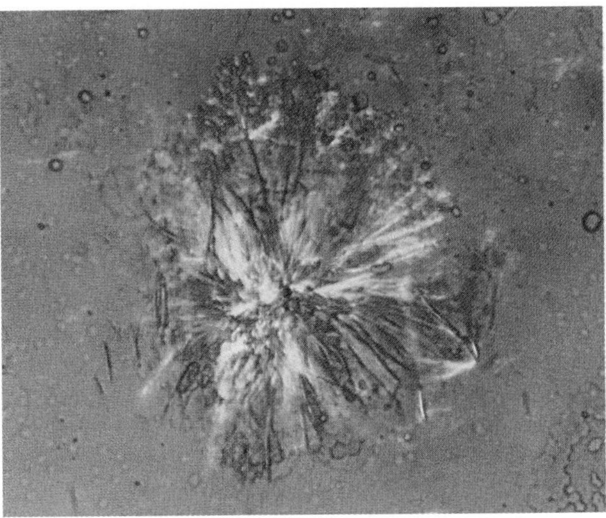

FIGURE 119.11. Strongly birefringent, needle-like lipid crystals with positive elongation observed in a patient with hemarthrosis. Compensated polarized light (×200). (From Reginato AJ, Kurnik B. Calcium oxalate and other crystals associated with kidney diseases and arthritis. *Semin Arthritis Rheum* 1989;18:198–224, with permission.)

Fabry's Disease

Fabry's disease is a rare, sex-linked, inborn error of glycosphingolipid metabolism, which results from an enzymic deficiency of lysosomal α-galactosidase (132). Glycosphingolipid accumulates in endothelial cells and a variety of tissues including heart, kidney, nerves, cornea, and synovium (132). The gene responsible for the expression of the enzyme is localized on the long arm of the X chromosome at Xq22 (132–134). Heterozygous females present with mild manifestations when compared with hemizygous males and can be recognized by characteristic corneal opacities by slit-lamp microscopy (whorl-like epithelial dystrophy) (132).

Skin manifestations are characterized by the presence of blue or red angiokeratomas or telangiectasias localized around the buttocks, thigh, penis, scrotum, or lower abdomen, and hypohydrosis (132–136). Kidney involvement is characterized by proteinuria and abnormal urinary sediment with birefringent lipid liquid crystal or Maltase crosses (132). Diagnosis is usually suspected by renal biopsy on the basis of the presence of lipid vacuoles in tubular and glomerular cells (132). Vascular changes occur in the brain, retina, heart, and bowel, and may result in stroke (135), myocardial infarction, myocardiopathy, valvular changes, arrhythmia and sudden death, and chronic ischemic bowel disease (136,137).

Musculoskeletal manifestations occur in many patients (132,137–141). These manifestations include Raynaud's phenomenon, lymphedema, and painful crises of burning paresthesias of palms and soles, usually exacerbated by warm weather. These crises can be associated with high fever and increased sedimentation rate. Polyarthritis associated with flexion contractures mainly of the distal interphalangeal joints, noncharacteristic bone pain, with or without aseptic bone necrosis (head of the femur and ankle bone infarcts), multiple enthesopathies, and acromegalic-like facies have also been reported. The clinical manifestations of Fabry's disease can be confused with those of several connective tissue diseases and syndromes, including systemic lupus erythematosus, CREST syndrome, and scleroderma. The association of Fabry's disease with SLE has been described in four patients (142).

The diagnosis of Fabry's disease can be confirmed by measurement of the α-galactosidase activity in plasma, serum, leukocytes, and fibroblasts (132,133).

Paresthesias can be managed with phenytoin or carbamazepine, and antiplatelet medications may decrease vascular symptoms (143). Renal transplantation provides only transitory improvement; enzymatic and gene therapy are good prospects (137).

CRYOGLOBULIN CRYSTALS

Paraprotein and cryoglobulins can crystallize within plasma cells of patients with multiple myeloma (1–3) (Fig. 119.12).

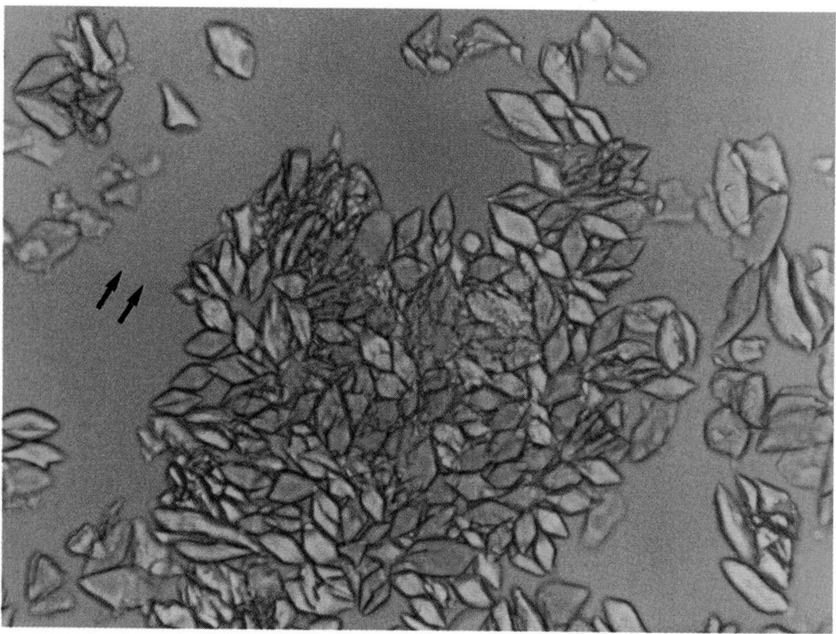

FIGURE 119.12. Cryoglobulin crystals. Polygonal birefringent crystals with positive elongation of serum cryoprecipitate of a patient with multiple myeloma. Compensated polarized light (×200). (From Reginato AJ, Kurnik B. Calcium oxalate and other crystals associated with kidney diseases and arthritis. *Semin Arthritis Rheum* 1989;18: 198–224, with permission.)

Similar crystals can be seen independent of plasma cells in the renal glomeruli, tubules, lungs, skin, liver, spleen, lymph nodes, adrenals, testis, and cornea (1,35–39,41). These deposits can be associated with variable degrees of organ failure (1–3,36). They may also occur in coronary and renal arteries and induce thrombosis and infarction (36). Similar crystalline deposits have been observed in peripheral vessels of patients with essential cryoglobulinemia with purpuric and necrotic skin lesions (2,37,38), as well as in the synovial membrane in association with synovitis (1–3,37,38).

Crystallographic Features

Paraprotein crystals are characterized by their large size, ranging from 3 to 60 µm or more, and their polymorphic shapes, which may vary with the cooling process used (1–3). They usually appear as hexagonal, diamond-shaped, or polygonal crystals, but may resemble squares, rectangles, rhomboids, or needles (35,36). They may show strong birefringency with either a positive or a negative elongation and stain with Giemsa and hematoxylin and eosin. Transmission and electron microscopic studies of amorphous, gelatinous, and crystalline cryoglobulins have shown the ability of these crystals to form macromolecular nets and trap cells (41). These morphologic properties of cryoglobulin crystals may explain their ability to induce vascular occlusion, and inflammation (37,35,41).

Clinical Features

Episodic joint pain followed by an erosive, chronic, symmetric polyarthritis involving joints of the hands and feet, and one ankle has been observed in one patient with cryoprecipitable immunoglobulin G in his serum and cryoglobulin crystals in joint fluid and synovium (35). Another patient with erosive polyarthritis and crystallized monoclonal cryoglobulin also has been reported (1), and in two reports patients presented with polyarthritis and vasculitis mimicking rheumatoid disease (38,45). Two patients with multiple myeloma and corneal paraprotein crystalline deposits have been described with foot arthritis, including podagra (2). Arthritis associated with cryoglobulinemia but without paraprotein crystals in synovial fluid has also been reported (40).

CHARCOT-LEYDEN CRYSTALS

Charcot-Leyden crystals are formed in the cytoplasm of disrupted eosinophils and are found in eosinophils in the sputum of asthmatic patients; in the tissue of patients with hypereosinophilia and eosinophilic disease processes such as eosinophilic bone granulomas; in the stools of patients with parasitic infections; in the infiltrates of granulocytic leukemia; and in the synovial fluid of patients with eosinophilic synovitis (46–49) (Fig. 119.13). Circulating Charcot-Leyden crystals (144) have been observed in patients with hypereosinophilic syndrome, and crystalline deposits were found in thrombosed vessels and in the renal glomeruli. Immunotactoid crystalline material also have been found in the glomeruli of these patients (49).

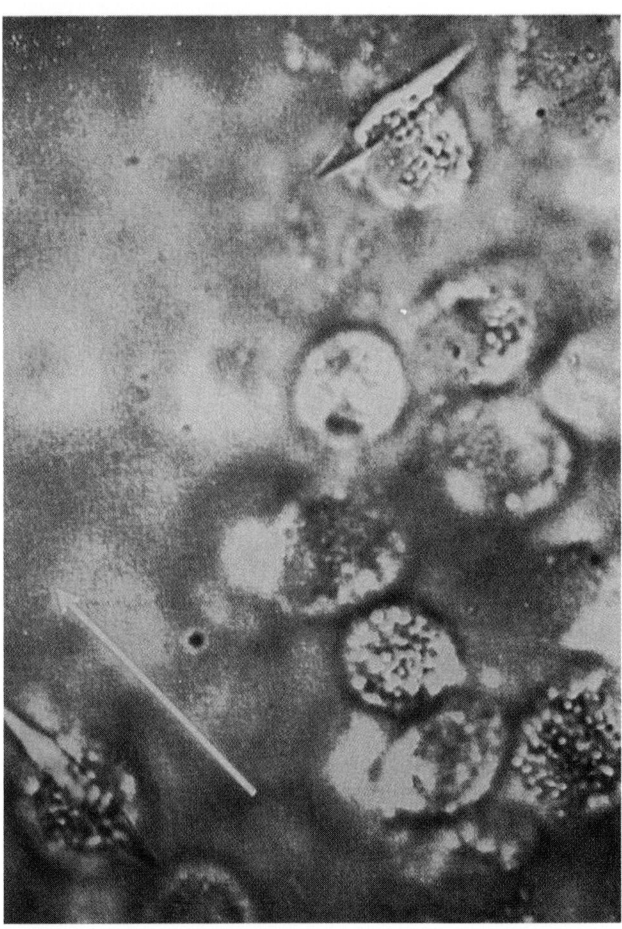

FIGURE 119.13. Charcot-Leyden crystals in synovial fluid of a patient with eosinophilic synovitis. Compensated polarized light (×350). *Arrow* indicates compensator axis. (Courtesy of Dr. R. DeMedicis.)

Crystallographic Features

Charcot-Leyden crystals are bipyramidal, hexagonal-shaped crystals formed by a lysophospholipase or phospholipase B and show mild to strong birefringency with positive or negative elongation. (45,143) (Fig. 119.13). Crystal sizes range from 17 to 25 μm. With hematoxylin and eosin stain, they appear eosinophilic; with Giemsa stain, they appear light purple or pink under fluorescent microscopy. These crystals appear as bright yellow-green fluorescent needles (45,143). The fluorescent technique seems to be more sensitive than light micropsy for the detection of Charcot-Leyden crystals (143).

Clinical Features

Eosinophilic synovitis associated with Charcot-Leyden crystals on wet synovial fluid preparation has been documented in seven patients with a history of allergic reactions and dermatographism (45–48). These patients developed painless monarthritis after minor trauma without concurrent allergic symptoms. Joint swelling was seen in the knee of seven patients and in the first metatarsophalangeal joint of another patient. Each episode subsided within 1 to 2 weeks without therapy; three patients had recurrent episodes. Synovial fluid was mildly inflammatory, with leukocyte counts of 10,850 ± 3,665/μL and up to 46% eosinophils. Charcot-Leyden crystals were seen inside cells on wet preparations.

CYSTINOSIS

Cystinosis is an autosomal-recessive inborn error of metabolism characterized by excessive accumulation of cystine in reticuloendothelial cells of liver, spleen, lymph nodes, and bone marrow resulting from defective carrier-mediated transport of cystine across the lysosomal membrane (146). The most severe type is infantile cystinosis (nephrogenic), and is characterized by polydipsia, polyuria, crystalline deposits in renal tubule and glomeruli, Fanconi's syndrome, and progressive renal failure. These patients also present with conjunctivitis, retinopathy, vitamin D–resistant rickets, and myopathy (2,146–149).

Crystallographic Features

Cystine crystals have a characteristic hexahedral shape with a weak-to-intense birefringence (2,3). Typical crystals are rarely seen in tissue deposits, where they appear polymorphic, assuming square, rectangular, lozenge, and even acicular (needle-like) shapes. These crystals are seen inside cells, surrounded by membrane-bound structures, and intracellular crystals may form *in situ* rather than by phagocytosis of preformed crystals (1–3,146).

Clinical Features

Symptomatic crystal deposits in bone were described in a single patient and correlated with focal demineralization (3,50). In another patient, cystinosis of bone was associated with acute knee and wrist synovitis and with polyarthralgias of larger joints (51), but no cystine crystals were found in the synovial fluid. Radiographs revealed coarse bone trabeculation with diffuse demineralization and flattening of one of the metacarpal heads with punctiform, periarticular, calcific deposits. Cystine crystalline deposits in muscle have been found in patients with long-standing cystinosis and generalized muscle weakness and wasting (3,52,148,149). Also, patients with cystinosis and Fanconi's syndrome may develop plasma and muscle carnitine deficiency. Carnitine tubular reabsorption is decreased in Fanconi syndrome due to cystinosis, and the failure to reabsorb carnitine results in serum and muscle carnitine deficiency (148). As a consequence of muscle carnitine deficiency, free fatty acids fail to be degraded and accumulate as fat droplets in the muscles of patients with cystinosis (52,148,149). After renal transplantation, cystine accumulation continues in nonrenal tissues with crystalline deposits in eyes, testicles, skin, muscles, and thyroid (53,54). Of the 36 patients with nephropathic cystinosis studied at the National Institutes of Health who underwent renal transplantation, 14% were legally blind, a substantial number of patients had delayed bone ages, 33% of the patients had signs of distal myopathy with swallowing dysfunction, and more than 85% required thyroid replacement therapy (149).

Management

Management of patients with cystinosis includes adequate fluid intake and correction of metabolic acidosis, hypokalemia, and rickets (149–151). End-stage renal failure can be managed with dialysis or renal transplantation (150). Oral administration of cysteamine has been shown to stabilize renal function, improve growth, and decrease cystine crystalline corneal deposits (151).

XANTHINE CRYSTALS

Xanthinuria is an uncommon, hereditary disorder of purine metabolism resulting from a deficiency of the enzyme xanthine oxidase (152). It is characterized by hypouricemia; decreased uric acid excretion in the urine; and the presence of xanthinuria, hypoxanthinuria, and xanthine kidney stones. Hypoxanthine and xanthine crystals have been identified in the muscle of three patients with xanthinuria and tender muscles (55–57). Muscle pain was crampy and increased by walking. Two other patients presented with acute arthritis mimicking gout; unfortunately, no synovial fluid was obtained (1). Xanthine, hypoxanthine, and oxypurinol crystals also have been identified in muscles of a patient with Lesch-Nyhan syndrome and another with lymphoma managed with allopurinol (2). Deposits of xanthine, hypoxanthine, and oxypurinol crystals have been described in skeletal muscle in the absence of muscle pain or weakness in ten patients with gout treated with allopurinol (1,56,152).

Crystallographic Features

Xanthine crystals are plate-like or rhomboidal in shape, measure up to 2.5 μm, and are strongly birefringent (1). Hypoxanthine crystals are more polymorphic, although they may also appear as large plates or rhomboidal crystals. They range in size from 9.5 to 50 μm and show strong negative birefringence. Exact identification of these crystals requires electron or x-ray diffraction analysis (1).

ALUMINUM

In hemodialyzed patients, aluminum intoxication has been associated with a mineralization defect of bone matrix, resulting in osteomalacia, adynamic bone disease, bone pain, and fractures (2,60). Transmission electron microscopy and x-ray elemental microdispersive analysis have shown amorphous deposits of aluminum phosphate inside mitochondria of bone cells as well as extracellular, hexagonal crystals measuring 200 to 1000 Å at the mineralization front (60). Aluminum levels in synovial fluid, synovium, and articular cartilage of patients undergoing chronic dialysis are higher than normal (58,59,61,62). A large proportion of dialysis patients may also have amyloid and iron deposits in the synovium, as well as secondary hyperparathyroidism (153). It has been difficult to separate such conditions from possible articular aluminum deposition (59–63). Intraarticular injections of crystalline and amorphous aluminum phosphate in rabbits induced acute and chronic synovitis (62,154), but these results cannot be extrapolated directly to humans. Aluminum intoxication in patients with chronic dialysis has been suspected as one of the pathogenic factors leading to soft tissue calcification and osteosclerosis (63). In a case report, aluminum containing particles were observed in a patient with chondrocalcinosis receiving aluminum hydroxyde antiacid (63).

HEMOGLOBIN CRYSTALS

Hemoglobin crystals have been described in stored normal human blood, the blood of patients with sickle cell anemia, and the blood of rats and white deer (1–3). Hemoglobin and hematoidin crystals may be found occasionally in synovial fluid of patients with hemarthrosis (65,66) and sickle cell arthropathy (67,68). Rat hemoglobin crystals injected into rat skin air pouches induced mild acute inflammation (1).

Crystallographic Features

Human hemoglobin crystals are rectangular and measure 10 to 12 μm in length and are usually found inside red cells or extracellularly (Fig. 119.14A). They are weakly birefringent with either positive or negative elongation (1,65,66).

HEMATOIDIN CRYSTALS

Hematoidin crystals, formed as a by-product of hemoglobin degradation under reduced oxygen tension, have been found in hematomas and hemarthrosis (1,65,66). Possible hematoidin crystals have been found in the synovial fluid of four patients with hemarthrosis (65,66) and in one patient with sickle cell disease and pseudoseptic arthritis (67), and also as artifactual crystals in bloody fluid kept in the refrigerator for several weeks (66).

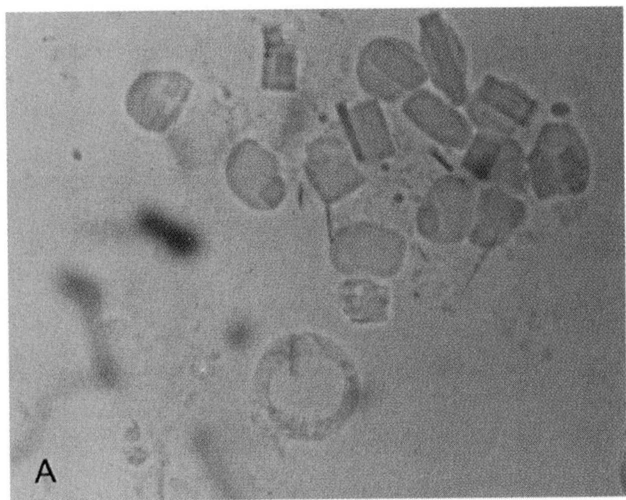

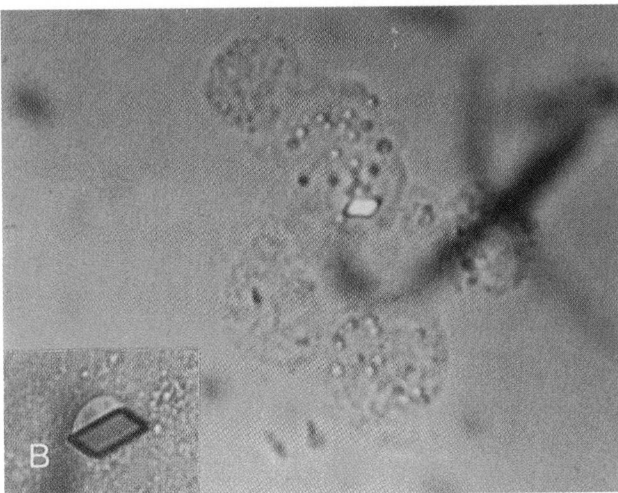

FIGURE 119.14. A: Weakly birefringent rectangular hemoglobin crystals and characteristic monosodium urate crystals in a patient with gout and bloody fluid. Compensated polarized light (×400) (From Tate G, Schumacher HR, Reginato AJ, et al. Synovial fluid crystals derived from hemoglobin crystals. J Rheumatol 1992;19:111–114, with permission.) **B:** Rhomboid golden brown colored crystals (suspected hematoidin crystals) observed in a patient with hemarthrosis due to septic arthritis. Ordinary light (×400). (From Reginato AJ. *Manual para el estudio del liquido synovial, bursal y identificacion de cristales.* Barcelona: Imprenta Rapida, 1993:87, with permission.)

Crystallographic Features

Hematoidin-like crystals described in synovial fluid are rhomboid, measure 8 to 10 μm in length, and are bright gold or brown under ordinary light (Fig. 119.14B). In other cytologic preparations, they may resemble needles forming cockleburr arrays of various sizes, ranging from 2 to 25 μm, but occasionally reaching 100 μm. Under compensated polarized light they show intense birefringence with positive and negative elongation (1,65,66).

The role of these hemoglobin-derived crystals in inducing articular inflammation is uncertain (1,65), but knowledge of their presence in synovial fluid is important to avoid confusion with CPPD or other pathologic crystals (2).

FOREIGN-BODY SYNOVITIS

The introduction of hard penetrating particles into joints, tendon sheaths, and periarticular soft tissues can induce monarticular synovitis, tenosynovitis, or cellulitis by causing infection or sterile inflammatory foreign-body reaction (71–73,75–80,157–168). Materials most commonly associated with foreign-body synovitis are shown in Table 119.6. Similar chronic granulomatous reaction of synovium can be induced by wear particles from articular implants such as metals (75,158,167,168), silicones (76,80), polyethylene (75,158,162), and methylmethacrylate (158,162,167). Bullet fragments, when lodged inside major joints, may induce mild synovitis and

TABLE 119.6. PARTICLES ASSOCIATED WITH FOREIGN BODY SYNOVITIS

- Vegetable
  - Plant thorns
    - Date and sentinel plants
    - Blackthorn bushes
    - Roses, yuccas, hawthorns
    - Mesquites, bougainvilleas
    - *Ulex europeus* (Tojo)
    - Burning bush
  - Wood splinters
  - Starch
- Marine
  - Sea urchin spine
  - Chitin spines (crab, seamouse)
  - Fish bone
- Mineral
  - Stone, gravel, silica
  - Brick fragments
- Metals
  - Vitalium
  - Stainless steel
  - Lead
- Miscellaneous
  - Silicone
  - Glass
  - Fiberglass
  - Polyethylene
  - Methylmethacrylate
  - Plastic
  - Rubber
  - Lace fabric
  - Grease[a]
  - Paint[a]

[a]High-pressure injection gun.

cause systemic manifestations of lead toxicity (159,165,166). High-pressure injection injury of fingers with paint or grease guns usually induces a delayed necrotizing dactylitis, which requires emergency surgical drainage and debridement (2).

Clinical Features

Clinical presentation of foreign-body synovitis is characterized by the sudden onset of pain at the site of the injury. Acute synovitis usually appears several days after the injury. Inflammation at the site of the penetrating injury may subside completely or become chronic with a steady or relapsing clinical course (71). Frequently, the initial injury is forgotten by the patient or overlooked by the examiner. Joints most commonly involved are those of the hands and knees. Joint involvement is characterized by a variable degree of periarticular inflammatory swelling and synovial thickening of small joints (71), while larger joints may have large and persistent joint effusions. Fever, myalgias, lymph node enlargement, and synovitis of other noninjured joints have been reported in patients with sea urchin synovitis (71,73). In patients with high-pressure injection gun injury, the only initial clinical finding may be a painless puncture wound in the fingertip. After a few hours, however, signs of rapidly necrotizing dactylitis become apparent.

Diving and other marine recreational activities, farming, and gardening are well-recognized risk factors (157). Intravenous drug abuse also may be a possible risk factor (158). Foreign-body synovitis must be differentiated from other conditions associated with acute, recurrent, or chronic monarticular synovitis such as infectious arthritis, gout, pseudogout, and monarticular juvenile rheumatoid arthritis (71,157), or other causes of dactylitis. These conditions include typical and atypical mycobacterial infections (tuberculous dactylitis or spina ventosa), erysipeloid, seal finger (staphylococcal dactylitis of seal hunters), sarcoidosis, psoriasis, tophaceous gout, and giant cell tumor of flexor tendon sheaths of fingers.

Laboratory Findings

The white blood cell count and erythrocyte sedimentation rate are usually normal (71). Synovial fluid can be cloudy or bloody; in those patients with detritic synovitis resulting from metallic loose joint prostheses, it may be brownish and contain abundant dark metallic debris (71,66). Synovial fluid leukocyte counts range from 10,000 to 60,000/μL, with predominance of neutrophils (71). Fresh preparations of synovial fluid may reveal birefringent fragments of plant thorns, polyethylene, or polymethyl methacrylate (75), or nonbirefringent particles such as needle-shape fiberglass and metallic particles (63). Metallic particles appear as black rods or dots (63).

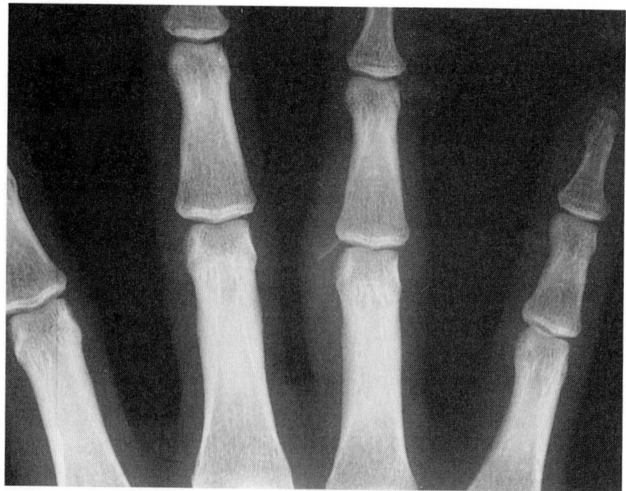

FIGURE 119.15. Soft tissue swelling surrounding a radiopaque sea urchin spine in a patient with foreign-body synovitis. (From Ferreiro-Seoane JL. *Foreign body synovitis. Primer on the rheumatic diseases.* Atlanta: Arthritis Foundation, 1993:294, with permission.)

Radiographic Features

Radiographs are useful to detect radiodense particles of metals, fish bones, and sea urchin spines (Fig. 119.15), but wood, plastic, and plant thorn particles are usually missed. Radiographs may reveal only soft tissue swelling when obtained early. In patients with a chronic or relapsing course, however, periarticular demineralization, areas of localized osteolysis, osteosclerosis, periosteal new bone formation and pathologic fractures can be seen (71,155). These changes may mimic those of osteomyelitis or primary bone tumors (71). Dense fish bone seen inside joints can be confused with synovial osteochondromatosis and faint lead deposits in articular cartilage can mimic chondrocalcinosis (71), but usually present a greater metallic density. Ultrasonography (169), computed tomography (CT) (170,171), and nuclear magnetic resonance imaging (NMRI) (172–175) may be helpful in detecting small pieces of nonmetallic, wood splinter, or plastic foreign bodies when radiographs are unrevealing. In an experimental model, ultrasound and NMRI were shown to be more sensitive than CT scans for detection and localization of wood splinters embedded in muscle. Plant thorns are difficult to identify with any of these methods (172).

Pathologic Features

Excisional biopsy and synovectomy with bacteriologic studies of synovium, synovial fluid, and periarticular tissues are usually required for diagnosis and successful management of patients with a chronic or relapsing course

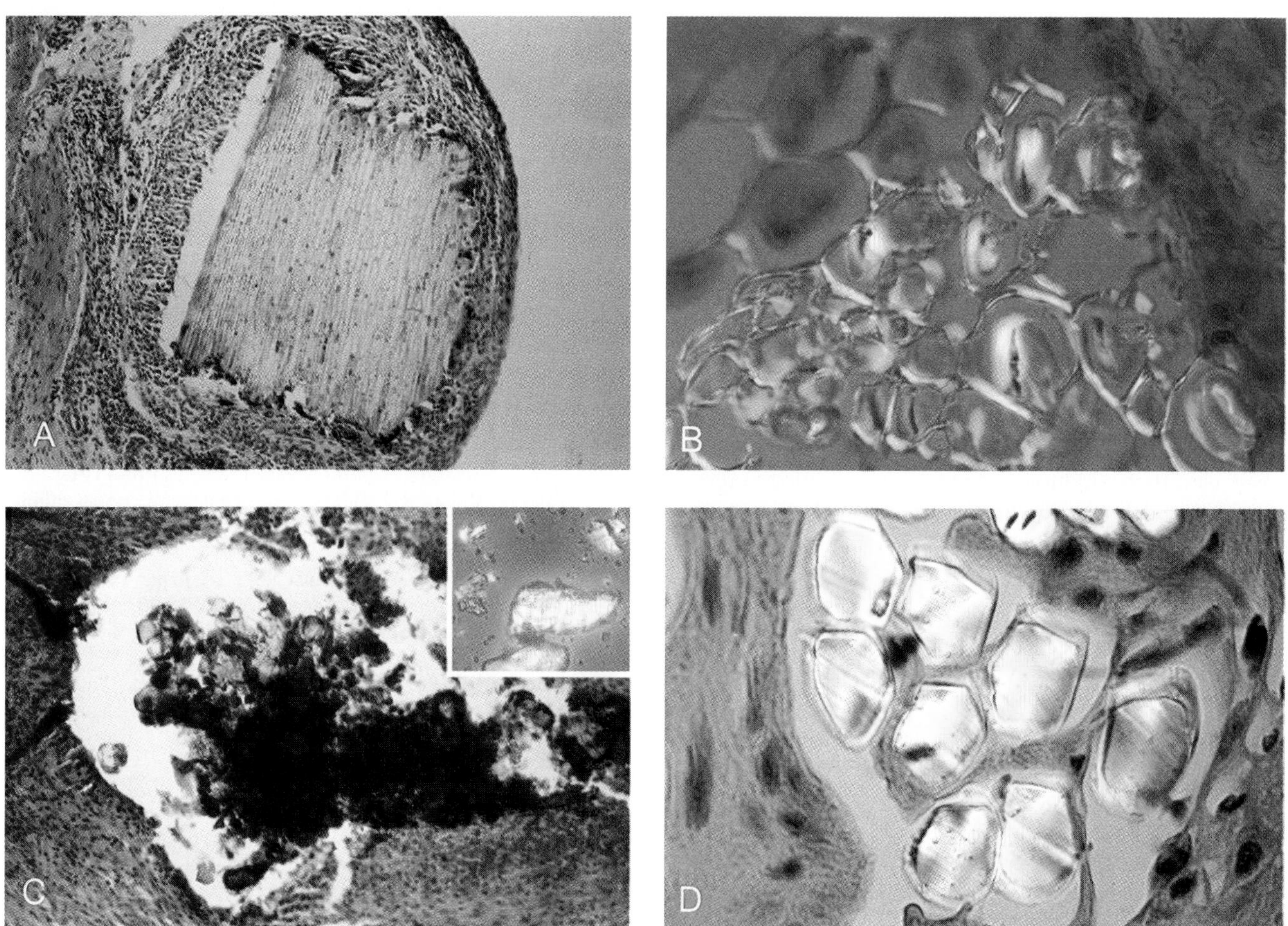

FIGURE 119.16. Pathologic findings in foreign body synovitis. **A:** Plant thorn showing multiple cells separated by thin septa (H&E, ×10). **B:** Birefringent cell septum of a similar plant thorn. Compensated polarized light (×300). **C:** Deeply stained sea urchin spine fragment found in synovium. Insert shows sea urchin birefringent fragments (H&E, ×200). **D:** Highly birefringent pleomorphic plastic fragments. Compensated polarized light (×200). (From Reginato AJ, Ferreiro JL, O'Connor CR, et al. Clinical and pathologic studies of twenty-six patients with penetrating foreign body injury to the joints, bursae, and tendon sheaths. Arthritis Rheum 1990;33:1753–1762, with permission.)

(71). Synovium usually reveals synovial cell proliferation and diffuse infiltrates of lymphocytes and plasma cells with focal collections of polymorphonuclear cells. Giant cell formation in synovium is usually striking in those patients in whom foreign bodies are found inside the joint, but may be minimal or absent in patients in whom foreign particles are located in periarticular tissues or skin (63). Granulomas identical to those seen in sarcoidosis have been found in association with sea urchin synovitis (71,73). Polarized light microscopy is useful in detecting birefringent fragments of plant thorn (Fig. 119.16A,B), polyethylene, polymethyl methacrylate, sea urchin spines (calcium carbonate crystals) (Fig. 119.16C) and plastic fragments (Fig. 119.16D). Elemental dispersive microprobe analysis may allow precise identification of metal particles, silica, silicon, and fiberglass (62).

Mechanisms of Inflammation

Mechanisms mediating foreign-body synovitis are not well understood, but several have been postulated including associated low-grade infection; the presence of toxins, alkaloid, mitogens, or other proteins on the surface of foreign bodies; and crystalline or paracrystalline structures with a negative surface charge (71). Few experimental studies of foreign-body effects on synovium and skin of animals have been performed. In one study, minimal acute inflammation was induced by the injection of sterilized ground plant thorns or sea urchin spines into rabbit knees and into the rat skin air pouch model of synovium (71), but 1 to 4 weeks later, both synovium and skin showed prominent chronic inflammation with lymphocytes, plasma cells, and giant cells. In another study, the inflammatory reaction induced by plant thorns injected into rat paws and human forearm skin, correlated with the surface charge of the thorns (71).

Therapy

In about one-third of patients with foreign-body synovitis, the inflammatory changes subside spontaneously. The remaining patients with a chronic or relapsing course usually require an excisional biopsy with complete synovectomy and articular lavage (71). Occasionally, recurrent joint swelling with periosteal new bone formation can be seen after removal of the foreign body and synovectomy.

Arthroscopy has been performed in a few patients with knee plant thorn–induced synovitis, but has failed to reveal the suspected foreign bodies by direct visualization or by histologic studies of the small amount of synovium obtained (71).

REFERENCES

1. Reginato AJ, Kurnik B. Calcium oxalate and other crystals associated with kidney diseases and arthritis. *Semin Arthritis Rheum* 1989;18:198–224.
2. Reginato AJ, Falasca GF, Usmani Q. Do we really need to pay attention to the less common crystals? *Curr Opin Rheumatol* 1999;11:446–452.
3. Reginato AJ, Falasca GF. Calcium oxalate an other miscellaneous crystal related arthropathies. In: Smith ChJ, Holers V, eds. *Gout, hyperuricemia and other crystal-associated arthropathies.* New York: Marcel Dekker, 1999:369–393.
4. Reginato AJ, Ferreiro J, Barbazan C, et al. Arthropathy and cutaneous calcinosis in hemodialysis oxalosis. *Arthritis Rheum* 1986:29:1387–1396.
5. Benhamou CL, Rouchon JP, Geslin N, et al. Arthropathie microcristalline a oxalate de calcium au cours d'une oxalose primitive. *Rev Rhum Med Osteoartic* 1985;52:267–270.
6. Schumacher HR, Reginato AJ, Pullman S. Synovial fluid oxalate deposition complicating rheumatoid arthritis with amyloidosis and renal failure: demonstration of intracellular oxalate crystals. *J Rheumatol* 1987;4:361–366.
7. Rosenthal A, Ryan LM, McCarty DJ. Arthritis associated with calcium oxalate crystals in an nephritic patient treated with peritoneal dialysis. *JAMA* 1988;260:1290–1292.
8. Verbruggen LA, Bourgain C, Berbeelen D. Late presentation and microcrystalline arthropathy in primary hyperoxaluria. *Clin Exp Rheumatol* 1989;7:631–633.
9. Coral A, Van Holsbeeck M, Hegg C. Secondary oxalosis complicating chronic renal failure (oxalate gout). *Skeletal Radiol* 1990;19:147–149.
10. Benhamou CL, Bardin T, Tourliere D, et al. Atteinte osseuse de l'oxalose primitive. Etude de 20 cas. (Bone involvement in primary oxalosis. Study of 20 cases). *Rev Rhum Mal Osteoartic* 1991;58:763–769.
11. Voisin L, Bardin T, Bueni CL, et al. The arthropathy of primary oxalosis. *Arthritis Rheum* 1991;34:S145(abst).
12. Schnitzler CM, Korja-Jacobs DW. Skeletal manifestations of primary oxalosis. *Pediatr Nephrol* 1991;5:193–199.
13. Abuelo G, Schwartz ST, Reginato AJ. Cutaneous oxalosis after long term hemodialysis. *Arch Intern Med* 1992;152:1517–1520.
14. Hoffman G, Schumacher HR, Paul H, et al. Calcium oxalate microcrystalline associated arthritis in end stage renal disease. *Ann Intern Med* 1982;97:36–42.
15. Ring E, Wendler H, Ratschek M, et al. Bone disease of primary hyperoxaluria. *Infancy Pediatr Radiol* 1989;20:131–133.
16. Desmond P, Hennessy D. Skeletal abnormalities in primary oxalosis. *Aust Radiol* 1993;37:83–85.
17. Wise CM, White RE, Agudelo C. Synovial fluid lipid abnormalities in various disease states; review and classification. *Semin Arthritis Rheum* 1987;16:222–230.
18. Schumacher HR, Michaelis R. Recurrent tendinitis and Achilles tendon nodule with positively birefringent crystals in a patient with hyperlipoproteinemia. *J Rheumatol* 1989;16: 1387–1389.
19. Fam AG, Pritzker KPH, Cheng P-T, et al. Cholesterol crystals in osteoarthritic joint effusions. *J Rheumatol* 1981;8:273–280.
20. Fam AG. Subcutaneous cholesterol crystal deposition and tophus formation. *Arthritis Rheum* 1989;32:1190–1191.
21. Sax PA, Altman RD. Subcutaneous cholesterol crystals mimicking calcinosis cutis in systemic sclerosis. *J Rheumatol* 1991; 18:743–745.
22. Pritzker KPH, Fam AG, Omar SA, et al. Experimental cholesterol crystal arthropathy. *J Rheumatol* 1981;8:281–290.
23. Riordan JW, Dieppe PA. Cholesterol crystals in shoulder synovial fluid. *Br J Rheumatol* 1987;26:430–432.
24. Van Offel JF, De Clerck LS, Kersschot IE. Cholesterol crystals and IgE-containing immune complexes in rheumatoid pericarditis. *Clin Rheumatol* 1991;10:78–80.
25. Fishel B, Weiss S, Eventov E, et al. Chylous cyst of shoulder joint in a patient with rheumatoid arthritis. *Clin Exp Rheumatol* 1988;6:79–80.
26. Lazarevic MB, Skosey JL, Vintic J, et al. Cholesterol crystals in synovial and bursal fluids. *Semin Arthritis Rheum* 1993;23: 99–103.
27. Reginato, AJ, Schumacher HR, Allan DA, et al. Acute monarthritis associated with lipid liquid crystals. *Ann Rheum Dis* 1985;44:537–643.
28. Trostle DC, Schumacher HR, Medsger TA, et al. Microspherule associated acute monarticular arthritis. *Arthritis Rheum* 1986; 29:1166–1168.
29. Schlesinger PA, Stillman MT, Peterson L. Polyarthritis with birefringent lipid within synovial fluid macrophages: case report and ultrastructural study. *Arthritis Rheum* 1986;25:1365–1368.
30. Gardner GC, Terkeltaub RA. Acute monarthritis associated with intracellular positively birefringent maltese cross appearing spherules. *J Rheumatol* 1989;16:294–396.
31. Ugai K, Kurosaka M, Hirohata K. Lipid microspherules in synovial fluid of patients with pigmented villonodular synovitis. *Arthritis Rheum* 1988;31:1442–1446.
32. Rivest CH, Hazeltine M, Gilles G, et al. Acute polyarthritis associated with birefringent lipid microspherules occurring in a patient with long standing rheumatoid arthritis. *J Rheumatol* 1992;19:617–620.
33. Choi SJ, Schumacher HR, Clayburne G, et al. Liposome-induced synovitis in rabbits. *Arthritis Rheum* 1986;29:889–896.
34. Choi SJ, Schumacher HR, Clayburne G. Experimental hemarthrosis produces mild inflammation associated with intracellular maltese crosses. *Ann Rheum Dis* 1986;459: 1025–1028.
35. Langlands DR, Dawkins RL, Matz LR, et al. Arthritis associated with crystallizing cryoprecipitable IG paraprotein. *Am J Med* 1980;68:461–465.
36. Dornan TL, Blundell JW, Morgan AG, et al. Widespread crystallization of paraprotein in myelomatosis. *Q J Med* 1985;222: 659–667.
37. Stone GC, Bruce AW, Oppliger IR, et al. A vasculopathy with

deposition of lambda light chain crystals. *Ann Intern Med* 1989;110:275–276.
38. Papot T, Musset L, Bardin T, et al. Cryocrystalglobulinemia as a cause of systemic vasculopathy and widespread erosive arthropathy. *Arthritis Rheum* 1996;39:335–340.
39. Nishi S. Glomerulonephritis with various crystalline deposits. *Am J Nephrol* 1993;13:471–474.
40. An HS, Namey TC, Kim H. Essential cryoglobulinemia associated with intense and persistent synovitis of the knees. *Clin Orthop* 1987;215:173–178.
41. Hasegawa H, Ozawa T, Tada N, et al. Multiple myeloma-associated systemic vasculopathy due to crystal globulin or polyarteritis nodosa. *Arthritis Rheum* 1996;39:330–334.
42. Denko CW. Cryoglobulin induced inflammation. *Agents Actions* 1985;17:92–96.
43. Albert L, Inman DA, Gordon A, et al. Cryocrystalglobulinemia mimicking rheumatoid arthritis and vasculitis. *J Rheumatol* 1996;23:1272–1277
44. Requena L, Sarasa JL, Masilorens F, et al. Follicular spicules of the nose: a peculiar cutaneous manifestation of multiple myeloma with cryoglobulinemia. *J Am Acad Dermatol* 1995;32: 834–839.
45. Brown JP, Rola-Pleszcynski M, Menard HA. Eosinophilic synovitis: clinical observations on a newly recognized subset of patients with dermatographism. *Arthritis Rheum* 1986;29: 1147–1150.
46. Weller PF, Bach D, Austen KF. Human eosinophil lysophospholipase: the sole protein component of Charcot Leyden crystal. *J Immunol* 1982;128:1346–1350.
47. Dougados M, Benhamod L, Amor B. Charcot-Leyden crystals in synovial fluid [letter]. *Arthritis Rheum* 1983;26:1416.
48. Menard HA, DeMedicis R, Lussier A, et al. Charcot-Leyden crystals in synovial fluid. *Arthritis Rheum* 1981;14:1591–1593.
49. Choi Y, Lee JD, Yang KH, et al. Immunotactoid glomerulopathy associated with idiopathic hypereosinophilic syndrome. *Am J Nephrol* 1998;18:337–343.
50. Antoci B, Gherlinzoni G. Cystinosis of bone. *Ital J Orthop Traumatol* 1975;1:81–97.
51. Stephan J, Pitrova S, Pazderka V. Cystinosis with crystal-induced synovitis and arthropathy. *Z Rheumatol* 1976;35: 347–355.
52. Charnas LR, Luciano CA, Dalakas M, et al. Distal vacular myopathy in nephrotic cystinosis. *Ann Neurol* 1994;35: 181–188.
53. Hillenbrabd M, Stropahl G, Seiter H. Massive tumor-like testicular cystine tophaceous deposits in patients with infantile cystinosis. *Br J Urol* 1998;81:331–332.
54. Guillet G, Sassaolas B, Fromentoux S, et al. Skin storage of cystine and premature skin ageing in cystinosis. *Lancet* 1998; 352:1444–1445.
55. Berman L, Salomon L. Xanthine gout, crystal deposition in skeletal muscle in a case of xanthinuria. *Rheumatologie* 1975;5: 253–256.
56. Isaacs A, Heffron IH, Berman L. Xanthine, hypoxanthine and muscle pain: histochemical and biochemical observations. *S Afr Med J* 1975;49:1035–1038.
57. Chalmers RA, Watts RWE, Bitenski L, et al. Microscopic studies on crystals in skeletal muscle in two cases of xanthinuria. *J Pathol* 1969;99:45–65.
58. Netter P. Does aluminum have a pathogenic role in dialysis associated arthropathy? *Ann Rheum Dis* 1990;49:573–575.
59. Netter P, Kessler M, Burnel D, et al. Aluminum in the joint tissues of chronic renal failure patients treated with regular hemodialysis and aluminum compounds. *J Rheumatol* 1984;11: 66–70.
60. Plachot J, Gournot-Witmer G, Halpern S, et al. Bone Ultrastructure and x-rays microanalysis of aluminum-intoxicated hemodialyzed patients. *Kidney Int* 1984;25:796–803.
61. Chaussidon M, Ketter P, Kessler M, et al. Dialysis associate arthropathy: secondary ion mass spectrometry evidence of aluminum silicate in α2-microglobulin amyloid synovial tissue and articular cartilage. *Nephron* 1993;65:559–563.
62. Netter P, Fener P, Steinmetz J. Amorphous alumino-silicates in synovial fluid in dialysis associated arthropathy [letter]. *Lancet* 1991;337:554–555.
63. Zins B, Zingraff J, Basile C, et al. Tumoral calcification in hemodialysis patients; possible role of aluminum intoxication. *Nephron* 1992;60:260–267.
64. Mora GF, Legua AG, Benyacar MA, et al. Aluminum-containing particles in synovial fluid of a patient with normal rneal function and chondrocalcinosis. *J Clin Rheumatol* 1999;5: 83–88.
65. Tate G, Schumacher HR, Reginato AJ, et al. Synovial fluid crystals derived from hemoglobin crystals. *J Rheumatol* 1992;19: 111–114.
66. Reginato AJ. *Manual para el estudio del liquido synovial, bursal y identificacion de cristales.* Barcelona: Imprenta Rapida, 1993:87.
67. Mann D, Schumacher HR. Pseudo septic inflammatory knee effusion caused by phagocytosis of sickled erythrocyte after fracture into the knee joint. *Arthritis Rheum* 1995;38:284–287.
68. Shumacher HR, Van Linthoudt D, Manno CS, et al. Diffuse chondrolytic arthritis in sickle cell disease. *J Rheumatol* 1993; 20:385–389.
69. Freemont AJ, Denton J. Synovial fluid findings in early traumatic arthritis. *J Rheumatol* 1989;15:881–882.
70. Freemont AJ. What is the significance of synovial fluid lipid crystals in an isolated monarthritis? *Br J Rheumatol* 1992; 31:183–184.
71. Reginato AJ, Ferreriro S, O'Connor CR, et al. Clinical and pathologic studies of twenty-six patients with penetrating foreign body injury to the joints, bursae, and tendon sheaths. *Arthritis Rheum* 1990;33:1753–1762.
72. Wilson GE, Curry JK, Kennaugh JH, et al. Severe granulomatous arthritis due to spinous injury by a "sea mouse" annelid worm. *J Clin Pathol* 1990;43:291–294.
73. Cracchiolo A, Goldberg L. Local and systemic reactions to puncture injuries by the sea urchin spine and the date palm thorn. *Arthritis Rheum* 1977;30:1306–1313.
74. Rosai J. Peritoneum, retroperitoneum and related structures. Foreign body granulomas. In: Rosai J, ed. *Ackerman's surgical pathology.* New York: CV Mosby, 1996:2136–2137.
75. Crugnola A, Schiller A, Radin E. Polymeric debris in synovium after total joint replacement. Histological identification. *J Bone Joint Surg* 1977;59A:860–862.
76. Khoo CT. Silicone synovitis. The current role of silicone elastomer implant in joint reconstruction. *J Hand Surg* 1993;18: 679–686.
77. Luiz CP, Ramanathan EB, Buhi L, et al. A case of date palm thorn induced extra-articular synovitis with rice bodies. *Br J Rheumatol* 1994;33:1190–1191.
78. Kehir MM, Snoussi H, Kochbati S, et al. Synovitis caused by plant thorn and chronic polyarthritis. A propos of a case and review of literature. *Rev Rheum* 1994;61:48–50.
79. Goupille P, Fouguet B, Fauard L, et al. Two cases of plant thorn synovitis difficulties in diagnosis and treatment. *J Rheumatol* 1990;17:252–254.
80. Christie A, Pierret G, Levitan J. Silicone synovitis. *Semin Arthritis Rheum* 1989;19:166–171.
81. Arbus GS, Sniderman S. Oxalosis with peripheral gangrene. *Arch Pathol* 1974;97:107–110.
82. Lewis RD, Lowenstam HA, Rossman GR. Oxalate nephrosis and crystalline myocarditis. Case report with postmortem and

crystallographic studies. *Arch Pathol Lab Med* 1974;98: 149–155.

83. West RR, Salyer WR, Hutchins GM. Adult onset primary oxalosis with complete heart block. *Johns Hopkins Med J* 1973;133:195–200.
84. Hricik DE, Hussain R. Pancytopenia and hepatosplenomegaly in oxalosis. *Arch Intern Med* 1984;144:167–168.
85. Watts RWE. Primary hyperoxaluria type I. *Q J Med* 1994; 97:593–600.
86. McKusic VA. *Mendellian inheritance in man. Catalogs of autosomal dominant, autosomal recessive and x-linked phenotypes,* 10th ed. Baltimore: John Hopkins University Press, 1992:1618–1621.
87. Danpure CJ, Jennings PR, Watts RWE. Enzymological diagnosis of primary hyperoxaluria by measurement of hepatic alanine: glyoxylate aminotransferase activity. *Lancet* 1987;1:289–293.
88. Hillman RE. Primary hyperoxaluria. In: Scriver CR, ed. *The metabolic basis of inherited diseases. Primary hyperoxalurias,* 6th ed. New York: McGraw-Hill, 1989:933–944.
89. Wise PJ, Danpure CJ, Jennings PR. Immunological heterogeneity of hepatic alanine-glyoxylate aminotransferase in primary hyperoxaluria type I. *FEBS Lett* 1987;222:17–20.
90. Danpure CJ. Molecular clinical heterogeneity in primary hyperoxaluria type I. *Am J Kidney Dis* 1991;17:364–369.
91. Danpure CJ. Primary hyperoxaliuria type I and peroxisome to mitochondrion mistargeting of alanine: glyoxylate amino transferase. *Biochimie* 1993;75:309–315.
92. Danpure CJ. The molecular basis of alanine glyoxylate aminotransferase mistargeting: the most common cause of primary hyperoxaliuria type 1. *J Nephrol* 1998;11(suppl 1):8–12.
93. Takada Y, Kaneko N, Esumi H, et al. Human peroxisomal l-alanine: glyoxylate aminotransferase: evolutionary loss of a mitochondrial targeting signal by point mutation of the initiation codon. *Biochem J* 1990;268:517–520.
94. Purdue PE, Lumb MJ, Fox M, et al. Characterization and chromosomal mapping of a genomic clone encoding human alanine: glyoxylate aminotransferase. *Genomics* 1991;10:34–42.
95. Purdue PE, Lumb MJ, Allsop J, et al. An intronic duplication in the alanine: glyoxylate aminotransferase gene facilitates identification mutations in compound heterozygote patients with primary hyperoxaluria type I. *Hum Genet* 1991;87:394–396.
96. Danpure CJ, Birdney GM, Rumsby G, et al. Molecular characterization and clinical use of a polymorphic tandem repeat in an intron of the human alanine: glyoxylate amino transferase gene. *Hum Genet* 1994;94:55–64.
97. Purdue PE, Lumb MJ, Fox M, et al. Characterization and chromosomal mapping of a genomic clone encoding human alanine: glyoxylate aminotransferase. *Genomics* 1991;10:34–42.
98. Williams HE, Smith LH Jr. L-Glyceric aciduria, a new genetic variant of primary oxaluria. *N Engl J Med* 1968;278:233–239.
99. Chalmers RA, Tracey BM, Mistry J, et al. L-Glyceric aciduria (primary hyperoxaluria type 2) in siblings in two unrelated families. *J Inherit Metab Dis* 1984;7(suppl 2):133–134.
100. Kemper MJ, Conrad S, Muller-Wiefel DE. Primary hyperoxaliuria type 2. *Eur J Pediatr* 1997;156:509–512.
101. Chlebeck PT, Milliner DS, Smith LH, et al. Long-term prognosis in primary hyperoxaluria type 2 (L-glyceric aciduria). *Am J Kidney Dis* 1994;23:255–259.
102. Smith LH. Diet and hyperoxaluria in the syndrome of idiopathic calcium oxalate urolithiasis. *Am J Kidney Dis* 1991; 17:370–375.
103. Sanz P, Reig R. Clinical and pathological findings in fatal plant oxalosis. *Am J Forensic Med Pathol* 1992;13:342–345.
104. Chedwick VS, Modha K, Durling RH. Mechanism for hyperoxaluria in patients with ileal dysfunction. *N Engl J Med* 1973; 289:172–176.
105. Hage MC, Streem SB, Hall PM. Enteric hyperoxaluria associated with external biliary drainage. *J Urol* 1994;151:396–397.
106. Allen A, Clutterbuck E, Maidment G, et al. Enteric hyperoxaliuria and renal failure associated with lymphangiectasia. *Nephrol Dial Transplant* 1997;12:802–806.
107. Louthrenco W, Park YS, Phillipe L, et al. Localized peripheral calcium oxalate crystal deposition caused by aspergillus niger infection. *J Rheumatol* 1990;17:407–412.
108. Worcester EM, Nakagawa Y, Bushinsky DA, et al. Evidence that serum calcium oxalate supersaturation is a consequence of oxalate retention in patients with chronic renal failure. *J Clin Invest* 1986;77:1888–1896.
109. Symmans PJ, Brady K, Keen E. Calcium oxalate crystal deposition in epitheloid histiocytes of granulomatous lymphadenitis: analysis by light and electron microscopy. *Histopathology* 1995; 27:423–429.
110. Pecorrlla I, McCartney AC, Lucas S, et al. Histological study of oxalosis in the eye and anexa of AIDS patients. Histopathology 1995;27:431–438.
111. Canaverse C, Salomone M, Massara C, et al. Primary oxalosis mimicking hyperparathyroidism diagnosed after long-term hemodialysis. *Am J Nephrol* 1990;10:344–349.
112. Brady HR, Meema HE, Rabinovich S, et al. Oxalate bone disease-an emerging form of renal osteodystrophy. *Int J Artif Organ* 1989;12:715–719.
113. Julian BA, Faugere MC, Malluche HH. Oxalosis in bone causing a radiographical mimicry of renal osteodystrophy. *Am J Kidney Dis* 1987;9:438–440.
114. Gherardi G, Poggie A, Sisca S, et al. Bone oxalosis and renal osteodystrophy. *Arch Pathol Lab Med* 1980;104:105–111.
115. Jahn H, Franck RM, Voegel JC, et al. Scanning electron microscopy and x-ray diffraction studies of human bone oxalosis. *Calcif Tissue Int* 1980;30:109–119.
116. Hasselbacher P. Stimulation of synovial fibroblasts by calcium oxalate and monosodium urate monohydrate. A mechanism of connective tissue degradation in oxalosis and gout. *J Lab Clin Med* 1982;100:977–981.
117. Ramsay AG, Reed RG. Oxalate removal by hemodialysis stage renal disease. *Am J Kidney Dis* 1984;4:123–127.
118. Balcke P, Schmidt P, Zazgornik J, et al. Ascorbic acid aggravates secondary hyperoxalemia in patients on chronic hemodialysis. *Ann Intern Med* 1984;10:344–345.
119. Ott SW, Andress DL, Sherrard DJ. Bone oxalate in long term hemodialysis patients who ingested high doses of vitamin C. *Am J Kidney Dis* 1986;113:450–454.
120. Pru C, Eaton JR, Kjellstrand C. Vitamin C intoxication and hyperoxalemia in chronic hemodialysis patients. *Nephron* 1985; 39:112–116.
121. Milliner DS, Eickholt JT, Bergstralh EJ, et al. Results of long-term treatment with orthophosphate and pyridoxine in patients with primary hyperoxaluria. *N Engl J Med* 1994;331: 1553–1558.
122. Leumann E, Hoppe B, Neuhaus T. Management of primary hyperoxaluria: efficacy or oral citrate administration. *Pediatr Nephrol* 1993;7:207–211.
123. Holmes RP. Pharmacological approaches in the treatment of primary hyperoaluria. *J Nephrol* 1998;11(suppl 1):32–35.
124. Toussaint C. Pyridoxine responsive Ph1: Treatment. *J Nephrol* 1998;11(suppl 1):49–50.
125. Broyer M, Brunner FP, Brynger H. Kidney transplantation in primary oxalosis: data from the EDTA registry. *Nephrol Dial Transplant* 1990;5:332–336.
126. McDonald JC, Landrenea MD, Rohr MS, et al. Reversal by liver transplantation of the complications of primary hyperoxaluria as well as the metabolic defect. *N Engl J Med* 1989;321:1100–1103.

127. Uribarri J, Miller Ch, Burrow L. Combined liver-kidney transplantation for the genetic disorder primary hyperoxaluria type I. *Mt Sinai J Med* 1994;61:32–36.
128. Kemper MJ, Nokelmper D, Rogiers X, et al. Pre-emptive liver transplantation in primary hyperoxaluria type I, timing and preliminary results. *J Nephrol* 1998;119(suppl 1):46–48.
129. Corts J, Castellanos J, Reginato AJ, et al. Tumoral calcinosis containing hydroxyapatite and cholesterol crystals associated with dermatomyositis. *Arthritis Rheum* 1992;35:S76(abst).
130. Smith MC, Chose MK, Henry AR. The clinical spectrum of renal cholesterol embolization. *Am J Med* 1981;11:174–180.
131. Pritzker KPH, Fam AG, Omar SA, et al. Experimental cholesterol crystal arthropathy. *J Rheumatol* 1981;8:281–290.
132. Desnick RJ, Bishop DF. α-Galactosidase deficiency: Fabry disease. In: Scriver CR, Resnick RJ, Ioannou YA, et al., eds. *The metabolic basis of inherited disease.* 7th ed. New York: McGraw-Hill, 1995:2741–2784.
133. Kirkilionis AJ, Riddell DC, Spence MW, et al. Fabry disease in a large Nova Scotia kindred: carrier detection using leucocyte alphagalactosidase activity and an NcoI polymorphism detected by an alpha-galactosidase cDNA clone. *J Med Genet* 1991; 28:232–240.
134. Eng CM, Desnick RJ. Molecular basis of Fabry disease: mutations and polymorphisms in the human alpha-galactosidase A gene. *Hum Mutat* 1994;3:103–111.
135. Grewal RP. Stroke in Fabry's disease. *J Neurol* 1994;241: 153–156.
136. Jardine DL, Fitzpatrick MA, Troughton WD, et al. Small bowel ischaemia in Fabry's disease. *J Gastroenterol Hepatol* 1994;9: 201–205.
137. Wise D, Wallace HL, Jellink EH. Angiokeratoma corporis diffusum: a clinical study of 8 affected families. *Q J Med* 1962; 31:177–206.
138. Sheth KJ, Bernhard GC. The arthropathy of Fabry's disease. *Arthritis Rheum* 1979;22:781–783.
139. Faira SO, Roverano S, Iribas JL, et al. Joint manifestations of Fabry's disease. *Clin Rheumatol* 1992;11:562–565.
140. Dubost JJ, Sauvezie B, Galtier J, et al. La maladic de Fabry etiologie rare de syndrome inflammatoire au long cours. *Rev Rhum* 1986;53:525–528.
141. Kato H, Sato K, Hattori S, et al. Fabry's disease. *Intern Med* 1992;31:682–685.
142. Rahman P, Gladman DD, Wither J, et al. Coexistence of Fabry's disease and systemic lupus erythematosus. *Clin Exp Rheumatol* 1998;16:475–478.
143. Lockman LA, Hunninghake DB, Krivit W, et al. Relief of pain of Fabry's disease by diphenylhydantoin. *Neurology* 1973;23: 871–875.
144. Honsoon P, Burton TJ, Van der Bel-Kahn JM. Circulating Charcot-Leyden crystals in hypereosinophilic syndrome. *Am J Clin Pathol* 1981;75:236–242.
145. Carson HJ, Buschmann RJ, Weisz-Carrington P, et al. Identification of Charcot-Leyden crystals by electron microscopy. *Ultrastruct Pathol* 1992;16:403–411.
146. Gahl WA, Schneider JA, Aula PP, et al. Lysosomal transport disorders. Cystinosis and sialic acid storage disorders. In: Scriver CR, Beudet AL, Sly WS, et al., eds. *The metabolic basis of inherited diseases,* 7th ed. New York: McGraw-Hill, 1995: 3763–3787.
147. Gahl WA, Tietze F, Bashan N, et al. Defective cystine exodus from isolated lysosome-rich fractions of cystinotic leucocytes. *J Biol Chem* 1982;257:9570–9575.
148. Gahl WA, Dalakas MC, Charnas L, et al. Myopathy and cystine storage in muscles in a patient with nephropathic cystinosis. *N Engl J Med* 1988;319:1461–1464.
149. Gahl WA, Thoeme JG, Schneider JR, et al. Cystinosis progress in a prototypic disease. *Ann Intern Med* 1988;109:557–569.
150. Almond PS, Matas AJ, Nakhleh RE, et al. Renal transplantation for infantile cystinosis: long term follow-up. *J Pediatr Surg* 1993;28:232–238.
151. Kaiser-Kupfer ML, Gazzo MA, Datiles MB, et al. A randomized placebo-controlled trial of cysteamine eye drops in nephropathiccistinosis. *Arch Ophthalmol* 1990;108:689–693.
152. Simmonds A, Reiter S, Nishin O. Hereditary Xanthinuria. In: Scriver CR, Beaudet AL, Sly WS, et al., eds. *The metabolic basis of inherited diseases,* 7th ed. New York: McGraw-Hill, 1995: 1781–1797.
153. Kessler ML, Netter PA, Azoulay E, et al. Dialysis associated arthropathy: a multicenter survey of 171 patients receiving hemodialysis for over 10 years. *Br J Rheumatol* 1992;31: 157–162.
154. Netter P, Delongeas JL, Faure G, et al. Inflammatory effect of aluminum phosphate. *Ann Rheum Dis* 1983;42:114–118.
155. Krpan D, Milutinovic S, Tomicic D, et al. Oxalosis associated with aluminum bone disease: a new type of mixed renal osteodystrophy. *Nephron* 1994;66:99–101.
156. Zins B, Zingraff J, Petitcleree T, et al. Tumoral calcification in hemodialysis patients possible role of aluminum intoxication. *Nephron* 1992;60:260–267.
157. O'Connor CR, Reginato AJ, DeLong W. Foreign body reaction simulating acute septic arthritis. *J Rheumatol* 1988;15: 1568–1571.
158. Peimer CA, Taleisnik J, Sherwin FS. Pathologic fractures: a complication of microparticulate synovitis. *J Hand Surg (Am)* 1991;16:835–843.
159. Windler EC, Smith RB, Bryan WJ, et al. Lead intoxication and traumatic arthritis of hip secondary to retained bullet fragments. A case report. *J Bone Joint Surg* 1978;60:254–255.
160. Ponge T, Caumon JP, Friol JP, et al. Plant thorn synovitis caused by pyracantha coccinea (burning bush) [letter]. *Presse Med* 1993;18:1279–1280.
161. Goupille P, Fouquet B, Favard L, et al. Two cases of plant thorn synovitis. Difficulties in diagnosis and treatment. *J Rheumatol* 1990;17:252–254.
162. Kaufman RL, Tong I, Beardmore TD. Prosthetic synovitis: clinical and histologic characteristics. *J Rheumatol* 1985;12: 1066–1074.
163. Khoo CT. Silicone synovitis. The current role of silicone elastomer implants in joint reconstruction. Review article. *J Hand Surg* 1993;18:679–686.
164. Raimbeau G, Fondimare A. Late flexor synovitis induced by the use of a fabric lace. *Ann Chir Main Memb Super* 1994;13:56–59.
165. Scalfani SJA, Vuletin JC, Twersty J. Lead arthropathy: arthritis caused by retained intra-articular bullets. *Radiology* 1985;156: 299–302.
166. Janzen DL, Tirenan PFJ, Rabassa AE, et al. Lead "bursogram" and focal synovitis secondary to a retained intra-articular bullet fragment. *Skeletal Radiol* 1995;4:142–144.
167. Bostman OM. Osteoarthritis of the ankle after foreign-body reaction to absorbable pins and screws: a three to nine-year follow up study. *J Bone Joint Surg* 1988;80B:333–338.
168. Fasano FJ Jr, Hansen RH. Foreign body granuloma and synovitis of the finger:a hazard of ring removal by the sawing technique. *J Hand Surg* 1987;12:621–623.
169. Little CL, Parker MG, Callowich MC, et al. The ultrasonic detection of soft tissue foreign bodies. *Invest Radiol* 1986;21: 275–277.
170. Bauer AR, Yutani D. Computed tomography localization of wooden foreign bodies in children's extremities. *Arch Surg* 1983; 118:1084–1086.

171. Klein B, McGahan JP. Thorn synovitis: CT diagnosis. *J Comput Assist Tomogr* 1985;9:1135–1136.
172. Russel RC, Williamson DA, Sullivan JW, et al. Detection of foreign body in the hand. *J Hand Surg* 1991;16:2–11.
173. Maillot F, Goupille P, Valat JP. Plant thorn synovitis diagnosed by magnetic resonance imaging. *Scand J Rheumatol* 1994;23:154–155.
174. Mizel MS, Steinmetz ND, Trepman E. Detection of wooden foreign bodies in muscle tissue: experimental comparison of computed tomography, magnetic resonance imaging, and ultrasonography. *Foot Ankle Int* 1994;15:437–442.
175. Chan M, Chowchuen P, Workman T, et al. Silicone synovitis: MR imaging in five patients. *Skeletal Radiol* 1998;27:13–17.

120

METABOLIC DISEASES OF MUSCLE

ROBERT L. WORTMANN

A wide variety of conditions can be classified as metabolic diseases of muscle. These have in common an underlying abnormality in muscle glycogen, lipid, or adenosine triphosphate (ATP) metabolism. The study of metabolic muscle disease is relatively new. Myophosphorylase deficiency, the first described metabolic myopathy, was predicted in 1951 (1) and the biochemical defect identified in 1959 (2). Subsequently, additional defects of glycogen metabolism and disorders of lipid and purine metabolism in muscle have been recognized. The sequencing of mitochondrial DNA just over a decade ago has resulted in the discovery of and better understanding of a wide number of metabolic myopathies. Other metabolic diseases of muscle surely await discovery.

Clinically, metabolic myopathies must be considered in the differential diagnosis of individuals with proximal muscle weakness, myoglobinuria, or exercise intolerance as a result of fatigue, myalgias, or cramps. The evaluation of such patients requires an awareness of potential diagnoses, an understanding of energetics in normal muscle, and an acceptance that much remains to be learned about this general area before more successful therapies will be available.

SKELETAL MUSCLE FIBERS

Skeletal muscle contains multinucleated cells called fibers, functionally grouped in motor units. A motor unit consists of all the fibers innervated by an individual motor neuron. The fibers within each motor unit have common histochemical and electrophysiologic properties and can be classified based on those characteristics (Table 120.1). Type 1 (red) fibers respond to stimulation slowly, but are relatively resistant to fatigue. They are rich in lipids, mitochondria, and oxidative enzymes. In contrast, type 2B (white) fibers respond to stimulation briskly and with greater force, but fatigue rapidly. Their glycogen content and myophosphorylase activity are greater. The properties of type 2A fibers share some properties with each of the other types and respond to stimulation in an intermediate fashion.

Individual human muscles are composed of mixtures of all fiber types. Approximately half of fibers are type 1 and half type 2 in populations of sampled individuals. However, considerable variation exists among individuals. Highly trained muscle is composed of type 1 and type 2A fibers. Type 2B fibers predominate in muscle of obese and deconditioned individuals.

TABLE 120.1. PROPERTIES OF MUSCLE FIBER TYPES

Fiber Type Designation	1	2A	2B
Color	Red	Red	White
Twitch type	SO	FOG	FG
Motor unit properties			
Twitch speed	Slow	Intermediate	Fast
Tetanic force	Small	Large	Largest
Fatigue resistance	Highest	High	Low
Histochemical properties			
ATPase (pH 4.4)	High	Low	Low
ATPase (pH 10.6)	Low	High	High
Glycogen	Low	High	High
Lipid	High	Variable	Low
Myophosphorylase	Low	High	High
NADH dehydrogenase	High	Intermediate	Low

SO, slow twitch oxidative; FOG, fast twitch oxidative glycolytic; FG, fast twitch glycolytic; ATPase, adenosine triphosphatase; NADH, reduced nicotinamide adenine dinucleotide.

CONTRACTION AND RELAXATION

Muscular activity can be initiated by electric, chemical, and mechanical stimulation to produce an action potential transmitted along the cell membrane. An action potential moves along a motor neuron to a presynaptic nerve terminal, where depolarization causes the release of acetylcholine, which diffuses to the postsynaptic membrane of the muscle cell and binds to specific receptors. Such binding causes conformational changes, opening channels permeable to sodium and potassium. As a consequence, sodium moves into the cell and potassium moves out, depolarizing the muscle fiber and generating a signal called an *end-plate potential.* As the wave of depolarization spreads, the resting state of the membrane is restored and maintained, in part by an active sodium potassium exchanger [Na-K–dependent adenosine triphosphatase (ATPase)]. The wave of depolarization spreads from the membrane to the interior of the muscle fiber through the system of T tubules, connecting the cell surface with the sarcoplasmic reticulum (Fig. 120.1). When the signal reaches the sarcoplasmic reticulum, calcium is released from the lateral sacs to diffuse among the fibrils, initiating contraction.

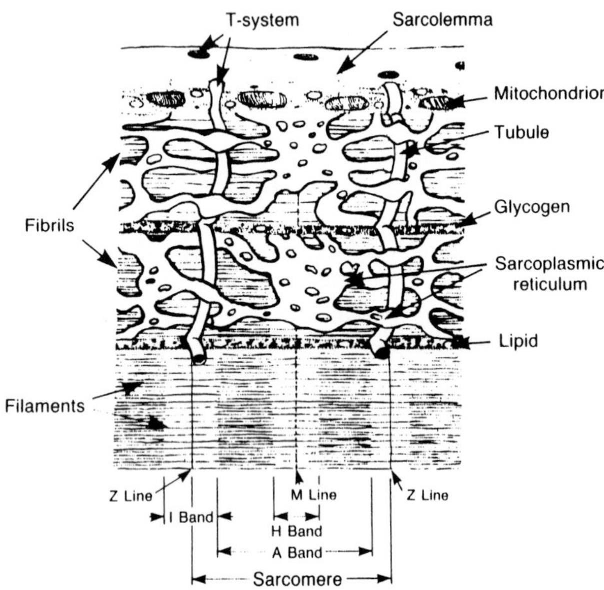

FIGURE 120.1. Structure of a skeletal muscle fiber. Each muscle fiber is a multinucleated cell composed of fibrils that contain filaments of contractile proteins surrounded by a plasma membrane, the sarcolemma. Communication between the plasma membrane and fibrils is provided by the T-system of tubules that runs along the border of the sarcomeres and connects to the sarcoplasmic reticulum that invests the fibrils. The varying refractile indices of the filaments give skeletal muscle its characteristic cross-striated appearance by electron microscopy (see Fig. 120.8). The functional contractile unit of the muscle cell is the sarcomere and is defined as the area between two Z lines. The A band is composed of the thick filaments (myosin), and the M line is due to bulges in the centers of the thick filaments. At rest, the I band is the area occupied by thin filaments (troponin, tropomyosin, and actin) not overlapped by myosin. With contraction, cross-bridges are formed between thick and thin filaments, Z lines move toward the M line, and the I bands become smaller.

Contraction in muscle occurs as a consequence of a magnesium-dependent actomyosin ATPase. The activity of this enzyme results in the formation of cross-bridges between actin and myosin and the sliding of filaments. At rest, actomyosin ATPase is inhibited and there are no cross-bridges between the thick filaments (myosin) and thin filaments (troponin, tropomyosin, and actin). Troponin, along with tropomyosin, and protein that connects troponin to actin, inhibits the interaction of actin and myosin. As calcium concentrations around myofibrils increase, calcium binds to troponin causing conformational changes that release the inhibition of actomyosin ATPase. With the hydrolysis of ATP, actin-containing filaments bridge with and slide along myosin, shortening the fiber.

Muscle fiber relaxation is also the result of an active process. Shortly after calcium is released, it is pumped back into the sarcoplasmic reticulum by a calcium-dependent ATPase. Once the concentration of calcium around the fibrils is lowered, calcium is displaced from troponin and the interaction between actin and myosin stops, cross-links are broken, and fiber lengthening occurs.

ENERGY METABOLISM IN SKELETAL MUSCLE

Energy necessary for muscle contraction is provided by the hydrolysis of ATP. Intracellular concentrations of ATP are maintained by the action of enzymes such as creatine phosphokinase (CPK), adenylate cyclase, and myoadenylate deaminase. The energy needed to replenish ATP when it is consumed during muscle contraction is provided by the intermediary metabolism of carbohydrate and lipid by the pathways of glycolysis, the citric acid cycle, β-oxidation, and oxidative phosphorylation (3–5).

The immediate source of energy for skeletal muscle during work is found in preformed organic compounds containing high-energy phosphate such as ATP and creatine phosphate. At rest, the terminal phosphate of ATP is transferred to creatine, forming creatine phosphate and adenosine diphosphate (ADP) in a reaction catalyzed by CPK. Creatine phosphate thus acts as a reservoir of high-energy phosphate immediately available to reform ATP, and CPK acts to buffer cytoplasmic changes in ATP concentration. CPK and its products, creatine and creatine phosphate, also play a significant role in the transport of energy from mitochondria to myofibrils. This latter action is referred to as the creatine-creatine phosphate shuttle (Fig. 120.2) (6).

During rest and less strenuous exercise, the activity of CPK renders the concentration of ATP within cells con-

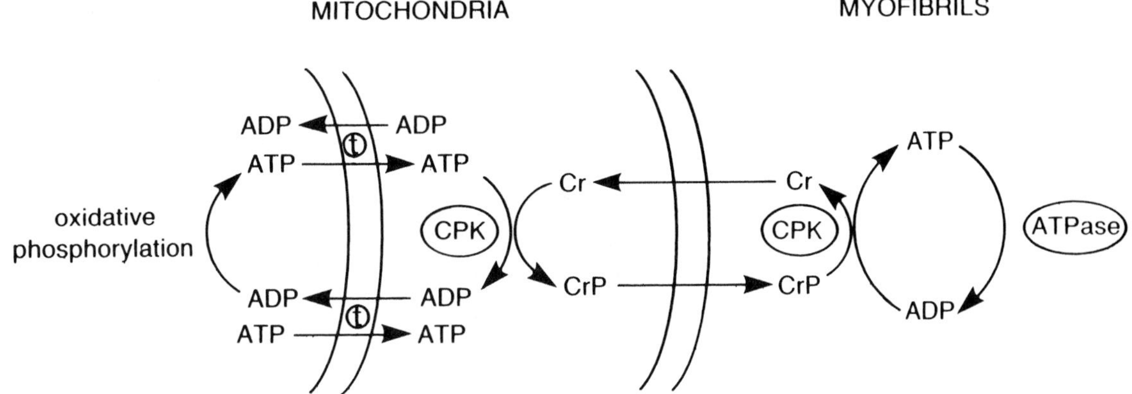

FIGURE 120.2. Scheme of the creatine-creatine phosphate shuttle. Creatine phosphokinase (CPK) is located on the inner mitochondrial membrane, on myofibrils, and in the cytoplasm. It provides a buffer mechanism for maintaining homeostatic concentrations of intracellular adenine nucleotides and plays an important role in the energy transfer within the cell after adenosine triphosphate (ATP) is produced in mitochondria. CPK also buffers adenosine diphosphate (ADP) and inorganic phosphate levels. The cytosolic ADP concentration is a regulator of glycolysis. Cr, creatine; CrP, creatine phosphate; t, adenine nucleotide translocase.

stant at the expense of creatine phosphate. When metabolic requirements, such as those that occur during prolonged contraction and muscle fatigue, exceed the capacity of oxidative phosphorylation to regenerate ATP, creatine phosphate is used to replenish ATP. When approximately 50% of the creatine phosphate has been converted to creatine, ATP levels begin to fall and inosine monophosphate (IMP) accumulates. ATP is hydrolyzed to ADP and then to adenosine monophosphate (AMP) by adenylate kinase, and the AMP is converted to IMP by myoadenylate deaminase. During recovery from exercise, IMP is converted back to AMP by a two-step process. The conversion of AMP to IMP and back to AMP has been called the purine nucleotide cycle (Fig. 120.3). The reactions of the purine nucleotide cycle (a) reduce AMP levels, which are inhibitory to ATP generating reactions; (b) generate ammonia, which stimulates glycolysis; and (c) release fumarate, which is converted to malate, an intermediate of the citric acid cycle and promoter of oxidative phosphorylation.

The majority of cellular energy is produced in mitochondria by degradation of metabolites through the citric acid cycle and respiratory (cytochrome) chain. Products of the aerobic degradation of carbohydrate (pyruvate) and fatty acids enter the Krebs cycle, generating reducing equivalents. The respiratory chain, a series of enzymes and coenzymes that function as hydrogen carriers, transfers reducing equivalents to molecular oxygen (Fig. 120.4 and Table 120.2). The large amount of free energy released is captured and conserved in the form of ATP by a process called oxidative phosphorylation. Factors that influence the relative amounts of carbohydrate and lipids used for ATP production include the oxygen concentration of blood and muscle blood flow, the number of

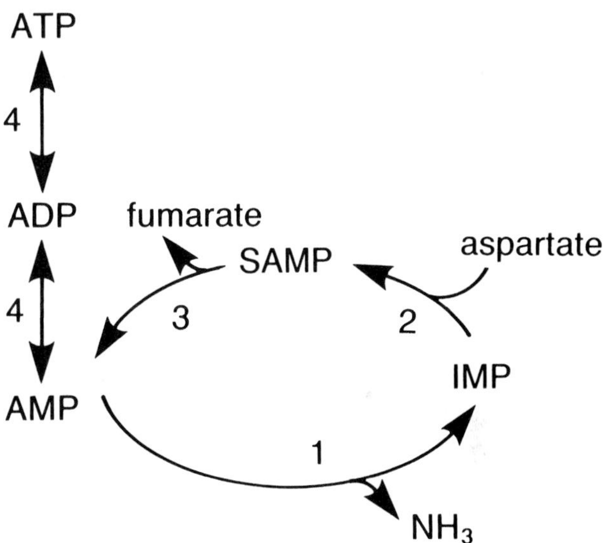

FIGURE 120.3. The purine nucleotide cycle. When muscle contraction is sufficient to exceed the buffering capacity of creatine phosphate and deplete adenosine triphosphate (ATP), adenosine diphosphate (ADP), and adenosine monophosphate (AMP) are formed by the activity of adenylate kinase. Under these conditions, glycolysis becomes the major route for regeneration of ATP, and the enzymes of the purine nucleotide cycle play a critical regulatory role. The conversion of AMP to inosine monophosphate (IMP) by myoadenylate deaminase causes ammonia release and changes in nucleotide concentrations that stimulate glycolysis. IMP accumulates until muscle activity decreases and recovery occurs. Oxidative conditions are restored and AMP is regenerated by a two-step process with the liberation of fumarate. Fumarate is converted to malate, which is an intermediate in the Krebs cycle. The increased levels of malate drive the citric acid cycle, causing efficient resynthesis of ATP by oxidative phosphorylation. 1, myoadenylate deaminase; 2, adenylsuccinate synthetase; 3, adenylsuccinate lyase; 4, adenylate kinase; NH_3, ammonia; SAMP, adenylsuccinate.

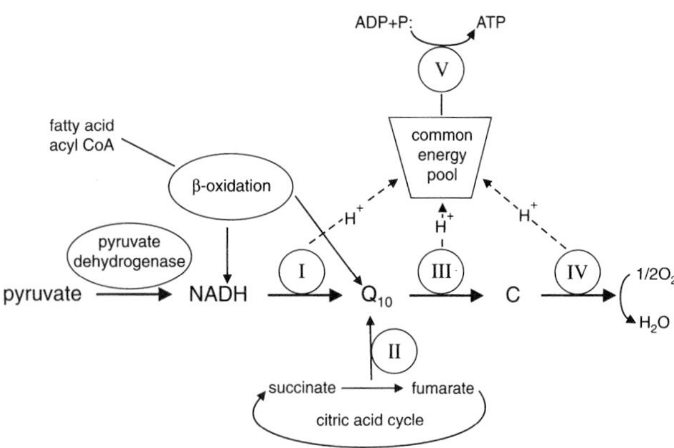

FIGURE 120.4. Scheme of respiratory chain-linked oxidative phosphorylation. Oxidative phosphorylation takes place in mitochondria. This process generates ATP by means of five multiple subunit enzyme complexes (I–V). These are located within the mitochondrial inner membrane. Reduced nicotinamide adenine dinucleotide (NADH) is oxidized by complex I and succinate is oxidized by complex II with electrons transferred to cytochrome Q_{10} (also called ubiquinone). From cytochrome Q_{10}, the electrons are transferred to complex III, cytochrome C, complex IV, and oxygen, sequentially. The energy released is used to pump hydrogen ions out of the mitochondrial inner membrane through complexes I, III, and IV, producing an electrochemical gradient that allows complex V (ATP synthase) to condense ADP and inorganic phosphate (Pi) to form ATP. Both ATP and ADP are exchanged across the mitochondrial inner membrane by an adenine nucleotide translocator.

mitochondria and glycogen stores in muscle, and plasma free fatty acid levels.

Intracellular glycogen stores provide the major source of carbohydrate available for energy production in skeletal muscle. Most glucose entering the fibers from the blood is converted to glycogen, although glucose itself can be metabolized directly to pyruvate under certain conditions. On demand, glucose units are enzymatically split from glycogen and are degraded through a series of reactions to pyruvate (Fig. 120.5). Under aerobic conditions, pyruvate enters the Krebs cycle and is metabolized by that cycle and by oxidative phosphorylation to carbon dioxide and water. In the process, large amounts of energy are liberated to form ATP. The metabolism of one molecule of glucose by aerobic glycolysis yields a net gain of 38 molecules of ATP.

During exercise of short duration and high intensity, the major source of energy is glycogen, not glucose. Glycogen, a branched homopolymer of glucose, is a major storage form of carbohydrate in the body and is distributed evenly between slow- and fast-twitch muscle fibers at rest. Although glycogen products can enter the aerobic pathways previously described, they can also be metabolized anaerobically. In anaerobic glycolysis, pyruvate does not enter the Krebs cycle but is converted to lactate instead. This process produces smaller quantities of ATP (two ATPs per molecule of glucose or three ATPs per glucose unit from glycogen) compared to aerobic metabolism. Muscle glycogen stores are limited and can be depleted after 90 minutes of exercise at an intensity of 70% maximum oxygen uptake. In contrast, the supply of lipid is plentiful.

Lipids in the form of fatty acids constitute the major substrates for energy production for muscles at rest, during contraction, and during recovery. The speed at which free fatty acids can be mobilized and the rate of energy production from them is slow compared to glycogen (7). Plasma free fatty acids provide the largest source of lipids; intracellular stores provide very small contributions. Long chain fatty acids move through the bloodstream from adipose tissue bound to albumin. These, plus smaller fatty acids, move across endothelial cells and into muscle cells, where they are available for energy production, storage, or synthesis into membrane components. Each of these processes requires activation of the fatty acids to acyl–coenzyme A (CoA) derivatives. The resulting activated fatty acids can undergo oxidation following carnitine-mediated transport into mitochondria catalyzed

TABLE 120.2. COMPOSITION OF RESPIRATORY CHAIN COMPLEXES

Complex	Enzyme Activity	Prosthetic Groups
I.	NADH-CoQ reductase (NADH dehydrogenase)	Flavin mononucleotide (FMA) Iron sulfur proteins
II.	Succinate-CoQ reductase (succinate dehydrogenase)	Flavin adenine dinucleotide (FAD) Cytochrome b_{560} Iron sulfur proteins
III.	CoQH2-cytochrome c reductase (cytochrome Q dehydrogenase)	Cytochrome b_{562} Cytochrome b_{566} Iron sulfur protein center Cytochrome c_1
IV.	Cytochrome c oxidase	Cytochrome a Cytochrome a_3 Copper
V.	ATP synthase	Magnesium

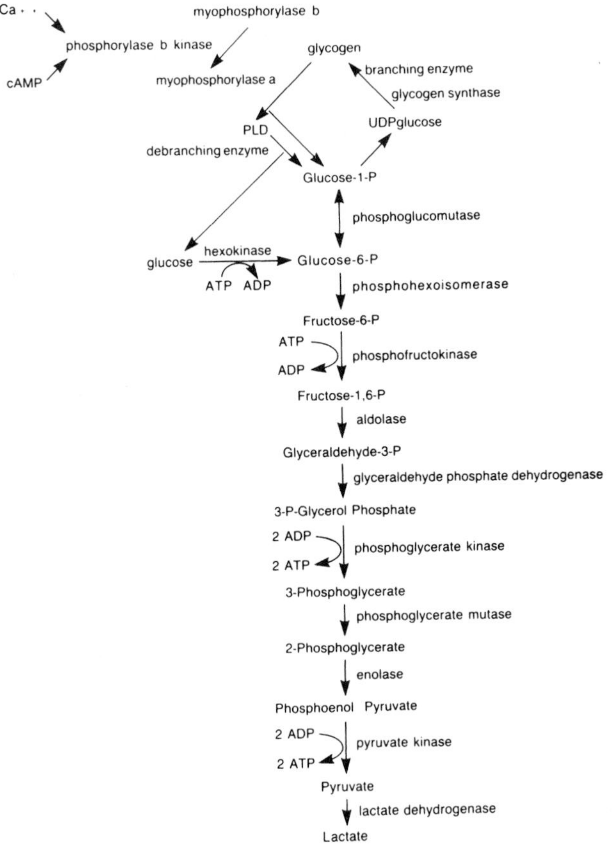

FIGURE 120.5. Pathways for glycogen metabolism and glycolysis. Glucose moves across the sarcoplasmal membrane into the cell, where it is phosphorylated by hexokinase. The resulting glucose-6-phosphate is then converted to glucose-1-phosphate by phosphoglucomutase and then to uridinediphosphoglucose (UDPG) by UDPG pyrophosphorylase. Glycogen synthesis then proceeds by a combination of reactions catalyzed by glycogen-synthase, transferring glucose molecules from UDPG to a preexisting polymeric chain of other glucose molecules, which are linked by β-1,4-glucosidic bonds in a linear fashion, and branching enzyme, which results in the formation of new outer side chains by forming β-1,6-glucosyl bonds. Glycogen remains in reserve until metabolic demands lead to the activation of myophosphorylase. Myophosphorylase exists in active (phosphorylase a) and inactive (phosphorylase b) forms. Conversion of the inactive to the active form is regulated by the enzyme phosphorylase b kinase, which is stimulated either by calcium release from the sarcoplasmic reticulum or by 3′,5′-cyclic adenosine monophosphate (cAMP)-dependent protein kinase. Active phosphorylase can degrade only about 35% of a glycogen molecule to glucose-1-phosphate. In the process, it leaves phosphorylase-limit dextrans (PLDs), containing terminal β-1,6-glucosidically bound glucose units each covered by three β-1,4-glucosidically bound units. Further degradation of PLD requires the action of debranching enzyme (amylo-1,6-glucosidase). The glucose-1-phosphate formed is then available for entry into the glycolytic pathway. Under anaerobic conditions it is converted in ten steps to lactate. For each glucose unit entering the pathway, one ATP molecule is hydrolyzed but four ATP molecules are generated and two lactate molecules result. Under aerobic conditions, the end product of glycolysis is pyruvate. Pyruvate molecules can enter the Krebs cycle and proceed through oxidative phosphorylation. Rate-limiting steps in glycolysis are those catalyzed by phosphofructokinase, glyceraldehyde phosphate dehydrogenase, and phosphoglycerate kinase.

by carnitine palmitoyltransferase (CPT) (Fig. 120.6) or esterification leading to the formation of cytosolic triglyceride droplets that provide a depot of lipid for future use. Once in the mitochondria, fatty acyl-CoA units are converted to acetyl-CoA by the process of β-oxidation, and acetyl-CoA is processed through the citric acid cycle.

DISORDERS OF GLYCOGEN METABOLISM

The discovery in 1959 of myophosphorylase deficiency in muscle was the first report of a biochemical abnormality in an inherited myopathy (2). This observation occurred 8 years after McArdle (1) had deduced that "a gross failure of the breakdown in muscle of glycogen to lactate acid" was responsible for lifelong exercise intolerance in a 30-year-old man. Subsequently, additional inborn errors of glycogen metabolism associated with muscle symptoms have been reported (8,9) (Table 120.3), and undoubtedly more remain to be described. Individuals with a glycogen storage disease are well at rest and perform mild exercise without difficulty, because free fatty acids are the major source of energy under those conditions. The enzymatic block that interferes with the use of carbohydrate to generate ATP causes problems only when exercise reaches a level that produces anaerobic conditions. The inability to replenish depleted high-energy phosphate stores then results in pain, contracture, and muscle necrosis.

DEFECTS OF GLYCOGENOLYSIS

Myophosphorylase Deficiency (McArdle's Disease)

Myophosphorylase deficiency is the prototypic muscle glycogenosis defect. It has an autosomal-recessive pattern of inheritance and is attributed to a variety of defects in the gene for the muscle isoform of the enzyme (11). The most common inborn error is a nonsense mutation at codon 49 of exon 1 for the myophosphorylase gene (11). Some individuals are homozygous; others are compound heterozygotes for different mutations (11,12).

The cardinal clinical manifestation of myophosphorylase deficiency is exercise intolerance associated with pain, fatigue, stiffness, or weakness. The degree of exercise intolerance varies among affected individuals. Symptoms always resolve with rest and can follow activities of high intensity and short duration or activities that require less intense effort for longer intervals. In fact, affected individuals function well, provided they adjust their activities to a level below their individual threshold for symptoms. When they exceed their exercise tolerance, they become symptomatic. In addition to stiffness and weakness, painful muscle cramps are sometimes associated with muscle necrosis, myoglobinuria, and potentially reversible renal failure.

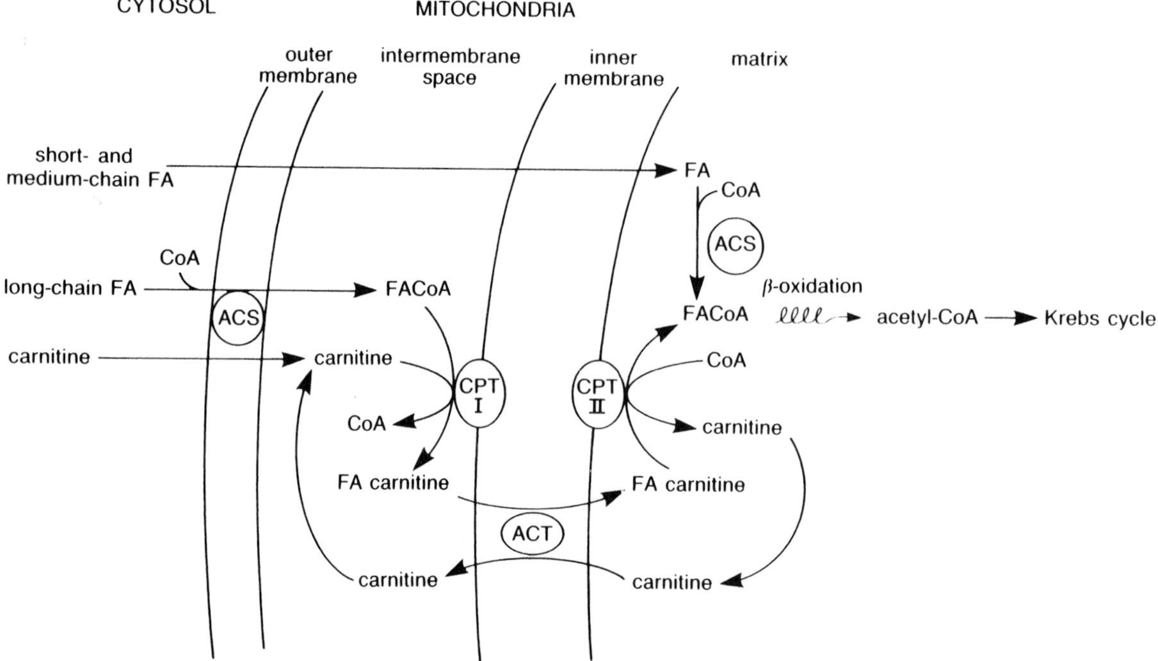

FIGURE 120.6. Scheme of fatty acid metabolism in mitochondria. Short- and medium-chain fatty acids cross the mitochondrial membrane by diffusion, but the process for long-chain fatty acids is more complex, requiring four steps. First, the long-chain fatty acids must be activated, a reaction catalyzed by acyl-CoA synthetase (ACS) in the outer mitochondrial membrane. The acyl-CoA products formed are substrate for the second step, the formation of acylcarnitine by the action of carnitine palmitoyltransferase 1 (CPT I). L-Carnitine is ubiquitous and has the primary function of transferring long-chain fatty acids across the inner mitochondrial membrane by ACT. Finally, the long-chain acylcarnitine is converted to the corresponding acyl-CoA structure by carnitine palmitoyltransferase 2 (CPT II), which is located on the matrix side of the inner mitochondrial membrane. Once in the mitochondrial matrix, the fatty acids are converted to acetyl-CoA by a repetitive process called β-oxidation. The β-oxidation process nets five molecules of adenosine triphosphate for each acetyl-CoA molecule generated, and each acetyl-CoA molecule formed is available for combustion through the Krebs cycle. Accordingly, the degradation of one molecule of palmityl-CoA requires seven β-oxidation cycles, yields eight acetyl-CoA molecules, and produces 131 molecules of ATP. ACT, acylcarnitine translocase; FA, fatty acid.

TABLE 120.3. INBORN ERRORS OF GLYCOGEN METABOLISM THAT AFFECT MUSCLE

Enzyme Deficiency	Eponym	Symptoms
Acid maltase	Pompe's disease	Proximal weakness
Brancher enzyme	Andersen's disease	Hypotonia, weakness
Debrancher enzyme	Cori-Forbes' disease	Proximal weakness
Phosphorylase b kinase	—	Exercise intolerance, cramps, myoglobulinuria
Myophosphorylase	McArdle's disease	Exercise intolerance, cramps, myoglobulinuria
Phosphofructokinase	Tarui's disease	Exercise intolerance, cramps, myoglobulinuria
Phosphoglycerate kinase	—	Exercise intolerance, myoglobulinuria
Phosphoglycerate mutase	—	Exercise intolerance, myoglobulinuria
Lactate dehydrogenase	—	Exercise intolerance, cramps, myoglobulinuria

Individuals typically become symptomatic between the ages of 10 and 25 years. Although some symptoms usually are noted in childhood, many are often overlooked and recognized only in retrospect. For unknown reasons, severe cramps and myoglobulinuria are rare before adolescence. The late development of significant symptoms accounts for the rarity of the diagnosis before age 10. Another reason is the clinical heterogeneity of the disease. Some individuals complain only of being tired and having poor stamina, but others develop progressive muscle weakness that tends to be proximal and may initially be misdiagnosed as polymyositis (13). The development of fixed proximal muscle weakness later in life is attributed to recurrent, exertional muscle injury (14). These symptoms may develop so insidiously that the diagnosis is not made until after age 75 (15).

Magnetic resonance spectroscopy confirms the muscle biochemistry predicted by the known enzymatic block (16). Concentrations of ATP and creatine phosphate are normal at rest. With exercise, however, pH does not decrease and the recovery of energy-rich metabolites to normal levels is delayed. The intolerance for aerobic exercise is attributed to limited pyruvate availability interfering with normal oxidative metabolism (17). Exercise studies demonstrate low maximum oxygen consumption and small arteriovenous oxygen differences reflecting a defect in oxidative metabolism due to impaired substrate availability (18). Some individuals experience a "second wind" phenomenon; if they stop their activities at the onset of myalgia or stiffness and rest briefly, they can then resume exercising with increased tolerance. This ability to tolerate gradually increasing workloads is probably due to the combination of increased blood flow in exercising muscles and mobilization of fatty acids (19).

Elevated levels of serum CPK are a common finding in myophosphorylase deficiency, helping to distinguish it from the other significant metabolic myopathy that causes myoglobulinuria, namely carnitine palmitoyltransferase deficiency. Electromyographic (EMG) studies are usually normal unless myoglobinuria is present, although nonspecific abnormalities including increased insertional activity and an increased number of polyphasic potentials, as well as evidence of muscular irritability with fibrillations and positive waves (changes that can also be seen in inflammatory muscle disease), have been reported. The cramps that follow voluntary activity or ischemic exercise are electrically silent (1).

TABLE 120.4. PROTOCOL FOR FOREARM ISCHEMIC EXERCISE TESTING

A blood sample for analysis of baseline lactate and ammonia concentration is drawn through an indwelling needle in an antecubital vein preferably without use of a tourniquet.

A sphygmomanometer cuff is placed on the upper arm and inflated to, and maintained at, a level at least 20 mm Hg above systolic pressure while the subject squeezes a tennis ball, or like object, vigorously at a rate of one squeeze every 2 seconds for 90 seconds.

After 90 seconds, the cuff is deflated and additional venous samples are obtained 1, 3, 5, and 10 minutes thereafter.

In normal individuals, lactate and ammonia concentrations increase at least threefold from baseline values. The major reason for a false-positive result is insufficient work by the subject while exercising (21). More work is required to increase ammonia levels than lactate levels. When an abnormal result is obtained, the putative diagnosis should always be confirmed by muscle biopsy.

A useful, but nonspecific, tool used to study individuals suspected of being deficient in myophosphorylase is the forearm ischemic exercise test (Table 120.4). This test exploits the abnormal biochemistry that results from the absence of myophosphorylase activity. Normal muscle generates lactate from the degradation of glycogen when it exercises intensely under ischemic or anaerobic conditions (Fig. 120.5). This pathway is blocked when myophosphorylase activity is absent, and consequently no lactate is released into the circulation under anaerobic conditions. Additionally, ammonia, inosine, and hypoxanthine concentrations increase significantly, providing evidence of excessive purine nucleotide breakdown (20). Similarly, other defects in the glycogenolytic and glycolytic pathways can interfere with lactate production during ischemic exercise and provide similar results.

In normal individuals, venous lactate levels increase three- to sixfold shortly after ischemic exercise; in myophosphorylase-deficient individuals, levels do not change (Table 120.5. The test can be painful if performed

TABLE 120.5. RESULTS OF FOREARM ISCHEMIC EXERCISE TESTING

	Normal		Myophosphorylase Deficiency		Myoadenylate Deaminase Deficiency	
Sample	Lactate	NH_3	Lactate	NH_3	Lactate	NH_3
Baseline	0.8	15	0.9	20	1.2	26
1 minute			0.8	94	3.8	26
3 minute	5.9	106	0.9	82	2.4	29
5 minute	3.8	91	0.9	40	1.6	30
10 minute	1.2	30	0.9	25	1.4	27

Lactate in mEq/L; NH_3 (ammonia) in M/L.

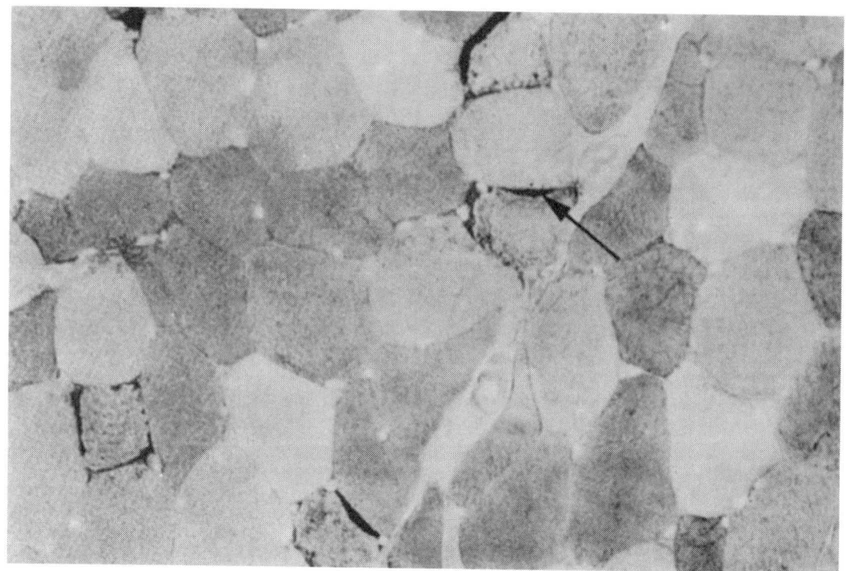

FIGURE 120.7. Muscle biopsy specimen from a patient with myophosphorylase deficiency. The periodic acid-Schiff–positive material *(arrow)*, seen at the periphery of the cells and as lines within the cells, is excess glycogen.

correctly. Some normal individuals cannot exercise more than a minute under ischemic conditions and find they are unable to fully flex or extend their fingers. The pain completely clears and full function is regained immediately after restoring the circulation. Painful persistent cramping, contracture, and even myoglobinuria can occur in an individual with McArdle's disease. The major limitation of the test is that some individuals cannot or will not exercise with enough intensity to raise lactate concentrations above baseline, and thus give false-positive results (21). Thus, if lactate concentrations do rise after ischemic exercise, myophosphorylase deficiency is excluded, but if lactate levels do not rise after ischemic exercise, the diagnosis is a possibility.

The definitive diagnosis is made by analysis of muscle tissue. Classic changes observed with light microscopy include thick deposits of glycogen at the periphery and thinner, linear deposits within cells (Fig. 120.7). The amount of variation is wide, and in milder cases deposits may not be obvious, even with periodic acid-Schiff (PAS) staining. The deposition is readily appreciated using the electron microscope (Fig. 120.8). Specific histochemical staining for myophosphorylase activity secures the diagnosis. False-positive results can be seen in patients with low residual activity or when they are regenerating fibers after rhabdomyolysis. Regenerating fibers in immature muscle cells express a different isoenzyme.

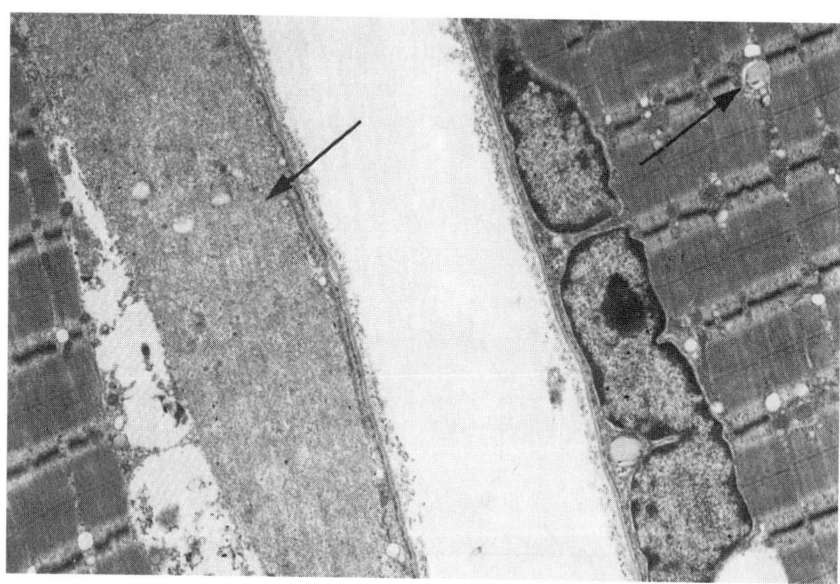

FIGURE 120.8. Electron micrograph demonstrating increased glycogen deposition beneath the sarcolemma and between filaments *(arrows)*. These changes could be seen in all glycogen storage diseases.

Although no specific treatment is available for myophosphorylase deficiency, some believe aerobic exercise training and a high-protein diet are useful (22,23). Vitamin B_6 supplementation may also improve exercise performance (24). Nonetheless, simply making the diagnosis is useful in establishing the basis for the patient's symptoms and for counseling concerning activities of daily living and prognosis.

Other Defects in Glycogen Metabolism

Deficiencies of brancher and debrancher enzymes have been reported but are rare. Brancher enzyme deficiency causes fatal hepatic failure in childhood, which can be associated with hypotonia and contractures or exercise intolerance and cardiomyopathy (25). It is characterized histologically by deposition of an abnormal PAS-positive polysaccharide. Brancher enzyme deficiency has been reported in an adult with muscle involvement and adult polyglucosan body disease (26). Debrancher enzyme splits the terminal glucose residues from phosphorylase-limit dextran that remains after the action of myophosphorylase. The deficiency is inherited as an autosomal-recessive trait, localized to chromosome 1 (27). Deficiency of debrancher enzyme results in phosphorylase-limit dextran accumulation and deposition in muscle, liver, and blood cells. This defect presents in childhood and commonly causes hepatomegaly, fasting hypoglycemia, and failure to thrive. Less frequently, individuals may develop slowly progressive muscle weakness with exercise intolerance and distal muscle wasting, beginning after age 20. There may also be associated neuropathy. These individuals have elevated CPK levels (28).

Phosphorylase b kinase helps regulate glycogen metabolism through the activation of myophosphorylase and inhibition of glycogen synthetase. The enzyme consists of four subunits and is under complex regulation, allowing for the variable inheritance and heterogeneous clinical pictures. These include an X-linked deficiency that causes hepatomegaly, fasting hypoglycemia, and growth retardation, and an autosomal-recessive disease that presents with various combinations of myopathy, hepatomegaly, and fetal/infantile cardiomegaly. Exercise intolerance with or without exertional myoglobulinuria, mimicking McArdle's disease, can be seen in adults (29,30). In contrast to McArdle's disease, however, CPK levels are not uniformly elevated and the lactate response to forearm ischemic exercise is usually normal or only blunted.

DEFECTS IN GLYCOLYSIS

Phosphofructokinase Deficiency (Tarui's Disease)

The clinical manifestations of phosphofructokinase deficiency can be identical to McArdle's disease. However, phosphofructokinase deficiency can also cause hemolytic anemia that may be seen with or without myopathy, depending on the genetic defect. Isoenzymes of phosphofructokinase vary in subunit composition. Generally, the muscle enzyme consists of M subunits, and the erythrocyte enzyme contains M and L subunits. Phosphofructokinase deficiency is inherited as an autosomal-recessive trait, with the M subunit mapped to chromosome 1. The L subunit is mapped to chromosome 21. Defects in the L subunit cause only hemolysis, but defects involving M subunits can affect both muscle and red cells. Considerable heterogeneity exists at molecular and clinical levels (31–33).

Most patients with the muscle form of Tarui's disease are diagnosed as adults, but in retrospect report having had problems with either exercise intolerance or cramps in their youth (33). Phosphofructokinase-deficient individuals differ from myophosphorylase-deficient individuals in that the "second wind" phenomenon is less common and exercise intolerance is likely to be associated with nausea and vomiting. The lack of a second wind is attributed to a block in oxidative metabolism that prevents lipolysis and prevents release of free fatty acid (34). Indeed, in these individuals, glucose lowers exercise and oxidative capacity by this mechanism, depriving them of their major source of energy. Carbohydrates may actually induce an "out-of-wind" phenomenon (35).

About one-third of patients develop myoglobinuria, and most have elevated serum CPK levels at rest. EMG is either normal or provides nonspecific results, suggesting myopathy or inflammation. Predictably, venous lactate levels fail to increase after forearm ischemic exercise, and, during exercise, ^{31}P magnetic resonance spectroscopy demonstrates an absence of pH change and the appearance of a phosphomonoester peak representing the hexose phosphates that accumulate because of the metabolic block (36). Histochemical analysis of muscle tissue is needed to confirm the diagnosis. In addition to increased glycogen deposition and decreased phosphofructokinase activity, deficient muscle also contains an abnormal polysaccharide similar to that seen in brancher enzyme deficiency (28). Hemolysis associated with myopathic disease may be subclinical, causing only an increased reticulocyte count, or severe, causing jaundice and gallstones. Hyperuricemia and gout are common in these individuals, perhaps because of the high levels of purines released with hemolysis and during exercise (37,38). Therapeutic recommendations are similar to those for myophosphorylase deficiency, plus avoidance of exercise after high-carbohydrate meals (39).

Other Defects in Glycolysis

Deficiencies of phosphoglycerate kinase (40), phosphoglycerate mutase (41), and lactate dehydrogenase (LDH) (42) have been described in individuals whose symptoms began during adolescence or later and included exercise intolerance, myalgias, and exercise-induced myoglobinuria. These genetic defects all cause a failure of lactate release after ischemic exercise and require histochemical studies for diagnosis.

Acid Maltase Deficiency

Acid maltase is an enzyme, found in lysosomes, that catalyzes the release of glucose from maltose, oligosaccharides, and glycogen. Its precise role in cellular metabolism is not known. The gene for this enzyme is localized on chromosome 17, and the deficiency is transmitted by autosomal-recessive inheritance (43), producing three clinical syndromes. These differ in age of presentation, organ involvement, and prognosis (44). The infantile form (Pompe's disease) causes symptoms of muscle weakness, hypotonia, and congestive heart failure that begin shortly after birth and progress to death within the first 2 years of life. This form is characterized by massive glycogen deposits in cardiac, hepatic, neural, and muscular tissues. The second variety presents in early childhood with muscle weakness that is more proximal than distal and may affect respiratory muscles. It tends not to involve the heart or liver and progresses slowly. Death, usually a result of respiratory failure, occurs before age 30. The adult form causes few problems before age 20 and typically manifests as muscle weakness beginning in the third and fourth decade (45). Although diaphragmatic involvement and respiratory failure dominate the clinical picture in about one-third of cases, most develop a slowly progressive myopathy that is easily confused with polymyositis or limb-girdle muscular dystrophy. The weakness tends to occur in proximal muscles and the torso. Individual muscles or even parts of muscles can be affected, but craniobulbar muscles are spared.

CPK is almost always elevated. EMG is always abnormal, though variably. The characteristic changes include an unusually intense electrical irritability in response to movement of the needle electrode and myotonic discharges in the absence of clinical myotonia. In some individuals, however, the changes are indistinguishable from those observed in some cases of polymyositis. Acid maltase–deficient subjects have no block in anaerobic glycolysis or nonlysosomal glycogenolysis; thus, venous lactate concentrations increase normally after forearm ischemic exercise. A high-protein diet, nocturnal respiratory support, and resistive respiratory muscle exercise may be helpful (44,46). This difference readily distinguishes these patients from individuals with other recognized forms of glycogen storage disease.

Acid maltase deficiency causes a vacuolar myopathy. The vacuoles have a high glycogen content and stain for acid phosphatase. Small foci of acid phosphatase activity may also be found in muscle fibers that do not contain vacuoles. Glycogen is readily seen in involved muscle by electron microscopy, but the excess glycogen is not confined just to vacuolar structures. It is unclear why this nonlysosomal glycogen accumulates and why it is not degraded by cytosolic enzymes, nor is it clear what causes the muscular symptoms, because the pathways of glycogen and glucose metabolism for energy production are intact.

TABLE 120.6. VACUOLAR MYOPATHIES

Metabolic	Acid maltase deficiency
	Carnitine deficiency
Dystrophic	Acute lesions of Duchenne's
	Oculopharyngeal
Inflammatory	Inclusion body myositis
Toxic	Alcohol
	Chloroquine
	Colchicine
	Zidovudine (AZT)
Infections	Echovirus
Miscellaneous	Distal myopathy
	Lafara's disease
	Periodic paralysis

Biochemical studies are necessary to prove the diagnosis. Although characteristic EMG changes in the presence of typical vacuolar changes on biopsy from a patient with weakness involving respiratory muscles are strongly suggestive, they are not specific. Furthermore, these abnormalities tend to be less widespread and less striking in many adult cases and other causes of vacuolar myopathy must be excluded (Table 120.6). Assay of acid maltase in muscle, lymphocytes, cultured fibroblasts, or urine can be performed, but measurement of acid β-glucosidase activity in muscle and histopathologic analysis of muscle tissue appear to provide no additional value when the enzyme activity is clearly lacking in leukocytes (47).

DISORDERS OF METABOLISM WITHIN MITOCHONDRIA

Plasma free fatty acids are the major source of energy while fasting, at rest, and while exercising at low intensity and for long duration. The disorders of lipid metabolism (9) could be included within the classification of mitochondrial myopathies because the defects all involve processes that occur within these organelles. However, the term *mitochondrial myopathy* is used to designate a specific subset of disorders. Abnormalities involving the processing of long-chain fatty acids for energy lead to lipid storage myopathies, conditions in which the predominant pathologic alteration is the accumulation of abnormal amounts of lipid droplets between myofibrils (Fig. 120.9). Carnitine deficiency is the classic example of such a myopathy. Deficiencies of carnitine palmitoyltransferase or fatty acid acyl-CoA dehydrogenases are the other major biochemical defects in the use of fatty acids for energy that cause human disease (Fig. 120.6). The term *mitochondrial myopathy* is applied to cases of muscle disease in which the major morphologic abnormalities

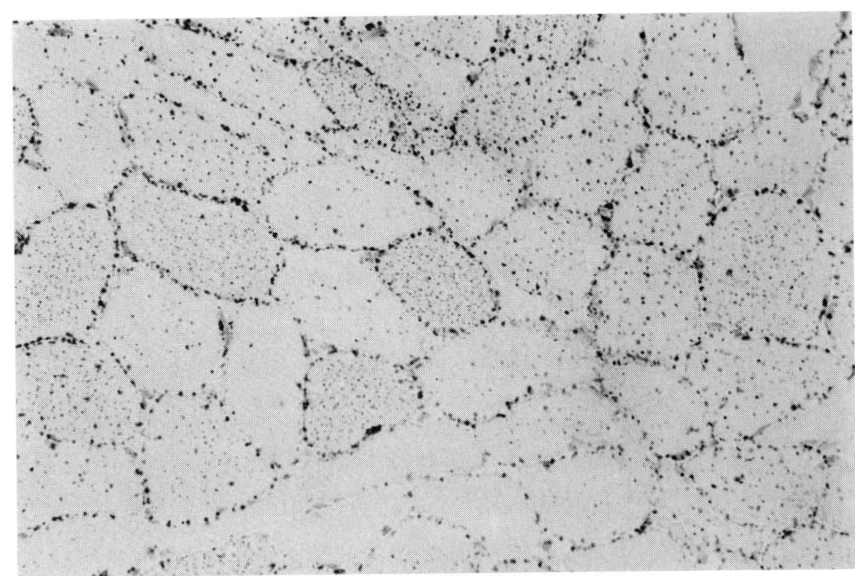

FIGURE 120.9. Muscle tissue stained with oil red O. Lipid droplets of varying size are deposited between myofibrils. Large collections appear as vacuoles. The increased staining is typical of lipid storage myopathy but by itself is a nonspecific finding.

are alterations in the number, size, and structure of mitochondria. These changes are nonspecific and are associated with widely varying clinical syndromes. Today, it is also meaningful to consider mitochondrial myopathies as disorders in muscle that result from disruption of the pathways of oxidative metabolism and energy transfer. Deficiencies of carnitine, carnitine palmitoyltransferase, or enzymes of β-oxidation have not usually been included under this classification because there are no associated changes in mitochondrial structure. The classification of these diseases will undoubtedly change as more is learned about them.

Carnitine Deficiency States

L-Carnitine is essential for the transfer of long-chain fatty acids across the inner mitochondrial membrane and helps regulate CoA/acyl-CoA ratios in mitochondria. Sources of carnitine include the diet, with red meat and dairy products containing large quantities, and de novo synthesis from lysine and methionine in liver, brain, and kidney. Carnitine is transported from the blood by an active saturable process into muscle, which contains 98% of the body stores. The major route of elimination from the body is in the urine.

In 1973, Engel and Angelini (48) reported the first recognized case of muscle carnitine deficiency in an individual with lipid storage myopathy. In 1975, Karpati et al. (49) reported another form of carnitine deficiency, a systemic variety. Carnitine deficiencies are now classified as either primary or secondary. Primary deficiencies have a genetic basis and can be further divided into myopathic and systemic forms. Secondary deficiencies are those that result from other disorders or from genetic defects in other pathways of intermediary metabolism.

Primary Carnitine Deficiencies

The syndrome of myopathic carnitine deficiency is characterized by progressive muscle weakness that generally begins in childhood (50,51). The weakness is of the limb-girdle variety, but facial and pharyngeal muscle involvement is observed. Less common features are exertional myalgias, myoglobinuria, and cardiomyopathy. At least half the patients have high CPK levels, and most have myopathic changes (polyphasic motor unit potentials of small amplitude and short duration) on EMG. Serum carnitine concentrations are usually normal, a finding consistent with the evidence indicating that a defect in carnitine transport into muscle cells underlies this form of the disease. The only histologic abnormality in muscle is the nonspecific finding of increased lipid (Fig. 120.9). Similar changes can occur with ischemia and obesity. The diagnosis is made by biochemical analysis of muscle tissue. Carnitine replacement therapy provides variable results.

The first reported patient with systemic carnitine deficiency was an 11-year-old boy with progressive muscle weakness and a history of recurrent attacks that resembled Reye's syndrome (49). The attacks began with vomiting and were followed by coma, hepatosplenomegaly, liver function abnormalities, and hypoglycemia. This defect results from inheritance of nonfunctional high-affinity carnitine receptors (52). Onset of this autosomal-recessive disorder is almost always in early childhood, with the attack preceding the onset of muscle weakness in the majority of cases. A lipid storage myopathy is seen on muscle biopsy (53). Cardiac muscle involvement, manifested by congestive heart failure, is common. Carnitine concentrations are reduced in skeletal muscle, heart, liver, and serum, and dramatic improvement can be seen with dietary carnitine supplementation. Attacks resembling Reye's syndrome also occur in acyl-CoA dehydrogenase deficiency states, and exercise intolerance occurs with defects in oxidative phosphorylation (see Mitochondrial Myopathies, below). In fact, many individuals previously believed to have primary carnitine deficiencies have been found to have a secondary deficiency resulting from another metabolic defect (53,54).

Secondary Carnitine Deficiencies

Carnitine deficiency can be secondary to genetic defects in other reactions in intermediary metabolism or to other disorders. The histologic features of lipid storage myopathy are present in these inborn errors of metabolism. Other disorders in which carnitine deficiency has been observed include renal failure requiring chronic hemodialysis (but not chronic peritoneal dialysis), end-stage cirrhosis with cachexia, valproic acid therapy for seizure disorders, myxedema, adrenal insufficiency, hypopituitarism, and pregnancy (55,56).

TREATMENT

In theory, all types of carnitine deficiency should be effectively treated with L-carnitine dietary supplementation. In reality, however, the response to this therapy is variable. Attempts at treatment should include a diet rich in carbohydrates and medium-chain fatty acids and avoidance of fasting. During acute attacks, therapy should be designed to prevent hypoglycemia and to correct any electrolyte and acid-base imbalances that develop.

Dietary supplementation with L-carnitine has sometimes been successful in improving each form of deficiency. The dose for children is 100 mg/kg/day (57); adults require 2 to 4 g in divided doses. Preparations containing the DL-isomer of carnitine should not be used, because it is not effective and can actually cause muscle weakness (58). Some patients benefit from steroid therapy and propranolol. Intravenous infusion of L-carnitine (20 mg/kg) at the end of dialysis treatment decreases postdialysis symptoms, improves exercise capacity and sense of well-being, and possibly increases muscle mass in patients requiring chronic hemodialysis (59). Additionally, treatment with riboflavin alone or in combination with L-carnitine has proven beneficial in individual patients with low acyl-CoA dehydrogenase activities (60), carnitine palmitoyltransferase deficiency (61), and other mitochondrial myopathies (62).

Carnitine Palmitoyltransferase Deficiency

In 1973, DiMauro and Melis-DiMauro (63) first reported a deficiency of the muscle form of carnitine palmitoyltransferase in two brothers with recurrent myoglobinuria. Approximately 80% of those with this inborn error who are symptomatic are male.

Molecular heterogeneity exists in this autosomal-receive trait, although some heterozygotes may be at risk for clinical symptoms (64). Patients typically experience attacks of myalgias, cramps, stiffness, or tenderness, with myoglobulinuria. Attacks usually develop following prolonged exercise, fasting, or other metabolic stress. This is not surprising since carnitine palmitoyltransferase is necessary for transport of long-chain fatty acids into mitochondria for energy production. Cold exposure, infection, high fat intake, and emotional stress may also be important contributing and precipitating factors. Use of ibuprofen or diazepam, general anesthesia, surgery, and pregnancy may also be factors (64–66). Mild attacks may be experienced in childhood, but severe attacks usually do not occur until the teenage years or later. About 25% of individuals develop renal failure with episodes of myoglobinuria, but this is reversible. Respiratory failure may result during severe attacks.

The clinical picture of carnitine palmitoyltransferase differs in several ways from that of the glycogen storage diseases that also cause myoglobinuria. Carnitine palmitoyltransferase–deficient patients can perform brief intervals of intense exercise and do not experience warning signs or a second "out-of-wind" phenomenon, and cannot abort attacks with rest. CPK is usually normal, except during episodes of rhabdomyolysis, or with prolonged fasting, and the increase in serum lactate concentration after forearm ischemic exercise is normal. Electrophysiologic studies and muscle tissue are entirely normal between attacks. Lipid accumulation is rarely observed in carnitine palmitoyltransferase–deficient muscle, and the diagnosis is made by measuring carnitine palmitoyltransferase activity in muscle (67). Based on the known biochemistry, it would be predicted that carnitine palmitoyltransferase deficiency and carnitine deficiency would cause similar abnormalities, but this is not the case. Fixed weakness is quite unusual (66). Carnitine palmitoyltransferase deficiency may present in adulthood with features characteristic of some mitochondrial myopathies. These include exercise intolerance associated with external ophthalmoplegia and ragged red fibers in skeletal muscle (68). Why the clinical and histologic features of this deficiency differ from carnitine deficiency is not understood.

Management consists primarily of education, although the combination of oral supplementation of L-carnitine and riboflavin may be of some benefit (61). Avoidance of both prolonged strenuous exercise and fasting will prevent most attacks. Infection may not be preventable, but the need for adequate rest during an infection must be emphasized. Myoglobinuria constitutes a medical emergency. Interestingly, the development of renal failure does not correlate well with the amount of myoglobin in the urine. Treatment consists of hydration and use of an osmotic diuretic, such as mannitol, to force excretion of a dilute urine (69). Alkalinizing the urine may also be prudent, but its necessity has not been clearly established.

Defects in β-Oxidation

Fatty acids are metabolized in mitochondria through β-oxidation. The acyl-CoA dehydrogenases are flavoproteins that catalyze the first step of this process. There are four distinct straight-chain acyl-CoA dehydrogenases with specificity for acyl-CoA esters of different chain length. Genetic deficiencies of these enzymes most commonly mimic primary systemic carnitine deficiency (52). Typically they present as fasting intolerance with either hepatic, cardiomyopathic, or myopathic disease. The biochemical abnormalities noted during attacks may include hypoketotic hypoglycemia, hypocarnitinemia, and dicarboxylic aciduria (70).

The myopathic presentations of short-chain acyl-CoA dehydrogenase deficiency include neonatal hypotonia, skeletal muscle weakness and hypotonia in infancy, and severe muscle wasting with scoliosis in a 16-year-old girl (71). Long-chain acyl-CoA dehydrogenase deficiency can present in infancy or adulthood. Infants and children may develop muscle weakness and hypotonia, experience episodes of muscle pain and fatigue associated with high serum CPK levels, and have attacks of myoglobulinuria. Adults present with weakness of limb-girdle, cervical, and masticatory muscle weakness (72). Deficiencies of all three fatty acid acyl-CoA dehydrogenase activities have been reported in a 38-year-old man who presented with a 2-year history of neck pain and proximal muscle weakness, elevated serum CK levels, myopathic EMG changes, and abnormal accumulation of lipid on muscle biopsy (73). Treatment with riboflavin resulted in normalization of muscle histology and improved strength.

Muscle Coenzyme Q_{10} Deficiency

Coenzyme Q is an obligatory receptor of electrons derived from β-oxidation of fatty acids. A deficiency of muscle coenzyme Q_{10} has been reported in two sisters with increased fatigability and progressive proximal and trunk muscle weakness that began in childhood (74). Subsequently, each developed ataxia, dysarthria, and tremor. Histology revealed abnormal accumulations of lipid. Additionally, all type 1 fibers were ragged-red with Gomori trichrome staining. Therapy with oral coenzyme Q_{10} yielded improvement in all symptoms.

Mitochondrial Myopathies

Oxidative phosphorylation and energy transfer (Fig. 120.4) take place in mitochondria. Mitochondria are unique organelles that contain their own DNA. Mitochondrial DNA (mtDNA) encodes for 13 structural proteins. All are components of oxidative phosphorylation systems, including seven subunits of complex I, one of complex III, three of complex IV, and two of ATP synthase. The components of complex II are encoded by nuclear DNA. In contrast to nuclear DNA, mtDNA is circular and is derived totally from the mother's oocyte. Multiple mitochondria are present in every cell and each contains multiple genomes. Mitochondrial DNA is subject to frequent spontaneous mutations, presumably because it is constantly exposed to oxygen free radicals leaked from the electron transport chain and lacks a DNA repair system.

In normal tissues, all mtDNA molecules are identical, a state termed *homoplasmy.* If mutations are inherited, homoplasmy is maintained. If spontaneous mutations occur, different populations, mutant and wild types, exist within the same cells. This state is termed *heteroplasmy.* The phenotypic expression of a pathogenic mutation is largely determined by the relative properties of mutant versus wild types. With heteroplasmy at cell division, the proportion of mutant mitochondrial genomes may shift, leading to phenotypic changes. Consequently, mitochondrial diseases can be inherited or develop later in life (9,75–77).

The most typical morphologic change in mitochondrial diseases is the "ragged-red" fiber, a distorted-appearing fiber that contains large peripheral and intermyofibrillar aggregates of abnormal mitochondria (Fig. 120.10). These appear as red deposits with the modified Gomori trichrome stain, primarily in type 1 and to a lesser degree in type 2A fibers. Most ragged-red fibers fail to stain for cytochrome oxidase activity (78). An occasional ragged-red fiber is not diagnostic of a mitochondrial myopathy, but the presence of these fibers does indicate the possibility of one of those diseases. On the other hand, many diseases that result from mitochondrial defects do not manifest this change. Additional changes, such as increased amounts of lipid or glycogen, intramitochondrial inclusions, or changes in mitochondrial size or shape, can be seen at the ultrastructural level.

Mitochondrial diseases are associated with a variety of clinical manifestations (Table 120.7). Even though the biochemical abnormalities are expressed and can be identical in

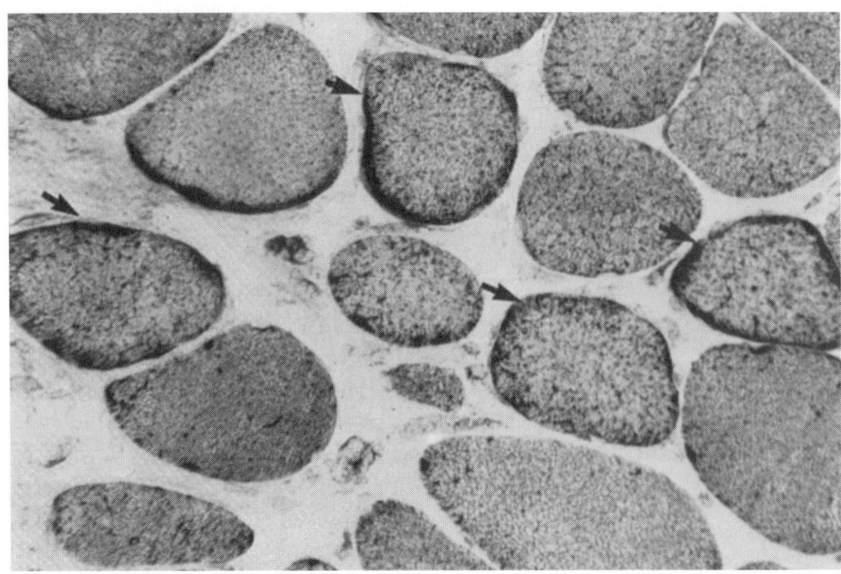

FIGURE 120.10. Typical-appearing ragged-red fiber is strongly suggestive, but not diagnostic, of a mitochondrial myopathy.

skeletal muscle, myopathy may not be apparent clinically. In general, the abnormalities can be divided into the syndromes that cause limb myopathy, with or without ophthalmoplegia, and those in which central nervous system manifestations predominate. The former cause problems primarily affecting muscle, with manifestations such as exercise intolerance, muscle weakness that may have limb-girdle or fascioscapulohumeral distributions, or extraocular muscle dysfunction with or without bulbar and limb involvement. Hypermetabolism, salt craving, and peripheral neuropathy have been reported in other cases, indicating extreme heterogeneity. Although most of these diseases affect infants, some cause symptoms in childhood that are recognized to be the result of a disease only retrospectively, after the diagnosis is made later in adult life (78–83).

Adult-onset mitochondrial myopathies most commonly cause exercise intolerance, proximal or generalized weakness, and, rarely, myoglobulinemia. Individuals may even present in their 70s (80–83). CK values may be normal or elevated, and electrophysiologic studies are not particularly distinctive. The most characteristic features on muscle biopsy are increased numbers of ragged-red fibers with increased activity of succinate dehydrogenase and decreased cytochrome C oxidase. Electron microscopy may show increased numbers of mitochondria, larger mitochondria, or decreased numbers of the organelle. Magnetic resonance spectroscopy reveals reduced phosphocreatine to inorganic phosphate ratios (84).

Mitochondrial syndromes can result from a variety of changes at the molecular level. The Kearns-Sayre syndrome, Pearson's syndrome, and the syndrome of chronic progressive external ophthalmoplegia are associated with a variety of defects affecting all respiratory chain complexes and attributed to large deletions of mitochondrial DNA. Mito-

TABLE 120.7. MITOCHONDRIAL DISEASES

Syndrome	Defect
Early onset	
Alper's (progressive infantile poliodystrophy)	I, IV, PDC
Leigh's (subacute necrotizing encephalomyelopathy)	I, IV, PDC
Pearson's (bone marrow/pancreas syndrome)	I
Childhood or adult onset	
Kearns-Sayre	I, II, III, IV, I + VI
MELAS (myopathy, encephalopathy, lactic acidosis, strokes)	IV
MERRF (myoclonic epilepsy with ragged-red fibers)	I, II, III, IV, I + IV
MNGIE (myoneurogastrointestinal encephalopathy)	IV
Dementia, ataxia, deafness, myopathy	I, I + IV
NARP (neurogenic weakness, ataxia, retinitis pigmentation)	IV
Proximal weakness and exercise intolerance	I, I–III
Exercise intolerance and myoglobinuria	III

I, cytochrome complex I; II, cytochrome complex II; III, cytochrome complex III; IV, cytochrome complex IV; PDC, pyruvate dehydrogenase complex.

chondrial encephalopathy, lactic acidosis, and stroke-like (MELAS) syndrome and the myoclonus epilepsy, ragged red fiber (MERRF) disease are caused by single mutations of mitochondrial genes. Multiple deletions have been described in three more cases of familial myopathy and late-onset mitochondrial myopathy in the elderly (80,81,84,85). In contrast, mutations at a single locus of nuclear genes that encode for proteins in complex I and IV underlie syndromes of pure limb myopathies and fulminant infantile lactic acidosis. Finally, mitochondrial DNA depletion can cause childhood myopathy (86).

Whereas the diseases described here are inherited, acquired mitochondrial syndromes can also occur. Mitochondrial myopathy has resulted from toxic effects of zidovudine (AZT) therapy in patients infected with the human immunodeficiency virus (HIV) (87), clofibrate-induced myopathy (88), and selenium deficiency (89). Mitochondrial abnormalities have also been found as part of the aging process (90) and in muscle of some patients with polymyositis, inclusion body myositis, and polymyalgia rheumatica (91–94).

Although results are anecdotal to date, individuals with any type of mitochondrial myopathy may benefit with the oral use of L-carnitine, riboflavin, ascorbate, ubiquinone (coenzyme Q_{10}), menadione, or creatine (74,79,95,96). Moderate-intensity aerobic exercise training may also benefit some patients with these disorders (97).

DISORDERED PURINE METABOLISM

Myoadenylate Deaminase Deficiency

Myoadenylate deaminase, a distinct isoenzyme of adenylate deaminase found only in skeletal muscle, catalyzes the irreversible deamination of AMP to IMP and plays an important role in the purine nucleotide cycle (Fig. 120.3). This deficiency first reported in 1978, is probably the most common metabolic change in muscle recognized today. Approximately 2% of a large series of muscle biopsy specimens were deficient in myoadenylate deaminase activity (98).

Myoadenylate deaminase deficiency exists in both primary (inherited) and secondary (acquired) forms (99,100). The secondary deficiencies are associated with a wide variety of other neuromuscular diseases including periodic paralysis, influenza-like illness, Kugelberg-Welander disease, amyotrophic lateral sclerosis, spinal muscular atrophy, facial and limb-girdle myopathies, polymyositis, dermatomyositis, systemic lupus erythematosus, systemic sclerosis, diabetes, hyperthyroidism, and gout (98). Serum enzymes such as CPK and aldolase are usually normal in primary myoadenylate deaminase deficiency and vary according to the associated condition in secondary deficiencies. Results of EMG are also normal or nonspecific. The measurement of venous lactate and ammonia concentrations following forearm ischemic exercise is effective for screening for myoadenylate deaminase deficiency (Table 120.5). However, submaximal exercise performance because of weakness, pain, or poor effort can be responsible for false-positive results (21). Consequently, failure to generate ammonia after exercise does not indicate myoadenylate deaminase deficiency unless an adequate effort is documented. An abnormal result from forearm ischemic exercise testing should be followed by a muscle biopsy to confirm the putative enzyme deficiency. The structure of muscle tissue is usually normal. Histochemical techniques are useful in establishing the deficiency state. Myoadenylate deaminase deficiency has also been found to coexist with myophosphorylase deficiency (101).

The myoadenylate deaminase gene (*AMPD1*) is located on the short arm of chromosome 1 (102). A single mutant allele appears to be responsible for most, if not all, cases of primary deficiency (103). This nonsense mutation in exon 2 results in normal abundance of myoadenylate deaminase transcripts but deficient (generally less than 2% of normal) enzyme protein. In contrast, higher residual activities of immunoreactive enzyme protein occur in the secondary deficiencies, and reductions occur in other muscle enzymes such as CPK and adenylate kinase (99). Furthermore, the reduction in enzyme activity occurs in conjunction with a parallel decrease in myoadenylate deaminase messenger RNA (100). The factors responsible for the molecular changes underlying the secondary deficiency states are not understood, although myonecrosis appears to play a significant role in the secondary myoadenylate deaminase deficiency associated with polymyositis.

The precise relationship between myoadenylate deaminase deficiency and muscular symptoms is unknown, as approximately 2% of Caucasians and African Americans are homozygous for the nonsense mutation. Although over 100 cases of myoadenylate deaminase deficiency have been reported to have symptoms of myopathy, clearly the majority of myoadenylate deaminase–deficient individuals are asymptomatic. The disparity between the frequency of the mutant *AMPD1* allele and the prevalence of myopathic symptoms suggests that either the deficiency is not the major cause of the myopathy in individuals with the inherited defect or some compensatory mechanism protects them from the harmful effects of the mutation.

A potential molecular explanation for amelioration of symptoms secondary to this nonsense mutation in exon 2 of the *AMPD1* gene has been proposed (104). The primary transcript of the *AMPD1* gene is subject to alternative splicing. In that process, the only exon that is alternatively removed is exon 2. Consequently, if a fraction of *AMPD1* transcripts in individuals with this inherited defect have exon 2 deleted and these transcripts encode a functional peptide, the defect could be at least partially corrected.

ENDOCRINE MYOPATHIES

A variety of endocrine diseases can cause symptoms of neuromuscular dysfunction. These include disorders of either hyperfunction or hypofunction of the adrenal, parathyroid, pituitary, and thyroid glands. A major mechanism responsible for the symptoms involves electrolyte imbalance. This should not be surprising because muscle contraction requires transmembrane shifts in sodium, potassium, and calcium; inorganic phosphate is critical to the maintenance of high-energy compounds; and magnesium is an essential cofactor for ATPase activity. Thus, any hormonal change (or disease, drug, or other factor) that raises or lowers the concentrations of these ions can cause myopathic symptoms by altering surface membrane excitability, excitation-contraction coupling, or actin-myosin bridging. Endocrine disorders also cause skeletal muscle dysfunction through the effects of hormones on protein and carbohydrate metabolism. The rheumatic aspects and myopathic syndromes associated with endocrinopathies are discussed in Chapter 124.

CLINICAL EVALUATION

The evaluation of patients with suspected metabolic muscle disease begins with a careful history and a thorough physical examination. Myopathies typically cause weakness, exercise intolerance as a result of fatigue, and postexertional myalgias, cramps, and stiffness. The weakness develops insidiously and is therefore ignored until it becomes truly limiting. The actual onset of the symptoms is often difficult to determine even in retrospect. Everyone experiences cramps, stiffness, and pain after certain exercise. Thus, the patient may deny the significance of his problems, and physicians may disregard the patient's complaints for many years. Distinguishing between normal and abnormal exercise intolerance can be difficult.

The problem of diagnosing a metabolic muscle disease is confounded because patients are often completely asymptomatic at rest and have no abnormal physical findings. The most significant complaints are severe, prolonged cramps and red wine–colored urine indicating myoglobinuria. Although these findings can hardly be ignored, special attention and questioning are required to determine the significance of the less dramatic symptoms. The weakness of a metabolic myopathy is proximal and symmetrically distributed. Initial complaints include difficulty climbing stairs or reaching a high shelf. Physical examination may be entirely normal and at most may show only weakness in a limb-girdle distribution. The prime importance of the physical examination in a neuromuscular disease may be to rule out evidence of a neurologic component.

Measurement of muscle enzymes and electrodiagnostic studies are indicated if the patient's complaints are suspicious for myopathy or severe enough to alter his lifestyle. Increased levels of CPK, aldolase, serum glutamic-oxaloacetic transaminase (SGOT), serum glutamic-pyruvic transaminase (SGPT), and LDH may be observed in the blood of patients with muscle disease. Of these, the CPK is the most sensitive. In metabolic diseases of muscle, however, the presence of an elevated CPK is variable. Levels are usually increased in patients with glycogen storage diseases but are usually normal in the other diseases such as carnitine palmitoyltransferase or myoadenylate deaminase deficiency. An isolated elevation of the CPK should be interpreted with caution. In normal individuals, spurious elevations can result from fever, blunt trauma, intramuscular injection, aerobic exercise, EMG, muscle biopsy, and the use of medications such as morphine and barbiturates, which retard the excretion of the enzyme in the urine (105). The patient's race and sex must also be considered in the interpretation of CPK levels. CPK values are significantly higher in healthy asymptomatic blacks than in whites or Hispanics and in males compared to females (106,107). CPK levels are always raised in patients who have rhabdomyolysis. The MB isoenzyme fraction, which is usually considered to be derived from cardiac muscle, may be increased under these conditions because regenerating skeletal muscle also expresses this form.

Nerve conduction studies are entirely normal in metabolic myopathies. Finding normal nerve conduction in a patient with symptoms of muscle dysfunction defines the process as a myopathy by exclusion. The EMG may also be normal in these individuals. Exceptions include deficiencies of acid maltase, debrancher enzyme, and carnitine. But even in these conditions, the finding of abnormal motor unit potential and fibrillations is variable and nondiagnostic (44). The electromyogram, however, may be useful in clearly demonstrating myopathic changes and indicating preferential sites for muscle biopsy on the opposite side of the body.

Measurement of venous lactate and ammonia before and after forearm ischemic exercise provides a useful tool for ruling out myoadenylate deaminase deficiency and all myopathic forms of glycogen storage disease except acid maltase deficiency. Individuals with myoadenylate deaminase deficiency exhibit little ammonia compared to normal amounts of lactate under these conditions, whereas patients with the glycogenic and glycolytic defects exhibit the opposite result (Tables 120.4 and 120.5). Valid results from the forearm ischemic exercise test require an appropriate exercise effort on the part of the individual because false-positive results can result from poor subject performance (21,108). A positive result must be confirmed by tissue analysis.

A muscle biopsy produces the most important diagnostic information in the evaluation of a patient with a suspected metabolic muscle disease. It is, however, the final step in the clinical evaluation and should not be performed until a preliminary diagnosis has been made. Selection of the muscle for biopsy is important. A clinically weak muscle that has not been traumatized (by intramuscular injection, EMG needle, or previous biopsy) is ideal. If weakness is not obvious, the biopsy site may be guided by EMG abnormalities on the opposite side of the body. Severely involved muscle, as seen acutely in rhabdomyolysis, should be avoided. The tissue can be severely distorted, and the biochemical features of regenerating muscle can provide confusing information.

Magnetic resonance imaging (MRI) provides a noninvasive means of identifying the patterns of distribution and severity of muscle involvement and may also be used to determine a biopsy site (109,110). Both MRI and computed tomography (CT) can also be used to demonstrate areas of fat infiltration, muscle degeneration, or atrophy in glycogen storage diseases and mitochondrial myopathies (110,111).

Routine muscle histology can be helpful primarily in ruling out other conditions that can cause symptoms of muscle dysfunction such as inflammatory muscle diseases and muscular dystrophies. Histochemical studies can provide critically important information. The increased glycogen storage of disorders of glycogen metabolism can be detected with PAS staining (Fig. 120.7). Increased lipid accumulation, indicative of lipid storage myopathy, can be identified with Sudan or oil red O stains (Fig. 120.9). The Gomori modified trichrome stain reveals changes in mitochondria and the ragged-red fiber (Fig. 120.10). Acid phosphatase stains demonstrate increased lysosomal enzyme activity indicative of acid maltase deficiency. Abnormal staining with reduced nicotinamide adenine dinucleotide (NADH) dehydrogenase, and other oxidative enzyme stains, suggests mitochondrial defects. Specific enzyme defects can be diagnosed with stains for myophosphorylase, phosphofructokinase, LDH, cytochrome oxidase, and myoadenylate deaminase (Fig. 120.11). Carnitine concentration and carnitine

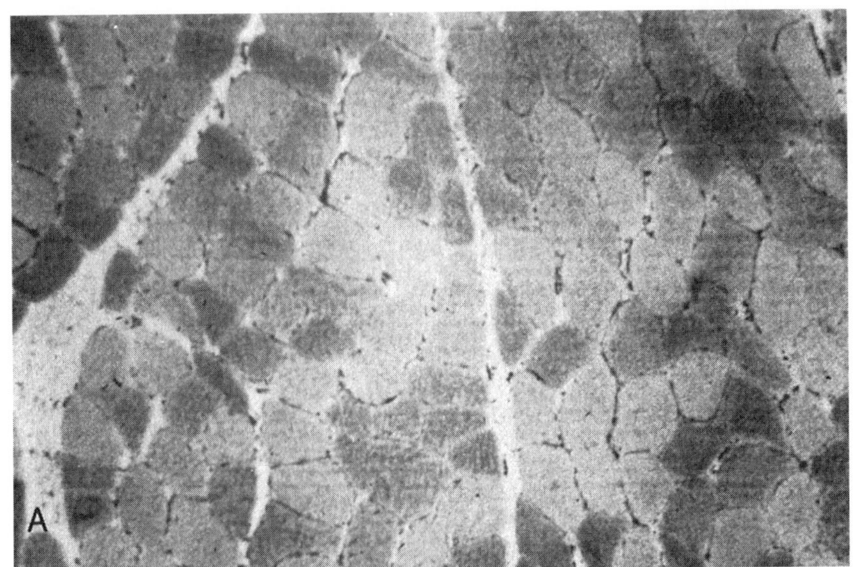

FIGURE 120.11. A: Muscle stained for myoadenylate deaminase activity with normal results. **B:** Muscle from an individual with myoadenylate deaminase deficiency stained by the same method as the tissue in **A**.

palmitoyltransferase activity can be determined on muscle homogenate by radiochemical techniques.

Ultrastructural analysis by electron microscopy is clearly more sensitive than light microscopy in identifying glycogen (Fig. 120.8) and lipid deposition and reveals morphologic changes in mitochondria, membranes, and sarcoplasmic reticulum. This technique will play an increased role in the evaluation of metabolic muscle diseases.

In the future, the evaluation of patients with symptoms of muscle dysfunction will include ^{31}P magnetic resonance spectroscopy. Presently, this technique is used primarily for research purposes. Magnetic resonance spectroscopy can be used to measure tissue contents of ATP, creatine phosphate, and inorganic phosphate (112). This technique can be used to follow the shifts in these metabolites during exercise and to determine the pH of the tissue studied. It is noninvasive and harmless. Magnetic resonance spectroscopy has been applied to patients with McArdle's disease (16,22), confirming the predicted rapid decreases in creatine phosphate and lack of pH change during ischemic exercise. At least four different patterns of metabolic change have been identified in muscle of patients with mitochondrial myopathies (113). Additional studies with this technique will help elucidate normal patterns of muscle metabolism and altered states in various diseases and will provide a valuable tool in following the effects of therapies.

REFERENCES

1. McArdle B. Myopathy due to a defect in muscle glycogen breakdown. *Clin Sci* 1951;24:13–35.
2. Mommaerts WFHM, Illingworth B, Pearson CM, et al. A functional disorder of muscle associated with the absence of phosphorylase. *Proc Natl Acad Sci U S A* 1959;45:791–797.
3. Kushmerick MJ. Patterns in mammalian muscle energetics. *J Exp Biol* 1985;115:165–177.
4. Layzer RB. How muscles use fuel. *N Engl J Med* 1991;324: 411–412.
5. Lee CP, Martens ME. Mitochondrial respiration and energy metabolism in muscle. In: Engel AG, Franzini-Armstrong C, eds. *Myology,* 2nd ed. New York: McGraw-Hill, 1994:624–647.
6. Bessman SP, Carpenter CL. The creatine-creatine phosphate shuttle. *Annu Rev Biochem* 1985;54:831–862.
7. Haller RG, Bertocci LA. Exercise evaluation of metabolic myopathies. In: Engel AG, Franzini-Armstrong C, eds. *Myology,* 2nd ed. New York: McGraw-Hill, 1994:807–821.
8. DiMauro S, Tsujino S. Non-lysosomal glycogenoses. In: Engel AG, Franzini-Armstrong C, eds. *Myology,* 2nd ed. New York: McGraw-Hill, 1986:1554–1576.
9. Wortmann RL. Metabolic diseases of muscle. In: Wortmann RL, ed. *Diseases of skeletal muscle.* Philadelphia: Lippincott, Williams & Wilkins, 2000;157-187.
10. Bartram C, Edwards R, Clague J, et al. McArdle's disease: a nonsense mutation in exon 1 of the muscle glycogen phosphorylase gene explains some but not all cases. *Hum Mol Genet* 1993;2:1291–1293.
11. Tsujino S, Shanske S, DiMauro S. Molecular heterogeneity of myophosphorylase deficiency. *N Engl J Med* 1993;329: 241–245.
12. Tsujino S, Shanske S, Martinuzzi A, et al. Two novel nonsense mutations in Caucasian patients with myophosphorylase deficiency (McArdle's disease). *Hum Mutat* 1995;6:276–277.
13. Wortmann RL. Myositis or myopathy. *J Rheumatol* 1989;16: 1525–1527.
14. Fleckenstein JL, Peshock RM, Lewis SF, et al. Magnetic resonance imaging of muscle injury and atrophy in glycolytic myopathies. *Muscle Nerve* 1989;12:849–855.
15. Felice KJ, Schneebaum AB, Royden-Jones J Jr. McArdle's disease with late-onset symptoms: case report and review of the literature. *J Neurol Neurosurg Psychiatry* 1992; 55:407–408.
16. Bendahan D, Confort-Gouny S, Kozak-Ribbens C, et al. ^{31}P NMR characterization of the metabolic abnormalities associated with the lack of glycogen phosphorylase activity in human forearm muscle. *Biochem Biophys Res Commun* 1992; 185:16–21.
17. Sahlin K, Areskoa NH, Haller RG, et al. Impaired oxidative metabolism increases adenine nucleotide breakdown in McArdle's disease. *J Appl Physiol* 1990;69:1231–1235.
18. Haller RG, Lewis SF, Cook JD, et al. Myophosphorylase deficiency impairs muscle oxidative metabolism. *Ann Neurol* 1985; 17:196–199.
19. Braakhakke JP, de Bruin MI, Stegeman DF, et al. The second wind phenomenon in McArdle's disease. *Brain* 1986;109: 1087–1101.
20. Mineo I, Kono N, Hara N, et al. Myogenic hyperuricemia. A common pathophysiologic feature of glycogenosis types III, V, and VII. *N Engl J Med* 1987;317:75–80.
21. Valen PA, Nakayama DA, Veum J, et al. Myoadenylate deaminase deficiency and forearm ischemic exercise testing. *Arthritis Rheum* 1987;30:661–668.
22. Jensen KE, Jakobsen J, Thomsen C, et al. Improved energy kinetics following high-protein diet in McArdle's syndrome: a ^{31}P magnetic resonance spectroscopy study. *Acta Neurol Scand* 1990;81:499–503.
23. MacLean D, Vissing J, Vissing SF, et al. Oral branched-chain amino acids do not improve exercise capacity in McArdle's disease. *Neurology* 1998;51:1456–1459.
24. Beyon RJ, Bartrum C, Hopkins P, et al. McArdle's disease: molecular genetics and metabolic consequences of the phenotype. *Muscle Nerve* 1995;3:S18–S22.
25. Sernella S, Riepe RE, Langston C, et al. Severe cardiomyopathy in branching enzyme deficiency. *J Pediatr* 1987;111:51–56.
26. Bruno C, Servidei S, Shanske S, et al. Glycogen branching enzyme deficiency in adult polyglucosan body disease. *Ann Neurol* 1993;33:88–93.
27. Yang-Feng TL, Zhena K, Yu J, et al. Assignment of the human glycogen debrancher gene to chromosome 1P21. *Genomics* 1992;13:931–934.
28. Coleman R, Winters H, Wolf B, et al. Glycogen debranching enzyme deficiency: long-term study of serum enzyme activities and clinical features. *J Inherit Metab Dis* 1992;15:869–881.
29. Clemens P, Yamamoto M, Engel AG. Adult phosphorylase b kinase deficiency. *Ann Neurol* 1990;28:529–538.
30. Wilkinson D, Tonin P, Shanske S, et al. Clinical and biochemical features of 10 adult patients with muscle phosphorylase kinase deficiency. *Neurology* 1994;44:461–466.
31. Sherman JB, Raben N, Nicastri C, et al. Common mutations in the phosphofructokinase-M gene in Ashkenazi Jewish patients with glycogenosis VII (Tarui's disease) and their population frequency. *Am J Hum Genet* 1994;55:305–313.
32. Raben N, Nichols RC, Boerkoel C, et al. Various classes of mutations in patients with phosphofructokinase deficiency (Tarui's disease). *Muscle Nerve* 1995;3(suppl):S39–S44.
33. Sivakumar J, Vasconeelos O, Goldfarb L, et al. Late-onset muscle weakness in partial phosphofructokinase deficiency: a unique myopathy with vacuolar, abnormal mitochondria, and

an absence of the common exon 5/intron 5 junction point mutation. *Neurology* 1996;46:1337–1342.
34. Lewis SF, Vora S, Haller RG. Abnormal oxidative metabolism and O_2 transport in phosphofructokinase deficiency. *J Appl Physiol* 1991;70:391–398.
35. Haller RG, Lewis SF. Glucose-induced exertional fatigue in muscle phosphofructokinase deficiency. *N Engl J Med* 1991;324:364–369.
36. Bertocci LA, Haller RG, Lewis SF, et al. Abnormal high energy phosphate metabolism in human muscle phosphofructokinase deficiency. *J Appl Physiol* 1991;70:1201–1207.
37. Kono N, Mineo I, Shimizu T, et al. Increased plasma uric acid after exercise in muscle phosphofructokinase deficiency. *Neurology* 1986;36:106–108.
38. Minco I, Tarui S. Myogenic hyperuricemia: what can we learn from metabolic myopathies? *Muscle Nerve* 1995;3(suppl): S75–S81.
39. Wortmann RL. Metabolic myopathies. In: Johnson RT, Griffin JW, eds. *Current therapy in neurologic disease.* St. Louis: Mosby-Year Book, 1993:397–402.
40. Tonin P, Shanske S, Miranda AF, et al. Phosphoglycerate kinase deficiency: biochemical and molecular genetic studies in a new myopathic variant (PGK Alberta). *Neurology* 1993;43:387–391.
41. Tsujino S, Shanske S, Sakoda S, et al. The molecular genetic basis of muscle phosphoglycerate mutase (PGAM) deficiency. *Am J Hum Genet* 1993;54:472–477.
42. Kanno T, Mackawa M. Lactate dehydrogenase M-subunit deficiencies: clinical features, metabolic background, and genetic heterogeneities. *Muscle Nerve* 1995;3(suppl):S54–S60.
43. Martiniuk F, Bodkin M, Tzall S, et al. Isolation and partial characterization of the structural gene for human acid α-glucosidase. *DNA Cell Biol* 1991;10:283–292.
44. Engel AG, Hirschhorn R. Acid maltese deficiency. In: Engel DG, Franzini-Armstrong C, eds. *Myology,* 2nd ed. New York: McGraw-Hill, 1994:1533–1553.
45. Barohn RJ, McVey AL, DiMauro S. Adult acid maltase deficiency. *Muscle Nerve* 1993;16:672–676.
46. Issacs H, Savage N, Badenhorst M, et al. Acid maltase deficiency: a case study and review of the pathophysiological changes and proposed therapeutic measures. *J Neurol Neurosurg Psychiatry* 1986;49:1011–1018.
47. Ausems MGEM, Lochman P, vanDiggelen OP, et al. A diagnostic protocol for adult-onset glycogen storage disease type II. *Neurology* 1999;52:851–853.
48. Engel AG, Angelini C. Carnitine deficiency of skeletal muscle associated with lipid storage myopathy: a new syndrome. *Science* 1973;179:899–902.
49. Karpati G, Carpenter S, Engel AG, et al. The syndrome of systemic carnitine deficiency: clinical, morphologic, biochemical and pathophysiologic features. *Neurology* 1975;25:16–24.
50. Carrier HM, Berthillier G. Carnitine levels in normal children and adults and in patients with diseased muscle. *Muscle Nerve* 1990;3:326–334.
51. Rebouche CJ, Paulson DJ. Carnitine metabolism and function in humans. *Annu Rev Nutr* 1986;6:41–66.
52. Treem WR, Stanley CA, Finegold DN, et al. Primary carnitine deficiency due to a failure of carnitine transport in kidney, muscle, and fibroblasts. *N Engl J Med* 1988;319:1331–1336.
53. DiDonato S. Disorders of lipid metabolism affecting skeletal muscle: carnitine deficiency syndromes, defects in the catabolic pathway, and Chanarin disease. In: Engel AG, Franzini-Armstrong C, eds. *Myology,* 2nd ed. New York: McGraw-Hill, 1994: 1587–1609.
54. Row PC, Valle D, Brusilow SW. Inborn errors of metabolism referred with Reye's syndrome. A changing pattern. *JAMA* 1988;260:3167–3170.
55. Laub MC, Paetzke-Brunner I, Jaeger G. Serum carnitine during valproic acid therapy. *Epilepsia* 1986;27:559–562.
56. Cederblad G, Fahraeus L, Lindgren K. Plasma carnitine and renal-carnitine clearance during pregnancy. *Am J Clin Nutr* 1986;44:379–383.
57. Strumpf DA, Parker WD, Angelini C. Carnitine deficiency, organic acidemias, and Reye's syndrome. *Neurology* 1985;35: 1041–1045.
58. Keith RE. Symptoms of carnitine-like deficiency in a trained runner taking DL-carnitine supplements. *JAMA* 1986;255:1137.
59. Ahmed S, Robertson HT, Golper TA, et al. Multicenter trial of L-carnitine in maintenance hemodialysis patients: II. Clinical and biochemical effects. *Kidney Int* 1990;38:912–918.
60. Turnbull DM, Shepherd IM, Ashworth B, et al. Lipid storage myopathy associated with low acyl-CoA dehydrogenase activities. *Brain* 1988;111:815–828.
61. Lindsley HB, Kepes JJ, Tekkanat KK, et al. Treatment of carnitine palmityltransferase (CPT) deficiency with L-carnitine and riboflavin. *Arthritis Rheum* 1990;33(suppl):S70.
62. Bersen PL, Gabreëls FJM, Ruitenbeck W, et al. Successful treatment of pure myopathy, associated with complex I deficiency, with riboflavin and carnitine. *Arch Neurol* 1991;48:334–338.
63. DiMauro S, DiMauro P. Muscle carnitine palmitoyltransferase deficiency and myoglobinuria. *Science* 1973;182:929–931.
64. Taggart RT, Smail D, Apolito C, et al. Novel mutations associated with carnitine palmitoyltransferase II deficiency. *Hum Mutual* 1999;13:210–220.
65. Ross NS, Hoppel CL. Partial muscle carnitine palmitoyltransferase-A deficiency. Rhabdomyolysis associated with transiently decreased muscle carnitine content after ibuprofen therapy. *JAMA* 1987;257:62–65.
66. Kieval RI, Sotrel A, Weinblatt ME. Chronic myopathy with a partial deficiency of the carnitine palmitoyltransferase enzyme. *Arch Neurol* 1989;46:575–576.
67. Zierz S, Engel AG. Regulatory properties of a mutant carnitine palmitoyltransferase in human skeletal muscle. *Eur J Biochem* 1985;149:207–214.
68. Carey MP, Poulton K, Hawkins C, et al. Carnitine palmitoyltransferase deficiency with an atypical presentation and ultrastructural mitochondrial abnormalities. *J Neurol Neurosurg Psychiatry* 1987;50:1060–1070.
69. Gabow PA, Kaehny WD, Kelleher SP. The spectrum of rhabdomyolysis. *Medicine* 1982;61:141–152.
70. Roe CR, Coates PM. Mitochondrial fatty acid oxidation disorders. In Scriver CR, Beaudet AL, Sly WS, et al., eds. *The metabolic and molecular bases of inherited disease,* 7th ed. New York: McGraw-Hill, 1995:1501–1533.
71. Ribes A, Riudor, Garavaglia B, et al. Mild or absent clinical signs in twin sisters with short-chain acyl-CoA dehydrogenase deficiency. *Eur J Pediatr* 1998;157:317–320.
72. DiDonato S, Taroni F, Gellera C, et al. Long-chain acyl-CoA dehydrogenase deficiency in muscle in an adult with lipid myopathy. *Neurology* 1988;38:269A–271A.
73. Turnbull DM, Shepherd IM, Ashworth B, et al. Lipid storage myopathy associated with low acyl-CoA dehydrogenase activities. *Brain* 1988;111:815–828.
74. Ogasahara S, Engel AG, Frens D, et al. Muscle coenzyme Q10 deficiency in familial mitochondrial encephalopathy. *Proc Natl Acad Sci U S A* 1989;86:2379–2387.
75. Morgan-Hughes JA. Mitochondrial diseases. In: Engel AG, Franzini-Armstrong C, eds. *Myology,* 2nd ed. New York: McGraw-Hill, 1994:1610–1660.
76. Shanske S, DiMauro S. Diagnosis of mitochondrial encephalomyopathies. *Curr Opin Rheumatol* 1997;9:496–503.
77. Zeviani M, Tiranti V, Piantades C. Mitochondrial disorders. *Medicine* 1998; 77:59–72.

78. Morgan-Hughes JA, Cooper JM, Holt IJ, et al. Mitochondrial myopathies: clinical defects. *Biochem Soc Trans* 1990;18:523–526.
79. Bouzidi MF, Schagger H, Collombet JM, et al. Decreased expression of ubiquinol-cytochrome C reductase subunits in patients exhibiting mitochondrial myopathy with progressive exercise intolerance. *Neuromusc Disord* 1993;3:599–604.
80. Johnson W, Karpati G, Carpenter S, et al. Late-onset mitochondrial myopathy. *Ann Neurol* 1995;37:16–23.
81. Austin SA, Vriscsendrop FJ, Thandroyen FT, et al. Expanding the phenotype of the 8344 transfer RNAlysine mitochondrial DNA mutation. *Neurology* 1998;51:1447–1450.
82. Vissing J, Salamon MB, Arlien-Sborg P, et al. A new mitochondrial tRNAMet gene mutation in a patient with dystrophic muscle and exercise intolerance. *Neurology* 1998;50:1875–1878.
83. Andreu AL, Brano C, Dunne TC, et al. A nonsense mutation (G15059A) in the cytochrome b gene in a patient with exercise intolerance and myoglobinuria. *Ann Neurol* 1999; 45:127–130.
84. Genge A, Karpati G, Arnold D, et al. Familial myopathy with conspicuous depletion of mitochondria in muscle fibers: a morphologically distinct disease. *Neuromusc Disord* 1995;5: 139–144.
85. Kawashima S, Ohta S, Kagawa Y, et al. Widespread tissue distribution of multiple mitochondrial DNA deletions in familial mitochondrial myopathy. *Muscle Nerve* 1994;17:741–746.
86. VuTH, Sciacco M, Tanji K, et al. Clinical manifestations of mitochondrial DNA depletion. *Neurology* 1998; 1783–1790.
87. Chariot P, Monnet I, Mouchet M, et al. Determination of the blood lactate: pyruvate ratio as a noninvasive test for the diagnosis of zidovudine myopathy. *Arthritis Rheum* 1994;37:583–586.
88. Bardosi A, Scheidt P, Goebel H. Mitochondrial myopathy: a result of clofibrate/etiofibrate treatment? *Acta Neurolopathol* 1985;68:164–168.
89. Osaki Y, Nichino I, Murakami N, et al. Mitochondrial abnormalities in selenium-deficient myopathy. *Muscle Nerve* 1998;21: 637–639.
90. Wallace DC. Mitochondrial genetics: a paradigm for aging and degenerative diseases? *Science* 1992;256:628–632.
91. Rifai Z, Welle S, Kamp C, et al. Ragged red fibers in normal aging and inflammatory myopathy. *Ann Neurol* 1995;37:24–29.
92. Blume G, Peesstronk A, Frank B, et al. Polymyositis with cytochrome oxidase negative muscle fibers: early quadriceps weakness and poor response to immunosuppressive therapy. *Brain* 1997;120:39–45.
93. Levine TD, Pestronk A. Inflammatory myopathy with cytochrome oxidase negative fibers: methotrexate treatment. *Muscle Nerve* 1998;21:1724–1728.
94. Harle JR, Pellissier JJ. Polymyalgia rheumatica and mitochondrial myopathy: clinicopathologic and biochemical studies in five cases. *Am J Med* 1992;92:167–172.
95. Campos Y, Huertas R, Lorenzo G, et al. Plasma carnitine insufficiency and effectiveness of L-carnitine therapy in patients with mitochondrial myopathy. *Muscle Nerve* 1993;16:150–153.
96. Tarnopolsky M, Martin J. Creatine monohydrate increases strength in patients with neuromuscular disease. *Neurology* 1999;52:854–857.
97. Taivassalo T, DeStefano N, Argon Z. Effects of aerobic training in patients with mitochondrial myopathies. *Neurology* 1998;50: 1055–1060.
98. Sabina RL, Holmes EW. Myoadenylate deaminase deficiency. In: Scriver CR, Beaudet AL, Sly WS, et al., eds. *The metabolic basis of inherited disease,* 7th ed. New York: McGraw-Hill, 1995:1769–1780.
99. Fishbein WN. Myoadenylate deaminase deficiency: inherited and acquired forms. *Biochem Med* 1985;33:158–169.
100. Sabina RL, Sulaiman AR, Wortmann RL. Molecular analysis of acquired myoadenylate deaminase deficiency in polymyositis (idiopathic inflammatory myopathy). *Adv Exp Biol Med* 1991;309B:203–205.
101. Tsujino S, Shanske S, Carroll JE, et al. Double trouble: combined myophosphorylase and AMP deaminase deficiency in a child homozygous for nonsense mutations at both loci. *Neuromusc Disord* 1995;5:263–266.
102. Sabina RL, Morisaki T, Clarke P, et al. Characterization of the human and rat myoadenylate deaminase genes. *J Biol Chem* 1990;265:9423–9433.
103. Morisaki T, Gross M, Morisaki H, et al. Molecular basis of AMP deaminase deficiency in skeletal muscle. *Proc Natl Acad Sci U S A* 1992;89:6457–6461.
104. Morisaki H, Morisaki T, Newby LK, et al. Alternative splicing: a mechanism for phenotypic rescue of a common inherited defect. *J Clin Invest* 1993;91:2275–2280.
105. Hood D, Van Lente F, Estes M. Serum enzyme alterations in chronic muscle disease. A biopsy-based diagnostic assessment. *Am J Clin Pathol* 1991;95:402–407.
106. Black HR, Quallich H, Gareleck CB. Racial differences in serum creatine kinase levels. *Am J Med* 1986;81:497–487.
107. Worrall JG, Phongasthorn V, Hooper RJL, et al. Racial variation in serum creatine kinase unrelated to lean body mass. *Br J Rheumatol* 1990;29:371–373.
108. Sinkeler SPT, Daanen HAM, Wevers RA, et al. The relation between blood lactate and ammonia in ischemic handgrip exercise. *Muscle Nerve* 1985;8:523–527.
109. Lamminen AE. Magnetic resonance imaging of primary skeletal muscle diseases: patterns of distribution and severity of involvement. *Br J Radiol* 1990;63:946–950.
110. Park JH, Olsen NJ. Imaging of skeletal muscle. In Wortmann RL, ed. *Diseases of skeletal muscle.* Philadelphia: Lippincott, Williams & Wilkins, 1999.
111. De Jager AE, van der Vleit TM, van der Ree TC, et al. Muscle computed tomography in adult-onset acid maltase deficiency. *Muscle Nerve* 1998;21:398–400.
112. Kent-Braun JA, Miller RG, Weiner MW. Magnetic resonance spectroscopy studies of human muscle. *Radiol Clin North Am* 1994;32:313–335.
113. Matthews PM, Allaire C, Shoubridge EA, et al. In vivo muscle magnetic resonance spectroscopy in the clinical investigation of mitochondrial disease. *Neurology* 1991;41:114–120.

121

OCHRONOSIS, HEMOCHROMATOSIS, AND WILSON'S DISEASE

H. RALPH SCHUMACHER, JR.

ALKAPTONURIA AND OCHRONOSIS

Alkaptonuria is a hereditary disorder characterized by homogentisic acid in the urine, which, when oxidized, imparts a brownish black color to the urine. The term *alkaptonuria,* denoting an avidity for oxygen in alkaline solution, was coined by Boedeker in 1859 and is derived from fusion of an Arabic word meaning "alkali" and a Greek word *(kaptein)* meaning "to suck up avidly." When freshly voided urine is alkalinized, polymerization of homogentisic acid is accelerated, and the urine turns black. Ochronosis denotes a bluish-black pigmentation of connective tissue in patients with alkaptonuria, usually apparent clinically in the cartilage of the ear, in the skin, and in the sclera. This term was originated by Virchow in 1866, who described the microscopic appearance of this pigmentation as "ochre" or dark yellow.

Alkaptonuria itself is a symptomless condition. Clinical signs and symptoms develop when pigment is deposited in cartilage and other connective tissues (ochronosis). The relationship between alkaptonuria and ochronosis was first recognized in 1902 by Albrecht. Table 121.1 lists features of these diseases and the related musculoskeletal conditions.

Historical Overview

The earliest clinical observation, that of a boy who passed dark urine, was made by Scribonius in 1584. Boedeker, in 1859, was the first to isolate homogentisic acid from the urine of a patient with alkaptonuria. In 1891, Wolkow and Bauman established the chemical structure of this compound as 2,5-dihydroxyphenyl-acetic acid and named it homogentisic acid. In 1958, LaDu and his collaborators (1) demonstrated the absence of the enzyme homogentisic acid oxidase in the liver of a patient with alkaptonuria, ochronotic spondylosis, and peripheral arthropathy.

Nature of the Biochemical Lesion

Alkaptonuria results from a defect in the metabolic pathway for the aromatic amino acid tyrosine. Normally, the benzene ring of homogentisic acid is cleaved by the enzyme homogentisic acid oxidase, and maleylacetoacetic acid is formed. LaDu et al. (1) assayed liver homogenates from ochronotic patients and control subjects and demonstrated that the pattern of enzyme activities in the alkaptonuric liver was essentially the same as in the control liver, with the

TABLE 121.1. DIAGNOSTIC FEATURES OF ALKAPTONURIA, OCHRONOSIS, OCHRONOTIC SPONDYLITIS, AND PERIPHERAL ARTHROPATHY

- Alkaptonuria
  - Urine turns black
    - On alkalinization
    - On standing
    - When tested for sugar by Benedict's reagent; in addition, yellow-orange precipitate forms
  - Positive family history
- Ochronosis
  - Pigmentation of cartilage and skin:
    - Pinna of ear, eardrum, and cerumen
    - Sclera
    - Skin over malar area, nose, axilla, and groin
  - Prostatic calculi
- Ochronotic spondylosis
  - Calcification and ossification of intervertebral discs
  - Disproportionately little osteophytosis
  - Sarcoiliac joints not fused and no "bamboo" spine
  - Loss of lumbar lordosis
  - Spine rigid and stooped, knees flexed, stance typical
- Ochronotic peripheral arthropathy
  - Knees, shoulders, and hips most commonly affected
  - Synovial fluid contains small amounts of homogentisic acid and is noninflammatory, except with occasional calcium pyrophosphate crystal-associated inflammation
  - Brittle cartilage fragments and pigmented "chards" in the synovium
  - Osteochrondral joint bodies common
  - Small joints of hands and feet usually not affected

exception of homogentisic acid oxidase activity, which was completely absent in the alkaptonuric patient. Of interest is the presence of the enzyme maleylacetoacetic acid isomerase in the alkaptonuric liver despite the apparent absence of the substrate maleylacetoacetic acid, which could be derived only from the metabolism of homogentisic acid. The presence of this enzyme in the absence of its substrate demonstrates that the expression of this enzyme is not dependent on its substrate.

Genetic Factors

Alkaptonuria appears to be transmitted by a single recessive autosomal gene. In four families, the gene has been mapped to chromosome 3q2 (2). The occasional occurrence of this disorder in successive generations of certain families may be the result of consanguineous marriages in which homozygotes mate with heterozygotes. The present concept of the mode of transmission of alkaptonuria, originally advanced by Garrod and challenged at times, has been substantiated by several careful family studies in which complete pedigrees were available (3). One family carried human leukocyte antigen HLA-B27 in eight of ten members with alkaptonuria (4).

Laboratory Aspects of Alkaptonuria

The freshly voided urine of an alkaptonuric patient is of normal color and does not darken immediately unless it is alkaline or contains less than a normal concentration of vitamin C or other reducing agents. On standing, it may turn brownish black as the homogentisic acid becomes oxidized. If Benedict's reagent is used to test the urine for sugar, the yellowish orange precipitate that is formed as the result of the reduction of copper by homogentisic acid can be misinterpreted as indicating glucosuria. The color of the supernatant solution in these cases is always brownish black, which is diagnostic for alkaptonuria.

With the use of copper-reduction tablets (Clinitest), a black supernatant may also be seen in patients with malignant melanoma and after intravenous urography with sodium diatrizoate (Hypaque) and other x-ray contrast media (5). Specific glucose oxidase tapes (Clinistix) may not detect urine glucose in diabetics with ochronosis because of interference with the peroxidase-indicator chromogen reaction by homogentisic acid (6). Spuriously increased serum and urinary uric acid determinations have been described in ochronosis when colorimetric methods were used, but values were normal by the uricase spectrophotometric technique (6).

Diagnostic Tests for Alkaptonuria

Several presumptive, but nonspecific, tests for alkaptonuria are available. These tests are color reactions based on the reducing properties of homogentisic acid. Thus, in the Briggs test, molybdate is reduced and a deep blue color is obtained. When a drop of urine is placed on photographic paper, a black spot indicates reduction of silver. When sodium hydroxide is added to the freshly passed urine, homogentisic acid is rapidly oxidized, and the urine promptly darkens. A specific enzymatic method for quantitative determination of homogentisic acid in urine and blood has been developed (7). Thin-layer chromatography can also be used.

Pathologic Features of Ochronosis

The lesions of ochronosis result from the intercellular or intracellular deposition of pigment in many tissues. The exact chemical composition of the pigment has not yet been defined, although it is believed to be a polymer derived from homogentisic acid. Benzoquinone acetic acid may be an intermediate compound that, when bound to connective tissue, may participate in a polymerization process leading to the final pigment formation (8). Homogentisic acid is concentrated preferentially by connective tissue, but this process is reversible until after polymerization (8). Homogentisic acid has been shown to inhibit hydroxylysine formation *in vitro* (9). The predilection of ochronosis for cartilage that contains hydroxylysine-rich collagen may be in part related to this. A deleterious effect of homogentisic acid on growth of cultured chondrocytes has been demonstrated (10). The typical pathologic findings include granules of insoluble, melanin-like pigment, which are usually found in the skin and subcutis, cartilage of joints, intervertebral discs including the annulus fibrosus as well as the nucleus pulposus, tracheal cartilage, epithelial cells of the renal tubules, and the islets of the pancreas. Pigment granules impregnate the walls of large and medium-sized arteries and arterioles, including the aorta and the pulmonary, coronary, and renal arteries.

Clinical Picture of Ochronosis

Patients with alkaptonuria who live to the fourth decade almost invariably develop ochronosis. The cartilage of the ear, especially the concha and anthelix, is frequently involved and takes on a slate-blue discoloration while becoming irregularly thickened and inflexible. When the pinna is transilluminated, the opaque pigmented area is prominent. The cerumen in the external canal is often black, and the periphery of the tympanic membrane is grayish black. Many patients with long-standing ochronosis exhibit impaired hearing. Pigmentation of the sclera is usually localized to a small area midway between the limbus of the cornea and the inner or outer canthus. The skin over the malar areas, nose, axilla, and groin is often pigmented.

Deposition of pigment in the intervertebral discs and articular cartilage of the large joints leads to spondylosis and peripheral arthropathy. Loud cardiac murmurs, mostly systolic, have been noted in approximately 15% to 20% of patients with ochronosis (11). Pigment deposits in the mitral and aortic valves may be associated with deformity of the leaflets or cusps. Clinically significant aortic stenosis has been successfully treated by aortic valve replacement (12).

Prostatic calculi occur in a large proportion of men with ochronosis and are readily palpable on rectal examination. Dysuria and frequency of urination may be present. Calculi may be passed spontaneously or removed surgically. These calculi have a characteristic black color and contain ochronotic pigment and calcium phosphate salts.

Ochronotic Spondylosis

The majority of patients with ochronosis past the age of 30 develop spondylosis. Symptoms usually consist of stiffness and discomfort in the lower back. In approximately 10% to 15% of patients with ochronosis, the onset of spondylosis occurs with herniation of a nucleus pulposus (11). In such instances, the symptoms and signs are indistinguishable from those in typical cases of herniated disc without alkaptonuria. The earliest site of spondylosis is the lumbar spine; years later, the dorsal, and finally the cervical, spine become involved. Stiffness of the lower back slowly progresses to rigidity and obliteration of normal lumbar lordosis. In many cases, lumbar kyphosis develops. Symptoms may be minimal despite prominent radiographic changes. Spinal stenosis may occur.

The earliest change apparent in radiographs of the spine consists of a wafer of calcification, and actual ossification, in the intervertebral disc of the lumbar spine (Fig. 121.1). Crystallographic study has shown the calcium in these discs to be hydroxyapatite (13). Radiographic evidence of calcified intervertebral discs in adults is characteristic of ochronosis, but this is not diagnostic because similar changes can also be seen in pseudogout, hemochromatosis, chronic respiratory paralytic poliomyelitis, spinal fusion of any origin, and occasionally other disorders, and in the absence of detectable associated disease. Secondary narrowing of the intervertebral spaces occurs. Osteophytes are usually small. Splits in disc material appear to account for radiolucencies in the discs that have been termed "vacuum discs" (14). In contrast to ankylosing spondylitis, the sacroiliac joints in ochronotic spondylosis are not fused, although they may show degenerative changes; the interfacetal articulations retain a normal radiographic appearance, and annular ossification with a "bamboo" pattern does not appear. The marked narrowing of multiple intervertebral spaces results in a loss of several inches in height. The spinal deformity and forward stoop cause the patient to stand with knees flexed and with a broad base. This posture imparts to the patient with ochronotic spondylosis a stance and gait similar to that of a patient with ankylosing spondylitis (Fig. 121.2).

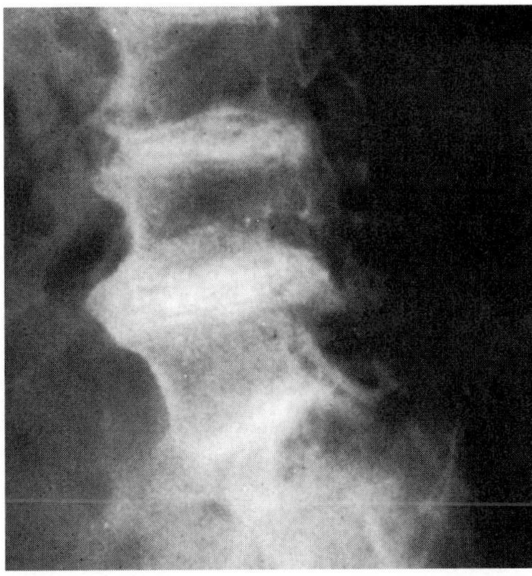

FIGURE 121.1. Radiograph of the lumbar spine of a 55-year-old man with ochronotic spondylosis. Note the calcification of intervertebral discs. The osteophytes are of only moderate size.

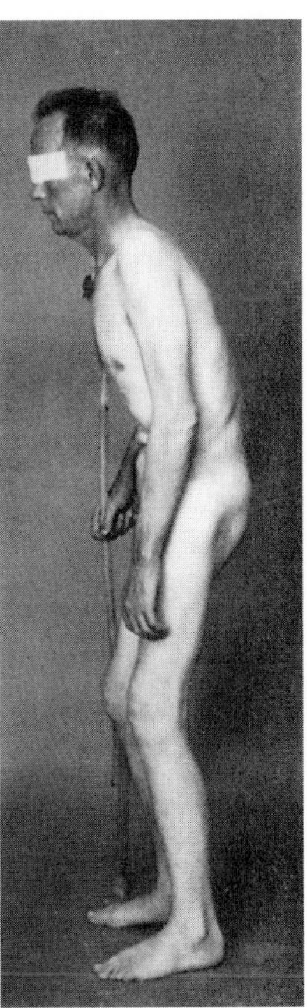

FIGURE 121.2. Typical posture and stance of a patient with ochronotic spondylosis: forward stoop, loss of lumbar lordosis, flexed hips and knees, and wide-based stance. This 40-year-old man lost 6 inches in height.

Ochronotic Peripheral Arthropathy

Degenerative arthritis of the peripheral joints also occurs, although it is less frequent and develops later than spondylosis. The joints most commonly affected are the knees, shoulders, and hips, in descending order of frequency. The knees are involved in the majority of cases of peripheral arthritis. Pain, stiffness, crepitation, flexion contractures, and limitation of motion are the most common features. In the peripheral joints, symptoms often antedate any visible radiographic changes. Effusion occurs in about half of these cases. Synovial fluid is generally clear, viscous, and yellow, without darkening on exposure to alkali. Although homogentisic acid can be demonstrated, its concentration is much lower than in the urine. Occasionally, black specks of ochronotic cartilage are seen suspended in the fluid (15,16). Leukocyte counts in a large series reported by Hüttl (17) ranged from 112 to 700/mm^3 with predominantly mononuclear cells. Occasional cells have dark inclusions that appear to be phagocytosed cartilage containing ochronotic pigment (Fig. 121.3). Synovial effusions or membrane can contain calcium pyrophosphate crystals without inflammation (16–19) (see also Chapters 4 and 117), or the patient may have typical acute episodes of pseudogout with increased synovial fluid leukocyte counts (20).

Pigmentation of the articular cartilage occurs initially in the deeper layers, with relative sparing of the surface. It is seen predominantly in the matrix of the tangential zone but also in chondrocytes. Necrosis of chondrocytes occurs. Pigment appears by electron microscopy to be associated with the surface of collagen fibers in cartilage but not in synovium (18,21). The pigmented articular cartilage is brittle; minute fragments are broken off and are displaced into the synovial tissue (Fig. 121.4). Shards can be phagocytosed (22) and may evoke a foreign-body reaction and induce formation of new bone tissue called osteochondral bodies (Fig. 121.5) (23). These bodies may be several centimeters in diameter and are readily palpable in and around the knee joint. They are often not tender and may be freely movable. Surgical removal may be necessary when the bodies interfere with motion.

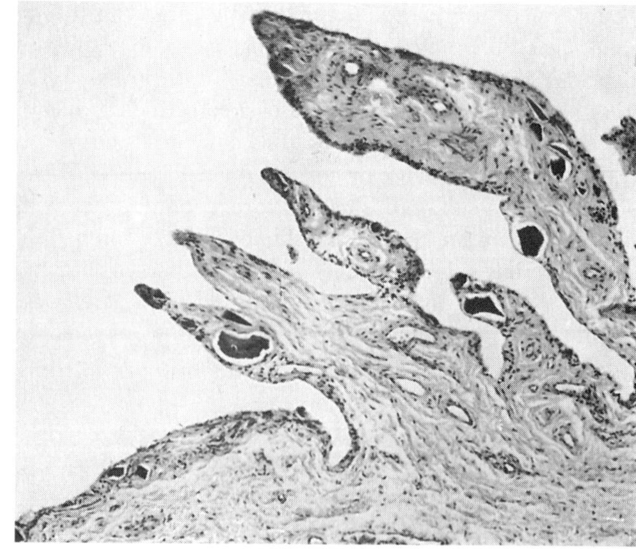

FIGURE 121.4. Synovial tissue in ochronotic arthropathy. Minute fragments of darkly pigmented cartilage lie within the superficial portion of the tissue. The sharp edges of the "shards" are characteristic. A foreign-body cell reaction is present at the margins of a few and is accompanied by mild synovial fibrosis. Associated infiltration of lymphocytes and plasma cells may also be present (hematoxylin and eosin stain, ×90).

The radiographic appearance of the large peripheral joints in ochronotic arthritis, virtually indistinguishable from that of primary osteoarthritis (OA), demonstrates narrowing of the joint space, small marginal osteophytes, and eburnation. Rarely, the diagnosis is first suggested at knee arthroscopy or surgery when the black pigmentation is encountered unexpectedly (24). Protrusio acetabuli may be seen (18). Ossifica-

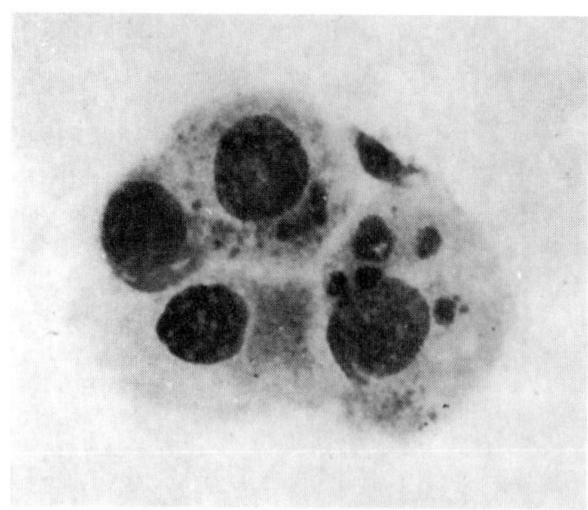

FIGURE 121.3. Synovial fluid mononuclear cells in ochronotic arthropathy. The dark cytoplasmic inclusions appear to be phagocytized pigmented debris (Giemsa stain, ×1,250). (From Huttl S. Synovial effusion. A nosographic and diagnostic study. Part I. *Acta Rheum Baln Pistiniana* 1970;5:1–100, with permission.)

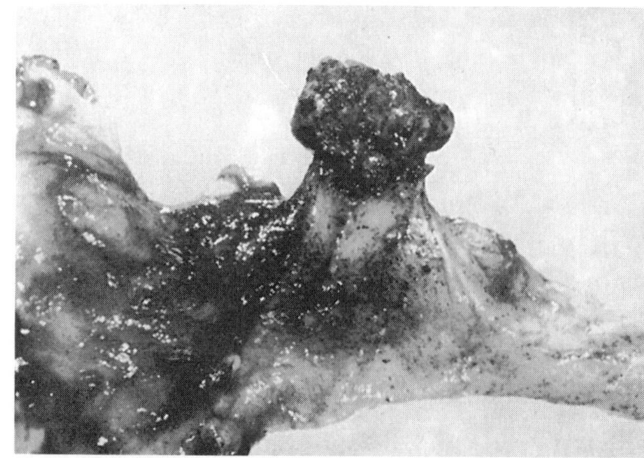

FIGURE 121.5. Synovial tissue in ochronotic arthropathy. Numerous pigmented deposits are present. A polypoid nodule has formed in the central portion as an osteochondroid reaction of the displaced cartilage fragments.

tion or calcification of the ligaments and tendons near the joints may be present (25). Rupture of deeply pigmented ochronotic Achilles tendons has been reported.

In contrast to rheumatoid arthritis (RA) and OA, the small joints of the hands and feet are rarely affected in ochronosis.

Experimental and Nonalkaptonuric Production of Ochronosis

Rats fed 8% L-tyrosine for 18 to 24 months develop pigment deposition in joint capsules and cartilages and a degenerative arthritis similar to that in spontaneous human alkaptonuria (26). The cartilage pigment is melanin-like and includes phenolic derivatives such as homogentisic acid or its metabolite benzoquinone acetic acid. Mice have been described with a mutation causing high levels of urinary homogentisic acid but no ochronosis (27).

A grossly bluish black connective tissue pigmentation associated with degenerative arthritis also has been described following prolonged administration of quinacrine in the absence of alkaptonuria. Ochronosis-like skin pigmentation attributed to enormous elastotic fibers has occurred in some African-Americans using hydroquinone bleaching creams (28). Application of phenol dressings has been reported to produce ochronosis with alkaptonuria and arthropathy. Cartilage pigmentation does not occur in metastatic malignant melanoma. Black pigmented costal cartilages have been reported after methyldopa therapy (29).

Treatment

It is not yet feasible to use gene therapy or to compensate for the deficiency of homogentisic acid oxidase. Attempts have been made to treat patients with a diet low in phenylalanine and tyrosine that is, unfortunately, unpalatable. Urinary excretion of homogentisic acid can be decreased, but clinical change was minimal in patients with advanced joint disease. Initiation of this diet at an early age, before massive ochronosis develops, has not been tried. Reduced protein intake can also decrease urinary homogentisic acid levels, but this regimen is impractical for routine treatment. Although high doses of ascorbic acid do not decrease total urine homogentisic acid levels, they have been reported to reduce binding to connective tissue in experimental alkaptonuria of rats and to reverse homogentisic acid–induced chondrocyte growth inhibition *in vitro* (30). Despite this, long-term use of ascorbic acid has not been useful in limited trials in human ochronosis.

Symptomatic measures are of most practical value. Analgesics, braces, a program limiting joint overuse, and weight reduction have all provided some help. Adrenal corticosteroids, X-irradiation, tyrosinase, insulin, various vitamins, and phenylbutazone are among the measures tried without benefit. Total joint replacements of hips and knees have been successful (31).

HEMOCHROMATOSIS

Hemochromatosis is a chronic disease first recognized by Trousseau in 1865 and characterized pathologically by excessive iron deposition and fibrosis in many organs and tissues with ultimate functional impairment in untreated patients. This disorder occurs in a clinically detectable form in at least 1 in 250 people in various populations of European origin. Clinical disease occurs five times more often in men than in women. Frequent clinical manifestations include hepatomegaly and cirrhosis; skin pigmentation, mostly from increased melanin; diabetes; other endocrine dysfunction; and heart failure (32,33). Sicca syndrome has been reported, possibly adding to confusion with other rheumatic diseases (34). Arthropathy occurs in 20% to 40% of patients. Hemochromatosis is often idiopathic, with a definite increased familial incidence first recognized by Sheldon (33) in 1935. It is inherited as an autosomal-recessive trait. A gene on chromosome 6 termed HLA-H or HFE has now been identified that exhibits a mutation resulting in the substitution of a tyrosine for cysteine at position 282 of the encoded proteins. At least 80% of hemochromatosis patients in several studies have been homozygous for this mutation (35). At least one other less common mutation has also been found. The encoded protein resembles class I major histocompatibility complex (MHC) proteins and has been proposed to possibly modify β_2-microglobulin binding. β_2-microglobulin knockout mice interestingly develop iron overload. Hemochromatosis can also occasionally be a late result of alcoholic cirrhosis or occasionally of multiple transfusions, refractory anemia, or long-term excessive oral iron ingestion. In all instances, iron absorption is excessive. Significant overload occurs only after many years, so the onset of symptoms is most common between 40 and 60 years. A form of hemochromatosis occurring before age 30 is often associated with hypogonadism and cardiac involvement. This is not obviously familial but may be associated with arthropathy as occurs in older patients (36). Tables 121.2 and 121.3

TABLE 121.2. DIAGNOSTIC FEATURES OF HEMOCHROMATOSIS

Cirrhosis with iron deposition, predominantly in parenchymal cells
Iron deposition in other organs causing cardiomyopathy, diabetes, or other endocrine deficiencies
Increased skin pigmentation, largely by melanin
Elevated serum iron concentration and saturated iron-binding capacity

TABLE 121.3. DIAGNOSTIC FEATURES OF ARTHROPATHY OF HEMOCHROMATOSIS

Degenerative arthropathy
Prominent involvement of metacarpophalangeal and proximal and distal interphalangeal joints, hips, and knees
Chondrocalcinosis
Iron deposition in synovial lining cells

list diagnostic features of hemochromatosis and its related arthropathy.

Pathologic Features and Pathogenesis

Iron as hemosiderin can be identified histologically in symptomatically affected tissues, as well as elsewhere. The largest iron deposits are in the liver, and diagnosis is most frequently established by liver biopsy. Large amounts of hemosiderin are seen in parenchymal cells in the liver and in other organs. Iron confined to reticuloendothelial tissues is termed *hemosiderosis* and does not produce the clinical picture seen in hemochromatosis. Although suspected, iron has not been proven to be the cause of the tissue damage. Organ fibrosis, as in hemochromatosis, has not yet been produced by experimental iron overload alone. Iron may act in an additive fashion with nutritional deficiencies, alcohol, or other, still unidentified, hereditary factors.

Diagnosis

The most important simple diagnostic laboratory tests is the determination of serum iron concentration and the percentage saturation of the total iron-binding capacity. Both values are elevated in hemochromatosis, but they can also be elevated in hemolytic anemia and other situations. Greater than 50% saturation of iron-binding capacity should raise consideration of hemochromatosis; greater than 62% saturation should virtually always be investigated further with liver biopsy (37). Serum ferritin concentrations are often elevated but may be normal in precirrhotic disease (38) and may be nonspecifically elevated by inflammation. Polymerase chain reaction (PCR) testing for HLA-H can identify homozygotes or heterozygotes, with the latter not likely to be affected. Magnetic resonance imaging showing reduced signal intensity can suggest liver iron overload (39). Liver biopsy is needed to determine the extent of tissue iron deposition and the degree of tissue damage. One case of hemochromatosis with associated hypoxanthine-guanine phosphoribosyltransferase deficiency has been reported in which serum-iron concentrations and transferrin saturation were normal (40).

Osteopenia

Diffuse demineralization of bone can be seen, but its frequency and relationship to the hemochromatosis are difficult to ascertain. In one study 9 of 32 patients had osteoporosis. Severity correlated with degree of iron overload (41). A diffuse osteopenia of the hands, without the periarticular demineralization observed in RA, is most common. Hypogonadism is probably an important contributing factor (42). Serum calcium, phosphorus, and alkaline phosphatase levels are normal. Biopsy specimens have shown osteoporosis rather than osteomalacia. Experimental acute iron overload can produce iron deposits in osteoblasts and trabeculae with decreased osteoblast numbers and activity (43). Because osteopenia is also seen in alcoholic cirrhosis, a direct relation to the defect in iron metabolism is not always necessary.

Degenerative Arthropathy and Chondrocalcinosis

An arthropathy associated with hemochromatosis was first described in 1964 (44), and since then more than 300 cases have been reported (45–50). The most frequent joint involvement is degenerative, occurring in 20% to as high as 81% of patients with hemochromatosis (41,47). The age of onset varies from 20 to 70, but it is most common in the sixth decade. The onset of arthropathy is usually close in time to the onset of other symptoms of hemochromatosis, but joint symptoms and findings may antedate other clinical manifestations of hemochromatosis and may thus be the first clue to diagnosis (46,51,52). Joint symptoms occasionally are first noted many years later, even after completion of phlebotomy therapy.

Hands, knees, and hips are most frequently involved, although other joints including the ankles and feet can be affected. Characteristic hand findings are a firm, only mildly tender, enlargement of the metacarpophalangeal and the proximal and distal interphalangeal joints. The second and third metacarpophalangeal joints are most often affected (Fig. 121.6). These joints are stiff and have limited motion but no increased warmth or erythema. Ulnar deviation is not seen. Involvement is generally symmetric. Pain, when present, is accentuated on use. Morning stiffness usually lasts less than half an hour. This arthropathy is gradually progressive. Acute inflammation has occasionally been described, and whether it is always due to associated chondrocalcinosis and crystal-induced synovitis is not certain. Test results for rheumatoid factor are typically negative. Sedimentation rates are only occasionally elevated. Serum uric acid levels are generally normal and occasionally low (40).

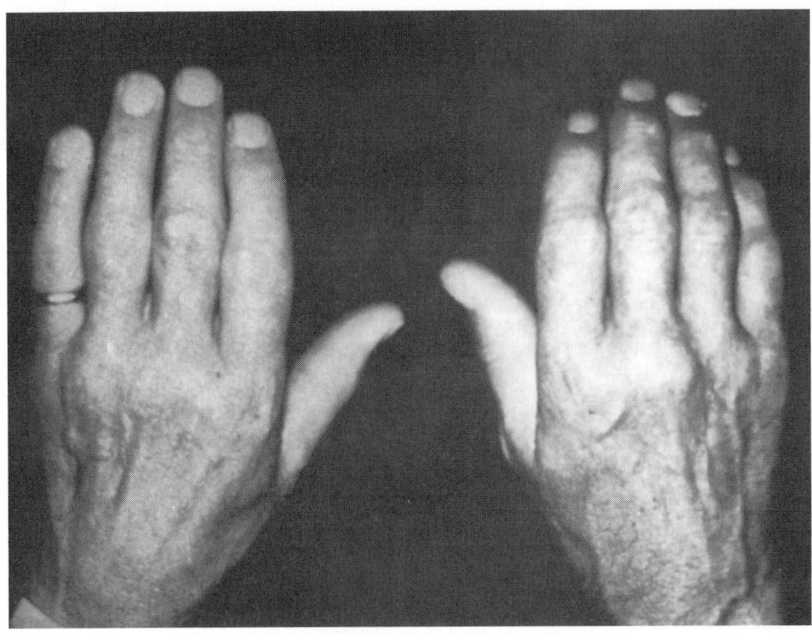

FIGURE 121.6. Photograph of the hands of a 45-year-old man with hemochromatosis. Note the knobby enlargement at the metacarpophalangeal, proximal interphalangeal, and distal interphalangeal joints. He is unable to extend these joints fully.

Radiographs often show the characteristic involvement of the metacarpophalangeal, proximal, and distal interphalangeal joints. Narrowing of the joint space, subchondral cysts, joint-space irregularity, subchondral sclerosis, and moderate bony proliferation with frequent hook-like osteophytes are seen (44,53) (Fig. 121.7). In 30% to 60% of those with arthropathy, especially older patients, chondrocalcinosis is also seen. Radiographs of other joints show changes similar to those in the hands and are often indistinguishable from OA and idiopathic chondrocalcinosis. Involvement of the fourth and fifth metacarpophalangeal joints is rare in idiopathic chondrocalcinosis and is most suggestive of underlying hemochromatosis. In one study, hip radiographs showed an unusual stripping of the cartilage from the bone (54).

Synovial fluid is usually noninflammatory, with low leukocyte counts and predominantly mononuclear cells, adequate viscosity, and a pale yellow color. Iron levels in synovial fluid are comparable to serum levels (48). Synovial tissue shows a striking deposition of iron, mostly in the syn-

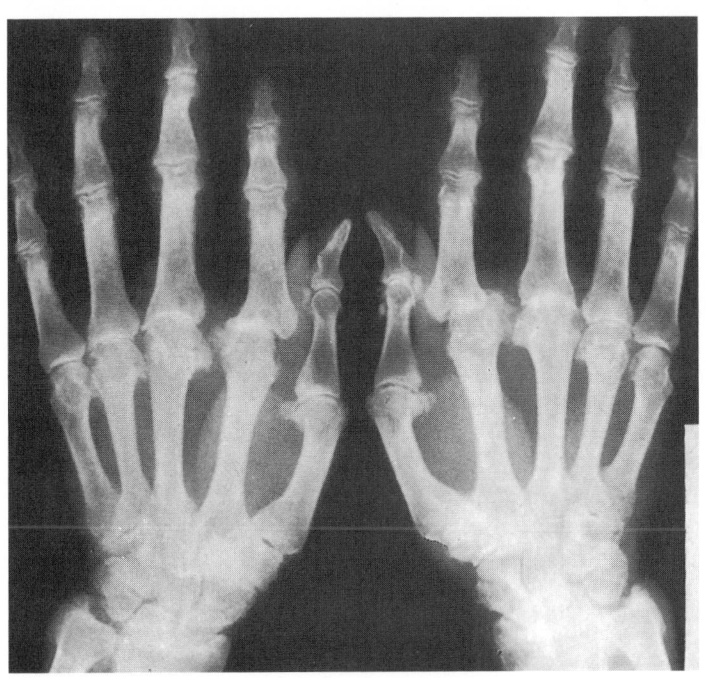

FIGURE 121.7. Radiograph of hands showing involvement of the metacarpophalangeal and the proximal and distal interphalangeal joints, with characteristic joint-space narrowing, cystic subchondral lesions, joint-space irregularity, subluxation, some osteophytosis, and areas of bony sclerosis. Multiple periarticular calcifications are also present in the interphalangeal joint of the left thumb, and probable chondrocalcinosis is seen at the right ulnocarpal joint. Osteopenia is minimal in these hands.

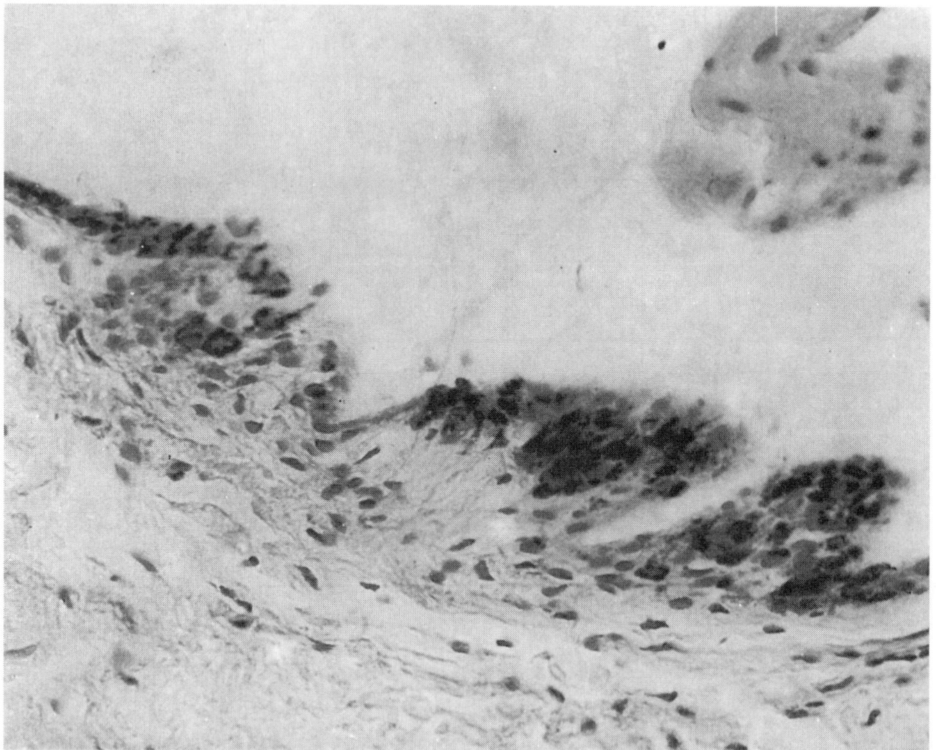

FIGURE 121.8. Synovium in hemochromatosis with dark Prussian blue-stained iron granules in the synovial lining cells (×400).

ovial lining cells, but also in some deeper cells. On hematoxylin and eosin staining, golden-brown hemosiderin granules are seen. The iron can also be stained with Prussian blue (Fig. 121.8). By electron microscopy, the iron is principally seen in type B or synthetic (fibroblastic) lining cells (Fig. 121.9) (55). This distribution of synovial iron differs from that in hemarthrosis, RA, and other diseases in which iron is presumably derived from gross or microscopic bleeding into the joint. In these conditions, the iron is mostly found in deeper cells and macrophages. In addition to the iron, most synovial membranes in hemochromatosis show only mild lining-cell proliferation, fibrosis, and scattered chronic inflammatory cells. Biopsies of synovium during bouts of acute inflammation have not been reported.

Chondrocalcinosis with hemochromatosis, although usually associated with degenerative arthropathy, can also be an isolated joint finding (51). Calcification is most commonly detected in menisci and articular cartilages at the knee, but it can also be seen at the wrists, fingers, elbows, shoulders, hips, ankles, toes, symphysis pubis, intervertebral discs, and the periarticular soft tissues and bursae.

Iron staining of cartilage has also been noted, but this is seen in chondrocytes and at the line of ossification, not at the site of crystal deposits (55,56). Similarly, x-ray diffraction and chemical studies have shown no iron at the sites of cartilage calcification (47,56). Periarticular and bursal calcifications have not been studied to determine the type of calcium salt. Crystals resembling hydroxyapatite have been identified in hemochromatotic synovium and cartilage by electron microscopy (see also Chapter 4) (55,56). Even when no calcification is radiographically visible, cartilage calcium pyrophosphate crystals or apatite are often identifiable by light and electron microscopy (56).

Possible Mechanisms for Arthropathy

It is appealing to speculate that the iron directly or indirectly causes the osteoarthropathy, but such has not been demonstrated. Arthropathy has only occasionally been reported in patients with transfusion siderosis (57,58), which suggests that factors other than iron deposition are required. Patients with spherocytosis appear to develop iron overload only when they are also heterozygous for the hemochromatosis gene (59). Many patients with iron-loading anemias do not survive long enough to develop tissue damage. Aseptic necrosis and osteopenia, but no other arthropathy, have been reported in Bantu siderosis. That experimental iron loading of rabbits produces cartilage degeneration only when initiated early in life suggests the importance of early initiation of the toxic effect of iron

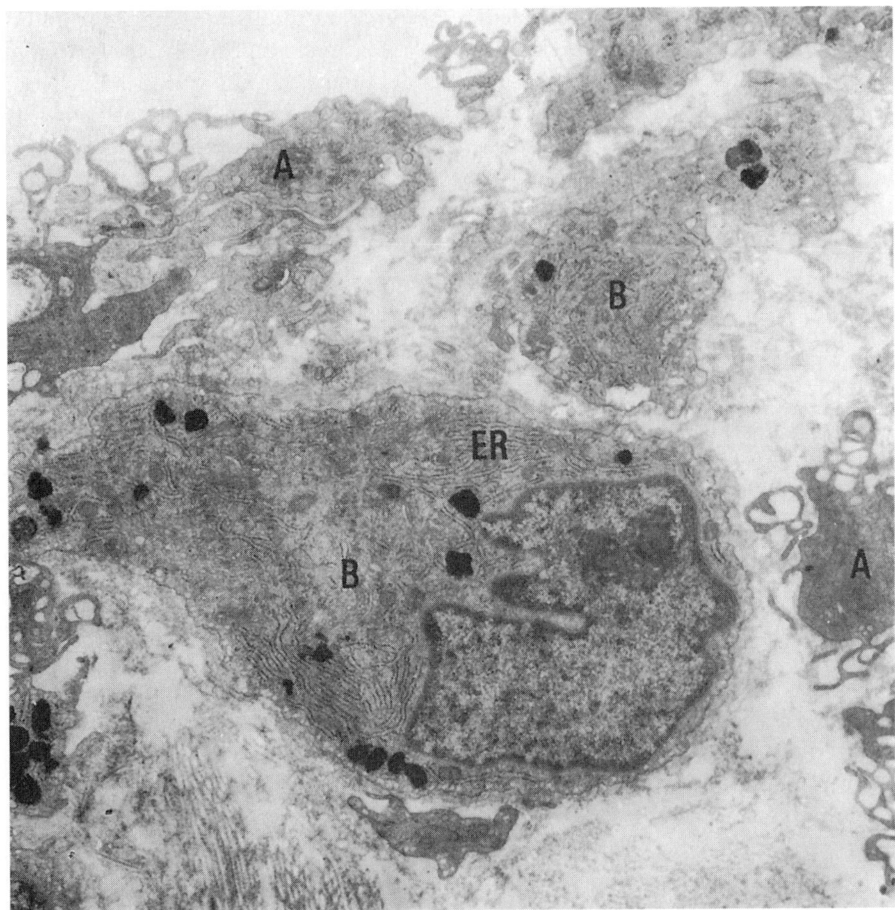

FIGURE 121.9. Electron micrograph of electron-dense iron deposits in type B synovial lining cells *(B)* in hemochromatosis. Type B cells are primarily synthetic in function and have profuse rough endoplasmic reticulum (ER). The type A cells *(A)* often have prominent filopodia and vacuoles and are believed to be more active in phagocytosis. Here they contain no identifiable iron (×13,000).

(60). Localized predominantly in synthetic-type cells in cartilage or synovium, iron might cause joint damage by altering the proteins, polysaccharide, or collagen produced by such cells. Ferric citrate *in vitro* stimulated synovial fibroblast proliferation at least in part by downregulating prostaglandin E_2 (PGE_2) production (61). Iron can injure chondrocytes or other cells by lipid peroxidation of membranes. Several possible ways that iron or transferrin saturation can affect the immune system have been reviewed (62). Ferric ion can irreversibly oxidize ascorbic acid and can impair hydroxylation of proline and thus allow deficient collagen formation (60). Iron might produce damage by binding to connective tissue protein polysaccharides as it does *in vitro* in the Hale's stain for protein polysaccharide. Some iron is present in lysosomes, and it could increase the release of lysosomal enzymes.

In vitro, iron inhibits pyrophosphatase and might in this manner help to allow the deposition of the calcium pyrophosphate of chondrocalcinosis (63). Experimental synovial siderosis also inhibited clearance of calcium pyrophosphate crystals from rabbit joints (64). Increased levels of parathyroid hormone have been described in patients with arthropathy (65). The primary site of joint damage is not established. Cartilage is most suspect in this degenerative process, but subchondral bone or synovial involvement may also be important because cartilage depends on both of these tissues for nutrition. No correlation has been found between the presence of advanced liver disease, generalized osteopenia, diabetes, or other endocrine disease and the arthropathy. Classic RA has been reported to coexist in several cases, so the arthropathy is not an iron-altered rheumatoid disease.

Treatment

The present therapy of hemochromatosis is directed at prompt removal of the excess iron by phlebotomy, and this approach appears to reverse cardiac failure, improve liver function, and ameliorate diabetes. Improvement depends largely on the amount of existing tissue damage. Prevention certainly would be preferable, so serum iron concentrations of relatives should be checked, and prophylactic phlebotomy should be considered. Phlebotomy of 450 mL per week, until the development of mild iron deficiency anemia or demonstrable depletion of liver iron, is usual. Maintenance phlebotomy every 2 to 3 months is usually required. Alcohol and excessive vitamin C ingestion can increase iron absorption and should be avoided. Supportive treatment of the diabetes, liver disease, and heart failure is pursued as needed. Phlebotomy has not had any consistent beneficial effect on the arthritis; arthritis and chondrocalcinosis may progress (47) and clinical arthritis has even developed after therapeutic phlebotomy. One *in vitro* study showed that ferrous iron inhibited de novo formation of calcium pyrophosphate crystals and suggested that depletion of ferrous ions by phlebotomy could remove an inhibitor of calcium pyrophosphate crystal formation (66). Irreversible connective tissue and joint change may well become established long before arthritis can be clinically or radiographically detected. Treatment of the arthritis is symptomatic; analgesics, nonsteroidal antiinflammatory drugs, and systematic range-of-motion exercises are sometimes helpful. However, treatment is also frustrating. Anecdotal attempts at therapy with colchicine, antimalarial drugs, or tetracyclines have not shown any promising trends. Studies are needed. Prosthetic hip and knee arthroplasties have been successfully performed in patients with advanced disease, although further breakdown after 18 months has occurred in a knee after prosthetic arthroplasty.

WILSON'S DISEASE

Hepatolenticular degeneration (Wilson's disease), described by Wilson (67) in 1912, is an uncommon familial disease characterized by a ring of golden brown pigment at the corneal margin, known as the Kayser-Fleischer ring, sometimes visible only on slit-lamp examination; basal ganglion degeneration; and cirrhosis. The disease is inherited as an autosomal-recessive trait. The gene has now been mapped to chromosome 13q14.3. A variety of mutations have been found. The most frequent mutation results in a change from histidine to glutamine at amino acid position 1069. A rapid PCR test has been developed to test for this mutation (68). The function of the gene product is not yet known (69). Symptoms may first appear between the ages of 4 and 50. Neurologic symptoms are usually earliest and include tremor, rigidity, dysarthria, incoordination, and personality change. Liver involvement can mimic chronic hepatitis or can cause fulminant hepatic failure. Many patients also develop renal tubular disease manifested by aminoaciduria, proteinuria, glucosuria, renal stones, phosphaturia, defective urine acidification, or uricosuria. Uricosuria often results in low serum uric acid levels. Hemolytic anemia can occur. Untreated disease is invariably fatal (70).

Characteristic disorders of copper metabolism are present (71). Copper concentrations are increased in liver, brain, and other tissues, urine copper excretion is increased, and the serum copper-binding protein ceruloplasmin as well as total serum copper are almost always decreased. Measurement of the hepatic copper concentration appears to be the most reliable test. Although the basic underlying defect is not known, increased absorption of copper can be demonstrated. Copper may cause the tissue damage. Mobilization of copper from the body seems to produce an improvement in many patients. Although seen in at least 95% of patients, Kayser-Fleischer rings are not entirely specific and may be seen in other diseases (72). Table 121.4 lists osseous and articular changes in Wilson's disease.

Osteopenia

Radiographic evidence of demineralization of bone has long been recognized in Wilson's disease and occurs in 25% to 50% of patients (73,74). Osteopenia is seen at all ages and usually is asymptomatic. Occasional patients have pathologic fractures. Others have definite rickets (75), or osteomalacia that can be attributed to the renal tubular disease.

Arthropathy

Boudin et al. (76) first described articular involvement in Wilson's disease in 1957. Joint changes are rare in childhood but are seen in up to 50% of adults. Most patients studied have been 20 to 40 years old. Articular involvement

TABLE 121.4. BONE AND JOINT CHANGES IN WILSON'S DISEASE

Bone demineralization
Occasionally, rickets or osteomalacia attributable to renal tubular disease
Premature degenerative arthritis with prominent subchondral bone fragmentation
Prominent involvement of wrists, knees, and less often, other joints
Periarticular calcifications and bone fragments

ranges from premature OA with pronounced symptoms to asymptomatic radiographic findings (73,74,77–82). Scattered subchondral bone fragmentations, cortical irregularity, and sclerosis at the margin of wrist, hand, elbow, shoulder, hip, and knee joints are seen (Fig. 121.10). The cartilage space is often narrowed. Early age of onset and prominent involvement of wrists suggest a difference from the usual OA. Tiny periarticular cysts (74), vertebral wedging and marginal irregularity (82), osteochondritis dissecans, and chondromalacia patellae (77) have been seen in several patients and may be related to Wilson's disease. Periarticular calcifications are common; many such calcifications occur in ligaments, tendons, and capsule insertions. Other calcifications seem to represent bone fragments. There is occasional radiographic evidence of chondrocalcinosis (77,78,82). The cause of the chondrocalcinosis has not been well studied. Although copper has been identified in some cartilages by elemental analysis, calcium crystals were not found in one light and electron microscopic study (74). Calcium pyrophosphate crystals were reported earlier in an intervertebral disc. Joint effusions are usually small, with clear, viscous fluid and 200 to 300 cells/mm^3, predominantly mononuclear cells (77,79). Synovial fluid copper and ceruloplasmin levels have not been studied. Only mild lining-cell hyperplasia and small numbers of chronic inflammatory cells have been noted on synovial biopsies (79,80). In one case, copper and iron were reported in the synovium by elemental analysis (80).

No correlation has been found between the severity of the disease, spasticity and tremors, osteopenia, liver or renal disease, and the arthropathy. The primary defect may occur in the cartilage or subchondral bone, but no histologic or chemical studies of these tissues have been conducted. Although the joint involvement in Wilson's disease is generally milder, an analogy can be made with that of hemochromatosis. In both diseases, the metal excess is a possible mechanism for direct or

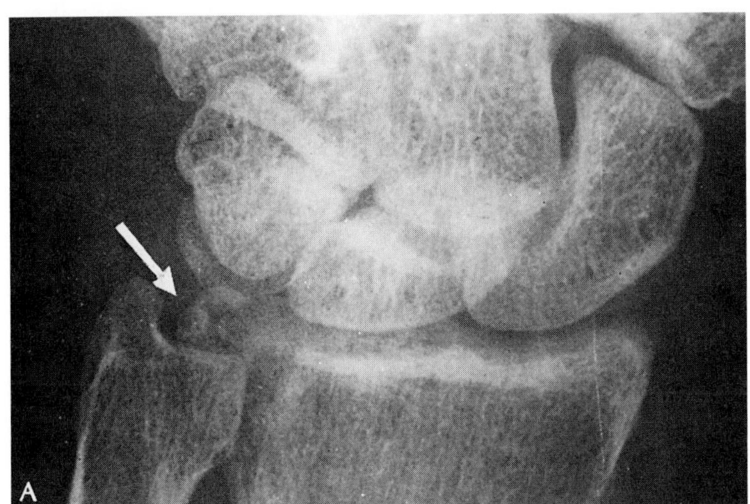

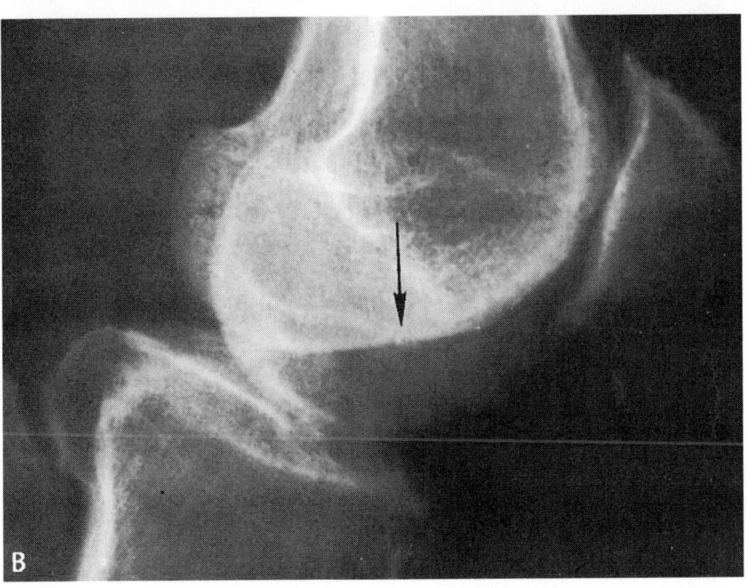

FIGURE 121.10. Arthropathy in a 30-year-old woman with Wilson's disease. **A:** Wrist. Note the bony ossicles *(arrow)* suggested to be a result of cortical fragmentation. Some sclerosis is also present at the distal radius. **B:** Knee. Ossicles are seen near the tibiofibular articulation. Significant chondromalacia patellae with spurs is present on the posterior surface of the patella. The articular cortex of the lateral femoral condyle is irregular, with a suggestion of fragmentation (arrow).

indirect production of the arthropathy. Short-term experimental copper loading has not produced arthropathy. McCarty and Pepe (63) have shown *in vitro* inhibition of inorganic cytosolic pyrophosphatase by cupric as well as by ferrous ions and have suggested this inhibition as a possible mechanism for deposition of calcium pyrophosphate producing chondrocalcinosis in Wilson's disease and hemochromatosis. Hepatic hypertrophic osteoarthropathy has been reported to complicate Wilson's disease (83).

Treatment

D-Penicillamine, 1 to 4 g/day orally, is the most successful chelating agent for mobilizing copper from the tissue and has produced definite clinical improvement in mental and neurologic changes in many patients. Treatment must be continued for life. Low-copper diets and potassium sulfide may also be used to decrease copper absorption. Symptomatic disease may be preventable by early D-penicillamine treatment of asymptomatic persons with biochemical abnormalities only (84). Occasional patients treated with penicillamine still develop arthropathy. Whether early and long-term treatment will decrease the bone and joint disease is not yet known. Occasionally, penicillamine appears to cause polymyositis or lupus-like syndromes (see Chapter 33). Acute polyarthritis complicated penicillamine therapy in five patients with Wilson's disease (78). There is some controversy about the safety of penicillamine in pregnancy (85,86). Zinc (87), trientine, a newer chelating agent (86), or tetrathiomolybdate may be considered as alternative therapies in patients who cannot tolerate penicillamine. Liver transplants have been used successfully.

REFERENCES

1. LaDu BN, Zannoni VG, Laster L, et al. The nature of the defect in tyrosine metabolism in alcaptonuria. *J Biol Chem* 1958;230:251–260.
2. Pollak MR, Chou YH, Cerda JJ, et al. Homozygosity mapping of the gene for alkaptonuria to chromosome 3q2. *Nat Genet* 1993;5:201–204.
3. Knox WE. Sir Archibald Garrod's inborn errors of metabolism. II. Alkaptonuria. *Am J Hum Genet* 1958;10:95–124.
4. Gaucher A, Pourel J, Raffoux C, et al. HLA antigens and alkaptonuria. *J Rheumatol* 1977;3(suppl):97–100.
5. Lee S, Schoen I. Black copper reduction reaction simulating alkaptonuria—occurrence after intravenous urography. *N Engl J Med* 1966;275:266–267.
6. Kelley WN, Fox IH, Feldman JM, et al. Significant laboratory artifacts in alkaptonuria. *Arthritis Rheum* 1969;12:673.
7. Seegmiller JE, Zannoni VG, Laster L, et al. An enzymatic spectrophotometric method for the determination of homogentisic acid in plasma and urine. *J Biol Chem* 1961;236:774–777.
8. Zannoni VG, Malawista SE, LaDu BN. Studies on ochronosis. II. Studies on benzoquinoneacetic acid, a probable intermediate in the connective tissue pigmentation of alcaptonuria. *Arthritis Rheum* 1962;5:547–556.
9. Murray JC, Lindberg KA, Pinnell SR. In vitro inhibition of chick embryo lysyl hydroxylase by homogentisic acid. *J Clin Invest* 1977;59:1071–1079.
10. Angeles AP, Badger R, Gruber H, et al. Chondrocyte growth inhibition induced by homogentisic acid and its partial prevention with ascorbic acid. *J Rheumatol* 1989;16:512–517.
11. O'Brien WM, LaDu DN, Bunim JJ. Biochemistry pathologic and clinical aspects of alcaptonuria, ochronosis and ochronotic arthropathy. *Am J Med* 1963;34:813–838.
12. Levine HD, Paris AF, Holdworth DE, et al. Aortic valve replacement for ochronosis of the aortic valve. *Chest* 1978;74:466–467.
13. Bywaters EGL, Dorling J, Sutor J. Ochronosis densification. *Arthritis Rheum Dis* 1970;29:563(abst).
14. Deeb Z, Frayha R. Multiple vacuum disks, an early sign of ochronosis: radiologic findings in 2 biopsies. *J Rheumatol* 1976;3:82–87.
15. Hunter T, Gordon DA, Ogryzlo MA. The ground pepper sign of synovial fluid: a new diagnostic feature of ochronosis. *J Rheumatol* 1974;1:45–53.
16. Reginato AJ, Schumacher HR, Martinez VA. Ochronotic arthropathy with calcium pyrophosphate crystal deposition. *Arthritis Rheum* 1973;16:705–714.
17. Huttl S. Synovial effusion. A nosographic and diagnostic study. Part I. *Acta Rheum Baln Pistiniana* 1970;5:1–100.
18. Schumacher HR, Holdsworth DE. Ochronotic arthropathy. 1. Clinicopathologic studies. *Semin Arthritis Rheum* 1977;6:207–246.
19. McClure J, Smith PS, Gramp AA. Calcium pyrophosphate dihydrate (CPPD) deposition in ochronotic arthropathy. *J Clin Pathol* 1983;36:894–902.
20. Rynes RJ, Sosman JL, Holdsworth DE. Pseudogout in ochronosis: report of a case. *Arthritis Rheum* 1975;18:21–25.
21. Mohr W, Wessinghage D, Lendschaw E. Die Ultrastruktur von Hyalinem Knorpel und Gelenkkapsel-gewebe bei der alkaptonurischen Ochronose. *Z Rheumatol* 1980;39:55–73.
22. Gaines JJ, Tom GD, Khankhaniam N. An ultrastructural and light microscopic study of the synovium in ochronotic arthropathy. *Hum Pathol* 1987;18:1160–1164.
23. O'Brien WM, Banfield WG, Sokoloff L. Studies on the pathogenesis of ochronotic arthropathy. *Arthritis Rheum* 1961;4:137–152.
24. Lurie DP, Musil D. Knee arthropathy in ochronosis: diagnosis by arthroscopy with ultrastructural features. *J Rheumatol* 1984;11:101–103.
25. MacKenzie CR, Major P, Hunter T. Tendon involvement in a case of ochronosis. *J Rheumatol* 1982;9:634–636.
26. Blivaiss BB, Rosenberg EF, Katuzov H, et al. Experimental ochronosis: induction in rats by long-term feeding of L-tyrosine. *Arch Pathol* 1966;82:45–53.
27. Montagutelli X, Laloutette A, Coude M, et al. AKU, a mutation of the mouse homologous to human alkaptonuria, maps to chromosome 16. *Genomics* 1994;19:9–11.
28. Horshaw RA, Zimmerman KG, Menter A. Ochronosis-like pigmentation from hydroquinone bleaching creams in American blacks. *Arch Dermatol* 1985;121:105–108.
29. Rausing A, Rosen U. Black cartilage after therapy with levodopa and methyldopa. *Arch Pathol Lab Med* 1994;118:531–535.
30. Lustberg TJ, Schulman JD, Seegmiller JE. Decreased binding of 14C-homogentisic acid induced by ascorbic acid in connective tissue of rats with experimental alcaptonuria. *Nature* 1970;222:770–771.
31. Carrier DA, Harris CM. Bilateral hip and bilateral knee arthroplasties in a patient with ochronotic arthropathy. *Orthop Rev* 1990;19:1005–1009.

32. Finch SC, Finch CA. Idiopathic hemochromatosis: an iron storage disease. *Medicine* 1955;34:381–430.
33. Sheldon JH. *Haemochromatosis.* London: Oxford University Press, 1935.
34. Blandford RL, Dowdle JR, Stephens MR, et al. Sicca syndrome associated with idiopathic hemochromatosis. *Br Med J* 1979; 1(6174):1323.
35. Puéchal X. Genetic hemochromatosis: Why is discovery of the HLA-H gene of interest to rheumatologists. *Rev Rhum* (English Edition) 1997;64:527–529.
36. Goldschmidt H, Spiera H, Schumacher HR Jr, et al. Idiopathic hemochromatosis presenting as arthropathy and amenorrhea in a young woman. *Am J Med* 1987;82:1057–1059.
37. Baer DM, Simons JL, Staples RL, et al. Hemochromatosis screening in asymptomatic ambulatory men 30 years of age and older. *Am J Med* 1995;98:464–468.
38. Wands JR, Rowe JA, Mezey SE, et al. Normal serum ferritin concentrations in precirrhotic hemochromatosis. *N Engl J Med* 1976;294:302–305.
39. Murphy FB, Bernardino ME. MR imaging of focal hemochromatosis. *J Comput Assist Tomogr* 1986;10:1044–1046.
40. Rosner IA, Askari AD, McLaren GD, et al. Arthropathy, hypouricemia, and normal serum iron studies in hereditary hemochromatosis. *Am J Med* 1981;70:870–874.
41. Sinigaglia L, Fargian S, Fracanzani AL, et al. Bone and joint involvement in genetic hemochromatosis: role of cirrhosis and iron overload. *J Rheumatol* 1997;24:1809–1813.
42. Diamond T, Stiel D, Posen S. Osteoporosis in hemochromatosis; iron excess, gonadal deficiency or other factors. *Ann Intern Med* 1989;110:430–436.
43. deVernejoul MC, Pointillart A, Golenzer CC, et al. Effects of iron overload on bone remodelling on pigs. *Am J Pathol* 1984; 116:377–383.
44. Schumacher HR. Hemochromatosis and arthritis. *Arthritis Rheum* 1964;7:41–50.
45. Delbarre F. Les manifestations ostéo-articulaires de l'hémochromatose. *Presse Med* 1964;72:2973–2978.
46. Dymock IW, Hamilton EB, Laws JW, et al. Arthropathy of hemochromatosis. *Ann Rheum Dis* 1970;29:469–476.
47. Hamilton EB, Bomford AB, Laws JW, et al. The natural history of arthritis in idiopathic hemochromatosis: progression of the clinical and radiological features over 10 years. *Q J Med* 1981; 50:321–329.
48. Kra SJ, Hollingsworth JW, Finch SC. Arthritis with synovial iron deposition in a patient with hemochromatosis. *N Engl J Med* 1965;272:1268–1271.
49. Mitrovic D, Mazabraud A, Jaffres R, et al. Etude histologique et histoclinique des lésion articulaires de la chondrocalcinose survenant au cous d'une hémochromatose. *Arch Anat Pathol* 1966; 14:264–270.
50. Faraawi R, Harth M, Kertesz A, et al. Arthritis in hemochromatosis. *J Rheumatol* 1993;20:448–452.
51. Gordon DA, Clarke PV, Ogryzlo MA. The chondrocalcific arthropathy of iron overload. *Arch Intern Med* 1974;134:21–28.
52. Tanglao EC, Stern MA, Adudelo CA. Case report: arthropathy as the presenting symptom in hereditary hemochromatosis. *Am J Med Sci* 1996;312:306–309.
53. Adamson TC, Resnik CS, Guerra J Jr, et al. Hand and wrist arthropathies of hemochromatosis and calcium pyrophosphate deposition disease: distinct radiographic features. *Radiology* 1983;147:377–381.
54. Axford JS, Bomford A, Revell P, et al. Hip arthropathy in genetic hemochromatosis. Radiographic and histologic features. *Arthritis Rheum* 1991;34:357–361.
55. Schumacher HR. Ultrastructural characteristics of the synovial membrane in idiopathic hemochromatosis. *Ann Rheum Dis* 1972;31:465–473.
56. Schumacher HR. Articular cartilage in the degenerative arthropathy of hemochromatosis. *Arthritis Rheum* 1982;25:1460–1468.
57. Abbott DF, Gresham DF. Arthropathy in transfusional hemosiderosis. *Br Med J* 1972;1:418–419.
58. Sella EJ, Goodman AH. Arthropathy secondary to transfusion hemochromatosis. *J Bone Joint Surg* 1973;55A:1077–1081.
59. Mohler DN, Wheby MS. Case report: hemochromatosis heterozygotes may have significant iron overload when they also have hereditary spherocytosis. *Am J Med Sci* 1986;292: 320–324.
60. Brighton CT, Bigley EC, Smolenski BI. Iron induced arthritis in immature rabbits. *Arthritis Rheum* 1970;13:849–857.
61. Hisakawa N, Nishiva K, Tahara K, et al. Down regulation by iron of prostaglandin E2 production by human synovial fibroblasts. *Ann Rheum Dis* 1998;57:742–746.
62. DeSousa M, Breedvelt F, Dynesius-Trentham R, et al. Iron, iron binding proteins and immune system cells. *Ann NY Acad Sci* 1988;526:310–322.
63. McCarty DJ, Pepe PF. Erythrocyte neutral inorganic pyrophosphatase in pseudogout. *J Lab Clin Med* 1972;79:277–284.
64. McCarty DJ, Palmer DW, Garancis JC. Clearance of calcium pyrophosphate dihydrate crystals in vivo. III. Effects of synovial hemosiderosis. *Arthritis Rheum* 1981;24:706–710.
65. Pawlotsky Y. Hémochromatose génétique: arthropathres et fonction parathyroidienne. *Presse Med* 1993;22:1988–1990.
66. Cheng PT, Pritzker KP. Ferrous but not ferric ions inhibit de novo formation of calcium pyrophosphate dihydrate crystals: possible relationships to chondrocalcinosis and hemochromatosis. *J Rheumatol* 1988;15:321–324.
67. Wilson SAK. Progressive lenticular degeneration: a familial nervous disease associated with cirrhosis of the liver. *Brain* 1912; 34:295–509.
68. Maier-Dobersberger T, Ferenci P, Polli C, et al. Detection of the His 1069 Gln mutation in Wilson's disease by rapid polymerase chain reaction. *Ann Intern Med* 1997;127:21–26.
69. Yarze JC, Martin P, Munoz SJ, et al. Wilson's disease: current status. *Am J Med* 1992;92:643–654.
70. Dobyns WB, Goldstein NP, Gordon H. Clinical spectrum of Wilson's disease. *Mayo Clin Proc* 1979;54:35–42.
71. Perman JA, Werlin SL, Grand RJ, et al. Laboratory measurements of copper metabolism in the differentiation of chronic active hepatitis and Wilson disease in children. *J Pediatr* 1979; 94:564–568.
72. Weinberg LM, Brasitus TA, Leskowitch JH. Fluctuating Kayser-Fleischer-like rings in a jaundiced patient. *Arch Intern Med* 1981; 142:246–247.
73. Finby N, Bearn AG. Roentgenographic abnormalities of the skeletal system in Wilson's disease (hepatolenticular degeneration). *AJR* 1958;79:603–611.
74. Mindelzun R, Elkin M, Scheinberg IH, et al. Skeletal changes in Wilson's disease: a radiological study. *Radiology* 1970;94:127–132.
75. Cavallino R, Grossman H. Wilson's disease presenting with rickets. *Radiology* 1968;90:493–494.
76. Boudin G, Pépin B, Barbizet J, et al. Altérations ostéoarticulaires au cours de la dégénérescence hépatolenticulaire. *Bull Soc Méd Hôp Paris* 1957;73:756–761.
77. Feller E, Schumacher HR. Osteoarticular changes in Wilson's disease. *Arthritis Rheum* 1972;15:259–266.
78. Golding DN, Walshe JM. Arthropathy of Wilson's disease: study of clinical and radiological features in 32 patients. *Ann Rheum Dis* 1977;36:99–111.
79. Kaklamanis P, Spengos M. Osteoarticular change and synovial

biopsy findings in Wilson's disease. *Ann Rheum Dis* 1973;32: 422–427.
80. Kramer U, Weinberger A, Yarom R, et al. Synovial copper deposition as a possible explanation of arthropathy in Wilson's disease. *Bull Hosp Jt Dis* 1993;52:46–49.
81. Menerey K, Eider W, Brewer GJ, et al. The arthropathy of Wilson's disease. *J Rheumatol* 1988;15:331–337.
82. Zakraoui L, Amara N, Hamza M, et al. Les atteintes articulaires au cours de la maladie de Wilson. *Rev Rhum* 1986;53:345–348.
83. Pitt P, Mowat A, Williams R, et al. Hepatic hypertrophic osteoauthroathy and liver transplantation. *Ann Rheum Dis* 1994; 53:338–390.
84. Sternlieb I, Scheinberg IH. Prevention of Wilson's disease in asymptomatic patients. *N Engl J Med* 1968;278:352–359.
85. Endres W. Penicillamine in pregnancy—to ban or not to ban. *Klin Wochenschr* 1981;59:535–537.
86. Walshe JM. The management of pregnancy in Wilson's disease treated with trientine. *Q J Med* 1986;58:81–87.
87. Brewer GJ, Prasad AS, Cossack Z, et al. Treatment of Wilson's disease with oral zinc. *Clin Res* 1981;29:578A.

122

OSTEOPENIC BONE DISEASES

SARAH L. MORGAN
KENNETH G. SAAG
BRUCE A. JULIAN
HARRY BLAIR

This chapter discusses the pathogenesis, prevalence, diagnosis, and therapy of osteopenic bone diseases.

BONE BIOLOGY

This section describes the cellular processes that produce and degrade bone, key physical properties of the bone matrix, and changes in bone structure with major disease states.

Bone Cells and Bone Architecture

With the exception of necrosis or fracture, the bone surface is cellular. Exposed extracellular matrix, such as in articular cartilage, is subject to direct physical or chemical damage, while bone formation and destruction are controlled by cellular activity. The balance between bone synthesis by osteoblasts and bone degradation by osteoclasts determines bone mass. Focal or generalized skeletal problems including bone erosions in arthritis, osteomalacia in renal failure, and osteoporosis are mediated by abnormalities in cellular activity.

Bone adapts to stress, undergoes repair, and is periodically replaced. Its mineral content maintains serum calcium and pH. In keeping with this role in mineral homeostasis, the skeleton is broken down and re-formed at a rate vastly exceeding the replacement of other connective tissues. Reflecting this, the modified amino acid of collagen, hydroxyproline, is a urine marker for bone turnover, even though collagens are abundant elsewhere and dietary intake also affects hydroxyproline excretion. Because bone is involved in multiple activities that may oppose one another, the control of cellular activity in bone is complex.

Skeletal Modeling and Cartilage

Skeletal development depends on embryonic segmentation (formation of somites) that is reflected in the vertebral column. Genes in the master-regulatory transcription factor family Hox are important to this early embryologic bone formation including induction of limb buds. These master-regulatory genes affect the downstream responses of cartilage and bone cells (1). Primitive segmentation-related genes including sonic hedgehog and the proliferation-promoting protein fibroblast growth factor (FGF), along with the helix-loop helix transcription factor Twist, are involved in limb growth and condensation of the mesenchymal bone precursors. FGF function is controlled by expression of several FGF receptors. These segmentation, growth, and condensation genes begin functioning in advance of expression of genes including bone morphogenetic protein (BMP) genes (2) that are critical to later phases of skeletal differentiation, which control duplication of bones, formation of joint spaces, and participate in regulation of further cellular differentiation.

Hox genes encode for conserved DNA-binding proteins that regulate major blocks of genes in the early differentiation process. Sonic hedgehog (also called *shh*) is a secreted ligand that activates Gli nuclear-transcription factors, which mediate major aspects of mesenchymal patterning including segmentation and tissue separation. BMPs belong to the transforming growth factor-β (TGF-β) superfamily; further confusion is added by another acronym, *Gdf,* used for some of the BMPs. BMP genes are expressed in highly specific patterns that determine details of the skeletal structure; this is reflected in stripes of BMP expression such as that of Gdf 5 in developing joints in the arm and hand (3). In adults, skeletal modeling genes are relevant to tumor development and as causes of severe inherited diseases, which are, for the most part, beyond the scope of this chapter; however, many genes involved, including FGF, BMPs, parathyroid hormone–related peptide (PTHrp), and osteoblast/chondrocyte specific growth factors, are produced throughout life, and may be related to development of diseases, including arthritides, for which the etiology is unclear.

Most of the primitive skeleton is formed as hyaline cartilage; the major exceptions are flat bones of the skull and parts of the clavicles, which form as mesenchymal condensations without a cartilaginous stage (some bone formation in animals also skips the cartilage phase). Cartilage in most locations is replaced by bone during later development; key exceptions include joints, where cartilage is retained (or added, in the case of calvarial sutures). Cartilage-forming cells, chondrocytes, differentiate from primitive mesenchyme, but remain capable of cell division in processes such as continued growth of epiphyseal and articular cartilages. Chondrocytes exist as isolated cells within a nonmineralized, avascular matrix consisting of type II collagen, which provides strength, and hydrophilic glycoproteins (Table 122.1), which resist compressive forces, a combination that produces a strong, elastic tissue. Cartilage is not important in calcium homeostasis.

Cartilage is a model, or scaffold, on which bone forms in embryogenesis and at growth plates. In the adult skeleton, cartilage is retained mainly as the low-friction lining for joints and in specialized structures. The conversion of cartilage to bone is a multistage process. In the initial stages, the cartilage cells increase in size, secrete specialized proteins, and mineralize the surrounding matrix. This process requires 1,25-dihydroxyvitamin D. Cartilage mineralization is followed by degradation of the matrix by osteoclasts; after this, bone is deposited by osteoblasts (described in the next subsection). Only mineralized cartilage is degraded by osteoclasts. Retention of mineralized cartilage in bone is a hallmark of osteopetrosis, a group of diseases with deficient osteoclastic activity. Because cartilage is nonvascular, it is metabolically sluggish and heals slowly, although chondrocytes, including those in articular cartilages, are replaced. During fracture healing, a callus composed of fibrocartilage is formed. The fibrocartilage in callus has properties similar to hyaline cartilage, but contains larger amounts of collagen consisting of type I collagen in addition to the type II collagen that is characteristic of hyaline cartilage.

Conversion of cartilage to bone involves complex interactions between FGF and BMPs (which maintain cartilage proliferation and phenotype) with Indian hedgehog and PTHrp (4). Abnormalities of FGF receptors underlie many important growth disorders including craniosynostosis and several types of abnormalities of hand and foot development (5). Indian hedgehog (also called *ihh*) is a conserved drosophila segmentation gene that is downstream of the most primitive signals and that interacts with many other genes that regulate cartilage and bone cell proliferation, including PTHrp (6). PTHrp is an important extracellular signal that regulates both osteoblast and chondrocyte proliferation, formerly known as the humoral hypercalcemic factor of malignancy.

Several transcription factors are important in chondrocyte differentiation. The nuclear transcription factor Sox 9 is required for chondrocyte differentiation; its absence causes campomelic dysplasia (7). Campomelic dysplasia is a lethal disorder of skeletal development with severe dwarfism, indi-

TABLE 122.1. KEY CHARACTERISTICS OF SKELETAL CELLS

Chondrocyte
- *Products: Structural:* type II collagen, aggrecan, type XI collagen, and other glycoproteins
  - Regulatory: chondromodulins
- *Developmental factors:* Hoxa2, Sox9, Indian hedgehog; transforming growth factor-β (TGF-β) and related cytokines, the bone morphogenic proteins
- *Regulatory signals:* Systemic: 1,25 vitamin D (required for calcification)
  - Local: PTHrp, TGF-β, chondromodulins
- *Clinical markers:* Various glycoprotein markers are proposed, none are in general use

Osteoblast
- *Products:* Structural: type I collagen, osteocalcin (also called bone gla protein; it contains the posttranslationally modified amino acid τ-carboxyglutamate, which functions in calcium binding)
  - Regulatory: RANK-ligand (RANKL, TRANCE, ODF, OPGL), osteoprotegerin (OPG, OIF)
  - Mineralization: alkaline phosphatase; gap junctions (connexin 43)
- *Developmental factors:* Cbfa1 (osf2) and upstream cartilage-differentiation signals
- Regulatory signals: Systemic: PTH; 1,25 dihydroxyvitamin D
  - Local: numerous cytokines with uncertain physiologic roles
- *Clinical markers:* An alkaline phosphatase isoform (serum), osteocalcin (tissue and fluids)

Osteoclast
- *Products:* Enzymes: V-type H^+-ATPase; cathepsin K; tartrate-resistant acid phosphatase
  - Regulatory: Numerous cytokines, none specific
- *Developmental factors:* Colony-stimulating factor-1 (CSF-1) (fms-ligand) is required for precursor (monocyte) formation
  - Tumor necrosis factor superfamily receptors, particularly the RANK-ligand (OPGL) are key differentiation factors
  - OPG (osteoprotegerin) is a soluble decoy receptor that opposes RANK-ligand function
- *Regulatory signals:* Systemic: PTH; 1,25 dihydroxyvitamin D
  - Local: RANK-ligand; numerous other cytokines whose physiologic roles are not defined
- *Clinical markers:* Tartrate-resistant acid phosphatase (tissue), terminal collagen fragments containing cross-links (urine or serum), hydroxyproline (urine; less specific)

cating that chondrocyte differentiation is absolutely required for skeletal development. The transcription factor cbfa1, a key factor in bone development and the most specific single transcription factor for bone (described in the next subsection), is also required for completely normal cartilage differentiation, reflecting the close relationship of cartilage and bone cells (8). Its action is downstream of Hoxa2 and Sox 9 (1). Chondrocytes elaborate many of the same proteins made by osteoblasts, and during embryologic development many of the same factors are involved in regulation. The qualitative signals separating chondrocyte growth from that of osteoblasts depends in large part on TGF-β and related BMPs (9).

Development of Bone

Bone is produced by osteoblasts and degraded by osteoclasts, both of which are terminally differentiated cell types. Tumors that have features of osteoblasts or osteoclasts, osteosarcoma or giant tumor of bone, respectively, occur clinically. Normally, however, new generations of osteoblasts and osteoclasts form from precursor cells in response to the need to make or destroy bone. Osteoblasts divide during differentiation, but then form sheets connected by gap junctions that secrete type I collagen, bone mineral, and accessory proteins (Table 122.1). After osteoblasts bury themselves within matrix (and then are called osteocytes), they remain alive, connected to the bone surface by thin channels (canaliculi). Synthetic osteoblasts may undergo apoptosis when bone synthesis is downregulated; osteocytes are destroyed when this part of the matrix is recycled. Similarly, osteoclasts are formed to degrade a segment of the bone surface, and then undergo apoptosis (Fig. 122.1).

Mineralized bone is impervious, and the bone surface in living bone is cellular. Thus, humoral flow of water through bone, or of mineral into and out of bone, is of no importance. Occasionally, the theory of humoral deposition and degradation of bone, which was developed prior to the

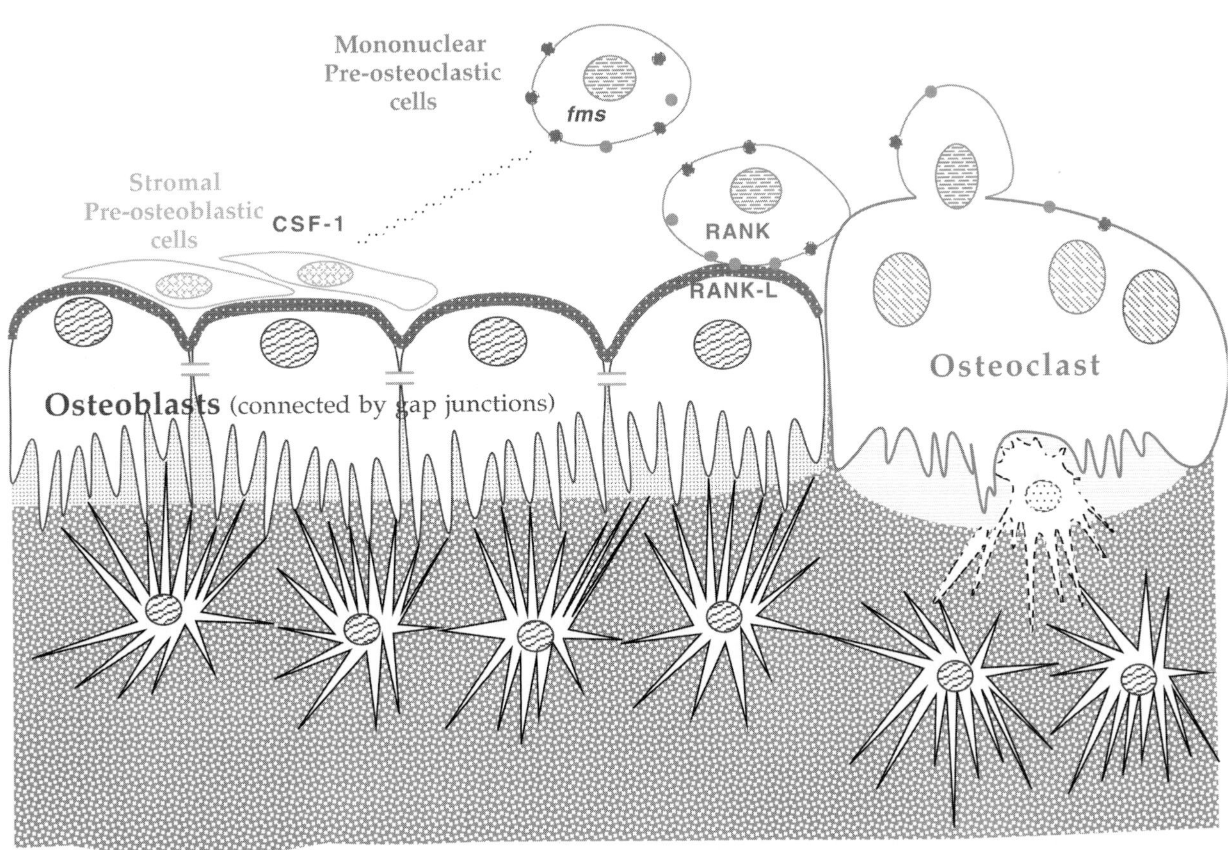

FIGURE 122.1. Osteoblasts differentiate from mesenchymal precursors, and produce factors including colony-stimulating factor 1 (CSF-1) (the ligand for *fms,* which supports macrophage development) and a cell-surface ligand that activates the receptor activator of nuclear factor κB (RANK), a powerful osteoclast-differentiation signal. Osteoblasts are connected by gap junctions during active bone synthesis, and act as a syncytium; there is also an inactive phase (normally about 80% of the bone surface is usually inactive). Osteoblasts secrete matrix that includes large amounts of type I collagen, and make osteocalcin and a characteristic alkaline phosphatase that are important for mineralization. Osteoblasts then secrete mineral and become buried in their matrix, connected to each other only by thin processes (canaliculi). Osteoclasts differentiate from monocytic precursors, with CSF-1 and RANK-ligand as predominant signals during normal turnover.

understanding of the cellular basis of bone, is still cited. However, it should be understood that the processes underlying bone pathology, including periarticular bone destruction and osteoporosis, are active and cell-mediated processes. By contrast, diffusion of toxins and enzymatic digestion are believed to be important in cartilage degradation.

Osteoblasts differentiate from pleuripotential stromal cells that also form fibroblasts, myocytes, and adipocytes (10). Osteoblastic differentiation is dependent on the master-regulatory transcription factors that are required for cartilage formation, but the particular differentiation of the osteoblast is largely controlled by the cbfa1 transcription factor (also called osf2, osteoblast-specific factor-2) (11). Defects in cbfa1 are one cause of osteopenia (12). Transcriptional control by PTH and vitamin D are also well-characterized and important elements guiding terminal osteoblastic differentiation and activity (13,14). In particular, it should be noted that PTH stimulates osteoblast proliferation and bone synthesis to a degree similar to the (largely indirect) PTH stimulation of bone degradation and calcium release. The difference between bone formation and bone degradation with PTH stimulus, and the consequent increase in serum calcium are reflected in the amount of nonmineralized bone (osteoid). This is the mineralization lag, which must be distinguished from osteomalacia due to bone mineralization defects such as those due to vitamin D deficiency. Secretory osteoblasts are connected by gap junctions, forming electrically connected groups of cells in which the secretory activity is coupled together (15,16). This allows synthesis of sheets of bone in a coordinated fashion. Pleuripotential osteoblast-forming cells occur throughout the body, but differentiation is limited to the skeleton except in inherited disorders such as fibrodysplasia ossificans progressiva in which BMP-4 or *fos* are ectopically expressed (17).

The osteoid produced by osteoblasts is mainly type I collagen. Collagens include long repeats of helical gly-pro-x triplets; nonhelical telopeptides in procollagen are removed from type I collagen during synthesis. "Telopeptide" refers to the amino acids at the end of a protein molecule, and here we are speaking of procollagen rather than collagen. The telopeptides of procollagen, cleaved off during collagen synthesis to form the mature collagen molecule, are entirely different from the telopeptide fragments of collagen, the terminal peptides of the mature molecule, which contain cross-links that are detected as markers of bone collagen degradation (vide infra). About half of the proline in collagen is posttranslationally modified to produce hydroxyproline by prolyl hydroxylase, an ascorbic acid–requiring enzyme. Because of this, hydroxyproline, which is largely excreted in the urine, is a marker of collagen catabolism; however, it is infrequently used because it has been superseded by immune assays of collagen degradation fragments. Individual collagen proteins are cross-linked at lysine or hydroxylysine residues by the lysyl oxidase system, creating insoluble fibers. Bone collagen is very highly cross-linked, and these collagen cross-links are poorly metabolized. These fragments circulate during collagen degradation, and these cross-links are good markers of bone resorption activity (Table 122.1). These fragments are frequently referred to as telopeptides without further specification.

Osteoblasts deposit hydroxyapatite-based mineral onto the osteoid via a process dependent on vitamin D and enzymes including an alkaline phosphatase. Mineral deposition is incompletely understood, although accessory proteins including osteocalcin appear to function in this process. Osteocalcin is a calcium-binding protein that contains γ-carboxy glutamic acid (18), and is therefore sensitive to coumadin. Bone mineralization defects with prolonged coumadin use have not emerged as a major clinical problem, however, and numerous reports suggest that heparin, which accumulates on bone, poses a much greater threat to bone density, although the mechanisms involved in heparin-induced osteoporosis are unclear.

Mineralization is a multistep process that includes a poorly characterized maturation process that normally results in a uniform, well-oriented, and dense mineralized matrix. Defects in the maturation process result in accumulation of immature woven bone, normally seen as the "primary spongiosa"; the initial bone forms on the cartilage model at the growth plate. Woven bone is easily distinguished in polarized light by a disordered pattern of collagen bundles relative to the regular pattern in normal mature bone. Woven bone is a prominent feature in high-turnover states such as hyperparathyroidism and Paget's disease.

Osteoclasts form by fusion of circulating monocyte-family precursors (19), and characteristically express massive amounts of a cell-surface vacuolar-like H^+–adenosine triphosphatase (ATPase) (20) that produces mineral-degrading acid. Osteoclasts secrete a tartrate-resistant acid phosphatase (TRAP) (21) and thiol proteinases including a recently discovered thiol proteinase required for efficient bone collagen degradation, cathepsin K (Table 122.1) (22,23). Deficiency of cathepsin K causes Toulouse-Lautrec disease (24). Osteoclast differentiation can be driven by various combinations of cytokines (25), although, under typical physiologic conditions, the ligand for receptor-activation of nuclear factor κB (RANK ligand, also called ODF or TRANCE, produced by lymphocytes and osteoblasts) and colony-stimulating factor 1 (CSF-1) (the *fms* ligand) are of particular significance (26). A natural soluble decoy receptor for RANK, OPG, also exists, the absence of which leads to severe osteoporosis in animal models (27).

Several other osteoclast- and osteoblast-produced signals and receptors, including interleukin-1β (IL-1β), IL-6, tumor necrosis factor-α (TNF-α), *hep*, epidermal growth factor (EGF), and *fms* affect osteoclastic formation or activity, are expressed in bone, and almost certainly affect some aspects of bone turnover, but the circumstances in which they are physiologically important are unclear. The RANK ligand and CSF-1 are sufficient for osteoclast formation *in vitro* and important *in vivo*, but they appear to function in a basal process of osteoclast formation that can be modified by numerous related signals, and TNF-α and IL-1β may be particularly important, replacing or augmenting RANK ligand under some circumstances. Similarly, tyrosine-kinase receptors other than *fms* may replace or augment CSF-1 signaling. Bone turnover is clearly driven by multiple forces, including hypocalcemia, fracture, acidosis, and skeletal flexion under load (21). Thus, it is likely that the cytokines that delimit bone turnover may vary somewhat due to local signals and special circumstances, while CSF-1 and RANK ligand are key factors important in mediating the overall balance of osteoblastic and osteoclastic activity in response to PTH and vitamin D.

Bone Turnover, Bone Mineral, and the Genesis of Osteoporosis

Bone mineral is a complex calcium salt with stoichiometry roughly approximating hydroxyapatite, 7(Ca^{2+}): 6(PO_4^{3-}): 2(OH^-) (21). Consequently, the deposition of mineral consumes many equivalents of calcium and inorganic bases; conversely, dissolving mineral absorbs acid and releases calcium. This is important to the cellular processes that make and degrade bone, in that the formation and dissolution of bone require remarkable ion transport processes. Hydroxyapatite forms in alkaline environments; the requirement of alkaline phosphatase for bone mineralization is one reflection of the active transport of the bone-producing osteoblasts. Conversely, osteoclasts are extremely active HCl-secreting cells, processing an acid load similar to that of the kidney.

The mineral content of bone also makes it a unique source of calcium and base equivalents for management of calcium and pH homeostasis. It has long been appreciated that bone mineral is exploited for the control of serum calcium, but it is also used to manage metabolic acid loads, a significant factor in the development of osteoporosis that is often overlooked (e.g., in renal disease). Experimental feeding of acid was noted to cause calciuria (28). Further, menopause is associated with increased circulating inorganic acids (such as sulfate, reflected in the anion gap), and experimental feeding of base reverses the calciuria associated with postmenopausal bone loss (29), although this has not been developed as a practical long-term treatment except in the case of renal tubular acidosis (30). It is likely that the decline with age in renal H^+-secretion capacity contributes to the development of osteoporosis with advanced age in both men and women, and any chronic metabolic acidosis will predispose the patient to bone loss. On the other hand, there is no consistent evidence that minor differences in dietary acid load, such as due to the amount of meat consumed, significantly reduce the bone mass of healthy people.

Hydroxyapatite is a good affinity substrate for many anions, including tetracyclines, which are fluorescent (31). Thus, the bone turnover process can be visualized by dosing a patient with tetracycline before and after a period of about 2 weeks, and by performing a bone biopsy 2 to 3 days after the second dose. Biopsies are typically performed on the iliac crest, and must be processed without decalcification to allow mineral to be evaluated. Tetracycline labels are observed in ultraviolet light (Fig. 122.2).

The properties of the bone mineral surface are relevant to the activity of bisphosphonates and group 13 (formerly group IIIa, the aluminum group) metals, which inhibit bone degradation. These compounds have considerable toxicity in cell culture, but in the living organism they are concentrated on the surface of the bone, directing their antimetabolic functions mainly to the cells that degrade bone, the osteoclasts (32). Many high-activity nitrogen-containing bisphosphonates, such as alendronate, inhibit posttranslational processing of guanosine triphosphate (GTP)-binding proteins that are important for normal cellular function (33). Although the bisphosphonates are also inorganic pyrophosphate (PPi) analogues and interfere with

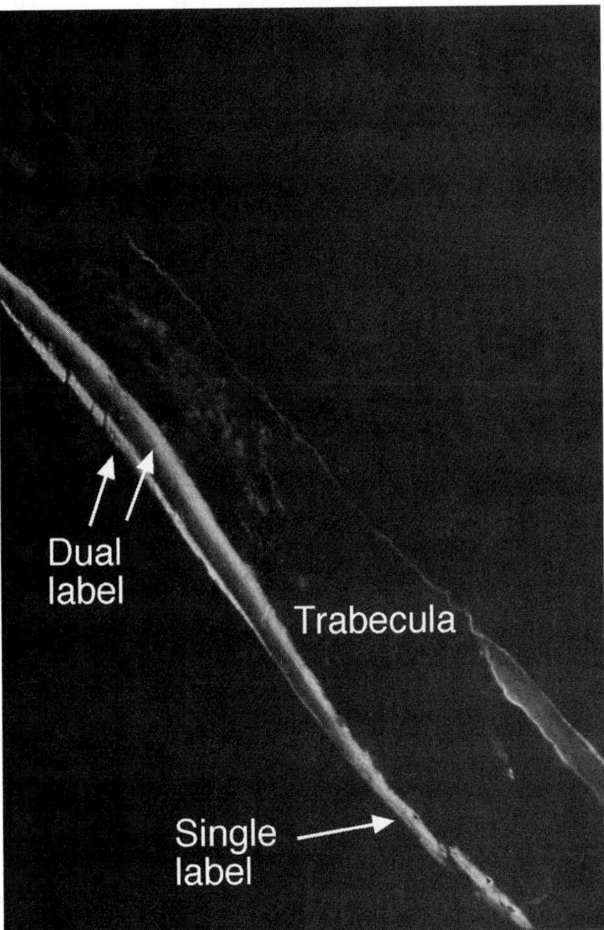

FIGURE 122.2. Dual tetracycline-labeled trabecular bone from an iliac crest biopsy of a 48-year-old woman. Approximately 10% of the trabecular surface has been formed in the 2-week period between labels. This suggests a turnover interval of the trabecular mass at this site of about 2 years. This rate is normal for a patient of this age and gender. (Magnification is ×400 diameters.)

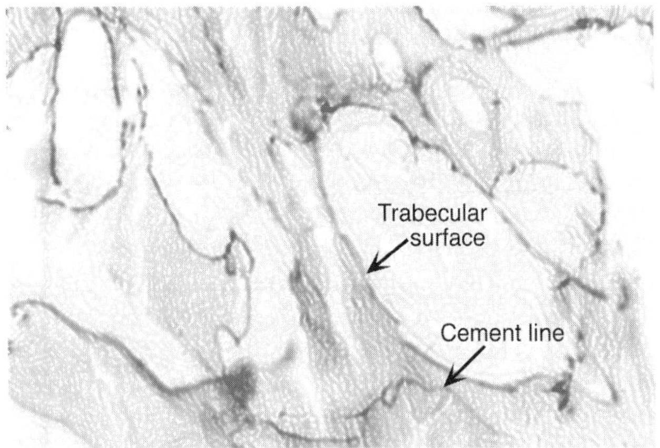

FIGURE 122.3 Aluminum deposition demonstrated with aurintricarbocylate, a red dye that chelates this metal. Undecalcified bone section from a dialysis patient. Note that the trabecular surfaces and cement lines *(arrows)* have adsorbed aluminum. (×400 diameters.)

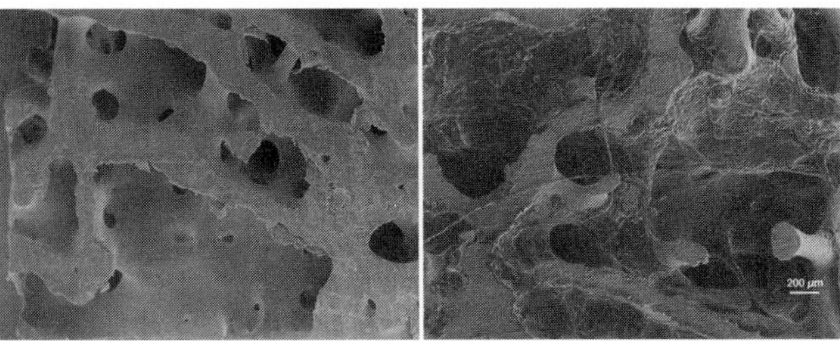

FIGURE 122.4. Scanning electron micrographs of subarticular bone showing that the trabeculae are thin plates of bone. **Left:** Normal bone. **Right:** In osteoporosis, the trabecular surface is particularly subject to erosion by osteoclasts, and the trabecular structure may be weakened to the point that collapse occurs.

a wide variety of other metabolic processes, the relative physiologic significance of this finding is unknown. The group 13 metals react with thiol groups and also interfere with metalloproteins. They also are metabolic inhibitors of broad specificity, and compounds such as Ga $(NO_3)_3$ affect many enzymes including the osteoclastic V-type H^+-ATPase (34). The physiologic mechanisms of their activity are not known with certainty, but Ga(III) compounds have found clinical use in hypercalcemia. Aluminum is a group 13 metal, but has relatively weak affinity for hydroxyapatite and therefore is not pharmacologically useful. However, in renal failure, where it cannot be excreted by renal filtration, aluminum may accumulate on the bone surface and cause osteomalacia (Fig. 122.3). Other substances that can accumulate on hydroxyapatite include heparins, which may be related to the adverse long-term effects of heparin administration on bone mass, although the detailed biochemical effects are not characterized in this case.

Relation of Regional Variations in Bone Architecture to Occurrence of Disorders

Much of the skeletal mass is composed of cortical bone, dense plates of solid bone at the surface that support loads along the axis of the bone. Cortical bone is remodeled at a fraction of the rate for trabecular bone. This tubular structure is strong and lightweight, and works well when the loading force is mainly along the axis; consequently, the shafts of the long bones are almost entirely cortex. In contrast, in subarticular sites and the vertebral bodies, which oppose loading forces that occur at a variety of angles, most of the bone mass is trabecular. This amounts to a series of thin plates of bone that are orthogonal to loads that occur at different angles depending on the joint position. In the subarticular sites, this trabecular bone comprises a series of interlocking arches that direct the load to the diaphyseal cortex. The trabecular bone has a very high ratio of surface to volume, and since only the surface of bone is active, the trabecular bone is mainly responsible for the metabolic functions of the skeleton and is remodeled rapidly (Fig. 122.2). This high remodeling rate, and the complex structure required to maintain strength, make the trabecular bone particularly sensitive to metabolic disorders and osteoporosis (Fig. 122.4). The highest ratio of trabecular to cortical bone in weight-bearing regions occurs in the spine and the junctions of long bones with complex joints, of which the femoral head is a particularly important example.

In the mature skeleton, only the joint surfaces retain a cartilaginous component. In accord with traditional nomenclature, the ends of the long bones are called the epiphyses; in joints, these are lined by the epiphyseal cartilages, which are tough, slick, and have a limited shock-absorbing ability. However, cartilage heals slowly and is sensitive to damage, with wear or inflammatory processes; if severely damaged, the epiphyseal cartilage will not recover. The regions with the most complex articular surfaces, such as the hands, are the most problematic regions in rheumatoid diseases. During skeletal growth, the epiphyses are separated from the swellings of the shafts, called the metaphyses, by cartilaginous growth plates. These plates are necessary for longitudinal growth, and injuries that cause premature fusion may result in deformities. The central shafts of the long bones are called the diaphyses.

The frequency of occurrence of many pathologic processes, including tumors, varies among regions of bone, reflecting in many cases the physiologic stresses that are active in specific regions. Bone cells respond to multiple signals that function to meet demands for growth/modeling, resistance to force, and systemic calcium homeostasis. The relative importance of these varies with location. For example, in order for growth of long bones to occur, the metaphysis is continually degraded as it is transformed from the broad epiphysis into the narrower shaft of the lengthening bone (Fig. 122.5), and, not surprisingly, this is the site where giant cell tumors of bone (constitutive osteoclast-promoting stromal cells) typically occur.

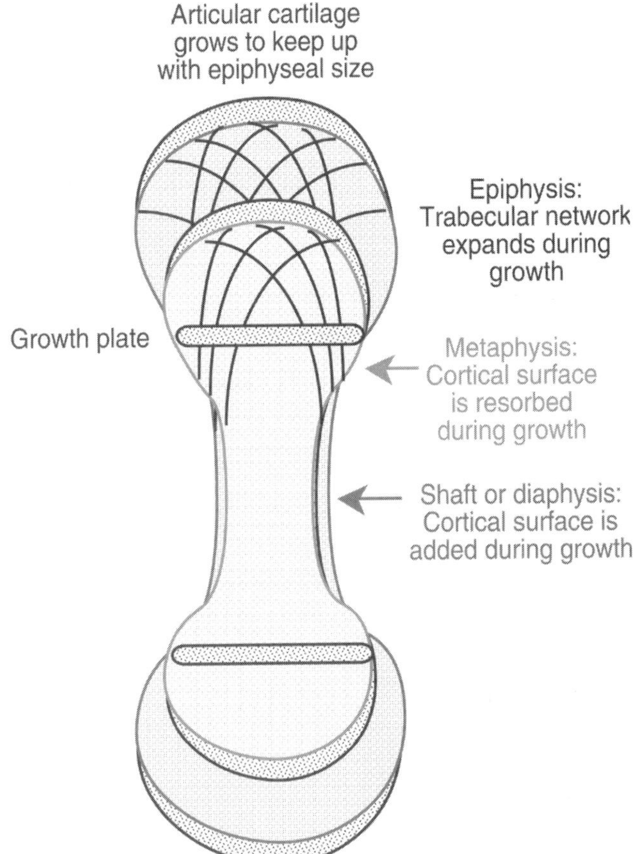
Articular cartilage grows to keep up with epiphyseal size
Epiphysis: Trabecular network expands during growth
Growth plate
Metaphysis: Cortical surface is resorbed during growth
Shaft or diaphysis: Cortical surface is added during growth

FIGURE 122.5. Regional variation in bone metabolism. In growing long bone, the surface of the metaphysis is degraded as the bone elongates and bone is added inside. Elsewhere, the cortex and epiphyses undergo appositional growth, and matrix is removed from the inner surfaces. The trabecular bone has a complex structure of interlocking arches, and it is also the main substrate used for systemic mineral homeostasis. Because of this, trabecular bone is remodeled frequently and is susceptible to failure in osteoporosis. Growth is modified by physical strain and systemic hormones, although the overall pattern is programmed. Defects in bone modeling and tumors occur at variable locations, reflecting the regional differences in the control of bone formation and resorption. Complex local control processes modify bone formation and degradation to produce these differences.

Relation of Systemic Factors to Cellular Activity and Bone Pathology

The major physiologic influences regulating the bone turnover rate are PTH and 1,25-dihydroxyvitamin D, the control of which are outside the focus of this chapter. However, there is no significant direct response of bone to calcium or phosphorus. Even the response to acidosis may, in large part, be mediated by PTH.

Osteoblasts contain abundant PTH receptors, and the response to PTH is 3′,5′-cyclic adenosine monophosphate (cAMP) dependent (13,35). Osteoblastic activity directly increases in parallel with osteoclast formation after PTH stimulation, and the osteoclastic effects are probably mediated mainly by osteoblast-produced cell-surface cytokines including RANK ligand (also called OPGL). A direct response of osteoclasts to PTH, not secondary to osteoblastic products, is not established and may not exist. Increased PTH is a factor in net bone loss in some circumstances, but this hormone is not specific for bone removal, but rather increases bone turnover with consequent mineral (calcium) mobilization. Because of the relation of PTH to bone turnover, PTH has been proposed to be useful in some cases of advanced osteoporosis despite its traditional description as a catabolic factor (36). The PTH response should not be oversimplified, however, and there are differential effects of the PTHrp and PTH (36) that are not fully characterized. PTHrp and PTH appear to have developed by gene duplication as they have similar N-terminal regions, both of which activate one type of PTH receptor (the type 1 receptor, the key PTH receptor involved in cartilage/bone development) (37), while a second type of receptor (the type 2 receptor) is PTH specific. The type 1 and type 2 receptors are homologous and are believed to have similar functional effects, although characterization is incomplete. PTHrp appears to be an important and conserved developmental protein, while PTH has both regulatory and developmental functions.

Because PTH increases bone formation and bone degradation in parallel, the net effect of mineral removal depends on a mineralization lag, in which PTH-stimulated osteoblasts do not mineralize newly formed bone, resulting in increased osteoid. In renal failure, the parathyroid glands often perceive a low effective calcium (calcium activity in formal chemical terms) because phosphate is retained, and phosphate complexes calcium. Thus, despite high total serum calcium concentrations, PTH directs further removal of mineral from the skeleton, resulting in a vicious cycle of degradation and rapid bone formation with poor mineralization. This process can be driven to the point that paratrabecular fibrous-like tissue forms, which has been termed "osteitis fibrosa" (Fig. 122.6A). This is not inflammatory or fibrous tissue; the process reverses entirely when the phosphate/PTH status is normalized, such as after renal transplantation. In addition, since the kidney performs the final hydroxylation to make calcitriol (the 1-hydroxylation), calcitriol is frequently deficient in chronic renal failure, leading to abnormalities in calcium absorption and mineralization, which, in the absence of adequate replacement, contribute to renal osteomalacia.

Both osteoblasts and osteoclasts respond to 1,25-dihydroxyvitamin D (38). Vitamin D is required for mineralization of cartilage and bone. While nutritional rickets in children is now rare because of improved diet and vitamin D supplementation, vitamin D deficiency can cause problems in the adult population. In addition to defects in vitamin D hydroxylation that accompany renal failure, vitamin D deficiency occurs in adults secondarily to drugs including some neuroleptics and antibiotics, and can be caused by vitamin D–consuming tumors (oncogenic osteomalacia). In older adults with poor nutrition, dietary deficiency is also a common problem. Insufficient vitamin D is reflected in accumulation of nonmineralized bone matrix (osteoid), or osteomalacia. If long-standing, osteomalacia reduces the bone turnover rate and may lead to microfrac-

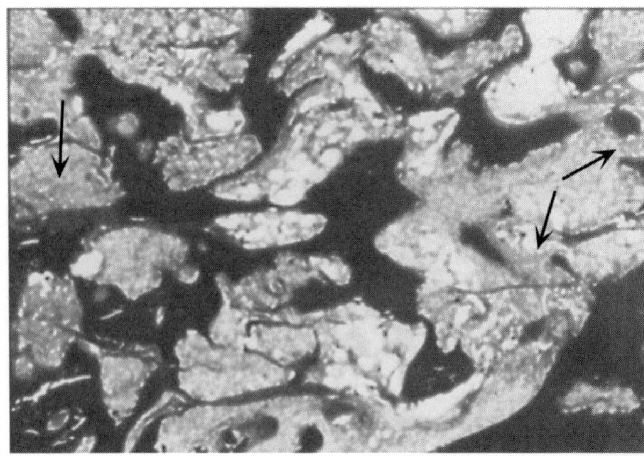
A

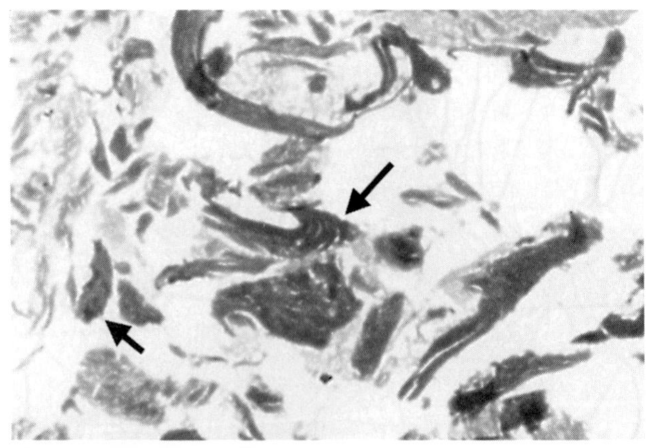
B

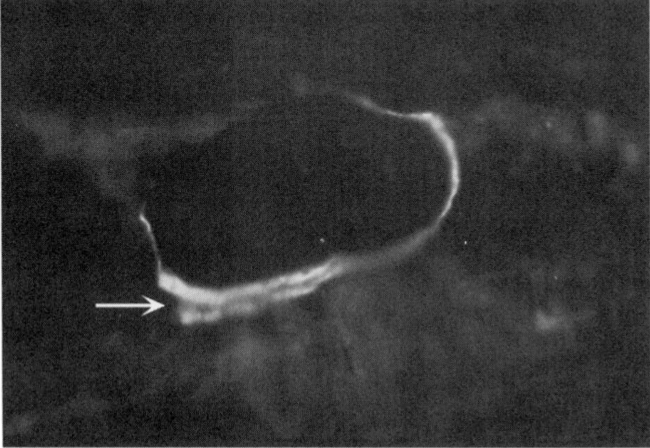
C

FIGURE 122.6. Histology of some major metabolic bone diseases. **A:** Hyperparathyroidism. High-turnover bone disease in a dialysis patient. There is greatly increased paratrabecular tissue (light red; *arrows*), and the trabeculae *(dark red)* are irregular due to increased osteoclastic activity. Marrow spaces *(yellow)* are decreased. The paratrabecular tissue in hyperparathyroidism is traditionally called osteitis fibrosa, but it is neither inflammatory nor fibrotic. It is stromal tissue that produces increased osteoblasts for the rapid bone turnover. This tissue disappears when the hyperparathyroidism resolves. (Von Kossa stain, ×125.) **B:** Osteomalacia due to vitamin D deficiency. Curettings from the fractured femoral head of a 40-year-old woman who received phenytoin for a seizure disorder, and suffered bilateral femoral head fractures. Phenytoin interferes with 25-hydroxylation of vitamin D. The severe osteomalacia as shown by Goldner-trichrome stain; osteoid is orange *(arrows)* and mineralized bone is blue-green (×250 diameters). **C:** Reduced activity of bone formation and degradation due to osteoporosis (low-turnover osteoporosis). Epifluorescence photograph of a dual-tetracycline labeled specimen as in Fig. 122.2. Note the thin and closely spaced double labels (×400 diameters).

tures, bone pain, and severe skeletal pathology including femoral fractures (Fig. 122.6B). Steroid hormones that have profound effects on bone metabolism include estrogens, androgens, and corticosteroids (39,40). Despite the importance of these steroids, the mechanisms of their effects on bone remain controversial. Osteoblasts and preosteoclastic cells contain receptors for both estrogens and corticosteroids, and these cells produce numerous steroid-responsive proteins. However, the detailed mechanisms responsible for the major physiologic effects of these hormones remain to be defined.

Weight bearing causes measurable flexion of the skeleton, and under normal circumstances has a positive effect on the function of the bone-forming cells, reflected in the dense bone observed in heavier patients and athletes. The mechanism of this effect is mainly attributed to the stretch response in osteoblasts (41). This gain is reversible, however, since the skeletal mass will turn over many times during life; an excellent example of this is the profound osteopenia that occurs with prolonged bed rest or in the lower extremities of paraplegics.

Following severe bone loss, the skeleton typically shows reduced bone formation and resorption, the so-called low-turnover osteoporosis (Fig. 122.6C). This may reflect in part an escape mechanism, where cellular activity is somehow inhibited by the weakened state of the skeleton, presumably mediated by excessive flexion under load, but the precise mechanism has not been defined. In some cases the condition will respond to exogenous PTH stimulation (36).

MEASUREMENT OF BONE MASS

This section discusses methodologies for the assessment of bone mass and fracture risk.

Analysis of the Skeleton

There are two basic types of bone in the human skeleton. Cortical bone makes up approximately 80% of the skeleton. It is dense and is the major component of long bones. The metabolic activity of cortical bone is fairly low. Trabecular or cancellous bone makes up 20% of the skeleton. Trabecular bone has an interlacing strut network structure and high metabolic activity (42). Table 122.2 shows the relative cortical and trabecular composition of the skeleton (43). The skeleton can be further classified by a variety of other methods: axial (spine) and appendicular (extremities), weight bearing and non–weight bearing, and central (spine and proximal femur) and peripheral (43). Therefore, assessment of bone mineral content in several sites provides varying information on differing types of bone (i.e., trabecular vs. cortical).

Conventional Radiography

Plain radiographs are an inaccurate method to assess bone mineral density (BMD). Bone loss must exceed 30% to 40% before it is visible by radiograph (44).

TABLE 122.2. THE RELATIVE PERCENTAGES OF CORTICAL AND TRABECULAR BONE AT VARIOUS SKELETAL SITES[A]

Region of Interest	Trabecular Bone (%)	Cortical Bone (%)
AP spine (DPA/DXA)	66	34
AP spine (QCT)	100	
Lateral spine (DXA)[b]	++++	
Femoral neck	25	75
Ward's area[b]	++++	
Trochanteric region	50	50
Os calcis	95	5
Midradius	1	99
Distal radius	20	80
8-mm radius	25	75
5-mm radius	40	60
Ultradistal radius	66	34
Phalanges	40	60
Total body	20	80

[a]The exact composition of some of these skeletal sites is controversial. These are considered clinically useful characterizations of the percentages of cortical and trabecular bone.
[b]This site is highly trabecular, but the exact composition is not defined in the literature.
AP, anteroposterior; DPA, dual-photon absorptiometry; DXA, dual-energy x-ray absorptiometry; QCT, quantitative computed tomography.
From Bonnick SL. *Bone densitometry in clinical practice.* Totawa, NJ: Humana, 1998:34, with permission.

The Singh index, which classifies five different trabecular patterns in the hip (45), has been reported to correlate with histologic grading of the iliac crest. However, other authors have concluded that the Singh index does not predict BMD of the proximal femur accurately (46–48) and has a low sensitivity but a relatively high specificity in the characterization of low BMD (46–48). Other radiographic measurements, such as hip axis length, can help predict hip fracture (49,50). Reduced thickness of the femoral shaft and neck cortex, a reduction in the index of tensile trabeculae, a wide trochanteric region, and a combination of these measurements predicted hip fracture as well as BMD of the femoral neck in one study (51). Vertebral fractures are identified by plain radiographs. Morphometrically, vertebral fractures can be classified as end-plate, anterior wedge, and crush fractures (Fig. 122.7).

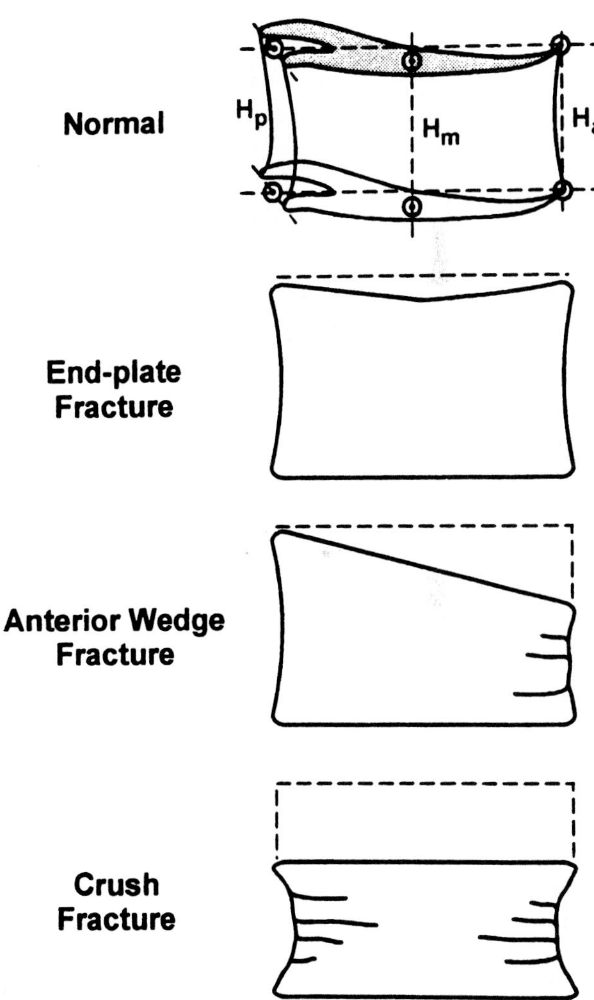

FIGURE 122.7. Vertebral morphometry measurements are typically based on placement of six points that define the anterior (H_a), middle (H_m), and posterior (H_p) heights of the vertebral body. Crush, wedge, and end-plate fractures are illustrated. (From Rosen CJ, ed. *Osteoporosis:* diagnostic and therapeutic principles. Totowa, NJ: Humana Press, 1996:86, with permission.)

Radiographic Absorptiometry

Radiographic absorptiometry assesses BMD by comparing the bone density on a plain hand radiograph with a standardized aluminum wedge that is calibrated in arbitrary units (52,53). The use of computed image processing has improved precision and reduced operator error (52,53). BMD of the phalanges measured by radiographic absorptiometry was significantly correlated with dual-energy x-ray absorptiometry of the radius, spine, and femoral neck as well as quantitative computed tomography (QCT) of the spine (54). Phalangeal bone density by radiographic absorptiometry has been shown to predict nonspine, vertebral, hip, and overall fracture risk (55,56).

Single-Photon Absorptiometry (SPA) and Single-Energy X-Ray Absorptiometry (SXA)

These methods use a highly collimated photon beam (^{125}I) or a radiograph source to measure attenuation at peripheral skeletal sites (57) and are most applicable to peripheral sites that contain cortical bone (44,58). The difference in absorption between the bone and soft tissues allows calculation of bone mineral content (58,59). Hip and spine bone mass by dual-energy x-ray absorptiometry (DXA) and BMD of the calcaneus, distal radius, and proximal radius by single photon absorptiometry were each inversely related to risk of fracture (60). No method was significantly better as a predictor of fracture.

Dual-Photon Absorptiometry (DPA)

Dual-photon absorptiometry is a modification of the single-energy technique that uses a radioisotope source, such as gadolinium 153, that emits photons at two energy levels. A constant soft tissue mass is not required, and central areas of the body such as the spine can be scanned (58,61).

Dual-Energy X-Ray Absorptiometry (DXA)

Overview

Dual-energy x-ray absorptiometry (DXA) has largely replaced DPA and SXA as the most widely used bone mass measurement technique in the United States (62,63). Although many modern measures of bone mass provide fracture risk prediction (64), DXA affords a fast, reliable, and accurate measurement of bone mass with very limited radiation exposure (Table 122.3). It is currently the gold standard for both patient care and osteoporosis clinical investigation (65).

TABLE 122.3. COMPARISON OF CURRENTLY USED TECHNIQUES FOR MEASURING BONE MINERAL DENSITY

	Precision in Vivo (%)	Accuracy Error (%)	Effective Dose Equivalent[a] (μSv)
Single-photon absorptiometry			
Distal third radius	1–2	4–6	<1
Os calcis	1–2	4–6	<1
Dual-photon absorptiometry			
Lumbar spine	2–4	5–10	5
Proximal femur	3–5	5–10	3
Total body	2–3	1–2	3
Dual x-ray absorptiometry (pencil beam)			
Lumbar spine			
PA	1	4–8	1
Lateral	2–3	5–10	3
Proximal femur	1–2	4–8	1
Total body	1	1–2	3
Quantitative computed tomography			
Single energy spine	2–4	5–15	50
Dual energy spine	4–6	3–6	100
Peripheral quantitative computed tomography (pQCT)	0.5–1	2–8	<1
Quantitative ultrasound			
Ultrasound transmission velocity (UTV)	0.2–5	2–4	0
Broadband ultrasound attenuation (BUA)	1.3–3.8	?	0

[a]Does not include dose due to localization radiographs such as spine films and computed radiographs. The effective dose equivalent, introduced in 1977 by the International Radiological Protection, permits estimates of the radiologic risk of partial-body radiation exposures, to be compared with whole body radiation exposure. For comparison, radiograph, depending on the technique, has an effective dose of 100 to 150 μSv.

From Lane NE, Jergas M, Genant HK. Osteoporosis and bone mineral assessment. In: Koopman WJ, ed., *Arthritis and Allied Conditions,* 13th ed. with permission.

DXA uses high and low x-ray energies to account for soft tissue attenuation. Compared to DPA, the examination is shorter and has both greater accuracy and precision. Both pencil-beam and fan-beam devices are currently in use with faster scan times on newer instruments (66). DXA is a two-dimensional measure of BMD. It does not measure true volume density but rather area density calculated as the quotient of bone mineral content and area. On DXA, bone mass is reported as an absolute value in g/cm^2, a comparison to age- and sex-matched reference range (the Z-score), and a comparison to mean bone mass of young adult normal individuals (the T-score or young adult Z-score) (Fig. 122.8). T-scores are used to both predict fracture risk and classify disease status (see above). A change of one standard deviation (SD) in either the T- or Z-score correlates to a change of approximately 0.06 g/cm^2 or about 10% of BMD. Although the Z-score is of less clinical value than the T-score, Z-scores significantly deviating from normal may be indicative of secondary causes of a metabolic bone disease other than osteoporosis. Modern DXAs also produce a density-based image useful in interpreting scan quality (Fig. 122.8) (see below).

Normative manufacturer-specific databases have historically been used to determine age- and sex-matched BMD parameters, but most major DXA manufacturers have recently switched to the National Health and Nutrition Examination Survey (NHANES) III database. In a large clinical referral population, this change from manufacturers' to NHANES III databases resulted in a 21% reduction in osteoporosis diagnosis at the femoral neck and 20% reduction using the total hip measurement (67). DXA results vary between and within manufacturers' different machines. An effort to standardize DXA values has been undertaken (68), and it is possible to convert values between manufacturers' machines (69). To maintain quality control, the DXA operator should use a standard phantom and the application of the multirule Shewart chart and cumulative sum chart (CUSUM) (43). DXA precision studies also should be done at least once for all scan types on each machine and if a new technician is hired or if there is a major change in equipment (70).

DXA can be used to measure bone mass at central and peripheral sites. Results are highly correlated (r >.9) with DPA measurements at these locations (71,72). The choice of site(s) scanned should depend on the anticipated rates of change in bone mass within these skeletal locations and the precision of the testing device at these various sites. The central DXA sites of the hip and spine, followed by peripheral sites of the wrist and heel, are the most desired imaging locations. Central DXA of the spine and hip has excellent precision and good accuracy (Table 122.3). Central DXA is generally preferred because the quantity of cancellous bone of central sites is highly indicative of the osteoporosis burden and fracture risk (73). In osteoporosis, the earliest bone loss begins in the cancellous bone. A higher proportion of early postmenopausal women have lower cancellous BMD than cortical BMD (74). Approximately 33% of the spongy trabecular bone of the hip and spine remodels each year as opposed to only 3% turnover of compact cortical bone found more often in the peripheral skeleton. At the spine, DXA reports BMD of individual vertebra as well as total BMD of L1-L4 (Fig. 122.8). The femoral neck, the trochanter, and the total hip are the three measurement sites of greatest clinical interest at the hip. Ward's triangle, the site of lowest BMD that is nearly exclusively trabecular bone, is an area with less predictive value and reproducibility than other locations. Total body BMD also can be obtained with newer machines and can be used to calculate total body bone mineral content. Central measurements are used to diagnose osteoporosis, assess fracture risk, and follow up the response to antiosteoporotic therapies.

The ability to detect significant serial changes in DXA depends on the rate of change in BMD at a particular site (Fig. 122.8). A 2.77% change is required between two successive DXA studies to achieve a statistically significant difference with 95% confidence. This change value is multiplied by the precision error (coefficient of variation) of the measuring device to determine the amount of BMD change that is needed to indicate a significant improvement or worsening in BMD at the 95% confidence level. For example, if the device has a 2% precision error, a change in BMD of about 5.6% is needed to be confident that this is not due to chance or precision error.

Peripheral DXA of the forearm correlates well with peripheral SXA, and thus can be expected to predict fracture risk with good precision (75). Heel DXA correlates well with other heel imaging technologies and adequately discriminates osteoporotic from normal young subjects (76). However, the much slower rate of bone remodeling at sites such as the heel limits this technology for monitoring response to therapies. The enhanced portability of dedicated peripheral DXA instruments and their lower cost renders them increasingly attractive for community osteoporosis screening.

Fracture Risk Prediction

BMD measured by DXA is the strongest known predictive factor for risk of hip and spinal fractures (77,78). Spinal fracture is inversely proportional to bone mineral content (79). For each decline of approximately 1 SD of bone mass, there is a 1.3- to 2.5-fold increase in fracture risk at any site (60,78,80–84). In the Study of Osteoporotic Fractures, the risk of hip fracture was inversely related to BMD in the calcaneus or proximal and distal radius measured by SPA (85).

The Kirklin Clinic

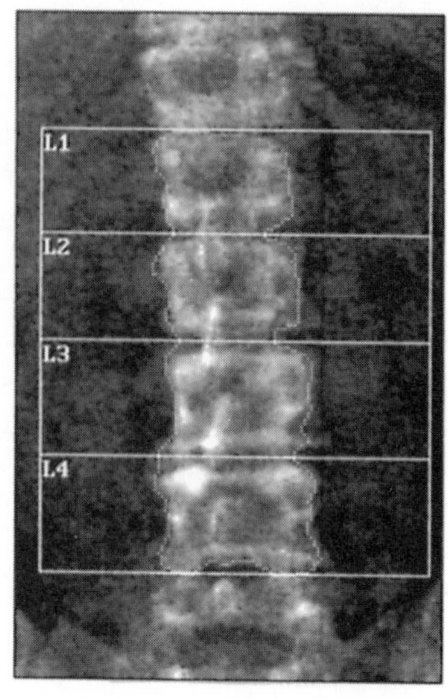

A

011109917 Wed Nov 10 15:28 1999
Name: PRINT OUT
Comment: osteoporosis
I.D.: Sex: F
S.S.#: 00 Ethnic: W
ZIP Code: 35209 Height: 5' 1"
Operator: BA Weight: 111
BirthDate: 12/06/28 Age: 70

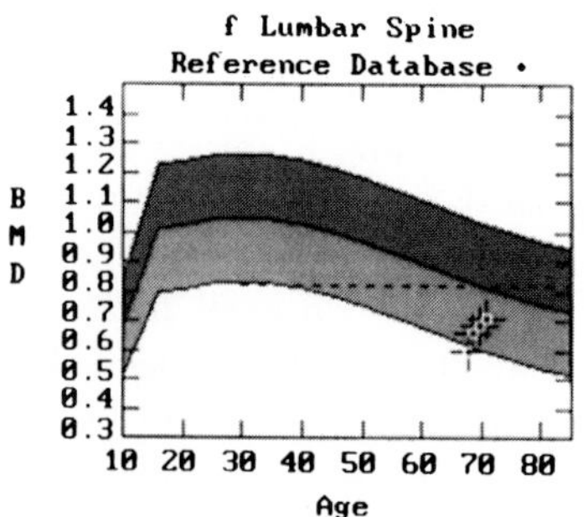

Region	Est.Area (cm^2)	Est.BMC (grams)	BMD (gms/cm^2)
L1	10.32	6.20	0.601
L2	11.46	8.00	0.698
L3	12.91	9.73	0.753
L4	14.39	10.67	0.741
TOTAL	49.08	34.59	0.705

BMD(L1-L4) = 0.705 g/cm^2

Region	BMD	T(30.0)		Z	
L1	0.601	-2.94	65%	-1.03	84%
L2	0.698	-3.00	68%	-0.87	88%
L3	0.753	-3.01	69%	-0.77	90%
L4	0.741	-3.41	66%	-1.10	86%
L1-L4	0.705	-3.11	67%	-0.95	87%

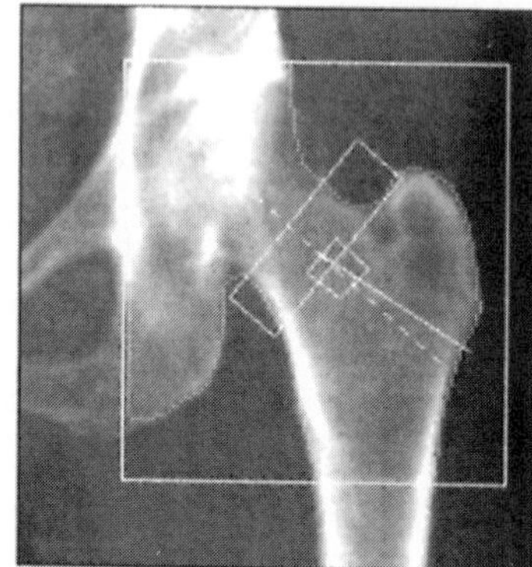

B

Region	Est.Area (cm^2)	Est.BMC (grams)	BMD (gms/cm^2)
Neck	4.88	2.66	0.546
Troch	9.71	4.73	0.487
Inter	14.55	9.55	0.657
TOTAL	29.14	16.95	0.582
Ward's	1.24	0.50	0.403

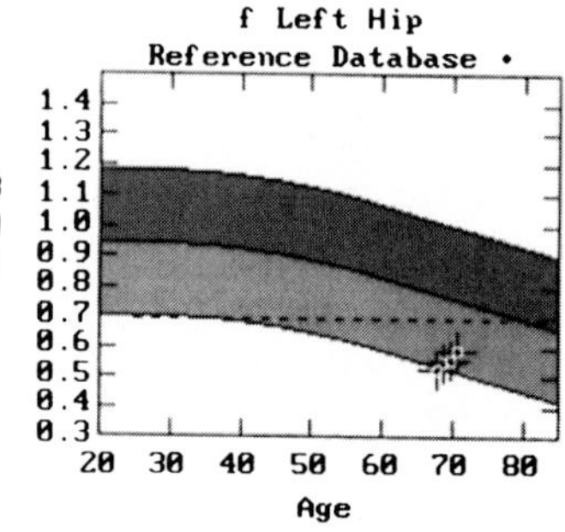

BMD(Total[L]) = 0.582 g/cm^2

Region	BMD	T		Z	
Neck	0.546	-2.73 (25.0)	64%	-0.88	85%
Troch	0.487	-2.13 (25.0)	69%	-0.77	86%
Inter	0.657	-2.86 (35.0)	60%	-1.55	73%
TOTAL	0.582	-2.95 (25.0)	62%	-1.40	77%
Ward's	0.403	-2.83 (25.0)	55%	-0.23	94%

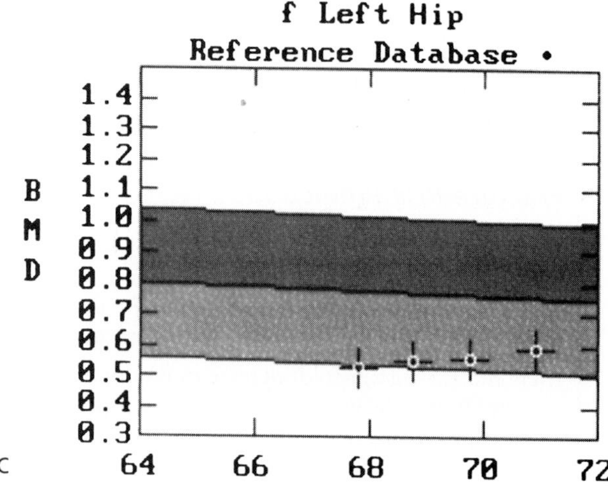

C

Total[L]

	09/25/96	09/17/97
09/17/97	4.1%	
09/23/98	5.3%*	1.2%
11/10/99	11.7%*	7.3%*

TABLE 122.4. INCREASE IN AGE-ADJUSTED RELATIVE RISK FOR SPINE OR HIP FRACTURE PER SD DECREASE IN BONE MASS, MEASURED AT VARIOUS SKELETAL SITES

Site	Spine Fracture RR	Hip Fracture RR
AP lumbar spine	2.2[b]	1.6[b]
Total femur		2.7[b]
Femoral neck	2.0[b]	2.6[b], 2.8[b]
Ward's		2.8[b]
Trochanter	1.7[b]	2.7[b], 2.4[b]
Distal radius		1.6[b], 3.1[b]
Midradius	2.5[a]	1.5[b], 1.9[a]
Calcaneus		2.0[b]
Phalanges	3.4[c]	1.8[c]
Metacarpals	1.9[c]	

SD, Standard deviation.
[a]Per SD decrease in bone mineral content.
[b]Per SD decrease in bone mineral density.
[c]Per SD decrease in radiographic absorptiometry units.
RR, relative risk; SD, standard deviation.
From Bonnick SL. *Bone densitometry in clinical practice.* Totawa, NJ: Humana, 1998:117, with permission.

Women with femoral neck BMD in the lowest quartile had an 8.5-fold greater risk of hip fracture than individuals in the highest quartile (78). Each SD decrement in femoral neck BMD raised the age-adjusted risk of fractures 2.6-fold [95% confidence interval (CI) = 1.9–3.6] (78). Although fracture risk at any site can be accurately assessed using a variety of noninvasive bone mass measurements (Table 122.4), BMD at the femoral neck is a better predictor of hip fracture than BMD at the spine, radius, and calcaneus (78). Decreases of 2 SD in radial and calcaneal bone mass are associated with four- to sixfold increases in risk for vertebral fracture (81). Increasing age and decreasing BMD of the radius predict subsequent nonspinal fractures (82). It is estimated that a 50-year-old woman has a 19% lifetime risk of fracture if radial bone mass is in the 10th percentile and an 11% lifetime risk if bone mass is in the 90th percentile (86).

Population-based studies show that hip fractures are uncommon among women with femoral neck BMD greater than 1.0 g/cm^2 (87). Libanati and co-workers (88) found that a 30% loss of BMD from peak BMD at the hip was necessary before hip fractures occurred after moderate trauma.

Potential Pitfalls in DXA Measurement

Osteoporosis occurs inhomogeneously throughout the body, dependent on age and underlying cause of bone loss. A 15% or greater discordance between sites, particularly in the elderly, means that imaging only one site, particularly using a peripheral device, may be misleading (62,89,90). Measurement at multiple sites increases the chances of successfully detecting osteoporosis (91,92). Due to the high prevalence of facet and posterior element spinal osteoarthritis among adults over 65, measurement of spinal DXA in the posterior-anterior projection may be falsely elevated (92–95). In older adults, measurement of the hip or lateral DXA imaging of the spine may circumvent this problem and has a better correlation with QCT measurements of the spine (92,96–99). Lateral imaging may also be of greater sensitivity in glucocorticoid-induced osteoporosis (100). Precision of a lateral scan may be slightly inferior due to greater thickness and nonuniformity of soft tissues in this projection (101–103). Precision of lateral DXA also varies depending on whether the scan is done with the patient in the decubitus or the supine position (96). Newer machines with a rotatable C-arm allow easier supine positioning with better imaging precision.

The visual image of the regions of interest allows the DXA reader to screen for artifacts (i.e., calcium pills in the gut, metal objects on clothing, objects in pockets, etc.), positioning errors (wrong vertebra imaged, hip malrotated, etc.), and anatomic deformities or changes [severe scoliosis, calcified aorta (104), vertebral crush fractures, etc.] that may limit scan precision and accuracy.

FIGURE 122.8. Dual x-ray absorptiometry (DXA) printout for a 70-year-old Caucasian woman. **A:** DXA of this patient's lumbar spine showing imaging windows for vertebrae L1–L4. Estimated vertebral areas, bone mineral content (BMC), and bone mineral density (BMD) are shown *(middle)*. BMD is plotted against a lumbar spine reference database showing the patient's current value as well as previous readings indicated by *crosses (right, top)*. The *dark (top) bar* of the graph indicates 2 standard deviations above normal and the *lighter (bottom) bar* 2 standard deviations below normal for age. The *dashed line* corresponds to 2 standard deviations below peak bone mass. T-scores (peak bone mass matched) show that the patient is well below the World Health Organization definition of osteoporosis (T-score <–2.5) at each vertebral level and for the lumbar spine overall. The Z-score is an age-matched measurement. **B:** Similar parameters are shown for the left hip and, based on T-scores, there is osteoporosis at both the femoral neck and total hip. **C:** At both the hip and lumbar spine, there has been significant 3-year improvement in BMD. The serial plot *(left)* and table shows a nearly 12% increases at the left hip. The asterisk (*) signifies a significant increase or decline between two values. An 18.4% increase in BMD was also seen at the lumbar spine (data not shown).

Quantitative Computed Tomography (QCT)

Similar to DXA, QCT provides an accurate assessment of fracture risk and measurement of bone loss (98,105,106). In contrast to DXA, QCT gives a true three-dimensional view of BMD and accurately discriminates trabecular bone from cortical bone with good precision (Table 122.3). Using standard computed tomography (CT) imaging equipment, QCT is most often performed at the spine. Marrow fat increases with age and glucocorticoid use. Thus, QCT may overestimate the extent of bone loss in these two clinical settings by up to 5% (106–108). External bone mineral reference phantoms (commonly K_2HPO_4 solution) are used to calibrate the CT measurements to bone-equivalent values (typically expressed in milligrams of hydroxyapatite per cubic centimeter) (63). QCT software automatically places regions of interest inside the vertebral body (109). In addition to the slightly higher radiation exposure (although significantly less than a routine CT examination) (Table 122.3), reliance on an imaging device that is heavily used for other clinical applications and the higher cost of QCT have limited the widespread adoption of this modality. Advances in QCT include the use of volumetric CT to produce three-dimensional images and the advent of high-resolution CT to define bone morphometry (63). In addition to central QCT devices, peripheral QCT of the wrist (ultradistal radius) and heel are sometimes used (110,111).

Ultrasound

Quantitative ultrasound was approved in the United States in 1998 as a complementary technique to measure bone mass. Compared to DXA or QCT, this method has desirable attributes of lower cost, less complicated instrumentation, portability, and absence of ionizing radiation. Proponents of quantitative ultrasound claim that, in addition to bone density, it provides information about structure and mechanical properties of bone, but this point remains somewhat controversial.

Although early experiments to determine material properties of bone were completed more than 30 years ago, ultrasound has only recently been applied to detection of osteoporosis. Better hardware and software have significantly improved precision of measurements and ease of use. A variety of terms have been used to describe ultrasonic properties of bone, but without uniform convention. Measurements include velocity of sound and attenuation. Some instruments use an empirical algorithm to combine these two parameters in a single term, *stiffness* or *quantitative ultrasound index,* but they do not reflect a biochemical property of bone. Ultrasound studies are usually performed of the calcaneus because it has two nearly plane-parallel sides, is surrounded only by a thin layer of soft tissue, consists mainly of trabecular bone, and is an easily accessible, weight-bearing bone. Tibia, patella, distal radius, and proximal phalanges are examined less often.

Velocity of sound is a function of the time required for a sound wave to travel from one transducer to another. In the clinical setting, measurement at the heel includes transit times through several materials—calcaneal bone, fat, and soft tissue—the latter two of which may have clinically important effects, depending on their relative size. Velocity of sound through bone assesses travel from one bone surface to the other, and is calculated as the quotient of the transit time of an ultrasound wave through bone and the diameter of the bone. This measurement is a function of mass density and elastic modulus, which may be influenced by bone mass, distribution of trabecular and cortical bone, trabecular orientation, and composition of organic and inorganic components. Accordingly, bone mass and quantitative characteristics of bone may alter this measurement. Several studies have demonstrated that this velocity depends on how the ultrasound beam is oriented to the principal direction of the trabeculae (112). Normal bone will have a higher value than osteoporotic bone. Three different calculations for the speed of sound (SOS) have been reported, dependent on the manufacturer: heel velocity (calcaneus plus soft tissue, as with contact instruments that use pads or gel pressed against the skin), bone velocity (calcaneus only), and time of flight velocity (transit time between transducers at fixed separation, as in water-bath instruments; this measurement assumes a constant heel thickness). These three calculations yield slightly different values that correlate strongly with each other (113). Velocities range from 1,400 to 2,300 m/sec for trabecular bone to 3,000 to 3,600 m/sec for cortical bone.

Attenuation of ultrasound waves is less well understood than velocity and is strongly affected by reflection and absorption of the energy, as well as frequency of the wave. Trabecular separation, connectivity, orientation, compressive strength, and hardness influence ultrasonic attenuation in bone. In contrast, BMD is not affected by spatial relationships of the trabeculae. Factors contributing to attenuation include beam spreading (diffraction), scattering, absorption, and mode conversion; scattering is the predominant mechanism in trabecular bone, whereas absorption is more important in cortical bone. Normal bone has higher attenuation than osteoporotic bone.

When a low-frequency range is used, about 100 to 1,000 kHz, total attenuation (expressed on a logarithmic scale) is linearly proportional to frequency (reviewed in ref. 114). With higher frequencies, the attenuation is greater and nonlinear. In quantitative ultrasound techniques, attenuation of ultrasound is measured using the low-frequency range and is termed *broadband ultrasound attenuation* (BUA). The slope of the resultant regression line is the BUA value and is reported in units of dB/MHz (decibels/megahertz). Unfortunately, frequency ranges used in this measurement differ between manufacturers, rendering comparisons between instruments difficult.

There are no universally accepted criteria for an ultrasonic diagnosis of osteoporosis. Because ultrasound and x-ray fundamentally differ regarding the bone properties each technique measures, it may be inappropriate to use DXA criteria for diagnosis by ultrasound. Most ultrasound instruments express the BUA and SOS values as SD unit differences from the mean values for healthy young adults (T-scores). The risk of fracture roughly doubles for a 1 SD reduction in BUA or SOS.

There is controversy over whether ultrasound is simply a surrogate for bone densitometry or whether ultrasound provides different, potentially clinically more important, information. In a study of 64 Caucasian women, BUA and SOS correlated with heel BMD, measured by DXA (r = .73 and .68, respectively) (115). In recent studies, site-specific measurements of BUA and BMD correlated with r values of about .8. Even so, it is not possible to predict BMD by ultrasound measurements. This discrepancy may reflect imprecision or arise because the two techniques measure different properties of bone. Correlations between BUA and BMD differ related to the relative composition of the bone (cortical versus trabecular) and direction of the sound wave. Compared to bone densitometry, ultrasound may provide additional information about bone quality (116). Concerns have arisen about the precision of ultrasound measurements. The precision of *in vivo* SOS measurements is about 0.19% to 0.30% and for BUA is about 1.0% to 3.8%. Although these ranges are two- to threefold larger than precision errors for measurement of BMD by DXA, they are significantly smaller than differences between osteoporotic individuals and healthy controls. Very fast digital signal processors calculate averaged amplitude, BUA, and SOS. This imaging allows the operator to define a region of interest and has improved precision. The posterior part of the calcaneus has an area with minimal attenuation; this localization method is better than using fixed coordinates (117). The technique ensures that, in different patients and in repeated measurements of a patient, the same area of bone is assessed, independently of the overall heel size. The ultrasound values vary by about 7.5% between the right and left heel, so it is important to measure the same site in longitudinal studies. In addition, some instruments have shown significant drift, so that recalibration with a phantom is necessary. Addressing these issues has increased the suitability of ultrasound technology for screening populations at risk for osteoporosis and improved the feasibility of follow-up studies.

The ultrasonic properties of bone change with age. The fall in BUA of the calcaneus after menopause parallels the decrement in vertebral BMD. Population values for BUA and SOS in Caucasian, Greek, and Spanish women are similar at a given age (118), whereas African Americans have slightly higher values for both (119).

Ultrasound can identify older postmenopausal women with osteoporosis in cross-sectional retrospective studies. BUA values were significantly decreased in older women with osteoporosis, or those with vertebral, hip, or Colles' (wrist) fractures (65) compared to unaffected subjects. In several studies, discrimination by ultrasound was as strong as by DXA BMD (reviewed in ref. 116). Even after adjusting for BMD, ultrasound measurements differentiated patients with hip fractures from healthy controls (120). In elderly women, ultrasound of the calcaneus was as good as or better than BMD of the hip as a predictor of hip fracture (121). In general, ultrasonic measurements of the calcaneus are better for identifying patients with fracture of the hip than patients with fracture of the spine.

Quantitative ultrasound can prospectively predict vertebral fracture, hip fracture, and stress fracture in the lower extremities (reviewed in ref. 65). In one study, new vertebral fractures in 130 postmenopausal women were assessed over a 2-year interval (122). Women with transmission velocity measurements of the patella more than 1 SD below the mean for the group had a 3.3- to 4.6-fold greater likelihood of sustaining a vertebral fracture. In a study of 6,183 women followed prospectively for 1.4 years, low calcaneal BUA and low femoral neck BMD values were associated with an increased risk of subsequent hip and nonvertebral fracture (123). In a study of 7,598 women older than 75 years, SOS and BUA of the calcaneus were as good as dual-photon x-ray absorptiometry femoral-neck BMD for predicting hip fractures (124).

Results for younger women are less consistent. Some investigators found ultrasound insufficient to identify early postmenopausal women with low BMD in the hip and spine, as measured by DXA (reviewed in ref. 125). In contrast, calcaneal SOS and BUA predicted stress fracture during United States Army basic training in young white women, but not in young African American women (126).

Few studies have assessed change in ultrasound measurements of bone during long-term therapy. Because of lower precision of the measurement relative to DXA, such studies will require longer intervals of observation. In addition to concerns about slightly inferior precision, the very slow rate of bone mass change at the calcaneus requires that a much greater interval elapse between ultrasound measurements in order to observe a significant difference. Nonetheless, treatment with calcitonin (127) or intermittent slow-release sodium fluoride with continuous calcium citrate (128) showed positive changes in ultrasound parameters that agreed with improved BMD. Further studies are needed before ultrasound can be generally used to assess skeletal responses to therapy.

Indications for Bone Mass Measurement

The National Osteoporosis Foundation (NOF) and the Osteoporosis Society of Canada have issued guidelines for bone mass testing of postmenopausal Caucasian women (129). According to the NOF, bone mass testing is suggested only when the results would influence a treatment decision. Such testing is indicated in all postmenopausal women under age 65 with one or more additional risk factors for osteoporosis besides menopause and in all older women regardless of additional risk factors (129). In addition, measurement of the bone mass of the hip and spine should be considered in postmenopausal women who present with fractures, in women considering therapy for osteoporosis if the testing would facilitate a decision, and in women who have had prolonged therapy with hormone replacement therapy (129). Lastly, it should be noted that women are more likely to initiate estrogen and other osteoporosis therapy if they know their bone mass is below normal (130).

Payment Indications for Bone Mass Measurement in the United States

The Balanced Budget Act of 1997 established bone mass measurement as a screening benefit effective July 1, 1998 (131,132). Individuals falling into one of five categories are covered:

An estrogen-deficient woman at clinical risk of osteoporosis, as determined by a physician or a qualified nonphysician practitioner, based on her medical history and other findings.

A person with vertebral abnormalities, as demonstrated by radiograph, indicative of osteoporosis, osteopenia, or vertebral fracture.

A person receiving, or expecting to receive, long-term glucocorticoid therapy (equivalent to >7.5 mg of prednisone per day for 3 months).

A person with primary hyperparathyroidism.

A person being monitored to assess the response to, or efficacy of, a Food and Drug Administration (FDA)-approved osteoporosis drug therapy.

The technologies covered include all central and peripheral radiologic procedures, and ultrasound. In general, follow-up bone mass measurements are limited to one every 2 years. However, they may be covered more frequently than every 2 years when medically necessary. Examples include monitoring individuals on glucocorticoids for more than 3 months and a confirmatory baseline measurement if the initial test was done with a method different from what will be used to follow the therapeutic response.

OSTEOPOROSIS

Definition

"Osteoporosis is a systemic skeletal disease characterized by low bone mass and microarchitectural deterioration of bone tissue with a consequent increase in bone fragility and susceptibility to fracture" (133).

The World Health Organization (WHO) defines osteoporosis as BMD more than 2.5 SD below the peak BMD of gender- and ethnicity-matched 30-year-old healthy Caucasian women (T-score) (134,135). Severe osteoporosis is a BMD more than 2.5 SD below the mean value of peak bone mass and the presence of fractures. Osteopenia is defined as a BMD between −1 and −2.5 SD below the mean value of peak bone mass in young Caucasian normal women. Normal bone density is defined as a BMD between +1 and −1 SD from the mean value of peak bone mass. The WHO criteria are based on epidemiologic data that relate fracture incidence to BMD in Caucasian women. There is controversy regarding proper cutoff values in other ethnic and gender groups (136,172). These are densitometric criteria only and do not provide a differential diagnosis of the causes of bone loss. Because BMD is a continuous measure of fracture risk, the chosen cutoffs are arbitrary; however, other diseases such as hypertension and hypercholesterolemia also use arbitrary cutoffs for diagnosis and therapeutic decisions (74,134,137). Other definitions of osteoporosis restrict the diagnosis to individuals with nonviolent fractures (134). However, from the standpoint of prevention, this latter definition may be too restrictive.

Patterns, Prevalence, Incidence, and Impact of Osteoporosis and Fractures

Prevalence of Low BMD/Fractures

By definition, from the WHO criteria, approximately 15% of non-Hispanic white American young adults have osteopenia and about 0.6% have osteoporosis (138). By age 60 to 70 years, one of three non-Hispanic white women will have osteoporosis and the remainder osteopenia; by age 80 years, 70% will have osteoporosis (138). Based on examination of femoral bone density in NHANES III (1988–1994), an estimated 13% to 18% of non-Hispanic white American women (4 to 6 million) have osteoporosis and 37% to 50% (13 to 17 million) have osteopenia (136). Using the T-score cutoffs applied to women, it is estimated that 1% to 4% of American non-Hispanic white men (280,000 to 1 million) have osteoporosis and 15% to 33% (4 to 9 million) have osteopenia (136). Figure 122.9 shows the prevalence of osteoporosis and osteopenia at the femoral-neck in non-Hispanic white, non-Hispanic black, and Mexican-American men and women.

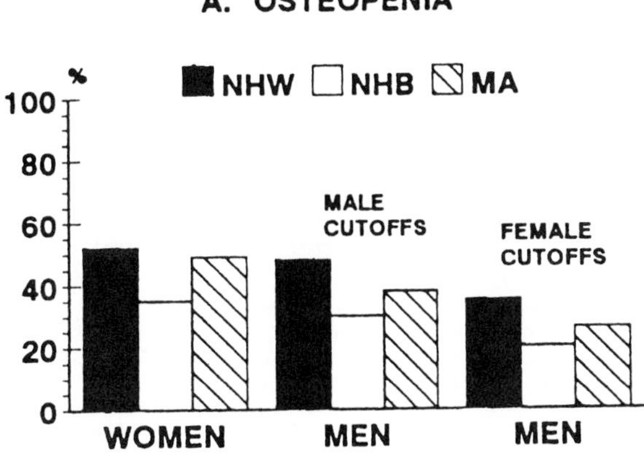

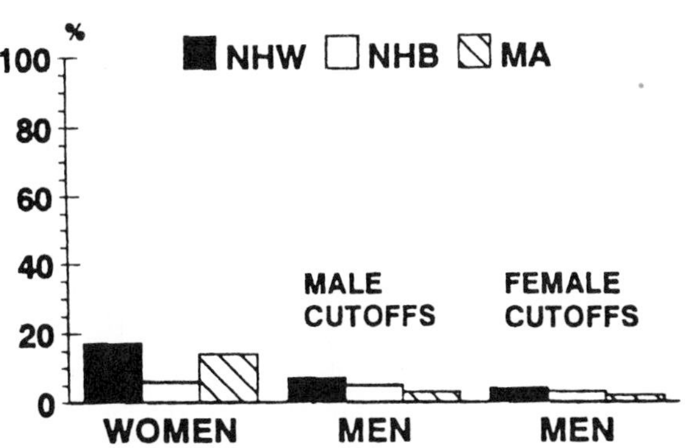

FIGURE 122.9. Age-adjusted prevalence of low femur neck bone mineral density by race or ethnicity, ages 50+ years. NHW, non-Hispanic white; NHB, non-Hispanic black; MA, Mexican American. (From Looker AC, Orwoll ES, Johnston CC, et al. Prevalence of low femoral bone density in older US adults from NHANES III. *J Bone Miner Res* 1997;12:1761–1768, with permission.)

Patterns of Fracture with Low Bone Mass

Fracture is the ultimate undesirable clinical manifestation of low bone mass and most often involves the wrist, femoral neck, and vertebral bodies. Fractures of the metatarsals, humerus, ribs, toes, leg, pelvis, hand, and clavicle have also been related to low BMD (139,140). Figure 122.10 shows the incidence of fractures in various sites stratified by age (141).

Incidence and Prevalence of Fracture

The number of fractures in a population depends not only on fracture incidence but also on population size (142). Hip fracture is less common among Asians than Caucasians, but because of the larger worldwide Asian population, 33% of all osteoporotic fractures occur in Asia (143). By the year 2050, three-quarters of all elderly individuals will live in Asia, Latin America, and Africa, and over half of all hip fractures will occur in Asia. In addition, growth and aging of the world's population will further increase the incidence and prevalence of fractures (143,144). The estimated number of fractures among North American women was >200,000 in 1990 and is estimated to increase to 469,000 in 2025 and be >500,000 in 2050 (143). The percentage of fractures attributable to osteoporosis is less for nonwhites than whites, and less for men than women.

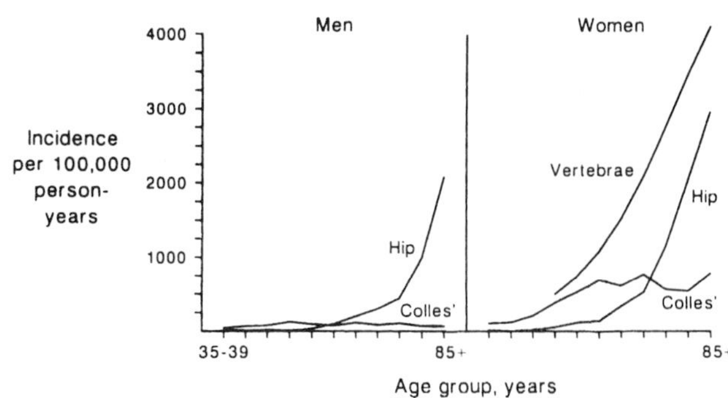

FIGURE 122.10. Incidence rates for the three common osteoporotic fractures (Colles', hip, and vertebral) in men and women, plotted as a function of age at the time of the fracture. (From Riggs BL, Melton LJ III. Involutional osteoporosis. *N Engl J Med* 1986;314:1676–1684, with permission.)

The incidence rate for hip fractures is approximately 2 per 1,000 patient-years at age 65 to 69 in Caucasian and non–Caucasian women, and increases to about 26 per 1,000 patient-years at age 80 to 84 (145). The incidence and prevalence of vertebral fractures is low prior to age 50 years and rises almost exponentially thereafter (79,141, 146,147) (Fig. 122.10). Cooper and colleagues (148) reported that vertebral fractures among Caucasian women in Minnesota increased with age, with an incidence of 145 per 100,000 person-years. Ninety percent of all hip and spinal fractures are related to osteoporosis (149). Among American women, the incidence of wrist fractures increases rapidly at the time of menopause and plateaus at about 700 per 100,000 person-years after age 60 (141,146).

Lifetime Risk of Fractures

The lifetime risk of any fracture in the hip, spine, or distal forearm is about 40% in Caucasian women over 50 years of age and 13% in Caucasian men of similar age (74). The estimated lifetime risk for fracture at various sites in 50-year-old Caucasian men and women is shown in Table 122.5 (74).

TABLE 122.5. ESTIMATED LIFETIME FRACTURE RISK IN 50-YEAR-OLD WHITE WOMEN AND MEN[A,B]

Site	Women %, (95% Confidence Interval)	Men %, (95% Confidence Interval)
Proximal femur	17.5 (16.8, 18.2)	6.0 (5.6, 6.5)
Vertebral fracture	15.6 (14.8, 16.3)	5.0 (4.6, 5.4)
Distal forearm fracture	16.0 (15.2, 16.7)	2.5 (2.2, 3.1)
Any fracture	39.7 (38.7, 40.6)	13.1 (12.4, 13.7)

[a]Age 50 years was chosen because this is about the average age of menopause in women.
[b]Using incidence of clinically diagnosed fractures only.
From Melton LJ, Chrischilles EA, Cooper C, et al. Perspective: How many women have osteoporosis? *J Bone Miner Res* 1992;7:1005–1010, with permission.

Impact of Osteoporosis

Osteoporosis and consequent fractures are major public health concerns in the United States. The economic costs of osteoporotic fractures are large and somewhat difficult to assess because the total includes expenses for surgery and hospitalization, rehabilitation, long-term care costs, loss of productivity, and medications (142,144). Phillips and co-workers (150), using national databases, estimated annual direct medical costs in 1986 of all types of fractures and complications related to osteoporosis as $2.8 billion for inpatient care, $2.1 billion for nursing home care, and $0.2 billion for outpatient care (150). Other investigators have estimated annual costs of up to $14 billion (151,153). It is possible that within 50 years the cost of hip fractures alone in the United States could exceed $16 billion in 1984 dollars (154). Other burdens associated with fracture include poor resultant functional status, pain, a diminished quality of life, loss of independence, and fear and depression (138,144).

Hip fractures result in more than 7 million days of restricted activity and 6,000 admissions to nursing homes annually in the United States; 74% of all nursing home admissions are related to osteoporosis (142,150–152,155). For hip fractures, about half of the health care costs reflect nursing home expenses. There is an increased mortality within 1 year of hip fracture (156,157), and 50% of survivors never fully recover (133). In the Study of Osteoporotic Fractures, 14% of the deaths after pelvic or hip fracture were directly caused by the fracture, 17% were related to chronic underlying conditions, and 69% were not related to the fracture (157). The authors concluded that most of the increased mortality was due to underlying poor health and comorbidities. The mortality associated with vertebral fractures was also greater than expected in the general population (156,157), while the mortality of patients with wrist fractures was similar (156,157).

Patterns of Acquisition and Loss of BMD

Figure 122.11 shows the lifetime accrual and loss of BMD in men and women. Peak BMD is the maximum possible with normal growth and represents a genetically and environmentally determined apex from which future losses occur (158). A cross-sectional study of premenopausal Caucasian women aged 8 to 50 years, using DXA, found that from about age 8 until the end of the second decade, bone size and bone mass increase rapidly (158). Most skeletal density (both trabecular and cortical) is accumulated by age 18. Some skeletal sites, such as the skull, increase in density until menopause (158). In cortical bone, a slow phase of loss begins at age 40, ranging from 0.3% to 0.5% per year in both men and women (141). At menopause in women not taking hormone replacement therapy, losses average about 1% per year but may approach 3% to 5% per year (133). After this accelerated loss for about 8 to 10 years, the rate decreases in another slow phase (141). A longitudinal population-based study in Australia of men and women ≥60 years reported a loss in the femoral neck of 0.9% per year in women and 0.82% per year in men. The rate increased with age in both genders (159), never reaching a plateau. The cumulative lifetime losses of bone may be as much as 30% to 40% of peak BMD in women and 20% to 30% in men (133,144).

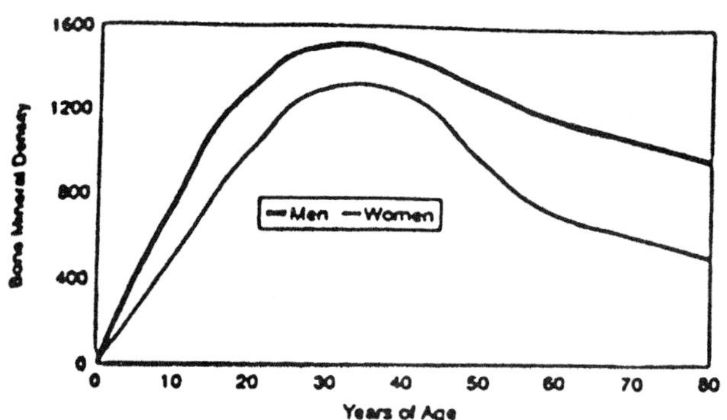

FIGURE 122.11. Age-related bone mineral density for men and women. (From Christenson RH. Biochemical markers of bone metabolism: an overview. *Clin Biochem* 1997;30:573–593, with permission.)

Genetics

BMD at any particular age is an interplay of endogenous factors, including genetics, and exogenous environmental factors (158). It is estimated that 46% to 62% of BMD is attributable to inherited factors (160). Seeman and co-workers (161) concluded that postmenopausal osteoporosis may result from a low peak bone mass, because daughters of women with osteoporosis had relatively low BMD in the lumbar spine and femoral neck. Tylavsky and co-workers (162) determined that radial bone mass in post-adolescent daughters of women with osteoporosis was lower compared to individuals with no maternal history of osteoporosis. Other investigators have suggested that 70% to 85% of the individual variance in bone mass is genetically determined (163,164). Twin and family studies support the importance of genetic influences in accrual of BMD (160–162,165,166).

Current evidence suggests that allelic variations of many genes alter bone mass and likely contribute to the pathogenesis of osteoporosis (163). Candidates include genes for the vitamin D receptor, the estrogen receptor, TGF-β, IL-6, collagen type I, and collagenase (164). Polymorphisms in the vitamin D receptor have been associated with BMD, but the significance is controversial (167–169). Lifestyle risk factors modify the genetic influence on BMD. For example, among individuals with a vitamin D receptor genotype associated with low spinal BMD (a restriction site within the vitamin D receptor designated as bb), greater calcium intake and weight-bearing physical activity appeared to improve BMD (169). In addition, specific genes that regulate bone mass, bone turnover, and bone loss likely play roles in determining BMD (170). Studies have shown the importance of genetic influences on type I collagen synthesis (170); a COL1A1 gene polymorphism was associated with a lower BMD and an increased fracture rate (171).

Epidemiologic Risk Factors for Low BMD and Fracture

Many factors have been identified as risk factors for low BMD and fracture, and the following sections review some of them.

Bone Mineral Density

BMD is one of the strongest predictors of fracture, and 40% to 80% of the variance in bone strength is attributed to BMD (172). The strong association of BMD and fracture risks was discussed above. Below we review the interactive effects of previous fractures and BMD on future fracture risk. Studies have correlated BMD and multiple risk factors with hip fracture. Figure 122.12relates calcaneal bone density and number of prevalent risk factors to the annual risk of hip fracture (173). For a woman with normal calcaneal bone density and two risk factors, the fracture incidence was 1.1 per 1,000 woman-years. In contrast, a calcaneal bone density in the lowest tertile and five risk factors increased the incidence of hip fracture to 27 per 1,000 woman-years. This study demonstrates that numerous factors, independent of BMD, increase the risk of fracture. Black and co-workers (60) found that non-spine and wrist fracture risk in the same population was inversely related to bone density measurement at the proximal femur and spine. The combination of low BMD and previous fracture also predicts future fracture (174,175) (Fig. 122.13). Women in the lowest tertile for BMD, with two fractures, have a 75-fold greater risk of fracture than individuals in the highest tertile with no fractures. A history of vertebral fracture alone also predicted a subsequent fracture. One crush or wedge vertebral fracture increased the risk of an additional vertebral fracture by 4.1- to 5.3-fold. The presence of more than two wedge or crush vertebral fractures increased the risk by about 12-fold.

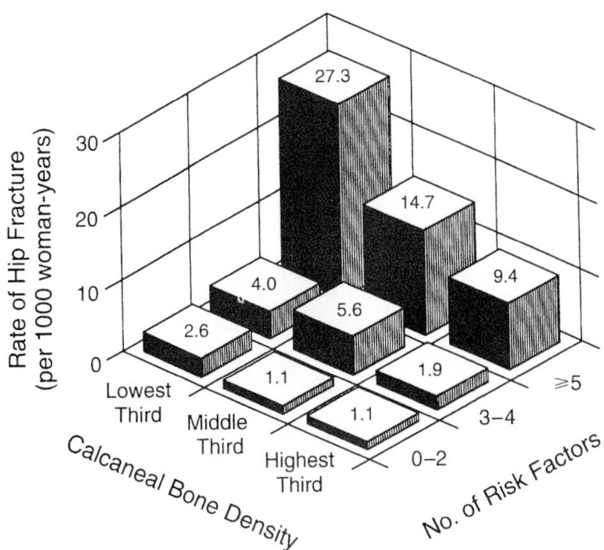

FIGURE 122.12. Annual risk of hip fracture according to the number of risk factors and the age-specific calcaneal bone density. The risk factors are as follows: age ≥80; maternal history of hip fracture; any fracture (except hip fracture) since the age of 50; fair, poor, or very poor health; previous hyperthyroidism; anticonvulsant therapy; current long-acting benzodiazepine therapy; current weight less than at the age of 25; height at the age of 25 ≥168 cm; caffeine intake more than the equivalent of two cups of coffee per day; on feet ≤4 hours a day; no walking for exercise; inability to rise from chair without using arms; lowest quartile (standard deviation >2.44) of depth perception; lower quartile (≤0.70 unit) of contrast sensitivity; and pulse rate >80 per minute. (From Cummings S, Nevitt MC, Browner WS, et al. Risk factors for hip fracture in white women. Study of Osteoporotic Fractures Research Group. *N Engl J Med* 1995;332: 767–773, with permission.)

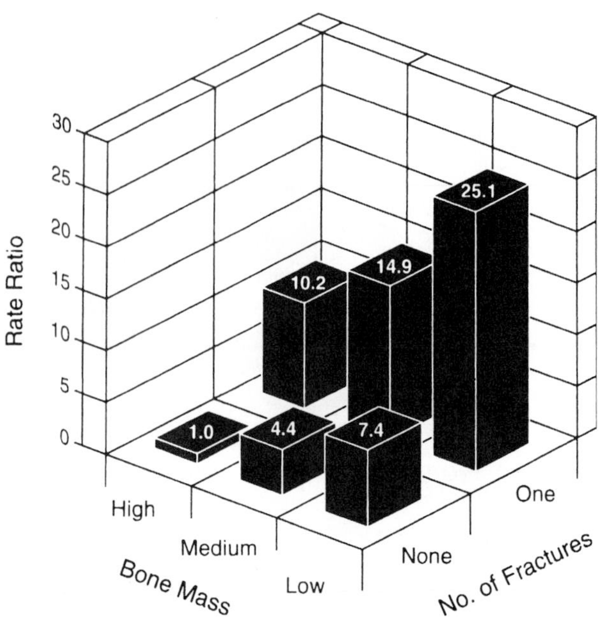

FIGURE 122.13. Influence of bone mass and previous fractures on fracture rate. Bone mass was categorized into three groups (high, medium, low) of equal numbers of subjects. Number at *top* of each *bar* indicates rate of new vertebral fractures relative to rate among women in highest bone mass category without any previous fractures. Women with low bone mass and one previous fracture at baseline develop new fractures 25 times faster than women with high bone mass and no previous fracture. (From Deal CL. Osteoporosis, diagnosis and management. *Am J Med* 1997;102:35S–39S, with permission.)

Gender, Age, and Ethnicity

BMD decreases with age in both men and women (133). The lifetime risk of fracture is approximately twofold greater in women than men (144). After menopause, although the risk of distal forearm and vertebral fracture increases, the incidence of Colles' fracture plateaus. The incidence of hip fractures sharply rises later in life (141) (Fig. 122.10). In a study of osteoporotic fractures, appendicular bone mass in women decreased by about 5% every 5 years after age 65 (176). In addition, after adjusting for bone density at the femoral neck, the risk of hip fracture doubled with each decade of life [relative risk (RR) = 2.0, 1.3, 3.0) (78). The rate of bone loss in the hip increases with age, increasing the risk of hip fracture by 21% per 5 years in women 80 years and older (177). Rates of calcaneal loss also increase in older women (177).

Axial and appendicular bone mass are greater in African American than Caucasian women before and after menopause (178,179). The incidences of osteopenia and osteoporosis are higher in Hispanic whites than in non-Hispanic blacks and Mexican Americans (136) as shown by the NHANES III data set. Bhudhikanok and co-workers (180) compared BMD and bone mineral content in healthy Asian and Caucasian-American men and women and found no significant differences in BMD in youths through midpuberty. BMD is lower in Asian men at maturity and is attributed to smaller bone size. Fractures occur approximately twofold more frequently in Caucasians of North European ancestry than African Americans or Asians (144). Caucasian women are 1.5- to 4-fold more likely to have a hip fracture after age 40 than African American women (145).

Body Weight/Composition and BMD

Body weight is strongly and positively associated with BMD (181). In the Study of Osteoporotic Fractures, body mass was responsible for most of the effect. At non–weight-bearing sites, adiposity appears to have more important effects than body mass (181). In addition, smaller body size and weight are predictive of fracture because of lower hip BMD (182). In non–African American women who are 65 years of age, involuntary weight loss is a strong predictor of fragility fracture at sites including the hip. Voluntary weight loss was not predictive of hip fracture (183); however, a cohort of women who voluntarily modified their lifestyle to lose weight had a higher rate of loss of BMD at the hip and lumbar spine than a weight-stable group (184).

Reproductive Factors/Sex Hormones and BMD and Fracture

The use of oral contraceptives for 6 years or longer is associated with higher BMD at the lumbar spine and femoral neck, but not at the ultradistal wrist or radius in postmenopausal women, compared to women who had never used oral contraceptives (185). Women using an oral contraceptive pill with ≥50 μg of ethinylestradiol had a 44% lower risk of hip fracture than women who had never taken them (186).

Tubal ligation has been associated with estrogen deficiency and dysfunctional uterine bleeding, but not low BMD or fractures (187). The use of depot medroxyprogesterone for pelvic pain or contraception in young women was associated with low BMD at the spine and femoral neck, likely because the users were partially estrogen deficient (188,189).

Amenorrheic athletes and individuals with anorexia nervosa have decreased BMD (186,190–193). The pathogenesis is probably related to a variety of factors, including low body mass, estrogen deficiency (amenorrhea), and cortisol excess (190). In retired female elite ballet dancers compared with nonathletic age-matched controls, menstrual disturbance (>2 months between menses) was negatively associated with lumbar spine and ultradistal radial BMD, but not with BMD loss at the femur (194).

It has been difficult to find a relationship between number of pregnancies, BMD, and fractures later in life (195). While bone mass decreases during pregnancy, in most women it recovers by 6 months postpartum. In the Study of Osteoporotic Fractures, breast-feeding or the number of pregnancies was not associated with BMD (176). Perhaps pregnancy unmasks, rather than causes, low BMD (196).

In the Study of Osteoporotic Fractures, each 5-year delay in menopause was associated with a 1.3% higher bone mass in the distal radius (176). After adjusting for age and duration of estrogen use, radial and calcaneal BMD was greater in women using estrogen alone than in those reporting no current estrogen use or concurrent use of estrogen and progesterone. There was no association between progesterone use and BMD (176). In the cross-sectional Rancho Bernardo study, estrogen replacement initiated early and continued late in life was associated with the maintenance of high BMD (197). In addition, late estrogen use (after age 60) has a beneficial effect similar to estrogen begun in early menopause (197). Current estrogen use, compared to no estrogen use, decreased the risk of fractures of the wrist and all nonspine sites in non–African American women older than 64. There was a trend toward a lower risk of hip fracture in current users of estrogen compared to women never on estrogen. Estrogen therapy to lower fracture risk appears to be most effective when initiated within 5 years of menopause and continued for more than 10 years (198).

Endogenous hormone concentrations are related to BMD and fractures. In the Study of Osteoporotic Fractures, in elderly women with estradiol concentrations between 10 to 25 pg/mL, BMD was higher than in women with estradiol concentrations <5 pg/mL (199,200). Estradiol concentrations <5 pg/mL and sex hormone binding globulin concentrations ≥1.0 μg/dL are associated with a higher risk of vertebral and hip fracture (199). Higher concentrations of sex hormone binding globulin are associated with greater loss of bone at the hip and calcaneus (201).

Medications and BMD/Fracture

Chronic treatment with several medications may significantly decrease BMD (Table 122.6). Some antiepileptic agents (such as phenobarbital, primidone, and phenytoin, in contrast to valproic acid, which has no effect) may induce hyperparathyroidism by accelerating metabolism of vitamin D through stimulation of hepatic microsomal enzymes. As a result, these agents may contribute to the genesis of rickets and osteomalacia (202). Doses of vitamin D as large as 4,000 IU weekly may be required to maintain normal serum 25-hydroxyvitamin D levels. In children on valproate or carbamazepine for treatment of seizures, valproate, but not carbamazepine, significantly reduced both axial and appendicular BMD (203).

Anticoagulants

Prolonged therapy with heparin, as used in treatment or prophylaxis for thrombophlebitis in pregnant women to avoid fetal toxicity secondary to warfarin, causes osteoporosis. Fractures developed in 2% of pregnant women treated with a mean daily dose of 19,000 IU heparin for 25 weeks (204). Another study found that one-third of pregnant women treated with 12,000 to 50,000 IU daily lost at least 10% of BMD in the proximal femur, and this loss persisted 6 months after delivery (205). Histomorphometric studies in experimental animals showed that heparin decreased bone formation and increased bone resorption (206), and that heparin was retained in bone at an undefined site for at least 8 weeks after stopping treatment (207). No parameter has been shown to identify women at greatest risk for developing heparin-induced osteoporosis (208). Two other factors contribute to the genesis of bone loss in this setting, pregnancy itself and breast-feeding, so it has been difficult to determine the effect of heparin alone (209). There is no evidence that treatment with calcium or vitamin D supplement, or both, prevents this skeletal complication (205). Low-molecular-weight heparin may exhibit less skeletal toxicity than standard heparin, although this opinion is somewhat controversial (reviewed in ref. 208). Short-term intravenous high-dose heparin to treat acute thromboembolism has not been associated with osteoporosis.

The effect of the vitamin K antagonist warfarin on BMD is variable (203,210,211). In the Study of Osteoporotic Fractures, warfarin use was not associated with low BMD, but it was associated with poor health, involuntary weight loss, nonthiazide diuretic use, and frailty (211). In another study, men taking warfarin were matched to control subjects with similar medical conditions who were not on warfarin. Lumbar spine BMD was significantly lower in the warfarin-treated group than in the control group (210).

Thiazide Diuretics

Thiazide diuretic use is associated with relatively higher levels of BMD (212–216). A cross-sectional study of women using thiazide diuretics for more than 10 years demonstrated higher radial bone mass compared to those untreated (215). Furthermore, among thiazide users, nonsignificant trends of lower fracture risk for nonspinal fractures, including the hip and wrist, were observed (215). The incidence of falls was similar among thiazide and nonthiazide users.

Antidepressant Drugs

In a case-controlled study of women older than 66 years of age, the use of selective serotonin reuptake inhibitors, secondary tricyclics, or tertiary tricyclic antidepressants conferred higher risks of hip fracture. Current use was associated with a higher risk of fracture than past use (217).

Glucocorticoids

Glucocorticoid use has been associated with low BMD and fractures. Low-dose prednisone therapy causes rapid loss of axial BMD in patients with rheumatoid arthritis (RA) (218–220). Glucocorticoid-associated bone disease is discussed in more detail below.

TABLE 122.6. DISEASES AND DRUG THERAPIES ASSOCIATED WITH OSTEOPENIA AND FRACTURE

Unique to women	Immobilization or microgravity
Natural menopause	Low calcium or vitamin D intake
Pregnancy	Sedentary lifestyle
Hypogonadism	Smoking
Agonist for gonadotropin-releasing hormone or Depo-Provera	Malignancy
Gonadal dysgenesis (e.g., Turner's syndrome)	Lymphoproliferative and myeloproliferative diseases (lymphoma and leukemia)
Endometriosis	Multiple myeloma
Unique to men	Systemic mastocytosis
Hypogonadism	Tumor secretion of parathyroid hormone–related peptide
Constitutional delay of puberty	Nutritional disorders
Hemochromatosis (due either to infiltration of testes (hypergonadotropic) or pituitary (hypgonadotropic)	Eating disorders such as anorexia nervosa
Kallman's syndrome (isolated gonadotropin deficiency)	Osteomalacia
Klinefelter's syndrome (genotype XXY)	Malabsorption syndromes
Orchitis, viral	Parenteral nutrition
Men and women	Pernicious anemia
Age-related bone loss	Other diseases
Connective tissue diseases	Chronic obstructive pulmonary disease (often secondary to glucocorticoid usage)
Ankylosing spondylitis	Chronic renal failure
Osteogenesis imperfecta	Congenital porphyria
Rheumatoid arthritis	Epidermolysis bullosa
Spinal cord injury	Hemochromatosis
Endocrine causes	Hemophilia
Acromegaly	Homocystinuria
Adrenal trophy and Addison's disease	Hypophosphatasia
Cushing's syndrome	Idiopathic scoliosis
Diabetes mellitus type 1	Multiple sclerosis
Glucocorticoid excess (endogenous and exogenous)	Sarcoidosis
Gonadotroph cell adenoma	Thalassemia
Hyperparathyroidism (primary and secondary)	*Medications*
Hyperprolactinemia (as a cause of hypogonadism)	Aluminum
Hyperthyroidism	Antiepileptics (some)
Hypocalcitoninemia?	Chemotherapeutic agents that cause chemical castration
Hypogonadism (primary, secondary, or surgical)	Cyclosporin A and tacrolimus
Panhypopituitarism	Cytotoxic drugs
Thyrotoxicosis	Glucocorticoids and adrenocorticotropin
Gastrointestinal diseases	Heparin (perhaps less severe with low molecular weight compounds)
Cholestatic liver disease (especially primary biliary cirrhosis)	Lithium
Gastrectomy	Methotrexate
Inflammatory bowel disease (especially regional enteritis)	Tamoxifen (premenopausal use)
Postgastrectomy	Thyroid hormone (in excess)
Lifestyle/genetic factors	Warfarin?
Excessive alcohol	
Excessive caffeine?	
Excessive exercise (impairment of hypothalamic-pituitary axis)	
Excessive protein intake	

Smoking and Alcohol Use

The lifestyle habits of smoking and chronic alcohol usage increase the risk of osteoporosis. Studies of twins have shown that cigarette smoking decreases bone mass; women who smoked at least one pack per day had a 5% to 10% deficit in perimenopausal bone mass compared to their nonsmoking twin (221). In the Study of Osteoporotic Fractures, current smokers had a 4.3% decrease in distal radial bone mass and past smokers had a 1.177% decrease in bone mass compared with individuals who had never smoked (176). No dose response was demonstrated in smokers regarding amount of tobacco used over a lifetime. Postulated mechanisms of the adverse effects of smoking on bone metabolism include enhanced hepatic 2-hydroxylation of estradiol with a decrease in bioactive estrogens and decreased production of endogenous estrogen (222). Furthermore, smoking may reverse the protective effect of oral estrogen on the risk of a hip fracture (223).

Chronic alcohol abuse has long been associated with bone loss and fractures. Ethanol directly inhibits osteoblast proliferation (224), decreasing bone formation and mineralization; bone resorption may be normal or decreased (225). Long-term ethanol use also exerts indirect toxic effects on bone metabolism, by inducing hypogonadism (226). Alcohol usage during adolescence may permanently reduce peak bone mass in young men (227). Abstinence from alcohol for several years may significantly increase BMD, but not to normal (228).

Caffeine Consumption

In the Study of Osteoporotic Fractures, 10 cups of caffeinated coffee daily for 30 years was associated with a 1.1% decrease in distal radial bone mass (176). In the Rancho Bernardo study, lifetime caffeine consumption, equivalent to two cups per day, was inversely associated with BMD at the hip and spine (229). This relationship is independent of age, body mass index, alcohol intake, exercise, and estrogen or thiazide diuretic use. In contrast, in women drinking ≥1 glass of milk per day, there was no significant relationship between BMD and caffeine intake.

Calcium

Calcium is one of the numerous nutritional factors that affect BMD. Adequate calcium intake is important in achieving peak BMD. Johnston and co-workers (230) supplemented 70 pairs of female twins aged 6 to 14 years with either placebo or calcium citrate malate for 3 years. The calcium-supplemented twin developed a higher BMD. The increases in BMD were most pronounced in individuals who were prepubertal at the start of the trial. Nieves and co-workers (231) evaluated food-frequency questionnaires in women aged 30 to 39 years that estimated prior calcium intake during adolescence; calcium and phosphorus intakes were positively correlated with hip BMD. An increase in teenage calcium consumption from 800 to 1,200 mg/day was estimated to increase hip BMD by 6%. From dietary recalls in the Rancho Bernardo study, higher teenage milk intake was associated with higher BMD at the spine and midradius (232). Higher milk consumption in adulthood was associated with higher BMD in the midradius, spine, total hip, and trochanter. Calcium's role in osteoporosis prevention and treatment, particularly among older women is discussed below.

Vitamin D

Vitamin D deficiency reduces BMD. Among general populations of North America and Western Europe, vitamin D deficiency may be commonplace. This is particularly true among the elderly, the institutionalized, and individuals who have little sun exposure (233,234). Vitamin D deficiency, coupled with low calcium intake leads to relative secondary hyperparathyroidism and subsequent bone resorption. Calcium supplemented at 1,000 mg/day may be useful in suppressing PTH increases seen in the winter among elderly women (235). In the Study of Osteoporotic Fractures, women with serum 1,25-dihydroxyvitamin D <23 pg/mL had a significantly increased risk of fracture (RR = 2.1, 95% CI = 1.2–2.5) (199). In a study comparing postmenopausal community-dwelling women admitted for hip fracture or elective hip replacement, the fracture group had lower serum 25-hydroxyvitamin D concentrations and higher PTH concentrations. Indeed, 50% of patients with hip fractures had low 25-hydroxyvitamin D concentrations (236).

Vitamin D excess is also associated with low BMD. Occult vitamin D intoxication has been detected in patients using nonprescription dietary supplements containing vitamin D (237). Patients using active vitamin D metabolites, in particular, should be counseled on cautious use of nutritional supplements. If vitamin D intoxication occurs, the symptoms are nausea, weakness, constipation, and somnolence. It is also deleterious to bone (237). In a case series, discontinuation of large supplements of vitamin D lowered 25-hydroxyvitamin D concentrations to normal and increased BMD at the lumbar spine and femoral neck (237,238).

Activity/Weight-Bearing Exercise

Immobilization results in loss of bone mass. Injuries to extremities are associated with rapid bone loss that reflects the severity of the injury (239). Later, the magnitude of chronic loss of bone corresponds to the degree of functional impairment and whether significant pain persists. Early weight-bearing activity is recommended to minimize this bone loss.

Weight-bearing exercise is associated with increased BMD. In the Study of Osteoporotic Fractures, after adjustment for age and weight, a 2,000-kcal increase in vigorous activity per week for the previous 12 months was associated with a 2% increase in distal radial bone mass and a 3.9% increase in the calcaneus (176). In the same cohort, more leisure-time exercise or sports activity significantly reduced the risk for hip fracture (240). Moderate to vigorously active women had significantly lower risks of hip (42% reduction) and vertebral fractures (33% reduction) compared to non-active women. High-impact exercise regimens that load axial and leg bones improve muscular power and dynamic balance, which lowers risk for falls and fracture (241).

Falls and Fractures

Factors predisposing to falls such as lower limb dysfunction, neurologic conditions, barbiturate use, and visual impairment are important in the risk of fracture (146,242,243). In some populations, the rate of fall-related injuries is increasing (244). In a longitudinal, epidemiologic population-based survey in residents of Finland >60 years of age, postural instability and muscular weakness were predictors of fracture (245). In a prospective study, slower gait, difficulty performing tandem walk, and reduced visual acuity were independent risk factors for hip fracture (246).

While BMD is an important predictor of whether a fracture will occur after a fall, the direction of a fall influences the site of fracture (247). The force of a fall and factors that may attenuate the force at the point of impact also determine whether a bone breaks. Falling to the side or straight down near the hip increases the risk of hip fracture, while falling on an outstretched hand or backward increases the risk of a wrist fracture. Breaking the momentum of a fall by grabbing onto or hitting an object slows the momentum of the hip and wrist, whereas falling on a hard surface increases the risk of hip fracture. Triceps weakness is an independent risk factor for hip fracture, suggesting that arm extension is a less effective defense during a fall in individuals with weak arms. One intriguing physical medicine approach to fracture prevention is the use of hip padding. In a randomized controlled trial, external hip protectors significantly lowered the risk of hip fractures in nursing home residents by over 50% (248). Long-term adherence and large-scale study of this strategy in noninstitutionalized populations are needed to determine if this approach is generalizable.

Bone Morphometric Factors and Fracture Risk

Bone geometry is also a predictor of fracture risk. Hip axis length (defined as the distance from the greater trochanter to the pelvic brim) is positively associated with hip fracture (49,50). For each SD increase in length, the risk of fracture doubles. A greater length is associated with more fractures of the femoral neck and trochanter. Gluer and co-workers (51) showed four other measurements independently predicted fracture risk: diminished thickness of the femoral shaft cortex, diminished thickness of the femoral neck cortex, reduced tensile trabecular index, and wider trochanteric region. In contrast, there is no relationship between hip fracture and femoral neck width or neck/shaft angle.

Clinical Evaluation

The clinical evaluation of osteoporosis is directed toward identifying lifestyle risk factors and pertinent physical findings and assessing secondary causes of osteopenia. Table 122.6 lists conditions associated with osteopenia/osteoporosis.

History

A careful evaluation of osteoporosis includes identification of a family history of metabolic bone disease, lifestyle risk factors, a history of change in height and weight, history of previous fractures, a reproductive history (evidence of hypogonadism), an endocrine history, dietary factors (including lifetime and current calcium consumption, vitamin D, sodium, caffeine), a smoking history, alcohol intake, exercise, history of renal or hepatic failure, and past and current medications and supplements. In addition, factors that increase the risk of falls such as neuromuscular disease and unsafe living conditions should also be sought. A history of bone pain is useful; however, osteoporosis is not painful unless fractures develop. Further, a large proportion of vertebral fractures may occur without overt symptoms.

Physical Examination

Height measurement is a vital part of the physical examination at each visit (249–251). Comparison of current height with that on the driver's license is helpful in identifying height loss. Loss of 2 inches is a fairly sensitive indicator of vertebral compression (175). The spine should be examined for conformation, and spinal and paraspinous tenderness. If kyphosis is present, the possibility of pulmonary compromise should be considered. A "buffalo hump," easy bruisability, and striae suggest Cushing's syndrome. Blue sclerae indicate osteogenesis imperfecta. The number of missing teeth has been correlated with losses in BMD (252–254). A joint assessment may suggest rheumatologic causes of low BMD. The neurologic examination is important because muscular weakness predisposes for falls, and an underlying neurologic problem may be discovered. A gynecologic examination or prostatic examination should be included if hormone replacement therapy is considered (255).

Laboratory Evaluation

The laboratory assessment seeks possible secondary causes of loss of BMD. Table 122.7 lists laboratory tests that may be appropriate. Many are not cost-effective if ordered for

TABLE 122.7. LABORATORY EVALUATION OF DECREASED BONE MASS

Test	Diagnosis Ruled In or Ruled Out
Serum protein electrophoresis/complete blood count	Multiple myeloma
Hyperparathyroidism	Serum calcium and phosphorus
Serum intact parathyroid hormone	Hyperparathyroidism
Serum creatinine	Renal failure
Liver enzymes	Liver failure
24-hour urine free cortisol or dexamethasone suppression test	Cushing's syndrome
Thyroid-stimulating hormone	Hyperthyroidism
Follicle-stimulating hormone	Menopause
Free testosterone	Male hypogonadism
Urine calcium/creatinine ratio	Hypercalciuria
25-monohydroxy vitamin D_3 and alkaline phosphatase	Vitamin D deficiency or osteomalacia

every patient. An intact PTH concentration, for example, should be obtained if the calcium concentration is elevated and the phosphorus concentration is low, or if clinical suspicion is high for hyperparathyroidism.

Bone Turnover Markers

Biochemical markers of bone turnover are sometimes used in the management of osteoporosis. While bone formation and resorption are usually coupled, net imbalances can be evaluated with these assays. Table 122.8 lists bone turnover markers that can be classified as indices of bone formation or resorption (256). Bone balance would theoretically be the net difference between formation and resorption.

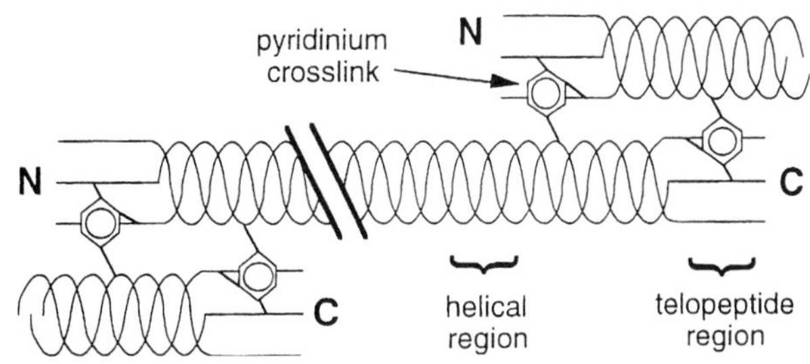

FIGURE 122.14. Fibrils of collagen showing the nonhelical carboxyterminal and aminoterminal ends bonding to the helical areas of adjacent fibrils by pyridinium cross-links. (From Christenson RH. Biochemical markers of bone metabolism: an overview. *Clin Biochem* 1997;30:573–593, with permission.)

Bone Formation Markers

The markers of bone formation reflect synthesis by osteoblasts or the postrelease metabolism of procollagen (42). Bone-specific alkaline phosphatase is produced by osteoblasts. Osteocalcin is a vitamin K–dependent calcium-binding protein synthesized by osteoblasts and its production is also controlled by 1,25-dihydroxyvitamin D. Serum concentrations of osteocalcin reflect the relative activity of osteoblasts. Bone disorders with increases in bone-specific alkaline phosphatase and osteocalcin include Paget's disease, primary hyperparathyroidism, rickets, metastatic carcinoma, osteomalacia, and renal osteodystrophy. There may be mild increases in the markers in osteoporosis. Collagen precursor proteins are released during collagen formation, and serum carboxyterminal and aminoterminal peptides of type I procollagen can be measured. The carboxyterminal propeptide of type I collagen is less sensitive than bone-specific alkaline phosphatase or osteocalcin, and may also be elevated in individuals with impaired hepatic function (256).

Bone Resorption Markers

Resorptive markers indicate the activity of osteoclasts and collagen degradation (42). Tartrate-resistant acid phosphatase is produced by osteoclasts and mostly reflects increased bone resorptive activity. Figure 122.14 shows the collagen molecule with telopeptide regions and pyridinium cross-links. Pyridinium cross-links include pyridinoline and deoxypyridinoline. These fragments are released into the circulation and ultimately excreted in urine. Of the two cross-links, deoxypyridinoline is more specific for collagen breakdown. The collagen telopeptides are composed of short nonhelical regions with pyridinoline cross-links, and may be measured in serum or urine. Urinary hydroxyproline may originate from other tissues and dietary sources and is now rarely used to gauge bone resorption.

Bone markers provide an assessment of dynamic aspects of skeletal metabolism as opposed to the more static assessment by bone densitometry (42,256). Bone markers are useful to categorize an individual as having fast or slow bone turnover. Fracture risk appears to be related to faster bone turnover (256). Bone markers also predict response to therapy, and are helpful in monitoring compliance with antiresorptive therapies.

Shane and co-workers (257,258) showed elevated urinary concentrations of bone resorption markers 3 months after cardiac transplantation. However, loss of BMD at the femoral neck did not predict fracture in women 6 months after engraftment (259); therefore, bone markers may better reflect the rapid bone loss that occurs within the first

TABLE 122.8. BIOCHEMICAL MARKERS OF BONE TURNOVER

Formation	Resorption
From osteoblasts, in serum	From osteoclasts
Bone alkaline phosphatase	Tartrate-resistant acid phosphatase
Osteocalcin	
From bone matrix, in serum	
Procollagen I carboxyterminal propeptide	Aminoterminal telopeptide of type I collagen
Procollagen I aminoterminal propeptide	Carboxyterminal telopeptide of type I collagen
From bone matrix, in Urine	
	Pyridinoline and deoxypyridinoline crosslinks
	Aminoterminal telopeptide of type I collagen
	Hydroxyproline from collagen degradation

From Rosalki SB. Biochemical markers of bone turnover. *Int J Clin Pract* 1998;52:255–256, with permission.

year after surgery. Higher rates of bone loss, documented by densitometry, have been associated with higher concentrations of resorptive markers (257).

Bone turnover markers predict BMD changes and fractures. In elderly women >75 years of age, urinary amino and carboxy telopeptides of type I collagen and free deoxypyridinoline predicted hip fractures, independently of BMD (260). Increased excretion of undercarboxylated osteocalcin was also an independent predictor in the same cohort (261). The predictive value of bone markers in measuring fracture risk and bone loss has been recently reviewed (262).

Schneider and co-workers (263) measured urinary *N*-telopeptide concentrations of type I collagen in a cross-sectional study of ambulatory older adults. There was a significant decrease in BMD at the hip and spine by increasing quintile of aminoterminal telopeptide of type I collagen in the urine (263). The concentrations discriminated between normal/osteopenic and osteoporotic T-scores in men in all sites except the spine. For women on estrogen versus women not on therapy, this assay discriminated between normal/osteopenia and osteoporosis at all sites.

Bone turnover markers may be useful to monitor the efficacy of therapy and patient compliance with antiresorptive medications. Greenspan and co-workers (264) demonstrated that decreases in urinary collagen cross-links after 6 months on alendronate therapy were associated with increases in BMD at the hip and spine after 2.5 years of treatment. The minimal or absent decrements in urinary *N*-telopeptide concentrations suggested poor compliance with the dosing regimen or impaired drug absorption. Similar results have been shown with estrogen therapy. Prestwood and co-workers (265) found that urinary bone resorptive markers decreased during a short-term course of estrogen replacement and increased after stopping therapy. Chesnut and colleagues (266) evaluated changes in urinary *N*-telopeptide of type I collagen in recently postmenopausal women receiving hormone replacement and calcium supplements over a 1-year interval. Decreases in the telopeptide were associated with significant increases in BMD at the hip and spine. Sustained elevations of resorptive markers in women on calcium only were associated with loss of BMD. The most significant association between BMD and response to hormone replacement therapy at 1 year was with urinary *N*-telopeptide of type I collagen. In summary, bone markers are biochemical tests that can help to monitor effectiveness of therapy and to evaluate fracture risk. Further work is necessary to determine which patients benefit from the use of formation and resorption markers and which particular markers are of greatest clinical value.

PREVENTION AND TREATMENT OF OSTEOPENIC BONE DISEASES

There has been a revolution in the management of osteoporosis due, in part, to the availability of an increasing array of new and effective pharmacotherapeutic options (137,267). Although changes in BMD may accurately predict fracture risk, when evaluating prevention and treatment studies, the effect of an intervention on fracture incidence is most critical.

Treatment Guidelines

Numerous general medical and specialty societies have promulgated guidelines for osteoporosis treatment (255,268–273). In 1998, the NOF issued guidelines in collaboration with ten multidisciplinary medical organizations. The therapeutic recommendations were based on the age of the person under consideration, the BMD T-score, and the presence of accompanying risk factors. The NOF guidelines advocates pharmacologic intervention to reduce the risk of fractures in the following:

Women with BMD T-scores below −2 in the absence of risk factors (see above).

Women with BMD T-scores below −1.5 if other risk factors are present.

Women over age 70 with multiple risk factors (especially those with previous non-hip, non-spine fractures), as they are at high enough risk to initiate treatment without BMD testing.

Older guidelines by the American College of Physicians advised that postmenopausal women who have had a hysterectomy and women at risk for coronary heart disease might benefit specifically from estrogen replacement therapy (ERT) (274).

Physical Modalities

Despite a paucity of objective data to support its efficacy, bracing of the spine for osteoporosis pain control is commonplace (275). In addition to limited data on effectiveness, excessive reliance on bracing can adversely lead to muscular weakness and loss of postural support. Patient concerns about the cost, aesthetics, and discomfort of certain braces and corsets limit even short-term adherence to many devices (276). One type of brace, a posture training support systems that has been developed to help strengthen back musculature, has good anecdotal efficacy for pain control based on a small uncontrolled trial (277).

Exercise

Impaired functional and physical status is strongly associated with a heightened risk of vertebral compression fractures (278) (also see the above risk factors). Accordingly, weight-bearing exercise and general physical conditioning have long been considered important elements of osteoporosis management. There are longitudinal data and an increasing number of randomized controlled trials demonstrating that moderate to intensive weight-bearing exercise can lead to modest increases of about 1% to 3% in bone mineral content (BMC) for both men and premenopausal women (241,279–282). An exception is the loss of BMD seen among competitive female athletes or other women who experience oligomenorrhea or amenorrhea due to excessive training (283,284). For an exercise to be effective in altering BMD, it appears it must strain the skeletal site (285). Exercise-induced bone mass gains are particularly notable in weight-bearing sites such as the tibia, particularly in runners, and in the spine among weight lifters (286). In the postmenopausal woman, the effects of exercise on bone mass, particularly in the hip and distal radius, are more modest in most studies, (285,287–292). One study among older women demonstrated a 5% lumbar BMD gain in 9 months associated with vigorous weight-bearing activity three times per week (293). Continued physical activity is required to maintain observed BMD gains (293,294). Spinal extension exercises are preferred over flexion maneuvers (which may lead to spinal compression deformities) and may be weakly linked to fewer compression deformities (295). At least one prospective trial has demonstrated that back strengthening exercises decrease kyphosis (296). Due to variations in populations evaluated, different exercise programs studied, and variable bone sites measured, no conclusions can be drawn about the effects of exercise on fracture prevention. However, through its additional benefits on muscle strengthening, coordination, and balance, physical activity leads to fracture prevention in ways other than just through an increase in BMD (241).

Pain Control

Acute vertebral compression fractures result in considerable pain that may become chronic (81,297). Some patients progress to a syndrome of crescendo vertebral collapse resulting in chronic back (298). Postural changes of kyphosis and rare neurologic compromise may further increase back discomfort. The use of braces and corsets (discussed above) is one approach to help transiently alleviate this discomfort. Nonsteroidal antiinflammatory medications, nonnarcotic analgesics (acetaminophen, tramadol, etc.), and the judicious use of narcotic pain relievers may all be justifiable when symptoms necessitate pain control. Low-dose tricyclic antidepressants (e.g., amitriptyline 10 to 25 mg/day) and other neurotropic agents (such as tegretol and gabapentum) can provide adjunctive assistance in chronic pain management. Localized nerve blocks and other anesthetic injections are yet another option in refractory situations. Transcutaneous electrical nerve stimulation (TENS) units, applications of heat and cold, and the use of therapeutic ultrasound have all been suggested, but largely without rigorously conducted randomized controlled trials to support their efficacy. Calcitonin and certain bisphosphonate medications have been promulgated for perceived effects on pain associated with acute compression deformities (see below).

Percutaneous vertebroplasty with polymethylmethacrylate impregnation into the vertebral body has been explored for the treatment of painful vertebral compression deformities. A case report (299) and an open-label study of 26 patients (300) describe acute pain relief in the vast majority of recipients. The mechanism of pain relief of this proposed technique and its long-term efficacy and safety merit further investigation.

Calcium and Vitamin D

The ability to absorb calcium diminishes with aging (301), and the average American diet includes less than 600 mg/day of calcium. Thus, conscientious calcium intake is a recommendation for older persons, in particular. In contrast to prescription antiresorptive agents, calcium alone may somewhat reduce but not fully prevent bone loss (302,303). In postmenopausal women, sufficient calcium provided through dietary and exogenous sources effectively decreases appendicular skeletal bone loss by 1% to 3% compared to women who do not consume adequate calcium (302,304–310). In a 4-year study of calcium treatment (1 g/day), BMD gains were most prominent during year 1 and declined during follow-up (although the calcium group continued to do better than placebo) (304). There was borderline reduction in the rate of symptomatic fracture in this study as well. The predominantly short-term effects of calcium may relate to their effects on transient remodeling, particularly the space of bone that is undergoing rapid turnover and that responds most rapidly to antiresorptive agents (311). Calcium may be most beneficial for women further out from menopause (307,312). However, even among younger women, calcium supplementation prevents bone loss at various skeletal sites (313,314). Bone loss in men may be less likely to be prevented by calcium and vitamin D (315). In a meta-analysis of trials using calcium with ERT versus ERT alone, there was a substantially larger increases in BMD at all sites using the combination (316).

Despite negative results from some observational studies (317–319), other observational (320,321) and a few interventional (304,322–324) investigations suggest that calcium may lower vertebral fracture rate by about 10%. The small size of these studies and the differences in populations limit our ability to form a meaningful conclusion about the effects of calcium on fracture rate. A meta-analysis of four randomized controlled trials (304,323–325) found a 24% risk reduction for hip fractures (326). However, the study by Chapuy et al. (325) showing a 30% hip fracture reduction also included 800 IU of vitamin D_3 in the intervention group.

Varying amounts of elemental calcium are found in different food groups and nutritional supplements (Table 122.9). Calcium is equally well absorbed (25–30%) from either milk products or from calcium carbonate (327).

TABLE 122.9. FOOD SOURCES OF BIOAVAILABLE CALCIUM

Food	Serving Size (g)	Calcium Content[a] (mg)	Fractional Absorption[b] (%)	Estimated Absorbable Ca/Serving (mg)	Servings Needed to Equal 1 Glass of Milk
Milk (or 1 glass yogurt or 1½ oz. cheddar cheese)	240	300	32.1	96.3	1.0
Beans, dried	177	50	15.6	7.8	12.3
Broccoli	71	35	61.3	21.5	4.5
Cabbage	85	79	52.7	41.6	2.3
Kale	65	47	58.8	27.6	3.5
Spinach	90	122	5.1	6.2	15.5
Tofu, calcium set	126	258	31.0	80.0	1.2

[a]Adjusted for load; for milk, this is fractional absorption (Fx abs) = 0.889 – 0.0964 in load; for low-oxalate vegetables, after adjusting by the ratio of fractional absorption determined for kale relative to milk at the same load, the equation becomes Fx abs = 0.959 – 0.0964 in load.
[b]Calcium content (mg) × Fx abs.
From Weaver CM, Heaney RP. Shils ME, Olson JA, Shike S, et al., eds. *Modern nutrition in health and disease,* 9th ed. Baltimore: Williams & Wilkins, 1999:147, with permission.

However, calcium is not equally bioavailable in all foods; certain leafy vegetables (e.g., spinach) have poor calcium bioavailability due to high oxalate content. Although some studies suggest that calcium citrate has slightly higher absorption than other preparations (328,329), other investigations indicate that they are equally well absorbed (330).

One area of controversy concerns the safe use of calcium supplements in patients with a history of nephroureterolithiasis. High intake of dietary calcium appears to decrease the risk of stones, whereas intake of high doses of supplemental calcium may modestly increase risk (331,332). Dietary calcium may beneficially bind oxalate, the primary ingredient in most renal stones.

Although calcium supplements are well tolerated by many, constipation (in about 10% of users) and dyspepsia limit long-term adherence. Trials of different preparations and times of administration may maximize patient satisfaction. Consensus recommendations for daily doses of elemental calcium range from 1,200 to 1,500 mg per day in postmenopausal women not on hormone replacement therapy (HRT) and 1,000 to 1,200 mg in premenopausal women, men, and postmenopausal women on HRT (268,333,334). The increasing variety of food and beverage products available in the United States that are calcium fortified have made heavy reliance on exogenous calcium salt supplements less necessary to achieve daily requirements.

Vitamin D is a group of fat-soluble sterols that includes ergocalciferol (vitamin D_2) and cholecalciferol (vitamin D_3). Most potent among vitamin D analogues are the active metabolites calcitriol and α-calcidol. Calcitriol is 1,25-dihydroxyvitamin D_3, a synthetic active metabolite of vitamin D. 1-α-hydroxyvitamin D_3 (α-calcidol), a synthetic precursor of calcitriol, is not available in the United States. Both active agents may increase calcium absorption and prevent spinal bone loss, particularly among older women (335–339). Despite BMD gains, several studies have not shown a beneficial effect of active vitamin D metabolites on fracture rate (340–342). A study of 622 women followed over a 3-year period showed a 69% reduction in vertebral fracture incidence on 0.5 μg daily of calcitriol (341). Of note, this study also showed an unexplained increase in fractures in the group receiving calcium alone. Furthermore, the potential for hypercalciuria and hypercalcemia with active vitamin D preparations limit their routine use and require careful serum and urine monitoring. If calcitriol is used, it is important to moderate calcium supplementation.

Inactivated vitamin D analogues also have been studied for their effects on bone. Vitamin D given as a large annual injection of 150,000 to 300,000 IU decreased nonvertebral fractures (343). In a large randomized placebo-controlled study of 3,270 institutionalized women in France, cholecalciferol 800 IU/day significantly decreased PTH levels, increased femoral BMD by 2.7%, and lowered the risk of hip and other nonvertebral fractures among elderly women (322,325). Another study of 389 men and women ages 65 and older who were supplemented with 500 mg of calcium plus 700 IU of vitamin D_3 confirmed a protective effect including both reduced bone loss and decreased incidence of nonvertebral fractures (344). In contrast, in a large Dutch study of over 2,500 older women, calcium plus 400 IU of vitamin D failed to demonstrate a protective effect against hip fracture (345). A final conclusion is confounded by differences in patient characteristics as well as doses and preparations of vitamin D among different studies. Because of the variability of serum vitamin D level assays, the high frequency of relative vitamin D deficiency among older adults, and accumulating data of vitamin D's direct benefits on bone, it is recommended that older adults be supplemented with 400 to 800 IU of vitamin D_3, the amount found in many multivitamins (268). In individuals with documented vitamin D deficiency or calcium malabsorption, higher vitamin D levels are needed.

Drug Therapies

The majority of pharmacologic therapies useful for the prevention and treatment of osteoporosis affect bone remodeling by either inhibiting bone resorption or enhancing bone formation. The majority of the agents currently licensed in the United States and other countries inhibit bone resorption. Reported below are the results of observational studies and clinical trials examining pharmacologic agents for primary prevention (before low bone mass), secondary prevention (after low bone mass but before fractures), and tertiary prevention (after fractures or in patients with very low bone mass) of osteoporosis.

Estrogen

Due to the accelerated rate of bone loss that occurs at the time of menopause, ERT has been commonly used in postmenopausal women to prevent osteoporosis. ERT has a direct effect on bone mass through receptors on osteoclasts and other bone cells, and it results in lowered bone turnover and resorption. In addition to its alleviation of menopausal symptoms, such as hot flashes and urogenital atrophy, ERT has long been advocated as a protective agent for postmenopausal bone loss. ERT is most effective in decreasing bone mass when initiated soon after menopause and used continuously. Prospective studies have demonstrated lumbar spine BMD increases of 1% to 4% at 1 year in women receiving conjugated estrogen at 0.3 to 0.625 mg/day in combination with calcium (346–352). One of the few primary prevention studies showed that 100 oophorectomized women treated with mestranol had gains of up to 29% in lumbar BMD over 10 years. There was also preservation of bone at the radius and metacarpal regions during the first 8 years of therapy followed by slow bone loss thereafter (353). More recently, the Postmenopausal Estrogen/Progestin Intervention (PEPI) trial showed about a 2% increase in hip BMD after 1 year in patients randomized to one of the treatment arms containing conjugated estrogen 0.625 mg/day (351). Of interest, 98% of women on ERT lost less than 1% per year, the median bone loss in the placebo group. BMD changes are paralleled by significant declines in biochemical markers of bone turnover such as urinary *N*-teleopeptide of type I collagen (266).

Observational studies suggest a 25% to 70% risk reduction for fractures associated with the use of ERT (198, 321,354–362). In addition to PEPI, Lufkin et al. (363) conducted one of the very few randomized controlled trials of ERT to show a significant effect on fractures. Use of the transdermal patch resulted in a 5.3% increase in lumbar BMD and a 61% reduction in vertebral fractures among older women with documented osteoporosis. This study additionally confirmed potential benefits of ERTs in older women who are at higher risk of fractures (364–367). Despite these data on spinal fractures, no clinical trial has been large enough to assess the risk of appendicular fractures.

In addition to their modest beneficial effects on bone, ERT raises high-density lipoproteins (HDL) and lowers low-density lipoproteins (LDL) in postmenopausal women (368,369). ERT affects climacteric symptoms, relieves vaginal dryness, and may improve female sexual function. ERT may decrease levels of plasminogen-activator inhibitor type 1, a potential partial explanation for its cardioprotective effects among some patients (370). A number of observational studies report a 35% to 80% reduction in cardiovascular events and prolonged survival among women with coronary heart disease (CHD) compared with nonusers (359,371–379). If women who chose to take ERT are healthier and have a more favorable CHD profile, it is possible that the cardiovascular risk reduction seen with ERT might be attributable to selection bias (377,380,381). Indeed, results from the Heart and Estrogen/Progestin Replacement Study (HERS), a randomized, blinded, placebo-controlled study of secondary cardiovascular prevention among women with prior vascular disease, identified an increase in CHD events in the first 2 years of therapy. This increase in CHD events occurred despite an [illegible]1% lowering of LDL and 10% rise in mean HDL level. S[illegible]ly more encouraging, there was a reduction in CHD e[illegible] year 4 and 5 of the trial (377). Since it is pos[illegible] women who have already experienced a vascular e[illegible] be preselected for a heightened prevalence of hyp[illegible] bility, it is unknown whether this deleterious effe[illegible] in secondary cardiovascular prevention carries o[illegible] mary prevention among the general public. Provo[illegible] liminary work suggests that estrogen may reduce [illegible] colorectal cancer (382) and be protective against [illegible] (383,384).

Beyond the heart disease controversy, three sig[illegible] concerns with ERT are an increased risk of thromboe[illegible] events (partially discussed above), hyperplastic effects [illegible] the endometrium potentially leading to endometrial cancer, and a heightened risk for breast cancer. Venous thromboembolic events are three to four times more common among estrogen users than nonusers (absolute risk of about 4 per 1,000) (377,385–388). Smoking may further heighten this risk and can also attenuate the effects of estrogen on bone (360). Estrogen causes endometrial thickening, an effect that is offset by the concomitant administration of progestin in women with an intact uterus. Estrogen and progestin can be administered in a cyclical fashion, although this will lead to some endometrial hyperplasia and women may experience menstrual-type bleeding. Alternatively, daily administration of estrogen with continuous low-dose progestin (e.g., medroxyprogesterone 2.5 mg/day) is generally well tolerated with rare breakthrough bleeding and no documented increase in the endometrial thickness. Although progestin may attenuate the estrogen-induced increase in serum HDL (351), it does not significantly impede bone benefits

(198,351). Indeed, progestin, like estrogen, decreases bone turnover, although to a lesser extent (389). Although many studies have failed to find an increased breast cancer risk with ERT (390,391), a combined analysis of 51 studies indicated that a relative risk of 1.35 for breast cancer is attributable to 5 years of estrogen compared with never-users (392,393). Invasive breast cancers that may develop among estrogen users appears to have a more favorable histologic prognosis (394). Data awaited from the ongoing Women's Health Initiative may further clarify the breast cancer controversy. ERT in women with a family history of breast cancer was not associated with increased breast cancer incidence in one large population-based cohort study (378), although a strong family history of breast cancer continues to be a major reservation to the recommendation of estrogen use for both patients and physicians.

Less life-threatening but more symptomatic concerns with estrogen use includes breast tenderness, weight gain, headaches, and hypertension. A major impediment to ERT is long-term adherence. A high proportion of estrogen prescriptions are never filled and less than 50% of women who initiate therapy are still using it 5 years later (395,396). Transdermal estrogens may be better tolerated with fewer side effects and improved adherence (397). Of note, for discontinuous users, withdrawal of estrogen results in accelerated bone loss ("catch-up") in some but not in all studies (361,398,399). Ultimately, the decision to initiate ERT needs to be individualized and based on a balanced assessment of risk and benefits by the physician and patient (274,400). Risk for breast cancer, potential for hypercoagulability, cardiovascular risk/benefit assessment, menopausal symptoms, and suitability for the use of alternative bone protective agents are among key considerations to balance in making a decision (359,401,402).

Selective Estrogen Receptor Modulators

An increasing array of mixed tissue-specific estrogen agonists/antagonists have been or are being developed for use in osteoporosis. Selective estrogen receptor modulators (SERMs) are nonsteroidal synthetic compounds that have estrogen-like properties on the bone and cardiovascular systems yet are estrogen antagonists to the breast and, in some cases, the endometrium. The first SERM, tamoxifen, has been used mostly as a preventative and therapeutic agent for breast cancer. It has a weak antiresorptive effect on vertebral BMD, although its uterine stimulatory effects and absence of amelioration of menopausal symptoms have markedly limited its use as an antiosteoporosis drug (403–405). The first SERM developed both for breast cancer prevention and for osteoporosis, raloxifene, is now licensed in many countries for osteoporosis (406). Raloxifene is a benzothipene derivative with antiestrogenic effects on the breast and uterus and estrogenic effects on the skeleton and lipid profile. It significantly lowers biochemical markers of bone remodeling to levels equivalent to conjugated estrogens (407). In postmenopausal women, after 6 months of raloxifene 60 mg/day, bone mass in the lumbar spine and total increased significantly by 2.4%. LDL, total cholesterol, and triglycerides all declined, and HDL increased (408). After 3 years of follow-up in the Multiple Outcomes of Raloxifene Evaluation (MORE), a multicenter study of over 7,700 postmenopausal women with at least one vertebral fracture or osteoporosis on the basis of a T-score ≤–2.5, 60 mg/day of raloxifene increased BMD of the spine by 2.6%, femoral neck BMD by 2.1%, and reduced vertebral fracture risk by 30% (409). To date, raloxifene has not been proven to prevent fractures at nonvertebral sites. Similar to tamoxifen, the risk of invasive breast cancer was decreased by 76% during the MORE study (410). Hot flashes and other menopausal symptoms may recur on raloxifene, but potentially less commonly than noted with tamoxifen. Similar to estrogen, with raloxifene there is an increase in lower extremity edema, as well as a roughly threefold increased risk of deep venous thrombosis (409). Additional SERMs, such as droloxifene, have preliminary data (411) and are now in final phases of clinical testing or under development.

Calcitonin

Calcitonin is a naturally occurring peptide hormone produced by the parafollicular C cells in the thyroid gland. Calcitonin binds to high-affinity receptors and directly inhibits osteoclasts leading to mild antiresorptive effects. Salmon calcitonin is a synthetic preparation that is 40 to 50 times more potent than human calcitonin and has the longest half-life of all synthetic preparations (412). When used for prevention or treatment of osteoporosis, salmon calcitonin is administered either subcutaneously (up to 100 IU daily for osteoporosis), or more commonly intranasally (200 IU daily). Nasal calcitonin results in sustained plasma levels, although its biologic activity is only 25% to 50% of that seen with parenteral administration. Calcitonin can also be administered rectally with reasonable absorption (413). Calcitonin should be administered with adequate calcium (at least 1 g) and vitamin D (400 IU day). Up to half of patients administered salmon calcitonin long-term develop calcitonin-specific antibodies. Although the significance of these antibodies on treatment effectiveness is not fully certain, neutralizing antibodies may retard the long-term effects of this agent (414). Some investigations have attempted to circumvent this problem by administering the agent intermittently (415). Randomized controlled trials of both injectable (416–419) and intranasal (420–423) calcitonin for treatment of established postmenopausal osteoporosis have consistently shown either stabilization of BMD or small but significant increases in vertebral BMD of approximately 1% to 3%. Beneficial BMD effects at the hip have not yet been reported. Modest increases in vertebral BMD with intranasal calcitonin are accompanied by significant declines in biochemical measures of bone resorption (424). Injectable calcitonin may work better for high turnover osteoporosis (425).

Two older studies have suggested but not confirmed a vertebral fracture protective effect of either injectable or nasal calcitonin (416,426). Preliminary results from a 5-year multicenter study designed to assess whether calcitonin nasal spray reduced vertebral fractures among postmenopausal women with established osteoporosis and at least one prevalent fracture showed a 36% reduction in vertebral fractures in the 200 IU group, but not in the 100 or 400 IU groups. Interpretation of study results was limited by an approximately 50% dropout rate (427).

Based on the results of several small controlled trials, calcitonin may also have analgesic efficacy for acute compression fracture pain (428–430). The exact mechanism of this analgesic effect is not well understood but may relate to increases in central nervous system effects on plasma endorphins (431).

Nasal calcitonin is generally well tolerated with occasional rhinitis minimized by alternating nostrils each day. Headache, flushing, nausea, and diarrhea have been reported more commonly with subcutaneous rather than with intranasal calcitionin.

Bisphosphonates

The bisphosphonates are a class of antiresorptive agents characterized by a phosphorus-carbon-phosphorus bond. Bisphosphonates are being increasingly recognized as potent inhibitors of bone resorption and fractures when administered orally or by intravenous infusion (432,433). Variations in the structure of the amino side chains of these drugs affects their pharmacologic activity (see comparative structures in Fig. 122.15). All oral bisphosphonates are poorly absorbed, with bioavailability of less than 1%. Thus, they must be taken on an empty stomach to maximize absorption. Bisphosphonates are rapidly cleared renally, with only 20% to 60% remaining in the bone. In bone, these agents bind tightly to hydroxyapatite crystals in the resorption lacunae of bone where they have a long skeletal retention (about 10 years for alendronate). Only bisphosphonates present on the bone surface exert an antiresorptive effect. After prolonged administration, a regional paracrine effect of continuously deposited bisphosphonates may account for a lack of rapid loss of BMD gains seen when these agents are discontinued (434). The mechanism of action of bisphosphonates is incompletely understood but it appears that the nitrogen-containing bisphosphonates (i.e., alendronate and risedronate) serve as antiresporptive agents by impairing cholesterol metabolism of the osteoclast, leading to cytoskeletal alterations and premature osteoclast cell death via apoptosis (435–437). Bisphosphonates may also have poorly defined anabolic effects that could correlate with

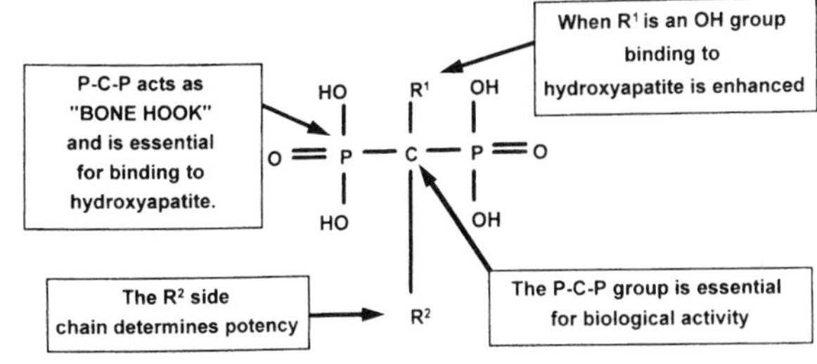

BISPHOSPHONATE	R1	R2
Etidronate*	OH	CH_3
Clodronate*	Cl	Cl
Pamidronate*	OH	$CH_2CH_2\ NH_2$
Alendronate*	OH	$(CH_2)_3\ NH_2$
Risedronate*	OH	CH_2-3-pyridine
Tiludronate*	H	CH_2-S-phenyl-Cl
Ibandronate*	OH	$CH_2CH_2\ N(CH_3)$ (pentyl)
Zoledronate	OH	CH_2-imidazole
YH529	OH	CH_2-2-imidazo-pyridinyl
Incadronate (YM175)	H	N-(cyclo-heptyl)
Olpadronate	OH	$CH_2CH_2\ N(CH_3)_2$
Neridronate	OH	$(CH_2)_5\ NH_2$
EB-1053	OH	CH_2-1-pyrrolidinyl

* indicates bisphosphonates already approved for one or more indications in one or more countries. Pamidronate is the most extensively used for Pagets Disease.

FIGURE 122.15. Structures of bisphosphonates used in clinical studies and under development. (From Graham R, Russell G, Rogers MJ, et al. The pharmacology of biphosphonates and new insights into their mechanisms of action. *J Bone Miner Res* 1999; 14:53–65, with permission.)

the persistent increase in BMD seen beyond the first year of therapy when the remodeling space is filled-in.

As a class, bisphosphonates may cause gastrointestinal intolerance, particularly at low pH (438). There have been rare reports of severe esophagitis (439). Recommendations to reduce gastrointestinal symptoms and maximize absorption (bisphosphonates are bound by divalent cations) include ingesting pills with 8 oz water, remaining upright for at least 30 minutes after swallowing the tablet, and having nothing to eat or drink for 30 to 60 minutes before and after ingesting each pill. Achalasia and esophageal strictures are contraindications to bisphosphonate therapy. Some studies suggest that gastrointestinal safety may be better for particular agents (440).

Four bisphosphonates—etidronate, alendronate, risedronate, and pamidronate—are licensed in many countries for osteoporosis, Paget's disease, myositis ossificans progressiva, heterotopic ossification, and/or hypercalcemia. Three additional agents—clodronate, tiludronate, and ibandronate—are available in at least one country but are less commonly used than the other agents used for osteoporosis.

Etidronate, a first-generation medicinal bisphosphonate, was originally developed as a detergent additive to soften hard water (441). Because of its lower potency and the need for higher doses, continuous administration of etidronate may impair osteoblast function and lead to bone mineralization abnormalities such as osteomalacia. Etidronate is thus administered cyclically, typically 400 mg/day 2 weeks out of every 3 months. Etidronate reduces bone turnover to levels seen in premenopausal women. In postmenopausal women with one to four osteoporotic compression fractures and radiologic evidence of osteopenia, cyclically administered etidronate increased BMD by 4% over 2 years (442). A slight reduction in vertebral fractures, predominately in high-risk groups, has been noted in some studies (442–444). Fracture reduction at nonvertebral sites has not been demonstrated with etidronate. Beneficial effects have been seen in both fracture-free patients (445) and in early menopausal women (446). Etidronate combined with estrogen resulted in more BMD gain than with either agent alone (11% increase in lumbar BMD with the combination) (447).

Pamidronate has been used most commonly for the treatment of lytic bone metastases and Paget's disease (448,449). It is used uncommonly for osteoporosis treatment. For patients with postmenopausal or idiopathic osteoporosis, oral pamidronate (150 mg/day in conjunction with other antiosteoporotic therapy) significantly increased and sustained a 3% gain in vertebral bone mineral content over 1 year (450). Intravenous pamidronate at 60 mg every 3 months for 1 year also alleviated chronic back pain associated with vertebral fractures (451). In clinical practice, many start with 30 mg every 3 months and increase the dose based on response to therapy. Side effects with intravenous administration included malaise, nausea, fever, and skeletal pain. Intravenous pamidronate is a therapeutic alternative for patients with severe osteoporosis who cannot tolerate oral bisphosphonates.

Alendronate, a second-generation bisphosphonate, was the first aminobisphosphonate approved by the FDA for the treatment and prevention of osteoporosis. Human and primate work indicate that alendronate is a potent inhibitor of bone resorption without detrimental effects on mineralization (452–454). Multiple studies of postmenopausal women receiving 10 mg alendronate daily showed a lumbar spine BMD increase of 7% to nearly 9% over a 2-year period (455,456). Smaller significant changes were seen at the femoral neck and trochanter. In early postmenopausal women, 5 mg/day of alendronate prevented the loss of BMD at the spine, hip, and total body (457). In a separate study, the 5-mg dose prevented bone loss to nearly the same extent as an estrogen-progestin combination (estrogen effect was 1% to 2% greater than 5 mg) (458). Among over 2,027 older women with at least one prior vertebral fracture and low femoral neck BMD in the Fracture Intervention Trial (FIT), alendronate led to a significant 47% and 51% reduction in morphometric vertebral and hip fractures, respectively (459). In FIT subjects without prevalent vertebral fractures, alendronate 10 mg/day decreased radiographic vertebral fractures by 44% (460). A multinational study of alendronate similarly identified a 47% risk reduction for nonvertebral fractures (461). In a meta-analysis of all published and proprietary data (five studies), the relative risk of a nonvertebral fractures was 0.71 (462). In postmenopausal women with low BMD despite ongoing ERT, the addition of alendronate significantly increased BMD in the lumbar spine and hip trochanter (463). A residual decrease in bone turnover may be found for up to 2 years after discontinuation of alendronate (434,464). Safety has been acceptable in clinical trials with no significant increases in serious adverse effects or significant gastrointestinal adverse effects between treatment groups or placebo. In a study of glucocorticoid-induced osteoporosis, there was a small increase in nonserious upper gastrointestinal adverse effects on those taking alendronate 10 mg but not 5 mg or placebo (465). Results of bone histomorphometry indicate that alendronate increases bone turnover in a dose-dependent manner but does not impair mineralization (452,454).

Risedronate is a third-generation pyridinyl bisphosphonate that increases bone mass and prevents fractures (466). Treatment with 5 mg of risedronate significantly lowered the risk of both new vertebral (41% reduction) and nonvertebral (39% reduction) over a 3-year period in women with at least one prior vertebral fracture (467). Preliminary data suggest a potential beneficial effect of risedronate 5 mg daily on hip fractures among women with very low bone mass. Risedronate is generally well tolerated with no significant differences in upper gastrointestinal adverse events between those receiving placebo and risedronate (467). Tiludronate has also been shown to prevent postmenopausal bone loss (468).

There are an increasing number of studies documenting the effectiveness of several bisphosphonates both in terms of BMD gains and, of more importance, with regard to reduction of both vertebral and nonvertebral fractures. It appears that from a bone perspective, newer bisphosphonates are the most consistently effective antiresporptive agents currently available. Despite an increasing duration of significant worldwide experience with bisphosphonates, questions remain on the exact mechanism by which these agents work, the necessary duration of therapy, long-term safety among women of child-bearing potential, and safety and efficacy in children.

Sodium Fluoride

Fluoride is an anabolic agent approved in many countries for the treatment of osteoporosis. It has not gained widespread acceptance in the United States due in part to its narrow therapeutic window and studies reporting higher fracture rates despite increased vertebral BMD. Fluoride is a potent stimulator of new bone via a mitogenic effect on the osteoblast, and it typically leads to a rapid increase in axial BMD (469). Increased vertebral BMD of up to 8% may occur, potentially at the expense of BMD loss in peripheral bones (such as the midradius).

Despite the BMD effects, there has been either no protective effect or a heightened risk of both vertebral and nonvertebral fractures (470–475). A randomized trial of 25 mg of monofluorophosphate in 460 elderly men and women in Finland showed a trend toward more fractures in those getting treatment rather than placebo (476). Fluoride appears to increase trabecular width, but it does not form new trabeculae (477). Stress fractures of weight-bearing bones (leading to a lower extremity pain syndrome) (478,479), osteomalacia (480), and an increased risk of femoral neck fractures (481) have been observed.

Fluoride may result in arthralgias/arthritis and numerous gastrointestinal side effects (dyspepsia, nausea, vomiting) in about 30% of users, although gastrointestinal symptoms appear less frequent with the slow-release preparation.

Fluoride's variable effect on bone is likely influenced by differences in dose, preparation, treatment regimen, duration of therapy, and variable populations treated. In patients with established osteoporosis, the beneficial effects of fluoride on both BMD and vertebral fracture end points may be potentially achieved by administering sodium fluoride at moderate doses [20 mg/day (475) or 50 mg/day (482)], using it in patients with milder osteoporosis (475), and choosing a slow-release preparation combined with calcium citrate (483,484). Intermittent use of slow-release fluoride is associated with few bone histologic abnormalities (485). Since slow release fluoride is not available in the United States and the other preparations have a very narrow therapeutic window with mixed beneficial and deleterious results, the routine use of fluoride cannot be recommended.

Androgens

Use of androgens for male osteoporosis is discussed below. In women, synthetic androgens such as nandrolone decanoate and stanazol have been tried with small increases in BMD (486–490). Virilizing side effects, lowering of HDL, hepatotoxicity, and the need for parenteral administration minimize the enthusiasm for androgens.

Thiazide Diuretics

Observational investigations suggesting that thiazide diuretics may maintain BMD and prevent fractures are discussed under Epidemiology Risk Factors for Low BMD and Fracture (see above) (212,213,215,216,491). Additionally, in men with osteoporosis, correction of hypercalciuria with low-dose thiazides can lead to a significant increase in BMD (492). In addition to their effects on lowering blood pressure, thiazides have adverse effects on lipid and electrolyte profiles and are generally not well tolerated by the normotensive patient. Given their relatively weak effects on bone in nonhypercalciuric patients, they are not a first-line therapy.

Potential Future Therapies

Parathyroid Hormone (PTH)

In contrast to its perceived catabolic action on bone, exogenously administered PTH can increase bone turnover and lead to in an elevated BMD in both rodent models and, more recently, in human studies (493–495). Estrogen-deficient perimenopausal women receiving PTH (amino acids 1–34) had less bone loss from the proximal femur and experienced increased BMD in the spine (496,497). Osteoporotic men getting PTH and 1,25-$(OH)_2$ vitamin D also had improved spinal bone mass (498). In postmenopausal women on estrogen, PTH (1–34) given as subcutaneous injections significantly increased BMD by 13% at the lumbar spine and decreased incident vertebral fractures of the spine (499). A small study of postmenopausal women with osteoporosis also showed significant increases in lumbar BMD (500). The effects of PTH appear to be preserved even in the presence of potent antiresorptive agents such as alendronate (501). Selective parathyroid receptor agonists and antagonists are under investigation and may play a future role in osteoporosis (502). Although many questions remain about the dose, mode of administration, potential toxicity, and selective effects on different skeletal sites, PTH retains promise as a bone anabolic agent.

Growth Factors

Use in osteoporosis of growth hormone (GH), insulin-like growth factor I (IGF-1), and TGF-β stems from the benefits of GH supplementation for children with significant growth retardation (503), the known reduction in IGF levels with aging and osteoporosis (504), and the prominent role that TGF-β plays in bone development. In men with low IGF-1 levels, three times per week administration of biosynthetic GH resulted in a significant 1.6% increase in lumbar BMD at 6 months (505). GH given cyclically, either alone or with calcitonin for 2 years, achieved a significant 2.7% increase in BMD of the lumbar spine and hip in postmenopausal women (506). This effect, however, was not significantly different from calcitonin alone. Recombinant growth factors have been used short-term in women with osteoporosis (503,507). IGF-1 may enhance formation of type I collagen more than GH in men with idiopathic osteoporosis (508). Modest BMD gains are associated with a relatively high incidence of adverse experiences such as gynecomastia and edema. Of even greater concern, growth factors are mitogenic and high levels of IGF-1 may potentate prostate and breast cancer.

Tibolone

Tibolone is a synthetic steroid with estrogenic, androgenic, and progesterogenic properties (509). Unlike estrogen, it does not stimulate the endometrium, yet it may be effective in treating climacteric symptoms. A number of small and moderate-sized trials have evaluated its effects on bone with increases in lumbar BMD (510–512), particularly notable in early postmenopausal women (513). In one study, there was less perimenopausal bleeding in comparison with a combined estrogen/progestin regimen (514). Fracture data are not yet available, and further studies are needed to assess long-term safety and effectiveness.

Ipriflavone

Ipriflavone is a synthetic flavenoid that may have a beneficial effect on BMD of the radius and spine in established and early osteoporosis (515–517). It is already licensed in some countries.

SPECIAL TOPICS

Glucocorticoid-Induced Osteoporosis

Epidemiology

For several decades, osteoporosis has been a well-recognized complication of supraphysiologic levels of glucocorticoids (518–520). Glucocorticoid-induced osteoporosis (GIOP) is second in frequency only to the osteoporosis that occurs after menopause and is the commonest form of drug-induced osteoporosis. Based on community surveys, glucocorticoids are used by an estimated 0.2% to 0.5% of the general population (521–523). Patients with RA, polymyalgia rheumatica, temporal arteritis, and other chronic rheumatic disorders compose over half of glucocorticoid users in some populations (521).

During the first 6 to 12 months of glucocorticoid therapy, there is an initial rapid loss of 3% to 27% of BMD (107,524–527). Trabecular bone is preferentially affected followed ultimately by losses in cortical bone (528). The literature is divided, however, on whether trabecular bone is lost most rapidly from the trochanter (529–533) or the lumbar spine (219,534). Among RA patients receiving steroids, the hands and forearms may be partially spared from bone loss (107,535). Bone loss may be potentially reversible by lowering or cessation of the glucocorticoid (107). Cumulative steroid dose is the most important predictor of bone loss (528,531,532,536). Alternate-day dosing does not spare bone (537). Early in the course of GIOP there is a generalized thinning of trabeculae, and, in contrast to idiopathic osteoporosis, it is not until later that trabecular disconnections occur (538). Following approximately 2 years of glucocorticoid therapy, there is a slowed rate of bone loss in many patients. However, BMD continues to be lost at a rate higher than with normal aging.

In addition to older women, significant bone loss may occur in both men (219,539–541) and in premenopausal women (542). However, people who already have very low bone mass (such as postmenopausal women who have not taken hormone replacement therapy) are more likely to reach a fracture threshold sooner (Fig. 122.16). Certain dis-

A 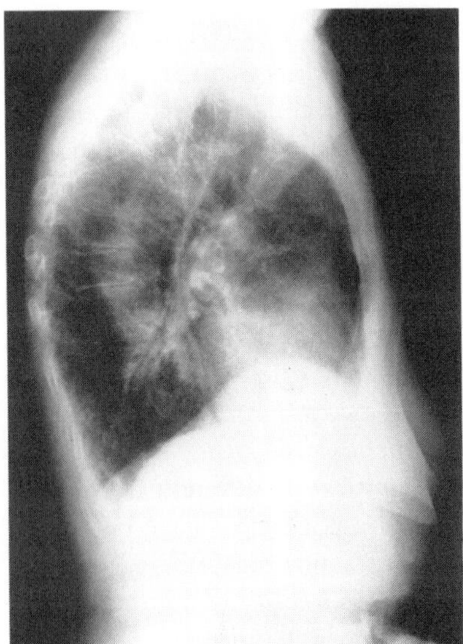

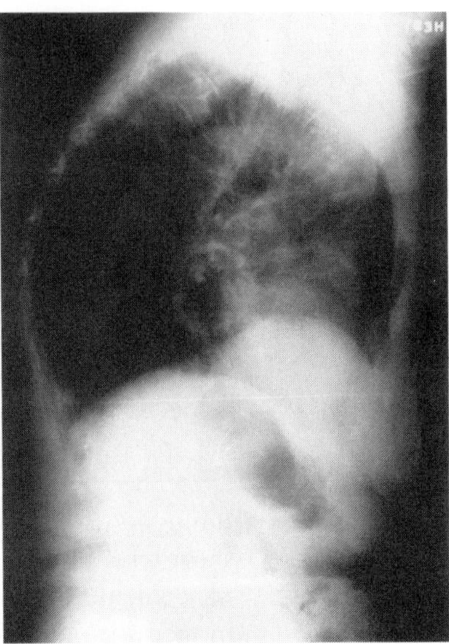 B

FIGURE 122.16. A: Lateral chest radiograph of a 70-year old woman recently begun on 60 mg of prednisone for temporal arteritis *(left).* Although radiographs do not demonstrate osteoporosis until 30% of bone mass has already been lost, it appears she already has low bone mass. **B:** Lateral chest radiograph 1 year after having received an average dosage of 20 mg/day of prednisone *(right).* She has developed an accentuated thoracic kyphosis due to multiple painful compression deformities.

eases and treatments concomitantly accelerate bone loss. RA causes both regional and generalized bone loss (531, 533,543–547). Similar bone effects have been noted with polymyalgia rheumatica (548). Independent of glucocorticoids, RA patients are at higher risk for fracture (549,550). Glucocorticoids are associated with significant bone loss and fractures in populations of predominantly younger women with systemic lupus erythematosis (551,552). A large literature also confirms the negative effects of glucocorticoids on bone in other inflammatory diseases very commonly requiring glucocorticoids (522) such as asthma (553–556), chronic obstructive pulmonary disease (541), inflammatory bowel disease (557–559), nephrotic syndrome (560), sarcoidosis (561), and organ transplantation (see below).

Controversy exists about whether a safe glucocorticoid dose exists, particularly in the context of RA treatments (520). A number of cross-sectional and even some longitudinal investigations have failed to identify an adverse effect of low-dose glucocorticoids on bone in RA patients (529,543, 544,562–564). Some authors have proposed that glucocorticoids do not adversely effect bone and may even protect bone in RA patients by improving functional status and reducing circulating proinflammatory cytokines that are deleterious to bone (543,564). Observational studies have suggested that prednisone doses below 5 mg/day may have fewer negative effects on bone among RA patients (534,565). However, several of these studies were small, and the possibility of missing an important effect due to a type II statistical error exists. A meta-analysis concluded that the effect of glucocorticoids on bones among RA patients was at worst modest (566). However, one of the included studies reported improved BMD at the lumbar spine, but paradoxically showed bone loss at all other locations measured (530). When the authors pooled only randomized controlled trials (n = 2), they observed a deleterious effect of glucocorticoids on bone. Notwithstanding, a single dose of only 2.5 mg of prednisone has almost immediate effects on serum osteocalcin levels, a measure of bone formation (567).

Since glucocorticoids may affect both bone quantity and quality (568), fractures are the outcome measure of greatest importance. Indeed, glucocorticoid-treated patients may experience fractures at a higher BMD threshold than nonusers (569). Studies of steroid dose effects are confounded by the variable timing of glucocorticoid administration, differing disease process, variable alternative osteoporosis risk factors (independent of glucocorticoid use), and the fact that fracture risk is ultimately determined by factors other than just BMD. Case control studies of general populations show that glucocorticoids lead to a roughly twofold increased risk of fractures independent of age, gender, and the presence of RA (550,570). Among RA patients, an increased rate of fractures has been observed in both cross-sectional and longitudinal studies (525,565,571–573). A large observational study of RA patients indicated that a woman taking an average dosage of 8.6 mg of prednisone has a nearly 33% chance of a self-reported clinical fracture after 5 years of follow-up (572). Other observational studies suggest that over 40% of long-term users will ultimately fracture (528,574). At least two retrospective studies identify fractures as one of the most commonly documented complication of supraphysiologic glucocorticoid use (565, 573). However, observational studies of this type may be prone to selection bias and confounding by indication, whereby sicker RA patients are more likely to have an adverse outcome. Placebo arms of randomized controlled trials document about a 15% incidence of morphometrically defined vertebral fractures after only 1 year in patients on median doses of less than 10 mg/day (465,575). Although safer for bone than oral or enteral glucocorticoids, even nonsystemically administered glucocorticoids may have biologic effects on bone (576–579).

To further explore whether a safe dose exists, a large review of administrative data from the United Kingdom identified over 240,000 glucocorticoid users who were matched by age, gender, and clinical practice to a similar-sized cohort of nonsystemic (topical, opthalmic, aural, or nasal) glucocorticoid users. The relative risk of both hip and spine fractures increased in a dosage-dependent fashion, with a trend toward increased risk seen even below the physiologic range of 2.5 to 7.5 mg/d of prednisolone. This study, taken in context of the other investigations, provides further evidence that a safe dose of glucocorticoid for bone may not truly exist (Fig. 122.17) (580).

Pathogenesis

The etiology of GIOP is multifactorial and occurs, in many cases, concomitantly with normal age and menopause-associated bone loss. There are two major pathways by which patients on glucocorticoids develop abnormalities in bone

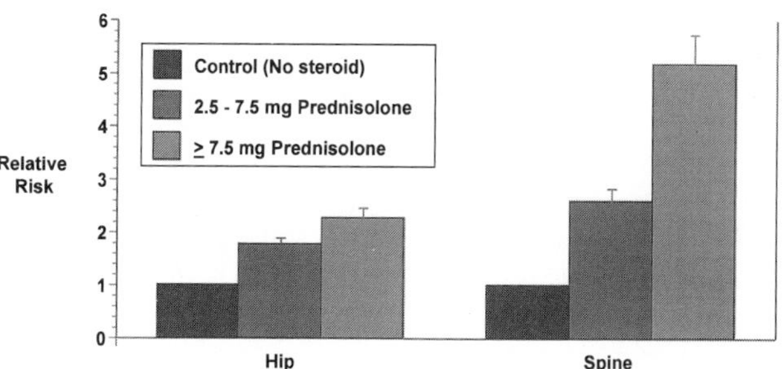

FIGURE 122.17. Effects of low-dose prednisolone on bone. The relative risk of both hip and spine fracture increases in a dosage-dependent fashion, with a trend toward increased risk seen even below the physiologic replacement range of 2.5 to 7.5 mg/day of prednisolone. (From Van Staa TP, Leufkens HGM, Abenhaim L, et al. Use of oral corticosteroids and risk of fractures. *J Bone Miner Res* 2000;15:993–1000, with permission.)

metabolism: first, a reduction in bone formation, and second, an increase in bone resorption (581–583). Controversy exists surrounding the relative importance of these mechanisms on bone loss among glucocorticoid users.

Glucocorticoids increase bone resorption by decreasing calcium absorption (584,585) and increasing urinary calcium excretion (586,587). These effects on calcium may be partially mediated by direct effects of glucocorticoids on vitamin D or its receptors (588). As reported by some but not by all investigators, reduced serum levels of ionized calcium may lead to a relative secondary hyperparathyroidism and increased bone resorption (586). Glucocorticoids also enhance the responsiveness of the osteoblasts, which potentiates bone resorption (589). Glucocorticoids reduce circulating levels of sex hormones that normally inhibit bone resorption (590–592).

Of potentially greatest importance, glucocorticoids adversely affect bone formation (593). Histologically, this is indicated by reduced trabecular wall thickness (594). Glucocorticoids cause both a decrease in absolute number of osteoblasts and their premature death by apoptosis. Glucocorticoids modulate the response of osteoblasts to skeletal growth factors such as IGF-1, IGF-2 and cytokines such as TGF-β and platelet-derived growth factor-B (PDGF-B) (583). Osteoblast inhibition is evident by decreases in serum osteocalcin levels (588,595). Osteoblast dysfunction results in incomplete repair of the bone remodeling lacunae (596) (Fig. 122.18).

Diagnostic Evaluation of the Patient on Glucocorticoids

There should be a high suspicion for potential bone loss among all patients initiating or chronically using glucocorticoids. The most effective way to determine a person's osteoporosis status and risk for future bone loss is to assess BMD by DXA or an alternate bone mass measurement technique. Current recommendations for bone mass measurement of patients on glucocorticoids have been proposed by the U.S. Bone Mass Measurement Act and by different medical societies and federal agencies (129,131,597,598). Most guidelines suggest a BMD test if the patient will receive treatment with >7.5 mg of prednisone or its equivalent and treatment for at least 1 to 6 months. The lumbar spine and trochanter demonstrate rapid bone loss with glucocorticoids and respond reliably to effective GIOP interventions, and thus are sensitive imaging sites. Peripheral BMD measurements in the wrist, fingers, and heels, while generally valid and predictive of fracture risk, might be influenced by the localized effects of arthritis, or limited by positioning difficulties due to joint deformities. If only a single site can be measured in an older arthritis patient on glucocorticoids, a hip DXA is preferred.

It is also important to consider gonadal status in chronic glucocorticoid users. In perimenopausal women, measurement of the follicle-stimulating hormone (FSH) and estradiol levels may provide further clarification. Premenopausal

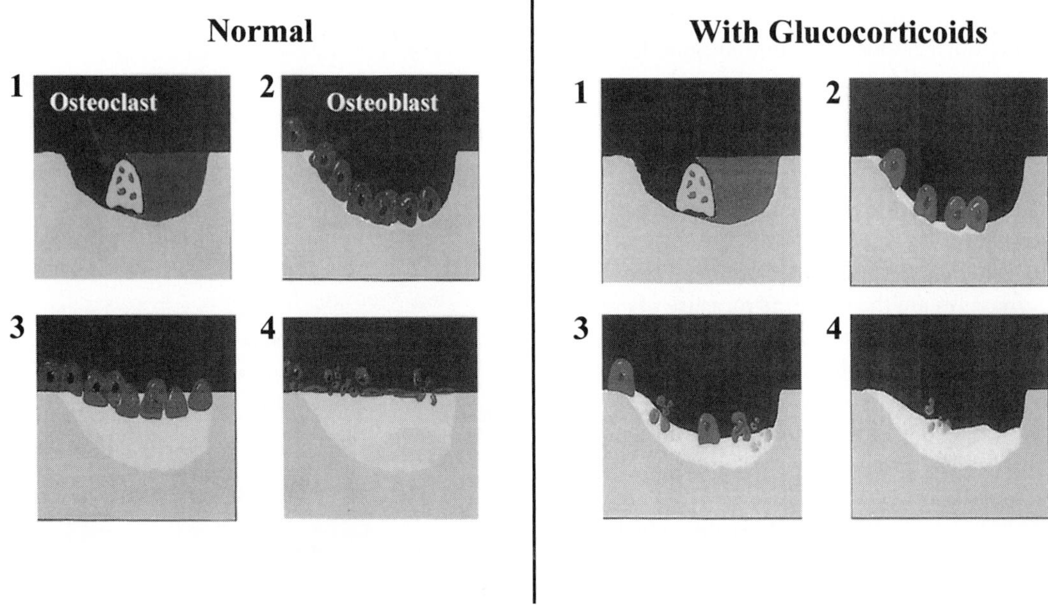

FIGURE 122.18. Normal cycle of bone remodeling shown **(left)** with an abnormal one caused by glucocorticoid excess **(right)**. Glucocorticoid-associated osteoporosis is caused by both a decrease in absolute number of osteoblasts and their premature death by apoptosis. Osteoblast dysfunction results in the incomplete repair of bone remodeling lacunae. (From Manolagas SC, Weinstein RS. New developments in the pathogenesis and treatment of steroid-induced osteoporosis. *J Bone Miner Res* 1999;14:1061–1066, with permission)

women with severe RA also may be estrogen deficient, often manifested by oligomenorrhea or amenorrhea. Given a well-defined association between RA and male hypogonadism (599,600), measurement of free testosterone in men on chronic glucocorticoids, or those with symptoms of gonadal insufficiency, is warranted.

A very high value of a bone resorption marker (such as urinary *N*-telopeptides or deoxypyridinoline cross-links) may identify patients with particularly rapid bone turnover or substantiate a lack of response to antiresorptive agents. An elevated 24-hour urinary calcium to creatinine ratio (greater that 250 mg for women or 300 mg for men) is also indicative of rapid bone turnover, such as seen among patients newly using glucocorticoid.

Even in patients who are assumed to have osteoporosis on the basis of severe RA, chronic glucocorticoid use, or their postmenopausal status, selective screening for other causes of bone loss should be considered. Hyperparathyroidism, hyperthyroidism, osteomalacia (due to poor dietary vitamin D intake and inadequate sun exposure), or multiple myeloma can all contribute to low bone mass among patients on glucocorticoids. Although not indicated in all glucocorticoid users with low BMD, laboratory evaluation for these and other conditions should be undertaken based on clinical suspicion.

Prevention and Treatment

The most effective intervention for prevention of bone loss and fractures among glucocorticoid users is glucocorticoid discontinuation or, at a minimum, dose reduction (601). Practically, this is not always possible due to the severity of many chronic inflammatory diseases. Putative bone-sparing glucocorticoids such as deflazacort have been identified (530,602) but are not available in the United States and may not be truly safer than conventional glucocorticoids at an equipotent dose. Based on an understanding of the pathogenesis of GIOP, a number of the agents used in postmenopausal osteoporosis have particular relevance for GIOP. As discussed below, vitamin D and calcium may increase gastrointestinal calcium absorption and limit renal losses, thiazide diuretics may decrease urinary calcium excretion, estrogen and testosterone supplements may help offset gonadal deficiency, bisphosphonates and calcitonin may prevent bone resorption, and fluoride and PTH might stimulate osteoblastic bone formation.

Calcium and Vitamin D

Calcium decreases bone resorption as measured by urinary hydroxyproline (603). However, calcium alone may not prevent bone loss, particularly in patients prone to poor absorption (604). In accord with the American College of Rheumatology GIOP guidelines (605), elemental calcium at 1,200 to 1,500 mg/d is necessary, although generally not sufficient as a sole therapy for most patients on glucocorticoids.

Vitamin D can be administered in a variety of formulations that have been investigated for GIOP prevention and treatment (528,606–608). In a prevention study, calcium, calcitriol, and calcitonin used in varying combinations were given to patients for 1 year, and then patients were followed for an additional second year off therapy. At the lumbar spine, those subjects randomized to receive a combination containing calcitriol experienced significantly less bone loss than those receiving calcium alone. In year 2, a slight lumbar spine BMD increase was seen among those subjects who received calcitonin. No differential effects between the three treatment arms was observed at the femoral neck, where bone loss occurred in all three treatment groups (606). Indicative of the need to carefully monitor serum and urinary calcium in patients receiving 0.5 to 1.0 μg of calcitriol (when used in combination with calcium), nearly 25% of those patients receiving calcitriol developed hypercalcemia. Other studies of active D metabolites, particularly α-calcidol, have shown efficacy in several (607,608), but not all, studies (528).

Inactivated vitamin D preparations may also have merit in GIOP. In a 2-year trial of RA patients on chronic low doses of glucocorticoids, 1,000 mg of calcium carbonate and 500 IU of vitamin D prevented bone loss in the lumbar spine and trochanter (609). An earlier study of smaller doses of both vitamin D and calcium did not demonstrate a significant differential effect of calcium alone, although a small increase in BMD was noted in both groups (610). Data are more equivocal with respect to ergocalciferol, typically administered orally as 50,000 units once weekly (611). A meta-analysis of different formulations of vitamin D, including its active metabolites and analogues, demonstrated a moderate pooled effect size at the lumbar spine of 0.6 (95% CI = 0.34–0.85) (612). The meta-analysis conclusions did not vary if only active vitamin D metabolites were analyzed or if the analysis was restricted only to prevention studies. Due to the impairment in calcium absorption mediated by glucocorticoids and the common occurrence of vitamin D deficiency among housebound patients suffering with chronic inflammatory conditions, vitamin D should be supplemented in all glucocorticoid users (613,614). This can be simply and efficaciously accomplished by providing 800 IU/day of vitamin D_3, available through a multivitamin, and the additional D contained in many calcium supplements. Provided that there is careful use of exogenous calcium and monitoring of urine and serum calcium, vitamin D might alternatively be administered as calcitriol.

Thiazide Diuretics

Only one study has specifically examined the efficacy of thiazides agent in glucocorticoid-treated patients. In combination with dietary sodium restriction, hydrochlorthiazide 50 mg twice a day improved total body calcium economy (615). Despite this paucity of evidence, thiazides may make pathophysiologic sense during the early phase of glucocorticoid use when there is profound hypercalciuria. On the other hand, the side effects of thiazides substantially moderate enthusiasm.

Calcitonin

When bone mass is measured at the lumbar spine, calcitonin is weakly effective at both preventing and treating GIOP. In addition to the Sambrook et al. (606) prevention trial discussed above, Adachi and colleagues (616) found that spinal bone density declined on placebo (5%), while the calcitonin-treated group had a nonsignificant decline of 1.3% over 1 year. Although less lumbar bone was lost in an observational study of sarcoid patients who received calcitonin for GIOP prevention (617), a randomized controlled prevention study in polymyalgia rheumatica patients did not show greater bone preservation with injectable calcitonin (618). In one of three treatment studies, placebo patients lost 7.8% BMD over 2 years, while the nasal calcitonin–treated group had an increase of 2.8% (619). An asthma treatment study of subcutaneous calcitonin showed similar levels of BMD gain in the forearm (620). However, at a lower dose, 100 IU/day, nasal calcitonin was not efficacious in treating the spine (621). For glucocorticoid-induced osteoporosis, calcitonin is a relatively weak antiresorptive agent. It potentially maintains bone mass but, in most studies, calcitonin does not lead to a marked increase in BMD. There has not been a documented benefit of its effects on fracture reduction in GIOP.

Estrogen and Testosterone

In the only randomized controlled trial of ERT in GIOP, postmenopausal women with RA received either ERT (transdermal estradiol 50 μ/d) or calcium supplementation (400 mg/d) (622). At the end of 2 years, women on ERT had higher bone density in the spine than those receiving calcium alone. There were no significant differences at the femur. Two small observational studies of ERT demonstrated reduced bone loss in the spine among chronic glucocorticoid users (623,624).

A randomized crossover trial of testosterone in the treatment of GIOP examined men with asthma (625). All hypogonadal men were also given calcium supplements (1,000 mg/d). The results of the study indicate that BMD of the lumbar spine increased significantly on testosterone, whereas it decreased with placebo. In men with low serum testosterone, intermittent administration of medroxyprogesterone also may help maintain bone mass (626). No primary prevention studies of estrogen have been completed and fracture data are similarly unavailable. Hormonally deficient women and men should be offered replacement for bone as well as other potential health benefits. Hormone replacement therapy is not indicated just in older women but also in premenopausal women who are oligomenorrheic or amenorrheic associated with their chronic inflammatory diseases and men who are hypogonadal (both on the basis of their underlying disorders and/or glucocorticoid effects). SERMs may offer an as yet unproven therapeutic option in glucocorticoid-induced osteoporosis.

Bisphosphonates

When administered over 1 or 2 years to patients on glucocorticoids for a variety of chronic inflammatory disorders, etidronate, pamidronate, alendronate, and risedronate are efficacious in preventing and/or treating bone loss at the spine and in regions of the hip. A number of observational or open-label studies (627–634) and at least seven randomized controlled clinical trials (611,628,635–639) have examined the effects of etidronate on GIOP. Of the randomized studies, most have demonstrated either increased (611,635,637) or preserved (628,636) lumbar BMD compared with placebo, which often included calcium. In the largest prevention trial, cyclical etidronate was instituted within 100 days of prednisone initiation in 141 men and women, beginning prednisone therapy for a variety of conditions (611). The placebo group had a decrease in lumbar BMD of 3.2%, while the treatment group had an increase of 0.6% at 1 year. Similar effects were seen at the trochanter. Bone density at the femoral neck did not differ significantly between groups. A trend toward a significant fracture reduction was seen in the postmenopausal women in this study. The largest treatment study with etidronate also confirmed that etidronate, when administered with calcium and vitamin D, resulted in a significant 4.5% increase in lumbar BMD (635).

Alendronate has proven efficacy in both preventing and treating bone loss associated with glucocorticoid use and in preventing vertebral fractures (465,640,641). In the combined report from two multinational studies, 477 new and chronic glucocorticoid users were studied, including postmenopausal women, premenopausal women, and men. At the spine, there was a significant increase in BMD of 2.9% on 10 mg of alendronate, and a slight loss of 0.4% on placebo. Similar effects were seen at the trochanter, and smaller but significant gains in BMD were noted at the femoral neck (465). A second-year extension to this study among 208 (37%) of the original subjects who continued to take >7.5 mg of prednisone (or equivalent glucocorticoid) documented similar beneficial effects at the spine, trochanter, and femoral neck (642). A significant 90% reduction in an overall small number of incident vertebral fractures was also observed. Of note, 5 mg of alendronate was statistically equivalent to 10 mg, except among postmenopausal women not receiving estrogen, where 10 mg resulted in significantly greater increases in lumbar BMD.

Risedronate at either 2.5 or 5.0 mg per day maintained or increased bone mass at the lumbar spine, trochanter, and femoral neck in patients beginning glucocorticoids (575). At the lumbar spine, bone mass was maintained with an increase of 0.6% in the group receiving 5 mg of risedronate compared to a loss of 2.8% in the control group. Similar effects were seen at the trochanter. At the femoral neck, bone mass increased 0.8% in those given 5 mg of risedronate with a loss of 3.1% in the control group. In patients already on long-term glucocorticoids, that 2.5 and 5.0 mg of risedronate maintained or increased bone mass at the lumbar spine, trochanter, and femoral neck (643,644). Risedronate studies demonstrated a 70% reduction in vertebral fracture rate in chronic glucocorticoid users (644).

Intravenous pamidronate may afford another effective therapeutic alternative for highly selected individuals who are not candidates for oral bisphosphonate therapy (450,645–647). As measured by QCT, a technique that may give high values for trabecular bone mass, a >19% increase in lumbar BMD at 1 year was seen in a randomized controlled study (646).

In all large randomized controlled trials of bisphosphonate (450,645–647), bone mass was either maintained or increased with bisphosphonate therapy, while a decline was generally seen in the control group in the prevention studies. In the treatment studies, a bisphosphonate was always more effective than control therapy, although the control groups did not always lose bone at a significant rate. A Cochrane review further concluded that bisphosphonates are effective in preventing and treating glucocorticoid-associated bone loss both at the lumbar spine and the femoral neck (614).

Fluoride, Parathyroid Hormone, and Other Anabolic Agents

Since a primary pathologic defect of glucocorticoid-associated bone disease occurs in the osteoblast, there has been considerable interest in the use of anabolic agents. Different preparations of fluoride either alone (648–651) or in combination with a bisphosphonate agents (652) were potentially efficacious in GIOP. However, the absence from the U.S marketplace of the more effective slow-release fluoride preparation and the narrow therapeutic window and poor tolerability of the currently available preparations keep fluoride out of the standard GIOP armamentarium. Anabolic steroids have been investigated in a limited fashion with increased BMD noted in the forearm in one study (653). Limited investigative work with cyclically administered PTH also has been encouraging with 1-year increases in lumbar BMD of 11% reported (654). Lastly, preliminary animal work with growth hormone and other growth factors suggests another possible avenue of therapeutic approach (655).

Despite accumulating data on the effectiveness of antiosteoporotic therapies in GIOP, only 5% to 30% of patients on glucocorticoids in the United States and Great Britain receive therapies to prevent or treat GIOP (521,522, 656–659). Although there are many reasons for the low use of GIOP interventions and significant practice pattern variation in GIOP management, it appears that symptomatic glucocorticoid toxicities such as mood changes, weight gain, insomnia, hypertension, and hyperglycemia may receive more attention from some patients and physicians (660).

Treatment Approach

A treatment algorithm is proposed (Fig. 122.19) (661). Given the accumulating data on the efficacy of bisphosphonates for both preventing and treating GIOP, some authori-

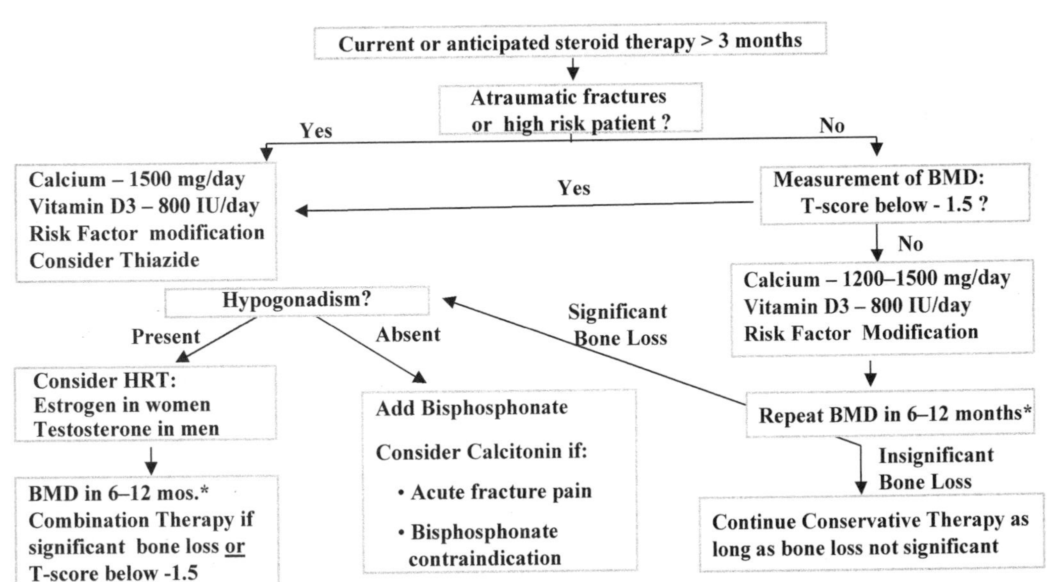

FIGURE 122.19. Treatment algorithm for the management of glucocorticoid-associated bone disease. (Adapted from Rosen HN, Rosenblatt M. Prevention and treatment of glucocorticoid-induced osteoporosis. In: Rose B, ed. UpToDate, vol 6, no. 3. Wellesley, MA: UpToDate, 1998, with permission.)

ties add a bisphosphonate immediately in all high-risk pati ents. While the algorithm represents a rational approach, this is a rapidly changing area and it is anticipated that GIOP mar agement will be further refined, based on emerging literatur e as well as societal cost-effectiveness considerations.

Ma e Osteoporosis

Ost eoporosis in men is common, as about 20% of all osteoporotic fractures occur in men. However, because its clinical nportance has been recognized only recently, this disorder has received modest research attention, and no consensus has been reached about the approach to treatment. As the population ages, osteoporosis in men will become an even greater public health problem.

Epidemiology

I rast to the studies of relationships between fractures, ass, propensity for falls, and other risk factors in the epidemiologic study of male osteoporosis has erally limited to the frequency and distribution of . The incidence of fracture in young adults is n men than women, presumably due to a greater e to trauma. At about age 50, the trend reverses. I er, the frequency of fracture associated with minimal tra a increases with age in older men, as in women. In No h America, men age 50 had a lifetime risk for fracture of t e hip, spine, or forearm of 13.1% (74). In the United Stat s, the incidence of hip fracture in men older than 65 yea is 4 to 5 in 1,000 (662), about half that in women of sim ar age. This 1:2 gender ratio has been observed in several countries around the world (143). In many geographic are , age-adjusted incidence of hip fractures has increased in r cent years for both genders, but more so for men (663). Inci lence of hip fracture in men may differ between different thnic groups. African American men have a rate about half that of Caucasians (664), and Japanese men living in Jap n or Hawaii may have a lower frequency than Caucasi n men in the United States (665).

hip fracture causes significant morbidity and carries a sub antial risk for mortality. In men age ≥75 years, 21% to 30% die within 6 months (662,664,666), a rate two- to thre fold higher than for women (667,668). This higher risk may reflect more severe concomitant illnesses. Unfortun tely, among survivors at 1 year, fewer than half of the sur vors resume prefracture activity levels.

steoporotic vertebral fractures in men are not as uncommo as had been assumed previously. In the United States and several European countries, the rates are about half those in v omen (reviewed in refs. 669,670). However, in women the ise in prevalence of vertebral fracture with age markedly exce ds that in men (670). Fractures are more common in the ow thoracic region in men, but may occur at any level (rev ewed in ref. 669). Elderly men less often fracture more thar one vertebral body (671). Most fractures are the anterior compression type; crush fractures occur less commonly than in women, thereby accounting for less kyphosis in men (672).

The incidence of fracture of an upper extremity in men does not significantly change with increasing age. This finding may reflect gender differences in the type of falls or the site of bone loss. Men lose cortical bone at a slower rate than women, whereas the rate of loss of trabecular bone is similar for the two genders. A fracture of the distal forearm in a man portends a significant risk for hip fracture, since it is indicative of decreased bone mass, a greater risk for falling, or both (673).

Pathogenesis

Men with osteoporotic fractures of the vertebrae and hip have lower BMD than individuals without a fracture (reviewed in ref. 671). This lower BMD is the culmination of a multitude of influences on bone metabolism, including genetic and environmental factors affecting attainment of peak bone density, strength and interconnectivity of trabeculae, and rate and distribution of bone loss during aging. Determinants of peak bone mass include various hormonal effects, diet, exercise, and genetic factors. The greater bone mass in men than women is mostly related to body size, with the exception of a few sites such as the radius (674). After attaining peak bone mass, men maintain a stable BMD during middle age, and then lose bone at an accelerating rate into old age (675). This rate may reach 5% to 10% per decade, and is greater in trabecular than cortical bone. The basis for this bone loss is not always clear, but hypogonadism and vitamin D deficiency of mild renal insufficiency may play important roles (663,676,677). Lower bone fragility in men than women may reflect not only higher peak bone mass and preservation of cortical bone, but also thinning rather than perforation of trabeculae with consequent loss of connectivity, and less severe intracortical porosity (reviewed in ref. 671).

The cellular mechanism of bone loss in men with primary osteoporosis may significantly differ from that in postmenopausal women. In contrast to an accelerated rate of bone resorption in women, men apparently lose bone due to reduced bone formation (671). Biochemical markers of bone formation, including serum osteocalcin and carboxy-terminal propeptide of type 1 collagen, decrease with increasing age. These results agree with a decreased percentage of double-labeled trabecular surfaces in iliac crest biopsy specimens (678). On the other hand, markers of bone resorption increased a little or not at all (679). The cellular basis for the decreased bone formation is uncertain, but some studies have shown decreased osteoblastic proliferative activity, whereas synthetic activity, measured by osteocalcin responsiveness to vitamin D, was normal (680). The biochemical basis for bone loss in older men remains enigmatic. Investigators have suggested reduced activity of growth hormone and IGF-1 (reviewed in ref. 671), perhaps through interactions with androgens.

Androgens may directly increase bone mass by binding to receptors on osteoblasts and chondrocytes to stimulate their proliferation (681), and indirectly by stimulating synthesis of growth factors, cytokines, and bone-matrix protein (682,683). The cellular mechanism is unknown. Osteoblasts have androgen receptors at densities consistent with other androgen-sensitive tissues, and with similar binding affinities (149,684,685). Androgen deficiency before puberty leads to low BMD in cortical and trabecular bone (686), whereas bone loss due to hypogonadism in later life is more pronounced at trabecular sites (687,688). Androgen deficiency has been found in 5% to 20% of younger men with vertebral fracture and in up to 50% of older men with femoral neck fracture (reviewed in ref. 686). Loss of bone mass is rapid after treatment with antiandrogens (689) or orchiectomy (690) for prostatic cancer. Testosterone replacement significantly increases bone mass in men with established gonadal failure (691). Serum testosterone levels decrease with age due to decreased Leydig cell number, changes in hypothalamic-pituitary function, and coexistent illness, such as RA (600) and lung cancer (671,692). This change is not always accompanied by a rise in serum gonadotropin levels (671,693) and hypogonadism may not be clinically apparent. The circulating level of testosterone that defines male hypogonadism in regard to bone health is unknown, and it is unclear if a particular level is a biologic threshold. A clinically important observation is the absence of bone loss after vasectomy (694).

Androgens may not be the only gonadal hormone important for bone health in men (reviewed in ref. 695). Osteoblasts express the cytochrome-P450 enzyme aromatase (estrogen synthetase) that converts testosterone to estradiol, and these cells have estrogen receptors (696). In healthy men, serum estradiol levels are comparable to those in postmenopausal women, but a greater fraction is in the free form due to competition with androgen for binding to sex hormone binding globulin (696). In a case-controlled study, men with vertebral fractures had estradiol levels significantly lower than unaffected controls (697). Case reports described a man with defective aromatase activity (556) and another with nonfunctioning estrogen receptors (682); both had markedly reduced BMD despite normal or increased serum testosterone levels and normal androgen receptors. Another 28-year-old man with an inactivating mutation of his aromatase gene presented with an eunuchoid habitus and nonclosure of the epiphyses, below-average BMD, and a bone age of 15 years (698). Treatment with serial intramuscular injections of testosterone was not beneficial, but therapy with transdermal estradiol produced skeletal maturation, marked increase in vertebral BMD, and epiphyseal closure. In a cross-sectional study of healthy older men with no history of bone disease, BMD of the lumbar spine and hip correlated with serum estradiol levels, but not serum testosterone levels (699). Treatment of men with osteoporotic vertebral fracture with pharmacologic doses of testosterone was associated with proportionate increases in estradiol levels. Increases in vertebral BMD correlated more closely with changes in serum estradiol levels than with changes in serum testosterone levels (700). An inability to undergo aromatization may explain why some androgens, such as nandrolone, do not sustain an early increase in BMD (699). Some investigators postulate that estrogens have a role, equivalent to testosterone, in the maintenance of the normal male skeleton (40).

As many as 20% to 40% of men with an osteoporotic fracture have no identifiable medical condition or risk factor associated with osteoporosis; they are designated as having primary osteoporosis to distinguish them from men who have lost substantial bone mass secondary to any of various conditions (reviewed in ref. 682) (Table 122.6). The most prominent of these are glucocorticoid therapy, alcoholism, solid-organ transplantation, gastrointestinal and thyroid/parathyroid disorders, and malignancy.

Evaluation

In men with clinical features or findings suggestive of metabolic bone disease, such as radiographic osteopenia, low-trauma fractures, or disorders associated with bone loss, measurement of BMD should be considered. These measurements may be used to confirm low bone mass, gauge its severity, and serve as a baseline to assess the progression of disease or therapeutic response. Criteria to define osteoporosis in men are not as clear as for women. The average young man has greater total bone mineral content than the average young woman, although volumetric BMD is similar. Estimates of fracture risk derived from measurements of women may not apply to men. Measurements obtained by DXA are vulnerable to differences in bone size because results are expressed as areal density (mineral content per unit area) rather than volumetric density. The number of observations is relatively limited, compared to those for women, and there is no consensus for the densitometric criteria for osteoporosis. Nonetheless, lower bone density is associated with an increased risk for fracture, and measurements can be used to monitor serial changes in bone mass.

The initial history and physical examination should be undertaken with knowledge of conditions associated with osteoporosis. Special attention should be given to signs of genetic, nutritional, and lifestyle (alcohol or tobacco) factors, systemic illness, and medication usage. Laboratory tests should include a complete blood count, serum calcium, phosphorus, alkaline phosphatase, liver enzymes, creatinine, 25-hydroxyvitamin D, and free testosterone (some investigators prefer bioavailable testosterone, which is the sum of free testosterone and that bound weakly to albumin; reviewed in ref. 701). Measurement of luteinizing hormone (LH), FSH, and prolactin levels will assess whether a pituitary tumor is present. Pituitary magnetic resonance imaging is generally limited to men younger than 50 years, and those with visual disturbance or recent onset of headaches, hyperprolactinemia without antidopaminergic drugs, and very low serum gonadotropin or bioavailable testosterone (701). If the cause of osteoporosis remains undefined, measurement of serum thyroid-stimulating hormone, and 24-hour urinary calcium and cortisol, and perhaps serum estradiol, should be considered.

Measurement of biochemical markers of bone turnover is controversial. Studies of the correlation of various markers with histologic features of bone metabolism or risk of fracture in men are not yet available (669). Nonetheless, an increase in biochemical indices may indicate a condition associated with greater bone turnover, such as thyrotoxicosis, hyperparathyroidism, hypogonadism, or mastocytosis. A transiliac bone biopsy is generally performed only in special circumstances because of its cost and invasiveness, but may be undertaken to identify unusual causes of osteoporosis diagnosed only by histologic studies (such as mastocytosis) or to ensure that osteomalacia is not present.

Treatment

To achieve maximal adult bone mass, adolescent boys should be encouraged to ingest 1,200 to 1,500 mg of calcium daily in their diets, participate in regular weight-bearing exercise, maintain ideal body weight, and avoid use of tobacco and excessive alcohol. Extending this approach into adulthood, it is recommended that men ages 25 to 65 consume 1,000 mg of calcium daily and that men over the age of 65 years consume 1,500 mg daily.

Few clinical trials have directly addressed therapy of men with osteoporosis. Current approaches incorporate several recommendations derived from treatment of osteoporotic women, although underlying pathogenic mechanisms differ between the genders.

Testosterone increases BMD in hypogonadal men (702,703) or those on glucocorticoid therapy (625), and has been used empirically in eugonadal men, albeit in short-term trials. The most effective, safe, practical, and inexpensive supplements are intramuscular testosterone enanthate or cyprionate. The usual dose is 200 mg every 14 days, but this may be tailored for individual patients to range from 100 mg weekly to 300 mg every 3 weeks. Some patients dislike the variations in well-being, sexual activity, and emotional stability that parallel swings in testosterone levels. Transdermal patches can be applied to nongenital or shaved scrotal skin. Oral testosterone undecanoate entails the inconvenience of three daily doses. Treatment with subdermal implants is more difficult to reverse if side effects develop. The goal of therapy is a physiologic testosterone profile (701). Side effects generally are not serious (671). Excessive libido is uncommon. Weight may increase due to anabolic effects on lean mass or salt and water retention, particularly in men with cardiac disease, cirrhosis, or nephrotic syndrome. Urinary retention is uncommon in the absence of prostatic cancer, and there is generally no significant effect on serum prostatic-specific antigen or prostatic volume. Whether the likelihood for prostatic cancer increases must await large clinical trials. Some men develop erythrocytosis due to augmented erythropoiesis. Levels of total and HDL-cholesterol frequently decrease. Gynecomastia may develop due to aromatization of testosterone to estradiol. 17α-alkylated androgens should be avoided because of greater risks for increased liver enzymes, cholestasis, and liver tumors. Contraindications to androgen therapy include prostatic cancer, prostatic hypertrophy, sleep apnea, inappropriate sexual behavior, and breast cancer.

Among other therapies, bisphosphonates currently offer substantial promise, although experience is limited. Intermittent cyclical treatment with etidronate increased lumbar BMD over a 2-year interval in an unselected group of men with osteoporotic vertebral fractures (704). Preliminary data from trials with pamidronate, alone (450) or with fluoride (705), have been encouraging. Furthermore, pamidronate was beneficial for men with glucocorticoid-induced osteoporosis (646). Calcitonin reduced loss of bone mass after orchiectomy (reviewed in ref. 671) and in another small study prevented bone loss when combined with calcium supplements (706). Correction of hypercalciuria with hydrochlorothiazide 25 mg twice daily can significantly increase bone mass (492). Treatment of elderly men with vitamin D and calcium supplementation for 3 years increased BMD at the femoral neck and lumbar spine compared to men given placebo, and the rate of nonvertebral fractures was lower (344). Supplementation with vitamin D and calcium are relatively inexpensive and safe, and may potentiate other therapeutic interventions (316). Treatment with fluoride has been generally avoided because of concerns that fracture rates have not decreased, despite increases in BMD. A prospective, controlled, randomized 3-year trial showed that intermittent, low-dose fluoride combined with continuous calcium supplementation increased BMD in the spine, hip, and radius, and significantly reduced the incidence of vertebral fracture (707). Evaluation of other therapies, including PTH, growth hormone, other anabolic agents, or estrogen combined with testosterone, must await clinical trials.

Organ Transplantation

In recent years, solid-organ transplantation has become established as the best therapy for patients with end-stage renal, hepatic, cardiac, and pulmonary disease. Bone marrow transplantation has been increasingly used for patients with hematopoietic and breast malignancies. From 1990 to 1998, a total of 142,743 patients underwent solid-organ transplantation in the United States alone, about 59% of whom received a renal allograft (708). With improving efficacy of immunosuppressive medications, 1-year allograft survival ranges from 75% for cadaveric lung allografts to 94% for living-donor renal allografts, and 5-year survival rates range from 41% to 77%, respectively. Thus, many patients survive their organ failure, but suffer adverse consequences of immunosuppression, peripheral effects of their disease, or increasing age. Unfortunately, transplant recipients frequently are afflicted with symptomatic osteoporosis and other musculoskeletal complications that reduce their quality of life and potential for rehabilitation.

Pathogenesis and Clinical Presentation

Osteoporosis after organ transplantation develops from a complex interplay of skeletal toxicities of immunosuppressants, complications unique to failure of the particular organ, and other factors that contribute to bone loss in the general population. Glucocorticoids continue to be an integral component of most long-term immunosuppressive regimens and are the cornerstone for treatment of acute rejection. Although the calcineurin-phosphatase inhibitors cyclosporine and tacrolimus have permitted use of lower doses, glucocorticoids significantly contribute to bone loss after engraftment. Areas of the skeleton rich in trabecular bone (e.g., vertebrae, ribs, and distal ends of long bones) and the cortical rim of vertebrae are most severely affected. Glucocorticoids have a wide range of effects that reduce bone mass: decreased intestinal absorption of calcium and hypercalciuria that lead to secondary hyperparathyroidism; suppression of adrenocorticotropic and gonadotropin hormones that causes secondary hypogonadism; decreased bone formation due to reduced recruitment and differentiation of osteoblasts, and inhibited synthesis of type 1 collagen; and increased bone resorption by osteoclasts (reviewed in ref. 709). Cyclosporine and tacrolimus greatly accelerate bone turnover in experimental animals, and the amount of trabecular bone lost within a month is substantial. Some of this effect may be mediated by IL-1, a cytokine that stimulates bone resorption. In animals given cyclosporine, bone loss can be prevented by antiresorptive agents, including bisphosphonates, estrogen, and calcitonin (reviewed in ref. 710). The bone loss of transplant recipients taking a calcineurin inhibitor in combination with glucocorticoids, and sometimes a third immunosuppressant, is less striking. Other immunosuppressants either have no clinically important skeletal toxicity (azathioprine) or have not been sufficiently evaluated (mycophenolate mofetil and sirolimus).

The relative risks and clinical manifestations of loss of BMD posttransplant vary greatly by the organ engrafted. Patients with severe renal insufficiency are at increased risk for decreased bone mass (711) and may have any of several histologic derangements, including hyperparathyroidism, osteomalacia, adynamic (aplastic) bone disease, or more than one disorder. These patients are frequently hypogonadal, and may have been treated with medications that alter bone metabolism and reduce bone mass, including glucocorticoids and cyclosporine for treatment of glomerulonephritis and loop diuretics for hypertension. Caucasian patients with end stage renal disease have a higher prevalence of osteoporosis than African Americans, independent of the type of renal osteodystrophy (712). The loss of bone mass after renal transplantation is greatest in the first 6 months, during which time it may average 7%. This occurs even in the setting of mild pretransplant hyperparathyroidism, relatively modest doses of glucocorticoids, and excellent allograft function (713). Fractures may occur in atypical locations such as the metatarsals, and less commonly in long bones; vertebral fractures are relatively uncommon in at least one study (714) and in our clinical experience. The highest fracture rate is in patients with diabetic renal disease who comprise about a third of newly transplanted patients in many centers. Bone loss after renal engraftment may contribute to osteonecrosis of the hips, knees, or humeral heads, a complication detectable by magnetic resonance imaging in 5% to 10% of recipients within 3 to 6 months of engraftment. Osteonecrosis is quite rare among recipients of other solid-organ allografts. Recipients of hepatic, cardiac, lung, and bone marrow transplants have a higher prevalence of osteoporosis before engraftment than renal allograft recipients. Some cholestatic hepatic disorders, e.g., primary biliary cirrhosis, are especially associated with severe osteoporosis, presumably due to accumulation of toxins (possibly bilirubin) that markedly impair osteoblastic activity (715). Bone marrow recipients frequently have undergone treatment with radiation or alkylating agents that render them hypogonadal.

Prevention and Treatment

Bone loss is a common complication for many potential recipients awaiting organ transplantation. Measurement of bone mass by DXA identifies patients who will benefit from therapy designed to maintain or improve bone mass and, it is hoped, reduce risk for osteoporotic fracture after engraftment. All patients should ingest 1,000 to 1,500 mg calcium daily (depending on age, use of glucocorticoids, and menopausal status) and 400 to 800 IU vitamin D. A regular walking exercise program and abstinence from smoking and excessive ethanol should be encouraged. Hormonal replacement therapy is reasonable for hypogonadal men and women. Patients with osteoporosis awaiting transplantation may be treated with a bisphosphonate (not currently approved by the FDA if creatinine clearance is less than 30 mL/min) or calcitonin.

Few studies have directly examined treatment of solid-organ transplant recipients, and the current approaches have been extrapolated from experiences with glucocorticoid-induced bone losses (see above). Continuing hormonal replacement therapy in hypogonadal patients and the general approach outlined above for transplantation candidates seems reasonable. Preliminary data from the treatment of liver, heart, and renal allograft recipients with bisphosphonates have been encouraging (709,716–718). Some cardiac allograft recipients benefited from calcium and gonadal hormonal replacement (719), while for others, vitamin D analogues reduced bone loss (720). The results with calcitonin have been less conclusive (709,721,722). Reports of treatment with sodium fluoride are limited and recommendations must await further experience.

Osteomalacia

Normal bone growth and mineralization require adequate vitamin D, calcium, and phosphorus. A prolonged deficiency of any of these leads to accumulation of unmineralized bone matrix, or osteoid, and slow bone formation. Decreased mineralization in young patients causes rickets due to damage of growth plates (epiphyses) and newly formed trabecular and cortical bone. Strength of the bone matrix is decreased, leading to structural deformities in weight-bearing bones such as bowing. In older individuals in whom epiphyses have closed and only bone is affected, this defective mineralization is called osteomalacia. Osteoid normally mineralizes in 5 to 10 days; in patients with osteomalacia, the interval may be as long as 3 months. Bone histomorphometry shows an increased ratio of unmineralized matrix to bone, low bone formation rates, inactive osteoblasts, and markedly diminished uptake of tetracycline labeling consistent with slow bone turnover. BMD is variable; it may be significantly decreased in patients with secondary hyperparathyroidism, but normal or increased in patients with chronic hypophosphatemia and normal serum calcium levels.

Rickets may develop in infants. Circumstances have included breast-feeding in the absence of a vitamin D or phosphorus supplement, use of formulas containing less than 20 mg calcium per deciliter, total parenteral nutrition with solutions without adequate calcium and vitamin D, and high-phytate diets that bind calcium in the gut. Genetically determined abnormalities of vitamin D metabolism, such as vitamin D–dependent-rickets type I (deficient renal 25-hydroxyvitamin D 1α-hydroxylase activity) and type II (abnormal intracellular receptor for 1,25-dihydroxyvitamin D) and hypophosphatemic vitamin D–resistant rickets, affect a few infants (723). Insufficient mineralization of bone may develop because of hypovitaminosis D due to chronic dietary intake less than 70 IU (rare in the United States due to supplementation of food products such as milk); decreased synthesis due to minimal exposure to sunlight (bed-bound institutionalized patients); reduced vitamin D absorption due to biliary, pancreatic, proximal small bowel mucosal disease, or bile acid-binding resins; increased urinary excretion of vitamin D metabolites in patients with nephrotic syndrome and normal renal clearance function (724); and increased vitamin D catabolism by medications that activate hepatic drug-metabolizing enzymes (such as phenytoin, barbiturates, and rifampin). Clinically significant chronic hypophosphatemia may result from renal wasting due to Fanconi's syndrome (secondary to many conditions, including systemic lupus, Sjögren's syndrome, or amyloidosis), renal tubular acidosis (more frequently with type II than type I), monoclonal gammopathy, "phosphotonin" (a humoral substance secreted by some tumors, most commonly mesenchymal in origin), decreased intestinal absorption due to antacid abuse, or chronic total parenteral nutrition if inadequate phosphorus is provided. Defective mineralization of osteoid may result from aluminum toxicity due to treatment with aluminum-containing antacids (especially in chronic renal failure) or aluminum-containing solutions for total parenteral nutrition, first-generation bisphosphonate (etidronate), or fluoride (aggravated by low intake of calcium), or from hypophosphastasia or fibrogenesis imperfecta ossium.

Clinical and Diagnostic Features

Patients with rickets may have hypotonia, weakness, and, in severe cases, tetany (reviewed in ref. 725). The costochondral junctions may be prominent, a deformity termed the rachitic rosary. Bowing of long bones in the legs, and kyphosis and lordosis in the back, can cause a waddling gait. Fractures may occur. The skull may show frontal bossing and flattening of parietal bones. Clinical manifestations of osteomalacia may mimic rheumatic disorders with generalized aching bone pain, easy fatigue, proximal weakness, and periarticular tenderness. These symptoms promptly resolve with treatment to correct the mineralization defect. Radiographs of patients with rickets may show general demineralization with thinning of cortical surfaces of long bones, widening, fraying, and cupping of distal ends of the shaft, and loss of the zone of provisional cartilaginous calcification. Some patients with osteomalacia exhibit thin cortical radiolucent lines (stress fractures) perpendicular to the bone shaft that are often symmetrical and bilateral (called Looser zones); other patients may have multiple old rib fractures with poor callus formation.

Laboratory features of vitamin D–deficiency osteomalacia are low or normal serum calcium level, hypophosphatemia, increased serum alkaline phosphatase level, normal serum osteocalcin level, increased serum PTH level (if hypocalcemia is present), and a low serum 25-hydroxyvitamin D level. Secondary hyperparathyroidism and hypophosphatemia stimulate renal synthesis of 1,25-dihydroxyvitamin D to maintain normal serum levels. Urinary calcium excretion is decreased. In calcium-deficiency osteomalacia, PTH levels are increased, 1,25-dihydroxyvitamin D levels are normal, and serum phosphorus levels may be low or normal. In osteomalacia due to hyperphosphaturia, levels of serum calcium, osteocalcin, PTH, and

25-hydroxyvitamin D are normal, serum alkaline phosphatase levels are usually increased, serum phosphorus and 1,25-dihydroxyvitamin D levels are low, and urinary phosphorus excretion is very high. Patients with type II renal tubular acidosis have defective reabsorption of bicarbonate and manifest hyperchloremic hypokalemic acidosis with hypophosphatemia due to augmented phosphaturia. Low serum 1,25-dihydroxyvitamin D levels in some patients may be the consequence of abnormal proximal tubular metabolism. Patients with renal tubular acidosis and Fanconi's syndrome may also excrete excessive amounts of calcium, magnesium, and potassium, as well as uric acid, glucose, amino acids, and citrate. Nephrocalcinosis may reduce glomerular filtration rate. Aluminum-associated osteomalacia in patients with chronic renal failure is much less common since curtailment of the widespread usage of aluminum-containing phosphate binders to control hyperphosphatemia and improved methods to prepare dialysate solutions. Afflicted patients manifest hypercalcemia with modest doses of vitamin D or calcium supplements, low serum PTH levels, and normal 25-hydroxyvitamin D levels. Hypophosphatasia is a rare autosomal-dominant disorder with decreased serum bone alkaline phosphatase level; serum calcium, phosphorus, 25-hydroxyvitamin D and 1,25-dihydroxyvitamin D levels are not reduced. No treatment is available. Fibrogenesis imperfecta ossium is a very rare, apparently acquired, disorder of collagen for which there is no therapy.

Treatment

Patients with nutritional rickets due to vitamin D deficiency may be treated with 600,000 IU vitamin D_2 (100,000 IU orally every 2 hours for six doses). Improvement in the serum calcium, phosphorus, alkaline phosphatase, and 25-hydroxyvitamin D levels within 4 to 7 days distinguishes nutritional rickets from genetic metabolic bone disease (726). Breast-fed infants require 400 IU vitamin D_2 per day orally to prevent rickets, while infants on chronic total parenteral nutrition need 20 to 25 IU (0.5 µ/kg) daily in the solution (reviewed in ref. 727). Adults consuming diets low in vitamin D–fortified foods may take 1,500 to 5,000 IU vitamin D_2 daily orally until serum chemistries and urinary calcium excretion return to normal, after which 400 IU daily will suffice. In patients with intestinal fat malabsorption, treatment should include control of the primary disease and use of a more polar vitamin D compound such as 25-hydroxyvitamin D, 20 to 30 µg per day, or 1,25-dihydroxyvitamin D, 0.15 to 0.50 µg per day, given orally, or ergocalciferol 10,000 to 50,000 IU given intramuscularly and titrated to the response in serum chemistries. Supplemental calcium, 1,000 to 2,000 mg per day, should also be provided. Treatment for several months may be necessary for the serum chemistries to return to normal. Patients should be carefully monitored for toxicity of vitamin D therapy, generally manifested as hypercalcemia or hypercalciuria. To prevent vitamin D deficiency in settings other than malabsorption or prematurity, daily 30-minute exposure to sunlight (728), ultraviolet B irradiation of the back with a suberythemal dosage for 3 to 7 minutes three times a week (729), consumption of 400 IU per day in fortified foods, or a dietary supplement is recommended.

Rickets due to chronic calcium deficiency markedly improved after increasing daily oral calcium intake to 700 mg in an infant (730) or to 2,000 mg in older children (731). Solutions for chronic total parenteral nutrition of infants and young children should contain calcium in a concentration of 20 to 60 mg/dL to prevent osteomalacia (727). Phosphorus treatment of phosphate-deficient breast-fed infants is 25 mg per kg body weight per day and 120 mg per kg body weight per day orally in premature infants (727). Total parenteral nutrition for these young patients should use solutions with phosphorus in a concentration of 15 to 47 mg/dL. Total parenteral nutrition solutions with synthetic amino acids rather than casein hydrolysates reduce the risk of aluminum-induced osteomalacia, but other additives may contain significant amounts of the metal (727).

In patients with renal tubular acidosis, restoration of the serum bicarbonate level to normal using sodium bicarbonate supplements or Shohl's solution reverses bone resorption and hypercalciuria. Patients with osteomalacia due to hyperphosphaturia in Fanconi's syndrome need oral phosphate supplements, generally 1 to 4 g per day given in four to six doses and many also benefit from treatment with 1,25-dihydroxyvitamin D, 0.5 to 1.5 µg per day (reviewed in ref. 732). Calcium supplements may be necessary to avoid symptomatic hypocalcemia, but should not be taken concomitantly with a phosphorus supplement. Once the bone disease has healed, the vitamin D can be discontinued.

Hyperparathyroidism

Primary

Primary hyperparathyroidism and malignancy are the two most common causes of hypercalcemia, accounting for more than 90% of patients with hypercalcemia (733). The prevalence of primary hyperparathyroidism ranges from 1 in 400 to 1 in 1,000, and has increased severalfold in the last 25 years due to the more common use of multichannel autoanalyzers for blood tests. Primary hyperparathyroidism can occur at any age, but most individuals are between 40 and 60 years and the female to male ratio is about 3:1. A parathyroid adenoma is the cause in about 80% of patients, whereas hyperplasia of all glands is found in about 15% to 20% of patients and parathyroid carcinoma in fewer than 0.5%. If the disorder appears in childhood, a familial hyperparathyroid syndrome such as a multiple endocrine neoplasia should be considered.

Oversecretion of PTH primarily affects the skeleton and kidneys. Pronounced osseous manifestations, such as subperiosteal resorption of the middle phalanges (radial aspect, in particular) and distal clavicle, "salt-and-pepper" skull, and bone cysts are now relatively uncommon, and affect less than 5% of patients. More frequent is loss of bone mass, preferentially in sites rich in cortical bone such as the distal third of the forearm or femoral neck. Although some studies found that fractures were more common in women with primary hyperparathyroidism (734), others have not (735,736). Nephrolithiasis develops in about 5% of patients, a frequency much less than three decades ago. Diffuse deposition of calcium-phosphate complexes may cause nephrocalcinosis that can lead to interstitial fibrosis and reduce renal clearance. About 25% to 30% of patients have hypercalciuria. Complications due to severe hypercalcemia, such as proximal weakness in the legs, weight loss, nausea, constipation, pancreatitis, and band keratopathy, are now rare. Most patients are asymptomatic and are discovered after routine laboratory screening shows a serum calcium concentration not more than 1 mg/dL above normal.

The diagnosis is generally established by an increased serum intact PTH concentration in a patient with hypercalcemia. Occasionally a patient with familial hypocalciuric hypercalcemia has an increased serum PTH level, but the very low urinary calcium/creatinine ratio, less than 0.01, distinguishes this condition from primary hyperparathyroidism. The serum phosphorus concentration is low-normal or low, and some patients exhibit a mild non-anion-gap hyperchloremic metabolic acidosis. Patients with significant bone disease may have increased levels of markers of bone formation (serum bone-specific alkaline phosphatase and osteocalcin) and bone resorption (urinary calcium and collagen cross-links). Patients with humoral hypercalcemia of malignancy have low serum PTH concentrations; the increased PTHrp does not cross-react in assays for intact PTH.

The cure for hyperparathyroidism is surgical removal of the parathyroid adenoma or carcinoma, or most of the hyperplastic tissue, after which bone mass often increases for several years (737). The general guidelines for recommending surgery in patients without carcinoma are a serum calcium concentration more than 1 mg/dL above the upper limit of normal, a significant complication (overt bone disease, nephrolithiasis), marked hypercalciuria (more than 400 mg daily), BMD Z-score of the distal radius worse than −2.0, and age less than 50 years. Postoperatively, hypocalcemia may develop due to increased skeletal uptake, the "hungry bone" syndrome. For preoperative management or for patients deemed unable to undergo parathyroid surgery, medical management includes adequate hydration and moderate intake of calcium, avoidance of thiazide diuretics that may increase serum calcium concentrations, and regular ambulatory exercise. Ultrasonography-guided percutaneous injection of ethanol into a parathyroid adenoma has been recommended by some investigators (738), but requires further study. Calcitonin offers substantial benefit for management of acute hypercalcemia, but resistance to the drug limits long-term therapy. Estrogen supplements for postmenopausal women and bisphosphonates also can be considered. Bisphosphonates may be more effective when given cyclically rather than continuously; with the latter therapy, a compensatory increase in PTH raises the serum calcium concentration back to pretreatment levels after about 3 months. Treatment in the future may include calcimimetic agents acting on the calcium-sensing receptor to suppress synthesis of PTH.

Secondary

Secondary hyperparathyroidism is relatively common in the elderly and may cause enough bone loss to contribute to the genesis of osteoporosis. The major factor in the regulation of the secretion of PTH is the concentration of ionized calcium in extracellular fluid; calcitriol deficiency and phosphate retention are also important, and the three are not mutually exclusive. Glucocorticoid therapy, fat malabsorption, loop diuretic therapy, and renal insufficiency may cause secondary hyperparathyroidism. The laboratory findings include low-normal to mildly decreased serum calcium level, decreased serum phosphorus level, mild metabolic acidosis, decreased urinary calcium excretion, and mildly increased serum PTH level. Treatment generally includes calcium supplements and small doses of calcitriol to increase intestinal absorption of calcium, and is monitored by serial measurements of serum PTH.

In renal insufficiency, secondary hyperparathyroidism becomes histologically apparent when the creatinine clearance decreases to 50 to 60 mL/min (739). With worsening renal dysfunction, hyperparathyroid bone disease frequently includes paratrabecular tissue (composed of mesenchymal cells) and osteoclast-mediated scalloping and tunneling of trabeculae—sometimes termed "osteitis fibrosis cystica." In patients with severe renal insufficiency, parathyroid cells not only increase in size but also proliferate. Some cells partially escape normal control by regulatory factors, and portions of enlarged glands become nodular and may exhibit a monoclonal growth pattern (740). These patients are resistant to treatment with calcitriol and calcium supplements and normalization of serum phosphorus levels, and often require parathyroid reduction surgery. The choice of the surgical procedure, subtotal parathyroidectomy or total parathyroidectomy with autotransplantation of a portion of one gland, depends largely on the surgeon. Several new agents, including calcimimetics and nonhypercalcemic derivatives of vitamin D, will soon be available.

Hyperthyroidism

Bone disease of hyperthyroidism is a type of high-turnover osteoporosis. Serum triiodothyronine levels inversely correlate with bone mass (741). Patients may have bone pain and fracture, in addition to other features of hyperthyroidism. Bone loss in patients with thyrotoxicosis may be worse in women than men (173). Although the disease is often endogenous, prolonged treatment with exogenous thyroid hormone in doses sufficient to suppress thyroid-stimulating hormone may reduce BMD. Radiographs may show diffuse osteopenia; abnormal striations of cortical bone are observed occasionally. Biochemical parameters usually include normal or mildly increased serum calcium levels and increased serum alkaline phosphatase levels. Urinary excretion of calcium and collagen breakdown fragments are often increased.

Thyroid hormone increases bone turnover. While osteoblasts have thyroid hormone receptors, and are required for the skeletal effects of thyroid hormone, the net stimulatory effect on bone formation is less than that on bone resorption. Calcium released during accelerated bone resorption decreases secretion of PTH, which in turn decreases renal excretion of phosphorus and may increase serum phosphorus levels. These changes decrease the activity of renal 1α-hydroxylase and lower serum 1,25-dihydroxyvitamin D levels. Histomorphometric measurements generally show increased bone turnover, with increased osteoclasts and osteoclastic surface and increased osteoid formation surfaces involving cortical and trabecular bone. Despite low serum 1,25-dihydroxyvitamin D levels, the mineralization rate is normal.

Correction of the hyperthyroid state often restores bone mass (742,743). Estrogen for women or bisphosphonates may be considered if an accelerated rate of bone loss or decreased bone mass is present.

Osteogenesis Imperfecta Tarda

Occasionally an adult with multiple fractures, especially in the long bones of the legs, and radiographic osteopenia has osteogenesis imperfecta. A genetically determined inability to form quantitatively or qualitatively normal collagen characterizes this group of disorders. Several mutations in the gene for type 1 procollagen have been identified; all result in formation of unstable collagen helices (744). Most patients develop fractures in childhood. One prenatal form is lethal. Some individuals are deaf or have blue sclera, but others have only osseous manifestations. If the disease begins in childhood, bones may grow abnormally. Extremities are short, legs are bowed, and saber shins occur. Pectus excavatum or carinatum can appear, as well as a dome-shaped forehead and lateral widening of the skull. Fractures usually diminish in frequency at puberty, but increase in the perimenopausal period in women and at a similar age in men.

If no phenotypic characteristic of osteogenesis imperfecta is present except for fragile bones, diagnosis can be difficult. A positive family history and a history of multiple fractures in childhood are suggestive. Radiographs show thinning of cortical and trabecular areas of bones, especially metacarpals and metatarsals. Platybasia of the skull and bone islands in the cranium suggest osteogenesis imperfecta. Bone biopsy shows diminished quantities of osteoid and excessive osteocyte numbers. Therapy with sodium fluoride, calcitonin, or gonadal hormones has been advocated, but it is not clear that any intervention reduces fracture rates.

Other Causes of Bone Loss

As shown in Table 122.6, many other disorders may reduce bone mass to the degree sufficient to satisfy the WHO's bone densitometry criterion for osteoporosis. About 20% of women with osteoporosis attributed to natural menopause, and 50% to 60% of younger women and men with osteoporosis have identifiable secondary causes for bone loss (reviewed in refs. 724 and 745). While not all of these disorders have been associated with an increased rate of fracture, a few warrant comment.

Gastrointestinal Disease

Patients afflicted with the gastrointestinal disorders in Table 122.6 may develop a spectrum of bone disease, ranging from osteoporosis to osteomalacia (reviewed in ref. 745). Several pathogenic mechanisms contribute: (a) calcium malabsorption, alone or combined with malabsorption of vitamin D, leading to secondary hyperparathyroidism; (b) impaired absorption of vitamin D, altered metabolism of vitamin D, or reduced enterohepatic circulation of vitamin D metabolites; and (c) glucocorticoid treatment of inflammatory bowel disease. Although early reports suggested that the bone disorder in patients with primary biliary cirrhosis was predominantly osteomalacia, subsequent histomorphometric studies showed that osteoporosis was more common (746). Some investigators proposed that bilirubin has a direct toxicity on bone metabolism by impairing osteoblastic function (715). Bone disease after gastrectomy is also more commonly osteoporosis than osteomalacia. Calcium malabsorption is more likely due to loss of duodenal absorptive surface than achlorhydria (747). Celiac sprue has long been known to cause rickets in children and osteomalacia in adults (748). Some patients with gluten-sensitive enteropathy develop secondary hyperparathyroidism, presumably due to calcium malabsorption (749). These skeletal complications develop even without steatorrhea or frequent bowel movements (750). In one study, biopsy-confirmed celiac sprue was tenfold more common in patients with osteoporosis than in controls (751). Patients with inflammatory bowel disease may have decreased BMD due to osteomalacia or osteoporosis, and the risk is greater for Crohn's disease than ulcerative colitis (559). The risk for osteoporosis in Crohn's disease may be greater in men than women, and in patients with jejunal involvement or previous bowel resection (752).

Malignancy

In malignancy, osteoporosis can develop due to skeletal effects of various cytokines, rather than localized bone destruction due to metastatic disease. In multiple myeloma, abnormal plasma cells secrete several osteoclast-stimulating factors, including IL-1, IL-6, lymphotoxin, and PTHrp (reviewed in ref. 753). Biochemical markers for bone resorption are often increased, whereas serum alkaline phosphatase, a marker for bone formation, may not be (754). In some patients with advanced disease, lower serum levels of another marker for bone formation, osteocalcin, correlated with longer survival (755). Decreased osteoblastic function may be due to IL-1β (756). Other neoplasms also may produce hormones that alter bone metabolism and cause hypercalcemia, most commonly PTHrp in solid malignancies (757), 1,25-dihydroxyvitamin D in lymphomas and benign granulomas (758), and, rarely, PTH (reviewed in ref. 757). However, the prevalence of osteoporosis in these settings is uncertain.

ACKNOWLEDGMENTS

This work was supported by grants 1R29 AR42674, 1R03 AR46432-01, 1R01 AR47700, 1R01 AG 12951, and M01-RR-00032 from the National Institutes of Health and the Office of Dietetic Supplements and the Department of Veterans Affairs.

REFERENCES

1. Kanzler B, Kuschert SJ, Liu YH, et al. Hoxa-2 restricts the chondrogenic domain and inhibits bone formation during development of the branchial area. *Development* 1998;125: 2587–2597.
2. Iwasaki M, Le AX, Helms JA. Expression of indian hedgehog, bone morphogenetic protein 6 and gli during skeletal morphogenesis. *Mech Dev* 1997;69:197–202.
3. Storm EE, Kingsley DM. GDF5 coordinates bone and joint formation during digit development. *Dev Biol* 1999;209:11–27.
4. Kronenberg HM, Lanske B, Kovacs CS, et al. Functional analysis of the PTH/PTHrP network of ligands and receptors. *Recent Prog Hormone Res* 1998;53:283–301.
5. Wilkie AO. Craniosynostosis: genes and mechanisms. *Hum Mol Genet* 1997;6:1647–1656.
6. Suda N. Parathyroid hormone-related protein (PTHrP) as a regulating factor of endochondral bone formation. *Oral Dis* 1997;3:229–231.
7. Lefebvre V, de Crombrugghe B. Toward understanding SOX9 function in chondrocyte differentiation. *Matrix Biol* 1998;16: 529–540.
8. Ferguson CM, Miclau T, Hu D, et al. Common molecular pathways in skeletal morphogenesis and repair. *Ann NY Acad Sci* 1998;857:33–42.
9. Moses HL, Serra R. Regulation of differentiation by TGF-beta. *Curr Opin Genet Dev* 1996;6:581–586.
10. Rickard DJ, Kassem M, Hefferan TE, et al. Isolation and characterization of osteoblast precursor cells from human bone marrow. *J Bone Miner Res* 1996;11:312–324.
11. Ducy P, Karsenty G. Genetic control of cell differentiation in the skeleton. *Curr Opin Cell Biol* 1998;10:614–619.
12. Ducy P, Starbuck M, Priemel M, et al. A cbfa1-dependent genetic pathway controls bone formation beyond embryonic development. *Genes Dev* 1999;13:1025–1036.
13. Partridge NC, Bloch SR, Pearman AT. Signal transduction pathways mediating parathyroid hormone regulation of osteoblastic gene expression. *J Cell Biochem* 1994;55:321–327.
14. Meszaros JG, Karin NJ, Akanbi K, et al. Down-regulation of L-type Ca2+ channel transcript levels by 1,25-dihydroxyvitamin D3. Osteoblastic cells express L-type alpha1C Ca2+ channel isoforms. *J Biol Chem* 1996;271:32981–32985.
15. Jones SJ, Gray C, Sakamaki H, et al. The incidence and size of gap junctions between the bone cells in rat calvaria. *Anat Embryol* 1993;187:343–352.
16. Donahue HJ, McLeod KJ, Rubin CT, et al. Cell-to-cell communication in osteoblastic networks: cell line-dependent hormonal regulation of gap junction function. *J Bone Miner Res* 1995;10:881–889.
17. Kaplan FS, Shore EM. Bone morphogenetic proteins and c-fos: early signals in endochondral bone formation. *Bone* 1996;19: 13S–21S.
18. Aubin JE, Liu F, Malaval L, et al. Osteoblast and chondroblast differentiation. *Bone* 1995;17:77S–83S.
19. Suda T, Udagawa N, Nakamura I, et al. Modulation of osteoclast differentiation by local factors. *Bone* 1995;17:87S–91S.
20. Blair HC, Teitelbaum SL, Ghiselli R, et al. Osteoclastic bone resorption by a polarized vacuolar proton pump. *Science* 1989; 245:855–857.
21. Blair HC. How the osteoclast degrades bone. *Bioessays* 1998;20: 837–846.
22. Tezuka K, Tezuka Y, Maejima A, et al. Molecular cloning of a possible cysteine proteinase predominantly expressed in osteoclasts. *J Biol Chem* 1994;269:1106–1109.
23. Bossard MJ, Tomaszek TA, Thompson SK, et al. Proteolytic activity of human osteoclast cathepsin K. Expression, purification, activation, and substrate identification. *J Biol Chem* 1996; 271:12517–12524.
24. Gelb BD, Shi GP, Chapman A, et al. Pycnodysostosis, a lysosomal disease caused by cathepsin K deficiency. *Science* 1996; 273:1236–1238.
25. Matayoshi A, Brown C, DiPersio JF, et al. Human blood mobilized hematopoietic precursors differentiate into osteoclasts in the absence of stromal cells. *Proc Natl Acad Sci U S A* 1996;93:10785–10790.
26. Lacey DL, Timms E, Tan H-L, et al. Osteoprotegerin ligand is a cytokine that regulates osteclast differentiation and activation. *Cell* 1998;93:165–176.
27. Mizuno A, Amizuka N, Irie K, et al. Severe osteoporosis in mice lacking osteoclastogenesis inhibitory factor/osteoprotegerin. *Biochem Biophys Res Commun* 1998;247:610–615.
28. Fitz R, Alsberg CL, Henderson J. Concerning the excretion of phosphoric acid during experimental acidosis in rabbits. *Am J Physiol* 1997;18:113.
29. Sebastian A, Harris ST, Ottaway JH, et al. Improved mineral balance and skeletal metabolism in postmenopausal women treated with potassium bicarbonate. *N Engl J Med* 1994;330: 1776–1781.

30. Heering P, Degenhardt S, Grabensee B. Tubular dysfunction following kidney transplantation. *Nephron* 1996;74:501–511.
31. Frost HM. Tetracycline labeling of bone and the zone of demarcation of osteoid seams. *Can J Biochem Pharmacol* 1962;40: 485–490.
32. Carano A, Teitelbaum SL, Konsek JD, et al. Bisphosphonates directly inhibit bone resorption activity of isolated avian osteoclasts in vitro. *J Clin Invest* 1990;85:456–461.
33. Luckman SP, Hughes DE, Coxon FP, et al. Nitrogen-containing bisphosphonates inhibit the mevalonate pathway and prevent post-translational phenylation of GTP-binding proteins, including Ras. *J Bone Miner Res* 1998;13:581–589.
34. Blair HC, Teitelbaum SL, Tan H-L, et al. Reversible inhibition of osteoclastic activity by bone-bound gallium (III). *J Cell Biochem* 1992;48:401–410.
35. Watrous DA, Andrews BS. The metabolism and immunology of bone. *Semin Arthritis Rheum* 1989;19:45–65.
36. Mierke DF, Pellegrini M. Parathyroid hormone and parathyroid hormone-related protein: model systems for the development of an osteoporosis therapy. *Curr Pharm Design* 1999;5:21–36.
37. Verheijen MH, Karperien M, Chung U, et al. Parathyroid hormone-related peptide (PTHrP) induces parietal endoderm formation exclusively via the type I PTH/PTHrP receptor. *Mech Dev* 1999;81:151–161.
38. Haussler MR, Haussler CA, Jurutka PW, et al. The vitamin D hormone and its nuclear receptor: molecular actions and disease states. *J Endocrinol* 1997;154S:S57–S73.
39. Picado C, Luengo M. Corticosteroid-induced bone loss. Prevention and management. *Drug Safety* 1996;15:347–359.
40. Riggs BL, Khosla S, Melton LJ. A unitary model for involutional osteoporosis: estrogen deficiency causes both type I and type II osteoporosis in postmenopausal womoen and contributes to bone loss in aging men. *J Bone Miner Res* 1998; 13:763–773.
41. Duncan RL, Hruska KA, Misler S. Parathyroid hormone activation of stretch-activated cation channels in osteosarcoma cells (UMR-106.01). *FEBS Lett* 1992;307:219–223.
42. Christenson RH. Biochemical markers of bone metabolism: an overview. *Clin Biochem* 1997;30:573–593.
43. Bonnick SL. *Bone densitometry in clinical practice.* Totowa, NJ: Humana, 1998.
44. Johnston CC, Epstein S. Clinical, biochemical, radiographic, epidemiologic, and economic features of osteoporosis. *Orthopedic Clin North Am* 1981;12:559–569.
45. Singh M, Nagrath AR, Maini PS. Changes in trabecular pattern of the upper end of the femur as an index of osteoporosis. *J Bone Joint Surg* 1970;52:457–467.
46. Hubsch P, Kocanda H, Youssefzadeh S, et al. Comparison of dual energy x-ray absorptiometry of the proximal femur with morphological data. *Acta Radiol* 1992;33:477–481.
47. Masud T, Jawed S, Doyle DV, et al. A population study of the screening potential of assessment of trabecular pattern of the femoral neck (Singh index): the Chingford study. *Br J Radiol* 1995;68:389–393.
48. Koot KV, Kesselaer SM, Clevers GJ, et al. Evaluation of the Singh index for measuring osteoporosis. *J Bone Joint Surg* 1996; 78:831–834.
49. Faulkner KG, Cummings SR, Black D, et al. Simple measurement of femoral geometry predicts hip fracture: the Study of Osteoporotic Fractures. *J Bone Miner Res* 1993;8:1211–1217.
50. Duboeuf F, Hans D, Schott AM, et al. Different morphometric and densitometric parameters predict cervical and trochanteric hip fracture: the EPIDOS study. *J Bone Miner Res* 1997;12: 1895–1902.
51. Gluer C-C, Cummings SR, Pressman A, et al. Prediction of hip fractures from pelvic radiographs: the Study of Osteoporotic Fractures. *J Bone Miner Res* 1994;9:671–677.
52. Yang S-O, Hagiwara S, Engelke K, et al. Radiographic absorptiometry for bone mineral assessment of the phalanges: precision and accuracy study. *Radiology* 1994;192:857–859.
53. Yates AJ, Ross PD, Lydick E, et al. Radiographic absorptiometry in the diagnosis of osteoporosis. *Am J Med* 1995;98:2A-41S–2A-47S.
54. Kleerekoper M, Nelson DA, Flynn MJ, et al. Comparison of radiographic absorptiometry with dual-energy-x-ray absorptiometry and quantitative computer tomography in normal older white and black men. *J Bone Miner Res* 1994;9:1745–1749.
55. Mussolino ME, Looker AC, Madans JH, et al. Phalangeal bone density and hip fracture risk. *Arch Intern Med* 1997;157: 433–438.
56. Huang C, Russ PD, Yates AJ, et al. Prediction of fracture risk by radiographic absorptiometry and quantitative ultrasound: a prospective study. *Calcif Tissue Int* 1998;1998:380–384.
57. Genant HK, Engelke K, Fuerst T, et al. Noninvasive assessment of bone mineral and structure: state of the art. *J Bone Miner Res* 1996;11:707–730.
58. Kimmel PL. Radiologic methods to evaluate bone mineral content. *Ann Intern Med* 1984;100:908–911.
59. Cameron JR, Sorenson J. Measurement of bone mineral in vivo: an improved method. *Science* 1963;142:230–232.
60. Black DM, Cummings SR, Genant HK, et al. Axial and appendicular bone density predict fractures in older women. *J Bone Miner Res* 1992;7:633--638.
61. Bohr H, Schaadt O. Bone mineral content of femoral bone and the lumbar spine measured in women with fracture of the femoral neck by dual photon absorptiometry. *Clin Orthop Rel Res* 1983;179:240–245.
62. Miller PD, Bonnick SL, Rosen CJ. Consensus of an international panel on the clinical utility of bone mass measurements in the detection of low bone mass in the adult population. *Calcif Tissue Int* 1996;58:207–214.
63. Genant H, Lang T, Engelke K, et al. Advances in the noninvasive assessment of bone density, quality, and structure. *Calcif Tissue Int* 1996;59(suppl 1):S10–S15.
64. Kleerekoper M, Nelson DA. Which bone density measurement? *J Bone Miner Res* 1997;12(5):712–714.
65. Baran DT, Faulkner KG, Genant HK, et al. Diagnosis and management of osteoporosis: guidelines for the utilization of bone densitometry. *Calcif Tissue Int* 1997;61:433–440.
66. Mazess R, Chesnut CH III, McClung M, et al. Enhanced precision with dual-energy x-ray absorptiometry. *Calcif Tissue Int* 1992;51:14–17.
67. Chen Z, Maricic M, Lund P, et al. How the new hologic hip normal reference values affect the densitometric diagnosis of osteoporosis. *Osteoporos Int* 1998;8:423–427.
68. Genant HK, Grampp S, Gluer CC, et al. Universal standardization for dual x-ray absorptiometry: patient and phantom cross-calibration results. *J Bone Miner Res* 1994;9:1503–1514.
69. Faulkner KG, Roberts LA, McClung MR. Discrepancies in normative data between lunar and hologic DXA systems. *Osteoporosis Int* 1996;6:432–436.
70. Gluer CC, Blake G, Lu Y, et al. Accurate assessment of precision errors: how to measure the reproducibility of bone densitometry techniques. *Osteoporosis Int* 1995;5:262–270.
71. Gluer CC, Steiger P, Selvidge R, et al. Comparative assessment of dual-photon-absorptiometry and dual-energy-radiography. *Radiology* 1990;174:223–228.
72. Mazess RB, Collick B, Trempe J, et al. Performance evaluation of a dual energy x-ray bone densitometer. *Calcif Tissue Int* 1989;44:228–232.

73. Christiansen C. Postmenopausal bone loss and the risk of osteoporosis. *Osteoporosis Int* 1994;S1:S47–S51.
74. Melton LJ III, Chrischilles EA, Cooper C, et al. Perspective: how many women have osteoporosis? *J Bone Miner Res* 1992;7:1005–1010.
75. Faulkner KG, McClung MR, Schmeer MS, et al. Densitometry of the radius using single and dual energy absorptiometry. *Calcif Tissue Int* 1994;54:208–211.
76. Greenspan S, Bouxsein M, Melton M, et al. Precision and discriminatory ability of calcaneal bone assessment technologies. *J Bone Miner Res* 1997;12(8):1303–1312.
77. Melton LJ III, Atkinson EJ, O'Fallon WM, et al. Long-term fracture prediction by bone mineral assessed at different skeletal sites. *J Bone Miner Res* 1993;8(10):1227–1233.
78. Cummings SR, Black DM, Nevitt MC, et al. Bone density at various sites for prediction of hip fractures. *Lancet* 1993;341:72–75.
79. Ross PD, Wasnich RD, Vogel JM. Detection of prefracture spinal osteoporosis using bone mineral absorptiometry. *J Bone Miner Res* 1988;3:1–11.
80. Melton LJ III, Atkinson EJ, O'Fallon WM, et al. Long-term fracture risk prediction with bone mineral measurements made at various skeletal sites. *J Bone Miner Res* 1991;6(S1):S136.
81. Ross PD, Ettinger B, Davis JW, et al. Evaluation of adverse health outcomes associated with vertebral fractures. *Osteoporosis Int* 1991;1:134–140.
82. Hui SL, Slemenda CW, Johnston CC. Age and bone mass as predictors of fracture in a prospective study. *J Clin Invest* 1988;81:1804–1809.
83. Ross PD, Genant HK, Davis JW, et al. Predicting vertebral fracture incidence from prevalent fractures and bone density among non-black, osteoporotic women. *Osteoporosis Int* 1993;3:120–126.
84. Wasnich RD, Ross PD, Davis JW, et al. A comparison of single and multi-site BMC measurements for assessment of spine fracture probability. *J Nucl Med* 1989;30:1166–1171.
85. Cummings SR, Black DM, Nevitt MC, et al. Appendicular bone density and age predict hip fracture in women. *JAMA* 1990;263:665–668.
86. Black DM, Cummings SR, Melton LJ III. Appendicular bone mineral and a woman's lifetime risk of hip fractures. *J Bone Miner Res* 1992;7:639–646.
87. Melton LJ III, Wahner HW, Richelson LS, et al. Osteoporosis and risk of hip fracture. *Am J Epidemiol* 1986;124:254–261.
88. Libanati CR, Schulz EE, Shook JE, et al. Hip mineral density in females with a recent hip fracture. *J Clin Endocrinol Metab* 1992;74:351–356.
89. Davis JW, Ross PD, Wasnich RD. Evidence for both generalized and regional low bone mass among elderly women. *J Bone Miner Res* 1994;9:305–309.
90. Miller PD, Bonnick SL, Johnston CC Jr, et al. The challenges of peripheral bone density Testing: Which patients need additional central density skeletal measurements? *J Clin Densitometry* 1998;1(3):211–217.
91. Pouilles JM, Tremollieres R, Ribot C. Spine and femur densitometry at the menopause: Are both sites necessary in the assessment of the risk of osteoporosis? *Calcif Tissue Int* 1993;52:344–347.
92. Greenspan SL, Maitland-Ramsey L, Myers E. Classification of osteoporosis in the elderly is dependent on site specific analysis. *Calcif Tissue Int* 1996;58:409–414.
93. Reid IR, Evans MC, Ames R, et al. The influence of osteophytes and aortic calcification on spinal mineral density in postmenopausal women. *J Clin Endocrinol Metab* 1991;72:1372–1374.
94. Rizzoli R, Slosman D, Bonjour JP. The role of dual energy x-ray absorptiometry of lumbar spine and proximal femur in the diagnosis and follow-up of osteoporosis. *Am J Med* 1995;98(suppl 2A):33S–36S.
95. Lafferty FW, Rowland DY. Correlations of dual-energy x-ray absorptiometry, quantitative computed tomography, and single photon absorptiometry with spinal and non-spinal fractures. *Osteoporosis Int* 1996;6:407–415.
96. Mazess RB, Gifford AA, Bisek JP, et al. DEXA measurement of spine density in the lateral projection. I: Methodology. *Calcif Tissue Int* 1991;49:235–239.
97. Duboeuf F, Pommet R, Meunier PJ, et al. Dual-energy x-ray absorptiometry of the spine in anteroposterior and lateral projections. *Osteoporosis Int* 1994;4:110–116.
98. Yu W, Gluer CC, Grampp S, et al. Spinal bone mineral assessment in postmenopausal women: a comparison between dual x-ray absorptiometry and quantitative computed tomography. *Osteoporosis Int* 1995;5:433–439.
99. Finkelstein J, Cleary RL, Butler J, et al. A comparison of lateral versus anterior-posterior spine dual energy x-ray absorptiometry for the diagnosis of osteopenia. *J Clin Endocrinol Metab* 1994;78:724–730.
100. Reid IR, Evans MC, Stapleton J. Lateral spine densitometry is a more sensitive indicator of glucocorticoid-induced bone loss. *J Bone Miner Res* 1992;7:1221–1225.
101. Engelke K, Gluer CC, Genant HK. Factors influencing short-term precision of dual x-ray bone absorptiometry (DXA) of spine and femur. *Calcif Tissue Int* 1995;56:19–25.
102. Hangartner TN, Johnston CC. Influence of fat on bone measurements with dual-energy absorptiometry. *Bone Miner* 1990;9:71–81.
103. Lanarch TA, Boyd SJ, Smart RC, et al. Reproducibility of lateral spine scans using dual energy x-ray absorptiometry. *Calcif Tissue Int* 1992;51:255–258.
104. Frye MA, Melton LJ III, Bryant SC, et al. Osteoporosis and calcification of the aorta. *Bone Miner* 1992;19:185–194.
105. Pacifici R, Rupich R, Griffin M, et al. Dual energy radiography versus quantitative computer tomography for the diagnosis of osteoporosis. *J Clin Endocrinol Metab* 1990;70:705–710.
106. Genant HK, Steiger P, Block JE, et al. Quantitative computed tomography: update 1987. *Calcif Tissue Int* 1987;41:179–186.
107. Laan RFJM, Buijs WCAM, van Erning LJT, et al. Differential effects of glucocorticoids on cortical appendicular and cortical vertebral bone mineral content. *Calcif Tissue Int* 1993;52:5–9.
108. Gluer CC, Genant HK. Impact of marrow fat on accuracy of quantitative CT. *J Comput Assist Tomogr* 1989;13:1023–1035.
109. Kalendar WA, Brestowsky H, Felsenberg D. Bone mineral measurements: automated determination of the midvertebral CT section. *Radiology* 1988;168:219–221.
110. Schneider P, Borner W, Mazess RB, et al. The relationship of peripheral to axial bone density. *Bone Miner* 1988;4:279–287.
111. Takada M, Engelke K, Hagiwara S, et al. Accuracy and precision study in vitro for peripheral quantitative computed tomography. *Osteoporosis Int* 1996;6:207–212.
112. Lang TF. Summary of research issues in imaging and noninvasive bone measurement. *Bone* 1998;22:S159–S160.
113. Njeh CF, Boivin CM, Langston CM. The role of ultrasound in the assessment of osteoporosis: a review. *Osteoporosis Int* 1997;7:7–22.
114. Gluer C, Jergas M, Hans D. Peripheral measurement of techniques for the assessment of osteoporosis. *Semin Nucl Med* 1997;27:229–247.
115. Waud CE, Lew R, Baran DT. The relationship between ultrasound and densitometric measurements of bone mass at the calcaneus in women. *Calcif Tissue Int* 1992;51:415–418.
116. Prins SH, Jorgensen HL, Jorgensen LV, et al. The role of quantitative ultrasound in the assessment of bone: a review. *Clin Physiol* 1998;18:3–17.

117. Damilakis J, Perisinakis K, Vagios E, et al. Effect of region of interest location on ultrasound measurements of the calcaneus. *Calcif Tissue Int* 1998;63:300–305.
118. Agren M, Karellas A, Leahey D, et al. Ultrasound attenuation of the calcaneus: a sensitive and specific discriminator of osteopenia in postmenopausal women. *Calcif Tissue Int* 1991;48240–244.
119. Sowers M, Jannausch M, Scholl T, et al. The reproducibility of ultrasound bone measures in a triethnic population of pregnant adolescents and adult women. *J Bone Miner Res* 1998;13: 1768–1774.
120. Turner CH, Peacock M, Timmerman L, et al. Calcaneal ultrasonic measurements discriminate hip fracture independently of bone mass. *Osteoporos Int* 1995;5:130–135.
121. Gluer CC, Cummings SR, Bauer DC, et al. Associations between quantitative ultrasound and recent fractures. *J Bone Miner Res* 1994;9:S153(abst).
122. Heaney RP, Avioli LV, Chesnut HI, et al. Ultrasound velocity through bone predicts incident vertebral deformity. *J Bone Miner Res* 1995;10:341–345.
123. Bauer DC, Gluer CC, Cauley JA, et al. Broadband ultrasound attenuation predicts fractures strongly and independently of densitometry in older women. A prospective study. *Arch Intern Med* 1997;157:629–634.
124. Hans D, Dargent-Molina P, Schott AM, et al. Ultrasonographic heel measurements to predict hip fracture in elderly women: the EPIDOS prospective study. *Lancet* 1996;348:511–514.
125. Cheng S, Tylavsky F, Carbone L. Utility of ultrasound to assess risk of fracture. *J Am Geriatr Soc* 1997;45:1382–1394.
126. Laurin ML, Kimmel DB, Lappe JM, et al. Differences in stress fracture during basic training in black and white female soldiers. *J Bone Miner Res* 1996;suppl 1:S363(abst).
127. Gonnelli S, Cepollaro C, Pondrelli C, et al. Ultrasound parameters in osteoporotic patients treated with salmon calcitonin: a longitudinal study. *Osteoporosis Int* 1996;7:303–307.
128. Zerwekh JE, Antich PP, Mehta S, et al. Reflection ultrasound velocities and histomorphometric and connectivity analyses: correlations and effect of slow-release sodium fluoride. *J Bone Miner Res* 1997;12:2068–2075.
129. Sturtridge W, Lentle B, Hanley DA. The use of bone density measurement in the diagnosis and management of osteoporosis. *Can Med Assoc J* 1996;155(7):924–992.
130. Rubin SM, Cummings SR. Results of bone densitometry affect women's decisions about taking measures to prevent fractures. *Ann Intern Med* 1992;116:990–995.
131. Health Care Financing Administration. 42 CFR Part 410, et al. Medicare program coverage of and payment for bone mass measurements. *Fed Reg* 1998;63(121):34320–34328.
132. Watts NB. Understanding the bone mass measurement act. *J Clin Densitometry* 1999;2:211–217.
133. Conference Report. Consensus Development Conference: diagnosis, prophylaxis and treatment of osteoporosis. *Am J Med* 1993;94:646–650.
134. Kanis JA. Osteoporosis and osteopenia. *J Bone Miner Res* 1990;5:209–211.
135. Kanis JA, Melton LJ III, Christiansen C, et al. The diagnosis of osteoporosis. *J Bone Miner Res* 1994;9:1137–1141.
136. Looker AC, Orwoll ES, Johnston CC, et al. Prevalence of low femoral bone density in older US adults from NHANES III. *J Bone Miner Res* 1997;12:1761–1768.
137. Raisz LG. The osteoporosis revolution. *Ann Intern Med* 1997;5: 458–462.
138. Ross PD. Osteoporosis: frequency, consequences, and risk factors. *Arch Intern Med* 1996;156:1399–1411.
139. Cummings SR, Kelsey JL, Nevitt MC, et al. Epidemiology of osteoporosis and osteoporotic fractures. *Epidemiol Rev* 1985;7: 178–208.
140. Seeley DG, Browner WS, Nevitt MC, et al. Which fractures are associated with low appendicular bone mass in elderly women? *Ann Intern Med* 1991;115:837–842.
141. Riggs LB, Melton LJ III. Involutional osteoporosis. *N Engl J Med* 1986;341:1676–1686.
142. Lindsay R. The burden of osteoporosis: cost. *Am J Med* 1995; 98:9S–11S.
143. Cooper C, Campion G, Melton LJ III. Hip fractures in the elderly: a world-wide projection. *Osteoporosis Int* 1992;2:285–289.
144. Barrett-Connor E. The economic and human costs of osteoporotic fracture. *Am J Med* 1995;98:2S–8S.
145. Farmer ME, White LR, Brody JA, et al. Race and sex differences in hip fracture incidence. *Am J Public Health* 1984;74: 1374–1830.
146. Melton LJ, Cummings SR. Heterogeneity of age-related fractures: implications for epidemiology. *Bone* 1987;2:321–331.
147. Ross PD, Fujiwara S, Huang C, et al. Vertebral fracture prevalence in women in Hiroshima compared to Caucasians or Japanese in the US. *Int J Epidemiol* 1995;24:1171–1177.
148. Cooper C, Atkinson EJ, O'Fallon WM, et al. Incidence of clinically diagnosed vertebral fractures: a population-based study in Rochester, Minnesota. *J Bone Miner Res* 1992;7:221–227.
149. Melton LJ, Thamer J, Ray NF, et al. Fractures attributable to osteoporosis: report from the National Osteoporosis Foundation. *J Bone Miner Res* 1997;12:16–23.
150. Phillips S, Fox N, Jacobs J, et al. The direct medical costs of osteoporosis for American women aged 45 and older. *Bone* 1986;9:271–279.
151. Chrischilles EA, Butler CD, Davis CS, et al. A model of lifetime osteoporosis impact. *Arch Intern Med* 1991;151:2026–2032.
152. Chrischilles E, Shireman T, Wallace R. Costs and health effects of osteoporotic fractures. *Bone* 1994;15:377–386.
153. Ray NF, Chan JK, Thamer M, et al. Medical expenditures for the treatment of osteoporotic fractures in the United States in 1995: report from the National Osteoporosis Foundation. *J Bone Miner Res* 1997;12:24–35.
154. Cummings SR, Rubin SM, Black D. The future of hip fractures in the United States. *Clin Orthop* 1990;252:163–166.
155. Melton LJ III. Hip fractures: a worldwide problem today and tomorrow. *Bone* 1993;13(suppl):1–8.
156. Cooper C, Atkinson EJ, Jacobsen SJ, et al. Population-based survival after osteoporotic fractures. *Am J Epidemiol* 1993;137: 1001–1005.
157. Browner WS, Pressman AR, Nevitt MC, et al. Mortality following fractures in older women: the Study of Osteoporotic Fractures. *Arch Intern Med* 1996;156:1521–1525.
158. Matkovic V, Jelic T, Wardlaw GM, et al. Timing of peak bone mass in Caucasian females and its implication for the prevention of osteoporosis: inference from a cross-sectional model. *J Clin Invest* 1994;93:799–808.
159. Jones G, Nguyen T, Sambrook P, et al. Progressive loss of bone in the femoral neck in elderly people: longitudinal findings from the Dubbo osteoporosis epidemiology study. *Br J Med* 1994;309:691–695.
160. Krall EA, Dawson-Hughes B. Heritable and life-style determinants of bone mineral density. *J Bone Miner Res* 1993;8:1–8.
161. Seeman E, Hopper JL, Bach LA, et al. Reduced bone mass in daughters of women with osteoporosis. *N Engl J Med* 1989; 320::554–558.
162. Tylavsky PA, Bortz AD, Hancock RL, et al. Familial resemblance of radial bone mass between premenopausal mothers and their college-age daughters. *Calcif Tissue Int* 1989;45:265–272.
163. Ralston SH. Sciences, medicine, and the future: osteoporosis. *Br Med J* 1997;315:469–472.
164. Ralston SH. The genetics of osteoporosis. *Q Med J* 1997;90: 247–251.

165. Dequeker J, Nijs J, Verstraeten A, et al. Genetics of bone mineral content at the spine and radius: a twin study. *Bone* 1987; 8:207–209.
166. Gueguen R, Jouanny P, Guillemin F, et al. Segregation analysis and variance components analysis of bone mineral density in healthy families. *J Bone Miner Res* 1995;10:2017–2022.
167. Eisman JA. Vitamin D receptors gene alleles and osteoporosis: an affirmative view. *J Bone Miner Res* 1995;10:1289–1293.
168. Peacock M. Vitamin D receptor gene alleles and osteoporosis: a contrasting view. *J Bone Miner Res* 1995;10:1249–1297.
169. Salamone LM, Glynn NW, Black DM, et al. Determinants of premenopausal bone mineral density. The interplay of genetic and lifestyle factors. *J Bone Miner Res* 1996;11:1557–1565.
170. Tokita A, Kelly PJ, Nguyen TV, et al. Genetic influence of type I collagen synthesis and degradation: further evidence for genetic regulation of bone turnover. *J Clin Endocrinol Metab* 1994;78:1461–1466.
171. Keen RW, Woodford-Richens KL, Grants SFA, et al. Association of polymorphism at the type I collagen (COL1A1) locus with reduced bone mineral density, increased fracture risk, and increased collagen turnover. *Arthritis Rheum* 1999;42:285–290.
172. Cummings SR. Bone mass measurements and risk of fracture in Caucasian women: a review of findings from prospective studies. *Am J Med* 1995;98:24S–28S.
173. Cummings S, Nevitt MC, Browner WS, et al. Risk factors for hip fracture in white women. Study of Osteoporotic Fractures Research Group. *N Engl J Med* 1995;332:767–773.
174. Ross PD, Davis JW, Epstein RS, et al. Preexisting fractures and bone mass predict vertebral fracture incidence in women. *Ann Intern Med* 1991;114:919–923.
175. Deal CL. Osteoporosis, diagnosis and management. *Am J Med* 1997;102:35S–39S.
176. Bauer DC, Browner WS, Cauley JA, et al. Factors associated with appendicular bone mass in older women. *Ann Intern Med* 1993;118:657–665.
177. Ensrud KE, Palmero L, Black DM, et al. Hip and calcaneal bone loss increases with advancing age. Longitudinal results form the Study of Osteoporotic Fractures. *J Bone Miner Res* 1995;10:1778–1787.
178. Liel Y, Edwards J, Shary J, et al. The effect of race and body habitus on bone mineral density of the radius, hip, and spine in premenopausal women. *J Clin Endocrinol Metab* 1988;66: 1247–1250.
179. DeSimone DP, Steven J, Edwards J, et al. Influence of body habitus and race on bone mineral density of the midradius, hip, spine in aging women. *J Bone Miner Res* 1989;4:827–830.
180. Bhudhikanok GS, Wang M-C, Eckert K, et al. Difference in bone mineral in young Asian and Caucasian Americans may reflect difference in bone size. *J Bone Miner Res* 1996;11: 1545–1556.
181. Glauber HS, Vollmer WM, Nevitt MC, et al. Body weight versus body fat distribution, adiposity, and frame size as predictors of bone density. *J Clin Endocrinol Metab* 1995;80:1118–1123.
182. Ensrud KE, Lipschutz RC, Cauley JA, et al. Body size and hip fracture risk in older women: a prospective study. *Am J Med* 1997;103:274–280.
183. Ensrud KE, Cauley J, Lipschutz R, et al. Weight change and fractures in older women. *Arch Intern Med* 1997;157:857–863.
184. Salamone LM, Cauley JA, Black DM, et al. Effect of a lifestyle intervention on bone mineral density in premenopausal women: a randomized trial. *Am J Clin Nutr* 1999;70:97–103.
185. Kritz-Silverstein D, Barrett-Connor E. Bone mineral density in postmenopausal women as determined by prior oral contraceptive use. *Am J Public Health* 1993;83:100–102.
186. Michaelsson K, Baron JA, Farahmand BY, et al. Oral-contraceptive use and risk of hip fracture: a case-control study. *Lancet* 1999;353:1481–1484.
187. Fox KM, Cummings SR. Gynecology: Is tubal ligation a risk factor for low bone mineral density and increased risk of fracture? *Am J Obstet Gynecol* 1995;172:101–105.
188. Cundy T, Evans M, Roberts H, et al. Bone density in women receiving depot medroxyprogesterone acetate for contraception. *Br Med J* 1991;303:13–16.
189. Cundy T, Cornish J, Evans MC, et al. Recovery of bone density in women who stop using depot medroxyprogesterone acetate. *Br Med J* 1993;308:247–248.
190. Biller BMK, Saxe V, Herzog DB, et al. Mechanisms of osteoporosis in adult and adolescent women with anorexia nervosa. *J Clin Endocrinol Metab* 1989;68:548–554.
191. Rigotti NA, Neer RM, Skates SU, et al. The clinical course of osteoporosis in anorexia nervosa. A longitudinal study of cortical bone mass. *JAMA* 1991;265:1133–1138.
192. Carmichael KA, Carmichael DA. Bone metabolism and osteopenia in eating disorders. *Medicine* 1995;74:254–267.
193. Rencken ML, Chesnut CH III, Drinkwater BL. Bone mineral density at multiple skeletal sites in amenorrheic athletes. *JAMA* 1996;276:238–340.
194. Khan KM, Green RM, Saul A, et al. Retired elite female ballet dancers and nonathletic controls have similar bone mineral density at weight-bearing sites. *J Bone Miner Res* 1996;11:1566–1574.
195. Kritz-Silverstein D, Barrett-Connor E, Hollenbach KA. Pregnancy and lactation as determinants of bone mineral density in postmenopausal women. *Am J Epidemiol* 1992;136:1052–1059.
196. Rizzoli R, Bonjour JP. Pregnancy-associated osteoporosis. *Lancet* 1996;347:1274–1276.
197. Schneider DL, Barrett-Connor EL, Morton DJ. Timing of postmenopausal estrogen for optimal bone mineral density. The Rancho Bernardo Study. *JAMA* 1997;277:543–547.
198. Cauley JA, Seeley DG, Ensrud K, et al. Estrogen replacement therapy and fractures in older women. *Ann Intern Med* 1995; 122:9–16.
199. Cummings SR, Browner WS, Bauer D, et al. Endogenous hormones and the risk of hip and vertebral fractures in older women. *N Engl J Med* 1998;339:733–738.
200. Ettinger B, Pressman A, Sklarin P, et al. Associations between low levels of serum estradiol, bone density, and fractures among elderly women: the study of osteoporotic fractures. *J Clin Endocrinol Metab* 1998;38:2239–2243.
201. Stone K, Bauer DC, Black DM, et al. Hormonal factors of bone loss in elderly women: a prospective study. *J Bone Miner Res* 1998;13:1167–1174.
202. Winnacker J, Yeager H, Saunders JA, et al. Rickets in children receiving anticonvulsant drugs: biochemical and hormonal markers. *Am J Dis Child* 1977;131:286—290.
203. Sheth R, Wesolowski CA, Jacob JC, et al. Effect of carbamazepine and valproate on bone mineral density. *J Pediatr* 1995;127:256–262.
204. Dahlman TC. Osteoporotic fractures and the recurrence of thromboembolism during pregnancy and the puerperium in 184 women undergoing thromboprophylaxis with heparin. *Am J Obstet Gynecol* 1993;168:1265–1270.
205. Barbour LA, Kick SD, Steiner JF, et al. A prospective study of heparin-induced osteoporosis in pregnancy using bone densitometry. *Am J Obstet Gynecol* 1994;170:862–869.
206. Muir JM, Andrew M, Hirsh J, et al. Histomorphometric analysis of the effects of standard heparin on trabecular bone in vivo. *Blood* 1996;88:1314–1320.
207. Shaughnessy SG, Hirsh J, Bhandari M, et al. A histomorphometric evaluation of heparin-induced bone loss after discontinuation of heparin treatment in rats. *Blood* 1999;93:1231–1236..

208. Nelson-Piercy C. Heparin-induced osteoporosis. *Scand J Rheumatol* 1998;27:68–71.
209. Smith R, Phillips AJ. Osteoporosis during pregnancy and its management. *Scand J Rheumatol* 1998;27:66–67.
210. Philip WJU, Martin JC, Richardson JM, et al. Decreased axial and peripheral bone density in patients taking long-term warfarin. *Q J Med* 1995;88:635–640.
211. Jamal SA, Browner WS, Bauer DC, et al. Warfarin use and risk for osteoporosis in elderly women. *Ann Intern Med* 1998;128: 829–832.
212. Jones G, Nguyen T, Sambrook PN, et al. Thiazide diuretics and fractures: can meta-analysis help? *J Bone Miner Res* 1995;10: 106–111.
213. Feskanich D, Willet WC, Stampfer MJ, et al. A prospective study of thiazide use and fractures in women. *Osteoporosis Int* 1997;7:79–84.
214. Wasnich R, Davis J, Ross P, et al. Effect of thiazides on rates of bone mineral loss: a longitudinal study. *Br Med J* 1990;301: 1303–1305.
215. Cauley JA, Cummings SR, Seeley DG, et al. Effects of thiazide diuretic therapy on bone mass, fractures, and falls. The Study of Osteoporotic Fractures Research Group. *Ann Intern Med* 1993;118:666–673.
216. LaCroix AZ, Wienpahl J, White LR, et al. Thiazide diuretic agents and the incidence of hip fracture. *N Engl J Med* 1990; 322:286.
217. Liu B, Anderson G, Mittmann N, et al. Use of selective serotonin receptor uptake inhibitors or tricyclic antidepressants and risk of hip fractures in elderly people. *Lancet* 1998;351:1303–1307.
218. Laan RFJM, van Riel PLCM, van Erning TJTO, et al. Vertebral osteoporosis in rheumatoid arthritis patients: effect of low dose prednisone therapy. *Br J Rheumatol* 1992;31:91–96.
219. Garton MJ, Reid DM. Bone mineral density of the hip and of the anteroposterior and lateral dimensions of the spine in men with rheumatoid arthritis. Effects of low-dose corticosteroids. *Arthritis Rheum* 1993;36:222–228.
220. Laan RFJM, van Riel PLCM, van de Putte LBA, et al. Low dose prednisone induces rapid reversible axial bone loss in patients with rheumatoid arthritis. *Ann Intern Med* 1993;119:963–968.
221. Hopper JL, Seeman E. The bone density of female twins discordant for tobacco use. *N Engl J Med* 1994;330:387–392.
222. Michnovicz JJ, Hershcopf RJ, Naganuma H, et al. Increased 2-hydroxylation of estradiol as a possible mechanism for the anti-estrogenic effect of cigarette smoking. *N Engl J Med* 1986;315: 1305–1309.
223. Kiel DP, Baron JA, Anderson JJ, et al. Smoking eliminates the protective effect of oral estrogens on the risk for hip fracture among women. *Ann Intern Med* 1992;116:716–721.
224. Diamond T, Stiel D, Lunzer M, et al. Ethanol reduces bone formation and may cause osteoporosis. *Am J Med* 1989;86:282–288.
225. Diez A, Puig J, Serrano S, et al. Alcohol-induced bone disease in the absence of severe chronic liver damage. *J Bone Miner Res* 1994;9:825–831.
226. Van Thiel DH, Lester R, Sheerins RJ. Hypogonadism in alcoholic liver disease: evidence for a double defect. *Gastroenterology* 1974;67:1188–1199.
227. Klein RF. Alcohol-induced bone disease: impact of ethanol on osteoblast proliferation. *Alcoholism Clin Exp Res* 1997;21: 392–399.
228. Peris P, Pares A, Guanabens N, et al. Bone mass improves in alcoholics after 2 years of abstinence. *J Bone Miner Res* 1994;9: 1607–1612.
229. Barrett-Connor E, Chang JC, Edelstein SL. Coffee-associated osteoporosis offset by daily milk consumption. The Rancho Bernardo Study. *JAMA* 1994;271:280–283.
230. Johnston CC, Miller JZ, Slemenda CW, et al. Calcium supplementation and increases in bone mineral density in children. *N Engl J* Med 1992;327:82–87.
231. Nieves JW, Golden AL, Siris E, et al. Teenage and current calcium intake are related to bone mineral density of the hip and forearm in women aged 30–39 years. *Am J Epidemiol* 1995; 141:342–351.
232. Soroko SH, Holbrook TL, Edelstein S, et al. Lifetime milk consumptions and bone mineral density in older women. *Am J Public Health* 1994;84:1319–1322.
233. Bell NH. Vitamin D metabolism, aging and bone loss. *J Clin Endocrinol Metab* 1995;80:1051.
234. Chapuy MC, Preziosi P, Maamer M, et al. Prevalence of vitamin D insufficiency in an adult normal population. *Osteoporosis Int* 1997;7(5):439–443.
235. Storm D, Eslin R, Porter ES, et al. Calcium supplementation prevents seasonal bone loss and changes in biochemical markers of bone turnover in elderly New England women: a randomized placebo-controlled trial. *J Clin Endocrinol Metab* 1998;83: 3817–3825.
236. LeBoff MS, Kohlmeier L, Hurwitz S, et al. Occult vitamin D deficiency in postmenopausal US women with acute hip fracture. *JAMA* 1999;281:1505–1511.
237. Adams JS, Lee G. Gains in bone mineral density with resolution of vitamin D intoxication. *Ann Intern Med* 1997;127:203–206.
238. Marriott BM. Vitamin D supplementation: a word of caution. *Ann Intern Med* 1997;127:231–233.
239. Jarvinen M, Kannus P. Injury of an extremity as a risk factor for the development of osteoporosis. *J Bone Joint Surg* 1997;79: 263–276.
240. Gregg EW, Cauley JA, Seeley DG, et al. Physical activity and osteoporotic fracture risk in older women. *Ann Intern Med* 1998;129:81–88.
241. Heinonen A, Kannus P, Sievanen H, et al. Randomised controlled trial of effect of high-impact exercise on selected risk factors for osteoporotic fractures. *Lancet* 1996;348: 1343–1347.
242. Grisso JA, Kelsey JL, Strom BL, et al., and the Northeast hip fractures study group. Risk factors for falls as a cause of hip fracture in women. *N Engl J Med* 1991;324:1326–1331.
243. Greenspan SL, Myers ER, Maitland LA, et al. Fall severity and bone mineral density as risk factors for hip fracture in ambulatory elderly. *JAMA* 1994;271:128–133.
244. Kannus P, Parkkari J, Koskinen S, et al. Fall-induced injuries and deaths among older adults. *JAMA* 1999;281:1895–1899.
245. Nguyen T, Sambrook P, Kelly P, et al. Prediction of osteoporotic fractures by postural instability and bone density. *Br Med J* 1993;307:1111–1115.
246. Dargent-Molina P, Favier F, Grandjean H, et al. Fall-related factors and risk of hip fracture: the EPIDOS prospective study. *Lancet* 1996;348:145–149.
247. Nevitt MC, Cummings SR. Types of fall and risk of hip and wrist fractures: the Study of Osteoporotic Fractures. *J Am Geriatr Soc* 1993;41:1226–1234.
248. Lauritzen JB, Petersen MM, Lund B. Effect of external hip protectors on hip fractures. *Lancet* 1993;341:11–13.
249. Nicholson PHF, Haddaway MJ, Davie MWJ, et al. Vertebral deformity, bone mineral density, back pain and height loss in unscreened women over 50 years. *Osteoporosis Int* 1993;3: 303–307.
250. Coles RJ, Clements DG, Evans WD. Measurement of height: practical considerations for the study of osteoporosis. *Osteoporosis Int* 1994;4:353–356.
251. Hunt AH. The relationship between height change and bone mineral density. *Orthop Nursing* 1996;15:57–71.

252. Taguchi A, Tanimoto K, Suei Y, et al. Tooth loss and mandibular osteopenia. *Oral Surg Oral Med* 1995;79:127–132.
253. Wactawski-Wende J, Grossi SG, Trevisan M, et al. The role of osteopenia in oral bone loss and periodontal disease. *J Periodontol* 1996;67:1076–1084.
254. Jeffcoat M. Osteoporosis: a possible modifying factor in oral bone loss. *Ann Periodontol* 1998;3:312–321.
255. Hodgson SF, Johnston CC. AACE clinical practice guidelines for the prevention and treatment of postmenopausal osteoporosis. *Endocr Pract* 1996;2:155–181.
256. Rosalki SD. Biochemical markers of bone turnover. *Int J Clin Pract* 1998;42:255–256.
257. Shane E, Rivas M, McMahon DJ, et al. Bone loss and turnover after cardiac transplant. *J Clin Endocrinol Metab* 1997;82: 1497–1506.
258. Shane E, Rodino MA, McMahon DJ, et al. Prevention of bone loss after heart transplantation with antiresorptive therapy: a pilot study. *J Heart Lung Transplant* 1998;17:1089–1096.
259. Shane E, Rivas M, Staron RB, et al. Fracture after cardiac transplantation: a prospective longitudinal study. *J Clin Endocrinol Metab* 1996;81:1740–1746.
260. Garnero PHE, Chapuy M-C, Marcelli C, et al. Markers of bone resorption predict hip fracture in elderly women: the EPIDOS prospective study. *J Bone Miner Res* 1996;11:1531–1538.
261. Vergnaud P, Garnero P, Meunier PJ, et al. Undercarboxylated osteocalcin measured with a specific immunoassay precits hip fracture in elderly women: the EPIDOS study. *J Clin Endocrinol Metab* 1997;82:719–724.
262. Ross PD. Predicting bone loss and fracture risk with biochemical markers. *J Clin Densitometry* 1999;2:285–294.
263. Schneider DL, Barrett-Connor E. Urinary N-telopeptide levels discriminate normal, osteopenic, and osteoporotic bone mineral density. *Arch Intern Med* 1997;157:1241–1245.
264. Greenspan SL, Parker RA, Ferguson L, et al. Early changes in biochemical markers on bone turnover predict the long-term response to alendronate therapy in representative elderly women: a randomized clinical trial. *J Bone Miner Res* 1998;13: 1431–1438.
265. Prestwood KM, Pilbeam CC, Burleson JA, et al. The short term effects of conjugated estrogen on bone turnover in older women. *J Clin Endocrinol Metab* 1994;79:366–371.
266. Chesnut CH, Bell NH, Clark GS, et al. Hormone replacement therapy in postmenopausal women: urinary N-telopeptide of type I collagen monitors therapeutic effect and predicts response of bone mineral density. *Am J Med* 1997;102:29–37.
267. Eastell R. Treatment of postmenopausal osteoporosis. *N Engl J Med* 1998;338:736–746.
268. National Osteoporosis Foundation. *Physician's guide to the prevention and treatment of osteoporosis.* Belle Mead, NJ: Excerpta Medica, 1998.
269. Amarshi N, Scoggin A, Ensworth S. Osteoporosis: review of guidelines and consensus statements. *Am J Managed Care* 1997; 3(7):1077–1084.
270. Jones G, Hogan DB, Yendt E, et al. Vitamin D metabolites and analogs in the treatment of osteoporosis. *Can Med Assoc J* 1996; 155(7):955–961.
271. Siminoski K, Josse RG. Calcitonin in the treatment of osteoporosis. *Can Med Assoc J* 1996;155(7):962–965.
272. Murray TM. Calcium nutrition and osteoporosis. *Can Med Assoc J* 1996;155:935–939.
273. Prior JC, Barr SI, Chow R, et al. Physical activity as therapy for osteoporosis. *Can Med Assoc J* 1996;155:940–944.
274. Keating NL, Cleary PD, Rossi AS, et al. Use of hormone replacement therapy by postmenopausal women in the United States. *Ann Intern Med* 1999;130:545–553.
275. Perry J. The use of external support in the treatment of low-back pain. *J Bone Joint Surg* 1970;52A:1440–1442.
276. Ahlgren SA, Hansen T. The use of lumbosacral corsets prescribed for low back pain. *Prosthet Orthot Int* 1978;2:101–104.
277. Kaplan RS, Sinaki M, Hameister MD. Effect of back supports on back strength in patients with osteoporosis: a pilot study. *Mayo Clin Proc* 1996;71:235–241.
278. Lyles KW, Gold DT, Shipp KM, et al. Association of osteoporotic vertebral compression fractures with impaired functional status. *Am J Med* 1993;94:595–601.
279. Friedlander AL, Genant HK, Sadowsky S, et al. A two-year program of aerobics and weight training enhances bone mineral density of young women. *J Bone Miner Res* 1995;10:574–585.
280. Snow-Harter C, Bouxsein ML, Lewis BT, et al. Effects of resistance and endurance exercise on bone mineral status of young women: a randomized exercise intervention trial. *J Bone Miner Res* 1992;7:761–769.
281. Forwood MR, Burr DB. Physical activity and bone mass: exercises in futility? *Bone Miner* 1993;21:89–112.
282. Block JE. Interpreting studies of exercise and osteoporosis: a call for rigor. *Controlled Clin Trials* 1997;18:54–57.
283. Prior JC, Vigna YM, Schechter MT, et al. Spinal bone loss and ovulatory disturbances. *N Engl J Med* 1990;323:1221–1227.
284. Snow CM. Exercise and bone mass in young and premenopausal women. *Bone* 1996;18:51S–55S.
285. Grove KA, Londeree BR. Bone density in postmenopausal women: high impact vs low impact exercise. *Med Sci Sports Exerc* 1992;24:1190–1194.
286. Karlsson MK, Johnell O, Obrant KJ. Bone mineral density in weight lifters. *Calcif Tissue Int* 1993;52:212–215.
287. Chow R, Harrison JE, Notarius C. Effect of two randomised exercise programmes on bone mass of healthy postmenopausal women. *Br Med J* 1987;295:1441–1444.
288. Hatori M, Hasegawa A, Adachi H, et al. The effects of walking at the anaerobic threshold level on vertebral bone loss in postmenopausal women. *Calcif Tissue Int* 1993;52:411–414.
289. Lohman T, Going S, Pameter R, et al. Effects of resistance training on regional and total bone mineral density in premenopausal women: a randomized prospective study. *J Bone Miner Res* 1995;10:1015–1024.
290. Pruitt LA, Jackson RD, Bartels RL, et al. Weight-training effects on bone mineral density in early postmenopausal women. *J Bone Miner Res* 1992;7:179–185.
291. Aloia JF, Cohn SH, Ostuni JA, et al. Prevention of involutional bone loss by exercise. *Ann Intern Med* 1978;89:356–358.
292. Nelson ME, Fiatarone MA, Morganti CM, et al. Effects of high-intensity strength training on multiple risk factors for osteoporotic fractures: a randomized controlled trial. *JAMA* 1994;272:1909–1914.
293. Dalsky GP, Stocke KS, Ehsani AA, et al. Weight-bearing exercise training and lumbar bone mineral content in postmenopausal women. *Ann Intern Med* 1988;108:824–828.
294. Karlsson MK, Johnell O, Obrant KJ. Is bone mineral density advantage maintained long-term in previous weight lifters? *Calcif Tissue Int* 1995;57:325–328.
295. Sinaki M, Mikkelsen BA. Postmenopausal spinal osteoporosis: flexion versus extension exercises. *Arch Phys Med Rehabil* 1984; 65:593–596.
296. Itoi E, Sinaki M. Effect of back-strengthening exercise on posture in healthy women 49 to 65 years of age. *Mayo Clin Proc* 1994;69:1054–1059.
297. Cook DH, Guyatt GH, Adachi JD, et al. Quality of life issues in women with vertebral fractures due to osteoporosis. *Arthritis Rheum* 1993;36:750–756.
298. Kaplan FS, Scherl JD, Wisneski R, et al. The cluster phenome-

non in patients who have multiple vertebral compression fractures. *Clin Orthop Rel Res* 1993;297:161–167.
299. Mathis JM, Petri M, Naff N. Percutaneous vertebroplasty treatment of steroid-induced osteoporotic compression fractures. *Arthritis Rheum* 1998;41:171–175.
300. Jensen ME, Evans AJ, Mathis JM, et al. Percutaneous polymethylmethacrylate vertebroplasty in the treatment of osteoporotic vertebral body compression fractures: technical aspects. *Am J Neuroradiol* 1997;18:1897–1904.
301. Bullamore JR, Gallagher JC, Wilkinson R, et al. Effect of age on calcium absorption. *Lancet* 1970;2:535.
302. Riis B, Thomsen K, Christiansen C. Does calcium supplementation prevent postmenopausal bone loss? A double-blind controlled clinical study. *N Engl J Med* 1987;316:173–177.
303. Davis JW, Ross PD, Johnson NE, et al. Estrogen and calcium supplement use among Japanese-American women: effects upon bone loss when used singly and in combination. *Bone* 1995;17(4):369–373.
304. Reid IR, Ames W, Evans MC, et al. Long-term effects of calcium supplementation on bone loss and fractures in postmenopausal women: a randomized controlled trial. *Am J Med* 1995;98:331–335.
305. Aloia JF, Vaswani A, Yeh JK, et al. Calcium supplementation with and without hormone replacement therapy to prevent postmenopausal bone loss. *Ann Intern Med* 1994;120:97–103.
306. Smith EL, Gilligan C, Smith PE, et al. Calcium supplementation and bone loss in middle-aged women. *Am J Clin Nutr* 1989;50:833–842.
307. Dawson-Hughes B, Dallal GE, Krall EA, et al. A controlled trial of the effect of calcium supplementation on bone density in postmenopausal women. *N Engl J Med* 1990;323:878–883.
308. Prince RL, Smith M, Dick IM, et al. Prevention of postmenopausal osteoporosis. A comparative study of exercise, calcium supplementation, and hormone-replacement therapy. *N Engl J Med* 1991;325:1189–1195.
309. Elders PJM, Netelenbos JC, Lips P, et al. Calcium supplementation reduces vertebral bone loss in perimenopausal women: a controlled trial in 248 women between 46 and 55 years of age. *J Clin Endocrinol Metab* 1991;73:533–540.
310. Reid IR, Ames RW, Evans MC, et al. Effect of calcium supplementation on bone loss in postmenopausal women. *N Engl J Med* 1993;328:460–464.
311. Heaney RP. The bone remodeling transient: implications for the interpretation of clinical studies of bone mass change. *J Bone Miner Res* 1994;9:1515–1523.
312. Cumming RG. Calcium intake and bone mass: a quantitative review of the evidence. *Calcif Tissue Int* 1990;47:194–210.
313. Recker RR, Davies KM, Hinders SM, et al. Bone gain in young adult women. *JAMA* 1992;268:2403–2408.
314. Baran D, Sorensen A, Grimes J, et al. Dietary modification with diary products for preventing vertebral bone loss in premenopausal women: a three-year prospective study. *J Clin Endocrinol Metab* 1990;70:264–270.
315. Orwoll ES, Oviatt SK, McClung MR, et al. The rate of bone mineral loss in normal men and the effects of calcium and cholecalciferol supplementation. *Ann Intern Med* 1990;112:29–34.
316. Nieves JW, Komar L, Cosman F, et al. Calcium potentiates the effect of estrogen and calcitonin on bone mass: review and analysis. *Am J Clin Nutr* 1998;67:18–24.
317. Cooper C, Barker DJP, Wickham C. Physical activity, muscle strength, and calcium intake in fracture of the proximal femur in Britain. *Br Med J* 1988;297:1443–1446.
318. Wickham CAC, Walsh K, Cooper C, et al. Dietary calcium, physical activity and risk of hip fracture: a prospective study. *Br Med J* 1989;299:889–892.
319. Cumming RG, Cummings SR, Nevitt MC, et al. Calcium intake and fracture risk: results from the Study of Osteoporotic Fractures. *Am J Clin Epidemiol* 1997;145:926–934.
320. Holbrook TL, Barrett-Connor E, Wingard DL. Dietary calcium and risk of hip fracture: a prospective population study. *Lancet* 1988;2:1046–1049.
321. Kanis JA, Johnell O, Gullberg B, et al. Evidence for efficacy of drugs affecting bone metabolism in preventing hip fracture. *Br Med J* 1992;305:1124–1128.
322. Chapuy MC, Arlot ME, Delmas PD, et al. Effect of calcium and cholecalciferol treatment for three years on hip fractures in elderly women. *Br Med J* 1994;308:1081–1082.
323. Chevalley T, Rizzoli R, Nydegger V, et al. Effects of calcium supplements on femoral bone mineral density and vertebral fracture rate in vitamin-D replete elderly patients. *Osteoporosis Int* 1994;4:245–252.
324. Recker RR, Hinders S, Davies KM, et al. Correcting calcium nutrition deficiency prevents spine fractures in elderly women. *J Bone Miner Res* 1996;11:1961–1966.
325. Chapuy MC, Arlot ME, Duboeuf F, et al. Vitamin D3 and calcium to prevent hip fractures in elderly women. *N Engl J Med* 1992;327:1637–1642.
326. Cumming RG, Nevitt MC. Calcium for prevention of osteoporotic fractures in postmenopausal women. *J Bone Miner Res* 1997;12:1321–1329.
327. Recker RR, Bammi A, Barger-Lux MJ, et al. Calcium absorbability from milk products, an imitation milk, and calcium carbonate 1–3. *Am J Clin Nutr* 1988;47:93–95.
328. Harvey JA, Zobitz MM, Pak CYC. Dose dependency of calcium absorption: a comparison of calcium carbonate and calcium citrate. *J Bone Miner Res* 1988;3:253–258.
329. Hansen C, Werner E, Erbes HJ, et al. Intestinal calcium absorption from different calcium preparations: influence of anion and solubility. *Osteoporosis Int* 1996;6:386–393.
330. Heaney RP, Dowell MS, Barger-Lux MJ. Absorption of calcium as the carbonate and citrate salts, with some observations on method. *Osteoporosis Int* 1999;9:19–23.
331. Curhan GC, Willett WC, Speizer FE, et al. Comparison of dietary calcium with supplemental calcium and other nutrients as factors affecting the risk for kidney stones in women. *Ann Intern Med* 1997;126:497–504.
332. Curhan GC, Willett WC, Rimm EB, et al. A prospective study of dietary calcium and other nutrients and the risk of symptomatic kidney stones. *N Engl J Med* 1993;328:833–838.
333. NIH Consensus Development Conference. Optimal calcium intake. *JAMA* 1994;272:1942–1948.
334. Institute of Medicine. *Dietary reference intakes: calcium, phosphorus, magnesium, vitamin D, and fluoride.* New York: Academy Press, 1997.
335. Aloia JF, Vaswani A, Yeh JK, et al. Calcitriol in the treatment of postmenopausal osteoporosis. *Am J Med* 1988;84:401–408.
336. Gallagher JC, Goldgar D. Treatment of postmenopausal osteoporosis with high doses of synthetic calcitriol: a randomized controlled study. *Ann Intern Med* 1990;113:649–655.
337. Orimo H, Shiraki M, Hayashi T, et al. Reduced occurrence of vertebral crush fractures in senile osteoporosis treated with 1 alpha(OH)D3. *Bone Miner* 1987;3:47–52.
338. Orimo H, Shiraki M, Hayashi Y, et al. Effects of 1 alpha-hydroxyvitamin D3 on lumbar bone mineral density and vertebral fractures in patients with postmenopausal osteoporosis. *Calcif Tissue Int* 1994;54:370–376.
339. Shiraki M, Itoh H, Orimo H. The ultra long-term treatment of senile osteoporosis with 1 alpha-hydroxyvitamin D3. *Bone Miner* 1993;20:223–234.
340. Gallagher JC, Riggs BL, Recker RR, et al. The effect of calcitriol

on patients with postmenopausal osteoporosis with special reference to fracture frequency. *Proc Soc Exp Biol Med* 1989;191: 287–292.

341. Tilyard MW, Spears GFS, Thomson J, et al. Treatment of postmenopausal osteoporosis with calcitriol or calcium. *N Engl J Med* 1992;326:357–362.
342. Ott SM, Chesnut CH III. Calcitriol treatment is not effective in postmenopausal osteoporosis. *Ann Intern Med* 1989;110:267–274.
343. Heikinheimo RJ, Knkovaara JA, Harju EJ, et al. Annual injection of vitamin D and fractures of aged bones. *Calcif Tissue Int* 1992;51:105–110.
344. Dawson-Hughes B, Harris SS, Krall EA, et al. Effect of calcium and vitamin D supplementation on bone density in men and women 65 years of age and older. *N Engl J Med* 1997;337: 670–676.
345. Lips P, Graafmans WC, Ooms ME, et al. Vitamin D supplementation and fracture incidence in elderly people. A randomized, placebo-controlled clinical trial. *Ann Intern Med* 1996; 124:400–406.
346. Lindsay R, Hart DM, Aitken JM, et al. Long-term prevention of postmenopausal osteoporosis by oestrogen. *Lancet* 1976;1: 1038–1041.
347. Recker RR, Saville PD, Heaney RP. Effect of estrogens and calcium carbonate on bone loss in postmenopausal women. *Ann Intern Med* 1977;87:649–655.
348. Horsman A, Gallagher JC, Simpson M, et al. Prospective trial of oestrogen and calcium in postmenopausal women. *Br Med J* 1977;2:789–792.
349. Nachtigall LE, Nachtigall RH, Nachtigall RD, et al. Estrogen replacement therapy 1: a 10-year prospective study in the relationship to osteoporosis. *Obstet Gynecol* 1979;53:277.
350. Ettinger B, Genant HK, Cann EE. Postmenopausal bone loss is prevented by treatment with low-dosage estrogen with calcium. *Ann Intern Med* 1987;106:40–45.
351. The PEPI Writing Group. Effects of hormone therapy on bone mineral density: results from the postmenopausal estrogen/progestin interventions (PEPI) trial. *JAMA* 1996;275:1380–1396.
352. Recker RR, Davies M, Dowd RM, et al. The effect of low-dose continuous estrogen and progesterone therapy with calcium and vitamin D on bone in elderly women. A randomized, controlled trial. *Ann Intern Med* 1999;130:897–904.
353. Lindsay R, Hart DM, Forrest C, et al. Prevention of spinal osteoporosis in oophorectomized women. *Lancet* 1980;2:1151–1157.
354. Weiss NS, Ure CL, Ballard JH, et al. Decreased risks of fractures of the hip and lower forearm with postmenopausal use of estrogen. *N Engl J Med* 1980;303:1195–1198.
355. Paganini-Hill A, Ross RK, Gerkins VR, et al. Menopausal estrogen therapy and hip fractures. *Ann Intern Med* 1981;95:28–31.
356. Hutchinson TA, Polansky SM, Feinstein AR. Post-menopausal estrogens protect against fractures of hip and distal radius. A case-control study. *Lancet* 1979;2:705–709.
357. Ettinger B, Genant HK, Cann CE. Long-term estrogen replacement therapy prevents bone loss and fractures. *Ann Intern Med* 1985;102:319–324.
358. Naessen T, Persson I, Adami HO, et al. Hormone replacement therapy and the risk for the first hip fracture. A prospective, population-based cohort study. *Ann Intern Med* 1990;113:95–103.
359. Grady D, Rubin SM, Petitti DB, et al. Hormone therapy to prevent disease and prolong life in postmenopausal women. *Ann Intern Med* 1992;117:1016–1037.
360. Kiel DP, Felson DT, Anderson JJ, et al. Hip fracture and the use of estrogens in postmenopausal women: the Framingham study. *N Engl J Med* 1987;317:1169–1174.
361. Felson DT, Zhang Y, Hannan MT, et al. The effect of postmenopausal estrogen therapy on bone density in elderly women. *N Engl J Med* 1993;329:1141–1146.
362. Maxim P, Ettinger B, Spitalny GM. Fracture protection provided by long-term estrogen treatment. *Osteoporosis Int* 1995;5:23–29.
363. Lufkin EG, Whaner HW, O'Fallon WM, et al. Treatment of postmenopausal osteoporosis with transdermal estrogen. *Ann Intern Med* 1992;117:1–9.
364. Christiansen C, Riis BJ. 17-beta-estradiol and continuous norethisterone: a unique treatment of established osteoporosis in elderly women. *J Clin Endocrinol Metab* 1990;71:836–841.
365. Lindsay R, Tohme JF. Estrogen treatment of patients with established postmenopausal osteoporosis. *Obstet Gynecol* 1990;72: 290–295.
366. Marx CW, Dailey GED, Cheney C, et al. Do estrogens improve bone mineral density in osteoporotic women over age 65? *J Bone Miner Res* 1992;7:1275–1279.
367. Quigley ME, Martin PL, Burnier AM, et al. Estrogen therapy arrests bone loss in elderly women. *Am J Obstet Gynecol* 1987; 156:1516–1523.
368. Hazzard WR. Estrogen replacement and cardiovascular disease: serum lipids and blood pressure effects. *Am J Obstet Gynecol* 1989;161:1847–1853.
369. Walsh BW, Schiff I, Rosner B, et al. Effects of postmenopausal estrogen replacement on the concentrations and metabolism of plasma lipoproteins. *N Engl J Med* 1991;325:1196–1204.
370. Koh KK, Mincemoyer R, Bui MN, et al. Effects of hormone-replacement therapy on fibrinolysis in postmenopausal women. *N Engl J Med* 1997;336:683–690.
371. Bush TL, Barrett-Connor E, Cowan LD, et al. Cardiovascular mortality and noncontraceptive use of estrogen in women: results from the Lipid Research Clinics Program Follow-up Study. *Circulation* 1987;75:1102–1109.
372. Sullivan JM, Vander Zwaag R, Hughes JP, et al. Estrogen replacement and coronary artery disease. *Arch Intern Med* 1990; 150:2557–2562.
373. O'Brien JE, Peterson ED, Keeler GP, et al. Relation between estrogen replacement therapy and restenosis after percutaneous coronary interventions. *J Am Coll Cardiol* 1996;28:1111–1118.
374. Newton KM, LaCroix AZ, McKnight B, et al. Estrogen replacement therapy and prognosis after first myocardial infarction. *Am J Epidemiol* 1997;145:269–277.
375. Sullivan JM, El-Zeky F, Vander Zwaag R, et al. Effect on survival of estrogen replacement therapy after coronary artery bypass grafting. *Am J Cardiol* 1997;79:847–850.
376. O'Keefe JH, Kim SC, Hall RR, et al. Estrogen replacement therapy after coronary angioplasty in women. *J Am Coll Cardiol* 1997;29:1–5.
377. Hulley S, Grady D, Busch T, et al. Randomized trial of estrogen plus progestin for secondary prevention of coronary heart disease in postmenopausal women. *JAMA* 1998;280:605–613.
378. Sellers TA, Mink PJ, Cerhan JR, et al. The role of hormone replacement therapy in the risk for breast cancer and total mortality in women with a family history of breast cancer. *Ann Intern Med* 1997;127:973–980.
379. Grodstein F, Stampfer MJ, Colditz GA, et al. Postmenopausal hormone therapy and mortality. *N Eng J Med* 1997;336(25): 1769–1775.
380. Barrett-Connor E. Postmenopausal estrogen and prevention bias. *Ann Intern Med* 1991;115:455–456.
381. Grodstein F, Stampfer MJ, Manson JE, et al. Postmenopausal estrogen and progestin use and the risk of cardiovascular disease. *N Engl J Med* 1996;335:453–461.
382. Grodstein F, Martinez E, Platz E, et al. Postmenopausal hormone use and risk for colorectal cancer and adenoma. *Ann Intern Med* 1998;128:705–712.
383. Tang MX, Jacobs D, Stern Y, et al. Effect of oestrogen during menopause on risk and age at onset of Alzheimer's disease. *Lancet* 1996;348:429–432.

384. Yaffe K, Sawaya G, Lieberburg I, et al. Estrogen therapy in postmenopausal women: effects of cognitive function and dementia. *JAMA* 1998;279:688–695.
385. Jick H, Derby LE, Myers MW, et al. Risk of hospital admission for idiopathic venous thromboembolism among users of postmenopausal oestrogens. *Lancet* 1996;348:981–983.
386. Daly E, Vessey MP, Hawkins MM, et al. Risk of venous thromboembolism in users of hormone replacement therapy. *Lancet* 1996;348:977–980.
387. Grodstein F, Stampfer MJ, Goldhaber SZ, et al. Prospective study of exogenous hormones and risk of pulmonary embolism in women. *Lancet* 1996;348:983–987.
388. Gutthann SP, Rodriguez LAG, Castellsague J, et al. Hormone replacement therapy and risk of venous thromboembolism: population based case-control study. *Br Med J* 1997;314:796–800.
389. Breslau NA. Calcium, estrogen, and progestin in the treatment of osteoporosis. *Rheum Dis Clin North Am* 1994;20:691–716.
390. Steinberg KK, Thacker SB, Smith J, et al. A meta-analysis of the effect of estrogen replacement therapy on the risk of breast cancer. *JAMA* 1991;265:1985–1990.
391. Bergkvist L, Adami HO, Persson I, et al. The risk of breast cancer after estrogen and estrogen-progestin replacement. *N Engl J Med* 1989;321:293–297.
392. Colditz GA, Hankinson SE, Hunter DJ, et al. The use of estrogens and progestins and the risk of breast cancer in postmenopausal women. *N Engl J Med* 1995;332:1589–1593.
393. Collaborative Group on Hormonal Factors in Breast Cancer. Breast cancer and hormone replacement therapy. *Lancet* 1997; 350:1047–1059.
394. Gapstur SM, Morrow M, Sellers TA. Hormone replacement therapy and risk of breast cancer with a favorable histology: results of the Iowa Women's Health Study. *JAMA* 1999;281:2091–2097.
395. Ravnikar VA. Compliance with hormone therapy. *Am J Obstet Gynecol* 1987;156:1332–1334.
396. Hahn RG. Compliance considerations with estrogen replacement: withdrawal bleeding and other factors. *Am J Obstet Gynecol* 1989;161(6 pt 2):1854–1858.
397. Chetkowski RJ, Meldrum DR, Steingold KA, et al. Biologic effects of transdermal estradiol. *N Engl J Med* 1986;314:1615–1620.
398. Lindsay R, Hart DM, Fogelman I. Bone mass after withdrawal of oestrogen replacement. *Lancet* 1981;1:729.
399. Christiansen C, Christensen MS, Transbol IB. Bone mass in postmenopausal women after withdrawal of oestrogen/gestagen replacement therapy. *Lancet* 1981;1:459–461.
400. Col NF, Eckman MH, Karas RH, et al. Patient-specific decisions about hormone replacement therapy in post-menopausal women. *JAMA* 1997;277:1140–1147.
401. Daley J. Medical uncertainty and practice variation get personal: What should I do about hormone replacement therapy? (editorial). *Ann Intern Med* 1999;130(7):602–604.
402. O'Connor AM, Tugwell P, Wells GA, et al. Randomized trial of a portable, self-administered decision aid for postmenopausal women considering long-term preventive hormone therapy. *Med Decis Making* 1998;18:295–303.
403. Love RR, Mazess RB, Bardens HS, et al. Effects of tamoxifen on uterus and ovaries of postmenopausal women in a randomised breast cancer prevention trial. *N Engl J Med* 1995;311:977–980.
404. Wright CDP, Compston JE. Tamoxifen; oestrogen or antioestrogen in bone. *Q J Med* 1995;88:307–310.
405. Grey AB, Stapleton JP, Evans MC, et al. The effect of the antioestrogen tamoxifen on bone mineral density in normal late postmenopausal women. *Am J Med* 1995;99:636–641.
406. Khovidhunkit W, Shoback DM. Clinical effects of raloxifene hydrochloride in women. *Ann Intern Med* 1999;130:431–439.
407. Draper MW, Flowers DE, Huster WJ, et al. A controlled trial of raloxifene (LY139481) HCl: impact on bone turnover and serum lipid profile in healthy postmenopausal women. *J Bone Miner Res* 1996;11:835–842.
408. Delmas PD, Bjarnason NH, Mitlak BH, et al. Effects of raloxifene on bone mineral density, serum cholesterol concentrations, and uterine endometrium in postmenopausal women. *N Engl J Med* 1997;337(23):1641–1647.
409. Ettinger B, Black DM, Mitlak BH, et al. Reduction of vertebral fracture risk in postmenopausal women with osteoporosis treated with raloxifene: results from a 3-year randomized clinical trial. *JAMA* 1999;282(7):637–645.
410. Cummings SR, Eckert S, Krueger KA, et al. The effect of raloxifene on risk of breast cancer in postmenopausal women: results from the MORE randomized trial. *JAMA* 1999;281(23):2189–2197.
411. Ke HZ, Simmons HA, Pirie CM, et al. Droloxifene, a new estrogen antagonist/agonist, prevents bone loss in ovariectomized rats. *Endocrinology* 1995;136:2435–2441.
412. Plosker GL, McTavish D. Intranasal salcatonin (salmon calcitonin): a review of its pharmacological properties and role in the management of postmenopausal osteoporosis. *Drugs Aging* 1996;8:378–399.
413. Overgaard K, Agnusdei D, Hansen MA, et al. Dose-response bioactivity and bioavailability of salmon calcitonin in premenopausal and postmenopausal women. *J Clin Endocrinol Metab* 1991;72:344–349.
414. Muff R, Dambacher MA, Fischer JA. Formation of neutralizing antibodies during intranasal synthetic salmon calcitonin treatment of postmenopausal osteoporosis. *Osteoporosis Int* 1991;1:72–75.
415. Overgaard K, Hansen MA, Nelsen V-A, et al. Discontinuous calcitonin treatment of established osteoporosis-effects of withdrawal of treatment. *Am J Med* 1990;89:1–7.
416. Gennari C, Chierichetti SM, Bigazzi S, et al. Comparative effects on bone mineral content of calcium and calcium plus salmon calcitonin given in two different regimens in postmenopausal osteoporosis. *Curr Ther Res* 1985;38:455–464.
417. Ljunghall S, Gardsell P, Johnell O, et al. Synthetic human calcitonin and postmenopausal osteoporosis: a placebo-controlled, double-blind study. *Calcif Tissue Int* 1991;49:17–19.
418. MacIntyre I, Stevenson JC, Whitehead BI, et al. Calcitonin for prevention of postmenopausal bone loss. *Lancet* 1988;1: 1900–1902.
419. Mazzuoli GF, Passeri M, Gennari C, et al. Effects of salmon calcitonin in postmenopausal osteoporosis: a controlled double-blind clinical study. *Calcif Tissue Int* 1986;38:3–8.
420. Ellerington MC, Hillard TC, Whitcroft SIJ, et al. Intranasal salmon calcitonin for the prevention and treatment of postmenopausal osteoporosis. *Calcif Tissue Int* 1996;59:6–11.
421. Overgaard K, Riis BJ, Christiansen C, et al. Effect of salcotonin given intranasally on early postmenopausal bone loss. *Br Med J* 1989;299:477–479.
422. Reginster JY, Deroisy R, Lecart MP, et al. A double-blind, placebo-controlled, dose-finding trial of intermittent nasal salmon calcitonin for prevention of postmenopausal lumbar spine bone loss. *Am J Med* 1995;98:452–458.
423. Thamsborg G, Storm TL, Sykulski R, et al. Effect of different doses of nasal salmon calcitonin on bone mass. *Calcif Tissue Int* 1991;48:302–307.
424. Nielsen NM, von der Recke P, Hansen MA, et al. Estimation of the effect of salmon calcitonin in established osteoporosis by biochemical bone markers. *Calcif Tissue Int* 1994;55:8–11.
425. Civitelli R, Gonnelli S, Zacchei F, et al. Bone turnover in postmenopausal osteoporosis. Effect of calcitonin treatment. *J Clin Invest* 1988;82:1268–1274.
426. Overgaard K, Hansen MA, Jensen SB, et al. Effect of salcatonin given intranasally on bone mass and fracture rates in established osteoporosis: a dose response study. *Br Med J* 1992;305: 556–559.

427. Silverman SL, Chesnut C, Andriano K, et al. Salmon calcitonin nasal spray (NS-CT) reduces risk of vertebral fracture(s) (VF) in established osteoporosis and has continuous efficacy with prolonged treatment: accrued 5 year worldwide data of the PROOF study. *J Bone Miner Res* 1998;23(suppl 5):S174.
428. Lyritis GP, Tsakalabos S, Magiasis B, et al. Analgesic effect of salmon calcitonin on osteoporotic vertebral fractures. Double-blind, placebo-controlled study. *Calcif Tissue Int* 1991;49: 369–372.
429. Lyritis GP, Paspati I, Karachalios T, et al. Pain relief from nasal salmon calcitonin in osteoporositc vertebral crush fractures. A double blind, placebo controlled clinical study. *Acta Orthop Scand Suppl* 1997;275:112–114.
430. Pun KK, Chan LWL. Analgesic effect of intranasal salmon calcitonin in the treatment of osteoporotic vertebral fractures. *Clin Ther* 1989;11(2):205–209.
431. Laurin L, Overman Z, Graf E, et al. Calcitonin-induced increase in ACTH, b-endorphin and cortical secretion. *Horm Metab Res* 1986;18:268–271.
432. Fleisch H. New bisphosphonates in osteoporosis. *Osteoporosis Int* 1993;2(suppl):S15–22.
433. McClung MR. Current bone mineral density data on bisphosphonates in postmenopausal osteoporosis. *Bone* 1996;19:195S–198S.
434. Stock JL, Bell NH, Chesnut CH III, et al. Increments in bone mineral density of the lumbar spine and hip and suppression of bone turnover are maintained after discontinuation of alendronate on postmenopausal women. *Am J Med* 1997;103:291–297.
435. Rodan GA. Mechanisms of action of bisphosphonates. *Annu Rev Pharmacol Toxicol* 1998;38:375–388.
436. Hughes DE, Wright KR, Uy HL, et al. Bisphosphonates promote apoptosis in murine osteoclasts in vitro and in vivo. *J Bone Miner Res* 1995;10:1478–1487.
437. Graham R, Russell G, Rogers MJ, et al. The pharmacology of bisphosphonates and new insights into their mechanisms of action. *J Bone Miner Res* 1999;14(suppl 2):53–65.
438. Peter CP, Handt LK, Smith SM. Esophageal irritation due to alendronate sodium tablets: possible mechanisms. *Dig Dis Sci* 1998;43(9):1998–2002.
439. De Groen PC, Lubbe DF, Hirsch LJ, et al. Esophagitis associated with the use of alendronate. *N Engl J Med* 1996;335: 1016–1021.
440. van Staa T, Abenhaim L, Cooper C. Upper gastrointestinal adverse events and cyclical etidronate. *Am J Med* 1997;103: 462–467.
441. Francis MD, Centner RL. The development of diphosphonates as significant health care product. *J Chem Educ* 1978;55: 760–766.
442. Watts NB, Harris ST, Genant HK, et al. Intermittent cyclical etidronate treatment of postmenopausal osteoporosis. *N Engl J Med* 1990;323:73–79.
443. Storm T, Thamsborg G, Steiniche T, et al. Effect of intermittent cyclical etidronate therapy on bone mass and fracture in women with postmenopausal osteoporosis. *N Engl J Med* 1990;322: 1265–1271.
444. Harris ST, Watts NB, Jackson RD, et al. Four year study of intermittent cyclic etidronate treatment of postmenopausal osteoporosis: three years of blinded therapy followed by one year of therapy. *Am J Med* 1993;95:557.
445. Fairney A, Kyd P, Thomas E, et al. The use of cyclical etidronate in osteoporosis: changes after completion of 3 years treatment. *J Rheumatol* 1998;37:51–56.
446. Herd RJM, Balena R, Blake GM, et al. The prevention of early postmenopausal bone loss by cyclical etidronate therapy: a 2-year, double-blind, placebo-controlled study. *Am J Med* 1997; 103:92–99.
447. Wimalawansa SJ. Combined therapy with estrogen and etidronate has an additive effect on bone mineral density in the hip and vertebrae: four-year randomized study. *Am J Med* 1995; 99:36–42.
448. Hortobagyl GN, Terhiault RL, Porter L, et al. Efficacy of pamidronate in reducing skeletal complications in patients with breast and lytic bone metastases. *N Engl J Med* 1996;335: 1785–1791.
449. Fitton A, McTavish D. Pamidronate: a review of its pharmacological properties and therapeutic efficacy in resorptive bone disease. *Drugs* 1991;41:289–318.
450. Valkema R, Vismans F-JE, Papapoulos SE, et al. Maintained improvement in calcium balance and bone mineral content in patients with osteoporosis treated with the bisphosphonate APD. *Bone Miner* 1989;5:183–192.
451. Gangji V, Appelboom T. Analgesic effect of intravenous pamidronate on chronic back pain due to osteoporotic vertebral fractures. *Clin Rheumatol* 1999;18:266–267.
452. Balena R, Toolan BC, Shea M, et al. The effects of 2-year treatment with the aminobisphosphonate alendronate on bone metabolism, bone histomorphometry, and bone strength in ovariectomized nonhuman primates. *J Clin Invest* 1993;92: 2577–2586.
453. Schenk KR, Eggli P, Fleisch H, et al. Quantitative morphometric evaluation of the inhibition activity of new aminobisphosphonates on bone resorption in the rat. *Calcif Tissue Int* 1986; 38:342–349.
454. Chavassieux PM, Arlot ME, Reda C, et al. Histomorphometric assessment of the long-term effects of alendronate on bone quality and remodeling in patients with osteoporosis. *J Clin Invest* 1997;100:1475–1480.
455. Liberman UA, Weiss SR, Bröll J, et al. Effect of oral alendronate on bone mineral density and the incidence of fractures in postmenopausal osteoporosis. *N Engl J Med* 1995;333:1437–1443.
456. Chesnut CH, McClung MR, Ensrud KE, et al. Alendronate treatment of the postmenopausal osteoporotic woman: effect of multiple dosages on bone mass and bone remodeling. *Am J Med* 1995;99:144–152.
457. McClung M, Clemmesen B, Daifotis A, et al. Alendronate prevents postmenopausal bone loss in women without osteoporosis: a double-blind, randomized, controlled trial. *Ann Intern Med* 1998;128:253–261.
458. Hosking D, Chilvers CED, Christiansen C, et al. Prevention of bone loss with alendronate in postmenopausal women under 60 years of age. *N Engl J Med* 1998;338:485–492.
459. Black DM, Cummings SR, Karpf DB, et al. Randomised trial of effect of alendronate on risk of fracture in women with existing vertebral fractures. *Lancet* 1996;348:1535–1541.
460. Cummings SR, Black DM, Thompson DE, et al. Effect of alendronate on risk of fracture in women with low bone density but without vertebral fractures. *JAMA* 1998;280:2077–2082.
461. Pols HAP, Felsenberg D, Hanley DA, et al. Multinational, placebo-controlled, randomized trial of the effects of alendronate on bone density and fracture risk in postmenopausal women with low bone mass: results of the FOSIT study. *Osteoporosis Int* 1999;9:461–468.
462. Karpf DB, Shapiro DR, Seeman E, et al. Prevention of nonvertebral fractures by alendronate: a meta-analysis. *JAMA* 1997; 277:1159–1164.
463. Lindsay R, Cosman F, Lobo RA, et al. Addition of alendronate to ongoing hormone replacement therapy in the treatment of osteoporosis: a randomized, controlled clinical trial. *J Clin Endocrinol Metab* 1999;84:3076–3081.
464. Rossini M, Gatti D, Zamberlan N, et al. Long-term effects of a treatment course with oral alendronate of postmenopausal osteoporosis. *J Bone Miner Res* 1994;9:1833–1837.
465. Saag KG, Emkey R, Schnitzer T, et al. Alendronate for the treat-

ment and prevention of glucocorticoid-induced osteoporosis. *N Engl J Med* 1998;339:292–299.

466. Mortensen L, Charles P, Bekker PJ, et al. Risedronate increases bone mass in an early postmenopausal population: two years of treatment plus one year of follow-up. *J Clin Endocrinol Metab* 1998;83:396–402.
467. Harris ST, Watts NB, Genant HK, et al. Effects of risedronate treatment on vertebral and nonvertebral fractures in women with postmenopausal osteoporosis: a randomized controlled trial. *JAMA* 1999;282:1344–1352.
468. Reginster JY, Deroisy R, Denis D, et al. Prevention of postmenopausal bone loss by tiludronate. *Lancet* 1989;2:1469.
469. Heaney RP, Baylink DJ, Johnston CC Jr, et al. Fluoride therapy for the vertebral crush fracture syndrome. A status report. *Ann Intern Med* 1989;111:678–680.
470. Dambacher MA, Ittner J, Ruegsegger P. Long-term fluoride therapy of postmenopausal osteoporosis. *Bone* 1986;7:199–205.
471. Riggs BL, Hodgson SF, O'Fallon MW, et al. Effect of fluoride treatment on the fracture rate in postmenopausal women with osteoporosis. *N Engl J Med* 1990;322:802–809.
472. Kleerekoper M, Peterson EL, Nelson DA, et al. A randomized trial of sodium fluoride as a treatment for postmenopausal osteoporosis. *Osteoporosis Int* 1991;1:155–161.
473. Hodsman AB, Drost DJ. The response of vertebral bone mineral density during the treatment of osteoporosis with sodium fluoride. *J Clin Endocrinol Metab* 1989;69:932–938.
474. Meunier PJ, Sebert JL, Reginster JY, et al. Fluoride salts are no better prevention at preventing new vertebral fractures than calcium-vitamin D in postmenopausal osteoporosis: the FAVOS study. *Osteoporosis Int* 1998;8:4–12.
475. Reginster JY, Meurmans L, Zegels B, et al. The effect of sodium monofluorophosphate plus calcium on vertebral fracture rate in postmenopausal women with moderate osteoporosis: a randomized, controlled trial. *Ann Intern Med* 1998;129:1–8.
476. Inkovaara JA, Heikinheimo R, Jarvinen K, et al. Prophylactic fluoride treatment on aged bones. *Br Med J* 1975;3:73–74.
477. Aaron JE, Vernejoul MCd, Kanis JA. The effect of sodium fluoride on trabecular architecture. *Bone* 1991;12:307–310.
478. Schnitzler CM, Solomon I. Trabecular stress fractures during fluoride therapy for osteoporosis. *Skeletal Radiol* 1985;14: 276–279.
479. Orcel P, Vernejoul MCd, Prier A, et al. Stress fractures of the lower limbs in osteoporotic patients treated with fluoride. *J Bone Miner Res* 1990;5(suppl):S191–S194.
480. Briancon D, Meunier PJ. Treatment of osteoporosis with fluoride, calcium and vitamin D. *Orthop Clin North Am* 1981;12: 629–648.
481. Gerster JC, Charhon SA, Jaeger F, et al. Bilateral fractures of femoral neck in patients with moderate renal failure receiving fluoride for spinal osteoporosis. *Br Med J* 1983;287:723–725.
482. Mamelle N, Meunier PJ, Dusan R, et al. Risk-benefit ratio of sodium fluoride treatment in primary vertebral osteoporosis. *Lancet* 1988;2:361–365.
483. Pak CYC, Sakhaee K, Piziak V, et al. Slow-release sodium fluoride in the management of postmenopausal osteoporosis. A randomized controlled trial. *Ann Intern Med* 1994;120:625–632.
484. Pak CYC, Sakhaee K, Adams-Huet B, et al. Treatment of postmenopausal osteoporosis with slow-release sodium fluoride. Final report of a randomized controlled trial. *Ann Intern Med* 1995;123:401–408.
485. Schnitzler CM, Wing JR, Raal FJ, et al. Fewer bone histomorphometric abnormalities with intermittent than with continuous slow-release sodium fluoride therapy. *Osteoporosis Int* 1997; 7:376–389.
486. Need HG, Horowitz M, Bridges A, et al. Effects of nandrolene decanoate and antiresorptive therapy on vertebral density in osteoporotic postmenopausal women. *Arch Intern Med* 1989; 149:57–60.
487. Riggs BL. Formation-stimulating regimens other than sodium fluoride. *Am J Med* 1993;95:62S–68S.
488. Johansen JS, Hassager C, Podenphant J. Treatment of postmenopausal osteoporosis: is the anabolic steroid nandrolone decanoate a candidate? *Bone Miner* 1989;6:77–86.
489. Chesnut CH III, Ivey JL, Gruber HE, et al. Stanazol in the postmenopausal osteoporosis: therapeutic efficacy and possible mechanisms of action. *Metabolism* 1983;32:571–580.
490. Hassager C, Riis BJ, Podenphat J, et al. Nadrolene decanoate treatment of postmenopausal osteoporosis for 2 years and effects of withdrawal. *Maturitas* 1989;11:305–317.
491. Wasnich RD, Benfante J, Yano K, et al. Thiazide effect on the mineral content of bone. *N Engl J Med* 1983;309:344–347.
492. Adams JS, Song CF, Kantorovich V. Rapid recovery of bone mass in hypercalciuric, osteoporotic men treated with hydrochlorothiazide. *Ann Intern Med* 1999;130:658–660.
493. Reeve J, Meunier PJ, Parsons JA, et al. Anabolic effect of human parathyroid hormone fragment on trabecular bone in involutional osteoporosis: a multicentre trial. *Br Med J* 1980;280: 1340–1344.
494. Dempster DW, Cosman F, Parisien M, et al. Anabolic actions of parathyroid hormone on bone. *Endocr Rev* 1993;14:690–709.
495. Reginster JY, Taquet AN, Fraikin G, et al. Parathyroid hormone in the treatment of involutional osteoporosis: back to the future. *Osteoporosis Int* 1997;7(suppl 3):S163–S168.
496. Finkelstein JS, Klibanski A, Schaefer EH, et al. Parathyroid hormone for the prevention of bone loss induced by estrogen deficiency. *N Engl J Med* 1994;331(24):1618–1623.
497. Finkelstein JS, Klibanski A, Arnold AL, et al. Prevention of estrogen deficiency-related bone loss with human parathyroid hormone-(1–34): a randomized controlled trial. *JAMA* 1998; 280(12):1067–1073.
498. Slovik DM, Rosenthal DI, Doppelt SH, et al. Restoration of spinal bone in osteoporotic men by treatment with human parathyroid hormone (1–34) and 1,25-dihydroxyvitamin D. *J Bone Miner Res* 1986;1(4):377–381.
499. Lindsay R, Nieves J, Formica C, et al. Randomized controlled study of effect of parathyroid hormone on vertebral bone mass and fracture incidence among postmenopausal women on oestrogen with osteoporosis. *Lancet* 1997;350:550–556.
500. Hodsman AB, Fraher LJ, Watson PH, et al. A randomized controlled trial to compare the efficacy of cyclical parathyroid hormone versus cyclical parathyroid hormone and sequential calcitonin to improve bone mass in postmenopausal women with osteoporosis. *J Clin Endocrinol Metab* 1997;82(2):620–628.
501. Cosman F, Nieves J, Woelfert L, et al. Alendronate does not block the anabolic effect of PTH in postmenopausal osteoporotic women. *J Bone Miner Res* 1998;13(6):1051–1055.
502. Stewart AF. PTHrP(1-36) as a skeletal anabolic agent for the treatment of osteoporosis. *Bone* 1996;19:303–306.
503. Marcus R. Recombinant human growth hormone as potential therapy for osteoporosis. *Baillieres Clin Endocrinol Metab* 1998;12(2):251–260.
504. Ljunghall S, Johansson AG, Burman P, et al. Low plasma levels of insulin-like growth factor 1 (IGF-1) in male patients with idiopathic osteoporosis. *J Intern Med* 1992;232:59–64.
505. Rudman D, Feller AG, Nagraj HS, et al. Effects of human growth hormone in men over 60 years old. *N Engl J Med* 1990;323(1):1–6.
506. Holloway L, Kohlmeier L, Kent K, et al. Skeletal effects of cyclic recombinant human growth hormone and salmon calcitonin in osteopenic postmenopausal women. *J Clin Endocrinol Metab* 1997;82(4):1111–1117.
507. Ebeling PR, Jones JD, O'Fallon WM, et al. Short-term effects

of recombinant human insulin-like growth factor I on bone turnover in normal women. *J Clin Endocrinol Metab* 1993;77: 1384–1387.

508. Johansson AG, Lindh E, Blum WF, et al. Effects of growth hormone and insulin-like growth factor I in men with idiopathic osteoporosis. *J Clin Endocrinol Metab* 1996;81:44–48.
509. Moore RA. Livial: a review of clinical studies. *Br J Obstet Gynaecol* 1999;106(suppl 19):1–21.
510. Bjarnason NH, Bjarnason K, Haarbo J, et al. Tibolone: prevention of bone loss in late postmenopausal women. *J Clin Endocrinol Metab* 1996;81:2419–2422.
511. Studd J, Arnala I, Kicovic PM, et al. A randomized study of tibolone on bone mineral density in osteoporotic postmenopausal women with previous fractures. *Obstet Gynecol* 1998;92:574–579.
512. Beardsworth SA, Kearney CE, Purdie DW. Prevention of postmenopausal bone loss at lumbar spine and upper femur with tibolone: a two-year randomised controlled trial. *Br J Obstet Gynaecol* 1999;106:678–683.
513. Berning B, Kuik CV, Kuiper JW, et al. Effects of two doses of tibolone on trabecular and cortical bone loss in early postmenopausal women: a two-year randomized, placebo-controlled study. *Bone* 1996;19:395–399.
514. Hammar M, Christau S, Nathorst-Boos J, et al. A double-blind, randomised trial comparing the effects of tibolone and continuous combined hormone replacement therapy in postmenopausal women with menopausal symptoms. *Br J Obstet Gynaecol* 1998;105:904–911.
515. Brandi ML. Flavonoids: biochemical effects and therapeutic application. *Bone Miner* 1992;S3:S3–S14.
516. Reginster JY. Ipriflavone: pharmacological properties and usefulness in postmenopausal osteoporosis. *Bone Miner* 1993;23: 223–232.
517. Kovacs AB. Efficacy of ipriflavone in the prevention and treatment of postmenopausal osteoporosis. *Agents Actions* 1994;41:86–87.
518. Sambrook PN, Jones G. Corticosteroid osteoporosis. *Br J Rheumatol* 1995;34:8–12.
519. Adachi J, Ioannidis G. *Primer on corticosteroid-induced osteoporosis*, 1st ed, vol 1. Philadelphia: Lippincott Williams & Wilkins, 1999.
520. Saag KG. Osteoporosis in rheumatoid arthritis: the role of glucocorticoids. *Rheum Arthritis Ind Rev* 1999;11(2):3–5.
521. Walsh LJ, Wong CA, Pringle M, et al. Use of oral corticosteroids in the community and the prevention of secondary osteoporosis: a cross sectional study. *Br Med J* 1996;313:344–346.
522. Mudano A, Allison J, Hill J, et al. Glucocorticoid-induced osteoporosis: process of care and patient outcomes in a managed care population. *Arthritis Rheum* 1999;42(suppl 9):S73.
523. Christensen PM, Kristiansen IS, Brosen K, et al. Use of prednisolone and concurrent pharmacological prevention of osteoporosis. *Arthritis Rheum* 1999;42(suppl 9):S289.
524. Reid IR, Evans MC, Wattie DJ, et al. Bone mineral density of the proximal femur and lumbar spine in glucocorticoid-treated asthmatic patients. *Osteoporosis Int* 1992;2:103–105.
525. Verstraeten A, Dequeker J. Vertebral and peripheral bone mineral content and fracture incidence in postmenopausal patients with rheumatoid arthritis: effect of low dose corticosteroids. *Ann Rheum Dis* 1986;45:852–857.
526. LoCascio V, Bonnucci E, Imbimbo B, et al. Bone loss in response to long-term glucocorticoid therapy. *Bone Miner* 1990; 8:39–51.
527. LoCascio V, Bonnucci E, Imbimbo B, et al. Bone loss after glucocorticoid therapy. *Calcif Tissue Int* 1984;36:435–438.
528. Dykman TR, Gluck OS, Murphy WA, et al. Evaluation of factors associated with glucocorticoid-induced osteopenia in patients with rheumatic diseases. *Arthritis Rheum* 1985;28:361–368.
529. Sambrook PN, Eisman JA, Yeates MG, et al. Osteoporosis in rheumatoid arthritis: safety of low dose corticosteroids. *Ann Rheum Dis* 1986;45:950–953.
530. Messina OD, Barreira JC, Zanchetta JR, et al. Effect of low doses of deflazacort vs prednisone on bone mineral content in premenopausal rheumatoid arthritis. *J Rheumatol* 1992;19: 1520–1526.
531. Hall GM, Spector TD, Griffin JA, et al. The effect of rheumatoid arthritis and steroid therapy on bone density in postmenopausal women. *Arthritis Rheum* 1993;36:1510–1516.
532. Kroger H, Honaken R, Saarikoski S, et al. Decreased axial bone mineral density in perimenopausal women with rheumatoid arthritis—a population based study. *Ann Rheum Dis* 1994;53: 18–23.
533. Lane NE, Pressman AR, Star VL, et al. Rheumatoid arthritis and bone mineral density in elderly women. *J Bone Miner Res* 1995;10:257–263.
534. Buckley LM, Leib ES, Cartularo KS, et al. Effects of low dose glucocorticoids on the bone mineral density of patients with rheumatoid arthritis. *J Rheumatol* 1995;22:1055–1059.
535. Hansen M, Podenphant J, Florescu A, et al. A randomised trial of differentiated prednisolone treatment in active rheumatoid arthritis. Clinical benefits and skeletal side effects. *Ann Rheum Dis* 1999;58:713–718.
536. Reid IR, Heap SW. Determinants of vertebral mineral density in patients receiving long-term glucocorticoid therapy. *Arch Intern Med* 1990;150:2545–2548.
537. Gluck OS, Murphy WA, Hahn TJ, et al. Bone loss in adults receiving alternate day glucocorticoid therapy. *Arthritis Rheum* 1981;24:892–898.
538. Aaron JE, Francis RM, Peacock M, et al. Contrasting microanatomy of idiopathic and corticosteroid-induced osteoporosis. *Clin Orthop Rel Res* 1989;243:294–305.
539. Saito JK, Davis JW, Wasnich RD, et al. Users of low-dose glucocorticoids have increased bone loss rates: a longitudinal study. *Calcif Tissue Int* 1995;57:115–119.
540. Pearce G, Tabensky A, Delmas PD, et al. Corticosteroid-induced bone loss in men. *J Clin Endocrinol Metab* 1998;83: 801–806.
541. McEvoy CE, Ensrud KE, Bender E, et al. Association between corticosteroid use and vertebral fractures in older men with chronic obstructive pulmonary disease. *Am J Respir Crit Care Med* 1998;157:704–709.
542. Als OS, Gotfredsen A, Christiansen C. The effect of glucocorticoids on bone mass in rheumatoid arthritis patients. *Arthritis Rheum* 1985;28:369–375.
543. Gough KS, Lilley J, Eyre S, et al. Generalised bone loss in patients with early rheumatoid arthritis. *Lancet* 1994;344:23–27.
544. Hansen M, Florescu A, Stoltenberg M, et al. Bone loss in rheumatoid arthritis. Influence of disease activity, duration of the disease, functional capacity, and corticosteroid treatment. *Scand J Rheumatol* 1996;25:367–376.
545. Gough A, Sambrook P, Devlin J, et al. Osteoclastic activation is the principal mechanism leading to secondary osteoporosis in rheumatoid arthritis. *J Rheumatol* 1998;25:1282–1289.
546. Suzuki Y, Mizushima Y. Osteoporosis in rheumatoid arthritis. *Osteoporosis Int* 1997;(suppl 7):S217–S222.
547. Towheed TE, Brouillard D, Yendt E, et al. Osteoporosis in rheumatoid arthritis: findings in the metacarpal, spine, and hip and a study of the determinants of both localized and generalized osteopenia. *J Rheumatol* 1995;22:440–443.
548. Dolan AL, Moniz C, Dasgupta B, et al. Effects of inflammation and treatment on bone turnover and bone mass in polymyalgia rheumatica. *Arthritis Rheum* 1997;40:2022–2029.
549. Spector TD, Hall GM, McCloskey EV, et al. Risk of vertebral fracture in women with rheumatoid arthritis. *Br Med J* 1993; 306:558.

550. Cooper C, Coupland C, Mitchell M. Rheumatoid arthritis, corticosteroid therapy and hip fracture. *Ann Rheum Dis* 1995; 54:49–52.
551. Kipen Y, Buchbinder R, Forbes A, et al. Prevalence of reduced bone mineral density in systemic lupus erythematosus and the role of steroids. *J Rheumatol* 1997;24:1922–1929.
552. Ramsey-Goldman R, Dunn JE, Huang C-F, et al. Frequency of fractures in women with systemic lupus erythematosus: comparison with United States population data. *Arthritis Rheum* 1999;42:882–890.
553. Ruegsegger P, Medici TC, Anliker M. Corticosteroid-induced bone loss. A longitudinal study of alternate day therapy in patients with bronchial asthma using quantitative computed tomography. *Eur J Clin Pharmacol* 1983;25:615–620.
554. Schatz M, Dudl J, Zeiger RS, et al. Osteoporosis in corticosteroid-treated asthmatic patients: clinical correlates. *Allergy Proc* 1993;14:341–345.
555. Ebeling PR, Erbas B, Hopper JL, et al. Bone mineral density and bone turnover in asthmatics treated with long-term inhaled or oral glucocorticoids. *J Bone Miner Res* 1998;13:1283–1289.
556. Villareal MS, Klaustermeyer WB, Hahn TJ, et al. Osteoporosis in steroid-dependent asthma. *Ann Allergy Asthma Immunol* 1996;76:369–372.
557. Compston JE, Judd D, Crawley EO, et al. Osteoporosis in patients with inflammatory bowel disease. *Gut* 1987;28:410–415.
558. Bernstein CN, Seeger LL, Sayre JW, et al. Decreased bone density in inflammatory bowel disease is related to corticosteroid use and not disease diagnosis. *J Bone Miner Res* 1995;10:250–256.
559. Andreassen H, Rungby J, Dahlerup JF, et al. Inflammatory bowel disease and osteoporosis. *Scand J Gastroenterol* 1997;32: 1247–1255.
560. Olgaard K, Storm T, van Wowern N, et al. Glucocorticoid-induced osteoporosis in the lumbar spine, forearm and mandible of nephrotic patients: a double-blind study on the high-dose, long-term effects of prednisone versus deflazacort. *Calcif Tissue Int* 1992;50:490–494.
561. Rizzato G, Tosi G, Mella C, et al. Prednisone-induced bone loss in sarcoidosis: a risk especially frequent in postmenopausal women. *Sarcoidosis* 1988;5:93–96.
562. Leboff MS, Wade JP, Mackowiak S, et al. Low dose prednisone does not affect calcium homeostasis or bone density in postmenopausal women with rheumatoid arthritis. *J Rheumatol* 1991;18:339–344.
563. Sambrook PN, Cohen ML, Eisman JA, et al. Effects of low dose corticosteroids on bone mass in rheumatoid arthritis: a longitudinal study. *Ann Rheum Dis* 1989;48:535–538.
564. Sambrook PN, Eisman J, Champion GD, et al. Determinants of axial bone loss in rheumatoid arthritis. *Arthritis Rheum* 1987; 30:721–728.
565. Saag KG, Koehnke R, Caldwell JR, et al. Low dose long-term corticosteroid therapy in rheumatoid arthritis: an analysis of serious adverse events. *Am J Med* 1994;96:115–123.
566. Verhoeven MC, Boers M. Limited bone loss due to corticosteroids; a systematic review of prospective studies in rheumatoid arthritis and other diseases. *J Rheumatol* 1997;24:1495–1503.
567. Nielsen HK, Charles P, Mosekilde L. The effect of single oral doses of prednisone on the circadian rhythm of serum ostecalcin in normal subjects. *J Clin Endocrinol Metab* 1988;67:1025.
568. Peel NFA, Moore DJ, Barrington NA, et al. Risk of vertebral fracture and relationship to bone mineral density in steroid treated rheumatoid arthritis. *Ann Rheum Dis* 1995;54:801–806.
569. Luengo M, Picado C, Del Rio L, et al. Vertebral fractures in steroid dependent asthma and involutional osteoporosis: a comparative study. *Thorax* 1991;46:803–806.
570. Baltzan MA, Suissa S, Bauer DC, et al. Hip fractures attributable to corticosteroid use. *Lancet* 1999;353:1327.
571. Lems WF, Jahangier ZN, Jacobs JWG, et al. Vertebral fractures in patients with rheumatoid arthritis treated with corticosteroids. *Clin Exp Rheumatol* 1995;13:293–297.
572. Michel BA, Bloch DA, Wolfe F, et al. Fractures in rheumatoid arthritis: an evaluation of associated risk factors. *J Rheumatol* 1993;20:1666–1669.
573. McDougall R, Sibley J, Haga M, et al. Outcome in patients with rheumatoid arthritis receiving prednisone compared to matched controls. *J Rheumatol* 1994;21:1207–1213.
574. Adinoff AD, Hollister JR. Steroid-induced fractures and bone loss in patients with asthma. *N Engl J Med* 1983;309:265–268.
575. Cohen S, Levy RM, Keller M, et al. Risedronate therapy prevents corticosteroid-induced bone loss: a twelve-month, multicenter, randomized, double-blind, placebo-controlled, parallel-group study. *Arthritis Rheum* 1999;42(11):2309–2318.
576. Emkey RD, Lindsay R, Lyssy J, et al. The systemic effect of intraarticular administration of corticosteroid on markers on bone formation and bone resorption in patients with rheumatoid arthritis. *Arthritis Rheum* 1996;39:277–282.
577. Teelucksingh S, Padfield PL, Tibi L, et al. Inhaled corticosteroids, bone formation, and osteocalcin. *Lancet* 1991;338 (8758):60–61.
578. Marystone JF, Barrett-Connor EL, Morton DJ. Inhaled and oral corticosteroids: their effects on bone mineral density in older adults. *Am J Public Health* 1995;85:1693–1695.
579. Toogood JH, Baskerville JC, Markov AE, et al. Bone mineral density and the risk of fracture in patients receiving long-term inhaled steroid therapy for asthma. *J Allergy Clin Immunol* 1995;96:157–166.
580. van Staa TP, Leufkens HGM, Abenahim L, et al. Use of oral corticosteroids and risk of fractures. *J Bone Miner Res Suppl* 2000;15:993–1000.
581. Adachi JD, Bensen WG, Hodsman AB. Corticosteroid-induced osteoporosis. *Semin Arthritis Rheum* 1993;22(6):375–384.
582. Lukert BP, Raisz LG. Glucocorticoid-induced osteoporosis. *Rheum Dis Clin North Am* 1994;20:629–650.
583. Canalis E. Mechanisms of glucocorticoid action in bone: implications to glucocorticoid-induced osteoporosis. *J Clin Endocrinol Metab* 1996;81:3441–3447.
584. Hahn TJ, Halstead LR, Baran DT. Effects of short-term glucocorticoid administration on intestinal calcium absorption and circulating vitamin D metabolite concentrations in man. *J Clin Endocrinol Metab* 1981;52:111.
585. Morris HA, Need AG, O'Loughlin PD, et al. Malabsorption of calcium in corticosteroid-induced osteoporosis. *Calcif Tissue Int* 1990;46:305–308.
586. Suzuki Y, Ichikawa Y, Saito E, et al. Importance of increased urinary calcium excretion in the development of secondary hyperparathyroidism of patients under glucocorticoid therapy. *Metabolism* 1983;32:151–156.
587. Nielsen HK, Thomsen K, Eriksen EF, et al. The effects of high-dose glucocorticoid administration on serum bone gamma carboxyglutamic acid containing protein, serum alkaline phosphatase and vitamin D metabolites in normal subjects. *Bone Miner* 1988;4:105.
588. Godschalk M, Levy J, Downs RW. Glucocorticoids decrease vitamin D receptor numbers and gene expression in human osteosarcoma cells. *J Bone Miner Res* 1992;7:21.
589. Urena P, Iida-Klein A, Kong X-F, et al. Regulation of parathyroid hormone (PTH)/PTH-related peptide receptor messenger ribonucleic acid by glucocorticoids and PTH in ROS17/2.8 and OK cells. *Endocrinology* 1994;134:451–456.
590. Sakakura M, Takebe K, Nakagawa S. Inhibition of luteinizing hormone secretion induced by synthetic LRH by long-term treatment with glucocorticoids in human subjects. *J Clin Endocrinol Metab* 1975;40:774.

591. Doerr P, Pirke KM. Cortisol-induced suppression of plasma testosterone in normal adult males. *J Clin Endocrinol Metab* 1976;43:622.
592. MacAdams MR, White RH, Chipps BE. Reduction of serum testosterone levels during chronic glucocorticoid therapy. *Ann Intern Med* 1986;104:648–654.
593. Ishida Y, Heersche JNM. Glucocorticoid-induced osteoporosis: both in vivo and in vitro concentrations of glucocorticoids higher than physiological levels attenuate osteoblast differentiation. *J Bone Miner Res* 1998;13:1822–1826.
594. Dempster DW, Arlot MA, Meunier PJ. Mean wall thickness and formation periods of trabecular bone packets in corticosteroid-induced osteoporosis. *Calcif Tissue Int* 1983;61:173.
595. Kotowicz MA, Hall S, Hunder GG, et al. Relationship of glucocorticoid dosage to serum bone gla-protein concentration in patients with rheumatologic disorders. *Arthritis Rheum* 1990; 33:1487.
596. Manolagas SC, Weinstein RS. New developments in the pathogenesis and treatment of steroid-induced osteoporosis. *J Bone Miner Res* 1999;14:1061–1066.
597. Foundation NO. *Physician's guide to prevention and treatment of osteoporosis.* Belle Mead, NJ: Excerpta Medica, 1998.
598. Eastell R, Reid DM, Compston J, et al. A UK consensus group on management of glucocorticoid-induced osteoporosis: an update. *J Intern Med* 1998;244:271–292.
599. Martens HF, Sheets PK, Tenover JS, et al. Decreased testosterone levels in men with rheumatoid arthritis: effect of low dose prednisone therapy. *J Rheumatol* 1994;21:1427–1431.
600. Spector TD, Perry LA, Tubb G, et al. Low free testosterone levels in rheumatoid arthritis. *Ann Rheum Dis* 1988;47:65–68.
601. Pocock NA, Eisman JA, Dunstan CR, et al. Recovery from steroid-induced osteoporosis. *Ann Intern Med* 1987;107:319.
602. Gray R, Doherty SM, Galloway J, et al. A double-blind study of deflazacort and prednisone in patients with chronic inflammatory disorders. *Arthritis Rheum* 1991;34:287–295.
603. Reid IR, Ibbertson HK. Calcium supplements in the prevention of steroid-induced osteoporosis. *Am J Clin Nutr* 1986;44: 287–290.
604. Bernstein CN, Seeger LL, Anton PA, et al. A randomized, placebo-controlled trial of calcium supplementation for decreased bone density in corticosteroid-using patients with inflammatory bowel disease: a pilot study. *Aliment Pharmacol Ther* 1996;10:777–786.
605. ACR. ACR Task Force on Rheumatology Guidelines. Recommendations for the prevention and treatment of glucocorticoid-induced osteoporosis. *Arthritis Rheum* 1996;39:1791–1801.
606. Sambrook P, Birmingham J, Kelly P, et al. Prevention of corticosteroid osteoporosis. A comparison of calcium, calcitriol, and calcitonin. *N Engl J Med* 1993;328:1747–1752.
607. Braun JJ, Birkenhager-Frenkel DH, Rietvoeld AH, et al. Influence of 1 alpha-(OH)D3 administration on bone and bone mineral metabolism in patients on chronic glucocorticoid treatment; A double blind controlled study. *Clin Endocrinol* 1983;18:265–273.
608. Reginster JY, Kuntz D, Verdickt W, et al. Prophylactic use of alfacalcidol in corticosteroid-induced osteoporosis. *Osteoporosis Int* 1999;9:75–81.
609. Buckley LM, Leib ES, Cartularo KS, et al. Calcium and vitamin D3 supplementation prevents bone loss in the spine secondary to low-dose corticosteroids in patients with rheumatoid arthritis. *Ann Intern Med* 1996;125:961–968.
610. Bijlsma JWJ, Raymakers JA, Mosch C, et al. Effect of oral calcium and vitamin D on glucocorticoid-induced osteopenia. *Clin Exp Rheumatol* 1988;6:113–119.
611. Adachi JD, Bensen WG, Brown J, et al. Intermittent etidronate therapy to prevent corticosteroid-induced osteoporosis. *N Engl J Med* 1997;337:382–387.
612. Amin S, LaValley MP, Simms RW, et al. The role of vitamin D in corticosteroid-induced osteoporosis. *Arthritis Rheum* 1999; 42(8):1740–1751.
613. American College of Rheumatology Task Force on Osteoporosis Guidelines. Recommendations for the prevention and treatment of glucocorticoid-induced osteoporosis. *Arthritis Rheum* 1986;39:1791–1801.
614. Homik J, Suarez-Almazor M, Shea B, et al. *Calcium and vitamin D for corticosteroid-induced osteoporosis* (Cochrane Review). The Cochrane Library, issue 1. Oxford: Update Software, 1999.
615. Adams JS, Wahl TO, Lukert BP. Effects of hydrochlorothiazide and dietary sodium restriction on calcium metabolism in corticosteroid treated patients. *Metabolism* 1981;30:217–221.
616. Adachi J, Bensen WG, Bell MJ, et al. Salmon calcitonin nasal spray in the prevention of corticosteroid-induced osteoporosis. *Br J Rheumatol* 1997;36(2):255–257.
617. Montemurro L, Schiraldi G, Fraioli P, et al. Prevention of corticosteroid-induced osteoporosis with salmon calcitonin in sarcoid patients. *Calcif Tissue Int* 1991;49:71–76.
618. Healey JH, Paget SA, Williams-Russo P, et al. A randomized controlled trial of salmon calcitonin to prevent bone loss in corticosteroid-treated temporal arteritis and polymyalgia rheumatica. *Calcif Tissue Int* 1996;58:73–80.
619. Luengo M, Pons F, Martinez de Osaba MJ, et al. Prevention of further bone mass loss by nasal calcitonin in patients on long term glucocorticoid therapy for asthma: a two year follow up study. *Thorax* 1994;49:1099.
620. Ringe J-D, Welzel D. Salmon calcitonin in the therapy of corticosteroid-induced osteoporosis. *Eur J Clin Pharmacol* 1987; 33:35–39.
621. Kotaniemi A, Piirainen H, Paimela L, et al. Is continuous intranasal salmon calcitonin effective in treating axial bone loss in patients with active rheumatoid arthritis receiving low dose glucocorticoid therapy? *J Rheumatol* 1996;23:1875–1879.
622. Hall GM, Daniels M, Doyle DV, et al. Effect of hormone replacement therapy on bone mass in rheumatoid arthritis patients treated with and without steroids. *Arthritis Rheum* 1994;37:1499–1505.
623. Lukert BP, Johnson BE, Robinson RG. Estrogen and progesterone replacement therapy reduces glucocorticoid-induced bone loss. *J Bone Miner Res* 1992;7:1063–1069.
624. Sambrook P, Birmingham J, Champion D, et al. Postmenopausal bone loss in rheumatoid arthritis: effect of estrogens and androgens. *J Rheumatol* 1992;19:357–361.
625. Reid IR, Wattie DJ,Evans MC, et al. Testosterone therapy in glucocorticoid-treated men. *Arch Intern Med* 1996;156: 1173–1177.
626. Grecu EO, Weinshelbaum A, Simmons R. Effective therapy of glucocorticoid-induced osteoporosis with medroxyprogesterone acetate. *Calcif Tissue Int* 1990;46:294–299.
627. Bird HA, Hill J, Sitton NG, et al. A clinical and biochemical assessment of etidronate disodium in patients with active rheumatoid arthritis. *Clin Rheumatol* 1988;7:91–94.
628. Wolfhagen FH, vanBuuren HR, denOuden JW, et al. Cyclic etidronate in the prevention of bone loss in corticosteroid-treated primary biliary cirrhosis. *J Hepatol* 1997;26:325–330.
629. Mulder H, Struys A. Intermittent cyclical etidronate in the prevention of corticosteroid-induced bone loss. *Br J Rheumatol* 1994;33:348–350.
630. Adachi JD, Cranney A, Goldsmith CH, et al. Intermittent cyclic therapy with etidronate in the prevention of corticosteroid induced bone loss. *J Rheumatol* 1994;21:1922–1926.
631. Sebaldt RJ, Ioannidis G, Adachi JD, et al. 36 month intermittent cyclical etidronate treatment in patients with established corticosteroid induced osteoporosis. *J Rheumatol* 1999;26:1545–1549.
632. Diamond T, McGuigan L, Barbagallo S, et al. Cyclical etidronate

plus ergocalciferol prevents glucocorticoid-induced bone loss in postmenopausal women. *Am J Med* 1995;98:459–463.
633. Riemens SC, Oostdijk A, van Doormaal JJ, et al. Bone loss after liver transplantation is not prevented by cyclical etidronate, calcium and alphacalcidol. *Osteoporosis Int* 1996;6:213–218.
634. Struys A, Snelder AA, Mulder H. Cyclical etidronate reverses bone loss of the spine and proximal femur in patients with established corticosteroid-induced osteoporosis. *Am J Med* 1995;99:235–242.
635. Pitt P, Todd P, Webber D, et al. A double blind placebo controlled study to determine the effects of intermittent cyclical etidronate on bone mineral density in patients on long term oral corticosteroid treatment. *Thorax* 1998;53:351–356.
636. Roux C, Oriente P, Laan R, et al. Randomized trial of effect of cyclical etidronate in the prevention of corticosteroid-induced bone loss. *J Clin Endocrinol Metab* 1998;83:1128–1133.
637. Geusens P, Dequeker J, Vanhoof J, et al. Cyclical etidronate increases bone density in the spine and hip of postmenopausal women receiving long term corticosteroid treatment. A double blind, randomised placebo controlled study. *Ann Rheum Dis* 1998;57:724–727.
638. Jenkins EA, Walker-Bone KE, Wood A, et al. The prevention of corticosteroid-induced bone loss with intermittent cyclical etidronate. *Scand J Rheumatol* 1999;28:152–156.
639. Skingle SJ, Crisp AJ. Increased bone density in patients on steroids with etidronate. *Lancet* 1994;344:543.
640. Gonnelli S, Rottoli P, Cepollaro C, et al. Prevention of corticosteroid-induced osteoporosis with alendronate in sarcoid patients. *Calcif Tissue Int* 1997;6:382–385.
641. Falcini F, Trapani S, Ermini M, et al. Intravenous administration of alendronate counteracts the in vivo effects of glucocorticoids on bone remodeling. *Calcif Tissue Int* 1996;58: 166–169.
642. Saag K, Emkey R, Cividino A, et al. Effects of Alendronate for two years on BMD and fractures in patients receiving glucocorticoids. *J Bone Miner Res* 1998;23(suppl 5):S182.
643. Devogelaer JP, Hughes R, Laan R, et al. Residronate is effective and well-tolerated in patients on chronic corticosteroid therapy. *J Bone Miner Res* 1998;23(suppl 5):S480.
644. Reid DM, Hughes RA, Laan RFSM, et al. Efficacy and safety of daily risedronote in the treatment of corticosteroid-induced osteoporosis in man and woman: a randomized trial. *J Bone Miner* 2000;15:1006–1013.
645. Gallacher SJ, Fenner JAK, Anderson K, et al. Intravenous pamidronate in the treatment of osteoporosis associated with corticosteroid dependent lung disease: an open pilot study. *Thorax* 1992;47:932–936.
646. Reid IR, King AR, Alexander CJ, et al. Prevention of steroid-induced osteoporosis with (3-amino-1-hydroxypropylidene)-1, 1-bisphosphonate (APD). *Lancet* 1988;1:143–146.
647. Boutsen Y, Jamart J, Esselinckx W, et al. Primary prevention of glucocorticoid-induced osteoporosis with intermittent intravenous pamidronate: a randomized trial. *Calcif Tissue Int* 1997; 61:266–271.
648. Rizzoli R, Chevalley T, Slosman DO, et al. Sodium monofluorophosphate increases vertebral bone mineral density in patients with corticosteroid-induced osteoporosis. *Osteoporosis Int* 1995;5:39–46.
649. Greenwald M, Brandli D, Spector S, et al. Corticosteroid-induced osteoporosis: effects of a treatment with slow-release sodium fluoride. *Osteoporosis Int* 1992;2:303–304.
650. Lems WF, Jacobs WG, Bijlsma JWJ, et al. Effect of sodium fluoride on the prevention of corticosteroid-induced osteoporosis. *Osteoporosis Int* 1997;7:575–582.
651. Guaydier-Souquires G, Kotzi PO, Sabatier JP, et al. In corticosteroid-treated respiratory diseases, monofluorophosphate increases lumbar bone density: a double-masked randomized study. *Osteoporosis Int* 1996;6:171.
652. Lems WF, Jacobs JWG, Bijlsma JWJ, et al. Is addition of sodium fluoride to cyclical etidronate beneficial in the treatment of corticosteroid induced osteoporosis? *Ann Rheum Dis* 1997;56:357–363.
653. Adami S, Fossaluzza V, Rossini M. Prevention of corticosteroid-induced osteoporosis with nandrolone decanoate. *Bone Miner* 1991;15:73.
654. Lane NE, Sanchez S, Modin GW, et al. Parathyroid hormone treatment can reverse corticosteroid-induced osteoporosis. Results of a randomized controlled clinical trial. *J Clin Invest* 1998;102(8):1627–1633.
655. Tanaka H, Seino Y. Does growth hormone treatment prevent corticosteroid-induced osteoporosis? *Bone* 1996;18:493–494.
656. Peat ID, Healy S, Reid DM, et al. Steroid induced osteoporosis: an opportunity for prevention? *Ann Rheum Dis* 1995;54: 66–68.
657. Aagaard EM, Lin P, Modin GW, et al. Prevention of glucocorticoid-induced osteoporosis: provider practice at an urban county hospital. *Am J Med* 1999;107:456–460.
658. Nair B, Sibley J, Haga M. Osteoporosis (OP) prevention in patients on continuous oral corticosteroid therapy among internal medicine specialists. *Arthritis Rheum* 1997;40(suppl):S309.
659. Buckley LM, Marquez M, Hudson JO, et al. Variations in physician perceptions of the risk of osteoporosis in corticosteroid users by physician specialty. *J Rheumatol* 1998;25:2195–2202.
660. Buckley LM, Marquez M, Feezor R, et al. Prevention of corticosteroid-induced osteoporosis. *Arthritis Rheum* 1999;42(8): 1736–1739.
661. Rosen HN, Rosenblatt M. Prevention and treatment of glucocorticoid-induced osteoporosis. In: Rose B, ed. *UpToDate,* vol 6, no. 3. Wellesley, MA: UpToDate, 1998.
662. Bacon WE, Smith GS, Baker SP. Geographic variation in the occurrence of hip fractures among the elderly white US population. *Am J Public Health* 1989;79:1556–1558.
663. Anderson FH. Osteoporosis in men. *Int J Clin Pract* 1998;52: 176–180.
664. Jacobsen SJ, Goldberg J, Miles TP, et al. Hip fracture incidence among the old and very old: a population-based study of 745,435 cases. *Am J Public Health* 1990;80:871–873.
665. Ross PD, Norimatsu H, Davis JW, et al. A comparison of hip fracture incidence among native Japanese, Japanese Americans, and American Caucasians. *Am J Epidemiol* 1991;133:801–809.
666. Poor G, Atkinson EJ, Lewallen DG, et al. Age-related hip fractures in men: clinical spectrum and short-term outcomes. *Osteoporosis Int* 1995;5:419–426.
667. Melton LJI, Riggs BL. Epidemiology of age-related fractures. In: Avioli LV, ed. *The osteoporotic syndrome.* New York: Grune & Stratton, 1983:45–72.
668. Myers AH, Robinson EG, Van Natta ML, et al. Hip fractures among the elderly: factors associated with in-hospital mortality. *Am J Epidemiol* 1991;134:1128–1137.
669. Orwoll ES. Osteoporosis in men. *Endocrinol Metab Clin North Am* 1998;27:349–367.
670. Seeman E. Osteoporosis in men: epidemiology, pathophysiology, and treatment possibilities. *Am J Med* 1993;95:22S–28S.
671. Seeman E. Osteoporosis in men. *Baillieres Clin Rheumatol* 1997; 11:613–629.
672. Mann T, Oviatt SK, Wilson D, et al. Vertebral deformity in men. *J Bone Miner Res* 1992;7:1259–1265.
673. Mallmin H, Ljunghall S, Persson I, et al. Fracture of the distal forearm as a forecaster of subsequent hip fracture: a population-based cohort study with 24 years follow-up. *Calcif Tissue Int* 1993;52:269–272.
674. Reeve J, Kroger H, Nijs J, et al. Radial cortical and trabecular

bone densities of men and women standardized with the European forearm phantom. *Calcif Tissue Int* 1996;58:135–143.

675. Tobin J, Fox KM, Cejku ML, et al. Bone density changes in normal men: a 4–19 year longitudinal study. *J Bone Miner Res* 1993;8:S142(abst).
676. Diamond T, Smerdely P, Kormas N, et al. Hip fracture in elderly men: the importance of subclinical vitamin D deficiency and hypogonadism. *Med J Aust* 1998;169:138–141.
677. Orwoll ES, Meier DE. Alterations in calcium, vitamin D, and parathyroid hormone physiology in men with aging: relationship to the development of senile osteopenia. *Clin Endocrinol Metab* 1986;63:1262–1269.
678. Clarke BL, Ebeling PR, Jones JD, et al. Changes in quantitative bone histomorphometry in aging healthy men. *J Clin Endocrinol Metab* 1996;81:2264–2270.
679. Tsai K, Twu S, Chieng P, et al. Prevalence of vertebral fractures in men and women in urban Taiwanese communities. *Calcif Tissue Int* 1996;59:249–253.
680. Marie PJ, de Vernejoul MC, Connes D, et al. Decreased DNA synthesis by cultured osteoblastic cells in eugonadal osteoporotic men with defective bone formation. *J Clin Invest* 1991;88:1167–1172.
681. Abu EO, Horner A, Kusec V, et al. The localization of androgen receptors in human bone. *J Clin Endocrinol Metab* 1997; 82:3493–3497.
682. Eastell R, Boyle IT, Compston J, et al. Management of corticosteroid-induced osteoporosis. *J Intern Med* 1995;237:439–447.
683. Bellido T, Jilka RL, Boyce BF, et al. Regulation of interleukin-6, osteoclastogenesis, and bone mass by androgens the role of the androgen receptor. *J Clin Invest* 1995;95:2886–2895.
684. Diaz MN, O'Neill TW, Silman AJ. The influence of family history of hip fracture on the risk of vertebral deformity in men and women: the European Vertebral Osteoporosis Study. *Bone* 1997;20:145–149.
685. Morishima A, Grumbach MM, Simpson ER, et al. Aromatase deficiency in male and female siblings caused by a novel mutation and the physiological role of estrogens. *J Clin Endocrinol Metab* 1995;80:3689–3698.
686. Anderson FH, Francis RM, Selby PL, et al. Sex hormones and osteoporosis in men. *Calcif Tissue Int* 1998;62:185–188.
687. Silman AJ, O'Neill TW, Cooper C, et al. Influence of physical activity on vertebral deformity in men and women: results from the European Vertebral Osteoporosis Study. *J Bone Miner Res* 1997;12:813–819.
688. Kiel DP, Zhang Y, Hannan MT, et al. The effect of smoking at different life stages on bone mineral density in elderly men and women. *Osteoporosis Int* 1996;6:240–248.
689. Daniell HW. Osteoporosis after orchiectomy for prostate cancer. *J Urol* 1997;157:439–444.
690. Collinson MP, Tyrrel CJ, Hutton C. Osteoporosis occurring in two patients receiving LHRH analogs for carcinoma of the prostate. *Calcif Tissue Int* 1994;54:327–328.
691. Guo C-Y, Jones H, Eastell R. Treatment of isolated hypogonadotropic hypogonadism: effect on bone mineral density and bone turnover. *J Clin Endocrinol Metab* 1997;82:658–665.
692. Aasebo U, Bremnes RM, de Jong FH, et al. Pituitary-gonadal dysfunction in male patients with lung cancer: association with serum inhibin levels. *Acta Oncol* 1994;33:177–180.
693. Morley JE, Kaiser FE, Sih R, et al. Testosterone and frailty. *Clin Geriatr Med* 1997;13:685–694.
694. Byrne PAC, Evans WD, Rajan KT. Does vasectomy predispose to osteoporosis? *Br J Urol* 1997;79:599–601.
695. Vanderschueren D, Boonen S, Bouillon R. Action of androgens versus estrogens in male skeletal homeostasis. *Bone* 1998;23: 391–400.
696. Roa-Pena L, Zreik T, Harada N, et al. Human osteoblast-like cells express aromatase immunoreactivity. *Menopause* 1994;1:73–77.
697. Bernecker PM, Willvonseder R, Resch H. Decreased estrogen levels in patients with primary osteoporosis. *J Bone Miner Res* 1995;10(suppl 1):364(abst.
698. Adachi JD, Bensen WG, Bianchi F, et al. Vitamin D and calcium in the prevention of corticosteroid-induced osteoporosis: a 3-year followup. *J Rheumatol* 1996;23:995–1000.
699. Anderson FH. Male osteoporosis. *Curr Opin Orthop* 1997;8: 80–85.
700. Van Slyck EJ, Kleerekoper M, Abraham JP, et al. Case report: non-secretary multiple myeloma with osteoporosis: immunocytologic and bone resorptive studies. *Am J Med Sci* 1986;291:347–351.
701. Bhasin S, Bagatell CJ, Bremner WJ, et al. Issues in testosterone replacement in older men. *J Clin Endocrinol Metab* 1998;83: 3435–3448.
702. Anderson FH, Francis RM, Faulkner K. Androgen supplementation in eugonadal men with osteoporosis-effects of 6 months of treatment on bone mineral density and cardiovascular risk factors. *Bone* 1996;18:171–177.
703. Leifke E, Korner H-C, Link TM, et al. Effects of testosterone replacement therapy on cortical and trabecular bone mineral density, vertebral body area and paraspinal muscle area in hypogonadal men. *Eur J Endocrinol* 1998;138:51–58.
704. Anderson FH, Francis RM, Bishop JC, et al. Effect of intermittent cyclical disodium etidronate therapy on bone mineral density in men with vertebral fractures. *Age Ageing* 1997;26:359–365.
705. Devogelaer JP, Nagant de Deuxchaisnes C, Stein F. Bioavailability of enteric-coated sodium fluoride tablets as affected by the administration of calcium supplements at different time intervals. *J Bone Miner Res* 1990;5:S75–S79.
706. Erlacher L, Kettenbach J, Kiener H, et al. Salmon calcitonin and calcium in the treatment of male osteoporosis: the effects on bone mineral density. *Wien Klin Wochenschr* 1997;109:270–274.
707. Ringe JD, Dorst A, Kipshoven C, et al. Avoidance of vertebral fractures in men with idiopathic osteoporosis by a three year therapy with calcium and low-dose intermittent monofluorophosphate. *Osteoporosis Int* 1998;8:47–52.
708. United Network for Organ Sharing. *The U.S. scientific registry of transplant recipients and the organ procurement and transplantation network 1998.* Washington, DC: Department of Health and Human Services Health Resources and Services Administration, 1998.
709. Rodino MA, Shane E. Osteoporosis after organ transplantation. *Am J Med* 1998;104::459–469.
710. Epstein S, Shane E, Bilezikian JP. Organ transplantation and osteoporosis. *Curr Opin Rheumatol* 1995;7:255–261.
711. Rix M, Andreassen H, Eskildsen P, et al. Bone mineral density and biochemical markers of bone turnover in patients with predialysis chronic renal failure. *Kidney Int* 1999;56:1084–1093.
712. Stehman-Breen CO, Sherrard D, Walker A, et al. Racial differences in bone mineral density and bone loss among end-stage renal disease patients. *Am J Kidney Dis* 1999;33:941–946.
713. Julian BA, Laskow DA, Dubovsky J, et al. Rapid loss of vertebral mineral density after renal transplantation. *N Engl J Med* 1991;325:544–550.
714. Ramsey-Goldman R, Dunn JE, Dunlop DD, et al. Increased risk of fracture in patients receiving solid organ transplants. *J Bone Miner Res* 1999;14:456–463.
715. Janes C, Dickson E, Bonde S, et al. Role of hyperbilirubinemia in inhibition of osteoblast proliferation in patients with chronic cholestatic jaundice. *J Bone Miner Metab* 1992; 7(suppl):S98(abst).
716. Fan S, Almond MK, Ball E, et al. Pamidronate therapy as prevention of bone loss following renal transplantation. *Kidney Intl* 2000;57:684–690.
717. Reeves HL, Francis RM, Manas DM, et al. Intravenous bisphosphonate prevents symptomatic osteoporotic vertebral

collapse in patients after liver transplantation. *Liver Transplant Surg* 1998;4:404–409.

718. Shane E. Transplantation osteoporosis. In: Favus MJ, ed. *Primer on the metabolic bone diseases and disorders of mineral metabolism,* 4th ed. Chicago: Lippincott Williams & Wilkins, 1999:296–301.
719. Stempfle H-U, Werner C, Echtler S, et al. Prevention of osteoporosis after cardiac transplantation. *Transplantation* 1999;68: 523–530.
720. Van Cleemput J, Daenen W, Geusens P, et al. Prevention of bone loss in cardiac transplant recipients. A comparison of bisphosphonates and vitamin D. *Transplantation* 1996;61:1495–1499.
721. Grotz WH, Rump LC, Niessen A, et al. Treatment of osteopenia and osteoporosis after kidney transplantation. *Transplantation* 1998;66:1004–1008.
722. Valero MA, Loinaz C, Larrodera L, et al. Calcitonin and bisphosphonate treatment and bone loss after liver transplantation. *Calcif Tissue Int* 1995;57:15–19.
723. Liberman UA, Marx S. Vitamin D-dependent rickets. In: Favus MJ, ed. *Primer on the metabolic bone diseases and disorders of mineral metabolism,* 4th ed. Chicago: Lippincott Williams & Wilkins, 1999:323–328.
724. Mittal SK, Dash SC, Tiwari SC, et al. Bone histology in patients with nephrotic syndrome and normal renal function. *Kidney Int* 1999;55:1912–1919.
725. Klein GL. Metabolic bone disease of total parenteral nutrition. In: Favus MJ, ed. *Primer on the metabolic bone diseases and disorders of mineral metabolism,* 4th ed. Chicago: Lippincott Williams & Wilkins, 1999:319–323.
726. Shah BR, Finberg L. Single-day therapy for nutritional vitamin D-deficiency rickets: a preferred method. *J Pediatr* 1994;125: 487–492.
727. Klein GL. Nutritional rickets and osteomalacia. In: Favus MJ, ed. *Primer on the metabolic bone diseases and disorders of mineral metabolism,* 4th ed. Chicago: Lippincott Williams & Wilkins, 1999:315–319.
728. Reid IR, Gallagher DJA, Bosworth J. Prophylaxis against vitamin D deficiency by elderly by regular sunlight exposure. *Age Ageing* 1986;15:35–40.
729. Chel VG, Ooms ME, Popp-Snijders C, et al. Ultraviolet irradiation corrects vitamin D deficiency and suppresses secondary hyperparathyroidism in the elderly. *J Bone Miner Res* 1998; 13:1238–1242.
730. Kooh SW, Fraser D, Reilly B.J, et al. Rickets due to calcium deficiency. *N Engl J Med* 1977;297:1264–1266.
731. Marie PJ, Pettifor JM, Ross FP, et al. Histological osteomalacia due to dietary calcium deficiency in children. *N Engl J Med* 1982;307:584–588.
732. Chesney RW. Fanconi syndrome and renal tubular acidosis. In: Favus MJ, ed. *Primer on the metabolic bone diseases and disorders of mineral metabolism,* 4th ed. Chicago: Lippincott Williams & Wilkins, 1999:340–343.
733. Bilezikian JP. Primary Hyperparathyroidism. In: Favus MJ, ed. *Primer on the metabolic bone diseases and disorders of mineral metabolism,* 4th ed. Chicago: Lippincott Williams & Wilkins, 1999:187–192.
734. Peacock M, Horsman A, Aaron JE, et al. The role of parathyroid hormone in bone loss. In: Christiansen C, ed. *Osteoporosis.* Glostrup, Denmark: Department of Clinical Chemistry, Glostrup Hospital, 1984:463–467.
735. Parfitt AM, Rao DS, Kleerekoper M. Asymptomatic hyperparathyroidism discovered by multichannel biochemical screening: clinical course and considerations bearing on the need for surgical intervention. *J Bone Miner Res* 1991;6:S97–S101.
736. Wilson RJ, Rao S, Ellis B, et al. Mild asymptomatic primary hyperparathyroidism is not a risk factor for vertebral fractures. *Ann Intern Med* 1988;109:959–962.
737. Silverberg SJ, Gartenberg F, Jacobs TP, et al. Increased bone density after parathyroidectomy in primary hyperparathyroidism. *J Clin Endocrinol Metab* 1995;80:729–734.
738. Karstrup S, Hegedus L, Holm HH. Acute change in parathyroid function in primary hyperparathyroidism following ultrasonically guided ethanol injection into solitary parathyroid adenomas. *Acta Endocrinol* 1993;129:377–380.
739. Malluche HH, Ritz E, Lange HP, et al. Bone histology in incipient and advanced renal failure. *Kidney Int* 1976;9:355–362.
740. Hory B, Drueke TB. The parathyroid-bone axis in uremia: new insights into old questions. *Curr Opin Nephrol Hypertens* 1997; 6:40–48.
741. Schoutens A, Laurent E, Markowicz E, et al. Serum triiodothyronine, bone turnover, and bone mass changes in euthyroid pre- and postmenopausal women. *Calcif Tissue Int* 1991;49:95–100.
742. Rosen CJ, Adler RA. Longitudinal changes in lumbar bone density among thyrotoxic patients after attainment of euthyroidism. *J Clin Endocrinol Metab* 1992;75:1531–1534.
743. Diamond T, Vine J, Smart R, et al. Thyrotoxic bone disease in women: a potentially reversible disorder. *Ann Intern Med* 1994; 120:8–11.
744. Dalgeish R. The human type I collagen mutation database. *Nucleic Acids Res* 1997;25:181–187.
745. Harper KD, Weber TJ. Secondary osteoporosis; diagnostic conditions. *Endocrinol Metab Clin North Am* 1998;27:325–348.
746. Stellon AJ, Webb A, Compston J, et al. Lack of osteomalacia in chronic cholestatic liver disease. *Bone* 1986;7:181–185.
747. Nilas L, Christiansen C. Influence of PTH and 1,25(OH)2D on calcium homeostatis and bone mineral content after gastric surgery. *Calcif Tissue Int* 1985;37:461–466.
748. Caraceni MP, Molteni N, Bardella MT, et al. Bone and mineral metabolism in adult celiac disease. *Am J Gastroenterol* 1988; 83:274–277.
749. Selby PL, Davies M, Adams JE, et al. Bone loss in celiac disease is related to secondary hyperparathyroidism. *J Bone Miner Res* 1999;14:652–657.
750. Moss AJ, Waterhouse C, Terry R. Gluten-sensitive enteropathy with osteomalacia but without steatorrhea. *N Engl J Med* 1965; 272:825–830.
751. Lindh E, Ljunghall S, Larsson K, et al. Screening for antibodies against gliadin in patients with osteoporosis. *J Intern Med* 1992; 231:403–406.
752. Robinson RJ, Al Azzawi F, Iqbal SJ, et al. Osteoporosis and determinants of bone density in patients with Crohn's disease. *Dig Dis Sci* 1998;43:2500–2506.
753. Mundy GR, Yoneda T, Guise TA. Hypercalcemia in hematologic malignancies and in solid tumors associated with extensive localized bone destruction. In: Favus MJ, ed. *Primer on the metabolic bone diseases and disorders of mineral metabolism,* 4th ed. Chicago: Lippincott Williams & Wilkins, 1999:208–211.
754. Pecherstorfer M, Zimmer-Roth I, Schililng T, et al. The diagnostic value of urinary pyridinium crosslinks of collagen, serum total alkaline phosphatase, and urinary calcium excretion in neoplastic bone disease. *J Clin Endocrinol Metab* 1995;80:97–103.
755. Carlson K, Ljunghall S, Simonsson B, et al. Serum osteocalcin concentrations in patients with multiple myeloma—correlation with disease stage and survival. *J Intern Med* 1992;231:133–137.
756. Stashenko P, Dewhirst FE, Rooney ML, et al. Interleukin-1β is a potent inhibitor of bone formation in vitro. *J Bone Miner Res* 1987;2:559–565.
757. Adams JS. Hypercalcemia due to granuloma-forming disorders. In: Favus MJ, ed. *Primer on the metabolic bone diseases and disorders of mineral metabolism,* 4th ed. Chicago: Lippincott Williams & Wilkins, 1999:212–214.
758. Roberts MM, Stewart AF. Humoral hypercalcemia of malignancy. In: Favus MJ, ed. *Primer on the metabolic bone diseases and disorders of mineral metabolism,* 4th ed. Chicago: Lippincott Williams & Wilkins, 1999:203–207.

123

PAGET'S DISEASE OF BONE

ROY D. ALTMAN

Paget's disease of bone, or osteitis deformans, is a chronic disorder of the adult skeleton characterized by an accelerated turnover of parts of the skeleton resulting in localized softened, disorganized, and enlarged bone.

Although there are early descriptions suggesting what is now called Paget's disease of bone, Sir James Paget (1) clarified the condition with the assistance of (Sir) Henry Butlin in a presentation to the Royal Medical Chirurgical Society of London in 1876. Paget's disease of bone should be differentiated from several other conditions that bear his name, such as Paget's disease of the breast, Paget's disease of the anus, Paget van Schrotter syndrome, Paget's abscess, and Paget's quiet necrosis. Paget has also been credited with the description of carpal tunnel syndrome, *Trichina spiralis,* metastatic tumors to ovaries, dermatofibrosarcoma protuberans, and toxic shock syndrome.

That Paget's disease of bone has early origins is suggested by paleopathologic evidence from medieval skeletons (2), American-Indian skeletons (3), and an Egyptian mummy (4).

EPIDEMIOLOGY

Paget's disease is more prevalent with increasing age and affects men more than women by a ratio of 3:2 (5,6). While the incidence is unknown, wide variations exist in prevalence around the world. The highest prevalence is in Europe, exclusive of Scandinavia and Switzerland (7), with the next highest prevalence occurring among emigrants from high-prevalence areas in other parts of the world, such as Argentina, Australia, and New Zealand. There are only isolated case reports in native African blacks, Orientals, and Asian-Indians.

Early radiographic studies place the prevalence at 3.5% to 4.5% of the adult population in England, with a high of 8.3% in a part of Lancashire (8). After 20 years, a repeat study in Lancashire estimates the prevalence at 2% (6). Initial studies in the United States place the prevalence higher in New York than in Georgia, Kentucky, or Rhode Island (9,10). A review of pelvic radiographs from the U.S. Department of Health and Human Services (National Health and Nutrition Survey I) found the prevalence to be about 1% of the general population in the United States (5). There is a suggestion that there is a decrease in the prevalence of Paget's disease worldwide because of increased prevalence with older age groups, a reduction in the prevalence when compared to prior studies, and a decrease in the severity of disease in newly diagnosed patients (11).

Paget's disease is present in about 13% of relatives (siblings and successive generations of relatives) of those with Paget's disease (12). Nonfamilial cases tend to have a later onset of disease than familial cases.

Only 21% of patients with Paget's disease responding to a questionnaire felt that quality of life was very good or excellent (13). Feelings of depression (47%) and fair/poor health (42%) were common. Survival is normal, with most deaths due to malignancy (14).

ETIOLOGY

A genetic predisposition for Paget's disease is suggested by the persistence of the disease with migration of subpopulations to other parts of the world (e.g., England to Australia and New Zealand; Italy to Argentina), and the increased prevalence found among first-degree relatives. This familial form appears to be based on an autosomal-dominant inheritance, but represents a minority of those with Paget's disease. It may be that there are "familial" and "sporadic" forms of the disease with different modes of inheritance (15). There is a suggestion of linkage of the diseases with the human leukocyte antigen (HLA) locus on chromosome 6 (now labeled PDB1) (16,17). Familial expansile osteolysis is an autosomal-dominant disease with some similarities to Paget's disease of bone, linked to chromosome 18q21-22 (also labeled PDB2) (18); however, PDB2 is not always present in families with Paget's disease and may require an additional gene for expression of Paget's disease (19).

A viral etiology was first suspected because bone electron microscopic studies demonstrated nuclear and cytoplasmic inclusions (20). Evidence of a viral etiology of Paget's disease includes electron microscopy, immunohistochemistry of bone and cultured osteoclasts, identification of paramyxovirus by *in situ* hybridization and reverse-transcriptase polymerase chain reaction, potential association of dogs to people with Paget's disease, the demonstration that the canine distemper virus can infect bone cells and replicate in human tissue, overexpression of the antiapoptotic oncogene *Bcl-2* in pagetic bone, increased serum levels of interleukin-6 (IL-6) (osteoclast precursor recruitment), and the proto-oncogene *c-fos* (increases osteoclast activity) (21–24). The hypothesis is that a paramyxovirus (e.g., respiratory syncytial virus or canine distemper virus) enters a susceptible host and localizes to isolated areas of the skeleton. The virus stimulates oncogenes to increase osteoclastic recruitment and activity, with a reduction in osteoclastic programmed cell death. However, there are persuasive arguments against a viral etiology (25,26), and the viral etiology fails to explain why Paget's disease localizes to certain parts of the skeleton, whether there is a latent period, and why there is a latent period if it is present.

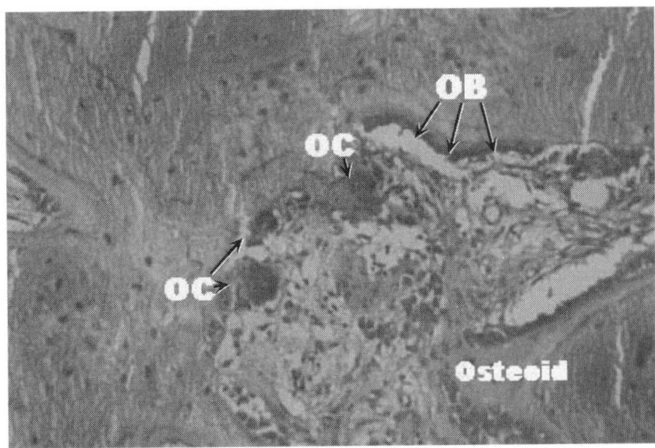

FIGURE 123.1. Light microscopic examination of Paget's bone from an iliac crest biopsy. Scalloped edges indicate active osteoclastic activity. There are multiple large osteoclasts (OC), numerous osteoblasts (OB), and irregular osteoid seams—some of which are poorly calcified (osteoid). The remaining marrow is fibrotic (x400).

ANATOMY AND PATHOPHYSIOLOGY

Gross Anatomy

Flat bones become broadened and thickened. Vertebral bodies become enlarged in all spheres and may have deforming fractures. The skull becomes enlarged, often unevenly, with flattening of its base. Inner and outer tables become thickened and enlarged. There is bowing of long bones, related to gravity or at sites related to the pull of muscles. The cortex of the long bones thickens and extends outward as well as inward, compromising the marrow cavity. Bones become heavy and vary from friable to very hard, and may fracture.

Microanatomy

The initial phase of Paget's disease involves an increase in osteoclastic activity. There is an increased birth rate of the basic multicellular bone units (27). Active bone metabolism is reflected by increases in (a) the number of osteoclasts, (b) resorption surface, and (c) depth of the resorption areas up to seven times normal (Fig. 123.1). Resorption of existing bone by the basic multicellular units are greater than normal, creating larger spaces.

Osteoclasts are derived from monocyte/macrophage precursors of the bone marrow. Pagetic osteoclasts generally contain many more than the normal three to four nuclei and become quite large (may exceed 200 μm in diameter). It has been suggested that these abnormal cells may result from an increase of IL-6, *c-fos*, and/or *Bcl-2*. There is no increase in tumor necrosis factor (TNF), fibroblast growth factor (FGF), transforming growth factor (TGF), or insulin-like growth factor (IGF) (28). Under electron microscopy, osteoclasts otherwise have mostly normal characteristics. However, the nuclei are abnormal, containing nuclear inclusions in various size and arrangements, suggesting a viral configuration (20,29). The individual nuclear microfilament inclusions average 15 nm in diameter and are in a hexagonal arrangement, tightly packed in a paracrystalline array. In the cytoplasm, the inclusions are found in random strands or loose bundles.

The normal coupling of resorption and formation of bone matrix is maintained in Paget's disease (30). The repair is characterized by an increase in number of osteoblasts, osteoid, and deposition surfaces. The quantities of osteoid synthesized are often not adequate to fill the tunneled cavities; alternatively, the osteoblasts may synthesize and secrete collagen into cavities with markedly irregular surfaces, followed by deposition of woven rather than lamellar bone. The resultant bone is disorganized, with thickened trabeculae and a haphazard appearance of woven bone with shortened lamellar collagen fibrils. The trabeculae often contain unmineralized osteoid (Fig. 123.1). It appears that pagetic osteoblasts produce an excess of collagen matrix that is synthesized in an anarchic fashion to produce a woven bone in a typical mosaic that can be easily visualized under polarizing light. Gaps in lamellar and woven bone are filled with fibrous connective tissue. Remaining bone becomes heavily calcified and sclerotic.

Quantitative bone histomorphometry shows increased trabecular bone area, forming surfaces, and osteoid area. The linear rate of matrix formation is elevated. Trabeculae are thick and numerous (27). There is poor definition of the boundary between cortical and medullary bone, and trabecular bone volume is more than twice normal. Both endosteal and epiphyseal bone units are involved, which causes the bone to become thick as well as long.

There is enlargement of the haversian canals with open communication to the medullary canal, an increase in arterial capillaries, increase in arterial blood flow, and enlargement of the marrow sinuses, with venous stasis. In later phases, the resorption decreases, with less vascularity.

With the heavily calcified osteoid, total body calcium is often increased. However, the alternating heavily calcified and fibrotic areas of long bone produce the characteristic radiographic appearance of coarse trabeculation.

Uninvolved bone from patients with Paget's disease may show characteristics of increased remodeling, suggestive of secondary increased parathyroid activity (27).

Teeth may be involved with a mosaic pattern similar to the adjacent pagetic bone. Teeth may loosen as the lamina dura is often thinned. The histologic (and radiographic) appearance of bone from the pagetic mandible or maxilla may be confused with fibrous dysplasia of bone. In contrast, fibrous dysplasia is usually unilateral and uncommonly expands the adult skeleton.

CLINICAL SYNDROME

It is estimated that 80% of those with Paget's disease are asymptomatic and without overt clinical findings. The clinical relevance of Paget's disease derives from its potential complications (31) (Table 123.1).

A common scenario for Paget's disease involves its discovery in an individual over the age of 50 as an incidental finding from a laboratory test or radiograph. The disease progresses slowly, with little influence on quality of life. Eventually, there may be changes in the size and shape of the involved bones, including enlargement of the skull, but this rarely causes any changes in mentation. There is a tendency to involvement of the right side of the body, where the long bones become enlarged and bowed. The spine becomes shortened, accentuating kyphosis. Pain develops from the involved bones or associated arthritis. Paget felt that those portions of the skeleton most subject to stress and strain show the greatest evidence of involvement (32). Paget's disease may involve a single bone or nearly the entire skeleton.

General symptoms may include dizziness, stiffness, weakness, and fatigability. There may be a tendency to somnambulance, limitation of joint motion, flattening of the chest with kyphosis, shortened torso, and prominence of the pelvis (Fig. 123.2).

Pain from Paget's disease is aching, poorly described, and occasionally continuous at night. The cause of the pain is not clear in most patients, but may be related to unmineralized osteoid (similar to osteomalacia) (Fig. 123.1), venous congestion (similar to bone ischemia), or stretching of the periosteum (i.e., bowed long bone pain with weight bearing). Pressure on the periosteum of a pagetic bone may precipitate pain; for instance, heel pain with calcaneal Paget's disease commonly occurs upon weight bearing (33). In addition to the above, pain in patients with Paget's disease is commonly related to osteoarthritis (34). Rapidly increasing bone pain should alert one to the possibility of malignancy in the pagetic bone or an impending fracture.

Skull deformity includes local knobby deformity, frontal bossing, and diffuse enlargement. There may be associated dilated scalp veins, which should not be confused with temporal arteries or temporal arteritis (35). Focal enlargement of the zygoma, mandible, or maxilla may give the face a grotesque appearance. Maxillary disease exceeds mandibular involvement by a ratio of 2:1; rarely, both bones are involved in the same patient. Gums may become swollen and infected. The skull may become thickened, softened, and enlarged, and may have the gross appearance of an inverted triangle.

TABLE 123.1. CLINICAL FINDINGS IN PATIENTS WITH PAGET'S DISEASE OF BONE

Findings	Pathophysiology
Bone pain	Periosteal, ischemic bone, unmineralized osteoid
Deformity of bone	Structurally softened bone bending to gravity or muscular pull
Fracture	Transverse fracture of structurally weakened bone, osteolysis, microfracture of bowed extremity, vertebral compression fracture
Osteoarthritis	Secondary to juxtaarticular Paget's disease, change in joint congruity, altered gait dynamics
Increased cardiac demand	Highly metabolic bone
Malignancy	Sarcoma of pagetic bone; metastatic disease from other malignancies to pagetic bone
Reduced auditory acuity	Pagetic petrous bony invasion of the cochlea
Altered mental status	Platybasia with high-pressure hydrocephalus
Paraparesis/paraplegia	Spinal cord ischemia, cord compression
Low back pain	Vertebral enlargement with altered spinal dynamics, vertebral and facet osteoarthritis, spinal stenosis, active spinal Paget's disease, unrelated osteoarthritis
Hypercalcemia	Primary or secondary hyperparathyroidism, active Paget's disease with immobilization, immobilization from fracture
Altered visual acuity	Rupture of angioid streak, optic nerve entrapment

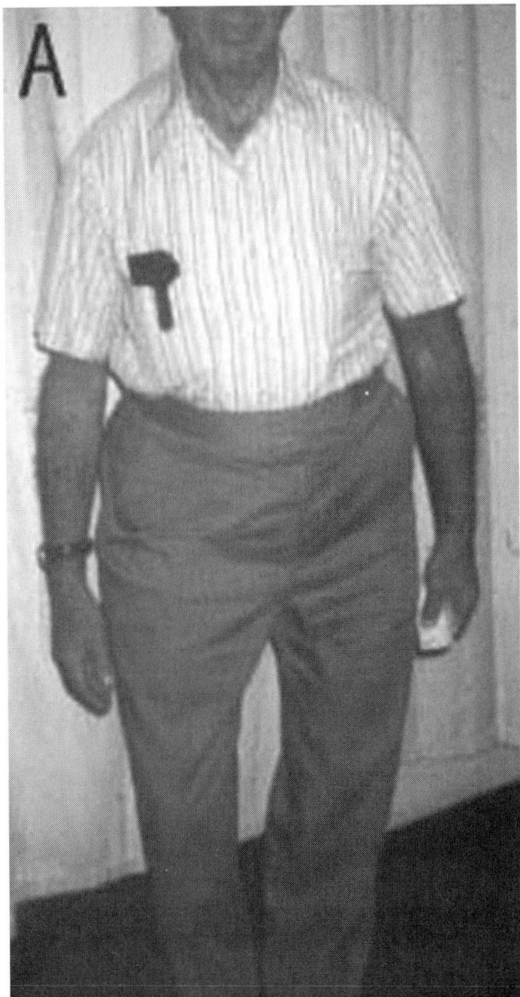

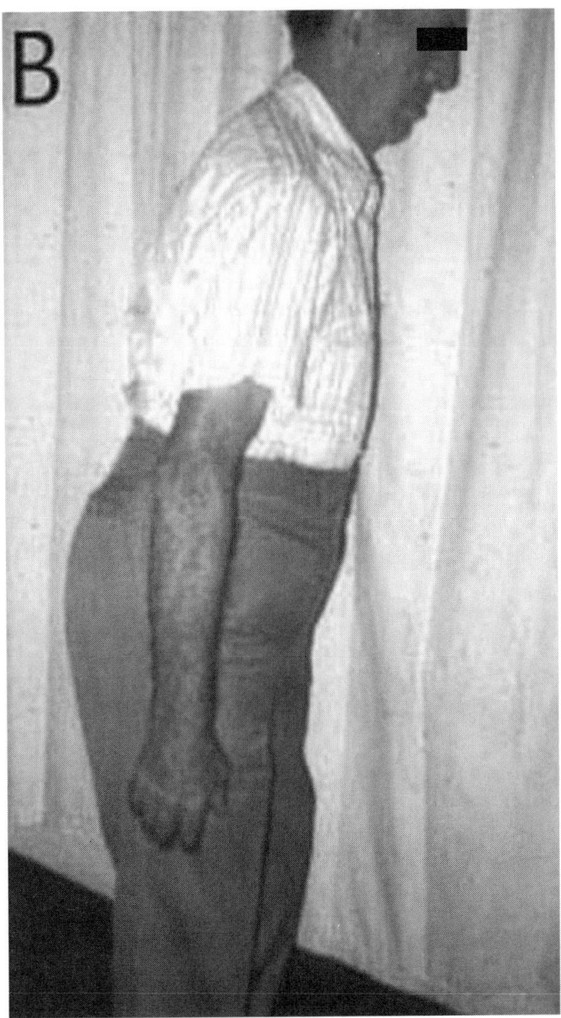

FIGURE 123.2. A, anterior and **B**, side view. Photographs of a patient with severe Paget's disease demonstrate an anthropoid appearance with simian posturing. The trunk is shortened with a flared pelvis and forward posturing. The spine is fixed and inflexible, suggesting ankylosing spondylitis. There is a functional flexion contracture at the hips with bowed extremities.

Deformity of the spine, usually from both spinal enlargement and compression fractures, may result in a short stature, simian posturing, and the tendency to bend forward while standing (Fig. 123.2). The patient may develop scoliosis, an accentuated dorsal kyphosis, and straightening or reversal of the normal lumbar lordosis, giving the patient an anthropoid appearance.

Pelvic Paget's disease causes a weight-bearing–induced axial (or medial) migration of the hips (protusio acetabuli), producing a functional flexion contracture at the hips, thereby accentuating the forward flexion of the trunk. Reduced spinal mobility and functional flexion contractures of the hips result in a distinct limp that simulates the gait of a patient with ankylosing spondylitis and accentuates the simian posture.

The softened long bones become bowed, from stress of weight bearing and/or pull at the insertion of ligaments. The thigh or leg develops an anterior and lateral bow that produces a functional flexion contracture at the knee and a varus or bowed knee appearance, despite the elongation of the involved bone and an often hyperextended knee of 5 to 10 degrees. If only one of the lower extremities is bowed, the ipsilateral heel may not touch the ground, resulting in a "roller coaster" gait. If the lateral bow is severe, the ankle becomes everted on contact with the ground. Both conditions may be partially corrected by orthotics. Gait analysis may reveal a decrease in velocity and cadence and an increase in stride time and double-limb support time (36). A bowed forearm or arm produces a functional extension contracture at the elbow, reducing the ability to feed oneself, comb one's hair, etc.

Fractures were the reason for the diagnosis in 8% (37) of patients with Paget's disease and were present in 18% of 1,339 patients in a literature review (38). Fractures may be incomplete, complete, or compression. Spinal compression fractures are increased because of coexistent osteoporosis with the softened bone of Paget's disease. Pagetic ribs may fracture with little or no detectable trauma. Horizontal or incomplete fractures of long bones are only occasionally symptomatic, and uncommonly advance to completion. Long bone completed fractures are generally perpendicular or transverse to the external cortex, whereas spiral fractures are the usual fractures of nonpagetic long bones. Often, there is wide separation of fragments without comminution. The most common fracture sites are the femur, tibia, lumbar spine, humerus, and dorsal spine, in decreasing frequency (38). Femoral fractures commonly occur through the shaft just below the lesser trochanter. Tibial fractures tend to occur in the upper one-third of the shaft. The resulting callus calcifies but is often pagetic. Early fixation of the fracture is encouraged as a means of reducing the risk of nonunion. Fractures may be the herald of sarcoma, and careful review of the radiographs is appropriate.

Osteoarthritis is related to Paget's disease by the following proposed mechanisms (39):

1. Uniform bony enlargement. Enlarged pagetic bone alters the congruity between joint surfaces. For example, enlargement of the femoral head exceeds the confined acetabular space, causing cartilage compression and atrophy. Enlargement of the bone along the ileopectineal line also impinges upon the joint space, resulting in axial (or medial) joint space narrowing; this is in contrast to idiopathic osteoarthritis of the hip, which is most often narrowed superiorly (Fig. 123.3).
2. Uneven bony enlargement. There is an uneven expansion of the pagetic subchondral bony plate, creating an uneven base for the articular cartilage. The high peaks of cartilage may undergo pressure necrosis, while the lower peaks may undergo disuse atrophy.
3. Altered joint biodynamics. The bowed extremity alters the contact areas of the articular cartilage, hence changing joint congruity and altering cartilage biodynamics.
4. Softened pelvis. The entire pagetic bone softens and tends to migrate axially (protrusio acetabuli). This results in a functional flexion contracture of the hips, causing forward bending while standing or walking. These altered dynamics often result in osteoarthritis of the hips and/or low back pain.

Although low back pain accounts for the clinical presentation in 30% of patients with Paget's disease, the presence of lumbosacral Paget's disease could explain the pain in only 12%, whereas osteoarthritis was present in the remainder (40). Paget's disease seemed to be directly or indirectly involved with spinal osteoarthritis by the mechanisms above. Lumbar canal stenosis correlates with the degree of symptoms and findings (41,42).

Active Paget's disease increases the blood flow to the involved bone and creates a state of high cardiac output. There is an associated increase in blood flow to the surrounding tissues, including the skin. Commonly, the involved extremity is palpably warm. Degree of bone turnover (as reflected by chemistries) is a better reflection of demand for blood than the area of skeletal Paget's disease (42). However, involvement of more than 15% of the skeleton correlates with cardiac enlargement and depressed myocardial contractility (43). When the serum alkaline phosphatase increases to four times the upper normal value, skeletal blood flow doubles from 300 mL/min, or 6% of the blood volume per minute, to about 12% (42). Uncommonly, the demand for blood by the pagetic bone precipitates congestive heart failure.

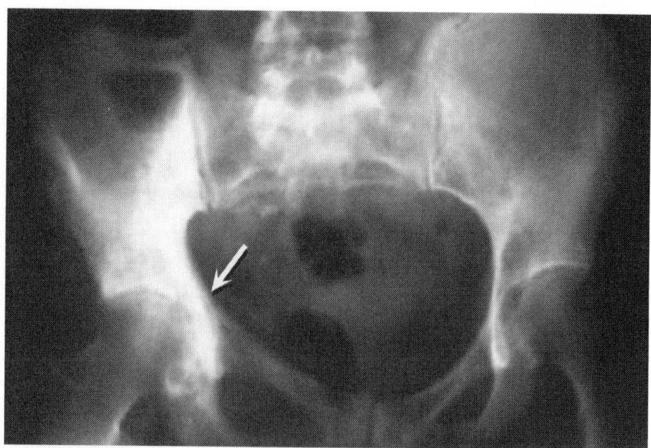

FIGURE 123.3. Radiograph of the pelvis shows diffuse Paget's disease of the right hemipelvis with sclerotic changes of the iliac bones and thickening with heavy calcification of the ileopectineal line (brim sign) *(arrow)*. Paget's disease also involves the proximal right femur. The diameter of the right proximal femoral head is 0.4 cm wider than the left. The radiographic joint space is narrowed in the axial plane, and there is an axial migration of the hip (protrusio acetabulum). Although not obvious from the radiograph, the Paget's disease also involves the left hemipelvis.

Sarcomas in pagetic bone are often insidious but may be suspected because of increasing pain, rapid development of neurologic deficit, or fracture. The plain radiograph may need to be supplemented by computed tomography (CT) or magnetic resonance imaging (MRI) to clarify the diagnosis. Suspicion of pagetic sarcoma or metastatic disease to a pagetic lesion is the major justification for bone biopsy. Bone sarcoma occurs in fewer than 1% of patients with Paget's disease. This is a 40-fold increase in bone sarcomas over the general population, and causes approximately 100 deaths in the United States each year. The mean survival time from diagnosis is 9 months, as these tumors are resistant to therapy, often metastatic to the lung upon discovery, and often multifocal in origin (44). Most sarcomas occur in patients with oligo-ostotic Paget's disease. Sarcomas most frequently occur in the spine, skull, pelvis, femur (Fig. 123.4), tibia, and humerus. Pagetic sarcomas are derived from five cell types: osteoblast, chondroblast, osteocyte, undifferentiated cell (stem-cell type), and myofibroblast (45). Pagetic sarcomas are often nonosteoblastic,

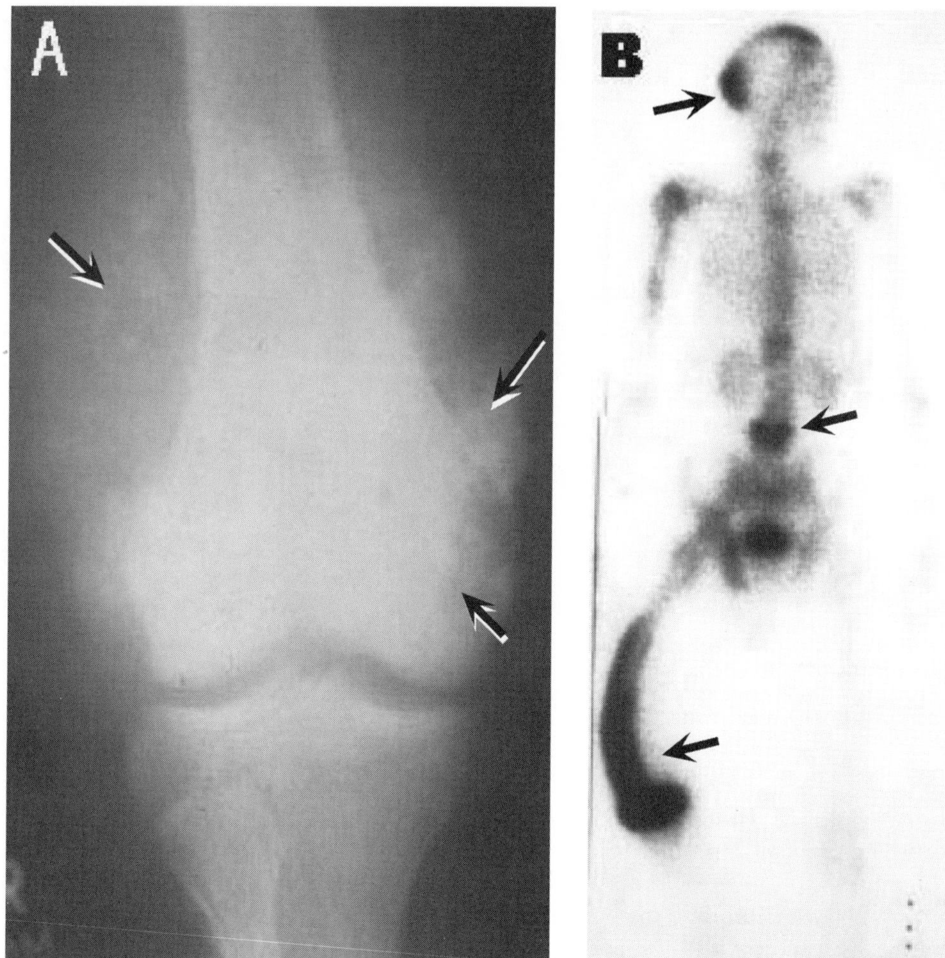

FIGURE 123.4. A: Anteroposterior radiograph of a knee demonstrating disruption of the cortex with bony deposits in the soft tissues *(arrows)*. This mass effect is strongly suspicious of sarcomatous changes of Paget's disease. **B:** A technetium ^{99m}Tc-labeled bisphosphonate bone scan of the same patient shows intense uptake of the nuclide by the sarcoma involving the distal right femur and right zygoma. The ^{99m}Tc-labeled bisphosphonate also localizes to the body of a pagetic vertebra *(wide arrow)*, involving the superior facets of the posterior neural arch in a Y-like configuration. Paget's disease is also present in the right hemipelvis, sacrum, and proximal right humerus.

which may also account for the frequent lack of localization in the nuclide on bone scan. There may be a reduction in the number of pagetic sarcomas over the last 20 years that is unexplained, but potentially related to the new therapies for Paget's disease of bone. However, this morbid complication of Paget's disease still exists (46).

Giant-cell tumors can occur in pagetic bone and are sometimes familial (47). Numerous tumors may metastasize to pagetic bone, presumably because of high perfusion and abnormal structure of the pagetic lesion.

A variety of skull symptoms include headaches, "noise," tinnitus, vertigo, and "rushing" sensations. Invasion of the cochlea by pagetic bone causes hearing loss and may cause vertigo with an unsteady gait and loss of balance. Skull enlargement can be followed by a change in hat size or in regular measurements of the circumference of the skull. The heavy and soft pagetic skull appears to settle around the top of the neck (Fig. 123.5), causing platybasia. Platybasia sometimes causes refractory occipital headaches or obstruction to flow of spinal fluid through the fourth ventricle (48). The hydrocephalis dementia complex of communication hydrocephalus that may develop from platybasia often responds to ventriculoatrial shunt (48).

Maxillary or mandibular involvement may disrupt the lamina dura and loosen teeth. Patients with Paget's disease suffer greater difficulty with dental extraction and experience more postextraction complications than is normally expected (49,50). Mouth pain from gingivitis may be superimposed on loosened teeth.

Hearing loss is common with Paget's disease of the skull, is sensorineural, and results from invasion of the cochlea from the pagetic petrous ridge (51).

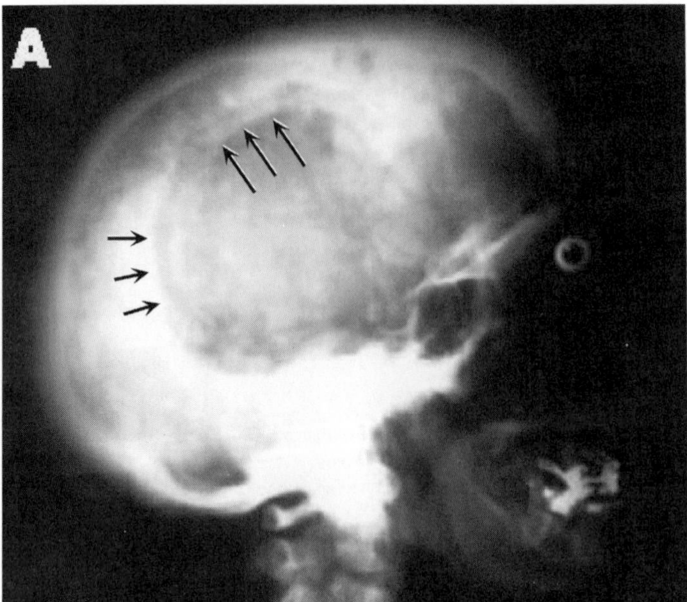

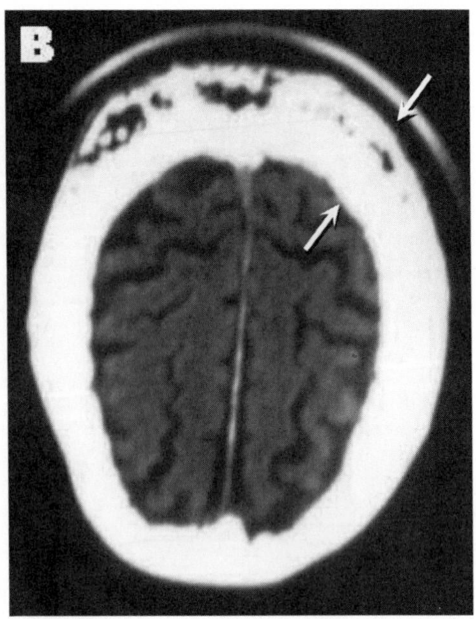

FIGURE 123.5. A: Lateral radiograph of the skull shows the thickened skull and osteoporosis circumscripta of both lateral temporal bones *(short arrows, right; long arrows, left)*. Platybasia is present. **B:** Axial section of the skull by computed tomography (CT) of the skull demonstrates cortical atrophy, and a wide, thick skull mostly composed of wide diploic areas *(arrows)*.

Sudden partial or complete visual loss may be due to rupture of angioid streaks. Angioid streaks on funduscopic examination are fibrovascular changes of the superficial (Bruch's) membrane of the eye. They occur in about 15% of pagetic patients, mostly in those with Paget's disease of the skull (52). Visual loss can also occur from pagetic bony impingement of the optic nerve. Pagetic enlargement of the orbit may interfere with muscular function to the eye. Facial nerve paralysis with "crocodile tears" may also develop (53).

A variety of neurologic complications can occur (54). The most serious is paraparesis/paraplegia. When present, it is related to Paget's disease of dorsal or cervical vertebrae. Rather than cord compression, this complication is theorized to be secondary to a spinal artery steal syndrome (55). Since these patients often respond to medication, improvement is felt to be related to decreased perfusion of the pagetic vertebrae, with resultant improved blood flow to the small vessels of the spinal cord.

Hypercalcemia may be related to coexistent Paget's disease and hyperparathyroidism (56), immobilization with active disease, or immobilization from fracture.

Forms of miscellaneous conditions and nonarticular complications that can be seen include inflammatory periarthritis or shoulder-hand syndrome with humoral or scapular Paget's disease, fibrosing syndromes such as Peyronie's disease in as many as 31% of men (57), and Paget's disease in the enthesopathy of diffuse idiopathic skeletal hyperostosis (DISH) (37,58). There is limited evidence of an increased prevalence of gout with Paget's disease.

LABORATORY ANALYSIS

Metabolically, turnover of bone is active in Paget's disease and may be reflected in the laboratory evaluation.

Anabolic bone activity in Paget's disease is assessed by the serum alkaline phosphatase, which may be extremely elevated. The levels of the serum alkaline phosphatase are a function of the activity of the Paget's disease. Spontaneous decreases in the serum alkaline phosphatase can occur over prolonged periods of time and are related to the natural history of Paget's disease moving into a healed, sclerotic, inactive phase. Rapid rises in serum alkaline phosphatase may be due to sarcomatous degeneration of a pagetic bone; however, pagetic sarcomas are also commonly associated with low levels of serum alkaline phosphatase.

The bone-specific alkaline phosphatase isoenzyme is helpful in identifying active Paget's disease in patients with a normal total serum alkaline phosphatase and in differentiating alkaline phosphatase of bone versus hepatic origin. In patients with Paget's disease and a normal total serum alkaline phosphatase, the bone-specific alkaline phosphatase isoenzyme is elevated in 60% of patients (59). The bone-specific alkaline phosphatase has a sensitivity of 86% and specificity of 100% for Paget's disease of bone (60). However, in most patients with Paget's disease, there is no advantage of routinely following the bone-specific alkaline phosphatase isoenzyme. Other markers of anabolic bone activity have not been as useful in Paget's disease of bone.

Catabolic activity of bone can be determined by measuring several urinary peptides that are derived almost exclusively from bone collagen, and that correlate with the serum alkaline phosphatase. The urinary fragments that correlate best are the pyridinoline cross-links (59,60) and the amino-terminal telopeptide of type I collagen (61). These have replaced the urine hydroxyproline because of the ease of collecting a second morning specimen with rapid analysis (hydroxyproline requires a 24-hour specimen on a gelatin-free diet and 2 days for the analysis). These tests are of value in selected patients with Paget's disease.

Suppressive therapy for Paget's disease decreases resorption before it suppresses formation as reflected by a reduction in hydroxyproline excretion prior to a decrease in serum alkaline phosphatase (30,62).

There are normal values of serum (bound or unbound) calcium and inorganic phosphate. Calcium accumulates in the bone, and total body calcium is elevated. As above, hypercalcemia can occur, most often related to coincident hyperparathyroidism.

IMAGING

Radiography and Magnetic Resonance Imaging

The pelvis is involved in approximately 80% of patients with Paget's disease, with the skull, spine, and femur following in frequency. Sequential radiographs suggest that Paget's disease begins in the end of the diaphysis of long bones, extending from that site (63) with a yearly progression of 9.4 mm in the tibia and 8.5 mm in the skull (64).

The radiographic appearances of Paget's disease include osteolytic, osteoblastic, fibrotic, and sclerotic phases that roughly correlate with the morbid anatomy (65). However, the radiographic appearance of the lesion and the site involved does not correlate with symptoms.

Skull involvement may be reflected by diffuse cortical thickening, spotty osteoblastic "cotton-wool" lesions, osteoporosis circumscripta (Fig. 123.5), and platybasia. Early changes include diminished density of the diploe and thinning of the outer table of bone from within (66). Age-related cerebral cortical atrophy is commonly seen on CT or MRI. Disruption of the inner or outer table of the cortex suggests malignancy. Paget's disease invasion of the cochlea is demonstrated by CT (67). Platybasia with change in mental status can be best evaluated by MRI and magnetic resonance angiography (MRA). Paget's disease rarely involves both the maxilla and mandible and must be differentiated from fibrous dysplasia of bone.

Vertebral changes include enlarged vertebral bodies in all planes, increased radiodensity (ivory vertebra), osteoporosis, or a thickened cortex combined with trabecular osteoporosis ("picture-frame vertebra") (Fig. 123.6). Prox-

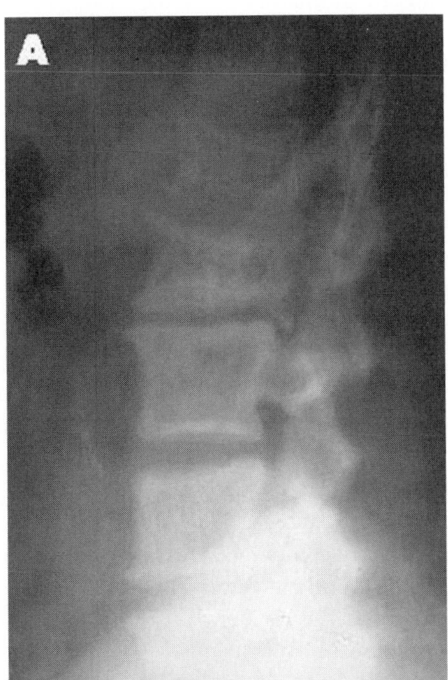

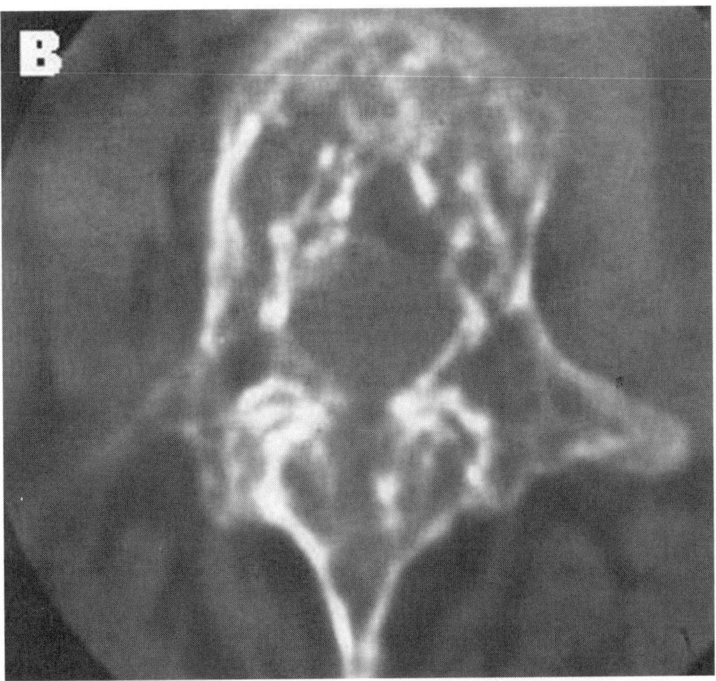

FIGURE 123.6. A: Lateral radiograph of the lumbar spine shows Paget's disease of all lumbar vertebrae. There are compression fractures of the second and third lumbar vertebra. The fourth and fifth lumbar vertebrae are enlarged in the anteroposterior and superior-inferior planes. The thick cortices of the fourth lumbar vertebra surround mixed changes of the body of the vertebrae, giving it a "picture-frame" appearance. **B:** Axial view of the fourth lumbar vertebra by CT demonstrates dramatic osteoporosis, coarse trabeculation, and enlargement of the neural arch.

imal-distal widening of the vertebrae leads to loss of the normal curvature of the spine. Posterior widening of the vertebra leads to spinal canal impingement. Central collapse of porotic vertebrae gives a "codfish vertebra" pattern. Facets become enlarged and develop secondary osteoarthritis.

Pelvic changes are most often diffuse and bilateral, involving the adjacent sacrum (Fig. 123.3). The sacroiliac joints are often disrupted or fused but rarely symptomatic. The ilei may be porotic, diffusely radiodense, or have whorls of coarse trabeculation. The ileopectineal line is often thickened and sclerotic in appearance (brim sign) (Fig. 123.3) (68). The softened pelvis migrates axially, giving the pelvic brim a triangular appearance or triradiate deformity (69). Patchy sclerotic areas may cause difficulty in separating blastic tumors (e.g., metastatic prostate cancer) from coexistent Paget's disease.

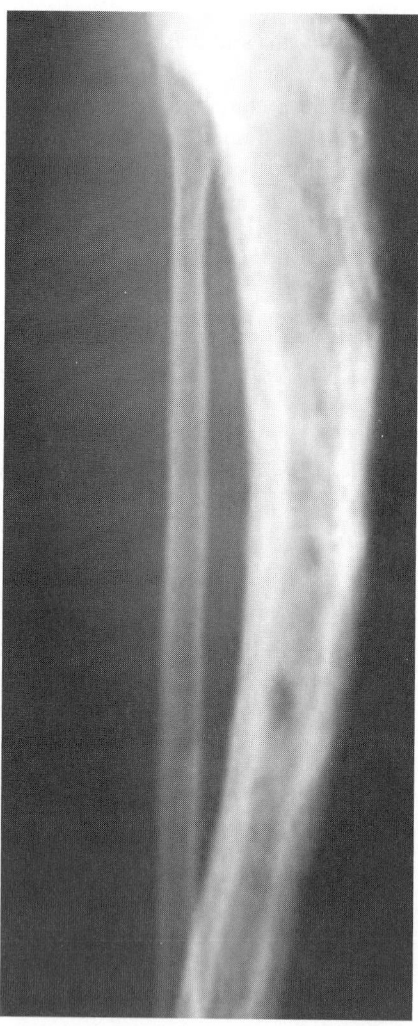

FIGURE 123.7. Lateral radiograph of leg demonstrating a marked anterior bow to the tibia with a thickened proximal cortex, and areas of fibrosis.

Long bones may demonstrate homogeneous sclerosis, trabecular coarsening, cortical thickening, and lysis (70). Tubular bones demonstrate a thickened cortex with subperiosteal bone and narrowing of the medullary canal (Fig. 123.7). The shaft of the long bone can demonstrate a "flame sign." Proximal or distal areas of long bones are thickened and demonstrate coarse trabeculation. Long bones are often bowed, and stress microfractures may be present on the convex surface.

Pagetic sarcomas are suspected when there is disruption of the cortex and fluffy calcifications with a soft tissue mass effect surrounding the involved bone (Fig. 123.4). Osteolysis rather than osteosclerosis is the major radiographic characteristic of sarcoma (71). When present, giant-cell tumors of the skull or facial bones in elderly patients with polyostotic Paget's disease are benign in appearance. Radiographically, giant-cell tumors are lytic expansile lesions with a soft tissue mass. Pagetic fat-filled marrow spaces can simulate tumor (72).

Completed fractures of the femur are commonly subtrochanteric in location (73). In contrast to traumatic fractures of long bones that are most often spiral, fractures through pagetic bone are most often transverse.

Bone Scanning

Bone scanning is based on a pertechnetate-labeled bisphosphonate with a strong tendency to localize at sites of blastic activity of bone, inflammatory or damaged soft tissue, and blood flow. The unique diffuse cortical uptake separates the bone scan of Paget's disease from other diseases (Fig. 123.8). All pagetic sites do not accumulate the radionuclide equally, and there are differences in scintigraphic activity at each anatomic site. Recurrent active disease recurrence can be detected by nuclear scan prior to an increase in alkaline phosphatase (74).

As many as 20% of pagetic sites are not detected radiographically but are detected by bone scan (65,75). Evidence of the lack of development of new lesions comes from bone scans on patients followed for over 15 years (76). Bisphosphonate bone scanning continues to be of value for patients receiving bisphosphonates as suppressive therapy (77). However, the nuclide is less evenly distributed to sites of Paget's disease in patients having received pagetic suppressive therapy. Not all sites of Paget's disease on the bone scan change, or change equally with therapy, and treated Paget's disease may suggest metastatic malignancy (78). Pinhole bone scintigraphy better identifies the cortical and rim uptake of Paget's disease (79).

Gallium readily localizes to active Paget's disease. Reduction of activity of bone was better demonstrated by radiolabeled gallium than by radiolabeled bisphosphonates, perhaps because gallium uptake more specifically reflects cellular activity (80). If an area of expected active

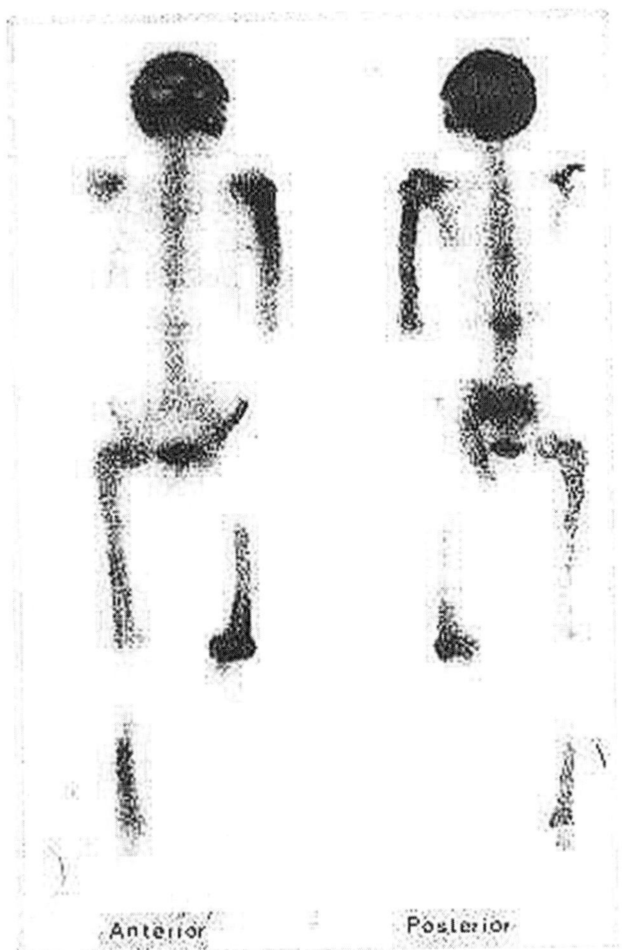

FIGURE 123.8. A ^{99m}Tc-labeled bisphosphonate bone scan localizes to areas of active bone deposition of Paget's disease. There is intense localization of the nuclide to the skull, left humerus, eighth dorsal vertebra, second lumbar vertebra, sacrum, left more than right hemipelvis, proximal right femur, distal left femur, and distal right tibia. The diffuse uptake of the individual bones is typical of Paget's disease.

Paget's disease fails to accumulate the nuclide, sarcomatous change may be suspected. In such cases TI-201 scanning may be of value (81). Nevertheless, photon deficiency in Paget's disease may be present early in the disease even without sarcoma.

DIAGNOSIS

Clinical Features

Symptoms may be present for a period of years before the diagnosis. The majority of patients have no apparent clinical abnormalities. The diagnosis is occasionally apparent from clinical examination, such as finding a large skull with frontal bossing and dilated scalp veins, short stature with simian posturing, and lateral/anterior bow to an extremity.

To differentiate osteoarthritis from Paget's disease, lidocaine can be injected into the suspected joint, such as a hip or a knee. If there is prompt relief of pain, the symptoms are most likely osteoarthritic in origin.

Serum Alkaline Phosphatase Measurement

The diagnosis of Paget's disease is often suggested by a serum alkaline phosphatase elevation (see Laboratory Analysis, above).

Radiograph

The roentgenographic features of Paget's disease are characteristic and most often diagnostic. Only rarely will the initial lytic phase of Paget's disease present some difficulty. Only bones potentially involved with Paget's disease should be radiographed. Bone surveys are not recommended.

Pelvic Paget's disease can mimic osteoblastic metastases. However, the accentuated trabecular pattern, enlargement of the involved bone, thickening of the iliopectineal line, a triangular appearance of the pelvic brim, and diffuse distribution of Paget's disease in the pelvis are characteristic.

The picture frame vertebra with condensation of the vertebral cortex, ivory vertebra, and the coarse trabecular pattern differentiate Paget's disease from vertebral hemangioma, the "rugger-jersey" spine of renal osteodystrophy, or osteoporosis. The ivory vertebra may mimic blastic skeletal metastases and lymphoma. Long-bone epiphyseal involvement, widespread sclerosis, bony enlargement, thickened cortex, bowing, sharply demarcated bone lysis, and an advancing osteolytic wedge are characteristic of Paget's disease.

However, increased skeletal density may be seen in blastic bone metastases (e.g., breast, prostatic carcinoma), myelofibrosis, fluorosis, malignant mastocytosis, renal osteodystrophy, fibrous dysplasia of bone, the Weismann-Netter-Stuhl syndrome, and tuberous sclerosis. Examination and laboratory testing may be needed to distinguish these diseases. Axial osteomalacia, osteogenesis imperfecta osseum, familial idiopathic hyperphosphatasia, and hyperostosis frontalis may on occasion be difficult to distinguish from Paget's disease.

Bone Scan

The bone scan is helpful in outlining the extent of bony involvement in Paget's disease. Because Paget's disease, once discovered, rarely adds new bone, repeat bone scan is rarely needed. Spread within the involved bone does occur; this can be evaluated by radiograph and occasionally by bone scan.

Bone Biopsy

In Paget's disease, the radiograph is characteristic and most often confirms diagnosis. However, bone biopsy may be needed if malignant transformation or another tumor metastatic to bone is suspected. Biopsy of the osteolytic wedge is unnecessary and should be avoided because of increased risk of fracture (82).

TREATMENT

General Measures

Paget's disease is rarely a serious illness, and therapy, though very effective, is not always needed. Most often symptoms in Paget's disease are mild and readily suppressed by a therapeutic program. In patients with symptomatic disease, an array of physical, medicinal, and surgical measures are often effective. Death from Paget's disease is rare and probably limited to those developing sarcoma of the pagetic lesion.

Orthopedic Measures

Symptoms related to bowed lower extremities or pelvic deformity can often be mitigated by mechanical devices such as orthotics (e.g., a heel lift, a medial wedge to the heel and sole). Surgical procedures for Paget's disease may include osteotomy for tibial or femoral deformity, open or closed reduction for fracture, joint arthroplasty for secondary osteoarthritis, and spinal decompression for symptoms and signs of cord compression.

Pagetic bone may be hard and difficult to cut, or may be soft and bleed excessively. The latter is reduced by suppressive medications prior to surgery. Total joint replacement for hip or knee is effective (83). However, loosening is more common than in the nonpagetic population, perhaps due to the mechanical problems induced by softened bone and bowed extremities.

Antiinflammatory Drugs

Antiinflammatory drugs reduce skeletal vascularity and possibly bone resorption (84). However, their value in Paget's disease may be related to reducing the pain from secondary osteoarthritis.

Guidelines for Suppressive Medicinal Therapy

There are now potent and generally safe suppressive agents of bone metabolism. This has changed the philosophy regarding suppressive therapy for Paget's disease (Table 123.2). The indications for suppressive therapy for Paget's disease of bone now include active Paget's disease, including an asymptomatic serum alkaline phosphatase twice the upper limit of the normal range. Although not proven, it is felt that suppressive therapy will prevent or retard progression of complications of Paget's disease. However, this is with the understanding that suppressive therapies will not correct existing complications of Paget's disease (e.g., hearing loss, deformity, osteoarthritis).

Although back pain is common in patients with Paget's disease, it is uncommonly a direct cause of symptoms. Back pain in patients with Paget's disease is often due to an arthritic process that may or may not have resulted from the Paget's disease. Therapy for Paget's disease should be administered with caution and without unrealistic expectations.

Paraparesis or paraplegia is an uncommon complication of Paget's disease of the dorsal or cervical spine. Paraparesis and paraplegia have often been reversed, at least in part, by medicinal therapy, which is often considered because these patients are often poor candidates for surgical decompression.

Treatment before a surgical procedure will decrease the vascularity of the pagetic bone, resulting in reduced blood loss and more rapid healing.

The osteolytic phase of long bones is uncommon, occurring in about 10% of radiographs. Among the bisphosphonates, only etidronate should not be used. Calcitonin induces radiographic healing, but withdrawal of calcitonin is often followed by rapid progression of osteolysis (82).

Patient follow-up should be at 3-month intervals while the Paget's disease is active. While inactive, the follow-up can occur at intervals of 6 to 12 months. Follow-up should include a history and physical examination, with determination of the total serum alkaline phosphatase. Repeat radiographs are needed for following an osteolytic region, but otherwise are only occasionally necessary. Repeat bone scans are rarely needed.

Bisphosphonates

The agents of choice for Paget's disease are the bisphosphonates, which are pyrophosphate analogues that replace the central oxygen of pyrophosphate with a carbon. They are resistant to enzyme degradation, and have a prolonged half-life in bone. Perhaps of more relevance in Paget's disease, bisphosphonates are also potent osteoclast inhibitors (85). The antiresorptive properties of the bisphosphonates are more potent when they contain a nitrogen atom in an alkyl side chain extending from the central carbon, and even more potent when the side chain contains a tertiary nitrogen. The bisphosphonate hydroxyl group binds to mineral surfaces, while the interaction with osteoclast molecular targets is determined by the side chain from the central carbon (86). Exposed apatite concentrates the bisphosphonate in the space beneath the osteoclast (87). Ingestion of calcium from the bone that contains the bisphosphonate leads to osteoclast apoptosis (88). Bisphosphonates may affect the osteoclasts by other mechanisms. Some of the bisphosphonates bind to adenosine triphosphate to form a nonhy-

TABLE 123.2. MEDICINAL THERAPY FOR PAGET'S DISEASE OF BONE

Purpose of therapy
- Normalize the serum alkaline phosphatase and/or other markers of bone turnover in order to
  - control symptoms and
  - reduce risk of complications

Indications for therapy
- Control or reduce complications
  - Pagetic bone pain
  - Paraparesis/paraplegia from spinal Paget's disease
  - Nonunion fracture of pagetic bone[a]
  - Paget's disease of the skull such as headache or dizziness[b]
  - High-output cardiac failure
- Asymptomatic Paget's disease
  - Serum alkaline phosphatase or other bone turnover marker twice the limits of the upper limit of normal
  - Paget's disease in a high-risk location such as skull, spine, long bones, juxtaarticular
  - Preoperative orthopedic surgery to reduce operative hemorrhage; immobilization hypercalcemia[c]
  - Osteolytic Paget's disease[d]

Duration of therapy
- Normalize the serum alkaline phosphatase and/or other markers of bone turnover

  or
- Until maximum recommended duration of therapy

Therapy agent (preference of U.S. FDA-approved agents in descending order)
1. Nitrogen containing biphosphonate: e.g. (alphabetic order),
   - Alendronate
   - Pamidronate
   - Risedronate
   - Tiludronate
2. Other bisphosphonate
   - Etidronate
3. Calcitonin
   - Parenteral synthetic salmon calcitonin

Note: Do not treat for reversal of existing defects, such as hearing loss, osteoarthritis, deformity

Monitoring
- Every 3 months during and immediately following therapy until stable
- Every 6 to 12 months to monitor for exacerbation
- Retreatment indications are the same as for initial treatment indications

[a]Etidronate.
[b]Not symptoms of platybasia.
[c]Parenteral salmon calcitonin.
[d]Agents other than etidronate.

drolyzable complex that is cytotoxic (this includes the non–nitrogen-containing bisphosphonates), and others prevent protein prenylation in osteoclasts (this includes the nitrogen-containing bisphosphonates).

Only about 1% (range 0.6% to 3.0%) of orally ingested bisphosphonates are absorbed. Absorption is dose dependent and is decreased by intraluminal binding to calcium or food contents. Several of the bisphosphonates can cause an erosive esophagitis, particularly in patients with esophageal reflux. Esophagitis with etidronate is uncommon; it has been reported with alendronate, pamidronate, and tiludronate, and may be less common with risedronate. Following absorption, 50% of the bisphosphonates are excreted by the kidneys within 20 minutes. The plasma half-life is about 3 hours, and 20% to 50% of the absorbed bisphosphonates are bound to bone by 72 hours. The elimination half-life of bisphosphonates from recently formed crystals is 90 to 300 days.

At the recommended doses, all of the bisphosphonates have been shown to be effective in suppressing the clinical and laboratory manifestations of Paget's disease. All have demonstrated short- and long-term clinical and laboratory effectiveness. As above, there is greater potency of the nitrogen-containing bisphosphonates, particularly those containing a tertiary nitrogen.

The response to repeat therapy with disodium etidronate is variable, and there is often increasing resistance to repeated treatments. There is less information available on the other bisphosphonates, but it appears that reduced effectiveness with retreatment occurs with them all. However, most patients with Paget's disease will respond to a different bisphosphonate when resistance has developed to one of the bisphosphonates.

In general, the bisphosphonates should be administered as a single dose upon rising in the morning on an empty stomach with at least 8 ounces of water, followed by a fast for at least 30 minutes (perhaps up to 1 hour). The patient should stay in the upright position. In addition to esophagitis, there are only occasional skin rashes, transient increases in bone pain, and other uncommon and less certain adverse effects.

Disodium etidronate (Didronel) was the first of the bisphosphonates to be used in Paget's disease (89,90). The usual dose of etidronate for Paget's disease is 5 mg/kg per day or 400 mg daily for a 40-kg (88-lb) to 80-kg (176-lb) patient for 6 months. The drug is supplied in 200- and 400-mg tablets. The absence of esophagitis allows dosing midway between meals or at night before bed on an empty stomach. An unusual adverse effect, seemingly unique to etidronate, is asymptomatic hyperphosphatemia. Hyperphosphatemia appears to be due to a direct renal effect of disodium etidronate in humans and does not occur in other animals. Another unique adverse effect of etidronate among the presently used bisphosphonates is increasing bone pain due to unmineralized osteoid (osteomalacia-like). Although the fracture rate with etidronate may not be increased (91), etidronate should be discontinued if increasing bone pain occurs.

Clodronate is the second bisphosphonate to be used in Paget's disease and is available in many parts of the world (92,93). Hyperparathyroidism has been found in patients treated with clodronate and seems to be prevented by dietary supplements of vitamin D (94).

Pamidronate (APD, Aredia) is a potent inhibitor of bone resorption. It is 100 times more potent than disodium etidronate in its effect on osteoclasts, yet has little effect on calcium deposition at therapeutic doses (95,96). Unique adverse reactions to pamidronate include transient fever (usually less than 39.2°C), transient lymphopenia, mild and transient nausea, and uveitis (95). Pamidronate should be administered intravenously in 60- to 90-mg infusions with normal saline or dextrose/water. A variety of regimens have been used effectively, including a set of daily infusions for 3 to 5 days, once weekly for 3 to 5 weeks, once with reevaluation monthly, and so forth.

Alendronate (Fosamax) is a potent nitrogen-containing bisphosphonate. Benefit has been demonstrated in several clinical trials without evidence of abnormal mineralization on bone biopsy (97–99). Alendronate should be administered at a dose of 40 mg/day for 6 months. The author feels that alendronate can be administered for only 3 months if the alkaline phosphatase has normalized at that time.

Risedronate (Actonel) is a potent tertiary nitrogen-containing bisphosphonate with demonstrated efficacy as an oral agent in Paget's disease (100–103). Risedronate should be administered at a dose of 30 mg/day for 2 months. The potency of this agent is demonstrated by the short administration time.

Tiludronate (Skelid) is a nitrogen-containing bisphosphonate, effective in suppression of Paget's disease and with potential antiinflammatory properties (104–106).

Other bisphosphonates include ibandronate (2 mg intravenously), Olpadronate (dimethyl APD; oral dose 100 to 200 mg/day for 3.5 ± 2.4 months or given intravenously) (107), and zoledronate (effective in 7 to 10 days after a single infusion of 200 or 400 μg) (106,109).

Calcitonin had been the most commonly utilized therapy for Paget's disease for many years (110,111). It is now rarely used because of the effectiveness and safety of the newer bisphosphonates. During calcitonin therapy, there may be a reduction of symptoms by the end of the first month of therapy, sometimes occurring dramatically in the first few weeks, sometimes reversing Paget's disease-induced paraparesis or paraplegia (112,113). Salmon calcitonin has homology to calcitonin gene-related peptide, providing an analgesia that is independent of its effects on bone turnover. Nasal calcitonin can be used successfully in some patients, but is inconsistently of benefit when the patient has been exposed to other forms of therapy for Paget's disease (114). Parenteral synthetic salmon calcitonin (Calcimar, Miacalcin) should be administered as 100 Medical Research Council (MRC) or International Units (IU) or 0.5 mL subcutaneously or intramuscularly daily for the first month. The dose can be decreased or the interval between doses increased depending on the severity of disease and response to therapy. Salmon calcitonin should be refrigerated. It is supplied as 400 units per 2-mL vial. Synthetic human calcitonin is no longer readily available. When used, salmon calcitonin (Miacalcin) by nasal spray should be used as 400 units in each nostril once daily, alternating sides of the nose.

Adverse reactions to calcitonin are most common during the initial period of therapy and include gastrointestinal (nausea, vomiting, abdominal pain, cramps, diarrhea); vascular symptoms (flushing of face, tingling of hands and feet); local reactions at the injection sites (pain, erythema, pruritis); and other reactions, such as urinary frequency, rash, unpleasant metallic taste, rhinorrhea, and occasional angioedema.

Plicamycin (Mithramycin) was the first effective therapeutic agent used in Paget's disease. Because of its potential adverse reactions, plicamycin has been relegated to a backup role in the treatment of Paget's disease (115).

Oral or intravenous gallium nitrate has demonstrated a modest effect in Paget's disease (116). The major adverse event was mild anemia with retreatment.

CONCLUSION

Paget's disease of bone involves a change in the structure of isolated areas of the skeleton. Histologically, Paget's disease demonstrates rapid bone turnover with activated, large, distorted osteoclasts and excessively active osteoblasts leading to a disorganized, heavily calcified, fibrotic, enlarged, and softened bone. There is as yet no uniform opinion that Paget's disease is triggered by or originates from a virus (although some evidence favors this view), and there is increasing evidence of a genetic predisposition to the disease. The prevalence of Paget's disease in the United States is estimated to be around 1% of the adult population. There appears to be more men than women with Paget's disease, and there is an increasing prevalence with age.

Paget's disease uncommonly causes symptoms, and those with Paget's disease are not generally very ill, though somewhat impaired. When present, symptoms include bone pain, osteoarthritis, hearing loss, skull symptoms, hypercalcemia, or, rarely, sarcoma of pagetic bone. The best laboratory test for detection and follow-up patients with Paget's disease is the total serum alkaline phosphatase test. Other measures of bone turnover are also elevated. Radiographs are characteristic, and findings are rarely confused with other diseases. The bone scan helps determine the extent of bony involvement and often localizes active areas before a radiograph. Bone biopsy is only needed if malignancy is suspected.

Therapy includes physical (e.g., heel lift) and orthopedic measures (e.g., hip or knee prosthesis). New and safe medications reduce the activity of disease and probably alter the course of disease. Several bisphosphonates are available and should be used in the presence of active disease.

REFERENCES

1. Paget J. On a form of chronic inflammation of bones (osteitis deformans). *Med Chir Trans* 1877;60:37–63.
2. Aaron JE, Rogers J, Kanis JA. Paleohistology of Paget's disease in two medieval skeletons. *Am J Phys Anthropol* 1992;89:325–331.
3. Denninger HS. Paleopathological evidence of Paget's disease. *Ann Med Hist* 1933;5:73–81.
4. Hutchinson J. On osteitis deformans. *Illus Med News* 1889;2:169.
5. Altman RD, Bloch DA, Hochberg MC, et al. Prevalence of pelvic Paget's disease in the United States. *J Bone Miner Res* 2000;15:461–465.
6. Cooper C, Schafheutle K, Dennison E, et al. The epidemiology of Paget's disease in Britain: is the prevalence decreasing? *J Bone Miner Res* 1999;14:192–197.
7. Detheridge FM, Guyer PB, Barker DJP. European distribution of Paget's disease of bone. *Br Med J* 1982;285:1005–1008.
8. Barker DJP, Chamberlain AT, Guyer PB, et al. Paget's disease of bone: the Lancashire focus. *Br Med J* 1980;4:1105–1107.
9. Guyer PB, Chamberlain AT. Paget's disease of bone in two American cities. *Br Med J* 1980;281:985.
10. Rosenbaum HD, Hanson DJ. Geographic variation in the prevalence of Paget's disease of bone. *Radiology* 1969;92:959–963.
11. Cundy T, McAnulty K, Wattie D, et al. Evidence for secular change in Paget's disease. *Bone* 1997;20:69–71.
12. Siris ES, Ottman R, Flaster E, et al. Familial aggregation of Paget's disease of bone. *J Bone Miner Res* 1991;6:495–500.
13. Gold DT, Boisture J, Shipp KM, et al. Paget's disease of bone and quality of life. *J Bone Miner Res* 1996;11:1897–1904.
14. Barker DJP. The epidemiology of Paget's disease of bone. *Br Med Bull* 1984;40(4):396–400.
15. Van Hul H. Paget's disease from a genetic perspective. *Bone* 1999;24(suppl):29S–30S.
16. Fotino M, Haymovits A, Falk CT. Evidence for linkage between HLA and Paget's disease. *Transplant Proc* 1977;9:1867–1868.
17. Tilyard MW, Gardner RJM, Milligan L, et al. A probable linkage between familial Paget's disease and the HLA loci. *Aust NZ J Med* 1982;12:498–500.
18. Cody JD, Singer FR, Roodman GD, et al. Genetic linkage of Paget's disease of the bone to chromosome 18q. *Am J Hum Genet* 1997;61:1117–1122.
19. Haslam SJ, Van Hul W, Morales-Piga A, et al. Paget's disease of bone: evidence for a susceptibility locus on chromosome 18 and for genetic heterogeneity. *J Bone Miner Res* 1998;13:911–917.
20. Rebel A, Malkani K, Basle M, et al. Particularites ultrastructuales des osteoclastes de la maladie de Paget. *Rev Rhum* 1974; 41:767–771.
21. Reddy SV, Singer FR, Mallette L, et al. Detection of measles virus nucleocapsid transcripts in circulating blood cells from patients with Paget's disease. *J Bone Min Res* 1996;11:1602–1607.
22. Mee AP, Dixon JA, Hoyland JA, et al. Detection of canine distemper virus in 100% of Paget's disease samples by in situ-reverse transcriptase-polymerase chain reaction. *Bone* 1998; 23:171–175.
23. Hoyland JA, Freemont AJ, Sharpe PT. Interleukin-6, IL-6 receptor and IL-6 nuclear factor gene expression in Paget's disease. *J Bone Miner Res* 1994;9:75–80.
24. Hoyland JA, Sharpe PT. Up-regulation of cFos proto-oncogene expression in pagetic osteoclasts. *J Bone Miner Res* 1994;9: 1191–1194.
25. Ralston SH, Helfrich MH. Are paramyxoviruses involved in Paget's disease? A negative view. *Bone* 1999;5(suppl):17S–18S.
26. Rima BK. Paramyxoviruses and chronic human disease. *Bone* 1999;5(suppl):23S–26S.
27. Meunier PJ, Coindre JM, Edouard CM, et al. Bone histomorphometry in Paget's disease. *Arthritis Rheum* 1980;23:1095–1103.
28. Ralston SH, Hoey SA, Gallacher SJ, et al. Cytokine and growth factor expression in Paget's disease: analysis by reverse-transcription/polymerase chain reaction. *Br J Rheumatol* 1994;33:620–625.
29. Mills BG, Singer FR. Nuclear inclusions in Paget's disease of bone. *Science* 1976;194:201–202.
30. Krane SM. Skeletal metabolism in Paget's disease of bone. *Arthritis Rheum* 1980;23:1087–1094.
31. Barry HC. *Paget's disease of bone.* London: E&S Livingstone, 1969:82.
32. Bhardwaj OP. Monostotic Paget's disease of bone. *J Indian Med Assoc* 1964;43:341.
33. Lichniak JE. The heel in systemic disease. *Clin Podiatr Med Surg* 1990;7:225–241.
34. Hamdy RC, Moore S, LeRoy J. Clinical presentation of Paget's disease of the bone in older patients. *South Med J* 1993;86: 1097–1100.
35. Altman RD, Gray RG. Scalp vein sign in Paget's disease of bone. *J Rheumatol* 1982;9:624–626.
36. Gainey JC, Kadaba MP, Wootten ME, et al. Gait analysis of patients who have Paget disease. *J Bone Joint Surg* 1989;71A(4): 568–579.
37. Altman RD, Collins B. Musculoskeletal manifestations of Paget's disease of bone. *Arthritis Rheum* 1980;23:1121–1127.
38. Altman RD, Ciliberti E. Orthopedic events in Paget's disease of bone. [Unpublished report].
39. Helliwell PS. Osteoarthritis and Paget's disease. *Br J Rheumatol* 1995;34:1061–1063.
40. Altman RD, Brown M, Gargano F. Low back pain in Paget's disease of bone. *Clin Orthop* 1987;217:152–161.
41. Weisz GM. Lumbar spinal canal stenosis in Paget's disease. *Spine* 1983;8:192–198.

42. Wootton R, Reeve J, Veall N. The clinical measurement of skeletal blood flow. *Clin Sci Mol Med* 1976;50:261–268.
43. Arnalich F, Plaza I, Sobrino JA, et al. Cardiac size and function in Paget's disease of bone. *Int J Cardiol* 1984;5:491–505.
44. Choquette D, Haraoui B, Altman RD, et al. Simultaneous multifocal sarcomatous degeneration in Paget's disease of bone. *Clin Orthop* 1983;179:308–311.
45. Reddick RL, Michelitch HJ, Levine AM, et al. Osteogenic sarcoma. *Cancer* 1980;45:64–71.
46. Jattiot F, Goupille P, Azias I, et al. Fourteen cases of sarcomatous degeneration in Paget's disease. *J Rheumatol* 1999;26:150–155.
47. Jacobs TP, Michelsen T, Polay JS, et al. Giant cell tumor in Paget's disease: familial and geographic clustering. *Cancer* 1979; 44:742.
48. Goldhammer Y, Braham J, Kosary IZ. Hydrocephalic dementia in Paget's disease of the skull: treatment by ventriculoatrial shunt. *Neurology* 1979;29:513–516.
49. Smith BJ, Eveson JW. Paget's disease of bone with particular reference to dentistry. *J Oral Pathol* 1981;10:233–247.
50. Sofaer JA. Dental extractions in Paget's disease of bone. *Int J Oral Surg* 1984;13:79–84.
51. Bone HG, Cody DD, Monsell EM. Application of quantitative CT to Paget's disease of bone. *Semin Arthritis Rheum* 1994;23: 244–247.
52. Clarkson JG, Altman RD. Angioid streaks. *Surv Ophthalmol* 1982;25:235–246.
53. Downey R, Siris ES, Antunes JL. "Crocodile tears" and Paget's disease: ca se report. *Neurosurgery* 1980;7(6):621–622.
54. Schmidek HH. Neurologic and neurosurgical sequelae of Paget's disease of bone. *Clin Orthop Rel Res* 1977;127:70–77.
55. Herzberg L, Bayliss E. Spinal-cord syndrome due to noncompressive Paget's disease of bone: a spinal-artery steal phenomenon reversible with calcitonin. *Lancet* 1980;2:13–15.
56. Avramides A, Leonidas J-R, Chen C-K, et al. Coexistence of Paget's disease and hyperparathyroidism. *NY State J Med* 1981; 81:660–662.
57. Lyles KW, Gold DT, Newton RA, et al. Peyronie's disease is associated with Paget's disease of bone. *J Bone Miner Res* 1997; 12:929–934.
58. Morales AA, Valdazo P, Corres J, et al. Coexistence of Paget's bone disease and diffuse idiopathic skeletal hyperostosis in males. *Clin Exp Rheumatol* 1993;11:361–365.
59. Delmas PD, Gineyts E, Bertholin A, et al. Immunoassay of pyridinoline crosslink excretion in normal adults and in Paget's disease. *J Bone Miner Res* 1993;8:643–648.
60. Alvarez L, Guanabens N, Peris P, et al. Discriminative value of biochemical markers of bone turnover in assessing the activity of Paget's disease. *J Bone Miner Res* 1995;10:458–465.
61. Alvarez L, Peris P, Pons F, et al. Relationship between biochemical markers of bone turnover and bone scintigraphic indices in assessment of Paget's disease activity. *Arthritis Rheum* 1997;40:461–468.
62. Russell RGG, Beard DJ, Cameron EC, et al. Biochemical markers of bone turnover in Paget's disease. *Metab Bone Dis Rel Res* 1981;4/5:255–262.
63. Renier J-C, Leroy E, Audran M. The initial site of bone lesions in Paget's disease: a review of two hundred cases. *Rev Rhum* (English edition) 1996;63:823–829.
64. Renier, J-C, Audrian M. Progression in length and width of pagetic lesions, and estimation of age at disease onset. *Rev Rhum* (English edition) 1997;64:35–42.
65. Buchoff HS, Altman RD. Paget's disease: correlation of pain, x-rays and bone scans. *Arthritis Rheum* 1981;24(suppl):572.
66. Olmstead WW. Some skeletogenic lesions with common calvarial manifestations. *Radiol Clin North Am* 1981;19:703–713.
67. Tjon-a-Tham RTO, Bloem JL, Falke THM, et al. Magnetic resonance imaging in Paget disease of the skull. *AJNR* 1985;6: 879–881.
68. Marshall TR, Ling JT. The brim sign: a new sign found in Paget's disease (osteitis deformans) of the pelvis. *Am J Roentgenol Rad Ther Nucl Med* 1963;90:1267–1270.
69. Chakravorty NK. Triradiate deformity of the pelvis in Paget's disease of bone. *Postgrad Med J* 1980;56:213–215.
70. Friedman AC, Orcutt J, Madewell JE. Paget's disease of the hand: radiographic spectrum. *AJR* 1982;138:691–693.
71. Price CHG, Goldie W. Paget's sarcoma of bone. *J Bone Joint Surg* 1967;51B:205.
72. Jaffe HL. Paget's disease of bone. *Arch Pathol* 1933;15:83.
73. Grundy M. Fractures of the femur in Paget's disease of bone, their etiology, and treatment. *J Bone Joint Surg* 1970;52B:252.
74. Vellenga CJLR, Pauwels EKJ, Bijvoet OLM, et al. Bone scintigraphy in Paget's disease treated with combined calcitonin and diphosphonate (EHDP). *Metab Bone Dis Rel Res* 1982;4:103–111.
75. Fogelman I, Carr D. A comparison of bone scanning and radiology in the assessment of patients with symptomatic Paget's disease. *Eur J Nucl Med* 1980;5:417–421.
76. Renier J-C, Audran M. Polyostotic Paget's disease. *Rev Rhum* (English edition) 1997;64:233–242.
77. Vellenga CJLR, Pauwels EKJ, Bijvoet OLM, et al. Untreated Paget disease of bone studied by scintigraphy. *Radiology* 1984; 153:799–805.
78. Ryan WG, Fordham EW, Ali A. Treated Paget's disease of bone mimicking metastatic cancer. *Clin Nucl Med* 1995;20:69–85.
79. Bahk YW, Park YH, Chung SK, et al. Bone pathologic correlation of multimodality imaging in Paget's disease. *J Nucl Med* 1995;36:1421–1426.
80. Waxman AD, McKee D, Siemsen JK, et al. Gallium scanning in Paget's disease of bone: effect of calcitonin. *AJR* 1980;134: 303–306.
81. Colarinha P, Fonseca AT, Salfado L, et al. Diagnosis of malignant change in Paget's disease by TI-201. *Clin Nucl Med* 1996; 21:299–301.
82. Eisman JA, Martin TJ. Osteolytic Paget's disease. *J Bone Joint Surg* 1986;68A(1):112–117.
83. Kaplan FS. Severe orthopaedic complications of Paget's disease. *Bone* 1999;24(suppl):43–46.
84. Baran DT, Jaffe BM, Avioli LV. Plasma prostaglandin E levels in Paget's disease: effect of indomethacin. *Calcif Tissue Int* 1979; 29:5–6.
85. Basle MF, Rebel A, Renier JC, et al. Bone tissue in Paget's disease treated with ethane-1, hydroxy-1,1 diphosphonate (EHDP) (structure, ultrastructure and immunocytology). *Clin Orthop Rel Res* 1984;184:281–288.
86. Van Beck E, Hoekstra M, van der Ruit M, et al. Structural requirements for bisphosphonate actions in vitro. *J Bone Miner Res* 1994;9:1875–1882.
87. Sato M, Grasser W, Endo N, et al. Bisphosphonate action. Alendronate localisation in rat bone and effects on osteoclast ultrastructure. *J Clin Invest* 1991;88:2095–2105.
88. Rogers MJ, Frith JC, Luckman SP, et al. Molecular mechanisms of action of bisphosphonates. *Bone* 1998;5(suppl):73–79.
89. Altman RD, Johnston CC, Khairi MRA, et al. Influence of disodium etidronate on clinical and laboratory manifestations of Paget's disease of bone (osteitis deformans). *N Engl J Med* 1973; 289:1379–1384.
90. Altman RD. Long-term follow-up therapy with intermittent etidronate disodium in Paget's disease of bone. *Am J Med* 1985; 79:583–590.
91. Johnston CC Jr, Altman RD, Canfield RE, et al. Review of fracture experience during treatment of Paget's disease of bone with etidronate disodium (EHDP). *Clin Orthop* 1983;172:186–194.

92. Arboleya LR, Sanchez J, Iglesias G, et al. Tratamiento de la enfermedad osea de Paget con clodronato en infusion intraveosa. *Rev Esp Reumatol* 1998;25:13–17.
93. Khan SA, McCloskey EV, Eyres KS, et al. Comparison of three intravenous regimens of clodronate in Paget's disease of bone. *J Bone Miner Res* 1996;11:178–182.
94. Delmas PD, Chapuy MC, Vignon E, et al. Long term effects of dichloromethylene diphosphonates in Paget's disease of bone. *J Clin Endocrinol Metab* 1982;54:837–844.
95. Mazieres B, Ahmed I, Moulinier L, et al. Pamidronate infusions for the treatment of Paget's disease of bone. *Rev Rhum* (English edition) 1996;63:36–43.
96. Cundy T. Wattie D, King AR. High-dose pamidronate in the management of resistant Paget's disease. *Calcif Tissue Int* 1996; 58:6–8.
97. Reid, Nicholson GC, Weinstein RS, et al. Biochemical and radiologic improvement in Paget's disease of bone treated with alendronate: a randomized placebo-controlled trial. *Am J Med* 1996;171:341–348.
98. Khan SA, Vasikaran S, McCloskey EV, et al. Alendronate in the treatment of Paget's disease of bone. *Bone* 1997;20:263–271.
99. Siris E, Weinstein RS, Altman R, et al. Comparative study of alendronate versus etidronate for the treatment of Paget's disease of bone. *J Clin Endocrinol Metab* 1996;81:961–967.
100. Siris, ES, Chines AA, Altman RD, et al. Risedronate in the treatment of Paget's disease of bone: an open label, multicenter trial. *J Bone Miner Res* 1998;13:1032–1038.
101. Hosking DJ, Eusebio RA, Chines AA. Paget's disease of bone: reduction of disease activity with oral risedronate. *Bone* 1998; 22:51–55.
102. Miller PD, Brown JP, Siris ES, et al., for the Paget's Risedronate/Etidronate Study Group. A randomized, double-blind comparison of risedronate and etidronate in the treatment of Paget's disease of bone. *Am J Med* 1999;106:513–520.
103. Brown JP, Hosking DJ, Ste-Marie L, et al. Risedronate, a highly effective, short-term oral treatment for Paget's disease: a dose response study. *Calcif Tissue Int* 1999;64:93–99.
104. Monkkonen J, Simila J, Rogers MJ. Effects of tiludronate and ibandronate on the secretion of proinflammatory cytokines and nitric oxide from macrophages in vitro. *Life Sci* 1998;62: PL95–102.
105. Fraser WD, Stamp TC, Creek RA, et al. A double-blind, multicentre, placebo-controlled study of tiludronate in Paget's disease of bone. *Postgrad Med J* 1997;73:496–502.
106. Dovogelaer JP, Malghem J, Stasse P, et al. Biological and radiological responses to oral etidronate and tiludronate in Paget's disease of bone. *Bone* 1997;20:259–261.
107. Gonzalez D, Pastrana M, Mautalen C. Treatment of Paget's disease with olpadronate. Its efficacy in partial responders to oral pamidronate. *Midicina (B Aires)* 1997;57(suppl 1):25–31.
108. Garnero P, Gineyts E, Schaffer AV, et al. Measurement of urinary excretion of nonisomerized and beta-isomerized forms of type I collagen breakdown products to monitor the effects of the bisphosphonate zoledronate in Paget's disease. *Arthritis Rheum* 1998;41:354–360.
109. Arden-Cordone M, Siris ES, Lyles KW, et al. Antiresorptive effect of a single infusion of microgram quantities of zoledronate in Paget's disease of bone. *Calcif Tissue Int* 1997;60:415–418.
110. MacIntyre I, Evans IMA, Hobitz HHG. Chemistry, physiology, and therapeutic applications of calcitonin. *Arthritis Rheum* 1980;23:1139–1147.
111. El Sammaa M, Linthicum F Jr, House HP, et al. Calcitonin as treatment for hearing loss in Paget's disease. *Am J Otol* 1986; 7(4):241–243.
112. Melick RA, Eberling P, Hjhorth RJ. Improvement in paraplegia in vertebral Paget's disease treated with calcitonin. *Br Med J* 1976;1(6010):627–628.
113. Walpin LA, Singer FR. Paget's disease: reversal of severe paraparesis using calcitonin. *Spine* 1979;4(3):213–219.
114. Reginster JY, Jeugmans-Huynen AM, Wouters M, et al. The effect of nasal hCT on bone turnover in Paget's disease of bone-implications for the treatment of other metabolic bone diseases. *Br J Rheumatol* 1992;31:35–39.
115. Ryan WG, Fordham EW. Mithramycin and Paget's disease revisited. *Ann Intern Med* 1984;100:771.
116. Bockman RS, Bosco B. Treatment of patients with advanced Paget's disease of bone with two cycles of gallium nitrate. *Semin Arthritis Rheum* 1994;23:268–269.

124

RHEUMATIC ASPECTS OF ENDOCRINOPATHIES

MARY E. CRONIN

Hormonal excess or deprivation can lead to a variety of syndromes with musculoskeletal manifestations. Awareness of their features can suggest the appropriate diagnosis. Their recognition is important because they are often treatable. Such states of altered hormonal balance, including pregnancy, have shed light on the pathogenesis of some rheumatic disorders and promise new insights into their treatment. These relationships are described in this chapter. The role of the neuroendocrine system in immunity is a relatively new area of research, but it is now well recognized that the neuroendocrine system has both direct and indirect regulatory functions affecting the immune system. The study of the clinical implications of these systems to rheumatic diseases is still in an early stage but merits close attention. An excellent review of this area can be found in Chapter 40.

ACROMEGALY

Pituitary adenomas may produce excessive quantities of growth hormone, resulting in acromegaly. The resulting anabolic and bone metabolism effects can lead to significant changes in connective tissues. In older persons, in whom epiphyseal closure has already taken place, acromegaly occurs, whereas the result is *gigantism* if the adenoma occurs before puberty. Acromegaly, a rare disease with a prevalence of 50 to 70 cases per million, is generally diagnosed 10 to 15 years after the presumed onset of hormone hypersecretion (1). Although many anabolic influences derive from the direct action of this hormone, stimulation of chondroitin sulfate and collagen synthesis by articular chondrocytes is due to insulin-like growth factors induced by growth hormone (2–4). Insulin-like growth factor I (IGF-I), also known as somatomedin C, and IGF-II (somatomedin A) are synthesized predominantly in the liver, and also in chondrocytes, kidney, muscle, pituitary, and the gastrointestinal tract. IGF-I in particular is a potent stimulus of cellular proliferation and is further discussed in Chapter 20 (2–4).

Growth hormone and IGF-I act synergistically to stimulate the proliferation of soft tissues including bursae, joint capsules, synovium, cartilage (Fig. 124.1), and bone. Soft tissue changes include coarse, thickened digits; bursal thickening caused by noninflammatory fibrous hyperplasia, particularly of the prepatellar, olecranon, and subacromial bursae; and joint capsular hypertrophy and laxity permitting hypermobility. Synovial thickening, villous and usually noninflammatory, is explained by increased adipose and fibrous tissue rather than by synoviocyte hyperplasia. An abnormally thickened heel pad can be found in 35% of acromegalic patients.

Most endochondral tissues in adults are not so susceptible to growth hormone as they are in the prepubertal state. Some cartilage remains responsive, such as the

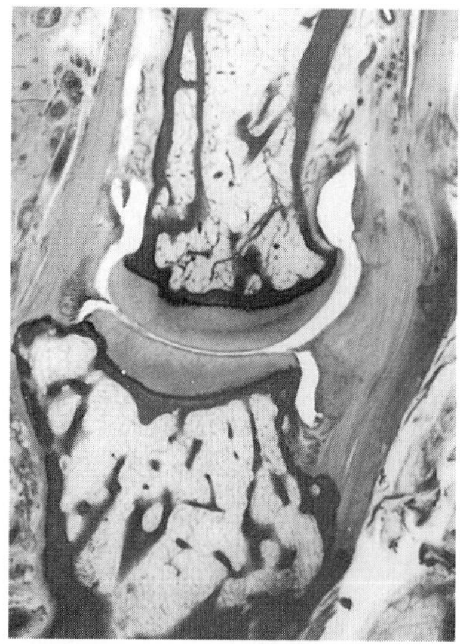

FIGURE 124.1. Midsagittal section through the distal toe of a 50-year-old acromegalic man; irregular hypertrophy and hyperplasia of the cartilage, and bony overgrowth at the joint margins with sparse, thickened trabeculae has occurred. (Courtesy of Dr. R.T. McCluskey, Department of Pathology, Massachusetts General Hospital, Boston.)

mandibular condyle, so that the jaw may actually lengthen, and the costochondral junctions, resulting in fusiform enlargement associated with a beading pattern and rib lengthening. This process results in an increased anteroposterior diameter of the chest. Cartilaginous overgrowth may also occur in the larynx, interfering with speech and, rarely, with respiratory function. Bony thickening results in a thickened calvarium, enlarged mandible, and *hyperostosis frontalis interna.* Another characteristic finding is widening of the distal ungual tufts, seen in 67% of patients (4). This can lead to an appearance of the hands similar to that of clubbing. The sesamoid bones are enlarged in approximately half these patients, and even the stapedial footplate of the ear may be affected, causing auditory symptoms.

The rheumatologic manifestations of acromegaly listed in Table 124.1 are found frequently if sought by careful medical history, physical examination, and laboratory testing. They are a major cause of morbidity and disability. Their presence correlates more with the duration of disease than with absolute levels of growth hormone. Rheumatic complaints, however, may arise early in the disease and can be the presenting manifestation. With the exception of soft tissue thickening, carpal tunnel symptoms, and paresthesias, many of these rheumatologic consequences of prolonged exposure to growth hormone may not remit with ablative pituitary therapy, but earlier recognition and treatment of this endocrine disorder may change this pessimistic view (1,4–6). Newer studies evaluating patients after longer periods of treatment suggest that cartilage overgrowth can be partially reversed (7).

TABLE 124.1. RHEUMATIC MANIFESTATIONS OF ACROMEGALY

- Tissue overgrowth
  - Bursal hyperplasia
  - Capsular thickening
  - Synovial proliferation and edema
  - Cartilage hyperplasia
  - Bony proliferation
- Arthropathy
  - Hypermobility of joints
  - Cartilage degeneration
  - Bony remodeling with osteophytosis and periosteal reaction
  - Intermittent (crystal-induced?) synovitis
- Muscle abnormalities
  - Increased muscle mass
  - Proximal weakness, fatigue, myalgias, cramps
- Neuropathy
  - Palpable peripheral nerves
  - Peripheral neuropathy
  - Carpal tunnel syndrome
- Others
  - Back pain and hypermobility
  - Kyphosis
  - Raynaud's phenomenon

Arthropathy

The usual manifestations of acromegalic arthropathy resemble those of osteoarthritis (OA), with cartilaginous thickening and hypermobility as important distinguishing features. Involvement of large and small peripheral joints may occur in as many as 75% of patients. The arthropathy consists of a noninflammatory proliferation of articular and periarticular structures, with osteophytosis and degenerative changes of the articular cartilage. The arthropathy has been divided into an early form consisting of hypermobility, recurrent effusions, and widened joint spaces, and an advanced form with bony hypertrophy, loss of motion, and deformities. Human necropsy studies and animal experimentation using exogenous growth hormone to produce polyarticular lesions have shed light on the pathogenesis of these changes (4,8). The cartilaginous matrix, although massively thickened in acromegaly, is laid down in a random manner, and degenerative changes arise in the middle and basal layers, leading to friability, fissuring, and ulceration. Joint hypermobility caused by capsular hypertrophy and redundancy accelerates this degenerative process. It is interesting that elderly patients with growth hormone deficiency have fewer radiographic changes of OA than do age- and sex-matched controls (9).

Such OA-like changes may be monoarticular or polyarticular, and can involve the knees, shoulders, hips, or hands; the elbows and ankles are involved less frequently. In some patients, intermittent episodes of joint pain last weeks or months. The exact mechanism responsible for these episodes and the possible role of calcium pyrophosphate dihydrate (CPPD) crystals remain to be determined (4). Less commonly, patients complain initially of joint pain and morning stiffness. This presentation, together with the elevated erythrocyte sedimentation rate seen in some patients, can cause confusion with rheumatoid arthritis (RA).

Physical examination often reveals many of the characteristics of OA, but the pronounced degree of joint crepitation, attributed to cartilaginous thickening and joint hypermobility, help to differentiate acromegalic arthropathy from primary OA. Palpable dorsal phalangeal ridging just distal to the proximal interphalangeal joints also may be useful diagnostically. Thickened synovium and periarticular tissues may have a swollen appearance, but effusions are relatively rare, and when present are noninflammatory, contain no crystals, and have low leukocyte counts, as in OA.

The radiographic features of acromegaly include widened cartilage spaces, enlarged bones with periosteal remodeling and increased density along the shaft, marginal osteophyte formation, and calcified tendinous and capsular insertions (4). The cartilage space can be quantitated easily by measuring the second metacarpophalangeal joint space on an anteroposterior radiogram. The normal space in men is less than 3 mm, and in women, is less than 2 mm. Approximately one third of acromegalic individuals have

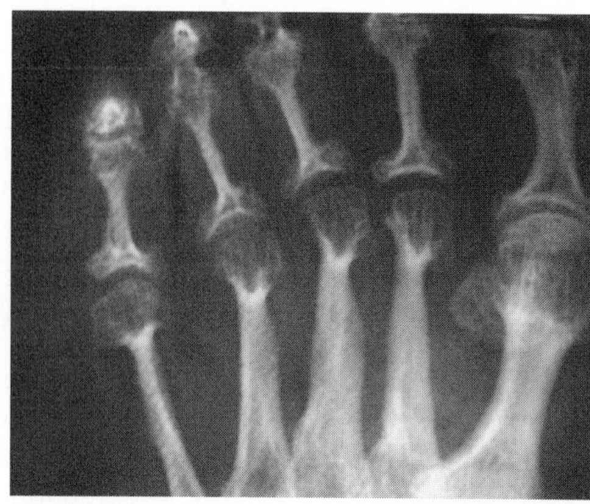

FIGURE 124.2. Radiograph of an acromegalic foot showing widened joint spaces, periosteal proliferation, dense diaphyses with pipe-stem configuration, and thickened and widely spaced trabeculae, giving a porotic appearance of the metatarsal heads.

increased joint spaces (5). Exostoses at the sites of ligamentous attachments produce a "squared-off" appearance at the bone ends. Although thickening of the trabeculae at the epiphyses occurs, their simultaneous widening may lead to an osteoporotic appearance while the diaphyses remain dense; this is especially common at the metacarpal and metatarsal heads (Fig. 124.2). The humeral and femoral heads may develop a mushroom configuration along with joint-space widening. Hypertrophic spurring with flaring of the femoral and tibial condyles may be found on knee films.

Troublesome symptoms can be treated with nonsteroidal antiinflammatory agents and other conservative measures, as in OA (see Chapter 112). Although intraarticular corticosteroids are reported to be ineffective, no controlled studies are available. Advanced degenerative changes may be treated surgically; preoperative corticosteroids may be required in a previously treated acromegalic patient with pituitary insufficiency.

McCune–Albright syndrome is a rare, nonheritable condition consisting of polyostotic fibrous dysplasia, *café au lait* spots, and endocrinopathies including acromegaly, hyperthyroidism, and hyperparathyroidism. The fibrous dysplasia occurs early in life with variable onset of the endocrinopathies, so patients can have either gigantism or acromegaly (4).

Myopathy

In up to 50% of acromegalic patients with long-standing disease, a proximal myopathy may develop. Growth hormone preferentially increases proximal muscle mass in experimental animals, but the muscle is functionally inefficient. Muscle biopsies from patients with acromegaly have shown both hypertrophic and atrophic changes occurring separately or concurrently. Type I fiber hypertrophy and type IIa and type IIb muscle fiber atrophy predominate. The atrophy is not that of disuse, which affects type I fibers primarily. Disease duration, but not growth hormone levels, correlated with biopsy findings (10). Ultrastructurally, glycogen and lipofuscin deposits, coiled membranous bodies (probably phospholipid), and pleomorphic mitochondria with abnormal cristae and vacuolization have been found, consistent with the known influence of growth hormone on glycogen uptake in skeletal muscle and its stimulation of ribonucleic acid (RNA) turnover. A causal relation between the mitochondrial disruption and the decreased muscle strength noted clinically has not been established.

Proximal weakness and decreased exercise tolerance are the usual manifestations of myopathy, followed by myalgias, cramps, and muscle twitching. The muscles may feel flabby, with weakness out of proportion to muscle mass. The serum creatine kinase (CK) and aldolase levels, although usually normal, may be increased as a reflection of patchy necrosis. The electromyogram (EMG) is abnormal in most untreated acromegalic patients with myopathy, even those without demonstrable weakness, but the findings of low-amplitude, short-duration, and polyphasic potentials are nonspecific myopathic findings (11). In treated patients, the EMGs and CK levels are usually normal, although muscle biopsies might still show myopathic changes (12). Return of normal strength after pituitary ablative therapy is gradual and may be incomplete even after 2 years (11).

Neuropathy

As noted in Table 124.1, several forms of neuropathy are associated with acromegaly. These neuropathies do not correlate with increased growth hormone levels, may be independent of carpal tunnel syndrome, and may occur without concomitant diabetes mellitus. Their pathogenesis is varied and consists of the following: (a) possible metabolic effects on the neuron directly or indirectly related to growth hormone; (b) compression of the spinal cord secondary to bony (foramen magnum, vertebral body) and paraspinal connective tissue overgrowth; and (c) ischemic neuropathy secondary to proliferation of endoneural and perineural tissues. Vague paresthesias involving several peripheral nerves may be the earliest symptoms, and these resolve after treatment. Five of 11 acromegalic patients had palpable enlargement of the ulnar or popliteal nerves with paresthesias, decreased or absent deep tendon reflexes, distal wasting, and even footdrop (13). Decreased vibratory and position sense also has been described. Microscopic studies of peripheral nerves revealed a decrease in both myelinated and unmyelinated fibers, with segmental demyelination and remyelination, and occasional axonal degeneration. The supporting neural tissues were increased, with significant proliferation, particularly in the hypertrophic form (13).

In as many as 50% of patients with acromegaly, typical carpal tunnel syndrome, usually bilateral, develops (4).

Although encroachment on the carpal tunnel by enlarging bone and soft tissue is a major part of the pathogenesis of this disorder, local swelling and hypertrophy of the median nerve itself also may contribute. Edema has been observed beneath the transverse carpal ligament at operation. The disappearance of this soft tissue swelling after pituitary therapy can account for the rapid improvement in symptoms after surgery, but the return to normal of nerve-conduction velocities is more prolonged.

Back Pain

Nearly half of acromegalic patients complain of back pain during the course of their disease. Although most symptoms are in the lumbosacral spine, cervical and thoracic involvement also may occur. Despite severe pain and sometimes advanced radiographic changes, patients may exhibit hypermobility of the spine. This striking finding may be a key in distinguishing between this and other spinal disorders and is presumably due to the enlarged intervertebral discs, which retain their resiliency and turgor (4,8). Such mobility may accelerate spinal degeneration and osteophyte formation. Radiographically, disc spaces are normal or increased, and occasionally calcified. Hypertrophic spurring develops at the anterior vertebral margin, mimicking diffuse idiopathic skeletal hyperostosis. Posteriorly, exaggeration of the normal concavity of the vertebral body is probably caused by remodeling or pressure from paraspinal tissues. Kyphosis is frequently observed, possibly resulting from the barrel-chest deformity secondary to rib elongation.

Raynaud's Phenomenon

Raynaud's phenomenon occurred in 14 of 25 acromegalic patients in one series. Although the exact mechanism is uncertain, thickening of the blood vessel walls may contribute to its development.

Gigantism

The accelerated endochondral ossification and lengthening of tubular bone that occurs in prepubertal patients with a pituitary adenoma is termed gigantism. The disorder is rare, and the true incidence of rheumatic manifestations is not known. The arthropathy, myopathy, and hypertrophic neuropathy noted in acromegaly also may occur in gigantism. The incidence of carpal tunnel syndrome may be less frequent. Bony and soft tissue growth occur in tandem, and thus the carpal tunnel may not be compromised.

GROWTH HORMONE DEFICIENCY

The rheumatic effects of growth hormone deficiency appear to be limited to reduced bone mineral content, although the majority of studies are restricted to children. There is recent interest in the study of adults with relative deficiencies of growth hormone. These studies have revealed less OA in adults with growth hormone deficiency (9). The study of the effects of growth hormone deficiency as well as the replacement of this hormone will likely reveal interesting new insights for rheumatologists.

HYPOTHYROIDISM

In primary hypothyroidism, hyaluronic acid and other mucoproteins deposit in many organs and tissues. Many of the numerous rheumatic syndromes associated with this disorder are probably secondary to such deposits in connective tissues and basement membranes (Table 124.2). The stimulus for the synthesis of the excess hyaluronic acid may be thyroid-stimulating hormone (TSH) (14). If this hypothesis is correct, it would account for the apparent paucity of musculoskeletal syndromes in secondary

TABLE 124.2. RHEUMATIC MANIFESTATIONS OF THYROID DISORDERS

- Hypothyroidism
  - Peripheral neuropathy: carpal tunnel syndrome
  - Arthropathy: noninflammatory viscous effusions, chondrocalcinosis (calcium pyrophosphate crystals), Charcot-like joint destruction, hyperuricemia and gout, flexor tenosynovitis, epiphyseal dysplasia, adhesive capsulitis, avascular necrosis
  - Myopathy: aches, pain, stiffness, cramping, weakness, myoedema, hypertrophy
- Hyperthyroidism
  - Thyroid acropachy: clubbing, periosteal proliferation, soft tissue swelling, pretibial myxedema, exophthalmos, LATS (long-acting thyroid stimulator)
  - Periarthritic osteoporosis
  - Myopathy: atrophy, exophthalmic ophthalmoplegia, myasthenia gravis, periodic paralysis
  - Adhesive capsulitis
- Autoimmune (Hashimoto's) thyroiditis
  - Fibrositis syndrome
  - Chest-wall pains
  - Association with connective tissue diseases

hypothyroidism, in which concentrations of TSH are low. Other possible reasons for the infrequency of rheumatologic problems in secondary hypothyroidism include its rarity and its association with other endocrine deficiencies, which might mask musculoskeletal symptoms.

Neuropathy

Neurologic features, although frequent in myxedema, are easily overlooked. Hypothyroid patients have few spontaneous complaints, and the neurologic examination is difficult to perform, owing to the patient's inability to cooperate. Several authors have emphasized the generalized nature of the *peripheral neuropathy* (15,16). Originally believed to be caused by nerve compression by mucinous deposits, it is now thought to be due to a neuronal metabolic dysfunction secondary to the hypothyroid state. Segmental demyelination of nerve fibers has been detected with a proliferation of Schwann cells, together with mucinous infiltration of the endoneurium and perineurium. The neuropathy is primarily sensory; slowed sensory conductive velocities have been found in the ulnar, median, and posterior tibial nerves. Abnormalities of conduction in the motor fibers have been found also, although the reported frequency is variable. All 25 patients with myxedema in one series complained of paresthesias, and 60% had diminished peripheral sensation. Sensory loss involved primarily pain and light touch; decreased vibratory sensation was less common. One of the best recognized neurologic complications of hypothyroidism is *carpal tunnel syndrome.* Approximately 10% of all patients with carpal tunnel syndrome have myxedema. Conversely, median nerve compression can be documented in from 5% to 80% of those with hypothyroidism. Symptoms of carpal tunnel syndrome can occur before clinical hypothyroidism is apparent. This association is important because treatment with thyroid replacement is followed by complete relief of the neuropathy, thus avoiding surgery.

In addition to the effects of hypothyroidism on peripheral nerves, the cerebral cortex, cerebellum, and cranial nerves also may be involved. In hypothyroid patients, the cerebrospinal fluid protein concentration averages 115% above normal, with γ-globulin levels more than 3 times normal (16). With rare exceptions, all neurologic manifestations of hypothyroidism disappear completely after treatment.

Arthropathy

The initial studies of Bland and Frymoyer (14), and the subsequent clinical pathologic study by Dorwart and Schumacher (17), have defined a joint disorder distinctive for myxedema. Characteristic features are listed in Table 124.2. Joint involvement usually develops concurrent with the onset of hypothyroidism, but occasionally antedates the development of clinical myxedema. Approximately one third of hypothyroid patients have symptomatic synovial effusions. Inflammation is neither common nor severe, and there is minimal pain, and tenderness and only slight warmth and erythema. The arthritis is usually bilateral, most often affecting the knees; the ankles, metacarpophalangeal joints, and small joints of the hands and feet are less frequently involved. Although the hip and the epiphysis of the femoral head are more commonly involved in children, cases have been reported in adults (18). Periarticular tissues appear thickened, and the increased intraarticular fluid is reflected in a sluggish "bulge" sign. This finding, caused by hyperviscosity, is secondary to an increased concentration of synovial fluid hyaluronic acid (17). The synovial fluid otherwise is generally noninflammatory, with a leukocyte count of less than 1,000/mm^3.

Radiographs are characteristically normal except for signs of effusions. Occasionally a hypothyroid patient will have an erosive arthropathy of the fingers that may be responsive to therapy with thyroxine (19,20).

Additionally, although Frymoyer and Bland (14) excluded patients with hyaline cartilage calcification from their series, they commented that radiographs in three cases showed destructive lesions of the tibial plateau and what appeared to be pathologic compression fractures. Because a Charcot-like destructive arthropathy has been associated with chondrocalcinosis (see Chapter 117), these three patients may have had associated CPPD crystal deposition. Dorwart and Schumacher (17) found chondrocalcinosis of the knee in seven of 12 myxedematous patients; nine patients had knee effusions, with CPPD crystals demonstrable in six. Conversely, an increased incidence of hypothyroidism (10.5%) was found in a study of 105 patients with chondrocalcinosis (21). Both intraleukocytic and extracellular calcium pyrophosphate and sodium urate crystals were noted, but without an associated inflammatory response. However, others have not demonstrated an association between the two (22–24).

The frequent failure of patients with myxedema to manifest intense inflammatory joint effusions in response to either sodium urate or calcium pyrophosphate crystals is of interest. Two findings may provide the explanation. First, neutrophil functions are reduced in hypothyroidism, an abnormality corrected after treatment with thyroxine (25). Second, the high intrinsic viscosity and elevated concentration of hyaluronic acid in synovial fluid impedes the chemotactic movement of leukocytes and diminishes the rate of crystal endocytosis (26). After treatment with thyroid hormone, several patients have developed typical crystal-induced inflammatory joint attacks, in contrast to the resolution of non–crystal-related joint pain and effusions.

Asymptomatic hyperuricemia often occurs in hypothyroid men, but not women (23). The increased incidence of clinical myxedema in patients with gout is small but significant (27). A prospective study evaluated the prevalence of hypothyroidism in 54 patients with crystal-proven gout as compared with age-, sex-, and weight-controlled patients. The women with gout were 2.5 times as likely to have an elevated TSH as compared with controls, whereas male patients with gout were 6 times as likely. A group of patients with gout identified retrospectively showed an even higher prevalence of hypothyroidism (28).

Wrist-flexor tenosynovitis associated with hypothyroidism was reported not to respond to thyroid therapy, but to subside promptly after injections of corticosteroid into the tendon sheaths (17). Although biopsies were not performed, hyaluronate deposition was believed to be responsible for the thickened, tender, and boggy palmar sheaths.

Ligamentous laxity occurs in approximately one third of patients with myxedema. The synovial effusions with edematous, lax joint capsules, ligaments, and tendons resemble the changes seen in an animal model of hypothyroidism thought to be due to increased concentrations of hyaluronate in the involved tissues. Myxedematous joint disease has been described only in primary hypothyroidism, in which levels of TSH are increased. This hormone may increase synovial synthesis of hyaluronate, which may result in the changes described.

Both the congenital and the acquired forms of hypothyroidism in children can delay epiphyseal closure and retard maturation and ossification. This phenomenon, most often seen in the femoral head, may cause slipped capital femoral epiphysis. Helpful diagnostic features in such children include hip pain, limping, and an elevated serum CK level (29).

Myopathy

Myopathic features may accompany many endocrinopathies, but numerically their occurrence in hypothyroidism is probably the most important. Besides the slow movement and delayed muscle contraction and relaxation classically seen in hypothyroidism, about half of these patients complain of *weakness* and *muscle cramps, aches* and *pains,* or *stiffness.* Muscle hypertrophy occurs in about 12% of patients. Pain and stiffness may be present during rest and are exacerbated on exposure to cold, thus resembling primary fibromyalgia. Such muscular symptoms may be the presenting complaints in many patients without overt clinical hypothyroidism. Like the neuropathy and arthropathy, myopathy can antedate the diagnosis of hypothyroidism by several months. The various muscle symptoms of hypothyroidism probably constitute a continuous spectrum, beginning with aches and pains and progressing to muscle cramping, proximal weakness, and even hypertrophy in association with severe, longstanding hypothyroidism. The myopathy can even precede laboratory evidence of hypothyroidism, so repeated thyroid testing in unexplained myopathies may be warranted (30). A case of rhabdomyolysis with hypothyroidism has been reported (31).

On physical examination, weakness usually is not severe. The proximal muscles are principally affected. Muscle contraction and relaxation are slowed, owing more often to muscle disease than to altered nerve conduction or to defective neuromuscular transmission. Direct percussion of the muscle with a reflex hammer leads to an interesting sign, termed the "mounding phenomenon" or *myoedema.* This transient focal ridging seen in response to striking or pinching the muscle persists for several seconds and also can be present in patients with hypoalbuminemia. Muscles are usually of normal bulk; atrophy is rare in hypothyroidism. Generalized hypertrophy of muscles, when observed in infants and children, is called the *Kocher–Debré–Sémélaigne* syndrome, and in adults, *Hoffman's syndrome.* This unusual finding, producing an athletic or "herculean" appearance, disappears with therapy. Percussion of hypertrophic muscles produces prolonged contractions resembling myotonia, although EMG studies have shown muscle responses to be electrically silent.

The activities of most "muscle" enzymes are increased in the serum of patients with hypothyroidism. CK has been best studied, and its concentrations correlate well with the severity of hypothyroidism. The exact contribution of the cardiac muscle isoenzyme to the serum CK level in hypothyroidism remains to be resolved. The CK level returns to normal within 2 months after restoration of the euthyroid state. In the few studies of patients with hypopituitarism and secondary hypothyroidism, myopathy was not a clinical feature, and serum CK levels were normal, suggesting a role for TSH in the pathogenesis of hypothyroid myopathy.

EMG changes are independent of muscle bulk. Approximately half the patients demonstrate increased needle insertional activity and hyperirritability. An equal number manifest polyphasic motor unit action potentials. Frequently, chains of repetitive discharges are observed after reflex motion. These changes are nonspecific indicators of myopathy and not pathognomonic of hypothyroid muscle disease.

Although biopsies may be normal, light microscopy reveals evidence of muscle degeneration in many patients, as well as areas of focal necrosis, regeneration, and basophilia with vacuolization of fibers. Fiber size varies, and the sarcolemmal nuclei are numerous, enlarged, and centrally positioned. Mucoprotein deposits, widespread in multiple organs in hypothyroidism, are found in the muscles of one third of patients. Histochemical staining has demonstrated a decrease in type II fibers proportional to the severity of the hypothyroidism. This lower percentage of type II fibers correlates with the severity of the disease and with the elevation of CK levels. With treatment, the ratios of the fiber types return to normal (32). The pathophysiology of myopathy in hypothyroidism is poorly understood. A study of the effects of L-thyroxine on muscle bioenergetics in humans and rodents using ^{31}P magnetic resonance spectroscopy suggests a hormone-dependent mitochondrial disorder that is reversible with therapy. Such changes were not present in patients or rodents with hyperthyroidism (33).

Although most cases of connective tissue disease have occurred in patients with autoimmune thyroiditis, a case of hypothyroidism secondary to panhypopituitarism with Raynaud's phenomenon has been reported; all symptoms resolved after thyroid hormone replacement (34).

Osteoporosis Associated with L-Thyroxine Treatment

Thyroid hormone activates osteoclasts and accelerates remodeling of bone. Excess hormone, whether endogenous or exogenous, causes more rapid resorption than does formation of bone, with resulting osteoporosis (35). A number of studies have measured bone mineral density in women with Grave's disease or in women receiving replacement therapy for hypothyroidism. Some revealed a loss of bone mineral density as great as 9% or more as compared with age-matched control patients without thyroid disease, whereas others have not confirmed this finding (36,37). Some studies have suggested that osteoporosis might be accelerated in patients with low serum concentrations of TSH, indicating overreplacement despite clinical euthyroidism; others have not found this correlation. The association between TSH levels and osteoporosis remains ill defined thus far, but the information available argues for replacement therapy with the lowest adequate dose possible of L-thyroxine in the hope of preventing accelerated rates of bone loss.

HYPERTHYROIDISM

Thyroid Acropachy

This extraordinary rheumatic manifestation of hyperthyroidism usually follows treatment for thyrotoxicosis (38). Thyroid acropachy, or thickening of small parts, occurs in approximately 1% of patients with past or present thyroid disease and usually develops approximately 1 year after either thyroidectomy or radioablation. The fingers and toes become *clubbed,* and patients develop *periostitis* of the digits and distal extremities with swelling of soft tissues. Usually these patients also have *exophthalmos* and *pretibial myxedema.* These features, in addition to the presence in the serum of long-acting thyroid stimulator (LATS), help to differentiate thyroid acropachy from other causes of hypertrophic osteoarthropathy. When this syndrome appears, patients are often clinically hypothyroid. Signs of inflammation are not prominent, although the syndrome is *painful,* especially on palpation over the periosteal new bone. Partial improvement, with incomplete resolution of pains in the extremities and digits and subsidence of the periosteal new bone proliferation, occurs in some patients after treatment with thyroid hormone or prednisone (see also Chapter 96).

Immune factors appear to participate in the pathogenesis of Graves' disease and possibly in its extrathyroidal manifestations, including acropachy (39). Patients with Graves' disease have circulating thyroid-stimulating immunoglobulins, considered to be antibodies to the TSH receptor on thyroid cell membranes. The presence of other thyroid autoantibodies suggests a close relation between Graves' disease and Hashimoto's thyroiditis. Evidence indicates an antigen-specific defect in suppressor T-cell function with genetic predisposition. Interferon-γ can induce the expression of major histocompatibility complex (MHC) class II antigens on the surface of thyrocytes. Thyrocytes could then function as antigen-presenting cells, thereby facilitating autoimmune responses to "self" or altered self antigens (39). Additional evidence linking these disorders includes the development of acropachy in both, their occurrence in the same families, and their histopathologic coexistence within the same thyroid gland. The significant excess of the histocompatibility antigens human leukocyte antigen (HLA)-B8 and HLA-DR3 in patients with Graves' disease is evidence of a genetic association. The precise role of organ-specific autoantibodies or sensitized leukocytes in the production of either of these thyroid disorders or of the acropachy remains unclear.

Another rheumatic association of uncertain pathogenesis is periarthritis of the shoulder, which is said to coexist with hyperthyroidism and to respond to restoration of the euthyroid state (40). Marked osteoporosis, with subsequent fractures, also is frequently seen in thyrotoxicosis and is due to bone resorption stimulated by thyroid hormone, possibly by osteoclast-activating factor, or interleukin-1β (IL-1β), with subsequent elevation of serum calcium and phosphorus levels. Both parathyroid hormone and 1,25 dihydroxyvitamin D_3 concentrations are decreased (35). Osteoporosis also is reversible when the thyroid disorder is treated.

Thyrotoxic Myopathy

Clinical evidence of weakness can be found in almost all thyrotoxic patients. The myopathy of thyrotoxicosis can be mild, characterized by weakness, fatigability, and minimal atrophy, or it can be extreme, characterized by proximal wasting and severe weakness, resembling polymyositis. Unlike polymyositis, acute inflammatory changes are not evident, and laryngeal and pharyngeal muscles are usually not involved. Atrophy and infiltration by fat cells and lymphocytes occur. "Muscle" enzymes are generally not increased in the serum, although creatinuria is present. EMG abnormalities include short-duration motor unit potentials and an increased percentage of polyphasic potentials. Full recovery of muscle strength occurs as patients become euthyroid. There is controversy over the possible beneficial effect of β-adrenergic blockade on thyrotoxic myopathy (41).

Three other forms of myopathy are less common. *Exophthalmic ophthalmoplegia* usually parallels the severity of exophthalmos. Associated findings include swelling of the eyelid and conjunctiva and sometimes of the optic nerve head. A second form is the coexistence of Graves' disease in 5% of patients with *myasthenia gravis.* The association of these disorders has a distinct female sex preponderance. Patients respond to neostigmine, but improvement is incomplete, owing to the thyrotoxicosis. *Thyrotoxic periodic paralysis* is the third of the rarer forms of skeletal muscle involvement in thyrotoxicosis. It is similar to the periodic paralysis of primary hypokalemia. This syndrome has the cardinal features of flaccid paralysis of the extremities, with absent reflexes and diminished electrical excitability. Precipitating factors are thought to be exercise, a high carbohydrate intake, and the administration of insulin or epinephrine. This disorder is rare in white persons and is more common in Asian male patients. Serum potassium concentrations are usually low, and the administration of potassium salts can prevent or abort attacks. Restoration of the euthyroid state leads to resolution of the paralytic attacks.

Autoimmune (Hashimoto's) Thyroiditis

Early in the course of autoimmune thyroiditis, as the thyroid gland gradually enlarges, most patients are euthyroid, and some are hyperthyroid. With progressive lymphocytic infiltration, fibrosis, and obliteration of thyroid follicles, hypothyroidism develops in nearly half of these patients. This common cause of diffuse goiter, with a female predilection, is frequently associated with musculoskeletal symptoms. The most common rheumatic syndrome resembles *fibromyalgia;* patients complain of stiffness of the joints and muscles, exacerbated by cold or dampness, and worse on arising in the morning or after any period of immobility. This syndrome resembles that seen in hypothyroidism and can be present in autoimmune thyroiditis even in the absence of thyroid deficiency. Another rheumatic symptom is unusual chest-wall pains of intermittent nature. Described in 12% of patients with Hashimoto's disease, these thoracic and shoulder-girdle pains, lasting for several minutes to hours, are relieved by changes of position or by mild exercises (42). Half of the patients with Hashimoto's disease have an *elevated erythrocyte sedimentation rate,* with or without rheumatic symptoms.

Most patients with Hashimoto's disease have high serum titers of thyroid antibodies, both to thyroglobulin and to microsomal antigens. Cellular immunity also may be important in the pathogenesis of the disease (39). Biologic false-positive tests for syphilis, rheumatoid factors, and antinuclear antibodies also are common. Hashimoto's disease coexists with other autoimmune disorders, especially pernicious anemia and hemolytic anemia, and possibly with RA, systemic lupus erythematosus (SLE), and Sjögren's syndrome. These disorders appear in family members of patients with autoimmune thyroiditis too frequently to be coincidental.

The frequency of thyroid disease in patients with rheumatic disorders also has been examined. Although patients with connective tissue diseases, notably SLE and RA, have a high incidence of antibodies to thyroid antigens, the majority are euthyroid and do not have detectable goiters. Prospective studies showed frequent thyroid-function test abnormalities, including elevated TSH, in patients with SLE or RA. The most common abnormalities were consistent with incipient or true hypothyroidism. Mild-to-moderate hypothyroidism may be missed because of the similarity of some of its symptoms with those of rheumatic disorders (43,44). Despite this and other uncontrolled series, the coexistence of either hyperthyroidism or hypothyroidism with RA, polymyositis, scleroderma, or SLE may be coincidental and deserves further investigation. Two other situations associated with thyroid disorders are known: (a) the administration of antithyroid drugs may be followed by syndromes resembling either RA or SLE, especially in women (45); and (b) falsely low values of serum thyroxine can be seen in patients treated either with salicylates or with corticosteroid hormones.

PARATHYROID DISORDERS

Hyperparathyroidism

A number of rheumatic findings are associated with parathyroid hormone excess (Table 124.3). A more detailed discussion of the osseous consequences of increased levels of

TABLE 124.3. RHEUMATIC MANIFESTATIONS OF PARATHYROID DISORDERS

Hyperparathyroidism
Asymptomatic hypercalcemia and osteoporosis
Osteitis fibrosa cystica
Subperiosteal resorption
Bony erosions
Joint laxity
Tendon avulsions/ruptures
Back abnormalities
Degenerative arthritis
Chondrocalcinosis and pseudogout
Charcot-like joints
Hyperuricemia and gout
Ectopic calcifications
Neuromyopathy
Hypoparathyroidism and pseudohypoparathyroidism
Subcutaneous calcifications; myopathy
Paraspinal ligament calcifications (spondylitis without sacroiliitis)

this hormone, including osteitis fibrosa cystica, may be found in Chapter 122.

Most patients are diagnosed with hyperparathyroidism before the development of osteitis fibrosa cystica because of findings of hypercalcemia by automated biochemical screening tests. Varying degrees of osteoporosis may improve after surgical removal of the adenoma. These patients, however, never achieve normal bone mineral density after their operations and might require further medical management of osteoporosis (46,47).

The resorptive effects of parathyroid hormone on bone may lead to the characteristic subperiosteal erosive radiographic appearance, particularly at the radial aspect of the middle phalanges, the medial aspect of the proximal femur or tibia, and the inferior aspect of the distal third of the clavicle. Erosions also may occur in juxtaarticular sites, especially at the interphalangeal, metacarpophalangeal, carpal, and acromioclavicular joints. These lesions can be found in the absence of subperiosteal resorption, may be symmetric, and may be associated with morning stiffness, thus mimicking RA. Several features distinguish parathyroid disorders: (a) the erosions may have a shaggy appearance; (b) they often occur at the distal interphalangeal joints and spare the proximal interphalangeal joints; (c) joint-space narrowing in association with these erosions is uncommon because parathyroid hormone does not directly induce inflammatory synovitis or cartilage dissolution; and (d) concurrent articular calcification is common.

Parathyroid hormone increases collagenase activity, which may account for the *laxity of capsular and ligamentous structures* seen in this disorder. Tendon ruptures and avulsions have been reported (48). Tendon rupture in patients with SLE also can be associated with hyperparathyroidism. These patients almost invariably have chronic renal failure and elevated levels of parathyroid hormone (49). *Vertebral subluxation* occurs, especially in the cervical spine; dorsal kyphosis is present, with anterior bowing of the sternum, and the lumbar spine is hypermobile. Additional changes include *sacroiliac erosions* and *intervertebral disc calcifications.* The laxity leads to joint trauma, which contributes to the back pain, disc protrusion, and degenerative joint changes seen in hyperparathyroidism.

Chondrocalcinosis has been reported in 18% to 25% of patients with hyperparathyroidism (49,50) (see also Chapter 117). CPPD crystal deposition may cause attacks of pseudogout, which can precede the recognition of parathyroid hormone excess and may thus be an initial manifestation of this disease. *Pseudogout* attacks may flare within 2 to 3 days of parathyroidectomy, or they may occur later, often coincident with the postoperative nadir of the serum calcium level (51). Once chondrocalcinosis is present, it usually persists in spite of parathyroidectomy, and the frequency of episodes of pseudogout continues unabated or even increases. Bywaters et al. (52) have described subchondral cyst formation with subsequent destructive joint changes in 15 of 19 patients with hyperparathyroidism. More than half of their patients had chondrocalcinosis. Because similar joint changes with severe destruction and the development of Charcot-like joints have been described in association with chondrocalcinosis *per se,* the relative contribution of CPPD crystals and parathyroid hormone to this type of arthropathy remains to be elucidated. The presence of severe OA should prompt a search for CPPD crystals, and if these are found, for the metabolic diseases associated with them, including hyperparathyroidism.

The persistently elevated serum calcium levels in primary hyperparathyroidism may result in nephrocalcinosis and a nephropathy characterized by an impaired tubular-concentrating mechanism. Some hyperparathyroid patients have a decreased uric acid clearance, which may explain the finding of hyperuricemia. The incidence of actual gouty attacks in hyperparathyroidism varies from 3% to 45% (27). Because hyperuricemia and gout do not seem to occur without underlying renal changes, they may persist after parathyroidectomy. Elevated levels of parathyroid hormone were found in about 70% of patients with CPPD crystal deposits and in age- and sex-matched control subjects with OA of the knee (22). Chemical hyperparathyroidism occurred in patients in both groups. Serum levels of parathyroid hormone correlated directly with serum calcium levels, female patients having the most severe OA, and with bone density. These findings have not been confirmed.

In secondary hyperparathyroidism, as well as in other disorders in which metastatic calcifications are found, deposits of amorphous and crystalline basic calcium phosphate salts may occur in periarticular or articular tissues. Their presence can induce a local inflammatory reaction with pain and swelling (see also Chapter 119). Treatment consists of prophylaxis with aluminum hydroxide gels and the use of antiinflammatory agents or intraarticular corticosteroids during acute episodes.

Fatigue, generalized weakness, and other neuromuscular complaints occur in the majority of patients with primary or secondary hyperparathyroidism. Weakness, usually in the *proximal muscles* and often only in the lower extremities, is now rare because of earlier detection of the disorder (53). Other neurologic findings include abnormalities of the cranial nerves, long-tract signs, and decreased vibratory sensation. Muscle enzyme levels are not elevated, and nerve-conduction velocities are reported to be normal despite other EMG findings, suggesting a neuropathic process. Muscle biopsy reveals neurogenic atrophy of both fiber types, with type II atrophy predominating. Parathyroidectomy usually rapidly reverses the symptoms. Other causes of neuromuscular symptoms in hyperparathyroid patients are a polymyositis-like myopathy and an ischemic myopathy caused by intravascular calcifications that occurs in the secondary hyperparathyroidism associated with uremia. Cutaneous and digital vasculopathy, secondary to the vascular calcifications, also have been described (54).

Hypoparathyroidism

In addition to the bony features of hypoparathyroidism, pseudohypoparathyroidism, and pseudopseudohypoparathyroidism, *subcutaneous* and *ectopic calcifications* may be seen. *Spondylitis without sacroiliitis,* with extensive paraspinal calcifications in hypoparathyroidism and pseudohypoparathyroidism, has been reported (55). Myopathy, in association with elevated serum levels of CK and normal muscle biopsy, also has been seen in hypoparathyroidism (56).

DIABETES MELLITUS

The musculoskeletal complications of diabetes mellitus, both articular and periarticular, are listed in Table 124.4. Some of these, such as destructive arthropathy, reflex sympathetic dystrophy, carpal tunnel syndrome, interosseous muscle wasting, and proximal weakness, may be primarily the result of neuropathic changes. Ischemic vascular disease also may contribute to their genesis. Complications that appear to be related to a proliferation of fibrous tissue include the increased incidence of capsulitis of the shoulder, Dupuytren's contractures, flexor tenosynovitis, and flexion contractures. The collagen from skin and tendon samples of young diabetics is stiff and stabilized, similar to samples from normal control subjects 50 to 65 years older. Improved glycemic control will not reverse the changes that have occurred but can slow progression (57). Possible reasons for excessive fibrosis and accelerated aging of collagen are discussed in Chapter 104.

The association between diabetes and hyperuricemia or gout remains controversial. Joslin et al. (58) reported only one case of gout in 1,500 diabetic patients, and studies of patients with hyperuricemia compared with age- and weight-matched controls showed no difference in results of glucose tolerance tests. Nonobese, type II diabetic patients have no greater incidence of gout than the normal population. Similarly, there is a consensus that there is no increase in the incidence of diabetes in gout (27). Less clearly defined is the putative association with ankylosing hyperostosis. Controlled studies have failed to support an association of diabetes mellitus with CPPD crystal deposition (59) (see Chapter 117).

Neuropathy

Diabetic neuropathy may take several forms: (a) a peripheral symmetric sensory or sensorimotor loss; (b) a mononeuropathy multiplex with an increased frequency of cranial nerve involvement; (c) a neuropathy resulting in proximal muscle weakness, termed diabetic amyotrophy; (d) a radiculopathy leading to lancinating pains in a dermatomal distribution; (e) an autonomic neuropathy; and (f) carpal tunnel syndrome. With *peripheral neuropathic* involvement, patients frequently have a stocking-glove distribution of sensory loss, with decreased vibratory and position sense and decreased or absent deep-tendon reflexes. Wasting of the interosseous muscles of the hands and feet may give a claw-hand or hammer-toe appearance.

Mononeuropathies most commonly affect the third and sixth cranial nerves, and occasionally the fourth and seventh as well. Mononeuropathy involving the motor supply of the proximal hip and leg muscles, and less often of the upper extremities, occurs more in men, often in those with only mild diabetes. This so-called *diabetic amyotrophy* is usually bilateral but asymmetric. Muscle biopsy shows a predominance of type I fibers, with type II atrophy and no evidence of significant necrosis or inflammation. Muscle enzyme levels are normal, and the EMG shows some fibrillation potentials. The weakness may spontaneously remit. Control

TABLE 124.4. RHEUMATIC MANIFESTATIONS OF DIABETES MELLITUS

- Neuropathy
  - Distal sensory and sensorimotor disorders
  - Mononeuropathy multiplex
  - Diabetic amyotrophy
  - Radiculopathy
  - Autonomic neuropathy
- Neuroarthropathy
  - Osteolysis
  - Osteoporosis
  - Charcot joint
  - Reflex sympathetic dystrophy
  - Coexistent osteomyelitis
  - Periarthritis of the shoulder (adhesive capsulitis)
- Other associations
  - Hyperuricemia and gout?
  - Ankylosing hyperostosis (DISH)
  - Flexion contractures (Dupuytren's contractures, limited joint mobility)
  - Tenosynovitis
  - Osteoporosis?

of hyperglycemia contributes to recovery. *Diabetic radiculopathy* may occur secondary to infarction of a nerve root, with resultant lancinating pains. These pains are sometimes confused with the symptoms of a herniated disc. When proprioceptive loss and ataxia accompany this shooting pain, it is called "diabetic pseudotabes."

Involvement of the *autonomic nervous system* results in orthostatic hypotension, impotence, dyshidrosis, and diarrhea. Autonomic dysfunction may be related to unilateral or bilateral reflex sympathetic dystrophy and to the apparently increased shoulder pain seen in diabetes. *Periarthritis (adhesive capsulitis) of the shoulder*, often bilateral, was found in 11% of a large group of diabetic patients (60). Conversely, in another study, approximately 25% of patients with periarthritis were diabetic (61). This entity occurs more commonly in women on the nondominant side of the body and produces aching with limitation of shoulder motion. Calcific bursitis and tendinitis may be present. The natural course of the disorder varies, but spontaneous remissions may occur. Physical therapy, antiinflammatory drugs, and local corticosteroid injections are helpful. Although 5% to 17% of patients with carpal tunnel syndrome have diabetes, systematic, controlled observations have not demonstrated a significant association (62).

Arthropathy

As a consequence of sensory neuropathy, severe arthropathy with Charcot-like changes develops in approximately 0.1% of long-standing diabetes (59,63). The tarsometatarsal and metatarsophalangeal joints are by far the most common sites of involvement, but changes may rarely affect joints above the ankle. A combination of microfragmentation from trauma, ischemia from small blood vessel disease, and superimposed infection can contribute to the clinical and radiographic changes of neuroarthropathy. Vasodilatation and increased blood flow due to autonomic neuropathy results in osteoporosis. This leads to an increase in bone fragility, predisposing to microfractures with little or no history of trauma (64). All patients with diabetic neuroarthropathy have peripheral neuropathy. In advanced disease, the longitudinal arch of the foot collapses, leading to an unstable gait and a "rocker-sole" appearance. Ulcerations and plantar callosities occur over hypoesthetic pressure points. Osteolysis of bone can develop, with periosteal reaction and remodeling, whittling of the metatarsal bones, cupping deformities, and telescoping of the phalanges (59,63). Fractures may be the initial lesion in a Charcot joint or may simply contribute to more extensive joint damage. In all involved joints, the discrepancy between pain, which is minimal or absent, and the destructive radiographic appearance, which is severe, is striking. Establishing the diagnosis of coexistent osteomyelitis in patients with Charcot joints can be difficult. Combined three-phase bone scanning and ^{111}In-labeled WBC scan can be helpful in this setting (65). The mainstay of therapy of Charcot arthropathy is rest of the involved area until the inflammatory phase resolves, attention to care of the feet including proper shoes, treatment of concomitant osteomyelitis, and amputation if required (see Chapter 91) (66).

OA is more common in patients with type II diabetes than in controls. In addition, it tends to be more severe with an earlier presentation. Obesity is more common in diabetic patients, however, and the contribution of diabetes, insulin, or IGF-I to OA is unknown. Horn et al. (67) compared type II diabetic patients with weight- and age-matched controls and found no difference in the severity of degenerative disease of the knee, but osteophytes were less common in the diabetic patients. They hypothesized that lack of insulin at the cellular level or diabetic microvascular disease contributes to the diminution of reactive bone formation. Likewise, ankylosing hyperostosis (DISH) has been reported as more prevalent in patients with diabetes, but a recent case–control study suggests that glucoregulation in patients with DISH is no different from that in patients matched for age, sex, and weight/height index (68).

A group of disorders of more obscure pathogenesis has in common excessive proliferation of fibroblastic tissue. Fibrous palmar nodules with subsequent Dupuytren's contractures have been reported in as many as 21% of diabetic patients; diabetes was found in 10% of those with Dupuytren's contractures (see Chapter 104) (69). Diabetes also has been described in 10% to 30% of all adult cases of trigger finger or flexor tenosynovitis (70). The syndrome of limited joint mobility (cheiroarthropathy) was first described in the hands of insulin-dependent, juvenile-onset diabetic patients. It is now recognized that the syndrome is not limited to insulin-dependent or juvenile-onset diabetics and can be seen in the shoulders, wrists, elbows, hips, knees, and feet, as well as the hands (59). The stiffness and limited mobility appear to be related to a thick, tight, waxy skin. Simple screening tests for limited joint mobility of the hands consist of asking the patient to appose the palmar aspects of the hands ("prayer sign") or place both hands on a table palm down with fingers fanned. The entire palmar surface of the fingers makes contact in normal persons. Originally, limited joint mobility was thought to correlate with the presence of retinopathy, nephropathy, or neuropathy, but more recent studies suggest that no relation exists (59). The clinical signs and the presence of microvascular disease are reminiscent of scleroderma, but nailfold capillaroscopy is normal (71). It has recently been proposed that the syndrome of limited joint mobility and trigger finger are interrelated manifestations of tenosynovitis. Corticosteroid injections of the tendon sheaths in 25 diabetic patients with trigger finger and 14 with limited joint mobility resulted in a 90% response rate at 1 month (72).

Insulin-resistant diabetes mellitus secondary to insulin receptor antibodies has been associated with multiple rheumatic complaints suggestive of SLE, Sjögren's syndrome, or progressive systemic sclerosis. Fourteen such patients developed features of an autoimmune disease; eight of the 14 met the American Rheumatism Association criteria for SLE, and in four, glomerulonephritis histologically consistent with lupus nephritis developed (73). Whenever a patient has extremely insulin-resistant diabetes mellitus and features of a systemic rheumatic disease, the possibility of circulating antibodies to insulin receptors should be considered.

Osteoporosis

Patients with type I, or insulin-dependent, diabetes mellitus are reported to have osteoporosis. This is frequently true in patients with poor control of their disease (74). Osteoporosis in non–insulin-dependent diabetes is controversial. There are reports of low bone mineral density and increased bone mineral density, as well as normal bone mineral density (75–77). A large, well-controlled prospective study of patients with type II diabetes mellitus concluded that both men and women with non–insulin-dependent diabetes have increased bone mineral density as measured by dual-energy x-ray absorptiometry of the lumbar spine and proximal femur. This result correlated with fewer reported fractures in women. These findings could not be explained by age, obesity, smoking, use of medications such as estrogens or thiazide diuretics, or OA. The increase in bone density may be the result of hyperinsulinemia (78).

CORTICOSTEROID EXCESS AND DEFICIENCY

Corticosteroid excess due to adrenal hyperproduction or secondary to exogenous administration can profoundly affect the musculoskeletal system. Generalized osteoporosis and pathologic fractures are consequences in bone. Osteonecrosis is observed with exogenous corticosteroid excess, but rarely in Cushing's disease. Changes in the vertebral column can cause severe pain, kyphosis, and loss of height. In children, growth is retarded, and, if not corrected, results in permanently short stature. A polyarthropathy associated with Cushing's disease has been reported in a single patient (79). A noninflammatory proximal myopathy may progress from the pelvic to the shoulder girdle and, ultimately, to the distal musculature. Serum muscle enzyme levels are usually normal in states of corticosteroid excess, but urinary creatine excretion is increased (80). After correction of hypercortisolism, creatinuria subsides. This dissociation between serum and urine laboratory tests may help to differentiate corticosteroid-related versus inflammatory myopathies. The EMG in corticosteroid myopathy has yielded confusing results and is not helpful diagnostically. Muscle biopsy reveals type II atrophy without inflammatory change. Although some recovery of muscle strength occurs within days after reduction of corticosteroid dose, complete resolution usually takes 1 to 4 months.

Adrenal insufficiency after corticosteroid discontinuation may be associated with constitutional symptoms of weakness, fatigue and lassitude, and arthralgias. Addison's disease is generally associated with weakness, but flexion contractures caused by progressive stiffening of the pelvic girdle and thigh muscles can occur. This painful condition, also seen in patients with hypopituitarism, responds to therapy with corticosteroids but not mineralocorticoids (81). A number of articles have reported an association between Addison's disease and antiphospholipid antibodies as well as the development of hypoadrenalism secondary to thrombosis, hemorrhage, or both in patients with primary antiphospholipid antibody syndrome. The possibility of a clotting disorder related to these antibodies should not be overlooked in patients with acute adrenal insufficiency (82).

CARCINOID ARTHROPATHY

Distinctive rheumatologic findings occur in at least 10% of carcinoid patients. Arthralgias of the wrists and hands, constant stiffness and pain on movement, and marked intensification of pain after a sustained grip are characteristic complaints. Because the arthralgias can be rapidly reversed with parachlorophenylalanine, which blocks serotonin synthesis, serotonin is believed to be responsible for these symptoms. Bradykinin and histamine also may be involved. One may detect juxtaarticular demineralization and erosions of the metacarpophalangeal joints and of the proximal and distal interphalangeal joints, with subchondral cystic changes (83).

ECTOPIC HORMONAL SYNDROMES

Tumor cells can synthesize polypeptide hormones, such as adrenocorticotropic hormone, growth hormone, TSH, and parathyroid hormone, with structural and functional characteristics similar or identical to those of normal hormones (84). Because the bony, myopathic, and neuropathic changes associated with endocrinopathies require prolonged hormonal exposure, these syndromes are not seen with ectopic hormone production by malignant tissues. Several cases of *hypertrophic pulmonary osteoarthropathy* have been reported in patients with *acromegalic* physical features and increases in growth hormone or similar substances that resolved when the tumor was removed, suggesting a possible relation (85). The periosteal proliferation seen in this osteoarthropathy may resemble the periosteal remodeling of acromegaly, but further clarification is needed to determine whether any hormonal substance mediates this syndrome.

PREGNANCY

The symptoms of RA frequently remit during pregnancy. Because of Hench's description in 1938 of the beneficial action of pregnancy in RA, improvement has been reported in numerous other rheumatic disorders as well (Table 124.5). Many of these reports have dealt with a few patients or even a single patient, however, and, with rare exception, the observations have been retrospective and anecdotal.

The most complete data have been accumulated regarding the course of RA during gestation and in the postpartum period. Improvement of disease was not noted in all pregnancies. Only 74% had some degree of subsidence of arthritis activity during gestation. Fifty percent of patients with RA had some degree of improvement of disease activity during the first trimester of pregnancy. Thereafter, an additional 24% experienced relief of symptoms throughout the second and third trimesters, some even waiting until the last month of gestation for improvement. In 23% of published cases, patients failed to note an amelioration of arthritis (86). Some even experienced worsening of symptoms; still others experienced the onset of their disease during pregnancy. There are no factors to predict a patient's response to pregnancy, including presence or absence of rheumatoid factor, disease duration, or functional class, but whatever response the patient had with her first pregnancy is predictive for subsequent ones. A recent prospective nationwide study in the United Kingdom confirmed these previous observations. Approximately two thirds reported improvement. Only 27 of 140 women had clinical remission. Four of these patients continued to receive some therapy. Thirty-seven of the 140 had significant disability during pregnancy, although only 16% had more swelling, and 19%, more pain (87).

TABLE 124.5. DISORDERS REPORTED TO BE AMELIORATED BY PREGNANCY

Rheumatoid arthritis
Psoriatic arthropathy (and psoriasis)
Fibrositis
Intermittent hydrarthrosis
Erythema nodosum
Sarcoidosis
Raynaud's phenomenon
Gout (possibly)
Cutaneous anaphylaxis
Angioneurotic edema
Experimental animal diseases
Experimental vasculitis (dogs)
Adjuvant arthritis (rats)
Carrageenan inflammation (rats)
Allergic thyroiditis (guinea pigs)
Disorders with variable course
Systemic lupus erythematosus
Scleroderma
Myasthenia gravis
Inflammatory bowel disease
Necrotizing cutaneous vasculitis
Ankylosing spondylitis
Polyarteritis nodosa
Polymyositis/dermatomyositis
Behçet's disease
Juvenile rheumatoid arthritis
Wegener's: relapses

After delivery, the symptoms of RA recurred in more than 90% of patients, although complete data are not available. Information has been published on the postpartum experience of 189 patients (84). All had an exacerbation after parturition; 64% noted a return of symptoms by the eighth week after delivery. Thirty-six percent had no joint inflammation until more than 8 weeks after delivery. These data indicate that the benefits of pregnancy are temporary, lasting an average of 6 weeks after delivery. The return of symptoms can be abrupt or insidious and is not related to the resumption of menstruation or to the termination of lactation. A careful quantitation of disease activity has not been performed, but it is generally stated that postpartum RA is at least as severe as that before gestation (84).

There are few studies of the effect of RA on fertility or on the fetus. One retrospective study found that the fertility rate of patients with RA was normal, although the rate of spontaneous abortion was slightly higher, but in general, patients with RA have successful pregnancies with normal babies (88).

Considerable clinical experience during pregnancy has been accumulated also with SLE. Most authors have noted a high spontaneous abortion rate in pregnancies occurring before the onset of the first recognizable manifestation of this disease, as well as in pregnancies after the onset of clinical disease. Spontaneous abortions may be related to antiphospholipid antibodies, particularly antibodies to cardiolipin (89). The occurrence of heart block in offspring of mothers with SLE is now well known and is related to anti-Ro (SSA) antibody. Mothers of babies born with complete heart block should be monitored for signs of rheumatic disease, because the diagnosis may not be apparent before delivery. The disease did not develop in one mother until 16 years after the birth of the first of three children with congenital heart block. The risk for congenital heart block in additional pregnancies is low but still present. The heart block is not reversible. Up to one third of children born with this problem will die in the neonatal period, and the majority of those that survive will require permanent pacemakers (90). Neonatal lupus also has been described in the infants of women with antibodies to U1RNP (91).

Less certain is the relation between disease activity and pregnancy, including the progression of renal or other organ dysfunction. As with RA, exacerbations of SLE have been documented frequently in the postpartum period. Less frequent exacerbations, usually of minor consequence, have been noted in more recent studies. Renal function deterioration is not frequent and usually reversible (92,93). These apparently conflicting results may be due to more aggressive therapy or differences in the definition of a lupus flare. It can be difficult to differentiate changes caused only by pregnancy from true disease exacerbation. Serum hemolytic complement levels may be helpful, because these are usually high in normal pregnancies. A high ratio of CH_{50} to complement cleavage fragment Ba may be particularly helpful in differentiating preeclampsia from active SLE (94). Because of these uncertainties, a number of investigators have suggested that pregnancies be delayed in patients with SLE until their disease has been inactive for 6 months or more before conception. The same risks during pregnancy have been reported in patients with mixed connective tissue disease (95) (see Chapter 73).

Factors Responsible for Amelioration

The factors responsible for improvement of RA during pregnancy are not yet known. The increased susceptibility of pregnant women to certain infectious diseases and the specific suppression of normal immune responses during pregnancy might be relevant. During gestation, women are believed to have increased morbidity and mortality from certain infectious agents, chiefly viruses and fungi (96). The virulence of these intracellular microorganisms may be related to impaired cell-mediated immunity. Skin-graft rejection is delayed, and in vitro T-lymphocyte responses are depressed, effects believed to be mediated by the serum or plasma of pregnancy. The ameliorating substances may be responsible for all the clinical alterations associated with gestation (86,96).

Hench suggested that blood cortisol increases during pregnancy explain the suppression of rheumatoid activity. Subsequent studies have shown, however, that the increased corticosteroid concentrations alone were not fully responsible for the observed improvement. Measurement of plasma cortisol levels did not correlate with disease activity during pregnancy. Plasma cortisol levels decrease to normal by 48 hours after delivery, and yet RA remains suppressed after delivery for more than 6 weeks in 50% of patients. The hormone is mostly transcortin bound during gestation and is therefore not biologically active. Thus despite the original enthusiasm for cortisol, other factors responsible for improvement during gestation have been sought (96).

A variety of other products of pregnancy, including placental extracts, umbilical cord serum, and blood or urine fractions, have been used to treat RA without reproducible improvement. The concentrations of many plasma proteins are increased during gestation, including (a) carrier proteins, such as transcortin, thyroxin-binding globulin, testosterone-binding globulin, estrogen-binding globulin, transferrin, and ceruloplasmin; (b) coagulation proteins, including fibrinogen and factors VII, VIII, and IX; (c) plasminogen; (d) α_2-macroglobulin; (e) C-reactive protein and other so-called "acute phase" proteins; and (f) pregnancy-associated plasma proteins. Furthermore, ovarian and placental hormones influence the expression of multiple cytokines including increased production of IL-1, IL-2, and IL-6 (97).

Of these proteins, studies on the biologic activities of the pregnancy-associated α_2-glycoprotein have been the most promising. This glycoprotein is found at low concentrations in the serum of women who are not pregnant and increases during gestation in most individuals (98). After delivery, the level decreases at a slower rate than the other pregnancy-associated plasma proteins. The timing of changes in the concentration of plasma pregnancy-associated α_2-glycoprotein paralleled both remissions and postpartum exacerbations of RA. Additionally, approximately 25% of women have only minimal elevations of this protein in the plasma during gestation; this finding may explain the failure of this percentage of patients to experience clinical improvements (96). Pregnancy-associated α2-glycoprotein affects a variety of *in vitro* parameters of inflammation and acts on the membranes of isolated organelles, polymorphonuclear leukocytes, and lymphocytes as well (96). Unlike previous observations with corticosteroid hormones, pregnancy-associated α_2-glycoprotein is effective *in vitro* in physiologic concentrations.

The dramatic changes in the metabolism of the sex hormones during pregnancy are well known. Estrogens reduce the metabolic activity of neutrophils, alter delayed skin-test reactivity in experimental animals, and suppress the development and severity of adjuvant arthritis in rats. Progesterone also has been shown *in vitro* to suppress leukocyte functions. Most of these effects have resulted from large, nonphysiologic amounts of these sex hormones, however (86). Despite original enthusiasm, the beneficial effects of sex hormones on patients with RA have not been substantiated by clinical trials, but carefully controlled studies have not been performed. Because estrogenic hormones are known to induce a variety of serum protein changes similar to those in pregnancy, their effect on serum concentrations of pregnancy-associated α_2-glycoprotein has been studied. Significant increases in this protein were observed during the administration of either a combination of estrogen and progesterone or estrogen alone. Serum concentrations of pregnancy-associated α_2-glycoprotein induced by exogenous sex hormone administration reached only one tenth the levels usually found during pregnancy (96), however, and this may account for the failure of estrogens to produce the clinical response observed during gestation. Thus sex hormones, corticosteroids, and pregnancy-associated α_2-glycoprotein, the plasma constituents increased during pregnancy, have been demonstrated *in vitro* and in some animal models to possess antiinflammatory activity. Other potential ameliorating factors in patients with RA include (a) the carbohydrate composition of immunoglobulin G molecules, which is altered in RA and partially corrected in the pregnant state; (b) a defect in suppressor T lymphocytes; (c) antibodies to HLA-DR molecules that inhibit a cell-mediated reaction in RA; and (d) maternal–fetal disparities for HLA-DQA present in 78% of patients with RA who experienced pregnancy-related remission versus 25% in those who continued to have active disease (99). No single theory for amelioration of disease stands out. It is likely that the interaction of multiple systems is involved.

SEX HORMONES IN AUTOIMMUNE DISORDERS

Many although not all autoimmune diseases are more common in women than in men (100). In SLE, the best example, the female-to-male ratio can be as high as 15:1. The ratio varies with age. In premenarchal or postmenopausal women, the ratio decreases to 2:1. This change in ratio suggests hormonal influence. Metabolism of estrogens and androgens in patients with lupus has been investigated. Patients with SLE showed an elevation of 16-hydroxylated metabolites with increased estrogenic activity. First-degree relatives of these patients also had higher levels of 16-hydroxylated metabolites; a genetic predisposition to altered estrogen metabolism is implied. A recent study reported that the incidence of disease flare in patients who developed cyclophosphamide-induced ovarian failure was significantly less than that in those patients who did not have ovarian failure (101). Because of these hormonal effects, the use of oral contraceptives in SLE has been controversial. In older studies, oral contraceptive agents either exacerbated latent SLE or induced the formation of antibodies to nuclear antigens. Patients with antinuclear antibodies believed to be secondary to oral contraceptive use had rheumatic complaints of arthralgias, myalgias, and morning stiffness, and two had synovitis. The newer, low-dose estrogen agents appear to be a safe alternative in patients with SLE. Studies have shown no difference in flare rates in patients taking oral contraceptives as compared with a control group. Because of the increased risk of thrombosis, these agents should not be used in patients with the antiphospholipid syndrome and should be used with caution when active renal disease is present (102,103).

The use of estrogens in postmenopausal women carries some risk for the development of SLE. A recent study examined the incidence of SLE in the Nurses' Health Study cohort. This cohort consists of 69,435 women aged 30 to 55 years in 1976 who have been followed up with biennial questionnaires regarding diagnoses, exposures, and health practices. The age-adjusted relative risk for SLE was 2.5 for current users and 1.8 for past users. Duration of use was associated with the level of incidence (104). However, postmenopausal estrogen therapy in patients with SLE does not seem to alter the course of their disease (105).

The study of the relation between menstrual cycle phase and the symptoms of RA has yielded conflicting reports, but a patient with recurring inflammatory polyarthritis during menses has been reported (106). In addition to the exacerbating effects of estrogens, it is postulated that androgens play a protective role in autoimmune disease. Indeed, there is a higher incidence of SLE in patients with Klinefelter's syndrome. Treatment of these patients with testosterone may have a therapeutic effect on their autoimmune disease as well, but studies with more potent androgens have had conflicting results. More recently, dehydroepiandrosterone (DHEA) a weaker androgenic steroid, has been used to treat SLE. Although this hormone has not been shown to improve very active lupus, there are encouraging reports in milder disease, allowing reduction in corticosteroid use (107). The effect of androgen therapy in RA is controversial. An uncontrolled study of seven male patients showed a favorable response with such therapy, and ongoing studies in animal models support the role of androgen suppression of inflammation, most likely through the modulation of cytokine production, particularly IL-10 (108,109).

The effects of sex steroid hormones on autoimmune disease have been studied in murine lupus models. Androgens suppressed murine lupus, and estrogens accelerated the disease. The estrogen antagonist, tamoxifen, has been reported to have a positive therapeutic effect in a murine model of SLE. Estrogen receptor–like binding has been found in mouse thymus tissue, and estrogens may inhibit the clearance of immune complexes; these findings reflect the probable influence of sex hormones on the immune system by means of thymus epithelium and the reticuloendothelial system. Thymic hormones also are influenced by sex hormones. T cells, however, appear to be the primary target for hormones. Hormonal manipulation has a profound effect on T cells, with effects on B cells probably orchestrated indirectly through T cells. Additionally, the observation that androgens preserved IL-2 activity in some mice with lupus suggests a relation between IL-2 expression and sex hormones. Antiinflammatory cytokine levels can be affected by changes in hormone levels. IL-10 in particular is affected by pregnancy. Studies in this area may help explain the reason disease remits and/or exacerbates during pregnancy in the autoimmune diseases (109).

Expression of class II MHC antigens on "nontraditional" antigen-presenting cells such as thyroid epithelium or pancreatic islet cells has been proposed as a mechanism for autoimmunity involving these organs. Interferon-γ produced by T lymphocytes can upregulate major histocompatibility antigens on a variety of cell types and might contribute to autoimmunity in general. Other cytokines such as tumor necrosis factor-α are involved as well. Sex hormones modulate many of these cytokines. Subsets of T cells have estrogen receptors; mice treated with estrogens produce increased levels of IL-1. IL-1 also is elevated during the luteal phase of the menstrual cycle. Estrogen stimulation of T lymphocytes from female mice resulted in a greater production of interferon-γ. The promoter for the interferon-γ gene in transgenic mice can be upregulated by estrogen, and this is probably a normal control mechanism. IL-2 production by lymphocytes is diminished by treatment with estrogens. All of these changes could have profound effects on autoimmunity (110).

The results of these and other studies suggest an important role for hormonal modulation of the immune system in autoimmune disorders, in particular SLE, and is leading to novel therapeutic techniques (see Chapters 40 and 43).

Autoimmunity and the Hypothalamic–Pituitary–Adrenal Axis

The role of the central nervous system (CNS) and the hypothalamic–pituitary–adrenal (HPA) axis in autoimmunity has not been defined, but the observation that RA does not develop on the affected side after a cerebrovascular accident or polio has been noted for years. Stress has long been clinically associated with exacerbations of autoimmune diseases and suspected as a component in their initiation, but no objective data support these observations. New information about the interactions between the CNS, HPA axis, and immune system includes the observation that cytokines elaborated by immune cells have direct effects on the HPA axis. IL-1 can stimulate the hypothalamus to secrete corticotropin-releasing factor (CRF), which triggers the whole HPA axis with the result of secretion of adrenal corticosteroids. IL-2 stimulates the pituitary to release adrenocorticotropic hormone (ACTH) and thus also stimulates the adrenal glands. Corticosteroids have many immunomodulating effects, including inhibition of the secretion of both IL-1 and -2, thus providing feedback inhibition of the immune system as well as of the HPA axis. IL-6 has been found to have similar activities (110–112).

Cells of the immune system have receptors for ACTH, prolactin, and endorphins as a possible additional link to the HPA axis. They also secrete a number of neuropeptides including ACTH, endorphins, thyrotropin, prolactin, and others. These substances are secreted in response to virus infections, mitogens, and to hypothalamic-releasing factor (110–112).

A few studies have had more direct implications for autoimmune diseases. Sternberg et al. (113) found that a strain of rats considered "high stress" do not develop streptococcal cell wall–induced arthritis unless treated with a corticosteroid-receptor antagonist, whereas "low-stress" Lewis rats do develop arthritis. The Lewis rats have smaller adrenal glands, and treatment of them with low doses of corticosteroids decreased the intensity of the arthritis. Studies of adjuvant-induced arthritis in rats revealed higher concentrations of substance P in the joints that become inflamed. Through immunohistochemical staining, a decreased level of substance P was detected in rheumatoid versus normal synovium. Substance P might be involved in the onset of disease and might be depleted at later times. Substance P has direct *in vitro* effects, including increased synoviocyte proliferation and increased release of prostaglandin E_2 and collagenase, all of which could have profound effects on the development of pannus and cartilage destruction (114) (see Chapter 40).

It is obvious from these and many other studies that the interactions between the immune and the central neuroendocrine systems are being explored diligently. Future studies will undoubtedly have important effects on our knowledge of the pathogenesis of autoimmune states and on treatment strategies to interrupt or modulate the process.

REFERENCES

1. Acromegaly Therapy Consensus Development Panel. Consensus statement: benefits versus risks of medical therapy for acromegaly. *Am J Med* 1994;97:468–473.
2. Melmed S. Acromegaly. *N Engl J Med* 1990;322:966–977.
3. W¸ster C. Growth hormone and bone metabolism. *Acta Endocrinol* 1933;128(suppl 2):14–18.
4. Lieberman SA, Björkengren AG, Hoffman AR. Rheumatologic and skeletal changes in acromegaly. *Endocrinol Metab Clin North Am* 1992;21:615–631.
5. Anton HC. Hand measurements in acromegaly. *Clin Radiol* 1972;23:445–450.
6. Lacks S, Jacobs RP. Acromegalic arthropathy: a reversible rheumatic disease. *J Rheumatol* 1986;13:634–636.
7. Colao A, Marzullo P, Vallone G, et al. Reversibility of joint thickening in acromegalic patients: an ultrasonography study. *J Clin Endocrinol Metab* 1998;83:2121–2125.
8. Barkan A. Acromegalic arthropathy and sleep apnea. *J Endocrinol* 1997;155:S41–S44.
9. Bagge E, Eden S, Rosen T, et al. The prevalence of radiographic osteoarthritis is low in elderly patients with growth hormone deficiency. *Acta Endocrinol* 1993;129:296–300.
10. Nagulesparen M, Trickey R, Davies MJ, et al. Muscle changes in acromegaly. *Br Med J* 1976;2:914–915.
11. Pickett JBE III, Layzer RB, Levin SR, et al. Neuromuscular complications of acromegaly. *Neurology* 1975;25:638–645.
12. Khaleeli AA, Levy RD, Edwards RHT, et al. The neuromuscular features of acromegaly: a clinical and pathological study. *J Neurol Neurosurg Psychiatry* 1984;47:1009–1015.
13. Low PA, McLeod JR, Turtle JR, et al. Peripheral neuropathy in acromegaly. *Brain* 1974;97:139–152.
14. Bland JH, Frymoyer JW. Rheumatic syndromes of myxedema. *N Engl J Med* 1970;282:1171–1174.
15. Rao SN, Katiyar BC, Nair KR, et al. Neuromuscular status in hypothyroidism. *Acta Neurol Scand* 1980;61:167–177.
16. Swanson JW, Kelly JD, McConahey WM. Neurologic aspects of thyroid dysfunction. *Mayo Clin Proc* 1981;56:504–512.
17. Dorwart BB, Schumacher HR. Joint effusions, chondrocalcinosis and other rheumatic manifestations in hypothyroidism: a clinicopathologic study. *Am J Med* 1975;59:780–790.
18. McLean RM, Podell DN. Bone and joint manifestations of hypothyroidism. *Semin Arthritis Rheum* 1995;24:282–290.
19. Neeck G, Riedel W, Schmidt KL. Neuropathy myopathy and destructive arthropathy in primary hypothyroidism. *J Rheumatol* 1990;17:1697–1700.
20. Gerster JC, Valceschine P. Destructive arthropathy of fingers in

primary hypothyroidism without chondrocalcinosis: report of 3 cases. *J Rheumatol* 1992;19:637–641.
21. Dieppe PA, Alexander GJ, Jones HE, et al. Pyrophosphate arthropathy: a clinical and radiological study of 105 cases. *Ann Rheum Dis* 1982;41:371–376.
22. McCarty DJ, Silcox DC, Coe F, et al. Diseases associated with calcium pyrophosphate dihydrate crystal deposition: a controlled study. *Am J Med* 1974;56:704–714.
23. Komatireddy GR, Ellman MH, Brown NL. Lack of association between hypothyroidism and chondrocalcinosis. *J Rheumatol* 1989;16:807–808.
24. Job-Deslandre C, Menkes CJ, Quinot M, et al. Does hypothyroidism increase the prevalence of chondrocalcinosis? *Br J Rheumatol* 1993;32:197–198.
25. Farid NR, Woodford G, Au B, et al. Polymorphonuclear leukocyte function in hypothyroidism. *Horm Res* 1976;7:247–253.
26. Brandt KD. The effect of synovial hyaluronate on the ingestion of monosodium urate crystals by leukocytes. *Clin Chim Acta* 1974;55:307–315.
27. Newcombe DS. Endocrinopathies and uric acid metabolism. *Semin Arthritis Rheum* 1973;2:281–300.
28. Erickson AR, Enzenauer RJ, Nordstrom DM, et al. The prevalence of hypothyroidism in gout. *Am J Med* 1994;97:231–234.
29. Hirano T, Stamelos S, Harris V, et al. Association of primary hypothyroidism and slipped capital femoral epiphysis. *J Pediatr* 1978;93:262–264.
30. Rodolico C, Toscano A, Benvenga S, et al. Skeletal muscle disturbances may precede clinical and laboratory evidence of autoimmune hypothyroidism. *J Neurol* 1998;245:555–556.
31. Halverson PB, Kozin F, Ryan LM, et al. Rhabdomyolysis and renal failure in hypothyroidism. *Ann Intern Med* 1979;91:57–58.
32. McKeran RO, Slavin G, Andrews TM, et al. Muscle fibre type changes in hypothyroid myopathy. *J Clin Pathol* 1975;28: 659–663.
33. Argov Z, Rehshaw PF, Boden B, et al. Effects of thyroid hormones on skeletal muscle bioenergetics: in vivo phosphorus-31 magnetic resonance spectroscopy study of humans and rats. *J Clin Invest* 1988;81:1695–1701.
34. Shagan BP, Friedman SA. Raynaud's phenomenon and thyroid deficiency. *Arch Intern Med* 1980;140:831–832.
35. Auwerx J, Bouillon R. Mineral and bone metabolism in thyroid disease: a review. *Q J Med* 1986;60:737–752.
36. Stall GM, Harris S, Sokoll LJ, et al. Accelerated bone loss in hypothyroid patients overtreated with L-thyroxine. *Ann Intern Med* 1990;113:265–269.
37. Franklyn JA, Betteridge J, Daykin J, et al. Long-term thyroxine treatment and bone mineral density. *Lancet* 1992;340:9–13.
38. Gimlette TMD. Thyroid acropachy. *Lancet* 1960;1:22–24.
39. Volpé R. Autoimmunity causing thyroid dysfunction. *Endocrinol Metab Clin North Am* 1991;20:565–587.
40. Wohlgethan JR. Frozen shoulder in hyperthyroidism. *Arthritis Rheum* 1987;30:936–939.
41. Miller JL, Ismail F, Waligora JK, et al. Modulating influence of *d,l*-propranolol on triiodothyronine-induced skeletal muscle protein degradation. *Endocrinology* 1985;117:869–871.
42. Becker KL, Ferguson RH, McConahey WM. The connective tissue diseases and symptoms associated with Hashimoto's thyroiditis. *N Engl J Med* 1963;268:277–280.
43. Miller FW, Moore GF, Weintraub BD, et al. Prevalence of thyroid disease and thyroid function test abnormalities in patients with systemic lupus erythematosus. *Arthritis Rheum* 1987;30:1124–1131.
44. Shiroky JB, Cohen M, Ballachey ML, et al. Thyroid dysfunction in rheumatoid arthritis: a controlled prospective study. *Ann Rheum Dis* 1993;52:454–456.
45. Bajaj S, Bell MJ, Shumak S, et al. Antithyroid arthritis syndrome. *J Rheumatol* 1998;25:1235–1239.
46. Wishart J, Horowitz M, Need A, et al. Relationship between forearm and vertebral mineral density in postmenopausal women with primary hyperparathyroidism. *Arch Intern Med* 1990;150:1329–1331.
47. Martin P, Bergmann P, Gillet C, et al. Long-term irreversibility of bone loss after surgery for primary hyperparathyroidism. *Arch Intern Med* 1990;150:1495–1497.
48. Preston ET. Avulsion of both quadriceps tendons in hyperparathyroidism. *JAMA* 1972;221:406–407.
49. Babini SM, Maldonado Cocco JA, de la Sota M, et al. Tendinous laxity and Jaccoud's syndrome in patients with systemic lupus erythematosus: possible role of secondary hyperparathyroidism. *J Rheumatol* 1989;16:494–498.
50. Hamilton EBD. Diseases associated with CPPD deposition disease. *Arthritis Rheum* 1976;19:353–357.
51. Bilezikian JP, Connor TB, Aptekar R, et al. Pseudogout after parathyroidectomy. *Lancet* 1973;1:445–446.
52. Bywaters EGL, Dixon A St J, Scott JT. Joint lesions of hyperparathyroidism. *Ann Rheum Dis* 1963;22:171–184.
53. Turken SA, Cafferty M, Silverberg SJ, et al. Neuromuscular involvement in mild asymptomatic primary hyperparathyroidism. *Am J Med* 1989;87:553–557.
54. Wilkinson H, Iveson JM. Digital vasculopathy associated with hyperparathyroidism. *Br J Rheumatol* 1993;32:86.
55. Chaykin LB, Frame B, Sigler JW. Spondylitis: a clue to hypoparathyroidism. *Ann Intern Med* 1969;70:995–1000.
56. Kruse K, Scheunemann W, Baier W, et al. Hypocalcemic myopathy in idiopathic hypoparathyroidism. *Eur J Pediatr* 1982;138:280–282.
57. Lyons TJ, Bailie KE, Dyer DG, et al. Decrease in skin collagen glycation with improved glycemic control in patients with insulin-dependent diabetes mellitus. *J Clin Invest* 1991;87: 1910–1915.
58. Joslin EP, Root HF, White P, et al., eds. *Treatment of diabetes mellitus.* 9th ed. Philadelphia: Lea & Febiger, 1952.
59. Rothschild BM. Diabetes and arthritis. *Comp Ther* 1994;20: 347–350.
60. Bridgeman JE. Periarthritis of the shoulder and diabetes mellitus. *Ann Rheum Dis* 1972;31:69–71.
61. Lequesne M, Dang N, Bensasson M, et al. Increased association of diabetes mellitus with capsulitis of the shoulder and shoulder hand syndrome. *Scand J Rheumatol* 1977;6:53–56.
62. Pastan RS, Cohen AS. The rheumatologic manifestations of diabetes mellitus. *Med Clin North Am* 1978;62:829–839.
63. Sinha S, Munichoodappa CS, Kozak GP. Neuropathy (Charcot joints) in diabetes mellitus. *Medicine* 1972;51:191–210.
64. Shaw JE, Boulton AJM. The pathogenesis of diabetic foot problems: an overview. *Diabetes* 1997;46(suppl 2):S58–S61.
65. Lipman BT, Collier BD, Carrera GF, et al. Detection of osteomyelitis in the neuropathic foot: nuclear medicine, MRI, and conventional radiography. *Clin Nucl Med* 1998;23: 77–82.
66. Newman LG, Waller J, Palestro, CJ, et al. Unsuspected osteomyelitis in diabetic foot ulcers. *JAMA* 1991;266:1246–1251.
67. Horn CA, Bradley JD, Brandt KD, et al. Impairment of osteophyte formation in hyperglycemic patients with type II diabetes mellitus and knee osteoarthritis. *Arthritis Rheum* 1992;35: 336–342.
68. Daragon A, Mejjad O, Czernichow P, et al. Vertebral hyperostosis and diabetes mellitus: a case-control study. *Ann Rheum Dis* 1995;54:375–378.
69. Viljanto JA. Dupuytren's contracture: a review. *Semin Arthritis Rheum* 1973;3:155–176.

70. Strom L. Trigger finger in diabetes. *J Med Soc N J* 1977;74: 951–954.
71. Trapp RG, Soler NG, Spencer-Green G. Nailfold capillaroscopy in type I diabetes with vasculopathy and limited joint mobility. *J Rheumatol* 1986;13:917–920.
72. Sibbett WL, Eaton RP. Corticosteroid responsive tenosynovitis is a common pathway for limited joint mobility in the diabetic hand. *J Rheumatol* 1997;24:931–936.
73. Tsokos GC, Gorden P, Antonovych T, et al. Lupus nephritis and other autoimmune features in patients with diabetes mellitus due to autoantibody to insulin receptors. *Ann Intern Med* 1985; 102:176–181.
74. McNair P. Bone mineral metabolism in human type I (insulin dependent) diabetes mellitus. *Dan Med Bull* 1988;35:109–121.
75. Bauer DC, Browner WS, Cauley JA, et al. Factors associated with appendicular bone mass in older women: the Study of Osteoporotic Fractures research group. *Ann Intern Med* 1993; 118:657–665.
76. Levin ME, Boisseau VC, Avioli LV. Effects of diabetes mellitus on bone mass in juvenile and adult-onset diabetes. *N Engl J Med* 1976;294:241–245.
77. Wakasugi M, Wakao, R, Tawata M, et al. Bone mineral density measured by dual energy x-ray absorptiometry in patients with non-insulin-dependent diabetes mellitus. *Bone* 1993;14: 29–33.
78. van Daele PLA, Stolk RP, Burger H, et al. Bone density in non-insulin-dependent diabetes mellitus: the Rotterdam study. *Ann Intern Med* 1995;122:409–414.
79. Kingsley GH, Hickling P. Polyarthropathy associated with Cushing's disease. *Br Med J* 1986;292:1363.
80. Askari A, Vignos PJ, Moskowitz RW. Steroid myopathy in connective tissue disease. *Am J Med* 1976;61:485–492.
81. Ebinger G, Six R, Bruyland M, Somers G. Flexion contractures: a forgotten symptom in Addison's disease and hypopituitarism. *Lancet* 1986;2:858.
82. Asherson RA, Hughes GRV. Hypoadrenalism, Addison's disease and antiphospholipid antibodies. *J Rheumatol* 1991;18:1–3.
83. Plonk JW, Feldman JM. Carcinoid arthropathy. *Arch Intern Med* 1974;134:651–654.
84. Odell WD, Wolfsen AR. Humoral syndromes associated with cancer. *Annu Rev Med* 1978;29:379–406.
85. DuPont B, Hoyer I, Borgeskov S, et al. Plasma growth hormone and hypertrophic osteoarthropathy in carcinoma of the bronchus. *Acta Med Scand* 1970;188:25–30.
86. DaSilva JAP, Spector TD. The role of pregnancy in the course and aetiology of rheumatoid arthritis. *Clin Rheumatol* 1992;11: 189–194.
87. Barrett JH, Brennan P, Fiddler M, et al. Does rheumatoid arthritis remit during pregnancy and relapse postpartum? Results from a nationwide study in the United Kingdom performed prospectively from late pregnancy. *Arthritis Rheum* 1999;42:1219–1227.
88. Kaplan D. Fetal wastage in patients with rheumatoid arthritis. *J Rheumatol* 1986;13:875–877.
89. Lockshin MD, Druzin ML, Goei S, et al. Antibody to cardiolipin as a predictor of fetal distress or death in pregnant patients with systemic lupus erythematosus. *N Engl J Med* 1985;313:152–156.
90. Waltuck J, Buyon JP. Autoantibody-associated congenital heart block: outcome in mothers and children. *Ann Intern Med* 1994; 120:544–551.
91. Provost TT, Watson R, Gammon WR, et al. The neonatal lupus syndrome associated with U1 RNP (nRNP) antibodies. *N Engl J Med* 1987;316:1135–1138.
92. Petri M. Clinical features of systemic lupus erythematosus. *Curr Opin Rheumatol* 1994;6:481–486.
93. Petri M. Lupus and pregnancy. *Bull Rheum Dis* 1995;44:1–3.
94. Abramson SB, Buyon JP. Activation of the complement pathway: comparison of normal pregnancy, preeclampsia, and systemic lupus erythematosus. *Am J Reprod Immunol* 1992;28:183–187.
95. Kaufman RL, Kitridou RC. Pregnancy in mixed connective tissue disease: comparison with systemic lupus erythematosus. *J Rheumatol* 1982;9:549–555.
96. Persellin RH. Inhibitors of inflammatory and immune responses in pregnancy serum. *Clin Rheum Dis* 1981;7:769–780.
97. Buyon JP, Yaron M, Lockshin MD. First International Conference on Rheumatic Diseases in Pregnancy. *Arthritis Rheum* 1993;36:59–64.
98. Von Schoultz B. A quantitative study of the pregnancy zone protein in the sera of pregnant and puerperal women. *Am J Obstet Gynecol* 1974;119:792–797.
99. Nelson JL, Ostensen M. Pregnancy and rheumatoid arthritis. *Rheum Dis Clin North Am* 1997;23:195–212.
100. Beeson PB. Age and sex associations of 40 autoimmune diseases. *Am J Med* 1994;96:457–462.
101. Mok CC, Wong RWS, Lau CS. Ovarian failure and flares of systemic lupus erythematosus. *Arthritis Rheum* 1999;42:1274–1280.
102. Julkunen HA, Kaaja R, Friman C. Contraceptive practice in women with systemic lupus erythematosus. *Br J Rheumatol* 1993;32:227–230.
103. Bruce IN, Laskin CA. Sex hormones in systemic lupus erythematosus: a controversy for modern times. *J Rheumatol* 1997;24: 1461–1463.
104. Sánchez-Guerrero J, Liang MH, Karlson EW, et al. Postmenopausal estrogen therapy and the risk for developing systemic lupus erythematosus. *Ann Intern Med* 1995;122:430–433.
105. Arden NK, Lloyd ME, Spector TD, et al. Safety of hormone replacement therapy in systemic lupus erythematosus. *Lupus* 1994;3:11–13.
106. McDonagh JE, Singh MM, Griffiths ID. Menstrual arthritis. *Ann Rheum Dis* 1993;52:65–66.
107. Van Vollerhoven RF, Engelman EG, McGuire JL. Dehydroepiandrosterone in systemic lupus erythematosus: results of a double-blind, placebo controlled randomized clinical trial. *Arthritis Rheum* 1995;38:1826–1831.
108. DaSilva JAP, Larbre J, Seed MP, et al. Sex differences in inflammation induced cartilage damage in rodents: the influence of sex steroids. *J Rheumatol* 1994;21:330–337.
109. Cutolo M. The roles of steroid hormones in arthritis. *Br J Rheumatol* 1998;37:597–601.
110. Sarvetnick N, Fox HS. Interferon-gamma and the sexual dimorphism of autoimmunity. *Mol Biol Med* 1990;7:323–331.
111. Chrousos GP. The hypothalamic-pituitary-adrenal axis and immune-mediated inflammation. *N Engl J Med* 1995;332: 1351–1362.
112. Walker S, Jara L, eds. Prolactin in SLE. *Lupus* 1998;7:371–427.
113. Sternberg EM, Hill JM, Chrousos GP, et al. Inflammatory mediator-induced hypothalamic-pituitary-adrenal axis activation is defective in streptococcal cell wall arthritis-susceptible Lewis rats. *Proc Natl Acad Sci U S A* 1989;86:2374–2378.
114. Mapp P, Kidd B. The role of substance P in rheumatic disease. *Semin Arthritis Rheum* 1994;23(suppl):3–9.

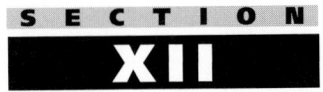

INFECTIOUS ARTHRITIS

125

PRINCIPLES OF DIAGNOSIS AND TREATMENT OF JOINT INFECTIONS

ARA H. DIKRANIAN
MICHAEL H. WEISMAN

It is sobering to reflect that septic arthritis remains an almost identical challenge to the clinician today as it was 20 years ago. The prognosis for the patient has not changed appreciably over these past two decades (1,2). This seems paradoxical in light of advances in the spectrum and availability of antibiotics and the increasing utilization of an almost infinite array of diagnostic imaging techniques. We really do not know why this has occurred. It is possible to speculate that the phenomenon must relate to risk factors for the development of septic arthritis in the current decade. The patients that we see in our practices and those that are reported in the literature commonly have severe chronic illnesses such as acquired immunodeficiency syndrome (AIDS), and receive heroic treatments such as vital organ and bone marrow transplants, renal dialysis, and immunosuppressive and steroid treatment of chronic illnesses. For example, in virtually every series in the literature, there are a substantial number of patients with rheumatoid arthritis (RA), and this population is generally the nodular, seropositive subgroup with long-standing disease and a poor prognosis. As these RA patients will receive experimental chemotherapeutic procedures designed to deplete or dysregulate lymphocytes, macrophages, and their associated cytokines, the prognosis for septic arthritis is not likely to change in the near future.

The diagnosis and treatment of septic arthritis are intertwined, as they have been for the past 20 years, because the most important prognostic factor in septic arthritis is the speed with which the diagnosis is recognized and antibiotics are instituted. For a rule of thumb, if patients are treated within 1 week from the onset of symptoms, they usually do well; conversely, if their disease lasts for a month before treatment, they almost always do poorly. What happens in between will be proportional to the speed with which treatment is instituted. Therefore the recognition of septic arthritis is probably the single most important therapeutic modality available to the clinician.

We have organized this chapter as a framework and overview of the clinical problem of septic arthritis. The following chapters are the building blocks to complete the structure. They are written along the lines of the specific infectious agents that cause arthritis (bacteria, fungi, mycobacteria, viruses, and spirochetes) and contain necessary and important details; they should be consulted in relevant cases. This chapter consists of six sections: epidemiology of septic arthritis, pathogenesis of joint infection, diagnosis (including imaging studies and joint fluid examination), treatment (including drainage of infected joints), outcome, and special circumstances. Each section begins with an introduction summarizing the important and relevant information from the previous edition of this textbook (3). This is followed by a discussion of recent information, generally from the past 5 years, pertinent to the topic. Specific recommendations and "clinical pearls" are highlighted throughout in tables, figures, and in the text. The reader is further referred to two excellent recent reviews on this topic (4,5).

EPIDEMIOLOGY

Recent reviews have placed the yearly incidence of bacterial arthritis from 2 to 10 per 100,000 in the general population to 30 to 40 per 100,000 in patients with RA and 40 to 68 per 100,0000 in patients with joint prostheses (4,6). The mortality rate ranges from 5% to 25%, essentially unchanged in the past 25 years (4). The predominance of *Staphylococcus aureus* has also remained unchanged over the past 40 years, and is now complicated by antibiotic-resistant organisms (5). *Staphylococcus aureus* causes 80% of joint infections in patients with concurrent RA and diabetes mellitus (4); it is the primary pathogen in hip infections (7) and is the primary pathogen in polyarticular septic arthritis, found in 70% to 80% of such patients (8,9). Gram-negative bacilli are common causes of bacterial arthritis in intravenous drug users, in the elderly, and in seriously immunocompromised hosts (10). Gram-negative bacilli, especially

TABLE 125.1. BACTERIAL ISOLATES IN SEPTIC ARTHRITIS (%)

Bacterium	Weston (10) (N = 199)	Kaandorp (11) (N = 188)	Ryan (12) (N = 1,158)	Peters (13) (N = 72)	Morgan (7) (N = 167)	Le Dantec (14) (N = 179)
S. aureus	54	41	39	52	37	56
All streptococci	18	18	28	n.a.	21	10
β-Hemolytic	12	5	7	11	16	9
S. pneumoniae	5.5	3.5	9.7	0	1	0
Gram-negative bacilli	7.5	15	19	8	5	16
H. influenzae	7.5	4	6	n.a.	1	0
N. gonorrheae	4.5	0	0.6	3	12	3
Mixed flora	3	n.a.	n.a.	1	10	n.a.
M. tuberculosis	0.5	2.5	7.7	3	0	n.a.
Unknown	18	12	n.a.	0	13	n.a.

Adapted from Goldenberg DL. Septic arthritis. *Lancet* 1998;351:197–202, with permission.

Haemophilus influenzae are the most common pathogens in the newborn and in all children younger than 5 years (4). Table 125.1 tabulates the prevalence of organisms involved in septic arthritis from several series. The knee, hip, and ankle are the most commonly involved joints in septic arthritis (Table 125.2). It is open to speculation why certain joints are involved more frequently than others; variables such as size of the joint and trauma are likely to play a role.

Analogous to what has been observed regarding the pathogenesis of crystal deposition diseases, joints previously affected by osteoarthritis (OA), trauma, or surgery are predisposed toward infection. However, in contrast to the observed rarity of gout attacks in patients with RA, septic arthritis occurring with RA or other inflammatory arthritides does occur and may be particularly difficult to diagnose and treat. Traditionally, RA, extremes of age, and diseased joints have been regarded as significant risk factors for developing septic arthritis (6,10,13). Many other risk factors have been proposed in reviews of the subject, but proof is lacking. In a prospective study of patients with joint disease attending a rheumatology clinic in Amsterdam, 37 patients with septic arthritis were identified with risk factors of age older than 80 years [odds ratio (OR) 3.5], diabetes mellitus (OR 3.3), RA (OR 4), recent joint surgery (OR 5), hip or knee prosthesis (OR 15), and skin infection (OR 27); the presence of skin infection in a person with a hip or knee prosthesis increased the risk of septic arthritis 73 times (15). It seems clear that once infection does occur in the patient with risk factors such as RA or diabetes, it is notoriously more difficult to diagnose and treat, and unusual organisms may be responsible.

PATHOGENESIS OF SEPTIC ARTHRITIS

It is axiomatic that infections of the joint come from the bloodstream. In fact, the source in 67% of cases of septic arthritis is hematogenous, whereas in 33% of cases, it is due to direct extension from a contiguous source (6). However, the joint must have an extensive capacity to protect itself from colonization and bacterial growth considering the countless bacteremias and superficial cutaneous infections in humans, but the few instances of associated septic arthritis. The reasons for this discrepancy are largely unknown, although there has been speculation about the importance of temperature, host factors including immune responses, and the unique characteristics of specific organisms. This appears to be especially true for gram-negative organisms, which are common causes of septicemia and yet invade the joint only when there has been either preexisting joint damage or host immune compromise; staphylococci and other gram-positive cocci seem to have a special affinity for syn-

TABLE 125.2. FREQUENCY OF JOINTS AFFECTED (%) IN SEPTIC ARTHRITIS

Joint	Peters (13) (N = 72)	Morgan (7) (N = 167)	Kaandorp (11) (N = 188)	Weston(10) (N = 199)
Knee	42	54	48	30
Hip	13	13	21	16
Ankle	12	8	12	6
Shoulder	10	5	5	8
Wrist	7	5	7	4
Elbow	6	5	9	9
Hand	1	5	4	8

ovial structures independent of the vagaries of the host, as discussed later.

Infection in a joint space must be considered different from infections in soft tissues (such as cellulitis) largely due to the characteristics of the space itself causing retarded movement of solutes into the surrounding vascular network. These factors will diminish bacterial growth and actually keep it dormant, allowing microorganisms to survive even in the presence of appropriate concentrations of antibiotic in the fluid. Therefore drainage of pus, fluid, and other debris, as well as decompressing joint pressure, will speed the healing process and clear the infection more rapidly (3).

Why Does Septic Arthritis Occur?

Addressing the concept that a joint must have an extensive capacity to protect itself from colonization and bacterial growth, it has been shown that the joint space itself causes a slowing of solute movement into the surrounding vascular network. However, once the process takes place and bacteria are "trapped," extensive cellular and molecular changes occur as demonstrated in a variety of animal models (16,17). Additionally, host factors in the pathogenesis of infectious arthritis have been reviewed (18), covering both the direct effects of bacterial disease ("classic" septic arthritis) and the indirect, associated arthritis (so-called "reactive" arthritis). Koopman (18) stressed the pivotal role of T cells and the fact that only T and B lymphocytes possess surface recognition structures [T-cell and immunoglobulin (Ig) receptors, respectively] that are capable of interacting with a wide and diverse group of foreign and self antigens. He pointed to the salient features of immune recognition of foreign antigens, focusing on the potential importance of major histocompatibility molecules, antigen processing, the T-cell receptor, heterogeneity of T cells based on cytokine elaboration, and microbial superantigens. However, there are important gaps in our knowledge and in our ability to connect these bench observations to the observed clinical phenomena. Despite clear evidence that major immunodeficiencies create patterns of host susceptibility to infection (e.g., AIDS, agammaglobulinemia), there is no straightforward explanation as to exactly how this happens. Further, it is still unclear how host immune responses induce and perpetuate injury from a septic process in otherwise immunocompetent individuals.

An animal model of *S. aureus* septic arthritis exhibits striking histologic and immunohistochemical changes in the joint (19,20). Synovial proliferation occurs in association with $CD4^+$ T-cell infiltration at 48 hours, and major histocompatibility class II molecules are expressed on the synovial cells. Additionally, as the process proceeds, macrophage-like cells in the synovium express interleukin-1 (IL-1) and tumor necrosis factor-α (TNF-α). Experimental *in vivo* depletion of $CD4^+$ cells results in a considerably milder course of *S. aureus* arthritis. It is possible to speculate that the observed high prevalence and aggressive nature of *S. aureus* septic arthritis in patients with RA may relate not only to the organism itself, but also to the functions of the $CD4^+$ cells that are modified by the rheumatoid disease process.

A mouse model has provided additional insight into the pathogenesis of *S. aureus* septic arthritis (21,22). Mutations of two loci in a signal-transduction system that regulates the expression of at least 15 virulence genes were identified in *S. aureus.* An intravenous inoculation of 10^7 colony-forming units of wild-type or mutant bacterial strains into Swiss mice induced either arthritis or osteitis within 3 weeks in 80% to 90% of the animals; the same strain was then later recovered from the joints. Mutant strains displayed less frequent and clinically milder forms of arthritis. The wild-type strain exhibited arthritis in 60% of the animals and erosive changes in 40%; in contrast, fewer than 30% of the selected mutant strains developed arthritis, and none had erosive changes.

Two studies have suggested that adherence to collagen may be a factor in the pathogenesis of *S. aureus* septic arthritis. *S. aureus* with a mutated collagen receptor gene induced arthritis in only 27% of mice compared with 70% with the wild-type strain, and bacterial adherence to collagen was reduced in organisms with the mutant gene (23). In experiments using a collagen receptor–positive strain of *S. aureus,* the strain adhered to both cartilage and collagen and was blocked by collagen receptor–specific antibodies (24). Although it has been demonstrated that other organisms causing arthritis have collagen-binding components, this may prove to be an important pathogenic step, potentially amenable to preventive measures or even to an interventional strategy.

A more recently described potential bacterial virulence factor is the polysaccharide capsule, especially serotype 5 (CP5). When CP5 expressing *S. aureus* were inoculated intravenously in a mouse model, not only was mortality greater than in the group inoculated with CP(–) strains (55% vs. 18%), but a higher frequency and more severe form of arthritis were seen; this was postulated to be due to the decreased ability of macrophages to ingest and intracellularly kill the CP(+) bacteria (25).

A discussion of the pathogenesis of septic arthritis in the 21st century cannot be complete without a discussion of AIDS, arthroscopy, pregnancy, and septic arthritis of the hip in children. Sepsis as a cause of arthritis in human immunodeficiency virus (HIV) infection is surprisingly uncommon. The organisms that typically affect HIV patients in general also induce septic arthritis. In a 1992 review of nine cases of AIDS-associated septic arthritis, of which seven were culture positive, four grew *S. aureus,* and three harbored atypical organisms (26). Disseminated sporotrichosis, cryptococcus, and *Mycobacterium avium intracellulare* (MAI) have been reported as causes of infected joints (27–29). A newly recognized pathogen, *Mycobacterium haemophilum,* has been isolated in 13 patients with AIDS and other immunodeficiencies; nine of these 13 had arthritis (30). If the HIV patient is also an intravenous drug abuser, the nature of the organisms follows the drug-abuse pattern, independent of HIV status.

Organisms typically found in these cases include *S. aureus, Candida, Pseudomonas* species, and group A streptococcus. The most frequently involved joints are the hip and knee, and the typical presentation is a monoarticular arthritis in 86% of cases. Characteristic target joints for infection in drug abusers, such as the sternoclavicular and sacroiliac joints, also may be involved (31,32).

More common causes of arthritis in HIV patients, which may be confused with septic arthritis, aside from the well-known associations of psoriatic arthritis and Reiter's syndrome, are AIDS-associated arthritis and the painful articular syndrome, both described in the early 1990s, and rarely reported since in the literature (33,34). AIDS-associated arthritis is a subacute oligoarthritis typically affecting the knees and ankles, with incapacitating pain, noninflammatory synovial fluid, and good response to nonsteroidal anti-inflammatory drugs and intraarticular steroids; it usually remits within 6 weeks. The second type of acute arthritis mimicking sepsis in HIV patients is the painful articular syndrome, characterized by severe, sharp joint pain without attendant synovitis, usually involving the knees, shoulders, and elbows and lasting 2 to 24 hours. The cause of both these syndromes is unknown.

Direct inoculation of the joint, producing a septic arthritis, remains an extremely uncommon occurrence. However, two reported conditions, arthroscopy and pregnancy, have been highlighted as being associated with septic arthritis, resulting from direct inoculation. In a retrospective analysis of 4,245 arthroscopies of the knee over a 4-year period, 18 instances of septic arthritis were observed, a complication rate of 0.42% (35). The major medical risk factor for this complication was the use of long-acting intraoperative corticosteroids; the usual surgical risk factors (longer operative time, increased number of procedures) also were noted. Almost all cases were caused by *S. aureus.* In a retrospective study of 2,500 anterior cruciate ligament arthroscopic reconstructions done at the Hospital for Special Surgery between 1988 and 1993, seven (0.3%) experienced postoperative (2 weeks to 2 months) septic knees; six of seven had concomitant open procedures performed. All patients were treated with antibiotics, and after a mean follow-up of 29 months, six of seven had minimal to no pain in the operated-on knee. This study points to the infrequency of complications with arthroscopic surgery and the additional risk of open procedures; however, it is reassuring to realize that the complications were recognized promptly and that almost all patients did well with antibiotic therapy (36). Only one case of septic arthritis was observed after 335 office-based rheumatology-related knee arthroscopies (37). This low complication rate occurred despite a high prevalence (27.5%) of patients undergoing the procedure who had inflammatory rheumatic diseases or who were taking corticosteroids and immunosuppressive agents. The one case of septic arthritis occurred in a patient who had OA and received an intraarticular steroid injection after the procedure. In these and other observational analyses, it is always difficult to identify the individual contributions of patient risk (why was the procedure done in the first place?), or whether the steroid injection made a local or a systemic contribution. In the same regard, the incidence of septic complications from total joint arthroplasty has been reduced in recent years by several factors: greater surgical experience of the operator, shorter operation time, perioperative parenteral prophylactic antibiotics, and aggressive pretreatment of infection foci before the arthroplasty is performed (3).

The recognition that a postpartum septic hip may be due to direct inoculation as a result of retrograde flow warrants concern. During labor, increased abdominal pressure is believed to force blood through the ligamentum teres into the hip joint via the valveless iliac veins, in similar fashion as retrograde flow from the sacral veins into the internal vertebral plexus of Batson and the sacroiliac joint (38).

Finally, childhood septic arthritis of the hip is a special case for a variety of reasons: (a) the process may occur secondary to adjacent metaphyseal osteomyelitis because part of the femoral neck is intraarticular; (b) the mechanism of spread to the joint from the bone will depend on the age of the patient because the vascular anatomy changes with age; (c) a rapid build-up of articular pressure can cause bone and cartilage destruction as well as secondary avascular necrosis of the femoral head; (d) hip pain may be referred to the groin, thigh, buttocks, or knee, causing initial confusion in differential diagnosis and delay in recognition; and (e) there exists an inflammatory condition termed transient synovitis of the hip or "irritable hip" in children, which may be mistaken for septic arthritis.

DIAGNOSIS

Recognition of infection is the key to its management. This is especially true in deeply situated axial joints such as the hip, shoulder, symphysis pubis, and sacroiliac where treatment is often delayed because inflammation is clinically masked and the problem is ascribed to noninfectious causes.

Imaging studies are notoriously unreliable in the initial stages of a septic joint and usually will not be able to distinguish among the various inflammatory causes of an acute arthritis. Changes in the conventional plain radiograph and computerized tomography scan lag behind the process, although they may be helpful in establishing a baseline for further comparisons. A magnetic resonance imaging (MRI) scan will be able to differentiate among muscles, fibrous structures, and blood vessels in the early stages of inflammation and add to the precision with which extensions of infection can be identified, although specificity for infection is not possible.

Scintigraphic studies using technetium or gallium are positive in early stages of infection and may be useful in evaluating deeper structures such as the spine, hip, and shoulder for the presence of an abnormality. However, inflammatory conditions of any kind, as well as some degenerative processes, may give similar images. Further, we do not have a clear idea of the correlation between the image and the putative physiologic process, such as blood flow, bone formation, and bone resorption. It is possible that the variability in studies examining the sensitivity and specificity of scanning may be due to the timing of the procedure in what is clearly a dynamic process. However, scintigraphy does appear to be able to distinguish between underlying articular and overlying soft-tissue inflammation.

Principles of Diagnosis

It is clear that the time-honored, traditional "index of suspicion" remains the most important diagnostic tool for septic arthritis. In the 21st century, this axiom may even be more important because the classic concept of a patient with a septic joint is changing. More often today, the patients will be elderly, with minimal signs or symptoms of inflammation. They often are immunocompromised, possess multiple infected joints, and have synovial fluid total white cell counts far less than the typical 100,000/mm^3 or even less than 50,000/mm^3. The importance of the synovial fluid examination is summarized in Table 125.3.

A number of attempts have been made in the past decade to establish the utility of clinical findings, ancillary laboratory tests, and synovial fluid analyses in the correct diagnosis of septic arthritis. In 72 patients with septic arthritis, the peripheral blood leukocyte count was normal in 55% of the patients, and in 13% of cases, the erythrocyte sedimentation rate (ESR) was less than 20 mm/h (13). However, blood leukocytosis, sedimentation rate, and synovial fluid leukocytosis are extremely variable in septic arthritis, as seen in Fig. 125.1. The presence of fever and rigors is even less sensitive; frequencies of temperature greater than 38°C have been reported in as few as 40% of patients with septic arthritis (Fig. 125.2). In children with hip pain and a differential diagnosis between septic hip and transient synovitis, an ESR greater than 20 mm/h or a body temperature greater than 37.5°C correctly identified 97% of the cases of septic arthritis with a false-positivity rate of 47% (39). It is a reasonable conclusion that all children with an "irritable" hip who have an elevated ESR or a temperature greater than 37.5°C should have the hip aspirated for culture and sensitivity.

If the gold standard remains the culture of synovial fluid, and the platinum standard is a synovial biopsy for culture (although rarely used, except for fungal or mycobacterial disease), the silver standard has been the synovial fluid white blood cell count and percentage of polymorphonuclear leukocytes. Traditionally we have taught residents and

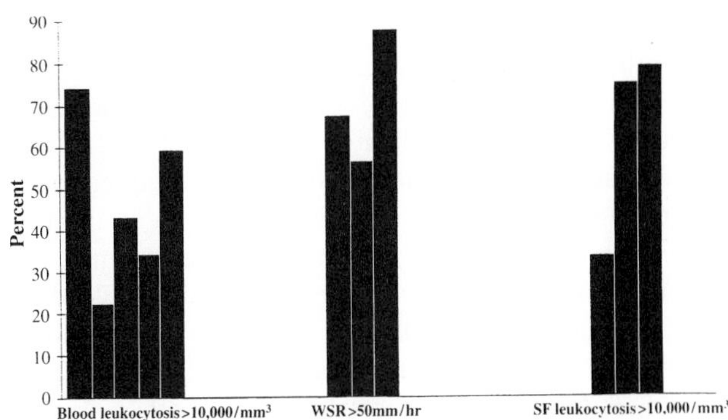

FIGURE 125.1. Reported frequencies of leukocytosis and increased sedimentation in septic arthritis. (Reproduced and adapted from Pioro MH, Mandell BF. Septic arthritis. *Rheum Dis Clin North Am* 1997;23:239–258, with permission.)

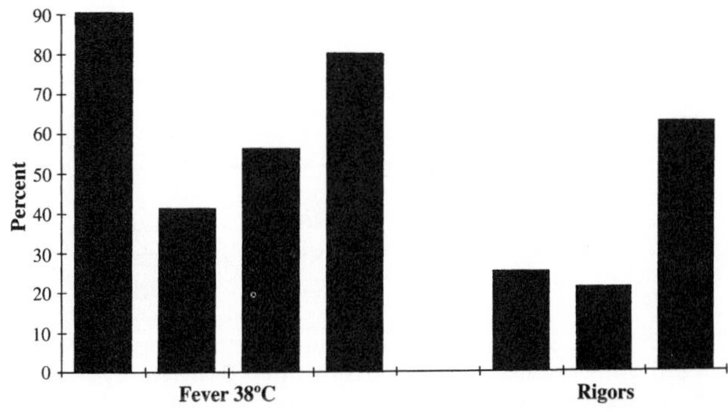

FIGURE 125.2. Reported frequencies of fever and rigors in septic arthritis. (Reproduced and adapted from Pioro MH, Mandell BF. Septic arthritis. *Rheum Dis Clin North Am* 1997;23:239–258, with permission.)

TABLE 125.3. JOINT FLUID EXAMINATION: THE SEVEN DEADLY SINS OF OMISSION AND COMMISSION

1. Never defer aspiration and examination of joint fluid once infection is considered
2. The needle should be introduced through clinically uninvolved skin and subcutaneous tissue
3. The old-fashioned method of using dilute acetic acid to lyse red cells in a hemocytometer may falsely reduce synovial fluid white blood cell counts because of trapping of cells by coagulated hyaluronate
4. If it is uncertain that the fluid is blood or bloody synovial fluid, perform a Ropes' test: drop the fluid in dilute acetic acid. If it clumps, it contains hyaluronate; if it disperses, it is blood
5. Synovial fluid lactate, glucose, pH, and complement studies do not differentiate infection from other inflammatory conditions. A culture does this
6. We have been taught in the past that the higher the synovial fluid white blood cell (WBC) count and the greater the percentage of polymorphonuclear cells, the more likely the process is infectious. This may no longer be true. The diagnostic value of the synovial fluid leukocyte count in an individual case is poor. Counts <50,000/mm^3 and even <25,000/mm^3 are commonly seen in infectious arthritis
7. Crystals and infection may coexist in the same joint. Finding crystals does not rule out an infectious process. A culture will do that

primary care physicians according to the maxim that the higher the synovial white cell count, the more likely that the joint is infected. Given the concept of "pseudoseptic" arthritis (to be discussed later), the very large overlap between infected and noninfected synovial fluid leukocyte counts (Fig. 125.3) (40), and the apparent decrease in mean synovial fluid white blood cell counts in recent times, this statement may be not only incorrect, but also misleading. In 1990, Shmerling et al. (41) evaluated the diagnostic importance of synovial fluid chemistries (lactate, glucose, protein, etc.) and found them lacking in both sensitivity and specificity, confirming clinical experience.

However, a fundamental change that has occurred in the last decade is a revised notion of what a typical synovial fluid white cell count is in a septic joint. In the 1950s, Ropes and Bauer (42) published their guidelines for the separation between infectious and inflammatory synovial white blood cell counts; their threshold was close to 50,000 cells/mm^3. Their classic treatise described 29 fluids in patients with "specific infectious arthritis-positive culture" containing a mean total leukocyte count of 73,370 cells/mm^3 with a range from 7,800 to 266,000. When this was reexamined in the late 1970s by Krey and Bailen (43), 30% of their patients with septic arthritis had counts less than 50,000 cells/mm^3 (Fig. 125.4), although the percentage of polymorphonuclear leukocytes was always more than 90%. When Krey and Bailen examined these same patients by repeated aspirations over several days, large increases in synovial white cell counts were noted in the infected patients compared with stability in the chronic inflammatory cases, further adding to the separation (Table 125.4). A more recent study of synovial fluid leukocytosis in bacterial and other forms of arthritis revealed mean leukocyte counts of 36,000/mm^3 in bacterial arthritis compared with 28,800/mm^3 in probable bacterial arthritis, 19,000/mm^3 in reactive arthritis, and 12,300/mm^3 in RA (44). In patients with RA and a septic joint, the median white blood cell count was 118,600/mm^3. By 1992, 40 years later, the reported mean synovial fluid leukocyte count in septic arthritis has decreased from the original 73,370 cells/mm^3 of Ropes and Bauer to 36,000 cells/mm^3 in the most recent series (44).

The culture establishes the presence of an infected joint. In situations in which the culture is negative (as in a patient already taking antibiotics), the diagnosis is a clinical one,

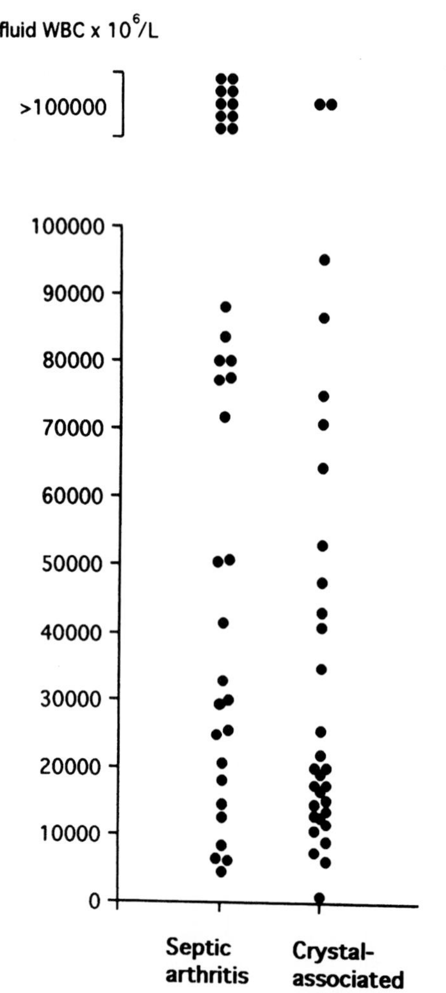

FIGURE 125.3. Synovial fluid leukocyte counts in septic arthritis (n = 33) and crystal-associated arthritis (n = 31). Twenty-six percent of patients with crystal-associated arthritis had counts greater than 50,000 × 10^3/mL. (Reproduced from Söderquist B, Jones I, Fredlund H, et al. Bacterial or crystal-associated arthritis? Discriminating ability of serum inflammatory markers. *Scand J Infect Dis* 1998:30:591–596, with permission.)

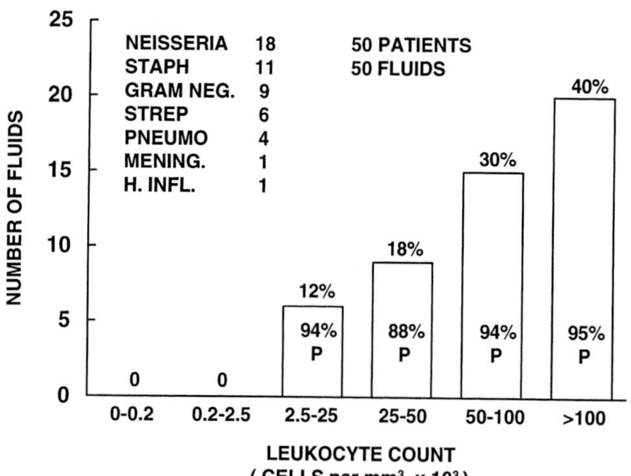

FIGURE 125.4. Synovial fluid leukocyte counts in cases with septic arthritis. These fluids are grouped by synovial fluid leukocyte count per cubic millimeter × 10^3. P, Percentage of polymorphonuclear leukocytes. Thirty percent of fluids had total leukocyte counts less than 50,000/mm^3, and 30% were between 50,000 and 100,000/mm^3. (Reproduced and adapted from Krey PR, Bailen DA. Synovial fluid leukocytosis. *Am J Med* 1979;67:436–442, with permission.)

TABLE 125.4. SEQUENTIAL LEUKOCYTE COUNTS AT THE TIME OF REPEATED ARTHROCENTESIS IN 20 PATIENTS WITH VARIOUS DIAGNOSES, ILLUSTRATING THE INCREASES IN SEPTIC ARTHRITIS COMPARED WITH RELATIVE STABILITY IN NONINFECTIOUS INFLAMMATORY CONDITIONS

	Leukocyte Count/mm^3		
Case No.	From	To	Interval in Days
Infectious arthritis[a]			
1 (*pneumococcus*)	12,900	59,000	1
2 (*gonococcus*)	8,100	31,000	2
3 (*gonococcus*)	61,700	80,000	0.5
4 (*streptococcus*)	153,000	300,000	2
5 (*Escherichia coli*)[b]	71,800	220,000	7
Gout			
6	2,000	3,500	1
7	16,100	16,600	3
8	31,800	9,800	2
9	4,600	15,500	4
10	28,500	1,100	6
Pseudogout			
11	3,500	4,600	1
12	29,600	10,000	2
13	13,900	9,500	2
14	54,500	5,000	4
15	75,000	35,000	2
Rheumatoid arthritis			
16	19,100	26,300	2
17	6,000	9,000	2
18	8,200	9,800	2
19	11,000	7,600	3
20	13,700	33,000	5

[a]Before antibiotic treatment, except [b].
Adapted from Krey PR, Bailen DA. Synovial fluid leukocytosis. *Am J Med* 1979;67:436–442, with permission.

and the patient is treated as if he or she has the disease, according to principles enumerated later and discussed in more detail in Chapter 126. Goldenberg (4) noted that the synovial fluid culture is positive in 90% of cases of nongonococcal bacterial arthritis and 50% of those of gonococcal arthritis; the Gram stains are positive in only 50% and 25%, respectively. Blood cultures are positive in 50% to 70% of patients with nongonococcal bacterial arthritis (12). Genitourinary cultures are positive in 70% to 90% of patients with disseminated gonococcal infection. The reported frequencies of positive synovial or blood cultures vary according to the organisms involved, as seen in Table 125.5. A common misconception in diagnosing septic arthritis is to assume that a positive blood culture with culture-negative synovial fluid establishes the diagnosis. As Kortekangas et al. (45) pointed out, this is not necessarily

TABLE 125.5. REPORTED FREQUENCIES OF POSITIVE SYNOVIAL FLUID AND BLOOD GRAM STAIN AND CULTURES, BY ORGANISM

Organism	Positive Synovial Fluid Gram Stain (%)	Positive Synovial Fluid Cultures (%)	Positive Blood Cultures (%)
Nongonococcal arthritis	11–80	66–95	24–76
Bacteria			
Gram-positive	75–80	—	—
Gram-negative	50–58	—	—
Neisseria gonorrheae	25–30	25–50	10–50

Reproduced and adapted from Pioro MH, Mandell BF. Septic arthritis. *Rheum Dis Clin North Am* 1997;23:239–258, with permission.

correct because most bacteremic patients do not get arthritis of any kind (as only 1% of patients symptomatic with *S. aureus* bacteremia get septic arthritis). In an attempt to justify routine cultures of synovial fluid, or perhaps to discover occult infection, two recent large-scale audits in Britain and Scotland showed that the routine culture of synovial fluid is unnecessary if septic arthritis is not clinically suspected (46,47). In an attempt to increase the yield of true-positive cultures and specifically to examine whether certain blood-culture methods contributed to a microbiologic diagnosis, Kortekangas et al. (45) examined three different culture approaches in 90 patients; they concluded that the choice of culture method was not critical. In patients already taking antibiotics, though, synovial fluid culture in blood-culture bottles has been shown to be superior to culture in conventional solid media (48). Polymerase chain reaction (PCR) increases the yield in culture-negative, clinical *Neisseria gonorrheae* infection; however, the practical clinical utility of this method remains to be established (49,50). A recent report of a patient with RA and prosthetic knee joints casts further questions on the clinical use of PCR; the patient had *S. aureus* DNA detected by PCR from his knee joints even after 10 weeks of therapy, despite adequate antibiotic treatment and a sterile synovial fluid (51).

The finding of crystals in a joint or the presence of chondrocalcinosis on radiographs should not dissuade the clinician from the diagnosis of septic arthritis. The coexistence of crystal disease and septic arthritis has been reported in 31 case reports published in the English literature since 1969 (52). Experimental animal studies propose a mechanism for this coexistence; infection in a joint lowers the pH and raises the intraarticular temperature, factors that decrease the solubility of urate and favor the precipitation of urate crystals (53).

Imaging Studies

Radiographic studies have a limited role at the time of the initial diagnosis of septic arthritis because of the lag time required to yield an image demonstrating damage to hard tissues. Contrast arthrography at the time of diagnostic aspiration has important utility because of its role in confirming the position of the needle with respect to the joint (54). Scintigraphy may be useful in identifying a "hot" joint that is deep or clinically inaccessible such as the hip or sacroiliac, but specificity is lacking and, in addition, there may be false negatives at times for no apparent reason. A study comparing the use of technetium-99m with positive synovial fluid culture reported a sensitivity of 100% and specificity of 85% (55).

It is clear that one should make a diagnosis and certainly begin treatment well before the plain radiograph reveals any features of septic arthritis. However, if there is a substantial delay in recognition of a septic joint, patients may have radiographic features of infection on the plain film. Resnick and Niwayama (56) have stressed that the indistinct margins of erosions and the poorly defined nature of the bony destruction are the most characteristic aspects of a septic process. In contrast, erosions or cysts that appear in gout, RA, OA, and calcium pyrophosphate deposition disease are sharply marginated. In Table 125.6, indications and limitations to be considered when ordering imaging studies for septic arthritis are summarized (56–58).

TABLE 125.6. INDICATION FOR IMAGING STUDIES AND THEIR LIMITATIONS

1. Plain film: Of all the radiographic features of infection, the poorly defined nature of the bony destruction (the presence of "fuzzy" osseous margins) is most characteristic
2. Computed tomography: This technique will delineate the extent of the osseous and soft tissue processes, especially in areas of complex and overlapping anatomy such as the vertebral column
3. Arthrography: Contrast opacification of the joint will outline the extent of synovial inflammation and delineate the presence of capsular, tendinous, and soft tissue injury. This is especially true for deep or inaccessible joints such as the hip, shoulder, or sacroiliac. Removal of fluid for analysis should take place before injecting any contrast agent
4. Ultrasonography: This technique can detect effusions in the hips of children and in adults. It may be used to detect fluid in superficially located joints, synovial cysts, bursae, and tendon sheaths
5. Scintigraphy: Bone-seeking radiopharmaceutic agents have major diagnostic limitations because of the changing patterns of scintigraphic activity on initial and subsequent images, largely caused by the evolving nature of the process over time
6. Magnetic resonance: This technique appears quite sensitive in the imaging of musculoskeletal processes, but the different choices of MR protocols (such as enhancement and suppression techniques, and contrast agents) are still in a process of evolution and are critical to the specificity and precision of the image. Clearly, the specificity of this technique will continue to improve, and MR will likely replace all existing modalities except for the plain film

Reproduced from Resnick D, Niwayama G. Osteomyelitis, septic arthritis, and soft tissue infection: axial skeleton; mechanisms and situations; organisms. In: Resnick D, ed. *Diagnosis of bone and joint disorders.* Philadelphia: WB Saunders, 1995:2315–2558, with permission.

TREATMENT

Principles of management of patients with septic arthritis are summarized in Table 125.7. It is useful to conceptualize three elements in the initial management of such a patient: (a) choice of antibiotics; (b) method of drainage; and (c) guidelines for monitoring success or failure.

Antibiotics

Treatment with parenteral antibiotics should begin immediately when a septic joint is suspected and continue well past initial clinical improvement, although there are no controlled studies that have established exactly how long this should be. Guidelines have been suggested for duration of parenteral antibiotic therapy in uncomplicated cases, recognizing the large variability in prognostic factors from patient to patient: 2 weeks for *H. influenzae, Streptococcus,* or gram-negative cocci, and 3 weeks for *Staphylococcus* and gram-negative bacilli. These guidelines are quite reasonable and appear standard across many sources (59).

The duration of treatment may be confused by the presence of postinfectious synovitis, a culture-negative inflammatory synovitis lasting days to weeks after the joint is sterile. This phenomenon is thought to result from residual microbial products still present in either the joint cavity or the synovial membrane. Although this entity has not been formally studied, it is recognized by experienced clinicians. It can be safely treated with nonsteroidal antiinflammatory agents.

The choice of initial antibiotic coverage should be guided primarily by host factors such as the age of the patient, the presumed source of the infection, the patient's own infection profile and experience with certain organisms, and the presence of immunosuppression. Cost and availability specific to an institution formulary also play a role. Culture results and sensitivity testing will guide changes in therapy. The reader should consult Chapter 126 as well as recent reviews (60,61) for a more detailed discussion of choice of antibiotics in specific situations. However, recent published guidelines (59) have general applicability:

1. Initial therapy should consist of a cephalosporin or semisynthetic penicillin to cover gram-positive cocci including staphylococci.
2. If the patient is allergic to penicillin, vancomycin or clindamycin can be used.
3. Infections of the hand after human or animal bites should be treated with antibiotics that cover mouth flora.
4. Initial therapy for suspected gram-negative bacteria should include a third-generation cephalosporin, adjusted later for culture results and susceptibility testing.

Although the clinical presentation of *Neisseria gonorrheae* arthritis has not changed recently, the frequency of penicillin resistance has reached clinical significance. In a review of 41 cases of gonococcal arthritis occurring from 1985 to 1991, Wise et al. (62) found penicillin resistance in 5% of isolates. Therefore the correct recommendations for a case of suspected gonococcal arthritis should consist of a third-generation cephalosporin as the initial agent of choice until sensitivities are known.

Antibiotic-Delivery Systems

With the advent of simpler parenteral antibiotic-delivery systems and the increasing use of home healthcare, hospitalization is not an absolute requirement for the treatment

TABLE 125.7. PRINCIPLES OF ANTIBIOTIC TREATMENT OF INFECTIOUS ARTHRITIS

1. Treatment with parenteral antibiotics should begin immediately when a septic joint is suspected. The choice of antibiotic should be based on the patient's age and the suspected pathogenetic organism. Changes can be made later when cultures are available. There is no role for direct instillation of antibiotics into the joint
2. Parenteral antibiotics should be maintained until clinical signs of infection improve and synovial white blood cell (WBC) counts revert toward normal. With at-home parenteral therapy available, hospitalization is not always required
3. A rapid decrease or progressive decline in synovial fluid leukocyte count and sterility on culture suggests control of the infection. The converse means that there is a need to reassess the choice of antibiotic, the method of drainage, or both
4. There is a wide variation in the treatment response time for patients with a septic joint. Causes for this variation include the type of organism, specific host factors such as an underlying comorbid condition, the particular joint involved, and the promptness with which therapy had been instituted. Two weeks' duration of parenteral antibiotic therapy is the "rule of thumb" for the usual uncomplicated septic joint in a normal host; however, the treatment period may last ≤6 weeks. The role of oral antibiotics as a follow-on to parenteral treatment has not been examined critically
5. Postinfectious synovitis, a persistent inflammatory response likely caused by residual microbial products in the synovial membrane or the joint cavity, may lead to confusion about adequacy of antibiotic treatment or treatment duration. This condition can be safely treated with nonsteroidal antiinflammatory agents

of patients with septic arthritis once all of the other therapeutic principles (adequate drainage, mobilization, pain control) are met. Mauceri et al. (63) reported an 83% success rate in 18 patients with a computer-controlled pump system compared with success rates of 83% to 86% for inpatients treated conventionally. These patients had a variety of bone and joint infections with six older than 60 years, and two of the six diabetic. Five of the six high-risk patients did extremely well. The published results of the use of orally administered antibiotics in septic arthritis are quite limited, and there simply are not enough data to assess this mode of antibiotic delivery critically.

Prophylaxis and Prevention of Prosthetic Joint Infections

With respect to dental procedures that are considered routine, prosthetic joints have not been identified as high risk compared weith prosthetic cardiac valves; guidelines for prophylaxis of cardiac valves have been published (64). Both the American Dental Association and the Academy of Oral Medicine have stated that there is little evidence to support an increased risk of prosthetic joint infection with common dental procedures (65). Nevertheless, most practitioners appear to treat patients with prosthetic joints as they would treat patients with artificial cardiac valves. In a nationwide survey of 1,666 orthopedic surgeons published in 1985, 57% of the respondents did not believe that there was a relation between transient bacteremia from dental procedures and prosthetic joint infections. Nevertheless, 93% of these same respondents, in their practice, recommended that antibiotic prophylaxis be given to patients with prosthetic joints undergoing dental procedures (65). Bacteremia, if documented or strongly suspected by signs or symptoms, most assuredly deserves aggressive antibiotic therapy in patients with prosthetic joints. This was amply illustrated in two patients in whom septic arthritis developed in their prosthetic joints 7 and 10 months after documented bacteremia occurring in association with an extraarticular infection; in one of these patients, transient joint pain occurred in the prosthetic joint at the time of the bacteremia (66).

Treatment of Infected Prosthetic Joints

Treatment of infected prosthetic joints in the 21st century remains an ordeal for the patient and a nightmare for the orthopedic surgeon. The literature seems quite clear on this subject; the best results seem to come from aggressive resection arthroplasties and reimplantation. In a retrospective review of 24 infected total knee arthroplasties, Ivey et al. (67) observed that in only three of 10 knees treated conservatively at the outset with debridement and antibiotics was the infection controlled; complete control of the infection was achieved in 13 of 13 knees treated initially with resection arthroplasty. In all of these cases, treatment with antibiotics was begun within 1 week of the onset of symptoms, and the results were not influenced by whether the infections were considered early or late. Ivey et al. stated, with apparently good justification, that resection arthroplasty is the most reliable treatment option for infection control, but that an unstable, painful joint will result. Reimplantation appears to be the best subsequent management option for pain-free ambulation. Further support for this suggestion comes from the observations of Tsukayama et al. (68); 13 instances of chronic prosthetic joint infections were treated with debridement and long-term parenteral antibiotics followed by oral antibiotics. Only three patients were able to retain their prostheses with this approach. These authors emphasized the frequent and disabling adverse reactions that occurred with long-term antibiotics; 38% of patients experienced events that led to changes in antibiotic regimens. Furthermore, Peters et al. (13) looked at nine patients with 11 infected prosthetic joints, four with removal before initiation of antibiotics, and the other five with seven infected prosthetic joints receiving treatment with long-term antibiotics; all five patients had relapse of bacterial arthritis within 10 days of stopping therapy successfully administered for 6 to 24 months.

Drainage of Infected Joints

There is established consensus as well as intuitive reasoning that drainage of an infected joint space will speed healing and permit antibiotics to be effective. It is less clear, however, what factors mediate the response to the drainage: is it reduction in pressure, removal of fluid, break-up of adhesions and loculations, or combinations thereof? Further, it is not known if the primary or the secondary location of infection (the synovium, synovial fluid, cartilage, or subchondral bone) is the rate-limiting step in the healing process. Each of these questions and the absence of answers fuel an ongoing debate (and sometimes disagreement) between rheumatologists and orthopedic surgeons: what is the proper method of initial drainage of an infected joint, what are the guidelines for moving on from a conservative to an operative approach, and which operative approach should be undertaken? In the absence of definitive answers from controlled clinical trials, information from relevant case series, expert opinion and consensus, and animal studies contribute to the basis of current practice.

There are advantages and disadvantages to both medical and surgical approaches, and these issues should be weighed in each decision. It is generally agreed that surgical drainage is indicated in septic arthritis of the hip (especially in children), poorly accessible joints (e.g., sacroiliac and sternoclavicular) that are difficult to monitor for adequacy of drainage, suspected soft-tissue extension of infection, and inadequate clinical response to antibiotic therapy after 5 to

TABLE 125.8. GUIDELINES FOR INITIAL SURGICAL DRAINAGE OF SEPTIC JOINTS

Children with a septic hip, to avoid rapid build up of pressure and compromise to the vascular supply of the femoral head

Joints that are deeply situated or difficult to drain repeatedly with a needle, such as the shoulder, the hip in adults, or the sacroiliac

Extraarticular extension of infection (such as the sternoclavicular or sternomanubrial joints)

Infection has been present for some time, and adhesions or secondary osteomyelitis is expected

Septic arthritis is superimposed on rheumatoid arthritis or another underlying joint disease

7 days (Table 125.8). If there is little or no clinical improvement during the initial 5 to 7 days of parenteral antibiotics and needle drainage, as gauged by evaluation of serial synovial fluid leukocyte counts and cultures, the efficacy of the ongoing antibiotic and drainage regimen should be questioned and reevaluated. This scenario usually means that drainage is not adequate, and a surgical approach should be considered. From the seminal series of 59 patients with nongonococcal septic arthritis published by Goldenberg and Cohen in 1976 (69), the demonstration of a significant decrease in serial synovial fluid leukocyte counts between days 5 and 7 in those patients with eventual recovery remains a landmark observation (Table 125.9). Surgical drainage also should be considered when a previously damaged (e.g., rheumatoid) joint becomes infected, because the data on infected rheumatoid joints indicate a particularly poor outcome with medical therapy (11).

Although no truly controlled study has been performed and only case observations are available for assistance, no series has demonstrated an advantage of initial open arthrotomy over deferred open arthrotomy drainage in the uncomplicated case. Conversely, there are distinct advantages of closed needle drainage over open arthrotomy—serial synovial leukocyte counts can be performed, as well as serial cultures, to guide assessment of treatment adequacy. Additionally, a closed-space infection from a community-acquired organism will not be turned into an open surgical wound with the possibility of a secondary wound infection caused by hospital-acquired organisms. Once the joint is approached surgically, it is often unclear how much tissue to remove or how to continue to drain the joint once the initial adhesions are lysed. Finally, the issue of medical versus surgical management is now even more complicated with the advent of an aggressive medical (tidal irrigation) and a less morbid surgical (arthroscopy) approach to drainage.

TABLE 125.9. SERIAL CHANGES IN SYNOVIAL FLUID LEUKOCYTE COUNT

	Mean Leukocyte Count (cells/mm^3)	
Hospital Day	Complete Recovery	Poor Outcome
1	86,000 (38)	88,000 (12)
3	56,000	68,000 (8)
5	32,000 (16)	59,000 (8)
7	20,000 (12)	55,000 (6)
9	4,800 (8)	60,000 (3)
12	1,700 (3)	57,000 (2)

Compares patients with eventual complete recovery with those with poor results. A substantial decrease is demonstrated by 5 days; however, 5 to 7 days is the usual benchmark for success.
Figures in parentheses indicate number of synovial fluid specimens.
Adapted from Goldenberg DL, Cohen AS. Active infectious arthritis. *Am J Med* 1976;60:369–377, with permission.

Tidal Irrigation

Repeated irrigation and distention of a joint at the bedside, with saline under local anesthesia, has been described by Ike (70) in a series of 11 septic knees that were treated after needle aspirations no longer contained purulent material. Under normal circumstances, it could be assumed that these 11 cases would have gone directly to arthrotomy. Instead, four of 11 did not require surgery and responded to tidal irrigation alone. Predictors of a good response to irrigation were a decrease in synovial fluid leukocyte count (>25%) or decrease in synovial fluid volume (>50%) after the first irrigation. The patients who did not respond to irrigation and went to surgery had extensive adhesions and synovitis. Although Ike's observations are uncontrolled, it does seem reasonable to assume that tidal irrigation can be added to medical therapy and potentially avoid an unnecessary operation in selected cases. The success of the procedure also appears to be operator dependent and time consuming; additional experience in the knee as well as in other joints is needed to assess the proper role for tidal irrigation.

Arthroscopy

Arthroscopy has almost completely replaced open arthrotomy as the treatment of choice for exploring the infected joint, lavaging its contents, and removing detritus. Surgical and medical morbidity is lower, and the procedure can be repeated. However, technical advances will be necessary to bring this procedure beyond its current utility for larger joints. There have been no direct comparisons between arthroscopy and open arthrotomy for drainage of an infected joint. It is unlikely that there will ever be a clinical trial, because arthroscopy has become an accepted mode of treatment in anticipation of data. Parisien and Shaffer (71) reviewed 16 patients with septic arthritis (of 13 knees, two shoulders, and one ankle) treated arthroscopically during the period 1976 to 1987. None of the patients was given a trial of conservative medical treatment, and all were treated within a few days from the onset of symptoms. The patients appeared to do well, although we do not know what would have happened with an alternate approach. The outcome measures were not explicitly stated, and it is difficult to follow all of the patients described in the report. It is not possible to determine from this study how to drain these arthroscopically treated joints after the initial procedure has been conducted. More information is needed, especially regarding joints other than the knee.

Lane et al. (72) have cast doubt on the initial conservative management of septic arthritis of the knee. Needle drainage was not successful as the only mode of drainage in patients with specific risk factors such as a delay in treatment greater than 3 days, underlying illnesses, and infection with either *S. aureus* or gram-negative enteric organisms. Lane et al. used formal arthrotomy with incision and drainage; six knees treated primarily with open drainage had successful resolution of the infection. The 23 knees for which repeated closed aspiration failed had to be managed by secondary incision and drainage. Although Lane et al. recognized the role of arthroscopy in the treatment of septic arthritis of the knee, they thought that the presence of loculations, adhesions, and thick viscous fluid make debridement difficult and less likely to be successful with arthroscopy. This view is not shared by Jackson (73) from Baylor University, who has stated that the arthroscope, or "minimally invasive surgery," is quite successful in debriding necrotic tissue, draining purulent material, and breaking down loculations. Additionally, the arthroscope provides a mechanism for repeated distention and irrigation of the joint with sterile saline, akin to tidal irrigation.

Given the controversy and the lack of data to support a definitive position about which drainage procedure to use and when to use it, such decisions must be guided by clinical judgment and a patient-centered approach. Ho (74) examined the four drainage approaches available: needle aspiration, tidal irrigation, arthroscopy, and arthrotomy. These techniques represent a continuum or a spectrum of approaches, and their use should be guided by the known prognostic factors for a poor outcome in septic arthritis. The young healthy person with gonococcal arthritis should be managed with aspiration and antibiotics alone, and the RA patient with a delay in diagnosis, multiple joint sepsis, and an infected hip should proceed to arthrotomy. Further study must determine the proper role of tidal irrigation. Arthroscopy avoids many of the morbidities associated with open incision and drainage, yet not all joints are accessible. Ho stated explicitly that open, formal arthrotomy will continue to be needed infrequently in the management of patients with septic arthritis, reserving its role for urgent decompression because of compromised blood supply, joints inaccessible to other means of drainage, the possibility of osteomyelitis, or when other means of drainage have failed to eradicate the infection.

Finally, a goat model of septic arthritis with *S. aureus* was developed to determine if antibiotics alone or in combination with arthroscopy, arthroscopy with debridement, arthrotomy, or needle drainage was more effective in eradicating infection and preventing damage (assessed by biochemical–histologic ratings). The investigators found indistinguishable results in all five treatment arms, including antibiotics alone. The authors concluded that if infection is treated early with antibiotics, all drainage modalities (including none) result in minimal damage to the cartilage (75). However, it seems clear that the model was not very sensitive to change, as the control arm (antibiotics alone) showed only minimal damage. Additional studies are needed with an animal model that provides an assay system more relevant to human disease.

OUTCOME IN SEPTIC ARTHRITIS

It remains unexplained and paradoxic that the outcome in patients with septic arthritis has not changed over the past two decades. Analogous to the situation with septic shock, the number of patients who die and the number of joints that sustain permanent damage are remarkably stable in spite of advances in medical technology, therapeutics, and diagnostic skill and accuracy. Who are the patients that continue to have a poor outcome? As in the past, patients with a poor outcome experience a delay in diagnosis, often have polyarticular septic arthritis, possess positive blood cultures, and have RA as an underlying disease.

In two recent large surveys, the mortality rate for septic arthritis was 10%, and morbidity (defined as osteomyelitis and poor functional outcome) was 31% (10,13). Multivariate risk factors for morbidity were identified as age older than 65 years, diabetes mellitus, surgery, and infection with gram-positive bacteria; risk factors for mortality were identified as age younger than 65 years, confusion, and polyarticular septic arthritis. Open surgical drainage was associated with reduced mortality compared with medical management in this study; however, in the absence of randomization, it is not possible to determine whether the patients taken to surgery were overall healthier than those managed medically. In a recent prospective Dutch community survey of 154 patients with 174 septic joints, half with preexisting joint disease, and a third with synthetic joints monitored over a 2-year period, 21% of patients had a poor outcome (defined as death or severe overall functional deterioration), and 33% of joints had a poor outcome (amputation, arthrodesis, prosthetic surgery, or severe functional deterioration). Older age, preexisting joint disease, and the presence of synthetic joint material were poor prognostic factors. There was no association in this study of poor outcome with *S. aureus* infection, treatment delay, or polyarticular disease (11).

Pioro (5), in her review, wrote, "Septic arthritis in rheumatoid arthritis patients has a significantly worse outcome than in non–rheumatoid arthritis patients. Mortality and morbidity rates have remained unchanged in the past 40 years." Mortality rates for RA patients with monoarticular infection are 15% to 22% and 47% to 56% with polyarticular septic arthritis. Functional outcome also is poor, with 33% to 35% of RA patients achieving complete recovery of the infected joint compared with 70% in the general population. A retrospective review of 181 RA patients reported 16% to 22% of patients had recurrence of infection in nonprosthetic joints (76).

Traditionally in nonpolyarticular septic arthritis cases, the delay in initiating treatment remains an important factor in determining outcome, as it has for the past 20 years. Studahl et al. (77), by using a standardized scoring system to assess long-term results 2 to 11 years after the acute event in 65 septic knees, noted that treatment delay longer than 5 days was associated with significant mobility loss superimposed on a background of 79% good to excellent long-term results. From a retrospective review of 72 adults with septic arthritis, if a diagnosis was made and treatment initiated at a mean of 10 days from the onset of symptoms, there was little or no deterioration in joint function, compared with a mean of 30 days, in which case, there invariably was severe deterioration (13). Although half of the cases were patients who had RA, patients with such preexisting joint disease had the same functional outcome as those without it. A mean of 10 days' disease duration before treatment appears to be longer than expected for patients with a good outcome. These authors pointed out that the primary focus of infection appears to be the skin; they recommend aggressive antibiotic treatment of RA patients with skin infections, especially if infections occur on the legs or feet. In RA, the relation between septic arthritis with staphylococci and skin infections, polyarticular presentation, delay in diagnosis, and poor prognosis appears to be a theme that is interwoven in many series and reports (76).

Polyarticular Septic Arthritis

Supporting evidence for the concept of polyarticular septic arthritis as an important clinical entity with a poor prognosis comes from Yu et al. (78), who retrospectively reviewed 230 adult patients with nongonococcal septic arthritis from 1985 to 1989. The major predictor of mortality was a polyarticular presentation. If patients had four or more joints involved, all died. Additional factors affecting mortality were small-joint involvement and positive blood cultures. Duration of disease before initiation of therapy was not an independent factor altering prognosis. Pitkin and Eykyn (79) emphasized that the lack of joint signs and the prominent systemic features in polyarticular septic arthritis may contribute to a delay in diagnosis; they reported 100% mortality in six cases of RA with multifocal staphylococcal arthritis. These patients did not have overt signs of joint inflammation. Many joints were frankly purulent even when they appeared clinically unaffected. Twenty-five cases of polyarticular septic arthritis, observed over a period of 13 years, were retrospectively reviewed, compared with previously described cases, and contrasted to 95 cases of monoarticular arthritis seen in the same hospital (8). Their characteristics are presented in Table 125.10. Many of these patients had associated infected skin nodules and ulcers. Polyarticular septic arthritis represented 16.6% of septic arthritis from the same hospital, compared with 15% on average in the literature. The outcome of polyarticular septic arthritis was poor; 32% died compared with 31% to 42% of polyarticular septic arthritis cases from previous series reported in the literature and 4% among cases of monoarticular septic arthritis. The investigators noted, once again, the paradoxic situation of a death rate exactly the same as it was 40 years ago, a phenomenon that could not be explained by a different distribution of bacterial species. Death occurred in four of 11 patients with *S. aureus* polyarticular septic arthritis and RA and in three of nine cases of *S. aureus* polyarticular septic arthritis without RA. These authors noted that the prognosis of monoarticular septic arthritis in association with RA has improved over the past 20 years (death rate

TABLE 125.10. CHARACTERISTICS OF 25 CASES OF POLYARTICULAR SEPTIC ARTHRITIS

Male predominance
Knee the most frequent location, followed by elbow, shoulder, and hip
Average of four joints involved
Causative organisms was *Staphylococcus aureus* in 20 of 25 cases
Blood culture positive in 19 of 22 cases
Fever and severe leukocytosis absent in 10 of 25 cases
Rheumatoid arthritis present in 10 of 25 cases
30% mortality (eight of 25 cases died) compared with 4% in monoarticular cases

Reproduced from Dubost J-J, Fis I, Denis P, et al. Polyarticular septic arthritis. *Medicine* 1993;72:296–310, with permission.

declined from 21% to 12%); however, the mortality for rheumatoid patients with polyarticular septic arthritis remained quite high, up to 50% in some series.

Shoulder

Septic arthritis of the shoulder represents a special situation worth emphasizing because of the difficulty in making a diagnosis in this joint (80,81). A delay in diagnosis is common, leading to poor functional long-term outcome. In a series of 18 septic shoulder cases, only five regained forward flexion to 90 degrees or more after treatment; eight regained no active motion in the glenohumeral joint, and two died. All but one had a delay in diagnosis, and one third were not correctly diagnosed for 1 month or more. The authors pointed out that although pain and diminished motion may be present, few patients have local signs of infection, perhaps leading to alternative noninfectious diagnoses. Intraarticular corticosteroid injections may have contributed to staphylococcal infection in seven of eight patients (81).

DIAGNOSTIC AND THERAPEUTIC DILEMMAS ASSOCIATED WITH SEPTIC ARTHRITIS

Three conditions often pose a problem for the diagnostician and a conundrum to the person directing the therapy because of their resemblance to septic arthritis. Antibiotics are frequently given to these patients, and later an index of suspicion is raised when the patients fail to respond to the antimicrobial therapy or when laboratory results point to other diagnoses. These diagnoses include pseudoseptic arthritis, "reactive" arthritis, and poststreptococcal arthritis. Because of the confusing and overlapping clinical features of each of these conditions with septic arthritis and the controversial nature of treating reactive arthritis with antibiotics, they are discussed in this chapter.

Pseudoseptic Arthritis

Pseudoseptic arthritis occurs in otherwise typical chronic inflammatory polyarthritis, and the synovial cultures are negative. By definition, patients have fever, chills, and a monoarticular arthritis clearly out of proportion to the rest of the joint disease. Call et al. (82) first described this phenomenon in 1985 with RA in which the synovial fluid white blood cell count was greater than 50,000 cells/mm^3; one patient's fluid contained 395,000 cells/mm^3. The fluid differential count contained a predominance of polymorphonuclear cells, ranging from 77% to 97%. Antibiotics were stopped after cultures remained negative, and patients experienced a rapid resolution of their signs and symptoms. The authors proposed that in this clinical setting, one may consider withholding antibiotics if no organisms are seen on smear, no portal of entry is identified on physical examination, and no concomitant infection is present. Singleton et al. (83) suggested that poorly controlled RA or recent discontinuation of a disease-modifying drug usually contributes to this process. Most of their patients had a polyarticular presentation, were taking prednisone, and later improved with an increase in prednisone dosage. An abrupt discontinuation of a corticosteroid was suggested as causal in another case (84). In the Singleton et al. (83) review of 328 cases of RA seen over a 4-year period, pseudoseptic arthritis was more common than septic arthritis; six of the former were seen compared with four of the latter.

Ho has proposed an expansion of the definition of pseudoseptic arthritis to include fever and acute arthritis in a variety of diseases including juvenile rheumatoid arthritis (JRA), crystal deposition diseases, and reactive arthritis (85). The definition could include any acute arthritis (either mono- or polyarthritis) superimposed on a chronic rheumatic disease associated with fever and a synovial fluid leukocytosis of greater than 50,000 cells/mm^3 with a negative bacterial culture. The problem for the clinician is that the patient does not come to the doctor with a known negative synovial fluid culture. Further, it must be reiterated that an increasing proportion of septic arthritis patients are now being seen without fever or chills and possessing synovial fluid white blood cell counts far less than 50,000/mm^3. Even if it is statistically more likely that the patient with fever, chills, and synovial fluid leukocytosis will have pseudoseptic arthritis, it is difficult to justify withholding antibiotics for the 24 to 48 hours necessary to rule out an infectious process. Thus in RA, seronegative spondyloarthropathy, or juvenile-onset RA, if a patient has an equal likelihood of either a septic or a pseudoseptic arthritis, it should be presumed septic until proven otherwise. Fewer serious errors will be made if this rule is followed.

Reactive Arthritis

Most recent published studies related to septic arthritis actually deal with reactive arthritis. Recent studies have evaluated the link between bacterial triggers of reactive arthritis and the arthritis itself, focusing on the transport of microbial antigen from the primary infection site to the joint (86). If the bacteria are in a form that can be eradicated by antimicrobial agents, it is extremely important to determine whether antibiotic therapy can influence the degree of arthritis and the prognosis of the patient. Factors that must be considered to interpret the data regarding antibiotic treatment include the specific offending organism, route of infection, timing and length of treatment, and potential for additional mechanisms of action of the antimicrobials. It would also be extremely interesting to determine whether the extraarticular manifestations of the spondyloarthropathies are influenced by antimicrobial therapy. Many unanswered questions remain—does reactive arthritis represent an autoimmune process or a subclinical or clinically undetectable infectious process; what is the role of molecular mimicry; and how does human leukocyte antigen (HLA)-B27 confer disease susceptibility?

Differences have long been recognized between postenteric- and postgenital-infection reactive arthritis. Prognosis is generally thought to be better after enteric infections than after sexually acquired disease. However, as a recent review by Leirisalo-Repo et al. (87) shows that despite the initial complete resolution noted in at least 80% of postenteric cases, some post–*Salmonella* arthritis becomes chronic or recurrent; only 20% of their cases of inpatient *Salmonella* arthritis were completely normal at a mean of 11 years. Sacroiliitis is a common complication of reactive arthritis; 20% of patients after *Yersinia* and *Shigella* infections developed sacroiliitis after 5 to 10 years, with this being more common in patients with HLA-B27 (88). HLA-B27 does not correlate in this case with the peripheral arthritis found in conjunction with sacroiliitis, as is typical of spondyloarthropathies (89). In another series, the incidence of sacroiliitis in *Chlamydia*-associated arthritis was 33% and 54% in HLA-B27–negative and –positive patients, respectively (90).

Recent reports of finding bacterial particles or DNA have blurred the distinction between reactive arthritis and actual infectious arthritis. Schumacher, in a recent excellent review (91), noted that *Chlamydia* may be viable but difficult to culture from reactive joints, with many published reports of finding antigen, DNA, RNA, and even structures that look like *Chlamydia trachomatis* by electron microscopy in the joint. However, Wilkinson et al. (92) could not correlate *C. trachomatis* DNA presence in the synovial fluid of patients with undifferentiated oligoarthritis (including four with sexually acquired reactive arthritis) with a *Chlamydia*-specific synovial T-cell response or a serologic response; in other words, *C. trachomatis* was detected in approximately 30% of patients with undifferentiated oligoarthritis in synovial fluid. An inverse correlation was found between the detection of *Chlamydia* and specific lymphocyte proliferation, indicating that a weak T-cell response contributes to bacterial persistence. In a series of 411 synovial biopsies and synovial fluid samples, *Chlamydia* DNA was detected in 48 of 98 samples from patients with Reiter's syndrome and reactive arthritis; however, 16 of 75 specimens from RA patients also demonstrated *Chlamydia* DNA (93). PCR has had its most encouraging application in *Chlamydia*-induced arthritis (94,95), although recent reports of positive *Chlamydia* PCR in unexpected clinical circumstances raise again the question of the clinical relevance of such findings (96).

A prospective, placebo-controlled, randomized study of 40 patients treated with short-term (10–14 days) antibiotic therapy early in the course of reactive arthritis was reported by Fryden in 1990 (97). The patients had a variety of enteric infections, and the majority in the treatment group (13 of 20 cases) were positive for *Yersinia*; 58% of all patients were HLA-B27 positive. No difference was observed between treatment and control groups with respect to duration of arthritis, sedimentation rates, or serum antibody levels. In none of the patients did a chronic arthritis develop. An outbreak of *Salmonella* enterocolitis at a radiology symposium allowed an additional observational study of short-term antibiotics in early reactive arthritis (98); 58% of the subjects received short-term (mean, 9.1 days) antibiotics for the enterocolitis. Neither joint symptoms nor duration of arthritis was influenced by antibiotic treatment at the 6-month follow-up point.

The use of antibiotics in reactive arthritis after genitourinary infection may be more effective. In Greenland, 109 Inuit subjects were analyzed retrospectively for episodes of arthritis after antibiotic therapy for urethritis or cervicitis caused by *N. gonorrheae, Chlamydia trachomatis,* or presumed nonspecific urethral infection (99). In patients treated with erythromycin or tetracycline, there were fewer subsequent instances of reactive arthritis compared with untreated or penicillin-treated episodes. The data appear to support the use of antibacterials to prevent the onset and recurrence of reactive arthritis induced by *Chlamydia.* In a more recent double-blind study, 104 patients diagnosed with either reactive arthritis or undifferentiated oligoarthritis were treated for 3 months with 1,000 mg/day of ciprofloxacin or placebo. Ciprofloxacin was not superior to placebo in reactive arthritis or undifferentiated oligoarthritis patients; this also was true for patients in whom enterobacteria could be identified as the triggering bacterium. In contrast, ciprofloxacin seemed to be superior to placebo in patients with *Chlamydia*-induced arthritis; however, this difference was not statistically significant because of the small number of patients in this group (100). A probable beneficial result of antibiotic treatment for *Clamydia*-induced reactive arthritis and nonbeneficial result for enteric-induced reactive arthritis is in line with an earlier study by Lauhio et al. (101), in which longer term (3 months) antibiotic treatment with lymecycline in reactive arthritis induced by *Chlamydia, Yersinia,* or *Campylobacter* was undertaken. There were no differences in outcome between treated and placebo groups; however, when the *Chlamydia*-induced group was analyzed separately, the lymecycline-treated group had 50% recovery at 15 weeks, and all patients recovered by 30 weeks; the placebo group recovered by 40 weeks. These studies support the contention that treatment with tetracyclines shortens the duration of arthritis if triggered by *C. trachomatis.* In contrast, Wollenhaupt et al. (102) did not note an effect of doxycycline therapy over a 4-month period in patients with *Chlamydia*-induced arthritis; the disease duration was longer than 6 months in this investigation. Furthermore, *C. trachomatis* can persist in the synovial membrane despite treatment with adequate antibiotics, as has recently been demonstrated (103). In established, chronic, reactive arthritis, a placebo-controlled trial of a fluoroquinolone administered for 3 months showed no difference between treatment arms; most of the patients had *Yersinia*-induced disease (104).

Poststreptococcal Reactive Arthritis

If indeed there is an entity called poststreptococcal reactive arthritis, it consists of a chronic, recurrent arthritis primarily of the lower extremity, weight-bearing joints (105). The anti-streptolysin O (ASO) titer is elevated, and the disease is readily distinguishable from acute rheumatic fever by its chronicity and the absence of carditis. Gutierrez-Urena (106) described six patients with arthritis, sore throat, elevated ASO titers, and other serologic evidence of streptococcal infection. Skin involvement in three patients proved to be a leukocytoclastic vasculitis. No evidence of cardiac disease was noted. In contrast to acute rheumatic fever, these patients did not respond to high-dose aspirin, and their signs and symptoms lasted from 3 to 6 months. In a recent Dutch study, in a series of 23 patients with a mean age of 42 years, arthritis developed after throat infection with group A β-hemolytic *Streptococcus;* 17% of them had positive throat cultures, and all had increasing titers of ASO and anti-DNAaseB. Thirty percent had erythema nodosum, 22% had erythema multiforme, and none had evidence of carditis. These authors concluded that differentiating characteristics of poststreptococcal arthritis and acute rheumatic fever are older age at onset, female predominance, nonmigratory nature of arthritis, higher frequency of erythema nodosum, and most important, absence of carditis (107). The question of the need for prophylactic penicillin remains unsettled in this group of patients. Using similar reasoning, a Finnish study supported the notion that there may be a symptom complex that is triggered by a streptococcal infection, yet is distinct from acute rheumatic fever (108). These investigators evaluated 76 adult patients admitted to the hospital for an acute arthritis accompanied by an elevated ASO titer (>500 Todd units). Twenty-six had known rheumatic disease, 25 displayed nonspecific arthralgias, 20 had otherwise typical reactive arthritis, and five had septic arthritis; none possessed criteria for acute rheumatic fever. The authors concluded that acute rheumatic fever is rare in this population. However, the interpretation of the meaning of the ASO titer with these conditions is problematic. The authors speculated that a streptococcal infection may trigger a known rheumatic disease. It is safer to conclude that the ASO titer elevation is coincidental because no observations of ASO titers were made in a control or comparative population. Evidence for the existence of a condition called poststreptococcal reactive arthritis distinct from acute rheumatic fever remains unconvincing at this time, and certainly one cannot justify antibiotic prophylaxis in this population.

CONCLUSIONS

For the third millennium, whereas several aspects of septic arthritis remain unchanged from the past, much is different. What remains constant is the concept that the diagnosis and treatment of an infected joint are really the same issue, only viewed in different ways. That is, the single most important factor that determines prognosis is the speed with which the diagnosis is made and treatment initiated. Other issues that remain constant are the presence of *S. aureus* as the most frequent offending organism, and the fact that we still have not resolved the problem of the best way to drain an infected joint. Conversely, the patient with septic arthritis may now be more difficult to diagnose. No longer is it advisable to rely on the synovial fluid white blood cell count to separate infectious from noninfectious causes of acute arthritis. The synovial fluid leukocyte count, on the average, is less than 50,000 cells/mm^3, with many counts less than 25,000 cells/mm^3. Today's patient often has a polyarticular presentation, and in certain subsets (infectious arthritis in RA, for example), polyarticular septic arthritis may be the rule rather than the exception. Finally, and regrettably, what appears to remain the same is the prognosis of the patient, largely based on who gets septic arthritis: patients with immunosuppression, transplanted organs, malignancies, and other serious underlying diseases.

REFERENCES

1. Goldenberg DL. Bacterial arthritis. *Curr Opin Rheumatol* 1994; 6:394–400.
2. Goldenberg DL. Bacterial arthritis. *Curr Opin Rheumatol* 1995; 7:310–314.
3. Javors JM, Weisman MH. Principles of diagnosis and treatment of joint infections. In: Koopman WJ, ed. *Arthritis and allied conditions.* Philadelphia: Lea & Febiger, 1997:2253–2266.
4. Goldenberg DL. Septic arthritis. *Lancet* 1998;351:197–202.
5. Pioro MH, Mandell BF. Septic arthritis. *Rheum Dis Clin North Am* 1997;23:239–258.
6. Kaandorp CJE, Dinant HJ, van de Laar MAFJ, et al. Incidence and sources of native and prosthetic joint infection: a community based prospective survey. *Ann Rheum Dis* 1997;56:470–475.
7. Morgan DS, Fisher D, Merianos A, et al. An 18 year clinical review of septic arthritis from tropical Australia. *Epidemiol Infect* 1996;117:423–428.
8. Dubost JJ, Fis I, Denis P, et al. Polyarticular septic arthritis. *Medicine* 1993;72:296–310.
9. Epstein JH, Zimmermann B, Ho G. Polyarticular septic arthritis. *J Rheumatol* 1986;13:1105–1107.
10. Weston VC, Jones AC, Bradbury N, et al. Clinical features and outcome of septic arthritis in a single UK health district 1982-1991. *Ann Rheum Dis* 1999;58:214–219.
11. Kaandorp CJE, Krijnen P, Bernelot Moens HJ, et al. The outcome of bacterial arthritis: a prospective community-based study. *Arthritis Rheum* 1997;40:884–892.
12. Ryan MJ, Kavanagh R, Wall PG, et al. Bacterial joint infections in England and Wales: analysis of bacterial isolates over a four year period. *Br J Rheumatol* 1997;36:370–373.

13. Peters RHJ, Rasker JJ, Jacobs JWG, et al. Bacterial arthritis in a district hospital. *Clin Rheumatol* 1992;11:351–355.
14. Le Dantec L, Maury F, Flipo RM, et al. Peripheral pyogenic arthritis: a study of one hundred seventy nine cases. *Rev Rheum* 1996;63:103–110.
15. Kaandorp CJE, van Schaardenburg D, Krijnen P, et al. Risk factors for septic arthritis in patients with joint disease: a prospective study. *Arthritis Rheum* 1995;38:1819–1825.
16. Mikhail IS, Alarcón GS. Nongonococcal bacterial arthritis. *Rheum Dis Clin North Am* 1993;19:311–331.
17. Bremell T, Abdelnour A, Tarkowski A. Histopathological and serological progression of experimental *Staphylococcus aureus* arthritis. *Infect Immun* 1992;60:2976–2985.
18. Koopman WJ. Host factors in the pathogenesis of arthritis triggered by infectious organisms. *Rheum Dis Clin North Am* 1993; 19:279–292.
19. Abdelnour A, Bremell T, Holmdahl R, et al. Role of T lymphocytes in experimental *Staphylococcus aureus* arthritis. *Scand J Immunol* 1994;39:403–408.
20. Bremell T, Lange S, Holmdahl R, et al. Immunopathological features of rat *Staphylococcus aureus* arthritis. *Infect Immun* 1994;62:2334–2344.
21. Abdelnour A, Arvidson S, Bremell T, et al. The accessory gene regulator (agr) controls *Staphylococcus aureus* virulence in a murine arthritis model. *Infect Immun* 1993;61:3879–3885.
22. Bremell T, Lange S, Yacoub A, et al. Experimental *Staphylococcus aureus* arthritis in mice. *Infect Immun* 1991;59:2615–2623.
23. Patti JM, Bremell T, Krajewska-Pietrasik D, et al. The *Staphylococcus aureus* collagen adhesin is a virulence determinant in experimental septic arthritis. *Infect Immun* 1994;62: 152–161.
24. Switalski LM, Patti JM, Butcher W, et al. A collagen receptor in *Staphylococcus aureus* strains isolated from patients with septic arthritis mediates adhesion to cartilage. *Mol Microbiol* 1993; 7:99–107.
25. Nilsson IM, Lee JC, Bremell T, et al. The role of staphylococcal polysaccharide microcapsule expression in septicemia and septic arthritis. *Infect Immun* 1997;65:4216–4221.
26. Hughes RA, Rowe IF, Shanson D, et al. Septic bone, joint and muscle lesions associated with human immunodeficiency virus infection. *Br J Rheumatol* 1992;31:381–388.
27. Heller HM, Fuhrer J. Disseminated sporotrichosis in patients with AIDS: case report and review of the literature. *AIDS* 1991; 5:1243–1246.
28. Ricciardi DD, Sepkowitz DV, Berkowitz LB, et al. Cryptococcal arthritis in a patient with acquired immune deficiency syndrome: case report and review of the literature. *J Rheumatol* 1986;13:455–458.
29. Ventura G, Gasparini G, Lucia MB, et al. Osteoarticular bacterial infections are rare in HIV-infected patients. *Acta Orthop Scand* 1997;68:554–558.
30. Straus WL, Ostroff SM, Jernigan DB, et al. Clinical and epidemiologic characteristics of *Mycobacterium haemophilum,* an emerging pathogen in immunocompromised patients. *Ann Intern Med* 1994;120:118–125.
31. Fernandez SM, Quiralte J, Del Arco A, et al. Osteoarticular infection associated with the human immunodeficiency virus. *Clin Exp Rheumatol* 1991;9:489–493.
32. Rivera J, Montaegudo I, Lopez-Longo J, et al. Septic arthritis in patients with acquired immunodeficiency syndrome with human immunodeficiency virus infection. *J Rheumatol* 1992; 19:1960–1962.
33. Berman A, Espinoza LR, Diaz JD, et al. Rheumatic manifestations of human immunodeficiency virus infection. *Am J Med* 1988;85:59–64.
34. Rynes RI, Goldenberg DL, DiGiacomo R, et al. Acquired immunodeficiency syndrome-associated arthritis. *Am J Med* 1988;84:810–816.
35. Armstrong RW, Bolding F, Joseph R. Septic arthritis following arthroscopy: clinical syndromes and analysis of risk factors. *J Arthrosc Rel Surg* 1992;8:213–223.
36. Williams RJ, Laurencin CT, Warren RF, et al. Septic arthritis after arthroscopic anterior cruciate ligament reconstruction: diagnosis and management. *Am J Sports Med* 1997;25:261–267.
37. Szachnowski P, Wei N, Arnold WJ, et al. Complications of office based arthroscopy of the knee. *J Rheumatol* 1995;22:1722–1725.
38. Howell JD, Sheddon RJ. Septic arthritis of the hip complicating pregnancy. *Postgrad Med J* 1995;71:316–317.
39. Del Beccaro MA, Champoux AN, Bockers T, et al. Septic arthritis versus transient synovitis of the hip: the value of screening laboratory tests. *Ann Emerg Med* 1992;21:1418–1422.
40. Soderquist B, Jones I, Fredlund H, et al. Bacterial or crystal-associated arthritis? Discriminating ability of serum inflammatory markers. *Scand J Infect Dis* 1998;30:591–596.
41. Shmerling AH, Delbanco TL, Tosteson ANA, et al. Synovial fluid tests: what should be ordered? *JAMA* 1990;264:1009–1014.
42. Ropes MW, Bauer W, eds. *Synovial fluid changes in joint disease.* Cambridge: Harvard University Press, 1953.
43. Krey PR, Bailen DA. Synovial fluid leukocytosis. *Am J Med* 1979;67:436–442.
44. Kortekangas P, Aro HT, Tuominen J, et al. Synovial fluid leukocytosis in bacterial arthritis vs. reactive arthritis and rheumatoid arthritis in the adult knee. *Scand J Rheumatol* 1992;21:283–288.
45. Kortekangas P, Aro HT, Lehtonen O-P. Synovial fluid culture and blood culture in acute arthritis: a multi-case report of 90 patients. *Scand J Rheumatol* 1995;24:44–47.
46. Gupta MN, Gemmell C, Kelly B, et al. Can the routine culture of synovial fluid be justified? *Br J Rheumatol* 1998;37:798–799.
47. Pal B, Nash EJ, Oppenheim B, et al. Routine synovial fluid culture: is it necessary? Lessons from an audit. *Br J Rheumatol* 1997;36:1116–1117.
48. von Essen R. Culture of joint specimens in bacterial arthritis. *Scand J Rheumatol* 1997;26:293–300.
49. Liebling MR, Arkfeld DG, Michelini GA, et al. Identification of *Neisseria gonorrhoeae* in synovial fluid using the polymerase chain reaction. *Arthritis Rheum* 1994;37:702–709.
50. Muralidhar B, Rumore PM, Steinman CR. Use of the polymerase chain reaction to study arthritis due to *Neisseria gonorrhoeae. Arthritis Rheum* 1994;37:710–717.
51. Canvin JMG, Goutcher SC, Hagig M, et al. Persistence of *Staphylococcus aureus* as detected by polymerase chain reaction in the synovial fluid of a patient with septic arthritis. *Br J Rheumatol* 1997;36:203–206.
52. Ilahi OA, Swarma U, Hamill RJ, et al. Concomitant crystal and septic arthritis. *Orthopedics* 1996;19:613–617.
53. Dorwart BB, Hansell JR, Schumacher HR. Effects of cold and heat on urate crystal-induced synovitis in the dog. *Arthritis Rheum* 1974;17:563–571.
54. Goldman AB. Arthrography for rheumatic disease. *Rheum Dis Clin North Am* 1991;17:505–542.
55. Mudun A, Unal S, Aktay R, et al. Tc-99m nanocolloid and Tc-99m three-phase bone imaging in osteomyelitis and septic arthritis: a comparative study. *Clin Nucl Med* 1995;20:772–778.
56. Resnick D, Niwayama G. Osteomyelitis, septic arthritis, and soft tissue infection: axial skeleton. In: Resnick D, ed. *Diagnosis of bone and joint disorders.* Philadelphia: WB Saunders, 1995: 2419–2447.
57. Resnick D, Niwayama G. Osteomyelitis, septic arthritis, and soft tissue infection: mechanisms and situations. In: Resnick D, ed. *Diagnosis of bone and joint disorders.* Philadelphia: WB Saunders, 1995:2325–2418.
58. Resnick D, Niwayama G. Osteomyelitis, septic arthritis, and

soft tissue infection: organisms. In: Resnick D, ed. *Diagnosis of bone and joint disorders.* Philadelphia: WB Saunders, 1995: 2448–2558.

59. Smith JW, Piercy EA. State-of-the-art clinical article: infectious arthritis. *Clin Infect Dis* 1995;20:225–231.
60. Fung MF, Louie JS. Infectious agent arthritis. In: Weisman MH, Weinblatt ME, eds. *Treatment of the rheumatic diseases.* Philadelphia: WB Saunders, 1995:321–334.
61. Smith JW, Piercy EA. Infectious arthritis. In: Mandell GL, Bennett JE, Dolin R, eds. *Principles and practice of infectious diseases.* New York: Churchill Livingston, 1995:1032–1055.
62. Wise CM, Morris CR, Wasilauskas BL, et al. Gonococcal arthritis in an era of increasing penicillin resistance: presentations and outcomes in 41 recent cases (1985-1991). *Arch Intern Med* 1994;154:2690–2695.
63. Mauceri AA, HIAT Study Group. Treatment of bone and joint infections utilizing a third-generation cephalosporin with an outpatient drug delivery device. *Am J Med* 1994;97:14–22.
64. Dajani AS, Taubert KA, Wilson W, et al. Prevention of bacterial endocarditis: recommendations by the American Heart Association. *JAMA* 1997;277:1794–1801.
65. Little JW, Falace DA. Prosthetic implants. In: Little JW, Falace DA, eds. *Dental management of the medically compromised patient.* St. Louis: CV Mosby, 1993:533–542.
66. Maniloff G, Greenwald R, Laskin R, et al. Delayed postbacteremic prosthetic joint infection. *Clin Orthop* 1987;223:194–197.
67. Ivey FM, Hicks CA, Calhoun JH, et al. Treatment options for infected knee arthroplasties. *Rev Infect Dis* 1990;12:468–478.
68. Tsukayama DT, Wicklund B, Gustilo RB. Suppressive antibiotic therapy in chronic prosthetic joint infections. *Orthopedics* 1991;14:841–844.
69. Goldenberg DL, Cohen AS. Acute infectious arthritis. *Am J Med* 1976;60:369–377.
70. Ike RW. Tidal irrigation in septic arthritis of the knee: a potential alternative to surgical drainage. *J Rheumatol* 1993;20:2104–2111.
71. Parisien JS, Shaffer B. Arthroscopic management of pyarthrosis. *Clin Orthop* 1992;275:243–247.
72. Lane JG, Falahee MH, Wojtys EM, et al. Pyarthrosis of the knee. *Clin Orthop* 1990;252:198–204.
73. Jackson RJ. The minimally invasive treatment of septic arthritis. *J Rheumatol* 1993;20:2004.
74. Ho G. How best to drain an infected joint: will we ever know for certain? *J Rheumatol* 1993;20:2001–2003.
75. Nord KD, Dore DD, Deeney VF, et al. Evaluation of treatment modalities for septic arthritis with histological grading and analysis of levels of uronic acid, neutral protease, and interleukin-1. *J Bone Joint Surg Am* 1995;77:258–265.
76. Gardner GC, Weisman MH. Pyarthrosis in patients with rheumatoid arthritis: a report of 13 cases and a review of the literature from the past 40 years. *Am J Med* 1990;88:503–511.
77. Studahl M, Bergman B, Kalebo P, et al. Septic arthritis of the knee: a 10-year review and long-term follow-up using a new scoring system. *Scand J Infect Dis* 1994;26:85–93.
78. Yu LP, Bradley JD, Hugenberg ST, et al. Predictors of mortality in non-post-operative patients with septic arthritis. *Scand J Rheumatol* 1992;21:142–144.
79. Pitkin AD, Eykyn SJ. Covert multi-focal infective arthritis. *J Infect* 1993;27:297–300.
80. Gelberman RH, Menon J, Austerlitz MS, et al. Pyogenic arthritis of the shoulder in adults. *J Bone Joint Surg Am* 1980;62: 550–553.
81. Leslie BM, Harris JM, Driscoll D. Septic arthritis of the shoulder in adults. *J Bone Joint Surg Am* 1989;71:1516–1522.
82. Call RS, Ward JR, Samuelson CO. "Pseudoseptic" arthritis in patients with rheumatoid arthritis. *West J Med* 1985;143: 471–473.
83. Singleton JD, West SG, Nordstrom DM. "Pseudoseptic" arthritis complicating rheumatoid arthritis: a report of six cases. *J Rheumatol* 1991;18:1319–1322.
84. Satoh M, Ajmani AK. Acute exacerbation mimicking "pseudoseptic" arthritis in rheumatoid arthritis could be caused by abrupt discontinuation of glucocorticoid. *J Rheumatol* 1993;20: 1441–1442.
85. Ho G. Pseudoseptic arthritis. *Rhode Island Med* 1994;77:7–9.
86. Hughes RA, Keat AC. Reiter's syndrome and reactive arthritis: a current view. *Semin Arthritis Rheum* 1994;24:190–210.
87. Leirisalo-Repo M, Helenius P, Hannu T, et al. Long-term prognosis of reactive *Salmonella* arthritis. *Ann Rheum Dis* 1997;56: 516–520.
88. Amor B. Reiter's syndrome: long term follow up data. *Ann Rheum Dis* 1979;38:32–33.
89. Leirisalo-Repo M, Suoranta H. Ten-year follow-up study of patients with *Yersinia* arthritis. *Arthritis Rheum* 1988;31:533–537.
90. Wollenhaupt J, Kolbus F, Weissbrodt H, et al. Manifestations of *Chlamydia* induced arthritis in patients with silent versus symptomatic urogenital chlamydial infection. *Clin Exp Rheumatol* 1995;13:453–458.
91. Schumacher HR. Reactive arthritis. *Rheum Dis Clin North Am* 1998;24:261–273.
92. Wilkinson NZ, Kingsley GH, Sieper J, et al. Lack of correlation between the detection of *Chlamydia trachomatis* DNA in synovial fluid from patients with a range of rheumatic diseases and the presence of an antichlamydial immune response. *Arthritis Rheum* 1998;41:845–854.
93. Schumacher HR, Arayssi T, Branigan P, et al. Surveying for evidence of synovial *Chlamydia trachomatis* by polymerase chain reaction: a study of 411 synovial biopsies and synovial fluids. *Arthritis Rheum* 1997;40(suppl):270.
94. Bas S, Griffais R, Kvien TK, et al. Amplification of plasmid and chromosome *Chlamydia* DNA in synovial fluid of patients with reactive arthritis and undifferentiated seronegative oligoarthropathies. *Arthritis Rheum* 1995;38:1005–1013.
95. Taylor-Robinson D, Gilroy CB, Thomas BJ, et al. Detection of *Chlamydia trachomatis* DNA in joints of reactive arthritis patients by polymerase chain reaction. *Lancet* 1992;340:81–82.
96. Schumacher HR, Arayssi T, Crane M, et al. *Chlamydia trachomatis* nucleic acids can be found in the synovium of some asymptomatic subjects. *Arthritis Rheum* 1999;42:1281–1284.
97. Fryden A, Bengtsson A, Foberg U, et al. Early antibiotic treatment of reactive arthritis associated with enteric infections: clinical and serological study. *BMJ* 1990;301:1299–1302.
98. Locht H, Kihlstrom E, Lindstrom FD. Reactive arthritis after *Salmonella* among medical doctors: study of an outbreak. *J Rheumatol* 1993;20:845–848.
99. Bardin T, Enel C, Cornelis F, et al. Antibiotic treatment of venereal disease and Reiter's syndrome in a Greenland population. *Arthritis Rheum* 1992;35:190–194.
100. Sieper J, Fendler C, Laitko S, et al. No benefit of long-term ciprofloxacin treatment in patients with reactive arthritis and undifferentiated oligoarthritis. *Arthritis Rheum* 1999;42:1386–1396.
101. Lauhio A, Leirisalo-Repo M, Lahdevirta J, et al. Double-blind, placebo-controlled study of three-month treatment with lymecycline in reactive arthritis, with special reference to *Chlamydia* arthritis. *Arthritis Rheum* 1991;34:6–14.
102. Wollenhaupt J, Hammer M, Pott HG, et al. A double-blind, placebo controlled comparison of 2 weeks versus 4 months treatment with doxycycline in *Chlamydia*-induced reactive arthritis. *Arthritis Rheum* 1997;40(suppl):143.
103. Beutler AM, Hudson AP, Whittum-Hudson JA. *Chlamydia trachomatis* can persist in joint tissue after antibiotic treatment in chronic Reiter's syndrome/reactive arthritis. *J Clin Rheumatol* 1997;3:125–130.

104. Toivanen A, Yli-Kerttula T, Luukkainen R, et al. Effect of antimicrobial treatment on chronic reactive arthritis. *Clin Exp Rheumatol* 1993;11:301–307.
105. Deighton C. β-Haemolytic streptococci and reactive arthritis in adults. *Ann Rheum Dis* 1993;52:475–482.
106. Gutierrez-Urena S, Molina J, Molina JF, et al. Poststreptococcal reactive arthritis, clinical course, and outcome in 6 adult patients. *J Rheumatol* 1995;22:1710–1713.
107. Jansen TLTA, Janssen M, de Jong AJL, et al. Post-streptococcal reactive arthritis: a clinical and serological description, revealing its distinction from acute rheumatic fever. *J Intern Med* 1999; 245:261–267.
108. Valtonen JMO, Koskimies S, Miettinen A, et al. Various rheumatic syndromes in adult patients associated with high antistreptolysin O titers and their differential diagnosis with rheumatic fever. *Ann Rheum Dis* 1993;52:527–530.

126

BACTERIAL ARTHRITIS

ROBERT W. IKE

The general principles of septic arthritis are discussed in Chapter 125. The characteristics of causative microorganisms, the host, and the clinical setting in which bacterial arthritis occurs are the subject of this chapter.

PATHOGENS CAUSING BACTERIAL ARTHRITIS

Musculoskeletal syndromes accompanying acute infection with *Neisseria gonorrhoeae* account for about 20% of all bacterial infections causing arthritis (see Chapter 127). Remaining joint infections are caused by an array of bacterial species distributed among staphylococci, streptococci, gram-negative organisms, and anaerobic species in proportions that have not changed substantially over several decades (Fig. 126.1) (1–8).

Gram-positive Cocci

The gram-positive cocci of the Micrococcaceae and Streptococcaceae families cause most cases (50–90%) of nongonococcal bacterial arthritis (1,3,7,9,10). *Staphylococcus* species, mainly *Staphylococcus aureus* but sometimes coagulase-negative staphylococci, and rarely, *Micrococcus* species (11), represent the Micrococcaceae family. The Streptococcaceae include the hemolytic streptococci, different groups of viridans streptococci including *Pneumococcus* and *Aerococcus* species.

Staphylococci are the predominant organisms causing septic arthritis. *S. aureus* causes 43% to 64% of all cases in the elderly (Table 126.1) and 77% of reported joint infections in patients with rheumatoid arthritis (RA; Table 126.2). Staphylococci compose 75% to 90% of the gram-positive bacteria found in infected prosthetic joints, with *S. epidermidis* being more common than *S. aureus.* In the neonate, staphylococci cause 25% of the community-acquired joint infections and 62% of the nosocomial cases. Overall, 13% to 44% of all cases of childhood septic arthritis are due to *S. aureus* (Table 126.3).

The microbiologic, clinical, therapeutic, and preventive aspects of diseases caused by *S. aureus* have been reviewed (12). Methicillin-resistant staphylococci (MRSA: more appropriately considered "multiply resistant" *S. aureus*) deserve special therapeutic consideration that includes empiric use of vancomycin in areas where methicillin-resistant staphylococci are prevalent (4) while culture and antibiotic-sensitivity results are pending. The fluoroquinolones show *in vitro* activity against methicillin-resistant staphylococci, multiple antibiotic-resistant gram-negative bacilli, and β-lactamase-producing *N. gonorrhoeae* (13). This class of antimicrobial agents might be considered in patients with serious infections caused by MRSA when vancomycin cannot be used, or when β-lactams or aminoglycosides are contraindicated (14). Rifampin can be used adjunctively to treat *S. aureus* joint infections that persist in the face of antibiotics that kill the isolate *in vitro*; persistent intracellular organisms are killed by rifampin, which can penetrate leukocyte membranes (15).

S. aureus produces a number of extracellular and cell-associated factors, but it is unclear how these affect virulence *in vivo.* Surface factors that may be important in pathogenesis include the cell wall (activates complement and stimulates cytokine release), capsular polysaccharide (promotes adhesion to host cell surfaces), and fibronectin-binding protein (16). Collagen receptors are not more prevalent among *S. aureus* strains from septic joints when compared with other isolates, indicating that specific collagen binding is not a major tropic factor (17). Staphylococcal toxic shock syndrome toxin and the enterotoxins are superantigens and have the potential to suppress plasma cell differentiation and antibody responsiveness. Staphylococcal toxins sometimes complicate septic arthritis, shown by the occasional case of septic arthritis with toxic shock syndrome (18).

Streptococci account for 15% to 30% of all cases of nongonococcal bacterial arthritis. In large surveys of septic arthritis, cases due to streptococci (mainly *S. pyogenes* group A) seem to follow a benign course. Infections caused by non-A Lancefield serotypes tend to be more complicated, however (19). Joint infections caused by group B strepto-

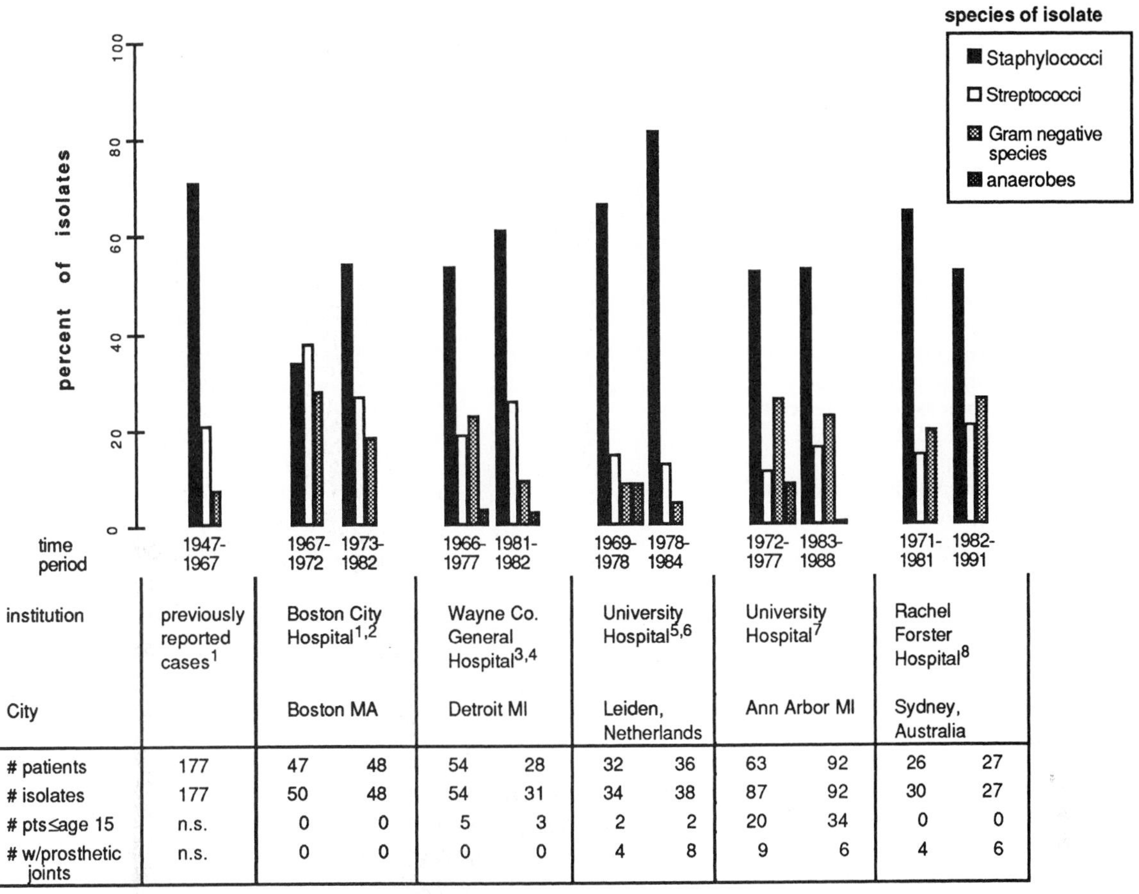

FIGURE 126.1. Distribution of isolates from synovial fluid of patients with bacterial septic arthritis: changes over different periods at five institutions.

TABLE 126.1. SEPTIC ARTHRITIS IN THE ELDERLY

	Vincent and Amirault, 1990 (167)	Cooper and Cawley, 1986 (168)	McGuire and Kauffman, 1985 (169)	Ho and Su, 1982 (170)	Willkens, et al., 1960 (171)
Study period	1979–1988	1973–1982	1973–1983	1975–1980	1954–1959
No. of patients	21	21	23	1111	13
Mean age	72.3	73.8	67.7	66.7	63.9
Age range	60–92	60–85	60–87	60–78	60–82
With underlying joint disease	71%	71%	65%	55%	23%
With knee infections	38%	48%	43%	55%	54%
Next most frequent site of infection	Shoulder (24%)	Hip (38%)	Wrist (17%)	Shoulder (27%)	Shoulder (38%)
Infected with *Staphylococcus aureus*	67%	43%	52%	64%	62%
Infected with gram-negative bacilli	—	14%	35%	18%	—
Poor functional outcome	—	52%	—	40%	46%
In-hospital mortality	29%	33%	22%	9%	—

TABLE 126.2. BACTERIAL ARTHRITIS IN RHEUMATOID ARTHRITIS PATIENTS

Number of patients	238
Patient characteristics	
Age in years (range)	59.4 (27–82)
>60 years	53% (125/238)
Mean duration of rheumatoid arthritis in years (range)	14 (1–55)
Systemic corticosteroid therapy	53% (89/168)
Clinical features	
Time to diagnosis >7 days	41% (37/91)
Fever	42% (50/118)
Hypothermia (T < 37°C)	22% (16/72)
Leukocytosis >10,000 cells/mm^3	48% (76/100)
ESR >100 mm/hr	49% (33/67)
Synovial fluid leucocyte count (mean)	126,000 (n = 76)
Prosthetic joint	8% (38/455)[b]
Fistulization	5% (22/455)[b]
Polyarticular infection	34% (80/238)
Microbiology of 238 bacterial isolates[a]	
Gram-positive cocci	
Staphylococci	58%
Hemolytic *Streptococci*	11%
Pneumococcus	7%
Hemophilus	1%
Gram-negative bacilli	16%
Positive blood cultures	60% (70/116)
Portal of entry	
Skin	62/115
Intraarticular injection	17/115
Outcome	
Surgical treatment	52% (95/183)
Deaths	
Overall	27% (58/215)
Polyarticular disease	49% (36/74)
Monarticular disease	19% (22/114)

Data from Dubost JJ, Fis I, Sorbrier M, et al. Septic arthritis in patients with rheumatoid arthritis. A review of twenty-four cases and of the medical literature. *Rev Rheum [Engl Ed]* 1994;61:143–156.
[a]See text for other bacteria responsible for septic arthritis in patients with rheumatoid arthritis.
[b]Denominator of 455 represents total number of joints infected in 238 patients.

TABLE 126.3. SEPTIC ARTHRITIS IN CHILDREN

	Luhmann and Luhmann, 1999	Fink and Nelson, 1986 (72)	Sequeira, et al., 1985 (141)	Wilson and Dipaola, 1986 (142)	Speiser et al., 1985 (143)	Welkon et al. et al., 1986 (144)	Jackson et al. 1992
Study period	1991–1997	1955–1984	1972–1981	1974–1983	1974–1983	1975–1985	1980–1990
Location	St. Louis	Dallas	Chicago	Glasgow	St. Louis	Philadelphia	Kansas
Total cases	64	591	32	61	86	95	96
Percentage of patients with confirmed bacterial diagnosis	59	66	100	92	84	64	67
Among those with proven bacterial cause							
Positive Gram's stain of synovial fluid	8	33	—	—	10–54[a]	—	—
Positive culture of synovial fluid	71	79	97	71–80[b]	36–70[a]	84	—
Positive blood culture	18	33	—	41	46	46	—
Site of infection (%)							
Knee	20	40	37	29	30	49	40
Hip	42	23	27	40	29	27	30
Ankle		13	15	22	17	17	12
(Total)	62	76	79	91	76	93	82
More than 1 affected joint	5	7	—	5	7	8	—
Coexistimg osteomyelitis (%)	—	—	—	—	—	13	16
Infecting agent (%)							
Staphylococcus aureus	26	17	25	44	37	13	19
Hemophilus influenza	3	25	37	16	17	29	25
Others	71	25	38	32	29	22	25
Culture-negative specimens	41	33	—	8	16	36	29

[a]The lower percentages reflect results of patients receiving antibiotics; the higher values are from studies of patients not treated with antibiotics.
[b]Arthrotomy yielded a 71% positivity rate versus 80% for aspirated samples.

cocci (*S. agalactiae*) have been further elucidated. Diabetes mellitus predisposes to group B streptococcal septic arthritis (20,21). Twenty percent of adults with group B streptococcal joint infection have polyarticular disease (22,23); joints of the axial skeleton (21) and prosthetic joints (20) are commonly involved, and an aggressive course is common (20,21). Metastatic infections can include endophthalmitis (19). Group B streptococcus also is a major cause of community-acquired septic arthritis in neonates (24).

Serious group G streptococcal infection occurs in patients with malignancy, alcoholism, and diabetes mellitus (25). Septic arthritis caused by group G streptococcus is often polyarticular (26% of 38 cases) (26). More than one third of the patients reported had underlying RA, and more than one fourth of the infections affected a prosthetic joint. Polymicrobial infection, frequently associated with *S. aureus,* implicates the skin as the common portal of entry (25,26). Although the presumed source of infection is usually cellulitis, the gastrointestinal tract harbors group G streptococci and at least two cases of group G streptococcal arthritis have been described in which the search for the source of infection has disclosed an occult colon carcinoma (27,28).

Joint infection by group C streptococcus is rare. Polyarticular sepsis (in seven of 16 patients), high mortality (four of 16), requirement for drainage beyond needle aspiration (eight of 16), and poor functional outcome (four of 12) characterized the 16 reported cases (29–32). Group D enterococcus is another rare cause of septic arthritis, with both reported cases requiring surgical excision of the affected joints for cure (33). Unlike other streptococcal joint infections for which penicillin is still considered the drug of choice, enterococcal disease requires a combined regimen of ampicillin and gentamicin similar to that used in enterococcal endocarditis (33). A similar antibiotic regimen has been recommended for septic arthritis due to other nongroup A streptococci (26,30). A woman with septic arthritis of a hip caused by *Aerococcus viridans* responded to treatment with penicillin and open drainage (34). This microorganism is similar to other viridans streptococci, but can be confused with enterococci. Other viridans streptococci that have caused septic arthritis include *S. sanguis* (35), *S. milleri* (36), *S. anginosus-constellatus* (37), and *S. mitis* (38).

S. pneumoniae has remained an uncommon cause of joint infection. Predispositions include alcoholism, hypogammaglobulinemia (39), and underlying joint disease such as RA (40), gout (41), and joint prostheses (42). Pneumococci often infect joints by seeding from a primarily infected site, such as pneumonia, meningitis, or rarely, endocarditis; however, one or more joints can be the sole site(s) of infection (39). Polyarticular pneumococcal infection is common (22,43). Septic arthritis due to penicillin-resistant pneumococci (treated with vancomycin) has been described (44). Invasive pneumococcal disease in children only rarely involves bones or joints, and the emergence of antibiotic resistance has not changed clinical presentation or response to treatment (45).

Gram-positive Bacilli

Gram-positive bacillary septic arthritis is extremely rare. *Listeria monocytogenes* can cause meningitis and bacteremia in hosts compromised by alcoholism, hematologic or lymphoproliferative malignancy, or immunosuppressive treatment for nonmalignant disease (46). Bone and joint infections due to *L. monocytogenes* occur in similarly compromised patients (47), with septic arthritis reported in patients with RA (48,49), gout (50), and in prosthetic joints of patients with RA (51–53), or with other systemic disorders such as renal transplantation (54) or diabetes mellitus (55). Other gram-positive bacilli that have caused septic arthritis include *Corynebacterium pyogenes* (56), *C. kutscheri* (57), *Bacillus cereus* (58), and other Bacillus species (59). The two most important gram-negative cocci that infect joints are *N. gonorrhoeae* and *N. meningitidis,* as discussed in Chapter 127. *Propionibacterium acnes,* an anaerobic gram-positive rod, can cause septic arthritis in joint prostheses (60) and in joints affected by RA (61).

Gram-negative Cocci and Coccobacilli

The two most important gram-negative cocci that infect joints are *N. gonorrhoeae* and *N. meningitidis,* as discussed in Chapter 127. Other members of the family Neisseriaceae that have caused joint infection include Branhamella, Moraxella, and Kingella species. *Moraxella (Branhamella) catarrhalis* has been implicated in pyogenic sacroiliitis in a 15-year-old girl with an upper respiratory tract infection (62), septic arthritis of the hip in a 23-year-old Navajo man (63), and septic knee arthritis with bacteremia in a 41-year-old man (64).

Joint infections caused by Moraxella or Kingella species usually follow an indolent course (65). Infants and young children (younger than 4 years) appear especially vulnerable to bone and joint infections caused by *K. kingae* (65,66). Among 25 Israeli children with invasive Kingella infections seen over a 5-year period, 16 had septic arthritis, with a clear trend to seasonal onset (during warmer months) (67). Adult cases of *K. kingae* septic arthritis include a 49-year-old alcoholic (68), a 51-year-old woman with RA and Felty's syndrome (69), and a 76-year-old man with chronic lung disease (70).

Haemophilus influenzae is an aerobic, pleomorphic, gram-negative coccobacillus. Of the typable strains, type B is the major pathogen in humans. In adults, it is an important cause of pneumonia, meningitis, epiglottitis, and acute sinusitis (71). *Haemophilus* rarely infects diarthrodial joints, causing less than 1% of all bacterial septic arthritis in adults (9). In children, *H. influenzae* can cause bacteremia, meningitis, pneumonia, epiglottitis, pericarditis, cellulitis, osteomyelitis, and arthritis (about 8% of all infections) (72). Among bacteria that cause septic arthritis in children, *H. influenzae* once rivaled *S. aureus* as a major pathogen (see Bacterial Arthritis in Children); incidence of these bone and joint infections has declined considerably with widespread use of *H. influenzae* type b vaccine (73).

H. influenzae arthritis is most common in children aged 6 months to 2 years. The disease in children is usually monoarticular, predominantly affecting the hips, knees, or ankles (72), and often follows an upper respiratory tract infection or otitis media with bacteremia (74,75). Concurrent meningitis (8–30%) and osteomyelitis (12–22%) are not uncommon (74,75).

The much more rare adult disease has some different clinical features. Nearly three fourths of 29 reported cases had a systemic or local predisposition to infection (76). About half the cases were polyarticular, with over a quarter accompanied by tenosynovitis, bursitis, or both. Thus adult *H. influenzae* arthritis can mimic the polyarthritis and tenosynovitis of gonococcal infection, resemble *S. aureus* septic olecranon bursitis (77), or involve a prosthetic joint (76). Because of prevalent β-lactamase–positive strains, amoxicillin/clavulanate has replaced ampicillin as the antibiotic regimen of choice for *H. influenzae*; chloramphenicol or cefuroxime are alternatives.

Gram-negative Bacilli

Gram-negative bacilli account for 7% to 26% of cases of adult nongonococcal septic arthritis (78). Analysis of data from three periods (before 1960, the 1960s, and the 1970s) showed frequencies of gram-negative bacillary arthritis of 6%, 14%, and 27%, respectively. This trend was thought to reflect the apparent increasing frequency of gram-negative bacteremia (79), but has not been sustained beyond the 1970s (Fig. 126.1). Gram-negative bacilli account for one fourth of all joint infections in the elderly (Table 126.2) and about 10% of those in RA patients. Intravenous drug users are especially prone to bone and joint infections from Pseudomonas (80), Serratia (81,82), and Staphylococcus. Gram-negative bacilli caused fewer than 10% of joint infections among children older than 2 years, but accounted for more than one fourth of the joint infections in younger children (78) and were an important nosocomial pathogen in neonates (24). Aerobic gram-negative rods have been reported in 10% to 20% of prosthetic joint infections.

Host factors influence many of the clinical features including the microbiology, the particular joint(s) infected, and treatment outcome. In a series of 13 older patients from Boston (mean age, 56 years) with serious underlying systemic diseases, preexisting joint disease, or both, *Escherichia coli* or *Proteus mirabilis* septic arthritis developed secondary to hematogenous spread from the urinary or biliary tract (78). *S. marcescens, P. aeruginosa,* and Salmonella species were less common isolates. The patients often had been receiving antibiotics, corticosteroids, or both, and the infection was monoarticular, most commonly affecting a knee. Many patients failed to respond to medical treatment alone and required subsequent surgical debridement. Mortality was high, and the cure rate low. In contrast, a series of 21 otherwise healthy younger patients (mean age, 29 years) whose primary predisposition was intravenous drug use, had infections localized to the sternal articulations often caused by *P. aeruginosa* (83). *E. coli* and *P. mirabilis* were less common isolates, with single cases due to *Enterobacter aerogenes, E. liquefaciens, Klebsiella pneumoniae, Eikenella corrodens, Acinetobacter anitratus,* and *Bacteroides fragilis.* Despite frequent juxtaarticular osteomyelitis, periarticular abscess requiring surgery, or both, the cure rate was 90%, and the mortality only 5%. In another elderly rural population (mean age, 61 years) of 22 patients infected with a range of bacilli comparable to that in the Boston series, mortality was only 5%, and good outcomes were achieved in 68% (84). Prompt diagnosis, early treatment, and more effective antibiotics might have been responsible for the better results.

Among Enterobacteriaceae, *E. coli* and *P. mirabilis* are the most frequent isolates from septic joints, followed by *Klebsiella, Enterobacter, Serratia,* and *Morganella* sp. *Salmonella* sp. (85,86), *Arizona hinshawii* (87), *Yersinia enterocolitica* (88,89), *Campylobacter fetus* (90), and *C. jejuni* (91) have been isolated from synovial fluids. For *Salmonella, Yersinia, Shigella flexneri,* or *C. jejuni,* reactive arthritis after gastrointestinal infection is the more common association, however (see Chapter 67).

P. aeruginosa, a member of the Pseudomonadaceae family, is an important cause of gram-negative septic arthritis in chronically debilitated older patients with serious systemic illnesses, and in younger parenteral drug users. Chronic joint infection with *Pseudomonas* is possible, as illustrated by a reported case in which the bacterial cause of migratory polyarthritis, which developed after a surgical wound infection, was not found for 2 years because synovitis was mild and systemic features were absent (92). *P. aeruginosa* also is the most common etiologic agent associated with osteochondritis of the foot from puncture wounds seen in children (93) and in adults (94). Treatment requires adequate debridement and drainage of the infected site, an aminoglycoside, and an antipseudomonal semisynthetic penicillin given for 4 to 6 weeks (95). One exception: a knee infected with *P. aeruginosa* failed to respond to gentamicin and azlocillin (96), but responded to ceftazidime given intravenously and intraarticularly. Other reported exceptions include a septic knee caused by *P. cepacia* (97) and a case of osteochondritis of the foot caused by *P. maltophilia* (98). Typically resistant to aminoglycosides, antipseudomonal penicillins, and first- and second-generation cephalosporins, these *Pseudomonas* sp proved difficult to eradicate even with third-generation cephalosporins.

The spectrum of gram-negative bacillary septic arthritis is constantly expanding with reports of new isolations. Examples of such occurrences include joint infections caused by *Capnocytophaga ochracea* (99), *Plesiomonas shigelloides* (100), and *Aeromonas hydrophila* (101).

Anaerobic Bacteria

Anaerobic bacteria account for less than 1% of all cases of acute hematogenous septic arthritis affecting native joints. Use of improved methods to collect, transport, cultivate, and identify anaerobic bacteria may prove this to be an underestimation. Furthermore, anaerobic bacteria can be recovered mixed with facultative or aerobic species (102). A review that included data from the preantibiotic era found that more than one third of 180 anaerobic joint infections were caused by *Fusobacterium necrophorum* (103). *Fusobacterium* infections of joints have reemerged, usually complicating oropharyngeal infections (102). Anaerobic cocci, *B. fragilis,* and other *Fusobacterium, Bacteroides,* and *Clostridium* species accounted for most of the other cases. *Propionobacterium acnes,* an anaerobic organism once considered a contaminant when found in synovial fluid, has been recognized as a legitimate joint pathogen (104) and accounted for 36% of all isolates in one recent series of anaerobic septic arthritis (102). Foul odor of synovial fluid [found in 37% of all cases in one series (102)] provides a clue to anaerobic joint infection.

Anaerobes are found in infected joint prostheses 5% to 10% of the time (105,106). Anaerobic bacteria caused joint infection in two different clinical settings at the Mayo Clinic (107); most cases occurred after joint surgery—53% after reconstructive surgery, and 28% after trauma—with anaerobic cocci, such as *Peptococcus* and *Peptostreptococcus* sp, as major pathogens. *B. fragilis* was the most frequent cause (19%) of a second type of infection, occurring in patients with chronic illnesses such as inflammatory bowel disease, RA, psoriatic arthritis, and chronic osteomyelitis. The anaerobic bacteria seeding the joints arrived hematogenously from intraabdominal sources, decubitus ulcers, or by direct extension from adjacent chronic osteomyelitis. Patients with anaerobic septic arthritis not related to surgery had 50% mortality, with poor outcome attributed to their debilitated antecedent condition. Anaerobic septic arthritis can occasionally develop in younger patients after trauma without surgery, usually involving *P. acnes* or *Clostridium* sp (102). Because *Clostridium* species reside in the gut, the reported discovery of an occult colon carcinoma in the search for source of infection in a patient with *Clostridium* septic arthritis should come as no surprise (108).

Treatment of anaerobic septic arthritis should include management of the underlying disease, antimicrobial therapy directed against all major isolates based on their individual susceptibility, and removal of infected prostheses or internal fixation devices. Surgical drainage or debridement to remove necrotic tissue that can sustain the anaerobic conditions may be necessary. Antimicrobials that provide adequate coverage for resistant *Bacteroides* sp as well as most other anaerobic bacteria include clindamycin, metronidazole (excluding *P. acnes*), imipenem, and the combination of a β-lactamase inhibitor (e.g., clavulanic acid) and a penicillin.

Microorganisms Acquired from Animals

Pasteurella multocida

Pasteurella multocida is a small, aerobic, facultatively anaerobic, gram-negative coccobacillus found in the normal oral flora of many domestic and wild animals (109). Human infections can result from casual contact with cats or dogs or more commonly from their bites and scratches. Sites affected in 446 cases of human infection by *P. multocida* included skin (48%), oral and respiratory tract (14%), cardiovascular system (13%), bones and joints (13%), central nervous system (5%), gastrointestinal tract (4%), genitourinary tract (4%), and the eye (1%) (109). Bone and joint infections comprise three categories: osteomyelitis, septic arthritis with osteomyelitis, and septic arthritis alone (110). Osteomyelitis, commonly affecting forearm, leg, hand, or wrist, ensues from wound infection that extends to adjacent bone or by direct inoculation of *P. multocida* into the periosteum by a bite. Almost all the cases of septic arthritis with osteomyelitis affect the small joints and bones of the hand after cat bites, and nearly always occur in otherwise healthy people.

In sharp contrast, septic arthritis caused by *P. multocida* without osteomyelitis rarely occurs in a host who is not immunocompromised or in a joint not previously damaged. Chronic RA receiving corticosteroid treatment is the most common underlying joint disease. Here, bacteria disseminate hematogenously rather than by local extension or direct penetration. Bacteremia and polyarticular infection might be noted (111–113), but the infection is usually monoarticular, with the knee most commonly affected. The interval between animal contact and onset of joint symptoms can range from days to months, and a specific bite or scratch might not be recalled (114). Almost a third of the reported cases have involved total knee replacements (110), usually in patients with RA. *P. multocida* infection of bilateral knee prostheses in a patient with osteoarthritis (OA) also has been reported, however (111). Joint infection with *P. multocida* has been reported along with *S. aureus* in a prosthetic knee (12), with *S. sanguis* in a sternoclavicular joint (35), and with *P. aeruginosa* in a patient with bilateral knee prostheses (111).

Penicillin is the agent of choice for treatment of *P. multocida* septic arthritis. Drainage of the infected joint is necessary. Some patients with infected knee prostheses were able to retain the artificial joint (112), but removal was eventually required in others (111). Prophylactic antibiotic treatment of animal bites can prevent systemic infection, but penicillin-allergic patients should receive trimethoprim/sulfamethoxazole or ciprofloxacin, as septic arthritis has been reported despite erythromycin prophylaxis after a cat bite (115).

Rat-bite Fever

Two microorganisms, *Streptobacillus moniliformis,* a pleomorphic gram-negative rod, and *Spirillum minus,* a spirochete, can cause rat-bite fever. Both are normal flora in the oropharynx of many rodents. *Streptobacillus* infection presents with fever, morbilliform or petechial rash, and polyarticular pain 2 to 10 days after a rodent bite. Rarely, streptobacilli have been isolated from joint fluid (116). *S. moniliformis* septic arthritis has developed in patients who had no history of rodent bite but worked or resided in rat-infested areas (117). *S. minus* causes a febrile illness after an incubation period of more than 10 days. Joint symptoms are rare, but regional adenopathy draining the site of the bite is common. Treatment is with penicillin for both causative agents.

Brucellosis

Brucellosis has a worldwide distribution, but the pathogenic species encountered depends on the geographic location. The four species causing human disease (and respective common animal source) are *Brucella melitensis* (sheep and goats), *B. abortus* (cattle), *B. suis* (pigs), and *B. canis* (dogs). The clinical manifestations and the severity of disease vary according to the responsible species and the host (118,119). Humans acquire the disease from infected animals. Ingestion of raw milk or dairy products made from unpasteurized milk, inhalation of aerosolized bacteria, or contact with contaminated animals through broken skin or conjunctiva are the known routes of infection. Examples of ingestion-acquired, laboratory-acquired, and abattoir-acquired disease are well documented. Patterns of joint involvement suggest a spondyloarthropathy, with axial fibrocartilaginous joints and lower extremity diarthrodial joints predominating. A comprehensive review of 304 cases of human infection by *B. melitensis* from Lima, Peru, found joint involvement in one third (33.8%) of patients (119). Sacroiliitis (46.6%), peripheral arthritis (38.8%), or a combination of the two (7.8%) accounted for 93.2% of musculoskeletal involvement, tending to occur in young patients with acute infection. Spondylitis (6.8%) was most common in the lumbosacral region, generally affecting older patients with more chronic infection. Paraspinal abscesses may complicate vertebral brucellosis and can be the cause of antibiotic resistance until found and drained (120). Sacroiliitis is usually unilateral and nondestructive, and responds to antibiotic treatment. Peripheral arthritis also responds to antibiotic treatment, but can remit spontaneously, raising the possibility of a reactive form of brucellar arthritis (119). Recovery of the microorganisms from the sacroiliac joint, sternoclavicular joint, or other peripheral joints is uncommon but well documented (118,119). Proof of chronic infection with *Brucella* species can be difficult, as antibody tests measure immunoglobulin M (IgM) responses, whereas IgG responses predominate in chronic infection (119).

Most recent reports of skeletal brucellosis come from South America (119–121), the Iberian peninsula (122), and the Middle East (123,124). In the United States, *B. melitensis* infections are uncommon relative to *B. abortus* and *B. suis. B. canis* has been responsible for at least two cases of septic arthritis in children (118,125). Effective antibiotic regimens against brucellosis consist of tetracycline or doxycycline plus streptomycin, but trimethoprim/sulfamethoxazole, rifampin, and third-generation cephalosporins have all been used with some success (118,125,126). A prospective study that compared treatment of brucellosis with doxycycline and either rifampin or streptomycin found similar outcomes for both regimens, although therapeutic failure among patients with spondylitis was more common with the doxycycline–rifampin regimen (127).

Spirochetes

S. minus is a rare cause of rat-bite fever in the U.S. Lyme arthritis, caused by *Borrelia burgdorferi,* is the subject of Chapter 129. Another spirochete, *Treponema pallidum,* is responsible for syphilitic joint disease (128). Chronic arthritis in primary or secondary syphilis is rare. In tertiary syphilis, arthritis can result from gummata located in the juxtaarticular tissue, cartilage, or bone. Large, usually painless effusions with little evidence of limitation of motion are characteristic of gummatous arthritis. Chronic syphilitic polyarthritis can mimic RA and has been described as the presenting feature in a patient with human immunodeficiency virus (HIV) infection (129). Syphilitic spondylitis is an osteitis caused by the invasion of bone and periosteum by *T. pallidum.* Charcot's joint secondary to syphilis occurs in 5% of patients with tabes dorsalis and primarily involves the weight-bearing articulations (see Chapter 91).

Congenital syphilis has been associated with several musculoskeletal syndromes. Parrot's pseudoparalysis is an osteochondritis affecting the epiphysis and articular cartilage of the humerus or the tibia of neonates and infants within the first 3 months of life. Clutton's joint is a late sequela of congenital syphilis manifested by chronic hydrarthrosis of one or both knees in children aged between 6 and 16 years.

Mycoplasma

Mycoplasmas as agents of human disease have been reviewed by Cassell and Cole (130). Septic arthritis has resulted from infection with *Mycoplasma hominis, M. pneumoniae,* and *Ureaplasma urealyticum.* In some patients with hypogammaglobulinemia, polyarthritis resembling RA develops, whereas in others, acute septic arthritis developed; mycoplasmas and ureaplasmas have been cultured from their joint fluids (131,132). Mycoplasma joint infection is responsive to antibiotic treatment; tetracycline or erythromycin are used most frequently. Involvement of *Mycoplasma* species in arthritis-associated illnesses affecting several animal species (133)—including primates—has fueled speculation regarding the role of mycoplasmas in chronic human arthritides; sensitive and specific tests for molecular traces of mycoplasma in synovial tissue should help to settle this question (134). Prosthetic joint infection with *M. hominis* has been reported in two patients with RA (135,136), and in another patient with systemic lupus erythematosus (137). All three patients retained their joint prostheses with antibiotic treatment and joint drainage, debridement, or both.

Nocardia

Nocardia are aerobic, gram-positive, partially acid-fast bacteria that form branching filaments. *Nocardia asteroides* and *N. brasiliensis* are the major pathogens causing human disease. Septic arthritis from either organism is rare. The reported cases are usually in patients who are immunocompromised from corticosteroids, other immunosuppressive drugs (138,139), or HIV infection (140). However, described Nocardia synovial infections in otherwise healthy patients include a case of olecranon bursitis in a 44-year-old man (141) and knee pyoarthrosis that followed a thorn puncture in an 11-year-old boy (142). Trimethoprim and sulfamethoxazole is the antibiotic combination of choice. Treatment duration is usually prolonged, from months to a year.

CLINICAL FEATURES OF BACTERIAL ARTHRITIS: HOST ASPECTS

Bacterial Arthritis in Children

Clinical Features

Because acute joint dysfunction and systemic sepsis appear differently in infants and children than in adults, clinical presentations of bacterial arthritis in the pediatric age group do not usually mirror those seen in adults. The pathophysiology and principles of management are basically the same, however. Table 126.3 summarizes seven series from the past two decades, with 1,005 patients available for analysis. The largest study comes from Dallas, comprising 591 cases collected over 30 years, which found no significant increase in the incidence of septic arthritis between 1955 and 1984 (74). In the seven series, bacteriologic confirmation varied from 59% to 100%, in part reflecting the nonuniform inclusion criteria used by the different authors (74,143–148). Overall, a causative bacterium could be identified in 716 (71%) of 1,005 children with septic arthritis.

Cultures of the synovial fluid were positive in only 70% to 97% of the cases of septic arthritis with bacteriologic confirmation (Table 126.3). When antibiotics had been given before joint aspiration, the yield from synovial fluid cultures decreased to 36% (145). Similarly, microorganisms were found on the gram-stained smear of the synovial fluid more often in those who had not received antibiotics (54%) than in those who had (19%) (145). Overall, bacteria were seen on one third of all synovial fluid Gram stains (74). At least some "culture-negative" episodes could be due to fastidious organisms not captured by routine culture methods; for example, 93% of all positive cases due to *K. kingea* (a fastidious gram-negative coccobacillus) were detected only when the initial synovial fluid specimen was inoculated into a blood-culture bottle (149).

Blood cultures were positive in 18% to 46% of children with septic arthritis, and were often the only clue in identifying the responsible pathogen. Cultures of other extraarticular sites of infection also enhanced the likelihood of bacteriologic confirmation.

In two series, instances of septic arthritis accompanied by contiguous acute osteomyelitis were actively sought and accounted for about 15% of all cases (146,147). Almost all were neonates or children younger than 2 years. In a neonate, infection of bone and joint space is common because the transphysial blood supply facilitates rapid spread from the metaphysis to the epiphysis and into the joint (150). In a child, the metaphysis of the proximal femur, proximal humerus, proximal radius, and distal–lateral tibia is intraarticular; thus infection can spread easily from bone into the joint space. Bony tenderness near the affected joint is an important clue to diagnosis. Joints affected by concurrent septic arthritis and osteomyelitis are much more prone to sequelae than are those affected by septic arthritis alone. Children with septic arthritis whose symptoms have lasted more than 7 days or who have received prior antibiotics are at risk for concurrent osteomyelitis (147).

Pathogens causing septic arthritis vary according to age of the patient. In neonates, staphylococci, group B streptococci [usually acquired *in utero* or during birth (150)], and Enterobacteriaceae are the most common isolates (151,152). In children between 6 months and 2 years of age, *H. influenzae* was once most common (74,143,146). Widespread use of vaccine against *Haemophilus* B strains has reduced this incidence, with *K. kingea* emerging as a more common gram-negative pathogen (148,153). Among children older than 5 years, and in neonates or infants younger than 6 months, *S. aureus* is the major pathogen.

The bacteria that cause septic arthritis in the neonatal and early infancy periods can be further subdivided according to where the infection was acquired (24). Pathogens in community-acquired joint infections include group B streptococci (52%), staphylococci (25%), gonococci (17%), and gram-negative bacilli (5%). In sharp contrast, the relative frequencies of hospital-acquired pathogens are staphylococci (62%), Candida (17%), gram-negative enteric bacilli (13%), and streptococcus and *H. influenzae* (4% each). Nosocomial outbreaks of multiply resistant staphylococci are not uncommon, and can be complicated by bone and joint infection (154). Risk factors for septic arthritis in neonates include prematurity, respiratory distress syndrome, and umbilical artery catheterization (155).

Joint infections in children favor the large joints of the lower extremities. In a review of infections in 1,023 joints,

39% affected the knee; 26%, the hip; and 13%, the ankle (74). These three joint sites accounted for 79% of the joint infections in 948 patients. Data from other studies (Table 126.3) confirm this joint distribution. Aspiration of both hips of any neonate who has a bone or joint infection at another site has been recommended. In the neonate, the hip is a difficult joint to examine and is the most common joint to be infected. Multifocal skeletal infection is common, and the sequelae of a missed hip infection are severe (150).

Therapy

The following factors must all be taken into account when planning drug treatment: the age-dependent vulnerability to a specific pathogen, the circumstances under which the joint infection is acquired, regional trends in the bacterial causes of septic arthritis, local antibiotic susceptibility patterns, and realization that bacteriologic confirmation may elude 30% of the cases of presumed bacterial arthritis in children. The most efficacious, specific, least toxic, and least expensive drug should be chosen. A positive Gram-stained smear of the synovial fluid and the results of the laboratory investigation of extraarticular sites of infection (i.e., cerebrospinal fluid, sputum, and urine) are used to determine the most appropriate antibiotic treatment before culture confirmation. When the Gram-stained smear shows no microorganisms, broad-spectrum antimicrobial agents with optimal activity against the most likely pathogens should be chosen. For example, in the neonate with hospital-acquired bacterial arthritis, the antibiotic regimen must be directed at *S. aureus* as well as gram-negative enteric bacilli. Empiric treatment of community-acquired infection should be directed against group B streptococci, staphylococci, and gonococci. In children between ages 6 months and 5 years in whom *K. kingea* is suspected but *S. aureus* cannot be ruled out, initial treatment should be a penicillinase-resistant penicillin (154) or cefuroxime alone (145). In the child older than 5 years and in the adolescent, the initial antibiotic treatment should be directed at *S. aureus* for monoarthritis. Vancomycin should be chosen as the initial antistaphylococcal drug in areas where the prevalence of methicillin resistance is high. Polyarticular disease in a sexually active adolescent warrants treatment directed at *N. gonorrhoeae.*

The duration of antibiotic therapy and the mode of joint drainage have not been studied in a controlled, prospective fashion. Recommendations concerning the duration of antibiotic treatment vary between 2 and 4 weeks for uncomplicated bacterial arthritis caused by less virulent pathogens and 4 and 6 weeks for joint sepsis caused by *S. aureus* or gram-negative bacilli and for joint infections complicated by osteomyelitis. The length of hospitalization may be reduced by using home intravenous therapy (156) or substituting oral antibiotics (157) in carefully controlled situations.

General consensus on draining a child's infected joint recognizes the need for prompt surgical decompression of hip infections and for open drainage of other joints when repeated needle aspirations show persistent infection or are technically difficult to accomplish. The morbidity of arthrotomy must be weighed against the benefits of initial open drainage. One study showed that infections of joints other than the hip had an excellent chance of responding to nonoperative treatment when there was minimal delay in diagnosis and treatment (158).

The outcome of treated bacterial arthritis in children is a function of the patient's age, the joint infected, the infecting microorganism, and the promptness of diagnosis and treatment. Because infection occurs in areas of growth, deformity and local growth retardation are common consequences with lifelong effects. Overall, about 25% of children with bacterial arthritis had some degree of residual abnormality on long-term follow-up (159,160). Infants, especially those with infected hips, did worse (144). Outcome of hip infection was generally less favorable than that of the knee or ankle (159,160). Knee joint infection during the first 2 years of life is often followed by significant deformity, however (161). Of the two most common causes of childhood septic arthritis, *S. aureus* was more likely to lead to residual impairment than was *H. influenzae* (145), although this finding was not invariable (160). Finally, delay in diagnosis and treatment was clearly detrimental to the outcome of treatment (158).

Bacterial Arthritis in the Elderly

In 1900, barely 4% of the total population of the U.S., or 3 million people, were 65 years and older. In 1990, 12% of the population of the U.S., or 32 million people, are 65 or older. By the year 2050, 64 million Americans will be 65 years and older (162). Although the incidence of septic arthritis in adults has not changed significantly over the last several decades (163), a British study spanning 30 years showed that the percentage of patients older than 60 had increased from 19% between 1954 and 1963 to 45% in the following decade (164). These observations suggest that a larger percentage of septic arthritis cases from the geriatric population can be expected. Of 402 adults with septic arthritis reported from 1960 to 1986, 163 (41%) were older than 60 years (165).

The older patient is more likely to display some of the systemic diseases that impair host defense. The most common comorbidities among adults with septic arthritis are diabetes mellitus, cirrhosis, chronic renal failure, RA, and neoplastic disease (2). Two other major risk factors for infectious complications are associated with the management of these chronic illnesses: invasive diagnostic procedures and surgical interventions, and use of immunosuppressive drugs. Even in the absence of overt systemic illness, the aging process can lead to the decline of immune function and increased susceptibility to infectious diseases (166).

Table 126.1 summarizes data from five retrospective studies of nongonococcal bacterial arthritis in 89 elderly patients (167–171). Their mean age was 70.3 years. Underlying joint disease was common, affecting 23% to 71% (mean, 61%). OA and RA were the most common of these diseases, but gout, systemic lupus erythematosus, and hemophiliac arthropathy also were noted. Many patients had an antecedent history of joint trauma. The knee was the most commonly affected joint, followed by the hip, shoulder, and wrist.

The microbiology of acute bacterial joint infection in the elderly is not different from that of adult nongonococcal septic arthritis in general. *S. aureus* was the predominant microorganism, responsible for 43% to 67% of the cases of septic arthritis in the elderly (Table 126.1). Other, less common, gram-positive coccal causes included various streptococci, pneumococci, and *S. epidermidis,* in that order. *N. gonorrhoeae* was much less frequent in the elderly, but when it occurred, its features were similar to those seen in younger persons with gonococcal arthritis (see Chapter 127) (172).

Gram-negative bacilli have emerged as a significant cause of septic arthritis in the last three decades (78) because of the increased incidence of bacteremia caused by gram-negative bacillary organisms (79) and because of the septic arthritis caused by *P. aeruginosa* (80) and *S. marcescens* (82) in intravenous drug users (less likely in a geriatric population than among young adults). The percentages of the elderly with septic arthritis caused by gram-negative bacilli were 14%, 18%, and 35% in three series (Table 126.1). These figures are similar to the 23% rate among 97 adults seen between 1965 and 1982 at the Boston University Medical Center (2).

Septic Arthritis Complicating Rheumatoid Arthritis

Clinical Features

Bacterial infection of a joint already affected by RA is "dangerous, not only to limb but to life" (173). Kellgren et al. (174), in 1958, were the first to report that a joint previously damaged by RA is prone to bacterial invasion, a phenomenon since confirmed by others (175–177). This serious complication of RA is frequently updated and reviewed (178–181), most recently in 1994 (182). Factors that might promote joint infection in RA include the therapeutic use of corticosteroids, cytotoxic drugs, or both, as well as intrinsic defects in RA patients that impair normal host defenses including decreased chemotaxis (183) and phagocytosis by synovial fluid neutrophils (184), depressed hemolytic complement levels, and decreased bacteriolytic activity of synovial fluid (185).

Typically, the patient is older, with long-standing seropositive disease and significant functional impairment and debility (Table 126.2). Nearly half of the patients (45%) were receiving systemic corticosteroids. Thus the clinical expression of joint infection can be blunted, with an insidious rather than abrupt onset. Fever and toxicity are often absent (Table 126.3); only 56% of cases had peripheral blood leukocytosis. Increased pain in one or more joints can easily be mistaken for an RA flare, thus delaying the true diagnosis and subjecting the patient to treatment at a more advanced stage of infection. A high index of suspicion must be maintained, and joint fluid must be studied if septic arthritis complicating RA is suspected. One series of cases showed periarticular manifestations (e.g., sinus tract formation, concomitant septic bursitis, and infected synovial cysts) associated with joint infection, sometimes heralding its onset (179). A flare of RA accompanied by fever and sterile but purulent fluid from one or several joints—"pseudosepsis"—must be treated presumptively as infection until Gram stains and cultures prove negative (186); unusually prompt improvement is common and permits empiric discontinuation of antibiotics.

Table 126.2 provides the relative frequencies of the various bacteria found in infections of the rheumatoid joint. Gram-positive cocci caused 76% of the infections, and *S. aureus* was the major pathogen. Gram-negative bacilli were responsible for the remaining cases, with Enterobacteriaceae accounting for most of them. Polymicrobial infection was extremely rare (175). The spectrum of bacterial causes continues to broaden with reports of cases caused by uncommon and opportunistic pathogens, including *Plesiomonas shigelloides* (100), *P. multocida* (187), *K. kingae* (69), *Listeria monocytogenes* (48), *Micrococcus luteus* (11), *Bacteroides melaninogenicus* (188), and *B. fragilis* (189). *Mycobacterium tuberculosis* was found in two of 11 patients with RA and joint infection encountered over a 9-year period at a center in Spain, where the tuberculosis infection rate is relatively high (181). Polyarticular infection, to which rheumatoid patients are predisposed because of damage to multiple joints, occurs in 25% of cases. Some microorganisms have a predilection to infect multiple joints, for example, *B. fragilis* (189), pneumococci (40), and group G streptococci (26). Polyarticular infection can be subtle, and in some cases is documented only by a vigilant survey of all joints in a patient with septic RA (190). Large joints, especially the knee, are affected most commonly, but unusual sites such as the temporomandibular joint (188,191) and the cricoarytenoid joint can be involved (192).

The source of infection can be identified in a majority of cases. Cutaneous infections—cellulitis, infected skin ulcers, ulcerated rheumatoid nodules, wound infections—were the most common portal in 115 reviewed cases, particularly when *S. aureus* was the responsible agent (63% of cases) (193). Previous intraarticular injections contributed to infection in more than one fourth of cases due to *S. aureus,* but less than 2% of cases involving other organisms; some consider injections given within 3 months of infection as contributory (180), indicating that several mechanisms may underlie this relation.

Therapy

Treatment of septic arthritis superimposed on RA adheres to the principles of therapy for acute bacterial arthritis in general. Systemic antibiotic administration and adequate drainage of the purulent synovial fluid are necessary. Whether the infected rheumatoid joint is better served by immediate open surgical drainage and debridement is debatable (176,179). In 104 RA patients with septic arthritis in which the initial mode of therapy and outcome could be determined, those who were managed medically had poor joint outcome more often when compared with patients initially subjected to surgery (39% vs. 17%) (179). Arthrotomy or arthroscopy might be indicated when the diagnosis of infection is uncertain or delayed and when joint aspiration is difficult because of intrasynovial adhesions and debris (rice bodies). The deleterious effect of delayed diagnosis on outcome is illustrated by a study showing that patients with full recovery had an average delay of 6.6 days between onset of symptoms and diagnosis, whereas in those with a poor outcome, the average delay was 18.0 days (177).

Acute septic arthritis complicating RA carries a mortality of 27% (Table 126.2), much higher than the overall rate of 9% in adults with nongonococcal septic arthritis (22). This partly reflects the extremely poor outcome (mortality of 49%) of RA patients with polyarticular septic arthritis (22). Only half of surviving patients recover their preinfection level of function.

Bacterial Arthritis in Systemic Lupus Erythematosus

Despite recognition that (a) arthritis is a common feature of systemic lupus erythematosus and (b) infection is an important complication of systemic lupus erythematosus, the development of bacterial arthritis in systemic lupus erythematosus remains an underappreciated phenomenon (194,195). In an exhaustive review of the literature seeking all cases of polyarticular septic arthritis (196), 16 cases of polyarticular sepsis in systemic lupus erythematosus were uncovered along with 19 systemic lupus erythematosus patients with monoarticular infection for comparison. Most patients (80%) were receiving immunosuppressive drugs at the time of diagnosis. In contrast to RA patients with septic arthritis, systemic lupus erythematosus was of relatively recent onset, averaging 4 to 6 years in duration. In a few cases, septic arthritis developed at a site of osteonecrosis, but in many others, a previously normal joint was involved. Gram-negative bacteria—most often Salmonella—accounted for infection in 75% of polyarticular cases and more than half the monoarticular cases. The majority underwent surgery, but the fatality rate was nearly half that for RA polyarticular sepsis (25% vs. 49%), and only one monarticular case proved fatal. Of 11 lupus patients with Salmonella septic arthritis seen over a 6-year period at one center, all had nephritis and were receiving corticosteroids (197).

Septic arthritis accompanying disseminated infection with *Neisseria* species [*meningitidis* (198) and *gonorrhoeae* (199)] and the pneumococci (200) have been reported. The risk for serious infections by encapsulated bacteria in patients with systemic lupus erythematosus derives in part from low circulating complement levels and functional hyposplenism. Immunization against these organisms, when possible, has been recommended (198).

Bacterial Arthritis in Immunodeficient Patients

Humoral Immunodeficiency

Hypogammaglobulinemia predisposes patients to recurrent infections of the respiratory tract with encapsulated organisms (e.g., *Hemophilus, Streptococcus*). Acute pyarthrosis can occasionally arise in such patients, however, and is almost always due to organisms of the family Mycoplasmataceae: *Mycoplasma* (201) or *Ureaplasma* (132). The syndrome is not uncommon; of 91 patients followed up over a 20-year period at Middlesex, 21 (23%) had at least one episode of acute pyarthrosis involving one or more joints (202). The arthritis that ensues is not always associated with abundant synovial fluid, but follows an erosive destructive course typical of unrecognized septic arthritis (203) (Fig. 126.2). A chronic erosive arthritis with rheumatoid features also can develop (204). Each of these scenarios contrasts to the frequent polyarticular synovitis seen in hypogammaglobulinemic patients that seems to subside with gammaglobulin replacement but is never destructive (205). Isolation of these organisms requires the use of special broth media (206), and "culture-negative" cases have been confirmed by polymerase chain reaction techniques (207). Treatment requires parenteral antibiotics to which the organisms prove susceptible, usually a macrolide and sometimes streptomycin, along with adequate gammaglobulin replacement. Use of serum with enhanced activity against these organisms has been proposed for refractory cases (208). Reasons for the peculiar susceptibility of hypogammaglobulinemic patients to joint infection with these organisms have yet to be satisfactorily explained. However, absence of a specific antibody against Mycoplasmataceae seems to permit colonization of respiratory and urogenital mucosal surfaces (209); furthermore, Mycoplasmataceae phagocytized in the absence of specific antibody are not killed and may be transported to distant sites (210). Risk for joint infection by Mycoplasmataceae seems to be independent of the etiology for hypogammaglobulinemia, as cases have been reported in Bruton's X-linked agammaglobulinemia (202), common variable immunodeficiency (211), treatment-induced hypogammaglobulinemia (210), and hypogammaglobulinemia associated with systemic lupus ery-

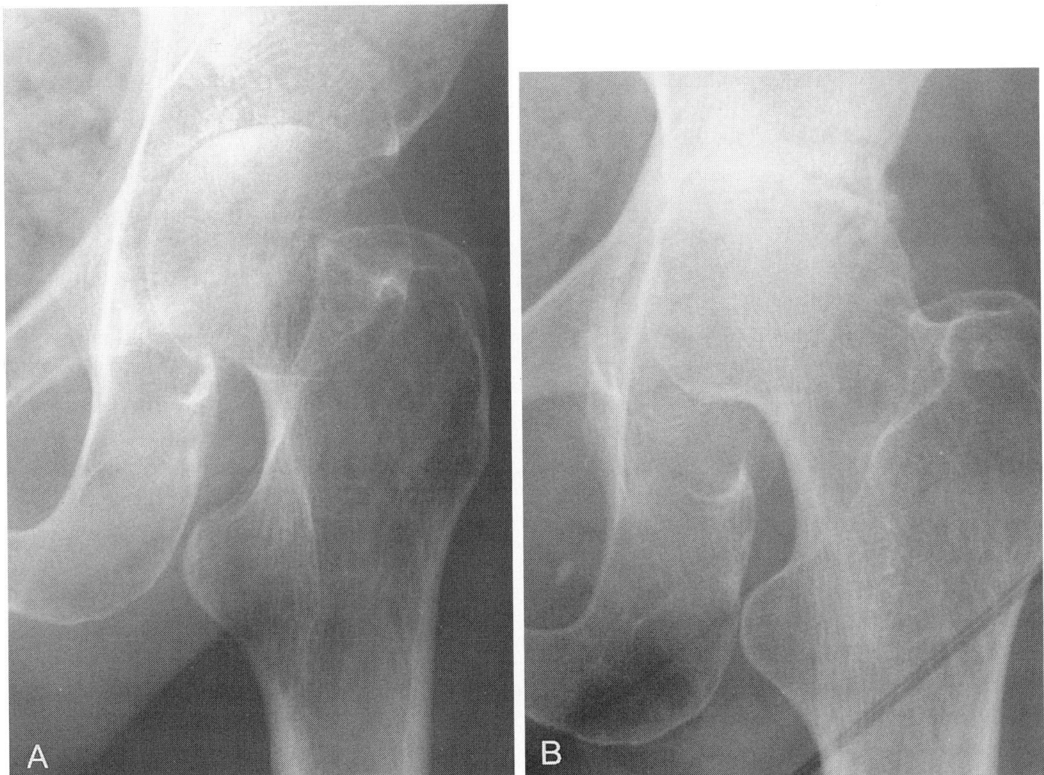

FIGURE 126.2. Left hip joint infection due to Mycoplasma in a hypogammaglobulinemic patient. **A:** Radiograph taken on admission. In a 49-year-old woman with common variable immunodeficiency treated with monthly gammaglobulin infusions, generalized arthralgia, fever, and left leg edema developed 3 months previously. Symptoms improved somewhat after empiric treatment with corticosteroids, antibiotics (ciprofloxacin), and intensification of the gammaglobulin regimen. Hip pain returned and rendered the patient unable to walk for 1 month. Aspiration of the hip yielded 10 mL of purulent synovial fluid from which Mycoplasmae were identified 11 days later. Pain, fever, and effusion resolved with open drainage and doxycycline. However, radiographic features of secondary osteoarthritis progressed, shown on radiographs taken 6 months after presentation **(B)**.

thematosus (212). From data in the U.K. registry of patients with humoral immunodeficiency, it is estimated that such patients have a 1:20 to 1:55 chance of developing mycoplasma arthritis sometime in their lives (204). Other organisms reported to cause septic arthritis in hypogammaglobulinemic patients include *S. aureus* (201) and *H. influenzae* (76,213).

CELLULAR IMMUNODEFICIENCY (INCLUDING HIV INFECTION)

Septic arthritis is an uncommon complication of HIV infection (214,215) (Chapter 131). Although no prospective or cohort studies of the incidence and prevalence of septic arthritis in HIV-infected individuals are available, several studies suggested that this complication is uncommon. In a longitudinal study of 170 HIV-positive patients followed up at the Cleveland Clinic for a mean of 24.6 months, one case of septic arthritis was observed (216). Among 4,023 HIV-infected patients admitted to a large Italian university hospital over a 12-year period, five patients had septic arthritis (217). However, seven cases of septic arthritis were seen over a 3-year period by London-based rheumatologists serving two hospitals that followed up a population of approximately 3,000 HIV-positive patients, of whom 800 had acquired immunodeficiency syndrome (AIDS) (218). Admissions over a 5-year period to three major Atlanta hospitals serving nearly 4,000 HIV-infected patients included 10 cases of septic arthritis (219). In developing countries with endemic HIV infection, concurrent septic arthritis and HIV infection is seen more frequently. A 19-month study of acute arthritis cases admitted to the central hospital in Kigali, Rwanda—which admits more than 3,000 HIV-infected patients each year—included 24 cases of septic arthritis; 19 occurred in HIV-positive patients (79%), compared with the HIV seroprevalence of 30% in the local adult population (215).

Clinical syndromes and causative agents of septic arthritis differ somewhat according to the risk factors for HIV infection. Among homosexual men, approximately one fifth of reported septic arthritis cases have involved *N. gonorrhoeae* (215,220). Because none of these cases occurred in severely immunosuppressed individuals, the occurrence of gonococcal arthritis may be more closely related to shared behavioral risk factors for HIV and gonococcal infection rather than to the degree of immunosuppression. Nongonococcal pyogenic bacteria account for the majority of septic arthritis in this group, with *S. aureus* the most commonly identified organism. *Salmonella* species, common causes of bacteremia in AIDS patients, have been identified in several cases of septic arthritis (221,222). Other unusual pyogenic bacteria reported to cause septic arthritis in AIDS include species of *Nocardia* (140) and *Helicobacter* (223). Despite the frequency of fungal and mycobacterial infections in HIV-positive homosexual patients, only a few cases of joint infections with these organisms have appeared, and no predominant species has emerged (215,224,225), although atypical mycobacteria are more common than *M. tuberculosis* (226). Generally, septic arthritis presentation is typical—with fever, acute arthritis, and purulent joint fluid—and favorable outcome is expected. Cultures of joint fluid and blood help differentiate septic arthritis from the acute reactive arthritis syndromes that can occur in these patients (227). Reported cases in which bacterial infection of a joint takes a rather indolent course (228), or is discovered only by Gram stain and culture of bland synovial fluid obtained from an AIDS patient with unexplained fever (218), illustrate the clinical vigilance sometimes required to identify septic arthritis in the HIV-infected patient.

The emergence of HIV infection in persons with hemophilia has changed the clinical approach to new joint symptoms in these patients. Before HIV, only 15 cases of septic arthritis had been reported in hemophiliacs, with an estimated incidence of less than 0.15% (229). These cases most commonly affected the knee, with *S. aureus* as the causative organism. Since 1987, more than 40 cases of septic arthritis have been reported complicating hemophilia, although HIV status was not always noted (229–233). Reported infections have involved only those joints previously affected by hemophilic arthropathy and may be accompanied by fever but seldom show peripheral blood leukocytosis (233). Salmonella and *S. pneumonia* are important pathogens that were not seen in the pre-HIV era. The presentation of septic arthritis can be indistinguishable from a spontaneous hemarthrosis in a hemophiliac patient; thus septic arthritis should be considered in a patient with a painful and swollen joint that does not respond readily to factor replacement (229–231). Intravenous drug users are at risk for septic arthritis and HIV infection. However, it appears that the clinical spectrum of septic arthritis that arises in the HIV-positive intravenous drug user is not dissimilar to that recognized in intravenous drug users before the HIV era: fibrocartilaginous joints seem particularly prone to infection, and staphylococci, gram-negatives, and fungi (especially Candida) are common causative agents (234). A study that examined septic arthritis affecting intravenous drug users, comparing features of HIV-positive and HIV-negative cases, found that HIV-positive patients sometimes had sites involved other than the hip, knee, sacroiliac, and sternocostal joints (seven of 27 cases) and organisms isolated other than *S. aureus, C. albicans,* and *M. tuberculosis* (235). The mean age and sex distribution was similar across groups, however, and most HIV-positive patients did not have profound immunodeficiency at the time of septic arthritis.

Whereas developing countries contain the largest number of HIV-positive patients, only one report has examined the characteristics of septic arthritis occurring in HIV-positive patients (236). Although most patients with septic arthritis were HIV positive, the range of joint infections seen was similar to those usually encountered at the hospital where the study was conducted.

Congenital deficiencies in cellular immunity (ataxia telangiectasia, severe combined immunodeficiency, and the syndromes of Wiskott–Aldrich, Nezeloff, and DiGeorge) can occasionally be complicated by joint disease, usually of a noninfectious nature. Infections tend to be fungal, protozoal, or viral, rather than bacterial (237).

MISCELLANEOUS IMMUNODEFICIENCY STATES

Skeletal infection can be the presenting feature of an immunodeficiency state in early childhood. An immunologic and clinical study of 15 children with bone or joint infections found nine with an abnormality of immunoglobulins, complement, or phagocytes (238). Patients with phagocytic defects in the setting of chronic granulomatous disease or hyperimmunoglobulinemia E are susceptible to infection with several organisms, especially staphylococci (239,240); in one series of 21 patients with hyperimmunoglobulinemia E, four had joint infections (241). Patients deficient in one of the early components of complement tend to have autoimmune disorders; however, septic arthritis due to *H. influenzae* or *S. pneumoniae* has been described in persons with C2 deficiency (242). Joint involvement may complicate meningococcemia in 12% of cases occurring in (late component) complement deficiency states, or it may be a part of disseminated gonococcal infection, to which these patients are also susceptible (243).

Infection in Previously Invaded Joints

Prosthetic Joint Infections

Clinical Features

Bacterial infection of a prosthetic joint is a rare, but devastating and costly event. Hip and knee replacements, which account for most of the more than 430,000 joint-replacement operations performed in the U.S. each year, harbor a

1% to 2% chance of becoming infected over the life of the patient or replacement (244,245). Shoulder, elbow, and ankle prostheses do not fare so well. Reported infection rates for elbow prostheses are as high as 6% (244) and 9% (60), similar to the rates for hip and knee prostheses when they were first performed (241).

Nearly all infected prosthetic joints are painful (106). The constant nature of the pain can help differentiate prosthetic sepsis from other causes of new pain in a prosthetic joint (e.g., loosening, fracture), wherein pain tends to be use related (246). Other symptoms from the infected prosthesis can differ according to timing of the onset of infection. Infection that begins immediately after surgery usually causes fever, constitutional symptoms, and gross alterations in the surgical wound, such as purulent discharge from the incompletely healed incision or development of a sinus tract once the wound has healed. Infections occurring later can be quite indolent, with few systemic signs and local findings of only swelling or tenderness. Prosthetic joint infections have been classified according to route of bacterial infection (local vs. hematogenous) (247) and timing of infection onset (early, within 12 weeks of implantation; subacute, within the first year after implantation; late, >1 year from implantation) (248). Neither classification approach is entirely satisfactory, because mechanisms of infection and timing of presentation can overlap.

Several aspects of the indwelling prosthesis and host response promote susceptibility to infection regardless of source or timing. The prosthesis and binding cement (usually methylmethacrylate) present a relatively avascular expanse on which pathogens may persist and be sequestered from circulating immunologic defenses and from systemic antibiotics (249,250). In the presence of prosthetic devices, many bacteria elaborate a fibrous exopolysaccharide (glycocalyx) in which organisms can grow and form thick biofilms that further impair host defenses (246,251). Bacteria adherent to biomaterials are less sensitive to antibiotics both *in vitro* and *in vivo* (252,253). Fastidious measures to minimize implantation of bacteria into the operative field (laminar flow rooms, negative pressure exhaust suits for operating room personnel, prophylactic antibiotics) are now routine and have considerably cut the rates of postoperative infection, but have not eliminated the problem entirely. Perioperative factors associated with septic arthritis developing within a year after arthroplasty were determined in a prospective multicenter study of 362 knee and 2,651 hip arthroplasties (254); for both knee and hip cases, wound infection and wound-healing problems conferred the greatest risk for subsequent prosthetic infection. Risk for prosthetic hip infection also was greater with diabetes, failed healing of a fracture around a new prosthesis, urinary tract infection, or a slow recovery. For knee prostheses, enhanced risk for infection also was conferred by RA, wound problems requiring antibiotics, and persistent pain with limited function in the operated-on knee. Prior joint arthroplasty and presence of malignancy also increase risk for prosthetic joint infection (255).

Early infections that arise from adjacent soft tissues generally are caused by a single pathogen, usually a coagulase-negative staphylococcus (106), but polymicrobial sepsis with as many as five different organisms has been described (245,248). Rarely, latent foci of osteomyelitis can be reactivated at surgery; postoperative recrudescence of *S. aureus* and *M. tuberculosis,* with negative intraoperative bone cultures, has been described (256,257).

Any bacteremia can infect a joint prosthesis (258). Dentogingival infections and manipulations can cause viridans streptococcal and anaerobic (*Peptococcus, Peptostreptococcus*) infection of a prosthesis. Pyogenic skin infections can lead to staphylococcal (*S. aureus, S. epidermidis*) and streptococcal (groups A, B, C, and G) prosthetic infections. Genitourinary and gastrointestinal tract procedures have been associated with gram-negative, enterococcal, and anaerobic infection of prostheses. Twenty percent to 40% of prosthetic joint infections arise by the hematogenous route, with the remainder being locally introduced. Prosthetic joint infection can be caused by aerobic gram-positive cocci (75–80%), aerobic gram-negative rods (10–20%), and anaerobic microorganisms (5–10%) (105,106). Staphylococci account for 75% to 90% of the gram-positive coccal infections. *S. epidermidis* might be more common than *S. aureus* in prosthetic joint infections (106), in contrast with septic arthritis in natural joints, where *S. aureus* predominates. The presence of a foreign body might play a permissive role in infections caused by the less virulent microorganisms (252). Among the gram-negative bacilli, *E. coli, P. mirabilis,* and *P. aeruginosa* are the major culprits (253). Anaerobic bacteria, accounting for 5% to 10% of infections, include *Peptococcus* sp., *Peptostreptococcus* sp., *Clostridium perfringens,* and *B. fragilis* (248,259). However, the spectrum of microbial agents capable of causing prosthetic joint infections is unlimited and includes organisms ordinarily considered "contaminants" of cultures such as *Corynebacteria, Propionobacteria,* and *Bacillus* sp. Polymicrobial infections range from 6% (248) to 25% (245), and usually occur early.

Suspected prosthetic joint infection can be absolutely confirmed only by demonstrating a microorganism in a specimen taken from tissue or fluid adjacent to the prosthesis. Infection can be presumed when a painful prosthesis is accompanied by fever, purulent drainage, or a positive blood culture. In most cases, however, suspected infection must be differentiated from the various aseptic and mechanical problems that more commonly cause pain in these patients. Several findings on plain radiographs raise suspicion of infection: (a) abnormal lucencies in the bone–cement interface, (b) changes in position of prosthetic components, (c) cement fractures, (d) periosteal reaction, and (e) motion of components on stress views (258). Arthrography can show abnormal communications between the joint space and multiple defects in the bone–cement interface. These abnormalities can be found in about half of all septic prostheses and are related to duration of infection. Because these changes also can be seen with aseptic prostheses, they cannot be considered diagnostic of infection. To determine whether a loosened prosthesis has failed because of infection, at least five specimens should be obtained for culture at the time of revision arthroplasty; isolation of the same organism from three or more specimens is highly predictive of infection (260).

The commonly used radionuclide scanning methods neither reliably detect all infected prostheses nor exclude aseptic cases. The increased vascularity and enhanced metabolic activity detected by technetium diphosphonate occur routinely in prostheses for 6 months after operation; thereafter, uptake is considered abnormal, but can reflect inflammation and possible loosening without infection. Sequential scanning with technetium followed by gallium is 60% to 70% sensitive and 81% to 89% specific for infection (261). Scanning that uses indium-labeled autologous white blood cells also has been used. Unfortunately, this technique has not proven to be as accurate as first reports indicated (262). Ultrasonography, which can be useful in localizing periarticular fluid for aspiration, may delineate features that suggest an infected prosthesis. In one study, 48 patients (33 with pain) with hip prostheses underwent ultrasound examinations; the six patients (all painful) ultimately shown to be infected had a significantly larger joint effusion, and five of six had extracapsular fluid collections (263).

Blood studies that reflect systemic inflammation, such as elevated leukocyte count and sedimentation rate, have been used to evaluate patients with suspected prosthetic infection, but are inadequate to diagnose clinical sepsis. Other more sensitive measures of the acute-phase response have been evaluated; plasma viscosity and C-reactive protein both increase immediately after joint replacement, but C-reactive protein decreases to normal levels within 2 weeks (264). Thus an elevated C-reactive protein level could be useful in detecting the acute inflammation that would accompany a prosthetic joint infection.

Aspiration of painful joint replacements has a high reported sensitivity and specificity in the several studies that have compared fluid culture with culture of tissues obtained at operative exploration of the affected joint (261,265). With radiographic guidance, about one third to one half of all taps will be "dry"; sterile saline injected into a dry joint cannot always be retrieved. With ultrasensitive radiometric culture techniques (^{14}C-labeled substrate in bottles, with release of $^{14}CO_2$ into the head gas of the bottle taken as evidence of bacterial growth), needle aspiration of painful hip prostheses was 87% sensitive and 95% specific for infection (266). Hence aspiration is a generally sound method that identifies most infected arthroplasties, but still fails to diagnose a small number. Therefore open exploration and biopsy of several sites remains the standard method for diagnosis of an infected arthroplasty. When samples taken from suggestive areas show more than five neutrophils in five different fields (×50), infection is highly likely (267).

Therapy

Once the infecting organism has been identified, the patient undergoes exploration and meticulous debridement of the joint. The implant is removed, and all sinuses, infected tissues, cement, and cement–bone membrane are excised. For whatever joint is infected, three basic approaches may be followed (261,268). The patient may be left with an excision arthroplasty, or the joint may be revised (exchanged) in one or two stages. An excision arthroplasty will function differently, with some residual pain and instability. A one-stage revision may be undertaken safely if a single infecting organism has been identified and is of low virulence (269). The patient should be in good general health with no systemic toxicity and should have sufficient bone stock so as not to require grafting. Methylmethacrylate cement impregnated with antibiotics to which the infecting organism is sensitive is used in reimplantation (270,271). If the organism is of high virulence or has not been identified, a two-stage revision is appropriate, with 4 to 6 weeks of antibiotics given between time of removal and time of placement of the new implant. Success rates for reimplantation with antibiotic-impregnated cement range from 39% to 91% in six retrospective series reporting one-stage procedures and 73% to 100% in three series examining two-stage procedures (261). Debridement with retention of prosthesis followed by continuous antistaphylococcal therapy is sometimes successful (69% failure rate within 2 years), particularly if done soon after onset of symptoms (272). In a prospective randomized trial of 33 patients with staphylococcal infection of stable orthopedic implants (including 15 prosthetic joints), all those treated with ciprofloxacin and rifampin were cured of infection compared with 58% of those receiving ciprofloxacin alone (273). Long-term suppression of prosthetic joint infection with oral antibiotics has been attempted in cases in which the medical condition of the patient makes definitive surgical management risky. At the University of Michigan, nine of 19 patients with infected hip prostheses showed no deterioration after a mean of 4.1 years (274); however, two other centers have reported far less success, with 8% and 23% effectively suppressed for less than 2 years, and 38% experiencing adverse effects from antibiotics at one center (275,276). Suppressive oral antibiotic therapy as sole treatment should be considered only for patients who fulfill the following five criteria: (a) prosthesis removal not possible, (b) relatively avirulent pathogen, (c) pathogen sensitive to oral antibiotic, (d) chosen oral antibiotic tolerated by patient, and (e) prosthesis not loose.

Efforts to prevent prosthetic joint infection begin in the preoperative period and continue for the life of the patient. Patients receiving methotrexate for RA should discontinue the medication a week before surgery and resume taking it a week after; in a prospective trial, no infection occurred in any of 19 patients randomized to this protocol, whereas four of 13 patients who continued taking methotrexate became infected (277). Early recognition and prompt therapy for any infection are critical to reduce the risk for hematogenous seeding of the joint implant. The use of prophylactic antibiotics in anticipation of bacteremic events (i.e., oral surgery, cystoscopy, colonoscopy with biopsy, surgical procedures on infected or contaminated tissues) has been suggested on the same empiric basis on which endocarditis prophylaxis (278) has been recommended (279,280). However, no data are available with which the cost-effectiveness of these measures can be analyzed, and the approach to prevention remains controversial. Routine antibiotic prophylaxis before all dental procedures would lead to more substantial costs from morbidity due to antibiotic reactions than would be saved from reduction of a presumed low-level risk for prosthetic joint infection (281). Nevertheless, antibiotic prophylaxis before dental procedures on infected areas (gingivitis, tooth abscesses, gross caries) is recommended by those who are skeptical about wider-ranging predental prophylaxis, particularly when the patient has risk factors for deep infection (e.g., RA, diabetes mellitus, immunosuppressive therapy) (281,282).

Infection after Arthrocentesis

Prior arthrocentesis is considered a risk factor for septic arthritis, particularly if corticosteroids are instilled afterward. Rates for this occurrence are extremely low, ranging from 1:1,000 to 1:16,000 in older series (283–285). Because many arthrocenteses are performed in clinical practice, this rare complication accounts for a substantial number of joint infections. In five series in which prior corticosteroid injections were mentioned as a potential cause for septic arthritis, 20% of all cases of septic arthritis could be linked to this risk factor (196,286). This figure may be specious, because most series of bacterial arthritis either contain no cases of postinjection infection or fail to distinguish them. Four possible mechanisms account for joint infection after arthrocentesis: (a) contamination of the injected drug preparation, (b) introduction of bacteria from the skin, (c) hematogenous colonization of the puncture track, and (d) corticosteroid activation of previously quiescent infection (286). Of these, only the first can be formally proven, as has been done in two reports in which the species of bacteria isolated from the joint also was found in the vial of corticosteroids used previously on the patients affected (287,288). Unusual gram-negative isolates (*S. marcescens, P. cepacia*) were involved in both instances. Resident skin flora (e.g., *S. epidermidis, S. albus,* Propionobacteria) are rarely found to be the cause of postinjection infection. Nevertheless, skin cleansing before arthrocentesis and attention to aseptic technique during the procedure are still warranted (289). Most cases of infection that follow arthrocentesis probably arise when transient bacteremia colonizes the needle track, where capillary integrity has been disrupted, thereby providing a locus of least resistance. Latent infection reactivated by corticosteroids often involves mycobacteria (286). Clinical features of postinjection joint infection resemble typical bacterial septic arthritis in most respects, with similar distribution of microorganisms, affected joints, and concurrent conditions. Delay in diagnosis is common, confounded by the underlying joint disease and its treatment as well as consideration of "postinjection flare" as a cause of the persistent joint signs.

Infection after Arthroscopy

Joint infection is an uncommon but serious complication of arthroscopy. Large surveys for postarthroscopy complications place the infection rate at 0.04% to 0.3% (290–292). Knee arthroscopies predominate in these surveys, and infection after arthroscopy of other joints may occur more frequently. A 1988 survey of 10,282 arthroscopies by 21 experienced arthroscopists included 14 hip arthroscopies, of which one was complicated by septic arthritis (292). In general, the chances for infection increase in proportion to the extent of joint invasion and tissue manipulation during the procedures; one practice—tying the sutures of a meniscal repair over an external button (292)—has been abandoned because of the high rate of infectious complications. Other risk factors for infection include corticosteroid injection after arthroscopy [which increased the infection risk more than 27-fold in one series (293)], incomplete disinfection of the arthroscope between cases, excessive foot traffic through the arthroscopy suite, and proximity of nonsterile materials to the joint being arthroscoped (e.g., cardiac monitoring cables lying near the shoulder) (294). Two clinical syndromes have been described (293), both within 1 to 10 days of arthroscopy. Infection due to virulent microorganisms, usually *S. aureus,* appears as typical septic arthritis, with acute onset of pain and fever, peripheral leukocytosis, and purulent joint fluid with positive Gram stains. Nearly as many cases are due to coagulase-negative staphylococcus and occur in a more indolent fashion. Because of the low or absent fever, lack of joint erythema, and joint fluid with "inflammatory" rather than "purulent" characteristics, these cases can be mistakenly ascribed to benign postarthroscopy effusion or activity of the underlying joint disease. Detection of these cases also is confounded by the tendency to accept a low-grade fever for 24 to 48 hours after arthroscopy and to disregard as contaminants any "skin flora" grown from synovial fluid.

Infection of Fibrocartilaginous Joints

Bacterial infection of an axial skeleton fibrocartilaginous joint usually does not have the cardinal signs of swelling, warmth, and limited motion that raise suspicion for infection in appendicular diarthrodial joints. Thus infection of the fibrocartilaginous joints of the pelvis (sacroiliac joint, symphysis pubis) and thoracic cage (sternoclavicular, acromioclavicular, and sternomanubrial joints) is often slow to be detected. The patient populations prone to infections in these structures differ somewhat from those in whom infections in diarthrodial joints develop, and the infections cause characteristic clinical syndromes.

The *sacroiliac joint* is an amphiarthrodial structure with an inferior portion composed of a synovium-lined cavity and opposed hyaline cartilage surfaces and a superior portion in which fibrocartilage is interposed between sacrum and ilium, stabilized by broad, strong ligaments (295). Infection of the sacroiliac joint accounts for 1% to 2% of all cases of septic arthritis (296,297). Reported cases of sacroiliac infection are notable for the panoply of (incorrect) diagnoses initially proposed to explain the clinical presentation, ranging from appendicitis to sciatica and septic hip (62,298). Because any motion of the pelvis relative to the spine irritates the sacroiliac joint, patients with sacroiliac infection prefer to lie very still in bed and are averse to any movement. Consequently, maneuvers that stress the sacroiliac joint are usually not part of the initial examination.

The sacroiliac joint is innervated by most or all of the major nerve trunks passing near it, including the superior gluteal, obturator, and first two sacral nerves (295). Thus anterior thigh pain is common, as is a "positive" straight leg–raising test, leading to the erroneous consideration of lumbar disc pathology in many patients. The thin anterior capsule of an infected sacroiliac joint may rupture early on, allowing purulent drainage to fill the iliac fossa and travel along the tendons of the short external rotators to enter the buttock (299). Such patients complain of buttock pain on the side of the affected sacroiliac joint and may have a palpable mass in the buttock. Pus that tracks from the sacroiliac joint to the iliac fossa can cause retroperitoneal irritation and lower quadrant tenderness, mimicking an intraabdominal process that can be mistaken for appendicitis.

Most patients have sudden onset of fever and continuous pain exacerbated by weight bearing. About 25% of reported patients had subacute illnesses with slight or no fever, and less intense pain (300). The erythrocyte sedimentation rate (ESR) is almost always elevated. Blood cultures are positive in about half the reported cases, although much time can pass before the sacroiliac joint is confirmed as the primary site of infection. Physical examination maneuvers that stress the sacroiliac joint—direct palpation, pelvic compression, Gaenslen's maneuver, the FABERE test (flexion, abduction, external rotation, and extension of the ipsilateral hip)—seldom were performed at presentation in reported cases, but nearly always raised suspicion for sacroiliac joint pathology when finally done (299). Initial plain radiographs of the sacroiliac joint are usually normal (300,301). Bone scan, with attention to the early perfusion phase (296), usually localizes the affected sacroiliac joint, but can be normal in the first few days after onset of symptoms (62). Computed tomography (CT) can show joint-space widening, subchondral bony changes, and abnormalities in adjacent soft tissue (swelling, abscess formation) that suggest pathology in the sacroiliac joint (300,302) (Fig. 126.3). Use of magnetic resonance imaging (MRI) with gadolinium-DPTA enhancement in five cases of septic sacroiliitis showed abnormalities before any other imaging modality, including sacroiliac joint effusions, bone edema, and adjacent soft tissue abscesses (303); however, others have reported cases in which MRI did not identify sacroiliac joint pathology that was later shown by other imaging modalities (299).

The combination of positive blood cultures and an abnormal sacroiliac joint is sufficient to make the diagnosis of septic sacroiliitis. For blood culture–negative cases, several methods have been described to obtain tissue or fluid from the affected sacroiliac joint to confirm infection and identify the responsible agent. Aspiration of the joint at the bedside is extremely difficult (301,304); chances for successful aspiration are enhanced by use of general anesthesia (62) and confirming entry of the space, using fluoroscopy (301) or CT (302). When cultures are negative or nondiagnostic, or when empiric antibiotics have not effected clinical improvement, open biopsy is indicated to provide multiple tissue samples and drainage (300). Resolution without surgical drainage is usual, but surgery is occasionally needed to drain abscesses or debride bone and cartilage that may be dead or sequestered (297).

Distant sites of infection sometimes develop. The case of a 3.5-year-old girl with concomitant meningitis and sacroiliitis due to *S. aureus* illustrated a situation that could be more common than appreciated, because the meninges are directly opposed to the sacroiliac joint (305). Most isolates from blood or sacroiliac joint in reported cases have been due to *S. aureus.* Intravenous drug users show a propensity for infection with multiply resistant staphylococci (including *S. epidermidis*) and *Pseudomonas* (62,82). Treatment with parenteral antibiotics directed against staphylococci (and *Pseudomonas* in patients at risk), with adjustment according to sensitivities of the isolate, is required for at least 4 weeks (299,304); most authors recommended 6 weeks

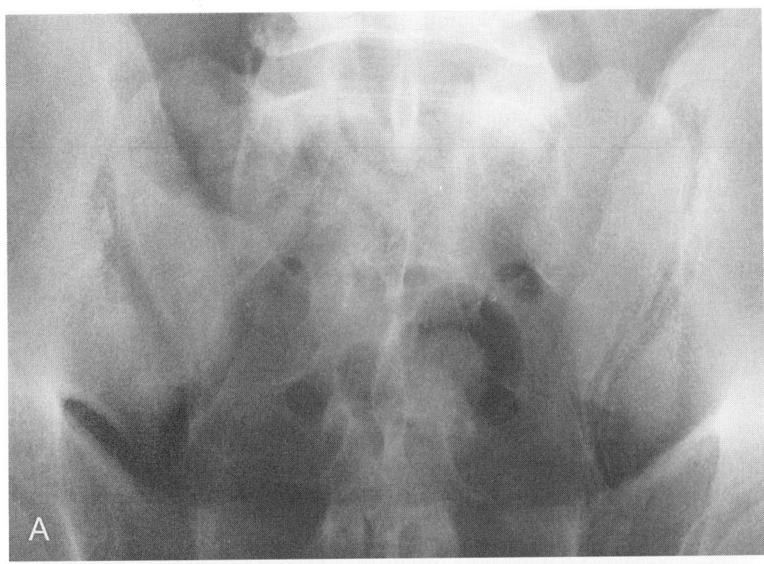

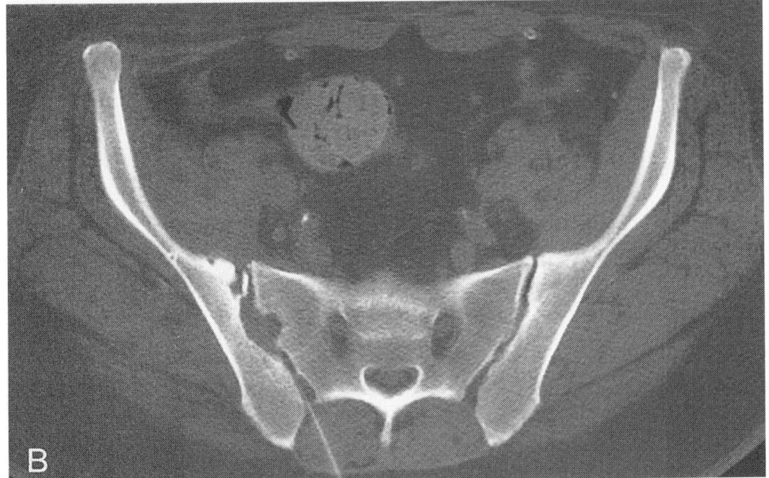

FIGURE 126.3. Sacroiliac joint infection due to coagulase-positive Staphylococcus in a hemodialysis patient. Radiograph of sacroiliac joints **(A)** shows joint widening and indistinct cortical margins at the right sacroiliac joint. CT scan **(B)** shows bony erosion, fragmentation of bone, and a small iliac sequestrum. Soft tissue anterior to right sacroiliac joint appears more prominent with less distinct septation of iliacus muscle from adjacent pelvic tissues when compared with normal left side, suggesting inflammation or abscess. A CT scan was used to guide needle aspiration of the joint. Pain had developed in the region of the right hip 10 weeks previously; a concomitant positive blood culture was ascribed at the time to line sepsis and treated with a single intravenous dose of vancomycin and removal of Sorenson catheter.

(62,300), with a longer course if osteomyelitis is present. Bacteriologic and clinical cure is the rule, with a rare patient experiencing persistent pain arising from a damaged sacroiliac joint (297).

The *pubic symphysis* is an amphiarthrodial joint in which hyaline cartilage lining the two opposing pubic bones is separated by a thick fibrocartilaginous disc but no synovium (306). Infection of the pubic symphysis nearly always involves bone as well as joint space, and has been given several names: pyogenic (or infectious) osteitis pubis, osteomyelitis of the symphysis pubis, pubic osteomyelitis, and pyogenic infection of the symphysis pubis (307). The condition is rare, occurring as an uncommon complication of urologic (308) or gynecologic (309) operations and an occasional consequence of intravenous drug use (310). Most patients have suprapubic pain worsened with walking. Some patients develop a waddling gate due to spasm of the rectus abdominis and adductor muscles (308). Other locations and radiation of pain—to hips, thigh, and groin—can confound diagnostic efforts. Constitutional and systemic features (including fever) often are not present, and a prolonged smoldering course is common. Pubic tenderness is usually present, but pain exacerbated by other maneuvers can divert attention to the structures being examined (310). Hence pain on hip motion may suggest a primary process involving the hip and pain with pelvic compression may implicate the sacroiliac joint. The leukocyte count is usually normal, but the ESR has been elevated in all reported cases. Initial radiographs are frequently normal, but joint-space widening, irregularity of the pubic margins, and separation of the joint can be seen, particularly if there has been a long delay in diagnosis. Bone scans are positive in all but the most acute cases. Blood cultures are seldom positive. Aspiration of the pubic symphysis joint space is feasible, particularly with CT guidance (311). However, open biopsy of bone and fibrocartilage has a much higher yield, and is usually required to establish a bacteriologic diagnosis (310). *P. aeruginosa* has been responsible for nearly all cases in intravenous drug users (310), and is the next most common isolate after staphylococci in pubic symphysis infections acquired after pelvic operations (312). Some patients who undergo open debridement for presumed pubic symphysis infections do not grow organisms from tissue specimens, yet have histopathologic features of osteomyelitis and respond clinically to antibiotics (309). Pubic symphysis infections share many features with "osteitis pubis," a painful but self-limited condition that can cause pubic pain and haziness of the pubic symphysis after pelvic procedures; pain persisting more than 6 weeks and not responding to antiinflammatory treatment should prompt search for pubic symphysis infection (313).

Bacterial infection of the *sternoclavicular joint* accounts for 5% to 10% of all septic arthritis cases (314,315). Intravenous drug users are particularly prone to sternoclavicular joint infection; in one report of septic arthritis in intravenous heroin users, 37% had an infected sternoclavicular joint (316). Upper extremity septic thrombophlebitis can affect the sternoclavicular joint by contiguous extension, and probably is the mechanism by which sternoclavicular joint infection occasionally develops in patients receiving hemodialysis (317) or those with central venous subclavian catheters (318). Older reports of septic arthritis in RA patients suggested that sternoclavicular joint infection occurred more often than in nonselected patient populations with septic arthritis (174), but more recent studies have not shown this (182). Several patients have developed sternoclavicular joint infection with no identifiable predisposition other than a recent median sternotomy (315). Healthy adults rarely can develop sternoclavicular joint infection (319).

The unique anatomy of the sternoclavicular joint and its relation to adjacent structures help explain various modes of presentation, complications, and problems in diagnosis and management (314). The sternoclavicular joint is the only direct connection of the shoulder girdle apparatus to the axial skeleton. The joint is composed of a biconcave fibrocartilaginous meniscus interposed between the sternum and the clavicle, with cavities on either side of the meniscus lined by synovium, and a dense ligamentous capsule surrounding all. The interclavicular ligament connects the two sternoclavicular joint menisci to each other, and each meniscus is attached inferiorly to the first rib where it meets the sternum. The sternohyoid muscles, trachea, and large vessels of the neck are just posterior to the sternoclavicular joint.

Presenting symptoms of sternoclavicular joint infection vary (36,314,320). Pain in the shoulder region, neck, or chest usually precedes detectable joint swelling. Fever is common, but not universal, and constitutional symptoms of malaise and weight loss can predominate. In a series of five patients in which details from 60 previously reported cases were added, correct diagnosis was often delayed, with duration of preceding complaints ranging from 1 day to 2 months (320). Because shoulder movement is almost always quite painful when the sternoclavicular joint is inflamed, an erroneous consideration of septic shoulder can ensue. Swelling often extends beyond the sternoclavicular joint, with swelling over the medial clavicle (suggesting tumor) and induration of soft tissues of the chest wall or neck in some cases. Soft tissue shadows of the sternoclavicular joint overlying the lung apex can evoke the clinical diagnosis of apical lung tumor or pneumonia (320).

Although the sternoclavicular joint is easily assessed by direct palpation, its orientation and structure make arthrocentesis difficult (314). Exploratory arthrotomy is indicated for diagnosis when suspected sternoclavicular joint infection cannot be confirmed by cultures of synovial fluid or blood. Open drainage and debridement also is indicated for extraarticular abscess, if clinically suspected or shown by imaging studies, and for extensive sternal or clavicular osteomyelitis. The sternoclavicular joint is poorly seen on plain radiographs (314), and sternoclavicular joint inflammation is unreliably demonstrated by bone scans, which can be normal early in the course and sometimes show uptake due to other processes, such as sternoclavicular joint OA (314,315). CT has been advocated for all suspected cases, as it delineates the sternoclavicular joint and can show extension of the infection to involve the first costochondral junction, or the mediastinum, whether as mediastinitis (with increased soft tissue attenuation of subjacent mediastinal fat and obliteration of normal fat planes surrounding the brachiocephalic vessels) or as frank mediastinal abscess (321). Abscess formation in sternoclavicular joint infection is common, complicating 20% of cases in a 1988 review in which most abscesses were found without sophisticated imaging (320). Osteomyelitis, usually of the clavicle, was shown radiographically or pathologically in more than half the reported cases in the same review (320).

The most common organisms causing sternoclavicular joint infection are *S. aureus* and *P. aeruginosa,* the latter causing most cases in intravenous drug users, and the former affecting most others with sternoclavicular joint infection (320,322). Other organisms, including groups B and G streptococcus, *E. coli, H. influenzae, S. marcescens,* and *B. melitensis,* and other pathogens have been isolated (35,320,322). *Fusobacterium necrophorum,* a member of the anaerobic gram-negative family Bacteroidaceae and part of the resident normal flora of oral cavity and gastrointestinal and female urogenital tracts, was a common cause of sternoclavicular joint infection in the preantibiotic era and was found as the cause of sternoclavicular joint infection in an otherwise healthy young man reported in 1993 (323).

Treatment of sternoclavicular joint infection requires high-dose intravenous antibiotics given at least 2 to 3 weeks for nonresistant *S. aureus* and 4 to 6 weeks for *Pseudomonas.* If osteomyelitis is present, the antibiotic course should be lengthened at least 2 weeks. Surgery is required for eradication of abscesses, mediastinitis, and extensive osteomyelitis (318). Clavicular osteomyelitis that persists despite intensive antibiotic therapy and debridement can be cured by resection of the medial clavicular head (320). Prognosis is excellent for patients whose infection is eradicated, even if surgery is required. However, deaths due to endocarditis and uncontrolled sepsis have occurred in patients with sternoclavicular joint infection in whom recognition and treatment were delayed (315). The medial border of the acromion process and distal clavicle are connected by a short taut joint capsule to comprise the acromioclavicular joint. Articular surfaces are mainly fibrocartilaginous, and a pad of fibrocartilage may project into the joint from above, sometimes partitioning the joint completely. Bacterial infection of the acromioclavicular joint is extremely rare, with only four cases of bacterial septic arthritis reported (30,228, 324,325). Shoulder pain and limited motion can be severe. All but one case had an abnormal radiograph, and all had abnormal bone scans. Surgical management is appropriate for most cases, as the acromioclavicular joint space is small and sometimes complex, and acromioclavicular joint infections tend to involve bone early on; three fourths of reported cases underwent arthrotomy and clavicular debridement or resection.

The manubriosternal joint is an amphiarthrodial joint similar in construction to the symphysis pubis. The articulating ends of the sternum and manubrium are covered by hyaline cartilage, connected by fibrocartilage and ligaments. A true joint space, lined by oval synovium-like cells, exists in 30% to 45% of individuals (326). Only six cases of manubriosternal joint infection have been reported (327–332). Each had fever and anterior chest pain [mistaken for myocardial ischemia in one case (332)]. All but two had a tender anterior chest mass overlying the sternal angle. Radiographic appearance of the manubriosternal joint, which can be demonstrated on a lateral chest radiograph if the patient's arms are held above the horizontal (326), was abnormal in four of six cases. Responsible organisms (*S. aureus,* five; *Pseudomonas,* one) were found in synovial fluid in the four cases where it was obtained (one by arthrotomy), bone (one case), or blood (four cases). In one case, an adjacent thymus abscess shown by CT was surgically drained (332).

Septic Arthritis Associated with Crystal-induced Arthritis

Acute arthritis due to an inflammatory response to microcrystalline material within the joint can mimic septic arthritis, particularly when the patient has fever and constitutional symptoms, and the synovial fluid is opaque (group III) and has a very high leukocyte count (333). Awareness that features of sepsis can accompany acute crystalline arthritis guides the clinician to consider the diagnosis of occult crystal arthritis in patients with unexplained fever (334), and demands that crystals be sought in patients with acute pyarthrosis before committing to medical or surgical management of septic arthritis (335). Bacterial infection can occasionally coexist with acute crystal arthritis, however.

Simultaneous gout and septic arthritis is so uncommon that it was once postulated that preexisting gout somehow "protected" joints against bacterial infection (336). However, 22 cases of coexistent gout and septic arthritis had been reported before 1997 (337–346). Most patients had preexisting polyarticular gout and several acutely swollen joints. Monoarticular presentations involved the knee (six of 11 cases) more often than the metatarsophalangeal (two of nine cases). Tophi, seen in 10 of 22 cases, were considered to be a risk factor for concomitant infection (345). Other comorbidities considered as risk factors for septic arthritis (diabetes, chronic renal insufficiency, alcoholism) were common in these patients. However, in some otherwise healthy patients, concomitant gout and septic arthritis was the first manifestation of gout (341,342). In most cases, acute arthritis was initially ascribed to gout based on synovial fluid findings, and then treated as infection when bacteriologic results emerged (cultures of blood or synovial fluid). None of these cases responded to conventional medical therapy for gout, although none had received intraarticular or systemic corticosteroids. In two cases, gout became evident during the course of treatment for established bacterial arthritis (339,342). Addition of treatment directed at gout led to resolution of persistent inflammatory effusions in two otherwise "cured" patients (332). Many cases (14 of 22) required surgical drainage, perhaps because of delayed recognition of joint infection. Poor functional outcome was common, and five patients died. Causative bacteria ran the usual gamut (staphylococci, 11; streptococci, six; gram-negative, five), although several cases involved strains of *Streptococcus* usually considered as rare pathogens in bacterial septic arthritis: *Pneumococcus,* three cases; and *Streptococcus* group C, two cases. None of the cases described could be considered a "typical" gouty flare. For each case identified, at least one of the after scenarios applied: worsening of synovitis despite conventional medical treatment of gout, fever accompanying polyarthritis or grossly purulent joint fluid, acute arthritis developing during or shortly after treatment of an infection at another site, polyarthritis that included a joint not previously affected by gout, or monoarthritis with very high fever (>40°C). Although it is not standard practice to submit synovial fluid from all gouty joints for Gram stain and culture, any of the aforementioned situations should raise sufficient suspicion for infection that such additional testing is performed.

Acute arthritis with synovial fluid exhibiting leukocytes engulfing calcium pyrophosphate dihydrate (CPPD) crystals—the pseudogout syndrome—can mimic septic arthritis but sometimes accompanies frank joint infection. Of 314 patients with proven pseudogout seen over a 16-year period at the Mayo Clinic, five had concomitant septic arthritis; Gram stain of synovial fluid showed organisms in only one case (347). Although this association is reported only about as often as gout and sepsis, it is probably much more common. Of reported cases, nearly all were monoarticular, and most involved the knee (342,347). Patients tend to be older. Chondrocalcinosis was seen in about half the joints reported. Gram stain showed organisms less than half the time. Unlike many cases of pseudogout, in which identification of crystals may require a dedicated search, CPPD crystals tend to be abundant in synovial fluid later shown to be infected (348). Because risk for concomitant infection cannot reliably be predicted in patients with pseudogout, synovial fluid should be cultured in all patients.

Several patients have been reported with acute bacterial infection of a joint accompanied by crystals of both monosodium urate and CPPD (342,349–351). In two cases, crystals appeared in joint fluid only after bacterial infection was identified and treatment begun (349,350). These cases support the proposed mechanism for appearance of crystals in an infected joint: liberation of crystals embedded in cartilage and synovium by hydrolytic enzymes released from leukocytes phagocytizing bacteria in the joint. This phenomenon has been demonstrated in an animal air-pouch model; CPPD introduced into the air pouch (with a structure similar to a simple synovium-lined joint) becomes embedded in the joint lining and then becomes degraded and released after live bacteria introduced into the pouch elicited an inflammatory reaction (349).

Arthritis associated with basic calcium phosphate crystals (apatite) can take several forms, the most common being a rapidly progressive destructive arthropathy of large joints (shoulder, hip, knee) (352). Presence of apatite in synovial fluid is not readily confirmed, because it is suggested only by special staining, does not have a distinctive appearance under the polarizing light microscope, and is confirmed only by electron microscopy. Four cases of apatite-associated destructive arthropathy have been reported in which accelerated destruction of the joint (and in two cases, death of the patient) was due to an infection superimposed on the previously documented arthropathy (353,354). All patients complained of sudden increases in already severe joint pain, but only one had fever. Antemortem diagnoses made in three cases led to effective treatment of the joint infection. As for other patients with preexisting joint damage, sudden worsening of symptoms in patients with apatite arthropathy should prompt a search for infection.

Other Predispositions to Septic Arthritis

Two uncommon underlying joint diseases sometimes complicated by septic arthritis are hemophiliac arthropathy and Charcot (neuropathic) joints. *S. aureus* has caused infection of a "target" joint of hemophiliacs with prior recurrent hemarthroses (355). Many hemophiliacs are infected by HIV, which can further increase the risk of developing septic arthritis (230,355). Traumatic hemarthrosis in elderly patients with OA can become secondarily infected by *S. aureus* (356). Charcot joints caused by tabes dorsalis, syringomyelia, or congenital insensitivity to pain have been sites of bacterial infection, usually gram-positive cocci affecting the knee (357), shoulder (358), or ankle (359). A change in chronic symptoms from a Charcot joint, particularly if accompanied by inflammatory synovial fluid, should prompt a search for infection; however, a case has been described in which bilateral neuropathic shoulders yielded inflammatory synovial fluid for which no infectious or crystalline etiology could be found (360).

Other specific examples of increased host susceptibility to bacterial infections of bone and joint are illustrated by patients with chronic renal failure (361), renal transplant (362), and sickle cell anemia (363). Bacterial infections are a major cause of morbidity and mortality among patients with sickle cell anemia (364,365). These patients and those with related hemoglobinopathies are at increased risk of bacterial meningitis, pneumococcal bacteremia, and Salmonella osteomyelitis. The musculoskeletal manifestations of sickle cell disease are protean and result from different pathogenic mechanisms ranging from ischemic necrosis of the bone to synovitis, hemarthrosis, and secondary gout (53) (see Chapter 94). The predilections of Salmonella species to cause osteomyelitis, and of *S. pneumoniae* to cause septic arthritis, are noteworthy (363). The differentiation of ischemic bone infarcts from multifocal bacterial osteomyelitis is often difficult, and the exclusion of a bacterial cause of inflammatory joint fluid must be made.

A report from a renal unit detailed the varied presentations and the difficulties in diagnosis and management of serious bone and joint infections among patients with chronic renal failure (361). Extradural abscess in the lumbar region and discitis with vertebral osteomyelitis and paravertebral abscess of the thoracic spine were commonly caused by *S. aureus.* Infections of the sternoclavicular joint, and the large peripheral joints and long bones by *S. aureus, Pseudomonas, Serratia,* and *Proteus* sp, are reminiscent of the skeletal infections seen in intravenous drug users. The spectrum of infectious arthritis among renal transplant patients illustrates some consequences of antirejection immunosuppression, which leaves the patient vulnerable to bacterial agents and opportunistic microorganisms (362). In addition to *S. aureus* and the more common gram-negative bacilli, other causes included *Nocardia asteroides, Cryptococcus neoformans, M. tuberculosis, M. chelonei, M. fortuitum, M. kansasii, M. scrofulaceum, M. gordonae,* and cytomegalovirus.

Polyarticular Septic Arthritis

Although acute bacterial arthritis is most often monoarticular, polyarticular infection occurs in 5% to 8% of pediatric cases (Table 126.3) and in 10% to 19% of nongonococcal adult cases (22,196). Bacteria with predilections for polyarticular involvement include *N. gonorrhoeae* (2), *B. fragilis* (189), *S. pneumoniae,* group G streptococcus, and *H. influenzae* (22), but *S. aureus* accounts for at least half of all cases (196). Prior disease in multiple joints predisposes to polyarticular sepsis; 18% to 35% of RA patients with joint infections have polyarticular involvement (182). Joint infections are uncommon in systemic lupus erythematosus or gout, but tend to be polyarticular when they occur (196,342). Polyarticular sepsis can occur without florid systemic or local features (196), and sometimes can be documented only by a careful survey of all joints in a clinically septic patient (190). Poor prognosis of polyarticular sepsis is conferred by older age (older than 50 years), RA, or staphylococcal infection; the overall mortality rate (30%) has not changed appreciably over several decades (196).

Polymicrobial Septic Arthritis

Polymicrobial septic arthritis (two or more bacterial species) is rare in a normal joint unless penetrating trauma has occurred or surgery has been recently performed. Combinations of gram-positive, gram-negative, mixed gram-positive and gram-negative, aerobic, and anaerobic microorganisms have all been encountered (366–368). Most instances of polymicrobic infection involve two different microorganisms, but cases with three or four microbes have been reported (366,368). In one review, hip infections were most common among the 12 adults, many resulting from a communication of a retroperitoneal or pelvic abscess directly with the hip (366). In prosthetic joint infections, 6% to 25% of the cases were polymicrobial (245,248), and early postoperative wound infections accounted for most of these infections.

THERAPY FOR BACTERIAL ARTHRITIS

Suggested antimicrobial therapy has been discussed in the sections dealing with specific organisms. The principles of diagnosis and management are summarized in Chapter 125. Draining with repeated needle aspiration must produce repeated success in decompressing local pus accumulation. A serial decrease in the total joint fluid leukocyte count and sterility of the aspirate are good omens, correlating with a good outcome (170).

A summary of recommended antimicrobials and alternative drugs is provided in Table 126.4 for most of the microor-

TABLE 126.4. ANTIBIOTIC THERAPY REGIMENS FOR BACTERIAL ARTHRITIS

Microorganism	Antibiotic of choice	Alternative drugs
Staphylococcus aureus	Nafcillin (plus Rifampin, if persistent infection)	Cefazolin
Methicillin-resistant staphylococcus	Vancomycin	Trimethoprim/Sulfamethoxazole Clindamycin
Streptococcus		
Group A	Penicillin G	Cefazolin
Non-Group A	Penicillin plus an aminoglycoside	Cefazolin plus an aminoglycoside
Pneumococcus	Penicillin G	Vancomycin (if PCN resistant)
Enterococcus	Penicillin or ampicillin plus gentamicin	Vancomycin plus an aminoglycoside
Neisseria gonorrhoeae	A third-generation cephalosporin (ceftriaxone)	Ciprofloxacin or Ofloxacin Spectinomycin
Hemophilus influenzae	Amoxicillin plus clavulanate	A third-generation cephalosporin Cefuroxime Chloramphenicol
Enterobacteriaceae	A third-generation cephalosporin (cefotaxime, ceftizoxime, or ceftriaxone)	Imipenem Aztreonam Ampicillin An aminoglycoside (not alone)
Pseudomonas aeruginosa	Antipseudomonal penicillin plus an aminoglycoside	An aminoglycoside plus ceftazidime, imipenem, or aztreonam
Bacteroides fragilis	Metronidazole	Clindamycin
Mycoplasma/ureaplasma	Doxycycline (parenteral)	Erythromycin (parenteral) Ciprofloxacin or Ofloxacin Azithromycin

Table prepared with the assistance of Carol Chenoweth, M.D., of the Division of Infectious Diseases at the University of Michigan Medical Center.

ganisms causing bacterial arthritis. Drug dosages and duration of treatment must be determined for each case.

REFERENCES

1. Goldenberg DL, Cohen AS. Acute infectious arthritis: a review of patients with nongonococcal joint infections (with emphasis on therapy and prognosis). *Am J Med* 1976;60:369–377.
2. Goldenberg DL, Reed JI. Bacterial arthritis. *N Engl J Med* 1985;312:764–771.
3. Manshady BM, Thompson GR, Weiss JJ. Septic arthritis in a general hospital 1966-1977. *J Rheumatol* 1980;7:523–530.
4. Ang-Fonte GZ, Rozboril MB, Thompson GR. Changes in nongonococcal septic arthritis: drug abuse and methicillin-resistant *Staphylococcus aureus. Arthritis Rheum* 1985;28:210–213.
5. Meijers KAE, Cats A, van den Broek PJ, et al. (Sub)acute microbial arthritis. *Ned Tijdschr Geneeskd* 1980;124:2084–2089.
6. Meijers KAE, Dijkmans BAC, Hermans J, et al. Non-gonococcal infectious arthritis: a retrospective study. *J Infect* 1987;14:13–20.
7. Rosenthal J, Bole GG, Robinson WD. Acute nongonococcal infectious arthritis: evaluation of risk factors, therapy, and outcome. *Arthritis Rheum* 1980;23:889–897.
8. Youssef PP, York JR. Septic arthritis: a second decade of experience. *Aust N Z J Med* 1994;24:307–311.
9. Sharp JT, Lidksy MD, Duffy J, et al. Infectious arthritis. *Arch Intern Med* 1979;139:1125–1130.
10. Cooper C, Cawley MID. Bacterial arthritis in an English health district: a 10 year review. *Ann Rheum Dis* 1986;45:458–463.
11. Wharton M, Rice JR, McCallum R, et al. Septic arthritis due to *Micrococcus luteus. J Rheumatol* 1986;13:659–660.
12. Sheagren JN. *Staphylococcus aureus: the persistent pathogen.* N Engl J Med 1984;310:1368–1373, 1437–1442.
13. Wolfson JS, Hooper DC. The fluoroquinolones: structures, mechanisms of action and resistance, and spectra of activity in vitro. *Antimicrob Agents Chemother* 1985;28:581–586.
14. Hooper DC, Wolfson JS. The fluoroquinolones: pharmacology, clinical uses, and toxicities in humans. *Antimicrob Agents Chemother* 1985;28:716–721.
15. Beam TR Jr. Sequestration of staphylococci at an inaccessible focus. *Lancet* 1979;2:227–228.
16. Cunningham R, Cockayne A, Humphreys H. Clinical and molecular aspects of the pathogenesis of *Staphylococcus aureus* bone and joint infections. *J Med Microbiol* 1996;44:157–164.
17. Thomas MG, Peacock S, Daenke S, et al. Adhesion of *Staphylococcus aureus* to collagen is not a major virulence determinant for septic arthritis, osteomyelitis, or endocarditis. *J Infect Dis* 1999;179:291–293.
18. Thompson TD, Friedman AL. Simultaneous occurrence of *Staphylococcus aureus*-associated septic arthritis and toxic shock syndrome. *Clin Pediatr (Phila)* 1994;33:243–245.
19. Deighton C. Beta haemolytic streptococci and musculoskeletal sepsis in adults. *Ann Rheum Dis* 1993;52:483–487.
20. Small CB, Slater LN, Lowy FD, et al. Group B streptococcal arthritis in adults. *Am J Med* 1984;76:367–375.
21. Pischel KD, Weisman MH, Cone RO. Unique features of group B streptococcal arthritis in adults. *Arch Intern Med* 1985;145:97–102.
22. Epstein JH, Zimmermann B, Ho G Jr. Polyarticular septic arthritis. *J Rheumatol* 1986;13:1105–1107.
23. Laster AJ, Michels ML. Group B streptococcal arthritis in adults. *Am J Med* 1984;76:910–915.
24. Dan M. Septic arthritis in young infants: clinical and microbiologic correlations and therapeutic implications. *Rev Infect Dis* 1984;6:147–155.
25. Vartian C, Lerner PI, Shlaes DM, et al. Infections due to Lancefield group G streptococci. *Medicine (Baltimore)* 1985;64:75–88.
26. Schattner A, Vosti KL. Bacterial arthritis due to beta-hemolytic streptococci of serogroups A, B, C, F, and G. *Medicine (Baltimore)* 1998;77:122–139.
27. Lyon LJ, Nevin MA. Carcinoma of the colon presenting as pyogenic arthritis. *JAMA* 1979;241:2060.
28. Trenker SW, Braunstein EM, Lynn MD, et al. Group G streptococcal arthritis and bowel disease; a rare enteric arthropathy. *Gastrointest Radiol* 1987;12:265–267.
29. Ike RW. Septic arthritis due to group C streptococcus: report and review of the literature. *J Rheumatol* 1990;17:1230–1236.
30. Sobrino J, Bosch X, Wennberg J, et al. Septic arthritis secondary to group C streptococcus typed as *Streptococcus equisimilis. J Rheumatol* 1991;18:485–486.
31. Collazos J, Echevarria MJ, Ayarza R, et al. *Streptococcus zooepidemicus* septic arthritis: case report and review of group C streptococcal arthritis. *Clin Infect Dis* 1992;15:744–746.
32. Cook MA, Bloomfield DA. Group C streptococcal arthritis. *J Am Osteopath Assoc* 1993;93:508–509.
33. Zwillich SH, Hamory BH, Walker SE. Enterococcus: an unusual cause of septic arthritis. *Arthritis Rheum* 1984;27:591–595.
34. Taylor PW, Trueblood MC. Septic arthritis due to *Aerococcus viridans. J Rheumatol* 1985;12:1004–1005.
35. Nitsche JF, Vaughan JH, Williams G, et al. Septic sternoclavicular arthritis with *Pasteurella multocida* and *Streptococcus sanguis. Arthritis Rheum* 1982;25:467–469.
36. Seviour PW, Dieppe PA. Sternoclavicular joint infection as a cause of chest pain. *Br Med J* 1984;288:133–134.
37. Hynd RF, Klofkorn RW, Wong JK. *Streptococcus anginosus-constellatus* infection of the sternoclavicular joint. *J Rheumatol* 1984;11:713–715.
38. Catto BA, Jacobs MR, Shlaes DM. *Streptococcus mitis: a cause of serious infection in adults.* Arch Intern Med 1987;147:885–888.
39. Kauffman CA, Watanakunakorn C, Phair JP. Pneumococcal arthritis. *J Rheumatol* 1976;3:409–419.
40. Good AE, Gayes JM, Kauffman CA, et al. Multiple pneumococcal pyarthrosis complicating rheumatoid arthritis. *South Med J* 1978;71:502–504.
41. Edwards GS Jr, Russell IJ. Pneumococcal arthritis complicating gout. *J Rheumatol* 1980;7:907–910.
42. Mallory TH. Sepsis in total hip replacement following pneumococcal pneumonia. *J Bone Joint Surg Am* 1973;55:1753–1754.
43. Andersen BR, Mayer ME, Geiseler PJ, et al. Multi-joint pneumococcal pyarthrosis in a patient with a chemotactic defect. *Arthritis Rheum* 1983;26:1160–1162.
44. Fullerton RC, McNabb PC. Community-acquired pneumonia and septic arthritis caused by penicillin-resistant pneumococci. *J Tenn Med Assoc* 1989;82:13–14.
45. Bradley JS, Kaplan SL, Tan TQ, et al. Pediatric pneumococcal bone and joint infections: the Pediatric Multicenter Pneumococcal Surveillance Study Group (PMPSSG). *Pediatrics* 1998;102:1376–1382.
46. Nieman RE, Lorber B. Listeriosis in adults: a changing pattern. *Rev Infect Dis* 1980;2:207–227.
47. Louthrenoo W, Schumacher HR Jr. *Listeria monocytogenes* osteomyelitis complicating leukemia: report and literature review of listeria osteoarticular infections. *J Rheumatol* 1990;17:107–110.
48. Wilson APR, Prouse PJ, Gumpel JM. *Listeria monocytogenes* septic arthritis following intra-articular yttrium-90 therapy. *Ann Rheum Dis* 1984;43:518–519.
49. Newman JH, Waycott S, Cooney LM Jr. Arthritis due to *Listeria monocytogenes. Arthritis Rheum* 1979;22:1139–1140.

50. Breckenridge RL Jr, Buck L, Tooley E, et al. *Listeria monocytogenes* septic arthritis. *Am J Clin Pathol* 1980;73:140–141.
51. Curosh NA, Perednia DA. *Listeria monocytogenes* septic arthritis: a case report and review of the literature. *Arch Intern Med* 1989;149:1207–1208.
52. Booth LV, Walters MT, Tuck AC, et al. *Listeria monocytogenes* infection in a prosthetic knee joint in rheumatoid arthritis. *Ann Rheum Dis* 1990;49:58–59.
53. Massarotti EM, Dinerman H. Septic arthritis due to *Listeria monocytogenes: report and review of the literature.* J Rheumatol 1990;17:111–113.
54. Abadie SM, Dalovisio JR, Pankey GA, et al. *Listeria monocytogenes* arthritis in a renal transplant recipient. *J Infect Dis* 1987; 156:413–414.
55. Weiler PJ, Hastings DE. *Listeria monocytogenes,* an unusual cause of late infection in a prosthetic hip joint. *J Rheumatol* 1990;17:705–707.
56. Norenberg DD, Bigley DV, Virata RL, et al. *Corynebacterium pyogenes* septic arthritis with plasma cell synovial infiltrate and monoclonal gammopathy. *Arch Intern Med* 1978;138:810–811.
57. Messina OD, Maldonado-Cocco JA, Pescio A, et al. *Corynebacterium kutscheri* septic arthritis. *Arthritis Rheum* 1989;32:1053.
58. Robinson SC. *Bacillus cereus* septic arthritis following arthrography. *Clin Orthop* 1979;145:237–238.
59. Morrison VA, Chia JKS. Septic arthritis due to *Bacillus. South Med J* 1986;79:522–523.
60. Morrey BF, Bryan RS. Infection after total elbow arthroplasty. *J Bone Joint Surg Am* 1983;65:330–338.
61. Kooijmans-Coutinho MF, Markusse HM, Dijkmans BAC. Infectious arthritis caused by *Propionibacterium acnes: a report of two cases.* Ann Rheum Dis 1989;48:85–852.
62. Gordon G, Kabins SA. Pyogenic sacroiliitis. *Am J Med* 1980;69: 50–56.
63. Craig DB, Wehrle PA. *Branhamella catarrhalis* septic arthritis. *J Rheumatol* 1983;10:985–986.
64. Melendez PR, Johnson RH. Bacteremia and septic arthritis caused by *Moraxella catarrhalis. Rev Infect Dis* 1991;13:428–429.
65. Patel NJ, Moore TL, Weiss TD, et al. *Kingella kingae* infectious arthritis: case report and review of literature of *Kingella* and *Moraxella* infections. *Arthritis Rheum* 1983;26:557–559.
66. de Groot R, Glover D, Clausen C, et al. Bone and joint infections caused by *Kingella kingae: six cases and review of the literature.* Rev Infect Dis 1988;10:998–1004.
67. Yagupsky P, Dagan R, Howard CB, et al. Clinical features and epidemiology of invasive *Kingella kingae* infections in southern Israel. *Pediatrics* 1993;92:800–804.
68. Vincent J, Podewell C, Frankin GW, et al. Septic arthritis due to *Kingella (Moraxella) kingii. J Rheumatol* 1981;8:501–503.
69. Lewis DA, Settas L. *Kingella kingae* causing septic arthritis in Felty's syndrome. *Postgrad Med J* 1983;59:525–526.
70. Salminen I, Von Essen R, Koota K, et al. A pitfall in purulent arthritis brought out in *Kingella kingae* infection of the knees. *Ann Rheum Dis* 1984;43:656–657.
71. Hirschmann JV, Everett ED. *Haemophilus influenzae* infections in adults: report of nine cases and a review of the literature. *Medicine (Baltimore)* 1979;58:80–94.
72. Dajani AS, Asmar BI, Thirumoorthi MC. Systemic *Hemophilus influenzae* disease: an overview. *J Pediatr* 1979;94:355–364.
73. Bowerman SG, Green NE, Mencio GA. Decline of bone and joint infections attributable to *Haemophilus influenzae* type B. *Clin Orthop* 1997;341:128–133.
74. Fink CW, Nelson JD. Septic arthritis and osteomyelitis in children. *Clin Rheum Dis* 1986;12:423–435.
75. Rotbart HA, Glode MP. *Haemophilus influenzae* type B septic arthritis in children: report of 23 cases. *Pediatrics* 1985;75: 254–259.
76. Borenstein DG, Simon GL. *Hemophilus influenzae* septic arthritis in adults: a report of four cases and a review of the literature. *Medicine (Baltimore)* 1986;65:191–201.
77. Ho G Jr, Tice AD, Kaplan SR. Septic bursitis in the prepatellar and olecranon bursae. *Ann Intern Med* 1978;89:21–27.
78. Goldenberg DL, Cohen AS. Arthritis due to gram-negative bacilli. *Clin Rheum Dis* 1978;4:197–210.
79. Kreger BE, Craven DE, Carling PC, et al. Gram-negative bacteremia. III. Reassessment of etiology, epidemiology and ecology in 612 patients. *Am J Med* 1980;68:332–343.
80. Miskew DB, Lorenz MA, Pearson RL, et al. *Pseudomonas aeruginosa* bone and joint infection in drug abusers. *J Bone Joint Surg Am* 1983;65:829–832.
81. Donovan TL, Chapman MW, Harrington KD, et al. *Serratia* arthritis: report of seven cases. *J Bone Joint Surg Am* 1976;58: 1009–1011.
82. Ross GN, Baraff LJ, Quismorio FP. *Serratia* arthritis in heroin users. *J Bone Joint Surg Am* 1975;57:1158–1160.
83. Bayer AS, Chow AW, Louie JS, et al. Gram-negative bacillary septic arthritis: clinical, radiographic, therapeutic, and prognostic features. *Semin Arthritis Rheum* 1977;7;123–132.
84. Newman ED, Davis DE, Harrington TM. Septic arthritis due to gram negative bacilli: older patients with good outcome. *J Rheumatol* 1988;15:659–662.
85. David JR, Black RL. *Salmonella* arthritis. *Medicine (Baltimore)* 1960;39:385–403.
86. Brodie TD, Ehresmann GR. *Salmonella dublin* arthritis: an initial case presentation. *J Rheumatol* 1983;10:144–146.
87. Quismorio FP Jr, Jakes JT, Zarnow AJ, et al. Septic arthritis due to *Arizona hinshawii. J Rheumatol* 1983;10:147–150.
88. Spira TJ, Kabins SA. *Yersinia enterocolitica* septicemia with septic arthritis. *Arch Intern Med* 1976;36:1305–1308.
89. Taylor BG, Zafarzai MZ, Humphreys DW, et al. Nodular pulmonary infiltrates and septic arthritis associated with *Yersinia enterocolitica* bacteremia. *Am Rev Respir Dis* 1977;116:525–529.
90. Kilo C, Hagemann PO, Marzi J. Septic arthritis and bacteremia due to *Vibrio fetus. Am J Med* 1965;38:962–971.
91. Pasticci MB, Baratta E, Del Favero A, et al. *Campylobacter jejuni: an unusual cause of infectious arthritis.* Postgrad Med J 1992;68:151–152.
92. Van Heereveld HA, Van Riel PL, Meis JF, et al. Chronic polyarthritis due to *Pseudomonas aeruginosa. Br J Rheumatol* 1993; 32:1021–1022.
93. Niall DM, Murphy PG, Fogarty EE, et al. Puncture wound related pseudomonas infections of the foot in children. *Ir J Med Sci* 1997;166:98–101.
94. Siebert WT, Dewan S, Williams TW. *Pseudomonas* puncture wound osteomyelitis in adults. *Am J Med Sci* 1982;283:83–88.
95. Schmid FR. Routine drug treatment of septic arthritis. *Clin Rheum Dis* 1984;10:293–311.
96. Walton K, Hilton RC, Sen RA. *Pseudomonas* arthritis treated with parenteral and intra-articular ceftazidime. *Ann Rheum Dis* 1985;44:499–500.
97. Matteson EL, McCune WJ. Septic arthritis caused by treatment resistant *Pseudomonas cepacia. Ann Rheum Dis* 1990;49:258–259.
98. Baltimore RS, Jenson HB. Puncture wound osteochondritis of the foot caused by *Pseudomonas maltophilia. Pediatr Infect Dis J* 1990;9:143–144.
99. Winn RE, Chase WF, Lauderdale PW, et al. Septic arthritis involving *Capnocytophaga ochracea. J Clin Microbiol* 1984;19:538–540.
100. Gordon DL, Philpot CR, McGuire C. *Plesiomonas shigelloides* septic arthritis complicating rheumatoid arthritis. *Aust N Z J Med* 1983;13:275–276.
101. Chmel H, Armstrong D. Acute arthritis caused by *Aeromonas hydrophila: clinical and therapeutic aspects.* Arthritis Rheum 1976;19:169–172.

102. Brook I, Frazier EH. Anaerobic osteomyelitis and arthritis in a military hospital: a 10-year experience. *Am J Med* 1993;94: 21–28.
103. Finegold SM. *Anaerobic bacteria in human disease.* New York: Academic Press, 1977:443–454.
104. Yocum RC, McArthur J, Petty BG, et al. Septic arthritis caused by *Propionibacterium acnes. JAMA* 1982;248:1740–1741.
105. Hunter G, Dandy D. The natural history of the patient with an infected total hip replacement. *J Bone Joint Surg Br* 1977; 59:293–297.
106. Brause BD. Infections associated with prosthetic joints. *Clin Rheum Dis* 1986;12:523–536.
107. Finegold RH Jr, Rosenblatt JE, Tenney JH, et al. Anaerobic septic arthritis. *Clin Orthop* 1982;164:141–148.
108. Hovenden JL, Murdoch GE, Evans AT. Non-traumatic *Clostridium septicum* arthritis in a patient with caecal carcinoma. *Br J Rheumatol* 1992;3:571–572.
109. Weber DJ, Wolfson JS, Swartz MN, et al. *Pasteurella multocida* infections: report of 34 cases and review of the literature. *Medicine (Baltimore)* 1984;63:133–154.
110. Ewing R, Fainstein V, Musher DM, et al. Articular and skeletal infections caused by *Pasteurella multocida. South Med J* 1980; 73:1349–1352.
111. Orton DW, Fulcher WH. *Pasteurella multocida: bilateral septic joint prostheses from a distant cat bite.* Ann Emerg Med 1984; 13:1065–1067.
112. Mellors JW, Schoen RT. *Pasteurella multocida* septic arthritis. *Conn Med* 1984;48:221–223.
113. Baker GL, Oddis CV, Medsger TA. *Pasteurella multocida* polyarticular septic arthritis. *J Rheumatol* 1987;14:355–357.
114. Chevalier X, Martigny J, Avouac B, et al. Report of 4 cases of *Pasturella multocida* septic arthritis. *J Rheumatol* 1991;18: 1890–1892.
115. Levin JM, Talan DA. Erythromycin failure with subsequent *Pasteurella multocida* meningitis and septic arthritis in a cat-bite victim. *Ann Emerg Med* 1990;19:1458–1461.
116. Holroyd KJ, Reiner AP, Dick JD. *Streptobacillus moniliformis* polyarthritis mimicking rheumatoid arthritis: an urban case of rat bite fever. *Am J Med* 1988;85:711–714.
117. Fordham JN, McKay-Ferguson E, Davies A, et al. Rat bite fever without the bite. *Ann Rheum Dis* 1992;51:411–412.
118. Young EJ. Human brucellosis. *Rev Infect Dis* 1983;5:821–842.
119. Gotuzzo E, Alarcon GS, Bocanegra TS, et al. Articular involvement in human brucellosis: a retrospective analysis of 304 cases. *Semin Arthritis Rheum* 1982;12:245–255.
120. Ariza J, Gudiol F, Valverde J, et al. Brucellar spondylitis: a detailed analysis based on current findings. *Rev Infect Dis* 1985; 7:656–664.
121. Gotuzzo E, Seas C, Guerra JG, et al. Brucellar arthritis: a study of 39 Peruvian families. *Ann Rheum Dis* 1987;46:506–509.
122. Colmenero JD, Reguera JM, Fernandez-Nebro A, et al. Osteoarticular complications of brucellosis. *Ann Rheum Dis* 1991;50:23–26.
123. Khateeb MI, Araj GF, Majeed SA, et al. Brucella arthritis: a study of 96 cases in Kuwait. *Ann Rheum Dis* 1990;49:994–998.
124. Tekkok IH, Berker M, Ozcan OE, et al. Brucellosis of the spine. *Neurosurgery* 1993;33:838–844.
125. Tosi MF, Nelson TJ. *Brucella canis* infection in a 17-month-old child successfully treated with moxalactam. *J Pediatr* 1982;101: 725–727.
126. Gomez-Reino FJ, Mateo I, Fuertes A, et al. Brucellar arthritis in children and its successful treatment with trimethoprim-sulphamethoxazole. *Ann Rheum Dis* 1986;5:256–258.
127. Ariza J, Gudiol F, Pallares R, et al. Treatment of human brucellosis with doxycycline plus rifampin or doxycycline plus streptomycin: a randomized, double-blind study. *Ann Intern Med* 1992;117:25–30.
128. Reginato AJ. Syphilitic arthritis and osteitis. *Rheum Dis Clin North Am* 1993;19:379–398.
129. Burgoyne M, Agudelo C, Pisko E. Chronic syphilitic polyarthritis mimicking systemic lupus erythematosus/rheumatoid arthritis as the initial presentation of human immunodeficiency virus infection. *J Rheumatol* 1992;19:313–315.
130. Cassell GH, Cole BC. Mycoplasma as agents of human disease. *N Engl J Med* 1981;304:80–89.
131. Taylor-Robinson D, Gumpel JM, Hill A, et al. Isolation of *Mycoplasma pneumoniae* from synovial fluid of a hypogammaglobulinemic patient in a survey of patients with inflammatory polyarthritis. *Ann Rheum Dis* 1978;37:180–182.
132. Vogler LB, Waites KB, Wright PF, et al. *Ureaplasma urealyticum* polyarthritis in agammaglobulinemia. *Pediatr Infect Dis* 1985;4: 687–691.
133. Hakkarainen K, Turunen H, Miettinen A, et al. Mycoplasmas and arthritis. *Ann Rheum Dis* 1992;51:1170–1172.
134. Blanchard A, Hamrick W, Duffy L, et al. Use of the polymerase chain reaction for detection of *Mycoplasma fermentans* and *Mycoplasma genitalium* in the urogenital tract and amniotic fluid. *Clin Infect Dis* 1993;17(suppl 1):S272–S279.
135. Sneller M, Wellborne F, Barile MF, et al. Prosthetic joint infection with *Mycoplasma hominis. J Infect Dis* 1986;153:174–175.
136. Madoff S, Hooper DC. Nongenitourinary infections caused by *Mycoplasma hominis* in adults. *Rev Infect Dis* 1988;10:602–613.
137. Nylander N, Tan M, Newcombe DS. Successful management of *Mycoplasma hominis* septic arthritis involving a cementless prosthesis. *Am J Med* 1989;87:348–352.
138. Rao KV, O'Brien TJ, Andersen RC. Septic arthritis due to *Nocardia asteroides* after successful kidney transplantation. *Arthritis Rheum* 1981;24:99–101.
139. Ostrum RF. *Nocardia* septic arthritis of the hip with associated avascular necrosis: a case report. *Clin Orthop* 1993;288: 282–286.
140. Ray TD, Nimityongskul P, Ramsey KM. Disseminated *Nocardia asteroides* infection presenting as septic arthritis in a patient with AIDS. *Clin Infect Dis* 1994;18:256–257.
141. Chowdhary G, Wormser GP, Mascarenhas BR. *Nocardia* bursitis. *J Rheumatol* 1988;15:139–140.
142. Freiberg AA, Herzenberg JE, Sangeorzan JA. Thorn synovitis of the knee joint with *Nocardia* pyarthrosis. *Clin Orthop* 1993; 287:233–236.
143. Sequeira W, Swedler WI, Skosey JL. Septic arthritis in childhood. *Ann Emerg Med* 1985;14:1185–1187.
144. Wilson NIL, Di Paola M. Acute septic arthritis in infancy and childhood: 10 years' experience. *J Bone Joint Surg Br* 1986;68: 584–587.
145. Speiser JC, Moore TL, Osborn TG, et al. Changing trends in pediatric septic arthritis. *Semin Arthritis Rheum* 1985;15: 132–138.
146. Welkon CJ, Long SS, Fisher MC, et al. Pyogenic arthritis in infants and children: a review of 95 cases. *Pediatr Infect Dis* 1986;5:669–676.
147. Jackson MA, Burry VF, Olson LC. Pyogenic osteomyelitis associated with adjacent osteomyelitis: identification of the sequelaprone child. *Pediatr Infect Dis J* 1992;11:9–13.
148. Luhmann JD, Luhmann SJ. Etiology of septic arthritis in children: an update for the 1990s. *Pediatr Emerg Care* 1999;15: 40–42.
149. Yagupsky P, Dagan R, Howard CW, et al. High prevalence of *Kingella kingae* in joint fluid from children with septic arthritis revealed by the BACTEC blood culture system. *J Clin Microbiol* 1992;30:1278–1281.

150. Morrissy RT. Bone and joint infection in the neonate. *Pediatr Ann* 1989;18:33–34, 36–38, 40, 42–44.
151. Pittard WB III, Thullen JD, Fanaroff AA. Neonatal septic arthritis. *J Pediatr* 1976;88:621–624.
152. Fink CW, Dech VQ, Howard JR Jr, et al. Infection of bones and joints in children. *Arthritis Rheum* 1977;20:578–583.
153. Lundy DW, Kehl DK. Increasing prevalence of *Kingella kingae* in osteoarticular infections in young children. *J Pediatr Orthop* 1998;18:262–267.
154. Ish-Horowitz MR, McIntyre P, Nade S, et al. Bone and joint infections caused by multiply resistant *Staphylococcus aureus* in a neonatal intensive care unit. *Pediatr Infect Dis J* 1992;11:82–87.
155. Frederiksen B, Christiansen P, Knudsen FU. Acute osteomyelitis and septic arthritis in the neonate: risk factors and outcome. *Eur J Pediatr* 1993;152:577–580.
156. Rehm SJ, Weinstein AJ. Home intravenous antibiotic therapy: a team approach. *Ann Intern Med* 1983;99:388–392.
157. Syrogiannopoulos GA, Nelson JD. Duration of antimicrobial therapy for acute suppurative osteoarticular infections. *Lancet* 1988;1:37–40.
158. Herndon WA, Knauer S, Sullivan JA, et al. Management of septic arthritis in children. *J Pediatr Orthop* 1986;6:576–578.
159. Gillspie R. Septic arthritis in childhood. *Clin Orthop* 1973;96: 152–159.
160. Howard JB, Highgenboten CL, Nelson JD. Residual effects of septic arthritis in infancy and childhood. *JAMA* 1976;236: 932–935.
161. Strong M, Lejman T, Michno P, et al. Sequelae from septic arthritis of the knee during the first two years of life. *J Pediatr Orthop* 1994;14:743–751.
162. U.S. Dept. of Commerce Economics and Statistics Administration Bureau of the Census, Dept. of Health and Human Services Administration on Aging. *Census of population and housing (1990). Special tabulation on aging.* Washington, DC: U.S. Government Printing Office, 1994.
163. Kelly PJ. Bacterial arthritis in the adult. *Orthop Clin North Am* 1975;6:973–981.
164. Newman JH. Review of septic arthritis throughout the antibiotic era. *Ann Rheum Dis* 1976;35:198–200.
165. Lalley EV, Ho G Jr., Mitrane M. Rheumatologic disorders in the elderly. In: Gambert SE, ed. *Contemporary geriatric medicine.* Vol III. New York: Plenum Medical Book Co., 1988:189–198.
166. Schneider EL. Infectious diseases in the elderly. *Ann Intern Med* 1983;98:395–400.
167. Vincent GM, Amirault JD. Septic arthritis in the elderly. *Clin Orthop* 1990;251:241–245.
168. Cooper C, Cawley MID. Bacterial arthritis in the elderly. *Gerontology* 1986;32:222–227.
169. McGuire NM, Kauffman CA. Septic arthritis in the elderly. *J Am Geriatr Soc* 1985;33:170–174.
170. Ho G Jr, Su EY. Therapy of septic arthritis. *JAMA* 1982;247: 797–800.
171. Willkens RF, Healey LA, Decker JL. Acute infectious arthritis in the aged and chronically ill. *Arch Intern Med* 1960;106:354–364.
172. Geelhoed-Duyvestijn PH, van der Meer JW, Lichtendahl-Bernards AT, et al. Disseminated gonococcal infection in the elderly patients. *Arch Intern Med* 1986;146:1739–1740.
173. Septic arthritis in rheumatoid disease. *Br Med J* 1976;2: 1089–1090.
174. Kellgren JH, Ball J, Fairbrother RW, et al. Suppurative arthritis complicating rheumatoid arthritis. *Br Med J* 1958;1:1193–1200.
175. Karten I. Septic arthritis complicating rheumatoid arthritis. *Ann Intern Med* 1969;70:1147–1158.
176. Gristina AG, Rovere GD, Shoji H. Spontaneous septic arthritis complicating rheumatoid arthritis. *J Bone Joint Surg Am* 1974;56:1180–1184.
177. Blackburn WD Jr, Dunn TL, Alarcon GS. infection versus disease activity in rheumatoid arthritis: eight years' experience. *South Med J* 1986;79:1238–1241.
178. Goldenberg DL. Infectious arthritis complicating rheumatoid arthritis and other chronic rheumatic disorders. *Arthritis Rheum* 1989;32:496–502.
179. Gardner GC, Weisman MH. Pyarthrosis in patients with rheumatoid arthritis: a report of 13 cases and a review of the literature from the past 40 years. *Am J Med* 1990;88:503–511.
180. Östensson A, Geborek P. Septic arthritis as a non-surgical complication in rheumatoid arthritis: relation to disease severity and therapy. *Br J Rheumatol* 1991;30:35–38.
181. Spria LM, SolΘ MN, Sacanell AR, et al. Infectious arthritis in patients with rheumatoid arthritis. *Ann Rheum Dis* 1992;51: 402–404.
182. Dubost JJ, Fis I, Sorbrier M, et al. Septic arthritis in patients with rheumatoid arthritis: a review of twenty-four cases and of the medical literature. *Rev Rhum Engl Ed* 1994;61:143–156.
183. Mowat AG, Baum J. Chemotaxis of polymorphonuclear leukocytes from patients with rheumatoid arthritis. *J Clin Invest* 1971;50:2541–2549.
184. Turner RA, Shumacher HR, Myers AR. Phagocytic function of polymorphonuclear leukocytes in rheumatic diseases. *J Clin Invest* 1973;52:1632–1635.
185. Pruzanski W, Leers WD, Wardlaw AC. Bacteriolytic and bactericidal activity of sera and synovial fluids in rheumatoid arthritis and in osteoarthritis. *Arthritis Rheum* 1974;17:207–218.
186. Singleton JD, West SG, Nordstrom DM. "Pseudoseptic" arthritis complicating rheumatoid arthritis: a report of six cases. *J Rheumatol* 1991;18:1319–1322.
187. Barth WF, Healey LA, Decker JL. Septic arthritis due to *Pasteurella multocida* complicating rheumatoid arthritis. *Arthritis Rheum* 1968;11:394–399.
188. Dodd MJ, Griffiths ID, Freeman R. Pyogenic arthritis due to Bacteroides complicating rheumatoid arthritis. *Ann Rheum Dis* 1982;41:248–249.
189. Rosenkranz P, Lederman MM, Gopalakrishna KV, et al. Septic arthritis caused by *Bacteroides fragilis. Rev Infect Dis* 1990;12: 20–30.
190. Pitkin AD, Eykyn SJ. Covert multi-focal infective arthritis. *J Infect* 1993;27:297–300.
191. Trimble LD, Schoenaers JAH, Stoelinga PJW. Acute suppurative arthritis of the temporomandibular joint in a patient with rheumatoid arthritis. *J Maxillofac Surg* 1983;11:92–95.
192. Berger AJ, Calcaterra VE. Septic cricoarytenoid arthritis. *Otolaryngol Head Neck Surg* 1983;91:211–213.
193. Peters RHJ, Rasker JJ, Jacobs JWG, et al. Bacterial arthritis in a district hospital. *Clin Rheumatol* 1992;11:351–355.
194. Quismorio FP, Dubois EL. Septic arthritis in systemic lupus erythematosus. *J Rheumatol* 1975;2:73–82.
195. Hunter T, Plummer FA. Infectious arthritis complicating systemic lupus erythematosus. *Can Med Assoc J* 1980;122:791–793.
196. Dubost JJ, Fis I, Denis P, et al. Polyarticular septic arthritis. *Medicine (Baltimore)* 1993;72:296–310.
197. Chen JY, Luo SF, Wu YJ, Wang CM, et al. *Salmonella* septic arthritis in systemic lupus erythematosus and other systemic diseases. *Clin Rheumatol* 1998;17:282–287.
198. Mitchell SR, Nguyen PQ, Katz P. Increased risk of neisserial infections in systemic lupus erythematosus. *Semin Arthritis Rheum* 1990;20:174–184.
199. Edelen JS, Lockshin MD, LeRoy EC. Gonococcal arthritis in two patients with active lupus erythematosus: a diagnostic problem. *Arthritis Rheum* 1971;14:557–559.

200. Webster J, Williams BD, Smith AP, et al. Systemic lupus erythematosus presenting as pneumococcal septicaemia and septic arthritis. *Ann Rheum Dis* 1990;49:181–183.
201. Hansel TT, Haeney MR, Thompson RA. Primary hypogammaglobulinemia and arthritis. *Br Med J* 1987;295:174–175.
202. Furr PM, Taylor-Robinson D, Webster AD. Mycoplasmas and ureaplasmas in patients with hypogammaglobulinaemia and their role in arthritis: microbiological observations over twenty years. *Ann Rheum Dis* 1994;53:183–187.
203. Forgacs P, Kundsin RB, Margles SW, et al. A case of *Ureaplasma urealyticum* septic arthritis in a patient with hypogammaglobulinemia. *Clin Infect Dis* 1993;16:293–294.
204. Franz A, Webster AD, Furr PM, et al. Mycoplasmal arthritis in patients with primary immunoglobulin deficiency: clinical features and outcome in 18 patients. *Br J Rheumatol* 1997;36: 661–668.
205. Webster ADB, Loewi G, Dourmashkin RD, et al. Polyarthritis in adults with hypogammaglobulinemia and its rapid response to immunoglobulin treatment. *Br Med J* 1976;1:1314–1316.
206. Taylor-Robinson D, Furr PM. Recovery and identification of human genital tract mycoplasma. *Isr J Med Sci* 1981;7: 648–653.
207. Lee AH, Ramanujam T, Ware P, et al. Molecular diagnosis of *Ureaplasma urealyticum* septic arthritis in a patient with hypogammaglobulinemia. *Arthritis Rheum* 1992;35:443–448.
208. Gelfand EW. Unique susceptibility of patients with antibody deficiency to mycoplasma infection. *Clin Infect Dis* 1993; 17(suppl 1):250–253.
209. Webster ADR, Furr PM, Hughes-Jones NC, et al. Critical dependence on antibody for defence against mycoplasmas. *Clin Exp Immunol* 1988;71:383–387.
210. Taylor-Robinson D, Furr PM, Webster ADB. *Ureaplasma urealyticum* in the immunocompromised host. *Pediatr Infect Dis* 1986;5:S236–S238.
211. Kraus VB, Baraniuk JN, Hill GB, et al. *Ureaplasma urealyticum* septic arthritis in hypogammaglobulinemia. *J Rheumatol* 1988; 15:369–371.
212. Clough W, Cassell GH, Duffy LB, et al. Septic arthritis and bacteremia due to Mycoplasma resistant to antimicrobial therapy in a patient with systemic lupus erythematosus. *Clin Infect Dis* 1992;15:402–407.
213. Hawkins RE, Malone JD, Ebbeling WL. Common variable hypogammaglobulinemia presenting as nontypable *Haemophilus influenzae* septic arthritis in an adult. *J Rheumatol* 1991;18:775–776.
214. Goldenberg DL. Septic arthritis and other infections of rheumatologic significance. *Rheum Dis Clin North Am* 1991;17: 149–156.
215. Saraux A, Taelman H, Blanche P, et al. HIV infection as a risk factor for septic arthritis. *Br J Rheumatol* 1997;36:333–337.
216. Calabrese LH. The rheumatic manifestations of infection with the human immunodeficiency virus. *Semin Arthritis Rheum* 1989;18:225–239.
217. Ventura G, Gasparini G, Lucia MB, et al. Osteoarticular bacterial infections are rare in HIV-infected patients: 14 cases found among 4,023 HIV-infected patients. *Acta Orthop Scand* 1997;68:554–558.
218. Hughes RA, Rowe IF, Shanson A, et al. Septic bone, joint and muscle lesions associated with human immunodeficiency virus infection. *Br J Rheumatol* 1992;31:381–388.
219. Vassilopoulos D, Chalasani P, Jurado R, et al. Musculoskeletal infections in patients with human immunodeficiency virus infection. *Medicine (Baltimore)* 1997;76:284–294.
220. Strongin IS, Kale SA, Raymond MK, et al. An unusual presentation of gonococcal arthritis in an HIV positive patient. *Ann Rheum Dis* 1991;50:572–573.
221. Lothrenoo W. *Salmonella* septic arthritis in patients with human immunodeficiency virus infection. *J Rheumatol* 1993;20: 1454–1455.
222. Stein M, Houston S, Pozniak A, et al. HIV infection and *Salmonella* septic arthritis. *Clin Exp Rheumatol* 1993;11:187–189.
223. Husmann M, Gries C, Jehnichen P, et al. *Helicobacter* sp. strain Mainz isolated from an AIDS patient with septic arthritis: case report and nonradioactive analysis of 16S rRNA sequence. *J Clin Microbiol* 1994;32:3037–3039.
224. Friedman AW, Ike RW. *Mycobacterium kansasii* septic arthritis in a patient with the acquired immunodeficiency syndrome. *Arthritis Rheum* 1993;36:1631–1632.
225. Gallant JE, Alwood K, Chaisson R. Osteomyelitis due to *Mycobacterium kansasii* and *Mycobacterium avium* complex in an HIV-infected patient. *Infect Dis Clin Pract* 1994;3:297–299.
226. Hirsch R, Miller SM, Kazi S, et al. Human immunodeficiency virus-associated atypical mycobacterial skeletal infections. *Semin Arthritis Rheum* 1996;25:347–356.
227. Calabrese LH. Human immunodeficiency virus (HIV) infection and arthritis. *Rheum Dis Clin North Am* 1993;19:477–488.
228. Zimmermann B III, Erickson AD, Mikolich DJ, et al. Septic acromioclavicular arthritis and osteomyelitis in a patient with acquired immunodeficiency syndrome. *Arthritis Rheum* 1989; 32:1175–1178.
229. Bleasel JF, York JR, Rickard KA. Septic arthritis in human immunodeficiency virus infected haemophiliacs. *Br J Rheumatol* 1990;29:494–496.
230. Ragni MV, Hanley EN. Septic arthritis in hemophilic patients and infection with human immunodeficiency virus (HIV). *Ann Intern Med* 1989;110:168–169.
231. Merchan EC, Magallon M, Manso F, et al. Septic arthritis in HIV positive haemophiliacs: four cases and a literature review. *Int Orthop* 1992;16:302–306.
232. Gregg-Smith SJ, Pattison RM, Dodd CA, et al. Septic arthritis in haemophilia. *J Bone Joint Surg Br* 1993;75:368–370.
233. Barzilai A, Varon D, Martinowitz U, et al. Characteristics of septic arthritis in human immunodeficiency virus-infected haemophiliacs versus other risk groups. *Rheumatol Oxford* 1999; 38:139–142.
234. Rivera J, Monteagudo I, Lopez-Longo J, et al. Septic arthritis in patients with acquired immunodeficiency syndrome with human immunodeficiency virus infection. *J Rheumatol* 1992; 19:1960–1962.
235. Munoz-Fernandez S, Macia MA, Pantoja L, et al. Osteoarticular infection in intravenous drug abusers: influence of HIV infection and differences with non drug abusers. *Ann Rheum Dis* 1993;52:570–574.
236. Blanche P, Taelman H, Saraux A, et al. Acute arthritis and human immunodeficiency virus infection in Rwanda. *J Rheumatol* 1993;20:2123–2127.
237. Iyer M, Gorevic PD. Reactive arthropathy and autoimmunity in non-HIV-associated immunodeficiency. *Curr Opin Rheumatol* 1993;5:475–482.
238. Kuo KN, Lloyd-Roberts GC, Orme IM, et al. Immunodeficiency and infantile bone and joint infection. *Arch Dis Child* 1975;50:51–56.
239. Donabedian H, Gakllin JI. The hyperimmunoglobulinemia E recurrent infection (Job's) syndrome. *Medicine (Baltimore)* 1983;62:195–208.
240. Tauber AI, Borregaard N, Simons E, et al. Chronic granulomatous disease: a syndrome of phagocyte oxidase deficiencies. *Medicine (Baltimore)* 1983;62:286–309.
241. Buckley RH, Sampson HA. The hyperimmunoglobulinemia E syndrome. In: Franklin EC, ed. *Clinical immunology update:* reviews for physicians. New York: Elsevier, 1981: 147–167.

242. Ruddy S. Complement deficiencies: the second component. *Prog Allergy* 1986;39:250–266.
243. Ross SC, Densen P. Complement deficiency states and infection: epidemiology, pathogenesis, and consequences of neisserial and other infections in an immune deficiency. *Medicine (Baltimore)* 1984;63:243–273.
244. Total hip joint replacement in the United States [Consensus Conferences]. *JAMA* 1982;248:1817–1821.
245. Poss R, Thornhill TS, Ewald FC, et al. Factors influencing the incidence and outcome of infection following total joint arthroplasty. *Clin Orthop* 1984;182:117–126.
246. Gristina AG, Kolkin J. Total joint replacement and sepsis. *J Bone Joint Surg Am* 1983;65:128–134.
247. Ainscow DAP, Denham RA. The risk of haematogenous infection in total joint replacements. *J Bone Joint Surg Br* 1984;66: 580–582.
248. Inman RD, Gallegos KV, Brause BD, et al. Clinical and microbial features of prosthetic joint infection. *Am J Med* 1984;77:47–53.
249. Petty W. The effect of methylmethacrylate on bacterial inhibiting properties of normal human serum. *Clin Orthop* 1978; 132:266–277.
250. Petty W. The effect of methylmethacrylate on bacterial phagocytosis and killing by human polymorphonuclear leukocytes. *J Bone Joint Surg Am* 1978;60:752–757.
251. Costerton JW, Irwin RT, Cheng K-J. The bacterial glycocalyx in nature and disease. *Annu Rev Microbiol* 1981;35:299–324.
252. Gristina AG, Costerton JW, Hobgood CD, et al. Bacterial adhesion, biomaterials, the foreign body effect, and infection from natural ecosystems to infections in man: a brief review. *Contemp Orthop* 1987;14:27–35.
253. Widmer AF, Frei R, Rajacic Z, et al. Correlation between in vivo and in vitro efficacy of antimicrobial agents against foreign body infections. *J Infect Dis* 1990;162:96–102.
254. Wymenga AB, van Horn JR, Theeuwes A, et al. Perioperative factors associated with septic arthritis after arthroplasty. *Acta Orthop Scand* 1992;63:665–671.
255. Berbari EF, Hanssen AD, Duffy MC, et al. Risk factors for prosthetic joint infection: case-control study. *Clin Infect Dis* 1998; 27:1247–1254.
256. Prince A, Neu HC. Microbiology of infections of the prosthetic joint. *Orthop Rev* 1979;8:91–96.
257. Brause BD. Prosthetic joint infections. *Curr Opin Rheumatol* 1989;1:194–198.
258. Brause BD. Infections with prostheses in bones and joints. In: Mandell GL, Douglas RG Jr, Bennett JE, eds. *Mandell, Douglas and Bennett's principles and practice of infectious diseases.* 4th ed. New York: Churchill Livingstone, 1995:1051–1055.
259. Eftekhar NS. Wound infection complicating total hip joint arthroplasty. *Orthop Rev* 1979;8:49–64.
260. Atkins BL, Athanasou N, Deeks JJ, et al. Prospective evaluation of criteria for microbiological diagnosis of prosthetic-joint infection at revision arthroplasty: the OSIRIS Collaborative Study Group. *J Clin Microbiol* 1998;36:2932–2939.
261. Cuckler JM, Star AM, Alavi A, et al. Diagnosis and management of the infected total joint arthroplasty. *Orthop Clin North Am* 1991;22:523–530.
262. Glithero PR, Grogoris P, Harding LK, et al. White cell scans and infected joint replacements: failure to detect chronic infection. *J Bone Joint Surg Br* 1993;75:371–374.
263. van Holsbeeck MT, Eyler WR, Sherman LS, et al. Detection of infection in loosened hip prostheses: efficacy of sonography. *AJR Am J Roentgenol* 1994;163:381–384.
264. Choudry RR, Rice RPO, Triffitt PD, et al. Plasma viscosity and C-reactive protein after total hip and knee arthroplasty. *J Bone Joint Surg Br* 1992;74:523–524.
265. Tigges S, Stiles RG, Meli RJ, et al. Hip aspiration: a cost-effective and accurate methop of evaluating the potentially infected hip prosthesis. *Radiology* 1993;189:485–488.
266. Roberts P, Walters AJ, McMinn DJW. Diagnosing infection in hip replacements. *J Bone Joint Surg Br* 1992;74:265–269.
267. Felman DS. The role of intra-operative frozen section in revision total joint arthroplasty. *J Bone Joint Surg Am* 1995;77: 1807–1813.
268. Rand JA. Alternatives to reimplantation for salvage of the total knee arthroplasty complicated by infection. *J Bone Joint Surg Am* 1993;75:282–289.
269. Turner RH, Miley GD, Fremont-Smith P. Septic total hip replacement and revision arthroplasty. In: Turner RH, Schiller AD, eds. *Revision total hip arthroplasty.* New York: Grune & Stratton, 1982:291–314.
270. Buchholz HW, Elson RA, Engelbrecht E, et al. Management of deep infection of total hip replacement. *J Bone Joint Surg Br* 1981;63:342–353.
271. Wroblewski BM. One-stage revision of infected cemented total hip arthroplasty. *Clin Orthop* 1986;211:103–107.
272. Brandt CM, Sistrunk WW, Duffy MC, et al. *Staphylococcus aureus* prosthetic joint infection treated with debridement and prosthesis retention. *Clin Infect Dis* 1997;24:914–919.
273. Zimmerli W, Widmer AF, Blatter M, et al. Role of rifampin for treatment of orthopedic implant-related staphylococcal infections: a randomized controlled trial: Foreign-Body Infection (FBI) Study Group. *JAMA* 1998;279:1537–1541.
274. Goulet JA, Pelici PM, Brause BD, et al. Prolonged suppression of infection in total hip arthroplasty. *J Arthroplasty* 1988;3: 109–116.
275. Johnson DP, Bannister GC. The outcome of infected arthroplasty of the knee. *J Bone Joint Surg Br* 1986;63:289–291.
276. Tsukayama DT, Wickland B, Gustilo RB. Suppressive antibiotic therapy in prosthetic joint infections. *Orthopedics* 1991;14: 841–844.
277. Carpenter MT, West SG, Vogelgesang SA, et al. Postoperative joint infections in rheumatoid arthritis patients on methotrexate therapy. *Orthopedics* 1996;19:207–210.
278. Dajani AS, Bisno AL, Chung KJ, et al. Prevention of bacterial endocarditis: recommendations by the American Heart Association. *JAMA* 1990;264:2919–2922.
279. Blackburn WD Jr, Alarcon GS. Prosthetic joint infections: a role for prophylaxis. *Arthritis Rheum* 1991;34:110–117.
280. Nelson JP, Fitzgerald RH Jr, Jaspers MT, et al. Prophylactic antimicrobial coverage in arthroplasty patients. *J Bone Joint Surg Am* 1990;72:1.
281. Field EA, Martin MV. Prophylactic antibiotics for patients with artificial joints undergoing oral and dental surgery: necessary or not? *Br J Oral Maxillofac Surg* 1991;29:341–346.
282. Waldman BJ, Mont MA, Hungerford DS. Total knee arthroplasty infections associated with dental procedures. *Clin Orthop* 1997;343:164–172.
283. Kendall PH. Untoward effects following local hydrocortisone injection. *Ann Phys Med* 1958;4:170–175.
284. Gedda PO. Septic arthritis from cortisone. *JAMA* 1960;172: 1675–1676.
285. Hollander JL. Arthrocentesis and intrasynovial therapy. In: McCarty DJ, ed. *Arthritis and allied conditions.* 9th ed. Philadelphia: Lea & Febiger, 1979:402–414.
286. von Essen R, Savolainen HA. Bacterial infection following intra-articular injection. *Scand J Rheumatol* 1989;18:7–12.
287. Nakashima AK, McCarthy MA, Martone WJ, et al. Epidemic septic arthritis caused by *Serratia marcescens* and associated with a benzalkonium chloride antiseptic. *J Clin Microbiol* 1987;25: 1014–1018.
288. Kothari T, Reyes MP, Brooks M. *Pseudomonas cepacia* septic

arthritis due to intraarticular injections of methylprednisolone. *Can Med Assoc J* 1977;116:1230–1235.

289. Smith RW, Campbell MJ, O'Connell SO, et al. Methods of skin preparation prior to intra-articular injection. *Br J Rheumatol* 1993;32:648.
290. Sherman OH, Fox JM, Snyder SJ, et al. Arthroscopy: "no problem surgery." *J Bone Joint Surg Am* 1986;68:256–265.
291. Committee on Complications of the Arthroscopy Association of North America. Complications in arthroscopy: the knee and other joints. *Arthroscopy* 1986;2:253–258.
292. Small NC. Complications in arthroscopic surgery performed by experienced arthroscopists. *Arthroscopy* 1988;4:215–221.
293. Armstrong RW, Bolding F, Joseph R. Septic arthritis following arthroscopy: clinical syndromes and risk factors. *Arthroscopy* 1992;8:213–222.
294. Armstrong RW, Bolding F. Septic arthritis after arthroscopy: the contributing roles of intraarticular steroids and environmental factors. *Am J Infect Control* 1994;22:16–18.
295. Bellamy N, Park W, Rooney PJ. What do we know about the sacroiliac joint? *Semin Arthritis Rheum* 1983;2:282–313.
296. Shanahan MDG, Ackroyd CE. Pyogenic infection of the sacroiliac joint. *J Bone Joint Surg Br* 1985;67:605–608.
297. Zimmermann B III, Mikolich DJ, Lally EV. Septic sacroiliitis. *Semin Arthritis Rheum* 1996;26:592–604.
298. Moyer RA, Bross JE, Harrington TM. Pyogenic sacroiliitis in a rural population. *J Rheumatol* 1990;17:1364–1368.
299. Bohay DR, Gray JM. Sacroiliac joint pyarthrosis. *Orthop Rev* 1993;22:817–823.
300. Vyskocil JJ, McIlroy MA, Brennan TA, et al. Pyogenic infection of the sacroiliac joint. *Medicine (Baltimore)* 1991;70:188–197.
301. Miskew DB, Block RA, Witt PF. Aspiration of infected sacroiliac joints. *J Bone Joint Surg Am* 1979;61:1071–1072.
302. Bankoff MS, Sarno RC, Carter BL. CT scanning in septic sacroiliac arthritis or periarticular osteomyelitis. *Comput Radiol* 1984;8:165–170.
303. Sandrasegaran K, Saifuddin A, Coral A, et al. Magnetic resonance imaging of septic sacroiliitis. *Skeletal Radiol* 1994;23: 289–292.
304. Kerr R. Pyogenic sacroiliitis. *Orthopedics* 1985;8:1030–1034.
305. Cieslak TJ, Ottolini MG, O'Neill KM, et al. *Staphylococcus aureus* meningitis associated with pyogenic infection of the sacroiliac joint. *South Med J* 1993;86:1175–1178.
306. Gamble JG, Simmons SC, Freedman M. The symphysis pubis: anatomic and pathologic considerations. *Clin Orthop* 1986; 203:261–272.
307. Sequeira W. Diseases of the pubic symphysis. *Semin Arthritis Rheum* 1986;16:11–21.
308. Burns JR, Gregory JG. Osteomyelitis of the symphysis pubis after urologic surgery. *J Urol* 1977;12:663–669.
309. Rosenthal RE, Spickard WA, Markham RD, et al. Osteomyelitis of the symphysis pubis: a separate disease from osteitis pubis: report of three cases and review of the literature. *J Bone Joint Surg Am* 1982;64:123–128.
310. Sequeira W, Jones E, Siegel ME, et al. Pyogenic infections of the pubic symphysis. *Ann Intern Med* 1982;96:604–606.
311. Nitsche A, Mogni GO, Gorostiaga PE. Septic arthritis of the pubic symphysis. *Clin Exp Rheumatol* 1989;7:421–422.
312. Bouza E, Winston DL, Hewitt WL. Infectious osteitis pubis. *Urology* 1978;12:663–669.
313. Sexton DJ, Heskestad L, Lambeth WR, et al. Postoperative pubic osteomyelitis misdiagnosed as osteitis pubis: report of four cases and review. *Clin Infect Dis* 1993;17:695–700.
314. Yood RA, Goldenberg DL. Sternoclavicular joint arthritis. *Arthritis Rheum* 1980;23:232–239.
315. Tomford JW. Septic sternoclavicular arthritis: diagnostic clues and management. *Cleve Clin J Med* 1990;57:15–16.
316. Lopez-Longo F-J, Ménard H-A, Carreno L, et al. I. Primary septic arthritis in heroin users: early diagnosis by radioisotopic imaging and geographic variations in the causative agents. *J Rheumatol* 1987;14:991–994.
317. Renoult E, Lataste A, Jonon B, et al. Sternoclavicular joint infection in hemodialysis patients. *Nephron* 1990;56:212–213.
318. Aglas F, Gretler J, Rainer F, et al. Sternoclavicular septic arthritis: a rare but serious complication of subclavian venous catheterization. *Clin Rheumatol* 1994;13:507–512.
319. Gillis S, Friedman B, Caraco Y, et al. Septic arthritis of the sternoclavicular joint in healthy adults. *J Intern Med* 1990;228: 275–278.
320. Wohlgethan JR, Newberg AH, Reed JI. The risk of abscess from sternoclavicular septic arthritis. *J Rheumatol* 1988;15:1302–1306.
321. Pollack MS. Staphylococcal mediastinitis due to sternoclavicular pyarthrosis: CT appearance. *J Comput Assist Tomogr* 1990; 14:924–927.
322. Bayer AS, Chow AW, Louie JS, et al. Sternoarticular pyoarthrosis due to gram-negative bacilli: report of eight cases. *Arch Intern Med* 1977;137:1036–1040.
323. Lau ES, Shuckett R. Fusobacterium septic arthritis of the sternoclavicular joint. *J Rheumatol* 1993;20:1979–1981.
324. Griffith PH III, Boyadjis TA. Acute pyarthrosis of the acromioclavicular joint. *Orthopedics* 1984;7:1727–1728.
325. Blankstein A, Amsallem JL, Rubinstein E, et al. Septic arthritis of the acromioclavicular joint. *Arch Orthop Trauma Surg* 1985; 103:417–418.
326. Parker VS, Malhotra CM, Ho G Jr, et al. Radiographic appearance of the sternomanubrial joint in arthritis and related conditions. *Radiology* 1984;153:343–347.
327. Glushakow AS Carlson D, DePalma AF. Pyarthrosis of the manubriosternal joint. *Clin Orthop* 1976;114:214–215.
328. Borgmeier PJ, Kalovidouris AE. Septic arthritis of the sternomanubrial joint due to *Pseudomonas pseudomallei. Arthritis Rheum* 1980;23:1057–1059.
329. Gruber BL, Kaufman LD, Gorevic PD. Septic arthritis involving the manubriosternal joint. *J Rheumatol* 1985;12: 803–804.
330. Lopez-Longo FJ, Monteagudo I, Vaquero FJ, et al. Primary septic arthritis of the manubriosternal joint in a heroin user. *Clin Orthop* 1986;202:230–231.
331. Van Linthoudt D, De Torrente A, Humair L, et al. Septic manubriosternal arthritis in a patient with Reiter's disease. *Clin Rheumatol* 1987;6:293–295.
332. Rubinstien E, Slavin J. Thymic abscess with bacteremia and manubriosternal pyarthrosis in a geriatric patient. *Chest* 1993; 103:962–964.
333. Frischnecht J, Steigerwald JC. High synovial fluid white blood cell counts in pseudogout: possible confusion with septic arthritis. *Arch Intern Med* 1975;135:298–299.
334. Rahman MU, Shenberger KN, Schumacher HR Jr. Initially unrecognized calcium pyrophosphate dihydrate deposition disease as a cause of fever. *Am J Med* 1990;89:115–116.
335. Radcliffe K, Pattrick M, Doherty M. Complications resulting from misdiagnosing pseudogout as sepsis. *Br Med J* 1986;93: 440–441.
336. Kuzell WC, Schaffarzick RW, Naugler WE, et al. Some observations on 520 gouty patients. *J Chronic Dis* 1955;2:645–669.
337. Hess RJ, Martin JH. Pyarthrosis complicating gout. *JAMA* 1971;218:592–593.
338. McConville JH, Pototsky RS, Calia FM, et al. Septic and crystalline joint disease: a simultaneous occurrence. *JAMA* 1975; 231:841–842.
339. Hamilton ME, Parris TM, Gibson RS, et al. Simultaneous gout and pyarthrosis. *Arch Intern Med* 1980;140:917–919.
340. Edwards GS Jr, Russell IJ. Pneumococcal arthritis complicating

gout: case report and literature review. *J Rheumatol* 1980;7: 907–910.

341. Heinicke M, Gomez-Reino JJ, Gorevic PD. Crystal arthropathy as a complication of septic arthritis. *J Rheumatol* 1981;8: 529–531.
342. Baer PA, Tenebaum J, Fam AG, et al. Coexistent septic and crystal arthritis: report of four cases and literature review. *J Rheumatol* 1986;13:604–607.
343. O'Connell PG, Milburn BM, Nashel DJ. Coexistent gout and septic arthritis: a report of two cases and literature review. *Clin Exp Rheumatol* 1985;3:265–267.
344. Salvi A, Rossi M, Balestrieri GP, et al. Septic polyarthritis in chronic tophaceous gout. *Recent Prog Med* 1991;8:527–528.
345. Holland NW, Gonzalez EB, Agudelo CA. Coexistence of gout and septic arthritis. *Arthritis Rheum* 1994;37:S236(abst).
346. Ilahi OA, Swarna U, Hamill RJ, et al. Concomitant crystal and septic arthritis. *Orthopedics* 1996;19:613–617.
347. Zyskowski LP, Silverfield JC, O'Duffy JD. Pseudogout masking other arthritides. *J Rheumatol* 1983;10:449–453.
348. Jobanputra P, Gibson T. Diagnosis of pseudogout and septic arthritis. *Br J Rheumatol* 1987;6:379–380.
349. Gordon TP, Reid C, Rozenbilds MAM, et al. Crystal shedding in septic arthritis: case reports and in vivo evidence in an animal model. *Aust N Z J Med* 1986;16:336–340.
350. Smith JR, Phelps P. Septic arthritis, gout, pseudogout and osteoarthritis in the knee of a patient with multiple myeloma. *Arthritis Rheum* 1972;15:89–96.
351. Jarrett MP, Grayzel AI. Simultaneous gout, pseudogout, and septic arthritis. *Arthritis Rheum* 1980;23:128–129.
352. Schumacher HR, Somlyo AP, Tse RL, et al. Arthritis associated with apatite crystals. *Ann Intern Med* 1977;87:411–416.
353. Jones A, Henderson MJ, Berman P, et al. Septic arthritis complicating apatite associated destructive arthropathy. *Ann Rheum Dis* 1990;49:1005–1007.
354. Bendall RP, Jacobson SK, Adebajo A. Septic arthropathy complicating apatite associated destructive arthritis. *Ann Rheum Dis* 1991;50:967.
355. Scott JP, Maurer HS, Dias L. Septic arthritis in two teenaged hemophiliacs. *J Pediatr* 1985;107:748–751.
356. Helliwell M. *Staphylococcus aureus* infection complicating haemarthroses in elderly patients. *Clin Rheumatol* 1985;4:90–92.
357. Martin JR, Root HS, Kim SO, et al. Staphylococcus suppurative arthritis occurring in neuropathic knee joints. *Arthritis Rheum* 1965;8:389–402.
358. Goodman MA, Swartz W. Infection in a Charcot joint. *J Bone Joint Surg Am* 1985;67:642–643.
359. Ascuitto R, Drennan J, Fitzgerald V. Group C streptococcal arthritis an osteomyelitis in an adolescent with a hereditary sensory neuropathy. *Pediatr Infect Dis* 1985;4:553–554.
360. Louthrenoo W, Ostrov BE, Park YS, et al. Pseudoseptic arthritis: an unusual presentation of neuropathic arthropathy. *Ann Rheum Dis* 1991;50:717–721.
361. Spencer JD. Bone and joint infection in a renal unit. *J Bone Joint Surg Br* 1986;68:489–493.
362. Bomalaski JS, Williamson PK, Goldstein CS. Infectious arthritis in renal transplant patients. *Arthritis Rheum* 1986;29:227–232.
363. Syrogiannopoulos GA, McCracken GH, Nelson JD. Osteoarticular infections in children with sickle cell disease. *Pediatrics* 1986;78:1019–1096.
364. Barrett-Connor E. Bacterial infection and sickle cell anemia. *Medicine (Baltimore)* 1971;50:97–112.
365. Espinoza LR, Spilberg I, Osterland CK. Joint manifestations of sickle cell disease. *Medicine (Baltimore)* 1974;53:295–305.
366. Esposito AL, Gleckman RA. Acute polymicrobic septic arthritis in adult: case report and literature review. *Am J Med Sci* 1974; 267:251–254.
367. Petty BG, Sowa DT, Charache P. Polymicrobial polyarticular septic arthritis. *JAMA* 1983;249:2069–2072.
368. Mikolich DJ, Schlaeffer F, Ryter RJ. Polymicrobial polyarticular arthritis. *J Rheumatol* 1994;21:971–972.

127

GONOCOCCAL ARTHRITIS AND OTHER NEISSERIAL INFECTIONS

DON L. GOLDENBERG

The incidence of gonococcal arthritis and disseminated gonococcal infection (DGI) appears to be decreasing. In the three largest series of bacterial arthritis reported in 1996 through 1997, the incidence of gonococcal arthritis varied from 0.6% to 12% of cases (1–3). This is related to the decrease in the incidence of gonorrhea in most parts of the world during the past few decades. For example, the incidence of gonorrhea in the United States was 468 per 100,000 in 1975 and decreased to 149 per 100,000 in 1995 (4). However, gonococcal arthritis is still the most common form of septic arthritis in young, sexually active individuals.

MICROBIOLOGY AND EPIDEMIOLOGY OF DISSEMINATED GONOCOCCAL INFECTION

Neisseria gonorrhoeae are fastidious aerobic or facultative anaerobic gram-negative cocci that grow best on selective media (4). Specific typing methods to identify gonococcal strains have been based on outer membrane antigens, nutritional requirements, and plasmid and antibiotic sensitivity. Certain microbial and host factors are important determinants in the dissemination of gonococcal infections. The microbial factors include cell-surface structures that can be modified to increase virulence.

Gonococcal cell-wall structural components that help to determine bacterial virulence include the pili, the trilaminar outer membrane containing proteins I, II, and III, as well as lipopolysaccharide and peptidoglycan (4,5). Gonococcal pili are long, hair-like protein filaments. Pili facilitate attachment to epithelial cells. Once they are attached to the mucosal surface, endocytosis allows the gonococci to pass through epithelial cells with subsequent release into subepithelial tissues. Pili also impede phagocytosis by polymorphonuclear leukocytes. Strains that express pili are more virulent than are strains that do not contain pili. Strains can switch between P^+ (presence of pilus) and P^-. Gonococcal strains also can shift the antigenic type of pilus that they express.

Protein I is the predominant outer membrane protein and is important in attachment and endocytosis (4,5). It functions as a porin, providing aqueous anion channels through the hydrophobic gonococcal membrane. Protein I is genetically stable and therefore used for gonococcal serotyping. It also has been used for vaccine development. Protein II consists of a group of eight heat-labile proteins that are important in gonococcal attachment, intergonococcal adhesion, and susceptibility to the bactericidal activity of normal human sera. Protein II is associated with colony morphology. Colonies containing protein II are opaque, whereas those lacking protein II are transparent. Protein III, present in all strains of *N. gonorrhoeae,* is closely associated with Protein I and is important in generating blocking antibodies. Gonococcal lipopolysaccharide contributes to local cytotoxicity and systemic toxicity, including fever. A single gonococcal strain can express up to six lipopolysaccharide variants. Gonococcal peptidoglycan has arthropathic properties (6). This arthropathic property might be potentiated by the persistence of hydrolase-resistant peptidoglycan.

Gonococcal typing has led to a greater understanding of the clinical manifestations and virulence factors underlying disseminated gonococcal infection (4,5,7–9). Classification has relied primarily on serotyping and auxotyping. Gonococci expressing the low-molecular-weight protein IA are more likely to disseminate than are those expressing high-molecular-weight protein IB. Serum resistance also is strongly associated with protein IA. Local inflammation is linked to the ability of a gonococcal strain to resist the complement-dependent bactericidal action of normal human serum (7,8). Differences in C3b processing *in vitro* matched *in vivo* cervical findings (9). The stable nutritional requirements for growth (termed *auxotype*) of gonococcal colonies isolated from patients with disseminated gonococcal infection differ from those of colonies isolated from patients with uncomplicated gonorrhea. Strains requiring arginine, hypoxanthine, and uracil for growth (AHU strains) are commonly isolated from patients with disseminated gonococcal infection. The AHU auxotype is resistant to the natural bactericidal activity of normal human serum and has a unique sensitivity to antibiotics.

Microbial phenotypic characteristics not only may determine virulence and ability to disseminate but also may influence the clinical features of disseminated gonococcal infection. Seventy-five percent of the *N. gonorrhoeae* isolates from patients with tenosynovitis and dermatitis were resistant to the bactericidal activity of normal human sera, whereas only 47% of strains isolated from patients with suppurative arthritis demonstrated similar resistance (8). In sixty-nine percent of those patients with suppurative arthritis, but only in 17% of those with dermatitis–tenosynovitis, did a significant increase in serum bactericidal antibody activity develop. The serotypes of gonococci vary from one region of the country to another, explaining the greater prevalence of DGI in some geographic locations.

Disseminated gonococcal infection is four times more common in female patients (4,7). This relates to the fact that gonorrhea is more often asymptomatic in women and therefore may be more often untreated. Host virulence factors that predispose to gonorrhea and DGI include prior antibiotics, any high-risk sexual practices such as multiple partners and prostitution, and sexual activity after recent menstruation and during the immediate postpartum period (4,7). Women who acquire postpartum gonococcal infections or at certain phases of their menstrual cycle harbor strains of *N. gonorrhoeae* that are more resistant to killing by normal human sera and have a transparent colonial morphology.

Congenital or acquired complement deficiencies also predispose patients to neisserial infections as a result of the absence of complement-dependent serum bactericidal activity (4,7,9). Patients with systemic lupus erythematosus also are at increased risk for DGI (10). In a review of 41 cases of DGI from 1985 to 1991, comorbid conditions were common, including parenteral drug use in eight, systemic lupus erythematosus in three, and human immunodeficiency virus (HIV) infection in one (10).

There are two mechanisms of gonococcal antibiotic resistance, chromosomal mutation and the acquisition of plasmids (4,5,7). These mechanisms either decrease the permeability of the gonococcal membrane to antibiotics, decrease the affinity of penicillin-binding proteins for β-lactams, or increase the concentration of penicillin-binding proteins. The prevalence of antibiotic-resistant gonococci varies from one community to the next. Eighteen (56%) of the 32 gonococcal isolates from the synovial fluid of South Africans with gonococcal arthritis were penicillinase-producing strains (11). In contrast to the usual AHU auxotype disseminated gonococcal infection strains, most of these isolates were prototrophic ("wild type"). Testing for penicillinase-producing strains of *N. gonorrhoeae* is simple, inexpensive, and widely available. However, other types of antimicrobial resistance, such as chromosomally mediated resistance, can be detected only with expensive and technically difficult methods and are often not well standardized. Antimicrobial susceptibility testing of all gonococcal isolates should be routinely performed.

CLINICAL MANIFESTATIONS OF DISSEMINATED GONOCOCCAL INFECTION

Only about 25% of patients with DGI recall a history of urethritis or cervicitis (4,7,10,12). Therefore, DGI generally develops after untreated mucosal infections. Reports of the last sexual encounter before the onset of the initial symptoms of DGI have varied from 1 day to several weeks.

The most common symptoms in DGI are migratory polyarthralgias, tenosynovitis, dermatitis, and fever (Table 127.1) (4,7,10,12). Tenosynovitis is an important clue in the diagnosis of DGI because it is rare in most other forms of septic arthritis. Often multiple tendons are simultaneously inflamed, especially around the dorsum of the wrists, fingers, ankles, and toes. The concurrent presence of dermatitis and tenosynovitis, which has been designated the acute arthritis–dermatitis syndrome, is highly suggestive of DGI.

Dermatitis occurs in 40% to 70% of patients with DGI (Table 127.1). Skin lesions usually are multiple and most often occur on the extremities or the trunk, but rarely on the face, palms, or soles (Fig. 127.1). These lesions are often painless, and patients may be unaware of their existence, although some skin lesions are painful. The most common skin lesions are hemorrhagic macules or papules, but pustules, vesicles, bullae, erythema nodosum, or erythema multiforme also have been described. New skin lesions may develop during the initial 24 to 48 hours of antibiotic therapy.

Frank, purulent arthritis occurs in 40% to 80% of patients (4,7,10,12). Usually more than one joint is involved, and knees, wrists, and ankles are affected most commonly.

TABLE 127.1. INITIAL SYMPTOMS AND SIGNS IN DISSEMINATED GONOCOCCAL INFECTION

Symptom, Sign	Percentage of Patients
Migratory polyarthralgias	70
Tenosynovitis	67
Dermatitis	55
Fever	55
Purulent arthritis	55
(Monoarthritis)	(20)
(Polyarthritis)	(35)
Genitourinary symptoms	25

From references 4, 7, 10, and 12, with permission.

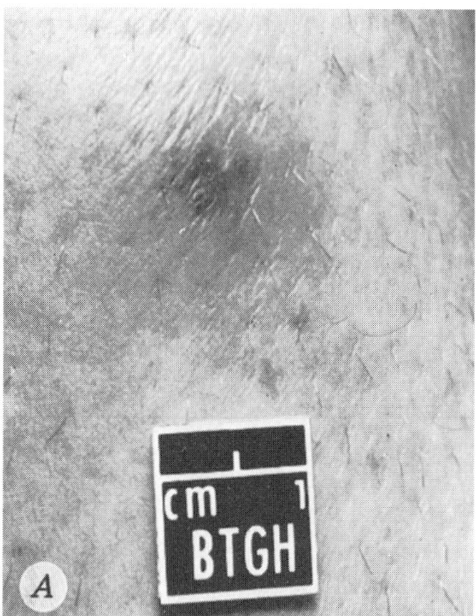

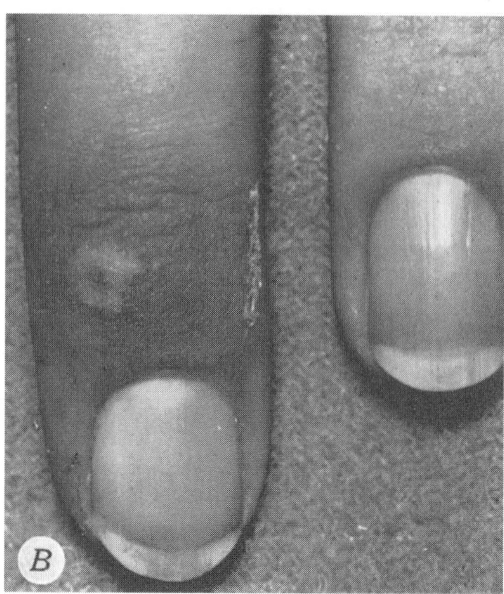

FIG. 127.1. Skin lesions characteristic of septicemia due to *Neisseria gonorrhoeae*. **A:** Hemorrhagic spot 5 to 6 mm in diameter on the upper arm; the gray area 1 to 2 mm in diameter in the center indicates necrosis. **B:** Pustulovesicular lesion on the finger of the same patient; the necrotic center is evident as a gray area.

Sometimes a relatively transient effusion with an unimpressive synovial fluid leukocytosis is present, but most often the clinical and synovial fluid characteristics are similar to those of other forms of bacterial arthritis. The mean synovial fluid leukocyte count in gonococcal arthritis is approximately 50,000 cells/mm^3. Although chronic gonococcal arthritis was common in the preantibiotic era, it is now rare, but should be still included in the differential diagnosis of inflammatory arthritis lasting several weeks or even months.

Most patients are febrile, although the average temperature is usually only moderately elevated (4,7,10,12). A modest peripheral blood leukocytosis is common, with a recent report of a mean peripheral blood leukocyte count of 11,700 cells/mm^3 (10). Transiently elevated liver-function studies have been described, probably representing subclinical hepatitis during bacteremia (4). Gonococcal meningitis and endocarditis have been reported rarely in the antibiotic era.

Some investigators have proposed that DGI progresses sequentially from a bacteremic phase, characterized by chills, tenosynovitis, and skin lesions, to a joint localized phase manifested by purulent arthritis (4,7,10,12). The diagnostic utility of such a classification is suspect, however, because of the significant clinical overlap and the inconsistent temporal sequence of the articular manifestations.

DIAGNOSIS

The diagnosis of DGI should be suspected in any young, sexually active patient who has acute arthritis and dermatitis (4,7,10,12). Although tenosynovitis can occur with other types of arthritis, the presence of tenosynovitis or arthritis in association with a skin rash is sufficient clinical grounds for a presumptive diagnosis of DGI. Most patients are febrile, demonstrate peripheral blood leukocytosis, and have an elevated erythrocyte sedimentation rate and other acute-phase reactants, but such nonspecific findings are not always present. If synovial fluid can be aspirated, the leukocyte count is generally 30,000 to 100,000 cell/mm^3, although the range is wider than in the joint effusions of nongonococcal bacterial arthritis. Some fluids are relatively acellular.

The definitive diagnosis of neisserial infections requires Gram's stain identification of typical gram-negative intracellular diplococci or recovery of *N. gonorrhoeae* on culture. However, synovial fluid Gram's stain have been positive in fewer than 25% of patients with gonococcal arthritis, and synovial fluid cultures positive in only 30% to 60% (4,6,7,12,13). The urethra should be swabbed to obtain a specimen for culture because most men do not have a urethral discharge. In women, a specimen should be obtained directly from the cervix. Rectal and pharyngeal cultures should be obtained, particularly the latter, because pharyngeal gonorrhea may more often predispose to disseminated infection. Genitourinary cultures are positive in 70% to 86% of patients with DGI.

Optimal culture yield requires rapid transfer of specimens to the microbiology laboratory and incubation in a moist environment of 5% CO_2 at 34°C to 37°C (4). Ideally, specimens from normally sterile sites, including synovial fluid and blood, should be inoculated on chocolate agar at the bedside. The chocolate agar should be prewarmed to at least room temperature. However, specimens from sites with normal bacteria flora, such as the cervix, rectum, and pharynx, should be inoculated on selective media that incorporate antibiotics to suppress the growth of the normal flora, but not *N. gonorrhoeae.* Thayer-Martin media incorporates vancomycin, colistin, and nystatin into chocolate agar, but there are now other selective media including modified Thayer-Martin, Martin-Lewis, and New York media. *N. gonorrhoeae* may be differentiated from other *Neisseria* species by its ability to use glucose but not maltose, sucrose, or lactose and by its ability to reduce nitrates (the oxidase test).

The polymerase chain reaction has been used for the detection of specific nucleic acids to identify bacteria, including *N. gonorrhoeae,* in clinical specimens (14). Polymerase chain reaction involves amplification of specific DNA sequences, as defined by two oligonucleotide primers complementary to the relevant target DNA base sequences, allowing detection of very small amounts of specific DNA. With the nested polymerase chain reaction, *N. gonorrhoeae* was detected in 11 of 14 patients with clinically typical, but culture-negative, gonococcal arthritis (15). Three patients had positive genitourinary cultures, and all responded quickly to antibiotics. In contrast, none of the 11 patients tested with Reiter's syndrome and only one of 16 with other forms of arthritis were positive by polymerase chain reaction, providing a specificity of 96% and sensitivity of 79%. In a similar study, the synovial fluid of five of eight patients with DGI was positive by polymerase chain reaction (16). All specimens that were culture positive had a positive polymerase chain reaction, but two culture-negative specimens also were polymerase chain reaction positive (Fig. 127.2). In samples in which polymerase chain reaction was performed before and after treatment, weaker signal strength corresponding to 100-fold decreases in *N. gonorrhoeae* DNA were found after antimicrobial therapy (Fig. 127.2).

Therefore wider availability of the polymerase chain reaction may prove to be of significant importance in the diagnosis, treatment, and understanding of DGI (14). Its most useful indication would be to confirm or exclude the diagnosis in patients with suspected DGI but negative synovial fluid cultures. It may also have some utility in predicting treatment response in those patients with persistent joint effusions. Polymerase chain reaction also may help to shed light on the debate regarding the importance of viable organisms in the joint of patients with gonococcal arthritis. The presence of gonococcal DNA, even in culture-negative synovial fluid, indicates that bacteria were, or still are, present in the joint and required to induce the synovitis associated with DGI. The extreme sensitivity of polymerase chain reaction makes contamination with DNA from other bacteria problematic. Furthermore, current methods cannot differentiate DNA from *N. gonorrhoeae* and that from *N. meningitidis.*

Currently a presumptive diagnosis of DGI is still often made on the basis of a positive genitourinary culture and a characteristic clinical presentation (4,7,10,12). Most patients, especially those without large, purulent effusions and with a short duration of symptoms, will respond to antibiotics within 24 to 48 hours. This rapid therapeutic response is very helpful in confirming the diagnosis in suspected cases of DGI that are culture negative. However, such a therapeutic response to antibiotics may not occur in cases caused by penicillin-resistant strains. Antibiotic-resistant organisms may be more difficult to eradicate, therefore causing chronic synovitis and possible irreversible joint destruction. Unusual clinical presentations and failure to initiate appropriate antibiotics has resulted in delays of treatment in such situations.

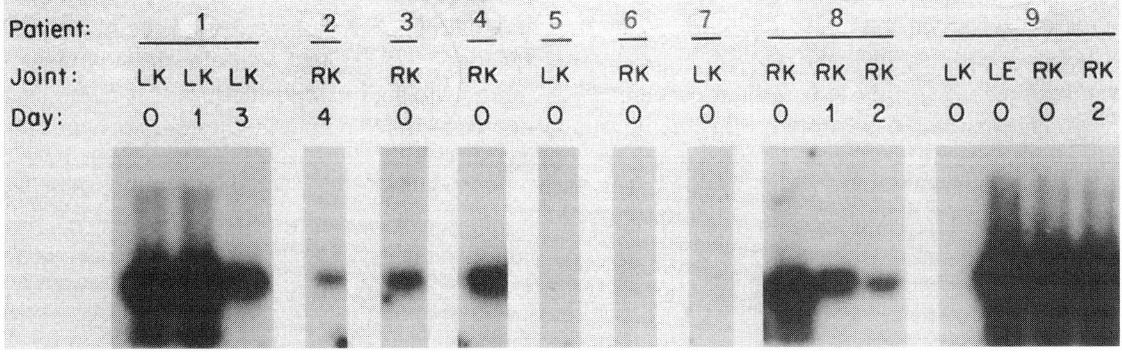

FIG. 127.2. The results of polymerase chain reaction in synovial fluid of nine patients with gonococcal arthritis. Six of the nine fluids demonstrate *N. gonorrhoeae* DNA by polymerase chain reaction. Serial samples at day 0 (pretreatment) and after antibiotic treatment are positive by polymerase chain reaction in patients 1, 8, and 9. (Reproduced from Muralidhar B, Rumore PM, Steinman CR. Use of the polymerase chain reaction to study arthritis due to *Neisseria gonorrhoeae. Arthritis Rheum* 1994;37:713, with permission.)

DIFFERENTIAL DIAGNOSIS

The most important differential diagnostic category is other forms of bacterial arthritis (4,7,10,12). Meningococcal arthritis is the most difficult to distinguish from DGI. However, most other forms of bacterial arthritis present as monoarthritis and occur in young children, elderly patients, or patients with compromised host defense mechanisms or prior arthritis. Tenosynovitis and dermatitis are rare in nonneisserial forms of bacterial arthritis.

Because of the similar associated risk factors, rheumatic manifestations of HIV infection should be considered in patients with possible DGI (17,18). Furthermore, patients with DGI may be HIV positive (17). Arthralgias or noninflammatory joint effusions occur in HIV disease, whereas purulent effusions have not been reported with HIV infection unless there is coexistent bacterial arthritis. Secondary syphilis also may be confused with DGI, although the rash associated with syphilis is generally a diffuse maculopapular dermatitis. Diagnostic testing for *Chlamydia,* HIV, and syphilis is appropriate in selected patients with suspected DGI.

Other major differential diagnostic considerations include hepatitis B, Reiter's syndrome, acute rheumatic fever, bacterial endocarditis, other bacteremias, and other connective tissue diseases. Polyarthritis, tenosynovitis, and skin rash are common in hepatitis; the rash and arthritis generally occur in the anicteric phase. The skin rash is usually urticarial, and the synovial fluid leukocyte count is usually lower than that in DGI. The most helpful diagnostic features of hepatitis B–associated arthritis are elevated hepatocellular enzymes and the identification of hepatitis B surface antigen in the blood, along with negative blood and synovial fluid cultures. Reiter's syndrome also may cause arthritis, tenosynovitis, and urethritis. In classic Reiter's syndrome, the urethritis is not due to *N. gonorrhoeae,* but rather to other organisms, particularly *Chlamydia trachomatis.* Other differentiating clinical features of Reiter's syndrome include the presence of conjunctivitis, characteristic mucocutaneous lesions, circinate balanitis, and keratoderma blennorrhagica. Clinical and radiologic evidence of sacroiliitis and the presence of human leukocyte antigen (HLA)-B27 also are characteristic of Reiter's syndrome. Acute rheumatic fever, or more often poststreptococcal arthritis, may cause polyarthritis in young adults, usually without carditis, chorea, or subcutaneous nodules. If a skin rash is present, it usually is transient (erythema marginatum). The diagnosis relies on evidence of a recent streptococcal throat infection, confirmed by culture or by serologic testing of blood, and a rapid response to salicylates or other antiinflammatory agents.

Many bacteremias or other systemic infections can cause musculoskeletal and dermatologic manifestations that mimic DGI. It is especially important to differentiate bacterial endocarditis from DGI. Purulent arthritis is not common in bacterial endocarditis unless hematogenous spread to the synovium occurs, such as is occasionally seen in endocarditis caused by *Staphylococcus aureus.* Myalgias, arthralgias, tendonitis, and back pain are common musculoskeletal manifestations associated with bacterial endocarditis, particularly in subacute disease that already has been present for several weeks. Viral diseases including measles and rubella, as well as various arboviral infections not commonly seen in the United States, also can cause skin lesions and arthritis. Rarely infections caused by herpesviruses are accompanied by a skin rash and arthralgias. The characteristic erythema chronicum migrans rash and the development of clinical manifestations, such as neurologic symptoms, should easily differentiate patients with Lyme disease from those with DGI.

As described earlier, patients with systemic lupus erythematosus may be predisposed to neisserial infections. Therefore it is very important to consider DGI or meningococcal infection in the lupus patient with an acute febrile illness that may mimic an exacerbation of systemic lupus erythematosus.

PATHOGENESIS

Suppurative arthritis caused by *N. gonorrhoeae* is generally considered to follow bacteremic spread of the organisms to the synovium, with local replication of bacteria and subsequent release of proteolytic enzymes from synovial lining cells and from extravasated polymorphonuclear leukocytes (4,7,10,12). Eventually, cartilage is destroyed, as in most other types of bacterial arthritis. Gonococcal bacteremia is more likely to cause arthritis or tenosynovitis than is infection with pneumococci or other common bacteria. Microscopically, the synovial membrane initially reveals lining-cell hyperplasia and infiltration by polymorphonuclear leukocytes (19). Gram-stained smears of the synovial membrane are sometimes initially positive. If a second synovial membrane specimen is obtained 5 to 7 days after treatment, most of the acute infiltrate will have subsided, but chronic inflammatory cells will be prominent. Rarely a chronic synovitis persists despite appropriate antibiotic therapy (4,7,10,12). This sterile synovitis may be responsible for persistent pain and joint effusions despite eradication of the acute infection, a phenomenon termed postinfectious arthritis (19).

Clinical and laboratory evidence indicates that the arthralgias, tenosynovitis, dermatitis, and the "sterile" arthritis associated with DGI could be due to immune-mediated mechanisms or hypersensitivity (19). The initial presentation of DGI often resembles that of serum sickness, with tenosynovitis and migratory polyarthralgias that are usually transient and often disappear without antimicrobial therapy. Similar musculoskeletal symptoms are common in immune complex–related infections such as hepatitis, but they are absent in nonneisserial bacterial arthritis. Furthermore, as discussed earlier, *N. gonorrhoeae* is recovered from fewer than 50% of purulent synovial effusions, in contrast with nongonococcal bacterial arthritis. Positive blood cultures are found in fewer than one third of patients with DGI, and positive blood and synovial fluid cultures are rare (Table 127.2). Skin lesions are almost always sterile. The frequent absence of

TABLE 127.2. CULTURE RESULTS IN DISSEMINATED GONOCOCCAL INFECTION

Site	Isolation of *N. gonorrheae* (%)
Genitourinary	83
Synovial fluid	35
Rectum	27
Pharynx	8
Blood	8
Skin	0

From references 4, 7, 10, and 12, with permission.

positive blood, skin, and synovial fluid cultures may be a result of the fastidious growth requirements of *N. gonorrhoeae,* yet the organisms are easily recovered from the genitourinary tract or other local sites in most cases of DGI. Therefore some investigators have suggested a role for immune-mediated phenomena or hypersensitivity in the synovitis and dermatitis associated with DGI (4,7,10,12).

Noninfectious dermatitis such as erythema nodosum, erythema multiforme, and vasculitis have been reported in DGI. Gonococcal cell wall components, gonococcal antibody, and complement have been demonstrated in the skin lesions. Circulating immune complexes also have been detected in patients with DGI. In animal models of gonococcal arthritis, intraarticular injections of nonviable *N. gonorrhoeae* or gonococcal lipopolysaccharide isolated from the cell wall of *N. gonorrhoeae* caused an initially acute and then chronic, persistent synovitis (19). A lipopolysaccharide concentration as low as 5 μg (10^{-6} g dry weight) caused arthritis, whereas much larger concentrations of another gonococcal antigenic component, the outer membrane protein, did not cause synovitis. Therefore clinical and laboratory evidence indicate that, in some circumstances, the synovitis, tenosynovitis, and dermatitis associated with DGI may not require viable *N. gonorrhoeae.* The studies using polymerase chain reaction to demonstrate gonococcal DNA in the synovial fluid of suspected gonococcal arthritis suggest that organisms initially do enter the synovial cavity in DGI (15,16). Whether gonococcal arthritis requires viable organisms to persist in the joint has not been resolved.

TREATMENT

The initial antibiotic of choice for DGI is a third-generation β-lactamase–resistant cephalosporin (4,13). Ceftriaxone, 1 g parenterally every 24 hours, or ceftizoxime or cefotaxime, 1 g parenterally every 8 hours, usually is recommended. Antibiotic-resistant strains may cause a chronic arthritis that requires hospitalization for appropriate susceptibility testing and for longer courses of parenteral antibiotics and joint drainage. Therefore older DGI treatment recommendations that included modest doses of multiple antibiotics and outpatient, oral regimens, may no longer be appropriate.

Parenteral therapy should be continued until there is marked clinical improvement, at which time, patients can usually be switched to oral antibiotics and discharged from the hospital. Another full week of oral therapy with ciprofloxacin, 500 mg twice daily, or cefixime, 400 mg twice daily, is recommended. In penicillin-allergic patients, initial treatment should be spectinomycin, 2 g parenterally every 12 hours. Unless appropriate tests for concurrent *Chlamydia* infection are negative, patients should also be given doxycycline, 100 mg every 12 hours for 7 days. If the patient is pregnant, erythromycin should be used instead of doxycycline. If cultures indicate that the strain of *N. gonorrhoeae* is sensitive to penicillin, ampicillin or amoxicillin and clavulanic acid can be substituted (Fig. 127.3).

Patients with joint effusions should be hospitalized and the joint effusions drained by repeated needle aspiration. Although open surgical drainage or arthroscopy is rarely required in DGI, any joint not responding adequately must be evaluated for more definitive drainage. The mean duration of hospitalization for DGI is 5.8 days. The length of hospitalization correlates with higher synovial fluid leukocyte counts, higher erythrocyte sedimentation rate, presence of positive synovial fluid cultures, and presence of comorbid conditions (10).

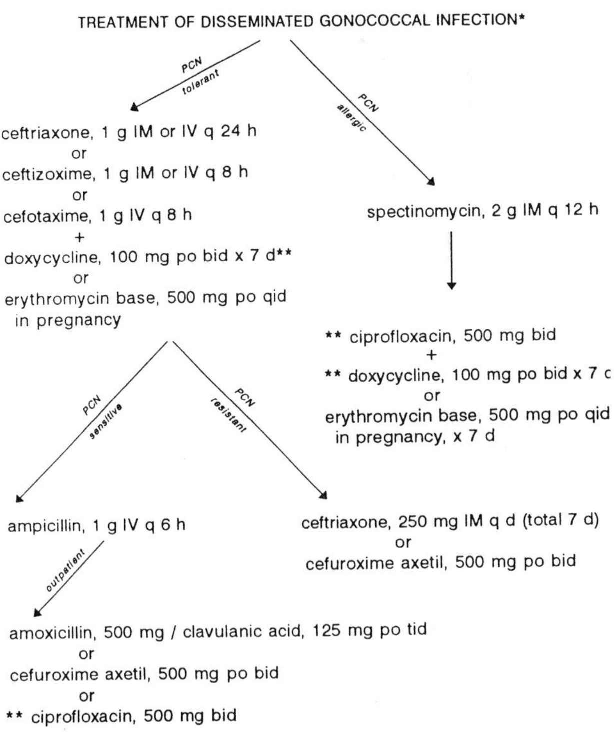

FIG. 127.3. An algorithmic approach to the antimicrobial therapy of disseminated gonococcal infection. (Reproduced from Scopelitis E, Martinez-Osuna P. Gonococcal arthritis. *Rheum Dis Clin North Am* 1993;19:372, with permission.)

MENINGOCOCCAL AND OTHER NEISSERIAL ARTHRITIS

N. meningitidis can be differentiated from *N. gonorrhoeae* microbiologically because the former ferments both dextrose and maltose, whereas the latter ferments only dextrose. Only *N. meningitidis* has an immunizing polysaccharide capsule. Most other microbial characteristics, however, are identical. Furthermore, although traditionally it has been thought that *N. meningitidis* was acquired via the respiratory tract and *N. gonorrhoeae* via the genitourinary tract, either organism can cause disease by venereal transmission and be recovered from joint fluid, blood, cerebrospinal fluid, conjunctiva, or pharynx.

The articular and dermatologic manifestations of disseminated meningococcal infection are virtually identical to those of DGI (20,21). Arthritis occurs in 2% to 10% of acute meningococcal infections. Three distinct types have been described: (a) an acute polyarthritis, usually associated with acute meningococcemia and meningitis; (b) a monoarthritis or oligoarthritis that usually begins 5 to 7 days after septicemia; and (c) a primary acute pyogenic arthritis, not associated with meningitis or classic signs of meningococcemia. However, as noted in DGI, the notion of distinct articular syndromes can be alternatively interpreted as an evolution from one clinical phase to the next. The proposed pathogenesis of the articular manifestations of meningococcal arthritis is similar to that of DGI. Direct bacterial invasion of the synovium and recovery of *N. meningitidis* from synovial fluid is most common in chronic, primary meningococcal arthritis. In most cases of acute, polyarticular arthritis associated with meningococcemia, however, the synovial fluid is sterile. A postinfectious arthritis or immune-mediated synovitis has been postulated to account for this disorder. Classic meningococcal purpura associated with severe meningococcemia might be present, but the dermatitis often resembles that of DGI. Tenosynovitis is common, especially in association with acute polyarthritis. The polymerase chain reaction has been used to identify *N. meningitidis* in the synovial membrane (22).

The acute arthritis–dermatitis syndrome of meningococcal infections may be as common as DGI in certain areas of the country (20,21). These data strengthen the case for hospitalization of all patients with the arthritis–dermatitis syndrome. Treatment includes antimeningococcal antibiotics and joint drainage when necessary.

Nongonococcal, nonmeningococcal *Neisseria,* such as *N. sicca,* may rarely cause joint disease (23). These organisms are often saprophytic inhabitants of the upper respiratory tract and are usually considered to be nonpathogenic. Thus positive cultures may be considered as contaminants. Many of these organisms are resistant to penicillin, and antimicrobial choice should be guided by the results of antibiotic susceptibility tests.

REFERENCES

1. Le Dantec L, Maury F, Flipo RM, et al. Peripheral pyogenic arthritis: a study of one hundred seventy-nine cases. *Rev Rheum Eng* 1996;63:103–110.
2. Ryan MJ, Kavanaugh R, Wall PG, et al. Bacterial joint infections in England and Wales: analysis of bacterial isolates over a four year period. *Br J Rheumatol* 1997;36:370–373.
3. Morgan DS, Fisher D, Merianos A, et al. An 18 year clinical review of septic arthritis from tropical Australia. *Epidemiol Infect* 1996;117:423–428.
4. Cucurull E, Espinoza LR. Gonococcal arthritis. *Rheum Dis Clin North Am* 1998;24:305–322.
5. Naumann M. Host cell interactions and signalling with *Neisseria gonorrhoeae. Curr Opin Microbiol* 1999;2:62–70.
6. Fleming TJ. Arthropathic properties of gonococcal peptidoglycan fragments: implications for the pathogenesis of disseminated gonococcal disease. *Infect Immun* 1986;52:600–608.
7. O'Brien JP, Goldenberg DL, Rice PA. Disseminated gonococcal infection: a prospective analysis of 49 patients and a review of pathophysiology and immune mechanisms. *Medicine* 1983;62: 395–406.
8. Rice PA, Goldenberg DL. Clinical manifestations of disseminated infection caused by *Neisseria gonorrhoeae* are linked to differences in bacterial reactivity of infecting strains. *Ann Intern Med* 1981;95:175–178.
9. McQuillen DP. Complement processing and immunoglobulin binding to *Neisseria gonorrhoeae* determined in vitro simulates in vivo effects. *J Infect Dis* 1999;179:124–135.
10. Wise CM, Morris CR, Wasilauskas BL, et al. Gonococcal arthritis in an era of increasing penicillin resistance: presentations and outcomes in 41 recent cases (1985-1991). *Arch Intern Med* 1994;154:2690–2695.
11. Hoosen AA, Mody GM, Goga IE, et al. Prominence of penicillinase-producing strains of *Neisseria gonorrhoeae* in gonococcal arthritis: experience in Durban, South Africa. *Br J Rheumatol* 1994;33:840–841.
12. Angulo JM. Gonococcal arthritis. *Compr Ther* 1999;25:155–162.
13. Lewis DA. Acute gonococcal arthritis: an unusual host and pathogen combination. *J Clin Pathol* 1995;48:86–88.
14. Louie JS, Liebling MR. The polymerase chain reaction in infectious and post-infectious arthritis. *Rheum Dis Clin North Am* 1998;24:227–236.
15. Liebling MR, Arkfeld DG, Michelini GA, et al. Identification of *Neisseria gonorrhoeae* in synovial fluid using the polymerase chain reaction. *Arthritis Rheum* 1994;37:702–709.
16. Muralidhar B, Rumore PM, Steinman CR. Use of the polymerase chain reaction to study arthritis due to *Neisseria gonorrhoeae. Arthritis Rheum* 1994;37:710–717.
17. Saraux A, Taelman H, Blanche P, et al. HIV infections as a risk factor for septic arthritis. *Br J Rheumatol* 1997;36:333–337.
18. Vassilopoulos D, Chalasani P, Jurado RL, et al. Musculoskeletal infections in patients with human immunodeficiency virus infection. *Medicine* 1997;76:284–294.
19. Goldenberg DL, Reed JI, Rice PA. Arthritis in rabbits induced by killed *Neisseria gonorrhoeae* and gonococcal lipopolysaccharide. *J Rheumatol* 1984;11:3–8.
20. Wells M, Gibbons RB. Primary meningococcal arthritis: case report and review of the literature. *Milit Med* 1997;162: 769–772.
21. Dillon M, Nourse C, Dowling F, et al. Primary meningococcal arthritis. *Pediatr Infect Dis J* 1997;16:331–332.
22. Edgeworth TJ. Diagnosis of primary meningococcal arthritis using the polymerase chain reaction. *J Infect* 1998;37:199.
23. Geisler WM, Markovitz DM. Septic arthritis caused by *Neisseria sicca. J Rheumatol* 1998;25:826–828.

128

ARTHRITIS DUE TO MYCOBACTERIA, FUNGI, AND PARASITES

MAREN LAWSON MAHOWALD

Tuberculous, fungal, and parasitic infections of the musculoskeletal system pose a diagnostic challenge because the clinical presentation and results of initial diagnostic studies are similar to those of noninfectious chronic inflammatory musculoskeletal disorders. Mycobacterial and fungal infections are increasing in nonendemic areas because of immigration and travel to, from, and within developing countries. The clinical importance of fungal infections is increasing because of the increasing numbers of immunocompromised patients as a result of human immunodeficiency virus (HIV) infection, malignancy (especially leukemia), chemotherapy, immunosuppressive therapy (especially in organ transplantation), and an expanding population of elderly patients with chronic debilitating diseases. Timely diagnosis requires a high index of suspicion based on the knowledge of the typical features as well as unusual clinical presentations of fungal infections. These infections should be considered in patients with chronic monoarticular or pauciarticular arthritis and in various other situations, including spondylitis, spondylodiscitis, tendonitis, and erythema nodosum (Table 128.1). Definitive diagnosis depends on identification of the organism in synovial fluid, synovial tissue, abscesses, or osseous tissue.

MYCOBACTERIA

Mycobacterium tuberculosis

Epidemiology

An estimated 8 million people worldwide are infected with *Mycobacterium tuberculosis* (*M. tuberculosis*), and 2 million deaths were attributed to tuberculosis (TB) in 1998 (1). In some developing countries, 75% to 85% of adults have *M. tuberculosis* infection (2). In the second half of the twentieth century, tuberculosis in the United States declined from 84,304 cases in 1952 to 22,201 cases in 1985, followed by a resurgence until 1992 (26,673 cases) that was associated with the HIV epidemic; increased immigration from TB-endemic countries; increased TB transmission in nursing homes, hospitals, and prisons, and among the homeless; and the emergence of multidrug-resistant strains (3). During this period of resurgence, active TB developed in many recently infected individuals, which indicated increased transmission of TB rather than increased reactivation of latent TB. From 1992 to 1998, the number of TB cases in the U.S. declined 31% to 18,361 (case rate, 6.8 per 100,000), largely because of more effective TB-control programs (4) (Fig. 128.1). Nevertheless, approximately 15 million persons in the U.S. have latent TB infection and are at risk of future disease. Overall, the decline in TB cases represents a substantial decrease in cases among U.S.-born persons and a small increase in the number of cases among foreign-born persons (Fig. 128.1). Since the mid-1980s, the proportion of TB cases increased among foreign-born residents from Asia, Africa, and Latin America, where TB rates are 5 to 30 times higher than U.S. rates (5). HIV-infected persons are at much higher risk of active TB disease from reactivation or primary *M. tuberculosis* infection and have higher rates of infection with multidrug-resistant strains (6,7). During 1998, 8.1% of TB cases involved strains resistant to isoniazide, and 1.1% were multidrug resistant (8).

Extrapulmonary tuberculosis has a broad spectrum of clinical manifestations involving almost any organ system (Fig. 128.2) and remains a cause of fever of unknown origin (9,10). In recent years, both the total number of TB cases and the number of extrapulmonary TB cases has declined. In 1996 there were 4,142 cases of extrapulmonary TB (19.4% of 21,337 total TB cases), and in 1997, there were 3,554 cases of extrapulmonary TB (17.9% of 19,851 total TB cases) (11). Approximately 11% of extrapulmonary TB involves bones and joints (approximately 2% of all TB cases). Extrapulmonary TB occurs more often in racial and ethnic minorities, persons with HIV infection, immigrants from high-prevalence countries, the elderly, children younger than 15 years, and others who are immunocompromised. In persons with HIV infection, the incidence of TB is 500 times that in the general population, and 25% to 50% of new TB patients are HIV positive (12,13). The proportion of extrapulmonary TB is increased

TABLE 128.1. TYPICAL CLINICAL PRESENTATIONS OF OSTEOARTICULAR INFECTIONS DUE TO MYCOBACTERIA AND FUNGI

Tuberculosis
Spondylitis or spondylodiscitis with paraspinal abscesses
Monoarticular disease of large weight-bearing joints
Dactylitis in a child
Poncet's disease
Nontuberculous mycobacteria
Arthritis or tendonitis in hand or wrist
Multifocal bone, joint, and tendon with HIV infection
Leprosy
Polyarthritis with erythema nodosum leprosum
Destruction of small bones and joints of hands and feet
Neuropathic Charcot joints at wrists or ankles
Coccidioidomycosis
Migratory polyarthritis with erythema nodosum/multiforme and fever
Indolent monoarticular arthritis of knee with low-grade fever
Blastomycosis
Acute monoarticular arthritis of large weight-bearing joints associated with lung and skin involvement
Spondylitis
Painless osseous lesions
Cryptococcosis
Monarticular arthritis secondary to osseous infection
Spondylitis with paraspinal abscess
Progressive lytic bone lesions
Histoplasmosis
Additive polyarthritis with erythema nodosum
Tenosynovitis at the wrist
Sporotrichosis
Monoarticular or oligoarticular arthritis of knee, wrist, or hand
Polyarthritis with disseminated skin lesions
Chronic arthritis of one or both knees
Candidiasis
Acute monoarticular arthritis of the knee in a patient with serious concurrent illness
Indolent monoarticular arthritis after intraarticular corticosteroid injection
Actinomycosis
Spondylitis with paraspinal abscess
Madura foot

HIV, human immunodeficiency virus.

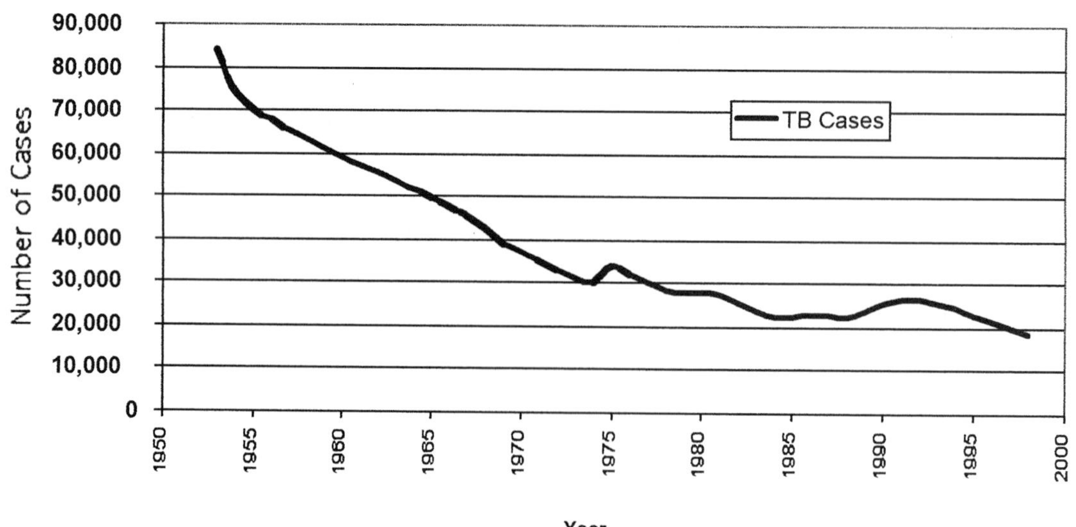

FIGURE 128.1. Cases of tuberculosis in the United States. (From Anonymous. Progress toward the elimination of tuberculosis: United States, 1998. *MMWR* 1999;48:732–736, and Summary of notifiable diseases, United States, 1997. *MMWR* 1998;46:1–87, with permission.)

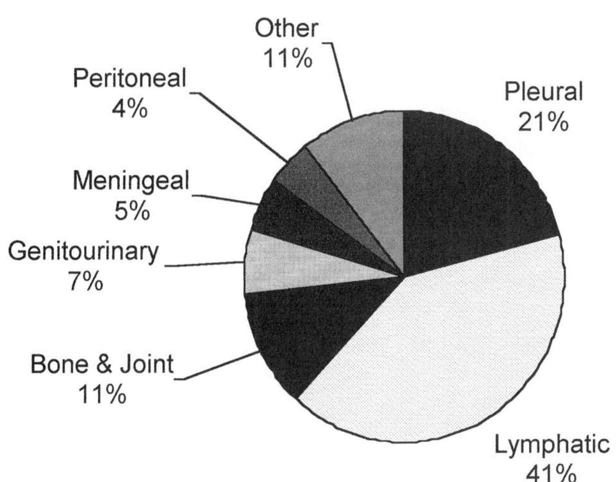

FIGURE 128.2. Extrapulmonary tuberculosis in the United States. (From Division of TB Elimination, CDC Surveillance Reports. *Reported tuberculosis in the US 1996 and 1997, June 21, 1999 update.* Atlanta: Centers for Disease Control, 1999, with permission.)

in this group of patients, and the time from infection to disease is decreased. The control of TB is further complicated by the emergence of multiple drug–resistant organisms. Most new infections with multiple drug–resistant TB are seen in individuals from developing countries and those who also are infected with HIV (14).

There are 50 species in the genus *Mycobacterium.* All are obligate anaerobes, tend to grow slowly, and are intracellular parasites. Infection with *M. tuberculosis* occurs through inhalation of aerosolized bacteria from the index case with pulmonary TB. *De novo* infection in the nonimmunized host depends on the number of organisms that survive phagocytosis by alveolar macrophages. Mycobacteria multiply intracellularly and rupture the alveolar macrophage. Free organisms are then phagocytosed by other macrophages; stimulate secretion of cytokines such as interferons, growth factors, and tumor necrosis factor; and upregulate human leukocyte antigen (HLAs) and T-cell receptors. Hematogenous dissemination to distant organs may produce metastatic foci capable of recrudescence of active infection at later times. Other organisms reach the lymphatic system and regional lymph nodes where cellular immunity is generated. $CD4^+$ T cells provide protective immune responses in the lung, help B cells and $CD8^+$ cytotoxic suppressor cells, and produce cytokines that recruit more monocytes, which participate in granuloma formation (Ghon's lesion). Cell-wall components are important in the host response. Muramyl dipeptide is a potent adjuvant that enhances both humoral and cellular immunity and elicits granuloma formation. Lipoarabinomannan, a cell-wall glycolipid, inhibits macrophage effector functions, thus acting as a virulence factor. Humoral immunity plays a negligible protective role against TB, but genetic susceptibility to infection appears to be real. In nursing homes and prisons, the TB infection rate is twofold greater in blacks than in whites (15).

Clinical TB represents failure of the local immune defense. If the initial lesion is not contained by the inflammatory response, tuberculous pneumonia develops. Three percent to 10% of initial infections develop clinical disease within 2 years and at a rate of 0.05% to 0.10% per year thereafter. In purified protein derivative (PPD)-positive patients, clinical disease results from reactivation rather than reinfection. Trauma or local factors appear to play a role in the reactivation of disease (16,17), and rates of reactivation are higher in immunocompromised individuals (18,19). Osteoarticular tuberculosis tends to be a disease of children in developing countries and a disease of the elderly and immunocompromised individuals in Western countries. Skeletal infection can develop either by hematogenous or lymphatic spread from chronic pleural, renal, or lymph node foci, or by reactivation of latent infection at sites seeded in the primary illness (20,21). In the U.S., osteoarticular tuberculosis usually results from recrudescence of latent infection. The rarity of bone and joint tuberculosis in Western countries has lowered the index of suspicion in the medical community, often resulting in unfortunate delays in diagnosis for many months or years (22), or misdiagnosis as osteoarthritis (OA), rheumatoid arthritis (RA), or bone metastases.

Peripheral Osteoarticular Tuberculosis

Tuberculous infection of diarthrodial joints produces chronic low-grade pain, swelling, and stiffness with slowly progressive loss of function, and eventual abscess formation (23). Articular tuberculosis typically develops when a focus of osteomyelitis in adjacent subchondral epiphyseal bone erodes through the articular surface into the joint space. Rarely the synovium may be seeded directly via the bloodstream. An initial inflammatory reaction in the synovium is followed by formation of granulation tissue, effusion, and production of a pannus. Mycobacteria do not themselves produce collagenase, so that the articular surface is not rapidly destroyed, as in pyogenic infections. The proliferative synovial pannus destroys the cartilage at the periphery of the joint, erodes into subchondral cancellous bone, and produces demineralization and necrosis, destroying the support structure of the articular cartilage. Ultimately, the process results in severe destruction of bone, formation of paraarticular cold abscesses, and spontaneous external fistulation. Healing takes place by the formation of fibrous tissue, which often produces fibrous ankylosis of the joint (24).

In regions in which it is endemic, the weight-bearing joints are most commonly affected (60–90%), whereas in nonendemic areas, upper extremity joints may be almost as frequently involved as lower extremity joints. The arthritis occurs as chronic monoarticular disease in approximately 85% of patients. Involvement of three or more joints is very rare (25,26). The peak incidence of peripheral arthritis is in the fourth and fifth decades in developed countries, where it is rare in patients in the first decade of life, and the incidence in male subjects and nonwhites is much higher than in female subjects and whites. Tuberculous arthritis in children may be difficult to distinguish from juvenile inflammatory arthritis, resulting in delayed diagnosis, unless a tuberculin skin test is performed during the evaluation of chronic monoarthritis (27,28). A polyarticular or oligoarticular pattern of TB may be seen in the elderly, immunocompromised individuals, those taking corticosteroids, or after trauma (29,30). Cases with multifocal osteoarticular TB may be misdiagnosed as having malignant disease, especially in nonendemic areas (31). Half the patients may have no evidence for pulmonary TB and may have a negative tuberculin skin test (32). The most common presentation is chronic progressive joint pain and swelling without warmth or erythema, loss of motion, and often periarticular abscess formation and spontaneous drainage. Systemic symptoms that may occur include fever, night sweats, weight loss, anorexia, cough, and dyspnea. However, as many as 42% may be afebrile, and a third of patients may have no systemic symptoms (33). In one large series, Garrido et al. (20) reported radiographic changes in peripheral TB infection that included soft-tissue swelling (90%), osteopenia (72%), joint-space narrowing (66%), erosions (64%), cysts (66%), bony sclerosis (20%), periostitis (15%), and calcifications (5%).

In the hip, tubercle bacilli may localize in the synovium, acetabulum, or proximal femur. Bony destruction is seen most commonly in the acetabulum. The femoral neck and head and trochanteric epiphysis, or trochanteric bursa, also may be involved (34,35). Symptoms include mild-to-moderate pain in the groin, knee, or thigh, and limitation of motion. A limp is the most common presenting complaint in children. Atrophy of the gluteal muscles and tenderness in the groin often are present. At rest, the hip is held in flexion and abduction. Later severe destruction of the femoral neck and acetabulum occurs with formation of a cold abscess and sinus tract, which usually points to the outer thigh.

In the knee, pain is insidious in onset and may be present for years before the patient seeks medical attention. About 20% of patients describe swelling, and 10% have stiffness as the initial complaint. Localized heat and muscular wasting are usually present on examination. A limp, synovial swelling, and limitation of motion are common. Although pure synovial infection does occur, most patients have involvement of both synovium and bone (36). In the ankle, elbow, and wrist, joint damage results in marked joint instability that usually requires arthrodesis or spontaneous fusion for functional restoration after antituberculous therapy (37).

TB infection of prosthetic joints is usually due to reactivation of previous osteoarticular infection and occurs years after implantation or may be identified at the time of arthroplasty. Clinically, joint pain is slowly progressive, and joint aspiration usually does not yield fluid. Multiple samples of tissue should be obtained for histologic and culture studies. Infection may be eradicated without removing the prosthesis but requires prolonged multidrug therapy (38–40).

Tuberculosis infection involving soft tissue sites (tenosynovium, bursa, muscle, or deep fascia) is uncommon but may mimic common local inflammatory disorders and is therefore likely to be misdiagnosed (41). Soft tissue infections cause focal swelling that may or may not be painful and often coexist with involvement of adjacent bony structures. [In reported cases, patients often had a history of rheumatic diseases, had been treated with corticosteroids and immunosuppressive drugs, or were receiving dialysis (42).] A history of antecedent local trauma may be obtained (43). Diagnosis may be delayed because a bursal injection of corticosteroid may produce a temporary decrease in the swelling or pain. Tuberculosis involving tendons in the hand and wrist may cause a carpal tunnel syndrome (44). Infection of the trochanteric bursa and subdeltoid bursa has also been reported.

Tuberculous rheumatism or Poncet's disease was reported in 1887. Poncet described inflammatory polyarthritis of the hands and feet in 12 patients with a past or current history of visceral tuberculosis. He called it tuberculous rheumatism; however, there was no evidence of bacteriologic involvement of the joints themselves. The course of the arthritis was usually chronic, producing deformity without suppuration or caseation, and was associated with cachexia or disseminated TB within several years. Other authors have reported symmetric polyarthritis in patients with TB whose symptoms abated with antituberculous therapy but not with antiinflammatory therapy and who had no mycobacteria in their joints. The concept of a reactive arthritis to tuberculosis has remained controversial because the rigor with which foci of TB infection were sought in these cases has been variable (45–48).

Tuberculosis of the Spine

In the early twentieth century, TB of the spine was common and caused severe disability (49). Since the advent of antituberculous drugs, characteristic spinal deformities and neurologic damage have declined. However, in developing countries, TB remains a serious health problem. For example, in Somalia, 54% of those older than 15 years are tuberculin test positive (50). Spinal TB accounts for 50% of skeletal TB and recently, in the United Kingdom and France, up to 70% of patients with spinal TB were foreign-born patients from developing countries (51).

Pathogenic mechanisms leading to spinal TB include (a) hematogenous dissemination during the initial infection, which produces granulomas in bone causing bone destruction; (b) spread of infection to bone via lymphatic drainage from another focus of tuberculosis (e.g., from pleural or kidney via paraaortic lymph nodes to erode into the vertebral body); or (c) recrudescence of an old pulmonary infection with hematogenous spread to the spine, in which case the patient will also have signs of pulmonary TB infection (52). Patterns of tuberculous spinal involvement include paradiscal, anterior, and central (53). In the paradiscal or spondylodiscitis form, infection typically starts in the anterior portion of the vertebral bodies and invades the disc space early. As the disc and anterior vertebrae are destroyed, the characteristic anterior wedging of two adjacent vertebrae with disc-space loss produces kyphotic gibbus deformity. Anterior lesions develop under the anterior spinal ligament to involve several vertebrae. Central lesions (spondylitis without disk involvement) involve the entire vertebral body, resulting in significant deformity. Abscesses are common and may dissect for long distances along fascial planes to form abscesses remote from the spinal infection. There are several mechanisms of neurologic injury in spinal TB. Paraspinal abscesses may exert ischemic pressure on the subjacent spinal cord, whereas posterior extrusion of caseous or granulation tissue may cause anterior cord compression or inflammatory vasculitis with thrombosis of the spinal vessels. Sudden cord transection with severe spinal instability may occur rarely. Spinal root compression may occur with arachnoiditis or extension of paraosseous abscess through the dura.

In regions in which TB is endemic, spinal tuberculosis (Pott's disease) is seen primarily in children and young adults. In the U.S. and Europe, cases in the first decade of life have almost disappeared, and most patients are older than 20 years (mean, 49 years; range, 24–76 years). The thoracic spine is most commonly involved, followed by the lumbar spine and cervical spine. More than one vertebral body (average, 2.5; range, 1–5) and the disc space are usually involved. Skip areas with radiographically normal vertebrae in between occur in about 10% of patients. Paraspinous abscesses are common (50–96%) and may involve the neck, groin, chest wall, or sternum. The incidence of neurologic symptoms caused by cord compression in spinal TB (Pott's paraplegia) varies from 12% to 50% in different series. Epidural compression of the cord or the cauda equina syndrome may occur, and coexistent cord and root compression may cause both upper and lower motor neuron weakness. In the U.S., patients with spinal TB are predominantly men (70%), 50% are immigrants, 45% homeless, 25% HIV-infected, and 25% i.v. drug users. The tuberculin test is positive in 95% of patients, and the erythrocyte sedimentation rate (ESR) elevated in most (mean, 65; range, 30–122). Approximately one third of patients with spinal TB have no evidence of extraspinal TB, but two thirds have pulmonary TB, and half of these have disseminated disease (54).

The clinical presentation is usually that of insidious pain with a history of weight loss, fever, malaise associated with neurologic deficits, abscesses, or sinus tracts. Patients also may have symptoms from affected organ systems such as the urinary, pulmonary, and lymphatic systems. Peripheral white blood cell count is usually normal, the ESR is usually elevated, and the tuberculin skin test is positive in 86% of patients with spinal lesions.

Definitive diagnosis of spinal TB is made by computed tomography (CT)-guided biopsy to demonstrate a positive acid-fast smear, positive *M. tuberculosis* culture, or granulomatous inflammation on histologic examination (55,56). The CT scan also defines the anatomy of the bony damage and paraspinal masses. Magnetic resonance imaging (MRI) is needed to evaluate compression of neural elements. If MRI is not available, a CT myelogram can be used. Plain radiographs are used to localize lesions and measure alignment and deformity. Spinal deformity is present in most patients with thoracic and cervical lesions and is less common in lumbar lesions (57,58). Bone scans may be negative in approximately one third of cases.

Treatment options for spinal TB are selected based on the presence or absence of spinal instability, neurologic deficits, and the level of surgical expertise available. In the preantibiotic era, spinal TB was treated with prolonged immobilization and body casting. The mortality was 20%, and 20% to 30% had recurrence of infection. The initial success with chemotherapy in the 1960s prompted use of surgery to drain abscesses and markedly decreased the period of immobilization (59). In 1963, the Medical Research Council of Great Britain (MRC) began a multinational, clinical trial of five types of mechanical therapy combined with two chemotherapeutic regimens [pyrazinamide (PAS) and isoniazid (INH) for 18 months with or without streptomycin for the first 3 months]. The five types of mechanical treatment included (a) no restraints; (b) body cast in ambulant patients; (c) bed rest for 6 months; (d) minimal debridement; and (e) radical anterior excision with bone grafting (the "Hong Kong operation"). A recent report summarizes the 20-year experience (60). Eighteen months of INH and PAS in ambulant outpatients was successful in the majority of patients. The addition of streptomycin did not improve results, nor did casting or initial bed rest. The minimal-debridement operation did not add any benefit to medical treatment alone. The radical resection of diseased bone and repair of the defect with bone grafts resulted in earlier bony fusion and less increase in kyphosis. This favorable initial outcome was sustained up to the 20-year report. The MRC trial did not include patients with paraplegia or involvement of more than three vertebrae. The patients were younger and had a relatively acute disease course. In nonendemic areas, ambulant chemotherapy alone has had poorer results than those in the MRC Trial. In the U.S., indications for surgery include a neurologic deficit, spinal instability, spinal deformity with more than 50% vertebral collapse or deformity of more than 5 degrees, nonresponse or noncompliance with medical therapy, or a nondiagnostic needle biopsy (61,62).

There is general agreement that Pott's paraplegia should be treated with combined medical and surgical treatment. Spinal instability and angulation, once present, are likely to progress without surgery. In patients with neurologic deficits, debridement removes necrotic tissue, preventing progression, and results in resolution of neurologic deficits (63). If surgical resources are limited, medical treatment alone may still be effective. A large study from Korea demonstrated that treatment with two drugs (INH, ethambutol, or PAS) and physical therapy resulted in resolution of paraplegia in 78% of cases within 6 months (64).

Other notable sites of TB involvement of the axial skeleton are the sacroiliac joints and the ribs. Rib lesions are often associated with a local soft tissue mass and pain. They generally occur in patients with other skeletal involvement, particularly in the spine. Sacroiliac joint involvement, usually unilateral, occurs in about 7% of patients with skeletal TB. With sacroiliac joint infection, the chief complaint is buttock and low back pain for 2 weeks to more than 1 year, described as continuous and severe enough to awaken the patient from sleep at night. Most patients have constitutional symptoms and tenderness to direct palpation of the sacroiliac joint (65,66). Multifocal TB of bone is rare and tends to be seen in individuals from endemic areas who are immunosuppressed, taking long-term corticosteroid treatment, alcoholic, or elderly. The lesions often have mild periosteal reaction, bone sclerosis, and severe bone destruction. Imaging with ^{99m}Tc is usually abnormal. The initial diagnosis is often malignancy, with correct diagnosis made on the biopsy. A mycotic aneurysm of the aorta, created when a paraspinous abscess penetrates the vessel wall, may occasionally complicate spinal TB. The resulting hematoma walls off to form a false aneurysm. Penetration of the abscess into the arterial blood may lead to secondary hematogenous spread and miliary disease (67).

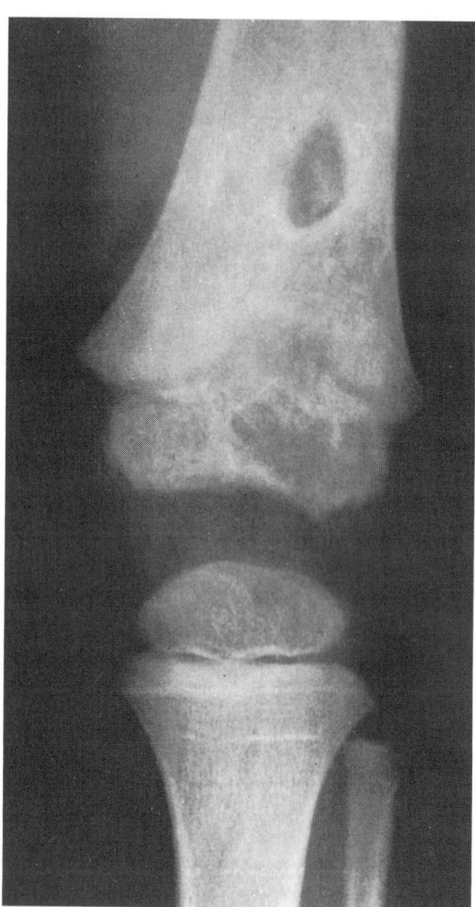

FIGURE 128.3. Tuberculosis of the knee and femur in a child.

Radiographic Signs

There are no pathognomonic radiographic signs of skeletal TB (68,69). In general, TB causes destruction of bone without stimulating much reactive new bone formation. Destructive osseous lesions adjacent to joints are often oval with clear margins (Fig. 128.3). As they expand and erode the cortex, some periosteal reaction occurs. A sequestrum of necrotic cancellous bone may occur. When the joint itself is involved, local osteopenia and soft tissue swelling are early signs. Later, small subchondral erosions appear at the margins of the joint (Fig. 128.4). The cartilage space tends to be preserved until extensive destruction of adjacent cortical bone has occurred (Fig. 128.5). With advanced disease, total destruction of the joint can occur. Destruction is not accompanied by osteophyte formation, but the shadow of a cold abscess containing calcified debris may be seen. Juxtaarticular osteopenia and cortical cyst formation may be complicated by spontaneous fractures.

In the spine, the classic picture is narrowing of the disc space with vertebral collapse and a paraspinous abscess. Scalloping of the anterior vertebral surface is common. Occasional infection of the central portion of the vertebrae may cause extensive bone destruction without disc space invasion. In about 10% of patients, productive or sclerotic changes, which are difficult to see radiographically, may occur in infected vertebrae. In the sacroiliac joint, TB infection produces joint-space widening as a result of bony ero-

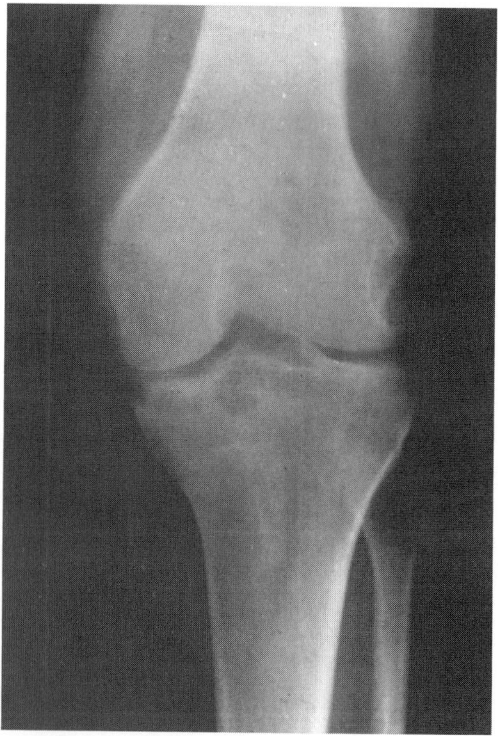

FIGURE 128.4. Tuberculosis of the knee in an adult. (Courtesy of Donald Resnick, M.D.)

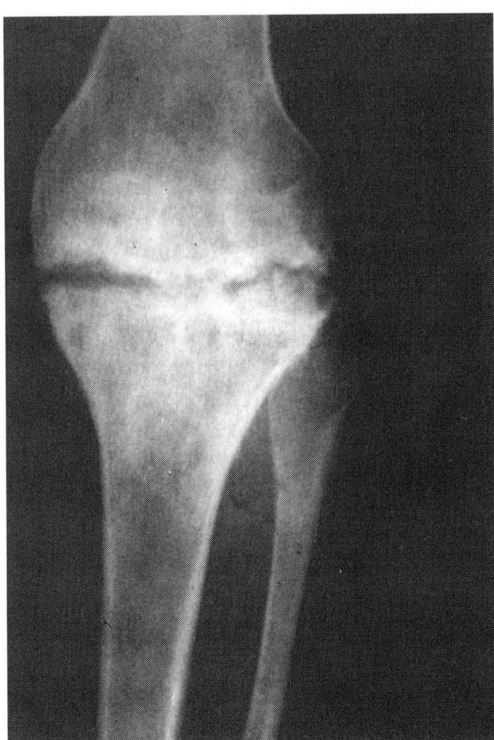

FIGURE 128.5. Advanced tuberculosis of the knee. (Courtesy of Donald Resnick, M.D.)

sions in the sacral and iliac joint margins. Juxtaarticular sclerosis or osteopenia are equally prevalent. Bone scans may show increased uptake of ^{99m}Tc-pyrophosphate in early lesions; however, imaging may be insensitive with low-grade indolent or severely destructive lesions. Therefore a negative bone scan does not rule out the diagnosis of tuberculous bone infection. CT scanning is useful in delineating the extent of bone destruction and adjacent soft tissue masses and in guiding percutaneous needle biopsy and drainage. MRI is useful in delineating the extent of disease, especially along the spinal cord.

Diagnostic Tests

Diagnosis of tuberculous arthritis requires a high index of suspicion and acquisition of material for histologic examination and culture. Microbiologic and histologic studies are complementary for maximal diagnostic yield. The quickest and most reliable method of diagnosis is biopsy. A positive diagnosis can be made by either histology or culture of synovial tissue in more than 90% of specimens. Synovial fluid culture is positive in approximately 25% to 80%, and a positive smear is obtained in 20% to 40% of cases. Synovial fluid protein is always elevated, and 60% of patients have fluid with low glucose levels. The synovial white blood cell count varies widely but is usually between 10,000 and 20,000/mm^3 with more than 75% polymorphonuclear leukocytes. In the case of spinal disease, material for culture is best obtained with a needle biopsy guided by fluoroscopy or CT.

The tuberculin skin test with PPD (5-TU) may be helpful. A positive reaction of greater than 10 mm induration at 48 hours occurs in 50% to 90% of individuals infected with *M. tuberculosis.* Reactions of 5 to 10 mm may be seen with other mycobacterial infections, prior bacillus Calmette–Guérin (BCG) immunization, and in HIV-infected patients who are infected with *M. tuberculosis.* False-negative tuberculin tests are seen in 15% to 20% of patients with active infection who are elderly, immunocompromised, or malnourished. Two-step testing can be carried out if the initial test is negative, and a second test is administered 1 to 3 weeks later. A positive second test is likely due to a boosted reaction from TB infection that occurred a long time ago (70).

Major advances have been made in TB diagnostics including methods to detect growth of *M. tuberculosis* more rapidly in specimens and rapid-detection methods using nucleic acid amplification techniques that provide results in hours (71). The BACTEC radiometric culture system contains radioactive palmitate as the sole carbon source and can detect the organism's metabolism in 2 to 6 days, thus reducing the time to detection of mycobacterial growth. Two new tests can identify *M. tuberculosis* ribosomal RNA (MTD; Gen-Probe, San Diego, CA, U.S.A.) and DNA (Amplicor; Roche Molecular Systems, Branchburg, NJ, U.S.A.) in clinical specimens within 24 hours (72) and have high sensitivity and specificity (73,74). However, these rapid tests do not replace acid-fast staining and culture of the tissues. Culture of the organism is necessary for drug-susceptiblity testing. Restriction fragment length polymorphism analyses are used to identify specific strains in localized outbreaks of infection (75). Direct amplification tests based on the polymerase chain reaction (PCR) have not had extensive testing with osteoarticular tissues (76). False-positive results can occur with contamination, and false-negative results can occur if PCR inhibitors are present in infected tissues. PCR-based approaches also have been used to detect other mycobacterial and fungal infections.

Medical Treatment of Tuberculosis

For children with bone and joint TB, treatment should last at least 12 months. For adults, treatment should be of 6 months' duration; however, if the response is inadequate or slow, treatment should be prolonged to 12 months. The initial phase of treatment should be 8 weeks with four drugs: INH (5 mg/kg, up to 300 mg orally daily), rifampin (10 mg/kg, up to 600 mg orally daily), PAS (15–30 mg/kg, up to 2 g daily), and ethambutol (5–15 mg/kg) or streptomycin (15 mg/kg up to 1 g daily) until susceptibility to INH and rifampin is shown. The continuation phase of treatment includes INH and rifampin daily for 16 to 44 weeks. If the incidence of multidrug-resistant TB is less than 4%, ethambutol or streptomycin may not be necessary for patients with no individual risk factors for drug resistance (77,78). Updated recommendations for drug therapy can be readily obtained from the CDC World Wide Web site for the Morbidity and Mortality Weekly Reports: htp://www.cdc.gov/ [go to Publications and Scientific Data, then Morbidity and Mortality Weekly Report (MMWR)]. The major contraindication to the combined use of INH and rifampin is the presence of active liver disease. PAS and streptomycin should not be given to pregnant women. The optimal duration of treatment of osseous tuberculosis has not been defined. Response to treatment must be evaluated in each case (79). In articular TB with absent or minimal bone involvement, drug therapy alone may be effective (80). Immobilization should be used early to relieve pain and prevent deformity or hip dislocation, especially in the young child. Joints should be repeatedly aspirated to remove purulent effusion, and joint lavage or arthroscopy used to ensure adequate drainage. If periarticular bone involvement is extensive, debridement of the foci of bone infection may hasten healing. Synovectomy with curettage may be important in children with hip disease (81). When articular destruction is extensive in weight-bearing joints, arthrodesis has been the procedure of choice to restore function in those too young for arthroplasty or in joints such as ankles and wrists. In developing countries where sitting cross-legged and squatting are important, Girdlestone's excision arthroplasty has been used effectively for hip disease. Total joint arthroplasty may be successful if the active infection is controlled (82).

Mycobacterium bovis and *Bacillus* Calmette–Guérin

In the first half of the twentieth century, *M. bovis* accounted for 11% of osteoarticular TB. *M. bovis* in milk from infected cows enters humans through the tonsils or the intestinal mucosa, produces lesions in cervical and abdominal lymph nodes, and has an affinity for bone. During World War II, as much as 25% of TB was caused by *M. bovis.* With elimination of bovine TB and widespread pasteurization of milk, infection with *M. bovis* has become rare, usually occurring in elderly individuals exposed to infected milk as children or those immigrating from regions in which bovine TB is still endemic, such as Mexico (83).

BCG is an *M. bovis* attenuated by subculture, which is used for vaccination against tuberculosis and as an adjuvant immunostimulator for bladder cancer and other malignancies. Tuberculous osteomyelitis may occur in children who were immunized as infants (84). Several rheumatic syndromes have been reported in association with BCG immunotherapy (85,86). Intravesicular BCG for superficial bladder cancer is associated with granulomatous cystitis, dysuria, hematuria, malaise, fever, and transient arthritis or migratory arthralgias in up to 3% of patients. The symptoms occur after the first few treatments, increase in severity with additional treatments, and can be prevented with INH prophylaxis (BCG is resistant to PAS). Rarely BCG vaccination or immunotherapy can be complicated by progressive systemic BCG infection, including monoarthritis with positive synovial cultures for *M. bovis,* infection of a joint prosthesis (87,88), or vertebral osteomyelitis (89). Additionally, a seronegative, asymmetric oligoarthritis with morning stiffness, local inflammation, and elevated ESR can occur (90,91). Some of these patients are HLA-B27$^+$, suggesting a reactive form of arthritis similar to adjuvant disease in rodents (92).

Nontuberculous Mycobacteria

Nontuberculous mycobacteria (NTM) are ubiquitous worldwide and are cultured from human and nonhuman hosts, as well as reservoirs in soil, water, vegetables, and dust (93). The nontuberculous mycobacteria are classified by pigment production. Formerly regarded as harmless saprophytic organisms with low pathogenicity for humans (94), nontuberculous mycobacteria have become opportunistic pathogens in immunocompromised individuals. They produce pulmonary disease resembling typical TB and can infect joints, tendons, bursae, and bones (Table 128.2). Patients with arthritis rarely have active pulmonary disease. Common sites of infection

TABLE 128.2. OSTEOARTICULAR TUBERCULOUS AND NONTUBERCULOUS MYCOBACTERIAL INFECTIONS

Organism	Bone	Joint	Tenosynovium or Soft Tissues	Comments
Mycobacterium tuberculosis	Usual	Uncommon	Rare	Can infect prostheses Can disseminate
M. kansasii	Uncommon	Usual	Usual	Can be multifocal in the immunoincompetent
M. marinum	Very rare	Usual	Most common	Very rare dissemination
M. avium intracellulare	Rare	Uncommon	Uncommon	Dissemination with HIV infection
M. fortuitum; M. chelonei	Uncommon	Usual	Rare	Can infect prostheses
M. haemophilum	Usual	Usual	Rare	Dissemination in the immunoincompetent
M. leprae	Uncommon	Usual	Rare	Erythema nodosum leprosum Swollen hand and forearm

HIV, human immunodeficiency virus.

include the hand (53%), wrist (19%), and knee (18%). Infection of the hip, elbow, ankle, and prepatellar and olecranon bursae, as well as periarticular tissue simulating arthritis, also have been described, and 17% of cases are polyarticular. Several patents with flexor tendonitis at the wrist have had carpal tunnel syndrome. A history of prior trauma or operation has been obtained in about half the patients, and 36% to 58% have had prior intraarticular injection of corticosteroids. About one fourth of patients with nontuberculous mycobacteria infections have an underlying illness such as HIV infection (95) or another form of arthritis, such as degenerative joint disease, RA, or systemic lupus erythematosus. Approximately one half of musculoskeletal infections in patients with HIV infection are due to nontuberculous mycobacteria. The infections are indolent, causing an insidious onset of joint pain and swelling, often with periarticular cystic masses or chronically draining wounds. Constitutional symptoms are present in only 8%, and fewer than 15% of joints are red and warm.

Pathologic changes in nontuberculous mycobacteria infections are indistinguishable from *M. tuberculosis* infections (96). Synovial and osseous tissue cultures for acid-fast bacilli may be positive when synovial fluid cultures are negative. Radiographic changes in nontuberculous mycobacteria infections demonstrate preservation of central joint spaces with sclerotic borders of marginal erosions. Patchy lytic lesions and periosteal new bone formation indicate osteomyelitis (97). In children, skin testing with PPDs prepared from nontuberculous mycobacteria correlates well with culture results. In adults, cross-reactivity between various PPDs can lead to confusion. Microscopic examination of synovial fluid or biopsy material may reveal granuloma and acid-fast bacilli, but definitive diagnosis of the type of infection requires culture. Although data are not as plentiful on atypical infections, it appears that the yield of positive cultures from biopsies and synovial fluid will be similar to that obtained with *M. tuberculosis.*

These organisms are often resistant to the standard antituberculosis drug regimen, and recurrence of infection is common. Selection of therapy for nontuberculous mycobacteria infections should be based on species identified, host immunocompetence, and extent of infection. Interpretation of *in vitro* sensitivity testing of nontuberculous mycobacteria isolates is controversial and may not accurately predict clinical efficacy (98). A combination of four or five drugs and synovectomy may be necessary (99). Generally, surgical debridement or excision is needed for extensive or deep infections, and amputation may be required to control infection. Empiric treatments recommended later must be modified based on both sensitivity tests and the clinical response.

There are more than 50 species of nontuberculous mycobacteria, but only a few of them are important human pathogens (100). The group I photochromogens (produce yellow pigment after exposure to light), *M. kansasii* and *M. marinum,* are the most frequent organisms causing osteoarticular nontuberculous mycobacteria infections (56%), followed by the group III nonphotochromogens (17%) including the *M. avium* and *M. intracellularis* complex (MAC) (101,102). The group II scotochromogens (produce yellow pigment when grown in the dark; 9%; *M. gordonae, M. scrofulaceum, M. szulgae, M. xenopi*) are usually disregarded as contaminants, but sporadic cases of osteomyelitis, bursal, tendon sheath, and prosthesis infections have been reported (103,104). The group IV rapid growers (*M. chelonae* and *M. fortuitum*) cause 11% of nontuberculous mycobacteria osteoarticular infections and are found in water taps. These organisms are from human sources (*M. chelonae*), animals, soil, or water (*M. fortuitum*), and have been recovered from postoperative slow-healing wounds, sinus tracts, and joints.

M. kansasii is found in milk, meat, and water supplies. It can occasionally cause an indolent and often nondestructive arthritis or tenosynovitis in the hand, wrist, knee, ankle, or elbow in healthy individuals. In those with comorbid conditions (transplants, RA, systemic lupus erythematosus, or taking steroids) bone infection and joint destruction are more frequent (105). In immunocompromised patients, pulmonary disease is often interstitial with endobronchitis, and dissemination with multifocal osteoarticular disease may occur (106). Treatment with INH, ethambutol, and rifampin for 18 to 24 months is recommended.

M. marinum causes tuberculosis in fish. Human infection occurs as a superficial nodule, ulcerated skin plaque (swimming-pool granuloma), synovitis, or tenosynovitis in fingers (61%) and hands (14%) or the knee (18%) (107). Predilection for the extremities is thought to be related to cooler body temperature. A history of penetrating trauma during occupational or recreational exposure to salt or fresh water or timber splinters is often present. Delay in diagnosis is common (mean, 5 months), and infections are often misdiagnosed as RA or gout. More than half the patients are initially given intraarticular steroid treatment before diagnosis. Local spread occurs in 20% to 25% of cases, but the infection rarely disseminates (2%). There is a single case report of *M. marinum* as a cause of osteoarticular infection in an immunocompromised patient, associated with severe bone and joint involvement (108). Treatment with rifampin and ethambutol or sulfonamide with trimethoprim is recommended for 3 to 6 months or longer, based on clinical response. Surgical debridement is recommended for joint infection.

Individuals with chronic pulmonary disease or immunosuppression due to corticosteroids are at risk for disseminated MAC infection. MAC also is the most common systemic bacterial infection among HIV-infected patients (109). In HIV-infected patients with very low $CD4^+$ T-cell counts, intermittent MAC bacteremias may infect every organ and tissue including bone, tendon sheath, bursa, and joint, producing a clinical picture with insidious onset and progression (110). Patients develop night sweats, wasting, diarrhea and abdominal pain, hepatosplenomegaly, anemia, and elevated alkaline phosphatase. Bone lesions cause localized pain, focal abnormalities on radiographs, and abnormal bone scans (111). Surgical debridement and multidrug therapy are needed, but are often limited by side effects and drug interactions. MAC strains are resistant to first-line antituberculosis drugs. A multidrug-treatment regimen that includes ethambutol plus rifampin (cannot use rifampin with protease inhibitors) or rifabutin; ciprofloxacin, amikacin or clofazimine, and clarithromycin or azithromycin is recommended for 1 year after cultures become negative in HIV-negative patients and for life in HIV-infected patients.

M. fortuitum, a group IV rapid grower, is found in soil, water, and fish, and can cause pulmonary disease, corneal ulcerations, and infection of bones, joints, and prosthetic joints. It causes joint infection by direct penetration and was reported in an iatrogenic outbreak caused by contaminated needles used for joint injections, as well as in a joint infection after a dog bite (112). *M. fortuitum* is resistant to antituberculous drugs. Treatment requires both surgical debridement and chemotherapy with amikacin and cefoxitin or a combination of two drugs including ofloxacin or ciprofloxacin, doxycycline, sulfamethoxazole, or clarithromycin (113).

M. haemophilum is a slow-growing, fastidious organism requiring low culture temperature and iron-supplemented medium. It is a rare but emerging human pathogen, primarily in immunoincompetent hosts (114). It can cause painful ulcerating cutaneous lesions, bacteremia, and infection of lung, bone, and joints (ankles, knees, and wrists). Skin lesions may masquerade as Kaposi's sarcoma. More than half the patients have osteoarticular sites of infection. The optimal drug regimen is currently uncertain, but resistance to INH and ethambutol has been reported (115).

Leprosy

During the past decade, there have been dramatic changes in the prevalence of leprosy since the introduction of multidrug therapy and widespread BCG immunization of children in endemic areas (BCG immunization induces 50% protective efficacy). The number of patients registered for treatment has decreased from 12 million to 1 million, with approximately 600,000 new cases per year. Of the total disease burden, 81% occurs in five countries: India (57%), Brazil, Indonesia, Myanmar, and Nigeria (116,117). In the U.S., there are about 7,000 patients, with 200 new cases diagnosed annually, mostly in immigrants and in some armadillo handlers (118). Leprosy occurs as a spectrum between lepromatous leprosy (LL), with a high bacillary load and defective cellular immunity, and tuberculoid leprosy (TL), with a small bacillary load and effective cellular immunity. Intermediate between LL and TL are forms of borderline leprosy (BL), borderline LL, and borderline TL. The indolent course of leprosy is punctuated by reactions wherein inflammation develops at sites of infection, often after therapy has started. Joint involvement can be subdivided into several distinct rheumatic syndromes (119,120).

In LL, absence of specific cellular immunity results in a systemic disease with bacteremia and widespread organ infiltration, including a skin infiltration, erythema nodosum leprosum (Lepra type 2), in which inflamed subcutaneous nodules develop in crops. This reaction is a vasculitis or panniculitis and may be accompanied by fever and arthralgias, pitting edema of the hands from the metacarpal joints to the midforearm, or RA-like polyarthritis in proximal interphalangeal joints, metacarpophalangeal joints, wrists, metatarsophalangeal joints, ankles, and knees. The ESR is elevated, anemia common, and rheumatoid factor (RF) tests have been reported positive in 15% to 35% of LL cases, and erosions may be seen in radiographs of the small joints (121). Synovial biopsy reveals an acute inflammatory reaction. In most patients, lepra organisms are not detected in the synovium, and the synovial fluid is a transudate. It has been postulated that this form of arthritis has an immunologic basis.

In TL or BL, a vigorous cellular immunity localizes the bacilli and produces asymmetric macules or skin plaques and involvement of cutaneous nerves. TL may be accompanied by swelling of hands, knees, and ankles, and BL, by a subacute symmetric polyarthritis of the small joints of the hands. RF is positive in only 5% of TL patients. Antinuclear antibodies (ANAs) are usually negative in all patients. True septic arthritis, with purulent synovial fluid containing lepra cells with ingested organisms and high synovial fluid complement values, also may occasionally occur in these patients. Additionally, infection of the nasal mucosa and cartilage may lead to septal collapse and a "saddle nose deformity" (122).

Another type of chronic arthritis with recurrent swelling of large and small joints is independent of the type of leprosy (123). This arthritis begins insidiously months to years after the first symptoms of leprosy and involves the wrists, small joints of the hands and feet, and the knees. It is associated with morning stiffness and erosions on radiographs (124). It responds poorly to nonsteroidal antiinflammatory drugs, but improves with treatment of the underlying disease (125). During LL, hypergammaglobulinemia may be associated with positive autoantibody tests (RF, ANA). It is not known if these are true autoantibodies or represent cross-reactions with components of the lepra organism.

The most common joint deformities in leprosy occur secondary to disease in the peripheral nerves. Neurotrophic changes lead to bone absorption, especially in the distal ends of the metatarsals. Sensory loss and repeated trauma are responsible for degenerative changes and aseptic necrosis of bone. These changes, accompanied by infection in soft tissue and bone, are responsible for loss of terminal digits and severe deformities of the hands and feet. The claw hand that occurs secondary to nerve damage can further compound the disability. True neuropathic joints with complete disorganization of the weight-bearing surfaces and supporting bone also may occur. Charcot joints are most frequently seen at the wrist and ankle. Another form of arthritis occurs secondary to bone disease. Direct infection of bone occurs most commonly in the distal ends of the phalanges. Subchondral bone may collapse and cause destruction of the adjacent joint. In addition to arthritis, a necrotizing vasculitis, the Lucio phenomenon, may manifest as large recurrent ulcerations in the lower legs.

The diagnosis of leprosy rests on demonstration of acid-fast bacilli in skin smears, histologic evidence of lepra organisms, and involvement of peripheral nerves on skin biopsy. From a clinical standpoint, the cardinal sign is anesthesia of the skin. Typically, thermal and tactile senses are lost before the ability to sense pain and pressure. The ulnar and peroneal nerves frequently are involved early. Treatment of leprosy requires a coordinated effort that includes attention to the social needs of the patient as well as specialized drug therapy and physical measures to protect the skin and joints and to reduce contractures. In response to the increasing incidence of primary and secondary dapsone resistance, the World Health Organization now recommends the use of three drugs for 2 to 5 years in patients with multibacillary disease (dapsone, rifampin, and clofazimine, minocycline, or newer fluoroquinolones). Dapsone and rifampin for 6 months are recommended for those with paucibacillary disease. In the U.S., patients with leprosy are entitled to treatment by the U.S. Public Health Service.

FUNGAL DISEASES

Coccidioidomycosis

Coccidioidomycosis is caused by a fungus found in the soil throughout the semiarid areas of southern California, Arizona, New Mexico, western Texas, northern Mexico, Argentina, and other scattered areas in Central and South America (Table 128.3). The fungus multiplies in the soil after the winter rains, resulting in a higher incidence of disease in the summer months. Primary infection occurs 1 to 3 weeks after inhalation of spores; however, most patients are asymptomatic. Some develop self-limited clinical signs that include fever, malaise, cough, or chest pain. Up to 20% of those with primary infection develop erythema nodosum or erythema multiforme lesions that are very painful, last for 1 week, and indicate a strong immune reaction with a good prognosis. In approximately 1% of patients, disseminated disease and/or a progressive pulmonary infection closely resembling TB develops. Dissemination is more common in certain racial groups: Filipinos, African Americans, Latin Americans, and Native Americans. Patients with collagen vascular diseases or lymphomas who are taking corticosteroids or who are pregnant may be at greater risk, and patients HIV infection appear to be more susceptible to severe disease. Increased pathogenicity is related to high antibody titers and circulating immune complexes (126).

Arthritis occurs in both the benign primary illness and the chronic disseminated form. In primary disease, the arthritis is polyarticular and often migratory ("desert rheumatism"). It may be related to circulating immune complexes, is usually associated with erythema nodosum/erythema multiforme, and clears without residual deformity in 2 to 4 weeks (127,128). In 10% to 50% of those with disseminated disease, arthritis may occur alone or secondary to penetration from adjacent bone infection (129,130). The most common presentation is chronic monoarticular arthritis of the knee with low-grade fever. The typical patient is in the mid-30s and otherwise in good health. Male outnumber female patients by 4 to 1. A history of antecedent arthritis or joint injury is rare, and only

TABLE 128.3. OSTEOARTICULAR FUNGAL INFECTIONS

Organism	Bone	Joint	Tenosynovium or Soft Tissues	Comments
Coccidiodomycosis	Occasional; can be multifocal	Usual	Rare	"Desert rheumatism" or "valley fever"; *erythema nodosum*/multiforme; can cause fistulas
Blastomycosis	Usual	Occasional	Uncommon	Soil and decaying matter; skin lesions; occasional fistulization
Cryptococcosis	Usual; often multifocal	Rare	Very rare	Pigeon droppings, dissemination increased by immunosuppression
Histoplasmosis	Rare	Uncommon	Rare	*Erythema nodosum*/multiforme; chicken, starling, bat excrement; African *duboisii* strain has predilection for bone
Sporotrichosis	Occasional	Usual	Usual	Soil, sphagnum moss; ulcerating subcutaneous nodules and lymphatic spread; can fistulate
Candidiasis	Uncommon	Usual	Rare	Can infect prosthesis and follow intra-articular steroid injection or i.v. drug abuse
Actinomycosis	Usual	Usual	Usual	Madura foot, tissue destructive, grains in draining pus

10% of patients have evidence of coccidioidal infection in extraarticular sites. If the organisms seed directly to synovium, symptoms of an indolent synovitis with effusion, stiffness, and mild pain dominate the early course. If infection begins in adjacent bone with later penetration into the joint, the early signs are pain and loss of motion without effusion. In either case, untreated synovial infection gradually progresses to villous hypertrophy and pannus formation, often leading to subchondral bone erosion later in the course. The indolent nature of this process is reflected in the long interval from onset of symptoms to diagnosis, a mean of 4.5 years. Its destructive nature is clear; about 40% of patients show destructive changes and/or adjacent osteomyelitis at diagnosis. The knee is involved in 70% of cases. The wrist and hand (11%) and the ankle (7%) are the next most commonly affected sites.

Infection of bone occurs in 10% to 20% of patients with disseminated disease. Sites most often involved are the ends of the long bones, the skull, vertebrae, and ribs. Approximately 60% of patients have involvement of a single site. Radionucleotide scans may identify lesions not apparent on radiographs. Bone lesions involving more than three sites occur in 20% of patients and are associated with rapid dissemination and a poor prognosis. In the more indolent forms of disseminated disease, solitary bone lesions are common. The course of these solitary lesions is one of slow destruction of bone that may progress to involve adjacent joints.

Most joint infections are diagnosed by culture or histologic examination of synovial tissue, which may reveal noncaseating granulomas with spherules containing endospores. The characteristic spherules found in purulent material are best seen after digestion with 20% potassium hydroxide. *Coccidioides immitis* can be cultured on Sabouraud's agar. Synovial fluid has a moderate leukocytosis with predominance of lymphocytes, elevated protein, and normal glucose. Fewer than 5% of synovial fluid cultures are positive. Although most patients with disseminated coccidioidomycosis are anergic, 80% of those with coccidioidal arthritis have a positive skin test to coccidioidin. Serologic tests are helpful with diagnosis and in monitoring response to treatment. The latex agglutination test or immunodiffusion tests are useful for detecting IgM antibodies in early primary disease. It is positive within 1 to 3 weeks of infection in 80% of cases, reverts to negative after 6 months, but becomes positive again with relapse or reinfection. In disseminated disease, complement fixation titers (IgG) are more than 1:16, and titers more than 1:128 are associated with bone and joint involvement. Ninety percent of patients with coccidioidal arthritis have positive complement fixation tests.

Treatment should include surgical drainage and debridement plus systemic antifungal agents such as itraconazole, fluconazole (131), ketoconazole, or amphotericin B (132, 133). .About 80% of patients with osteoarticular disease have shown a good initial response to ketoconazole, but half relapsed. In severely immunocompromised patients with rapidly progressive disseminated disease, stabilization with amphotericin B followed by fluconazole may be needed.

Blastomycosis

Blastomyces dermatitidis is found in the Ohio and Mississippi River valleys, Middle Atlantic states, the southeastern states with the exception of Florida, and also in southern Africa, Israel, Lebanon, Mexico, and Venezuela. Peak incidence of infection is in the 30- to 60-year age group. The organism exists in the soil, in geographically restricted microfoci associated with decaying organic material (134). Male are affected more often than female subjects, presumably owing to their greater exposure through outdoor activities. Infection begins in the lungs after inhalation of spores and may be asymptomatic or produce an acute self-limited respiratory illness with cough, chest pain, and high fever. In some patients, a chronic cavitary pulmonary infection may develop, and in others, dissemination from the lungs to skin, bone, joints, central nervous system, genitourinary tract, and spleen may occur. Extrapulmonary infection spreads from the lungs by lymphatic or hematogenous routes. Skin and bone are the most frequently involved sites. Skeletal involvement occurs in half of patients, and approximately 5% will present with joint pain. Immunocompromised individuals, especially those with HIV infection, are more susceptible to blastomycosis, and the disease is more aggressive in these individuals (135).

Articular blastomycosis is different from other fungal infections, as it usually occurs as an acute monoarticular synovitis in a patient who is systemically ill with active pulmonary and multifocal extrapulmonary disease. The knee is the most frequently involved joint, followed by the ankle, elbow, wrist, and hand. In approximately 70% of patients, joint infection results from hematogenous seeding to synovium; in 30%, it is a consequence of extension of an underlying osteomyelitis. Osseous blastomycosis is frequently painless and is most common in the vertebrae, ribs, tibia, tarsus, and skull, although involvement of almost every site in bone has been reported. Direct extension into the joint is most often seen at the knee. Spinal infection is associated with destruction of disc spaces, erosion of anterior vertebral bodies, involvement of paraspinal soft tissue, and dissection of the infection beneath the anterior longitudinal ligament. Vertebral infection usually occurs in the thoracic or lumbar areas, but is rare in the cervical spine.

Blastomyces dermatitidis organisms are usually seen on potassium hydroxide–treated smears of synovial fluid, sputum, or material from abscesses. Cytologic analysis may reveal the organisms when routine smears are negative (136). Definitive diagnosis is made on culture. An immunodiffusion test using the A antigen of the yeast phase is reasonably specific (92%), but not very sensitive (77%). Amphotericin B, ketoconazole, and itraconazole all are effective in blastomycotic arthritis, but the low incidence of side effects and high rate of cure make itraconazole the drug of choice for uncomplicated disease. Immunocompromised individuals and patients with HIV infection may require more aggressive therapy with amphotericin B followed by itraconazole. Although the role of operative treatment has not been fully defined, debridement of devitalized bone or synovium may benefit patients who fail to respond to antifungal drugs, and loculated purulent synovial fluid may need surgical drainage (137).

Cryptococcosis

Cryptococcosis is one of the more common systemic fungal infections. The organism is widely distributed in nature. Pigeon droppings appear to be a particularly dangerous source of infection. Predisposing factors for susceptibility to this disease include HIV infection, organ transplantation, corticosteroid treatment, lymphoma, and sarcoidosis. Infection with *Cryptococcus neoformans* begins in the lungs with inhalation of spores and spreads to other organs, especially the central nervous system. Bone infection occurs in about 10% of patients and follows a slowly progressive course. Radiographic changes consist of lytic lesions with sharply scalloped margins and little reaction in adjacent bone or periosteum. These lesions may be found in the metaphyses of long bones, in the flat bones or vertebrae, the ribs, tarsal bones, or carpal bones. Vertebral infection resulting in paraspinal abscess formation can mimic TB. Joint infection is rare, only a few detailed reports of cryptococcal arthritis exist in the literature (138,139). Half involved the knee, and three fourths were monoarticular. About three fourths of these patients were immunosuppressed or had an identifiable underlying illness. The synovial fluid of some patients was grossly purulent, whereas others had a relatively low white blood cell count of about 2,000 cells/mm^3.

Cryptococcal antigens can be detected in sera or synovial fluid by agglutination of latex particles coated with anticryptococcal antibody in a high percentage of cases. RFs can give a false-positive test. Serologic tests for antibody to cryptococcal antigens are not helpful. Amphotericin B given in combination with 5-fluorocytosine is the recommended treatment. Although debridement of joints also may be advisable, the data are insufficient to conclude whether medical or combined medical–surgical treatment is more effective (140). In nonimmunocompromised individuals with limited disease, fluconazole may be a reasonable alternate therapy.

Histoplasmosis

Histoplasmosis is the most prevalent pulmonary fungal infection in humans and animals. *Histoplasma capsulatum* grows in mycelial form in soil with high nitrogen content, where it produces spores that infect humans when inhaled. It thrives in ground contaminated with chicken, bird (especially starlings), or bat excreta. it is endemic in the valleys of the Mississippi, Ohio, St. Lawrence, and Rio Grande rivers, and areas in South America, southern Mexico, Indonesia, the Philippines, Turkey, and Africa. In these areas, up to 60% to 90% of young men have positive skin tests. Pulmonary infection may be acute or chronic in individuals with underlying chronic lung disease. Fortunately, both primary infection and reinfection are usually benign self-limited diseases. Symptoms range from a transient flu-like illness with pneumonitis to more generalized disease characterized by fever, night sweats, malaise, chest pain, dyspnea, and weight loss. In approximately 10% of patients, an acute additive polyarthralgia/polyarthritis may occur with or without erythema nodosum and/or erythema multiforme. The joint involvement clears without residual deformity. Disseminated histoplasmosis may be asymptomatic or acute and progressive, with fulminant disease that is often fatal. Disseminated histoplasmosis occurs in fewer than 0.1% of infections, usually in older or immunocompromised persons (141). Chronic arthritis is an unusual clinical problem occurring as an indolent infection of the knee (both unilateral and bilateral) and as tenosynovitis of the wrist, causing carpal tunnel syndrome.

The diagnosis depends on demonstration of *Histoplasma capsulatum* in histologic sections or culture of involved tissues. Immunologic tests play a minor role in diagnosis. In sensitized persons, the histoplasmin skin test may induce antibodies that will influence serologic tests drawn more than a few days after the skin test. The complement fixation test is quite sensitive, but cross-reactions may occur with other fungal diseases. Most reported cases of histoplasma arthritis have been treated with amphotericin B and surgical debridement. Ketoconazole or itraconazole appear to be reasonable alternatives (142), and in one case, treatment of an infected knee with fluconazole alone was successful (143).

Sporotrichosis

Sporotrichosis is a rare cause of chronic granulomatous arthritis. The organism is a ubiquitous fungus that lives on plants, sphagnum moss, or in the soil. Most reported cases are from the North American continent, but the infection also is endemic in South America, South Africa, and Southeast Asia. Infection with this organism is usually limited to the skin, where it begins as a painful red nodule at the site of a scratch or a thorn prick; however, pulmonary infection may occur through inhalation. Cutaneous sporotrichosis may spread proximally by the lymphatics to form multiple necrotic secondary satellite lesions, or it may penetrate directly into adjacent tissues. Only a small percentage of people exposed to the fungus develop the systemic form of infection.

Two forms of extracutaneous sporotrichosis have been described, unifocal and multifocal (144). Osteoarticular infection is the most common form of unifocal or localized extracutaneous disease. It occurs primarily in men aged 40 years or older who are involved in outdoor occupations or hobbies. It has been associated with alcohol abuse and diseases or drugs that compromise the immune system (145), but most patients have no underlying disease and are not systemically ill. It occurs as a chronic monoarthritis or oligoarthritis. Morning stiffness and fever are absent, but the ESR is usually elevated. A history of transient improvement with intraarticular steroids but poor response to oral steroids or aspirin may be obtained. The knee is most often involved, followed in decreasing frequency by the wrist, small joints of the hand, ankle, and elbow. Tenosynovitis may occur in the hand or wrist. Unifocal systemic sporotrichosis may also present in the lungs as cavitary disease resembling tuberculosis or rarely as an indolent meningitis.

Multifocal or disseminated systemic sporotrichosis typically involves simultaneous infection of the skin, joints, and bones. Many of these patients have a compromised immune system and are systemically ill on presentation (146). Skin lesions after dissemination differ from those in typical cutaneous sporotrichosis. Dusty red nodules up to several centimeters in diameter develop randomly any place on the body except the palms and soles. The lesions eventually ulcerate and may heal while new ones appear. They commonly occur around joints, on the face, and scalp, and usually precede joint symptoms. In this form of the disease, the arthritis is polyarticular in about two thirds of patients. As in the unifocal form, tendonitis may be present, and fistulas may develop after surgical procedures on the joints if proper antifungal therapy is not given. Infection of bones spares the vertebrae, ribs, and jaw, but involves long bones near the joints. Joint infection is rarely related to extension of osseous infection. Pulmonary involvement occurs in fewer than 20% of patients with multifocal disease. It differs from unifocal lung disease in that nodules are smaller and do not cavitate. Central nervous system involvement may also occur.

Diagnosis of sporotrichosis arthritis rests on culture of *Sporothrix schenckii* from joint fluid or synovial tissue because the organism is difficult to see on direct examination of pus or tissue. The percentage of positive tests is higher with cultures of tissue. The best yield occurs with culture of both tissue and fluid. Joint fluid shows the pattern of low-grade inflammation with cell counts of 8,000 to 20,000/mm^3 and decreased glucose concentration. Two serologic tests, a latex slide test and an enzyme-linked immunosorbent assay (ELISA) can be used for diagnosis and to follow treatment. Soft tissue swelling, osteoporosis, decreased joint space, and erosions similar to those occurring in RA may be seen radiographically.

Potassium iodide remains the treatment of choice for cutaneous sporotrichosis because of ease of administration and low cost; however, intolerance of side effects is frequent. Treatment with amphotericin B alone or in combination with surgical debridement of infected joints has been effective (147). Intraarticular amphotericin B also has been used successfully in some cases. Recent evidence indicates that itraconazole is as effective as amphotericin B in nonmeningeal, extrapulmonary disease. Results of treatment of unifocal disease are usually excellent. Oral ketoconazole has given poor results. The main cause of poor results is a long delay between onset of disease and diagnosis. The outcome of multifocal sporotrichosis is less certain.

Candidal Arthritis

Candida species that are pathogenic for humans are also commensal organisms. Since the introduction of antibiotics in the 1940s, there has been a sharp increase in candidal infections. With the introduction of antifungal agents, non-*albicans Candida* species resistant to these drugs are increasing. Nosocomial candidemia most often arises from an endogenous source because of previous colonization. Neutrophils rather than macrophages are the first line of defense against *Candida* organisms; hence, the increased risk for systemic candidiasis in neutropenic patients. In contrast, impaired cellular immunity is associated with a chronic mucocutaneous form of infection. Additional risk factors for candidemia include indwelling catheters, prolonged antibiotic use, parenteral hyperalimentation, extensive burns, major surgery, previous colonization of mucosal sites, i.v. drug abuse, corticosteroids, bone marrow transplantation, cancer chemotherapy, diabetes, and very low birth weight in neonates (148).

In recent case series, *Candida* species were found in approximately 5% of septic arthritis cases in children (149) and they account for less than 1% of septic arthritis cases in adults. Although osteoarticular infections caused by *Candida* species are rare, there appears to be an increasing frequency of these infections, and they are almost always associated with an underlying illness or direct predisposing cause. In adults, several distinct clinical syndromes have been described, including chronic monoarthritis, prosthetic joint infection, and an acute or subacute monoarthritis or polyarthritis (150). An indolent chronic monoarticular arthritis occurs after direct inoculation of *Candida* organisms into the joint. This may occur after repeated joint aspiration or intraarticular injection of corticosteroids. These patients have a mean age of 62 years, are almost always afebrile, and usually have underlying OA or RA. The knee is the most frequently involved joint, and the positive synovial fluid culture is often a surprise.

Fungal infections of joint prostheses are extremely rare (fewer than 30 cases thus far reported); however, the majority have been due to non-*albicans Candida* species (151, 152). Most of these patients have no evidence of disseminated fungal infection and are in their 60s. About half have additional risk factors such as treatment with antibiotics or immunosuppressive drugs. The average interval between surgery and onset of symptoms is 14 months. Pain and limited range of motion are more frequent presenting symptoms in the patients with joint replacement, perhaps because of the frequent association with loosening of the prosthesis. In both of these groups, uncommon species of *Candida* are more likely to be isolated from the joint than is *C. albicans* (153,154).

Candida arthritis may also occur secondary to hematogenous spread. In these cases, endogenous *C. albicans,* originating in the gastrointestinal or genital tracts, is the usual infecting agent. Common exogenous sources are hyperalimentation and i.v. drug abuse. Most of the adults have a serious underlying illness, such as cancer, renal failure, sepsis, or a connective tissue disease. Antibiotics, chemotherapy, immunosuppressive treatment, or indwelling intravenous catheters are frequently involved. The arthritis is monoarticular in 75% and polyarticular in 25% of the cases. The knee is the most common site followed by other large joints, the spine, and bursae. The majority of patients (two thirds) have an acute onset of their arthritis with a painful course. Contaminated heroin also has been noted as a predisposing cause. A distinctive syndrome of follicular and nodular lesions of the scalp, beard, and pubis with ocular infection or multiple osteoarticular lesions of the intervertebral discs, knee, or chondrocostal junctions has been noted in this group of individuals (155). *Candida* arthritis has occurred in fewer than 1% of HIV-infected patients. It usually occurs in those patients with a history of i.v. drug abuse and follows a pattern similar to that in drug abusers who are HIV negative.

Most children with candidal arthritis have been younger than 1 year old. All have had a serious underlying illness, and most were critically ill at the time the arthritis was diagnosed. As in adults, antibiotics, immunosuppression, and catheters were frequently implicated as predisposing causes. Candidal arthritis may occur in as many as 2% of infants receiving hyperalimentation (156,157). Only one case has been reported in association with chronic mucocutaneous candidiasis. Multiple joint infections occur about twice as often in infants as in adults (35% vs. 15%), and coexistent metaphyseal osteomyelitis is more common in infants. Joint infection may follow fungal septicemia by intervals of 2 to 12 weeks. Symptoms include pain, tenderness, synovial thickening, and effusion, but red-hot joints are infrequent.

The synovial fluid contains a mean of 38,000 leukocytes/mm^3 with 80% polymorphonuclear leukocytes, but lower counts may be found in patients with leukemia. Synovial fluid glucose levels have been low in 70% of reported cases. Culture of synovial fluid is a highly reliable method for identifying *Candida* species. A new method to detect fungi more rapidly in blood and body fluid cultures are the BACTEC and BacT/Alert systems, which should be specifically requested when fungal infection is suspected. Gram's stain is not reliable, being negative in 80% of culture-positive samples. Serologic tests for anticandidal antibodies do not clearly differentiate local infection or colonization from systemic disease. Utility of fungal metabolites such as D-arabinitol, enzymes such as enolase, and cell wall components (mannoprotein and mannans) are under study as diagnostic tools. Recognition of the dermal manifestations that occur in about 10% of disseminated candidiasis patients may help in the diagnosis. A variety of lesions have been described including multiple discreet erythematous papules and nodules of varying size, purpuric lesions with pale centers, necrotic eschars, and nodular subcutaneous abscesses. A triad of fever, erythematous papules, and severe, diffuse muscle tenderness also has been reported with disseminated disease. Biopsy of a dermal lesion may provide a definitive diagnosis (158).

The relatively small number of reported cases makes it difficult to draw firm conclusions regarding optimal treatment. Amphotericin B alone has resulted in eradication of the infection in about 60% of cases in which it has been used. The failure rate appears to be less if it is combined with surgical debridement or removal of the prosthesis. The combined use of intraarticular and intravenous amphotericin B has succeeded when intravenous treatment alone has failed. 5-Fluorocytosine should not be used alone, but may be useful as a supplement to amphotericin B (159). Recent reports indicated that fluconazole (400 mg/day) alone can be as effective as amphotericin B and is less toxic (160). Ketoconazole has had varying success (161); more encouraging results have been obtained with fluconazole (162,163). If fluconazole has been used as prophylaxis in a neutropenic patient, the species causing candidiasis is likely to be a relatively resistant *C. krusei* or *C. glabrata.* Unfortunately, the utility of fungal antibiotic sensitivity testing is not yet fully established. In both neutropenic and nonneutropenic patients, the cytokine granulocyte-(macrophage)—colony stimulating factor (GM-CSF) appears to be a useful adjunct for invasive candidiasis.

MYCETOMA (MADURA FOOT)

Mycetoma is a slowly progressive, chronic suppurative infection that is endemic in tropical and semitropical climates of Africa, India, southern Asia, Central and South America, Mexico, western Texas, and parts of California (164). Occasional cases occur in temperate climates such as humid mountain regions of Latin America and in Romania. The largest number of patients with mycetoma live between the Tropic of Cancer and the Tropic of Capricorn. The infection involves skin, subcutaneous tissue, and bone, usually in the hands or feet. It is caused by several species of actinomycetes (actinomycetoma) or true fungi (eumycetoma) that are saprophytes in the soil or on vegetation. In arid regions, most frequent etiologic agents include *Madurella mycetomatis* (most common cause in Africa and India), *Actinomadura madurae, A. pelletieri,* and *Streptomyces somaliensis.* In the occasional case in temperate climates, most frequent etiologic agents include *Pseudallescheria boydii* (most common cause in North America), *Nocardia brasiliensis* (most common cause in Mexico and South America), *M. grisea, M. mycetomatis, A. madurae,* and *N. asteroides* (most common cause in Japan).

Mycetoma develops after soil contamination of a penetrating skin wound; thus, it commonly involves the foot, where it invades subcutaneous tissue, bone, and ligaments (165). The clinical features are rather uniform regardless of the etiologic agent (166,167). The initial site of inoculation develops a small, hard, painless nodule(s) that later ulcerates and drains. Spontaneous fistulation and drainage of pus with granules (sclerotia) is followed by gradual closing of sinus tracts as the deeper infection broadens and deepens, extending along fascial planes, destroying tendons, muscle, and bone. In long-standing cases, the foot becomes swollen and nodular, with multiple sinus tracts producing a characteristic tumefaction of the foot. A similar process may involve the hand. Systemic symptoms and regional lymphadenopathy are uncommon. Histologically, the granules are surrounded by eosinophilic material and a granulomatous tissue reaction with chronic inflammatory cells, epithelioid cells, and multinucleated giant cells. Effective treatment requires accurate identification of the infecting organism, prolonged high-dose administration of the appropriate antimicrobial agent, and surgical debridement. Clues to the specific etiologic agent are found on microscopic examination of the grains, but definitive diagnosis requires culture of the grains on a selective medium. Radiographic changes include periosteal reactions, sclerosis, cortical erosions, and joint destruction. CT scanning is useful to define the extent of the lesion.

Prognosis depends to some extent on the causative organism and is better with actinomycotic than with eumycotic (true fungi) mycetoma. The treatment of choice for actinomycetomas is streptomycin sulfate, 1,000 mg/day i.m., plus amikacin, trimethoprim-sulfamethoxazole, dapsone, rifampin, sulfadoxine, or pyrimethamine if response is slow or poor. Treatment takes months to years and must be continued for as long as it takes for resolution. Treatment of eumycetomas with antifungal agents is problematic because these organisms are resistant to amphotericin B and 5-fluocytosine, requiring long-term administration of ketoconazole or itraconazole (168), or fluconazole for *P. boydii.* Surgical excision of smaller lesions is recommended, and amputation is often necessary (169).

OTHER FORMS OF FUNGAL ARTHRITIS

Actinomyces Arthritis

Actinomycosis is caused by an anaerobic, bacteria-like, obligate parasite, *Actinomyces israelii,* which is a normal resident of the human mouth. Endogenous infection occurs through direct extension from the teeth, particularly after dental procedures or injury to the mouth and jaw. Intraabdominal infection after ingestion of the organism often spreads from the appendix to muscle, bone, or other organs. It also may follow aspiration into an atelectatic portion of the lung. Infection of the spine is usually secondary to abscesses in adjacent tissues and typically involves several vertebrae, but not the intervening discs. Adjacent pedicles, transverse processes, and the heads of contiguous ribs may be eroded. In the vertebrae, channels of infection surrounded by sclerotic bone cause a "honeycomb" or "soap bubble" radiographic appearance. Long, dense, longitudinal spurs and sclerotic changes in the lateral portions of the vertebrae are sometimes seen when infection spreads from the abdomen to the spine by way of the psoas muscle. Dense trabeculae and sclerosis make vertebral collapse uncommon. Any level of the spine may be affected. Symptoms vary from mild local pain to severe restriction of motion, radicular pain, or weakness accompanied by fever, weight loss, and malaise. Extension of the infection into the spinal canal may result in meningitis. Diagnosis is made by identification of sulfur granules on Gram stain of pus from the abscesses and is confirmed by growth of the organism in anaerobic culture. Blood cultures are rarely positive. No serologic test is currently available for actinomycosis. Treatment with tetracycline has been successful, but penicillin is the drug of choice.

In addition to Madura foot, *P. boydii,* a soil and polluted water saprophyte, can rarely cause an indolent monoarticular or oligoarthritis in peripheral joints (knee, foot, wrist, and small joints of the hand and fingers). There are no systemic signs of infection, and there is often an antecedent history of minor trauma (170,171). Treatment is problematic because the organism is resistant to standard antifungal drugs except for miconazole, which is no longer available, and ketoconazole. Synoviectomy and debridement are recommended, and amputation is often necessary. No information regarding treatment with the newer triazoles is available.

Nocardia species are found in the soil of composting vegetation worldwide. Most cases of infection occur in immunocompromised individuals by inhalation. Hematogenous dissemination from the pulmonary infection to the central nervous system, skin, and subcutaneous tissues occurs most commonly. *N. brasiliensis* infection of joints by contiguous spread has occurred with mycetoma. *N. asteroides* is a very rare cause of monoarticular arthritis after hematogenous dissemination, occurring in a few patients treated with corticosteroids or immunosuppressive drugs (172).

PARASITES

Parasitic infections may cause arthritis by direct invasion of the joints or through secondary immune mechanisms. They may also involve periarticular tissues and produce soft tissue rheumatic syndromes (Table 128.4). These mechanisms are

TABLE 128.4. TYPICAL RHEUMATOLOGIC SYNDROMES ASSOCIATED WITH PARASITES

Filariasis
- Chylous effusion of the knee
- Monoarthritis or oligoarthritis of large joints
- Myalgias and back pain

Trichinosis
- Myositis with fever, periorbital edema, and headache
- Eosinophilia

Cysticercosis
- Myalgias, fever, skin and muscle nodules, and eosinophilia

Echinococcosis
- Bone cysts
- Muscle cysts

Dracunculosis
- Monoarthritis with periarticular ulcers in the legs
- Acute arthritis with worm in the joint

Schistosomiasis
- Polyarthritis with myalgias
- Pauciarticular arthritis with sacroiliitis, and enthesopathy
- Acute myeloradiculopathy with low back pain and rapidly progressive weakness and autonomic dysfunction

Giardiasis
- Seronegative arthritis of knees, ankles, and feet with fever, abdominal pain, diarrhea, and headache

not mutually exclusive (173). Joint involvement is relatively rare in these diseases, but a large number of people in developing countries have parasitic infections. For example, 600 million people are estimated to have schistosomiasis or filariasis. Thus even a low incidence of arthritis may result in significant morbidity in these populations.

Filariasis

The lymphatic-dwelling, filarial parasite *Wuchereria bancrofti* is transmitted by mosquitoes and is found in tropic and subtropic areas. The adult worms live in the lymphatics where they first cause reversible and then irreversible damage to lymph flow, resulting in brawny edema and elephantiasis. An acute inflammatory arthritis of the knee may occur, associated with fever and inguinal lymphadenopathy. The initial episode typically lasts only 7 to 10 days, but recurrent, less inflammatory effusions may follow. Later, an insidious mono- or oligoarthritis develops in hip, knee, or ankle with mildly inflammatory and chylous synovial fluid (microfilariae may be observed). There are few, if any, constitutional symptoms. The ESR is often normal, and the serum RF is usually negative. Resolution of the arthritis is seen with treatment of the underlying filariasis.

Infection with the guinea worm *Dracunculus medinensis* can involve the joints by several mechanisms. The adult female worm, which infects millions of people on the Indian subcontinent and in West Africa, migrates into the subcutaneous tissues, usually of the lower leg, ankle, or foot, where it emerges from the base of a cutaneous ulcer to discharge its larvae. A septic arthritis may occur secondary to bacterial infection of periarticular ulcers. In other cases, a mild synovitis occurs in joints adjacent to deep-seated worms. The most dramatic form of arthritis occurs when the worm enters the synovial space and discharges its larvae. An intense inflammation results, probably from the toxic effects of the uterine secretions. The synovial fluid is exudative, and the diagnosis can be confirmed by the finding of the larvae in the fluid. Surgical removal of the worm and irrigation of the joint cavity results in prompt relief of symptoms. Other filaria may cause arthritis through direct invasion of the joint. In both loa loa and onchocerciasis, microfilaria have been found in the synovial fluid of patients with inflammatory arthritis of the knee. Musculoskeletal pain, particularly back pain, is a frequent early symptom of onchocerciasis (174). A symmetric polyarthritis, possibly caused by deposition of immune complexes, also has been described in this disease.

Dirofilaria, a species of animal parasites that includes the dog heartworm, rarely infects humans and does not survive to complete the life cycle in humans. Clinically these infections usually occur as a subcutaneous nodule or solitary pulmonary nodule. An associated self-limited, intermittent, oligoarticular arthritis has been reported. The duration of symptoms can be shortened by surgical removal of the subcutaneous nodule containing the worm (175).

Trichinosis

Trichinella spiralis is a tissue-dwelling round worm that is transmitted directly from host to host by eating contaminated meat. The adult worm causes few if any symptoms in the intestine. In contrast, systemic invasion by the larvae, which occurs about 2 weeks after infection, typically results in myositis, with myalgia, weakness, and muscle swelling associated with fever, periorbital edema, and headache. Muscle enzymes are elevated in the serum, but the ESR is usually normal. Frequent involvement of the extraocular muscles and eosinophilia helps to distinguish trichinosis from polymyositis. A definitive diagnosis can be made with serologic testing or finding eosinophilic myositis and larvae on muscle biopsy.

Schistosomiasis

Schistosomes are blood flukes that parasitize the venous channels of the human host. They are endemic in Africa, Asia, South America, and the Caribbean islands. Infection is usually acquired in childhood. Like other helminths, schistosomes do not multiply in humans. They do, however, produce eggs that release enzymes to facilitate their exit from the body. The immune response to the eggs and their products results in granuloma formtion and subsequent disruption of the function of the tissues in which they form. Two types of arthritis have been described. In the acute phase, a symmetric polyarthralgia/arthritis with myalgias often involves the metacarpophalangeal and metatarsophalangeal joints, the wrists, the knees, and the ankles. It is associated with morning stiffness and gelling. This type of arthritis often begins within days of the onset of systemic symptoms of schistosomiasis, resolves within a month of initiation of treatment for the underlying disease, and might be immune complex mediated, In the chronic phase, a pauciarticular arthritis is associated with enthesopathy, thought to be a form of reactive arthritis. The reactive type usually occurs as low-back, thigh, knee, or heel pain. In one series of 124 patients with joint complaints, radiographs of the sacroiliac joints and heels were each abnormal in 40% of the cases (176). None of the patients had morning stiffness or symptoms in the hands. Tests for RF were negative. In three of 11 biopsies of the knee, ova were identified in the synovium, but the other biopsies showed chronic synovitis with lymphocytic plasma cell infiltrates and no ova or adult worms. Some patients show features of both (177). A little known syndrome of schistosomal myeloradiculopathy occurs with radicular low back pain that rapidly progresses to leg weakness and autonomic dysfunction (178). Diagnosis is made on imaging, demonstrating a filling defect due to expansion of the spinal cord where the eggs were deposited. Cerebrospinal fluid exhibits increased protein, predominantly lymphocytic pleocytosis, and anti-*Schistosoma* antibodies in 85% of cases. Corticosteroids and antischistosomotic drugs exert a favorable effect.

Cestode Infection

Infection with the pork tapeworm *Taenia solium* may cause fever, eosinophilia, and myalgias during the invasive phase. Late in the disease, cysticerci are frequently found in subcutaneous tissue or muscle, where they form painless nodules. Actual joint involvement is extremely rare. In echinococcosis, the embryos are freed from the eggs in the intestine and enter the bloodstream, where they are usually filtered out in the capillary beds of the liver or lung. Occasionally they may lodge in bone, where the formation of the bladder-like cyst results in an enlarging mass that may cause chronic bone pain or spontaneous fracture. The cyst rarely may involve a joint.

Other Helminthic Infections

Reactive arthritis or "parasitic rheumatism" has been described with *Strongyloides stercoralis, Taenia saginata,* and *Toxocara canis* infections. Patients have symmetric polyarthritis, asymmetric oligoarthritis, and also muscle pain and stiffness reminiscent of polymyalgia rheumatica. Most, but not all, have had osinophilia. The ESR is usually elevated, and the RF is usually negative. In all reported cases, the joint symptoms have resolved with treatment of the underlying infection. In most cases, synovial biopsies or synovial fluid analyses have failed to reveal the organism. Immune complexes were found in serum and synovial fluid in two patients, and in one case, immunoglobulin and complement deposits were found in the synovium. These cases may represent a reactive arthritis or immune complex–mediated disease, but in one instance, direct joint infection was documented through the identification of *S. stercoralis* worms in the joints. Joint symptoms resolved after treatment with thiabendazole.

Protozoan Infection

A seronegative reactive-type arthritis involving primarily the knees, ankles, and feet may occur with *Giardia, Amoebae, Trichomonas,* and *Toxoplasma* infections. In some children with *Giardia lamblia,* the arthritis is associated with fever, abdominal pain, diarrhea, and headache, whereas in a few, it is the only symptom. Synovial biopsy does not reveal organisms. More than one course of treatment with metronidazole may be needed to eliminate the parasite and thus alleviate the joint symptoms. *Cryptosporidium* has been associated with a reactive polyarthritis in upper and lower extremities after the self-limited gastroenteritis. An RA-like symmetric polyarthritis has been noted in a few patients with toxoplasmosis.

REFERENCES

1. World Health Organization. *The world health report 1999:* making a difference. Geneva: World Health Organization, 1999:116.
2. Snider GL. Tuberculosis then and now: a personal perspective on the last 50 years. *Ann Intern Med* 1997;126:237–243.
3. O'Brien RJ, Simone PM. Tuberculosis elimination revisited: obstacles, opportunities and a renewed commitment: advisory council for the elimination of tuberculosis. *MMWR* 1999; 48:RR-9.
4. Gasner MR, Maw KL, Feldman GE, et al. The use of legal action in New York city to ensure treatment of tuberculosis. *N Engl J Med* 1999;340:359–366.
5. Wilberschied L. Foreign born tuberculosis cases exceed US-born tuberculosis cases: New York City, *J Urban Health* 1997; 76:143–144.
6. Havlir DV, Barnes PF. Tuberculosis in patients with human immunodeficiency virus infection. *N Engl J Med* 1999;340: 367–373.
7. Pablos-Mendez A, Raviglione MC, Lazlo A, et al. Global surveillance of antituberculosis-drug resistance 1994-1997. *N Engl J Med* 1998;338:1641–1649.
8. Anonymous. Progress toward the elimination of tuberculosis: United States. *MMWR* 1999;48:732–736.
9. Puttick MPE, Stein HB, Chan RMT, et al. Soft tissue tuberculosis: a series of 11 cases. *J Rheumatol* 1995;22:1321–1325.
10. Alvarez S, McCabe WR. Extrapulmonary tuberculosis revisited: a review of experience at Boston city and other hospitals. *Medicine* 1984;63:25–55.
11. Division of TB Elimination, CDC Surveillance Reports. *Reported tuberculosis in the US 1996 and 1997.* Atlanta: Centers for Disease Control and Prevention, 1998.
12. Weissler JC. Tuberculosis: immunopathogenesis and therapy. *Am J Med Sci* 1993;305:52–65.

13. Frieden TR, Fujiwara PI, Washko RM, et al. Tuberculosis in New York City: turning the tide. *N Engl J Med* 1995;333: 229–233.
14. Huebner RE, Castro KG. The changing face of tuberculosis. *Annu Rev Med* 1995;46:47–55.
15. Haas DW, Des Prez RM. *Mycobacterium tuberculosis.* In: Mandell GL, Bennett JE, Dolin R, eds. *Principles and practice of infectious diseases.* 4th ed. New York: Churchill Livingston, 1995:2213–2242.
16. Evanchick CC, Davis DE, Harrington TM. Tuberculosis of peripheral joints: an often missed diagnosis. *J Rheumatol* 1986;13:187–189.
17. Newton P, Sharp J, Barnes KL. Bone and joint tuberculosis in greater Manchester 1969-79. *Ann Rheum Dis* 1982;41:1–6.
18. Chaisson RE, Schecter GF, Theuer LP, et al. Pulmonary tuberculosis in patients with AIDS. *Am Rev Respir Dis* 1987;136: 570–574.
19. Rieder HL, Snider DE, Cauthen GM. Extrapulmonary TB in the US. *Am Rev Respir Dis* 1990;141:347–351.
20. Garrido G, Gomez-Reino JJ, Fernandez-Dapica P, et al. A review of peripheral tuberculous arthritis. *Semin Arthritis Rheum* 1988;18:142–149.
21. Grosskopf I, Ben David A, Charach G, et al. Bone and joint tuberculosis: a 10-year review. *Isr J Med Sci* 1994;30:278–283.
22. Ellis ME, El-Ramahi KM, Al-Dalaan AN. Tuberculosis of peripheral joints: a dilemma in diagnosis. *Tuber Lung Dis* 1993;74:399–404.
23. Vohra R, Kang HS. Tuberculosis of the elbow. *Acta Orthop Scand* 1995;66:57–58.
24. Kutzbach GA. Tuberculous arthritis. In: Spinoza LR, ed. *Infections in the rheumatic diseases.* Orlando: Grune & Stratton, 1988:131–138.
25. Valdazo JP, Perez-Ruiz F, Albarracin A, et al. Tuberculous arthritis: report of a case with multiple joint involvement and periarticular tuberculous abscesses. *J Rheumatol* 1990;17:399–401.
26. Linares LF, Valcarcel A, Mesa Del Castilla J, et al. Tuberculous arthritis with multiple joint involvement. *J Rheumatol* 1991;18: 635–636.
27. ZahraaJ, Johnson D, Lim-Dunham JE, et al. Unusual features of osteoarticular tuberculosis in children. *J Pediatr* 1996;129: 597–602.
28. Ruggieri M, Pavone V, Polizzi A, et al. Tuberculosis of the ankle in childhood: clinica, roentgenographic and computed tomography findings. *Clin Pediatr (Phila)* 1997;36:529–534.
29. Garrido, G, Gomez-Reinao J, Fernandez-Dapacia P, et al. A review of peripheral tuberculous arthritis. *Semin Arthritis Rheum* 1988;18:142–149.
30. Valdazo J, Perez-Ruiz F, Albarracin A, et al. Tuberculous arthritis: report of a case with multiple joint involvement and periarticular tuberculous abscesses. *J Rheumatol* 1990;17:399–401.
31. Muradali D, Gold WL, Vellend H, et al. Multifocal osteoarticular tuberculosis: report of four cases and review of management. *Clin Infect Dis* 1993;17:204–209.
32. Fancourt GJ, Ebden P, Garner P, et al. Bone tuberculosis: results and experience in Leicestershire. *Br J Dis Chest* 1986;80: 265–272.
33. Grosskopf I, Ben David A, Charach G, et al. Bone and joint tuberculosis: a 10 year review. *Isr J Med Sci* 1994;30:278–283.
34. Olive A, Gonzalez-Ustes J, Fuiz J. On tuberculosis of the bones and joints. *J Rheumatol* 1998;25:11.
35. King AD, Griffith J, Rushton A, et al. Tuberculosis of the greater trochanter and the trochanteric bursa. *J Rheumatol* 1998;25:391–393.
36. Kulshrestha A, Misra RN, Agarwal P, et al. Magnetic resonance appearance of tuberculosis of the knee joint with ruptured Baker's cyst. *Australas Radiol* 1995;39:80–83.
37. Tsai YH, Ueng SW, Shih CH. Tuberculosis of the ankle: report of four cases. *Chang-Keng I Hsueh Tsa Chih* 1998;21:481–486.
38. Spinner RJ, Sexton DJ, Goldner RD, et al. Periprosthetic infections due to *Mycobacterium tuberculosis* in patients with no prior history of tuberculosis [Review]. *J Arthroplasty* 1996;11:217–222.
39. Gravallese EM, Weissman BN, Brodsky G, et al. Loosening of a revision total hip replacement in a 60 year old woman with longstanding rheumatoid arthritis. *Arthritis Rheum* 1995;38:1315–1327.
40. Berbari EF, Hanssen AD, Duffy MC, et al. Prosthetic joint infection due to *Mycobacterium tuberculosis: a case series and review of the literature.* Am J Orthop 1998;27:219–227.
41. Chen WS, Eng HL. Tuberculous tenosynovitis of the wrist mimicking de Quervains's disease. *J Rheumatol* 1994;21:763–765.
42. Roverano S, Freyre H, Paira S. Soft tissue tuberculosis in systemic lupus erythematosus: presentation of two cases. *J Clin Rheumatol* 1999;5:107–109.
43. Puttick MPE, Stein HB, Chan RMT, et al. Soft tissue tuberculosis: a series of 11 cases. *J Rheumatol* 1995;22:1321–1325.
44. Cramer K, Swiler JG, Milek MA. Tuberculous tenosynovitis of the wrist: two case reports. *Clin Orthop* 1991;262:137–140.
45. Southwood TR, Hancock EJ, Petty RE, et al. Tuberculous rheumatism (Poncet's disease) in a child. *Arthritis Rheum* 1988; 31:1311–1313.
46. Dall L, Long L. Stanford Poncet's disease: tuberculous rheumatism. *Rev Infect Dis* 1989;11:105–107.
47. Southwood TR, Gaston JS. The molecular basis of Poncet's disease? *Br J Rheumatol* 1990;29:72–74.
48. DeHart DJ. Poncet's disease: case report. *Clin Infect Dis* 1992; 15:560.
49. Mankin H. Weekly clinicopathological exercise. *N Engl J Med* 1996;334:784–790.
50. Peltola H, Mohamed ON, Kataja M, et al. Risk of infection of *M. tuberculosis* among children and mothers in Somalia. *Clin Infect Dis* 1991;18:106–111.
51. Pertuiset E, Beaudreuil J, Liote F, et al. Spinal tuberculosis in adults: a study of 103 cases in a developed country, 1980-1994. *Medicine* 1999;78:309–320.
52. Mitchison DA, Chalmers J. Musculoskeletal tuberculosis. In: Hughes SPF, Fitzgerald RH, eds. *Musculoskeletal infections.* Chicago: Year Book Medical, 1986:186–215.
53. Boachie-Adjei O, Squllante RG. Tuberculosis of the spine. *Orthop Clin North Am* 1996;27:95–103.
54. Rezai AR, Lee M, Cooper PR, et al. Modern management of spinal tuberculosis. *Neurosurgery* 1995;36:87–97.
55. Silverman JF, Larkin EW, Carney M, et al. Fine needle aspiration cytology of tuberculosis of the lumbar vertebrae (Pott's disease). *Acta Cytol* 1986;30:538–542.
56. Mondal A. Cytological diagnosis of vertebral tuberculosis with fine needle aspiration biopsy. *J Bone Joint Surg* 1994;76:181–184.
57. Stanley DJ. Tuberculosis of the spine: imaging features. *AJR Am J Roentgenol* 1995;164:659–664.
58. Kim NH, Lee HM, Suh JS. Magnetic resonance imaging for the diagnosis of tuberculous spondylitis. *Spine* 1994;19:2451–2455.
59. Martini M, Adjrad A, Boudjemaa A. Tuberculous osteomyelitis: a review of 125 cases. *Int Orthop* 1986;10:201–207.
60. Upadhyay SS, Sahi MJ, Sell P, et al. Longitudinal changes in spinal deformity after anterior spinal surgery for tuberculosis of the spine in adults. *Spine* 1994;19:542–549.
61. Louw JA. Spinal tuberculosis with neurological deficit: treatment with anterior vascularised rib grafts, posterior osteotomies, and fusion. *J Bone Joint Surg Br* 1990;72:686–693.
62. Omari B, Robertson JM, Nelson RJ, et al. Pott's disease: a resurgent challenge to the thoracic surgeon. *Chest* 1989;9:145–150.
63. Colmenero JD, Jimenez-Mejias ME, Sanchez-Lora FJ, et al. Pyogenic, tuberculous, and brucellar vertebral osteomyelitis: a

descriptive and comparative study of 219 cases. *Ann Rheum Dis* 1997;56:709–715.
64. Pattisson PRM. Pott's paraplegia: an account of the treatment of 89 consecutive patients. *Paraplegia* 1986;24:77–91.
65. Pouchot J, Vinceneux P, Barge J, et al. Tuberculosis of the sacroiliac joint: clinical features, outcome and evaluation of closed needle biopsy in 11 consecutive cases. *Am J Med* 1988; 84:622–628.
66. Kim NH, Lee HM, Yoo JD, et al. Sacroiliac joint tuberculosis: classification and treatment. *Clin Orthop* 1999;358:215–222.
67. Felson B, Akers PV, Hall GS, et al. Mycotic tuberculous aneurysm of the thoracic aorta. *JAMA* 1977;237:1104–1108.
68. Haygood TM, Williamson SL. Radiographic findings of extremity tuberculosis in childhood: back to the future? *Radiographics* 1994;14:561–570.
69. Buchelt M, Lack W, Kutschera HP, et al. Comparison of tuberculous and pyogenic spondylitis. *Clin Orthop* 1993;296:192–199.
70. Friedland JS. Tuberculosis. In: Armstron D, Cohen J, eds. *Infectious diseases.* London: Mosby, 1999:1–30.
71. Centers for Disease Control, Advisory Council for the Elimination of Tuberculosis (ACET). Tuberculosis elimination revisited: obstacles, opportunities, and a renewed commitment. *MMWR* 1999;48(no.RR-9):1–13.
72. Havlir DV, Barnes PF. Tuberculosis in patients with the human immunodeficiency virus infection. *N Engl J Med* 1999;340: 367–373.
73. Witebsky FG, Conville PS. The laboratory diagnosis of mycobacterial diseases. *Infect Dis Clin North Am* 1993;7:359–376.
74. Miller N, Hernandez SG, Cleary TJ. Evaluation of Gen-Probe amplified *Mycobacterium tuberculosis* direct test and PCR for direct detection of *Mycobacterium tuberculosis* in clinical specimens. *J Clin Microbiol* 1994;32:393–397.
75. Agerton TB, Valway SE, Blinkhorn RJ, et al. Spread of strain W, a highly drug-resistant strain of *Mycobacterium tuberculosis* across the United States. *Clin Infect Dis* 1999;29:85–92.
76. Berk RH, Yazici M, Atabgey N, et al. Detection of *Mycobacterium tuberculosis* in formaldehyde solution fixed paraffin-imbedded tissue by polymerase chain reaction in Pott's disease. *Spine* 1996;21:1991–1995.
77. National Center for HIV, STD and TB Prevention, Division of Tuberculosis Elimination. *Self-study modules on tuberculosis.* www.cdc.gov/phtn/tbmodules/ April 23, 1999.
78. Drugs for tuberculosis. *Med Lett Drugs Ther* 1995:37:67–70.
79. American Thoracic Society. Treatment of tuberculosis and tuberculosis infection in adults and children. *Am J Respir Crit Care Med* 1994;149:1359–1374.
80. Lee AS, Campbell JA, Hoffman EB. Tuberculosis of the knee in children. *J Bone Joint Surg Br* 1995;77:313–318.
81. Negusse W. Bone and joint tuberculosis in childhood in a children's hospital. *Ethiop Med J* 1993;31:51–61.
82. Laforgia R, Murphy JCM, Redfern TR. Low friction arthroplasty for old quiescent infection of the hip. *J Bone Joint Surg Br* 1988;70:373–376.
83. Dankner WM, Waecker NJ, Essey MA, et al. *Mycobacterium bovis* infections in San Diego: a clinicoepidemiologic study of 73 patients and a historical review of a forgotten pathogen. *Medicine* 1993;72:11–37.
84. Wang MN, Chen WM, Lee KS, et al. Tuberculous osteomyelitis in young children. *J Pediatr Orthop* 1999;19:151–155.
85. Lamm DL, Stodgill VD, Stodgdill BJ, et al. Complications of bacillus Calmette-Guérin immunotherapy in 1278 patients with bladder cancer. *J Urol* 1986;135:272–274.
86. Ochsenkuhn T, Weber MM, Caselmann WH. Arthritis after *Mycobacterium bovis* immunotherapy for bladder cancer. *Ann Intern Med* 1990;112:882.
87. Chazerain P, Desplaces N, Mamoudy P, et al. Prosthetic total knee infection with a bacillus Calmette Guérin strain after BCG therapy for bladder cancer. *J Rheumatol* 1993;20:2171–2172.
88. Guerra CE, Betts RF, O'Keefe RJ, et al. *Mycobacterium bovis* osteomyelitis involving a hip arthroplasty after intravesicular bacille Calmette-Guerin for bladder cancer. *Clin Infect Dis* 1998;27:639–640.
89. Aljada IS, Crane JK, Corriere N, et al. *Mycobacterium bovis* BCG causing vertebral osteomyelitis (Pott's disease) following intravesical BCG therapy. *J Clin Microbiol* 1999;37:2106–2108.
90. Xerri B, Chretien Y, Le Parc JM. Reactive polyarthritis induced by intravesical BCG therapy for carcinoma of the bladder. *Eur J Med* 1993;2:503–505.
91. Belmatoug N, Levy-Djebbour S, Appelbom T, et al. Polyarthritis in four patients treated with intravesical bacillus of Calmette-Guérin for bladder carcinoma. *Rev Rhum Engl* 1993;60:130–134.
92. Buchs N, Chevrel G, Miossec Pl. Bacillus Calmette-Guerin induced aseptic arthritis: an experimental model of reactive arthritis [Editorial]. *J Rheumatol* 1998;25:1662–1665.
93. Yangco BG, Espinoza CG, Germain BF. Nontuberculous mycobacterial joint infections. In: Espinoza L, Goldenberg D, Arnett F, et al., eds. *Infections in the rheumatic diseases.* Orlando: Grune & Stratton, 1988:139–157.
94. Woods GL, Washington JA. Mycobacteria other than *Mycobacterium tuberculosis: review of microbiological and clinical aspects.* Rev Infect Dis 1987;9:275–294.
95. Butt AA, Janney A. Arthritis due to *Mycobacterium fortuitum. Scand J Infect Dis* 1998.30:525–527.
96. Travis WD, Travis LB, Robert GD, et al. The histopathologic spectrum in *Mycobacterium marinum* infection. *Arch Pathol Lab Med* 1985;109:1109–1113.
97. Schnadig VJ, Quadri SF, Boyvat F, et al. *Mycobacterium kansasii* osteomyelitis presenting as a solitary lytic lesion of the ulna: fine-needle aspiration finding and morphologic comparison with other mycobacteria. *Diagn Cytopathol* 1998;19:94–97.
98. Iredell J, Whitby M, Blacklock Z. *Mycobacterium marinum* infection: epidemiology and presentation in Queensland 1971-1990. *Med J Aust* 1992;157:596–598.
99. Horsburgh CR. *Mycobacterium avium* complex infection in the acquired immunodeficiency syndrome. *N Engl J Med* 1991;324:1332–1338.
100. Griffith DE. Nontuberculosis mycobacteria. In: Armstrong D, Cohen J, eds. *Infectious diseases.* Vol 10. London: Mosby, 1999: 1–31.
101. Ekerot L, Jacobsson L, Forsgren A. *Mycobacterium marinum* wrist arthritis: local and systemic dissemination caused by concomitant immunosuppressive therapy. *Scand J Infect Dis* 1998. 30:84–87.
102. Blumenthal DR, Zucker JR, Hawkins CC. *Mycobacterium avium* complex induces septic arthritis and osteomyelitis in a patient with the acquired immunodeficiency syndrome [Letters]. *Arthritis Rheum* 1990;33:757–758.
103. Yuen K, Fam AG, Simor A. *Mycobacterium xenopi* arthritis [Review]. *J Rheumatol* 1998;25:1016–1018.
104. Hurr H, Sorg T. *Mycobacterium szulgai* osteomyelitis. *J Infect* 1998;37:191–192.
105. Glickstein S, Nashel DJ. *Mycobacterium kansasii* septic arthritis complicating rheumatic disease. *Semin Arthritis Rheum* 1987; 16:231–235.
106. Sherer Rl, Sable R, Sonnenberg M, et al. Disseminated infection with *Mycobacterium kansasii* in the acquired immunodeficiency syndrome. *Ann Intern Med* 1986;105:710–712.
107. Alloway JA, Evangelisti SM, Sartin JS. *Mycobacterium marinum* arthritis. *Semin Arthritis Rheum* 1995;24:382–390.
108. Barton A, Bernstein RM, Struthers JK, et al. *Mycobacterium marinum* infection causing septic arthritis and osteomyelitis. *Br J Rheumatol* 1997;36:1207–1209.

109. Benson CA, Ellner JJ. *Mycobacterium avium* complex infection and AIDS: advances in theory and practice. *Clin Infect Dis* 1993;17:7–20.
110. Sheppard DC, sullam PM. Primary septic arthritis and osteomyelitis due to *Mycobacterium avium* complex in a patient with AIDS. *Clin Infect Dis* 1997;25:925–926.
111. Mahowald ML, Messner RP. Chronic infective arthritis. In: Schlossberg D, ed. *Orthopedic infection.* New York: Springer-Verlag, 1988:76–91.
112. Ip FK, Chow SP. *Mycobacterium fortuitum* infections of the hand. *J Hand Surg [Br]* 1992;17:675–677.
113. Samuels LE, Sharma S, Morris RJ, et al. *Mycobacterium fortuitum* infection of the sternum: review of the literature and case illustration. *Arch Surg* 1996;131:1344–1346.
114. Hirsch R, Miller SM, Kazi S, et al. Human immunodeficiency virus-associated atypical mycobacterial skeletal infections. *Semin Arthritis Rheum* 1996;25:347–356.
115. Straus WL, Ostroff SM, Hernigan DB, et al. Clinical and epidemiologic characteristics of *Mycobacterium haemophilum,* an emerging pathogen in immunocompromised patients. *Ann Intern Med* 1994;120:118–125.
116. Britton WJ. Leprosy. In: Armstron D, Cohen J, eds. *Infectious diseases.* London: Mosby, 1999:1–16.
117. Barbosa LSG, Scheinberg MA. Articular manifestations of leprosy. In: Espinosa L, Goldenberg D, Arnett F, et al., eds. *Infections in the rheumatic diseases.* Orlando: Grune & Stratton, 1988:159–163.
118. Gelber RH. Leprosy (Hansen's disease). In: Mandell GL, Bennett JE, Dolin R, eds. *Principles and practice of infectious diseases.* New York: Churchill Livingston, 1995:2243–2250.
119. Gibson T, Ahsan Q, Hussein K. Arthritis of leprosy. *Br J Rheumatol* 1994;33:963–966.
120. Pernambuco JC, Cossermelli-Messina W. Rheumatic manifestations of leprosy: clinical aspects. *J Rheumatol* 1993;20:897–899.
121. Chavez-Legaspi M, Gomez-Vazquez A, Garcia-de la Torre I. Study of rheumatoid manifestations and serologic abnormalities in patients with lepromatous leprosy. *J Rheumatol* 1985;12: 738–741.
122. Garcia-de la Torre I. Autoimmune phenomena in leprosy, particularly antinuclear antibodies and rheumatoid factor. *J Rheumatol* 1993;20:900–903.
123. Atkin SL, EL-Ghobarey, Kamel M, et al. Clinical and laboratory studies of arthritis in leprosy. *Br Med J* 1989;298:1423–1425.
124. Carpintero P, Logrono C, Carreto A, et al. Progression of bone lesions in cured leprosy patients. *Acta Leprol* 1998;11:21–24.
125. Terreri MTA, Lutti D, Len C, et al. Leprosy: an unusual cause of arthritis in children. *J Trop Pediatr* 1997;24:184–186.
126. Mitchelll TG. Systemic fungi. In: Armstrong D, Cohen J, eds. *Infectious diseases.* London: Mosby, 1999:1–27.
127. Cuellar ML, Silveira LH, Citera G, et al. Other fungal arthritides. *Rheum Dis Clin North Am* 1993;19:439–455.
128. Kushwaha VP, Shaw BA, Gerardi JA, et al. Musculoskeletal coccidioidomycosis: a review of 25 cases. *Clin Orthop* 1996;332: 190–199.
129. Bayer AS, Guze LB. Fungal arthritis II: coccidioidal synovitis: clinical, diagnostic, therapeutic and prognostic considerations. *Semin Arthritis Rheum* 1979;8:200–211.
130. Lund PJ, Chan KM, Unger EC, et al. Magnetic resonance imaging in coccidioidal arthritis. *Skeletal Radiol* 1996;25:661–665.
131. Sarosi GA, Davies SF. Therapy for fungal infections. *Mayo Clin Proc* 1994;69:1111–1117.
132. Perez-Gomez A, Prieto A, Torresano M, et al. Role of the new azoles in the treatment of fungal osteoarticular infections. *Semin Arthritis Rheum* 1998 27:226–244.
133. Bried JM, Galgiani JN. *Coccidioides immitis* infection in bones and joints. *Clin Orthop* 1985;211:235–243.
134. Klein BS, Vergeront JM, Week RJ, et al. Isolation of *Blastomyces dermatitidis* in soil associated with a large outbreak of blastomycosis in Wisconsin. *N Engl J Med* 1986;314:529–534.
135. Pappas PG, Threlkeld MG, Bedsole GD, et al. Blastomycosis in immunocompromised patients. *Medicine* 1993;72:311–325.
136. George AL, Hays JT, Graham BS. Blastomycosis presenting as monoarticular arthritis: the role of synovial fluid cytology. *Arthritis Rheum* 1985;28:516–521.
137. Abril A, Campbell MD, Cotton VR Jr, et al. Polyarticular blastomycotic arthritis. *J Rheumatol* 1998;25:1019–1021.
138. Ricciardi DD, Sepkowitz DV, Berkowitz LB, et al. Cryptococcal arthritis in a patient with acquired immune deficiency syndrome: case report and review of the literature. *J Rheumatol* 1986;13:455–458.
139. Stead KJ, Klugman KP, Painter ML, et al. Septic arthritis due to *Cryptococcus neoformans. Br J Infect* 1988;17:139–145.
140. Raftopoulos I, Meller JL, Harris V, et al. Cryptococcal rib osteomyelitis in a pediatric patient [Review]. *J Pediatr Surg* 1998;33:771–773.
141. Hansen K, St. Clair EW. Disseminated histoplasmosis in systemic lupus erythematosus: case report and review of the literature. *Semin Arthritis Rheum* 1998;28:193–199.
142. Como JA, Dismukes WE. Oral azole drugs as systemic antifungal therapy. *N Engl J Med* 1994;330:263–272.
143. Darouche RO, Cadle RM, Zenon GJ, et al. Articular histoplasmosis. *J Rheumatol* 1992;19:1991–1993.
144. Rex JH. *Sporothrix schenckii.* In: Mandel GL, Bennett JE, Dolin R, eds. *Principles and practice of infectious diseases.* 4th ed. New York: Churchill Livingston, 1995:2321–2324.
145. Gullberg RM, Quintanilla A, Levin ML, et al. Sporotrichosis: recurrent cutaneous, articular and central nervous system infection in a renal transplant recipient. *Rev Infect Dis* 1987;9:369–375.
146. Lipstein-Kresch E, Isenberg HD, Singer C, et al. Disseminated *Sporothrix schenckii* infection with arthritis in a patient with acquired immune deficiency syndrome. *J Rheumatol* 1985;12: 805–808.
147. Zachiaris J, Crosby LA. Sporotrichal arthritis of the knee. *Am J Knee Surg* 1997;10:171–174.
148. Lipovsky MM, Hoepelman AIM. Opportunistic fungi. In: Armstrong D, Cohen J, eds. *Infectious diseases.* London: Mosby, 1999:1–26.
149. Luhmann JD, Luhmann SJ. Etiology of septic arthritis in children: an update for the 1990s. *Pediatr Emerg Care* 1999;15:40–42.
150. Cuende E, Barbadillo C, E-Mazzucchelli R, et al. Candida arthritis in adult patients who are not intravenous drug addicts. *Semin Arthritis Rheum* 1993;22:224–341.
151. Brooks DH, Pupparo F. Successful salvage of a primary total knee arthroplasty infected with *Candida parapsilosis* [Review]. *J Arthroplasty* 1998;13:707–712.
152. Tunkel AR, Thomas CY, Wispelwey B. Candida prosthetic arthritis. *Am J Med* 1993;94:100–103.
153. Silvera LH, Cuellar ML, Citera G, et al. Candida arthritis. *Rheum Dis Clin North Am* 1993;19:427–437.
154. Weems JJ. *Candida parapsilosis: epidemiology, pathogenicity, clinical manifestations, and antimicrobial susceptibility.* Clin Infect Dis 1992;14:756–766.
155. Dupont B, Drouket E. Cutaneous, ocular, and osteoarticular candidiasis in heroin addicts: new clinical and therapeutic aspects in 38 patients. *J Infect Dis* 1985;152:577–591.
156. Murphy O, Gray J, Wagget J, et al. Candida arthritis complicating long term total parenteral nutrition. *Pediatr Infect Dis J* 1997;16:329.
157. Yousefzadeh DK, Jackson JH. Neonatal and infantile candidal arthritis with or without osteomyelitis: a clinical and radiographic review of 21 cases. *Skeletal Radiol* 1980;5:77–90.

158. Marcus J, Grossman ME, Yunakov MJ, et al. Disseminated candidiasis, candida arthritis and unilateral skin lesions. *J Am Acad Dermatol* 1992;26:295–297.
159. Patel R. Antifungal agents. Part I. Amphotericin B preparations and flucytosine [Review]. *Mayo Clin Proc* 1998;73:1205–1225.
160. Weers-Pothoff G, Havermans JF, Kamphuis J, et al. *Candida tropicalis* arthritis in a patient with acute myeloid leukemia successfully treated with fluconazole: case report and review of the literature. *Infection* 1997;25:109–111.
161. Terrell CL. Anti-fungal agents. Part II. The azoles [Review]. *Mayo Clin Proc* 1999;74:78–100.
162. Flanagan PG, Barnes RA. Hazards of inadequate fluconazole dosage to treat deep-seated or systemic *Candida albicans* infection. *J Infect* 1997;35:295–297.
163. Barson WJ, Marcon MJ. Successful therapy of *Candida albicans* arthritis with a sequential intravenous amphotericin B and oral fluconazole regimen. *Pediatr Infect Dis J* 1996;23:1179–1180.
164. Ten Broeke R, Walenkamp G. The Madura foot: an "innocent foot mycosis." *Acta Orthop Belg* 1998;64:248–248.
165. McGinnis MR. Mycetoma. *Dermatol Clin* 1996:14:97–104.
166. Hazra B, Bandyopadhyay s, Saha SK, et al. A study of mycetoma in eastern India. *J Commun Dis* 1998;30:7–11.
167. Riviti EA, Aoki V. Deep fungal infections in tropical countries. *Clin Dermatol* 1999;17:171–190.
168. Paugam A, Tourte-Schaefer C, Deita A, et al. Clinical cure of fungal madura foot with oral itraconazole. *Cutis* 1997;60:191–193.
169. Richardson MD. Subcutaneous mycoses. In: Armstrong D, Cohen J, eds. *Infectious diseases.* London: Mosby, 1999:1–28.
170. Dinulos JG, Darmstadt GL, Wilson CB, et al. *Nocardia asteroides* septic arthritis in a healthy child. *Pediatr Infect Dis J* 1999;18:308–310.
171. Dellestable F, Kures K, Mainard D, et al. Fungal arthritis due to *Pseudallescheria boydii* (*Scedosporium apiospermum*). *J Rheumatol* 1994;21:766–768.
172. Ostrum RF. Nocardia septic arthritis of the hip with associated avascular necrosis. *Clin Orthop* 1993;288:282–286.
173. Bocanegra TS, Vasey FB. Musculosleletal syndromes in parasitic diseases. *Rheum Dis Clin North Am* 1993;19:505–513.
174. Nwoke BEB. Musculoskeletal pain in onchocerciasis. *Angew Parasitol* 1992;33:133–138.
175. Corman LC. Acute arthritis occurring in association with subcutaneous *Dirofilaria tenuis* infection. *Arthritis Rheum* 1987; 30:1431–1434.
176. Bassiouni M, Kamel M. Bilharzial arthropathy. *Ann Rheum Dis* 1984;43:806–809.
177. Atkin SL, Kamel M, el-Hady AM, et al. Schistosomiasis and inflammatory polyarthritis: a clinical, radiological, and laboratory study of 96 patients infected by *S. mansoni* with particular reference to the diarthrodial joint. *Q J Med* 1986;59: 479–487.
178. Ferrari TC. Spinal cord schistosomiasis: a report of 2 cases and review emphasizing clinical aspects. *Medicine* 1999;78:176–190.

129

LYME DISEASE

STEPHEN E. MALAWISTA

Lyme disease is a tick-borne inflammatory disorder caused by a spirochete, *Borrelia burgdorferi.* Its clinical hallmark is an early expanding skin lesion, *erythema migrans* (EM), which may be followed weeks to months later by neurologic, cardiac, or joint abnormalities. Symptoms may refer to any one of these four systems alone or in combination. Other organ systems rarely may be affected. All stages of Lyme disease may respond to antibiotics, but treatment of early disease is the most successful. Endemic foci of Lyme disease are widely distributed throughout the United States and Europe.

HISTORICAL OVERVIEW

"Lyme arthritis" was recognized in November 1975 because of an unusual geographic cluster of children with inflammatory arthropathy in the region of Lyme, Connecticut (1). Its early elucidation—natural history (1–6), immunopathogenesis (7–11), epidemiology (12–15), pathology (2,4,11), and therapy (16–19)—was carried out primarily at Yale University by Steere, Malawista, and their colleagues. It soon became clear that this was a multisystem disorder (*Lyme disease*) (2–6) occurring at any age, in both sexes, and often preceded by a characteristic expanding skin lesion, *erythema chronicum migrans* (20), a term now shortened by convention to EM. In Europe, EM had been associated with the bite of the sheep tick, *Ixodes ricinus* (21), and with tick-borne meningopolyneuritis (22,23); these syndromes are now subsumed under the names Lyme disease or *Lyme borreliosis.* In the Lyme region, a closely related deer tick, *Ixodes scapularis* (a member of the so-called *I. ricinus* complex; also called for a time, *I. dammini*), was implicated as the principal disease vector on epidemiologic grounds (12–15).

In 1982, Burgdorfer et al. (24) isolated the spirochete that bears his name from *Ixodes scapularis* ticks collected on Shelter Island, New York, and linked it serologically to patients with Lyme disease. Within months, this organism had been cultured from blood, skin, and cerebrospinal fluid (CSF) of patients, and specific immunoglobulin M (IgM) and IgG antibody responses had been delineated (25,26). Because it is infectious in origin but inflammatory in expression, Lyme disease, beyond its intrinsic interest as a new nosologic entity, presents a unique well-characterized human model for an infectious etiology of rheumatic disease (27). During 25 years of study, much has been learned about the etiology, pathogenesis, clinical spectrum, and treatment of Lyme disease, but many questions remain unanswered, particularly related to the pathogenesis of chronically persistent symptoms experienced by some patients.

CAUSATIVE AGENT: *BORRELIA BURGDORFERI*

Of the three spirochetes pathogenic for humans, Treponemes, Leptospires, and Borrelia, the etiologic agent for Lyme disease has been classified as Borrelia based on immunochemical and molecular criteria. *B. burgdorferi* (Fig. 129.1) is 10 to 30 μm long and 0.2 to 0.25 μm wide and, unlike *T. pallidum,* can be cultivated in artificial media (28). Its generation time *in vitro* is on the order of 12 to 20 hours. It resembles other *Borrelia* in that it has an outer membrane with three layers that surrounds a periplasmic space that contains a variable number of endoflagella and a protoplasmic cylinder (28). *B. burgdorferi* has a linear chromosome and both linear and circular plasmids. Its entire genomic sequence has been determined (29). Immunodominant, species-specific, outer-surface lipoproteins are encoded in plasmids and are immunologically variable; recombinant forms of one of them, outer-surface protein A (OspA), have been successful as vaccines (30,31). Non–species-specific antigens of importance are flagellin (41 kd) and a heat-shock protein (60 kd).

Three different genospecies have been described: *B. burgdorferi sensu stricto, B. garinii,* and group VS461 (32); the last is now called *B. afzelii.* At least seven serotypes have been described based on expression of different serologically defined epitopes of OspA (33). North American isolates have been relatively homogeneous antigenically; European isolates have shown much greater variability, particularly of OspA and OspB (34,35). It has been speculated that differences in the clinical manifestations of European and North American Lyme disease may reflect variation in the organotropism and

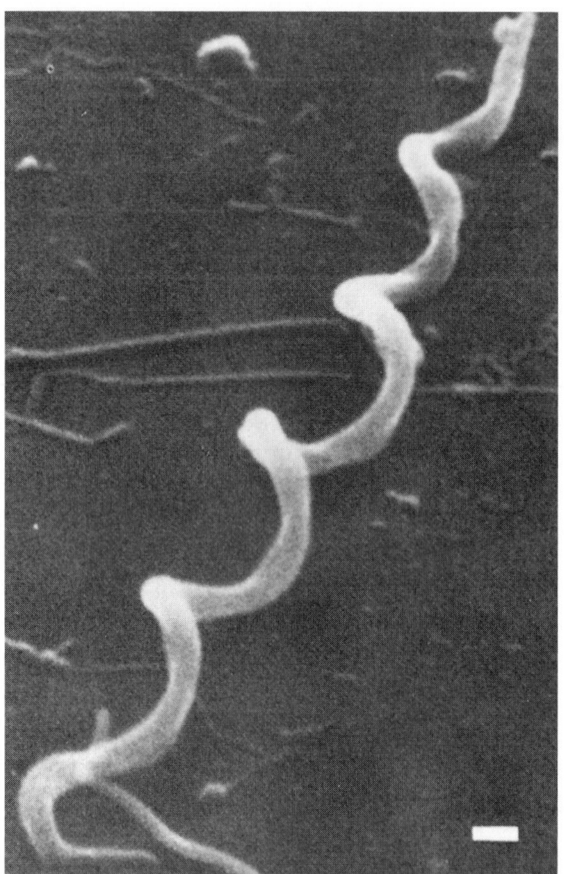

FIGURE 129.1. Scanning electron micrograph of *Borrelia burgdorferi* isolated from the spinal fluid of a patient with meningoencephalitis (25) whose Lyme disease had begun 2 1/2 months earlier with erythema chronicum migrans. Bar, 0.5 μm. (Reproduced from Johnson RC, Hyde FW, Rumpel CM. Taxonomy of the Lyme disease spirochetes. *Yale J Biol Med* 1984;57; 529–527, with permission.)

virulence of different strains of *B. burgdorferi.* In particular, *B. afzelii* seems to be the primary genospecies that causes the chronic skin lesion *acrodermatitis chronica atrophicans,* whereas the other species have a greater tendency for dissemination (36,37). The molecular bases for these differences in pathogenic potential are yet to be elucidated.

PATHOGENESIS

Lyme disease behaves like a rheumatic disorder (27) because the generally rather unaggressive causative organism, *B. burgdorferi,* is both powerful antigenically and apparently able periodically to gain access to immunologically privileged sites (i.e., to hide in tissue). Initially, disease develops after inoculation of skin with *B. burgdorferi* from an infected tick, leading to the herald skin lesion, EM. In addition to EM, *B. burgdorferi* causes another early skin lesion, benign lymphocytoma (38), and a late one, *acrodermatitis chronica atrophicans* (38–40), both of which are seen primarily in Europe.

Recovery of *B. burgdorferi* is straightforward from infected ticks but difficult from patients, except from EM lesions (39,41), where the clinical diagnosis is usually obvious, in part because of the relative paucity of organisms in human specimens. Nevertheless, rare positive cultures are reported at all stages of the illness, from blood (early) (25,26,42,43), secondary annular lesions (39), meningitic CSF (25), joint fluid (44), iris (45), ligamentous tissue (46), and even from an *acrodermatitis chronica atrophicans* that had been present for more than 10 years (39). Spirochetes have been identified by silver stain or by immunofluorescence in some histologic sections of EM (47), usually peripherally, and rarely of secondary annular lesions (48), synovium (49), brain (50), eye (51), heart (50,52), spleen (53), liver (54), kidney, bone marrow (55), skeletal muscle (56), and ligamentous tissue (45).

From these data, combined with the known clinical and epidemiologic features of Lyme disease (see later), the following pathogenetic sequence is likely. *B. burgdorferi* is transmitted to the skin of the host by the tick vector, but generally only after at least 48 hours of engorgement (57,58). Within 3 to 32 days (6), EM appears, and replicating organisms that survive the inflammatory response migrate outward in the skin, spread in lymph (regional adenopathy), and disseminate in blood to secondary skin sites (secondary annular lesions) and other organs [e.g., central nervous system (CNS), liver, spleen, eye, skeletal muscle, and heart]. Maternal–fetal transmission (55,59,60) is distinctly uncommon.

In the clinical laboratory, characteristic immune abnormalities are found. At disease onset (EM), almost all patients have evidence of circulating immune complexes (9,10). At that time, the findings of elevated serum IgM levels and cryoglobulins containing IgM predict, in untreated patients, subsequent nervous system, heart, or joint involvement (7,8) (i.e., early humoral findings have prognostic significance). These abnormalities tend to persist during neurologic or cardiac involvement. Later in the illness, when arthritis is present, serum IgM levels are more often normal. By then, immune complexes are usually lacking in serum but are present uniformly in joint fluid (10), where their titers correlate positively with the local concentration of polymorphonuclear leukocytes (61). Mononuclear cells from blood exhibit an antigen-specific proliferative response during infection, but the greatest reactivity to antigen is seen in cells from inflamed joints. Adjacent to that joint fluid, on biopsy, a proliferative synovium is seen, often replete with lymphocytes and plasma cells that are presumably capable of producing immunoglobulin locally (2). Thus an initially disseminated, immune-mediated inflammatory disorder becomes localized and propagated in joints in some patients. Similarly, local production of antibody in the CSF is a hallmark of CNS involvement (62,63).

Although *B. burgdorferi* seems not to destroy tissue directly, histologically one sees an amplified, nonspecific immune-cell component—macrophages, neutrophils, and natural killer cells—as well as infiltration of tissues with specific immune cells—B and T lymphocytes—often associated with vasculopathic changes. The spirochetes appear to activate complement (64) and contain lipopolysaccharide-like molecules that nonspecifically activate monocytes, macrophages, synovial lining cells, and B cells (65,66). Spirochetes interact with both neutrophils and macrophages *in vitro,* and macrophages ingest them by both Fc-dependent and -independent mechanisms (67–70). The induction of proinflammatory cytokines [especially interleukin-1 (IL-1), tumor necrosis factor-α (TNFα), and IL-6], by activation of these cells, no doubt serves to amplify the immune/inflammatory response (71). Lipidated outer-surface proteins (Osps) are themselves potent stimulators of cytokine production and can cause localized inflammation *in vivo* (72–74). Such cytokines also activate endothelial cells, inducing the expression of adhesion molecules including E-selectin, vascular cell adhesion molecule-1 (VCAM-1), and intercellular adhesion molecule-1 (ICAM-1), facilitating the egress of innate immune cells to sites of inflammation (75). The spirochetes also upregulate cytokines from endothelial (76–78), glial (71), and synovial cells (79). They adhere to plasminogen (80), to several extracellular matrix proteins (81–83), and to epithelial as well as to endothelial cells. They penetrate endothelial monolayers primarily by passing through intracellular junctions (84–86), and the induction of cytokines may help them bridge the blood–brain barrier. They can bind neural glycolipid; they adhere to galactocerebroside, a sphingolipid located on the surface of myelin-producing cells in the CNS and peripheral nervous system (87) with associated inflammatory damage (85). They can induce the production of cross-reactive antibodies and of specific immune B and T lymphocytes that may be associated histologically with endarteritic microvascular occlusive changes (e.g., in nervous tissue, hearts, joints), but it is not clear that these phenomena persist in the absence of live spirochetes (85,88,89). Synoviocytes cultured from a patient with Lyme disease spontaneously secreted collagenase and prostaglandin E_2, both of which may contribute to joint injury (11).

Chronic manifestations of Lyme disease are limited largely to the nervous system (3,62,63,90–92), joints (4,93,94), and skin (39). Although organisms are hard to find in later stages of this disorder, it is entirely possible that persistent live spirochetes or their undegraded antigens are driving the illness throughout its course. Evidence for this interpretation includes the responsiveness of most patients to antibiotics, the rare sightings of spirochetes in affected tissues, the variable recovery from affected tissues and fluids of spirochetal DNA amplified by the polymerase chain reaction (PCR; see later), and an expansion of the antibody response to additional spirochetal antigens over time (95). If live spirochetes are invariably present, it is not yet clear how they occasionally remain out of harm's way in the face of both antibiotic therapy and the body's usual phagocytic and other immune clearance mechanisms. *B. burgdorferi* may express different surface antigens *in vivo* than in culture (96–98). However, unlike *B. hermsii* in relapsing fever (99), it is not clear that *B. burgdorferi* stays ahead of the immune response by spontaneous expression of alternative forms of a variable major Osp and downregulation of others throughout the course of infection (100,101). Other possible mechanisms of evasion include becoming invisible to the immune system by stripping itself of exposed foreign antigen or by coating itself with host protein [indeed, IgM appears to bind nonspecifically to *B. burgdorferi* (102)] and persistence inside cells. In regard to this last possibility, there is evidence that *B. burgdorferi* can survive in association with macrophages, fibroblasts, and endothelial and synovial cells (68,84,103–105), but the situation *in vivo* requires further study.

Antibodies to the spirochete that cross-react with host tissue may serve to amplify the immune response (106–108). Two candidates for such activity are the 41-kd spirochetal protein flagellin and a heat-shock protein. IgM antibodies from patients with neurologic Lyme disease bind to normal human axons. A monoclonal antibody binds to human myelinated fibers of peripheral and CNS tissue, to synovial cells, and to cardiac muscle (106). Other antibodies to self protein that may be found in patients with Lyme disease are directed against myelin and myelin basic protein, cardiolipin, and IgG (as rheumatoid factor). Patients with Lyme radiculomyelitis have yielded autoimmune T cells that are stimulated by myelin, myelin basic protein, cardiolipin, and galactocerebroside (107), and T cells reactive with *B. burgdorferi*–specific heat-shock proteins have been identified (108). Persistent arthritis is often associated with human leukocyte antigen (HLA)-DR4 or with antibody reactive with OspA (109), and OspA was preferentially recognized by T cells from patients with treatment-resistant Lyme arthritis (110). Indeed, it is proposed but not proven that Lyme arthritis may persist by an autoimmune mechanism, triggered by OspA, after the spirochete is gone (111). However, even chronic Lyme arthritis generally resolves within 4 years (112), and it remains to be seen whether any putatively autoimmune phenomena persist when the last spirochetes have been killed and their antigens degraded (89).

EPIDEMIOLOGY

Lyme disease is widespread in temperate climates of the northern hemisphere in the U.S. and across Europe and Asia (113–116). Although it has been reported in 48 of the United States, there are three distinct foci (14): the Northeast from southern Maine to Maryland, the upper Midwest, and the West in northern California. Of more than 10,000 new cases currently being reported each year, more than 90% come from only eight states: Connecticut, Maryland, Massachusetts, New Jersey, New York, Pennsylvania, Minnesota, and Wisconsin (116). It has been estimated that the ratio of unreported to reported cases may be as high as 5:1.

Lyme disease accounts for more than 95% of U.S. vector-borne infectious diseases. The primary vectors are tiny, hard-bodied ticks of the *Ixodes ricinus* complex: major foci of disease correspond to the distribution of *I. scapularis* (Northeast and Midwest United States) (14,113), *I. pacificus* (West) (14,117), *I. ricinus* (Europe and Western Soviet Union) (113,114), and *I. persulcatus* (Soviet Union, China, and Japan) (115). [*I. scapularis* in the Northeast United States had been thought to be a separate species, *I. dammini,* but is now considered conspecific with *I. scapularis,* its current designation (118)]. Other ticks, including the lone star tick, *Amblyomma americanum,* may be vectors in some areas of the U.S. (119,120). Biting insects are possible secondary vectors, but laboratory evidence supporting their ability to transmit *B. burgdorferi* is lacking (121,122).

In one early U.S. study, only 31% of 314 patients recalled a tick bite at the skin site where EM developed days to weeks later; thus most patients were unaware of having been bitten (6). In that study, the six ticks that were saved were all nymphal *I. scapularis,* whose peak questing period is May through July, and which is now known to be the stage primarily responsible for transmission of the infecting organism to humans. This tick has a life cycle (larva, nymph, and adult) spanning 2 years. Both the larval and nymphal stages feed preferentially on a variety of small mammals, especially the white-footed mouse (*Peromyscus leucopus*), which appears to be the most important reservoir of *B. burgdorferi* (13,123,124). Infected nymphs transmit spirochetes to mice from which previously uninfected larval ticks subsequently acquire infection (Fig. 129.2). Adult ticks feed primarily on larger mammals, especially white-tailed deer. In areas in which

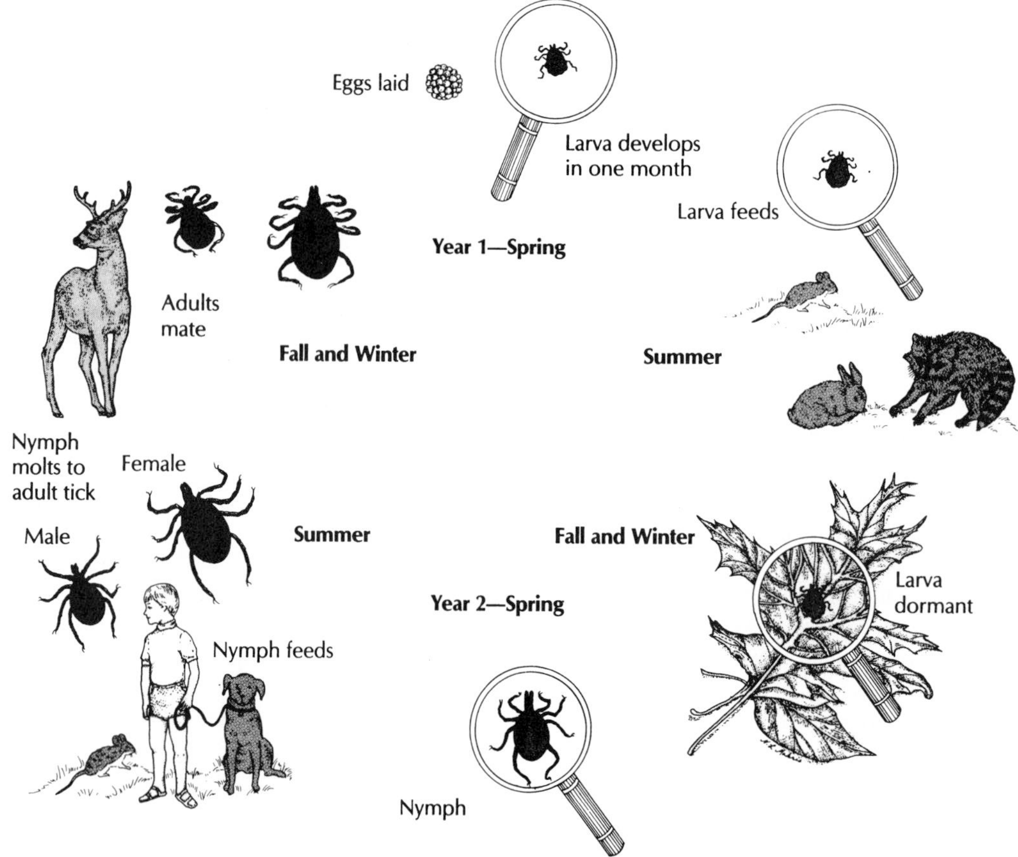

FIGURE 129.2. Life cycle of *Ixodes scapularis* spans 2 years. In the spring of the first year (**top**), eggs hatch, and six-legged larvae develop. In the summer, the larvae feed once. From their preferred host, the white-footed mouse, they acquire *Borrelia burgdorferi,* the spirochete that causes Lyme disease. Next spring (**bottom**), the larvae molt into eight-legged nymphs, which feed once. Again, mice are the preferred host; humans to whom the ticks transmit Lyme disease are not necessary for maintenance of the ticks' life cycle. The nymphs molt into adult male and female ticks. Mating often occurs while the female is feeding on deer. The male might remain on the deer; the female drops off and subsequently lays her eggs. This figure is based on research by Andrew Spielman and colleagues. (Reproduced from Rahn DW, Malawista SE. Clinical judgement in Lyme disease. *Hosp Pract* 1990;25:39–56, with permission.)

Lyme disease is endemic, the prevalence of *B. burgdorferi* in nymphal *I. scapularis* ranges from about 20% to more than 60% (116). This can be compared with an infection rate of 1% to 2% in *I. pacificus,* which feed preferentially on lizards that are incompetent reservoirs of *B. burgdorferi* and thus act as zooprophylactic hosts (117). A complex, two-tick enzootic cycle has been elucidated to explain how *B. burgdorferi* is maintained in nature in California (125). An epidemiologically silent focus involving *Neotoma mexicana* (a wood rat) and *Ixodes spinipalpis* has been described in northern Colorado (126).

B. burgdorferi has been isolated, or specific antibody found, in blood and tissues of a wide variety of large and small animals, including domestic dogs, which can develop arthritis, and birds, which provide a natural means of distributing infected and uninfected ticks to new locales (127–131). Indiscriminate feeding on a variety of animals by infected immature *I. scapularis* may favor the spread of infection.

The earliest known cases in the U.S. occurred on Cape Cod in 1962 and in Lyme, Connecticut, in 1965 (14), but studies using PCR have indicated the presence of *B. burgdorferi* DNA in museum specimens of ticks from the region of Montauk, Long Island, New York, as early as the 1940s (132) and in ear specimens from two mice collected on Cape Cod, Massachusetts, in 1894 (133). The increasing incidence of Lyme disease in the U.S. in recent decades may be explained by multiple factors, including an increase in the number of ixodid ticks, the outward migration of residential areas into previously rural woodlands (habitats favored by ixodid ticks and their hosts), an exploding deer population, and increased recognition.

Disease can occur at any age and in either sex, but the highest incidence is generally in children younger than 15 years and in middle-aged adults, probably because of activities that place these groups at higher risk for contacting an infected tick vector (15). Onset of illness is generally between May 1 and November 30 in temperate climates, with the peak in June and July (6). Limited studies have shown a significant prevalence of asymptomatic seropositivity in high-risk populations (134).

A variety of public health approaches have been proposed to control the spread of Lyme disease. The most important measure is education of individuals at risk of exposure to infected ticks. Prompt removal of (even embedded) ticks suffices to prevent infection in the vast majority of exposed individuals (135). Eliminating deer, which are important as hosts for adult *I. scapularis* ticks, can reduce the total tick population, but is impractical in all but special closed environments such as islands. Permethrin-impregnated cotton balls distributed in the nesting environment of mice have been shown to reduce the rate of tick infestation in the mouse population, which in turn can reduce the risk of human exposure. This approach has obvious practical limitations, not the least of which is the expense of treating all but very small environments such as one's own yard (136).

CLINICAL CHARACTERISTICS

Lyme disease can present itself at different clinical stages: early, localized, cutaneous involvement (EM); or early disseminated disease characterized by multiple secondary skin lesions, headache, and musculoskeletal, flu-like symptoms (stage 1); a period weeks to months later during which cardiac or acute neurologic manifestations may occur (stage 2); and, weeks to a year or two after EM, intermittent attacks of frank arthritis that may sometimes become chronic (i.e., last >1 year), or CNS involvement (stage 3). Chronic skin involvement also may occur years after onset (acrodermatitis chronica atrophicans), predominantly in Europe. This staging system is convenient but somewhat overcategoric, as stages may overlap or be skipped entirely; seroconversion can occur without any symptoms at all having been recognized (119,137). As a guide to clinical decision making, it is most useful to characterize patients as having early localized (EM), acute disseminated with or without neurologic involvement, or chronic disease.

Early Manifestations

EM, the clinical hallmark of early Lyme disease, begins as a red macule or papule at the site of a tick bite (2,6). Only a minority of affected individuals are aware of having been bitten. After an incubation period of a few days to a month, the area of redness expands to a mean diameter of 15 cm or more (range, 3–68 cm), usually with partial central clearing (Fig. 129.3). (Five centimeters is the minimal defining diameter required in surveillance studies by the Centers for Disease Control.) The outer border is red, generally flat, and without scale. The center is occasionally indurated, vesicular, or necrotic. Variations may occur—multiple rings, for example. The thigh, groin, and axilla are particularly common sites. The lesion is warm to touch and minimally tender, although cutaneous hypersensitivity is common. Lesions are easily missed if out of sight, so a careful skin examination is essential when Lyme disease is suspected clinically. Its actual incidence in a study of children with Lyme disease was 90% (138), although the absence of EM might have made the diagnosis less easily appreciated. Routine histology is nonspecific: a heavy dermal infiltrate of mononuclear cells, without epidermal change except at the site of the tick bite. *B. burgdorferi* can usually be isolated by culture of EM lesions in BSK medium (139).

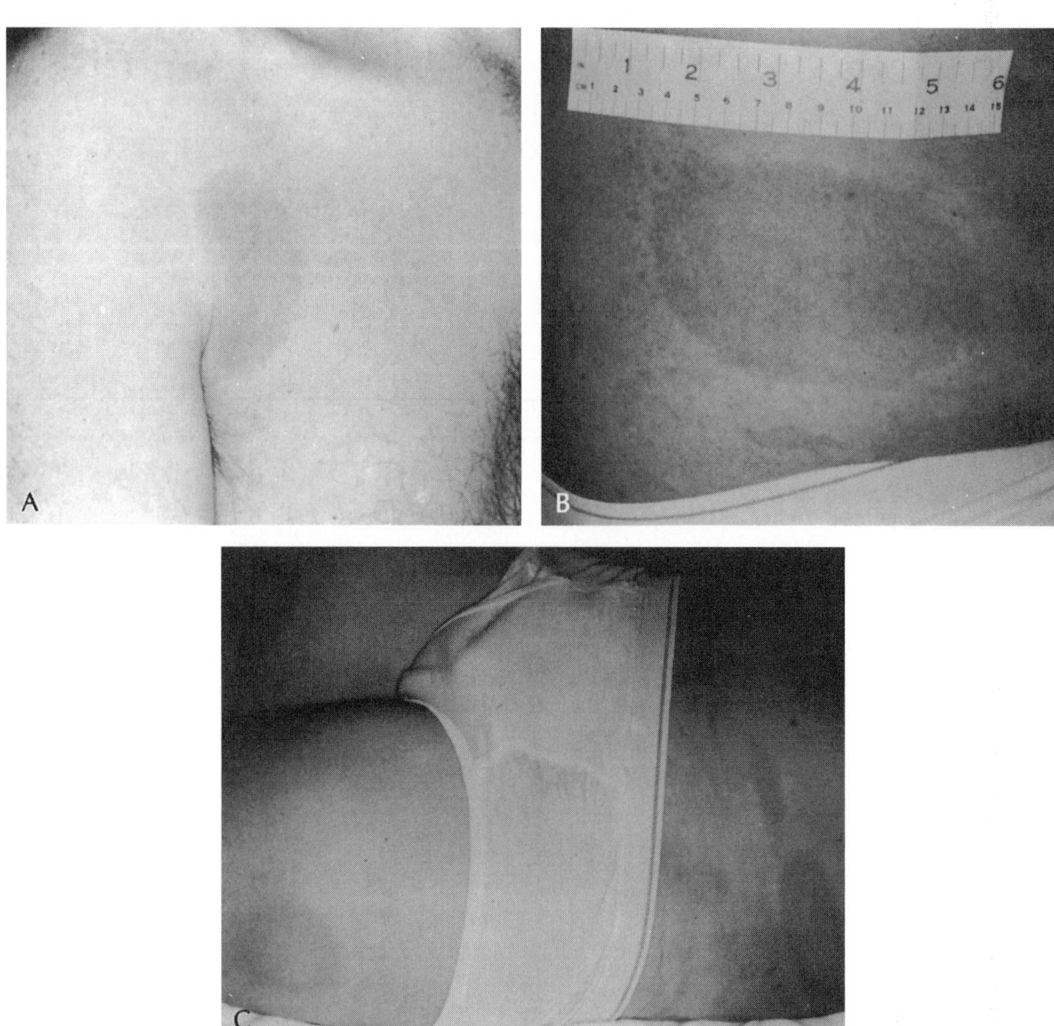

FIGURE 129.3. Dermatologic manifestations of Lyme disease. **A:** Erythema migrans *(EM).* An early lesion is seen 4 days after detection. **B:** In a 10-day lesion of EM, the red outer ring has expanded, and central clearing is beginning. **C:** Eight days after onset of EM, similar secondary lesions have appeared, and several of their borders have merged. (Reproduced from Steere AC, Bartenhagen NH, Craft JE, et al. The early clinical manifestations of Lyme disease. *Ann Intern Med* 1983;99:76–82, with permission.)

In an early prospective study (6), within days of onset of EM, almost half of U.S. patients developed multiple annular secondary lesions signaling early dissemination of the spirochete (Fig. 129.3; Table 129.1); *B. burgdorferi* have been cultured from these lesions (39). The percentage of such patients is less in recent years—23% in a large study of children (138)—perhaps in part because of early antibiotic therapy. Secondary lesions resemble primary ones, but are generally smaller, expand less, and lack indurated centers. Individual lesions may come and go, and their borders sometimes merge. Additionally, benign lymphocytoma cutis has been reported in Europe (39). EM and secondary lesions fade even without treatment in 3 to 4 weeks (range, 1 day–14 months), although spirochetes are still present locally in untreated patients (140). EM may recur.

EM is often accompanied by acute, flu-like symptoms: malaise and fatigue, headache, fever and chills, myalgias, and arthralgias (Table 129.2) (2, 6). However, a respiratory component is distinctly unusual. Some patients have brief (hours) episodic attacks of excruciating headache and neck pain or stiffness, suggesting meningeal irritation, or difficulty concentrating, suggesting mild encephalopathy. Although spinal fluid within the first few weeks of illness is generally normal, these symptoms may reflect early neurologic dissemination (3,141,142). Except for fatigue and lethargy, which are often constant, the early signs and symptoms are typically intermittent and changing. A patient may have headache and neck stiffness for several days, to be replaced by migratory musculoskeletal pain involving one to a few joints (generally without swelling), tendons, bursae, muscles, or bone. Pain

TABLE 129.1. EARLY SIGNS OF LYME DISEASE

Signs	No. of Patients N = 314	(%)
Erythema migrans[a]	314	(100)
Multiple annular lesions	150	(48)
Lymphadenopathy		
Regional	128	(41)
Generalized	63	(20)
Pain on neck flexion	52	(17)
Malar rash	41	(13)
Erythematous throat	38	(12)
Conjunctivitis	35	(11)
Right upper quadrant tenderness	24	(8)
Splenomegaly	18	(6)
Hepatomegaly	16	(5)
Muscle tenderness	12	(4)
Periorbital edema	10	(3)
Evanescent skin lesions	8	(3)
Abdominal tenderness	6	(2)
Testicular swelling	2	(1)

[a]Erythema migrans was required for inclusion in this study.
Reproduced from Steere AC, Bartenhagen NH, Craft JE, et al. The early clinical manifestations of Lyme disease. *Ann Intern Med* 1983;99:79, with permission.

TABLE 129.2. EARLY SYMPTOMS OF LYME DISEASE

Symptoms	No. of Patients N = 314	(%)
Malaise, fatigue, and lethargy	251	(80)
Headache	200	(64)
Fever and chills	185	(59)
Stiff neck	151	(48)
Arthralgias	150	(48)
Myalgias	135	(43)
Backache	81	(26)
Anorexia	73	(23)
Sore throat	53	(17)
Nausea	53	(17)
Dysesthesia	35	(11)
Vomiting	32	(10)
Abdominal pain	24	(8)
Photophobia	19	(6)
Hand stiffness	16	(5)
Dizziness	15	(5)
Cough	15	(5)
Chest pain	12	(4)
Ear pain	12	(4)
Diarrhea	6	(2)

Reproduced from Steere AC, Bartenhagen NH, Craft JE, et al. The early clinical manifestations of Lyme disease. *Ann Intern Med* 1983;99:79, with permission.

often lasts a few hours to several days in a given location. These symptoms may begin before or after EM appears (or without it) and last for months (especially fatigue and lethargy) after the skin lesions have disappeared.

In Europe, untreated EM more commonly has a prolonged, indolent course, and is less commonly associated with multiple secondary lesions, systemic symptoms, laboratory abnormalities, or subsequent arthritis (143).

Later Manifestations

Neurologic Involvement

Within several weeks to months of the onset of illness, in a minority of untreated patients [15% in one series (3)], definite neurologic abnormalities develop, involving either the CNS (62,91) or peripheral nervous system (92). The most common acute abnormalities are meningitis with or without an accompanying encephalopathy, cranial neuritis most commonly involving the facial nerve, which may be affected bilaterally (144), and motor or sensory radiculoneuritis (Fig. 129.4) (3,90). Less common syndromes, which occur much later in disease, include chorea, focal demyelinating encephalopathy or myelopathy, chronic encephalopathy, peripheral polyneuropathy, and transverse myelitis (3,62,63,92,145). Any of these manifestations may occur as the sole manifestation of Lyme disease (90).

Lyme meningitis causes a lymphocytic pleocytosis (generally a few to a few hundred cells per cubic millimeter) and

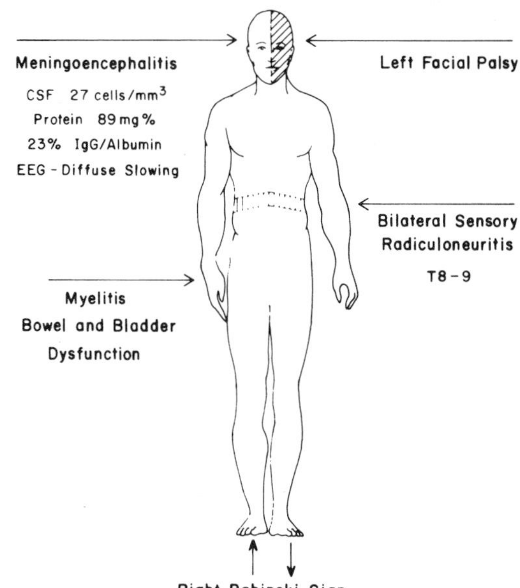

FIGURE 129.4. Neurologic abnormalities of Lyme disease that occurred in a 58-year-old man. Three weeks after the onset of erythema migrans, the patient developed meningoencephalitis, left facial palsy, and bilateral sensory radiculoneuritis. Although long-tract signs are unusual in Lyme disease, this patient had bowel and bladder dysfunction and a right Babinski sign, suggestive of myelitis.

mild protein elevation in the CSF, but glucose usually remains normal. Headache may be excruciating and frequently fluctuates from day to day or even hour to hour. Neck stiffness is not prominent, and Kernig's and Brudzinski's signs are absent. Encephalopathy is usually subtle, with mild impairment of mentation or memory accompanied by diffuse slowing on electroencephalogram. These relatively acute neurologic manifestations will resolve spontaneously but often only after persisting for months (3). *B. burgdorferi* has been cultured rarely from the CSF of individuals with acute neurologic Lyme disease. Studies with PCR have supported the hypothesis that acute neurologic abnormalities result from direct infection of the CNS (146).

Chronic neurologic disease may first appear years after onset of Lyme disease, is typically subtle and difficult to diagnose definitively, and does not remit spontaneously (63,147). Cognitive deficits, particularly affecting short-term memory, and sensory polyneuropathy with distal paresthesias and abnormalities on electromyography or nerve-conduction testing, may occur as late neurologic manifestations of Lyme disease (62,63). "Progressive Borrelia encephalomyelitis" (148) has been seen more frequently in Europe than in the U.S.

CNS Lyme disease is often associated with local synthesis of immunoglobulin within the CSF, resulting in oligoclonal bands or hyperconcentration of specific antibody, findings that reflect the presence of local antigen, and presumably active infection; they are helpful in diagnosis (62,63). The PCR is much less likely to be positive in CSF than in joint fluid of untreated patients with Lyme disease (see later).

Carditis

Carditis occurs within weeks to months of onset in up to 8% of untreated patients (5). The most common clinical manifestation is fluctuating atrioventricular block (first degree, Wenckebach, or complete heart block). Occasionally the heart is affected more diffusely with electrocardiographic changes compatible with acute myopericarditis, radionuclide or cardiac ultrasound evidence of contractile dysfunction, or rarely, cardiomegaly on chest radiograph (5). Biopsy-proven endomyocarditis (149,150), and, in one fatal case, spirochete-positive pancarditis (52) have been reported. No patients have had significant valvular lesions [cf. acute rheumatic fever (see Chapter 86)] (5). Carditis is usually brief and self-limited (3 days to 6 weeks). Although clinical manifestations are usually limited to the conduction system, subclinical myocardial involvement may be more extensive (50). Carditis, like other symptoms of disseminated disease, may be the presenting manifestation of Lyme disease (151).

Patients typically have palpitations, lightheadedness, or syncope. The electrocardiogram (ECG) shows variable degrees of atrioventricular block and often nonspecific ST-T wave changes. With improved recognition of EM and early Lyme disease and prompt institution of antibiotic therapy, carditis has become less common. Most individuals with carditis today have cardiac manifestations without having noted a preceding EM. Once resolved, carditis does not recur. This diagnosis should be suspected in individuals (adult or children) in endemic areas with new cardiac conduction-system disturbances without other explanations for organic heart disease.

Arthritis

From weeks to as long as 2 years after the onset of illness, frank arthritis develops in about 60% of untreated patients (2,4,11), usually characterized by intermittent attacks of inflammation in one or two large joints. Involvement is classically asymmetric and not very painful. The knee is by far the most commonly affected joint. The onset of overt arthritis may be preceded by months or even years of intermittent migratory myalgias, arthralgias, and periarticular pain. Attacks typically begin suddenly with the rapid development of effusions. Joint fluid accumulation may be massive and lead to the formation of Baker's cysts, which may dissect into the calf and rupture. Although this pattern of inflammatory monoarthritis of the knee is most common in Lyme arthritis, both large and small joints may be affected, and a few patients have had symmetric polyarthritis. Individual attacks of arthritis generally last a few weeks to a few months, followed by spontaneous remission. Attacks usually recur in the same or another joint for several years but decrease in frequency by 10% to 20% per year and ultimately cease in most patients, even without antibiotic therapy (93). Fatigue commonly accompanies active joint involvement, but fever or other systemic symptoms are unusual.

Joint fluid white cell counts vary widely from 500 to 110,000 cells/mm^3 and average about 25,000 cells/mm^3 with a predominance of polymorphonuclear leukocytes (2). Total protein has ranged from 3 to 8 g/dL. C3 and C4 levels are usually greater than one third serum levels, and glucose levels usually greater than two thirds those of serum glucose. Tests for rheumatoid factor and antinuclear antibody are generally negative. Culture of joint fluid has been almost invariably negative for *B. burgdorferi* (44). However, by PCR, *B. burgdorferi* DNA is found in joint fluid of most untreated patients with arthritis, suggesting the presence of spirochetes nearby; such DNA may not be detectable after antibiotic therapy (152–154).

In about 10% of patients with arthritis, especially those with HLA class II antigen DR4, involvement in large joints may become chronic, with pannus formation and erosion of cartilage and bone, despite antibiotic therapy that is curative in other patients (Fig. 129.5A) (4,11,93,94). The development of a humoral immune response against OspA and B has been statistically associated with the development of chronic arthritis in this patient group (155). The synovial lesion mimics the histopathology of rheumatoid arthritis (RA): as noted earlier, there are surface deposits of fibrin, villous hypertrophy, vascular proliferation, and a heavy infiltration

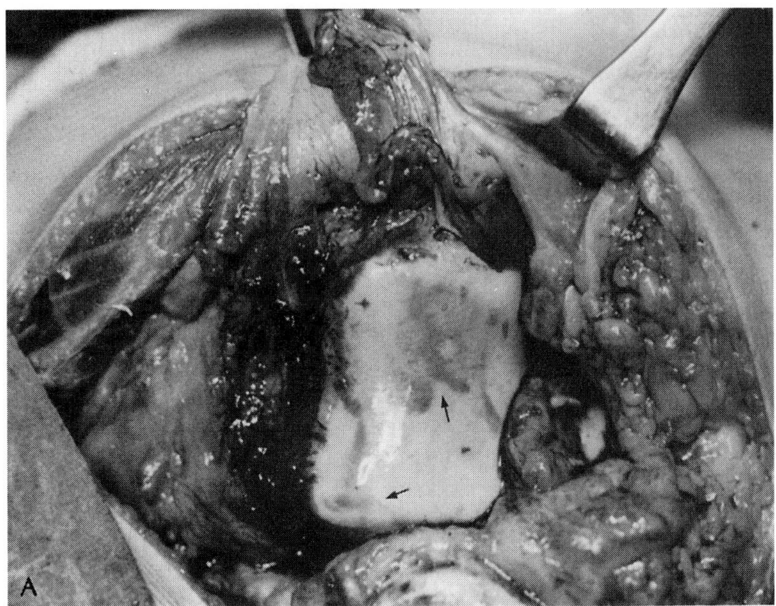

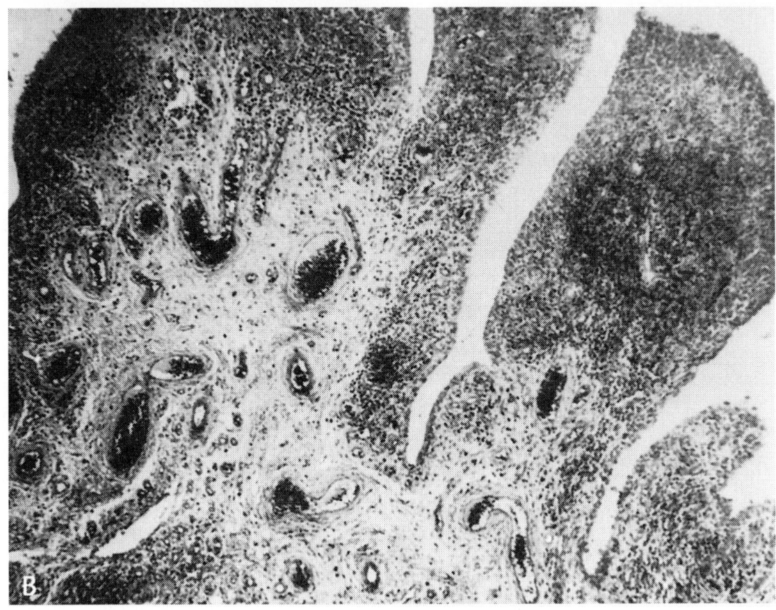

FIGURE 129.5. A: The knee of a patient with Lyme disease at the time of synovectomy. The patient had typical erythema migrans in June 1974, followed by intermittent migratory polyarthritis. Two years later, persistent swelling of the right knee developed. After 7 months, he underwent synovectomy. The articular surface of the femur can be seen; the arrows show what was the advancing border of pannus, now stripped away from the underlying eroded cartilage. **B:** Tissue structure of affected synovium. Individual polypoid stalks show central edema and vascular proliferation. Surrounding the central core is a rim of predominantly mononuclear cells. In one area, an aggregate resembling a lymphoid follicle is seen. (Reproduced from Steere AC, Malawista SE, Hardin JH, et al. Erythema chronicum migrans and Lyme arthritis: the enlarging clinical spectrum. *Ann Intern Med* 1977;86:693, with permission.)

of mononuclear cells (Fig. 129.5B) (2,4,11). Additionally, there may be an obliterative endarteritis and, rarely, demonstrable nearby spirochetes by monoclonal antibody or silver staining (49,85). Taken with generation of the proinflammatory materials described under Pathogenesis, we appear to have in chronic Lyme arthritis the joint fluid cell counts, the immune reactants (except for rheumatoid factor), the synovial histology, the amounts of inflammatory mediators released, and sometimes the resulting destruction of cartilage and bone that are characteristic of RA. However, to call persistent Lyme arthritis "chronic" is something of a misnomer because, although by definition it is present for more than 1 year, the inflammation generally resolves within 4 years, even without further antibiotic therapy (89,112).

Acrodermatitis chronica atrophicans

Another late finding (years) associated with *B. burgdorferi* infection is a chronic skin lesion, *acrodermatitis chronica atrophicans* (38,39), well known in Europe but rare in the U.S. (155). Lesions begin as violaceous infiltrated plaques or nodules, especially on extensor surfaces of acral areas of extremities. Eventually epidermal and dermal atrophy develop. This lesion appears to result from chronic persistence of infection in skin and has been particularly associated with *B. afzelii,* which is prevalent in Europe (36,37,157). There may be underlying joint changes in regions near involved skin. *Acrodermatitis chronica atrophicans* also seems to have a predilection for limbs previously affected by radiculoneuropathy.

LABORATORY TESTS

The diagnosis of Lyme disease is primarily clinical. Culture of *B. burgdorferi* from patients permits definitive diagnosis, but is rarely successful (25,42,43) except from skin biopsies (25,39,41), in which recovery can approach 80% (139), but for which the diagnosis is usually obvious. Culture of skin becomes important when a lesion suggesting EM occurs in a patient from a region in which Lyme disease was not previously endemic (158,159). Spirochetes are not often seen by direct examination of blood, plasma, plasma pellets, or skin transudate specimens of EM (25), and special tissue-staining techniques (47–49) are of low yield and not readily available.

Determination of specific antibody titers is the most helpful adjunctive diagnostic test for Lyme disease in routine clinical settings. When determined by immunofluorescence or enzyme-linked immunosorbent assay (ELISA), specific IgM antibody titers against *B. burgdorferi* usually reach a peak between the third and sixth week after the onset of disease; specific IgG titers increase more slowly and are generally highest months later when arthritis is present (Fig. 129.6) (25,160). They are particularly useful in differentiating Lyme arthritis from other rheumatic syndromes, especially when EM was missed, forgotten, or absent.

Many commercially available serologic tests for Lyme disease have performed poorly, having unacceptably low sensitivity and specificity and inconsistency of results (161–163). Additionally, indiscriminate use of Lyme serologies when the pretest likelihood of Lyme disease has been very low has led to test results with very low positive predictive value. Even a highly specific test will have a low positive predictive value when the likelihood of Lyme disease is less than 5% (164–166). The most important clinical caveat is that a positive serologic test increases the likelihood that a patient has Lyme disease after the first few weeks of illness, but does not by itself confirm the diagnosis, particularly in questionable epidemiologic and clinical circumstances. Questionable positive results should be con-

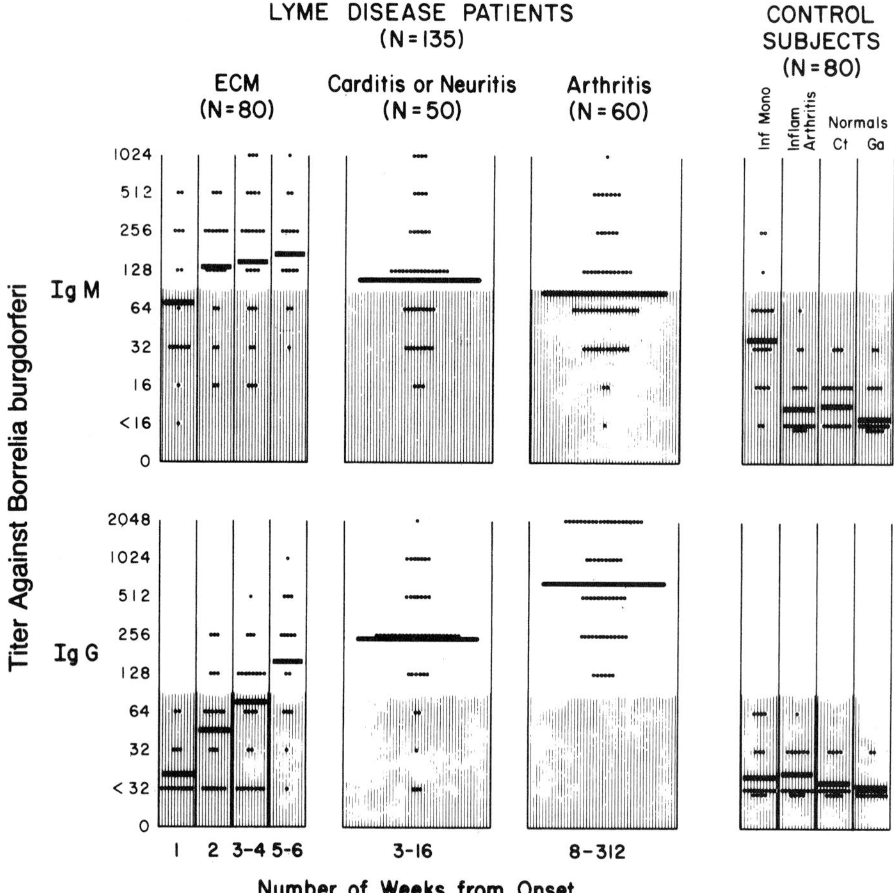

FIGURE 129.6. Antibody titers against *Borrelia burgdorferi* in serum samples from 135 patients with different clinical manifestations of Lyme disease, from 40 control patients with infectious mononucleosis or inflammatory arthritis, and from 40 normal control subjects, as determined by indirect immunofluorescence. *Heavy bar,* Geometric mean titer for each group; *shaded areas,* the range of titers generally observed in control subjects. Note that all patients with Lyme arthritis have elevated immunoglobulin G antibody titers. (Reproduced from Steere AC, Grodzicki RL, Kornblatt AN, et al. The spirochetal etiology of Lyme disease. *N Engl J Med* 1983;308:733–740, with permission.)

firmed by Western blot analysis; some workers have suggested that all positive results should be confirmed except for highly positive ones in individuals who have typical clinical manifestations and have had an opportunity for exposure in a known endemic area (167).

Certain sources of false positivity and negativity have been well studied. *B. burgdorferi* contains epitopes that are cross-reactive with other spirochetes, including *T. pallidum*, but patients with Lyme disease do not have positive VDRL tests, and those with other spirochetal illnesses have negative Lyme Western blots (6,167). A few cases of true seronegative Lyme disease have been reported (168), but they are rare. The typical clinical setting for seronegative Lyme disease is in a partially treated patient with persistent symptoms, in whom the antigenic load is presumed to be small, with persistence of infection in privileged sites, particularly the CNS. The best safeguard against this circumstance is to ensure that patients have received antibiotic therapy appropriate for their disease, and that, regardless of serologic status, they be monitored clinically after treatment until symptoms have resolved.

The determination of specific CSF antibody levels is a useful adjunct in the diagnosis of neurologic involvement in Lyme disease (62,63). When infection involves the CNS, specific antibody is secreted by B cells locally, leading to increased concentrations relative to serum (when corrected for total immunoglobulin). Such hyperconcentration of specific antibody is the best laboratory evidence of CNS Lyme disease (62,169). Both IgG and IgA antibody levels have been reported to be predictive of CNS Lyme disease (63,169). Positive CSF antibody tests are confirmatory of CNS Lyme disease, but the absence of a positive test does not rule out CNS involvement.

The PCR has been applied to human fluids as an adjunct in the diagnosis of Lyme disease and as a means of elucidating sites of nearby active infection with *B. burgdorferi* (43,142,146,152–154,170), with variable success. It appears most helpful in Lyme arthritis. Despite a general inability to culture the Lyme spirochete from synovial fluid, DNA belonging to it [particularly from plasmidic targets (152)] was amplified from almost all joint fluids of patients with untreated Lyme arthritis (153). After treatment the fluids often became negative, suggesting either cure or at least reduction in the burden of spirochetal DNA (and presumably of spirochetes) to below the level of detection. Positivity in CSF of patients with putative neurologic Lyme disease has been more variable, but it is useful when positive (142,146,154,170). PCR on plasma during dissemination of spirochetes is of low yield (18% in one study) (43). Warning: false positivity is a constant threat; PCR should be limited to specimens processed and amplified under stringent conditions, always with appropriate positive and negative controls.

Tests of the T-cell blastogenic response to *B. burgdorferi* antigens have demonstrated that a cell-mediated immune response occurs early after onset of infection, but such tests have not been useful in routine clinical practice because of their technical difficulty and because of the rarity of positive T-cell tests when serologies are negative (168,171).

The most common nonspecific laboratory abnormalities, particularly early in the illness, are a high erythrocyte sedimentation rate, an elevated total serum IgM level, and a transiently increased serum glutamic oxaloacetic transaminase (SGOT) level (Table 129.3) (2,7,172). As expected, each of these findings is more common in individuals with disseminated early disease than with localized disease.

TABLE 129.3. LABORATORY FINDINGS IN EARLY LYME DISEASE

Laboratory Test	No. of Patients with Abnormal Values N = 314	(%)	Median (Range) of Abnormal Values
Hematology			
Hematocrit	37	(12)	35 (36–81)
Leukocytes >10^4/mm^3	24	(8)	12 (11–18)
Erythrocyte sedimentation rate (ESR) >20 mm/h	166	(53)	35 (21–58)
Immunoglobulins			
IgM >250 mg/dL	104	(33)	310 (252–930)
IgG >1,500 mg/dL	10	(3)	1,550 (1,520–1,760)
IgA >400 mg/dL	12	(4)	440 (410–580)
Liver function			
Aspartate aminotransferase (SGOT) >35 U/mL	59	(18)	71 (36–251)
Alamine aminotransferase (SGPT) >32 U/mL[a]	47	(15)	125 (42–491)
Lactate dehydrogenase (LDH) >600 U/mL[a]	49	(16)	775 (608–1,080)
Renal function			
Microscopic hematuria (red cells/hpf)	18	(6)	15 (10–25)

[a]Tested only in the 55 patients with abnormal SGOT; creatine phosphokinase (CPK) was normal in all these patients. Reproduced from Steers AC, Bartenhagen NH, Craft JE, et al. The early clinical manifestations of Lyme disease. *Ann Intern Med* 1983;99:80, with permission.

Patients may be mildly anemic early in the illness and occasionally have elevated white cell counts with shifts to the left in the differential count. A few patients have had microscopic hematuria, sometimes with mild proteinuria (dipstick); values for creatinine and blood urea nitrogen have been normal. Throughout the illness, serum C3 and C4 levels are generally normal or elevated. Rheumatoid factor and antinuclear antibodies are usually absent. A few patients have had antibodies to phospholipid, but Lyme disease is not associated with a coagulopathy. There are no examples of positive urine cultures in patients with Lyme disease, and positive tests on urine for specific antigen or for spirochetal DNA have not been validated.

DIFFERENTIAL DIAGNOSIS

EM is the herald lesion of Lyme disease (Fig. 129.3). When present in its classic form in individuals with exposure in endemic areas, it is virtually diagnostic. However, some patients are not aware of having had EM, and in others, its appearance is not always characteristic. A lesion suggesting EM occurring in a patient from a previously nonendemic region for Lyme disease (158,159) should be suspect. Secondary lesions might suggest *erythema multiforme,* but blistering of skin, mucosal lesions, and involvement of the palms and soles are not features of Lyme disease. Malar rash may suggest systemic lupus erythematosus; an urticarial rash, hepatitis B infection or serum sickness. Evanescent blotches and circles may resemble *erythema marginatum,* but those of Lyme disease do not expand.

Early musculoskeletal flu-like symptoms may be misinterpreted, especially when EM is absent or missed or is not the first manifestation. In patients with particularly severe constitutional symptoms, consider possible concomitant infection with two other emerging illnesses whose causative agents are transmitted by the same tick: the rickettsia-like disorder, human granulocytic ehrlichiosis (HGE; watch for leukopenia, thrombocytopenia, elevated transaminases, occasional inclusions in granulocytes) (173,174) or the malaria-like disorder, babesiosis (occasional inclusions in erythrocytes) (175).

Severe headache and stiff neck may resemble; aseptic or viral meningitis; abdominal symptoms, hepatitis, and generalized tender lymphadenopathy and splenomegaly, infectious mononucleosis. As in the last infection, fatigue may be a major and persistent complaint. However, initial presentations of an isolated chronic fatigue syndrome or of fibromyalgia-like complaints (diffuse aching, trigger points, sleep disturbance) are not characteristic of Lyme disease (164,176–179). An isolated facial weakness may mimic Bell's-like palsy of other causes, but in an area in which Lyme disease is endemic, a bilateral facial palsy may be more likely to signal this disorder than Guillain–Barré syndrome or granulomatous disease.

In later stages, Lyme disease may mimic other immune-mediated disorders. Like rheumatic fever, Lyme disease may be associated with sore throat followed by migratory polyarthritis (more often, polyarthralgias) and carditis, but without evidence of valvular involvement or of a preceding streptococcal infection. Migratory pain in tendons and joints also may suggest disseminated gonococcal disease. Late neurologic involvement may suggest multiple sclerosis (transverse myelitis), Guillain–Barré syndrome (symmetric peripheral neuropathy), a major mood disorder with disturbed sleep and energy depletion, a process leading to dementia with cognitive deficits, or brain tumor. A distinguishing feature of neurologic Lyme disease is that it may affect all levels of the neuraxis: peripheral and cranial nerves, meninges, nerve roots, spinal cord, and the brain itself (90). In adults with Lyme arthritis, the large knee effusions can resemble those in Reiter's syndrome, and the occasional symmetric polyarthritis, that of RA. In children, the attacks of arthritis, although generally shorter, may be identical to those seen in the oligoarticular form of juvenile rheumatoid arthritis (JRA), but without iridocyclitis.

A major source of diagnostic confusion has emerged regarding the relation between Lyme disease and fibromyalgia. Fibromyalgia constitutes up to 25% of the consultative practice in rheumatology. Lyme disease can be one of many triggers of this common syndrome, and its appearance is not an indication of persistent infection (176–179). Failure to recognize fibromyalgia leads to gross overdiagnosis of Lyme disease, particularly when there is inappropriate reliance on low-level, nondiagnostic serologic results (164,165,177,179). The characteristic trigger points, fatigue, and sleep disturbance that characterize fibromyalgia must be distinguished from the joint and neurologic involvement of Lyme disease, because the treatments for the two disorders are different (see later).

TREATMENT

All stages of Lyme disease respond to properly chosen antibiotic therapy, although the response is most likely to be definitive early in the disease, and certain late manifestations may respond incompletely or inconsistently. Nevertheless, late treatment, even on the order of months, is better than very late treatment: in one study (180), the delay in therapy for patients with long-term sequelae averaged 34.5 months, compared with a delay of 2.7 months in those without such sequelae.

Current antibiotic recommendations represent a distillation of published studies, practical considerations, and clinical experience, and will doubtless be modified in the future. Antibiotic choices must be made with attention to the extent of disease as well as to the stage of illness. The leading cause of failure of antibiotic therapy for Lyme disease is incorrect diagnosis; there is no substitute for careful clinical evaluation. At all stages, resolution may be slow and lag behind therapy.

The appropriate therapeutic end point is therefore often difficult to determine, which has led to some degree of upward creep in the recommended durations of therapy, without formal study. Patients must be observed after treatment until resolution is complete or has ceased, before determinations are made about the need for more therapy. No clinical trials have determined the need for, or effectiveness of, courses longer than 4 weeks for any stage of Lyme disease (longer courses for persistent symptoms are under study). Current recommendations are summarized in Table 129.4.

Early Disease

Early Lyme disease responds promptly to oral antibiotic therapy, particularly when localized to a single skin lesion with minimal or no associated systemic symptoms. EM resolves in days, and subsequent major sequelae (myocarditis, meningoencephalitis, or recurrent arthritis) are generally prevented (17,181,182). Signs of early dissemination (multiple secondary skin lesions, myalgias, arthralgias, fever, headache, stiff neck, or photophobia) reflect more pervasive infection and have been thought to carry a greater likelihood of recurrence after oral antibiotics, particularly when neurologic symptoms are present (17,182). However, with meningitis excluded, a large group of patients with early disseminated disease had excellent and essentially equal responses to 3 weeks of oral doxycycline or 2 weeks of intravenous ceftriaxone (183), and over several months, the two regimens were equally effective in preventing the late manifestations of disease. Careful evaluation for subtle CNS involvement, including lumbar puncture in patients with memory impairment or difficulty in concentrating, as well as prominent headache or facial palsy, and electrodiagnostic studies in those with dysesthesias should be undertaken in all patients before antibiotic

TABLE 129.4. TREATMENT RECOMMENDATIONS

Early Lyme disease[a]
- Doxycycline, 100 mg twice daily for 21 days
- Amoxicillin, 500 mg 3 times daily for 21 days[b]
- Cefuroxime axetil, 500 mg twice daily for 21 days
- Azithromycin, 500 mg daily for 7 days[c] (less effective than other regimens)

Neurologic manifestations
- Bell's-like palsy (no other neurologic abnormalities)
  - Oral regimens for early disease suffice
- Meningitis (with or without radiculoneuropathy or encephalitis)[d]
  - Ceftriaxone, 2 g daily for 14–28 days
  - Penicillin G, 20 million units daily for 14–28 days
  - Doxycycline, 100 mg twice daily (oral or intravenous) for 14–28 days[e]
  - Chloramphenicol, 1 g 4 times daily for 14–28 days

Arthritis[f]
- Doxycycline, 100 mg twice daily for 30 days
- Amoxicillin and probenecid, both at 500 mg 3 times daily for 30 days[g]
- Ceftriaxone, 2 g daily for 14–28 days
- Penicillin G, 20 million units daily for 14–28 days

Carditis
- Ceftriaxone, 2 g daily for 14 days
- Penicillin G, 20 million units daily for 14 days
- Doxycycline, 100 mg orally twice daily for 21 days[h]
- Amoxicillin, 500 mg 3 times daily for 21 days[h]

Pregnancy
- Localized early disease
  - Amoxicillin, 500 mg 3 times daily for 21 days
- Any manifestation of disseminated disease
  - Penicillin G, 20 million units daily for 14–28 days
- Asymptomatic seropositivity
  - No treatment necessary

[a]Without neurologic, cardiac, or joint involvement. For early Lyme disease limited to single erythema migrans lesion, 10 days is sufficient.
[b]Some experts advise addition of probenecid, 500 mg, 3 times daily.
[c]Experience with this agent is limited; optimal duration of therapy is unclear.
[d]Optimal duration of therapy has not been established. There are no controlled trials of therapy longer than 4 weeks for any manifestation of Lyme disease.
[e]No published experience in the United States.
[f]An oral regimen should be selected only if there is no neurologic involvement.
[g]Amoxicillin is generally administered 3 times daily, but the only trial of this agent for Lyme arthritis used a 4-times-daily regimen.
[h]Oral regimens have been reserved for mild carditis limited to first-degree heart block with PR 0.30 seconds and normal ventricular function.

selection. Because of the potential for early neurologic spread, patients with abnormal electrodiagnostic studies or spinal fluids, or even prominent neurologic complaints with normal spinal fluid, should be considered for intravenous antibiotic therapy (141,142,184). Patients treated early may not mount a systemic immune response and may be susceptible to reinfection (185,186).

For adults, preferred regimens include oral doxycycline (100 mg twice a day) or amoxicillin (500 mg three times a day), to which some recommend the addition of probenecid (500 mg three times a day) (182) (pediatric dose, 30 mg/kg/day each for 21 days). The former antibiotic is the drug of choice if concomitant HGE, which does not respond to the penicillins, is suspected. Although many patients with localized disease have been treated successfully with shorter courses (10–14 days), 3 weeks of therapy may be safer. Certainly all patients with prominent systemic symptoms and secondary skin lesions should be given the longer course of therapy. In the case of penicillin allergy, cefuroxime axetil (500 mg twice a day) or erythromycin (250 mg four times a day) represent current alternatives for those who cannot take doxycycline (pregnant or lactating women or children younger than 9 years) with appropriate pediatric dosage adjustments) (187). Outcomes with erythromycin or the newer macrolide, azithromycin, have been less satisfactory than with the other antibiotics (17,181,188).

Rare, isolated instances of maternal–fetal transmission of *B. burgdorferi* infection have occurred when Lyme disease has been untreated (55) or inadequately treated (60) during pregnancy. Epidemiologic surveys have failed to demonstrate congenital anomalies clearly attributable to maternal Lyme disease (189), however, and there is no evidence of risk to a developing fetus ascribable to maternal seropositivity alone in the absence of clinical evidence of active infection (190). Nevertheless, the available data provide additional impetus for early treatment with amoxicillin, cefuroxime, or erythromycin for localized early Lyme disease occurring during pregnancy, and consideration should be given to intravenous therapy for more advanced stages of infection.

About 10% of patients experience a Jarisch–Herxheimer-like reaction (higher fever, redder rash, or greater pain) during the first 24 hours of therapy (17). Regardless of which drug is selected and the duration of administration, many patients with disseminated early disease have brief (hours to days) recurrent episodes of pain in joints, tendons, bursae, or muscles, often with ongoing fatigue, which may continue for 3 months or longer after completion of antibiotic therapy (17,182). These symptoms seem not to reflect continuing infection and do not respond to further antibiotic therapy (they may reflect the persistence of residual undegraded antigen); they eventually resolve spontaneously in almost all cases. Persistent neurologic complaints may, however, reflect inadequately treated neurologic involvement that may progress over time even in seronegative individuals. This last point should serve to emphasize the importance of careful neurologic evaluation before institution of oral antibiotic therapy for early disease.

Later Disease

Optimal therapy for specific major organ involvement is still being defined. The most significant problem in arriving at recommendations for therapy lies in determining proper end points, because there are no definitive means of establishing microbiologic cure, and symptoms often resolve slowly or incompletely.

Neurologic Disease

Acute neurologic manifestations including meningitis, cranial neuropathies, and radiculoneuritis have been shown to respond to intravenous penicillin G (20 million IU a day in six divided doses for 10 days) (18), although longer courses (14–21 days) are generally recommended at present (191). Ceftriaxone (192) and cefotaxime (193) have both been found effective when given intravenously for 14 days and may be superior to penicillin (192). Meningitic symptoms usually begin to subside by the second day of therapy and disappear by 7 to 10 days. Radicular pain and motor deficits frequently require 7 to 8 weeks for recovery and do not always resolve completely (18). Because of this delayed or incomplete resolution, some experts routinely recommend 4 weeks of therapy for CNS Lyme disease; courses longer than 4 weeks have not been studied systematically.

Doxycycline (100 mg twice a day for 14 days) has been used successfully in Europe for the treatment of radiculoneuropathy (194) but has not been studied in the U.S. The recently recognized genetic differences and variation in dissemination between European and North American *B. burgdorferi* isolates (32,33,157) have suggested that results from clinical trials on the two continents may not be directly comparable.

Chronic neurologic manifestations including encephalopathy and peripheral neuropathy are less uniformly responsive to antibiotic therapy, but they do usually respond, albeit slowly, to 4 weeks of intravenous ceftriaxone (62,63,92,195). Not unexpectedly, some patients have persistent, nonprogressive deficits after antibiotic therapy.

Many individuals with subtle neurologic complaints such as forgetfulness, sleep disturbance, energy depletion, chronic headaches, and impaired concentrating ability have been assumed to have neurologic Lyme disease, often without a convincing epidemiologic history, a clearly defined neurologic lesion, or serologic confirmation. The costs and risks associated with misdiagnosis and inappropriate intravenous antibiotic therapy are considerable (164,196). As in most ill-defined circumstances, it is best to withhold therapy until an accurate assessment has been made; therapeutic trials for vague symptoms often contribute more confusion than clarity. The American College of Rheumatology has published a guideline recommending against intravenous therapy for nonspecific symptoms in seropositive individuals (165).

Carditis

Carditis responds rapidly (in days) to intravenous antibiotic therapy with one of the above agents (151), but it has also been treated successfully with oral antibiotics, salicylates, or glucocorticoids (5). In any case, spontaneous resolution is the rule, but because carditis appears to result from direct myocardial invasion by spirochetes (149), and because there is a high correlation of untreated carditis with other system involvement, all cases should be treated with antibiotics for a minimum of 2 weeks. Prednisone (40–60 mg/day in divided doses) produced a rapid resolution of heart block (5), but may possibly interfere with attempts to cure the illness definitively and therefore should be used for brief courses (less than 7 days) or be avoided entirely. For patients with allergy to penicillin and cephalosporins, doxycycline (100 mg twice a day for 30 days) is reasonable but unevaluated. Temporary pacing may be required; permanent pacing, rarely (5,151).

Arthritis

For established Lyme arthritis, even with unremitting involvement, oral doxycycline (100 mg twice a day for 4 weeks) or amoxicillin/probenecid (500 mg each four times a day) each cured the large majority of patients (109). Intravenous ceftriaxone is probably as effective when given for at least 2 weeks and has the advantage of treating concomitant neurologic involvement, which may not be treated adequately with oral agents (109,192). Parenteral penicillin has been shown to be effective for some patients but is probably less effective than oral doxycycline or amoxicillin (19).

Antibiotic failures occur with all regimens, particularly in individuals of the HLA-DR4 phenotype (94). During treatment, the affected joint should be rested, and accumulated synovial fluid removed by needle aspiration (19). Optimal therapy for arthritis, as for the later neurologic complications of Lyme disease, is not yet clear. In difficult cases, longer periods of the highest tolerated oral doses of amoxicillin (with probenecid), a tetracycline, or longer intravenous therapy with ceftriaxone or penicillin may be considered but still require formal study. The PCR may prove useful for defining when infection has been eradicated from the joint (197) (or at least reduced to below the level of detection). Arthroscopic synovectomy is useful for antibiotic treatment failures, particularly those involving the knee (198); this procedure is often curative.

Fibromyalgia

The relation of Lyme disease to fibromyalgia—the former may be one of many triggers of the latter—is discussed in the section on differential diagnosis. The treatment of fibromyalgia (see Chapter 90) is the same whether or not there is a history of Lyme disease or positive Lyme serology and does not include antibiotics.

Acrodermatitis Chronica Atrophicans

Rarely seen in the U.S., the infiltrative lesions of acrodermatitis chronica atrophicans are usually cured by 4 weeks of oral regimens, either penicillin V, 1.5 million IU t.i.d., or doxycycline, 100 mg b.i.d. (40,199).

Tick Bites

The recommended approach to tick bites in endemic areas is to remove the tick and observe the bite site for the development of EM. In one randomized, controlled trial in Connecticut, the risk of acquiring Lyme disease after a tick bite was less than the risk of adverse reaction to antibiotics administered prophylactically (135). In this trial, no individual seroconverted silently, and no individual developed manifestations of disseminated disease, so the only risk of watchful waiting appeared to be that of developing EM. This risk was approximately 1%, even though the tick infection rate was approximately 20%. A separate cost-effectiveness analysis, which assumed that one third of infected individuals would have later disease and require intravenous therapy, recommended prophylactic therapy only if the risk of acquiring Lyme disease after a tick bite exceeded 3% (200). Thus the current evidence does not favor the administration of prophylactic antibiotics. A watched tick bite allows very early treatment of EM in the small minority of patients in whom it will develop, and this is the stage of disease most amenable to therapy.

Vaccine

Two vaccines against Lyme disease, both containing one of the outer surface lipoproteins (OspA) of *B. burgdorferi* as a recombinant protein, appear to be safe and effective (30,31), and one of them is available as of this writing. Recipients were given three injections: the first two, 1 month apart in the spring, and a booster dose a year later. Efficacy during the first year was 49% in one study and 68% in the other (probably not significantly different); efficacy increased after the third injection to 76% and 92%, respectively. The elderly were generally less well protected. Side effects were mild to moderate and typically self-limited.

Their mechanism of action is unique: spirochetes are killed in the midgut of the tick by the antibody-laden blood meal, before they ever reach the host (97). A potential disadvantage of this out-of-body protection is that the host's immune system may never see the spirochete again and is thereby deprived of anamnesis. Current studies are directed at the duration of protection (i.e., the need for further booster injections); the degree of cross-strain protection (201); and the longer-term safety of the vaccine.

REFERENCES

1. Steere AC, Malawista SE, Snydman DR, et al. Lyme arthritis: an epidemic of oligoarticular arthritis in children and adults in three Connecticut communities. *Arthritis Rheum* 1977;20:7–17.
2. Steere AC, Malawista SE, Hardin JA, et al. Erythema chronicum migrans and Lyme arthritis: the enlarging clinical spectrum. *Ann Intern Med* 1977;86:685–698.
3. Reik L, Steere AC, Bartenhagen NH, Shope RE, Malawista SE. Neurologic abnormalities of Lyme disease. *Medicine (Baltimore)* 1979;58:281–294.
4. Steere AC, Gibofsky A, Patarroyo ME, Winchester RJ, Hardin JA, Malawista SE. Chronic Lyme arthritis: clinical and immunogenetic differentiation from rheumatoid arthritis. *Ann Intern Med* 1979;90:896–901.
5. Steere AC, Batsford WP, Weinberg M, Alexander J, Berger HJ, Wolfson S, Malawista SE. Lyme carditis: cardiac abnormalities of Lyme disease. *Ann Intern Med* 1980;93:8–16.
6. Steere AC, Bartenhagen NH, Craft JE, Hutchinson GJ, Newman JH, Rahn SW, Sigal LH, Spieler PN, Stenn KS, Malawista SE. The early clinical manifestations of Lyme disease. *Ann Intern Med* 1983;99:76–82.
7. Steere AC, Hardin JA, Malawista SE. Erythema chronicum migrans and Lyme arthritis: cryoimmunoglobulins and clinical activity of skin and joints. *Science* 1977;196:1121–1122.
8. Steere AC, Hardin JA, Ruddy S, Mummaw JG, Malawista SE. Lyme arthritis: correlation of serum and cryoglobulin IgM with activity, and serum IgG with remission. *Arthritis Rheum* 1979;22:471–483.
9. Hardin JA, Walker LC, Steere AC, Trumble TC, Tung KS, Williams RC Jr, Ruddy S, Malawista SE. Circulating immune complexes in Lyme arthritis: detection by the ^{125}I-C1q binding, C1q solid phase, and Raji cell assays. *J Clin Invest* 1979;63: 468–477.
10. Hardin JA, Steere AC, Malawista SE. Immune complexes and the evolution of Lyme arthritis: dissemination and localization of abnormal C1q binding activity. *N Engl J Med* 1979;301: 1358–1363.
11. Steere AC, Brinckerhoff CE, Miller DJ, Drinker H, Harris ED Jr, Malawista SE. Elevated levels of collagenase and prostaglandin E_2 from synovium associated with erosion of cartilage and bone in a patient with chronic Lyme arthritis. *Arthritis Rheum* 1980;23:591–599.
12. Steere AC, Broderick TF, Malawista SE. Erythema chronicum migrans and Lyme arthritis: epidemiologic evidence for a tick vector. *Am J Epidemiol* 1978;108:312–321.
13. Wallis RC, Brown SE, Kloter KO, et al. Erythema chronicum migrans and lyme arthritis: field study of ticks. *Am J Epidemiol* 1978;108:322–327.
14. Steere AC, Malawista SE. Cases of Lyme disease in the United States: locations correlated with distribution of *Ixodes dammini. Ann Intern Med* 1979;91:730–733.
15. Steere AC, Malawista SE. *The epidemiology of Lyme disease.* New York: Gower Medical Publishing, 1983:33–42.
16. Steere AC, Malawista SE, Newman JH, et al. Antibiotic therapy in Lyme disease. *Ann Intern Med* 1980;93:1–8.
17. Steere AC, Hutchinson GJ, Rahn DW, Sigal LH, Craft JE, De Sanna ET, Malawista SE. Treatment of the early manifestations of Lyme disease. *Ann Intern Med* 1983;99:22–26.
18. Steere AC, Pachner AR, Malawista SE. Neurologic abnormalities of Lyme disease: successful treatment with high-dose intravenous penicillin. *Ann Intern Med* 1983;99:767–772.
19. Steere AC, Green J, Schoen RT, Taylor E, Hutchinson GJ, Rahn DW, Malawista SE. Successful parenteral penicillin therapy of established Lyme arthritis. *N Engl J Med* 1985;312:869–874.
20. Afzelius A. Verhandlungen der Dermatologischen Gesellschaft zu Stockholm on October 29, 1909. *Arch Dermatol Syph* 1910; 101:404.
21. Thone A. *Ixodes ricinus* and erythema chronicum migrans (Afzelius). *Dermatologica* 1968;136:57–60.
22. Garin-Bujadoux C. Paralysie par les tiques. *J Med Lyon* 1922; 71:765–767.
23. Bannwarth A. Zur Klinik und Pathogenese der "chronischen lymphozytaren Meningitis." *Arch Psychiatry Nervenkr* 1944; 117:161–185.
24. Burgdorfer W, Barbour AG, Hayes SF, et al. Lyme disease: a tick-borne spirochetosis? *Science* 1982;216:1317–1319.
25. Steere AC, Grodzicki RL, Kornblatt AN, Craft JE, Barbour AG, Burgdorfer W, Schmid GP, Johnson E, Malawista SE. The spirochetal etiology of Lyme disease. *N Engl J Med* 1983;308: 733–740.
26. Benach JL, Bosler EM, Hanrahan JP, et al. Spirochetes isolated from the blood of two patients with Lyme disease. *N Engl J Med* 1983;308:740–742.
27. Malawista SE, Steere AC, Hardin JA. Lyme disease: a unique human model for an infectious etiology of rheumatic disease. *Yale J Biol Med* 1984;57:473–477.
28. Hayes S, Burgdorfer W. Ultrastructure of Borrelia burgolorperi. In: Weber K, *Prospects of Lyme borreliosis.* Berlin: Springer-Verlag, 1993:20–43.
29. Fraser CM, Casjens S, Huang WM, et al. Genomic sequence of a Lyme disease spirochaete, *Borrelia burgdorferi. Nature* 1997; 390:580–586.
30. Sigal LH, Zahradnik JM, Lavin P, Patella SJ, Bryant G, Haselby R, Hilton E, Kunkel M, Adler-Klein D, Doherty T, Evans J, Molloy PJ, Seidner AL, Sabetta JR, Simon HJ, Klempner MS, Mays J, Marks D, Malawista SE. A vaccine consisting of recombinant *Borrelia burgdorferi* outer-surface protein A to prevent Lyme disease: recombinant outer-surface protein A Lyme disease vaccine Study consortium [published erratum appears in *N Engl J Med* 1998;339:571]. *N Engl J Med* 1998;339:216–222.
31. Steere AC, Sikand VK, Meurice F, et al. Vaccination against Lyme disease with recombinant *Borrelia burgdorferi* outer-surface lipoprotein A with adjuvant: Lyme Disease Vaccine Study Group. *N Engl J Med* 1998;339:209–215.
32. Baranton G, Postic D, Saint Girons I, et al. Delineation of *Borrelia burgdorferi* sensu stricto, *Borrelia garinii* sp. nov., and group VS461 associated with Lyme borreliosis. *Int J Syst Bacteriol* 1992;42:378–383.
33. Wilske B, Preac-Mursic V, Gobel UB, et al. An OspA serotyping system for *Borrelia burgdorferi* based on reactivity with monoclonal antibodies and OspA sequence analysis. *J Clin Microbiol* 1993;31:340–350.
34. Barbour AG, Heiland RA, Howe TR. Heterogeneity of major proteins in Lyme disease Borreliae: a molecular analysis of North American and European isolates. *J Infect Dis* 1985;152:478–484.
35. Barbour AG. Plasmid analysis of *Borrelia burgdorferi,* the Lyme disease agent. *J Clin Microbiol* 1988;26:475–478.
36. Wienecke R, Zochling N, Neubert U, et al. Molecular subtyping of *Borrelia burgdorferi* in erythema migrans and acrodermatitis chronica atrophicans. *J Invest Dermatol* 1994;103:19–22.
37. van Dam AP, Kuiper H, Vos K, et al. Different genospecies of *Borrelia burgdorferi* are associated with distinct clinical manifestations of Lyme borreliosis. *Clin Infect Dis* 1993;17:708–717.
38. Weber K, Schierz G, Wilske B, et al. European erythema migrans disease and related disorders. *Yale J Biol Med* 1984;57:463–471.
39. Asbrink E, Hovmark A. Successful cultivation of spirochetes from skin lesions of patients with erythema chronicum migrans Afzelius and acrodermatitis chronica atrophicans. *Acta Pathol Microbiol Immunol Scand B* 1985;93:161–163.

40. Asbrink E, Hovmark A, Hederstedt B. Serological studies of erythema chronicum migrans Afzelius and acrodermatitis chronica atrophicans with indirect immunofluorescence and enzyme-linked immunosorbent assays. *Acta Derm Venereol (Stockh)* 1985;65:509–514.
41. Berger BW, Kaplan MH, Rothenberg IR, et al. Isolation and characterization of the Lyme disease spirochete from the skin of patients with erythema chronicum migrans. *J Am Acad Dermatol* 1985;13:444–449.
42. Nadelman RB, Pavia CS, Magnarelli LA, et al. Isolation of *Borrelia burgdorferi* from the blood of seven patients with Lyme disease. *Am J Med* 1990;88:21–26.
43. Goodman JL, Bradley JF, Ross AE, et al. Bloodstream invasion in early Lyme disease: results from a prospective, controlled, blinded study using the polymerase chain reaction [published erratum appears in *Am J Med* 1996;101:239]. *Am J Med* 1995; 99:6–12.
44. Snydman DR, Schenkein DP, Berardi VP, et al. *Borrelia burgdorferi* in joint fluid in chronic Lyme arthritis. *Ann Intern Med* 1986;104:798–800.
45. Haupl T, Hahn G, Rittig M, et al. Persistence of *Borrelia burgdorferi* in ligamentous tissue from a patient with chronic Lyme borreliosis. *Arthritis Rheum* 1993;36:1621–1626.
46. Preac-Mursic V, Pfister HW, Spiegel H, et al. First isolation of *Borrelia burgdorferi* from an iris biopsy. *J Clin Neuroophthalmol* 1993;13:155–161; discussion 162.
47. Berger BW, Clemmensen OJ, Ackerman AB. Lyme disease is a spirochetosis: a review of the disease and evidence for its cause. *Am J Dermatopathol* 1983;5:111–124.
48. Berger BW. Erythema chronicum migrans of Lyme disease. *Arch Dermatol* 1984;120:1017–1021.
49. Johnston YE, Duray PH, Steere AC, Kashgarian M, Buza J, Malawista SE, Askenase PW. Lyme arthritis: spirochetes found in synovial microangiopathic lesions. *Am J Pathol* 1985; 118:26–34.
50. MacDonald AB. Borrelia in the brains of patients dying with dementia [Letter]. *JAMA* 1986;256:2195–2196.
51. Steere AC, Duray PH, Kauffmann DJ, et al. Unilateral blindness caused by infection with the Lyme disease spirochete, *Borrelia burgdorferi. Ann Intern Med* 1985;103:382–384.
52. Marcus LC, Steere AC, Duray PH, et al. Fatal pancarditis in a patient with coexistent Lyme disease and babesiosis: demonstration of spirochetes in the myocardium. *Ann Intern Med* 1985;103:374–376.
53. Rank EL, Dias SM, Hasson J, et al. Human necrotizing splenitis caused by *Borrelia burgdorferi. Am J Clin Pathol* 1989;91: 493–498.
54. Goellner MH, Agger WA, Burgess JH, et al. Hepatitis due to recurrent Lyme disease. *Ann Intern Med* 1988;108:707–708.
55. Schlesinger PA, Duray PH, Burke BA, et al. Maternal-fetal transmission of the Lyme disease spirochete, *Borrelia burgdorferi. Ann Intern Med* 1985;103:67–68.
56. Atlas E, Novak SN, Duray PH, et al. Lyme myositis: muscle invasion by *Borrelia burgdorferi. Ann Intern Med* 1988;109:245–246.
57. Shih CM, Pollack RJ, Telford SRd, et al. Delayed dissemination of Lyme disease spirochetes from the site of deposition in the skin of mice. *J Infect Dis* 1992;166:827–831.
58. Sood SK, Salzman MB, Johnson BJ, et al. Duration of tick attachment as a predictor of the risk of Lyme disease in an area in which Lyme disease is endemic. *J Infect Dis* 1997;175:996–999.
59. MacDonald AB. Human fetal borreliosis, toxemia of pregnancy, and fetal death. *Zentralbl Bakteriol Mikrobiol Hyg A* 1986;263: 189–200.
60. Weber K, Bratzke HJ, Neubert U, et al. *Borrelia burgdorferi* in a newborn despite oral penicillin for Lyme borreliosis during pregnancy. *Pediatr Infect Dis J* 1988;7:286–289.
61. Hardin JA, Steere AC, Malawista SE. The pathogenesis of arthritis in Lyme disease: humoral immune responses and the role of intra-articular immune complexes. *Yale J Biol Med* 1984; 57:589–593.
62. Halperin JJ, Luft BJ, Anand AK, et al. Lyme neuroborreliosis: central nervous system manifestations. *Neurology* 1989;39: 753–759.
63. Logigian EL, Kaplan RF, Steere AC. Chronic neurologic manifestations of Lyme disease. *N Engl J Med* 1990;323:1438–1444.
64. Benach JL, Coleman JL, Garcia-Monco JC, et al. Biological activity of *Borrelia burgdorferi* antigens. *Ann N Y Acad Sci* 1988; 539:115–125.
65. Habicht G. Cytokines in *Borrelia burgdorferi* infection. In: Schutzer SE, ed. *Lyme disease:* molecular and immunologic approaches. Cold Spring Harbor, NY: Cold Spring Harbor Laboratory Press, 1992:149–167.
66. Yang L, Ma Y, Schoenfeld R, et al. Evidence for B-lymphocyte mitogen activity in *Borrelia burgdorferi*-infected mice. *Infect Immun* 1992;60:3033–3041.
67. Peterson PK, Clawson CC, Lee DA, et al. Human phagocyte interactions with the Lyme disease spirochete. *Infect Immun* 1984;46:608–611.
68. Montgomery RR, Nathanson MH, Malawista SE. The fate of *Borrelia burgdorferi,* the agent for Lyme disease, in mouse macrophages: destruction, survival, recovery. *J Immunol* 1993; 150:909–915.
69. Montgomery RR, Nathanson MH, Malawista SE. Fc- and non-Fc-mediated phagocytosis of *Borrelia burgdorferi* by macrophages. *J Infect Dis* 1994;170:890–893.
70. Montgomery RR, Malawista SE. Entry of *Borrelia burgdorferi* into macrophages is end-on and leads to degradation in lysosomes. *Infect Immun* 1996;64:2867–2872.
71. Habicht GS, Katona LI, Benach JL. Cytokines and the pathogenesis of neuroborreliosis: *Borrelia burgdorferi* induces glioma cells to secrete interleukin-6. *J Infect Dis* 1991;164:568–574.
72. Ma Y, Weis JJ. *Borrelia burgdorferi* outer surface lipoproteins OspA and OspB possess B-cell mitogenic and cytokine-stimulatory properties. *Infect Immun* 1993;61:3843–3853.
73. Radolf JD, Norgard MV, Brandt ME, et al. Lipoproteins of *Borrelia burgdorferi* and *Treponema pallidum* activate cachectin/tumor necrosis factor synthesis: analysis using a CAT reporter construct. *J Immunol* 1991;147:1968–1974.
74. Norgard MV, Riley BS, Richardson JA, et al. Dermal inflammation elicited by synthetic analogs of *Treponema pallidum* and *Borrelia* burgdorferi lipoproteins. *Infect Immun* 1995;63: 1507–1515.
75. Sellati TJ, Burns MJ, Ficazzola MA, et al. *Borrelia burgdorferi* upregulates expression of adhesion molecules on endothelial cells and promotes transendothelial migration of neutrophils in vitro. *Infect Immun* 1995;63:4439–4447.
76. Wooten RM, Modur VR, McIntyre TM, et al. *Borrelia burgdorferi* outer membrane protein A induces nuclear translocation of nuclear factor-kappa B and inflammatory activation in human endothelial cells. *J Immunol* 1996;157:4584–4590.
77. Ebnet K, Simon MM, Shaw S. Regulation of chemokine gene expression in human endothelial cells by proinflammatory cytokines and *Borrelia burgdorferi. Ann N Y Acad Sci* 1996;797: 107–117.
78. Burns MJ, Sellati TJ, Teng EI, et al. Production of interleukin-8 (IL-8) by cultured endothelial cells in response to *Borrelia burgdorferi* occurs independently of secreted [corrected] IL-1 and tumor necrosis factor alpha and is required for subsequent transendothelial migration of neutrophils [published erratum appears in *Infect Immun* 1997;65:2508]. *Infect Immun* 1997;65: 1217–1222.
79. Straubinger RK, Straubinger AF, Summers BA, et al. *Borrelia*

burgdorferi induces the production and release of proinflammatory cytokines in canine synovial explant cultures. *Infect Immun* 1998;66:247–258.

80. Hu LT, Perides G, Noring R, et al. Binding of human plasminogen to *Borrelia burgdorferi. Infect Immun* 1995;63:3491–3496.
81. Leong JM, Morrissey PE, Ortega-Barria E, et al. Hemagglutination and proteoglycan binding by the Lyme disease spirochete, *Borrelia burgdorferi. Infect Immun* 1995;63:874–883.
82. Guo BP, Norris SJ, Rosenberg LC, et al. Adherence of *Borrelia burgdorferi* to the proteoglycan decorin. *Infect Immun* 1995;63:3467–3472.
83. Grab DJ, Givens C, Kennedy R. Fibronectin-binding activity in *Borrelia burgdorferi. Biochim Biophys Acta* 1998;1407:135–145.
84. Comstock LE, Thomas DD. Penetration of endothelial cell monolayers by *Borrelia burgdorferi. Infect Immun* 1989;57:1626–1628.
85. Duray P. Target organs of *Borrelia burgdorferi* infection: functional responses and histology. In: Schutzer SE, ed. *Lyme disease:* molecular and immunologic approaches. Cold Spring Harbor, NY: Cold Spring Harbor Laboratory Press, 1992:11–30.
86. Szczepanski A, Furie MB, Benach JL, et al. Interaction between *Borrelia burgdorferi* and endothelium in vitro. *J Clin Invest* 1990;85:1637–1647.
87. Garcia Monco JC, Wheeler CM, Benach JL, et al. Reactivity of neuroborreliosis patients (Lyme disease) to cardiolipin and gangliosides. *J Neurol Sci* 1993;117:206–214.
88. Aberer E, Brunner C, Suchanek G, et al. Molecular mimicry and Lyme borreliosis: a shared antigenic determinant between *Borrelia burgdorferi* and human tissue [see comments]. *Ann Neurol* 1989;26:732–737.
89. Malawista SE, Resolution of Lyme arthritis, acute or prolonged: A new look. *Inflammation* 2000;24:493–503.
90. Pachner AR, Steere AC. The triad of neurologic manifestations of Lyme disease: meningitis, cranial neuritis, and radiculoneuritis. *Neurology* 1985;35:47–53.
91. Pachner AR, Duray P, Steere AC. Central nervous system manifestations of Lyme disease. *Arch Neurol* 1989;46:790–795.
92. Halperin JJ, Little BW, Coyle PK, et al. Lyme disease: cause of a treatable peripheral neuropathy. *Neurology* 1987;37:1700–1706.
93. Steere AC, Schoen RT, Taylor E. The clinical evolution of Lyme arthritis. *Ann Intern Med* 1987;107:725–731.
94. Steere AC, Dwyer E, Winchester R. Association of chronic Lyme arthritis with HLA-DR4 and HLA-DR2 alleles [published erratum appears in *N Engl J Med* 1991;324:129] [see comments]. *N Engl J Med* 1990;323:219–223.
95. Craft JE, Fischer DK, Shimamoto GT, et al. Antigens of *Borrelia burgdorferi* recognized during Lyme disease: appearance of a new immunoglobulin M response and expansion of the immunoglobulin G response late in the illness. *J Clin Invest* 1986;78:934–939.
96. Montgomery RR, Malawista SE, Feen KJ, et al. Direct demonstration of antigenic substitution of *Borrelia burgdorferi* ex vivo: exploration of the paradox of the early immune response to outer surface proteins A and C in Lyme disease. *J Exp Med* 1996;183:261–269.
97. de Silva AM, Telford SR III, Brunet LR, et al. *Borrelia burgdorferi* OspA is an arthropod-specific transmission-blocking Lyme disease vaccine. *J Exp Med* 1996;183:271–275.
98. de Silva AM, Fikrig E. Arthropod- and host-specific gene expression by *Borrelia burgdorferi. J Clin Invest* 1997;99:377–379.
99. Meier JT, Simon MI, Barbour AG. Antigenic variation is associated with DNA rearrangements in a relapsing fever Borrelia. *Cell* 1985;41:403–409.
100. Bundoc VG, Barbour AG. Clonal polymorphisms of outer membrane protein OspB of *Borrelia burgdorferi. Infect Immun* 1989;57:2733–2741.
101. Zhang JR, Hardham JM, Barbour AG, et al. Antigenic variation in Lyme disease borreliae by promiscuous recombination of VMP-like sequence cassettes. *Cell* 1997;89:275–285.
102. Dorward DW, Huguenel ED, Davis G, et al. Interactions between extracellular *Borrelia burgdorferi* proteins and non-Borrelia-directed immunoglobulin M antibodies. *Infect Immun* 1992;60:838–844.
103. Klempner MS, Noring R, Rogers RA. Invasion of human skin fibroblasts by the Lyme disease spirochete, *Borrelia burgdorferi. J Infect Dis* 1993;167:1074–1081.
104. Girschick HJ, Huppertz HI, Russmann H, et al. Intracellular persistence of *Borrelia burgdorferi* in human synovial cells. *Rheumatol Int* 1996;16:125–132.
105. Chary-Valckenaere I, Jaulhac B, Champigneulle J, et al. Ultrastructural demonstration of intracellular localization of *Borrelia burgdorferi* in Lyme arthritis [Letter]. *Br J Rheumatol* 1998;37:468–470.
106. Sigal LH. Cross-reactivity between *Borrelia burgdorferi* flagellin and a human axonal 64,000 molecular weight protein. *J Infect Dis* 1993;167:1372–1378.
107. Martin R, Ortlauf J, Sticht-Groh V, et al. *Borrelia burgdorferi: specific and autoreactive T-cell lines from cerebrospinal fluid in Lyme radiculomyelitis.* Ann Neurol 1988;24:509–516.
108. Shanafelt MC, Hindersson P, Soderberg C, et al. T cell and antibody reactivity with the *Borrelia burgdorferi* 60-kDa heat shock protein in Lyme arthritis. *J Immunol* 1991;146:3985–3992.
109. Steere AC, Levin RE, Molloy PJ, et al. Treatment of Lyme arthritis. *Arthritis Rheum* 1994;37:878–888.
110. Lengl-Janssen B, Strauss AF, Steere AC, et al. The T helper cell response in Lyme arthritis: differential recognition of *Borrelia burgdorferi* outer surface protein A in patients with treatment-resistant or treatment-responsive Lyme arthritis. *J Exp Med* 1994;180:2069–2078.
111. Gross DM, Forsthuber T, Tary-Lehmann M, et al. Identification of LFA-1 as a candidate autoantigen in treatment- resistant Lyme arthritis. *Science* 1998;281:703–706.
112. Steere AC. Musculoskeletal features of Lyme disease. In: Rahn DW, Evans J, eds. *Lyme disease.* Philadelphia: American College of Physicians, 1998:107–122.
113. Schmid GP. The global distribution of Lyme disease. *Rev Infect Dis* 1985;7:41–50.
114. Dekonenko EJ, Steere AC, Berardi VP, et al. Lyme borreliosis in the Soviet Union: a cooperative US-USSR report. *J Infect Dis* 1988;158:748–753.
115. Burgdorfer W. Vector/host relationships of the Lyme disease spirochete, *Borrelia burgdorferi. Rheum Dis Clin North Am* 1989;15:775–787.
116. Dennis DT. Epidemiology, ecology, and prevention of Lyme disease. In: Rahn DW, Evans J, eds. *Lyme disease.* Philadelphia: American College of Physicians, 1998:7–34.
117. Burgdorfer W, Lane RS, Barbour AG, et al. The western black-legged tick, *Ixodes pacificus: a vector of* Borrelia burgdorferi. *Am J Trop Med Hyg* 1985;34:925–930.
118. Oliver JH Jr, Owsley MR, Hutcheson HJ, et al. Conspecificity of the ticks *Ixodes scapularis* and *I. dammini* (Acari: Ixodidae). *J Med Entomol* 1993;30:54–63.
119. Schulze TL, Bowen GS, Bosler EM, et al. *Amblyomma americanum: a potential vector of Lyme disease in New Jersey.* Science 1984;224:601–603.
120. Magnarelli LA, Anderson JF, Apperson CS, et al. Spirochetes in ticks and antibodies to *Borrelia burgdorferi* in white-tailed deer from Connecticut, New York State, and North Carolina. *J Wildl Dis* 1986;22:178–188.
121. Magnarelli LA, Anderson JF, Barbour AG. The etiologic agent of Lyme disease in deer flies, horse flies, and mosquitoes. *J Infect Dis* 1986;154:355–358.

122. Luger SW. Lyme disease transmitted by a biting fly [Letter]. *N Engl J Med* 1990;322:1752.
123. Spielman A, Wilson ML, Levine JF, et al. Ecology of *Ixodes dammini*-borne human babesiosis and Lyme disease. *Annu Rev Entomol* 1985;30:439–460.
124. Mather TN, Wilson ML, Moore SI, et al. Comparing the relative potential of rodents as reservoirs of the Lyme disease spirochete (*Borrelia burgdorferi*). *Am J Epidemiol* 1989;130:143–150.
125. Brown RN, Lane RS. Lyme disease in California: a novel enzootic transmission cycle of *Borrelia burgdorferi. Science* 1992; 256:1439–1442.
126. Maupin GO, Gage KL, Piesman J, et al. Discovery of an enzootic cycle of *Borrelia burgdorferi* in *Neotoma mexicana* and *Ixodes spinipalpis* from northern Colorado, an area where Lyme disease is nonendemic. *J Infect Dis* 1994;170:636–643.
127. Bosler EM, Coleman JL, Benach JL, et al. Natural distribution of the *Ixodes dammini* spirochete. *Science* 1983;220:321–322.
128. Magnarelli LA, Anderson JF, Burgdorfer W, et al. Parasitism by *Ixodes dammini* (Acari: Ixodidae) and antibodies to spirochetes in mammals at Lyme disease foci in Connecticut, USA. *J Med Entomol* 1984;21:52–57.
129. Anderson JF, Johnson RC, Magnarelli LA, et al. Identification of endemic foci of Lyme disease: isolation of *Borrelia burgdorferi* from feral rodents and ticks (*Dermacentor variabilis*). *J Clin Microbiol* 1985;22:36–38.
130. Kornblatt AN, Urband PH, Steere AC. Arthritis caused by *Borrelia burgdorferi* in dogs. *J Am Vet Med Assoc* 1985;186:960–964.
131. Anderson JF, Johnson RC, Magnarelli LA, et al. Involvement of birds in the epidemiology of the Lyme disease agent *Borrelia burgdorferi. Infect Immun* 1986;51:394–396.
132. Persing DH, Telford SR III, Rys PN, Dodge DE, White TJ, Malawista SE, Spielman A. Detection of *Borrelia burgdorferi* DNA in museum specimens of *Ixodes dammini* ticks. *Science* 1990;249:1420–1423.
133. Marshall WF III, Telford SR III, Rys PN, Rutledge BJ, Mathiesen D, Malawista SE, Spielman A, Persing DH. Detection of *Borrelia burgdorferi* DNA in museum specimens of *Peromyscus leucopus. J Infect Dis* 1994;170:1027–1032.
134. Steere AC, Taylor E, Wilson ML, et al. Longitudinal assessment of the clinical and epidemiological features of Lyme disease in a defined population. *J Infect Dis* 1986;154:295–300.
135. Shapiro ED, Gerber MA, Holabird NB, et al. A controlled trial of antimicrobial prophylaxis for Lyme disease after deer-tick bites. *N Engl J Med* 1992;327:1769–1773.
136. Ginsberg H. *Ecology and environmental management of Lyme disease.* Newark, NJ: Rutgers University Press, 1993:126–156.
137. Hanrahan JP, Benach JL, Coleman JL, et al. Incidence and cumulative frequency of endemic Lyme disease in a community. *J Infect Dis* 1984;150:489–496.
138. Gerber MA, Shapiro ED, Burke GS, et al. Lyme disease in children in southeastern Connecticut: Pediatric Lyme Disease Study Group [see comments]. *N Engl J Med* 1996;335:1270–1274.
139. Berger BW, Johnson RC, Kodner C, et al. Cultivation of *Borrelia burgdorferi* from erythema migrans lesions and perilesional skin. *J Clin Microbiol* 1992;30:359–361.
140. Kuiper H, van Dam AP, Spanjaard L, et al. Isolation of *Borrelia burgdorferi* from biopsy specimens taken from healthy-looking skin of patients with Lyme borreliosis. *J Clin Microbiol* 1994; 32:715–720.
141. Garcia-Monco JC, Villar BF, Alen JC, et al. *Borrelia burgdorferi* in the central nervous system: experimental and clinical evidence for early invasion. *J Infect Dis* 1990;161:1187–1193.
142. Luft BJ, Steinman CR, Neimark HC, et al. Invasion of the central nervous system by *Borrelia burgdorferi* in acute disseminated infection [published erratum appears in *JAMA* 1992;268:872]. *JAMA* 1992;267:1364–1367.
143. Asbrink E, Olsson I. Clinical manifestations of erythema chronicum migrans Afzelius in 161 patients: a comparison with Lyme disease. *Acta Derm Venereol* 1985;65:43–52.
144. Clark JR, Carlson RD, Sasaki CT, et al. Facial paralysis in Lyme disease. *Laryngoscope* 1985;95:1341–1345.
145. Ackermann R, Rehse-Kupper B, Gollmer E, et al. Chronic neurologic manifestations of erythema migrans borreliosis. *Ann N Y Acad Sci* 1988;539:16–23.
146. Keller TL, Halperin JJ, Whitman M. PCR detection of *Borrelia burgdorferi* DNA in cerebrospinal fluid of Lyme neuroborreliosis patients. *Neurology* 1992;42:32–42.
147. Reik L Jr, Smith L, Khan A, et al. Demyelinating encephalopathy in Lyme disease. *Neurology* 1985;35:267–269.
148. Ackermann R, Gollmer E, Rehse-Kupper B. [Progressive Borrelia encephalomyelitis: chronic manifestation of erythema chronicum migrans disease of the nervous system]. *Dtsch Med Wochenschr* 1985;110:1039–1042.
149. de Koning J, Hoogkamp-Korstanje JA, van der Linde MR, et al. Demonstration of spirochetes in cardiac biopsies of patients with Lyme disease. *J Infect Dis* 1989;160:150–153.
150. Stanek G, Klein J, Bittner R, et al. Isolation of *Borrelia burgdorferi* from the myocardium of a patient with longstanding cardiomyopathy. *N Engl J Med* 1990;322:249–252.
151. McAlister HF, Klementowicz PT, Andrews C, et al. Lyme carditis: an important cause of reversible heart block. *Ann Intern Med* 1989;110:339–345.
152. Persing DH, Rutledge BJ, Rys PN, Podzorski DS, Mitchell PD, Reed KD, Liu B, Fikrig E, Malawista SE. Target imbalance: disparity of *Borrelia burgdorferi* genetic material in synovial fluid from Lyme arthritis patients. *J Infect Dis* 1994;169:668–672.
153. Nocton JJ, Dressler F, Rutledge BJ, et al. Detection of *Borrelia burgdorferi* DNA by polymerase chain reaction in synovial fluid from patients with Lyme arthritis. *N Engl J Med* 1994330 229–234.
154. Bradley JF, Johnson RC, Goodman JL. The persistence of spirochetal nucleic acids in active Lyme arthritis. *Ann Intern Med* 1994;120:487–489.
155. Kalish RA, Leong JM, Steere AC. Association of treatment-resistant chronic Lyme arthritis with HLA-DR4 and antibody reactivity to OspA and OspB of *Borrelia burgdorferi. Infect Immun* 1993;61:2774–2779.
156. Kaufman LD, Gruber BL, Phillips ME, et al. Late cutaneous Lyme disease: acrodermatitis chronica atrophicans. *Am J Med* 1989;86:828–830.
157. Canica MM, Nato F, du Merle L, et al. Monoclonal antibodies for identification of *Borrelia afzelii* sp. nov. associated with late cutaneous manifestations of Lyme borreliosis. *Scand J Infect Dis* 1993;25:441–448.
158. Masters E, Granter S, Duray P, et al. Physician-diagnosed erythema migrans and erythema migrans-like rashes following Lone Star tick bites. *Arch Dermatol* 1998;134:955–960.
159. Barbour AG, Maupin GO, Teltow GJ, et al. Identification of an uncultivable Borrelia species in the hard tick *Amblyomma americanum: possible agent of a Lyme disease-like illness.* J Infect Dis 1996;173:403–409.
160. Craft JE, Grodzicki RL, Steere AC. Antibody response in Lyme disease: evaluation of diagnostic tests. *J Infect Dis* 1984;149: 789–795.
161. Schwartz BS, Goldstein MD, Ribeiro JM, et al. Antibody testing in Lyme disease: a comparison of results in four laboratories [see comments]. *JAMA* 1989;262:3431–3434.
162. Luger SW, Krauss E. Serologic tests for Lyme disease: interlaboratory variability. *Arch Intern Med* 1990;150:761–763.
163. Magnarelli LA, Miller JN, Anderson JF, et al. Cross-reactivity of nonspecific treponemal antibody in serologic tests for Lyme disease. *J Clin Microbiol* 1990;28:1276–1279.

164. Lightfoot RW Jr, Luft BJ, Rahn DW, et al. Empiric parenteral antibiotic treatment of patients with fibromyalgia and fatigue and a positive serologic result for Lyme disease: a cost-effectiveness analysis [see comments]. *Ann Intern Med* 1993;119:503–509.
165. Britton MC, Gardner P, Kaufman RL. Appropriateness of parenteral antibiotic treatment for patients with presumed Lyme disease: a joint statement of the American College of Rheumatology and the Council of the Infectious Diseases Society of America [Comment]. *Ann Intern Med* 1993;119:518.
166. Sigal LH. Pitfalls in the diagnosis and management of Lyme disease. *Arthritis Rheum* 1998;41:195–204.
167. Dressler F, Whalen JA, Reinhardt BN, et al. Western blotting in the serodiagnosis of Lyme disease. *J Infect Dis* 1993;167:392–400.
168. Dattwyler RJ, Volkman DJ, Luft BJ, et al. Seronegative Lyme disease: dissociation of specific T- and B-lymphocyte responses to *Borrelia burgdorferi*. *N Engl J Med* 1988;319:1441–1446.
169. Halperin JJ, Krupp LB, Golightly MG, et al. Lyme borreliosis-associated encephalopathy. *Neurology* 1990;40:1340–1343.
170. Pachner AR, Delaney E. The polymerase chain reaction in the diagnosis of Lyme neuroborreliosis. *Ann Neurol* 1993;34:544–550.
171. Zoschke DC, Skemp AA, Defosse DL. Lymphoproliferative responses to *Borrelia burgdorferi* in Lyme disease. *Ann Intern Med* 1991;114:285–289.
172. Horowitz HW, Dworkin B, Forseter G, et al. Liver function in early Lyme disease. *Hepatology* 1996;23:1412–1417.
173. Goodman JL, Nelson C, Vitale B, et al. Direct cultivation of the causative agent of human granulocytic ehrlichiosis [see comments] [published erratum appears in *N Engl J Med* 1996; 335:361]. *N Engl J Med* 1996;334:209–215.
174. Nadelman RB, Horowitz HW, Hsieh TC, et al. Simultaneous human granulocytic ehrlichiosis and Lyme borreliosis. *N Engl J Med* 1997;337:27–30.
175. Krause PJ, Telford SR III, Spielman A, et al. Concurrent Lyme disease and babesiosis: evidence for increased severity and duration of illness. *JAMA* 1996;275:1657–1660.
176. Dinerman H, Steere A. Fibromyalgia following Lyme disease: association with neurologic involvement and lack of response to antibiotic therapy. *Arthritis Rheum* 1990;33:S136.
177. Hsu VM, Patella SJ, Sigal LH. "Chronic Lyme disease" as the incorrect diagnosis in patients with fibromyalgia [see comments]. *Arthritis Rheum* 1993;36:1493–1500.
178. Sigal LH. Summary of the first 100 patients seen at a Lyme disease referral center. *Am J Med* 1990;88:577–581.
179. Steere AC, Taylor E, McHugh GL, et al. The overdiagnosis of Lyme disease. *JAMA* 1993;269:1812–1816.
180. Shadick NA, Phillips CB, Logigian EL, et al. The long-term clinical outcomes of Lyme disease: a population-based retrospective cohort study. *Ann Intern Med* 1994;121:560–567.
181. Massarotti EM, Luger SW, Rahn DW, et al. Treatment of early Lyme disease. *Am J Med* 1992;92:396–403.
182. Dattwyler RJ, Volkman DJ, Conaty SM, et al. Amoxycillin plus probenecid versus doxycycline for treatment of erythema migrans borreliosis. *Lancet* 1990;336:1404–1406.
183. Dattwyler RJ, Luft BJ, Kunkel MJ, et al. Ceftriaxone compared with doxycycline for the treatment of acute disseminated Lyme disease. *N Engl J Med* 1997;337:289–294.
184. Pfister HW, Preac-Mursic V, Wilske B, et al. Latent Lyme neuroborreliosis: presence of *Borrelia burgdorferi* in the cerebrospinal fluid without concurrent inflammatory signs. *Neurology* 1989;39:1118–1120.
185. Shrestha M, Grodzicki RL, Steere AC. Diagnosing early Lyme disease. *Am J Med* 1985;78:235–240.
186. Aguero-Rosenfeld ME, Nowakowski J, McKenna DF, et al. Serodiagnosis in early Lyme disease [published erratum appears in *J Clin Microbiol* 1994;32:860]. *J Clin Microbiol* 1993;31: 3090–3095.
187. Nadelman RB, Luger SW, Frank E, et al. Comparison of cefuroxime axetil and doxycycline in the treatment of early Lyme disease. *Ann Intern Med* 1992;117:273–280.
188. Luft BJ, Dattwyler RJ, Johnson RC, et al. Azithromycin compared with amoxicillin in the treatment of erythema migrans: a double-blind, randomized, controlled trial [see comments]. *Ann Intern Med* 1996;124:785–791.
189. Markowitz LE, Steere AC, Benach JL, et al. Lyme disease during pregnancy. *JAMA* 1986;255:3394–3396.
190. Strobino BA, Williams CL, Abid S, et al. Lyme disease and pregnancy outcome: a prospective study of two thousand prenatal patients. *Am J Obstet Gynecol* 1993;169:367–374.
191. Rahn D, Malawista S. *Treatment of Lyme disease.* St. Louis: Mosby, 1994.
192. Dattwyler RJ, Halperin JJ, Volkman DJ, et al. Treatment of late Lyme borreliosis: randomised comparison of ceftriaxone and penicillin. *Lancet* 1988;1:1191–1194.
193. Pfister HW, Preac-Mursic V, Wilske B, et al. Cefotaxime vs penicillin G for acute neurologic manifestations in Lyme borreliosis: a prospective randomized study. *Arch Neurol* 1989;46: 1190–1194.
194. Dotevall L, Alestig K, Hanner P, et al. The use of doxycycline in nervous system *Borrelia burgdorferi* infection. *Scand J Infect Dis Suppl* 1988;53:74–79.
195. Logigian EL, Kaplan RF, Steere AC. Successful treatment of Lyme ancephalopathy with intravenous ceftriaxons. *J Infect Dis* 1999;180:377–383.
196. Centers for Disease Control and Prevention. Ceftriaxone-associated biliary complications of treatment of suspected disseminated Lyme disease—New Jersey, 1990-1992. *JAMA* 1993;269: 979–980.
197. Malawista SE, Barthold SW, Persing DH. Fate of *Borrelia burgdorferi* DNA in tissues of infected mice after antibiotic treatment [see comments]. *J Infect Dis* 1994;170:1312–1316.
198. Schoen RT, Aversa JM, Rahn DW, et al. Treatment of refractory chronic Lyme arthritis with arthroscopic synovectomy. *Arthritis Rheum* 1991;34:1056–1060.
199. Aberer E, Breier F, Stanek G, et al. Success and failure in the treatment of acrodermatitis chronica atrophicans. *Infection* 1996;24:85–87.
200. Magid D, Schwartz B, Craft J, et al. Prevention of Lyme disease after tick bites: a cost-effectiveness analysis. *N Engl J Med* 1992; 327:534–541.
201. Lovrich SD, Callister SM, Lim LC, et al. Seroprotective groups of Lyme borreliosis spirochetes from North America and Europe. *J Infect Dis* 1994;170:115–121.

130

VIRAL ARTHRITIS

STANLEY J. NAIDES

The immune response serves to protect the host from external attack by infectious agents and regulates itself to avoid self-annihilation. Failure to differentiate self from foreign antigens may result in autoimmunity. The ability of viruses to subvert the immune system's surveillance to become persistent in the host, and the ability of viral genes to interact with host cell regulatory systems, render viruses attractive etiologic candidates for various idiopathic diseases. Autoimmune or autoimmune-like responses to known infections further fuels speculation that viruses may act as etiologic agents or triggers in some rheumatic disease. Arthralgias and frank arthritis are often features of known viral infections. For example, Togaviruses regularly cause epidemics of acute febrile arthritis affecting thousands of individuals. In some individuals, acute illness becomes prolonged or chronic. Whether viral arthritis results from a single initial event during acute infection that modifies the immune response, which leads to molecular mimicry with breaking of tolerance (1), or rather an ongoing interaction between virus and the immune system is required for chronic disease remains to be determined. Viral latency suggests that triggering virus may play a role in perpetuating disease. Given chronic exposure to virus or viral antigen, the immune response may broaden to target self-antigen through epitope spreading (2). Alternatively, virus may interact with host cell regulatory genes to alter growth patterns or eliminate cell populations through cytopathic effects or induction of apoptosis. Selective enhancement or elimination of target populations could lead to immune dysregulation. Immune responses to specific pathogens may not be narrowly targeted, causing nonspecific immune-mediated destruction of host tissues. Describing the mechanisms by which specific viruses cause arthritis may provide insights into mechanisms of idiopathic disease as well as identify specific etiologic agents for subsets of idiopathic autoimmune disease.

PARVOVIRUS B19

Virology

Human parvovirus B19 was discovered in 1975 in a human serum coded "number 19, panel B" used as a control for hepatitis B surface antigen (HBsAg) testing (3,4). An antigen with nonidentity to HBsAg was detected on Ouchterlony gels (5). Electron microscopy of the serum revealed spherical virions and empty shells typical of the Parvoviridae. Parvo derives from the Latin *parvus,* meaning small. In the current Sixth Report of the International Committee on Taxonomy of Viruses, the family Parvoviridae, comprising small, nonenveloped, single-stranded DNA viruses, is composed of two subfamilies, Parvovirinae and Densovirinae. Parvovirinae comprises three genera: *Parvovirus, Erythrovirus,* and *Dependovirus* (6). The *Erythrovirus* genus consists of those members of the family that replicate autonomously in erythroid mammalian host cells, and cause "red" rashes. The genus *Dependovirus* consists of those members of the family that require the presence of a helper virus, such as adenovirus or herpesvirus, to replicate and include the adeno-associated viruses (AAVs) used as gene therapy vectors.

B19 icosahedral particles may appear as intact or hollow spherical particles on electron microscopy. The B19 genome is a 5.6-kb, single-stranded DNA molecule characterized by imperfect palindromes at both the 3′ and 5′ ends, which form terminal hairpin loops (7–9). The 3′ terminus allows self-priming during viral DNA replication (10–12). B19 packages both positive and negative sense DNA strands in equal numbers, but only a single genome copy is enclosed per capsid. B19 integration into host genome has not been demonstrated to date. B19 uses a single strong promoter, which initiates transcription of both a left-handed, nonstructural protein gene, and a right-handed structural gene region (13). The nonstructural protein, NS1, is a helicase of approximately 74,000 daltons (14–16). Because B19 replicates using a modified rolling hairpin model characteristic of the autonomous parvoviruses; monomeric and dimeric replicative forms generated during replication containing two and four copies, respectively, of progeny strands are reduced by NS1 to a packagable genome (17). NS1 may play a role in assembly of viral DNA into mature viral capsids, as it may be found covalently bound to intact virions (18). It is suspected that NS1 may also cut host DNA and/or upregulate cellular gene expression [e.g., interleukin-6 (IL-6) and tumor necrosis factor-α (TNF-α)] (19,20). Mutations in the nucleotide-binding domain of NS1 prevent NS1-associated cell toxicity (21). Anti-NS1 antibodies have been reported in chronic B19 arthropathy, but sensitivity and specificity for arthropathy have been questioned (22,23).

Structural proteins VP1 and VP2 are 84,000 and 58,000 daltons, respectively (15,16). Both structural proteins are encoded in the same open reading frame, but VP2 transcription is initiated at an alternate downstream splice site (24). Therefore, VP1 and VP2 are identical except for the N-terminal 227 amino acids of VP1. Precipitation of recombinant empty B19 capsids containing VP1 and VP2, as well as whole infectious virions, by antibody to unique VP1 region fusion protein suggests that the unique VP1 region is exposed on the external surface of the virion. The ability of antibodies to the unique N-terminal portion of VP1 to neutralize B19 replication in bone marrow suspension cultures suggests that this region of VP1 plays a role in cell attachment and cell entry (25). The receptor for B19 consists of the P blood group antigen, or globoside (Gb4), and related neutral glycosphingolipids (26,27). Gb4 is the major constituent of erythrocyte plasma membranes, as well as a component of cell membranes in other tissues (27, 28). B19, like other parvoviruses, replicates and assembles in the cell nucleus. Identification of intranuclear inclusions around the inner aspect of the nuclear membrane with condensation of chromatin material seen on examination of bone marrow or other tissues suggests the possibility of B19 infection (29–32).

Epidemiology

Experimental infections in normal volunteers helped define the natural history of B19 infection (33). B19 viremic plasma was inoculated into the nostrils of seronegative normal volunteers. Virus was detected in serum after 6 days and peaked on days 8 and 9 after inoculation. B19 DNA could be detected in nasal and oropharyngeal secretions during viremia. Shedding in urine or feces did not occur. Viremia cleared with the appearance of high-titer anti-B19 IgM antibody on days 11 to 12 after inoculation, and anti-B19 IgG antibody appeared by the end of the second week after inoculation, or shortly thereafter. Subjects with preexistent anti-B19 antibodies usually did not develop viremia, except for one individual with trace amounts of anti-B19 IgG before inoculation; he developed a transient low-titer IgM response and increased levels of anti-B19 IgG antibody. None of the volunteers with significant titers of preinoculation anti-B19 IgG developed anti-B19 IgM. The resulting illness was biphasic. Although some subjects were asymptomatic during the viremia, others had a flu-like illness with malaise, myalgia, transient fever, headache, pruritus, and/or chills. Onset of anti-B19 IgM antibody was associated with clearance of viremia and a second phase of illness characterized by rash, arthralgia, and arthritis. Hemoglobin also decreased, but the decrease in hemoglobin was not clinically significant in these normal individuals. Neutropenia, lymphopenia, and thrombocytopenia occurred in several subjects. Absolute areticulocytosis occurred from peak viremia until several days after appearance of IgM antibody, after which there was a rebound reticulocytosis.

In natural infection, the usual incubation period until onset of symptoms ranges from 6 to 18 days. Individuals are infectious during viremia when they shed virus in nasal and oral secretions. As onset of rash, arthralgia, or arthritis is temporally associated with the appearance of anti-B19 IgM antibody, which clears viremia, most patients seen by the rheumatologist for rash or joint symptoms will no longer be infectious. Anti-B19 IgM antibody may be present for up to 2 to 3 months after an acute infection, but declines thereafter. Thus there is a brief window of opportunity in which to make a diagnosis of B19 infection by IgM serology. Anti-B19 IgG antibody response is long-lived but is usually not diagnostically helpful, because seroprevalence in the adult population ranges between 40% to 80%. Individuals begin acquiring anti-B19 IgG antibody after entering school, when their risk of exposure to infected children increases (34).

B19 infection is common and geographically widespread. A large proportion of B19 infections in community outbreaks remain asymptomatic or as undiagnosed nonspecific viral illnesses (35–37). Outbreaks occur in late winter and spring, although epidemics have also been reported in summer and fall. In a given community, outbreaks tend to cycle every 3 to 5 years, representing the interval between accumulation in local schools of fresh cohorts of susceptible children. Because the seroprevalence of anti-B19 IgG antibodies is only approximately 50% in adults, outbreaks often involve susceptible adults as well. The risk of infection in adults with multiple exposures may be as high as 50% (38). School teachers, day-care workers, hospital personnel, and others with frequent occupational exposure to children have increased risk of infection (38,39). Sporadic cases occur between outbreaks. Transmission is presumed to be through respiratory tract secretions.

Clinical Features

Both common and less common presentations of B19 infection are listed in Table 130.1. Transient aplastic crisis was the first clinical syndrome associated with B19 infection (40). Transient aplastic crisis is a well-known entity first described in 1950 as an acute decrease in hemoglobin associated with cessation of reticulocyte production in chronic hemolytic anemia. The areticulocytosis associated with the viremic phase of B19 infection renders the patient with a variety of chronic hemolytic anemias unable to maintain baseline hemoglobin and hematocrit levels in the

TABLE 130.1. CLINICAL PRESENTATIONS OF B19 INFECTION[a]

Common
Asymptomatic infection
Transient aplastic crisis
Erythema infectiosum
Hydrops fetalis
Acute and chronic arthropathy
Chronic or recurrent bone marrow suppression in immunocompromised hosts
Less common
Skin
Vesiculopustular eruption
Henoch–Schönlein purpura
Thrombotic thrombocytopenic purpura
"Gloves and socks" syndrome
Hematologic
Anemia
Thrombocytopenia
Leukopenia
Benign acute lymphadenopathy
Hemophagocytic syndrome
Vasculitis
Polyarteritis nodosa
Wegener's granulomatosis
Liver
Hepatocellular enzyme elevations
Non-A, non-B, non-C fulminant liver failure
Nervous system
Parasthesias
Meningitis
Sensorineural hearing loss

[a]Additional clinical presentations attributed to B19 are discussed in the text.

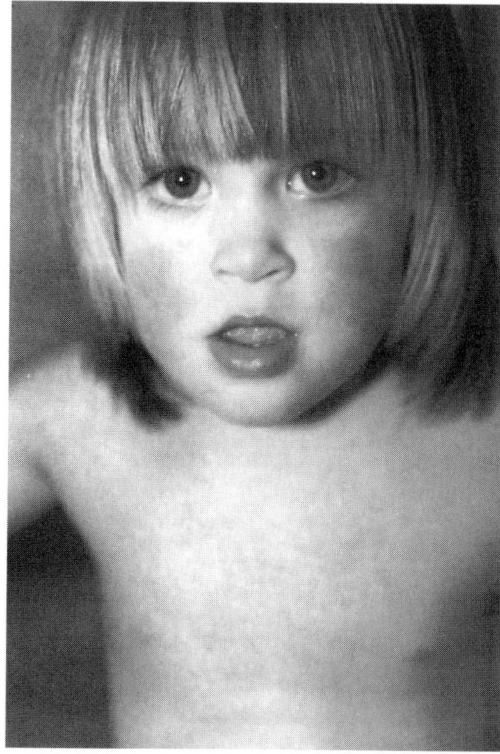

FIGURE 130.1. Classic "slapped cheeks" of a child with erythema infectiosum, or fifth disease, caused by parvovirus B19. A lacy macular erythematous eruption also is present on the trunk but not in focus. (From Feder HM Jr. Fifth disease. *N Engl J Med* 1994;331:1062, with permission.)

face of chronic peripheral destruction of erythrocytes (40–67). Erythrocyte growth arrest in these patients occurs at the giant pronormoblast stage of development. Marginal intranuclear inclusions may be seen in these cells (30,68–70). In immunocompromised patients, B19 infection may become persistent and lead to chronic or recurrent episodes of anemia, leukopenia, and/or thrombocytopenia (71–80). B19-induced thrombocytopenia and leukopenia presumably result from nonpermissive infection in precursors in these two hematopoietic lineages (81). B19 infection is the leading cause of pure red cell aplasia in patients with acquired immunodeficiency syndrome (74).

Healthy children may have erythema infectiosum, or fifth disease, as enumerated among major childhood rash illnesses at the end of the nineteenth century. Anderson et al. (82) first associated B19 with erythema infectiosum during a typical outbreak in a North London school. Approximately 85% of the children had bright red "slapped cheeks," the classic facial rash of erythema infectiosum (Fig. 130.1). The rash may occur on the torso and extremities as an erythematous, lacy or reticular, macular or maculopapular eruption (82,83). It rarely causes a vesicular or hemorrhagic eruption (84). Pruritus occurs in approximately 50% of the patients. A majority of children have recurrent rash, with sun exposure, hot bath, or physical activity, lasting weeks or months after infection. Constitutional symptoms, when they do occur, tend to be mild in children, and include fever, headache, sore throat, cough, anorexia, vomiting, diarrhea, and arthralgia. Recurrent rash is not associated with recurrent viremia or viral shedding, and children are not infectious during the recurrent rash or in the interval between eruptions (36,84–95). In susceptible adults, the rash tends to be subtler than in children, or is absent. Constitutional and articular symptoms in adults tend to be more severe, often occurring as a flu-like illness with prominent arthralgias and joint swellings. Adults also may have sudden-onset polyarthralgias/polyarthritis, without rash or flu-like prodrome. Ager et al. (96) described an outbreak of erythema infectiosum in 1961 through 1962 in Port Angeles, Washington. Diagnosis was made on the basis of a typical rash. Arthralgia was reported in 5.1%, and joint swelling in 2.8% of children younger than 10 years; in 11.5% and 5.3%, respectively, in adolescents; but in 77.2% and 59.6%, respectively, in adults 20 years or older (96).

White et al. (97) demonstrated that B19 could cause a chronic rheumatoid-like arthropathy. Nineteen of 153 patients with "early synovitis" tested retrospectively had anti-B19 IgM antibodies in acute phase sera. Although approximately one third of the cohort were men, all 19 patients with evidence of B19 infection were women, reflecting a female predominance. Typically, patients have acute, moderately severe, symmetric polyarthritis. Only a few joints may be involved initially, but additional joints become involved within 24 to 48 hours, demonstrating a rheumatoid pattern, including the finger proximal interphalangeal joints, metacarpophalangeal joints, wrists, elbows, shoulders, feet, ankles, knees, and hips. Cervical spine, occasionally, and lumbosacral spine, rarely, are affected. Patients complain of joint pain, stiffness, and variable swelling. Joint symptoms may last for a few days to weeks, usually improving within 2 weeks. In the initial report of White et al. (97), only two of 19 patients experienced complete resolution. The remaining 17 patients had symptoms for longer than 2 months, and 3 for more than 4 years. Two thirds had episodic flares with worsening of morning stiffness and joint pain, but remained symptomatic between flares. One third had episodic flares, but were symptom free between flares. Subsequent case reports and series described a similar pattern of joint involvement in adults (98–101).

Despite the clinical similarity to rheumatoid arthritis (RA) in terms of distribution and symmetry of joint involvement and the occurrence of morning stiffness, patients with documented acute anti-B19 IgM antibody and arthropathy followed up over time do not develop marginal erosions, joint destruction, or rheumatoid nodules, except for the occasional case report in which concurrent classic, seropositive erosive RA cannot be ruled out (97,100–102). About 50% of patients whose symptoms become chronic meet American Rheumatism Association criteria for a diagnosis of RA (101,103,104). Patients typically have morning stiffness that lasts for more than an hour; symmetric involvement of proximal interphalangeal, metacarpophalangeal, and wrist joints; and at least three hand joints involved. Usually the entire proximal interphalangeal and metacarpophalangeal joint tier is involved (101,104,105). Transient expression of low to moderate titer autoantibodies during acute infection, including rheumatoid factor, anti-DNA, antilymphocyte, and antinuclear antibodies may suggest seropositive RA or systemic lupus erythematosus (106–108). Although an initial report suggested that chronic B19 arthropathy may be associated with human leukocyte antigen (HLA) DR4 positivity, as in classic erosive RA, subsequent studies by the same group demonstrated no increased association with DR4 (109,110). Absence of rheumatoid nodules and joint destruction in B19 arthropathy helps differentiate B19 disease from classic, erosive RA (103). Serologic surveys of RA populations for evidence of B19 virus or increased prevalence of anti-B19 IgG antibody have not demonstrated a role for B19 in classic RA (111–117). Chronic B19 arthropathy patients followed up over time do not develop thickened synovium (101). Arthroscopic examination of knee joints of patients with chronic B19 arthropathy identified B19 DNA in synovium but did not detect morphologic or histologic changes (118). In the absence of inflammation in B19 arthropathy, direct viral effects on joint tissues is an attractive alternative mechanism for joint symptoms. The presence of chronic synovial inflammation or thickening in a patient with previously documented B19 infection should lead to consideration of a second concurrent process to account for synovitis. The clinical presentation of B19 arthropathy may suggest a diagnosis of early classic RA, either seropositive or seronegative for rheumatoid factor. Failure to obtain parvovirus B19 serology at initial presentation may leave the diagnostic IgM antibody response undetected and result in failure to diagnosis B19 arthropathy in those patients who subsequently have persistent joint symptoms. Transiently elevated serum liver enzymes, which may occur in acute B19 infection, may be incorrectly attributed to nonsteroidal antiinflammatory agents and militate against their use (119).

In immune-competent individuals with chronic B19 arthropathy, B19 DNA has been found in bone marrow aspirates and synovium (103,118,120). The diagnostic utility of detecting B19 DNA in tissues from patients with chronic arthritis suspected to have B19 arthropathy, however, is questionable because B19 DNA has also been detected by using sensitive nested polymerase chain reaction (PCR) techniques in synovium from healthy military recruits undergoing arthroscopy for trauma, suggesting that B19 may persist in a latent state even in healthy individuals (121). The difference between a virally induced disease state and asymptomatic carriage of a latent virus may depend on viral load and the interactions between virus and host. In adult fifth disease and chronic B19 arthropathy patients, IgG antibodies to the N-terminal of the VP1 capsid protein, known to contain neutralizing epitopes, are absent (122). Absence of neutralizing antibody to B19 may allow a greater B19 load during persistence. Antibodies to the NS1 nonstructural protein have been reported in some patients with chronic B19 arthropathy (123–125). However, anti-NS1 antibodies have not been consistently identified in chronic B19 arthropathy patients nor does the presence of anti-NS1 antibodies have any apparent effect on the course of B19 infection in pregnancy (23,125,126). It is more likely that the presence of anti-NS1 antibody reflects immune responses to either NS1 on the surface of B19 virions or NS1 liberated during cell death, rather than the antibodies themselves playing a pathogenic role. There is evidence to suggest that overexpression of B19 NS1 *in vitro* is cytotoxic (19,21). NS1 protein, however, could play a pathogenic role in perpetuating chronic B19 arthropathy through its interaction with cellular genes. NS1 has been shown to upregulate transcription, for example, of the IL-6 promotor and the HIV LTR in the presence of *tat* and an intact *tar* element (127,128). A recent study reported B19 DNA and proteins with a high prevalence in RA synovium and concluded that B19 was responsible for upregulation of IL-6 and TNF-α (20). These findings remain to be confirmed. NS1 induced apoptosis in erythroid series cells (129). NS1 also may induce apoptosis in liver-derived cells nonpermissive for B19 replication (130). Similar mechanisms in synoviocyte subpopulations might induce autoimmunity by disrupting normal patterns of cell interactions and intercellular regulation.

UNCOMMON MANIFESTATIONS OF B19 INFECTION

Rash in adults may include a vesiculopustular eruption with features of morbilliform and vesiculopustular lesions. Extravasation of erythrocytes into the dermis eventually gives the vesiculopustules a hemorrhagic appearance (84). Purpura or petechiae may be seen in the absence of thrombocytopenia, although some patients may have purpura or petechiae as a result of thrombocytopenia (131–135). Henoch–Schönlein purpura has also been described (136,137). A "gloves and socks" syndrome of acral erythema with sharp demarcation at the wrists and ankles, respectively, has been described and may include edema and pruritis of the affected parts. Resolution may occur with desquamation (138–141). This presentation is not specific for B19, as other viral infections also may trigger the gloves-and-socks syndrome (142–145).

Finger and toe paresthesias have been described, as has progressive arm weakness with mild slowing of nerve-conduction velocities and decreased amplitudes of motor and sensory potentials in brachial nerve plexes (146–149). Encephalopathy and aseptic meningitis may occur (71,150–152). Carpal tunnel syndrome can result from wrist swelling (153). B19 infection may trigger fibromyalgia, but this appears to represent a nonspecific viral trigger (154). There is no evidence that B19 causes chronic fatigue syndrome (155). B19 infection may occur as isolated neutropenia, thrombocytopenia, anemia, or as idiopathic thrombocytopenic purpura (131,132,156,157). Self-limited benign acute lymphadenopathy has been reported in one series (158), and several cases of hemophagocytic syndrome have been associated with B19 infection (159–162). Hemophagocytic syndrome in association with lymphadenopathy resembling necrotizing lymphadenitis (Kikuchi's disease) also has been seen (163). Transiently abnormal liver enzymes have been observed in healthy adults with acute B19 arthropathy, and in neonates surviving anemia and nonimmune hydrops secondary to B19 infection *in utero* (119,164). B19 infection has been associated with acute hepatitis and some cases of non-A, non-B, non-C acute fulminant liver failure with or without associated aplastic anemia (131,165–167). Associations of cutaneous vasculitis, polyarteritis nodosa, or Wegener's granulomatosis with B19 infection have been observed in small series (168–172). However, screening larger series of patients with polyarteritis nodosa or Wegener's granulomatosis for evidence of B19 infection has failed to demonstrate a significant prevalence of B19 infection (173,174). B19 infection may be misdiagnosed as new-onset systemic lupus erythematosus (175,176). Antiphospholipid antibodies, when seen in acute B19 infection, may have the same specificity and cofactor dependence as antiphospholipids associated with systemic lupus erythematosus (177). A role for B19 infection in juvenile rheumatoid arthritis (JRA) has been suggested, but the described monoarticular or pauciarticular presentation in the children is in contrast to the arthritis pattern in adults, suggesting that either the disease presentation in children is different, or age is a confounding factor in that JRA occurs at a time when children acquire B19 infection (178).

Diagnosis

Most patients with B19 arthropathy with recent-onset joint symptoms are anti-B19 IgM antibody positive (179,180). Both radioimmunoassays (RIAs) and enzyme-linked immunosorbent assays (ELISAs) have been used to detect B19 antigen and specific antibody to B19 capsid (34,101,181,182). Wild-type virus, recombinant viral capsid, fusion proteins, and peptides have been used as reagent antigens (34,94,101,134,181–197). The antibody-capture tests are highly sensitive and specific (34,101,181). Early reports of cross-reactivity between anti-B19 and antirubella antibodies were based on use of counter immunoelectrophoresis, but cross-reactivity has not been observed with RIA and ELISA methods (198–200). By using the antibody-capture ELISA with whole virus or recombinant empty capsid as an antigen source, tested in parallel with B19 virus–negative serum as a background control, we have failed to identify interference from rheumatoid factor or autoantibodies in sera from patients with systemic lupus erythematosus. Deoxyribonucleic acid (DNA) hybridization in dot-blot and Southern formats, PCR, and immune adherence PCR have all been used to detect B19 DNA in serum and tissues (76,166,183,201–208). Direct or PCR *in situ* hybridization has allowed morphologic characterization of infected tissues and cellular localization of viral DNA (209,210). Combinations of methods (e.g., hybridization, antibody capture, and peroxidase or luminescent labeling) allow amplification of detection signal and have been used in a number of research and diagnostic laboratories (211,212). Electron microscopy allows morphologic identification of B19 as well as species confirmation by immunoaggregation with specific antisera or by immunogold labeling, but is labor intensive and is not clinically practical (70,209,213).

Treatment

B19 persistence in chronic B19 arthropathy with a selective deficit in neutralizing antibodies would suggest that patients with chronic arthropathy may be treated with intravenous immunoglobulin, analogous to treatment of B19 persistence in more globally immunocompromised patients (74). A preliminary study of treatment of chronic B19 arthropathy patients with intravenous immunoglobulin, however, showed no long-term impact on B19 persistence or symptoms (214). As a nonenveloped virus, B19 is not removed by standard solvent detergent decontamination of pooled blood products (215–223). Assuming that repletion of anti-B19 neutralizing antibodies is adequate to clear a B19 infection may be too simplistic. Chronic mink infection with Aleutian disease virus, another autonomous parvovirus, is associated with persistent circulating immune complexes containing viral antigen. Passive antibody transfer to infected mink only exacerbates disease (224,225). Nonsteroidal antiinflammatory drugs appear adequate to control symptoms of chronic B19 arthropathy. Acetaminophen and low-dose tricyclic antidepressants may be useful adjuncts for pain control.

RUBELLA VIRUS

The Togaviridae family consists of spherical enveloped single-stranded positive sense RNA viruses. The Togaviridae family consists of two genera: rubiviruses and alphaviruses (226). Rubella virus is the sole member of the genus rubivirus. Rubella measures 50 to 70 nm in diameter with a 30-nm dense core (227). The envelope is acquired during budding at vesicles or the cell surface. Hemagglutinin activity is located in the spike-like projections on the envelope measuring 5 to 6 nm. The hemagglutinin mediates agglutination of erythrocytes from a variety of animal species (228).

Epidemiology

Rubella naturally infects only humans. Transmission is by nasopharyngeal secretions, with peak incidence in late winter and spring. Approximately 50% of rubella infections are subclinical (229–231). Before widespread rubella vaccination, infection occurred mostly in children in outbreaks occurring in 6- to 9-year cycles. With vaccination, young adults primarily are affected, but with risk of infection reduced to 10% to 20% of the pre–vaccine era risk (232,233).

The incubation period to onset of rash is 14 to 21 days (234). Viremia occurs 6 to 7 days before eruption, peaks immediately before eruption, and clears within 48 hours of the rash (235). Nasopharyngeal secretions may contain virus from 7 days before rash until 14 days after. Shedding is maximal just before onset of the rash until 5 to 6 days later (223,236).

Clinical Features

Clinical manifestations in children and adults range from asymptomatic infection to the classic syndrome of low-grade fever, rash, coryza, malaise, and prominent posterior cervical, postauricular, and occipital lymphadenopathy (223,236,237). Constitutional symptoms may precede rash by 5 days. The rash may first appear morbilliform on the face before spreading to the torso, and upper and then lower extremities over a 2- to 3-day period. The facial rash may clear as the extremities become involved. In some cases, the rash may be limited to a transient blush (223).

Joint symptoms are common in adults, especially women, occurring 1 week before or 1 week after onset of the rash. Joint involvement is usually symmetric. It may be migratory, resolving over a few days to 2 weeks. Arthralgias are more common than frank arthritis. Stiffness is prominent. The proximal interphalangeal joints, metacarpophalangeal joints, knees, wrists, ankles, and elbows are most frequently affected (238–242). Periarthritis, tenosynovitis, and carpal tunnel syndrome also occur. In some patients, symptoms may persist for several months or years (240–243).

Live attenuated vaccines have been used for rubella vaccination with a high frequency of postvaccination arthralgia, myalgia, arthritis, and neuropathies (244–250). The pattern of joint involvement is similar to that of natural infection. Arthritis usually occurs 2 weeks after inoculation and lasts less than a week. However, symptoms may persist in some patients for more than a year. HPV77 series and Cendehill vaccine strains were all found to have unacceptable levels of postvaccination arthralgia and arthritis (244–251). The currently used vaccine RA27/3 was thought to have a markedly reduced incidence of postvaccination joint symptoms, but more recent studies report joint symptoms in as many as 15% or more of recipients (251–254).

In children, two postvaccination neuropathic syndromes occur. In the "arm syndrome," a brachial radiculoneuropathy causes arm and hand pain and dysesthesias that are worse at night. The second syndrome is a lumbar radiculoneuropathy characterized by popliteal fossa pain on arising in the morning. Those affected assume a "catcher's crouch" position, hence the term catcher's crouch syndrome. The pain subsides through the day. Both syndromes occur 1 to 2 months after vaccination. The initial episode may last up to 2 months and may recur for up to 1 year, but recurrences are usually shorter in duration. There is no permanent damage (255).

Diagnosis

Rubella may be cultured from tissues and body fluids, including throat swabs (256). Antirubella IgM and IgG are usually positive at onset of joint symptoms (257–259). Because antirubella IgM antibody peaks 8 to 21 days after symptom onset and then wanes over the next 4 to 5 weeks, detection of antirubella IgM indicates recent infection, usually in the last 1 to 2 months (260). Antirubella IgG increases over days 7 to 21 after symptom onset. The presence of IgG in a single serum sample documents only immunity (261). Diagnosis based on IgG serology requires paired acute and convalescent sera.

Pathogenesis

Failure to mount an adequate immune response to specific epitopes may allow rubella virus to persist in patients with rubella arthritis (262–269). Virus can be detected in synovial fluid during arthritis flares and in lymphocytes years after symptom resolution (270,271). Onset of rash and arthritis is coincident with the appearance of antibodies, including neutralizing antibodies to whole virus, suggesting a role for antibody or immune complex deposition in synovitis (223).

Management

Nonsteroidal antiinflammatory agents are used for symptom control. Low to moderate doses of steroids have been used by some investigators to control symptoms and viremia (272).

HEPATITIS B VIRUS

Hepatitis B virus (HBV) is a member of the family Hepadnaviridae, genus Orthohepadnavirus. It is an enveloped icosahedral virus, measuring 42 nm in diameter. The genome is a double-stranded circular DNA with sections of single strandedness (273,274).

Epidemiology

HBV is transmitted by parenteral and sexual routes (275–277). HBV infection occurs worldwide, but the prevalence of hepatitis B surface antigen (Australian antigen) is higher in Asia, the Middle East, and sub-Sahara Africa. The prevalence in China may be as high as 10%, compared with 0.01% in the United States (278). Most acute infections in regions in which it is endemic occur asymptomatically at an early age, many perinatally from infected mothers. Childhood infection rates may be as high as 5% annually. Carriage rates and specific antibody gradually decline with advanced age. In industrialized countries, most infections occur in adulthood during sexual or needle exposures. Infection in adults is more often associated with acute hepatitis. Persistent infection follows acute hepatitis in 5% to 10%. HBV is a common cause of chronic liver disease and a leading cause of hepatocellular carcinoma in regions where it is endemic (279,280).

Clinical Features

The incubation period before hepatitis ranges from 45 to 120 days (280–283). Several days to a month before icterus appears, patients may experience fever, myalgia, malaise, anorexia, nausea, and vomiting. Significant viremia occurs early in infection; soluble immune complexes with circulating HBsAg are formed as anti–hepatitis B surface antigen antibodies (HBsAb) are produced. HBV-containing immune complexes cause sudden and often severe arthritis that is usually symmetric with simultaneous involvement of several joints, but arthritis may be migratory or additive. The small joints of the hands may have fusiform swelling. Knees often are involved. Wrists, ankles, elbows, shoulders, and other large joints may be affected as well. Morning stiffness is common. Arthritis and urticaria may precede jaundice by days to weeks and usually subside soon after the onset of clinical jaundice. However, in some patients, arthritis and rash may persist several weeks after the onset of jaundice (284–287). Patients in whom chronic active hepatitis or chronic HBV viremia develops may have recurrent arthralgias or arthritis (288). Polyarteritis nodosa (PAN) may be associated with chronic hepatitis B viremia (289).

Diagnosis

Urticaria in the presence of polyarthritis should raise the possibility of HBV infection. Acute hepatitis may be asymptomatic, but elevated bilirubin and transaminases are usually present when the arthritis appears. At the time of arthritis onset, peak levels of serum HBsAg are detectable. Virions, viral DNA, polymerase, and hepatitis B e antigen may be detectable in serum. IgM anti–hepatitis B core antigen antibodies are present and indicate acute HBV infection, as opposed to past or chronic infection (290–294). Joint fluid examination is not diagnostic.

Management

Management is limited to supportive measures including nonsteroidal antiinflammatory agents.

HEPATITIS C VIRUS

HCV is a member of the family Flaviviridae. HCV is an enveloped spherical virus measuring 38 to 50 nm in diameter. The genome is a single-stranded positive sense RNA (295).

Epidemiology

HCV occurs worldwide. Seroprevalence is highest in Africa and Asia, where it may cause 25% of acute and chronic hepatitis. In Japan, this figure may reach 50% (296). Estimates of carriage in the general population in the U.S. range from 2.7 to 4 million (297,298). HCV is transmitted by parenteral and sexual routes, although the latter may not be significant (299–302). HCV is responsible for 95% of posttransfusion hepatitis in countries routinely screening donated blood for HBV. More than 50% of all cases of non-A, non-B hepatitis are attributable to HCV infection (303). Eleven HCV genotypic variants exist and differ in their geographic distribution and pathogenicity, including severity of disease and response to interferon-α (IFN-α) (303,304).

Clinical Features

Acute HCV infection is usually benign, with up to 80% of posttransfusion infections being asymptomatic. Liver enzyme elevations, when present, are usually minimal (305–307). Patients in the community with jaundice represent acquired cases with more symptomatic illness and more significant enzyme elevations. Fulminant HCV hepatitis is rare (308). HCV is strongly associated with HBV-negative hepatocellular carcinoma, especially in Africa and Japan (309–312).

Acute-onset polyarthritis in a rheumatoid distribution, involving the small joints of the hand, wrists, shoulders, knees, and hips, has been reported in acute HCV infection (313,314). HCV infection is often associated with type II cryoglobulins and rheumatoid factor. Patients may have essential mixed cryoglobulinemia, a triad of arthritis, palpable purpura, and cryoglobulinemia. The majority of patients with essential mixed cryoglobulinemia have HCV infection (315,316). HCV infection also is seen in nonessential secondary cryoglobulinemia, although less commonly. The presence of anti-HCV antibodies in essential mixed cryoglobulinemia is associated with more severe cutaneous involvement (e.g., Raynaud's phenomena, purpura, livedo, distal ulcers, and gangrene). HCV RNA may be found in 75% of cryoprecipitates from patients with essential mixed cryoglobulinemia and anti-HCV antibodies (317). Cryoglobulinemia is discussed further in Chapters 70 and 82.

Diagnosis

Serologic tests use an array of antigens in an enzyme immunoassay. A recombinant strip immunoblot assay (RIBA) is confirmatory. Second-generation RIBA-2 tests for reactivity to four viral antigens: c22-3, c33c, c100-3, and 5-1-1. A positive RIBA-2, especially to c22-3 and c33c, is a sensitive assay for HCV infection. C33c positivity is associated with viremia (318). A minority of patients may have HCV RNA detectable by PCR amplification methods in the absence of a positive serology (319,320). Because the liver enzymes do not reflect liver histology, a liver biopsy for staging of liver disease is warranted in patients who are anti-HCV antibody or HCV RNA positive, even in the face of normal liver enzymes.

Pathogenesis

Chronic HCV infection leads to cirrhosis, end-stage liver failure, and hepatocellular carcinoma, but the frequency of these sequelae and the mechanisms by which they occur are not known (312). HCV infection persists despite vigorous antibody response to an array of viral epitopes. A high rate of mutation in the envelope protein is responsible for emergence of neutralization escape mutants and quasispecies (321). HCV may elicit cryoglobulins because the HCV virus surface has IgG Fc–binding properties. Presumably, the anti-HCV immune response also targets adjacent bound IgG Fc through epitope spreading (J.T. Stapleton, personal communication, 1999).

Management

IFN-α has been shown to be useful in the treatment of chronic HCV hepatitis and HCV-associated cryoglobulinemia. IFN-α2b at a dose of 3 million units thrice weekly for 6 months suppresses viral titers and ameliorates clinical disease in about 50% of patients (322). Relapse after completion of the initial course of therapy is common. High doses of IFN-α or combination therapy with IFN α and ribaviran have reduced recurrence rates (323,324). Those with symptomatic cryoglobulinemia, after IFN therapy fails, may require immunosuppressive therapy. There is controversy whether IFN therapy precipitates autoimmune disease, such as autoimmune thyroiditis (325,326).

RETROVIRUSES

Retroviruses are discussed in Chapter 131.

ALPHAVIRUSES

The genus alphaviruses are arthropod-borne members of the Togaviridae family of spherical, enveloped, single-stranded positive sense RNA viruses. Several alphaviruses cause acute arthropathy, whereas others cause encephalopathy. Our discussion is limited to the former.

CHIKUNGUNYA VIRUS

Chikungunya virus was first isolated during an epidemic of febrile arthritis in Tanzania in 1952 to 1953. The local tribal word, *Chikungunya,* "that which twists or bends up," was applied to the virus and the disease. Similar epidemics likely occurred in Indonesia, Africa, India, Asia, and possibly the southern U.S. from 1779 to 1828 (327,328). The reinfestation of *Aedes aegypti* and the introduction of *Aedes albopictus* into the Western hemisphere raises the specter of an emergence in new geographic areas (329–331).

Epidemiology

Chikungunya virus is transmitted from its reservoir hosts (baboons, monkeys, and in Senegal, scotophilus bat species) to humans by *Aedes* mosquitoes in south and west-central

Africa, Thailand, Vietnam, and India. Humans may serve as a reservoir during outbreaks. *Mansonia africana* and mosquitoes from other genera also may act as vectors (332). Communities without recent exposure are at risk for high attack rates. In a 1964 epidemic in Bangkok, Thailand, an estimated 40,000 patients in an urban area of 2 million were infected. The seroconversion rate to Chikungunya virus antibody positivity was 31% (333).

Clinical Features

After an incubation period that ranges from 1 to 12 days, but is usually 2 to 3 days, Chikungunya fever has explosive onset associated with fever and severe arthralgia (334). Fever to 39°C to 40°C is accompanied by rigors. The acute illness ranges from 1 to 7 days. After the acute illness, fever may resolve for 1 to 2 days before recrudescence. A migratory polyarthralgia of the small joints of the hands, wrists, feet, and ankles occurs with less prominent involvement of the large joints. Previously injured joints may be more severely affected. Stiffness and swelling may occur, but large effusions are uncommon. Facial and neck flushing is typical. A macular or maculopapular rash appears on the torso, extremities, and occasionally the face, palms, and soles at 1 to 10 days into the illness. Typically rash is associated with defervescence. The rash may last 1 to 5 more days, recurs with fever, and may be pruritic. Isolated petechiae and mucosal bleeding occur, and in some patients, the skin desquamates (335). Myalgias and back and shoulder pain are common. Suffusion of the conjunctiva is prominent. Sore throat, pharyngitis, headache, photophobia, retroorbital pain, anorexia, nausea, vomiting, and abdominal pain may be present. Tender lymphadenopathy is usually not massive. Those with more severe symptoms at presentation may have symptom persistence for months before resolution. Approximately 10% of patients have arthralgias or arthritis at 1 year after infection.

Symptoms in children tend to be milder. In symptomatic children, nausea and vomiting, pharyngitis, and facial flushing are prominent features, but rash, arthralgias, and arthritis are uncommon. Children may have a mild dengue-like hemorrhagic fever, headache, pharyngeal injection, vomiting, diarrhea, constipation, abdominal pain, cough, or lymphadenopathy. Arthralgia and arthritis in children are milder and of shorter duration. A destructive arthropathy may occur in occasional adults, with chronic symptoms (336). Low-titer rheumatoid factor may be found in those with long-standing symptoms (337).

Diagnosis

Chikungunya fever should be considered in any febrile patient resident in or returning from areas in which it is endemic. A history of epidemic occurrence should be sought. Synovial fluid shows decreased viscosity, poor mucin clot, and 2,000 to 5,000 white cells/mm^3. Virus may be isolated during days 2 through 4. In some patients with more intensive acute viremia, viral antigen may be detected in sera by hemagglutination assay. As viremia is cleared, hemagglutination-inhibition antibodies develop. Complement fixation antibodies are positive by the third week and slowly decrease over the subsequent year. Neutralizing antibody production parallels agglutination inhibition activity. Chikungunya virus–specific IgM antibodies may be found for 6 months or longer (338).

Pathogenesis

After mosquito bite, intense viremia occurs within 48 hours. Viremia begins to wane around day 3. The appearance of hemagglutination-inhibition activity and neutralizing antibody is associated with the viremia. Involved skin shows erythrocyte extravasation from superficial capillaries and perivascular cuffing. Skin hemorrhage may result from platelet aggregation caused by agglutination of virus adsorbed to platelets (337). Synovitis in Chikungunya fever probably results from direct viral infection of synovium (327).

Management

Management is supportive. During the acute attack, range-of-motion exercises ameliorate stiffness. Nonsteroidal anti-inflammatory agents are useful. Chloroquine phosphate (250 mg per day) has been used when nonsteroidal antiinflammatory agents failed (339).

O'NYONG-NYONG VIRUS

O'nyong-nyong virus was first described in the Acholi province of northwestern Uganda in February 1959. Within 2 years, it spread through Uganda and the surrounding region, with attack rates of 50% to 60% and local case rates of 9% to 78%, ultimately affecting 2 million people. Disease spread at a rate of 2 to 3 km daily (340,341). After the epidemic, the virus was not detected again until it was isolated from *Anopheles funestus* mosquitoes in Kenya in 1978 (342). Beginning in 1996, another outbreak in northwestern Uganda occurred (343,344). *Anopheles gambiae* also may serve as a vector. Despite the absence of diagnosed cases, serologic surveys indicate that O'nyong-nyong virus is endogenous (345). The nonhuman vertebrate reservoir for O'nyong-nyong virus is unknown.

Clinical Features

O'nyong-nyong fever is clinically similar to Chikungunya infections (346). *O'nyong-nyong* means "joint breaker" in the Acholi dialect of northwestern Uganda. After a minimum of an 8-day incubation period, polyarthralgia/polyarthritis begins abruptly. As joint symptoms improve, usually 4 days after onset, a uniform rash appears for 4 to 7 days and clears by fading. Fever may not be prominent, but postcervical lymphadenopathy may be marked. There are no long-term sequelae, although residual joint pain often persists.

Diagnosis

Hemagglutination-inhibition or complement fixation tests identify the virus (340). Intracerebral injection of virus-containing body fluids into suckling mice produces runting, rash, and alopecia (347). O'nyong-nyong virus is serologically related to Chikungunya virus. Mouse antisera raised against Chikungunya virus or O'nyong-nyong virus react equally well with O'nyong-nyong virus, but O'nyong-nyong antisera do not react well with Chikungunya virus (348). The mechanisms of O'nyong-nyong virus pathogenesis are unknown.

Management is symptomatic. Patients recover without sequelae.

IGBO ORA VIRUS

Igbo Ora virus is related to Chikungunya and O'nyong-nyong viruses (349). In 1984, an epidemic of fever, myalgias, rash, and arthralgias occurred in four villages in the Ivory Coast. *Igbo Ora* was coined as "the disease that breaks your wings." The virus was isolated from *Anopheles funestus* and *Anopheles gambiae* mosquitoes and from affected individuals.

ROSS RIVER VIRUS (EPIDEMIC POLYARTHRITIS)

Epidemics of a febrile illness characterized by rash and arthritis have been observed in Australia since 1928. Epidemics occurred among non-Australian soldiers stationed there during World War II. Ross River virus was initially isolated from mosquitoes, and then serologically associated with epidemic polyarthritis, and isolated from epidemic polyarthritis patients in Australia (350). Weber's line is a hypothetical line separating the Australian geographic zone from the Asiatic zone. West of Weber's line, antibodies to Ross River virus are not found. East of Weber's line, Ross River virus infection has been seen in New South Wales, Papua New Guinea, West New Guinea, the Bismarck Archipelago, Rossel Island, and the Solomon Islands (351). From 1979 to 1980, a major epidemic of febrile polyarthritis occurred in the Fiji Islands, affecting more than 40,000 individuals (352). Serologic surveys suggested that a low level of Ross River virus infection was present throughout the Fiji Islands before 1979. After the epidemic, seroprevalence was as high as 90% in some communities. A similar epidemic occurred in the Cook Islands early in 1980.

In Australia, both endemic cases and epidemics occur in tropical and temperate regions annually. Significant numbers of cases are reported in Queensland and New South Wales, where local climate and topography favor mosquito populations. However, cases and outbreaks occur in other regions as well. Infection rates range from 0.2% to 3.5% per year. Seroprevalence is 27% to 39% in the plains of the Murray Valley river and 6% to 15% in temperate coastal zones (353). Epidemic periods are preceded by high rainfall, which increases mosquito populations. Cases occur from spring through autumn. The salt marsh *Aedes vigilax* is the dominant vector on Australia's eastern coast. *Aedes camptorhynchus* breeds in salt marshes of southern Australia. *Culex annulirostris* is a fresh-water–breeding vector. Other Australian *Aedes* sp and *Mansonia uniformus* also serve as vectors. Domestic animals, rodents, and marsupials serve as intermediate hosts. In the Pacific islands outbreaks, *Aedes polynesiensis, Aedes aegypti, Aedes vigilax,* and *Culex annulirostris* have served as vectors. During epidemics in Fiji and New South Wales, the majority of those infected were symptomatic (354). Male and female infection rates were similar, but a female predominance occurs in presenting cases. The case-to-infection ratio is lower in children than in adults.

Clinical Features

A 7- to 11-day incubation period ends abruptly with arthralgias (355). A sometimes pruritic, macular, papular, or maculopapular rash typically follows onset of arthralgia by 1 to 2 days, but in some cases precedes the joint symptoms by 11 days or follows by 15 days. Vesicles, papules, or petechiae may be seen. The typical rash involves the trunk and extremities, but palms, soles, and face also may be involved. The rash resolves by fading to a brownish discoloration or by desquamation. Approximately 50% of patients have no fever, and in those who do, fevers may be modest, lasting only 1 to 3 days. Headache, nausea, and myalgias are common. Mild photophobia, respiratory symptoms, and lymphadenopathy may occur.

In a majority of patients, an asymmetric and migratory arthralgia is incapacitating. Finger interphalangeal joints, metacarpophalangeal joints, wrists, knees, and ankles are commonly involved. Shoulders, elbows, and toes may be involved, and less commonly. axial, hip, and temporomandibular joints. Arthralgias are worse in the morning and after periods of inactivity. Mild exercise helps alleviate arthralgias. One third of patients have synovitis on examination. Polyarticular swelling and tenosynovitis are common. Up to one third have paresthesias and palm or sole pain. Classic carpal tunnel syndrome may be encountered. Whereas residual polyarthralgia may be present at 1 month, 50% of affected patients can return to activities of daily living by then. Joint symptoms may recur, but recurrences gradually resolve. A few patients still have joint symptoms 3 years later (355).

Diagnosis

Ross River virus infection should be considered in the differential diagnosis in anyone with a febrile arthritis living in or traveling from the appropriate geographic setting. Synovial fluid cell counts reportedly range from 1,500 to 13,800 cells/mm^3, with predominantly monocytes and vacuolated macrophages and a few neutrophils. Virus has been isolated only from antibody-negative sera. In Australian epidemics before 1979, patients were antibody positive at presentation. In the Pacific Island epidemics of 1979 to 1980, patients were viremic and seronegative for up to 1 week after illness (356). Virus is stable in serum at 0°C to −10°C for up to 1 month. Ross River virus antigen is detectable by fluorescent antibody staining of infected tissue culture cells inoculated with acute patient serum (357).

Pathogenesis

Ross River viral antigen is detectable early in disease by immunofluorescence in monocytes and tissue macrophages, but intact virus is not identifiable by electron microscopy or cell culture (358). Dermal vessels in both the erythematous and purpuric rash show mild perivascular mononuclear cell, mostly T lymphocytic, infiltrates. Extravasation of erythrocytes is seen in the purpuric form of rash. Viral antigen may be found in epithelial cells and the perivascular zone in erythematous lesions. In the purpuric skin lesions, viral antigen is found in epithelial cells but not in the perivascular zone (359).

Management

Management is symptomatic. Aspirin or nonsteroidal antiinflammatory drugs provide relief for joint pain, although nonsteroidal antiinflammatory drugs are preferred, given the associated purpura in some patients. In occasional patients, prolonged joint symptoms develop, but eventual full recovery occurs (360,361).

BARMAH FOREST VIRUS

Barmah Forest virus, a newly described alphavirus in Australia, may occur in a fashion similar to epidemic febrile polyarthritis (362).

SINDBIS VIRUS

Sindbis virus was isolated from *Culex* mosquitoes in the Egyptian village of the same name in 1952. It has become the prototype alphavirus used in studies of alphavirus molecular virology.

Epidemiology

Sindbis virus infection occurs in the forested areas of Scandinavia: Sweden, Finland, and the neighboring Karelian isthmus of Russia. Local names for infection are Okelbo disease, Pogosta disease, and Karelian fever, respectively (334). *Aedes, Culex,* and *Culiseta* species transmit the virus to humans. Birds serve as an intermediate host (363). Individuals involved in outdoor activities or forestry-related occupations are at risk. Sporadic cases and small outbreaks of Sindbis virus infection have been reported in Uganda, Zimbabwe, Central Africa, South Africa, and Australia (327).

Clinical Features

Patients have rash and arthralgia, although one may precede the other by a few days. Constitutional symptoms including fever, fatigue, malaise, headache, nausea, vomiting, pharyngitis, and paresthesias may be present but are usually not severe. A macular rash typically begins on the torso, spreading to the arms, legs, palms, soles, and occasionally head. The macules evolve to papules, which have a tendency to vesiculate. Vesiculation is particularly prominent on pressure points, including palms and soles, where it may become hemorrhagic. The rash fades to a brownish discoloration. Rash may recur during convalescence (334).

Arthralgias and arthritis involve the small joints of the hands and feet, wrists, elbows, ankles, and knees. Occasionally the axial skeleton becomes involved. Tendonitis of the extensor tendons of the hand and the Achilles tendon is common. Chronic nonerosive arthropathy is present in as many as one third of patients 2 or more years after onset. A small number have symptoms 5 to 6 years after initial infection (363).

Diagnosis

Antibodies appear during the first week of illness and may be detected by hemagglutination inhibition and complement fixation tests (364).

Pathogenesis

Dermal lesions have perivascular edema, lymphocytic infiltrates, hemorrhage, and areas of necrosis. Sindbis virus has been isolated from a skin vesicle in the absence of viremia. Persistence of antiviral IgM antibody years after Sindbis virus infection raises the possibility that the arthritis is associated with viral persistence with direct viral effect on the synovium (363).

Management

Management is supportive.

MAYARO VIRUS

Mayaro virus was first recognized in Trinidad in 1954. It is endemic in the forested areas of Peru, Bolivia, and Brazil and is known to have caused epidemics of febrile arthritis in Bolivia and Brazil. *Haemogogus* mosquitoes feeding in the tropical rain forest transmit Mayaro virus from a monkey reservoir to humans. In an outbreak in Belterra, Brazil, in 1988, 800 of 4,000 exposed latex gatherers were infected, with a clinical attack rate of 80%. Illness was characterized by sudden onset of fever, headache, dizziness, chills, and arthralgias in the fingers, wrists, ankles, and toes. One fifth had joint swelling. Some patients had prominent unilateral inguinal lymphadenopathy. Leukopenia was common. Viremia was present during the first 2 days of illness. On day 2 to 5 of illness, the fever resolved, but maculopapular truncal and extremity rash appeared, lasting 3 days. Recovery was complete, although some patients had persistent arthralgias at 2-month follow-up (365–367).

Mayaro virus has been isolated from a bird in Louisiana (368). American volunteer workers returning from Peru have been seen by local physicians in the U.S. with acute Mayaro virus illness (369). Despite the occurrence of alphavirus infections outside of North America, it is important that physicians and health care workers in the U.S. and Canada be knowledgeable about these diseases. The importance of being prepared for viral infections emerging in new geographic ranges was underscored by the recent fatal outbreak of West Nile fever virus, mosquito-borne flavivirus, in the New York City area in 1999 (370).

OTHER VIRUSES

Joint symptoms are seen in a variety of viral syndromes in addition to those noted earlier, in which arthralgia and arthritis are prominent characteristic features. Children with varicella have been reported rarely to develop brief monoarticular or pauciarticular arthritis thought to be viral in origin (371). Arthritis may be associated with mumps; small- or large-joint synovitis lasts up to several weeks. Arthritis may precede or follow parotitis by up to 4 weeks (372). Adenovirus and coxsackievirus A9, B2, B3, B4, and B6 infections have been associated with recurrent episodes of polyarthritis, pleuritis, myalgia, rash, pharyngitis, myocarditis, and leukocytosis (373,374). Echovirus 9 infection causes polyarthritis, fever, and myalgias in a few cases (375). Mononucleosis from Epstein–Barr virus is frequently accompanied by polyarthralgia. Monoarticular arthritis of the knee also has been reported (376,377). Arthritis associated with cytomegalovirus infections is rare. However, a severe polyarthritis in bone marrow transplant recipients due to cytomegalovirus has been reported; abundant cytomegalovirus may be visualized on electron microscopy of synovial fluid aspirated from affected joints (378). Herpes hominis occasionally causes arthritis of the knee, dubbed "herpes gladiatorum" because it is seen in wrestlers (379). Vaccinia virus has been associated with postvaccination knee arthritis in two cases (380).

REFERENCES

1. Albert LJ, Inman RD. Molecular mimicry and autoimmunity. *N Engl J Med* 1999;341:2068–2074.
2. Vanderlugt CL, Begolka WS, Neville KL, et al. The functional significance of epitope spreading and its regulation by co-stimulatory molecules. *Immunol Rev* 1998;164:63–72.
3. Pattison JR. The discovery of human parvovirus. In: Pattison JR, ed. *Parvoviruses and human disease.* Boca Raton: CRC Press, 1988:1–4.
4. Vandervelde EM, Goffin C, Megson B, et al. User's guide to some new tests for hepatitis-B antigen. *Lancet* 1974;2:1066.
5. Cossart YE, Field AM, Cant B, et al. Parvovirus-like particles in human sera. *Lancet* 1975;1:72–73.
6. Murphy FA, Fauquet CM, Bishop DHL, et al. *Virus taxonomy:* the classification and nomenclature of viruses: *the sixth report of the International Committee on Taxonomy of Viruses.* Vienna: Springer-Verlag, 1995. Online http://www.ncbi.nlm.nih.gov/ict/viruslist/ssdna_viruses.pdf.
7. Astell CR, Blundell MC. Sequence of the right hand terminal palindrome of the human B19 parvovirus genome has the potential to form a "stem plus arms" structure. *Nucleic Acids Res* 1989;17:5857.
8. Cotmore SF, Tattersall P. Characterization and molecular cloning of a human parvovirus genome. *Science* 1984;226:1161–1165.
9. Summers J, Jones SE, Anderson MJ. Characterization of the genome of the agent of erythrocyte aplasia permits its classification as a human parvovirus. *J Gen Virol* 1983;64:2527–2532.
10. Astell CR. Terminal hairpins of parvovirus genomes and their role in DNA replication. In: Tijssen P, ed. *Handbook of parvoviruses.* Vol I. Boca Raton: CRC Press, 1990:59–79.
11. Tattersall P, Ward DC. Rolling hairpin model for replication of parvovirus and linear chromosomal DNA. *Nature* 1976;263:106–109.
12. Deiss V, Tratschin JD, Weitz M, et al. Cloning of the human parvovirus B19 genome and structural analysis of its palindromic termini. *Virology* 1990;175:247–254.
13. Blundell MC, Beard C, Astell CR. In vitro identification of a B19 parvovirus promoter. *Virology* 1987;157:534–538.
14. Beard C, St. Amand J, Astell CR. Transient expression of B19 parvovirus gene products in COS-7 cells transfected with B19-SV40 hybrid vectors. *Virology* 1989;172:659–664.
15. Cotmore SF, McKie VC, Anderson LJ, et al. Identification of the major structural and nonstructural proteins encoded by human parvovirus B19 and mapping of their genes by procaryotic expression of isolated genomic fragments. *J Virol* 1986;60:548–557.
16. Ozawa K, Young N. Characterization of capsid and noncapsid proteins of B19 parvovirus propagated in human erythroid bone marrow cell cultures. *J Virol* 1987;61:2627–2630.
17. Astell CR, Luo WX, Brunstein J, et al. B19 parvovirus: biochemical and molecular features. *Monogr Virol* 1997;20:16–41.
18. Cotmore SF, Tattersall P. A genome-linked copy of the NS-1 polypeptide is located on the outside of infectious parvovirus particles. *J Virol* 1989;63:3902–3911.
19. Ozawa K, Ayub J, Kajigaya S, et al. The gene encoding the nonstructural protein of B19 (human) parvovirus may be lethal in transfected cells. *J Virol* 1988;62:2884–2889.

20. Takahashi Y, Murai C, Shibata S, et al. Human parvovirus B19 as a causative agent for rheumatoid arthritis. *Proc Natl Acad Sci U S A* 1998;95:8227–8232.
21. Momoeda M, Wong S, Kawase M, et al. A putative nucleoside triphosphate-binding domain in the nonstructural protein of B19 parvovirus is required for cytotoxicity. *J Virol* 1994;68: 8443–8446.
22. Von Poblotzki A, Hemauer A, Gigler A, et al. Antibodies to the nonstructural protein of parvovirus B19 in persistently infected patients: implications for pathogenesis. *J Infect Dis* 1995;172: 1346–1359.
23. Jones LP, Erdman DD, Anderson LJ. Prevalence of antibodies to parvovirus B19 nonstructural protein in persons with various clinical outcomes following B19 infection. *J Infect Dis* 1999; 180:500–504.
24. Ozawa K, Ayub J, Hao YS, et al. Novel transcription map for the B19 (human) pathogenic parvovirus. *J Virol* 1987;61:2395–2406.
25. Rosenfeld SJ, Yoshimoto K, Kajigaya S, et al. Unique region of the minor capsid protein of human parvovirus B19 is exposed on the virion surface. *J Clin Invest* 1992;89:2023–2029.
26. Brown KE, Anderson SM, Young NS. Erythrocyte P antigen: cellular receptor for B19 parvovirus. *Science* 1993;262:114–117.
27. Cooling LLW, Koerner TAW, Naides SJ. Multiple glycosphingolipids determine the tissue tropism of parvovirus B19. *J Infect Dis* 1995;172:1198–1205.
28. Issitt PD. The P blood group system, In: Issitt PD, ed. *Applied blood group serology.* 3rd ed. Miami: Montgomery Scientific Publications, 1985:203–218.
29. Knisely AS, O'Shea PA, McMillan P, et al. Electron microscopic identification of parvovirus virions in erythroid-line cells in fatal hydrops fetalis. *Pediatr Pathol* 1988;8:163–170.
30. Morey AL, Ferguson DJ, Leslie DO, et al. Intracellular localization of parovirus B19 nucleic acid at the ultracellular level by in situ hybridization with digoxigenin-labelled probes. *Histochem J* 1993;25:421–429.
31. Krause JR, Penchansky L, Knisely AS. Morphological diagnosis of parvovirus B19 infection: a cytopathic effect easily recognized in air-dried, formalin-fixed bone marrow smears stained with hematoxylin-eosin or Wright-Giemsa. *Arch Pathol Lab Med* 1992;116:178–180.
32. Palmer EL, Martin ML. Parvoviridae. In: Palmer EL, Martin ML, eds. *Electron microscopy in viral diagnosis.* Boca Raton: CRC Press, 1988:149–152.
33. Anderson MJ, Higgins PG, Davis LR, et al. Experimental parvoviral infection in humans. *J Infect Dis* 1985;152:257–265.
34. Anderson LJ, Tsou RA, Chorba TL, et al. Detection of antibodies and antigens of human parvovirus B19 by enzyme-linked immunosorbent assay. *J Clin Microbiol* 1986;24:522–526.
35. Plummer FA, Hammond GW, Forward K, et al. An erythema infectiosum-like illness caused by human parvovirus infection. *N Engl J Med* 1985;313:74–79.
36. Chorba T, Coccia P, Holman RC, et al. The role of parvovirus B19 in aplastic crisis and erythema infectiosum (fifth disease). *J Infect Dis* 1986;154:383–393.
37. Goldfarb J. Parvovirus infection in children. *Adv Pediatr Infect Dis* 1989;4:211–222.
38. Gillespie SM, Cartter ML, Asch S, et al. Occupational risk of human parvovirus B19 infection for school and day-care personnel during an outbreak of erythema infectiosum. *JAMA* 1990;263:2061–2065.
39. Bell LM, Naides SJ, Stoffman P, et al. Human parvovirus B19 infection among hospital staff members after contact with infected patients. *N Engl J Med* 1989;321:485–491.
40. Pattison JR, Jones SE, Hodgson J, et al. Parvovirus infections and hypoplastic crisis in sickle-cell anaemia. *Lancet* 1981;1: 664–665.
41. Bertrand Y, Lefrere JJ, Leverger G, et al. Autoimmune haemolytic anaemia revealed by human parvovirus linked erythroblastopenia. *Lancet* 1985;2:382–383.
42. Davidson RJ, Brown T, Wiseman D. Human parvovirus infection and aplastic crisis in hereditary spherocytosis. *J Infect* 1984; 9:298–300.
43. Duncan JR, Potter CB, Cappellini MD, et al. Aplastic crisis due to parvovirus infection in pyruvate kinase deficiency. *Lancet* 1983;2:14–16.
44. Evans JP, Rossiter MA, Kumaran TO, et al. Human parvovirus aplasia: case due to cross infection in a ward. *Br Med J* 1984; 288:681.
45. Goldman F, Rotbart H, Gutierrez K, et al. Parvovirus-associated aplastic crisis in a patient with red blood cell glucose-6-phosphate dehydrogenase deficiency. *Pediatr Infect Dis J* 1990;9: 593–594.
46. Green DH, Bellingham AJ, Anderson MJ. Parvovirus infection in a family associated with aplastic crisis in an affected sibling pair with hereditary spherocytosis. *J Clin Pathol* 1984;37:1144–1146.
47. Hanada T, Koike K, Takeya T, et al. Human parvovirus B19-induced transient pancytopenia in a child with hereditary spherocytosis. *Br J Haematol* 1988;70:113–115.
48. Kelleher JF Jr, Luban NL, Cohen BJ, et al. Human serum parvovirus as the cause of aplastic crisis in sickle cell disease. *Am J Dis Child* 1984;138:401–403.
49. Lefrere JJ, Bourgeois H. Human parvovirus associated with erythroblastopenia in iron deficiency anaemia. *J Clin Pathol* 1986; 39:1277–1278.
50. Lefrere JJ, Courouce AM, Bertrand Y, et al. Human parvovirus and aplastic crisis in chronic hemolytic anemias: a study of 24 observations. *Am J Hematol* 1986;23:271–275.
51. Lefrere JJ, Courouce AM, Boucheix C, et al. Aplastic crisis and erythema infectiosum (fifth disease) revealing a hereditary spherocytosis in a familial human parvovirus infection. *Nouv Rev Fr Hematol* 1986;28:7–9.
52. Lefrere JJ, Courouce AM, Girot R, et al. Six cases of hereditary spherocytosis revealed by human parvovirus infection. *Br J Haematol* 1986;62:653–658.
53. Lefrere JJ, Courouce AM, Girot R, et al. Human parvovirus and thalassaemia. *J Infect* 1986;13:45–49.
54. Lefrere JJ, Girot R, Courouce AM, et al. Familial human parvovirus infection associated with anemia in siblings with heterozygous beta-thalassemia. *J Infect Dis* 1986;153:977–979.
55. Mabin DC, Chowdhury V. Aplastic crisis caused by human parvovirus in two patients with hereditary stomatocytosis. *Br J Haematol* 1990;76:153–154.
56. Mehta J, Singhal S, Mehta BC. Aplastic crisis and leg ulceration: two rare complications of hereditary sideroblastic anaemia. *J Assoc Phys India* 1992;40:466–467.
57. Negami T, Ohta M, Okuda K, et al. Parvovirus B19-induced aplastic crisis in a patient with iron deficiency anemia. *Rinsho Ketsueki* 1994;35:670–675.
58. Rao KR, Patel AR, Anderson MJ, et al. Infection with parvovirus-like virus and aplastic crisis in chronic hemolytic anemia. *Ann Intern Med* 1983;98:930–932.
59. Rappaport ES, Quick G, Ransom D, et al. Aplastic crisis in occult hereditary spherocytosis caused by human parvovirus (HPV B19). *South Med J* 1989;82:247–251.
60. Rechavi G, Vonsover A, Manor Y, et al. Aplastic crisis due to human B19 parvovirus infection in red cell pyrimidine-5′-nucleotidase deficiency. *Acta Haematol* 1989;82:46–49.
61. Saarinen UM, Chorba TL, Tattersall P, et al. Human parvovirus B19-induced epidemic acute red cell aplasia in patients with hereditary hemolytic anemia. *Blood* 1986;67:1411–1417.
62. Summerfield GP, Wyatt GP. Human parvovirus infection revealing hereditary spherocytosis. *Lancet* 1985;2:1070.

63. Takahashi M, Koike T, Moriyama Y, et al. Inhibition of erythropoiesis by human parvovirus-containing serum from a patient with hereditary spherocytosis in aplastic crisis. *Scand J Haematol* 1986;37:118–124.
64. Tsukada T, Koike T, Koike R, et al. Epidemic of aplastic crisis in patients with hereditary spherocytosis in Japan. *Lancet* 1985; 1:1401.
65. West NC, Meigh RE, Mackie M, et al. Parvovirus infection associated with aplastic crisis in a patient with HEMPAS. *J Clin Pathol* 1986;39:1019–1020.
66. Rao SP, Miller ST, Cohen BJ. Transient aplastic crisis in patients with sickle cell disease: B19 parvovirus studies during a 7-year period. *Am J Dis Child* 1992;146:1328–1330.
67. Serjeant GR, Topley JM, Mason K, et al. Outbreak of aplastic crises in sickle cell anaemia associated with parvovirus-like agent. *Lancet* 1981;2:595–597.
68. Burton PA. Intranuclear inclusions in marrow of hydropic fetus due to parvovirus infection. *Lancet* 1986;2:1155.
69. Caul EO, Usher MJ, Burton PA. Intrauterine infection with human parvovirus B19: a light and electron microscopy study. *J Med Virol* 1988;24:55–66.
70. Naides SJ, Weiner CP. Antenatal diagnosis and palliative treatment of non-immune hydrops fetalis secondary to fetal parvovirus B19 infection. *Prenat Diagn* 1989;9:105–114.
71. Cassinotti P, Schultze D, Schlageter P, et al. Persistent human parvovirus B19 infection following an acute infection with meningitis in an immunocompetent patient. *Eur J Clin Microbiol Infect Dis* 1993;12:701–704.
72. Chrystie IL, Almeida JD, Welch J. Electron microscopic detection of human parvovirus (B19) in a patient with HIV infection. *J Med Virol* 1990;30:249–252.
73. de Mayolo JA, Temple JD. Pure red cell aplasia due to parvovirus B19 infection in a man with HIV infection. *South Med J* 1990;83:1480–1481.
74. Frickhofen N, Abkowitz JL, Safford M, et al. Persistent B19 parvovirus infection in patients infected with human immunodeficiency virus type 1 (HIV-1): a treatable cause of anemia in AIDS. *Ann Intern Med* 1990;113:926–933.
75. Frickhofen N, Young NS. Persistent parvovirus B19 infections in humans. *Microb Pathog* 1989;7:319–327.
76. Frickhofen N, Young NS. Polymerase chain reaction for detection of parvovirus B19 in immunodeficient patients with anemia. *Behring Inst Mitt* 1990;85:46–54.
77. Kurtzman G, Frickhofen N, Kimball J, et al. Pure red-cell aplasia of 10 years' duration due to persistent parvovirus B19 infection and its cure with immunoglobulin therapy. *N Engl J Med* 1989;321:519–523.
78. Kurtzman GJ, Cohen B, Meyers P, et al. Persistent B19 parvovirus infection as a cause of severe chronic anaemia in children with acute lymphocytic leukaemia. *Lancet* 1988;2:1159–1162.
79. Rao SP, Miller ST, Cohen BJ. Severe anemia due to B19 parvovirus infection in children with acute leukemia in remission. *Am J Pediatr Hematol Oncol* 1990;12:194–197.
80. Kurtzman GJ, Ozawa K, Cohen B, et al. Chronic bone marrow failure due to persistent B19 parvovirus infection. *N Engl J Med* 1987;317:287–294;
81. Potter CG, Potter AC, Hatton CS, et al. Variation of erythroid and myeloid precursors in the marrow and peripheral blood of volunteer subjects infected with human parvovirus (B19). *J Clin Invest* 1987;79:1486–1492.
82. Anderson MJ, Lewis E, Kidd IM, et al. An outbreak of erythema infectiosum associated with human parvovirus infection. *J Hyg (Lond)* 1984;93:85–93.
83. Anderson MJ, Jones SE, Fisher Hoch SP, et al. Human parvovirus: the cause of erythema infectiosum (fifth disease)? *Lancet* 1983;1:1378.
84. Naides SJ, Piette W, Veach LA, et al. Human parvovirus B19-induced vesiculopustular skin eruption. *Am J Med* 1988; 84:968–972.
85. Andrews M, Martin RWY, Duff AR, et al. Fifth disease: report of an outbreak. *J R Coll Gen Pract* 1984;34:573–574.
86. Brandrup F, Larsen PO. Erythema infectiosum (fifth disease). *Br Med J* 1976;1:47–48.
87. Clarke HC. Erythema infectiosum: an epidemic with a probable posterythema phase. *Can Med Assoc J* 1984;130:603–604.
88. Cramp HE, Armstrong BDJ. Erythema infectiosum: an outbreak of "slapped cheek" disease in north Devon. *Br Med J* 1976;1:885–886.
89. Lauer BA, MacCormack JN, Wilfert C. Erythema infectiosum: an elementary school outbreak. *Am J Dis Child* 1976;130:252–254.
90. LeFebvre RB, Berns KI. Unique events in parvovirus replication. *Microbiol Sci* 1984;1:163–167.
91. Mansfield F. Erythema infectiosum: slapped face disease. *Aust Fam Physician* 1988;17:737–738.
92. Mynott MJ. An epidemic of erythema infectiosum in a school. *Practitioner* 1985;229:767–768.
93. Nunoue T, Okochi K, Mortimer PP, et al. Human parvovirus (B19) and erythema infectiosum. *J Pediatr* 1985;107:38–40.
94. Okabe N, Koboyashi S, Tatsuzawa O, et al. Detection of antibodies to human parvovirus in erythema infectiosum (fifth disease). *Arch Dis Child* 1984;59:1016–1019.
95. Shneerson JM, Mortimer PP, Vandervelde EM. Febrile illness due to a parvovirus. *Br Med J* 1980;280:1580.
96. Ager EA, Chin TDY, Poland JD. Epidemic erythema infectiosum. *N Engl J Med* 1966;275:1326–1331.
97. White DG, Woolf AD, Mortimer PP, et al. Human parvovirus arthropathy. *Lancet* 1985;1:419–421.
98. Smith CA, Woolf AD, Lenci M. Parvoviruses: infections and arthropathies. *Rheum Dis Clin North Am* 1987;13:249–263.
99. Stoll T, Brühlmann P, Brunner U, et al. Parvovirus-B19-induced arthritis/arthropathy and its importance in differential diagnosis of rheumatoid arthritis. *Schweiz Med Wochenschr* 1995;125:347–354.
100. Woolf AD, Campion GV, Chishick A, et al. Clinical manifestations of human parvovirus B19 in adults. *Arch Intern Med* 1989;149:1153–1156.
101. Naides SJ, Scharosch LL, Foto F, et al. Rheumatologic manifestations of human parvovirus B19 infection in adults: initial two-year clinical experience. *Arthritis Rheum* 1990;33:1297–1309.
102. Reid DM, Reid TM, Brown T, et al. Human parvovirus-associated arthritis: a clinical and laboratory description. *Lancet* 1985;1:422–425.
103. Naides SJ. Rheumatic manifestations of parvovirus B19 infection. *Rheum Dis Clin North Am* 1998;24:375–401.
104. Silman AJ. The 1987 revised American Rheumatism Association criteria for rheumatoid arthritis [Editorial]. *Br J Rheumatol* 1988;27:341–343.
105. Naides SJ, Field EH. Transient rheumatoid factor positivity in acute human parvovirus B19 infection. *Arch Intern Med* 1988; 148:2587–2589.
106. Sasaki T, Takahashi Y, Yoshinaga K, et al. An association between human parvovirus B-19 infection and autoantibody production. *J Rheumatol* 1989;16:708–709.
107. Semble EL, Agudelo CA, Pegram PS, Human parvovirus B19 arthropathy in two adults after contact with childhood erythema infectiosum. *Am J Med* 1987;83:560–562.
108. Klouda PT, Corbin SA, Bradley BA, et al. HLA and acute arthritis following human parvovirus infection. *Tissue Antigens* 1986;28:318–319.
109. Woolf AD, Campion GV, Klouda PT, et al. HLA and the manifestations of human parvovirus B19 infection. *Arthritis Rheum* 1987;30:S52.

110. Hajeer AH, MacGregor AJ, Rigby AS, et al. Influence of previous exposure to human parvovirus B19 infection in explaining susceptibility to rheumatoid arthritis: an analysis of disease discordant twin pairs. *Ann Rheum Dis* 1994;53:137–139.
111. Nikkari S, Luukkainen R, Mottonen T, et al. Does parvovirus B19 have a role in rheumatoid arthritis? *Ann Rheum Dis* 1994; 53:106–111.
112. Nikkari S, Toivanen P. Parvovirus B19 in rheumatoid arthritis: comment on the article by Kerr et al. [Letter; comment]. *Br J Rheumatol* 1996;35:494.
113. Nikkari S, Roivainen A, Hannonen P, et al. Persistence of parvovirus B19 in synovial fluid and bone marrow. *Ann Rheum Dis* 1995;54:597–600.
114. Harrison B, Silman A, Barrett E, et al. Low frequency of recent parvovirus infection in a population-based cohort of patients with early inflammatory polyarthritis. *Ann Rheum Dis* 1998;57: 375–377.
115. Saal JG, Steidle M, Einsele H, et al. Persistence of B19 parvovirus in synovial membranes of patients with rheumatoid arthritis. *Rheumatol Int* 1992;12:147–151.
116. Altschuler EL. Parvovirus B19 and the pathogenesis of rheumatoid arthritis: a case for historical reasoning. *Lancet* 1999;354: 1026–1027.
117. Naides SJ, Foto F, Marsh JL, et al. Synovial tissue analysis in patients with chronic parvovirus B19 arthropathy. *Clin Res* 1991;39:733A.
118. Naides SJ. Transient liver enzyme abnormalities in acute human parvovirus (HPV) infection. *Clin Res* 1987;35:859A.
119. Foto F, Saag KG, Scharosch LL, et al. Parvovirus B19-specific DNA in bone marrow from B19 arthropathy patients: evidence for B19 viral persistence. *J Infect Dis* 1993;167:744–748.
120. Soderlund M, von Essen R, Haapasaari J, et al. Persistence of parvovirus B19 DNA in synovial membranes of young patients with and without chronic arthropathy. *Lancet* 1997;349:1063–1065.
121. Naides SJ, Scharosch LL, Hays-Goldsmith S, et al. Defective parvovirus B19 capsid protein epitope recognition in B19 arthropathy. *Arthritis Rheum* 1992;35:S36.
122. Von Poblotzki A, Gigler A, Lang B, et al. Antibodies to parvovirus B19 NS-1 protein in infected individuals. *J Gen Virol* 1995;76:519–527.
123. Gareus R, Gigler A, Hemauer A, et al. Characterization of cis-acting and NS1 protein-responsive elements in the p6 promoter of parvovirus B19. *J Virol* 1998;72:609–616.
124. Hemauer A, Gigler A, Searle K, et al. Seroprevalence of parvovirus B19 NS1-specific IgG in B19-infected and uninfected individuals and in infected pregnant women. *J Med Virol* 2000; 60:48–55.
125. Searle K, Schalasta G, Enders G. Development of antibodies to the nonstructural protein NS1 of parvovirus B19 during acute symptomatic and subclinical infection in pregnancy: implications for pathogenesis doubtful. *J Med Virol* 1998;56:192–198.
126. Moffatt S, Tanaka N, Tada K, et al. A cytotoxic nonstructural protein, NS1, of human parvovirus B19 induces activation of interleukin-6 gene expression. *J Virol* 1996;70:8485–8491.
127. Sol N, Morinet F, Alizon M, et al. Trans-activation of the long terminal repeat of human immunodeficiency virus type 1 by the parvovirus B19 NS1 gene product. *J Gen Virol* 1993;74:2011–2014.
128. Moffatt S, Yaegashi N, Tada K, et al. Human parvovirus B19 nonstructural (NS1) protein induces apoptosis in erythroid lineage cells. *J Virol* 1998;72:3018–3028.
129. Karetnyi YV, Beck PR, Markin RS, et al. Human parvovirus B19 infection in acute fulminant liver failure. *Arch Virol* 1999; 144:1713–1724.
130. Heegaard ED, Rosthoj S, Petersen B, et al. Role of parvovirus B19 infection in childhood idiopathic thrombocytopenic purpura. *Acta Paediatr* 1999;88:614–617.
131. Lefrere JJ, Courouce AM, Kaplan C. Parvovirus and idiopathic thrombocytopenic purpura. *Lancet* 1989;1:279.
132. Lefrere JJ, Courouce AM, Muller JY, et al. Human parvovirus and purpura. *Lancet* 1985;1:730.
133. Mortimer PP, Cohen BJ, Rossiter MA, et al. Human parvovirus and purpura. *Lancet* 1985;1:730–731.
134. Shiraishi H, Umetsu K, Yamamoto H, et al. Human parvovirus (HPV/B19) infection with purpura. *Microbiol Immunol* 1989; 33:369–372.
135. Lefrere JJ, Courouce AM, Soulier JP, et al. Henoch-Schonlein purpura and human parvovirus infection. *Pediatrics* 1986;78: 183–184.
136. Challine-Lehmann D, Mauberquez S, Pawlotsky J, et al. Parvovirus B19 and Schonlein-Henoch purpura in adults [Letter]. *Nephron* 1999;83:172.
137. Etienne A, Harms M. Cutaneous manifestations of parvovirus B19 infection. *Presse Med* 1996;25:1162–1165.
138. Garcia-Bermejo, Auffray P, Jimenez-Reyes J, et al. "Gloves and socks" purpura syndrome caused by human parvovirus B19 [Letter]. [Spanish]. *Enferm Infecc Microbiol Clin* 1996;14: 398–399.
139. Sotto A, Bessis D, Jourdan J. Gloves and socks edema disclosing parvovirus B19 infection [Letter]. [French]. *Presse Med* 1997;26:421.
140. Stone MS, Murph JR. Papular-purpuric gloves and socks syndrome: a characteristic viral exanthem. *Pediatrics* 1993;92: 864–865.
141. Carrascosa JM, Bielsa I, Ribera M, et al. Papular-purpuric gloves-and-socks syndrome related to cytomegalovirus infection. *Dermatology* 1995;191:269–270.
142. Drago F, Parodi A, Rebora A. Gloves-and-socks syndrome in a patient with Epstein-Barr virus infection. *Dermatology* 1997; 194:374.
143. Guibal F, Buffet P, Mouly F, et al. Papular-purpuric gloves and socks syndrome with hepatitis B infection [Letter]. *Lancet* 1996;347:473.
144. Perez-Ferriols A, Martinez-Aparicio A, Aliaga-Boniche A. Papular-purpuric "gloves and socks" syndrome caused by measles virus [Letter]. *J Am Acad Dermatol* 1994;30:291–292.
145. Denning DW, Amos A, Rudge P, et al. Neuralgic amyotrophy due to parvovirus infection. *J Neurol Neurosurg Psychiatry* 1987; 50:641–642.
146. Faden H, Gary GW Jr, Anderson LJ. Chronic parvovirus infection in a presumably immunologically healthy woman. *Clin Infect Dis* 1992;15:595–597.
147. Faden H, Gary GW Jr, Korman M. Numbness and tingling of fingers associated with parvovirus B19 infection. *J Infect Dis* 1990;161:354–355.
148. Walsh KJ, Armstrong RD, Turner AM. Brachial plexus neuropathy associated with human parvovirus infection. *Br Med J* 1988;296:896.
149. Tabak F, Mert A, Ozturk R, et al. Prolonged fever caused by parvovirus B19-induced meningitis: case report and review. *Clin Infect Dis* 1999;29:446–447.
150. Suzuki N, Terada S, Inoue M. Neonatal meningitis with human parvovirus B19 infection. *Arch Dis Child Fetal Neonatal* 1995; 73:F196–F197.
151. Umene K, Nunoue T. A new genome type of human parvovirus B19 present in sera of patients with encephalopathy. *J Gen Virol* 1995;76:2645–2651.
152. Samli K, Cassinotti P, de Freudenreich J, et al. Acute bilateral carpal tunnel syndrome associated with human parvovirus B19 infection. *Clin Infect Dis* 1996;22:162–164.
153. Samii K, Cassinotti P, De Freudenreich J, et al. Acute bilateral carpal tunnel syndrome associated with human parvovirus B19 infection. *Clin Infect Dis* 1996;22:162–164.

154. Berg AM, Naides SJ, Simms RW. Established fibromyalgia syndrome and parvovirus B19 infection. *J Rheumatol* 1993;20: 1941–1943.
155. Ilaria RL Jr, Komaroff AL, Fagioli LR, et al. Absence of parvovirus B19 infection in chronic fatigue syndrome. *Arthritis Rheum* 1995;38:638–641.
156. Anonymous. Human parvovirus B19 infections in United Kingdom 1984-86. *Lancet* 1987;1:738–739.
157. Van Elsacker-Niele AMW, Weiland HT, Kroes ACM, et al. Parvovirus B19 infection and idiopathic thrombocytopenic purpura. *Ann Hematol* 1996;72:141–144.
158. Tsuda H, Maeda Y, Nakagawa K. Parvovirus B19-related lymphadenopathy. *Br J Haematol* 1993;85:631–632.
159. Boruchoff SE, Woda BA, Pihan GA, et al. Parvovirus B19-associated hemophagocytic syndrome. *Arch Intern Med* 1990;150: 897–899.
160. Muir K, Todd WTA, Watson WH, et al. Viral-associated haemophagocytosis with parvovirus-B19-related pancytopenia. *Lancet* 1992;339:1139–1140.
161. Shirono K, Tsuda H. Parvovirus B19-associated haemophagocytic syndrome in healthy adults. *Br J Haematol* 1995;89: 923–926.
162. Watanabe M, Shimamoto Y, Yamaguchi M, et al. Viral-associated haemophagocytosis and elevated serum TNF-α with parvovirus-B19-related pancytopenia in patients with hereditary spherocytosis. *Clin Lab Haematol* 1994;16:179–182.
163. Yufu Y, Matsumoto M, Miyamura T, et al. Parvovirus B19-associated haemophagocytic syndrome with lymphadenopathy resembling histiocytic necrotizing lymphadenitis (Kikuchi's disease). *Br J Haematol* 1997;96:868–871.
164. Tsuda H. Liver dysfunction caused by parvovirus B19. *Am J Gastroenterol* 1993;88:1463.
165. Yoto Y, Kudoh T, Haseyama K, et al. Human parvovirus B19 infection associated with acute hepatitis. *Lancet* 1996;347: 868–869.
166. Langnas AN, Markin RS, Cattral MS, et al. Parvovirus B19 as a possible causative agent of fulminant liver failure and associated aplastic anemia. *Hepatology* 1995;22:1661–1665.
167. Longo G, Luppi M, Bertesi M, et al. Still's disease, severe thrombocytopenia, and acute hepatitis associated with acute parvovirus B19 infection. *Clin Infect Dis* 1998;26:994–995.
168. Andres E, Grunenberger F, Schlienger JL, et al. Cutaneous vasculitis disclosing parvovirus B19 infection [Letter]. *Ann Med Intern* 1997;148:107–108.
169. Corman LC, Dolson DJ. Polyarteritis nodosa and parvovirus B19 infection. *Lancet* 1992;339:491.
170. Corman LC, Staud R. Association of Wegener's granulomatosis with parvovirus B19 infection: comment on the concise communication by Nikkari et al. [Letter; comment]. *Arthritis Rheum* 1995;38:1174–1175.
171. Finkel TH, Torok TJ, Ferguson PJ, et al. Chronic parvovirus B19 infection and systemic necrotizing vasculitis: opportunistic infection or aetiological agent? *Lancet* 1994;343:1255–1258.
172. Nikkari S, Mertsola J, Korvenranta H, et al. Wegener's granulomatosis and parvovirus B19 infection. *Arthritis Rheum* 1994;37:1707–1708.
173. Leruez-Ville M, Lauge A, Morinet F, et al. Polyarteritis nodosa and parvovirus B19 [Letter; comment]. *Lancet* 1994;344:263–264.
174. Nikkari S, Vainionpaa R, Toivanen P, et al. Association of Wegener's granulomatosis with parvovirus B19 infection: comment on the concise communication by Nikkari et al. [Reply]. *Arthritis Rheum* 1997;38:1175.
175. Fawaz-Estrup F. Human parvovirus infection: rheumatic manifestations, angioedema, C1 esterase inhibitor deficiency, ANA positivity, and possible onset of systemic lupus erythematosus. *J Rheumatol* 1996;3:1180–1185.
176. Vigeant P, MΘnard H-A, Boire G. Chronic modulation of the autoimmune response following parvovirus B19 infection. *J Rheumatol* 1994;1:1165–1167.
177. Loizou S, Cazabon JK, Walport MJ, et al. Similarities of specificity and cofactor dependence in serum antiphospholipid antibodies from patients with human parvovirus B19 infection and from those with systemic lupus erythematosus. *Arthritis Rheum* 1997;40:103–108.
178. Nocton JJ, Miller LC, Tucker LB, et al. Human parvovirus B19-associated arthritis in children. *J Pediatr* 1993;122: 186–190.
179. Bruu A-L, Nordbo SA. Evaluation of five commercial tests for detection of immunoglobulin M antibodies to human parvovirus B19. *J Clin Microbiol* 1995;33:1363–1365.
180. Patou G, Ayliffe U. Evaluation of commercial enzyme linked immunosorbent assay for detection of B19 parvovirus IgM and IgG. *J Clin Pathol* 1991;44:831–834.
181. Bell LM, Naides SJ, Stoffman P, et al. Human parvovirus B19 infection among hospital staff members after contact with infected patients. *N Engl J Med* 1989;321:485–491.
182. Cohen BJ, Mortimer PP, Pereira MS. Diagnostic assays with monoclonal antibodies for the human serum parvovirus-like virus (SPLV). *J Hyg* 1983;91:113–130.
183. Anderson MJ, Jones SE, Minson AC. Diagnosis of human parvovirus infection by dot-blot hybridization using cloned viral DNA. *J Med Virol* 1985;15:163–172.
184. Anderson MJ, Pattison JR. The human parvovirus: brief review. *Arch Virol* 1984;82:137–148.
185. Brown KE, Buckley MM, Cohen BJ, et al. An amplified ELISA for the detection of parvovirus B19 IgM using monoclonal antibody to FITC. *J Virol Methods* 1989;26:189–198.
186. Brown CS, Van Lent JWM, Vlak JM, et al. Assembly of empty capsids by using baculovirus recombinants expressing human parvovirus B19 structural proteins. *J Virol* 1991;65:2702–2706.
187. Cubie HA, Leslie EE, Smith S, et al. Use of recombinant human parvovirus B19 antigens in serological assays. *J Clin Pathol* 1993;46:840–845.
188. Fridell E, Trojnar J, Mehlin H, et al. A cyclized peptide for studies of human parvovirus B19 infection. *J Immunol Methods* 1991;138:125–128.
189. Koch WC. A synthetic parvovirus B19 capsid protein can replace viral antigen in antibody-capture enzyme immunoassays. *J Virol Methods* 1995;55:67–82.
190. Morinet F, D'Auriol L, Tratschin JD, et al. Expression of the human parvovirus B19 protein fused to protein A in *Escherichia coli: recognition by IgM and IgG antibodies in human sera.* J Gen Virol 1989;70:3091–3097.
191. Salimans MMM, van Bussel MJAWM, Brown CS, et al. Recombinant parvovirus B19 capsids as a new substrate for detection of B19-specific IgG and IgM antibodies by an enzyme-linked immunosorbent assay. *J Virol Methods* 1992; 39:247–258.
192. Soderlund M, Brown CS, Spaan WJ, et al. Epitope type-specific IgG responses to capsid proteins VP1 and VP2 of human parvovirus B19. *J Infect Dis* 1995;172:1431–1436.
193. Tsao EI, Mason MR, Cacciuttolo MA, et al. Production of parvovirus B19 vaccine in insect cells co-infected with double baculoviruses. *Biotechnol Bioeng* 1996;49:130–138.
194. Wang Q-Y, Erdman DD. Development and evaluation of capture immunoglobulin G and M hemadherence assays by using human type O erythrocytes and recombinant parvovirus B19 antigen. *J Clin Microbiol* 1995;33:2466–2467.
195. Fridell E, Trojnar J, Wahren B. A new peptide for human parvovirus B19 antibody detection. *Scand J Infect Dis* 1989;21: 597–603.
196. Sato H, Hirata J, Furukawa M, et al. Identification of the region

including the epitope for a monoclonal antibody which can neutralize human parvovirus B19. *J Virol* 1991;65:1667–1672.
197. Sato H, Hirata J, Kuroda N, et al. Identification and mapping of neutralizing epitopes of human parvovirus B19 by using human antibodies. *J Virol* 1991;65:5485–5490.
198. Cohen BJ, Shirley JA. Dual infection with rubella and human parvovirus. *Lancet* 1985;2:662–663.
199. Cohen BJ, Supran EM. IgM serology for rubella and human parvovirus B19. *Lancet* 1987;1:393.
200. Kurtz JB, Anderson MJ. Cross-reactions in rubella and parvovirus specific IgM tests. *Lancet* 1985;2:1356.
201. Clewley JP, Cohen BJ. Investigation of human parvovirus B19 infection using PCR. In: Clewley JP, ed. *The polymerase chain reaction (PCR) for human viral diagnosis.* Boca Raton: CRC Press, 1995:205–215.
202. Koch WC, Adler SP. Detection of human parvovirus B19 DNA by using the polymerase chain reaction. *J Clin Microbiol* 1990; 28:65–150.
203. Naides SJ, Howard EJ, Swack NS, et al. Parvovirus B19 as a cause of anemia in human immunodeficiency virus-infected patients. *J Infect Dis* 1994;169:939–940.
204. Clewley JP. Detection of human parvovirus using a molecularly cloned probe. *J Med Virol* 1985;15:173–181.
205. Clewley JP. Polymerase chain reaction assay of parvovirus B19 DNA in clinical specimens. *J Clin Microbiol* 1989;27:2647–2651.
206. Hassam S, Briner J, Tratschin JD, et al. In situ hybridization for the detection of human parvovirus B19 nucleic acid sequences in paraffin-embedded specimens. *Virchows Arch B* 1990;59: 257–261.
207. Mori J, Field AM, Clewley JP, et al. Dot blot hybridization assay of B19 virus DNA in clinical specimens. *J Clin Microbiol* 1989;27:459–464.
208. Gibellini D, Zerbini M, Musiani M, et al. Microplate capture hybridization of amplified parvovirus B19 DNA fragment labeled with digoxigenin. *Mol Cell Probes* 1993;7:453–458.
209. Schwarz TF, Nerlich A, Hottenträger B, et al. Parvovirus B19 infection of the fetus: histology and in situ hybridization. *Am J Clin Pathol* 1991;96:121–126.
210. Field AM, Cohen BJ, Brown KE, et al. Detection of B19 parvovirus in human fetal tissues by electron microscopy. *J Med Virol* 1991;35:85–95.
211. Hicks KE, Beard S, Cohen BJ, et al. A simple and sensitive DNA hybridization assay used for the routine diagnosis of human parvovirus B19 infection. *J Clin Microbiol* 1995;33: 2473–2475.
212. Zerbini M, Gibellini D, Musiani M, et al. Automated detection of digoxigenin-labelled B19 parvovirus amplicons by a capture hybridization assay. *J Virol Methods* 1995;55:1–9.
213. Zerbini M, Musiani M, Gibellini D, et al. Evaluation of strand-specific RNA probes visualized by colorimetric and chemiluminescent reactions for the detection of B19 parvovirus DNA. *J Virol Methods* 1993;45:169–178.
214. Zerbini M, Musiani M, Gibellini D, et al. Evaluation of strand-specific RNA probes visualized by colorimetric and chemiluminescent reactions for the detection of B19 parvovirus DNA. *J Virol Methods* 1993;45:169–178.
215. Fritz B, Moore K, Naides SJ. A combined pseudoreplica-immunochemical technique for research and diagnostic virology. *J Microsc Res Tech* 1992;21:59–64.
216. Saag KG, True CA, Naides SJ. Intravenous immunoglobulin treatment of chronic parvovirus B19 arthropathy. *Arthritis Rheum* 1993;36(suppl):S67.
217. McOmish F, Yap PL, Jordan A, et al. Detection of parvovirus B19 in donated blood: a model system for screening by polymerase chain reaction. *J Clin Microbiol* 1993;31:323–328.
218. Mosley JW. Should measures be taken to reduce the risk of human parvovirus (B19) infection by transfusion of blood com ponents and clotting factor concentrates? *Transfusion* 1994;34: 744–746.
219. Moor AC, Dubbelman TM, Van Steveninck J, et al. Transfusion-transmitted diseases: risks, prevention and perspectives. *Eur J Haematol* 1999;62:1–18.
220. Prowse C, Ludlam CA, Yap PL. Human parvovirus B19 and blood products. *Vox Sang* 1997;72:1–10.
221. Wakamatsu C, Takakura F, Kojima E., et al. Screening of blood for human parvovirus B19 and characterization of the results. *Vox Sang* 1999;76:14–21.
222. Sayers MH. Transfusion-transmitted viral infections other than hepatitis and human immunodeficiency virus infection: cytomegalovirus, Epstein-Barr virus, human herpesvirus 6, and human parvovirus B19. *Arch Pathol Lab Med* 1994;118:346–349.
223. Azzi A, Morfini M, Mannucci PM. The transfusion-associated transmission of parvovirus B19. *Transfus Med Rev* 1999;13: 194–204.
224. Yee TT, Cohen BJ, Pasi KJ, et al. Transmission of symptomatic parvovirus B19 infection by clotting factor concentrate. *Br J Haematol* 1996;93:457–459.
225. Solheim BG, Rollag H, Svennevig JL, et al. Viral safety of solvent/detergent-treated plasma. *Transfusion* 2000;40:84–90.
226. Wolinsky JS. Rubella. In: Fields BN, Knipe DM, Howley PM, et al., eds. *Fields virology.* 3rd ed. Philadelphia: Lippincott-Raven Press, 1996:899–929.
227. Porter DD, Larsen AE, Porter HG. The pathogenesis of Aleutian disease of mink. II. Enhancement of tissue lesions following the administration of a killed virus vaccine or passive antibody. *J Immunol* 1972;109:1–7.
228. Porter DD, Larsen AE, Porter HG. The pathogenesis of Aleutian disease of mink. 3. Immune complex arteritis. *Am J Pathol* 1973;71:331–344.
229. Murphy FA, Fauquet CM, Bishop DHL, et al. *Virus taxonomy: the classification and nomenclature of viruses: the Sixth Report of the International Committee on Taxonomy of Viruses.* Vienna: Springer-Verlag, 1995. Online, http://www.ncbi.nlm.nih.gov/ict/viruslist/+strandedssrna_viruses.pdf.
230. Oshiro LS, Schmidt NJ, Lennette EH. Electron microscopic studies of rubella virus. *J Gen Virol* 1969;5:205–210.
231. Frey TK. Molecular biology of rubella virus. *Adv Virus Res* 1994;44:69–160.
232. Horstmann DM. The rubella story, 1881-1985. *S Afr Med J* 1986;11(suppl):60–63.
233. Horstmann DM, Pajot TG, Liebhaber H. Epidemiology of rubella: subclinical infection and occurrence of reinfection. *Am J Dis Child* 1969;118:133–136.
234. Fogel A, Handsher R, Barnea B. Subclinical rubella in pregnancy: occurrence and outcome. *Isr J Med Sci* 1985;21:133–138.
235. Centers for Disease Control and Prevention. Reported vaccine-preventable diseases—United States, 1993, and the childhood immunization initiative. *JAMA* 1994;271:651–652.
236. Anonymous. Rubella and congenital rubella syndrome—United States, January 1, 1991-May 7, 1994. *MMWR* 1994;43:397–401.
237. Heggie AD, Robbins FC. Natural rubella acquired after birth: clinical features and complications. *Am J Dis Child* 1969;118: 12–17.
238. Davis WJ, Larson HE, Simsarian JP, et al. A study of rubella immunity and resistance to infection. *JAMA* 1971;215:600–608.
239. Green RH, Balsamo MR Giles JP, et al. Studies of the natural history and prevention of rubella. *Am J Dis Child* 1965;110: 348–365.
240. Sever JL, Hardy JB, Nelson KB, et al. Rubella in the collaborative perinatal research study. II. Clinical and laboratory findings in children through 3 years of age. *Am J Dis Child* 1969;118: 123.

241. Ford DK. The microbiological causes of rheumatoid arthritis [Editorial]. *J Rheumatol* 1991;18:1441–1442.
242. Grahame R, Armstrong R, Simmons N, et al. Chronic arthritis associated with the presence of intrasynovial rubella virus. *Ann Rheum Dis* 1983;42:2–13.
243. Smith CA, Petty RE, Tingle AJ. Rubella virus and arthritis. *Rheum Dis Clin North Am* 1987;13:265–274.
244. Polk BF, Modlin JF, White JA, et al. A controlled comparison of joint reactions among women receiving one of two rubella vaccines. *Am J Epidemiol* 1982;115:19–25.
245. Tingle AJ, Chantler JK, Pot KH, et al. Postpartum rubella immunization: association with development of prolonged arthritis, neurological sequelae, and chronic rubella viremia. *J Infect Dis* 1985;152:606–612.
246. Ueno Y. Rubella arthritis: an outbreak in Kyoto. *J Rheumatol* 1994;21:874–876.
247. Austin SM, Altman R, Barnes EK, et al. Joint reactions in children vaccinated against rubella. I. Comparison of two vaccines. *Am J Epidemiol* 1972;95:53–58.
248. Benjamin CM, Chew GC, Silman AJ. Joint and limb symptoms in children after immunisation with measles, mumps, and rubella vaccine. *BMJ* 1992;304:1075–1078.
249. Chantler JK, Tingle AJ, Petty RE. Persistent rubella virus infection associated with chronic arthritis in children. *N Engl J Med* 1985;313:1117–1123.
250. Miki NP, Chantler JK. Differential ability of wild-type and vaccine strains of rubella virus to replicate and persist in human joint tissue. *Clin Exp Rheumatol* 1992;10:3–12.
251. Preblud SR. Some current issues relating to rubella vaccine. *JAMA* 1985;254:253–256.
252. Tingle AJ, Ford DK, Price GE, et al. Prolonged arthritis in identical twins after rubella immunization. *Ann Intern Med* 1979; 90:203–204.
250. Tingle AJ, Allen M, Petty RE, et al. Rubella-associated arthritis. I. Comparative study of joint manifestations associated with natural rubella infection and RA 27/3 rubella immunisation. *Ann Rheum Dis* 1986;45:110–114.
251. Howson CP, Fineberg HV. Adverse events following pertussis and rubella vaccines: summary of a report to the Institute of Medicine. *JAMA* 1992;267:392–396.
252. Mitchell LA, Tingle AJ, Shukin R, et al. Chronic rubella vaccine-associated arthropathy. *Arch Intern Med* 1993;153:2268–2274.
253. Balfour HH Jr, Balfour CL, Edelman CK, et al. Evaluation of Wistar RA27/3 rubella virus vaccine in children. *Am J Dis Child* 1976;130:1089–1091.
254. Benjamin CM, Chew GC, Silman AJ. Joint and limb symptoms in children after immunisation with measles, mumps, and rubella vaccine. *BMJ* 1992;304:1075–1078.
255. Schaffner W, Fleet WF, Kilroy AW, et al. Polyneuropathy following rubella immunization: a follow-up study and review of the problem. *Am J Dis Child* 1974;127:684–688.
256. Davis WJ, Larson HE, Simsarian JP, et al. A study of rubella immunity and resistance to infection. *JAMA* 1971;215:600–608.
257. Wittenburg RA, Roberts MA, Elliott LB, et al. Comparative evaluation of commercial rubella virus antibody kits. *J Clin Microbiol* 1985;21:161–163.
258. Stewart GL, Parkman PD, Hopps HE, et al. Rubella-virus hemagglutination-inhibition test. *N Engl J Med* 1967;276:554–557.
259. Herrmann KL. Available rubella serologic tests. *Rev Infect Dis* 1985;7(suppl 1):S108–S112.
260. Chernesky MA, Wyman L, Mahony JB, et al. Clinical evaluation of the sensitivity and specificity of a commercially available enzyme immunoassay for detection of rubella virus-specific immunoglobulin M. *J Clin Microbiol* 1984;20:400–404.
261. Meurman OH. Persistence of immunoglobulin G and immunoglobulin M antibodies after postnatal rubella infection determined by solid-phase radioimmunoassay. *J Clin Microbiol* 1978;7:1–34.
262. Chaye H, Ou D, Chong P, et al. Human T- and B-cell epitopes of E1 glycoprotein of rubella virus. *J Clin Immunol* 1993;13: 93–100.
263. Chaye H, Chong P, Tripet B, et al. Localization of the virus neutralizing and hemagglutinin epitopes of E1 glycoprotein of rubella virus. *Virology* 1992;189:482–492.
264. Marttila J, Ilonen J, Lehtinen M, et al. Definition of three minimal T helper cell epitopes of rubella virus E1 glycoprotein. *Clin Exp Immunol* 1996;104:394–397.
265. Mauracher CA, Mitchell LA, Tingle AJ. Selective tolerance to the E1 protein of rubella virus in congenital rubella syndrome. *J Immunol* 1993;151:2041–2049.
266. Ou D, Chong P, Tripet B, et al. Analysis of T- and B-cell epitopes of capsid protein of rubella virus by using synthetic peptides. *J Virol* 1992;66:1674–1681.
267. Ou D, Chong P, Choi Y, et al. Identification of T-cell epitopes on E2 protein of rubella virus, as recognized by human T-cell lines and clones. *J Virol* 1992;66:6788–6793.
268. Ou D, Chong P, Tingle AJ, et al. Mapping T-cell epitopes of rubella virus structural proteins E1, E2, and C recognized by T-cell lines and clones derived from infected and immunized populations. *J Med Virol* 1993;40:175–183.
269. Wolinsky JS, Sukholutsky E, Moore WT, et al. An antibody- and synthetic peptide-defined rubella virus E1 glycoprotein neutralization domain. *J Virol* 1993;67:961–968.
270. Cunningham AL, Fraser JR. Persistent rubella virus infection of human synovial cells cultured in vitro. *J Infect Dis* 1985;151: 638–645.
271. Rawls WE, Melnick JL. Rubella virus carrier cultures derived from congenitally infected infants. *J Exp Med* 1966;123:795–816.
272. Mitchell LA, Tingle AJ, Shukin R, et al. Chronic rubella vaccine-associated arthropathy. *Arch Intern Med* 1993;153: 2268–2274.
273. Hollinger FB. Hepatitis B virus. In: Fields BN, Knipe DM, Chanock RM, et al., eds. *Fields virology.* 2nd ed. New York: Raven Press, 1990:2171–2236.
274. Seeger C. Hepatitis B virus. In: Webster RG, Granoff A, eds. *Encyclopedia of virology.* San Diego: Academic Press, 1994: 560–564.
275. Alter HJ, Purcell RH, Gerin JL, et al. Transmission of hepatitis B virus to chimpanzees by hepatitis B surface antigen-positive saliva and semen. *Hepatology* 1997;16:928–933.
276. Scott RM, Snitbhan R, Bancroft WH, et al. Experimental transmission of hepatitis B virus by semen and saliva. *J Infect Dis* 1980;142:67–71.
277. Bancroft WH, Snitbhan R, Scott RM, et al. Transmission of hepatitis B virus to gibbons by exposure to human saliva containing hepatitis B surface antigen. *J Infect Dis* 1977;135:79–85.
278. Mast EE, Alter MJ. Epidemiology of viral hepatitis: an overview. *Semin Virol* 1993;4:273–283.
279. Robinson WS. Hepatitis B viruses. In: Webster RG, Granoff A, eds. *Encyclopedia of virology.* San Diego: Academic Press, 1994: 554–559.
280. Hollinger FB. Hepatitis B virus. In: Fields BN, Knipe DM, Howley PM, et al., eds. *Fields virology.* 3rd ed. Philadelphia: Lippincott-Raven Press, 1996:2739–2807.
281. Allen JG, Sayman WA. Serum hepatitis from transfusions of blood. *JAMA* 1962;180:1079–1085.
282. Barker LF, Murray R. Relationship of virus dose to incubation time of clinical hepatitis and time of appearance of hepatitis-associated antigen. *Am J Med Sci* 1972;263:27–33.
283. Havens WP Jr, Ward R, Drill VA, et al. Experimental production of hepatitis by feeding icterogenic materials. *Proc Soc Exp Biol Med* 1944;57:206–208.

284. Alpert E, Jackson D. Besides the liver, what does the virus of hepatitis attack? *Heart Lung* 1982;11:177–180.
285. Caroli J. Serum-sickness-like prodromata in viral hepatitis: Caroli's triad. *Lancet* 1972;1:964–965.
286. Gocke DJ. Extrahepatic manifestations of viral hepatitis. *Am J Med Sci* 1975;270:49–52.
287. Veyre B, Brette R. Hepatitis B at the premonitory stage: incidence of articular and cutaneous manifestations, apropos of 100 cases. *Nouv Press Med* 1975;4:1349–1352.
288. Csepregi A, Rojkovich B, Nemesanszky E, et al. Chronic seropositive polyarthritis associated with hepatitis B virus-induced chronic liver disease: a sequel of virus persistence. *Arthritis Rheum* 2000;43:232–323.
289. Guillevin L, Lhote F, Cohen P, et al. Polyarteritis nodosa related to hepatitis B virus: a prospective study with long-term observation of 41 patients. *Medicine* 1995;74:238–253.
290. Brzosko WJ, Mikulska B, Cianciara J, et al. Immunoglobulin classes of antibody to hepatitis B core antigen. *J Infect Dis* 1975;132:1–5.
291. Cohen BJ. The IgM antibody responses to the core antigen of hepatitis B virus. *J Med Virol* 1978;3:141–149.
292. Kryger P, Mathiesen LR, Moller AM, et al. Enzyme-linked immunosorbent assay for detection of immunoglobulin M antibody to hepatitis B core antigen. *J Clin Microbiol* 1981;13:405–409.
293. Rimland D, Parkin WE, Miller GB Jr, et al. Hepatitis B outbreak traced to an oral surgeon. *N Engl J Med* 1977;296:953–958.
294. Hoofnagle JH. Serologic markers of hepatitis B virus infection. *Annu Rev Med* 1981;32:1–11.
295. Purcell RH. Hepatitis C virus. In: Webster RG, Granoff A, eds. *Encyclopedia of virology*. San Diego: Academic Press, 1994:569–574.
296. Kuboki M, Shinzawa H, Shao L, et al. A cohort study of hepatitis C virus (HCV) infection in an HCV epidemic area of Japan: age and sex-related seroprevalence of anti-HCV antibody, frequency of viremia, biochemical abnormality and histological changes. *Liver* 1999;19:88–96.
297. Williams I. Epidemiology of hepatitis C in the United States. *Am J Med* 1999;107:2S–9S.
298. Alter MJ. Hepatitis C virus infection in the United States. *J Hepatol* 1999;31(suppl 1):88–91.
299. Chiaramonte M, Stroffolini T, Lorenzoni U, et al. Risk factors in community-acquired chronic hepatitis C virus infection: a case-control study in Italy. *J Hepatol* 1996;24:129–134.
300. Pereira BJ, Wright TL, Schmid CH, et al. A controlled study of hepatitis C transmission by organ transplantation: the New England Organ Bank Hepatitis C Study Group [published errata appear in *Lancet* 1995;345:662 and 1995;345:662] *Lancet* 1995;345:484–487.
301. Salleras L, Bruguera M, Vidal J, et al. Importance of sexual transmission of hepatitis C virus in seropositive pregnant women: a case-control study. *J Med Virol* 1997;52:164–167.
302. Neumayr G, Propst A, Schwaighofer H, et al. Lack of evidence for the heterosexual transmission of hepatitis C. *Q J Med* 1999;92:505–508.
303. Bhandari BN, Wright TL. Hepatitis C: an overview. *Annu Rev Med* 1995;46:309–317.
304. Davis GL. Hepatitis C virus genotypes and quasispecies. *Am J Med* 1999;107:21S–26S.
305. Seeff LB. Natural history of hepatitis C. *Am J Med* 1999;107:10S–15S.
306. Alberti A, Chemello L, Benvegnu L. Natural history of hepatitis C. *J Hepatol* 1999;31(suppl 1):17–24.
307. Marcellin P. Hepatitis C: the clinical spectrum of the disease. *J Hepatol* 1999;31(suppl 1):9–16.
308. Liddle C. Hepatitis C. *Anaesth Intens Care* 1996;24:180–183.
309. Hoshiyama A, Kimura A, Fujisawa T, et al. Clinical and histologic features of chronic hepatitis C virus infection after blood transfusion in Japanese children. *Pediatrics* 2000;105:62–65.
310. Kato Y, Nakata K, Omagari K, et al. Risk of hepatocellular carcinoma in patients with cirrhosis in Japan: analysis of infectious hepatitis viruses. *Cancer* 1994;74:2234–2238.
311. Omagari K, Komatsu K, Kato Y, et al. Clinical manifestations of HBsAg and anti-HCV negative chronic liver disease in Nagasaki Prefecture, Japan. *Intern Med* 1996;35:600–604.
312. Seeff LB, Miller RN, Rabkin CS, et al. 45-year follow-up of hepatitis C virus infection in healthy young adults. *Ann Intern Med* 2000;132:105–111.
313. Siegel LB, Cohn L, Nashel D. Rheumatic manifestations of hepatitis C infection. *Semin Arthritis Rheum* 1993;3:49–154.
314. Ueno Y, Kinoshita R, Kishimoto I, et al. Arthritis associated with hepatitis C virus infection. *Br J Rheumatol* 1994;33:289–291.
315. Bichard P, Ounanian A, Girard M, et al. High prevalence of hepatitis C virus RNA in the supernatant and the cryoprecipitate of patients with essential and secondary type II mixed cryoglobulinemia. *J Hepatol* 1994;21:58–63.
316. Misiani R, Bellavita P, Fenili D, et al. Hepatitis C virus infection in patients with essential mixed cryoglobulinemia. *Ann Intern Med* 1992;117:573–577.
317. Zapico R, Quevedo E, Arribas JR, et al. Evidence of hepatitis C virus antibodies in the cryoprecipitate of patients with mixed cryoglobulinemia. *J Rheumatol* 1994;21:229–233.
318. Van der Poel C L. Hepatitis C virus: into the fourth generation. *Vox Sang* 1994;67(suppl 3):95–98.
319. Stapleton JT, Klinzman D, Schmidt WN, et al. Prospective comparison of whole-blood- and plasma-based hepatitis C virus RNA detection systems: improved detection using whole blood as the source of viral RNA. *J Clin Microbiol* 1999;37:484–489.
320. Schmidt WN, Wu P, Cederna J, et al. Surreptitious hepatitis C virus (HCV) infection detected in the majority of patients with cryptogenic chronic hepatitis and negative HCV antibody tests. *J Infect Dis* 1997;176:27–33.
321. Shimizu YK, Hijikata M, Iwamoto A, et al. Neutralizing antibodies against hepatitis C virus and the emergence of neutralization escape mutant viruses. *J Virol* 1994;68:1494–1500.
322. Jenkins PJ, Cromie SL, Bowden DS, et al. Chronic hepatitis C and interferon alfa therapy: predictors of long term response. *Med J Aust* 1996;164:150–152.
323. Bacon BR. Available options for treatment of interferon nonresponders. *Am J Med* 1999;107:67S–70S.
324. Jacobson I. Management of interferon relapsers. *Am J Med* 1999;107:62S–66S.
325. Bell TM, Bansal AS, Shorthouse C, et al. Low-titre auto-antibodies predict autoimmune disease during interferon-alpha treatment of chronic hepatitis C. *J Gastroenterol Hepatol* 1999;14:419–422.
326. Fernandez-Soto L, Gonzalez A, Escobar-Jimenez F, et al. Increased risk of autoimmune thyroid disease in hepatitis C vs hepatitis B before, during, and after discontinuing interferon therapy. *Arch Intern Med* 1998;158:1445–1448.
327. Peters CJ, Dalrymple JM. Alphaviruses. In: Fields BN, Knipe DM, Chanock RM, et al., eds. *Fields virology.* 2nd ed. New York: Raven Press, 1990:713–761.
328. Ross RW. The Newala epidemic. III. The virus: isolation, pathogenic properties and relationship to the epidemic. *J Hyg* 1956;54:177–191.
329. Moore CG. *Aedes albopictus* in the United States: current status and prospects for further spread. *J Am Mosq Control Assoc* 1999;15:221–227.
330. Fink TM, Hau B, Baird BL, et al. *Aedes aegypti* in Tucson, Arizona. *Emerg Infect Dis* 1998;4:703–704.

331. Engelthaler DM, Fink TM, Levy CE, et al. The reemergence of *Aedes aegypti* in Arizona. *Emerg Infect Dis* 1997;3:241–242.
332. Jupp PG, McIntosh BM. *Aedes furcifer* and other mosquitoes as vectors of Chikungunya virus at Mica, northeastern Transvaal, South Africa. *J Am Mosq Control Assoc* 1990;6:415–420.
333. Halstead SB, Nimmannitya S, Margiotta MR. Dengue and Chikungunya virus infection in man in Thailand, 1962-1964. II. Observations on disease in outpatients. *Am J Trop Med Hyg* 1969;18:972–983.
334. Tesh RB. Arthritides caused by mosquito-borne viruses. *Annu Rev Med* 1998;233:31–40.
335. Halstead SB, Udomsakdi S, Singharaj P, et al. Dengue and Chikungunya virus infection in man in Thailand, 1962-1964. III. Clinical, epidemiologic, and virologic observations on disease in non-indigenous white persons. *Am J Trop Med Hyg* 1969;18:984–996.
336. Brighton SW, Simson IW. A destructive arthropathy following Chikungunya virus arthritis: a possible association. *Clin Rheumatol* 1984;3:253–258.
337. Fourie ED, Morrison JG. Rheumatoid arthritic syndrome after Chikungunya fever. *S Afr Med J* 1979;56:130–132.
338. Nakitare GW, Bundo K, Igarashi A. Enzyme-linked immunosorbent assay (ELISA) for antibody titers against Chikungunya virus of human serum from Kenya. *Trop Med* 1983;25:119–128.
339. Brighton SW. Chloroquine phosphate treatment of chronic Chikungunya arthritis: an open pilot study. *S Afr Med J* 1984; 66:217–218.
340. Williams MC, Woodall JP, Porterfield JS. O'Nyong-nyong fever: an epidemic virus disease in east Africa. V. Human antibody studies by plaque inhibition and other serological tests. *Trans R Soc Trop Med Hyg* 1962;56:166–172.
341. Williams MC, Woodall JP, Gillett JD. O'nyong-nyong fever: an epidemic in East Africa. VII. Virus isolations from man and serological studies up to July 1961. *Trans R Soc Trop Med Hyg* 1965;59:186–197.
342. Johnson BK, Gichogo A, Gitau G, et al. Recovery of O'nyong-nyong virus from *Anopheles funestus* in western Kenya. *Trans R Soc Trop Med Hyg* 1981;75:239–241.
343. Kiwanuka N, Sanders EJ, Rwaguma EB, et al. O'nyong-nyong fever in south-central Uganda, 1996-1997: clinical features and validation of a clinical case definition for surveillance purposes. *Clin Infect Dis* 1999;29:1243–1250.
344. Sanders EJ, Rwaguma EB, Kawamata J, et al. O'nyong-nyong fever in south-central Uganda, 1996-1997: description of the epidemic and results of a household-based seroprevalence survey. *J Infect Dis* 1999;180:1436–1443.
345. Marshall TF, Keenlyside RA, Johnson BK, et al. The epidemiology of O'nyong-nyong in the Kano Plain, Kenya. *Ann Trop Med Parasitol* 1982;76:153–158.
346. Shore H. O'Nyong-nyong fever: an epidemic virus disease in east Africa. III. Some clinical and epidemiological observations in the northern province. *Trans R Soc Trop Med Hyg* 1961;55: 361–373.
347. Williams MC, Woodall JP, Porterfield JS. O'nyong-nyong fever: an epidemic virus disease in East Africa. *Trans R Soc Trop Med Hyg* 1962;56:166–172.
348. Blackburn NK, Besselaar TG, Gibson G. Antigenic relationship between Chikungunya virus strains and O'nyong nyong virus using monoclonal antibodies. *Res Virol* 1995;146: 69–73.
349. Moore DL, Causey OR, Carey DE, et al. Arthropod-borne viral infections of man in Nigeria, 1964-1970. *Ann Trop Med Parasitol* 1975;69:49–64.
350. Aaskov JG, Ross PV, Harper JJ, et al. Isolation of Ross River virus from epidemic polyarthritis patients in Australia. *Aust J Exp Biol Med Sci* 1985;63:587–597.
351. Scrimgeour EM, Matz LR, Aaskov JG. A study of arthritis in Papua New Guinea. *Aust N Z J Med* 1987:17:51–54.
352. Bennett NM, Cunningham AL, Fraser JR, et al. Epidemic polyarthritis acquired in Fiji. *Med J Aust* 1980;1:316–317.
353. Boughton CR, Hawkes RA, Naim HM, et al. Arbovirus infections in humans in New South Wales: seroepidemiology of the alphavirus group of togaviruses. *Med J Aust* 1984;141;700–704.
354. Hawkes RA, Boughton CR, Naim HM, et al. A major outbreak of epidemic polyarthritis in New South Wales during the summer of 1983/1984. *Med J Aust* 1985;143:330–333.
355. Fraser JRE. Epidemic polyarthritis and Ross River virus disease. *Clin Rheum Dis* 1986;12:369–388.
356. Aaskov JG, Mataika JU, Lawrence GW, et al. An epidemic of Ross River virus infection in Fiji, 1979. *Am J Trop Med Hyg* 1981;30:1053–1059.
357. Tesh RB, McLean RG, Shroyer DA, et al. Ross River virus (Togaviridae: Alphavirus) infection (epidemic polyarthritis) in American Samoa. *Trans R Soc Trop Med Hyg* 1981;75:426–431.
358. Fraser JR, Cunningham AL, Clarris BJ, et al. Cytology of synovial effusions in epidemic polyarthritis. *Aust N Z J Med* 1981; 11:168–173.
359. Fraser JR, Ratnamohan VM, Dowling JP, et al. The exanthem of Ross River virus infection: histology, location of virus antigen and nature of inflammatory infiltrate. *J Clin Pathol* 1983;36: 1256–1263.
360. Stocks N, Selden S, Cameron S. Ross River virus infection: diagnosis and treatment by general practitioners in South Australia. *Aust Fam Physician* 1997;26:710–717.
361. Watson DA, Ross SA. Corticosteroids for the complications of Ross River virus infection [Letter retracted in: *Med J Aust* 1998;169:64] *Med J Aust* 1998;168:92.
362. Lindsay MDA, Johansen CA, Broom AK, et al. Emergence of Barmah Forest virus in western Australia. *Emerg Infect Dis* (online) 1995;1:1–6.
363. Niklasson B, Espmark A, Lundstrom J. Occurrence of arthralgia and specific IgM antibodies three to four years after Ockelbo disease. *J Infect Dis* 1988;157:832–835.
364. Carter IW, Smythe LD, Fraser JR, et al. Detection of Ross River virus immunoglobulin M antibodies by enzyme-linked immunosorbent assay using antibody class capture and comparison with other methods. *Pathology* 1985;17:503–508.
365. Hoch AL, Peterson NE, LeDuc JW, et al. An outbreak of Mayaro virus disease in Belterra, Brazil. III. Entomological and ecological studies. *Am J Trop Med Hyg* 1981;30:689–698.
366. LeDuc JW, Pinheiro FP, Travassos da Rosa AP. An outbreak of Mayaro virus disease in Belterra, Brazil. II. Epidemiology. *Am J Trop Med Hyg* 1981;30:682–688.
367. Pinheiro FP, Freitas RB, Travassos da Rosa JF, et al. An outbreak of Mayaro virus disease in Belterra, Brazil. I. Clinical and virological findings. *Am J Trop Med Hyg* 1981;30:674–681.
368. Calisher CH, Gutierrez E, Maness KS, et al. Isolation of Mayaro virus from a migrating bird captured in Louisiana in 1967. *Bull Pan Am Health Org* 1974;8:243–248.
369. Tesh RB, Watts DM, Russell K, et al. Mayaro virus disease: an emerging mosquito-borne zoonosis in tropical South America. *Clin Infect Dis* 1999;28:67–73.
370. Anderson JF, Andreadis TG, Vossbrinck CR, et al. Isolation of West Nile virus from mosquitoes, crows, and a Cooper's hawk in Connecticut. *Science* 1999;286:2331–2333.
371. Chen MK, Wang CC, Lu JJ, et al. Varicella arthritis diagnosed by polymerase chain reaction. *J Formos Med Assoc* 1999;98:519–521.
372. Harel L, Amir J, Reish O, et al. Mumps arthritis in children. *Pediatr Infect Dis J* 1990;9:928–929.

373. Bayer AS. Arthritis associated with common viral infections: mumps, coxsackievirus, and adenovirus. *Postgrad Med* 1980;68: 55–58, 60, 63–4.
374. Rahal JJ, Millian SJ, Noriega ER. Coxsackievirus and adenovirus infection: association with acute febrile and juvenile rheumatoid arthritis. *JAMA* 1976;235:2496–2501.
375. Blotzer JW, Myers AR. Echovirus-associated polyarthritis: report of a case with synovial fluid and synovial histologic characterization. *Arthritis Rheum* 1978;21:978–981.
376. Berger RG, Raab-Traub N. Acute monoarthritis from infectious mononucleosis. *Am J Med* 1999;107:177–178.
377. Bonneville M, Scotet E, Peyrat MA, et al. Epstein-Barr virus and rheumatoid arthritis [Editorial]. *Rev Rhum Engl Ed* 1998; 65:365–368.
378. Burns LJ, Gingrich RD. Cytomegalovirus infection presenting as polyarticular arthritis following autologous BMT. *Bone Marrow Transplant* 1993;11:77–79.
379. Shelley WB. Herpetic arthritis associated with disseminate herpes simplex in a wrestler. *Br J Dermatol* 1980;103:209–212.
380. Nitzkin JL, Anderson L, Skaggs JW, et al. Complications of smallpox vaccination in Kentucky in 1968: results of a statewide survey. *J Ky Med Assoc* 1971;69:184–189.

131

RETROVIRUS-ASSOCIATED RHEUMATIC DISORDERS

LUIS R. ESPINOZA
MARTA L. CUÉLLAR

The association of retroviral infection with a variety of rheumatic disorders is well established (1–9). In recent years, a number of reports have described the identification of particles resembling retroviruses in affected tissue from patients with psoriasis (10), Sjögren's syndrome (SS) (11,12), rheumatoid arthritis (RA) (13), and systemic lupus erythematosus (SLE) (14). Furthermore, a human endogenous retrovirus genome (HERV-K) has been implicated in the pathogenesis of certain autoimmune disorders such as insulin-dependent diabetes mellitus (IDDM) (15), and a retrovirus related to the endogenous element ERV-9 has been identified in multiple sclerosis (16). This association is further strengthened by the occurrence of a variety of rheumatic syndromes and autoimmune phenomena during retroviral infections in humans and animals (17–20). Caprine arthritis–encephalitis virus (CAEV) induces an inflammatory articular process in goats, which closely resembles RA (21). Similarly, rhesus monkeys experimentally infected with simian immunodeficiency virus develop inflammatory polyarthritis (22). The most important association, however, between retroviral infection and inflammatory musculoskeletal manifestations occurs with human immunodeficiency virus type 1 (HIV-1) and also with human T-cell leukemia virus-1 (HTLV-1) infections (1–4,23,24). Because of the great importance and relevance of HIV-1 infection worldwide, we describe and discuss its associated musculoskeletal manifestations in more detail.

HUMAN IMMUNODEFICIENCY VIRUS INFECTION

The epidemic of HIV infection continues to spread worldwide, with developing countries being the areas of most rapid expansion. In the 12 months ending on December 1, 1998, 5.8 million newly infected cases of HIV infection occurred worldwide, bringing the total of infected individuals to 33.4 million. The number of deaths worldwide reached 2.5 million. The most striking aspect of the pandemic is that nearly 70% of new infections occurred in sub-Saharan Africa, with several African countries in this region having more than 20% of adults infected. South Africa is an area of concern, with the epidemic growing explosively. Another world area of great concern is India, with a reported HIV-seropositive prevalence of 2%.

Overall, the incidence of HIV infection in the United States is declining. The total number of new cases during the 12 months preceding December 1, 1998, reached 44,000 in North America. HIV infection data, however, should be interpreted with caution. HIV surveillance reports may not be representative of all persons infected with HIV because not all infected persons have been tested. In addition, many HIV-reporting states offer anonymous HIV testing, and home collection HIV test kits are widely available in the U.S. (25).

During 1998, 48,269 persons were reported with acquired immunodeficiency syndrome (AIDS), more than half (57%) from the states of New York, Florida, New Jersey, California, and Texas. A total of 688,200 persons has been reported in the U.S. with AIDS since the beginning of the epidemic. In 1997, the most recent full year for which estimates are available, an estimated 270,841 persons were living with AIDS, a 12% increase from 1996. The number of persons living with AIDS increased as a result of improved survival, thanks to the availability of newer antiretroviral treatments and substantial decreases in the number of deaths in 1997. This reported decline in the AIDS incidence applies to all regions in the U.S., all racial/ethnic groups, and all exposure groups (25).

Among geographic regions of the U.S., the South has experienced the smallest decline (12%) in number of new AIDS cases. Among racial/ethnic groups, the decrease is smaller in blacks (9%) than in whites or Hispanics. Additionally, data from prevalence surveys show a higher prevalence of HIV in non-Hispanic blacks than in other racial/ethnic groups in most populations surveyed (25).

Among exposure groups, men who have sex with men continue to compose the largest proportion of new AIDS cases. Although men who have sex with men have seen the sharpest decline in AIDS incidence (19%), this group still experiences the highest HIV prevalence rates among populations at risk for HIV nationwide (25).

Infection with HIV results in a wide spectrum of clinical manifestations that ranges from the asymptomatic state to AIDS (26–29). The acute retroviral stage begins after initial exposure and is characterized by the appearance of an HIV-specific antibody response, high levels of viremia with evidence of immunologic activation, decline in CD4$^+$ cell counts, inversion of the CD4$^+$:CD8$^+$ ratio, and absolute increase of CD8$^+$ lymphocytes. Symptoms develop within 5 to 30 days after exposure, and seroconversion occurs from 1 to 10 weeks after the acute illness, lasts 4 to 6 weeks, and leads into the second phase of the disease, in which the level of viremia declines, eventually reaching a "set point." This phase, which may last up to 10 years, is further characterized by a gradual decline in the numbers of CD4$^+$ T lymphocytes. The third phase is characterized by a marked decline in the number of CD4$^+$ T lymphocytes, increase in the levels of circulating virus and infected cells, and the development of the constellation of signs and symptoms characteristic of AIDS.

Musculoskeletal manifestations may develop at any phase of the infection, being more prevalent in later stages in Western populations and in early stages in African populations. A variety of rheumatic syndromes can occur, ranging from isolated symptoms including arthralgias and myalgias to well-defined or distinct disorders such as Reiter's syndrome, psoriatic arthritis, vasculitis, and polymyositis (1–4).

Etiopathogenic Considerations

Retroviruses

Retroviruses have the ability to copy their RNA genome into DNA by using reverse transcriptase. Human retroviruses belong to the family Retroviridae and are classified into three subfamilies (Table 131.1): oncovirus (HTLV); lentivirus (HIV); and spumavirus (30–32). They also can be classified into simple or complex, depending on their genome organization, that is, *gag, pol,* and *env* genes, with or without extra nonstructural genes with regulatory or auxiliary functions. The *gag* and *env* genes encode the core nucleocapsid polypeptides (e.g., p-24) and surface-coat proteins of the virus (e.g., gp-120), respectively, whereas the *pol* gene gives rise to the viral reverse transcriptase and other enzymatic activities. The glycoprotein gp-120 recognizes the receptor for the virus on target cells (CD4$^+$ lymphocytes and macrophages) and is also the target for neutralizing antibodies. The *pol* gene products are located in the core of the virion and function to replicate the viral genomic RNA, which is reverse-transcribed into double-stranded DNA by the viral DNA polymerase. The persistence and replication of the HIV genome in CD4$^+$ T lymphocytes leads to dysfunction and depletion of these lymphocytes, development of a profound state of immunosuppression, and eventual occurrence of the opportunistic infections and malignancies characteristic of AIDS (28). HIV attachment and fusion with target cells requires CD4 molecules and one of two other accessory receptors designated CCR5 and CXCR4. Resistance to HIV primary infection is evident in individuals who are homozygous for a deletion in the CCR5 gene (33).

Worldwide, most AIDS patients are infected with HIV-1, whereas a second virus, HIV-2, is responsible for some cases of a milder form of the disease in West Africa. HIV-1 itself is further subdivided into two genetically distinct subgroups, group M and group O, each of which is further subdivided into numerous subtypes. A new HIV variant, designated YBF30, appears to be a member of an entirely separate third HIV group. The M ("major") group accounts for the overwhelming majority of infections with HIV, and the O ("outlier") group is found almost exclusively in Cameroon, West Africa. Interestingly, YBF30, designated the N group, is highly homologous to a strain of SIV—the simian version of HIV—isolated earlier from a chimpanzee in neighboring Gabon. The similarities between YBF30 and chimpanzee SIV suggest that the evolutionary ancestors of N group viruses might have been transmitted to humans from nonhuman primates. A similar scenario is thought to be responsible for the evolution of HIV-2, which is genetically similar to SIV strains.

TABLE 131.1. RETROVIRUSES (RETROVIRIDAE)

Human	Disease
Oncovirus	
HTLV-1	Adult T-cell leukemia
HTLV-2	Tropical spastic paraparesis
	Hairy cell leukemia
Lentivirus	
HIV-1	AIDS
HIV-2	AIDS
Spumavirus	

HTLV, Human T-cell leukemia virus; HIV, human immunodeficiency virus; AIDS, acquired immunodeficiency syndrome.

HIV-induced Immunodeficiency

The mechanisms underlying the development of HIV-induced immunodeficiency are complex and not completely understood. Although the key defect leading to immune deficiency is diminished levels of CD4$^+$ lymphocytes, multiple factors may play a role (Table 131.2) (35). Direct CD4$^+$ lymphocyte lysis by HIV or indirect cytotoxic effects through host immune mechanisms against infected cells have been proposed but are not well documented. In recent years, it has become clearly established that HIV replication is an active process throughout all phases of the HIV infection, and more important, the number of infected CD4$^+$ lymphocytes explains, in part, the loss of CD4$^+$ cells in all stages of the disease process. This virus replication occurs not only in peripheral blood, but also in lymphoid tissue including peripheral lymph nodes, bone

TABLE 131.2. MECHANISMS OF HIV-INDUCED IMMUNODEFICIENCY

Direct effect
Viral replication in hematopoietic organs (thymus, bone marrow, and peripheral lymph nodes)
Disruption of the microarchitecture of the immune system
Indirect effect
Immune activation: production of proinflammatory cytokines
Enhanced apoptosis
Syncytium formation
Cytokine dysregulation
Miscellaneous
Shortened telomeres
Facilitation of HIV replication by opportunistic infections

HIV, human immunodeficiency virus.

marrow, and thymus. This results eventually in disruption of the microarchitecture of the immune system and leads to an immunosuppressive effect.

A decreased number of circulating CD4+ lymphocytes and an expansion in the number of CD8+ cells characterizes the early stages of HIV infection, whereas all circulating lymphoid populations, including CD8+ lymphocytes, B lymphocytes, and natural killer cells, decrease in number in later stages of HIV infection (36). Selective depletion of certain functional subsets of CD4+ lymphocytes, particularly naive CD4+ cells, is characteristic of HIV infection (37). Functional studies reveal losses in antigen-specific responses mediated by memory cells (38). Sequential loss of antigen, alloantigen, and mitogen reactivity occurs as HIV progresses. This inexorably leads to a depletion of reactive cell clones, resulting in holes in the repertoire of responsiveness and a failure of host defenses.

CD8+ lymphocytes are major effectors of cell-mediated cytotoxicity, produce β-chemokines and other soluble factors, and may prevent HIV propagation through the inhibition of virus binding to cellular co-receptors. Furthermore, the development of a CD8+ cytolytic response plays a critical role in the host defense against HIV infection because it is associated with downregulation of HIV propagation in the early stages of HIV infection (39). Accumulated evidence suggests that the preservation of CD4+ and CD8+ cell responses to HIV is associated with a better outcome (40).

Immune activation, especially in early stages of HIV infection, has been demonstrated. Both the CD4+ and CD8+ lymphocytes of HIV-infected patients express activation markers such as CD38 and class II human leukocyte antigen DR (HLA-DR) major histocompatibility antigens (41). Furthermore, monocyte activation in HIV infection also occurs, and results in production of high levels of tumor necrosis factor-α (TNF-α) and interleukin-6 (IL-6). These proinflammatory cytokines can upregulate HIV expression and may drive HIV production *in vivo*. Dysregulation in the production of IL-12 and γ-interferon (IFN-γ) may play an important role in the increased susceptibility of HIV patients to infection with intracellular microorganisms, particularly *Mycobacterium tuberculosis* or atypical mycobacteria. Both IL-12 and IFN-γ seem to be essential for the development of protective cell-mediated immunity to mycobacterial pathogens in mice and humans.

Other potential mechanisms underlying immunodeficiency in HIV infection include dysregulation in cytokine production with Th1 to Th2 switch, syncytium formation, shortened telomere, enhanced apoptosis, and superantigen-mediated destruction of CD4+ cells.

T-cell deficiency is almost always accompanied by deficient humoral immunity. This may, in part, explain the increased prevalence of bacterial infections in patients with T-cell deficiency.

HIV-Associated Rheumatic Disease: Pathogenic Considerations

A variety of mechanisms by which retroviruses including HIV-1 might influence the immune system and lead to the development of autoimmune abnormalities and rheumatic manifestations have been described. To date, however, the pathogenic mechanisms have not yet been definitively established. It is likely that the responsible mechanisms are complex and multifactorial (Table 131.3).

Direct Effect of Retrovirus

Experimental animal models of retrovirus-induced disease, such as CAEV, and the Rhesus monkey infected with SIV, provide support for primary retroviral infection within joints (20–22). In these models, intact virions can be detected in synovial and also muscle tissue. In addition, specific viral proteins may directly stimulate the immune system by upregulating proinflammatory cytokines through nuclear factor-κB. This has been demonstrated

TABLE 131.3. MECHANISMS UNDERLYING HIV-ASSOCIATED RHEUMATIC MANIFESTATIONS

Direct effect
Viral replication in affected tissue (i.e., synovium, endothelium, muscle)
Indirect effect
Immune activation resulting in
a) Increased serum immunoglobulins
b) Circulating immune complexes
c) Elevated circulating levels of proinflammatory cytokines
d) Multiple autoantibodies
Switch from Th1 to Th2 functional predominance
Genetic factors: HLA-B27, HLA-DR5, -DR6, and -DR7; non-HLA factors
Environmental factors: comorbid infections

HIV, human immunodeficiency virus; HLA, human leukocyte antigen.

for the Tax protein of HTLV-1 *in vitro* in transfected human cells and *in vivo* in transgenic mice (42). It also has been shown that the HIV *tat* gene induces skin lesions in transgenic mice resembling the psoriasiform lesions described in association with HIV-1 infection (43). In humans with retrovirus-associated rheumatic disorders, only a few reports have identified HIV in synovial fluid aspirates. HIV DNA also has been identified by *in situ* hybridization within dendritic cells isolated from both synovium and peripheral blood of HIV-infected individuals with arthritis. HIV-related p-24 antigen was localized in synovial tissue of individuals with arthritis, but viral particles were not identified in the same specimen by electron microscopy or culture (44). Several other HIV-related antigens including gp-41 and gp-120 have been identified in tissues of HIV-infected individuals.

Strong circumstantial evidence providing support for a direct role of HIV infection in the triggering of reactive arthritis or spondyloarthropathy is the striking increase in the prevalence of these disorders in Central Africa. Before the advent of HIV infection, spondyloarthropathy (SpA) disorders were rare in sub-Saharan Africa (45). This was thought to be due to the extremely low prevalence of HLA-B27 in the population (46). The prevalence of SpA has dramatically increased by severalfold since the advent of HIV infection and is not correlated with gastrointestinal Gram-negative infection, which is highly prevalent in the area (46,47).

Indirect Effects of HIV Infection

HIV infection leads to dysregulation of the production of a variety of cytokines, resulting in an increased production of certain proinflammatory cytokines such as IL-1, IL-6, and TNF-α, which can stimulate *in vivo* replication of HIV (48,49). The proinflammatory cytokines may play a role in tissue damage associated with opportunistic infections, and in some of the clinical manifestations including cachexia, encephalopathy, and arthritis. In some HIV-infected patients, the switch from a functional T-helper type 1 (Th-1) to a T-helper type 2 (Th-2) phenotype may facilitate further progression of the disease, including the appearance of rheumatic manifestations (50).

Furthermore, IL-1 and TNF-α, have been identified in the muscle of HIV-infected patients. IL-1β mRNA has been shown in muscle fibers by *in situ* hybridization, suggesting that IL-1 was produced in the affected muscle cells (51). HIV infection of CD4$^+$ lymphocytes and also macrophages may result in the release of growth factors (e.g., endothelial cell growth factors), which may also contribute to some of the clinical manifestations (52).

Reactive Immune Mechanisms in HIV Infection

Immune-mediated mechanisms may play a role in the pathogenesis of HIV disease, including rheumatic syndromes. A state of immune activation exists in the early stages of HIV infection, and both B- and T-cell hyperresponsiveness can be demonstrated (41,53). Elevated levels of serum immunoglobulins, circulating immune complexes, and of multiple autoantibodies including antinuclear antibodies (ANA), antiphospholipid antibodies, and antilymphocyte, antiplatelet, antithyroid, antisperm, antibrain, and several other tissue-specific autoantibodies have been demonstrated in the serum of HIV-infected patients.

Molecular mimicry between ribonucleoprotein (RNP) antigens and retroviral core proteins exists, and this has been suggested as a possible mechanism for the induction of autoimmunity in SLE and SS. This also may be present in HIV infection and potentially contributes to the increased expression of autoantibodies observed in the disease. Retroviruses encode superantigens that can lead to the expansion or deletion of certain subsets of T cells.

An important role for CD4$^+$ lymphocytes in the pathogenesis of synovitis is suggested by spontaneous amelioration or frank remission of joint inflammation in African patients with the onset of full-blown AIDS and exceptionally low CD4$^+$ counts (47).

Genetic Factors: Role of the HLA System

Participation of HLA-B27 antigen in the pathogenesis of HIV-associated spondyloarthropathy is indicated by the finding that the prevalence of HLA-B27 in white HIV patients with Reiter's syndrome is similar to that found in the idiopathic form (1,4). A strong association of HLA-B27 with psoriasis alone and psoriatic arthritis (PsA) in the presence of HIV infection was recently reported (54). As previously noted, these data do not apply to African blacks in whom HIV-associated reactive arthritis–spondyloarthropathy does not correlate with a high prevalence of HLA-B27 (47).

The class II HLA antigen HLA-DR5 is prevalent in African-American patients with HIV and diffuse infiltrative lymphocytosis syndrome (DILS), suggesting a pathogenic role for a host immune response(s) to HIV-derived peptides (55).

Infection with Arthritogenic and Other Microorganisms

Infections with a multitude of microorganisms, including arthritogenic organisms, may occur in HIV-infected individuals (56–58). An increased frequency of *Yersinia*-induced reactive arthritis in HIV-positive individuals has been reported (57). Low titers of antibodies specific for *Chlamydia* were found in 60% and high-titer antibodies in 33% of HIV-positive individuals, compared with 8% and 1.7%, respectively, in normal controls (56). It should be stressed that these studies were conducted in white populations in whom HLA-B27 is known to be highly prevalent.

Studies in Central Africa do not provide support for a significant role of gram-negative microorganisms such as *Shigella* in the reactive arthritis seen in this population (47). The prevalence of *Shigella* infection was similar in HIV-positive and -negative individuals.

Some opportunistic infections including *Giardia lamblia,* syphilis, and viruses including cytomegalovirus; hepatitis B, A, and C; and Epstein–Barr virus also may contribute to some of the rheumatic manifestations seen in HIV patients.

The existence of inflammatory musculoskeletal disorders with profound immunodeficiency secondary to HIV infection is well established. It is likely that complex interactions among environmental factors (the retroviruses, arthritogenic pathogens, and other opportunistic microorganisms), genetic factors such as HLA-B27 and HLA-DR5, and immune-mediated responses participate in the pathogenesis of rheumatic syndromes associated with retrovirus infection.

Epidemiologic Considerations

Epidemiologic studies have provided conflicting data regarding the prevalence of HIV-associated rheumatic disorders. Early reports from selected HIV-infected cohorts indicated a high prevalence of spondyloarthropathy ranging from 0.5% to 11% for Reiter's syndrome, psoriatic arthritis, and undifferentiated spondyloarthropathy (59). A major flaw, however, with these data was the lack of meaningful control groups, although for the most part, data were consistent and comparable across studies. Some of the subsequently observed differences may have been due to the referral bias and terminology used by the different groups. For example, Berman et al. (60) reported a prevalence of 11.2% for Reiter's syndrome and 2.2% for undifferentiated spondyloarthropathy, whereas Calabrese et al. (6) reported nearly opposite findings: 1.7% prevalence for Reiter's syndrome and 11.1% for undifferentiated spondyloarthropathy. Considering that most HIV-associated Reiter's syndrome is seen in an incomplete form, it is probable that some of these patients may have had undifferentiated spondyloarthropathy or *vice versa.*

In contrast, epidemiologic studies conducted by questionnaires and chart reviews and by using a broad definition for Reiter's syndrome, without any criteria for undifferentiated spondyloarthropathy, have reported a prevalence identical to that seen in the general population. Recently published data from Central Africa may shed light on and further clarify previously reported discrepancies in the prevalence of HIV-associated spondyloarthropathy (47). In the late 1980s, several countries in this region of the world began to experience an increased prevalence of spondyloarthropathy including psoriatic arthritis. A study by Njobvu et al. (47) is perhaps the most informative because of its prospective nature and the large number of patients involved. It was performed (1994–1996) in Lusaka, Zambia, a city of 1.3 million people in which the prevalence of HIV positivity is 30% of the adult population. Furthermore, the prevalence of HIV positivity is 70% among inpatients compared with 50% in the outpatient population. The overall prevalence found for spondyloarthropathy was 180 in 100,000 in HIV-positive individuals versus 15 in 100,000 in the non–HIV patient population.

Most patients diagnosed with a spondyloarthropathy were HIV positive; in other words, 87% of those with reactive arthritis, 98% of those with undifferentiated arthritis, and 92% of patients with psoriatic arthritis. In contrast, none of the 30 patients diagnosed with RA during that time were HIV positive, and only 18% of osteoarthritis (OA) patients had HIV positivity.

These data provide strong support for earlier studies demonstrating an increased frequency of spondyloarthropathy in HIV-infected individuals and strengthen the notion of a direct etiologic role for HIV infection in the inflammatory articular involvement seen. This is further supported by the lack of association between spondyloarthropathy and gram-negative microorganisms such as *Shigella* in the same population (47).

The prevalence of rheumatic disorders in Western countries is decreasing as a result of the development of more effective antiretroviral therapeutic regimens.

RHEUMATIC MANIFESTATIONS

A wide spectrum of clinical musculoskeletal manifestations is associated with HIV infection, ranging from arthralgias and reactive arthritis at one end of the spectrum to more severe clinical disorders such as systemic necrotizing vasculitis at the other end (Table 131.4). Geographic variation in disease expression has been noted (e.g., a higher fre-

TABLE 131.4. HIV-ASSOCIATED MUSCULOSKELETAL DISORDERS

Spondyloarthropathies
Reiter's syndrome or reactive arthritis
Psoriatic arthritis
Undifferentiated spondyloarthropathy
HIV-associated arthritis
Connective tissue disorders
Polymyositis–dermatomyositis
SLE-like syndrome
Sjögren's-like syndrome
Vasculitis
Septic arthritis
Miscellaneous
Avascular bone necrosis
Fibromyalgia
Raynaud's phenomenon
Behçet's syndrome

HIV, human immunodeficiency virus; SLE, systemic lupus erythematosus.

quency of SS in certain parts of the country), as well as an association of certain clinical manifestations with specific extrinsic factors (e.g., a higher frequency of septic arthritis in intravenous drug users).

Arthralgias and Painful Articular Syndrome

Arthralgias are the most common rheumatic manifestation associated with HIV infection (3). They occur at any stage of HIV infection in approximately 12% to 45% of patients and are generally of mild to moderate intensity, transient or intermittent, and oligoarticular. Large joints such as knees, shoulders, and elbows are most commonly involved, although small joints can be affected.

Painful articular syndrome also may occur, and it was more commonly observed before the introduction of newer and more specific antiretroviral therapy (3). It is characterized by severe intermittent pain, usually involving fewer than four joints and without evidence of synovitis; is of short duration (less than 24 hours), and requires analgesic therapy, often including narcotics. This manifestation usually occurs in late stages of the disease. Other pain syndromes also may occur in HIV-infected individuals.

Spondyloarthropathy

Clinical manifestations consistent with a diagnosis of spondyloarthropathy are frequently described in patients with HIV infection (1,3,4). Reiter's syndrome or reactive arthritis, PsA, undifferentiated spondyloarthropathy, SAPHO syndrome (synovitis, acne, pustulosis, hyperostosis, osteomyelitis), enthesitis, and uveitis have been reported (5–9).

Reiter's Syndrome

Reiter's syndrome and reactive arthritis were the first rheumatic disorders to be recognized in HIV-infected individuals and represent the most common arthritides seen in this group (1). Both disorders seem to be preferentially associated with homosexuality as a risk factor and are less prevalent in HIV-infected intravenous drug users. HIV-associated Reiter's syndrome has been described after dysentery with positive serology for *Yersinia,* or in association with positive culture for *Shigella* and *Salmonella* (3).

The onset of Reiter's syndrome may precede the diagnosis of HIV, but most commonly follows the development of clinical evidence of immunosuppression in Western countries. It may feature involvement of large or small peripheral joints and may be the reason for the first presentation to the hospital. Fever, weight loss, diarrhea, and generalized lymphadenopathy may be present. Reiter's syndrome also may occur concomitant with the development of clinical immunosuppression.

In most patients with HIV infection and Reiter's syndrome, the incomplete form develops, but the classic triad of urethritis, conjunctivitis, and arthritis also may occur. Joint involvement tends to be asymmetric and oligoarticular, but erosive polyarthritis, severe enthesopathy, and poor response to treatment may be seen in about one third of affected patients. The remaining two thirds exhibit a mild and self-limiting course. Extraarticular manifestations, including enthesitis, nail involvement with subungual hyperkeratosis, circinate balanitis, keratoderma hemorrhagica, oral ulcers, and uveitis are commonly seen. Constitutional complaints including fever, fatigue, and weight loss often are present and, when associated with generalized lymphadenopathy, rapid progression of articular complaints, as well as the presence of leukopenia or lymphopenia, should raise the suspicion of underlying HIV infection. Radiographic evidence of sacroiliac involvement and a high prevalence of HLA-B27 in white individuals also may be seen.

HIV-associated Reiter's syndrome in Africans exhibits certain clinical characteristics that are strikingly different from those seen in Western countries (47). In Africans, disease appears clinically to be more aggressive, frequently polyarticular, more persistent, and remission takes longer to occur. Erosive arthritis, enthesitis, and joint fusion in the ankle–foot/hand–wrist complex occur more frequently. Most patients (80%) were in World Health Association (WHO) stage 1 of their HIV disease. Of interest, patients in stage 4 were generally in remission with regard to their Reiter's signs and symptoms. HLA-B27 negativity was found in all patients tested (47).

Undifferentiated Spondyloarthropathy

Undifferentiated spondyloarthropathy is also recognized to be associated with HIV infection. Its prevalence was reported to be 2.2% to 11.1%, and probably much higher in nonwhite populations (59). Njobvu et al. (47) found a frequency of almost 30% in the HIV-associated inflammatory arthropathy, similar to the frequency of HIV-associated arthritis and Reiter's syndrome. Patients with HIV-associated undifferentiated spondyloarthropathy exhibit low back pain, enthesitis, conjunctivitis, oligoarthritis, plantar fasciitis, diarrhea, and radiologic evidence of sacroiliitis, but lack the presence of spondylitis. In African HIV patients, undifferentiated spondyloarthropathy also tends to be more aggressive than in whites, very similar to the manner in which Reiter's syndrome behaves in this population. HLA-27 is usually negative. Arthropathy affects joints of both upper and lower extremities in the majority of patients (77%), and affects upper limbs only in 2%, and lower limbs in 21%. Arthritogenic microorganisms, especially *Shigella,* do not seem to play an important role (47). In this group of patients, it may be difficult to distinguish incomplete Reiter's syndrome from undifferentiated spondyloarthropathy.

Psoriatic Arthritis

Psoriasis and PsA occur with increased prevalence in HIV-infected individuals (62–65). The fact that some HIV-1 transgenic animal models experience a psoriasiform skin lesion, with increase in the epidermal layer thickness, along with hyperkeratosis and parakeratosis, supports a direct effect of retroviral infection in the lesions described in humans in association with HIV infection (43). A variety of skin disorders have been described in association with HIV infection, especially in the advanced stages. These include seborrheic dermatitis and benign and malignant forms of psoriasis. New onset or exacerbation of underlying psoriasis in high-risk individuals should alert clinicians to the possible presence of underlying HIV infection.

The prevalence of psoriasis in HIV infection ranges from 1% to 20%, and the prevalence of PsA in this group varies between 1% and 32% (9). Psoriasis and PsA can precede or follow the clinical onset of immunodeficiency. Psoriasis vulgaris is the most common form of skin involvement noted, but more severe forms such as pustular and exfoliative erythrodermia may occur. PsA affects male homosexuals more

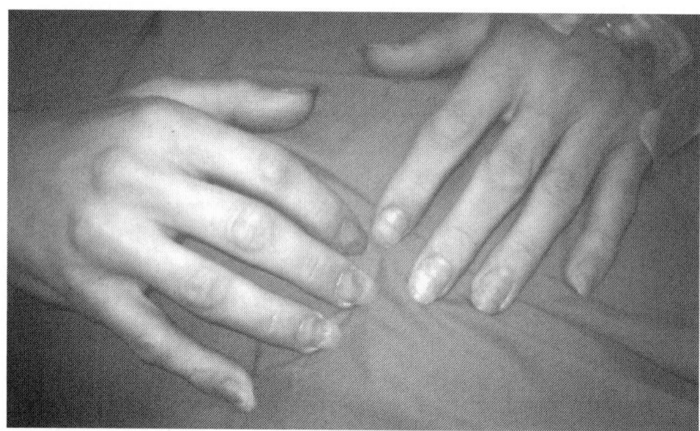

FIGURE 131.1. Asymmetric polyarthritis involving right wrist, some metacarpophalangeal and proximal and distal interphalangeal involvement. Nail involvement also is present.

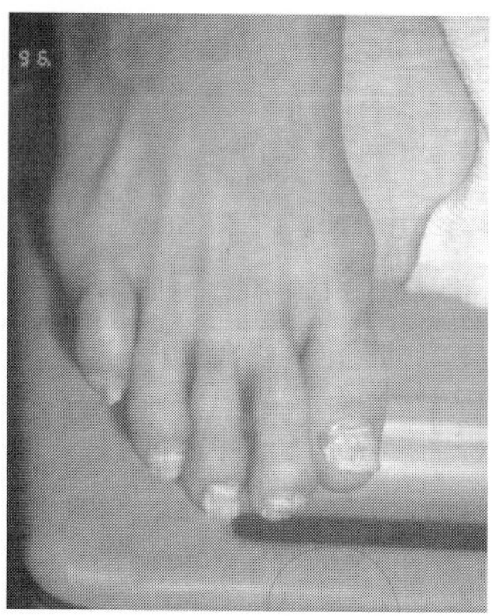

FIGURE 131.2. Dactylitis and sausage-toe deformities, accompanied by dystrophic nail changes.

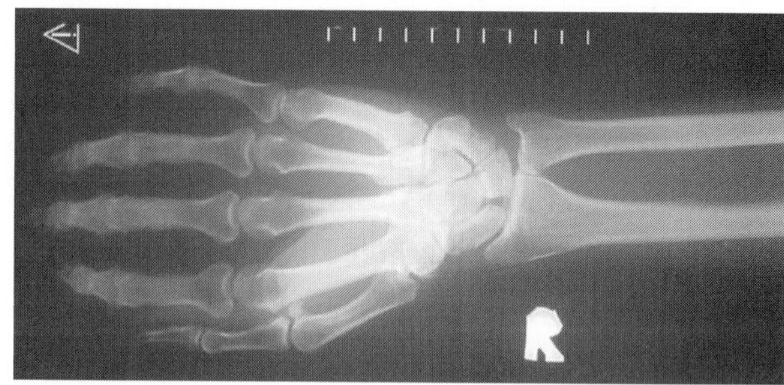

FIGURE 131.3. Right hand radiograph showing significant paraarticular osteopenia.

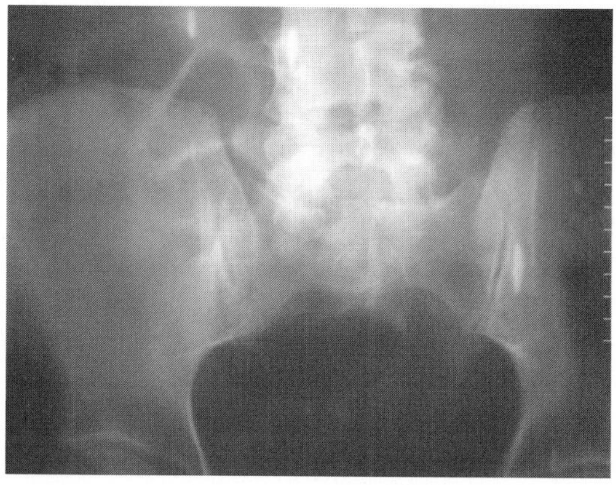

FIGURE 131.4. Sacroiliac joint radiograph demonstrating unilateral sacroiliitis: sclerosis and erosive changes.

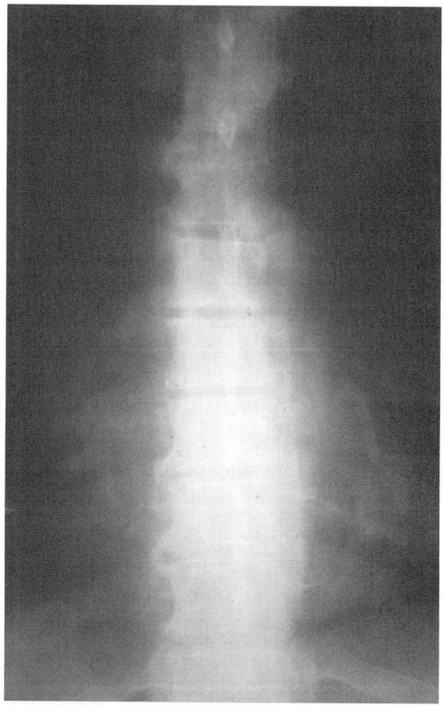

FIGURE 131.5. Thoracic spine radiograph showing asymmetric spondylitis. Notice chunky syndesmophytes.

commonly, and the articular pattern is more frequently polyarticular and asymmetric, large and small joint (Fig. 131.1), accompanied by enthesopathy and dactylitis (Fig. 131.2). Nail involvement occurs in more than half of the patients (Figs. 131.1 and 131.2). Paraarticular osteopenia also can be seen (Fig. 131.3). Sacroiliitis, usually asymmetric and/or unilateral (Fig. 131.4), and characteristic findings of psoriatic spondylitis (Fig. 131.5) are seen in patients with chronic disease, usually more than 5 years in duration. In our own experience, up to 30% of PsA exhibits spondylitis, and this seems to be directly related to longer survival due to antiretroviral therapy. These changes were not seen during the early years of the epidemic, in which most patients died sooner. Rapidly progressive spondyloarthropathy of the cervical spine may develop, with atlantodental subluxation requiring spondylodesis (65).

The clinical course of PsA is variable, ranging from mild to a rapidly progressive, deforming form of the disease despite the use of aggressive therapy.

In general, there is no clear association of psoriasis and PsA occurring in HIV-infected patients with particular HLA antigens. Preliminary evidence, however, suggests HLA-B27 might be a risk factor. From a clinical point of view, it is often difficult to distinguish PsA from Reiter's syndrome with arthritis and keratodermia blenorrhagica, with or without HIV positivity.

HIV-associated Arthritis

Oligoarticular and asymmetric peripheral arthritis is frequently reported in association with HIV infection (3,9). We recently reported our findings in a large group of HIV-infected patients (n = 270) who were prospectively evaluated for the presence of rheumatic complaints (67). The main objective of the study was to define the frequency and characteristics of HIV-associated arthritis. A total of 21 (7.8%) patients was diagnosed as having HIV-associated arthritis. Fourteen (66%) patients were homosexuals, four (19%) IV drug users, and three (14%) heterosexuals. Twelve (57%) were in stage IV, five (23%) in stage III, and four (19%) in stage II. Ten (47%) patients had oligoarticular involvement, eight (38%) monoarticular, two (9%) asymmetric polyarthritis, and one (4%) symmetric polyarthritis. Rheumatoid factor (RF) and HLA-B27 antigen were negative in all patients studied. The mean duration of arthritis was 2 weeks (range, 1–24 weeks). No radiographic erosive changes were noted. It was concluded that the pattern of joint involvement of HIV-associated arthritis is similar to that of other viral disorders: acute onset, short duration, no recurrences, no HLA association, and no destructive disease. In addition, patients exhibiting this syndrome lack extraarticular clinical manifestations associated with Reiter's syndrome. It should be noted that there appear to be clinical differences between HIV-associated arthropathy [both spondyloarthropathy and HIV-associated arthritis (67)] among whites and African blacks (Table 131.5).

TABLE 131.5. HIV-ASSOCIATED ARTHROPATHY

	Whites	African Blacks
Frequency	+	+++
Severity	+ to ++	+++
WHO stage	III – IV	I
CD4 count	<250	≥250
AIDS effect	Flare	Remission
HLA-B27	++	—
Spondylitis	+	—
Gram-infection	+	—

AIDS, acquired immunodeficiency syndrome; WHO, World Health Organization; HIV, human immunodeficiency virus; HLA, human leukocyte antigen.

CONNECTIVE TISSUE DISORDERS

Muscle Involvement

Muscle involvement was one of the earliest manifestations recognized in the course of HIV infection, and in the past several years, a wide spectrum of manifestations has been clearly established (Table 131.6) (68–72). Myalgias, usually generalized and indistinguishable from fibromyalgia but occasionally localized, are the most common muscular complaints, transient in nature, and readily responsive to analgesics.

Significant muscle weakness may be the presenting complaint in HIV diseases. In general, HIV-associated polymyositis and, to a lesser extent, dermatomyositis also may occur. In the latter two, the clinical course and laboratory and electromyographic findings are similar to those of the idiopathic forms. Histopathologic findings in skin and muscle tissues show various degrees of cell necrosis, vacuolization, fibrosis, and mononuclear cell infiltration with predominantly $CD8^+$ cells, although $CD4^+$ cells, B lymphocytes, and macrophages also are present. HIV-infected individuals also may exhibit muscle weakness in association with nemaline rod bodies and muscle fiber necrosis but

TABLE 131.6. HIV-ASSOCIATED MUSCLE INVOLVEMENT

Myalgias
Inflammatory myopathy
Polymyositis
Dermatomyositis
Nemaline rod myopathy
Subclinical neuromuscular involvement
HIV/HTLV-1 polymyositis
Zidovudine (AZT) toxic myopathy
Pyomyositis

HIV, human immunodeficiency virus; HTLV, human T-cell leukemia virus.

without inflammatory cell infiltrates. This myopathic disorder also may be seen in older patients with polymyositis.

By far, however, the most common cause of proximal muscle weakness in HIV-infected patients is secondary to zidovudine (azidothymidine; AZT) therapy. It usually appears after several months of therapy. Muscle biopsy reveals a multifocal necrotizing myopathy with characteristic "ragged-red" fibers, indicative of abnormal mitochondria, and with minimal or no inflammation. Electron microscopy reveals abnormal mitochondria with paracrystalline inclusions. The clinical manifestations rapidly resolve after drug discontinuation.

Muscle weakness associated with disuse or muscle atrophy usually has multiple causes including neurologic disease, wasting syndrome, infection, and/or antiretroviral therapy.

Pyomyositis is increasingly recognized in HIV-infected individuals. Etiologic agents are often gram-positive organisms, but *Mycobacterium avium* also may be seen. In some African countries, more than 30% of patients with pyomyositis are HIV positive, and the great majority (85%) meet criteria for AIDS (73). Diagnosis requires confirmation of the causative organism with needle aspiration under ultrasound guidance. Magnetic resonance imaging (MRI) studies are particularly helpful to localize the soft tissue abnormalities.

Sjögren's-like Syndrome

Symptoms of dry eyes and dry mouth, with positive Schirmer's test, are frequently reported in HIV-infected patients including children (74–78). Enlargement, at times massive, of the major salivary glands or symptoms of dry mouth are characteristic of the so-called *HIV-associated salivary gland disease,* also designated *DILS.* Labial salivary gland biopsy reveals lymphocytic infiltrates, mostly $CD8^+$ cells in focal and other patterns. Other distinguishing features from the idiopathic form include negative SS-A, SS-B, and RF autoantibodies, age younger than 40 years, male sex, and the presence of generalized lymphadenopathy. The lymphoid infiltrate resembles morphologically the features of persistent generalized lymphadenopathy. High prevalence of HLA-DR5 in affected African-American patients and HLA-DR6 and DR7 in white patients has been reported. Some patients with DILS may have a positive SS-A antibody associated with HLA-DR3 (78).

Vasculitis

A variety of vasculitic syndromes have been reported in association with HIV infection (3,79–82). Whether these cases represent a direct consequence of retroviral infection or reflect secondary causes, such as co-infection with multiple microorganisms and/or drug therapies, remains to be established (83,84).

Primary angiitis of the central nervous system (CNS), systemic necrotizing angiitis or periarteritis nodosa, Henoch–Schönlein purpura, and leukocytoclastic vasculitis have been described in association with HIV infection (80–82). The HIV antigen and genome have been identified in endothelial vessel walls of patients with necrotizing vasculitis. Cytomegalovirus and/or immune complexes also have been identified. Affected patients usually have involvement of the neuromuscular system and skin, and constitutional complaints such as fever and weight loss may not be present. Hypertension, livedo reticularis, testicular pain, and kidney, CNS, and gastrointestinal tract involvement are found less frequently. Antineutrophil cytoplasm antibodies (ANCA) may occur occasionally.

A high prevalence of cryoglobulins has recently been reported in HIV-infected patients (85).

HIV Infection and Coexistent Connective Tissue Disorders

Full-blown HIV infection may have an array of clinical manifestations that can mimic some of the idiopathic forms of connective tissue disease, especially SLE, RA, and polymyositis (3,74). Complicating this issue is the presence of false-positive HIV antibody tests both by enzyme-linked immunosorbent assay (ELISA) and Western blot techniques in some patients, particularly those with SLE.

Furthermore, disease activity in these disorders can be altered or ameliorated by concomitant HIV-related immunosuppression. Disease activity in SLE is exacerbated after antiretroviral treatment (86).

Musculoskeletal Infection

A wide spectrum of clinical manifestations secondary to infection may be seen in HIV-infected patients (Table 131.7).

Septic Arthritis

Septic arthritis is a rare event (0.3% to 3.5%) in patients with HIV infection, but represents the most common mus-

TABLE 131.7. MUSCULOSKELETAL INFECTIONS IN HIV INFECTION

Septic arthritis
Pyomyositis
Osteomyelitis
Miscellaneous
Cellulitis
Septic tenosynovitis
Bursitis
Soft tissue abscesses

culoskeletal infectious process in this population (87–92). The natural history of septic arthritis in HIV-infected individuals is identical to that occurring in nonimmunosuppressed individuals (90). The majority of patients are young men, with intravenous drug abuse and hemophilia as the main risk factors. The clinical picture is predominantly monoarticular, with the large, weight-bearing joints of the lower extremities (knees and hips) being most commonly involved. Involvement of the sternoclavicular joint is common, especially in intravenous drug users. Most patients exhibit constitutional symptoms and signs, including chills, fever, and night sweats. Leukocytosis is seen in only half of the patients.

Staphylococcus aureus is the agent most commonly isolated, although numerous other microorganisms, including *Streptococcus pneumoniae, Salmonella, Mycobacterium tuberculosis, Morganella morganii,* and opportunistic fungal infections may be found (93–96).

In general, there is not a good correlation between septic arthritis and $CD4^+$ cell counts when a pyogenic microorganism is involved, and most patients exhibiting this association have a $CD4^+$ cell count greater than $250/mm^3$. In contrast, HIV-infected patients with opportunistic infection as the causative agent usually have $CD4^+$ cell counts less than $100/mm^3$. The clinical response to conventional antibiotic therapy is excellent, and the mortality rate associated with septic arthritis is less than 3% (90).

Osteomyelitis

Bone infection represents the most common musculoskeletal septic complication after septic arthritis (88,90,97). In almost half of all cases, no risk factors can be identified. Young male homosexuals and i.v. drug users overall appear at increased risk. A characteristic feature is the association of osteomyelitis with very low $CD4^+$ cell counts, usually less than $50/mm^3$.

Numerous microorganisms, including opportunistic ones, have been isolated including *Streptococcus* sp., *Candida albicans, Histoplasma capsulatum, Nocardia, Salmonella* sp. and *Toruplosis glabrata.* Bone biopsy and culture is often needed for diagnosis. Blood and synovial fluid cultures allow identification of the causative organism in 20% to 35% of cases. The presence of osteomyelitis is a poor prognostic sign and is associated with a mortality rate exceeding 20% (90).

Other Septic Musculoskeletal Complications

Pyomyositis, cellulitis, septic tenosynovitis and bursitis, and soft tissue abscesses also may occur. Gram-positive microorganisms, particularly *Staphylococcus aureus* and *Streptococcus pyogenes,* are the most common etiologic agents, although any other gram-positive and/or gram-negative microorganisms may be involved (90).

MISCELLANEOUS RHEUMATIC DISORDERS

A variety of common and uncommon rheumatic disorders may be seen in association with HIV infection, including fibromyalgia, relapsing polychondritis, immune complex glomerulonephritis, Raynaud's phenomenon, aseptic bone necrosis, hypertrophic osteoarthropathy, Sweet's syndrome, Behçet's syndrome, enthesitis, and regional pain syndromes. Whether this is a true or chance association remains to be elucidated. The prevalence of these disorders has not been clearly established (97–102).

MUSCULOSKELETAL MANIFESTATIONS ASSOCIATED WITH OTHER RETROVIRAL INFECTIONS

HTLV-1 Infection

Human T-cell leukemia virus type 1 (HTLV-1) is a type C human retrovirus implicated in adult T-cell leukemia and in a variety of autoimmune clinical disorders including lymphocytic alveolitis, SS, myelopathy or tropical spastic paraparesis (HAM/TSP), polymyositis, uveitis, and polyarthritis (103,104).

The clinical picture of SS and polymyositis is identical to that seen in idiopathic or HIV-associated disease.

HTLV-1–associated arthropathy is characterized by oligoarticular large-joint involvement, usually involving the knees. Polyarthritis preferentially involving shoulders, wrists, and knees can occur, and in this situation, differentiation from RA is difficult because of the presence of an elevated erythrocyte sedimentation rate (ESR) and positive RF in approximately half of the patients (24). Anti-HTLV antibodies are detected in both sera and synovial fluid in all patients. Adult T-cell leukemia cells or "flower" cells constitute about 12% of synovial fluid lymphocytes (24).

Proliferation of the synovial lining cells and of subsynovial vascular endothelium occurs. Villus formation also may occur. Activated $CD4^+$ and $CD8^+$ T cells and B cells, and upregulation of HLA-DR antigen are seen. HTLV-1 proviral DNA, as well as IL-1 and IL-6 mRNA, has been detected in synovial cell lines.

Radiographic findings include narrowing of the joint space, small bony erosions, and minimal osteoporosis.

Anticardiolipin antibodies have been reported in 32% of HLTV-1–associated HAM/TSP, but their significance is uncertain (105).

A pathogenic role for HTLV-1 is suggested by induction of chronic arthritis in mice transgenic for the HTLV-1 *tax* gene and also the development of autoimmune diseases and autoantibodies including anticardiolipin in rats transgenic for the HTLV-1 *env-pox* gene.

HIV-II Infection

Enthesopathy of the Achilles and triceps tendon insertions in a young woman with HIV-II infection has been described (106).

Other Retroviruses

Particles resembling retroviruses have been detected in affected tissue from patients with SS and RA (10–16).

More recently, a new human retrovirus genome, designated human retrovirus 5 (HRV-5), genetically related to simian D-type retroviruses, rodent intracisternal A-type particles, and murine mammary tumor virus, and with little sequence similarity to HIV or HTLV, has been detected in 53% of synovial samples from inflammatory fluids, in 12% of blood samples from RA, and in 16% of blood samples from SLE patients (107). Preliminary data suggest the possible involvement of HRV-5 in autoimmune and rheumatic disease.

LABORATORY FINDINGS

Laboratory abnormalities are common but nonspecific for the most part. Elevated levels of serum immunoglobulins, moderate elevation of the ESR, circulating immune complexes, low-grade complement activation, low-titer ANA, RF, false-positive tests for syphilis, and multiple other autoantibodies including anticardiolipin antibodies and lupus anticoagulants are seen in the majority of patients (108,109). Other acute-phase reactants also may be elevated. Synovial effusions, when present, tend to be small, transient, and are of inflammatory character. Leukocyte counts range from 2,000 to 14,500/cm^3 in synovial fluid, and p-24 antigen can be demonstrated in synoviocytes and mononuclear subsynovial cells. A gamut of radiologic findings is seen including soft tissue swelling, erosions, ankylosis, joint-space narrowing, whittling, osteolytic lesions, periostitis, sacroiliac joint-space widening and erosions, and syndesmophyte formation (47,110).

THERAPY

Therapeutic management of HIV infection–associated rheumatic complaints can be very challenging oftentimes because of the profound state of immunosuppression exhibited by the patients. Fortunately, with the advent of newer antiretroviral agents and combination therapy, there is growing evidence that treated patients experience a recovery of immune function that allows a more aggressive therapeutic approach for their rheumatic manifestations (90).

In general, most patients with HIV infection exhibit mild to moderately severe, self-limiting rheumatic disorders. Many patients experience a good response to a combination of analgesics and nonsteroidal antiinflammatory drugs (NSAIDs).

Second-line antiinflammatory agents administered at conventional doses, including sulfasalazine and methotrexate, are indicated and proven to be safe for patients refractory to NSAIDs (111). Other immunosuppressive agents, including moderate doses of prednisone, cyclosporine, D-penicillamine, antimalarials, and etretinate, have been successfully used in patients with polymyositis, recalcitrant forms of Reiter's syndrome and PsA, SS, and vasculitis.

Antiretroviral therapy and the prophylactic use of antimicrobial agents, including pentamidine and trimethoprim/sulfamethoxazole or cotrimazole, are accompanied by improvement of psoriasis and associated rheumatic complaints. The use of intravenous immune globulin in HIV infection as well as certain cytokines including IL-12, IL-2, IFN-γ, and granulocyte–macrophage/colony-stimulating factor (GM-CSF) has resulted in a significant decrease in the morbidity related to infections (112). It also is possible that this therapeutic approach may be of benefit for some HIV patients exhibiting arthritis refractory to conventional therapy.

Whereas immunosuppressive agents in an HIV patient should be used with caution because of the possibility of precipitating immunodeficiency and Kaposi's sarcoma, we have not seen this in our experience (111).

Intraarticular steroids can be very useful in the management of severely inflamed joints. Thalidomide has been claimed to be effective in the management of oral aphthous ulcerations.

The therapeutic management of HIV patients exhibiting rheumatic complaints often poses a challenge, and should involve a team approach including primary care physicians and nurses, a nutritionist, a social worker, occupational and physical therapists, and HIV specialists and rheumatologists (113). With newer antiretroviral and other therapeutic approaches, HIV patients have experienced improvements in both survival and quality of life.

REFERENCES

1. Winchester R, Bernstein DH, Fisher HD, et al. The co-occurrence of Reiter's syndrome and acquired immunodeficiency. *Ann Intern Med* 1987;106:19–26.
2. Withrington RH, Cornes P, Harris JRN, et al. Isolation of human immunodeficiency virus from synovial fluid of a patient with reactive arthritis. *Br Med J* 1987;294:484–486.
3. Berman A, Espinoza LR, Diaz J, et al. Rheumatic manifestations of human immunodeficiency virus infection. *Am J Med* 1988;85:59–64.
4. Espinoza LR, Aguilar JL, Berman A, et al. Rheumatic manifestations associated with human immunodeficiency virus infection. *Arthritis Rheum* 1989;32:1615–1622.

5. Buskila D, Gladman DD, Langevitz P, et al. Rheumatologic manifestations of infection with the human immunodeficiency virus (HIV). *Clin Exp Rheumatol* 1990;8:567–572.
6. Calabrese LH, Kelley DM, Myers A, et al. Rheumatic symptoms and human immunodeficiency virus infection: the influence of clinical and laboratory variables in a longitudinal cohort study. *Arthritis Rheum* 1991;34:257–261.
7. Davis P, Stein M. Human immunodeficiency virus-related connective tissue diseases: a Zimbabwean perspective. *Rheum Dis Clin North Am* 1991;17:89–98.
8. Medina-Rodriguez F, Guzman C, Jara LJ, et al. Rheumatic manifestations in human immunodeficiency virus positive and negative individuals: a study of 2 populations with similar risk factors. *J Rheumatol* 1993;20:1880–1885.
9. Cuellar ML. HIV-infection-associated inflammatory musculoskeletal disorders. *Rheum Dis Clin North Am* 1998;24:403–421.
10. Iversen C-J. The expression of retrovirus-like particles in psoriasis. *J Invest Dermatol* 1990;90:41S–43S.
11. Garry RF, Fermin CD, Hart DJ, et al. Detection of a human intracisternal A-type retroviral particle antigenically related to HIV. *Science* 1990;250:1127–1129.
12. Yamano S, Renard JN, Mizuno F, et al. Retrovirus in salivary glands from patients with Sjögren's syndrome. *J Clin Pathol* 1997;50:223–230.
13. Stransky G, Vernon J, Aicher WK, et al. Virus-like particles in synovial fluids from patients with rheumatoid arthritis. *Br J Rheumatol* 1993;32:1044–1048.
14. Talal N, Dauphinee MJ, Dang H, et al. A conserved idiotype and antibodies to retroviral proteins in systemic lupus erythematosus. *J Clin Invest* 1990;85:1866–1871.
15. Conrad B, Weissmahr RN, Boni J, et al. A human endogenous retroviral superantigen as candidate autoimmune gene in type I diabetes. *Cell* 1997;90:303–313.
16. Perron H, Garson JA, Bedin F, et al. Molecular identification of a novel retrovirus repeatedly isolated from patients with multiple sclerosis. *Proc Natl Acad Sci U S A* 1997;94:7583–7588.
17. Narayan O, Zink MC, Gorrell M, et al. The lentiviruses of sheep and goats. In: Levy JA, ed. *The retroviridae.* Vol 2. New York: Plenum Press, 1993:229–255.
18. Garry RF, Krieg AM, Cheevers WP, et al. Retroviruses and their roles in chronic inflammatory diseases and autoimmunity. In: Levy JA, ed. *The retroviridae.* Vol 4. New York: Plenum Press, 1995:491–603.
19. Nakagawa K, Brusic V, McColl G, et al. Direct evidence for the expression of multiple endogenous retroviruses in the synovial compartment in rheumatoid arthritis. *Arthritis Rheum* 1997;40: 627–638.
20. Urnovitz HB, Murphy WH. human endogenous retroviruses: nature, occurrence, and clinical implications in clinical disease. *Clin Microbiol Rev* 1996;9:72–99.
21. Michaels FH, Banks KL, Reitz MS. Lessons from caprine and bovine retrovirus infections. *Rheum Dis Clin North Am* 1991; 17:5–23.
22. Roberts E, Martin L. Arthritis in Rhesus monkeys experimentally infected with simian immunodeficiency virus. *Lab Invest* 1991;65:637–643.
23. Bowness P, Davies KA, Tosswill J, et al. Autoimmune disease and HTLV-1 infection. *Br J Rheumatol* 1991;30:141–143.
24. Nishioka K, Nakajima T, Hasunuma T, et al. Rheumatic manifestations of human leukemia virus infection. *Rheum Dis Clin North Am* 1993;19:489–503.
25. Centers for Disease Control. U.S. HIV and AIDS cases reported through December 1998. *Hiv Aids Surveill Rep* 1999; 10:1–43.
26. Siegal FP, Lopez C, Hammer GS, et al. Severe acquired immunodeficiency in male homosexuals, manifested by chronic perianal ulcerative herpes simplex lesions. *N Engl J Med* 1981;305: 1439–1444.
27. Weiss RA. How does HIV cause AIDS? *Science* 1993;260: 1273–1279.
28. Fauci AS. Multifactorial nature of human immunodeficiency virus disease: implications for therapy. *Science* 1993;262: 1011–1018.
29. Coffin JM. HIV populations dynamics in vivo: implications for genetic variation, pathogenesis, and therapy. *Science* 1995;267: 483–487.
30. Subarao S, Schochetman G. Genetic variability of HIV-1. *AIDS* 1996;10(suppl A):S13.
31. Barre-Sinoussi F, Chermann JC. Isolation of a T lymphocyte retrovirus from a patient at risk for acquired immunodeficiency syndrome (AIDS). *Science* 1983;220:868–871.
32. Gallo RC, Saluhuddin SZ, Popovic M, et al. Frequent detection and isolation of cytopathic retrovirus (HLTV). *Science* 1984; 224:500–503.
33. Dean M, Carrington M, Winkler C, et al. Genetic restriction of HIV-1 infection and progression to AIDS by a deletion allele of CKR5 structural gene. *Science* 1996;273:1856–1859.
34. Balter M. New HIV strain could pose health threat. *Science* 1998;281:1425–1426.
35. Powderly WG, Landay A, Lederman MM. Recovery of the immune system with antiretroviral therapy. *JAMA* 1998;280: 72–77.
36. Mildvan D, Mathur U, Enlow RW, et al. Opportunistic infections and immune deficiency in homosexual men. *Ann Intern Med* 1982;96:700–704.
37. Roederer M, Dubs JG, Anderson MT, et al. CD8 naive T cell count decreases progressively in HIV-infected adults. *J Clin Invest* 1995;95:2061–2066.
38. Schnittman SM, Lane HC, Greenhouse J, et al. Preferential infection of CD4$^+$ memory T cells by human immunodeficiency virus type 1: evidence for a role in the selective T-cell functional defects observed in infected individuals. *Proc Natl Acad Sci U S A* 1990;87:6058–6062.
39. Walker CM, Moody DJ, Stites DP, et al. CD8$^+$ lymphocytes can control HIV infection in vitro by suppressing virus replication. *Science* 1986;234:1563–1566.
40. Rosenberg ES, Billingsley JM, Caliendo AM, et al. Vigorous HIV-1 specific CD4$^+$ T cell responses associated with control of viremia. *Science* 1997;278:1447–1450.
41. Liu Z, Cumberland WG, Hultin LE, et al. Elevated CD38 antigen expression on CD8$^+$ T cells is a stronger marker for the risk of chronic HIV disease progression to AIDS and death in the multicenter AIDS cohort study than CD4$^+$ cell count, soluble immune activation markers, or combination of HLA-DR and CD38 expression. *J Acquir Immune Defic Syndr Hum Retrovirol* 1997;16:83–92.
42. Iwakura Y, Tosu M, Yoshida E, et al. Induction of inflammatory arthropathy resembling rheumatoid arthritis in mice transgenic for HTLV-1. *Science* 1991;253:1026–1028.
43. Vogel J, Hinrichs SH, Reynolds RK, et al. The HIV *tat* gene induces dermal lesions resembling Kaposi's sarcoma in transgenic mice. *Nature* 1996;335:606–608.
44. Espinoza LR, Aguilar JL, Espinoza CG, et al. HIV-associated arthropathy: HIV antigen demonstration in the synovial membrane. *J Rheumatol* 1990;17:1195–1199.
45. Adebajo AO. Epidemiology and community studies in Africa. *Baillieres Clin Rheumatol* 1995;9:21–30.
46. Lowe RF. The distribution of blood groups and HLA antigens of Zimbabwean Africans. *Centr Afr J Med* 1981;(suppl 1):19.
47. Njobvu P, McGill P, Kerr H, et al. Spondyloarthropathy and human immunodeficiency virus infection in Zambia. *J Rheumatol* 1998;25:1553–1559.

48. Folks TM, Justement J, Kinter A, et al. Cytokine-induced expression of HIV-1 in a chronically infected promonocyte cell line. *Science* 1987;238:800–802.
49. Poli G, Fauci AS. The effect of cytokines and pharmacologic agents on chronic HIV infection. *AIDS Res Hum Retrovir* 1992; 8:191–197.
50. Romagnani S, Maggi E. Th1 versus Th2 responses in AIDS. *Curr Opin Immunol* 1994;6:616–622.
51. Gherardi RK, Florea-Strat A, Fromont G, et al. Cytokine expression in the muscle of HIV-infected patients: evidence for interleukin-1 alpha accumulation in mitochondria of AZT fibers. *Ann Neurol* 1994;36:752–758.
52. Nakamura S, Salahuddin SZ, Riberfield P, et al. Kaposi's sarcoma cells long-term culture with growth factor from retrovirus-infected CD4+ cells. *Science* 1988;242:426–430.
53. Groux H, Torpier G, Monte D, et al. Activation induced death by apoptosis in CD4+ T cells from human immunodeficiency virus-infected asymptomatic individuals. *J Exp Med* 1992;175: 331–340.
54. Reveille JD, Conan MA, Duvic M. Human immunodeficiency virus associated psoriasis, psoriatic arthritis and Reiter's syndrome: a disease continuum. *Arthritis Rheum* 1990;33:1574–1578.
55. Itescu S. Diffuse infiltrative lymphocytosis syndrome in human immunodeficiency virus infection: a Sjögren's-like disease. *Rheum Dis Clin North Am* 1991;17:99–105.
56. Gutierrez F, Espinoza LR, Nelson R, et al. Serologic evidence for *Chlamydia* infection in human immunodeficiency virus-infected patients. *Rev Mex Rheumatol* 1990;5(suppl):62.
57. Hughes RA, Keats ACS. *Yersinia* reactive arthritis and human immunodeficiency virus infection. *Arthritis Rheum* 1990;33:558.
58. Burgoyne M, Agudelo C, Pisko E. Chronic syphilitic polyarthritis mimicking systemic lupus erythematosus/rheumatoid arthritis as the initial presentation of human immunodeficiency virus infection. *J Rheumatol* 1992;19:313–315.
59. Espinoza LR, Jara LJ, Espinoza CG, et al. There is an association between human immunodeficiency virus infection and spondyloarthropathies. *Rheum Dis Clin North Am* 1992;17:257–266.
60. Berman A, Reboredo G, Spindler A, et al. Rheumatic manifestations in populations at risk for HIV infection: the added effect of HIV. *J Rheumatol* 1991;18:1564–1568.
61. Clark MR, Solinger AM, Hochberg MC. Human immunodeficiency virus infection is not associated with Reiter's syndrome. *Rheum Dis Clin North Am* 1991;18:267–276.
62. Cuellar ML, Espinoza LR. HIV-associated spondyloarthropathy: lessons from the third world. *J Rheumatol* 1999;26:2071–2073.
63. Espinoza LR, Berman A, Vasey FB, et al. Psoriatic arthritis and acquired immunodeficiency syndrome. *Arthritis Rheum* 1988; 31:1034–1040.
64. Arnett FC, Reveille JD, Duvic M. Psoriasis and psoriatic arthritis associated with human immunodeficiency virus infection. *Rheum Dis Clin North Am* 1991;17:59–78.
65. Schewe CK, Kellner H. Rapidly progressive seronegative spondyloarthropathy with atlantodental subluxation in a patient with moderately advanced HIV infection. *Clin Exp Rheumatol* 1996;14:83–85.
66. Rynes RI, Goldenberg DL, DiGiacomo R, et al. Acquired immunodeficiency syndrome-associated arthritis. *Am J Med* 1988;84:810–812.
67. Berman A, Cahn P, Perez H, et al. HIV infection associated arthritis: clinical characteristics. *J Rheumatol* 1999;26:1158–1162.
68. Snider WD, Simpson DM, Nielsen S, et al. Neurologic complications of acquired immunodeficiency syndrome: analysis of 50 patients. *Ann Neurol* 1983;14:403–418.
69. Dalakas MC, Pezeshkpour GH, Gravell M, et al. Polymyositis associated with AIDS retrovirus. *JAMA* 1986;256:2381–2383.
70. Espinoza LR, Aquilar JR, Espinoza CG, et al. Characteristics and pathogenesis of myositis in human immunodeficiency virus infection: distinction from azidothymidine-induced myopathy. *Rheum Dis Clin North Am* 1991;17:117–129.
71. Gresh J, Aguilar JL, Espinoza LR. Human immunodeficiency virus (HIV) infection-associated dermatomyositis. *J Rheumatol* 1989;31:1034–1040.
72. Dalakas MC, Pezeshkpour GH, Flakerty M. Progressive nemaline (rod) myopathy associated with HIV infection. *N Engl J Med* 1987;317:1602–1603.
73. Ansaloni L, Acaye GL, Re MC. Case-control comparison of HIV and pyomyositis. *Trop Med Int Health* 1996;1:210–217.
74. DeClerk LS, Couthenye MM, DeBroe ME, et al. Acquired immunodeficiency syndrome mimicking Sjögren's syndrome and systemic lupus erythematosus. *Arthritis Rheum* 1988;31:272–275.
75. Itescu S, Brancato LJ, Buxbaum J, et al. A diffuse infiltrative CD8 lymphocytosis syndrome in human immunodeficiency virus (HIV) infection: a host immune response associated with HLA-DR5. *Ann Intern Med* 1990;112:3–10.
76. Schiodt M. HIV-associated salivary gland disease: a review. *Oral Surg Oral Med Pathol* 1992;73:164–167.
77. Ulirsch RC, Jaffe ES. Sjögren's syndrome-like illness associated with the acquired immunodeficiency syndrome-related complex. *Hum Pathol* 1987;18:1063–1068.
78. Hansen A, Feist E, Hiepe F, et al. Diffuse infiltrative lymphocytosis syndrome in a patient with anti-52-kd Rol SSA and human immunodeficiency virus type 1. *Arthritis Rheum* 1999; 42:578–580.
79. Calabrese LH. Vasculitis and infection with the human immunodeficiency virus. *Rheum Dis Clin North Am* 1991;17:131–147.
80. Cooper LM, Patterson JAK. Allergic granulomatosis and angiitis of Churg-Strauss: case report in a patient with antibodies to human immunodeficiency virus and hepatitis B virus. *Int J Dermatol* 1989;28:597–599.
81. Yanker BA, Skolnik PR, Shoukimas GM, et al. Cerebral granulomatous angiitis associated with isolation of human T lymphotrophic virus type III from the central nervous system. *Ann Neurol* 1986;20:362–366.
82. Velji AM. Leukocytoclastic vasculitis associated with positive HTLV-III serological findings. *JAMA* 1986;256:2196–2198.
83. Huang TE, Chou SM. Occlusion hypertrophic arteritis as the cause of discrete necrosis in CNS toxoplasmosis in the acquired immunodeficiency syndrome. *Hum Pathol* 1988;19:1210–1212.
84. Gherardi R, Belec L, Mhiri C, et al. The spectrum of vasculitis in human immunodeficiency virus-infected patients: a clinicopathologic evaluation. *Arthritis Rheum* 1993;36:1164–1174.
85. Dimitra Kapoulos AN, Kordossis T, Hatzakis A, et al. Mixed cryoglobulinemia in HIV-1 infection: the role of HIV-1. *Ann Intern Med* 1999;130:226–230.
86. Molina JF, Citera G, Rosler D, et al. Coexistence of human immunodeficiency virus infection and systemic lupus erythematosus. *J Rheumatol* 1995:22:347–352.
87. Muñoz P, Miranda ME, Llancaqueo A, et al. Hemophilus species bacteremia in adults: the importance of the human immunodeficiency virus epidemic. *Arch Intern Med* 1997;157: 1869–1873.
88. Vassilopoulos D, Chalasani P, Jurado RL, et al. Musculoskeletal infections in patients with human immunodeficiency virus infection. *Medicine* 1997;76:284–294.
89. Ventura G, Gasparini G, Lucia MB, et al. Osteoarticular bacterial infections are rare in HIV-infected patients: fourteen cases among 4023 HIV-infected patients. *Acta Orthop Scand* 1997; 68:554–558.
90. Espinoza LR, Berman A. Soft-tissue and osteoarticular infections in HIV-infected patients and other immunodeficiency states. *Baillieres Clin Rheumatol* 1999;13:115–128.
91. Corelli M, Lapadula G, Pipitone N, et al. Isolated sternoclavic-

ular joint arthritis in heroin addicts and/or HIV positive patients: three cases. *Clin Rheumatol* 1993;12:422–425.
92. Saraux A, Taelman H, Blanche P, et al. HIV infection as risk factor for septic arthritis. *Br J Rheumatol* 1997;36:333–337.
93. Trivalle C, Cremieux AC, Carbon C. Pneumococcal septic arthritis in HIV infection. *Presse Med* 1995;24:1566–1568.
94. Fernandez Guerrero ML, Ramos JM, Nunez A, et al. Focal infection due to non-typhi Salmonella in patients with AIDS: report of 10 cases and review. *Clin Infect Dis* 1997;25: 690–697.
95. Gutierrez C, Cruz L, Olive A, et al. Salmonella septic arthritis in HIV patients. *Br J Rheumatol* 1993;32:88.
96. Hirsch R, Miller SM, Kazi S, et al. Human immunodeficiency virus-associated atypical mycobacterial skeletal infections. *Semin Arthritis Rheum* 1996;25:347–356.
97. Benbouazza K, Allali F, Bezza A, et al. Pubic tuberculous osteoarthritis. *Rev Chir Orthop Rep l'App Mot* 1997;83: 670–672.
98. Gerster JC, Rossetti G. Aseptic avascular osteonecrosis mimicking arthritis in HIV infection. *J Rheumatol* 1998;25:604–605.
99. Bileckot R, Mouaya A, Makuwa M. Prevalence and clinical presentation of arthritis in HIV-positive patients seen at a rheumatology department in Congo-Brazzaville. *Rev Rheum Engl Ed* 1998;65:549–554.
100. Olive A, Fuente MJ, Veny A, et al. Vasculitis and oral and genital ulcers: Behcet's syndrome or HIV infection. *Clin Exp Rheumatol* 1999;17:124.
101. Cuellar ML, Espinoza LR. HIV infection and Behcet's syndrome. *Clin Exp Rheumatol* 1999;17:633–634.
102. Belzunegui J, Cangio J, Pego JM, et al. Relapsing polychondritis and Behcet's syndrome in a patient with HIV infection. *Ann Rheum Dis* 1994;53:780–782.
103. Hollsberg P, Hafler DA. Pathogenesis of diseases induced by human lymphotropic virus type 1 infection. *N Engl J Med* 1993;328:1173–1182.
104. Nakamura H, Eguchi K, Nakamura T, et al. High prevalence of Sjögren's syndrome in patients with HTLV-1 associated myelopathy. *Ann Rheum Dis* 1997;56:167–172.
105. Faghiri Z, Wilson WA, Taheri F, et al. Antibodies to cardiolipin and β2-glycoprotein-1 in HTLV-1 associated myelopathy/tropical spastic paraparesis. *Lupus* 1999;8:210–214.
106. Boissier MC, Lefrere JJ, Freyfus P. Rheumatic manifestations in a patient with human immunodeficiency virus type 2 infection. *Arthritis Rheum* 1991;34:790.
107. Griffiths DJ, Cooke SP, Hervé C, et al. Detection of human retrovirus 5 in patients with arthritis and systemic lupus erythematosus. *Arthritis Rheum* 1999;42:448–454.
108. Rubbert A, Bock E, Schwab J, et al. Anticardiolipin antibodies in HIV infection: association with cerebral perfusion defects as detected by ^{99m}Tc-HMPAO SPECT. *Clin Exp Immunol* 1994; 98:361–368.
109. Massabki PS, Accetturi C, Nishie IA, et al. Clinical implications of autoantibodies in HIV infection. *AIDS* 1997;11:1845–1850.
110. Eustace SJ, Lan HH, Katz J, et al. HIV arthritis. *Radiol Clin North Am* 1996;34:450–453.
111. Maurer TA, Zacklein HS, Tuffanelli L, et al. The use of methotrexate for treatment of psoriasis in patents with HIV infection. *J Am Acad Dermatol* 1994;31:372–375.
112. Spector SA, Gelber RD, McGrath N, et al. A controlled trial of intravenous immune globulin for the prevention of serious bacterial infection in children. *N Engl J Med* 1994;331: 1181–1187.
113. Gutierrez FJ, Martinez-Ossna P, Seleznick MJ, et al. Rheumatologic rehabilitation for patients with HIV. In: Mukand J, ed. *Rehabilitation for patients with HIV disease.* New York: McGraw-Hill, 1991:77–93.

SUBJECT INDEX

Note: Page numbers followed by f indicate figures; those followed by t indicate tables.

C

D

F

G

H

L

M

N

O

P

Q

R

S

T

U